DRUG INFORMATION HANDBOOK for ADVANCED PRACTICE NURSING

A Comprehensive Resource for Nurse Practitioners, Nurse Midwives and Clinical Specialists, including Selected Disease Management Guidelines

12th Edition

Senior Editors:

Beatrice B. Turkoski, RN, PhD
Brenda R. Lance, RN, MSN
Elizabeth A. Tomsik, PharmD, BCPS

Foreword By:

Margaret A. Fitzgerald, DNP, FNP-BC, NP-C, FAANP, CSP

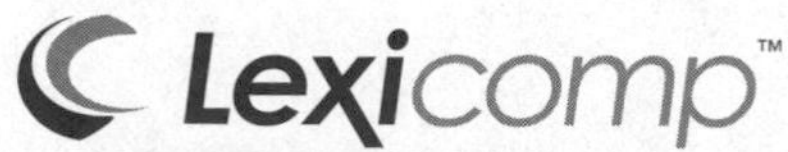

DRUG INFORMATION HANDBOOK for ADVANCED PRACTICE NURSING

A Comprehensive Resource for Nurse Practitioners, Nurse Midwives, and Clinical Specialists, including Selected Disease Management Guidelines

Beatrice B. Turkoski, RN, PhD
Senior Editor
Associate Professor, Graduate Faculty,
Pharmacology for Advanced Practice Nurses
College of Nursing
Kent State University
Kent, Ohio

Brenda R. Lance, RN, MSN
Senior Editor
Program Development Director
NorthCoast HealthCare Management Services
NorthCoast Infusion Network
Beachwood, Ohio

Elizabeth A. Tomsik, PharmD, BCPS
Senior Editor
Manager
Adverse Drug Reactions Group
Lexi-Comp, Inc
Hudson, Ohio

Foreword by:
Margaret A. Fitzgerald, DNP, FNP-BC, NP-C, FAANP, CSP

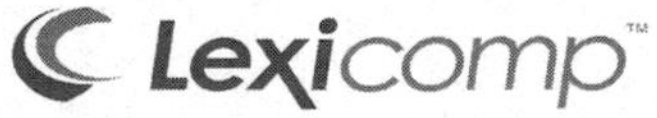

NOTICE

This data is intended to serve the user as a handy reference and not as a complete drug information resource. It does not include information on every therapeutic agent available. The publication covers over 1000 commonly used drugs and is specifically designed to present important aspects of drug data in a more concise format than is typically found in medical literature or product material supplied by manufacturers.

The nature of drug information is that it is constantly evolving because of ongoing research and clinical experience and is often subject to interpretation. While great care has been taken to ensure the accuracy of the information and recommendations presented, the reader is advised that the authors, editors, reviewers, contributors, and publishers cannot be responsible for the continued currency of the information or for any errors, omissions, or the application of this information, or for any consequences arising therefrom. Therefore, the author(s) and/or the publisher shall have no liability to any person or entity with regard to claims, loss, or damage caused, or alleged to be caused, directly or indirectly, by the use of information contained herein. Because of the dynamic nature of drug information, readers are advised that decisions regarding drug therapy must be based on the independent judgment of the clinician, changing information about a drug (eg, as reflected in the literature and manufacturer's most current product information), and changing medical practices. Therefore, this data is designed to be used in conjunction with other necessary information and is not designed to be solely relied upon by any user. The user of this data hereby and forever releases the authors and publishers of this data from any and all liability of any kind that might arise out of the use of this data. The editors are not responsible for any inaccuracy of quotation or for any false or misleading implication that may arise due to the text or formulas as used or due to the quotation of revisions no longer official.

Certain of the authors, editors, and contributors have written this book in their private capacities. No official support or endorsement by any federal or state agency or pharmaceutical company is intended or inferred.

The publishers have made every effort to trace any third party copyright holders, if any, for borrowed material. If they have inadvertently overlooked any, they will be pleased to make the necessary arrangements at the first opportunity.

If you have any suggestions or questions regarding any information presented in this data, please contact our drug information pharmacists at (330) 650-6506. Book revisions are available at our website at http://www.lexi.com/home/revisions/.

This manual was produced using Lexi-Comp's Information Management System™ (LIMS) — A complete publishing service of Lexi-Comp Inc

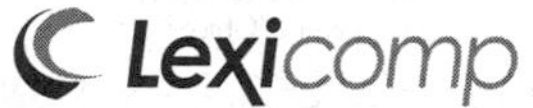

1100 Terex Road • Hudson, Ohio 44236
(330) 650-6506

ISBN 978-1-59195-295-4

TABLE OF CONTENTS

FOREWORD

Nationwide, there are now more than 270,000 advanced practice nurses (APNs). As our ranks grow, so do our practice responsibilities. We write thousands of prescriptions daily as we provide care, often to the most vulnerable members of society. As with all busy clinicians, the APN needs ready references that help guide care, especially in the fast-changing field of pharmacotherapeutics.

During the course of APN practice, prescribing questions need to be answered quickly and precisely. When the question is about drug therapy, often the answer is hard to find:

- *Where can you find information on both FDA-approved and unlabeled uses of a drug?*
- *When prescribing a certain medication, is there a food, herbal, alcohol, or drug interaction?*
- *How should the drug be started?*
- *How should the dose be adjusted?*
- *How long until a therapeutic dose is reached and therapeutic effect realized?*
- *What is the critical information the prescriber needs to convey to the patient and family in order to ensure safety and facilitate an optimum outcome?*

The *Drug Information Handbook for Advanced Practice Nursing* provides this valuable information and much more, in a clear, concise format. Seldom has so much rich information been found in a single source. A section on pharmacokinetics, pharmacodynamics, and therapeutics sets the stage in this helpful handbook. Each drug monograph features a clear guide to safe prescribing, highlighting important issues, such as information on prescribing for children, adults, geriatrics, and during pregnancy and lactation. All generic drug names and cross-references are highlighted in red, a helpful feature in an information-intensive text. There are 60 fields of pertinent data that can appear in each monograph, including effects on laboratory values, as well as, information on monitoring for adverse reactions and required ongoing monitoring. Features of this 12th edition include improved patient education and physical assessment fields; the addition of numerous new drug monographs and updates for previously-approved medications.

This edition includes new immunization administration recommendations, as well as information on renal function estimation for both adult and pediatric patients. Given the current focus on evidence-based healthcare, a ready-reference for this type of information is critically-important. The section on preventing prescribing errors is particularly welcome, given the current complexity of care.

The publication of the *Drug Information Handbook for Advanced Practice Nursing* comes at an exciting and challenging time. The increasing complexity of clinical care and development of new therapies contribute to the challenges of prescriptive practice. The need for quality references to enhance APN practice continues. In this regard, the *Drug Information Handbook for Advanced Practice Nursing* is a valuable asset.

Margaret A. Fitzgerald, DNP, FNP-BC, NP-C, FAANP, CSP

Dr Fitzgerald is the Founder, President, and Principal Lecturer with Fitzgerald Health Education Associates, an international provider of NP Certification Preparation and ongoing continuing education for NPs and other healthcare providers. An internationally recognized presenter, she has provided more than 1000 programs for numerous professional organizations, universities, national, and state healthcare professional associations on a wide variety of clinical topics. In addition, she is a family nurse practitioner at the Greater Lawrence Family Health Center in Lawrence, Massachusetts, where her clinical practice focuses on the primary care of multigenerational Latino families and is adjunct faculty to the Health Center's Family Practice Residency Program.

ABOUT THE EDITORS

Beatrice B. Turkoski, RN, PhD

Dr Turkoski received her BSN from Alverno College in Wisconsin, an MS in Community Health Nursing from the University of Wisconsin-Milwaukee School of Nursing, and a PhD from the University of Wisconsin. She also earned an MA in bioethics from Case Western Reserve University in Cleveland, Ohio. Her extensive professional nursing experience includes several years as a clinician in critical care in Wisconsin and Israel, Director of Nursing, clinician, and researcher in gerontology and chronic adult illness in Wisconsin and Ohio.

In her graduate faculty role at Kent State University College of Nursing, Dr Turkoski developed and teaches the Advanced Pharmacology course for graduate students in the Nurse Practitioner and Clinical Nurse Specialist programs. Her expertise in this area is highly regarded by both students and faculty. She also conducts continuing education programs and workshops in pharmacology and nursing practice.

Dr Turkoski is an active member and past officer in several national and international professional organizations. She has made presentations at scientific conferences in the United States, Europe, China, Korea, Canada, and Israel. Dr Turkoski is also a frequent contributor to professional journals.

Brenda R. Lance, RN, MSN

Ms Lance received a diploma in nursing from Methodist Hospital School of Nursing in Lubbock, Texas. She also has earned bachelor's and master's degrees in nursing from Kent State University, Kent, Ohio.

Ms Lance's nursing experiences and expertise are numerous and varied. Her nursing career spans over 35 years, having worked in intensive care, emergency room, ambulatory care clinics, home health, and home infusion. She is currently the Program Development Director for NorthCoast HealthCare Management Services and NorthCoast Infusion Network located in Beachwood, Ohio.

In addition to many years of direct patient care experience, she is also certified in risk management, has extensive experience in Joint Commission on Accreditation of Healthcare Organizations standards and Medicare regulations for home health, and has been a military nurse for the past 30 years. She retired with the rank of Captain (0-6) from the U.S. Naval Reserve Nurse Corps.

Ms Lance is a member of the Sigma Theta Tau (National Honor Society of Nursing) and National Home Infusion Association.

Elizabeth A Tomsik, PharmD, BCPS

Dr Tomsik received her bachelor's degree in pharmacy from the Albany College of Pharmacy and her Doctor of Pharmacy degree from the University of Sciences in Philadelphia. She completed a one-year residency at Truman Medical Center in Kansas City and went on to work at Hahnemann University Hospital for 2 years in the field of nutrition. She continued her work at Louis Stokes Veterans Affairs Medical Center in Cleveland for 12 years. Her areas of practice included intensive care, coronary care, nutrition support, and anticoagulation. She was actively involved in residency training and was in charge of the pharmacy residency program for many years. She held faculty appointments from Case Western Reserve University, College of Medicine and The University of Toledo, College of Pharmacy. She has been a Board Certified Pharmacotherapy Specialist since 1999.

Dr Tomsik has been with Lexi-Comp, Inc since 1999. She is actively involved in enhancing Lexi-Comp's database with a focus in the area of poisonings. She is currently the manager of the adverse drug reaction section within the content division at Lexi.

Dr Tomsik is a member of the Ohio College of Clinical Pharmacy, the American Academy of Clinical Toxicology, the American College of Clinical Pharmacy, and the Society of Critical Care Medicine.

EDITORIAL ADVISORY PANEL

Tom Palma, MS, RPh
Medical Science Pharmacist
Lexi-Comp, Inc
Hudson, Ohio

Susie H. Park, PharmD, BCPP
Assistant Professor of Clinical Pharmacy
University of Southern California
Los Angeles, California

Alpa Patel, PharmD
Antimicrobial Clinical Pharmacist
University of Louisville Hospital
Louisville, Kentucky

Gayle Pearson, BSPharm, MSA
Drug Information Pharmacist
Peter Lougheed Centre,
Alberta Health Services
Calgary, Alberta, Canada

James A. Ponto, MS, RPh, BCNP
Chief Nuclear Pharmacist
Department of Radiology
University of Iowa, Hospitals and Clinics
Professor of Clinical Pharmacy
Department of Pharmacy Practice and Science
University of Iowa College of Pharmacy
Iowa City, Iowa

James Reissig, PharmD
Assistant Director, Clinical Services
Akron General Medical Center
Akron, Ohio

A.J. (Fred) Remillard, PharmD
Assistant Dean, Research and Graduate Affairs
College of Pharmacy and Nutrition
University of Saskatchewan
Saskatoon, Saskatchewan

Curtis M. Rimmermann, MD, MBA, FACC
Gus P. Karos Chair, Clinical Cardiovascular Medicine
Department of Cardiovascular Medicine
Cleveland Clinic Foundation
Cleveland, Ohio

P. David Rogers, PharmD, PhD, FCCP
Professor and Associate Dean for Translational Research
University of Tennessee College of Pharmacy
Memphis, Tennessee

Martha Sajatovic, MD
Professor of Psychiatry
Case Western Reserve University
Cleveland, Ohio
Department of Psychiatry
University Hospitals of Cleveland
Cleveland, Ohio

Jennifer K. Sekeres, PharmD, BCPS
Infectious Diseases Clinical Specialist
The Cleveland Clinic Foundation
Cleveland, Ohio

Todd P. Semla, MS, PharmD, BCPS, FCCP, AGSF
Clinical Pharmacy Specialist
Department of Veterans Affairs
Pharmacy Benefits Management Services
Associate Professor, Clinical
Department of Medicine and Psychiatry and Behavioral Health
Feinberg School of Medicine
Northwestern University
Chicago, Illinois

Joseph Snoke, RPh, BCPS
Manager
Core Pharmacology Group
Lexi-Comp, Inc
Hudson, Ohio

Joni Lombardi Stahura, BS, PharmD, RPh
Pharmacotherapy Specialist
Lexi-Comp, Inc
Hudson, Ohio

Stephen Marc Stout, PharmD, MS, BCPS
Pharmacotherapy Specialist
Lexi-Comp, Inc
Hudson, Ohio

Dan Streetman, PharmD, RPh
Pharmacotherapy Specialist
Lexi-Comp, Inc
Hudson, Ohio

Darcie-Ann Streetman, PharmD, RPh
Clinical Pharmacist
University of Michigan Health System
Ann Arbor, Michigan

Carol K. Taketomo, PharmD
Director of Pharmacy and Nutrition Services
Children's Hospital Los Angeles
Los Angeles, California

Mary Temple-Cooper, PharmD
Pediatric Clinical Research Specialist
Hillcrest Hospital
Mayfield Heights, Ohio

Elizabeth A. Tomsik, PharmD, BCPS
Manager
Adverse Drug Reactions Group
Lexi-Comp, Inc
Hudson, Ohio

Dana Travis, RPh
Pharmacotherapy Specialist
Lexi-Comp, Inc
Hudson, Ohio

Jennifer Trofe-Clark, PharmD
Clinical Transplant Pharmacist
Hospital of The University of Pennsylvania
Philadelphia, Pennsylvania

Beatrice B. Turkoski, RN, PhD
Associate Professor, Graduate Faculty, Pharmacology for Advanced Practice Nurses
College of Nursing
Kent State University
Kent, Ohio

Amy Van Orman, PharmD, BCPS
Pharmacotherapy Specialist
Lexi-Comp, Inc
Hudson, Ohio

Heather L. VandenBussche, PharmD
Professor of Pharmacy, Pediatrics
Pharmacy Practice
Ferris State University College of Pharmacy
Kalamazoo, Michigan

David M. Weinstein, PhD, RPh
Manager
Metabolism, Interactions, and Genomics Group
Lexi-Comp, Inc
Hudson, Ohio

Anne Marie Whelan, PharmD
College of Pharmacy
Dalhouise University
Halifax, Nova Scotia

Nathan Wirick, PharmD
Infectious Disease and Antibiotic Management Clinical Specialist
Hillcrest Hospital
Cleveland, Ohio

Richard L. Wynn, BSPharm, PhD
Professor of Pharmacology
Baltimore College of Dental Surgery
Dental School
University of Maryland Baltimore
Baltimore, Maryland

Sallie Young, PharmD, BCPS, AQ Cardiology
Clinical Pharmacy Specialist, Cardiology
Penn State Milton S. Hershey Medical Center
Hershey, Pennsylvania

Jennifer Zimmer-Young, PharmD, CCRP
Educator, Clinical Pharmacist
ThedaCare
Appleton, Wisconsin

DESCRIPTION OF SECTIONS AND FIELDS

Introduction

This and other documents in this section provide guidelines for the use of the handbook including descriptions of Preventing Prescribing Errors and Basic Pharmacotherapeutic Concepts (Pharmacokinetics, Pharmacodynamics, Patient Factors That Influence Drug Therapy, and Pharmacotherapeutics).

Individual Drug Monographs

Medications are arranged alphabetically by generic name. U.S. brand names and index terms are cross-referenced between monographs.

Monograph Fields

Generic Name — U.S. adopted name.

Pronunciation — Phonetic pronunciation of generic name.

U.S. Brand Names — Trade names (manufacturer-specific) found in the United States. The symbol [DSC] appears after trade names that have been recently discontinued.

Index Terms — Includes names or accepted abbreviations of the generic drug; may include common brand names no longer available; this field is used to create cross-references to monographs.

Generic Availability (U.S.) — Indicates availability of generic products in the United States.

Pharmacologic Category — Indicates one or more systematic classifications of the drug.

Medication Safety Issues — In an effort to promote the safe use of medications, this field is intended to highlight possible sources of medication errors such as look-alike/sound-alike drugs or highly concentrated formulations which require vigilance on the part of healthcare professionals. In addition, medications which have been associated with severe consequences in the event of a medication error are also identified in this field.

Medication Guide Available — Identifies drugs that have an FDA-approved Medication Guide.

Prescribing and Access Restrictions — Provides information on any special requirements regarding the prescribing, obtaining or dispensing of drugs, including access restrictions pertaining to drugs with REMS elements and those drugs whose access restrictions are not REMS-related.

Pregnancy Risk Factor — Five categories established by the FDA to indicate the potential of a systemically absorbed drug for causing risk to fetus.

Lactation — Indicates if the drug listed in the monograph is present in breast milk and the manufacturers' recommendation for use while breast-feeding (where recommendation of American Academy of Pediatrics differs, notation is made).

Use — Description of FDA-approved indications of the drug

Unlabeled/Investigational Use — Information pertaining to non-FDA-approved and investigational indications of the drug.

Mechanism of Action/Effect — How the drug works in the body to elicit a response.

Contraindications — Information pertaining to inappropriate use of the drug as dictated by approved labeling.

Warnings/Precautions — Precautionary considerations, hazardous conditions related to use of the drug, and disease states or patient populations in which the drug should be cautiously used. Boxed warnings, when present, are clearly identified and are adapted from the FDA-approved labeling. Consult the product labeling for the black box warning through the manufacturer's or the FDA website.

Drug Interactions — Agents that, when combined with the drug, may affect therapy; may include the following:

Metabolism/Transport Effects	If a drug has demonstrated involvement with cytochrome P450 enzymes, or other metabolism or transport proteins, this field will identify the drug as an inhibitor, inducer, or substrate of the specific enzyme(s) (eg, CYP1A2 or UGT1A1). CYP450 isoenzymes are identified as substrates (minor or major), inhibitors (weak, moderate, or strong), and inducers (weak or strong).
Avoid Concomitant Use	Designates drug combinations which should not be used concomitantly, due to an unacceptable risk:benefit assessment. Frequently, the concurrent use of the agents is explicitly prohibited or contraindicated by the product labeling.
Decreased Effect	Drug combinations that result in a decreased therapeutic effect between the drug listed in the monograph and other drugs or drug classes.
Increased Effect/Toxicity	Drug combinations that result in an increased or toxic therapeutic effect between the drug listed in the monograph and other drugs or drug classes.
Nutritional/Ethanol Interactions	Presents a description of the interaction between the drug listed in the monograph and ethanol, food, or herb/nutraceuticals.
Lab Interactions	Listing of assay interferences when relevant.
Adverse Reactions	Only side effects >1% are included and are grouped by percentage of incidence (if known) and/or body system.
Pharmacodynamics/Kinetics	
Onset of Action	The time after drug administration when therapeutic effect is observed; may also include time for peak therapeutic effect.
Duration of Action	Length of therapeutic effect.
Absorption	The amount of absorbed drug, including rate and route for the drug listed.
Bioavailability	Fraction of administered drug dose that enters systemic circulation.
Time to Peak	Describes the relative time after ingestion when concentration achieves the highest serum concentration
Protein Binding	The percent of drug listed in the monograph bound to circulating proteins (ie, albumin, etc)
Half-Life Elimination	The reported half-life of elimination for the parent or metabolites of the drug
Metabolism	Describes the site of metabolism and may include the percentage of active metabolites.
Excretion	Route of drug elimination
Pharmacokinetic Note	Provides additional pharmacokinetic information when needed.
Product Availability	Provides availability information on products that have been approved by the FDA, but not yet available for use. Estimates for when a product may be available are included, when this information is known. May also provide any unique or critical drug availability issues.
Controlled Substance	The controlled substance classification from the Drug Enforcement Agency (DEA); U.S. schedules are I-V; schedules vary by country and sometimes state (ie, Massachusetts uses I-VI).
Available Dosage Forms	Information with regard to form, strength, and availability of the drug in the United States. **Note:** Additional formulation information (eg, excipients, preservatives) is included when available. Please consult product labeling for further information.
Dosing	The amount of drug to be typically given or taken during therapy; may include the following:
Adult	The recommended amount of drug to be given to adult patients
Adult and Geriatric	This combined field is only used to indicate that no specific adjustments for elderly patients were identified. However, other issues should be considered (eg, renal or hepatic impairment). Also refer to Geriatric Considerations for additional information related to the elderly.

Geriatric	A suggested amount of drug to be given to elderly patients; may include adjustments from adult dosing (lack of information in the monograph may imply that the drug is not used in the elderly patient or no specific adjustments could be identified)
Pediatric	Suggested amount of drug to be given to neonates, infants, and children
Renal Impairment	Suggested dosage adjustments based on compromised renal function; may include dosing instructions for patients on dialysis
Hepatic Impairment	Suggested dosage adjustments based on compromised liver function
Adjustment for Toxicity	Suggested dosage adjustments in the event specific toxicities related to therapy are noted, such as hematologic toxicities related to cancer chemotherapy
Administration	
Oral I.M. I.V. Inhalation Topical Other	The administration field contains subfields by route regarding issues relative to appropriately giving a medication; includes suggestions on final drug concentrations and/or rates of infusion for parenteral medications and comments regarding the timing of drug administration relative to meals.
Stability	
Reconstitution	Includes comments on solution choice with time or conditions for the mixture to maintain full potency before administration
Storage	Information relating to appropriate storage of the medication prior to opening the manufacturer's original packaging; information is only given if recommendations are for storage at other than room temperature; includes storage requirements for reconstituted products
Monitoring and Teaching Issues	
Laboratory Monitoring	Suggested laboratory tests to monitor for safety and efficacy of the drug
Physical Assessment	Monitoring guidelines
Patient Education	Suggested items to discuss with the patient or caregiver when taking the medication; may include issues regarding contraception, self-monitoring, precautions, and administration
Dietary Considerations	Includes information on how the medication should be taken relative to meals or food
Geriatric Considerations	Comments or suggestions of drug use in elderly patients; may include monitoring, dose adjustments, precautions, or comments on appropriateness of use
Breast-Feeding Considerations	Information pertinent to or associated with the human use of the drug as it relates to clinical effects on the nursing infant or postpartum woman.
Pregnancy Considerations	Comments related to safe drug administration during pregnancy, if appropriate
Other Issues	Additional pertinent information regarding nursing issues
Additional Information	Information about sodium content and/or pertinent information about specific brands
Related Information	Cross-reference to other pertinent drug information in this handbook

Pharmacologic Category Index

Lists all drugs by their unique pharmacologic category and includes cross-references to the monographs

Appendix

The last section is an extensive appendix of useful information that includes conversion laboratory information, comparison charts for selected classes of drugs, therapy guidelines, and treatment guidelines for selected therapy.

PREGNANCY CATEGORIES

Pregnancy Categories (sometimes referred to as pregnancy risk factors) are a letter system currently required under the *Teratogenic Effects* subsection of the product labeling. The system was initiated in 1979. The categories are required to be part of the package insert for prescription drugs that are systemically absorbed.

The categories are defined as follows:

A Adequate and well-controlled studies in pregnant women have not shown that the drug increases the risk of fetal abnormalities.

B Animal reproduction studies show no evidence of impaired fertility or harm to the fetus; however, no adequate and well-controlled studies have been conducted in pregnant women.
or
Animal reproduction studies have shown adverse events; however, studies in pregnant women have not shown that the drug increases the risk of abnormalities.

C Animal reproduction studies have shown an adverse effect on the fetus. There are no adequate and well-controlled studies in humans and the benefits from the use of the drug in pregnant women may be acceptable, despite its potential risks.
or
Animal reproduction studies have not been conducted.

D Based on human data, the drug can cause fetal harm when administered to pregnant women, but the potential benefits from the use of the drug may be acceptable, despite its potential risks.

X Studies in animals or humans have demonstrated fetal abnormalities (or there is positive evidence of fetal risk based on reports and/or marketing experience) and the risk of using the drug in pregnant women clearly outweighs any possible benefit (for example, safer drugs or other forms of therapy are available).

The categories do not take into consideration nonteratogenic effects (that information is currently presented separately). In 2008, the Food and Drug Administration (FDA) proposed new labeling requirements which would eliminate the use of the pregnancy category system and replace it with scientific data and other information specific to the use of the drug in pregnant women. These proposed changes were suggested because the current category system may be misleading. For instance, some practitioners may believe that risk increases from category A to B to C to D to X, which is not the intent. In addition, practitioners may not be aware that some medications are categorized based on animal data, while others are based on human data. When the new labeling requirements are approved, product labeling will contain pregnancy and lactation subsections, each describing a risk summary, clinical considerations, and section for specific data.

For full descriptions of the current and proposed labeling requirements, refer to the following websites:

Labeling Requirements for Prescription Drugs and/or Insulin (Code of Federal Regulations, Title 21, Volume 4, Revised April 1, 2010). Available at: http://www.accessdata.fda.gov/scripts/cdrh/cfdocs/cfCFR/CFRSearch.cfm?fr=201.57.

Content and Format of Labeling for Human Prescription Drug and Biological Products; Requirements for Pregnancy and Lactation Labeling (Federal Register, May 29, 2008). Available at: http://frwebgate.access.gpo.gov/cgi-bin/getdoc.cgi?dbname=2008_register&docid=fr29my08-33.pdf.

PREVENTING PRESCRIBING ERRORS

Prescribing errors account for the majority of reported medication errors and have prompted healthcare professionals to focus on the development of steps to make the prescribing process safer. Prescription legibility has been attributed to a portion of these errors and legislation has been enacted in several states to address prescription legibility. However, eliminating handwritten prescriptions and ordering medications through the use of technology [eg, computerized prescriber order entry (CPOE)] has been the primary recommendation. Whether a prescription is electronic, typed, or hand-printed, additional safe practices should be considered for implementation to maximize the safety of the prescribing process. Listed below are suggestions for safer prescribing:

- Ensure correct patient by using at least 2 patient identifiers on the prescription (eg, full name, birth date, or address). Review prescription with the patient or patient's caregiver.
- If pediatric patient, document patient's birth date or age and most recent weight. If geriatric patient, document patient's birth date or age.
- Prevent drug name confusion:
  - Use TALLman lettering (eg, buPROPion, busPIRone, predniSONE, prednisoLONE). For more information see: http://www.fda.gov/Drugs/DrugSafety/MedicationErrors/ucm164587.htm.
  - Avoid abbreviated drug names (eg, MSO_4, $MgSO_4$, MS, HCT, 6MP, MTX), as they may be misinterpreted and cause error.
  - Avoid investigational names for drugs with FDA approval (eg, FK-506, CBDCA).
  - Avoid chemical names such as 6-mercaptopurine or 6-thioguanine, as sixfold overdoses have been given when these were not recognized as chemical names. The proper names of these drugs are mercaptopurine or thioguanine.
  - Use care when prescribing drugs that look or sound similar (eg, look- alike, sound-alike drugs). Common examples include: Celebrex® vs Celexa®, hydroxyzine vs hydralazine, Zyprexa® vs Zyrtec®.
- Avoid dangerous, error-prone abbreviations (eg, regardless of letter-case: U, IU, QD, QOD, µg, cc, @). Do not use apothecary system or symbols. Additionally, text messaging abbreviations (eg, "2Day") should never be used.
  - For more information see: http://www.ismp.org/Tools/errorproneabbreviations.pdf
- Always use a leading zero for numbers less than 1 (0.5 mg is correct and .5 mg is **incorrect**) and never use a trailing zero for whole numbers (2 mg is correct and 2.0 mg is **incorrect**).
- Always use a space between a number and its units as it is easier to read. There should be no periods after the abbreviations mg or mL (10 mg is correct and 10mg is **incorrect**).
- For doses that are greater than 1,000 dosing units, use properly placed commas to prevent 10-fold errors (100,000 units is correct and 100000 units is **incorrect**).
- Do not prescribe drug dosage by the type of container in which the drug is available (eg, do not prescribe "1 amp", "2 vials", etc).
- Do not write vague or ambiguous orders which have the potential for misinterpretation by other healthcare providers. Examples of vague orders to avoid: "resume pre-op medications," "give drug per protocol," or "continue home medications."
- Review each prescription with patient (or patient's caregiver) including the medication name, indication, and directions for use.
- Take extra precautions when prescribing *high alert drugs* (drugs that can cause significant patient harm when prescribed in error). Common examples of these drugs include: Anticoagulants, chemotherapy, insulins, opiates, and sedatives.
  - For more information see: http://www.ismp.org/Tools/highalertmedications.pdf

To Err is Human: Building a Safer Health System, Kohn LT, Corrigan JM, and Donaldson MS, eds, Washington, D.C.: National Academy Press, 2000.

A Complete Outpatient Prescription[1]

A complete outpatient prescription can prevent the prescriber, the pharmacist, and/or the patient from making a mistake and can eliminate the need for further clarification. The complete outpatient prescription should contain:

- Patient's full name
- Medication indication
- Allergies
- Prescriber name and telephone or pager number
- For pediatric patients: Their birth date or age and current weight
- For geriatric patients: Their birth date or age
- Drug name, dosage form and strength
- For pediatric patients: Intended daily weight-based dose so that calculations can be checked by the pharmacist (ie, mg/kg/day or units/kg/day)
- Number or amount to be dispensed

- Complete instructions for the patient or caregiver, including the purpose of the medication, directions for use (including dose), dosing frequency, route of administration, duration of therapy, and number of refills.
- Dose should be expressed in convenient units of measure.
- When there are recognized contraindications for a prescribed drug, the prescriber should indicate knowledge of this fact to the pharmacist (ie, when prescribing a potassium salt for a patient receiving an ACE inhibitor, the prescriber should write "K serum leveling being monitored").

Upon dispensing of the final product, the pharmacist should ensure that the patient or caregiver can effectively demonstrate the appropriate administration technique. An appropriate measuring device should be provided or recommended. Household teaspoons and tablespoons should not be used to measure liquid medications due to their variability and inaccuracies in measurement; oral medication syringes are recommended.

For additional information see: http://www.ppag.org/attachments/files/111/Guidelines_Peds.pdf

[1]Levine SR, Cohen MR, Blanchard NR, et al, "Guidelines for Preventing Medication Errors in Pediatrics," *J Pediatr Pharmacol Ther*, 2001, 6:426-42.

ABBREVIATIONS, ACRONYMS, AND SYMBOLS

Abbreviations Which May Be Used in This Reference

Abbreviation	Meaning
5-HT	5-hydroxytryptamine
AAP	American Academy of Pediatrics
ABG	arterial blood gases
ABW	adjusted body weight
AACT	American Academy of Clinical Toxicology
ACC	American College of Cardiology
ACE	angiotensin converting enzyme
ACLS	advanced cardiac life support
ACOG	American College of Obstetricians and Gynecologists
ACTH	adrenocorticotrophic hormone
ADH	alcohol dehydrogenase
ADHD	attention-deficit/hyperactivity disorder
ADLs	activities of daily living
AED	antiepileptic drug
AHA	American Heart Association
AIDS	acquired immune deficiency syndrome
AIMS	Abnormal Involuntary Movement Scale
ALS	amyotrophic lateral sclerosis
ALT	alanine aminotransferase
AMA	American Medical Association
ANC	absolute neutrophil count
aPTT	activated partial thromboplastin
ARB	angiotensin receptor blocker
ARDS	acute respiratory distress syndrome
AST	aspartate aminotransferase
AUC	area under the curve
BDI	Beck Depression Inventory
BEC	blood ethanol concentration
BLS	basic life support
BMI	body mass index
BMT	bone marrow transplant
BP	blood pressure
BPH	benign prostatic hyperplasia
BPRS	Brief Psychiatric Rating Scale
BSA	body surface area
BUN	blood urea nitrogen
CABG	coronary artery bypass graft
CAD	coronary artery disease
CAN	Canadian
CAPD	continuous ambulatory peritoneal dialysis
CAS	chemical abstract service
CBC	complete blood count
CBT	cognitive behavioral therapy
Cl_{cr}	creatinine clearance
CDC	Centers for Disease Control and Prevention
CF	cystic fibrosis
CGI	Clinical Global Impression
CHD	coronary heart disease
CHF	congestive heart failure; chronic heart failure
CIE	chemotherapy-induced emesis
C-II	schedule two controlled substance

Abbreviations Which May Be Used in This Reference *(continued)*

Abbreviation	Meaning
C-III	schedule three controlled substance
C-IV	schedule four controlled substance
C-V	schedule five controlled substance
CIV	continuous I.V. infusion
C_{max}	maximum plasma concentration
C_{min}	minimum plasma concentration
CMV	cytomegalovirus
CNS	central nervous system or coagulase negative staphylococcus
COLD	chronic obstructive lung disease
COPD	chronic obstructive pulmonary disease
COX	cyclooxygenase
CPK	creatine phosphokinase
CRF	chronic renal failure
CRP	C-reactive protein
CRRT	continuous renal replacement therapy
CSF	cerebrospinal fluid
CSII	continuous subcutaneous insulin infusion
CT	computed tomography
CVA	cerebrovascular accident
CVVH	continuous venovenous hemofiltration
CVVHD	continuous venovenous hemodialysis
CVVHDF	continuous venovenous hemodiafiltration
CYP	cytochrome
D_5W	dextrose 5% in water
DBP	diastolic blood pressure
DEHP	di(3-ethylhexyl)phthalate
DIC	disseminated intravascular coagulation
DM	diabetes mellitus
DMARD	disease modifying antirheumatic drug
DSC	discontinued
DSM-IV	Diagnostic and Statistical Manual
DVT	deep vein thrombosis
EBV	Epstein-Barr virus
ECG	electrocardiogram
ECMO	extracorporeal membrane oxygenation
ECT	electroconvulsive therapy
ED	emergency department
EEG	electroencephalogram
EF	ejection fraction
EG	ethylene glycol
EGA	estimated gestational age
EIA	enzyme immunoassay
ELISA	enzyme-linked immunosorbent assay
EPS	extrapyramidal side effects
ESR	erythrocyte sedimentation rate
ESRD	end stage renal disease
EtOH	alcohol
FDA	Food and Drug Administration
FTT	failure to thrive
GABA	gamma-aminobutyric acid
GAD	generalized anxiety disorder
GERD	gastroesophageal reflux disease
GFR	glomerular filtration rate
GGT	gamma-glutamyltransferase
GI	gastrointestinal
GU	genitourinary
GVHD	graft versus host disease

Abbreviations Which May Be Used in This Reference *(continued)*

Abbreviation	Meaning
HAM-A	Hamilton Anxiety Scale
HAM-D	Hamilton Depression Scale
HDL	high density lipoprotein
HF	heart failure
HFSA	Heart Failure Society of America
HIV	human immunodeficiency virus
HMG-CoA	3-hydroxy-3-methylglutaryl-coenzyme A
HOCM	hypertrophic obstructive cardiomyopathy
HPA	hypothalamic-pituitary-adrenal
HSV	herpes simplex virus
HTN	hypertension
HUS	hemolytic uremic syndrome
IBD	inflammatory bowel disease
IBS	irritable bowel syndrome
IBW	ideal body weight
ICD	implantable cardioverter defibrillator
ICH	intracranial hemorrhage
ICP	intracranial pressure
IDDM	insulin dependent diabetes mellitus
IDSA	Infectious Diseases Society of America
IHSS	idiopathic hypertrophic subaortic stenosis
I.M.	intramuscular
INR	international normalized ration
Int. unit	international unit
IOP	intraocular pressure
IUGR	intrauterine growth retardation
I.V.	intravenous
IVP	intravenous push
IVPB	intravenous piggyback
JIA	juvenile idiopathic arthritis
JNC	Joint National Committee
KIU	kallikrein inhibitor unit
LAMM	L-α-acetyl methadol
LDH	lactate dehydrogenase
LDL	low density lipoprotein
LFT	liver function test
LGA	large for gestational age
LR	lactated ringers
LVEF	left ventricular ejection fraction
LVH	left ventricular hypertrophy
MADRS	Montgomery Asbery Depression Rating Scale
MAOIs	monamine oxidase inhibitors
MDD	major depressive disorder
MDRD	modification of diet in renal disease
MDRSP	multidrug resistant *streptococcus pneumoniae*
mEq	milliequivalent
mg	milligram
MI	myocardial infarction
mL	milliliter
mm	millimeter
mM	millimolar
mm Hg	millimeters of mercury
MMSE	mini mental status examination
M/P	milk to plasma ratio
MPS I	mucopolysaccharidosis I
MRHD	maximum recommended human dose
MRI	magnetic resonance imaging

Abbreviations Which May Be Used in This Reference *(continued)*

Abbreviation	Meaning
MUGA	multiple gated acquisition scan
NAS	neonatal abstinence syndrome
NF	National Formulary
NFD	Nephrogenic fibrosing dermopathy
ng	nanogram
NIDDM	Noninsulin dependent diabetes mellitus
NKA	no known allergies
NKDA	No known drug allergies
NMDA	n-methyl-d-aspartic acid
NMS	neuroleptic malignant syndrome
NNRTI	non-nucleoside reverse transcriptase inhibitor
NRTI	nucleoside reverse transcriptase inhibitor
NS	normal saline
NSAID	nonsteroidal anti-inflammatory drug
NSF	nephrogenic systemic fibrosis
NSTEMI	Non-ST-elevation myocardial infarction
OA	osteoarthritis
OCD	obsessive-compulsive disorder
OHSS	ovarian hyperstimulation syndrome
OTC	over-the-counter
PAT	paroxysmal atrial tachycardia
PD	Parkinson's disease; peritoneal dialysis
PDA	patent ductus arteriosus
PDE-5	phosphodiesterase-5
PE	pulmonary embolus
PEG tube	percutaneous endoscopic gastrostomy tube
PHN	post-herpetic neuralgia
PID	pelvic inflammatory disease
PMDD	premenstrual dysphoric disorder
PONV	postoperative nausea and vomiting
PPN	peripheral parenteral nutrition
PROM	premature rupture of membranes
PSVT	paroxysmal supraventricular tachycardia
PT	prothrombin time
PTSD	post-traumatic stress disorder
PTT	partial thromboplastin time
PUD	peptic ulcer disease
PVD	peripheral vascular disease
QT_c	corrected QT interval
QT_c-F	corrected QT interval by Fredricia's formula
RA	rheumatoid arthritis
REM	rapid eye movement
RPLS	reversible posterior leukoencephalopathy syndrome
SA	sinoatrial
SAD	seasonal affective disorder
SAH	subarachnoid hemorrhage
SBE	subacute bacterial endocarditis
SBP	systolic blood pressure
S_{Cr}	serum creatinine
SERM	selective estrogen receptor modulator
SGA	small for gestational age
SGOT	serum glutamic oxaloacetic aminotransferase
SGPT	serum glutamic pyruvate transaminase
SI	International System of Units or Systeme international d'Unites
SIADH	syndrome of inappropriate antidiuretic hormone secretion
SLE	systemic lupus erythematosus
SNRI	serotonin norepinephrine reuptake inhibitor

Abbreviations Which May Be Used in This Reference *(continued)*

Abbreviation	Meaning
SSKI	saturated solution of potassium iodide
SSRIs	selective serotonin reuptake inhibitors
STD	sexually transmitted disease
STEM I	ST-elevation myocardial infarction
SubQ	subcutaneous
supp	suppository
SVT	supraventricular tachycardia
SWFI	sterile water for injection
syr	syrup
$T_{1/2}$	half-life
tab	tablet
TB	tuberculosis
TC	total cholesterol
TCA	tricyclic antidepressant
TD	tardive dyskinesia
TG	triglyceride
TIA	transient ischemic attack
TMA	thrombotic microangiopathy
T_{max}	time to maximum observed concentration, plasma
TNF	Tumor necrosis factor
TPN	total parenteral nutrition
tr, tinct	tincture
tsp	teaspoonful
UC	ulcerative colitis
ULN	upper limits of normal
URI	upper respiratory infection
USAN	United States Adopted Names
USP	United States Pharmacopeia
UTI	urinary tract infection
UV	ultraviolet
V_d	volume of distribution
VEGF	vascular endothelial growth factor
VF	ventricular fibrillation
VT	ventricular tachycardia
VTE	venous thromboembolism
vWD	von Willebrand disease
VZV	varicella zoster virus
YBOC	Yale Brown Obsessive-Compulsive Scale
YMRS	Young Mania Rating Scale

Common Weights, Measures, or Apothecary Abbreviations

Abbreviation	Meaning
<[1]	less than
>[1]	greater than
≤	less than or equal to
≥	greater than or equal to
ac	before meals or food
ad	to, up to
ad lib	at pleasure
AM	morning
AMA	against medical advice
amp	ampul
amt	amount
aq	water
aq. dest.	distilled water

Common Weights, Measures, or Apothecary Abbreviations *(continued)*

Abbreviation	Meaning
ASAP	as soon as possible
a.u.[1]	each ear
bid	twice daily
bm	bowel movement
C	Celsius, centigrade
cal	calorie
cap	capsule
cc[1]	cubic centimeter
cm	centimeter
comp	compound
cont	continue
d	day
d/c[1]	discharge
dil	dilute
disp	dispense
div	divide
dtd	give of such a dose
Dx	diagnosis
elix, el	elixir
emp	as directed
et	and
ex aq	in water
F	Fahrenheit
f, ft	make, let be made
g	gram
gr	grain
gtt	a drop
h	hour
hs[1]	at bedtime
kcal	kilocalorie
kg	kilogram
L	liter
liq	a liquor, solution
M	molar
mcg	microgram
m. dict	as directed
mEq	milliequivalent
mg	milligram
microL	microliter
mL	milliliter
mm	millimeter
mM	millimolar
mm Hg	millimeters of mercury
ng	nanogram
no.	number
noc	in the night
non rep	do not repeat, no refills
NPO	nothing by mouth
NV	nausea and vomiting
O, Oct	a pint
o.d.[1]	right eye
o.l.	left eye
o.s.[1]	left eye
o.u.[1]	each eye
pc, post cib	after meals
PM	afternoon or evening
P.O.	by mouth

Common Weights, Measures, or Apothecary Abbreviations *(continued)*

Abbreviation	Meaning
P.R.	rectally
prn	as needed
pulv	a powder
q	every
qad	every other day
qd[1,2]	every day, daily
qh	every hour
qid	four times a day
qod[1,2]	every other day
qs	a sufficient quantity
qs ad	a sufficient quantity to make
Rx	take, a recipe
SL	sublingual
stat	at once, immediately
SubQ	subcutaneous
supp	suppository
syr	syrup
tab	tablet
tal	such
tid	three times a day
tr, tinct	tincture
trit	triturate
tsp	teaspoon
u.d.	as directed
ung	ointment
v.o.	verbal order
w.a.	while awake
x3	3 times
x4	4 times

[1]ISMP error-prone abbreviation.

[2]JCAHO Do Not Use list.

Additional abbreviations used and defined within a specific monograph or text piece may only apply to that text.

REFERENCES

The Institute for Safe Medication Practices (ISMP) list of Error-Prone Abbreviations, Symbols, and Dose Designations. Available at http://www.ismp.org/Tools/errorproneabbreviations.pdf

The Joint Commission Official "Do Not Use" list. Available at http://www.jointcommission.org/Do_Not_Use_List_of_Abbreviations/

BASIC PHARMACOTHERAPEUTIC CONCEPTS

Safe and effective drug therapy requires an understanding of the basic principles of pharmacokinetics and pharmacodynamics and an awareness of how individual patient traits and lifestyles influence the actions and effects of drugs. A brief overview of basic concepts is discussed on the following pages.

1. Pharmacokinetics and Pharmacodynamics
2. Patient Factors That Influence Drug Therapy (pregnancy, age, weight, lifestyle)
3. Pharmacotherapeutics

PHARMACOKINETICS

The pharmacokinetics principles of absorption, distribution, and elimination govern how quickly a drug becomes available to the target organ and how long the drug will remain available.

Absorption

Absorption refers to how a drug progresses from the dosage form given into one bodily compartment into the blood stream to be distributed to the target site of action. The rate and degree of absorption depends on the formulation of the drug, the route of drug administration, and physiological variables. Drugs administered by the I.V. route require no absorption since they enter the circulatory system directly. Intramuscularly or subcutaneously administered drugs involve differing degrees of absorption. For instance, formulations in oil or microfine crystals (long-acting) have longer absorption times than other formulations and drugs administered into the deltoid muscle are absorbed faster than those administered into the gluteus muscle because of the increased blood flow in the deltoid muscle.

The oral route of drug administration is the preferred route for most drug therapy because it is more comfortable for the patient and usually safer and easier to use. The enteral route however, has a longer absorption time than other routes of absorption. This is, in part, related to the particular drug formulation (compressed tablet, extended release, repeat action). Anything that reduces systemic blood flow can reduce absorption rates, strenuous exercise decreases splanchnic blood flow as more blood is diverted to the muscles; pain and stress can also reduce blood flow in this area. Prolonged intestinal transit time (experienced with high-fat meals, solid food, anticholinergic drugs) may delay absorption rate, but increase the amount of total drug absorption. In addition, drug-drug interactions or drug-food interactions can reduce absorption; substances that significantly alter the gastric pH (eg, H_2-blockers, such as famotidine or proton pump inhibitors such as omeprazole, etc) can, in turn effect the absorption rates of some drugs. Absorption from the gastrointestinal tract may involve active transport across membranes. Some enzymes actually "pump" drug back into the GI lumen, opposing their absorption. One such enzyme is p-glycoprotein. Drugs which inhibit p-glycoprotein abolish this "pumping" action, and may lead to dramatic increases in the absorption of some drugs.

Orally administered drugs must pass through the portal system before they enter the systemic circulation. Many drugs undergo metabolic changes as they pass through the liver prior to reaching the systemic circulation. This means a substantial portion of the dose will never reach its target tissue (first-pass effect). The orally administered dose required to achieve a specific therapeutic response may, therefore be much larger than the dose for a route that bypasses portal circulation (parenteral or transdermal). Enterohepatic recycling (reabsorption) may occur with some drugs and may be a particular concern in some cases of toxicity. A few drugs (eg, digoxin, leflunomide, levothyroxine) re-enter the gastrointestinal tract (via excretion in the bile) from the bloodstream. They are then reabsorbed from the intestine and re-enter the circulatory system. Administration of substances, such as charcoal or cholestyramine resin (Questran®) or sodium polystyrene sulfonate (Kayexalate®), that bind the recycled drug in the GI tract, may be necessary to rapidly reduce the toxic serum levels of the recycled drug.]

Other routes of drug administration (eg, vaginal, rectal, topical, buccal, inhalation) all have positive and negative aspects of absorption. Advantages of drug absorption via these alternative sites include the ability to establish relatively high local concentrations of drugs at target tissues as well as the ability to bypass the "first-pass" metabolism of orally administered drugs. Drugs administered by inhalation must be formulated in microsized particles and are typically administered by nebulization or aerosolization in order to reach the terminial airways. Rectal absorption for systemic drugs is generally slow and administration of these drugs is often uncomfortable or painful. However, for some drugs and for some patients (for example, in severe nausea where oral medications cannot be administered), this is either the only route available or may be the route of choice. Topical absorption has the advantage of continuous absorption, although onset of action is generally slower than other forms of administration and degree of absorption may differ considerably depending on patient characteristics. Transdermal formulations have been designed to work together with the absorptive properties of the skin and may allow the delivery of a consistent rate of drug absorption for several days. Drugs for ophthalmic and otic administration are highly specific and are designed to produce high local concentrations, however healthcare professionals should also take the absorption properties and systemic effects of drugs administered by these routes into consideration.

Distribution

Distribution of an absorbed drug is dependent on several physical and/or chemical characteristics of the drug, including affinity for lipid or aqueous tissue and ability to permeate various tissue barriers (sometimes through the assistance of specific transport proteins), pH differences, blood flow, and degree of protein binding. The size and charge of the drug molecules will also help determine to which bodily compartment they are distributed. Drugs localize to specific tissues according to the combined properties of both drug and tissue. Drug concentrations can vary considerably between organs.

Drugs enter the system by one or another means of absorption, circulate (distribute) through the body via the circulatory system, interact with target receptors, and are excreted from the body in due course. When blood flow is impeded, the distribution of any substance in the blood is also impeded. Anything that alters the concentration of blood (eg, dehydration or edema) may also impact the distribution of drug molecules to the target site.

Albumin levels may also influence the distribution of some drugs that have a potential for binding to large proteins. Usually, the degree to which any drug binds to albumin remains predictable (eg, gentamicin <30% bound and warfarin >97% bound). Dosing recommendations are predicated on the idea that a certain level of unbound molecules remain "free" in the circulation when albumin levels are "normal." When disease states, nutritional status, or other drugs significantly change the amount of albumin available for binding or the ability to bind to this "carrier" protein, toxic serum levels of free (unbound) drug may occur.

Physiological barriers also influence distribution. One example is the blood-brain barrier that is a continuous network of cells with tight junctions that make the brain impermeable to some drugs according to their degree of water or lipid solubility. This makes the brain less accessible to drugs that are able to accumulate in other tissues (eg, many chemotherapeutic drugs and many antibiotics). In addition to this physical barrier, a substantial part of the ability of the brain to exclude certain chemicals is related to the presence of specialized transport proteins which actively "pump" these chemicals out of the CSF. Drugs which inhibit transport enzymes may influence the ability of drug to accumulate in tissues such as the brain.

Elimination via Metabolism

Elimination via metabolism is the process of biotransformation that occurs when a drug changes from its parent form to a more water-soluble form.

Some drugs are not metabolized and are excreted from the body unchanged (aminoglycosides, gabapentin). However, most drugs are metabolized in the liver, in tissues, in the gastric system, or in the lungs. The metabolites are most often inactive forms of the parent that are more water soluble than the parent drug and can therefore be excreted in the urine. In some instances, metabolism is required to convert a biologically inactive drug (prodrug) to an active form. Dopamine does not cross the blood-brain barrier; however, levodopa, an inactive precursor of dopamine, does cross the blood-brain barrier where it is metabolized to dopamine. In other cases, metabolism results in active metabolites (imipramine metabolizes to desipramine).

Hepatic metabolism is a result of specific enzymes and can be influenced by other drugs. In particular, enzymes belonging to the cytochrome P450 family are frequently involved in drug metabolism. Some drugs stimulate an increase in specific enzyme activity which increases the metabolism breakdown of other drugs; thereby decreasing the availability of the second drug (eg, phenobarbital induces the enzyme that metabolizes theophylline). Conversely, when a drug inhibits the enzyme activity necessary for metabolism of a second drug, toxic levels of the second drug can result (eg, cimetidine inhibits the enzyme that metabolizes theophylline; theophylline metabolism is inhibited thereby causing an elevated theophylline level). Much has been learned about the specific pathways by which certain drugs are metabolized, allowing more accurate prediction of potential interactions. Knowing that a drug is either an enzyme inhibitor or an enzyme inducer should cause a nurse monitoring drug effects to be alert for the effects of any other drugs that may be potentially affected.

Elimination via Excretion

Elimination via excretion is the process by which a drug or its metabolites is removed from the body.

Drugs can be eliminated through the lungs, kidneys, liver, skin, intestinal tract, or via excretory glands – in sweat, tears, saliva, or breast milk. Peritoneal dialysis or hemodialysis may also be used to remove drugs from the body.

Half-life is the time required for the blood levels of a drug to be diminished by one-half. This can be expressed as the percentage of the original concentration over time (eg, after one half-life 50% remains, after the second half-life 25%, third half-life 12.5%, etc). With normal functioning excretion, the half-life of a drug will help to determine spacing of dosing schedules. While a true half-life of a drug is specific to its persistence in an individual patient, it is a common practice to express this value as a population average measured in clinical trials. Because of this, it is important to recognize that the half-life in an individual patient can vary considerably, and may be substantially different in patients with organ dysfunction or deficiencies in metabolizing enzymes. For example, in the presence of decreased kidney function, elimination is slowed or delayed and more of the drug remains in the body than half-life figures from an otherwise healthy population would indicate. The actual half-life in these persons may be several times longer than the population average. Extended half-lives may result in higher drug accumulation. Elderly persons frequently have decreased kidney function as a part of the aging process – drugs excreted primarily via the kidneys thereby hold the potential for toxic levels for elderly persons when given in "normal" doses.

PHARMACODYNAMICS

Pharmacodynamics refers to the time course and relationships which determine how a drug brings about biophysical or biochemical changes.

Drug molecules must interact with specific receptors on target cell membranes in order to effect some biochemical or biophysical action. The drug-receptor interaction may alter or modify cellular function, at times activating new responses and/or previously unexpressed potential of the cell; however, drugs do not cause a new function in a cell or tissue. Action at the cellular level then impacts the tissue function in measurable or observable ways. For instance, insulin interacts with receptors to facilitate glucose transport across cellular membranes, this in turn causes a measurable decrease in serum glucose levels; atropine blocks acetylcholine receptors, which results in a decrease in the effects of acetylcholine (anticholinergic response; see Pharmacologic Category Index). The effects of drug and receptor interactions may be desired (beneficial) or nonbeneficial (adverse or side effects).

Most drug molecules can only interact with specific receptors. These may be located within the cell or on cellular membranes for which they have an affinity in a "lock-and-key" type bond. Following interaction with a receptor, a sequence of events may occur within the cell. Pathways in the cell may be activated to alter the production or activity of the cellular enzymes. In some cases, this involves the activation of specific genes. Drugs that stimulate receptor actions are called agonists. Drugs that fit to receptors and prevent or inhibit cellular responses to other drugs or endogenous compounds are called antagonists. In some instances, antagonist action is desirable (eg, naloxone competes with opioids for opioid receptors and may be used to reverse an opioid overdose).

Some drugs are extremely specific for one kind of receptor and some drugs are less specific so that they nonselectively stimulate all of a particular class of receptors. For instance, epinephrine will stimulate all beta-adrenergic receptors resulting in stimulation of both cardiac tissue and pulmonary smooth muscle tissue whereas terbutaline is more selective for beta$_2$ adrenergic receptors and resulting action is primarily on the smooth muscle of the lungs.

Several factors may also influence the number of specific receptors (up-regulation or down-regulation) and their ability to couple with other drugs or endogenous substances. The changes in number of receptors (increase or decrease) or sensitivity may result in drug tolerance (eg, biogenic amines [antidepressants]). The rebound phenomena that follows abrupt withdrawal of some drugs is related to an increase in the availability of receptor sites as the drug is released from the receptor (ie, clonidine). Disease states can influence number and responsiveness of receptors (eg, thyroid hormones can increase the number of beta receptors and their sensitivity to catecholamines in cardiac muscle, which may account for the tachycardia of thyrotoxicosis). Age can decrease responsiveness to insulin. Pharmacodynamics are normally associated with changes in drug concentrations (pharmacokinetics). In other words, the concentration of available drug in systemic circulation as determined by pharmacokinetic properties (bioavailability, metabolism, and excretion) have direct influence on the degree of biophysical or biochemical changes effected by drugs or pharmacodynamics.

Ideally, the dose of a drug should achieve the desired response without the occurrence of adverse effects. Unfortunately, with some drugs, the onset of adverse effects occurs before therapeutic dosage levels can be reached. This precludes the use of this drug. Fortunately, many drugs have a fairly wide window of safety (eg, the relationship between effective dosing levels and adverse effects is wide enough so that adverse or toxic responses can be minimalized). Some drugs, however, have a very narrow therapeutic index (TI); the range between therapeutic effect and toxic response is very small. Drugs with a narrow TI should be monitored (physical assessment and/or serum drug levels) on a regular basis (eg, lithium, digoxin, phenytoin, theophylline, etc).

PATIENT FACTORS THAT INFLUENCE DRUG THERAPY

Many factors related to an individual patient, or a group of similar patients, can impact the pharmacokinetics of drugs and relate to adverse reactions.

Pregnancy / Lactation

The changes that occur during pregnancy may necessitate dosage changes for some drugs. Decreased gastric tract motility, increased blood volume, decreased protein binding sites, and increased glomerular filtration rates may alter the degree of anticipated pharmacotherapeutic response.

Primarily, the concern about drugs during pregnancy is the effect of drugs on the fetus, either teratogenic (causing birth defects) or systemic (causing addiction). Although many drugs cross the placenta, the type of drug, the concentration of that drug, and the gestational age at time of exposure of the fetus are primary determinants of fetal reaction. When prescribing or administering drugs to any childbearing age female, it is vital to ask when her last menstrual period was and, if necessary, to wait for the results of a pregnancy test before starting any drug therapy. Of course, it is best to avoid all drugs during pregnancy, however, in some cases, the physiological context (ie, cardiac output, renal blood flow, etc) may be altered enough to require the use of drugs that are not needed by the same woman when not pregnant.

Most systematically absorbed drugs have been assigned a pregnancy risk factor based on the drugs potential to cause birth defects. This permits an evaluation of the risk:benefit ratio when prescribing or administering drugs becomes necessary. Drugs in the risk factor class "A" are generally considered to be safe for use during pregnancy, class "X" drugs are never safe and are known to be positively teratogenic. See Pregnancy Categories on page 12.

Contraception note: Many drugs will interact with and decrease the effect of oral contraceptives (eg, barbiturates, protease inhibitors, rifampin, and carbamazepine). When a second drug will decrease the effect of oral contraceptives, the patient needs to be educated about the necessity for using a "barrier" (nonhormonal) form of contraception. Barrier contraception (alone or in combination with some form of oral contraception) is often recommended for the patient who must take selected drugs with pregnancy risk factors "D" (idarubicin) or class "X" (isotretinoin).

Because many drugs and substances used by a mother appear in breast milk, care must be taken to evaluate the drug effects on the lactating woman and the infant. Some drugs are identified as being clearly contraindicated during lactation, others may cross into breast milk but adverse side effects on the fetus have not been identified, and for some drugs the administration times should be distanced from nursing time. Nurses should advise lactating women about the effects that drugs may have on the infant.

Age

All pharmacokinetics (absorption, distribution, metabolism, and excretion) are different in infants, young adults, and elderly patients. Elderly patients may have mildly decreased or severely decreased blood flow to all organs, gastric motility may be slowed, kidney function may be reduced, decreased nutrition may result in decreased albumin, and sedentary lifestyles may have an impact on drug response. Slower gastric motility means that absorption is slowed, resulting in longer time periods to clinical response. Decreased blood flow means that distribution is altered, resulting in decreased response or longer response time. Excretion may be altered with decreased glomerular filtration rates or slower gastric emptying which can result in increased levels of drug remaining in the system.

The ratio between total body water and total body fat also changes with age; older persons have decreased amounts of total body water and higher body fat. This aspect of aging also influences the blood concentration of some drugs. In a person with increased body fat, fat-soluble drugs are distributed to tissues more than to plasma; resulting in a longer response time as the drug must then be redistributed from tissue to plasma. The idiosyncratic response incidence also increases with an aging population. Responses to drugs may be both more exaggerated or diminished with the "usual" doses of some drugs.

In addition, and of major concern with elderly patients, is the incidence of poly-pharmacy; the increased numbers of drugs the patient may be taking. Older patients may have 2, 3, 4, or 5 (or more) chronic conditions for which they are taking medication. In addition, they may be seeing a different prescriber for each of these conditions. Often, it is a nurse who identifies and coordinates the care of these elderly patients, and the nurse must be aware of the possibility for increased incidence of adverse effects.

Body Weight / Build

Most "recommended" dosages of drugs are based on the average size, young or middle aged adult (usually males). Extremely obese or extremely thin patients may be prone to adverse effects as a result of "nonindividualized" prescribing. Serum creatinine is a breakdown product of skeletal muscle and its levels in the serum are frequently used to estimate renal function. Decreased muscle mass can result in reduced creatinine from muscle breakdown, leading to a serum creatinine, which is artificially low or appears normal. When dosing is based on estimated creatinine clearance (which is calculated based on the serum creatinine) rather than "actual" creatinine clearance, normal doses may be administered to patients with a diminished capacity for excretion, potentially leading to accumulation and toxicity. This is a particular problem in elderly and/or debilitated patients.

Smoking, Alcohol, Nutrition, and Hydration

Smoking has a direct impact on liver enzyme activity, blood flow, and the central nervous system. Excessive alcohol intake impacts liver enzymes, renal function, and has an additive effect with most antipsychotic, sedative, or anxiolytic medications, as well as altering responses to many other medications. Nutrition and hydration also play an important part in drug responses and possible adverse reactions. Poor hydration may result in reduced blood flow and excretion. Decreased or prolonged gastric motility can result in slowed excretion and/or prolonged absorption. Poor or inadequate nutrition may result in decreased protein available for binding.

It is vital that a patient's current habits are considered when prescribing, administering, or monitoring drug therapy, but in addition, patients must be aware of the need to inform their professional care provider that they have changed their smoking, alcohol, or dietary patterns. When dosage of theophylline is based on the fact that the patient is a smoker, the theophylline dosage must be adjusted to prevent overdose, if the patient quits smoking. When a patient is on warfarin, drastic increases in the amount of vitamin K intake through increased green leafy vegetables can dramatically alter the dose of warfarin.

Other Patient Factors That Influence Drug Response

- Genetic variations
- Differences in circadian patterns
- Disease states
- Psychological temperament

Genetic differences in enzymes may influence the effectiveness of therapy or the incidence of adverse effects (fast acetylators or slow acetylators). The emerging science of pharmacogenomics is devoted to the investigation of these genetic differences in drug response, and offers the hope of truly individualized therapy. Circadian rhythms differ among individuals and have an impact on absorption patterns, hormone secretion, or urinary excretion patterns. Disease states can and do change all aspects of pharmacokinetics. Cirrhosis can impair liver enzyme metabolism rate. Kidney disease will reduce excretion rates for many drugs. Abnormal thyroid function can influence drug metabolism. Diseases which affect blood circulation (eg, hypertension, CHF, Raynaud's phenomena, malignancies, etc) can have an impact on absorption, distribution, and excretion. Diabetes impacts the response to many drugs. Malnutrition, commonly associated with disease, can drastically reduce albumin levels.

PHARMACOTHERAPEUTICS

Drug therapy is used for treatment of disease or symptoms of diseases (empiric, supportive, maintenance, or palliative), for prevention (immunization), and for diagnosis (iodine, barium). In some cases, drugs may be used to correct imbalances or improve regulation of excessive physiological responses.

Optimal drug therapy should be both effective and safe. It needs to be tailored to the patient and the problem (see Patient Factors That Influence Drug Therapy). Assessing the problem is the first step, this involves identifying the problem (eg, etiology, laboratory confirmation, subjective and objective symptoms, urgency, severity, and prognosis) and determining what is the goal of therapy. Identifying and assessing the various options require knowledge of what drug therapy is appropriate. These steps lead to clinical decision-making (eg, selecting the drug regimen that is appropriate to meet the goal for this patient).

While professionals responsible for prescribing medications usually select therapy, the implementing of therapy is often a responsibility of nurses, in collaboration with pharmacists. Implementing therapy includes not only the preparation and dispensing of the drug, but also the education of those individual(s) who will administer the drug: nurses, patients, and family members. A major aspect of the education of patients includes how to administer the drug, when to administer the drug, and any dietary or drug-related precautions.

Monitoring the results of that therapy is a major responsibility that involves the prescriber, pharmacist, nurse, patient, and other healthcare providers. A major aspect of monitoring is communicating the subjective and objective responses to the responsible prescriber. Patients, nurses, and other caregivers must know the anticipated results of drug therapy and how to assess and report possible adverse effects.

The design, implementation, and monitoring of drug therapy in an individual patient is a complex and time-consuming task, requiring participation of many members of the healthcare team. Several common types of problems may be encountered in drug therapy. These include omissions of potentially beneficial drugs from the regimen, duplications in therapy, selection/titration to the appropriate dosage, the identification and management of drug interactions, and the identification and management of adverse reactions. An awareness of these potential problems is essential to enhance the safety of drug therapy.

Drug Interactions

Drug interactions are a major concern in drug therapy. Interactions may occur between food and drugs or between different drugs (ie, over-the-counter drugs, herbals, home remedies, and prescription drugs). Careful assessment of **ALL** substances patients are using to treat themselves is imperative for safe drug therapy. Patients may not consider some of the substances they use to treat themselves as drugs and nurses may need to be highly sensitive and very aware when they discuss this subject with the patient.

The potential for drug interactions increases exponentially with the number of drugs a person is taking. Thus, the more illnesses a patient has, the more likely it is he/she will be taking multiple drugs, and the more likely he/she will be to experience drug interactions.

Drugs can interact with other drugs to produce additive effects (when combined they produce similar cumulative effects with a lesser dose of either drug than they would alone), synergistic effects (the combination produces a greater response than either alone), or antagonistic effect (one drug negates or reverses the effect of the other drug). Such interactions can be a result of altering the pharmacokinetics of the drugs involved; increasing or decreasing either the rate or the quantity in absorption, altering the distribution through competitive receptor binding, changing the metabolism by inducing or reducing actions of liver enzymes, altering blood flow, or excretion by altering renal clearance.

Food, alcohol, and cigarette smoking can interact with drugs. Absorption of some drugs is enhanced with high fat meals (griseofulvin) or by low protein or high carbohydrate meals (theophylline). Whereas, absorption of some drugs is slowed, rather than blocked, when the stomach is full and gastric transport is slowed. Other drugs can bind with food to impair or prevent absorption of food byproducts such as carbohydrates or vitamins (eg, cholestyramine, mineral oil). Some drugs, such as isotretinoin, are isomers of vitamins and dietary intake of vitamin A can cause overdose reactions.

Other foods can produce pharmacologic activity on their own and when the patient is also taking a medication that is designed to result in that same pharmacologic activity the result may be life-threatening. For instance, patients using a monoamine oxidase (MAO) inhibitor should avoid foods containing tyramines or tryptophan to prevent excess release of catecholamines resulting in severe potentially life-threatening effects.

Drugs can also impact the results of laboratory tests. This is the basis for instructions from the laboratory to "hold" certain medications prior to some laboratory tests.

Adverse Drug Reactions

Adverse reactions to drug therapy can range from mild to debilitating and life-threatening. Mild reactions may either be not severe enough to discontinue the drug or will disappear when the drug is discontinued. Severe or life-threatening reactions may require immediate discontinuance, treatment with other drugs, or dialysis. Adverse reactions may be related to the dosing, they may be inherent in the drug's primary actions, they may be iatrogenic to the drug, or they may be related to individual patient sensitivity or genetics.

Dose-related side effects can be addressed through careful dosage adjustment. Adverse effects associated with inherent properties of the drugs (constipation with opiates or some pain medications) can be addressed through appropriate interventions (ie, increasing fluids, fiber in diets, increased exercise, or stool softeners). Iatrogenic effects (ie, GI irritation and bleeding from aspirin or indomethacin, orthostatic hypotension from antihypertensives) can be reduced by taking a complete patient history, by patient administration and precaution education (eg, safe dose, time, diet, activity, etc), by prescribing another drug to address the anticipated iatrogenic response, or by choosing another drug for treatment. Thorough knowledge of the possible adverse effects, coupled with anticipatory action, will reduce the incidence of adverse side effects.

True allergic responses usually result from previous exposure to one drug or drugs with related chemical composition that sensitizes the patient's immune system. Careful drug histories and assessment of a patient's reported previous adverse responses will help in averting allergic reactions. Idiosyncratic responses are those that are specific to that patient and are generally unpredictable, although many times these are genetically determined.

ALPHABETICAL LISTING OF DRUGS

- **A-200® Lice Treatment Kit [OTC]** *see* Pyrethrins and Piperonyl Butoxide *on page 1530*
- **A-200® Maximum Strength [OTC]** *see* Pyrethrins and Piperonyl Butoxide *on page 1530*

Abacavir (a BAK a veer)

U.S. Brand Names Ziagen®

Index Terms Abacavir Sulfate; ABC

Generic Availability (U.S.) No

Pharmacologic Category Antiretroviral Agent, Reverse Transcriptase Inhibitor (Nucleoside)

Medication Guide Available Yes

Pregnancy Risk Factor C

Lactation Excretion in breast milk unknown/contraindicated

Use Treatment of HIV infections in combination with other antiretroviral agents

Mechanism of Action/Effect Nucleoside reverse transcriptase inhibitor which interferes with HIV viral RNA-dependent DNA polymerase resulting in inhibition of viral replication

Contraindications Hypersensitivity to abacavir or any component of the formulation (do not rechallenge patients who have experienced hypersensitivity to abacavir regardless of *HLA-B*5701* status); moderate-to-severe hepatic impairment

Warnings/Precautions Abacavir should always be used as a component of a multidrug regimen. **[U.S. Boxed Warning]: Serious and sometimes fatal hypersensitivity reactions have occurred.** Patients testing positive for the presence of the *HLA-B*5701* allele are at an increased risk for hypersensitivity reactions. Screening for *HLA-B*5701* allele status is recommended prior to initiating therapy or reinitiating therapy in patients of unknown status, including patients who previously tolerated therapy. Therapy is **not** recommended in patients testing positive for the *HLA-B*5701* allele. An allergy to abacavir should be reported in the patient's medical record (DHHS, 2011). Reactions usually occur within 9 days of starting abacavir; ~90% occur within 6 weeks. Patients exhibiting symptoms from two or more of the following: Fever, skin rash, constitutional symptoms (malaise, fatigue, aches), respiratory symptoms (eg, pharyngitis, dyspnea, cough), and GI symptoms (eg, abdominal pain, diarrhea, nausea, vomiting) should discontinue therapy immediately and call for medical attention. Abacavir should be permanently discontinued if hypersensitivity cannot be ruled out, even when other diagnoses are possible and regardless of *HLA-B*5701* status. Abacavir SHOULD NOT be restarted because more severe symptoms may occur within hours, including LIFE-THREATENING HYPOTENSION AND DEATH. Fatal hypersensitivity reactions have occurred following the reintroduction of abacavir in patients whose therapy was interrupted (ie, interruption in drug supply, temporary discontinuation while treating other conditions). In some cases, signs of hypersensitivity may have been previously present, but attributed to other medical conditions (eg, acute onset respiratory diseases, gastroenteritis, reactions to other medications). If abacavir is restarted following an interruption in therapy, evaluate the patient for previously unsuspected symptoms of hypersensitivity. To report these events on abacavir hypersensitivity, a registry has been established (1-800-270-0425).

[U.S. Boxed Warning]: Lactic acidosis and severe hepatomegaly with steatosis (sometimes fatal) have occurred with antiretroviral nucleoside analogues. Female gender, prior liver disease, obesity, and prolonged treatment may increase the risk of hepatotoxicity. May be associated with fat redistribution. Immune reconstitution syndrome may develop; further evaluation and treatment may be required. Use has been associated with an increased risk of myocardial infarction (MI) in observational studies; however, based on a meta-analysis of 26 randomized trials, the FDA has concluded there is not an increased risk. Consider using with caution in patients with risks for coronary heart disease and minimizing modifiable risk factors (eg, hypertension, hyperlipidemia, diabetes mellitus, and smoking) prior to use. Products may contain propylene glycol. Safety and efficacy in children <3 months of age have not been established.

Drug Interactions

Avoid Concomitant Use There are no known interactions where it is recommended to avoid concomitant use.

Decreased Effect

The levels/effects of Abacavir may be decreased by: Protease Inhibitors

Increased Effect/Toxicity

The levels/effects of Abacavir may be increased by: Ganciclovir-Valganciclovir; Ribavirin

Nutritional/Ethanol Interactions Ethanol: Ethanol may increase the risk of toxicity.

Adverse Reactions Hypersensitivity reactions (which may be fatal) occur in ~5% of patients (see Warnings/Precautions). Symptoms may include anaphylaxis, fever, rash (including erythema multiforme), fatigue, diarrhea, abdominal pain; respiratory symptoms (eg, pharyngitis, dyspnea, cough, adult respiratory distress syndrome, or respiratory failure); headache, malaise, lethargy, myalgia, myolysis, arthralgia, edema, paresthesia, nausea and vomiting, mouth ulcerations, conjunctivitis, lymphadenopathy, hepatic failure, and renal failure.

Note: Rates of adverse reactions were defined during combination therapy with other antiretrovirals (lamivudine and efavirenz **or** lamivudine and zidovudine). Only reactions which occurred at a higher frequency in adults (except where noted) than in the comparator group are noted. Adverse reaction rates attributable to abacavir alone are not available.

>10%:

Central nervous system: Headache (7% to 13%)

Gastrointestinal: Nausea (7% to 19%, children 9%)

1% to 10%:

Central nervous system: Depression (6%), fever/chills (6%, children 9%), anxiety (5%)

Dermatologic: Rash (5% to 6%, children 7%)
Endocrine & metabolic: Triglycerides increased (2% to 6%)
Gastrointestinal: Diarrhea (7%), vomiting (children 9%), amylase increased (2%)
Hematologic: Thrombocytopenia (1%)
Hepatic: AST increased (6%)
Neuromuscular & skeletal: Musculoskeletal pain (5% to 6%)
Miscellaneous: Hypersensitivity reactions (2% to 9%; may include reactions to other components of antiretroviral regimen), infection (ENT 5%)

Pharmacodynamics/Kinetics

Absorption Rapid and extensive absorption

Bioavailability 83%

Time to Peak 0.7-1.7 hours

Protein Binding 50%

Half-Life Elimination 1.5 hours

Metabolism Hepatic via alcohol dehydrogenase and glucuronyl transferase to inactive carboxylate and glucuronide metabolites

Excretion Primarily urine (as metabolites, 1.2% as unchanged drug); feces (16% total dose)

Available Dosage Forms

Solution, oral:
Ziagen®: 20 mg/mL (240 mL)

Tablet, oral:
Ziagen®: 300 mg

Dosing

Adult & Geriatric HIV treatment: Oral: 300 mg twice daily or 600 mg once daily in combination with other antiretroviral agents

Pediatric HIV treatment: Oral: 3 months to 16 years: 8 mg/kg body weight twice daily (maximum: 300 mg twice daily) in combination with other antiretroviral agents

Hepatic Impairment
Mild dysfunction (Child-Pugh score 5-6): 200 mg twice daily (oral solution is recommended)
Moderate-to-severe dysfunction (Child-Pugh score >6): Use is contraindicated by the manufacturer.

Administration

Oral May be administered with or without food.

Stability

Storage Store oral solution and tablets at controlled room temperature of 20°C to 25°C (68°F to 77°F). Oral solution may be refrigerated; do not freeze.

Monitoring and Teaching Issues

Laboratory Monitoring CBC with differential, serum creatine kinase, CD4 count, HIV RNA plasma levels, serum transaminases, triglycerides, serum amylase; *HLA-B*5701* genotype status prior to initiation of therapy and prior to reinitiation of therapy in patients of unknown *HLA-B*5701* status

Physical Assessment Assess closely for any previous exposure/allergy to abacavir and evaluate risk factors for heart disease prior to beginning treatment. Patient must be closely monitored for any sign of hypersensitivity reaction, which can occur within hours or at any time and may be fatal (can also occur at reintroduction with patients who have no history of previous reaction). Assess decrease in infections and progression of disease, viral load, and CD4 count.

Patient Education You will be provided with a medication guide to help educate you about the medication and a warning card summarizing symptoms of hypersensitivity. This drug will not cure HIV, nor has it been found to reduce transmission of HIV; use appropriate precautions to prevent spread to other persons. This drug is prescribed as one part of a multidrug combination; take exactly as directed for full course of therapy. Maintain adequate hydration, unless instructed to restrict fluids. Avoid alcohol. Frequent blood tests may be required. May cause dizziness, weakness, nausea, and vomiting. Seek immediate emergency care if you experience unusual chest pain, palpitations, or if you suspect you are having a heart attack. Stop drug and report immediately symptoms of hypersensitivity (eg, fever; rash; fatigue, malaise, lethargy; persistent nausea, vomiting, diarrhea, abdominal pain; mouth sores; sore throat, cough, difficulty breathing; headache; swelling of face, mouth or throat; numbness or loss of sensation; pain, tingling, or numbness in toes, feet, muscles or joints; swollen glands; alterations in urinary pattern; swelling of extremities or weight gain). Do not restart without specific instruction by your prescriber.

Dietary Considerations May be taken with or without food.

Breast-Feeding Considerations In infants born to mothers who are HIV positive, HAART while breast-feeding may decrease postnatal infection. However, maternal or infant antiretroviral therapy does not completely eliminate the risk of postnatal HIV transmission. In addition, multiclass-resistant virus has been detected in breast-feeding infants despite maternal therapy.

In the United States where formula is accessible, affordable, safe, and sustainable, complete avoidance of breast-feeding by HIV-infected women is recommended to decrease potential transmission of HIV.

Pregnancy Considerations Adverse events have been observed in some animal reproduction studies. It is not known if abacavir crosses the human placenta. No increased risk of overall birth defects has been observed following first trimester exposure according to data collected by the antiretroviral pregnancy registry. Cases of lactic acidosis/hepatic steatosis syndrome related to mitochondrial toxicity have been reported in pregnant women receiving nucleoside analogues. It is not known if pregnancy itself potentiates this known side effect;

however, women may be at increased risk of lactic acidosis and liver damage. In addition, these adverse events are similar to other rare but life-threatening syndromes which occur during pregnancy (eg, HELLP syndrome). Hepatic enzymes and electrolytes should be monitored frequently during the third trimester of pregnancy in women receiving nucleoside analogues and clinicians should watch for early signs of the syndrome. The pharmacokinetics of abacavir are not significantly changed by pregnancy and dose adjustment is not needed for pregnant women. The Perinatal HIV Guidelines Working Group considers abacavir to be an alternative NRTI in dual nucleoside combination regimens.

Healthcare providers are encouraged to enroll pregnant women exposed to antiretroviral medications in the Antiretroviral Pregnancy Registry (1-800-258-4263 or www.APRegistry.com). Healthcare providers caring for HIV-infected women and their infants may contact the National Perinatal HIV Hotline (888-448-8765) for clinical consultation.

Additional Information A high rate of early virologic nonresponse was observed when abacavir, lamivudine, and tenofovir were used as the initial regimen in treatment-naive patients. Use of this combination is not recommended; patients currently on this regimen should be closely monitored for modification of therapy. Use regimens of abacavir and nevirapine with caution; both agents cause hypersensitivity reactions early in therapy (DHHS, 2011).

Hypersensitivity testing (*HLA-B*5701*): Prevalence of hypersensitivity reactions has been estimated at 5% to 8% in Caucasians and 2% to 3% in African-Americans. Pretherapy identification of *HLA-B*5701*-positive patients, and subsequent avoidance of abacavir therapy in these patients has been shown to reduce the occurrence of abacavir-mediated hypersensitivity reactions. An allergy to abacavir should be reported in the patient's medical record (DHHS, 2011). A skin patch test is in development for clinical screening purposes; however, only PCR-mediated genotyping methods are currently in clinical practice use for documentation of this susceptibility marker.

Abacavir and Lamivudine (a BAK a veer & la MI vyoo deen)

U.S. Brand Names Epzicom®

Index Terms Abacavir Sulfate and Lamivudine; Lamivudine and Abacavir

Generic Availability (U.S.) No

Pharmacologic Category Antiretroviral Agent, Reverse Transcriptase Inhibitor (Nucleoside)

Medication Guide Available Yes

Pregnancy Risk Factor C

Lactation See individual agents.

Use Treatment of HIV infections in combination with other antiretroviral agents

Available Dosage Forms

Tablet:

Epzicom®: Abacavir 600 mg and lamivudine 300 mg

Dosing

Adult HIV: Oral: One tablet (abacavir 600 mg and lamivudine 300 mg) once daily

Renal Impairment Cl_{cr} <50 mL/minute: Use not recommended

Hepatic Impairment Use contraindicated.

Administration

Oral May be administered with or without food.

Monitoring and Teaching Issues

Laboratory Monitoring Amylase, bilirubin, blood glucose, serum creatine kinase, liver enzymes, hematologic parameters, triglycerides, viral load, and CD4 count, *HLA-B*5701* genotype status prior to initiation of therapy and prior to reinitiation of therapy in patients of unknown *HLA-B*5701* status

Physical Assessment See individual agents.

Patient Education See individual agents.

Abacavir, Lamivudine, and Zidovudine
(a BAK a veer, la MI vyoo deen, & zye DOE vyoo deen)

U.S. Brand Names Trizivir®

Index Terms 3TC, Abacavir, and Zidovudine; Azidothymidine, Abacavir, and Lamivudine; AZT, Abacavir, and Lamivudine; Compound S, Abacavir, and Lamivudine; Lamivudine, Abacavir, and Zidovudine; ZDV, Abacavir, and Lamivudine; Zidovudine, Abacavir, and Lamivudine

Generic Availability (U.S.) No

Pharmacologic Category Antiretroviral Agent, Reverse Transcriptase Inhibitor (Nucleoside)

Medication Guide Available Yes

Pregnancy Risk Factor C

Lactation See individual agents.

Use Treatment of HIV infection (either alone or in combination with other antiretroviral agents) in patients whose regimen would otherwise contain the components of Trizivir®

Available Dosage Forms

Tablet, oral:

Trizivir®: Abacavir 300 mg, lamivudine 150 mg, and zidovudine 300 mg

Dosing

Adult HIV treatment: Oral: 1 tablet twice daily. **Note:** Not recommended for patients <40 kg.

Geriatric Use with caution.

Pediatric HIV treatment: Adolescents: Refer to adult dosing (not recommended for patients <40 kg).

Renal Impairment Cl_{cr} ≤50 mL/minute: Avoid use.

Hepatic Impairment Use contraindicated.

Administration

Oral Administer without regard to food or water.

Monitoring and Teaching Issues

Laboratory Monitoring Blood glucose, CBC with differential, serum creatine kinase, CD4 count, HIV RNA plasma levels, bilirubin, serum transaminases, triglycerides, serum amylase; *HLA-B*5701* genotype status prior to initiation of therapy and prior to reinitiation of therapy in patients of unknown *HLA-B*5701* status

Physical Assessment See individual agents.

Patient Education See individual agents.

Related Information

Abacavir *on page 30*

LamiVUDine *on page 1054*

Zidovudine *on page 1890*

◆ **Abacavir Sulfate** *see* Abacavir *on page 30*

◆ **Abacavir Sulfate and Lamivudine** *see* Abacavir and Lamivudine *on page 32*

Abatacept (ab a TA sept)

U.S. Brand Names Orencia®

Index Terms BMS-188667; CTLA-4Ig

Generic Availability (U.S.) No

Pharmacologic Category Antirheumatic, Disease Modifying

Medication Safety Issues

Sound-alike/look-alike issues:

Orencia® may be confused with Oracea®

Pregnancy Risk Factor C

Lactation Excretion in breast milk unknown/not recommended

Use

Treatment of moderately- to severely-active adult rheumatoid arthritis (RA); may be used as monotherapy or in combination with other DMARDs

Treatment of moderately- to severely-active juvenile idiopathic arthritis (JIA); may be used as monotherapy or in combination with methotrexate

Note: Abatacept should **not** be used in combination with anakinra or TNF-blocking agents

Mechanism of Action/Effect Prevents activation of T cells

Contraindications There are no contraindications listed within the FDA-approved labeling.

Warnings/Precautions Caution should be exercised when considering the use of abatacept in patients with a history of recurrent infections, with conditions that predispose them to infections, or with chronic, latent, or localized infections. Patients who develop a new infection while undergoing treatment should be monitored closely. If a patient develops a serious infection, abatacept should be discontinued. Screen patients for latent tuberculosis infection prior to initiating abatacept; safety in tuberculosis-positive patients has not been established. Treat patients testing positive according to standard therapy prior to initiating abatacept. Adult patients receiving abatacept in combination with TNF-blocking agents had higher rates of infections (including serious infections) than patients on TNF-blocking agents alone. The manufacturer does not recommend concurrent use with anakinra or TNF-blocking agents. Monitor for signs and symptoms of infection when transitioning from TNF-blocking agents to abatacept. Due to the affect of T-cell inhibition on host defenses, abatacept may affect immune responses against infections and malignancies; impact on the development and course of malignancies is not fully defined.

Use caution with chronic obstructive pulmonary disease (COPD), higher incidences of adverse effects (COPD exacerbation, cough, rhonchi, dyspnea) have been observed; monitor closely. Rare cases of hypersensitivity, anaphylaxis, or anaphylactoid reactions have been reported; medications for the treatment of hypersensitivity reactions should be available for immediate use. Patients should be screened for viral hepatitis prior to use; antirheumatic therapy may cause reactivation of hepatitis B. Patients should be brought up to date with all immunizations before initiating therapy. Live vaccines should not be given concurrently or within 3 months of discontinuation of therapy; there is no data available concerning secondary transmission of live vaccines in patients receiving therapy. May contain maltose, which may result in falsely-elevated serum glucose readings on the day of infusion. Higher incidences of infection and malignancy were observed in the elderly; use with caution.

Drug Interactions

Avoid Concomitant Use

Avoid concomitant use of Abatacept with any of the following: Anti-TNF Agents; BCG; Belimumab; Natalizumab; Pimecrolimus; Roflumilast; Tacrolimus (Topical); Vaccines (Live)

Decreased Effect

Abatacept may decrease the levels/effects of: BCG; Sipuleucel-T; Vaccines (Inactivated); Vaccines (Live)

The levels/effects of Abatacept may be decreased by: Echinacea

Increased Effect/Toxicity

Abatacept may increase the levels/effects of: Belimumab; Leflunomide; Natalizumab; Vaccines (Live)

The levels/effects of Abatacept may be increased by: Anti-TNF Agents; Denosumab; Pimecrolimus; Roflumilast; Tacrolimus (Topical); Trastuzumab

Nutritional/Ethanol Interactions Herb/Nutraceutical: Avoid echinacea (has immunostimulant properties; consider therapy modifications).

Lab Interactions Contains maltose; may result in falsely elevated blood glucose levels with dehydrogenase pyrroloquinolinequinone or glucose-dye-oxidoreductase testing methods on the day of infusion. Glucose monitoring methods which utilize glucose dehydrogenase nicotine adenine dinucleotide (GDH-NAD), glucose oxidase, or glucose hexokinase are recommended.

Adverse Reactions Note: Percentages not always reported; COPD patients experienced a higher frequency of COPD-related adverse reactions (COPD exacerbation, cough, dyspnea, pneumonia, rhonchi)

>10%:

Central nervous system: Headache (≤18%)
Gastrointestinal: Nausea
Respiratory: Nasopharyngitis (12%), upper respiratory tract infection
Miscellaneous: Infection (adults 54%; children 36%), antibody formation (2% to 41%)

1% to 10%:

Cardiovascular: Hypertension (7%)
Central nervous system: Dizziness (9%), fever
Dermatologic: Rash (4%)
Gastrointestinal: Dyspepsia (6%), abdominal pain, diarrhea
Genitourinary: Urinary tract infection (6%)
Neuromuscular & skeletal: Back pain (7%), limb pain (3%)
Respiratory: Cough (8%), bronchitis, pneumonia, rhinitis, sinusitis
Miscellaneous: Infusion-related reactions (2% to 9%), herpes simplex, influenza

Pharmacodynamics/Kinetics

Half-Life Elimination 8-25 days

Available Dosage Forms

Injection, powder for reconstitution [preservative free]:
Orencia®: 250 mg

Dosing

Adult Rheumatoid arthritis: I.V.: Dosing is according to body weight. Repeat dose at 2 weeks and 4 weeks after initial dose, and every 4 weeks thereafter:

<60 kg: 500 mg
60-100 kg: 750 mg
>100 kg: 1000 mg

Geriatric Refer to adult dosing. Due to potential for higher rates of infections and malignancies, use caution.

Pediatric JIA: I.V.:

Children ≥6 years and <75 kg: 10 mg/kg, repeat dose at 2 and 4 weeks after initial infusion, and every 4 weeks thereafter

Children ≥6 years and >75 kg: **Note:** Dosage is according to body weight. Repeat dose at 2 weeks and 4 weeks after initial dose and every 4 weeks thereafter:

75-100 kg: 750 mg
>100 kg: 1000 mg

Adjustment for Toxicity Withhold therapy for patients with serious infections.

Administration

I.V. Infuse over 30 minutes. Administer through a 0.2-1.2 micron low protein-binding filter

Stability

Reconstitution Reconstitute each vial with 10 mL SWFI using the provided silicone-free disposable syringe (discard solutions accidentally reconstituted with siliconized syringe as they may develop translucent particles). Inject SWFI down the side of the vial to avoid foaming. The reconstituted solution contains 25 mg/mL abatacept. Further dilute (using a silicone-free syringe) in 100 mL NS to a final concentration of ≤10 mg/mL. Prior to adding abatacept to the 100 mL bag, the manufacturer recommends withdrawing a volume of NS equal to the abatacept volume required, resulting in a final volume of 100 mL. Mix gently; do not shake.

Storage Prior to reconstitution, store at 2°C to 8°C (36°F to 46°F). Protect from light. After dilution, may be stored for up to 24 hours at room temperature or refrigerated at 2°C to 8°C (36°F to 46°F). Must be used within 24 hours of reconstitution.

Monitoring and Teaching Issues

Laboratory Monitoring Hepatitis and TB screening prior to therapy initiation

Physical Assessment Perform testing for tuberculosis prior to initiating therapy. Assess for infection prior to initiating infusion.

Patient Education This drug can only be administered by infusion. You may be more susceptible to infections. Report signs of infection. May cause falsely elevated blood glucose readings on day of infusion. You may experience headache, sore throat, and nausea. Report immediately respiratory difficulty, hives, dizziness, nausea, flushing, cough, or wheezing.

Geriatric Considerations The number of elderly (≥65 years of age) were insufficient to draw significant clinical conclusions. The studies to date have not demonstrated any differences in safety and efficacy between young adults and elderly. However, the frequency of infections and malignancy was higher in those >65 years of age than those <65 years. Since elderly experience a higher incidence of infections and malignancies, use abatacept with caution in this population.

Breast-Feeding Considerations Due to the potential for adverse reactions and possible effects on the developing immune system, breast-feeding is not recommended.

Pregnancy Considerations Teratogenic effects were not observed in animal studies. There are no adequate and well-controlled studies in pregnant women. Due to the potential risk for development of autoimmune disease in the fetus, use during pregnancy only if clearly needed. A pregnancy registry has been established to monitor outcomes of women exposed to abatacept during pregnancy (1-877-311-8972).

◆ **Abbott-43818** *see* Leuprolide *on page* 1082

◆ **ABC** *see* Abacavir *on page* 30

◆ **ABCD** *see* Amphotericin B Cholesteryl Sulfate Complex *on page* 115

◆ **Abelcet®** *see* Amphotericin B (Lipid Complex) *on page* 119

◆ **ABI-007** *see* Paclitaxel (Protein Bound) *on page* 1390

◆ **Abilify®** *see* Aripiprazole *on page* 143

◆ **Abilify Discmelt®** *see* Aripiprazole *on page* 143

◆ **Ablavar™** *see* Gadofosveset *on page* 845

◆ **ABLC** *see* Amphotericin B (Lipid Complex) *on page* 119

◆ **Abraxane®** *see* Paclitaxel (Protein Bound) *on page* 1390

◆ **Abstral®** *see* FentaNYL *on page* 744

◆ **ABT-335** *see* Fenofibric Acid *on page* 742

◆ **ABX-EGF** *see* Panitumumab *on page* 1403

◆ **AC 2993** *see* Exenatide *on page* 726

Acamprosate (a kam PROE sate)

U.S. Brand Names Campral®

Index Terms Acamprosate Calcium; Calcium Acetylhomotaurinate

Generic Availability (U.S.) No

Pharmacologic Category GABA Agonist/Glutamate Antagonist

Pregnancy Risk Factor C

Lactation Excretion in breast milk unknown/use caution

Use Maintenance of alcohol abstinence

Mechanism of Action/Effect Mechanism not fully defined. Structurally similar to GABA, acamprosate appears to restore balance to GABA and glutamate activities which are disrupted in alcohol dependence. During therapeutic use, alcohol intake is reduced, but does not cause a disulfiram-like reaction following alcohol ingestion.

Contraindications Hypersensitivity to acamprosate or any component of the formulation; severe renal impairment (Cl_{cr} <30 mL/minute)

Warnings/Precautions Should be used as part of a comprehensive program to treat alcohol dependence. Treatment should be initiated as soon as possible following the period of alcohol withdrawal, when the patient has achieved abstinence. Acamprosate does not eliminate or diminish the symptoms of alcohol withdrawal. Use caution in moderate renal impairment (Cl_{cr} 30-50 mL/minute). Suicidal ideation, attempted and completed suicides have occurred in acamprosate-treated patients; monitor for depression and/or suicidal thinking. Traces of sulfites may be present in the formulation.

Drug Interactions

Avoid Concomitant Use There are no known interactions where it is recommended to avoid concomitant use.

Decreased Effect There are no known significant interactions involving a decrease in effect.

Increased Effect/Toxicity There are no known significant interactions involving an increase in effect.

Nutritional/Ethanol Interactions

Ethanol: Abstinence is required during treatment. Ethanol does not affect the pharmacokinetics of acamprosate; however, the continued use of ethanol will decrease desired efficacy of acamprosate.

Food: Food decreases absorption of acamprosate (not clinically significant).

Adverse Reactions Note: Many adverse effects associated with treatment may be related to alcohol abstinence; reported frequency range may overlap with placebo.

>10%: Gastrointestinal: Diarrhea (10% to 17%)

1% to 10%:

Cardiovascular: Syncope, palpitation, edema (peripheral)

Central nervous system: Insomnia (6% to 9%), anxiety (5% to 8%), depression (4% to 8%), dizziness (3% to 4%), pain (2% to 4%), paresthesia (2% to 3%), headache, somnolence, amnesia, tremor, chills

Dermatologic: Pruritus (3% to 4%), rash

Endocrine & metabolic: Weight gain, libido decreased

Gastrointestinal: Anorexia (2% to 5%), flatulence (1% to 3%), nausea (3% to 4%), abdominal pain, dry mouth (1% to 3%), vomiting, dyspepsia, constipation, appetite increased, taste perversion
Genitourinary: Impotence
Neuromuscular & skeletal: Weakness (5% to 7%), back pain, myalgia, arthralgia
Ocular: Abnormal vision
Respiratory: Rhinitis, dyspnea, pharyngitis, bronchitis
Miscellaneous: Diaphoresis (2% to 3%), suicide attempt

Pharmacodynamics/Kinetics

Bioavailability 11%

Protein Binding Negligible

Half-Life Elimination 20-33 hours

Metabolism Not metabolized

Excretion Urine (as unchanged drug)

Available Dosage Forms

Tablet, delayed release, enteric coated, oral:
Campral®: 333 mg

Dosing

Adult & Geriatric Alcohol abstinence: Oral: 666 mg 3 times/day (a lower dose may be effective in some patients).

Adjustment in patients with low body weight (unlabeled): A lower dose (4 tablets/day) may be considered in patients with low body weight (eg, <60 kg).

Note: Treatment should be initiated as soon as possible following the period of alcohol withdrawal, when the patient has achieved abstinence.

Renal Impairment

Cl_{cr} 30-50 mL/minute: Initial dose should be reduced to 333 mg 3 times/day.
Cl_{cr} <30 mL/minute: Contraindicated in severe renal impairment.

Administration

Oral May be administered without regard to meals. Tablet should be swallowed whole; do not crush or chew.

Stability

Storage Store at 25°C (77°F); excursions permitted to 15°C to 30°C (59°F to 86°F).

Monitoring and Teaching Issues

Physical Assessment May cause depression. Monitor for suicide ideation.

Patient Education Taking this medication helps maintain abstinence only when used as part of a treatment program that includes counseling and support. Swallow tablet whole. Do not chew or crush. Can cause drowsiness. You may experience diarrhea, peripheral edema, insomnia, anxiety, depression, and generalized weakness. Report persistent diarrhea, excessive or sudden weight gain, swelling of extremities, respiratory difficulties, fainting, or thoughts of suicide.

Dietary Considerations Abstinence is required during treatment. May be taken without regard to meals. Each 333 mg tablet contains 33 mg of elemental calcium.

Geriatric Considerations Initial studies did not include sufficient geriatric patients to be able to derive sufficient data to compare elderly to younger adults. Only 41 out of 4234 patients in clinical trials were ≥65 years of age with none ≥75 years. However, since this medication is cleared renally exclusively, caution should be used since many elderly have Cl_{cr} 30-50 mL/minute where dosage reduction is required (see Dosing).

Pregnancy Considerations Teratogenic in animal studies. No adequate or well-controlled studies in pregnant women; use only if potential benefit outweighs possible risk to the fetus.

- **Acamprosate Calcium** *see* Acamprosate *on page* 35
- **Acanya®** *see* Clindamycin and Benzoyl Peroxide *on page* 401

Acarbose (AY car bose)

U.S. Brand Names Precose®

Generic Availability (U.S.) Yes

Pharmacologic Category Antidiabetic Agent, Alpha-Glucosidase Inhibitor

Medication Safety Issues

Sound-alike/look-alike issues:
Precose® may be confused with PreCare®

International issues:
Precose® [U.S., Malaysia] may be confused with Precosa brand name for *Saccharomyces boulardii* [Finland, Sweden]

Pregnancy Risk Factor B

Lactation Excretion in breast milk unknown/not recommended

Use Adjunct to diet and exercise to lower blood glucose in patients with type 2 diabetes mellitus (noninsulin dependent, NIDDM)

Mechanism of Action/Effect Delays glucose absorption and lowers postprandial hyperglycemia.

Contraindications Hypersensitivity to acarbose or any component of the formulation; patients with diabetic ketoacidosis or cirrhosis; patients with inflammatory bowel disease, colonic ulceration, partial intestinal obstruction, or in patients predisposed to intestinal obstruction; patients who have chronic intestinal diseases associated with marked disorders of digestion or absorption, and in patients who have conditions that may deteriorate as a result of increased gas formation in the intestine

Warnings/Precautions Acarbose given in combination with a sulfonylurea or insulin will cause a further lowering of blood glucose and may increase the hypoglycemic potential of the sulfonylurea or insulin. Treatment-emergent elevations of serum transaminases (AST and/or ALT) occurred in up to 14% of acarbose-treated patients in long-term studies. These serum transaminase elevations appear to be dose related and were asymptomatic, reversible, more common in females, and, in general, were not associated with other evidence of liver dysfunction. Fulminant hepatitis has been reported rarely. It may be necessary to discontinue acarbose and administer insulin if the patient is exposed to stress (ie, fever, trauma, infection, surgery). Use not recommended in patients with significant impairment (S_{cr} >2 mg/dL); use with caution in other patients with renal impairment.

Drug Interactions

Avoid Concomitant Use There are no known interactions where it is recommended to avoid concomitant use.

Decreased Effect

Acarbose may decrease the levels/effects of: Digoxin

The levels/effects of Acarbose may be decreased by: Corticosteroids (Orally Inhaled); Corticosteroids (Systemic); Luteinizing Hormone-Releasing Hormone Analogs; Somatropin; Thiazide Diuretics

Increased Effect/Toxicity

Acarbose may increase the levels/effects of: Hypoglycemic Agents

The levels/effects of Acarbose may be increased by: Herbs (Hypoglycemic Properties); Pegvisomant

Nutritional/Ethanol Interactions Ethanol: Limit ethanol.

Adverse Reactions >10%:

Gastrointestinal: Diarrhea (31%) and abdominal pain (19%) tend to return to pretreatment levels over time; frequency and intensity of flatulence (74%) tend to abate with time

Hepatic: Transaminases increased (≤4%)

Pharmacodynamics/Kinetics

Absorption <2% as active drug, ~35% as metabolites

Bioavailability Low systemic bioavailability of parent compound; acts locally in GI tract

Time to Peak Active drug: ~1 hour

Half-Life Elimination ~2 hours

Metabolism Exclusively via GI tract, principally by intestinal bacteria and digestive enzymes; 13 metabolites identified (major metabolites are sulfate, methyl, and glucuronide conjugates)

Excretion Urine (~34% as inactive metabolites, <2% parent drug and active metabolite); feces (~51% as unabsorbed drug)

Available Dosage Forms

Tablet, oral: 25 mg, 50 mg, 100 mg

Precose®: 25 mg, 50 mg, 100 mg

Dosing

Adult & Geriatric Type 2 diabetes: Oral:

Initial: 25 mg 3 times/day with the first bite of each main meal; to reduce GI effects, some patients may benefit from initiating at 25 mg once daily with gradual titration to 25 mg 3 times/day as tolerated

Maintenance dose: Should be adjusted at 4- to 8-week intervals based on 1-hour postprandial glucose levels and tolerance until maintenance dose is reached; maintenance dose: 50-100 mg 3 times/day. Dosage must be individualized on the basis of effectiveness and tolerance while not exceeding the maximum recommended dose.

Maximum:

≤60 kg: 50 mg 3 times/day

>60 kg: 100 mg 3 times/day

Patients receiving sulfonylureas or insulin: Acarbose given in combination with a sulfonylurea or insulin will cause a further lowering of blood glucose and may increase the hypoglycemic potential of the sulfonylurea or insulin. If hypoglycemia occurs, appropriate adjustments in the dosage of these agents should be made.

Renal Impairment

Cl_{cr} <25 mL/minute: Peak plasma concentrations were 5 times higher and AUCs were 6 times larger than in volunteers with normal renal function.

Significant renal dysfunction (S_{cr} >2 mg/dL): Use is not recommended.

Administration

Oral Should be **administered with the first bite of each main meal.**

Stability

Storage Store at <25°C (77°F). Protect from moisture.

Monitoring and Teaching Issues

Laboratory Monitoring Postprandial glucose, glycosylated hemoglobin levels, and serum transaminase levels should be checked every 3 months during the first year of treatment and periodically thereafter, renal function (serum creatinine)

Physical Assessment Teach patient importance of diabetic control.

Patient Education Take this medication with the first bite of each main meal. Do not take other medications with or within 2 hours of this medication unless advised by prescriber. Avoid alcohol. It is important to follow dietary and lifestyle recommendations of prescriber. You will be instructed in signs of hyper-/hypoglycemia. If combining acarbose with other diabetic medication (eg, sulfonylureas, insulin), keep source of glucose in the form of dextrose (NOT table sugar, candy, or cookies) on hand in case hypoglycemia occurs. May cause mild side effects during first weeks of acarbose therapy (eg, bloating, flatulence, diarrhea, abdominal discomfort); these should diminish over time. Report severe or persistent side effects, fever, extended vomiting or flu, or change in color of urine or stool.

Dietary Considerations Take with food (first bite of meal).

Geriatric Considerations No specific trials in older adults have been conducted; mean age in clinical trials has been <60 years; monitor change in preprandial blood glucose concentrations to account for potential age-related changes in postprandial glucose. In clinical trials, elderly had serum concentrations 1.5 times those of younger adults. Patients with Cl_{cr} <25 mL/minute had serum concentrations 5 times those with normal renal clearance. No clinical significance can be attributed to this at this time. No adjustments in dose are recommended. Intensive glucose control (Hb A_{1c} <6.5%) has been linked to increased all cause and cardiovascular mortality, hypoglycemia requiring assistance, and weight gain in adult type 2 diabetes. For elderly patients with diabetes who are relatively healthy, attaining target goals for aspirin use, blood pressure, lipids, smoking cessation, and diet and exercise may be more important than normalized glycemic control.

Breast-Feeding Considerations It is not known if acarbose is found in breast milk; however, low amounts of acarbose are absorbed systemically in adults, which may limit the amount that could distribute into breast milk. Breast-feeding is not recommended by the manufacturer.

Pregnancy Considerations Adverse events have not been reported in animal reproduction studies; therefore, acarbose is classified as pregnancy category B. Low amounts of acarbose are absorbed systemically which should limit fetal exposure. Maternal hyperglycemia can be associated with adverse effects in the fetus, including macrosomia, neonatal hyperglycemia, and hyperbilirubinemia; the risk of congenital malformations is increased when the Hb A_{1c} is above the normal range. Diabetes can also be associated with adverse effects in the mother. Poorly-treated diabetes may cause end-organ damage that may in turn negatively affect obstetric outcomes. Physiologic glucose levels should be maintained prior to and during pregnancy to decrease the risk of adverse events in the mother and the fetus. Acarbose has been studied for its potential role in treating GDM; however, only limited information is available describing pregnancy outcomes. Until additional safety and efficacy data are obtained, the use of oral agents is generally not recommended as routine management of GDM or type 2 diabetes mellitus during pregnancy. Insulin is the drug of choice for the control of diabetes mellitus during pregnancy.

Related Information

Diabetes Mellitus Management, Adults *on page 2026*

- **Accolate®** *see* Zafirlukast *on page 1882*
- **AccuNeb®** *see* Albuterol *on page 58*
- **Accupril®** *see* Quinapril *on page 1538*
- **Accuretic®** *see* Quinapril and Hydrochlorothiazide *on page 1540*
- **ACE** *see* Captopril *on page 284*
- **Aceon®** *see* Perindopril Erbumine *on page 1442*
- **Acephen™ [OTC]** *see* Acetaminophen *on page 38*

Acetaminophen (a seet a MIN oh fen)

U.S. Brand Names Acephen™ [OTC]; APAP 500 [OTC]; Aspirin Free Anacin® Extra Strength [OTC]; Cetafen® Extra [OTC]; Cetafen® [OTC]; Excedrin® Tension Headache [OTC]; Fever-all® [OTC]; Genebs Extra Strength [OTC] [DSC]; Infantaire [OTC]; Little Fevers™ [OTC]; Mapap® Arthritis Pain [OTC]; Mapap® Children's [OTC]; Mapap® Extra Strength [OTC]; Mapap® Infant's [OTC]; Mapap® Junior Rapid Tabs [OTC]; Mapap® [OTC]; Nortemp Children's [OTC]; Ofirmev™; Pain & Fever Children's [OTC]; Pain Eze [OTC]; Silapap Children's [OTC]; Silapap Infant's [OTC]; Triaminic™ Children's Fever Reducer Pain Reliever [OTC]; Tylenol® 8 Hour [OTC]; Tylenol® Arthritis Pain Extended Relief [OTC]; Tylenol® Children's Meltaways [OTC]; Tylenol® Children's [OTC]; Tylenol® Extra Strength [OTC]; Tylenol® Infant's Concentrated [OTC]; Tylenol® Jr. Meltaways [OTC]; Tylenol® [OTC]; Valorin Extra [OTC]; Valorin [OTC]

Index Terms APAP; N-Acetyl-P-Aminophenol; Paracetamol

Generic Availability (U.S.) Yes: Excludes extended release products; injectable formulation

Pharmacologic Category Analgesic, Miscellaneous

Medication Safety Issues

Sound-alike/look-alike issues:

Acephen® may be confused with AcipHex®

FeverALL® may be confused with Fiberall®

Triaminic™ Children's Fever Reducer Pain Reliever may be confused with Triaminic® cough and cold products

Tylenol® may be confused with atenolol, timolol, Tuinal®, Tylenol® PM, Tylox®

International issues:

Depon [Greece] may be confused with Depen brand name for penicillamine [U.S.]; Depin brand name for nifedipine [India]; Dipen brand name for dilitazem [Greece]

Duorol [Spain] may be confused with Diuril brand name for chlorothiazide [U.S., Canada] and furosemide [Philippines]

Paralen [Czech Republic] may be confused with Aralen brand name for chloroquine [U.S., Mexico, and Philippines]

Duplicate therapy issues: This product contains acetaminophen, which may be a component of combination products. Do not exceed the maximum recommended daily dose of acetaminophen.

Pregnancy Risk Factor C

Lactation Enters breast milk/use caution (AAP rates "compatible"; AAP 2001 update pending)

Use Treatment of mild-to-moderate pain and fever (analgesic/antipyretic)

I.V.: Additional indication: Management of moderate-to-severe pain when combined with opioid analgesia

Mechanism of Action/Effect Reduces fever by acting on the hypothalamus to cause vasodilatation and sweating

Contraindications Hypersensitivity to acetaminophen or any component of the formulation; severe hepatic impairment or severe active liver disease (Ofirmev™)

Warnings/Precautions Limit dose to <4 g/day. May cause severe hepatotoxicity on acute overdose; in addition, chronic daily dosing in adults has resulted in liver damage in some patients. Use with caution in patients with alcoholic liver disease; consuming ≥3 alcoholic drinks/day may increase the risk of liver damage. Use caution in patients with hepatic impairment or active liver disease. Use of intravenous formulation is contraindicated in patients with severe hepatic impairment or severe active liver disease. Use caution in patients with known G6PD deficiency; rare reports of hemolysis have occurred. Use caution in patients with chronic malnutrition and hypovolemia (intravenous formulation). Use caution in patients with severe renal impairment; consider dosing adjustments. Hypersensitivity and anaphylactic reactions have been reported; discontinue immediately if symptoms of allergic or hypersensitivity reactions occur.

OTC labeling: When used for self-medication, patients should be instructed to contact healthcare provider if used for fever lasting >3 days or for pain lasting >10 days in adults or >5 days in children.

Drug Interactions

Metabolism/Transport Effects Substrate (minor) of CYP1A2, 2A6, 2C9, 2D6, 2E1, 3A4; **Inhibits** CYP3A4 (weak)

Avoid Concomitant Use There are no known interactions where it is recommended to avoid concomitant use.

Decreased Effect

The levels/effects of Acetaminophen may be decreased by: Anticonvulsants (Hydantoin); Barbiturates; CarBAMazepine; Cholestyramine Resin; Peginterferon Alfa-2b

Increased Effect/Toxicity

Acetaminophen may increase the levels/effects of: Dasatinib; Imatinib; SORAfenib; Vitamin K Antagonists

The levels/effects of Acetaminophen may be increased by: Conivaptan; Dasatinib; Imatinib; Isoniazid; Metyrapone; Probenecid; SORAfenib

Nutritional/Ethanol Interactions

Ethanol: Excessive intake of ethanol may increase the risk of acetaminophen-induced hepatotoxicity. Avoid ethanol or limit to <3 drinks/day.

Food: Rate of absorption may be decreased when given with food.

Herb/Nutraceutical: St John's wort may decrease acetaminophen levels.

Adverse Reactions Oral, Rectal: Frequency not defined:

Dermatologic: Rash

Endocrine & metabolic: May increase chloride, uric acid, glucose; may decrease sodium, bicarbonate, calcium

Hematologic: Anemia; blood dyscrasias (neutropenia, pancytopenia, leukopenia)

Hepatic: Bilirubin increased, alkaline phosphatase increased

Renal: Ammonia increased, nephrotoxicity with chronic overdose, analgesic nephropathy

Miscellaneous: Hypersensitivity reactions (rare)

I.V.:

>10%: Gastrointestinal: Nausea (adults 34%; children ≥5%), vomiting (adults 15%; children ≥5%)

1% to 10%:

Cardiovascular: Edema (peripheral), hypervolemia, hypo/hypertension, tachycardia

Central nervous system: Headache (adults 10%; children ≥1%), insomnia (adults 7%; children ≥1%), agitation (children ≥5%), anxiety, fatigue

Dermatologic: Pruritus (children ≥5%), rash

Endocrine & metabolic: Hypoalbuminemia, hypokalemia, hypomagnesemia, hypophosphatemia

Gastrointestinal: Constipation (children ≥5%), abdominal pain, diarrhea

Hematologic: Anemia

Hepatic: Transaminases increased

Local: Infusion site pain

Neuromuscular & skeletal: Muscle spasms, pain in extremity, trismus

Ocular: Periorbital edema

Renal: Oliguria (children ≥1%)

Respiratory: Atelectasis (children ≥5%), breath sounds abnormal, dyspnea, hypoxia, pleural effusion, pulmonary edema, stridor, wheezing

Pharmacodynamics/Kinetics

Onset of Action

Oral: <1 hour

I.V.: Analgesia: 5-10 minutes; Antipyretic: Within 30 minutes

Peak effect: I.V.: Analgesic: 1 hour

Duration of Action
I.V., Oral: Analgesia: 4-6 hours
I.V.: Antipyretic: ≥6 hours

Absorption Primarily absorbed in small intestine (rate of absorption dependent upon gastric emptying); minimal absorption from stomach; varies by dosage form

Time to Peak Serum: Oral: Immediate release: 10-60 minutes (may be delayed in acute overdoses); I.V.: 15 minutes

Protein Binding 10% to 25% at therapeutic concentrations; 8% to 43% at toxic concentrations

Half-Life Elimination Prolonged following toxic doses
Neonates: 7 hours (range: 4-10 hours)
Infants: ~4 hours (range: 1-7 hours)
Children: 3 hours (range: 2-5 hours)
Adolescents: ~3 hours (range: 2-4 hours)
Adults: ~2 hours (range: 2-3 hours); may be slightly prolonged in severe renal insufficiency (Cl_{cr}<30 mL/minute): 2-5.3 hours

Metabolism At normal therapeutic dosages, primarily hepatic metabolism to sulfate and glucuronide conjugates, while a small amount is metabolized by CYP2E1 to a highly reactive intermediate, N-acetyl-p-benzoquinone imine (NAPQI), which is conjugated rapidly with glutathione and inactivated to nontoxic cysteine and mercapturic acid conjugates. At toxic doses (as little as 4 g daily) glutathione conjugation becomes insufficient to meet the metabolic demand causing an increase in NAPQI concentrations, which may cause hepatic cell necrosis. Oral administration is subject to first pass metabolism.

Excretion Urine (<5% unchanged; 60% to 80% as glucuronide metabolites; 20% to 30% as sulphate metabolites; ~8% cysteine and mercapturic acid metabolites)

Available Dosage Forms For available OTC formulations, consult specific product labeling.

Dosing

Adult & Geriatric Note: No dose adjustment required if converting between different acetaminophen formulations.

Pain or fever:
Oral, rectal: 325-650 mg every 4-6 hours or 1000 mg 3-4 times/day; do **not** exceed 4 g/day
I.V.:
<50 kg: 15 mg/kg every 6 hours or 12.5 mg/kg every 4 hours; maximum single dose: 750 mg/dose; maximum daily dose: 75 mg/kg/day (≤3.75 g/day)
≥50 kg: 650 mg every 4 hours or 1000 mg every 6 hours; maximum single dose: 1000 mg/dose; maximum daily dose: 4 g/day

Pediatric Note: No dose adjustment required if converting between different acetaminophen formulations.

Pain or fever:
Oral, rectal: Children <12 years: 10-15 mg/kg/dose every 4-6 hours as needed; do **not** exceed 5 doses (2.6 g) in 24 hours; alternatively, the following age-based doses may be used; see table.

Acetaminophen Dosing (Oral and Rectal Formulations)

Age	Dosage (mg)	Age	Dosage (mg)
0-3 mo	40	4-5 y	240
4-11 mo	80	6-8 y	320
1-2 y	120	9-10 y	400
2-3 y	160	11 y	480

Note: Higher rectal doses have been studied for use in preoperative pain control in children. However, specific guidelines are not available and dosing may be product dependent. The safety and efficacy of alternating acetaminophen and ibuprofen dosing has not been established.

I.V.:
Children 2-12 years: 15 mg/kg every 6 hours **or** 12.5 mg/kg every 4 hours; maximum single dose: 15 mg/kg/dose; maximum daily dose: 75 mg/kg/day (≤3.75 g/day)
Adolescents >12 years: Refer to adult dosing.

Renal Impairment
Oral (Aronoff, 2007):
Children:
Cl_{cr} <10 mL/minute: Administer every 8 hours.
Intermittent hemodialysis or peritoneal dialysis: Administer every 8 hours.
CRRT: No adjustments necessary.
Adults:
Cl_{cr} 10-50 mL/minute: Administer every 6 hours.
Cl_{cr} <10 mL/minute: Administer every 8 hours.
Intermittent hemodialysis or peritoneal dialysis: No adjustment necessary.
CRRT: Administer every 8 hours.
I.V.: Cl_{cr} ≤30 mL/minute: Use with caution; consider decreasing daily dose and extending dosing interval.

Hepatic Impairment Use with caution. Limited, low-dose therapy is usually well tolerated in hepatic disease/cirrhosis. However, cases of hepatotoxicity at daily acetaminophen dosages <4 g/day have been reported. Avoid chronic use in hepatic impairment.

Administration

Oral Shake suspension well before pouring dose.

I.V. For I.V. infusion only. May administer undiluted over 15 minutes.

Doses <1000 mg (<50 kg): Withdraw appropriate dose from vial and place into separate empty, sterile container prior to administration. Small volume pediatric doses (up to 60 mL) may be placed in a syringe and infused over 15 minutes via syringe pump.

Doses of 1000 mg (≥50 kg): Insert vented I.V. set through vial stopper.

Stability

Reconstitution Injectable solution may be administered directly from the vial without further dilution. For doses <1000 mg, withdraw the appropriate volume and transfer to a separate sterile container (eg, glass bottle, plastic I.V. container, syringe) for administration.

Storage

Injection: Store intact vials at room temperature of 20°C to 25°C (68°F to 77°F); do not refrigerate or freeze. Use within 6 hours of opening vial or transferring to another container. Discard any unused portion; single use vials only.

Oral formulations: Store at controlled room temperature.

Suppositories: Store at <27°C (80°F); do not freeze.

Monitoring and Teaching Issues

Laboratory Monitoring Serum APAP levels with long-term use in patients with hepatic disease

Physical Assessment Assess patient for history of liver disease or ethanol abuse (acetaminophen and excessive ethanol may have adverse liver effects).

Patient Education Take with food or milk. While using this medication, avoid or limit alcohol to <3 drinks/day and avoid other prescription or OTC medications that contain acetaminophen. Maintain adequate hydration, unless instructed to restrict fluid intake. This medication will not reduce inflammation; consult prescriber for anti-inflammatory, if needed. Report unusual bleeding (stool, mouth, urine) or bruising, unusual fatigue and weakness, change in elimination patterns, or change in color of urine or stool.

Dietary Considerations Some products may contain phenylalanine.

Breast-Feeding Considerations Low concentrations of acetaminophen are excreted into breast milk and can be detected in the urine of nursing infants. Adverse reactions have generally not been observed; however, a rash caused by acetaminophen exposure was reported in one breast-feeding infant.

Pregnancy Considerations Animal reproduction studies have not been conducted with intravenous acetaminophen. Acetaminophen crosses the placenta and can be detected in cord blood, newborn serum, and urine immediately after delivery. An increased risk of teratogenic effects has not been observed following maternal use of acetaminophen during pregnancy. Prenatal constriction of the ductus arteriosus has been noted in case reports following maternal use during the third trimester. The use of acetaminophen in normal doses during pregnancy is not associated with an increased risk of miscarriage or still birth; however, an increase in fetal death or spontaneous abortion may be seen following maternal overdose if treatment is delayed. Frequent maternal use of acetaminophen during pregnancy may be associated with wheezing and asthma in early childhood. The absorption may be delayed and the bioavailability of acetaminophen may be decreased in some women during pregnancy due to delayed gastric emptying.

◆ **Acetaminophen and Butalbital** *see* Butalbital and Acetaminophen *on page 261*

Acetaminophen and Codeine (a seet a MIN oh fen & KOE deen)

U.S. Brand Names Capital® and Codeine; Tylenol® with Codeine No. 3; Tylenol® with Codeine No. 4

Index Terms Codeine and Acetaminophen; Tylenol #2; Tylenol #3; Tylenol Codeine

Generic Availability (U.S.) Yes

Pharmacologic Category Analgesic, Opioid

Medication Safety Issues

Sound-alike/look-alike issues:

Capital® may be confused with Capitrol®

Tylenol® may be confused with atenolol, timolol, Tuinal®, Tylox®

International issues:

Codex: Brand name for acetaminophen/codeine [Brazil], but also the brand name for *saccharomyces boulardii* [Italy]

Codex [Brazil] may be confused with Cedax brand name for ceftibuten [U.S. and multiple international markets]

T3 is an error-prone abbreviation (mistaken as liothyronine)

High alert medication: The Institute for Safe Medication Practices (ISMP) includes this medication among its list of drug classes which have a heightened risk of causing significant patient harm when used in error.

Duplicate therapy issues: This product contains acetaminophen, which may be a component of other combination products. Do not exceed the maximum recommended daily dose of acetaminophen.

Pregnancy Risk Factor C

Lactation Enters breast milk/use caution

Use Relief of mild-to-moderate pain

Controlled Substance C-III; C-V

Available Dosage Forms

Solution, oral [C-V]: Acetaminophen 120 mg and codeine 12 mg per 5 mL

Suspension, oral [C-V]: Acetaminophen 120 mg and codeine 12 mg per 5 mL

Capital® and Codeine [C-V]: Acetaminophen 120 mg and codeine 12 mg per 5 mL

Tablet [C-III]: Acetaminophen 300 mg and codeine 15 mg; acetaminophen 300 mg and codeine 30 mg; acetaminophen 300 mg and codeine 60 mg

Tylenol® with Codeine No. 3: Acetaminophen 300 mg and codeine 30 mg

Tylenol® with Codeine No. 4: Acetaminophen 300 mg and codeine 60 mg

Dosing

Adult Doses should be adjusted according to severity of pain and response of the patient. Adult doses ≥60 mg codeine fail to give commensurate relief of pain but merely prolong analgesia and are associated with an appreciably increased incidence of side effects.

Cough (Antitussive): Oral: Based on codeine (15-30 mg/dose) every 4-6 hours (maximum: 360 mg/24 hours based on codeine component)

Pain (Analgesic): Oral: Based on codeine (30-60 mg/dose) every 4-6 hours (maximum: 4000 mg/24 hours based on acetaminophen component)

1-2 tablets every 4 hours to a maximum of 12 tablets/24 hours

Geriatric Doses should be titrated to appropriate analgesic effect.

One Tylenol® No. 3 tablet every 4 hours; do **not** exceed 4 g/day acetaminophen.

Pediatric

Analgesic: Oral:

Codeine: 0.5-1 mg codeine/kg/dose every 4-6 hours

Acetaminophen: 10-15 mg/kg/dose every 4 hours up to a maximum of 2.6 g/24 hours for children <12 years; alternatively, the following can be used:

3-6 years: 5 mL 3-4 times/day as needed of elixir

7-12 years: 10 mL 3-4 times/day as needed of elixir

Children >12 years: 15 mL every 4 hours as needed of elixir

Renal Impairment See individual agents.

Hepatic Impairment Use with caution. Limited, low-dose therapy is usually well tolerated in hepatic disease/cirrhosis; however, cases of hepatotoxicity at daily acetaminophen dosages <4 g/day have been reported. Avoid chronic use in hepatic impairment.

Administration

Oral May be administered with food.

Monitoring and Teaching Issues

Physical Assessment See individual agents.

Patient Education See individual agents.

Related Information

Acetaminophen *on page* 38

Codeine *on page* 421

◆ **Acetaminophen and Hydrocodone** *see* Hydrocodone and Acetaminophen *on page* 915

◆ **Acetaminophen and Oxycodone** *see* Oxycodone and Acetaminophen *on page* 1383

◆ **Acetaminophen, Butalbital, and Caffeine** *see* Butalbital, Acetaminophen, and Caffeine *on page* 260

◆ **Acetaminophen, Caffeine, Codeine, and Butalbital** *see* Butalbital, Acetaminophen, Caffeine, and Codeine *on page* 261

◆ **Acetasol® HC** *see* Acetic Acid, Propylene Glycol Diacetate, and Hydrocortisone *on page* 43

AcetaZOLAMIDE (a set a ZOLE a mide)

U.S. Brand Names Diamox® Sequels®

Generic Availability (U.S.) Yes

Pharmacologic Category Anticonvulsant, Miscellaneous; Carbonic Anhydrase Inhibitor; Diuretic, Carbonic Anhydrase Inhibitor; Ophthalmic Agent, Antiglaucoma

Medication Safety Issues

Sound-alike/look-alike issues:

AcetaZOLAMIDE may be confused with acetoHEXAMIDE

Diamox® Sequels® may be confused with Diabinese®, Dobutrex®, Trimox®

International issues:

Diamox [Canada and multiple international markets] may be confused with Zimox brand name for amoxicillin [Italy] and carbidopa/levodopa [Greece]

Pregnancy Risk Factor C

Lactation Enters breast milk/not recommended (AAP rates "compatible"; AAP 2001 update pending)

Use Treatment of glaucoma (chronic simple open-angle, secondary glaucoma, preoperatively in acute angle-closure); drug-induced edema or edema due to congestive heart failure (adjunctive therapy); centrencephalic epilepsies (immediate release dosage form); prevention or amelioration of symptoms associated with acute mountain sickness

Unlabeled/Investigational Use Metabolic alkalosis; respiratory stimulant in COPD; urine alkalinization

Available Dosage Forms

Capsule, extended release, oral: 500 mg

Capsule, sustained release, oral:

Diamox® Sequels®: 500 mg

Injection, powder for reconstitution: 500 mg

Tablet, oral: 125 mg, 250 mg

Dosing

Adult Note: I.M. administration is not recommended.

Glaucoma:

Chronic simple (open-angle): Oral: 250 mg 1-4 times/day or 500 mg extended release capsule twice daily

Secondary, acute (closed-angle): I.V.: 250-500 mg, may repeat in 2-4 hours to a maximum of 1 g/day

Edema: Oral, I.V.: 250-375 mg once daily

Epilepsy: Oral: 8-30 mg/kg/day in 1-4 divided doses, not to exceed 1 g/day. **Note:** Extended release capsule is not recommended for treatment of epilepsy.

Metabolic alkalosis (unlabeled use): I.V. 250 mg every 6 hours for 4 doses or 500 mg single dose; reassess need based upon acid-base status

Mountain sickness: Oral: Manufacturer's labeling: 500-1000 mg daily, in divided doses every 8-12 hours (immediate release tablets) or divided every 12-24 hours (extended release capsules). Alternative recommendations suggest use of lower doses to reduce side effects: 125-250 mg twice daily for prevention or treatment of mild sickness, and 250 mg twice daily for treatment of moderate sickness (Hackett, 2001). Therapy should begin 24-48 hours before and continue during ascent and for at least 48 hours after arrival at the high altitude. **Note:** In situations of rapid ascent (such as rescue or military operations), 1000 mg/day is recommended (manufacturer's labeling).

Urine alkalinization (unlabeled use): Oral: 5 mg/kg/dose repeated 2-3 times over 24 hours

Respiratory stimulant in COPD (unlabeled use): Oral, I.V.: 250 mg twice daily

Geriatric Oral: Initial: 250 mg once or twice daily; use lowest effective dose possible.

Pediatric Note: I.M. administration is not recommended.

Glaucoma:

Oral: 8-30 mg/kg/day or 300-900 mg/m^2/day divided every 8 hours

I.V.: 20-40 mg/kg/24 hours divided every 6 hours, not to exceed 1 g/day

Edema: Oral, I.V.: 5 mg/kg or 150 mg/m^2 once every day

Epilepsy: Oral: Refer to adult dosing.

Renal Impairment

Cl_{cr} 10-50 mL/minute: Administer every 12 hours.

Cl_{cr} <10 mL/minute: Avoid use (ineffective).

Moderately dialyzable (20% to 50%)

Administration

Oral May be administered with food. May cause an alteration in taste, especially carbonated beverages. Short-acting tablets may be crushed and suspended in cherry or chocolate syrup to disguise the bitter taste of the drug; do not use fruit juices. Alternatively, submerge tablet in 10 mL of hot water and add 10 mL honey or syrup.

I.M. I.M. administration is painful because of the alkaline pH of the drug; use by this route is not recommended.

I.V. I.V.: No specific guidance given by manufacturer, but I.V. push at a rate of up to 500 mg over 3 minutes has been reported in a clinical trial (Mazur, 1999); a study to assess cerebrovascular reserve has used rapid I.V. push of up to 1 g over ≤1 minute (Piepgras, 1990)

Monitoring and Teaching Issues

Laboratory Monitoring Intraocular pressure; serum electrolytes, periodic CBC with differential

Physical Assessment Assess allergy history prior to beginning therapy. Monitor for signs of excessive dosing and acidosis (especially in elderly). Measure intraocular pressure at the beginning of therapy and periodically throughout. Monitor growth in pediatric patients. Monitor blood glucose levels closely if patients have diabetes.

Patient Education Do not chew or crush long-acting capsule (contents may be sprinkled on soft food). May be administered with food to decrease GI upset. You will need periodic ophthalmic examinations while taking this medication. You may experience drowsiness, dizziness, weakness, nausea, loss of appetite, or altered taste. Monitor serum glucose closely (may cause altered blood glucose in some patients with diabetes or unusual response to some forms of glucose testing). You may experience increased sensitivity to sunlight. Report unusual and persistent tiredness; numbness, burning, or tingling of extremities or around mouth, lips, or anus; muscle weakness; black stool; or excessive depression.

◆ **Acetic Acid, Hydrocortisone, and Propylene Glycol Diacetate** *see* Acetic Acid, Propylene Glycol Diacetate, and Hydrocortisone *on page* 43

Acetic Acid, Propylene Glycol Diacetate, and Hydrocortisone

(a SEE tik AS id, PRO pa leen GLY kole dye AS e tate, & hye droe KOR ti sone)

U.S. Brand Names Acetasol® HC; VoSol® HC

Index Terms Acetic Acid, Hydrocortisone, and Propylene Glycol Diacetate; Hydrocortisone, Acetic Acid, and Propylene Glycol Diacetate; Propylene Glycol Diacetate, Acetic Acid, and Hydrocortisone

Generic Availability (U.S.) Yes

Pharmacologic Category Otic Agent, Anti-infective

Medication Safety Issues
Sound-alike/look-alike issues:
VoSol® may be confused with Vexol®

Use Treatment of superficial infections of the external auditory canal caused by organisms susceptible to the action of the antimicrobial, complicated by swelling

Available Dosage Forms
Solution, otic [drops]: Acetic acid 2%, propylene glycol diacetate 3%, and hydrocortisone 1% (10 mL)
Acetasol® HC, VoSol® HC: Acetic acid 2%, propylene glycol diacetate 3%, and hydrocortisone 1% (10 mL)

Dosing
Adult & Geriatric Otitis externa (superficial): Otic: Instill 3-5 drops in ear(s) every 4-6 hours
Pediatric Children ≥3 years: Refer to adult dosing.

Administration
Other After removing cerumen and debris, solution may be applied by inserting a cotton wick into the ear canal and saturating with the solution. Wick may remain in place for 24 hours and then removed; however, drops should continue to be instilled into ear canal as long as indicated.

Monitoring and Teaching Issues
Physical Assessment See individual agents.
Patient Education See individual agents.

- **Acetoxymethylprogesterone** *see* MedroxyPROGESTERone *on page 1154*
- **Acetylsalicylic Acid** *see* Aspirin *on page 155*
- **Achromycin** *see* Tetracycline *on page 1744*
- **Aciclovir** *see* Acyclovir (Systemic) *on page 44*
- **Aciclovir** *see* Acyclovir (Topical) *on page 48*
- **AcipHex®** *see* Rabeprazole *on page 1544*
- **Aclaro®** *see* Hydroquinone *on page 927*
- **Aclaro PD®** *see* Hydroquinone *on page 927*
- **ACT-D** *see* DACTINomycin *on page 455*
- **ActHIB®** *see Haemophilus* b Conjugate Vaccine *on page 893*
- **Actigall®** *see* Ursodiol *on page 1827*
- **Actimmune®** *see* Interferon Gamma-1b *on page 1007*
- **Actinomycin** *see* DACTINomycin *on page 455*
- **Actinomycin D** *see* DACTINomycin *on page 455*
- **Actinomycin CI** *see* DACTINomycin *on page 455*
- **Actiq®** *see* FentaNYL *on page 744*
- **Activase®** *see* Alteplase *on page 86*
- **Activated Ergosterol** *see* Ergocalciferol *on page 650*
- **Activated Protein C, Human, Recombinant** *see* Drotrecogin Alfa *on page 594*
- **Activella®** *see* Estradiol and Norethindrone *on page 674*
- **Actonel®** *see* Risedronate *on page 1585*
- **Actoplus Met®** *see* Pioglitazone and Metformin *on page 1463*
- **Actoplus Met® XR** *see* Pioglitazone and Metformin *on page 1463*
- **Actos®** *see* Pioglitazone *on page 1460*
- **Acular®** *see* Ketorolac (Ophthalmic) *on page 1046*
- **Acular LS®** *see* Ketorolac (Ophthalmic) *on page 1046*
- **Acuvail®** *see* Ketorolac (Ophthalmic) *on page 1046*
- **ACV** *see* Acyclovir (Systemic) *on page 44*
- **ACV** *see* Acyclovir (Topical) *on page 48*
- **Acycloguanosine** *see* Acyclovir (Systemic) *on page 44*
- **Acycloguanosine** *see* Acyclovir (Topical) *on page 48*

Acyclovir (Systemic) (ay SYE kloe veer)

U.S. Brand Names Zovirax®
Index Terms Aciclovir; ACV; Acycloguanosine
Generic Availability (U.S.) Yes
Pharmacologic Category Antiviral Agent
Medication Safety Issues
Sound-alike/look-alike issues:
Acyclovir may be confused with ganciclovir, Retrovir®, valacyclovir
Zovirax® may be confused with Doribax®, Valtrex®, Zithromax®, Zostrix®, Zyloprim®, Zyvox®
Pregnancy Risk Factor B
Lactation Enters breast milk/use with caution (AAP rates "compatible"; AAP 2001 update pending)

Use Treatment of genital herpes simplex virus (HSV) and HSV encephalitis

Unlabeled/Investigational Use Prevention of HSV reactivation in HIV-positive patients; prevention of HSV reactivation in hematopoietic stem cell transplant (HSCT); prevention of HSV reactivation during periods of neutropenia in patients with cancer; prevention of varicella zoster virus (VZV) reactivation in allogenic HSCT; prevention of CMV reactivation in low-risk allogeneic HSCT; treatment of disseminated HSV or VZV in immunocompromised patients with cancer; empiric treatment of suspected encephalitis in immunocompromised patients with cancer

Mechanism of Action/Effect Inhibits DNA synthesis and viral replication

Contraindications Hypersensitivity to acyclovir, valacyclovir, or any component of the formulation

Warnings/Precautions Use with caution in immunocompromised patients; thrombocytopenic purpura/hemolytic uremic syndrome (TTP/HUS) has been reported. Use caution in the elderly, pre-existing renal disease (may require dosage modification), or in those receiving other nephrotoxic drugs. Renal failure (sometimes fatal) has been reported. Maintain adequate hydration during oral or intravenous therapy. Use I.V. preparation with caution in patients with underlying neurologic abnormalities, serious hepatic or electrolyte abnormalities, or substantial hypoxia.

Varicella-zoster: Treatment should begin within 24 hours of appearance of rash; oral route not recommended for routine use in otherwise healthy children with varicella, but may be effective in patients at increased risk of moderate-to-severe infection (>12 years of age, chronic cutaneous or pulmonary disorders, long-term salicylate therapy, corticosteroid therapy).

Drug Interactions

Avoid Concomitant Use

Avoid concomitant use of Acyclovir (Systemic) with any of the following: Zoster Vaccine

Decreased Effect

Acyclovir (Systemic) may decrease the levels/effects of: Zoster Vaccine

Increased Effect/Toxicity

Acyclovir (Systemic) may increase the levels/effects of: Mycophenolate; Tenofovir; Zidovudine

The levels/effects of Acyclovir (Systemic) may be increased by: Mycophenolate

Nutritional/Ethanol Interactions Food: Does not affect absorption of oral acyclovir.

Adverse Reactions

Oral:

>10%: Central nervous system: Malaise (≤12%)

1% to 10%:

Central nervous system: Headache (≤2%)

Gastrointestinal: Nausea (2% to 5%), vomiting (≤3%), diarrhea (2% to 3%)

Parenteral:

1% to 10%:

Dermatologic: Hives (2%), itching (2%), rash (2%)

Gastrointestinal: Nausea/vomiting (7%)

Hepatic: Liver function tests increased (1% to 2%)

Local: Inflammation at injection site or phlebitis (9%)

Renal: BUN increased (5% to 10%), creatinine increased (5% to 10%), acute renal failure

Pharmacodynamics/Kinetics

Absorption Oral: 15% to 30%

Bioavailability Oral: 10% to 20% with normal renal function (bioavailability decreases with increased dose)

Time to Peak Serum: Oral: Within 1.5-2 hours

Protein Binding 9% to 33%

Half-Life Elimination Terminal: Neonates: 4 hours; Children 1-12 years: 2-3 hours; Adults: 3 hours

Metabolism Converted by viral enzymes to acyclovir monophosphate, and further converted to diphosphate then triphosphate (active form) by cellular enzymes

Excretion Urine (62% to 90% as unchanged drug and metabolite)

Available Dosage Forms

Capsule, oral: 200 mg

Zovirax®: 200 mg

Injection, powder for reconstitution: 500 mg, 1000 mg

Injection, solution [preservative free]: 50 mg/mL (10 mL, 20 mL)

Suspension, oral: 200 mg/5 mL (473 mL)

Zovirax®: 200 mg/5 mL (473 mL)

Tablet, oral: 400 mg, 800 mg

Zovirax®: 400 mg, 800 mg

Dosing

Adult & Geriatric Note: Obese patients should be dosed using ideal body weight

Genital herpes simplex virus (HSV) infection:

I.V.: Immunocompetent: Initial episode, severe: 5 mg/kg/dose every 8 hours for 5-7 days **or** 5-10 mg/kg/dose every 8 hours for 2-7 days, follow with oral therapy to complete at least 10 days of therapy (CDC, 2010)

Oral:

Initial episode: 200 mg every 4 hours while awake (5 times/day) for 10 days **or** 400 mg 3 times/day for 7-10 days (CDC, 2010)

Recurrence: 200 mg every 4 hours while awake (5 times/day) for 5 days (per manufacturer's labeling; begin at earliest signs of disease)

Alternatively, the following regimens are also recommended by the CDC: 400 mg 3 times/day for 5 days; 800 mg twice daily for 5 days; 800 mg 3 times/day for 2 days (CDC, 2010)

Chronic suppression: 400 mg twice daily or 200 mg 3-5 times/day, for up to 12 months followed by re-evaluation (per manufacturer's labeling)

Herpes zoster (shingles):

Oral: Immunocompetent: 800 mg every 4 hours (5 times/day) for 7-10 days

I.V.: Immunocompromised: 10 mg/kg/dose or 500 mg/m^2/dose every 8 hours for 7 days

HSV encephalitis: I.V.: 10 mg/kg/dose every 8 hours for 10 days (per manufacturer's labeling); 10-15 mg/kg/dose every 8 hours for 14-21 days also reported

Mucocutaneous HSV:

I.V.: Immunocompromised: 5 mg/kg/dose every 8 hours for 7 days (per manufacturer's labeling); dosing for up to 14 days also reported

Oral: Immunocompromised (unlabeled use): 400 mg 5 times a day for 7-14 days

Varicella-zoster (chickenpox): Begin treatment within the first 24 hours of rash onset:

Oral: >40 kg (immunocompetent): 800 mg/dose 4 times a day for 5 days

I.V.:

Manufacturer's labeling (immunocompromised): 10 mg/kg/dose every 8 hours for 7 days

CDC HIV guidelines (immunocompromised): 10-15 mg/kg/dose every 8 hours for 7-10 days

Prevention of HSV reactivation in HIV-positive patients (unlabeled use): Oral: 400-800 mg 2-3 times/day (CDC, 2010)

Prevention of HSV reactivation in HSCT (unlabeled use): *CDC recommendation:* **Note:** Start at the beginning of conditioning therapy and continue until engraftment or until mucositis resolves (~30 days)

Oral: 200 mg 3 times/day

I.V.: 250 mg/m^2/dose every 12 hours

Prevention of VZV reactivation in allogeneic HSCT (unlabeled use): *NCCN guidelines:* Oral: 800 mg twice a day

Prevention of CMV reactivation in low-risk allogeneic HSCT (unlabeled use): *NCCN guidelines:* **Note:** Requires close monitoring (due to weak activity); not for use in patients at high risk for CMV disease: Oral: 800 mg 4 times/day

Treatment of disseminated HSV or VZV or empiric treatment of suspected encephalitis in immunocompromised patients with cancer: (unlabeled use): *NCCN guidelines:* I.V.: 10-12 mg/kg/dose every 8 hours

Treatment of episodic HSV infection in HIV-positive patient (unlabeled use): Oral: 400 mg 3 times/day for 5-10 days (CDC, 2010)

Pediatric Note: Obese patients should be dosed using ideal body weight

Genital herpes simplex virus (HSV) infection:

I.V.: Children ≥12 years: Refer to adult dosing.

Oral:

Immunocompetent:

Initial episode (unlabeled use): 40-80 mg/kg/day divided into 3-4 doses for 5-10 days (maximum: 1 g/day)

Chronic suppression (unlabeled use; limited data): 80 mg/kg/day in 3 divided doses (maximum: 1 g/day), re-evaluate after 12 months of treatment

Immunocompromised (unlabeled use; CDC, 2009): Initial episode:

Children <45 kg: 60 mg/kg/day divided into 3 doses for 5-14 days (maximum: 1.2 g/day)

Adolescents: 400 mg twice daily for 5-14 days

Herpes zoster (shingles): I.V.:

Children <12 years (immunocompromised): 20 mg/kg/dose every 8 hours for 7 days

Children ≥12 years: Refer to adult dosing.

HSV encephalitis: I.V.:

Children 3 months to 12 years: 20 mg/kg/dose every 8 hours for 10 days (per manufacturer's labeling); dosing for 14-21 days also reported

Children ≥12 years: Refer to adult dosing.

Mucocutaneous HSV: I.V.:

Children <12 years (immunocompromised): 10 mg/kg/dose every 8 hours for 7 days

Children ≥12 years: Refer to adult dosing.

Neonatal HSV: I.V.: Neonate: Birth to 3 months: 10 mg/kg/dose every 8 hours for 10 days (manufacturer's labeling); 20 mg/kg/dose every 8 hours for 14 (skin and mucous membrane disease) to 21 days (CNS disease) (CDC, 2010)

Varicella-zoster (chickenpox): Begin treatment within the first 24 hours of rash onset:

Oral: **Note:** The CDC HIV guidelines recommended duration of therapy is 7-10 days or until no new lesions for 48 hours (for patients with mild varicella and no or moderate immune suppression).

Children ≥2 years and ≤40 kg (immunocompetent): 20 mg/kg/dose (up to 800 mg/dose) 4 times/day for 5 days

Children >40 kg: Refer to adult dosing.

I.V.:

Manufacturer's labeling (immunocompromised):

Children <12 years: 20 mg/kg/dose every 8 hours for 7 days

Children ≥12 years: 10 mg/kg/dose every 8 hours for 7 days

CDC HIV guidelines (immunocompromised):

Children <1 year: 10 mg/kg/dose every 8 hours for 7-10 days or until no new lesions for 48 hours

Children ≥1 year: 10 mg/kg/dose or 500 mg/m^2/dose every 8 hours for 7-10 days or until no new lesions for 48 hours

Adolescents: Refer to adult dosing.

Varicella-zoster acute retinal necrosis infection in HIV-exposed/-positive patients (unlabeled use; CDC, 2009): I.V.: Infants and Children: 10-15 mg/kg/dose every 8 hours for 10-14 days, followed by valacyclovir for 4-6 weeks

Prevention of HSV reactivation in HIV-exposed/-positive patients (unlabeled use; CDC, 2009): Oral: 20 mg/kg/dose twice daily (maximum: 400 mg/dose)

Prevention of HSV reactivation in HSCT (unlabeled use): *CDC recommendation:* **Note:** Start at the beginning of conditioning therapy and continue until engraftment or until mucositis resolves (~30 days): I.V.: 250 mg/m^2/dose every 8 hours or 125 mg/m^2/dose every 6 hours

Renal Impairment

Oral:

Cl_{cr} 10-25 mL/minute/1.73 m^2: Normal dosing regimen 800 mg every 4 hours: Administer 800 mg every 8 hours

Cl_{cr} <10 mL/minute/1.73 m^2:

Normal dosing regimen 200 mg every 4 hours or 400 mg every 12 hours: Administer 200 mg every 12 hours

Normal dosing regimen 800 mg every 4 hours: Administer 800 mg every 12 hours

I.V.:

Cl_{cr} 25-50 mL/minute/1.73 m^2: Administer recommended dose every 12 hours

Cl_{cr} 10-25 mL/minute/1.73 m^2: Administer recommended dose every 24 hours

Cl_{cr} <10 mL/minute/1.73 m^2: Administer 50% of recommended dose every 24 hours

Hemodialysis: Administer dose after dialysis

Continuous ambulatory peritoneal dialysis (CAPD): Administer 50% of normal dose once daily; no supplemental dose needed

Continuous renal replacement therapy (CRRT): Drug clearance is highly dependent on the method of renal replacement, filter type, and flow rate. Appropriate dosing requires close monitoring of pharmacologic response, signs of adverse reactions due to drug accumulation, as well as drug levels in relation to target trough (if appropriate). The following are general recommendations only (based on dialysate flow/ultrafiltration rates of 1 L/hour) and should not supersede clinical judgment:

CVVH or CVVHD/CVVHDF: 5-7.5 mg/kg every 24 hours

Note: The higher dose of 7.5 mg/kg is recommended for infections with CNS involvement (Trotman, 2005).

Administration

Oral May be administered with or without food.

I.V. For I.V. infusion only. Avoid rapid infusion. Infuse over 1 hour to prevent renal damage. Maintain adequate hydration of patient. Check for phlebitis and rotate infusion sites. Avoid I.M. or SubQ administration.

Stability

Reconstitution Powder for injection: Reconstitute acyclovir 500 mg powder with SWFI 10 mL; do not use bacteriostatic water containing benzyl alcohol or parabens. For intravenous infusion, dilute in D_5W, D_5NS, $D_5{}^1/_4NS$, $D_5{}^1/_2NS$, LR, or NS to a final concentration ≤7 mg/mL. Concentrations >10 mg/mL increase the risk of phlebitis.

Storage

Capsule, tablet: Store at controlled room temperature of 15°C to 25°C (59°F to 77°F); protect from moisture.

Injection: Store powder at controlled room temperature of 15°C to 25°C (59°F to 77°F). Reconstituted solutions remain stable for 12 hours at room temperature. Do not refrigerate reconstituted solutions or solutions diluted for infusion as they may precipitate as they may precipitate. Once diluted for infusion, use within 24 hours.

Monitoring and Teaching Issues

Laboratory Monitoring Urinalysis, BUN, serum creatinine, liver enzymes, CBC

Physical Assessment Assess carefully for use cautions. Patient should be adequately hydrated during I.V. therapy and monitored closely during intravenous administration.

Patient Education This is not a cure for herpes, nor will this medication reduce the risk of transmission to others when lesions are present; avoid sexual intercourse when visible lesions are present. Oral doses may be taken with food. Maintain adequate hydration, unless instructed to restrict fluid intake. May cause nausea, vomiting, lightheadedness, dizziness, headache, fever, or muscle pain. Report any change in urination (difficulty urinating, dark colored or concentrated urine), persistent lethargy, acute headache, severe nausea or vomiting, confusion or hallucinations, rash, or respiratory difficulty.

Dietary Considerations May be taken with or without food. Some products may contain sodium.

Geriatric Considerations For herpes zoster, acyclovir should be started within 72 hours of the appearance of the rash to be effective. Dose adjustment may be necessary depending on creatinine clearance.

Breast-Feeding Considerations Nursing mothers with herpetic lesions near or on the breast should avoid breast-feeding. Limited data suggest exposure to the nursing infant of ~0.3 mg/kg/day following oral administration of acyclovir to the mother.

Pregnancy Considerations Teratogenic effects were not observed in animal studies. Acyclovir has been shown to cross the human placenta. There are no adequate and well-controlled studies in pregnant women. Results from a pregnancy registry, established in 1984 and closed in 1999, did not find an increase in the number of birth defects with exposure to acyclovir when compared to those expected in the general population. However, due to the small size of the registry and lack of long-term data, the manufacturer recommends using during pregnancy with caution and only when clearly needed. Data from the pregnancy registry may be obtained from GlaxoSmithKline.

Acyclovir (Topical) (ay SYE kloe veer)

U.S. Brand Names Zovirax®

Index Terms Aciclovir; ACV; Acycloguanosine

Generic Availability (U.S.) No

Pharmacologic Category Antiviral Agent, Topical

Medication Safety Issues

Sound-alike/look-alike issues:

Acyclovir may be confused with ganciclovir, Retrovir®, valacyclovir

Zovirax® may be confused with Doribax®, Valtrex®, Zithromax®, Zostrix®, Zyloprim®, Zyvox®

International issues:

Opthavir [Mexico] may be confused with Optivar brand name for azelastine [U.S.]

Pregnancy Risk Factor B

Use Treatment of herpes labialis (cold sores), mucocutaneous HSV in immunocompromised patients

Available Dosage Forms

Cream, topical:

Zovirax®: 5% (2 g, 5 g)

Ointment, topical:

Zovirax®: 5% (15 g, 30 g)

Dosing

Adult & Geriatric

Genital HSV: Topical: Immunocompromised: Ointment: Initial episode: 1/2" ribbon of ointment for a 4" square surface area every 3 hours (6 times/day) for 7 days

Herpes labialis (cold sores): Topical: Apply 5 times/day for 4 days

Mucocutaneous HSV: Topical: Ointment: Non-life-threatening, immunocompromised: 1/2" ribbon of ointment for a 4" square surface area every 3 hours (6 times/day) for 7 days

Pediatric Herpes labialis (cold sores): Topical: Children ≥12 years: Refer to adult dosing.

Administration

Topical Not for use in the eye. Apply using a finger cot or rubber glove to avoid transmission to other parts of the body or to other persons.

Monitoring and Teaching Issues

Patient Education Use gloves or finger cot when applying. This is not a cure for herpes, nor will this medication reduce the risk of transmission to others when lesions are present; avoid sexual intercourse when visible lesions are present.

Acyclovir and Hydrocortisone (ay SYE kloe veer & hye droe KOR ti sone)

U.S. Brand Names Xerese™

Index Terms Hydrocortisone and Acyclovir; ME-609; Xerclear

Generic Availability (U.S.) No

Pharmacologic Category Antiviral Agent, Topical; Corticosteroid, Topical

Pregnancy Risk Factor B

Lactation Excretion in breast milk unknown/use caution

Use Treatment of recurrent herpes labialis (cold sores)

Dosing

Adult Herpes labialis (cold sores): Topical: Apply 5 times/day for 5 days

Geriatric Refer to adult dosing.

Pediatric Herpes labialis (cold sores): Topical: Children ≥12 years: Refer to adult dosing.

Administration

Topical For external use only; not for use in the eye, inside the mouth or nose, or on the genitals. Apply to clean, dry area using a finger cot or rubber glove to avoid transmission to other parts of the body or to other persons. Use sufficient amount to cover the affected area(s), including the outer margin of cold sore; do not rub affected area. Initiate therapy early (ie, during the prodrome or when lesions appear).

◆ **AD32** *see* Valrubicin *on page* 1836

◆ **Adacel®** *see* Diphtheria and Tetanus Toxoids, and Acellular Pertussis Vaccine *on page* 552

◆ **Adalat® CC** *see* NIFEdipine *on page* 1313

Adalimumab (a da LIM yoo mab)

U.S. Brand Names Humira®; Humira® Pen

Index Terms Antitumor Necrosis Factor Apha (Human); D2E7; Human Antitumor Necrosis Factor Alpha

Generic Availability (U.S.) No

Pharmacologic Category Antirheumatic, Disease Modifying; Gastrointestinal Agent, Miscellaneous; Monoclonal Antibody; Tumor Necrosis Factor (TNF) Blocking Agent

Medication Safety Issues

Sound-alike/look-alike issues:

Humira® may be confused with Humulin®, Humalog®

Humira® Pen may be confused with HumaPen® Memoir®

Medication Guide Available Yes

Pregnancy Risk Factor B

Lactation Excretion in breast milk unknown/not recommended

Use

Treatment of active rheumatoid arthritis (moderate-to-severe) and active psoriatic arthritis; may be used alone or in combination with disease-modifying antirheumatic drugs (DMARDs); treatment of ankylosing spondylitis

Treatment of moderately- to severely-active Crohn's disease in patients with inadequate response to conventional treatment, or patients who have lost response to or are intolerant of infliximab

Treatment of moderate-to-severe plaque psoriasis

Treatment of moderately- to severely-active juvenile idiopathic arthritis

Mechanism of Action/Effect Adalimumab decreases signs and symptoms of psoriatic arthritis, rheumatoid arthritis, Crohn's disease, and ankylosing spondylitis; inhibits progression of structural damage in rheumatoid and psoriatic arthritis

Contraindications There are no contraindications listed within the FDA-approved labeling.

Canadian labeling: Additional contraindications (not in U.S. labeling): Hypersensitivity to adalimumab or any component of the formulation; severe infection (eg, sepsis, tuberculosis, opportunistic infection)

Warnings/Precautions **[U.S. Boxed Warnings]: Patients should be evaluated for latent tuberculosis infection with a tuberculin skin test prior to therapy. Treatment of latent tuberculosis should be initiated before adalimumab is used. Tuberculosis (disseminated or extrapulmonary) has been reactivated while on adalimumab.** Most cases have been reported within the first 8 months of treatment. Doses higher than recommended are associated with an increased risk for tuberculosis reactivation. **Patients with initial negative tuberculin skin tests should receive continued monitoring for tuberculosis throughout treatment; active tuberculosis has developed in this population during treatment.** Rare reactivation of hepatitis B virus (HBV) has occurred in chronic virus carriers; evaluate prior to initiation, during, and for several months after treatment. Evaluate patients at risk for HBV infection prior to therapy to determine HBV status. Adalimumab may affect defenses against infections and malignancies.

[U.S. Boxed Warning]: Serious and potential fatal infections (including invasive fungal and other opportunistic infections) have been reported in patients receiving TNF-blocking agents, including adalimumab. Cases of unrecognized invasive fungal infections (eg, histoplasmosis, blastomycosis, coccidioidomycosis) have also been reported with anti-TNF agent use. Use caution with chronic infection, history of recurrent infection, or predisposition to infection (eg, diabetes or residence/travel from areas of endemic mycoses). Do not give to patients with an active chronic or localized infection. Many of the serious infections have occurred in patients on concomitant immunosuppressive therapy. Other opportunistic infections included *Aspergillus* and *Nocardia*. Use caution in patients who have resided in regions where histoplasmosis and tuberculosis are endemic. Patients who develop a new infection while undergoing treatment with adalimumab should be monitored closely. If a patient develops a serious infection or sepsis, adalimumab should be discontinued. **[U.S. Boxed Warning]: Lymphoma and other malignancies have been reported in children and adolescent patients receiving other TNF-blocking agents.** Half the cases are lymphomas (Hodgkin's and non-Hodgkin's) and the other cases are varied, but include malignancies not typically observed in this population. Most patients were receiveing concomitant immunosuppressants. Rare cases of lymphoma have also been reported in association with adalimumab. A higher incidence of nonmelanoma skin cancers was noted in adalimumab treated patients, when compared to the control group. Impact on the development and course of malignancies is not fully defined.

May exacerbate pre-existing or recent-onset demyelinating CNS disorders. Worsening and new-onset heart failure (HF) has been reported; use caution in patients with decreased left ventricular function. Use caution in patients with HF. Patients should be brought up to date with all immunizations before initiating therapy. No data are available concerning the effects of adalimumab on vaccination. Live vaccines should not be given concurrently. No data are available concerning secondary transmission of live vaccines in patients receiving adalimumab. Rare cases of pancytopenia (including aplastic anemia) have been reported with TNF-blocking agents; with significant hematologic abnormalities, consider discontinuing therapy. Positive antinuclear antibody titers have been detected in patients (with negative baselines) treated with adalimumab. Rare cases of autoimmune disorder, including lupus-like syndrome, have been reported; monitor and discontinue adalimumab if symptoms develop. May cause hypersensitivity reactions, including anaphylaxis; monitor. The packaging (needle cover of prefilled syringe) may contain latex. Product may contain polysorbate 80.

Drug Interactions

Avoid Concomitant Use

Avoid concomitant use of Adalimumab with any of the following: Abatacept; Anakinra; BCG; Belimumab; Canakinumab; Certolizumab Pegol; Natalizumab; Pimecrolimus; Rilonacept; Roflumilast; Tacrolimus (Topical); Vaccines (Live)

Decreased Effect
Adalimumab may decrease the levels/effects of: BCG; Sipuleucel-T; Vaccines (Inactivated); Vaccines (Live)

The levels/effects of Adalimumab may be decreased by: Echinacea

Increased Effect/Toxicity
Adalimumab may increase the levels/effects of: Abatacept; Anakinra; Belimumab; Canakinumab; Certolizumab Pegol; Leflunomide; Natalizumab; Rilonacept; Vaccines (Live)

The levels/effects of Adalimumab may be increased by: Abciximab; Denosumab; Pimecrolimus; Roflumilast; Tacrolimus (Topical); Trastuzumab

Nutritional/Ethanol Interactions Herb/nutraceutical: Echinacea may decrease the therapeutic effects of adalimumab; avoid concurrent use.

Adverse Reactions
>10%:
Central nervous system: Headache (12%)
Dermatologic: Rash (6% to 12%)
Local: Injection site reaction (12% to 20%; includes erythema, itching, hemorrhage, pain, swelling)
Neuromuscular & skeletal: CPK increased (15%)
Respiratory: Upper respiratory tract infection (17%), sinusitis (11%)
Miscellaneous: Antibodies to adalimumab (3% to 26%; significance unknown), positive ANA (12%)

5% to 10%:
Cardiovascular: Hypertension (5%)
Endocrine & metabolic: Hyperlipidemia (7%), hypercholesterolemia (6%)
Gastrointestinal: Nausea (9%), abdominal pain (7%)
Genitourinary: Urinary tract infection (8%)
Hepatic: Alkaline phosphatase increased (5%)
Local: Injection site reaction (8%; other than erythema, itching, hemorrhage, pain, swelling)
Neuromuscular & skeletal: Back pain (6%)
Renal: Hematuria (5%)
Miscellaneous: Accidental injury (10%), flu-like syndrome (7%)

<5%:
Cardiovascular: Arrhythmia, atrial fibrillation, chest pain, CHF, coronary artery disorder, heart arrest, MI, palpitation, pericardial effusion, pericarditis, peripheral edema, syncope, tachycardia, thrombosis (leg), vascular disorder
Central nervous system: Confusion, fever, hypertensive encephalopathy, multiple sclerosis, subdural hematoma
Dermatologic: Cellulitis, erysipelas
Endocrine & metabolic: Dehydration, menstrual disorder, parathyroid disorder
Gastrointestinal: Diverticulitis, esophagitis, gastroenteritis, gastrointestinal hemorrhage, vomiting
Genitourinary: Cystitis, pelvic pain
Hematologic: Agranulocytosis, granulocytopenia, leukopenia, pancytopenia, paraproteinemia, polycythemia
Hepatic: Cholecystitis, cholelithiasis, hepatic necrosis
Neuromuscular & skeletal: Arthralgia, arthritis, bone fracture, bone necrosis, joint disorder, muscle cramps, myasthenia, pain in extremity, paresthesia, pyogenic arthritis, synovitis, tendon disorder, tremor
Ocular: Cataract
Renal: Kidney calculus, pyelonephritis
Respiratory: Asthma, bronchospasm, dyspnea, lung function decreased, pleural effusion, pneumonia
Miscellaneous: Adenoma, allergic reactions (1%), carcinoma (including breast, gastrointestinal, skin, urogenital), healing abnormality, herpes zoster, ketosis, lupus erythematosus syndrome, lymphoma, melanoma, postsurgical infection, sepsis, tuberculosis (reactivation of latent infection; miliary, lymphatic, peritoneal and pulmonary)

Pharmacodynamics/Kinetics
Bioavailability Absolute: 64%
Time to Peak Serum: SubQ: 131 ± 56 hours
Half-Life Elimination Terminal: ~2 weeks (range: 10-20 days)
Excretion Clearance increased in the presence of antiadalimumab antibodies; decreased in patients ≥40 years of age

Available Dosage Forms
Injection, solution [preservative free]:
Humira®: 20 mg/0.4 mL (0.4 mL); 40 mg/0.8 mL (0.8 mL)
Humira® Pen: 40 mg/0.8 mL (0.8 mL)

Dosing
Adult & Geriatric
Rheumatoid arthritis: SubQ: 40 mg every other week; may be administered with other DMARDs; patients not taking methotrexate may increase dose to 40 mg every week
Ankylosing spondylitis, psoriatic arthritis: SubQ: 40 mg every other week
Crohn's disease: SubQ: Initial: 160 mg given as 4 injections on day 1 or over 2 days, then 80 mg 2 weeks later (day 15); Maintenance: 40 mg every other week beginning day 29. **Note:** Some patients may require 40 mg every week as maintenance therapy (Lichtenstein, 2009).
Plaque psoriasis: SubQ: Initial: 80 mg as a single dose; maintenance: 40 mg every other week beginning 1 week after initial dose

Pediatric

Juvenile idiopathic arthritis (JIA): Children ≥4 years: SubQ:
15 kg to <30 kg: 20 mg every other week
≥30 kg: 40 mg every other week

Administration

Other For SubQ injection; rotate injection sites. Do not use if solution is discolored. Do not administer to skin which is red, tender, bruised, or hard; rotate injection sites. Needle cap of the prefilled syringe may contain latex.

Stability

Storage Store under refrigeration at 2°C to 8°C (36°F to 46°F); do not freeze. Protect from light.

Monitoring and Teaching Issues

Laboratory Monitoring CBC may be monitored during therapy for hematologic effects.

Physical Assessment Perform tuberculin skin test prior to initiating therapy. Monitor for signs of tuberculosis throughout therapy. Do not initiate therapy if active infection is present. Monitor for signs and symptoms of infection, enlarged lymph nodes, or skin lesions/eruptions. Assess for liver dysfunction. Assess results of PDD at regular intervals during treatment. Teach patient proper injection technique and syringe/needle disposal. Latex-sensitive patients: Needle cap of prefilled syringe contains latex.

Patient Education Inform prescriber of any allergies, history of tuberculosis, or any kind of infection you have. If self-administered, follow directions for injection and needle/syringe disposal exactly. You may be more susceptible to infection. May cause headache or dizziness; if persistent, consult prescriber. Report persistent fever, increased bruising or bleeding, respiratory tract infection, unhealed or infected wounds, urinary tract infection, flu-like symptoms, unexplained weight loss, persistent cough, enlarged lymph nodes, new skin lesions or eruptions, or unusual bump or sore that does not heal. Stop drug and report immediately persistent nausea or abdominal pain; numbness or tingling; problems with vision; weakness in legs; chest pains, respiratory difficulty; weight gain; swelling of extremities; joint pain; skin rash; or redness, swelling, or pain at injection site.

Breast-Feeding Considerations It is not known whether adalimumab is secreted in human milk. Because many immunoglobulins are secreted in milk and the potential for serious adverse reactions exists, a decision should be made whether to discontinue nursing or discontinue the drug, taking into account the importance of the drug to the mother.

Pregnancy Considerations Teratogenic effects were not observed in animal studies, however, there are no adequate and well-controlled studies in pregnant women. Use during pregnancy only if clearly needed. A pregnancy registry has been established to monitor outcomes of women exposed to adalimumab during pregnancy (877-311-8972).

◆ **Adamantanamine Hydrochloride** *see* Amantadine *on page 91*

Adapalene (a DAP a leen)

U.S. Brand Names Differin®

Generic Availability (U.S.) Yes

Pharmacologic Category Acne Products; Topical Skin Product, Acne

Pregnancy Risk Factor C

Lactation Excretion in breast milk unknown/use caution

Use Treatment of acne vulgaris

Mechanism of Action/Effect Retinoid-like compound which is a modulator of cellular differentiation, keratinization, and inflammatory processes, all of which represent important features in the pathology of acne vulgaris

Contraindications Hypersensitivity to adapalene or any component in the vehicle gel

Warnings/Precautions Use with caution in patients with eczema. Avoid excessive exposure to sunlight and sunlamps. Avoid contact with abraded skin, mucous membranes, eyes, mouth, angles of the nose.

Certain cutaneous signs and symptoms such as erythema, dryness, scaling, burning, or pruritus may occur during treatment; these are most likely to occur during the first 2-4 weeks and will usually lessen with continued use. Safety and efficacy have not been established in children <12 years of age.

Drug Interactions

Avoid Concomitant Use There are no known interactions where it is recommended to avoid concomitant use.

Decreased Effect

Adapalene may decrease the levels/effects of: Contraceptives (Progestins)

Increased Effect/Toxicity

The levels/effects of Adapalene may be increased by: Vitamin A

Adverse Reactions >10%: Dermatologic: Erythema, scaling, dryness, pruritus, burning, pruritus or burning immediately after application

Pharmacodynamics/Kinetics

Absorption Topical: Minimal

Excretion Bile

Available Dosage Forms

Cream, topical: 0.1% (45 g)

Differin®: 0.1% (45 g)

Gel, topical: 0.1% (45 g)

Differin®: 0.1% (45 g); 0.3% (45 g)

Dosing

Adult & Geriatric Acne: Topical: Apply once daily before bedtime; results appear after 8-12 weeks of therapy.

Pediatric Children >12 years: Refer to adult dosing.

Monitoring and Teaching Issues

Patient Education Apply with gloves in thin film at night to thoroughly clean/dry skin; avoid area around eyes or mouth. Do not apply occlusive dressing. Results may take 8-12 weeks to appear. You may experience transient burning or stinging immediately after applying. Report worsening of condition or skin redness, dryness, peeling, or burning that persists between applications. Avoid excessive exposure to sunlight or sunlamps.

Pregnancy Considerations There are no adequate and well-controlled studies in pregnant women. Use only if benefit outweighs the potential risk to fetus.

Adapalene and Benzoyl Peroxide (a DAP a leen & BEN zoe il peer OKS ide)

U.S. Brand Names Epiduo®

Index Terms Benzoyl Peroxide and Adapalene

Generic Availability (U.S.) No

Pharmacologic Category Acne Products; Topical Skin Product; Topical Skin Product, Acne

Pregnancy Risk Factor C

Lactation Excretion in breast milk unknown/use caution

Use Topical treatment of acne vulgaris

Available Dosage Forms

Gel, topical:

Epiduo®: Adapalene 0.1% and benzoyl peroxide 2.5% (45 g)

Dosing

Adult & Geriatric Acne vulgaris: Topical: Apply once daily to affected areas after skin has been cleaned and dried

Pediatric Children ≥12 years: Refer to adult dosing.

Administration

Topical Apply a pea-sized amount for each area of the face (eg, forehead, chin, each cheek). Skin should be clean and dry before applying. For external use only; avoid applying to eyes and mucous membranes.

Monitoring and Teaching Issues

Physical Assessment See individual agents.

Patient Education See individual agents.

◆ **Adcirca®** *see* Tadalafil *on page* 1700

◆ **ADD 234037** *see* Lacosamide *on page* 1051

◆ **Addaprin [OTC]** *see* Ibuprofen *on page* 938

◆ **Adderall®** *see* Dextroamphetamine and Amphetamine *on page* 510

◆ **Adderall XR®** *see* Dextroamphetamine and Amphetamine *on page* 510

Adefovir (a DEF o veer)

U.S. Brand Names Hepsera®

Index Terms Adefovir Dipivoxil; Bis-POM PMEA

Generic Availability (U.S.) No

Pharmacologic Category Antiretroviral Agent, Reverse Transcriptase Inhibitor (Nucleotide)

Pregnancy Risk Factor C

Lactation Excretion in breast milk unknown/not recommended

Use Treatment of chronic hepatitis B with evidence of active viral replication (based on persistent elevation of ALT/AST or histologic evidence), including patients with lamivudine-resistant hepatitis B

Mechanism of Action/Effect Acyclic nucleotide reverse transcriptase inhibitor (adenosine analog) which interferes with HBV viral DNA polymerase resulting in inhibition of viral replication

Contraindications Hypersensitivity to adefovir or any component of the formulation

Warnings/Precautions **[U.S. Boxed Warning]: Use with caution in patients with renal dysfunction or in patients at risk of renal toxicity (including concurrent nephrotoxic agents or NSAIDs).** Chronic administration may result in nephrotoxicity. Dosage adjustment is required in adult patients with renal dysfunction or in patients who develop renal dysfunction during therapy; no data available for use in children ≥12 years or adolescents with renal impairment. Not recommended as first line therapy of chronic HBV due to weak antiviral activity and high rate of resistance after first year. May be more appropriate as second-line agent in treatment-naïve patients. Combination therapy with lamivudine in nucleoside-naïve patients has not been shown to provide synergistic antiviral effects. In patients with lamivudine-resistant HBV, switching to adefovir monotherapy was associated with a higher risk of adefovir resistance compared to adding adefovir to lamivudine therapy (Lok, 2009).

Calculate creatinine clearance before initiation of therapy. Consider alternative therapy in patients who do not respond to adefovir monotherapy treatment. **[U.S. Boxed Warning]: May cause the development of HIV resistance in patients with unrecognized or untreated HIV infection.** Determine HIV status prior to initiating treatment with adefovir. **[U.S. Boxed Warning]: Fatal cases of lactic acidosis and severe hepatomegaly with steatosis have been reported with the use of nucleoside analogues alone or in combination with other antiretrovirals.** Female gender, obesity, and prolonged treatment may increase the risk of hepatotoxicity. Treatment should be discontinued in patients with lactic acidosis or signs/symptoms of hepatotoxicity (which may occur without marked transaminase elevations). **[U.S. Boxed Warning]: Acute exacerbations of hepatitis may occur (in up to 25% of patients) when antihepatitis therapy is discontinued.** Exacerbations typically occur within 12 weeks and may be self-limited or resolve upon resuming treatment; risk may be increased with advanced liver disease or cirrhosis. Monitor patients following discontinuation of therapy. Safety and efficacy in children <12 years of age have not been established. Do not use concurrently with tenofovir (Viread®) or any product containing tenofovir (eg, Truvada®, Atripla®).

Drug Interactions

Avoid Concomitant Use There are no known interactions where it is recommended to avoid concomitant use.

Decreased Effect

Adefovir may decrease the levels/effects of: Tenofovir

Increased Effect/Toxicity

The levels/effects of Adefovir may be increased by: Ganciclovir-Valganciclovir; Ribavirin; Tenofovir

Nutritional/Ethanol Interactions

Ethanol: Should be avoided in hepatitis B infection due to potential hepatic toxicity.

Food: Does not have a significant effect on adefovir absorption.

Adverse Reactions

>10%:

Central nervous system: Headache (24% to 25%)

Gastrointestinal: Abdominal pain (15%), diarrhea (up to 13%)

Hepatic: Hepatitis exacerbation (up to 25% within 12 weeks of adefovir discontinuation)

Neuromuscular & skeletal: Weakness (up to 25%)

Renal: Hematuria (grade ≥3: 11%)

1% to 10%:

Dermatologic: Rash, pruritus

Endocrine & metabolic: Hypophosphatemia (<2 mg/dL: 1% and 3% in pre-/post-liver transplant patients, respectively)

Gastrointestinal: Flatulence (up to 8%), dyspepsia (5% to 9%), nausea, vomiting

Neuromuscular & skeletal: Back pain (up to 10%)

Renal: Serum creatinine increased (≥0.5 mg/dL: 2% to 3% in compensated liver disease; incidence may be higher in patients with decompensated cirrhosis or in liver transplant recipients), renal failure

Note: In liver transplant patients with baseline renal dysfunction, frequency of increased serum creatinine has been observed to be as high as 32% to 51% at 48 and 96 weeks post-transplantation, respectively; considering the concomitant use of other potentially nephrotoxic medications, baseline renal insufficiency, and predisposing comorbidities, the role of adefovir in these changes could not be established.

Respiratory: Cough (6% to 8%), rhinitis (up to 5%)

Pharmacodynamics/Kinetics

Bioavailability 59%

Time to Peak 1.75 hours

Protein Binding ≤4%

Half-Life Elimination 7.5 hours; prolonged in renal impairment

Metabolism Prodrug; rapidly converted to adefovir (active metabolite) in intestine

Excretion Urine (45% as active metabolite within 24 hours)

Available Dosage Forms

Tablet, oral:

Hepsera®: 10 mg

Dosing

Adult & Geriatric Hepatitis B (chronic): Oral: 10 mg once daily

Treatment duration (AASLD practice guidelines): Adults:

Hepatitis Be antigen (HBeAg) positive chronic hepatitis: Treat ≥1 year until HBeAg seroconversion and undetectable serum HBV DNA; continue therapy for ≥6 months after HBeAg seroconversion

HBeAg negative chronic hepatitis: Treat >1 year until hepatitis B surface antigen (HBsAg) clearance

Note: Patients achieving a <2 log decrease in serum HBV DNA after at least 6 months of therapy should either receive additional treatment or be switched to an alternative therapy (Lok, 2009).

Pediatric Hepatitis B (chronic): Children ≥12 years: Oral: 10 mg once daily

Renal Impairment Adult recommendations only (no dosage adjustment recommendations available for patients <18 years with renal impairment):

Cl_{cr} ≥50 mL/minute: No dosage adjustment necessary

Cl_{cr} 20-49 mL/minute: 10 mg every 48 hours

Cl_{cr} 10-19 mL/minute: 10 mg every 72 hours

Hemodialysis: 10 mg every 7 days (following dialysis)

Hepatic Impairment No adjustment required.

Administration

Oral May be administered without regard to food.

Stability

Storage Store controlled room temperature of 25°C (77°F).

Monitoring and Teaching Issues

Laboratory Monitoring HIV status (prior to initiation of therapy); serum creatinine (prior to initiation and during therapy; every 3 months in patients with medical conditions which predispose to renal insufficiency and in all patients treated for >1 year; more frequent monitoring required if pre-existing real insufficiency detected [Lok, 2009]); LFTs for several months following discontinuation of adefovir; HBV DNA (every 3-6 months during therapy); HBeAg and anti-HBe

Physical Assessment Use with caution in presence of renal dysfunction or risk of renal toxicity. Assess viral load. Monitor for lactic acidosis and altered hepatic status on a regular basis throughout therapy.

Patient Education Use appropriate precautions to prevent spread to other persons. You will require frequent blood tests; follow recommended schedule. Maintain adequate hydration, unless instructed to restrict fluid intake. May cause headache, abdominal pain, diarrhea, or weakness. Report unusual bleeding (blood in urine, tarry stools, or easy bruising), unresolved diarrhea, signs of infection (eg, fever, chills, sore throat, burning urination, flu-like symptoms), persistent fatigue, muscle weakness, or changes in urinary pattern.

Dietary Considerations May be taken without regard to food.

Pregnancy Considerations Teratogenic effects were not observed in animal studies. There are no adequate and well-controlled studies in pregnant women. Use in pregnancy only when clearly needed. Pregnant women exposed to adefovir should be registered with the pregnancy registry (800-258-4263).

Additional Information Adefovir dipivoxil is a prodrug, rapidly converted to the active component (adefovir). It was previously investigated as a treatment for HIV infections (at dosages substantially higher than the approved dose for hepatitis B). The NDA was withdrawn, and no further studies in the treatment of HIV are anticipated (per manufacturer).

◆ **Adefovir Dipivoxil** *see* Adefovir *on page* 52

◆ **Adenocard® IV** *see* Adenosine *on page* 54

◆ **Adenoscan®** *see* Adenosine *on page* 54

Adenosine (a DEN oh seen)

U.S. Brand Names Adenocard® IV; Adenoscan®

Index Terms 9-Beta-D-Ribofuranosyladenine

Generic Availability (U.S.) Yes

Pharmacologic Category Antiarrhythmic Agent, Miscellaneous; Diagnostic Agent

Medication Safety Issues

High alert medication: The Institute for Safe Medication Practices (ISMP) includes this medication among its list of drugs which have a heightened risk of causing significant patient harm when used in error.

Pregnancy Risk Factor C

Lactation Excretion in breast milk unknown

Use

Adenocard®: Treatment of paroxysmal supraventricular tachycardia (PSVT) including that associated with accessory bypass tracts (Wolff-Parkinson-White syndrome); when clinically advisable, appropriate vagal maneuvers should be attempted prior to adenosine administration; **not effective for conversion of atrial fibrillation, atrial flutter, or ventricular tachycardia**

Adenoscan®: Pharmacologic stress agent used in myocardial perfusion thallium-201 scintigraphy

Unlabeled/Investigational Use

ACLS/PALS Guidelines (2010): Stable, narrow-complex regular tachycardias; unstable narrow-complex regular tachycardias while preparations are made for synchronized direct-current cardioversion; stable regular monomorphic, wide-complex tachycardia as a therapeutic (if SVT) and diagnostic maneuver

Adenoscan®: Acute vasodilator testing in pulmonary artery hypertension

Available Dosage Forms

Injection, solution [preservative free]: 3 mg/mL (2 mL, 4 mL)

Adenocard® IV: 3 mg/mL (2 mL, 4 mL)

Adenoscan®: 3 mg/mL (20 mL, 30 mL)

Dosing

Adult

Paroxysmal supraventricular tachycardia (Adenocard®): I.V. (rapid, over 1-2 seconds, via peripheral line; see **Note**): Initial: 6 mg; if not effective within 1-2 minutes, 12 mg may be given; may repeat 12 mg bolus if needed (maximum single dose: 12 mg). Follow each dose with 20 mL normal saline flush. **Note:** Initial dose of adenosine should be reduced to 3 mg if patient is currently receiving carbamazepine or dipyridamole, has a transplanted heart or if adenosine is administered via central line (ACLS, 2010).

Pharmacologic stress testing (Adenoscan®): I.V.: Continuous I.V. infusion via peripheral line: 140 mcg/kg/minute for 6 minutes using syringe or columetric infusion pump; total dose: 0.84 mg/kg. Thallium-201 is injected at midpoint (3 minutes) of infusion.

Acute vasodilator testing in pulmonary artery hypertension (unlabeled use) (Adenoscan®): I.V.: Initial: 50 mcg/kg/minute increased by 50 mcg/kg/minute every 2 minutes to a maximum dose of 500 mcg/kg/minute (Schrader, 1992) **or** to a maximum dose of 250 mcg/kg/minute (McLaughlin, 2009); acutely assess vasodilator response

Geriatric Refer to adult dosing. Elderly may be more sensitive to effects of adenosine.

Pediatric Rapid I.V. push (over 1-2 seconds) via peripheral line, followed by a normal saline flush:

Paroxysmal supraventricular tachycardia (Adenocard®): Infants and Children: I.V.:

Manufacturer's recommendation:

Children <50 kg: Initial: 0.05-0.1 mg/kg (maximum initial dose: 6 mg). If conversion of PSVT does not occur within 1-2 minutes, may increase dose by 0.05-0.1 mg/kg. May repeat until sinus rhythm is established or to a maximum single dose of 0.3 mg/kg or 12 mg. Follow each dose with normal saline flush.

Children ≥50 kg: Refer to adult dosing.

Pediatric advanced life support (PALS, 2010): Treatment of SVT: I.V., I.O.: Initial: 0.1 mg/kg (maximum initial dose: 6 mg); if not effective within 1-2 minutes, administer 0.2 mg/kg (maximum single dose: 12 mg). Follow each dose with ≥5 mL normal saline flush.

Administration

I.V.

Adenocard®: For rapid bolus I.V. use only; administer I.V. push over 1-2 seconds at a peripheral I.V. site as proximal as possible to trunk (not in lower arm, hand, lower leg, or foot); follow each bolus with a rapid normal saline flush (infants and children ≥5 mL; adults 20 mL). Use of 2 syringes (one with adenosine dose and the other with NS flush) connected to a T-connector or stopcock is recommended. If administered via **central line** in adults, reduce initial dose (ACLS, 2010).

Adenoscan®: For I.V. infusion only via peripheral line

Monitoring and Teaching Issues

Physical Assessment Requires use of infusion pump and continuous cardiac and hemodynamic monitoring during infusion. Emergency resuscitation equipment should be immediately available. Monitor for adverse reactions. Adenosine could produce bronchoconstriction in patients with asthma.

Patient Education Adenosine is administered in emergencies; patient education should be appropriate to the situation. May cause facial flushing. Report chest pain or pressure or difficulty breathing immediately.

Related Information

Antiarrhythmic Drugs *on page 1978*

- ◆ **ADH** *see* Vasopressin *on page 1851*
- ◆ **ADL-2698** *see* Alvimopan *on page 90*
- ◆ **Adoxa®** *see* Doxycycline *on page 586*
- ◆ **Adoxa® Pak™ 1/75** *see* Doxycycline *on page 586*
- ◆ **Adoxa® Pak™ 1/150** *see* Doxycycline *on page 586*
- ◆ **Adrenaclick™ [DSC]** *see* EPINEPHrine (Systemic, Oral Inhalation) *on page 629*
- ◆ **Adrenalin®** *see* EPINEPHrine (Nasal) *on page 633*
- ◆ **Adrenalin®** *see* EPINEPHrine (Systemic, Oral Inhalation) *on page 629*
- ◆ **Adrenaline** *see* EPINEPHrine (Nasal) *on page 633*
- ◆ **Adrenaline** *see* EPINEPHrine (Systemic, Oral Inhalation) *on page 629*
- ◆ **ADR (error-prone abbreviation)** *see* DOXOrubicin *on page 579*
- ◆ **Adria** *see* DOXOrubicin *on page 579*
- ◆ **Adriamycin®** *see* DOXOrubicin *on page 579*
- ◆ **Adrucil®** *see* Fluorouracil (Systemic) *on page 787*
- ◆ **Advair Diskus®** *see* Fluticasone and Salmeterol *on page 804*
- ◆ **Advair® HFA** *see* Fluticasone and Salmeterol *on page 804*
- ◆ **Advate** *see* Antihemophilic Factor (Recombinant) *on page 133*
- ◆ **Advil® [OTC]** *see* Ibuprofen *on page 938*
- ◆ **Advil® Children's [OTC]** *see* Ibuprofen *on page 938*
- ◆ **Advil® Infants' [OTC]** *see* Ibuprofen *on page 938*
- ◆ **Advil® Migraine [OTC]** *see* Ibuprofen *on page 938*
- ◆ **AeroBid® [DSC]** *see* Flunisolide (Oral Inhalation) *on page 783*
- ◆ **AeroBid®-M [DSC]** *see* Flunisolide (Oral Inhalation) *on page 783*
- ◆ **Afeditab® CR** *see* NIFEdipine *on page 1313*
- ◆ **Afinitor®** *see* Everolimus *on page 720*
- ◆ **Afluria®** *see* Influenza Virus Vaccine (Inactivated) *on page 978*
- ◆ **Aggrastat®** *see* Tirofiban *on page 1774*
- ◆ **Aggrenox®** *see* Aspirin and Dipyridamole *on page 160*
- ◆ **AGN 1135** *see* Rasagiline *on page 1559*
- ◆ **Agriflu®** *see* Influenza Virus Vaccine (Inactivated) *on page 978*

- ◆ **AHF (Human)** *see* Antihemophilic Factor (Human) *on page 132*
- ◆ **AHF (Human)** *see* Antihemophilic Factor/von Willebrand Factor Complex (Human) *on page 134*
- ◆ **AHF (Recombinant)** *see* Antihemophilic Factor (Recombinant) *on page 133*
- ◆ **A-hydroCort** *see* Hydrocortisone (Systemic) *on page 917*
- ◆ **A-Hydrocort®** *see* Hydrocortisone (Systemic) *on page 917*
- ◆ **A-hydroCort** *see* Hydrocortisone (Topical) *on page 920*
- ◆ **AICC** *see* Anti-inhibitor Coagulant Complex *on page 136*
- ◆ **AK-Dilate™** *see* Phenylephrine (Ophthalmic) *on page 1452*
- ◆ **Akne-mycin®** *see* Erythromycin (Topical) *on page 661*
- ◆ **Ala-Cort** *see* Hydrocortisone (Topical) *on page 920*
- ◆ **Alagesic [DSC]** *see* Butalbital, Acetaminophen, and Caffeine *on page 260*
- ◆ **Alagesic LQ** *see* Butalbital, Acetaminophen, and Caffeine *on page 260*
- ◆ **Ala-Scalp** *see* Hydrocortisone (Topical) *on page 920*
- ◆ **Alavert® Allergy 24 Hour [OTC]** *see* Loratadine *on page 1128*
- ◆ **Alavert™ Allergy and Sinus [OTC]** *see* Loratadine and Pseudoephedrine *on page 1129*
- ◆ **Alavert® Children's Allergy [OTC]** *see* Loratadine *on page 1128*

Albendazole (al BEN da zole)

U.S. Brand Names Albenza®

Generic Availability (U.S.) No

Pharmacologic Category Anthelmintic

Medication Safety Issues

Sound-alike/look-alike issues:

Albenza® may be confused with Aplenzin™, Relenza®

International issues:

Albenza [U.S.] may be confused with Avanza brand name for mirtazapine [Australia]

Pregnancy Risk Factor C

Lactation Excretion in breast milk unknown/use caution

Use Treatment of parenchymal neurocysticercosis caused by *Taenia solium* and cystic hydatid disease of the liver, lung, and peritoneum caused by *Echinococcus granulosus*

Unlabeled/Investigational Use Albendazole has activity against *Ascaris lumbricoides* (roundworm); *Ancylostoma caninum*; *Ancylostoma duodenale* and *Necator americanus* (hookworms); cutaneous larva migrans; *Enterobius vermicularis* (pinworm); *Giardia duodenalis* (giardiasis); *Gnathostoma spinigerum*; *Gongylonema* sp; *Mansonella perstans* (filariasis); *Oesophagostomum bifurcum*; *Opisthorchis sinensis* (liver fluke); *Trichinella spiralis* (Trichinellosis); visceral larva migrans (toxocariasis); activity has also been shown against the liver fluke *Clonorchis sinensis*, *Giardia lamblia*, *Cysticercus cellulosae*, and *Echinococcus multilocularis*. Albendazole has also been used for the treatment of intestinal microsporidiosis (*Encephalitozoon intestinalis*), disseminated microsporidiosis (*E. hellem*, *E. cuniculi*, *E. intestinalis*, *Pleistophora* sp, *Trachipleistophora* sp, *Brachiola vesicularum*), and ocular microsporidiosis (*E. hellem*, *E. cuniculi*, *Vittaforma corneae*).

Available Dosage Forms

Tablet, oral:

Albenza®: 200 mg

Dosing

Adult & Geriatric

Neurocysticercosis: Oral:

<60 kg: 15 mg/kg/day in 2 divided doses (maximum: 800 mg/day) for 8-30 days

≥60 kg: 800 mg/day in 2 divided doses for 8-30 days

Note: Give concurrent anticonvulsant and steroid therapy during first week.

Hydatid: Oral:

<60 kg: 15 mg/kg/day in 2 divided doses (maximum: 800 mg/day)

≥60 kg: 800 mg/day in 2 divided doses

Note: Administer dose for three 28-day cycles with a 14-day drug-free interval in between each cycle.

***Ancylostoma caninum*, *Ascaris lumbricoides* (roundworm), *Ancylostoma duodenale* (hookworm), and *Necator americanus* (hookworm) (unlabeled use):** Oral: 400 mg as a single dose

***Clonorchis sinensis* (Chinese liver fluke) (unlabeled use):** Oral: 10 mg/kg/day for 7 days

Cutaneous larva migrans (unlabeled use): Oral: 400 mg once daily for 3 days

***Enterobius vermicularis* (pinworm) (unlabeled use):** Oral: 400 mg as a single dose; repeat in 2 weeks

***Giardia duodenalis* (giardiasis) (unlabeled use):** Oral: 400 mg once daily for 5 days

***Gnathostoma spinigerum* (unlabeled use):** Oral: 800 mg/day in 2 divided doses for 21 days

Gongylonemiasis (unlabeled use): Oral: 400 mg once daily for 3 days

***Mansonella perstans* (unlabeled use):** Oral: 800 mg/day in 2 divided doses for 10 days

***Oesophagostomum bifurcum* (unlabeled use):** Oral: 400 mg as a single dose (Ziem, 2004)

***Trichinella spiralis* (Trichinellosis) (unlabeled use):** Oral: 800 mg/day in 2 divided doses for 8-14 days plus steroids for severe symptoms

Visceral larva migrans (toxocariasis) (unlabeled use): Oral: 800 mg/day in 2 divided doses for 5 days

Cysticercus cellulosae **(unlabeled use):** Oral: 800 mg/day in 2 divided doses for 8-30 days; may be repeated as necessary

Disseminated microsporidiosis (unlabeled use): Oral: 800 mg/day in 2 divided doses

Echinococcus granulosus **(tapeworm) (unlabeled use):** Oral: 800 mg/day in 2 divided doses for 1-6 months

Intestinal microsporidiosis (*E. intestinalis*) (unlabeled use): Oral: 800 mg/day in 2 divided doses for 21 days

Ocular microsporidiosis (unlabeled use): Oral: 800 mg/day in 2 divided doses, in combination with fumagillin

Pediatric

Neurocysticercosis: Oral: Refer to adult dosing.

Hydatid: Oral: Refer to adult dosing.

Cysticercus cellulosae **(unlabeled use):** Oral: 15 mg/kg/day (maximum: 800 mg/day) in 2 divided doses for 8-30 days; may be repeated as necessary

Echinococcus granulosus **(tapeworm) (unlabeled use):** Oral: 15 mg/kg/day (maximum: 800 mg) divided twice daily for 1-6 months

Giardia duodenalis **(giardiasis) (unlabeled use):** Oral: 10 mg/kg/day for 5 days (Yereli, 2004)

Microsporidiosis (other than *Enterocytozoon bienuesi or* or *V. corneae*), disseminated or intestinal infection (HIV-positive, unlabeled use): Oral: Infants and Children: 15 mg/kg/day (maximum: 800 mg/day) in 2 divided doses continued until immune reconstitution after HAART initiation (CDC, 2009)

For the following unlabeled uses, refer to adult dosing: *Ancylostoma caninum*, *Ascaris lumbricoides* (roundworm), *Ancylostoma duodenale* (hookworm), *Clonorchis sinensis*, (Chinese liver fluke), cutaneous larva migrans, *Enterobius vermicularis* (pinworm), *Gnathostoma spinigerum*, gongylonemiasis, *Mansonella perstans*, *Necator americanus* (hookworm), *Oesophagostomum bifurcum*, *Trichinella spiralis* (Trichinellosis), visceral larva migrans (toxocariasis)

Administration

Oral Should be administered with a high-fat meal. Administer anticonvulsant and steroid therapy during first week of neurocysticercosis therapy. If patients have difficulty swallowing, tablets may be crushed or chewed, then swallowed with a drink of water.

Monitoring and Teaching Issues

Laboratory Monitoring Monitor fecal specimens for ova and parasites for 3 weeks after treatment; if positive, retreat; LFTs and CBC with differential at start of each 28-day cycle and every 2 weeks during therapy (more frequent monitoring for patients with liver disease); pregnancy test

Physical Assessment Dosing based on identification of parasite. Assess laboratory results for reduction or elimination of ova and parasites. Monitor for elevated LFTs and leukopenia.

Patient Education Laboratory tests may be required; maintain recommended schedule. Take with a high-fat meal. Follow prescriber's suggestions to prevent reinfection. May cause loss of hair (reversible), nausea, vomiting, dizziness, or headaches. Report unusual fever, persistent or unresolved abdominal pain, vomiting, yellowing of skin or eyes, darkening of urine, or light colored stools.

◆ **Albenza®** *see* Albendazole *on page 56*

Albumin (al BYOO min)

U.S. Brand Names Albuminar®-25; Albuminar®-5; AlbuRx® 25; AlbuRx® 5; Albutein®; Buminate; Flexbumin 25%; Human Albumin Grifols® 25%; Plasbumin®-25; Plasbumin®-5

Index Terms Albumin (Human); Normal Human Serum Albumin; Normal Serum Albumin (Human); Salt Poor Albumin; SPA

Generic Availability (U.S.) Yes: Excludes low aluminum formulation

Pharmacologic Category Blood Product Derivative; Plasma Volume Expander, Colloid

Medication Safety Issues

Sound-alike/look-alike issues:

Albutein® may be confused with albuterol

Buminate® may be confused with bumetanide

Pregnancy Risk Factor C

Lactation Excretion in breast milk unknown/compatible

Use Plasma volume expansion and maintenance of cardiac output in the treatment of certain types of shock or impending shock; may be useful for burn patients, ARDS, and cardiopulmonary bypass; other uses considered by some investigators (but not proven) are retroperitoneal surgery, peritonitis, and ascites; unless the condition responsible for hypoproteinemia can be corrected, albumin can provide only symptomatic relief or supportive treatment

Note: Nutritional supplementation is not an appropriate indication.

Unlabeled/Investigational Use In cirrhotics, administered with diuretics to help facilitate diuresis; large volume paracentesis; volume expansion in dehydrated, mildly-hypotensive cirrhotics; to prevent renal impairment and reduce mortality associated with spontaneous bacterial peritonitis (SBP) in patients with cirrhosis

Available Dosage Forms

Injection, solution [preservative free]: 5% [50 mg/mL] (250 mL, 500 mL); 20% [200 mg/mL] (50 mL, 100 mL); 25% [250 mg/mL] (50 mL, 100 mL)
Albuminar®-5: 5% [50 mg/mL] (250 mL, 500 mL)
Albuminar®-25: 25% [250 mg/mL] (50 mL, 100 mL)
AlbuRx® 5: 5% [50 mg/mL] (250 mL, 500 mL)
AlbuRx® 25: 25% [250 mg/mL] (50 mL, 100 mL)
Albutein®: 5% [50 mg/mL] (250 mL, 500 mL); 25% [250 mg/mL] (50 mL, 100 mL)
Buminate: 5% [50 mg/mL] (250 mL, 500 mL); 25% [250 mg/mL] (20 mL)
Flexbumin 25%: 25% [250 mg/mL] (50 mL, 100 mL)
Human Albumin Grifols® 25%: 25% [250 mg/mL] (50 mL, 100 mL)
Plasbumin®-5: 5% [50 mg/mL] (50 mL, 250 mL)
Plasbumin®-25: 25% [250 mg/mL] (20 mL, 50 mL, 100 mL)

Dosing

Adult & Geriatric

Note: Use **5%** solution in hypovolemic patients or intravascularly-depleted patients. Use **25%** solution in patients in whom fluid and sodium intake is restricted.

Usual dose: 25 g; initial dose may be repeated in 15-30 minutes if response is inadequate; no more than 250 g should be administered within 48 hours.

Hypoproteinemia: I.V.: 0.5-1 g/kg/dose; repeat every 1-2 days as calculated to replace ongoing losses.

Hypovolemia: 5% albumin: 0.5-1 g/kg/dose; repeat as needed. **Note:** May be considered after inadequate response to crystalloid therapy and when nonprotein colloids are contraindicated. The volume administered and the speed of infusion should be adapted to individual response.

Large-volume paracentesis (>5 L): 25% albumin: 5-8 g for every liter removed (Garcia-Compeán, 1993; Moore, 2003) **or** 50 g total for paracentesis >5 L (ATS, 2004). **Note:** Administer soon after the procedure to avoid postprocedural complications (eg, hypovolemia, hyponatremia, renal impairment) (Moore, 2003).

SBP in patients with cirrhosis: 25% albumin: Initial: 1.5 g/kg, followed by 1 g/kg on day 3 (in conjunction with appropriate antimicrobial therapy) (Sort, 1999; ATS, 2004). **Note:** Clinical trial employed albumin 20%; however, the difference in concentration compared with 25% albumin is deemed to be clinically inconsequential.

Pediatric

Note: 5% should be used in hypovolemic patients or intravascularly-depleted patients. **25%** should be used in patients in whom fluid and sodium intake must be minimized.

Dose depends on condition of patient: Hypovolemia: I.V.: 0.5-1 g/kg/dose (10-20 mL/kg/dose of albumin 5%); maximum dose: 6 g/kg/day

Administration

I.V. For I.V. administration only. Use within 4 hours after opening vial; discard unused portion. In emergencies, may administer as rapidly as necessary to improve clinical condition. After initial volume replacement:

5%: Do not exceed 2-4 mL/minute in patients with normal plasma volume; 5-10 mL/minute in patients with hypoproteinemia

25%: Do not exceed 1 mL/minute in patients with normal plasma volume; 2-3 mL/minute in patients with hypoproteinemia

Monitoring and Teaching Issues

Laboratory Monitoring Hematocrit

Physical Assessment Asses patient for hepatic or renal failure. Patient should be monitored closely for pulmonary edema and cardiac failure (assess vital signs and central venous pressure) during administration. Monitor frequently for hypovolemia or fluid overload. If fever, tachycardia, hypotension, or dyspnea occurs, infusion should be stopped and prescriber notified.

Patient Education This medication can only be administered intravenously. You will be monitored closely during the infusion. Report immediately any pain or bruising at infusion site, acute headache, difficulty breathing, chills, chest pain or tightness, palpitations, or sudden pain.

- ◆ **Albuminar®-5** *see* Albumin *on page* 57
- ◆ **Albuminar®-25** *see* Albumin *on page* 57
- ◆ **Albumin-Bound Paclitaxel** *see* Paclitaxel (Protein Bound) *on page* 1390
- ◆ **Albumin (Human)** *see* Albumin *on page* 57
- ◆ **Albumin-Stabilized Nanoparticle Paclitaxel** *see* Paclitaxel (Protein Bound) *on page* 1390
- ◆ **AlbuRx® 5** *see* Albumin *on page* 57
- ◆ **AlbuRx® 25** *see* Albumin *on page* 57
- ◆ **Albutein®** *see* Albumin *on page* 57

Albuterol (al BYOO ter ole)

U.S. Brand Names AccuNeb®; ProAir® HFA; Proventil® HFA; Ventolin® HFA; VoSpire ER®

Index Terms Albuterol Sulfate; Salbutamol; Salbutamol Sulphate

Generic Availability (U.S.) Yes

Pharmacologic Category $Beta_2$-Adrenergic Agonist

Medication Safety Issues

Sound-alike/look-alike issues:

Albuterol may be confused with Albutein®, atenolol

Proventil® may be confused with Bentyl®, PriLOSEC®, Prinivil®

Salbutamol may be confused with salmeterol

Ventolin® may be confused with phentolamine, Benylin®, Vantin

Pregnancy Risk Factor C

Lactation Excretion in breast milk unknown/use caution

Use Treatment or prevention of bronchospasm in patients with reversible obstructive airway disease; prevention of exercise-induced bronchospasm

Mechanism of Action/Effect Relaxes bronchial smooth muscle by action on beta$_2$-receptors with little effect on heart rate

Contraindications Hypersensitivity to albuterol or any component of the formulation

Injection formulation (Canadian labeling; product not available in U.S.): Hypersensitivity to albuterol or any component of the formulation; tachyarrhythmias; risk of abortion during first or second trimester

Warnings/Precautions Optimize anti-inflammatory treatment before initiating maintenance treatment with albuterol. Do not use as a component of chronic therapy without an anti-inflammatory agent. Only the mildest forms of asthma (Step 1 and/or exercise-induced) would not require concurrent use based upon asthma guidelines. Patient must be instructed to seek medical attention in cases where acute symptoms are not relieved or a previous level of response is diminished. The need to increase frequency of use may indicate deterioration of asthma, and treatment must not be delayed.

Use caution in patients with cardiovascular disease (arrhythmia or hypertension or HF), convulsive disorders, diabetes, glaucoma, hyperthyroidism, or hypokalemia. Beta-agonists may cause elevation in blood pressure, heart rate, and result in CNS stimulation/excitation. Beta$_2$-agonists may increase risk of arrhythmia, increase serum glucose, or decrease serum potassium.

Immediate hypersensitivity reactions (urticaria, angioedema, rash, bronchospasm) have been reported. Do not exceed recommended dose; serious adverse events, including fatalities, have been associated with excessive use of inhaled sympathomimetics. Rarely, paradoxical bronchospasm may occur with use of inhaled bronchodilating agents; this should be distinguished from inadequate response. All patients should utilize a spacer device or valved holding chamber when using a metered-dose inhaler; in addition, face masks should be used in children <4 years of age.

Patient response may vary between inhalers that contain chlorofluorocarbons and those which are chlorofluorocarbon-free.

Drug Interactions

Avoid Concomitant Use

Avoid concomitant use of Albuterol with any of the following: Iobenguane I 123

Decreased Effect

Albuterol may decrease the levels/effects of: Iobenguane I 123

The levels/effects of Albuterol may be decreased by: Alpha-/Beta-Blockers; Beta-Blockers (Beta1 Selective); Beta-Blockers (Nonselective); Betahistine

Increased Effect/Toxicity

Albuterol may increase the levels/effects of: Loop Diuretics; Sympathomimetics

The levels/effects of Albuterol may be increased by: Atomoxetine; Cannabinoids; MAO Inhibitors; Tricyclic Antidepressants

Nutritional/Ethanol Interactions

Food: Avoid or limit caffeine (may cause CNS stimulation).

Herb/Nutraceutical: Avoid ephedra, yohimbe (may cause CNS stimulation). Avoid St John's wort (may decrease the levels/effects of albuterol).

Lab Interactions Increased renin (S), aldosterone (S)

Adverse Reactions Incidence of adverse effects is dependent upon age of patient, dose, and route of administration.

Cardiovascular: Angina, atrial fibrillation, arrhythmias, chest discomfort, chest pain, extrasystoles, flushing, hyper-/hypotension, palpitation, supraventricular tachycardia, tachycardia

Central nervous system: CNS stimulation, dizziness, drowsiness, headache, insomnia, irritability, lightheadedness, migraine, nervousness, nightmares, restlessness, seizure

Dermatologic: Angioedema, rash, urticaria

Endocrine & metabolic: Hyperglycemia, hypokalemia, lactic acidosis

Gastrointestinal: Diarrhea, dry mouth, dyspepsia, gastroenteritis, nausea, unusual taste, vomiting

Genitourinary: Micturition difficulty

Local: Injection: Pain, stinging

Neuromuscular & skeletal: Muscle cramps, musculoskeletal pain, tremor, weakness

Otic: Otitis media, vertigo

Respiratory: Asthma exacerbation, bronchospasm, cough, epistaxis, laryngitis, oropharyngeal drying/irritation, oropharyngeal edema, pharyngitis, rhinitis, upper respiratory inflammation, viral respiratory infection

Miscellaneous: Allergic reaction, anaphylaxis, diaphoresis, lymphadenopathy

Pharmacodynamics/Kinetics

Onset of Action Peak effect:

Nebulization/oral inhalation: 0.5-2 hours

CFC-propelled albuterol: 10 minutes

Ventolin® HFA: 25 minutes

Oral: 2-3 hours

Duration of Action Nebulization/oral inhalation: 3-4 hours; Oral: 4-6 hours

Half-Life Elimination Inhalation: 3.8 hours; Oral: 3.7-5 hours

Metabolism Hepatic to an inactive sulfate

Excretion Urine (30% as unchanged drug)

Available Dosage Forms

Aerosol, for oral inhalation:

ProAir® HFA: 90 mcg/inhalation (8.5 g)

Proventil® HFA: 90 mcg/inhalation (6.7 g)

Ventolin® HFA: 90 mcg/inhalation (8 g, 18 g)

Solution, for nebulization: 0.5% [100 mg/20 mL] (1s); 0.083% [2.5 mg/3 mL] (25s, 30s)

Solution, for nebulization [preservative free]: 0.021% [0.63 mg/3 mL] (25s); 0.042% [1.25 mg/3 mL] (25s, 30s); 0.083% [2.5 mg/3 mL] (10s, 24s, 25s, 30s, 60s); 0.5% [2.5 mg/0.5 mL] (10s, 30s)

AccuNeb®: 0.021% [0.63 mg/3 mL] (25s); 0.042% [1.25 mg/3 mL] (25s)

Syrup, oral: 2 mg/5 mL (473 mL, 480 mL)

Tablet, oral: 2 mg, 4 mg

Tablet, extended release, oral: 4 mg, 8 mg

VoSpire ER®: 4 mg, 8 mg

Dosing

Adult

Bronchospasm:

Metered-dose inhaler: 2 puffs every 4-6 hours as needed (NIH Guidelines, 2007):

Solution for nebulization: 2.5 mg 3-4 times daily as needed; Quick relief: 1.25-5 mg every 4 to 8 hours as needed (NIH Guidelines, 2007)

Oral: 2-4 mg/dose 3-4 times/day; maximum dose not to exceed 32 mg/day (divided doses)

Extended release: 8 mg every 12 hours; maximum dose not to exceed 32 mg/day (divided doses). A 4 mg dose every 12 hours may be sufficient in some patients, such as adults of low body weight.

I.V. continuous infusion (Canadian labeling; product not available in U.S.]): Severe bronchospasm and status asthmaticus: Initial: 5 mcg/minute; may increase up to 10-20 mcg/minute at 15- to 30-minute intervals if needed

Exacerbation of asthma (acute, severe) (NIH Guidelines, 2007):

Metered-dose inhaler: 4-8 puffs every 20 minutes for up to 4 hours, then every 1-4 hours as needed

Solution for nebulization: 2.5-5 mg every 20 minutes for 3 doses, then 2.5-10 mg every 1-4 hours as needed, **or** 10-15 mg/hour by continuous nebulization

Exercise-induced bronchospasm (prevention): *Metered-dose inhaler:* 2 puffs 5-30 minutes prior to exercise

Geriatric

Inhalation: Refer to adult dosing.

Bronchospasm (treatment): Oral: 2 mg 3-4 times/day; maximum: 8 mg 4 times/day

Pediatric

Bronchospasm:

Oral, regular release:

Children 2-6 years: 0.1-0.2 mg/kg/dose 3 times/day (maximum: 12 mg/day)

Children 6-12 years: 2 mg/dose 3-4 times/day (maximum: 24 mg/day)

Children >12 years: 2-4 mg/dose 3-4 times/day (maximum: 32 mg/day)

Oral, extended release:

Children 6-12 years: 4 mg every 12 hours (maximum: 24 mg/day)

Children >12 years: 8 mg every 12 hours (maximum: 32 mg/day)

Metered-dose inhaler (90 mcg/puff): NIH Guidelines, 2007: Quick relief:

Children ≤4 years: 2 puffs every 4-6 hours as needed

Children 5-11 years: 2 puffs every 4-6 hours as needed

Children ≥12 years: 2 puffs every 4-6 hours as needed

Solution for nebulization:

Manufacturer's recommendations:

Children 2-12 years (AccuNeb®): 0.63-1.25 mg 3-4 times daily as needed

Children ≥12 years: 2.5 mg 3-4 times daily as needed

NIH Guidelines, 2007: Quick relief:

Children ≤4 years: 0.63-2.5 mg every 4-6 hours as needed

Children ≥5 years: 1.25-5 mg every 4-8 hours as needed

Exacerbation of asthma (acute, severe) (NIH Guidelines, 2007):

Metered-dose inhaler (90 mcg/puff):

Children <12 years: 4-8 puffs every 20 minutes for 3 doses, then every 1-4 hours as needed

Children ≥12 years: 4-8 puffs every 20 minutes for up to 4 hours, then every 1-4 hours as needed

Solution for nebulization:

Children <12 years: 0.15 mg/kg (minimum: 2.5 mg) every 20 minutes for 3 doses, then 0.15-0.3 mg/kg (maximum: 10 mg) every 1-4 hours as needed, **or** 0.5 mg/kg/hour by continuous nebulization

Children ≥12 years: 2.5-5 mg every 20 minutes for 3 doses, then 2.5-10 mg every 1-4 hours as needed, **or** 10-15 mg/hour by continuous nebulization

Exercise-induced bronchospasm (prevention): *Metered-dose inhaler (90 mcg/puff):*

Children ≤4 years: 1-2 puffs 5 minutes prior to exercise (NIH Guidelines, 2007)

Children >4 years: 2 puffs 5-30 minutes prior to exercise

Renal Impairment Use with caution in patients with renal impairment. No dosage adjustment required (including patients on hemodialysis, peritoneal dialysis, or CRRT; Aronoff, 2007).

Administration

Oral Do not crush or chew extended release tablets.

I.V. Infusion solution (Canadian labeling; product not available in U.S.): Do not inject undiluted. Reduce concentration by at least 50% before infusing. Administer as a continuous infusion via infusion pump.

Inhalation

Metered-dose inhaler: Shake well before use; prime prior to first use, and whenever inhaler has not been used for >2 weeks or when it has been dropped, by releasing 3-4 test sprays into the air (away from face). HFA inhalers should be cleaned with warm water at least once per week; allow to air dry completely prior to use. A spacer device or valved holding chamber is recommended for use with metered-dose inhalers.

Solution for nebulization: Concentrated solution should be diluted prior to use. Blow-by administration is not recommended, use a mask device if patient unable to hold mouthpiece in mouth for administration.

Stability

Reconstitution Solution for nebulization: To prepare a 2.5 mg dose, dilute 0.5 mL of solution to a total of 3 mL with normal saline; also compatible with cromolyn or ipratropium nebulizer solutions.

Storage

HFA aerosols: Store at 15°C to 25°C (59°F to 77°F).

Ventolin® HFA: Discard when counter reads 000 or 12 months after removal from protective pouch, whichever comes first. Store with mouthpiece down.

Infusion solution (Canadian labeling; product not available in U.S.): Ventolin® I.V.: Store at 15°C to 30°C (59°F to 86°F). Protect from light. After dilution, discard unused portion after 24 hours.

Solution for nebulization (0.5%): Store at 2°C to 25°C (36°F to 77°F).

AccuNeb®: Store at 2°C to 25°C (36°F to 77°F). Do not use if solution changes color or becomes cloudy. Use within 1 week of opening foil pouch.

Syrup: Store at 20°C to 25°C (68°F to 77°F).

Tablet: Store at 20°C to 25°C (68°F to 77°F).

Tablet, extended release: Store at 20°C to 25°C (68°F to 77°F)

Monitoring and Teaching Issues

Laboratory Monitoring Arterial or capillary blood gases (if patients condition warrants); FEV_1, peak flow, and/or other pulmonary function tests; serum potassium, serum glucose (in selected patients)

Physical Assessment For inpatient care, monitor vital signs at beginning of therapy and periodically throughout. Evaluate effectiveness of therapy (relief of airway obstruction).

Patient Education Maintain adequate hydration, unless instructed to restrict fluid intake. You may experience nervousness, dizziness, dry mouth, unpleasant taste, or stomach upset. Report unresolved GI upset, dizziness, chest pain or palpitations, nervousness or insomnia, muscle cramping or tremor, or respiratory difficulty.

Self-administered inhalation: Shake canister before using. Sit when using medication. Close eyes when administering albuterol to avoid spraying into eyes. Exhale slowly and completely through nose; inhale deeply through mouth while administering aerosol. Hold breath for 5-10 seconds after inhalation. Wait at least 1 full minute between inhalations. Wash mouthpiece between use. If more than one inhalation medication is used, use albuterol first and wait 5 minutes between medications. Prime inhaler prior to first use, and whenever the inhaler has not been used for more than 2 weeks.

Self-administered nebulizer: Wash hands before and after treatment. Wash and dry nebulizer after each treatment. Twist open the top of one unit-dose vial and squeeze contents into nebulizer reservoir. Connect nebulizer reservoir to the mouthpiece or face mask. Connect nebulizer to compressor. Sit in comfortable, upright position. Place mouthpiece in your mouth or put on face mask and turn on compressor. If face mask is used, avoid leakage around the mask to avoid mist getting into eyes, which may cause vision problems. Breathe calmly and deeply until no more mist is formed in nebulizer (about 5 minutes).

Dietary Considerations Oral forms should be taken with water 1 hour before or 2 hours after meals.

Geriatric Considerations Because of its minimal effect on $beta_1$-receptors and its relatively long duration of action, albuterol is a rational choice in elderly when a beta-agonist is indicated. Elderly patients may find it beneficial to utilize a spacer device when using a metered dose inhaler. Oral use should be avoided due to adverse effects.

Pregnancy Considerations Albuterol crosses the placenta; tocolytic effects, fetal tachycardia, fetal hypoglycemia secondary to maternal hyperglycemia with oral or intravenous routes reported. Available evidence suggests safe use as an inhalation during pregnancy, and albuterol is the preferred short-acting beta agonist for use in asthma according to the NHLBI 2007 Guidelines for the Diagnosis and Management of Asthma.

Additional Information The 2007 National Heart, Lung, and Blood Institute Guidelines for the Diagnosis and Management of Asthma do not recommend the use of oral systemic albuterol as a quick-relief medication and do not recommend regularly scheduled daily, chronic use of inhaled beta-agonists for long-term control of asthma.

◆ **Albuterol and Ipratropium** *see* Ipratropium and Albuterol *on page* 1011

◆ **Albuterol Sulfate** *see* Albuterol *on page* 58

Alcaftadine (al KAF ta deen)

U.S. Brand Names Lastacaft™

Generic Availability (U.S.) No

Pharmacologic Category Histamine H_1 Antagonist; Histamine H_1 Antagonist, Second Generation; Mast Cell Stabilizer

Pregnancy Risk Factor B

Lactation Excretion in breast milk unknown/use caution

Use Prevention of itching associated with allergic conjunctivitis

Available Dosage Forms

Solution, ophthalmic:

Lastacaft™: 0.25% (3 mL)

Dosing

Adult & Geriatric Allergic conjunctivitis: Ophthalmic: Instill 1 drop into each eye once daily.

Pediatric Allergic conjunctivitis: Ophthalmic: Children ≥2 years: Refer to adult dosing.

Administration

Other For topical ophthalmic use only. Contact lenses should be removed prior to application, and may be reinserted 10 minutes after administration. Do not insert contacts if eyes are red. Avoid contaminating the applicator tip with affected eye(s).

◆ **Aldactazide®** *see* Hydrochlorothiazide and Spironolactone *on page* 914

◆ **Aldactone®** *see* Spironolactone *on page* 1678

◆ **Aldara®** *see* Imiquimod *on page* 959

Aldesleukin (al des LOO kin)

U.S. Brand Names Proleukin®

Index Terms IL-2; Interleukin 2; Interleukin-2; Lymphocyte Mitogenic Factor; Recombinant Human Interleukin-2; T-Cell Growth Factor; TCGF; Thymocyte Stimulating Factor

Generic Availability (U.S.) No

Pharmacologic Category Antineoplastic Agent, Miscellaneous; Biological Response Modulator

Medication Safety Issues

Sound-alike/look-alike issues:

Aldesleukin may be confused with oprelvekin

Proleukin® may be confused with oprelvekin

High alert medication: The Institute for Safe Medication Practices (ISMP) includes this medication among its list of drug classes which have a heightened risk of causing significant patient harm when used in error.

Pregnancy Risk Factor C

Lactation Excretion in breast milk unknown/not recommended

Use Treatment of metastatic renal cell cancer, metastatic melanoma

Unlabeled/Investigational Use Treatment of acute myeloid leukemia (AML)

Mechanism of Action/Effect Aldesleukin is a human recombinant interleukin-2 product which promotes proliferation, differentiation, and recruitment of T and B cells, natural killer (NK) cells, and thymocytes; causes cytolytic activity in a subset of lymphocytes and subsequent interactions between the immune system and malignant cells; can stimulate lymphokine-activated killer (LAK) cells and tumor-infiltrating lymphocytes (TIL) cells.

Contraindications Hypersensitivity to aldesleukin or any component of the formulation; patients with abnormal thallium stress or pulmonary function tests; patients who have had an organ allograft. **Retreatment is contraindicated** in patients who have experienced sustained ventricular tachycardia (≥5 beats), uncontrolled or unresponsive cardiac arrhythmias, chest pain with ECG changes consistent with angina or MI, cardiac tamponade, intubation >72 hours, renal failure requiring dialysis for >72 hours, coma or toxic psychosis lasting >48 hours, repetitive or refractory seizures, bowel ischemia/perforation, or GI bleeding requiring surgery.

Warnings/Precautions Hazardous agent - use appropriate precautions for handling and disposal.

[U.S. Boxed Warning]: High-dose aldesleukin therapy has been associated with capillary leak syndrome (CLS), characterized by vascular tone loss and extravasation of plasma proteins and fluid into extravascular space. CLS results in significant hypotension and reduced organ perfusion which may be severe and can result in death; CLS onset is immediately after treatment initiation. Cardiac arrhythmia, angina, MI, respiratory insufficiency (requiring intubation), gastrointestinal bleeding or infarction, renal insufficiency, edema and mental status changes are also associated with CLS. Monitor fluid status and organ perfusion status carefully; consider fluids and/or pressor agents to maintain organ perfusion. **[U.S. Boxed Warning]: Therapy should be restricted to patients with normal cardiac and pulmonary**

functions as defined by thallium stress and formal pulmonary function testing. Extreme caution should be used in patients with a history of prior cardiac or pulmonary disease and in patients who are fluid-restricted or where edema may be poorly tolerated. Withhold treatment for signs of organ hypoperfusion, including altered mental status, reduced urine output, systolic BP <90 mm Hg or cardiac arrhythmia. Once blood pressure is normalized, may consider diuretics for excessive weight gain/edema. Recovery from CLS generally begins soon after treatment cessation. Perform a thorough clinical evaluation prior to treatment initiation; exclude patients with significant cardiac, pulmonary, renal, hepatic, or central nervous system impairment from treatment. Patients with a more favorable performance status prior to treatment initiation are more likely to respond to aldesleukin treatment, with a higher response rate and generally lower toxicity.

[U.S. Boxed Warning]: Should be administered under the supervision of an experienced cancer chemotherapy physician in a facility with cardiopulmonary or intensive specialists and intensive care facilities available. Adverse effects are frequent and sometimes fatal. May exacerbate pre-existing or initial presentation of autoimmune diseases and inflammatory disorders; exacerbation and/or new onset have been reported with aldesleukin and interferon alfa combination therapy. Patients should be evaluated and treated for CNS metastases and have a negative scan prior to treatment; new neurologic symptoms and lesions have been reported in patients without pre-existing evidence of CNS metastases (symptoms generally improve upon discontinuation, however, cases with permanent damage have been reported). Mental status changes (irritability, confusion, depression) can occur and may indicate bacteremia, sepsis, hypoperfusion, CNS malignancy, or CNS toxicity. May cause seizure; use with caution in patients with seizure disorder.

[U.S. Boxed Warning]: Impaired neutrophil function is associated with treatment; patients are at risk for disseminated infection (including sepsis and bacterial endocarditis), and central line-related gram-positive infections. Treat pre-existing bacterial infection appropriately prior to treatment initiation. Monitor for signs of infection or sepsis during treatment. Antibiotic prophylaxis which has been associated with a reduced incidence of staphylococcal infections in aldesleukin studies includes the use of oxacillin, nafcillin, ciprofloxacin, or vancomycin.

[U.S. Boxed Warning]: Withhold treatment for patients developing moderate-to-severe lethargy or somnolence; continued treatment may result in coma. Standard prophylactic supportive care during high-dose aldesleukin treatment includes acetaminophen to relieve constitutional symptoms and an H_2 antagonist to reduce the risk of GI ulceration and/or bleeding. May impair renal or hepatic function; patients must have a serum creatinine ≤1.5 mg/dL prior to treatment. Concomitant nephrotoxic or hepatotoxic agents may increase the risk of renal or hepatic toxicity. Enhancement of cellular immune function may increase the risk of allograft rejection in transplant patients. An acute array of symptoms resembling aldesleukin adverse reactions (fever, chills, nausea, rash, pruritus, diarrhea, hypotension, edema, and oliguria) were observed within 1-4 hours after iodinated contrast media administration, usually when given within 4 weeks after aldesleukin treatment, although has been reported several months after aldesleukin treatment. The incidence of dyspnea and severe urogenital toxicities is potentially increased in elderly patients.

Drug Interactions

Avoid Concomitant Use

Avoid concomitant use of Aldesleukin with any of the following: Corticosteroids

Decreased Effect

The levels/effects of Aldesleukin may be decreased by: Corticosteroids

Increased Effect/Toxicity

Aldesleukin may increase the levels/effects of: Hypotensive Agents

The levels/effects of Aldesleukin may be increased by: Contrast Media (Non-ionic); Interferons (Alfa)

Nutritional/Ethanol Interactions Ethanol: May increase CNS adverse effects.

Adverse Reactions

>10%:

- Cardiovascular: Hypotension (71%; grade 4: 3%), peripheral edema (28%), tachycardia (23%), edema (15%), vasodilation (13%), supraventricular tachycardia (12%; grade 4: 1%), cardiovascular disorder (11%; includes blood pressure changes, HF and ECG changes)
- Central nervous system: Chills (52%), confusion (34%; grade 4: 1%), fever (29%; grade 4: 1%), malaise (27%), somnolence (22%), anxiety (12%), pain (12%), dizziness (11%)
- Dermatologic: Rash (42%), pruritus (24%), exfoliative dermatitis (18%)
- Endocrine & metabolic: Acidosis (12%; grade 4: 1%), hypomagnesemia (12%), hypocalcemia (11%)
- Gastrointestinal: Diarrhea (67%; grade 4: 2%), vomiting (19% to 50%; grade 4: 1%), nausea (19% to 35%), stomatitis (22%), anorexia (20%), weight gain (16%), abdominal pain (11%)
- Hematologic: Thrombocytopenia (37%; grade 4: 1%), anemia (29%), leukopenia (16%)
- Hepatic: Hyperbilirubinemia (40%; grade 4: 2%), AST increased (23%; grade 4: 1%)
- Neuromuscular & skeletal: Weakness (23%)
- Renal: Oliguria (63%; grade 4: 6%), creatinine increased (33%; grade 4: 1%)
- Respiratory: Dyspnea (43%; grade 4: 1%), lung disorder (24%; includes pulmonary congestion, rales, and rhonchi), cough (11%), respiratory disorder (11%; includes acute respiratory distress syndrome, infiltrates and pulmonary changes)
- Miscellaneous: Infection (13%; grade 4: 1%)

1% to 10%:

Cardiovascular: Arrhythmia (10%), cardiac arrest (grade 4: 1%), MI (grade 4: 1%), ventricular tachycardia (grade 4: 1%)

Central nervous system: Coma (grade 4: 2%), stupor (grade 4: 1%), psychosis (grade 4: 1%)

Gastrointestinal: Abdomen enlarged (10%)

Hematologic: Coagulation disorder (grade 4: 1%)

Hepatic: Alkaline phosphatase increased (10%)

Renal: Anuria (grade 4: 5%), acute renal failure (grade 4: 1%)

Respiratory: Rhinitis (10%), apnea (grade 4: 1%)

Miscellaneous: Sepsis (grade 4: 1%)

Pharmacodynamics/Kinetics

Half-Life Elimination I.V.: Initial: 6-13 minutes; Terminal: 80-120 minutes

Metabolism Renal (metabolized to amino acids)

Excretion Urine (primarily as metabolites)

Available Dosage Forms

Injection, powder for reconstitution:

Proleukin®: 22 x 10^6 int. units

Dosing

Adult & Geriatric Consider premedication with an antipyretic to reduce fever, an H_2 antagonist for prophylaxis of gastrointestinal irritation/bleeding, antiemetics, and antidiarrheals; continue for 12 hours after the last aldesleukin dose. Antibiotic prophylaxis is recommended to reduce the incidence of infection.

Renal cell carcinoma: I.V.: 600,000 int. units/kg every 8 hours for a maximum of 14 doses; repeat after 9 days for a total of 28 doses per course; retreat if tumor shrinkage observed (and if no contraindications) at least 7 weeks after hospital discharge date

or

Unlabeled dosing: 720,000 int. units/kg every 8 hours for up to 12 doses; repeat with a second cycle 10-15 days later (Klapper, 2008)

Melanoma: I.V.:

Single-agent use: 600,000 int. units/kg every 8 hours for a maximum of 14 doses; repeat after 9 days for a total of 28 doses per course; retreat if tumor shrinkage observed (and if no contraindications) at least 7 weeks after hospital discharge date

or

Unlabeled dosing: 720,000 int. units/kg every 8 hours for 12-15 doses; repeat with a second cycle ~14 days after the first dose of the initial cycle (Smith, 2008)

Combination biochemotherapy (unlabeled use): 9 million int. units/m²/day continuous infusion over 24 hours for 4 days every 3 weeks for up to 4 cycles (Atkins, 2008) **or** 9 million int. units/m²/day continuous infusion over 24 hours days 5 to 8, 17 to 20, and 26 to 29 every 42 days for up to 5 cycles (Eton, 2002) **or** 9 million int. units/m²/day continuous infusion over 24 hours for 4 days every 3 weeks for 6 cycles (Legha, 1998)

Pediatric Consider premedication with an antipyretic to reduce fever, an H_2 antagonist for prophylaxis of gastrointestinal irritation/bleeding, antiemetics, and antidiarrheals; continue for 12 hours after the last aldesleukin dose. Antibiotic prophylaxis is recommended to reduce the incidence of infection.

AML (unlabeled use): I.V.: 9 million int. units (9 x 10^6 int. units)/m²/day continuous infusion over 24 hours daily for 4 days; repeat 4 days later with 1.6 million int. units (1.6 x 10^6 int. units)/m²/day continuous infusion over 24 hours daily for 10 days (Lange, 2008)

Renal Impairment No specific recommendations by manufacturer. Use with caution.

Adjustment for Toxicity Withhold or interrupt a dose for toxicity; do not reduce the dose.

Cardiovascular toxicity:

Atrial fibrillation, supraventricular tachycardia or bradycardia that is persistent, recurrent or requires treatment: Withhold dose; may resume when asymptomatic with full recovery to normal sinus rhythm.

Systolic BP <90 mm Hg (with increasing pressor requirements): Withhold dose; may resume treatment when systolic BP ≥90 mm Hg and stable or pressor requirements improve.

Any ECG change consistent with MI, ischemia or myocarditis (with or without chest pain), or suspected cardiac ischemia: Withhold dose; may resume when asymptomatic, MI/myocarditis have been ruled out, suspicion of angina is low, or there is no evidence of ventricular hypokinesia.

CNS toxicity: Mental status change, including moderate confusion or agitation: Withhold dose; may resume when resolved completely.

Dermatologic toxicity: Bullous dermatitis or marked worsening of pre-existing skin condition: Withhold dose; may treat with antihistamines or topical products (do not use topical steroids); may resume with resolution of all signs of bullous dermatitis.

Gastrointestinal: Stool guaiac repeatedly >3-4+: Withhold dose; may resume with negative stool guaiac.

Hepatotoxicity: Signs of hepatic failure, encephalopathy, increasing ascites, liver pain, hypoglycemia: Withhold dose and discontinue treatment for balance of cycle; may initiate a new course if indicated only after at least 7 weeks past resolution of all signs of hepatic failure (including hospital discharge).

Infection: Sepsis syndrome, clinically unstable: Withhold dose; may resume when sepsis syndrome has resolved, patient is clinically stable, and infection is under treatment.

Renal toxicity:

Serum creatinine >4.5 mg/dL (or ≥4 mg/dL with severe volume overload, acidosis or hyperkalemia): Withhold dose; may resume when <4 mg/dL and fluid/electrolyte status is stable.

Persistent oliguria or urine output <10 mL/hour for 16-24 hours with rising serum creatinine: Withhold dose; may resume when urine output >10 mL/hour with serum creatinine decrease of >1.5 mg/dL or normalization.

Respiratory toxicity: Oxygen saturation <90%: Withhold dose; may resume when >90%.

Retreatment with aldesleukin is contraindicated with the following toxicities: Sustained ventricular tachycardia (≥5 beats), uncontrolled or unresponsive cardiac arrhythmias, chest pain with ECG changes consistent with angina or MI, cardiac tamponade, intubation >72 hours, renal failure requiring dialysis for >72 hours, coma or toxic psychosis lasting >48 hours, repetitive or refractory seizures, bowel ischemia/perforation, or GI bleeding requiring surgery

Administration

I.V. Infuse over 15 minutes. Allow solution to reach room temperature prior to administration. Do not administer with an inline filter. Flush before and after with D_5W, particularly if maintenance I.V. line contains sodium chloride.

Other May be administered by SubQ injection (unlabeled route).

Stability

Reconstitution Reconstitute vials with 1.2 mL SWFI (preservative free) to a concentration of 18 million units (1.1 mg)/1 mL (sterile water should be injected towards the side of the vial). Gently swirl; do not shake. Further dilute with 50 mL of D_5W. Smaller volumes of D_5W should be used for doses ≤1.5 mg; avoid concentrations <30 mcg/mL and >70 mcg/mL (an increased variability in drug delivery has been seen). Plastic (polyvinyl chloride) bags result in more consistent drug delivery and are recommended. Filtration may result in loss of bioactivity. Addition of 0.1% albumin has been used to increase stability and decrease the extent of sorption if low final concentrations cannot be avoided.

Storage Store intact vials under refrigeration at 2°C to 8°C (36°F to 46°F). Protect from light. Plastic (polyvinyl chloride) bags result in more consistent drug delivery and are recommended. According to the manufacturer, reconstituted vials and solutions diluted for infusion are stable for 48 hours at room temperature or refrigerated although refrigeration is preferred because they do not contain preservatives. Do not freeze. Solution diluted with D_5W to a concentration of 220 mcg/mL and repackaged into tuberculin syringes was reported to be stable for 14 days refrigerated.

Monitoring and Teaching Issues

Laboratory Monitoring Baseline and periodic: CBC with differential and platelets, blood chemistries including electrolytes, renal and hepatic function tests; pulmonary function tests and arterial blood gases (baseline); thallium stress test (prior to treatment)

Physical Assessment Infusion site should be monitored for extravasation. Vital signs; cardiac, respiratory, and CNS status; fluid balance; signs of systemic sepsis, changes in mental status, and laboratory reports should be assessed daily prior to beginning infusion and for 2 hours following infusion.

Patient Education Avoid alcohol. Maintain adequate hydration, unless instructed to restrict fluid intake. Can cause hypotension. You will be susceptible to infection. May cause increased sensitivity to sunlight, nausea, vomiting, stomatitis, anorexia, malaise, or weakness. This drug may result in many side effects; you will be monitored and assessed closely during therapy. Report any changes in urination, swelling of extremities, weight gain, unusual bruising or bleeding, chest pain or palpitations, acute dizziness, respiratory difficulty, fever or chills, changes in cognition or mental status, rash, feelings of pain or numbness in extremities, severe or persistent GI upset or diarrhea, vaginal discharge or mouth sores, yellowing of eyes or skin, or changes in color of urine or stool.

Breast-Feeding Considerations Due to the potential for serious adverse reactions in the nursing infant, breast-feeding should be discontinued during treatment.

Pregnancy Considerations Maternal toxicity and embryocidal effects were noted in animal studies. There are no adequate and well-controlled studies in pregnant women; use during pregnancy only if benefits to the mother outweigh potential risk to the fetus. Contraception is recommended for fertile males or females using this medication.

Additional Information 18 x 10^6 int. units = 1.1 mg protein

◆ **Aldex® CT** *see* Diphenhydramine and Phenylephrine *on page 546*

◆ **Aldomet** *see* Methyldopa *on page 1200*

Alefacept (a LE fa sept)

U.S. Brand Names Amevive®

Index Terms B 9273; BG 9273; Human LFA-3/IgG(1) Fusion Protein; LFA-3/IgG(1) Fusion Protein, Human

Generic Availability (U.S.) No

Pharmacologic Category Monoclonal Antibody

Prescribing and Access Restrictions Alefacept will be distributed directly to physician offices or to a specialty pharmacy; injections are intended to be administered in the physician's office. Contact Amevive® Start Assistance Program (ASAP) at 1-800-477-6472 to initiate treatment.

Pregnancy Risk Factor B

Lactation Excretion in breast milk unknown/not recommended

Use Treatment of moderate-to-severe chronic plaque psoriasis in adults who are candidates for systemic therapy or phototherapy

Mechanism of Action/Effect Alefacept is a monoclonal antibody against a specific receptor on T lymphocytes, and reduces the number of both $CD4^+$ and $CD8^+$ T lymphocytes. It improves symptoms of psoriasis by decreasing the number of activated T lymphocytes, and their production of inflammatory mediators such as interferon gamma.

Contraindications Hypersensitivity to alefacept or any component of the formulation; history of severe malignancy; patients with HIV infection or other clinically-important infections

Warnings/Precautions Hazardous agent - use appropriate precautions for handling and disposal. Has been associated with hypersensitivity reactions; rare anaphylaxis also reported. Alefacept induces a decline in circulating T-lymphocytes ($CD4^+$ and $CD8^+$); $CD4^+$ lymphocyte counts should be monitored every 2 weeks throughout therapy. Do not initiate in pre-existing depression of $CD4^+$ lymphocytes and withhold treatment in any patient who develops a depressed $CD4^+$ lymphocyte count (<250 cells/µL) during treatment; permanently discontinue if $CD4^+$ lymphocyte counts remain <250 cells/µL for 1 month.

Alefacept may increase the risk of malignancies; use caution in patients at high risk for malignancy. Discontinue if malignancy develops during therapy. Alefacept may increase the risk of infection and may reactivate latent infection; monitor for new infections. Avoid use in patients receiving other immunosuppressant drugs or phototherapy. In post-marketing reports, significant transaminase elevations, as well as rare cases of hepatitis, fatty liver, decompensation of cirrhosis, and acute hepatic failure (a causal relationship not established). Discontinue if signs and symptoms of hepatic injury occur. Safety and efficacy of live or attenuated vaccines have not been evaluated. Safety and efficacy have not been established in pediatric patients.

Drug Interactions

Avoid Concomitant Use

Avoid concomitant use of Alefacept with any of the following: BCG; Belimumab; Natalizumab; Pimecrolimus; Roflumilast; Tacrolimus (Topical); Vaccines (Live)

Decreased Effect

Alefacept may decrease the levels/effects of: BCG; Sipuleucel-T; Vaccines (Inactivated); Vaccines (Live)

The levels/effects of Alefacept may be decreased by: Echinacea

Increased Effect/Toxicity

Alefacept may increase the levels/effects of: Belimumab; Leflunomide; Natalizumab; Vaccines (Live)

The levels/effects of Alefacept may be increased by: Denosumab; Pimecrolimus; Roflumilast; Tacrolimus (Topical); Trastuzumab

Nutritional/Ethanol Interactions Ethanol: Avoid ethanol (may increase risk of liver toxicity).

Adverse Reactions

≥10%:

Hematologic: Lymphopenia (up to 10% of patients required temporary discontinuation, up to 17% during a second course of therapy)

Local: Injection site reactions (up to 16% of patients; includes pain, inflammation, bleeding, edema, or other reaction)

1% to 10%:

Central nervous system: Chills (6%; primarily during intravenous administration), dizziness (≥2%)

Dermatologic: Pruritus (≥2%)

Gastrointestinal: Nausea (≥2%)

Neuromuscular & skeletal: Myalgia (≥2%)

Respiratory: Pharyngitis (≥2%), cough increased (≥2%)

Miscellaneous: Malignancies (1% vs 0.5% in placebo), antibodies to alefacept (3%; significance unknown), infection (1% requiring hospitalization)

Pharmacodynamics/Kinetics

Bioavailability 63% (following I.M. administration)

Half-Life Elimination 270 hours (following I.V. administration)

Excretion Clearance: 0.25 mL/hour/kg

Available Dosage Forms

Injection, powder for reconstitution:

Amevive®: 15 mg

Dosing

Adult & Geriatric Psoriasis (moderate-to-severe chronic plaque psoriasis):

I.M.: 15 mg once weekly; usual duration of treatment: 12 weeks

Second course: A second course of treatment may be initiated at least 12 weeks after completion of the initial course of treatment, provided $CD4^+$ T-lymphocyte counts are within the normal range.

Note: $CD4^+$ T-lymphocyte counts should be monitored before initiation of treatment and every 2 weeks during therapy. Dosing should be withheld if $CD4^+$ counts are <250 cells/µL, and dosing should be permanently discontinued if $CD4^+$ lymphocyte counts remain at <250 cells/µL for longer than 1 month.

Renal Impairment No dosage adjustment required.

Administration

I.M. I.M. injections should be administered at least 1 inch from previous administration sites.

Stability

Reconstitution Reconstitute 15 mg vial for I.M. solution with 0.6 mL of SWFI (supplied); 0.5 mL of reconstituted solution contains 15 mg of alefacept. Gently swirl to avoid foaming. Do not filter reconstituted solutions. Do not mix with other medications or solutions.

Storage Store under refrigeration at 2°C to 8°C (36°F to 46°F). Protect from light. Following reconstitution, may be stored for up to 4 hours at 2°C to 8°C (36°F to 46°F). Discard any unused solution after 4 hours.

Monitoring and Teaching Issues

Laboratory Monitoring Baseline CD4$^+$ T-lymphocyte counts prior to initiation and every 2 weeks during treatment course

Physical Assessment Monitor closely for the development of malignancies or infections.

Patient Education This medication can only be administered by injection. Report immediately any pain or irritation at injection site; chills; rash; difficulty swallowing or breathing; or feelings of tightness in chest. Avoid alcohol. You will need weekly blood tests while receiving this medication. May cause nausea or muscle pain. Report unusual feelings of fatigue or weakness, signs of infection (eg, cough, runny nose, sore throat, swollen glands, mouth sores, burning on urination, fever, chills), abdominal pain, jaundice, easy bruising, dark urine, or pale stools.

Dietary Considerations Some products may contain sucrose.

Breast-Feeding Considerations It is not known whether alefacept is excreted in breast milk. Since alefacept is an immunosuppressant, and transfer of proteins into breast milk may occur, breast-feeding women are cautioned to discontinue breast-feeding or to discontinue use of the drug while breast-feeding (recommendations per manufacturer).

Pregnancy Considerations Effects in pregnancy are not known. Teratogenic effects have not been observed in animal studies. Patients who become pregnant during therapy or within 8 weeks of treatment are advised to enroll in pregnancy registry (866-263-8483).

Alendronate (a LEN droe nate)

U.S. Brand Names Fosamax®

Index Terms Alendronate Sodium; Alendronic Acid Monosodium Salt Trihydrate; MK-217

Generic Availability (U.S.) Yes: Tablet

Pharmacologic Category Bisphosphonate Derivative

Medication Safety Issues

Sound-alike/look-alike issues:

Alendronate may be confused with risedronate

Fosamax® may be confused with Flomax®, Fosamax Plus D®, fosinopril, Zithromax®

International issues:

Fosamax [U.S., Canada, and multiple international markets] may be confused with Fisamox brand name for amoxicillin [Australia]

Medication Guide Available Yes

Pregnancy Risk Factor C

Lactation Excretion in breast milk unknown/use caution

Use Treatment and prevention of osteoporosis in postmenopausal females; treatment of osteoporosis in males; Paget's disease of the bone in patients who are symptomatic, at risk for future complications, or with alkaline phosphatase ≥2 times the upper limit of normal; treatment of glucocorticoid-induced osteoporosis in males and females with low bone mineral density who are receiving a daily dosage ≥7.5 mg of prednisone (or equivalent)

Mechanism of Action/Effect A bisphosphonate which inhibits bone resorption via actions on osteoclasts or on osteoclast precursors; decreases the rate of bone resorption, leading to an indirect increase in bone mineral density. In Paget's disease, characterized by disordered resorption and formation of bone, inhibition of resorption leads to an indirect decrease in bone formation; but the newly-formed bone has a more normal architecture.

Contraindications Hypersensitivity to alendronate, other bisphosphonates, or any component of the formulation; hypocalcemia; abnormalities of the esophagus which delay esophageal emptying such as stricture or achalasia; inability to stand or sit upright for at least 30 minutes; oral solution should not be used in patients at risk of aspiration

Warnings/Precautions Use caution in patients with renal impairment (not recommended for use in patients with Cl_{cr} <35 mL/minute); hypocalcemia must be corrected before therapy initiation; ensure adequate calcium and vitamin D intake. May cause irritation to upper gastrointestinal mucosa. Esophagitis, dysphagia, esophageal ulcers, esophageal erosions, and esophageal stricture (rare) have been reported; risk increases in patients unable to comply with dosing instructions. Use with caution in patients with dysphagia, esophageal disease, gastritis, duodenitis, or ulcers (may worsen underlying condition). Discontinue use if new or worsening symptoms develop.

Osteonecrosis of the jaw (ONJ) has been reported in patients receiving bisphosphonates. Risk factors include invasive dental procedures (eg, tooth extraction, dental implants, boney surgery); a diagnosis of cancer, with concomitant chemotherapy or corticosteroids; poor oral hygiene, ill-fitting dentures; and comorbid disorders (anemia, coagulopathy, infection, preexisting dental disease). Most reported cases occurred after I.V. bisphosphonate therapy; however, cases have been reported following oral therapy. A dental exam and preventative dentistry should be performed prior to placing patients with risk factors on chronic bisphosphonate therapy. The manufacturer's labeling states that discontinuing bisphosphonates in patients requiring invasive dental procedures may reduce the risk of ONJ. However, other experts suggest that there is no evidence that discontinuing therapy reduces the risk of developing ONJ (Assael, 2009). The benefit/risk must be assessed by the treating physician and/or dentist/surgeon prior to any invasive dental procedure. Patients developing ONJ while on bisphosphonates should receive care by an oral surgeon.

Atypical femur fractures have been reported in patients receiving bisphosphonates for treatment/prevention of osteoporosis. The fractures include subtrochanteric femur (bone just below the hip joint) and diaphyseal femur (long segment of the thigh bone). Some patients experience prodromal pain weeks or months before the fracture occurs. It is unclear if bisphosphonate therapy is the cause for these fractures, although the majority have been reported in patients taking bisphosphonates. Patients receiving long-term (>3-5 years) therapy may be at an increased risk. Discontinue bisphosphonate therapy in patients who develop a femoral shaft fracture.

Severe (and occasionally debilitating) bone, joint, and/or muscle pain have been reported during bisphosphonate treatment. The onset of pain ranged from a single day to several months. Consider discontinuing therapy in patients who experience severe symptoms; symptoms usually resolve upon discontinuation. Some patients experienced recurrence when rechallenged with same drug or another bisphosphonate; avoid use in patients with a history of these symptoms in association with bisphosphonate therapy.

Drug Interactions

Avoid Concomitant Use There are no known interactions where it is recommended to avoid concomitant use.

Decreased Effect

The levels/effects of Alendronate may be decreased by: Antacids; Calcium Salts; Iron Salts; Magnesium Salts; Proton Pump Inhibitors

Increased Effect/Toxicity

Alendronate may increase the levels/effects of: Phosphate Supplements

The levels/effects of Alendronate may be increased by: Aminoglycosides; Aspirin; Nonsteroidal Anti-Inflammatory Agents

Nutritional/Ethanol Interactions

Ethanol: Avoid ethanol (may increase risk of osteoporosis and gastric irritation).

Food: All food and beverages interfere with absorption. Coadministration with caffeine may reduce alendronate efficacy. Coadministration with dairy products may decrease alendronate absorption. Beverages (especially orange juice and coffee) and food may reduce the absorption of alendronate as much as 60%.

Lab Interactions Bisphosphonates may interfere with diagnostic imaging agents such as technetium-99m-diphosphonate in bone scans.

Adverse Reactions Note: Incidence of adverse effects (mostly GI) increases significantly in patients treated for Paget's disease at 40 mg/day.

>10%: Endocrine & metabolic: Hypocalcemia (transient, mild, 18%); hypophosphatemia (transient, mild, 10%)

1% to 10%:

Central nervous system: Headache (up to 3%)

Gastrointestinal: Abdominal pain (1% to 7%), acid reflux (1% to 4%), dyspepsia (1% to 4%), nausea (1% to 4%), flatulence (up to 4%), diarrhea (1% to 3%), gastroesophageal reflux disease (1% to 3%), constipation (up to 3%), esophageal ulcer (up to 2%), abdominal distension (up to 1%), gastritis (up to 1%), vomiting (up to 1%), dysphagia (up to 1%), gastric ulcer (1%), melena (1%)

Neuromuscular & skeletal: Musculoskeletal pain (up to 6%), muscle cramps (up to 1%)

Pharmacodynamics/Kinetics

Bioavailability Fasting: 0.6%; reduced up to 60% with food or drink

Protein Binding ~78%

Half-Life Elimination Exceeds 10 years

Metabolism None

Excretion Urine; feces (as unabsorbed drug)

Available Dosage Forms

Tablet, oral: 5 mg, 10 mg, 35 mg, 40 mg, 70 mg

Fosamax®: 10 mg, 70 mg

Dosing

Adult & Geriatric Note: Patients should receive supplemental calcium and vitamin D if dietary intake is inadequate.

Osteoporosis in postmenopausal females: Oral:

Prophylaxis: 5 mg once daily **or** 35 mg once weekly

Treatment: 10 mg once daily **or** 70 mg once weekly

Osteoporosis in males: Oral: 10 mg once daily **or** 70 mg once weekly

Osteoporosis secondary to glucocorticoids in males and females: Oral: Treatment: 5 mg once daily; a dose of 10 mg once daily should be used in postmenopausal females who are not receiving estrogen

Paget's disease of bone in males and females: Oral: 40 mg once daily for 6 months

Retreatment: Relapses during the 12 months following therapy occurred in 9% of patients who responded to treatment. Specific retreatment data are not available. Following a 6-month post-treatment evaluation period, treatment with alendronate may be considered in patients who have relapsed based on increases in serum alkaline phosphatase, which should be measured periodically. Retreatment may also be considered in those who failed to normalize their serum alkaline phosphatase.

Renal Impairment

Cl_{cr} 35-60 mL/minute: None necessary.

Cl_{cr} <35 mL/minute: Alendronate is not recommended due to lack of experience.

Hepatic Impairment No adjustment necessary.

Administration

Oral Alendronate must be taken with plain water (tablets 6-8 oz; oral solution follow with 2 oz) first thing in the morning and ≥30 minutes before the first food, beverage, or other medication of the day. Do not take with mineral water or with other beverages. Patients should be instructed to stay upright (not to lie down) for at least 30 minutes **and** until after first food of the day (to reduce esophageal irritation).

Stability

Storage Store tablets and oral solution at room temperature of 15°C to 30°C (59°F to 86°F). Keep in well-closed container.

Monitoring and Teaching Issues

Laboratory Monitoring

Osteoporosis: Bone mineral density as measured by central dual-energy x-ray absorptiometry (DXA) of the hip or spine (prior to initiation of therapy and at least every 2 years; after 6-12 months of combined glucocorticoid and alendronate treatment); serum calcium and 25(OH)D

Paget's disease: Alkaline phosphatase, serum calcium and 25(OH)D

Physical Assessment Assess history for any previous adverse response to bisphosphonate therapy and ability to comply with administration instructions. Use caution with renal impairment. Correct any hypocalcemia prior to beginning treatment. Patients at risk for osteonecrosis of the jaw (eg, chemotherapy, corticosteroids, poor oral hygiene) should have dental exams; necessary preventive dentistry should be done before beginning bisphosphonate therapy. Monitor for immediate or long-term musculoskeletal pain. Teach patient specific administration directions. Instruct patient in lifestyle and dietary changes that will have a beneficial impact.

Patient Education Take first thing in the morning, at least 30 minutes before the first food or beverage of the day. Take tablets with a full 6- to 8-ounce glass of water; follow solution with 2 ounces of water. Wait at least 30 minutes after taking alendronate before eating or drinking anything else. Stay in sitting or standing position for 30 minutes following administration and until after the first food of the day to reduce potential for esophageal irritation. Consult prescriber to determine necessity of lifestyle changes (eg, decreased smoking, decreased alcohol intake). Consult prescriber before having any dental procedures; inform dentist that you are taking this medication. You may experience flatulence, bloating, nausea, acid regurgitation, temporary bone pain, or muscle cramps. Report persistent muscle or bone pain or leg cramps; persistent unresolved GI pain or upset; unusual fever or chills; or pain in mouth, jaws, or teeth.

Dietary Considerations Ensure adequate calcium and vitamin D intake; women and men >50 years of age should consume 1200-1500 mg/day of elemental calcium and 800-1000 int. units/day of vitamin D. Wait at least 30 minutes after taking alendronate before taking any supplement. Alendronate must be taken with plain water first thing in the morning and at least 30 minutes before the first food or beverage of the day. Do not take with mineral water or with other beverages.

Geriatric Considerations Since many elderly patients receive diuretics, evaluation of electrolyte status (calcium, phosphate, magnesium, potassium) may need to be done periodically due to the drug class (bisphosphonate). The elderly are frequently treated long-term for osteoporosis and patients should be advised to report any lower extremity pain that cannot be explained or lasts for more than a week.

Pregnancy Considerations Safety and efficacy have not been established in pregnant women. Animal studies have shown delays in delivery and fetal/neonatal death (secondary to hypocalcemia). Bisphosphonates are incorporated into the bone matrix and gradually released over time. Theoretically, there may be a risk of fetal harm when pregnancy follows the completion of therapy. Based on limited case reports with pamidronate, serum calcium levels in the newborn may be altered if administered during pregnancy.

Related Information

Osteoporosis Management *on page 2067*

◆ **Alendronate Sodium** *see* Alendronate *on page 67*

◆ **Alendronic Acid Monosodium Salt Trihydrate** *see* Alendronate *on page 67*

◆ **Aler-Cap [OTC]** *see* DiphenhydrAMINE (Systemic) *on page 543*

◆ **Aler-Dryl [OTC]** *see* DiphenhydrAMINE (Systemic) *on page 543*

◆ **Aler-Tab [OTC]** *see* DiphenhydrAMINE (Systemic) *on page 543*

◆ **Aleve® [OTC]** *see* Naproxen *on page 1289*

Alfuzosin (al FYOO zoe sin)

U.S. Brand Names Uroxatral®

Index Terms Alfuzosin Hydrochloride

Generic Availability (U.S.) No

Pharmacologic Category Alpha$_1$ Blocker

Pregnancy Risk Factor B

Lactation Not indicated for use in women

Use Treatment of the functional symptoms of benign prostatic hyperplasia (BPH)

Mechanism of Action/Effect An antagonist of alpha$_1$-adrenoreceptors in the lower urinary tract. Blockade of these adrenoreceptors can cause smooth muscles in the bladder neck and prostate to relax, resulting in an improvement in urine flow rate and a reduction in BPH symptoms.

Contraindications Hypersensitivity to alfuzosin or any component of the formulation; moderate or severe hepatic insufficiency (Child-Pugh class B and C); concurrent use with potent CYP3A4 inhibitors (eg, itraconazole, ketoconazole, ritonavir)

Warnings/Precautions Not intended for use as an antihypertensive drug. May cause significant orthostatic hypotension and syncope, especially with first dose; anticipate a similar effect if therapy is interrupted for a few days, if dosage is rapidly increased, or used with antihypertensives (particularly vasodilators), PDE-5 inhibitors, nitrates or other medications which may result in hypotension. Discontinue if symptoms of angina occur or worsen. Alfuzosin has been shown to prolong the QT interval alone (minimal) and with other drugs with comparable effects on the QT interval (additive); use with caution in patients with known QT prolongation (congenital or acquired). Patients should be cautioned about performing hazardous tasks when starting new therapy or adjusting dosage upward. Discontinue if symptoms of angina occur or worsen. Rule out prostatic carcinoma before beginning therapy. Use caution with severe renal or mild hepatic impairment; contraindicated in moderate-to-severe hepatic impairment. Intraoperative floppy iris syndrome has been observed in cataract surgery patients who were on or were previously treated with alpha$_1$-blockers. Causality has not been established and there appears to be no benefit in discontinuing alpha-blocker therapy prior to surgery. May cause priapism. Contraindicated in patients taking strong CYP3A4 inhibitors.

Drug Interactions

Metabolism/Transport Effects Substrate of CYP3A4 (major)

Avoid Concomitant Use

Avoid concomitant use of Alfuzosin with any of the following: Alpha1-Blockers; CYP3A4 Inhibitors (Strong); Protease Inhibitors

Decreased Effect

The levels/effects of Alfuzosin may be decreased by: CYP3A4 Inducers (Strong); Deferasirox; Herbs (CYP3A4 Inducers)

Increased Effect/Toxicity

Alfuzosin may increase the levels/effects of: Alpha1-Blockers; Calcium Channel Blockers; QTc-Prolonging Agents

The levels/effects of Alfuzosin may be increased by: Beta-Blockers; CYP3A4 Inhibitors (Moderate); CYP3A4 Inhibitors (Strong); MAO Inhibitors; Phosphodiesterase 5 Inhibitors; Protease Inhibitors

Nutritional/Ethanol Interactions

Food: Food increases the extent of absorption.

Herb/Nutraceutical: Avoid St John's wort (may decrease alfuzosin levels).

Adverse Reactions

1% to 10%:

Central nervous system: Dizziness (6%), fatigue (3%), headache (3%), pain (1% to 2%)

Gastrointestinal: Abdominal pain (1% to 2%), constipation (1% to 2%), dyspepsia (1% to 2%), nausea (1% to 2%)

Genitourinary: Impotence (1% to 2%)

Respiratory: Upper respiratory tract infection (3%), bronchitis (1% to 2%), pharyngitis (1% to 2%), sinusitis (1% to 2%)

Pharmacodynamics/Kinetics

Absorption Decreased 50% under fasting conditions

Bioavailability 49% following a meal

Time to Peak Plasma: 8 hours following a meal

Protein Binding 82% to 90%

Half-Life Elimination 10 hours

Metabolism Hepatic, primarily via CYP3A4; metabolism includes oxidation, O-demethylation, and N-dealkylation; forms metabolites (inactive)

Excretion Feces (69%); urine (24%; 11% as unchanged drug)

Available Dosage Forms

Tablet, extended release, oral:

Uroxatral®: 10 mg

Dosing

Adult & Geriatric Benign prostatic hyperplasia (BPH): Oral: 10 mg once daily

Renal Impairment Bioavailability and maximum serum concentrations are increased by ~50% with mild (Cl_{cr} 60-80 mL/minute), moderate (Cl_{cr} 30-59 mL/minute), or severe (Cl_{cr} <30 mL/minute) renal impairment.

Note: Safety data is limited in patients with severe renal impairment (Cl_{cr} <30 mL/minute). Use with caution.

Hepatic Impairment

Mild hepatic impairment: Use has not been studied; use caution.

Moderate or severe hepatic impairment (Child-Pugh class B and C): Clearance is decreased 1/3 to 1/4 and serum concentration is increased three- to fourfold; use is contraindicated.

Administration

Oral Tablet should be swallowed whole; do not crush or chew. Administer once daily (immediately following a meal); should be taken at the same time each day.

Stability

Storage Store at room temperature of 25°C (77°F); excursions permitted to 15°C to 30°C (59°F to 86°F). Protect from light and moisture.

Monitoring and Teaching Issues

Physical Assessment Prostatic carcinoma should be ruled out before beginning therapy. Monitor for improved urine flow and hypotension prior to treatment and on a regular basis.

Patient Education Take at the same time each day. Swallow tablet whole; do not crush or chew. May cause drowsiness, dizziness, headache, or postural hypotension. Report chest pain or severe dizziness.

Dietary Considerations Take immediately following a meal at the same time each day.

Geriatric Considerations Alfuzosin is a functionally uroselective alpha-blocker, therefore, having minimal effects on the cardiovascular system. Alfuzosin has been available in Europe for many years and appears to be well tolerated in elderly. In one study, orthostatic changes were minimal and not influenced by age.

Pregnancy Considerations Teratogenic effects were not observed in animal studies; however, alfuzosin is not indicated for use in women.

Related Information

Pharmacotherapy of Urinary Incontinence *on page 2071*

- **Alfuzosin Hydrochloride** *see* Alfuzosin *on page 69*
- **Alimta®** *see* Pemetrexed *on page 1429*
- **Alinia®** *see* Nitazoxanide *on page 1324*

Aliskiren (a lis KYE ren)

U.S. Brand Names Tekturna®

Index Terms Aliskiren Hemifumarate; SPP100

Generic Availability (U.S.) No

Pharmacologic Category Renin Inhibitor

Medication Safety Issues

Sound-alike/look-alike issues:

Tekturna® may be confused with Valturna®

International issues:

Aliskiren may be confused with Aliseum which is a brand name for diazepam in Italy

Pregnancy Risk Factor C (1st trimester); D (2nd and 3rd trimesters)

Lactation Excretion in breast milk unknown/not recommended

Use Treatment of hypertension, alone or in combination with other antihypertensive agents

Unlabeled/Investigational Use Treatment of persistent proteinuria in patients with type 2 diabetes mellitus, hypertension, and nephropathy despite administration of optimized recommended renoprotective therapy (eg, angiotensin II receptor blocker)

Mechanism of Action/Effect Aliskerin is a direct renin inhibitor, resulting in blockade of the conversion of angiotensinogen to angiotensin I. Angiotensin I suppression decreases the formation of angiotensin II (Ang II), resulting in blood pressure reduction.

Contraindications

U.S. labeling: There are no contraindications listed in manufacturer's labeling.

Canada labeling: Hypersensitivity to aliskiren or any component of the formulation

Warnings/Precautions [U.S. Boxed Warning]: Based on human data, drugs that act on the renin-angiotensin system can cause injury and death to the developing fetus when used in the second and third trimesters. Aliskiren should be discontinued as soon as possible once pregnancy is detected. Since the effect of aliskiren on bradykinin levels is unknown, the risk of kinin-mediated etiologies of angioedema occurring is also unknown. Use with caution in any patient with a history of angioedema (of any etiology) as angioedema, some cases necessitating hospitalization and intubation, has been observed (rarely) with aliskiren use. Discontinue immediately following any signs and symptoms of angioedema; do not readminister. Prolonged frequent monitoring may be required especially if tongue, glottis, or larynx are involved as they are associated with airway obstruction. Patients with a history of airway surgery may have a higher risk of airway obstruction. Early, aggressive, and appropriate management is critical. Hyperkalemia may occur (rarely) during monotherapy; risk may increase in patients with predisposing factors (eg, renal dysfunction, diabetes mellitus or concomitant use with ACE inhibitors, potassium-sparing diuretics, potassium supplements, and/or potassium-containing salts). Symptomatic hypotension may occur (rarely) during the initiation of therapy, particularly in patients with an activated renin-angiotensin system (ie, volume or salt-depleted patients). Use with caution in patients with severe renal impairment; not studied in patients with severe renal impairment (eGFR <30 mL/minute and/or S_{cr} ≥1.7 mg/dL [women]; S_{cr} ≥2 mg/dL [men]), history of dialysis, nephrotic syndrome, or renovascular hypertension. Use with caution or avoid in patients with deteriorating renal function or renal artery stenosis (bilateral or unilateral). Concurrent use with strong inhibitors of P-glycoprotein (eg, cyclosporine, itraconazole) is not recommended.

Drug Interactions

Metabolism/Transport Effects Substrate of CYP3A4 (minor), P-glycoprotein

Avoid Concomitant Use

Avoid concomitant use of Aliskiren with any of the following: CycloSPORINE; CycloSPORINE (Systemic)

Decreased Effect

Aliskiren may decrease the levels/effects of: Furosemide

The levels/effects of Aliskiren may be decreased by: Grapefruit Juice; Herbs (Hypertensive Properties); Methylphenidate; P-Glycoprotein Inducers; Yohimbine

Increased Effect/Toxicity

Aliskiren may increase the levels/effects of: Amifostine; Antihypertensives; Hypotensive Agents; RiTUXimab

The levels/effects of Aliskiren may be increased by: Atorvastatin; Conivaptan; CycloSPORINE; CycloSPORINE (Systemic); Diazoxide; Herbs (Hypotensive Properties); Itraconazole; Ketoconazole; Ketoconazole (Systemic); MAO Inhibitors; Pentoxifylline; P-Glycoprotein Inhibitors; Phosphodiesterase 5 Inhibitors; Prostacyclin Analogues; Verapamil

Nutritional/Ethanol Interactions

Food: High-fat meals decrease absorption.

Herb/Nutraceutical: Avoid herbs with *hypertensive* properties (bayberry, blue cohosh, cayenne, ephedra, ginger, ginseng [American], kola, licorice). Avoid herbs with *hypotensive* properties (black cohosh, California poppy, coleus, garlic, goldenseal, hawthorn, mistletoe, periwinkle, quinine, shepherd's purse).

Adverse Reactions 1% to 10%:

Dermatologic: Rash (1%)

Endocrine & metabolic: Hyperkalemia (monotherapy ≤1%; concurrent with ACE inhibitor in patients with diabetes 6%)

Gastrointestinal: Diarrhea (2%)

Hematologic: Creatine kinase increased (>300%: 1%)

Renal: BUN increased (≤7%), serum creatinine increased (≤7%)

Respiratory: Cough (1%)

Pharmacodynamics/Kinetics

Onset of Action Maximum antihypertensive effect: Within 2 weeks

Absorption Poor; absorption decreased by high-fat meal. Aliskiren is a substrate of P-glycoprotein; concurrent use of P-glycoprotein inhibitors may increase absorption.

Bioavailability ~3%

Time to Peak 1-3 hours

Half-Life Elimination ~24 hours (range: 16-32 hours)

Metabolism Extent of metabolism unknown; *in vitro* studies indicate metabolism via CYP3A4

Excretion Urine (~25% of absorbed dose excreted unchanged in urine); feces (unchanged via biliary excretion)

Available Dosage Forms

Tablet, oral:

Tekturna®: 150 mg, 300 mg

Dosing

Adult Hypertension: Initial: 150 mg once daily; may increase to 300 mg once daily (maximum: 300 mg/day). **Note:** Prior to initiation, correct hypovolemia and/or closely monitor volume status in patients on concurrent diuretics during treatment initiation.

Geriatric Refer to adult dosing. No initial dosage adjustment required.

Renal Impairment

Mild-to-moderate impairment (eGFR ≥30 mL/minute and/or S_{cr} <1.7 mg/dL [women]; S_{cr} <2 mg/dL [men]): No dose adjustment required

Severe impairment (eGFR <30 mL/minute and/or S_{cr} ≥1.7 mg/dL [women]; S_{cr} ≥2 mg/dL [men]): Use caution; not studied in severe renal impairment

Hepatic Impairment No dosage adjustment required.

Administration

Oral Administer at the same time daily; may take with or without a meal, but consistent administration with regards to meals is recommended.

Stability

Storage Store at 25°C (77°F); excursions permitted to 15°C to 30°C (59°F to 86°F). Protect from moisture.

Monitoring and Teaching Issues

Laboratory Monitoring Serum potassium, BUN, serum creatinine

Physical Assessment Evaluate renal status prior to beginning therapy. Assess BUN, serum potassium, and serum creatinine. Monitor for angioedema and hypotension at beginning of therapy, when changing dose, and on a regular basis throughout.

Patient Education Take at same time each day; may be taken with meals. This drug does not eliminate the need for diet or exercise regimen. May cause dizziness or hypotension. Report immediately any unusual swelling of eyes, face, lips, mouth, throat, or any difficulty swallowing of breathing; changes in urinary pattern; or palpitations or irregular heartbeat.

Dietary Considerations May be taken with or without food; however, a high-fat meal reduces absorption. Consistent administration with regards to meals is recommended.

Geriatric Considerations The pharmacokinetic studies in elderly (≥65 years of age) demonstrated an increased AUC; however, adjustments in starting dose are not necessary. Blood pressure response and adverse effects were similar to younger adults in studies where 19% of patients were >65 years of age.

Pregnancy Considerations Medications which act on the renin-angiotensin system are reported to have the following fetal/neonatal effects: Hypotension, neonatal skull hypoplasia, anuria, renal failure, and death; oligohydramnios is also reported. These effects are reported to occur with exposure during the second and third trimesters. There are no adequate and well-controlled studies in pregnant women. Women who use aliskiren during pregnancy or become pregnant during therapy should be warned of the potential risks to the fetus. **[U.S. Boxed Warning]: Based on human data, drugs that act on the renin-angiotensin system can cause injury and death to the developing fetus when used in the second and third trimesters. Aliskiren should be discontinued as soon as possible once pregnancy is detected.**

Related Information

Angiotensin Agents *on page 1974*

Aliskiren, Amlodipine, and Hydrochlorothiazide

(a lis KYE ren, am LOE di peen, & hye droe klor oh THYE a zide)

U.S. Brand Names Amturnide™

Index Terms Aliskiren, Hydrochlorothiazide, and Amlodipine; Amlodipine Besylate, Aliskiren Hemifumarate, and Hydrochlorothiazide; Amlodipine, Aliskiren, and Hydrochlorothiazide; Amlodipine, Hydrochlorothiazide, and Aliskiren; Hydrochlorothiazide, Aliskiren, and Amlodipine; Hydrochlorothiazide, Amlodipine, and Aliskiren

Generic Availability (U.S.) No

Pharmacologic Category Calcium Channel Blocker; Calcium Channel Blocker, Dihydropyridine; Diuretic, Thiazide; Renin Inhibitor

Medication Safety Issues

Sound-alike/look-alike issues:

Amturnide™ may be confused with AMILoride

Pregnancy Risk Factor D

Lactation Excretion in breast milk unknown/not recommended

Use Treatment of hypertension (not for initial therapy)

Available Dosage Forms

Tablet, oral:

Amturnide™: Aliskiren 150 mg, amlodipine 5 mg, and hydrochlorothiazide 12.5 mg; Aliskiren 300 mg, amlodipine 5 mg, and hydrochlorothiazide 12.5 mg; Aliskiren 300 mg, amlodipine 5 mg, and hydrochlorothiazide 25 mg; Aliskiren 300 mg, amlodipine 10 mg, and hydrochlorothiazide 12.5 mg; Aliskiren 300 mg, amlodipine 10 mg, and hydrochlorothiazide 25 mg

Dosing

Adult Note: Not for initial therapy. Dose is individualized; combination product may be substituted for individual components in patients currently maintained on all three agents separately, used to switch a patient on any dual combination of the components who is experiencing dose-limiting adverse reactions from an individual component (to a lower dose of that component), or used as add-on therapy in patients not adequately controlled with any two of the following: Aliskiren, dihydropyridine calcium channel blockers, and thiazide diuretics.

Hypertension: Oral: *Add-on/switch therapy/replacement therapy:* Aliskiren 150-300 mg and amlodipine 5-10 mg and hydrochlorothiazide 12.5-25 mg once daily; dose may be titrated after 2 weeks of therapy. Maximum recommended daily dose: Aliskiren 300 mg; amlodipine 10 mg; hydrochlorothiazide 25 mg

Geriatric Hypertension: Oral:

Patients ≥65 and <75 years: Refer to adult dosing.

Patients ≥75 years: Initial: Amlodipine 2.5 mg (strength not available in combination product)

Renal Impairment Cl_{cr} ≤30 mL/minute: Use of combination product is not recommended.

Hepatic Impairment Severe hepatic impairment: Initial: Amlodipine 2.5 mg daily (strength not available in combination product).

Administration

Oral Administer at the same time daily. May take with or without a meal, but consistent administration with regard to meals is recommended.

Monitoring and Teaching Issues

Laboratory Monitoring Serum electrolytes, BUN, serum creatinine

Physical Assessment See individual agents.

Patient Education See individual agents.

Aliskiren and Amlodipine

(a lis KYE ren & am LOE di peen)

U.S. Brand Names Tekamlo™

Index Terms Aliskiren Hemifumarate and Amlodipine Besylate; Amlodipine and Aliskiren

Generic Availability (U.S.) No

Pharmacologic Category Calcium Channel Blocker; Calcium Channel Blocker, Dihydropyridine; Renin Inhibitor

Medication Safety Issues An FDA-approved patient medication guide, which is available with the product information and at http://www.pharma.us.novartis.com/product/pi/pdf/tekamlo_pmg.pdf, must be dispensed with this medication for each new outpatient prescription and refill.

Medication Guide Available Yes

Pregnancy Risk Factor D

Lactation Excretion in breast milk unknown/not recommended

Use Treatment of hypertension, alone or in combination with other antihypertensive agents, including use as initial therapy in patients likely to need multiple antihypertensives for adequate control

Available Dosage Forms

Tablet, oral:

Tekamlo™: 150/5: Aliskiren 150 mg and amlodipine 5 mg, 300/5: Aliskiren 300 mg and amlodipine 5 mg, 150/10: Aliskiren 150 mg and amlodipine 10 mg, 300/10: Aliskiren 300 mg and amlodipine 10 mg

Dosing

Adult

Hypertension: Oral: Dosage must be individualized. Combination product may be used as initial therapy or substituted for individual components in patients currently maintained on both agents separately or in patients not adequately controlled with monotherapy (using one of the agents or an agent within same antihypertensive class).

Initial therapy: Aliskiren 150 mg and amlodipine 5 mg once daily; dose may be titrated at 2- to 4-week intervals; maximum recommended daily doses: Aliskiren 300 mg; amlodipine 10 mg

Add-on therapy: Initiate by adding the lowest available dose of the alternative component (aliskiren 150 mg or amlodipine 5 mg); dose may be titrated at 2- to 4-week intervals; maximum recommended daily doses: Aliskiren 300 mg; amlodipine 10 mg

Replacement therapy: Substitute for the individually titrated components

Note: Prior to initiation, correct hypovolemia and/or closely monitor volume status in patients on concurrent diuretics during treatment initiation.

Geriatric Refer to adult dosing. No initial dosage adjustment required.

Renal Impairment

Mild-to-moderate impairment (eGFR ≥30 mL/minute and/or S_{cr} <1.7 mg/dL [women]; S_{cr} <2 mg/dL [men]): No dose adjustment required

Severe impairment (eGFR <30 mL/minute and/or S_{cr} ≥1.7 mg/dL [women]; S_{cr} ≥2 mg/dL [men]): Use caution; not studied in severe renal impairment

Hepatic Impairment Use caution; no dosage adjustment required; titrate slowly.

Administration

Oral Administer at the same time daily. May take with or without a meal, but consistent administration with regards to meals is recommended.

Monitoring and Teaching Issues

Laboratory Monitoring Serum potassium, BUN, serum creatinine

Physical Assessment See individual agents.

Patient Education See individual agents.

Aliskiren and Hydrochlorothiazide (a lis KYE ren & hye droe klor oh THYE a zide)

U.S. Brand Names Tekturna HCT®

Index Terms Aliskiren Hemifumarate and Hydrochlorothiazide; Hydrochlorothiazide and Aliskiren

Generic Availability (U.S.) No

Pharmacologic Category Diuretic, Thiazide; Renin Inhibitor

Pregnancy Risk Factor D

Lactation Enters breast milk/not recommended

Use Treatment of hypertension, including use as initial therapy in patients likely to need multiple antihypertensives for adequate control

Available Dosage Forms

Tablet:

Tekturna HCT®: 150/12.5: Aliskiren 150 mg and hydrochlorothiazide 12.5 mg; 150/25: Aliskiren 150 mg and hydrochlorothiazide 25 mg; 300/12.5: Aliskiren 300 mg and hydrochlorothiazide 12.5 mg; 300/25: Aliskiren 300 mg and hydrochlorothiazide 25 mg

Dosing

Adult Note: Dosage must be individualized. Combination product may be used as initial therapy or substituted for individual components in patients currently maintained on both agents separately or in patients not adequately controlled with monotherapy (using one of the agents or an agent within same antihypertensive class).

Hypertension: Oral:

Initial therapy: Aliskiren 150 mg and hydrochlorothiazide 12.5 mg once daily, dose may be titrated at 2- to 4-week intervals; maximum recommended daily doses: Aliskiren 300 mg; hydrochlorothiazide 25 mg

Add-on therapy: Initiate by adding the lowest available dose of the alternative component (aliskiren 150 mg or hydrochlorothiazide 12.5 mg); titrate to effect; maximum recommended daily doses: Aliskiren 300 mg; hydrochlorothiazide 25 mg

Replacement therapy: Substitute for the individually titrated components

Geriatric Refer to adult dosing. No initial dosage adjustment required.

Renal Impairment

Mild-to-moderate impairment (Cl_{cr} >30 mL/minute): No adjustment required.

Severe impairment (Cl_{cr} ≤30 mL/minute): Use not recommended.

Hepatic Impairment No initial dosage adjustment required; titrate slowly.

Administration

Oral Administer at the same time daily; may take with or without a meal, but consistent administration with regards to meals is recommended.

Monitoring and Teaching Issues

Laboratory Monitoring Serum electrolytes, BUN, serum creatinine

Physical Assessment See individual agents.

Patient Education See individual agents.

Aliskiren and Valsartan (a lis KYE ren & val SAR tan)

U.S. Brand Names Valturna®

Index Terms Aliskiren Hemifumarate and Valsartan; Valsartan and Aliskiren

Generic Availability (U.S.) No

Pharmacologic Category Angiotensin II Receptor Blocker; Renin Inhibitor

Medication Safety Issues

Sound-alike/look-alike issues:

Valturna® may be confused with Tekturna®, valsartan

Pregnancy Risk Factor D

Lactation Excretion in breast milk unknown/not recommended

Use Treatment of hypertension, including use as initial therapy in patients likely to need multiple antihypertensives for adequate control

Available Dosage Forms

Tablet:

Valturna®: 150/160: Aliskiren 150 mg and valsartan 160 mg; 300/320: Aliskiren 300 mg and valsartan 320 mg

Dosing

Adult & Geriatric Hypertension: Oral: Dose is individualized; combination product may be used as initial therapy or substituted for individual components in patients currently maintained on both agents separately or in patients not adequately controlled with monotherapy (using one of the agents or an agent within same antihypertensive class). Titrate at 2- to 4-week intervals as necessary.

Initial therapy: Aliskiren 150 mg and valsartan 160 mg once daily; titrate to effect (maximum daily aliskiren dose: 300 mg; maximum daily valsartan dose: 320 mg)

Patients not controlled with single-agent therapy: Aliskiren 150 mg and valsartan 160 mg once daily; titrate to effect (maximum daily aliskiren dose: 300 mg; maximum daily valsartan dose: 320 mg)

Renal Impairment

Mild-to-moderate impairment (Cl_{cr} ≥30 mL/minute): No dose adjustment required.

Severe impairment (Cl_{cr} <30 mL/minute): Use caution; not studied in severe renal impairment.

Hepatic Impairment In mild-to-moderate liver disease no adjustment is needed. Use caution in patients with severe hepatic impairment; clinical experience is limited.

Administration

Oral Administer at the same time daily; may take with or without a meal, but consistent administration with regards to meal is recommended. Avoid taking with high-fat meals.

Monitoring and Teaching Issues

Laboratory Monitoring Baseline and periodic electrolyte panels, renal and liver function, urinalysis; in HF, serum potassium during dose escalation and periodically thereafter

Physical Assessment See individual agents.

Patient Education See individual agents.

- **Aliskiren Hemifumarate** *see* Aliskiren *on page 71*
- **Aliskiren Hemifumarate and Amlodipine Besylate** *see* Aliskiren and Amlodipine *on page 73*
- **Aliskiren Hemifumarate and Hydrochlorothiazide** *see* Aliskiren and Hydrochlorothiazide *on page 74*
- **Aliskiren Hemifumarate and Valsartan** *see* Aliskiren and Valsartan *on page 75*
- **Aliskiren, Hydrochlorothiazide, and Amlodipine** *see* Aliskiren, Amlodipine, and Hydrochlorothiazide *on page 73*

Alitretinoin (a li TRET i noyn)

U.S. Brand Names Panretin®

Generic Availability (U.S.) No

Pharmacologic Category Antineoplastic Agent, Miscellaneous; Retinoic Acid Derivative

Medication Safety Issues

Sound-alike/look-alike issues:

Panretin® may be confused with pancreatin

High alert medication: The Institute for Safe Medication Practices (ISMP) includes this medication among its list of drugs which have a heightened risk of causing significant patient harm when used in error.

Pregnancy Risk Factor D

Lactation Excretion in breast milk unknown/not recommended

Use Orphan drug: Topical treatment of cutaneous lesions in AIDS-related Kaposi's sarcoma

Unlabeled/Investigational Use Cutaneous T-cell lymphomas

Available Dosage Forms

Gel, topical:

Panretin®: 0.1% (60 g)

Dosing

Adult & Geriatric

Kaposi's sarcoma: Topical: Apply gel twice daily to cutaneous lesions.

T-cell lymphomas (unlabeled use): Topical: Apply gel twice daily to cutaneous lesions.

Administration

Topical Do not use occlusive dressings.

Monitoring and Teaching Issues

Physical Assessment Teach patient appropriate use/application and need to avoid DEET-containing insect repellents.

Patient Education For external use only. Avoid use of any product containing DEET, such as insect repellent. Wear protective clothing and/or avoid exposure to direct sun or sunlamps. Wash hands thoroughly before applying. Avoid applying skin products that contain alcohol or harsh chemicals during treatment. Do not apply occlusive dressings. Stop treatment and inform prescriber if rash, skin irritation, redness, scaling, or excessive dryness appears.

- ◆ **Alka-Seltzer® P.M. [OTC]** *see* Aspirin and Diphenhydramine *on page* *159*
- ◆ **Alkeran®** *see* Melphalan *on page* *1162*
- ◆ **All Day Allergy [OTC]** *see* Cetirizine *on page* *351*
- ◆ **Allegra®** *see* Fexofenadine *on page* *757*
- ◆ **Allegra-D® 12 Hour** *see* Fexofenadine and Pseudoephedrine *on page* *759*
- ◆ **Allegra-D® 24 Hour** *see* Fexofenadine and Pseudoephedrine *on page* *759*
- ◆ **Allegra® Allergy 12 Hour [OTC]** *see* Fexofenadine *on page* *757*
- ◆ **Allegra® Allergy 24 Hour [OTC]** *see* Fexofenadine *on page* *757*
- ◆ **Allegra® Children's Allergy [OTC]** *see* Fexofenadine *on page* *757*
- ◆ **Allegra® Children's Allergy ODT [OTC]** *see* Fexofenadine *on page* *757*
- ◆ **Allegra® ODT [DSC]** *see* Fexofenadine *on page* *757*
- ◆ **AllerMax® [OTC]** *see* DiphenhydrAMINE (Systemic) *on page* *543*
- ◆ **Allfen [OTC]** *see* GuaiFENesin *on page* *890*
- ◆ **Allfen CD** *see* Guaifenesin and Codeine *on page* *891*
- ◆ **Allfen CDX** *see* Guaifenesin and Codeine *on page* *891*
- ◆ **Alli™ [OTC]** *see* Orlistat *on page* *1365*

Allopurinol (al oh PURE i nole)

U.S. Brand Names Aloprim®; Zyloprim®

Index Terms Allopurinol Sodium

Generic Availability (U.S.) Yes

Pharmacologic Category Xanthine Oxidase Inhibitor

Medication Safety Issues

Sound-alike/look-alike issues:

Allopurinol may be confused with Apresoline

Zyloprim® may be confused with Xylo-Pfan®, ZORprin®, Zovirax®

Pregnancy Risk Factor C

Lactation Enters breast milk/use caution (AAP rates "compatible"; AAP 2001 update pending)

Use

Oral: Prevention of attack of gouty arthritis and nephropathy; treatment of secondary hyperuricemia which may occur during treatment of tumors or leukemia; prevention of recurrent calcium oxalate calculi

I.V.: Treatment of elevated serum and urinary uric acid levels when oral therapy is not tolerated in patients with leukemia, lymphoma, and solid tumor malignancies who are receiving cancer chemotherapy

Mechanism of Action/Effect Allopurinol inhibits xanthine oxidase, the enzyme responsible for the conversion of hypoxanthine to xanthine to uric acid. Allopurinol is metabolized to oxypurinol which is also an inhibitor of xanthine oxidase; allopurinol acts on purine catabolism, reducing the production of uric acid without disrupting the biosynthesis of vital purines.

Contraindications Hypersensitivity to allopurinol or any component of the formulation

Warnings/Precautions Do not use to treat asymptomatic hyperuricemia. Has been associated with a number of hypersensitivity reactions, including severe reactions (vasculitis and Stevens-Johnson syndrome); discontinue at first sign of rash. Reversible hepatotoxicity has been reported; use with caution in patients with pre-existing hepatic impairment. Bone marrow suppression has been reported; use caution with other drugs causing myelosuppression. Caution in renal impairment, dosage adjustments needed. Use with caution in patients taking diuretics concurrently. Risk of skin rash may be increased in patients receiving amoxicillin or ampicillin. The risk of hypersensitivity may be increased in patients receiving thiazides, and possibly ACE inhibitors. Use caution with mercaptopurine or azathioprine; dosage adjustment necessary.

Drug Interactions

Avoid Concomitant Use

Avoid concomitant use of Allopurinol with any of the following: Didanosine

Decreased Effect

The levels/effects of Allopurinol may be decreased by: Antacids

Increased Effect/Toxicity

Allopurinol may increase the levels/effects of: Amoxicillin; Ampicillin; Anticonvulsants (Hydantoin); AzaTHIOprine; CarBAMazepine; ChlorproPAMIDE; Cyclophosphamide; Didanosine; Mercaptopurine; Theophylline Derivatives; Vitamin K Antagonists

The levels/effects of Allopurinol may be increased by: ACE Inhibitors; Loop Diuretics; Thiazide Diuretics

Nutritional/Ethanol Interactions

Ethanol: May decrease effectiveness.

Iron supplements: Hepatic iron uptake may be increased.

Vitamin C: Large amounts of vitamin C may acidify urine and increase kidney stone formation.

Adverse Reactions

Dermatologic: Rash

Endocrine & metabolic: Gout (acute)

Gastrointestinal: Diarrhea, nausea

Hepatic: Alkaline phosphatase increased, liver enzymes increased

Pharmacodynamics/Kinetics

Onset of Action Peak effect: 1-2 weeks

Absorption Oral: ~80%; Rectal: Poor and erratic

Bioavailability 49% to 53%

Time to Peak Plasma: Oral: 30-120 minutes

Protein Binding <1%

Half-Life Elimination

Normal renal function: Parent drug: 1-3 hours; Oxypurinol: 18-30 hours

End-stage renal disease: Prolonged

Metabolism ~75% to active metabolites, chiefly oxypurinol

Excretion Urine (76% as oxypurinol, 12% as unchanged drug)

Allopurinol and oxypurinol are dialyzable

Available Dosage Forms

Injection, powder for reconstitution: 500 mg (base)

Aloprim®: 500 mg (base)

Tablet, oral: 100 mg, 300 mg

Zyloprim®: 100 mg, 300 mg

Dosing

Adult Doses >300 mg should be given in divided doses.

Gout: Oral: Mild: 200-300 mg/day; Severe: 400-600 mg/day; to reduce the possibility of acute gouty attacks, initiate dose at 100 mg/day and increase weekly to recommended dosage. Maximum daily dose: 800 mg/day.

Secondary hyperuricemia associated with chemotherapy:

Oral: 600-800 mg/day in 2-3 divided doses for prevention of acute uric acid nephropathy for 2-3 days starting 1-2 days before chemotherapy

I.V.: 200-400 mg/m^2/day (maximum: 600 mg/day)

Note: Intravenous daily dose can be given as a single infusion or in equally divided doses at 6-, 8-, or 12-hour intervals. A fluid intake sufficient to yield a daily urinary output of at least 2 L in adults and the maintenance of a neutral or, preferably, slightly alkaline urine are desirable.

Recurrent calcium oxalate stones: 200-300 mg/day in single or divided doses

Geriatric Oral: Initial: 100 mg/day; increase until desired uric acid level is obtained. Refer to adult dosing.

Pediatric

Gout: Children >10 years: Refer to adult dosing.

Recurrent calcium oxalate stones: Children >10 years: Refer to adult dosing.

Secondary hyperuricemia associated with chemotherapy:

Oral: Children ≤10 years: 10 mg/kg/day in 2-3 divided doses **or** 200-300 mg/m^2/day in 2-4 divided doses, maximum: 800 mg/24 hours, for prevention of acute uric acid nephropathy (begin 1-2 days before chemotherapy)

Alternative (manufacturer labeling):

<6 years: 150 mg/day in 3 divided doses

6-10 years: 300 mg/day in 2-3 divided doses

>10 years: Refer to adult dosing.

I.V.:

Children ≤10 years: Starting dose: 200 mg/m^2/day

Note: Intravenous daily dose can be given as a single infusion or in equally divided doses at 6-, 8-, or 12-hour intervals. Adequate fluid intake and the maintenance of a neutral or, preferably, slightly alkaline urine are desirable.

Children >10 years: Refer to adult dosing.

Renal Impairment

Oral: Must be adjusted due to accumulation of allopurinol and metabolites; see table.

Adult Maintenance Doses of Allopurinol[1]

Creatinine Clearance (mL/min)	Maintenance Dose of Allopurinol (mg)
140	400 daily
120	350 daily
100	300 daily
80	250 daily
60	200 daily
40	150 daily
20	100 daily
10	100 every 2 days
0	100 every 3 days

[1]This table is based on a standard maintenance dose of 300 mg of allopurinol per day for a patient with a creatinine clearance of 100 mL/min.

I.V.:

Cl_{cr} 10-20 mL/minute: Administer 200 mg/day.

Cl_{cr} 3-10 mL/minute: Administer 100 mg/day.

Cl_{cr} <3 mL/minute: Administer 100 mg/day at extended intervals.

Hemodialysis: Administer dose after hemodialysis or administer 50% supplemental dose.

Administration

Oral Should be administered after meals with plenty of fluid.

I.V. Infuse over 15-60 minutes. The rate of infusion depends on the volume of the infusion. Whenever possible, therapy should be initiated at 24-48 hours before the start of chemotherapy known to cause tumor lysis (including adrenocorticosteroids). I.V. daily dose can be administered as a single infusion or in equally divided doses at 6-, 8-, or 12-hour intervals.

Stability

Reconstitution Further dilution with NS or D_5W (50-100 mL) to ≤6 mg/mL is recommended.

Storage

Powder for injection: Store at controlled room temperature of 15°C to 30°C (59°F to 86°F). Following reconstitution, intravenous solutions should be stored at 20°C to 25°C. Do not refrigerate reconstituted and/or diluted product. Must be administered within 10 hours of solution preparation.

Tablet: Store at controlled room temperature of 15°C to 25°C (59°F to 77°F).

Monitoring and Teaching Issues

Laboratory Monitoring CBC, serum uric acid levels, hepatic and renal function, especially at start of therapy

Patient Education Maintain adequate hydration, unless instructed to restrict fluid intake. Do not use alcohol. You may experience drowsiness, nausea, vomiting, heartburn, or hair loss (reversible). Report immediately skin rash or lesions; painful urination or blood in urine or stool; pain or irritation of the eyes; swelling of lips, mouth, or tongue; unusual fatigue; easy bruising or bleeding; yellowing of skin or eyes; any change in color of urine or stool; unresolved nausea or vomiting; or numbness of extremities.

Dietary Considerations Should take oral forms after meals with plenty of fluid. Fluid intake should be administered to yield neutral or slightly alkaline urine and an output of ~2 L (in adults).

Geriatric Considerations Adjust dose based on renal function.

Pregnancy Considerations There are few reports describing the use of allopurinol during pregnancy; no adverse fetal outcomes attributable to allopurinol have been reported in humans; use only if potential benefit outweighs the potential risk to the fetus.

◆ **Allopurinol Sodium** *see* Allopurinol *on page* 76

Almotriptan (al moh TRIP tan)

U.S. Brand Names Axert®

Index Terms Almotriptan Malate

Generic Availability (U.S.) No

Pharmacologic Category Antimigraine Agent; Serotonin 5-$HT_{1B, 1D}$ Receptor Agonist

Medication Safety Issues

Sound-alike/look-alike issues:

Axert® may be confused with Antivert®

Pregnancy Risk Factor C

Lactation Excretion in breast milk unknown/use caution

Use Acute treatment of migraine with or without aura in adults (with a history of migraine) and adolescents (with a history of migraine lasting ≥4 hours when left untreated)

Mechanism of Action/Effect Selective agonist for serotonin receptor in cranial arteries; causes vasoconstriction and relief of migraine.

Contraindications Hypersensitivity to almotriptan or any component of the formulation; hemiplegic or basilar migraine; known or suspected ischemic heart disease (eg, angina pectoris, MI, documented silent ischemia, coronary artery vasospasm, Prinzmetal's variant angina); cerebrovascular syndromes (eg, stroke, transient ischemic attacks); peripheral vascular disease (eg, ischemic bowel disease); uncontrolled hypertension; use within 24 hours of another 5-HT_1 agonist; use within 24 hours of ergotamine derivatives and/or ergotamine-containing medications (eg, dihydroergotamine, ergotamine)

Warnings/Precautions Almotriptan is only indicated for the treatment of acute migraine headache; not indicated for migraine prophylaxis, or the treatment of cluster headaches, hemiplegic migraine, or basilar migraine. If a patient does not respond to the first dose, the diagnosis of acute migraine should be reconsidered.

Almotriptan should not be given to patients with documented ischemic or vasospastic CAD. Patients with risk factors for CAD (eg, hypertension, hypercholesterolemia, smoker, obesity, diabetes, strong family history of CAD, menopause, male >40 years of age) should undergo adequate cardiac evaluation prior to administration; if the cardiac evaluation is "satisfactory," the first dose of almotriptan should be given in the healthcare provider's office. All patients should undergo periodic evaluation of cardiovascular status during treatment. Cardiac events (coronary artery vasospasm, transient ischemia, myocardial infarction, ventricular tachycardia/fibrillation, cardiac arrest, and death), cerebral/subarachnoid hemorrhage, stroke, peripheral vascular ischemia, and colonic ischemia have been reported with 5-HT_1 agonist administration. Significant elevation in blood pressure, including hypertensive crisis, has also been reported on rare occasions following 5-HT_1 agonist administration in patients with and without a history of hypertension.

Transient and permanent blindness and partial vision loss have been reported (rare) with 5-HT_1 agonist administration. Almotriptan contains a sulfonyl group which is structurally different from a sulfonamide. Cross-reactivity in patients with sulfonamide allergy has not been evaluated; however, the manufacturer recommends that caution be exercised in this patient population. Use with caution in liver or renal dysfunction. Symptoms of agitation, confusion, hallucinations, hyper-reflexia, myoclonus, shivering, and tachycardia (serotonin syndrome) may occur with concomitant proserotonergic drugs (ie, SSRIs/SNRIs or triptans) or agents which reduce almotriptan's metabolism. Efficacy has not been demonstrated in improvement of migraine-associated symptoms (eg, phonophobia, nausea, photophobia) in patients aged 12-17 years (Linder, 2008).

Drug Interactions

Metabolism/Transport Effects Substrate (minor) of CYP2D6, 3A4

Avoid Concomitant Use

Avoid concomitant use of Almotriptan with any of the following: Ergot Derivatives; MAO Inhibitors; Sibutramine

Decreased Effect

The levels/effects of Almotriptan may be decreased by: Peginterferon Alfa-2b

Increased Effect/Toxicity

Almotriptan may increase the levels/effects of: Ergot Derivatives; Serotonin Modulators

The levels/effects of Almotriptan may be increased by: CYP3A4 Inhibitors (Strong); Ergot Derivatives; MAO Inhibitors; Sibutramine

Adverse Reactions 1% to 10%:

Central nervous system: Somnolence (≤5%), dizziness (≤4%), headache (≤2%)
Gastrointestinal: Nausea (1% to 3%), vomiting (≤2%), xerostomia (1%)
Neuromuscular & skeletal: Paresthesia (≤1%)

Pharmacodynamics/Kinetics

Absorption Well absorbed

Bioavailability ~70%

Time to Peak Plasma: 1-3 hours

Protein Binding ~35%

Half-Life Elimination 3-4 hours

Metabolism Via MAO type A oxidative deamination (~27% of dose) and CYP3A4 and 2D6 (~12% of dose) to inactive metabolites

Excretion Urine (~75%; ~40% of total dose as unchanged drug); feces (~13% of total dose as unchanged drug and metabolites)

Available Dosage Forms

Tablet, oral:

Axert®: 6.25 mg, 12.5 mg

Dosing

Adult & Geriatric Migraine: Oral: Initial: 6.25-12.5 mg in a single dose; if the headache returns, repeat the dose after 2 hours; no more than 2 doses (maximum daily dose: 25 mg)
Note: The safety of treating more than 4 migraines/month has not been established.

Dosage adjustment with concomitant use of an enzyme inhibitor:

Patients receiving a potent CYP3A4 inhibitor: Initial: 6.25 mg in a single dose; maximum daily dose: 12.5 mg
Patients with renal impairment and concomitant use of a potent CYP3A4 inhibitor: Avoid use
Patients with hepatic impairment and concomitant use of a potent CYP3A4 inhibitor: Avoid use

Pediatric Migraine: Oral: Children ≥12 years: Refer to adult dosing.

Renal Impairment Severe renal impairment (Cl_{cr} ≤30 mL/minute): Initial: 6.25 mg in a single dose; maximum daily dose: 12.5 mg

Hepatic Impairment Initial: 6.25 mg in a single dose; maximum daily dose: 12.5 mg

Administration

Oral Administer without regard to meals.

Stability

Storage Store at 25°C (77°F); excursions permitted to 15°C to 30°C (59°F to 86°F).

Monitoring and Teaching Issues

Physical Assessment Clear diagnosis of migraines should be determined before beginning treatment. Cardiovascular status should be evaluated prior to initiating medication and periodically thereafter. Assess risk for coronary artery disease, liver or renal dysfunction, or sulfonamide allergy. Assess potential for interactions with ergot-containing drugs, SSRIs, and MAO inhibitors patient may be taking. Teach patient proper use (treatment of acute migraine; not prevention of migraine).

Patient Education This drug is to be used to reduce your migraine, not to prevent or reduce the number of attacks. Do not use more than two doses in 24 hours and do not take within 24 hours of any other migraine medication without consulting prescriber. May cause dizziness, fatigue, or drowsiness. Report immediately any chest pain or palpitations, feelings of tightness or pressure in jaw or throat, dizziness, or skin rash.

Dietary Considerations May be taken without regard to meals.

Geriatric Considerations Use cautiously in elderly, particularly since many have cardiovascular disease, which would put them at risk for cardiovascular adverse effects. Safety and efficacy in elderly patients >65 years of age have not been established.

Pregnancy Considerations There are no adequate and well-controlled studies in pregnant women. Use in pregnancy should be limited to situations where benefit outweighs risk to fetus. In some (but not all) animal studies, administration was associated with embryolethality, fetal malformations, and decreased pup weight.

Related Information

Antimigraine Drugs: 5-HT_1 Receptor Agonists *on page 1985*

- **Almotriptan Malate** *see* Almotriptan *on page 78*
- **Alodox™** *see* Doxycycline *on page 586*
- **Aloe Vesta® Antifungal [OTC]** *see* Miconazole (Topical) *on page 1224*
- **Alomide®** *see* Lodoxamide *on page 1125*
- **Aloprim®** *see* Allopurinol *on page 76*
- **Alora®** *see* Estradiol (Systemic) *on page 670*
- **Aloxi®** *see* Palonosetron *on page 1396*
- **Alphagan® P** *see* Brimonidine *on page 230*
- **1α-Hydroxyergocalciferol** *see* Doxercalciferol *on page 579*
- **Alphanate®** *see* Antihemophilic Factor/von Willebrand Factor Complex (Human) *on page 134*
- **Alphaquin HP®** *see* Hydroquinone *on page 927*

ALPRAZolam (al PRAY zoe lam)

U.S. Brand Names Alprazolam Intensol™; Niravam™; Xanax XR®; Xanax®

Generic Availability (U.S.) Yes: Excludes oral solution

Pharmacologic Category Benzodiazepine

Medication Safety Issues

Sound-alike/look-alike issues:

ALPRAZolam may be confused with alprostadil, LORazepam, triazolam

Xanax® may be confused with Fanapt®, Lanoxin®, Tenex®, Tylox®, Xopenex®, Zantac®, ZyrTEC®

Beers Criteria medication: This drug may be inappropriate for use in geriatric patients (high severity risk).

Pregnancy Risk Factor D

Lactation Enters breast milk/not recommended (AAP rates "of concern"; AAP 2001 update pending)

Use Treatment of anxiety disorder (GAD); panic disorder, with or without agoraphobia; anxiety associated with depression

Unlabeled/Investigational Use Anxiety in children

Mechanism of Action/Effect Binds to stereospecific benzodiazepine receptors on the postsynaptic GABA neuron at several sites within the central nervous system, including the limbic system, reticular formation. Enhancement of the inhibitory effect of GABA on neuronal excitability results by increased neuronal membrane permeability to chloride ions. This shift in chloride ions results in hyperpolarization (a less excitable state) and stabilization.

Contraindications Hypersensitivity to alprazolam or any component of the formulation (cross-sensitivity with other benzodiazepines may exist); narrow-angle glaucoma; concurrent use with ketoconazole or itraconazole; pregnancy

Warnings/Precautions Rebound or withdrawal symptoms, including seizures, may occur 18 hours to 3 days following abrupt discontinuation or large decreases in dose (more common in patients receiving >4 mg/day or prolonged treatment). Breakthrough anxiety may occur at the end of dosing interval. Use with caution in patients receiving concurrent CYP3A4 inhibitors. Use with caution in renal impairment or predisposition to urate nephropathy. Use with caution in elderly or debilitated patients, patients with hepatic disease (including alcoholics), renal impairment, or obese patients.

Causes CNS depression (dose related) which may impair physical and mental capabilities. Patients must be cautioned about performing tasks that require mental alertness (eg, operating machinery or driving). Effects with other sedative drugs or ethanol may be potentiated. Benzodiazepines have been associated with falls and traumatic injury and should be used with extreme caution in patients who are at risk of these events. Due to increased sensitivity in the elderly, smaller doses of benzodiazepines may be safer and as effective. Avoid using doses >2 mg daily of alprazolam (Beers Criteria). Use with caution in patients with respiratory disease or impaired gag reflex.

Use caution in patients with depression, particularly if suicidal risk may be present. Episodes of mania or hypomania have occurred in depressed patients treated with alprazolam. May cause physical or psychological dependence. Acute withdrawal may be precipitated in patients after administration of flumazenil.

Benzodiazepines have been associated with anterograde amnesia. Paradoxical reactions have been reported with benzodiazepines, particularly in adolescent/pediatric or psychiatric patients. Does not have analgesic, antidepressant, or antipsychotic properties.

Drug Interactions

Metabolism/Transport Effects **Substrate** of CYP3A4 (major)

Avoid Concomitant Use

Avoid concomitant use of ALPRAZolam with any of the following: Indinavir; OLANZapine

Decreased Effect

The levels/effects of ALPRAZolam may be decreased by: CarBAMazepine; CYP3A4 Inducers (Strong); Deferasirox; Rifamycin Derivatives; St Johns Wort; Theophylline Derivatives; Yohimbine

Increased Effect/Toxicity

ALPRAZolam may increase the levels/effects of: Alcohol (Ethyl); CloZAPine; CNS Depressants; Methotrimeprazine

The levels/effects of ALPRAZolam may be increased by: Antifungal Agents (Azole Derivatives, Systemic); Aprepitant; Calcium Channel Blockers (Nondihydropyridine); Cimetidine; Conivaptan; Contraceptives (Estrogens); Contraceptives (Progestins); CYP3A4 Inhibitors (Moderate); CYP3A4 Inhibitors (Strong); Dasatinib; Droperidol; Fluconazole; Fosaprepitant; Grapefruit Juice; Indinavir; Isoniazid; Macrolide Antibiotics; Methotrimeprazine; Nefazodone; OLANZapine; Protease Inhibitors; Proton Pump Inhibitors; Selective Serotonin Reuptake Inhibitors

Nutritional/Ethanol Interactions

Cigarette smoking: May decrease alprazolam concentrations up to 50%.

Ethanol: Avoid ethanol (may increase CNS depression).

Food: Alprazolam serum concentration is unlikely to be increased by grapefruit juice because of alprazolam's high oral bioavailability. The C_{max} of the extended release formulation is increased by 25% when a high-fat meal is given 2 hours before dosing. T_{max} is decreased 30% when food is given immediately prior to dose. T_{max} is increased by 30% when food is given ≥1 hour after dose.

Herb/Nutraceutical: St John's wort may decrease alprazolam levels. Avoid valerian, St John's wort, kava kava, gotu kola (may increase CNS depression).

Lab Interactions Increased with alkaline phosphatase

Adverse Reactions

>10%:

Central nervous system: Abnormal coordination, cognitive disorder, depression, drowsiness, fatigue, irritability, lightheadedness, memory impairment, sedation, somnolence

Gastrointestinal: Appetite increased/decreased, constipation, salivation decreased, weight gain/loss, xerostomia

Genitourinary: Micturition difficulty

Neuromuscular & skeletal: Dysarthria

1% to 10%:

Cardiovascular: Hypotension

Central nervous system: Agitation, attention disturbance, confusion, depersonalization, derealization, disorientation, disinhibition, dizziness, dream abnormalities, fear, hallucinations, hypersomnia, nightmares, seizure, talkativeness

Dermatologic: Dermatitis, pruritus, rash

Endocrine & metabolic: Libido decreased/increased, menstrual disorders

Gastrointestinal: Salivation increased

Genitourinary: Incontinence

Hepatic: Bilirubin increased, jaundice, liver enzymes increased

Neuromuscular & skeletal: Arthralgia, ataxia, myalgia, paresthesia

Ocular: Diplopia

Respiratory: Allergic rhinitis, dyspnea

Pharmacodynamics/Kinetics

Onset of Action Immediate release and extended release formulations: 1 hour

Duration of Action Immediate release: 5.1 ± 1.7 hours; Extended release: 11.3 ± 4.2 hours

Absorption Extended release: Slower relative to immediate release formulation resulting in a concentration that is maintained 5-11 hours after dosing

Bioavailability 90%

Time to Peak Immediate release: 1-2 hours; Extended release: ~9 hours; decreased by 1 hour following bedtime dosing compared to morning dosing

Protein Binding 80%; primarily to albumin

Half-Life Elimination
Adults (healthy): 11.2 hours (immediate release range: 6.3-26.9 hours; extended release range: 10.7-15.8 hours)
Elderly: 16.3 hours (range: 9-26.9 hours)
Alcoholic liver disease: 19.7 hours (range: 5.8-65.3 hours)
Obesity: 21.8 hours (range: 9.9-40.4 hours)

Metabolism Hepatic via CYP3A4; forms two active metabolites (4-hydroxyalprazolam and α-hydroxyalprazolam)

Excretion Urine (as unchanged drug and metabolites)

Controlled Substance C-IV

Available Dosage Forms

Solution, oral:
Alprazolam Intensol™: 1 mg/mL (30 mL)

Tablet, oral: 0.25 mg, 0.5 mg, 1 mg, 2 mg
Xanax®: 0.25 mg, 0.5 mg, 1 mg, 2 mg

Tablet, extended release, oral: 0.5 mg, 1 mg, 2 mg, 3 mg
Xanax XR®: 0.5 mg, 1 mg, 2 mg, 3 mg

Tablet, orally disintegrating, oral: 0.25 mg, 0.5 mg, 1 mg, 2 mg
Niravam™: 0.25 mg, 0.5 mg, 1 mg, 2 mg

Dosing

Adult Note: Treatment >4 months should be re-evaluated to determine the patient's continued need for the drug

Anxiety: Oral: *Immediate release:* Effective doses are 0.5-4 mg/day in divided doses; the manufacturer recommends starting at 0.25-0.5 mg 3 times/day; titrate dose upward; usual maximum: 4 mg/day. Patients requiring doses >4 mg/day should be increased cautiously. Periodic reassessment and consideration of dosage reduction is recommended.

Anxiety associated with depression: Oral: *Immediate release:* Average dose required: 2.5-3 mg/day in divided doses

Ethanol withdrawal (unlabeled use): Oral: *Immediate release:* Usual dose: 2-2.5 mg/day in divided doses

Panic disorder: Oral:

Immediate release: Initial: 0.5 mg 3 times/day; dose may be increased every 3-4 days in increments ≤1 mg/day. Mean effective dosage: 5-6 mg/day; many patients obtain relief at 2 mg/day, as much as 10 mg/day may be required

Extended release: 0.5-1 mg once daily; may increase dose every 3-4 days in increments ≤1 mg/day (range: 3-6 mg/day)

Switching from immediate release to extended release: Patients may be switched to extended release tablets by taking the total daily dose of the immediate release tablets and giving it once daily using the extended release preparation.

Preoperative sedation: Oral: 0.5 mg in evening at bedtime and 0.5 mg 1 hour before procedure

Dose reduction: Abrupt discontinuation should be avoided. Daily dose may be decreased by 0.5 mg every 3 days, however, some patients may require a slower reduction. If withdrawal symptoms occur, resume previous dose and discontinue on a less rapid schedule.

Geriatric Initial: 0.125-0.25 mg twice daily; increase by 0.125 mg/day as needed. The smallest effective dose should be used.
Immediate release: Initial 0.25 mg 2-3 times/day
Extended release: Initial: 0.5 mg once daily

Pediatric

Anxiety (unlabeled use): Oral: Immediate release: Initial: 0.005 mg/kg/dose or 0.125 mg/dose 3 times/day; increase in increments of 0.125-0.25 mg, up to a maximum of 0.02 mg/kg/dose or 0.06 mg/kg/day (0.375-3 mg/day). See "Dose Reduction" comment in adult dosing.

Note: Treatment >4 months should be re-evaluated to determine the patient's continued need for the drug.

Renal Impairment No guidelines for adjustment; use caution.

Hepatic Impairment Oral: Reduce dose by 50% to 60% or avoid in cirrhosis.

Administration

Oral

Immediate release preparations: Can be administered sublingually with comparable onset and completeness of absorption.

Extended release tablet: Should be taken once daily in the morning; do not crush, break, or chew.

Orally-disintegrating tablets: Using dry hands, place tablet on top of tongue. If using one-half of tablet, immediately discard remaining half (may not remain stable). Administration with water is not necessary.

Stability

Storage Orally-disintegrating tablet: Store at room temperature of 20°C to 25°C (68°F to 77°F). Protect from moisture. Seal bottle tightly and discard any cotton packaged inside bottle.

Monitoring and Teaching Issues

Physical Assessment Assess for signs of CNS depression. Assess for history of addiction; long-term use can result in dependence, abuse, or tolerance; periodically evaluate need for continued use. For inpatient use, institute safety measures to prevent falls. Taper dosage slowly when discontinuing.

Patient Education Drug may cause physical and/or psychological dependence. Avoid alcohol. You may experience drowsiness, lightheadedness, impaired coordination, dizziness, blurred vision, nausea, vomiting, dry mouth, constipation, altered sexual drive or ability (reversible), or photosensitivity. Report persistent CNS effects (eg, confusion, depression, increased sedation, excitation, headache, agitation, insomnia or nightmares, dizziness, fatigue, impaired coordination, changes in personality, or changes in cognition); changes in urinary pattern; muscle cramping, weakness, tremors, or rigidity; ringing in ears or visual disturbances; chest pain, palpitations, or rapid heartbeat; excessive perspiration; excessive GI symptoms (eg, cramping, constipation, vomiting, anorexia); or worsening of condition.

Dietary Considerations Extended release tablet should be taken once daily in the morning.

Geriatric Considerations This medication is considered to be potentially inappropriate in this patient population (Beers Criteria severity: High).

Breast-Feeding Considerations In a study of eight postpartum women, peak concentrations of alprazolam were found in breast milk ~1 hour after the maternal dose and the half-life was ~14 hours. Samples were obtained over 36 hours following a single oral dose of alprazolam 0.5 mg. Metabolites were not detected in breast milk. In this study, the estimated exposure to the breast-feeding infant was ~3% of the weight-adjusted maternal dose. Drowsiness, lethargy, or weight loss in nursing infants have been observed in case reports following maternal use of some benzodiazepines.

Pregnancy Considerations Benzodiazepines have the potential to cause harm to the fetus. Alprazolam and its metabolites cross the human placenta. Teratogenic effects have been observed with some benzodiazepines; however, additional studies are needed. The incidence of premature birth and low birth weights may be increased following maternal use of benzodiazepines; hypoglycemia and respiratory problems in the neonate may occur following exposure late in pregnancy. Neonatal withdrawal symptoms may occur within days to weeks after birth and "floppy infant syndrome" (which also includes withdrawal symptoms) has been reported with some benzodiazepines.

Additional Information Not intended for management of anxieties and minor distresses associated with everyday life. Treatment longer than 4 months should be re-evaluated to determine the patient's need for the drug. Patients who become physically dependent on alprazolam tend to have a difficult time discontinuing it; withdrawal symptoms may be severe. To minimize withdrawal symptoms, taper dosage slowly; do not discontinue abruptly. Abrupt discontinuation after sustained use (generally >10 days) may cause withdrawal symptoms.

Related Information

Benzodiazepines *on page 1988*

◆ **Alprazolam Intensol™** *see* ALPRAZolam *on page 80*

Alprostadil (al PROS ta dill)

U.S. Brand Names Caverject Impulse®; Caverject®; Edex®; Muse®; Prostin VR Pediatric®

Index Terms PGE_1; Prostaglandin E_1

Generic Availability (U.S.) Yes: Solution for injection

Pharmacologic Category Prostaglandin; Vasodilator

Medication Safety Issues

Sound-alike/look-alike issues:

Alprostadil may be confused with alPRAZolam

Pregnancy Risk Factor X/C (Muse®)

Lactation Not indicated for use in women

Use

Prostin VR Pediatric®: Temporary maintenance of patency of ductus arteriosus in neonates with ductal-dependent congenital heart disease until surgery can be performed. These defects include cyanotic (eg, pulmonary atresia, pulmonary stenosis, tricuspid atresia, Fallot's tetralogy, transposition of the great vessels) and acyanotic (eg, interruption of aortic arch, coarctation of aorta, hypoplastic left ventricle) heart disease.

Caverject®: Treatment of erectile dysfunction of vasculogenic, psychogenic, or neurogenic etiology; adjunct in the diagnosis of erectile dysfunction

Edex®, Muse®: Treatment of erectile dysfunction of vasculogenic, psychogenic, or neurogenic etiology

Unlabeled/Investigational Use Investigational: Treatment of pulmonary hypertension in infants and children with congenital heart defects with left-to-right shunts

Mechanism of Action/Effect

Erectile dysfunction: Causes vasodilation by dilation of cavernosal arteries when injected along the penile shaft, allowing blood flow to, and entrapment in, the lacunar spaces of the penis (ie, corporeal veno-occlusive mechanism)

Neonate: Has direct effects on smooth muscle of ductus arteriosus.

Contraindications Hypersensitivity to alprostadil or any component of the formulation; hyaline membrane disease or persistent fetal circulation and when a dominant left-to-right shunt is present; respiratory distress syndrome; conditions predisposing patients to priapism (sickle cell anemia, multiple myeloma, leukemia); patients with anatomical deformation of the penis, penile implants; use in men for whom sexual activity is inadvisable or contraindicated; pregnancy

Warnings/Precautions Use cautiously in neonates with bleeding tendencies. **[U.S. Boxed Warning]: Apnea may occur in 10% to 12% of neonates with congenital heart defects, especially in those weighing <2 kg at birth.** Apnea usually appears during the first hour of drug infusion. When used for patency of ductus arteriosus infuse for the shortest time at the lowest dose consistent with good patient care. Use for >120 hours has been associated with antral hyperplasia and gastric outlet obstruction.

When used in erectile dysfunction, priapism may occur; treat proloonged priapism (erection persisting for >4 hours) immediately to avoid penile tissue damage and permanent loss of potency; discontinue therapy if signs of penile fibrosis develop (penile angulation, cavernosal ▶

fibrosis, or Peyronie's disease). When used in erectile dysfunction (Muse®), syncope occurring within 1 hour of administration has been reported. The potential for drug-drug interactions may occur when Muse® is prescribed concomitantly with antihypertensives.

Drug Interactions

Avoid Concomitant Use There are no known interactions where it is recommended to avoid concomitant use.

Decreased Effect There are no known significant interactions involving a decrease in effect.

Increased Effect/Toxicity There are no known significant interactions involving an increase in effect.

Nutritional/Ethanol Interactions Ethanol: Avoid concurrent use (vasodilating effect).

Adverse Reactions

Intraurethral:

>10%: Genitourinary: Penile pain, urethral burning

2% to 10%:

- Central nervous system: Headache, dizziness, pain
- Genitourinary: Vaginal itching (female partner), testicular pain, urethral bleeding (minor)

Intracavernosal injection:

>10%: Genitourinary: Penile pain

1% to 10%:

- Cardiovascular: Hypertension
- Central nervous system: Headache, dizziness
- Genitourinary: Prolonged erection (>4 hours, 4%), penile fibrosis, penis disorder, penile rash, penile edema
- Local: Injection site hematoma and/or bruising

Intravenous:

>10%:

- Cardiovascular: Flushing
- Central nervous system: Fever
- Respiratory: Apnea

1% to 10%:

- Cardiovascular: Bradycardia, hyper-/hypotension, tachycardia, cardiac arrest, edema
- Central nervous system: Seizure, headache, dizziness
- Endocrine & metabolic: Hypokalemia
- Gastrointestinal: Diarrhea
- Hematologic: Disseminated intravascular coagulation
- Neuromuscular & skeletal: Back pain
- Respiratory: Upper respiratory infection, flu syndrome, sinusitis, nasal congestion, cough
- Miscellaneous: Sepsis, localized pain in structures other than the injection site

Pharmacodynamics/Kinetics

Onset of Action Rapid

Duration of Action <1 hour

Protein Binding Plasma: 81% to albumin

Half-Life Elimination 5-10 minutes

Metabolism ~75% by oxidation in one pass via lungs

Excretion Urine (90% as metabolites) within 24 hours

Available Dosage Forms

Injection, powder for reconstitution:

- Caverject Impulse®: 10 mcg, 20 mcg
- Caverject®: 20 mcg, 40 mcg
- Edex®: 10 mcg, 20 mcg, 40 mcg

Injection, solution: 500 mcg/mL (1 mL)

- Prostin VR Pediatric®: 500 mcg/mL (1 mL)

Pellet, urethral:

- Muse®: 250 mcg (6s); 500 mcg (6s); 1000 mcg (6s)

Dosing

Adult

Erectile dysfunction:

Intracavernous (Caverject®, Edex®): Individualize dose by careful titration; doses >40 mcg (Edex®) or >60 mcg (Caverject®) are not recommended: Initial dose must be titrated in physician's office. Patient must stay in the physician's office until complete detumescence occurs; if there is no response, then the next higher dose may be given within 1 hour; if there is still no response, a 1-day interval before giving the next dose is recommended; increasing the dose or concentration in the treatment of impotence results in increasing pain and discomfort.

Vasculogenic, psychogenic, or mixed etiology: Initiate dosage titration at 2.5 mcg, increasing by 2.5 mcg to a dose of 5 mcg and then in increments of 5-10 mcg depending on the erectile response until the dose produces an erection suitable for intercourse, not lasting >1 hour; if there is absolutely no response to initial 2.5 mcg dose, the second dose may be increased to 7.5 mcg, followed by increments of 5-10 mcg

Neurogenic etiology (eg, spinal cord injury): Initiate dosage titration at 1.25 mcg, increasing to a dose of 2.5 mcg and then 5 mcg; increase further in increments 5 mcg until the dose is reached that produces an erection suitable for intercourse, not lasting >1 hour

Maintenance: Once appropriate dose has been determined, patient may self-administer injections at a frequency of no more than 3 times/week with at least 24 hours between doses

Intraurethral (Muse® Pellet):

Initial: 125-250 mcg

Maintenance: Administer as needed to achieve an erection; duration of action is about 30-60 minutes; use only two systems per 24-hour period

Geriatric Elderly patients may have a greater frequency of renal dysfunction; lowest effective dose should be used. In clinical studies with Edex®, higher minimally effective doses and a higher rate of lack of effect were noted.

Pediatric

Patent ductus arteriosus I.V.:

Prostin VR Pediatric®: I.V. continuous infusion into a large vein, or alternatively through an umbilical artery catheter placed at the ductal opening: 0.05-0.1 mcg/kg/minute with therapeutic response, rate is reduced to lowest effective dosage. With unsatisfactory response, rate is increased gradually; maintenance: 0.01-0.4 mcg/kg/minute.

Note: PGE_1 is usually given at an infusion rate of 0.1 mcg/kg/minute, but it is often possible to reduce the dosage to 1/2 or even 1/10 without losing the therapeutic effect.

Note: Therapeutic response is indicated by increased pH in those with acidosis or by an increase in oxygenation (PO_2) usually evident within 30 minutes.

Administration

I.V. Patent ductus arteriosus (Prostin VR Pediatric®): I.V. continuous infusion into a large vein or alternatively through an umbilical artery catheter placed at the ductal opening; manufacturer recommended maximum concentration for I.V. infusion: 20 mcg/mL

Other Erectile dysfunction: Use a 1/2 inch, 27- to 30-gauge needle. Inject into the dorsolateral aspect of the proximal third of the penis, avoiding visible veins; alternate side of the penis for injections.

Stability

Reconstitution

Caverject® Impulse™: Provided as a dual-chamber syringe with diluent in one chamber. To mix, hold syringe with needle pointing upward and turn plunger clockwise; turn upside down several times to mix. Device can be set to deliver specified dose, each device can be set at various increments.

Caverject® powder: Use only the supplied diluent for reconstitution (ie, bacteriostatic/sterile water with benzyl alcohol 0.945%).

Edex®: Reconstitute with NS.

Storage

Caverject® Impulse™: Store at controlled room temperature of 15°C to 30°C (59°F to 86°F). Following reconstitution, use within 24 hours and discard any unused solution.

Caverject® powder: The 5 mcg, 10 mcg, and 20 mcg vials should be stored at or below 25°C (77°F); The 40 mcg vial should be stored at 2°C to 8°C until dispensed. After dispensing, stable for up to 3 months at or below 25°C. Following reconstitution, all strengths should be stored at or below 25°C (77°F); do not refrigerate or freeze; use within 24 hours.

Caverject® solution: Prior to dispensing, store frozen at -20°C to -10°C (-4°F to -14°F). Once dispensed, may be stored frozen for up to 3 months, or under refrigeration at 2°C to 8°C (36°F to 46°F) for up to 7 days. Do not refreeze. Once removed from foil wrap, solution may be allowed to warm to room temperature prior to use. If not used immediately, solution should be discarded. Shake well prior to use.

Edex®: Store at controlled room temperature of 15°C to 30°C (59°F to 86°F); following reconstitution, use immediately and discard any unused solution.

Muse®: Refrigerate at 2°C to 8°C (36°F to 46°F); may be stored at room temperature for up to 14 days

Prostin VR Pediatric®: Refrigerate at 2°C to 8°C (36°F to 46°F). The following stability information has also been reported: May be stored at 20°C for up to 34 days or 30°C for up to 26 days (Cohen, 2007). Prior to infusion, dilute with D_5W or NS; use within 24 hours.

Monitoring and Teaching Issues

Physical Assessment Neonate: Monitor closely; apnea has occurred during first hour after administration. **Erectile dysfunction:** After individual dose titration is determined, the Caverject® injection (or Muse®) is generally self-administered. Teach patient appropriate injection technique and syringe/needle disposal.

Patient Education Use no more than 3 times/week, allowing 24 hours between injections. Avoid alcohol. Use alternate sides of penis with each injection. The risk of transmitting blood-borne disease is increased with use of alprostadil injections since a small amount of bleeding at injection site is possible. Stop using and contact prescriber immediately if erections last more than 4 hours, or you experience moderate to severe penile pain. Report penile problems (eg, nodules, new penile pain, rash, bruising, numbness, swelling, signs of infection, abnormal ejaculations); cardiac symptoms (hyper-/hypotension, chest pain, palpitations, irregular heartbeat); flushing, fever, or flu-like symptoms; or respiratory difficulty.

Geriatric Considerations Elderly may have concomitant diseases which would contraindicate the use of alprostadil. Other forms of attaining penile tumescence are recommended.

Pregnancy Considerations Alprostadil is embryotoxic in animal studies. It is not indicated for use in women. The manufacturer of Muse® recommends a condom barrier when being used during sexual intercourse with a pregnant women.

◆ **Alrex®** *see* Loteprednol *on page* 1136

◆ **Alsuma™** *see* SUMAtriptan *on page* 1691

◆ **Altace®** *see* Ramipril *on page* 1552

◆ **Altafrin** *see* Phenylephrine (Ophthalmic) *on page* 1452

◆ **Altaryl [OTC]** *see* DiphenhydrAMINE (Systemic) *on page* 543

Alteplase (AL te plase)

U.S. Brand Names Activase®; Cathflo® Activase®

Index Terms Alteplase, Recombinant; Alteplase, Tissue Plasminogen Activator, Recombinant; tPA

Generic Availability (U.S.) No

Pharmacologic Category Thrombolytic Agent

Medication Safety Issues

Sound-alike/look-alike issues:

Activase® may be confused with Cathflo® Activase®, TNKase®

Alteplase may be confused with Altace®

"tPA" abbreviation should not be used when writing orders for this medication; has been misread as TNKase (tenecteplase)

High alert medication: The Institute for Safe Medication Practices (ISMP) includes this medication (I.V.) among its list of drugs which have a heightened risk of causing significant patient harm when used in error.

Pregnancy Risk Factor C

Lactation Excretion in breast milk unknown/use caution

Use Management of ST-elevation myocardial infarction (STEMI) for the lysis of thrombi in coronary arteries; management of acute ischemic stroke (AIS); management of acute pulmonary embolism (PE)

Recommended criteria for treatment:

STEMI: Chest pain ≥20 minutes duration, onset of chest pain within 12 hours of treatment (or within prior 12-24 hours in patients with continuing ischemic symptoms), and ST-segment elevation >0.1 mV in at least two contiguous precordial leads or two adjacent limb leads on ECG or new or presumably new left bundle branch block (LBBB)

AIS: Onset of stroke symptoms within 3 hours of treatment

Acute pulmonary embolism: Age ≤75 years: Documented massive PE (defined as acute PE with sustained hypotension [SBP <90 mm Hg for ≤15 minutes or requiring inotropic support], persistent profound bradycardia [HR <40 bpm with signs or symptoms of shock], or pulselessness); alteplase may be considered for submassive PE with clinical evidence of adverse prognosis (eg, new hemodynamic instability, worsening respiratory insufficiency, severe RV dysfunction, or major myocardial necrosis) and low risk of bleeding complications. **Note:** Not recommended for patients with low-risk PE (eg, normotensive, no RV dysfunction, normal biomarkers) or submassive acute PE with minor RV dysfunction, minor myocardial necrosis, and no clinical worsening (Jaff, 2011).

Cathflo® Activase®: Restoration of central venous catheter function

Unlabeled/Investigational Use Acute ischemic stroke presenting 3-4.5 hours after symptom onset; acute peripheral arterial occlusive disease

Mechanism of Action/Effect Dissolves thrombus (clot)

Contraindications Hypersensitivity to alteplase or any component of the formulation

Treatment of STEMI or PE: Active internal bleeding; history of CVA; ischemic stroke within 3 months (Antman, 2004; Jaff, 2011); recent intracranial or intraspinal surgery or trauma; intracranial neoplasm; prior intracranial hemorrhage (Antman, 2004; Jaff, 2011); arteriovenous malformation or aneurysm; known bleeding diathesis; severe uncontrolled hypertension (listed as a relative contraindication in STEMI [Antman, 2004] and PE [Jaff, 2011] guidelines); suspected aortic dissection (Antman, 2004; Jaff, 2011); significant closed head or facial trauma (Antman, 2004; Jaff, 2011) within 3 months with radiographic evidence of bony fracture or brain injury (Jaff, 2011)

Treatment of acute ischemic stroke: Evidence of intracranial hemorrhage or suspicion of subarachnoid hemorrhage on pretreatment evaluation; intracranial or intraspinal surgery within 3 months; stroke or serious head injury within 3 months; history of intracranial hemorrhage; uncontrolled hypertension at time of treatment (eg, >185 mm Hg systolic or >110 mm Hg diastolic); seizure at the onset of stroke; active internal bleeding; intracranial neoplasm; arteriovenous malformation or aneurysm; multilobar cerebral infarction (hypodensity >$^1/_3$ cerebral hemisphere; Adams, 2007); clinical presentation suggesting post-MI pericarditis; known bleeding diathesis including but not limited to current use of oral anticoagulants producing an INR >1.7, an INR >1.7, administration of heparin within 48 hours preceding the onset of stroke with an elevated aPTT at presentation, platelet count <100,000/mm^3.

Additional exclusion criteria within clinical trials:

Presentation <3 hours after initial symptoms (NINDS, 1995): Time of symptom onset unknown, rapidly improving or minor symptoms, major surgery within 2 weeks, GI or urinary tract hemorrhage within 3 weeks, aggressive treatment required to lower blood pressure, glucose level <50 or >400 mg/dL, and arterial puncture at a noncompressible site or lumbar puncture within 1 week.

Presentation 3-4.5 hours after initial symptoms (ECASS-III; Hacke, 2008): Age >80 years, time of symptom onset unknown, rapidly improving or minor symptoms, current use of anticoagulants regardless of INR, glucose level <50 or >400 mg/dL, aggressive intravenous treatment required to lower blood pressure, major surgery or severe trauma within 3 months, baseline National Institutes of Health Stroke Scale (NIHSS) score >25, and history of both stroke and diabetes.

Warnings/Precautions Concurrent heparin anticoagulation may contribute to bleeding. In the treatment of acute ischemic stroke, concurrent use of anticoagulants was not permitted during the initial 24 hours of the <3 hour window trial (NINDS, 1995). Initiation of SubQ heparin (≤10,000 units) or equivalent doses of low molecular weight heparin for prevention of DVT during the first 24 hours of the 3-4.5 hour window trial was permitted and did not increase the incidence of intracerebral hemorrhage (Hacke, 2008). For acute PE, withhold heparin during the 2-hour infusion period. Monitor all potential bleeding sites. Do not use doses >150 mg; associated with increased risk of intracranial hemorrhage. Intramuscular injections and non-essential handling of the patient should be avoided. Venipunctures should be performed carefully and only when necessary. If arterial puncture is necessary, use an upper extremity vessel that can be manually compressed. If serious bleeding occurs, the infusion of alteplase and heparin should be stopped. Avoid aspirin for 24 hours following administration of alteplase; administration within 24 hours increases the risk of hemorrhagic transformation.

For the following conditions, the risk of bleeding is higher with use of thrombolytics and should be weighed against the benefits of therapy: Recent major surgery (eg, CABG, obstetrical delivery, organ biopsy, pregnancy, previous puncture of noncompressible vessels), prolonged CPR with evidence of thoracic trauma, lumbar puncture within 1 week, cerebrovascular disease, recent gastrointestinal or genitourinary bleeding, recent trauma, hypertension (systolic BP >175 mm Hg and/or diastolic BP >110 mm Hg), high likelihood of left heart thrombus (eg, mitral stenosis with atrial fibrillation), acute pericarditis, subacute bacterial endocarditis, hemostatic defects including ones caused by severe renal or hepatic dysfunction, significant hepatic dysfunction, pregnancy, diabetic hemorrhagic retinopathy or other hemorrhagic ophthalmic conditions, septic thrombophlebitis or occluded AV cannula at seriously infected site, advanced age (eg, >75 years), any other condition in which bleeding constitutes a significant hazard or would be particularly difficult to manage because of location. When treating acute MI or pulmonary embolism, use with caution in patients receiving oral anticoagulants. In the treatment of acute ischemic stroke within 3 hours of stroke symptom onset, the current use of oral anticoagulants producing an INR >1.7 is contraindicated.

Coronary thrombolysis may result in reperfusion arrhythmias. Patients who present **within 3 hours** of stroke symptom onset should be treated with alteplase unless contraindications exist. A longer time window (**3-4.5 hours** after symptom onset) has now been formally evaluated and shown to be safe and efficacious for select individuals (del Zoppo, 2009; Hacke, 2008). Treatment of patients with minor neurological deficit or with rapidly improving symptoms is not recommended. Follow standard management for STEMI while infusing alteplase.

Cathflo® Activase®: When used to restore catheter function, use Cathflo® cautiously in those patients with known or suspected catheter infections. Evaluate catheter for other causes of dysfunction before use. Avoid excessive pressure when instilling into catheter.

Drug Interactions

Avoid Concomitant Use There are no known interactions where it is recommended to avoid concomitant use.

Decreased Effect

The levels/effects of Alteplase may be decreased by: Aprotinin; Nitroglycerin

Increased Effect/Toxicity

Alteplase may increase the levels/effects of: Anticoagulants; Drotrecogin Alfa

The levels/effects of Alteplase may be increased by: Antiplatelet Agents; Herbs (Anticoagulant/Antiplatelet Properties); Nonsteroidal Anti-Inflammatory Agents; Salicylates

Nutritional/Ethanol Interactions Herb/Nutraceutical: Avoid cat's claw, dong quai, evening primrose, feverfew, red clover, horse chestnut, garlic, green tea, ginseng, ginkgo (all have additional antiplatelet activity).

Lab Interactions Altered results of coagulation and fibrinolytic agents

Adverse Reactions As with all drugs which may affect hemostasis, bleeding is the major adverse effect associated with alteplase. Hemorrhage may occur at virtually any site. Risk is dependent on multiple variables, including the dosage administered, concurrent use of multiple agents which alter hemostasis, and patient predisposition. Rapid lysis of coronary artery thrombi by thrombolytic agents may be associated with reperfusion-related atrial and/or ventricular arrhythmia. **Note:** Lowest rate of bleeding complications expected with dose used to restore catheter function.

1% to 10%:

- Cardiovascular: Hypotension
- Central nervous system: Fever
- Dermatologic: Bruising (1%)
- Gastrointestinal: GI hemorrhage (5%), nausea, vomiting
- Genitourinary: GU hemorrhage (4%)
- Hematologic: Bleeding (0.5% major, 7% minor: GUSTO trial)
- Local: Bleeding at catheter puncture site (15.3%, accelerated administration)

Additional cardiovascular events associated **with use in STEMI:** AV block, cardiogenic shock, heart failure, cardiac arrest, recurrent ischemia/infarction, myocardial rupture, electromechanical dissociation, pericardial effusion, pericarditis, mitral regurgitation, cardiac tamponade, thromboembolism, pulmonary edema, asystole, ventricular tachycardia, bradycardia, ruptured intracranial AV malformation, seizure, hemorrhagic bursitis, cholesterol crystal embolization

Additional events associated **with use in pulmonary embolism:** Pulmonary re-embolization, pulmonary edema, pleural effusion, thromboembolism

Additional events associated **with use in stroke:** Cerebral edema, cerebral herniation, seizure, new ischemic stroke

Pharmacodynamics/Kinetics

Duration of Action >50% present in plasma cleared ~5 minutes after infusion terminated, ~80% cleared within 10 minutes

Excretion Clearance: Rapidly from circulating plasma (550-650 mL/minute), primarily hepatic; >50% present in plasma is cleared within 5 minutes after the infusion is terminated, ~80% cleared within 10 minutes

Available Dosage Forms

Injection, powder for reconstitution:

Activase®: 50 mg, 100 mg

Cathflo® Activase®: 2 mg

Dosing

Adult & Geriatric

ST-elevation myocardial infarction (STEMI): I.V. (Activase®): Front loading dose (weight-based):

Patients >67 kg: Total dose: 100 mg over 1.5 hours; infuse 15 mg over 1-2 minutes. Infuse 50 mg over 30 minutes. Infuse remaining 35 mg of alteplase over the next hour. See **"Note."**

Patients ≤67 kg: Infuse 15 mg I.V. bolus over 1-2 minutes, then infuse 0.75 mg/kg (not to exceed 50 mg) over next 30 minutes, followed by 0.5 mg/kg over next 60 minutes (not to exceed 35 mg). See **"Note."**

Note: All patients should receive 162-325 mg of chewable nonenteric coated aspirin as soon as possible and then daily. Administer concurrently with heparin 60 units/kg bolus (maximum: 4000 units) followed by continuous infusion of 12 units/kg/hour (maximum: 1000 units/hour) and adjust to aPTT target of 50-70 seconds (or 1.5-2 times the upper limit of control).

Acute massive or submassive pulmonary embolism (PE): I.V. (Activase®): 100 mg over 2 hours. **Note:** Not recommended for submassive PE with minor RV dysfunction, minor myocardial necrosis, and no clinical worsening or low-risk PE (ie, normotensive, no RV dysfunction, normal biomarkers) (Jaff, 2011).

Acute ischemic stroke: I.V. (Activase®): Within 3 hours of the onset of symptom onset (labeled use) **or** within 3-4.5 hours of symptom onset (unlabeled use; del Zoppo, 2009; Hacke, 2008): **Note:** Initiation of anticoagulants (eg, heparin) or antiplatelet agents (eg, aspirin) within 24 hours after starting alteplase is not recommended; however, initiation of aspirin between 24-48 hours after stroke onset is recommended (Adams, 2007). Initiation of SubQ heparin (≤10,000 units) or equivalent doses of low molecular weight heparin for prevention of DVT during the first 24 hours of the 3-4.5 hour window trial did not increase incidence of intracerebral hemorrhage (Hacke, 2008).

Recommended total dose: 0.9 mg/kg (maximum total dose: 90 mg)

Patients ≤100 kg: Load with 0.09 mg/kg (10% of 0.9 mg/kg dose) as an I.V. bolus over 1 minute, followed by 0.81 mg/kg (90% of 0.9 mg/kg dose) as a continuous infusion over 60 minutes.

Patients >100 kg: Load with 9 mg (10% of 90 mg) as an I.V. bolus over 1 minute, followed by 81 mg (90% of 90 mg) as a continuous infusion over 60 minutes.

Central venous catheter clearance: Intracatheter (Cathflo® Activase® 1 mg/mL):

Patients <30 kg: 110% of the internal lumen volume of the catheter, not to exceed 2 mg/2 mL; retain in catheter for 0.5-2 hours; may instill a second dose if catheter remains occluded

Patients ≥30 kg: 2 mg (2 mL); retain in catheter for 0.5-2 hours; may instill a second dose if catheter remains occluded

Acute peripheral arterial occlusive disease (unlabeled use): Intra-arterial: 0.02-0.1 mg/kg/hour for up to 36 hours

Advisory Panel to the Society for Cardiovascular and Interventional Radiology on Thrombolytic Therapy recommendation: ≤2 mg/hour and subtherapeutic heparin (aPTT <1.5 times baseline)

Pediatric Central venous catheter clearance: Intracatheter: Patients <30 kg: 110% of the internal lumen volume of the catheter, not to exceed 2 mg/2 mL; retain in catheter for 0.5-2 hours; may instill a second dose if catheter remains occluded

Administration

I.V.

Activase®: ST-elevation MI: Accelerated infusion: Bolus dose may be prepared by one of three methods:

1) Removal of 15 mL reconstituted (1 mg/mL) solution from vial
2) Removal of 15 mL from a port on the infusion line after priming
3) Programming an infusion pump to deliver a 15 mL bolus at the initiation of infusion

Activase®: Acute ischemic stroke: Bolus dose (10% of total dose) may be prepared by one of three methods:

1) Removal of the appropriate volume from reconstituted solution (1 mg/mL)
2) Removal of the appropriate volume from a port on the infusion line after priming
3) Programming an infusion pump to deliver the appropriate volume at the initiation of infusion

Note: Remaining dose for STEMI, AIS, or total dose for acute pulmonary embolism may be administered as follows: Any quantity of drug not to be administered to the patient must be removed from vial(s) prior to administration of remaining dose.

50 mg vial: Either PVC bag or glass vial and infusion set

100 mg vial: Insert spike end of the infusion set through the same puncture site created by transfer device and infuse from vial

If further dilution is desired, may be diluted in equal volume of 0.9% sodium chloride or D_5W to yield a final concentration of 0.5 mg/mL.

Other Cathflo® Activase®: Intracatheter: Instill dose into occluded catheter. Do not force solution into catheter. After a 30-minute dwell time, assess catheter function by attempting to aspirate blood. If catheter is functional, aspirate 4-5 mL of blood in patients ≥10 kg or 3 mL in patients <10 kg to remove Cathflo® Activase® and residual clots. Gently irrigate the catheter with NS. If catheter remains nonfunctional, let Cathflo® Activase® dwell for another 90 minutes (total dwell time: 120 minutes) and reassess function. If catheter function is not restored, a second dose may be instilled.

Stability

Reconstitution

Activase®:

50 mg vial: Use accompanying diluent (50 mL sterile water for injection); do not shake. Final concentration: 1 mg/mL.

100 mg vial: Use transfer set with accompanying diluent (100 mL vial of sterile water for injection); no vacuum is present in 100 mg vial. Final concentration: 1 mg/mL.

Cathflo® Activase®: Add 2.2 mL SWFI to vial; do not shake. Final concentration: 1 mg/mL.

Storage

Activase®: The lyophilized product may be stored at room temperature (not to exceed 30°C/86°F), or under refrigeration. Once reconstituted, it should be used within 8 hours.

Cathflo® Activase®: Store lyophilized product under refrigeration. The following stability information has also been reported: Intact vials may be stored at room temperature for up to 4 months (Cohen, 2007). Once reconstituted, it should be used within 8 hours.

Monitoring and Teaching Issues

Laboratory Monitoring CBC, PTT

Physical Assessment Assess vital signs and ECG prior to, during, and after therapy. Arrhythmias may occur; treatment should be immediately available. Infusion site (and any other potential bleeding sites) should be monitored and patient assessed for hemorrhage during therapy and for 1 hour following therapy. Strict bedrest should be maintained and bleeding precautions should be instituted.

Patient Education This medication can only be administered by infusion; you will be monitored closely during and after treatment. You will have a tendency to bleed easily; use caution to prevent injury. Follow instructions for strict bedrest to reduce the risk of injury. If bleeding occurs, report immediately. Report unusual pain (acute headache, joint pain, chest pain); unusual bruising or bleeding; blood in urine, stool, or vomit; bleeding gums; or change in mentation.

Geriatric Considerations No specific changes in use in elderly patients are necessary.

Pregnancy Considerations Teratogenic effects were not observed in animal studies. There are no adequate and well-controlled studies in pregnant women. The risk of bleeding may be increased in pregnant women. Use during pregnancy is limited; administer to pregnant women only if the potential benefits justify the risk to the fetus.

◆ **Alteplase, Recombinant** *see* Alteplase *on page 86*

◆ **Alteplase, Tissue Plasminogen Activator, Recombinant** *see* Alteplase *on page 86*

◆ **Altoprev®** *see* Lovastatin *on page 1138*

Altretamine (al TRET a meen)

U.S. Brand Names Hexalen®

Index Terms Hexamethylmelamine; HEXM; HMM; HXM; NSC-13875

Generic Availability (U.S.) No

Pharmacologic Category Antineoplastic Agent, Miscellaneous

Medication Safety Issues

High alert medication: The Institute for Safe Medication Practices (ISMP) includes this medication among its list of drugs which have a heightened risk of causing significant patient harm when used in error.

International issues:

Hexalen®: Brand name for hexetidine in Greece

Pregnancy Risk Factor D

Lactation Excretion in breast milk unknown/not recommended

Use Palliative treatment of persistent or recurrent ovarian cancer

Available Dosage Forms

Gelcap, oral:

Hexalen®: 50 mg

Dosing

Adult & Geriatric Refer to individual protocols.

Ovarian cancer: Oral: 260 mg/m²/day in 4 divided doses for 14 or 21 days of a 28-day cycle

Alternatively (unlabeled use): 4-12 mg/kg/day in 3-4 divided doses for 21-90 days

Alternatively (unlabeled use): 240-320 mg/m²/day in 3-4 divided doses for 21 days, repeated every 6 weeks

Alternatively (unlabeled use): 150 mg/m²/day in 3-4 divided doses for 14 days of a 28-day cycle

Adjustment for Toxicity Temporarily withhold for 14 days or longer, and resume dose at 200 mg/m²/day for any of the following:

Platelet count <75,000/mm³

White blood cell count <2000/mm³ or granulocyte count <1000/mm³

Progressive neurotoxicity

Gastrointestinal intolerance not responsive to antiemetic regimens

Administration

Oral Administer total daily dose as 3-4 divided doses after meals and at bedtime.

Monitoring and Teaching Issues

Laboratory Monitoring CBC with differential, liver function tests

Physical Assessment Use with caution in patients previously treated with other myelosuppressive drugs, with pre-existing neurotoxicity, or with renal or hepatic dysfunction. Monitor for neuropathy, gastrointestinal upset, and anemia.

Patient Education Take preferably after meals. Avoid alcohol. May cause nausea or vomiting. You will be more susceptible to infection. Report any numbness, tingling, or pain in extremities; unrelieved nausea or vomiting; tremors; yellowing of skin or eyes; fever; chills; easy bruising or unusual bleeding; extreme weakness; or increased fatigue.

◆ **Aluminum Sucrose Sulfate, Basic** *see* Sucralfate *on page 1684*

◆ **Alvesco®** *see* Ciclesonide (Oral Inhalation) *on page 366*

Alvimopan (al VI moe pan)

U.S. Brand Names Entereg®

Index Terms ADL-2698; LY246736

Generic Availability (U.S.) No

Pharmacologic Category Gastrointestinal Agent, Miscellaneous; Opioid Antagonist, Peripherally-Acting

Medication Safety Issues

Sound-alike/look-alike issues:

Alvimopan may be confused with almotriptan

Prescribing and Access Restrictions As a requirement of the REMS program, access to this medication is restricted. Only hospitals enrolled in the ENTEREG Access Support and Education (E.A.S.E.™) Program may administer this medication. Hospital staff must be educated on the need to limit to short-term (no more than 15 doses) and inpatient use. Hospitals may contact the E.A.S.E.™ program at 1-866-423-6567 (1-866-4ADOLOR).

Pregnancy Risk Factor B

Lactation Excretion in breast milk unknown/use caution

Use Accelerate the time to upper and lower GI recovery following partial large or small bowel resection surgery with primary anastomosis

Mechanism of Action/Effect An opioid receptor antagonist which blocks opioid binding at the mu receptor; alvimopan has restricted ability to cross the blood-brain barrier at therapeutic doses. It selectively and competitively binds to the GI tract mu opioid receptors and antagonizes the peripheral effects of opioids on gastrointestinal motility and secretion. Does not affect opioid analgesic effects or induce opioid withdrawal symptoms.

Contraindications Patients who have taken therapeutic doses of opioids for more than 7 consecutive days immediately prior to alvimopan

Warnings/Precautions [U.S. Boxed Warning]: For short-term (≤15 doses) hospital use only. Only hospitals that have registered through the ENTEREG Access Support and Education (E.A.S.E.™) Program and met all requirements may use. It will not be dispensed to patients who have been discharged from the hospital. Use not recommended in patients with complete bowel obstruction. Use with caution in patients with hepatic or renal impairment; use not recommended in patients with severe hepatic impairment or ESRD. Use with caution is patients recently exposed to opioids; may be more sensitive to gastrointestinal adverse effects (eg, abdominal pain, diarrhea, nausea and vomiting). Contraindicated in patients who have received therapeutic opioids for >7 consecutive days immediately prior to use. A trend towards an increased incidence of MI was observed in alvimopan (low dose) treated patients compared to placebo in a 12-month study in patients treated with opioids for chronic pain. MI was generally observed more frequently in the initial 1-4 months of treatment. Other studies have not observed this trend and a causal relationship has not been found. Patients of Japanese descent should be monitored closely for gastrointestinal side effects (eg, abdominal pain, cramping, diarrhea) due to possibility of greater drug exposure; discontinue use if side effects occur.

Drug Interactions

Metabolism/Transport Effects Substrate of P-glycoprotein

Avoid Concomitant Use There are no known interactions where it is recommended to avoid concomitant use.

Decreased Effect There are no known significant interactions involving a decrease in effect.

Increased Effect/Toxicity

The levels/effects of Alvimopan may be increased by: Analgesics (Opioid)

Nutritional/Ethanol Interactions Food: When administered with a high-fat meal, extent and rate of absorption may be reduced (C_{max} and AUC decreased by ~38% and 21%, respectively).

Adverse Reactions 1% to 10%: **Note:** Incidence reported limited to bowel resection patients only.

Endocrine & metabolic: Hypokalemia (10%)

Gastrointestinal: Dyspepsia (7%)

Genitourinary: Urinary retention (3%)
Hematologic: Anemia (5%)
Neuromuscular & skeletal: Back pain (3%)

Pharmacodynamics/Kinetics

Bioavailability ~6% (range: 1% to 19%)

Time to Peak Plasma: Parent drug: ~2 hours; Metabolite: 36 hours

Protein Binding Parent drug: 80%; metabolite: 94% (both primarily to albumin)

Half-Life Elimination 10-17 hours

Metabolism Hydrolyzed to an amide hydrolysis compound (active metabolite) by gut microflora; further metabolism of active metabolite to glucuronide conjugates and other minor metabolites

Excretion Urine (~35% as unchanged drug and metabolites); feces (via biliary excretion)

Available Dosage Forms

Capsule, oral:
Entereg®: 12 mg

Dosing

Adult & Geriatric Note: For hospital use only.

Management of postoperative ileus: Oral:
Initial: 12 mg administered 30 minutes to 5 hours prior to surgery
Maintenance: 12 mg twice daily beginning the day after surgery for a maximum of 7 days or until discharged from hospital (maximum total treatment: 15 doses)

Renal Impairment
Mild-to-severe impairment: No adjustment needed; use caution.
ESRD: Use not recommended.

Hepatic Impairment
Mild-to-moderate impairment (Child-Pugh class A and B): No adjustment needed; use caution.
Severe impairment (Child-Pugh class C): Use not recommended.

Administration

Oral Patient must be hospitalized. Initial dose should be administered 30 minutes to 5 hours prior to surgery. May be administered with or without food.

Stability

Storage Store at 25°C (77°F); excursions permitted to 15°C to 30°C (59°F to 86°F).

Monitoring and Teaching Issues

Physical Assessment For restricted in-hospital use only for patients with an ileus.

Patient Education This medication is used to improve bowel function after surgery. Report any gastrointestinal upset, difficulty passing urine, or unusual back pain.

Dietary Considerations Take with or without food; high-fat meals may decrease the rate and extent of absorption

Pregnancy Considerations Animal studies have not shown teratogenic effects to the fetus. However, there are no adequate and well-controlled studies in pregnant women; use during pregnancy only if clearly needed.

Amantadine (a MAN ta deen)

Index Terms Adamantanamine Hydrochloride; Amantadine Hydrochloride; Symmetrel

Generic Availability (U.S.) Yes

Pharmacologic Category Anti-Parkinson's Agent, Dopamine Agonist; Antiviral Agent; Antiviral Agent, Adamantane

Medication Safety Issues

Sound-alike/look-alike issues:
Amantadine may be confused with ranitidine, rimantadine
Symmetrel may be confused with Synthroid®

Pregnancy Risk Factor C

Lactation Enters breast milk/not recommended

Use Prophylaxis and treatment of influenza A viral infection (per manufacturer labeling; also refer to current ACIP guidelines for recommendations during current flu season); treatment of parkinsonism; treatment of drug-induced extrapyramidal symptoms

Available Dosage Forms

Capsule, oral: 100 mg
Capsule, softgel, oral: 100 mg
Solution, oral: 50 mg/5 mL (473 mL)
Syrup, oral: 50 mg/5 mL (10 mL, 473 mL, 480 mL)
Tablet, oral: 100 mg

Dosing

Adult

Influenza A treatment/prophylaxis: Note: Due to issues of resistance, amantadine is no longer recommended for the treatment or prophylaxis of influenza A. Please refer to the current ACIP recommendations. The following is based on the manufacturer's labeling:

Influenza A treatment: Oral: 200 mg once daily **or** 100 mg twice daily (may be preferred to reduce CNS effects); **Note:** Initiate within 24-48 hours after onset of symptoms; continue for 24-48 hours after symptom resolution (duration of therapy is generally 3-5 days).

Influenza A prophylaxis: Oral: 200 mg once daily **or** 100 mg twice daily (may be preferred to reduce CNS effects). **Note:** Continue prophylaxis throughout the peak influenza activity in the community or throughout the entire influenza season in patients who cannot be vaccinated. Development of immunity following vaccination takes ~2 weeks; amantadine therapy should be considered for high-risk patients from the time of vaccination until immunity has developed.

Drug-induced extrapyramidal symptoms: Oral: 100 mg twice daily; may increase to 300 mg/day in divided doses, if needed

Parkinson's disease: Oral: Usual dose: 100 mg twice daily as monotherapy; may increase to 400 mg/day in divided doses, if needed, with close monitoring. **Note:** Patients with a serious concomitant illness or those receiving high doses of other anti-parkinson drugs should be started at 100 mg/day; may increase to 100 mg twice daily, if needed, after one to several weeks.

Geriatric Patients ≥65 years: Adjust dose based on renal function; some patients tolerate the drug better when it is given in 2 divided daily doses (to avoid adverse neurologic reactions). Influenza A treatment/prophylaxis: 100 mg once daily

Pediatric

Influenza A treatment/prophylaxis: Oral: **Note:** Due to issues of resistance, amantadine is no longer recommended for the treatment or prophylaxis of influenza A. Please refer to the current ACIP recommendations.

Influenza A treatment:

1-9 years: 5 mg/kg/day in 2 divided doses (manufacturer's range: 4.4-8.8 mg/kg/day); maximum dose: 150 mg/day

≥10 years and <40 kg: 5 mg/kg/day in 2 divided doses (CDC, 2011)

≥10 years and ≥40 kg: 100 mg twice daily (CDC, 2011)

Note: Initiate within 24-48 hours after onset of symptoms; continue for 24-48 hours after symptom resolution (duration of therapy is generally 3-5 days)

Influenza A prophylaxis: Refer to "Influenza A treatment" dosing. **Note:** Continue prophylaxis throughout the peak influenza activity in the community or throughout the entire influenza season in patients who cannot be vaccinated. Development of immunity following vaccination takes ~2 weeks; amantadine therapy should be considered for high-risk patients from the time of vaccination until immunity has developed. For children <9 years receiving influenza vaccine for the first time, amantadine prophylaxis should continue for 6 weeks (4 weeks after the first dose and 2 weeks after the second dose).

Renal Impairment

Cl_{cr} 30-50 mL/minute: Administer 200 mg on day 1, then 100 mg/day

Cl_{cr} 15-29 mL/minute: Administer 200 mg on day 1, then 100 mg on alternate days

Cl_{cr} <15 mL/minute: Administer 200 mg every 7 days

Hemodialysis: Administer 200 mg every 7 days

Peritoneal dialysis: No supplemental dose is needed

Continuous arteriovenous or venous-venous hemofiltration: No supplemental dose is needed

Monitoring and Teaching Issues

Laboratory Monitoring Renal function

Physical Assessment Recommendations for antiviral susceptibility and effectiveness may change. Validate with the CDC recommendations for use prior to prescribing. Monitor renal function at beginning of therapy and periodically throughout. Assess blood pressure; monitor for signs of fluid retention. When treating Parkinson's disease, taper slowly when discontinuing.

Patient Education Maintain adequate hydration, unless instructed to restrict fluid intake, and void before taking medication. Take last dose of day in the afternoon to reduce incidence of insomnia. May cause dizziness or lightheadedness. Avoid alcohol. You may experience decreased mental alertness or coordination, loss of impulse control (possibly manifested as pathological gambling, libido increases, and/or binge eating), nausea, or dry mouth. Report unusual swelling of extremities, respiratory difficulty or shortness of breath, change in vision, change in gait or increased tremors, suicide ideation, changes in the appearance of skin moles or other unusual skin changes, or changes in mentation (eg, depression, anxiety, irritability, hallucination, slurred speech).

◆ **Amantadine Hydrochloride** *see* Amantadine *on page 91*

◆ **Amaryl®** *see* Glimepiride *on page 870*

Ambenonium (am be NOE nee um)

U.S. Brand Names Mytelase®

Index Terms Ambenonium Chloride

Generic Availability (U.S.) No

Pharmacologic Category Cholinergic Agonist

Pregnancy Risk Factor C

Lactation Excretion in breast milk unknown/not recommended

Use Treatment of myasthenia gravis

Mechanism of Action/Effect Action increases acetylcholine concentration at transmission sites in parasympathetic neurons and skeletal muscles by inhibiting acetylcholinesterase

Contraindications Routine administration of atropine or other belladonna alkaloids with ambenonium is contraindicated because they may suppress the muscarinic symptoms of excessive gastrointestinal stimulation, leaving only the more serious symptoms of muscle fasciculations and paralysis as signs of overdosage; should not be administered to patients receiving mecamylamine

Warnings/Precautions Prolonged action after cholinergics; drug should be discontinued until the patient is stabilized. Use with caution in patients with asthma, epilepsy, bradycardia, hyperthyroidism, Parkinson's disease, urinary obstruction, or peptic ulcer. Differentiation of cholinergic/myasthenia crisis is critical; use edrophonium and clinical judgment. Anticholinergic insensitivity may develop for brief or prolonged periods. Reduce or withhold dosages until the patient becomes sensitive again. May require respiratory support. Safety and efficacy have not been established in children.

Drug Interactions

Avoid Concomitant Use There are no known interactions where it is recommended to avoid concomitant use.

Decreased Effect There are no known significant interactions involving a decrease in effect.

Increased Effect/Toxicity

The levels/effects of Ambenonium may be increased by: Acetylcholinesterase Inhibitors

Lab Interactions Increased aminotransferase [ALT/AST] (S), amylase (S)

Adverse Reactions Frequency not defined.

Cardiovascular: Arrhythmias (especially bradycardia), hypotension, carbon monoxide decreased, tachycardia, AV block, nodal rhythm, ECG changes (nonspecific), cardiac arrest, syncope, flushing

Central nervous system: Convulsions, dysarthria, dysphonia, dizziness, loss of consciousness, drowsiness, headache

Dermatologic: Skin rash, thrombophlebitis (I.V.), urticaria

Gastrointestinal: Hyperperistalsis, nausea, vomiting, salivation, diarrhea, stomach cramps, dysphagia, flatulence

Genitourinary: Urinary urgency

Neuromuscular & skeletal: Weakness, fasciculations, muscle cramps, spasms, arthralgia

Ocular: Small pupils, lacrimation

Respiratory: Bronchial secretions increased, laryngospasm, bronchiolar constriction, respiratory muscle paralysis, dyspnea, respiratory depression, respiratory arrest, bronchospasm

Miscellaneous: Diaphoresis increased, anaphylaxis, allergic reactions

Available Dosage Forms

Caplet, oral:

Mytelase®: 10 mg

Dosing

Adult & Geriatric Myasthenia gravis: Oral: 5-25 mg 3-4 times/day

Monitoring and Teaching Issues

Physical Assessment Assess bladder and sphincter adequacy prior to administering medication. Monitor for cholinergic crisis.

Patient Education This drug will not cure myasthenia gravis, but it may reduce the symptoms. Maintain adequate hydration, unless instructed to restrict fluid intake. May cause dizziness, drowsiness, postural hypotension, vomiting, loss of appetite, or diarrhea. Report persistent abdominal discomfort; significantly increased salivation, sweating, tearing, or urination; flushed skin; chest pain or palpitations; acute headache; unresolved diarrhea; excessive fatigue, insomnia, dizziness, or depression; increased muscle, joint, or body pain; vision changes or blurred vision; or shortness of breath or wheezing.

◆ **Ambenonium Chloride** *see* Ambenonium *on page 92*

◆ **Ambien®** *see* Zolpidem *on page 1905*

◆ **Ambien CR®** *see* Zolpidem *on page 1905*

◆ **AmBisome®** *see* Amphotericin B (Liposomal) *on page 121*

Ambrisentan (am bri SEN tan)

U.S. Brand Names Letairis®

Index Terms BSF208075

Generic Availability (U.S.) No

Pharmacologic Category Endothelin Antagonist; Vasodilator

Medication Guide Available Yes

Prescribing and Access Restrictions As a requirement of the REMS program, access to this medication is restricted. Ambrisentan (Letairis®) is only available through Letairis Education and Access Program (LEAP). Only prescribers and pharmacies registered with LEAP may prescribe and dispense ambrisentan. Further information may be obtained from the manufacturer, Gilead Sciences, Inc (1-866-664-5327).

Pregnancy Risk Factor X

Lactation Excretion in breast milk unknown/not recommended

Use Treatment of pulmonary artery hypertension (PAH) World Health Organization (WHO) Group I to improve exercise ability and decrease the rate of clinical deterioration

Mechanism of Action/Effect Decreases symptoms of pulmonary artery hypertension and slows progression of the disease by causing vasodilation of the pulmonary arteries.

Contraindications Pregnancy

Canadian labeling: Additional contraindications (not in U.S. labeling): Hypersensitivity to ambrisentan or any component of the formulation

Warnings/Precautions [U.S. Boxed Warning]: Use in pregnancy is contraindicated; may cause birth defects. Exclude pregnancy prior to initiation of therapy and monthly thereafter. Two reliable methods of contraception must be used in women of childbearing potential during therapy and for one month after stopping treatment except in patients with tubal ligation or an implanted IUD (Copper T 380A or LNg 20). No other contraceptive measures are required for these patients. A missed menses should be reported to healthcare provider and prompt immediate pregnancy testing. Women should also be educated on the appropriate use of emergency contraception if failure of contraceptive is known or suspected or in the event of unprotected sex.

[U.S. Boxed Warning]: Because of the high likelihood of teratogenic effects, ambrisentan is only available through the LEAP restricted distribution program. Patients, prescribers, and pharmacies must be registered with and meet conditions of LEAP. Call 1-866-664-5327 for more information.

Use caution in patients with low hemoglobin levels. May cause decreases in hemoglobin and hematocrit (monitoring of hemoglobin is recommended. Use not recommended in patients with clinically significant anemia. Development of peripheral edema due to treatment and/or disease state (pulmonary arterial hypertension) may occur; a higher incidence is seen in elderly patients. Sperm count may be reduced in men during treatment (as observed with bosentan). No changes in sperm function or hormone levels have been noted. Fertility issues may require discussion with patient. Increases in serum liver aminotransferases have been reported during postmarketing use; however, in the majority of the cases, alternative causes of hepatotoxicity could be identified. Perform liver enzyme testing only when clinically indicated. Discontinue therapy if signs/symptoms of hepatic injury appear, if serum liver aminotransferases >5 times ULN are observed, or if aminotransferases are increased in the presence of bilirubin >2 times ULN. Hepatotoxicity has been reported with other endothelin receptor antagonists (eg, bosentan); however, ambrisentan may be tried in patients that have experienced asymptomatic increases in liver enzymes caused by another endothelin receptor antagonist after the liver enzymes have returned to normal. Use caution in patients with mild hepatic impairment; use not recommended in patients with moderate-to-severe impairment. There have also been post-marketing reports of fluid retention requiring treatment (eg, diuretics, fluid management, hospitalization). Further evaluation may be necessary to determine cause and appropriate treatment or discontinuation of therapy. Discontinue in any patient with pulmonary edema suggestive of pulmonary veno-occlusive disease (PVOD).

Drug Interactions

Metabolism/Transport Effects Substrate of CYP3A4 (minor), 2C19 (minor); UGT1A3, 1A9, 2B7; P-glycoprotein

Avoid Concomitant Use There are no known interactions where it is recommended to avoid concomitant use.

Decreased Effect There are no known significant interactions involving a decrease in effect.

Increased Effect/Toxicity

The levels/effects of Ambrisentan may be increased by: Conivaptan; CycloSPORINE; CycloSPORINE (Systemic)

Nutritional/Ethanol Interactions

Food: Grapefruit/grapefruit juice may increase levels/effects of ambrisentan.

Herb/Nutraceutical: Avoid St John's wort (concurrent use may decrease levels/effects of ambrisentan).

Adverse Reactions

>10%:

Cardiovascular: Peripheral edema (17%)

Central nervous system: Headache (15%)

1% to 10%:

Cardiovascular: Palpitation (5%), flushing (4%)

Gastrointestinal: Constipation (4%), abdominal pain (3%)

Hematologic: Hemoglobin decreased (7% to 10%)

Respiratory: Nasal congestion (6%), dyspnea (4%), nasopharyngitis (3%), sinusitis (3%)

Pharmacodynamics/Kinetics

Time to Peak ~2 hours

Protein Binding 99%

Half-Life Elimination ~9 hours

Metabolism Hepatic via CYP3A4, CYP2C19, and uridine 5'-diphosphate glucuronosyltransferases (UGTs) 1A9S, 2B7S, and 1A3S; *in vitro* studies also suggest it is a substrate of organic anion transport protein (OATP) and P-glycoprotein (P-gp)

Excretion Primarily nonrenal

Available Dosage Forms

Tablet, oral:

Letairis®: 5 mg, 10 mg

Dosing

Adult & Geriatric

Pulmonary arterial hypertension: Oral: Initial: 5 mg once daily; if tolerated, may increase to maximum 10 mg once daily

Coadministration with cyclosporine: Oral: Ambrisentan dose should not exceed 5 mg/day

Renal Impairment

Mild-to-moderate renal impairment: No dosage adjustment required

Severe renal impairment: There is no data available for use in severe renal impairment.

Hepatic Impairment

Mild hepatic impairment: There is no data available for use in mild hepatic impairment; exposure may be increased.

Moderate-to-severe hepatic impairment: Use not recommended.

Administration

Oral Swallow tablet whole. Do not split, crush, or chew tablets. May be administered with or without food.

Stability

Storage Store in original packaging at 25°C (77°F); excursions permitted to 15°C to 30°C (59°F to 86°F).

Monitoring and Teaching Issues

Laboratory Monitoring Liver enzyme testing when clinically appropriate. A woman of childbearing potential must have a negative pregnancy test prior to the initiation of therapy and monthly thereafter. Hemoglobin and hematocrit should be measured at baseline, at 1 month, and periodically thereafter (generally stabilizes after the first few weeks of treatment).

Physical Assessment Assess for symptoms of hepatic problems and fluid retention.

Patient Education Pregnancy must be excluded prior to initiation and monthly thereafter. Two forms of contraception must be used during therapy (except in patients with tubal ligation or an implanted IUD). Avoid grapefruit or grapefruit juice. You may experience headache, nasal congestion, fatigue, or constipation. Report signs of fluid retention (unusual weight gain, swelling of the extremities), shortness of breath, unusual bleeding or bruising, change in color of urine or stool, loss of appetite, abdominal pain, yellowing of skin or eyes, or unusual fatigue.

Dietary Considerations May be taken with or without food. Avoid grapefruit and grapefruit juice.

Pregnancy Considerations [U.S. Boxed Warning]: Use in pregnancy is contraindicated. Based on animal studies, ambrisentan is likely to produce major birth defects if used by pregnant women. Pregnancy must be excluded prior to initiation of therapy and follow-up pregnancy tests should be obtained monthly. Two reliable methods of contraception must be used throughout treatment and for one month after stopping treatment unless the patient has undergone a tubal ligation or the insertion of an intrauterine device (Copper T 380A or LNg 20). No other contraceptive measures are required for these patients.

- **AMD3100** *see* Plerixafor *on page 1468*
- **Amerge®** *see* Naratriptan *on page 1291*
- **A-Methapred** *see* MethylPREDNISolone *on page 1208*
- **A-Methapred®** *see* MethylPREDNISolone *on page 1208*
- **Amethopterin** *see* Methotrexate *on page 1193*
- **Amevive®** *see* Alefacept *on page 65*
- **Amfepramone** *see* Diethylpropion *on page 527*
- **AMG 073** *see* Cinacalcet *on page 373*
- **AMG-162** *see* Denosumab *on page 486*

Amikacin (am i KAY sin)

Index Terms Amikacin Sulfate

Generic Availability (U.S.) Yes

Pharmacologic Category Antibiotic, Aminoglycoside

Medication Safety Issues

Sound-alike/look-alike issues:

Amikacin may be confused with Amicar®, anakinra

Amikin® may be confused with Amicar®, Kineret®

Pregnancy Risk Factor D

Lactation Enters breast milk/not recommended

Use Treatment of serious infections (bone infections, respiratory tract infections, endocarditis, and septicemia) due to organisms resistant to gentamicin and tobramycin, including *Pseudomonas*, *Proteus*, *Serratia*, and other gram-negative bacilli; documented infection of mycobacterial organisms susceptible to amikacin

Unlabeled/Investigational Use Bacterial endophthalmitis

Available Dosage Forms

Injection, solution: 50 mg/mL (2 mL); 250 mg/mL (2 mL, 4 mL)

Dosing

Adult & Geriatric Individualization is critical because of the low therapeutic index

Note: Use of ideal body weight (IBW) for determining the mg/kg/dose appears to be more accurate than dosing on the basis of total body weight (TBW)

In morbid obesity, dosage requirement may best be estimated using a dosing weight of IBW + 0.4 (TBW - IBW)

Initial and periodic peak and trough plasma drug levels should be determined, particularly in critically-ill patients with serious infections or in disease states known to significantly alter aminoglycoside pharmacokinetics (eg, cystic fibrosis, burns, or major surgery). Manufacturer recommends a maximum daily dose of 15 mg/kg/day (or 1.5 g/day in heavier patients). Higher doses may be warranted based on therapeutic drug monitoring or susceptibility information.

Usual dosage range:

I.M., I.V.: 5-7.5 mg/kg/dose every 8 hours; **Note:** Some clinicians suggest a daily dose of 15-20 mg/kg for all patients with normal renal function. This dose is at least as efficacious with similar, if not less, toxicity than conventional dosing.

Intrathecal/intraventricular (unlabeled route): Meningitis (susceptible gram-negative organisms): 5-50 mg/day

Indication-specific dosing:

Endophthalmitis, bacterial (unlabeled use): Intravitreal: 0.4 mg/0.1 mL NS in combination with vancomycin

Hospital-acquired pneumonia (HAP): I.V.: 20 mg/kg/day with antipseudomonal beta-lactam or carbapenem (American Thoracic Society/ATS guidelines)

Meningitis (susceptible gram-negative organisms):

I.V.: 5 mg/kg every 8 hours (administered with another bacteriocidal drug)

Intrathecal/intraventricular (unlabeled route): Usual dose: 30 mg/day (IDSA, 2004); Range: 5-50 mg/day (with concurrent systemic antimicrobial therapy) (Gilbert, 1986; Guardado, 2008; IDSA, 2004; Kasiakou, 2005)

Mycobacterium fortuitum, M. chelonae, or M. abscessus: I.V.: 10-15 mg/kg daily for at least 2 weeks with high dose cefoxitin

Pediatric Usual dosage range: Infants and Children: I.M., I.V.: 5-7.5 mg/kg/dose every 8 hours

Note: Individualization is critical because of the low therapeutic index

Use of ideal body weight (IBW) for determining the mg/kg/dose appears to be more accurate than dosing on the basis of total body weight (TBW)

In morbid obesity, dosage requirement may best be estimated using a dosing weight of IBW + 0.4 (TBW - IBW)

Initial and periodic peak and trough plasma drug levels should be determined, particularly in critically-ill patients with serious infections or in disease states known to significantly alter aminoglycoside pharmacokinetics (eg, cystic fibrosis, burns, or major surgery). Manufacturer recommends a maximum daily dose of 15 mg/kg/day (or 1.5 g/day in heavier patients). Higher doses may be warranted based on therapeutic drug monitoring or susceptibility information.

Renal Impairment Some patients may require larger or more frequent doses if serum levels document the need (ie, cystic fibrosis or febrile granulocytopenic patients).

Cl_{cr} ≥60 mL/minute: Administer every 8 hours

Cl_{cr} 40-60 mL/minute: Administer every 12 hours

Cl_{cr} 20-40 mL/minute: Administer every 24 hours

Cl_{cr} <20 mL/minute: Loading dose, then monitor levels

Dialyzable (50% to 100%)

Administer dose postdialysis or administer $^2/_3$ normal dose as a supplemental dose postdialysis and follow levels.

Peritoneal dialysis effects: Dose as for Cl_{cr} <20 mL/minute: Follow levels.

Continuous arteriovenous or venovenous hemodiafiltration effects: Dose as for Cl_{cr} 10-40 mL/minute: Follow levels.

Administration

I.M. Administer I.M. injection in large muscle mass. Administer around-the-clock to promote less variation in peak and trough serum levels. Do not mix with other drugs, administer separately.

I.V. Infuse over 30-60 minutes.

Some penicillins (eg, carbenicillin, ticarcillin, and piperacillin) have been shown to inactivate *in vitro*. This has been observed to a greater extent with tobramycin and gentamicin, while amikacin has shown greater stability against inactivation. Concurrent use of these agents may pose a risk of reduced antibacterial efficacy *in vivo*, particularly in the setting of profound renal impairment. However, definitive clinical evidence is lacking. If combination penicillin/aminoglycoside therapy is desired in a patient with renal dysfunction, separation of doses (if feasible), and routine monitoring of aminoglycoside levels, CBC, and clinical response should be considered.

Other Intrathecal/Intraventricular (unlabeled route): Reserved solely for meningitis due to susceptible gram-negative organisms. Available formulation contains sodium metabisulfite. If possible, consider alternative therapy with gentamicin or tobramycin as both of theses agents are available as preservative-free formulations.

Monitoring and Teaching Issues

Laboratory Monitoring Perform culture and sensitivity testing prior to initiating therapy. Urinalysis, BUN, serum creatinine, appropriately timed peak and trough concentrations. Initial and periodic peak and trough plasma drug levels should be determined, particularly in critically-ill patients with serious infections or in disease states known to significantly alter aminoglycoside pharmacokinetics (eg, cystic fibrosis, burns, or major surgery). Aminoglycoside levels measured from blood taken from Silastic® central catheters can sometimes give falsely high readings (draw levels from alternate lumen or peripheral stick, if possible). Some penicillin derivatives may accelerate the degradation of aminoglycosides.

Physical Assessment Assess allergy history prior to beginning therapy. Monitor for ototoxicity, nephrotoxicity, and neurotoxicity. Hearing and renal status should be assessed before, during, and after therapy.

Patient Education This drug can only be administered by I.V. or I.M. injection. It is important to maintain adequate hydration, unless instructed to restrict fluid intake. Report immediately any change in hearing acuity, ringing or roaring in ears, alteration in balance, vertigo, feeling of fullness in head; pain, tingling, or numbness of any body part; or change in urinary pattern or decrease in urine. Report signs of opportunistic infection (eg, white plaques in mouth, vaginal discharge, unhealed sores, sore throat, unusual fever, chills); persistent diarrhea; or pain, redness, or swelling at injection site.

Related Information

Antimicrobial Drugs of Choice *on page* 2008

Peak and Trough Guidelines *on page* 1958

◆ **Amikacin Sulfate** *see* Amikacin *on page* 95

AMILoride (a MIL oh ride)

Index Terms Amiloride Hydrochloride

Generic Availability (U.S.) Yes

Pharmacologic Category Diuretic, Potassium-Sparing

Medication Safety Issues

Sound-alike/look-alike issues:

AMILoride may be confused with amiodarone, amLODIPine, amrinone

Pregnancy Risk Factor B

Lactation Excretion in breast milk unknown/not recommended

Use Counteracts potassium loss induced by other diuretics in the treatment of hypertension or edematous conditions including CHF, hepatic cirrhosis, and hypoaldosteronism; usually used in conjunction with more potent diuretics such as thiazides or loop diuretics

Unlabeled/Investigational Use Investigational: Cystic fibrosis; reduction of lithium-induced polyuria; pediatric hypertension

Mechanism of Action/Effect Inhibits sodium reabsorption in the distal tubule, cortical collecting tubule, and collecting duct subsequently reducing both potassium and hydrogen excretion resulting in weak natriuretic, diuretic, and antihypertensive activity; increases sodium loss; increases potassium retention; decreases calcium excretion; decreases magnesium loss

Contraindications Hypersensitivity to amiloride or any component of the formulation; presence of elevated serum potassium levels (>5.5 mEq/L); if patient is receiving other potassium-conserving agents (eg, spironolactone, triamterene) or potassium supplementation (medicine, potassium-containing salt substitutes, potassium-rich diet); anuria; acute or chronic renal insufficiency; evidence of diabetic nephropathy. Patients with evidence of renal impairment or diabetes mellitus should not receive this medicine without close, frequent monitoring of serum electrolytes and renal function.

Warnings/Precautions [U.S. Boxed Warning]: Hyperkalemia can occur; patients at risk include those with renal impairment, diabetes, the elderly, and the severely ill. Serum potassium levels must be monitored at frequent intervals especially when dosages are changed or with any illness that may cause renal dysfunction. Excess amounts can lead to profound diuresis with fluid and electrolyte loss; close medical supervision and dose evaluation are required. Watch for and correct electrolyte disturbances; adjust dose to avoid dehydration. In cirrhosis, avoid electrolyte and acid/base imbalances that might lead to hepatic encephalopathy. Use with extreme caution in patients with diabetes mellitus; monitor closely. Discontinue amiloride 3 days prior to glucose tolerance testing. Use with caution in patients who are at risk for metabolic or respiratory acidosis (eg, cardiopulmonary disease, uncontrolled diabetes). Safety and efficacy have not been established in children.

Drug Interactions

Avoid Concomitant Use

Avoid concomitant use of AMILoride with any of the following: Tacrolimus

Decreased Effect

AMILoride may decrease the levels/effects of: Cardiac Glycosides; QuiNIDine

The levels/effects of AMILoride may be decreased by: Herbs (Hypertensive Properties); Methylphenidate; Nonsteroidal Anti-Inflammatory Agents; Yohimbine

Increased Effect/Toxicity

AMILoride may increase the levels/effects of: ACE Inhibitors; Amifostine; Ammonium Chloride; Antihypertensives; Cardiac Glycosides; Hypotensive Agents; RiTUXimab; Tacrolimus

The levels/effects of AMILoride may be increased by: Angiotensin II Receptor Blockers; Diazoxide; Drospirenone; Eplerenone; Herbs (Hypotensive Properties); MAO Inhibitors; Nonsteroidal Anti-Inflammatory Agents; Pentoxifylline; Phosphodiesterase 5 Inhibitors; Potassium Salts; Prostacyclin Analogues; Tolvaptan

Nutritional/Ethanol Interactions Food: Hyperkalemia may result if amiloride is taken with potassium-containing foods.

Lab Interactions Increased potassium (S)

Adverse Reactions 1% to 10%:

Central nervous system: Headache, fatigue, dizziness

Endocrine & metabolic: Hyperkalemia (up to 10%; risk reduced in patients receiving kaliuretic diuretics), hyperchloremic metabolic acidosis, dehydration, hyponatremia, gynecomastia

Gastrointestinal: Nausea, diarrhea, vomiting, abdominal pain, gas pain, appetite changes, constipation

Genitourinary: Impotence

Neuromuscular & skeletal: Muscle cramps, weakness

Respiratory: Cough, dyspnea

Pharmacodynamics/Kinetics

Onset of Action 2 hours

Duration of Action 24 hours

Absorption ~15% to 25%

Time to Peak Serum: 6-10 hours

Protein Binding 23%

Half-Life Elimination Normal renal function: 6-9 hours; End-stage renal disease: 8-144 hours

Metabolism No active metabolites

Excretion Urine and feces (equal amounts as unchanged drug)

Available Dosage Forms

Tablet, oral: 5 mg

Dosing

Adult Hypertension, edema (to limit potassium loss): Oral: Initial: 5-10 mg/day (up to 20 mg)
Hypertension (JNC 7): 5-10 mg/day in 1-2 divided doses

Geriatric Oral: Initial: 5 mg once daily or every other day

Pediatric Hypertension (unlabeled use): Children 1-17 years: Oral: 0.4-0.625 mg/kg/day (maximum: 20 mg/day)

Renal Impairment Oral:
Cl_{cr} 10-50 mL/minute: Administer 50% of normal dose.
Cl_{cr} <10 mL/minute: Avoid use.

Administration

Oral Administer with food or meals to avoid GI upset.

Monitoring and Teaching Issues

Laboratory Monitoring Serum electrolytes, renal function

Physical Assessment Assess whether patient is at risk for hyperkalemia. Assess electrolytes and fluid status. Monitor for hyperkalemia.

Patient Education Take early in day with food. Do not increase dietary intake of potassium unless instructed by prescriber. Report muscle cramping or weakness, unresolved nausea or vomiting, palpitations, or respiratory difficulty.

Dietary Considerations Take with food or meals to avoid GI upset. Do not use salt substitutes or low salt milk without checking with healthcare provider.

Geriatric Considerations Use lower initial dose, and adjust dose for renal impairment.

Pregnancy Considerations Teratogenic effects were not observed in animal studies.

Additional Information Medication should be discontinued if potassium level exceeds 6.5 mEq/L. Combined with hydrochlorothiazide as Moduretic®. Amiloride is considered an alternative to triamterene or spironolactone.

Related Information

Heart Failure (Systolic) *on page 2040*

Amiloride and Hydrochlorothiazide (a MIL oh ride & hye droe klor oh THYE a zide)

Index Terms Hydrochlorothiazide and Amiloride

Generic Availability (U.S.) Yes

Pharmacologic Category Diuretic, Combination

Pregnancy Risk Factor B

Lactation Enters breast milk/contraindicated

Use Potassium-sparing diuretic; antihypertensive

Available Dosage Forms

Tablet: 5/50: Amiloride 5 mg and hydrochlorothiazide 50 mg

Dosing

Adult Hypertension, edema: Oral: Initial: 1 tablet/day; may be increased to 2 tablets/day if needed; usually given in a single dose

Geriatric Oral: Initial: 1/2 to 1 tablet/day

Renal Impairment See individual agents.

Administration

Oral May administer with food.

Monitoring and Teaching Issues

Physical Assessment See individual agents.

Patient Education See individual agents.

Related Information

AMILoride *on page 97*
Hydrochlorothiazide *on page 912*

◆ **Amiloride Hydrochloride** *see* AMILoride *on page 97*
◆ **2-Amino-6-Mercaptopurine** *see* Thioguanine *on page 1752*
◆ **2-Amino-6-Trifluoromethoxy-benzothiazole** *see* Riluzole *on page 1582*
◆ **Aminobenzylpenicillin** *see* Ampicillin *on page 124*
◆ **4-aminopyridine** *see* Dalfampridine *on page 458*
◆ **5-Aminosalicylic Acid** *see* Mesalamine *on page 1177*
◆ **Aminoxin® [OTC]** *see* Pyridoxine *on page 1532*

Amiodarone (a MEE oh da rone)

U.S. Brand Names Cordarone®; Pacerone®

Index Terms Amiodarone Hydrochloride; Nexterone®

Generic Availability (U.S.) Yes

Pharmacologic Category Antiarrhythmic Agent, Class III

Medication Safety Issues

Sound-alike/look-alike issues:
Amiodarone may be confused with aMILoride, amrinone
Cordarone® may be confused with Cardura®, Cordran®

High alert medication: The Institute for Safe Medication Practices (ISMP) includes this medication among its list of drugs which have a heightened risk of causing significant patient harm when used in error.

Beers Criteria medication: This drug may be inappropriate for use in geriatric patients (high severity risk).

International issues:

Ambyen [Great Britain] may be confused with Ambien® which is a brand name for zolpidem in the U.S.

Medication Guide Available Yes

Pregnancy Risk Factor D

Lactation Enters breast milk/not recommended (AAP rates "of concern"; AAP 2001 update pending)

Use Management of life-threatening recurrent ventricular fibrillation (VF) or hemodynamically-unstable ventricular tachycardia (VT) refractory to other antiarrhythmic agents or in patients intolerant of other agents used for these conditions

Unlabeled/Investigational Use

Cardiac arrest with persistent ventricular tachycardia (VT) or ventricular fibrillation (VF) if defibrillation, CPR, and vasopressor administration have failed (ACLS/PALS guidelines)

Control of hemodynamically-stable monomorphic VT, polymorphic VT with a normal baseline QT interval, or wide-complex tachycardia of uncertain origin (ACLS/PALS guidelines)

Control of rapid ventricular rate due to accessory pathway conduction in pre-excited atrial arrhythmias (ACLS guidelines)

Control of stable narrow-complex tachycardia (ACLS guidelines)

Heart rate control in patients with atrial fibrillation and heart failure [no accessory pathway] (ACC/AHA/ESC Practice Guidelines)

Paroxysmal supraventricular tachycardia (SVT) (not initial drug of choice)

Prevention of postoperative atrial fibrillation associated with cardiothoracic surgery

Pharmacologic adjunct to ICD therapy to suppress symptomatic ventricular tachyarrhythmias in otherwise optimally-treated patients with heart failure (ACC/AHA/ESC Practice Guidelines)

Pharmacologic conversion of atrial fibrillation to normal sinus rhythm; maintenance of normal sinus rhythm

Mechanism of Action/Effect Class III antiarrhythmic agent which inhibits adrenergic stimulation, prolongs the action potential and refractory period in myocardial tissue; decreases AV conduction and sinus node function. Amiodarone shows beta-blocker-like and calcium channel blocker-like effects on SA and AV nodes.

Contraindications Hypersensitivity to amiodarone, iodine, or any component of the formulation; severe sinus-node dysfunction; second- and third-degree heart block (except in patients with a functioning artificial pacemaker); bradycardia causing syncope (except in patients with a functioning artificial pacemaker); cardiogenic shock

Warnings/Precautions [U.S. Boxed Warning]: Only indicated for patients with life-threatening arrhythmias because of risk of toxicity. Alternative therapies should be tried first before using amiodarone. Patients should be hospitalized when amiodarone is initiated. Currently, the 2005 ACLS guidelines recommend I.V. amiodarone as the preferred antiarrhythmic for the treatment of pulseless VT/VF, both life-threatening arrhythmias. In patients with non-life-threatening arrhythmias (eg, atrial fibrillation), amiodarone should be used only if the use of other antiarrhythmics has proven ineffective or are contraindicated.

[U.S. Boxed Warning]: Lung damage (abnormal diffusion capacity) may occur without symptoms. Monitor for pulmonary toxicity. Evaluate new respiratory symptoms; pre-existing pulmonary disease does not increase risk of developing pulmonary toxicity, but if pulmonary toxicity develops then the prognosis is worse. The lowest effective dose should be used as appropriate for the acuity/severity of the arrhythmia being treated. **[U.S. Boxed Warning]: Liver toxicity is common, but usually mild with evidence of increased liver enzymes. Severe liver toxicity can occur and has been fatal in a few cases.**

[U.S. Boxed Warning]: Amiodarone can exacerbate arrhythmias, by making them more difficult to tolerate or reverse; other types of arrhythmias have occurred, including significant heart block, sinus bradycardia new ventricular fibrillation, incessant ventricular tachycardia, increased resistance to cardioversion, and polymorphic ventricular tachycardia associated with QT_c prolongation (torsade de pointes [TdP]). Risk may be increased with concomitant use of other antiarrhythmic agents or drugs that prolong the QT_c interval. Proarrhythmic effects may be prolonged.

Monitor pacing or defibrillation thresholds in patients with implantable cardiac devices (eg, pacemakers, defibrillators). Use very cautiously and with close monitoring in patients with thyroid or liver disease. May cause hyper- or hypothyroidism. Hyperthyroidism may result in thyrotoxicosis and may aggravate or cause breakthrough arrhythmias. If any new signs of arrhythmia appear, hyperthyroidism should be considered. Thyroid function should be monitored prior to treatment and periodically thereafter.

May cause optic neuropathy and/or optic neuritis, usually resulting in visual impairment. Corneal microdeposits occur in a majority of patients, and may cause visual disturbances in some patients (blurred vision, halos); these are not generally considered a reason to discontinue treatment. Corneal refractive laser surgery is generally contraindicated in amiodarone users. Avoid excessive exposure to sunlight; may cause photosensitivity.

Amiodarone is a potent inhibitor of CYP enzymes and transport proteins (including p-glycoprotein), which may lead to increased serum concentrations/toxicity of a number of medications. Particular caution must be used when a drug with QT_c-prolonging potential relies on metabolism via these enzymes, since the effect of elevated concentrations may be additive with the effect of amiodarone. Carefully assess risk:benefit of coadministration of other drugs which may prolong QT_c interval. Patients may still be at risk for amiodarone–related drug interactions after the drug has been discontinued. The pharmacokinetics are complex (due to prolonged duration of action and half-life) and difficult to predict. Correct electrolyte disturbances, especially hypokalemia or hypomagnesemia, prior to use and throughout therapy. Use caution when initiating amiodarone in patients on warfarin. Cases of increased INR with or without bleeding have occurred in patients treated with warfarin; monitor INR closely after initiating amiodarone in these patients.

May cause hypotension and bradycardia (infusion-rate related). Caution in surgical patients; may enhance hemodynamic effect of anesthetics; associated with increased risk of adult respiratory distress syndrome (ARDS) postoperatively. May be inappropriate in the elderly due to a risk of QT_c-interval prolongation, torsade de pointes, and lack of efficacy in the elderly (Beers Criteria). Injection contains benzyl alcohol, which has been associated with "gasping syndrome" in neonates. Safety and efficacy of amiodarone in children has not been fully established.

Drug Interactions

Metabolism/Transport Effects Substrate of CYP1A2 (minor), CYP2C8 (major at low concentration), CYP2C19 (minor), CYP2D6 (minor), CYP3A4 (major), P-glycoprotein; **Inhibits** CYP1A2 (weak), CYP2A6 (moderate), CYP2B6 (weak), CYP2C9 (moderate), CYP2C19 (weak), CYP2D6 (moderate), CYP3A4 (moderate), P-glycoprotein

Avoid Concomitant Use

Avoid concomitant use of Amiodarone with any of the following: Agalsidase Beta; Artemether; Dronedarone; Grapefruit Juice; Lumefantrine; Nilotinib; Pimozide; Protease Inhibitors; QuiNINE; Silodosin; Tetrabenazine; Thioridazine; Tolvaptan; Topotecan; Toremifene; Vandetanib; Ziprasidone

Decreased Effect

Amiodarone may decrease the levels/effects of: Agalsidase Beta; Clopidogrel; Codeine; Sodium Iodide I131; TraMADol

The levels/effects of Amiodarone may be decreased by: Bile Acid Sequestrants; CYP2C8 Inducers (Highly Effective); CYP3A4 Inducers (Strong); Deferasirox; Etravirine; Grapefruit Juice; Herbs (CYP3A4 Inducers); Orlistat; Peginterferon Alfa-2b; P-Glycoprotein Inducers; Phenytoin; Rifamycin Derivatives

Increased Effect/Toxicity

Amiodarone may increase the levels/effects of: Antiarrhythmic Agents (Class Ia); Beta-Blockers; Cardiac Glycosides; Colchicine; CycloSPORINE; CycloSPORINE (Systemic); CYP2A6 Substrates; CYP2C9 Substrates (High risk); CYP2D6 Substrates; CYP3A4 Substrates; Dabigatran Etexilate; Dronedarone; Eplerenone; Everolimus; FentaNYL; Fesoterodine; Flecainide; HMG-CoA Reductase Inhibitors; Lidocaine; Lidocaine (Systemic); Lidocaine (Topical); Loratadine; Lurasidone; P-Glycoprotein Substrates; Phenytoin; Pimecrolimus; Pimozide; QTc-Prolonging Agents; QuiNINE; Rivaroxaban; Salmeterol; Saxagliptin; Silodosin; Tamoxifen; Tetrabenazine; Thioridazine; Tolvaptan; Topotecan; Toremifene; Vandetanib; Vilazodone; Vitamin K Antagonists; Ziprasidone

The levels/effects of Amiodarone may be increased by: Alfuzosin; Artemether; Azithromycin; Azithromycin (Systemic); Calcium Channel Blockers (Nondihydropyridine); Chloroquine; Cimetidine; Ciprofloxacin; Ciprofloxacin (Systemic); Conivaptan; CYP2C8 Inhibitors (Moderate); CYP2C8 Inhibitors (Strong); CYP3A4 Inhibitors (Moderate); CYP3A4 Inhibitors (Strong); Deferasirox; Eribulin; Fingolimod; Gadobutrol; Grapefruit Juice; Lumefantrine; Nilotinib; P-Glycoprotein Inhibitors; Protease Inhibitors; QuiNINE

Nutritional/Ethanol Interactions

Food: Increases the rate and extent of absorption of amiodarone. Grapefruit juice increases bioavailability of oral amiodarone by 50% and decreases the conversion of amiodarone to N-DEA (active metabolite); altered effects are possible; use should be avoided during therapy.

Herb/Nutraceutical: St John's wort may decrease amiodarone levels or enhance photosensitization. Avoid ephedra (may worsen arrhythmia). Avoid dong quai.

Adverse Reactions In a recent meta-analysis, patients taking lower doses of amiodarone (152-330 mg daily for at least 12 months) were more likely to develop thyroid, neurologic, skin, ocular, and bradycardic abnormalities than those taking placebo (Vorperian, 1997). Pulmonary toxicity was similar in both the low dose amiodarone group and in the placebo group but there was a trend towards increased toxicity in the amiodarone group. Gastrointestinal and hepatic events were seen to a similar extent in both the low dose amiodarone group and placebo group. As the frequency of adverse events varies considerably across studies as a function of route and dose, a consolidation of adverse event rates is provided by Goldschlager, 2000.

>10%:

Cardiovascular: Hypotension (I.V. 16%, refractory in rare cases)

Central nervous system (3% to 40%): Abnormal gait/ataxia, dizziness, fatigue, headache, malaise, impaired memory, involuntary movement, insomnia, poor coordination, peripheral neuropathy, sleep disturbances, tremor

Dermatologic: Photosensitivity (10% to 75%)

Endocrine & Metabolic: Hypothyroidism (1% to 22%)

Gastrointestinal: Nausea, vomiting, anorexia, and constipation (10% to 33%)

Hepatic: AST or ALT level >2x normal (15% to 50%)

Ocular: Corneal microdeposits (>90%; causes visual disturbance in <10%)

1% to 10%:

Cardiovascular: CHF (3%), bradycardia (3% to 5%), AV block (5%), conduction abnormalities, SA node dysfunction (1% to 3%), cardiac arrhythmia, flushing, edema. Additional effects associated with I.V. administration include asystole, atrial fibrillation, cardiac arrest, electromechanical dissociation, pulseless electrical activity (PEA), ventricular tachycardia, and cardiogenic shock.

Dermatologic: Slate blue skin discoloration (<10%)

Endocrine & metabolic: Hyperthyroidism (3% to 10%; more common in iodine-deficient regions of the world), libido decreased

Gastrointestinal: Abdominal pain, abnormal salivation, abnormal taste (oral), diarrhea, nausea (I.V.)

Hematologic: Coagulation abnormalities

Hepatic: Hepatitis and cirrhosis (<3%)

Local: Phlebitis (I.V., with concentrations >3 mg/mL)

Ocular: Visual disturbances (2% to 9%), halo vision (<5% occurring especially at night), optic neuritis (1%)

Respiratory: Pulmonary toxicity has been estimated to occur at a frequency between 2% and 7% of patients (some reports indicate a frequency as high as 17%). Toxicity may present as hypersensitivity pneumonitis; pulmonary fibrosis (cough, fever, malaise); pulmonary inflammation; interstitial pneumonitis; or alveolar pneumonitis. ARDS has been reported in up to 2% of patients receiving amiodarone, and postoperatively in patients receiving oral amiodarone.

Miscellaneous: Abnormal smell (oral)

Pharmacodynamics/Kinetics

Onset of Action Oral: 2 days to 3 weeks; I.V.: May be more rapid; Peak effect: 1 week to 5 months

Duration of Action After discontinuing therapy: 7-50 days

Note: Mean onset of effect and duration after discontinuation may be shorter in children than adults

Absorption Slow and variable

Bioavailability Oral: 35% to 65%

Time to Peak Serum: 3-7 hours

Protein Binding 96%

Half-Life Elimination Terminal: 40-55 days (range: 26-107 days); shorter in children

Metabolism Hepatic via CYP2C8 and 3A4 to active N-desethylamiodarone metabolite; possible enterohepatic recirculation

Excretion Feces; urine (<1% as unchanged drug)

Product Availability

Nexterone®: FDA approved January 2009; expected availability first quarter 2011; consult prescribing information for additional information

Nexterone® is an injection formulation that is free of polysorbate 80 and free of benzyl alcohol.

Available Dosage Forms

Injection, solution: 50 mg/mL (3 mL, 9 mL, 18 mL)

Tablet, oral: 200 mg, 400 mg

Cordarone®: 200 mg

Pacerone®: 100 mg, 200 mg, 400 mg

Dosing

Adult Note: Lower loading and maintenance doses are preferable in women and all patients with low body weight.

Atrial fibrillation pharmacologic cardioversion (ACC/AHA/ESC Practice Guidelines) (unlabeled use):

Oral: *Inpatient:* 1.2-1.8 g/day in divided doses until 10 g total, then 200-400 mg/day maintenance. *Outpatient:* 600-800 mg/day in divided doses until 10 g total, then 200-400 mg/day maintenance; although not supported by clinical evidence, a maintenance dose of 100 mg/day is commonly used especially for the elderly or patients with low body mass (Fuster, 2006; Zimetbaum, 2007). **Note:** Other regimens have been described and may be used clinically:

400 mg 3 times/day for 5-7 days, then 400 mg/day for 1 month, then 200 mg/day

or

10 mg/kg/day for 14 days, followed by 300 mg/day for 4 weeks, followed by maintenance dosage of 200 mg/day (Roy, 2000)

I.V.: 5-7 mg/kg over 30-60 minutes, then 1.2-1.8 g/day continuous infusion or in divided oral doses until 10 g total. Maintenance: See oral dosing.

Atrial fibrillation prophylaxis following open heart surgery (unlabeled use): Note: A variety of regimens have been used in clinical trials, including oral and intravenous regimens:

Oral: Starting in postop recovery, 400 mg twice daily for up to 7 days. Alternative regimen of amiodarone: 600 mg/day for 7 days prior to surgery, followed by 200 mg/day until hospital discharge, has also been shown to decrease the risk of postoperative atrial fibrillation.

I.V.: Starting at postop recovery, 1000 mg infused over 24 hours for 2 days has been shown to reduce the risk of postoperative atrial fibrillation.

Recurrent atrial fibrillation (unlabeled use): No standard regimen defined; examples of regimens include: Oral: Initial: 10 mg/kg/day for 14 days; followed by 300 mg/day for 4 weeks, followed by maintenance dosage of 200 mg/day (Roy, 2000). Other regimens have been described and are used clinically (ie, 400 mg 3 times/day for 5-7 days, then 400 mg/day for 1 month, then 200 mg/day).

Ventricular arrhythmias: Oral: 800-1600 mg/day in 1-2 doses for 1-3 weeks, then when adequate arrhythmia control is achieved, decrease to 600-800 mg/day in 1-2 doses for 1 month; maintenance: 400 mg/day; lower doses are recommended for supraventricular arrhythmias.

Pulseless VT or VF (ACLS, 2010): I.V. push, I.O.: Initial: 300 mg; if pulseless VT or VF continues after subsequent defibrillation attempt or recurs, administer supplemental dose of 150 mg. **Note:** *Handbook of Emergency Cardiovascular Care* (AHA, 2005) recommends dilution in 20-30 mL D_5W (ACLS guidelines do not specify); however, in this setting, administering **undiluted** is preferred (Dager, 2006; Skrifvars, 2004). **Note:** Limited experience with I.O. administration of amiodarone (ACLS, 2010).

Upon return of spontaneous circulation, follow with an infusion of 1 mg/minute for 6 hours, then 0.5 mg/minute for 18 hours (mean daily doses >2.1 g/day have been associated with hypotension).

Stable VT or SVT (unlabeled use): First 24 hours: 1050 mg according to following regimen

Step 1: 150 mg (100 mL) over first 10 minutes (mix 3 mL in 100 mL D_5W)

Step 2: 360 mg (200 mL) over next 6 hours (mix 18 mL in 500 mL D_5W): 1 mg/minute

Step 3: 540 mg (300 mL) over next 18 hours: 0.5 mg/minute

Note: After the first 24 hours: 0.5 mg/minute utilizing concentration of 1-6 mg/mL

Breakthrough stable VT or SVT: 150 mg supplemental doses in 100 mL D_5W or NS over 10 minutes (mean daily doses >2.1 g/day have been associated with hypotension)

I.V. to oral therapy conversion: Use the following as a guide:

<1 week I.V. infusion: 800-1600 mg/day

1- to 3-week I.V. infusion: 600-800 mg/day

>3 week I.V. infusion: 400 mg

Note: Conversion from I.V. to oral therapy has not been formally evaluated. Some experts recommend a 1-2 day overlap when converting from I.V. to oral therapy especially when treating ventricular arrhythmias.

Recommendations for conversion to intravenous amiodarone after oral administration: During long-term amiodarone therapy (ie, ≥4 months), the mean plasma-elimination half-life of the active metabolite of amiodarone is 61 days. Replacement therapy may not be necessary in such patients if oral therapy is discontinued for a period <2 weeks, since any changes in serum amiodarone concentrations during this period may **not** be clinically significant.

Geriatric Refer to adult dosing. No specific guidelines available. Dose selection should be cautious, at low end of dosage range, and titration should be slower to evaluate response. Although not supported by clinical evidence, a maintenance dose of 100 mg/day is commonly used especially for the elderly or patients with low body mass (Fuster, 2006; Zimetbaum, 2007).

Pediatric

Arrhythmias (unlabeled use):

Loading dose: Oral: 10-20 mg/kg/day in 1-2 doses for 4-14 days or until adequate control of arrhythmia or prominent adverse effects occur; alternative loading dose in children <1 year: 600-800 mg/1.73 m^2/day in 1-2 divided doses/day.

Maintenance dose: Oral: Dose may be reduced to 5 mg/kg/day for several weeks (or 200-400 mg/1.73 m^2/day given once daily); if no recurrence of arrhythmia, dose may be further reduced to 2.5 mg/kg/day; maintenance doses may be given 5-7 days/week.

Arrhythmias (unlabeled use, dosing based on limited data):

Loading dose: I.V.: 5 mg/kg over 30 minutes; may repeat up to 3 times if no response.

Maintenance dose: I.V.: Continuous infusion: 10-20 mg/kg/day followed by conversion to oral therapy as appropriate

Note: I.V. administration at low flow rates (potentially associated with use in pediatrics) may result in leaching of plasticizers (DEHP) from intravenous tubing. DEHP may adversely affect male reproductive tract development. Alternative means of dosing and administration (1 mg/kg aliquots) may need to be considered.

Pulseless VT or VF (PALS dosing): I.V.: 5 mg/kg (maximum: 300 mg/dose) rapid I.V. bolus or I.O.; repeat up to a maximum daily dose of 15 mg/kg. (**Note:** Maximum recommended daily dose in adolescents is 2.2 g.)

Perfusing tachycardias (PALS dosing): I.V.: Loading dose: 5 mg/kg (maximum: 300 mg/dose) I.V. over 20-60 minutes or I.O.; may repeat up to maximum dose of 15 mg/kg/day. (**Note:** Maximum recommended daily dose in adolescents is 2.2 g.)

Renal Impairment No dosage adjustment necessary.

Hemodialysis: Not dialyzable (0% to 5%); supplemental dose is not necessary

Peritoneal dialysis: Not dialyzable (0% to 5%); supplemental dose is not necessary

Hepatic Impairment Dosage adjustment is probably necessary in substantial hepatic impairment. No specific guidelines available. If hepatic enzymes exceed 3 times normal or double in a patient with an elevated baseline, consider decreasing the dose or discontinuing amiodarone.

Administration

Oral Administer consistently with regard to meals. Take in divided doses with meals if GI upset occurs or if taking large daily dose. If GI intolerance occurs with single-dose therapy, use twice daily dosing.

I.V. For infusions >1 hour, use concentrations ≤2 mg/mL unless a central venous catheter is used. Use only volumetric infusion pump; use of drop counting may lead to underdosage. Administer through an I.V. line located as centrally as possible. During pulseless VT/VF, the *Handbook of Emergency Cardiovascular Care* (AHA, 2005) recommends dilution in 20-30 mL D_5W; however, in this setting, administering **undiluted** is preferred (Dager, 2006; Skrifvars, 2004).

Adjust administration rate to urgency (give more slowly when perfusing arrhythmia present). Slow the infusion rate if hypotension or bradycardia develops. Infusions >2 hours must be administered in a non-PVC container (eg, glass or polyolefin). PVC tubing is recommended for administration regardless of infusion duration. **Note:** I.V. administration at lower flow rates (potentially associated with use in pediatrics) and higher concentrations than recommended may result in leaching of plasticizers (DEHP) from intravenous tubing. DEHP may adversely affect male reproductive tract development. Alternative means of dosing and administration (1 mg/kg aliquots) may need to be considered.

Stability

Storage Store at room temperature. Protect from light. When admixed in D_5W to a final concentration of 1-6 mg/mL, the solution is stable at room temperature for 24 hours in polyolefin or glass, or for 2 hours in PVC. Infusions >2 hours must be administered in a non-PVC container (eg, glass or polyolefin). Do not use evacuated glass containers; buffer may cause precipitation.

Monitoring and Teaching Issues

Laboratory Monitoring Thyroid function before initiation of treatment and then periodically thereafter (some experts suggest every 3-6 months), pulmonary function, liver enzymes (semiannually), serum electrolytes (potassium, magnesium)

Physical Assessment Eye examinations should be performed periodically. Monitor cardiac status closely and assess for CNS changes. Monitor for signs of pulmonary toxicity (eg, nonproductive cough, dyspnea, pleuritic pain, weight loss, fever, malaise). **I.V.:** Requires continuous cardiac/hemodynamic monitoring and observation for adverse reactions.

Patient Education

I.V.: Emergency use: Patient condition will determine amount of patient education required.

Oral: May be taken with food to reduce GI disturbance, but be consistent. Always take with food or always take without food. Avoid grapefruit juice. Regular blood work, ophthalmic exams, and cardiac assessment will be necessary while taking this medication on a long-term basis. You may experience dizziness, weakness, insomnia, hypotension, nausea, vomiting, loss of appetite, stomach discomfort, abnormal taste, photosensitivity, or decreased libido (reversible). Report persistent dry cough or shortness of breath; chest pain, palpitations, irregular or slow heartbeat; unusual bruising or bleeding; blood in urine or feces (black stool); warmth, swelling, pain in calves; heat or cold intolerance; weight loss or gain; restlessness; hair thinning; changes in menses; sweating; swelling in neck; muscle tremor, weakness, numbness, or changes in gait; fever; malaise; skin rash (bluish-gray color) or irritation; visual disturbances; or changes in urinary patterns.

Dietary Considerations Take consistently with regard to meals. Amiodarone is a potential source of large amounts of inorganic iodine; ~3 mg of inorganic iodine per 100 mg of amiodarone is released into the systemic circulation. Recommended daily allowance for iodine in adults is 150 mcg.

Grapefruit juice is not recommended.

Geriatric Considerations Information describing the clinical use and pharmacokinetics in elderly is lacking; however, elderly may be predisposed to toxicity. Half-life may be prolonged due to decreased clearance; monitor closely. It is recommended to start dosing at the lower end of dosing range.

This medication is considered to be potentially inappropriate in this patient population (Beers Criteria severity: High).

Breast-Feeding Considerations Hypothyroidism may occur in nursing infants. Both amiodarone and its active metabolite are excreted in human milk. Breast-feeding may lead to significant infant exposure and potential toxicity.

Pregnancy Considerations May cause fetal harm when administered to a pregnant woman, leading to congenital goiter and hypo- or hyperthyroidism.

Related Information

Antiarrhythmic Drugs *on page 1978*

◆ **Amiodarone Hydrochloride** *see* Amiodarone *on page 98*

◆ **Amitiza®** *see* Lubiprostone *on page 1139*

Amitriptyline (a mee TRIP ti leen)

Index Terms Amitriptyline Hydrochloride; Elavil

Generic Availability (U.S.) Yes

Pharmacologic Category Antidepressant, Tricyclic (Tertiary Amine)

Medication Safety Issues

Sound-alike/look-alike issues:

Amitriptyline may be confused with aminophylline, imipramine, nortriptyline

Elavil® may be confused with Aldoril®, Eldepryl®, enalapril, Equanil®, Mellaril®, Plavix®

Beers Criteria medication: This drug may be inappropriate for use in geriatric patients (high severity risk).

Medication Guide Available Yes

Pregnancy Risk Factor C

Lactation Enters breast milk/not recommended (AAP rates "of concern"; AAP 2001 update pending)

Use Relief of symptoms of depression

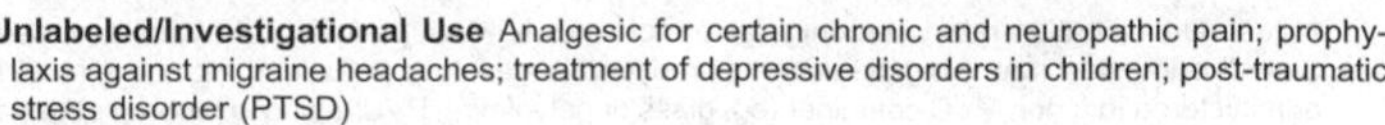

Unlabeled/Investigational Use Analgesic for certain chronic and neuropathic pain; prophylaxis against migraine headaches; treatment of depressive disorders in children; post-traumatic stress disorder (PTSD)

Available Dosage Forms

Tablet, oral: 10 mg, 25 mg, 50 mg, 75 mg, 100 mg, 150 mg

Dosing

Adult

Depression: Oral: 50-150 mg/day single dose at bedtime or in divided doses; dose may be gradually increased up to 300 mg/day.

Chronic pain management (unlabeled use): Oral: Initial: 25 mg at bedtime; may increase as tolerated to 100 mg/day.

Migraine prophylaxis (unlabeled use): Oral: Initial: 10-25 mg at bedtime; usual dose: 150 mg; reported dosing ranges: 10-400 mg/day

Post-traumatic stress disorder (PTSD) (unlabeled use): Oral: 75-200 mg/day

Geriatric Depression: Oral: Initial: 10-25 mg at bedtime; dose should be increased in 10-25 mg increments every week if tolerated; dose range: 25-150 mg/day. See Renal/Hepatic Impairment.

Pediatric

Chronic pain management (unlabeled use): Oral: Initial: 0.1 mg/kg at bedtime, may advance as tolerated over 2-3 weeks to 0.5-2 mg/kg at bedtime

Depressive disorders:

Children (unlabeled use): Oral: Initial doses of 1 mg/kg/day given in 3 divided doses with increases to 1.5 mg/kg/day have been reported in a small number of children (n=9) 9-12 years of age; clinically, doses up to 3 mg/kg/day (5 mg/kg/day if monitored closely) have been proposed

Adolescents: Initial: 25-50 mg/day; may administer in divided doses; increase gradually to 100 mg/day in divided doses.

Migraine prophylaxis (unlabeled use): Oral: Initial: 0.25 mg/kg/day, given at bedtime; increase dose by 0.25 mg/kg/day to maximum 1 mg/kg/day. Reported dosing ranges: 0.1-2 mg/kg/day; maximum suggested dose: 10 mg.

Renal Impairment Nondialyzable

Hepatic Impairment Use with caution and monitor plasma levels and patient response.

Monitoring and Teaching Issues

Physical Assessment Assess for suicidal tendencies or unusual changes in behavior before beginning therapy and periodically thereafter. Caution patients with diabetes; may alter serum glucose levels. Taper dosage slowly when discontinuing.

Patient Education It may take several weeks to achieve desired results. Restrict use of alcohol. Maintain adequate hydration, unless instructed to restrict fluid intake. If you have diabetes, monitor glucose levels closely; this medication may alter glucose levels. May cause drowsiness, lightheadedness, impaired coordination, dizziness, blurred vision, constipation, urinary retention, postural hypotension, altered sexual drive or ability (reversible), or photosensitivity. Report persistent CNS effects (eg, nervousness, restlessness, insomnia, headache, agitation, impaired coordination, changes in cognition); suicide ideation; muscle cramping, weakness, tremors, or rigidity; ringing in ears or visual disturbances; chest pain, palpitations, or irregular heartbeat; blurred vision; or worsening of condition.

Related Information

Antidepressant Agents *on page 1982*

Peak and Trough Guidelines *on page 1958*

◆ **Amitriptyline Hydrochloride** *see* Amitriptyline *on page 103*

AmLODIPine (am LOE di peen)

U.S. Brand Names Norvasc®

Index Terms Amlodipine Besylate

Generic Availability (U.S.) Yes

Pharmacologic Category Calcium Channel Blocker; Calcium Channel Blocker, Dihydropyridine

Medication Safety Issues

Sound-alike/look-alike issues:

AmLODIPine may be confused with aMILoride

Norvasc® may be confused with Navane®, Norvir®, Vascor®

Pregnancy Risk Factor C

Lactation Excretion in breast milk unknown/not recommended

Use Treatment of hypertension; treatment of symptomatic chronic stable angina, vasospastic (Prinzmetal's) angina (confirmed or suspected); prevention of hospitalization due to angina with documented CAD (limited to patients without heart failure or ejection fraction <40%)

Mechanism of Action/Effect Inhibits calcium ion from entering the "slow channels" or select voltage-sensitive areas of vascular smooth muscle and myocardium during depolarization; a peripheral arterial vasodilator that causes a reduction in blood pressure

Contraindications Hypersensitivity to amlodipine or any component of the formulation

Warnings/Precautions Increased angina and/or MI has occurred with initiation or dosage titration of calcium channel blockers. Symptomatic hypotension with or without syncope can rarely occur; blood pressure must be lowered at a rate appropriate for the patient's clinical condition. Use caution in severe aortic stenosis and/or hypertrophic cardiomyopathy with outflow tract obstruction. Use caution in patients with hepatic impairment; may require lower starting dose; titrate slowly with severe hepatic impairment. The most common side effect is peripheral edema; occurs within 2-3 weeks of starting therapy. Reflex tachycardia may occur with use. Peak antihypertensive effect is delayed; dosage titration should occur after 7-14 days on a given dose. Initiate at a lower dose in the elderly.

Drug Interactions

Metabolism/Transport Effects Substrate of CYP3A4 (major); **Inhibits** CYP1A2 (moderate), 2A6 (weak), 2B6 (weak), 2C8 (weak), 2C9 (weak), 2D6 (weak), 3A4 (weak)

Avoid Concomitant Use There are no known interactions where it is recommended to avoid concomitant use.

Decreased Effect

AmLODIPine may decrease the levels/effects of: Clopidogrel; QuiNIDine

The levels/effects of AmLODIPine may be decreased by: Barbiturates; Calcium Salts; CarBAMazepine; CYP3A4 Inducers (Strong); Deferasirox; Herbs (CYP3A4 Inducers); Herbs (Hypertensive Properties); Methylphenidate; Nafcillin; Rifamycin Derivatives; Yohimbine

Increased Effect/Toxicity

AmLODIPine may increase the levels/effects of: Amifostine; Antihypertensives; Calcium Channel Blockers (Nondihydropyridine); CYP1A2 Substrates; Hypotensive Agents; Magnesium Salts; Neuromuscular-Blocking Agents (Nondepolarizing); Nitroprusside; Phenytoin; RiTUXimab; Tacrolimus; Tacrolimus (Systemic)

The levels/effects of AmLODIPine may be increased by: Alpha1-Blockers; Antifungal Agents (Azole Derivatives, Systemic); Calcium Channel Blockers (Nondihydropyridine); Conivaptan; CycloSPORINE; CycloSPORINE (Systemic); CYP3A4 Inhibitors (Moderate); CYP3A4 Inhibitors (Strong); Dasatinib; Diazoxide; Fluconazole; Grapefruit Juice; Herbs (Hypotensive Properties); Macrolide Antibiotics; Magnesium Salts; MAO Inhibitors; Pentoxifylline; Phosphodiesterase 5 Inhibitors; Prostacyclin Analogues; Protease Inhibitors

Nutritional/Ethanol Interactions

Food: Grapefruit juice may modestly increase amlodipine levels.

Herb/Nutraceutical: St John's wort may decrease amlodipine levels. Avoid herbs with *hypertensive* properties (bayberry, blue cohosh, cayenne, ephedra, ginger, ginseng [American], kola, licorice). Avoid herbs with *hypotensive* properties (black cohosh, California poppy, coleus, garlic, goldenseal, hawthorn, mistletoe, periwinkle, quinine, shepherd's purse).

Adverse Reactions

>10%: Cardiovascular: Peripheral edema (2% to 15% dose related; HF patients: 27% [Packer, 1996])

1% to 10%:

Cardiovascular: Flushing (1% to 5% dose related), palpitation (1% to 5% dose related)

Central nervous system: Dizziness (1% to 3% dose related), fatigue (5%), somnolence (1% to 2%)

Dermatologic: Rash (1% to 2%), pruritus (1% to 2%)

Endocrine & metabolic: Male sexual dysfunction (1% to 2%)

Gastrointestinal: Nausea (3%), abdominal pain (1% to 2%), dyspepsia (1% to 2%)

Neuromuscular & skeletal: Muscle cramps (1% to 2%), weakness (1% to 2%)

Respiratory: Dyspnea (1% to 2%), pulmonary edema (HF patients: 27% [Packer, 1996])

Pharmacodynamics/Kinetics

Duration of Action Antihypertensive effect: 24 hours

Absorption Oral: Well absorbed

Bioavailability 64% to 90%

Time to Peak Plasma: 6-12 hours

Protein Binding 93% to 98%

Half-Life Elimination Terminal: 30-50 hours; increased with hepatic dysfunction

Metabolism Hepatic (>90%) to inactive metabolites

Excretion Urine (10% of total dose as unchanged drug, 60% of total dose as metabolites)

Available Dosage Forms

Tablet, oral: 2.5 mg, 5 mg, 10 mg

Norvasc®: 2.5 mg, 5 mg, 10 mg

Dosing

Adult

Hypertension: Oral: Initial dose: 5 mg once daily; maximum dose: 10 mg once daily. In general, titrate in 2.5 mg increments over 7-14 days. Usual dosage range (JNC 7): 2.5-10 mg once daily.

Angina: Oral: Usual dose: 5-10 mg; most patients require 10 mg for adequate effect.

Geriatric Dosing should start at the lower end of dosing range due to possible increased incidence of hepatic, renal, or cardiac impairment. Elderly patients also show decreased clearance of amlodipine.

Hypertension: Oral: 2.5 mg once daily

Angina: Oral: 5 mg once daily

Pediatric Hypertension: Oral: Children 6-17 years: 2.5-5 mg once daily

Renal Impairment Dialysis: Hemodialysis and peritoneal dialysis do not enhance elimination. Supplemental dose is not necessary.

Hepatic Impairment

Hypertension: Administer 2.5 mg once daily

Angina: Administer 5 mg once daily

Administration

Oral May be administered without regard to meals.

Stability

Storage Store at room temperature of 15°C to 30°C (59°F to 86°F).

Monitoring and Teaching Issues

Physical Assessment Assess therapeutic effectiveness (blood pressure, angina pattern, weight, and peripheral edema).

Patient Education May cause headache or constipation. Report unrelieved headache, severe constipation, peripheral or facial swelling, weight gain, respiratory changes, or worsening of chest pain or pressure.

Dietary Considerations May be taken without regard to meals.

Geriatric Considerations Elderly may experience a greater hypotensive response. Constipation may be more of a problem in elderly. Calcium channel blockers are no more effective in elderly than other therapies, however, they do not cause significant CNS effects which is an advantage over some antihypertensive agents.

Pregnancy Considerations Embryotoxic effects have been demonstrated in animal studies. No well-controlled studies have been conducted in pregnant women. Use in pregnancy only when clearly needed and when the benefits outweigh the potential hazard to the fetus.

Related Information

Calcium Channel Blockers *on page 1993*

- **Amlodipine, Aliskiren, and Hydrochlorothiazide** *see* Aliskiren, Amlodipine, and Hydrochlorothiazide *on page 73*
- **Amlodipine and Aliskiren** *see* Aliskiren and Amlodipine *on page 73*

Amlodipine and Atorvastatin (am LOW di peen & a TORE va sta tin)

U.S. Brand Names Caduet®

Index Terms Atorvastatin and Amlodipine; Atorvastatin Calcium and Amlodipine Besylate

Generic Availability (U.S.) No

Pharmacologic Category Antilipemic Agent, HMG-CoA Reductase Inhibitor; Calcium Channel Blocker; Calcium Channel Blocker, Dihydropyridine

Pregnancy Risk Factor X

Lactation Excretion in breast milk unknown/contraindicated

Use For use when treatment with both amlodipine and atorvastatin is appropriate:

Amlodipine: Treatment of hypertension; treatment of chronic stable angina, vasospastic (Prinzmetal's) angina (confirmed or suspected); prevention of hospitalization or to decrease coronary revascularization procedure due to angina with documented CAD (limited to patients without heart failure or ejection fraction <40%)

Atorvastatin: Treatment of dyslipidemias or primary prevention of cardiovascular disease (atherosclerotic) as detailed here:

Primary prevention of cardiovascular disease (high-risk for CVD): To reduce the risk of MI or stroke in patients without evidence of coronary heart disease who have multiple CVD risk factors or type 2 diabetes; also reduces the risk for angina or revascularization procedures in patients with multiple CVD risk factors without evidence of coronary heart disease

Secondary prevention of cardiovascular disease: To reduce the risk of MI, stroke, revascularization procedures, angina, and hospitalization for heart failure

Treatment of dyslipidemias: To reduce elevations in total cholesterol, LDL-C, apolipoprotein B, and triglycerides in patients with elevations of one or more components, and/or to increase low HDL-C as present in heterozygous familial/nonfamilial hypercholesterolemia and mixed dyslipidemia (Fredrickson type IIa and IIb hyperlipidemias); treatment of primary dysbetalipoproteinemia (Fredrickson type III), elevated serum TG levels (Fredrickson type IV), and homozygous familial hypercholesterolemia

Treatment of heterozygous familial hypercholesterolemia (HeFH) in adolescent patients (10-17 years of age, females >1 year postmenarche) having LDL-C ≥190 mg/dL or LDL-C ≥160 mg/dL with positive family history of premature cardiovascular disease (CVD) or with two or more CVD risk factors.

Available Dosage Forms

Tablet:

Caduet®:

2.5/10: Amlodipine 2.5 mg and atorvastatin 10 mg; 2.5/20: Amlodipine 2.5 mg and atorvastatin 20 mg; 2.5/40: Amlodipine 2.5 mg and atorvastatin 40 mg

5/10: Amlodipine 5 mg and atorvastatin 10 mg; 5/20: Amlodipine 5 mg and atorvastatin 20 mg; 5/40: Amlodipine 5 mg and atorvastatin 40 mg; 5/80: Amlodipine 5 mg and atorvastatin 80 mg

10/10: Amlodipine 10 mg and atorvastatin 10 mg; 10/20: Amlodipine 10 mg and atorvastatin 20 mg; 10/40: Amlodipine 10 mg and atorvastatin 40 mg; 10/80: Amlodipine 10 mg and atorvastatin 80 mg

Dosing

Adult Note: Dose is individualized; combination product may be used as initial therapy or substituted for individual components in patients currently maintained on both agents separately or in patients not adequately controlled with monotherapy (using one of the agents or an agent within same pharmacologic class).

Hypertension, angina, and hyperlipidemia: Oral:

Initial therapy: Amlodipine 5 mg and atorvastatin 10-20 mg once daily; dose may be titrated after 1-2 weeks (amlodipine component) and after 2-4 weeks (atorvastatin component) to a maximum daily dose: Amlodipine 10 mg; atorvastatin 80 mg

Add-on therapy/replacement therapy: Amlodipine 5-10 mg and atorvastatin 10-80 mg once daily; dose may be titrated after 1-2 weeks (amlodipine component) and after 2-4 weeks (atorvastatin component) to a maximum daily dose: Amlodipine 10 mg; atorvastatin 80 mg

Dosage adjustment for atorvastatin with concomitant medications:

Cyclosporine: Atorvastatin dose should not exceed 10 mg/day

Clarithromycin, itraconazole, ritonavir plus saquinavir, or lopinavir plus ritonavir when atorvastatin dose >20 mg: Ensure that the lowest dose necessary of atorvastatin is used

Geriatric Refer to adult dosing. Consider starting amlodipine at the lower end of dosing range due to increased incidence of hepatic, renal, or cardiac impairment. Elderly patients also show decreased clearance of amlodipine.

Pediatric Note: Dose is individualized; combination product may be used as initial therapy or substituted for individual components in patients currently maintained on both agents separately or in patients not adequately controlled with monotherapy (using one of the agents or an agent within same pharmacologic class).

Hypertension and hyperlipidemia: 10-17 years (females >1 year postmenarche): Oral:

Initial therapy: Amlodipine 2.5 mg and atorvastatin 10 mg once daily; dose may be titrated after 1-2 weeks (amlodipine component) and after 2-4 weeks (atorvastatin component) to a maximum daily dose: Amlodipine 5 mg; atorvastatin 20 mg

Add-on therapy/replacement therapy: Amlodipine 2.5-5 mg and atorvastatin 10-20 mg once daily; dose may be titrated after 1-2 weeks (amlodipine component) and after 2-4 weeks (atorvastatin component) to a maximum daily dose: Amlodipine 5 mg; atorvastatin 20 mg

Dosage adjustment for atorvastatin with concomitant medications: Refer to adult dosing.

Renal Impairment No dosage adjustment is necessary.

Hepatic Impairment Contraindicated in patients with active liver disease.

Administration

Oral May be administered without regard to meals.

Monitoring and Teaching Issues

Laboratory Monitoring See individual agents.

Physical Assessment See individual agents.

Patient Education See individual agents.

Amlodipine and Benazepril (am LOE di peen & ben AY ze pril)

U.S. Brand Names Lotrel®

Index Terms Benazepril Hydrochloride and Amlodipine Besylate

Generic Availability (U.S.) Yes

Pharmacologic Category Angiotensin-Converting Enzyme (ACE) Inhibitor; Calcium Channel Blocker; Calcium Channel Blocker, Dihydropyridine

Pregnancy Risk Factor D

Lactation

Amlodipine: Excretion in breast milk unknown/not recommended

Benazepril: Enters breast milk

Use Treatment of hypertension

Available Dosage Forms

Capsule: 2.5/10: Amlodipine 2.5 mg and benazepril 10 mg; 5/10: Amlodipine 5 mg and benazepril 10 mg; 5/20: Amlodipine 5 mg and benazepril 20 mg; 5/40: Amlodipine 5 mg and benazepril hydrochloride 40 mg; 10/20: Amlodipine 10 mg and benazepril 20 mg; 10/40: Amlodipine 10 mg and benazepril hydrochloride 40 mg

Lotrel®: 2.5/10: Amlodipine 2.5 and benazepril 10 mg; 5/10: Amlodipine 5 mg and benazepril 10 mg; 5/20: Amlodipine 5 mg and benazepril 20 mg; 5/40: Amlodipine 5 mg and benazepril 40 mg; 10/20: Amlodipine 10 mg and benazepril 20 mg; 10/40: Amlodipine 10 mg and benazepril 40 mg

Dosing

Adult Note: Dose is individualized; combination product may be substituted for individual components in patients currently maintained on both agents separately or in patients not adequately controlled with monotherapy (using one of the agents or an agent within same antihypertensive class).

Hypertension: Oral: 2.5-10 mg (amlodipine) and 10-40 mg (benazepril) once daily; maximum: Amlodipine: 10 mg/day; benazepril: 80 mg/day

Geriatric Initial dose: 2.5 mg (based on amlodipine component). Refer to adult dosing.

Renal Impairment Cl_{cr} ≤30 mL/minute: Use of combination product is not recommended.

Hepatic Impairment Initial dose: 2.5 mg based on amlodipine component.

Monitoring and Teaching Issues

Laboratory Monitoring BUN, electrolytes, and serum creatinine; in patients with renal impairment and/or collagen vascular disease, monitor CBC with differential periodically

Physical Assessment See individual agents.

Patient Education See individual agents.

Related Information

AmLODIPine *on page 104*

Benazepril *on page 195*

Amlodipine and Olmesartan (am LOE di peen & olme SAR tan)

U.S. Brand Names Azor™

Index Terms Amlodipine Besylate and Olmesartan Medoxomil; Olmesartan and Amlodipine

Generic Availability (U.S.) No

Pharmacologic Category Angiotensin II Receptor Blocker; Calcium Channel Blocker; Calcium Channel Blocker, Dihydropyridine

Pregnancy Risk Factor C/D (2nd and 3rd trimesters)

Lactation Excretion in breast milk unknown/not recommended

Use Treatment of hypertension, including initial treatment in patients who will require multiple antihypertensives for adequate control

Available Dosage Forms

Tablet:

Azor™: 5/20: Amlodipine 5 mg and olmesartan medoxomil 20 mg; 5/40: Amlodipine 5 mg and olmesartan medoxomil 40 mg; 10/20: Amlodipine 10 mg and olmesartan medoxomil 20 mg; 10/40: Amlodipine 10 mg and olmesartan medoxomil 40 mg

Dosing

Adult Dose is individualized; combination product may be substituted for individual components in patients currently maintained on both agents separately or in patients not adequately controlled with monotherapy (using one of the agents or an agent within the same antihypertensive class). May also be used as initial therapy in patients who are likely to need >1 antihypertensive to control blood pressure.

Hypertension: Oral:

Initial therapy (antihypertensive naive): Amlodipine 5 mg/olmesartan 20 mg once daily; dose may be increased after 1-2 weeks of therapy. Maximum recommended dose: Amlodipine 10 mg/day; olmesartan 40 mg/day.

Add-on/replacement therapy: Amlodipine 5-10 mg and olmesartan 20-40 mg once daily depending upon previous doses, current control, and goals of therapy; dose may be titrated after 2 weeks of therapy. Maximum recommended dose: Amlodipine 10 mg/day; olmesartan 40 mg/day.

Geriatric Initial therapy is not recommended in patients ≥75 years of age.

Renal Impairment No specific guidelines for dosage adjustment.

Hepatic Impairment Initial therapy is not recommended.

Administration

Oral Administer with or without food.

Monitoring and Teaching Issues

Laboratory Monitoring Baseline and periodic electrolyte panels, renal and liver function, urinalysis

Physical Assessment See individual agents.

Patient Education See individual agents.

Related Information

AmLODIPine *on page 104*

Olmesartan *on page 1349*

◆ **Amlodipine and Telmisartan** *see* Telmisartan and Amlodipine *on page 1719*

Amlodipine and Valsartan (am LOE di peen & val SAR tan)

U.S. Brand Names Exforge®

Index Terms Amlodipine Besylate and Valsartan; Valsartan and Amlodipine

Generic Availability (U.S.) No

Pharmacologic Category Angiotensin II Receptor Blocker; Calcium Channel Blocker; Calcium Channel Blocker, Dihydropyridine

Pregnancy Risk Factor D

Lactation Excretion in breast milk unknown/not recommended

Use Treatment of hypertension

Available Dosage Forms

Tablet:

Exforge®: 5/160: Amlodipine 5 mg and valsartan 160 mg; 5/320 mg: Amlodipine 5 mg and valsartan 320 mg; 10/160: Amlodipine 10 mg and valsartan 160 mg; 10/320: Amlodipine 10 mg and valsartan 320 mg

Dosing

Adult Note: Dose is individualized; combination product may be used as initial therapy or substituted for individual components in patients currently maintained on both agents separately or in patients not adequately controlled with monotherapy (using one of the agents or an agent within same antihypertensive class).

Hypertension: Oral:

Initial therapy: Amlodipine 5 mg and valsartan 160 mg once daily, dose may be titrated after 1-2 weeks of therapy. Maximum recommended doses: Amlodipine 10 mg/day; valsartan 320 mg/day

Add-on/replacement therapy: Amlodipine 5-10 mg and valsartan 160-320 mg once daily; dose may be titrated after 3-4 weeks of therapy. Maximum recommended doses: Amlodipine 10 mg/day; valsartan 320 mg/day

Geriatric Refer to adult dosing. Initiate amlodipine at 2.5 mg/day; due to decreased clearance.

Renal Impairment

Cl_{cr} >10 mL/minute: No dosage adjustment necessary.

Cl_{cr} ≤10 mL/minute: Use caution; titrate slowly.

Hepatic Impairment Mild-to-moderate hepatic impairment: No initial dosage adjustment required, titrate slowly. Amlodipine and valsartan exposure increased in presence of hepatic impairment.

Amlodipine: Use caution in severe hepatic impairment; lower initial doses may be required.

Valsartan: Mild-to-moderate hepatic impairment: No dosage adjustment required; however, patients with mild-to-moderate chronic disease have twice the exposure as healthy volunteers.

Administration

Oral Administer with or without food.

Monitoring and Teaching Issues

Laboratory Monitoring Baseline and periodic electrolyte panels, renal and liver function, urinalysis; in CHF, serum potassium during dose escalation and periodically thereafter

Physical Assessment See individual agents.

Patient Education See individual agents.

Related Information

AmLODIPine *on page 104*

Valsartan *on page 1838*

- **Amlodipine Besylate** *see* AmLODIPine *on page 104*
- **Amlodipine Besylate, Aliskiren Hemifumarate, and Hydrochlorothiazide** *see* Aliskiren, Amlodipine, and Hydrochlorothiazide *on page 73*
- **Amlodipine Besylate and Olmesartan Medoxomil** *see* Amlodipine and Olmesartan *on page 108*
- **Amlodipine Besylate and Telmisartan** *see* Telmisartan and Amlodipine *on page 1719*
- **Amlodipine Besylate and Valsartan** *see* Amlodipine and Valsartan *on page 108*
- **Amlodipine Besylate, Valsartan, and Hydrochlorothiazide** *see* Amlodipine, Valsartan, and Hydrochlorothiazide *on page 109*
- **Amlodipine, Hydrochlorothiazide, and Aliskiren** *see* Aliskiren, Amlodipine, and Hydrochlorothiazide *on page 73*
- **Amlodipine, Hydrochlorothiazide, and Valsartan** *see* Amlodipine, Valsartan, and Hydrochlorothiazide *on page 109*

Amlodipine, Valsartan, and Hydrochlorothiazide

(am LOE di peen, val SAR tan, & hye droe klor oh THYE a zide)

U.S. Brand Names Exforge HCT®

Index Terms Amlodipine Besylate, Valsartan, and Hydrochlorothiazide; Amlodipine, Hydrochlorothiazide, and Valsartan; Hydrochlorothiazide, Amlodipine, and Valsartan; Valsartan, Hydrochlorothiazide, and Amlodipine

Generic Availability (U.S.) No

Pharmacologic Category Angiotensin II Receptor Blocker; Calcium Channel Blocker; Calcium Channel Blocker, Dihydropyridine; Diuretic, Thiazide

Pregnancy Risk Factor D

Lactation Enters breast milk/not recommended

Use Treatment of hypertension (not for initial therapy)

Available Dosage Forms

Tablet, oral:

Exforge HCT®: Amlodipine 5 mg, valsartan 160 mg, and hydrochlorothiazide 12.5 mg; Amlodipine 5 mg, valsartan 160 mg, and hydrochlorothiazide 25 mg; Amlodipine 10 mg, valsartan 160 mg, and hydrochlorothiazide 12.5 mg; Amlodipine 10 mg, valsartan 160 mg, and hydrochlorothiazide 25 mg; Amlodipine 10 mg, valsartan 320 mg, and hydrochlorothiazide 25 mg

Dosing

Adult & Geriatric Note: Not for initial therapy. Dose is individualized; combination product may be substituted for individual components in patients currently maintained on all three agents separately or in patients not adequately controlled with any two of the following antihypertensive classes: calcium channel blockers, angiotensin II receptor blockers, and diuretics.

Hypertension: Oral: Add-on/switch/replacement therapy: Amlodipine 5-10 mg and valsartan 160-320 mg and hydrochlorothiazide 12.5-25 mg once daily; dose may be titrated after 2 weeks of therapy. Maximum recommended daily dose: Amlodipine 10 mg/valsartan 320 mg/hydrochlorothiazide 25 mg

Renal Impairment

Cl_{cr} >30 mL/minute: No adjustment needed.

Cl_{cr} ≤30 mL/minute: Use of combination not recommended; contraindicated in patients with anuria.

Hepatic Impairment Use of combination is not recommended in severe hepatic impairment. Use with caution in mild-to-moderate hepatic impairment; monitor for worsening of hepatic or renal function and adverse reactions.

Administration

Oral Administer with or without food.

Monitoring and Teaching Issues

Laboratory Monitoring Serum electrolytes, renal function

Physical Assessment See individual agents.

Patient Education See individual agents.

◆ **AMN107** *see* Nilotinib *on page* 1316

◆ **Amnesteem®** *see* Isotretinoin *on page* 1030

◆ **Amoclan** *see* Amoxicillin and Clavulanate Potassium *on page* 113

Amoxicillin (a moks i SIL in)

U.S. Brand Names Moxatag™

Index Terms *p*-Hydroxyampicillin; Amoxicillin Trihydrate; Amoxil; Amoxycillin

Generic Availability (U.S.) Yes: Excludes extended-release formulation

Pharmacologic Category Antibiotic, Penicillin

Medication Safety Issues

Sound-alike/look-alike issues:

Amoxicillin may be confused with amoxapine, Augmentin®

Amoxil may be confused with amoxapine

International issues:

Fisamox [Australia] may be confused with Fosamax brand name for alendronate [U.S., Canada, and multiple international markets] and Vigamox brand name for moxifloxacin [U.S., Canada, and multiple international markets]

Limoxin [Mexico] may be confused with Lanoxin brand name for digoxin [U.S., Canada, and multiple international markets]; Lincocin brand name for lincomycin [U.S., Canada, and multiple international markets]

Zimox: Brand name for amoxicillin [Italy], but also the brand name for carbidopa/levodopa [Greece]

Zimox [Italy] may be confused with Diamox which is the brand name for acetazolamide [Canada and multiple international markets]

Pregnancy Risk Factor B

Lactation Enters breast milk/use caution (AAP rates "compatible"; AAP 2001 update pending)

Use Treatment of otitis media, sinusitis, and infections caused by susceptible organisms involving the upper and lower respiratory tract, skin, and urinary tract; prophylaxis of infective endocarditis in patients undergoing surgical or dental procedures; as part of a multidrug regimen for *H. pylori* eradication

Unlabeled/Investigational Use Postexposure prophylaxis for anthrax exposure with documented susceptible organisms

Mechanism of Action/Effect Interferes with bacterial cell wall synthesis during active multiplication, causing cell wall death and resultant bactericidal activity against susceptible bacteria

Contraindications Hypersensitivity to amoxicillin, penicillin, other beta-lactams, or any component of the formulation

Warnings/Precautions In patients with renal impairment, doses and/or frequency of administration should be modified in response to the degree of renal impairment; in addition, use of certain dosage forms (eg, extended release 775 mg tablet and immediate release 875 mg tablet) should be avoided in patients with Cl_{cr} <30 mL/minute or patients requiring hemodialysis. A high percentage of patients with infectious mononucleosis have developed rash during therapy with amoxicillin; ampicillin-class antibiotics not recommended in these patients. Serious and occasionally severe or fatal hypersensitivity (anaphylactoid) reactions have been reported in patients on penicillin therapy, especially with a history of beta-lactam hypersensitivity, history of sensitivity to multiple allergens, or previous IgE-mediated reactions (eg, anaphylaxis, angioedema, urticaria). Use with caution in asthmatic patients. Prolonged use may result in fungal or bacterial superinfection, including *C. difficile*-associated diarrhea (CDAD) and pseudomembranous colitis; CDAD has been observed >2 months postantibiotic treatment. Chewable tablets contain phenylalanine.

Drug Interactions

Avoid Concomitant Use

Avoid concomitant use of Amoxicillin with any of the following: BCG

Decreased Effect

Amoxicillin may decrease the levels/effects of: BCG; Mycophenolate; Typhoid Vaccine

The levels/effects of Amoxicillin may be decreased by: Fusidic Acid; Tetracycline Derivatives

Increased Effect/Toxicity

Amoxicillin may increase the levels/effects of: Methotrexate

The levels/effects of Amoxicillin may be increased by: Allopurinol; Probenecid

Lab Interactions Altered response to Benedict's reagent in Clinitest®

Some penicillin derivatives may accelerate the degradation of aminoglycosides *in vitro*, leading to a potential underestimation of aminoglycoside serum concentration.

Adverse Reactions Frequency not defined.

Central nervous system: Agitation, anxiety, behavioral changes, confusion, dizziness, headache, hyperactivity (reversible), insomnia, seizure

Dermatologic: Acute exanthematous pustulosis, erythematous maculopapular rash, erythema multiforme, exfoliative dermatitis, hypersensitivity vasculitis, mucocutaneous candidiasis, Stevens-Johnson syndrome, toxic epidermal necrolysis, urticaria

Gastrointestinal: Black hairy tongue, diarrhea, hemorrhagic colitis, nausea, pseudomembranous colitis, tooth discoloration (brown, yellow, or gray; rare), vomiting

Hematologic: Agranulocytosis, anemia, eosinophilia, hemolytic anemia, leukopenia, thrombocytopenia, thrombocytopenia purpura

Hepatic: Acute cytolytic hepatitis, ALT increased, AST increased, cholestatic jaundice, hepatic cholestasis

Renal: Crystalluria

Miscellaneous: Anaphylaxis, serum sickness-like reaction

Pharmacodynamics/Kinetics

Absorption Oral: Rapid and nearly complete; food does not interfere

Extended-release tablet: Rate of absorption is slower compared to immediate-release formulations; food decreases the rate but not extent of absorption

Time to Peak Capsule: 2 hours; Extended-release tablet: 3.1 hours; Suspension: 1 hour

Protein Binding 17% to 20%

Half-Life Elimination

Neonates, full-term: 3.7 hours

Infants and Children: 1-2 hours

Adults: Normal renal function: 0.7-1.4 hours

Cl_{cr} <10 mL/minute: 7-21 hours

Metabolism Partially hepatic

Excretion Urine (60% as unchanged drug); lower in neonates

Pharmacokinetic Note Extended-release tablets: In healthy volunteers, serum drug concentrations were below 0.25 mcg/mL and undetectable at 16 hours following dosing.

Available Dosage Forms

Capsule, oral: 250 mg, 500 mg

Powder for suspension, oral: 125 mg/5 mL (80 mL, 100 mL, 150 mL); 200 mg/5 mL (50 mL, 75 mL, 100 mL); 250 mg/5 mL (80 mL, 100 mL, 150 mL); 400 mg/5 mL (50 mL, 75 mL, 100 mL)

Tablet, oral: 500 mg, 875 mg

Tablet, chewable, oral: 125 mg, 200 mg, 250 mg, 400 mg

Tablet, extended release, oral:

Moxatag™: 775 mg

Dosing

Adult & Geriatric

Usual dosage range: Oral: 250-500 mg every 8 hours or 500-875 mg twice daily **or** extended-release tablet 775 mg once daily

Anthrax exposure (CDC guidelines): Oral: **Note:** Postexposure prophylaxis in pregnant or nursing women only with documented susceptible organisms: 500 mg every 8 hours

Chlamydial infection during pregnancy (unlabeled use): Oral: 500 mg 3 times/day for 7 days (CDC, 2010)

Ear, nose, throat, genitourinary tract, or skin/skin structure infections:

Mild-to-moderate: Oral: 500 mg every 12 hours **or** 250 mg every 8 hours

Severe: Oral: 875 mg every 12 hours **or** 500 mg every 8 hours

Tonsillitis and/or pharyngitis: Oral: Extended release tablet: 775 mg once daily

***Helicobacter pylori* eradication:** Oral: 1000 mg twice daily; requires combination therapy with at least one other antibiotic and an acid-suppressing agent (proton pump inhibitor or H_2 blocker)

Lower respiratory tract infections: Oral: 875 mg every 12 hours **or** 500 mg every 8 hours

Lyme disease: Oral: 500 mg every 6-8 hours (depending on size of patient) for 21-30 days

Prophylaxis against infective endocarditis: Oral: 2 g 30-60 minutes before procedure. **Note:** American Heart Association (AHA) guidelines now recommend prophylaxis only in patients undergoing invasive procedures and in whom underlying cardiac conditions may predispose to a higher risk of adverse outcomes should infection occur. As of April 2007, routine prophylaxis for GI/GU procedures is no longer recommended by the AHA.

Prophylaxis in total joint replacement patients undergoing dental procedures which produce bacteremia: 2 g 1 hour prior to procedure

Pediatric

Usual dosage range:

Children ≤3 months: Oral: 20-30 mg/kg/day divided every 12 hours

Children >3 months and <40 kg: Oral: 20-50 mg/kg/day in divided doses every 8-12 hours

Children ≥12 years: Oral: Extended-release tablet: 775 mg once daily

Acute otitis media: Children >3 months and <40 kg: Oral: 80-90 mg/kg/day divided every 12 hours

Anthrax exposure (CDC guidelines): Children >3 months and <40 kg: Oral: **Note:** Post-exposure prophylaxis only with documented susceptible organisms: 80 mg/kg/day in divided doses every 8 hours (maximum: 500 mg/dose)

Community-acquired pneumonia:

4 months to <5 years: 80-100 mg/kg/day divided every 8 hours

5-15 years: 100 mg/kg/day divided every 8 hours; **Note:** Treatment with a macrolide or doxycycline (if age >8 years) is preferred due to higher prevalence of atypical pathogens in this age group

Ear, nose, throat, genitourinary tract, or skin/skin structure infections: Children >3 months and <40 kg: Oral:

Mild-to-moderate: 25 mg/kg/day in divided doses every 12 hours **or** 20 mg/kg/day in divided doses every 8 hours

Severe: 45 mg/kg/day in divided doses every 12 hours **or** 40 mg/kg/day in divided doses every 8 hours

Tonsillitis and/or pharyngitis: Children ≥12 years: Extended release tablet: 775 mg once daily

Lower respiratory tract infections: Children >3 months and <40 kg: Oral: 45 mg/kg/day in divided doses every 12 hours **or** 40 mg/kg/day in divided doses every 8 hours

Lyme disease: Children >3 months and <40 kg: Oral: 25-50 mg/kg/day divided every 8 hours (maximum: 500 mg)

Prophylaxis against infective endocarditis: Children >3 months and <40 kg: Oral: 50 mg/kg 1 hour before procedure. **Note:** American Heart Association (AHA) guidelines now recommend prophylaxis only in patients undergoing invasive procedures and in whom underlying cardiac conditions may predispose to a higher risk of adverse outcomes should infection occur. As of April 2007, routine prophylaxis for GI/GU procedures is no longer recommended by the AHA.

Renal Impairment

Use of certain dosage forms (eg, extended-release 775 mg tablet and immediate-release 875 mg tablet) should be avoided in patients with Cl_{cr} <30 mL/minute or patients requiring hemodialysis

Cl_{cr} 10-30 mL/minute: 250-500 mg every 12 hours

Cl_{cr} <10 mL/minute: 250-500 mg every 24 hours

Moderately dialyzable (20% to 50%) by hemodialysis or peritoneal dialysis; approximately 50 mg of amoxicillin per liter of filtrate is removed by continuous arteriovenous or venovenous hemofiltration. Dose as per Cl_{cr} <10 mL/minute guidelines.

Administration

Oral Administer around-the-clock to promote less variation in peak and trough serum levels. The appropriate amount of suspension may be mixed with formula, milk, fruit juice, water, ginger ale, or cold drinks; administer dose immediately after mixing.

Moxatag™ extended release tablet: Administer within 1 hour of finishing a meal.

Some penicillins (eg, carbenicillin, ticarcillin, and piperacillin) have been shown to inactivate aminoglycosides *in vitro*. This has been observed to a greater extent with tobramycin and gentamicin, while amikacin has shown greater stability against inactivation. Concurrent use of these agents may pose a risk of reduced antibacterial efficacy *in vivo*, particularly in the setting of profound renal impairment. However, definitive clinical evidence is lacking. If combination penicillin/aminoglycoside therapy is desired in a patient with renal dysfunction, separation of doses (if feasible), and routine monitoring of aminoglycoside levels, CBC, and clinical response should be considered.

Stability

Storage

Amoxil®: Oral suspension remains stable for 14 days at room temperature or if refrigerated (refrigeration preferred). Unit-dose antibiotic oral syringes are stable at room temperature for at least 72 hours (Tu, 1988).

Moxatag™: Store at 25°C (77°F); excursions permitted to 15°C to 30°C (59°F to 86°F).

Monitoring and Teaching Issues

Laboratory Monitoring Perform culture and sensitivity testing prior to initiating therapy.

Physical Assessment Assess culture and sensitivity report and patient allergy history prior to starting therapy. Monitor for opportunistic infection.

Patient Education Multiple daily doses should be taken at equal intervals around-the-clock. May be taken with milk, juice, or food. Maintain adequate hydration, unless instructed to restrict fluid intake. May cause nausea, vomiting, or diarrhea. Report respiratory difficulty; rash, itching, or hives; easy bruising or bleeding; persistent diarrhea; signs of opportunistic infection (eg, unusual sore throat, fever, chills, fatigue, thrush, vaginal discharge); CNS changes (confusion, agitation, dizziness, insomnia); or if condition being treated worsens or does not improve by time prescription is completed.

Dietary Considerations May be taken with food.

Moxatag™: Take within 1 hour of finishing a meal.

Geriatric Considerations Resistance to amoxicillin has been a problem in patients on frequent antibiotics or in nursing homes. Alternative antibiotics may be necessary in these populations. Consider renal function.

Breast-Feeding Considerations Very small amounts of amoxicillin are excreted in breast milk. The manufacturer recommends that caution be exercised when administering amoxicillin to nursing women. Nondose-related effects could include modification of bowel flora and allergic sensitization of the infant.

Pregnancy Considerations Adverse events have not been observed in animal studies; therefore, amoxicillin is classified as pregnancy category B. There is no documented increased risk of adverse pregnancy outcome or teratogenic effects caused by amoxicillin. It is the drug of choice for the treatment of chlamydial infections in pregnancy and for anthrax prophylaxis when penicillin susceptibility is documented.

Due to pregnancy-induced physiologic changes, amoxicillin clearance is increased during pregnancy resulting in lower concentrations and smaller AUCs. Oral ampicillin-class antibiotics are poorly-absorbed during labor.

Related Information

Antimicrobial Drugs of Choice *on page 2008*
Community-Acquired Pneumonia in Adults *on page 2021*
Helicobacter pylori Treatment *on page 2045*

Amoxicillin and Clavulanate Potassium

(a moks i SIL in & klav yoo LAN ate poe TASS ee um)

U.S. Brand Names Amoclan; Augmentin ES-600®; Augmentin XR®; Augmentin®

Index Terms Amoxicillin and Clavulanic Acid; Clavulanic Acid and Amoxicillin

Generic Availability (U.S.) Yes

Pharmacologic Category Antibiotic, Penicillin

Medication Safety Issues

Sound-alike/look-alike issues:

Augmentin® may be confused with amoxicillin, Azulfidine®

Pregnancy Risk Factor B

Lactation Enters breast milk/use caution

Use Treatment of otitis media, sinusitis, and infections caused by susceptible organisms involving the lower respiratory tract, skin and skin structure, and urinary tract; spectrum same as amoxicillin with additional coverage of beta-lactamase producing *B. catarrhalis*, *H. influenzae*, *N. gonorrhoeae*, and *S. aureus* (not MRSA). The expanded coverage of this combination makes it a useful alternative when amoxicillin resistance is present and patients cannot tolerate alternative treatments.

Available Dosage Forms

Powder for oral suspension: 200: Amoxicillin 200 mg and clavulanate potassium 28.5 mg per 5 mL; 400: Amoxicillin 400 mg and clavulanate potassium 57 mg per 5 mL; 600: Amoxicillin 600 mg and clavulanate potassium 42.9 mg per 5 mL

Amoclan:

200: Amoxicillin 200 mg and clavulanate potassium 28.5 mg per 5 mL
400: Amoxicillin 400 mg and clavulanate potassium 57 mg per 5 mL
600: Amoxicillin 600 mg and clavulanate potassium 42.9 mg per 5 mL

Augmentin®:

125: Amoxicillin 125 mg and clavulanate potassium 31.25 mg per 5 mL
250: Amoxicillin 250 mg and clavulanate potassium 62.5 mg per 5 mL

Augmentin ES-600®: Amoxicillin 600 mg and clavulanate potassium 42.9 mg per 5 mL

Tablet: 250: Amoxicillin 250 mg and clavulanate potassium 125 mg; 500: Amoxicillin 500 mg and clavulanate potassium 125 mg; 875: Amoxicillin 875 mg and clavulanate potassium 125 mg

Augmentin®:

500: Amoxicillin 500 mg and clavulanate potassium 125 mg
875: Amoxicillin 875 mg and clavulanate potassium 125 mg

Tablet, chewable: 200: Amoxicillin 200 mg and clavulanate potassium 28.5 mg; 400: Amoxicillin 400 mg and clavulanate potassium 57 mg

Tablet, extended release: Amoxicillin 1000 mg and clavulanate acid 62.5 mg

Augmentin XR®: 1000: Amoxicillin 1000 mg and clavulanate acid 62.5 mg

Dosing

Adult & Geriatric Note: Dose is based on the amoxicillin component; see "Augmentin® Product-Specific Considerations" table.

Susceptible infections: Children >40 kg and Adults: Oral: 250-500 mg every 8 hours or 875 mg every 12 hours

Augmentin® Product-Specific Considerations

Strength	Form	Consideration
125 mg	S	q8h dosing
	S	For adults having difficulty swallowing tablets, 125 mg/5 mL suspension may be substituted for 500 mg tablet.
200 mg	CT, S	q12h dosing
	CT	Contains phenylalanine
	S	For adults having difficulty swallowing tablets, 200 mg/5 mL suspension may be substituted for 875 mg tablet.
250 mg	S, T	q8h dosing
	T	Not for use in patients <40 kg
	S	For adults having difficulty swallowing tablets, 250 mg/5 mL suspension may be substituted for 500 mg tablet.
400 mg	CT, S	q12h dosing
	CT	Contains phenylalanine
	S	For adults having difficulty swallowing tablets, 400 mg/5 mL suspension may be substituted for 875 mg tablet.
500 mg	T	q8h or q12h dosing
600 mg	S	q12h dosing
		Not for use in adults or children ≥40 kg
		600 mg/5 mL suspension is not equivalent to or interchangeable with 200 mg/5 mL or 400 mg/5 mL due to differences in clavulanic acid.
875 mg	T	q12h dosing; not for use in Cl_{cr} <30 mL/minute
1000 mg	XR	q12h dosing
		Not for use in children <16 years of age
		Not interchangeable with two 500 mg tablets
		Not for use if Cl_{cr} <30 mL/minute or hemodialysis

Legend: CT = chewable tablet, S = suspension, T = tablet, XR = extended release.

Acute bacterial sinusitis: Oral: Extended release tablet: Two 1000 mg tablets every 12 hours for 10 days

Bite wounds (animal/human): Oral: 875 mg every 12 hours **or** 500 mg every 8 hours

Chronic obstructive pulmonary disease: Oral: 875 mg every 12 hours **or** 500 mg every 8 hours

Diabetic foot: Oral: Extended release tablet: Two 1000 mg tablets every 12 hours for 7-14 days

Diverticulitis, perirectal abscess: Oral: Extended release tablet: Two 1000 mg tablets every 12 hours for 7-10 days

Erysipelas: Oral: 875 mg every 12 hours **or** 500 mg every 8 hours

Febrile neutropenia: Oral: 875 mg every 12 hours

Pneumonia:

Aspiration: Oral: 875 mg every 12 hours

Community-acquired: Oral: Extended release tablet: Two 1000 mg tablets every 12 hours for 7-10 days

Pyelonephritis (acute, uncomplicated): Oral: 875 mg every 12 hours **or** 500 mg every 8 hours

Skin abscess: Oral: 875 mg every 12 hours

Pediatric Note: Dose is based on the amoxicillin component; see "Augmentin® Product-Specific Considerations" table.

Susceptible infections: Infants <3 months: Oral: 30 mg/kg/day divided every 12 hours using the 125 mg/5 mL suspension

Lower respiratory tract infections, severe infections, sinusitis: Children ≥3 months and <40 kg: Oral: 45 mg/kg/day divided every 12 hours **or** 40 mg/kg/day divided every 8 hours

Mild-to-moderate infections: Children ≥3 months and <40 kg: Oral: 25 mg/kg/day divided every 12 hours or 20 mg/kg/day divided every 8 hours

Otitis media (Augmentin ES-600®): Children ≥3 months and <40 kg: Oral: 90 mg/kg/day divided every 12 hours for 10 days in children with severe illness and when coverage for β-lactamase positive *H. influenzae* and *M. catarrhalis* is needed.

Children >40 kg: Refer to adult dosing.

Renal Impairment

Cl_{cr} <30 mL/minute: Do not use 875 mg tablet or extended release tablets.

Cl_{cr} 10-30 mL/minute: 250-500 mg every 12 hours

Cl_{cr} <10 mL/minute: 250-500 every 24 hours

Hemodialysis: Moderately dialyzable (20% to 50%)

250-500 mg every 24 hours; administer dose during and after dialysis. Do not use extended release tablets.

Peritoneal dialysis: Moderately dialyzable (20% to 50%)

Amoxicillin: Administer 250 mg every 12 hours

Clavulanic acid: Dose for Cl_{cr} <10 mL/minute

Continuous arteriovenous or venovenous hemofiltration effects:

Amoxicillin: ~50 mg of amoxicillin/L of filtrate is removed

Clavulanic acid: Dose for Cl_{cr} <10 mL/minute

Administration

Oral Administer around-the-clock to promote less variation in peak and trough serum levels. Administer with food to increase absorption and decrease stomach upset; shake suspension well before use. Extended release tablets should be administered with food.

Some penicillins (eg, carbenicillin, ticarcillin, and piperacillin) have been shown to inactivate aminoglycosides *in vitro*. This has been observed to a greater extent with tobramycin and gentamicin, while amikacin has shown greater stability against inactivation. Concurrent use of these agents may pose a risk of reduced antibacterial efficacy *in vivo*, particularly in the setting of profound renal impairment. However, definitive clinical evidence is lacking. If combination penicillin/aminoglycoside therapy is desired in a patient with renal dysfunction, separation of doses (if feasible), and routine monitoring of aminoglycoside levels, CBC, and clinical response should be considered.

Monitoring and Teaching Issues

Laboratory Monitoring Renal, hepatic, and hematologic function periodically with prolonged therapy. Perform culture and sensitivity testing prior to initiating therapy.

Physical Assessment See individual agents.

Patient Education See individual agents.

Related Information

Amoxicillin *on page 110*

Community-Acquired Pneumonia in Adults *on page 2021*

◆ **Amoxicillin and Clavulanic Acid** *see* Amoxicillin and Clavulanate Potassium *on page 113*

◆ **Amoxicillin, Clarithromycin, and Lansoprazole** *see* Lansoprazole, Amoxicillin, and Clarithromycin *on page 1064*

◆ **Amoxicillin Trihydrate** *see* Amoxicillin *on page 110*

◆ **Amoxil** *see* Amoxicillin *on page 110*

◆ **Amoxycillin** *see* Amoxicillin *on page 110*

◆ **Amphetamine and Dextroamphetamine** *see* Dextroamphetamine and Amphetamine *on page 510*

◆ **Amphotec®** *see* Amphotericin B Cholesteryl Sulfate Complex *on page 115*

Amphotericin B Cholesteryl Sulfate Complex

(am foe TER i sin bee kole LES te ril SUL fate KOM plecks)

U.S. Brand Names Amphotec®

Index Terms ABCD; Amphotericin B Colloidal Dispersion

Generic Availability (U.S.) No

Pharmacologic Category Antifungal Agent, Parenteral

Medication Safety Issues

Safety issues:

Lipid-based amphotericin formulations (Amphotec®) may be confused with conventional formulations (Amphocin®, Fungizone®)

Large overdoses have occurred when conventional formulations were dispensed inadvertently for lipid-based products. Single daily doses of conventional amphotericin formulation never exceed 1.5 mg/kg.

High alert medication: The Institute for Safe Medication Practices (ISMP) includes this medication among its list of drugs which have a heightened risk of causing significant patient harm when used in error.

Pregnancy Risk Factor B

Lactation Excretion in breast milk unknown/contraindicated

Use Treatment of invasive aspergillosis in patients who have failed amphotericin B deoxycholate treatment, or who have renal impairment or experience unacceptable toxicity which precludes treatment with amphotericin B deoxycholate in effective doses.

Unlabeled/Investigational Use Effective in patients with serious *Candida* species infections

Mechanism of Action/Effect Binds to ergosterol altering cell membrane permeability in susceptible fungi and causing leakage of cell components with subsequent cell death

Contraindications Hypersensitivity to amphotericin B or any component of the formulation

Warnings/Precautions Anaphylaxis has been reported with amphotericin B-containing drugs. If severe respiratory distress occurs, the infusion should be immediately discontinued. During the initial dosing, the drug should be administered under close clinical observation. Infusion reactions, sometimes severe, usually subside with continued therapy - manage with decreased rate of infusion and pretreatment with antihistamines/corticosteroids.

Drug Interactions

Avoid Concomitant Use

Avoid concomitant use of Amphotericin B Cholesteryl Sulfate Complex with any of the following: Gallium Nitrate

Decreased Effect

Amphotericin B Cholesteryl Sulfate Complex may decrease the levels/effects of: Saccharomyces boulardii

The levels/effects of Amphotericin B Cholesteryl Sulfate Complex may be decreased by: Antifungal Agents (Azole Derivatives, Systemic)

Increased Effect/Toxicity

Amphotericin B Cholesteryl Sulfate Complex may increase the levels/effects of: Aminoglycosides; Colistimethate; CycloSPORINE; CycloSPORINE (Systemic); Flucytosine; Gallium Nitrate

The levels/effects of Amphotericin B Cholesteryl Sulfate Complex may be increased by: Corticosteroids (Orally Inhaled); Corticosteroids (Systemic)

Adverse Reactions

>10%: Central nervous system: Chills, fever

1% to 10%:

Cardiovascular: Hypotension, tachycardia
Central nervous system: Headache
Dermatologic: Rash
Endocrine & metabolic: Hypokalemia, hypomagnesemia
Gastrointestinal: Nausea, diarrhea, abdominal pain
Hematologic: Thrombocytopenia
Hepatic: LFT change
Neuromuscular & skeletal: Rigors
Renal: Creatinine increased
Respiratory: Dyspnea

Note: Amphotericin B colloidal dispersion has an improved therapeutic index compared to conventional amphotericin B, and has been used safely in patients with amphotericin B-related nephrotoxicity; however, continued decline of renal function has occurred in some patients.

Pharmacodynamics/Kinetics

Half-Life Elimination 28-29 hours; prolonged with higher doses

Available Dosage Forms

Injection, powder for reconstitution:

Amphotec®: 50 mg, 100 mg

Dosing

Adult & Geriatric

Note: Premedication: For patients who experience chills, fever, hypotension, nausea, or other nonanaphylactic infusion-related immediate reactions, premedicate with the following drugs 30-60 minutes prior to drug administration: A nonsteroidal (eg, ibuprofen, choline magnesium trisalicylate) with or without diphenhydramine **or** acetaminophen with diphenhydramine **or** hydrocortisone 50-100 mg. If the patient experiences rigors during the infusion, meperidine may be administered.

Usual dosage: I.V.: 3-4 mg/kg/day (infusion of 1 mg/kg/hour); maximum: 7.5 mg/kg/day

A regimen of 6 mg/kg/day has been used for treatment of life-threatening invasive mold infections in immunocompromised patients; maximum: 7.5 mg/kg/day

Initially infuse at 1 mg/kg/hour. Rate of infusion may be increased with subsequent doses to 3 mg/kg/hour as patient tolerance allows. Treatment should continue as patient tolerance allows, until complete resolution of microbiologic and clinical evidence of fungal disease.

Pediatric Refer to adult dosing.

Administration

I.V. For a patient who experiences chills, fever, hypotension, nausea, or other nonanaphylactic infusion-related reactions, premedicate with the following drugs 30-60 minutes prior to drug administration: A nonsteroidal (eg, ibuprofen, choline magnesium trisalicylate) with or without diphenhydramine **or** acetaminophen with diphenhydramine **or** hydrocortisone 50-100 mg. If the patient experiences rigors during the infusion, meperidine may be administered. If severe respiratory distress occurs, the infusion should be immediately discontinued.

Stability

Reconstitution Reconstitute 50 mg and 100 mg vials with 10 mL and 20 mL of SWI, respectively. The reconstituted vials contain 5 mg/mL of amphotericin B. Shake the vial gently by hand until all solid particles have dissolved. Further dilute amphotericin B colloidal dispersion with D_5W.

Storage Store intact vials under refrigeration. After reconstitution, the solution should be refrigerated at 2°C to 8°C (36°F to 46°F) and used within 24 hours. Concentrations of 0.1-2 mg/mL in D_5W are stable for 14 days at 4°C and 23°C if protected from light, however, due to the occasional formation of subvisual particles, solutions should be used within 48 hours.

Monitoring and Teaching Issues

Laboratory Monitoring Monitor serum electrolytes (especially potassium and magnesium), liver function, and CBC. Perform culture and sensitivity testing prior to initiating therapy.

Physical Assessment Assess culture and sensitivity report and patient's previous exposure to amphotericin B prior to starting therapy. Assess potential for interactions with other nephrotoxic drugs patient may be taking. Patient should be monitored closely for infusion related reactions (eg, anaphylaxis, chills, fever, nausea, vomiting, rigors, hypotension, acute respiratory distress) and cardiopulmonary resuscitation should be available. If acute respiratory distress occurs, infusion should be stopped and prescriber notified.

Patient Education This medication can only be administered by infusion and therapy may last several weeks. You will be monitored closely during and after infusion; report immediately any pain or swelling at infusion site, chills, nausea, chest pain, swelling of face or mouth, difficulty breathing, muscle cramping, acute anxiety, or other infusion reactions. Maintain adequate hydration, unless instructed to restrict fluid intake. May cause postural hypotension, nausea, or vomiting. Report chest pain or palpitations; CNS disturbances; skin rash; unusual chills or fever; persistent nausea, vomiting, or abdominal pain; sore throat; excessive fatigue; swelling of extremities or unusual weight gain; difficulty breathing; pain at infusion site; muscle cramping; or weakness.

Geriatric Considerations The pharmacokinetics and dosing of amphotericin have not been studied in the elderly. It appears that use is similar to young adults. Caution should be exercised and renal function and desired effect monitored closely.

Breast-Feeding Considerations Due to limited data, consider discontinuing nursing during therapy.

Additional Information Controlled trials which compare the original formulation of amphotericin B to the newer liposomal formulations (ie, Amphotec®) are lacking. Thus, comparative data discussing differences among the formulations should be interpreted cautiously. Although the risk of nephrotoxicity and infusion-related adverse effects may be less with Amphotec®, the efficacy profiles of Amphotec® and the original amphotericin formulation are comparable. Consequently, Amphotec® should be restricted to those patients who cannot tolerate or fail a standard amphotericin B formulation.

◆ **Amphotericin B Colloidal Dispersion** *see* Amphotericin B Cholesteryl Sulfate Complex *on page 115*

Amphotericin B (Conventional) (am foe TER i sin bee con VEN sha nal)

Index Terms Amphotericin B Deoxycholate; Amphotericin B Desoxycholate

Generic Availability (U.S.) Yes

Pharmacologic Category Antifungal Agent, Parenteral

Medication Safety Issues

Safety issues:

Conventional amphotericin formulations (Amphocin®, Fungizone®) may be confused with lipid-based formulations (AmBisome®, Abelcet®, Amphotec®).

Large overdoses have occurred when conventional formulations were dispensed inadvertently for lipid-based products. Single daily doses of conventional amphotericin formulation never exceed 1.5 mg/kg.

High alert medication: The Institute for Safe Medication Practices (ISMP) includes this medication (intrathecal administration) among its list of drugs which have a heightened risk of causing significant patient harm when used in error.

Pregnancy Risk Factor B

Lactation Excretion in breast milk unknown/contraindicated

Use Treatment of severe systemic and central nervous system infections caused by susceptible fungi such as *Candida* species, *Histoplasma capsulatum*, *Cryptococcus neoformans*, *Aspergillus* species, *Blastomyces dermatitidis*, *Torulopsis glabrata*, and *Coccidioides immitis*; fungal peritonitis; irrigant for bladder fungal infections; used in fungal infection in patients with bone marrow transplantation, amebic meningoencephalitis, ocular aspergillosis (intraocular injection), candidal cystitis (bladder irrigation), chemoprophylaxis (low-dose I.V.), immunocompromised patients at risk of aspergillosis (intranasal/nebulized), refractory meningitis (intrathecal), coccidioidal arthritis (intra-articular/I.M.).

Low-dose amphotericin B has been administered after bone marrow transplantation to reduce the risk of invasive fungal disease.

Available Dosage Forms

Injection, powder for reconstitution: 50 mg

Dosing

Adult & Geriatric Note: Premedication: For patients who experience infusion-related immediate reactions, premedicate with the following drugs 30-60 minutes prior to drug administration: NSAID (with or without diphenhydramine) **or** acetaminophen with diphenhydramine **or** hydrocortisone 50-100 mg. If the patient experiences rigors during the infusion, meperidine may be administered.

Test dose: I.V.: 1 mg infused over 20-30 minutes. Many clinicians believe a test dose is unnecessary.

Susceptible fungal infections: I.V.: Adults: 0.05-1.5 mg/kg/day; 1-1.5 mg/kg over 4-6 hours every other day may be given once therapy is established; aspergillosis, rhinocerebral mucormycosis, often require 1-1.5 mg/kg/day; do not exceed 1.5 mg/kg/day

Aspergillosis, disseminated: I.V.: 0.6-0.7 mg/kg/day for 3-6 months

Bone marrow transplantation (prophylaxis): I.V.: Low-dose amphotericin B 0.1-0.25 mg/kg/day has been administered after bone marrow transplantation to reduce the risk of invasive fungal disease.

Candidemia (neutropenic or non-neutropenic): I.V.: 0.5-1 mg/kg/day until 14 days after first negative blood culture and resolution of signs and symptoms (Pappas, 2009)

Candidiasis, chronic, disseminated: I.V.: 0.5-0.7 mg/kg/day for 3-6 months and resolution of radiologic lesions (Pappas, 2009)

Dematiaceous fungi: I.V.: 0.7 mg/kg/day in combination with an azole

Endocarditis: I.V.: 0.6-1 mg/kg/day (with or without flucytosine) for 6 weeks after valve replacement; **Note:** If isolates susceptible and/or clearance demonstrated, guidelines recommend step-down to fluconazole; also for long-term suppression therapy if valve replacement is not possible (Pappas, 2009)

Endophthalmitis, fungal:

Intravitreal (unlabeled use): 10 mcg in 0.1 mL (in conjunction with systemic therapy)

I.V.: 0.7-1 mg/kg/day (with or without flucytosine) for at least 4-6 weeks (Pappas, 2009)

Esophageal candidiasis: I.V.: 0.3-0.7 mg/kg/day for 14-21 days after clinical improvement (Pappas, 2009)

Histoplasmosis: Chronic, severe pulmonary or disseminated: I.V.: 0.5-1 mg/kg/day for 7 days, then 0.8 mg/kg every other day (or 3 times/week) until total dose of 10-15 mg/kg; may continue itraconazole as suppressive therapy (lifelong for immunocompromised patients)

Meningitis:

Candidal: I.V.: 0.7-1 mg/kg/day (with or without flucytosine) for at least 4 weeks; **Note:** Liposomal amphotericin favored by IDSA guidelines based on decreased risk of nephrotoxicity and potentially better CNS penetration (Pappas, 2009)

Cryptococcal or Coccidioides: I.T.: Initial: 0.01-0.05 mg as single daily dose; may increase daily in increments of 0.025-0.1 mg as tolerated (maximum: 1.5 mg/day; most patients will tolerate a maximum dose of ~0.5 mg/treatment). Once titration to a maximum tolerated dose is achieved, that dose is administered daily. Once CSF improvement noted, may decrease frequency on a weekly basis (eg, 5 times/week, then 3 times/week, then 2 times/week, then once weekly, then once every other week, then once every 2 weeks, etc) until administration occurs once every 6 weeks. Typically, concurrent oral azole therapy is maintained (Stevens, 2001). **Note:** IDSA notes that the use of I.T. amphotericin for cryptococcal meningitis is generally discouraged and rarely necessary (Perfect, 2010).

Histoplasma: I.V.: 0.5-1 mg/kg/day for 7 days, then 0.8 mg/kg every other day (or 3 times/week) for 3 months total duration; follow with fluconazole suppressive therapy for up to 12 months

Meningoencephalitis, cryptococcal (Perfect, 2010): I.V.:

HIV positive: Induction: 0.7-1 mg/kg/day (plus flucytosine 100 mg/kg/day) for 2 weeks, then change to oral fluconazole for at least 8 weeks; alternatively, amphotericin (0.7-1 mg/kg/day) may be continued uninterrupted for 4-6 weeks; maintenance: amphotericin 1 mg/kg/week for ≥1 year may be considered, but inferior to use of azoles

HIV negative: Induction: 0.7-1 mg/kg/day (plus flucytosine 100 mg/kg/day) for 2 weeks (low-risk patients), ≥4 weeks (non-low-risk, but without neurologic complication, immunosuppression, underlying disease, and negative CSF culture at 2 weeks), >6 weeks (neurologic complication or patients intolerant of flucytosine) Follow with azole consolidation/maintenance treatment.

Oropharyngeal candidiasis: I.V.: 0.3 mg/kg/day for 7-14 days (Pappas, 2009)

Osteoarticular candidiasis: I.V.: 0.5-1 mg/kg/day for several weeks, followed by fluconazole for 6-12 months (osteomyelitis) or 6 weeks (septic arthritis) (Pappas, 2009)

Penicillium marneffei: I.V.: 0.6 mg/kg/day for 2 weeks

Pneumonia: Cryptococcal (mild-to-moderate): I.V.:

HIV positive: 0.5-1 mg/kg/day

HIV negative: 0.5-0.7 mg/kg/day (plus flucytosine) for 2 weeks

Sporotrichosis: Pulmonary, meningeal, osteoarticular or disseminated: I.V.: Total dose of 1-2 g, then change to oral itraconazole or fluconazole for suppressive therapy

Urinary tract candidiasis (Pappas, 2009):

Fungus balls: I.V.: 0.5-0.7 mg/kg/day with or without flucytosine 25 mg/kg 4 times daily

Pyelonephritis: I.V.: 0.5-0.7 mg/kg/day with or without flucytosine 25 mg/kg 4 times daily for 2 weeks

Symptomatic cystitis: I.V.: 0.3-0.6 mg/kg/day for 1-7 days

Bladder irrigation: Irrigate with 50 mcg/mL solution instilled periodically or continuously for 5-10 days or until cultures are clear for fluconazole-resistant *Candida*

Pediatric Note: Premedication: For patients who experience infusion-related immediate reactions, premedicate with the following drugs 30-60 minutes prior to drug administration: NSAID (with or without diphenhydramine) **or** acetaminophen with diphenhydramine **or** hydrocortisone 50-100 mg. If the patient experiences rigors during the infusion, meperidine may be administered.

Test dose: I.V.: Infants and Children: 0.1 mg/kg/dose to a maximum of 1 mg; infuse over 30-60 minutes. Many clinicians believe a test dose is unnecessary.

Susceptible fungal infections: I.V.: Infants and Children: Maintenance dose: 0.25-1 mg/kg/day given once daily; infuse over 2-6 hours. Once therapy has been established, amphotericin B can be administered on an every-other-day basis at 1-1.5 mg/kg/dose; cumulative dose: 1.5-2 g over 6-10 weeks

Note: Duration of therapy varies with nature of infection: Usual duration is 4-12 weeks or cumulative dose of 1-4 g.

Indication-specific dosing: Infants and Children:

Aspergillosis (HIV-exposed/-positive): I.V.: 1-1.5 mg/kg/day once daily (CDC, 2009)

Candidiasis (HIV-exposed/-positive):

Invasive: I.V.: 0.5-1.5 mg/kg/day once daily (CDC, 2009)

Esophageal: I.V.: 0.3-0.5 mg/kg/day once daily (CDC, 2009)

Oropharyngeal, refractory: I.V.: 0.3-0.5 mg/kg/day (CDC, 2009)

Coccidioidomycosis (HIV-exposed/-positive): I.V.: 0.5-1 mg/kg/day (CDC, 2009)

***Cryptococcus,* CNS disease (HIV-exposed/-positive):** I.V.: 0.7-1 mg/kg/day plus flucytosine; **Note:** Minimum 2 week induction followed by consolidation and chronic suppressive therapy; may increase amphotericin dose to 1.5 mg/kg/day if flucytosine is not tolerated.

***Cryptococcus*, Disseminated (non-CNS disease) or severe pulmonary disease (HIV-exposed/-positive):** I.V.: 0.7-1 mg/kg/day once daily with or without flucytosine

Histoplasma, CNS or severe disseminated: I.V.: 1 mg/kg/day once daily (CDC, 2009)

Renal Impairment

If renal dysfunction is due to the drug, the daily total can be decreased by 50% or the dose can be given every other day. I.V. therapy may take several months.

Poorly dialyzed; no supplemental dose is necessary when using hemo- or peritoneal dialysis or continuous renal replacement therapy (CRRT).

Administration in dialysate: 1-2 mg/L of peritoneal dialysis fluid either with or without low-dose I.V. amphotericin B (a total dose of 2-10 mg/kg given over 7-14 days). Precipitate may form in ionic dialysate solutions.

Administration

I.V. May be infused over 4-6 hours. For a patient who experiences chills, fever, hypotension, nausea, or other nonanaphylactic infusion-related reactions, premedicate with the following drugs 30-60 minutes prior to drug administration: A nonsteroidal (eg, ibuprofen, choline magnesium trisalicylate) with or without diphenhydramine **or** acetaminophen with diphenhydramine **or** hydrocortisone 50-100 mg. If the patient experiences rigors during the infusion, meperidine may be administered. Bolus infusion of normal saline immediately preceding, or immediately preceding and following amphotericin B may reduce drug-induced nephrotoxicity. Risk of nephrotoxicity increases with amphotericin B doses >1 mg/kg/day. Infusion of admixtures more concentrated than 0.25 mg/mL should be limited to patients absolutely requiring volume contraction.

Monitoring and Teaching Issues

Laboratory Monitoring BUN and serum creatinine levels should be determined every other day when therapy is increased and at least weekly thereafter. Monitor serum electrolytes (especially potassium and magnesium), liver function, and CBC. Perform culture and sensitivity testing prior to initiating therapy.

Physical Assessment Assess culture and sensitivity report and patient's previous exposure to amphotericin B prior to starting therapy. Assess potential for interactions with other nephrotoxic drugs patient may be taking. Patient should be monitored closely for infusion-related reactions (eg, anaphylaxis, chills, fever, nausea, vomiting, rigors, hypotension, acute respiratory distress) and cardiopulmonary resuscitation should be available. If acute respiratory distress occurs, infusion should be stopped and prescriber notified.

Patient Education I.V.: You will be monitored closely during and after infusion; report immediately any pain or swelling at infusion site, chills, nausea, chest pain, swelling of face or mouth, difficulty breathing, muscle cramping, acute anxiety, or other infusion reactions. May cause nausea, vomiting, anorexia, generalized muscle or joint pain, or hypotension. Report severe muscle cramping or weakness; chest pain or palpitations; CNS disturbances; skin rash; change in urinary patterns or difficulty voiding; unusual bruising or bleeding; or pain, redness, or swelling at infusion site.

- **Amphotericin B Deoxycholate** *see* Amphotericin B (Conventional) *on page 117*
- **Amphotericin B Desoxycholate** *see* Amphotericin B (Conventional) *on page 117*

Amphotericin B (Lipid Complex) (am foe TER i sin bee LIP id KOM pleks)

U.S. Brand Names Abelcet®

Index Terms ABLC

Generic Availability (U.S.) No

Pharmacologic Category Antifungal Agent, Parenteral

Medication Safety Issues

Safety issues:

Lipid-based amphotericin formulations (Abelcet®) may be confused with conventional formulations (Amphocin®, Fungizone®)

Large overdoses have occurred when conventional formulations were dispensed inadvertently for lipid-based products. Single daily doses of conventional amphotericin formulation never exceed 1.5 mg/kg.

High alert medication: The Institute for Safe Medication Practices (ISMP) includes this medication among its list of drugs which have a heightened risk of causing significant patient harm when used in error.

Pregnancy Risk Factor B

Lactation Enters breast milk/contraindicated

Use Treatment of aspergillosis or any type of progressive fungal infection in patients who are refractory to or intolerant of conventional amphotericin B therapy

Unlabeled/Investigational Use Effective in patients with serious *Candida* species infections

Mechanism of Action/Effect Mechanism is like amphotericin - includes binding to ergosterol altering cell membrane permeability in susceptible fungi and causing leakage of cell components with subsequent cell death.

Contraindications Hypersensitivity to amphotericin or any component of the formulation

Warnings/Precautions Anaphylaxis has been reported with amphotericin B-containing drugs. If severe respiratory distress occurs, the infusion should be immediately discontinued. During the initial dosing, the drug should be administered under close clinical observation. Acute reactions (including fever and chills) may occur 1-2 hours after starting an intravenous infusion. These reactions are usually more common with the first few doses and generally diminish with subsequent doses.

Drug Interactions

Avoid Concomitant Use

Avoid concomitant use of Amphotericin B (Lipid Complex) with any of the following: Gallium Nitrate

Decreased Effect

Amphotericin B (Lipid Complex) may decrease the levels/effects of: Saccharomyces boulardii

The levels/effects of Amphotericin B (Lipid Complex) may be decreased by: Antifungal Agents (Azole Derivatives, Systemic)

Increased Effect/Toxicity

Amphotericin B (Lipid Complex) may increase the levels/effects of: Aminoglycosides; Colistimethate; CycloSPORINE; CycloSPORINE (Systemic); Flucytosine; Gallium Nitrate

The levels/effects of Amphotericin B (Lipid Complex) may be increased by: Corticosteroids (Orally Inhaled); Corticosteroids (Systemic)

Lab Interactions Increased BUN (S), serum creatinine, alkaline phosphate, bilirubin; decreased magnesium, potassium (S)

Adverse Reactions Nephrotoxicity and infusion-related hyperpyrexia, rigor, and chilling are reduced relative to amphotericin deoxycholate.

>10%:

Central nervous system: Chills, fever
Renal: Serum creatinine increased
Miscellaneous: Multiple organ failure

1% to 10%:

Cardiovascular: Hypotension, cardiac arrest
Central nervous system: Headache, pain
Dermatologic: Rash
Endocrine & metabolic: Bilirubinemia, hypokalemia, acidosis
Gastrointestinal: Nausea, vomiting, diarrhea, gastrointestinal hemorrhage, abdominal pain
Renal: Renal failure
Respiratory: Respiratory failure, dyspnea, pneumonia

Pharmacodynamics/Kinetics

Half-Life Elimination ~24 hours

Excretion Clearance: Increases with higher doses (5 mg/kg/day): 400 mL/hour/kg

Available Dosage Forms

Injection, suspension [preservative free]:

Abelcet®: 5 mg/mL (20 mL)

Dosing

Adult & Geriatric Note: Premedication: For patients who experience infusion-related immediate reactions, premedicate with the following drugs 30-60 minutes prior to drug administration: A nonsteroidal anti-inflammatory agent ± diphenhydramine **or** acetaminophen with diphenhydramine **or** hydrocortisone 50-100 mg. If the patient experiences rigors during the infusion, meperidine may be administered.

Usual dosage range: I.V.: 2.5-5 mg/kg/day as a single infusion

Pediatric Note: Premedication: For patients who experience infusion-related immediate reactions, premedicate with the following drugs 30-60 minutes prior to drug administration: A nonsteroidal anti-inflammatory agent ± diphenhydramine **or** acetaminophen with diphenhydramine **or** hydrocortisone 50-100 mg. If the patient experiences rigors during the infusion, meperidine may be administered.

Usual dosage range: I.V.: 2.5-5 mg/kg/day as a single infusion

Aspergillosis, coccidioidomycosis (non-CNS), *Cryptococcus* (non-CNS), or invasive candidiasis (HIV-exposed/-positive): I.V.: 5 mg/kg/dose once daily; may consider addition of flucytosine for severe candidal or cryptococcal disease (CDC, 2009)

Renal Impairment The effects of renal impairment on drug pharmacokinetics or pharmacodynamics are currently unknown. The dose of amphotericin B lipid complex may be adjusted or drug administration may have to be interrupted in patients with acute kidney dysfunction to reduce the magnitude of renal impairment.

Hemodialysis: Supplemental dose is not necessary.
Peritoneal dialysis: Supplemental dose is not necessary.
Continuous renal replacement therapy (CRRT): No supplemental dosage necessary

Administration

I.V. For patients who experience nonanaphylactic infusion-related reactions, premedicate 30-60 minutes prior to drug administration with a nonsteroidal anti-inflammatory agent ± diphenhydramine **or** acetaminophen with diphenhydramine **or** hydrocortisone 50-100 mg. If the patient experiences rigors during the infusion, meperidine may be administered.

Administer at an infusion rate of 2.5 mg/kg/hour (over 2 hours). Invert infusion container several times prior to administration and every 2 hours during infusion if it exceeds 2 hours.

Stability

Reconstitution Shake vial gently to disperse yellow sediment at bottom of container. Dilute with D_5W to 1-2 mg/mL.

Storage Intact vials should be stored at 2°C to 8°C (35°F to 46°F); do not freeze. Protect intact vials from exposure to light. Solutions for infusion are stable for 48 hours under refrigeration and 6 hours at room temperature. Protect from light. Following reconstitution, protect from light.

Monitoring and Teaching Issues

Laboratory Monitoring BUN and serum creatinine levels should be determined every other day while therapy is increased and at least weekly thereafter. Monitor serum electrolytes (especially potassium and magnesium), liver function, and CBC. Perform culture and sensitivity testing prior to initiating therapy.

Physical Assessment Assess culture and sensitivity report and patient's previous exposure to amphotericin B prior to starting therapy. Assess potential for interactions with other nephrotoxic drugs patient may be taking. Patient should be monitored closely for infusion related reactions (eg, anaphylaxis, chills, fever, nausea, vomiting, rigors, hypotension, acute respiratory distress) and cardiopulmonary resuscitation should be available. If acute respiratory distress occurs, infusion should be stopped and prescriber notified.

Patient Education This medication can only be administered by infusion and therapy may last several weeks. May cause postural hypotension, nausea, or vomiting. Report chest pain or palpitations; CNS disturbances; skin rash; chills or fever; persistent nausea, vomiting, or abdominal pain; sore throat; excessive fatigue; swelling of extremities or unusual weight gain; respiratory difficulty; pain at infusion site; or muscle cramping or weakness.

Geriatric Considerations The pharmacokinetics and dosing of amphotericin have not been studied in elderly. It appears that use is similar to young adults; caution should be exercised and renal function and desired effect monitored closely.

Breast-Feeding Considerations Due to limited data, consider discontinuing nursing during therapy.

Additional Information As a modification of dimyristoyl phosphatidylcholine:dimyristoyl phosphatidylglycerol 7:3 (DMPC:DMPG) liposome, amphotericin B lipid-complex has a higher drug to lipid ratio and the concentration of amphotericin B is 33 M. ABLC is a ribbon-like structure, not a liposome.

Controlled trials which compare the original formulation of amphotericin B to the newer liposomal formulations (ie, Abelcet®) are lacking. Thus, comparative data discussing differences among the formulations should be interpreted cautiously. Although the risk of nephrotoxicity and infusion-related adverse effects may be less with Abelcet®, the efficacy profiles of Abelcet® and the original amphotericin formulation are comparable. Consequently, Abelcet® should be restricted to those patients who cannot tolerate or fail a standard amphotericin B formulation.

Amphotericin B (Liposomal) (am foe TER i sin bee lye po SO mal)

U.S. Brand Names AmBisome®

Index Terms L-AmB

Generic Availability (U.S.) No

Pharmacologic Category Antifungal Agent, Parenteral

Medication Safety Issues

Safety issues:

Lipid-based amphotericin formulations (AmBisome®) may be confused with conventional formulations (Amphocin®, Fungizone®) or with other lipid-based amphotericin formulations (Abelcet®, Amphotec®)

Large overdoses have occurred when conventional formulations were dispensed inadvertently for lipid-based products. Single daily doses of conventional amphotericin formulation never exceed 1.5 mg/kg.

High alert medication: The Institute for Safe Medication Practices (ISMP) includes this medication among its list of drugs which have a heightened risk of causing significant patient harm when used in error.

Pregnancy Risk Factor B

Lactation Excretion in breast milk unknown/not recommended

Use Empirical therapy for presumed fungal infection in febrile, neutropenic patients; treatment of patients with *Aspergillus* species, *Candida* species, and/or *Cryptococcus* species infections refractory to amphotericin B desoxycholate (conventional amphotericin), or in patients where renal impairment or unacceptable toxicity precludes the use of amphotericin B desoxycholate; treatment of cryptococcal meningitis in HIV-infected patients; treatment of visceral leishmaniasis

Unlabeled/Investigational Use Treatment of systemic *Histoplasmosis* infection

Mechanism of Action/Effect Amphotericin B, the active ingredient, binds to the sterol component of a cell membrane leading to alterations in cell permeability and cell death. While amphotericin B has a higher affinity for the ergosterol component of the fungal cell membrane, it can also bind to the cholesterol component of the mammalian cell leading to cytotoxicity. AmBisome®, the liposomal preparation of amphotericin B, has been shown to penetrate the cell wall of both extracellular and intracellular forms of susceptible fungi.

Contraindications Hypersensitivity to amphotericin B deoxycholate or any component of the formulation

Warnings/Precautions Patients should be under close clinical observation during initial dosing. As with other amphotericin B-containing products, anaphylaxis has been reported. Facilities for cardiopulmonary resuscitation should be available during administration. Acute infusion reactions (including fever and chills) may occur 1-2 hours after starting infusions; reactions are more common with the first few doses and generally diminish with subsequent doses. Immediately discontinue infusion if severe respiratory distress occurs; the patient should not receive further infusions. Concurrent use of amphotericin B with other nephrotoxic drugs may enhance the potential for drug-induced renal toxicity. Concurrent use with antineoplastic

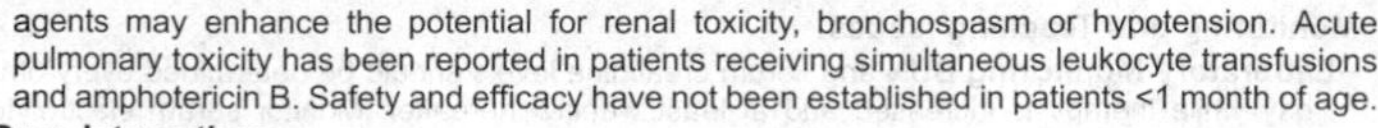

agents may enhance the potential for renal toxicity, bronchospasm or hypotension. Acute pulmonary toxicity has been reported in patients receiving simultaneous leukocyte transfusions and amphotericin B. Safety and efficacy have not been established in patients <1 month of age.

Drug Interactions

Avoid Concomitant Use

Avoid concomitant use of Amphotericin B (Liposomal) with any of the following: Gallium Nitrate

Decreased Effect

Amphotericin B (Liposomal) may decrease the levels/effects of: Saccharomyces boulardii

The levels/effects of Amphotericin B (Liposomal) may be decreased by: Antifungal Agents (Azole Derivatives, Systemic)

Increased Effect/Toxicity

Amphotericin B (Liposomal) may increase the levels/effects of: Aminoglycosides; Colistimethate; CycloSPORINE; CycloSPORINE (Systemic); Flucytosine; Gallium Nitrate

The levels/effects of Amphotericin B (Liposomal) may be increased by: Corticosteroids (Orally Inhaled); Corticosteroids (Systemic)

Adverse Reactions Percentage of adverse reactions is dependent upon population studied and may vary with respect to premedications and underlying illness. Incidence of decreased renal function and infusion-related events are lower than rates observed with amphotericin B deoxycholate.

>10%:

- Cardiovascular: Peripheral edema (15%), edema (12% to 14%), tachycardia (9% to 19%), hypotension (7% to 14%), hypertension (8% to 20%), chest pain (8% to 12%), hypervolemia (8% to 12%)
- Central nervous system: Chills (29% to 48%), insomnia (17% to 22%), headache (9% to 20%), anxiety (7% to 14%), pain (14%), confusion (9% to 13%)
- Dermatologic: Rash (5% to 25%), pruritus (11%)
- Endocrine & metabolic: Hypokalemia (31% to 51%), hypomagnesemia (15% to 50%), hyperglycemia (8% to 23%), hypocalcemia (5% to 18%), hyponatremia (9% to 12%)
- Gastrointestinal: Nausea (16% to 40%), vomiting (11% to 32%), diarrhea (11% to 30%), abdominal pain (7% to 20%), constipation (15%), anorexia (10% to 14%)
- Hematologic: Anemia (27% to 48%), blood transfusion reaction (9% to 18%), leukopenia (15% to 17%), thrombocytopenia (6% to 13%)
- Hepatic: Alkaline phosphatase increased (7% to 22%), bilirubinemia (≤18%), ALT increased (15%), AST increased (13%), liver function tests abnormal (not specified) (4% to 13%)
- Local: Phlebitis (9% to 11%)
- Neuromuscular & skeletal: Weakness (6% to 13%), back pain (12%)
- Renal: Nephrotoxicity (14% to 47%), creatinine increased (18% to 40%), BUN increased (7% to 21%), hematuria (14%)
- Respiratory: Dyspnea (18% to 23%), lung disorder (14% to 18%), cough (2% to 18%), epistaxis (9% to 15%), pleural effusion (13%), rhinitis (11%)
- Miscellaneous: Infusion reactions (4% to 21%), sepsis (7% to 14%), infection (11% to 13%)

2% to 10%:

- Cardiovascular: Arrhythmia, atrial fibrillation, bradycardia, cardiac arrest, cardiomegaly, facial swelling, flushing, postural hypotension, valvular heart disease, vascular disorder, vasodilation
- Central nervous system: Agitation, abnormal thinking, coma, depression, dysesthesia, dizziness (7% to 9%), hallucinations, malaise, nervousness, seizure, somnolence
- Dermatologic: Alopecia, bruising, cellulitis, dry skin, maculopapular rash, petechia, purpura, skin discoloration, skin disorder, skin ulcer, urticaria, vesiculobullous rash
- Endocrine & metabolic: Acidosis, fluid overload, hypernatremia (4%), hyperchloremia, hyperkalemia, hypermagnesemia, hyperphosphatemia, hypophosphatemia, hypoproteinemia, lactate dehydrogenase increased, nonprotein nitrogen increased
- Gastrointestinal: Abdomen enlarged, amylase increased, dyspepsia, dysphagia, eructation, fecal incontinence, flatulence, gastrointestinal hemorrhage (10%), hematemesis, hemorrhoids, gum/oral hemorrhage, ileus, mucositis, rectal disorder, stomatitis, ulcerative stomatitis, xerostomia
- Genitourinary: Vaginal hemorrhage
- Hematologic: Coagulation disorder, hemorrhage, prothrombin decreased
- Hepatic: Hepatocellular damage, hepatomegaly, veno-occlusive liver disease
- Local: Injection site inflammation
- Neuromuscular & skeletal: Arthralgia, bone pain, dystonia, myalgia, neck pain, paresthesia, rigors, tremor
- Ocular: Conjunctivitis, dry eyes, eye hemorrhage
- Renal: Abnormal renal function, acute renal failure, dysuria, renal failure, toxic nephropathy, urinary incontinence
- Respiratory: Asthma, atelectasis, dry nose, hemoptysis, hyperventilation, pharyngitis, pneumonia, pulmonary edema, respiratory alkalosis, respiratory insufficiency, respiratory failure, sinusitis, hypoxia (6% to 8%)
- Miscellaneous: Allergic reaction, cell-mediated immunological reaction, flu-like syndrome, graft-versus-host disease, herpes simplex, hiccup, procedural complication (8% to 10%), diaphoresis (7%)

Pharmacodynamics/Kinetics

Half-Life Elimination Terminal: 174 hours

Available Dosage Forms

Injection, powder for reconstitution:

AmBisome®: 50 mg

Dosing

Adult & Geriatric

Usual dosage range: I.V.: 3-6 mg/kg/day; **Note:** Higher doses (15 mg/kg/day) have been used clinically (Walsh, 2001)

Note: Premedication: For patients who experience nonanaphylactic infusion-related immediate reactions, premedicate with the following drugs 30-60 minutes prior to drug administration: A nonsteroidal anti-inflammatory agent ± diphenhydramine; **or** acetaminophen with diphenhydramine; **or** hydrocortisone 50-100 mg. If the patient experiences rigors during the infusion, meperidine may be administered.

Indication-specific dosing: I.V.:

Cryptococcal meningitis (HIV-positive): 6 mg/kg/day or 4-6 mg/kg/day in combination with addition of oral flucytosine 25 mg/kg 4 times daily (unlabeled combination; (unlabeled combination; CDC, 2009)

Empiric candidiasis therapy: 3-5 mg/kg/day (Pappas, 2009)

Endocarditis: I.V.: 3-5 mg/kg/day (with or without flucytosine 25 mg/kg 4 times daily) for 6 weeks after valve replacement; **Note:** If isolates susceptible and/or clearance demonstrated, guidelines recommend step-down to fluconazole; also for long-term suppression therapy if valve replacement is not possible (Pappas, 2009)

Fungal sinusitis: Limited data in immunocompromised patients have shown efficacy with 3-10 mg/kg/day (Barron, 2005; Pagano, 2004; Rokicka, 2006). **Note:** An azole antifungal is recommended if causative organism is *Aspergillus* spp or *Pseudallescheria boydii* (*Scedosporium* sp).

Osteoarticular candidiasis: I.V.: 3-5 mg/kg/day for several weeks, followed by fluconazole for 6-12 months (osteomyelitis) or 6 weeks (septic arthritis)

Systemic fungal infections *(Aspergillus, Candida, Cryptococcus):* 3-5 mg/kg/day

General invasive Candidal disease: 3-5 mg/kg/day with oral flucytosine 25 mg/kg 4 times daily (unlabeled combination; Pappas, 2009)

Candidal meningitis: 3-5 mg/kg/day with oral flucytosine 25 mg/kg 4 times daily (unlabeled combination; Pappas, 2009)

Histoplasmosis (unlabeled use): 3-5 mg/kg/day (CDC, 2009)

Visceral leishmaniasis:

Immunocompetent: 3 mg/kg/day on days 1-5, and 3 mg/kg/day on days 14 and 21; a repeat course may be given in patients who do not achieve parasitic clearance

Note: Alternate regimen of 2 mg/kg/day for 5 days has been reportedly effective.

Immunocompromised: 4 mg/kg/day on days 1-5, and 4 mg/kg/day on days 10, 17, 24, 31, and 38

Pediatric

Usual dosage range: Children ≥1 month: I.V.: 3-6 mg/kg/day

Note: Premedication: For patients who experience nonanaphylactic infusion-related immediate reactions, premedicate with the following drugs 30-60 minutes prior to drug administration: A nonsteroidal anti-inflammatory agent ± diphenhydramine; **or** acetaminophen with diphenhydramine; **or** hydrocortisone 50-100 mg. If the patient experiences rigors during the infusion, meperidine may be administered.

Indication-specific dosing: Children ≥1 month: I.V.:

Empiric therapy: 3 mg/kg/day

Systemic fungal infections *(Aspergillus, Candida, Cryptococcus):* 3-5 mg/kg/day

Systemic fungal infections (HIV-exposed/-positive [CDC, 2009; unlabeled use]):

Aspergillosis: 5 mg/kg/day once daily

Candida, invasive: 5 mg/kg/day once daily (may consider addition of oral flucytosine for severe disease)

Cryptococcal meningitis: 4-6 mg/kg/day once daily plus oral flucytosine

Cryptococcus, disseminated (non-CNS): 3-5 mg/kg/day (may consider addition of oral flucytosine)

Histoplasmosis: 3-5 mg/kg/day once daily

Visceral leishmaniasis:

Immunocompetent: 3 mg/kg/day on days 1-5, and 3 mg/kg/day on days 14 and 21; a repeat course may be given in patients who do not achieve parasitic clearance

Note: Alternate regimen of 10 mg/kg/day for 2 days has been reportedly effective.

Immunocompromised: 4 mg/kg/day on days 1-5, and 4 mg/kg/day on days 10, 17, 24, 31, and 38

Renal Impairment None necessary; effects of renal impairment are not currently known.

Hemodialysis: Supplemental dose is not necessary.

Peritoneal dialysis effects: Supplemental dose is not necessary.

Continuous renal replacement therapy (CRRT): No supplemental dosage necessary

Administration

I.V. Intravenous infusion, over a period of approximately 2 hours. Infusion time may be reduced to approximately 1 hour in patients in whom the treatment is well-tolerated. If the patient experiences discomfort during infusion, the duration of infusion may be increased. Discontinue if severe respiratory distress occurs.

For a patient who experiences chills, fever, hypotension, nausea, or other nonanaphylactic infusion-related reactions, premedicate with the following drugs, 30-60 minutes prior to drug administration: A nonsteroidal (eg, ibuprofen, choline magnesium trisalicylate) with or without diphenhydramine **or** acetaminophen with diphenhydramine **or** hydrocortisone 50-100 mg. If the patient experiences rigors during the infusion, meperidine may be administered.

Stability

Reconstitution Reconstitute with 12 mL SWFI to a concentration of 4 mg/mL. The use of any solution other than those recommended, or the presence of a bacteriostatic agent in the solution, may cause precipitation. **Shake the vial vigorously** for 30 seconds, until dispersed into a translucent yellow suspension.

Filtration and dilution: The 5-micron filter should be on the syringe used to remove the reconstituted AmBisome®. Dilute to a final concentration of 1-2 mg/mL (0.2-0.5 mg/mL for infants and small children).

Storage Store intact vials at ≤25°C (≤77°F). Reconstituted vials are stable refrigerated at 2°C to 8°C (36°F to 46°F) for 24 hours. Do not freeze. Manufacturer's labeling states infusion should begin within 6 hours of dilution with D_5W; data on file with Astellas Pharma shows extended formulation stability when admixed in D_5W at 0.2-2 mg/mL (in polyolefin or PVC bags) for up to 11 days when stored refrigerated at 2°C to 8°C (36°F to 46°F).

Monitoring and Teaching Issues

Laboratory Monitoring BUN and serum creatinine levels should be determined every other day while therapy is increased and at least weekly thereafter. Serum potassium and magnesium should be monitored closely. Monitor electrolytes, liver function, hematocrit, and CBC regularly.

Physical Assessment Assess culture and sensitivity report and patient's previous exposure to Amphotericin B prior to starting therapy. Assess other nephrotoxic drugs patient may be taking for potential interactions or toxicity. Patient should be monitored closely for infusion-related reactions (eg, anaphylaxis, chills, fever, nausea, vomiting, rigors, hypotension, acute respiratory distress); facilities for cardiopulmonary resuscitation should be available during infusion. If acute respiratory distress occurs, infusion should be stopped and prescriber notified.

Patient Education This medication can only be administered by infusion and therapy may last several weeks. You will be monitored closely during and after infusion; report immediately any pain or swelling at infusion site, difficulty breathing or chest pain, chills, nausea, swelling of face or mouth, muscle cramping, acute anxiety, or other infusion reactions. You may experience dizziness, anxiety, confusion, nausea, vomiting, or loss of appetite. Report chest pain or palpitations; CNS disturbances; skin rash; unusual chills or fever; persistent nausea, vomiting, or abdominal pain; sore throat; excessive fatigue; swelling of extremities or unusual weight gain; difficulty breathing; muscle cramping; or weakness.

Breast-Feeding Considerations Due to the potential for serious adverse reactions in the nursing infant, breast-feeding is not recommended.

Pregnancy Considerations Animal studies did not demonstrate teratogenicity. There are no adequate and well-controlled studies in pregnant women. Conventional amphotericin B has been used successfully to treat systemic fungal infection in a limited number (case reports) of pregnant women.

Additional Information Amphotericin B (liposomal) is a true single bilayer liposomal drug delivery system. Liposomes are closed, spherical vesicles created by mixing specific proportions of amphophilic substances such as phospholipids and cholesterol so that they arrange themselves into multiple concentric bilayer membranes when hydrated in aqueous solutions. Single bilayer liposomes are then formed by microemulsification of multilamellar vesicles using a homogenizer. Amphotericin B (liposomal) consists of these unilamellar bilayer liposomes with amphotericin B intercalated within the membrane. Due to the nature and quantity of amphophilic substances used, and the lipophilic moiety in the amphotericin B molecule, the drug is an integral part of the overall structure of the amphotericin B liposomal liposomes. Amphotericin B (liposomal) contains true liposomes that are <100 nm in diameter.

Ampicillin (am pi SIL in)

Index Terms Aminobenzylpenicillin; Ampicillin Sodium; Ampicillin Trihydrate

Generic Availability (U.S.) Yes

Pharmacologic Category Antibiotic, Penicillin

Medication Safety Issues

Sound-alike/look-alike issues:

Ampicillin may be confused with aminophylline

Pregnancy Risk Factor B

Lactation Enters breast milk/use caution

Use Treatment of susceptible bacterial infections (nonbeta-lactamase-producing organisms); treatment or prophylaxis of infective endocarditis; susceptible bacterial infections caused by streptococci, pneumococci, nonpenicillinase-producing staphylococci, *Listeria*, meningococci; some strains of *H. influenzae*, *Salmonella*, *Shigella*, *E. coli*, *Enterobacter*, and *Klebsiella*

Mechanism of Action/Effect Interferes with bacterial cell wall synthesis during active multiplication, causing cell wall death and resultant bactericidal activity against susceptible bacteria

Contraindications Hypersensitivity to ampicillin, any component of the formulation, or other penicillins

Warnings/Precautions Dosage adjustment may be necessary in patients with renal impairment. Serious and occasionally severe or fatal hypersensitivity (anaphylactoid) reactions have been reported in patients on penicillin therapy, especially with a history of beta-lactam hypersensitivity, history of sensitivity to multiple allergens, or previous IgE-mediated reactions (eg, anaphylaxis, angioedema, urticaria). Use with caution in asthmatic patients. High percentage of patients with infectious mononucleosis have developed rash during therapy with ampicillin; ampicillin-class antibiotics not recommended in these patients. Appearance of a rash should be carefully evaluated to differentiate a nonallergic ampicillin rash from a hypersensitivity reaction. Ampicillin rash occurs in 5% to 10% of children receiving ampicillin and is a generalized dull red, maculopapular rash, generally appearing 3-14 days after the start of therapy. It normally begins on the trunk and spreads over most of the body. It may be most intense at pressure areas, elbows, and knees. Prolonged use may result in fungal or bacterial superinfection, including *C. difficile*-associated diarrhea (CDAD) and pseudomembranous colitis; CDAD has been observed >2 months postantibiotic treatment.

Drug Interactions

Avoid Concomitant Use

Avoid concomitant use of Ampicillin with any of the following: BCG

Decreased Effect

Ampicillin may decrease the levels/effects of: Atenolol; BCG; Mycophenolate; Typhoid Vaccine

The levels/effects of Ampicillin may be decreased by: Chloroquine; Fusidic Acid; Tetracycline Derivatives

Increased Effect/Toxicity

Ampicillin may increase the levels/effects of: Methotrexate

The levels/effects of Ampicillin may be increased by: Allopurinol; Probenecid

Nutritional/Ethanol Interactions Food: Food decreases ampicillin absorption rate; may decrease ampicillin serum concentration.

Lab Interactions Increased protein, positive Coombs' [direct]; alters result of urinary glucose (Benedict's solution, Clinitest®)

Some penicillin derivatives may accelerate the degradation of aminoglycosides *in vitro*, leading to a potential underestimation of aminoglycoside serum concentration.

Adverse Reactions Frequency not defined.

Central nervous system: Fever, penicillin encephalopathy, seizure

Dermatologic: Erythema multiforme, exfoliative dermatitis, rash, urticaria

Note: Appearance of a rash should be carefully evaluated to differentiate (if possible) nonallergic ampicillin rash from hypersensitivity reaction. Incidence is higher in patients with viral infection, *Salmonella* infection, lymphocytic leukemia, or patients that have hyperuricemia.

Gastrointestinal: Black hairy tongue, diarrhea, enterocolitis, glossitis, nausea, oral candidiasis, pseudomembranous colitis, sore mouth or tongue, stomatitis, vomiting

Hematologic: Agranulocytosis, anemia, hemolytic anemia, eosinophilia, leukopenia, thrombocytopenia purpura

Hepatic: AST increased

Renal: Interstitial nephritis (rare)

Respiratory: Laryngeal stridor

Miscellaneous: Anaphylaxis, serum sickness-like reaction

Pharmacodynamics/Kinetics

Absorption Oral: 50%

Time to Peak Oral: Within 1-2 hours

Protein Binding 15% to 25%

Half-Life Elimination

Children and Adults: 1-1.8 hours

Anuria/end-stage renal disease: 7-20 hours

Excretion Urine (~90% as unchanged drug) within 24 hours

Available Dosage Forms

Capsule, oral: 250 mg, 500 mg

Injection, powder for reconstitution: 125 mg, 250 mg, 500 mg, 1 g, 2 g, 10 g

Powder for suspension, oral: 125 mg/5 mL (100 mL, 200 mL); 250 mg/5 mL (100 mL, 200 mL)

Dosing

Adult

Usual dosage range:

Oral: 250-500 mg every 6 hours

I.M., I.V.: 250-500 mg every 6 hours

Actinomycosis: I.V.: 50 mg/kg/day for 4-6 weeks then oral amoxicillin

Cholangitis (acute): I.V.: 2 g every 4 hours with gentamicin

Diverticulitis: I.M., I.V.: 2 g every 6 hours with metronidazole

Endocarditis:

Infective: I.V.: 12 g/day via continuous infusion or divided every 4 hours

Prophylaxis: Dental, oral, or respiratory tract procedures: I.M., I.V.: 2 g within 30-60 minutes prior to procedure in patients not allergic to penicillin and unable to take oral amoxicillin. Intramuscular injections should be avoided in patients who are receiving anticoagulant therapy. In these circumstances, orally administered regimens should be given whenever possible. Intravenously administered antibiotics should be used for patients who are unable to tolerate or absorb oral medications. **Note:** American Heart Association (AHA) guidelines now recommend prophylaxis only in patients undergoing invasive procedures and in whom underlying cardiac conditions may predispose to a higher risk of adverse outcomes should infection occur.

Prophylaxis in total joint replacement patient: I.M., I.V.: 2 g 1 hour prior to the procedure

Genitourinary and gastrointestinal tract procedures: I.M., I.V.:

High-risk patients: 2 g within 30 minutes prior to procedure, followed by ampicillin 1 g (or amoxicillin 1 g orally) 6 hours later; must be used in combination with gentamicin. **Note:** As of April 2007, routine prophylaxis for GI/GU procedures is no longer recommended by the AHA.

Moderate-risk patients: 2 g within 30 minutes prior to procedure

Group B strep prophylaxis (intrapartum): I.V.: 2 g initial dose, then 1 g every 4 hours until delivery

***Listeria* infections:** I.V.: 2 g every 4 hours (consider addition of aminoglycoside)

Sepsis/meningitis: I.M., I.V.: 150-250 mg/kg/day divided every 3-4 hours (range: 6-12 g/day)

Urinary tract infections (*Enterococcus* suspected): I.V.: 1-2 g every 6 hours with gentamicin

Geriatric Administer usual adult dose unless renal function is markedly reduced.

Pediatric

Usual dosage range: Infants and Children:

Oral: 50-100 mg/kg/day in doses divided every 6 hours (maximum: 2-4 g/day)

I.M., I.V.: 100-400 mg/kg/day in divided doses every 6 hours (maximum: 12 g/day)

Endocarditis prophylaxis: Infants and Children: I.M., I.V.:

Dental, oral, or respiratory tract procedures: 50 mg/kg within 30-60 minutes prior to procedure in patients not allergic to penicillin and unable to take oral amoxicillin. Intramuscular injections should be avoided in patients who are receiving anticoagulant therapy. In these circumstances, orally administered regimens should be given whenever possible. Intravenously administered antibiotics should be used for patients who are unable to tolerate or absorb oral medications.

Note: American Heart Association (AHA) guidelines now recommend prophylaxis only in patients undergoing invasive procedures and in whom underlying cardiac conditions may predispose to a higher risk of adverse outcomes should infection occur.

Genitourinary and gastrointestinal tract procedures:

High-risk patients: 50 mg/kg (maximum: 2 g) within 30 minutes prior to procedure, followed by ampicillin 25 mg/kg (or amoxicillin 25 mg/kg orally) 6 hours later; must be used in combination with gentamicin. **Note:** As of April 2007, routine prophylaxis for GI/GU procedures is no longer recommended by the AHA.

Moderate-risk patients: 50 mg/kg within 30 minutes prior to procedure.

Mild-to-moderate infections: Infants and Children:

Oral: 50-100 mg/kg/day in doses divided every 6 hours (maximum: 2-4 g/day)

I.M., I.V.: 100-150 mg/kg/day in divided doses every 6 hours (maximum: 2-4 g/day)

Severe infections/meningitis: Infants and Children: I.M., I.V.: 200-400 mg/kg/day in divided doses every 6 hours (maximum: 6-12 g/day)

Renal Impairment

Cl_{cr} >50 mL/minute: Administer every 6 hours

Cl_{cr} 10-50 mL/minute: Administer every 6-12 hours

Cl_{cr} <10 mL/minute: Administer every 12-24 hours

Hemodialysis: Moderately dialyzable (20% to 50%); administer dose after dialysis

Peritoneal dialysis: Moderately dialyzable (20% to 50%)

Administer 250 mg every 12 hours

Continuous arteriovenous or venovenous hemofiltration effects: Dose as for Cl_{cr} 10-50 mL/minute; ~50 mg of ampicillin per liter of filtrate is removed

Administration

Oral Administer around-the-clock to promote less variation in peak and trough serum levels. Administer on an empty stomach (ie, 1 hour prior to, or 2 hours after meals) to increase total absorption.

I.V. Administer around-the-clock to promote less variation in peak and trough serum levels. Administer over 3-5 minutes (125-500 mg) or over 10-15 minutes (1-2 g). More rapid infusion may cause seizures. Ampicillin and gentamicin should not be mixed in the same I.V. tubing.

Some penicillins (eg, carbenicillin, ticarcillin, and piperacillin) have been shown to inactivate aminoglycosides *in vitro*. This has been observed to a greater extent with tobramycin and gentamicin, while amikacin has shown greater stability against inactivation. Concurrent use of these agents may pose a risk of reduced antibacterial efficacy *in vivo*, particularly in the setting of profound renal impairment. However, definitive clinical evidence is lacking. If combination penicillin/aminoglycoside therapy is desired in a patient with renal dysfunction, separation of doses (if feasible), and routine monitoring of aminoglycoside levels, CBC, and clinical response should be considered.

Stability

Reconstitution I.V.: Minimum volume: Concentration should not exceed 30 mg/mL due to concentration-dependent stability restrictions. Standard diluent: 500 mg/50 mL NS; 1 g/50 mL NS; 2 g/100 mL NS.

Storage

Oral: Oral suspension is stable for 7 days at room temperature or for 14 days under refrigeration.

I.V.:

Solutions for I.M. or direct I.V. should be used within 1 hour. Solutions for I.V. infusion will be inactivated by dextrose at room temperature. If dextrose-containing solutions are to be used, the resultant solution will only be stable for 2 hours versus 8 hours in the 0.9% sodium chloride injection. D_5W has limited stability.

Stability of parenteral admixture in NS at room temperature (25°C) is 8 hours.

Stability of parenteral admixture in NS at refrigeration temperature (4°C) is 2 days.

Monitoring and Teaching Issues

Laboratory Monitoring Perform culture and sensitivity testing prior to initiating therapy.

Physical Assessment Assess results of culture and sensitivity tests and patient's allergy history prior to starting therapy. Monitor for opportunistic infection (fever, chills, unhealed sores, white plaques in mouth or vagina, purulent vaginal discharge).

Patient Education Take at equal intervals around-the-clock; preferably on an empty stomach (1 hour before or 2 hours after meals). Maintain adequate hydration, unless instructed to restrict fluid intake. May cause nausea, vomiting, or diarrhea. Report immediately any rash; persistent diarrhea; swelling of face, tongue, mouth, or throat; or chest tightness. Report if condition being treated worsens or does not improve by the time prescription is completed.

Dietary Considerations Take on an empty stomach 1 hour before or 2 hours after meals. Some products may contain sodium.

Geriatric Considerations Adjust dose for renal function.

Breast-Feeding Considerations Ampicillin is excreted in breast milk. The manufacturer recommends that caution be exercised when administering ampicillin to nursing women. Due to the low concentrations in human milk, minimal toxicity would be expected in the nursing infant. Nondose-related effects could include modification of bowel flora and allergic sensitization.

Pregnancy Considerations Adverse events have not been observed in animal studies; therefore, ampicillin is classified as pregnancy category B. Ampicillin crosses the human placenta, providing detectable concentrations in the cord serum and amniotic fluid. Most studies have not identified a teratogenic potential for ampicillin use during pregnancy. Two possible associations (congenital heart disease and cleft palate) have been noted; each of these was observed in a single study, was not substantiated by other studies, and may have been chance associations. Ampicillin is recommended for use in pregnant women for the management of premature rupture of membranes. Ampicillin is considered an acceptable alternative to penicillin for the prevention of early-onset Group B Streptococcal (GBS) disease in newborns.

The volume of distribution of ampicillin is increased during pregnancy and the half-life is decreased. As a result, serum concentrations in pregnant patients are approximately 50% of those in nonpregnant patients receiving the same dose. Higher doses may be needed during pregnancy. Although oral absorption is not altered during pregnancy, oral ampicillin is poorly-absorbed during labor.

Related Information

Antimicrobial Drugs of Choice *on page 2008*

Community-Acquired Pneumonia in Adults *on page 2021*

I.V. to Oral Conversion *on page 1956*

Ampicillin and Sulbactam (am pi SIL in & SUL bak tam)

U.S. Brand Names Unasyn®

Index Terms Sulbactam and Ampicillin

Generic Availability (U.S.) Yes

Pharmacologic Category Antibiotic, Penicillin

Pregnancy Risk Factor B

Lactation Enters breast milk/use caution

Use Treatment of susceptible bacterial infections involved with skin and skin structure, intra-abdominal infections, gynecological infections; spectrum is that of ampicillin plus organisms producing beta-lactamases such as *S. aureus*, *H. influenzae*, *E. coli*, *Klebsiella*, *Acinetobacter*, *Enterobacter*, and anaerobes

Available Dosage Forms

Injection, powder for reconstitution: 1.5 g [ampicillin 1 g and sulbactam 0.5 g]; 3 g [ampicillin 2 g and sulbactam 1 g]; 15 g [ampicillin 10 g and sulbactam 5 g]

Unasyn®: 1.5 g [ampicillin 1 g and sulbactam 0.5 g]; 3 g [ampicillin 2 g and sulbactam 1 g]; 15 g [ampicillin 10 g and sulbactam 5 g]; 15 g [ampicillin 10 g and sulbactam 5 g

Dosing

Adult & Geriatric Doses expressed as ampicillin/sulbactam combination.

Susceptible infections: I.M., I.V.: 1.5-3 g every 6 hours (maximum: Unasyn® 12 g)

Amnionitis, cholangitis, diverticulitis, endometritis, endophthalmitis, epididymitis/orchitis, liver abscess, osteomyelitis (diabetic foot), peritonitis: I.V.: 3 g every 6 hours; **Note:** Due to high rates of *E. coli* resistance, not recommended for the treatment of community-acquired intra-abdominal infections (Solomkin, 2010)

Endocarditis: I.V.: 3 g every 6 hours with gentamicin or vancomycin for 4-6 weeks

Orbital cellulitis: I.V.: 1.5 g every 6 hours

Parapharyngeal space infections: I.V.: 3 g every 6 hours

***Pasteurella multocida* (human, canine/feline bites):** I.V.: 1.5-3 g every 6 hours

Pelvic inflammatory disease: I.V.: 3 g every 6 hours with doxycycline

Peritonitis (CAPD): Intraperitoneal:

Anuric, intermittent: 3 g every 12 hours

Anuric, continuous: Loading dose: 1.5 g; maintenance dose: 150 mg

Pneumonia:

Aspiration, community-acquired: I.V.: 1.5-3 g every 6 hours

Hospital-acquired: I.V.: 3 g every 6 hours

Urinary tract infections, pyelonephritis: I.V.: 3 g every 6 hours for 14 days

Pediatric

Susceptible infections: Children ≥1 year: I.V.: 100-400 mg ampicillin/kg/day divided every 6 hours (maximum: 8 g ampicillin/day, 12 g Unasyn®). **Note:** The American Academy of Pediatrics recommends a dose of up to 300 mg/kg/day for severe infection in infants >1 month of age.

Epiglottitis: Children ≥1 year: I.V.: 100-200 mg ampicillin/kg/day divided in 4 doses

Mild-to-moderate infections: Children ≥1 year: I.V.: 100-200 mg ampicillin/kg/day (150-300 mg Unasyn®) divided every 6 hours (maximum: 8 g ampicillin/day, 12 g Unasyn®)

Peritonsillar and retropharyngeal abscess: Children ≥1 year: I.V.: 50 mg ampicillin/kg/dose every 6 hours

Severe infections: Children ≥1 year: I.V.: 200-400 mg ampicillin/kg/day divided every 6 hours (maximum: 8 g ampicillin/day, 12 g Unasyn®)

Renal Impairment

Cl_{cr} 15-29 mL/minute: Administer every 12 hours

Cl_{cr} 5-14 mL/minute: Administer every 24 hours

Hemodialysis: Give dose after hemodialysis

Continuous ambulatory peritoneal dialysis (CAPD): 3 g every 24 hours

Continuous renal replacement therapy (CRRT): Drug clearance is highly dependent on the method of renal replacement, filter type, and flow rate. Appropriate dosing requires close monitoring of pharmacologic response, signs of adverse reactions due to drug accumulation, as well as drug levels in relation to target trough (if appropriate). The following are general recommendations only (based on dialysate flow/ultrafiltration rates of 1 L/hour) and should not supersede clinical judgment:

CVVH: 3 g every 12 hours

CVVHD/CVVHDF: 3 g every 8 hours

Administration

I.V. Administer around-the-clock to promote less variation in peak and trough serum levels. Administer by slow injection over 10-15 minutes or I.V. over 15-30 minutes. Ampicillin and gentamicin should not be mixed in the same I.V. tubing.

Some penicillins (eg, carbenicillin, ticarcillin, and piperacillin) have been shown to inactivate aminoglycosides *in vitro*. This has been observed to a greater extent with tobramycin and gentamicin, while amikacin has shown greater stability against inactivation. Concurrent use of these agents may pose a risk of reduced antibacterial efficacy *in vivo*, particularly in the setting of profound renal impairment. However, definitive clinical evidence is lacking. If combination penicillin/aminoglycoside therapy is desired in a patient with renal dysfunction, separation of doses (if feasible), and routine monitoring of aminoglycoside levels, CBC, and clinical response should be considered.

Monitoring and Teaching Issues

Laboratory Monitoring Hematologic, renal, and hepatic function with prolonged therapy. Perform culture and sensitivity testing prior to initiating therapy.

Physical Assessment See individual agents.

Patient Education See individual agents.

Related Information

Ampicillin *on page 124*

Antimicrobial Drugs of Choice *on page 2008*

I.V. to Oral Conversion *on page 1956*

◆ **Ampicillin Sodium** *see* Ampicillin *on page 124*

◆ **Ampicillin Trihydrate** *see* Ampicillin *on page 124*

◆ **Ampyra™** *see* Dalfampridine *on page 458*

◆ **Amrix®** *see* Cyclobenzaprine *on page 432*

◆ **Amturnide™** *see* Aliskiren, Amlodipine, and Hydrochlorothiazide *on page 73*

◆ **Amylase, Lipase, and Protease** *see* Pancrelipase *on page 1400*

◆ **AN100226** *see* Natalizumab *on page 1292*

◆ **Anafranil®** *see* ClomiPRAMINE *on page 403*

◆ **Anaprox®** *see* Naproxen *on page 1289*

◆ **Anaprox® DS** *see* Naproxen *on page 1289*

Anastrozole (an AS troe zole)

U.S. Brand Names Arimidex®

Index Terms ICI-D1033; ZD1033

Generic Availability (U.S.) Yes

Pharmacologic Category Antineoplastic Agent, Aromatase Inhibitor

Medication Safety Issues

Sound-alike/look-alike issues:

Anastrozole may be confused with anagrelide, letrozole

Arimidex® may be confused with Aromasin®

Pregnancy Risk Factor X

Lactation Excretion in breast milk unknown/not recommended

Use First-line treatment of locally-advanced or metastatic breast cancer (hormone receptor-positive or unknown) in postmenopausal women; treatment of advanced breast cancer in postmenopausal women with disease progression following tamoxifen therapy; adjuvant treatment of early hormone receptor-positive breast cancer in postmenopausal women

Unlabeled/Investigational Use Treatment of recurrent or metastatic endometrial or uterine cancers, treatment of recurrent ovarian cancer

Mechanism of Action/Effect Potent and selective nonsteroidal aromatase inhibitor. By inhibiting aromatase, the conversion of androstenedione to estrone, and testosterone to estradiol, is prevented, thereby decreasing tumor mass or delaying progression in patients with tumors responsive to hormones. Anastrozole causes an 85% decrease in estrone sulfate levels.

Contraindications Hypersensitivity to anastrozole or any component of the formulation; use in women who are or may become pregnant

Warnings/Precautions Hazardous agent - use appropriate precautions for handling and disposal. Use is contraindicated in women who are or may become pregnant. Anastrozole offers no clinical benefit in premenopausal women with breast cancer. Patients with pre-existing ischemic cardiac disease have an increased risk for ischemic cardiovascular events.

Due to decreased circulating estrogen levels, anastrozole is associated with a reduction in bone mineral density (BMD); decreases (from baseline) in total hip and lumbar spine BMD have been reported. Patients with pre-existing osteopenia are at higher risk for developing osteoporosis (Eastell, 2008). When initiating anastrozole treatment, follow available guidelines for bone mineral density management in postmenopausal women with similar fracture risk; concurrent use of bisphosphonates may be useful in patients at risk for fractures.

Elevated total cholesterol levels (contributed to by LDL cholesterol increases) have been reported in patients receiving anastrozole; use with caution in patients with hyperlipidemias; cholesterol levels should be monitored/managed in accordance with current guidelines for patients with LDL elevations. Plasma concentrations in patients with stable hepatic cirrhosis were within the range of concentrations seen in normal subjects across all clinical trials; use has not been studied in patients with severe hepatic impairment. Safety and efficacy in children have not been established.

Drug Interactions

Metabolism/Transport Effects Inhibits CYP1A2 (weak), 2C8 (weak), 2C9 (weak), 3A4 (weak)

Avoid Concomitant Use

Avoid concomitant use of Anastrozole with any of the following: Estrogen Derivatives

Decreased Effect

The levels/effects of Anastrozole may be decreased by: Estrogen Derivatives; Tamoxifen

Increased Effect/Toxicity There are no known significant interactions involving an increase in effect.

Adverse Reactions

>10%:

Cardiovascular: Vasodilatation (25% to 36%), ischemic cardiovascular disease (4%; 17% in patients with pre-existing ischemic heart disease), hypertension (2% to 13%), angina (2%; 12% in patients with pre-existing ischemic heart disease)

Central nervous system: Mood disturbance (19%), fatigue (19%), pain (11% to 17%), headache (9% to 13%), depression (5% to 13%)

Dermatologic: Rash (6% to 11%)

Endocrine & metabolic: Hot flashes (12% to 36%)

Gastrointestinal: Nausea (11% to 19%), vomiting (8% to 13%)

Neuromuscular & skeletal: Weakness (16% to 19%), arthritis (17%), arthralgia (2% to 15%), back pain (10% to 12%), bone pain (6% to 11%), osteoporosis (11%)

Respiratory: Pharyngitis (6% to 14%), cough increased (8% to 11%)

1% to 10%:

Cardiovascular: Peripheral edema (5% to 10%), chest pain (5% to 7%), edema (7%), venous thromboembolic events (2% to 4%), ischemic cerebrovascular events (2%), MI (1%)

Central nervous system: Insomnia (2% to 10%), dizziness (6% to 8%), anxiety (2% to 6%), fever (2% to 5%), malaise (2% to 5%), confusion (2% to 5%), nervousness (2% to 5%), somnolence (2% to 5%), lethargy (1%)

Dermatologic: Alopecia (2% to 5%), pruritus (2% to 5%)

Endocrine & metabolic: Hypercholesterolemia (9%), breast pain (2% to 8%)

Gastrointestinal: Diarrhea (8% to 9%), constipation (7% to 9%), abdominal pain (7% to 9%), weight gain (2% to 9%), anorexia (5% to 7%), xerostomia (6%), dyspepsia (7%), weight loss (2% to 5%)

Genitourinary: Urinary tract infection (2% to 8%), vulvovaginitis (6%), pelvic pain (5%), vaginal bleeding (1% to 5%), vaginitis (4%), vaginal discharge (4%), vaginal hemorrhage (2% to 4%), leukorrhea (2% to 3%), vaginal dryness (2% to 5%)

Hematologic: Anemia (2% to 5%), leukopenia (2% to 5%)

Hepatic: Liver function tests increased (1% to 10%), alkaline phosphatase increased (1% to 10%), gamma GT increased (≤5%)

Local: Thrombophlebitis (2% to 5%)

Neuromuscular & skeletal: Fracture (1% to 10%), arthrosis (7%), paresthesia (5% to 7%), joint disorder (6%), myalgia (2% to 6%), neck pain (2% to 5%), carpal tunnel syndrome (3%), hypertonia (3%)

Ocular: Cataracts (6%)

Respiratory: Dyspnea (8% to 10%), sinusitis (2% to 6%), bronchitis (2% to 5%), rhinitis (2% to 5%)

Miscellaneous: Lymphedema (10%), infection (2% to 9%), flu-like syndrome (2% to 7%), diaphoresis (2% to 5%), cyst (5%), neoplasm (5%), tumor flare (3%)

Pharmacodynamics/Kinetics

Onset of Action Onset of estradiol reduction: 70% reduction after 24 hours; 80% after 2 weeks therapy

Duration of Action Duration of estradiol reduction: 6 days

Absorption Well absorbed; extent of absorption not affected by food

Time to Peak Plasma: ~2 hours without food; 5 hours with food
Protein Binding Plasma: 40%
Half-Life Elimination ~50 hours
Metabolism Extensively hepatic (~85%) via N-dealkylation, hydroxylation, and glucuronidation; primary metabolite (triazole) inactive
Excretion Feces; urine (urinary excretion accounts for ~10% of total elimination, mostly as metabolites)

Available Dosage Forms
Tablet, oral: 1 mg
Arimidex®: 1 mg

Dosing
Adult & Geriatric Females: Postmenopausal:
Breast cancer, advanced: Oral: 1 mg once daily; continue until tumor progression
Breast cancer, early (adjuvant treatment): Oral: 1 mg once daily; optimal duration unknown, duration in clinical trial is 5 years
Renal Impairment Dosage adjustment is not necessary.
Hepatic Impairment
Mild-to-moderate impairment or stable hepatic cirrhosis: Dosage adjustment is not required.
Severe hepatic impairment: Has not been studied in this population.

Administration
Oral May be administered with or without food.

Stability
Storage Store at 20°C to 25°C (68°F to 77°F).

Monitoring and Teaching Issues
Laboratory Monitoring Bone mineral density; total cholesterol and LDL
Physical Assessment Assess carefully for use cautions. Evaluate bone mineral density and cholesterol levels.
Patient Education Maintain adequate hydration, unless instructed to restrict fluid intake. Anastrozole may cause or worsen osteoporosis; discuss ways to decrease this risk with prescriber. You may experience dizziness or fatigue; nausea, vomiting, or loss of appetite; increased pelvic, bone, or tumor pain; hot flashes; rash; or loss of hair. Report chest pain, palpitations, persistent headache, or dizziness; unresolved nausea or vomiting; pain or burning on urination; unusual or persistent nervousness, confusion, or anxiety; flu-like symptoms; or respiratory difficulty.
Dietary Considerations May be taken with or without food.
Geriatric Considerations No age-related changes in pharmacokinetics were noted in clinical trials.
Pregnancy Considerations Fetotoxicity was observed in animal studies. Anastrozole is contraindicated in women who are or may become pregnant (may cause fetal harm if administered during pregnancy). Use in premenopausal women with breast cancer does not provide any clinical benefit.

Additional Information Oncology Comment: The American Society of Clinical Oncology (ASCO) guidelines for adjuvant endocrine therapy in postmenopausal women with HR-positive breast cancer (Burstein, 2010) recommend considering aromatase inhibitor (AI) therapy at some point in the treatment course (primary, sequentially, or extended). Optimal duration at this time is not known; however, treatment with an AI should not exceed 5 years in primary and extended therapies, and 2-3 years if followed by tamoxifen in sequential therapy (total of 5 years). If initial therapy with AI has been discontinued before the 5 years, consideration should be taken to receive tamoxifen for a total of 5 years. The optimal time to switch to an AI is also not known, but data supports switching after 2-3 years of tamoxifen (sequential) or after 5 years of tamoxifen (extended). If patient becomes intolerant or has poor adherence, consideration should be made to switch to another AI or initiate tamoxifen.

- **Ancef** *see* Cefazolin *on page 312*
- **Ancobon®** *see* Flucytosine *on page 775*
- **Androderm®** *see* Testosterone *on page 1739*
- **AndroGel®** *see* Testosterone *on page 1739*
- **Android®** *see* MethylTESTOSTERone *on page 1212*
- **AneCream™ [OTC]** *see* Lidocaine (Topical) *on page 1107*
- **Anectine®** *see* Succinylcholine *on page 1683*
- **Anestafoam™ [OTC]** *see* Lidocaine (Topical) *on page 1107*
- **Aneurine Hydrochloride** *see* Thiamine *on page 1751*
- **Angeliq®** *see* Drospirenone and Estradiol *on page 594*

Anidulafungin (ay nid yoo la FUN jin)

U.S. Brand Names Eraxis™
Index Terms LY303366
Generic Availability (U.S.) No
Pharmacologic Category Antifungal Agent, Parenteral; Echinocandin
Pregnancy Risk Factor C
Lactation Excretion in breast milk unknown/use caution

Use Treatment of candidemia and other forms of *Candida* infections (including those of intra-abdominal, peritoneal, and esophageal locus)

Unlabeled/Investigational Use Treatment of infections due to *Aspergillus* spp.

Mechanism of Action/Effect Noncompetitive inhibitor of 1,3-beta-D-glucan synthase resulting in reduced formation of 1,3-beta-D-glucan, an essential polysaccharide comprising 30% to 60% of *Candida* cell walls (absent in mammalian cells); decreased glucan content leads to osmotic instability and cellular lysis

Contraindications Hypersensitivity to anidulafungin, other echinocandins, or any component of the formulation

Warnings/Precautions Histamine-mediated reactions (eg, urticaria, flushing, hypotension) have been observed; these may be related to infusion rate. Elevated liver function tests, hepatitis, and worsening hepatic failure have been reported. Monitor for progressive hepatic impairment if increased transaminase enzymes noted. Safety and efficacy in pediatric patients, neutropenic patients, or other *Candida* infections (eg, endocarditis, osteomyelitis, meningitis) have not been established.

Drug Interactions

Avoid Concomitant Use There are no known interactions where it is recommended to avoid concomitant use.

Decreased Effect

Anidulafungin may decrease the levels/effects of: Saccharomyces boulardii

Increased Effect/Toxicity There are no known significant interactions involving an increase in effect.

Adverse Reactions 2% to 10%:

Endocrine & metabolic: Hypokalemia (3%)
Gastrointestinal: Diarrhea (3%)
Hepatic: Transaminase increased (<1% to 2%)

Pharmacodynamics/Kinetics

Protein Binding 84%

Half-Life Elimination 27 hours

Metabolism No hepatic metabolism observed; undergoes slow chemical hydrolysis to open-ring peptide lacking antifungal activity

Excretion Feces (30%, 10% as unchanged drug); urine (<1%)

Available Dosage Forms

Injection, powder for reconstitution:
Eraxis™: 50 mg, 100 mg

Dosing

Adult & Geriatric

Candidemia, intra-abdominal or peritoneal candidiasis: I.V.: 200 mg loading dose on day 1, followed by 100 mg daily for at least 14 days after last positive culture

Esophageal candidiasis: I.V.: 100 mg loading dose on day 1, followed by 50 mg daily for at least 14 days and for at least 7 days after symptom resolution

Renal Impairment No adjustment necessary, including dialysis patients.

Hepatic Impairment No adjustment necessary.

Administration

I.V. For intravenous use only; infusion rate should not exceed 1.1 mg/minute

Stability

Reconstitution Aseptically add 15 mL (50 mg vial) or 30 mL (100 mg vial) of sterile water for injection to each vial. Swirl to dissolve; do not shake. Further dilute 50 mg, 100 mg, or 200 mg in 50 mL, 100 mL, or 200 mL, respectively, of D_5W or NS.

Storage Store vials at 2°C to 8°C (36°F to 46°F); do not freeze. The reconstituted solution can be stored for up to 1 hour at 2°C to 8°C (36°F to 46°F) prior to dilution into the infusion solution; do not freeze. If the infusion solution is not used immediately, it should be stored in a refrigerator at 2°C to 8°C (36°F to 46°F) and administered within 24 hours of preparation; do not freeze.

Monitoring and Teaching Issues

Laboratory Monitoring Liver function tests

Physical Assessment Assess results of liver function tests on a regular basis.

Patient Education This medication can only be administered by infusion. Report immediately any pain, burning, or swelling at infusion site, or any signs of allergic reaction (eg, respiratory difficulty or swallowing, back pain, chest tightness, rash, hives, or swelling of lips or mouth). Report diarrhea and muscle cramps or weakness.

Pregnancy Considerations Skeletal teratogenic effects were noted in animal studies. There are no adequate and well-controlled studies in pregnant women. Use only if benefit outweighs risk.

- ◆ **Anolor 300** *see* Butalbital, Acetaminophen, and Caffeine *on page* *260*
- ◆ **Ansamycin** *see* Rifabutin *on page* *1576*
- ◆ **Antabuse®** *see* Disulfiram *on page* *557*
- ◆ **Antagon** *see* Ganirelix *on page* *851*
- ◆ **Antara®** *see* Fenofibrate *on page* *739*
- ◆ **Anti-4 Alpha Integrin** *see* Natalizumab *on page* *1292*
- ◆ **Anti-CD20 Monoclonal Antibody** *see* RITUXimab *on page* *1596*
- ◆ **anti-c-erB-2** *see* Trastuzumab *on page* *1804*
- ◆ **Anti-Diarrheal [OTC]** *see* Loperamide *on page* *1126*

◆ **Antidigoxin Fab Fragments, Ovine** *see* Digoxin Immune Fab *on page 533*

◆ **Antidiuretic Hormone** *see* Vasopressin *on page 1851*

◆ **anti-ERB-2** *see* Trastuzumab *on page 1804*

Antihemophilic Factor (Human) (an tee hee moe FIL ik FAK tor HYU man)

U.S. Brand Names Hemofil M; Koāte®-DVI; Monarc-M™; Monoclate-P®

Index Terms AHF (Human); Factor VIII (Human)

Generic Availability (U.S.) Yes

Pharmacologic Category Antihemophilic Agent; Blood Product Derivative

Medication Safety Issues

Sound-alike/look-alike issues:

Factor VIII may be confused with Factor XIII

Pregnancy Risk Factor C

Lactation Excretion in breast milk unknown/use caution

Use Prevention and treatment of hemorrhagic episodes in patients with hemophilia A (classic hemophilia); perioperative management of hemophilia A; can be of significant therapeutic value in patients with acquired factor VIII inhibitors not exceeding 10 Bethesda units/mL

Available Dosage Forms

Injection, powder for reconstitution:

Hemofil M: Vial labeled with international units

Koāte®-DVI: ~250 int. units, ~500 int. units, ~1000 int. units

Monarc-M™: Vial labeled with international units

Monoclate-P®: ~250 int. units, ~500 int. units, ~1000 int. units, ~1500 int. units

Dosing

Adult & Geriatric Hemophilia: I.V.: Individualize dosage based on coagulation studies performed prior to treatment and at regular intervals during treatment. In general, administration of factor VIII 1 int. unit/kg will increase circulating factor VIII levels by ~2 int. units/dL. (General guidelines presented; consult individual product labeling for specific dosing recommendations.)

Dosage based on desired factor VIII increase (%):

To calculate dosage needed based on desired factor VIII increase (%):

Body weight (kg) x 0.5 int. units/kg x desired factor VIII increase (%) = int. units factor VIII required

For example:

50 kg x 0.5 int. units/kg x 30 (% increase) = 750 int. units factor VIII

Dosage based on expected factor VIII increase (%):

It is also possible to calculate the **expected** % factor VIII increase:

(# int. units administered x 2%/int. units/kg) divided by body weight (kg) = expected % factor VIII increase

For example:

(1400 int. units x 2%/int. units/kg) divided by 70 kg = 40%

General guidelines:

Minor hemorrhage: 10-20 int. units/kg as a single dose to achieve FVIII plasma level ~20% to 40% of normal. Mild superficial or early hemorrhages may respond to a single dose; may repeat dose every 12-24 hours for 1-3 days until bleeding is resolved or healing achieved.

Moderate hemorrhage/minor surgery: 15-25 int. units/kg to achieve FVIII plasma level 30% to 50% of normal. If needed, may continue with a maintenance dose of 10-15 int. units/kg every 8-12 hours.

Major to life-threatening hemorrhage: Initial dose 40-50 int. units/kg, followed by a maintenance dose of 20-25 int. units/kg every 8-12 hours until threat is resolved, to achieve FVIII plasma level 80% to 100% of normal.

Major surgery: 50 int. units/kg given preoperatively to raise factor VIII level to 100% before surgery begins. May repeat as necessary after 6-12 hours initially and for a total of 10-14 days until healing is complete. Intensity of therapy may depend on type of surgery and postoperative regimen.

Bleeding prophylaxis: May be administered on a regular basis for bleeding prophylaxis. Doses of 24-40 int. units/kg 3 times/week have been reported in patients with severe hemophilia to prevent joint bleeding.

If bleeding is not controlled with adequate dose, test for presence of inhibitor. It may not be possible or practical to control bleeding if inhibitor titers are >10 Bethesda units/mL.

Pediatric Refer to adult dosing.

Administration

I.V. Over 5-10 minutes (maximum: 10 mL/minute). Infuse Monoclate-P® at 2 mL/minute.

Monitoring and Teaching Issues

Laboratory Monitoring In patients with circulating inhibitors, the inhibitor level should be monitored; hematocrit

Physical Assessment Patient should be monitored closely during and after infusion for any change in vital signs, cardiac and CNS status, or hypersensitivity reactions (eg, chills, fever, chest pain, respiratory difficulty). Assess results of hematocrit and coagulation studies. Monitor bleeding and coagulation status. Monitor for anemia.

Patient Education This medication can only be given intravenously. Report immediately any sudden-onset headache, rash, chest or back pain, wheezing or respiratory difficulties, hives, itching, low-grade fever, stomach pain, or nausea/vomiting to prescriber. Wear identification indicating that you have a hemophilic condition.

Antihemophilic Factor (Recombinant)

(an tee hee moe FIL ik FAK tor ree KOM be nant)

U.S. Brand Names Advate; Helixate® FS; Kogenate® FS; Recombinate; Xyntha™
Index Terms AHF (Recombinant); Factor VIII (Recombinant); rAHF
Generic Availability (U.S.) No
Pharmacologic Category Antihemophilic Agent
Medication Safety Issues
Sound-alike/look-alike issues:
Factor VIII may be confused with Factor XIII

Confusion may occur due to the omitting of "Factor VIII" from some product labeling. Review product contents carefully prior to dispensing any antihemophilic factor.

Pregnancy Risk Factor C
Lactation Excretion in breast milk unknown/use caution
Use Prevention and treatment of hemorrhagic episodes in patients with hemophilia A (classic hemophilia or congenital factor VIII deficiency); perioperative management of hemophilia A; prophylaxis of joint bleeding and to reduce risk of joint damage in children with hemophilia A with no pre-existing joint damage; can be of significant therapeutic value in patients with acquired factor VIII inhibitors ≤10 Bethesda units/mL

Available Dosage Forms
Injection, powder for reconstitution:
Recombinate: 2000 int. units
Injection, powder for reconstitution [preservative free]:
Advate: 250 int. units, 500 int. units, 1000 int. units, 1500 int. units, 2000 int. units, 3000 int. units
Helixate® FS: 250 int. units, 500 int. units, 1000 int. units, 2000 int. units, 3000 int. units
Kogenate® FS: 250 int. units, 500 int. units, 1000 int. units, 2000 int. units, 3000 int. units
Recombinate: 250 int. units, 500 int. units, 1000 int. units, 1500 int. units
Xyntha™: 250 int. units, 500 int. units, 1000 int. units, 2000 int. units

Dosing
Adult & Geriatric Hemophilia: I.V.: Individualize dosage based on coagulation studies performed prior to treatment and at regular intervals during treatment. In general, administration of factor VIII 1 int. unit/kg will increase circulating factor VIII levels by ~2 int. units/dL. (General guidelines presented; consult individual product labeling for specific dosing recommendations.)

Dosage based on desired factor VIII increase (%):
To calculate dosage needed based on desired factor VIII increase (%):
[Body weight (kg) x desired factor VIII increase (%)] divided by 2%/int. units/kg = int. units factor VIII required
For example:
50 kg x 30 (% increase) divided by 2%/int. units/kg = 750 int. units factor VIII
Dosage based on expected factor VIII increase (%):
It is also possible to calculate the **expected** % factor VIII increase:
(# int. units administered x 2%/int. units/kg) divided by body weight (kg) = expected % factor VIII increase
For example:
(1400 int. units x 2%/int. units/kg) divided by 70 kg = 40%
General guidelines:
Minor hemorrhage: 10-20 int. units/kg as a single dose to achieve FVIII plasma level ~20% to 40% of normal. Mild superficial or early hemorrhages may respond to a single dose; may repeat dose every 12-24 hours for 1-3 days until bleeding is resolved or healing achieved.
Moderate hemorrhage/minor surgery: 15-30 int. units/kg to achieve FVIII plasma level 30% to 60% of normal. May repeat 1 dose at 12-24 hours if needed. Some products suggest continuing for ≥3 days until pain and disability are resolved.
Major to life-threatening hemorrhage: Initial dose 40-50 int. units/kg followed by a maintenance dose of 20-25 int. units/kg every 8-24 hours until threat is resolved, to achieve FVIII plasma level 60% to 100% of normal.
Major surgery: 50 int. units/kg given preoperatively to raise factor VIII level to 100% before surgery begins. May repeat as necessary after 6-12 hours initially and for a total of 10-14 days until healing is complete. Intensity of therapy may depend on type of surgery and postoperative regimen.
Bleeding prophylaxis: May be administered on a regular basis for bleeding prophylaxis. Doses of 24-40 int. units/kg 3 times/week have been reported in patients with severe hemophilia to prevent joint bleeding.

If bleeding is not controlled with adequate dose, test for presence of inhibitor. It may not be possible or practical to control bleeding if inhibitor titers >10 Bethesda units/mL.

Pediatric
Hemophilia: Refer to adult dosing.
Joint bleeding prophylaxis (Helixate® FS, Kogenate® FS): 25 int. units/kg every other day

Administration
I.V. I.V. infusion over 5-10 minutes (maximum: 10 mL/minute).
Advate: Infuse over ≤5 minutes (maximum: 10 mL/minute)
Helixate® FS, Kogenate® FS: Infuse over 1-15 minutes; based on patient tolerability
Xyntha™: Infuse over several minutes; adjust based on patient comfort. Do not admix or administer in same tubing as other medications.

Monitoring and Teaching Issues

Laboratory Monitoring Plasma factor VIII activity; development of factor VIII inhibitors; hemoglobin, hematocrit

Physical Assessment Patient should be monitored closely during and after infusion for any change in vital signs, cardiac and CNS status, or hypersensitivity reactions (eg, chills, fever, chest pain, respiratory difficulty). Assess results of hematocrit and coagulation studies. Monitor bleeding and coagulation status. Monitor for anemia.

Patient Education This medication can only be given intravenously. Report immediately any sudden-onset headache, rash, chest or back pain, wheezing or respiratory difficulties, hives, itching, low-grade fever, stomach pain, or nausea/vomiting to prescriber. Wear identification indicating that you have a hemophilic condition.

Antihemophilic Factor/von Willebrand Factor Complex (Human)

(an tee hee moe FIL ik FAK tor von WILL le brand FAK tor KOM plex HYU man)

U.S. Brand Names Alphanate®; Humate-P®; Wilate®

Index Terms AHF (Human); Factor VIII (Human); Factor VIII Concentrate; FVIII/vWF; von Willebrand Factor/Factor VIII Complex; VWF/FVIII Concentrate; VWF:RCo; vWF:RCof

Generic Availability (U.S.) No

Pharmacologic Category Antihemophilic Agent; Blood Product Derivative

Medication Safety Issues

Sound-alike/look-alike issues:

Factor VIII may be confused with Factor XIII

Pregnancy Risk Factor C

Lactation Excretion in breast milk unknown/use caution

Use

Factor VIII deficiency: Alphanate®, Humate-P®: Prevention and treatment of hemorrhagic episodes in patients with hemophilia A (classical hemophilia) or acquired factor VIII deficiency (Alphanate® only); **Note:** Wilate® is not approved for use in patients with hemophilia A or acquired factor VIII deficiency

von Willebrand disease (VWD):

Alphanate®: Prophylaxis with surgical and/or invasive procedures in patients with VWD when desmopressin is either ineffective or contraindicated; **Note:** Not indicated for patients with severe VWD undergoing major surgery

Humate-P®: Treatment of spontaneous or trauma-induced bleeding, as well as prevention of excessive bleeding during and after surgery in patients with severe VWD, including mild or moderate disease where use of desmopressin is known or suspected to be inadequate; **Note:** Not indicated for the prophylaxis of spontaneous bleeding episodes

Wilate®: Treatment of spontaneous and trauma-induced bleeding in patients with severe VWD, including mild or moderate disease where use of desmopressin is known or suspected to be inadequate or contraindicated; **Note:** Not indicated for prophylaxis of spontaneous bleeding or prevention of excessive bleeding during and after surgery)

Available Dosage Forms

Injection, powder for reconstitution [human derived]:

Alphanate®:

250 int. units [Factor VIII and VWF:RCo ratio varies by lot]
500 int. units [Factor VIII and VWF:RCo ratio varies by lot]
1000 int. units [Factor VIII and VWF:RCo ratio varies by lot]
1500 int. units [Factor VIII and VWF:RCo ratio varies by lot]

Humate-P®:

FVIII 250 int. units and VWF:RCo 600 int. units
FVIII 500 int. units and VWF:RCo 1200 int. units
FVIII 1000 int. units and VWF:RCo 2400 int. units

Dosing

Adult & Geriatric

Factor VIII deficiency: General guidelines (consult specific product labeling for Alphanate® or Humate-P®): I.V.:

Individualize dosage based on coagulation studies performed prior to treatment and at regular intervals during treatment; in general, administration of factor VIII 1 int. unit/kg will increase circulating factor VIII levels by ~2 int. units/dL.

Minor hemorrhage: Loading dose: FVIII:C 15 int. units/kg to achieve FVIII:C plasma level ~30% of normal. If second infusion is needed, half the loading dose may be given once or twice daily for 1-2 days.

Moderate hemorrhage: Loading dose: FVIII:C 25 int. units/kg to achieve FVIII:C plasma level ~50% of normal; Maintenance: FVIII:C 15 int. units/kg every 8-12 hours for 1-2 days in order to maintain FVIII:C plasma levels at 30% of normal. Repeat the same dose once or twice daily for up to 7 days or until adequate wound healing.

Life-threatening hemorrhage/major surgery: Loading dose: FVIII:C 40-50 int. units/kg; Maintenance: FVIII:C 20-25 int. units/kg every 8-12 hours to maintain FVIII:C plasma levels at 80% to 100% of normal for 7 days. Continue same dose once or twice daily for another 7 days in order to maintain FVIII:C levels at 30% to 50% of normal.

von Willebrand disease (VWD): Treatment:

Humate-P®: I.V.: Individualize dosage based on coagulation studies performed prior to treatment and at regular intervals during treatment; in general, administration of factor VIII 1 int. unit/kg would be expected to raise circulating VWF:RCo ~5 int. units/dL

Type 1, mild VWD: Minor hemorrhage (if desmopressin is not appropriate) or major hemorrhage:
Loading dose: VWF:RCo 40-60 int. units/kg
Maintenance dose: VWF:RCo 40-50 int. units/kg every 8-12 hours for 3 days, keeping VWF:RCo nadir >50%; follow with 40-50 int. units/kg daily for up to 7 days
Type 1, moderate or severe VWD:
Minor hemorrhage: VWF:RCo 40-50 int. units/kg for 1-2 doses
Major hemorrhage:
Loading dose: VWF:RCo 50-75 int. units/kg
Maintenance dose: VWF:RCo 40-60 int. units/kg every 8-12 hours for 3 days to keep the VWF:RCo nadir >50%, then 40-60 int. units/kg daily for a total of up to 7 days
Types 2 and 3 VWD:
Minor hemorrhage: VWF:RCo 40-50 int. units/kg for 1-2 doses
Major hemorrhage:
Loading dose: VWF:RCo 60-80 int. units/kg
Maintenance dose: VWF:RCo 40-60 int. units/kg every 8-12 hours for 3 days, keeping the VWF:RCo nadir >50%; follow with 40-60 int. units/kg daily for a total of up to 7 days

Wilate®: I.V.:
Minor hemorrhage:
Loading dose: VWF:RCo: 20-40 int. units/kg
Maintenance dose: 20-30 int. units/kg every 12-24 hours for ≤3 days, keeping the VWF: RCo nadir >30%
Major hemorrhage:
Loading dose: VWF:RCo: 40-60 int. units/kg
Maintenance dose: 20-40 int. units/kg every 12-24 hours for 5-7 days, keeping the VWF: RCo nadir >50%

von Willebrand disease (VWD): Prophylaxis: I.V.:

Alphanate®: *Surgery/procedure prophylaxis (except patients with type 3 undergoing major surgery):*
Preoperative dose: VWF:RCo: 60 int. units/kg 1 hour prior to surgery
Maintenance dose: VWF:RCo: 40-60 int. units/kg every 8-12 hours as clinically needed. May reduce dose after third postoperative day; continue treatment until healing is complete. For minor procedures, maintain VWF of 40% to 50% during postoperative days 1-3; for major procedures maintain VWF of 40% to 50% for ≥3-7 days.

Humate-P®: *Surgery/procedure prevention of bleeding:*
Emergency surgery: Administer VWF:RCo 50-60 int. units/kg; monitor trough coagulation factor levels for subsequent doses
Surgical management (nonemergency):
Loading dose calculation based on baseline target VWF:RCo: (Target peak VWF:RCo - Baseline VWF:RCo) x weight (in kg) / IVR = int. units VWF:RCo required. Administer loading dose 1-2 hours prior to surgery. **Note:** If *in vivo* recovery (IVR) not available, assume 2 int. units/dL per int. units/kg of VWF:RCo product administered.
Target concentrations for VWF:RCo following loading dose:
Major surgery: 100 int. units/dL
Minor surgery: 50-60 int. units/dL
Maintenance dose: Initial: One-half loading dose, followed by subsequent dosing determined by target trough concentrations, generally every 8-12 hours. Patients with shorter half-lives may require dosing every 6 hours.
Target maintenance trough VWF:RCo concentrations:
Major surgery: >50 int. units/dL for up to 3 days, followed by >30 int. units/dL for a minimum total treatment of 72 hours
Minor surgery: ≥30 int. units/dL for a minimum duration of 48 hours
Oral surgery: ≥30 int. units/dL for a minimum duration of 8-12 hours

Pediatric

Factor VIII deficiency: Refer to adult dosing.
von Willebrand disease (VWD): Treatment: Refer to adult dosing.
von Willebrand disease (VWD): Prophylaxis:
Surgery/procedure prophylaxis (except patients with type 3 undergoing major surgery) (Alphanate®): I.V.:
Preoperative dose: VWF:RCo: 75 int. units/kg 1 hour prior to surgery
Maintenance dose: VWF:RCo: 50-75 int. units/kg every 8-12 hours as clinically needed. May reduce dose after third postoperative day; continue treatment until healing is complete.
Surgery/procedure prevention of bleeding (Humate-P®): Refer to adult dosing.

Administration

I.V.

Alphanate®: Infuse slowly (maximum rate 10 mL/minute)
Humate-P®: Infuse slowly (maximum rate 4 mL/minute)
Wilate®: Infuse slowly at a rate of 2-4 mL/minute

Monitoring and Teaching Issues

Laboratory Monitoring AHF levels prior to and during treatment; in patients with circulating inhibitors, the inhibitor level should be monitored; hematocrit; monitor for signs and symptoms of intravascular hemolysis; bleeding; VWF activity (circulating levels of functional VWF are measured as ristocetin cofactor activity [VWF:RCo]). In surgical patients, monitor VWF:RCo at baseline and after surgery, trough VWF:RCo and FVIII:C at least daily.

Physical Assessment Patient should be monitored closely during and after infusion for any change in vital signs, cardiac and CNS status, or hypersensitivity reactions (eg, chills, fever, chest pain, respiratory difficulty). Assess results of hematocrit and coagulation studies. Monitor bleeding and coagulation status. Monitor for anemia.

Patient Education This medication can only be given intravenously. Report immediately any sudden-onset headache, rash, chest or back pain, wheezing or respiratory difficulties, hives, itching, low-grade fever, stomach pain, or nausea/vomiting to prescriber. Wear identification indicating that you have a hemophilic condition.

◆ **Anti-Hist [OTC]** *see* DiphenhydrAMINE (Systemic) *on page 543*

Anti-inhibitor Coagulant Complex (an TEE in HI bi tor coe AG yoo lant KOM pleks)

U.S. Brand Names Feiba NF; Feiba VH [DSC]

Index Terms AICC; aPCC; Coagulant Complex Inhibitor

Generic Availability (U.S.) No

Pharmacologic Category Activated Prothrombin Complex Concentrate (aPCC); Antihemophilic Agent; Blood Product Derivative

Pregnancy Risk Factor C

Use Hemophilia A & B patients with inhibitors who are to undergo surgery or those who are bleeding

Unlabeled/Investigational Use Acquired hemophilia with factor VIII or factor IX inhibitor titers >5 Bethesda units (BU)

Available Dosage Forms

Injection, powder for reconstitution:

Feiba NF: ~500 units, ~1000 units, ~2500 units

Dosing

Adult & Geriatric Control of bleeding: I.V.: **Note:** Considered a first-line treatment when factor VIII inhibitor titer is >5 Bethesda units (BU) (antihemophilic factor may be preferred when titer <5 BU)

General dosing guidelines: 50-100 units/kg (maximum: 200 units/kg/day)

Joint hemorrhage: 50 units/kg every 12 hours; may increase to 100 units/kg every 12 hours; continue until signs of clinical improvement occur (maximum: 200 units/kg/day)

Mucous membrane bleeding: 50 units/kg every 6 hours; may increase to 100 units/kg every 6 hours up to 2 doses only (maximum: 200 units/kg/day)

Soft tissue hemorrhage (eg, retroperitoneal bleed): 100 units/kg every 12 hours (maximum: 200 units/kg/day)

Other severe hemorrhage (eg, intracranial hemorrhage): 100 units/kg every 12 hours; may be used every 6 hours if needed; continue until clinical improvement (maximum: 200 units/kg/day unless severity of hemorrhage justifies higher doses). **Note:** If total single dose exceeds 100 units/kg or total daily dose exceeds 200 units/kg/day, monitor closely for DIC and/or coronary ischemia.

Pediatric Refer to adult dosing.

Administration

I.V. For I.V. injection or drip infusion only; maximum infusion rate: 2 units/kg/minute. Following reconstitution, complete infusion within 3 hours.

Monitoring and Teaching Issues

Laboratory Monitoring Monitor for control of bleeding; signs and symptoms of DIC (blood pressure changes, pulse rate changes, chest pain/cough, fibrinogen decreased, platelet count decreased, fibrin-fibrinogen degradation products, significantly-prolonged thrombin time, PT, or partial thromboplastin time); hemoglobin and hematocrit; hypotension; have epinephrine ready to treat hypersensitivity reactions. **Note:** Tests used to control efficacy such as aPTT, WBCT, and TEG do not correlate with clinical improvement. Dosing to normalize these values may result in DIC.

Physical Assessment Assess potential for interactions with other pharmacological agents patient may be taking that may affect coagulation or platelet function. Patient should be monitored closely during and after infusion for any change in vital signs, cardiac and CNS status, or hypersensitivity reactions (chills, fever, chest pain, respiratory difficulty). If hypotension develops, the rate of infusion should be slowed and prescriber notified.

Patient Education This medication can only be administered by infusion; you will be monitored during and after infusion. Report immediately any sudden-onset headache, rash, chest or back pain, wheezing or respiratory difficulties, hives, itching, low-grade fever, stomach pain, or nausea/vomiting to prescriber. Wear identification indicating that you have a hemophilic condition.

◆ **anti-Tac Monoclonal antibody** *see* Daclizumab *on page 453*

Antithymocyte Globulin (Equine) (an te THY moe site GLOB yu lin E kwine)

U.S. Brand Names Atgam®

Index Terms Antithymocyte Immunoglobulin; ATG; Horse Antihuman Thymocyte Gamma Globulin; Lymphocyte Immune Globulin

Generic Availability (U.S.) No

Pharmacologic Category Immune Globulin; Immunosuppressant Agent; Polyclonal Antibody

Medication Safety Issues

Sound-alike/look-alike issues:

Antithymocyte globulin equine (Atgam®) may be confused with antithymocyte globulin rabbit (Thymoglobulin®)

Atgam® may be confused with Ativan®

Pregnancy Risk Factor C

Lactation Excretion in breast milk unknown/use caution

Use Prevention and treatment of acute renal allograft rejection; treatment of moderate-to-severe aplastic anemia in patients not considered suitable candidates for bone marrow transplantation

Unlabeled/Investigational Use Prevention and treatment of other solid organ allograft rejection; prevention or treatment of graft-versus-host disease (GVHD) following allogeneic stem cell transplantation; treatment of myelodysplastic syndrome (MDS)

Available Dosage Forms

Injection, solution:

Atgam®: 50 mg/mL (5 mL)

Dosing

Adult & Geriatric Note: An intradermal skin test is recommended prior to administration of the initial dose of ATG; use 0.1 mL of a fresh 1:1000 dilution of ATG in normal saline; observe every 15-20 minutes for 1 hour. A positive skin reaction consists of a wheal ≥10 mm in diameter. If a positive skin test occurs, the first infusion should be administered in a controlled environment with intensive life support immediately available. A systemic reaction precludes further administration of the drug. The absence of a reaction does **not** preclude the possibility of an immediate sensitivity reaction.

Note: Premedication with diphenhydramine, hydrocortisone, and acetaminophen is recommended prior to first dose.

Aplastic anemia protocol: I.V.: 10-20 mg/kg/day for 8-14 days, then give every other day for 7 more doses for a total of 21 doses in 28 days **or**

Unlabeled dosing: 40 mg/kg/day for 4 days (Rosenfeld, 1995).

Renal allograft rejection, prevention: I.V.: 15 mg/kg/day for 14 days, then give every other day for 7 more doses for a total of 21 doses in 28 days; the initial dose should be administered within 24 hours before or after transplantation.

Renal allograft rejection, treatment: I.V.: 10-15 mg/kg/day for 14 days, then administer every other day for 7 more doses for a total of 21 doses in 28 days.

Acute GVHD treatment (unlabeled use): I.V.: 30 mg/kg/dose every other day for 6 doses (MacMillan, 2007) **or** 15 mg/kg/dose twice daily for 10 doses (MacMillan, 2002)

Myelodysplastic syndrome (unlabeled use): I.V.: 40 mg/kg/dose once daily for 4 days; an intradermal test dose was administered prior to treatment (Molldrem, 2002)

Pediatric Note: See adult dosing for notes on intradermal skin testing and premedication.

Aplastic anemia protocol: I.V.: 10-20 mg/kg/day for 8-14 days; then administer every other day for 7 more doses; additional doses may be given every other day for 21 total doses in 28 days **or**

Unlabeled dosing: Children >10 kg: 40 mg/kg/day for 4 days (Rosenfeld, 1995).

Renal allograft: I.V.: 5-25 mg/kg/day

Acute GVHD treatment (unlabeled use): I.V.: 30 mg/kg/dose every other day for 6 doses (MacMillan, 2007) **or** 15 mg/kg/dose twice daily for 10 doses (MacMillan, 2002)

Adjustment for Toxicity

Anaphylaxis: Stop infusion immediately; administer epinephrine. May require corticosteroids, respiration assistance, and/or other resuscitative measures. Do not resume infusion.

Hemolysis (severe and unremitting): May require discontinuation of treatment.

Administration

I.V. Infuse dose over at least 4 hours. Any severe systemic reaction to the skin test, such as generalized rash, tachycardia, dyspnea, hypotension, or anaphylaxis, should preclude further therapy. Epinephrine and resuscitative equipment should be nearby. Patient may need to be pretreated with an antipyretic, antihistamine, and/or corticosteroid. Mild itching and erythema can be treated with antihistamines. May cause vein irritation (chemical phlebitis) if administered peripherally. Infuse into a vascular shunt, arterial venous fistula, or high-flow central vein through a 0.2-1 micron in-line filter.

First dose: Premedicate with diphenhydramine orally 30 minutes prior to and hydrocortisone I.V. 15 minutes prior to infusion and acetaminophen 2 hours after start of infusion.

Monitoring and Teaching Issues

Laboratory Monitoring Lymphocyte profile, CBC with differential, platelet count

Physical Assessment Assess for history of previous allergic reactions. Intradermal skin testing and premedication are recommended with the first dose. Treatment for hypersensitivity should be available. Monitor vital signs during infusion and observe for adverse or allergic reactions closely. Monitor for signs of infection.

Patient Education This medication can only be administered by infusion. You will be closely monitored during the infusion. Ask for assistance if you must get up or change position. Do not have any vaccinations for the next 3 months without consulting prescriber. Immediately report chills; persistent dizziness or nausea; itching or stinging; acute back pain; flank pain; chest pain, tightness, or rapid heartbeat; or respiratory difficulty.

- ◆ **Antithymocyte Immunoglobulin** *see* Antithymocyte Globulin (Equine) *on page 136*
- ◆ **Antitumor Necrosis Factor Apha (Human)** *see* Adalimumab *on page 48*
- ◆ **Anti-VEGF Monoclonal Antibody** *see* Bevacizumab *on page 211*
- ◆ **Anti-VEGF rhuMAb** *see* Bevacizumab *on page 211*

- ◆ **Antivert®** *see* Meclizine *on page 1153*
- ◆ **Anucort-HC™** *see* Hydrocortisone (Topical) *on page 920*
- ◆ **Anu-med HC** *see* Hydrocortisone (Topical) *on page 920*
- ◆ **Anusol-HC®** *see* Hydrocortisone (Topical) *on page 920*
- ◆ **Anzemet®** *see* Dolasetron *on page 567*
- ◆ **4-AP** *see* Dalfampridine *on page 458*
- ◆ **APAP** *see* Acetaminophen *on page 38*
- ◆ **APAP 500 [OTC]** *see* Acetaminophen *on page 38*
- ◆ **aPCC** *see* Anti-inhibitor Coagulant Complex *on page 136*
- ◆ **Apidra®** *see* Insulin Glulisine *on page 988*
- ◆ **Apidra® SoloStar®** *see* Insulin Glulisine *on page 988*
- ◆ **Aplenzin™** *see* BuPROPion *on page 252*
- ◆ **Aplonidine** *see* Apraclonidine *on page 139*
- ◆ **Apokyn®** *see* Apomorphine *on page 138*

Apomorphine (a poe MOR feen)

U.S. Brand Names Apokyn®

Index Terms Apomorphine Hydrochloride; Apomorphine Hydrochloride Hemihydrate

Generic Availability (U.S.) No

Pharmacologic Category Anti-Parkinson's Agent, Dopamine Agonist

Prescribing and Access Restrictions Apokyn® is only available through a select group of specialty pharmacies and cannot be obtained through a retail pharmacy. Apokyn® may be obtained from the following specialty pharmacies: Accredo Nova Factor or PharmaCare. To obtain the medication, contact the APOKYN Call Center at 1-877-7APOKYN (1-877-727-6596).

Pregnancy Risk Factor C

Lactation Excretion in breast milk unknown/contraindicated

Use Treatment of hypomobility, "off" episodes with Parkinson's disease

Unlabeled/Investigational Use Treatment of erectile dysfunction

Available Dosage Forms

Injection, solution:

Apokyn®: 10 mg/mL (3 mL)

Dosing

Adult & Geriatric Begin antiemetic therapy 3 days prior to initiation and continue for 2 months before reassessing need.

Parkinson's disease, "off" episode: SubQ: Initial test dose 2 mg, **medical supervision required; see "Note"**. Subsequent dosing is based on both tolerance and response to initial test dose.

If patient tolerates test dose and responds: Starting dose: 2 mg as needed; may increase dose in 1 mg increments every few days; maximum dose: 6 mg

If patient tolerates but does not respond to 2 mg test dose: Second test dose: 4 mg

If patient tolerates and responds to 4 mg test dose: Starting dose: 3 mg, as needed for "off" episodes; may increase dose in 1 mg increments every few days; maximum dose 6 mg

If patient does not tolerate 4 mg test dose: Third test dose: 3 mg

If patient tolerates 3 mg test dose: Starting dose: 2 mg as needed for "off" episodes; may increase dose in 1 mg increments to a maximum of 3 mg

If therapy is interrupted for >1 week, restart at 2 mg and gradually titrate dose.

Note: Medical supervision is required for all test doses with standing and supine blood pressure monitoring predose and 20-, 40-, and 60 minutes postdose. If subsequent test doses are required, wait >2 hours before another test dose is given; next test dose should be timed with another "off" episode. If a single dose is ineffective for a particular "off" episode, then a second dose should not be given. The average dosing frequency was 3 times/day in the development program with limited experience in dosing >5 times/day and with total daily doses >20 mg. Apomorphine is intended to treat the "off" episodes associated with levodopa therapy of Parkinson's disease and has not been studied in levodopa-naive Parkinson's patients.

Renal Impairment

Mild-to-moderate impairment: Reduce test dose and starting dose: 1 mg

Severe impairment: Has not been studied

Hepatic Impairment

Mild-to-moderate impairment: Use caution

Severe impairment: Has not been studied

Administration

I.V. Not for I.V. administration.

Other SubQ: Initiate antiemetic 3 days before test dose of apomorphine and continue for 2 months (if patient to be treated) before reassessment. Administer in abdomen, upper arm, or upper leg; change site with each injection. 3 mL cartridges are used with a manual, reusable, multidose injector pen. Injector pen can deliver doses up to 1 mL in 0.02 mL increments. Do not give intravenously; thrombus formation or pulmonary embolism may occur.

Monitoring and Teaching Issues

Physical Assessment Patient must be monitored closely for minimum of 90 minutes following each test dose. Monitor for orthostatic hypotension, nausea, vomiting, dyskinesias, and excessive sedation or somnolence. Teach patient or caregiver proper injection technique and needle disposal.

Patient Education Follow specific directions for administration with injection pen or syringe and needle disposal. Avoid alcohol. An antiemetic may be prescribed to reduce nausea or vomiting. May cause headache, drowsiness, dizziness, loss of impulse control (possibly manifested as pathological gambling, libido increases, and/or binge eating), postural hypotension, nausea, or vomiting. Report immediately any irregular or rapid heartbeat, chest pain, palpitations, difficulty breathing, or shortness of breath; unusual or sudden sleepiness; unusual muscle or skeletal movements or weakness, tremors, or altered gait; CNS changes (hallucinations, confusion, insomnia, anxiety, or depression); suicide ideation; redness, swelling, or irritation at injection site; changes in the appearance of skin moles; or other unusual skin changes.

◆ **Apomorphine Hydrochloride** *see* Apomorphine *on page 138*

◆ **Apomorphine Hydrochloride Hemihydrate** *see* Apomorphine *on page 138*

◆ **APPG** *see* Penicillin G Procaine *on page 1435*

Apraclonidine (a pra KLOE ni deen)

U.S. Brand Names Iopidine®

Index Terms Aplonidine; Apraclonidine Hydrochloride; p-Aminoclonidine

Generic Availability (U.S.) Yes

Pharmacologic Category $Alpha_2$ Agonist, Ophthalmic

Medication Safety Issues

Sound-alike/look-alike issues:

Iopidine® may be confused with indapamide, iodine, Lodine®

Pregnancy Risk Factor C

Lactation Excretion in breast milk unknown/use caution

Use Prevention and treatment of postsurgical intraocular pressure (IOP) elevation; short-term, adjunctive therapy in patients who require additional reduction of IOP

Available Dosage Forms

Solution, ophthalmic: 0.5% (5 mL, 10 mL)

Iopidine®: 0.5% (5 mL, 10 mL); 1% (0.1 mL)

Dosing

Adult & Geriatric Postsurgical intraocular pressure elevation (prevention/treatment): Ophthalmic:

0.5%: Instill 1-2 drops in the affected eye(s) 3 times/day

1%: Instill 1 drop in operative eye 1 hour prior to anterior segment laser surgery, second drop in eye immediately upon completion of procedure

Renal Impairment Although the topical use of apraclonidine has not been studied in renal failure patients, structurally-related clonidine undergoes a significant increase in half-life in patients with severe renal impairment. Close monitoring of cardiovascular parameters in patients with impaired renal function is advised.

Hepatic Impairment Close monitoring of cardiovascular parameters in patients with impaired liver function is advised because the systemic dosage form of clonidine is partially metabolized in the liver.

Administration

Other Wait 5 minutes between instillation of other ophthalmic agents to avoid washout of previous dose. After topical instillation, finger pressure should be applied to lacrimal sac to decrease drainage into the nose and throat and minimize possible systemic absorption.

Monitoring and Teaching Issues

Physical Assessment Monitor intraocular pressure.

Patient Education For use in eyes only. May sting on instillation, do not touch dropper to eye. Visual acuity may be decreased after administration. Night vision may be decreased. Distance vision may be altered.

◆ **Apraclonidine Hydrochloride** *see* Apraclonidine *on page 139*

Aprepitant (ap RE pi tant)

U.S. Brand Names Emend®

Index Terms L 754030; MK 869

Generic Availability (U.S.) No

Pharmacologic Category Antiemetic; Substance P/Neurokinin 1 Receptor Antagonist

Medication Safety Issues

Sound-alike/look-alike issues:

Aprepitant may be confused with fosaprepitant

Emend® (aprepitant) oral capsule formulation may be confused with Emend® for injection (fosaprepitant).

Pregnancy Risk Factor B

Lactation Excretion in breast milk unknown/not recommended

Use Prevention of acute and delayed nausea and vomiting associated with moderately- and highly-emetogenic chemotherapy (in combination with other antiemetics); prevention of postoperative nausea and vomiting (PONV)

Mechanism of Action/Effect Prevents acute and delayed vomiting at the substance P/neurokinin 1 (NK_1) receptor; augments the antiemetic activity of 5-HT_3 receptor antagonists and corticosteroids to inhibit acute and delayed phases of chemotherapy-induced emesis.

Contraindications Hypersensitivity to aprepitant or any component of the formulation; concurrent use with cisapride or pimozide

Warnings/Precautions Use caution with agents primarily metabolized via CYP3A4; aprepitant is a 3A4 inhibitor. Effect on orally administered 3A4 substrates is greater than those administered intravenously. Chronic continuous use is not recommended; however, a single 40 mg aprepitant oral dose is not likely to alter plasma concentrations of CYP3A4 substrates. Use caution with severe hepatic impairment; has not been studied in patients with severe hepatic impairment (Child-Pugh class C). Not studied for treatment of existing nausea and vomiting. Chronic continuous administration is not recommended.

Drug Interactions

Metabolism/Transport Effects Substrate of CYP1A2 (minor), 2C19 (minor), 3A4 (major); **Inhibits** CYP2C9 (weak), 2C19 (weak), 3A4 (moderate); **Induces** CYP2C9 (weak), 3A4 (weak)

Avoid Concomitant Use

Avoid concomitant use of Aprepitant with any of the following: Cisapride; Pimozide; Tolvaptan

Decreased Effect

Aprepitant may decrease the levels/effects of: Contraceptives (Estrogens); Contraceptives (Progestins); CYP2C9 Substrates (High risk); PARoxetine; Saxagliptin; TOLBUTamide; Warfarin

The levels/effects of Aprepitant may be decreased by: CYP3A4 Inducers (Strong); Deferasirox; Herbs (CYP3A4 Inducers); PARoxetine; Rifamycin Derivatives

Increased Effect/Toxicity

Aprepitant may increase the levels/effects of: Benzodiazepines (metabolized by oxidation); Cisapride; Colchicine; Corticosteroids (Systemic); CYP3A4 Substrates; Diltiazem; Eplerenone; Everolimus; FentaNYL; Halofantrine; Lurasidone; Pimecrolimus; Pimozide; Ranolazine; Salmeterol; Saxagliptin; Tolvaptan; Vilazodone

The levels/effects of Aprepitant may be increased by: Antifungal Agents (Azole Derivatives, Systemic); Conivaptan; CYP3A4 Inhibitors (Moderate); CYP3A4 Inhibitors (Strong); Dasatinib; Diltiazem

Nutritional/Ethanol Interactions

Food: Aprepitant serum concentration may be increased when taken with grapefruit juice; avoid concurrent use.

Herb/Nutraceutical: Avoid St John's wort (may decrease aprepitant levels).

Adverse Reactions Note: Adverse reactions reported as part of a combination chemotherapy regimen or with general anesthesia.

>10%:
- Central nervous system: Fatigue (≤18%)
- Gastrointestinal: Nausea (6% to 13%), constipation (9% to 10%)
- Neuromuscular & skeletal: Weakness (≤18%)
- Miscellaneous: Hiccups (11%)

1% to 10%:
- Cardiovascular: Hypotension (≤6%), bradycardia (≤4%)
- Central nervous system: Dizziness (≤7%)
- Endocrine & metabolic: Dehydration (≤6%)
- Gastrointestinal: Diarrhea (≤10%), dyspepsia (≤6%), abdominal pain (≤5%), epigastric discomfort (4%), gastritis (4%), stomatitis (3%)
- Hepatic: ALT increased (≤6%), AST increased (3%)
- Renal: Proteinuria (7%), BUN increased (5%)

Pharmacodynamics/Kinetics

Bioavailability ~60% to 65%

Time to Peak Plasma: ~3-4 hours

Protein Binding >95%

Half-Life Elimination Terminal: ~9-13 hours

Metabolism Extensively hepatic via CYP3A4 (major); CYP1A2 and CYP2C19 (minor); forms 7 metabolites (weakly active)

Available Dosage Forms

Capsule, oral:

Emend®: 40 mg, 80 mg, 125 mg

Combination package, oral:

Emend®: Capsule: 80 mg (2s) and Capsule: 125 mg (1s)

Dosing

Adult & Geriatric

Prevention of chemotherapy-induced nausea/vomiting: Oral: 125 mg 1 hour prior to chemotherapy on day 1, followed by 80 mg once daily on days 2 and 3 (in combination with a corticosteroid and 5-HT_3 antagonist antiemetic)

Prevention of PONV: Oral: 40 mg within 3 hours prior to induction

Renal Impairment No dose adjustment necessary in patients with renal disease or end-stage renal disease maintained on hemodialysis.

Hepatic Impairment

Mild-to-moderate impairment (Child-Pugh classes A and B): No adjustment necessary.

Severe impairment (Child-Pugh class C): Use caution; no data available.

Administration

Oral

Chemotherapy induced nausea/vomiting: Administer with or without food. First dose should be given 1 hour prior to antineoplastic therapy; subsequent doses should be given in the morning.

PONV: Administer within 3 hours prior to induction; follow healthcare providers instructions about food/drink restrictions prior to surgery.

Stability

Storage Store at room temperature of 20°C to 25°C (68°F to 77°F).

Monitoring and Teaching Issues

Physical Assessment Use with caution in presence of severe hepatic impairment. Monitor for fatigue, weakness, gastrointestinal disturbance, and dehydration.

Patient Education This medication is intended to prevent or treat nausea/vomiting; it may be prescribed in combination with other medications; follow directions and timing exactly. May by taken with or without food; do not take with grapefruit juice. Report unusual fatigue, weakness, dizziness, disorientation, abdominal discomfort, chest pain, or respiratory distress to prescriber.

Dietary Considerations May be taken with or without food.

Geriatric Considerations In two studies by the manufacturer, with a total of 544 patients, 31% were >65 years of age, while 5% were >75 years. No differences in safety and efficacy were noted between elderly subjects and younger adults. No dosing adjustment is necessary.

Pregnancy Considerations Teratogenic effects were not observed in animal studies. There are no adequate and well-controlled studies in pregnant women; use only if clearly needed. Efficacy of hormonal contraceptive may be reduced; alternative or additional methods of contraception should be used both during treatment with fosaprepitant or aprepitant and for at least 1 month following the last fosaprepitant/aprepitant dose.

Additional Information Oncology Comment: Aprepitant is recommended in the American Society of Clinical Oncology (ASCO) oncology antiemetic guidelines for use in combination with a serotonin receptor antagonist and dexamethasone for chemotherapy with high emetic risk and for chemotherapy regimens of moderate emetic risk which contain an anthracycline and cyclophosphamide (Kris, 2006). The National Comprehensive Cancer Network® (NCCN) Clinical Practice Guidelines in Oncology for Antiemesis (version 1.2011) recommend the same use of aprepitant as is in the ASCO recommendation. In addition to the moderately emetogenic chemotherapy listed above, the NCCN guidelines suggest that aprepitant may also be used for select moderately emetogenic regimens containing carboplatin, cisplatin, doxorubicin, epirubicin, ifosfamide, irinotecan and methotrexate. Either fosaprepitant 115 mg or aprepitant (125 mg orally) are administered on day 1; for day 2 and 3, patients should receive aprepitant 80 mg orally.

- **Aprepitant Injection** *see* Fosaprepitant *on page 826*
- **Apresazide [DSC]** *see* Hydralazine and Hydrochlorothiazide *on page 911*
- **Apresoline [DSC]** *see* HydrALAZINE *on page 909*
- **Apri®** *see* Ethinyl Estradiol and Desogestrel *on page 695*
- **Apriso™** *see* Mesalamine *on page 1177*
- **Aptivus®** *see* Tipranavir *on page 1771*
- **Aquanil HC® [OTC]** *see* Hydrocortisone (Topical) *on page 920*
- **Aqueous Procaine Penicillin G** *see* Penicillin G Procaine *on page 1435*
- **Ara-C** *see* Cytarabine *on page 445*
- **Arabinosylcytosine** *see* Cytarabine *on page 445*
- **Aralen®** *see* Chloroquine *on page 359*
- **Aranelle®** *see* Ethinyl Estradiol and Norethindrone *on page 701*
- **Aranesp®** *see* Darbepoetin Alfa *on page 463*
- **Aranesp® SingleJect®** *see* Darbepoetin Alfa *on page 463*
- **Arava®** *see* Leflunomide *on page 1068*
- **Arcalyst™** *see* Rilonacept *on page 1581*
- **Aredia®** *see* Pamidronate *on page 1397*

Arformoterol (ar for MOE ter ol)

U.S. Brand Names Brovana®

Index Terms (R,R)-Formoterol L-Tartrate; Arformoterol Tartrate

Generic Availability (U.S.) No

Pharmacologic Category $Beta_2$-Adrenergic Agonist; $Beta_2$-Adrenergic Agonist, Long-Acting

Medication Guide Available Yes

Pregnancy Risk Factor C

Lactation Excretion in breast milk unknown/use caution

Use Long-term maintenance treatment of bronchoconstriction in chronic obstructive pulmonary disease (COPD), including chronic bronchitis and emphysema

Available Dosage Forms

Solution, for nebulization:

Brovana®: 15 mcg/2 mL (30s, 60s)

Dosing

Adult & Geriatric COPD: Nebulization: 15 mcg twice daily; maximum: 30 mcg/day

Renal Impairment No adjustment required.

Hepatic Impairment No dosage adjustment required, but use caution; systemic drug exposure prolonged (1.3- to 2.4-fold).

Administration

Inhalation Nebulization: Remove each vial from individually sealed foil pouch immediately before use. Use with standard jet nebulizer connected to an air compressor, administer with mouthpiece or face mask. Administer vial undiluted and do not mix with other medications in nebulizer.

Monitoring and Teaching Issues

Laboratory Monitoring FEV_1, peak flow, and/or other pulmonary function tests; serum glucose, serum potassium

Physical Assessment Teach patient appropriate use and care of nebulizer.

Patient Education This drug is intended for long-term use. Do not mix with other medications in your nebulizer. Maintain adequate hydration, unless instructed to restrict fluid intake. You may experience nervousness, tremor, headache, muscle cramps, trouble sleeping, dizziness, or tiredness. Report rapid heart rate, chest pain, or palpitations; swelling of extremities or weight gain; back or leg pain; increased shortness of breath; or difficulty breathing.

◆ **Arformoterol Tartrate** *see* Arformoterol *on page 141*

Argatroban (ar GA troh ban)

Generic Availability (U.S.) No

Pharmacologic Category Anticoagulant, Thrombin Inhibitor

Medication Safety Issues

Sound-alike/look-alike issues:

Argatroban may be confused with Aggrastat®, Orgaran®

High alert medication: The Institute for Safe Medication Practices (ISMP) includes this medication among its list of drugs which have a heightened risk of causing significant patient harm when used in error.

Pregnancy Risk Factor B

Lactation Excretion in breast milk unknown/not recommended

Use Prophylaxis or treatment of thrombosis in patients with heparin-induced thrombocytopenia (HIT); adjunct to percutaneous coronary intervention (PCI) in patients who have or are at risk of thrombosis associated with HIT

Unlabeled/Investigational Use To maintain extracorporeal circuit patency (prefilter administration) of continuous renal replacement therapy (CRRT) in critically-ill patients with HIT

Available Dosage Forms

Injection, solution: 100 mg/mL (2.5 mL)

Dosing

Adult & Geriatric

Prophylaxis of thrombosis (heparin-induced thrombocytopenia): I.V.:

Initial dose: 2 mcg/kg/minute; **Note:** Use of actual body weight up to 130 kg (BMI up to 51 kg/m^2) is supported (Rice, 2007); weight range included in phase II and III clinical trials: 33-204 kg (actual body weight). A maximum initial dose in mcg/minute has not been determined; adjust maintenance dose based on aPTT results.

Maintenance dose: Patient may not be at steady-state but measure aPTT after 2 hours; adjust dose until the steady-state aPTT is 1.5-3 times the initial baseline value, not exceeding 100 seconds; dosage should not exceed 10 mcg/kg/minute

Note: Critically-ill patients with normal hepatic function have become excessively anticoagulated with FDA-approved or lower starting doses of argatroban. Doses between 0.15-1.3 mcg/kg/minute were required to maintain aPTTs in the target range (Reichert, 2003). In a prospective observational study of critically-ill patients with MODS and suspected or proven HIT, an initial infusion dose of 0.2 mcg/kg/minute was found to be sufficient and safe in this population (Beiderlinden, 2007). Consider reducing starting dose to 0.2 mcg/kg/minute in critically-ill patients with multiple organ dysfunction (MODS) defined as a minimum number of two organ failures. Another report of a cardiac patient with anasarca secondary to acute renal failure had a reduction in argatroban clearance similar to patients with hepatic dysfunction. Reduced clearance may have been due to reduced liver perfusion (de Denus, 2003). The American College of Chest Physicians has recommended an initial infusion rate of 0.5-1.2 mcg/kg/minute for patients with heart failure, MODS, severe anasarca, or postcardiac surgery (Hirsch, 2008).

Conversion to oral anticoagulant: Because there may be a combined effect on the INR when argatroban is combined with warfarin, loading doses of warfarin should not be used. Warfarin therapy should be started at the expected daily dose.

Patients receiving ≤2 mcg/kg/minute of argatroban: Argatroban therapy can be stopped when the combined INR on warfarin and argatroban is >4; repeat INR measurement in 4-6 hours; if INR is below therapeutic level, argatroban therapy may be restarted. Repeat procedure daily until desired INR on warfarin alone is obtained.

Patients receiving >2 mcg/kg/minute of argatroban: In order to predict the INR on warfarin alone, reduce dose of argatroban to 2 mcg/kg/minute; measure INR for argatroban and warfarin 4-6 hours after dose reduction; argatroban therapy can be stopped when the combined INR on warfarin and argatroban is >4. Repeat INR measurement in 4-6 hours; if INR is below therapeutic level, argatroban therapy may be restarted. Repeat procedure daily until desired INR on warfarin alone is obtained.

Note: The American College of Chest Physicians recommends monitoring chromogenic factor X assay when transitioning from argatroban to warfarin (Hirsh, 2008). Factor X levels <45% have been associated with INR values >2 after the effects of argatroban have been eliminated (Arpino, 2005).

Prefilter administration for continuous renal replacement therapy (CRRT) in critically-ill patients with HIT (unlabeled use; Link, 2009): 0.1-1.5 mcg/kg/minute. **Note:** Loading dose of 100 mcg/kg was administered during clinical trial; however, this may be unnecessary.

Percutaneous coronary intervention (PCI): I.V.:

Initial: Begin infusion of 25 mcg/kg/minute and administer bolus dose of 350 mcg/kg (over 3-5 minutes). ACT should be checked 5-10 minutes after bolus infusion; proceed with procedure if ACT >300 seconds. Following initial bolus:

ACT <300 seconds: Give an additional 150 mcg/kg bolus, and increase infusion rate to 30 mcg/kg/minute (recheck ACT in 5-10 minutes)

ACT >450 seconds: Decrease infusion rate to 15 mcg/kg/minute (recheck ACT in 5-10 minutes)

Once a therapeutic ACT (300-450 seconds) is achieved, infusion should be continued at this dose for the duration of the procedure.

If dissection, impending abrupt closure, thrombus formation during PCI, or inability to achieve ACT >300 seconds: An additional bolus of 150 mcg/kg, followed by an increase in infusion rate to 40 mcg/kg/minute may be administered.

Note: Post-PCI anticoagulation, if required, may be achieved by continuing infusion at a reduced dose of 2-10 mcg/kg/minute, with close monitoring of aPTT.

Pediatric Heparin-induced thrombocytopenia (dosing based on limited data from critically-ill patients): I.V.:

Initial dose: 0.75 mcg/kg/minute

Maintenance dose: Patient may not be at steady-state but measure aPTT after 2 hours; adjust dose until the steady-state aPTT is 1.5-3 times the initial baseline value, not exceeding 100 seconds; dosage may be adjusted in increments of 0.1-0.25 mcg/kg/minute. **Note:** Frequent dosage adjustments may be required to maintain desired anticoagulant activity.

Renal Impairment Removal during hemodialysis and continuous venovenous hemofiltration is clinically insignificant. No dosage adjustment required.

Hepatic Impairment Decreased clearance and increased elimination half-life are seen with hepatic impairment; dose should be reduced.

Children: Initial dose: 0.2 mcg/kg/minute; adjust dose in increments of ≤0.05 mcg/kg/minute

Adults: Initial dose for moderate hepatic impairment is 0.5 mcg/kg/minute. **Note:** During PCI, avoid use in patients with elevations of ALT/AST (>3 times ULN); the use of argatroban in these patients has not been evaluated.

Administration

I.V. Solution **must be diluted to 1 mg/mL** prior to administration.

Monitoring and Teaching Issues

Laboratory Monitoring Hemoglobin, hematocrit; baseline aPTT prior to start of therapy. Patient may not be at steady-state but check aPTT 2 hours after start of therapy to adjust dose, keeping the steady-state aPTT 1.5-3 times the initial baseline value (not exceeding 100 seconds).

Physical Assessment Assess patient for use cautions. Assess potential for interactions with drugs that affect platelet function or coagulation. Monitor for abnormal bleeding, GI pain, epistaxis, hematuria, and irritation at infusion site. Observe bleeding precautions.

Patient Education This medication can only be administered by intravenous infusion and you will be monitored with blood tests during therapy. You may have a tendency to bleed easily; use electric razor, brush teeth with soft brush, floss with waxed floss, avoid all scissors or sharp instruments (knives, needles, etc), and avoid injury or bruising. Report stomach cramping or pain, dark or bloody stools, blood in urine, acute headache or confusion, respiratory difficulty, nosebleed, or bleeding from gums.

- ◆ **8-Arginine Vasopressin** *see* Vasopressin *on page* 1851
- ◆ **Aricept®** *see* Donepezil *on page* 569
- ◆ **Aricept® ODT** *see* Donepezil *on page* 569
- ◆ **Aridol™** *see* Mannitol *on page* 1146
- ◆ **Arimidex®** *see* Anastrozole *on page* 128

Aripiprazole (ay ri PIP ray zole)

U.S. Brand Names Abilify Discmelt®; Abilify®

Index Terms BMS 337039; OPC-14597

Generic Availability (U.S.) No

Pharmacologic Category Antipsychotic Agent, Atypical

Medication Safety Issues

Sound-alike/look-alike issues:

Abilify® may be confused with Ambien®

ARIPiprazole may be confused with proton pump inhibitors (dexlansoprazole, esomeprazole, lansoprazole, omeprazole, pantoprazole, RABEprazole)

Medication Guide Available Yes

Pregnancy Risk Factor C

Lactation Excretion in breast milk unknown/not recommended

Use

Oral: Acute and maintenance treatment of schizophrenia; acute (manic and mixed episodes) and maintenance treatment of bipolar I disorder as monotherapy or as an adjunct to lithium or valproic acid; adjunctive treatment of major depressive disorder; treatment of irritability associated with autistic disorder

Injection: Agitation associated with schizophrenia or bipolar I disorder

Unlabeled/Investigational Use Depression with psychotic features; aggression (children); conduct disorder (children); Tourette syndrome (children); psychosis/agitation related to Alzheimer's dementia

Mechanism of Action/Effect Aripiprazole (quinolinone antipsychotic) is a dopamine-serotonin system stabilizer with activity at dopamine and serotonin receptors.

Contraindications Hypersensitivity to aripiprazole or any component of the formulation

Warnings/Precautions **[U.S. Boxed Warning]: Elderly patients with dementia-related psychosis treated with antipsychotics are at an increased risk of death compared to placebo.** Most deaths appeared to be either cardiovascular (eg, heart failure, sudden death) or infectious (eg, pneumonia) in nature. In addition, an increased incidence of cerebrovascular effects (eg, transient ischemic attack, cerebrovascular accidents) has been reported in studies of placebo-controlled trials of aripiprazole in elderly patients with dementia-related psychosis. Aripiprazole is not approved for the treatment of dementia-related psychosis.

[U.S. Boxed Warning]: Antidepressants increase the risk of suicidal thinking and behavior in children, adolescents, and young adults (18-24 years of age) with major depressive disorder (MDD) and other psychiatric disorders; consider risk prior to prescribing. The possibility of a suicide attempt is inherent in major depression and may persist until remission occurs. Patients treated with antidepressants should be observed for clinical worsening and suicidality, especially during the initial few months of a course of drug therapy, or at times of dose changes, either increases or decreases. Prescriptions should be written for the smallest quantity consistent with good patient care. The patient's family or caregiver should be alerted to monitor patients for the emergence of suicidality and associated behaviors; patients should be instructed to notify their healthcare provider if any of these symptoms or worsening depression or psychosis occur.

Leukopenia, neutropenia, and agranulocytosis (sometimes fatal) have been reported in clinical trials and postmarketing reports with antipsychotic use; presence of risk factors (eg, pre-existing low WBC or history of drug-induced leuko-/neutropenia) should prompt periodic blood count assessment. Discontinue therapy at first signs of blood dyscrasias or if absolute neutrophil count $<1000/mm^3$.

A medication guide concerning the use of antidepressants should be dispensed with each prescription. **Aripiprazole is not FDA approved for adjunctive treatment of depression in children.**

May cause extrapyramidal symptoms (EPS), including pseudoparkinsonism, acute dystonic reactions, akathisia, and tardive dyskinesia (risk of these reactions is very low relative to typical/conventional antipsychotics, frequencies reported are similar to placebo). Risk of dystonia (and probably other EPS) may be greater with increased doses, use of conventional antipsychotics, males, and younger patients. May be associated with neuroleptic malignant syndrome (NMS).

May be sedating, use with caution in disorders where CNS depression is a feature. May cause orthostatic hypotension (although reported rates are similar to placebo); use caution in patients at risk of this effect or those who would not tolerate transient hypotensive episodes (cerebrovascular disease, cardiovascular disease, or other medications which may predispose).

Use caution in patients with Parkinson's disease; predisposition to seizures; and severe cardiac disease. May alter cardiac conduction; life-threatening arrhythmias have occurred with therapeutic doses of antipsychotics. Esophageal dysmotility and aspiration have been associated with antipsychotic use; use caution in patients at risk of pneumonia (eg, Alzheimer's disease). May alter temperature regulation. Significant weight gain has been observed with antipsychotic therapy; incidence varies with product. Monitor waist circumference and BMI.

Atypical antipsychotics have been associated with development of hyperglycemia; in some cases, may be extreme and associated with ketoacidosis, hyperosmolar coma, or death. Reports of hyperglycemia with aripiprazole therapy have been few and specific risk associated with this agent is not known. Use caution in patients with diabetes or other disorders of glucose regulation; monitor for worsening of glucose control.

Abilify Discmelt®: Use caution in phenylketonuria; contains phenylalanine.

Drug Interactions

Metabolism/Transport Effects Substrate (major) of CYP2D6, 3A4

Avoid Concomitant Use

Avoid concomitant use of ARIPiprazole with any of the following: Metoclopramide

Decreased Effect

ARIPiprazole may decrease the levels/effects of: Amphetamines; Anti-Parkinson's Agents (Dopamine Agonist); Quinagolide

The levels/effects of ARIPiprazole may be decreased by: CarBAMazepine; CYP3A4 Inducers (Strong); Deferasirox; Herbs (CYP3A4 Inducers); Lithium formulations; Peginterferon Alfa-2b

Increased Effect/Toxicity

ARIPiprazole may increase the levels/effects of: Alcohol (Ethyl); CNS Depressants; Methotrimeprazine; Methylphenidate

The levels/effects of ARIPiprazole may be increased by: Acetylcholinesterase Inhibitors (Central); Conivaptan; CYP2D6 Inhibitors (Moderate); CYP2D6 Inhibitors (Strong); CYP3A4 Inhibitors (Moderate); CYP3A4 Inhibitors (Strong); Darunavir; Dasatinib; Droperidol; Lithium formulations; Methotrimeprazine; Methylphenidate; Metoclopramide; Tetrabenazine

Nutritional/Ethanol Interactions

Ethanol: Avoid ethanol (may increase CNS depression).

Food: Ingestion with a high-fat meal delays time to peak plasma level.

Herb/Nutraceutical: St John's wort may decrease aripiprazole levels. Avoid kava kava, gotu kola, valerian, St John's wort (may increase CNS depression).

Adverse Reactions Unless otherwise noted, frequency of adverse reactions is shown as reported for adult patients receiving oral administration. Spectrum and incidence of adverse effects similar in children; exceptions noted when incidence much higher in children.

>10%:

Central nervous system: Headache (27%; injection 12%), agitation (19%), insomnia (18%), anxiety (17%), EPS (dose related; 5% to 16%; children 6% to 26%), akathisia (dose related; 8% to 13%; injection 2%), sedation (dose related; 5% to 11%; children 8% to 24%; injection 3% to 9%)

Gastrointestinal: Weight gain (8% to 30%; highest frequency in patients with BMI <23), nausea (15%; injection 9%), constipation (11%), vomiting (11%; children 9% to 14%; injection 3%), dyspepsia (9%)

1% to 10%:

Cardiovascular: Orthostatic hypotension (1% to 4%; injection 1% to 3%), tachycardia (injection 2%), chest pain, hypertension, peripheral edema

Central nervous system: Dizziness (10%; injection 8%), pyrexia (children 5% to 9%), restlessness (5% to 6%), fatigue (dose related; 6%; children 8% to 17%; injection 2%), lethargy (children 2% to 5%), lightheadedness (4%), pain (3%), dystonia (children 1%), hypersomnia (1%), irritability (children 1%), coordination impaired, suicidal ideation

Dermatologic: Rash (children 2%), hyperhidrosis

Endocrine & metabolic: Dysmenorrhea (children 2%)

Gastrointestinal: Salivation increased (dose related; children 4% to 9%), appetite decreased (children 4% to 7%), appetite increased (children 7%), xerostomia (5%), toothache (4%), abdominal discomfort (3%), diarrhea (children 5%), weight loss

Local: Injection site reaction (injection)

Neuromuscular & skeletal: Tremor (dose related; 5% to 6%; children 6% to 10%), extremity pain (4%), stiffness (4%), myalgia (2%), spasm (2%), arthralgia (children 1%), dyskinesia (children 1%), CPK increased, weakness

Ocular: Blurred vision (3%; children 3% to 8%)

Respiratory: Nasopharyngitis (children 6%), pharyngolaryngeal pain (3%), cough (3%), rhinorrhea (children 2%), aspiration pneumonia, dyspnea, nasal congestion

Miscellaneous: Thirst (children 1%)

Pharmacodynamics/Kinetics

Onset of Action Initial: 1-3 weeks

Absorption Well absorbed

Bioavailability I.M.: 100%; Tablet: 87%

Time to Peak I.M.: 1-3 hours; Tablet: 3-5 hours

With high-fat meal: Aripiprazole: Delayed by 3 hours; dehydro-aripiprazole: Delayed by 12 hours

Protein Binding ≥99%, primarily to albumin

Half-Life Elimination

Aripiprazole: 75 hours; dehydro-aripiprazole: 94 hours

CYP2D6 poor metabolizers: Aripiprazole: 146 hours

Metabolism Hepatic, via CYP2D6, CYP3A4 (dehydro-aripiprazole metabolite has affinity for D_2 receptors similar to the parent drug and represents 40% of the parent drug exposure in plasma)

Excretion Feces (55%, ~18% of the total dose as unchanged drug); urine (25%, <1% of the total dose as unchanged drug)

Available Dosage Forms

Injection, solution:

Abilify®: 7.5 mg/mL (1.3 mL)

Solution, oral:

Abilify®: 1 mg/mL (150 mL)

Tablet, oral:

Abilify®: 2 mg, 5 mg, 10 mg, 15 mg, 20 mg, 30 mg

Tablet, orally disintegrating, oral:

Abilify Discmelt®: 10 mg, 15 mg

Dosing

Adult & Geriatric Note: Oral solution may be substituted for the oral tablet on a mg-per-mg basis, up to 25 mg. Patients receiving 30 mg tablets should be given 25 mg oral solution. Orally disintegrating tablets (Abilify Discmelt®) are bioequivalent to the immediate release tablets (Abilify®).

Acute agitation (schizophrenia/bipolar mania): I.M.: 9.75 mg as a single dose (range: 5.25-15 mg); repeated doses may be given at ≥2-hour intervals to a maximum of 30 mg/day. **Note:** If ongoing therapy with aripiprazole is necessary, transition to oral therapy as soon as possible.

Bipolar I disorder (acute manic or mixed episodes): Oral:

Stabilization:

Monotherapy: Initial: 15 mg once daily. May increase to 30 mg once daily if clinically indicated; safety of doses >30 mg/day has not been evaluated

Adjunct to lithium or valproic acid: Initial: 10-15 mg once daily. May increase to 30 mg once daily if clinically indicated; safety of doses >30 mg/day has not been evaluated.

Maintenance: Continue stabilization dose for up to 6 weeks; efficacy of continued treatment >6 weeks has not been established.

Depression (adjunctive with antidepressants): Oral: Initial: 2-5 mg/day (range: 2-15 mg/day); dose adjustments of up to 5 mg/day may be made in intervals of ≥1 week. **Note:** Dosing based on patients already receiving antidepressant therapy.

Schizophrenia: Oral: 10-15 mg once daily; may be increased to a maximum of 30 mg once daily (efficacy at dosages above 10-15 mg has not been shown to be increased). Dosage titration should not be more frequent than every 2 weeks.

Dosage adjustment with concurrent CYP450 inducer or inhibitor therapy: Oral:

CYP3A4 inducers (eg, carbamazepine): Aripiprazole dose should be doubled (20-30 mg/day); dose should be subsequently reduced (10-15 mg/day) if concurrent inducer agent discontinued.

CYP3A4 inhibitors (eg, ketoconazole): Aripiprazole dose should be reduced to 1/2 of the usual dose, and proportionally increased upon discontinuation of the inhibitor agent.

CYP2D6 inhibitors (eg, fluoxetine, paroxetine): Aripiprazole dose should be reduced to 1/2 of the usual dose, and proportionally increased upon discontinuation of the inhibitor agent.

Pediatric Note: Oral solution may be substituted for the oral tablet on a mg-per-mg basis, up to 25 mg. Patients receiving 30 mg tablets should be given 25 mg oral solution. Orally disintegrating tablets (Abilify Discmelt®) are bioequivalent to the immediate release tablets (Abilify®).

Aggression, conduct disorder, Tourette syndrome (unlabeled uses): Oral: 5-20 mg/day

Bipolar I disorder (acute manic or mixed episodes): Children ≥10 years: Oral: Initial: 2 mg daily for 2 days, followed by 5 mg daily for 2 days with a further increase to target dose of 10 mg daily as monotherapy or as adjunct to lithium or valproic acid; subsequent dose increases may be made in 5 mg increments, up to a maximum of 30 mg/day.

Irritability associated with autistic disorder: Children ≥6 years: Oral: Initial: 2 mg daily for 7 days, followed by an increase to target dose of 5 mg daily; subsequent dose increases may be made in 5 mg increments at intervals of ≥1 week as needed up to a maximum of 15 mg/day.

Schizophrenia: Adolescents ≥13 years: Oral: Initial: 2 mg daily for 2 days, followed by 5 mg daily for 2 days with a further increase to target dose of 10 mg daily; subsequent dose increases may be made in 5 mg increments up to a maximum of 30 mg/day (30 mg/day not shown to be more efficacious than 10 mg/day).

Renal Impairment No dosage adjustment required.

Hepatic Impairment No dosage adjustment required.

Administration

Oral May be administered with or without food. Tablet and oral solution may be interchanged on a mg-per-mg basis, up to 25 mg. Doses using 30 mg tablets should be exchanged for 25 mg oral solution. Orally disintegrating tablets (Abilify Discmelt®) are bioequivalent to the immediate release tablets (Abilify®).

Orally-disintegrating tablet: Remove from foil blister by peeling back (do not push tablet through the foil). Place tablet in mouth immediately upon removal. Tablet dissolves rapidly in saliva and may be swallowed without liquid. If needed, can be taken with liquid. Do not split tablet.

I.M. For I.M. use only; do not administer SubQ or I.V.; inject slowly into deep muscle mass

Stability

Storage

Injection solution: Store at controlled room temperature of 25°C (77°F); excursions permitted to 15°C to 30°C (59°F to 86°F). Protect from light.

Oral solution: Store at controlled room temperature of 25°C (77°F); excursions permitted to 15°C to 30°C (59°F to 86°F). Use within 6 months after opening.

Tablet: Store at controlled room temperature of 25°C (77°F); excursions permitted to 15°C to 30°C (59°F to 86°F).

Monitoring and Teaching Issues

Laboratory Monitoring Fasting lipid profile and fasting blood glucose/Hb A_{1c} (prior to treatment, at 3 months, then annually); BMI; CBC frequently during first few months of therapy in patients with pre-existing low WBC or a history of drug-induced leukopenia/neutropenia

Physical Assessment Assess personal/family history of diabetes, vital signs, blood pressure, mental status, thoughts of suicide ideation, abnormal involuntary movement scale (AIMS), and extrapyramidal symptoms (EPS). Weight and waist circumference should be assessed prior to treatment, at 4 weeks, 8 weeks, 12 weeks, and then at quarterly intervals. Consider titrating to a different antipsychotic agent for a weight gain ≥5% of the initial weight. This drug may alter glucose regulation and control; monitor closely. Assess for extrapyramidal symptoms prior to and during therapy.

Patient Education Take at the same time of day, without regard to meals. Do not alter dose; it may take some time to achieve desired results. Avoid alcohol. If you have diabetes, monitor blood glucose levels closely prior to treatment and periodically throughout; may cause hyperglycemia. You may be more vulnerable to overheating and dehydration while taking this medication; maintain adequate hydration. May cause headache, dizziness, problems sleeping, anxiety, nausea, vomiting, constipation, or orthostatic hypotension. Report chest pain or palpitations; persistent gastrointestinal effects; tremors; involuntary movements; altered gait; change in vision; change in mental status (especially suicide ideation); or weight gain.

Dietary Considerations May be taken with or without food. Some products may contain phenylalanine.

Geriatric Considerations Elderly patients have an increased risk of adverse response to side effects or adverse reactions to antipsychotics. Aripiprazole has been studied in elderly patients with psychosis associated with Alzheimer's disease. The package insert does not provide the outcomes of this study other than somnolence was more frequent with aripiprazole (8%) than placebo (1%). Clinical data have shown an increased incidence of serious cerebrovascular events in the elderly, some fatal. In light of significant risks and adverse effects in the elderly population (compared with limited data demonstrating efficacy in the treatment of dementia-related psychosis, aggression, and agitation), an extensive risk:benefit analysis should be performed prior to use. Aripiprazole's delayed onset of action and long half-life may limit its role in treating older persons with psychosis. Not approved for the treatment of patients with dementia-related psychosis.

Breast-Feeding Considerations Based on limited data from case reports, small amounts of aripiprazole have been detected in breast milk.

Pregnancy Considerations Aripiprazole demonstrated developmental toxicity and teratogenic effects in animal models. Antipsychotic use during the third trimester of pregnancy has a risk for abnormal muscle movements (extrapyramidal symptoms [EPS]) and withdrawal symptoms in newborns following delivery. Symptoms in the newborn may include agitation, feeding disorder, hypertonia, hypotonia, respiratory distress, somnolence, and tremor; these effects may be self-limiting or require hospitalization. Information specific to the use of aripiprazole in pregnancy is limited. Treatment algorithms have been developed by the ACOG and the APA for the management of depression in women prior to conception and during pregnancy (Yonkers, 2009). Healthcare providers are encouraged to enroll women 18-45 years of age exposed to aripiprazole during pregnancy in the Atypical Antipsychotics Pregnancy Registry (866-961-2388).

Related Information

Antipsychotic Agents *on page 1986*

◆ **Aristospan®** *see* Triamcinolone (Systemic) *on page 1812*

◆ **Arixtra®** *see* Fondaparinux *on page 817*

Armodafinil (ar moe DAF i nil)

U.S. Brand Names Nuvigil®

Index Terms R-modafinil

Generic Availability (U.S.) No

Pharmacologic Category Stimulant

Medication Guide Available Yes

Pregnancy Risk Factor C

Lactation Excretion in breast milk unknown/use caution

Use Improve wakefulness in patients with excessive daytime sleepiness associated with narcolepsy and shift work sleep disorder (SWSD); adjunctive therapy for obstructive sleep apnea/hypopnea syndrome (OSAHS)

Mechanism of Action/Effect Armodafinil is a stimulant with effects. The exact mechanism of action of armodafinil is unknown.

Contraindications Hypersensitivity to armodafinil, modafinil, or any component of the formulation

Warnings/Precautions For use following complete evaluation of sleepiness and in conjunction with other standard treatments (eg, CPAP). The degree of sleepiness should be reassessed frequently; some patients may not return to a normal level of wakefulness. Use is not recommended with a history of angina, cardiac ischemia, recent history of myocardial infarction, left ventricular hypertrophy, or patients with mitral valve prolapse who have developed mitral valve prolapse syndrome with previous CNS stimulant use. Blood pressure monitoring may be required in patients on armodafinil. New or additional antihypertensive therapy may be needed.

Serious and life-threatening rashes including Stevens-Johnson syndrome, toxic epidermal necrolysis, and drug rash with eosinophilia and systemic symptoms have been reported with modafinil, the racemate of armodafinil. In clinical trials of modafinil, these rashes were more likely to occur in children; however, in the postmarketing period, serious reactions have occurred in both adults and children. Most cases have been reported within the first 5 weeks of initiating therapy; however, rare cases have occurred after prolonged therapy.

Caution should be exercised when modafinil is given to patients with a history of psychosis; may impair the ability to engage in potentially hazardous activities. Stimulants may unmask tics in individuals with coexisting Tourette's syndrome. Use caution with renal or hepatic impairment (dosage adjustment in hepatic dysfunction is recommended). Use reduced doses in elderly patients. Safety and efficacy in children <17 years of age have not been established.

Drug Interactions

Metabolism/Transport Effects

Substrate of CYP3A4 (major); **Inhibits** CYP2C19 (moderate); **Induces** CYP1A2 (weak), 3A4 (moderate)

Avoid Concomitant Use

Avoid concomitant use of Armodafinil with any of the following: Clopidogrel; Iobenguane I 123

Decreased Effect

Armodafinil may decrease the levels/effects of: Clopidogrel; Contraceptives (Estrogens); CycloSPORINE; CycloSPORINE (Systemic); Iobenguane I 123; Saxagliptin

The levels/effects of Armodafinil may be decreased by: CYP3A4 Inducers (Strong); Deferasirox; Herbs (CYP3A4 Inducers)

Increased Effect/Toxicity

Armodafinil may increase the levels/effects of: CYP2C19 Substrates; Sympathomimetics

The levels/effects of Armodafinil may be increased by: Atomoxetine; Cannabinoids; Conivaptan; CYP3A4 Inhibitors (Moderate); CYP3A4 Inhibitors (Strong); Dasatinib

Nutritional/Ethanol Interactions

Ethanol: Avoid or limit ethanol.

Food: Delays absorption, but minimal effects on bioavailability. Food may affect the onset and time course of armodafinil.

Adverse Reactions

>10%: Central nervous system: Headache (14% to 23%; dose-related)

1% to 10%:

Cardiovascular: Palpitation (2%), increased heart rate (1%)

Central nervous system: Dizziness (5%), insomnia (4% to 6%; dose related), anxiety (4%), depression (1% to 3%; dose related), fatigue (2%), agitation (1%), attention disturbance (1%), depressed mood (1%), migraine (1%), nervousness (1%), pain (1%), pyrexia (1%), tremor (1%)

Dermatologic: Rash (1% to 4%; dose related), contact dermatitis (1%), hyperhidrosis (1%)

Gastrointestinal: Nausea (6% to 9%; dose related), xerostomia (2% to 7%; dose related), diarrhea (4%), abdominal pain (2%), dyspepsia (2%), anorexia (1%), appetite decreased (1%), constipation (1%), loose stools (1%), vomiting (1%)

Genitourinary: Polyuria (1%)

Hepatic: GGT increased (1%)

Neuromuscular & skeletal: Paresthesia (1%)

Respiratory: Dyspnea (1%)

Miscellaneous: Flu-like syndrome (1%), thirst (1%)

Pharmacodynamics/Kinetics

Absorption Readily absorbed

Time to Peak 2 hours (fasted)

Protein Binding ~60% (based on modafinil; primarily albumin)

Half-Life Elimination 15 hours; Steady state: ~7 days

Metabolism Hepatic, multiple pathways, including CYP3A4/5; metabolites include R-modafinil acid and modafinil sulfone; Clearance: 33 mL/minute, mainly via hepatic metabolism

Excretion Urine (80% predominantly as metabolites; <10% as unchanged drug)

Controlled Substance C-IV

Available Dosage Forms

Tablet, oral:

Nuvigil®: 50 mg, 150 mg, 250 mg

Dosing

Adult

Narcolepsy: Oral: 150-250 mg once daily in the morning

Obstructive sleep apnea/hypopnea syndrome (OSAHS): Oral: 150-250 mg once daily in the morning; 250 mg was not shown to have any increased benefit over 150 mg

Shift work sleep disorder (SWSD): Oral: 150 mg given once daily ~1 hour prior to work shift

Geriatric Refer to adult dosing. Consider lower initial dosage. Concentrations were almost doubled in clinical trials (based on modafinil).

Pediatric Not approved for use in children.

Renal Impairment Inadequate data to determine safety and efficacy in severe renal impairment.

Hepatic Impairment Severe hepatic impairment (Child-Pugh classes B and C): Based on modafinil, dose should be reduced by half.

Administration

Oral May be administered without regard to food.

Stability

Storage Store at 20°C to 25°C (68°F to 77°F).

Monitoring and Teaching Issues

Physical Assessment Monitor blood pressure at the beginning of therapy and periodically throughout.

Patient Education Avoid or limit alcohol. May cause headache, dizziness, dry mouth, or nausea. Report changes in thinking, persistent insomnia or headaches, rash, or chest pain or pressure.

Dietary Considerations Take with or without meals.

Geriatric Considerations There are no specific pharmacokinetic data for armodafinil, but the clearance of modafinil may be reduced in the elderly. Safety and effectiveness in persons >65 years of age have not been established.

Pregnancy Considerations There are no well-controlled studies of armodafinil in pregnant women. There have been reports of intrauterine growth retardation and spontaneous abortions in women using the both armodafinil and modafinil, but relationship to the drug is unknown.

Adverse events have been observed in animal studies. Armodafinil and modafinil have been studied in both rats and rabbits. Developmental toxicity (including visceral and skeletal abnormalities and decreased fetal weight) in rats (armodafinil and modafinil) and rabbits (modafinil) has been observed at doses correlating to those used clinically. Efficacy of steroidal contraceptives may be decreased; alternate means of contraception should be considered during therapy and for 1 month after modafinil is discontinued.

◆ **Armour® Thyroid** *see* Thyroid, Desiccated *on page 1757*

◆ **Aromasin®** *see* Exemestane *on page 724*

Arsenic Trioxide (AR se nik tri OKS id)

U.S. Brand Names Trisenox®

Index Terms As_2O_3

Generic Availability (U.S.) No

Pharmacologic Category Antineoplastic Agent, Miscellaneous

Medication Safety Issues

High alert medication: This medication is in a class the Institute for Safe Medication Practices (ISMP) includes among its list of drugs which have a heightened risk of causing significant patient harm when used in error.

Pregnancy Risk Factor D

Lactation Enters breast milk/not recommended

Use Remission induction and consolidation in patients with relapsed or refractory acute promyelocytic leukemia (APL) characterized by t(15;17) translocation or PML/RAR-alpha gene expression

Unlabeled/Investigational Use Initial treatment of APL, treatment of myelodysplastic syndrome (MDS)

Available Dosage Forms

Injection, solution [preservative free]:
Trisenox®: 1 mg/mL (10 mL)

Dosing

Adult

APL, relapsed or refractory: I.V.:

Induction: 0.15 mg/kg/day; administer daily until bone marrow remission; maximum induction: 60 doses

Consolidation: 0.15 mg/kg/day starting 3-6 weeks after completion of induction therapy; maximum consolidation: 25 doses over a period of up to 5 weeks

APL initial treatment (unlabeled use): I.V.:

Induction, consolidation, and maintenance (Mathews, 2006):

Induction: 10 mg/day; administer daily until bone marrow remission; maximum induction: 60 doses

Consolidation: 10 mg/day for 4 weeks, starting 4 weeks after completion of induction therapy

Maintenance: 10 mg/dose administered 10 days per month for 6 months, starting 4 weeks after completion of consolidation therapy

Consolidation therapy after remission induction with tretinoin, daunorubicin and cytarabine (Powell, 2007; Powell, 2010): Two consolidation courses (2 weeks apart): 0.15 mg/kg/day 5 days/week for 5 weeks

In combination with tretinoin (Estey, 2006; Ravandi, 2009):

Induction (beginning 10 days after initiation of tretinoin): 0.15 mg/kg/day until bone marrow remission; maximum induction: 75 doses

Consolidation: 0.15 mg/kg/day Monday through Friday for 4 weeks every 8 weeks for 4 cycles (weeks 1 to 4, 9 to 12, 17 to 20, and 25 to 28)

MDS (unlabeled uses): I.V.: 0.25 mg/kg/day 5 consecutive days/week for 2 weeks, followed by a 2-week rest period (Schiller, 2006)

Pediatric

APL, relapsed or refractory: I.V.: Children ≥4 years: Refer to adult dosing.

APL initial treatment (unlabeled use): I.V.: *Induction, consolidation, and maintenance (Mathews, 2006):*

Induction: 0.15 mg/kg/day (maximum dose: 10 mg); administer daily until bone marrow remission; maximum induction: 60 doses

Consolidation: 0.15 mg/kg/day (maximum dose: 10 mg) for 4 weeks, starting 4 weeks after completion of induction therapy

Maintenance: 0.15 mg/kg/dose (maximum dose: 10 mg) administered 10 days per month for 6 months, starting 4 weeks after completion of consolidation therapy

Renal Impairment

Severe renal impairment (Cl_{cr} <30 mL/minute): Use with caution (systemic exposure to metabolites may be higher); may require dosage reduction; monitor closely for toxicity.

Dialysis patients: Has not been studied.

Hepatic Impairment

Hepatic impairment: Use with caution.

Severe hepatic impairment (Child-Pugh class C): Monitor closely for toxicity.

Administration

I.V. I.V. infusion over 1-2 hours. If acute vasomotor reactions occur, infuse over a maximum of 4 hours. Does not require administration via a central venous catheter.

Monitoring and Teaching Issues

Laboratory Monitoring Baseline then weekly 12-lead ECG; monitor electrolytes, CBC with differential, and coagulation at baseline then at least twice weekly during induction and at least weekly during consolidation; more frequent monitoring may be necessary in unstable patients

Physical Assessment Assess cardiac and electrolyte status at beginning of and periodically during therapy.

Patient Education This medication can only be administered by intravenous infusion. Report immediately any redness, swelling, pain, or burning at infusion site. May cause dizziness, fatigue, blurred vision, nausea, vomiting, diarrhea, or decreased appetite. Report immediately unexplained fever; respiratory difficulty; chest pain or palpitations; confusion, lightheadedness, or fainting; unusual joint, back, or muscle pain; or tingling or loss of feeling.

◆ **Artane** *see* Trihexyphenidyl *on page 1818*
◆ **Arthrotec®** *see* Diclofenac and Misoprostol *on page 523*
◆ **Arzerra™** *see* Ofatumumab *on page 1342*
◆ **As_2O_3** *see* Arsenic Trioxide *on page 149*
◆ **ASA** *see* Aspirin *on page 155*
◆ **5-ASA** *see* Mesalamine *on page 1177*
◆ **ASA and Diphenhydramine** *see* Aspirin and Diphenhydramine *on page 159*
◆ **Asacol®** *see* Mesalamine *on page 1177*
◆ **Asacol® HD** *see* Mesalamine *on page 1177*
◆ **Ascomp® with Codeine** *see* Butalbital, Aspirin, Caffeine, and Codeine *on page 262*
◆ **Ascriptin® Maximum Strength [OTC]** *see* Aspirin *on page 155*
◆ **Ascriptin® Regular Strength [OTC]** *see* Aspirin *on page 155*

Asenapine (a SEN a peen)

U.S. Brand Names Saphris®

Pharmacologic Category Antimanic Agent; Antipsychotic Agent, Atypical

Medication Safety Issues

Sound-alike/look-alike issues:

Asenapine may be confused with Inapsine®

Pregnancy Risk Factor C

Lactation Excretion in breast milk unknown/not recommended

Use Acute and maintenance treatment of schizophrenia; treatment of acute mania or mixed episodes associated with bipolar I disorder (as monotherapy or in combination with lithium or valproate)

Mechanism of Action/Effect Atypical antipsychotic with high affinity for serotonin, dopamine, $alpha_1$- and $alpha_2$-adrenergic receptors, and histamine receptors; no affinity for muscarinic receptors. Results in improvement of psychotic symptoms and reduction of extrapyramidal and antimuscarinic side effects as compared to typical antipsychotics.

Contraindications There are no contraindications listed in the manufacturers labeling.

Warnings/Precautions **[U.S. Boxed Warning]: Elderly patients with dementia-related psychosis treated with atypical antipsychotics are at an increased risk of death compared to placebo.** Most deaths appeared to be either cardiovascular (eg, heart failure, sudden death) or infectious (eg, pneumonia) in nature. In addition, an increased incidence of cerebrovascular effects (eg, transient ischemic attack, cerebrovascular accidents) has been reported in studies of placebo-controlled trials of antipsychotics in elderly patients with dementia-related psychosis. Asenapine is not approved for the treatment of dementia-related psychosis.

Leukopenia, neutropenia, and agranulocytosis (sometimes fatal) have been reported in clinical trials and postmarketing reports with antipsychotic use; presence of risk factors (eg, pre-existing low WBC or history of drug-induced leuko/neutropenia) should prompt periodic blood count assessment. Discontinue therapy at first signs of blood dyscrasias or if absolute neutrophil count $<1000/mm^3$.

May be sedating; use with caution in disorders where CNS depression is a feature. Use with caution in Parkinson's disease. Use with caution in patients at risk of seizures, including those with a history of seizures, head trauma, brain damage, alcoholism, or concurrent therapy with medications which may lower seizure threshold. Use is not recommended in severe hepatic impairment; increased drug concentrations may occur. Esophageal dysmotility and aspiration have been associated with antipsychotic use; use with caution in patients at risk of aspiration pneumonia (ie, Alzheimer's disease). Elevates prolactin levels; use with caution in breast cancer or other prolactin-dependent tumors. May alter temperature regulation.

Use with caution in patients with cardiovascular diseases (eg, heart failure, history of myocardial infarction or ischemia, cerebrovascular disease, conduction abnormalities). May cause orthostatic hypotension; use with caution in patients at risk of this effect (eg, concurrent medication use which may predispose to hypotension/bradycardia or presence of hypovolemia) or in those who would not tolerate transient hypotensive episodes. May result in QT_c

prolongation. Risk may be increased by conditions or concomitant medications which cause bradycardia, hypokalemia, and/or hypomagnesemia. Avoid use in combination with QT_c-prolonging drugs and in patients with congenital long QT syndrome or patients with history of cardiac arrhythmia.

May cause extrapyramidal symptoms (EPS), including pseudoparkinsonism, acute dystonic reactions, akathisia, and tardive dyskinesia. Risk of dystonia (and probably other EPS) may be greater with increased doses, use of conventional antipsychotics, males, and younger patients. Risk of neuroleptic malignant syndrome (NMS) may be increased in patients with Parkinson's disease or Lewy body dementia. May cause hyperglycemia; in some cases may be extreme and associated with ketoacidosis, hyperosmolar coma, or death. Use with caution in patients with diabetes or other disorders of glucose regulation; monitor for worsening of glucose control. Significant weight gain has been observed with antipsychotic therapy; incidence varies with product. Monitor waist circumference and BMI.

The possibility of a suicide attempt is inherent in psychotic illness or bipolar disorder; use caution in high-risk patients during initiation of therapy. Prescriptions should be written for the smallest quantity consistent with good patient care. Use caution in elderly patients.

Drug Interactions

Avoid Concomitant Use

Avoid concomitant use of Asenapine with any of the following: Artemether; Dronedarone; Lumefantrine; Metoclopramide; Nilotinib; Pimozide; QuiNINE; Tetrabenazine; Thioridazine; Toremifene; Vandetanib; Ziprasidone

Decreased Effect

Asenapine may decrease the levels/effects of: Amphetamines; Anti-Parkinson's Agents (Dopamine Agonist); Quinagolide

The levels/effects of Asenapine may be decreased by: CYP1A2 Inducers (Strong); Lithium formulations; Peginterferon Alfa-2b

Increased Effect/Toxicity

Asenapine may increase the levels/effects of: Alcohol (Ethyl); CNS Depressants; Dronedarone; Methylphenidate; PARoxetine; Pimozide; QTc-Prolonging Agents; QuiNINE; Tetrabenazine; Thioridazine; Toremifene; Vandetanib; Ziprasidone

The levels/effects of Asenapine may be increased by: Acetylcholinesterase Inhibitors (Central); Alfuzosin; Artemether; Chloroquine; Ciprofloxacin; Ciprofloxacin (Systemic); Conivaptan; CYP1A2 Inhibitors (Moderate); CYP1A2 Inhibitors (Strong); FluvoxaMINE; Gadobutrol; Lithium formulations; Lumefantrine; MAO Inhibitors; Methylphenidate; Metoclopramide; Nilotinib; QuiNINE; Tetrabenazine

Nutritional/Ethanol Interactions Ethanol: Avoid ethanol (may increase CNS depression).

Adverse Reactions Actual frequency may be dependant upon dose and/or indication.

>10%:

Central nervous system: Somnolence (13% to 24%), insomnia (6% to 16%), extrapyramidal symptoms (6% to 12%), headache (12%), akathisia (4% to 11%; dose related), dizziness (3% to 11%)

Endocrine & metabolic: Hypertriglyceridemia (13% to 15%)

1% to 10%:

Cardiovascular: Peripheral edema (3%), hypertension (2% to 3%)

Central nervous system: Hypoesthesia (4% to 7%), fatigue (3% to 4%), anxiety (4%), depression (2%), irritability (1% to 2%)

Endocrine & metabolic: Cholesterol increased (8% to 9%), glucose increased (5% to 7%), hyperprolactinemia (2% to 3%)

Gastrointestinal: Constipation (4% to 7%), vomiting (4% to 7%), weight gain (2% to 5%), dyspepsia (3% to 4%), appetite increased (≤4%), salivation increased (≤4%), abnormal taste (3%), toothache (3%), abdominal discomfort (≤3%), xerostomia (1% to 3%)

Hematologic: Creatine kinase increased (6%)

Hepatic: Transaminases increased (<1% to 3%)

Neuromuscular & skeletal: Arthralgia (3%), extremity pain (2%)

Pharmacodynamics/Kinetics

Absorption Rapid

Bioavailability Sublingual: 35%; decreased if swallowed (<2%); decreased if administered with food or liquid

Time to Peak 0.5-1.5 hours

Protein Binding 95% (including albumin and α_1-acid glycoprotein)

Half-Life Elimination Terminal: ~24 hours

Metabolism Hepatic via CYP1A2 oxidation and UGT1A4 glucuronidation

Excretion Urine (~50%); feces (~40%)

Available Dosage Forms

Tablet, sublingual:

Saphris®: 5 mg, 10 mg

Dosing

Adult & Geriatric Note: Safety of doses >20 mg/day has not been evaluated:

Schizophrenia: Sublingual:

Acute treatment: Initial: 5 mg twice daily. Daily doses >20 mg/day in clinical trials did not appear to offer any additional benefits and increased risk of adverse effects.

Maintenance treatment: Initial: 5 mg twice daily; may increase to 10 mg twice daily after 1 week based on tolerability

Bipolar disorder: Sublingual:

Monotherapy: Initial: 10 mg twice daily; decrease to 5 mg twice daily if dose not tolerated

Combination therapy (with lithium or valproate): 5 mg twice daily; may increase to 10 mg twice daily based on tolerability

Renal Impairment No dosage adjustment is necessary.

Hepatic Impairment

Mild-to-moderate hepatic impairment (Child-Pugh class A or B): No dosage adjustment is necessary

Severe hepatic impairment (Child-Pugh class C): Use is not recommended

Administration

Oral Sublingual tablets should be placed under the tongue and allowed to disintegrate. Do not crush, chew, or swallow. Avoid eating or drinking for at least 10 minutes after administration.

Stability

Storage Store at 15°C to 30°C (59°F to 86°F).

Monitoring and Teaching Issues

Laboratory Monitoring Fasting lipid profile and fasting blood glucose/Hgb A_{1c} (baseline and periodically); CBC frequently during first few months of therapy in patients with pre-existing low WBC or a history of drug-induced leukopenia/neutropenia

Physical Assessment Monitor weight prior to treatment and periodically throughout. Be alert to the potential for orthostatic hypotension, especially during the titration phase. Initiate at lower doses and titrate to target dose. Taper dosage slowly when discontinuing.

Patient Education Sublingual tablets should be placed under tongue to dissolve. Avoid eating or drinking for at least 10 minutes. Avoid alcohol. Maintain adequate hydration. If you have diabetes, you may experience increased blood sugars; monitor blood sugars closely. You may experience excess sedation, drowsiness, problems sleeping, restlessness, dizziness, or blurred vision; dry mouth, nausea, or GI upset; postural hypotension; or urinary retention (void before taking medication). Report persistent CNS effects (eg, trembling fingers, altered gait or balance, excessive sedation, seizures, unusual muscle or skeletal movements, anxiety, abnormal thoughts [especially suicide ideation], confusion, personality changes); diaphoresis, chest pain, palpitations, rapid heartbeat, or severe dizziness; respiratory difficulty; or worsening of condition.

Dietary Considerations Avoid eating or drinking for at least 10 minutes after administration.

Geriatric Considerations Studies to date have not had sufficient numbers of patients to determine if elderly respond differently than younger adults. Given the high percentages of CNS adverse effects, patients should be monitored closely for somnolence, insomnia, EPS, akathisia, and dizziness. Elderly (with dementia-related psychosis) were determined, in initial studies with antipsychotics, to have an increased risk of death (1.6-1.7 times that seen in placebo groups). Asenapine is not approved for the treatment of dementia-related psychosis.

Pregnancy Considerations Animal studies indicate an increased risk of fetal mortality. Antipsychotic use during the third trimester of pregnancy has a risk for abnormal muscle movements (extrapyramidal symptoms [EPS]) and withdrawal symptoms in newborns following delivery. Symptoms in the newborn may include agitation, feeding disorder, hypertonia, hypotonia, respiratory distress, somnolence, and tremor; these effects may be self-limiting or require hospitalization. There are no adequate and well-controlled studies in pregnant women. Use during pregnancy only if the benefits justify the risk to the fetus.

Related Information

Antipsychotic Agents *on page 1986*

◆ **Asmanex® Twisthaler®** *see* Mometasone (Oral Inhalation) *on page 1252*

Asparaginase (a SPEAR a ji nase)

U.S. Brand Names Elspar®

Index Terms *E. coli* Asparaginase; *Erwinia* Asparaginase; L-asparaginase

Generic Availability (U.S.) No

Pharmacologic Category Antineoplastic Agent, Miscellaneous

Medication Safety Issues

Sound-alike/look-alike issues:

Asparaginase may be confused with pegaspargase

Elspar® may be confused with Elaprase™, Oncaspar®

High alert medication: This medication is in a class the Institute for Safe Medication Practices (ISMP) includes among its list of drug classes which have a heightened risk of causing significant patient harm when used in error.

Prescribing and Access Restrictions The *Erwinia* strain of asparaginase is no longer commercially available in the U.S., although may be obtained through clinical trials or on a compassionate use basis.

Pregnancy Risk Factor C

Lactation Excretion in breast milk unknown/not recommended

Use Treatment (in combination with other chemotherapy) of acute lymphoblastic leukemia (ALL)

Unlabeled/Investigational Use Treatment of lymphoblastic lymphoma

Mechanism of Action/Effect Asparaginase inhibits protein synthesis by hydrolyzing asparagine to aspartic acid and ammonia. Leukemia cells, especially lymphoblasts, require exogenous asparagine; normal cells can synthesize asparagine. Asparaginase is cycle-specific for the G_1 phase.

Contraindications History of serious allergic reaction to asparaginase or any *E. coli*-derived L-asparaginase; history of serious thrombosis, pancreatitis, or serious hemorrhagic events with prior L-asparaginase treatment

Warnings/Precautions Hazardous agent - use appropriate precautions for handling and disposal. Monitor for severe allergic reactions; immediate treatment for hypersensitivity reactions should be available during administration. May alter hepatic function; use caution with pre-existing liver impairment. Serious thrombosis, including sagittal sinus thrombosis may occur; discontinue with serious thrombotic events. Increased prothrombin time, partial thromboplastin time and hypofibrinogenemia may occur; cerebrovascular hemorrhage has been reported; monitor coagulation parameters; use cautiously in patients with an underlying coagulopathy. Monitor blood glucose; may cause hyperglycemia/glucose intolerance (possibly irreversible). May cause serious and possibly fatal pancreatitis; promptly evaluate patients with abdominal pain; discontinue permanently if pancreatitis develops. Appropriate measures must be taken to prevent tumor lysis syndrome and subsequent hyperuricemia and uric acid nephropathy; monitor, consider allopurinol, hydration and urinary alkalization.

Severe allergic reactions may occur; monitor; immediate treatment for hypersensitivity reactions should be available during administration. Risk factors for allergic reactions include: I.V. administration, doses >6000-12,000 units/m^2, patients who have received previous cycles of asparaginase, and intervals of even a few days between doses. Up to 33% of patients who have an allergic reaction to *E. coli* asparaginase will also react to the *Erwinia* form or pegaspargase. A test dose may be administered prior to the first dose of asparaginase, or prior to restarting therapy after a hiatus of several days. **False-negative rates of up to 80% to test doses of 2-50 units are reported.** Desensitization may be performed in patients found to be hypersensitive by the intradermal test dose or who have received previous courses of therapy with the drug.

Drug Interactions

Avoid Concomitant Use

Avoid concomitant use of Asparaginase with any of the following: BCG; Natalizumab; Pimecrolimus; Roflumilast; Tacrolimus (Topical); Vaccines (Live)

Decreased Effect

Asparaginase may decrease the levels/effects of: BCG; Sipuleucel-T; Vaccines (Inactivated); Vaccines (Live)

The levels/effects of Asparaginase may be decreased by: Echinacea

Increased Effect/Toxicity

Asparaginase may increase the levels/effects of: Dexamethasone; Dexamethasone (Systemic); Leflunomide; Natalizumab; Vaccines (Live)

The levels/effects of Asparaginase may be increased by: Denosumab; Pimecrolimus; Roflumilast; Tacrolimus (Topical); Trastuzumab

Lab Interactions Decreased thyroxine and thyroxine-binding globulin

Adverse Reactions Note: Immediate effects: Fever, chills, nausea, and vomiting occur in 50% to 60% of patients.

>10%:

Central nervous system: Fatigue, fever, chills, depression, agitation, seizure (10% to 60%), somnolence, stupor, confusion, coma (25%)

Endocrine & metabolic: Hyperglycemia/glucose intolerance (10%)

Gastrointestinal: Nausea, vomiting (50% to 60%), anorexia, abdominal cramps (70%), acute pancreatitis (15%, may be severe in some patients)

Hematologic: Hypofibrinogenemia and depression of clotting factors V and VIII, variable decrease in factors VII and IX, severe protein C deficiency and decrease in antithrombin III (may be dose limiting or fatal)

Hepatic: Transaminases, bilirubin, and alkaline phosphatase increased (transient)

Hypersensitivity: Acute allergic reactions (fever, rash, urticaria, arthralgia, hypotension, angioedema, bronchospasm, anaphylaxis (15% to 35%); may be dose limiting in some patients, may be fatal)

Renal: Azotemia (66%)

1% to 10%:

Endocrine & metabolic: Hyperuricemia

Gastrointestinal: Stomatitis

Miscellaneous: Allergic reaction (including anaphylaxis), antibody formation/immunogenicity (~25%)

Pharmacodynamics/Kinetics

Absorption I.M.: Produces peak blood levels 50% lower than those from I.V. administration

Time to Peak I.M.: 14-24 hours

Half-Life Elimination I.M.: 39-49 hours; I.V.: 8-30 hours

Metabolism Systemically degraded

Available Dosage Forms

Injection, powder for reconstitution:

Elspar®: 10,000 int. units

Dosing

Adult & Geriatric Refer to individual protocols. **Note:** Dose, frequency, number of doses, and start date may vary by protocol and treatment phase.

ALL:

I.V.:

6000 units/m^2/dose 3 times/week for ~6-9 doses **or**
1000 units/kg/day for 10 days **or**
High-dose therapy (unlabeled dose): 10,000 units/m^2/day for ~3-12 doses
Single-agent therapy (rare): 200 units/kg/day for 28 days

I.M.:

6000 units/m^2/dose 3 times/week for ~6-9 doses **or** 6000 units/m^2/dose every ~3 days for ~6-9 doses
High-dose therapy (unlabeled dose): 10,000 units/m^2/day for ~3-12 doses

Test dose: A test dose is often recommended prior to the first dose of asparaginase, or prior to restarting therapy after a hiatus of several days. Most commonly, 0.1 mL of a 20 units/mL (2 units) asparaginase dilution is injected intradermally, and the patient observed for at least 1 hour. False-negative rates of up to 80% to test doses of 2-50 units are reported.

Some practitioners recommend an asparaginase desensitization regimen for patients who react to a test dose, or are being retreated following a break in therapy. Doses are doubled and given every 10 minutes until the total daily dose for that day has been administered. One schedule begins with a total of 1 unit given I.V. and doubles the dose every 10 minutes until the total amount given is the planned dose for that day. For example, if a patient was to receive a total dose of 4000 units, he/she would receive injections 1 through 12 during the desensitization. See table.

Asparaginase Desensitization

Injection No.	Elspar Dose (int. units)	Accumulated Total Dose
1	1	1
2	2	3
3	4	7
4	8	15
5	16	31
6	32	63
7	64	127
8	128	255
9	256	511
10	512	1023
11	1024	2047
12	2048	4095
13	4096	8191
14	8192	16,383
15	16,384	32,767
16	32,768	65,535
17	65,536	131,071
18	131,072	262,143

Pediatric Refer to individual protocols. **Note:** Dose, frequency, number of doses, and start date may vary by protocol and treatment phase.

ALL:

I.V.:

6000 units/m^2/dose 3 times/week for ~6-9 doses **or**
1000 units/kg/day for 10 days **or**
High-dose therapy (unlabeled dose): 10,000 units/m^2/dose every ~3 days for ~4-8 doses

I.M.:

6000 units/m^2/dose 3 times/week **or** 6000 units/m^2/dose every ~3 days for ~6-9 doses
High-dose therapy (unlabeled dose): 10,000 units/m^2/dose every ~3 days for ~4-8 doses **or** 25,000 units/m^2/dose weekly for ~9 doses (generally used in high-risk continuation therapy)

Test dose: Refer to adult dosing.

Administration

I.M. Doses should be given as a deep intramuscular injection into a large muscle; volumes >2 mL should be divided and administered in 2 separate sites

I.V. Note: I.V. administration greatly increases the risk of allergic reactions and should be avoided if possible.

The following precautions should be taken when administering. Administer in 50-250 mL of D_5W over at least 30-60 minutes. The manufacturer recommends a test dose (0.1 mL of a dilute 20 unit/mL solution) prior to initial administration and when given after an interval of 7 days or more. Institutional policies vary. The skin test site should be observed for at least 1 hour for a wheal or erythema. Note that a negative skin test does not preclude the possibility of an allergic reaction. Desensitization may be performed in patients who have been found to be hypersensitive by the intradermal skin test or who have received previous courses of therapy with the drug. Have epinephrine, diphenhydramine, and hydrocortisone at the bedside. Have a running I.V. in place. A physician should be readily accessible.

Other Has been administered SubQ in specific protocols

Stability

Reconstitution For I.V. administration, reconstitute lyophilized powder with 5 mL sterile water for injection or NS. For I.M. administration, the manufacturer recommends reconstitution of the lyophilized powder with 2 mL NS to a concentration of 5000 units/mL; however, some institutions reconstitute with 1 mL NS for I.M. use, resulting in a concentration of 10,000 units/mL. Shake well, but not too vigorously. A 5 micron filter may be used to remove fiber-like particles in the solution (do not use a 0.2 micron filter; has been associated with loss of potency).

Standard I.M. dilution: 5000 units/mL (10,000 units/mL has been used by some institutions)
Standard I.V. dilution: Dilute in 50-250 mL NS or D_5W

Storage Intact vials of powder should be refrigerated at 2°C to 8°C (36°F to 48°F). Reconstituted solutions are stable 1 week refrigerated at 8°C (Stecher, 1999), although the manufacturer recommends use within 8 hours. Solutions for I.V. infusion are stable for 8 hours at room temperature or under refrigeration.

Monitoring and Teaching Issues

Laboratory Monitoring CBC with differential, serum amylase, blood glucose, uric acid, liver function prior to and frequently during therapy

Physical Assessment With each dose, patient should be monitored closely for acute hypersensitivity reactions (may occur in 10% to 35% of patients and can be fatal), hyperglycemia, CNS changes, nausea, or vomiting. In event of hypersensitivity or hyperglycemia, infusion should be stopped and prescriber notified immediately.

Patient Education This medication can only be given I.M. or I.V. Report immediately any pain or burning at infusion/injection site, rash, chest pain, respiratory difficulty or chest tightness, difficulty swallowing, or sharp back pain. It is vital to maintain adequate hydration, unless instructed to restrict fluid intake, and good nutritional status. May cause acute nausea or vomiting. Report unusual fever or chills, changes in mentation (confusion, agitation, depression, stupor, seizures), yellowing of skin or eyes, unusual bleeding or bruising, unhealed sores, or vaginal discharge.

Breast-Feeding Considerations Due to the potential for serious adverse reactions in the nursing infant, breast-feeding is not recommended.

Pregnancy Considerations Decreased weight gain, resorptions, gross abnormalities, and skeletal abnormalities were observed in animal studies. There are no adequate and well-controlled studies in pregnant women. Use during pregnancy only if clearly needed.

Additional Information Some institutions recommended the following precautions for asparaginase administration: Parenteral epinephrine, diphenhydramine, and hydrocortisone available at bedside; freely running I.V. in place; physician readily accessible; monitor the patient closely for 30-60 minutes; avoid administering at night.

The *E. coli* and the *Erwinia* strains of asparaginase differ slightly in their gene sequencing, and have slight differences in their enzyme characteristics. Both are highly specific for asparagine and have <10% activity for the D-isomer. The *E. coli* form is more commonly used. The *Erwinia* variety is no longer commercially available in the U.S., although may be obtained through clinical trials or on a compassionate use basis.

◆ **Aspart Insulin** *see* Insulin Aspart *on page 981*
◆ **Aspercin [OTC]** *see* Aspirin *on page 155*
◆ **Aspergum® [OTC]** *see* Aspirin *on page 155*

Aspirin (AS pir in)

U.S. Brand Names Ascriptin® Maximum Strength [OTC]; Ascriptin® Regular Strength [OTC]; Aspercin [OTC]; Aspergum® [OTC]; Aspir-low [OTC]; Aspirtab [OTC]; Bayer® Aspirin Extra Strength [OTC]; Bayer® Aspirin Regimen Adult Low Strength [OTC]; Bayer® Aspirin Regimen Children's [OTC]; Bayer® Aspirin Regimen Regular Strength [OTC]; Bayer® Genuine Aspirin [OTC]; Bayer® Plus Extra Strength [OTC]; Bayer® Women's Low Dose Aspirin [OTC]; Buffasal [OTC]; Bufferin® Extra Strength [OTC]; Bufferin® [OTC]; Buffinol [OTC]; Easprin®; Ecotrin® Arthritis Strength [OTC]; Ecotrin® Low Strength [OTC]; Ecotrin® [OTC]; Halfprin® [OTC]; St Joseph® Adult Aspirin [OTC]; Tri-Buffered Aspirin [OTC]; ZORprin® [DSC]

Index Terms Acetylsalicylic Acid; ASA; Baby Aspirin

Generic Availability (U.S.) Yes: Excludes gum

Pharmacologic Category Antiplatelet Agent; Salicylate

Medication Safety Issues

Sound-alike/look-alike issues:

Aspirin may be confused with Afrin®, Asendin®
Ascriptin® may be confused with Aricept®
Ecotrin® may be confused with Akineton®, Edecrin®, Epogen®
Halfprin® may be confused with Halfan®, Haltran®
ZORprin® may be confused with Zyloprim®

International issues:

Cartia [multiple international markets] may be confused with Cartia XT brand name for diltiazem [U.S.]

Lactation Enters breast milk (AAP recommends use "with caution"; AAP 2001 update pending)

Use Treatment of mild-to-moderate pain, inflammation, and fever; prevention and treatment of myocardial infarction (MI), acute ischemic stroke, and transient ischemic episodes; management of rheumatoid arthritis, rheumatic fever, osteoarthritis, and gout (high dose); adjunctive therapy in revascularization procedures (coronary artery bypass graft [CABG], percutaneous transluminal coronary angioplasty [PTCA], carotid endarterectomy), stent implantation

Unlabeled/Investigational Use Low doses have been used in the prevention of pre-eclampsia, complications associated with autoimmune disorders such as lupus or antiphospholipid syndrome; alternative therapy for prevention of thromboembolism associated with atrial fibrillation in patients not candidates for warfarin; pericarditis associated with MI; prosthetic valve thromboprophylaxis

Mechanism of Action/Effect Irreversibly inhibits cyclooxygenase-1 and 2 (COX-1 and 2) enzymes, which results in decreased formation of prostaglandin precursors; has antipyretic, analgesic, and anti-inflammatory properties

Contraindications Hypersensitivity to salicylates, other NSAIDs, or any component of the formulation; asthma; rhinitis; nasal polyps; inherited or acquired bleeding disorders (including factor VII and factor IX deficiency); do not use in children (<16 years of age) for viral infections (chickenpox or flu symptoms), with or without fever, due to a potential association with Reye's syndrome; pregnancy (3rd trimester especially)

Warnings/Precautions Use with caution in patients with platelet and bleeding disorders, renal dysfunction, dehydration, erosive gastritis, or peptic ulcer disease. Heavy ethanol use (>3 drinks/day) can increase bleeding risks. Avoid use in severe renal failure or in severe hepatic failure. Low-dose aspirin for cardioprotective effects is associated with a two- to fourfold increase in UGI events (eg, symptomatic or complicated ulcers); risks of these events increase with increasing aspirin dose; during the chronic phase of aspirin dosing, doses >81 mg are not recommended unless indicated (Bhatt, 2008).

Discontinue use if tinnitus or impaired hearing occurs. Caution in mild-to-moderate renal failure (only at high dosages). Patients with sensitivity to tartrazine dyes, nasal polyps, and asthma may have an increased risk of salicylate sensitivity. In the treatment of acute ischemic stroke, avoid aspirin for 24 hours following administration of alteplase; administration within 24 hours increases the risk of hemorrhagic transformation. Surgical patients should avoid ASA if possible, for 1-2 weeks prior to surgery, to reduce the risk of excessive bleeding (except in patients with cardiac stents that have not completed their full course of dual antiplatelet therapy [aspirin, clopidogrel]; patient-specific situations need to be discussed with cardiologist; AHA/ACC/SCAI/ACS/ADA Science Advisory provides recommendations). When used concomitantly with ≤325 mg of aspirin, NSAIDs (including selective COX-2 inhibitors) substantially increase the risk of gastrointestinal complications (eg, ulcer); concomitant gastroprotective therapy (eg, proton pump inhibitors) is recommended (Bhatt, 2008).

When used for self-medication (OTC labeling): Children and teenagers who have or are recovering from chickenpox or flu-like symptoms should not use this product. Changes in behavior (along with nausea and vomiting) may be an early sign of Reye's syndrome; patients should be instructed to contact their healthcare provider if these occur.

Drug Interactions

Metabolism/Transport Effects Substrate of CYP2C9 (minor)

Avoid Concomitant Use

Avoid concomitant use of Aspirin with any of the following: Influenza Virus Vaccine (Live/Attenuated); Ketorolac; Ketorolac (Systemic)

Decreased Effect

Aspirin may decrease the levels/effects of: ACE Inhibitors; Loop Diuretics; NSAID (Nonselective); Probenecid; Tiludronate

The levels/effects of Aspirin may be decreased by: Corticosteroids (Systemic); Nonsteroidal Anti-Inflammatory Agents; NSAID (Nonselective)

Increased Effect/Toxicity

Aspirin may increase the levels/effects of: Alendronate; Anticoagulants; Carbonic Anhydrase Inhibitors; Collagenase (Systemic); Corticosteroids (Systemic); Divalproex; Drotrecogin Alfa; Heparin; Ibritumomab; Methotrexate; PRALAtrexate; Salicylates; Sulfonylureas; Thrombolytic Agents; Tositumomab and Iodine I 131 Tositumomab; Valproic Acid; Varicella Virus-Containing Vaccines; Vitamin K Antagonists

The levels/effects of Aspirin may be increased by: Antidepressants (Tricyclic, Tertiary Amine); Antiplatelet Agents; Calcium Channel Blockers (Nondihydropyridine); Dasatinib; Ginkgo Biloba; Glucosamine; Herbs (Anticoagulant/Antiplatelet Properties); Influenza Virus Vaccine (Live/Attenuated); Ketorolac; Ketorolac (Systemic); Loop Diuretics; Nonsteroidal Anti-Inflammatory Agents; NSAID (Nonselective); Omega-3-Acid Ethyl Esters; Pentosan Polysulfate Sodium; Pentoxifylline; Prostacyclin Analogues; Selective Serotonin Reuptake Inhibitors; Serotonin/Norepinephrine Reuptake Inhibitors; Treprostinil

Nutritional/Ethanol Interactions

Ethanol: Avoid ethanol (may enhance gastric mucosal damage).

Food: Food may decrease the rate but not the extent of oral absorption.

Folic acid: Hyperexcretion of folate; folic acid deficiency may result, leading to macrocytic anemia.

Iron: With chronic aspirin use and at doses of 3-4 g/day, iron-deficiency anemia may result.

Sodium: Hypernatremia resulting from buffered aspirin solutions or sodium salicylate containing high sodium content. Avoid or use with caution in CHF or any condition where hypernatremia would be detrimental.

Benedictine liqueur, prunes, raisins, tea, and gherkins: Potential salicylate accumulation.

Fresh fruits containing vitamin C: Displace drug from binding sites, resulting in increased urinary excretion of aspirin.

Herb/Nutraceutical: Avoid cat's claw, dong quai, evening primrose, feverfew, garlic, ginger, ginkgo, red clover, horse chestnut, green tea, ginseng (all have additional antiplatelet activity). Limit curry powder, paprika, licorice; may cause salicylate accumulation. These foods contain 6 mg salicylate/100 g. An ordinary American diet contains 10-200 mg/day of salicylate.

Lab Interactions False-negative results for glucose oxidase urinary glucose tests (Clinistix®). Interferes with Gerhardt test, VMA determination; 5-HIAA, xylose tolerance test and T_3 and T_4.

Adverse Reactions As with all drugs which may affect hemostasis, bleeding is associated with aspirin. Hemorrhage may occur at virtually any site. Risk is dependent on multiple variables including dosage, concurrent use of multiple agents which alter hemostasis, and patient susceptibility. Many adverse effects of aspirin are dose related, and are rare at low dosages. Other serious reactions are idiosyncratic, related to allergy or individual sensitivity. Accurate estimation of frequencies is not possible. The reactions listed below have been reported for aspirin (frequency not defined).

Cardiovascular: Hypotension, tachycardia, dysrhythmias, edema

Central nervous system: Fatigue, insomnia, nervousness, agitation, confusion, dizziness, headache, lethargy, cerebral edema, hyperthermia, coma

Dermatologic: Rash, angioedema, urticaria

Endocrine & metabolic: Acidosis, hyperkalemia, dehydration, hypoglycemia (children), hyperglycemia, hypernatremia (buffered forms)

Gastrointestinal: Nausea, vomiting, dyspepsia, epigastric discomfort, heartburn, stomach pain, gastrointestinal ulceration (6% to 31%), gastric erosions, gastric erythema, duodenal ulcers

Hematologic: Anemia, disseminated intravascular coagulation (DIC), prothrombin times prolonged, coagulopathy, thrombocytopenia, hemolytic anemia, bleeding, iron deficiency anemia

Hepatic: Hepatotoxicity, transaminases increased, hepatitis (reversible)

Neuromuscular & skeletal: Rhabdomyolysis, weakness, acetabular bone destruction (OA)

Otic: Hearing loss, tinnitus

Renal: Interstitial nephritis, papillary necrosis, proteinuria, renal impairment, renal failure (including cases caused by rhabdomyolysis), BUN increased, serum creatinine increased

Respiratory: Asthma, bronchospasm, dyspnea, laryngeal edema, hyperpnea, tachypnea, respiratory alkalosis, noncardiogenic pulmonary edema

Miscellaneous: Anaphylaxis, prolonged pregnancy and labor, stillbirths, low birth weight, peripartum bleeding, Reye's syndrome

Pharmacodynamics/Kinetics

Duration of Action 4-6 hours

Absorption Rapid

Bioavailability 50% to 75% reaches systemic circulation

Time to Peak Serum: ~1-2 hours

Half-Life Elimination Parent drug: 15-20 minutes; Salicylates (dose dependent): 3 hours at lower doses (300-600 mg), 5-6 hours (after 1 g), 10 hours with higher doses

Metabolism Hydrolyzed to salicylate (active) by esterases in GI mucosa, red blood cells, synovial fluid, and blood; metabolism of salicylate occurs primarily by hepatic conjugation; metabolic pathways are saturable

Excretion Urine (75% as salicyluric acid, 10% as salicylic acid)

Available Dosage Forms

Caplet, oral:
- Ascriptin® Maximum Strength [OTC]: 500 mg
- Bayer® Aspirin Extra Strength [OTC]: 500 mg
- Bayer® Genuine Aspirin [OTC]: 325 mg
- Bayer® Plus Extra Strength [OTC]: 500 mg
- Bayer® Women's Low Dose Aspirin [OTC]: 81 mg

Caplet, enteric coated, oral:
- Bayer® Aspirin Regimen Regular Strength [OTC]: 325 mg

Gum, chewing, oral:
- Aspergum® [OTC]: 227 mg (12s)

Suppository, rectal: 300 mg (12s); 600 mg (12s)

Tablet, oral: 325 mg
- Ascriptin® Regular Strength [OTC]: 325 mg
- Aspercin [OTC]: 325 mg
- Aspirtab [OTC]: 325 mg
- Bayer® Genuine Aspirin [OTC]: 325 mg
- Buffasal [OTC]: 325 mg
- Bufferin® [OTC]: 325 mg
- Bufferin® Extra Strength [OTC]: 500 mg
- Buffinol [OTC]: 324 mg
- Tri-Buffered Aspirin [OTC]: 325 mg

Tablet, chewable, oral: 81 mg
- Bayer® Aspirin Regimen Children's [OTC]: 81 mg
- St Joseph® Adult Aspirin [OTC]: 81 mg

Tablet, delayed release, enteric coated, oral:
- Easprin®: 975 mg

Tablet, enteric coated, oral: 81 mg, 325 mg, 650 mg
- Aspir-low [OTC]: 81 mg
- Bayer® Aspirin Regimen Adult Low Strength [OTC]: 81 mg
- Ecotrin® [OTC]: 325 mg
- Ecotrin® Arthritis Strength [OTC]: 500 mg
- Ecotrin® Low Strength [OTC]: 81 mg
- Halfprin® [OTC]: 81 mg, 162 mg
- St Joseph® Adult Aspirin [OTC]: 81 mg

Dosing

Adult & Geriatric

Acute ischemic stroke: Oral: 150-325 mg once daily, initiated within 48 hours (in patients who are not candidates for alteplase and not receiving systemic anticoagulation)

Analgesic and antipyretic:
Oral: 325-650 mg every 4-6 hours up to 4 g/day
Rectal: 300-600 mg every 4-6 hours up to 4 g/day

Anti-inflammatory: Oral: Initial: 2.4-3.6 g/day in divided doses; usual maintenance: 3.6-5.4 g/day; monitor serum concentrations

Atrial fibrillation (in patients not candidates for warfarin or at low risk of ischemic stroke): Oral: 75-325 mg once daily

Bioprosthetic aortic valve: Oral: 50-100 mg once daily; usual dose: 81 mg once daily

Bioprosthetic mitral valve (following 3 months of anticoagulation): Oral: 50-100 mg once daily; usual dose: 81 mg once daily

CABG: Oral: 75-100 mg once daily (usual dose: 81 mg) initiated 6 hours following surgery; if bleeding prevents administration at 6 hours after CABG, initiate as soon as possible

CABG (internal mammary bypass graft): Oral: 75-162 mg once daily

Carotid artery stenting: Oral: 81-325 mg once daily beginning at least 24 hours (preferably 4 days) prior to procedure with concomitant clopidogrel

Carotid endarterectomy: Oral: 50-100 mg once daily preoperatively and daily thereafter; usual dose: 81 mg once daily

Infrainguinal arterial reconstruction/bypass: Oral: 75-100 mg once daily (begin preoperatively); usual dose: 81 mg once daily

Mechanical heart valve (with additional risk factors for thromboembolism): Oral: 50-100 mg once daily (in addition to warfarin); usual dose: 81 mg once daily

Mitral annular calcification (with documented stroke, TIA, or systemic embolism): Oral: 50-100 mg once daily; usual dose: 81 mg once daily

Mitral valve prolapse (with documented stroke or TIA): Oral: 50-100 mg once daily; usual dose: 81 mg once daily

Myocardial infarction (primary prevention): Oral: 75-162 mg once daily (Antman, 2004) **or** 75-100 mg (usual dose: 81 mg) once daily (Hirsh, 2008)

Non-ST-segment elevation myocardial infarction (NSTEMI): Oral: Initial: 162-325 mg; Maintenance: 75-100 mg once daily indefinitely; usual maintenance dose: 81 mg once daily

PCI: Oral: Initial: 75-325 mg (300-325 mg in aspirin naive patients) starting at least 2 hours (preferably 24 hours) before procedure; post procedure: 162-325 mg once daily (dose and duration varies with type of stent implanted); **Note:** Dose may be reduced to 75-162 mg once daily after appropriate duration based on stent-type is complete

Pericarditis associated with myocardial infarction: Oral: 162-325 mg once daily; doses as high as 650 mg every 4-6 hours may be required

Peripheral arterial disease: 75-100 mg once daily; usual dose: 81 mg once daily

Pre-eclampsia prevention (unlabeled use): 60-81 mg once daily (usual dose: 81 mg) during gestational weeks 13-26 (patient selection criteria not established)

Prosthetic valve thromboprophylaxis in pregnancy: 75-100 mg once daily; usual dose: 81 mg once daily

ST-segment elevation myocardial infarction (STEMI): Initial: 162-325 mg given on presentation (patient should chew nonenteric-coated aspirin especially if not taking before presentation); for patients unable to take oral, may use rectal suppository (300 mg). Maintenance (secondary prevention): 75-162 mg once daily indefinitely

Stroke (cardioembolic; anticoagulation contraindicated): Oral: 75-325 mg once daily

Stroke/TIA (noncardioembolic; secondary prevention): Oral: 50-325 mg once daily (Adams, 2008) **or** 50-100 mg once daily; usual dose: 81 mg once daily (Hirsh, 2008)

Pediatric

Analgesic and antipyretic: Oral, rectal: 10-15 mg/kg/dose every 4-6 hours, up to a total of 4 g/day

Anti-inflammatory: Oral: Initial: 60-90 mg/kg/day in divided doses; usual maintenance: 80-100 mg/kg/day divided every 6-8 hours; monitor serum concentrations

Antiplatelet effects: Oral: Adequate pediatric studies have not been performed; pediatric dosage is derived from adult studies and clinical experience and is not well established; suggested doses have ranged from 3-5 mg/kg/day to 5-10 mg/kg/day given as a single daily dose. Doses are rounded to a convenient amount (eg, 1/2 of 81 mg tablet).

Mechanical prosthetic heart valves: Oral: 6-20 mg/kg/day given as a single daily dose (used in combination with an oral anticoagulant in children who have systemic embolism despite adequate oral anticoagulation therapy (INR 2.5-3.5) and used in combination with low-dose anticoagulation (INR 2-3) and dipyridamole when full-dose oral anticoagulation is contraindicated)

Blalock-Taussig shunts: Oral: 1-5 mg/kg/day given as a single daily dose

Kawasaki disease: Oral: 80-100 mg/kg/day divided every 6 hours; monitor serum concentrations; after fever resolves: 3-5 mg/kg/day once daily; in patients without coronary artery abnormalities, give lower dose for at least 6-8 weeks or until ESR and platelet count are normal; in patients with coronary artery abnormalities, low-dose aspirin should be continued indefinitely

Antirheumatic: Oral: 60-100 mg/kg/day in divided doses every 4 hours

Renal Impairment

Cl_{cr} <10 mL/minute: Avoid use.
Dialyzable (50% to 100%)

Hepatic Impairment Avoid use in severe liver disease.

Administration

Oral Do not crush sustained release or enteric coated tablet. Administer with food or a full glass of water to minimize GI distress. For acute myocardial infarction, have patient chew tablet.

Stability

Storage Keep suppositories in refrigerator; do not freeze. Hydrolysis of aspirin occurs upon exposure to water or moist air, resulting in salicylate and acetate, which possess a vinegar-like odor. Do not use if a strong odor is present.

Monitoring and Teaching Issues

Physical Assessment Do not use for persons with allergic reaction to salicylate or other NSAIDs.

Patient Education Take with food or milk. Do not use aspirin with strong vinegar-like odor. Do not crush or chew extended release products. While using this medication, avoid alcohol, salicylate-containing foods, other medications containing aspirin or salicylate, or other NSAIDs without consulting prescriber. Maintain adequate hydration, unless instructed to restrict fluid intake. Inform prescribers and dentists that you are taking this medication prior to scheduling any surgery or dental procedure. You may experience nausea, vomiting, gastric discomfort, GI bleeding, ulceration, perforation (can occur with or without pain), or blood in stool. Stop taking aspirin and report ringing in ears, persistent stomach pain, unresolved nausea or vomiting, respiratory difficulty or shortness of breath, unusual bruising or bleeding (mouth, urine, stool), or skin rash.

Dietary Considerations Take with food or large volume of water or milk to minimize GI upset.

Geriatric Considerations Elderly are a high-risk population for adverse effects from nonsteroidal anti-inflammatory agents. As much as 60% of elderly with GI complications to NSAIDs can develop peptic ulceration and/or hemorrhage asymptomatically. The concomitant use of H_2 blockers and sucralfate is not effective as prophylaxis with the exception of NSAID-induced duodenal ulcers which may be prevented by the use of ranitidine. Misoprostol and proton pump inhibitors are the only prophylactic agents proven to help prevent the development of NSAID-induced ulcers. Also, concomitant disease and drug use contribute to the risk for GI adverse effects. Use lowest effective dose for shortest period possible. Consider renal function decline with age. Use of NSAIDs can compromise existing renal function especially when Cl_{cr} is ≤30 mL/minute. Tinnitus may be a difficult and unreliable indication of toxicity due to age-related hearing loss or eighth cranial nerve damage. CNS adverse effects such as confusion, agitation, and hallucination are generally seen in overdose or high dose situations, but elderly may demonstrate these adverse effects at lower doses than younger adults.

Breast-Feeding Considerations Low amounts of aspirin can be found in breast milk. Milk/plasma ratios ranging from 0.03-0.3 have been reported. Peak levels in breast milk are reported to be at ~9 hours after a dose. Metabolic acidosis was reported in one infant following an aspirin dose of 3.9 g/day in the mother. The WHO considers occasional doses of aspirin to be compatible with breast-feeding, but to avoid long-term therapy and consider monitoring the infant for adverse effects. Other sources suggest avoiding aspirin while breast-feeding due to the theoretical risk of Reye's syndrome.

Pregnancy Considerations Salicylates have been noted to cross the placenta and enter fetal circulation. Adverse effects reported in the fetus include mortality, intrauterine growth retardation, salicylate intoxication, bleeding abnormalities, and neonatal acidosis. Use of aspirin close to delivery may cause premature closure of the ductus arteriosus. Adverse effects reported in the mother include anemia, hemorrhage, prolonged gestation, and prolonged labor. Aspirin has been used for the prevention of pre-eclampsia; however, the ACOG currently recommends that it not be used in low-risk women. Low-dose aspirin is used to treat complications resulting from antiphospholipid syndrome in pregnancy (either primary or secondary to SLE). In general, low doses during pregnancy needed for the treatment of certain medical conditions have not been shown to cause fetal harm, however, discontinuing therapy prior to delivery is recommended. Use of safer agents for routine management of pain or headache should be considered.

◆ **Aspirin and Carisoprodol** *see* Carisoprodol and Aspirin *on page* 301

Aspirin and Diphenhydramine (AS pir in & dye fen HYE dra meen)

U.S. Brand Names Alka-Seltzer® P.M. [OTC]; Bayer® PM [OTC]

Index Terms ASA and Diphenhydramine; Aspirin and Diphenhydramine Citrate; Diphenhydramine and ASA; Diphenhydramine and Aspirin; Diphenhydramine Citrate and Aspirin

Generic Availability (U.S.) No

Pharmacologic Category Analgesic, Miscellaneous

Lactation See individual agents.

Use Aid in the relief of insomnia accompanied by minor pain or headache

Available Dosage Forms

Caplet:

Bayer® PM [OTC]: Aspirin 500 mg and diphenhydramine 38.3 mg

Tablet, effervescent:

Alka-Seltzer® P.M. [OTC]: Aspirin 325 mg and diphenhydramine 38 mg

Dosing

Adult & Geriatric

Pain-associated insomnia: Oral: Two tablets (650 mg aspirin/76 mg diphenhydramine citrate) **or** 2 caplets (1000 mg aspirin/76 mg diphenhydramine citrate) at bedtime or as directed by physician; do not exceed recommended dosage

Pediatric

Children ≥12 years: Refer to adult dosing.

Administration

Oral

Alka-Seltzer® PM: Dissolve tablets in 4 ounces of water before taking.

Bayer® PM: Administer each dose with a full glass of water.

Monitoring and Teaching Issues

Physical Assessment See individual agents.

Patient Education See individual agents.

Related Information

Aspirin *on page* 155

DiphenhydrAMINE (Systemic) *on page* 543

◆ **Aspirin and Diphenhydramine Citrate** *see* Aspirin and Diphenhydramine *on page* 159

Aspirin and Dipyridamole (AS pir in & dye peer ID a mole)

U.S. Brand Names Aggrenox®

Index Terms Aspirin and Extended-Release Dipyridamole; Dipyridamole and Aspirin

Generic Availability (U.S.) No

Pharmacologic Category Antiplatelet Agent

Medication Safety Issues

Sound-alike/look-alike issues:

Aggrenox® may be confused with Aggrastat®

Pregnancy Risk Factor D

Lactation Enters breast milk/use caution

Use Reduction in the risk of stroke in patients who have had transient ischemia of the brain or ischemic stroke due to thrombosis

Unlabeled/Investigational Use Hemodialysis graft patency

Mechanism of Action/Effect Antithrombotic action results from additive antiplatelet effects of aspirin and dipyridamole.

Contraindications Hypersensitivity to dipyridamole, aspirin, or any component of the formulation; allergy to NSAIDs; patients with the syndrome of asthma, rhinitis, and nasal polyps; children <16 years of age with viral infections; pregnancy (third trimester; aspirin)

Canadian labeling: Additional contraindications (not in U.S. labeling): Patients with hereditary fructose and/or galactose intolerance

Warnings/Precautions Patients who consume ≥3 alcoholic drinks per day may be at risk of bleeding. Use cautiously use in patients with inherited or acquired bleeding disorders, renal impairment, hypotension, unstable angina, recent MI or hepatic dysfunction. Avoid use in patients with a history of active peptic ulcer disease, severe hepatic failure, or severe renal impairment (Cl_{cr} <10 mL/minute). Monitor for signs and symptoms of GI ulcers and bleeding. Discontinue use if dizziness, tinnitus, or impaired hearing occurs. Discontinue use 24 hours prior to pharmacologic (I.V. dipyridamole) stress testing. Discontinue 1-2 weeks before elective surgical procedures to reduce the risk of bleeding. Use caution in the elderly who are at high risk for adverse events. Dose of aspirin in this combination may not be adequate to prevent for cardiac indications (eg, MI prophylaxis). Avoid use in children due to risk of Reye's syndrome in certain viral illness associated with aspirin component. Formulation may contain lactose and/or sucrose. Use in patients with fructose and/or galactose intolerance is contraindicated in the Canadian labeling.

Drug Interactions

Metabolism/Transport Effects

Aspirin: **Substrate** of CYP2C9 (minor)

Dipyridamole: **Inhibits** ABCG2, P-glycoprotein

Avoid Concomitant Use

Avoid concomitant use of Aspirin and Dipyridamole with any of the following: Influenza Virus Vaccine (Live/Attenuated); Ketorolac; Ketorolac (Systemic); Silodosin

Decreased Effect

Aspirin and Dipyridamole may decrease the levels/effects of: ACE Inhibitors; Loop Diuretics; NSAID (Nonselective); Probenecid; Tiludronate

The levels/effects of Aspirin and Dipyridamole may be decreased by: Corticosteroids (Systemic); Nonsteroidal Anti-Inflammatory Agents; NSAID (Nonselective)

Increased Effect/Toxicity

Aspirin and Dipyridamole may increase the levels/effects of: Adenosine; Alendronate; Anticoagulants; Beta-Blockers; Carbonic Anhydrase Inhibitors; Colchicine; Collagenase (Systemic); Corticosteroids (Systemic); Dabigatran Etexilate; Divalproex; Drotrecogin Alfa; Everolimus; Heparin; Hypotensive Agents; Ibritumomab; Methotrexate; P-Glycoprotein Substrates; PRALAtrexate; Regadenoson; Rivaroxaban; Salicylates; Silodosin; Sulfonylureas; Thrombolytic Agents; Topotecan; Tositumomab and Iodine I 131 Tositumomab; Valproic Acid; Varicella Virus-Containing Vaccines; Vitamin K Antagonists

The levels/effects of Aspirin and Dipyridamole may be increased by: Antidepressants (Tricyclic, Tertiary Amine); Antiplatelet Agents; Calcium Channel Blockers (Nondihydropyridine); Dasatinib; Ginkgo Biloba; Glucosamine; Herbs (Anticoagulant/Antiplatelet Properties); Influenza Virus Vaccine (Live/Attenuated); Ketorolac; Ketorolac (Systemic); Loop Diuretics; Nonsteroidal Anti-Inflammatory Agents; NSAID (Nonselective); Omega-3-Acid Ethyl Esters; Pentosan Polysulfate Sodium; Pentoxifylline; Prostacyclin Analogues; Selective Serotonin Reuptake Inhibitors; Serotonin/Norepinephrine Reuptake Inhibitors; Treprostinil

Nutritional/Ethanol Interactions Ethanol: Avoid ethanol (due to GI irritation).

Adverse Reactions

>10%:

Central nervous system: Headache (39%; tolerance usually develops)

Gastrointestinal: Abdominal pain (18%), dyspepsia (18%), nausea (16%), diarrhea (13%)

1% to 10%:

Cardiovascular: Cardiac failure (2%), syncope (1%)

Central nervous system: Fatigue (6%), pain (6%), amnesia (2%), malaise (2%), seizure (2%), confusion (1%), somnolence (1%)

Dermatologic: Purpura (1%)

Gastrointestinal: Vomiting (8%), GI bleeding (4%), melena (2%), rectal bleeding (2%), hemorrhoids (1%), GI hemorrhage (1%), anorexia (1%)

Hematologic: Hemorrhage (3%), anemia (2%)

Neuromuscular & skeletal: Arthralgia (6%), back pain (5%), weakness (2%), arthritis (2%), arthrosis (1%), myalgia (1%)

Respiratory: Cough (2%), epistaxis (2%), upper respiratory tract infection (1%)

Pharmacodynamics/Kinetics

Pharmacokinetic Note See individual agents.

Available Dosage Forms

Capsule:

Aggrenox®: Aspirin 25 mg (immediate release) and dipyridamole 200 mg (extended release)

Dosing

Adult & Geriatric

Stroke prevention: Oral: One capsule (dipyridamole 200 mg, aspirin 25 mg) twice daily

Alternative regimen for patients with intolerable headache: Oral: One capsule at bedtime and low-dose aspirin in the morning. Return to usual dose (1 capsule twice daily) as soon as tolerance to headache develops (usually within a week).

Hemodialysis graft patency (unlabeled use): Oral: One capsule (dipyridamole 200 mg, aspirin 25 mg) twice daily

Renal Impairment Avoid use in patients with severe renal dysfunction (Cl_{cr} <10 mL/minute).

Hepatic Impairment Avoid use in patients with severe hepatic impairment.

Administration

Oral Capsule should be swallowed whole; do not crush or chew. May be administered with or without food.

Stability

Storage Store at 25°C (77°F); excursions permitted to 15°C to 30°C (59°F to 86°F). Protect from excessive moisture.

Monitoring and Teaching Issues

Laboratory Monitoring Hemoglobin, hematocrit

Physical Assessment See individual agents.

Patient Education See individual agents.

Dietary Considerations May be taken with or without food.

Geriatric Considerations Plasma concentrations were 40% higher, but specific dosage adjustments have not been recommended. Some evidence suggests that the doses of dipyridamole commonly used are ineffective for prevention of platelet aggregation, however, the addition of aspirin will add substantial efficacy. The dose of aspirin is effective for platelet inhibition, but low enough to offer a low adverse drug reaction rate.

Breast-Feeding Considerations Both aspirin and dipyridamole are excreted in breast milk.

Pregnancy Considerations Animal reproduction studies have shown an increase in aspirin-related fetal toxicity with this combination. Refer to individual monographs.

Related Information

Aspirin *on page 155*

Dipyridamole *on page 556*

◆ **Aspirin and Extended-Release Dipyridamole** *see* Aspirin and Dipyridamole *on page 160*

◆ **Aspirin, Caffeine, and Butalbital** *see* Butalbital, Aspirin, and Caffeine *on page 262*

◆ **Aspirin, Caffeine, Codeine, and Butalbital** *see* Butalbital, Aspirin, Caffeine, and Codeine *on page 262*

◆ **Aspirin Free Anacin® Extra Strength [OTC]** *see* Acetaminophen *on page 38*

◆ **Aspir-low [OTC]** *see* Aspirin *on page 155*

◆ **Aspirtab [OTC]** *see* Aspirin *on page 155*

◆ **Astramorph®/PF** *see* Morphine (Systemic) *on page 1258*

◆ **Atacand®** *see* Candesartan *on page 278*

◆ **Atacand HCT®** *see* Candesartan and Hydrochlorothiazide *on page 280*

◆ **Atelvia™** *see* Risedronate *on page 1585*

Atenolol (a TEN oh lole)

U.S. Brand Names Tenormin®

Generic Availability (U.S.) Yes

Pharmacologic Category Beta Blocker, Beta-1 Selective

Medication Safety Issues

Sound-alike/look-alike issues:

Atenolol may be confused with albuterol, Altenol®, timolol, Tylenol®

Tenormin® may be confused with Imuran®, Norpramin®, thiamine, Trovan®

International issues:

Betanol® [Bangladesh] may be confused with Patanol® which is a brand name for olopatadine in the U.S.

Pregnancy Risk Factor D

Lactation Enters breast milk/use caution (AAP recommends "use with caution"; AAP 2001 update pending)

Use Treatment of hypertension, alone or in combination with other agents; management of angina pectoris; secondary prevention postmyocardial infarction

Unlabeled/Investigational Use Acute ethanol withdrawal, supraventricular and ventricular arrhythmias, and migraine headache prophylaxis

Mechanism of Action/Effect Competitively blocks response to beta-adrenergic stimulation, selectively blocks $beta_1$-receptors with little or no effect on $beta_2$-receptors except at high doses

Contraindications Hypersensitivity to atenolol or any component of the formulation; sinus bradycardia; sinus node dysfunction; heart block greater than first-degree (except in patients with a functioning artificial pacemaker); cardiogenic shock; uncompensated cardiac failure; pulmonary edema; pregnancy

Warnings/Precautions Consider pre-existing conditions such as sick sinus syndrome before initiating. Administer cautiously in compensated heart failure and monitor for a worsening of the condition (efficacy of atenolol in heart failure has not been established). **[U.S. Boxed Warning]: Beta-blocker therapy should not be withdrawn abruptly (particularly in patients with CAD), but gradually tapered to avoid acute tachycardia, hypertension, and/or ischemia.** Use caution with concurrent use of beta-blockers and either verapamil or diltiazem; bradycardia or heart block can occur. Beta-blockers should be avoided in patients with bronchospastic disease (asthma). Atenolol, with B_1 selectivity, has been used cautiously in bronchospastic disease with close monitoring. Use cautiously in peripheral arterial disease, especially if severe disease is present. Use cautiously in patients with diabetes - may mask hypoglycemic symptoms. Use cautiously in the renally impaired (dosage adjustment required). Use care with anesthetic agents which decrease myocardial function. Caution in myasthenia gravis or psychiatric disease (may cause CNS depression). Adequate alpha-blockade is required prior to use of any beta-blocker for patients with untreated pheochromocytoma. May induce or exacerbate psoriasis. Use caution with history of severe anaphylaxis to allergens; patients taking beta-blockers may become more sensitive to repeated challenges. Treatment of anaphylaxis (eg, epinephrine) in patients taking beta-blockers may be ineffective or promote undesirable effects.

Drug Interactions

Avoid Concomitant Use

Avoid concomitant use of Atenolol with any of the following: Methacholine

Decreased Effect

Atenolol may decrease the levels/effects of: Beta2-Agonists; Theophylline Derivatives

The levels/effects of Atenolol may be decreased by: Ampicillin; Herbs (Hypertensive Properties); Methylphenidate; Nonsteroidal Anti-Inflammatory Agents; Yohimbine

Increased Effect/Toxicity

Atenolol may increase the levels/effects of: Alpha-/Beta-Agonists (Direct-Acting); Alpha1-Blockers; Alpha2-Agonists; Amifostine; Antihypertensives; Bupivacaine; Cardiac Glycosides; Fingolimod; Hypotensive Agents; Insulin; Lidocaine; Lidocaine (Systemic); Lidocaine (Topical); Mepivacaine; Methacholine; Midodrine; RiTUXimab; Sulfonylureas

The levels/effects of Atenolol may be increased by: Acetylcholinesterase Inhibitors; Amiodarone; Anilidopiperidine Opioids; Calcium Channel Blockers (Nondihydropyridine); Diazoxide; Dipyridamole; Disopyramide; Dronedarone; Glycopyrrolate; Herbs (Hypotensive Properties); MAO Inhibitors; Pentoxifylline; Phosphodiesterase 5 Inhibitors; Prostacyclin Analogues; Reserpine

Nutritional/Ethanol Interactions

Food: Atenolol serum concentrations may be decreased if taken with food.

Herb/Nutraceutical: Avoid dong quai if using for hypertension (has estrogenic activity). Avoid ephedra, yohimbe, ginseng (may worsen hypertension). Avoid garlic (may have increased antihypertensive effect).

Lab Interactions Increased glucose; decreased HDL

Adverse Reactions 1% to 10%:

Cardiovascular: Persistent bradycardia, hypotension, chest pain, edema, heart failure, second- or third-degree AV block, Raynaud's phenomenon

Central nervous system: Dizziness, fatigue, insomnia, lethargy, confusion, mental impairment, depression, headache, nightmares

Gastrointestinal: Constipation, diarrhea, nausea

Genitourinary: Impotence

Miscellaneous: Cold extremities

Pharmacodynamics/Kinetics

Onset of Action Peak effect: Oral: 2-4 hours

Duration of Action Normal renal function: 12-24 hours

Absorption Oral: Rapid, incomplete (~50%)

Time to Peak Plasma: Oral: 2-4 hours

Protein Binding 6% to 16%

Half-Life Elimination Beta:

Neonates: ≤35 hours; Mean: 16 hours

Children: 4.6 hours; children >10 years may have prolonged half-life (>5 hours) compared to children 5-10 years (<5 hours)

Adults: Normal renal function: 6-7 hours, prolonged with renal impairment; End-stage renal disease: 15-35 hours

Metabolism Limited hepatic

Excretion Feces (50%); urine (40% as unchanged drug)

Available Dosage Forms

Tablet, oral: 25 mg, 50 mg, 100 mg

Tenormin®: 25 mg, 50 mg, 100 mg

Dosing

Adult & Geriatric

Hypertension: Oral: 25-50 mg once daily, may increase to 100 mg/day. Doses >100 mg are unlikely to produce any further benefit.

Angina pectoris: Oral: 50 mg once daily; may increase to 100 mg/day. Some patients may require 200 mg/day.

Postmyocardial infarction: Oral: 100 mg/day or 50 mg twice daily for 6-9 days postmyocardial infarction.

Pediatric Hypertension: Oral: Children: 0.5-1 mg/kg/dose given daily; range of 0.5-1.5 mg/kg/day; maximum dose: 2 mg/kg/day up to 100 mg/day

Renal Impairment

Cl_{cr} 15-35 mL/minute: Administer 50 mg/day maximum.

Cl_{cr} <15 mL/minute: Administer 50 mg every other day maximum.

Hemodialysis effects: Moderately dialyzable (20% to 50%) via hemodialysis. Administer dose postdialysis or administer 25-50 mg supplemental dose. Elimination is not enhanced with peritoneal dialysis. Supplemental dose is not necessary.

Administration

Oral When administered acutely for cardiac treatment, monitor ECG and blood pressure. May be administered without regard to meals.

Stability

Storage Protect from light.

Monitoring and Teaching Issues

Physical Assessment Assess blood pressure and heart rate prior to and following first dose and after any change in dosage. Assess for CHF, edema, new cough, dyspnea, or unresolved fatigue. Advise patients with diabetes to monitor glucose levels closely; beta-blockers may alter glucose tolerance. Taper dosage slowly when discontinuing. Teach patient hypotension precautions to report.

Patient Education Take with or without food. Take pulse daily (prior to medication) and follow prescriber's instruction about holding medication. If you have diabetes, monitor serum sugar closely; drug may alter glucose tolerance or mask signs of hypoglycemia. May cause fatigue, dizziness, postural hypotension, alteration in sexual performance (reversible), or constipation. Report unresolved swelling of extremities, respiratory difficulty or new cough, unresolved fatigue, unusual weight gain, or unresolved constipation.

Dietary Considerations May be taken without regard to meals.

Geriatric Considerations Due to alterations in the beta-adrenergic autonomic nervous system, beta-adrenergic blockade may result in less hemodynamic response than seen in younger adults. Studies indicate that despite decreased sensitivity to the chronotropic effects of beta-blockade with age, there appears to be an increased myocardial sensitivity to the negative inotropic effect during stress (ie, exercise). Controlled trials have shown the overall response rate for propranolol to be only 20% to 50% in the elderly. Therefore, all beta-adrenergic blocking drugs may result in a decreased response as compared to younger adults. Since many elderly have Cl_{cr} <35 mL/minute, creatinine clearance should be estimated or measured such that appropriate dose adjustment can be made.

Breast-Feeding Considerations Atenolol is excreted in breast milk and has been detected in the serum and urine of nursing infants. Peak concentrations in breast milk have been reported to occur between 2-8 hours after the maternal dose and in some cases are higher than the peak maternal serum concentration. Although most studies have not reported adverse events in nursing infants, avoiding maternal use while nursing infants with renal dysfunction or infants <44 weeks postconceptual age has been suggested. Beta-blockers with less distribution into breast milk may be preferred. The manufacturer recommends that caution be exercised when administering atenolol to nursing women.

Pregnancy Considerations Studies in pregnant women have demonstrated a risk to the fetus; therefore, the manufacturer classifies atenolol as pregnancy category D. Atenolol crosses the placenta and is found in cord blood. In a cohort study, an increased risk of cardiovascular defects was observed following maternal use of beta-blockers during pregnancy. Intrauterine growth restriction (IUGR), small placentas, as well as fetal/neonatal bradycardia, hypoglycemia, and/or respiratory depression have been observed following *in utero* exposure to beta-blockers as a class. Adequate facilities for monitoring infants at birth should be available. Untreated chronic maternal hypertension and pre-eclampsia are also associated with adverse events in the fetus, infant, and mother. The maternal pharmacokinetic parameters of atenolol during the second and third trimesters are within the ranges reported in nonpregnant patients. Although atenolol has shown efficacy in the treatment of hypertension in pregnancy, it is not the drug of choice due to potential IUGR in the infant.

Related Information

Beta-Blockers *on page 1990*

Atenolol and Chlorthalidone (a TEN oh lole & klor THAL i done)

U.S. Brand Names Tenoretic®

Index Terms Chlorthalidone and Atenolol

Generic Availability (U.S.) Yes

Pharmacologic Category Beta Blocker, Beta-1 Selective; Diuretic, Thiazide

Pregnancy Risk Factor D

Lactation Excretion in breast milk unknown/use caution

Use Treatment of hypertension with a cardioselective beta-blocker and a diuretic

Available Dosage Forms

Tablet:

50: Atenolol 50 mg and chlorthalidone 25 mg

100: Atenolol 100 mg and chlorthalidone 25 mg

Tenoretic®:

50: Atenolol 50 mg and chlorthalidone 25 mg

100: Atenolol 100 mg and chlorthalidone 25 mg

Dosing

Adult & Geriatric Hypertension: Oral: Initial (based on atenolol component): 1 (50 mg) tablet once daily, then individualize dose until optimal dose is achieved

Renal Impairment

Cl_{cr} 15-35 mL/minute: Administer 50 mg/day.

Cl_{cr} <15 mL/minute: Administer 50 mg every other day.

Administration

Oral May be administered without regard to meals.

Monitoring and Teaching Issues

Physical Assessment See individual agents.

Patient Education See individual agents.

Related Information

Atenolol *on page 161*

Chlorthalidone *on page 361*

- **ATG** *see* Antithymocyte Globulin (Equine) *on page 136*
- **Atgam®** *see* Antithymocyte Globulin (Equine) *on page 136*
- **Ativan®** *see* LORazepam *on page 1130*

Atomoxetine (AT oh mox e teen)

U.S. Brand Names Strattera®

Index Terms Atomoxetine Hydrochloride; LY139603; Methylphenoxy-Benzene Propanamine; Tomoxetine

Generic Availability (U.S.) No

Pharmacologic Category Norepinephrine Reuptake Inhibitor, Selective

Medication Safety Issues

Sound-alike/look-alike issues:

Atomoxetine may be confused with atorvastatin

Medication Guide Available Yes

Pregnancy Risk Factor C

Lactation Excretion in breast milk unknown/use caution

Use Treatment of attention deficit/hyperactivity disorder (ADHD)

Mechanism of Action/Effect Selectively inhibits the reuptake of norepinephrine (Ki 4.5nM) with little to no activity at the other neuronal reuptake pumps or receptor sites.

Contraindications Hypersensitivity to atomoxetine or any component of the formulation; use with or within 14 days of MAO inhibitors; narrow-angle glaucoma; current or past history of pheochromocytoma

Warnings/Precautions [U.S. Boxed Warning]: Use caution in pediatric patients; may be an increased risk of suicidal ideation. Closely monitor for clinical worsening, suicidality, or unusual changes in behavior; especially during the initial few months of a course of drug therapy, or at times of dose changes, either increases or decreases. The child's family or caregiver should be instructed to closely observe the patient and communicate condition with healthcare provider. New or worsening symptoms of hostility or aggressive behaviors have been associated with atomoxetine, particularly with the initiation of therapy. Use caution in patients with a history of psychotic illness or bipolar disorder; therapy may induce mixed/manic disorder or psychotic symptoms. Atomoxetine is not approved for major depressive disorder. Patients presenting with depressive symptoms should be screened for bipolar disorder. Recommended to be used as part of a comprehensive treatment program for attention deficit disorders. Atomoxetine does not worsen anxiety in patients with existing anxiety disorders or tics related to Tourette's disorder.

Use caution with hepatic disease (dosage adjustments necessary in hepatic impairment). Use may be associated with rare but severe hepatotoxicity; discontinue and do not restart if signs or symptoms of hepatotoxic reaction (eg, jaundice, pruritus, flu-like symptoms) or laboratory evidence of liver disease are noted. Use caution in patients who are poor metabolizers of CYP2D6 metabolized drugs ("poor metabolizers"), bioavailability increases.

Orthostasis can occur; use caution in patients predisposed to hypotension or those with abrupt changes in heart rate or blood pressure. CNS stimulant use has been associated with serious cardiovascular events including sudden death in patients with pre-existing structural cardiac abnormalities or other serious heart problems (sudden death in children and adolescents; sudden death, stroke, and MI in adults). These products should be avoided in patients with known serious structural cardiac abnormalities, cardiomyopathy, serious heart rhythm abnormalities, or other serious cardiac problems that could increase the risk of sudden death that these conditions alone carry. Patients should be carefully evaluated for cardiac disease prior to initiation of therapy. May cause increased heart rate or blood pressure; use caution with hypertension or other cardiovascular disease. Use caution with renal impairment. May cause urinary retention/hesitancy; use caution in patients with history of urinary retention or bladder outlet obstruction. Priapism has been associated with use (rarely). Allergic reactions (including angioneurotic edema, urticaria, and rash) may occur (rare).

Growth should be monitored during treatment. Height and weight gain may be reduced during the first 9-12 months of treatment, but should recover by 3 years of therapy. Safety and efficacy have not been evaluated in pediatric patients <6 years of age.

Drug Interactions

Metabolism/Transport Effects Substrate of CYP2C19 (minor), 2D6 (major)

Avoid Concomitant Use

Avoid concomitant use of Atomoxetine with any of the following: Iobenguane I 123; MAO Inhibitors

Decreased Effect

Atomoxetine may decrease the levels/effects of: Iobenguane I 123

The levels/effects of Atomoxetine may be decreased by: Peginterferon Alfa-2b

Increased Effect/Toxicity

Atomoxetine may increase the levels/effects of: Alcohol (Ethyl); Beta2-Agonists; CNS Depressants; Methotrimeprazine; Sympathomimetics

The levels/effects of Atomoxetine may be increased by: CYP2D6 Inhibitors (Moderate); CYP2D6 Inhibitors (Strong); Darunavir; Droperidol; MAO Inhibitors; Methotrimeprazine

Nutritional/Ethanol Interactions Ethanol: Avoid ethanol (may increase CNS depression).

Adverse Reactions Percentages as reported in children and adults; some adverse reactions may be increased in "poor metabolizers" (CYP2D6).

>10%:

- Central nervous system: Headache (2% to 19%), insomnia (2% to 15%), somnolence (4% to 11%)
- Gastrointestinal: Xerostomia (21%), nausea (7% to 21%), abdominal pain (7% to 18%), appetite decreased (11% to 16%), vomiting (3% to 11%)

1% to 10%:

- Cardiovascular: Systolic blood pressure increased (4% to 5%), diastolic pressure increased (≤4%), palpitation (3%), flushing (≥2%), tachycardia (≤2%), orthostatic hypotension (<2%)
- Central nervous system: Fatigue/lethargy (6% to 9%), dizziness (5% to 6%), irritability (≤6%), chills (3%), sleep disturbance (3%), mood swings (1% to 2%)
- Dermatologic: Hyperhidrosis (4%), rash (2%)
- Endocrine & metabolic: Hot flashes (8%), dysmenorrhea (6%), libido decreased (4%), menstruation disturbance (2%), orgasm abnormal (2%)
- Gastrointestinal: Constipation (1% to 9%), dyspepsia (4%), anorexia (<3%), weight loss (2% to 3%)
- Genitourinary: Erectile disturbance (9%), urinary hesitation/retention (7%), dysuria (3%), ejaculatory disturbance (3%), prostatitis (2%)
- Neuromuscular & skeletal: Paresthesia (3% adults; postmarketing observation in children), tremor (2%)
- Ocular: Mydriasis (≥2%)
- Respiratory: Sinus headache (3%)
- Miscellaneous: Jittery feeling (2%)

Pharmacodynamics/Kinetics

Absorption Rapid

Bioavailability 63% in extensive metabolizers; 94% in poor metabolizers

Time to Peak Plasma: 1-2 hours

Protein Binding 98%, primarily albumin

Half-Life Elimination Atomoxetine: 5 hours (up to 24 hours in poor metabolizers); Active metabolites: 4-hydroxyatomoxetine: 6-8 hours; N-desmethylatomoxetine: 6-8 hours (34-40 hours in poor metabolizers)

Metabolism Hepatic, via CYP2D6 and CYP2C19; forms metabolites (4-hydroxyatomoxetine, active, equipotent to atomoxetine; N-desmethylatomoxetine in poor metabolizers, limited activity)

Excretion Urine (80%, as conjugated 4-hydroxy metabolite); feces (17%)

Available Dosage Forms

Capsule, oral:

Strattera®: 10 mg, 18 mg, 25 mg, 40 mg, 60 mg, 80 mg, 100 mg

Dosing

Adult

Treatment of ADHD: Oral: Initial: 40 mg/day, increased after minimum of 3 days to ~80 mg/day; may administer as either a single daily dose or 2 evenly divided doses in morning and late afternoon/early evening. May increase to 100 mg/day in 2-4 additional weeks to achieve optimal response.

Dosage adjustment in patients receiving strong CYP2D6 inhibitors (eg, paroxetine, fluoxetine, quinidine) or patients known to be CYP2D6 poor metabolizers: Do not exceed 80 mg/day; dose adjustments should occur only after 4 weeks.

Note: Atomoxetine may be discontinued without the need for tapering dose.

Geriatric Use has not been evaluated in the elderly.

Pediatric Treatment of ADHD:

Children ≥6 years and ≤70 kg: Oral: Initial: 0.5 mg/kg/day, increase after minimum of 3 days to ~1.2 mg/kg/day; may administer as either a single daily dose or 2 evenly divided doses in morning and late afternoon/early evening. Maximum daily dose: 1.4 mg/kg or 100 mg, whichever is less.

Dosage adjustment in patients receiving strong CYP2D6 inhibitors (eg, paroxetine, fluoxetine, quinidine) or patients known to be CYP2D6 poor metabolizers: Do not exceed 1.2 mg/kg/day; dose adjustments should occur only after 4 weeks.

Children ≥6 years and >70 kg: Refer to adult dosing.

Note: Atomoxetine may be discontinued without the need for tapering dose.

Renal Impairment No adjustment needed.

Hepatic Impairment

Moderate hepatic insufficiency (Child-Pugh class B): All doses should be reduced to 50% of normal.

Severe hepatic insufficiency (Child-Pugh class C): All doses should be reduced to 25% of normal.

Administration

Oral May be administered with or without food. Swallow capsules whole; do not open capsules. Powder in capsules is an ocular irritant.

Stability

Storage Store at room temperature of 25°C (77°F).

Monitoring and Teaching Issues

Physical Assessment Use caution in presence of hepatic or renal impairment, hypertension, and cardiovascular disease. Pediatric patients should be screened/monitored for cardiovascular conditions prior to and during use. Observe closely during first few months of therapy and when dose is changed. Monitor growth regularly.

Patient Education Take at the same time of day, without regard for meals. You may experience CNS changes; fatigue or lethargy; irritability; sleep disturbances; nausea, vomiting, or decreased appetite; diarrhea; or constipation. Report immediately any chest pain, palpitations, or rapid heartbeat; suicide ideation; or persistent CNS changes (especially any increase in aggression or hostility). Inform prescriber of weight loss, fatigue, dizziness, or palpitations.

Dietary Considerations May be taken with or without food.

Pregnancy Considerations Decreased pup weight and survival were observed in animal studies. There are no adequate and well-controlled studies in pregnant women. Use only if potential benefit to the mother outweighs possible risk to fetus.

◆ **Atomoxetine Hydrochloride** *see* Atomoxetine *on page 164*

Atorvastatin (a TORE va sta tin)

U.S. Brand Names Lipitor®

Index Terms Atorvastatin Calcium

Generic Availability (U.S.) No

Pharmacologic Category Antilipemic Agent, HMG-CoA Reductase Inhibitor

Medication Safety Issues

Sound-alike/look-alike issues:

Atorvastatin may be confused with atomoxetine, lovastatin, nystatin, pitavastatin, pravastatin, rosuvastatin, simvastatin

Lipitor® may be confused with labetalol, Levatol®, lisinopril, Loniten®, Lopid®, Mevacor®, Zocor®, ZyrTEC®

Pregnancy Risk Factor X

Lactation Excretion in breast milk unknown/contraindicated

Use Treatment of dyslipidemias or primary prevention of cardiovascular disease (atherosclerotic) as detailed below:

Primary prevention of cardiovascular disease (high-risk for CVD): To reduce the risk of MI or stroke in patients without evidence of heart disease who have multiple CVD risk factors or type 2 diabetes. Treatment reduces the risk for angina or revascularization procedures in patients with multiple risk factors.

Secondary prevention of cardiovascular disease: To reduce the risk of nonfatal MI, nonfatal stroke, revascularization procedures, hospitalization for heart failure, and angina in patients with evidence of coronary heart disease.

Treatment of dyslipidemias: To reduce elevations in total cholesterol (C), LDL-C, apolipoprotein B, and triglycerides in patients with elevations of one or more components, and/or to increase low HDL-C as present in Fredrickson type IIa, IIb, III, and IV hyperlipidemias, heterozygous familial and nonfamilial hypercholesterolemia, and homozygous familial hypercholesterolemia

Treatment of heterozygous familial hypercholesterolemia (HeFH) in adolescent patients (10-17 years of age, females >1 year postmenarche) having LDL-C ≥190 mg/dL or LDL-C ≥160 mg/dL with positive family history of premature cardiovascular disease (CVD) or with two or more CVD risk factors.

Unlabeled/Investigational Use Secondary prevention in patients who have experienced a noncardioembolic stroke/TIA or following an ACS event regardless of baseline LDL-C using intensive lipid-lowering therapy

Mechanism of Action/Effect Inhibitor of 3-hydroxy-3-methylglutaryl coenzyme A (HMG-CoA) reductase, the rate-limiting enzyme in cholesterol synthesis (reduces the production of mevalonic acid from HMG-CoA); this then results in a compensatory increase in the expression of LDL receptors on hepatocyte membranes and a stimulation of LDL catabolism

Contraindications Hypersensitivity to atorvastatin or any component of the formulation; active liver disease; unexplained persistent elevations of serum transaminases; pregnancy; breast-feeding

Warnings/Precautions Secondary causes of hyperlipidemia should be ruled out prior to therapy. Atorvastatin has not been studied when the primary lipid abnormality is chylomicron elevation (Fredrickson types I and V). Liver function must be monitored by periodic laboratory assessment. May cause hepatic dysfunction. Use with caution in patients who consume large amounts of ethanol or have a history of liver disease; use is contraindicated in patients with active liver disease or unexplained persistent elevations of serum transaminases. Monitoring is recommended. Patients with a history of hemorrhagic stroke may be at increased risk for another hemorrhagic stroke with use.

Rhabdomyolysis with acute renal failure has occurred. Risk is dose related and is increased with concurrent use of lipid-lowering agents which may cause rhabdomyolysis (fibric acid derivatives or niacin at doses ≥1 g/day) or during concurrent use with potent CYP3A4 inhibitors (including amiodarone, clarithromycin, cyclosporine, erythromycin, itraconazole, ketoconazole, nefazodone, grapefruit juice in large quantities, verapamil, or protease inhibitors such as indinavir, nelfinavir, or ritonavir). Ensure patient is on the lowest effective atorvastatin dose. If concurrent use of clarithromycin or combination protease inhibitors (eg, lopinavir/ritonavir or ritonavir/saquinavir) is warranted consider dose adjustment of atorvastatin. Monitor closely if used with other drugs associated with myopathy. Weigh the risk versus benefit when combining any of these drugs with atorvastatin. Discontinue in any patient experiencing an acute or serious condition predisposing to renal failure secondary to rhabdomyolysis. Based upon current evidence, HMG-CoA reductase inhibitor therapy should be continued in the perioperative period unless risk outweighs cardioprotective benefit. Use with caution in patients with advanced age, these patients are predisposed to myopathy. Safety and efficacy have not been established in patients <10 years of age or in premenarcheal girls.

Drug Interactions

Metabolism/Transport Effects **Substrate** of CYP3A4 (major), P-glycoprotein; **Inhibits** CYP3A4 (weak), P-glycoprotein

Avoid Concomitant Use

Avoid concomitant use of Atorvastatin with any of the following: Red Yeast Rice; Silodosin; Topotecan

Decreased Effect

Atorvastatin may decrease the levels/effects of: Dabigatran Etexilate

The levels/effects of Atorvastatin may be decreased by: Antacids; Bosentan; CYP3A4 Inducers (Strong); Deferasirox; Efavirenz; Etravirine; P-Glycoprotein Inducers; Phenytoin; Rifamycin Derivatives; St Johns Wort

Increased Effect/Toxicity

Atorvastatin may increase the levels/effects of: Aliskiren; DAPTOmycin; Digoxin; Diltiazem; Everolimus; Midazolam; P-Glycoprotein Substrates; Rivaroxaban; Silodosin; Topotecan; Trabectedin; Verapamil

The levels/effects of Atorvastatin may be increased by: Amiodarone; Antifungal Agents (Azole Derivatives, Systemic); Colchicine; Conivaptan; CycloSPORINE; CycloSPORINE (Systemic); CYP3A4 Inhibitors (Moderate); CYP3A4 Inhibitors (Strong); Danazol; Dasatinib; Diltiazem; Dronedarone; Eltrombopag; Fenofibrate; Fenofibric Acid; Fluconazole; Fusidic Acid; Gemfibrozil; Grapefruit Juice; Macrolide Antibiotics; Nefazodone; Niacin; Niacinamide; P-Glycoprotein Inhibitors; Protease Inhibitors; QuiNINE; Red Yeast Rice; Rifamycin Derivatives; Sildenafil; Verapamil

Nutritional/Ethanol Interactions

Ethanol: Avoid excessive ethanol consumption (due to potential hepatic effects).

Food: Atorvastatin serum concentrations may be increased by grapefruit juice; avoid concurrent intake of large quantities (>1 quart/day). Red yeast rice contains an estimated 2.4 mg lovastatin per 600 mg rice.

Herb/Nutraceutical: St John's wort may decrease atorvastatin levels.

Adverse Reactions

>10%:

Gastrointestinal: Diarrhea (5% to 14%)

Neuromuscular & skeletal: Arthralgia (4% to 12%)

Respiratory: Nasopharyngitis (4% to 13%)

2% to 10%:

Central nervous system: Insomnia (1% to 5%)

Gastrointestinal: Nausea (4% to 7%), dyspepsia (3% to 6%)

Genitourinary: Urinary tract infection (4% to 8%)

Hepatic: Transaminases increased (2% to 3% with 80 mg/day dosing)

Neuromuscular & skeletal: Limb pain (3% to 9%), myalgia (3% to 8%), muscle spasms (2% to 5%), musculoskeletal pain (2% to 5%)

Respiratory: Pharyngolaryngeal pain (1% to 4%)

Additional class-related events or case reports (not necessarily reported with atorvastatin therapy): Cataracts, cirrhosis, dermatomyositis, eosinophilia, erectile dysfunction, extraocular muscle movement impaired, fulminant hepatic necrosis, gynecomastia, hemolytic anemia, interstitial lung disease, ophthalmoplegia, peripheral nerve palsy, polymyalgia rheumatica, positive ANA, renal failure (secondary to rhabdomyolysis), systemic lupus erythematosus-like syndrome, thyroid dysfunction, tremor, vasculitis, vertigo

Pharmacodynamics/Kinetics

Onset of Action Initial changes: 3-5 days; Maximal reduction in plasma cholesterol and triglycerides: 2 weeks

Absorption Rapid

Bioavailability ~14% (parent drug); ~30% (parent drug and equipotent metabolites)

Time to Peak Serum: 1-2 hours

Protein Binding ≥98%

Half-Life Elimination Parent drug: 14 hours; Equipotent metabolites: 20-30 hours

Metabolism Hepatic; forms active ortho- and parahydroxylated derivates and an inactive beta-oxidation product

Excretion Bile; urine (<2% as unchanged drug)

Available Dosage Forms

Tablet, oral:

Lipitor®: 10 mg, 20 mg, 40 mg, 80 mg

Dosing

Adult & Geriatric

Primary prevention: **Note:** Doses should be individualized according to the baseline LDL-cholesterol concentrations, the recommended goal of therapy, and patient response; adjustments should be made at intervals of 2-4 weeks

Hypercholesterolemia (heterozygous familial and nonfamilial) and mixed hyperlipidemia (Fredrickson types IIa and IIb): Oral: Initial: 10-20 mg once daily; patients requiring >45% reduction in LDL-C may be started at 40 mg once daily; range: 10-80 mg once daily

Homozygous familial hypercholesterolemia: Oral: 10-80 mg once daily

Secondary prevention:

Clinically-evident coronary heart disease: Oral: Initial: 80 mg once daily; adjust based on patient tolerability and recommended goal LDL-C (LaRosa, 2005)

Intensive lipid-lowering after an ACS event regardless of baseline LDL (unlabeled use): Oral: Initial: 80 mg once daily; adjust based on patient tolerability and recommended goal LDL-C (Cannon, 2004; Pederson, 2005; Schwartz, 2001). **Note:** Currently, the ACC/AHA guidelines for UA/NSTEMI do not specify which statin to use (Anderson, 2007).

Noncardioembolic stroke/TIA (unlabeled use): Oral: Initial: 80 mg once daily; adjust based on patient tolerability and recommended goal LDL-C (Adams, 2008; Amarenco, 2006)

Dosage adjustment for atorvastatin with concomitant medications:

Cyclosporine: Atorvastatin dose should not exceed 10 mg/day

Clarithromycin, itraconazole, ritonavir plus saquinavir, or lopinavir plus ritonavir when atorvastatin dose >20 mg: Ensure that the lowest dose necessary of atorvastatin is used.

Pediatric Note: Doses should be individualized according to the baseline LDL-cholesterol concentrations, the recommended goal of therapy, and patient response; adjustments should be made at intervals of 4 weeks

HeFH: Children 10-17 years (females >1 year postmenarche): Oral: 10 mg once daily (maximum: 20 mg/day)

Dosage adjustment for atorvastatin with concomitant medications:

Cyclosporine: Atorvastatin dose should not exceed 10 mg/day

Clarithromycin, itraconazole, ritonavir plus saquinavir, or lopinavir plus ritonavir when atorvastatin dose >20 mg: Ensure that the lowest dose necessary of atorvastatin is used.

Renal Impairment No adjustment is necessary.

Hepatic Impairment Contraindicated in active liver disease or in patients with unexplained persistent elevations of serum transaminases.

Administration

Oral May be administered with food if desired; may take without regard to time of day.

Stability

Storage Store at controlled room temperature of 20°C to 25°C (68°F to 77°F).

Monitoring and Teaching Issues

Laboratory Monitoring Monitor lipid levels after 2-4 weeks; LFTs prior to initiation and 12 weeks after initiation or first dose or dose elevation, and periodically (semiannually) thereafter; baseline CPK (recheck CPK in any patient with symptoms suggestive of myopathy). Monitor LDL-C at intervals no less than 4 weeks.

Physical Assessment Evaluate patient prior to use for history/existence of liver disease, large alcohol intake, or previous hemorrhagic stroke. Assess risk potential for interactions with other prescriptions or herbal products patient may be taking that may increase risk of rhabdomyolysis. Assess results of liver function tests, lipid levels, and CPK prior to initiation and at regular intervals.

Patient Education May take without regard to food; avoid large intake of grapefruit juice. You will need periodic laboratory evaluation during therapy. This drug does not eliminate the need for prescribed diet or exercise regimen. Avoid excessive alcohol. Report unusual muscle cramping or weakness, yellowing of skin or eyes, easy bruising or bleeding, or unusual fatigue.

Dietary Considerations May take with food if desired; may take without regard to time of day. Before initiation of therapy, patients should be placed on a standard cholesterol-lowering diet for 3-6 months and the diet should be continued during drug therapy. Red yeast rice contains an estimated 2.4 mg lovastatin per 600 mg rice. Atorvastatin serum concentration may be increased when taken with grapefruit juice; avoid concurrent intake of large quantities (>1 quart/day).

Geriatric Considerations Effective and well tolerated in elderly. The definition of and, therefore, when to treat hyperlipidemia in the elderly is a controversial issue. The National Cholesterol Education Program recommends that all adults maintain a plasma cholesterol <160 mg/dL. Elderly patients with one additional risk factor, goal LDL would be <130 mg/dL. It is the authors' belief that pharmacologic treatment be reserved for those who are unable to obtain a desirable plasma cholesterol concentration by diet alone and for whom the benefits of treatment are believed to outweigh the potential adverse effects, drug interactions, and cost of treatment.

Pregnancy Considerations Cholesterol biosynthesis may be important in fetal development. Contraindicated in pregnancy. Administer to women of childbearing potential only when conception is highly unlikely and patients have been informed of potential hazards.

Related Information

Hyperlipidemia Management *on page 2046*

◆ **Atorvastatin and Amlodipine** *see* Amlodipine and Atorvastatin *on page 106*

◆ **Atorvastatin Calcium** *see* Atorvastatin *on page 166*

◆ **Atorvastatin Calcium and Amlodipine Besylate** *see* Amlodipine and Atorvastatin *on page 106*

Atovaquone (a TOE va kwone)

U.S. Brand Names Mepron®

Generic Availability (U.S.) No

Pharmacologic Category Antiprotozoal

Pregnancy Risk Factor C

Lactation Excretion in breast milk unknown/use caution

Use Acute oral treatment of mild-to-moderate *Pneumocystis jirovecii* pneumonia (PCP) in patients who are intolerant to co-trimoxazole; prophylaxis of PCP in patients who are intolerant to co-trimoxazole

Unlabeled/Investigational Use Treatment of babesiosis; treatment/suppression of *Toxoplasma gondii* encephalitis; primary prophylaxis of HIV-infected persons at high risk for developing *Toxoplasma gondii* encephalitis

Available Dosage Forms

Suspension, oral:

Mepron®: 750 mg/5 mL (5 mL, 210 mL)

Dosing

Adult & Geriatric

Prevention of PCP: Oral: 1500 mg once daily with food

Treatment of mild-to-moderate PCP: Oral: 750 mg twice daily with food for 21 days

Babesiosis (unlabeled use): 750 mg twice daily with azithromycin for 7-10 days

***Toxoplasma gondii* encephalitis (unlabeled use; AIDS*info* guidelines):** Oral:

Prophylaxis: 1500 mg once daily with food

Treatment: 750 mg 4 times daily or 1500 mg twice daily with food for at least 6 weeks after resolution of signs and symptoms

Suppression after treatment: 750 mg 2-4 times/day with food

Pediatric

Children <13 years (unlabeled uses):

Prevention of PCP (CDC, 2009): Oral:

1-3 months: 30 mg/kg once daily with food

4-24 months: 45 mg/kg once daily with food

>24 months: 30 mg/kg once daily with food

Treatment of mild-to-moderate PCP (CDC, 2009): Oral:

Birth to 3 months: 30-40 mg/kg/day in 2 divided doses with food (maximum: 1500 mg/day)

3-24 months: 45 mg/kg/day in 2 divided doses with food (maximum: 1500 mg/day)

≥24 months: 30-40 mg/kg/day in 2 divided doses with food (maximum: 1500 mg/day)

Babesiosis: Oral: 40 mg/kg/day in 2 divided doses with food for 7-10 days

***Toxoplasma gondii* prophylaxis: (CDC, 2009):** Oral:
1-3 months: 30 mg/kg once daily with food
4-24 months: 45 mg/kg once daily with food
>24 months: 30 mg/kg once daily with food
Adolescents 13-16 years: Refer to adult dosing.

Administration

Oral Must be taken administered meals. Shake suspension gently before use. Once opened, the foil pouch can be emptied on a dosing spoon, in a cup, or directly into the mouth.

Monitoring and Teaching Issues

Physical Assessment Monitor for CNS and respiratory changes.

Patient Education Take with high-fat meals. You may experience dizziness or lightheadedness, problems sleeping, rash, weakness, cough, or flu-like symptoms. Report unresolved diarrhea, fever, mouth sores, unresolved headache, abdominal pain, shortness of breath, or vomiting.

Atracurium (a tra KYOO ree um)

Index Terms Atracurium Besylate

Generic Availability (U.S.) Yes

Pharmacologic Category Neuromuscular Blocker Agent, Nondepolarizing

Medication Safety Issues

High alert medication: The Institute for Safe Medication Practices (ISMP) includes this medication among its list of drugs which have a heightened risk of causing significant patient harm when used in error.

United States Pharmacopeia (USP) 2006: The Interdisciplinary Safe Medication Use Expert Committee of the USP has recommended the following:
- Hospitals, clinics, and other practice sites should institute special safeguards in the storage, labeling, and use of these agents and should include these safeguards in staff orientation and competency training.
- Healthcare professionals should be on high alert (especially vigilant) whenever a neuromuscular-blocking agent (NMBA) is stocked, ordered, prepared, or administered.

Pregnancy Risk Factor C

Lactation Excretion in breast milk unknown/use caution

Use Adjunct to general anesthesia to facilitate endotracheal intubation and to relax skeletal muscles during surgery; to facilitate mechanical ventilation in ICU patients; does not relieve pain or produce sedation

Mechanism of Action/Effect Blocks neural transmission at the myoneural junction by binding with cholinergic receptor sites

Contraindications Hypersensitivity to atracurium besylate or any component of the formulation

Warnings/Precautions Reduce initial dosage and inject slowly (over 1-2 minutes) in patients in whom substantial histamine release would be potentially hazardous (eg, patients with clinically-important cardiovascular disease). Maintenance of an adequate airway and respiratory support is critical. Certain clinical conditions may result in potentiation or antagonism of neuromuscular blockade:

Potentiation: Electrolyte abnormalities, severe hyponatremia, severe hypocalcemia, severe hypokalemia, hypermagnesemia, neuromuscular diseases, acidosis, acute intermittent porphyria, renal failure, hepatic failure

Antagonism: Alkalosis, hypercalcemia, demyelinating lesions, peripheral neuropathies, diabetes mellitus

Increased sensitivity in patients with myasthenia gravis, Eaton-Lambert syndrome; resistance in burn patients (>30% of body) for period of 5-70 days postinjury; resistance in patients with muscle trauma, denervation, immobilization, infection, chronic treatment with atracurium. Cross-sensitivity with other neuromuscular-blocking agents may occur; use extreme caution in patients with previous anaphylactic reactions. Use caution in the elderly. Bradycardia may be more common with atracurium than with other neuromuscular-blocking agents since it has no clinically-significant effects on heart rate to counteract the bradycardia produced by anesthetics. Should be administered by adequately trained individuals familiar with its use. Some dosage forms may contain benzyl alcohol which has been associated with "gasping syndrome" in neonates.

Drug Interactions

Avoid Concomitant Use

Avoid concomitant use of Atracurium with any of the following: QuiNINE

Decreased Effect

The levels/effects of Atracurium may be decreased by: Acetylcholinesterase Inhibitors; Loop Diuretics

Increased Effect/Toxicity

Atracurium may increase the levels/effects of: Cardiac Glycosides; Corticosteroids (Systemic); OnabotulinumtoxinA; RimabotulinumtoxinB

The levels/effects of Atracurium may be increased by: AbobotulinumtoxinA; Aminoglycosides; Calcium Channel Blockers; Capreomycin; Colistimethate; Inhalational Anesthetics; Ketorolac; Ketorolac (Systemic); Lincosamide Antibiotics; Lithium; Loop Diuretics; Magnesium Salts; Polymyxin B; Procainamide; QuiNIDine; QuiNINE; Spironolactone; Tetracycline Derivatives; Vancomycin

Adverse Reactions Mild, rare, and generally suggestive of histamine release

1% to 10%: Cardiovascular: Flushing

Causes of prolonged neuromuscular blockade: Excessive drug administration; cumulative drug effect, metabolism/excretion decreased (hepatic and/or renal impairment); accumulation of active metabolites; electrolyte imbalance (hypokalemia, hypocalcemia, hypermagnesemia, hypernatremia); hypothermia

Pharmacodynamics/Kinetics

Onset of Action Dose dependent: 2-3 minutes

Duration of Action Recovery begins in 20-35 minutes following initial dose of 0.4-0.5 mg/kg under balanced anesthesia; recovery to 95% of control takes 60-70 minutes

Half-Life Elimination Biphasic: Adults: Initial (distribution): 2 minutes; Terminal: 20 minutes

Metabolism Undergoes ester hydrolysis and Hofmann elimination (nonbiologic process independent of renal, hepatic, or enzymatic function); metabolites have no neuromuscular blocking properties; laudanosine, a product of Hofmann elimination, is a CNS stimulant and can accumulate with prolonged use. Laudanosine is hepatically metabolized.

Excretion Urine (<5%)

Available Dosage Forms

Injection, solution: 10 mg/mL (10 mL)

Injection, solution [preservative free]: 10 mg/mL (5 mL)

Dosing

Adult & Geriatric For I.V. administration only (not to be used I.M.): Dose to effect; doses must be individualized due to interpatient variability; use ideal body weight for obese patients.

Adjunct to surgical anesthesia (neuromuscular blockade):

I.V. (bolus): 0.4-0.5 mg/kg, then 0.08-0.1 mg/kg 20-45 minutes after initial dose to maintain neuromuscular block, followed by repeat doses of 0.08-0.1 mg/kg at 15- to 25-minute intervals

Initial dose after succinylcholine for intubation (balanced anesthesia): 0.2-0.4 mg/kg

Pretreatment/priming: I.V.: 10% of intubating dose given 3-5 minutes before initial dose

I.V. continuous infusion: Initial: 9-10 mcg/kg/minute at initial signs of recovery from bolus dose; block is usually maintained by a rate of 5-9 mcg/kg/minute under balanced anesthesia.

ICU neuromuscular blockade: I.V.: Initial (bolus) 0.4-0.5 mg/kg, followed by I.V. continuous infusion at an initial rate of 5-10 mcg/kg/minute; block is usually maintained by rate of 11-13 mcg/kg/minute (rates for pediatric patients may be higher).

Pediatric Adjunct to surgical anesthesia: I.V. (not to be used I.M.): Dose to effect; doses must be individualized due to interpatient variability; use ideal body weight for obese patients

Children 1 month to 2 years: Initial: 0.3-0.4 mg/kg followed by maintenance doses as needed to maintain neuromuscular blockade

Children >2 years: Refer to adult dosing.

Renal Impairment No adjustment is necessary.

Hepatic Impairment No adjustment is necessary.

Administration

I.M. Not for I.M. injection due to tissue irritation.

I.V. May be given undiluted as a bolus injection. Administration via infusion requires the use of an infusion pump. Use infusion solutions within 24 hours of preparation.

Stability

Reconstitution Atracurium should not be mixed with alkaline solutions.

Storage Refrigerate intact vials at 2°C to 8°C (36°F to 46°F); protect from freezing. Use vials within 14 days upon removal from the refrigerator to room temperature of 25°C (77°F). Dilutions of 0.2 mg/mL or 0.5 mg/mL in 0.9% sodium chloride, dextrose 5% in water, or 5% dextrose in sodium chloride 0.9% are stable for up to 24 hours at room temperature or under refrigeration.

Monitoring and Teaching Issues

Laboratory Monitoring Renal function (serum creatinine, BUN) and liver function when in ICU

Physical Assessment Dosage and rate of administration should be individualized and titrated to the desired effect, according to relevant clinical factors, premedication, concomitant medications, age, and general condition of the patient. Ventilatory support must be instituted and maintained until adequate respiratory muscle function and/or airway protection are assured. This drug is not an anesthetic or analgesic; pain must be treated with other agents. Continuous monitoring of vital signs, cardiac status, respiratory status, and degree of neuromuscular block (objective assessment with peripheral external nerve stimulator) is mandatory during infusion and until full muscle tone has returned. Safety precautions must be maintained until full muscle tone has returned. It may take longer for return of muscle tone in obese or elderly patients or patients with renal or hepatic disease, myasthenia gravis, myopathy, other neuromuscular disease, dehydration, electrolyte imbalance, or severe acid/base imbalance.

Long-term use: Monitor level of neuromuscular blockade, skeletal muscle movement, and respiratory effort. Reposition patient and provide appropriate skin care, mouth care, and care of patient's eyes every 2-3 hours while sedated. Provide appropriate emotional and sensory support (auditory and environmental).

Patient Education Patient will usually be unconscious prior to administration. Reassurance of constant monitoring and emotional support to reduce fear and anxiety should precede and follow administration. Following return of muscle tone, do not attempt to change position or rise from bed without assistance.

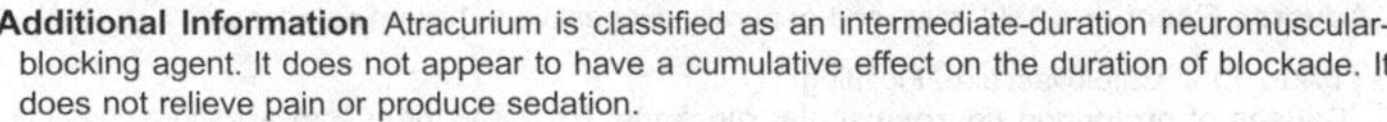

Additional Information Atracurium is classified as an intermediate-duration neuromuscular-blocking agent. It does not appear to have a cumulative effect on the duration of blockade. It does not relieve pain or produce sedation.

- **Atracurium Besylate** *see* Atracurium *on page 170*
- **Atralin™** *see* Tretinoin (Topical) *on page 1811*
- **Atripla®** *see* Efavirenz, Emtricitabine, and Tenofovir *on page 606*
- **AtroPen®** *see* Atropine *on page 172*

Atropine (A troe peen)

U.S. Brand Names AtroPen®; Atropine Care™; Isopto® Atropine; Sal-Tropine™

Index Terms Atropine Sulfate

Generic Availability (U.S.) Yes: Excludes tablet

Pharmacologic Category Anticholinergic Agent; Anticholinergic Agent, Ophthalmic; Antidote; Antispasmodic Agent, Gastrointestinal; Ophthalmic Agent, Mydriatic

Prescribing and Access Restrictions The AtroPen® formulation is available for use primarily by the Department of Defense.

Pregnancy Risk Factor B/C (manufacturer specific)

Lactation Enters breast milk/use caution (AAP rates "compatible"; AAP 2001 update pending)

Use

Injection: Preoperative medication to inhibit salivation and secretions; treatment of symptomatic sinus bradycardia, AV block (nodal level); antidote for acetylcholinesterase inhibitor poisoning (carbamate insecticides, nerve agents, organophosphate insecticides); adjuvant use with anticholinesterases (eg, edrophonium, neostigmine) to decrease their side effects during reversal of neuromuscular blockade

Note: Use is no longer recommended in the management of asystole or pulseless electrical activity (PEA) (ACLS, 2010).

Ophthalmic: Produce mydriasis and cycloplegia for examination of the retina and optic disc and accurate measurement of refractive errors; uveitis

Oral: Inhibit salivation and secretions

Mechanism of Action/Effect Blocks the action of acetylcholine at parasympathetic sites in smooth muscle, secretory glands, and the CNS; increases cardiac output, dries secretions. Atropine reverses the muscarinic effects of cholinergic poisoning. The primary goal in cholinergic poisonings is reversal of bronchorrhea and bronchoconstriction. Atropine has no effect on the nicotinic receptors responsible for muscle weakness, fasciculations, and paralysis.

Contraindications Hypersensitivity to atropine or any component of the formulation; narrow-angle glaucoma; adhesions between the iris and lens; tachycardia; obstructive GI disease; paralytic ileus; intestinal atony of the elderly or debilitated patient; severe ulcerative colitis; toxic megacolon complicating ulcerative colitis; hepatic disease; obstructive uropathy; renal disease; myasthenia gravis (unless used to treat side effects of acetylcholinesterase inhibitor); asthma; thyrotoxicosis; Mobitz type II block

Warnings/Precautions Use with caution in children with spastic paralysis; use with caution in elderly patients. Low doses cause a paradoxical decrease in heart rates. Heat prostration may occur in hot weather. Use with caution in patients with autonomic neuropathy, prostatic hyperplasia, hyperthyroidism, HF, cardiac arrhythmias, chronic lung disease, biliary tract disease; anticholinergic agents are generally not well tolerated in the elderly and their use should be avoided when possible. Atropine is rarely used except as a preoperative agent or in the acute treatment of bradyarrhythmias. In heart transplant recipients, atropine will likely be ineffective in treatment of bradycardia due to lack of vagal innervation of the transplanted heart; cholinergic reinnervation may occur over time (years), so atropine may be used cautiously; however, some may experience paradoxical slowing of the heart rate and high-degree AV block upon administration (ACLS, 2010; Bernheim, 2004).

Avoid relying on atropine for effective treatment of type II second-degree or third-degree AV block (with or without a new wide QRS complex). Asystole or bradycardic pulseless electrical activity (PEA): Although no evidence exists for significant detrimental effects, routine use is unlikely to have a therapeutic benefit and is no longer recommended (ACLS, 2010).

AtroPen®: There are no absolute contraindications for the use of atropine in severe organophosphate poisonings, however in mild poisonings, use caution in those patients where the use of atropine would be otherwise contraindicated. Formulation for use by trained personnel only.

Drug Interactions

Avoid Concomitant Use There are no known interactions where it is recommended to avoid concomitant use.

Decreased Effect

Atropine may decrease the levels/effects of: Acetylcholinesterase Inhibitors (Central); Secretin

The levels/effects of Atropine may be decreased by: Acetylcholinesterase Inhibitors (Central)

Increased Effect/Toxicity

Atropine may increase the levels/effects of: AbobotulinumtoxinA; Anticholinergics; Cannabinoids; OnabotulinumtoxinA; Potassium Chloride; RimabotulinumtoxinB

The levels/effects of Atropine may be increased by: Pramlintide

Adverse Reactions Severity and frequency of adverse reactions are dose related and vary greatly; listed reactions are limited to significant and/or life-threatening.

Cardiovascular: Arrhythmia, flushing, hypotension, palpitation, tachycardia

Central nervous system: Ataxia, coma, delirium, disorientation, dizziness, drowsiness, excitement, fever, hallucinations, headache, insomnia, nervousness

Dermatologic: Anhidrosis, urticaria, rash, scarlatiniform rash

Gastrointestinal: Bloating, constipation, delayed gastric emptying, loss of taste, nausea, paralytic ileus, vomiting, xerostomia, dry throat, nasal dryness

Genitourinary: Urinary hesitancy, urinary retention

Neuromuscular & skeletal: Weakness

Ocular: Angle-closure glaucoma, blurred vision, cycloplegia, dry eyes, mydriasis, ocular tension increased

Respiratory: Dyspnea, laryngospasm, pulmonary edema

Miscellaneous: Anaphylaxis

Pharmacodynamics/Kinetics

Onset of Action I.V.: Rapid

Absorption Complete

Half-Life Elimination 2-3 hours

Metabolism Hepatic

Excretion Urine (30% to 50% as unchanged drug and metabolites)

Available Dosage Forms

Injection, solution: 0.05 mg/mL (5 mL); 0.1 mg/mL (5 mL, 10 mL); 0.4 mg/mL (1 mL, 20 mL); 1 mg/mL (1 mL)

AtroPen®: 0.25 mg/0.3 mL (0.3 mL); 0.5 mg/0.7 mL (0.7 mL); 1 mg/0.7 mL (0.7 mL); 2 mg/0.7 mL (0.7 mL)

Injection, solution [preservative free]: 0.4 mg/0.5 mL (0.5 mL); 0.4 mg/mL (1 mL); 1 mg/mL (1 mL)

Ointment, ophthalmic: 1% (3.5 g)

Solution, ophthalmic: 1% (2 mL, 5 mL, 15 mL)

Atropine Care™: 1% (2 mL)

Isopto® Atropine: 1% (5 mL, 15 mL)

Tablet, oral:

Sal-Tropine™: 0.4 mg

Dosing

Adult Doses <0.5 mg have been associated with paradoxical bradycardia.

Inhibit salivation and secretions (preanesthesia):

I.M., I.V., SubQ: 0.4-0.6 mg 30-60 minutes preop and repeat every 4-6 hours as needed.

Oral: 0.4 mg; may repeat in 4 hours if necessary; 0.4 mg initial dose may be exceeded in certain cases and may repeat in 4 hours if necessary

Bradycardia (Note: Atropine may be ineffective in heart transplant recipients): *I.V.:* 0.5 mg every 3-5 minutes, not to exceed a total of 3 mg or 0.04 mg/kg (ACLS, 2010)

Neuromuscular blockade reversal: *I.V.:* 25-30 mcg/kg 30-60 seconds before neostigmine or 7-10 mcg/kg 30-60 seconds before edrophonium

Organophosphate or carbamate poisoning: Note: The dose of atropine required varies considerably with the severity of poisoning. Total amount of atropine used in carbamate poisoning is usually less. Severely poisoned patients may exhibit significant tolerance to atropine; ≥2 times the suggested doses may be needed. Titrate to pulmonary status (decreased bronchial secretions). Once patient is stable for a period of time, the dose/dosing frequency may be decreased. If atropinization occurs after 1-2 mg of atropine then re-evaluate working diagnosis.

I.V.: Initial: 1-5 mg; doses should be doubled every 5 minutes until signs of muscarinic excess abate (clearing of bronchial secretions, bronchospasm, and adequate oxygenation). Overly aggressive dosing may cause anticholinergic toxicity (eg, delirium, hyperthermia, and muscle twitching).

I.V. Infusion: 0.5-1 mg/hour or 10% to 20% of loading dose/hour

I.M.: AtroPen®: Mild symptoms: Administer 2 mg as soon as exposure is known or suspected. If severe symptoms develop after first dose, 2 additional doses should be repeated in 10 minutes; do not administer more than 3 doses. Severe symptoms: Immediately administer three 2 mg doses.

Nerve agent toxicity management: *I.M.:* See **Note**. Prehospital ("in the field") or hospital/emergency department: Mild-to-moderate symptoms: 2-4 mg; severe symptoms: 6 mg

Note: Pralidoxime is a component of the management of nerve agent toxicity; consult Pralidoxime for specific route and dose.

Prehospital ("in the field") management: Repeat atropine I.M. (2 mg) at 5-10 minute intervals until secretions have diminished and breathing is comfortable or airway resistance has returned to near normal.

Hospital management: Repeat atropine I.M. (2 mg) at 5-10 minute intervals until secretions have diminished and breathing is comfortable or airway resistance has returned to near normal.

Mydriasis, cycloplegia (preprocedure): *Ophthalmic* (1% solution): Instill 1-2 drops 1 hour before the procedure.

Uveitis: *Ophthalmic:*

1% solution: Instill 1-2 drops 4 times/day.

Ointment: Apply a small amount in the conjunctival sac up to 3 times/day. Compress the lacrimal sac by digital pressure for 1-3 minutes after instillation.

Geriatric Refer to adult dosing.

Nerve agent toxicity management (unlabeled use): See **Note**. I.M.: Elderly and frail patients:

Prehospital ("in the field"): Mild-to-moderate symptoms: 1 mg; severe symptoms: 2-4 mg

Hospital/emergency department: Mild-to-moderate symptoms: 1 mg; severe symptoms: 2 mg

Note: Pralidoxime is a component of the management of nerve agent toxicity.

Prehospital ("in the field") management: Repeat atropine I.M. (2 mg) at 5-10 minute intervals until secretions have diminished and breathing is comfortable or airway resistance has returned to near normal.

Hospital management: Repeat atropine I.M. (2 mg) at 5-10 minute intervals until secretions have diminished and breathing is comfortable or airway resistance has returned to near normal.

Pediatric Note: Doses <0.1 mg have been associated with paradoxical bradycardia.

Inhibit salivation and secretions (preanesthesia): Oral, I.M., I.V., SubQ: Neonates, Infants, and Children:

Children <5 kg: 0.02 mg/kg/dose 30-60 minutes preop then every 4-6 hours as needed. Use of a minimum dosage of 0.1 mg in neonates <5 kg will result in dosages >0.02 mg/kg. There is no documented minimum dosage in this age group.

Children >5 kg: 0.01-0.02 mg/kg/dose to a maximum 0.4 mg/dose 30-60 minutes preop; minimum dose: 0.1 mg

Alternate dosing:

3-7 kg (7-16 lb): 0.1 mg
8-11 kg (17-24 lb): 0.15 mg
11-18 kg (24-40 lb): 0.2 mg
18-29 kg (40-65 lb): 0.3 mg
>30 kg (>65 lb): 0.4 mg

Bradycardia:

I.V., I.O.: Neonates, Infants, and Children: 0.02 mg/kg, minimum dose 0.1 mg, maximum single dose: 0.5 mg; may repeat once in 3-5 minutes to a maximum total dose of 0.04 mg/kg or 1 mg (PALS, 2010). When treating bradycardia in neonates, reserve use for those patients unresponsive to improved oxygenation and epinephrine.

Intratracheal: Infants and Children: 0.04-0.06 mg/kg; may repeat once if needed (PALS, 2010)

Organophosphate or carbamate poisoning:

I.V.: Children: 0.03-0.05 mg/kg every 10-20 minutes until atropine effect, then every 1-4 hours for at least 24 hours

I.M. (AtroPen®): Children: Mild symptoms: Administer dose listed below as soon as exposure is known or suspected. If severe symptoms develop after first dose, 2 additional doses should be repeated in 10 minutes; do not administer more than 3 doses. Severe symptoms: Immediately administer 3 doses as follows:

<6.8 kg (15 lb): Use of **AtroPen® formulation not recommended**; administer atropine 0.05 mg/kg
6.8-18 kg (15-40 lb): 0.5 mg/dose
18-41 kg (40-90 lb): 1 mg/dose
>41 kg (>90 lb): 2 mg/dose

Nerve agent toxicity management: I.M.: Infants and Children: See following **Note**.

Prehospital ("in the field"):

Birth to <2 years: Mild-to-moderate symptoms: 0.05 mg/kg; severe symptoms: 0.1 mg/kg
2-10 years: Mild-to-moderate symptoms: 1 mg; severe symptoms: 2 mg
>10 years: Mild-to-moderate symptoms: 2 mg; severe symptoms: 4 mg

Hospital/emergency department:

Birth to <2 years: Mild-to-moderate symptoms: 0.05 mg/kg I.M. **or** 0.02 mg/kg I.V.; severe symptoms: 0.1 mg/kg I.M. **or** 0.02 mg/kg I.V.
2-10 years: Mild-to-moderate symptoms: 1 mg; severe symptoms: 2 mg
>10 years: Mild-to-moderate symptoms: 2 mg; severe symptoms: 4 mg

Note: Pralidoxime is a component of the management of nerve agent toxicity.

Prehospital ("in the field") management: Repeat atropine I.M. (0.05-0.1 mg/kg) at 5-10 minute intervals until secretions have diminished and breathing is comfortable or airway resistance has returned to near normal.

Hospital management: Repeat atropine I.M. (infants: 1 mg; all others: 2 mg) at 5-10 minute intervals until secretions have diminished and breathing is comfortable or airway resistance has returned to near normal.

Administration

I.M. AtroPen®: Administer to outer thigh. May be given through clothing as long as pockets at the injection site are empty. Hold autoinjector in place for 10 seconds following injection; massage the injection site.

I.V. Administer undiluted by rapid I.V. injection; slow injection may result in paradoxical bradycardia. In bradycardia, atropine administration should not delay treatment with external pacing.

Other Intratracheal: Dilute in NS or sterile water (absorption may be greater with sterile water). Spray drug quickly down tube. Follow immediately with several quick insufflations.

Stability

Storage Store injection at controlled room temperature of 15°C to 30°C (59°F to 86°F); avoid freezing. In addition, AtroPen® should be protected from light.

Monitoring and Teaching Issues

Physical Assessment Monitor for tachycardia and hypotension, especially if cardiac problems are present. Be alert to the potential of heat prostration in the presence of high temperatures.

Patient Education Maintain adequate hydration, unless instructed to restrict fluid intake. You may experience dizziness, blurred vision, sensitivity to light, dry mouth, nausea, vomiting, orthostatic hypotension, constipation, increased sensitivity to heat and decreased perspiration, or decreased milk supply if breast-feeding. Report hot, dry, flushed skin; blurred vision or vision changes; difficulty swallowing; chest pain, palpitations, or rapid heartbeat; painful or difficult urination; increased confusion, depression, or loss of memory; rapid or difficult respirations; muscle weakness or tremors; or eye pain.

Ophthalmic: Wash hands before using. Sit or lie down, open eye, look at ceiling, and instill prescribed amount of solution. Do not blink for 30 seconds. Close eye, roll eye in all directions, and apply gentle pressure to inner corner of eye for 1-2 minutes. Do not let tip of applicator touch eye; do not contaminate tip of applicator (may cause eye infection, eye damage, or vision loss). Temporary stinging or blurred vision may occur.

Geriatric Considerations Anticholinergic agents are generally not well tolerated in the elderly and their use should be avoided when possible. In elderly, anticholinergic agents should not be used as prophylaxis against extrapyramidal symptoms.

Breast-Feeding Considerations Trace amounts of atropine are excreted into breast milk. Anticholinergic agents may suppress lactation.

Pregnancy Considerations Animal reproduction studies have not been conducted. Atropine has been found to cross the human placenta.

◆ **Atropine and Difenoxin** *see* Difenoxin and Atropine *on page 528*

◆ **Atropine and Diphenoxylate** *see* Diphenoxylate and Atropine *on page 547*

◆ **Atropine Care™** *see* Atropine *on page 172*

◆ **Atropine Sulfate** *see* Atropine *on page 172*

◆ **Atrovent®** *see* Ipratropium (Nasal) *on page 1010*

◆ **Atrovent® HFA** *see* Ipratropium (Oral Inhalation) *on page 1009*

◆ **Augmentin®** *see* Amoxicillin and Clavulanate Potassium *on page 113*

◆ **Augmentin ES-600®** *see* Amoxicillin and Clavulanate Potassium *on page 113*

◆ **Augmentin XR®** *see* Amoxicillin and Clavulanate Potassium *on page 113*

◆ **Avage®** *see* Tazarotene *on page 1710*

◆ **Avakine** *see* InFLIXimab *on page 973*

◆ **Avalide®** *see* Irbesartan and Hydrochlorothiazide *on page 1014*

◆ **Avandamet®** *see* Rosiglitazone and Metformin *on page 1612*

◆ **Avandaryl®** *see* Rosiglitazone and Glimepiride *on page 1611*

◆ **Avandia®** *see* Rosiglitazone *on page 1609*

◆ **Avapro®** *see* Irbesartan *on page 1012*

◆ **Avapro® HCT** *see* Irbesartan and Hydrochlorothiazide *on page 1014*

◆ **Avastin®** *see* Bevacizumab *on page 211*

◆ **Avelox®** *see* Moxifloxacin (Systemic) *on page 1264*

◆ **Avelox® ABC Pack** *see* Moxifloxacin (Systemic) *on page 1264*

◆ **Avelox® I.V.** *see* Moxifloxacin (Systemic) *on page 1264*

◆ **Aviane™** *see* Ethinyl Estradiol and Levonorgestrel *on page 699*

◆ **Avian Influenza Virus Vaccine** *see* Influenza Virus Vaccine (H5N1) *on page 977*

◆ **AVINza®** *see* Morphine (Systemic) *on page 1258*

◆ **Avita®** *see* Tretinoin (Topical) *on page 1811*

◆ **Avodart®** *see* Dutasteride *on page 599*

◆ **Avonex®** *see* Interferon Beta-1a *on page 1003*

◆ **AVP** *see* Vasopressin *on page 1851*

◆ **Axert®** *see* Almotriptan *on page 78*

◆ **Axid®** *see* Nizatidine *on page 1332*

◆ **Axid® AR [OTC]** *see* Nizatidine *on page 1332*

◆ **Axiron®** *see* Testosterone *on page 1739*

◆ **Axiron®** *see* Testosterone *on page 1739*

◆ **AY-25650** *see* Triptorelin *on page 1824*

◆ **Aygestin®** *see* Norethindrone *on page 1334*

◆ **5-Aza-2'-deoxycytidine** *see* Decitabine *on page 476*

AzaCITIDine (ay za SYE ti deen)

U.S. Brand Names Vidaza®

Index Terms 5-Azacytidine; 5-AZC; AZA-CR; Azacytidine; Ladakamycin

Generic Availability (U.S.) No

Pharmacologic Category Antineoplastic Agent, DNA Methylation Inhibitor

Medication Safety Issues

Sound-alike/look-alike issues:

AzaCITIDine may be confused with azaTHIOprine

High alert medication: This medication is in a class the Institute for Safe Medication Practices (ISMP) includes among its list of drug classes which have a heightened risk of causing significant patient harm when used in error.

Pregnancy Risk Factor D

Lactation Excretion in breast milk unknown/not recommended

Use Treatment of myelodysplastic syndrome (MDS)

Unlabeled/Investigational Use Treatment of acute myelogenous leukemia (AML)

Mechanism of Action/Effect Antineoplastic effects may be a result of azacitidine's ability to promote hypomethylation of DNA leading to direct toxicity of abnormal hematopoietic cells in the bone marrow.

Contraindications Hypersensitivity to azacitidine, mannitol, or any component of the formulation; advanced malignant hepatic tumors

Warnings/Precautions Hazardous agent - use appropriate precautions for handling and disposal. Azacitidine may be hepatotoxic, use caution with hepatic impairment; use is contraindicated in patients with advanced malignant hepatic tumors. Progressive hepatic coma leading to death has been reported (rare) in patients with extensive tumor burden, especially those with a baseline albumin <30 g/L. Use caution with renal impairment; dose adjustment may be required. Serum creatinine elevations, renal tubular acidosis, and renal failure have been reported with combination chemotherapy; decrease or withhold dose for unexplained elevations in BUN or serum creatinine or reductions in serum bicarbonate to <20 mEq/L. Patients with renal and hepatic impairment were excluded from clinical studies. Neutropenia, thrombocytopenia, and anemia are common; may cause therapy delays and/or dosage reductions. Not FDA approved for use in children.

Drug Interactions

Avoid Concomitant Use

Avoid concomitant use of AzaCITIDine with any of the following: BCG; Natalizumab; Pimecrolimus; Roflumilast; Tacrolimus (Topical); Vaccines (Live)

Decreased Effect

AzaCITIDine may decrease the levels/effects of: BCG; Sipuleucel-T; Vaccines (Inactivated); Vaccines (Live)

The levels/effects of AzaCITIDine may be decreased by: Echinacea

Increased Effect/Toxicity

AzaCITIDine may increase the levels/effects of: Leflunomide; Natalizumab; Vaccines (Live)

The levels/effects of AzaCITIDine may be increased by: Denosumab; Pimecrolimus; Roflumilast; Tacrolimus (Topical); Trastuzumab

Adverse Reactions

>10%:

Cardiovascular: Peripheral edema (7% to 19%), chest pain (16%), pallor (16%), pitting edema (15%)

Central nervous system: Fever (30% to 52%), fatigue (13% to 36%), headache (22%), dizziness (19%), anxiety (5% to 13%), depression (12%), insomnia (9% to 11%), malaise (11%), pain (11%)

Dermatologic: Bruising (19% to 31%), petechiae (11% to 24%), erythema (7% to 17%), skin lesion (15%), rash (10% to 14%), pruritus (12%)

Endocrine & metabolic: Hypokalemia (6% to 13%)

Gastrointestinal: Nausea (48% to 71%), vomiting (27% to 54%), diarrhea (36%), constipation (34% to 50%), anorexia (13% to 21%), weight loss (16%), abdominal pain (11% to 16%), abdominal tenderness (12%)

Hematologic: Thrombocytopenia (66% to 70%; grades 3/4: 58%), anemia (51% to 70%; grades 3/4: 14%), neutropenia (32% to 66%; grades 3/4: 61%), leukopenia (18% to 48%; grades 3/4: 15%), febrile neutropenia (14% to 16%; grades 3/4: 13%), myelosuppression (nadir: days 10-17; recovery: days 28-31)

Local: Injection site reactions (14% to 29%): Erythema (35% to 43%; more common with I.V. administration), pain (19% to 23%; more common with I.V. administration), bruising (5% to 14%)

Neuromuscular & skeletal: Weakness (29%), rigors (26%), arthralgia (22%), limb pain (20%), back pain (19%), myalgia (16%)

Respiratory: Cough (11% to 30%), dyspnea (5% to 29%), pharyngitis (20%), epistaxis (16%), nasopharyngitis (15%), upper respiratory tract infection (9% to 13%), pneumonia (11%), crackles (11%)

Miscellaneous: Diaphoresis (11%)

5% to 10%:

Cardiovascular: Cardiac murmur (10%), hypertension (≤9%), tachycardia (9%), hypotension (7%), syncope (6%), chest wall pain (5%)

Central nervous system: Lethargy (7% to 8%), hypoesthesia (5%), postprocedural pain (5%)

Dermatologic: Cellulitis (8%), urticaria (6%), dry skin (5%), skin nodule (5%)

Gastrointestinal: Gingival bleeding (10%), oral mucosal petechiae (8%), stomatitis (8%), weight loss (≤8%), dyspepsia (6% to 7%), hemorrhoids (7%), abdominal distension (6%), loose stools (6%), dysphagia (5%), oral hemorrhage (5%), tongue ulceration (5%)

Genitourinary: Dysuria (8%), urinary tract infection (8% to 9%)

Hematologic: Hematoma (9%), postprocedural hemorrhage (6%)

Local: Injection site reactions: Pruritus (7%), hematoma (6%), rash (6%), granuloma (5%), induration (5%), pigmentation change (5%), swelling (5%)

Neuromuscular & skeletal: Muscle cramps (6%)

Renal: Hematuria (≤6%)

Respiratory: Rhinorrhea (10%), rales (9%), wheezing (9%), breath sounds decreased (8%), pharyngolaryngeal pain (6%), pleural effusion (6%), postnasal drip (6%), rhinitis (6%), rhonchi (6%), nasal congestion (6%), atelectasis (5%), sinusitis (5%)

Miscellaneous: Lymphadenopathy (10%), herpes simplex (9%), night sweats (9%), transfusion reaction (7%), mouth hemorrhage (5%)

Pharmacodynamics/Kinetics

Absorption SubQ: Rapid and complete

Bioavailability SubQ: ~89%

Time to Peak SubQ: 30 minutes

Half-Life Elimination I.V., SubQ: ~4 hours

Metabolism Hepatic; hydrolysis to several metabolites

Excretion Urine (50% to 85%); feces (minor)

Available Dosage Forms

Injection, powder for suspension:

Vidaza®: 100 mg

Dosing

Adult

MDS: I.V., SubQ: 75 mg/m^2/day for 7 days repeated every 4 weeks. Dose may be increased to 100 mg/m^2/day if no benefit is observed after 2 cycles and no toxicity other than nausea and vomiting have occurred. Treatment is recommended for at least 4 cycles; treatment may be continued as long as patient continues to benefit.

Note: Alternate (unlabeled) schedules (which have produced hematologic response) have been used for convenience in community oncology centers (Lyons, 2009):

75 mg/m^2/day for 5 days (Mon-Fri), 2 days rest (Sat, Sun), then 75 mg/m^2/day for 2 days (Mon, Tues); repeat cycle every 28 days **or**

50 mg/m^2/day for 5 days (Mon-Fri), 2 days rest (Sat, Sun), then 50 mg/m^2/day for 5 days (Mon-Fri); repeat cycle every 28 days **or**

75 mg/m^2/day for 5 days (Mon-Fri), repeat cycle every 28 days

AML (unlabeled use): SubQ: 75 mg/m2/day for 7 days repeated every 4 weeks (Sudan, 2006)

Dosage adjustment based on hematology: Adults: I.V., SubQ: MDS:

For baseline WBC ≥3.0 x 10^9/L, ANC ≥1.5 x 10^9/L, and platelets ≥75 x 10^9/L:

Nadir count: ANC <0.5 x 10^9/L or platelets <25 x 10^9/L: Administer 50% of dose during next treatment course

Nadir count: ANC 0.5-1.5 x 10^9/L or platelets 25-50 x 10^9/L: Administer 67% of dose during next treatment course

Nadir count: ANC >1.5 x 10^9/L or platelets >50 x 10^9/L: Administer 100% of dose during next treatment course

For baseline WBC <3 x 10^9/L, ANC <1.5 x 10^9/L, or platelets <75 x 10^9/L: Adjust dose as follows based on nadir counts and bone marrow biopsy cellularity at the time of nadir, unless clear improvement in differentiation at the time of the next cycle:

WBC or platelet nadir decreased 50% to 75% from baseline and bone marrow biopsy cellularity at time of nadir 30% to 60%: Administer 100% of dose during next treatment course

WBC or platelet nadir decreased 50% to 75% from baseline and bone marrow biopsy cellularity at time of nadir 15% to 30%: Administer 50% of dose during next treatment course

WBC or platelet nadir decreased 50% to 75% from baseline and bone marrow biopsy cellularity at time of nadir <15%: Administer 33% of dose during next treatment course

WBC or platelet nadir decreased >75% from baseline and bone marrow biopsy cellularity at time of nadir 30% to 60%: Administer 75% of dose during next treatment course

WBC or platelet nadir decreased >75% from baseline and bone marrow biopsy cellularity at time of nadir 15% to 30%: Administer 50% of dose during next treatment course

WBC or platelet nadir decreased >75% from baseline and bone marrow biopsy cellularity at time of nadir <15%: Administer 33% of dose during next treatment course

Note: If a nadir defined above occurs, administer the next treatment course 28 days after the start of the preceding course as long as WBC and platelet counts are >25% above the nadir and rising. If a >25% increase above the nadir is not seen by day 28, reassess counts every 7 days. If a 25% increase is not seen by day 42, administer 50% of the scheduled dose.

Dosage adjustment based on serum electrolytes: The manufacturer recommends that if serum bicarbonate falls to <20 mEq/L (unexplained decrease): Reduce dose by 50% for next treatment course

Geriatric Refer to adult dosing. Due to the potential for decreased renal function in the elderly, select dose carefully and closely monitor renal function.

Pediatric Refractory AML (unlabeled use): 250 mg/m^2/dose days 4 and 5 every 4 weeks (Steuber, 1996) **or** 300 mg/m^2/dose days 4 and 5 every 4 weeks (Hurwitz, 1995)

Renal Impairment Not studied in patients with renal impairment; select dose carefully (excretion is primarily renal; consider dose reduction); monitor closely for toxicity.

Hepatic Impairment Not studied in patients with hepatic impairment; use caution. Contraindicated in patients with advanced malignant hepatic tumors.

Adjustment for Toxicity Renal toxicity: If increases in BUN or serum creatinine (unexplained) occur, delay next cycle until values reach baseline or normal, then reduce dose by 50% for next treatment course.

Administration

I.V. Premedication for nausea and vomiting is recommended. Infuse over 10-40 minutes; infusion must be completed within 1 hour of (vial) reconstitution.

Other SubQ: Premedication for nausea and vomiting is recommended. The manufacturer recommends equally dividing volumes >4 mL into 2 syringes and injecting into 2 separate sites; however, policies for maximum SubQ administration volume may vary by institution; interpatient variations may also apply. Administer subsequent injections at least 1 inch from previous injection sites. Allow refrigerated suspensions to come to room temperature (up to 30 minutes) prior to administration. Resuspend by inverting the syringe 2-3 times and then rolling the syringe between the palms for 30 seconds. If azacitidine suspension comes in contact with the skin, immediately wash with soap and water.

Stability

Reconstitution Use appropriate precautions for handling and disposal.

SubQ: To prepare a 25 mg/mL suspension, slowly add 4 mL SWFI to each vial. Vigorously shake or roll vial until a suspension is formed (suspension will be cloudy).

I.V.: Reconstitute vial with 10 mL SWFI to form a 10 mg/mL solution; vigorously shake until solution is dissolved and clear. Mix in 50-100 mL of NS or lactated Ringer's injection for infusion.

Storage Prior to reconstitution, store powder at room temperature of 25°C (77°F); excursions permitted to 15°C to 30°C (59°F to 86°F).

SubQ: Following reconstitution, suspension may be stored at room temperature for up to 1 hour, or immediately refrigerated at 2°C to 8°C (36°F to 46°F) and stored for up to 8 hours.

I.V.: **Solutions for I.V. administration have very limited stability and must be prepared immediately prior to each dose.** Administration must be completed within 1 hour of (vial) reconstitution.

Monitoring and Teaching Issues

Laboratory Monitoring Liver function tests, electrolytes, CBC with differential and platelets, renal function tests (BUN and serum creatinine) should be obtained prior to initiation of therapy. Electrolytes, renal function (BUN and creatinine), CBC should be monitored prior to each cycle and periodically as needed to monitor response and toxicity.

Physical Assessment Use with caution in presence of hepatic or renal impairment (dose adjustment may be required). Pretreatment with antiemetic is recommended to reduce nausea and vomiting. Note specific administration, reconstitution, and storage instructions (I.V. and SubQ stability differs). Patient should be monitored closely for edema, chest pain, hypotension, CNS changes, gastrointestinal disturbances, and hematologic and hepatic effects.

Patient Education This medication can only be administered by injection or I.V.; report immediately any pain, burning, or swelling at injection/infusion site. Limit oral intake for 4-6 hours before therapy to reduce potential for nausea/vomiting. It is important that you maintain adequate nutrition between treatments and adequate hydration, unless instructed to restrict fluid intake. You may be susceptible to infection. May cause nausea, vomiting, abdominal tenderness, anorexia, mouth sores, or loss of hair (reversible). Report chest pain or palpitations; sore throat, fever, chills, unusual weakness or fatigue; unusual bruising/bleeding; change in color or frequency of urine or stool; itching or burning on urination; difficulty breathing; change in visual acuity; or pain, redness, or swelling at injection site.

Breast-Feeding Considerations Due to the potential for serious adverse reactions in the nursing infant, breast-feeding is not recommended.

Pregnancy Considerations Embryotoxicity, fetal death, and fetal abnormalities were observed in animal studies. There are no adequate and well-controlled studies in pregnant women. Women of childbearing potential should be advised to avoid pregnancy during treatment. In addition, males should be advised to avoid fathering a child while on azacitidine therapy.

Additional Information Oncology Comment: Azacitidine treatment for MDS is associated with an improvement in quality of life (including a reduction in transfusion requirements), a decrease in transformation to AML, and improved survival, when compared to best supportive care. Treatment should be continued for a minimum of 4-6 cycles (NCCN MDS guidelines v.2.2009).

- **AZA-CR** *see* AzaCITIDine *on page 175*
- **Azactam®** *see* Aztreonam *on page 185*
- **Azacytidine** *see* AzaCITIDine *on page 175*
- **5-Azacytidine** *see* AzaCITIDine *on page 175*
- **5-Aza-dCyd** *see* Decitabine *on page 476*
- **Azasan®** *see* AzaTHIOprine *on page 178*

AzaTHIOprine (ay za THYE oh preen)

U.S. Brand Names Azasan®; Imuran®

Index Terms Azathioprine Sodium

Generic Availability (U.S.) Yes

Pharmacologic Category Immunosuppressant Agent

Medication Safety Issues

Sound-alike/look-alike issues:

AzaTHIOprine may be confused with azaCITIDine, azatadine, azidothymidine, azithromycin, Azulfidine®

Imuran® may be confused with Elmiron®, Enduron®, Imdur®, Inderal®, Tenormin®

Azathioprine is metabolized to mercaptopurine; concurrent use of these commercially-available products has resulted in profound myelosuppression.

Pregnancy Risk Factor D

Lactation Enters breast milk/not recommended

Use Adjunctive therapy in prevention of rejection of kidney transplants; management of active rheumatoid arthritis (RA)

Unlabeled/Investigational Use Adjunct in prevention of rejection of solid organ (nonrenal) transplants; steroid-sparing agent for corticosteroid-dependent Crohn's disease (CD) and ulcerative colitis (UC); maintenance of remission in CD; fistulizing CD; dermatomyositis/polymyositis

Mechanism of Action/Effect Antagonizes purine metabolism and may inhibit synthesis of DNA, RNA, and proteins; may also interfere with cellular metabolism and inhibit mitosis; the 6-thioguanine nucleotides appear to mediate the majority of azathioprine's immunosuppressive and toxic effects

Contraindications Hypersensitivity to azathioprine or any component of the formulation; pregnancy (in patients with rheumatoid arthritis); patients with rheumatoid arthritis and a history of treatment with alkylating agents (eg, cyclophosphamide, chlorambucil, melphalan) may have a prohibitive risk of neoplasia with azathioprine treatment

Warnings/Precautions [U.S. Boxed Warning]: Chronic immunosuppression increases the risk of neoplasia and serious infections. Azathioprine has mutagenic potential to both men and women. Dose-related, delayed hematologic toxicities (leukopenia, thrombocytopenia, macrocytic anemia, pancytopenia) may occur; may be more severe with renal transplants undergoing rejection; dosage modification for hematologic toxicity may be necessary. Use with caution in patients with liver disease or renal impairment; monitor hematologic function closely. Azathioprine is metabolized to mercaptopurine; concomitant use may result in profound myelosuppression and should be avoided. Patients with genetic deficiency of thiopurine methyltransferase (TPMT) or concurrent therapy with drugs which may inhibit TPMT may be sensitive to myelosuppressive effects. Patients with intermediate TPMT activity may be at risk for increased myelosuppression; those with low or absent TPMT activity are at risk for developing severe myelotoxicity. TPMT genotyping or phenotyping may assist in identifying patients at risk for developing toxicity. TPMT testing does not substitute for CBC monitoring. Xanthine oxidase inhibitors may increase risk for hematologic toxicity; reduce azathioprine dose when used concurrently with allopurinol; patients with low or absent TPMT activity may require further dose reductions or discontinuation.

Hepatotoxicity (transaminase, bilirubin, and alkaline phosphatase elevations) may occur, usually in renal transplant patients and generally within 6 months of transplant; normally reversible with discontinuation; monitor liver function periodically. Rarely, hepatic veno-occlusive disease (VOD) has been reported; discontinue if hepatic VOD is suspected. Gastrointestinal toxicity may occur within the first several weeks of therapy and is reversible. Symptoms may include severe nausea, vomiting, diarrhea, rash, fever, malaise, myalgia, hypotension, and liver enzyme abnormalities. **[U.S. Boxed Warning]: Should be prescribed by physicians familiar with the risks, including hematologic toxicities and mutagenic potential.** Immune response to vaccines may be diminished. Hazardous agent - use appropriate precautions for handling and disposal.

Drug Interactions

Avoid Concomitant Use

Avoid concomitant use of AzaTHIOprine with any of the following: BCG; Febuxostat; Natalizumab; Pimecrolimus; Roflumilast; Tacrolimus (Topical)

Decreased Effect

AzaTHIOprine may decrease the levels/effects of: BCG; Sipuleucel-T; Vaccines (Inactivated); Vitamin K Antagonists

The levels/effects of AzaTHIOprine may be decreased by: Echinacea

Increased Effect/Toxicity

AzaTHIOprine may increase the levels/effects of: Leflunomide; Mercaptopurine; Natalizumab; Vaccines (Live)

The levels/effects of AzaTHIOprine may be increased by: 5-ASA Derivatives; ACE Inhibitors; Allopurinol; Denosumab; Febuxostat; Pimecrolimus; Ribavirin; Roflumilast; Sulfamethoxazole; Tacrolimus (Topical); Trastuzumab; Trimethoprim

Nutritional/Ethanol Interactions Herb/Nutraceutical: Avoid cat's claw, echinacea (have immunostimulant properties).

Lab Interactions TPMT phenotyping results will not be accurate following recent blood transfusions.

Adverse Reactions Frequency not always defined; dependent upon dose, duration, indication, and concomitant therapy.

Central nervous system: Fever, malaise

Gastrointestinal: Nausea/vomiting (RA: 12%), diarrhea

Hematologic: Leukopenia (renal transplant: >50%; RA: 28%), thrombocytopenia

Hepatic: Alkaline phosphatase increased, bilirubin increased, hepatotoxicity, transaminases increased

Neuromuscular & skeletal: Myalgia

Miscellaneous: Infection (renal transplant: 20%; RA: <1%; includes bacterial, fungal, protozoal, viral); neoplasia (other than lymphoma: 3%)

Pharmacodynamics/Kinetics

Absorption Oral: Well absorbed

Time to Peak Plasma: 1-2 hours (including metabolites)

Protein Binding ~30%

Half-Life Elimination Parent drug: 12 minutes; mercaptopurine: 0.7-3 hours; End-stage renal disease: Slightly prolonged

Metabolism Hepatic, to 6-mercaptopurine (6-MP), possibly by glutathione S-transferase (GST). Further metabolism of 6-MP (in the liver and GI tract), via three major pathways: Hypoxanthine guanine phosphoribosyltransferase (to 6-thioguanine-nucleotides, or 6-TGN), xanthine oxidase (to 6-thiouric acid), and thiopurine methyltransferase (TPMT), which forms 6-methylmercapotpurine (6-MMP).

Excretion Urine (primarily as metabolites)

Available Dosage Forms

Injection, powder for reconstitution: 100 mg

Tablet, oral: 50 mg

Azasan®: 75 mg, 100 mg

Imuran®: 50 mg

Dosing

Adult & Geriatric Note: Patients with intermediate TPMT activity may be at risk for increased myelosuppression; those with low or absent TPMT activity receiving conventional azathioprine doses are at risk for developing severe, life-threatening myelotoxicity. Dosage reductions are recommended for patients with reduced TPMT activity.

I.V. dose is equivalent to oral dose (dosing should be transitioned from I.V. to oral as soon as tolerated):

Renal transplantation (treatment usually started the day of transplant, however, has been initiated [rarely] 1-3 days prior to transplant): Oral, I.V.: Initial: 3-5 mg/kg/day usually given as a single daily dose, then 1-3 mg/kg/day maintenance

Rheumatoid arthritis: Oral:

Initial: 1 mg/kg/day given once daily or divided twice daily, for 6-8 weeks; increase by 0.5 mg/kg every 4 weeks until response or up to 2.5 mg/kg/day; an adequate trial should be a minimum of 12 weeks

Maintenance dose: Reduce dose by 0.5 mg/kg every 4 weeks until lowest effective dose is reached; optimum duration of therapy not specified; may be discontinued abruptly

Adjunctive management of severe recurrent aphthous stomatitis (unlabeled use): Oral: 50 mg once daily in conjunction with prednisone

Adjunctive management of dermatomyositis/polymyositis (unlabeled use): Oral: 50 mg/day in conjunction with prednisone; increase by 50 mg/week to total dose of 2-3 mg/kg/day (Briemberg, 2003); **Note:** Onset of beneficial effects may take 3-6 months; however, may be preferred over methotrexate in patients with pulmonary or hepatic toxicity.

Reduction of steroid use in CD or UC, maintenance of remission in CD or fistulizing disease (unlabeled uses): Oral: Initial: 50 mg once daily; may increase by 25 mg/day every 1-2 weeks as tolerated to target dose of 2-3 mg/kg/day

Dosage adjustment for concomitant use with allopurinol: Reduce azathioprine dose to one-third or one-fourth the usual dose when used concurrently with allopurinol. Patients with low or absent TPMT activity may require further dose reductions or discontinuation.

Pediatric Note: Patients with intermediate TPMT activity may be at risk for increased myelosuppression; those with low or absent TPMT activity receiving conventional azathioprine doses are at risk for developing severe, life-threatening myelotoxicity. Dosage reductions are recommended for patients with reduced TPMT activity.

Renal transplantation, rheumatoid arthritis (unlabeled uses): Refer to adult dosing.

Renal Impairment Although dosage reductions are recommended, specific guidelines are not available in the FDA-approved labeling; the following guidelines have been used by some clinicians (Aronoff, 2007):

Cl_{cr} >50 mL/minute: No adjustment recommended.

Cl_{cr} 10-50 mL/minute: Administer 75% of normal dose.

Cl_{cr} <10 mL/minute: Administer 50% of normal dose.

Hemodialysis (dialyzable; ~45% removed in 8 hours): Children: Administer 50% of normal dose; Adults: Supplement: 0.25 mg/kg

CAPD: Children: Administer 50% of normal dose; Adults: Unknown

CRRT: Children and Adults: Administer 75% of normal dose

Adjustment for Toxicity

Rapid WBC count decrease, persistently low WBC count, or serious infection: Reduce dose or temporarily withhold treatment.

Severe toxicity in renal transplantation: May require discontinuation.

Hepatic veno-occlusive disease: Permanently discontinue.

Administration

Oral Administering tablets after meals or in divided doses may decrease adverse GI events.

I.V. Can be administered IVP over 5 minutes at a concentration not to exceed 10 mg/mL **or** azathioprine can be further diluted with normal saline or D_5W and administered by intermittent infusion usually over 30-60 minutes; may be extended up to 8 hours.

Stability

Reconstitution Powder for injection: Reconstitute each vial with 10 mL sterile water for injection; may further dilute for infusion (in D_5W, ½NS, or NS). Use appropriate precautions for handling and disposal.

Storage

Tablet: Store at room temperature of 15°C to 25°C (59°F to 77°F); protect from light.

Powder for injection: Store intact vials at room temperature of 15°C to 25°C (59°F to 77°F). Protect from light. Reconstituted solution is stable for up to 2 weeks at room temperature or up to 4 days refrigerated; solutions diluted in D_5W, 1/2NS, or NS for infusion are stable at room temperature or refrigerated for up to 16 days; however, the manufacturer recommends use within 24 hours of reconstitution.

Monitoring and Teaching Issues

Laboratory Monitoring CBC with differential and platelets (weekly during first month, twice monthly for months 2 and 3, then monthly; monitor more frequently with dosage modifications), total bilirubin, liver function tests, TPMT genotyping or phenotyping

For use as immunomodulatory therapy in CD or UC, monitor CBC with differential weekly for 1 month, then biweekly for 1 month, followed by monitoring every 1-2 months throughout the course of therapy. LFT's should be assessed every 3 months.

Physical Assessment Monitor for opportunistic infection.

Patient Education May take in divided doses or with food if GI upset occurs. You will be susceptible to infection. You may experience nausea, vomiting, loss of appetite. Report abdominal pain and unresolved GI upset (eg, persistent vomiting or diarrhea); unusual fever or chills; bleeding or bruising; sore throat, unhealed sores, or signs of infection; yellowing of skin or eyes; or change in color of urine or stool. For rheumatoid arthritis, response may not occur for up to 3 months. For organ transplant, azathioprine will usually be prescribed with other antirejection medications.

Dietary Considerations May be taken with food.

Geriatric Considerations Toxicity to immunosuppressives is increased in elderly. Start with lowest recommended adult doses. Signs of infection, such as fever and WBC rise, may not occur. Lethargy and confusion may be more prominent signs of infection. In the elderly, adjust dose to creatinine clearance.

Breast-Feeding Considerations Due to risk of immunosuppression and serious adverse effects in the nursing infant, breast-feeding is not recommended.

Pregnancy Considerations Azathioprine was found to be teratogenic in animal studies; temporary depression in spermatogenesis and reduction in sperm viability and sperm count were also reported in mice. Azathioprine crosses the placenta in humans; congenital anomalies, immunosuppression, hematologic toxicities (lymphopenia, pancytopenia), and intrauterine growth retardation have been reported. There are no adequate and well-controlled studies in pregnant women. Azathioprine should not be used to treat arthritis during pregnancy. The potential benefit to the mother versus possible risk to the fetus should be considered when treating other disease states.

The National Transplantation Pregnancy Registry (NTPR, Temple University) is a registry for pregnant women taking immunosuppressants following any solid organ transplant. The NTPR encourages reporting of all immunosuppressant exposures during pregnancy in transplant recipients at 877-955-6877.

◆ **Azathioprine Sodium** *see* AzaTHIOprine *on page 178*

◆ **5-AZC** *see* AzaCITIDine *on page 175*

◆ **Azidothymidine** *see* Zidovudine *on page 1890*

◆ **Azidothymidine, Abacavir, and Lamivudine** *see* Abacavir, Lamivudine, and Zidovudine *on page 32*

◆ **Azilect®** *see* Rasagiline *on page 1559*

Azithromycin (Systemic) (az ith roe MYE sin)

U.S. Brand Names Zithromax®; Zithromax® TRI-PAK™; Zithromax® Z-PAK®; Zmax®

Index Terms Azithromycin Dihydrate; Azithromycin Hydrogencitrate; Azithromycin Monohydrate; Z-Pak; Zithromax TRI-PAK™; Zithromax Z-PAK®

Generic Availability (U.S.) Yes: Excludes extended release microspheres

Pharmacologic Category Antibiotic, Macrolide

Medication Safety Issues

Sound-alike/look-alike issues:

Azithromycin may be confused with azathioprine, erythromycin

Zithromax® may be confused with Fosamax®, Zinacef®, Zovirax®

Pregnancy Risk Factor B

Lactation Enters breast milk/use caution

Use Oral, I.V.: Treatment of acute otitis media due to *H. influenzae, M. catarrhalis*, or *S. pneumoniae*; pharyngitis/tonsillitis due to *S. pyogenes*; treatment of mild-to-moderate upper and lower respiratory tract infections, infections of the skin and skin structure, community-acquired pneumonia, pelvic inflammatory disease (PID), sexually-transmitted diseases (urethritis/cervicitis), pharyngitis/tonsillitis, and genital ulcer disease (chancroid) due to susceptible strains of *Chlamydophila pneumoniae, C. trachomatis, M. catarrhalis, H. influenzae, S. aureus, S. pneumoniae, Mycoplasma genitalium, Mycoplasma pneumoniae*, and *C. psittaci*; acute bacterial exacerbations of chronic obstructive pulmonary disease (COPD) due to *H. influenzae, M. catarrhalis*, or *S. pneumoniae*; acute bacterial sinusitis

Unlabeled/Investigational Use Prevention of (or to delay onset of) or treatment of MAC in patients with advanced HIV infection; prophylaxis of infective endocarditis in patients who are allergic to penicillin and undergoing surgical or dental procedures; pertussis

Mechanism of Action/Effect Inhibits RNA-dependent protein synthesis at the chain elongation step; binds to the 50S ribosomal subunit resulting in blockage of transpeptidation

Contraindications Hypersensitivity to azithromycin, other macrolide (eg, azalide or ketolide) antibiotics, or any component of the formulation

Warnings/Precautions Use with caution in patients with pre-existing liver disease; hepatic impairment, including hepatocellular and/or cholestatic hepatitis, with or without jaundice, has been observed. Discontinue if symptoms of malaise, nausea, vomiting, abdominal colic, and fever. Allergic reactions have been reported (rare); reappearance of allergic reaction may occur without further azithromycin exposure. May mask or delay symptoms of incubating gonorrhea or syphilis, so appropriate culture and susceptibility tests should be performed prior to initiating azithromycin. Prolonged use may result in fungal or bacterial superinfection, including *C. difficile*-associated diarrhea (CDAD) and pseudomembranous colitis; CDAD has been observed >2 months postantibiotic treatment. Use caution with renal dysfunction. Prolongation of the QT_c interval has been reported with macrolide antibiotics; use caution in patients at risk of prolonged cardiac repolarization. Use with caution in patients with myasthenia gravis. Safety and efficacy of systemically-administered azithromycin (oral, intravenous) have not been established in children <6 months of age with acute otitis media, acute bacterial sinusitis, or community-acquired pneumonia, or in children <2 years of age with pharyngitis/tonsillitis.

Oral suspensions (immediate release and extended release) are not interchangeable.

Drug Interactions

Metabolism/Transport Effects Substrate of CYP3A4 (minor); **Inhibits** CYP3A4 (weak)

Avoid Concomitant Use

Avoid concomitant use of Azithromycin (Systemic) with any of the following: Artemether; BCG; Dronedarone; Lumefantrine; Nilotinib; Pimozide; QuiNINE; Tetrabenazine; Thioridazine; Ziprasidone

Decreased Effect

Azithromycin (Systemic) may decrease the levels/effects of: BCG; Typhoid Vaccine

Increased Effect/Toxicity

Azithromycin (Systemic) may increase the levels/effects of: Amiodarone; Cardiac Glycosides; CycloSPORINE; CycloSPORINE (Systemic); Dronedarone; Pimozide; QTc-Prolonging Agents; QuiNINE; Tacrolimus; Tacrolimus (Systemic); Tacrolimus (Topical); Tetrabenazine; Thioridazine; Vitamin K Antagonists; Ziprasidone

The levels/effects of Azithromycin (Systemic) may be increased by: Alfuzosin; Artemether; Chloroquine; Ciprofloxacin; Ciprofloxacin (Systemic); Conivaptan; Gadobutrol; Lumefantrine; Nelfinavir; Nilotinib; QuiNINE

Nutritional/Ethanol Interactions Food: Rate and extent of GI absorption may be altered depending upon the formulation. Azithromycin suspension, not tablet form, has significantly increased absorption (46%) with food.

Adverse Reactions

>10%: Gastrointestinal: Diarrhea (4% to 9%; high single-dose regimens 12% to 14%), nausea (≤7%; high single-dose regimens 18%)

2% to 10%:

Dermatologic: Pruritus, rash

Gastrointestinal: Abdominal pain, anorexia, cramping, vomiting (especially with high single-dose regimens)

Genitourinary: Vaginitis

Local: (with I.V. administration): Injection site pain, inflammation

Pharmacodynamics/Kinetics

Absorption Oral: Rapid

Bioavailability Oral: 38%, decreased by 17% with extended release suspension; variable effect with food (increased with immediate or delayed release oral suspension, unchanged with tablet)

Time to Peak Oral: Serum: Immediate release: 2-3 hours; Extended release: 5 hours

Protein Binding Concentration dependent: Oral, I.V.: 7% to 51%

Half-Life Elimination Terminal: Oral, I.V.: Immediate release: 68-72 hours; Extended release: 59 hours

Metabolism Hepatic

Excretion Oral, I.V.: Biliary (major route); urine (6%)

Available Dosage Forms

Injection, powder for reconstitution: 500 mg

Zithromax®: 500 mg

Microspheres for suspension, extended release, oral:

Zmax®: 2 g/bottle (60 mL)

Powder for suspension, oral: 100 mg/5 mL (15 mL); 200 mg/5 mL (15 mL, 22.5 mL, 30 mL); 1 g/packet (3s, 10s)

Zithromax®: 100 mg/5 mL (15 mL); 200 mg/5 mL (15 mL, 22.5 mL, 30 mL); 1 g/packet (3s, 10s)

Tablet, oral: 250 mg, 500 mg, 600 mg

Zithromax®: 250 mg, 500 mg, 600 mg

Zithromax® TRI-PAK™: 500 mg

Zithromax® Z-PAK®: 250 mg

Dosing

Adult & Geriatric Note: Extended release suspension (Zmax®) is not interchangeable with immediate release formulations. Use should be limited to approved indications. All doses are expressed as immediate release azithromycin unless otherwise specified.

Bacterial sinusitis: Oral: 500 mg/day for a total of 3 days

Extended release suspension (Zmax®): 2 g as a single dose

Cat scratch disease (unlabeled use): Oral: >45.5 kg: 500 mg as a single dose, then 250 mg once daily for 4 days

Chancroid due to *H. ducreyi:* Oral: 1 g as a single dose (CDC, 2010)

Community-acquired pneumonia:

Oral: Extended release suspension (Zmax®): 2 g as a single dose

I.V.: 500 mg as a single dose for at least 2 days, follow I.V. therapy by the oral route with a single daily dose of 500 mg to complete a 7- to 10-day course of therapy.

Disseminated *M. avium* complex disease in patient with advanced HIV infection (unlabeled use): Oral:

Prophylaxis: 1200 mg once weekly (may be combined with rifabutin)

Treatment: 600 mg daily in combination with ethambutol 15 mg/kg

Gonococcal infection, uncomplicated (cervix, pharynx, rectum, urethra): Oral: 1 g as a single dose (in combination with a cephalosporin) (CDC, 2010)

Note: Monotherapy with azithromycin (1 g and 2 g) have been associated with resistance and/or treatment failure; use in combination with a cephalosporin (CDC, 2010). However, a single 2 g azithromycin dose is still an FDA-approved dose for gonococcal urethritis and cervicitis and also may be appropriate for treatment of a gonococcal infection in pregnant women who cannot tolerate a cephalosporin (CDC, 2010).

Granuloma inguinale (donovanosis): Oral: 1 g once a week for at least 3 weeks (and until lesions have healed) (CDC, 2010)

Mild-to-moderate respiratory tract, skin, and soft tissue infections: Oral: 500 mg in a single loading dose on day 1 followed by 250 mg/day as a single dose on days 2-5

Alternative regimen: Bacterial exacerbation of COPD: 500 mg/day for a total of 3 days

Pelvic inflammatory disease (PID): I.V.: 500 mg as a single dose for 1-2 days, follow I.V. therapy by the oral route with a single daily dose of 250 mg to complete a 7-day course of therapy.

Pertussis (CDC, 2005): Oral: 500 mg on day 1 followed by 250 mg/day on days 2-5 (maximum: 500 mg/day)

Prophylaxis against infective endocarditis (unlabeled use): Oral: 500 mg 30-60 minutes prior to the procedure. **Note:** American Heart Association (AHA) guidelines now recommend prophylaxis only in patients undergoing invasive procedures and in whom underlying cardiac conditions may predispose to a higher risk of adverse outcomes should infection occur. As of April 2007, routine prophylaxis for GI/GU procedures is no longer recommended by the AHA.

Prophylaxis against sexually-transmitted diseases following sexual assault: Oral: 1 g as a single dose (in combination with a cephalosporin and metronidazole) (CDC, 2010)

Urethritis/cervicitis: Oral: *Due to C. trachomatis or M. genitalium*: 1 g as a single dose

Pediatric Note: Extended release suspension (Zmax®) is not interchangeable with immediate release formulations. Use should be limited to approved indications. All doses are expressed as immediate release azithromycin unless otherwise specified.

Note: Adolescents ≥16 years: Refer to adult dosing.

Bacterial sinusitis: Children ≥6 months: Oral: 10 mg/kg once daily for 3 days (maximum: 500 mg/day)

Cat scratch disease (unlabeled use): Oral: <45.5 kg: 10 mg/kg as a single dose, then 5 mg/kg once daily for 4 days

Community-acquired pneumonia: Children ≥6 months: Oral: 10 mg/kg on day 1 (maximum: 500 mg/day) followed by 5 mg/kg/day once daily on days 2-5 (maximum: 250 mg/day)

Extended release suspension (Zmax®):

<75 lbs (34 kg): 60 mg/kg as a single dose; dose in mL is equal to the weight in lbs for patients <75 lbs (34 kg)

≥75 lbs (34 kg): Refer to adult dosing.

Disseminated *M. avium* (unlabeled use; CDC, 2009): Oral:

Treatment: 10-12 mg/kg/day (maximum: 500 mg)

Primary prophylaxis: 20 mg/kg (maximum: 1200 mg) once weekly (preferred) or alternatively, 5 mg/kg/day once daily (maximum: 250 mg/day)

Secondary prophylaxis: 5 mg/kg/day once daily (maximum: 250 mg/day) in combination with ethambutol, with or without rifabutin

Prophylaxis against infective endocarditis (unlabeled use): Oral: 15 mg/kg 30-60 minutes before procedure. **Note:** American Heart Association (AHA) guidelines now recommend prophylaxis only in patients undergoing invasive procedures and in whom underlying cardiac conditions may predispose to a higher risk of adverse outcomes should infection occur. As of April 2007, routine prophylaxis for GI/GU procedures is no longer recommended by the AHA.

Otitis media: Children ≥6 months: Oral:

1-day regimen: 30 mg/kg as a single dose (maximum dose: 1500 mg)

3-day regimen: 10 mg/kg once daily for 3 days (maximum: 500 mg/day)

5-day regimen: 10 mg/kg on day 1 (maximum: 500 mg/day) followed by 5 mg/kg/day once daily on days 2-5 (maximum: 250 mg/day)

Pharyngitis, tonsillitis: Children ≥2 years: Oral: 12 mg/kg/day once daily for 5 days (maximum: 500 mg/day)

Pertussis (CDC, 2005):

Children <6 months: 10 mg/kg/day for 5 day

Children ≥6 months: 10 mg/kg on day 1 (maximum: 500 mg/day) followed by 5 mg/kg/day once daily on days 2-5 (maximum: 250 mg/day)

Uncomplicated chlamydial urethritis or cervicitis (unlabeled use): Children ≥45 kg: 1 g as a single dose (CDC, 2010)

Renal Impairment Use caution in patients with GFR <10 mL/minute

Hepatic Impairment Use with caution due to potential for hepatotoxicity (rare). Specific guidelines for dosing in hepatic impairment have not been established.

Administration

Oral Immediate release suspension and tablet may be taken without regard to food; extended release suspension should be taken on an empty stomach (at least 1 hour before or 2 hours following a meal), within 12 hours of reconstitution.

I.V. Other medications should not be infused simultaneously through the same I.V. line.

Stability

Reconstitution Injection (Zithromax®): Prepare initiation solution by adding 4.8 mL of sterile water for injection to the 500 mg vial (resulting concentration: 100 mg/mL). Use of a standard syringe is recommended due to the vacuum in the vial (which may draw additional solution through an automated syringe).

The initial solution should be further diluted to a concentration of 1 mg/mL (500 mL) to 2 mg/mL (250 mL) in 0.9% sodium chloride, 5% dextrose in water, or lactated Ringer's. The diluted solution is stable for 24 hours at or below room temperature (30°C or 86°F) and for 7 days if stored under refrigeration (5°C or 41°F).

Storage

Injection (Zithromax®): Store intact vials of injection at room temperature. Reconstituted solution is stable for 24 hours when stored below 30°C (86°F).

Suspension, immediate release (Zithromax®): Store dry powder below 30°C (86°F). Following reconstitution, store at 5°C to 30°C (41°F to 86°F).

Suspension, extended release (Zmax®): Store dry powder ≤30°C (86°F). Following reconstitution, store at 25°C (77°F); excursions permitted to 15°C to 30°C (59°F to 86°F); do not refrigerate or freeze. Should be consumed within 12 hours following reconstitution.

Tablet (Zithromax®): Store between 15°C to 30°C (59°F to 86°F).

Monitoring and Teaching Issues

Laboratory Monitoring Liver function, CBC with differential. Perform culture and sensitivity testing prior to initiating therapy.

Physical Assessment Assess results of culture and sensitivity tests and patient's allergy history prior to beginning therapy. Evaluate results of LFTs and CBC with diff. Instruct patients being treated for STDs about preventing transmission.

Patient Education If administered by infusion, report immediately any redness, swelling, or pain at infusion site. Oral: Take extended release suspension 1 hour before or 2 hours after meals; immediate release suspension and tablets may be taken with or without food; tablet form may be taken with meals to decrease GI effects. Maintain adequate hydration, unless instructed to restrict fluid intake. If taken to treat a sexually-transmitted disease, follow advice of prescriber related to sexual intercourse and preventing transmission. May cause transient abdominal distress, diarrhea, and headache. Report signs of additional infections (eg, sores in mouth or vagina, vaginal discharge, unresolved fever, severe vomiting, or loose or foul-smelling stools).

Dietary Considerations

Some products may contain sodium and/or sucrose.

Oral suspension, immediate release, may be administered with or without food.

Oral suspension, extended release, should be taken on an empty stomach (at least 1 hour before or 2 hours following a meal).

Tablet may be administered with food to decrease GI effects.

Geriatric Considerations Dosage adjustment does not appear to be necessary in the elderly. Considered to be one of the drugs of choice in the outpatient treatment of community-acquired pneumonia in elderly.

Breast-Feeding Considerations Azithromycin is excreted in low amounts into breast milk. The manufacturer recommends that caution be exercised when administering azithromycin to breast-feeding women. Nondose-related effects could include modification of bowel flora.

Pregnancy Considerations Adverse events were not observed in animal studies; therefore, azithromycin is classified as pregnancy category B. Azithromycin crosses the placenta. Fetal malformations have not been observed following maternal use of azithromycin. The maternal serum half-life of azithromycin is unchanged in early pregnancy and decreased at term; however, high concentrations of azithromycin are sustained in the myometrium and adipose tissue. Azithromycin is recommended for the treatment of several infections, including chlamydia and *Mycobacterium avium* complex (MAC) in pregnant patients.

Additional Information Zithromax® tablets and immediate release suspension may be interchanged (eg, two Zithromax® 250 mg tablets may be substituted for one Zithromax® 500 mg tablet or the tablets may be substituted with the immediate release suspension); however, the extended release suspension (Zmax®) is not bioequivalent with Zithromax® and therefore should not be interchanged.

Related Information

Antimicrobial Drugs of Choice *on page 2008*
Community-Acquired Pneumonia in Adults *on page 2021*
Compatibility of Drugs *on page 1994*
I.V. to Oral Conversion *on page 1956*

- ◆ **Azithromycin Dihydrate** *see* Azithromycin (Systemic) *on page 181*
- ◆ **Azithromycin Hydrogencitrate** *see* Azithromycin (Systemic) *on page 181*
- ◆ **Azithromycin Monohydrate** *see* Azithromycin (Systemic) *on page 181*
- ◆ **Azo-Gesic™ [OTC]** *see* Phenazopyridine *on page 1446*
- ◆ **Azopt®** *see* Brinzolamide *on page 230*
- ◆ **Azor™** *see* Amlodipine and Olmesartan *on page 108*
- ◆ **AZO Standard® [OTC]** *see* Phenazopyridine *on page 1446*
- ◆ **AZO Standard® Maximum Strength [OTC]** *see* Phenazopyridine *on page 1446*
- ◆ **AZT + 3TC (error-prone abbreviation)** *see* Zidovudine and Lamivudine *on page 1894*
- ◆ **AZT, Abacavir, and Lamivudine** *see* Abacavir, Lamivudine, and Zidovudine *on page 32*
- ◆ **AZT (error-prone abbreviation)** *see* Zidovudine *on page 1890*
- ◆ **Azthreonam** *see* Aztreonam *on page 185*

Aztreonam (AZ tree oh nam)

U.S. Brand Names Azactam®; Cayston®

Index Terms Azthreonam

Generic Availability (U.S.) Yes: Injection (powder for reconstitution)

Pharmacologic Category Antibiotic, Miscellaneous

Medication Safety Issues

Sound-alike/look-alike issues:

Aztreonam may be confused with azidothymidine

Prescribing and Access Restrictions Cayston® (aztreonam inhalation solution) is only available through a select group of specialty pharmacies and cannot be obtained through a retail pharmacy. Because Cayston® may only be used with the Altera® Nebulizer System, it can only be obtained from the following specialty pharmacies: Cystic Fibrosis Services, Inc; IV Solutions; Foundation Care; and Pharmaceutical Specialties, Inc. This network of specialty pharmacies ensures proper access to both the drug and device. To obtain the medication and proper nebulizer, contact the Cayston Access Program at 1-877-7CAYSTON (1-877-722-9786) or at www.cayston.com.

Pregnancy Risk Factor B

Lactation Enters breast milk/not recommended (AAP rates "compatible"; AAP 2001 update pending)

Use

Injection: Treatment of patients with urinary tract infections, lower respiratory tract infections, septicemia, skin/skin structure infections, intra-abdominal infections, and gynecological infections caused by susceptible gram-negative bacilli

Inhalation: Improve respiratory symptoms in cystic fibrosis (CF) patients with *Pseudomonas aeruginosa*

Mechanism of Action/Effect Monobactam which is active only against gram-negative bacilli; inhibits bacterial cell wall synthesis during active multiplication, causing cell wall destruction

Contraindications Hypersensitivity to aztreonam or any component of the formulation

Warnings/Precautions Rare cross-allergenicity to penicillins and cephalosporins has been reported. Use caution in renal impairment; dosing adjustment required for the injectable formulation. Prolonged use may result in fungal or bacterial superinfection, including *C. difficile*-associated diarrhea (CDAD) and pseudomembranous colitis; CDAD has been observed >2 months postantibiotic treatment. Patients colonized with *Burkholderia cepacia* have not been studied. Safety and efficacy has not been established in patients with FEV_1 <25% or >75% predicted. To reduce the development of resistant bacteria and maintain efficacy reserve use for CF patients with known *Pseudomonas aeruginosa*. Bronchospasm may occur occur following nebulization; administer a bronchodilator prior to treatment.

Drug Interactions

Avoid Concomitant Use

Avoid concomitant use of Aztreonam with any of the following: BCG

Decreased Effect

Aztreonam may decrease the levels/effects of: BCG; Typhoid Vaccine

Increased Effect/Toxicity There are no known significant interactions involving an increase in effect.

Lab Interactions Urine glucose (Clinitest®), positive Coombs' test

Adverse Reactions

Injection: Adults: 1% to 10%:

Dermatologic: Rash

Gastrointestinal: Diarrhea, nausea, vomiting

Local: Thrombophlebitis, pain at injection site

Inhalation:

>10%:

Central nervous system: Pyrexia (13%; more often observed in children)

Respiratory: Cough (54%), nasal congestion (16%), pharyngeal pain (12%), wheezing (16%)

1% to 10%:

Cardiovascular: Chest discomfort (8%)

Dermatologic: Rash (2%)

Gastrointestinal: Abdominal pain (7%), vomiting (6%)

Respiratory: Bronchospasm (3%)

Pharmacodynamics/Kinetics

Absorption I.M.: Well absorbed; I.M. and I.V. doses produce comparable serum concentrations; Inhalation: Low systemic absorption

Time to Peak I.M., I.V. push: Within 60 minutes; I.V. infusion: 1.5 hours

Protein Binding 56%

Half-Life Elimination Injection:

Children 2 months to 12 years: 1.7 hours

Adults: Normal renal function: 1.7-2.9 hours

End-stage renal disease: 6-8 hours

Metabolism Injection: Hepatic (minor %)

Excretion Injection: Urine (60% to 70% as unchanged drug); feces (~13% to 15%)

Available Dosage Forms

Infusion, premixed iso-osmotic solution:

Azactam®: 1 g (50 mL); 2 g (50 mL)

Injection, powder for reconstitution: 1 g, 2 g

Azactam®: 1 g, 2 g

Powder for reconstitution, for oral inhalation [preservative free]:

Cayston®: 75 mg

Dosing

Adult & Geriatric

Urinary tract infection: I.M., I.V.: 500 mg to 1 g every 8-12 hours

Moderately severe systemic infections:

I.M.: 1 g every 8-12 hours

I.V.: 1-2 g every 8-12 hours

Severe systemic or life-threatening infections (especially caused by *Pseudomonas aeruginosa*): I.V.: 2 g every 6-8 hours; maximum: 8 g/day

Meningitis (gram-negative): I.V.: 2 g every 6-8 hours

***Pseudomonas aeruginosa* infection in cystic fibrosis:** Inhalation (nebulizer): 75 mg 3 times daily (at least 4 hours apart) for 28 days. Do not repeat for 28 days after completion.

Pediatric

Susceptible infections: I.M., I.V.: Children >1 month:

Mild-to-moderate infections: 30 mg/kg every 8 hours

Moderate-to-severe infections: 30 mg/kg every 6-8 hours; maximum: 120 mg/kg/day (8 g/day)

Infection in children with cystic fibrosis: I.V.: Children >1 month: 50 mg/kg/dose every 6-8 hours (ie, up to 200 mg/kg/day); maximum: 8 g/day

***Pseudomonas aeruginosa* infection in cystic fibrosis:** Inhalation (nebulizer): Children ≥7 years: 75 mg 3 times daily (at least 4 hours apart) for 28 days. Do not repeat for 28 days after completion.

Renal Impairment

Oral inhalation: Dosage adjustment not required for mild, moderate or severe renal impairment.

I.M., I.V.: Adults: Following initial dose, maintenance doses should be given as follows:

Cl_{cr} 10-30 mL/minute: 50% of usual dose at the usual interval

Cl_{cr} <10 mL/minute: 25% of usual dosage at the usual interval

Hemodialysis: Moderately dialyzable (20% to 50%); Loading dose of 500 mg, 1 g, or 2 g, followed by 25% of initial dose at usual interval; for serious/life-threatening infections, administer 1/8 of initial dose after each hemodialysis session (given in addition to the maintenance doses)

Continuous ambulatory peritoneal dialysis (CAPD): Administer as for Cl_{cr} <10 mL/minute

Continuous renal replacement therapy (CRRT): Drug clearance is highly dependent on the method of renal replacement, filter type, and flow rate. Appropriate dosing requires close monitoring of pharmacologic response, signs of adverse reactions due to drug accumulation, as well as drug levels in relation to target trough (if appropriate). The following are general recommendations only (based on dialysate flow/ultrafiltration rates of 1 L/hour) and should not supersede clinical judgment:

CVVH: 1-2 g every 12 hours

CVVHD/CVVHDF: 2 g every 12 hours

Administration

I.M. Administer by deep injection into large muscle mass, such as upper outer quadrant of gluteus maximus or the lateral part of the thigh. Doses >1 g should be administered I.V.

I.V. I.V. route is preferred for doses >1 g or in patients with severe life-threatening infections. Administer by slow I.V. push over 3-5 minutes or by intermittent infusion over 20-60 minutes.

Inhalation Administer using only an Altera® nebulizer system; **administer alone; do not mix with other nebulizer medications**. Administer a bronchodilator before administration of aztreonam (short-acting: 15 minutes to 4 hours before; long-acting: 30 minutes to 12 hours before). For patients on multiple inhaled therapies, administer bronchodilator first, then mucolytic, and lastly, aztreonam.

To administer Cayston®, pour reconstituted solution into the handset of the nebulizer system, turn unit on. Place the mouthpiece in the patient's mouth and encourage to breath normally through the mouth. Administration time is usually 2-3 minutes. Administer doses ≥4 hours apart.

Stability

Reconstitution

Inhalation: Reconstitute immediately prior to use. Squeeze diluent into opened glass vial. Replace rubber stopper and gently swirl vial until contents have completely dissolved.

I.M.: Reconstitute with at least 3 mL SWFI, sterile bacteriostatic water for injection, NS, or bacteriostatic sodium chloride.

I.V.:

Bolus injection: Reconstitute with 6-10 mL SWFI.

Infusion: Reconstitute to a final concentration ≤2%; the final concentration should not exceed 20 mg/mL.

Storage

Inhalation: Prior to reconstitution, store at 2°C to 8°C (36°F to 46°F). Once removed from refrigeration, aztreonam and the diluent may be stored at room temperature (up to 25°C [77°F]) for ≤28 days. Protect from light. Use immediately after reconstitution.

Injection: Prior to reconstitution, store at room temperature; avoid excessive heat. Reconstituted solutions are colorless to light yellow straw and may turn pink upon standing without affecting potency. Use reconstituted solutions and I.V. solutions (in NS and D_5W) within 48 hours if kept at room temperature (25°C) or 7 days under refrigeration (4°C).

Infusion: Solution for infusion may be frozen at less than -2°C (less than -4°F) for up to 3 months. Thawed solution should be used within 24 hours if thawed at room temperature or within 72 hours if thawed under refrigeration. **Do not refreeze.**

Monitoring and Teaching Issues

Laboratory Monitoring Obtain specimens for culture and sensitivity before the first dose.

Physical Assessment Assess results of culture and sensitivity tests and patient's allergy history before initiating therapy. I.V.: Infusion site should be monitored closely. Patient should be monitored closely during first dose for anaphylaxis. Bronchospasm may occur following inhalation administration; administer a bronchodilator prior to treatment.

Patient Education Report immediately any burning, pain, swelling, or redness at infusion or injection site; swelling of mouth or tongue; or chest pain or acute onset of difficulty breathing. May cause nausea or GI distress. Report any respiratory difficulty, coughing, wheezing, persistent diarrhea or vomiting, pain at injection site, unresolved fever, unhealed or new sores in mouth or vagina, or vaginal discharge.

Geriatric Considerations Injection: Adjust dose relative to renal function.

Breast-Feeding Considerations Very small amounts of aztreonam are excreted in breast milk. The poor oral absorption of aztreonam (<1%) may limit adverse effects to the infant. Nondose-related effects could include modification of bowel flora. Maternal use of aztreonam inhalation is not likely to pose a risk to breast-feeding infants.

Pregnancy Considerations Adverse events have not been observed in animal reproduction studies; therefore, the manufacturer classifies aztreonam as pregnancy category B. Aztreonam crosses the placenta and enters cord blood during middle and late pregnancy. Distribution to the fetus is minimal in early pregnancy. The amount of aztreonam available systemically following inhalation is significantly less in comparison to doses given by injection.

Additional Information Although marketed as an agent similar to aminoglycosides, aztreonam is a monobactam antimicrobial with almost pure gram-negative aerobic activity. It cannot be used for gram-positive infections.

Related Information

Antimicrobial Drugs of Choice *on page 2008*

Community-Acquired Pneumonia in Adults *on page 2021*

◆ **Azulfidine®** *see* Sulfasalazine *on page 1688*

◆ **Azulfidine EN-tabs®** *see* Sulfasalazine *on page 1688*

◆ **Azurette™** *see* Ethinyl Estradiol and Desogestrel *on page 695*

◆ **B6** *see* Pyridoxine *on page 1532*

◆ **B1939** *see* Eribulin *on page 652*

◆ **B2036-PEG** *see* Pegvisomant *on page 1428*

◆ **B 9273** *see* Alefacept *on page 65*

◆ **Baby Aspirin** *see* Aspirin *on page 155*

Baclofen (BAK loe fen)

U.S. Brand Names Gablofen®; Lioresal®

Generic Availability (U.S.) Yes: Tablets

Pharmacologic Category Skeletal Muscle Relaxant

Medication Safety Issues

Sound-alike/look-alike issues:

Baclofen may be confused with Bactroban®

Lioresal® may be confused with lisinopril, Lotensin®

High alert medication: The Institute for Safe Medication Practices (ISMP) includes this medication (intrathecal administration) among its list of drugs which have a heightened risk of causing significant patient harm when used in error.

Pregnancy Risk Factor C

Lactation Enters breast milk (small amounts)/compatible

Use Treatment of reversible spasticity associated with multiple sclerosis or spinal cord lesions

Orphan drug: Intrathecal: Treatment of intractable spasticity caused by spinal cord injury, multiple sclerosis, and other spinal disease (spinal ischemia or tumor, transverse myelitis, cervical spondylosis, degenerative myelopathy)

Unlabeled/Investigational Use Intractable hiccups, intractable pain relief, bladder spasticity, trigeminal neuralgia, cerebral palsy, short-term treatment of spasticity in children with cerebral palsy, Huntington's chorea

Mechanism of Action/Effect Inhibits the transmission of both monosynaptic and polysynaptic reflexes at the spinal cord level, possibly by hyperpolarization of primary afferent fiber terminals, with resultant relief of muscle spasticity

Contraindications Hypersensitivity to baclofen or any component of the formulation

Warnings/Precautions Use with caution in patients with seizure disorder or impaired renal function. **[U.S. Boxed Warning]: Avoid abrupt withdrawal of the drug; abrupt withdrawal of intrathecal baclofen has resulted in severe sequelae (hyperpyrexia, obtundation, rebound/exaggerated spasticity, muscle rigidity, and rhabdomyolysis), leading to organ failure and some fatalities.** Risk may be higher in patients with injuries at T-6 or above, history of baclofen withdrawal, or limited ability to communicate. May cause CNS depression, which may impair physical or mental abilities; patients must be cautioned about performing tasks which require mental alertness (eg, operating machinery or driving). Elderly are more sensitive to the effects of baclofen and are more likely to experience adverse CNS effects at higher doses.

Cases (most from pharmacy compounded preparations) of intrathecal mass formation at the implanted catheter tip have been reported; may lead to loss of clinical response, pain or new/worsening neurological effects. Neurosurgical evaluation and/or an appropriate imaging study should be considered if a mass is suspected.

Drug Interactions

Avoid Concomitant Use There are no known interactions where it is recommended to avoid concomitant use.

Decreased Effect There are no known significant interactions involving a decrease in effect.

Increased Effect/Toxicity

Baclofen may increase the levels/effects of: Alcohol (Ethyl); CNS Depressants; Methotrimeprazine

The levels/effects of Baclofen may be increased by: Droperidol; Methotrimeprazine

Nutritional/Ethanol Interactions

Ethanol: Avoid ethanol (may increase CNS depression).

Herb/Nutraceutical: Avoid valerian, St John's wort, kava kava, gotu kola.

Lab Interactions Increased alkaline phosphatase, AST, glucose, ammonia (B); decreased bilirubin (S)

Adverse Reactions

>10%:

Central nervous system: Drowsiness, vertigo, psychiatric disturbances, insomnia, slurred speech, ataxia, hypotonia

Neuromuscular & skeletal: Weakness

1% to 10%:

Cardiovascular: Hypotension

Central nervous system: Fatigue, confusion, headache

Dermatologic: Rash

Gastrointestinal: Nausea, constipation

Genitourinary: Polyuria

Pharmacodynamics/Kinetics

Onset of Action 3-4 days; Peak effect: 5-10 days

Absorption Oral: Rapid; dose dependent

Time to Peak Serum: Oral: Within 2-3 hours

Protein Binding 30%

Half-Life Elimination 3.5 hours

Metabolism Hepatic (15% of dose)

Excretion Urine and feces (85% as unchanged drug)

Available Dosage Forms

Injection, solution, intrathecal [preservative free]:

Gablofen®: 50 mcg/mL (1 mL); 500 mcg/mL (20 mL); 2000 mcg/mL (20 mL)

Lioresal®: 50 mcg/mL (1 mL); 500 mcg/mL (20 mL); 2000 mcg/mL (5 mL, 20 mL)

Tablet, oral: 10 mg, 20 mg

Dosing

Adult

Spasticity:

Oral: 5 mg 3 times/day, may increase 5 mg/dose every 3 days to a maximum of 80 mg/day

Intrathecal:

Test dose: 50-100 mcg, doses >50 mcg should be given in 25 mcg increments, separated by 24 hours. A screening dose of 25 mcg may be considered in very small patients. Patients not responding to screening dose of 100 mcg should not be considered for chronic infusion/implanted pump.

Maintenance: After positive response to test dose, a maintenance intrathecal infusion can be administered via an implanted intrathecal pump. Initial dose via pump: Infusion at a 24-hourly rate dosed at twice the test dose. Avoid abrupt discontinuation.

Hiccups (unlabeled use): Oral: 10-20 mg 2-3 times/day

Geriatric Oral (the lowest effective dose is recommended): Initial: 5 mg 2-3 times/day, increasing gradually as needed; if benefits are not seen withdraw the drug slowly.

Pediatric

Spasticity:

Oral (avoid abrupt withdrawal of drug) (unlabeled use): Caution: Pediatric dosing expressed as a daily amount, and NOT in mg/kg. Limited published data in children; the following is a compilation of small prospective studies (Albright, 1996; Milla, 1977; Scheinberg, 2006) and one large retrospective study (Lubsch, 2006):

<2 years: 10-20 mg daily divided every 8 hours; titrate dose every 3 days in increments of 5-15 mg/day to a maximum of 40 mg daily

2-7 years: Initial: 20-30 mg daily divided every 8 hours; titrate dose every 3 days in increments of 5-15 mg/day to a maximum of 60 mg daily

≥8 years: 30-40 mg daily divided every 8 hours; titrate dose every 3 days in increments of 5-15 mg/day to a maximum of 120 mg daily

Note: Baclofen dose may need to be increased over time. One retrospective analysis (Lubsch, 2006) suggested that increased doses were needed as the time increased from spasticity onset, as age increased, and as the number of concomitant antispasticity medications increased. A small number of patients required daily doses exceeding 200 mg.

Intrathecal: Refer to adult dosing.

Spasticity in cerebral palsy (unlabeled use): Oral: Initial: 5-10 mg/day in 3 divided doses (Delgado, 2010)

Renal Impairment May be necessary to reduce dosage; no specific guidelines have been established

Hemodialysis: Poor water solubility allows for accumulation during chronic hemodialysis. Low-dose therapy is recommended. There have been several case reports of accumulation of baclofen resulting in toxicity symptoms (organic brain syndrome, myoclonia, deceleration and steep potentials in EEG) in patients with renal failure who have received normal doses of baclofen.

Administration

Other Intrathecal: For screening dosages, dilute with preservative-free sodium chloride to a final concentration of 50 mcg/mL for bolus injection into the subarachnoid space. For maintenance infusions, concentrations of 500-2000 mcg/mL may be used.

Monitoring and Teaching Issues

Patient Education Abrupt discontinuation may cause hallucinations. Avoid alcohol use. You may experience transient drowsiness, lethargy, or dizziness. Intrathecal use: Keep scheduled pump refill visits; abrupt interruption can cause serious withdrawal symptoms. Report increased spasticity, itching, numbness, unresolved insomnia, painful urination, change in urinary patterns, constipation, high fever, or persistent confusion.

Geriatric Considerations The elderly are more sensitive to the effects of baclofen and are more likely to experience adverse CNS effects at higher doses. Two cases of encephalopathy were reported after inadvertent high doses (50 mg/day and 90 mg/day) were given to elderly patients.

- **Bactrim™** *see* Sulfamethoxazole and Trimethoprim *on page 1686*
- **Bactrim™ DS** *see* Sulfamethoxazole and Trimethoprim *on page 1686*
- **Baking Soda** *see* Sodium Bicarbonate *on page 1658*
- **Balziva™** *see* Ethinyl Estradiol and Norethindrone *on page 701*
- **Band-Aid® Hurt Free™ Antiseptic Wash [OTC]** *see* Lidocaine (Topical) *on page 1107*
- **Banophen™ [OTC]** *see* DiphenhydrAMINE (Systemic) *on page 543*
- **Banophen™ Anti-Itch [OTC]** *see* DiphenhydrAMINE (Topical) *on page 546*
- **Banzel®** *see* Rufinamide *on page 1617*
- **Baridium [OTC]** *see* Phenazopyridine *on page 1446*

Basiliximab (ba si LIK si mab)

U.S. Brand Names Simulect®

Generic Availability (U.S.) No

Pharmacologic Category Immunosuppressant Agent; Monoclonal Antibody

Pregnancy Risk Factor B

Lactation Excretion in breast milk unknown/not recommended

Use Prophylaxis of acute organ rejection in renal transplantation (in combination with cyclosporine and corticosteroids)

Unlabeled/Investigational Use Treatment of refractory acute graft-versus-host disease (GVHD); prevention of liver or cardiac transplant rejection

Mechanism of Action/Effect Chimeric (murine/human) immunosuppressant monoclonal antibody which blocks the alpha-chain of the interleukin-2 (IL-2) receptor complex; this receptor is expressed on activated T lymphocytes and is a critical pathway for activating cell-mediated allograft rejection

Contraindications Hypersensitivity to basiliximab or any component of the formulation

Warnings/Precautions To be used as a component of an immunosuppressive regimen which includes cyclosporine and corticosteroids. The incidence of lymphoproliferative disorders and/or opportunistic infections may be increased by immunosuppressive therapy. Severe hypersensitivity reactions, occurring within 24 hours, have been reported. Reactions, including anaphylaxis, have occurred both with the initial exposure and/or following re-exposure after several months. Use caution during re-exposure to a subsequent course of therapy in a patient who has previously received basiliximab; patients in whom concomitant immunosuppression was prematurely discontinued due to abandoned transplantation or early graft loss are at increased risk for developing a severe hypersensitivity reaction upon re-exposure. Discontinue permanently if a severe reaction occurs. Medications for the treatment of hypersensitivity reactions should be available for immediate use. Treatment may result in the development of human antimurine antibodies (HAMA); however, limited evidence suggesting the use of muromonab-CD3 or other murine products is not precluded. **[U.S. Boxed Warning]: Should be administered under the supervision of a physician experienced in immunosuppression therapy and organ transplant management.**

Drug Interactions

Avoid Concomitant Use

Avoid concomitant use of Basiliximab with any of the following: BCG; Belimumab; Natalizumab; Pimecrolimus; Roflumilast; Tacrolimus (Topical); Vaccines (Live)

Decreased Effect

Basiliximab may decrease the levels/effects of: BCG; Sipuleucel-T; Vaccines (Inactivated); Vaccines (Live)

The levels/effects of Basiliximab may be decreased by: Echinacea

Increased Effect/Toxicity

Basiliximab may increase the levels/effects of: Belimumab; Hypoglycemic Agents; Leflunomide; Natalizumab; Vaccines (Live)

The levels/effects of Basiliximab may be increased by: Abciximab; Denosumab; Herbs (Hypoglycemic Properties); Pimecrolimus; Roflumilast; Tacrolimus (Topical); Trastuzumab

Nutritional/Ethanol Interactions Herb/Nutraceutical: Echinacea may diminish the therapeutic effect of basiliximab. Avoid hypoglycemic herbs, including alfalfa, bilberry, bitter melon, burdock, celery, damiana, fenugreek, garcinia, garlic, ginger, ginseng, gymnema, marshmallow, and stinging nettle (may enhance the hypoglycemic effect of basiliximab).

Adverse Reactions Administration of basiliximab did not appear to increase the incidence or severity of adverse effects in clinical trials. Adverse events were reported in 96% of both the placebo and basiliximab groups.

>10%:

Cardiovascular: Hypertension, peripheral edema
Central nervous system: Fever, headache, insomnia, pain
Dermatologic: Acne, wound complications
Endocrine & metabolic: Hypercholesterolemia, hyperglycemia, hyper-/hypokalemia, hyperuricemia, hypophosphatemia
Gastrointestinal: Abdominal pain, constipation, diarrhea, dyspepsia, nausea, vomiting
Genitourinary: Urinary tract infection
Hematologic: Anemia
Neuromuscular & skeletal: Tremor
Respiratory: Dyspnea, infection (upper respiratory)
Miscellaneous: Viral infection

3% to 10%:

Cardiovascular: Abnormal heart sounds, angina, arrhythmia, atrial fibrillation, chest pain, generalized edema, heart failure, hypotension, tachycardia
Central nervous system: Agitation, anxiety, depression, dizziness, fatigue, hypoesthesia, malaise
Dermatologic: Cyst, hypertrichosis, pruritus, rash, skin disorder, skin ulceration
Endocrine & metabolic: Acidosis, dehydration, diabetes mellitus, fluid overload, glucocorticoids increased, hyper-/hypocalcemia, hyperlipemia, hypertriglyceridemia, hypoglycemia, hypomagnesemia, hyponatremia, hypoproteinemia
Gastrointestinal: Abdomen enlarged, esophagitis, flatulence, gastroenteritis, GI hemorrhage, gingival hyperplasia, melena, moniliasis, stomatitis (including ulcerative), weight gain
Genitourinary: Bladder disorder, dysuria, genital edema (male), impotence, ureteral disorder, urinary frequency, urinary retention
Hematologic: Hematoma, hemorrhage, leukopenia, polycythemia, purpura, thrombocytopenia, thrombosis
Neuromuscular & skeletal: Arthralgia, arthropathy, back pain, cramps, fracture, hernia, leg pain, myalgia, neuropathy, paresthesia, rigors, weakness
Ocular: Abnormal vision, cataract, conjunctivitis
Renal: Albuminuria, hematuria, nonprotein nitrogen increased, oliguria, renal function abnormal, renal tubular necrosis
Respiratory: Bronchitis, bronchospasm, cough, pharyngitis, pneumonia, pulmonary edema, sinusitis, rhinitis
Miscellaneous: Accidental trauma, cytomegalovirus (CMV) infection, herpes infection (simplex and zoster), infection, sepsis

Pharmacodynamics/Kinetics

Duration of Action Mean: 36 days (determined by IL-2R alpha saturation)

Half-Life Elimination Children 1-11 years: 9.5 days; Adolescents 12-16 years: 9.1 days; Adults: Mean: 7.2 days

Available Dosage Forms

Injection, powder for reconstitution [preservative free]:
Simulect®: 10 mg, 20 mg

Dosing

Adult & Geriatric Note: Patients previously administered basiliximab should only be re-exposed to a subsequent course of therapy with extreme caution.

Acute renal transplant rejection prophylaxis: I.V.: 20 mg within 2 hours prior to transplant surgery, followed by a second 20 mg dose 4 days after transplantation. The second dose should be withheld if complications occur (including severe hypersensitivity reactions or graft loss).

Acute cardiac transplant rejection prophylaxis (unlabeled use): I.V.: 20 mg on the day of transplant, followed by a second dose 4 days after transplantation (Mehra, 2005); usually given within the first hour postoperatively

Acute liver transplant rejection prophylaxis (unlabeled use): I.V.: 20 mg within 6 hours of organ reperfusion, followed by a second 20 mg dose 4 days after transplantation (Neuhaus, 2002)

Treatment of refractory acute GVHD (unlabeled use): I.V.: 20 mg on days 1 and 4; may repeat for recurrent acute GVHD (Schmidt-Hieber, 2005)

Pediatric Note: Patients previously administered basiliximab should only be re-exposed to a subsequent course of therapy with extreme caution.

Acute renal transplant rejection prophylaxis: I.V.:

Children <35 kg: 10 mg within 2 hours prior to transplant surgery, followed by a second 10 mg dose 4 days after transplantation; the second dose should be withheld if complications occur (including severe hypersensitivity reactions or graft loss)

Children ≥35 kg: Refer to adult dosing

Administration

I.V. For intravenous administration only. Infuse as a bolus or I.V. infusion over 20-30 minutes. (Bolus dosing is associated with nausea, vomiting, and local pain at the injection site.) For the treatment of acute GVHD (unlabeled use), the dose was diluted in 250 mL NS and administered over 30 minutes (Schmidt-Hieber, 2005).

Stability

Reconstitution Reconstitute with preservative-free sterile water for injection (reconstitute 10 mg vial with 2.5 mL, 20 mg vial with 5 mL). Shake gently to dissolve. May further dilute reconstituted solution with 25 mL (10 mg) or 50 mL (20 mg) 0.9% sodium chloride or dextrose 5% in water. When mixing the solution, gently invert the bag to avoid foaming. Do not shake solutions diluted for infusion.

Storage Store intact vials refrigerated at 2°C to 8°C (36°F to 46°F). Should be used immediately after reconstitution; however, if not used immediately, reconstituted solution may be stored at 2°C to 8°C for up to 24 hours or at room temperature for up to 4 hours. Discard the reconstituted solution if not used within 24 hours.

Monitoring and Teaching Issues

Physical Assessment Monitor cardiorespiratory and renal function during infusion and periodically following infusion. Allergic reactions, including anaphylaxis, have occurred both with the initial exposure and/or following re-exposure after several months. Equipment and medications for the treatment of hypersensitivity reactions should be available for immediate use. Be alert to opportunistic infections.

Patient Education This medication, which may help to reduce transplant rejection, can only be given by infusion. You will be monitored and assessed closely during infusion and thereafter. It is important that you report any changes or problems for evaluation. You will be susceptible to infection. You may experience trouble sleeping or headaches. Report any changes in urination; chest pain or palpitations; dizziness; respiratory difficulty; changes in cognition; rash; feelings of pain or numbness in extremities; weight gain; swelling of extremities; severe GI upset, pain, or diarrhea; unusual back or leg pain or muscle tremors; vision changes; or any sign of infection (eg, chills, fever, sore throat).

Breast-Feeding Considerations It is not known whether basiliximab is excreted in human milk. Because many immunoglobulins are secreted in milk and the potential for serious adverse reactions exists, a decision should be made whether to discontinue nursing or discontinue the drug, taking into account the importance of the drug to the mother.

Pregnancy Considerations Teratogenic effects were not observed in animal studies. IL-2 receptors play an important role in the development of the immune system. Use in pregnant women only when benefit exceeds potential risk to the fetus. Women of childbearing potential should use effective contraceptive measures before beginning treatment and for 4 months after completion of therapy with this agent. The National Transplantation Pregnancy Registry (NTPR, Temple University) is a registry for pregnant women taking immunosuppressants following any solid organ transplant. The NTPR encourages reporting of all immunosuppressant exposures during pregnancy in transplant recipients at 877-955-6877.

◆ **BAY 43-9006** *see* Sorafenib *on page 1670*

◆ **Baycadron™** *see* Dexamethasone (Systemic) *on page 499*

◆ **Bayer® Aspirin Extra Strength [OTC]** *see* Aspirin *on page 155*

◆ **Bayer® Aspirin Regimen Adult Low Strength [OTC]** *see* Aspirin *on page 155*

◆ **Bayer® Aspirin Regimen Children's [OTC]** *see* Aspirin *on page 155*

◆ **Bayer® Aspirin Regimen Regular Strength [OTC]** *see* Aspirin *on page 155*

◆ **Bayer® Genuine Aspirin [OTC]** *see* Aspirin *on page 155*

◆ **Bayer® Plus Extra Strength [OTC]** *see* Aspirin *on page 155*

◆ **Bayer® PM [OTC]** *see* Aspirin and Diphenhydramine *on page 159*

◆ **Bayer® Women's Low Dose Aspirin [OTC]** *see* Aspirin *on page 155*
◆ **Baza® Antifungal [OTC]** *see* Miconazole (Topical) *on page 1224*
◆ **BCNU** *see* Carmustine *on page 302*

Beclomethasone (Oral Inhalation) (be kloe METH a sone)

U.S. Brand Names QVAR®

Index Terms Vancenase

Generic Availability (U.S.) No

Pharmacologic Category Corticosteroid, Inhalant (Oral)

Medication Safety Issues

Sound-alike/look-alike issues:

Vanceril® may be confused with Vancenase

Pregnancy Risk Factor C

Lactation Excretion in breast milk unknown/use caution

Use Oral inhalation: Maintenance and prophylactic treatment of asthma; includes those who require corticosteroids and those who may benefit from a dose reduction/elimination of systemically-administered corticosteroids. Not for relief of acute bronchospasm.

Mechanism of Action/Effect Acts at cellular level to prevent or control inflammation

Contraindications Hypersensitivity to beclomethasone or any component of the formulation; status asthmaticus

Warnings/Precautions May cause hypercorticism or suppression of hypothalamic-pituitary-adrenal (HPA) axis, particularly in younger children or in patients receiving high doses for prolonged periods. HPA axis suppression may lead to adrenal crisis. Withdrawal and discontinuation of a corticosteroid should be done slowly and carefully. Particular care is required when patients are transferred from systemic corticosteroids to inhaled products due to possible adrenal insufficiency or withdrawal from steroids, including an increase in allergic symptoms. Patients receiving >20 mg per day of prednisone (or equivalent) may be most susceptible. Fatalities have occurred due to adrenal insufficiency in asthmatic patients during and after transfer from systemic corticosteroids to aerosol steroids; aerosol steroids do **not** provide the systemic steroid needed to treat patients having trauma, surgery, or infections.

Bronchospasm may occur with wheezing after inhalation; if this occurs, stop steroid and treat with a fast-acting bronchodilator. Supplemental steroids (oral or parenteral) may be needed during stress or severe asthma attacks. Not to be used in status asthmaticus or for the relief of acute bronchospasm. Corticosteroid use may cause psychiatric disturbances, including depression, euphoria, insomnia, mood swings, and personality changes. Pre-existing psychiatric conditions may be exacerbated by corticosteroid use. Prolonged use of corticosteroids may also increase the incidence of secondary infection, mask acute infection (including fungal infections), prolong or exacerbate viral infections, or limit response to vaccines. Exposure to chickenpox should be avoided; corticosteroids should not be used to treat ocular herpes simplex. Corticosteroids should not be used for cerebral malaria. Close observation is required in patients with latent tuberculosis and/or TB reactivity; restrict use in active TB (only in conjunction with antituberculosis treatment). Prolonged treatment with corticosteroids has been associated with the development of Kaposi's sarcoma (case reports); if noted, discontinuation of therapy should be considered.

Use with caution in patients with thyroid disease, hepatic impairment, renal impairment, cardiovascular disease, diabetes, glaucoma, cataracts, myasthenia gravis, patients at risk for osteoporosis, patients at risk for seizures, or GI diseases (diverticulitis, peptic ulcer, ulcerative colitis) due to perforation risk. Use caution following acute MI (corticosteroids have been associated with myocardial rupture). Because of the risk of adverse effects, systemic corticosteroids should be used cautiously in the elderly in the smallest possible effective dose for the shortest duration.

Orally-inhaled corticosteroids may cause a reduction in growth velocity in pediatric patients (~1 centimeter per year [range: 0.3-1.8 cm per year] and related to dose and duration of exposure). To minimize the systemic effects of orally-inhaled corticosteroids, each patient should be titrated to the lowest effective dose. Growth should be routinely monitored in pediatric patients. Safety and efficacy have not been established in children <5 years of age. There have been reports of systemic corticosteroid withdrawal symptoms (eg, joint/muscle pain, lassitude, depression) when withdrawing oral inhalation therapy.

Drug Interactions

Avoid Concomitant Use

Avoid concomitant use of Beclomethasone (Oral Inhalation) with any of the following: Aldesleukin; BCG; Natalizumab; Pimecrolimus; Roflumilast; Tacrolimus (Topical)

Decreased Effect

Beclomethasone (Oral Inhalation) may decrease the levels/effects of: Aldesleukin; Antidiabetic Agents; BCG; Corticorelin; Sipuleucel-T; Vaccines (Inactivated)

The levels/effects of Beclomethasone (Oral Inhalation) may be decreased by: Echinacea

Increased Effect/Toxicity

Beclomethasone (Oral Inhalation) may increase the levels/effects of: Amphotericin B; Leflunomide; Loop Diuretics; Natalizumab; Thiazide Diuretics

The levels/effects of Beclomethasone (Oral Inhalation) may be increased by: Denosumab; Pimecrolimus; Roflumilast; Tacrolimus (Topical); Trastuzumab

Adverse Reactions Frequency not defined.

Central nervous system: Agitation, depression, dizziness, dysphonia, headache, lightheadedness, mental disturbances

Dermatologic: Acneiform lesions, angioedema, atrophy, bruising, pruritus, purpura, striae, rash, urticaria

Endocrine & metabolic: Cushingoid features, growth velocity reduction in children and adolescents, HPA function suppression, weight gain

Gastrointestinal: Dry/irritated nose, throat and mouth, hoarseness, localized *Candida* or *Aspergillus* infection, loss of smell, loss of taste, nausea, unpleasant smell, unpleasant taste, vomiting

Ocular: Cataracts, glaucoma, intraocular pressure increased

Respiratory: Cough, paradoxical bronchospasm, pharyngitis, sinusitis, wheezing

Miscellaneous: Anaphylactic/anaphylactoid reactions, death (due to adrenal insufficiency, reported during and after transfer from systemic corticosteroids to aerosol in asthmatic patients), immediate and delayed hypersensitivity reactions

Pharmacodynamics/Kinetics

Onset of Action Therapeutic effect: 1-4 weeks

Absorption Readily; quickly hydrolyzed by pulmonary esterases to active metabolite (beclomethasone-17-monoproprionate [17-BMP]) prior to absorption

Time to Peak Plasma: Oral inhalation: BDP: 0.5 hours; 17-BMP: 0.7 hours

Protein Binding 17-BMP: 94% to 96%

Half-Life Elimination BDP: 0.5 hours; 17-BMP: 3 hours

Metabolism Pro-drug; undergoes rapid conversion to 17-BMP during absorption; followed by additional metabolism via CYP3A4 to other, less active metabolites (beclomethasone-21-monopropionate [21-BMP] and beclomethasone [BOH])

Excretion Feces (60%); urine (<10% to 12%)

Available Dosage Forms

Aerosol, for oral inhalation:

QVAR®: 40 mcg/inhalation (8.7 g); 80 mcg/inhalation (8.7 g)

Dosing

Adult & Geriatric Nasal inhalation and oral inhalation dosage forms are not to be used interchangeably.

Asthma: Inhalation, oral (doses should be titrated to the lowest effective dose once asthma is controlled) (QVAR®):

Patients previously on bronchodilators only: Initial dose 40-80 mcg twice daily; maximum dose 320 mcg twice day

Patients previously on inhaled corticosteroids: Initial dose 40-160 mcg twice daily; maximum dose 320 mcg twice daily

NIH Asthma Guidelines (NIH, 2007): HFA formulation (eg, QVAR®): Administer in divided doses:

"Low" dose: 80-240 mcg/day

"Medium" dose: >240-480 mcg/day

"High" dose: >480 mcg/day

Pediatric Nasal inhalation and oral inhalation dosage forms are not to be used interchangeably.

Asthma: Inhalation, oral (doses should be titrated to the lowest effective dose once asthma is controlled) (QVAR®):

Children 5-11 years: Initial: 40 mcg twice daily; maximum dose: 80 mcg twice daily

Children ≥12 years: Refer to adult dosing

NIH Asthma Guidelines (NIH, 2007): HFA formulation (eg, QVAR®): Administer in divided doses:

Children 5-11 years:

"Low" dose: 80-160 mcg/day

"Medium" dose: >160-320 mcg/day

"High" dose: >320 mcg/day

Children ≥12 years: Refer to adult dosing.

Administration

Inhalation QVAR®: Rinse mouth and throat after use to prevent *Candida* infection. Do not wash or put inhaler in water; mouth piece may be cleaned with a dry tissue or cloth. Prime canister before using.

Stability

Storage Do not store near heat or open flame. Do not puncture canisters. Store at 25°C (77°F); excursions permitted between 15°C to 30°C (59°F to 86°F). Rest QVAR® on concave end of canister with actuator on top.

Monitoring and Teaching Issues

Physical Assessment When changing from systemic steroids to inhalational steroids, taper reduction of systemic medication slowly. Growth should be routinely monitored in pediatric patients.

Patient Education It may take 1-4 weeks for you to realize full effects of treatment. Review use of inhaler with prescriber. Keep oral inhaler clean and unobstructed. Always rinse mouth after use of inhaler to prevent infection. If you are also using an inhaled bronchodilator, wait 10 minutes before using this steroid aerosol. Report skin rash, white plaques in mouth, unresolved headache, or worsening of condition or lack of improvement.

Inhalation: Sit when using. Take deep breaths for 3-5 minutes and clear nasal passages before administration. Hold breath for 5-10 seconds after use and wait 1-3 minutes between inhalations. If also using inhaled bronchodilator, use before beclomethasone. Rinse mouth after use to reduce aftertaste and prevent infection.

Geriatric Considerations Elderly patients may have difficulty with oral metered dose inhalers and may benefit from the use of a spacer or chamber device.

Breast-Feeding Considerations Other corticosteroids have been found in breast milk; however, information for beclomethasone is not available.

Pregnancy Considerations Teratogenic effects were observed in animal studies. No human data on beclomethasone crossing the placenta or effects on the fetus. A decrease in fetal growth has not been observed with inhaled corticosteroid use during pregnancy. Inhaled corticosteroids are recommended for the treatment of asthma (most information available using budesonide) and allergic rhinitis during pregnancy.

Additional Information Effects of inhaled steroids on growth have been observed in the absence of laboratory evidence of HPA axis suppression, suggesting that growth velocity is a more sensitive indicator of systemic corticosteroid exposure in pediatric patients than some commonly used tests of HPA axis function. The long-term effects of this reduction in growth velocity associated with orally-inhaled corticosteroids, including the impact on final adult height, are unknown. The potential for "catch up" growth following discontinuation of treatment with inhaled corticosteroids has not been adequately studied.

Related Information

Asthma *on page 2015*

Belimumab (be LIM yoo mab)

U.S. Brand Names Benlysta®

Pharmacologic Category Monoclonal Antibody

Medication Guide Available Yes

Pregnancy Risk Factor C

Lactation Excretion in breast milk unknown/not recommended

Use Treatment of autoantibody-positive (antinuclear antibody [ANA] and/or anti-double-stranded DNA [anti-ds-DNA]) systemic lupus erythematosus (SLE) in addition to standard therapy

Available Dosage Forms

Injection, powder for reconstitution:

Benlysta®: 120 mg, 400 mg

Dosing

Adult & Geriatric SLE: I.V.: Initial: 10 mg/kg every 2 weeks for 3 doses; Maintenance: 10 mg/kg every 4 weeks

Renal Impairment No dosage adjustment necessary for Cl_{cr} ≥15 mL/minute; has not been studied in Cl_{cr}<15 mL/minute

Hepatic Impairment Has not been studied.

Administration

I.V. Administer intravenously over 1 hour through a dedicated I.V. line. Do not give as an I.V. push or bolus. Discontinue infusion for severe hypersensitivity reaction (eg. anaphylaxis, angioedema). The infusion may be slowed or temporarily interrupted for minor reactions. Consider premedicating for prophylaxis against infusion reactions.

Monitoring and Teaching Issues

Patient Education This medication can only be administered by I.V. infusion. Report immediately any pain or irritation at injection site; chills; rash; difficulty swallowing or breathing; or feelings of tightness in chest. Avoid alcohol. May cause nausea, diarrhea, sore throat, and nasal irritation. Report unusual feelings of fatigue or weakness, signs of infection (eg, cough, runny nose, sore throat, swollen glands, mouth sores, burning on urination, fever, chills).

Belladonna and Opium (bel a DON a & OH pee um)

Index Terms B&O; Opium and Belladonna

Generic Availability (U.S.) Yes

Pharmacologic Category Analgesic Combination (Opioid); Antispasmodic Agent, Urinary

Medication Safety Issues

Sound-alike/look-alike issues:

B&O may be confused with beano®

Beers Criteria medication: This drug may be inappropriate for use in geriatric patients (high severity risk).

Pregnancy Risk Factor C

Lactation Excretion in breast milk unknown/use caution

Use Relief of moderate-to-severe pain associated with ureteral spasms not responsive to nonopioid analgesics and to space intervals between injections of opiates

Controlled Substance C-II

Available Dosage Forms

Suppository: Belladonna extract 16.2 mg and opium 30 mg; belladonna extract 16.2 mg and opium 60 mg

Dosing

Adult & Geriatric Pain: Rectal: 1 suppository 1-2 times/day, up to 4 doses/day

Pediatric Pain: Children >12 years: Refer to adult dosing.

Administration

Other Prior to rectal insertion, the finger and suppository should be moistened. Assist with ambulation.

Monitoring and Teaching Issues

Physical Assessment Monitor for signs of overdose. May cause physical and/or psychological dependence. For inpatients, implement safety measures to prevent falls.

Patient Education Drug may cause physical and/or psychological dependence. While using this medication, do not use alcohol. Maintain adequate hydration, unless instructed to restrict fluid intake. May cause hypotension, dizziness, or drowsiness; dry mouth or throat; constipation (if unresolved, consult prescriber about use of stool softeners); photosensitivity; or decreased perspiration. Report chest pain or palpitations, persistent dizziness, changes in mentation, changes in gait, blurred vision, shortness of breath, or respiratory difficulty.

Related Information

Opium Tincture *on page 1363*

- ◆ **Benadryl-D® Allergy & Sinus [OTC]** *see* Diphenhydramine and Phenylephrine *on page 546*
- ◆ **Benadryl-D® Children's Allergy & Sinus [OTC]** *see* Diphenhydramine and Phenylephrine *on page 546*
- ◆ **Benadryl® Allergy [OTC]** *see* DiphenhydrAMINE (Systemic) *on page 543*
- ◆ **Benadryl® Allergy Quick Dissolve [OTC]** *see* DiphenhydrAMINE (Systemic) *on page 543*
- ◆ **Benadryl® Children's Allergy [OTC]** *see* DiphenhydrAMINE (Systemic) *on page 543*
- ◆ **Benadryl® Children's Allergy FastMelt® [OTC]** *see* DiphenhydrAMINE (Systemic) *on page 543*
- ◆ **Benadryl® Children's Allergy Perfect Measure™ [OTC]** *see* DiphenhydrAMINE (Systemic) *on page 543*
- ◆ **Benadryl® Children's Dye Free Allergy [OTC]** *see* DiphenhydrAMINE (Systemic) *on page 543*
- ◆ **Benadryl® Dye-Free Allergy [OTC]** *see* DiphenhydrAMINE (Systemic) *on page 543*
- ◆ **Benadryl® Extra Strength Itch Stopping [OTC]** *see* DiphenhydrAMINE (Topical) *on page 546*
- ◆ **Benadryl® Itch Relief Extra Strength [OTC]** *see* DiphenhydrAMINE (Topical) *on page 546*
- ◆ **Benadryl® Itch Stopping [OTC]** *see* DiphenhydrAMINE (Topical) *on page 546*
- ◆ **Benadryl® Itch Stopping Extra Strength [OTC]** *see* DiphenhydrAMINE (Topical) *on page 546*

Benazepril (ben AY ze pril)

U.S. Brand Names Lotensin®

Index Terms Benazepril Hydrochloride

Generic Availability (U.S.) Yes

Pharmacologic Category Angiotensin-Converting Enzyme (ACE) Inhibitor

Medication Safety Issues

Sound-alike/look-alike issues:

Benazepril may be confused with Benadryl®

Lotensin® may be confused with Lioresal®, lovastatin

Pregnancy Risk Factor D

Lactation Enters breast milk

Use Treatment of hypertension, either alone or in combination with other antihypertensive agents

Mechanism of Action/Effect Competitive inhibitor of angiotensin-converting enzyme (ACE); prevents conversion of angiotensin I to angiotensin II, a potent vasoconstrictor; results in lower levels of angiotensin II which causes an increase in plasma renin activity and a reduction in aldosterone secretion

Contraindications Hypersensitivity to benazepril or any component of the formulation; patients with a history of angioedema (with or without prior ACE inhibitor therapy)

Warnings/Precautions Anaphylactic reactions may occur rarely with ACE inhibitors. At any time during treatment (especially following first dose) angioedema may occur rarely with ACE inhibitors. It may involve the head and neck (potentially compromising airway) or the intestine (presenting with abdominal pain). African-Americans and patients with idiopathic or hereditary angioedema may be at an increased risk. Prolonged frequent monitoring may be required especially if tongue, glottis, or larynx are involved as they are associated with airway obstruction. Patients with a history of airway surgery may have a higher risk of airway obstruction. Aggressive early and appropriate management is critical. Contraindicated in patients with history of angioedema with or without prior ACE inhibitor therapy. Hypersensitivity reactions may be seen during hemodialysis (eg, CVVHD) with high-flux dialysis membranes (eg, AN69), and rarely, during low density lipoprotein apheresis with dextran sulfate cellulose. Rare cases of anaphylactoid reactions have been reported in patients undergoing sensitization treatment with hymenoptera (bee, wasp) venom while receiving ACE inhibitors.

Symptomatic hypotension with or without syncope can occur with ACE inhibitors (usually with the first several doses); effects are most often observed in volume depleted patients; close monitoring of patient is required especially with initial dosing and dosing increases; blood pressure must be lowered at a rate appropriate for the patient's clinical condition. Initiation of therapy in patients with ischemic heart disease or cerebrovascular disease warrants close observation due to the potential consequences posed by falling blood pressure (eg, MI, stroke).

[U.S. Boxed Warning]: Based on human data, ACEIs can cause injury and death to the developing fetus when used in the second and third trimesters. ACEIs should be discontinued as soon as possible once pregnancy is detected. Use with caution in hypertrophic cardiomyopathy with outflow tract obstruction, severe aortic stenosis, or before, during, or immediately after major surgery.

Hyperkalemia may occur with ACE inhibitors; risk factors include renal dysfunction, diabetes mellitus, concomitant use of potassium-sparing diuretics, potassium supplements and/or potassium containing salts. Use cautiously, if at all, with these agents and monitor potassium closely. Cough may occur with ACE inhibitors. Other causes of cough should be considered (eg, pulmonary congestion in patients with heart failure) and excluded prior to discontinuation. Use with caution in patients with diabetes receiving insulin or oral antidiabetic agents; may be at increased risk for episodes of hypoglycemia.

May be associated with deterioration of renal function and/or increases in serum creatinine, particularly in patients with low renal blood flow (eg, renal artery stenosis, heart failure) whose glomerular filtration rate (GFR) is dependent on efferent arteriolar vasoconstriction by angiotensin II; deterioration may result in oliguria, acute renal failure, and progressive azotemia. Small increases in serum creatinine may occur following initiation; consider discontinuation only in patients with progressive and/or significant deterioration in renal function. Use with caution in patients with unstented unilateral/bilateral renal artery stenosis. When unstented bilateral renal artery stenosis is present, use is generally avoided due to the elevated risk of deterioration in renal function unless possible benefits outweigh risks. Concurrent use of angiotensin receptor blockers may increase the risk of clinically-significant adverse events (eg, renal dysfunction, hyperkalemia).

Rare toxicities associated with ACE inhibitors include cholestatic jaundice (which may progress to fulminant hepatic necrosis), agranulocytosis, neutropenia, or leukopenia with myeloid hypoplasia. Patients with collagen vascular diseases (especially with concomitant renal impairment) or renal impairment alone may be at increased risk for hematologic toxicity; periodically monitor CBC with differential in these patients.

Drug Interactions

Avoid Concomitant Use There are no known interactions where it is recommended to avoid concomitant use.

Decreased Effect

The levels/effects of Benazepril may be decreased by: Antacids; Aprotinin; Herbs (Hypertensive Properties); Methylphenidate; Nonsteroidal Anti-Inflammatory Agents; Salicylates; Yohimbine

Increased Effect/Toxicity

Benazepril may increase the levels/effects of: Allopurinol; Amifostine; Antihypertensives; AzaTHIOprine; CycloSPORINE; CycloSPORINE (Systemic); Ferric Gluconate; Gold Sodium Thiomalate; Hypotensive Agents; Iron Dextran Complex; Lithium; RiTUXimab

The levels/effects of Benazepril may be increased by: Angiotensin II Receptor Blockers; Diazoxide; DPP-IV Inhibitors; Eplerenone; Everolimus; Herbs (Hypotensive Properties); Loop Diuretics; MAO Inhibitors; Pentoxifylline; Phosphodiesterase 5 Inhibitors; Potassium Salts; Potassium-Sparing Diuretics; Prostacyclin Analogues; Sirolimus; Temsirolimus; Thiazide Diuretics; TiZANidine; Tolvaptan; Trimethoprim

Nutritional/Ethanol Interactions Herb/Nutraceutical: Avoid bayberry, blue cohosh, cayenne, ephedra, ginger, ginseng (American), kola, licorice (may worsen hypertension). Avoid black cohosh, California poppy, coleus, golden seal, hawthorn, mistletoe, periwinkle, quinine, shepherd's purse (may have increased antihypertensive effect).

Adverse Reactions

1% to 10%:

- Cardiovascular: Postural dizziness (2%)
- Central nervous system: Headache (6%), dizziness (4%), somnolence (2%)
- Renal: Serum creatinine increased (2%), worsening of renal function may occur in patients with bilateral renal artery stenosis or hypovolemia
- Respiratory: Cough (1% to 10%)

Eosinophilic pneumonitis, anaphylaxis, renal insufficiency, and renal failure have been reported with other ACE inhibitors. In addition, a syndrome including fever, myalgia, arthralgia, interstitial nephritis, vasculitis, rash, eosinophilia, and elevated ESR has been reported to be associated with ACE inhibitors.

Pharmacodynamics/Kinetics

Onset of Action

Reduction in plasma angiotensin-converting enzyme (ACE) activity: Peak effect: 1-2 hours after 2-20 mg dose

Reduction in blood pressure: Peak effect: Single dose: 2-4 hours; Continuous therapy: 2 weeks

Duration of Action Reduction in plasma angiotensin-converting enzyme (ACE) activity: >90% inhibition for 24 hours after 5-20 mg dose

Absorption Rapid (37%); food does not alter significantly; metabolite (benazeprilat) itself unsuitable for oral administration due to poor absorption

Time to Peak Parent drug: 0.5-1 hour

Protein Binding

Benazepril: ~97%

Benazeprilat: ~95%

Half-Life Elimination Benazeprilat: Effective: 10-11 hours; Terminal: Children: 5 hours, Adults: 22 hours

Metabolism Rapidly and extensively hepatic to its active metabolite, benazeprilat, via enzymatic hydrolysis; extensive first-pass effect

Excretion Urine (trace amounts as benazepril; 20% as benazeprilat; 12% as other metabolites)

Clearance: Nonrenal clearance (ie, biliary, metabolic) appears to contribute to the elimination of benazeprilat (11% to 12%), particularly patients with severe renal impairment; hepatic clearance is the main elimination route of unchanged benazepril

Dialysis: ~6% of metabolite removed within 4 hours of dialysis following 10 mg of benazepril administered 2 hours prior to procedure; parent compound not found in dialysate

Available Dosage Forms

Tablet, oral: 5 mg, 10 mg, 20 mg, 40 mg

Lotensin®: 5 mg, 10 mg, 20 mg, 40 mg

Dosing

Adult Hypertension: Oral: Initial: 10 mg/day in patients not receiving a diuretic; 20-80 mg/day as a single dose or 2 divided doses; the need for twice-daily dosing should be assessed by monitoring peak (2-6 hours after dosing) and trough responses.

Note: Patients taking diuretics should have them discontinued 2-3 days prior to starting benazepril. If they cannot be discontinued, then initial dose should be 5 mg; restart after blood pressure is stabilized if needed.

Geriatric Oral: Initial: 5-10 mg/day in single or divided doses; usual range: 20-40 mg/day; adjust for renal function. Also see "Note" in adult dosing.

Pediatric Hypertension: Children ≥6 years: Oral: Initial: 0.2 mg/kg/day (up to 10 mg/day) as monotherapy; dosing range: 0.1-0.6 mg/kg/day (maximum dose: 40 mg/day)

Renal Impairment

Cl_{cr} <30 mL/minute:

Children: Use is not recommended.

Adults: Administer 5 mg/day initially; maximum daily dose: 40 mg.

Hemodialysis: Moderately dialyzable (20% to 50%); administer dose postdialysis or administer 25% to 35% supplemental dose.

Peritoneal dialysis: Supplemental dose is not necessary.

Stability

Storage Store at ≤30°C (86°F). Protect from moisture.

Monitoring and Teaching Issues

Laboratory Monitoring Serum creatinine and potassium; if patient has collagen vascular disease and/or renal impairment, periodically monitor CBC with differential

Physical Assessment Blood pressure should be monitored after first doses and periodically throughout.

Patient Education Take first dose at bedtime. Do not take potassium supplements or salt substitutes containing potassium without consulting prescriber. This drug does not eliminate need for diet or exercise regimen as recommended by prescriber. May cause dizziness, fainting, lightheadedness, postural hypotension, nausea, vomiting, abdominal pain, dry mouth, or transient loss of appetite; report if these side effects persist. Report mouth sores; fever or chills; swelling of extremities, face, mouth, or tongue; or respiratory difficulty or unusual cough.

Geriatric Considerations Due to frequent decreases in glomerular filtration (also Cl_{cr}) with aging, elderly patients may have exaggerated responses to ACE inhibitors; differences in clinical response due to hepatic changes are not observed. ACE inhibitors may be preferred agents in elderly patients with congestive heart failure and diabetes mellitus. Diabetic proteinuria is reduced and insulin sensitivity is enhanced. In general, the side effect profile is favorable in elderly and causes little or no CNS confusion; use lowest dose recommendations initially. Many elderly may be volume depleted due to diuretic use and/or blunted thirst reflex resulting in inadequate fluid intake.

Benazepril and benazeprilat are substantially excreted by the kidney. Because elderly are more likely to have decreased renal function, care should be taken in dose selection, and it may be useful to monitor renal function.

Breast-Feeding Considerations Small amounts of benazepril and benazeprilat are found in breast milk.

Pregnancy Considerations Due to adverse events observed in humans, benazepril is considered pregnancy category D. Benazepril crosses the placenta. First trimester exposure to ACE inhibitors may cause major congenital malformations. An increased risk of cardiovascular and/or central nervous system malformations was observed in one study; however, an increased risk of teratogenic events was not observed in other studies. Second and third trimester use of an ACE inhibitor is associated with oligohydramnios. Oligohydramnios due to decreased fetal renal function may lead to fetal limb contractures, craniofacial deformation, and hypoplastic lung development. The use of ACE inhibitors during the second and third trimesters is also associated with anuria, hypotension, renal failure (reversible or irreversible), skull hypoplasia, and death in the fetus/neonate. Chronic maternal hypertension itself is also associated with adverse events in the fetus/infant. ACE inhibitors are not recommended during pregnancy to treat maternal hypertension or heart failure. Those who are planning a pregnancy should be considered for other medication options if an ACE inhibitor is currently prescribed or the ACE inhibitor should be discontinued as soon as possible once pregnancy is detected. The exposed fetus should be monitored for fetal growth, amniotic fluid volume, and organ formation. Infants exposed to an ACE inhibitor *in utero*, especially during the second and third trimester, should be monitored for hyperkalemia, hypotension, and oliguria.

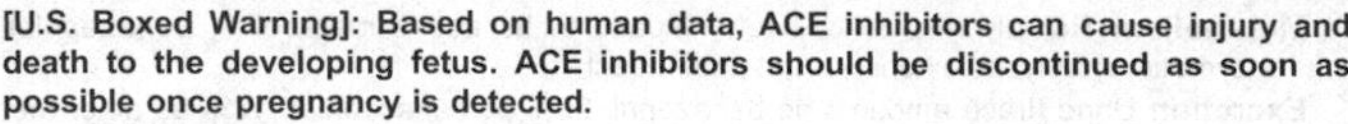

[U.S. Boxed Warning]: Based on human data, ACE inhibitors can cause injury and death to the developing fetus. ACE inhibitors should be discontinued as soon as possible once pregnancy is detected.

Related Information

Angiotensin Agents *on page 1974*

Benazepril and Hydrochlorothiazide

(ben AY ze pril & hye droe klor oh THYE a zide)

U.S. Brand Names Lotensin HCT®

Index Terms Benazepril Hydrochloride and Hydrochlorothiazide; Hydrochlorothiazide and Benazepril

Generic Availability (U.S.) Yes

Pharmacologic Category Angiotensin-Converting Enzyme (ACE) Inhibitor; Diuretic, Thiazide

Pregnancy Risk Factor D

Lactation Enters breast milk/not recommended

Use Treatment of hypertension

Available Dosage Forms

Tablet:

Generics:

5/6.25: Benazepril 5 mg and hydrochlorothiazide 6.25 mg
10/12.5: Benazepril 10 mg and hydrochlorothiazide 12.5 mg
20/12.5: Benazepril 20 mg and hydrochlorothiazide 12.5 mg
20/25: Benazepril 20 mg and hydrochlorothiazide 25 mg

Brands:

Lotensin HCT® 5/6.25: Benazepril 5 mg and hydrochlorothiazide 6.25 mg
Lotensin HCT® 10/12.5: Benazepril 10 mg and hydrochlorothiazide 12.5 mg
Lotensin HCT® 20/12.5: Benazepril 20 mg and hydrochlorothiazide 12.5 mg
Lotensin HCT® 20/25: Benazepril 20 mg and hydrochlorothiazide 25 mg

Dosing

Adult Note: Not for initial therapy; dose should be individualized.

Hypertension: Oral: Range: Benazepril: 5-20 mg; Hydrochlorothiazide: 6.25-25 mg/day

Add-on therapy:

Patients not adequately controlled on benazepril monotherapy: Initiate benazepril 10-20 mg/hydrochlorothiazide 12.5 mg; titrate to effect at 2- to 3-week intervals

Patients controlled on hydrochlorothiazide 25 mg/day but experience significant potassium loss with this regimen: Initiate benazepril 5 mg/hydrochlorothiazide 6.25 mg

Replacement therapy: Substitute for the individually titrated components

Geriatric Dose is individualized.

Renal Impairment Cl_{cr} ≤30 mL/minute: Not recommended; loop diuretics are preferred.

Monitoring and Teaching Issues

Laboratory Monitoring BUN, serum creatinine, and electrolytes; if patient has collagen vascular disease and/or renal impairment, periodically monitor CBC with differential

Physical Assessment See individual agents.

Patient Education See individual agents.

Related Information

Benazepril *on page 195*
Hydrochlorothiazide *on page 912*

◆ **Benazepril Hydrochloride** *see* Benazepril *on page 195*

◆ **Benazepril Hydrochloride and Amlodipine Besylate** *see* Amlodipine and Benazepril *on page 107*

◆ **Benazepril Hydrochloride and Hydrochlorothiazide** *see* Benazepril and Hydrochlorothiazide *on page 198*

Bendamustine (ben da MUS teen)

U.S. Brand Names Treanda®

Index Terms Bendamustine Hydrochloride; Cytostasan; SDX-105

Generic Availability (U.S.) No

Pharmacologic Category Antineoplastic Agent; Antineoplastic Agent, Alkylating Agent; Antineoplastic Agent, Alkylating Agent (Nitrogen Mustard)

Medication Safety Issues

Sound-alike/look-alike issues:

Bendamustine may be confused with carmustine, lomustine

High alert medication: This medication is in a class the Institute for Safe Medication Practices (ISMP) includes among its list of drug classes which have a heightened risk of causing significant patient harm when used in error.

Pregnancy Risk Factor D

Lactation Excretion in breast milk unknown/not recommended

Use Treatment of chronic lymphocytic leukemia (CLL); treatment of progressed indolent B-cell non-Hodgkin's lymphoma (NHL)

Unlabeled/Investigational Use Treatment of mantle cell lymphoma; salvage therapy for relapsed multiple myeloma; first-line therapy for follicular lymphoma; treatment of Waldenstrom's macroglobulinemia

Mechanism of Action/Effect Bendamustine is an alkylating agent (nitrogen mustard derivative) with a benzimidazole ring (purine analog) which causes cell death via several pathways. It is active against quiescent and dividing cells.

Contraindications Hypersensitivity to bendamustine, mannitol, or any component of the formulation

Warnings/Precautions Hazardous agent - use appropriate precautions for handling and disposal. Myelosuppression (neutropenia, thrombocytopenia, and anemia) is a common toxicity; may require therapy delay and/or dose reduction; monitor. Complications due to febrile neutropenia and severe thrombocytopenia have been reported. ANC should recover to ≥1000/mm^3 and platelets to ≥75,000/mm^3 prior to therapy/cycle initiation. Infections, including pneumonia and sepsis have been reported with use; may require hospitalization; septic shock and fatalities have occurred. Patients with myelosuppression are more susceptible to infection; monitor closely.

Infusion reactions, including chills, fever, pruritus, and rash are common; rarely, anaphylactic and anaphylactoid reactions have occurred, particularly with the second or subsequent cycle(s). In general, patients who experienced grade 3 or 4 allergic reactions were not rechallenged in CLL clinical trials. Consider premedication with antihistamines, antipyretics and/or corticosteroids for patients with a history of grade 1 or 2 infusion reaction. Discontinue for severe allergic reaction; consider discontinuation with grade 3 or 4 infusion reaction. Rash, toxic skin reactions and bullous exanthema have been reported with monotherapy and in combination with other antineoplastics; may be progressive or worsen with continued treatment; discontinue bendamustine treatment for severe or progressive skin reaction; monitor closely; discontinue bendamustine treatment for severe or progressive skin reaction. The risk for severe skin toxicity is increased with concurrent use of allopurinol and other medications known to cause skin toxicity; Stevens-Johnson syndrome and toxic epidermal necrolysis (TEN) have been reported. TEN has also been reported when used in combination with rituximab. Erythema, marked swelling, and pain have been reported with extravasation; monitor infusion site; avoid extravasation.

Tumor lysis syndrome may occur as a consequence of leukemia treatment, including treatment with bendamustine, usually occurring in the first treatment cycle. May lead to life threatening acute renal failure; adequate hydration and prophylactic allopurinol should be instituted prior to treatment in high-risk patients; monitor closely.

Use is not recommended in patients with moderate (AST or ALT 2.5-10 times ULN and total bilirubin 1.5-3 times ULN) or severe (total bilirubin >3 times ULN) hepatic impairment; use with caution in patients with mild hepatic impairment. Use is not recommended in patient with Cl_{cr} <40 mL/minute; use with caution in patients with mild-to-moderate renal impairment. Malignancies (including myelodysplastic syndrome, myeloproliferative disorders, acute myeloid leukemia and bronchial cancer) and premalignant diseases have been reported in patients who have received bendamustine. Safety and efficacy have not been established in children.

Drug Interactions

Metabolism/Transport Effects Substrate of CYP1A2; P-glycoprotein (ABCB1); BCRP (ABCG2)

Avoid Concomitant Use There are no known interactions where it is recommended to avoid concomitant use.

Decreased Effect

The levels/effects of Bendamustine may be decreased by: CYP1A2 Inducers (Strong)

Increased Effect/Toxicity

The levels/effects of Bendamustine may be increased by: CYP1A2 Inhibitors (Strong)

Adverse Reactions

>10%:

Cardiovascular: Peripheral edema (≤13%)

Central nervous system: Fatigue (9% to 57%), fever (24% to 34%), headache (≤21%), chills (6% to 14%), dizziness (≤14%), insomnia (≤13%)

Dermatologic: Rash (8% to 16%; grades 3/4: ≤3%)

Endocrine & metabolic: Dehydration (≤14%)

Gastrointestinal: Nausea (20% to 75%), vomiting (16% to 40%), diarrhea (9% to 37%), constipation (≤29%), anorexia (≤23%), weight loss (7% to 18%), stomatitis (≤15%), abdominal pain (5% to 13%), appetite loss (≤13%), dyspepsia (≤11%)

Hematologic: Myelosuppression (nadir: in week 3), lymphopenia (68% to 99%; grades 3/4: 47% to 94%), leukopenia (61% to 94%; grades 3/4: 28% to 56%), anemia (88% to 89%; grades 3/4: 11% to 13%), thrombocytopenia (77% to 86%; grades 3/4: 11% to 25%), neutropenia (75% to 86%; grades 3/4: 43% to 60%)

Hepatic: Bilirubin increased (≤34%; grades 3/4: 3%)

Neuromuscular & skeletal: Back pain (≤14%), weakness (8% to 11%)

Respiratory: Cough (4% to 22%), dyspnea (≤16%)

1% to 10%:

Cardiovascular: Tachycardia (≤7%), hypotension (≤6%), chest pain (≤6%), hypertension aggravated (≤3%)

Central nervous system: Anxiety (≤8%), depression (≤6%), pain (≤6%)

Dermatologic: Pruritus (5% to 6%), dry skin (≤5%)

Endocrine & metabolic: Hypokalemia (≤9%), hyperuricemia (≤7%; grades 3/4: 2%), hyperglycemia (grades 3/4: ≤3%), hypocalcemia (grades 3/4: ≤2%), hyponatremia (grades 3/4: ≤2%)

Gastrointestinal: Gastroesophageal reflux disease (≤10%), xerostomia (9%), taste alteration (≤7%), oral candidiasis (≤6%), abdominal distention (≤5%)
Genitourinary: Urinary tract infection (≤10%)
Hematologic: Febrile neutropenia (3% to 6%)
Hepatic: ALT increased (grades 3/4: ≤3%), AST increased (grades 3/4: ≤1%)
Local: Infusion site pain (≤6%), catheter site pain (≤5%)
Neuromuscular & skeletal: Arthralgia (≤6%), bone pain (≤5%), limb pain (≤5%)
Renal: Creatinine increased (grades 3/4: ≤2%)
Respiratory: Upper respiratory infection (10%), sinusitis (≤9%), pharyngolaryngeal pain (≤8%), pneumonia (≤8%), nasopharyngitis (6% to 7%), wheezing (≤5%), nasal congestion (≤5%)
Miscellaneous: Herpes infection (3% to 10%), infection (≤6%; grades 3/4: 2%), hypersensitivity (≤5%; grades 3/4: 1%), diaphoresis (≤5%), night sweats (≤5%)

Pharmacodynamics/Kinetics

Time to Peak At end of infusion

Protein Binding 94% to 96%

Half-Life Elimination Bendamustine: ~40 minutes; M3: ~3 hours; M4: ~30 minutes

Metabolism Hepatic, via CYP1A2 to active (minor) metabolites gamma-hydroxy bendamustine (M3) and N-desmethyl-bendamustine (M4)

Excretion Feces (~90%); urine (1% to 10%)

Available Dosage Forms

Injection, powder for reconstitution:
Treanda®: 25 mg, 100 mg

Dosing

Adult & Geriatric

Chronic lymphocytic leukemia (CLL): I.V.: 100 mg/m^2 on days 1 and 2 of a 28-day treatment cycle for up to 6 cycles

Non-Hodgkin's lymphoma (NHL), refractory: I.V.: 120 mg/m^2 on days 1 and 2 of a 21-day treatment cycle for up to 8 cycles

Follicular lymphoma, first-line (unlabeled use): I.V.: 90 mg/m^2 days 1 and 2 of a 28-day treatment cycle in combination with rituximab for up to 6 cycles (Rummel, 2009)

Mantle cell lymphoma (unlabeled use): I.V.: 90 mg/m^2 days 2 and 3 of a 28-day treatment cycle in combination with rituximab for up to 4 cycles (Rummel, 2005)

Multiple myeloma (unlabeled use): I.V.: 90-100 mg/m^2 on days 1 and 2 of a 28-day treatment cycle for at least 2 cycles (Knop, 2005)

Renal Impairment

Mild-to-moderate renal impairment: Use with caution.
Cl_{cr} <40 mL/minute: Use is not recommended.

Hepatic Impairment

Mild hepatic impairment: Use with caution.
Moderate hepatic impairment (AST or ALT 2.5-10 times ULN and total bilirubin 1.5-3 times ULN): Use is not recommended.
Severe hepatic impairment (total bilirubin >3 times ULN): Use is not recommended.

Adjustment for Toxicity

Infusion reactions:
Grade 1 or 2: Consider premedication with antihistamines, antipyretics, and corticosteroids in subsequent cycles
Grade 3 or 4: Consider discontinuing treatment

Treatment delay:
Hematologic toxicity ≥grade 4: Delay treatment until resolves (ANC ≥1000/mm^3, platelets ≥75,000/mm^3)
Nonhematologic toxicity ≥grade 2 (clinically significant): Delay treatment until resolves to ≤grade 1

Dose modification CLL:
Hematologic toxicity ≥grade 3: Reduce dose to 50 mg/m^2 on days 1 and 2 of each treatment cycle. For recurrent hematologic toxicity (≥grade 3), further reduce dose to 25 mg/m^2 on days 1 and 2 of the treatment cycle. May cautiously re-escalate dose in subsequent cycles.
Nonhematologic toxicity ≥grade 3 (clinically significant): Reduce dose to 50 mg/m^2 on days 1 and 2 of the treatment cycle with discretion. May cautiously re-escalate dose in subsequent cycles.

Dose modification in NHL:
Hematologic toxicity grade 4: Reduce dose to 90 mg/m^2 on days 1 and 2 of each treatment cycle. For recurrent hematologic toxicity (grade 4), further reduce dose to 60 mg/m^2 on days 1 and 2 of each treatment cycle.
Nonhematologic toxicity ≥grade 3: Reduce dose to 90 mg/m^2 on days 1 and 2 of the treatment cycle with discretion. For recurrent toxicity ≥grade 3, further reduce dose to 60 mg/m^2 on days 1 and 2 of each treatment cycle.

Administration

I.V. Infuse over 30 minutes for the treatment of CLL and over 60 minutes for NHL. Prophylactic treatment with allopurinol may be needed in patients at risk for tumor lysis syndrome. Consider premedication with antihistamines, antipyretics, and/or corticosteroids for patients with a previous grade 1 or 2 infusion reaction to bendamustine. Avoid extravasation; monitor I.V. site for redness, swelling, or pain.

Stability

Reconstitution Use appropriate precautions for handling and disposal. Reconstitute 25 mg vial with 5 mL and 100 mg vial with 20 mL of sterile water for injection to a concentration of 5 mg/mL; powder usually dissolves within 5 minutes. Prior to administration, dilute appropriate dose in 500 mL NS (or $D_{2.5}$$^1/_2$NS) to a final concentration of 0.2-0.6 mg/mL; mix thoroughly.

Storage Prior to reconstitution, store intact vials up to 25°C (77°F); excursions permitted up to 30°C (86°F). Protect from light. The solution in the vial (reconstituted with SWFI) is stable for 30 minutes (transfer to 500 mL infusion bag within that 30 minutes). The solution diluted in 500 mL for infusion is stable for 24 hours refrigerated or 3 hours at room temperature and room light. Infusion must be completed within these time frames.

Monitoring and Teaching Issues

Laboratory Monitoring CBC with differential (monitored weekly [initially] in clinical trials); serum creatinine (pretreatment); ALT, AST, and total bilirubin (pretreatment); monitor potassium and uric acid levels in patients at risk for tumor lysis syndrome

Physical Assessment Use with caution in presence of hepatic or renal impairment. Infusion site must be monitored closely to avoid extravasation. Monitor infusion reactions, including skin reactions; can occur with first or subsequent cycles and may require premedication or discontinuation.

Patient Education This medication can only be administered by I.V. Report immediately any pain, burning, or swelling at infusion site; sudden onset chest pain; respiratory difficulty; or difficulty swallowing. It is important that you maintain adequate nutrition between treatments and adequate hydration, unless instructed to restrict fluid intake. You will be susceptible to infection. May cause nausea, vomiting, weight loss, or diarrhea. Report immediately chills, fever, skin rash, persistent unusual fatigue, unusual bruising/bleeding, or signs of infection.

Breast-Feeding Considerations Due to the potential for serious adverse reactions in the nursing infant, breast-feeding is not recommended.

Pregnancy Considerations Teratogenic and nonteratogenic events were observed in animal studies following intraperitoneal dosing. There are no adequate and well-controlled studies in pregnant women. May cause fetal harm if administered during pregnancy. Effective contraception is recommended during and for 3 months after treatment for women and men of reproductive potential.

- ◆ **Bendamustine Hydrochloride** *see* Bendamustine *on page* *198*
- ◆ **Benemid [DSC]** *see* Probenecid *on page* *1508*
- ◆ **Benicar®** *see* Olmesartan *on page* *1349*
- ◆ **Benicar HCT®** *see* Olmesartan and Hydrochlorothiazide *on page* *1351*
- ◆ **Benlysta®** *see* Belimumab *on page* *194*
- ◆ **BenzaClin®** *see* Clindamycin and Benzoyl Peroxide *on page* *401*
- ◆ **Benzathine Benzylpenicillin** *see* Penicillin G Benzathine *on page* *1432*
- ◆ **Benzathine Penicillin G** *see* Penicillin G Benzathine *on page* *1432*
- ◆ **Benzene Hexachloride** *see* Lindane *on page* *1110*
- ◆ **Benzhexol Hydrochloride** *see* Trihexyphenidyl *on page* *1818*
- ◆ **Benzmethyzin** *see* Procarbazine *on page* *1510*

Benzonatate (ben ZOE na tate)

U.S. Brand Names Tessalon®; Zonatuss™

Index Terms Tessalon Perles

Generic Availability (U.S.) Yes: Capsule (softgel)

Pharmacologic Category Antitussive

Pregnancy Risk Factor C

Lactation Excretion in breast milk unknown/use caution

Use Symptomatic relief of nonproductive cough

Available Dosage Forms

Capsule, oral:

Zonatuss™: 150 mg

Capsule, softgel, oral: 100 mg, 200 mg

Tessalon®: 100 mg, 200 mg

Dosing

Adult & Geriatric Cough: Oral: 100 mg 3 times/day or every 4 hours up to 600 mg/day

Pediatric Children >10 years: Refer to adult dosing.

Administration

Oral Swallow capsule whole (do not break or chew).

Monitoring and Teaching Issues

Physical Assessment Assess effectiveness of therapy (relief of cough, lung sounds, and respiratory pattern). Monitor for CNS changes at beginning of therapy and periodically throughout.

Patient Education Do not break or chew capsule. Maintain adequate hydration, unless instructed to restrict fluid intake. You may experience drowsiness, impaired coordination, blurred vision, increased anxiety, upset stomach, or nausea. Report persistent CNS changes (dizziness, sedation, tremor, or agitation), numbness in chest or feeling of chill, visual changes or burning in eyes, numbness of mouth or difficulty swallowing, or lack of improvement or worsening or condition.

- ◆ **Benzoyl Peroxide and Adapalene** *see* Adapalene and Benzoyl Peroxide *on page* *52*
- ◆ **Benzoyl Peroxide and Clindamycin** *see* Clindamycin and Benzoyl Peroxide *on page* *401*

Benztropine (BENZ troe peen)

U.S. Brand Names Cogentin®

Index Terms Benztropine Mesylate

Generic Availability (U.S.) Yes

Pharmacologic Category Anti-Parkinson's Agent, Anticholinergic; Anticholinergic Agent

Medication Safety Issues

Sound-alike/look-alike issues:

Benztropine may be confused with bromocriptine

Pregnancy Risk Factor C

Lactation Excretion in breast milk unknown/use caution

Use Adjunctive treatment of Parkinson's disease; treatment of drug-induced extrapyramidal symptoms (except tardive dyskinesia)

Mechanism of Action/Effect Possesses both anticholinergic and antihistaminic effects. *In vitro* anticholinergic activity approximates that of atropine; *in vivo* it is only about half as active as atropine. Animal data suggest its antihistaminic activity and duration of action approach that of pyrilamine maleate. May also inhibit the reuptake and storage of dopamine, thereby prolonging the action of dopamine.

Contraindications Hypersensitivity to benztropine or any component of the formulation; pyloric or duodenal obstruction, stenosing peptic ulcers; bladder neck obstructions; achalasia; myasthenia gravis; children <3 years of age

Warnings/Precautions Use with caution in older children (dose has not been established). Use with caution in hot weather or during exercise. May cause anhydrosis and hyperthermia, which may be severe. The risk is increased in hot environments, particularly in the elderly, alcoholics, patients with CNS disease, and those with prolonged outdoor exposure.

Elderly patients frequently develop increased sensitivity and require strict dosage regulation - side effects may be more severe in elderly patients with atherosclerotic changes. Use with caution in patients with tachycardia, cardiac arrhythmias, hypertension, hypotension, glaucoma, prostatic hyperplasia (especially in the elderly), any tendency toward urinary retention, liver or kidney disorders, and obstructive disease of the GI or GU tract. When given in large doses or to susceptible patients, may cause weakness and inability to move particular muscle groups.

May be associated with confusion or hallucinations (generally at higher dosages). Intensification of symptoms or toxic psychosis may occur in patients with mental disorders. May cause CNS depression, which may impair physical or mental abilities; patients must be cautioned about performing tasks which require mental alertness (eg, operating machinery or driving). Benztropine does not relieve symptoms of tardive dyskinesia.

Drug Interactions

Metabolism/Transport Effects Substrate of CYP2D6 (minor)

Avoid Concomitant Use There are no known interactions where it is recommended to avoid concomitant use.

Decreased Effect

Benztropine may decrease the levels/effects of: Acetylcholinesterase Inhibitors (Central); Secretin

The levels/effects of Benztropine may be decreased by: Acetylcholinesterase Inhibitors (Central); Peginterferon Alfa-2b

Increased Effect/Toxicity

Benztropine may increase the levels/effects of: AbobotulinumtoxinA; Anticholinergics; Cannabinoids; OnabotulinumtoxinA; Potassium Chloride; RimabotulinumtoxinB

The levels/effects of Benztropine may be increased by: Pramlintide

Nutritional/Ethanol Interactions Ethanol: Avoid ethanol (may increase CNS depression).

Adverse Reactions Frequency not defined.

Cardiovascular: Tachycardia

Central nervous system: Confusion, disorientation, memory impairment, toxic psychosis, visual hallucinations

Dermatologic: Rash

Endocrine & metabolic: Heat stroke, hyperthermia

Gastrointestinal: Constipation, dry throat, ileus, nasal dryness, nausea, vomiting, xerostomia

Genitourinary: Urinary retention, dysuria

Ocular: Blurred vision, mydriasis

Miscellaneous: Fever

Pharmacodynamics/Kinetics

Onset of Action Oral: Within 1 hour; Parenteral: Within 15 minutes

Duration of Action 6-48 hours

Bioavailability 29%

Metabolism Hepatic (N-oxidation, N-dealkylation, and ring hydroxylation)

Available Dosage Forms

Injection, solution: 1 mg/mL

Cogentin®: 1 mg/mL

Tablet, oral: 0.5 mg, 1 mg, 2 mg

Dosing

Adult

Drug-induced extrapyramidal symptom: Oral, I.M., I.V.: 1-4 mg/dose 1-2 times/day

Acute dystonia: I.M., I.V.: 1-2 mg

Parkinsonism: Oral: 0.5-6 mg/day in 1-2 divided doses; if one dose is greater, give at bedtime. Titrate dose in 0.5 mg increments at 5- to 6-day intervals.

Geriatric Oral: Initial: 0.5 mg once or twice daily; titrate dose in 0.5 mg increments at every 5-6 days; maximum: 4 mg/day.

Pediatric Note: Use in children ≤3 years of age should be reserved for life-threatening emergencies.

Drug-induced extrapyramidal symptoms: Oral, I.M., I.V.: Children >3 years: 0.02-0.05 mg/kg/dose 1-2 times/day

Monitoring and Teaching Issues

Patient Education Take at the same time each day. Do not use alcohol. You may experience drowsiness, dizziness, confusion, blurred vision, increased susceptibility to heat stroke, decreased perspiration, or constipation. Report unresolved nausea, vomiting, or gastric disturbances; rapid or pounding heartbeat, chest pain, or palpitation; respiratory difficulty; CNS changes (hallucination, loss of memory, nervousness, etc); eye pain; prolonged fever; painful or difficult urination; unresolved constipation; increased muscle spasticity or rigidity; skin rash; or significant worsening of condition.

Geriatric Considerations Anticholinergic agents are generally not well tolerated in the elderly (often results in bowel, bladder, and CNS adverse effects) and their use should be avoided when possible. In the elderly, anticholinergic agents should not be used as prophylaxis against extrapyramidal symptoms.

Additional Information No significant difference in onset of I.M. or I.V. injection; therefore, there is usually no need to use the I.V. route. Improvement is sometimes noticeable a few minutes after injection.

- **Benztropine Mesylate** *see* Benztropine *on page 202*
- **Benzylpenicillin Benzathine** *see* Penicillin G Benzathine *on page 1432*
- **Benzylpenicillin Potassium** *see* Penicillin G (Parenteral/Aqueous) *on page 1433*
- **Benzylpenicillin Sodium** *see* Penicillin G (Parenteral/Aqueous) *on page 1433*

Benzylpenicilloyl Polylysine (BEN zil pen i SIL oyl pol i LIE seen)

U.S. Brand Names Pre-Pen®

Index Terms Benzylpenicilloyl-polylysine; Penicilloyl-polylysine; PPL

Generic Availability (U.S.) No

Pharmacologic Category Diagnostic Agent

Pregnancy Risk Factor C

Use Adjunct in assessing the risk of administering penicillin (penicillin G or benzylpenicillin) in patients suspected of clinical penicillin hypersensitivity

Unlabeled/Investigational Use Adjunct in assessment of hypersensitivity to other beta-lactam antibiotics (penicillins and cephalosporins) to determine the safety of penicillin administration in patients with a history of reaction to cephalosporins

Available Dosage Forms

Injection, solution:

Pre-Pen®: 6 x 10^{-5} M (0.25 mL)

Dosing

Adult & Geriatric Diagnostic aid for detection of penicillin allergy:

Note: Benzylpenicilloyl polylysine should always be applied first via the puncture technique. **Do not administer intradermally to patients who have a positive reaction to the puncture test.**

Puncture test: Apply a small drop of the skin test solution using a 22- to 28-gauge needle and make a single shallow puncture of the epidermis through the drop of solution. A positive reaction consists of a pale wheal surrounding the puncture site which develops within 10 minutes and ranges from 5-15 mm or more in diameter (wheal may be surrounded by erythema and variable degrees of itching). If a positive response is evident, the solution should be wiped off immediately. If the puncture test is negative or equivocal (<5 mm wheal, with little or no erythema and no itching) 15 minutes following the puncture test, an intradermal test may be performed.

Intradermal test: Using a 0.5-1 mL tuberculin syringe with a 3/8 to 5/8 inch, 26- to 30-gauge short bevel needle, inject a volume of skin test solution sufficient to raise a small intradermal bleb ~3 mm in diameter intradermally, in duplicate at least 2 cm apart. A control of 0.9% sodium chloride or allergen-diluting solution should be injected at least 5 cm from the antigen test site. Most skin responses to the intradermal test will develop within 5-15 minutes. A response to the skin test is read at 20 minutes.

Interpretation of intradermal test:

(-) Negative: No increase in size of original bleb or no greater reaction compared to the control site

(±) Ambiguous: Wheal only slightly larger than original bleb with or without erythematous flare and slightly larger than control site; OR discordance between duplicate test sites

(+) Positive: Itching and marked increase in size of original bleb to ≥5 mm. Wheal may exhibit pseudopods and be >20 mm in diameter.

Control site should be reactionless. If wheal >2-3 mm develops at control site, repeat the test. If same reaction occurs, consultation is necessary.

Pediatric Refer to adult dosing.

Administration

Other

Puncture test: Administer initially by puncture technique on the inner volar aspect of the forearm, followed by an intradermal injection only in patients with a negative reaction.

Intradermal: Do **not** administer intradermally to patients with a positive reaction (wheal of 5-15 mm or more in diameter). Administer the intradermal test on the upper, outer arm, below the deltoid muscle in the event a severe hypersensitivity reaction occurs and a tourniquet needs to be applied. During the skin test, immediate treatment with epinephrine should also be available.

◆ **Benzylpenicilloyl-polylysine** *see* Benzylpenicilloyl Polylysine *on page* 203

Bepotastine (be poe TAS teen)

U.S. Brand Names Bepreve™

Index Terms Bepotastine Besilate

Generic Availability (U.S.) No

Pharmacologic Category Histamine H_1 Antagonist; Histamine H_1 Antagonist, Second Generation; Mast Cell Stabilizer

Pregnancy Risk Factor C

Lactation Excretion in breast milk unknown/use caution

Use Treatment of itching associated with allergic conjunctivitis

Available Dosage Forms

Solution, ophthalmic:

Bepreve™: 1.5% (10 mL)

Dosing

Adult & Geriatric Allergic conjunctivitis: Ophthalmic: Instill 1 drop into the affected eye(s) twice daily

Pediatric Allergic conjunctivitis: Ophthalmic: Children ≥2 years: Refer to adult dosing.

Administration

Other For topical ophthalmic use only. Contact lenses should be removed prior to application, may be inserted after 10 minutes. Do not insert contacts if eyes are red. Avoid contaminating the applicator tip with affected eye(s).

Monitoring and Teaching Issues

Patient Education This medication is for external use only. You may experience mild headache or unusual taste after use. Contact prescriber if eye condition worsens or does not improve. Application: Wash hands thoroughly before applying. Remove contact lenses prior to administration and wait 10 minutes before reinserting. Apply this medication in the affected eye(s) as directed by prescriber. Tilt your head back and look up. Pull down lower lid, hold applicator directly over eye, and place 1 drop into lower lid. Close eyes for a minute. Apply gentle pressure with one finger at the corner of eye near the nose. Do not allow dropper to touch eye or any other surface. If you are using another kind of eye medication, wait several minutes before applying other medications.

◆ **Bepotastine Besilate** *see* Bepotastine *on page* 204

◆ **Bepreve™** *see* Bepotastine *on page* 204

Besifloxacin (be si FLOX a sin)

U.S. Brand Names Besivance™

Index Terms Besifloxacin Hydrochloride; BOL-303224-A; SS734

Generic Availability (U.S.) No

Pharmacologic Category Antibiotic, Ophthalmic; Antibiotic, Quinolone

Pregnancy Risk Factor C

Lactation Excretion in breast milk unknown/use caution

Use Treatment of bacterial conjunctivitis

Available Dosage Forms

Suspension, ophthalmic:

Besivance™: 0.6% (5 mL)

Dosing

Adult & Geriatric Bacterial conjunctivitis: Ophthalmic: Instill 1 drop into affected eye(s) 3 times/day (4-12 hours apart) for 7 days

Pediatric Bacterial conjunctivitis: Children ≥1 year: Ophthalmic: Refer to adult dosing.

Administration

Other Ophthalmic: Wash hands before and after instillation. Shake bottle once prior to each administration. Avoid contaminating the applicator tip with affected eye(s).

Monitoring and Teaching Issues

Patient Education Do not wear contact lenses while using this medication. Wash hands before applying; invert bottle and shake once before use. Remove cap and tilt head back; squeeze bottle gently and instill one drop into the affected eye(s). Avoid contaminating the tip; do not touch the tip with fingers or touch the tip to eye. You may experience eye redness or blurred vision. Discontinue immediately and contact prescriber if you experience a rash, pain, or allergic reaction.

◆ **Besifloxacin Hydrochloride** *see* Besifloxacin *on page* 204

◆ **Besivance™** *see* Besifloxacin *on page 204*

◆ **9-Beta-D-Ribofuranosyladenine** *see* Adenosine *on page 54*

◆ **Beta-HC® [OTC]** *see* Hydrocortisone (Topical) *on page 920*

Betamethasone (bay ta METH a sone)

U.S. Brand Names Beta-Val® [DSC]; Celestone®; Celestone® Soluspan®; Diprolene®; Diprolene® AF; Luxíq®

Index Terms Betamethasone Dipropionate; Betamethasone Dipropionate, Augmented; Betamethasone Sodium Phosphate; Betamethasone Valerate; Flubenisolone

Generic Availability (U.S.) Yes: Excludes aerosol, solution

Pharmacologic Category Corticosteroid, Systemic; Corticosteroid, Topical

Medication Safety Issues

Sound-alike/look-alike issues:

Luxiq® may be confused with Lasix®

International issues:

Beta-Val [U.S.] may be confused with Betanol brand name for metipranolol [Monaco]

Pregnancy Risk Factor C

Lactation Excretion in breast milk unknown/use caution

Use Inflammatory dermatoses such as seborrheic or atopic dermatitis, neurodermatitis, anogenital pruritus, psoriasis, inflammatory phase of xerosis

Unlabeled/Investigational Use Accelerate fetal lung maturation in patients with preterm labor

Mechanism of Action/Effect Binds to corticosteroid receptors in cell and acts to prevent or control inflammation

Contraindications Hypersensitivity to betamethasone, other corticosteroids, or any component of the formulation; systemic fungal infections; I.M. administration contraindicated in idiopathic thrombocytopenia purpura

Warnings/Precautions Very high potency topical products are not for treatment of rosacea, perioral dermatitis; not for use on face, groin, or axillae; not for use in a diapered area. Avoid concurrent use of other corticosteroids.

May cause hypercorticism or suppression of hypothalamic-pituitary-adrenal (HPA) axis, particularly in younger children or in patients receiving high doses for prolonged periods. HPA axis suppression may lead to adrenal crisis. Withdrawal and discontinuation of a corticosteroid should be done slowly and carefully. Particular care is required when patients are transferred from systemic corticosteroids to inhaled products due to possible adrenal insufficiency or withdrawal from steroids, including an increase in allergic symptoms. Patients receiving >20 mg per day of prednisone (or equivalent) may be most susceptible. Fatalities have occurred due to adrenal insufficiency in asthmatic patients during and after transfer from systemic corticosteroids to aerosol steroids; aerosol steroids do not provide the systemic steroid needed to treat patients having trauma, surgery, or infections. In stressful situations, HPA axis-suppressed patients should receive adequate supplementation with natural glucocorticoids (hydrocortisone or cortisone) rather than betamethasone (due to lack of mineralocorticoid activity).

Acute myopathy has been reported with high dose corticosteroids, usually in patients with neuromuscular transmission disorders; may involve ocular and/or respiratory muscles; monitor creatine kinase; recovery may be delayed. Corticosteroid use may cause psychiatric disturbances, including depression, euphoria, insomnia, mood swings, and personality changes. Pre-existing psychiatric conditions may be exacerbated by corticosteroid use. Prolonged use of corticosteroids may also increase the incidence of secondary infection, mask acute infection (including fungal infections), prolong or exacerbate viral infections, or limit response to vaccines. Exposure to chickenpox should be avoided; corticosteroids should not be used to treat ocular herpes simplex. Corticosteroids should not be used for cerebral malaria or viral hepatitis. Close observation is required in patients with latent tuberculosis and/or TB reactivity; restrict use in active TB (only in conjunction with antituberculosis treatment). Prolonged treatment with corticosteroids has been associated with the development of Kaposi's sarcoma (case reports); if noted, discontinuation of therapy should be considered. High-dose corticosteroids should not be used to manage acute head injury.

Use with caution in patients with thyroid disease, hepatic impairment, renal impairment, cardiovascular disease, diabetes, glaucoma, cataracts, myasthenia gravis, patients at risk for osteoporosis, patients at risk for seizures, or GI diseases (diverticulitis, peptic ulcer, ulcerative colitis) due to perforation risk. Use caution following acute MI (corticosteroids have been associated with myocardial rupture). Because of the risk of adverse effects, systemic corticosteroids should be used cautiously in the elderly in the smallest possible effective dose for the shortest duration. Do not use occlusive dressings on weeping or exudative lesions and general caution with occlusive dressings should be observed; adverse effects may be increased. Discontinue if skin irritation or contact dermatitis should occur; do not use in patients with decreased skin circulation. Withdraw therapy with gradual tapering of dose. May affect growth velocity; growth should be routinely monitored in pediatric patients. Topical use in patients ≤12 years of age is not recommended.

Drug Interactions

Metabolism/Transport Effects Inhibits CYP3A4 (weak)

Avoid Concomitant Use

Avoid concomitant use of Betamethasone with any of the following: Aldesleukin; BCG; Natalizumab; Pimecrolimus; Roflumilast; Tacrolimus (Topical)

Decreased Effect

Betamethasone may decrease the levels/effects of: Aldesleukin; Antidiabetic Agents; BCG; Calcitriol; Corticorelin; Isoniazid; Salicylates; Sipuleucel-T; Vaccines (Inactivated)

The levels/effects of Betamethasone may be decreased by: Aminoglutethimide; Antacids; Barbiturates; Bile Acid Sequestrants; Echinacea; Mitotane; Primidone; Rifamycin Derivatives

Increased Effect/Toxicity

Betamethasone may increase the levels/effects of: Acetylcholinesterase Inhibitors; Amphotericin B; Leflunomide; Loop Diuretics; Natalizumab; NSAID (COX-2 Inhibitor); NSAID (Nonselective); Thiazide Diuretics; Vaccines (Live); Warfarin

The levels/effects of Betamethasone may be increased by: Antifungal Agents (Azole Derivatives, Systemic); Aprepitant; Calcium Channel Blockers (Nondihydropyridine); Denosumab; Estrogen Derivatives; Fluconazole; Fosaprepitant; Macrolide Antibiotics; Neuromuscular-Blocking Agents (Nondepolarizing); Pimecrolimus; Quinolone Antibiotics; Roflumilast; Salicylates; Tacrolimus (Topical); Trastuzumab

Nutritional/Ethanol Interactions

Ethanol: Avoid ethanol (may enhance gastric mucosal irritation).

Food: Betamethasone interferes with calcium absorption.

Herb/Nutraceutical: Avoid cat's claw, echinacea (have immunostimulant properties).

Adverse Reactions

Systemic:

Cardiovascular: Congestive heart failure, edema, hyper-/hypotension

Central nervous system: Dizziness, headache, insomnia, intracranial pressure increased, lightheadedness, nervousness, pseudotumor cerebri, seizure, vertigo

Dermatologic: Ecchymoses, facial erythema, fragile skin, hirsutism, hyper-/hypopigmentation, perioral dermatitis (oral), petechiae, striae, wound healing impaired

Endocrine & metabolic: Amenorrhea, Cushing's syndrome, diabetes mellitus, growth suppression, hyperglycemia, hypokalemia, menstrual irregularities, pituitary-adrenal axis suppression, protein catabolism, sodium retention, water retention

Local: Injection site reactions (intra-articular use), sterile abscess

Neuromuscular & skeletal: Arthralgia, muscle atrophy, fractures, muscle weakness, myopathy, osteoporosis, necrosis (femoral and humeral heads)

Ocular: Cataracts, glaucoma, intraocular pressure increased

Miscellaneous: Anaphylactoid reaction, diaphoresis, hypersensitivity, secondary infection

Topical:

Dermatologic: Acneiform eruptions, allergic dermatitis, burning, dry skin, erythema, folliculitis, hypertrichosis, irritation, miliaria, pruritus, skin atrophy, striae, vesiculation

Endocrine and metabolic effects have occasionally been reported with topical use.

Pharmacodynamics/Kinetics

Time to Peak Serum: I.V.: 10-36 minutes

Protein Binding 64%

Half-Life Elimination 6.5 hours

Metabolism Hepatic

Excretion Urine (<5% as unchanged drug)

Available Dosage Forms

Aerosol, topical:
Luxíq®: 0.12% (50 g, 100 g)

Cream, topical: 0.05% (15 g, 45 g, 50 g); 0.1% (15 g, 45 g)
Diprolene® AF: 0.05% (15 g, 50 g)

Gel, topical: 0.05% (15 g, 50 g)

Injection, suspension: Betamethasone sodium phosphate 3 mg and betamethasone acetate 3 mg per 1 mL (5 mL)
Celestone® Soluspan®: Betamethasone sodium phosphate 3 mg and betamethasone acetate 3 mg per 1 mL (5 mL)

Lotion, topical: 0.05% (30 mL, 60 mL); 0.1% (60 mL)
Diprolene®: 0.05% (30 mL, 60 mL)

Ointment, topical: 0.05% (15 g, 45 g, 50 g); 0.1% (15 g, 45 g)
Diprolene®: 0.05% (15 g, 50 g)

Solution, oral:
Celestone®: 0.6 mg/5 mL (118 mL)

Dosing

Adult Base dosage on severity of disease and patient response

Inflammatory conditions:

Oral: 2.4-4.8 mg/day in 2-4 doses; range: 0.6-7.2 mg/day

I.M.: Betamethasone sodium phosphate and betamethasone acetate: 0.6-9 mg/day (generally, $^{1}/_{3}$ to $^{1}/_{2}$ of oral dose) divided every 12-24 hours

Psoriasis (scalp): Topical (foam): Apply to the scalp twice daily, once in the morning and once at night.

Rheumatoid arthritis/osteoarthritis:

Intrabursal, intra-articular, intradermal: 0.25-2 mL

Intralesional:

Very large joints: 1-2 mL
Large joints: 1 mL
Medium joints: 0.5-1 mL
Small joints: 0.25-0.5 mL

Steroid-responsive dermatoses: Therapy should be discontinued when control is achieved; if no improvement is seen, reassessment of diagnosis may be necessary.

Gel, augmented formulation: Apply once or twice daily; rub in gently. **Note:** Do not exceed 2 weeks of treatment or 50 g/week.

Lotion: Apply a few drops twice daily

Augmented formulation: Apply a few drops once or twice daily; rub in gently. **Note:** Do not exceed 2 weeks of treatment or 50 mL/week.

Cream/ointment: Apply once or twice daily

Augmented formulation: Apply once or twice daily. **Note:** Do not exceed 2 weeks of treatment or 45 g/week.

Geriatric Refer to adult dosing. Use the lowest effective dose.

Pediatric Base dosage on severity of disease and patient response.

Inflammatory conditions: Note: Use lowest dose listed as initial dose for adrenocortical insufficiency (physiologic replacement).

I.M.:

Children ≤12 years: 0.0175-0.125 mg base/kg/day divided every 6-12 hours **or** 0.5-7.5 mg base/m^2/day divided every 6-12 hours

Children >13 years: Refer to adult dosing.

Oral:

Children ≤12 years: 0.0175-0.25 mg/kg/day divided every 6-8 hours **or** 0.5-7.5 mg/m^2/day divided every 6-8 hours

Children >13 years: Refer to adult dosing.

Topical: Children ≥13 years (use in children ≤12 years is not recommended): Use minimal amount for shortest period of time to avoid HPA axis suppression

Steroid-responsive dermatoses: Topical: Refer to adult dosing

Hepatic Impairment Adjustments may be necessary in patients with liver failure because betamethasone is extensively metabolized in the liver

Administration

Oral Not for alternate day therapy; once daily doses should be given in the morning. May be administered with food to decrease GI distress.

I.M. Do **not** give injectable sodium phosphate/acetate suspension I.V.

Topical Apply topical sparingly to areas. Not for use on broken skin or in areas of infection. Do not apply to wet skin unless directed; do not cover with occlusive dressing. Do not apply very high potency agents to face, groin, axillae, or diaper area.

Foam: Invert can and dispense a small amount onto a saucer or other cool surface. Do not dispense directly into hands. Pick up small amounts of foam and gently massage into affected areas until foam disappears. Repeat until entire affected scalp area is treated.

Monitoring and Teaching Issues

Physical Assessment Growth should be routinely monitored in pediatric patients. With systemic administration, caution patients with diabetes to monitor glucose levels closely (corticosteroids may alter glucose levels).

Patient Education Take oral medication with or after meals. Avoid alcohol and limit intake of caffeine or stimulants. Prescriber may recommend increased dietary vitamins, minerals, or iron. If you have diabetes, monitor glucose levels closely (antidiabetic medication may need to be adjusted). Inform prescriber if you are experiencing greater-than-normal levels of stress (medication may need adjustment). You may be more susceptible to infection. Some forms of this medication may cause GI upset. Report promptly excessive nervousness or sleep disturbances, signs of infection (eg, sore throat, unhealed injuries), excessive growth of body hair or loss of skin color, vision changes, weight gain, swelling of face or extremities, respiratory difficulty, muscle weakness, change in color of stools (tarry) or persistent abdominal pain, or worsening of condition or failure to improve.

Topical: For external use only. Do not use for eyes, mucous membranes, or open wounds. Before using, wash and dry area gently. Apply in a thin layer (may rub in lightly). Apply light dressing (if necessary) to area being treated. Do not use occlusive dressing unless so advised by prescriber. Avoid prolonged or excessive use around sensitive tissues, genital, or rectal areas. Avoid exposing treated area to direct sunlight. Inform prescriber if condition worsens (redness, swelling, irritation, signs of infection, or open sores) or fails to improve.

Dietary Considerations May be taken with food to decrease GI distress.

Geriatric Considerations Because of the risk of adverse effects, systemic corticosteroids should be used cautiously in the elderly, in the smallest possible dose, and for the shortest possible time.

Breast-Feeding Considerations Corticosteroids are excreted in human milk. The onset of milk secretion after birth may be delayed and the volume of milk produced may be decreased by antenatal betamethasone therapy; this affect was seen when delivery occurred 3-9 days after the betamethasone dose in women between 28 and 34 weeks gestation. Antenatal betamethasone therapy did not affect milk production when birth occurred <3 days or >10 days of treatment. It is not known if systemic absorption following topical administration results in detectable quantities in human milk. Use with caution while breast-feeding; do not apply to nipples.

Pregnancy Considerations Adverse events have been observed with corticosteroids in animal reproduction studies. Betamethasone crosses the placenta; approximately 25% is metabolized by placental enzymes to an inactive metabolite. Due to its positive effect on stimulating fetal lung maturation, the injection is often used in patients with premature labor (24-34 weeks gestation). Topical products are not recommended for extensive use, in large quantities, or for long periods of time in pregnant women. Some studies have shown an association between first trimester systemic corticosteroid use and oral clefts; adverse events in the fetus/neonate have been noted in case reports following large doses of systemic corticosteroids during pregnancy. Women exposed to betamethasone during pregnancy for the treatment of an autoimmune disease may contact the OTIS Autoimmune Diseases Study at 877-311-8972.

Additional Information

Very high potency: Augmented betamethasone dipropionate ointment, lotion

High potency: Augmented betamethasone dipropionate cream, betamethasone dipropionate cream and ointment

Intermediate potency: Betamethasone dipropionate lotion, betamethasone valerate cream

Related Information

Corticosteroids *on page 1996*

Betamethasone and Clotrimazole (bay ta METH a sone & kloe TRIM a zole)

U.S. Brand Names Lotrisone®

Index Terms Clotrimazole and Betamethasone

Generic Availability (U.S.) Yes

Pharmacologic Category Antifungal Agent, Topical; Corticosteroid, Topical

Medication Safety Issues

Sound-alike/look-alike issues:

Clotrimazole may be confused with co-trimoxazole

Lotrisone® may be confused with Lotrimin®

Pregnancy Risk Factor C

Lactation Excretion in breast milk unknown/use caution

Use Topical treatment of various dermal fungal infections (including tinea pedis, cruris, and corpora in patients ≥17 years of age)

Available Dosage Forms

Cream: Betamethasone 0.05% and clotrimazole 1% (15 g, 45 g)

Lotrisone®: Betamethasone 0.05% and clotrimazole 1% (15 g, 45 g)

Lotion: Betamethasone 0.05% and clotrimazole 1% (30 mL)

Lotrisone®: Betamethasone 0.05% and clotrimazole 1% (30 mL)

Dosing

Adult

Allergic or inflammatory diseases: Topical: Apply to affected area twice daily, morning and evening

Tinea corporis, tinea cruris: Topical: Massage into affected area twice daily, morning and evening. Do not use for longer than 2 weeks; re-evaluate after 1 week if no clinical improvement. Do not exceed 45 g cream/week or 45 mL lotion/week.

Tinea pedis: Topical: Massage into affected area twice daily, morning and evening. Do not use for longer than 4 weeks; re-evaluate after 2 weeks if no clinical improvement. Do not exceed 45 g cream/week or 45 mL lotion/week.

Geriatric Refer to adult dosing. Use with caution. Skin atrophy and skin ulceration (rare) have been reported in patients with thinning skin. Do not use for diaper dermatitis or under occlusive dressings.

Pediatric

Children <17 years: Do not use.

Children ≥17 years: Refer to adult dosing.

Administration

Topical For external use only. Do not use on open wounds. Do not cover with occlusive dressings. Shake lotion well prior to use

Monitoring and Teaching Issues

Laboratory Monitoring Urinary free cortisol test, morning plasma cortisol test, and ACTH stimulation test may be used to evaluate HPA axis suppression

Physical Assessment See individual agents.

Patient Education See individual agents.

Related Information

Betamethasone *on page 205*

◆ **Betamethasone Dipropionate** *see* Betamethasone *on page 205*

◆ **Betamethasone Dipropionate and Calcipotriene Hydrate** *see* Calcipotriene and Betamethasone *on page 268*

◆ **Betamethasone Dipropionate, Augmented** *see* Betamethasone *on page 205*

◆ **Betamethasone Sodium Phosphate** *see* Betamethasone *on page 205*

◆ **Betamethasone Valerate** *see* Betamethasone *on page 205*

◆ **Betapace®** *see* Sotalol *on page 1673*

◆ **Betapace AF®** *see* Sotalol *on page 1673*

◆ **Betaseron®** *see* Interferon Beta-1b *on page 1005*

◆ **Beta-Val® [DSC]** *see* Betamethasone *on page 205*

Betaxolol (Systemic) (be TAKS oh lol)

U.S. Brand Names Kerlone®

Index Terms Betaxolol Hydrochloride

Generic Availability (U.S.) Yes

Pharmacologic Category Beta Blocker, Beta-1 Selective

Medication Safety Issues

Sound-alike/look-alike issues:

Betaxolol may be confused with bethanechol, labetalol

Pregnancy Risk Factor C

Lactation Enters breast milk/use caution

Use Management of hypertension

Unlabeled/Investigational Use Treatment of coronary artery disease

Mechanism of Action/Effect Competitively blocks beta$_1$-receptors, with little or no effect on beta$_2$-receptors

Contraindications Hypersensitivity to betaxolol or any component of the formulation; sinus bradycardia; heart block greater than first-degree (except in patients with a functioning artificial pacemaker); cardiogenic shock; uncompensated cardiac failure

Warnings/Precautions Consider pre-existing conditions (such as sick sinus syndrome) before initiating. Administer cautiously in compensated heart failure and monitor for a worsening of the condition. Beta-blocker therapy should not be withdrawn abruptly (particularly in patients with CAD), but gradually tapered to avoid acute tachycardia, hypertension, and/or ischemia. Use caution with concurrent use of beta-blockers, either verapamil or diltiazem, or digoxin; bradycardia or heart block can occur. Bradycardia may be observed more frequently in elderly patients (>65 years of age); dosage reductions may be necessary.

May precipitate or aggravate symptoms of arterial insufficiency in patients with peripheral vascular disease (PVD) and Raynaud's disease; use with caution; monitor for progression of arterial obstruction. In general, beta-blockers should be avoided in patients with bronchospastic disease. Betaxolol, with beta$_1$ selectivity, may be used cautiously in bronchospastic disease with the lowest possible dose (eg, 5-10 mg/day), availability of a bronchodilator, and close monitoring; if dosage increase is indicated, administer in divided doses. Use cautiously in patients with diabetes because it may potentiate and/or mask prominent hypoglycemic symptoms. May mask signs of hyperthyroidism (eg, tachycardia); use caution if hyperthyroidism is suspected, abrupt withdrawal may precipitate thyroid storm. May induce or exacerbate psoriasis. Use with caution in patients with cerebrovascular insufficiency; hypotension and decreased heart rate may reduce cerebral blood flow. Dosage adjustment required in severe renal impairment and in patients on dialysis. Use care with anesthetic agents which decrease myocardial function. Use with caution in patients with myasthenia gravis (may potentiate myasthenia-related muscle weakness, including diplopia and ptosis) or psychiatric disease (may cause CNS depression). Adequate alpha-blockade is required prior to use of any beta-blocker for patients with untreated pheochromocytoma. Use caution with history of severe anaphylaxis to allergens; patients taking beta-blockers may become more sensitive to repeated challenges. Treatment of anaphylaxis (eg, epinephrine) in patients taking beta-blockers may be ineffective or promote undesirable effects. Safety and efficacy of the oral formulation have not been established in children.

Drug Interactions

Metabolism/Transport Effects Substrate (major) of CYP1A2, 2D6; **Inhibits** CYP2D6 (weak)

Avoid Concomitant Use

Avoid concomitant use of Betaxolol (Systemic) with any of the following: Methacholine

Decreased Effect

Betaxolol (Systemic) may decrease the levels/effects of: Beta2-Agonists; Theophylline Derivatives

The levels/effects of Betaxolol (Systemic) may be decreased by: Barbiturates; CYP1A2 Inducers (Strong); Herbs (Hypertensive Properties); Methylphenidate; Nonsteroidal Anti-Inflammatory Agents; Peginterferon Alfa-2b; Rifamycin Derivatives; Yohimbine

Increased Effect/Toxicity

Betaxolol (Systemic) may increase the levels/effects of: Alpha-/Beta-Agonists (Direct-Acting); Alpha1-Blockers; Alpha2-Agonists; Amifostine; Antihypertensives; Antipsychotic Agents (Phenothiazines); Bupivacaine; Cardiac Glycosides; Fingolimod; Hypotensive Agents; Insulin; Lidocaine; Lidocaine (Systemic); Lidocaine (Topical); Mepivacaine; Methacholine; Midodrine; RiTUXimab; Sulfonylureas

The levels/effects of Betaxolol (Systemic) may be increased by: Acetylcholinesterase Inhibitors; Aminoquinolines (Antimalarial); Amiodarone; Anilidopiperidine Opioids; Antipsychotic Agents (Phenothiazines); Calcium Channel Blockers (Nondihydropyridine); CYP1A2 Inhibitors (Moderate); CYP1A2 Inhibitors (Strong); Diazoxide; Dipyridamole; Disopyramide; Dronedarone; Herbs (Hypotensive Properties); MAO Inhibitors; Pentoxifylline; Phosphodiesterase 5 Inhibitors; Propafenone; Propoxyphene; Prostacyclin Analogues; QuiNIDine; Reserpine

Nutritional/Ethanol Interactions Herb/Nutraceutical: Avoid bayberry; blue cohosh, cayenne, ephedra, ginger, ginseng (American), gotu kola, and licorice (may worsen hypertension). Avoid black cohosh, California poppy, coleus, golden seal, hawthorn, mistletoe, periwinkle, quinine, shepherd's purse (may have increased antihypertensive effects).

Lab Interactions Oral betaxolol may interfere with glaucoma screening tests.

Adverse Reactions 2% to 10%:

Cardiovascular: Bradycardia (6% to 8%; symptomatic bradycardia: <1% to 2%; dose-dependent), chest pain (2% to 7%), palpitation (2%), edema (≤2%; similar to placebo)

Central nervous system: Fatigue (3% to 10%), insomnia (1% to 5%), lethargy (3%)

Gastrointestinal: Nausea (2% to 6%), dyspepsia (4% to 5%), diarrhea (2%)

Neuromuscular & skeletal: Arthralgia (3% to 5%), paresthesia (2%)

Respiratory: Dyspnea (2%), pharyngitis (2%)
Miscellaneous: Antinuclear antibody positive (5%), cold extremities (2%)

Pharmacodynamics/Kinetics

Onset of Action 1-1.5 hours
Absorption ~100%
Bioavailability 89%
Time to Peak 1.5-6 hours
Protein Binding ~50%
Half-Life Elimination 14-22 hours; prolonged in hepatic disease and/or chronic renal failure
Metabolism Hepatic to multiple metabolites
Excretion Urine (>80%, as unchanged drug [15%] and inactive metabolites)

Available Dosage Forms

Tablet, oral: 10 mg, 20 mg
Kerlone®: 10 mg, 20 mg

Dosing

Adult Hypertension (labeled use), coronary artery disease (unlabeled use): Oral: 5-10 mg/day; may increase dose to 20 mg/day after 7-14 days if desired response is not achieved

Geriatric Hypertension: Oral: Refer to adult dosing. Initial: 5 mg/day.

Renal Impairment

Severe impairment: Initial dose: 5 mg/day; may increase every 2 weeks up to a maximum of 20 mg/day.

Hemodialysis: Initial dose: 5 mg/day; may increase every 2 weeks up to a maximum of 20 mg/day. Supplemental dose not required.

Administration

Oral Absorption is not affected by food.

Stability

Storage Avoid freezing. Store tablets at room temperature of 15°C to 25°C (59°F to 77°F).

Monitoring and Teaching Issues

Laboratory Monitoring Baseline renal function

Physical Assessment Advise patients with diabetes to monitor glucose levels closely; beta-blockers may alter glucose tolerance. Taper dosage slowly when discontinuing.

Patient Education May cause dizziness, fatigue, nausea, or vomiting. If you have diabetes, monitor serum sugar closely; drug may alter glucose tolerance or mask signs of hypoglycemia. Report chest pain, palpitations, or irregular heartbeat; persistent GI upset (eg, nausea, vomiting, diarrhea); unusual cough; respiratory difficulty; swelling or coolness of extremities; or depression.

Geriatric Considerations Due to alterations in the beta-adrenergic autonomic nervous system, beta-adrenergic blockade may result in less hemodynamic response than seen in younger adults. Studies indicate that despite decreased sensitivity to the chronotropic effects of beta-blockade with age, there appears to be an increased myocardial sensitivity to the negative inotropic effect during stress (ie, exercise). Controlled trials have shown the overall response rate for propranolol to be only 20% to 50% in elderly populations. Therefore, all beta-adrenergic blocking drugs may result in a decreased response as compared to younger adults.

Breast-Feeding Considerations Betaxolol is excreted into breast milk in amounts which may have a pharmacologic effect in the nursing infant. The manufacturer recommends that caution be exercised when administering betaxolol to nursing women.

Pregnancy Considerations Teratogenic were effects were not observed in animal reproduction studies; therefore, the manufacturer classifies betaxolol as pregnancy category C. Betaxolol crosses the placenta and can be detected in the amniotic fluid as well as umbilical cord blood. Measurable concentrations of betaxolol can also be found in the newborn blood and urine. In a cohort study, an increased risk of cardiovascular defects was observed following maternal use of beta-blockers during pregnancy. Intrauterine growth restriction (IUGR), small placentas, as well as fetal/neonatal bradycardia, hypoglycemia, and/or respiratory depression have been observed following *in utero* exposure to beta-blockers as a class. Following maternal use of betaxolol, the beta-blocker effects may persist in the neonate for several days after birth. Adequate facilities for monitoring infants at birth should be available. Untreated chronic maternal hypertension and pre-eclampsia are also associated with adverse events in the fetus, infant, and mother. The half-life and serum concentration of betaxolol immediately postpartum are not significantly different than what is observed in nonpregnant women. Betaxolol is currently not recommended for the initial treatment of hypertension in pregnancy.

Related Information

Beta-Blockers *on page 1990*

◆ **Betaxolol Hydrochloride** *see* Betaxolol (Systemic) *on page 208*

Bethanechol (be THAN e kole)

U.S. Brand Names Urecholine®
Index Terms Bethanechol Chloride
Generic Availability (U.S.) Yes
Pharmacologic Category Cholinergic Agonist

Medication Safety Issues

Sound-alike/look-alike issues:

Bethanechol may be confused with betaxolol

Pregnancy Risk Factor C

Lactation Excretion in breast milk unknown/not recommended

Use Treatment of acute postoperative and postpartum nonobstructive (functional) urinary retention; treatment of neurogenic atony of the urinary bladder with retention

Unlabeled/Investigational Use Gastroesophageal reflux

Available Dosage Forms

Tablet, oral: 5 mg, 10 mg, 25 mg, 50 mg

Urecholine®: 5 mg, 10 mg, 25 mg, 50 mg

Dosing

Adult

Urinary retention, neurogenic bladder: Oral: Initial: 10-50 mg 3-4 times/day (some patients may require dosages of 50-100 mg 4 times/day). To determine effective dose, may initiate at a dose of 5-10 mg, with additional doses of 5-10 mg hourly until an effective cumulative dose is reached. Cholinergic effects at higher oral dosages may be cumulative.

Gastroesophageal reflux (unlabeled): Oral: 25 mg 4 times/day

Geriatric Refer to adult dosing. Use the lowest effective dose.

Pediatric

Urinary retention (unlabeled use): Oral: 0.3-0.6 mg/kg/day in 3-4 divided doses

Gastroesophageal reflux (unlabeled use): Oral: 0.3-0.6 mg/kg/day in 3-4 divided doses

Administration

Oral Should be administered 1 hour before meals or 2 hours after meals.

Monitoring and Teaching Issues

Physical Assessment Assess bladder and sphincter adequacy prior to administering medication.

Patient Education Take on an empty stomach to avoid nausea or vomiting. Maintain adequate hydration, unless instructed to restrict fluid intake. May cause dizziness, hypotension, vomiting, or loss of appetite. Report persistent abdominal discomfort; significantly increased salivation, sweating, tearing, or urination; flushed skin; chest pain or palpitations; acute headache; unresolved diarrhea; excessive fatigue, insomnia, dizziness, or depression; increased muscle, joint, or body pain; vision changes or blurred vision; or respiratory difficulty or wheezing.

◆ **Bethanechol Chloride** *see* Bethanechol *on page 210*

◆ **Betimol®** *see* Timolol (Ophthalmic) *on page 1763*

Bevacizumab (be vuh SIZ uh mab)

U.S. Brand Names Avastin®

Index Terms Anti-VEGF Monoclonal Antibody; Anti-VEGF rhuMAb; rhuMAb-VEGF

Generic Availability (U.S.) No

Pharmacologic Category Antineoplastic Agent, Monoclonal Antibody; Vascular Endothelial Growth Factor (VEGF) Inhibitor

Medication Safety Issues

Sound-alike/look-alike issues:

Avastin® may be confused with Astelin®

Bevacizumab may be confused with cetuximab, riTUXimab

International issues:

Avastin [U.S., Canada, and multiple international markets] may be confused with Avaxim, a brand name for hepatitis A vaccine [Canada and multiple international markets]

High alert medication: This medication is in a class the Institute for Safe Medication Practices (ISMP) includes among its list of drug classes which have a heightened risk of causing significant patient harm when used in error.

Pregnancy Risk Factor C

Lactation Excretion in breast milk unknown/not recommended

Use Treatment of metastatic colorectal cancer; treatment of unresectable, locally advanced, recurrent or metastatic nonsquamous, nonsmall cell lung cancer; treatment of metastatic HER-2 negative breast cancer (who have not received chemotherapy for metastatic disease); treatment of progressive glioblastoma; treatment of metastatic renal cell cancer (not an approved use in Canada)

Note: For the treatment of metastatic breast cancer, effectiveness is based on improvement in progression-free survival; not indicated for the treatment of breast cancer with metastatic disease that has progressed following anthracycline and taxane treatment. For the treatment of glioblastoma, effectiveness is based on improvement in objective response rate.

Unlabeled/Investigational Use Treatment of recurrent ovarian cancer, recurrent cervical cancer, soft tissue sarcomas (angiosarcoma or hemangiopericytoma/solitary fibrous tumor), age-related macular degeneration (AMD)

Mechanism of Action/Effect Bevacizumab is a monoclonal antibody which binds to (and neutralizes) vascular endothelial growth factor (VEGF), preventing its association with endothelial receptors, Flt-1 and KDR. It blocks the formation of new blood vessels which in turn may slow the growth of all tissues (including metastatic tissue).

Contraindications There are no contraindications listed in the FDA-approved manufacturer's labeling.

Canadian labeling: Hypersensitivity to bevacizumab, any component of the formulation, Chinese hamster ovary cell products or other recombinant human or humanized antibodies; untreated CNS metastases

Warnings/Precautions [U.S. Boxed Warning]: Gastrointestinal perforation, fistula (including gastrointestinal, enterocutaneous, esophageal, duodenal, and rectal fistulas), intra-abdominal abscess, and wound dehiscence/wound healing complications have been reported in patients receiving bevacizumab for colorectal cancer and other cancers (not related to treatment duration). Most cases occur within 50 days of treatment initiation; may be fatal in some cases; monitor patients for signs/symptoms (eg, fever, abdominal pain with constipation and/or nausea/vomiting). Permanently discontinue in patients who develop these complications. Nongastrointestinal fistula formation (including tracheoesophageal, bronchopleural, biliary, vaginal, renal, and bladder fistulas) has been observed, most commonly within the first 6 months of treatment; permanently discontinue in patients who develop internal organ fistulas. The appropriate intervals between administration of bevacizumab and surgical procedures to avoid impairment in wound healing has not been established. Therapy should not be initiated within 28 days of major surgery and only following complete healing of the incision. Bevacizumab should be discontinued at least 28 days prior to elective surgery.

Bevacizumab is associated with an increased risk for arterial thromboembolic events (ATE), including cerebral infarction, stroke, MI, TIA, angina, and other ATEs, when used in combination with chemotherapy. History of ATE or ≥65 years of age may present an even greater risk; permanently discontinue with serious ATE; the safety of treatment reinitiation after ATE has not been studied. Although patients with cancer are at risk for venous thromboembolism (VTE), a meta-analysis of 15 controlled trials has demonstrated an increased risk for VTE in patients who received bevacizumab (Nalluri, 2008). Discontinue therapy in patients with severe arteriothrombotic event or life-threatening pulmonary embolism.

Use with caution in patients with cardiovascular disease. Among all approved indications, the incidence of heart failure (HF) and/or left ventricular dysfunction, is higher in patients receiving bevacizumab plus chemotherapy when compared to chemotherapy alone. Bevacizumab may potentiate the cardiotoxic effects of anthracyclines. HF is more common with prior anthracycline exposure and/or left chest wall irradiation. The safety of therapy resumption or continuation in patients with cardiac dysfunction has not been studied. In studies of patients with metastatic breast cancer, the incidence of grades 3 or 4 HF was increased in patients receiving bevacizumab plus paclitaxel, compared to the control arm. Patients with metastatic breast cancer who had received prior anthracycline therapy had a higher rate of HF compared to those receiving paclitaxel alone (3.8% vs 0.6% respectively). A meta-analysis of 5 studies which enrolled patients with metastatic breast cancer who received bevacizumab suggested an association with an increased risk of heart failure; all trials included in the analysis enrolled patients who either received prior or were receiving concurrent anthracycline therapy (Choueiri, 2011).

Bevacizumab may cause and/or worsen hypertension significantly; use caution in patients with pre-existing hypertension and monitor BP closely in all patients. Permanent discontinuation is recommended in patients who experience a hypertensive crisis or encephalopathy. Temporarily discontinue in patients who develop uncontrolled hypertension. Cases of reversible posterior leukoencephalopathy syndrome (RPLS) have been reported. Symptoms (which include headache, seizure, confusion, lethargy, blindness and/or other vision, or neurologic disturbances) may occur from 16 hours to 1 year after treatment initiation. Resolution of symptoms usually occurs within days after discontinuation; however, neurologic sequelae may remain. RPLS may be associated with hypertension; discontinue bevacizumab and begin management of hypertension, if present.

[U.S. Boxed Warning]: Severe or fatal hemorrhage, including hemoptysis, gastrointestinal bleeding, central nervous system hemorrhage, epistaxis, and vaginal bleeding have been observed. Avoid use in patients with serious hemorrhage or recent hemoptysis (≥2.5 mL blood). Serious pulmonary hemorrhage has been reported in patients receiving bevacizumab (primarily in patients with nonsmall cell lung cancer with squamous cell histology [not an FDA-approved indication]). Intracranial hemorrhage, including cases of grade 3 or 4 hemorrhage, has occurred in patients with previously treated glioblastoma. Treatment discontinuation is recommended in all patients with intracranial or other serious hemorrhage. Use with caution in patients with CNS metastases; once case of CNS hemorrhage was observed in an ongoing study of NSCLC patients with CNS metastases. Use in patients with CNS metastases is contraindicated in the Canadian labeling. Use with caution in patients at risk for thrombocytopenia.

Infusion reactions (eg, hypertension, hypertensive crisis, wheezing, oxygen desaturation, hypersensitivity [including anaphylactic/anaphylactoid reactions], chest pain, rigors, headache, diaphoresis) may occur with the first infusion (uncommon); interrupt therapy in patients experiencing severe infusion reactions; there are no data to address routine premedication use or reinstitution of therapy in patients who experience severe infusion reactions. Proteinuria and/or nephrotic syndrome have been associated with bevacizumab; risk may be increased in patients with a history of hypertension; thrombotic microangiopathy has been associated with bevacizumab-induced proteinuria. Withhold treatment for ≥2 g proteinuria/24 hours and resume when proteinuria is <2 g/24 hours; discontinue in patients with nephrotic syndrome. Elderly patients (≥65 years of age) are at higher risk for adverse events, including thromboembolic events and proteinuria; serious adverse events occurring more frequently in the elderly also include deep thrombophlebitis, sepsis, hyper-/hypotension, MI, CHF, leukopenia, anemia, dehydration, hypokalemia, and hyponatremia. Microangiopathic hemolytic anemia (MAHA) has been reported when bevacizumab has been used in combination with sunitinib. Concurrent therapy with sunitinib and bevacizumab is also associated with dose-limiting hypertension in patients with metastatic renal cell cancer. The incidence of hand-foot syndrome is increased in patients treated with bevacizumab plus sorafenib in comparison to those treated with sorafenib monotherapy. When used in combination with myelosuppressive chemotherapy, increased rates of severe or febrile neutropenia and neutropenic infection were reported. Bevacizumab, in combination with chemotherapy (or biologic therapy), is associated with an increased risk of treatment-related mortality; a higher risk of fatal adverse events was identified in a meta-analysis of 16 trials in which bevacizumab was used for the treatment of various cancers (breast cancer, colorectal cancer, non small cell lung cancer, pancreatic cancer, prostate cancer, and renal cell cancer) and compared to chemotherapy alone (Ranpora, 2011). When bevacizumab is used in combination with myelosuppressive chemotherapy, increased rates of severe or febrile neutropenia and neutropenic infection have been reported.

Drug Interactions

Avoid Concomitant Use

Avoid concomitant use of Bevacizumab with any of the following: SUNItinib

Decreased Effect There are no known significant interactions involving a decrease in effect.

Increased Effect/Toxicity

Bevacizumab may increase the levels/effects of: Antineoplastic Agents (Anthracycline); Irinotecan; SORAfenib; SUNItinib

The levels/effects of Bevacizumab may be increased by: SUNItinib

Adverse Reactions Percentages reported as monotherapy and as part of combination chemotherapy regimens. Some studies only reported hematologic toxicities grades ≥4 and non-hematologic toxicities grades ≥3.

>10%:

Cardiovascular: Hypertension (23% to 67%; grades 3/4: 5% to 18%), thromboembolic event (≤21%; grades 3/4: 15%; venous thrombus/embolus: 8%; grades 3/4: 5% to 7%; arterial thrombosis 6%; grades 3/4: 3%), hypotension (7% to 15%)

Central nervous system: Pain (31% to 62%), headache (24% to 37%; grades 3/4: 2% to 4%), dizziness (19% to 26%), fatigue (≤45%; grades 3/4: 4% to 19%), sensory neuropathy (grades 3/4: 1% to 17%; in combination with paclitaxel: 24%)

Dermatologic: Alopecia (6% to 32%), dry skin (7% to 20%), exfoliative dermatitis (3% to 19%), skin discoloration (2% to 16%)

Endocrine & metabolic: Hypokalemia (12% to 16%)

Gastrointestinal: Abdominal pain (50% to 61%; grades 3/4: 8%), vomiting (47% to 52%; grades 3/4: 6% to 11%), anorexia (35% to 43%), constipation (29% to 40%), diarrhea (grades 3/4: 1% to 34%), stomatitis (25% to 32%), gastrointestinal hemorrhage (19% to 24%), dyspepsia (17% to 24%), taste disorder (14% to 21%), flatulence (11% to 19%), weight loss (9% to 20%), nausea (grades 3/4: 4% to 12%)

Hematologic: Hemorrhage (≤40%; grades 3/4: 1% to 5%), leukopenia (grades 3/4: 37%), neutropenia (grade 4: 6% to 27%)

Neuromuscular & skeletal: Weakness (57% to 74%), myalgia (8% to 19%), back pain (≤12%)

Ocular: Tearing increased (6% to 18%)

Renal: Proteinuria (4% to 36%; grades 3/4: ≤7%; median onset: 5.6 months; median time to resolution: 6.1 months)

Respiratory: Upper respiratory infection (40% to 47%), epistaxis (16% to 35%), dyspnea (25% to 26%), rhinitis

Miscellaneous: Infection (≤55%; serious: 9% to 14%; pneumonia, catheter, or wound infections)

1% to 10%:

Cardiovascular: DVT (6% to 9%; grades 3/4: 9%), HF (grades 3/4: 1% to 4%), syncope (grades 3/4: 3%), intra-abdominal venous thrombosis (grades 3/4: 3%), cardio-/cerebrovascular arterial thrombotic event (2% to 4%), left ventricular dysfunction (grades 3/4: 1%)

Central nervous system: Confusion (1% to 6%), abnormal gait (1% to 5%); CNS hemorrhage (1% to 5%; grades 3/4: 1%), reversible posterior leukoencephalopathy syndrome ([RPLS] ≤1%)

Dermatologic: Nail disorder (2% to 8%), skin ulcer (≤6%), rash desquamation (grades 3/4: 3%), wound dehiscence (1% to 6%), acne (≤1%)

Endocrine & metabolic: Dehydration (grades 3/4: 3% to 10%), hyponatremia (grades 3/4: 4%)

Gastrointestinal: Xerostomia (4% to 7%), colitis (1% to 6%), ileus (grades 3/4: 4% to 5%), gingival bleeding (2% to 4%), fistula (1%), gastrointestinal perforation (≤4%), gastroesophageal reflux (≤2%), gingivitis (≤2%), mouth ulceration (≤2%), tooth abscess (≤2%), intra-abdominal abscess (1%), gastritis (≤1%), gingival pain (≤1%)

Genitourinary: Polyuria/urgency (3% to 6%), vaginal hemorrhage (4%)

Hematologic: Neutropenic fever/infection (5%; grades 3 and/or 4: 4% to 5%), thrombocytopenia (5%)

Hepatic: Bilirubinemia (1% to 6%)

Neuromuscular & skeletal: Bone pain (grades 3/4: 4%), neuropathy (other than sensory: grades 3/4: 1% to 5%)

Ocular: Blurred vision (≤2%)

Otic: Tinnitus (≤2%), deafness (≤1%)

Respiratory: Voice alteration (5% to 9%), pneumonitis/pulmonary infiltrates (grades 3/4: 5%), hemoptysis (nonsquamous histology 2%), pulmonary embolism (≤1%)

Miscellaneous: Infusion reactions (<3%)

Pharmacodynamics/Kinetics

Half-Life Elimination ~20 days (range: 11-50 days)

Excretion Clearance: 2.75-5 mL/kg/day

Available Dosage Forms

Injection, solution [preservative free]:

Avastin®: 25 mg/mL (4 mL, 16 mL)

Dosing

Adult & Geriatric Details concerning dosing in combination regimens should also be consulted.

Breast cancer, metastatic: I.V.: 10 mg/kg every 2 weeks (in combination with paclitaxel)

Colorectal cancer, metastatic: I.V.: 5 or 10 mg/kg every 2 weeks (in combination with fluorouracil-based chemotherapy)

Canadian labeling: 5 mg/kg every 2 weeks (in combination with fluorouracil-based chemotherapy)

Glioblastoma: 10 mg/kg every 2 weeks as monotherapy **or** in combination (unlabeled) with irinotecan (Vredenburgh, 2007)

Nonsmall cell lung cancer (nonsquamous cell histology): I.V.: 15 mg/kg every 3 weeks (in combination with carboplatin and paclitaxel) for 4-6 cycles followed by maintenance treatment (unlabeled use) of bevacizumab 15 mg/kg every 3 weeks as monotherapy until disease progression or unacceptable toxicity (Sandler, 2006)

Renal cell cancer, metastatic: 10 mg/kg every 2 weeks in combination with interferon alfa **or** (unlabeled) as monotherapy (Yang, 2003)

Age-related macular degeneration (unlabeled use): Intravitreal: 1.25 mg (0.05 mL) monthly until improvement/resolution, usually ~1-3 injections (Avery, 2006) or 2.5 mg (0.1 mL) every 4 weeks for 3 doses (Bashshur, 2006)

Ovarian cancer (unlabeled use): I.V.: 15 mg/kg every 3 weeks (Burger, 2007; Cannistra, 2007)

Adjustment for Toxicity I.V. administration (systemic): There are no recommended dosage reductions. Temporary suspension is recommended for severe infusion reactions, at least 4 weeks prior to elective surgery, in moderate-to-severe proteinuria (in most studies, treatment was withheld for ≥2 g proteinuria/24 hours), or in patients with severe hypertension which is not controlled with medical management. Permanent discontinuation is recommended (by the manufacturer) in patients who develop wound dehiscence requiring intervention, fistula (gastrointestinal and nongastrointestinal), gastrointestinal perforation, intra-abdominal abscess, hypertensive crisis, hypertensive encephalopathy, serious bleeding/hemorrhage, severe arterial thromboembolic event, nephrotic syndrome, or RPLS.

Administration

I.V.

I.V. infusion, usually after the other antineoplastic agents. Infuse the initial dose over 90 minutes. Infusion may be shortened to 60 minutes if the initial infusion is well tolerated. The third and subsequent infusions may be shortened to 30 minutes if the 60-minute infusion is well tolerated. Some institutions use a 10-minute infusion (0.5 mg/kg/minute) for bevacizumab dosed at 5 mg/kg (after tolerance at the 90-, 60-, and 30-minute infusion rates has been established; Reidy, 2007). Do not administer I.V. push.

Intravitreal injection (unlabeled use): Adequate anesthesia and a broad-spectrum antimicrobial agent should be administered prior to the procedure; administer topical antibiotics for 3 days after procedure.

Stability

Reconstitution Prior to infusion, dilute prescribed dose of bevacizumab in a total volume of 100 mL NS. Do not mix with dextrose-containing solutions.

Storage Store vials at 2°C to 8°C (36°F to 46°F); do not freeze. Protect from light; do not shake. Diluted solutions are stable for up to 8 hours under refrigeration. Discard unused portion of vial.

Monitoring and Teaching Issues

Laboratory Monitoring CBC with differential; urinalysis

Physical Assessment Assess patient for recent abdominal surgery, arterial thromboembolism, cardiovascular disease, hemoptysis, and CNS metastases prior to beginning treatment. Patient must be monitored closely during each infusion for infusion reaction (eg, hypertension, chest pain, wheezing, diaphoresis). In event of infusion reaction, infusion should be discontinued and patient assessed. Monitor for gastrointestinal perforation (abdominal pain, constipation, vomiting), serious bleeding, arterial thrombotic event, nephrotic syndrome, encephalopathy, and heart failure.

Patient Education This medication can only be administered by infusion; you will be closely monitored during infusion. Report immediately unusual back or abdominal pain; acute headache; difficulty breathing or chest tightness; difficulty swallowing; itching or rash; or redness, swelling, or pain at infusion site. Between treatments, maintain adequate nutrition and hydration, unless instructed to restrict fluid intake. You may experience loss of appetite, nausea, dry mouth, taste changes, loss of hair (will grow back when therapy is completed), or muscle or skeletal pain. Report immediately any unusual bleeding (blood in urine or tarry stool, nose bleeds, vaginal bleeding, bleeding from wound); abdominal pain, vomiting, constipation, or diarrhea; acute headache, dizziness, or confusion; seizure, vision changes, or unusual lethargy; changes in urinary pattern; pain, redness, swelling, or sudden loss of sensation in extremities; skin rash or hives; or unusual infection (fever or chills, cough, sore throat, pain or difficulty passing urine).

Geriatric Considerations Elderly patients ≥65 years of age had an increased incidence of arterial thromboembolic events; an increased risk for proteinuria; other serious adverse events occurring often include weakness, sepsis, hyper-/hypotension, CHF, constipation, anorexia, anemia, hyper-/hypokalemia, and diarrhea.

Breast-Feeding Considerations Immunoglobulins are excreted in breast milk, and it is assumed that bevacizumab may appear in breast milk. Due to concerns for effects on the infant, breast-feeding is not recommended. The half-life of bevacizumab is up to 50 days (average 20 days), and this should be considered when decisions are made concerning breast-feeding resumption.

Note: Canadian labeling recommends to discontinue breast-feeding during treatment and to avoid breast-feeding a minimum of 6 months following discontinuation of treatment.

Pregnancy Considerations There are no adequate or well-controlled studies in pregnant women; however, bevacizumab is teratogenic in animals. Angiogenesis is of critical importance to fetal development, and bevacizumab inhibits angiogenesis. Adequate contraception during therapy is recommended (and for ≥6 months following last dose of bevacizumab). Patients should also be counseled regarding prolonged exposure following discontinuation of therapy due to the long half-life of bevacizumab.

Based on animal studies, bevacizumab may disrupt normal menstrual cycles and impair fertility by several effects, including reduced endometrial proliferation and follicular developmental arrest. Some parameters do not recover completely, or recover very slowly following discontinuation.

Bexarotene (Systemic) (beks AIR oh teen)

U.S. Brand Names Targretin®

Generic Availability (U.S.) No

Pharmacologic Category Antineoplastic Agent, Miscellaneous

Medication Safety Issues

High alert medication: The Institute for Safe Medication Practices (ISMP) includes this medication among its list of drugs which have a heightened risk of causing significant patient harm when used in error.

Pregnancy Risk Factor X

Lactation Excretion in breast milk unknown/not recommended

Use Treatment of cutaneous manifestations of cutaneous T-cell lymphoma in patients who are refractory to at least one prior systemic therapy

Mechanism of Action/Effect Exact mechanism in is unknown. Acts to inhibit the growth of some tumor cell lines of hematopoietic and squamous cell origin.

Contraindications Hypersensitivity to bexarotene or any component of the formulation; pregnancy

Warnings/Precautions Hazardous agent - use appropriate precautions for handling and disposal. **[U.S. Boxed Warning]: Bexarotene is a retinoid, a drug class associated with birth defects in humans; do not administer during pregnancy.** Pregnancy test needed 1 week before initiation and every month thereafter. Effective contraception must be in place 1 month before initiation, during therapy, and for at least 1 month after discontinuation. Male patients with sexual partners who are pregnant, possibly pregnant, or who could become pregnant, must use condoms during sexual intercourse during treatment and for 1 month after last dose. Induces significant lipid abnormalities in a majority of patients (triglyceride, total cholesterol, and HDL); reversible on discontinuation. Use extreme caution in patients with underlying hypertriglyceridemia. Pancreatitis secondary to hypertriglyceridemia has been reported. Patients with risk factors for pancreatitis (eg, prior pancreatitis, uncontrolled hyperlipidemia, excess ethanol consumption, uncontrolled diabetes, biliary tract disease) should generally not receive bexarotene (oral). Monitor for liver function test abnormalities and discontinue drug if tests are three times the upper limit of normal values for AST, ALT, or bilirubin. Hypothyroidism occurs in about a third of patients. Monitor for signs and symptoms of infection about 4-8 weeks after initiation (leukopenia may occur). Any new visual abnormalities experienced by the patient should be evaluated by an ophthalmologist (cataracts can form, or worsen, especially in the geriatric population). May cause photosensitization. Safety and efficacy are not established in the pediatric population. Use only with extreme caution in patients with hepatic impairment. Limit additional vitamin A intake to <15,000 int. units/day. Use caution with diabetic patients.

Drug Interactions

Metabolism/Transport Effects Substrate of CYP3A4 (minor); **Induces** CYP3A4 (weak)

Avoid Concomitant Use

Avoid concomitant use of Bexarotene (Systemic) with any of the following: Tetracycline Derivatives; Vitamin A

Decreased Effect

Bexarotene (Systemic) may decrease the levels/effects of: Contraceptives (Estrogens); Contraceptives (Progestins); Saxagliptin

Increased Effect/Toxicity

Bexarotene (Systemic) may increase the levels/effects of: Vitamin A

The levels/effects of Bexarotene (Systemic) may be increased by: Conivaptan; Tetracycline Derivatives

Nutritional/Ethanol Interactions

Food: Bioavailability is increased when administered with a fat-containing meal. Bexarotene serum levels may be increased by grapefruit juice; avoid concurrent use.

Herb/Nutraceutical: Avoid dong quai, St John's wort (may also cause photosensitization). St John's wort may decrease bexarotene levels. Additional vitamin A supplements may lead to vitamin A toxicity (dry skin, irritation, arthralgias, myalgias, abdominal pain, hepatic changes).

Adverse Reactions First percentage is at a dose of 300 mg/m²/day; the second percentage is at a dose >300 mg/m²/day.

>10%:

Cardiovascular: Peripheral edema (13% to 11%)

Central nervous system: Headache (30% to 42%), chills (10% to 13%)

Dermatologic: Rash (17% to 23%), exfoliative dermatitis (10% to 28%)

Endocrine & metabolic: Hyperlipidemia (about 79% in both dosing ranges), hypercholesteremia (32% to 62%), hypothyroidism (29% to 53%)

Hematologic: Leukopenia (17% to 47%)

Neuromuscular & skeletal: Weakness (20% to 45%)

Miscellaneous: Infection (13% to 23%)

<10%:

Cardiovascular: Hemorrhage, hypertension, angina pectoris, right heart failure, tachycardia, cerebrovascular accident

Central nervous system: Fever (5% to 17%), insomnia (5% to 11%), subdural hematoma, syncope, depression, agitation, ataxia, confusion, dizziness, hyperesthesia

Dermatologic: Dry skin (about 10% for both dosing ranges), alopecia (4% to 11%), skin ulceration, acne, skin nodule, maculopapular rash, serous drainage, vesicular bullous rash, cheilitis

Endocrine & metabolic: Hypoproteinemia, hyperglycemia, weight loss/gain, breast pain

Gastrointestinal: Abdominal pain (11% to 4%), nausea (16% to 8%), diarrhea (7% to 42%), vomiting (4% to 13%), anorexia (2% to 23%), constipation, xerostomia, flatulence, colitis, dyspepsia, gastroenteritis, gingivitis, melena, pancreatitis, serum amylase increased

Genitourinary: Albuminuria, hematuria, urinary incontinence, urinary tract infection, urinary urgency, dysuria, kidney function abnormality

Hematologic: Hypochromic anemia (4% to 13%), anemia (6% to 25%), eosinophilia, thrombocythemia, coagulation time increased, lymphocytosis, thrombocytopenia

Hepatic: LDH increase (7% to 13%), hepatic failure

Neuromuscular & skeletal: Back pain (2% to 11%), arthralgia, myalgia, bone pain, myasthenia, arthrosis, neuropathy

Ocular: Dry eyes, conjunctivitis, blepharitis, corneal lesion, visual field defects, keratitis

Otic: Ear pain, otitis externa

Renal: Creatinine increased

Respiratory: Pharyngitis, rhinitis, dyspnea, pleural effusion, bronchitis, cough increased, lung edema, hemoptysis, hypoxia

Miscellaneous: Flu-like syndrome (4% to 13%), bacterial infection (1% to 13%)

Pharmacodynamics/Kinetics

Absorption Significantly improved by a fat-containing meal

Time to Peak ~2 hours

Protein Binding >99%

Half-Life Elimination ~7 hours

Metabolism Hepatic via CYP3A4 isoenzyme; four metabolites identified; further metabolized by glucuronidation

Excretion Primarily feces; urine (<1% as unchanged drug and metabolites)

Available Dosage Forms

Capsule, oral:

Targretin®: 75 mg

Dosing

Adult & Geriatric Cutaneous T-cell lymphoma: Oral: 300-400 mg/m²/day taken as a single daily dose.

Renal Impairment No studies have been conducted; however, renal insufficiency may result in significant protein binding changes and alter pharmacokinetics of bexarotene.

Hepatic Impairment No studies have been conducted; however, hepatic impairment would be expected to result in decreased clearance of bexarotene due to the extensive hepatic contribution to elimination.

Administration

Oral Administer capsule following a fat-containing meal.

Stability

Storage Store at 2°C to 25°C (36°F to 77°F). Protect from light.

Monitoring and Teaching Issues

Laboratory Monitoring If female, pregnancy test 1 week before initiation then monthly while on bexarotene; lipid panel before initiation, then weekly until lipid response established and then at 8-week intervals thereafter; baseline LFTs, repeat at 1, 2, and 4 weeks after initiation then at 8-week intervals thereafter if stable; baseline and periodic thyroid function tests; baseline CBC with periodic monitoring

Physical Assessment Assess pregnancy status, lipid panel, LFTs, thyroid function, and CBC prior to and during therapy. Monitor for CNS or cardiovascular effects, opportunistic infection, visual abnormalities, and hypoglycemia.

Patient Education It is preferable to take capsules after a fat-containing meal. Maintain adequate hydration, unless instructed to restrict fluid intake. Avoid grapefruit juice, St John's wort, or additional vitamin A supplements while using this medication. You may be more susceptible to infection. May cause nausea, vomiting, anorexia, flatulence, constipation, diarrhea, headache, back or muscle pain, or photosensitivity. Report chest pain, rapid heartbeat; unresolved GI effects, headache, back or muscle pain, skin dryness, skin rash or peeling, mucous membrane lesions, altered urinary patterns, flu syndrome or opportunistic infection (eg, weakness, fatigue, white plaques or sores in mouth, vaginal discharge, chills, fever), CNS disturbances (insomnia, dizziness, agitation, confusion, depression), or vision or hearing changes.

Dietary Considerations It is preferable to take the oral capsule following a fat-containing meal. Avoid grapefruit juice.

Breast-Feeding Considerations It is not known if bexarotene is excreted into breast milk. Due to the potential for serious adverse reactions in a nursing infant, the decision to continue or discontinue breast-feeding during therapy should take into account the risk of exposure to the infant and the benefits of treatment to the mother.

Pregnancy Considerations [U.S. Boxed Warning]: Bexarotene is a retinoid, a drug class associated with birth defects in humans; do not administer during pregnancy. Bexarotene caused birth defects when administered orally to pregnant rats. It must not be given to a pregnant woman or a woman who intends to become pregnant. If a woman becomes pregnant while taking the drug, it must be stopped immediately and appropriate counseling be given. In women of childbearing potential, therapy should be started on the second or third day of a normal menstrual period. Either abstinence or two forms of reliable contraception (one should be nonhormonal) must be used for at least 1 month before initiating therapy, during therapy, and for 1 month following discontinuation of bexarotene. A negative pregnancy test (sensitivity of at least 50 mIU/mL) within 1 week prior to beginning therapy, and monthly thereafter is required for women of childbearing potential. Male patients must use a condom during any sexual contact with women of childbearing age during therapy, and for 1 month following discontinuation of bexarotene.

Bexarotene (Topical) (beks AIR oh teen)

U.S. Brand Names Targretin®

Generic Availability (U.S.) No

Pharmacologic Category Antineoplastic Agent, Miscellaneous

Medication Safety Issues

High alert medication: The Institute for Safe Medication Practices (ISMP) includes this medication among its list of drugs which have a heightened risk of causing significant patient harm when used in error.

Pregnancy Risk Factor X

Lactation Excretion in breast milk unknown/not recommended

Use Treatment of cutaneous lesions in patients with refractory cutaneous T-cell lymphoma (stage 1A and 1B) or who have not tolerated other therapies

Available Dosage Forms

Gel, topical:

Targretin®: 1% (60 g)

Dosing

Adult & Geriatric Cutaneous lesions of T-cell lymphoma: Topical: Apply to lesions once every other day for first week, then increase on a weekly basis to once daily, 2 times/day, 3 times/day, and finally 4 times/day, according to tolerance.

Renal Impairment No studies have been conducted; however, renal insufficiency may result in significant protein binding changes and alter pharmacokinetics of bexarotene.

Hepatic Impairment No studies have been conducted; however, hepatic impairment would be expected to result in decreased clearance of bexarotene due to the extensive hepatic contribution to elimination.

Administration

Topical Allow gel to dry before covering with clothing. Avoid application to normal skin. Use of occlusive dressings is not recommended.

Monitoring and Teaching Issues

Laboratory Monitoring If female, pregnancy test 1 week before initiation then monthly while on bexarotene; lipid panel before initiation, then weekly until lipid response established and then at 8-week intervals thereafter; baseline LFTs, repeat at 1, 2, and 4 weeks after initiation then at 8-week intervals thereafter if stable; baseline and periodic thyroid function tests; baseline CBC with periodic monitoring

Patient Education Avoid applying to normal skin or mucous membranes. Do not use occlusive dressings.

◆ **Beyaz™** *see* Ethinyl Estradiol, Drospirenone, and Levomefolate *on page 706*

◆ **BG 9273** *see* Alefacept *on page 65*

◆ **Biaxin®** *see* Clarithromycin *on page 391*

◆ **Biaxin® XL** *see* Clarithromycin *on page 391*

Bicalutamide (bye ka LOO ta mide)

U.S. Brand Names Casodex®

Index Terms CDX; ICI-176334

Generic Availability (U.S.) Yes

Pharmacologic Category Antineoplastic Agent, Antiandrogen

Medication Safety Issues

Sound-alike/look-alike issues:

Casodex® may be confused with Kapidex™ [DSC]

International issues:
Casodex [U.S., Canada, and multiple international markets] may be confused with Capadex brand name for propoxyphene/acetaminophen [Australia, New Zealand]

Pregnancy Risk Factor X

Lactation Excretion in breast milk unknown/contraindicated

Use Treatment of metastatic prostate cancer (in combination with an LHRH agonist)

Unlabeled/Investigational Use Monotherapy for locally-advanced prostate cancer

Mechanism of Action/Effect Androgen receptor inhibitor; nonsteroidal antiandrogen that inhibits androgen uptake or inhibits binding of androgen in target tissues

Contraindications Hypersensitivity to bicalutamide or any component of the formulation; use in women, especially women who are or may become pregnant

Warnings/Precautions Hazardous agent - use appropriate precautions for handling and disposal. Rare cases of death or hospitalization due to hepatitis have been reported post-marketing. Use with caution in moderate-to-severe hepatic dysfunction. Hepatotoxicity generally occurs within the first 3-4 months of use; patients should be monitored for signs and symptoms of liver dysfunction. Bicalutamide should be discontinued if patients have jaundice or ALT is >2 times the upper limit of normal. Androgen-deprivation therapy may increase the risk for cardiovascular disease (Levine, 2010). May cause gynecomastia, breast pain, or lead to spermatogenesis inhibition. When used in combination with LHRH agonists, a loss of glycemic control and decrease in glucose tolerance has been reported in patients with diabetes; monitor. May cause gynecomastia or breast pain (at higher, unlabeled doses), or lead to spermatogenesis inhibition.

Drug Interactions

Avoid Concomitant Use

Avoid concomitant use of Bicalutamide with any of the following: Tolvaptan

Decreased Effect There are no known significant interactions involving a decrease in effect.

Increased Effect/Toxicity

Bicalutamide may increase the levels/effects of: Colchicine; CYP3A4 Substrates; Eplerenone; Everolimus; FentaNYL; Halofantrine; Lurasidone; Pimecrolimus; Ranolazine; Salmeterol; Saxagliptin; Tolvaptan; Vilazodone; Vitamin K Antagonists

Adverse Reactions Adverse reaction percentages reported as part of combination regimen with an LHRH analogue unless otherwise noted.

>10%:

Cardiovascular: Peripheral edema (13%)
Central nervous system: Pain (35%)
Endocrine & metabolic: Hot flashes (53%), breast pain (6%; monotherapy [150 mg]: 39% to 85%), gynecomastia (9%; monotherapy [150 mg]: 38% to 73%)
Gastrointestinal: Constipation (22%), nausea (15%), diarrhea (12%), abdominal pain (11%)
Genitourinary: Pelvic pain (21%), hematuria (12%), nocturia (12%)
Hematologic: Anemia (11%)
Neuromuscular & skeletal: Back pain (25%), weakness (22%)
Respiratory: Dyspnea (13%)
Miscellaneous: Infection (18%)

≥2% to 10%:

Cardiovascular: Chest pain (8%), hypertension (8%), angina pectoris (2% to <5%), cardiac arrest (2% to <5%), CHF (2% to <5%), edema (2% to <5%), MI (2% to <5%), coronary artery disorder (2% to <5%), syncope (2% to <5%)
Central nervous system: Dizziness (10%), headache (7%), insomnia (7%), anxiety (5%), depression (4%), chills (2% to <5%), confusion (2% to <5%), fever (2% to <5%), nervousness (2% to <5%), somnolence (2% to <5%)
Dermatologic: Rash (9%), alopecia (2% to <5%), dry skin (2% to <5%), pruritus (2% to <5%), skin carcinoma (2% to <5%)
Endocrine & metabolic: Hyperglycemia (6%), dehydration (2% to <5%), gout (2% to <5%), hypercholesterolemia (2% to <5%), libido decreased (2% to <5%)
Gastrointestinal: Dyspepsia (7%), weight loss (7%), anorexia (6%), flatulence (6%), vomiting (6%), weight gain (5%), dysphagia (2% to <5%), gastrointestinal carcinoma (2% to <5%), melena (2% to <5%), periodontal abscess (2% to <5%), rectal hemorrhage (2% to <5%), xerostomia (2% to <5%)
Genitourinary: Urinary tract infection (9%), impotence (7%), polyuria (6%), urinary retention (5%), urinary impairment (5%), urinary incontinence (4%), dysuria (2% to <5%), urinary urgency (2% to <5%)
Hepatic: LFTs increased (7%), alkaline phosphatase increased (5%)
Neuromuscular & skeletal: Bone pain (9%), paresthesia (8%), myasthenia (7%), arthritis (5%), pathological fracture (4%), hypertonia (2% to <5%), leg cramps (2% to <5%), myalgia (2% to <5%), neck pain (2% to <5%), neuropathy (2% to <5%)
Ocular: Cataract (2% to <5%)
Renal: BUN increased (2% to <5%), creatinine increased (2% to <5%), hydronephrosis (2% to <5%)
Respiratory: Cough (8%), pharyngitis (8%), bronchitis (6%), pneumonia (4%), rhinitis (4%), asthma (2% to <5%), epistaxis (2% to <5%), sinusitis (2% to <5%)
Miscellaneous: Flu-like syndrome (7%), diaphoresis (6%), cyst (2% to <5%), hernia (2% to <5%), herpes zoster (2% to <5%), sepsis (2% to <5%)

Pharmacodynamics/Kinetics

Absorption Rapid and complete; unaffected by food

Time to Peak Active enantiomer: ~31 hours

Protein Binding 96%

Half-Life Elimination Active enantiomer: ~6 days, ~10 days in severe liver disease

Metabolism Extensively hepatic; glucuronidation and oxidation of the R (active) enantiomer to inactive metabolites; the S enantiomer is inactive

Excretion Urine (36%, as inactive metabolites); feces (42%, as unchanged drug and inactive metabolites)

Available Dosage Forms

Tablet, oral: 50 mg

Casodex®: 50 mg

Dosing

Adult & Geriatric

Prostate cancer, metastatic: Oral: 50 mg once daily (in combination with an LHRH analogue)

Prostate cancer, locally-advanced (unlabeled use): Oral: 150 mg once daily (as monotherapy) (McLeod, 2006)

Renal Impairment No adjustment required

Hepatic Impairment No adjustment required for mild, moderate, or severe hepatic impairment; use caution with moderate-to-severe impairment. Discontinue if ALT >2 times ULN or patient develops jaundice.

Administration

Oral Dose should be taken at the same time each day with or without food. Treatment for metastatic cancer should be started concomitantly with an LHRH analogue.

Stability

Storage Store at room temperature of 20°C to 25°C (68°F to 77°F).

Monitoring and Teaching Issues

Laboratory Monitoring Liver function tests should be obtained at baseline and repeated regularly during the first 4 months of treatment, and periodically thereafter (in addition to monitoring signs/symptoms of liver dysfunction). Discontinue if jaundice is noted or ALT is >2 times the upper limit of normal. Periodically monitor CBC, ECG, echocardiograms, serum testosterone, luteinizing hormone, and prostate specific antigen (PSA). Monitor blood glucose in patients with diabetes. If initiating bicalutamide in patients who are on warfarin, closely monitor prothrombin time.

Physical Assessment Use caution in presence of hepatic impairment. Assess results of LFTs at baseline and periodically throughout. Advise patients with diabetes to monitor glucose levels closely (may induce hyperglycemia). Teach patient absolute need for barrier contraceptives.

Patient Education Take at the same time each day, with or without food. If you have diabetes, monitor serum glucose closely and notify prescriber of changes (this medication may alter glucose levels). May cause back, breast, or pelvic pain; hot flashes; dizziness, confusion, or drowsiness; nausea or vomiting; constipation; hair loss; impotence; or gynecomastia. Report unusual weight gain or swelling of extremities; easy bruising or bleeding; yellowing of skin or eyes; change in color of urine or stool; unresolved CNS changes (eg, nervousness, chills, insomnia, somnolence); skin rash, redness, or irritation; chest pain or palpitations; respiratory difficulty; urinary retention or inability to void; muscle weakness, tremors, or pain; or persistent gastrointestinal upset.

Dietary Considerations May be taken with or without food.

Geriatric Considerations Renal impairment has no clinically-significant changes in elimination of the parent compound or active metabolite; therefore, no dosage adjustment is needed in the elderly. In dosage studies, no difference was found between young adults and elderly with regard to steady-state serum concentrations for bicalutamide and its active R-enantiomer metabolite.

Breast-Feeding Considerations Bicalutamide is not indicated for use in women.

Pregnancy Considerations Animal studies have demonstrated teratogenicity. Bicalutamide use is contraindicated in women. Androgen receptor inhibition during pregnancy may affect fetal development.

◆ **Bicillin® L-A** *see* Penicillin G Benzathine *on page* 1432
◆ **Bicitra** *see* Sodium Citrate and Citric Acid *on page* 1660
◆ **BiCNU®** *see* Carmustine *on page* 302
◆ **Bidex®-400 [OTC]** *see* GuaiFENesin *on page* 890
◆ **Bidhist [DSC]** *see* Brompheniramine *on page* 234

Bimatoprost (bi MAT oh prost)

U.S. Brand Names Latisse®; Lumigan®

Generic Availability (U.S.) No

Pharmacologic Category Ophthalmic Agent, Antiglaucoma; Ophthalmic Agent, Miscellaneous; Prostaglandin, Ophthalmic

Pregnancy Risk Factor C

Lactation Excretion in breast milk unknown/use caution

Use Reduction of intraocular pressure (IOP) in patients with open-angle glaucoma or ocular hypertension; hypotrichosis treatment of the eyelashes

Mechanism of Action/Effect Decreases intraocular pressure by increasing outflow of aqueous humor. Increases the percent and duration of hairs in the growth phase, resulting in eyelash growth.

Contraindications

Latisse®: Hypersensitivity to bimatoprost or any component of the formulation

Lumigan®: There are no contraindications listed in the manufacturer's prescribing information.

Warnings/Precautions May cause permanent changes in eye color (increases the amount of brown pigment in the iris), the eyelid skin, and eyelashes. In addition, may increase the length and/or number of eyelashes (may vary between eyes). Use caution in patients with intraocular inflammation, aphakic patients, pseudophakic patients with a torn posterior lens capsule, or patients with risk factors for macular edema. Contains benzalkonium chloride (may be adsorbed by contact lenses). Safety and efficacy have not been determined for use in patients with angle-closure, inflammatory, or neovascular glaucoma. Not recommended for use in pediatrics <16 years of age due to potential concerns regarding long-term use and hyperpigmentation.

Latisse®: Additional warnings: Patients receiving medications to reduce intraocular pressure should consult their healthcare provider prior to using; may interfere with desired reduction of intraocular pressure. Unintentional hair growth may occur on skin that has repeated contact with solution; apply to upper eyelid only, blot away excess.

Drug Interactions

Avoid Concomitant Use There are no known interactions where it is recommended to avoid concomitant use.

Decreased Effect There are no known significant interactions involving a decrease in effect.

Increased Effect/Toxicity

The levels/effects of Bimatoprost may be increased by: Latanoprost

Adverse Reactions Adverse reactions and percentages are for Lumigan® unless noted:

>10%: Ocular: Conjunctival hyperemia (25% to 45%; Latisse®: <4%), growth of eyelashes, ocular pruritus (Latisse®: <4%)

1% to 10%:

Central nervous system: Headache (1% to 5%)

Dermatologic: Skin hyperpigmentation (Latisse®: <4%), abnormal hair growth

Hepatic: Liver function tests abnormal (1% to 5%)

Neuromuscular & skeletal: Weakness (1% to 5%)

Ocular: Dryness (Latisse®: <4%), erythema of the eyelid (Latisse®: <4%), irritation (Latisse®: <4%), allergic conjunctivitis, asthenopia, blepharitis, burning, cataract, conjunctival edema, conjunctival hemorrhage, discharge, eyelash darkening, foreign body sensation, iris pigmentation increased (may be delayed), pain, photophobia, pigmentation of periocular skin, superficial punctate keratitis, tearing, visual disturbance

Miscellaneous: Infections (10%; primarily colds and upper respiratory tract infections)

Pharmacodynamics/Kinetics

Onset of Action Reduction of IOP: ~4 hours; Peak effect: Maximum reduction of IOP: ~8-12 hours

Time to Peak ≤10 minutes

Protein Binding ~88%

Half-Life Elimination I.V.: ≤45 minutes

Metabolism Undergoes oxidation, N-deethylation, and glucuronidation after reaching systemic circulation; forms metabolites

Excretion Urine (67%); feces (25%)

Available Dosage Forms

Solution, ophthalmic:

Latisse®: 0.03% (3 mL)

Lumigan®: 0.01% (2.5 mL, 5 mL, 7.5 mL); 0.03% (2.5 mL, 5 mL, 7.5 mL)

Dosing

Adult & Geriatric

Open-angle glaucoma or ocular hypertension: Ophthalmic: Instill 1 drop into affected eye(s) once daily in the evening; do not exceed once-daily dosing (may decrease IOP-lowering effect). If used with other topical ophthalmic agents, separate administration by at least 5 minutes.

Hypotrichosis of the eyelashes: Ophthalmic, topical: Place one drop on applicator and apply evenly along the skin of the upper eyelid at base of eyelashes once daily at bedtime; repeat procedure for second eye (use a clean applicator).

Administration

Other

Latisse®: Remove make-up and contact lenses prior to application; ensure face is clean. Apply with the sterile applicator provided only; do not use other brushes or applicators. Use a tissue or cloth to blot any excess solution on the outside of the upper eyelid margin; do not apply to lower eyelash line. Do not reuse applicators; use new applicator for second eye. Applying more than once nightly will not increase eyelash growth; eyelash growth is expected to return to baseline when therapy is discontinued. May reinsert contacts 15 minutes after application.

Lumigan®: May be used with other eye drops to lower intraocular pressure. If using more than one ophthalmic product, wait at least 5 minutes in between application of each medication. Remove contact lenses prior to administration and wait 15 minutes before reinserting.

Stability

Storage Store between 2°C to 25°C (36°F to 77°F).

Monitoring and Teaching Issues

Patient Education For use in eyes only. Wash hands before instilling. Sit or lie down to instill. Open eye, look at ceiling, and instill prescribed amount of solution. Apply gentle pressure to inner corner of eye. Do not let tip of applicator touch eye; do not contaminate tip of applicator (may cause eye infection, eye damage, or vision loss). Contact prescriber concerning continued use of drops if eye infection develops, trauma occurs to the eye, and prior to eye surgery. This product contains benzalkonium chloride which may be adsorbed by contact lenses; remove contacts prior to administration and wait 15 minutes before reinserting. May cause permanent changes in eye color, eyelid, and eyelashes. May also increase the length and/or number of eyelashes. Changes may occur slowly (months to years). May be used with other eye drops to lower intraocular pressure. If using more than one eye drop medicine, wait at least 5 minutes in between application of each medication. Notify prescriber if conjunctivitis or eyelid reactions occur with use of this product.

Geriatric Considerations Evaluate patient's ability to self-administer eye drops

Pregnancy Considerations Decreased gestation, decreased body weight, increased late resorptions, and increased mortality were observed in animal studies with oral doses achieving serum levels >33 times human exposure. There are no adequate and well-controlled studies in pregnant women.

Additional Information The IOP-lowering effect was shown to be 7-8 mm Hg in clinical studies.

◆ **Bird Flu Vaccine** *see* Influenza Virus Vaccine (H5N1) *on page 977*

◆ **Bisacodyl and Polyethylene Glycol-Electrolyte Solution** *see* Polyethylene Glycol-Electrolyte Solution and Bisacodyl *on page 1475*

◆ **bis-chloronitrosourea** *see* Carmustine *on page 302*

◆ **Bismatrol** *see* Bismuth *on page 221*

◆ **Bismatrol [OTC]** *see* Bismuth *on page 221*

◆ **Bismatrol Maximum Strength [OTC]** *see* Bismuth *on page 221*

Bismuth (BIZ muth)

U.S. Brand Names Bismatrol Maximum Strength [OTC]; Bismatrol [OTC]; Diotame [OTC]; Kao-Tin [OTC]; Kaopectate® Extra Strength [OTC]; Kaopectate® [OTC]; Maalox® Total Relief® [OTC] [DSC]; Peptic Relief [OTC]; Pepto Relief [OTC]; Pepto-Bismol® Maximum Strength [OTC]; Pepto-Bismol® [OTC]

Index Terms Bismatrol; Bismuth Subsalicylate; Pink Bismuth

Generic Availability (U.S.) Yes

Pharmacologic Category Antidiarrheal

Medication Safety Issues

Sound-alike/look-alike issues:

Kaopectate® may be confused with Kayexalate®

Maalox® Total Relief® is a different formulation than other Maalox® liquid antacid products which contain aluminum hydroxide, magnesium hydroxide, and simethicone.

Note: Canadian formulation of Kaopectate® does not contain bismuth; the active ingredient in the Canadian formulation is attapulgite.

Pregnancy Risk Factor C/D (3rd trimester)

Lactation Excretion in breast milk unknown (salicylates enter breast milk)/use caution

Use Subsalicylate formulation: Symptomatic treatment of mild, nonspecific diarrhea; control of traveler's diarrhea (enterotoxigenic *Escherichia coli*); as part of a multidrug regimen for *H. pylori* eradication to reduce the risk of duodenal ulcer recurrence

Available Dosage Forms For available OTC formulations, consult specific product labeling.

Dosing

Adult & Geriatric

Treatment of nonspecific diarrhea, control/relieve traveler's diarrhea: Subsalicylate: Oral: 524 mg every 30 minutes to 1 hour as needed up to 8 doses/24 hours

***Helicobacter pylori* eradication:** Oral: Subsalicylate: 524 mg 4 times/day with meals and at bedtime; requires combination therapy

Pediatric

Nonspecific diarrhea, control/relieve traveler's diarrhea: Subsalicylate: Oral: Children >12 years: Refer to adult dosing.

Renal Impairment Bismuth has been associated with nephrotoxicity in overdose (Leussnik, 2002); although there are no specific recommendations by the manufacturer, consider using with caution in patients with renal impairment.

Administration

Oral Liquids must be shaken prior to use. Chewable tablets should be chewed thoroughly. Nonchewable caplets should be swallowed whole with a full glass of water.

Monitoring and Teaching Issues

Physical Assessment Assess patient allergy history prior to beginning treatment (contains ASA). Assess other drugs patient may be taking for potential interactions (eg, aspirin products). Monitor for CNS changes, impactions, and tinnitus.

Patient Education Chew tablet well or shake suspension well before using. Maintain adequate fluid intake to prevent dehydration unless instructed to restrict fluid intake. May darken stools and turn tongue black. If diarrhea persists for more than 2 days, consult healthcare provider. If tinnitus (ringing in the ears) occurs, this may indicate toxicity; discontinue use and notify healthcare provider.

Related Information

Helicobacter pylori Treatment *on page* 2045

◆ **Bismuth Subsalicylate** *see* Bismuth *on page* 221

Bisoprolol (bis OH proe lol)

U.S. Brand Names Zebeta®

Index Terms Bisoprolol Fumarate

Generic Availability (U.S.) Yes

Pharmacologic Category Beta Blocker, Beta-1 Selective

Medication Safety Issues

Sound-alike/look-alike issues:

Zebeta® may be confused with DiaBeta®, Zetia®

Pregnancy Risk Factor C

Lactation Excretion unknown/use caution

Use Treatment of hypertension, alone or in combination with other agents

Unlabeled/Investigational Use Chronic stable angina, supraventricular arrhythmias, PVCs, heart failure (HF)

Mechanism of Action/Effect Selective inhibitor of $beta_1$-adrenergic receptors; competitively blocks $beta_1$-receptors, with little or no effect on $beta_2$-receptors at doses ≤20 mg

Contraindications Cardiogenic shock; overt cardiac failure; marked sinus bradycardia; heart block greater than first-degree (except in patients with a functioning artificial pacemaker)

Warnings/Precautions Consider pre-existing conditions such as sick sinus syndrome before initiating. Use caution in patients with heart failure; use gradual and careful titration; monitor for symptoms of congestive heart failure. Use with caution in patients with myasthenia gravis, psychiatric disease (may cause CNS depression), bronchospastic disease, undergoing anesthesia; and in those with impaired hepatic function. Beta-blocker therapy should not be withdrawn abruptly (particularly in patients with CAD), but gradually tapered to avoid acute tachycardia, hypertension, and/or ischemia. Use caution in patients with PVD (can aggravate arterial insufficiency). Use caution with concurrent use of verapamil or diltiazem; bradycardia or heart block may occur. Bisoprolol, with $beta_1$-selectivity, may be used cautiously in bronchospastic disease with close monitoring. Use cautiously in patients with diabetes because it can mask prominent hypoglycemic symptoms. Use caution in hyperthyroidism since beta-blockade may mask signs of thyrotoxicosis. Dosage adjustment is required in patients with significant hepatic or renal dysfunction. Use care with anesthetic agents which decrease myocardial function. Adequate alpha-blockade is required prior to use of any beta-blocker for patients with untreated pheochromocytoma. May induce or exacerbate psoriasis. Use caution with history of severe anaphylaxis to allergens; patients taking beta-blockers may become more sensitive to repeated challenges. Treatment of anaphylaxis (eg, epinephrine) in patients taking beta-blockers may be ineffective or promote undesirable effects.

Drug Interactions

Metabolism/Transport Effects Substrate of CYP2D6 (minor), 3A4 (major)

Avoid Concomitant Use

Avoid concomitant use of Bisoprolol with any of the following: Methacholine

Decreased Effect

Bisoprolol may decrease the levels/effects of: Beta2-Agonists; Theophylline Derivatives

The levels/effects of Bisoprolol may be decreased by: Barbiturates; CYP3A4 Inducers (Strong); Deferasirox; Herbs (CYP3A4 Inducers); Herbs (Hypertensive Properties); Methylphenidate; Nonsteroidal Anti-Inflammatory Agents; Peginterferon Alfa-2b; Rifamycin Derivatives; Yohimbine

Increased Effect/Toxicity

Bisoprolol may increase the levels/effects of: Alpha-/Beta-Agonists (Direct-Acting); Alpha1-Blockers; Alpha2-Agonists; Amifostine; Antihypertensives; Antipsychotic Agents (Phenothiazines); Bupivacaine; Cardiac Glycosides; Fingolimod; Hypotensive Agents; Insulin; Lidocaine; Lidocaine (Systemic); Lidocaine (Topical); Mepivacaine; Methacholine; Midodrine; RiTUXimab; Sulfonylureas

The levels/effects of Bisoprolol may be increased by: Acetylcholinesterase Inhibitors; Aminoquinolines (Antimalarial); Amiodarone; Anilidopiperidine Opioids; Antipsychotic Agents (Phenothiazines); Calcium Channel Blockers (Nondihydropyridine); Conivaptan; CYP3A4 Inhibitors (Moderate); CYP3A4 Inhibitors (Strong); Dasatinib; Diazoxide; Dipyridamole; Disopyramide; Dronedarone; Herbs (Hypotensive Properties); MAO Inhibitors; Pentoxifylline; Phosphodiesterase 5 Inhibitors; Propafenone; Propoxyphene; Prostacyclin Analogues; QuiNIDine; Reserpine

Nutritional/Ethanol Interactions Herb/Nutraceutical: Avoid dong quai if using for hypertension (has estrogenic activity). Avoid ephedra, yohimbe, ginseng (may worsen hypertension). Avoid garlic (may have increased antihypertensive effect).

Adverse Reactions 1% to 10%:

Cardiovascular: Chest pain (1% to 2%)

Central nervous system: Fatigue (dose related; 6% to 8%), insomnia (2% to 3%), hypoesthesia (1% to 2%)

Gastrointestinal: Diarrhea (dose related; 3% to 4%), nausea (2%), vomiting (1% to 2%)

Neuromuscular & skeletal: Arthralgia, asthenia (dose related; ≤2%)

Respiratory: Upper respiratory infection (5%), rhinitis (3% to 4%), sinusitis (dose related; 2%), dyspnea (1% to 2%)

Pharmacodynamics/Kinetics

Onset of Action 1-2 hours

Absorption Rapid and almost complete

Bioavailability ~80%

Time to Peak 2-4 hours

Protein Binding ~30%

Half-Life Elimination Normal renal function: 9-12 hours; Cl_{cr} <40 mL/minute: 27-36 hours; Hepatic cirrhosis: 8-22 hours

Metabolism Extensively hepatic; significant first-pass effect (~20%)

Excretion Urine (50% as unchanged drug, remainder as inactive metabolites); feces (<2%)

Available Dosage Forms

Tablet, oral: 5 mg, 10 mg
Zebeta®: 5 mg, 10 mg

Dosing

Adult

Hypertension: Oral: 2.5-5 mg once daily; may be increased to 10 mg and then up to 20 mg once daily, if necessary; usual dose range (JNC 7): 2.5-10 mg once daily

HF (unlabeled use): Initial: 1.25 mg once daily; maximum recommended dose: 10 mg once daily. **Note:** Increase dose gradually and monitor for signs and symptoms of CHF.

Geriatric Oral: Initial: 2.5 mg/day; may be increased by 2.5-5 mg/day; maximum recommended dose: 20 mg/day

Renal Impairment
Cl_{cr} <40 mL/minute: Oral: Initial: 2.5 mg/day; increase cautiously
Not dialyzable

Administration

Oral May be administered without regard to meals.

Monitoring and Teaching Issues

Laboratory Monitoring Serum glucose regularly (if you have diabetes)

Physical Assessment Blood pressure and heart rate should be assessed prior to and following first dose and with any change in dosage. Taper dosage slowly when discontinuing. Advise patients with diabetes to monitor glucose levels closely; beta-blockers may alter glucose tolerance. Teach patient how to handle orthostatic hypotension.

Patient Education Take with or without food. Take pulse daily (prior to medication) and follow prescriber's instruction about holding medication. If you have diabetes, monitor serum sugar closely; drug may alter glucose tolerance or mask signs of hypoglycemia. May cause fatigue, dizziness, postural hypotension, alteration in sexual performance (reversible), or diarrhea. Report unresolved swelling of extremities, respiratory difficulty or new cough, unresolved fatigue, unusual weight gain, unresolved constipation, or unusual muscle weakness.

Dietary Considerations May be taken without regard to meals.

Geriatric Considerations Due to alterations in the beta-adrenergic autonomic nervous system, beta-adrenergic blockade may result in less hemodynamic response than seen in younger adults. Studies indicate that despite decreased sensitivity to the chronotropic effects of beta-blockade with age, there appears to be an increased myocardial sensitivity to the negative inotropic effect during stress (ie, exercise). Controlled trials have shown the overall response rate for propranolol to be only 20% to 50% in elderly populations. Therefore, all beta-adrenergic blocking drugs may result in a decreased response as compared to younger adults.

Breast-Feeding Considerations It is not known if bisoprolol is excreted into breast milk. The manufacturer recommends that caution be exercised when administering bisoprolol to nursing women.

Pregnancy Considerations Adverse events were observed in animal reproduction studies; therefore, the manufacturer classifies bisoprolol as pregnancy category C. In a cohort study, an increased risk of cardiovascular defects was observed following maternal use of beta-blockers during pregnancy. Intrauterine growth restriction (IUGR), small placentas, as well as fetal/neonatal bradycardia, hypoglycemia, and/or respiratory depression have been observed following *in utero* exposure to beta-blockers as a class. Adequate facilities for monitoring infants at birth should be available. Untreated chronic maternal hypertension and pre-eclampsia are also associated with adverse events in the fetus, infant, and mother. Limited information is available related to the use of bisoprolol for the treatment of hypertension in pregnancy; other agents may be more appropriate for use.

Related Information

Beta-Blockers *on page 1990*
Heart Failure (Systolic) *on page 2040*

Bisoprolol and Hydrochlorothiazide

(bis OH proe lol & hye droe klor oh THYE a zide)

U.S. Brand Names Ziac®

Index Terms Bisoprolol Fumarate and Hydrochlorothiazide; Hydrochlorothiazide and Bisoprolol

Generic Availability (U.S.) Yes

Pharmacologic Category Beta Blocker, Beta-1 Selective; Diuretic, Thiazide

Medication Safety Issues

Sound-alike/look-alike issues:
Ziac® may be confused with Tiazac®, Zerit®

Pregnancy Risk Factor C

Lactation Enters breast milk/not recommended

Use Treatment of hypertension

Unlabeled/Investigational Use Treatment of hypertension in the pediatric patient

Available Dosage Forms

Tablet, oral: 2.5/6.25: Bisoprolol 2.5 mg and hydrochlorothiazide 6.25 mg; 5/6.25: Bisoprolol 5 mg and hydrochlorothiazide 6.25 mg; 10/6.25: Bisoprolol 10 mg and hydrochlorothiazide 6.25 mg

Ziac®: 2.5/6.25: Bisoprolol 2.5 mg and hydrochlorothiazide 6.25 mg; 5/6.25: Bisoprolol 5 mg and hydrochlorothiazide 6.25 mg; 10/6.25: Bisoprolol 10 mg and hydrochlorothiazide 6.25 mg

Dosing

Adult & Geriatric Hypertension: Oral: Initial: Bisoprolol 2.5 mg and hydrochlorothiazide 6.25 mg once daily; dose may be titrated at ≥2-week intervals. Maximum dose (manufacturer recommended): Bisoprolol 20 mg/hydrochlorothiazide 12.5 mg once daily

Add-on/replacement therapy: Bisoprolol 2.5-20 mg and hydrochlorothiazide 6.25-12.5 mg once daily

Pediatric

Hypertension (unlabeled use): Oral: Initial: Bisoprolol 2.5 mg/hydrochlorothiazide 6.25 mg once daily; up to a maximum of bisoprolol 10 mg/hydrochlorothiazide 6.25 mg daily

Renal Impairment Caution should be used in dosing/titrating patients with renal impairment. Discontinue use with progressive renal impairment; use is contraindicated in patients with anuria.

Hepatic Impairment Caution should be used in dosing/titrating patients. Dosage adjustment necessary with severe impairment. Specific dosing recommendations are not provided in manufacturer labeling.

Administration

Oral May be administered without regard to meals.

Monitoring and Teaching Issues

Physical Assessment See individual agents.

Patient Education See individual agents.

Related Information

Bisoprolol *on page 222*

Hydrochlorothiazide *on page 912*

◆ **Bisoprolol Fumarate** *see* Bisoprolol *on page 222*

◆ **Bisoprolol Fumarate and Hydrochlorothiazide** *see* Bisoprolol and Hydrochlorothiazide *on page 223*

◆ **Bis-POM PMEA** *see* Adefovir *on page 52*

◆ **Bivalent Human Papillomavirus Vaccine** *see* Papillomavirus (Types 16, 18) Vaccine (Human, Recombinant) *on page 1409*

◆ **Blenoxane** *see* Bleomycin *on page 224*

◆ **Bleo** *see* Bleomycin *on page 224*

Bleomycin (blee oh MYE sin)

Index Terms Blenoxane; Bleo; Bleomycin Sulfate; BLM

Generic Availability (U.S.) Yes

Pharmacologic Category Antineoplastic Agent, Antibiotic

Medication Safety Issues

Sound-alike/look-alike issues:

Bleomycin may be confused with Cleocin®

High alert medication: This medication is in a class the Institute for Safe Medication Practices (ISMP) includes among its list of drugs which have a heightened risk of causing significant patient harm when used in error.

Pregnancy Risk Factor D

Lactation Excretion in breast milk unknown/not recommended

Use Treatment of squamous cell carcinomas of the head and neck, penis, cervix, or vulva, testicular carcinoma, Hodgkin's lymphoma, and non-Hodgkin's lymphoma; sclerosing agent for malignant pleural effusion

Unlabeled/Investigational Use Treatment of ovarian germ cell tumors

Mechanism of Action/Effect Inhibits synthesis of DNA; also inhibits (to a lesser degree) RNA and protein synthesis

Contraindications Hypersensitivity to bleomycin or any component of the formulation

Warnings/Precautions Hazardous agent - use appropriate precautions for handling and disposal. **[U.S. Boxed Warning]: Occurrence of pulmonary fibrosis (commonly presenting as pneumonitis; occasionally progressing to pulmonary fibrosis) is the most severe toxicity. Risk is higher in elderly patients or patients receiving >400 units total lifetime dose;** other possible risk factors include smoking and patients with prior radiation therapy or receiving concurrent oxygen. **A severe idiosyncratic reaction consisting of hypotension, mental confusion, fever, chills, and wheezing (similar to anaphylaxis) has been reported in 1% of lymphoma patients treated with bleomycin.** Since these reactions usually occur after the first or second dose, careful monitoring is essential after these doses. Use caution when administering O_2 during surgery to patients who have received bleomycin; the risk of bleomycin-related pulmonary toxicity is increased. Use caution with renal impairment (Cl_{cr} <50 mL/minute), may require dose adjustment. May cause renal or hepatic toxicity. **[U.S. Boxed Warning]: Should be administered under the supervision of an experienced cancer chemotherapy physician.**

Drug Interactions

Avoid Concomitant Use

Avoid concomitant use of Bleomycin with any of the following: BCG; Natalizumab; Pimecrolimus; Roflumilast; Tacrolimus (Topical); Vaccines (Live)

Decreased Effect

Bleomycin may decrease the levels/effects of: BCG; Cardiac Glycosides; Sipuleucel-T; Vaccines (Inactivated); Vaccines (Live)

The levels/effects of Bleomycin may be decreased by: Echinacea

Increased Effect/Toxicity

Bleomycin may increase the levels/effects of: Leflunomide; Natalizumab; Vaccines (Live)

The levels/effects of Bleomycin may be increased by: Denosumab; Filgrastim; Gemcitabine; Pimecrolimus; Roflumilast; Sargramostim; Tacrolimus (Topical); Trastuzumab

Adverse Reactions

>10%:

Dermatologic: Pain at the tumor site, phlebitis. About 50% of patients develop erythema, rash, striae, induration, hyperkeratosis, vesiculation, and peeling of the skin, particularly on the palmar and plantar surfaces of the hands and feet. Hyperpigmentation (50%), alopecia, nailbed changes may also occur. These effects appear dose related and reversible with discontinuation.

Gastrointestinal: Stomatitis and mucositis (30%), anorexia, weight loss

Respiratory: Tachypnea, rales, acute or chronic interstitial pneumonitis, and pulmonary fibrosis (5% to 10%); hypoxia and death (1%). Symptoms include cough, dyspnea, and bilateral pulmonary infiltrates. The pathogenesis is not certain, but may be due to damage of pulmonary, vascular, or connective tissue. Response to steroid therapy is variable and somewhat controversial.

Miscellaneous: Acute febrile reactions (25% to 50%)

1% to 10%:

Dermatologic: Skin thickening, diffuse scleroderma, onycholysis, pruritus

Miscellaneous: Anaphylactoid-like reactions (characterized by hypotension, confusion, fever, chills, and wheezing; onset may be immediate or delayed for several hours); idiosyncratic reactions (1% in lymphoma patients)

Pharmacodynamics/Kinetics

Absorption I.M. and intrapleural administration: 30% to 50% of I.V. serum concentrations; intraperitoneal and SubQ routes produce serum concentrations equal to those of I.V.

Time to Peak Serum: I.M.: Within 30 minutes

Protein Binding 1%

Half-Life Elimination Biphasic: Renal function dependent:

Normal renal function: Initial: 1.3 hours; Terminal: 9 hours

End-stage renal disease: Initial: 2 hours; Terminal: 30 hours

Metabolism Via several tissues including hepatic, GI tract, skin, pulmonary, renal, and serum

Excretion Urine (50% to 70% as active drug)

Available Dosage Forms

Injection, powder for reconstitution: 15 units, 30 units

Dosing

Adult The risk for pulmonary toxicity increases with age >70 years and cumulative lifetime dose of >400 units; 1 unit = 1 mg; details concerning dosage in combination regimens should also be consulted.

Test dose for lymphoma patients: I.M., I.V., SubQ: Because of the possibility of an anaphylactoid reaction, the manufacturer recommends administering 1-2 units of bleomycin before the first 1-2 doses; monitor vital signs every 15 minutes; wait a minimum of 1 hour before administering remainder of dose; if no acute reaction occurs, then the regular dosage schedule may be followed. **Note:** Test doses may not be predictive of a reaction (Lam, 2005) and/or may produce false-negative results.

Hodgkin's lymphoma (unlabeled dosing; combination regimens): I.V.:

ABVD: 10 units/m^2 days 1 and 15 of a 28-day treatment cycle (Straus, 2004)

BEACOPP: 10 units/m^2 day 8 of a 21-day treatment cycle (Dann, 2007; Diehl, 2003)

Stanford V: 5 units/m^2/dose in weeks 2, 4, 6, 8, 10 and 12 (Horning, 2002; Horning, 2000)

Testicular cancer (unlabeled dosing; combination therapy): I.V.: 30 units/dose days 1, 8, and 15 of a 21-day treatment cycle for 4 cycles (Culine, 2008; Nichols, 1998)

Ovarian germ cell cancer (unlabeled use; combination therapy): I.V.: 30 units/dose days 1, 8, and 15 of a 21-day treatment cycle for 3 cycles (Williams, 1994) **or** 15 units/m^2 day 1 of a 21-day treatment cycle for 4 cycles (Cushing, 2004)

Malignant pleural effusion: Intrapleural: 60 units as a single instillation; mix in 50-100 mL of NS

Pediatric The risk for pulmonary toxicity increases with cumulative lifetime dose of >400 units; 1 unit = 1 mg; details concerning dosage in combination regimens should also be consulted.

Test dose for lymphoma patients: I.M., I.V., SubQ: Because of the possibility of an anaphylactoid reaction, the manufacturer recommends administering 1-2 units of bleomycin before the first 1-2 doses; monitor vital signs every 15 minutes; wait a minimum of 1 hour before administering remainder of dose; if no acute reaction occurs, then the regular dosage schedule may be followed. **Note:** Test doses may not be predictive of a reaction (Lam, 2005) and/or may produce false-negative results.

Hodgkin's Lymphoma (unlabeled dosing; combination regimen): I.V.: ABVD: I.V.: 10 units/m^2 days 1 and 15 of a 28-day treatment cycle (Hutchinson, 1998)

Renal Impairment

The FDA-approved labeling recommends the following adjustments:

Cl_{cr} >50 mL/minute: No adjustment required
Cl_{cr} 40-50 mL/minute: Administer 70% of normal dose
Cl_{cr} 30-40 mL/minute: Administer 60% of normal dose
Cl_{cr} 20-30 mL/minute: Administer 55% of normal dose
Cl_{cr} 10-20 mL/minute: Administer 45% of normal dose
Cl_{cr} 5-10 mL/minute: Administer 40% of normal dose

The following guidelines have been used by some clinicians:

Aronoff, 2007: Adults: Continuous renal replacement therapy (CRRT): Administer 75% of dose

Kintzel, 1995:

Cl_{cr} 46-60 mL/minute: Administer 70% of dose
Cl_{cr} 31-45 mL/minute: Administer 60% of dose
Cl_{cr} <30 mL/minute: Consider use of alternative drug

Hepatic Impairment Not studied in patients with hepatic impairment; adjustment for hepatic impairment may be needed.

Administration

I.M. May cause pain at injection site.

I.V. I.V. doses should be administered slowly over 10 minutes.

Other

Intrapleural: 60 units in 50-100 mL NS; use of topical anesthetics or narcotic analgesia is usually not necessary

SubQ: May cause pain at injection site.

Stability

Reconstitution For I.V. use, reconstitute 15-unit vial with 5 mL with NS and the 30-unit vial with 10 mL NS; for I.M. or SubQ use, reconstitute 15-unit vial with 1-5 mL of SWFI, BWFI, or NS and the 30-unit vial with 2-10 mL of SWFI, BWFI, or NS. For intrapleural use, mix in 50-100 mL of NS. Use appropriate precautions for handling and disposal.

Storage Refrigerate intact vials of powder. Intact vials are stable for up to 4 weeks at room temperature. Solutions reconstituted in NS for are stable for up to 28 days refrigerated and 14 days at room temperature; however, the manufacturer recommends stability of 24 hours in NS at room temperature.

Monitoring and Teaching Issues

Laboratory Monitoring Pulmonary function (total lung volume, forced vital capacity, carbon monoxide diffusion), renal function, chest x-ray, liver function

Physical Assessment Evaluate results of pulmonary function tests prior to and at regular intervals during treatment. Pulmonary status should be evaluated for fine rales prior to each treatment (may be the first symptom of pulmonary toxicity). Lymphoma patients should be closely monitored (vital signs every 15 minutes) for 1 hour following test dose before remainder of dose is administered (for first and second dose). Infusion or injection site must be monitored closely to avoid extravasation. Monitor pulmonary, renal, and hepatic function regularly during therapy.

Patient Education This medication can only be administered by injection or infusion; report immediately any redness, burning, pain, or swelling at injection/infusion site. May cause loss of appetite, nausea, or vomiting; mouth sores; fever or chills (will usually resolve); rash, redness, peeling, or increased color of skin; or loss of hair (reversible after cessation of therapy). Report any change in respiratory status; respiratory difficulty; wheezing; air hunger; increased secretions; difficulty expectorating secretions; confusion; unresolved fever or chills; sores in mouth; vaginal itching, burning, or discharge; sudden onset of dizziness; acute headache; or burning, stinging, redness, or swelling at injection site.

Geriatric Considerations Pulmonary toxicity has been reported more frequently in geriatric patients (>70 years of age).

Breast-Feeding Considerations Due to the potential for serious adverse reactions in the nursing infant, breast-feeding is not recommended.

Pregnancy Considerations Animal studies have demonstrated teratogenic and abortifacient effects. There are no adequate and well-controlled studies in pregnant women. Women of childbearing potential should avoid becoming pregnant during treatment.

- **Bleomycin Sulfate** *see* Bleomycin *on page 224*
- **BLM** *see* Bleomycin *on page 224*
- **BMS-188667** *see* Abatacept *on page 33*
- **BMS 337039** *see* Aripiprazole *on page 143*
- **B&O** *see* Belladonna and Opium *on page 194*
- **BOL-303224-A** *see* Besifloxacin *on page 204*
- **Bonine® [OTC]** *see* Meclizine *on page 1153*
- **Boniva®** *see* Ibandronate *on page 936*
- **Boostrix®** *see* Diphtheria and Tetanus Toxoids, and Acellular Pertussis Vaccine *on page 552*

Bortezomib (bore TEZ oh mib)

U.S. Brand Names Velcade®

Index Terms LDP-341; MLN341; PS-341

Generic Availability (U.S.) No

Pharmacologic Category Antineoplastic Agent; Proteasome Inhibitor

Medication Safety Issues

High alert medication: This medication is in a class the Institute for Safe Medication Practices (ISMP) includes among its list of drug classes which have a heightened risk of causing significant patient harm when used in error.

Pregnancy Risk Factor D

Lactation Excretion in breast milk unknown/not recommended

Use Treatment of multiple myeloma; treatment of relapsed or refractory mantle cell lymphoma

Unlabeled/Investigational Use Treatment of Waldenström's macroglobulinemia, peripheral T-cell lymphoma, cutaneous T-Cell lymphomas (mycosis fungoides), systemic light-chain amyloidosis

Mechanism of Action/Effect Reversibly inhibits enzyme complexes (proteosomes) which control intracellular protein homeostasis. Inhibition leads to cell death (apoptosis).

Contraindications Hypersensitivity to bortezomib, boron, mannitol, or any component of the formulation

Warnings/Precautions Hazardous agent - use appropriate precautions for handling and disposal. May cause peripheral neuropathy (usually sensory but may be mixed sensorimotor); risk may be increased with previous use of neurotoxic agents or pre-existing peripheral neuropathy; adjustment of dose and schedule may be required; in a study of elderly patients receiving bortezomib with combination chemotherapy, the incidence of peripheral neuropathy was significantly reduced (when administered weekly) without an effect on outcome (Boccadoro, 2010; Palumbo, 2009). May cause hypotension (including postural and orthostatic); use caution with dehydration, history of syncope, or medications associated with hypotension (may require adjustment of antihypertensive medication, hydration, and mineralocorticoids and/or sympathomimetics). Has been associated with the development or exacerbation of heart failure (HF) and decreased left ventricular ejection fraction; monitor closely in patients with risk factors for HF or existing heart disease. Has also been associated with QT_c prolongation.

Pulmonary disorders including pneumonitis, interstitial pneumonia, lung infiltrates, and acute respiratory distress syndrome (ARDS) have been reported. Pulmonary hypertension (without left heart failure or significant pulmonary disease has been reported rarely). May cause tumor lysis syndrome; risk is increased in patients with high tumor burden prior to treatment. Reversible posterior leukoencephalopathy syndrome (RPLS) has been reported (rarely). Promptly evaluate with new or worsening cardiopulmonary symptoms. Symptoms of RPLS include confusion, headache, hypertension, lethargy, seizure, blindness and/or other vision, or neurologic disturbances; discontinue bortezomib if RPLS occurs. MRI is recommended for RPLS diagnosis. The safety of reinitiating bortezomib in patients previously experiencing RPLS is unknown. Herpes (zoster and simplex) reactivation has been reported with bortezomib; consider antiviral prophylaxis during therapy. Hematologic toxicity, including neutropenia and severe thrombocytopenia, may occur; risk is increased in patients with pretreatment platelet counts <75,000/µL; frequent monitoring is required throughout treatment; may require dosage adjustments; withhold treatment for platelets <30,000/µL. Hemorrhage (gastrointestinal and intracerebral) due to low platelet count has been observed. Acute liver failure has been reported (rarely) in patients receiving multiple concomitant medications and with serious underlying conditions. Hepatitis, transaminase increases, and hyperbilirubinemia have also been reported; may be reversible when discontinued. Use caution in patients with hepatic dysfunction; reduced initial doses are recommended for moderate and severe hepatic impairment (exposure is increased); closely monitor for toxicities. Hyper- and hypoglycemia may occur in diabetic patients receiving oral hypoglycemics; may require adjustment of diabetes medications. Nausea, vomiting, diarrhea or constipation may occur; may require antiemetics or antidiarrheals; ileus may occur; administer fluid and electrolytes to prevent dehydration.

Drug Interactions

Metabolism/Transport Effects Substrate of CYP1A2 (minor), 2C9 (minor), 2C19 (major), 2D6 (minor), 3A4 (major); **Inhibits** CYP1A2 (weak), 2C9 (weak), 2C19 (moderate), 2D6 (weak), 3A4 (weak)

Avoid Concomitant Use

Avoid concomitant use of Bortezomib with any of the following: Clopidogrel; Green Tea

Decreased Effect

Bortezomib may decrease the levels/effects of: Clopidogrel

The levels/effects of Bortezomib may be decreased by: Ascorbic Acid; CYP2C19 Inducers (Strong); CYP3A4 Inducers (Strong); Deferasirox; Green Tea; Herbs (CYP3A4 Inducers); Peginterferon Alfa-2b

Increased Effect/Toxicity

Bortezomib may increase the levels/effects of: CYP2C19 Substrates

The levels/effects of Bortezomib may be increased by: CYP2C19 Inhibitors (Moderate); CYP2C19 Inhibitors (Strong); CYP3A4 Inhibitors (Moderate); CYP3A4 Inhibitors (Strong); Dasatinib

Nutritional/Ethanol Interactions

Food: Avoid grapefruit juice (may increase bortezomib levels).

Herb/Nutraceutical: Avoid St John's wort (may decrease bortezomib levels). Avoid green tea and green tea extracts (may diminish the therapeutic effect of bortezomib) (Golden, 2009). Avoid ascorbic acid supplements, including multivitamins containing ascorbic acid (may diminish bortezomib activity) during treatment, especially 12 hours before and after bortezomib treatment (Perrone, 2009).

Adverse Reactions

>10%:

Cardiovascular: Edema (11% to 23%), cardiac disorder (treatment emergent: 15%), hypotension (13%; grades 3/4: 3%)

Central nervous system: Psychiatric disturbance (≤35%), fever (34%), dysesthesia (22%), headache (22%), insomnia (20%), dizziness (17%; excludes vertigo)

Dermatologic: Rash (18%)

Gastrointestinal: Nausea (55%), diarrhea (52%), constipation (41%), anorexia (36%), vomiting (33%), abdominal pain (15%), abnormal taste, dyspepsia

Hematologic: Thrombocytopenia (36%; grade 4: 5%; nadir: day 11; recovery: by day 21), anemia (29%; grade 4: <1%), neutropenia (17%; grade 4: 3%; nadir: day 11; recovery: by day 21)

Neuromuscular & skeletal: Weakness (64%; grades 3/4: 16%), peripheral neuropathy (39%; grade 3: 11%; grade 4: <1%), paresthesia (22%), arthralgia (17%), limb pain (15%), bone pain (14%), back pain (13%), myalgia (12%), muscle cramps (11%), rigors (≤11%)

Respiratory: Dyspnea (21%), cough (20%), respiratory tract infection (12% to 15%), nasopharyngitis (12%), pneumonia (12%)

Miscellaneous: Herpesvirus infections (12%)

1% to 10%:

Cardiovascular: Heart failure (5%; includes acute pulmonary edema, cardiac failure, congestive cardiac failure, cardiogenic shock, pulmonary edema)

Central nervous system: Anxiety (10%)

Endocrine & metabolic: Dehydration (10%), hypercalcemia (grade 4: 2%)

Hematologic: Bleeding events (≥grade 3: 4%)

Local: Injection site irritation (5%)

Frequency not defined (including postmarketing and/or case reports; limited to important or life-threatening): Acute diffuse infiltrative pulmonary disease, acute respiratory distress syndrome, alkaline phosphatase increased, amyloidosis, anaphylaxis, angina, angioedema, ascites, aspergillosis, atelectasis, atrial fibrillation, atrial flutter, AV block, bacteremia, bradycardia, cardiac amyloidosis, blurred vision, bronchitis, cardiac arrest, cardiac tamponade, cardiopulmonary arrest, cerebral hemorrhage, cerebrovascular accident, cholestasis, coma, confusion, conjunctival infection/irritation, cranial palsy, deep venous thrombosis, diplopia, disseminated intravascular coagulation (DIC), duodenitis (hemorrhagic), DVT, dysautonomia, dysphagia, encephalopathy, embolism, epistaxis, fecal impaction, fracture, gastritis (hemorrhagic), gastroenteritis, GGT increased, glomerular nephritis, hearing impairment, hematemesis, hematuria, hemoptysis, hemorrhagic cystitis, hepatic failure, hepatic hemorrhage, hepatitis, hepatocellular damage, herpes meningoencephalitis, hyperbilirubinemia, hyper-/hypoglycemia, hyper-/hypokalemia, hyper-/hyponatremia, hypersensitivity, hyperuricemia, hypocalcemia, hypoxia, ileus, immune complex hypersensitivity, inappropriate ADH secretion, injection site reaction, interstitial pneumonia, intestinal obstruction, intestinal perforation, intracerebral hemorrhage, ischemic colitis, ischemic stroke, laryngeal edema, left ventricular ejection fraction decreased, leukocytoclastic vasculitis, leukopenia, listeriosis, lymphopenia, melena, mental status change, MI, myocardial ischemia, neuralgia, neutropenic fever, ophthalmic herpes, oral candidiasis, pancreatitis, paralytic ileus, pericardial effusion, pericarditis, peritonitis, pleural effusion, pneumonitis, portal vein thrombosis, proliferative glomerular nephritis, pruritus, psychosis, pulmonary embolism, pulmonary hypertension, pulmonary infiltrate, QT_c prolongation, renal calculus, renal failure, respiratory failure, respiratory insufficiency, reversible posterior leukoencephalopathy syndrome (RPLS), seizure, septic shock, sepsis, sinus arrest, spinal cord compression, Stevens-Johnson syndrome, stomatitis, stroke (hemorrhagic), subarachnoid hemorrhage, subdural hematoma, suicidal ideation, Sweet's syndrome (acute febrile neutrophilic dermatosis), syncope, tachycardia, torsade de pointes, toxic epidermal necrolysis, toxoplasmosis, transaminases increased, transient ischemic attack, tumor lysis syndrome, urinary incontinence, urinary retention, urinary tract infection, urticaria, ventricular tachycardia

Pharmacodynamics/Kinetics

Protein Binding ~83%

Half-Life Elimination Single dose: 9-15 hours; multiple dosing: 1 mg/m^2: 40-193 hours; 1.3 mg/m^2: 76-108 hour

Metabolism Hepatic primarily via CYP2C19 and 3A4 and to a lesser extent CYP1A2; forms metabolites (inactive) via deboronization followed by hydroxylation

Available Dosage Forms

Injection, powder for reconstitution:

Velcade®: 3.5 mg

Dosing

Adult & Geriatric Details concerning dosing in combination regimens should also be consulted. **Note:** Consecutive doses should be separated by at least 72 hours.

Multiple myeloma (first-line therapy; in combination with melphalan and prednisone): I.V.: 1.3 mg/m^2 days 1, 4, 8, 11, 22, 25, 29, and 32 of a 42-day treatment cycle for 4 cycles, followed by 1.3 mg/m^2 days 1, 8, 22, and 29 of a 42-day treatment cycle for 5 cycles.

Alternative first-line therapy (studied in patients ≥65 years of age; unlabeled dosing): I.V.: 1.3 mg/m^2/dose days 1, 8, 15, and 22 of a 5-week treatment cycle, in combination with **either** melphalan and prednisone or melphalan, prednisone, and thalidomide (Boccadoro, 2010; Bringhen, 2010; Palumbo, 2009)

Relapsed multiple myeloma and mantle cell lymphoma: I.V.: 1.3 mg/m^2 twice weekly for 2 weeks on days 1, 4, 8, and 11 of a 21-day treatment cycle. Therapy extending beyond 8 cycles may be administered by the standard schedule or may be given once weekly for 4 weeks (days 1, 8, 15, and 22), followed by a 13-day rest (days 23 through 35).

Cutaneous or peripheral T-cell lymphoma (unlabeled use): I.V.: 1.3 mg/m^2 twice weekly for 2 weeks on days 1, 4, 8, and 11 of a 21-day treatment cycle (Zinzani, 2007).

Systemic light-chain amyloidosis (unlabeled use): I.V.: 1.3 mg/m^2 days 1, 4, 8, and 11 of a 21-day treatment cycle (with or without dexamethasone) (Kastritis, 2010)

Waldenström's macroglobulinemia (unlabeled use): I.V.: 1.3 mg/m^2 days 1, 4, 8, and 11 of a 21-day treatment cycle (Chen, 2007) **or** 1.3 mg/m^2 days 1, 4, 8, and 11 of a 21-day treatment cycle (in combination with dexamethasone and rituximab) (Treon, 2009) **or** 1.6 mg/m^2 days 1, 8, and 15 of a 28-day treatment cycle (in combination with rituximab) (Ghobrial, 2010)

Renal Impairment No dosage adjustment necessary. **Note:** Dialysis may reduce bortezomib concentrations; administer postdialysis.

Hepatic Impairment

Mild impairment (bilirubin ≤1 times ULN and AST >UNL or bilirubin >1-1.5 times ULN): No initial dose adjustment required

Moderate (bilirubin >1.5-3 times ULN) and severe impairment (bilirubin >3 times ULN): Reduce initial dose to 0.7 mg/m^2 in the first cycle; based on patient tolerance, may consider dose escalation to 1 mg/m^2 or further dose reduction to 0.5 mg/m^2 in subsequent cycles

Adjustment for Toxicity

Myeloma (first-line therapy):

Platelets should be ≥70,000/mm^3, ANC should be ≥1000/mm^3, and nonhematologic toxicities should resolve to grade 1 or baseline prior to therapy initiation.

Platelets ≤30,000/mm^3 or ANC ≤750/mm^3 on bortezomib day(s) (except day 1): Withhold bortezomib; if several bortezomib doses in consecutive cycles are withheld, reduce dose 1 level (1.3 mg/m^2/dose reduced to 1 mg/m^2/dose; 1 mg/m^2/dose reduced to 0.7 mg/m^2/dose)

Grade ≥3 nonhematological toxicity (other than neuropathy): Withhold bortezomib until toxicity resolves to grade 1 or baseline. May reinitiate bortezomib at 1 dose level reduction (1.3 mg/m^2/dose reduced to 1 mg/m^2/dose; 1 mg/m^2/dose reduced to 0.7 mg/m^2/dose).

Neuropathic pain and/or peripheral sensory or motor neuropathy: See "Neuropathic pain and/or peripheral sensory or motor neuropathy" toxicity adjustment guidelines below.

Relapsed multiple myeloma and mantle cell lymphoma:

Grade 3 nonhematological (excluding neuropathy) or Grade 4 hematological toxicity: Withhold until toxicity resolved; may reinitiate with a 25% dose reduction (1.3 mg/m^2/dose reduced to 1 mg/m^2/dose; 1 mg/m^2/dose reduced to 0.7 mg/m^2/dose)

Neuropathic pain and/or peripheral sensory or motor neuropathy:

Grade 1 without pain or loss of function: No action needed

Grade 1 with pain or Grade 2 interfering with function but not activities of daily living: Reduce dose to 1 mg/m^2

Grade 2 with pain or Grade 3 interfering with activities of daily living: Withhold until toxicity resolved, may reinitiate at 0.7 mg/m^2 once weekly

Grade 4: Discontinue therapy

Administration

I.V. Administer via rapid I.V. push (3-5 seconds).

Other SubQ (unlabeled administration route): Subcutaneous administration of bortezomib 1.3 mg/m^2 days 1, 4, 8, and 11 of a 21-day treatment cycle has been studied in a limited number of patients with relapsed multiple myeloma; doses were administered subcutaneously (concentration of 2.5 mg/mL) into the thigh or abdomen, rotating the injection site with each dose; release of data analysis is pending (Moreau, 2010).

Stability

Reconstitution Dilute each 3.5 mg vial with 3.5 mL NS to a final concentration of 1 mg/mL. Use appropriate precautions for handling and disposal.

Storage Prior to reconstitution, store at room temperature of 25°C (77°F); excursions permitted between 15°C to 30°C (59°F to 86°F). Protect from light. Once reconstituted, although the manufacturer recommends use within 8 hours, solution may be stored at room temperature for up to 3 days, or under refrigeration for up to 5 days, in vial or syringe (Andre, 2005). Protect from light.

Monitoring and Teaching Issues

Laboratory Monitoring CBC with differential and platelets (monitor frequently throughout therapy); liver function tests (in patients with existing hepatic impairment)

Physical Assessment Monitor for peripheral neuropathy, postural hypotension, dehydration, heart failure, and infections. Be alert to the potential for reactivation of herpes. Monitor for psychiatric disturbances.

Patient Education Avoid grapefruit juice, green tea, and ascorbic acid supplements. This medication can only be administered intravenously; you will be monitored during and following infusion. Maintain adequate hydration, unless instructed to restrict fluid intake. If you have diabetes, monitor blood sugars closely; may cause alterations in glycemic control. May cause headache, dizziness, anxiety, sleep disturbances, fever, fatigue, nausea, vomiting, loss of appetite, abnormal taste, constipation, or diarrhea. You may be more susceptible to infection. Report immediately any chest pain, respiratory difficulty, itching, rash, acute headache, throat tightness, pain, redness, or swelling at infusion site. Report swelling in extremities; weight gain; persistent headache; muscle, bone, or back pain; abdominal pain; cramping or loss of sensation or tingling of extremities; unusual bleeding; changes in vision; or psychiatric disturbances.

Dietary Considerations Green tea and green tea extracts may diminish the therapeutic effect of bortezomib and should be avoided (Golden, 2009). Avoid grapefruit juice. Avoid additional, nondietary sources of ascorbic acid supplements, including multivitamins containing ascorbic acid (may diminish bortezomib activity) during treatment, especially 12 hours before and after bortezomib treatment (Perrone, 2009).

Breast-Feeding Considerations Due to the potential for serious adverse reactions in the nursing infant, breast-feeding is not recommended.

Pregnancy Considerations Adverse effects (fetal loss and decreased fetal weight) were observed in animal studies. There are no adequate and well-controlled studies in pregnant women. Effective contraception is recommended for women of childbearing potential.

◆ **Brethaire [DSC]** *see* Terbutaline *on page* 1735

◆ **Brethine** *see* Terbutaline *on page* 1735

◆ **Brevibloc** *see* Esmolol *on page* 665

◆ **Brevicon®** *see* Ethinyl Estradiol and Norethindrone *on page* 701

◆ **Bricanyl [DSC]** *see* Terbutaline *on page* 1735

Brimonidine (bri MOE ni deen)

U.S. Brand Names Alphagan® P

Index Terms Brimonidine Tartrate

Generic Availability (U.S.) Yes

Pharmacologic Category $Alpha_2$ Agonist, Ophthalmic; Ophthalmic Agent, Antiglaucoma

Medication Safety Issues

Sound-alike/look-alike issues:

Brimonidine may be confused with bromocriptine

Pregnancy Risk Factor B

Lactation Excretion in breast milk unknown/not recommended

Use Lowering of intraocular pressure (IOP) in patients with open-angle glaucoma or ocular hypertension

Available Dosage Forms

Solution, ophthalmic: 0.15% (5 mL, 10 mL, 15 mL); 0.2% (5 mL, 10 mL, 15 mL)

Alphagan® P: 0.1% (5 mL, 10 mL, 15 mL); 0.15% (5 mL, 10 mL, 15 mL)

Dosing

Adult & Geriatric Glaucoma, ocular hypertension: Ophthalmic: Instill 1 drop in affected eye(s) 3 times/day (approximately every 8 hours)

Pediatric Children ≥2 years of age: Refer to adult dosing.

Administration

Other Remove contact lenses prior to administration; wait 15 minutes before reinserting if using products containing benzalkonium chloride. Separate administration of other ophthalmic agents by 5 minutes.

Monitoring and Teaching Issues

Physical Assessment Monitor intraocular pressure periodically.

Patient Education For use in eyes only. Wash hands before instilling. Remove contacts prior to administration and wait 15 minutes before reinserting. Sit or lie down to instill. Open eye, look at ceiling, and instill prescribed amount of solution. Apply gentle pressure to inner corner of eye. Do not let tip of applicator touch eyes; do not contaminate tip of applicator (may cause eye infection, eye damage, or vision loss). Brimonidine tartrate may cause fatigue or drowsiness in some patients. Avoid engaging in hazardous activities due to potential for decreased mental alertness until response known. Wait at least 15 minutes after instilling brimonidine tartrate before reinserting soft contact lenses.

◆ **Brimonidine Tartrate** *see* Brimonidine *on page* 230

Brinzolamide (brin ZOH la mide)

U.S. Brand Names Azopt®

Generic Availability (U.S.) No

Pharmacologic Category Carbonic Anhydrase Inhibitor; Ophthalmic Agent, Antiglaucoma

Pregnancy Risk Factor C

Lactation Excretion in breast milk unknown/not recommended

Use Lowers intraocular pressure in patients with ocular hypertension or open-angle glaucoma

Available Dosage Forms

Suspension, ophthalmic:

Azopt®: 1% (10 mL, 15 mL)

Dosing

Adult & Geriatric Glaucoma: Ophthalmic: Instill 1 drop in affected eye(s) 3 times/day

Administration

Other May be used concomitantly with other topical ophthalmic drug products to lower intraocular pressure. If more than one topical ophthalmic drug is being used, administer drugs at least 10 minutes apart.

Monitoring and Teaching Issues

Physical Assessment Measure intraocular pressure periodically.

Patient Education For use in eyes only. Tilt head back, place medication in conjunctival sac, and close eyes. Apply finger pressure at corner of eye for 1 minute following application. Do not let tip of applicator touch eye; do not contaminate tip of applicator (may cause eye infection, eye damage, or vision loss). If using other ophthalmic preparations, administer 10 minutes apart. May cause taste changes, runny nose, or vision changes (blurred vision, dry eye, foreign body sensation, eye discharge, temporary sensitivity to bright light, blurring or stinging, altered distance perception, reduced night vision acuity). Report skin rash or eye pain.

◆ **Brioschi® [OTC]** *see* Sodium Bicarbonate *on page* 1658

◆ **BRL 43694** *see* Granisetron *on page* 887

◆ **Bromax** *see* Brompheniramine *on page* 234

◆ **Bromday™** *see* Bromfenac *on page* 231

Bromfenac (BROME fen ak)

U.S. Brand Names Bromday™; Xibrom® [DSC]

Index Terms Bromfenac Sodium

Generic Availability (U.S.) No

Pharmacologic Category Nonsteroidal Anti-inflammatory Drug (NSAID), Ophthalmic

Pregnancy Risk Factor C

Lactation Excretion in breast milk unknown/use caution

Use Treatment of postoperative inflammation and reduction in ocular pain following cataract removal

Available Dosage Forms

Solution, ophthalmic:

Bromday™: 0.09% (1.7 mL)

Dosing

Adult & Geriatric

Bromday™: Ophthalmic: Instill 1 drop into affected eye(s) once daily beginning 1 day prior to surgery and continuing on the day of surgery and for 2 weeks postoperatively

Xibrom®: Ophthalmic: Instill 1 drop into affected eye(s) twice daily beginning 24 hours after surgery and continuing for 2 weeks postoperatively

Administration

Other Remove contact lenses prior to administration and wait 15 minutes before reinserting. Bromday™: May be used with other eye drops. If using more than 1 ophthalmic product, wait at least 5 minutes between application of each medication.

Monitoring and Teaching Issues

Physical Assessment Assess for intraocular bleeding. Evaluate allergy history with aspirin or other NSAIDs.

Patient Education Do not wear contact lenses while using this medication. Report any abnormal sensation in eye, redness, severe headache, or pain.

◆ **Bromfenac Sodium** *see* Bromfenac *on page* 231

Bromocriptine (broe moe KRIP teen)

U.S. Brand Names Cycloset®; Parlodel®; Parlodel® SnapTabs®

Index Terms Bromocriptine Mesylate; Cycloset®

Generic Availability (U.S.) Yes: Excludes Cycloset®

Pharmacologic Category Anti-Parkinson's Agent, Dopamine Agonist; Antidiabetic Agent, Dopamine Agonist; Ergot Derivative

Medication Safety Issues

Sound-alike/look-alike issues:

Bromocriptine may be confused with benztropine, brimonidine

Cycloset® may be confused with Glyset®

Parlodel® may be confused with pindolol, Provera®

Pregnancy Risk Factor B

Lactation Enters breast milk/contraindicated

Use Treatment of hyperprolactinemia associated with amenorrhea with or without galactorrhea, infertility, or hypogonadism; treatment of prolactin-secreting adenomas; treatment of acromegaly; treatment of Parkinson's disease

Cycloset®: Management of type 2 diabetes mellitus (noninsulin dependent, NIDDM) as an adjunct to diet and exercise

Unlabeled/Investigational Use Neuroleptic malignant syndrome

Mechanism of Action/Effect Semisynthetic ergot alkaloid derivative and a dopamine receptor agonist which activates postsynaptic dopamine receptors to decrease prolactin secretion (tuberoinfundibular pathway) and enhance coordinated motor control (nigrostriatal pathways).

In the treatment type 2 diabetes mellitus, bromocriptine's effect on improving glycemic control is unknown; however, when administered during the morning and released into the systemic circulation in a rapid, 'pulse-like' dose, it is believed to affect circadian rhythms thought to play a role in obesity and insulin resistance.

Contraindications Hypersensitivity to bromocriptine, ergot alkaloids, or any component of the formulation

Additional contraindications:

Parlodel®: Uncontrolled hypertension; pregnancy (risk to benefit evaluation must be performed in women who become pregnant during treatment for acromegaly, prolactinoma, or Parkinson's disease - hypertension during treatment should generally result in efforts to withdraw);

postpartum women with a history of coronary artery disease or other severe cardiovascular conditions (unless withdrawal of medication is medically contraindicated)

Cycloset®: Syncopal migraine; breast-feeding

Warnings/Precautions Complete evaluation of pituitary function should be completed prior to initiation of treatment of any hyperprolactinemia-associated dysfunction. Use caution in patients with a history of peptic ulcer disease, dementia, or cardiovascular disease (myocardial infarction, arrhythmia). Use with extreme caution or avoid in patients with psychosis. Symptomatic hypotension may occur in a significant number of patients. In addition, hypertension, seizures, MI, and stroke have been rarely associated with bromocriptine therapy. Severe headache or visual changes may precede events. The onset of reactions may be immediate or delayed (often may occur in the second week of therapy). Sudden sleep onset and somnolence have been reported with use, primarily in patients with Parkinson's disease. Patients must be cautioned about performing tasks which require mental alertness.

Use with caution in patients taking strong CYP3A4 inhibitors and/or major CYP3A4 substrates (includes protease inhibitors, azole antifungals, and some macrolide antibiotics); consider alternative agents that avoid or lessen the potential for CYP-mediated interactions. Concurrent antihypertensives or drugs which may alter blood pressure should be used with caution. Concurrent use with levodopa has been associated with an increased risk of hallucinations. Consider dosage reduction and/or discontinuation in patients with hallucinations. Hallucinations may require weeks to months before resolution.

Dopamine agonists have been associated with compulsive behaviors and/or loss of impulse control, which has manifested as pathological gambling, libido increases (hypersexuality), and/or binge eating. Causality has not been established, and controversy exists as to whether this phenomenon is related to the underlying disease, prior behaviors/addictions and/or drug therapy. Dose reduction or discontinuation of therapy has been reported to reverse these behaviors in some, but not all cases. Risk for melanoma development is increased in Parkinson's disease patients; drug causation or factors contributing to risk have not been established. Patients should be monitored closely and periodic skin examinations should be performed.

In the treatment of acromegaly, discontinuation is recommended if tumor expansion occurs during therapy. Digital vasospasm (cold sensitive) may occur in some patients with acromegaly; may require dosage reduction. Patients who receive bromocriptine during and immediately following pregnancy as a continuation of previous therapy (eg, acromegaly) should be closely monitored for cardiovascular effects. Should not be used postpartum in women with coronary artery disease or other cardiovascular disease. Use of bromocriptine to control or prevent lactation or in patients with uncontrolled hypertension is not recommended.

Monitoring and careful evaluation of visual changes during the treatment of hyperprolactinemia is recommended to differentiate between tumor shrinkage and traction on the optic chiasm; rapidly progressing visual field loss requires neurosurgical consultation. Discontinuation of bromocriptine in patients with macroadenomas has been associated with rapid regrowth of tumor and increased prolactin serum levels. Pleural and retroperitoneal fibrosis have been reported with prolonged daily use. Cardiac valvular fibrosis has also been associated with ergot alkaloids.

In the management of type 2 diabetes mellitus, Cycloset® ('quick-release' tablet) should not be interchanged with any other bromocriptine product due to formulation differences and resulting pharmacokinetics. Therapy is not appropriate in patients with diabetic ketoacidosis (DKA) or type 1 diabetes mellitus due to lack of efficacy in these patient populations. There is limited efficacy of use in combination with thiazolidinediones or in combination with insulin. Combination therapy with other hypoglycemic agents may increase risk for hypoglycemic events; dose reduction of concomitant hypoglycemics may be warranted.

Safety and efficacy have not been established in patients with hepatic or renal dysfunction. Safety and effectiveness in patients <11 years of age (for pituitary adenoma) have not been established. Safety has not been established for use >2 years in patients with Parkinson's disease.

Drug Interactions

Metabolism/Transport Effects Substrate of CYP3A4 (major); **Inhibits** CYP1A2 (weak), 3A4 (weak)

Avoid Concomitant Use

Avoid concomitant use of Bromocriptine with any of the following: Efavirenz; Itraconazole; Nitroglycerin; Posaconazole; Protease Inhibitors; Serotonin 5-HT1D Receptor Agonists; Sibutramine; Voriconazole

Decreased Effect

Bromocriptine may decrease the levels/effects of: Antipsychotics (Typical); Nitroglycerin

The levels/effects of Bromocriptine may be decreased by: Antipsychotics (Atypical); Metoclopramide

Increased Effect/Toxicity

Bromocriptine may increase the levels/effects of: CycloSPORINE; CycloSPORINE (Systemic); Serotonin 5-HT1D Receptor Agonists; Serotonin Modulators

The levels/effects of Bromocriptine may be increased by: Alpha-/Beta-Agonists; Antipsychotics (Typical); Conivaptan; CYP3A4 Inhibitors (Moderate); CYP3A4 Inhibitors (Strong); Dasatinib; Efavirenz; Itraconazole; Macrolide Antibiotics; MAO Inhibitors; Methylphenidate; Nitroglycerin; Posaconazole; Protease Inhibitors; Serotonin 5-HT1D Receptor Agonists; Sibutramine; Voriconazole

Nutritional/Ethanol Interactions

Ethanol: Avoid ethanol (may increase GI side effects or ethanol intolerance).

Herb/Nutraceutical: St John's wort may decrease bromocriptine levels.

Adverse Reactions Note: Frequency of adverse effects may vary by dose and/or indication.

>10%:

Central nervous system: Dizziness, fatigue, headache

Gastrointestinal: Constipation, nausea

Neuromuscular & skeletal: Weakness

Respiratory: Rhinitis

1% to 10%:

Cardiovascular: Hypotension (including postural/orthostatic), Raynaud's syndrome exacerbation, syncope

Central nervous system: Drowsiness, fatigue, lightheadedness, somnolence

Endocrine & metabolic: Hypoglycemia (4%; in combination with sulfonylureas or other antidiabetic agents: 7% to 9%)

Gastrointestinal: Abdominal cramps, anorexia, diarrhea, dyspepsia, GI bleeding, vomiting, xerostomia

Neuromuscular & skeletal: Digital vasospasm

Ocular: Amblyopia

Respiratory: Nasal congestion, sinusitis

Miscellaneous: Infection, flu-like syndrome

Pharmacodynamics/Kinetics

Onset of Action Parlodel®: Prolactin decreasing effect: 1-2 hours

Bioavailability Parlodel®: 28%; Cycloset®: 65% to 95%

Time to Peak Serum: Parlodel®: 1-3 hours; Cycloset®: 53 minutes

Protein Binding 90% to 96% (primarily albumin)

Half-Life Elimination Cycloset®: ~6 hours; Parlodel®: Biphasic: Terminal: 15 hours (range 8-20 hours)

Metabolism Primarily hepatic via CYP3A; extensive first-pass biotransformation (Cycloset®: ~93%)

Excretion Feces; urine (2% to 6% as unchanged drug and metabolites)

Available Dosage Forms

Capsule, oral: 5 mg

Parlodel®: 5 mg

Tablet, oral: 2.5 mg

Cycloset®: 0.8 mg

Parlodel® SnapTabs®: 2.5 mg

Dosing

Adult & Geriatric

Acromegaly: Oral: Initial: 1.25-2.5 mg daily increasing by 1.25-2.5 mg daily as necessary every 3-7 days; usual dose: 20-30 mg/day (maximum: 100 mg/day)

Hyperprolactinemia: Oral: Initial: 1.25-2.5 mg/day; may be increased by 2.5 mg/day as tolerated every 2-7 days until optimal response (range: 2.5-15 mg/day)

Parkinsonism: Oral: 1.25 mg twice daily, increased by 2.5 mg/day in 2- to 4-week intervals as needed (maximum: 100 mg/day)

Type 2 diabetes (Cycloset®): Oral: Initial: 0.8 mg once daily; may increase at weekly intervals in 0.8 mg increments as tolerated; usual dose: 1.6-4.8 mg/day (maximum: 4.8 mg/day)

Neuroleptic malignant syndrome (unlabeled use): Oral: 2.5 mg (orally or via gastric tube) every 8-12 hours, increased to a maximum of 45 mg/day, if needed; continue therapy until NMS is controlled, then taper slowly (Gortney, 2009; Strawn, 2007)

Pediatric

Hyperprolactinemia: Oral:

Children 11-15 years (based on limited information): Initial: 1.25-2.5 mg daily. Dosage may be increased as tolerated to achieve a therapeutic response (range 2.5-10 mg daily).

Children ≥16 years: Refer to adult dosing.

Hepatic Impairment No guidelines are available; however, adjustment may be necessary due to extensive hepatic metabolism.

Administration

Oral Administer with food to decrease GI distress.

Cycloset®: Administer within 2 hours of waking in the morning.

Stability

Storage Store at or below 25°C (77°F).

Monitoring and Teaching Issues

Laboratory Monitoring Pregnancy test during amenorrheic period; growth hormone (acromegaly) and prolactin levels; Hb A_{1C} and serum glucose (type 2 diabetes)

Physical Assessment Monitor blood pressure at beginning of therapy and periodically during course of treatment.

Patient Education May be prescribed in conjunction with levodopa/carbidopa. Therapeutic effects may take several weeks or months to achieve and you may need frequent monitoring during first weeks of therapy. Take with meals if GI upset occurs. Take at the same time each day. Maintain adequate hydration, unless instructed to restrict fluid intake. Do not use alcohol. Urine or perspiration may appear darker. You may experience drowsiness (can be sudden onset), dizziness, confusion, vision changes, loss of impulse control (possibly manifested as pathological gambling, libido increases, and/or binge eating), orthostatic hypotension, constipation, nasal congestion, nausea, vomiting, loss of appetite, or stomach discomfort. Report unresolved constipation or vomiting; chest pain or irregular heartbeat; acute headache or dizziness; CNS changes (eg, hallucination, loss of memory, seizures, acute headache, nervousness); suicide ideation; painful or difficult urination; increased muscle spasticity, rigidity, or involuntary movements; changes in the appearance of skin moles, skin rash, or other unusual skin changes; or significant worsening of condition.

Dietary Considerations Should be taken with food to decrease GI distress.

Geriatric Considerations No special considerations are recommended since drug is dosed to response; however, elderly may have concomitant diseases or drug therapy which may complicate therapy.

Breast-Feeding Considerations A previous indication for prevention of postpartum lactation was withdrawn voluntarily by the manufacturer following reports of serious adverse reactions, including stroke, MI, seizures, and severe hypertension. Use during breast-feeding is specifically contraindicated in the product labeling for Cycloset®. Use in postpartum women with a history of coronary artery disease or other severe cardiovascular conditions is specifically contraindicated in the product labeling for Parlodel® (unless withdrawal of medication is medically contraindicated). Based on the risk/benefit assessment, other treatments should be considered for lactation suppression.

Pregnancy Considerations No evidence of teratogenicity or fetal toxicity in animal studies. Bromocriptine is used for ovulation induction in women with hyperprolactinemia. In general, therapy should be discontinued if pregnancy is confirmed unless needed for treatment of macroprolactinoma. Data collected from women taking bromocriptine during pregnancy suggest the incidence of birth defects is not increased with use. However, the majority of women discontinued use within 8 weeks of pregnancy. Women not seeking pregnancy should be advised to use appropriate contraception.

Additional Information Usually used with levodopa or levodopa/carbidopa to treat Parkinson's disease. When adding bromocriptine, the dose of levodopa/carbidopa can usually be decreased.

In clinical trials in the treatment of type 2 diabetes, Cycloset® resulted in a mean change of Hb A_{1c} (%) from baseline of -0.1 when used as monotherapy, and a mean change from baseline of -0.1 to -0.4 when used in combination with sulfonylureas.

◆ **Bromocriptine Mesylate** *see* Bromocriptine *on page* 231

Brompheniramine (brome fen IR a meen)

U.S. Brand Names Bidhist [DSC]; Bromax; Lodrane® 24 [DSC]; LoHist-12; Respa®-BR [DSC]; TanaCof-XR [DSC]

Index Terms Brompheniramine Maleate; Brompheniramine Tannate

Generic Availability (U.S.) Yes: Chewable tablet

Pharmacologic Category Alkylamine Derivative; Histamine H_1 Antagonist; Histamine H_1 Antagonist, First Generation

Pregnancy Risk Factor C

Lactation Excretion in breast milk unknown/not recommended

Use Symptomatic relief of perennial and seasonal allergic rhinitis, vasomotor rhinitis, and other respiratory allergies

Available Dosage Forms

Tablet, extended release, oral:

Bromax: 11 mg

LoHist-12: 6 mg

Dosing

Adult Allergic rhinitis, allergic symptoms, vasomotor rhinitis: Oral:

Bromax, Respa®-BR: One tablet twice daily

Lodrane® 24: 1-2 capsules once daily

LoHist-12: 1-2 tablets every 12 hours (maximum: 4 tablets/day)

Pediatric Allergic rhinitis, allergic symptoms, vasomotor rhinitis: Oral:

Children 6-12 years:

Lodrane® 24: One capsule once daily

LoHist-12: One tablet every 12 hours (maximum: 2 tablets/day)

Children >12 years (Bromax, Lodrane® 24, LoHist-12, Respa®-BR): Refer to adult dosing.

Administration

Oral Extended release tablets are to be swallowed whole; do not crush or chew. Shake suspensions well before use.

Monitoring and Teaching Issues

Patient Education Follow dosing guidelines closely; measure dosage carefully, especially in pediatric patients. Avoid alcohol. You may experience drowsiness or dizziness. Report persistent sedation, confusion, agitation, blurred vision, or respiratory difficulty.

◆ **Brompheniramine Maleate** *see* Brompheniramine *on page* 234

◆ **Brompheniramine Tannate** *see* Brompheniramine *on page* 234

◆ **Brovana®** *see* Arformoterol *on page* 141

◆ **BSF208075** *see* Ambrisentan *on page* 93

◆ **B-type Natriuretic Peptide (Human)** *see* Nesiritide *on page* 1299

◆ **Budeprion XL®** *see* BuPROPion *on page* 252

◆ **Budeprion SR®** *see* BuPROPion *on page* 252

Budesonide (Systemic, Oral Inhalation) (byoo DES oh nide)

U.S. Brand Names Entocort® EC; Pulmicort Flexhaler®; Pulmicort Respules®

Generic Availability (U.S.) Yes: Suspension for nebulization

Pharmacologic Category Corticosteroid, Inhalant (Oral); Corticosteroid, Systemic

Pregnancy Risk Factor C (capsule)/B (inhalation)

Lactation Enters breast milk/use caution

Use

Nebulization: Maintenance and prophylactic treatment of asthma

Oral capsule: Treatment of active Crohn's disease (mild-to-moderate) involving the ileum and/or ascending colon; maintenance of remission (for up to 3 months) of Crohn's disease (mild-to-moderate) involving the ileum and/or ascending colon

Oral inhalation: Maintenance and prophylactic treatment of asthma; includes patients who require oral corticosteroids and those who may benefit from systemic dose reduction/elimination

Mechanism of Action/Effect Anti-inflammatory corticosteroid

Contraindications Hypersensitivity to budesonide or any component of the formulation; primary treatment of status asthmaticus, acute episodes of asthma; not for relief of acute bronchospasm

Canadian labeling: Additional contraindications (not in U.S. labeling): Moderate-to-severe bronchiectasis, pulmonary tuberculosis (active or quiescent), untreated respiratory infection (bacterial, fungal, or viral)

Warnings/Precautions May cause hypercorticism or suppression of hypothalamic-pituitary-adrenal (HPA) axis, particularly in younger children or in patients receiving high doses for prolonged periods. HPA axis suppression may lead to adrenal crisis. Withdrawal and discontinuation of a corticosteroid should be done slowly and carefully. Particular care is required when patients are transferred from systemic corticosteroids to inhaled products due to possible adrenal insufficiency or withdrawal from steroids, including an increase in allergic symptoms. Patients receiving >20 mg per day of prednisone (or equivalent) may be most susceptible. Fatalities have occurred due to adrenal insufficiency in asthmatic patients during and after transfer from systemic corticosteroids to aerosol steroids; aerosol steroids do not provide the systemic steroid needed to treat patients having trauma, surgery, or infections. Do not use this product to transfer patients directly from oral corticosteroid therapy.

Bronchospasm may occur with wheezing after inhalation; if this occurs stop steroid and treat with a fast-acting bronchodilator (eg, albuterol). Supplemental steroids (oral or parenteral) may be needed during stress or severe asthma attacks. Not to be used in status asthmaticus or for the relief of acute bronchospasm. Acute myopathy has been reported with high-dose corticosteroids, usually in patients with neuromuscular transmission disorders; may involve ocular and/or respiratory muscles; monitor creatine kinase; recovery may be delayed. Corticosteroid use may cause psychiatric disturbances, including depression, euphoria, insomnia, mood swings, and personality changes. Pre-existing psychiatric conditions may be exacerbated by corticosteroid use. Prolonged use of corticosteroids may also increase the incidence of secondary infection, mask acute infection (including fungal infections), prolong or exacerbate viral infections, or limit response to vaccines. Exposure to chickenpox should be avoided; corticosteroids should not be used to treat ocular herpes simplex. Corticosteroids should not be used for cerebral malaria or viral hepatitis. Close observation is required in patients with latent tuberculosis and/or TB reactivity; restrict use in active TB (only in conjunction with antituberculosis treatment). *Candida albicans* infections may occur in the mouth and pharynx; rinsing (and spitting) with water after inhaler use may decrease risk. Prolonged treatment with corticosteroids has been associated with the development of Kaposi's sarcoma (case reports); if noted, discontinuation of therapy should be considered.

Use with caution in patients with thyroid disease, hepatic impairment, renal impairment, cardiovascular disease, diabetes, glaucoma, cataracts, myasthenia gravis, patients at risk for osteoporosis, patients at risk for seizures, or GI diseases (diverticulitis, peptic ulcer, ulcerative colitis) due to perforation risk. Use caution following acute MI (corticosteroids have been associated with myocardial rupture). Because of the risk of adverse effects, systemic corticosteroids should be used cautiously in the elderly in the smallest possible effective dose for the shortest duration.

Orally-inhaled corticosteroids may cause a reduction in growth velocity in pediatric patients (~1 centimeter per year [range: 0.3-1.8 cm per year] and related to dose and duration of exposure). To minimize the systemic effects of orally-inhaled corticosteroids, each patient should be titrated to the lowest effective dose. Growth should be routinely monitored in pediatric patients. Withdraw systemic therapy with gradual tapering of dose. There have been reports of systemic corticosteroid withdrawal symptoms (eg, joint/muscle pain, lassitude, depression) when withdrawing oral inhalation therapy. Pulmicort Flexhaler™ contains lactose; very rare anaphylactic reactions have been reported in patients with severe milk protein allergy.

Drug Interactions

Metabolism/Transport Effects Substrate of CYP3A4 (major)

Avoid Concomitant Use

Avoid concomitant use of Budesonide (Systemic, Oral Inhalation) with any of the following: Aldesleukin; BCG; Natalizumab; Pimecrolimus; Roflumilast; Tacrolimus (Topical)

Decreased Effect

Budesonide (Systemic, Oral Inhalation) may decrease the levels/effects of: Aldesleukin; Antidiabetic Agents; BCG; Corticorelin; Sipuleucel-T; Vaccines (Inactivated)

The levels/effects of Budesonide (Systemic, Oral Inhalation) may be decreased by: Antacids; Bile Acid Sequestrants; Echinacea

Increased Effect/Toxicity

Budesonide (Systemic, Oral Inhalation) may increase the levels/effects of: Amphotericin B; Leflunomide; Loop Diuretics; Natalizumab; Thiazide Diuretics

The levels/effects of Budesonide (Systemic, Oral Inhalation) may be increased by: CYP3A4 Inhibitors (Moderate); CYP3A4 Inhibitors (Strong); Dasatinib; Denosumab; Pimecrolimus; Roflumilast; Tacrolimus (Topical); Trastuzumab

Nutritional/Ethanol Interactions Food: Grapefruit juice may double systemic exposure of orally-administered budesonide. Administration of capsules with a high-fat meal delays peak concentration, but does not alter the extent of absorption.

Adverse Reactions Reaction severity varies by dose and duration; not all adverse reactions have been reported with each dosage form.

>10%:

Central nervous system: Headache (≤21%)
Gastrointestinal: Nausea (≤11%)
Respiratory: Respiratory infection, rhinitis
Miscellaneous: Symptoms of HPA axis suppression and/or hypercorticism may occur in >10% of patients following administration of dosage forms which result in higher systemic exposure (ie, oral capsule), but may be less frequent than rates observed with comparator drugs (prednisolone). These symptoms may be rare (<1%) following administration via methods which result in lower exposures (topical).

1% to 10%:

Cardiovascular: Chest pain, edema, flushing, hypertension, palpitation, syncope, tachycardia
Central nervous system: Amnesia, dizziness, dysphonia, emotional lability, fatigue, fever, insomnia, malaise, migraine, nervousness, pain, sleep disorder, somnolence, vertigo
Dermatologic: Acne, alopecia, bruising, contact dermatitis, eczema, hirsutism, pruritus, pustular rash, rash, striae
Endocrine & metabolic: Adrenal insufficiency, hypokalemia, menstrual disorder
Gastrointestinal: Abdominal pain, anorexia, diarrhea, dyspepsia, flatulence, gastroenteritis (including viral), glossitis, intestinal obstruction, oral candidiasis, taste perversion, tongue edema, vomiting, weight gain, xerostomia
Genitourinary: Dysuria, hematuria, nocturia, pyuria
Hematologic: Cervical lymphadenopathy, leukocytosis, purpura
Hepatic: Alkaline phosphatase increased
Neuromuscular & skeletal: Arthralgia, back pain, fracture, hyperkinesis, hypertonia, myalgia, neck pain, paresthesia, weakness
Ocular: Conjunctivitis, eye infection
Otic: Earache, ear infection, external ear infection
Respiratory: Bronchitis, bronchospasm, cough, epistaxis, hoarseness, nasal congestion, nasal irritation, pharyngitis, sinusitis, stridor, throat irritation
Miscellaneous: Abscess, allergic reaction, C-reactive protein increased, erythrocyte sedimentation rate increased, fat distribution (moon face, buffalo hump); flu-like syndrome, herpes simplex, infection, moniliasis, viral infection, voice alteration

Pharmacodynamics/Kinetics

Onset of Action Pulmicort Respules®: 2-8 days; Inhalation: 24 hours

Peak effect: Pulmicort Respules®: 4-6 weeks; Inhalation: 1-2 weeks

Bioavailability Limited by high first-pass effect; Capsule: 9% to 21%; Pulmicort Respules®: 6%; Inhalation: 6% to 13%

Time to Peak Capsule: 0.5-10 hours (variable in Crohn's disease); Pulmicort Respules®: 10-30 minutes; Inhalation: 1-2 hours

Protein Binding 85% to 90%

Half-Life Elimination 2-3.6 hours

Metabolism Hepatic via CYP3A4 to two metabolites: 16 alpha-hydroxyprednisolone and 6 beta-hydroxybudesonide; minor activity

Excretion Urine (60%) and feces as metabolites

Available Dosage Forms

Capsule, enteric coated, oral:
Entocort® EC: 3 mg

Powder, for oral inhalation:
Pulmicort Flexhaler®: 90 mcg/inhalation (165 mg); 180 mcg/inhalation (225 mg)

Suspension, for nebulization: 0.25 mg/2 mL (30s); 0.5 mg/2 mL (30s)
Pulmicort Respules®: 0.25 mg/2 mL (30s); 0.5 mg/2 mL (30s); 1 mg/2 mL (30s)

Dosing

Adult & Geriatric

Asthma: *Oral inhalation:*

Pulmicort Flexhaler™: Initial: 360 mcg twice daily (selected patients may be initiated at 180 mcg twice daily); maximum: 720 mcg twice daily

NIH Asthma Guidelines (NIH, 2007) (administer in divided doses twice daily):
"Low" dose: 180-600 mcg/day
"Medium" dose: >600-1200 mcg/day
"High" dose: >1200 mcg/day

Pulmicort® Turbuhaler®: [CAN, not available in the U.S.]: Initial (during periods of severe asthma or when switching from oral corticosteroid therapy): 400-2400 mcg daily in 2-4 divided doses; Maintenance: 200-400 mcg twice daily (higher doses may be needed for short periods of time). **Note:** Patients taking 400 mcg/day may take as a single daily dose

Crohn's disease (active): *Oral:* 9 mg once daily in the morning for up to 8 weeks; recurring episodes may be treated with a repeat 8-week course of treatment. **Note:** Patients receiving CYP3A4 inhibitors should be monitored closely for signs and symptoms of hypercorticism; dosage reduction may be required. If switching from oral prednisolone, prednisolone dosage should be tapered while budesonide (Entocort™ EC) treatment is initiated.

Maintenance of remission: Following treatment of active disease (control of symptoms with CDAI <150), treatment may be continued at a dosage of 6 mg once daily for up to 3 months. If symptom control is maintained for 3 months, tapering of the dosage to complete cessation is recommended. Continued dosing beyond 3 months has not been demonstrated to result in substantial benefit.

Pediatric

Asthma:

Oral inhalation:

Pulmicort Flexhaler™: ≥6 years: Initial: 180 mcg twice daily (some patients may be initiated at 360 mcg twice daily); maximum: 360 mcg twice daily

NIH Asthma Guidelines (NIH, 2007) (administer in divided doses twice daily):

Children 5-11 years:

"Low" dose: 180-400 mcg/day

"Medium" dose: >400-800 mcg/day

"High" dose: >800 mcg/day

Children ≥12 years: Refer to adult dosing.

Pulmicort® Turbuhaler®: [CAN, not available in the U.S.]: Initial (during periods of severe asthma or when switching from oral corticosteroid therapy): 200-400 mcg daily in 2 divided doses; Maintenance: Individualized, lowest effective dose.

Nebulization: Children 12 months to 8 years: Pulmicort Respules®: Titrate to lowest effective dose once patient is stable; start at 0.25 mg/day or use as follows:

Previous therapy of bronchodilators alone: 0.5 mg/day administered as a single dose or divided twice daily (maximum daily dose: 0.5 mg)

Previous therapy of inhaled corticosteroids: 0.5 mg/day administered as a single dose or divided twice daily (maximum daily dose: 1 mg)

Previous therapy of oral corticosteroids: 1 mg/day administered as a single dose or divided twice daily (maximum daily dose: 1 mg)

NIH Asthma Guidelines (NIH, 2007):

Children 0-4 years:

"Low" dose: 0.25-0.5 mg/day

"Medium" dose: >0.5-1 mg/day

"High" dose: >1 mg/day

Children 5-11 years:

"Low" dose: 0.5 mg/day

"Medium" dose: 1 mg/day

"High" dose: 2 mg/day

Hepatic Impairment Monitor closely for signs and symptoms of hypercorticism; dosage reduction may be required.

Administration

Oral Oral capsule: Capsule should be swallowed whole; do not crush or chew.

Inhalation

Powder for inhalation:

Pulmicort Flexhaler™: Hold inhaler in upright position (mouthpiece up) to load dose. Do not shake prior to use. Unit should be primed prior to first use only. It will not need primed again, even if not used for a long time. Place mouthpiece between lips and inhale forcefully and deeply. Do not exhale through inhaler; do not use a spacer. Dose indicator does not move with every dose, usually only after 5 doses. Discard when dose indicator reads "0". Rinse mouth with water after each use to reduce incidence of candidiasis.

Pulmicort Turbuhaler® [CAN, not available in the U.S.]: Hold inhaler in upright position (mouthpiece up) to load dose. Do not shake inhaler after dose is loaded. Unit should be primed prior to first use. Place mouthpiece between lips and inhale forcefully and deeply; mouthpiece should face up. Do not exhale through inhaler; do not use a spacer. When a red mark appears in the dose indicator window, 20 doses are left. When the red mark reaches the bottom of the window, the inhaler should be discarded. Rinse mouth with water after use to reduce incidence of candidiasis.

Suspension for nebulization: Shake well before using. Use Pulmicort Respules® with jet nebulizer connected to an air compressor; administer with mouthpiece or facemask. Do not use ultrasonic nebulizer. Do not mix with other medications in nebulizer. Rinse mouth following treatments to decrease risk of oral candidiasis (wash face if using face mask).

Stability

Storage

Suspension for nebulization: Store upright at 20°C to 25°C (68°F to 77°F). Protect from light. Do not refrigerate or freeze. Once aluminum package is opened, solution should be used within 2 weeks. Continue to protect from light.

Oral inhaler (Pulmicort Flexhaler™): Store at controlled room temperature of 20°C to 25°C (68°F to 77°F). Protect from moisture.

Monitoring and Teaching Issues

Physical Assessment When changing from systemic steroids to inhalational steroids, taper reduction of systemic medication slowly (may take several months). Growth should be routinely monitored in pediatric patients.

Patient Education May take 1-2 weeks or longer before full effects are seen. Avoid grapefruit juice while taking this medication. May be more susceptible to infection; avoid exposure to chickenpox and measles unless immunity has been established. If exposure to measles or chickenpox occurs, notify your prescriber immediately. Report acute nervousness or inability to sleep; respiratory difficulty, sore throat, hoarseness, bronchitis, or bronchospasms; disturbed menstrual pattern; vision changes; loss of taste or smell perception; or worsening of condition or lack of improvement. Regular eye exams should be considered (risk of cataracts or glaucoma).

Oral capsule: Swallow whole; do not crush or chew capsule.

Inhalation/nebulization: This is not a bronchodilator and will not relieve acute asthma attacks. It may take several days for you to realize full effects of treatment. If you are also using an inhaled bronchodilator, wait 10 minutes before using this steroid aerosol. Take 5-10 deep breaths. Use inhaler on inspiration. Hold breath for 5-10 seconds after inhalation. Allow 1 full minute between inhalations. You may experience dizziness, anxiety, blurred vision, or taste disturbance or aftertaste. Rinse mouth with water following oral treatments to decrease risk of oral candidiasis (wash face if using a face mask).

Dietary Considerations Avoid grapefruit juice when using oral capsules.

Geriatric Considerations Ensure that patients can correctly use inhaler.

Breast-Feeding Considerations Following use of the powder for oral inhalation, ~0.3% to 1% of the maternal dose was found in breast milk. The maximum concentration appeared within 45 minutes of dosing. Plasma budesonide levels obtained from infants ~90 minutes after breast-feeding (~140 minutes after maternal dose) were below the limit of quantification. Concentrations of budesonide in breast milk are expected to be higher following administration of oral capsules than after an inhaled dose.

Pregnancy Considerations Adverse events have been observed with corticosteroids in animal reproduction studies. Studies of pregnant women using inhaled budesonide have not demonstrated an increased risk of abnormalities. Some studies have shown an association between first trimester systemic corticosteroid use and oral clefts; adverse events in the fetus/neonate have been noted in case reports following large doses of systemic corticosteroids during pregnancy. Budesonide is the preferred inhaled corticosteroid for the treatment of asthma in pregnant women.

Additional Information Effects of inhaled steroids on growth have been observed in the absence of laboratory evidence of HPA axis suppression, suggesting that growth velocity is a more sensitive indicator of systemic corticosteroid exposure in pediatric patients than some commonly used tests of HPA axis function. The long-term effects of this reduction in growth velocity associated with orally-inhaled corticosteroids, including the impact on final adult height, are unknown. The potential for "catch up" growth following discontinuation of treatment with inhaled corticosteroids has not been adequately studied.

Related Information

Asthma *on page* 2015

Budesonide (Nasal) (byoo DES oh nide)

U.S. Brand Names Rhinocort Aqua®

Generic Availability (U.S.) No

Pharmacologic Category Corticosteroid, Nasal

Pregnancy Risk Factor B

Lactation Enters breast milk/use caution

Use Management of symptoms of seasonal or perennial rhinitis

Canadian labeling: Additional use (not in U.S. labeling): Prevention and treatment of nasal polyps

Available Dosage Forms

Suspension, intranasal:

Rhinocort Aqua®: 32 mcg/inhalation (8.6 g)

Dosing

Adult & Geriatric

Nasal polyps: *Nasal inhalation:*

Canadian labeling:

Rhinocort® Aqua®: 256 mcg/day administered as a single 64 mcg spray in each nostril twice daily; maximum dose: 256 mcg/day

Rhinocort® Turbuhaler®: 100 mcg into each nostril twice daily; maximum: 400 mcg/day

Rhinitis: *Nasal inhalation:*

U.S. labeling (Rhinocort® Aqua®): 64 mcg/day as a single 32 mcg spray in each nostril. Some patients who do not achieve adequate control may benefit from increased dosage. A reduced dosage may be effective after initial control is achieved

Maximum dose: Children <12 years: 128 mcg/day; Adults: 256 mcg/day)

Canadian labeling:

Rhinocort® Aqua®: Initial: 256 mcg/day administered as two 64 mcg sprays in each nostril once daily or a single 64 mcg spray in each nostril twice daily; Maintenance: Individualize, lowest effective dose (maximum dose: 256 mcg/day)

Rhinocort® Turbuhaler®: Initial: 200 mcg into each nostril once daily; Maintenance: Individualize, lowest effective dose (maximum: 400 mcg/day)

Pediatric

Nasal polyps: *Nasal inhalation:*

Canadian labeling: Children ≥6 years: Refer to adult dosing.

Rhinitis: *Nasal inhalation:*

U.S. labeling (Rhinocort® Aqua®): Children ≥6 years: Refer to adult dosing.

Canadian labeling (Rhinocort® Aqua®, Rhinocort® Turbuhaler®): Children ≥6 years: Refer to adult dosing.

Hepatic Impairment Monitor closely for signs and symptoms of hypercorticism; dosage reduction may be required.

Administration

Inhalation

Powder for nasal inhalation: Rhinocort® Turbuhaler® [CAN, not available in the U.S.]: Hold inhaler in upright position and turn grey grip as far as it will go in one direction and then back to original position. Clicking sound means inhaler is loaded with dose and ready for use. Place nasal adapter into nostril and ensure firm fit. Cover opposite nostril with finger and inhale (sniff) quickly and forcefully. Do not exhale through inhaler. When a red mark appears in the dose indicator window, 20 doses are left. When the red mark reaches the bottom of the window, the inhaler should be discarded

Suspension for nasal inhalation: Shake gently before use. Prime before first use; discard after 120 sprays.

◆ **Budesonide and Eformoterol** *see* Budesonide and Formoterol *on page 239*

Budesonide and Formoterol (byoo DES oh nide & for MOH te rol)

U.S. Brand Names Symbicort®

Index Terms Budesonide and Eformoterol; Eformoterol and Budesonide; Formoterol and Budesonide; Formoterol Fumarate Dihydrate and Budesonide

Pharmacologic Category Beta$_2$-Adrenergic Agonist; Beta$_2$-Adrenergic Agonist, Long-Acting; Corticosteroid, Inhalant (Oral)

Medication Guide Available Yes

Pregnancy Risk Factor C

Lactation

Budesonide: Enters breast milk/use caution

Formoterol: Excretion in breast milk unknown/use caution

Use Treatment of asthma in patients ≥12 years of age where combination therapy is indicated; maintenance treatment of airflow obstruction associated with chronic obstructive pulmonary disease (COPD; including chronic bronchitis and emphysema)

Unlabeled/Investigational Use Treatment of asthma in children 5-11 years of age where combination therapy is indicated

Mechanism of Action/Effect Formoterol relaxes bronchial smooth muscle by selective action on beta$_2$ receptors with little effect on heart rate. Formoterol has a long-acting effect. Budesonide is a corticosteroid which controls the rate of protein synthesis, depresses the migration of polymorphonuclear leukocytes/fibroblasts, and reverses capillary permeability and lysosomal stabilization at the cellular level to prevent or control inflammation.

Contraindications Hypersensitivity to budesonide, formoterol, or any component of the formulation; need for acute bronchodilation in COPD or asthma (including status asthmaticus)

Canadian labeling: Additional contraindications (not in U.S. labeling): Hypersensitivity to inhaled lactose

Warnings/Precautions [U.S. Boxed Warning]: Long-acting beta$_2$-agonists (LABAs), such as formoterol, increase the risk of asthma-related deaths; budesonide and formoterol should only be used in patients not adequately controlled on a long-term asthma control medication (ie, inhaled corticosteroid) or whose disease severity requires initiation of two maintenance therapies. In a large, randomized, placebo-controlled U.S. clinical trial (SMART, 2006), salmeterol was associated with an increase in asthma-related deaths (when added to usual asthma therapy); risk is considered a class effect among all LABAs. Data are not available to determine if the addition of an inhaled corticosteroid lessens this increased risk of death associated with LABA use. Assess patients at regular intervals once asthma control is maintained on combination therapy to determine if step-down therapy is appropriate (without loss of asthma control), and the patient can be maintained on an inhaled corticosteroid only. LABAs are not appropriate in patients whose asthma is adequately controlled on low- or medium-dose inhaled corticosteroids. **[U.S. Boxed Warning]: LABAs may increase the risk of asthma-related hospitalization in pediatric and adolescent patients.**

Do **not** use for acute bronchospasm or acute symptomatic COPD. Short-acting beta$_2$-agonist (eg, albuterol) should be used for acute symptoms and symptoms occurring between treatments. Do **not** initiate in patients with significantly worsening or acutely deteriorating asthma or COPD. Increased use and/or ineffectiveness of short-acting beta$_2$-agonists may indicate rapidly deteriorating disease and should prompt re-evaluation of the patient's condition. Patients must be instructed to seek medical attention in cases where acute symptoms are not relieved by short-acting beta-agonist (not formoterol) or a previous level of response is diminished. Medical evaluation must not be delayed. Patients using inhaled, short acting beta$_2$-agonists should be instructed to discontinue routine use of these medications prior to beginning treatment with Symbicort®; short acting agents should be reserved for symptomatic relief of acute symptoms. Data are not available to determine if LABA use increases the risk of death in patients with COPD.

Immediate hypersensitivity reactions (urticaria, angioedema, rash, bronchospasm) have been reported. Do not exceed recommended dose; serious adverse events, including fatalities, have been associated with excessive use of inhaled sympathomimetics. Rarely, paradoxical bronchospasm may occur with use of inhaled bronchodilating agents; this should be distinguished from inadequate response. Pneumonia and other lower respiratory tract infections have been reported in patients with COPD following the use of inhaled corticosteroids; monitor COPD patients closely since pneumonia symptoms may overlap symptoms of exacerbations.

Use caution in patients with cardiovascular disease (arrhythmia or hypertension or HF), seizure disorders, diabetes, hepatic impairment, ocular disease, osteoporosis, thyroid disease, or hypokalemia. Beta agonists may cause elevation in blood pressure, heart rate, and result in CNS stimulation/excitation. Beta$_2$-agonists may increase risk of arrhythmia, increase serum glucose, or decrease serum potassium. Long-term use may affect bone mineral density in adults. Infections with *Candida albicans* in the mouth and throat (thrush) have been reported with use. Use with caution in patients taking strong CYP3A4 inhibitors (see Drug Interactions); consider alternative agents that avoid or lessen the potential for CYP-mediated interactions.

Budesonide may cause hypercorticism and/or suppression of hypothalamic-pituitary-adrenal (HPA) axis, particularly in younger children or in patients receiving high doses for prolonged periods. Caution is required when patients are transferred from systemic corticosteroids to products with lower systemic bioavailability (ie, inhalation). May lead to possible adrenal insufficiency or withdrawal symptoms, including an increase in allergic symptoms. Patients receiving prolonged therapy ≥20 mg per day of prednisone (or equivalent) may be most susceptible. Aerosol steroids do **not** provide the systemic steroid needed to treat patients having trauma, surgery, or infections.

Orally-inhaled and intranasal corticosteroids may cause a reduction in growth velocity in pediatric patients (~1 centimeter per year [range 0.3-1.8 cm per year] and related to dose and duration of exposure). To minimize the systemic effects of orally-inhaled and intranasal corticosteroids, each patient should be titrated to the lowest effective dose. Growth should be routinely monitored in pediatric patients.

Prolonged use of corticosteroids may also increase the incidence of secondary infection, mask acute infection (including fungal infections), prolong or exacerbate viral infections, or limit response to vaccines. Exposure to chickenpox should be avoided; corticosteroids should not be used to treat ocular herpes simplex. Corticosteroids should not be used for cerebral malaria. Close observation is required in patients with latent tuberculosis and/or TB reactivity restrict use in active TB (only in conjunction with antituberculosis treatment).

Some products available in Canada contain lactose; very rare anaphylactic reactions have been reported in patients with severe milk protein allergy. Withdraw systemic therapy with gradual tapering of dose. There have been reports of systemic corticosteroid withdrawal symptoms (eg, joint/muscle pain, lassitude, depression) when withdrawing oral inhalation therapy.

Drug Interactions

Metabolism/Transport Effects

Budesonide: **Substrate** (minor) of CYP3A4

Formoterol: **Substrate** (minor) of CYP2A6, 2C9, 2C19, 2D6

Avoid Concomitant Use

Avoid concomitant use of Budesonide and Formoterol with any of the following: Aldesleukin; BCG; Iobenguane I 123; Natalizumab; Pimecrolimus; Roflumilast; Tacrolimus (Topical)

Decreased Effect

Budesonide and Formoterol may decrease the levels/effects of: Aldesleukin; Antidiabetic Agents; BCG; Corticorelin; Iobenguane I 123; Sipuleucel-T; Vaccines (Inactivated)

The levels/effects of Budesonide and Formoterol may be decreased by: Alpha-/Beta-Blockers; Antacids; Beta-Blockers (Beta1 Selective); Beta-Blockers (Nonselective); Betahistine; Bile Acid Sequestrants; Echinacea

Increased Effect/Toxicity

Budesonide and Formoterol may increase the levels/effects of: Amphotericin B; Leflunomide; Loop Diuretics; Natalizumab; Sympathomimetics; Thiazide Diuretics

The levels/effects of Budesonide and Formoterol may be increased by: Atomoxetine; Caffeine; Cannabinoids; CYP3A4 Inhibitors (Moderate); CYP3A4 Inhibitors (Strong); Dasatinib; Denosumab; MAO Inhibitors; Pimecrolimus; Roflumilast; Tacrolimus (Topical); Theophylline Derivatives; Trastuzumab; Tricyclic Antidepressants

Adverse Reactions Note: Percentage of adverse events may be dose related; causation not established. Also see individual agents.

>10%:

Central nervous system: Headache (7% to 11%)

Respiratory: Nasopharyngitis (7% to 11%), upper respiratory tract infections (4% to 11%)

1% to 10%:

Central nervous system: Dizziness (<3%)

Gastrointestinal: Stomach discomfort (1% to 7%), oral candidiasis (1% to 6%), vomiting (1% to 3%)

Neuromuscular & skeletal: Back pain (2% to 3%)

Respiratory: Pharyngolaryngeal pain (6% to 9%), lower respiratory tract infection (3% to 8%), sinusitis (4% to 6%), bronchitis (5%), nasal congestion (3%)

Miscellaneous: Influenza (2% to 3%)

Pharmacodynamics/Kinetics

Onset of Action Asthma: 15 minutes; maximum benefit: May take ≥2 weeks

Pharmacokinetic Note See individual agents.

Available Dosage Forms

Aerosol for oral inhalation:

Symbicort® 80/4.5: Budesonide 80 mcg and formoterol fumarate dihydrate 4.5 mcg per actuation (6.9 g) [60 metered inhalations]; budesonide 80 mcg and formoterol fumarate dihydrate 4.5 mcg per actuation (10.2 g) [120 metered inhalations]

Symbicort® 160/4.5: Budesonide 160 mcg and formoterol fumarate dihydrate 4.5 mcg per actuation (6 g) [60 metered inhalations]; budesonide 160 mcg and formoterol fumarate dihydrate 4.5 mcg per actuation (10.2 g) [120 metered inhalations]

Dosing

Adult & Geriatric

Asthma: Oral inhalation:

U.S. labeling: Symbicort® 80/4.5, Symbicort® 160/4.5: Two inhalations twice daily (maximum: 4 inhalations/day). Recommended starting dose combination is determined according to asthma severity. In patients not adequately controlled on the lower combination dose following 1-2 weeks of therapy, consider the higher dose combination.

Canadian labeling:

Symbicort® 100 Turbuhaler® [CAN; not available in U.S.], Symbicort® 200 Turbuhaler® [CAN; not available in U.S.]:

Initial: 1-2 inhalations twice daily until symptom control, then titrate to lowest effective dosage to maintain control

Maintenance: 1-2 inhalations once or twice daily (maximum: 8 inhalations/day as temporary treatment in periods of worsening asthma)

Symbicort® Maintenance and Reliever Therapy (Symbicort® SMART): **Note:** Not approved in the U.S.:

Maintenance: Symbicort® 100 Turbuhaler® [CAN] **or** Symbicort® 200 Turbuhaler® [CAN]: 1-2 inhalations twice daily **or** 2 inhalations once daily

Reliever therapy: Symbicort® 100 Turbuhaler [CAN] **or** Symbicort® 200 Turbuhaler® [CAN]: 1 additional inhalation as needed, may repeat if no relief for up to 6 inhalations total (maximum: 8 inhalations/day)

COPD: Oral inhalation:

U.S. labeling: Symbicort® 160/4.5: Two inhalations twice daily (maximum: 4 inhalations/day)

Canadian labeling: Symbicort® 200 Turbuhaler® [CAN; not available in U.S.]: Two inhalations twice daily (maximum: 4 inhalations/day)

Pediatric Asthma: Oral inhalation:

Children 5-11 years (NIH Guidelines): Symbicort® 80/4.5: Two inhalations twice daily. Do not exceed 4 inhalations per day.

Children ≥12 years: Refer to adult dosing.

Hepatic Impairment Use of this combination has not been studied in patients with hepatic impairment; however, the manufacturer recommends close monitoring of patients with hepatic disease.

Administration

Inhalation

Symbicort® 80/4.5, Symbicort® 160/4.5: Prior to first use, inhaler must be primed by releasing 2 test sprays into the air; shake well for 5 seconds before each spray. Inhaler must be reprimed if not used for >7 days or if it has been dropped. Shake well for 5 seconds before each use. Discard inhaler after the labeled number of inhalations have been used or within 3 months after removal from foil pouch (do not use the "float test" to determine amount remaining in canister).

Symbicort® Turbuhaler® [CAN; not available in U.S.]:

To "load" inhaler: Turn grip on inhaler as far as it will move in one direction, then turn in opposite direction as far as it will go (inhaler is "loaded" with a dose, indicated by a "click"). Prior to first use, this procedure should be done twice, it does not need to be repeated with subsequent uses even when not used regularly.

Delivery of dose: Instruct patient to place mouthpiece gently between teeth, closing lips around inhaler. Instruct patient to inhale deeply and hold breath held for 5-10 seconds. The amount of drug delivered is small, and the individual will not sense the medication as it is inhaled. Remove mouthpiece prior to exhalation. Patient should not breathe out through the mouthpiece. After use of the inhaler, patient should rinse mouth/oropharynx with water and spit out rinse solution.

Stability

Storage

Symbicort® 80/4.5, Symbicort® 160/4.5: Store at room temperature of 20°C to 25°C (68°F to 77°F) with mouthpiece down. Do not puncture, incinerate, or store near heat or open flame. Discard inhaler after the labeled number of inhalations have been used or within 3 months after removal from foil pouch.

Symbicort® Turbuhaler®: Store at room temperature of 15°C to 30°C. Protect from heat and moisture.

Monitoring and Teaching Issues

Laboratory Monitoring FEV_1, peak flow meter; growth (in pediatric patients)

Physical Assessment See individual agents.

Patient Education See individual agents.

Pregnancy Considerations Teratogenic and embryocidal effects were observed in animal studies when administered by inhalation at doses less than the maximum equivalent human dose. Also see individual agents.

Additional Information Effects of inhaled/intranasal steroids on growth have been observed in the absence of laboratory evidence of HPA axis suppression, suggesting that growth velocity is a more sensitive indicator of systemic corticosteroid exposure in pediatric patients than some commonly used tests of HPA axis function. The long-term effects of this reduction in growth velocity associated with orally-inhaled and intranasal corticosteroids, including the impact on final adult height, are unknown. The potential for "catch up" growth following discontinuation of treatment with inhaled corticosteroids has not been adequately studied.

Related Information

Budesonide (Systemic, Oral Inhalation) *on page 235*

Formoterol *on page 820*

◆ **Buffasal [OTC]** *see* Aspirin *on page 155*

◆ **Bufferin® [OTC]** *see* Aspirin *on page 155*

◆ **Bufferin® Extra Strength [OTC]** *see* Aspirin *on page 155*

◆ **Buffinol [OTC]** *see* Aspirin *on page 155*

Bumetanide (byoo MET a nide)

Index Terms Bumex

Generic Availability (U.S.) Yes

Pharmacologic Category Diuretic, Loop

Medication Safety Issues

Sound-alike/look-alike issues:

Bumetanide may be confused with Buminate®

Bumex® may be confused with Brevibloc®, Buprenex®, Permax®

Pregnancy Risk Factor C

Lactation Excretion in breast milk unknown/not recommended

Use Management of edema secondary to heart failure or hepatic or renal disease (including nephrotic syndrome)

Unlabeled/Investigational Use Treatment of hypertension

Mechanism of Action/Effect Inhibits reabsorption of sodium and chloride in the ascending loop of Henle and proximal renal tubule, causing increased excretion of water, sodium, chloride, magnesium, phosphate, and calcium

Contraindications Hypersensitivity to bumetanide or any component of the formulation; anuria; patients with hepatic coma or in states of severe electrolyte depletion until the condition improves or is corrected

Warnings/Precautions [U.S. Boxed Warning]: Excessive amounts can lead to profound diuresis with fluid and electrolyte loss; close medical supervision and dose evaluation are required. Potassium supplementation and/or use of potassium-sparing diuretics may be necessary to prevent hypokalemia. In cirrhosis, initiate bumetanide therapy with conservative dosing and close monitoring of electrolytes; avoid sudden changes in fluid and electrolyte balance and acid/base status which may lead to hepatic encephalopathy. *In vitro* studies using pooled sera from critically-ill neonates have shown bumetanide to be a potent displacer of bilirubin; avoid use in neonates at risk for kernicterus. Coadministration of antihypertensives may increase the risk of hypotension.

Monitor fluid status and renal function in an attempt to prevent oliguria, azotemia, and reversible increases in BUN and creatinine; close medical supervision of aggressive diuresis required. Bumetanide-induced ototoxicity (usually transient) may occur with rapid I.V. administration, renal impairment, excessive doses, and concurrent use of other ototoxins (eg, aminoglycosides). Asymptomatic hyperuricemia has been reported with use.

Chemical similarities are present among sulfonamides, sulfonylureas, carbonic anhydrase inhibitors, thiazides, and loop diuretics (except ethacrynic acid); the manufacturer's labeling states that bumetanide may be used in patients allergic to furosemide. Use in patients with sulfonylurea allergy is not specifically contraindicated in product labeling; however, a risk of cross-reaction exists in patients with allergy to any of these compounds; avoid use when previous reaction has been severe. Discontinue if signs of hypersensitivity are noted.

Drug Interactions

Avoid Concomitant Use There are no known interactions where it is recommended to avoid concomitant use.

Decreased Effect

Bumetanide may decrease the levels/effects of: Lithium; Neuromuscular-Blocking Agents

The levels/effects of Bumetanide may be decreased by: Bile Acid Sequestrants; Herbs (Hypertensive Properties); Methylphenidate; Nonsteroidal Anti-Inflammatory Agents; Phenytoin; Probenecid; Salicylates; Yohimbine

Increased Effect/Toxicity

Bumetanide may increase the levels/effects of: ACE Inhibitors; Allopurinol; Amifostine; Aminoglycosides; Antihypertensives; CISplatin; Dofetilide; Hypotensive Agents; Lithium; Neuromuscular-Blocking Agents; RiTUXimab; Salicylates

The levels/effects of Bumetanide may be increased by: Beta2-Agonists; Corticosteroids (Orally Inhaled); Corticosteroids (Systemic); Diazoxide; Herbs (Hypotensive Properties); Licorice; MAO Inhibitors; Pentoxifylline; Phosphodiesterase 5 Inhibitors; Probenecid; Prostacyclin Analogues

Nutritional/Ethanol Interactions

Food: Bumetanide serum levels may be decreased if taken with food. It has been recommended that bumetanide be administered without food (Bard, 2004).

Herb/Nutraceutical: Avoid ephedra, yohimbe, ginseng (may worsen hypertension). Avoid dong quai if using for hypertension (has estrogenic activity). Avoid garlic (may have increased antihypertensive effect).

Adverse Reactions

>10%:

Endocrine & metabolic: Hyperuricemia (18%), hypochloremia (15%), hypokalemia (15%)

Renal: Azotemia (11%)

1% to 10%:

Central nervous system: Dizziness (1%)

Endocrine & metabolic: Hyponatremia (9%), hyperglycemia (7%), phosphorus altered (5%), CO_2 content altered (4%), bicarbonate altered (3%), calcium altered (2%)

Neuromuscular & skeletal: Muscle cramps (1%)

Renal: Serum creatinine increased (7%)

Miscellaneous: LDH altered (1%)

Pharmacodynamics/Kinetics

Onset of Action Oral, I.M.: 0.5-1 hour; I.V.: 2-3 minutes

Peak effect: Oral: 1-2 hours; I.V.: 15-30 minutes

Duration of Action 4-6 hours

Bioavailability 59% to 89% (median: 80%)

Protein Binding 95% to 96%

Half-Life Elimination Neonates: ~6 hours; Infants (1 month): ~2.4 hours; Adults: 1-1.5 hours

Metabolism Partially hepatic

Excretion Urine (81% of total dose; 45% of which is unchanged drug); feces (2% of total dose)

Available Dosage Forms

Injection, solution: 0.25 mg/mL (2 mL, 4 mL, 5 mL, 10 mL)

Tablet, oral: 0.5 mg, 1 mg, 2 mg

Dosing

Adult & Geriatric

Edema:

Oral: 0.5-2 mg/dose 1-2 times/day; if diuretic response to initial dose is not adequate, may repeat in 4-5 hours for up to 2 doses (maximum dose: 10 mg/day)

I.M., I.V.: 0.5-1 mg/dose; if diuretic response to initial dose is not adequate, may repeat in 2-3 hours for up to 2 doses (maximum dose: 10 mg/day)

Continuous I.V. infusion (unlabeled dose): Initial: 1 mg I.V. load then 0.5-2 mg/hour (Hunt, 2009)

Hypertension (unlabeled use): *Oral:* 0.5 mg daily (maximum dose: 5 mg/day); usual dosage range (JNC 7): 0.5-2 mg/day in 2 divided doses (Chobanian, 2003)

Pediatric Edema: *Oral, I.M., I.V.:* Infants and Children: 0.015-0.1 mg/kg/dose every 6-24 hours (maximum dose: 10 mg/day)

Administration

Oral An alternate-day schedule or a 3-4 daily dosing regimen with rest periods of 1-2 days in between may be the most tolerable and effective regimen for the continued control of edema.

I.V. Administer slowly, over 1-2 minutes.

Stability

Storage

I.V.: Store vials at 15°C to 30°C (59°F to 86°F). Infusion solutions should be used within 24 hours after preparation. Light sensitive; discoloration may occur when exposed to light.

Tablet: Store at 15°C to 30°C (59°F to 86°F).

Monitoring and Teaching Issues

Laboratory Monitoring Serum electrolytes, renal function

Physical Assessment Assess history of allergies and renal, electrolyte, hepatic, and pregnancy status prior to beginning treatment. Blood pressure, weight, and fluid status should be monitored at beginning of therapy and periodically during therapy. Assess electrolytes, renal function, and therapeutic effectiveness (reduced edema and cardiopulmonary symptoms). Monitor for hypotension, electrolyte imbalance, and ototoxicity.

Patient Education May be taken with food to reduce GI effects. If taking one dose daily, take single dose early in day; if taking twice daily, take last dose early in afternoon to prevent sleep interruptions. Include potassium-rich foods in your daily diet, but do not take supplemental potassium without consulting prescriber. May cause dizziness or weakness. Report palpitations or chest pain, swelling of ankles or feet, weight increase, increased fatigue, muscle cramps, trembling, and any changes in hearing.

Dietary Considerations Administration with food slows the rate and reduces the extent of absorption and may reduce diuretic efficacy (Bard, 2004). May require increased intake of potassium-rich foods.

Geriatric Considerations Loop diuretics are potent diuretics; excess amounts can lead to profound diuresis with fluid and electrolyte loss; close medical supervision and dose evaluation is required, particularly in the elderly. Severe loss of sodium and/or increases in BUN can cause confusion; for any change in mental status in patients on bumetanide, monitor electrolytes and renal function.

Pregnancy Considerations Adverse events have been observed in some animal studies.

Related Information

Heart Failure (Systolic) *on page* 2040

◆ **Bumex** *see* Bumetanide *on page* 242

◆ **Buminate** *see* Albumin *on page* 57

◆ **Bupap** *see* Butalbital and Acetaminophen *on page* 261

Bupivacaine (byoo PIV a kane)

U.S. Brand Names Bupivacaine Spinal; Marcaine®; Marcaine® Spinal; Sensorcaine®; Sensorcaine®-MPF; Sensorcaine®-MPF Spinal

Index Terms Bupivacaine Hydrochloride

Generic Availability (U.S.) Yes

Pharmacologic Category Local Anesthetic

Medication Safety Issues

Sound-alike/look-alike issues:

Bupivacaine may be confused with mepivacaine, ropivacaine

Marcaine® may be confused with Narcan®

High alert medication: The Institute for Safe Medication Practices (ISMP) includes this medication (epidural administration) among its list of drug classes which have a heightened risk of causing significant patient harm when used in error.

Pregnancy Risk Factor C

Lactation Enters breast milk/not recommended

Use Local or regional anesthesia; spinal anesthesia; diagnostic and therapeutic procedures; obstetrical procedures (only 0.25% and 0.5% concentrations)

0.25%: Local infiltration, peripheral nerve block, sympathetic block, caudal or epidural block

0.5%: Peripheral nerve block, caudal and epidural block

0.75% **(not for obstetrical anesthesia)**: Retrobulbar block, epidural block. **Note:** Reserve for surgical procedures where a high degree of muscle relaxation and prolonged effect are necessary

Mechanism of Action/Effect Blocks both the initiation and conduction of nerve impulses by decreasing the neuronal membrane's permeability to sodium ions, which results in inhibition of depolarization with resultant blockade of conduction

Contraindications Hypersensitivity to bupivacaine hydrochloride, amide-type local anesthetics, or any component of the formulation; obstetrical paracervical block anesthesia

Note: Use as intravenous regional anesthesia (Bier block) is considered contraindicated per accepted clinical practice.

Warnings/Precautions Do not use solutions containing preservatives for caudal or epidural block. Use with caution in patients with hepatic impairment. Local anesthetics have been associated with rare occurrences of sudden respiratory arrest; convulsions due to systemic toxicity leading to cardiac arrest have also been reported, presumably following unintentional intravascular injection. Intravenous regional anesthesia (Bier block) is **not** recommended; cardiac arrest and death have occurred with this method of administration. **[U.S. Boxed Warning]: The 0.75% concentration is not recommended for obstetrical epidural anesthesia; cardiac arrest with difficult resuscitation or death has occurred.** A test dose is recommended prior to epidural administration (prior to initial dose) and all reinforcing doses with continuous catheter technique. Use caution with cardiovascular dysfunction including patients with hypotension or heart block. Use caution in debilitated, elderly, or acutely ill patients; dose reduction may be required. Resuscitative equipment, oxygen, and other resuscitative drugs should be available for immediate use. Continuous intra-articular infusion of local anesthetics after arthroscopic or other surgical procedures is **not** an approved use; chondrolysis (primarily shoulder joint) has occurred following infusion, with some requiring arthroplasty or shoulder replacement.

Drug Interactions

Metabolism/Transport Effects Substrate (minor) of CYP1A2, 2C19, 2D6, 3A4

Avoid Concomitant Use There are no known interactions where it is recommended to avoid concomitant use.

Decreased Effect

The levels/effects of Bupivacaine may be decreased by: Peginterferon Alfa-2b

Increased Effect/Toxicity

The levels/effects of Bupivacaine may be increased by: Beta-Blockers; Conivaptan

Adverse Reactions Note: Incidence of adverse reactions is difficult to define. Most effects are dose related, and are often due to accelerated absorption from the injection site, unintentional intravascular injection, or slow metabolic degradation. The development of any central nervous system symptoms may be an early indication of more significant toxicity (seizure).

Cardiovascular: Hypotension, bradycardia, palpitation, heart block, ventricular arrhythmia, cardiac arrest

Central nervous system: Restlessness, anxiety, dizziness, seizure (0.1%); rare symptoms (usually associated with unintentional subarachnoid injection during high spinal anesthesia) include persistent anesthesia, paresthesia, paralysis, headache, septic meningitis, and cranial nerve palsies

Gastrointestinal: Nausea, vomiting; rare symptoms (usually associated with unintentional subarachnoid injection during high spinal anesthesia) include fecal incontinence and loss of sphincter control

Genitourinary: Rare symptoms (usually associated with unintentional subarachnoid injection during high spinal anesthesia) include urinary incontinence, loss of perineal sensation, and loss of sexual function

Neuromuscular & skeletal: Chondrolysis (continuous intra-articular administration), weakness

Ocular: Blurred vision, pupillary constriction

Otic: Tinnitus

Respiratory: Apnea, hypoventilation (usually associated with unintentional subarachnoid injection during high spinal anesthesia)

Miscellaneous: Allergic reactions (urticaria, pruritus, angioedema), anaphylactoid reactions

Pharmacodynamics/Kinetics

Onset of Action Anesthesia (route and dose dependent): 1-17 minutes

Duration of Action Route and dose dependent: 2-9 hours

Time to Peak Plasma: Caudal, epidural, or peripheral nerve block: 30-45 minutes

Protein Binding ~95%

Half-Life Elimination Age dependent: Neonates: 8.1 hours; Adults: 2.7 hours

Metabolism Hepatic; forms metabolite (pipecoloxylidine [PPX])

Excretion Urine (~6% unchanged)

Available Dosage Forms

Injection, solution: 0.25% [2.5 mg/mL] (50 mL); 0.5% [5 mg/mL] (50 mL)

Marcaine®: 0.5% [5 mg/mL] (50 mL)

Sensorcaine®: 0.25% [2.5 mg/mL] (50 mL); 0.5% [5 mg/mL] (50 mL)

Injection, solution [preservative free]: 0.25% [2.5 mg/mL] (10 mL, 20 mL, 30 mL, 50 mL); 0.5% [5 mg/mL] (10 mL, 20 mL, 30 mL); 0.75% [7.5 mg/mL] (10 mL, 20 mL, 30 mL)

Marcaine®: 0.25% [2.5 mg/mL] (10 mL, 30 mL, 50 mL); 0.5% [5 mg/mL] (10 mL, 30 mL); 0.75% [7.5 mg/mL] (10 mL, 30 mL)

Sensorcaine®-MPF: 0.25% [2.5 mg/mL] (10 mL, 30 mL); 0.5% [5 mg/mL] (10 mL, 30 mL); 0.75% [7.5 mg/mL] (10 mL, 30 mL)

Injection, solution, premixed in $D_{8.25}W$ [preservative free]:

Bupivacaine Spinal: 0.75% [7.5 mg/mL] (2 mL)

Marcaine® Spinal: 0.75% [7.5 mg/mL] (2 mL)

Sensorcaine®-MPF Spinal: 0.75% [7.5 mg/mL] (2 mL)

Dosing

Adult & Geriatric Note: Dose varies with procedure, depth of anesthesia, vascularity of tissues, duration of anesthesia, and condition of patient. Do not use solutions containing preservatives for caudal or epidural block.

Local anesthesia: Infiltration: 0.25% infiltrated locally; maximum: 175 mg

Caudal block (preservative free): 15-30 mL of 0.25% or 0.5%

Epidural block (other than caudal block; preservative free): Administer in 3-5 mL increments, allowing sufficient time to detect toxic manifestations of inadvertent I.V. or I.T. administration: 10-20 mL of 0.25% or 0.5%

Surgical procedures requiring a high degree of muscle relaxation and prolonged effects **only**: 10-20 mL of 0.75% (**Note:** Not to be used in obstetrical cases)

Peripheral nerve block: 5 mL of 0.25% or 0.5%; maximum: 400 mg/day

Sympathetic nerve block: 20-50 mL of 0.25%

Retrobulbar anesthesia: 2-4 mL of 0.75%

Spinal anesthesia: Preservative free solution of 0.75% bupivacaine in 8.25% dextrose:

Lower extremity and perineal procedures: 1 mL

Lower abdominal procedures: 1.6 mL

Normal vaginal delivery: 0.8 mL (higher doses may be required in some patients)

Cesarean section: 1-1.4 mL

Pediatric Note: Dose varies with procedure, depth of anesthesia, vascularity of tissues, duration of anesthesia, and condition of patient. Do not use solutions containing preservatives for caudal or epidural block.

Caudal block, epidural block, local anesthesia: Children >12 years: Refer to adult dosing.

Peripheral or sympathetic nerve block: Children >12 years: Refer to adult dosing.

Retrobulbar anesthesia: Children >12 years: Refer to adult dosing.

Administration

Other Solutions containing preservatives should not be used for epidural or caudal blocks.

Stability

Storage Store at controlled room temperature of 20°C to 25°C (68°F to 77°F).

Monitoring and Teaching Issues

Physical Assessment Monitor for return of sensation to area anesthetized. Teach patient appropriate interventions to promote safety.

Patient Education This medication is given to reduce sensation in the injected area. You will experience decreased sensation to pain, heat, or cold in the area and/or decreased muscle strength; use necessary caution to reduce incidence of possible injury until full sensation returns. If used in mouth, do not eat or drink until full sensation returns. Immediately report chest pain or palpitations; increased restlessness, anxiety, or dizziness; skeletal or muscle weakness; or respiratory difficulty.

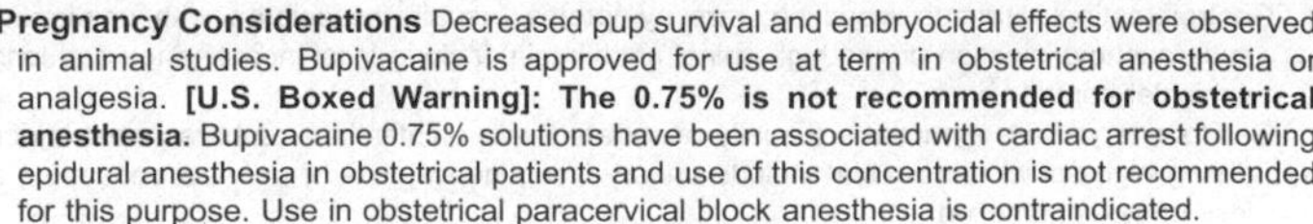

Pregnancy Considerations Decreased pup survival and embryocidal effects were observed in animal studies. Bupivacaine is approved for use at term in obstetrical anesthesia or analgesia. **[U.S. Boxed Warning]: The 0.75% is not recommended for obstetrical anesthesia.** Bupivacaine 0.75% solutions have been associated with cardiac arrest following epidural anesthesia in obstetrical patients and use of this concentration is not recommended for this purpose. Use in obstetrical paracervical block anesthesia is contraindicated.

◆ **Bupivacaine Hydrochloride** *see* Bupivacaine *on page 244*

◆ **Bupivacaine Spinal** *see* Bupivacaine *on page 244*

◆ **Buprenex®** *see* Buprenorphine *on page 246*

Buprenorphine (byoo pre NOR feen)

U.S. Brand Names Buprenex®; Butrans™; Subutex®

Index Terms Buprenorphine Hydrochloride

Generic Availability (U.S.) Yes: Excludes patch

Pharmacologic Category Analgesic, Opioid; Analgesic, Opioid Partial Agonist

Medication Safety Issues

Sound-alike/look-alike issues:

Buprenex® may be confused with Brevibloc®, Bumex®

High alert medication: The Institute for Safe Medication Practices (ISMP) includes this medication among its list of drug classes which have a heightened risk of causing significant patient harm when used in error.

Medication Guide Available Yes

Prescribing and Access Restrictions Prescribing of tablets for opioid dependence is limited to physicians who have met the qualification criteria and have received a DEA number specific to prescribing this product. Tablets will be available through pharmacies and wholesalers which normally provide controlled substances.

Pregnancy Risk Factor C

Lactation Enters breast milk/not recommended

Use

Injection: Management of moderate-to-severe pain

Sublingual tablet: Treatment of opioid dependence

Transdermal patch: Management of moderate-to-severe chronic pain in patients requiring an around-the-clock opioid analgesic for an extended period of time

Unlabeled/Investigational Use Injection: Management of opioid withdrawal in heroin-dependent hospitalized patients

Mechanism of Action/Effect Buprenorphine exerts its analgesic effect via high affinity binding to μ opiate receptors in the CNS; displays partial mu agonist and weak kappa antagonist activity

Contraindications Hypersensitivity to buprenorphine or any component of the formulation

Transdermal patch: Additional contraindications: Significant respiratory depression; severe asthma; known or suspected paralytic ileus; management of mild, acute, or intermittent pain; management of pain requiring short-term opioid analgesia; management of postoperative pain

Warnings/Precautions An opioid-containing analgesic regimen should be tailored to each patient's needs and based upon the type of pain being treated (acute versus chronic), the route of administration, degree of tolerance for opioids (naive versus chronic user), age, weight, and medical condition. The optimal analgesic dose varies widely among patients. Doses should be titrated to pain relief/prevention.

May cause CNS depression, which may impair physical or mental abilities. Effects with other sedative drugs or ethanol may be potentiated. Elderly may be more sensitive to CNS depressant and constipating effects. May cause respiratory depression - use caution in patients with respiratory disease or pre-existing respiratory depression. Hypersensitivity reactions, including bronchospasm, angioneurotic edema, and anaphylactic shock, have also been reported. Potential for drug dependency exists, abrupt cessation may precipitate withdrawal. Use caution in elderly, debilitated, pediatric patients, depression or suicidal tendencies. Tolerance, psychological and physical dependence may occur with prolonged use. Partial antagonist activity may precipitate acute narcotic withdrawal in opioid-dependent individuals.

Hepatitis has been reported with buprenorphine use; hepatic events ranged from transient, asymptomatic transaminase elevations to hepatic failure; in many cases, patients had preexisting hepatic dysfunction. Monitor liver function tests in patients at increased risk for hepatotoxicity (eg, history of alcohol abuse, pre-existing hepatic dysfunction, I.V. drug abusers) prior to and during therapy. Use with caution in patients with hepatic impairment; dosage adjustments are recommended in hepatic impairment.

Use with caution in patients with pulmonary or renal function impairment. Also use caution in patients with head injury or increased ICP, biliary tract dysfunction, patients with history of hyperthyroidism, morbid obesity, adrenal insufficiency, prostatic hyperplasia, urinary stricture, CNS depression, toxic psychosis, pancreatitis, alcoholism, delirium tremens, or kyphoscoliosis. May cause hypotension; use with caution in patients with hypovolemia, cardiovascular disease (including acute MI), or drugs which may exaggerate hypotensive effects (including phenothiazines or general anesthetics). May obscure diagnosis or clinical course of patients with acute abdominal conditions. Opioid therapy may lower seizure threshold; use caution in patients with a history of seizure disorders.

Transdermal patch: **[U.S. Boxed Warning]: Do not exceed one 20 mcg/hour transdermal patch due to the risk of QT_c-interval prolongation.** Avoid using in patients with history of long QT syndrome or in patients with predisposing factors increasing the risk of QT abnormalities (eg, concurrent medications such as antiarrhythmics, hypokalemia, unstable heart failure, unstable atrial fibrillation). **[U.S. Boxed Warning]: Healthcare provider should be alert to problems of abuse, misuse, and diversion.**

Sublingual tablets, which are used for induction treatment of opioid dependence, should not be started until effects of withdrawal are evident.

Drug Interactions

Metabolism/Transport Effects Substrate of CYP3A4 (major); **Inhibits** CYP1A2 (weak), 2A6 (weak), 2C19 (weak), 2D6 (weak)

Avoid Concomitant Use

Avoid concomitant use of Buprenorphine with any of the following: Atazanavir; MAO Inhibitors

Decreased Effect

Buprenorphine may decrease the levels/effects of: Analgesics (Opioid); Atazanavir; Pegvisomant

The levels/effects of Buprenorphine may be decreased by: Ammonium Chloride; CYP3A4 Inducers (Strong); Deferasirox; Efavirenz; Herbs (CYP3A4 Inducers); Mixed Agonist / Antagonist Opioids

Increased Effect/Toxicity

Buprenorphine may increase the levels/effects of: Alcohol (Ethyl); Alvimopan; CNS Depressants; Desmopressin; MAO Inhibitors; Selective Serotonin Reuptake Inhibitors; Thiazide Diuretics

The levels/effects of Buprenorphine may be increased by: Amphetamines; Antipsychotic Agents (Phenothiazines); Atazanavir; Conivaptan; CYP3A4 Inhibitors (Moderate); CYP3A4 Inhibitors (Strong); Dasatinib; Droperidol; Succinylcholine

Nutritional/Ethanol Interactions

Ethanol: Avoid ethanol (may increase CNS depression).

Herb/Nutraceutical: Avoid valerian, St John's wort, kava kava, gotu kola (may increase CNS depression).

Adverse Reactions

Injection:

>10%: Central nervous system: Sedation

1% to 10%:
- Cardiovascular: Hypotension
- Central nervous system: Respiratory depression, dizziness, headache
- Gastrointestinal: Vomiting, nausea
- Ocular: Miosis
- Otic: Vertigo
- Miscellaneous: Diaphoresis

Tablet:

>10%:
- Central nervous system: Headache (30%), pain (24%), insomnia (21% to 25%), anxiety (12%), depression (11%)
- Gastrointestinal: Nausea (10% to 14%), abdominal pain (12%), constipation (8% to 11%)
- Neuromuscular & skeletal: Back pain (14%), weakness (14%)
- Respiratory: Rhinitis (11%)
- Miscellaneous: Withdrawal syndrome (19%; placebo 37%), infection (12% to 20%), diaphoresis (12% to 13%)

1% to 10%:
- Central nervous system: Chills (6%), nervousness (6%), somnolence (5%), dizziness (4%), fever (3%)
- Gastrointestinal: Vomiting (5% to 8%), diarrhea (5%), dyspepsia (3%)
- Ocular: Lacrimation (5%)
- Respiratory: Cough (4%), pharyngitis (4%)
- Miscellaneous: Flu-like syndrome (6%)

Transdermal patch:

>10%:
- Central nervous system: Headache (16%), dizziness (16%), somnolence (14%),
- Gastrointestinal: Nausea (23%), constipation (14%), vomiting (11%)
- Local: Application site pruritus (15%)

1% to 10%:
- Cardiovascular: Peripheral edema (7%), chest pain, hypertension
- Central nervous system: Fatigue (5%), insomnia (3%), hypoesthesia (2%), anxiety, depression, fever, migraine
- Dermatologic: Pruritus (4%), rash (2%)
- Gastrointestinal: Xerostomia (7%), diarrhea (3%), abdominal discomfort (2%), anorexia (2%), upper abdominal pain
- Genitourinary: Urinary tract infection (3%)
- Local: Application site erythema (7%); application site rash (6%), application site irritation
- Neuromuscular & skeletal: Pain in extremity (3%), back pain (3%), joint swelling (3%), paresthesia (2%), tremor (2%), muscles spasms, musculoskeletal pain, myalgia, neck pain, weakness
- Respiratory: Dyspnea (3%), bronchitis, cough, nasopharyngitis, pharyngolaryngeal pain, sinusitis, upper respiratory tract infection
- Miscellaneous: Hyperhydrosis (4%), fall (4%), flu-like syndrome

Pharmacodynamics/Kinetics

Onset of Action Analgesic: I.M: Within 15 minutes; Peak effect: I.M.: ~1 hour; Transdermal patch: Steady state achieved by day 3

Duration of Action I.M.: ≥6 hours

Absorption I.M., SubQ: 30% to 40%

Bioavailability Relative to I.V. administration: I.M.: 70%; Sublingual tablet: 29%; Transdermal patch: ~15%

Time to Peak Plasma: Sublingual: 30 minutes to 1 hour (Kuhlman, 1996)

Protein Binding High (~96%, primarily to alpha- and beta globulin)

Half-Life Elimination I.V.: 2.2-3 hours; Apparent terminal half-life: Sublingual tablet: ~37 hours; Transdermal patch: ~26 hours. **Note:** Extended elimination half-life for sublingual administration may be due to depot effect (Kuhlman, 1996).

Metabolism Primarily hepatic via N-dealkylation by CYP3A4 to norbuprenorphine (active metabolite), and to a lesser extent via glucuronidation by UGT1A1 and 2B7 to buprenorphine 3-O-glucuronide; the major metabolite, norbuprenorphine, also undergoes glucuronidation via UGT1A3; extensive first-pass effect

Excretion Feces (~70%); urine (27% to 30%)

Controlled Substance C-III

Available Dosage Forms

Injection, solution: 0.3 mg/mL (1 mL)
Buprenex®: 0.3 mg/mL (1 mL)

Patch, transdermal:
Butrans™: 5 mcg/hour (4s); 10 mcg/hour (4s); 20 mcg/hour (4s)

Tablet, sublingual: 2 mg, 8 mg
Subutex®: 2 mg, 8 mg

Dosing

Adult

Acute pain (moderate-to-severe): Note: Long-term use is not recommended. The following recommendations are guidelines and do not represent the maximum doses that may be required in all patients. Doses should be titrated to pain relief/prevention. In high-risk patients (eg, elderly, debilitated, presence of respiratory disease) and/or concurrent CNS depressant use, reduce dose by one-half. Buprenorphine has an analgesic ceiling.

I.M.: Initial: Opiate-naive: 0.3 mg every 6-8 hours as needed; initial dose (up to 0.3 mg) may be repeated once in 30-60 minutes after the initial dose if needed; usual dosage range: 0.15-0.6 mg every 4-8 hours as needed

Slow I.V.: Initial: Opiate-naive: 0.3 mg every 6-8 hours as needed; initial dose (up to 0.3 mg) may be repeated once in 30-60 minutes after the initial dose if needed

Chronic pain (moderate-to-severe): Transdermal patch:

Opioid-naive patients: Initial: 5 mcg/hour applied once every 7 days

Opioid-experienced patients (conversion from other opioids to buprenorphine): Taper the current around-the-clock opioid for up to 7 days to ≤30 mg/day of oral morphine or equivalent before initiating therapy. Short-acting analgesics as needed may be continued until analgesia with transdermal buprenorphine is attained. There is a potential for buprenorphine to precipitate withdrawal in patients already receiving opioids.

Patients who were receiving daily dose of <30 mg of oral morphine equivalents: Initial: 5 mcg/hour applied once every 7 days

Patients who were receiving daily dose of 30-80 mg of oral morphine equivalents: Initial: 10 mcg/hour applied once every 7 days

Dose titration (opioid-naive or opioid-experienced patients): May increase dose, based on patient's supplemental short-acting analgesic requirements, with a minimum titration interval of 72 hours (maximum dose: 20 mcg/hour applied once every 7 days; risk for QT_c prolongation increases with doses ≥20 mcg/hour patch).

Discontinuation of therapy: Taper dose gradually to prevent withdrawal; consider initiating immediate-release opioids, if needed.

Opiate withdrawal in heroin-dependent hospitalized patients (unlabeled use): I.V. infusion: 0.3-0.9 mg (diluted in 50-100 mL of NS) over 20-30 minutes every 6-12 hours (Welsh, 2002)

Opioid dependence: Sublingual tablet: **Note:** The combination product, buprenorphine and naloxone, is preferred therapy over buprenorphine monotherapy for induction treatment (and stabilization/maintenance treatment) for short-acting opioid dependence (U.S. Department of Health and Human Services, 2005).

Manufacturer's labeling:

Induction: Day 1: 8 mg; Day 2 and subsequent induction days: 16 mg; usual induction dosage range: 12-16 mg/day (induction usually accomplished over 3-4 days). Treatment should begin at least 4 hours after last use of heroin or other short-acting opioids, preferably when first signs of withdrawal appear. Titrating dose to clinical effectiveness should be done as rapidly as possible to prevent undue withdrawal symptoms and patient drop-out during the induction period. There is little controlled experience with induction in patients on methadone or other long-acting opioids; consult expert physician experienced with this procedure.

Maintenance: Target dose: 16 mg/day; in some patients 12 mg/day may be effective; patients should be switched to the buprenorphine/naloxone combination product for maintenance and unsupervised therapy

Geriatric

Acute pain (moderate-to-severe): I.M., slow I.V.: 0.15 mg every 6 hours; elderly patients are more likely to suffer from confusion and drowsiness compared to younger patients. **Long-term use is not recommended.**

Chronic pain (moderate-to-severe): Transdermal patch: No specific dosage adjustments required; use caution due to potential for increased risk of adverse events.

Pediatric

Acute pain (moderate-to-severe):

Children 2-12 years: I.M., slow I.V.: 2-6 mcg/kg every 4-6 hours

Children ≥13 years: Refer to adult dosing.

Opioid dependence: Children ≥16 years: Refer to adult dosing.

Hepatic Impairment

Injection, sublingual tablet: Use caution due to extensive hepatic metabolism; dosage adjustments recommended although no specific recommendations are provided by the manufacturer.

Transdermal patch:

Mild-to-moderate impairment: Initial: 5 mcg/hour applied once every 7 days.

Severe impairment: Not studied; consider alternative therapy with more flexibility for dosing adjustments.

Administration

Oral Sublingual: Tablet should be placed under the tongue until dissolved; should not be swallowed. If two or more tablets are needed per dose, all may be placed under the tongue at once, or two at a time. To ensure consistent bioavailability, subsequent doses should always be taken the same way.

I.M. Administer via deep I.M. injection.

I.V. Administer slowly, over at least 2 minutes. Administration over 20-30 minutes preferred when managing opioid withdrawal in heroin-dependent hospitalized patients (Welsh, 2002).

Other Transdermal patch: Apply to patch to intact, nonirritated skin only. Apply to a hairless or nearly hairless skin site. If hairless site is not available, do not shave skin; hair at application site should be clipped. Prior to application, if the site must be cleaned, clean with clear water and allow to dry completely; do not use soaps, alcohol, lotions or abrasives due to potential for increased skin absorption. Do not use any patch that has been damaged, cut or manipulated in any way. Remove patch from protective pouch immediately before application. Remove the protective backing, and apply the sticky side of the patch to one of eight possible application sites (upper outer arm, upper chest, upper back, or the side of the chest [on either side of the body]). Firmly press patch in place and hold for ~15 seconds. Change patch every 7 days. Rotate patch application sites; wait ≥21 days before reapplying another patch to the same skin site. Avoid exposing application site to external heat sources (eg, heating pad, electric blanket, heat lamp, hot tub). If there is difficulty with patch adhesion, the edges of the system may be taped in place with first-aid tape. If the patch falls off during the 7-day dosing interval, dispose of the patch and apply a new patch to a different skin site.

Stability

Storage

Injection: Protect from excessive heat >40°C (>104°F). Protect from light.

Patch, tablet: Store at room temperature of 25°C (77°F).

Monitoring and Teaching Issues

Laboratory Monitoring LFTs (prior to initiation and during therapy)

Physical Assessment Monitor for effectiveness of pain relief. Monitor for possible respiratory depression prior to treatment and periodically throughout. For inpatients, implement safety measures to prevent falls. Assess patient's physical and/or psychological dependence. Discontinue slowly after prolonged use.

Patient Education Do not use alcohol, sedatives, tranquilizers, antihistamines, or pain medications without consulting prescriber. May cause dizziness, drowsiness, confusion, or blurred vision. You may experience nausea, vomiting, or constipation. If constipation is unresolved, consult prescriber about use of stool softeners and/or laxatives. Report unresolved nausea or vomiting, respiratory difficulty or shortness of breath, excessive sedation or unusual weakness, or rapid heartbeat or palpitations.

Geriatric Considerations One postmarketing study found that elderly patients were more likely to suffer from confusion and drowsiness after buprenorphine as compared to younger patients. Use transdermal system with caution in the elderly. Respiratory depression occurs more frequently in the elderly. In clinical trials, the incidence of adverse events was higher in older subjects.

Pregnancy Considerations Adverse effects have been observed in animal reproduction studies following buprenorphine subcutaneous and transdermal administration. In humans, withdrawal has been reported in infants of women receiving buprenorphine during pregnancy. Onset of symptoms ranged from day 1 to day 8 of life, most occurring on day 1.

Related Information

Opioid Analgesics *on page 2003*

Buprenorphine and Naloxone (byoo pre NOR feen & nal OKS one)

U.S. Brand Names Suboxone®

Index Terms Buprenorphine Hydrochloride and Naloxone Hydrochloride Dihydrate; Naloxone and Buprenorphine; Naloxone Hydrochloride Dihydrate and Buprenorphine Hydrochloride

Generic Availability (U.S.) No

Pharmacologic Category Analgesic, Opioid; Analgesic, Opioid Partial Agonist

Medication Safety Issues

High alert medication: The Institute for Safe Medication Practices (ISMP) includes this medication among its list of drug classes which have a heightened risk of causing significant patient harm when used in error.

Medication Guide Available Yes

Prescribing and Access Restrictions Prescribing of tablets for opioid dependence is limited to physicians who have met the qualification criteria and have received a DEA number specific to prescribing this product. Tablets will be available through pharmacies and wholesalers which normally provide controlled substances.

Pregnancy Risk Factor C

Lactation Buprenorphine: Enters breast milk/not recommended

Use Maintenance treatment for opioid dependence

Mechanism of Action/Effect See individual agents.

Contraindications Hypersensitivity to buprenorphine, naloxone, or any component of the formulation

Warnings/Precautions May cause respiratory depression - use caution in patients with respiratory disease or pre-existing respiratory depression. Potential for drug dependency exists, abrupt cessation may precipitate withdrawal. Hypersensitivity, including bronchospasm, angioneurotic edema, and anaphylactic shock, have been reported. Hepatitis has been reported with buprenorphine use; hepatic events ranged from transient, asymptomatic transaminase elevations to hepatic; in many cases, patients had preexisting hepatic dysfunction. Monitor liver function tests in all patients prior to and during therapy.

Use caution in elderly or debilitated patients. Use with caution in patients with hepatic or pulmonary function impairment. May cause CNS depression, which may impair physical or mental abilities. Patients must be cautioned about performing tasks which require mental alertness (eg, operating machinery or driving). Effects with other sedative drugs or ethanol may be potentiated. May cause orthostatic hypotension; use with caution in patients with hypovolemia, cardiovascular disease (including acute MI), or drugs which may exaggerate hypotension. Elderly may be more sensitive to CNS depressant and constipating effects. Use with caution in patients with head injury or increased ICP, biliary tract dysfunction, pancreatitis, patients with history of ileus or bowel obstruction, hyperthyroidism, adrenal insufficiency, prostatic hyperplasia, urinary stricture, CNS depression, psychosis, alcoholism, delirium tremens, kyphoscoliosis or morbidly obese patients. May obscure diagnosis or clinical course of patients with acute abdominal conditions. Partial antagonist activity of buprenorphine may precipitate acute narcotic withdrawal in opioid-dependent individuals upon rapid discontinuation. Naloxone may precipitate intense withdrawal symptoms in patients addicted to opiates when administered before the opioid effects have subsided, or if misused and administered parenterally by opioid-dependent individuals. Combination product is indicated for maintenance therapy for opioid dependence and should not be used for induction. Buprenorphine/naloxone is not appropriate for pain management; deaths have been reported in opioid-naive patients receiving oral buprenorphine for analgesia. Use caution with switching between formulations; potential for greater bioavailability with sublingual film compared to sublingual tablet; monitor closely for either over- or underdosing when switching patients from one formulation to another. Healthcare provider should be alert to problems of abuse, misuse, and diversion.

Drug Interactions

Avoid Concomitant Use

Avoid concomitant use of Buprenorphine and Naloxone with any of the following: Atazanavir; MAO Inhibitors

Decreased Effect

Buprenorphine and Naloxone may decrease the levels/effects of: Analgesics (Opioid); Atazanavir; Pegvisomant

The levels/effects of Buprenorphine and Naloxone may be decreased by: Ammonium Chloride; CYP3A4 Inducers (Strong); Deferasirox; Efavirenz; Herbs (CYP3A4 Inducers); Mixed Agonist / Antagonist Opioids

Increased Effect/Toxicity

Buprenorphine and Naloxone may increase the levels/effects of: Alcohol (Ethyl); Alvimopan; CNS Depressants; Desmopressin; MAO Inhibitors; Selective Serotonin Reuptake Inhibitors; Thiazide Diuretics

The levels/effects of Buprenorphine and Naloxone may be increased by: Amphetamines; Antipsychotic Agents (Phenothiazines); Atazanavir; Conivaptan; CYP3A4 Inhibitors (Moderate); CYP3A4 Inhibitors (Strong); Dasatinib; Droperidol; Succinylcholine

Adverse Reactions Also see individual agents.

>10%:

Central nervous system: Headache (36%), pain (22%)

Gastrointestinal: Vomiting (8%), erythema (oral mucosa; film), glossodynia (film), oral hypoesthesia (film)

Miscellaneous: Withdrawal syndrome (25%; placebo 37%), diaphoresis (14%)

1% to 10%:

Cardiovascular: Vasodilation (9%)

Gastrointestinal: Vomiting (7%)

Pharmacodynamics/Kinetics

Absorption Absorption is variable among patients following sublingual use, but variability within each individual patient is low.

Bioavailability Potential for greater bioavailability with sublingual film compared to sublingual tablet. Although pharmacokinetics were similar between the sublingual formulations, bioequivalence is variable

Half-Life Elimination Film: Buprenorphine: 24-42 hours; Naloxone: 2-12 hours

Controlled Substance C-III

Available Dosage Forms

Film, sublingual:

Suboxone®: Buprenorphine 2 mg and naloxone 0.5 mg; buprenorphine 8 mg and naloxone 2 mg

Tablet, sublingual:

Suboxone®: Buprenorphine 2 mg and naloxone 0.5 mg; buprenorphine 8 mg and naloxone 2 mg

Dosing

Adult & Geriatric

Opioid dependence: Sublingual: **Note:** Buprenorphine and naloxone combination product is not recommended for use during the induction period for long-acting opioids (eg, methadone); initial treatment should begin using buprenorphine oral sublingual tablets under supervision. Patients should be switched to the combination product for maintenance and unsupervised therapy. Doses provided based on buprenorphine content.

Manufacturer's labeling: Maintenance: Target dose: 16 mg/day as a single daily dose; dosage should be adjusted in increments of 2 mg or 4 mg to a level which maintains treatment and suppresses opioid withdrawal symptoms; usual range: 4-24 mg/day

Unlabeled dosing recommendations (U.S. Department of Health and Human Services, 2005):

Induction (only administer combination product for induction in patients who are dependent on **short-acting** opioids and whose last dose of opioids was >12-24 hours prior to induction):

Day 1 induction dose: Initial: 4 mg; may repeat dose after >2 hours if withdrawal symptoms not relieved; maximum daily dose on day 1: 8 mg/day

Day 2 induction dose: Previous dose from day 1 if no withdrawal symptoms present; if symptoms of withdrawal present, increase day 1 dose by 4 mg. If withdrawal symptoms not relieved after >2 hours, may administer 4 mg; maximum daily dose on day 2: 16 mg/day

Subsequent induction days: If withdrawal symptoms are not present, daily dose is established. If withdrawal symptoms are present, increase dose in increments of 2 mg or 4 mg each day as needed for symptom relief. Target daily dose by the end of the first week: 12 mg or 16 mg/day; maximum daily dose: 32 mg/day

Stabilization: Usual dose: 16-24 mg/day; maximum dose: 32 mg/day

Switching between sublingual tablets and sublingual film: Same dosage should be used as the previous administered product. **Note:** Potential for greater bioavailability with the sublingual film compared to the sublingual tablet; monitor closely for either over- or under-dosing when switching patients from one formulation to another.

Pediatric Opioid dependence: Children ≥16 years: Sublingual tablets: Refer to adult dosing.

Hepatic Impairment Moderate-to-severe impairment: Dosage adjustments recommended; however, no specific dosage adjustment recommendations provided by manufacturer.

Administration

Oral

Sublingual film: Film should be placed under the tongue. Keep under the tongue until film dissolves completely; film should not be chewed, swallowed or moved after placement. If more than one film is needed, the additional film should be placed under the tongue on the opposite side from the first film.

Sublingual tablet: Tablet should be placed under the tongue until dissolved; should not be swallowed. If two or more tablets are needed per dose, all may be placed under the tongue at once, or two at a time. To ensure consistent bioavailability, subsequent doses should always be taken the same way.

Stability

Storage Store at room temperature of 25°C (77°F).

Monitoring and Teaching Issues

Laboratory Monitoring Liver function tests (prior to initiation and during therapy)

Physical Assessment See individual agents.

Patient Education See individual agents.

Dietary Considerations

Ethanol: Avoid ethanol (may increase CNS depression).

Herb/Nutraceutical: Avoid valerian, St John's wort, kava kava, gotu kola (may increase CNS depression).

Pregnancy Considerations Withdrawal has been reported in infants of women receiving buprenorphine during pregnancy. Onset of symptoms ranged from day 1 to day 8 of life, most occurring on day 1.

Related Information

Buprenorphine *on page 246*

Naloxone *on page 1284*

◆ **Buprenorphine Hydrochloride** *see* Buprenorphine *on page 246*

◆ **Buprenorphine Hydrochloride and Naloxone Hydrochloride Dihydrate** *see* Buprenorphine and Naloxone *on page 249*

◆ **Buproban®** *see* BuPROPion *on page 252*

BuPROPion (byoo PROE pee on)

U.S. Brand Names Aplenzin™; Budeprion SR®; Budeprion XL®; Buproban®; Wellbutrin SR®; Wellbutrin XL®; Wellbutrin®; Zyban®

Index Terms Bupropion Hydrobromide; Bupropion Hydrochloride

Generic Availability (U.S.) Yes: Excludes bupropion hydrobromide tablet, sustained release hydrochloride tablet

Pharmacologic Category Antidepressant, Dopamine-Reuptake Inhibitor; Smoking Cessation Aid

Medication Safety Issues

Sound-alike/look-alike issues:

Aplenzin™ may be confused with Albenza®, Relenza®

BuPROPion may be confused with busPIRone

Wellbutrin SR® may be confused with Wellbutrin XL®

Wellbutrin XL® may be confused with Wellbutrin SR®

Zyban® may be confused with Zagam®, Diovan®

Medication Guide Available Yes

Pregnancy Risk Factor C

Lactation Enters breast milk/not recommended (AAP rates "of concern"; AAP 2001 update pending)

Use Treatment of major depressive disorder, including seasonal affective disorder (SAD); adjunct in smoking cessation

Unlabeled/Investigational Use Attention-deficit/hyperactivity disorder (ADHD); depression associated with bipolar disorder

Mechanism of Action/Effect Antidepressant structurally different from all other marketed antidepressants; like other antidepressants the mechanism of bupropion's activity is not fully understood; relatively weak inhibitor of the neuronal uptake of norepinephrine and dopamine

Contraindications Hypersensitivity to bupropion or any component of the formulation; seizure disorder; history of anorexia/bulimia; use of MAO inhibitors within 14 days; patients undergoing abrupt discontinuation of ethanol or sedatives (including benzodiazepines); patients receiving other dosage forms of bupropion

Warnings/Precautions [U.S. Boxed Warning]: Use in treating psychiatric disorders: Antidepressants increase the risk of suicidal thinking and behavior in children, adolescents, and young adults (18-24 years of age) with major depressive disorder (MDD) and other psychiatric disorders; consider risk prior to prescribing. Short-term studies did not show an increased risk in patients >24 years of age and showed a decreased risk in patients ≥65 years. All patients must be closely monitored for clinical worsening, suicidality, or unusual changes in behavior, especially during the initiation of therapy (generally first 1-2 months) or following an increase or decrease in dosage. The patient's family or caregiver should be instructed to closely observe the patient and communicate condition with healthcare provider. A medication guide should be dispensed with each prescription. **Bupropion is not FDA approved for use in children.**

[U.S. Boxed Warning]: Use in smoking cessation: Serious neuropsychiatric events, including depression, suicidal thoughts, and suicide, have been reported with use; some cases may have been complicated by symptoms of nicotine withdrawal following smoking cessation. Smoking cessation (with or without treatment) is associated with nicotine withdrawal symptoms and the exacerbation of underlying psychiatric illness; however, some of the behavioral disturbances were reported in treated patients who continued to smoke. These neuropsychiatric symptoms (eg, mood disturbances, psychosis, hostility) have occurred in patients with and without pre-existing psychiatric disease; many cases resolved following therapy discontinuation although in some cases, symptoms persisted. Monitor all patients for behavioral changes and psychiatric symptoms (eg, agitation, depression, suicidal behavior, suicidal ideation); inform patients to discontinue treatment and contact their healthcare provider immediately if they experience any behavioral and/or mood changes.

The possibility of a suicide attempt is inherent in major depression and may persist until remission occurs. Use caution in high-risk patients. Worsening depression and severe abrupt suicidality that are not part of the presenting symptoms may require discontinuation or modification of drug therapy. The patient's family or caregiver should be alerted to monitor patients for the emergence of suicidality and associated behaviors (such as agitation, irritability, hostility, impulsivity, and hypomania) and notify the healthcare provider.

May worsen psychosis in some patients or precipitate a shift to mania or hypomania in patients with bipolar disorder. Patients presenting with depressive symptoms should be screened for bipolar disorder. Monotherapy in patients with bipolar disorder should be avoided. **Bupropion is not FDA approved for bipolar depression.**

The risk of seizures is dose-dependent and increased in patients with a history of seizures, anorexia/bulimia, head trauma, CNS tumor, severe hepatic cirrhosis, abrupt discontinuation of sedative-hypnotics or ethanol, medications which lower seizure threshold (antipsychotics, antidepressants, theophyllines, systemic steroids), stimulants, or hypoglycemic agents. Risk of seizures may also be increased by chewing, crushing, or dividing long-acting products. Risk may be reduced by limiting the daily dose to bupropion hydrochloride ≤450 mg or bupropion hydrobromide 522 mg. Gradually increase dose incrementally to reduce risk. Discontinue and do not restart in patients experiencing a seizure.

May cause CNS stimulation (restlessness, anxiety, insomnia) or anorexia. May increase the risks associated with electroconvulsive therapy. Consider discontinuing, when possible, prior to elective surgery. May cause weight loss; use caution in patients where weight loss is not desirable. The incidence of sexual dysfunction with bupropion is generally lower than with SSRIs.

Use caution in patients with cardiovascular disease, history of hypertension, or coronary artery disease; treatment-emergent hypertension (including some severe cases) has been reported, both with bupropion alone and in combination with nicotine transdermal systems. All children diagnosed with ADHD who may be candidates for stimulant medications should have a thorough cardiovascular assessment to identify risk factors for sudden cardiac death prior to initiation of drug therapy. Use with caution in patients with hepatic or renal dysfunction and in elderly patients; reduced dose and/or frequency may be recommended. Elderly patients may be at greater risk of accumulation during chronic dosing. May cause motor or cognitive impairment in some patients; use with caution if tasks requiring alertness such as operating machinery or driving are undertaken. Arthralgia, myalgia, and fever with rash and other symptoms suggestive of delayed hypersensitivity resembling serum sickness have been reported.

Extended release tablet: Insoluble tablet shell may remain intact and be visible in the stool.

Drug Interactions

Metabolism/Transport Effects **Substrate** of CYP1A2 (minor), 2A6 (minor), 2B6 (major), 2C9 (minor), 2D6 (minor), 2E1 (minor), 3A4 (minor); **Inhibits** CYP2D6 (strong)

Avoid Concomitant Use

Avoid concomitant use of BuPROPion with any of the following: MAO Inhibitors; Tamoxifen; Thioridazine

Decreased Effect

BuPROPion may decrease the levels/effects of: Codeine; TraMADol

The levels/effects of BuPROPion may be decreased by: CYP2B6 Inducers (Strong); Lopinavir; Peginterferon Alfa-2b; Ritonavir

Increased Effect/Toxicity

BuPROPion may increase the levels/effects of: Alcohol (Ethyl); Atomoxetine; CNS Depressants; CYP2D6 Substrates; Fesoterodine; Methotrimeprazine; Nebivolol; Tamoxifen; Tetrabenazine; Thioridazine; Tricyclic Antidepressants

The levels/effects of BuPROPion may be increased by: Conivaptan; CYP2B6 Inhibitors (Moderate); CYP2B6 Inhibitors (Strong); Droperidol; MAO Inhibitors; Methotrimeprazine; Quazepam

Nutritional/Ethanol Interactions

Ethanol: Avoid ethanol (may increase CNS depression).

Herb/Nutraceutical: Avoid valerian, St John's wort, SAMe, gotu kola, kava kava (may increase CNS depression).

Lab Interactions May interfere with urine detection of amphetamine/methamphetamine (false-positive). Decreased prolactin levels.

Adverse Reactions Frequencies, when reported, reflect highest incidence reported with sustained release product.

>10%:

Cardiovascular: Tachycardia (11%)

Central nervous system: Headache (25% to 34%), insomnia (11% to 20%), dizziness (6% to 11%)

Gastrointestinal: Xerostomia (17% to 26%), weight loss (14% to 23%), nausea (1% to 18%)

Respiratory: Pharyngitis (3% to 13%)

1% to 10%:

Cardiovascular: Palpitation (2% to 6%), arrhythmias (5%), chest pain (3% to 4%), hypertension (2% to 4%; may be severe), flushing (1% to 4%), hypotension (3%)

Central nervous system: Agitation (2% to 9%), confusion (8%), anxiety (5% to 7%), hostility (6%), nervousness (3% to 5%), sleep disturbance (4%), sensory disturbance (4%), migraine (1% to 4%), abnormal dreams (3%), irritability (2% to 3%), somnolence (2% to 3%), pain (2% to 3%), memory decreased (≤3%), fever (1% to 2%), CNS stimulation (1% to 2%), depression

Dermatologic: Rash (1% to 5%), pruritus (2% to 4%), urticaria (1% to 2%)

Endocrine & metabolic: Menstrual complaints (2% to 5%), hot flashes (1% to 3%), libido decreased (3%)

Gastrointestinal: Constipation (5% to 10%), abdominal pain (2% to 9%), diarrhea (5% to 7%), flatulence (6%), anorexia (3% to 5%), appetite increased (4%), taste perversion (2% to 4%), vomiting (2% to 4%), dyspepsia (3%), dysphagia (≤2%)

Genitourinary: Polyuria (2% to 5%), urinary urgency (≤2%), vaginal hemorrhage (≤2%), UTI (≤1%)

Neuromuscular & skeletal: Tremor (3% to 6%), myalgia (2% to 6%), weakness (2% to 4%), arthralgia (1% to 4%), arthritis (2%), akathisia (≤2%), paresthesia (1% to 2%), twitching (1% to 2%), neck pain

Ocular: Blurred vision (2% to 3%), amblyopia (2%)

Otic: Tinnitus (3% to 6%), auditory disturbance (5%)

Respiratory: Upper respiratory infection (9%), cough increased (1% to 4%), sinusitis (1% to 5%)

Miscellaneous: Infection (8% to 9%), diaphoresis (5% to 6%), allergic reaction (including anaphylaxis, pruritus, urticaria)

Pharmacodynamics/Kinetics

Absorption Rapid

Time to Peak

Bupropion: Immediate release: Within 2 hours; Sustained release: Within 3 hours; Extended release: ~5 hours

Metabolite: Hydroxybupropion: Immediate release: ~3 hours; Extended release, sustained release: ~6-7 hours

Protein Binding 84%

Half-Life Elimination

Distribution: 3-4 hours

Elimination: 21 ± 9 hours; Metabolites: Hydroxybupropion: 20 ± 5 hours; Erythrohydrobupropion: 33 ± 10 hours; Threohydrobupropion: 37 ± 13 hours

Extended release (Aplenzin™): 21 ± 7 hours; Metabolites: Hydroxybupropion: 24 ± 5 hours; Erythrohydrobupropion: 31 ± 8 hours; Threohydrobupropion: 51 ± 9 hours

Metabolism Extensively hepatic via CYP2B6 to hydroxybupropion; non-CYP-mediated metabolism to erythrohydrobupropion and threohydrobupropion. Metabolite activity ranges from 20% to 50% potency of bupropion.

Excretion Urine (87%, primarily as metabolites); feces (10%, primarily as metabolites)

Available Dosage Forms

Tablet, oral: 75 mg, 100 mg

Wellbutrin®: 75 mg, 100 mg

Tablet, extended release, oral: 100 mg, 150 mg, 200 mg, 300 mg

Aplenzin™: 174 mg, 348 mg, 522 mg

Budeprion SR®: 100 mg, 150 mg

Budeprion XL®: 150 mg, 300 mg

Buproban®: 150 mg

Wellbutrin XL®: 150 mg, 300 mg

Tablet, sustained release, oral:

Wellbutrin SR®: 100 mg, 150 mg, 200 mg

Zyban®: 150 mg

Dosing

Adult

Depression: Oral:

Immediate release hydrochloride salt: 100 mg 3 times/day; begin at 100 mg twice daily; may increase to a maximum dose of 450 mg/day

Sustained release hydrochloride salt: Initial: 150 mg/day in the morning; may increase to 150 mg twice daily by day 4 if tolerated; target dose: 300 mg/day given as 150 mg twice daily; maximum dose: 400 mg/day given as 200 mg twice daily

Extended release:

Hydrochloride salt: Initial: 150 mg/day in the morning; may increase as early as day 4 of dosing to 300 mg/day; maximum dose: 450 mg/day

Hydrobromide salt (Aplenzin™): Target dose: 348 mg/day in the morning. Patients not previously on bupropion: Initial: 174 mg/day in the morning; may increase as early as day 4 of dosing to 348 mg/day; maximum dose: 522 mg/day. **Note:** 174 mg strength not currently available; 348 mg tablet cannot be split.

Switching from hydrochloride salt formulation (eg, Wellbutrin® immediate release, SR®, XL®) to hydrobromide salt formulation (Aplenzin™): **Note:** Patients being treated twice daily with bupropion hydrochloride would be switched to the equivalent once daily dose of bupropion hydrobromide.

Bupropion hydrochloride 150 mg is equivalent to bupropion hydrobromide 174 mg
Bupropion hydrochloride 300 mg is equivalent to bupropion hydrobromide 348 mg
Bupropion hydrochloride 450 mg is equivalent to bupropion hydrobromide 522 mg

SAD (Wellbutrin XL®): Oral: Initial: 150 mg/day in the morning; if tolerated, may increase after 1 week to 300 mg/day

Note: Prophylactic treatment should be reserved for those patients with frequent depressive episodes and/or significant impairment. Initiate treatment in the Autumn prior to symptom onset, and discontinue in early Spring with dose tapering to 150 mg/day for 2 weeks

Smoking cessation (Zyban®): Oral: Initiate with 150 mg once daily for 3 days; increase to 150 mg twice daily; treatment should continue for 7-12 weeks.

Note: Therapy should begin at least 1 week before target quit date. Target quit dates are generally in the second week of treatment. If patient successfully quits smoking after 7-12 weeks, may consider ongoing maintenance therapy based on individual patient risk: benefit. Efficacy of maintenance therapy (300 mg/day) has been demonstrated for up to 6 months. Conversely, if significant progress has not been made by the seventh week of therapy, success is unlikely and treatment discontinuation should be considered.

Dosing conversion between hydrochloride salt (eg, Wellbutrin®) immediate, sustained, and extended release products: Convert using same total daily dose (up to the maximum recommended dose for a given dosage form), but adjust frequency as indicated for sustained (twice daily) or extended (once daily) release products.

Geriatric

Depression: Oral (hydrochloride salt): Initial: 37.5 mg of immediate release tablets twice daily or 100 mg/day of sustained release tablets; increase by 37.5-100 mg every 3-4 days as tolerated. There is evidence that the elderly respond at 150 mg/day in divided doses, but some may require a higher dose. **Note:** Patients with Alzheimer's dementia-related depression may require a lower starting dosage of 37.5 mg once or twice daily (100 mg/day sustained release), increased as needed up to 300 mg/day in divided doses (300 mg/day for sustained release)

Smoking cessation: Refer to adult dosing.

Pediatric ADHD (unlabeled use): Oral (hydrochloride salt): Children and Adolescents: 1.4-6 mg/kg/day

Renal Impairment Use with caution and consider a reduction in dosing frequency; limited pharmacokinetic information suggests elimination of bupropion and/or the active metabolites may be reduced.

Moderate-to-severe renal impairment: Bupropion exposure was approximately twofold higher compared to normal subjects following a 150 mg single dose administration.

End-stage renal failure: Per the manufacturer, the elimination of hydroxybupropion and threohydrobupropion are reduced in patients with end-stage renal failure.

Hepatic Impairment

Mild-to-moderate hepatic impairment: Use with caution and/or reduced dose/frequency

Severe hepatic cirrhosis: Use with extreme caution; maximum dose:

Aplenzin™: 174 mg every other day

Wellbutrin®: 75 mg/day;

Wellbutrin SR®: 100 mg/day or 150 mg every other day

Wellbutrin XL®: 150 mg every other day

Zyban®: 150 mg every other day

Note: The mean AUC increased by ~1.5-fold for hydroxybupropion and ~2.5-fold for erythro/threohydrobupropion; median T_{max} was observed 19 hours later for hydroxybupropion, 31 hours later for erythro/threohydrobupropion; mean half-life for hydroxybupropion increased fivefold, and increased twofold for erythro/threohydrobupropion in patients with severe hepatic cirrhosis compared to healthy volunteers.

Administration

Oral May be taken without regard to meals. Zyban® and extended release tablets (hydrochloride and hydrobromide salt formulations) should be swallowed whole; do not crush, chew, or divide. The insoluble shell of the extended-release tablet may remain intact during GI transit and is eliminated in the feces. Data from the manufacturer states that dividing Wellbutrin SR® tablets resulted in an increased rate of release at 15 minutes: "However, the divided tablet retained its sustained-release characteristics with similar increases of released bupropion at each sampling point beyond 15 minutes when compared to the intact Wellbutrin SR® tablet..." Bupropion is hydroscopic and therefore should be stored in a dry place. Splitting of large quantities in advance of administration is not advised since loss of potency may result. If necessary, splitting should be done cleanly without crushing.

Stability

Storage Store at controlled room temperature of 20°C to 25°C (68°F to 77°F).

Aplenzin™, Wellbutrin XL®: Store at 15°C to 30°C (59°F to 86°F).

Monitoring and Teaching Issues

Physical Assessment Perform careful cardiovascular assessment prior to initiating therapy. Monitor blood pressure at beginning of therapy and periodically throughout. Monitor for clinical worsening; neuropsychiatric symptoms, such as changes in behavior, hostility, agitation, and depression; and suicidality, especially at the beginning of therapy or when dose changes occur. Taper dosage slowly when discontinuing.

Patient Education Be aware that bupropion is marketed under different names and should not be taken together; Zyban® is for smoking cessation. Excessive use or abrupt discontinuation of alcohol or sedatives may lower seizure threshold.

Depression: Take in equally divided doses. Do not use alcohol. May cause drowsiness, clouded sensorium, headache, restlessness, agitation, nausea, vomiting, dry mouth, weight loss, constipation, or impotence (reversible). Report persistent CNS effects (eg, agitation, confusion, anxiety, restlessness, insomnia, psychosis, hallucinations, seizures); suicide ideation; muscle weakness or tremor; skin rash or irritation; chest pain or palpitations, abdominal pain or blood in stools; yellowing of skin or eyes; or respiratory difficulty, bronchitis, or unusual cough.

Smoking cessation: May cause dry mouth and insomnia (these may resolve with continued use). Report any respiratory difficulty, unusual cough, dizziness, changes in behavior, agitation, anxiety, suicide ideation, seizures, or muscle tremors.

Geriatric Considerations Limited data available about the use of bupropion in the elderly; two studies have found it equally effective when compared to imipramine. Its side effect profile (minimal anticholinergic and blood pressure effects) may make it useful in persons who do not tolerate traditional cyclic antidepressants. A single and multiple dose pharmacokinetic study suggested that accumulation of bupropion and its metabolites may occur in the elderly.

Breast-Feeding Considerations Bupropion and its metabolites are excreted into breast milk, although neither bupropion nor its metabolites have been detected in the plasma of breast-fed infants. Adverse events have not been reported in older breast-fed infants; however, a seizure was noted in one 6-month old infant (a causal effect could not be confirmed). Breast-feeding is not recommended by the manufacturer.

Pregnancy Considerations Due to adverse events observed in some animal studies, bupropion is classified as pregnancy category C. A significant increase in major teratogenic effects has not been observed following exposure to bupropion during pregnancy; however, the risk of spontaneous abortions may be increased (additional studies are needed to confirm). The long-term effects on development and behavior have not been studied.

Pregnancy itself does not provide protection against depression. The ACOG recommends that therapy with antidepressants during pregnancy be individualized and should incorporate the clinical expertise of the mental health clinician, obstetrician, primary care provider, and pediatrician. If treatment is needed, consider gradually stopping antidepressants 10-14 days before the expected date of delivery to prevent potential withdrawal symptoms in the infant. If this is done and the woman is considered to be at risk of relapse from her major depressive disorder, the medication can be restarted following delivery, although the dose should be readjusted to that required before pregnancy. Bupropion has also been evaluated for smoking cessation during pregnancy; current recommendations suggest that pharmacologic treatments be considered only after other therapies have failed. Treatment algorithms have been developed by the ACOG and the APA for the management of depression in women prior to conception and during pregnancy (Yonkers, 2009).

Additional Information Risk of seizures: When using bupropion hydrochloride immediate release tablets, seizure risk is increased at total daily dosage >450 mg, individual dosages >150 mg, or by sudden, large increments in dose. Data for the immediate-release formulation of bupropion revealed a seizure incidence of 0.4% in patients treated at doses in the 300-450 mg/day range. The estimated seizure incidence increases almost 10-fold between 450 mg and 600 mg per day. Data for the sustained release dosage form revealed a seizure incidence of 0.1% in patients treated at a dosage range of 100-300 mg/day, and increases to ~0.4% at the maximum recommended dose of 400 mg/day.

Related Information

Antidepressant Agents *on page 1982*

◆ **Bupropion Hydrobromide** *see* BuPROPion *on page 252*

◆ **Bupropion Hydrochloride** *see* BuPROPion *on page 252*

◆ **Burn Jel® [OTC]** *see* Lidocaine (Topical) *on page 1107*

◆ **Burn Jel Plus [OTC]** *see* Lidocaine (Topical) *on page 1107*

◆ **BuSpar** *see* BusPIRone *on page 256*

BusPIRone (byoo SPYE rone)

Index Terms BuSpar; Buspirone Hydrochloride

Generic Availability (U.S.) Yes

Pharmacologic Category Antianxiety Agent, Miscellaneous

Medication Safety Issues

Sound-alike/look-alike issues:

BusPIRone may be confused with buPROPion

Pregnancy Risk Factor B

Lactation Excretion in breast milk unknown/not recommended

Use Management of generalized anxiety disorder (GAD)

Unlabeled/Investigational Use Management of aggression in mental retardation and secondary mental disorders; major depression; potential augmenting agent for antidepressants; premenstrual syndrome

Mechanism of Action/Effect The mechanism of action of buspirone is unknown. Buspirone has a high affinity for serotonin 5-HT_{1A} and 5-HT_2 receptors, without affecting benzodiazepine-GABA receptors. Buspirone has moderate affinity for dopamine D_2 receptors.

Contraindications Hypersensitivity to buspirone or any component of the formulation

Warnings/Precautions Use in severe hepatic or renal impairment is not recommended; does not prevent or treat withdrawal from benzodiazepines. Low potential for cognitive or motor impairment. Use with MAO inhibitors may result in hypertensive reactions. Restlessness syndrome has been reported in small number of patients; monitor for signs of any dopamine-related movement disorders. Buspirone does not exhibit cross-tolerance with benzodiazepines or other sedative/hypnotic agents. If substituting buspirone for any of these agents, gradually withdraw the drug(s) prior to initiating buspirone. Safety and efficacy of buspirone have not been established in children <6 years of age; no long-term safety/efficacy data available in children.

Drug Interactions

Metabolism/Transport Effects Substrate of CYP2D6 (minor), 3A4 (major)

Avoid Concomitant Use

Avoid concomitant use of BusPIRone with any of the following: MAO Inhibitors; Sibutramine

Decreased Effect

The levels/effects of BusPIRone may be decreased by: CYP3A4 Inducers (Strong); Deferasirox; Peginterferon Alfa-2b; Rifamycin Derivatives; Yohimbine

Increased Effect/Toxicity

BusPIRone may increase the levels/effects of: Alcohol (Ethyl); Antidepressants (Serotonin Reuptake Inhibitor/Antagonist); CNS Depressants; MAO Inhibitors; Methotrimeprazine; Selective Serotonin Reuptake Inhibitors; Serotonin Modulators

The levels/effects of BusPIRone may be increased by: Antifungal Agents (Azole Derivatives, Systemic); Calcium Channel Blockers (Nondihydropyridine); Conivaptan; CYP3A4 Inhibitors (Moderate); CYP3A4 Inhibitors (Strong); Dasatinib; Droperidol; Grapefruit Juice; Macrolide Antibiotics; Methotrimeprazine; Selective Serotonin Reuptake Inhibitors; Sibutramine

Nutritional/Ethanol Interactions

Ethanol: Ethanol (may increase CNS depression).

Food: Food may decrease the absorption of buspirone, but it may also decrease the first-pass metabolism, thereby increasing the bioavailability of buspirone. Grapefruit juice may cause increased buspirone concentrations; avoid intake of large quantities of grapefruit juice.

Herb/Nutraceutical: St John's wort may decrease buspirone levels or increase CNS depression. Avoid valerian, gotu kola, kava kava (may increase CNS depression).

Adverse Reactions

>10%: Central nervous system: Dizziness (12%)

1% to 10%:

Cardiovascular: Chest pain (≥1%)

Central nervous system: Drowsiness (10%), headache (6%), nervousness (5%), lightheadedness (3%), anger/hostility (2%), confusion (2%), excitement (2%), dream disturbance (≥1%)

Dermatologic: Rash (1%)

Gastrointestinal: Nausea (8%), diarrhea (2%)

Neuromuscular & skeletal: Numbness (2%), weakness (2%), musculoskeletal pain (1%), paresthesia (1%), incoordination (1%), tremor (1%)

Ocular: Blurred vision (2%)

Otic: Tinnitus (≥1%)

Respiratory: Nasal congestion (≥1%), sore throat (≥1%)

Miscellaneous: Diaphoresis (1%)

Pharmacodynamics/Kinetics

Absorption Rapid

Bioavailability ~4%

Time to Peak Serum: 40-90 minutes

Protein Binding 86% to 95%

Half-Life Elimination 2-3 hours

Metabolism Hepatic oxidation, primarily via CYP3A4; extensive first-pass effect

Excretion Urine: 29% to 63% (<0.1% dose excreted unchanged); feces: 18% to 38%

Available Dosage Forms

Tablet, oral: 5 mg, 7.5 mg, 10 mg, 15 mg, 30 mg

Dosing

Adult Anxiety disorders (GAD): Oral: 15 mg/day (7.5 mg twice daily); may increase in increments of 5 mg/day every 2-3 days to a maximum of 60 mg/day. Target dose for most people is 20-30 mg/day (10-15 mg twice daily).

Geriatric Oral: Initial: 5 mg twice daily, increase by 5 mg/day every 2-3 days as needed up to 20-30 mg/day; maximum daily dose: 60 mg/day

Pediatric Generalized anxiety disorder (GAD): Children ≥6 years and Adolescents: Oral: Initial: 5 mg daily; increase in increments of 5 mg/day at weekly intervals as needed, to a maximum dose of 60 mg/day divided into 2-3 doses

Renal Impairment Patients with impaired renal function demonstrated increased plasma levels and a prolonged half-life of buspirone. Use in patients with severe renal impairment not recommended.

Hepatic Impairment Patients with impaired hepatic function demonstrated increased plasma levels and a prolonged half-life of buspirone. Use in patients with severe hepatic impairment not recommended.

Stability

Storage Store at USP controlled room temperature of 25°C (77°F). Protect from light.

Monitoring and Teaching Issues

Patient Education May take 2-3 weeks to see full effect; do not discontinue this medicine without consulting prescriber. Avoid large quantities of grapefruit juice. Maintain adequate hydration, unless instructed to restrict fluid intake. You may experience drowsiness, lightheadedness, impaired coordination, dizziness, blurred vision; upset stomach, or nausea. Report persistent vomiting, chest pain or rapid heartbeat, persistent CNS effects (eg, confusion, restlessness, anxiety, insomnia, excitation, headache, dizziness, fatigue, impaired coordination); or worsening of condition.

Dietary Considerations Avoid large quantities of grapefruit juice.

Geriatric Considerations Because buspirone is less sedating than other anxiolytics, it may be a useful agent in geriatric patients when an anxiolytic is indicated.

Pregnancy Considerations No impairment of fertility or fetotoxic effects were noted in animal studies with doses 30 times maximum recommended human dose. There are no adequate and well-controlled studies in pregnant women.

Additional Information Has shown little potential for abuse; needs continuous use. Because of slow onset, not appropriate for "as needed" (prn) use or for brief, situational anxiety. Ineffective for treatment of benzodiazepine or ethanol withdrawal.

◆ **Buspirone Hydrochloride** *see* BusPIRone *on page* 256

Busulfan (byoo SUL fan)

U.S. Brand Names Busulfex®; Myleran®

Index Terms NSC-750

Generic Availability (U.S.) No

Pharmacologic Category Antineoplastic Agent, Alkylating Agent

Medication Safety Issues

Sound-alike/look-alike issues:

Busulfan may be confused with Butalan®

Myleran® may be confused with Alkeran®, Leukeran®, melphalan, Mylicon®

High alert medication: The Institute for Safe Medication Practices (ISMP) includes this medication among its list of drugs which have a heightened risk of causing significant patient harm when used in error.

Pregnancy Risk Factor D

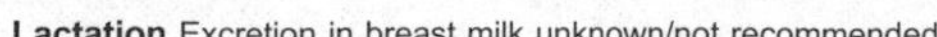

Lactation Excretion in breast milk unknown/not recommended

Use

Oral: Chronic myelogenous leukemia (CML); conditioning regimens for bone marrow transplantation

I.V.: Combination therapy with cyclophosphamide as a conditioning regimen prior to allogeneic hematopoietic progenitor cell transplantation for chronic myelogenous leukemia

Unlabeled/Investigational Use Oral: Bone marrow disorders, such as polycythemia vera and myeloid metaplasia; thrombocytosis

Mechanism of Action/Effect Interferes with DNA function; cytotoxic

Contraindications Hypersensitivity to busulfan or any component of the formulation; oral busulfan is contraindicated in patients without a definitive diagnosis of CML

Warnings/Precautions Hazardous agent - use appropriate precautions for handling and disposal. **[U.S. Boxed Warning]: May induce severe bone marrow suppression.** May result in severe neutropenia, thrombocytopenia and/or anemia. Seizures have been reported with use; use caution in patients predisposed to seizures; initiate prophylactic anticonvulsant therapy (eg, phenytoin) prior to treatment; use caution with history of seizures or head trauma. May cause delayed pulmonary toxicity (known as "busulfan lung" - bronchopulmonary dysplasia with pulmonary fibrosis); the average onset is 4 years (range: 4 months to 10 years). Cardiac tamponade as been reported in children with thalassemia treated with high-dose oral busulfan in combination with cyclophosphamide. Busulfan has been causally related to the development of secondary malignancies (tumors and acute leukemias). Busulfan has been associated with ovarian failure (including failure to achieve puberty).

High busulfan area under the concentration versus time curve (AUC) values (>1500 µM/minute) are associated with increased risk of hepatic veno-occlusive disease during conditioning for allogenic BMT; patients with of history of radiation therapy, prior chemotherapy (≥3 cycles) and prior stem cell transplantation are at increased risk. Oral busulfan doses above 16 mg/kg (based on IBW) and concurrent use with alkylating agents may also increase the risk for hepatic VOD. The solvent in I.V. busulfan, DMA, may impair fertility. DMA may also be associated with hepatotoxicity, hallucinations, somnolence, lethargy, and confusion. **[U.S. Boxed Warning]: Should be administered under the supervision of an experienced cancer chemotherapy physician.**

Drug Interactions

Metabolism/Transport Effects Substrate of CYP3A4 (major)

Avoid Concomitant Use

Avoid concomitant use of Busulfan with any of the following: BCG; Natalizumab; Pimecrolimus; Roflumilast; Tacrolimus (Topical); Vaccines (Live)

Decreased Effect

Busulfan may decrease the levels/effects of: BCG; Sipuleucel-T; Vaccines (Inactivated); Vaccines (Live); Vitamin K Antagonists

The levels/effects of Busulfan may be decreased by: CYP3A4 Inducers (Strong); Deferasirox; Echinacea; Herbs (CYP3A4 Inducers)

Increased Effect/Toxicity

Busulfan may increase the levels/effects of: Leflunomide; Natalizumab; Vaccines (Live); Vitamin K Antagonists

The levels/effects of Busulfan may be increased by: Antifungal Agents (Azole Derivatives, Systemic); Conivaptan; CYP3A4 Inhibitors (Moderate); CYP3A4 Inhibitors (Strong); Dasatinib; Denosumab; MetroNIDAZOLE; MetroNIDAZOLE (Systemic); Pimecrolimus; Roflumilast; Tacrolimus (Topical); Trastuzumab

Nutritional/Ethanol Interactions

Ethanol: Avoid ethanol due to GI irritation.

Food: No clear or firm data on the effect of food on busulfan bioavailability.

Herb/Nutraceutical: Avoid St John's wort (may decrease busulfan levels).

Adverse Reactions

I.V.:

>10%:

Cardiovascular: Tachycardia (44%), hypertension (36%; grades 3/4: 7%), edema (28% to 79%), thrombosis (33%), chest pain (26%), vasodilation (25%), hypotension (11%; grades 3/4: 3%)

Central nervous system: Insomnia (84%), fever (80%), anxiety (72% to 75%), headache (69%), chills (46%), pain (44%), dizziness (30%), depression (23%), confusion (11%)

Dermatologic: Rash (57%), pruritus (28%), alopecia (2% to 15%)

Endocrine & metabolic: Hypomagnesemia (77%), hyperglycemia (66%; grades 3/4: 15%), hypokalemia (64%), hypocalcemia (49%), hypophosphatemia (17%)

Gastrointestinal: Nausea (98%), mucositis/stomatitis (97%; grades 3/4: 26%), vomiting (43% to 95%), anorexia (85%), diarrhea (84%; grades 3/4: 5%), abdominal pain (72%), dyspepsia (44%), constipation (38%), xerostomia (26%), rectal disorder (25%), abdominal fullness (23%)

Hematologic: Myelosuppression (≤100%), neutropenia (100%; median recovery: 13 days), thrombocytopenia (98%; median onset: 5-6 days), lymphopenia (children: 79%), anemia (69%)

Hepatic: Hyperbilirubinemia (49%; grades 3/4: 30%), ALT increased (31%; grades 3/4: 7%), veno-occlusive disease (adults: 8% to 12%; children: 21%), jaundice (12%)

Local: Injection site inflammation (25%), injection site pain (15%)

Neuromuscular & skeletal: Weakness (51%), back pain (23%), myalgia (16%), arthralgia (13%)

Renal: Creatinine increased (21%), oliguria (15%)

Respiratory: Rhinitis (44%), lung disorder (34%), cough (28%), epistaxis (25%), dyspnea (25%), pneumonia (children: 21%), hiccup (18%), pharyngitis (18%)
Miscellaneous: Infection (51%), allergic reaction (26%)

1% to 10%:

Cardiovascular: Arrhythmia (5%), cardiomegaly (5%), atrial fibrillation (2%), ECG abnormal (2%), heart block (2%), heart failure (grade 3/4: 2%), pericardial effusion (2%), tamponade (children with thalassemia: 2%), ventricular extrasystoles (2%), hypervolemia
Central nervous system: Lethargy (7%), hallucination (5%), agitation (2%), delirium (2%), encephalopathy (2%), seizure (2%), somnolence (2%), cerebral hemorrhage (1%)
Dermatologic: Vesicular rash (10%), vesiculobullous rash (10%), skin discoloration (8%), maculopapular rash (8%), acne (7%), exfoliative dermatitis (5%), erythema nodosum (2%)
Endocrine & metabolic: Hyponatremia (2%)
Gastrointestinal: Ileus (8%), weight gain (8%), hematemesis (2%), pancreatitis (2%)
Hematologic: Prothrombin time increased (2%)
Hepatic: Hepatomegaly (6%)
Renal: Hematuria (8%), dysuria (7%), hemorrhagic cystitis (grade 3/4: 7%), BUN increased (3%)
Respiratory: Asthma (8%), alveolar hemorrhage (5%), hyperventilation (5%), hemoptysis (3%), pleural effusion (3%), sinusitis (3%), atelectasis (2%), hypoxia (2%)

Oral: Frequency not defined:

Central nervous system: Seizure
Dermatologic: Hyperpigmentation of skin (busulfan tan 5% to 10%), alopecia, rash, urticaria
Endocrine & metabolic: Amenorrhea, ovarian suppression
Hematologic: Myelosuppression (anemia, leukopenia, thrombocytopenia), pancytopenia

Pharmacodynamics/Kinetics

Duration of Action 28 days

Absorption Rapid and complete

Time to Peak Serum: Oral: Within 4 hours; I.V.: Within 5 minutes

Protein Binding 32% to plasma proteins and 47% to red blood cells

Half-Life Elimination After first dose: 3.4 hours; After last dose: 2.3 hours

Metabolism Extensively hepatic (may increase with multiple doses); glutathione conjugation followed by oxidation

Excretion Urine (10% to 50% as metabolites) within 24 hours (<2% as unchanged drug)

Available Dosage Forms

Injection, solution:

Busulfex®: 6 mg/mL (10 mL)

Tablet, oral:

Myleran®: 2 mg

Dosing

Adult Note: Premedicate with prophylactic anticonvulsant therapy (eg, phenytoin) prior to high-dose busulfan treatment.

CML remission induction: Oral: 60 mcg/kg/day or 1.8 mg/m^2/day; usual range: 4-8 mg/day (may be as high as 12 mg/day); Maintenance doses: 1-4 mg/day to 2 mg/week to maintain WBC 10,000-20,000 cells/mm^3

BMT marrow-ablative conditioning regimen:

Oral: 1 mg/kg/dose (ideal body weight) every 6 hours for 16 doses

I.V.: 0.8 mg/kg (ideal body weight or actual body weight, whichever is lower); for obese or severely-obese patients adjusted ideal body weight is recommended) every 6 hours for 4 days (a total of 16 doses)

Polycythemia vera (unlabeled use): Oral: 2-6 mg/day

Thrombocytosis (unlabeled use): Oral: 4-6 mg/day

Geriatric Oral (refer to individual protocols): Start with lowest recommended doses for adults.

Pediatric Note: Premedicate with prophylactic anticonvulsant therapy (eg, phenytoin) prior to high-dose busulfan treatment.

CML remission: Oral: Induction: 0.06-0.12 mg/kg/day **or** 1.8-4.6 mg/m^2/day; titrate dosage to maintain leukocyte count above 40,000/mm^3; reduce dosage by 50% if the leukocyte count reaches 30,000-40,000/mm^3; discontinue drug if counts fall to ≤20,000/mm^3.

BMT marrow-ablative conditioning regimen:

Oral: 1 mg/kg/dose (ideal body weight) every 6 hours for 16 doses

I.V.:

≤12 kg: 1.1 mg/kg/dose (ideal body weight) every 6 hours for 16 doses
>12 kg: 0.8 mg/kg/dose (ideal body weight) every 6 hours for 16 doses

Adjust dose to desired AUC [1125 μmol(min)] using the following formula:

Adjusted dose (mg) = Actual dose (mg) x [target AUC μmol(min) / actual AUC μmol(min)]

Renal Impairment I.V.: Has not been studied in patients with renal impairment per the FDA-approved labeling. Some clinicians suggest adjustment is not necessary (Aronoff, 2007).

Hepatic Impairment I.V.: Has not been administered in clinical studies in patients with hepatic impairment per the FDA-approved labeling. Busulfan has extensive hepatic metabolism and risk of hepatic veno-occlusive disease with high doses; dosage adjustment may be needed.

Administration

Oral BMT only: To facilitate ingestion of high oral doses, insert multiple tablets into gelatin capsules.

I.V. Intravenous busulfan should be administered as a 2-hour via central line.

Stability

Reconstitution Injection: Dilute (using manufacturer provided 5-micron filters for ampuls) in 0.9% sodium chloride injection or dextrose 5% in water. The dilution volume of busulfan injection, ensuring that the final concentration of busulfan is 0.5 mg/mL.

Storage

Injection: Store unopened ampuls and vials under refrigeration (2°C to 8°C). Final solution is stable for up to 8 hours at room temperature (25°C); the infusion must be completed within that 8-hour timeframe. Dilution of busulfan injection in 0.9% sodium chloride is stable for up to 12 hours at refrigeration (2°C to 8°C); the infusion must be completed within that 12-hour timeframe.

Tablet: Store at room temperature at 15°C to 30°C (59°F to 86°F).

Monitoring and Teaching Issues

Laboratory Monitoring CBC with differential and platelet count, liver function (evaluate transaminases, alkaline phosphatase, and bilirubin daily for at least 28 days post transplant)

Physical Assessment Identify any history of seizures, recent myelosuppressive therapy or radiation treatment, and pregnancy status prior to therapy. Dosing for obese patients should be based on adjusted ideal body weight. BMT: Phenytoin or clonazepam may be ordered prophylactically during and for at least 48 hours following completion of busulfan to reduce risk of seizures if patient is predisposed to seizures. Assess CBC with differential, platelet count, and LFTs. Monitor for adverse pulmonary effects (pulmonary fibrosis or toxicity; may be delayed 4 months to 10 years) or hematologic effects (pancytopenia, leukopenia, thrombocytopenia, anemia, and bone marrow suppression) during therapy and for several months following therapy.

Patient Education Maintain adequate nutrition and hydration, unless instructed to restrict fluid intake. Avoid excess alcohol and acidic or spicy foods (may increase gastrointestinal irritation). You will be more susceptible to infection. May cause dizziness, insomnia, or confusion; mouth sores; loss of hair or darkening of skin color (reversible when medication is discontinued); nausea, vomiting, or loss of appetite; constipation; diarrhea (consult prescriber if severe or persistent); amenorrhea; sterility; or skin rash. Report palpitations or chest pain, weight gain, CNS changes (anxiety, confusion, depression), unusual cough or difficulty breathing, numbness or tingling of extremities, unusual bruising or bleeding, or pain or changes in urination.

Geriatric Considerations Toxicity to immunosuppressives is increased in the elderly. Start with lowest recommended adult doses. Signs of infection, such as fever and rise in WBCs, may not occur. Lethargy and confusion may be more prominent signs of infection.

Breast-Feeding Considerations Due to the tumorigenicity potential and the potential for serious adverse reactions in the nursing infant, breast-feeding is not recommended.

Pregnancy Considerations Animal studies have demonstrated teratogenic effects. May cause fetal harm if administered during pregnancy. The solvent in I.V. busulfan, DMA, is associated with teratogenic effects and may impair fertility. There are no adequate and well-controlled studies in pregnant women. Women of childbearing potential should avoid pregnancy while receiving treatment.

Additional Information Oncology Comment: Low-dose monotherapy with oral busulfan for the palliative treatment of CML is no longer common. Treatment with imatinib or hematopoietic stem cell transplant (HSCT) are considered the primary treatments for CML (NCCN v1.2008).

◆ **Busulfex®** *see* Busulfan *on page* 257

Butalbital, Acetaminophen, and Caffeine

(byoo TAL bi tal, a seet a MIN oh fen, & KAF een)

U.S. Brand Names Alagesic LQ; Alagesic [DSC]; Anolor 300; Dolgic® Plus; Esgic-Plus™; Esgic®; Fioricet®; Margesic; Orbivan™; Repan®; Zebutal®

Index Terms Acetaminophen, Butalbital, and Caffeine

Generic Availability (U.S.) Yes: Tablet

Pharmacologic Category Barbiturate

Medication Safety Issues

Sound-alike/look-alike issues:

Fioricet® may be confused with Fiorinal®, Lorcet®

Repan® may be confused with Riopan®

Duplicate therapy issues: This product contains acetaminophen, which may be a component of other combination products. Do not exceed the maximum recommended daily dose of acetaminophen.

Pregnancy Risk Factor C

Lactation Enters breast milk/not recommended

Use Relief of the symptomatic complex of tension or muscle contraction headache

Available Dosage Forms

Capsule, oral:

Anolor 300, Esgic®, Margesic: Butalbital 50 mg, acetaminophen 325 mg, and caffeine 40 mg

Esgic-Plus™, Zebutal®: Butalbital 50 mg, acetaminophen 500 mg, and caffeine 40 mg

Orbivan™: Butalbital 50 mg, acetaminophen 300 mg, and caffeine 40 mg

Liquid, oral:

Alagesic LQ: Butalbital 50 mg, acetaminophen 325 mg, and caffeine 40 mg per 15 mL

Tablet, oral: Butalbital 50 mg, acetaminophen 325 mg, and caffeine 40 mg; butalbital 50 mg, acetaminophen 500 mg, and caffeine 40 mg
Dolgic® Plus: Butalbital 50 mg, acetaminophen 750 mg, and caffeine 40 mg
Esgic®, Fioricet®, Repan®: Butalbital 50 mg, acetaminophen 325 mg, and caffeine 40 mg
Esgic-Plus™: Butalbital 50 mg, acetaminophen 500 mg, and caffeine 40 mg

Dosing

Adult Tension or muscle contraction headache: Oral: 1-2 tablets or capsules (or 15-30 mL solution) every 4 hours; not to exceed 6 tablets or capsules (or 180 mL solution) daily

Geriatric Not recommended for use in the elderly.

Renal Impairment Dosage should be reduced.

Hepatic Impairment Dosage should be reduced.

Monitoring and Teaching Issues

Physical Assessment See individual agents.

Patient Education See individual agents.

Related Information

Acetaminophen *on page* 38

Butalbital, Acetaminophen, Caffeine, and Codeine

(byoo TAL bi tal, a seet a MIN oh fen, KAF een, & KOE deen)

U.S. Brand Names Fioricet® with Codeine

Index Terms Acetaminophen, Caffeine, Codeine, and Butalbital; Caffeine, Acetaminophen, Butalbital, and Codeine; Codeine, Acetaminophen, Butalbital, and Caffeine

Generic Availability (U.S.) Yes

Pharmacologic Category Analgesic Combination (Opioid); Barbiturate

Medication Safety Issues

Sound-alike/look-alike issues:

Fioricet® may be confused with Fiorinal®, Florinef®, Lorcet®, Percocet®
Phrenilin may be confused with Phenergan®, Trinalin®

High alert medication: The Institute for Safe Medication Practices (ISMP) includes this medication among its list of drug classes which have a heightened risk of causing significant patient harm when used in error.

Duplicate therapy issues: This product contains acetaminophen, which may be a component of other combination products. Do not exceed the maximum recommended daily dose of acetaminophen.

Pregnancy Risk Factor C (per manufacturer)

Lactation Enters breast milk/not recommended

Use Relief of symptoms of complex tension (muscle contraction) headache

Controlled Substance C-III

Available Dosage Forms

Capsule: Butalbital 50 mg, acetaminophen 325 mg, caffeine 40 mg, and codeine 30 mg
Fioricet® with Codeine: Butalbital 50 mg, acetaminophen 325 mg, caffeine 40 mg, and codeine 30 mg

Dosing

Adult & Geriatric Oral: Adults: 1-2 capsules every 4 hours. Total daily dosage should not exceed 6 capsules.

Hepatic Impairment Use with caution. Limited, low-dose therapy usually well tolerated in hepatic disease/cirrhosis. However, cases of hepatotoxicity at daily acetaminophen dosages <4 g/day have been reported. Avoid chronic use in hepatic impairment.

Monitoring and Teaching Issues

Laboratory Monitoring Hepatic and renal function tests (in patients with impairment)

Physical Assessment See individual agents.

Patient Education See individual agents.

Related Information

Acetaminophen *on page* 38
Codeine *on page* 421

Butalbital and Acetaminophen (byoo TAL bi tal & a seet a MIN oh fen)

U.S. Brand Names Bupap; Cephadyn; Phrenilin®; Phrenilin® Forte; Promacet; Sedapap®

Index Terms Acetaminophen and Butalbital

Generic Availability (U.S.) Yes

Pharmacologic Category Analgesic, Miscellaneous; Barbiturate

Medication Safety Issues

Duplicate therapy issues: This product contains acetaminophen, which may be a component of other combination products. Do not exceed the maximum recommended daily dose of acetaminophen.

Pregnancy Risk Factor C

Lactation Enters breast milk/not recommended

Use Relief of the symptomatic complex of tension or muscle contraction headache

Available Dosage Forms

Tablet:

Phrenilin®: Butalbital 50 mg and acetaminophen 325 mg

Bupap, Cephadyn, Promacet, Sedapap®: Butalbital 50 mg and acetaminophen 650 mg

Capsule:

Phrenilin® Forte: Butalbital 50 mg and acetaminophen 650 mg

Dosing

Adult Tension or muscle contraction headache: Oral: One tablet/capsule every 4 hours as needed (maximum dose: 6 tablets/day)

Phrenilin®: 1-2 tablets every 4 hours as needed (maximum: 6 tablets in 24 hours)

Geriatric Refer to adult dosing. Use with caution.

Renal Impairment Mild-to-moderate: Should decrease dose; in severe impairment, use with caution.

Hepatic Impairment Mild-to-moderate: Should decrease dose; in severe impairment, use with caution.

Monitoring and Teaching Issues

Physical Assessment See individual agents.

Patient Education See individual agents.

Related Information

Acetaminophen *on page 38*

PHENobarbital *on page 1447*

Butalbital, Aspirin, and Caffeine (byoo TAL bi tal, AS pir in, & KAF een)

U.S. Brand Names Fiorinal®

Index Terms Aspirin, Caffeine, and Butalbital; Butalbital Compound

Generic Availability (U.S.) Yes

Pharmacologic Category Barbiturate

Medication Safety Issues

Sound-alike/look-alike issues:

Fiorinal® may be confused with Fioricet®, Florical®, Florinef®

Pregnancy Risk Factor C/D (prolonged use or high doses at term)

Lactation Enters breast milk/use caution due to aspirin content

Use Relief of the symptomatic complex of tension or muscle contraction headache

Controlled Substance C-III

Available Dosage Forms

Capsule: Butalbital 50 mg, aspirin 325 mg, and caffeine 40 mg

Fiorinal®: Butalbital 50 mg, aspirin 325 mg, and caffeine 40 mg

Tablet: Butalbital 50 mg, aspirin 325 mg, and caffeine 40 mg

Dosing

Adult Tension or muscle contraction headache: Oral: 1-2 tablets or capsules every 4 hours; not to exceed 6 tablets or capsules/day

Geriatric Not recommended for use in the elderly.

Renal Impairment Dosage should be reduced.

Hepatic Impairment Dosage should be reduced.

Monitoring and Teaching Issues

Physical Assessment See individual agents.

Patient Education See individual agents.

Related Information

Aspirin *on page 155*

Butalbital, Aspirin, Caffeine, and Codeine
(byoo TAL bi tal, AS pir in, KAF een, & KOE deen)

U.S. Brand Names Ascomp® with Codeine; Fiorinal® with Codeine

Index Terms Aspirin, Caffeine, Codeine, and Butalbital; Butalbital Compound and Codeine; Codeine and Butalbital Compound; Codeine, Butalbital, Aspirin, and Caffeine

Generic Availability (U.S.) Yes

Pharmacologic Category Analgesic Combination (Opioid); Barbiturate

Medication Safety Issues

Sound-alike/look-alike issues:

Fiorinal® may be confused with Fioricet®, Florical®, Florinef®

High alert medication: The Institute for Safe Medication Practices (ISMP) includes this medication among its list of drug classes which have a heightened risk of causing significant patient harm when used in error.

Pregnancy Risk Factor C (per manufacturer)

Lactation Enters breast milk/not recommended

Use Relief of symptoms of complex tension (muscle contraction) headache

Controlled Substance C-III

Available Dosage Forms

Capsule: Butalbital 50 mg, aspirin 325 mg, caffeine 40 mg, and codeine 30 mg

Ascomp® with Codeine, Fiorinal® with Codeine: Butalbital 50 mg, aspirin 325 mg, caffeine 40 mg, and codeine 30 mg

Dosing

Adult Tension headache: Oral: 1-2 capsules every 4 hours as needed (maximum: 6 capsules/day)

Geriatric Use with caution; however, barbiturates (butalbital) are generally not recommended in the elderly.

Monitoring and Teaching Issues

Laboratory Monitoring Serial hepatic and renal function tests (in patients with impairment)

Physical Assessment See individual agents.

Patient Education See individual agents.

Related Information

Aspirin *on page 155*

Codeine *on page 421*

◆ **Butalbital Compound** *see* Butalbital, Aspirin, and Caffeine *on page 262*

◆ **Butalbital Compound and Codeine** *see* Butalbital, Aspirin, Caffeine, and Codeine *on page 262*

Butorphanol (byoo TOR fa nole)

Index Terms Butorphanol Tartrate; Stadol

Generic Availability (U.S.) Yes

Pharmacologic Category Analgesic, Opioid

Medication Safety Issues

Sound-alike/look-alike issues:

Stadol may be confused with Haldol®, sotalol

High alert medication: The Institute for Safe Medication Practices (ISMP) includes this medication among its list of drug classes which have a heightened risk of causing significant patient harm when used in error.

Pregnancy Risk Factor C

Lactation Enters breast milk (AAP rates "compatible"; AAP 2001 update pending)

Use

Parenteral: Management of moderate-to-severe pain; preoperative medication; supplement to balanced anesthesia; management of pain during labor

Nasal spray: Management of moderate-to-severe pain, including migraine headache pain

Controlled Substance C-IV

Available Dosage Forms

Injection, solution: 1 mg/mL (1 mL); 2 mg/mL (1 mL, 2 mL, 10 mL)

Injection, solution [preservative free]: 1 mg/mL (1 mL); 2 mg/mL (1 mL, 2 mL)

Solution, intranasal: 10 mg/mL (2.5 mL)

Dosing

Adult Note: These are guidelines and do not represent the maximum doses that may be required in all patients. Doses should be titrated to pain relief/prevention. Butorphanol has an analgesic ceiling.

Acute pain (moderate-to-severe):

I.M.: Initial: 2 mg, may repeat every 3-4 hours as needed; usual range: 1-4 mg every 3-4 hours as needed

I.V.: Initial: 1 mg, may repeat every 3-4 hours as needed; usual range: 0.5-2 mg every 3-4 hours as needed

Intranasal (spray) (includes use for migraine headache pain): Initial: 1 spray (~1 mg per spray) in 1 nostril; if adequate pain relief is not achieved within 60-90 minutes, an additional 1 spray in 1 nostril may be given; may repeat initial dose sequence in 3-4 hours after the last dose as needed

Alternatively, an initial dose of 2 mg (1 spray in each nostril) may be used in patients who will be able to remain recumbent (in the event drowsiness or dizziness occurs); additional 2 mg doses should not be given for 3-4 hours

Note: In some clinical trials, an initial dose of 2 mg (as 2 doses 1 hour apart or 2 mg initially - 1 spray in each nostril) has been used, followed by 1 mg in 1 hour; side effects were greater at these dosages

Migraine: *Nasal spray:* Refer to "moderate-to-severe pain" indication

Preoperative medication: *I.M.:* 2 mg 60-90 minutes before surgery

Supplement to balanced anesthesia: *I.V.:* 2 mg shortly before induction and/or an incremental dose of 0.5-1 mg (up to 0.06 mg/kg), depending on previously administered sedative, analgesic, and hypnotic medications

Pain during labor (fetus >37 weeks gestation and no signs of fetal distress):

I.M., I.V.: 1-2 mg; may repeat in 4 hours

Note: Alternative analgesia should be used for pain associated with delivery or if delivery is anticipated within 4 hours

Geriatric

I.M., I.V.: Initial dosage should generally be 1/2 of the recommended dose; repeated dosing must be based on initial response rather than fixed intervals, but generally should be at least 6 hours apart

Nasal spray: Initial dose should not exceed 1 mg; a second dose may be given after 90-120 minutes

Renal Impairment

I.M., I.V.: Initial dosage should generally be 1/2 of the recommended dose; repeated dosing must be based on initial response rather than fixed intervals, but generally should be at least 6 hours apart

Nasal spray: Initial dose should not exceed 1 mg; a second dose may be given after 90-120 minutes

Hepatic Impairment

I.M., I.V.: Initial dosage should generally be 1/2 of the recommended dose; repeated dosing must be based on initial response rather than fixed intervals, but generally should be at least 6 hours apart

Nasal spray: Initial dose should not exceed 1 mg; a second dose may be given after 90-120 minutes

Administration

Inhalation See Dosing.

Other Intranasal: Consider avoiding simultaneous intranasal migraine sprays; may want to separate by at least 30 minutes

Monitoring and Teaching Issues

Physical Assessment Monitor for effectiveness of pain relief prior to treatment and periodically throughout. For inpatients, implement safety measures to prevent falls. Assess patient's physical and/or psychological dependence. Discontinue slowly after prolonged use.

Patient Education May cause physical and/or psychological dependence. Do not use alcohol, sedatives, tranquilizers, antihistamines, or pain medications without consulting prescriber. May cause dizziness, drowsiness, confusion, or blurred vision; nausea or vomiting; or loss of appetite. Report unresolved nausea or vomiting; respiratory difficulty or shortness of breath; restlessness, insomnia, euphoria, or nightmares; excessive sedation or unusual weakness; facial flushing, rapid heartbeat, or palpitations; urinary difficulty; or vision changes.

Nasal administration: Do not use more frequently than prescribed. Blow nose prior to administering. Follow instructions on package insert. Insert nozzle of applicator gently into one nostril and exhale. With next breath, squeeze applicator once firmly and quickly once as you breath in. If adequate relief from headache is not achieved within 60-90 minutes, an additional 1 spray may be given. May be repeated in 3-4 hours following last dose, as needed. **Alternatively:** Two sprays may be given, one spray in each nostril, if you are able to remain lying down (in the event of drowsiness or dizziness). Additional doses should not be taken for 3-4 hours. Avoid using simultaneously with other intranasal migraine sprays. Separate by at least 30 minutes.

Related Information

Compatibility of Drugs *on page 1994*

Opioid Analgesics *on page 2003*

- **Butorphanol Tartrate** *see* Butorphanol *on page 263*
- **Butrans™** *see* Buprenorphine *on page 246*
- **BW-430C** *see* LamoTRIgine *on page 1057*
- **BW524W91** *see* Emtricitabine *on page 613*
- **Byetta®** *see* Exenatide *on page 726*
- **Bystolic®** *see* Nebivolol *on page 1295*
- **C2B8 Monoclonal Antibody** *see* RITUXimab *on page 1596*
- **311C90** *see* Zolmitriptan *on page 1903*
- **C225** *see* Cetuximab *on page 352*

Cabazitaxel (ca baz i TAKS el)

U.S. Brand Names Jevtana®

Index Terms RPR-116258A; XRP6258

Generic Availability (U.S.) No

Pharmacologic Category Antineoplastic Agent, Antimicrotubular; Antineoplastic Agent, Taxane Derivative

Medication Safety Issues

High alert medication: This medication is in a class the Institute for Safe Medication Practices (ISMP) includes among its list of drugs which have a heightened risk of causing significant patient harm when used in error.

Cabazitaxel requires a two-step dilution process prior to administration.

Pregnancy Risk Factor D

Lactation Excretion in breast milk unknown/not recommended

Use Treatment of hormone-refractory metastatic prostate cancer (in patients previously treated with a docetaxel-containing regimen)

Available Dosage Forms

Injection, solution:

Jevtana®: 40 mg/mL (1.5 mL)

Dosing

Adult Note: Premedicate at least 30 minutes prior to each dose of cabazitaxel with an antihistamine (eg, diphenhydramine I.V. 25 mg or equivalent), a corticosteroid (eg, dexamethasone 8 mg I.V. or equivalent), and an H_2 antagonist (eg, ranitidine 50 mg I.V. or equivalent). Antiemetic prophylaxis is also recommended. Details concerning dosing in combination regimens should also be consulted.

Prostate cancer: I.V.: 25 mg/m^2/dose once every 3 weeks (in combination with prednisone)

Renal Impairment Severe renal impairment (Cl_{cr} <30 mL/minute) or end-stage renal disease: Use with caution.

Hepatic Impairment Hepatic impairment (total bilirubin ≥ULN or AST and/or ALT ≥1.5 times ULN): Use is not recommended.

Adjustment for Toxicity

Hematologic toxicity:

Neutropenia ≥ grade 3 for > 1 week despite WBC growth factors: Delay treatment until ANC >1500/mm^3 and then reduce dose to 20 mg/m^2 with continued WBC growth factor secondary prophylaxis.

Neutropenic fever: Delay treatment until improvement/resolution and ANC >1500/mm^3 and then reduce dose to 20 mg/m^2 with continued WBC growth factor secondary prophylaxis.

Persistent hematologic toxicity (despite dosage reduction): Discontinue treatment.

Nonhematologic toxicity:

Severe hypersensitivity: Discontinue immediately.

Diarrhea ≥grade 3 or persistent despite appropriate medication, fluids, and electrolyte replacement: Delay treatment until improves or resolves and then reduce dose to 20 mg/m^2.

Persistent diarrhea (despite dosage reduction): Discontinue treatment.

Administration

I.V. Infuse over 1 hour using a 0.22 micron inline filter. Do not use polyurethane-containing infusion sets for administration. Allow to reach room temperature prior to infusion. Premedicate with an antihistamine, a corticosteroid, and an H_2 antagonist at least 30 minutes prior to infusion. Observe closely during infusion (for hypersensitivity). Antiemetic prophylaxis (oral or I.V.) is also recommended.

Monitoring and Teaching Issues

Laboratory Monitoring CBC with differential and platelets (weekly during first cycle, then prior to each treatment cycle)

Physical Assessment Assess carefully for contraindications or cautions (hepatic impairment, renal impairment, previous hypersensitivity reaction, increased risk for neutropenic complications). Premedicate 30 minutes prior to each dose (antihistamine, corticosteroid, and an H_2 antagonist). A prophylactic antiemetic is recommended. Patient must be monitored closely for hypersensitivity reaction (rash, erythema, hypotension, bronchospasm); discontinue and notify prescriber. Monitor for hypersensitivity, hypotension, myelosuppression, and GI irritation (including severe diarrhea) prior to, during, and between each infusion.

Patient Education This drug is only administered by intravenous infusion; you will be monitored closely during and following infusions. Immediately report any burning, pain, or swelling at infusion site; any unusual chest pain or tightness, rapid heartbeat, or palpitations; difficulty breathing; difficulty swallowing; or nausea or vomiting during infusion. You will be more susceptible to infection. It is important that you maintain adequate nutrition and fluid intake, unless instructed to restrict fluid intake. May cause fatigue, dizziness, headache, gastrointestinal upset, or loss of hair (will grow back after therapy). Report chest pain, palpitations, or swelling of extremities; difficult breathing; pain or decreased sensation in extremities; or unusual sign of weakness.

Cabergoline (ca BER goe leen)

Generic Availability (U.S.) Yes

Pharmacologic Category Ergot Derivative

Pregnancy Risk Factor B

Lactation Excretion in breast milk unknown/not recommended

Use Treatment of hyperprolactinemic disorders, either idiopathic or due to pituitary adenomas

Mechanism of Action/Effect Cabergoline is a long acting dopamine receptor agonist with a high affinity for D_2 receptors; prolactin secretion by the anterior pituitary is predominantly under hypothalamic inhibitory control exerted through the release of dopamine

Contraindications Hypersensitivity to ergot derivatives; uncontrolled hypertension; history of pulmonary, pericardial, cardiac valvular or retroperitoneal fibrotic disorders

Warnings/Precautions Initial doses >1 mg may cause orthostatic hypotension; concurrent use with antihypertensive agents may increase risk. Not indicated for the inhibition or suppression of physiologic lactation; other dopamine agonists are associated with cases of hypertension, stroke, and seizures. Use caution in patients with hepatic impairment; monitor LFTs. Should not be used in patients with pregnancy-induced hypertension unless benefit outweighs potential risk. In all patients, prolactin concentrations should be monitored monthly until normalized. Pleural effusion and pulmonary/retroperitoneal fibrosis have been reported with long-term use. Cardiac valvular disease (mitral, aortic, tricuspid regurgitation) has been associated with cabergoline (a potent 5-HT_{2B} agonist). Incidence may be higher for daily doses >2 mg and for duration of use ≥6 months. Following diagnosis of fibrosis/valvulopathy, discontinuation of

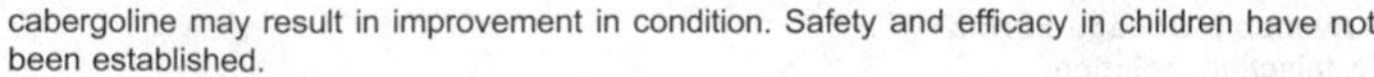

cabergoline may result in improvement in condition. Safety and efficacy in children have not been established.

Drug Interactions

Avoid Concomitant Use

Avoid concomitant use of Cabergoline with any of the following: Efavirenz; Itraconazole; Nitroglycerin; Posaconazole; Serotonin 5-HT1D Receptor Agonists; Sibutramine; Voriconazole

Decreased Effect

Cabergoline may decrease the levels/effects of: Nitroglycerin

Increased Effect/Toxicity

Cabergoline may increase the levels/effects of: Serotonin 5-HT1D Receptor Agonists; Serotonin Modulators

The levels/effects of Cabergoline may be increased by: Efavirenz; Itraconazole; MAO Inhibitors; Nitroglycerin; Posaconazole; Serotonin 5-HT1D Receptor Agonists; Sibutramine; Voriconazole

Nutritional/Ethanol Interactions Herb/Nutraceutical: Avoid products that enhance serotonin activity (includes SAMe [S-adenosylmethionine] and St John's wort); may increase the risk of serotonin syndrome.

Adverse Reactions

>10%:

Central nervous system: Headache (26%), dizziness (15% to 17%)

Gastrointestinal: Nausea (27% to 29%)

1% to 10%:

Cardiovascular: Postural hypotension (4%), hypotension (1%), dependent edema (1%), edema (peripheral 1%), palpitation (1%), syncope (1%)

Central nervous system: Fatigue (5% to 7%), vertigo (1% to 4%), depression (3%), somnolence (2% to 5%), nervousness (1% to 2%), anxiety (1%), insomnia (1%), concentration impaired (1%), malaise (1%)

Dermatologic: Acne (1%), pruritus (1%)

Endocrine: Hot flashes (1% to 3%), breast pain (1% to 2%), dysmenorrhea (1%)

Gastrointestinal: Constipation (7% to 10%), abdominal pain (5%), dyspepsia (2% to 5%), vomiting (2% to 4%), xerostomia (2%), diarrhea (2%), flatulence (2%), anorexia (1%), throat irritation (1%), toothache (1%)

Neuromuscular & skeletal: Weakness (6% to 9%), pain (2%), paresthesia (1% to 2%), arthralgia (1%)

Ocular: Abnormal vision (1%), periorbital edema (1%)

Respiratory: Rhinitis (1%)

Miscellaneous: Flu-like syndrome (1%)

Pharmacodynamics/Kinetics

Time to Peak 2-3 hours

Protein Binding 40% to 42%

Half-Life Elimination 63-69 hours

Metabolism Extensively hepatic via hydrolysis; minimal CYP mediated metabolism

Excretion Primarily feces (~60%); urine (~22%, <4% as unchanged drug)

Available Dosage Forms

Tablet, oral: 0.5 mg

Dosing

Adult Hyperprolactinemic disorders: Oral: Initial dose: 0.25 mg twice weekly; the dose may be increased by 0.25 mg twice weekly up to a maximum of 1 mg twice weekly according to the patient's serum prolactin level. Dosage increases should not occur more rapidly than every 4 weeks. Once a normal serum prolactin level is maintained for 6 months, the dose may be discontinued and prolactin levels monitored to determine if cabergoline is still required. The durability of efficacy beyond 24 months of therapy has not been established.

Geriatric Refer to adult dosing. No dosage recommendations suggested; however, start at the low end of the dosage range.

Renal Impairment No adjustment required.

Hepatic Impairment

Mild-to-moderate dysfunction (Child-Pugh Class B): No adjustment required

Severe dysfunction (Child-Pugh Class C): Use caution; significant increase in AUC

Stability

Storage Store at 20°C to 25°C (68°F to 77°F).

Monitoring and Teaching Issues

Laboratory Monitoring Serum prolactin level

Breast-Feeding Considerations Interferes with lactation and should not be given to women postpartum who are breast-feeding or who are planning to breast-feed. Not indicated for the suppression of physiologic lactation.

Pregnancy Considerations Teratogenic effects were not observed in most animal studies when administered in maternally nontoxic doses. Treatment of hyperprolactinemia may restore fertility in a previously infertile woman. Because information concerning the use of cabergoline in pregnancy is limited, bromocriptine is generally recommended to treat hyperprolactinemia in women who wish to conceive. Based on preliminary data, cabergoline has not been shown to increase the risk of congenital malformations or miscarriages when used early in pregnancy (treatment was generally stopped once pregnancy was diagnosed). Not recommended for use in patients with pregnancy-induced hypertension unless benefit outweighs potential risk.

Additional Information Bromocriptine and cabergoline are the only drugs indicated for the treatment of hyperprolactinemia. In the largest comparative clinical trial, prolactin levels normalized in 77% of patients treated with cabergoline compared to 59% of patients treated with bromocriptine. In that trial, 3% of patients discontinued treatment due to adverse effects in the cabergoline group versus 12% of patients in the bromocriptine group. In addition to the improved safety and efficacy profile, cabergoline (administered twice weekly) is more convenient than bromocriptine (administered 1-3 times/day) for patients to take.

◆ **Caduet®** *see* Amlodipine and Atorvastatin *on page* *106*
◆ **Cafcit®** *see* Caffeine *on page* *267*

Caffeine (KAF een)

U.S. Brand Names Cafcit®; Enerjets [OTC]; No Doz® Maximum Strength [OTC]; Vivarin® [OTC]

Index Terms Caffeine and Sodium Benzoate; Caffeine Citrate; Caffeine Sodium Benzoate; Sodium Benzoate and Caffeine

Generic Availability (U.S.) Yes: Tablet, caffeine and sodium benzoate injection, injection, oral solution

Pharmacologic Category Stimulant

Pregnancy Risk Factor C

Lactation Enters breast milk/use caution (AAP rates "compatible"; AAP 2001 update pending)

Use

Caffeine citrate: Treatment of idiopathic apnea of prematurity

Caffeine and sodium benzoate: Treatment of acute respiratory depression (not a preferred agent)

Caffeine [OTC labeling]: Restore mental alertness or wakefulness when experiencing fatigue

Unlabeled/Investigational Use Caffeine and sodium benzoate: Treatment of spinal puncture headache; CNS stimulant; diuretic; augmentation of seizure induction during electroconvulsive therapy (ECT)

Available Dosage Forms

Caplet:

No Doz® Maximum Strength [OTC], Vivarin® [OTC]: 200 mg

Injection, solution [preservative free]: 20 mg/mL (3 mL)

Cafcit®: 20 mg/mL (3 mL)

Lozenge:

Enerjets® [OTC]: 75 mg

Solution, oral [preservative free]: 20 mg/mL (3 mL)

Cafcit®: 20 mg/mL

Tablet: 200 mg

Vivarin® [OTC]: 200 mg

Dosing

Adult & Geriatric

Note: Caffeine citrate should not be interchanged with the caffeine sodium benzoate formulation.

Caffeine and sodium benzoate:

Electroconvulsive therapy: I.V.: 300-2000 mg

Respiratory depression: I.M., I.V.: 250 mg as a single dose; may repeat as needed. Maximum single dose should be limited to 500 mg; maximum amount in any 24-hour period should generally be limited to 2500 mg.

Spinal puncture headache (unlabeled use):

I.V.: 500 mg in 1000 mL NS infused over 1 hour, followed by 1000 mL NS infused over 1 hour; a second course of caffeine can be given for unrelieved headache pain in 4 hours.

Oral: 300 mg as a single dose

Stimulant/diuretic (unlabeled use): I.M., I.V.: 500 mg, maximum single dose: 1 g

OTC labeling (stimulant): Oral: 100-200 mg every 3-4 hours as needed

Pediatric

Note: Caffeine citrate should not be interchanged with the caffeine sodium benzoate formulation.

Caffeine citrate: Apnea of prematurity: Neonates: Oral, I.V.:

Loading dose: 10-20 mg/kg as caffeine citrate (5-10 mg/kg as caffeine base). If theophylline has been administered to the patient within the previous 3 days, a full or modified loading dose (50% to 75% of a loading dose) may be given.

Maintenance dose: 5 mg/kg/day as caffeine citrate (2.5 mg/kg/day as caffeine base) once daily starting 24 hours after the loading dose. Maintenance dose is adjusted based on patient's response and serum caffeine concentrations.

Caffeine and sodium benzoate: Stimulant:

I.M., I.V., SubQ: 8 mg/kg every 4 hours as needed

Oral: OTC labeling: Children ≥12 years: Refer to adult dosing.

Renal Impairment No dosage adjustment required.

Administration

Oral May be administered without regard to feedings or meals. May administer injectable formulation (caffeine citrate) orally.

I.M. Parenteral: **Caffeine and sodium benzoate:** May administer I.M. undiluted

I.V. Parenteral:

Caffeine citrate: Infuse loading dose over at least 30 minutes; maintenance dose may be infused over at least 10 minutes. May administer without dilution or diluted with D_5W to 10 mg caffeine citrate/mL.

Caffeine and sodium benzoate: I.V. as slow direct injection. For spinal headaches, dilute in 1000 mL NS and infuse over 1 hour. Follow with 1000 mL NS; infuse over 1 hour. May administer I.M. undiluted.

Monitoring and Teaching Issues

Patient Education You may experience excitability, flushing, dizziness, insomnia, or agitation. Report excessive excitability or nervousness, chest pain, or respiratory difficulty.

- **Caffeine, Acetaminophen, Butalbital, and Codeine** *see* Butalbital, Acetaminophen, Caffeine, and Codeine *on page 261*
- **Caffeine and Sodium Benzoate** *see* Caffeine *on page 267*
- **Caffeine Citrate** *see* Caffeine *on page 267*
- **Caffeine Sodium Benzoate** *see* Caffeine *on page 267*
- **Calan®** *see* Verapamil *on page 1858*
- **Calan® SR** *see* Verapamil *on page 1858*
- **Calciferol™ [OTC]** *see* Ergocalciferol *on page 650*
- **Calcijex®** *see* Calcitriol *on page 271*

Calcipotriene (kal si POE try een)

U.S. Brand Names Calcitrene™; Dovonex®

Generic Availability (U.S.) Yes: Excludes cream

Pharmacologic Category Topical Skin Product; Vitamin D Analog

Pregnancy Risk Factor C

Lactation Excretion in breast milk unknown/use caution

Use Treatment of plaque psoriasis; chronic, moderate-to-severe psoriasis of the scalp

Unlabeled/Investigational Use Vitiligo

Available Dosage Forms

Cream, topical:
Dovonex®: 0.005% (60 g, 120 g)

Ointment, topical:
Calcitrene™: 0.005% (60 g)

Solution, topical: 0.005% (60 mL)
Dovonex®: 0.005% (60 mL)

Dosing

Adult & Geriatric Psoriasis: Topical:
Cream: Apply a thin film to the affected skin twice daily for up to 8 weeks
Ointment: Apply a thin film to the affected skin once or twice daily
Solution: Apply to the affected scalp twice daily for up to 8 weeks

Administration

Topical For external use only.

Cream, ointment: Apply to affected skin; rub in gently and completely. Wash hands thoroughly before and after use.

Solution: Prior to using scalp solution, comb hair to remove debris; apply only to lesions. Rub in gently and completely. Avoid solution spreading or dripping onto forehead. Avoid contact with eyes. Wash hands thoroughly before and after use.

Monitoring and Teaching Issues

Laboratory Monitoring Serum calcium

Physical Assessment When applied to large areas of skin or for extensive periods of time, monitor for adverse skin or systemic reactions.

Patient Education For external use only. Before using, wash and dry area gently. Wear gloves to apply a thin film to affected area and rub in gently. If dressing is necessary, use a porous dressing. Avoid contact with eyes. Avoid exposing treated area to direct sunlight; sunburn can occur. Report increased swelling, redness, rash, itching, signs of infection, worsening of condition, or lack of healing.

Calcipotriene and Betamethasone (kal si POE try een & bay ta METH a sone)

U.S. Brand Names Taclonex Scalp®; Taclonex®

Index Terms Betamethasone Dipropionate and Calcipotriene Hydrate; Calcipotriol and Betamethasone Dipropionate

Generic Availability (U.S.) No

Pharmacologic Category Corticosteroid, Topical; Vitamin D Analog

Pregnancy Risk Factor C

Lactation Excretion in breast milk unknown/use caution

Use Treatment of psoriasis vulgaris

Unlabeled/Investigational Use Treatment of corticosteroid-responsive dermatoses

Available Dosage Forms

Ointment, topical:

Taclonex®: Calcipotriene 0.005% and betamethasone 0.064% (60 g, 100 g)

Suspension, topical:

Taclonex Scalp®: Calcipotriene 0.005% and betamethasone 0.064%

Dosing

Adult & Geriatric

Psoriasis vulgaris: Topical:

Gel (Xamiol® [CAN]): Apply to affected areas of scalp once daily for up to 4 weeks (maximum recommended dose: 15 g/day or 100 g/week). Application to >30% of body surface area is not recommended

Ointment: Apply to affected area once daily for up to 4 weeks (maximum recommended dose: 100 g/week). Application to >30% of body surface area is not recommended.

Suspension: Apply to affected area of the scalp once daily for 2 weeks or until clear; may continue for up to 8 weeks (maximum recommended dose: 100 g/week)

Renal Impairment Safety and efficacy have not been established with severe renal impairment.

Hepatic Impairment Safety and efficacy have not been established with severe hepatic impairment.

Administration

Topical Wash hands before and after use.

Gel (Xamiol® [CAN]): Shake well before use. Avoid use of occlusive dressings over treated areas.

Ointment: Rub into affected area gently and completely. Do not apply to face, axillae, or groin.

Suspension: Shake well before use. Do not apply within 12 hours of chemical hair treatment. Do not wash hair directly after use.

Monitoring and Teaching Issues

Laboratory Monitoring Baseline serum calcium levels and then periodically during treatment in patients at risk for hypercalcemia

Physical Assessment See individual agents.

Patient Education See individual agents.

Related Information

Betamethasone *on page 205*

Calcipotriene *on page 268*

◆ **Calcipotriol and Betamethasone Dipropionate** *see* Calcipotriene and Betamethasone *on page 268*

Calcitonin (kal si TOE nin)

U.S. Brand Names Fortical®; Miacalcin®

Index Terms Calcitonin (Salmon)

Generic Availability (U.S.) Yes: Intranasal solution

Pharmacologic Category Antidote; Hormone

Medication Safety Issues

Sound-alike/look-alike issues:

Calcitonin may be confused with calcitriol

Miacalcin® may be confused with Micatin®

Calcitonin nasal spray is administered as a single spray into **one** nostril daily, using alternate nostrils each day.

Pregnancy Risk Factor C

Lactation Excretion in breast milk unknown/not recommended

Use Treatment of Paget's disease of bone (osteitis deformans); adjunctive therapy for hypercalcemia; treatment of osteoporosis in women >5 years postmenopause

Mechanism of Action/Effect Peptide sequence similar to human calcitonin; functionally antagonizes the effects of parathyroid hormone. Directly inhibits osteoclastic bone resorption; promotes the renal excretion of calcium, phosphate, sodium, magnesium, and potassium by decreasing tubular reabsorption; increases the jejunal secretion of water, sodium, potassium, and chloride

Contraindications Hypersensitivity to calcitonin salmon or any component of the formulation

Warnings/Precautions A skin test should be performed prior to initiating therapy of calcitonin salmon in patients with suspected sensitivity; have epinephrine immediately available for a possible hypersensitivity reaction. A detailed skin testing protocol is available from the manufacturers. Temporarily withdraw use of nasal spray if ulceration of nasal mucosa occurs. Discontinue for ulcerations >1.5 mm or those that penetrate below the mucosa. Patients >65 years of age may experience a higher incidence of nasal adverse events with calcitonin nasal spray.

Drug Interactions

Avoid Concomitant Use There are no known interactions where it is recommended to avoid concomitant use.

Decreased Effect

Calcitonin may decrease the levels/effects of: Lithium

Increased Effect/Toxicity There are no known significant interactions involving an increase in effect.

Nutritional/Ethanol Interactions Ethanol: Avoid ethanol (may increase risk of osteoporosis).

Adverse Reactions Unless otherwise noted, frequencies reported are with nasal spray.

>10%: Respiratory: Rhinitis (≤12%, including ulcerative)

1% to 10%:

Cardiovascular: Flushing (nasal spray: <1%; injection: 2% to 5%), angina (1% to 3%), hypertension (1% to 3%)

Central nervous system: Depression (1% to 3%), dizziness (1% to 3%), fatigue (1% to 3%)

Dermatologic: Erythematous rash (1% to 3%)

Gastrointestinal: Nausea (injection: 10%; nasal spray: 2%), abdominal pain (1% to 3%), constipation (1% to 3%), diarrhea (1% to 3%), dyspepsia (1% to 3%)

Genitourinary: Cystitis (1% to 3%)

Local: Injection site reactions (injection: 10%)

Neuromuscular & skeletal: Back pain (5%), arthrosis (1% to 3%), myalgia (1% to 3%), paresthesia (1% to 3%)

Ocular: Conjunctivitis (1% to 3%), lacrimation abnormality (1% to 3%)

Respiratory: Nasal ulcerations (3%), bronchospasm (1% to 3%), sinusitis (1% to 3%), upper respiratory tract infection (1% to 3%)

Miscellaneous: Flu-like syndrome (1% to 3%), infection (1% to 3%), lymphadenopathy (1% to 3%)

Pharmacodynamics/Kinetics

Onset of Action

Hypercalcemia: I.M., SubQ: ~2 hours

Paget's disease: Within a few months; may take up to 1 year for neurologic symptom improvement

Duration of Action Hypercalcemia: I.M., SubQ: 6-8 hours

Bioavailability

I.M. 66%; SubQ: 71%; Nasal ~3-5% (relative to I.M.)

Time to Peak Plasma: SubQ ~23 minutes; Nasal: ~13 minutes

Half-Life Elimination Terminal: I.M. 58 minutes; SubQ 59-64 minutes; Nasal: ~18 minutes

Metabolism Metabolized in kidneys, blood and peripheral tissue

Excretion Urine (as inactive metabolites)

Available Dosage Forms

Injection, solution:

Miacalcin®: 200 int. units/mL (2 mL)

Solution, intranasal: 200 int. units/actuation (3.7 mL, 3.8 mL)

Fortical®: 200 int. units/actuation (3.7 mL)

Miacalcin®: 200 int. units/actuation (3.7 mL)

Dosing

Adult & Geriatric

Paget's disease *(Miacalcin®)*: I.M., SubQ: Initial: 100 units/day; maintenance: 50 units/day or 50-100 units every 1-3 days

Hypercalcemia *(Miacalcin®)*: Initial: I.M., SubQ: 4 units/kg every 12 hours; may increase up to 8 units/kg every 12 hours; if the response remains unsatisfactory, a further increase up to a maximum of 8 units/kg every 6 hours may be considered

Postmenopausal osteoporosis:

Miacalcin®: I.M., SubQ: 100 units/every other day

Fortical®, Miacalcin®: Intranasal: 200 units (1 spray) in one nostril daily

Administration

I.M. Injection solution: May be administered I.M. or SubQ; I.M route is preferred if the injection volume is >2 mL.

Inhalation Nasal spray: Before first use, allow bottle to reach room temperature, then prime pump by releasing at least 5 sprays until full spray is produced. To administer, place nozzle into nostril with head in upright position. Alternate nostrils daily. Do not prime pump before each daily use. Discard after 30 doses.

Other Injection solution: May be administered I.M. or SubQ. SubQ route is preferred for outpatient self-administration unless the injection volume is >2 mL.

Stability

Reconstitution Injection: NS has been recommended for the dilution to prepare a skin test in patients with suspected sensitivity.

Storage

Injection: Store under refrigeration at 2°C to 8°C (36°F to 46°F); protect from freezing. The following stability information has also been reported: May be stored at room temperature for up to 14 days (Cohen, 2007).

Nasal: Store unopened bottle under refrigeration at 2°C to 8°C (36°F to 46°F); do not freeze.

Fortical®: After opening, store for up to 30 days at 20°C to 25°C (68°F to 77°F); excursions permitted to 15°C to 30°C (59°F to 86°F). Store in upright position.

Miacalcin®: After opening, store for up to 35 days at room temperature of 15°C to 30°C (59°F to 86°F). Store in upright position.

Monitoring and Teaching Issues

Laboratory Monitoring Serum electrolytes and calcium, alkaline phosphatase and 24-hour urine collection for hydroxyproline excretion (Paget's disease), urinalysis (urine sediment); bone mineral density

Physical Assessment Skin test should be administered before initiating therapy if using calcitonin solution (increased erythema or skin wheal indicates positive reaction and allergy). If prescribing the nasal form, instruct patient to monitor for nasal irritation.

Patient Education If administered by injection, you will be instructed on how to give the injections and dispose of syringes/needles (follow directions exactly). May cause increased warmth and flushing (this should only last about 1 hour after administration; taking drug in evening may minimize these discomforts). Report significant nasal irritation if using nasal spray. Immediately report chest pain, depression, unresolved nausea or constipation, skin rash, palpitations, or respiratory difficulty.

Dietary Considerations Recommended amounts of vitamin D and calcium intake is essential for preventing/treating osteoporosis. Patients with Paget's disease and hypercalcemia should follow a low calcium diet as prescribed.

Geriatric Considerations Studies have shown calcitonin's effects on bone density and fracture rates are beneficial, particularly in women unable to tolerate estrogens. Calcium and vitamin D supplements should also be given. Calcitonin may also be effective in steroid-induced osteoporosis and other states associated with high bone turnover. Nasal spray may provide faster onset of analgesic effects than I.M.

Breast-Feeding Considerations Has been shown to decrease milk production in animals.

Pregnancy Considerations Decreased birth weight was observed in animal studies. Calcitonin does not cross the placenta.

Related Information

Osteoporosis Management *on page* 2067

◆ **Calcitonin (Salmon)** *see* Calcitonin *on page* 269

◆ **Calcitrene™** *see* Calcipotriene *on page* 268

Calcitriol (kal si TRYE ole)

U.S. Brand Names Calcijex®; Rocaltrol®; Vectical™

Index Terms 1,25 Dihydroxycholecalciferol

Generic Availability (U.S.) Yes: Excludes ointment

Pharmacologic Category Vitamin D Analog

Medication Safety Issues

Sound-alike/look-alike issues:

Calcitriol may be confused with alfacalcidol, calcifediol, Calciferol®, calcitonin, calcium carbonate, captopril, colestipol, paricalcitol, ropinirole

Dosage is expressed in mcg (micrograms), **not** mg (milligrams); rare cases of acute overdose have been reported

Pregnancy Risk Factor C

Lactation Enters breast milk/not recommended

Use

Oral, injection: Management of hypocalcemia in patients on chronic renal dialysis; management of secondary hyperparathyroidism in patients with chronic kidney disease (CKD); management of hypocalcemia in hypoparathyroidism and pseudohypoparathyroidism

Topical: Management of mild-to-moderate plaque psoriasis

Unlabeled/Investigational Use Decrease severity of psoriatic lesions in psoriatic vulgaris; vitamin D-dependent rickets

Mechanism of Action/Effect Calcitriol is a potent active metabolite of vitamin D. Vitamin D promotes absorption of calcium in the intestines and retention at the kidneys thereby increasing calcium levels in the serum; decreases excessive serum phosphatase levels, parathyroid hormone levels, and decreases bone resorption; increases renal tubule phosphate resorption

The mechanism by which calcitriol is beneficial in the treatment of psoriasis has not been established.

Contraindications Hypersensitivity to calcitriol or any component of the formulation; hypercalcemia, vitamin D toxicity

Topical: There are no contraindications listed in the manufacturer's labeling.

Warnings/Precautions

Oral, injection: Adequate dietary (supplemental) calcium is necessary for clinical response to vitamin D. Excessive vitamin D may cause severe hypercalcemia, hypercalciuria, and hyperphosphatemia; calcium-phosphate product (serum calcium times phosphorus) must not exceed 70 mg^2/dL^2. Other forms of vitamin D should be withheld during therapy. Immobilization may increase risk of hypercalcemia and/or hypercalciuria. Maintain adequate hydration. Use caution in patients with malabsorption syndromes (efficacy may be limited and/or response may be unpredictable). Use of calcitriol for the treatment of secondary hyperparathyroidism associated with CKD is not recommended in patients with rapidly worsening kidney function or in noncompliant patients. Increased serum phosphate levels in patients with renal failure may lead to calcification; the use of an aluminum-containing phosphate binder is recommended along with a low phosphate diet in these patients. Use with caution in patients taking cardiac glycosides; digitalis toxicity is potentiated by hypocalcemia. Products may contain coconut (capsule) or palm seed oil (oral solution). Some products may contain tartrazine.

Topical: May cause hypercalcemia; if alterations in calcium occur, discontinue treatment until levels return to normal. For external use only; not for ophthalmic, oral, or intravaginal use. Do not apply to facial skin, eyes, or lips. Absorption may be increased with occlusive dressings. Avoid or limit excessive exposure to natural or artificial sunlight, or phototherapy. The safety and effectiveness has not been evaluated in patients with erythrodermic, exfoliative, or pustular psoriasis.

Drug Interactions

Metabolism/Transport Effects Substrate of CYP3A4 (major); **Induces** CYP3A4 (weak)

Avoid Concomitant Use

Avoid concomitant use of Calcitriol with any of the following: Aluminum Hydroxide; Sucralfate; Vitamin D Analogs

Decreased Effect

Calcitriol may decrease the levels/effects of: Saxagliptin

The levels/effects of Calcitriol may be decreased by: Bile Acid Sequestrants; Corticosteroids (Systemic); CYP3A4 Inducers (Strong); Deferasirox; Herbs (CYP3A4 Inducers); Mineral Oil; Orlistat; Sevelamer

Increased Effect/Toxicity

Calcitriol may increase the levels/effects of: Aluminum Hydroxide; Cardiac Glycosides; Magnesium Salts; Sucralfate; Vitamin D Analogs

The levels/effects of Calcitriol may be increased by: Conivaptan; CYP3A4 Inhibitors (Moderate); CYP3A4 Inhibitors (Strong); Dasatinib; Thiazide Diuretics

Adverse Reactions

Oral, I.V.: Frequency not defined.

Cardiovascular: Cardiac arrhythmia, hypertension

Central nervous system: Apathy, headache, hypothermia, psychosis, sensory disturbances, somnolence

Dermatologic: Erythema multiforme, pruritus

Endocrine & metabolic: Dehydration, growth suppression, hypercalcemia, hypercholesterolemia, hypermagnesemia, hyperphosphatemia, libido decreased, polydipsia

Gastrointestinal: Abdominal pain, anorexia, constipation, metallic taste, nausea, pancreatitis, stomach ache, vomiting, weight loss, xerostomia

Genitourinary: Nocturia, urinary tract infection

Hepatic: ALT increased, AST increased

Local: Injection site pain (mild)

Neuromuscular & skeletal: Bone pain, myalgia, dystrophy, soft tissue calcification, weakness

Ocular: Conjunctivitis, photophobia

Renal: Albuminuria, BUN increased, creatinine increased, hypercalciuria, nephrocalcinosis, polyuria

Respiratory: Rhinorrhea

Miscellaneous: Allergic reaction

Topical:

>10%: Endocrine: Hypercalcemia (≤24%)

1% to 10%:

Dermatologic: Skin discomfort (3%), pruritus (1% to 3%)

Genitourinary: Urine abnormality (4%)

Renal: Hypercalciuria (3%)

Pharmacodynamics/Kinetics

Onset of Action Oral: ~2-6 hours

Duration of Action Oral, I.V.: 3-5 days

Absorption Oral: Rapid

Time to Peak Oral: 3-6 hours; Hemodialysis: 8-12 hours

Protein Binding 99.9%

Half-Life Elimination Children ~27 hours; Normal adults: 5-8 hours; Hemodialysis: 16-22 hours

Metabolism Primarily to 1,24,25-trihydroxycholecalciferol and 1,24,25-trihydroxy ergocalciferol

Excretion Primarily feces; urine

Available Dosage Forms

Capsule, softgel, oral: 0.25 mcg, 0.5 mcg

Rocaltrol®: 0.25 mcg, 0.5 mcg

Injection, solution: 1 mcg/mL (1 mL, 2 mL)

Calcijex®: 1 mcg/mL (1 mL)

Ointment, topical:

Vectical™: 3 mcg/g (100 g)

Solution, oral: 1 mcg/mL (15 mL)

Rocaltrol®: 1 mcg/mL (15 mL)

Dosing

Adult

Hypocalcemia in patients on chronic renal dialysis (manufacturer labeling):

Oral: 0.25 mcg/day or every other day (may require 0.5-1 mcg/day); increases should be made at 4- to 8-week intervals

I.V.: Initial: 1-2 mcg 3 times/week (0.02 mcg/kg) approximately every other day. Adjust dose at 2-4 week intervals; dosing range: 0.5-4 mcg 3 times/week

Hypocalcemia in hypoparathyroidism/pseudohypoparathyroidism (manufacturers labeling): Oral (evaluate dosage at 2- to 4-week intervals): Initial: 0.25 mcg/day, range: 0.5-2 mcg once daily

Secondary hyperparathyroidism associated with moderate-to-severe CKD in patients not on dialysis (manufacturer labeling): Oral: 0.25 mcg/day; may increase to 0.5 mcg/day

K/DOQI guidelines for vitamin D therapy in CKD:

CKD stage 3: Oral: 0.25 mcg/day. Treatment should only be started with serum 25(OH) D >30 ng/mL, serum iPTH >70 pg/mL, serum calcium <9.5 mg/dL and serum phosphorus <4.6 mg/dL

CKD stage 4: Oral: 0.25 mcg/day. Treatment should only be started with serum 25(OH) D >30 ng/mL, serum iPTH >110 pg/mL, serum calcium <9.5 mg/dL and serum phosphorus <4.6 mg/dL

CKD stage 5:

Peritoneal dialysis: Oral: Initial: 0.5-1 mcg 2-3 times/week or 0.25 mcg/day

Hemodialysis: **Note:** The following initial doses are based on plasma PTH and serum calcium levels for patients with serum phosphorus <5.5 mg/dL and Ca-P product <55. Adjust dose based on serum phosphate, calcium, and PTH levels. Intermittent I.V. administration may be more effective than daily oral dosing.

Plasma PTH 300-600 pg/mL and serum Ca <9.5 mg/dL: Oral, I.V.: 0.5-1.5 mcg

Plasma PTH 600-1000 pg/mL and serum Ca <9.5 mg/dL:

Oral: 1-4 mcg

I.V.: 1-3 mcg

Plasma PTH >1000 pg/mL and serum Ca <10 mg/dL:

Oral: 3-7 mcg

I.V.: 3-5 mcg

Psoriasis: Topical: Apply twice daily to affected areas (maximum: 200 g/week)

Vitamin D-dependent rickets (unlabeled use): Oral: 1 mcg once daily

Geriatric Refer to adult dosing. No dosage recommendations, but start at the lower end of the dosage range.

Pediatric

Hypocalcemia in hypoparathyroidism/pseudohypoparathyroidism (manufacturers labeling): Oral (evaluate dosage at 2- to 4-week intervals):

Children <1 year (unlabeled use): 0.04-0.08 mcg/kg once daily

Children 1-5 years: 0.25-0.75 mcg once daily

Children ≥6 years: Refer to adults dosing.

Secondary hyperparathyroidism associated with moderate-to-severe CKD in patients not on dialysis (manufacturer labeling): Oral:

Children <3 years: Initial dose: 0.01-0.015 mcg/kg/day

Children ≥3 years: Refer to adults dosing.

K/DOQI guidelines for vitamin D therapy in CKD:

CKD stage 2, 3: Oral:

<10 kg: 0.05 mcg every other day

10-20 kg: 0.1-0.15 mcg/day

>20 kg: 0.25 mcg/day

Note: Treatment should only be started with serum 25(OH) D >30 ng/mL, serum iPTH >70 pg/mL, serum calcium <10 mg/dL and serum phosphorus less than or equal to the age appropriate level.

CKD stage 4: Oral:

<10 kg: 0.05 mcg every other day

10-20 kg: 0.1-0.15 mcg/day

>20 kg: 0.25 mcg/day

Note: Treatment should only be started with serum 25(OH) D >30 ng/mL, serum iPTH >110 pg/mL, serum calcium <10 mg/dL and serum phosphorus less than or equal to the age appropriate level.

CKD stage 5: Oral, I.V.: **Note:** The following initial doses are based on plasma PTH and serum calcium levels for patients with serum phosphorus <5.5 mg/dL in adolescents or <6.5 in infants and children, and Ca-P product <55 in adolescents or <65 in infants and children <12 years. Adjust dose based on serum phosphate, calcium and PTH levels. Administer dose with each dialysis session (3 times/week). Intermittent I.V./oral administration is more effective than daily oral dosing.

Plasma PTH 300-500 pg/mL and serum Ca <10 mg/dL: 0.0075 mcg/kg (maximum: 0.25 mcg/day)

Plasma PTH >500-1000 pg/mL and serum Ca <10 mg/dL: 0.015 mcg/kg (maximum: 0.5 mcg/day)

Plasma PTH >1000 pg/mL and serum Ca <10.5 mg/dL: 0.025 mcg/kg (maximum: 1 mcg/day)

Vitamin D-dependent rickets (unlabeled use): Refer to adults dosing.

Adjustment for Toxicity K/DOQI guidelines: Children and Adults: CKD stage 3 and 4:

iPTH below target: Hold calcitriol until levels rise then resume treatment at half the previous dose. If the lowest dose was being used, switch to alternate day therapy.

Corrected total calcium >9.5 mg/dL (adults) or 10.2 mg/dL (children): Hold calcitriol until serum calcium returns to <9.5 mg/dL (adults) or <9.8 mg/dL (children) then resume treatment at half the previous dose. If the lowest dose was being used, switch to alternate day therapy.

Serum phosphorus >4.6 mg/dL (adults) or greater than the age appropriate limits in children: Hold calcitriol (or add/increase dose of phosphate binder) until levels of phosphorous decrease, then resume at half the prior dose.

Administration

Oral May be administered without regard to food. Administer with meals to reduce GI problems.

I.V. May be administered as a bolus dose I.V. through the catheter at the end of hemodialysis.

Topical Apply externally; not for ophthalmic, oral, or intravaginal use. Do not apply to eyes, lips, or facial skins. Rub in gently so that no medication remains visible. Limit application to only the areas of skin affected by psoriasis.

Stability

Storage

Injection: Store at room temperature of 15°C to 30°C (59°F to 86°F). Protect from light.

Oral capsule, solution: Store at room temperature of 20°C to 25°C (68°F to 77°F). Protect from light.

Topical: Store at room temperature of 25°C (77°F); excursions permitted to 15°C to 30°C (59°F to 86°F); do not refrigerate; do not freeze.

Monitoring and Teaching Issues

Laboratory Monitoring Alkaline phosphatase, serum creatinine

Serum calcium and phosphorus:

CKD stage 2-4: Every month for the first 3 months, then every 3 months

CKD stage 5: Every 2 weeks for 1 month, then monthly

Serum or plasma intact PTH (iPTH):

CKD stage 3 and 4: Every 3 months for 6 months, then every 3 months

CKD stage 5: Monthly for 3 months, then every 3 months

Physical Assessment Provide appropriate nutritional counseling.

Patient Education Maintain recommended diet and calcium supplementation. You may experience nausea, vomiting, loss of appetite, or metallic taste. Report CNS changes, unusual weakness or fatigue, or persistent nausea or vomiting.

Topical: Avoid or limit excessive exposure to sun or phototherapy. Protect skin with sunblock and protective clothing.

Dietary Considerations May be taken without regard to food. Give with meals to reduce GI problems. Adequate calcium intake should be maintained during therapy; dietary phosphorous may need to be restricted.

Geriatric Considerations Recommended daily allowances (RDA) have not been developed for persons >65 years of age; vitamin D, folate, and B_{12} (cyanocobalamin) have decreased absorption with age, but the clinical significance is yet unknown. Calorie requirements decrease with age and therefore, nutrient density must be increased to ensure adequate nutrient intake, including vitamins and minerals. Therefore, the use of a daily supplement with a multiple vitamin with minerals is recommended. Elderly consume less vitamin D, absorption may be decreased, and many elderly have decreased sun exposure; therefore, elderly should receive supplementation with 800 units of vitamin D (20 mcg)/day. This is a recommendation of particular need to those with high risk for osteoporosis.

Breast-Feeding Considerations Low levels are found in breast milk (~2 pg/mL)

Pregnancy Considerations Teratogenic effects have been observed in animal studies. Mild hypercalcemia has been reported in a newborn following maternal use of calcitriol during pregnancy. If calcitriol is used for the management of hypoparathyroidism in pregnancy, dose adjustments may be needed as pregnancy progresses and again following delivery. Vitamin D and calcium levels should be monitored closely and kept in the lower normal range.

◆ **Calcium Acetylhomotaurinate** *see* Acamprosate *on page* 35

Calcium Chloride (KAL see um KLOR ide)

Generic Availability (U.S.) Yes

Pharmacologic Category Calcium Salt; Electrolyte Supplement, Parenteral

Medication Safety Issues

Dosing issues:

Calcium chloride may be confused with calcium gluconate

Confusion with the different intravenous salt forms of calcium has occurred. There is a threefold difference in the primary cation concentration between calcium chloride (in which 1g = 13.6 mEq [270 mg] of elemental Ca++) and calcium gluconate (in which 1g = 4.65 mEq [90 mg] of elemental Ca++).

Prescribers should specify which salt form is desired. Dosages should be expressed either as mEq, mg, or grams of the salt form.

Pregnancy Risk Factor C

Use Treatment of acute symptomatic hypocalcemia; cardiac disturbances of hyperkalemia or hypocalcemia; emergent treatment of hypocalcemic tetany; treatment of severe hypermagnesemia

Unlabeled/Investigational Use Calcium channel blocker overdose; beta-blocker overdose; severe hyperkalemia (K+ >6.5 mEq/L with toxic ECG changes) [ACLS guidelines]; malignant arrhythmias (including cardiac arrest) associated with hypermagnesemia [ACLS guidelines]

Available Dosage Forms

Injection, solution: 10% (10 mL)

Injection, solution [preservative free]: 10% (10 mL)

Dosing

Adult & Geriatric Note: One gram of calcium chloride is equal to 270 mg of elemental calcium.

Dosages are expressed in terms of the calcium chloride salt based on a solution concentration of 100 mg/mL (10%) containing 1.4 mEq (27.3 mg)/mL elemental calcium.

Acute, symptomatic ionized hypocalcemia, hyperkalemia, or magnesium toxicity: Note: Routine use in cardiac arrest is not recommended due to the lack of improved survival (ACLS, 2010): I.V.: 500-1000 mg, may repeat as necessary

Beta-blocker overdose, refractory to glucagon and high-dose vasopressors (unlabeled use): I.V.: 1000 mg bolus via central line reported to quickly increase blood pressure (O'Grady, 2001)

Calcium channel blocker overdose (unlabeled use):

I.V.: 1000 mg every 10-20 minutes (total of 4 doses) **or** 1000 mg every 2-3 minutes until clinical effect is achieved; if favorable response obtained, consider I.V. infusion

I.V. infusion: 20-50 mg/kg/hour

Hypocalcemia secondary to citrated blood transfusion: I.V.: 200-500 mg per 500 mL of citrated blood (infused into another vein)

Note: Routine administration of calcium, in the absence of signs/symptoms of hypocalcemia, is generally not recommended. A number of recommendations have been published seeking to address potential hypocalcemia during massive transfusion of citrated blood; however, many practitioners recommend replacement only as guided by clinical evidence of hypocalcemia and/or serial monitoring of ionized calcium. In adults, clinically-significant hypocalcemia usually dose not occur until >5 units of packed red blood cells have been administered.

Hypocalcemic tetany: I.V.: 1000 mg over 10-30 minutes; may repeat after 6 hours

Pediatric Note: One gram of calcium chloride is equal to 270 mg of elemental calcium.

Dosages are expressed in terms of the calcium chloride salt based on a solution concentration of 100 mg/mL (10%) containing 1.4 mEq (27.3 mg)/mL elemental calcium.

Acute, symptomatic ionized hypocalcemia, hyperkalemia, or magnesium toxicity: Note: Routine use in cardiac arrest is not recommended due to the lack of improved survival (PALS, 2010): I.V.:

Neonates: 20 mg/kg; may repeat as necessary

Infants and Children: 20 mg/kg (maximum: 2000 mg/dose); may repeat as necessary (PALS, 2010)

Calcium channel blocker overdose (unlabeled use): Neonates, Infants, and Children (PALS, 2010):

I.V., I.O.: 20 mg/kg (maximum: 2000 mg/dose) over 5-10 minutes; if favorable response obtained, consider I.V. infusion

I.V. infusion: 20-50 mg/kg/hour

Hypocalcemic tetany: I.V.:

Neonates: 40-60 mg/kg/dose repeated every 6-8 hours

Infants and Children: 10 mg/kg over 5-10 minutes; may repeat after 6-8 hours or follow with an infusion with a maximum dose of 200 mg/kg/day; alternatively, higher doses of 35-50 mg/kg/dose repeated every 6-8 hours have been used

Hypocalcemia secondary to citrated blood transfusion: I.V.: Neonates, Infants, and Children: Give 32 mg (0.45 mEq elemental calcium) for each 100 mL citrated blood infused

Note: Routine administration of calcium, in the absence of signs/symptoms of hypocalcemia, is generally not recommended. A number of recommendations have been published seeking to address potential hypocalcemia during massive transfusion of citrated blood; however, many practitioners recommend replacement only as guided by clinical evidence of hypocalcemia and/or serial monitoring of ionized calcium.

Renal Impairment Cl_{cr} <25 mL/minute: Dosage adjustments may be necessary depending on the serum calcium concentration.

Administration

I.V. For I.V. administration only; avoid extravasation. Avoid rapid administration (do not exceed 100 mg/minute except in emergency situations). May be given over 2-5 minutes if rapid increase in serum calcium concentration is required. For I.V. infusion, dilute to a maximum concentration of 20 mg/mL and infuse over 1 hour or no greater than 45-90 mg/kg/hour (0.6-1.2 mEq/kg/hour); administration via a central or deep vein is preferred; do not use scalp, small hand or foot veins for I.V. administration since severe necrosis and sloughing may occur. Monitor ECG if calcium is infused faster than 2.5 mEq/minute; **stop the infusion if the patient complains of pain or discomfort.** Warm to body temperature. **Do not infuse calcium chloride in the same I.V. line as phosphate-containing solutions.**

Monitoring and Teaching Issues

Laboratory Monitoring Serum calcium and ionized calcium (normal: 8.5-10.2 mg/dL [total]; 4.5-5.0 mg/dL [ionized]), albumin, serum phosphate

Patient Education This medication can only be given intravenously. Do not make rapid postural changes while calcium is infusing. Report any feelings of excitation, chest pain, irregular or pounding heartbeat, vomiting, acute headache, or dizziness.

Calcium Gluconate (KAL see um GLOO koe nate)

U.S. Brand Names Cal-G [OTC]; Cal-GLU™ [OTC]

Generic Availability (U.S.) Yes

Pharmacologic Category Calcium Salt; Electrolyte Supplement, Oral; Electrolyte Supplement, Parenteral

Medication Safety Issues

Sound-alike/look-alike issues:

Calcium gluconate may be confused with calcium glubionate

Pregnancy Risk Factor C

Lactation Enters breast milk

Use Treatment and prevention of hypocalcemia; treatment of tetany, cardiac disturbances of hyperkalemia, cardiac resuscitation when epinephrine fails to improve myocardial contractions, hypocalcemia; calcium supplementation; hydrofluoric acid (HF) burns

Unlabeled/Investigational Use Calcium channel blocker overdose

Mechanism of Action/Effect As dietary supplement, used to prevent or treat negative calcium balance; in osteoporosis, it helps to prevent or decrease the rate of bone loss. The calcium in calcium salts moderates nerve and muscle performance and allows normal cardiac function.

Contraindications Hypersensitivity to calcium gluconate or any component of the formulation; ventricular fibrillation during cardiac resuscitation; digitalis toxicity or suspected digoxin toxicity; hypercalcemia

Warnings/Precautions Injection solution is for I.V. use only; do not inject SubQ or I.M. Avoid too rapid I.V. administration and avoid extravasation. Use with caution in digitalized patients, severe hyperphosphatemia, respiratory failure, or acidosis. May produce cardiac arrest. Hypercalcemia may occur in patients with renal failure; frequent determination of serum calcium is necessary. Use caution with renal disease. Use caution when administering calcium supplements to patients with a history of kidney stones. Solutions may contain aluminum; toxic levels may occur following prolonged administration in premature neonates or patients with renal dysfunction. Oral: Constipation, bloating, and gas are common with oral calcium supplements (especially carbonate salt). Taking calcium (≤500 mg) with food improves absorption. Calcium administration interferes with absorption of some minerals and drugs; use with caution. It is recommended to concomitantly administer vitamin D for optimal calcium absorption.

Drug Interactions

Avoid Concomitant Use There are no known interactions where it is recommended to avoid concomitant use.

Decreased Effect

Calcium Gluconate may decrease the levels/effects of: Bisphosphonate Derivatives; Calcium Channel Blockers; DOBUTamine; Eltrombopag; Estramustine; Phosphate Supplements; Quinolone Antibiotics; Thyroid Products; Trientine

The levels/effects of Calcium Gluconate may be decreased by: Trientine

Increased Effect/Toxicity

Calcium Gluconate may increase the levels/effects of: CefTRIAXone

The levels/effects of Calcium Gluconate may be increased by: Thiazide Diuretics

Lab Interactions Increased calcium (S); decreased magnesium

Adverse Reactions Frequency not defined.

I.V.:

Cardiovascular: Arrhythmia, bradycardia, cardiac arrest, hypotension, vasodilation, and syncope may occur following rapid I.V. injection

Central nervous system: Sense of oppression

Gastrointestinal: Chalky taste

Local: Abscess and necrosis following I.M. administration

Neuromuscular & skeletal: Tingling sensation

Miscellaneous: Heat waves

Oral: Gastrointestinal: Constipation

Pharmacodynamics/Kinetics

Absorption Requires vitamin D; calcium is absorbed in soluble, ionized form; solubility of calcium is increased in an acid environment

Protein Binding Primarily albumin

Excretion Primarily feces (as unabsorbed calcium); urine (20%)

Available Dosage Forms

Capsule, oral:

Cal-G [OTC]: 700 mg

Cal-GLU™ [OTC]: 515 mg

Injection, solution [preservative free]: 10% (10 mL, 50 mL, 100 mL)

Powder, oral: (480 g)

Tablet, oral: 500 mg, 648 mg

Dosing

Adult & Geriatric

Adequate Intake (as elemental calcium):

Adults, Male/Female:

19-50 years: 1000 mg/day

≥51 years: 1200 mg/day

Female: Pregnancy/Lactating: Same as for Adults, Male/Female

Dosage note: Calcium chloride has 3 times more elemental calcium than calcium gluconate. Calcium chloride is 27% elemental calcium; calcium gluconate is 9% elemental calcium. One gram of calcium chloride is equal to 270 mg of elemental calcium; 1 gram of calcium gluconate is equal to 90 mg of elemental calcium. The following dosages are expressed in terms of the calcium gluconate salt based on a solution concentration of 100 mg/mL (10%) containing 0.465 mEq (9.3 mg)/mL elemental calcium:

Hypocalcemia:

I.V.: 2-15 g/24 hours as a continuous infusion or in divided doses

Oral: 500 mg to 2 g 2-4 times/day

Hypocalcemia secondary to citrated blood infusion: I.V.: 500 mg to 1 g per 500 mL of citrated blood (infused into another vein). Single doses up to 2 g have also been recommended.

Note: Routine administration of calcium, in the absence of signs/symptoms of hypocalcemia, is generally not recommended. A number of recommendations have been published seeking to address potential hypocalcemia during massive transfusion of citrated blood; however, many practitioners recommend replacement only as guided by clinical evidence of hypocalcemia and/or serial monitoring of ionized calcium.

Hypocalcemic tetany: I.V.: 1-3 g/dose may be administered until therapeutic response occurs

Magnesium intoxication or cardiac arrest in the presence of hyperkalemia or hypocalcemia: I.V.: 500-800 mg/dose (maximum: 3 g/dose)

Maintenance electrolyte requirements for TPN: I.V.: Daily requirements: 1.7-3.4 g/1000 kcal/24 hours

Calcium channel blocker overdose (unlabeled use): I.V. infusion: 10% solution: 0.6-1.2 mL/kg/hour or I.V. 0.2-0.5 ml/kg every 15-20 minutes for 4 doses (maximum: 2-3 g/dose). In life-threatening situations, 1 g has been given every 1-10 minutes until clinical effect is achieved (case reports of resistant hypotension reported use of 12-18 g total).

Pediatric

Adequate Intake (as elemental calcium):

0-6 months: 210 mg/day
7-12 months: 270 mg/day
1-3 years: 500 mg/day
4-8 years: 800 mg/day
9-18 years: 1300 mg/day

Dosage note: Calcium chloride has 3 times more elemental calcium than calcium gluconate. Calcium chloride is 27% elemental calcium; calcium gluconate is (9% elemental calcium). One gram of calcium chloride is equal to 270 mg of elemental calcium; 1 gram of calcium gluconate is equal to 90 mg of elemental calcium. The following dosages are expressed in terms of the calcium gluconate salt based on a solution concentration of 100 mg/mL (10%) containing 0.465 mEq (9.3 mg)/mL elemental calcium:

Hypocalcemia:

I.V.:

Neonates: 200-800 mg/kg/day as a continuous infusion or in 4 divided doses (maximum: 1 g/dose)

Infants and Children: 200-500 mg/kg/day as a continuous infusion or in 4 divided doses (maximum: 2-3 g/dose)

Oral: Children: 200-500 mg/kg/day divided every 6 hours

Hypocalcemia secondary to citrated blood infusion: I.V.: Neonates, Infants, and Children: Give 98 mg (0.45 mEq **elemental** calcium) for each 100 mL citrated blood infused.

Note: Routine administration of calcium, in the absence of signs/symptoms of hypocalcemia, is generally not recommended. A number of recommendations have been published seeking to address potential hypocalcemia during massive transfusion of citrated blood; however, many practitioners recommend replacement only as guided by clinical evidence of hypocalcemia and/or serial monitoring of ionized calcium.

Hypocalcemic tetany: I.V.: Infants and Children: 100-200 mg/kg/dose over 5-10 minutes; may repeat every 6-8 hours **or** follow with an infusion of 500 mg/kg/day

Magnesium intoxication or cardiac arrest in the presence of hyperkalemia or hypocalcemia: I.V.: Infants and Children: 60-100 mg/kg/dose (maximum: 3 g/dose)

Renal Impairment Cl_{cr} <25 mL/minute: Dosage adjustments may be necessary depending on the serum calcium levels.

Administration

I.M. Not for I.M. or SubQ administration

I.V. For I.V. administration only; administer slowly (~1.5 mL calcium gluconate 10% per minute) through a small needle into a large vein in order to avoid too rapid increased in serum calcium and extravasation

Other Not for SubQ administration.

Stability

Storage

Do not refrigerate solutions. IVPB solutions/I.V. infusion solutions are stable for 24 hours at room temperature.

Standard diluent: 1 g/100 mL D_5W or NS; 2 g/100 mL D_5W or NS.

Maximum concentration in parenteral nutrition solutions is variable depending upon concentration and solubility (consult detailed reference).

Monitoring and Teaching Issues

Physical Assessment If administered I.V., monitor ECG, vital signs, and CNS. Observe infusion site closely. Avoid extravasation.

Patient Education Oral: Take with a full glass of water or juice, 1-3 hours after other medications and 1-2 hours before any iron supplements. May cause constipation or dry mouth. Report severe, unresolved GI disturbances and unusual emotional lability (mood swings).

Geriatric Considerations Constipation and gas can be significant in elderly, but are usually mild.

Breast-Feeding Considerations Endogenous calcium is excreted in breast milk.

Pregnancy Considerations Reproduction studies have not been completed.

Additional Information A topical 2.5% to 5% calcium gel for the treatment of hydrofluoric acid (HF) burns can be prepared by adding calcium gluconate to a surgical lubricant (water soluble such as K-Y® Jelly). Calcium chloride should not be used for this purpose. Use of injectable calcium gluconate (I.V., SubQ) has also been reported in the literature for the treatment of HF burns not amenable to topical treatment.

Related Information

Compatibility of Drugs *on page 1994*
Osteoporosis Management *on page 2067*

◆ **Calcium Leucovorin** *see* Leucovorin Calcium *on page 1080*

- **Calcium Levoleucovorin** *see* LEVOleucovorin *on page 1096*

Calcium Phosphate (Tribasic) (KAL see um FOS fate tri BAY sik)

U.S. Brand Names Posture® [OTC]
Index Terms Tricalcium Phosphate
Generic Availability (U.S.) No
Pharmacologic Category Calcium Salt
Use Dietary supplement
Available Dosage Forms For available OTC formulations, consult specific product labeling.
Dosing
Adult & Geriatric
Adequate Intake (as elemental calcium): Oral:
Male/Female:
19-50 years: 1000 mg/day
≥51 years: 1200 mg/day
Female: Pregnancy/Lactating: Same as for Adults, Male/Female
Dietary supplement: Oral: 2 tablets daily
Pediatric Adequate Intake (as elemental calcium): Oral:
0-6 months: 210 mg/day
7-12 months: 270 mg/day
1-3 years: 500 mg/day
4-8 years: 800 mg/day
9-18 years: 1300 mg/day
Renal Impairment Cl_{cr} <25 mL/minute: Dosage adjustments may be necessary depending on the serum calcium levels.
Monitoring and Teaching Issues
Patient Education Take with a full glass of water or juice, 1-3 hours after other medications and 1-2 hours before any iron supplements. May cause constipation or dry mouth. Report severe, unresolved GI disturbances and unusual emotional lability (mood swings).
Related Information
Osteoporosis Management *on page 2067*

- **Caldecort® [OTC]** *see* Hydrocortisone (Topical) *on page 920*
- **Caldolor™** *see* Ibuprofen *on page 938*
- **Cal-G [OTC]** *see* Calcium Gluconate *on page 275*
- **Cal-GLU™ [OTC]** *see* Calcium Gluconate *on page 275*
- **CaloMist™** *see* Cyanocobalamin *on page 431*
- **Cambia™** *see* Diclofenac (Systemic) *on page 518*
- **Camila®** *see* Norethindrone *on page 1334*
- **Camphorated Tincture of Opium (error-prone synonym)** *see* Paregoric *on page 1410*
- **Campral®** *see* Acamprosate *on page 35*
- **Camptosar®** *see* Irinotecan *on page 1015*
- **Camptothecin-11** *see* Irinotecan *on page 1015*
- **Canasa®** *see* Mesalamine *on page 1177*
- **Cancidas®** *see* Caspofungin *on page 307*

Candesartan (kan de SAR tan)

U.S. Brand Names Atacand®
Index Terms Candesartan Cilexetil
Generic Availability (U.S.) No
Pharmacologic Category Angiotensin II Receptor Blocker
Medication Safety Issues
Sound-alike/look-alike issues:
Atacand® may be confused with antacid
Pregnancy Risk Factor C (1st trimester); D (2nd and 3rd trimesters)
Lactation Enters breast milk/contraindicated
Use Alone or in combination with other antihypertensive agents in treating essential hypertension; treatment of heart failure (NYHA class II-IV)
Mechanism of Action/Effect Blocks the vasoconstrictor and aldosterone-secreting effects of angiotensin II by binding of angiotensin II at the AT1 receptor in many tissues, such as vascular smooth muscle and the adrenal gland. Independent of pathways for angiotensin II synthesis. Does not affect the response to bradykinin; does not bind to block other hormone receptors or ion channels known to be important in cardiovascular regulation.
Contraindications Hypersensitivity to candesartan or any component of the formulation; severe hepatic impairment and/or cholestasis; pregnancy; breast-feeding
Warnings/Precautions [U.S. Boxed Warning]: Based on human data, drugs that act on the angiotensin system can cause injury and death to the developing fetus when used in the second and third trimesters. Angiotensin receptor blockers should be discontinued as soon as possible once pregnancy is detected. May cause hyperkalemia; avoid potassium supplementation unless specifically required by healthcare provider. Avoid use or

use a smaller dose in patients who are volume depleted; correct depletion first. May be associated with deterioration of renal function and/or increases in serum creatinine, particularly in patients with low renal blood flow (eg, renal artery stenosis, heart failure) whose glomerular filtration rate (GFR) is dependent on efferent arteriolar vasoconstriction by angiotensin II. Use with caution in unstented unilateral/bilateral renal artery stenosis, pre-existing renal insufficiency, or significant aortic/mitral stenosis. Use with caution in patients with moderate hepatic impairment. Contraindicated with severe hepatic impairment and/or cholestasis. Use caution when initiating in heart failure; may need to adjust dose, and/or concurrent diuretic therapy, because of candesartan-induced hypotension. Hypotension may occur during major surgery and anesthesia; use cautiously before, during, and immediately after such interventions. Although concurrent therapy with an ACE inhibitor may be rational in select patients, concurrent use of ACE inhibitors may increase the risk of clinically-significant adverse events (eg, renal dysfunction, hyperkalemia).

Drug Interactions

Metabolism/Transport Effects Substrate of CYP2C9 (minor); **Inhibits** CYP2C8 (weak), 2C9 (weak)

Avoid Concomitant Use There are no known interactions where it is recommended to avoid concomitant use.

Decreased Effect

The levels/effects of Candesartan may be decreased by: Herbs (Hypertensive Properties); Methylphenidate; Nonsteroidal Anti-Inflammatory Agents; Yohimbine

Increased Effect/Toxicity

Candesartan may increase the levels/effects of: ACE Inhibitors; Amifostine; Antihypertensives; Hypotensive Agents; Lithium; Potassium-Sparing Diuretics; RiTUXimab

The levels/effects of Candesartan may be increased by: Diazoxide; Eplerenone; Herbs (Hypotensive Properties); MAO Inhibitors; Pentoxifylline; Phosphodiesterase 5 Inhibitors; Potassium Salts; Prostacyclin Analogues; Tolvaptan; Trimethoprim

Nutritional/Ethanol Interactions Herb/Nutraceutical: Avoid dong quai if using for hypertension (has estrogenic activity). Avoid ephedra, yohimbe, ginseng (may worsen hypertension). Avoid garlic (may have increased antihypertensive effect).

Adverse Reactions

Cardiovascular: Angina, hypotension (CHF 19%), MI, palpitation, tachycardia

Central nervous system: Dizziness, lightheadedness, drowsiness, headache, vertigo, anxiety, depression, somnolence, fever

Dermatologic: Angioedema, rash

Endocrine & metabolic: Hyperglycemia, hyperkalemia (CHF <1% to 6%), hypertriglyceridemia, hyperuricemia

Gastrointestinal: Dyspepsia, gastroenteritis

Genitourinary: Hematuria

Neuromuscular & skeletal: Back pain, CPK increased, myalgia, paresthesia, weakness

Renal: Serum creatinine increased (up to 13% in patients with CHF with drug discontinuation required in 6%)

Respiratory: Dyspnea, epistaxis, pharyngitis, rhinitis, upper respiratory tract infection

Miscellaneous: Diaphoresis increased

Pharmacodynamics/Kinetics

Onset of Action 2-3 hours; Peak effect: 6-8 hours

Duration of Action >24 hours

Bioavailability 15%

Time to Peak 3-4 hours

Protein Binding 99%

Half-Life Elimination Dose dependent: 5-9 hours

Metabolism To candesartan by the intestinal wall cells

Excretion Urine (26%)

Clearance: Total body: 0.37 mL/kg/minute; Renal: 0.19 mL/kg/minute

Available Dosage Forms

Tablet, oral:

Atacand®: 4 mg, 8 mg, 16 mg, 32 mg

Dosing

Adult

Hypertension: Oral: 4-32 mg once daily. Dosage must be individualized. Blood pressure response is dose related over the range of 2-32 mg. The usual recommended starting dose is 16 mg once daily when it is used as monotherapy in patients who are not volume depleted. It can be administered once or twice daily with total daily doses ranging from 8-32 mg; larger doses do not appear to have a greater effect and there is relatively little experience with such doses.

Congestive heart failure: Oral: Initial: 4 mg once daily; double the dose at 2-week intervals, as tolerated; target dose: 32 mg

Note: In selected cases, concurrent therapy with an ACE inhibitor may provide additional benefit.

Geriatric Refer to adult dosing. No initial dosage adjustment is necessary for elderly patients (although higher concentrations (C_{max}) and AUC were observed in these populations), for patients with mildly impaired renal function, or for patients with mildly impaired hepatic function.

Hepatic Impairment

Mild hepatic impairment: No initial dosage adjustment required.

Moderate hepatic impairment: Consider initiation at lower dosages (AUC increased by 145%).

Severe hepatic impairment and/or cholestasis: Contraindicated

Monitoring and Teaching Issues

Laboratory Monitoring Electrolytes, serum creatinine, BUN, urinalysis; in CHF, serum potassium during dose escalation and periodically thereafter

Physical Assessment Evaluate renal status and history prior to beginning treatment. Assess for potential interactions (eg, increased risk for hypotension, hyperkalemia). Assess results of laboratory tests (electrolytes, serum creatinine, BUN, urinalysis). Monitor for reduced hypertension. Monitor for tachycardia, CNS changes, hyperglycemia, and hypotension prior to treatment, when changing dose, and throughout therapy.

Patient Education Take with or without food. This drug does not eliminate need for diet or exercise regimen as recommended by prescriber. May cause dizziness, fainting, lightheadedness, postural hypotension, nausea, or vomiting. Report chest pain or palpitations; unusual weight gain or swelling of ankles and hands; persistent fatigue; unusual flu or cold symptoms or dry cough; respiratory difficulty; swelling of eyes, face, or lips; skin rash; muscle pain or weakness; or unusual bleeding (blood in urine).

Geriatric Considerations High concentrations occur in the elderly compared to younger subjects. AUC may be doubled in patients with renal impairment. No initial dose adjustment necessary since repeated dose did not demonstrate accumulation of drug or metabolites in elderly.

Pregnancy Considerations Medications which act on the renin-angiotensin system are reported to have the following fetal/neonatal effects: Hypotension, neonatal skull hypoplasia, anuria, renal failure, and death; oligohydramnios is also reported. These effects are reported to occur with exposure during the second and third trimesters. There are no adequate and well-controlled studies in pregnant women. **[U.S. Boxed Warning]: Based on human data, drugs that act on the angiotensin system can cause injury and death to the developing fetus when used in the second and third trimesters. Angiotensin receptor blockers should be discontinued as soon as possible once pregnancy is detected.**

Additional Information May have an advantage over losartan due to minimal metabolism requirements and consequent use in mild-to-moderate hepatic impairment

Related Information

Angiotensin Agents *on page 1974*

Heart Failure (Systolic) *on page 2040*

Candesartan and Hydrochlorothiazide

(kan de SAR tan & hye droe klor oh THYE a zide)

U.S. Brand Names Atacand HCT®

Index Terms Candesartan Cilexetil and Hydrochlorothiazide

Generic Availability (U.S.) No

Pharmacologic Category Angiotensin II Receptor Blocker; Diuretic, Thiazide

Pregnancy Risk Factor C/D (2nd and 3rd trimesters)

Lactation Enters breast milk/contraindicated

Use Treatment of hypertension; combination product should not be used for initial therapy

Available Dosage Forms

Tablet:

Atacand HCT®: 16/12.5: Candesartan 16 mg and hydrochlorothiazide 12.5 mg; 32/12.5: Candesartan 32 mg and hydrochlorothiazide 12.5 mg; 32/25: Candesartan 32 mg and hydrochlorothiazide 25 mg

Dosing

Adult & Geriatric Hypertension, replacement therapy: Oral: Combination product can be substituted for individual agents; maximum therapeutic effect would be expected within 4 weeks

Usual dosage range:

Candesartan: 16-32 mg/day, given once daily or twice daily in divided doses

Hydrochlorothiazide: 12.5-25 mg once daily

Renal Impairment Serum levels of candesartan are increased and the half-life of hydrochlorothiazide is prolonged in patients with renal impairment. Contraindicated with severe renal impairment (Cl_{cr} <30 mL/minute).

Hepatic Impairment Use with caution with moderate hepatic impairment. Contraindicated with severe hepatic impairment and/or cholestasis.

Administration

Oral May administer with or without food.

Monitoring and Teaching Issues

Laboratory Monitoring Serum electrolytes, BUN, creatinine

Physical Assessment See individual agents.

Patient Education See individual agents.

Related Information

Candesartan *on page 278*

Hydrochlorothiazide *on page 912*

◆ **Candesartan Cilexetil** *see* Candesartan *on page 278*

- **Candesartan Cilexetil and Hydrochlorothiazide** *see* Candesartan and Hydrochlorothiazide *on page 280*
- **CAPE** *see* Capecitabine *on page 281*

Capecitabine (ka pe SITE a been)

U.S. Brand Names Xeloda®

Index Terms CAPE

Generic Availability (U.S.) No

Pharmacologic Category Antineoplastic Agent, Antimetabolite; Antineoplastic Agent, Antimetabolite (Pyrimidine Analog)

Medication Safety Issues

Sound-alike/look-alike issues:

Xeloda® may be confused with Xenical®

High alert medication: This medication is in a class the Institute for Safe Medication Practices (ISMP) includes among its list of drug classes which have a heightened risk of causing significant patient harm when used in error.

Pregnancy Risk Factor D

Lactation Excretion in breast milk unknown/not recommended

Use Treatment of metastatic colorectal cancer; adjuvant therapy of Dukes' C colon cancer; treatment of metastatic breast cancer

Unlabeled/Investigational Use Treatment of gastric cancer, pancreatic cancer, esophageal cancer, ovarian cancer, metastatic renal cell cancer, neuroendocrine tumors, metastatic CNS lesions

Mechanism of Action/Effect Capecitabine is a prodrug of fluorouracil. It undergoes hydrolysis in the liver and tissues to form fluorouracil. It interferes with DNA (and to a lesser degree RNA) synthesis. Appears to be specific for G_1 and S phases of the cell cycle.

Contraindications Hypersensitivity to capecitabine, fluorouracil, or any component of the formulation; known deficiency of dihydropyrimidine dehydrogenase (DPD); severe renal impairment (Cl_{cr} <30 mL/minute)

Warnings/Precautions Hazardous agent - use appropriate precautions for handling and disposal. Use with caution in patients ≥80 years of age, or with renal or hepatic dysfunction. Patients with baseline moderate renal impairment require dose reduction. Patients with mild-to-moderate renal impairment require careful monitoring and subsequent dose reduction with any grade 2 or higher adverse event. Bone marrow suppression may occur, hematologic toxicity is more common when used in combination therapy; use with caution; dosage adjustments may be required. Canadian labeling recommends that patients with baseline platelets <100,000/mm^3 and/or neutrophils <1500/mm^3 not receive capecitabine therapy and also to withhold for grade 3 or 4 hematologic toxicity during treatment. Use with caution in patients who have received extensive pelvic radiation or alkylating therapy. Use cautiously with warfarin. Rare and unexpected severe toxicity may be attributed to dihydropyrimidine dehydrogenase (DPD) deficiency. Necrotizing enterocolitis (typhlitis) has been reported.

Capecitabine can cause severe diarrhea; median time to first occurrence is 34 days. Subsequent doses should be reduced after grade 3 or 4 diarrhea or recurrence of grade 2 diarrhea. Dehydration may occur rapidly in patients with diarrhea, nausea, vomiting, anorexia, and/or weakness; adequately hydrate prior to treatment initiation. Elderly patients may be a higher risk for dehydration. Note: the Canadian labeling recommends treatment interruption for dehydration requiring I.V. hydration lasting <24 hours and dosage reduction if I.V hydration required for ≥24 hours; correct precipitating factors and ensure rehydration prior to resuming therapy.

Hand-and-foot syndrome is characterized by numbness, dysesthesia/paresthesia, tingling, painless or painful swelling, erythema, desquamation, blistering, and severe pain. If grade 2 or 3 hand-and-foot syndrome occurs, interrupt administration of capecitabine until decreases to grade 1. Following grade 3 hand-and-foot syndrome, decrease subsequent doses of capecitabine. In patients with colorectal cancer, treatment with capecitabine immediately following 6 weeks of fluorouracil/leucovorin (FU/LV) therapy has been associated with an increased incidence of grade ≥3 toxicity, when compared to patients receiving the reverse sequence, capecitabine (two 3-week courses) followed by FU/LV (Hennig, 2008).

There has been cardiotoxicity associated with fluorinated pyrimidine therapy. May be more common in patients with a history of coronary artery disease. **[U.S. Boxed Warning]: Capecitabine may increase the anticoagulant effects of warfarin; monitor closely.**

Safety and efficacy in children <18 years of age have not been established.

Drug Interactions

Metabolism/Transport Effects Inhibits CYP2C9 (strong)

Avoid Concomitant Use

Avoid concomitant use of Capecitabine with any of the following: BCG; Natalizumab; Pimecrolimus; Roflumilast; Tacrolimus (Topical); Vaccines (Live)

Decreased Effect

Capecitabine may decrease the levels/effects of: BCG; Sipuleucel-T; Vaccines (Inactivated); Vaccines (Live)

The levels/effects of Capecitabine may be decreased by: Echinacea

Increased Effect/Toxicity

Capecitabine may increase the levels/effects of: Carvedilol; CYP2C9 Substrates (High risk); Leflunomide; Natalizumab; Phenytoin; Vaccines (Live); Vitamin K Antagonists

The levels/effects of Capecitabine may be increased by: Denosumab; Leucovorin Calcium-Levoleucovorin; Pimecrolimus; Roflumilast; Tacrolimus (Topical); Trastuzumab

Nutritional/Ethanol Interactions Food: Food reduced the rate and extent of absorption of capecitabine.

Adverse Reactions Frequency listed derived from monotherapy trials.

>10%:

Cardiovascular: Edema (9% to 15%)

Central nervous system: Fatigue (16% to 42%), fever (7% to 18%), pain (12%)

Dermatologic: Palmar-plantar erythrodysesthesia (hand-and-foot syndrome) (54% to 60%; grade 3: 11% to 17%; may be dose limiting), dermatitis (27% to 37%)

Gastrointestinal: Diarrhea (47% to 57%; may be dose limiting; grade 3: 12% to 13%; grade 4: 2% to 3%), nausea (34% to 53%), vomiting (15% to 37%), abdominal pain (7% to 35%), stomatitis (22% to 25%), appetite decreased (26%), anorexia (9% to 23%), constipation (9% to 15%)

Hematologic: Lymphopenia (94%; grade 4: 14%), anemia (72% to 80%; grade 4: <1% to 1%), neutropenia (2% to 26%; grade 4: 2%), thrombocytopenia (24%; grade 4: 1%)

Hepatic: Bilirubin increased (22% to 48%; grades 3/4: 11% to 23%)

Neuromuscular & skeletal: Paresthesia (21%)

Ocular: Eye irritation (13% to 15%)

Respiratory: Dyspnea (14%)

5% to 10%:

Cardiovascular: Venous thrombosis (8%), chest pain (6%)

Central nervous system: Headache (5% to 10%), lethargy (10%), dizziness (6% to 8%), insomnia (7% to 8%), mood alteration (5%), depression (5%)

Dermatologic: Nail disorder (7%), rash (7%), skin discoloration (7%), alopecia (6%), erythema (6%)

Endocrine & metabolic: Dehydration (7%)

Gastrointestinal: Motility disorder (10%), oral discomfort (10%), dyspepsia (6% to 8%), upper GI inflammatory disorders (colorectal cancer: 8%), hemorrhage (6%), ileus (6%), taste perversion (colorectal cancer: 6%)

Neuromuscular & skeletal: Back pain (10%), weakness (10%), neuropathy (10%), myalgia (9%), arthralgia (8%), limb pain (6%)

Ocular: Abnormal vision (colorectal cancer: 5%), conjunctivitis (5%)

Respiratory: Cough (7%)

Miscellaneous: Viral infection (colorectal cancer: 5%)

Pharmacodynamics/Kinetics

Absorption Rapid and extensive

Time to Peak 1.5 hours; Fluorouracil: 2 hours

Protein Binding <60%; ~35% to albumin

Half-Life Elimination 0.5-1 hour

Metabolism Hepatic: Inactive metabolites: 5′-deoxy-5-fluorocytidine, 5′-deoxy-5-fluorouridine; Tissue: Active metabolite: Fluorouracil

Excretion Urine (96%, 57% as α-fluoro-β-alanine); feces (<3%)

Available Dosage Forms

Tablet, oral:

Xeloda®: 150 mg, 500 mg

Dosing

Adult Note: Details concerning dosing in combination regimens should also be consulted. Capecitabine toxicities, particularly hand-foot syndrome, may be higher in North American populations (for the treatment of colorectal cancer); therapy initiation at doses of 1000 mg/m^2 twice daily (for 2 weeks every 21 days) may be considered (Haller, 2008; NCCN Colon Cancer Guidelines)

Metastatic breast cancer, metastatic colorectal cancer: Oral: 1250 mg/m^2 twice daily (morning and evening) for 2 weeks, every 21 days

Adjuvant therapy of Dukes' C colon cancer: Recommended for a total of 24 weeks (8 cycles of 2 weeks of drug administration and 1 week rest period).

Pancreatic cancer (unlabeled use): 1000 mg/m^2 twice daily for 2 weeks, every 21 days (NCCN Pancreatic Cancer Guidelines v.1.2009) **or** 1250 mg/m^2 twice daily for 2 weeks, every 21 days (Cartwright, 2002)

Geriatric The elderly may be more sensitive to the toxic effects of fluorouracil. Insufficient data are available to provide dosage modifications.

Renal Impairment

Cl_{cr} 51-80 mL/minute: No adjustment of initial dose.

Cl_{cr} 30-50 mL/minute: Administer 75% of normal dose.

Cl_{cr} <30 mL/minute: Use is contraindicated.

Hepatic Impairment

Mild-to-moderate impairment: No starting dose adjustment is necessary; however, carefully monitor patients.

Severe hepatic impairment: Patients have not been studied.

Adjustment for Toxicity

Dosage modification guidelines: See table.

Refer to package labeling for modifications when administered in combination with docetaxel.

Recommended Dose Modifications

Toxicity NCI Grades	During a Course of Therapy (Monotherapy)	Dose Adjustment for Next Cycle (% of starting dose)
Grade 1	Maintain dose level	Maintain dose level
Grade 2		
1st appearance	Interrupt until resolved to grade 0-1	100%
2nd appearance	Interrupt until resolved to grade 0-1	75%
3rd appearance	Interrupt until resolved to grade 0-1	50%
4th appearance	Discontinue treatment permanently	
Grade 3		
1st appearance	Interrupt until resolved to grade 0-1	75%
2nd appearance	Interrupt until resolved to grade 0-1	50%
3rd appearance	Discontinue treatment permanently	
Grade 4		
1st appearance	Discontinue permanently **or** If physician deems it to be in the patient's best interest to continue, interrupt until resolved to grade 0-1	50%

Dosage adjustments for hematologic toxicity in combination therapy with ixabepilone:

Neutrophils <500/mm^3 for ≥7 days or neutropenic fever: Hold for concurrent diarrhea or stomatitis until neutrophils recover to >1000/mm^3, then continue at same dose

Platelets <25,000/mm^3 (or <50,000/mm^3 with bleeding): Hold for concurrent diarrhea or stomatitis until platelets recover to >50,000/mm^3, then continue at same dose

Administration

Oral Usually administered in 2 divided doses taken 12 hours apart. Doses should be taken with water within 30 minutes after a meal.

Stability

Storage Store at room temperature of 25°C (77°F); excursions permitted between 15°C and 30°C (59°F and 86°F).

Monitoring and Teaching Issues

Laboratory Monitoring Renal function should be estimated at baseline to determine initial dose. During therapy, CBC with differential, hepatic function, and renal function should be monitored.

Physical Assessment Evaluate renal and hepatic function and CBC with differential at baseline and regularly during therapy. Assess all adverse reactions on a regular basis during therapy; dosage adjustments may be necessary. Teach sexually active female patients the necessity for contraception.

Patient Education Take within 30 minutes after a meal. Maintain adequate hydration, unless instructed to restrict fluid intake. You may be more susceptible to infection. May cause lethargy; dizziness; visual changes; confusion; anxiety; nausea; vomiting; loss of appetite; dry mouth; loss of hair (will grow back when treatment is discontinued); photosensitivity; dry, itchy skin; and dry or irritated eyes (avoid contact lenses). Report persistent or severe diarrhea, vomiting, or abdominal pain; skin rash, redness, tenderness, or peeling (especially hands and feet); respiratory difficulty; chest pain or palpitations; unusual bleeding or bruising; or vision changes.

Dietary Considerations Because current safety and efficacy data are based upon administration with food, it is recommended that capecitabine be administered with food. In all clinical trials, patients were instructed to take with water within 30 minutes after a meal.

Geriatric Considerations Patients ≥80 years of age may experience a greater incidence of grade 3 or 4 adverse events (diarrhea, hand-and-foot syndrome, nausea/vomiting).

Breast-Feeding Considerations It is not known if the drug is excreted in breast milk. Because of the potential for serious adverse reactions in nursing infants, it is recommended that nursing be discontinued when receiving capecitabine therapy.

Pregnancy Considerations Animal studies have demonstrated teratogenicity and fetal loss. There are no adequate and well-controlled studies in pregnant women; however, fetal harm may occur. Women of childbearing potential should avoid pregnancy.

Additional Information Oncology Comment: An investigational uridine prodrug, uridine triacetate (formerly called vistonuridine), has been studied in a limited number of cases of fluorouracil overdose. Of 17 patients receiving uridine triacetate beginning within 8-96 hours after fluorouracil overdose, all patients fully recovered (von Borstel, 2009). Updated data has described a total of 28 patients treated with uridine triacetate for fluorouracil overdose (including overdoses related to continuous infusions delivering fluorouracil at rates faster than prescribed), all of whom recovered fully (Bamat, 2010).

◆ **Capex®** *see* Fluocinolone (Topical) *on page* 785

◆ **Capital® and Codeine** *see* Acetaminophen and Codeine *on page 41*

◆ **Capozide®** *see* Captopril and Hydrochlorothiazide *on page 287*

Captopril (KAP toe pril)

Index Terms ACE

Generic Availability (U.S.) Yes

Pharmacologic Category Angiotensin-Converting Enzyme (ACE) Inhibitor

Medication Safety Issues

Sound-alike/look-alike issues:

Captopril may be confused with calcitriol, Capitrol®, carvedilol

International issues:

Acepril [Great Britain] may be confused with Accupril which is a brand name for quinapril in the U.S.

Acepril: Brand name for captopril [Great Britain], but also the brand name for enalapril [Hungary, Switzerland]; lisinopril [Malaysia]

Pregnancy Risk Factor C (1st trimester); D (2nd and 3rd trimesters)

Lactation Enters breast milk/not recommended (AAP rates "compatible"; AAP 2001 update pending)

Use Management of hypertension; treatment of heart failure, left ventricular dysfunction after myocardial infarction, diabetic nephropathy

Unlabeled/Investigational Use To delay the progression of nephropathy and reduce risks of cardiovascular events in hypertensive patients with type 1 or 2 diabetes mellitus; treatment of hypertensive crisis, rheumatoid arthritis; diagnosis of anatomic renal artery stenosis, hypertension secondary to scleroderma renal crisis; diagnosis of aldosteronism, idiopathic edema, Bartter's syndrome, postmyocardial infarction for prevention of ventricular failure; increase circulation in Raynaud's phenomenon, hypertension secondary to Takayasu's disease

Mechanism of Action/Effect Competitive inhibitor of angiotensin-converting enzyme (ACE); prevents conversion of angiotensin I to angiotensin II, a potent vasoconstrictor; results in lower levels of angiotensin II which causes an increase in plasma renin activity and a reduction in aldosterone secretion

Contraindications Hypersensitivity to captopril, any other ACE inhibitor, or any component of the formulation; angioedema related to previous treatment with an ACE inhibitor

Warnings/Precautions Anaphylactic reactions may occur rarely with ACE inhibitors. At any time during treatment (especially following first dose) angioedema may occur rarely with ACE inhibitors; may involve the head and neck (potentially compromising airway) or the intestine (presenting with abdominal pain). African-Americans and patients with idiopathic or hereditary angioedema may be at an increased risk. Prolonged frequent monitoring may be required especially if tongue, glottis, or larynx are involved as they are associated with airway obstruction. Patients with a history of airway surgery may have a higher risk of airway obstruction. Aggressive early and appropriate management is critical. Use in patients with previous angioedema associated with ACE inhibitor therapy is contraindicated. Severe anaphylactoid reactions may be seen during hemodialysis (eg, CVVHD) with high-flux dialysis membranes (eg, AN69), and rarely, during low density lipoprotein apheresis with dextran sulfate cellulose. Rare cases of anaphylactoid reactions have been reported in patients undergoing sensitization treatment with hymenoptera (bee, wasp) venom while receiving ACE inhibitors.

Symptomatic hypotension with or without syncope can occur with ACE inhibitors (usually with the first several doses); effects are most often observed in volume depleted patients; close monitoring of patient is required especially with initial dosing and dosing increases; blood pressure must be lowered at a rate appropriate for the patient's clinical condition. Initiation of therapy in patients with ischemic heart disease or cerebrovascular disease warrants close observation due to the potential consequences posed by falling blood pressure (eg, MI, stroke). Use with caution in hypertrophic cardiomyopathy with outflow tract obstruction, severe aortic stenosis, or before, during, or immediately after major surgery. **[U.S. Boxed Warning]: Based on human data, ACEIs can cause injury and death to the developing fetus when used in the second and third trimesters. ACEIs should be discontinued as soon as possible once pregnancy is detected.**

Hyperkalemia may occur with ACE inhibitors; risk factors include renal dysfunction, diabetes mellitus, concomitant use of potassium-sparing diuretics, potassium supplements and/or potassium containing salts. Use cautiously, if at all, with these agents and monitor potassium closely. Cough may occur with ACE inhibitors. Other causes of cough should be considered (eg, pulmonary congestion in patients with heart failure) and excluded prior to discontinuation.

May be associated with deterioration of renal function and/or increases in serum creatinine, particularly in patients with low renal blood flow (eg, renal artery stenosis, heart failure) whose glomerular filtration rate (GFR) is dependent on efferent arteriolar vasoconstriction by angiotensin II; deterioration may result in oliguria, acute renal failure, and progressive azotemia. Small increases in serum creatinine may occur following initiation; consider discontinuation only in patients with progressive and/or significant deterioration in renal function. Use with caution in patients with unstented unilateral/bilateral renal artery stenosis. When unstented bilateral renal artery stenosis is present, use is generally avoided due to the elevated risk of deterioration in renal function unless possible benefits outweigh risks. Concurrent use of angiotensin receptor blockers may increase the risk of clinically-significant adverse events (eg, renal dysfunction, hyperkalemia).

Rare toxicities associated with ACE inhibitors include cholestatic jaundice (which may progress to fulminant hepatic necrosis), agranulocytosis, neutropenia, or leukopenia with myeloid hypoplasia. Patients with collagen vascular diseases (especially with concomitant renal impairment) or renal impairment alone may be at increased risk for hematologic toxicity; closely monitor CBC with differential for the first 3 months of therapy and periodically thereafter in these patients.

Drug Interactions

Metabolism/Transport Effects Substrate of CYP2D6 (major)

Avoid Concomitant Use There are no known interactions where it is recommended to avoid concomitant use.

Decreased Effect

The levels/effects of Captopril may be decreased by: Antacids; Aprotinin; Herbs (Hypertensive Properties); Methylphenidate; Nonsteroidal Anti-Inflammatory Agents; Peginterferon Alfa-2b; Salicylates; Yohimbine

Increased Effect/Toxicity

Captopril may increase the levels/effects of: Allopurinol; Amifostine; Antihypertensives; AzaTHIOprine; CycloSPORINE; CycloSPORINE (Systemic); Ferric Gluconate; Gold Sodium Thiomalate; Hypotensive Agents; Iron Dextran Complex; Lithium; RiTUXimab

The levels/effects of Captopril may be increased by: Angiotensin II Receptor Blockers; CYP2D6 Inhibitors (Moderate); CYP2D6 Inhibitors (Strong); Darunavir; Diazoxide; DPP-IV Inhibitors; Eplerenone; Everolimus; Herbs (Hypotensive Properties); Loop Diuretics; MAO Inhibitors; Pentoxifylline; Phosphodiesterase 5 Inhibitors; Potassium Salts; Potassium-Sparing Diuretics; Prostacyclin Analogues; Sirolimus; Temsirolimus; Thiazide Diuretics; TiZANidine; Tolvaptan; Trimethoprim

Nutritional/Ethanol Interactions

Food: Captopril serum concentrations may be decreased if taken with food. Long-term use of captopril may result in a zinc deficiency which can result in a decrease in taste perception.

Herb/Nutraceutical: Avoid bayberry, blue cohosh, cayenne, ephedra, ginger, ginseng (American), kola, licorice (may worsen hypertension). Avoid black cohosh, california poppy, coleus, golden seal, hawthorn, mistletoe, periwinkle, quinine, shepherd's purse (may have increased antihypertensive effect).

Lab Interactions Positive Coombs' [direct]; may cause false-positive results in urine acetone determinations using sodium nitroprusside reagent

Adverse Reactions

1% to 10%:

Cardiovascular: Hypotension (1% to 3%), tachycardia (1%), chest pain (1%), palpitation (1%)

Dermatologic: Rash (maculopapular or urticarial) (4% to 7%), pruritus (2%); in patients with rash, a positive ANA and/or eosinophilia has been noted in 7% to 10%.

Endocrine & metabolic: Hyperkalemia (1% to 11%)

Hematologic: Neutropenia may occur in up to 4% of patients with renal insufficiency or collagen-vascular disease.

Renal: Proteinuria (1%), serum creatinine increased, worsening of renal function (may occur in patients with bilateral renal artery stenosis or hypovolemia)

Respiratory: Cough (<1% to 2%)

Miscellaneous: Hypersensitivity reactions (rash, pruritus, fever, arthralgia, and eosinophilia) have occurred in 4% to 7% of patients (depending on dose and renal function); dysgeusia - loss of taste or diminished perception (2% to 4%)

Frequency not defined:

Cardiovascular: Angioedema, cardiac arrest, cerebrovascular insufficiency, rhythm disturbances, orthostatic hypotension, syncope, flushing, pallor, angina, MI, Raynaud's syndrome, CHF

Central nervous system: Ataxia, confusion, depression, nervousness, somnolence

Dermatologic: Bullous pemphigus, erythema multiforme, Stevens-Johnson syndrome, exfoliative dermatitis

Endocrine & metabolic: Alkaline phosphatase increased, bilirubin increased, gynecomastia

Gastrointestinal: Pancreatitis, glossitis, dyspepsia

Genitourinary: Urinary frequency, impotence

Hematologic: Anemia, thrombocytopenia, pancytopenia, agranulocytosis, anemia

Hepatic: Jaundice, hepatitis, hepatic necrosis (rare), cholestasis, hyponatremia (symptomatic), transaminases increased

Neuromuscular & skeletal: Asthenia, myalgia, myasthenia

Ocular: Blurred vision

Renal: Renal insufficiency, renal failure, nephrotic syndrome, polyuria, oliguria

Respiratory: Bronchospasm, eosinophilic pneumonitis, rhinitis

Miscellaneous: Anaphylactoid reactions

Pharmacodynamics/Kinetics

Onset of Action Peak effect: Blood pressure reduction: 1-1.5 hours after dose

Duration of Action Dose related, may require several weeks of therapy before full hypotensive effect

Absorption 60% to 75%; reduced 30% to 40% by food

Time to Peak 1 hour

Protein Binding 25% to 30%

Half-Life Elimination Renal and cardiac function dependent: Adults: Healthy volunteers: 1.9 hours; Heart failure: 2.06 hours; Anuria: 20-40 hours

Metabolism 50%

Excretion Urine (>95%) within 24 hours (40% to 50% as unchanged drug)

Available Dosage Forms

Tablet, oral: 12.5 mg, 25 mg, 50 mg, 100 mg

Dosing

Adult & Geriatric Note: Titrate dose according to patient's response; use lowest effective dose.

Acute hypertension (urgency/emergency): Oral: 12.5-25 mg, may repeat as needed (may be given sublingually, but no therapeutic advantage demonstrated)

Heart failure: Oral:

Initial dose: 6.25-12.5 mg 3 times/day in conjunction with cardiac glycoside and diuretic therapy; initial dose depends upon patient's fluid/electrolyte status

Target dose: 50 mg 3 times/day

Hypertension: Oral: Initial: 12.5-25 mg 2-3 times/day; may increase by 12.5-25 mg/dose at 1- to 2-week intervals up to 50 mg 3 times/day. Maximum: 150 mg 3 times/day. Add diuretic before further dosage increases.

Usual dose range (JNC 7): 25-100 mg/day in 2 divided doses

LV dysfunction following MI: Oral: Initial: 6.25 mg; followed by 12.5 mg 3 times/day; increase to 25 mg 3 times/day over the next few days; followed by gradual increase to a goal of 50 mg 3 times/day (some dose schedules are more aggressive to achieve an increased goal dose within the first few days of initiation).

Diabetic nephropathy: Oral: 25 mg 3 times/day. May be taken with other antihypertensive therapy if required to further lower blood pressure

Pediatric Note: Titrate dose according to patient's response; use lowest effective dose.

Hypertension: Oral:

Infants: Initial: 0.15-0.3 mg/kg/dose; titrate dose upward to maximum of 6 mg/kg/day in 1-4 divided doses; usual required dose: 2.5-6 mg/kg/day

Children: Initial: 0.5 mg/kg/dose; titrate upward to maximum of 6 mg/kg/day in 2-4 divided doses.

Older Children: Initial: 6.25-12.5 mg/dose every 12-24 hours; titrate upward to maximum of 6 mg/kg/day.

Adolescents: Initial: 12.5-25 mg/dose given every 8-12 hours; increase by 25 mg/dose to maximum of 450 mg/day.

Renal Impairment

Cl_{cr} 10-50 mL/minute: Administer 75% of normal dose.

Cl_{cr} <10 mL/minute: Administer 50% of normal dose.

Note: Smaller dosages given every 8-12 hours are indicated in patients with renal dysfunction. Renal function and leukocyte count should be carefully monitored during therapy.

Hemodialysis effects: Moderately dialyzable (20% to 50%); administer dose postdialysis or administer 25% to 35% supplemental dose.

Peritoneal dialysis: Supplemental dose is not necessary.

Administration

Oral Unstable in aqueous solutions; to prepare solution for oral administration, mix prior to administration and use within 10 minutes.

Monitoring and Teaching Issues

Laboratory Monitoring BUN, electrolytes, serum creatinine; in patients with renal impairment and/or collagen vascular disease, closely monitor CBC with differential for the first 3 months of therapy and periodically thereafter

Physical Assessment Assess other pharmacological or herbal products patient may be taking that may impact renal function. When beginning therapy, patient should be closely monitored for anaphylactic reaction or severe angioedema. Assess results of renal function tests. Monitor blood pressure. Monitor for hypovolemia, angioedema, and postural hypotension when beginning therapy, adjusting dosage, and on a regular basis throughout.

Patient Education Do not use potassium supplement or salt substitutes without consulting prescriber. Take first dose at bedtime. Take all doses on an empty stomach, 1 hour before or 2 hours after meals. This drug does not eliminate need for diet or exercise regimen as recommended by prescriber. May cause dizziness, fainting, lightheadedness, postural hypotension, nausea, vomiting, abdominal pain, dry mouth, or transient loss of appetite. Report immediately swelling or numbness of face, mouth, or throat; unusual chest pain or palpitations; decreased urinary output; fever or chills; swelling of extremities; skin rash; numbness, tingling, or pain in muscles; or respiratory difficulty or unusual cough.

Dietary Considerations Should be taken at least 1 hour before or 2 hours after eating.

Geriatric Considerations Due to frequent decreases in glomerular filtration (also Cl_{cr}) with aging, elderly patients may have exaggerated responses to ACE inhibitors; differences in clinical response due to hepatic changes are not observed. ACE inhibitors may be preferred agents in elderly patients with congestive heart failure and diabetes mellitus. Diabetic proteinuria is reduced and insulin sensitivity is enhanced. In general, the side effect profile is favorable in the elderly and causes little or no CNS confusion; use lowest dose recommendations initially. Many elderly may be volume depleted due to diuretic use and/or blunted thirst reflex resulting in inadequate fluid intake.

Breast-Feeding Considerations Captopril is excreted in breast milk. Breast-feeding is not recommended by the manufacturer.

Pregnancy Considerations Due to adverse events observed in some animal studies, captopril is considered pregnancy category C during the first trimester. Based on human data, captopril is considered pregnancy category D if used during the second and third trimesters (per the manufacturer; however, one study suggests that fetal injury may occur at anytime during pregnancy). Captopril crosses the placenta and may affect ACE activity in the fetus. First trimester exposure to ACE inhibitors may cause major congenital malformations. An increased risk of cardiovascular and/or central nervous system malformations was observed in one study; however, an increased risk of teratogenic events was not observed in other studies. Second and third trimester use of an ACE inhibitor is associated with oligohydramnios. Oligohydramnios due to decreased fetal renal function may lead to fetal limb contractures, craniofacial deformation, and hypoplastic lung development. The use of ACE inhibitors during the second and third trimesters is also associated with anuria, hypotension, renal failure (reversible or irreversible), skull hypoplasia, and death in the fetus/neonate. Chronic maternal hypertension itself is also associated with adverse events in the fetus/infant. ACE inhibitors are not recommended during pregnancy to treat maternal hypertension or heart failure. Those who are planning a pregnancy should be considered for other medication options if an ACE inhibitor is currently prescribed or the ACE inhibitor should be discontinued as soon as possible once pregnancy is detected. The exposed fetus should be monitored for fetal growth, amniotic fluid volume, and organ formation. Infants exposed to an ACE inhibitor *in utero*, especially during the second and third trimester, should be monitored for hyperkalemia, hypotension, and oliguria.

[U.S. Boxed Warning]: Based on human data, ACE inhibitors can cause injury and death to the developing fetus when used in the second and third trimesters. ACE inhibitors should be discontinued as soon as possible once pregnancy is detected.

Related Information

Angiotensin Agents *on page 1974*

Heart Failure (Systolic) *on page 2040*

Captopril and Hydrochlorothiazide (KAP toe pril & hye droe klor oh THYE a zide)

U.S. Brand Names Capozide®

Index Terms Hydrochlorothiazide and Captopril

Generic Availability (U.S.) Yes

Pharmacologic Category Angiotensin-Converting Enzyme (ACE) Inhibitor; Diuretic, Thiazide

Medication Safety Issues

International issues:

Ecazide [France, Spain] may be confused with Eskazine, a brand name for trifluoperazine [Spain]

Pregnancy Risk Factor C/D (2nd and 3rd trimesters)

Lactation Enters breast milk/compatible

Use Management of hypertension

Available Dosage Forms

Tablet: 25/15: Captopril 25 mg and hydrochlorothiazide 15 mg; 25/25: Captopril 25 mg and hydrochlorothiazide 25 mg; 50/15: Captopril 50 mg and hydrochlorothiazide 15 mg; 50/25: Captopril 50 mg and hydrochlorothiazide 25 mg

Capozide® 25/15: Captopril 25 mg and hydrochlorothiazide 15 mg

Capozide® 25/25: Captopril 25 mg and hydrochlorothiazide 25 mg

Capozide® 50/15: Captopril 50 mg and hydrochlorothiazide 15 mg

Capozide® 50/25: Captopril 50 mg and hydrochlorothiazide 25 mg

Dosing

Adult Hypertension, CHF: May be substituted for previously titrated dosages of the individual components; alternatively, may initiate as follows: Oral:

Initial: Single tablet (captopril 25 mg/hydrochlorothiazide 15 mg) taken once daily; daily dose of captopril should not exceed 150 mg; daily dose of hydrochlorothiazide should not exceed 50 mg

Geriatric Refer to dosing in individual monographs.

Renal Impairment May respond to smaller or less frequent doses.

Monitoring and Teaching Issues

Laboratory Monitoring BUN, serum creatinine, and electrolytes; in patients with renal impairment and/or collagen vascular disease, closely monitor CBC with differential for the first 3 months of therapy and periodically thereafter.

Physical Assessment See individual agents.

Patient Education See individual agents.

Related Information

Captopril *on page 284*

Hydrochlorothiazide *on page 912*

◆ **Carafate®** *see* Sucralfate *on page 1684*

CarBAMazepine (kar ba MAZ e peen)

U.S. Brand Names Carbatrol®; Epitol®; Equetro®; TEGretol®; TEGretol®-XR

Index Terms CBZ; SPD417

Generic Availability (U.S.) Yes: Excludes capsule (extended release)

Pharmacologic Category Anticonvulsant, Miscellaneous

Medication Safety Issues

Sound-alike/look-alike issues:

CarBAMazepine may be confused with OXcarbazepine

Carbatrol® may be confused with Cartrol®

Epitol® may be confused with Epinal®

TEGretol®, TEGretol®-XR may be confused with Mebaral®, Toprol-XL®, Toradol®, TRENtal®

Medication Guide Available Yes

Pregnancy Risk Factor D

Lactation Enters breast milk/not recommended (AAP rates "compatible"; AAP 2001 update pending)

Use

Carbatrol®, Tegretol®, Tegretol®-XR: Partial seizures with complex symptomatology (psychomotor, temporal lobe), generalized tonic-clonic seizures (grand mal), mixed seizure patterns, trigeminal neuralgia

Equetro®: Acute manic and mixed episodes associated with bipolar 1 disorder

Unlabeled/Investigational Use Treatment of restless leg syndrome and post-traumatic stress disorders

Mechanism of Action/Effect In addition to anticonvulsant effects, carbamazepine has anticholinergic, antineuralgic, antidiuretic, muscle relaxant, antimanic, antidepressive, and and antiarrhythmic properties; may depress activity in the nucleus ventralis of the thalamus or decrease synaptic transmission or decrease summation of temporal stimulation leading to neural discharge by limiting influx of sodium ions across cell membrane or other unknown mechanisms; stimulates the release of ADH and potentiates its action in promoting reabsorption of water; chemically related to tricyclic antidepressants

Contraindications Hypersensitivity to carbamazepine, tricyclic antidepressants, or any component of the formulation; bone marrow depression; with or within 14 days of MAO inhibitor use; concurrent use of nefazodone

Warnings/Precautions **[U.S. Boxed Warning]: Potentially fatal blood cell abnormalities have been reported.** Patients with a previous history of adverse hematologic reaction to any drug may be at increased risk.

Antiepileptics are associated with an increased risk of suicidal behavior/thoughts with use (regardless of indication); patients should be monitored for signs/symptoms of depression, suicidal tendencies, and other unusual behavior changes during therapy and instructed to inform their healthcare provider immediately if symptoms occur.

Administer carbamazepine with caution to patients with history of cardiac damage, ECG abnormalities (or at risk for ECG abnormalities), hepatic or renal disease. When used to treat bipolar disorder, the smallest effective dose is suggested to reduce the risk for overdose/suicide; high-risk patients should be monitored for suicidal ideations. Prescription should be written for the smallest quantity consistent with good patient care. May activate latent psychosis and/or cause confusion or agitation; elderly patients may be at an increased risk for psychiatric effects. Potentially serious, sometimes fatal multiorgan hypersensitivity reactions have been reported with some antiepileptic drugs; monitor for signs and symptoms of possible disparate manifestations associated with lymphatic, hepatic, renal, and/or hematologic organ systems; gradual discontinuation and conversion to alternate therapy may be required.

Carbamazepine is not effective in absence, myoclonic, or akinetic seizures; exacerbation of certain seizure types have been seen after initiation of carbamazepine therapy in children with mixed seizure disorders. Abrupt discontinuation is not recommended in patients being treated for seizures. Dizziness or drowsiness may occur; caution should be used when performing tasks which require alertness until the effects are known. Effects with other sedative drugs or ethanol may be potentiated. Carbamazepine has a high potential for drug interactions; use caution in patients taking strong CYP3A4 inducers or inhibitors or medications significantly metabolized via CYP1A2, 2B6, 2C9, 2C19, and 3A4. Coadministration of carbamazepine and nefazodone may lead to insufficient plasma levels of nefazodone; combination is contraindicated. Carbamazepine has mild anticholinergic activity; use with caution in patients with increased intraocular pressure, or sensitivity to anticholinergic effects. Severe dermatologic reactions, including toxic epidermal necrolysis and Stevens-Johnson syndrome, although rarely reported, have resulted in fatalities. **[U.S. Boxed Warning]: Use caution and screen for the genetic susceptibility genotype (*HLA-B*1502* allele) in Asian patients. Patients with a positive result should not be started on carbamazepine.** Discontinue if there are any signs of hypersensitivity. Elderly patients may have an increased risk of SIADH-like syndrome.

Administration of the suspension will yield higher peak and lower trough serum levels than an equal dose of the tablet form; consider a lower starting dose given more frequently (same total daily dose) when using the suspension.

Drug Interactions

Metabolism/Transport Effects Substrate of CYP2C8 (minor), 3A4 (major); **Induces** CYP1A2 (strong), 2B6 (strong), 2C8 (strong), 2C9 (strong), 2C19 (strong), 3A4 (strong), P-glycoprotein

Avoid Concomitant Use

Avoid concomitant use of CarBAMazepine with any of the following: Dabigatran Etexilate; Dronedarone; Etravirine; Everolimus; Lurasidone; MAO Inhibitors; Nefazodone; Nilotinib; Pazopanib; Praziquantel; Ranolazine; Roflumilast; RomiDEPsin; Tolvaptan; Vandetanib; Voriconazole

Decreased Effect

CarBAMazepine may decrease the levels/effects of: Acetaminophen; ARIPiprazole; Bendamustine; Benzodiazepines (metabolized by oxidation); Calcium Channel Blockers (Dihydropyridine); Calcium Channel Blockers (Nondihydropyridine); Caspofungin; CloZAPine; Contraceptives (Estrogens); Contraceptives (Progestins); CycloSPORINE; CycloSPORINE (Systemic); CYP1A2 Substrates; CYP2B6 Substrates; CYP2C19 Substrates; CYP2C8 Substrates (High risk); CYP2C9 Substrates (High risk); CYP3A4 Substrates; Dabigatran Etexilate; Divalproex; Doxycycline; Dronedarone; Etravirine; Everolimus; Exemestane; Felbamate; Flunarizine; Gefitinib; GuanFACINE; Haloperidol; Imatinib; Irinotecan; Ixabepilone; Lacosamide; LamoTRIgine; Lopinavir; Lurasidone; Maraviroc; Mebendazole; Methadone;

Nefazodone; Nilotinib; Paliperidone; Pazopanib; P-Glycoprotein Substrates; Phenytoin; Praziquantel; Protease Inhibitors; Ranolazine; RisperiDONE; Roflumilast; RomiDEPsin; Rufinamide; Saxagliptin; Selective Serotonin Reuptake Inhibitors; SORAfenib; Tadalafil; Temsirolimus; Theophylline Derivatives; Thyroid Products; Tolvaptan; Topiramate; Treprostinil; Tricyclic Antidepressants; Ulipristal; Valproic Acid; Vandetanib; Vecuronium; Vitamin K Antagonists; Voriconazole; Ziprasidone; Zolpidem

The levels/effects of CarBAMazepine may be decreased by: CYP3A4 Inducers (Strong); Deferasirox; Divalproex; Felbamate; Herbs (CYP3A4 Inducers); Ketorolac; Ketorolac (Systemic); Mefloquine; Methylfolate; Phenytoin; Rufinamide; Theophylline Derivatives; Valproic Acid

Increased Effect/Toxicity

CarBAMazepine may increase the levels/effects of: Adenosine; Alcohol (Ethyl); ClomiPRAMINE; CNS Depressants; Desmopressin; Lithium; MAO Inhibitors; Methotrimeprazine; Phenytoin

The levels/effects of CarBAMazepine may be increased by: Allopurinol; Antifungal Agents (Azole Derivatives, Systemic); Calcium Channel Blockers (Nondihydropyridine); Carbonic Anhydrase Inhibitors; Cimetidine; Conivaptan; CYP3A4 Inhibitors (Moderate); CYP3A4 Inhibitors (Strong); Danazol; Darunavir; Dasatinib; Droperidol; Fluconazole; Grapefruit Juice; Isoniazid; LamoTRIgine; Macrolide Antibiotics; Methotrimeprazine; Nefazodone; Propoxyphene; Protease Inhibitors; Selective Serotonin Reuptake Inhibitors; Thiazide Diuretics; Zolpidem

Nutritional/Ethanol Interactions

Ethanol: Avoid ethanol (may increase CNS depression).

Food: Carbamazepine serum levels may be increased if taken with food. Carbamazepine serum concentration may be increased if taken with grapefruit juice; avoid concurrent use.

Herb/Nutraceutical: Avoid evening primrose (seizure threshold decreased). Avoid valerian, St John's wort, kava kava, gotu kola (may increase CNS depression).

Lab Interactions May cause false-positive serum TCA screen. May interact with some pregnancy tests; increased BUN, AST, ALT, bilirubin, alkaline phosphatase (S); decreased calcium, T_3, T_4, sodium (S)

Adverse Reactions Frequency not defined, unless otherwise specified.

Cardiovascular: Arrhythmias, AV block, bradycardia, chest pain (bipolar use), CHF, edema, hyper-/hypotension, lymphadenopathy, syncope, thromboembolism, thrombophlebitis

Central nervous system: Amnesia (bipolar use), anxiety (bipolar use), aseptic meningitis (case report), ataxia (bipolar use 15%), confusion, depression (bipolar use), dizziness (bipolar use 44%), fatigue, headache (bipolar use 22%), sedation, slurred speech, somnolence (bipolar use 32%)

Dermatologic: Alopecia, alterations in skin pigmentation, erythema multiforme, exfoliative dermatitis, photosensitivity reaction, pruritus (bipolar use 8%), purpura, rash, Stevens-Johnson syndrome, toxic epidermal necrolysis, urticaria

Endocrine & metabolic: Chills, fever, hyponatremia, syndrome of inappropriate ADH secretion (SIADH)

Gastrointestinal: Abdominal pain, anorexia, constipation, diarrhea, dyspepsia (bipolar use), gastric distress, nausea (bipolar use 29%), pancreatitis, vomiting (bipolar use 18%), xerostomia (bipolar use)

Genitourinary: Azotemia, impotence, renal failure, urinary frequency, urinary retention

Hematologic: Acute intermittent porphyria, agranulocytosis, aplastic anemia, bone marrow suppression, eosinophilia, leukocytosis, leukopenia, pancytopenia, thrombocytopenia

Hepatic: Abnormal liver function tests, hepatic failure, hepatitis, jaundice

Neuromuscular & skeletal: Back pain, pain (bipolar use 12%), peripheral neuritis, weakness

Ocular: Blurred vision, conjunctivitis, lens opacities, nystagmus

Otic: Hyperacusis, tinnitus

Miscellaneous: Diaphoresis, hypersensitivity (including multiorgan reactions, may include disorders mimicking lymphoma, eosinophilia, hepatosplenomegaly, vasculitis); infection (bipolar use 12%)

Pharmacodynamics/Kinetics

Absorption Slow

Bioavailability 85%

Time to Peak Unpredictable:

Immediate release: Suspension: 1.5 hour; tablet: 4-5 hours

Extended release: Carbatrol®, Equetro®: 12-26 hours (single dose), 4-8 hours (multiple doses); Tegretol®-XR: 3-12 hours

Protein Binding Carbamazepine: 75% to 90%, may be decreased in newborns; Epoxide metabolite: 50%

Half-Life Elimination Half-life is variable because of autoinduction which is usually complete 3-5 weeks after initiation of a fixed carbamazepine regimen.

Carbamazepine: Initial: 25-65 hours; Extended release: 35-40 hours; Multiple doses: Children: 8-14 hours; Adults: 12-17 hours

Epoxide metabolite: Initial: 25-43 hours

Metabolism Hepatic via CYP3A4 to active epoxide metabolite; induces hepatic enzymes to increase metabolism

Excretion Urine 72% (1% to 3% as unchanged drug); feces (28%)

Available Dosage Forms

Capsule, extended release, oral:

Carbatrol®: 100 mg, 200 mg, 300 mg

Equetro®: 100 mg, 200 mg, 300 mg

Suspension, oral: 100 mg/5 mL (5 mL, 10 mL, 450 mL)
TEGretol®: 100 mg/5 mL (450 mL)
Tablet, oral: 200 mg, 400 mg
Epitol®: 200 mg
TEGretol®: 200 mg
Tablet, chewable, oral: 100 mg
TEGretol®: 100 mg
Tablet, extended release, oral: 100 mg, 200 mg, 400 mg
TEGretol®-XR: 100 mg, 200 mg, 400 mg

Dosing

Adult & Geriatric Dosage must be adjusted according to patient's response and serum concentrations. Administer tablets (chewable or conventional) in 2-3 divided doses daily and suspension in 4 divided doses daily. Oral:

Epilepsy: Initial: 400 mg/day in 2 divided doses (tablets or extended release tablets) or 4 divided doses (oral suspension); increase by up to 200 mg/day at weekly intervals using a twice daily regimen of extended release tablets or capsules, or a 3-4 times/day regimen of other formulations until optimal response and therapeutic levels are achieved; usual dose: 800-1200 mg/day

Maximum recommended dose: 1600 mg/day; however, some patients have required up to 1.6-2.4 g/day

Trigeminal or glossopharyngeal neuralgia: Initial: 200 mg/day in 2 divided doses (tablets, extended release tablets, or extended release capsules) or 4 divided doses (oral suspension) with food, gradually increasing in increments of 200 mg/day as needed.

Maintenance: Usual: 400-800 mg daily in 2 divided doses (tablets, extended release tablets, or extended release capsules) or 4 divided doses (oral suspension); maximum dose: 1200 mg/day

Bipolar disorder: Initial: 400 mg/day in 2 divided doses (tablets, extended release tablets, or extended release capsules) or 4 divided doses (oral suspension), may adjust by 200 mg/day increments; maximum dose: 1600 mg/day.

Note: Equetro® is the only formulation specifically approved by the FDA for the management of bipolar disorder.

Pediatric Dosage must be adjusted according to patient's response and serum concentrations. Administer tablets (chewable or conventional) in 2-3 divided doses daily and suspension in 4 divided doses daily.

Epilepsy: Oral:

Children <6 years: Initial: 10-20 mg/kg/day divided twice or 3 times daily as tablets or 4 times/day as suspension; increase dose every week until optimal response and therapeutic levels are achieved

Maintenance dose: Divide into 3-4 doses daily (tablets or suspension); maximum recommended dose: 35 mg/kg/day

Children 6-12 years: Initial: 200 mg/day in 2 divided doses (tablets or extended release tablets) or 4 divided doses (oral suspension); increase by up to 100 mg/day at weekly intervals using a twice daily regimen of extended release tablets or 3-4 times daily regimen of other formulations until optimal response and therapeutic levels are achieved

Maintenance: Usual: 400-800 mg/day; maximum recommended dose: 1000 mg/day

Note: Children <12 years who receive ≥400 mg/day of carbamazepine may be converted to extended release capsules (Carbatrol®) using the same total daily dosage divided twice daily

Children >12 years: Refer to adult dosing.

Maximum recommended doses:
Children 12-15 years: 1000 mg/day
Children >15 years: 1200 mg/day

Renal Impairment Dosage adjustments are not required or recommended in the manufacturer's labeling; however, the following guidelines have been used by some clinicians (Aronoff, 2007):

Children and Adults:
GFR <10 mL/minute: Administer 75% of dose.
Hemodialysis, peritoneal dialysis: Administer 75% of dose.
Continuous renal replacement therapy (CRRT):
Children: Administer 75% of dose.
Adults: No dosage adjustment recommended.

Hepatic Impairment Use with caution in hepatic impairment; metabolized primarily in the liver.

Administration

Oral

Suspension: Must be given on a 3-4 times/day schedule versus tablets which can be given 2-4 times/day. Since a given dose of suspension will produce higher peak and lower trough levels than the same dose given as the tablet form, patients given the suspension should be started on lower doses given more frequently (same total daily dose) and increased slowly to avoid unwanted side effects. When carbamazepine suspension has been combined with chlorpromazine or thioridazine solutions, a precipitate forms which may result in loss of effect. Therefore, it is recommended that the carbamazepine suspension dosage form not be administered at the same time with other liquid medicinal agents or diluents. Should be administered with meals.

Extended release capsule (Carbatrol®, Equetro®): Consists of three different types of beads: Immediate release, extended-release, and enteric release. The bead types are combined in a ratio to allow twice daily dosing. May be opened and contents sprinkled over food such as a teaspoon of applesauce; may be administered with or without food; do not crush or chew.

Extended release tablet: Should be inspected for damage. Damaged extended release tablets (without release portal) should not be administered. Should be administered with meals; swallow whole, do not crush or chew.

Monitoring and Teaching Issues

Laboratory Monitoring CBC with platelet count, reticulocytes, serum iron, liver function tests, urinalysis, BUN, serum carbamazepine levels, thyroid function tests, serum sodium; pregnancy test; signs of rash; *HLA-B*1502* genotype screening prior to therapy initiation in patients of Asian descent.

Physical Assessment Taper dosage slowly when discontinuing. Teach patient safety and seizure precautions. Monitor for mental and CNS changes, excessive sedation (especially when initiating or increasing therapy), and suicide ideation. Baseline and periodic eye exams (slit lamp, funduscopy, and tonometry) are recommended.

Patient Education Do not use extended release tablets which have been damaged or crushed. While using this medication, do not use alcohol. Maintain adequate hydration, unless instructed to restrict fluid intake. You may experience drowsiness, dizziness, blurred vision, nausea, vomiting, loss of appetite, or dry mouth. Wear identification of epileptic status and medications. Report CNS changes, suicide ideation, mentation changes, depression, changes in cognition, muscle cramping, weakness, tremors, sore throat, mouth ulcers, swollen glands, fever, jaundice, changes in gait, persistent GI symptoms (cramping, constipation, vomiting, anorexia), rash or skin irritations, unusual bruising or bleeding (mouth, urine, stool), or worsening of seizure activity or loss of seizure control.

Dietary Considerations Drug may cause GI upset, take with large amount of water or food to decrease GI upset. May need to split doses to avoid GI upset.

Geriatric Considerations Elderly may have increased risk of SIADH-like syndrome. Elderly are more susceptible to carbamazepine-induced confusion and agitation, AV block, and bradycardia.

Breast-Feeding Considerations Carbamazepine and its metabolites are found in breast milk. The manufacturer does not recommend use while breast-feeding.

Pregnancy Considerations Adverse events were observed in animal reproduction studies and also in humans. Carbamazepine crosses the placenta and accumulates in fetal tissues. Dysmorphic facial features, cranial defects, cardiac defects, spina bifida, IUGR, and multiple other malformations are reported. Nausea, vomiting, and poor feeding have also been reported in the neonate following maternal carbamazepine use. Epilepsy itself, the number of medications, genetic factors, or a combination of these probably influences the teratogenicity of anticonvulsant therapy.

Contraceptives may be rendered less effective by the coadministration of carbamazepine; alternative methods of contraception should be considered to prevent pregnancy.

Patients exposed to carbamazepine during pregnancy are encouraged to enroll themselves into the AED Pregnancy Registry by calling 1-888-233-2334. Additional information is available at www.aedpregnancyregistry.org.

Other Issues

Timing of serum samples: Absorption is slow, peak levels occur 6-8 hours after ingestion of the first dose. The half-life ranges from 8-60 hours; therefore, steady-state is achieved in 2-5 days.

Therapeutic levels: 6-12 mcg/mL (SI: 25-51 µmol/L)

Toxic concentration: >15 mcg/mL. Patients who require higher levels of 8-12 mcg/mL (SI: 34-51 µmol/L) should be watched closely. Side effects including CNS effects occur commonly at higher dosage levels. If other anticonvulsants are given therapeutic range is 4-8 mcg/mL.

Related Information

Anticonvulsant Drugs of Choice *on page 1981*

Peak and Trough Guidelines *on page 1958*

◆ **Carbatrol®** *see* CarBAMazepine *on page 287*

Carbidopa and Levodopa (kar bi DOE pa & lee voe DOE pa)

U.S. Brand Names Parcopa®; Sinemet®; Sinemet® CR

Index Terms Levodopa and Carbidopa

Generic Availability (U.S.) Yes

Pharmacologic Category Anti-Parkinson's Agent, Decarboxylase Inhibitor; Anti-Parkinson's Agent, Dopamine Precursor

Medication Safety Issues

Sound-alike/look-alike issues:

Sinemet® may be confused with Serevent®

International issues:

Zimox: Brand name for carbidopa and levodopa [Greece], but also the brand name for amoxicillin [Italy]

Zimox [Greece] may be confused with Diamox which is a brand name for acetazolamide [Canada and multiple international markets]

Prescribing and Access Restrictions Duodopa™ intestinal gel (Canadian labeling; product not available in U.S.): In Canada, the Duodopa™ Education Program is a risk mitigation program established to provide safe and effective use of Duodopa™ in advanced Parkinson's patients. The program involves:

- Education of prescribing neurologists and other healthcare providers on suitable candidates for treatment, surgical procedures (PEG tube placement), and follow-up care including infusion device education.
- Distribution of educational materials to patients and caregivers describing Duodopa™ intestinal gel and its proper use, PEG tube placement, and complications associated with the mode of administration and/or PEG tube placement.

Pregnancy Risk Factor C

Lactation Excretion in breast milk unknown/use caution

Use Idiopathic Parkinson's disease; postencephalitic parkinsonism; symptomatic parkinsonism

Duodopa™ intestinal gel: Canadian labeling (not available in U.S.): Treatment of advanced levodopa-responsive Parkinson's disease in which severe motor symptoms are not controlled by other Parkinson's agents

Unlabeled/Investigational Use Restless leg syndrome

Mechanism of Action/Effect Parkinson's symptoms are due to a lack of striatal dopamine; levodopa circulates in the plasma to the blood-brain-barrier (BBB), where it crosses, to be converted by striatal enzymes to dopamine; carbidopa inhibits the peripheral plasma breakdown of levodopa by inhibiting its decarboxylation, and thereby increases available levodopa at the BBB

Contraindications Hypersensitivity to levodopa, carbidopa, or any component of the formulation; narrow-angle glaucoma; use of MAO inhibitors within prior 14 days (however, may be administered concomitantly with the manufacturer's recommended dose of an MAO inhibitor with selectivity for MAO type B); history of melanoma or undiagnosed skin lesions

Canadian labeling: Additional contraindications: Clinical or laboratory evidence of uncompensated cardiovascular, cerebrovascular, endocrine, renal, hepatic, hematologic or pulmonary disease; when administration of a sympathomimetic amine (eg, epinephrine, norepinephrine or isoproterenol) is contraindicated; intestinal gel therapy in patients with any condition preventing the required placement of a PEG tube for administration.

Warnings/Precautions Use with caution in patients with history of cardiovascular disease (including myocardial infarction and arrhythmias), pulmonary diseases (such as asthma), psychosis, wide-angle glaucoma, peptic ulcer disease, seizure disorder or prone to seizures, and in severe renal and hepatic dysfunction. Use with caution when interpreting plasma/urine catecholamine levels; falsely diagnosed pheochromocytoma has been rarely reported. Severe cases or rhabdomyolysis have been reported. Sudden discontinuation of levodopa may cause a worsening of Parkinson's disease. Elderly may be more sensitive to CNS effects of levodopa. May cause or exacerbate dyskinesias. Patients have reported falling asleep while engaging in activities of daily living; this has been reported to occur without significant warning signs. May cause orthostatic hypotension; Parkinson's disease patients appear to have an impaired capacity to respond to a postural challenge; use with caution in patients at risk of hypotension (such as those receiving antihypertensive drugs) or where transient hypotensive episodes would be poorly tolerated (cardiovascular disease or cerebrovascular disease). Observe patients closely for development of depression with concomitant suicidal tendencies.

Dopamine agonists have been associated with compulsive behaviors and/or loss of impulse control, which has manifested as pathological gambling, libido increases (hypersexuality), and/or binge eating. Causality has not been established, and controversy exists as to whether this phenomenon is related to the underlying disease, prior behaviors/addictions and/or drug therapy. Dose reduction or discontinuation of therapy has been reported to reverse these behaviors in some, but not all cases. Risk for melanoma development is increased in Parkinson's disease patients; drug causation or factors contributing to risk have not been established. Patients should be monitored closely and periodic skin examinations should be performed. Dopaminergic agents have been associated with a syndrome resembling neuroleptic malignant syndrome on abrupt withdrawal or significant dosage reduction after long-term use. Protein in the diet should be distributed throughout the day to avoid fluctuations in levodopa absorption.

Intestinal gel (available in Canada, not available in U.S.): Product should be prescribed only by neurologists experienced in the treatment of Parkinson's disease and who have completed the Duodopa™ Education Program. Response to levodopa/carbidopa intestinal gel therapy should be assessed with a test period (~3 days) of administration via a temporary nasoduodenal tube prior to placement of a percutaneous endoscopic gastrostomy (PEG) tube for permanent access and administration. Sudden deterioration in therapy response with recurring motor symptoms may indicate PEG tube complications (eg, displacement) or obstruction of the infusion device. Tube or infusion device complications may require initiation of oral levodopa/carbidopa therapy until complications are resolved. Discontinue therapy 2-3 hours prior to surgical procedures requiring general anesthesia, if possible. May resume therapy postoperatively when oral fluid intake is permitted.

Drug Interactions

Avoid Concomitant Use There are no known interactions where it is recommended to avoid concomitant use.

Decreased Effect

Carbidopa and Levodopa may decrease the levels/effects of: Antipsychotics (Typical)

The levels/effects of Carbidopa and Levodopa may be decreased by: Antipsychotics (Atypical); Glycopyrrolate; Iron Salts; Methionine; Metoclopramide; Phenytoin; Pyridoxine

Increased Effect/Toxicity

Carbidopa and Levodopa may increase the levels/effects of: MAO Inhibitors

The levels/effects of Carbidopa and Levodopa may be increased by: Antipsychotics (Typical); MAO Inhibitors; Methylphenidate; Sapropterin

Nutritional/Ethanol Interactions

Ethanol: Avoid ethanol (due to CNS depression).

Food: Avoid high protein diets due to potential for impaired levodopa absorption; levodopa competes with certain amino acids for transport across the gut wall or across the blood brain barrier.

Herb/Nutraceutical: Avoid kava kava (may decrease effects). Pyridoxine (vitamin B_6) in doses >10-25 mg (for levodopa alone) may decrease efficacy. Iron supplements or iron-containing multivitamins may reduce absorption of levodopa.

Lab Interactions False-positive reaction for urinary glucose with Clinitest®; false-negative reaction using Clinistix®; false-positive urine ketones with Acetest®, Ketostix®, Labstix®

Adverse Reactions Frequency not defined.

Cardiovascular: Arrhythmia, chest pain, edema, flushing, hypotension, hypertension, MI, orthostatic hypotension, palpitation, phlebitis, syncope

Central nervous system: Agitation, anxiety, ataxia, confusion, delusions, dementia, depression (with or without suicidal tendencies), disorientation, dizziness, dreams abnormal, EPS, euphoria, faintness, falling, fatigue, gait abnormalities, headache, hallucinations, impulse control symptoms, insomnia, malaise, memory impairment, mental acuity decreased, nervousness, neuroleptic malignant syndrome, nightmares, on-off phenomena, paranoid ideation, pathological gambling, psychosis, seizure (causal relationship not established), somnolence

Dermatologic: Alopecia, malignant melanoma, rash

Endocrine & metabolic: Hot flashes, hyperglycemia, hypokalemia, libido increased (including hypersexuality), uric acid increased

Gastrointestinal: Abdominal pain, abdominal distress, anorexia, bruxism, constipation, diarrhea, discoloration of saliva, duodenal ulcer, dyspepsia, dysphagia, flatulence, GI bleeding, heartburn, nausea, sialorrhea, taste alterations, tongue burning sensation, weight gain/loss, vomiting, xerostomia

Genitourinary: Discoloration of urine, glycosuria, urinary frequency, priapism, proteinuria, urinary incontinence, urinary retention, urinary tract infection

Hematologic: Agranulocytosis, anemia, Coombs' test abnormal, hematocrit decreased, hemoglobin decreased, hemolytic anemia, leukopenia

Hepatic: Alkaline phosphatase abnormal, ALT abnormal, AST abnormal, bilirubin abnormal, LDH abnormal

Neuromuscular & skeletal: Back pain, dyskinesias (including choreiform, dystonic and other involuntary movements), leg pain, muscle cramps, muscle twitching, numbness, paresthesia, peripheral neuropathy, shoulder pain, tremor increased, trismus, weakness

Ocular: Blepharospasm, blurred vision, diplopia, Horner's syndrome reactivation, mydriasis, oculogyric crises (may be associated with acute dystonic reactions)

Renal: Difficult urination

Respiratory: Cough, dyspnea, hoarseness, pharyngeal pain, upper respiratory infection

Miscellaneous: Discoloration of sweat, diaphoresis increased, hiccups, hypersensitivity reactions (angioedema, pruritus, urticaria, bullous lesions [including pemphigus-like reactions], Henoch-Schönlein purpura)

Pharmacodynamics/Kinetics

Bioavailability

Controlled release: Levodopa: Bioavailability is 70% to 75% relative to availability from immediate release formulation; Carbidopa: Bioavailability is ~58% relative to availability from immediate release formulation

Intestinal gel: Levodopa: Similar bioavailability relative to oral administration of tablet formulations (81% to 98%)

Time to Peak Immediate release: 0.5 hours; Controlled release: 2 hours; Intestinal gel: therapeutic plasma levels reached 10-30 minutes following morning bolus dose

Half-Life Elimination Immediate release: Levodopa (in presence of carbidopa): 1.5 hours; Half-life may be prolonged with controlled release formulations due to continuous absorption.

Metabolism Levodopa: Two major pathways (decarboxylation and O-methylation) and two minor pathways (transamination and oxidation) of metabolism; carbidopa inhibits the decarboxylation of levodopa to dopamine in the peripheral tissue to allow greater levodopa distribution into the CNS

Excretion Levodopa: Urine (as metabolites); Carbidopa: Urine (~50% of an oral dose)

Available Dosage Forms

Tablet: 10/100: Carbidopa 10 mg and levodopa 100 mg; 25/100: Carbidopa 25 mg and levodopa 100 mg; 25/250: Carbidopa 25 mg and levodopa 250 mg

Sinemet®:

10/100: Carbidopa 10 mg and levodopa 100 mg

25/100: Carbidopa 25 mg and levodopa 100 mg

25/250: Carbidopa 25 mg and levodopa 250 mg

Tablet, extended release: 25/100: Carbidopa 25 mg and levodopa 100 mg; 50/200: Carbidopa 50 mg and levodopa 200 mg

Tablet, orally disintegrating: 10/100: Carbidopa 10 mg and levodopa 100 mg; 25/100: Carbidopa 25 mg and levodopa 100 mg; 25/250: Carbidopa 25 mg and levodopa 250 mg
Parcopa®:
10/100: Carbidopa 10 mg and levodopa 100 mg [contains phenylalanine 3.4 mg/tablet; mint flavor]
25/100: Carbidopa 25 mg and levodopa 100 mg [contains phenylalanine 3.4 mg/tablet; mint flavor]
25/250: Carbidopa 25 mg and levodopa 250 mg [contains phenylalanine 8.4 mg/tablet; mint flavor]

Tablet, sustained release: 25/100: Carbidopa 25 mg and levodopa 100 mg; 50/200: Carbidopa 50 mg and levodopa 200 mg
Sinemet® CR:
25/100: Carbidopa 25 mg and levodopa 100 mg
50/200: Carbidopa 50 mg and levodopa 200 mg

Dosing

Adult & Geriatric

Parkinson's disease:
Oral:
Immediate release tablet, orally-disintegrating tablet:
Initial: Carbidopa 25 mg/levodopa 100 mg 3 times/day
Dosage adjustment: Alternate tablet strengths may be substituted according to individual carbidopa/levodopa requirements. Increase by 1 tablet every 1-2 days as necessary, except when using the carbidopa 25 mg/levodopa 250 mg tablets where increases should be made using ½-1 tablet every 1-2 days. Use of more than 1 dosage strength or dosing 4 times/day may be required (maximum: 8 tablets of any strength/day or 200 mg of carbidopa and 2000 mg of levodopa)
Controlled release tablet:
Patients not currently receiving levodopa: Initial: Carbidopa 50 mg/levodopa 200 mg 2 times/day, at intervals not <6 hours
Patients converting from immediate release formulation to controlled release: Initial: Dosage should be substituted at an amount that provides ~10% more of levodopa/day; total calculated dosage is administered in divided doses 2-3 times/day (or ≥3 times/day for patients maintained on levodopa ≥700 mg). Intervals between doses should be 4-8 hours while awake; when divided doses are not equal, smaller doses should be given toward the end of the day. Depending on clinical response, dosage may need to be increased to provide up to 30% more levodopa/day.
Dosage adjustment: May adjust every 3 days; intervals should be between 4-8 hours during the waking day (maximum dose: 8 tablets/day)
Intestinal infusion via PEG tube: Intestinal gel (Canadian labeling; not available in U.S.): **Note:** Conversion to/from oral levodopa tablet formulations and the intestinal gel formulation can be done on a 1:1 ratio. Total daily dose (expressed in terms of levodopa) consists of a morning bolus dose, a continuous maintenance dose, and additional bolus doses when necessary. Nighttime dosing may be necessary in certain rare situations (eg, nocturnal akinesia). Dosage adjustments should be carried out over a period of a few weeks.
Morning bolus dose (based on previous morning levodopa intake and volume to fill intestinal tubing): Usual: Levodopa 100-200 mg (5-10 mL); Maximum: Levodopa 300 mg (15 mL)
Continuous maintenance dose: Adjustable in increments of 2 mg/hour (0.1 mL/hour) and based on previous daily intake of levodopa: Usual: Levodopa 40-120 mg/hour (2-6 mL/hour) infused up to 16 hours; Range: Levodopa 20-200 mg/hour (1-10 mL/hour)
Additional bolus doses: Usual: Levodopa: 10-40 mg (0.5-2 mL), if needed for daytime hypokinesia; in patients requiring >5 additional boluses/day, the maintenance dose should be increased

Restless leg syndrome (RLS) (unlabeled use; Silber, 2004): Oral:
Immediate release tablet: Carbidopa 25 mg/levodopa 100 mg (0.5-1 tablet) given in the evening, at bedtime, or upon waking during the night with RLS symptoms
Controlled release tablet: Carbidopa 25 mg/levodopa 100 mg (1 tablet) before bedtime for RLS symptoms that awaken patient during the night

Renal Impairment Use with caution; manufacturer labeling makes no specific dosing recommendations.

Hepatic Impairment Use with caution; manufacturer labeling makes no specific dosing recommendations.

Administration

Oral Tablet formulations: Space doses evenly over the waking hours. Give with meals to decrease GI upset. Controlled release product should not be chewed or crushed. Orally-disintegrating tablets do not require water; the tablet should disintegrate on the tongue's surface before swallowing.

Other Intestinal gel (Canadian labeling; not available in U.S.): Gel is administered directly to the duodenum via a portable infusion pump (CADD-legacy Duodopa™ pump). Administer through a temporary nasoduodenal tube for at least 3 days to evaluate patient response and for dose optimization. Long-term administration requires placement of PEG tube for intestinal infusion. Continuous maintenance dose is infused throughout the day for up to 16 hours.

Stability

Storage

Tablet: Store at 20°C to 25°C (68°F to 77°F); excursions permitted between 15°C to 30°C (59°F to 86°F). Protect from light and moisture.
Intestinal gel (Canadian labeling; not available in U.S.): Store in refrigerator at 2°C to 8°C (36°F to 46°F). Keep in outer carton to protect from light. Cassettes are for single use only and should be discarded daily following infusion (up to 16 hours).

Monitoring and Teaching Issues

Laboratory Monitoring Periodic hepatic function tests, BUN, creatinine, and CBC

Patient Education Do not crush controlled release form. Therapeutic effects may take several weeks or months to achieve and you may need frequent monitoring during first weeks of therapy. Take with meals if GI upset occurs. Do not use alcohol. You may experience drowsiness, dizziness, confusion, vision changes, loss of impulse control (possibly manifested as pathological gambling, libido increases, and/or binge eating), orthostatic hypotension, constipation, dry skin, nausea, vomiting, or loss of appetite. Report unresolved constipation or vomiting, respiratory difficulty, dizziness, CNS changes (hallucination, loss of memory, nervousness, etc), suicide ideation, increased muscle spasticity or rigidity, changes in the appearance of skin moles, skin rash, or significant worsening of condition.

Dietary Considerations Avoid high protein diets (>2 g/kg) which may decrease the efficacy of levodopa via competition with amino acids in crossing the blood-brain barrier. Some products may contain phenylalanine.

Geriatric Considerations The elderly may be more sensitive to the CNS effects of levodopa.

Pregnancy Considerations Teratogenic effects were observed with levodopa and carbidopa in animal studies. There are case reports of levodopa crossing the placenta in humans.

Additional Information To block the peripheral conversion of levodopa to dopamine, ≥70 mg/day of carbidopa is needed. "On-off" (a clinical syndrome characterized by sudden periods of drug activity/inactivity), can be managed by giving smaller, more frequent doses of Sinemet® or adding a dopamine agonist or selegiline; when adding a new agent, doses of Sinemet® can usually be decreased. Protein in the diet should be distributed throughout the day to avoid fluctuations in levodopa absorption. Levodopa is the drug of choice when rigidity is the predominant presenting symptom.

Conversion from levodopa to carbidopa/levodopa: **Note:** Levodopa must be discontinued at least 12 hours prior to initiation of levodopa/carbidopa:

Initial dose: Levodopa portion of carbidopa/levodopa should be at least 25% of previous levodopa therapy.

Levodopa <1500 mg/day: Sinemet® or Parcopa™ (levodopa 25 mg/carbidopa 100 mg) 3-4 times/day

Levodopa ≥1500 mg/day: Sinemet® or Parcopa™ (levodopa 25 mg/carbidopa 250 mg) 3-4 times/day

Conversion from immediate release carbidopa/levodopa (Sinemet® or Parcopa™) to Sinemet® CR (50/200):

Sinemet® or Parcopa™ [total daily dose of levodopa]/Sinemet® CR:

Sinemet® or Parcopa™ (levodopa 300-400 mg/day): Sinemet® CR (50/200) 1 tablet twice daily

Sinemet® or Parcopa™ (levodopa 500-600 mg/day): Sinemet® CR (50/200) 1 1/2 tablets twice daily or 1 tablet 3 times/day

Sinemet® or Parcopa™ (levodopa 700-800 mg/day): Sinemet® CR (50/200) 4 tablets in 3 or more divided doses

Sinemet® or Parcopa™ (levodopa 900-1000 mg/day): Sinemet® CR (50/200) 5 tablets in 3 or more divided doses

Intervals between doses of Sinemet® CR should be 4-8 hours while awake; when divided doses are not equal, smaller doses should be given toward the end of the day

◆ **Carbidopa, Entacapone, and Levodopa** *see* Levodopa, Carbidopa, and Entacapone *on page 1091*

◆ **Carbidopa, Levodopa, and Entacapone** *see* Levodopa, Carbidopa, and Entacapone *on page 1091*

CARBOplatin (KAR boe pla tin)

Index Terms CBDCA; Paraplatin

Generic Availability (U.S.) Yes

Pharmacologic Category Antineoplastic Agent, Alkylating Agent; Antineoplastic Agent, Platinum Analog

Medication Safety Issues

Sound-alike/look-alike issues:

CARBOplatin may be confused with CISplatin, oxaliplatin

Paraplatin® may be confused with Platinol®

High alert medication: This medication is in a class the Institute for Safe Medication Practices (ISMP) includes among its list of drugs which have a heightened risk of causing significant patient harm when used in error.

Pregnancy Risk Factor D

Lactation Excretion in breast milk unknown/not recommended

Use Treatment of advanced ovarian cancer

Unlabeled/Investigational Use Treatment of bladder cancer, breast cancer (metastatic), central nervous system tumors, cervical cancer (recurrent or metastatic), endometrial cancer, esophageal cancer, head and neck cancer, Hodgkin's lymphoma (relapsed or refractory), malignant pleural mesothelioma, melanoma (advanced or metastatic), merkel cell carcinoma, neuroendocrine tumors (adrenal gland and carcinoid tumors), non-Hodgkin's lymphomas (relapsed or refractory), nonsmall cell lung cancer, prostate cancer, sarcomas (Ewing's sarcoma and osteosarcoma), small-cell lung cancer, testicular cancer, thymic malignancies, unknown primary adenocarcinoma, and as a conditioning regimen prior to hematopoietic stem cell transplantation

Mechanism of Action/Effect Carboplatin is an alkylating agent which covalently binds to DNA; possible cross-linking and interference with the function of DNA

Contraindications History of severe allergic reaction to cisplatin, carboplatin, other platinum-containing formulations, mannitol, or any component of the formulation; should not be used in patients with severe bone marrow depression or significant bleeding

Warnings/Precautions Hazardous agent - use appropriate precautions for handling and disposal. High doses have resulted in severe abnormalities of liver function tests. **[U.S. Boxed Warning]: Bone marrow suppression, which may be severe, is dose related;** reduce dosage in patients with bone marrow suppression; cycles should be delayed until WBC and platelet counts have recovered. Patients who have received prior myelosuppressive therapy and patients with renal dysfunction are at increased risk for bone marrow suppression. Anemia is cumulative.

When calculating the carboplatin dose using the Calvert formula and an estimated glomerular filtration rate (GFR), the laboratory method used to measure serum creatinine may impact dosing. Compared to other methods, standardized isotope dilution mass spectrometry (IDMS) may underestimate serum creatinine values in patients with low creatinine values (eg, ≤0.7 mg/dL) and may overestimate GFR in patients with normal renal function. This may result in higher calculated carboplatin doses and increased toxicities. If using IDMS, the Food and Drug Administration (FDA) recommends that clinicians consider capping estimated GFR at a maximum of 125 mL/minute to avoid potential toxicity.

[U.S. Boxed Warning]: Anaphylactic-like reactions have been reported with carboplatin; may occur within minutes of administration. Epinephrine, corticosteroids and antihistamines have been used to treat symptoms. The risk of allergic reactions (including anaphylaxis) is increased in patients previously exposed to platinum therapy. Skin testing and desensitization protocols have been reported (Confina-Cohen, 2005; Lee, 2004; Markman, 2003). When administered as sequential infusions, taxane derivatives (docetaxel, paclitaxel) should be administered before the platinum derivatives (carboplatin, cisplatin) to limit myelosuppression and to enhance efficacy. Clinically significant hearing loss has been reported to occur in pediatric patients when carboplatin was administered at higher than recommended doses in combination with other ototoxic agents (eg, aminoglycosides). Loss of vision (reversible) has been reported with higher than recommended doses. Peripheral neuropathy occurs infrequently, the incidence of peripheral neuropathy is increased patients >65 years of age and those who have previously received cisplatin treatment. Patients >65 years of age are more likely to develop severe thrombocytopenia. **[U.S. Boxed Warning]: Vomiting may occur;** may be severe in patients who have received prior emetogenic therapy. **[U.S. Boxed Warning]: Should be administered under the supervision of an experienced cancer chemotherapy physician.**

Drug Interactions

Avoid Concomitant Use

Avoid concomitant use of CARBOplatin with any of the following: BCG; Natalizumab; Pimecrolimus; Roflumilast; SORAfenib; Tacrolimus (Topical); Vaccines (Live)

Decreased Effect

CARBOplatin may decrease the levels/effects of: BCG; Sipuleucel-T; Vaccines (Inactivated); Vaccines (Live)

The levels/effects of CARBOplatin may be decreased by: Echinacea

Increased Effect/Toxicity

CARBOplatin may increase the levels/effects of: Leflunomide; Natalizumab; Taxane Derivatives; Topotecan; Vaccines (Live)

The levels/effects of CARBOplatin may be increased by: Aminoglycosides; Denosumab; Pimecrolimus; Roflumilast; SORAfenib; Tacrolimus (Topical); Trastuzumab

Nutritional/Ethanol Interactions Herb/Nutraceutical: Avoid black cohosh, dong quai in estrogen-dependent tumors.

Adverse Reactions Percentages reported with single-agent therapy.

>10%:

Central nervous system: Pain (23%)

Endocrine & metabolic: Hyponatremia (29% to 47%), hypomagnesemia (29% to 43%), hypocalcemia(22% to 31%), hypokalemia (20% to 28%)

Gastrointestinal: Vomiting (65% to 81%), abdominal pain (17%), nausea (without vomiting: 10% to 15%)

Hematologic: Myelosuppression (dose related and dose limiting; nadir at ~21 days; recovery by ~28 days), anemia (71% to 90%; grades 3/4: 21%), leukopenia (85%; grades 3/4: 15% to 26%), neutropenia (67%; grades 3/4: 16% to 21%), thrombocytopenia (62%; grades 3/4: 25% to 35%)

Hepatic: Alkaline phosphatase increased (24% to 37%), AST increased (15% to 19%)

Neuromuscular & skeletal: Weakness (11%)

Renal: Creatinine clearance decreased (27%), BUN increased (14% to 22%)

Miscellaneous: Hypersensitivity/allergic reaction (2% to 16%)

1% to 10%:

Central nervous system: Neurotoxicity (5%)

Dermatologic: Alopecia (2% to 3%)

Gastrointestinal: Constipation (6%), diarrhea (6%), stomatitis/mucositis (1%), taste dysgeusia (1%)

Hematologic: Bleeding (5%), hemorrhagic complications (5%)

Hepatic: Bilirubin increased (5%)

Neuromuscular & skeletal: Peripheral neuropathy (4% to 6%)
Ocular: Visual disturbance (1%)
Otic: Ototoxicity (1%)
Renal: Creatinine increased (6% to 10%)
Miscellaneous: Infection (5%)

Pharmacodynamics/Kinetics

Protein Binding Carboplatin: 0%; Platinum (from carboplatin): Irreversibly binds to plasma proteins

Half-Life Elimination Cl_{cr} >60 mL/minute: Carboplatin: 2.6-5.9 hours (based on a dose of 300-500 mg/m^2); Platinum (from carboplatin): ≥5 days

Metabolism Minimally hepatic to aquated and hydroxylated compounds

Excretion Urine (~70% as carboplatin within 24 hours; 3% to 5% as platinum within 1-4 days)

Available Dosage Forms

Injection, powder for reconstitution: 50 mg, 150 mg, 450 mg
Injection, solution: 10 mg/mL (5 mL, 15 mL, 45 mL, 60 mL)
Injection, solution [preservative free]: 10 mg/mL (5 mL, 15 mL, 45 mL)

Dosing

Adult Details concerning dosing in combination regimens should also be consulted. **Note:** Doses for adults are commonly calculated by the target AUC using the Calvert formula, where **Total dose (mg) = Target AUC x (GFR + 25)**. If estimating glomerular filtration rate (GFR) instead of a measured GFR, the Food and Drug Administration (FDA) recommends that clinicians consider capping estimated GFR at a maximum of 125 mL/minute to avoid potential toxicity.

Ovarian cancer, advanced: I.V.: 360 mg/m^2 every 4 weeks (as a single agent) **or** 300 mg/m^2 every 4 weeks (in combination with cyclophosphamide) **or** Target AUC 4-6 (single agent; in previously-treated patients)

Unlabeled dosing for advanced ovarian cancer: I.V.: Target AUC 5-7.5 every 3 weeks (in combination with paclitaxel) (Ozols, 2003; Parmar, 2003)

Bladder cancer (unlabeled use): I.V.: Target AUC 5 every 3 weeks (in combination with gemcitabine and paclitaxel) (Hainsworth, 2005) **or** Target AUC 5 every 3 weeks (in combination with gemcitabine) (Bamias, 2006) **or** Target AUC 6 every 3 weeks (in combination with paclitaxel) (Vaughn, 2002)

Breast cancer, metastatic (unlabeled use): I.V.: Target AUC 6 every 3 weeks (in combination with trastuzumab and paclitaxel) (Robert, 2006) **or** Target AUC 6 every 3 weeks (in combination with trastuzumab and docetaxel) (Pegram, 2004)

Cervical cancer, recurrent or metastatic (unlabeled use): I.V.: Target AUC 5 every 3 weeks (in combination with paclitaxel) (Pectasides, 2009) **or** Target AUC 5-6 every 4 weeks (in combination with paclitaxel) (Tinker, 2005) **or** 400 mg/m^2 every 28 days (as a single agent) (Weiss, 1990)

Endometrial cancer (unlabeled use): I.V.: Target AUC 5 every 3 weeks (in combination with paclitaxel) (Pectasides, 2008) **or** Target AUC 2 on days 1, 8, and 15 every 28 days (in combination with paclitaxel) (Secord, 2007)

Esophageal cancer (unlabeled use): I.V.: Target AUC 2 on days 1, 8, 15, 22, and 29 for 1 cycle (in combination with paclitaxel) (van Meerten, 2006) **or** Target AUC 5 every 3 weeks (in combination with paclitaxel) (El-Rayes, 2004)

Head and neck cancer (unlabeled use): I.V.: Target AUC 5 every 3 weeks (in combination with cetuximab) (Chan, 2005) **or** Target AUC 5 every 3 weeks (in combination with cetuximab and fluorouracil) (Vermorken, 2008) **or** 300 mg/m^2 every 4 weeks (in combination with fluorouracil) (Forastiere, 1992) **or** Target AUC 6 every 3 weeks (in combination with paclitaxel) (Clark, 2001)

Hodgkin's lymphoma, relapsed or refractory (unlabeled use): I.V.: Target AUC 5 (maximum dose 800 mg) for 2 cycles (in combination with ifosfamide and etoposide) (Moskowitz, 2001)

Malignant pleural mesothelioma (unlabeled use): I.V.: Target AUC 5 every 3 weeks (in combination with pemetrexed) (Castagneto, 2008; Ceresoli, 2006)

Melanoma, advanced or metastatic (unlabeled use): I.V.: Target AUC 2 days 1, 8, and 15 every 4 weeks (in combination with paclitaxel) (Rao, 2006)

Non-Hodgkin's lymphomas, relapsed or refractory (unlabeled use): I.V.: Target AUC 5 (maximum dose 800 mg) per cycle for 3 cycles (in combination with rituximab, ifosfamide and etoposide) (Kewalramani, 2004)

Nonsmall cell lung cancer (unlabeled use): I.V.: Target AUC 6 every 3 weeks (in combination with paclitaxel) (Schiller, 2002; Strauss, 2008) **or** Target AUC 6 every 3 weeks (in combination with bevacizumab and paclitaxel) (Sandler, 2006) **or** in combination with radiation therapy and paclitaxel (Belani, 2005):
Target AUC 6 every 3 weeks for 2 cycles **or**
Target AUC 6 every 3 weeks for 2 cycles; then target AUC 2 weekly for 7 weeks **or**
Target AUC 2 every week for 7 weeks; then target AUC 6 every 3 weeks for 2 cycles

Sarcomas: Ewing's sarcoma, osteosarcoma (unlabeled uses): I.V.: 400 mg/m^2/day for 2 days every 21 days (in combination with ifosfamide and etoposide) (van Winkle, 2005)

Small cell lung cancer (unlabeled use): I.V.: Target AUC 6 every 3 weeks (in combination with etoposide) (Skarlos, 2001) **or** Target AUC 5 every 3 weeks (in combination with irinotecan) (Hermes, 2008) **or** Target AUC 5 every 28 days (in combination with irinotecan) (Schmittel, 2006)

Thymic malignancies (unlabeled use): I.V.: Target AUC 5 every 3 weeks (in combination with paclitaxel) (Lemma, 2008)

Unknown primary adenocarcinoma (unlabeled use): I.V.: Target AUC 6 every 3 weeks (in combination with paclitaxel) (Briasoulis, 2000) **or** Target AUC 6 every 3 weeks (in combination with docetaxel) (Greco, 2000) **or** Target AUC 6 every 3 weeks (in combination with paclitaxel and etoposide) (Hainsworth, 2006) **or** Target AUC 5 every 3 weeks (in combination with paclitaxel and gemcitabine) (Greco, 2002)

Geriatric The Calvert formula should be used to calculate dosing for elderly patients.

Pediatric Details concerning dosing in combination regimens should also be consulted.

Glioma (unlabeled use): I.V.: 175 mg/m^2 weekly for 4 weeks every 6 weeks, with a 2-week recovery period between courses (in combination with vincristine) (Packer, 1997)

Sarcomas: Ewing's sarcoma, osteosarcoma (unlabeled uses): I.V.:400 mg/m^2/day for 2 days every 21 days (in combination with ifosfamide and etoposide) (van Winkle, 2005)

Renal Impairment Note: Dose determination with Calvert formula uses GFR and, therefore, inherently adjusts for renal dysfunction.

The FDA-approved labeling recommends the following dosage adjustment guidelines for single-agent therapy:

Baseline Cl_{cr} 41-59 mL/minute: Initiate at 250 mg/m^2 and adjust subsequent doses based on bone marrow toxicity

Baseline Cl_{cr} 16-40 mL/minute: Initiate at 200 mg/m^2 and adjust subsequent doses based on bone marrow toxicity

Baseline Cl_{cr} ≤15 mL/minute: No guidelines are available.

The following dosage adjustments have been used by some clinicians (Aronoff, 2007): Adults (for dosing based on mg/m^2):

Hemodialysis: Administer 50% of dose

Continuous ambulatory peritoneal dialysis (CAPD): Administer 25% of dose

Continuous renal replacement therapy (CRRT): 200 mg/m^2

Hepatic Impairment Minimal hepatic metabolism; dosage adjustment may not be needed. No specific dosage adjustment guidelines are available.

Adjustment for Toxicity Platelets <50,000 cells/mm^3 or ANC <500 cells/mm^3: Administer 75% of dose

Administration

I.V. Usually infused over 15-60 minutes, although some protocols may require infusions up to 24 hours. When administered as sequential infusions, taxane derivatives (docetaxel, paclitaxel) should be administered before platinum derivatives to limit myelosuppression and to enhance efficacy.

Stability

Reconstitution Reconstitute powder to yield a final concentration of 10 mg/mL. Reconstituted carboplatin 10 mg/mL should be further diluted to a final concentration of 0.5-2 mg/mL with D_5W or NS for administration. Use appropriate precautions for handling and disposal.

Storage Store intact vials at room temperature of 25°C (77°F); excursions permitted to 15°C to 30°C (59°F to 86°F). Protect from light. Further dilution to a concentration as low as 0.5 mg/mL is stable at room temperature (25°C) for 8 hours in NS; stable at room temperature or under refrigeration for at least 9 days in D_5W, although the manufacturer states to use within 8 hours due to lack of preservative.

Powder for reconstitution: Reconstituted to a final concentration of 10 mg/mL is stable for 5 days at room temperature (25°C).

Solution for injection: Multidose vials are stable for up to 14 days after opening when stored at room temperature.

Monitoring and Teaching Issues

Laboratory Monitoring CBC (with differential and platelet count), serum electrolytes, serum creatinine and BUN, creatinine clearance, liver function tests

Physical Assessment Assess patient allergy history prior to therapy and note specific use cautions (eg, bone marrow suppression and renal function). Assess other drugs patient may be taking for potential interactions (especially products that may be ototoxic or nephrotoxic and need for sequencing with taxane derivatives). Assess hematology, electrolytes, and renal and hepatic function tests prior to treatment and on a regular basis during therapy. Monitor for nausea and vomiting (pretreatment with antiemetic may be required), ototoxicity (audiometry may be advisable), bone marrow depression, anemia, bleeding, and peripheral neuropathy.

Patient Education This medicine can only be administered intravenously. Report immediately any redness, burning, pain, or swelling at infusion site. It is important that you maintain adequate nutrition and hydration, unless instructed to restrict fluid intake. You will be susceptible to infection. May cause nausea, vomiting, mouth sores, or loss of hair (reversible). Report chest pain or palpitations; sore throat, fever, chills, unusual fatigue; unusual bruising/bleeding; respiratory difficulty; numbness, pain, or tingling in extremities; muscle cramps or twitching; or change in hearing acuity.

Geriatric Considerations Peripheral neuropathy and severe thrombocytopenia are more frequent in patients >65 years of age.

Breast-Feeding Considerations Due to the potential for toxicity in nursing infants, breast-feeding is not recommended.

Pregnancy Considerations Embryotoxicity and teratogenicity have been observed in animal studies. There are no adequate and well-controlled studies in pregnant women. May cause fetal harm if administered during pregnancy. Women of childbearing potential should avoid becoming pregnant during treatment.

Other Issues Carboplatin is sometimes confused with cisplatin. Institute measures to prevent mix-ups.

◆ **Carboprost** *see* Carboprost Tromethamine *on page* 299

Carboprost Tromethamine (KAR boe prost tro METH a meen)

U.S. Brand Names Hemabate®

Index Terms Carboprost; Prostaglandin F_2

Generic Availability (U.S.) No

Pharmacologic Category Abortifacient; Prostaglandin

Pregnancy Risk Factor C

Lactation Excretion in breast milk unknown

Use Termination of pregnancy; treatment of refractory postpartum uterine bleeding

Unlabeled/Investigational Use Investigational: Hemorrhagic cystitis

Mechanism of Action/Effect Carboprost tromethamine is a prostaglandin similar to prostaglandin F_2. Carboprost tromethamine stimulates the gravid uterus to contract, which usually results in expulsion of the products of conception. Used to induce abortion between 13-20 weeks of pregnancy.

Contraindications Hypersensitivity to carboprost tromethamine or any component of the formulation; acute pelvic inflammatory disease; active cardiac, pulmonary, renal, or hepatic dysfunction

Warnings/Precautions **[U.S. Boxed Warning] Potent oxytocic agent; use with strict adherence to recommended dosing. Immediate intensive care and acute surgical facilities must be available.** Transient pyrexia and increased blood pressure may be observed with treatment. Use caution with history of asthma; hypotension or hypertension; cardiovascular, adrenal, renal, or hepatic disease; anemia; jaundice; diabetes; epilepsy; or compromised uteri. Concomitant use of antiemetic and antidiarrheal agents is recommended to decrease incidence of GI side effects. Safety and efficacy have not been established in pediatric patients.

Drug Interactions

Avoid Concomitant Use There are no known interactions where it is recommended to avoid concomitant use.

Decreased Effect There are no known significant interactions involving a decrease in effect.

Increased Effect/Toxicity There are no known significant interactions involving an increase in effect.

Adverse Reactions Frequency not defined. Effects due to increased smooth muscle contractility are most common.

Cardiovascular: Chest pain, flushing, hypertension, syncope, palpitation, tachycardia, tightness of chest

Central nervous system: Anxiety, chills/shivering, dizziness, drowsiness, dystonia, faintness, headache, lethargy, lightheadedness, nervousness, sleep disturbance, temperature elevation (may be drug induced or due to postabortion endometritis), vasovagal syndrome, vertigo

Dermatologic: Rash

Endocrine & metabolic: Breast tenderness, dysmenorrhea-like pain, endometritis, hot flashes, thyroid storm

Gastrointestinal: Choking sensation, diarrhea (~2/3 patients), dry throat, epigastric pain, gagging/retching, hematemesis, nausea (~1/3 patients), taste alteration, thirst, throat fullness, vomiting (~2/3 patients), xerostomia

Genitourinary: Perforated uterus, posterior cervical perforation, urinary tract infection, uterine bleeding (excessive), uterine rupture, uterine sacculation

Local: Injection site pain

Neuromuscular & skeletal: Backache, leg cramps, muscular pain, paresthesia, torticollis, weakness

Ocular: Blurred vision, eye pain, eyelid twitching

Otic: Tinnitus

Respiratory: Asthma, cough, bronchospasm, dyspnea, epistaxis, hyperventilation, pulmonary edema, respiratory distress, upper respiratory tract infection, wheezing

Miscellaneous: Diaphoresis, hiccups, retained placental fragment, septic shock

Pharmacodynamics/Kinetics

Excretion Urine

Available Dosage Forms

Injection, solution:

Hemabate®: Carboprost 250 mcg and tromethamine 83 mcg per mL (1 mL)

Dosing

Adult & Geriatric

Abortion: I.M.: 250 mcg, then 250 mcg at 1.5- to 3.5-hour intervals, depending on uterine response; a 500 mcg dose may be given if uterine response is not adequate after several 250 mcg doses; do not exceed 12 mg total dose or continuous administration for >2 days

Refractory postpartum uterine bleeding: I.M.: Initial: 250 mcg; if needed, may repeat at 15- to 90-minute intervals; maximum total dose: 2 mg (8 doses)

Hemorrhagic cystitis (unlabeled use): Bladder irrigation: [0.1-1.0 mg/dL as solution] 50 mL instilled into bladder 4 times/day for 1 hour

Administration

I.M. Give deep I.M.; rotate site if repeat injections are required.

I.V. Do not inject I.V.; may result in bronchospasm, hypertension, vomiting, or anaphylaxis.

Stability

Reconstitution Bladder irrigation: Dilute immediately prior to administration in NS; stability unknown.

Storage Store under refrigeration at 2°C to 8°C (36°F to 46°F).

Monitoring and Teaching Issues

Physical Assessment Premedication with an antiemetic should be considered. Assess for complete expulsion of uterine contents (fetal tissue).

Patient Education This medication is used to stimulate expulsion of uterine contents (fetal tissue) or stimulate uterine contractions to reduce uterine bleeding. Report increased blood loss, acute abdominal cramping, foul-smelling vaginal discharge, or persistent elevation of temperature. Increased temperature may occur 1-16 hours after therapy and last for several hours.

Pregnancy Considerations Teratogenic effects were not observed in animal studies. Carboprost tromethamine is not considered feticidal, but is used to terminate pregnancy due to its ability to stimulate uterine contractions. Use is not indicated if the fetus has reached a stage of viability *in utero*. Complete abortion may not be induced in ~20% of cases.

- **Cardene® I.V.** *see* NiCARdipine *on page 1309*
- **Cardene® SR** *see* NiCARdipine *on page 1309*
- **Cardizem®** *see* Diltiazem *on page 536*
- **Cardizem® CD** *see* Diltiazem *on page 536*
- **Cardizem® LA** *see* Diltiazem *on page 536*
- **Cardura®** *see* Doxazosin *on page 575*
- **Cardura® XL** *see* Doxazosin *on page 575*
- **Carimune® NF** *see* Immune Globulin *on page 961*
- **Carisoprodate** *see* Carisoprodol *on page 300*

Carisoprodol (kar eye soe PROE dole)

U.S. Brand Names Soma®

Index Terms Carisoprodate; Isobamate

Generic Availability (U.S.) Yes

Pharmacologic Category Skeletal Muscle Relaxant

Medication Safety Issues

Beers Criteria medication: This drug may be inappropriate for use in geriatric patients (high severity risk).

Pregnancy Risk Factor C

Lactation Enters breast milk/use caution

Use Short-term (2-3 weeks) treatment of acute musculoskeletal pain

Mechanism of Action/Effect Precise mechanism is not yet clear, but many effects have been ascribed to its central depressant actions. In animals, carisoprodol blocks interneuronal activity and depresses polysynaptic neuron transmission in the spinal cord and reticular formation of the brain. It is also metabolized to meprobamate, which has anxiolytic and sedative effects.

Contraindications Hypersensitivity to carisoprodol, meprobamate, or any component of the formulation; acute intermittent porphyria

Warnings/Precautions Can cause CNS depression, which may impair physical or mental abilities. Patients must be cautioned about performing tasks which require mental alertness (eg, operating machinery or driving); postmarketing reports of motor vehicle accidents have been associated with use. Effects with other CNS-depressant drugs or ethanol may be potentiated. Use with caution in patients with hepatic/renal dysfunction. Tolerance or drug dependence may result from extended use. Limit use to 2-3 weeks; use caution in patients who may be prone to addiction. May precipitate withdrawal after abrupt cessation of prolonged use.

Idiosyncratic reactions and/or severe allergic reactions may occur. Idiosyncratic reactions occur following the initial dose and may include severe weakness, transient quadriplegia, euphoria, or vision loss (temporary). Has been associated (rarely) with seizures in patients with and without seizure history. Carisoprodol should be used with caution in patients who are poor CYP2C19 metabolizers; poor metabolizers have been shown to have a fourfold increase in exposure to carisoprodol and a 50% reduced exposure to the metabolite meprobamate compared to normal metabolizers. This class of medication is poorly tolerated by the elderly due to anticholinergic effects, sedation, and weakness. Efficacy is questionable at dosages tolerated by elderly patients (Beers Criteria).

Drug Interactions

Metabolism/Transport Effects Substrate of CYP2C19 (major)

Avoid Concomitant Use There are no known interactions where it is recommended to avoid concomitant use.

Decreased Effect

The levels/effects of Carisoprodol may be decreased by: CYP2C19 Inducers (Strong)

Increased Effect/Toxicity

Carisoprodol may increase the levels/effects of: Alcohol (Ethyl); CNS Depressants; Methotrimeprazine

The levels/effects of Carisoprodol may be increased by: CYP2C19 Inhibitors (Moderate); CYP2C19 Inhibitors (Strong); Droperidol; Methotrimeprazine

Nutritional/Ethanol Interactions Ethanol: Avoid ethanol (may increase CNS depression).

Adverse Reactions

>10%: Central nervous system: Drowsiness (13% to 17%)

1% to 10%: Central nervous system: Dizziness (7% to 8%), headache (3% to 5%)

Pharmacodynamics/Kinetics

Onset of Action ~30 minutes

Duration of Action 4-6 hours

Time to Peak 1.5-2 hours

Half-Life Elimination ~2 hours; Meprobamate: 10 hours

Metabolism Hepatic, via CYP2C19 to active metabolite (meprobamate)

Excretion Urine, as metabolite

Available Dosage Forms

Tablet, oral: 350 mg

Soma®: 250 mg, 350 mg

Dosing

Adult Note: Carisoprodol should only be used for short periods (2-3 weeks) due to lack of evidence of effectiveness with prolonged use.

Acute musculoskeletal pain: Oral: 250-350 mg 3 times/day and at bedtime

Geriatric Not recommended for use in the elderly.

Pediatric Children ≥16 years: Refer to adult dosing.

Renal Impairment Use in renal impairment has not been studied; use with caution.

Dialysis: Removed by hemo- and peritoneal dialysis

Hepatic Impairment Use in hepatic impairment has not been studied; use with caution.

Administration

Oral Administer with or without food.

Stability

Storage Store at controlled room temperature of 20°C to 25°C (68°F to 77°F).

Monitoring and Teaching Issues

Physical Assessment Monitor for excessive drowsiness at beginning of therapy and periodically throughout. Do not discontinue abruptly; taper dosage slowly (withdrawal symptoms may occur).

Patient Education Do not use alcohol. You may experience drowsiness, dizziness, lightheadedness, nausea, vomiting, cramping, headache, or postural hypotension. Report excessive drowsiness or mental agitation; palpitations, rapid heartbeat, or chest pain; skin rash; muscle cramping or tremors; or respiratory difficulty.

Dietary Considerations May give with or without food.

Geriatric Considerations Avoid or use with caution in the elderly; not considered a drug of choice because of the risk of orthostatic hypotension and CNS depression; no data available on the use of skeletal muscle relaxants in the geriatric population.

This medication is considered to be potentially inappropriate in this patient population (Beers Criteria severity: High).

Breast-Feeding Considerations Carisoprodol levels in breast milk may be 2-4 times that of maternal plasma levels. The estimated dose to the infant was reported as 6.9% of the weight adjusted maternal dose in one case report and ~4% of the weight-adjusted maternal dose in another. In both cases, breast milk production was decreased requiring supplemental formula or cessation of breast-feeding. Other than slight sedation reported in one infant, no symptoms of withdrawal or other adverse events were noted in these 2 cases. Effects on long-term development are not known.

Pregnancy Considerations Animal data suggests that carisoprodol crosses placenta and adverse events have been observed in animal studies. Limited postmarketing data with meprobamate (the active metabolite) demonstrate a possible risk for congenital malformations. Use only if benefit outweighs the risk.

Carisoprodol and Aspirin (kar eye soe PROE dole & AS pir in)

U.S. Brand Names Soma® Compound

Index Terms Aspirin and Carisoprodol

Generic Availability (U.S.) Yes

Pharmacologic Category Skeletal Muscle Relaxant

Medication Safety Issues

Beers Criteria medication: This drug (carisoprodol) may be inappropriate for use in geriatric patients (high severity risk).

Pregnancy Risk Factor D

Lactation Enters breast milk/not recommended

Use Relief of discomfort associated with acute, painful skeletal muscle conditions

Available Dosage Forms

Tablet: Carisoprodol 200 mg and aspirin 325 mg

Soma® Compound: Carisoprodol 200 mg and aspirin 325 mg

Dosing

Adult Acute skeletal muscle pain: Oral: 1-2 tablets 4 times/day for 2-3 weeks (maximum: 8 tablets/24 hours)

Geriatric Avoid use in the elderly due to risk of orthostatic hypotension and CNS depression.

Pediatric Children ≥16 years: Refer to adult dosing.

Renal Impairment Use in renal impairment has not been studied; use with caution.

Hepatic Impairment Use in hepatic impairment has not been studied; use with caution.

Monitoring and Teaching Issues

Physical Assessment See individual agents.

Patient Education See individual agents.

Related Information

Aspirin *on page* 155

Carisoprodol *on page* 300

Carmustine (kar MUS teen)

U.S. Brand Names BiCNU®; Gliadel®

Index Terms BCNU; bis-chloronitrosourea; Carmustinum; WR-139021

Generic Availability (U.S.) No

Pharmacologic Category Antineoplastic Agent; Antineoplastic Agent, Alkylating Agent; Antineoplastic Agent, Alkylating Agent (Nitrosourea)

Medication Safety Issues

Sound-alike/look-alike issues:

Carmustine may be confused with bendamustine, lomustine

High alert medication: The Institute for Safe Medication Practices (ISMP) includes this medication among its list of drugs which have a heightened risk of causing significant patient harm when used in error.

Pregnancy Risk Factor D

Lactation Excretion in breast milk unknown/not recommended

Use

Injection: Treatment of brain tumors (glioblastoma, brainstem glioma, medulloblastoma, astrocytoma, ependymoma, and metastatic brain tumors), multiple myeloma, Hodgkin's disease (relapsed or refractory), non-Hodgkin's lymphomas (relapsed or refractory)

Wafer (implant): Adjunct to surgery in patients with recurrent glioblastoma multiforme; adjunct to surgery and radiation in patients with high-grade malignant glioma

Unlabeled/Investigational Use Treatment of metastatic melanoma

Mechanism of Action/Effect Interferes with the normal function of DNA and RNA by alkylation and cross-linking the strands of DNA and RNA, and by possible protein modification; may also inhibit enzyme processes by carbamylation of amino acids in protein

Contraindications Hypersensitivity to carmustine or any component of the formulation

Warnings/Precautions Hazardous agent - use appropriate precautions for handling and disposal. **[U.S. Boxed Warning]: Bone marrow suppression (thrombocytopenia, leukopenia) is the major toxicity and may be delayed; monitor blood counts weekly for at least 6 weeks after administration. Myelosuppression is cumulative; consider nadir blood counts from prior dose for dosage adjustment. May cause bleeding (due to thrombocytopenia) or infections (due to neutropenia); monitor closely.** Administer with caution to patients with depressed platelet, leukocyte, or erythrocyte counts; renal or hepatic impairment. Diluent contains significant amounts of ethanol; use caution with aldehyde dehydrogenase-2 deficiency or history of "alcohol-flushing syndrome."

[U.S. Boxed Warning]: Dose-related pulmonary toxicity may occur; patients receiving cumulative doses >1400 mg/m^2 are at higher risk. Baseline pulmonary function tests are recommended. **[U.S. Boxed Warning]: Delayed onset of pulmonary fibrosis has occurred up to 17 years after treatment** in children (1-16 years) who received carmustine in cumulative doses ranging from 770-1800 mg/m^2 combined with cranial radiotherapy for intracranial tumors. **[U.S. Boxed Warning]: Should be administered under the supervision of an experienced cancer chemotherapy physician.** Long-term use may be associated with the development of secondary malignancies. Safety and efficacy in children have not been established.

Drug Interactions

Avoid Concomitant Use

Avoid concomitant use of Carmustine with any of the following: BCG; Natalizumab; Pimecrolimus; Roflumilast; Tacrolimus (Topical); Vaccines (Live)

Decreased Effect

Carmustine may decrease the levels/effects of: BCG; Cardiac Glycosides; Sipuleucel-T; Vaccines (Inactivated); Vaccines (Live)

The levels/effects of Carmustine may be decreased by: Echinacea

Increased Effect/Toxicity

Carmustine may increase the levels/effects of: Leflunomide; Natalizumab; Vaccines (Live)

The levels/effects of Carmustine may be increased by: Cimetidine; Denosumab; Melphalan; Pimecrolimus; Roflumilast; Tacrolimus (Topical); Trastuzumab

Nutritional/Ethanol Interactions Ethanol: Diluent for infusion contains ethanol; avoid concurrent use of medications that inhibit aldehyde dehydrogenase-2 or cause disulfiram-like reactions.

Adverse Reactions

>10%:

Cardiovascular: Hypotension (with high-dose I.V. therapy, due to the alcohol content of the diluent)

Central nervous system: Ataxia, dizziness

Postoperatively: Seizure (wafer 5% to 54%), brain edema (wafer 4% to 23%)

Dermatologic: Burning (with skin contact), hyperpigmentation of skin (with skin contact)

Gastrointestinal: Severe nausea and vomiting, usually begins within 2-4 hours of drug administration and lasts for 4-6 hours; dose related. Patients should receive a prophylactic antiemetic regimen.

Hematologic: Myelosuppression (cumulative, dose related, delayed, and dose limiting), thrombocytopenia (onset: 28 days; recovery: 35-42 days), leukopenia (onset: 35-42 days; recovery: 42-56 days)

Hepatic: Reversible increases in bilirubin, alkaline phosphatase, and AST occur in 20% to 25% of patients

Local: Pain and burning at injection site, phlebitis

Neuromuscular & skeletal: Weakness (wafer 22%)

Ocular: Ocular toxicities (transient conjunctival flushing and blurred vision), retinal hemorrhages

Respiratory: Interstitial fibrosis occurs in up to 50% of patients receiving a cumulative dose >1400 mg/m^2, or bone marrow transplantation doses; may be delayed up to 3 years; rare in patients receiving lower doses. A history of lung disease or concomitant bleomycin therapy may increase the risk of this reaction. Patients with forced vital capacity (FVC) or carbon monoxide diffusing capacity of the lungs (DLCO) <70% of predicted are at higher risk.

Miscellaneous: Disease progression/performance deterioration (wafer 82%)

1% to 10%:

Cardiovascular: Chest pain, deep thrombophlebitis (wafer), facial edema (wafer), peripheral edema (wafer)

Central nervous system: Wafer: Amnesia, anxiety, aphasia, ataxia, brain abscess, confusion, convulsion, CSF leaks, depression, diplopia, dizziness, facial paralysis, headache, hemiplegia, hydrocephalus, hypoesthesia, insomnia, intracranial hypertension, meningitis, somnolence, speech disorder, stupor

Dermatologic: Facial flushing, probably due to the alcohol diluent; alopecia, rash (wafer), wound healing abnormal (wafer)

Gastrointestinal: Abdominal pain, anorexia, constipation, diarrhea, stomatitis

Hematologic: Anemia, hemorrhage (wafer)

Local: Abscess (wafer)

Neuromuscular & skeletal: Back pain

Pharmacodynamics/Kinetics

Half-Life Elimination Biphasic: Initial: 1.4 minutes; Secondary: 20 minutes (active metabolites: plasma half-life of 67 hours)

Metabolism Rapidly hepatic; forms active metabolites

Excretion Urine (~60% to 70%) within 96 hours; lungs (6% to 10% as CO_2)

Available Dosage Forms

Injection, powder for reconstitution:

BiCNU®: 100 mg

Wafer, for implantation:

Gliadel®: 7.7 mg (8s)

Dosing

Adult & Geriatric Refer to individual protocols.

Usual dosage (per manufacturer labeling): I.V.: 150-200 mg/m^2 every 6 weeks **or** 75-100 mg/m^2/day for 2 days every 6 weeks

Alternative regimens (unlabeled):

75-120 mg/m^2 days 1 and 2 every 6-8 weeks **or**

50-80 mg/m^2 days 1,2,3 every 6-8 weeks

Primary brain cancer: I.V.:

150-200 mg/m^2 every 6-8 weeks as a single dose **or**

75-120 mg/m^2 days 1 and 2 every 6-8 weeks **or**

20-65 mg/m^2 every 4-6 weeks **or**

0.5-1 mg/kg every 4-6 weeks **or**

40-80 mg/m^2/day for 3 days every 6-8 weeks

Autologous BMT: I.V.:

Combination therapy: Up to 300-900 mg/m^2

Single-agent therapy: Up to 1200 mg/m^2 (fatal necrosis is associated with doses >2 g/m^2)

Glioblastoma multiforme (recurrent), malignant glioma: Implantation (wafer): Up to 8 wafers may be placed in the resection cavity (total dose 62.6 mg); should the size and shape not accommodate 8 wafers, the maximum number of wafers allowed should be placed

Pediatric Refer to individual protocols: Children (unlabeled use): I.V.: 200-250 mg/m^2 every 4-6 weeks as a single dose

Renal Impairment I.V.: The FDA-approved labeling does not contain renal dosing adjustment guidelines. The following dosage adjustments have been used by some clinicians (Kintzel, 1995):

Cl_{cr} 46-60 mL/minute: Administer 80% of dose

Cl_{cr} 31-45 mL/minute: Administer 75% of dose

Cl_{cr} ≤30 mL/minute: Consider use of alternative drug.

Hepatic Impairment Dosage adjustment may be necessary; however, no specific guidelines are available.

Administration

I.V. Irritant (alcohol-based diluent). Injection: Significant absorption to PVC containers - should be administered in either glass or polyolefin containers. I.V. infusion over 1-2 hours is recommended; infusion through a free-flowing saline or dextrose infusion, or administration through a central catheter can alleviate venous pain/irritation.

High-dose carmustine: Maximum rate of infusion of ≤3 mg/m^2/minute to avoid excessive flushing, agitation, and hypotension; infusions should run over at least 2 hours; some investigational protocols dictate shorter infusions. **(High-dose carmustine is fatal if not followed by bone marrow or peripheral stem cell infusions.)**

Other Implant: Use appropriate precautions for handling and disposal; double glove before handling; outer gloves should be discarded as chemotherapy waste after handling wafers. Any wafer or remnant that is removed upon repeat surgery should be discarded as chemotherapy waste. The outer surface of the external foil pouch is not sterile. Open pouch gently; avoid pressure on the wafers to prevent breakage. Wafer that are broken in half may be used, however, wafers broken into more than 2 pieces should be discarded. Oxidized regenerated cellulose (Surgicel®) may be placed over the wafer to secure; irrigate cavity prior to closure.

Stability

Reconstitution Injection: Reconstitute initially with 3 mL of absolute alcohol; then further reconstitute with SWFI (27 mL) to a concentration of 3.3 mg/mL; protect from light; further dilute for infusion with D_5W or NS, using a non-PVC container.

Storage

Injection: Store intact vials under refrigeration at 2°C to 8°C (36°F to 46°F); provided diluent may be stored in refrigerator or at room temperature; intact vials are stable for 7 days at room temperature. Reconstituted solutions are stable for 24 hours refrigerated (2°C to 8°C) and protected from light. Solutions diluted to a concentration of 0.2 mg/mL in D_5W are stable for 8 hours at room temperature (25°C) in glass or polyolefin containers and protected from light.

Wafer: Store at or below -20°C (-4°F). Unopened foil pouches may be kept at room temperature for up to 6 hours.

Monitoring and Teaching Issues

Laboratory Monitoring CBC with differential, platelet count, pulmonary function, liver and renal function

Physical Assessment Administer antiemetic prior to therapy. Infusion site should be monitored closely to prevent extravasation. For BMT high-dose infusion: Patient must be monitored closely during and following infusion; supine (Trandelenburg position may be necessary), fluid support, and vasopressor support should be available. Assess results of hematology, pulmonary, hepatic, and renal function tests at baseline and periodically during therapy. Pulmonary function should be assessed for extended periods following high dose or BMT doses; acute lung injury can occur 1-3 months after treatment and pulmonary fibrosis may be delayed up to 3 years.

Patient Education This medication is usually administered by I.V. Report immediately any pain, burning, or swelling at infusion site; sudden onset chest pain; or difficulty breathing or swallowing. It is important that you maintain adequate nutrition between treatments and adequate hydration, unless instructed to restrict fluid intake. You will be susceptible to infection. May cause nausea, vomiting, anorexia, mouth sores, or hyperpigmentation of skin and loss of hair (reversible). Report immediately any dyspnea, cough, or fever; chest pain or palpitations; sore throat, chills, persistent or unusual fatigue; unusual bruising/bleeding; change in color of urine or stool; change in urinary pattern; change in visual acuity; seizure activity; or CNS changes.

Breast-Feeding Considerations Due to the potential for serious adverse reactions in the nursing infant, breast-feeding should be discontinued.

Pregnancy Considerations Teratogenicity and embryotoxicity have been demonstrated in animal studies. Carmustine can cause fetal harm if administered to a pregnant woman. There are no adequate and well-controlled studies in pregnant women. Women of childbearing potential should avoid becoming pregnant while on treatment.

Additional Information Accidental skin contact may cause transient burning and brown discoloration of the skin. Delayed onset pulmonary fibrosis occurring up to 17 years after treatment has been reported in patients who received cumulative doses >1400 mg/m^2.

◆ **Carmustinum** *see* Carmustine *on page* 302

◆ **Carrington® Antifungal [OTC]** *see* Miconazole (Topical) *on page* 1224

◆ **Cartia XT®** *see* Diltiazem *on page* 536

Carvedilol (KAR ve dil ole)

U.S. Brand Names Coreg CR®; Coreg®

Generic Availability (U.S.) Yes: Tablet

Pharmacologic Category Beta Blocker With Alpha-Blocking Activity

Medication Safety Issues

Sound-alike/look-alike issues:

Carvedilol may be confused with atenolol, captopril, carbidopa, carteolol

Coreg® may be confused with Corgard®, Cortef®, Cozaar®

Pregnancy Risk Factor C

Lactation Excretion in breast milk unknown/not recommended

Use Mild-to-severe heart failure of ischemic or cardiomyopathic origin (usually in addition to standard therapy); left ventricular dysfunction following myocardial infarction (MI) (clinically stable with LVEF ≤40%); management of hypertension

Unlabeled/Investigational Use Angina pectoris

Mechanism of Action/Effect Nonselective beta-adrenoreceptor and alpha-adrenergic blocking agent, lowers heart rate and blood pressure. Has been shown to lower risk of hospitalization and increase survival in patients with mild to severe heart failure.

Contraindications Serious hypersensitivity to carvedilol or any component of the formulation; decompensated cardiac failure requiring intravenous inotropic therapy; bronchial asthma or related bronchospastic conditions; second- or third-degree AV block, sick sinus syndrome, and severe bradycardia (except in patients with a functioning artificial pacemaker); cardiogenic shock; severe hepatic impairment

Warnings/Precautions Consider pre-existing conditions such as sick sinus syndrome before initiating. Heart failure patients may experience a worsening of renal function (rare); risk factors include ischemic heart disease, diffuse vascular disease, underlying renal dysfunction, and systolic BP <100 mm Hg. Initiate cautiously and monitor for possible deterioration in patient status (eg, symptoms of HF). Worsening heart failure or fluid retention may occur during upward titration; dose reduction or temporary discontinuation may be necessary. Adjustment of other medications (ACE inhibitors and/or diuretics) may also be required.

Symptomatic hypotension with or without syncope may occur with carvedilol (usually within the first 30 days of therapy); close monitoring of patient is required especially with initial dosing and dosing increases; blood pressure must be lowered at a rate appropriate for the patient's clinical condition. Initiation with a low dose, gradual up-titration, and administration with food may help to decrease the occurrence of hypotension or syncope. Patients should be advised to avoid driving or other hazardous tasks during initiation of therapy due to the risk of syncope. Beta-blocker therapy should not be withdrawn abruptly (particularly in patients with CAD), but gradually tapered to avoid acute tachycardia, hypertension, and/or ischemia.

In general, patients with bronchospastic disease should not receive beta-blockers; if used at all, should be used cautiously with close monitoring. May precipitate or aggravate symptoms of arterial insufficiency in patients with PVD and Raynaud's disease; use with caution and monitor for progression of arterial obstruction. Use caution with concurrent use of verapamil or diltiazem; bradycardia or heart block can occur. Use cautiously in patients with diabetes because it can mask prominent hypoglycemic symptoms. In patients with heart failure and diabetes, use of carvedilol may worsen hyperglycemia; may require adjustment of antidiabetic agents. May mask signs of hyperthyroidism (eg, tachycardia); if hyperthyroidism is suspected, carefully manage and monitor; abrupt withdrawal may exacerbate symptoms of hyperthyroidism or precipitate thyroid storm. May induce or exacerbate psoriasis. Use with caution in patients with myasthenia gravis or psychiatric disease (may cause CNS depression). Use with caution in patients with mild-to-moderate hepatic impairment; use is contraindicated in patients with severe impairment. Manufacturer recommends discontinuation of therapy if liver injury occurs (confirmed by laboratory testing). Adequate alpha-blockade is required prior to use of any beta-blocker for patients with untreated pheochromocytoma. Use caution with history of severe anaphylaxis to allergens; patients taking beta-blockers may become more sensitive to repeated challenges. Treatment of anaphylaxis (eg, epinephrine) in patients taking beta-blockers may be ineffective or promote undesirable effects. Use care with anesthetic agents that decrease myocardial function.

Drug Interactions

Metabolism/Transport Effects **Substrate** of CYP1A2 (minor), CYP2C9 (major), CYP2D6 (major), CYP2E1 (minor), CYP3A4 (minor), P-glycoprotein; **Inhibits** P-glycoprotein

Avoid Concomitant Use

Avoid concomitant use of Carvedilol with any of the following: Methacholine; Topotecan

Decreased Effect

Carvedilol may decrease the levels/effects of: Beta2-Agonists; Theophylline Derivatives

The levels/effects of Carvedilol may be decreased by: Barbiturates; Herbs (Hypertensive Properties); Methylphenidate; Nonsteroidal Anti-Inflammatory Agents; Peginterferon Alfa-2b; P-Glycoprotein Inducers; Rifamycin Derivatives; Yohimbine

Increased Effect/Toxicity

Carvedilol may increase the levels/effects of: Alpha-/Beta-Agonists (Direct-Acting); Alpha1-Blockers; Alpha2-Agonists; Amifostine; Antihypertensives; Antipsychotic Agents (Phenothiazines); Bupivacaine; Cardiac Glycosides; Colchicine; CycloSPORINE; CycloSPORINE (Systemic); Dabigatran Etexilate; Digoxin; Everolimus; Fingolimod; Hypotensive Agents; Insulin; Lidocaine; Lidocaine (Systemic); Lidocaine (Topical); Mepivacaine; Methacholine; Midodrine; P-Glycoprotein Substrates; RiTUXimab; Rivaroxaban; Sulfonylureas; Topotecan

The levels/effects of Carvedilol may be increased by: Acetylcholinesterase Inhibitors; Aminoquinolines (Antimalarial); Amiodarone; Anilidopiperidine Opioids; Antipsychotic Agents (Phenothiazines); Calcium Channel Blockers (Nondihydropyridine); Cimetidine; Conivaptan; CYP2C9 Inhibitors (Moderate); CYP2C9 Inhibitors (Strong); CYP2D6 Inhibitors (Moderate); CYP2D6 Inhibitors (Strong); Darunavir; Diazoxide; Dipyridamole; Disopyramide; Dronedarone; Herbs (Hypotensive Properties); MAO Inhibitors; Pentoxifylline; P-Glycoprotein Inhibitors; Phosphodiesterase 5 Inhibitors; Propafenone; Propoxyphene; Prostacyclin Analogues; QuiNIDine; Reserpine; Selective Serotonin Reuptake Inhibitors

Nutritional/Ethanol Interactions

Food: Food decreases rate but not extent of absorption. Administration with food minimizes risks of orthostatic hypotension.

Herb/Nutraceutical: Avoid herbs with hypertensive properties (bayberry, blue cohosh, cayenne, ephedra, ginger, ginseng [American], kola, licorice); may diminish the antihypertensive effect of carvedilol. Avoid herbs with hypotensive properties (black cohosh, California poppy, coleus, golden seal, hawthorn, mistletoe, periwinkle, quinine, shepherd's purse); may enhance the hypotensive effect of carvedilol.

Adverse Reactions Note: Frequency ranges include data from hypertension and heart failure trials. Higher rates of adverse reactions have generally been noted in patients with heart failure. However, the frequency of adverse effects associated with placebo is also increased in this population.

>10%:
- Cardiovascular: Hypotension (9% to 20%)
- Central nervous system: Dizziness (2% to 32%), fatigue (4% to 24%)
- Endocrine & metabolic: Hyperglycemia (5% to 12%)
- Gastrointestinal: Diarrhea (1% to 12%), weight gain (10% to 12%)
- Neuromuscular & skeletal: Weakness (7% to 11%)

1% to 10%:
- Cardiovascular: Bradycardia (2% to 10%), syncope (3% to 8%), peripheral edema (1% to 7%), generalized edema (5% to 6%), angina (1% to 6%), dependent edema (≤4%), AV block, cerebrovascular accident, hypertension, hyper-/hypovolemia, postural hypotension, palpitation
- Central nervous system: Headache (5% to 8%), depression, fever, hypoesthesia, hypotonia, insomnia, malaise, somnolence, vertigo
- Endocrine & metabolic: Hypercholesterolemia (1% to 4%), hypertriglyceridemia (1%), diabetes mellitus, gout, hyperkalemia, hyperuricemia, hypoglycemia, hyponatremia
- Gastrointestinal: Nausea (2% to 9%), vomiting (1% to 6%), abdominal pain, melena, periodontitis, weight loss
- Genitourinary: Impotence
- Hematologic: Anemia, prothrombin decreased, purpura, thrombocytopenia
- Hepatic: Alkaline phosphatase increased (1% to 3%), GGT increased, transaminases increased
- Neuromuscular & skeletal: Back pain (2% to 7%), arthralgia (1% to 6%), arthritis, muscle cramps, paresthesia
- Ocular: Blurred vision (1% to 5%)
- Renal: BUN increased (≤6%), nonprotein nitrogen increased (6%), albuminuria, creatinine increased, glycosuria, hematuria, renal insufficiency
- Respiratory: Cough (5% to 8%), nasopharyngitis (4%), rales (4%), dyspnea (>3%), pulmonary edema (>3%), rhinitis (2%), nasal congestion (1%), sinus congestion (1%)
- Miscellaneous: Injury (3% to 6%), allergy, flu-like syndrome, sudden death

Pharmacodynamics/Kinetics

Onset of Action 1-2 hours; Peak antihypertensive effect: ~1-2 hours

Absorption Rapid and extensive

Bioavailability Immediate release: 25% to 35% (due to significant first-pass metabolism); Extended release: 85% of immediate release

Time to Peak Extended release: 5 hours

Protein Binding >98%, primarily to albumin

Half-Life Elimination 7-10 hours

Metabolism Extensively hepatic, via CYP2D6, 2C9, 3A4, and 2C19 (2% excreted unchanged); three active metabolites (4-hydroxyphenyl metabolite is 13 times more potent than parent drug for beta-blockade); first-pass effect; plasma concentrations in the elderly and those with cirrhotic liver disease are 50% and 4-7 times higher, respectively

Excretion Primarily feces

Available Dosage Forms

Capsule, extended release, oral:
- Coreg CR®: 10 mg, 20 mg, 40 mg, 80 mg

Tablet, oral: 3.125 mg, 6.25 mg, 12.5 mg, 25 mg
- Coreg®: 3.125 mg, 6.25 mg, 12.5 mg, 25 mg

Dosing

Adult & Geriatric Reduce dosage if heart rate drops to <55 beats/minute.

Hypertension: Oral:

Immediate release: 6.25 mg twice daily; if tolerated, dose should be maintained for 1-2 weeks, then increased to 12.5 mg twice daily. If necessary, dosage may be increased to a maximum of 25 mg twice daily after 1-2 weeks.

Extended release: Initial: 20 mg once daily, if tolerated, dose should be maintained for 1-2 weeks then increased to 40 mg once daily if necessary; maximum dose: 80 mg once daily

Heart failure: Oral:

Immediate release: 3.125 mg twice daily for 2 weeks; if this dose is tolerated, may increase to 6.25 mg twice daily. Double the dose every 2 weeks to the highest dose tolerated by patient. (Prior to initiating therapy, other heart failure medications should be stabilized and fluid retention minimized.)

Maximum recommended dose:
- Mild-to-moderate heart failure:
  - <85 kg: 25 mg twice daily
  - >85 kg: 50 mg twice daily
- Severe heart failure: 25 mg twice daily

Extended release: Initial: 10 mg once daily for 2 weeks; if the dose is tolerated, increase dose to 20 mg, 40 mg, and 80 mg over successive intervals of at least 2 weeks. Maintain on lower dose if higher dose is not tolerated.

Left ventricular dysfunction following MI: Oral: **Note:** Should be initiated only after patient is hemodynamically stable and fluid retention has been minimized.

Immediate release: Initial 3.125-6.25 mg twice daily; increase dosage incrementally (ie, from 6.25-12.5 mg twice daily) at intervals of 3-10 days, based on tolerance, to a target dose of 25 mg twice daily.

Extended release: Initial: Extended release: Initial: 10-20 mg once daily; increase dosage incrementally at intervals of 3-10 days, based on tolerance, to a target dose of 80 mg once daily.

Angina pectoris (unlabeled use): Oral: *Immediate release:* 25-50 mg twice daily

Conversion from immediate release to extended release (Coreg CR®):

Current dose immediate release tablets 3.125 mg twice daily: Convert to extended release capsules 10 mg once daily

Current dose immediate release tablets 6.25 mg twice daily: Convert to extended release capsules 20 mg once daily

Current dose immediate release tablets 12.5 mg twice daily: Convert to extended release capsules 40 mg once daily

Current dose immediate release tablets 25 mg twice daily: Convert to extended release capsules 80 mg once daily

Renal Impairment None necessary

Hepatic Impairment Use is contraindicated in severe liver dysfunction.

Administration

Oral Administer with food to minimize the risk of orthostatic hypotension. Extended release capsules should not be crushed or chewed. Capsules may be opened and sprinkled on applesauce for immediate use.

Stability

Storage

Coreg®: Store at <30°C (<86°F). Protect from moisture.

Coreg CR®: Store at 25°C (77°F); excursions permitted to 15°C to 30°C (59°F to 86°F).

Monitoring and Teaching Issues

Laboratory Monitoring Renal studies, BUN, liver function

Physical Assessment Blood pressure and heart rate should be assessed prior to and following first dose and any change in dose. Caution patients with diabetes to monitor glucose levels closely (beta-blockers may alter glucose tolerance).

Patient Education Take pulse daily, prior to taking medication; follow prescriber's instruction about holding medication. If you have diabetes, monitor serum glucose closely (drug may alter glucose tolerance or mask signs of hypoglycemia). You may experience fatigue, dizziness, or postural hypotension. Report unresolved swelling of extremities; respiratory difficulty or new cough; unresolved fatigue; or unusual weight gain.

Dietary Considerations Should be taken with food to minimize the risk of orthostatic hypotension.

Geriatric Considerations Due to alterations in the beta-adrenergic autonomic nervous system, beta-adrenergic blockade may result in less hemodynamic response than seen in younger adults. In U.S. trials conducted by the manufacturer, hypertension patients who were elderly (>65%) had a higher incidence of dizziness (8.8% vs 6%) than seen in younger patients. No other differences noted between young and old in these trials.

Breast-Feeding Considerations It is not known if carvedilol is excreted into human milk. The manufacturer suggests that a decision should be made to either discontinue nursing or discontinue the medication.

Pregnancy Considerations Because adverse events were not observed in animal reproduction studies, carvedilol is classified as pregnancy category C. In a cohort study, an increased risk of cardiovascular defects was observed following maternal use of beta-blockers during pregnancy. Intrauterine growth restriction (IUGR), small placentas, as well as fetal/neonatal bradycardia, hypoglycemia, and/or respiratory depression have been observed following *in utero* exposure to beta-blockers as a class. Adequate facilities for monitoring infants at birth should be available. Untreated chronic maternal hypertension and pre-eclampsia are also associated with adverse events in the fetus, infant, and mother. Carvedilol is not currently recommended for the initial treatment of maternal hypertension during pregnancy.

Additional Information Fluid retention during therapy should be treated with an increase in diuretic dosage.

Related Information

Beta-Blockers *on page 1990*

Heart Failure (Systolic) *on page 2040*

◆ **Casodex®** *see* Bicalutamide *on page 217*

Caspofungin (kas poe FUN jin)

U.S. Brand Names Cancidas®

Index Terms Caspofungin Acetate

Generic Availability (U.S.) No

Pharmacologic Category Antifungal Agent, Parenteral; Echinocandin

Pregnancy Risk Factor C

Lactation Excretion in breast milk unknown/use caution

Use Treatment of invasive *Aspergillus* infections in patients who are refractory or intolerant of other therapy; treatment of candidemia and other *Candida* infections (intra-abdominal abscesses, esophageal, peritonitis, pleural space); empirical treatment for presumed fungal infections in febrile neutropenic patient

Mechanism of Action/Effect Blocks synthesis of a vital component of fungal cell wall, limiting its growth. The cell wall component is unique to specific fungi, limiting any potential for toxicity in mammals.

Contraindications Hypersensitivity to caspofungin or any component of the formulation

Warnings/Precautions Concurrent use of cyclosporine should be limited to patients for whom benefit outweighs risk, due to a high frequency of hepatic transaminase elevations observed during concurrent use. Use caution in hepatic impairment; increased transaminases and rare cases of liver impairment have been reported in pediatric and adult patients. Dosage reduction required in adults with moderate hepatic impairment; safety and efficacy have not been established in children with any degree of hepatic impairment and adults with severe hepatic impairment.

Drug Interactions

Avoid Concomitant Use There are no known interactions where it is recommended to avoid concomitant use.

Decreased Effect

Caspofungin may decrease the levels/effects of: Saccharomyces boulardii; Tacrolimus; Tacrolimus (Systemic)

The levels/effects of Caspofungin may be decreased by: Inducers of Drug Clearance; Rifampin

Increased Effect/Toxicity

The levels/effects of Caspofungin may be increased by: CycloSPORINE; CycloSPORINE (Systemic)

Adverse Reactions

>10%:

Cardiovascular: Hypotension (3% to 20%), peripheral edema (6% to 11%), tachycardia (4% to 11%)
Central nervous system: Fever (6% to 30%), chills (9% to 23%), headache (5% to 15%)
Dermatologic: Rash (4% to 23%)
Endocrine & metabolic: Hypokalemia (5% to 23%)
Gastrointestinal: Diarrhea (6% to 27%), vomiting (6% to 17%), nausea (4% to 15%)
Hematologic: Hemoglobin decreased (18% to 21%), hematocrit decreased (13% to 18%), WBC decreased (12%), anemia (2% to 11%)
Hepatic: Serum alkaline phosphatase increased (9% to 22%), transaminases increased (2% to 18%), bilirubin increased (5% to 13%)
Local: Phlebitis/thrombophlebitis (18%)
Renal: Serum creatinine increased (3% to 11%)
Respiratory: Respiratory failure (2% to 20%), cough (6% to 11%), pneumonia (4% to 11%)
Miscellaneous: Infusion reactions (20% to 35%), septic shock (11% to 14%)

5% to 10%:

Cardiovascular: Hypertension (5% to 6%; children 9% to 10%)
Dermatologic: Erythema (4% to 9%), pruritus (6% to 7%)
Endocrine & metabolic: Hypomagnesemia (7%), hyperglycemia (6%)
Gastrointestinal: Mucosal inflammation (4% to 10%), abdominal pain (4% to 9%)
Hepatic: Albumin decreased (7%)
Local: Infection (1% to 9%, central line)
Renal: Hematuria (10%), blood urea nitrogen increased (4% to 9%)
Respiratory: Dyspnea (9%), pleural effusion (9%), respiratory distress (≤8%), rales (7%)
Miscellaneous: Sepsis (5% to 7%)

Pharmacodynamics/Kinetics

Protein Binding ~97% to albumin

Half-Life Elimination Beta (distribution): 9-11 hours; Terminal: 40-50 hours

Metabolism Slowly, via hydrolysis and *N*-acetylation as well as by spontaneous degradation, with subsequent metabolism to component amino acids. Overall metabolism is extensive.

Excretion Urine (41%; primarily as metabolites, ~1% of total dose as unchanged drug); feces (35%; primarily as metabolites)

Available Dosage Forms

Injection, powder for reconstitution:

Cancidas®: 50 mg, 70 mg

Dosing

Adult & Geriatric Note: Duration of caspofungin treatment should be determined by patient status and clinical response. Empiric therapy should be given until neutropenia resolves. In patients with positive cultures, treatment should continue until 14 days after last positive culture. In neutropenic patients, treatment should be given at least 7 days after both signs and symptoms of infection **and** neutropenia resolve.

Aspergillosis, invasive: Initial dose: 70 mg on day 1; subsequent dosing: 50 mg/day. If clinical response inadequate, may increase up to 70 mg/day if tolerated, but increased efficacy not demonstrated. **Note:** Duration of therapy should be a minimum of 6-12 weeks or throughout period of immunosuppression.

Candidiasis: Initial dose: 70 mg on day 1; subsequent dosing: 50 mg/day; higher doses (150 mg once daily infused over ~2 hours) compared to the standard adult dosing regimen (50 mg once daily) have not demonstrated additional benefit or toxicity in patients with invasive candidiasis (Betts, 2009)

Esophageal: 50 mg/day; **Note:** The majority of patients studied for this indication also had oropharyngeal involvement.

Empiric therapy: Initial dose: 70 mg on day 1; subsequent dosing: 50 mg/day; if clinical response inadequate, may increase up to 70 mg/day if tolerated, but increased efficacy not demonstrated

Dosage adjustment with concomitant use of an enzyme inducer:

Patients receiving rifampin: 70 mg caspofungin daily

Patients receiving carbamazepine, dexamethasone, efavirenz, nevirapine, or phenytoin (and possibly other enzyme inducers) may require an increased daily dose of caspofungin (70 mg/day).

Pediatric

Aspergillosis, candidiasis, empiric therapy: Children >3 months to 17 years: I.V.: Initial dose: 70 mg/m^2 on day 1, subsequent dosing: 50 mg/m^2 once daily, may increase to 70 mg/m^2 once daily if clinical response inadequate (maximum dose: 70 mg)

Dosage adjustment with concomitant use of an enzyme inducer: Patients receiving carbamazepine, dexamethasone, efavirenz, nevirapine, phenytoin, or rifampin (and possibly other enzyme inducers): Consider 70 mg/m^2 once daily (maximum: 70 mg/day)

Renal Impairment No specific dosage adjustment is required; supplemental dose is not required following dialysis.

Hepatic Impairment

Children: Mild-to-severe hepatic insufficiency: No clinical experience

Adults:

Mild hepatic insufficiency (Child-Pugh score 5-6): No adjustment necessary.

Moderate hepatic insufficiency (Child-Pugh score 7-9): 70 mg on day 1 (where recommended), followed by 35 mg once daily.

Severe hepatic insufficiency (Child-Pugh score >9): No clinical experience.

Administration

I.V. Infuse slowly, over 1 hour

Stability

Reconstitution Bring refrigerated vial to room temperature. Reconstitute vials using 0.9% sodium chloride for injection, SWFI, or bacteriostatic water for injection. Mix gently until clear solution is formed; do not use if cloudy or contains particles. Solution should be further diluted with 0.9%, 0.45%, or 0.225% sodium chloride or LR (do not exceed final concentration of 0.5 mg/mL).

Storage Store vials at 2°C to 8°C (36°F to 46°F). Reconstituted solution may be stored at ≤25°C (≤77°F) for 1 hour prior to preparation of infusion solution. Infusion solutions may be stored at ≤25°C (≤77°F) and should be used within 24 hours; up to 48 hours if stored at 2°C to 8°C (36°F to 46°F).

Monitoring and Teaching Issues

Laboratory Monitoring Liver function

Physical Assessment Use caution in presence of hepatic impairment.

Patient Education This medication can only be administered by infusion. Report immediately any pain, burning, or swelling at infusion site or any signs of allergic reaction (eg, respiratory difficulty or swallowing, back pain, chest tightness, rash, hives, swelling of lips or mouth). Report gastrointestinal upset (nausea, vomiting, abdominal pain, diarrhea), swelling of extremities, chest pain or palpations, or unusual cough.

Geriatric Considerations The number of patients >65 years of age in clinical studies was not sufficient to establish whether a difference in response may be anticipated.

Pregnancy Considerations Adverse events have been observed in animal studies. There are no adequate and well-controlled studies in pregnant women. Should be used during pregnancy only if potential benefit justifies the potential risk to the fetus.

- **Caspofungin Acetate** *see* Caspofungin *on page 307*
- **Cataflam®** *see* Diclofenac (Systemic) *on page 518*
- **Catapres®** *see* CloNIDine *on page 408*
- **Catapres-TTS®-1** *see* CloNIDine *on page 408*
- **Catapres-TTS®-2** *see* CloNIDine *on page 408*
- **Catapres-TTS®-3** *see* CloNIDine *on page 408*
- **Catechins** *see* Sinecatechins *on page 1647*
- **Cathflo® Activase®** *see* Alteplase *on page 86*
- **Caverject®** *see* Alprostadil *on page 83*
- **Caverject Impulse®** *see* Alprostadil *on page 83*
- **Cayston®** *see* Aztreonam *on page 185*
- **Caziant®** *see* Ethinyl Estradiol and Desogestrel *on page 695*
- **CB-1348** *see* Chlorambucil *on page 357*
- **CBDCA** *see* CARBOplatin *on page 295*
- **CBZ** *see* CarBAMazepine *on page 287*
- **CC-5013** *see* Lenalidomide *on page 1071*
- **CCI-779** *see* Temsirolimus *on page 1723*
- **2-CdA** *see* Cladribine *on page 389*
- **CDB-2914** *see* Ulipristal *on page 1826*
- **CDCA** *see* Chenodiol *on page 356*
- **CDDP** *see* CISplatin *on page 384*
- **CDP870** *see* Certolizumab Pegol *on page 348*
- **CDX** *see* Bicalutamide *on page 217*
- **CE** *see* Estrogens (Conjugated/Equine, Systemic) *on page 682*

◆ **CE** *see* Estrogens (Conjugated/Equine, Topical) *on page 686*
◆ **Cedax®** *see* Ceftibuten *on page 334*
◆ **CEE** *see* Estrogens (Conjugated/Equine, Systemic) *on page 682*
◆ **CEE** *see* Estrogens (Conjugated/Equine, Topical) *on page 686*

Cefaclor (SEF a klor)

U.S. Brand Names Raniclor™
Generic Availability (U.S.) Yes: Excludes chewable tablet
Pharmacologic Category Antibiotic, Cephalosporin (Second Generation)
Medication Safety Issues
Sound-alike/look-alike issues:
Cefaclor may be confused with cephalexin
Pregnancy Risk Factor B
Lactation Enters breast milk/use caution
Use Treatment of susceptible bacterial infections including otitis media, lower respiratory tract infections, acute exacerbations of chronic bronchitis, pharyngitis and tonsillitis, urinary tract infections, skin and skin structure infections
Mechanism of Action/Effect Inhibits bacterial cell wall synthesis by binding to one or more of the penicillin-binding proteins (PBPs)
Contraindications Hypersensitivity to cefaclor, any component of the formulation, or other cephalosporins
Warnings/Precautions Modify dosage in patients with severe renal impairment. Prolonged use may result in fungal or bacterial superinfection, including *C. difficile*-associated diarrhea (CDAD) and pseudomembranous colitis; CDAD has been observed >2 months postantibiotic treatment. Use with caution in patients with a history of penicillin allergy, especially IgE-mediated reactions (eg, anaphylaxis, urticaria). Beta-lactamase-negative, ampicillin-resistant (BLNAR) strains of *H. influenzae* should be considered resistant to cefaclor. Extended release tablets are not approved for use in children <16 years of age. Some products may contain phenylalanine.

Drug Interactions

Avoid Concomitant Use
Avoid concomitant use of Cefaclor with any of the following: BCG

Decreased Effect
Cefaclor may decrease the levels/effects of: BCG; Typhoid Vaccine

Increased Effect/Toxicity
The levels/effects of Cefaclor may be increased by: Probenecid

Nutritional/Ethanol Interactions Food: Cefaclor serum levels may be decreased slightly if taken with food. The bioavailability of cefaclor extended release tablets is decreased 23% and the maximum concentration is decreased 67% when taken on an empty stomach.
Lab Interactions Positive direct Coombs', false-positive urinary glucose test using cupric sulfate (Benedict's solution, Clinitest®, Fehling's solution), false-positive serum or urine creatinine with Jaffé reaction

Adverse Reactions
1% to 10%:
Dermatologic: Rash (maculopapular, erythematous, or morbilliform) (1% to 2%)
Gastrointestinal: Diarrhea (3%)
Genitourinary: Vaginitis (2%)
Hematologic: Eosinophilia (2%)
Hepatic: Transaminases increased (3%)
Miscellaneous: Moniliasis (2%)
Reactions reported with other cephalosporins: Fever, abdominal pain, superinfection, renal dysfunction, toxic nephropathy, hemorrhage, cholestasis

Pharmacodynamics/Kinetics
Absorption Well absorbed, acid stable
Time to Peak Capsule: 60 minutes; Suspension: 45 minutes
Protein Binding 25%
Half-Life Elimination 0.5-1 hour; prolonged with renal impairment
Metabolism Partially hepatic
Excretion Urine (80% as unchanged drug)

Available Dosage Forms
Capsule, oral: 250 mg, 500 mg
Powder for suspension, oral: 125 mg/5 mL (75 mL, 150 mL); 250 mg/5 mL (75 mL, 150 mL); 375 mg/5 mL (50 mL, 100 mL)
Tablet, chewable, oral:
Raniclor™: 250 mg, 375 mg
Tablet, extended release, oral: 500 mg

Dosing
Adult & Geriatric Treatment of infections: Oral: Dosing range: 250-500 mg every 8 hours
Pediatric
Treatment of infections: Oral: Children >1 month: Dosing range: 20-40 mg/kg/day divided every 8-12 hours; maximum dose: 1 g/day
Otitis media: Oral: 40 mg/kg/day divided every 12 hours
Pharyngitis: Oral: 20 mg/kg/day divided every 12 hours

Renal Impairment

Cl_{cr} 10-50 mL/minute: Administer 50% to 100% of dose

Cl_{cr} <10 mL/minute: Administer 50% of dose

Hemodialysis: Moderately dialyzable (20% to 50%)

Administration

Oral Administer around-the-clock to promote less variation in peak and trough serum levels. Chewable tablet: Should be chewed before swallowing; should not be swallowed whole. Oral suspension: Shake well before using.

Stability

Storage Store at controlled room temperature. Refrigerate suspension after reconstitution. Discard after 14 days. Do not freeze.

Monitoring and Teaching Issues

Laboratory Monitoring Perform culture and sensitivity studies prior to initiating drug therapy; renal function

Physical Assessment Assess results of culture/sensitivity tests and patient's allergy history prior to therapy. Monitor for nephrotoxicity. Hypersensitivity can occur days after therapy is started. Advise patients with diabetes about use of Clinitest®. Teach patient to report hypersensitivity and opportunistic infection.

Patient Education Take at regular intervals around-the-clock, with or without food. Must chill after reconstitution. Do not chew or crush extended release tablets. Maintain adequate hydration, unless instructed to restrict fluid intake. May cause false test results with Clinitest®; use of another type of testing is preferable. May cause diarrhea. Report rash; breathing or swallowing difficulty; persistent diarrhea, nausea, vomiting, or abdominal pain; changes in urinary pattern or pain on urination; opportunistic infection (eg, vaginal itching or drainage, sores in mouth, blood in stool or urine, vaginal itching or drainage, unusual fever or chills); or CNS changes (eg, irritability, agitation, nervousness, insomnia, hallucinations).

Dietary Considerations Capsule, chewable tablet, and suspension may be taken with or without food. Some products may contain phenylalanine.

Geriatric Considerations Has not been studied in the elderly. Adjust dose for renal function in elderly. Considered to be one of the drugs of choice in the outpatient treatment of community-acquired pneumonia in elderly.

Breast-Feeding Considerations Small amounts of cefaclor are excreted in breast milk. The manufacturer recommends that caution be exercised when administering cefaclor to nursing women. Nondose-related effects could include modification of bowel flora.

Pregnancy Considerations Adverse events were not observed in animal reproduction studies; therefore, cefaclor is classified as pregnancy category B. It is not known if cefaclor crosses the placenta; other cephalosporins cross the placenta and are considered safe for use during pregnancy. An increased risk of teratogenic effects has not been observed following maternal use of cefaclor.

Cefadroxil (sef a DROKS il)

Index Terms Cefadroxil Monohydrate; Duricef

Generic Availability (U.S.) Yes

Pharmacologic Category Antibiotic, Cephalosporin (First Generation)

Pregnancy Risk Factor B

Lactation Enters breast milk (small amounts)/use caution (AAP rates "compatible"; AAP 2001 update pending)

Use Treatment of susceptible bacterial infections, including those caused by group A beta-hemolytic *Streptococcus*

Mechanism of Action/Effect Inhibits bacterial cell wall synthesis by binding to one or more of the penicillin-binding proteins (PBPs)

Contraindications Hypersensitivity to cefadroxil, any component of the formulation, or other cephalosporins

Warnings/Precautions Modify dosage in patients with severe renal impairment. Use with caution in patients with a history of penicillin allergy, especially IgE-mediated reactions (eg, anaphylaxis, angioedema, urticaria). Prolonged use may result in fungal or bacterial superinfection, including *C. difficile*-associated diarrhea (CDAD) and pseudomembranous colitis; CDAD has been observed >2 months postantibiotic treatment.

Drug Interactions

Avoid Concomitant Use

Avoid concomitant use of Cefadroxil with any of the following: BCG

Decreased Effect

Cefadroxil may decrease the levels/effects of: BCG; Typhoid Vaccine

Increased Effect/Toxicity

The levels/effects of Cefadroxil may be increased by: Probenecid

Nutritional/Ethanol Interactions Food: Concomitant administration with food, infant formula, or cow's milk does **not** significantly affect absorption.

Lab Interactions Positive direct Coombs', false-positive urinary glucose test using cupric sulfate (Benedict's solution, Clinitest®, Fehling's solution), false-positive serum or urine creatinine with Jaffé reaction

Adverse Reactions

1% to 10%: Gastrointestinal: Diarrhea

Reactions reported with other cephalosporins: Toxic epidermal necrolysis, abdominal pain, superinfection, renal dysfunction, toxic nephropathy, aplastic anemia, hemolytic anemia, hemorrhage, prothrombin time prolonged, BUN increased, creatinine increased, eosinophilia, pancytopenia, seizure

Pharmacodynamics/Kinetics

Absorption Rapid and well absorbed

Time to Peak Serum: 70-90 minutes

Protein Binding 20%

Half-Life Elimination 1-2 hours; Renal failure: 20-24 hours

Excretion Urine (>90% as unchanged drug)

Available Dosage Forms

Capsule, oral: 500 mg

Powder for suspension, oral: 250 mg/5 mL (50 mL, 100 mL); 500 mg/5 mL (75 mL, 100 mL)

Tablet, oral: 1 g

Dosing

Adult & Geriatric

Susceptible infections: Oral: 1-2 g/day in 2 divided doses

Orofacial infections: Oral: 250-500 mg every 8 hours

Pediatric Susceptible infections: Oral: 30 mg/kg/day divided twice daily up to a maximum of 2 g/day

Renal Impairment

Cl_{cr} 10-25 mL/minute: Administer every 24 hours.

Cl_{cr} <10 mL/minute: Administer every 36 hours.

Administration

Oral Administer around-the-clock to promote less variation in peak and trough serum levels.

Stability

Reconstitution Refrigerate suspension after reconstitution. Discard after 14 days.

Monitoring and Teaching Issues

Laboratory Monitoring Perform culture and sensitivity studies prior to initiating drug therapy; renal function

Physical Assessment Assess results of culture/sensitivity tests and patient's allergy history prior to therapy. Assess anticoagulants patient may be taking for potential interactions. Hypersensitivity can occur several days after therapy is started. Advise patients with diabetes about use of Clinitest®. Teach patient to report hypersensitivity, opportunistic infection, renal dysfunction, and anemia.

Patient Education Take at regular intervals around-the-clock, with or without food. Must be refrigerated for stability purposes. Maintain adequate hydration, unless instructed to restrict fluid intake. May cause false test results with Clinitest®; use of another type of glucose testing is preferable. May cause diarrhea. Report rash; breathing or swallowing difficulty; persistent diarrhea, nausea, vomiting, or abdominal pain; changes in urinary pattern or pain on urination; opportunistic infection (eg, vaginal itching or drainage, sores in mouth, blood in urine or stool, unusual fever or chills); or CNS changes (eg, irritability, agitation, nervousness, insomnia, hallucinations).

Geriatric Considerations Adjust dose for renal function in the elderly.

Breast-Feeding Considerations Very small amounts of cefadroxil are excreted in breast milk. The manufacturer recommends that caution be exercised when administering cefadroxil to nursing women. Nondose-related effects could include modification of bowel flora.

Pregnancy Considerations Adverse events were not observed in animal reproduction studies; therefore, cefadroxil is classified as pregnancy category B. Cefadroxil crosses the placenta. Limited data is available concerning the use of cefadroxil in pregnancy; however, adverse fetal effects were not noted in a small clinical trial. Adequate and well-controlled studies have been not completed in pregnant women.

◆ **Cefadroxil Monohydrate** *see* Cefadroxil *on page* 311

Cefazolin (sef A zoe lin)

Index Terms Ancef; Cefazolin Sodium

Generic Availability (U.S.) Yes

Pharmacologic Category Antibiotic, Cephalosporin (First Generation)

Medication Safety Issues

Sound-alike/look-alike issues:

CeFAZolin may be confused with cefoTEtan, cefOXitin, cefprozil, cefTAZidime, cefTRIAXone, cephalexin, cephalothin

Kefzol® may be confused with Cefzil®

Pregnancy Risk Factor B

Lactation Enters breast milk (small amounts)/use caution (AAP rates "compatible"; AAP 2001 update pending)

Use Treatment of respiratory tract, skin, genital, urinary tract, biliary tract, bone and joint infections, and septicemia due to susceptible gram-positive cocci (except *Enterococcus*); some gram-negative bacilli including *E. coli*, *Proteus*, and *Klebsiella* may be susceptible; surgical prophylaxis

Unlabeled/Investigational Use Prophylaxis against infective endocarditis

Mechanism of Action/Effect Inhibits bacterial cell wall synthesis by binding to one or more of the penicillin-binding proteins (PBPs)

Contraindications Hypersensitivity to cefazolin sodium, any component of the formulation, or other cephalosporins

Warnings/Precautions Modify dosage in patients with severe renal impairment. Use with caution in patients with a history of penicillin allergy, especially IgE-mediated reactions (eg, anaphylaxis, angioedema, urticaria). Prolonged use may result in fungal or bacterial superinfection, including *C. difficile*-associated diarrhea (CDAD) and pseudomembranous colitis; CDAD has been observed >2 months postantibiotic treatment. May be associated with increased INR, especially in nutritionally-deficient patients, prolonged treatment, hepatic or renal disease. Use with caution in patients with a history of seizure disorder; high levels, particularly in the presence of renal impairment, may increase risk of seizures.

Drug Interactions

Avoid Concomitant Use

Avoid concomitant use of CeFAZolin with any of the following: BCG

Decreased Effect

CeFAZolin may decrease the levels/effects of: BCG; Typhoid Vaccine

Increased Effect/Toxicity

CeFAZolin may increase the levels/effects of: Phenytoin; Vitamin K Antagonists

The levels/effects of CeFAZolin may be increased by: Probenecid

Lab Interactions Positive direct Coombs', false-positive urinary glucose test using cupric sulfate (Benedict's solution, Clinitest®, Fehling's solution), false-positive serum or urine creatinine with Jaffé reaction

Some penicillin derivatives may accelerate the degradation of aminoglycosides *in vitro*, leading to a potential underestimation of aminoglycoside serum concentration.

Adverse Reactions Frequency not defined.

Central nervous system: Fever, seizure

Dermatologic: Rash, pruritus, Stevens-Johnson syndrome

Gastrointestinal: Diarrhea, nausea, vomiting, abdominal cramps, anorexia, pseudomembranous colitis, oral candidiasis

Genitourinary: Vaginitis

Hepatic: Transaminases increased, hepatitis

Hematologic: Eosinophilia, neutropenia, leukopenia, thrombocytopenia, thrombocytosis

Local: Pain at injection site, phlebitis

Renal: BUN increased, serum creatinine increased, renal failure

Miscellaneous: Anaphylaxis

Reactions reported with other cephalosporins: Toxic epidermal necrolysis, abdominal pain, cholestasis, superinfection, toxic nephropathy, aplastic anemia, hemolytic anemia, hemorrhage, prothrombin time prolonged, pancytopenia

Pharmacodynamics/Kinetics

Time to Peak Serum: I.M.: 0.5-2 hours

Protein Binding 74% to 86%

Half-Life Elimination 90-150 minutes; prolonged with renal impairment

Metabolism Minimally hepatic

Excretion Urine (80% to 100% as unchanged drug)

Available Dosage Forms

Infusion, premixed iso-osmotic dextrose solution: 1 g (50 mL)

Injection, powder for reconstitution: 500 mg, 1 g, 10 g, 20 g, 100 g, 300 g

Dosing

Adult & Geriatric

Usual dosage range: I.M., I.V.: 1-1.5 g every 8 hours, depending on severity of infection; maximum: 12 g/day

Cholecystitis, mild-to-moderate: I.V.: 1-2 g every 8 hours for 4-7 days (provided source controlled)

Endocarditis due to MSSA (without prosthesis) (unlabeled use): I.V.: 2 g every 8 hours; **Note:** Recommended for penicillin-allergic (nonanaphylactoid) patients (Baddour, 2005)

Intra-abdominal infection, complicated, community-acquired, mild-to-moderate (in combination with metronidazole): I.V.: 1-2 g every 8 hours for 4-7 days (provided source controlled)

Moderate-to-severe infections: 500 mg to 1 g every 6-8 hours

Mild infection with gram-positive cocci: 250-500 mg every 8 hours

Perioperative prophylaxis: 1-2 g within 60 minutes prior to surgery (may repeat in 2-5 hours intraoperatively); followed by 500 mg to 1 g every 6-8 hours for 24 hours postoperatively

Cardiothoracic surgery: 1 g within 60 minutes prior to incision, followed by 1 g at sternotomy and 1 g after cardiopulmonary bypass; may continue 1 g every 6 hours for 24-48 hours postoperatively (Eagle, 2004)

Cholecystectomy: 1-2 g every 8 hours, discontinue within 24 hours unless infection outside gallbladder suspected

Total joint replacement: 1 g 1 hour prior to the procedure

Pneumococcal pneumonia: 500 mg every 12 hours

Severe infection: 1-1.5 g every 6 hours

Prophylaxis against infective endocarditis (unlabeled use): 1 g 30-60 minutes before procedure. **Note:** Intramuscular injections should be avoided in patients who are receiving anticoagulant therapy. In these circumstances, orally administered regimens should be given whenever possible. Intravenously administered antibiotics should be used for patients who are unable to tolerate or absorb oral medications.

Note: American Heart Association (AHA) guidelines now recommend prophylaxis only in patients undergoing invasive procedures and in whom underlying cardiac conditions may predispose to a higher risk of adverse outcomes should infection occur. As of April 2007, routine prophylaxis for GI/GU procedures is no longer recommended by the AHA.

UTI (uncomplicated): 1 g every 12 hours

Pediatric

Usual dosage range: I.M., I.V.: Children >1 month: 25-100 mg/kg/day divided every 6-8 hours; maximum: 6 g/day

Prophylaxis against infective endocarditis (unlabeled use): Infants and Children: 50 mg/kg 30-60 minutes before procedure; maximum dose: 1 g. Intramuscular injections should be avoided in patients who are receiving anticoagulant therapy. In these circumstances, orally administered regimens should be given whenever possible. Intravenously administered antibiotics should be used for patients who are unable to tolerate or absorb oral medications.

Note: American Heart Association (AHA) guidelines now recommend prophylaxis only in patients undergoing invasive procedures and in whom underlying cardiac conditions may predispose to a higher risk of adverse outcomes should infection occur. As of April 2007, routine prophylaxis for GI/GU procedures is no longer recommended by the AHA.

Renal Impairment

Cl_{cr} 35-54 mL/minute: Administer full dose in intervals of ≥8 hours

Cl_{cr} 11-34 mL/minute: Administer 1/2 usual dose every 12 hours

Cl_{cr} ≤10 mL/minute: Administer 1/2 usual dose every 18-24 hours

Hemodialysis: Moderately dialyzable (20% to 50%); administer dose postdialysis or administer supplemental dose of 0.5-1 g after dialysis

Continuous ambulatory peritoneal dialysis (CAPD): Administer 0.5 g every 12 hours

Continuous renal replacement therapy (CRRT): Drug clearance is highly dependent on the method of renal replacement, filter type, and flow rate. Appropriate dosing requires close monitoring of pharmacologic response, signs of adverse reactions due to drug accumulation, as well as drug levels in relation to target trough (if appropriate). The following are general recommendations only (based on dialysate flow/ultrafiltration rates of 1 L/hour) and should not supersede clinical judgment:

CVVH: 1-2 g every 12 hours

CVVHD/CVVHDF: 2 g every 12 hours

Administration

I.M. Inject deep I.M. into large muscle mass.

I.V. Inject direct I.V. over 5 minutes. Infuse intermittent infusion over 30-60 minutes.

Some penicillins (eg, carbenicillin, ticarcillin, and piperacillin) have been shown to inactivate aminoglycosides *in vitro*. This has been observed to a greater extent with tobramycin and gentamicin, while amikacin has shown greater stability against inactivation. Concurrent use of these agents may pose a risk of reduced antibacterial efficacy *in vivo*, particularly in the setting of profound renal impairment. However, definitive clinical evidence is lacking. If combination penicillin/aminoglycoside therapy is desired in a patient with renal dysfunction, separation of doses (if feasible), and routine monitoring of aminoglycoside levels, CBC, and clinical response should be considered.

Stability

Reconstitution Dilute 500 mg vial with 2 mL SWFI and 1 g vial with 2.5 mL SWFI; reconstituted solution may be directly injected after further dilution with 5 mL SWFI or further diluted for I.V. administration in 50-100 mL compatible solution; 10 g vial may be diluted with 45 mL to yield 1 g/5 mL or 96 mL to yield 1 g/10 mL.

Storage Store intact vials at room temperature and protect from temperatures exceeding 40°C. Reconstituted solutions of cefazolin are light yellow to yellow. Protection from light is recommended for the powder and for the reconstituted solutions. Reconstituted solutions are stable for 24 hours at room temperature and for 10 days under refrigeration. Stability of parenteral admixture at room temperature (25°C) is 48 hours. Stability of parenteral admixture at refrigeration temperature (4°C) is 14 days.

DUPLEX™: Store at 20°C to 25°C (68°F to 77°F); excursions permitted to 15°C to 30°C (59°F to 86°F) prior to activation. Following activation, stable for 24 hours at room temperature and for 7 days under refrigeration.

Monitoring and Teaching Issues

Laboratory Monitoring Perform culture and sensitivity studies prior to initiating drug therapy; renal function

Physical Assessment Assess results of culture/sensitivity tests and patient's allergy history prior to therapy. Assess anticoagulants (eg, warfarin) patient may be taking for potential interactions. Hypersensitivity can occur several days after therapy is started. Advise patients with diabetes about use of Clinitest®. Teach patient to report hypersensitivity, opportunistic infection, renal dysfunction, and anemia.

Patient Education This medication is administered by injection or infusion. Report immediately any redness, swelling, burning, or pain at injection/infusion site; rash or hives; or respiratory difficulty, chest pain, or difficulty swallowing. Maintain adequate hydration, unless instructed to restrict fluid intake. If you have diabetes, drug may cause false test results with Clinitest® urine glucose monitoring; use of another type of glucose monitoring is preferable. May cause diarrhea. Report rash; breathing or swallowing difficulty; persistent diarrhea, nausea, vomiting, or abdominal pain; changes in urinary pattern or pain on urination; opportunistic infection (eg, vaginal itching or drainage, sores in mouth, blood in stool or urine, unusual fever or chills); or CNS changes (eg, irritability, agitation, nervousness, insomnia, hallucinations).

Dietary Considerations Some products may contain sodium.

Geriatric Considerations Adjust dose for renal function.

Breast-Feeding Considerations Small amounts of cefazolin are excreted in breast milk. The manufacturer recommends that caution be exercised when administering cefazolin to nursing women. Nondose-related effects could include modification of bowel flora.

Pregnancy Considerations Adverse effects were not observed in animal reproduction studies; therefore, cefazolin is classified as pregnancy category B. Cefazolin crosses the placenta. Adverse events have not been reported in the fetus following administration of cefazolin prior to caesarean section. Cefazolin is recommended for group B streptococcus prophylaxis in pregnant patients with a nonanaphylactic penicillin allergy.

Due to pregnancy-induced physiologic changes, the pharmacokinetics of cefazolin are altered. The half-life is shorter and the AUC is smaller. The volume of distribution is unchanged.

Related Information

Compatibility of Drugs *on page 1994*

I.V. to Oral Conversion *on page 1956*

◆ **Cefazolin Sodium** *see* Cefazolin *on page 312*

Cefdinir (SEF di ner)

U.S. Brand Names Omnicef®

Index Terms CFDN

Generic Availability (U.S.) Yes

Pharmacologic Category Antibiotic, Cephalosporin (Third Generation)

Pregnancy Risk Factor B

Lactation Excretion in breast milk unknown

Use Treatment of community-acquired pneumonia, acute exacerbations of chronic bronchitis, acute bacterial otitis media, acute maxillary sinusitis, pharyngitis/tonsillitis, and uncomplicated skin and skin structure infections.

Mechanism of Action/Effect Inhibits bacterial cell wall synthesis by binding to one or more of the penicillin-binding proteins (PBPs) which in turn inhibits the final transpeptidation step of peptidoglycan synthesis in bacterial cell walls, thus inhibiting cell wall biosynthesis. Bacteria eventually lyse due to ongoing activity of cell wall autolytic enzymes (autolysins and murein hydrolases) while cell wall assembly is arrested.

Contraindications Hypersensitivity to cefdinir, any component of the formulation, other cephalosporins, or related antibiotics

Warnings/Precautions Administer cautiously to penicillin-sensitive patients, especially IgE-mediated reactions (eg, anaphylaxis, urticaria). Prolonged use may result in fungal or bacterial superinfection, including *C. difficile*-associated diarrhea (CDAD) and pseudomembranous colitis; CDAD has been observed >2 months postantibiotic treatment. Use caution with renal dysfunction (Cl_{cr} <30 mL/minute); dose adjustment may be required.

Drug Interactions

Avoid Concomitant Use

Avoid concomitant use of Cefdinir with any of the following: BCG

Decreased Effect

Cefdinir may decrease the levels/effects of: BCG; Typhoid Vaccine

The levels/effects of Cefdinir may be decreased by: Iron Salts

Increased Effect/Toxicity

The levels/effects of Cefdinir may be increased by: Probenecid

Lab Interactions False-positive reaction for urinary ketones may occur with nitroprusside- but not nitroferricyanide-based tests. False-positive urine glucose results may occur when using Clinitest®, Benedict's solution, or Fehling's solution; glucose-oxidase-based reaction systems (eg, Clinistix®, Tes-Tape®) are recommended. May cause positive direct Coombs' test.

Adverse Reactions

>10%: Gastrointestinal: Diarrhea (8% to 15%)

1% to 10%:

Central nervous system: Headache (2%)

Dermatologic: Rash (≤3%)

Endocrine & metabolic: Bicarbonate decreased (≤1%), hyperglycemia (≤1%), hyperphosphatemia (≤1%)

Gastrointestinal: Nausea (≤3%), abdominal pain (≤1%), vomiting (≤1%)

Genitourinary: Vaginal moniliasis (≤4%), urine leukocytes increased (≤2%), urine pH increased (≤1%), urine specific gravity increased (≤1%), vaginitis (≤1%)

Hematologic: Lymphocytes increased (≤2%), eosinophils increased (1%), lymphocytes decreased (1%), platelets increased (≤1%), PMN changes (≤1%), WBC decreased/increased (≤1%)

Hepatic: Alkaline phosphatase increased (≤1%), ALT increased (≤1%)

Renal: Proteinuria (1% to 2%), microhematuria (≤1%), glycosuria (≤1%)

Miscellaneous: GGT increased (≤1%), lactate dehydrogenase increased (≤1%)

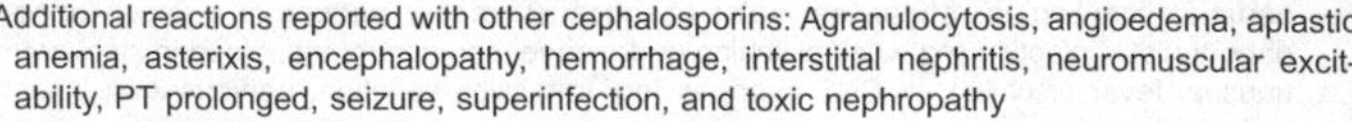

Additional reactions reported with other cephalosporins: Agranulocytosis, angioedema, aplastic anemia, asterixis, encephalopathy, hemorrhage, interstitial nephritis, neuromuscular excitability, PT prolonged, seizure, superinfection, and toxic nephropathy

Pharmacodynamics/Kinetics

Bioavailability Capsule: 16% to 21%; Suspension 25%

Time to Peak 3 hours

Protein Binding 60% to 70%

Half-Life Elimination ~100 minutes

Metabolism Minimal

Excretion Primarily urine (7% to 25% as unchanged drug)

Available Dosage Forms

Capsule, oral: 300 mg

Omnicef®: 300 mg

Powder for suspension, oral: 125 mg/5 mL (60 mL, 100 mL); 250 mg/5 mL (60 mL, 100 mL)

Omnicef®: 125 mg/5 mL (60 mL, 100 mL); 250 mg/5 mL (60 mL, 100 mL)

Dosing

Adult & Geriatric

Acute exacerbations of chronic bronchitis, pharyngitis/tonsillitis: Oral: 300 mg twice daily for 5-10 days **or** 600 mg once daily for 10 days

Acute maxillary sinusitis: Oral: 300 mg twice daily **or** 600 mg once daily for 10 days

Community-acquired pneumonia, uncomplicated skin and skin structure infections: Oral: 300 mg twice daily for 10 days

Pediatric

Children 6 months to 12 years:

Acute bacterial otitis media, pharyngitis/tonsillitis: Oral: 7 mg/kg/dose twice daily for 5-10 days **or** 14 mg/kg/dose once daily for 10 days (maximum: 600 mg/day)

Acute maxillary sinusitis: Oral: 7 mg/kg/dose twice daily **or** 14 mg/kg/dose once daily for 10 days (maximum: 600 mg/day)

Uncomplicated skin and skin structure infections: Oral: 7 mg/kg/dose twice daily for 10 days (maximum: 600 mg/day)

Children >12 years: Refer to adult dosing.

Renal Impairment

Cl_{cr} <30 mL/minute:

Children: 7 mg/kg once daily (maximum: 300 mg/day)

Adults: 300 mg once daily

Hemodialysis removes cefdinir; recommended initial dose: 300 mg (or 7 mg/kg/dose) every other day. At the conclusion of each hemodialysis session, 300 mg (or 7 mg/kg/dose) should be given. Subsequent doses (300 mg or 7 mg/kg/dose) should be administered every other day.

Hepatic Impairment No adjustment necessary.

Administration

Oral Twice daily doses should be given every 12 hours. May be administered with or without food. Manufacturer recommends administering at least 2 hours before or after antacids or iron supplements. Shake suspension well before use.

Stability

Reconstitution Oral suspension should be mixed with 38 mL water for the 60 mL bottle and 63 mL of water for the 100 mL bottle.

Storage Capsules and unmixed powder should be stored at 25°C (77°F); excursions permitted to 15°C to 30°C (59°F to 86°F). Oral suspension should be mixed with 38 mL water for the 60 mL bottle and 63 mL of water for the 100 mL bottle. After mixing, the suspension can be stored at room temperature of 25°C (77°F) for 10 days.

Monitoring and Teaching Issues

Laboratory Monitoring Perform culture and sensitivity studies prior to initiating drug therapy; renal function.

Physical Assessment Assess results of culture/sensitivity tests and patient's allergy history prior to therapy. Teach patient to report opportunistic infection and hypersensitivity.

Patient Education Take at regular intervals around-the-clock, with or without food. Chilling oral suspension improves flavor (do not freeze). Maintain adequate hydration, unless instructed to restrict fluid intake. May cause diarrhea, nausea, vomiting, or flatulence. Report rash; breathing or swallowing difficulty; persistent diarrhea, nausea, vomiting, or abdominal pain; changes in urinary pattern or pain on urination; opportunistic infection (eg, vaginal itching or drainage, sores in mouth, blood in stool or urine, unusual fever or chills); or CNS changes (eg, irritability, agitation, nervousness, insomnia, hallucinations).

Geriatric Considerations Cefdinir has not been studied exclusively in the elderly. Patients ≥65 years of age have been included in clinical. No information is available on their response or tolerance.

Breast-Feeding Considerations Cefdinir is not detectable in breast milk following a single cefdinir 600 mg dose. It is not known if it would be detectable after multiple doses. If present in breast milk, nondose-related effects could include modification of bowel flora.

Pregnancy Considerations Teratogenic events have not been observed in animal studies; therefore, cefdinir is classified as pregnancy category B. It is not known if cefdinir crosses the human placenta.

Cefditoren (sef de TOR en)

U.S. Brand Names Spectracef®

Index Terms Cefditoren Pivoxil

Generic Availability (U.S.) Yes

Pharmacologic Category Antibiotic, Cephalosporin (Third Generation)

Medication Safety Issues

International issues:

Spectracef [U.S., Great Britain, Mexico, Portugal, Spain] may be confused with Spectrocef brand name for cefotaxime [Italy]

Pregnancy Risk Factor B

Lactation Excretion in breast milk unknown/use caution

Use Treatment of acute bacterial exacerbation of chronic bronchitis or community-acquired pneumonia (due to susceptible organisms including *Haemophilus influenzae*, *Haemophilus parainfluenzae*, *Streptococcus pneumoniae*-penicillin susceptible only, *Moraxella catarrhalis*); pharyngitis or tonsillitis (*Streptococcus pyogenes*); and uncomplicated skin and skin-structure infections (*Staphylococcus aureus* - not MRSA, *Streptococcus pyogenes*)

Mechanism of Action/Effect Has bactericidal activity against susceptible gram-positive and gram-negative pathogens. Inhibits bacterial cell wall synthesis by binding to one or more of the penicillin-binding proteins (PBPs).

Contraindications Hypersensitivity to cefditoren, any component of the formulation, other cephalosporins, or milk protein; carnitine deficiency

Warnings/Precautions Use with caution in patients with a history of penicillin allergy, especially IgE-mediated reactions (eg, anaphylaxis, urticaria). Prolonged use may result in fungal or bacterial superinfection, including *C. difficile*-associated diarrhea (CDAD) and pseudomembranous colitis; CDAD has been observed >2 months postantibiotic treatment. Caution in individuals with seizure disorders; high levels, particularly in the presence of renal impairment, may increase risk of seizures. Use caution in patients with renal or hepatic impairment; modify dosage in patients with severe renal impairment. Cefditoren causes renal excretion of carnitine; do not use in patients with carnitine deficiency; not for long-term therapy due to the possible development of carnitine deficiency over time. May prolong prothrombin time; use with caution in patients with a history of bleeding disorder. Cefditoren tablets contain sodium caseinate, which may cause hypersensitivity reactions in patients with milk protein hypersensitivity; this does not affect patients with lactose intolerance.

Drug Interactions

Avoid Concomitant Use There are no known interactions where it is recommended to avoid concomitant use.

Decreased Effect

The levels/effects of Cefditoren may be decreased by: Antacids; H2-Antagonists; Proton Pump Inhibitors

Increased Effect/Toxicity

The levels/effects of Cefditoren may be increased by: Probenecid

Nutritional/Ethanol Interactions Food: Moderate- to high-fat meals increase bioavailability and maximum plasma concentration.

Lab Interactions May induce a positive direct Coomb's test. May cause a false-negative ferricyanide test. Glucose oxidase or hexokinase methods recommended for blood/plasma glucose determinations. False-positive urine glucose test when using copper reduction based assays (eg, Clinitest®).

Adverse Reactions

>10%: Gastrointestinal: Diarrhea (11% to 15%)

1% to 10%:

Central nervous system: Headache (2% to 3%)

Endocrine & metabolic: Glucose increased (1% to 2%)

Gastrointestinal: Nausea (4% to 6%), abdominal pain (2%), dyspepsia (1% to 2%), vomiting (1%)

Genitourinary: Vaginal moniliasis (3% to 6%)

Hematologic: Hematocrit decreased (2%)

Renal: Hematuria (3%), urinary white blood cells increased (2%)

Reactions reported with other cephalosporins: Anaphylaxis, aplastic anemia, cholestasis, hemorrhage, hemolytic anemia, renal dysfunction, reversible hyperactivity, serum sickness-like reaction, toxic nephropathy

Pharmacodynamics/Kinetics

Bioavailability ~14% to 16%; increased with moderate- to high-fat meal

Time to Peak 1.5-3 hours

Protein Binding 88% (*in vitro*), primarily to albumin

Half-Life Elimination 1.6 ± 0.4 hours

Metabolism Cefditoren pivoxil is hydrolyzed to cefditoren (active) and pivalate

Excretion Urine (as cefditoren and pivaloylcarnitine)

Available Dosage Forms

Tablet, oral: 200 mg, 400 mg

Spectracef®: 200 mg, 400 mg

Dosing

Adult & Geriatric

Acute bacterial exacerbation of chronic bronchitis: Oral: 400 mg twice daily for 10 days

Community-acquired pneumonia: Oral: 400 mg twice daily for 14 days

Dental infections (unlabeled use): Oral: 400 mg twice daily for 10 days

Pharyngitis, tonsillitis, uncomplicated skin and skin structure infections: Oral: 200 mg twice daily for 10 days

Pediatric Children ≥12 years: Refer to adult dosing.

Renal Impairment

Cl_{cr} 30-49 mL/minute/1.73 m^2: Maximum dose: 200 mg twice daily

Cl_{cr} <30 mL/minute/1.73 m^2: Maximum dose: 200 mg once daily

End-stage renal disease: Appropriate dosing not established

Hepatic Impairment

Mild-to-moderate impairment: Adjustment not required

Severe impairment (Child-Pugh class C): Specific guidelines not available

Administration

Oral Administer with meals.

Stability

Storage Store at controlled room temperature of 15°C to 30°C (59°F to 86°F). Protect from light and moisture.

Monitoring and Teaching Issues

Laboratory Monitoring Perform culture and sensitivity studies prior to initiating drug therapy; renal function

Physical Assessment Assess results of culture/sensitivity tests and patient's allergy history prior to therapy. Teach patient to report hypersensitivity, opportunistic infection, gastrointestinal upset, and diarrhea.

Patient Education Take at regular intervals around-the-clock, with food. Maintain adequate hydration, unless instructed to restrict fluid intake. If you have diabetes, monitor glucose levels closely. May cause diarrhea, nausea, or vomiting. Report rash; breathing or swallowing difficulty; persistent diarrhea, nausea, vomiting, or abdominal pain; opportunistic infection (eg, vaginal itching or drainage, sores in mouth, blood in stool or urine, or unusual fever or chills); or CNS changes (eg, irritability, agitation, nervousness, insomnia, hallucinations).

Dietary Considerations Cefditoren should be taken with meals. Plasma carnitine levels are decreased during therapy (39% with 200 mg dosing, 63% with 400 mg dosing); normal concentrations return within 7-10 days after treatment is discontinued.

Geriatric Considerations No dose adjustment is necessary for patients with normal age-adjusted renal function.

Breast-Feeding Considerations It is not known whether cefditoren is excreted in human milk. The manufacturer recommends caution when using cefditoren during breast-feeding. Other cephalosporins are considered safe during breast-feeding. If cefditoren reaches the breast milk, the limited oral absorption may minimize the effect on the nursing infant. Nondose-related effects could include modification of bowel flora.

Pregnancy Considerations Adverse events have not been observed in animal reproduction studies; therefore, the manufacturer classifies cefditoren as pregnancy category B. Other cephalosporins cross the placenta and are considered safe in pregnancy.

◆ **Cefditoren Pivoxil** *see* Cefditoren *on page* 317

Cefepime (SEF e pim)

U.S. Brand Names Maxipime®

Index Terms Cefepime Hydrochloride

Generic Availability (U.S.) Yes

Pharmacologic Category Antibiotic, Cephalosporin (Fourth Generation)

Medication Safety Issues

Sound-alike/look-alike issues:

Cefepime may be confused with cefixime, cefTAZidime

Pregnancy Risk Factor B

Lactation Enters breast milk/use caution

Use Treatment of uncomplicated and complicated urinary tract infections, including pyelonephritis caused by *Escherichia coli, Klebsiella pneumoniae*, or *Proteus mirabilis*; monotherapy for febrile neutropenia; uncomplicated skin and skin structure infections caused by *Streptococcus pyogenes* or methicillin-susceptible staphylococci; moderate-to-severe pneumonia caused by *Streptococcus pneumoniae, Pseudomonas aeruginosa, Klebsiella pneumoniae*, or *Enterobacter* species; complicated intra-abdominal infections (in combination with metronidazole) caused by *E. coli, P. aeruginosa, K. pneumoniae, Enterobacter* species, or *Bacteroides fragilis* against methicillin-susceptible staphylococci, *Enterobacter* sp, and many other gram-negative bacilli.

Children 2 months to 16 years: Empiric therapy of febrile neutropenia patients, uncomplicated skin/soft tissue infections, pneumonia, and uncomplicated/complicated urinary tract infections, including pyelonephritis.

Unlabeled/Investigational Use Brain abscess (postneurosurgical prevention); malignant otitis externa; septic lateral/cavernous sinus thrombosis

Mechanism of Action/Effect Inhibits bacterial cell wall synthesis by binding to one or more of the penicillin-binding proteins (PBPs)

Contraindications Hypersensitivity to cefepime, other cephalosporins, penicillins, other beta-lactam antibiotics, or any component of the formulation

Warnings/Precautions Modify dosage in patients with renal impairment (Cl_{cr} ≤60 mL/minute); may increase risk of encephalopathy, myoclonus, and seizures. Use with caution in patients with a history of penicillin or cephalosporin allergy, especially IgE-mediated reactions (eg, anaphylaxis, urticaria). Prolonged use may result in fungal or bacterial superinfection, including *C. difficile*-associated diarrhea (CDAD) and pseudomembranous colitis; CDAD has been observed >2 months postantibiotic treatment. Use with caution in patients with a history of gastrointestinal disease, especially colitis. May be associated with increased INR, especially in nutritionally-deficient patients, prolonged treatment, hepatic or renal disease. Use with caution in patients with a history of seizure disorder; high levels, particularly in the presence of renal impairment, may increase risk of seizures.

Drug Interactions

Avoid Concomitant Use

Avoid concomitant use of Cefepime with any of the following: BCG

Decreased Effect

Cefepime may decrease the levels/effects of: BCG; Typhoid Vaccine

Increased Effect/Toxicity

The levels/effects of Cefepime may be increased by: Probenecid

Lab Interactions Positive direct Coombs', false-positive urinary glucose test using cupric sulfate (Benedict's solution, Clinitest®, Fehling's solution), false-positive serum or urine creatinine with Jaffé reaction

Adverse Reactions

>10%: Hematologic: Positive Coombs' test without hemolysis (16%)

1% to 10%:

- Central nervous system: Fever (1%), headache (1%)
- Dermatologic: Rash (1% to 4%), pruritus (1%)
- Endocrine & metabolic: Hypophosphatemia (3%)
- Gastrointestinal: Diarrhea (≤3%), nausea (≤2%), vomiting (≤1%)
- Hematologic: Eosinophils (2%)
- Hepatic: ALT increased (3%), AST increased (2%), PTT abnormal (2%), PT abnormal (1%)
- Local: Inflammation, phlebitis, and pain (1%)

Reactions reported with other cephalosporins: Aplastic anemia, erythema multiforme, hemolytic anemia, hemorrhage, pancytopenia, PT prolonged, renal dysfunction, Stevens-Johnson syndrome, superinfection, toxic epidermal necrolysis, toxic nephropathy, vaginitis

Pharmacodynamics/Kinetics

Absorption I.M.: Rapid and complete

Time to Peak I.M.: 1-2 hours; I.V.: 0.5 hours

Protein Binding Plasma: ~20%

Half-Life Elimination 2 hours

Metabolism Minimally hepatic

Excretion Urine (85% as unchanged drug)

Available Dosage Forms

Infusion, premixed iso-osmotic dextrose solution: 1 g (50 mL); 2 g (100 mL)

Injection, powder for reconstitution: 1 g, 2 g

Maxipime®: 500 mg, 1 g, 2 g

Dosing

Adult & Geriatric

Brain abscess, postneurosurgical prevention (unlabeled use): I.V.: 2 g every 8 hours with vancomycin

Febrile neutropenia, monotherapy: I.V: 2 g every 8 hours for 7 days or until the neutropenia resolves

Intra-abdominal infections, complicated, severe (in combination with metronidazole): I.V.: 2 g every 12 hours for 7-10 days. **Note:** 2010 IDSA guidelines recommend 2 g every 8-12 hours for 4-7 days (provided source controlled). Not recommended for hospital-acquired intra-abdominal infections (IAI) associated with multidrug-resistant gram negative organisms or in mild-to-moderate community-acquired IAIs due to risk of toxicity and the development of resistant organisms (Solomkin, 2010).

Otitis externa, malignant (unlabeled use): I.V.: 2 g every 12 hours

Pneumonia: I.V.:

Nosocomial (HAP/VAP): 1-2 g every 8-12 hours; **Note:** Duration of therapy may vary considerably (7-21 days); usually longer courses are required if *Pseudomonas*. In absence of *Pseudomonas*, and if appropriate empiric treatment used and patient responsive, it may be clinically appropriate to reduce duration of therapy to 7-10 days (American Thoracic Society Guidelines, 2005).

Community-acquired (including pseudomonal): 1-2 g every 12 hours for 10 days

Septic lateral/cavernous sinus thrombosis (unlabeled use): I.V.: 2 g every 8-12 hours; with metronidazole for lateral

Skin and skin structure, uncomplicated: I.V.: 2 g every 12 hours for 10 days

Urinary tract infections, complicated and uncomplicated:

Mild-to-moderate: I.M., I.V.: 0.5-1 g every 12 hours for 7-10 days

Severe: I.V.: 2 g every 12 hours for 10 days

Pediatric

Febrile neutropenia: I.V.: 50 mg/kg/dose every 8 hours for 7 days or until neutropenia resolves

Skin and skin structure infections (uncomplicated) and pneumonia: I.V.: 50 mg/kg/dose every 12 hours for 10 days

Urinary tract infections, complicated and uncomplicated: I.V., I.M.: 50 mg/kg/dose every 12 hours for 7-10 days; **Note:** I.M. may be considered for mild-to-moderate infection only.

Renal Impairment

Cefepime Hydrochloride

Creatinine Clearance (mL/minute)	Recommended Maintenance Schedule			
>60 (normal recommended dosing schedule)	500 mg every 12 hours	1 g every 12 hours	2 g every 12 hours	2 g every 8 hours
30-60	500 mg every 24 hours	1 g every 24 hours	2 g every 24 hours	2 g every 12 hours
11-29	500 mg every 24 hours	500 mg every 24 hours	1 g every 24 hours	2 g every 24 hours
<11	250 mg every 24 hours	250 mg every 24 hours	500 mg every 24 hours	1 g every 24 hours

Hemodialysis: Initial: 1 g (single dose) on day 1. Maintenance: 500 mg once daily (1 g once daily in febrile neutropenic patients). Dosage should be administered after dialysis on dialysis days.

Continuous ambulatory peritoneal dialysis (CAPD): Removed to a lesser extent than hemodialysis; administer normal recommended dose every 48 hours

Continuous renal replacement therapy (CRRT) (Trotman, 2005): Drug clearance is highly dependent on the method of renal replacement, filter type, and flow rate. Appropriate dosing requires close monitoring of pharmacologic response, signs of adverse reactions due to drug accumulation, as well as drug levels in relation to target trough (if appropriate). The following are general recommendations only (based on dialysate flow/ultrafiltration rates of 1 L/hour) and should not supersede clinical judgment:

CVVH: 1-2 g every 12 hours

CVVHDF: 2 g every 12 hours

Note: Consider higher dosage of 4 g/day if treating *Pseudomonas* or life-threatening infections in order to maximize time above MIC.

Administration

I.M. Inject deep I.M. into large muscle mass.

I.V. Inject direct I.V. over 5 minutes (Garrelts, 1999). Infuse intermittent infusion over 30 minutes.

Stability

Storage

Vials: Store at 20°C to 25°C (68°F to 77°F). Protect from light. After reconstitution, stable in normal saline, D_5W, and a variety of other solutions for 24 hours at room temperature and 7 days refrigerated.

Premixed solution: Store frozen at -20°C (-4°F). Thawed solution is stable for 24 hours at room temperature or 7 days under refrigeration; do not refreeze.

Monitoring and Teaching Issues

Laboratory Monitoring Perform culture and susceptibility studies prior to initiating drug therapy; renal function

Physical Assessment Assess results of culture/sensitivity tests and patient's allergy history prior to therapy. Assess prothrombin time. Teach patient to report hypersensitivity, nephrotoxicity, and opportunistic infection.

Patient Education This medication is administered by infusion or injection. Report immediately any redness, swelling, burning, or pain at injection/infusion site; itching or hives; chest pain; or difficulty swallowing or breathing. Maintain adequate hydration, unless instructed to restrict fluid intake. May cause diarrhea, nausea, or vomiting. Report rash; breathing or swallowing difficulty; persistent diarrhea, nausea, vomiting, or abdominal pain; changes in urinary pattern or pain on urination; opportunistic infection (eg, vaginal itching or drainage, sores in mouth, blood in stool or urine, unusual fever or chills); or CNS changes (eg, irritability, agitation, nervousness, insomnia, hallucinations).

Geriatric Considerations Adjust dose for changes in renal function.

Breast-Feeding Considerations Small amounts of cefepime are excreted in breast milk. The manufacturer recommends that caution be exercised when administering cefepime to nursing women. Nondose-related effects could include modification of bowel flora.

Pregnancy Considerations Teratogenic effects were not observed in animal studies; therefore, cefepime is classified as pregnancy category B. It is not known if cefepime crosses the human placenta.

Related Information

Antimicrobial Drugs of Choice *on page* 2008

Community-Acquired Pneumonia in Adults *on page* 2021

◆ **Cefepime Hydrochloride** *see* Cefepime *on page* 318

Cefixime (sef IKS eem)

U.S. Brand Names Suprax®

Index Terms Cefixime Trihydrate

Generic Availability (U.S.) No

Pharmacologic Category Antibiotic, Cephalosporin (Third Generation)

Medication Safety Issues

Sound-alike/look-alike issues:

Cefixime may be confused with cefepime

Suprax® may be confused with Sporanox®, Surbex®

International issues:

Cefiton: Brand name for cefixime [Portugal] may be confused with Ceftim brand name for ceftazidime [Italy, Portugal]; Ceftime brand name for ceftazidime [Thailand]; Ceftin brand name for cefuroxime [U.S., Canada]

Pregnancy Risk Factor B

Lactation Excretion in breast milk unknown

Use Treatment of urinary tract infections, otitis media, respiratory infections due to susceptible organisms including *S. pneumoniae* and *S. pyogenes*, *H. influenzae*, and many Enterobacteriaceae; uncomplicated cervical/urethral gonorrhea due to *N. gonorrhoeae*

Mechanism of Action/Effect Inhibits bacterial cell wall synthesis by binding to one or more of the penicillin-binding proteins (PBPs)

Contraindications Hypersensitivity to cefixime, any component of the formulation, or other cephalosporins

Warnings/Precautions Prolonged use may result in fungal or bacterial superinfection, including *C. difficile*-associated diarrhea (CDAD) and pseudomembranous colitis; CDAD has been observed >2 months postantibiotic treatment. Modify dosage in patients with renal impairment. Use with caution in patients with a history of penicillin allergy, especially IgE-mediated reactions (eg, anaphylaxis, urticaria).

Drug Interactions

Avoid Concomitant Use

Avoid concomitant use of Cefixime with any of the following: BCG

Decreased Effect

Cefixime may decrease the levels/effects of: BCG; Typhoid Vaccine

Increased Effect/Toxicity

The levels/effects of Cefixime may be increased by: Probenecid

Nutritional/Ethanol Interactions Food: Delays cefixime absorption.

Lab Interactions Positive direct Coombs', false-positive urinary glucose test using cupric sulfate (Benedict's solution, Clinitest®, Fehling's solution), false-positive serum or urine creatinine with Jaffé reaction

Adverse Reactions

>10%: Gastrointestinal: Diarrhea (16%)

2% to 10%: Gastrointestinal: Abdominal pain, nausea, dyspepsia, flatulence, loose stools

Reactions reported with other cephalosporins: Interstitial nephritis, aplastic anemia, hemolytic anemia, hemorrhage, pancytopenia, agranulocytosis, colitis, superinfection

Pharmacodynamics/Kinetics

Absorption 40% to 50%

Time to Peak Serum: 2-6 hours; delayed with food

Protein Binding 65%

Half-Life Elimination Normal renal function: 3-4 hours; Renal failure: Up to 11.5 hours

Excretion Urine (50% of absorbed dose as active drug); feces (10%)

Available Dosage Forms

Powder for suspension, oral:

Suprax®: 100 mg/5 mL (50 mL, 100 mL); 200 mg/5 mL (50 mL, 75 mL)

Tablet, oral:

Suprax®: 400 mg

Dosing

Adult & Geriatric

Susceptible infections: Oral: 400 mg/day divided every 12-24 hours

***S. pyogenes* infections:** Treat for 10 days

Typhoid fever (unlabeled use): Oral: 20-30 mg/kg/day in 2 divided doses for 7-14 days after I.V. therapy

Uncomplicated cervical/urethral gonorrhea due to *N. gonorrhoeae*: Oral: 400 mg as a single dose

Pediatric

Susceptible infections: Oral:

Children ≥6 months: 8 mg/kg/day divided every 12-24 hours

Children >50 kg or >12 years: Refer to adult dosing.

***S. pyogenes* infections:** Treat for 10 days

Typhoid fever (unlabeled use): Oral: 20 mg/kg/day for 10-14 days; maximum 400 mg/day

Renal Impairment

Cl_{cr} 21-60 mL/minute: Administer 75% of the standard dose.

Cl_{cr} <20 mL/minute: Administer 50% of the standard dose.

10% removed by hemodialysis

Administration

Oral May be administered with or without food. Administer with food to decrease GI distress. Shake oral suspension well before use.

Stability

Storage After reconstitution, suspension may be stored for 14 days at room temperature or under refrigeration.

Monitoring and Teaching Issues

Laboratory Monitoring Perform culture and sensitivity studies prior to initiating drug therapy; renal function

Physical Assessment Assess results of culture/sensitivity tests and patient's allergy history prior to therapy. Monitor for anemia, hemorrhage, pancytopenia, agranulocytosis, and colitis during therapy. Teach patient to report hypersensitivity and opportunistic infection.

Patient Education Take at regular intervals around-the-clock, with or without food. Chilling oral suspension improves flavor (do not freeze); shake suspension thoroughly before using. Maintain adequate hydration, unless instructed to restrict fluid intake. May cause nausea, vomiting, or diarrhea. Report rash; breathing or swallowing difficulty; persistent diarrhea, nausea, vomiting, or abdominal pain; changes in urinary pattern or pain on urination; opportunistic infection (eg, vaginal itching or drainage, sores in mouth, blood in stool or urine, unusual fever or chills); or CNS changes (eg, irritability, agitation, nervousness, insomnia, hallucinations).

Dietary Considerations May be taken with food to decrease GI distress.

Geriatric Considerations Adjust dose for renal impairment.

Breast-Feeding Considerations It is not known if cefixime is excreted in breast milk. The manufacturer recommends that consideration be given to discontinuing nursing temporarily during treatment. Other cephalosporins are considered safe during breast-feeding. If present in breast milk, nondose-related effects could include modification of bowel flora.

Pregnancy Considerations Teratogenic effects were not observed in animal studies; therefore cefixime is classified as pregnancy category B. It is not known if cefixime crosses the human placenta; other cephalosporins cross the placenta and are considered safe in pregnancy. Congenital anomalies have not been associated with cefixime use during pregnancy (limited data). Cefixime is recommended for use in pregnant women for the treatment of gonococcal infections.

◆ **Cefixime Trihydrate** *see* Cefixime *on page 320*

◆ **Cefotan** *see* Cefotetan *on page 324*

Cefotaxime (sef oh TAKS eem)

U.S. Brand Names Claforan®

Index Terms Cefotaxime Sodium

Generic Availability (U.S.) Yes: Powder

Pharmacologic Category Antibiotic, Cephalosporin (Third Generation)

Medication Safety Issues

Sound-alike/look-alike issues:

Cefotaxime may be confused with cefOXitin, cefuroxime

International issues:

Spectrocef [Italy] may be confused with Spectracef brand name for cefditoren [U.S., Great Britain, Mexico, Portugal, Spain]

Pregnancy Risk Factor B

Lactation Enters breast milk/use caution (AAP rates "compatible"; AAP 2001 update pending)

Use Treatment of susceptible infection in respiratory tract, skin and skin structure, bone and joint, urinary tract, gynecologic as well as septicemia, and documented or suspected meningitis. Active against most gram-negative bacilli (not *Pseudomonas*) and gram-positive cocci (not enterococcus). Active against many penicillin-resistant pneumococci.

Mechanism of Action/Effect Inhibits bacterial cell wall synthesis by binding to one or more of the penicillin-binding proteins (PBPs)

Contraindications Hypersensitivity to cefotaxime, any component of the formulation, or other cephalosporins

Warnings/Precautions Modify dosage in patients with severe renal impairment. Prolonged use may result in superinfection. A potentially life-threatening arrhythmia has been reported in patients who received a rapid bolus injection via central line. Granulocytopenia and more rarely agranulocytosis may develop during prolonged treatment (>10 days). Minimize tissue inflammation by changing infusion sites when needed. Use with caution in patients with a history of penicillin allergy, especially IgE-mediated reactions (eg, anaphylaxis, urticaria). Prolonged use may result in fungal or bacterial superinfection, including *C. difficile*-associated diarrhea (CDAD) and pseudomembranous colitis; CDAD has been observed >2 months postantibiotic treatment.

Drug Interactions

Avoid Concomitant Use

Avoid concomitant use of Cefotaxime with any of the following: BCG

Decreased Effect

Cefotaxime may decrease the levels/effects of: BCG; Typhoid Vaccine

Increased Effect/Toxicity

The levels/effects of Cefotaxime may be increased by: Probenecid

Lab Interactions Positive direct Coombs', false-positive urinary glucose test using cupric sulfate (Benedict's solution, Clinitest®, Fehling's solution), false-positive serum or urine creatinine with Jaffé reaction

Adverse Reactions

1% to 10%:

Dermatologic: Rash, pruritus

Gastrointestinal: Diarrhea, nausea, vomiting, colitis

Local: Pain at injection site

Reactions reported with other cephalosporins: Agranulocytosis, aplastic anemia, cholestasis, hemolytic anemia, hemorrhage, nephropathy, pancytopenia, renal dysfunction, seizure, superinfection.

Pharmacodynamics/Kinetics

Time to Peak Serum: I.M.: Within 30 minutes

Half-Life Elimination

Cefotaxime: Premature neonates <1 week: 5-6 hours; Full-term neonates <1 week: 2-3.4 hours; Adults: 1-1.5 hours, prolonged with renal and/or hepatic impairment

Desacetylcefotaxime: 1.5-1.9 hours; prolonged with renal impairment

Metabolism Partially hepatic to active metabolite, desacetylcefotaxime

Excretion Urine (as unchanged drug and metabolites)

Available Dosage Forms

Infusion, premixed iso-osmotic solution:

Claforan®: 1 g (50 mL); 2 g (50 mL)

Injection, powder for reconstitution: 500 mg, 1 g, 2 g, 10 g, 20 g

Claforan®: 500 mg, 1 g, 2 g, 10 g

Dosing

Adult & Geriatric

Arthritis (septic): I.V.: 1 g every 8 hours

Brain abscess and meningitis: I.V.: 2 g every 4-6 hours

C-section: 1 g as soon as the umbilical cord is clamped, then 1 g I.M., I.V. at 6- and 12-hours intervals

Epiglottitis: I.V.: 2 g every 4-8 hours

Gonorrhea: I.M.: 1 g as a single dose; disseminated 1 g every 8 hours

Intra-abdominal infection, complicated, community-acquired, mild-to-moderate (in combination with metronidazole): I.V.: 1-2 g every 6 -8 hours for 4-7 days (provided source controlled)

Life-threatening infections: I.V.: 2 g every 4 hours

Liver abscess: I.V.: 1-2 g every 6 hours

Lyme disease:

Cardiac manifestations: I.V.: 2 g every 4 hours

CNS manifestations: I.V.: 2 g every 8 hours for 14-28 days

Moderate/severe infections: I.M., I.V.: 1-2 g every 8 hours

Orbital cellulitis: I.V.: 2 g every 4 hours

Peritonitis (spontaneous): I.V.: 2 g every 8 hours, unless life-threatening then 2 g every 4 hours

Septicemia: I.V.: 2 g every 6-8 hours

Skin and soft tissue:

Mixed, necrotizing: I.V.: 2 g every 6 hours, with metronidazole or clindamycin

Bite wounds (animal): I.V.: 2 g every 6 hours

Surgical prophylaxis: I.M., I.V.: 1 g 30-90 minutes before surgery

Uncomplicated infections: I.M., I.V.: 1 g every 12 hours

Pediatric

Infants and Children 1 month to 12 years:

Susceptible infections: I.M., I.V.: Infants and Children 1 month to 12 years: <50 kg: 50-200 mg/kg/day in divided doses every 6-8 hours

Epiglottitis: I.M., I.V.: 150-200 mg/kg/day in 4 divided doses with clindamycin for 7-10 days

Meningitis: I.M., I.V.: 200 mg/kg/day in divided doses every 6 hours

Pneumonia: I.V.: 200 mg/kg/day divided every 8 hours

Sepsis: I.V.: 150 mg/kg/day divided every 8 hours

Typhoid fever: I.M., I.V.: 150-200 mg/kg/day in 3-4 divided doses (maximum: 12 g/day); fluoroquinolone resistant: 80 mg/kg/day in 3-4 divided doses (maximum: 12 g/day)

Children >12 years: Refer to adult dosing.

Renal Impairment

Cl_{cr} 10-50 mL/minute: Administer every 8-12 hours.

Cl_{cr} <10 mL/minute: Administer every 24 hours.

Moderately dialyzable (20% to 50%)

Continuous ambulatory peritoneal dialysis (CAPD): Administer 0.5-1 g every 24 hours

Continuous renal replacement therapy (CRRT): Drug clearance is highly dependent on the method of renal replacement, filter type, and flow rate. Appropriate dosing requires close monitoring of pharmacologic response, signs of adverse reactions due to drug accumulation, as well as drug levels in relation to target trough (if appropriate). The following are general recommendations only (based on dialysate flow/ultrafiltration rates of 1 L/hour) and should not supersede clinical judgment:

CVVH: 1-2 g every 12 hours

CVVHD/CVVHDF: 2 g every 12 hours

Hepatic Impairment Moderate dosage reduction is recommended in severe liver disease.

Administration

I.M. Inject deep I.M. into large muscle mass.

I.V. Inject direct I.V. over 3-5 minutes. Infuse intermittent infusion over 30 minutes.

Stability

Reconstitution Reconstituted solution is stable for 12-24 hours at room temperature and 7-10 days when refrigerated and for 13 weeks when frozen. For I.V. infusion in NS or D_5W, solution is stable for 24 hours at room temperature, 5 days when refrigerated, or 13 weeks when frozen in Viaflex® plastic containers. Thawed solutions previously of frozen premixed bags are stable for 24 hours at room temperature or 10 days when refrigerated.

Monitoring and Teaching Issues

Laboratory Monitoring Perform culture and sensitivity studies prior to initiating drug therapy; CBC with differential (especially with long courses); renal function

Physical Assessment Assess results of culture/sensitivity tests and patient's allergy history prior to therapy. Evaluate CBC with differential. Monitor for diarrhea, nausea/vomiting, and nephrotoxicity regularly during therapy. Teach patient to report hypersensitivity and opportunistic infection.

Patient Education This medication is administered by injection or infusion. Report immediately any redness, swelling, burning, or pain at injection/infusion site; chest pain, palpitations, respiratory difficulty or swallowing; or itching or hives. Maintain adequate hydration, unless instructed to restrict fluid intake. May cause diarrhea, GI distress, or nausea. Report unresolved or persistent diarrhea, opportunistic infection (vaginal itching or drainage, sores in mouth, blood in stool or urine, easy bleeding or bruising, unusual fever or chills), or respiratory difficulty.

Dietary Considerations Some products may contain sodium.

Geriatric Considerations Adjust dose for renal impairment.

Breast-Feeding Considerations Very small amounts of cefotaxime are excreted in breast milk. The manufacturer recommends that caution be exercised when administering cefotaxime to nursing women. Nondose-related effects could include modification of bowel flora. The pregnancy-related changes in cefotaxime pharmacokinetics continue into the early postpartum period.

Pregnancy Considerations Teratogenic effects were not observed in animal studies; therefore, cefotaxime is classified as pregnancy category B. Cefotaxime crosses the placenta and can be found in fetal tissue. An increased risk of teratogenic effects has not been observed following maternal use. During pregnancy, peak cefotaxime serum concentrations are decreased and the serum half-life is shorter.

Related Information

Antimicrobial Drugs of Choice *on page 2008*

Community-Acquired Pneumonia in Adults *on page 2021*

◆ **Cefotaxime Sodium** *see* Cefotaxime *on page 322*

Cefotetan (SEF oh tee tan)

Index Terms Cefotan; Cefotetan Disodium

Generic Availability (U.S.) Yes

Pharmacologic Category Antibiotic, Cephalosporin (Second Generation)

Medication Safety Issues

Sound-alike/look-alike issues:

CefoTEtan may be confused with ceFAZolin, cefOXitin, cefTAZidime, Ceftin®, cefTRIAXone

CefoTEtan may be confused with Ceftin®

International issues:

Cefotan may be confused with Lexotan® which is a brand name for bromazepam in multiple international markets

Cefotan may be confused with Cefiton® which is a brand name for cefixime in Portugal

Pregnancy Risk Factor B

Lactation Enters breast milk (small amounts)/use caution

Use Surgical prophylaxis; intra-abdominal infections and other mixed infections; respiratory tract, skin and skin structure, bone and joint, urinary tract and gynecologic as well as septicemia; active against gram-negative enteric bacilli including *E. coli*, *Klebsiella*, and *Proteus*; less active against staphylococci and streptococci than first generation cephalosporins, but active against anaerobes including *Bacteroides fragilis*

Mechanism of Action/Effect Inhibits bacterial cell wall synthesis by binding to one or more of the penicillin-binding proteins (PBPs)

Contraindications Hypersensitivity to cefotetan, any component of the formulation, or other cephalosporins; previous cephalosporin-associated hemolytic anemia

Warnings/Precautions Modify dosage in patients with severe renal impairment. Although cefotetan contains the methyltetrazolethiol side chain, bleeding has not been a significant problem. Use with caution in patients with a history of penicillin allergy, especially IgE-mediated reactions (eg, anaphylaxis, urticaria). Cefotetan has been associated with a higher risk of hemolytic anemia relative to other cephalosporins (approximately threefold); monitor carefully during use and consider cephalosporin-associated immune anemia in patients who have received cefotetan within 2-3 weeks (either as treatment or prophylaxis). Prolonged use may result in fungal or bacterial superinfection, including *C. difficile*-associated diarrhea (CDAD) and pseudomembranous colitis; CDAD has been observed >2 months postantibiotic treatment. May be associated with increased INR, especially in nutritionally-deficient patients, prolonged treatment, hepatic or renal disease.

Drug Interactions

Avoid Concomitant Use

Avoid concomitant use of CefoTEtan with any of the following: BCG

Decreased Effect

CefoTEtan may decrease the levels/effects of: BCG; Typhoid Vaccine

Increased Effect/Toxicity

CefoTEtan may increase the levels/effects of: Alcohol (Ethyl); Vitamin K Antagonists

The levels/effects of CefoTEtan may be increased by: Probenecid

Nutritional/Ethanol Interactions Ethanol: Avoid ethanol (may cause a disulfiram-like reaction).

Lab Interactions Positive direct Coombs', false-positive urinary glucose test using cupric sulfate (Benedict's solution, Clinitest®, Fehling's solution), false-positive serum or urine creatinine with Jaffé reaction

Adverse Reactions

1% to 10%:

Gastrointestinal: Diarrhea (1%)

Hepatic: Transaminases increased (1%)

Miscellaneous: Hypersensitivity reactions (1%)

Reactions reported with other cephalosporins: Seizure, Stevens-Johnson syndrome, toxic epidermal necrolysis, renal dysfunction, toxic nephropathy, cholestasis, aplastic anemia, hemolytic anemia, hemorrhage, pancytopenia, agranulocytosis, colitis, superinfection

Pharmacodynamics/Kinetics

Time to Peak Serum: I.M.: 1.5-3 hours

Protein Binding 76% to 90%

Half-Life Elimination 3-5 hours

Excretion Primarily urine (as unchanged drug); feces (20%)

Available Dosage Forms

Injection, powder for reconstitution: 1 g, 2 g, 10 g

Dosing

Adult & Geriatric

Susceptible infections: I.M., I.V.: 1-6 g/day in divided doses every 12 hours; usual dose: 1-2 g every 12 hours for 5-10 days; 1-2 g may be given every 24 hours for urinary tract infection; **Note:** Due to high rates of *B. fragilis* group resistance, not recommended for the treatment of community-acquired intra-abdominal infections (Solomkin, 2010)

Orbital cellulitis, odontogenic infections: I.V.: 2 g every 12 hours

Pelvic inflammatory disease: I.V.: 2 g every 12 hours; used in combination with doxycycline

Preoperative prophylaxis: I.M., I.V.: 1-2 g 30-60 minutes prior to surgery; when used for cesarean section, dose should be given as soon as umbilical cord is clamped

Urinary tract infection: I.M., I.V.: 1-2 g may be given every 24 hours

Pediatric

Severe infections (unlabeled use): I.M., I.V.: 20-40 mg/kg/dose every 12 hours (maximum: 6 g/day)

Preoperative prophylaxis (unlabeled use): I.M., I.V.: 40 mg/kg 30-60 minutes prior to surgery

Pelvic inflammatory disease: Adolescents: I.V.: Refer to adult dosing.

Renal Impairment I.M., I.V.:

Cl_{cr} 10-30 mL/minute: Administer every 24 hours

Cl_{cr} <10 mL/minute: Administer every 48 hours

Hemodialysis: Dialyzable (5% to 20%); administer 1/4 the usual dose every 24 hours on days between dialysis; administer 1/2 the usual dose on the day of dialysis.

Continuous arteriovenous or venovenous hemodiafiltration effects: Administer 750 mg every 12 hours

Administration

I.M. Inject deep I.M. into large muscle mass.

I.V. Inject direct I.V. over 3-5 minutes. Infuse intermittent infusion over 30 minutes.

Stability

Reconstitution Reconstituted solution is stable for 24 hours at room temperature and 96 hours when refrigerated. For I.V. infusion in NS or D_5W solution and after freezing, thawed solution is stable for 24 hours at room temperature or 96 hours when refrigerated. Frozen solution is stable for 12 weeks.

Monitoring and Teaching Issues

Laboratory Monitoring Prothrombin time; perform culture and sensitivity studies prior to initiating drug therapy; renal function

Physical Assessment Assess results of culture/sensitivity tests and patient's allergy history prior to therapy. Assess prothrombin time. Advise patients with diabetes about use of Clinitest® (may cause false-positive test). Teach patient to report nephrotoxicity, opportunistic infection, and hypersensitivity reaction.

Patient Education This medication is administered by injection or infusion. Report immediately any redness, swelling, burning, or pain at injection/infusion site, or immediately report any itching, hives, difficulty swallowing, or respiratory difficulty. Maintain adequate hydration, unless instructed to restrict fluid intake. Avoid alcohol during therapy (may cause severe disulfiram-like reactions). May cause false test results with Clinitest®; use of another type of glucose testing is preferable. May cause diarrhea. Report rash; breathing or swallowing difficulty; persistent diarrhea, nausea, vomiting, or abdominal pain; changes in urinary pattern or pain on urination; opportunistic infection (eg, vaginal itching or drainage; sores in mouth; blood in stool or urine; unusual fever or chills); or CNS changes (eg, irritability, agitation, nervousness, insomnia, hallucinations).

Dietary Considerations Some products may contain sodium.

Geriatric Considerations Cefotetan has not been studied in the elderly. Adjust dose for renal function in the elderly.

Breast-Feeding Considerations Very small amounts of cefotetan are excreted in human milk. The manufacturer recommends caution when giving cefotetan to a breast-feeding mother. Nondose-related effects could include modification of bowel flora.

Pregnancy Considerations Adverse events have not been observed in animal reproduction studies; therefore, the manufacturer classifies cefotetan as pregnancy category B. Cefotetan crosses the placenta and produces therapeutic concentrations in the amniotic fluid and cord serum.

◆ **Cefotetan Disodium** *see* Cefotetan *on page* 324

Cefoxitin (se FOKS i tin)

U.S. Brand Names Mefoxin®
Index Terms Cefoxitin Sodium
Generic Availability (U.S.) Yes: Excludes infusion
Pharmacologic Category Antibiotic, Cephalosporin (Second Generation)
Medication Safety Issues
Sound-alike/look-alike issues:
CefOXitin may be confused with ceFAZolin, cefotaxime, cefoTEtan, cefTAZidime, cefTRIAXone, Cytoxan
Mefoxin® may be confused with Lanoxin®
Pregnancy Risk Factor B
Lactation Enters breast milk/use caution (AAP rates "compatible"; AAP 2001 update pending)
Use Less active against staphylococci and streptococci than first generation cephalosporins, but active against anaerobes including *Bacteroides fragilis*; active against gram-negative enteric bacilli including *E. coli*, *Klebsiella*, and *Proteus*; used predominantly for respiratory tract, skin, bone and joint, urinary tract and gynecologic as well as septicemia; surgical prophylaxis; intra-abdominal infections and other mixed infections; indicated for bacterial *Eikenella corrodens* infections
Mechanism of Action/Effect Inhibits bacterial cell wall synthesis by binding to one or more of the penicillin-binding proteins (PBPs)
Contraindications Hypersensitivity to cefoxitin, any component of the formulation, or other cephalosporins
Warnings/Precautions Modify dosage in patients with severe renal impairment. Prolonged use may result in superinfection. Use with caution in patients with a history of penicillin allergy, especially IgE-mediated reactions (eg, anaphylaxis, urticaria). Prolonged use may result in fungal or bacterial superinfection, including *C. difficile*-associated diarrhea (CDAD) and pseudomembranous colitis; CDAD has been observed >2 months postantibiotic treatment.
Drug Interactions

Avoid Concomitant Use
Avoid concomitant use of CefOXitin with any of the following: BCG

Decreased Effect
CefOXitin may decrease the levels/effects of: BCG; Typhoid Vaccine

Increased Effect/Toxicity
CefOXitin may increase the levels/effects of: Vitamin K Antagonists

The levels/effects of CefOXitin may be increased by: Probenecid

Lab Interactions Positive direct Coombs', false-positive urinary glucose test using cupric sulfate (Benedict's solution, Clinitest®, Fehling's solution), false-positive serum or urine creatinine with Jaffé reaction

Adverse Reactions
1% to 10%: Gastrointestinal: Diarrhea
Reactions reported with other cephalosporins: Agranulocytosis, aplastic anemia, cholestasis, colitis, erythema multiforme, hemolytic anemia, hemorrhage, pancytopenia, renal dysfunction, serum-sickness reactions, seizure, Stevens-Johnson syndrome, superinfection, toxic nephropathy, vaginitis

Pharmacodynamics/Kinetics
Time to Peak Serum: I.M.: 20-30 minutes
Protein Binding 65% to 79%
Half-Life Elimination 45-60 minutes; significantly prolonged with renal impairment
Excretion Urine (85% as unchanged drug)

Available Dosage Forms
Infusion, premixed iso-osmotic dextrose solution:
Mefoxin®: 1 g (50 mL); 2 g (50 mL)
Injection, powder for reconstitution: 1 g, 2 g, 10 g

Dosing
Adult & Geriatric
Susceptible infections: I.M., I.V.: 1-2 g every 6-8 hours (I.M. injection is painful); up to 12 g/day
Amnionitis and endomyometritis: I.M., I.V.: 2 g every 6-8 hours
Aspiration pneumonia, empyema, orbital cellulitis, parapharyngeal space, and human bites: I.M., I.V.: 2 g every 8 hours
Intra-abdominal infection, complicated, community acquired, mild-to-moderate: I.V.: 2 g every 6 hours for 4-7 days (provided source controlled)
Liver abscess: I.V.: 1 g every 4 hours
Mycobacterium species, not MTB or MAI: I.V.: 12 g/day with amikacin

Pelvic inflammatory disease:

Inpatients: I.V.: 2 g every 6 hours **plus** doxycycline 100 mg I.V. or 100 mg orally every 12 hours until improved, followed by doxycycline 100 mg orally twice daily to complete 14 days

Outpatients: I.M.: 2 g **plus** probenecid 1 g orally as a single dose, followed by doxycycline 100 mg orally twice daily for 14 days

Perioperative prophylaxis: I.M., I.V.: 1-2 g 30-60 minutes prior to surgery (may repeat in 2-5 hours intraoperatively) followed by 1-2 g every 6-8 hours for no more than 24 hours after surgery depending on the procedure

Pediatric

Perioperative prophylaxis: I.V.:

Infants >3 months and Children: 30-40 mg/kg 30-60 minutes prior to surgery followed by 30-40 mg/kg/dose every 6 hours for no more than 24 hours after surgery depending on the procedure

Adolescents: Refer to adult dosing.

Mild-to-moderate infection: I.M., I.V.: Infants >3 months and Children: 80-100 mg/kg/day in divided doses every 4-6 hours

Severe infection: I.M., I.V.: Infants >3 months and Children: 100-160 mg/kg/day in divided doses every 4-6 hours

Maximum dose: 12 g/day

Renal Impairment I.M., I.V.:

Cl_{cr} 30-50 mL/minute: Administer 1-2 g every 8-12 hours

Cl_{cr} 10-29 mL/minute: Administer 1-2 g every 12-24 hours

Cl_{cr} 5-9 mL/minute: Administer 0.5-1 g every 12-24 hours

Cl_{cr} <5 mL/minute: Administer 0.5-1 g every 24-48 hours

Hemodialysis: Moderately dialyzable (20% to 50%); administer a loading dose of 1-2 g after each hemodialysis; maintenance dose as noted above based on Cl_{cr}

Continuous arteriovenous or venovenous hemodiafiltration effects: Dose as for Cl_{cr} 10-50 mL/minute

Administration

I.M. Inject deep I.M. into large muscle mass.

I.V. Can be administered IVP over 3-5 minutes at a maximum concentration of 100 mg/mL or I.V. intermittent infusion over 10-60 minutes at a final concentration for I.V. administration not to exceed 40 mg/mL

Stability

Reconstitution Reconstitute vials with SWFI, bacteriostatic water for injection, NS, or D_5W. For I.V. infusion, solutions may be further diluted in NS, $D_5{}^1/_4NS$, $D_5{}^1/_2NS$, D_5NS, D_5W, $D_{10}W$, LR, D_5LR, mannitol 10%, or sodium bicarbonate 5%.

Storage Reconstituted solution is stable for 6 hours at room temperature or 7 days when refrigerated; I.V. infusion in NS or D_5W solution is stable for 18 hours at room temperature or 48 hours when refrigerated. Premixed frozen solution, when thawed, is stable for 24 hours at room temperature or 21 days when refrigerated.

Monitoring and Teaching Issues

Laboratory Monitoring Prothrombin times; perform culture and sensitivity studies prior to initiating drug therapy; renal function

Physical Assessment Assess results of culture/sensitivity tests and patient's allergy history prior to therapy. Monitor for nephrotoxicity. Evaluate prothrombin time and CBC with differential. Monitor for diarrhea, nausea, vomiting, and nephrotoxicity. Advise patients with diabetes about use of Clinitest®. Teach patient to report hypersensitivity and opportunistic infection.

Patient Education This medication is administered by injection or infusion. Report immediately any redness, swelling, burning, or pain at injection/infusion site; chest pain, palpitations, respiratory difficulty or swallowing; or itching or hives. Maintain adequate hydration, unless instructed to restrict fluid intake. May cause false test results with Clinitest®; use of another type of glucose testing is preferable. May cause diarrhea, GI distress, or nausea. Report rash; breathing or swallowing difficulty; persistent diarrhea, nausea, vomiting, or abdominal pain; changes in urinary pattern or pain on urination; opportunistic infection (eg, vaginal itching or drainage, sores in mouth, blood in stool or urine, unusual fever or chills); or CNS changes (eg, irritability, agitation, nervousness, insomnia, hallucinations).

Dietary Considerations Some products may contain sodium.

Geriatric Considerations Adjust dose for renal function in the elderly.

Breast-Feeding Considerations Very small amounts of cefoxitin are excreted in breast milk. The manufacturer recommends that caution be exercised when administering cefoxitin to nursing women. Nondose-related effects could include modification of bowel flora. Cefoxitin pharmacokinetics may be altered immediately postpartum.

Pregnancy Considerations Adverse events have not been observed in animal reproduction studies; therefore, cefoxitin is classified as pregnancy category B. Cefoxitin crosses the placenta and reaches the cord serum and amniotic fluid. Adequate well-controlled studies are not available in pregnant women.

Peak serum concentrations of cefoxitin during pregnancy may be similar to or decreased compared to nonpregnant values. Maternal half-life may be shorter at term. Pregnancy-induced hypertension increases trough concentrations in the immediate postpartum period.

◆ **Cefoxitin Sodium** *see* Cefoxitin *on page 326*

Cefpodoxime (sef pode OKS eem)

Index Terms Cefpodoxime Proxetil; Vantin

Generic Availability (U.S.) Yes

Pharmacologic Category Antibiotic, Cephalosporin (Third Generation)

Medication Safety Issues

Sound-alike/look-alike issues:

Vantin may be confused with Ventolin®

Pregnancy Risk Factor B

Lactation Enters breast milk (small amounts)/not recommended

Use Treatment of susceptible acute, community-acquired pneumonia caused by *S. pneumoniae* or nonbeta-lactamase producing *H. influenzae*; acute uncomplicated gonorrhea caused by *N. gonorrhoeae*; uncomplicated skin and skin structure infections caused by *S. aureus* or *S. pyogenes*; acute otitis media caused by *S. pneumoniae*, *H. influenzae*, or *M. catarrhalis*; pharyngitis or tonsillitis; and uncomplicated urinary tract infections caused by *E. coli*, *Klebsiella*, and *Proteus*

Mechanism of Action/Effect Inhibits bacterial cell wall synthesis by binding to one or more of the penicillin-binding proteins (PBPs)

Contraindications Hypersensitivity to cefpodoxime, any component of the formulation, or other cephalosporins

Warnings/Precautions Modify dosage in patients with severe renal impairment. Prolonged use may result in fungal or bacterial superinfection, including *C. difficile*-associated diarrhea (CDAD) and pseudomembranous colitis; CDAD has been observed >2 months postantibiotic treatment. Use with caution in patients with a history of penicillin allergy, especially IgE-mediated reactions (eg, anaphylaxis, urticaria).

Drug Interactions

Avoid Concomitant Use

Avoid concomitant use of Cefpodoxime with any of the following: BCG

Decreased Effect

Cefpodoxime may decrease the levels/effects of: BCG; Typhoid Vaccine

The levels/effects of Cefpodoxime may be decreased by: Antacids; H2-Antagonists

Increased Effect/Toxicity

The levels/effects of Cefpodoxime may be increased by: Probenecid

Nutritional/Ethanol Interactions Food: Food delays absorption; cefpodoxime serum levels may be increased if taken with food.

Lab Interactions Positive direct Coombs', false-positive urinary glucose test using cupric sulfate (Benedict's solution, Clinitest®, Fehling's solution), false-positive serum or urine creatinine with Jaffé reaction

Adverse Reactions

>10%:

Dermatologic: Diaper rash (12%)

Gastrointestinal: Diarrhea in infants and toddlers (15%)

1% to 10%:

Central nervous system: Headache (1%)

Dermatologic: Rash (1%)

Gastrointestinal: Diarrhea (7%), nausea (4%), abdominal pain (2%), vomiting (1% to 2%)

Genitourinary: Vaginal infection (3%)

Reactions reported with other cephalosporins: Seizure, Stevens-Johnson syndrome, toxic epidermal necrolysis, erythema multiforme, urticaria, serum-sickness reactions, renal dysfunction, interstitial nephritis toxic nephropathy, cholestasis, aplastic anemia, hemolytic anemia, hemorrhage, pancytopenia, agranulocytosis, colitis, vaginitis, superinfection

Pharmacodynamics/Kinetics

Absorption Rapid and well absorbed (50%), acid stable; enhanced in the presence of food or low gastric pH

Time to Peak Within 1 hour

Protein Binding 18% to 23%

Half-Life Elimination 2.2 hours; prolonged with renal impairment

Metabolism De-esterified in GI tract to active metabolite, cefpodoxime

Excretion Urine (80% as unchanged drug) in 24 hours

Available Dosage Forms

Granules for suspension, oral: 50 mg/5 mL (50 mL, 100 mL); 100 mg/5 mL (50 mL, 100 mL)

Tablet, oral: 100 mg, 200 mg

Dosing

Adult & Geriatric

Acute community-acquired pneumonia and bacterial exacerbations of chronic bronchitis: Oral: 200 mg every 12 hours for 14 days and 10 days, respectively

Acute maxillary sinusitis: Oral: 200 mg every 12 hours for 10 days

Pharyngitis/tonsillitis: Oral: 100 mg every 12 hours for 5-10 days

Skin and skin structure: Oral: 400 mg every 12 hours for 7-14 days

Uncomplicated gonorrhea (male and female) and rectal gonococcal infections (female): Oral: 200 mg as a single dose

Uncomplicated urinary tract infection: Oral: 100 mg every 12 hours for 7 days

Pediatric

Acute maxillary sinusitis: Oral: Children: 2 months to 12 years: 10 mg/kg/day divided every 12 hours for 10 days (maximum: 200 mg/dose)

Acute otitis media: Oral: Children:

2 months to 12 years: 10 mg/kg/day divided every 12 hours (400 mg/day) for 5 days (maximum: 200 mg/dose)

≥12 years: Refer to adult dosing.

Pharyngitis/tonsillitis: Oral: Children:

2 months to 12 years: 10 mg/kg/day in 2 divided doses for 5-10 days (maximum: 100 mg/dose)

≥12 years: Refer to adult dosing.

Renal Impairment

Cl_{cr} <30 mL/minute: Administer every 24 hours.

Hemodialysis: Dose 3 times/week following dialysis.

Hepatic Impairment Dose adjustment is not necessary in patients with cirrhosis.

Administration

Oral Administer around-the-clock to promote less variation in peak and trough serum levels.

Stability

Reconstitution Shake well before using. After mixing, keep suspension in refrigerator. Discard unused portion after 14 days.

Monitoring and Teaching Issues

Laboratory Monitoring Perform culture and sensitivity studies prior to initiating drug therapy; renal function

Physical Assessment Assess results of culture/sensitivity tests and patient's allergy history prior to therapy. Assess prothrombin time. Monitor for hemolytic anemia, hypoprothrombinemia, and bleeding. Teach patient to report nephrotoxicity, opportunistic infection, and hypersensitivity reaction.

Patient Education Take at regular intervals around-the-clock, with or without food. Shake suspension well before using. Maintain adequate hydration, unless instructed to restrict fluid intake. May cause nausea, vomiting, or diarrhea. Report rash; breathing or swallowing difficulty; persistent diarrhea, nausea, vomiting, or abdominal pain; changes in urinary pattern or pain on urination; opportunistic infection (eg, vaginal itching or drainage, sores in mouth, blood in stool or urine, unusual fever or chills); or CNS changes (eg, irritability, agitation, nervousness, insomnia, hallucinations).

Dietary Considerations May be taken with food.

Geriatric Considerations Considered one of the drugs of choice for outpatient treatment of community-acquired pneumonia in the elderly. Adjust dosage with renal impairment.

Breast-Feeding Considerations Very small amounts of cefpodoxime are excreted in breast milk. Breast-feeding is not recommended by the manufacturer. Other cephalosporins are considered safe during breast-feeding. Nondose-related effects could include modification of bowel flora.

Pregnancy Considerations Teratogenic events were not observed in animal studies; therefore, cefpodoxime is classified as pregnancy category B. It is not known if cefpodoxime crosses the human placenta. Other cephalosporins cross the placenta and are considered safe in pregnancy.

Related Information

Antimicrobial Drugs of Choice *on page 2008*

Community-Acquired Pneumonia in Adults *on page 2021*

◆ **Cefpodoxime Proxetil** *see* Cefpodoxime *on page 328*

Cefprozil (sef PROE zil)

Index Terms Cefzil

Generic Availability (U.S.) Yes

Pharmacologic Category Antibiotic, Cephalosporin (Second Generation)

Medication Safety Issues

Sound-alike/look-alike issues:

Cefprozil may be confused with ceFAZolin, cefuroxime

Cefzil may be confused with Cefol®, Ceftin®, Kefzol®

Pregnancy Risk Factor B

Lactation Enters breast milk/use caution (AAP rates "compatible"; AAP 2001 update pending)

Use Treatment of otitis media and infections involving the respiratory tract and skin and skin structure; active against methicillin-sensitive staphylococci, many streptococci, and various gram-negative bacilli including *E. coli*, some *Klebsiella*, *P. mirabilis*, *H. influenzae*, and *Moraxella*.

Mechanism of Action/Effect Inhibits bacterial cell wall synthesis by binding to one or more of the penicillin-binding proteins (PBPs)

Contraindications Hypersensitivity to cefprozil, any component of the formulation, or other cephalosporins

Warnings/Precautions Modify dosage in patients with severe renal impairment. Use with caution in patients with a history of penicillin allergy, especially IgE-mediated reactions (eg, anaphylaxis, urticaria). Prolonged use may result in fungal or bacterial superinfection, including *C. difficile*-associated diarrhea (CDAD) and pseudomembranous colitis; CDAD has been observed >2 months postantibiotic treatment. Some products may contain phenylalanine.

Drug Interactions

Avoid Concomitant Use

Avoid concomitant use of Cefprozil with any of the following: BCG

Decreased Effect

Cefprozil may decrease the levels/effects of: BCG; Typhoid Vaccine

Increased Effect/Toxicity

The levels/effects of Cefprozil may be increased by: Probenecid

Nutritional/Ethanol Interactions Food: Food delays cefprozil absorption.

Lab Interactions Positive direct Coombs', false-positive urinary glucose test using cupric sulfate (Benedict's solution, Clinitest®, Fehling's solution), false-positive serum or urine creatinine with Jaffé reaction

Adverse Reactions

1% to 10%:

Central nervous system: Dizziness (1%)
Dermatologic: Diaper rash (2%)
Gastrointestinal: Diarrhea (3%), nausea (4%), vomiting (1%), abdominal pain (1%)
Genitourinary: Vaginitis, genital pruritus (2%)
Hepatic: Transaminases increased (2%)
Miscellaneous: Superinfection

Reactions reported with other cephalosporins: Seizure, toxic epidermal necrolysis, renal dysfunction, interstitial nephritis, toxic nephropathy, aplastic anemia, hemolytic anemia, hemorrhage, pancytopenia, agranulocytosis, colitis, vaginitis, superinfection

Pharmacodynamics/Kinetics

Absorption Well absorbed (94%)

Time to Peak Serum: Fasting: 1.5 hours

Protein Binding 35% to 45%

Half-Life Elimination Normal renal function: 1.3 hours

Excretion Urine (61% as unchanged drug)

Available Dosage Forms

Powder for suspension, oral: 125 mg/5 mL (50 mL, 75 mL, 100 mL); 250 mg/5 mL (50 mL, 75 mL, 100 mL)

Tablet, oral: 250 mg, 500 mg

Dosing

Adult & Geriatric

Pharyngitis/tonsillitis: Oral: 500 mg every 24 hours for 10 days

Secondary bacterial infection of acute bronchitis or acute bacterial exacerbation of chronic bronchitis: Oral: 500 mg every 12 hours for 10 days

Uncomplicated skin and skin structure infections: Oral: 250 mg every 12 hours, or 500 mg every 12-24 hours for 10 days

Pediatric

Otitis media: Oral: Children >6 months to 12 years: 15 mg/kg every 12 hours for 10 days

Pharyngitis/tonsillitis: Oral: Children:

2-12 years: 7.5-15 mg/kg/day divided every 12 hours for 10 days (administer for >10 days if due to *S. pyogenes*); maximum: 1 g/day

≥13 years: Refer to adult dosing.

Uncomplicated skin and skin structure infections: Oral:

2-12 years: 20 mg/kg every 24 hours for 10 days; maximum: 1 g/day

≥13 years: Refer to adult dosing.

Renal Impairment

Cl_{cr} <30 mL/minute: Reduce dose by 50%.

Hemodialysis effects: 55% is removed by hemodialysis.

Administration

Oral Administer around-the-clock to promote less variation in peak and trough serum levels. Chilling the reconstituted oral suspension improves flavor (do not freeze).

Monitoring and Teaching Issues

Laboratory Monitoring Perform culture and sensitivity studies prior to initiating drug therapy; renal function

Physical Assessment Assess results of culture/sensitivity tests and patient's allergy history prior to therapy. Monitor for interstitial nephritis, hemolytic anemia, and hemorrhage. Advise patients with diabetes about use of Clinitest® (may cause false-positive test). Teach patient to report opportunistic infection and hypersensitivity reactions.

Patient Education Take at regular intervals around-the-clock, with or without food. Chilling oral suspension improves flavor (do not freeze). Maintain adequate hydration, unless instructed to restrict fluid intake. May cause false test results with Clinitest®; use of another type of glucose testing is preferable. May cause dizziness, nausea, vomiting, or diarrhea. Report rash; breathing or swallowing difficulty; persistent diarrhea, nausea, vomiting, or abdominal pain; changes in urinary pattern or pain on urination; opportunistic infection (eg, vaginal itching or drainage, sores in mouth, blood in stool or urine, unusual fever or chills); or CNS changes (eg, irritability, agitation, nervousness, insomnia, hallucinations).

Dietary Considerations May be taken with food. Oral suspension may contain phenylalanine; consult product labeling.

Geriatric Considerations Has not been studied exclusively in the elderly. Adjust dose for estimated renal function.

Breast-Feeding Considerations Small amounts of cefprozil are excreted in breast milk. The manufacturer recommends that caution be exercised when administering cefprozil to nursing women. Nondose-related effects could include modification of bowel flora.

Pregnancy Considerations Adverse events were not observed in animal reproduction studies; therefore, cefprozil is classified as pregnancy category B. It is not known if cefprozil crosses the human placenta. Other cephalosporins cross the placenta and are considered safe for use during pregnancy.

Related Information

Community-Acquired Pneumonia in Adults *on page 2021*

Ceftaroline Fosamil (sef TAR oh leen FOS a mil)

U.S. Brand Names Teflaro™

Index Terms PPI-0903; PPI-0903M; T-91825; TAK-599

Generic Availability (U.S.) No

Pharmacologic Category Antibiotic, Cephalosporin (Fifth Generation)

Pregnancy Risk Factor B

Lactation Excretion in breast milk unknown/use caution

Use Treatment of acute bacterial skin and skin structure infections (ABSSSI) caused by susceptible isolates of *Staphylococcus aureus* (including methicillin-susceptible and –resistant isolates), *Streptococcus pyogenes, Streptococcus agalactiae, Escherichia coli, Klebsiella pneumoniae*, and *Klebsiella oxytoca,* and community-acquired pneumonia (CAP) caused by *Streptococcus pneumoniae* (including cases with concurrent bacteremia), *Staphylococcus aureus* (methicillin-susceptible isolates only), *Haemophilus influenzae, Klebsiella pneumoniae, Klebsiella oxytoca,* and *Escherichia coli*

Mechanism of Action/Effect Inhibits bacterial cell wall synthesis by binding to 1 or more of the penicillin-binding proteins (PBPs)

Contraindications Hypersensitivity to ceftaroline, other cephalosporins, or any component of the formulation

Warnings/Precautions Use with caution in patients with a history of penicillin allergy, especially IgE-mediated reactions (eg, anaphylaxis, angioedema, urticaria). Prolonged use may result in fungal or bacterial superinfection, including *C. difficile*-associated diarrhea (CDAD) and pseudomembranous colitis; CDAD has been observed >2 months postantibiotic treatment. Use with caution in patients with renal impairment (Cl_{cr} ≤50 mL/minute); dosage adjustments recommended.

Drug Interactions

Avoid Concomitant Use

Avoid concomitant use of Ceftaroline Fosamil with any of the following: BCG

Decreased Effect

Ceftaroline Fosamil may decrease the levels/effects of: BCG; Typhoid Vaccine

Increased Effect/Toxicity

The levels/effects of Ceftaroline Fosamil may be increased by: Probenecid

Adverse Reactions

>10%: Hematologic: Positive Coombs' test without hemolysis (~11%)

2% to 10%:

Central nervous system: Headache (3% to 5%), insomnia (3% to 4%)
Dermatologic: Pruritus (3% to 4%), rash (3%)
Endocrine & metabolic: Hypokalemia (2%)
Gastrointestinal: Diarrhea (5%), nausea (4%), constipation (2%), vomiting (2%)
Hepatic: Transaminases increased (2%)
Local: Phlebitis (2%)

Pharmacodynamics/Kinetics

Time to Peak 1 hour

Protein Binding ~20%

Half-Life Elimination Normal renal function: 2.4 hours; Moderate renal impairment (Cl_{cr} 30-50 ml/minute): 4.5 hours

Metabolism Ceftaroline fosamil (inactive prodrug) undergoes rapid conversion to bioactive ceftaroline in plasma by phosphatase enzyme; ceftaroline is hydrolyzed to form inactive ceftaroline M-1 metabolite

Excretion Urine (~88%); feces (~6%)

Available Dosage Forms

Injection, powder for reconstitution:

Teflaro™: 600 mg

Dosing

Adult & Geriatric

Usual dosage range: I.V.: 600 mg every 12 hours

Indication-specific dosage: I.V.:

Pneumonia, community-acquired: 600 mg every 12 hours for 5-7 days
Skin and skin structure, complicated: 600 mg every 12 hours for 5-14 days

Renal Impairment

Cl_{cr} 31-50 mL/minute: Administer 400 mg every 12 hours
Cl_{cr} 15-30 mL/minute: Administer 300 mg every 12 hours
Cl_{cr} <15mL/minute and ESRD patients receiving hemodialysis: Administer 200 mg every 12 hours; should be given after hemodialysis, if applicable

Administration

I.V. Administer by slow I.V. infusion over 60 minutes.

Stability

Reconstitution Reconstitute 400 mg or 600 mg vial with 20 mL SWFI; mix gently; reconstituted solution should be further diluted for I.V. administration in >250 mL of a compatible solution (eg, D_5W, NS); use within 6 hours at room temperature or within 24 hours if refrigerated; color of infusion solutions ranges from clear and light to dark yellow depending on concentration and storage conditions.

Storage Store unused vials at 2°C to 8°C (36°F to 46°F).

Monitoring and Teaching Issues

Laboratory Monitoring Obtain specimen for culture and susceptibility prior to the first dose.

Geriatric Considerations Persons 65 years and older accounted for 30.5% of the participants (n=397) in the clinical trials leading to FDA's approval of ceftaroline. Similar cure rates for ABSSI and CABP were reported for those 65 years and older compared to younger adults. Adverse drug events were reported in 52.4% of older participants compared to 42.8% in patients less than 65 years of age. A 33% increase in ceftaroline's AUC was found in healthy older adults (65 and older) compared to younger adults. The increase in AUC was attributed to age-related decrease in kidney function.

Pregnancy Considerations Skeletal abnormalities have been observed in some but not all animal studies using maternally toxic doses. There are no adequate and well-controlled studies in pregnant women.

Additional Information Considered to be ineffective against *Pseudomonas aeruginosa*, *Enterococcus* species (including vancomycin-susceptible and -resistant isolates), extended-spectrum beta-lactamase (ESBL) producing or AmpC overexpressing Enterobacteriaceae.

Ceftazidime (SEF tay zi deem)

U.S. Brand Names Fortaz®; Tazicef®

Generic Availability (U.S.) Yes: Injection

Pharmacologic Category Antibiotic, Cephalosporin (Third Generation)

Medication Safety Issues

Sound-alike/look-alike issues:

CefTAZidime may be confused with ceFAZolin, cefepime, cefoTEtan, cefOXitin, cefTRIAXone
Ceptaz® may be confused with Septra®
Tazicef® may be confused with Tazidime®
Tazidime® may be confused with Tazicef®

International issues:

Ceftim [Italy, Portugual] and Ceftime [Thailand] brand names for ceftazidime may be confused with Ceftin brand name for cefuroxime [U.S., Canada]; Cefiton brand name for cefixime [Portugal]

Pregnancy Risk Factor B

Lactation Enters breast milk/use caution (AAP rates "compatible"; AAP 2001 update pending)

Use Treatment of documented susceptible *Pseudomonas aeruginosa* infection and infections due to other susceptible aerobic gram-negative organisms; empiric therapy of a febrile, granulocytopenic patient

Unlabeled/Investigational Use Bacterial endophthalmitis

Mechanism of Action/Effect Inhibits bacterial cell wall synthesis by binding to one or more of the penicillin-binding proteins (PBPs)

Contraindications Hypersensitivity to ceftazidime, any component of the formulation, or other cephalosporins

Warnings/Precautions Modify dosage in patients with severe renal impairment. Use with caution in patients with a history of penicillin allergy, especially IgE-mediated reactions (eg, anaphylaxis, urticaria). Prolonged use may result in fungal or bacterial superinfection, including *C. difficile*-associated diarrhea (CDAD) and pseudomembranous colitis; CDAD has been observed >2 months postantibiotic treatment. May be associated with increased INR, especially in nutritionally-deficient patients, prolonged treatment, hepatic or renal disease. Use with caution in patients with a history of seizure disorder; high levels, particularly in the presence of renal impairment, may increase risk of seizures.

Drug Interactions

Avoid Concomitant Use

Avoid concomitant use of CefTAZidime with any of the following: BCG

Decreased Effect

CefTAZidime may decrease the levels/effects of: BCG; Typhoid Vaccine

Increased Effect/Toxicity

The levels/effects of CefTAZidime may be increased by: Probenecid

Lab Interactions Positive direct Coombs', false-positive urinary glucose test using cupric sulfate (Benedict's solution, Clinitest®, Fehling's solution), false-positive serum or urine creatinine with Jaffé reaction

Adverse Reactions

1% to 10%:

Gastrointestinal: Diarrhea (1%)
Local: Pain at injection site (1%)
Miscellaneous: Hypersensitivity reactions (2%)

Reactions reported with other cephalosporins: Seizure, urticaria, serum-sickness reactions, renal dysfunction, interstitial nephritis, toxic nephropathy, BUN increased, creatinine increased, cholestasis, aplastic anemia, hemolytic anemia, pancytopenia, agranulocytosis, colitis, prolonged PT, hemorrhage, superinfection

Pharmacodynamics/Kinetics

Time to Peak Serum: I.M.: ~1 hour

Protein Binding 17%

Half-Life Elimination 1-2 hours, prolonged with renal impairment; Neonates <23 days: 2.2-4.7 hours

Excretion Urine (80% to 90% as unchanged drug)

Available Dosage Forms

Infusion, premixed iso-osmotic solution:

Fortaz®: 1 g (50 mL); 2 g (50 mL)

Injection, powder for reconstitution: 500 mg, 1 g, 2 g, 6 g

Fortaz®: 500 mg, 1 g, 2 g, 6 g

Tazicef®: 1 g, 2 g, 6 g

Dosing

Adult

Bacterial arthritis (gram negative bacilli): I.V.: 1-2 g every 8 hours

Bone and joint infections: I.V.: 2 g every 12 hours

Cystic fibrosis, lung infection caused by *Pseudomonas* spp: I.V.: 30-50 mg/kg every 8 hours (maximum: 6 g/day)

Endophthalmitis, bacterial (unlabeled use): Intravitreal: 2.25 mg/0.1 mL NS in combination with vancomycin

Intra-abdominal infection, severe (in combination with metronidazole): I.V.: 2 g every 8 hours for 4-7 days (provided source controlled). Not recommended for hospital-acquired intra-abdominal infections (IAI) associated with multidrug-resistant gram negative organisms or in mild-to-moderate community-acquired IAIs due to risk of toxicity and the development of resistant organisms (Solomkin, 2010).

Melioidosis: I.V.: 40 mg/kg every 8 hours for 10 days, followed by oral therapy with doxycycline or TMP/SMX

Otitis externa: I.V.: 2 g every 8 hours

Peritonitis (CAPD):

Anuric, intermittent: 1000-1500 mg/day

Anuric, continuous (per liter exchange): Loading dose: 250 mg; maintenance dose: 125 mg

Pneumonia: I.V.:

Uncomplicated: 500 mg to 1 g every 8 hours

Complicated or severe: 2 g every 8 hours

Skin and soft tissue infections: I.V., I.M.: 500 mg to 1 g every 8 hours

Severe infections, including meningitis, complicated pneumonia, endophthalmitis, CNS infection, osteomyelitis, gynecological, skin and soft tissue: I.V.: 2 g every 8 hours

Urinary tract infections: I.V., I.M.:

Uncomplicated: 250 mg every 12 hours

Complicated: 500 mg every 8-12 hours

Geriatric I.M., I.V.: Dosage should be based on renal function with a dosing interval not more frequent then every 12 hours.

Pediatric Susceptible infections: I.V.:

Children 1 month to 12 years: 30-50 mg/kg/dose every 8 hours; maximum dose: 6 g/day (higher doses reserved for immunocompromised patients, cystic fibrosis, or meningitis)

Children ≥12 years: Refer to adult dosing.

Renal Impairment

Cl_{cr} 30-50 mL/minute: Administer every 12 hours

Cl_{cr} 10-30 mL/minute: Administer every 24 hours

Cl_{cr} <10 mL/minute: Administer every 48-72 hours

Hemodialysis: Dialyzable (50% to 100%)

CAPD: Loading dose of 1 g, followed by 500 mg every 24 hours

Continuous renal replacement therapy (CRRT): Drug clearance is highly dependent on the method of renal replacement, filter type, and flow rate. Appropriate dosing requires close monitoring of pharmacologic response, signs of adverse reactions due to drug accumulation, as well as drug levels in relation to target trough (if appropriate). The following are general recommendations only (based on dialysate flow/ultrafiltration rates of 1 L/hour) and should not supersede clinical judgment:

CVVH: 1-2 g every 12 hours

CVVHD/CVVHDF: 2 g every 12 hours

Administration

I.M. Inject deep I.M. into large mass muscle.

I.V. Ceftazidime can be administered IVP over 3-5 minutes or I.V. intermittent infusion over 15-30 minutes.

Stability

Reconstitution

I.M.: Using SWFI, bacteriostatic water, lidocaine 0.5%, or lidocaine 1%, reconstitute the 500 mg vials with 1.5 mL or the 1 g vials with 3 mL; final concentration of *~280 mg/mL*

I.V.: Using SWFI, reconstitute as follows (**Note:** After reconstitution, may dilute further with a compatible solution to administer via I.V. infusion):

Fortaz®:

~100 mg/mL solution:

500 mg vial: 5.3 mL SWFI (withdraw 5 mL from the reconstituted vial to obtain a 500 mg dose)

1 g vial: 10 mL SWFI (withdraw 10 mL from the reconstituted vial to obtain a 1 g dose)

6 g vial: 56 mL SWFI (withdraw 10 mL from the reconstituted vial to obtain a 1 g dose)

~*170 mg/mL solution:* 2 g vial: 10 mL SWFI (withdraw 11.5 mL from the reconstituted vial to obtain a 2 g dose)

~*200 mg/mL solution:* 6 g vial: 26 mL SWFI (withdraw 5 mL from the reconstituted vial to obtain a 1 g dose)

Tazicef®:

~*95 mg/mL solution:* 1 g vial: 10 mL SWFI (withdraw 10.6 mL from the reconstituted vial to obtain a 1 g dose)

~*180 mg/mL solution:* 2 g vial: 10 mL SWFI (withdraw 11.2 mL from the reconstituted vial to obtain a 2 g dose)

Fortaz®, Tazicef®: ADD-Vantage® vials: Dilute in 50 or 100 mL of D_5W, NS, or 0.45% sodium chloride in an ADD-Vantage® flexible diluent container only.

Storage

Fortaz®: Store dry vials at 15°C to 30°C (59°F to 86°F). Protect from light. Reconstituted solution and solution further diluted for I.V. infusion are stable for 12 hours at room temperature, for 3 days when refrigerated, or for 12 weeks when frozen at -20°C (-4°F). After freezing, thawed solution in SWFI for I.M. administration is stable for 3 hours at room temperature or for 3 days when refrigerated; thawed solution in NS in a Viaflex® small volume container for I.V. administration is stable for 12 hours at room temperature or for 3 days when refrigerated; and thawed solution in SWFI in the original container is stable for 8 hours at room temperature or for 3 days when refrigerated.

Premixed frozen solution: Store frozen at -20°C (-4°F). Thawed solution is stable for 8 hours at room temperature or for 3 days under refrigeration; do not refreeze.

Fortaz®, Tazicef®: ADD-Vantage® vials: Following dilution, may be stored for up to 12 hours at room temperature or for 3 days under refrigeration. Freezing solutions in the ADD-Vantage® system is not recommended. Joined vials that have not been activated may be used within 14 days.

Tazicef® vials: Store dry vials at 20°C to 25°C (68°F to 77°F). Protect from light. Reconstituted vials and solution further diluted for I.V. infusion are stable for 24 hours at room temperature, for 7 days when refrigerated, or for 12 weeks when frozen at -20°C (-4°F). When thawed, solution is stable for 8 hours at room temperature and 4 days when refrigerated.

Monitoring and Teaching Issues

Laboratory Monitoring Perform culture and sensitivity studies prior to initiating drug therapy; renal function

Physical Assessment Monitor for nephrotoxicity. Assess prothrombin time. Monitor for hemolytic anemia, hypoprothrombinemia, and bleeding. Teach patient to report opportunistic infection and hypersensitivity reaction.

Patient Education This medication is administered by infusion or injection. Report immediately any redness, swelling, burning, or pain at injection/infusion site. Maintain adequate hydration, unless instructed to restrict fluid intake. May cause diarrhea. Report rash; breathing or swallowing difficulty; persistent diarrhea, nausea, vomiting, or abdominal pain; changes in urinary pattern or pain on urination; opportunistic infection (eg, vaginal itching or drainage, sores in mouth, blood in stool or urine, unusual fever or chills); or CNS changes (eg, irritability, agitation, nervousness, insomnia, hallucinations).

Dietary Considerations Some products may contain sodium.

Geriatric Considerations Changes in renal function associated with aging and corresponding alterations in pharmacokinetics result in every 12-hour dosing being an adequate dosing interval. Adjust dose based on renal function.

Breast-Feeding Considerations Very small amounts of ceftazidime are excreted in breast milk. The manufacturer recommends that caution be exercised when administering ceftazidime to nursing women. Ceftazidime in not absorbed when given orally; therefore, any medication that is distributed to human milk should not result in systemic concentrations in the nursing infant. Nondose-related effects could include modification of bowel flora.

Pregnancy Considerations Teratogenic effects were not observed in animal studies; therefore, ceftazidime is classified as pregnancy category B. Ceftazidime crosses the placenta and reaches the cord serum and amniotic fluid. Maternal peak serum concentration is unchanged in the first trimester. After the first trimester, serum concentrations decrease by approximately 50% of those in nonpregnant patients. Renal clearance is increased during pregnancy.

Additional Information With some organisms, resistance may develop during treatment (including *Enterobacter* spp and *Serratia* spp). Consider combination therapy or periodic susceptibility testing for organisms with inducible resistance.

Related Information

Antimicrobial Drugs of Choice *on page 2008*

Ceftibuten (sef TYE byoo ten)

U.S. Brand Names Cedax®

Generic Availability (U.S.) No

Pharmacologic Category Antibiotic, Cephalosporin (Third Generation)

Medication Safety Issues

Sound-alike/look-alike issues:

Cedax® may be confused with Cidex®

International issues:

Cedax [U.S. and multiple international markets] may be confused with Codex brand name for acetaminophen/codeine [Brazil] and *Saccharomyces boulardii* [Italy]

Pregnancy Risk Factor B

Lactation Excretion in breast milk unknown/use caution

Use Treatment of acute exacerbations of chronic bronchitis, acute bacterial otitis media, and pharyngitis/tonsillitis

Mechanism of Action/Effect Inhibits bacterial cell wall synthesis by binding to one or more of the penicillin-binding proteins (PBPs)

Contraindications Hypersensitivity to ceftibuten, any component of the formulation, or other cephalosporins

Warnings/Precautions Modify dosage in patients with moderate-to-severe renal impairment. Prolonged use may result in fungal or bacterial superinfection, including *C. difficile*-associated diarrhea (CDAD) and pseudomembranous colitis; CDAD has been observed >2 months postantibiotic treatment. Use with caution in patients with a history of colitis and other gastrointestinal diseases. Use with caution in patients with a history of penicillin allergy, especially IgE-mediated reactions (eg, anaphylaxis, urticaria). Oral suspension formulation contains sucrose.

Drug Interactions

Avoid Concomitant Use

Avoid concomitant use of Ceftibuten with any of the following: BCG

Decreased Effect

Ceftibuten may decrease the levels/effects of: BCG; Typhoid Vaccine

Increased Effect/Toxicity

The levels/effects of Ceftibuten may be increased by: Probenecid

Lab Interactions Positive direct Coombs', false-positive urinary glucose test using cupric sulfate (Benedict's solution, Clinitest®, Fehling's solution), false-positive serum or urine creatinine with Jaffé reaction

Adverse Reactions

1% to 10%:

Central nervous system: Headache (≤3%), dizziness (≤1%)

Gastrointestinal: Nausea (≤4%), diarrhea (3% to 4%), dyspepsia (≤2%), loose stools (≤2%), abdominal pain (1% to 2%), vomiting (1% to 2%)

Hematologic: Eosinophils increased (3%), hemoglobin decreased (1% to 2%), platelets increased (≤1%)

Hepatic: ALT increased (≤1%), bilirubin increased (≤1%)

Renal: BUN increased (2% to 4%)

Additional reactions reported with other cephalosporins: Allergic reaction, agranulocytosis, angioedema, aplastic anemia, anaphylaxis, asterixis, cholestasis, drug fever, encephalopathy, erythema multiforme, hemolytic anemia, hemorrhage, interstitial nephritis, neuromuscular excitability, neutropenia, pancytopenia, prolonged PT, renal dysfunction, seizure, superinfection, toxic nephropathy

Pharmacodynamics/Kinetics

Absorption Rapid; food decreases peak concentrations, delays T_{max}, and lowers AUC

Time to Peak 2-3 hours

Protein Binding 65%

Half-Life Elimination 2 hours; Cl_{cr} 30-49 mL/minute: 7 hours; Cl_{cr} 5-29 mL/minute: 13 hours; Cl_{cr} <5 mL/minute: 22 hours

Excretion Urine (~56%); feces (39%)

Available Dosage Forms

Capsule, oral:

Cedax®: 400 mg

Powder for suspension, oral:

Cedax®: 90 mg/5 mL (60 mL, 90 mL, 120 mL); 180 mg/5 mL (30 mL, 60 mL)

Dosing

Adult & Geriatric Susceptible infections: Oral: 400 mg once daily for 10 days

Pediatric Susceptible infections: Oral:

6 months to <12 years: 9 mg/kg/day for 10 days; maximum daily dose: 400 mg

≥12 years: Refer to adult dosing.

Renal Impairment

Cl_{cr} ≥50 mL//minute: No adjustment needed

Cl_{cr} 30-49 mL//minute: Administer 4.5 mg/kg or 200 mg every 24 hours.

Cl_{cr} 5-29 mL/minute: Administer 2.25 mg/kg or 100 mg every 24 hours.

Hemodialysis: Administer 400 mg or 9 mg/kg (maximum: 400 mg) after each hemodialysis session.

Administration

Oral

Capsule: Administer without regard to food.

Suspension: Administer 2 hours before or 1 hour after meals. Shake well before use.

Stability

Storage Store capsules and powder for suspension at 2°C to 25°C (36°F to 77°F). Reconstituted suspension is stable for 14 days when refrigerated at 2°C to 8°C (36°F to 46°F).

Monitoring and Teaching Issues

Laboratory Monitoring Renal, hepatic, and hematologic function periodically with prolonged therapy; perform culture and sensitivity studies prior to initiating drug therapy

Physical Assessment Assess results of culture/sensitivity tests and patient's allergy history prior to therapy. Monitor for nephrotoxicity, hemolytic anemia, hypoprothrombinemia, and bleeding. Teach patient to report opportunistic infection and hypersensitivity reaction.

Patient Education Take at regular intervals around-the-clock. Take capsules with or without food; take suspension 2 hours before or 1 hour after meals. Maintain adequate hydration, unless instructed to restrict fluid intake. May cause headache, dizziness, nausea, vomiting, or diarrhea. Report rash; breathing or swallowing difficulty; persistent diarrhea, nausea, vomiting, or abdominal pain; changes in urinary pattern or pain on urination; opportunistic infection (eg, vaginal itching or drainage, sores in mouth, blood in stool or urine, unusual fever or chills); or CNS changes (eg, irritability, agitation, nervousness, insomnia, hallucinations).

Dietary Considerations

Capsule: Take without regard to food.

Suspension: Take 2 hours before or 1 hour after meals.

Geriatric Considerations Has not been studied specifically in the elderly. Adjust dose for renal function.

Breast-Feeding Considerations Ceftibuten was not detectable in milk after a single 200 mg dose (limit of detection: 1 mcg/mL). It is not known if it would be detectable after a 400 mg dose or multiple doses. The manufacturer recommends that caution be exercised when administering ceftibuten to nursing women. If ceftibuten does reach the human milk, non-dose-related effects could include modification of bowel flora.

Pregnancy Considerations Teratogenic effects were not observed in animal studies; therefore, ceftibuten is classified as pregnancy category B. It is not know if ceftibuten crosses the placenta; other cephalosporins cross the placenta and are considered safe for use during pregnancy. Adequate and well-controlled studies have not been completed in pregnant women.

◆ **Ceftin®** *see* Cefuroxime *on page 340*

CefTRIAXone (sef trye AKS one)

U.S. Brand Names Rocephin®

Index Terms Ceftriaxone Sodium

Generic Availability (U.S.) Yes

Pharmacologic Category Antibiotic, Cephalosporin (Third Generation)

Medication Safety Issues

Sound-alike/look-alike issues:

CefTRIAXone may be confused with CeFAZolin, cefoTEtan, cefOXitin, cefTAZidime, Cetraxal®

Rocephin® may be confused with Roferon®

Pregnancy Risk Factor B

Lactation Enters breast milk/use caution (AAP rates "compatible"; AAP 2001 update pending)

Use Treatment of lower respiratory tract infections, acute bacterial otitis media, skin and skin structure infections, bone and joint infections, intra-abdominal and urinary tract infections, pelvic inflammatory disease (PID), uncomplicated gonorrhea, bacterial septicemia, and meningitis; used in surgical prophylaxis

Unlabeled/Investigational Use Treatment of chancroid, epididymitis, complicated gonococcal infections; sexually-transmitted diseases (STD); periorbital or buccal cellulitis; salmonellosis or shigellosis; atypical community-acquired pneumonia; epiglottitis, Lyme disease; used in chemoprophylaxis for high-risk contacts and persons with invasive meningococcal disease; sexual assault; typhoid fever, Whipple's disease

Mechanism of Action/Effect Inhibits bacterial cell wall synthesis by binding to one or more of the penicillin-binding proteins (PBPs)

Contraindications Hypersensitivity to ceftriaxone sodium, any component of the formulation, or other cephalosporins; **do not use in hyperbilirubinemic neonates**, particularly those who are premature since ceftriaxone is reported to displace bilirubin from albumin binding sites; concomitant use with intravenous calcium-containing solutions/products in neonates (≤28 days)

Warnings/Precautions Use with caution in patients with a history of penicillin allergy, especially IgE-mediated reactions (eg, anaphylaxis, urticaria). Abnormal gallbladder sonograms have been reported, possibly due to cetriaxone-calcium precipitates; discontinue in patients with signs and symptoms of gallbladder disease. Secondary to biliary obstruction, pancreatitis has been reported rarely. Use with caution in patients with a history of GI disease, especially colitis. Severe cases (including some fatalities) of immune-related hemolytic anemia have been reported in patients receiving cephalosporins, including ceftriaxone. Prolonged use may result in fungal or bacterial superinfection, including *C. difficile*-associated diarrhea (CDAD) and pseudomembranous colitis; CDAD has been observed >2 months postantibiotic treatment.

May be associated with increased INR (rarely), especially in nutritionally-deficient patients, prolonged treatment, hepatic or renal disease. No adjustment is generally necessary in patients with renal impairment; use with caution in patients with concurrent hepatic dysfunction and significant renal disease, dosage should not exceed 2 g/day. Ceftriaxone may complex with calcium causing precipitation. Fatal lung and kidney damage associated with calcium-ceftriaxone precipitates has been observed in premature and term neonates. Do not reconstitute, admix, or coadminister with calcium-containing solutions, even via separate infusion lines/sites or at different times in any neonatal patient. Ceftriaxone should not be diluted or administered simultaneously with any calcium-containing solution via a Y-site in any patient. However, ceftriaxone and calcium-containing solution may be administered sequentially of one another for use in patients **other than neonates** if infusion lines are thoroughly flushed, with a compatible fluid, between infusions

Drug Interactions

Avoid Concomitant Use

Avoid concomitant use of CefTRIAXone with any of the following: BCG

Decreased Effect

CefTRIAXone may decrease the levels/effects of: BCG; Typhoid Vaccine

Increased Effect/Toxicity

CefTRIAXone may increase the levels/effects of: Vitamin K Antagonists

The levels/effects of CefTRIAXone may be increased by: Calcium Salts (Intravenous); Probenecid; Ringer's Injection (Lactated)

Lab Interactions Positive direct Coombs', false-positive urinary glucose test using cupric sulfate (Benedict's solution, Clinitest®, Fehling's solution), false-positive serum or urine creatinine with Jaffé reaction

Adverse Reactions

>10%: Local: Induration (I.M. 5% to 17%), warmth (I.M.), tightness (I.M.)

1% to 10%:

Dermatologic: Rash (2%)

Gastrointestinal: Diarrhea (3%)

Hematologic: Eosinophilia (6%), thrombocytosis (5%), leukopenia (2%)

Hepatic: Transaminases increased (3%)

Local: Tenderness at injection site (I.V. 1%), pain

Renal: BUN increased (1%)

Reactions reported with other cephalosporins: Angioedema, allergic reaction, aplastic anemia, asterixis, cholestasis, encephalopathy, hemorrhage, hepatic dysfunction, hyperactivity (reversible), hypertonia, interstitial nephritis, LDH increased, neuromuscular excitability, pancytopenia, paresthesia, renal dysfunction, superinfection, toxic nephropathy

Pharmacodynamics/Kinetics

Absorption I.M.: Well absorbed

Time to Peak Serum: I.M.: 2-3 hours

Protein Binding 85% to 95%

Half-Life Elimination Normal renal and hepatic function: 5-9 hours; Renal impairment (mild-to-severe): 12-16 hours

Excretion Urine (33% to 67% as unchanged drug); feces (as inactive drug)

Available Dosage Forms

Infusion, premixed in D_5W: 1 g (50 mL); 2 g (50 mL)

Injection, powder for reconstitution: 250 mg, 500 mg, 1 g, 2 g, 10 g

Rocephin®: 500 mg, 1 g

Dosing

Adult & Geriatric

Dosage range: Usual dose: 1-2 g every 12-24 hours, depending on the type and severity of infection

Arthritis, septic (unlabeled use): I.V.: 1-2 g once daily

Brain abscess (unlabeled use): I.V.: 2 g every 12 hours with metronidazole

Cavernous sinus thrombosis (unlabeled use): I.V.: 2 g once daily with vancomycin or linezolid

Chancroid (unlabeled use): I.M.: 250 mg as single dose (CDC, 2010)

Chemoprophylaxis for high-risk contacts and persons with invasive meningococcal disease (unlabeled use): I.M.: 250 mg in a single dose

Cholecystitis, mild-to-moderate: 1-2 g every 12-24 hours for 4-7 days (provided source controlled)

Gonococcal infections (CDC, 2010):

Conjunctivitis, complicated (unlabeled use): I.M., I.V.: 1 g in a single dose

Disseminated (unlabeled use): I.M., I.V.: 1 g once daily for 24-48 hours may switch to cefixime (after improvement noted) to complete a total of 7 days of therapy

Endocarditis (unlabeled use): I.M., I.V.: 1-2 g every 24 hours for at least 28 days

Epididymitis, acute (unlabeled use): I.M.: 250 mg in a single dose with doxycycline

Meningitis: I.M., I.V.: 1-2 g every 12 hours for 10-14 days

Proctitis (unlabeled use): I.M.: 250 mg in a single dose with doxycycline

Prostatitis (unlabeled use): I.M.: 125-250 mg in a single dose with doxycycline

Uncomplicated cervicitis, pharyngitis, urethritis (unlabeled use): I.M.: 250 mg in a single dose with doxycycline or azithromycin

Infective endocarditis: I.M., I.V.:

Native valve: 2 g once daily for 2-4 weeks; **Note:** If using 2-week regimen, concurrent gentamicin is recommended

Prosthetic valve: I.M., I.V.: 2 g once daily for 6 weeks (with or without 2 weeks of gentamicin [dependent on penicillin MIC]); **Note:** For HACEK organisms, duration of therapy is 4 weeks

Enterococcus faecalis (resistant to penicillin, aminoglycoside, and vancomycin), native or prosthetic valve: 2 g twice daily for ≥8 weeks administered concurrently with ampicillin

Prophylaxis: I.M., I.V.: 1 g 30-60 minutes before procedure. Intramuscular injections should be avoided in patients who are receiving anticoagulant therapy. In these circumstances, orally administered regimens should be given whenever possible. Intravenously administered antibiotics should be used for patients who are unable to tolerate or absorb oral medications.

Note: American Heart Association (AHA) guidelines now recommend prophylaxis only in patients undergoing invasive procedures and in whom underlying cardiac conditions may predispose to a higher risk of adverse outcomes should infection occur. As of April 2007, routine prophylaxis for GI/GU procedures is no longer recommended by the AHA.

Intra-abdominal infection, complicated, community-acquired, mild-to-moderate (in combination with metronidazole): 1-2 g every 12-24 hours for 4-7 days (provided source controlled)

Lyme disease (unlabeled use): I.V.: 2 g once daily for 14-28 days

Mastoiditis (hospitalized; unlabeled use): I.V.: 2 g once daily; >60 years old: 1 g once daily

Meningitis: I.V.: 2 g every 12 hours for 7-14 days (longer courses may be necessary for selected organisms)

Orbital cellulitis (unlabeled use) and endophthalmitis: I.V.: 2 g once daily

Pelvic inflammatory disease: I.M.: 250 mg in a single dose plus doxycycline (with or without metronidazole) (CDC, 2010)

Pneumonia, community-acquired: I.V.: 1 g once daily, usually in combination with a macrolide; consider 2 g/day for patients at risk for more severe infection and/or resistant organisms (ICU status, age >65 years, disseminated infection)

Prophylaxis against sexually-transmitted diseases following sexual assault: I.M.: 250 mg as a single dose (in combination with azithromycin and metronidazole) (CDC, 2010)

Pyelonephritis (acute, uncomplicated): Females: I.V.: 1-2 g once daily (Stamm, 1993). Many physicians administer a single parenteral dose before initiating oral therapy (Warren, 1999).

Septic/toxic shock/necrotizing fasciitis (unlabeled use): I.V.: 2 g once daily; with clindamycin for toxic shock

Surgical prophylaxis: I.V.: 1 g 30 minutes to 2 hours before surgery

Cholecystectomy: 1-2 g every 12-24 hours, discontinue within 24 hours unless infection outside gallbladder suspected

Syphilis (unlabeled use): I.M., I.V.: 1 g once daily for 10-14 days; **Note:** Alternative treatment for early syphilis, optimal dose, and duration have not been defined (CDC, 2010)

Typhoid fever (unlabeled use): I.V.: 2 g once daily for 14 days

Whipple's disease (unlabeled use): Initial: 2 g once daily for 10-14 days, then oral therapy for ~1 year.

Pediatric

Dosage range: Infants and Children: Usual dose: I.M., I.V.:

Mild-to-moderate infections: 50-75 mg/kg/day in 1-2 divided doses every 12-24 hours (maximum: 2 g/day); continue until at least 2 days after signs and symptoms of infection have resolved

Serious infections: 80-100 mg/kg/day in 1-2 divided doses (maximum: 4 g/day)

Chemoprophylaxis for high-risk contacts and persons with invasive meningococcal disease (unlabeled use):

Children ≤15 years: I.M.: 125 mg in a single dose

Children >15 years: Refer to adult dosing.

Epididymitis, acute: Children >8 years (≥45 kg) and Adolescents (unlabeled use): I.M.: 125 mg in a single dose

Epiglottis (unlabeled use): I.M., I.V.: 50-100 mg/kg once daily; reported duration of treatment ranged from 2-14 days

Gonococcal infections:

Conjunctivitis, complicated (unlabeled use): I.M.:

<45 kg: 50 mg/kg in a single dose (maximum: 1 g)

≥45 kg: 1 g in a single dose

Disseminated (unlabeled use): I.M., I.V.:

Infants: 25-50 mg/kg/day as single daily dose for 7 days (10-14 days for meningitis) (CDC, 2010). **Note:** Use contraindicated in hyperbilirubinemic neonates.

Children <45 kg: 25-50 mg/kg once daily (maximum: 1 g)

Children ≥45 kg: 1 g once daily for 7 days

Endocarditis (unlabeled use):

<45 kg: I.M., I.V.: 50 mg/kg/day every 12 hours (maximum: 2 g/day) for at least 28 days

≥45 kg: I.V.: 1-2 g every 12 hours, for at least 28 days

Prophylaxis (due to maternal gonococcal infection): I.M., I.V.: 25-50 mg/kg as a single dose (maximum: 125 mg) (CDC, 2010)

Uncomplicated cervicitis, pharyngitis, proctitis, urethritis, vulvovaginitis (unlabeled use) (CDC, 2010):

≤45 kg: I.M.: 125 mg as a single dose

>45 kg: Refer to adult dosing.

Infective endocarditis: I.M., I.V.:

Native valve: 100 mg/kg once daily for 2-4 weeks; **Note:** If using 2-week regimen, concurrent gentamicin is recommended

Prosthetic valve: 100 mg/kg once daily for 6 weeks (with or without 2 weeks of gentamicin [dependent on penicillin MIC]); **Note:** For HACEK organisms, duration of therapy is 4 weeks

Enterococcus faecalis (resistant to penicillin, aminoglycoside, and vancomycin), native or prosthetic valve: 100 mg/kg once daily for ≥8 weeks administered concurrently with ampicillin

Prophylaxis: 50 mg/kg 30-60 minutes before procedure; maximum dose: 1 g. Intramuscular injections should be avoided in patients who are receiving anticoagulant therapy. In these circumstances, orally administered regimens should be given whenever possible. Intravenously administered antibiotics should be used for patients who are unable to tolerate or absorb oral medications.

Note: American Heart Association (AHA) guidelines now recommend prophylaxis only in patients undergoing invasive procedures and in whom underlying cardiac conditions may predispose to a higher risk of adverse outcomes should infection occur. As of April 2007, routine prophylaxis for GI/GU procedures is no longer recommended by the AHA.

Lyme disease, persistent arthritis (unlabeled use): I.M., I.V.: 75-100 mg/kg (maximum: 2 g) for 2-4 weeks

Meningitis: I.M., I.V.:

Uncomplicated: Loading dose of 100 mg/kg (maximum: 4 g), followed by 100 mg/kg/day divided every 12-24 hours (maximum: 4 g/day); usual duration of treatment is 7-14 days

Gonococcal, complicated:

<45 kg: 50 mg/kg/day given every 12 hours (maximum: 2 g/day); usual duration of treatment is 10-14 days

>45 kg: I.V.: 1-2 g every 12 hours; usual duration of treatment is 10-14 days

Ophthalmia neonatorum (unlabeled use): Infants: I.M., I.V.: 25-50 mg/kg as a single dose (maximum: 125 mg) (CDC, 2010)

Otitis media: I.M.:

Acute: 50 mg/kg in a single dose (maximum: 1 g)

Persistent or relapsing (unlabeled use): 50 mg/kg once daily for 3 days

Pneumonia: I.V.: 50-75 mg/kg once daily

Prophylaxis against sexually-transmitted diseases following sexual assault (unlabeled use):

≤45 kg: I.M.: 125 mg in a single dose (in combination with azithromycin and metronidazole) (CDC, 2010)

>45 kg: Refer to adult dosing.

Skin/skin structure infections: I.M., I.V.: 50-75 mg/kg/day in 1-2 divided doses (maximum: 2 g/day)

Typhoid fever (unlabeled use): I.V.: 75-80 mg/kg once daily for 5-14 days

Renal Impairment No adjustment is generally necessary; **Note:** Concurrent renal and hepatic dysfunction: Maximum dose: ≤2 g/day

Not dialyzable (0% to 5%)

Administer dose postdialysis.

Continuous ambulatory peritoneal dialysis (CAPD): Administer 1 g every 12 hours

Continuous renal replacement therapy (CRRT): Drug clearance is highly dependent on the method of renal replacement, filter type, and flow rate. Appropriate dosing requires close monitoring of pharmacologic response, signs of adverse reactions due to drug accumulation, as well as drug levels in relation to target trough (if appropriate). The following are general recommendations only (based on dialysate flow/ultrafiltration rates of 1 L/hour) and should not supersede clinical judgment:

CVVH or CVVHD/CVVHDF: 2 g every 12-24 hours

Hepatic Impairment No adjustment necessary unless there is concurrent renal dysfunction (see Renal Impairment).

Administration

I.M. Inject deep I.M. into large muscle mass; a concentration of 250 mg/mL or 350 mg/mL is recommended for all vial sizes except the 250 mg size (250 mg/mL is suggested); can be diluted with 1:1 water and 1% lidocaine for I.M. administration.

I.V. Do not reconstitute or coadminister with calcium-containing solutions. Infuse intermittent infusion over 30 minutes.

Stability

Reconstitution

I.M. injection: Vials should be reconstituted with appropriate volume of diluent (including D_5W, NS, SWFI, bacteriostatic water, or 1% lidocaine) to make a final concentration of 250 mg/mL or 350 mg/mL.

Volume to add to create a **250 mg/mL** solution:

250 mg vial: 0.9 mL
500 mg vial: 1.8 mL
1 g vial: 3.6 mL
2 g vial: 7.2 mL

Volume to add to create a **350 mg/mL** solution:

500 mg vial: 1.0 mL
1 g vial: 2.1 mL
2 g vial: 4.2 mL

I.V. infusion: Infusion is prepared in two stages: Initial reconstitution of powder, followed by dilution to final infusion solution.

Vials: Reconstitute powder with appropriate I.V. diluent (including SWFI, D_5W, $D_{10}W$, NS) to create an initial solution of ~100 mg/mL. Recommended volume to add:

250 mg vial: 2.4 mL
500 mg vial: 4.8 mL
1 g vial: 9.6 mL
2 g vial: 19.2 mL

Note: After reconstitution of powder, further dilution into a volume of compatible solution (eg, 50-100 mL of D_5W or NS) is recommended.

Piggyback bottle: Reconstitute powder with appropriate I.V. diluent (D_5W or NS) to create a resulting solution of ~100 mg/mL. Recommended initial volume to add:

1 g bottle:10 mL
2 g bottle: 20 mL

Note: After reconstitution, to prepare the final infusion solution, further dilution to 50 mL or 100 mL volumes with the appropriate I.V. diluent (including D_5W or NS) is recommended.

Storage

Powder for injection: Prior to reconstitution, store at room temperature ≤25°C (≤77°F). Protect from light.

Premixed solution (manufacturer premixed): Store at -20°C; once thawed, solutions are stable for 3 days at room temperature of 25°C (77°F) or for 21 days refrigerated at 5°C (41°F). Do not refreeze.

Stability of reconstituted solutions:

10-40 mg/mL: Reconstituted in D_5W, $D_{10}W$, NS, or SWFI: Stable for 2 days at room temperature of 25°C (77°F) or for 10 days when refrigerated at 4°C (39°F). Stable for 26 weeks when frozen at -20°C when reconstituted with D_5W or NS. Once thawed (at room temperature), solutions are stable for 2 days at room temperature of 25°C (77°F) or for 10 days when refrigerated at 4°C (39°F); does not apply to manufacturer's premixed bags. Do not refreeze.

100 mg/mL:

Reconstituted in D_5W, SWFI, or NS: Stable for 2 days at room temperature of 25°C (77°F) or for 10 days when refrigerated at 4°C (39°F).

Reconstituted in lidocaine 1% solution or bacteriostatic water: Stable for 24 hours at room temperature of 25°C (77°F) or for 10 days when refrigerated at 4°C (39°F).

250-350 mg/mL: Reconstituted in D_5W, NS, lidocaine 1% solution, bacteriostatic water, or SWFI: Stable for 24 hours at room temperature of 25°C (77°F) or for 3 days when refrigerated at 4°C (39°F).

Monitoring and Teaching Issues

Laboratory Monitoring Prothrombin times; perform culture and sensitivity studies prior to initiating drug therapy.

Physical Assessment Perform culture and sensitivity testing and assess patient's allergy history before initiating therapy. Assess for use precautions and contraindications. Assess prothrombin times.

Patient Education This medication can only be administered by injection or infusion. Report immediately any swelling, pain, burning, or redness at infusion/injection site; back pain; difficulty breathing or swallowing; rapid heartbeat; or chills. Maintain adequate hydration, unless instructed to restrict fluid intake. Report rash; breathing or swallowing difficulty; persistent diarrhea, nausea, vomiting, or abdominal pain; changes in urinary pattern or pain on urination; opportunistic infection (eg, vaginal itching or drainage, sores in mouth, blood in stool or urine, vaginal itching or drainage, unusual fever or chills); or CNS changes (eg, irritability, agitation, nervousness, insomnia, hallucinations).

Dietary Considerations Some products may contain sodium.

Geriatric Considerations No adjustment for changes in renal function necessary.

Breast-Feeding Considerations Small amounts of ceftriaxone are excreted in breast milk. The manufacturer recommends that caution be exercised when administering ceftriaxone to nursing women. Nondose-related effects could include modification of bowel flora.

Pregnancy Considerations Teratogenic effects have not been observed in animal studies; therefore, ceftriaxone is classified as pregnancy category B. The pharmacokinetics of ceftriaxone in the third trimester are similar to those of nonpregnant patients, with the possible exception of lower peak concentrations during labor. Ceftriaxone crosses the placenta and distributes to amniotic fluid. Ceftriaxone is recommended for use in pregnant women for the treatment of gonococcal infections.

Related Information

Antimicrobial Drugs of Choice *on page* 2008

Community-Acquired Pneumonia in Adults *on page* 2021

◆ **Ceftriaxone Sodium** *see* CefTRIAXone *on page* 336

Cefuroxime (se fyoor OKS eem)

U.S. Brand Names Ceftin®; Zinacef®

Index Terms Cefuroxime Axetil; Cefuroxime Sodium

Generic Availability (U.S.) Yes

Pharmacologic Category Antibiotic, Cephalosporin (Second Generation)

Medication Safety Issues

Sound-alike/look-alike issues:

Cefuroxime may be confused with cefotaxime, cefprozil, deferoxamine

Ceftin® may be confused with Cefzil®, Cipro®

Zinacef® may be confused with Zithromax®

International issues:

Ceftin [U.S., Canada] may be confused with Cefiton brand name for cefixime [Portugal]; Ceftim brand name for ceftazidime [Italy, Portugal]; Ceftime brand name for ceftazidime [Thailand]

Pregnancy Risk Factor B

Lactation Enters breast milk/use caution

Use Treatment of infections caused by staphylococci, group B streptococci, *H. influenzae* (type A and B), *E. coli*, *Enterobacter*, *Salmonella*, and *Klebsiella*; treatment of susceptible infections of the upper and lower respiratory tract, otitis media, urinary tract, uncomplicated skin and soft tissue, bone and joint, sepsis, uncomplicated gonorrhea, and early Lyme disease; surgical prophylaxis

Mechanism of Action/Effect Inhibits bacterial cell wall synthesis by binding to one or more of the penicillin-binding proteins (PBPs)

Contraindications Hypersensitivity to cefuroxime, any component of the formulation, or other cephalosporins

Warnings/Precautions Modify dosage in patients with severe renal impairment. Use with caution in patients with a history of penicillin allergy, especially IgE-mediated reactions (eg, anaphylaxis, urticaria). Prolonged use may result in fungal or bacterial superinfection, including *C. difficile*-associated diarrhea (CDAD) and pseudomembranous colitis; CDAD has been observed >2 months postantibiotic treatment. May be associated with increased INR, especially in nutritionally-deficient patients, prolonged treatment, hepatic or renal disease. Tablets and oral suspension are not bioequivalent (do not substitute on a mg-per-mg basis). Some products may contain phenylalanine.

Drug Interactions

Avoid Concomitant Use

Avoid concomitant use of Cefuroxime with any of the following: BCG

Decreased Effect

Cefuroxime may decrease the levels/effects of: BCG; Typhoid Vaccine

The levels/effects of Cefuroxime may be decreased by: Antacids; H2-Antagonists

Increased Effect/Toxicity

The levels/effects of Cefuroxime may be increased by: Probenecid

Nutritional/Ethanol Interactions Food: Bioavailability is increased with food; cefuroxime serum levels may be increased if taken with food or dairy products.

Lab Interactions Positive direct Coombs', false-positive urinary glucose test using cupric sulfate (Benedict's solution, Clinitest®, Fehling's solution); false-negative may occur with ferricyanide test. Glucose oxidase or hexokinase-based methods should be used.

Adverse Reactions

>10%: Gastrointestinal: Diarrhea (4% to 11%, duration-dependent)

1% to 10%:

Dermatologic: Diaper rash (3%)

Endocrine & metabolic: Alkaline phosphatase increased (2%), lactate dehydrogenase increased (1%)

Gastrointestinal: Nausea/vomiting (3% to 7%)

Genitourinary: Vaginitis (≤5%)

Hematologic: Eosinophilia (7%), hemoglobin and hematocrit decreased (10%)

Hepatic: Transaminases increased (2% to 4%)

Local: Thrombophlebitis (2%)

Reactions reported with other cephalosporins: Agranulocytosis, aplastic anemia, asterixis, encephalopathy, hemorrhage, neuromuscular excitability, serum-sickness reactions, superinfection, toxic nephropathy

Pharmacodynamics/Kinetics

Absorption Oral (cefuroxime axetil): Increases with food

Bioavailability Tablet: Fasting: 37%; Following food: 52%

Time to Peak Serum: I.M.: ~15-60 minutes; I.V.: 2-3 minutes; Oral: Children: 3-4 hours; Adults: 2-3 hours

Protein Binding 33% to 50%

Half-Life Elimination Children 1-2 hours; Adults: 1-2 hours; prolonged with renal impairment

Excretion Urine (66% to 100% as unchanged drug)

Available Dosage Forms

Infusion, premixed iso-osmotic solution:

Zinacef®: 750 mg (50 mL); 1.5 g (50 mL)

Injection, powder for reconstitution: 750 mg, 1.5 g, 7.5 g, 75 g

Zinacef®: 750 mg, 1.5 g, 7.5 g

Powder for suspension, oral: 125 mg/5 mL (100 mL); 250 mg/5 mL (50 mL, 100 mL)

Ceftin®: 125 mg/5 mL (100 mL); 250 mg/5 mL (50 mL, 100 mL)

Tablet, oral: 250 mg, 500 mg

Ceftin®: 250 mg, 500 mg

Dosing

Adult & Geriatric Note: Cefuroxime axetil film-coated tablets and oral suspension are not bioequivalent and are not substitutable on a mg/mg basis. All oral doses listed are for tablet formulation:

Bronchitis, acute (and exacerbations of chronic bronchitis):

Oral: 250-500 mg every 12 hours for 10 days

I.V.: 500-750 mg every 8 hours (complete therapy with oral dosing)

Cellulitis, orbital: I.V.: 1.5 g every 8 hours

Cholecystitis, mild-to-moderate: 1.5 g every 8 hours for 4-7 days (provided source controlled)

Gonorrhea:

Disseminated: I.M., I.V.: 750 mg every 8 hours

Uncomplicated:

Oral: 1 g as a single dose

I.M.: 1.5 g as single dose (administer in two different sites with probenecid)

Intra-abdominal infection, complicated, community-acquired, mild-to-moderate (in combination with metronidazole): 1.5 g every 8 hours for 4-7 days (provided source controlled)

Lyme disease (early): Oral: 500 mg twice daily for 20 days

Pharyngitis/tonsillitis and sinusitis: Oral: 250 mg twice daily for 10 days

Skin/skin structure infection, uncomplicated:

Oral: 250-500 mg every 12 hours for 10 days

I.M., I.V.: 750 mg every 8 hours

Pneumonia, uncomplicated: I.M., I.V.: 750 mg every 8 hours

Severe or complicated infections: I.M., I.V.: 1.5 g every 8 hours (up to 1.5 g every 6 hours in life-threatening infections)

Surgical prophylaxis: I.V.: 1.5 g 30 minutes to 1 hour prior to procedure (if procedure is prolonged can give 750 mg every 8 hours I.M.)

Cholecystectomy: I.V.: 1.5 g every 8 hours, discontinue within 24 hours unless infection outside gallbladder suspected

Open heart: I.V.: 1.5 g every 12 hours to a total of 6 g

Urinary tract infection, uncomplicated:

Oral: 125-250 mg twice daily for 7-10 days

I.V., I.M.: 750 mg every 8 hours

Pediatric Note: Cefuroxime axetil film-coated tablets and oral suspension are not bioequivalent and are not substitutable on a mg/mg basis.

Children 3 months to 12 years:

Epiglottitis: 150 mg/kg/day in 3 divided doses for 7-10 days

Acute otitis media, impetigo:

Oral:

Suspension: 30 mg/kg/day (maximum: 1 g/day) in 2 divided doses for 10 days

Tablet: 250 mg every 12 hours for 10 days

I.M., I.V.: 75-150 mg/kg/day divided every 8 hours (maximum dose: 6 g/day)

Acute bacterial maxillary sinusitis: Oral:

Suspension: 30 mg/kg/day in 2 divided doses for 10 days (maximum dose: 1 g/day)

Tablet: 250 mg twice daily for 10 days

Meningitis: NOT recommended (doses of 200-240 mg/kg/day divided every 6-8 hours have been used) (maximum dose: 9 g/day)

Pharyngitis, tonsillitis:

Oral:

Suspension: 20 mg/kg/day (maximum: 500 mg/day) in 2 divided doses for 10 days

Tablet: 125 mg every 12 hours for 10 days

I.M., I.V.: 75-150 mg/kg/day divided every 8 hours; maximum dose: 6 g/day

Children ≥13 years: Refer to adult dosing.

Renal Impairment

Cl_{cr} 10-20 mL/minute: Administer every 12 hours.

Cl_{cr} <10 mL/minute: Administer every 24 hours.

Hemodialysis: Dialyzable (25%)

Peritoneal dialysis: Dose every 24 hours

Continuous renal replacement therapy (CRRT): 1 g every 12 hours

Note: Cefuroxime axetil film-coated tablets and oral suspension are not bioequivalent and are not substitutable on a mg/mg basis.

Administration

Oral Administer with food. Shake well before use.

I.M. Inject deep I.M. into large muscle mass.

I.V. Inject direct I.V. over 3-5 minutes. Infuse intermittent infusion over 15-30 minutes.

Stability

Storage

Injection: Reconstituted solution is stable for 24 hours at room temperature and 48 hours when refrigerated. I.V. infusion in NS or D_5W solution is stable for 24 hours at room temperature, 7 days when refrigerated, or 26 weeks when frozen. After freezing, thawed solution is stable for 24 hours at room temperature or 21 days when refrigerated.

Oral suspension: Prior to reconstitution, store at 2°C to 30°C (36°F to 86°F). Reconstituted suspension is stable for 10 days at 2°C to 8°C (36°F to 46°F).

Tablet: Store at 15°C to 30°C (59°F to 86°F).

Monitoring and Teaching Issues

Laboratory Monitoring Perform culture and sensitivity studies prior to initiating therapy; renal function

Physical Assessment Assess results of culture/sensitivity tests and patient's allergy history prior to therapy. Monitor for nephrotoxicity. Assess prothrombin times. Monitor for hemolytic anemia, hypoprothrombinemia, and bleeding. Advise patients with diabetes about use of Clinitest® (may cause false-positive test). Teach patient to report opportunistic infection and hypersensitivity reaction.

Patient Education If administered by injection or infusion, report immediately any swelling, redness, or pain at injection/infusion site; respiratory difficulty or swallowing; chest pain; or rash. Oral tablets or suspension should be taken at regular intervals around-the-clock, with food. Shake well before using oral suspension. Maintain adequate hydration, unless instructed to restrict fluid intake. May cause false test results with Clinitest®; use of another type of glucose testing is preferable. Report rash; breathing or swallowing difficulty; persistent diarrhea, nausea, vomiting, or abdominal pain; changes in urinary pattern or pain on urination; opportunistic infection (eg, vaginal itching or drainage, sores in mouth, blood in stool or urine, unusual fever or chills); or CNS changes (eg, irritability, agitation, nervousness, insomnia, hallucinations).

Dietary Considerations Some products may contain phenylalanine and/or sodium.

Oral suspension: May be taken with food.

Geriatric Considerations Adjust dose for renal function in the elderly. Considered one of the drugs of choice for outpatient treatment of community-acquired pneumonia in the elderly.

Breast-Feeding Considerations Cefuroxime is excreted in breast milk. Manufacturer recommendations vary; caution is recommended if cefuroxime I.V. is given to a nursing woman and it is recommended to consider discontinuing nursing temporarily during treatment following oral cefuroxime. Nondose-related effects could include modification of bowel flora.

Pregnancy Considerations Adverse events were not observed in animal studies; therefore, cefuroxime is classified as pregnancy category B. Cefuroxime crosses the placenta and reaches the cord serum and amniotic fluid. Placental transfer is decreased in the presence of oligohydramnios. Several studies have failed to identify a teratogenic risk to the fetus from maternal cefuroxime use.

During pregnancy, mean plasma concentrations of cefuroxime are 50% lower, the AUC is 25% lower, and the plasma half-life is shorter than nonpregnant values. At term, plasma half-life is similar to nonpregnant values and peak maternal concentrations after I.M. administration are slightly decreased. Pregnancy does not alter the volume of distribution.

Related Information

Antimicrobial Drugs of Choice *on page 2008*

Community-Acquired Pneumonia in Adults *on page 2021*

I.V. to Oral Conversion *on page 1956*

◆ **Cefuroxime Axetil** *see* Cefuroxime *on page 340*

◆ **Cefuroxime Sodium** *see* Cefuroxime *on page 340*

◆ **Cefzil** *see* Cefprozil *on page 329*

◆ **CeleBREX®** *see* Celecoxib *on page 343*

Celecoxib (se le KOKS ib)

U.S. Brand Names CeleBREX®

Generic Availability (U.S.) No

Pharmacologic Category Nonsteroidal Anti-inflammatory Drug (NSAID), COX-2 Selective

Medication Safety Issues

Sound-alike/look-alike issues:

CeleBREX® may be confused with CeleXA®, cerebra, Cerebyx®, Cervarix®, Clarinex®

Medication Guide Available Yes

Pregnancy Risk Factor C (prior to 30 weeks gestation)/D (≥30 weeks gestation)

Lactation Enters breast milk/use caution

Use Relief of the signs and symptoms of osteoarthritis, ankylosing spondylitis, juvenile idiopathic arthritis (JIA), and rheumatoid arthritis; management of acute pain; treatment of primary dysmenorrhea

Mechanism of Action/Effect Inhibits prostaglandin synthesis by decreasing the activity of the enzyme, cyclooxygenase-2 (COX-2), which results in decreased formation of prostaglandin precursors; has antipyretic, analgesic, and anti-inflammatory properties. Celecoxib does not inhibit cyclooxygenase-1 (COX-1) at therapeutic concentrations.

Contraindications Hypersensitivity to celecoxib, sulfonamides, aspirin, other NSAIDs, or any component of the formulation; perioperative pain in the setting of coronary artery bypass graft (CABG) surgery

Canadian labeling: Additional contraindications (not in U.S. labeling): Pregnancy (third trimester); women who are breast-feeding; severe, uncontrolled heart failure; active gastrointestinal ulcer (gastric, duodenal, peptic) or bleeding; inflammatory bowel disease; cerebrovascular bleeding; severe liver impairment or active hepatic disease; severe renal impairment (Cl_{cr} <30 mL/minute) or deteriorating renal disease; known hyperkalemia; use in children

Warnings/Precautions [U.S. Boxed Warning]: NSAIDs are associated with an increased risk of serious (and potentially fatal) adverse cardiovascular thrombotic events, including MI and stroke. Risk may be increased with duration of use or pre-existing cardiovascular risk factors or disease. Carefully evaluate individual cardiovascular risk profiles prior to prescribing. New-onset or exacerbation of hypertension may occur (NSAIDS may impair response to thiazide or loop diuretics); may contribute to cardiovascular events; monitor blood pressure; use with caution in patients with hypertension. May cause sodium and fluid retention; use with caution in patients with edema, cerebrovascular disease, or ischemic heart disease. Avoid use in heart failure. Long-term cardiovascular risk in children has not been evaluated.

[U.S. Boxed Warning]: Celecoxib is contraindicated for treatment of perioperative pain in the setting of coronary artery bypass graft (CABG) surgery. Risk of MI and stroke may be increased with use following CABG surgery.

[U.S. Boxed Warning]: NSAIDs may increase risk of serious gastrointestinal ulceration, bleeding, and perforation (may be fatal). These events may occur at any time during therapy and without warning. Use caution with a history of GI disease (bleeding or ulcers), concurrent therapy with aspirin, anticoagulants and/or corticosteroids, smoking, use of alcohol, the elderly or debilitated patients. When used concomitantly with ≤325 mg of aspirin, a substantial increase in the risk of gastrointestinal complications (eg, ulcer) occurs; concomitant gastroprotective therapy (eg, proton pump inhibitors) is recommended (Bhatt, 2008).

Use the lowest effective dose for the shortest duration of time, consistent with individual patient goals, to reduce risk of cardiovascular or GI adverse events. Alternate therapies should be considered for patients at high risk.

NSAIDs may cause serious skin adverse events including exfoliative dermatitis, Stevens-Johnson syndrome (SJS), and toxic epidermal necrolysis (TEN); may occur without warning and in patients without prior known sulfa allergy. Anaphylactoid reactions may occur, even without prior exposure; patients with "aspirin triad" (bronchial asthma, aspirin intolerance, rhinitis) may be at increased risk. Do not use in patients who experience bronchospasm, asthma, rhinitis, or urticaria with NSAID or aspirin therapy. Use with caution in other forms of asthma.

Use with caution in patients with decreased hepatic (dosage adjustments are recommended for moderate hepatic impairment; not recommended for patients with severe hepatic impairment) or renal function. Transaminase elevations have been reported with use; closely monitor patients with any abnormal LFT. Severe hepatic reactions (eg, fulminant hepatitis, liver failure) have occurred with NSAID use, rarely; discontinue if signs or symptoms of liver disease develop, if systemic manifestations occur, or with persistent or worsening abnormal hepatic function tests. NSAID use may compromise existing renal function; dose-dependent decreases in prostaglandin synthesis may result from NSAID use, causing a reduction in renal blood flow which may cause renal decompensation (usually reversible). Patients with impaired renal function, dehydration, heart failure, liver dysfunction, those taking diuretics, ACE inhibitors, angiotensin II receptor blockers, and the elderly are at greater risk for renal toxicity. Rehydrate patient before starting therapy; monitor renal function closely. Not recommended for use in patients with advanced renal disease or severe renal insufficiency; discontinue use with persistent or worsening abnormal renal function tests. Long-term NSAID use may result in renal papillary necrosis. Should not be considered a treatment or replacement of corticosteroid-dependent diseases.

Anaphylactoid reactions may occur, even with no prior exposure to celecoxib. Use with caution in patients with known or suspected deficiency of cytochrome P450 isoenzyme 2C9; poor metabolizers may have higher plasma levels due to reduced metabolism; consider reduced initial doses. Alternate therapies should be considered in patients with JIA who are poor metabolizers of CYP2C9.

Anemia may occur with use; monitor hemoglobin or hematocrit in patients on long-term treatment. Celecoxib does not affect PT, PTT or platelet counts; does not inhibit platelet aggregation at approved doses.

When used for juvenile idiopathic arthritis (JIA), celecoxib is not FDA-approved in children <2 years of age or in children <10 kg. Use caution with systemic onset JIA (may be at risk for disseminated intravascular coagulation). Safety and efficacy have not been established for use in children for indications other than JIA.

Drug Interactions

Metabolism/Transport Effects **Substrate** of CYP2C9 (major), 3A4 (minor); **Inhibits** CYP2C8 (moderate), 2D6 (weak)

Avoid Concomitant Use

Avoid concomitant use of Celecoxib with any of the following: Ketorolac; Ketorolac (Systemic); Thioridazine

Decreased Effect

Celecoxib may decrease the levels/effects of: ACE Inhibitors; Angiotensin II Receptor Blockers; Antiplatelet Agents; Beta-Blockers; Codeine; Eplerenone; HydrALAZINE; Loop Diuretics; Potassium-Sparing Diuretics; Thiazide Diuretics; TraMADol

The levels/effects of Celecoxib may be decreased by: Bile Acid Sequestrants; CYP2C9 Inducers (Highly Effective); Peginterferon Alfa-2b

Increased Effect/Toxicity

Celecoxib may increase the levels/effects of: Aminoglycosides; Anticoagulants; Antiplatelet Agents; Bisphosphonate Derivatives; CycloSPORINE; CycloSPORINE (Systemic); CYP2C8 Substrates (High risk); CYP2D6 Substrates; Desmopressin; Digoxin; Eplerenone; Fesoterodine; Haloperidol; Lithium; Methotrexate; Nebivolol; Nonsteroidal Anti-Inflammatory Agents; Potassium-Sparing Diuretics; PRALAtrexate; Quinolone Antibiotics; Tamoxifen; Thioridazine; Thrombolytic Agents; Vancomycin; Vitamin K Antagonists

The levels/effects of Celecoxib may be increased by: Antidepressants (Tricyclic, Tertiary Amine); Conivaptan; Corticosteroids (Systemic); CYP2C9 Inhibitors (Moderate); CYP2C9 Inhibitors (Strong); Herbs (Anticoagulant/Antiplatelet Properties); Ketorolac; Ketorolac (Systemic); Probenecid; Selective Serotonin Reuptake Inhibitors; Treprostinil

Nutritional/Ethanol Interactions

Ethanol: Avoid ethanol (increased GI irritation).

Food: Peak concentrations are delayed and AUC is increased by 10% to 20% when taken with a high-fat meal.

Herb/Nutraceutical: Avoid concomitant use with herbs possessing anticoagulation/antiplatelet properties, including alfalfa, anise, bilberry, bladderwrack, bromelain, cat's claw, celery, chamomile, coleus, cordyceps, dong quai, evening primrose, fenugreek, feverfew, garlic, ginger, ginkgo biloba, ginseng (American, Panax, Siberian), grapeseed, green tea, guggul, horse chestnuts, horseradish, licorice, prickly ash, red clover, reishi, SAMe (S-adenosylmethionine), sweet clover, turmeric, white willow.

Adverse Reactions

≥2%

Cardiovascular: Peripheral edema

Central nervous system: Dizziness, fever, headache, insomnia

Dermatologic: Rash

Gastrointestinal: Abdominal pain, diarrhea, dyspepsia, flatulence, nausea, vomiting

Neuromuscular & skeletal: Arthralgia, back pain

Respiratory: Cough, nasopharyngitis, pharyngitis, rhinitis, sinusitis, upper respiratory tract infection

0.1% to 1.9%:

Cardiovascular: Angina, aortic valve incompetence, chest pain, coronary artery disorder, edema, facial edema, hypertension (aggravated), MI, palpitation, sinus bradycardia, tachycardia, ventricular hypertrophy

Central nervous system: Anxiety, depression, fatigue, hypoesthesia, migraine, nervousness, pain, somnolence, vertigo

Dermatologic: Alopecia, bruising, cellulitis, dermatitis, dry skin, photosensitivity, pruritus, rash (erythematous), rash (maculopapular), urticaria

Endocrine & metabolic: Hot flashes, hypercholesterolemia, hyperglycemia, hypokalemia, ovarian cyst, testosterone decreased

Gastrointestinal: Anorexia, appetite increased, constipation, diverticulitis, dysphagia, eructation, esophagitis, gastritis, gastroenteritis, gastroesophageal reflux, gastrointestinal ulcer, hemorrhoids, hiatal hernia, melena, stomatitis, tenesmus, weight gain, xerostomia

Genitourinary: Cystitis, dysuria, urinary frequency

Hematologic: Anemia, thrombocythemia

Hepatic: Alkaline phosphatase increased, transaminases increased

Neuromuscular & skeletal: Arthrosis, CPK increased, hypertonia, leg cramps, myalgia, paresthesia, synovitis, tendonitis

Ocular: Conjunctival hemorrhage, vitreous floaters

Otic: Deafness, labyrinthitis, tinnitus

Renal: Albuminuria, BUN increased, creatinine increased, hematuria, nonprotein nitrogen increased, renal calculi

Respiratory: Bronchitis, bronchospasm, dyspnea, epistaxis, laryngitis, pneumonia

Miscellaneous: Allergic reactions, allergy aggravated, cyst, diaphoresis, flu-like syndrome

Pharmacodynamics/Kinetics

Bioavailability Absolute bioavailability unknown

Time to Peak ~3 hours

Protein Binding ~97% primarily to albumin

Half-Life Elimination ~11 hours (fasted)

Metabolism Hepatic via CYP2C9; forms inactive metabolites

Excretion Feces (~57% as metabolites, <3% as unchanged drug); urine (27% as metabolites, <3% as unchanged drug)

Available Dosage Forms

Capsule, oral:

CeleBREX®: 50 mg, 100 mg, 200 mg, 400 mg

Dosing

Adult Note: Use the lowest effective dose for the shortest duration of time, consistent with individual patient treatment goals.

Osteoarthritis: Oral: 200 mg/day as a single dose or in divided doses twice daily

Ankylosing spondylitis: Oral: 200 mg/day as a single dose or in divided doses twice daily; if no effect after 6 weeks, may increase to 400 mg/day. If no response following 6 weeks of treatment with 400 mg/day, consider discontinuation and alternative treatment.

Canadian labeling; Recommended maximum dose: 200 mg/day

Rheumatoid arthritis: Oral: 100-200 mg twice daily

Acute pain or primary dysmenorrhea: Oral: Initial dose: 400 mg, followed by an additional 200 mg if needed on day 1; maintenance dose: 200 mg twice daily as needed

Canadian labeling; Recommended maximum dose for treatment of acute pain: 400 mg/day up to 7 days

Dosing adjustment in poor CYP2C9 metabolizers (eg, CYP2C9*3/*3): Consider reducing initial dose by 50%; consider alternative treatment in patients with JIA who are poor CYP2C9 metabolizers.

Canadian labeling: Recommended maximum dose: 100 mg/day.

Geriatric Refer to adult dosing. No specific adjustment based on age is recommended. However, the AUC in elderly patients may be increased by 50% as compared to younger subjects. Initiate at the lowest recommended dose in patients weighing <50 kg.

Pediatric Note: Use the lowest effective dose for the shortest duration of time, consistent with individual patient treatment goals.

Juvenile idiopathic arthritis (JIA): Oral: Children ≥2 years:

≥10 kg to ≤25 kg: 50 mg twice daily

>25 kg: 100 mg twice daily

*Dosing adjustment in poor CYP2C9 metabolizers (eg, CYP2C9*3/*3):* Consider alternative.

Renal Impairment

Advanced renal disease: Use is not recommended, however, if celecoxib treatment cannot be avoided, monitor renal function closely.

Severe renal insufficiency: Use is not recommended.

Canadian labeling: Cl_{cr} <30 mL/minute: Use is contraindicated.

Abnormal renal function tests (persistent or worsening): Discontinue use.

Hepatic Impairment

Moderate hepatic impairment (Child-Pugh class B): Reduce dose by 50%.

Severe hepatic impairment (Child-Pugh class C): Use is not recommended.

Canadian labeling: Use is contraindicated.

Abnormal liver function tests (persistent or worsening): Discontinue use.

Administration

Oral May be administered without regard to meals. Capsules may be swallowed whole or the entire contents emptied onto a teaspoon of cool or room temperature applesauce. The contents of the capsules sprinkled onto applesauce may be stored under refrigeration for up to 6 hours.

Stability

Storage Store at 25°C (77°F); excursions permitted to 15°C to 30°C (59°F to 86°F).

Monitoring and Teaching Issues

Laboratory Monitoring CBC, blood chemistry profile, periodic liver function tests; renal function (urine output, serum BUN and creatinine)

JIA: Monitor for development of abnormal coagulation tests with systemic onset JIA

Physical Assessment Evaluate cardiac risk and potential for GI bleeding prior to prescribing this medication. Assess allergy history (aspirin, NSAIDs, salicylates). Monitor blood pressure at the beginning of therapy and periodically during use.

Patient Education May be taken with food to reduce GI upset. Avoid alcohol. You may experience dizziness, confusion, blurred vision, anorexia, nausea, vomiting, taste disturbance, or gastric distress; GI bleeding, ulceration, or perforation can occur with or without pain. Stop taking medication and report immediately stomach pain or cramping, unusual bleeding or bruising (blood in vomitus, stool, or urine), chest pain, shortness of breath, weakness of extremities, or slurring of speech. Report skin rash, unusual fatigue, flu-like symptoms, jaundice, weakness, sudden weight gain or edema, changes in hearing (ringing in ears) or vision, changes in urination pattern, or respiratory difficulty.

Dietary Considerations May be taken without regard to meals.

Geriatric Considerations The elderly are at increased risk for adverse effects from NSAIDs. As many as 60% of elderly can develop peptic ulceration and/or hemorrhage asymptomatically; however, elderly patients may demonstrate these adverse effects at lower doses than younger adults. The elderly are also at increased risk of renal toxicity. Although celecoxib is associated with a decreased incidence of GI side effects, use the lowest recommended dose in patients weighing <50 kg.

Breast-Feeding Considerations Small amounts of celecoxib are found in breast milk. The manufacturer recommends that caution be exercised when administering celecoxib to nursing women.

Pregnancy Considerations Teratogenic effects have been observed in some animal studies; therefore, celecoxib is classified as pregnancy category C. Celecoxib is a NSAID that primarily inhibits COX-2 whereas other currently available NSAIDs are nonselective for COX-1 and COX-2. The effects of this selective inhibition to the fetus have not been well studied and limited information is available specific to celecoxib. NSAID exposure during the first trimester is not strongly associated with congenital malformations; however, cardiovascular anomalies and cleft palate have been observed following NSAID exposure in some studies. The use of a NSAID close to conception may be associated with an increased risk of miscarriage. Nonteratogenic effects have been observed following NSAID administration during the third trimester including: Myocardial degenerative changes, prenatal constriction of the ductus arteriosus, fetal tricuspid regurgitation, failure of the ductus arteriosus to close postnatally; renal dysfunction or failure, oligohydramnios; gastrointestinal bleeding or perforation, increased risk of necrotizing enterocolitis; intracranial bleeding (including intraventricular hemorrhage), platelet dysfunction with resultant bleeding; pulmonary hypertension. Because it may cause premature closure of the ductus arteriosus, the use of celecoxib is not recommended ≥30 weeks gestation. The chronic use of NSAIDs in women of reproductive age may be associated with infertility that is reversible upon discontinuation of the medication. A registry is available for pregnant women exposed to autoimmune medications including celecoxib. For additional information contact the Organization of Teratology Information Specialists, OTIS Autoimmune Diseases Study, at 877-311-8972.

Related Information

Nonsalicylate / Nonsteroidal Anti-Inflammatory Agents *on page* 2002

- **Celestone®** *see* Betamethasone *on page* 205
- **Celestone® Soluspan®** *see* Betamethasone *on page* 205
- **CeleXA®** *see* Citalopram *on page* 386
- **CellCept®** *see* Mycophenolate *on page* 1270
- **Cenestin®** *see* Estrogens (Conjugated A/Synthetic) *on page* 677
- **Cephadyn** *see* Butalbital and Acetaminophen *on page* 261

Cephalexin (sef a LEKS in)

U.S. Brand Names Keflex®

Index Terms Cephalexin Monohydrate

Generic Availability (U.S.) Yes

Pharmacologic Category Antibiotic, Cephalosporin (First Generation)

Medication Safety Issues

Sound-alike/look-alike issues:

Cephalexin may be confused with cefaclor, ceFAZolin, cephalothin, ciprofloxacin

Keflex® may be confused with Keppra®, Valtrex®

Pregnancy Risk Factor B

Lactation Enters breast milk (small amounts)/use caution

Use Treatment of susceptible bacterial infections including respiratory tract infections, otitis media, skin and skin structure infections, bone infections, and genitourinary tract infections, including acute prostatitis; alternative therapy for acute infective endocarditis prophylaxis

Mechanism of Action/Effect Inhibits bacterial cell wall synthesis by binding to one or more of the penicillin-binding proteins (PBPs)

Contraindications Hypersensitivity to cephalexin, any component of the formulation, or other cephalosporins

Warnings/Precautions Modify dosage in patients with severe renal impairment. Use with caution in patients with a history of penicillin allergy, especially IgE-mediated reactions (eg, anaphylaxis, urticaria). Prolonged use may result in fungal or bacterial superinfection, including *C. difficile*-associated diarrhea (CDAD) and pseudomembranous colitis; CDAD has been observed >2 months postantibiotic treatment. May be associated with increased INR, especially in nutritionally-deficient patients, prolonged treatment, hepatic or renal disease.

Drug Interactions

Avoid Concomitant Use

Avoid concomitant use of Cephalexin with any of the following: BCG

Decreased Effect

Cephalexin may decrease the levels/effects of: BCG; Typhoid Vaccine

Increased Effect/Toxicity

Cephalexin may increase the levels/effects of: MetFORMIN

The levels/effects of Cephalexin may be increased by: Probenecid

Nutritional/Ethanol Interactions Food: Peak antibiotic serum concentration is lowered and delayed, but total drug absorbed is not affected. Cephalexin serum levels may be decreased if taken with food.

Lab Interactions Positive direct Coombs', false-positive urinary glucose test using cupric sulfate (Benedict's solution, Clinitest®, Fehling's solution), false-positive serum or urine creatinine with Jaffé reaction, false-positive urinary proteins and steroids

Adverse Reactions Frequency not defined.

Central nervous system: Agitation, confusion, dizziness, fatigue, hallucinations, headache
Dermatologic: Angioedema, erythema multiforme (rare), rash, Stevens-Johnson syndrome (rare), toxic epidermal necrolysis (rare), urticaria
Gastrointestinal: Abdominal pain, diarrhea, dyspepsia, gastritis, nausea (rare), pseudomembranous colitis, vomiting (rare)
Genitourinary: Genital pruritus, genital moniliasis, vaginitis, vaginal discharge
Hematologic: Eosinophilia, hemolytic anemia, neutropenia, thrombocytopenia
Hepatic: ALT increased, AST increased, cholestatic jaundice (rare), transient hepatitis (rare)
Neuromuscular & skeletal: Arthralgia, arthritis, joint disorder
Renal: Interstitial nephritis (rare)
Miscellaneous: Allergic reactions, anaphylaxis

Pharmacodynamics/Kinetics

Absorption Rapid (90%); delayed in young children

Time to Peak Serum: ~1 hour

Protein Binding 6% to 15%

Half-Life Elimination Adults: 0.5-1.2 hours; prolonged with renal impairment

Excretion Urine (80% to 100% as unchanged drug) within 8 hours

Available Dosage Forms

Capsule, oral: 250 mg, 500 mg
Keflex®: 250 mg, 500 mg, 750 mg

Powder for suspension, oral: 125 mg/5 mL (100 mL, 200 mL); 250 mg/5 mL (100 mL, 200 mL)

Tablet, oral: 250 mg, 500 mg

Dosing

Adult & Geriatric

Dosing range: Oral: 250-1000 mg every 6 hours (maximum: 4 g/day)

Cellulitis and mastitis: Oral 500 mg every 6 hours

Furunculosis/skin abscess: Oral: 250 mg 4 times/day

Prophylaxis against infective endocarditis (dental, oral, or respiratory tract procedures): Oral: 2 g 30-60 minutes prior to procedure. **Note:** American Heart Association (AHA) guidelines now recommend prophylaxis only in patients undergoing invasive procedures and in whom underlying cardiac conditions may predispose to a higher risk of adverse outcomes should infection occur.

Prophylaxis in total joint replacement patients undergoing dental procedures which produce bacteremia: Oral: 2 g 1 hour prior to procedure

Streptococcal pharyngitis, skin and skin structure infections: Oral: 500 mg every 12 hours

Uncomplicated cystitis: Oral: 500 mg every 12 hours for 7-14 days

Pediatric

Usual dose: Oral: Children >1 year: Dosing range: 25-100 mg/kg/day in divided doses every 6-8 hours (maximum: 4 g/day)

Furunculosis: Oral: 25-50 mg/kg/day in 4 divided doses

Impetigo: Oral: 25 mg/kg/day in 4 divided doses

Otitis media: 75-100 mg/kg/day in 4 divided doses

Prophylaxis against infective endocarditis (dental, oral, or respiratory tract procedures):

Children >1-15 years: 50 mg/kg 30-60 minutes prior to procedure (maximum: 2 g). **Note:** American Heart Association (AHA) guidelines now recommend prophylaxis only in patients undergoing invasive procedures and in whom underlying cardiac conditions may predispose to a higher risk of adverse outcomes should infection occur.

Children >15 years: Refer to adult dosing.

Severe infections: Oral: 50-100 mg/kg/day in divided doses every 6-8 hours

Skin abscess: Oral: 50 mg/kg/day in 4 divided doses (maximum: 4 g)

Streptococcal pharyngitis, skin and skin structure infections: 25-50 mg/kg/day divided every 12 hours

Uncomplicated cystitis: Children >15 years: Refer to adult dosing.

Renal Impairment Adults:

Cl_{cr} 10-50 mL/minute: 500 mg every 8-12 hours

Cl_{cr} <10: 250-500 mg every 12-24 hours

Hemodialysis: 250 mg every 12-24 hours; moderately dialyzable (20% to 50%); give dose after dialysis session

Administration

Oral Take without regard to food. If GI distress, take with food. Give around-the-clock to promote less variation in peak and trough serum levels.

Stability

Storage

Capsule: Store at 15°C to 30°C (59°F to 86°F).

Powder for oral suspension: Refrigerate suspension after reconstitution; discard after 14 days.

Monitoring and Teaching Issues

Laboratory Monitoring Renal, hepatic, and hematologic function periodically with prolonged therapy; perform culture and sensitivity studies prior to initiating drug therapy.

Physical Assessment Assess results of culture/sensitivity tests and patient's allergy history prior to therapy. Monitor for nephrotoxicity. Advise patients with diabetes about use of Clinitest® (may cause false-positive test). Teach patient to report opportunistic infection and hypersensitivity reaction.

Patient Education Take at regular intervals around-the-clock, with or without food. Maintain adequate hydration, unless instructed to restrict fluid intake. May cause false test results with Clinitest®; use of another type of glucose testing is preferable. May cause diarrhea. Report rash; breathing or swallowing difficulty; persistent diarrhea, nausea, vomiting, or abdominal pain; changes in urinary pattern or pain on urination; opportunistic infection (eg, vaginal itching or drainage, sores in mouth, blood in stool or urine, unusual fever or chills); or CNS changes (eg, irritability, agitation, nervousness, insomnia, hallucinations).

Dietary Considerations Take without regard to food. If GI distress, take with food.

Geriatric Considerations Adjust dose for renal function.

Breast-Feeding Considerations Small amounts of cephalexin are excreted in breast milk. The manufacturer recommends that caution be exercised when administering cephalexin to nursing women. Maximum milk concentration occurs ~4 hours after a single oral dose and gradually disappears by 8 hours after administration. Nondose-related effects could include modification of bowel flora.

Pregnancy Considerations Adverse events were not observed in animal reproduction studies; therefore, cephalexin is classified as pregnancy category B. Cephalexin crosses the placenta and produces therapeutic concentrations in the fetal circulation and amniotic fluid. An increased risk of teratogenic effects has not been observed following maternal use of cephalexin; however, adequate and well-controlled studies have not been completed in pregnant women. Peak concentrations in pregnant patients are similar to those in non-pregnant patients. Prolonged labor may decrease oral absorption.

◆ **Cephalexin Monohydrate** *see* Cephalexin *on page* 346

◆ **Cerebyx®** *see* Fosphenytoin *on page* 834

Certolizumab Pegol (cer to LIZ u mab PEG ol)

U.S. Brand Names Cimzia®

Index Terms CDP870

Generic Availability (U.S.) No

Pharmacologic Category Antirheumatic, Disease Modifying; Gastrointestinal Agent, Miscellaneous; Tumor Necrosis Factor (TNF) Blocking Agent

Medication Guide Available Yes

Pregnancy Risk Factor B

Lactation Excretion in breast milk unknown/not recommended

Use Treatment of moderately- to severely-active Crohn's disease in patients who have inadequate response to conventional therapy; moderately- to severely-active rheumatoid arthritis (as monotherapy or in combination with nonbiological disease-modifying antirheumatic drugs [DMARDS])

Mechanism of Action/Effect Elevated levels of TNF-alpha have a role in the inflammatory process associated with Crohn's disease and in joint destruction associated with rheumatoid arthritis. Certolizumab pegol binds to and selectively neutralizes human TNF-alpha activity, inhibiting the role of TNF-alpha as a mediator in the inflammatory process.

Contraindications There are no contraindications listed within the manufacturer's labeling.

Warnings/Precautions **[U.S. Boxed Warning]: Patients receiving certolizumab are at increased risk for serious infections which may result in hospitalization and/or fatality; infections usually developed in patients receiving concomitant immunosuppressive agents (eg, methotrexate or corticosteroids). Active tuberculosis (or reactivation of latent tuberculosis), invasive fungal (including aspergillosis, blastomycosis, candidiasis, coccidioidomycosis, histoplasmosis, and pneumocystosis) and other opportunistic infections have been reported in patients receiving TNF-blocking agents, including certolizumab. Monitor closely for signs/symptoms of infection. Discontinue for serious infection or sepsis. Consider risks versus benefits prior to use in patients with a history of chronic or recurrent infection.** Caution should be exercised when considering the use in patients with concomitant immunosuppressive therapy or predisposition to infection (eg, diabetes or residence/travel from areas of endemic mycoses). Do not administer to patients with an active chronic or localized infection. Patients who develop a new infection while undergoing treatment should be monitored closely. If a patient develops a serious infection, therapy should be discontinued. **[U.S. Boxed Warning]: Lymphoma and other malignancies have been reported in children and adolescent patients receiving other TNF-blocking agents.** Use of TNF blockers may affect defenses against malignancies; impact on the development and course of malignancies is not fully defined. Lymphoma has been noted in clinical trials. Chronic immunosuppressant therapy use may be a predisposing factor for malignancy development; rheumatoid arthritis alone has been previously associated with an increased rate of lymphoma.

Tuberculosis has been reported with certolizumab treatment. **[U.S. Boxed Warnings]: Patients should be evaluated for tuberculosis risk factors and for latent tuberculosis infection (with a tuberculin skin test) prior to therapy. Treatment of latent tuberculosis should be initiated before use. Patients with initial negative tuberculin skin tests should receive continued monitoring for tuberculosis throughout treatment;** active tuberculosis has developed in this population during treatment. Use with caution in patients who have resided in regions where tuberculosis is endemic. If appropriate, antituberculosis therapy should be considered (prior to certolizumab treatment) in patients with several or with highly significant risk factors for tuberculosis development.

Rare and sometimes fatal reactivation of hepatitis B virus (HBV) has occurred in chronic virus carriers (usually in patients receiving concomitant immunosuppressive agents); evaluate prior to initiation, during, and for several months after treatment. Evaluate patients at risk for HBV infection prior to therapy to determine HBV status. Use with extreme caution in patients identified as HBV carriers, use has not been evaluated in this population. Discontinue certolizumab treatment (and initiate appropriate antiviral therapy) if HBV reactivation occurs if resumption of therapy is deemed necessary, use caution and monitor closely.

Hypersensitivity reactions, including angioedema, dyspnea, rash, serum sickness and urticaria have been reported (rarely) with treatment; discontinue and do not resume therapy if hypersensitivity occurs. Use with caution in patients who have experienced hypersensitivity with other TNF blockers. Use with caution in heart failure patients; worsening heart failure and new onset heart failure have been reported with TNF blockers, including certolizumab pegol; monitor closely. Rare cases of pancytopenia and other significant cytopenias, including aplastic anemia and have been reported with TNF-blocking agents. Leukopenia and thrombocytopenia have occurred with certolizumab; use with caution in patients with underlying hematologic disorders; consider discontinuing therapy with significant hematologic abnormalities. Autoantibody formation may develop; rarely resulting in autoimmune disorder, including lupus-like syndrome; monitor and discontinue if symptoms develop. A small number of patients (8%) develop antibodies to certolizumab during therapy. Antibody-positive patients may have an increased incidence of adverse events (including injection site pain/erythema, abdominal pain and erythema nodosum). Use with caution in patients with pre-existing or recent-onset CNS demyelinating disorders; rare cases of optic neuritis, seizure, peripheral neuropathy, and demyelinating disease (new onset or exacerbation) have been reported.

The manufacturer does not recommend concurrent use with anakinra or other tumor necrosis factor (TNF) blocking agents due to the risk of serious infections. Do not use in combination with biologic DMARDS. Patients should be up to date with all immunizations before initiating therapy; live vaccines should not be given concurrently. There is no data available concerning the effects of therapy on vaccination or secondary transmission of live vaccines in patients receiving therapy. Use has not been studied in patients with renal impairment; however, the pharmacokinetics of the pegylated (polyethylene glycol) component may be dependent on renal function. Use with caution in the elderly, may be at higher risk for infections.

Drug Interactions

Avoid Concomitant Use

Avoid concomitant use of Certolizumab Pegol with any of the following: Abatacept; Anakinra; Anti-TNF Agents; BCG; Canakinumab; Natalizumab; Pimecrolimus; Rilonacept; RiTUXimab; Roflumilast; Tacrolimus (Topical); Vaccines (Live)

Decreased Effect

Certolizumab Pegol may decrease the levels/effects of: BCG; Sipuleucel-T; Vaccines (Inactivated); Vaccines (Live)

The levels/effects of Certolizumab Pegol may be decreased by: Echinacea; Pegloticase

Increased Effect/Toxicity

Certolizumab Pegol may increase the levels/effects of: Abatacept; Anakinra; Canakinumab; Leflunomide; Natalizumab; Rilonacept; Vaccines (Live)

The levels/effects of Certolizumab Pegol may be increased by: Anti-TNF Agents; Denosumab; Pimecrolimus; RiTUXimab; Roflumilast; Tacrolimus (Topical); Trastuzumab

Nutritional/Ethanol Interactions Herb/Nutraceutical: Echinacea may decrease the therapeutic effects of certolizumab; avoid concurrent use.

Lab Interactions Tests for latent tuberculosis may be falsely negative while on certolizumab pegol treatment. Falsely elevated aPTT assays have been reported with PTT-Lupus Anticoagulant (LA) and Standard Target Activated Partial Thromboplastin time (STA-PTT) tests from Diagnostica Stago, and with HemosiL APTT-SP liquid and HemosiL lyophilized silica tests from Instrumentation Laboratories.

Adverse Reactions

>10%:

Central nervous system: Headache (5% to 18%)

Gastrointestinal: Nausea (≤11%)

Respiratory: Upper respiratory infection (6% to 20%), nasopharyngitis (4% to 13%)

Miscellaneous: Infection (14% to 38%; serious: 3%)

1% to 10%:

Cardiovascular: Hypertension (≤5%)

Central nervous system: Dizziness (≤6%), fever (≤5%), fatigue (≤3%)

Dermatologic: Rash (9%)

Gastrointestinal: Abdominal pain (≤6%), vomiting (5%)

Genitourinary: Urinary tract infection (≤8%)

Local: Injection site reactions (includes bleeding, burning, erythema, inflammation, pain, rash: ≤7%; incidence higher with placebo)

Neuromuscular & skeletal: Arthralgia (6% to 7%), back pain (≤4%)

Respiratory: Cough (≤6%), bronchitis (≤3%), pharyngitis (≤3%)

Miscellaneous: Antibody formation (7% to 8%), positive ANA (≤4%)

Pharmacodynamics/Kinetics

Bioavailability SubQ: ~80% (range: 76% to 88%)

Time to Peak Plasma: 54-171 hours

Half-Life Elimination ~14 days

Available Dosage Forms

Injection, powder for reconstitution [preservative free]:

Cimzia®: 200 mg

Injection, solution [preservative free]:

Cimzia®: 200 mg/mL (1 mL)

Dosing

Adult & Geriatric Note: Each 400 mg dose should be administered as 2 injections of 200 mg each

Crohn's disease: SubQ: Initial: 400 mg, repeat dose 2 and 4 weeks after initial dose; Maintenance: 400 mg every 4 weeks

Rheumatoid arthritis: SubQ: Initial: 400 mg, repeat dose 2 and 4 weeks after initial dose; Maintenance: 200 mg every other week. May consider maintenance dose of 400 mg every 4 weeks.

Renal Impairment Moderate-to-severe renal impairment: The pharmacokinetics of the pegylated (polyethylene glycol) component may be dependent on renal function; however, data is insufficient to provide a dosing recommendation.

Administration

Other SubQ: Bring to room temperature prior to administration. Total dose requires 2 vials **or** 2 prefilled syringes. After reconstitution (of vials), draw each vial into separate syringes (using 20-gauge needles).

Administer each syringe subcutaneously (using provided 23-gauge needle) to separate sites on abdomen or thigh. Rotate injections sites; do not administer to areas where skin is tender, bruised, red, or hard.

Stability

Reconstitution Vials: Allow to reach room temperature prior to reconstitution. Using aseptic technique, reconstitute each vial with 1 mL sterile water for injection (provided) to a concentration of ~200 mg/mL; the manufacturer recommends using a 20-gauge needle (provided). Gently swirl to facilitate wetting of powder; do not shake. Allow vials to set undisturbed (may take up to 30 minutes) until fully reconstituted. Reconstituted solutions should not contain visible particles or gels in the solution.

Storage Prior to reconstitution, store refrigerated at 2°C to 8°C (36°F to 46°F); do not freeze. Bring to room temperature prior to administration.

Prefilled syringe: Protect from light.

Vials: Reconstituted vials may be retained at room temperature for ≤2 hours or refrigerated (do not freeze) for ≤24 hours prior to administration.

Monitoring and Teaching Issues

Laboratory Monitoring Hepatitis B virus and TB screening prior to therapy initiation

Physical Assessment Perform tuberculin skin test prior to initiating therapy. Monitor for signs of tuberculosis and other infections throughout therapy. Do not initiate therapy if active infection is present. Assess results of PPD at regular intervals during treatment. Teach patient proper injection technique and syringe/needle disposal.

Patient Education Inform prescriber of allergies, history of tuberculosis, or any kind of infection you have. If self-administered, follow directions for injection and needle/syringe disposal exactly. You may be more susceptible to infection. May cause headache, nausea, or dizziness. Report persistent fever; respiratory tract infection; infected wounds; urinary tract infection; flu-like symptoms; signs of fluid retention (unusual weight gain, swelling of the extremities); shortness of breath; or redness, swelling, or pain at injection site.

Geriatric Considerations Studies to date have insufficient data to make conclusions for use in elderly. Anecdotal reports in clinical settings do not demonstrate any clinical difference between elderly and younger adults. Since elderly have a higher incidence of infection, use with caution and close monitoring.

Pregnancy Considerations Adverse effects were not observed in animal studies. There are no adequate and well-controlled studies in pregnant women.

◆ **Cerubidine®** *see* DAUNOrubicin Hydrochloride *on page* 474

◆ **Cervarix®** *see* Papillomavirus (Types 16, 18) Vaccine (Human, Recombinant) *on page* 1409

◆ **Cervidil®** *see* Dinoprostone *on page 540*
◆ **C.E.S.** *see* Estrogens (Conjugated/Equine, Systemic) *on page 682*
◆ **C.E.S.** *see* Estrogens (Conjugated/Equine, Topical) *on page 686*
◆ **Cesamet®** *see* Nabilone *on page 1274*
◆ **Cesia® [DSC]** *see* Ethinyl Estradiol and Desogestrel *on page 695*
◆ **Cetafen® [OTC]** *see* Acetaminophen *on page 38*
◆ **Cetafen® Extra [OTC]** *see* Acetaminophen *on page 38*

Cetirizine (se TI ra zeen)

U.S. Brand Names All Day Allergy [OTC]; ZyrTEC® Allergy [OTC]; ZyrTEC® Children's Allergy [OTC]; ZyrTEC® Children's Hives Relief [OTC]

Index Terms Cetirizine Hydrochloride; P-071; UCB-P071

Generic Availability (U.S.) Yes

Pharmacologic Category Histamine H_1 Antagonist; Histamine H_1 Antagonist, Second Generation; Piperazine Derivative

Medication Safety Issues

Sound-alike/look-alike issues:

ZyrTEC® may be confused with Lipitor©, Serax®, Xanax®, Zantac®, Zerit®, Zocor®, ZyPREXA®, ZyrTEC-D®

ZyrTEC® (cetirizine) may be confused with ZyrTEC® Itchy Eye (ketotifen)

Pregnancy Risk Factor B

Lactation Enters breast milk/not recommended

Use Perennial and seasonal allergic rhinitis and other allergic symptoms including urticaria; chronic idiopathic urticaria

Mechanism of Action/Effect Competes with histamine for H_1-receptor sites on effector cells in the GI tract, blood vessels, and respiratory tract

Contraindications Hypersensitivity to cetirizine, hydroxyzine, or any component of the formulation

Warnings/Precautions Cetirizine should be used cautiously in patients with hepatic or renal dysfunction; dosage adjustment recommended. Use with caution in the elderly; may be more sensitive to adverse effects. May cause drowsiness; use caution performing tasks which require alertness (eg, operating machinery or driving). Effects may be potentiated when used with other sedative drugs or ethanol.

Drug Interactions

Metabolism/Transport Effects Substrate of CYP3A4 (minor), P-glycoprotein

Avoid Concomitant Use There are no known interactions where it is recommended to avoid concomitant use.

Decreased Effect

Cetirizine may decrease the levels/effects of: Acetylcholinesterase Inhibitors (Central); Benzylpenicilloyl Polylysine; Betahistine

The levels/effects of Cetirizine may be decreased by: Acetylcholinesterase Inhibitors (Central); Amphetamines; P-Glycoprotein Inducers

Increased Effect/Toxicity

Cetirizine may increase the levels/effects of: Alcohol (Ethyl); Anticholinergics; CNS Depressants

The levels/effects of Cetirizine may be increased by: Conivaptan; Droperidol; P-Glycoprotein Inhibitors; Pramlintide

Nutritional/Ethanol Interactions Ethanol: Avoid ethanol (may increase CNS depression).

Lab Interactions May cause false-positive serum TCA screen.

Adverse Reactions

>10%: Central nervous system: Headache (children 11% to 14%, placebo 12%), somnolence (adults 14%, children 2% to 4%)

2% to 10%:

Central nervous system: Insomnia (children 9%, adults <2%), fatigue (adults 6%), malaise (4%), dizziness (adults 2%)

Gastrointestinal: Abdominal pain (children 4% to 6%), dry mouth (adults 5%), diarrhea (children 2% to 3%), nausea (children 2% to 3%, placebo 2%), vomiting (children 2% to 3%)

Respiratory: Epistaxis (children 2% to 4%, placebo 3%), pharyngitis (children 3% to 6%, placebo 3%), bronchospasm (children 2% to 3%, placebo 2%)

Pharmacodynamics/Kinetics

Onset of Action 15-30 minutes

Absorption Rapid

Time to Peak Serum: 1 hour

Protein Binding Plasma: Mean: 93%

Half-Life Elimination 8 hours

Metabolism Limited hepatic

Excretion Urine (70%); feces (10%)

Available Dosage Forms

Capsule, liquid gel, oral:

ZyrTEC® Allergy [OTC]: 10 mg

Syrup, oral: 5 mg/5 mL (5 mL, 118 mL, 120 mL, 473 mL, 480 mL)
ZyrTEC® Children's Allergy [OTC]: 5 mg/5 mL (118 mL)
ZyrTEC® Children's Hives Relief [OTC]: 5 mg/5 mL (118 mL)
Tablet, oral: 5 mg, 10 mg
All Day Allergy [OTC]: 10 mg
ZyrTEC® Allergy [OTC]: 10 mg
Tablet, chewable, oral: 5 mg, 10 mg
All Day Allergy [OTC]: 5 mg
ZyrTEC® Children's Allergy [OTC]: 5 mg, 10 mg

Dosing

Adult Perennial or seasonal allergic rhinitis, chronic urticaria: Oral: 5-10 mg once daily, depending upon symptom severity

Geriatric Oral: Initial: 5 mg once daily; may increase to 10 mg/day
Note: Manufacturer recommends 5 mg/day in patients ≥77 years of age.

Pediatric

Perennial allergic rhinitis, chronic urticaria: Oral:
6-12 months: 2.5 mg once daily
12 months to <2 years: 2.5 mg once daily; may increase to 2.5 mg every 12 hours if needed

Perennial or seasonal allergic rhinitis, chronic urticaria: Oral:
2-5 years: Initial: 2.5 mg once daily; may be increased to 2.5 mg every 12 hours **or** 5 mg once daily
≥6 years: Refer to adult dosing.

Renal Impairment
Children <6 years: Cetirizine use not recommended.
Children 6-11 years: <2.5 mg once daily
Children ≥12 and Adults:
Cl_{cr} 11-31 mL/minute or hemodialysis: Administer 5 mg once daily
Cl_{cr} <11 mL/minute, not on dialysis: Cetirizine use not recommended.

Hepatic Impairment
Children <6 years: Cetirizine use not recommended.
Children 6-11 years: <2.5 mg once daily
Children ≥12 and Adults: Administer 5 mg once daily

Administration

Oral May be administered with or without food.

Stability

Storage Store at room temperature.
Syrup: Store at room temperature of 15°C to 30°C (59°F to 86°F), or under refrigeration at 2°C to 8°C (36°F to 46°F).

Monitoring and Teaching Issues

Patient Education Avoid use of alcohol. You may experience drowsiness, dizziness, or dry mouth. Report persistent sedation, confusion, agitation, persistent nausea or vomiting, blurred vision, or lack of improvement or worsening of condition.

Dietary Considerations May be taken with or without food.

Geriatric Considerations Adjust dose for renal function.

Pregnancy Considerations Cetirizine was not shown to be teratogenic in animal studies; however, adequate studies have not been conducted in pregnant women. Use during pregnancy only if clearly needed.

◆ **Cetirizine Hydrochloride** *see* Cetirizine *on page* 351

◆ **Cetraxal®** *see* Ciprofloxacin (Otic) *on page* 380

Cetuximab (se TUK see mab)

U.S. Brand Names Erbitux®

Index Terms C225; IMC-C225; MOAB C225

Generic Availability (U.S.) No

Pharmacologic Category Antineoplastic Agent, Monoclonal Antibody; Epidermal Growth Factor Receptor (EGFR) Inhibitor

Medication Safety Issues
Sound-alike/look-alike issues:
Cetuximab may be confused with bevacizumab

Pregnancy Risk Factor C

Lactation Excretion in breast milk is unknown/not recommended

Use Treatment of metastatic colorectal cancer; treatment of squamous cell cancer of the head and neck

Note: Subset analyses (retrospective) in metastatic colorectal cancer trials have not shown a benefit with EGFR inhibitor treatment in patients whose tumors have codon 12 or 13 *KRAS* mutations; use is not recommended in these patients.

Unlabeled/Investigational Use Treatment of EGFR-expressing advanced nonsmall cell lung cancer (NSCLC)

Mechanism of Action/Effect Inhibits cell growth; induces apoptosis and decreases matrix metalloproteinase and vascular endothelial growth factor production.

Contraindications There are no contraindications listed in the manufacturer's labeling

Warnings/Precautions [U.S. Boxed Warning]: Severe infusion reactions (bronchospasm, stridor, hoarseness, urticaria, hypotension, loss of consciousness, shock, MI, cardiac arrest) have been reported in ~3% of patients; fatal outcome has been reported rarely. Approximately 90% of reactions occur with the first infusion despite the use of prophylactic antihistamines. **Note:** Although a 20 mg test dose was used in some studies, it did not reliably predict the risk of an infusion reaction, and is not recommended. In case of severe reaction, treatment should be stopped and permanently discontinued. Immediate treatment for anaphylactic/anaphylactoid reactions should be available during administration. The manufacturer recommends monitoring patients for at least 1 hour following completion of infusion, or longer if a reaction occurs. Mild-to-moderate infusion reactions are managed by slowing the infusion rate (by 50%) and administering antihistamines. Patients with pre-existing IgE antibody against cetuximab (specific for galactose-α-1,3-galactose) are reported to have a higher incidence of severe hypersensitivity reaction. Severe hypersensitivity reaction has been reported more frequently in patients living in the middle south area of the United States, including North Carolina and Tennessee (Chung, 2008; O'Neil, 2007).

[U.S. Boxed Warning]: Cardiopulmonary arrest has occurred in 2% of patients receiving radiation therapy in combination with cetuximab; closely monitor serum electrolytes during and after (for at least 8 weeks) cetuximab therapy; use caution with history of coronary artery disease, HF, and arrhythmias. Interstitial lung disease (ILD) has been reported; use caution with pre-existing lung disease; permanently discontinue with confirmed ILD. Acneiform rash has been reported in 76% to 88% of patients (severe in 1% to 17%), usually developing within the first 2 weeks of therapy; may require dose modification. Acneiform rash should be treated with topical and/or oral antibiotics; topical corticosteroids are not recommended. Other dermatologic toxicities, including dry skin, fissures, hypertrichosis, paronychial inflammation, and skin infections have been reported; related ocular toxicities (blepharitis, conjunctivitis, keratitis) may also occur. Sunlight may exacerbate skin reactions (limit sun exposure). Hypomagnesemia is common; the onset of electrolyte disturbance may occur within days to months after initiation of treatment; monitor during treatment and for at least 8 weeks after completion. Non-neutralizing anticetuximab antibodies were detected in 5% of evaluable patients. Safety and efficacy have not been established when used in combination with radiation therapy and cisplatin. Patients with colorectal cancer with tumors with a codon 12 or 13 *KRAS* mutation are unlikely to benefit from EGFR inhibitor therapy and should not receive cetuximab treatment. Safety and efficacy in children have not been established.

Drug Interactions

Avoid Concomitant Use There are no known interactions where it is recommended to avoid concomitant use.

Decreased Effect There are no known significant interactions involving a decrease in effect.

Increased Effect/Toxicity There are no known significant interactions involving an increase in effect.

Adverse Reactions Except where noted, percentages reported for cetuximab monotherapy.

>10%:

Central nervous system: Fatigue (89%), pain (17% to 51%), headache (26% to 33%), insomnia (10% to 30%), fever (27% to 30%), confusion (15%), anxiety (14%), chills/rigors (13%), depression (7% to 13%)

Dermatologic: Acneiform rash (76% to 90%; grades 3/4: 1% to 17%; onset: ≤14 days), rash (89%), dry skin (49%), pruritus (11% to 40%), nail changes/disorder (16% to 21%)

Endocrine & metabolic: Hypomagnesemia (55%; grades 3/4: 6% to 17%)

Gastrointestinal: Abdominal pain (26% to 59%), constipation (26% to 46%), diarrhea (25% to 39%), vomiting (25% to 37%), nausea (mild-to-moderate 29%), weight loss (7% to 27%), anorexia (23%), stomatitis (10% to 25%), xerostomia (11%)

Neuromuscular & skeletal: Weakness (45% to 48%), bone pain (15%)

Respiratory: Dyspnea (17% to 48%), cough (11% to 29%)

Miscellaneous: Infection (13% to 35%), infusion reaction (15% to 21%; grades 3/4: 2% to 5%; 90% of severe reactions occurred with first infusion)

1% to 10%:

Cardiovascular: Peripheral edema (10%), cardiopulmonary arrest (2%; with radiation therapy)

Dermatologic: Alopecia (4%), skin disorder (4%)

Endocrine & metabolic: Dehydration (2% to 10%)

Gastrointestinal: Dyspepsia (6%)

Hematologic: Anemia (9%)

Hepatic: Alkaline phosphatase increased (5% to 10%), transaminases increased (5% to 10%)

Neuromuscular & skeletal: Back pain (10%)

Ocular: Conjunctivitis (7%)

Renal: Renal failure (1%)

Respiratory: Pulmonary embolus (1%)

Miscellaneous: Sepsis (1% to 4%)

Pharmacodynamics/Kinetics

Half-Life Elimination ~112 hours (range: 63-230 hours)

Available Dosage Forms

Injection, solution [preservative free]:

Erbitux®: 2 mg/mL (50 mL, 100 mL)

Dosing

Adult & Geriatric Note: Premedicate with an H_1 antagonist (eg, diphenhydramine) I.V. 30-60 minutes prior to the first dose; premedication for subsequent doses is based on clinical judgement.

Colorectal cancer: I.V.:

Initial loading dose: 400 mg/m^2 infused over 120 minutes

Maintenance dose: 250 mg/m^2 infused over 60 minutes weekly

Biweekly administration (unlabeled dosing): 500 mg/m^2 every 2 weeks (initial dose infused over 120 minutes, subsequent doses infused over 60 minutes) (Pfeiffer, 2007)

Head and neck cancer: I.V.:

Initial loading dose: 400 mg/m^2 infused over 120 minutes

Maintenance dose: 250 mg/m^2 infused over 60 minutes weekly

Note: If given in combination with radiation therapy, administer loading dose 1 week prior to initiation of radiation course. Weekly maintenance dose should be completed 1 hour prior to radiation for the duration of radiation therapy (6-7 weeks).

NSCLC (unlabeled use): Initial loading dose: 400 mg/m^2, followed by maintenance dose: 250 mg/m^2 weekly (Pirker, 2009)

Adjustment for Toxicity

Infusion reactions, grade 1 or 2 and nonserious grades 3 or 4: Reduce the infusion rate by 50% and continue to use prophylactic antihistamines

Infusion reactions, severe: Immediately and permanently discontinue treatment

Pulmonary toxicity:

Acute onset or worsening pulmonary symptoms: Hold treatment

Interstitial lung disease: Permanently discontinue

Skin toxicity, mild-to-moderate: No dosage modification required

Acneiform rash, severe (grade 3 or 4):

First occurrence: Delay cetuximab infusion 1-2 weeks

If improvement, continue at 250 mg/m^2

If no improvement, discontinue therapy

Second occurrence: Delay cetuximab infusion 1-2 weeks

If improvement, continue at reduced dose of 200 mg/m^2

If no improvement, discontinue therapy

Third occurrence: Delay cetuximab infusion 1-2 weeks

If improvement, continue at reduced dose of 150 mg/m^2

If no improvement, discontinue therapy

Fourth occurrence: Discontinue therapy

Note: Dose adjustments are not recommended for severe **radiation** dermatitis.

Administration

I.V. I.V. infusion; loading dose over 2 hours, weekly maintenance dose over 1 hour. Do not administer as I.V. push or bolus. Do not shake or dilute. Administer via infusion pump or syringe pump. Following the infusion, an observation period (1 hour) is recommended; longer observation time (following an infusion reaction) may be required. Premedication with an H_1 antagonist prior to the initial dose is recommended. The maximum infusion rate is 10 mg/minute. Administer through a low protein-binding 0.22 micrometer in-line filter. Use 0.9% NaCl to flush line at the end of infusion.

For biweekly administration (unlabeled frequency and dose), the initial dose was infused over 120 minutes and subsequent doses infused over 60 minutes (Pfeiffer, 2007).

Stability

Reconstitution Reconstitution is not required. Appropriate dose should be added to empty sterile container; do not shake or dilute.

Storage Store unopened vials under refrigeration at 2°C to 8°C (36°F to 46°F); do not freeze. Preparations in infusion containers are stable for up to 12 hours under refrigeration at 2°C to 8°C (36°F to 46°F) and up to 8 hours at room temperature of 20°C to 25°C (68°F to 77°F).

Monitoring and Teaching Issues

Laboratory Monitoring Periodic monitoring of serum magnesium, calcium, and potassium are recommended to continue over an interval consistent with the half-life (8 weeks); monitor closely (during and after treatment) for cetuximab plus radiation therapy. *KRAS* genotyping of tumor tissue in patients with colorectal cancer.

Physical Assessment Use caution with pre-existing coronary or lung disease. Premedication with antihistamines is recommended. Patient must be monitored closely for airway obstruction, hives, and hypotension during and for 1 hour following infusion. Treatment for anaphylactic reactions should be available. In case of severe infusion reaction, treatment should be stopped and patient assessed. Dosing adjustment or permanent discontinuation may be necessary in event of infusion reaction. Instruct patient to report skin reactions, cough, dyspnea, gastrointestinal upset, and opportunistic infection.

Patient Education This medication can only be administered by infusion and you will be closely monitored during each infusion. Report immediately unusual chest tightness; difficulty breathing or swallowing; itching or skin rash; back pain or acute headache; or redness, swelling, or pain at infusion site. Maintain adequate nutrition and hydration, unless instructed to restrict fluid intake. You may experience feelings of weakness or fatigue, nausea, vomiting, loss of appetite, diarrhea, headache, back pain, skin rash or dryness, or loss of hair or nails (may grow back after therapy). Report immediately chest pain, irregular heart beat, or palpitations; difficulty breathing; persistent gastrointestinal disturbances (pain, constipation, diarrhea, vomiting); CNS changes (depression or insomnia); skin rash, dryness, or cracking; or any signs of infection.

Breast-Feeding Considerations Breast-feeding should be discontinued during treatment and for at least 60 days following the last dose.

Pregnancy Considerations In pregnant cynomolgus monkeys, cetuximab was detected in the amniotic fluid and in the serum of embryos. Although teratogenic effects were not observed in animal studies, increases in embryolethality and fetal loss were noted. There are no adequate and well-controlled studies in pregnant women. It is not known whether cetuximab can cause fetal harm or affect reproductive capacity. Because cetuximab inhibits epidermal growth factor (EGF), a component of fetal development, adverse effects on pregnancy would be expected. Cetuximab should only be given to a pregnant woman if the potential benefit justifies the potential risk to the fetus.

Additional Information Oncology Comment: EGFR expression is detected in nearly all patients with head and neck cancer; laboratory evidence of EGFR expression is not necessary for head and neck cancers.

The National Comprehensive Cancer Network® (NCCN) guidelines for colon cancer (v.2.2010) and the American Society of Clinical Oncology (ASCO) provisional clinical opinion (Allegra, 2009) recommend genotyping tumor tissue for *KRAS* mutation in all patients with metastatic colorectal cancer (genotyping may be done on archived specimens). Patients with known codon 12 or 13 *KRAS* gene mutations are unlikely to respond to EGFR inhibitors and should not receive cetuximab. Favorable progression-free survival and overall survival has been demonstrated with cetuximab in patients with *KRAS* wild-type (Karapetis, 2008; Van Cutsem, 2008). Because EGFR testing in colorectal tumors does not correlate with response, the NCCN guidelines do not recommend routine EGFR testing in colorectal cancer. Dermatologic toxicity with cetuximab is predictive for response; the presence of acneiform rash correlates with treatment response and prolonged survival (Cunningham, 2004).

The NCCN Non-Small Cell Lung cancer guidelines (v.2.2010) recommend cetuximab in combination with cisplatin and vinorelbine as a first-line therapy option in patients with advanced (stage IIIB or IV disease), with EGFR expression and a performance status of 0-2. Cetuximab maintenance therapy may be continued after 4-6 cycles of combination with chemotherapy.

Head and neck cancer guidelines from the NCCN (v.1.2009) recommend cetuximab with concurrent radiation therapy for squamous cell head and neck cancer. For advanced head and neck cancers, cetuximab may be used in combination with chemotherapy or as a single agent.

Cevimeline (se vi ME leen)

U.S. Brand Names Evoxac®

Index Terms Cevimeline Hydrochloride

Generic Availability (U.S.) No

Pharmacologic Category Cholinergic Agonist

Medication Safety Issues

Sound-alike/look-alike issues:

Cevimeline may be confused with Savella™

Evoxac® may be confused with Eurax®

Pregnancy Risk Factor C

Lactation Excretion in breast milk unknown/not recommended

Use Treatment of symptoms of dry mouth in patients with Sjögren's syndrome

Available Dosage Forms

Capsule, oral:

Evoxac®: 30 mg

Dosing

Adult Xerostomia (in Sjögren's syndrome): Oral: 30 mg 3 times/day

Geriatric Refer to adult dosing. No specific dosage adjustment is recommended; however, use caution when initiating due to potential for increased sensitivity.

Renal Impairment Not studied; no specific dosage adjustment is recommended

Hepatic Impairment Not studied; no specific dosage adjustment is recommended

Administration

Oral Administer with or without food.

Monitoring and Teaching Issues

Patient Education Take with or without food. You may experience decreased visual acuity, GI distress, nausea, diarrhea, or headache. Report unresolved diarrhea; abdominal pain; flatulence; anorexia; excessive salivation or sweating; unresolved respiratory distress; runny nose; cold or flu symptoms; joint, bone, or muscle weakness, pain, tremor, or cramping; chest pain or palpitations; swelling of extremities; or weight gain.

- **Cevimeline Hydrochloride** *see* Cevimeline *on page* *355*
- **CFDN** *see* Cefdinir *on page* *315*
- **CG** *see* Chorionic Gonadotropin (Human) *on page* *364*
- **CG5503** *see* Tapentadol *on page* *1708*
- **CGP 33101** *see* Rufinamide *on page* *1617*
- **CGP-39393** *see* Desirudin *on page* *490*
- **CGP-42446** *see* Zoledronic Acid *on page* *1899*
- **CGP-57148B** *see* Imatinib *on page* *951*
- **CGS-20267** *see* Letrozole *on page* *1078*

◆ **Chantix®** *see* Varenicline *on page 1848*

◆ **Chenodal™** *see* Chenodiol *on page 356*

◆ **Chenodeoxycholic Acid** *see* Chenodiol *on page 356*

Chenodiol (kee noe DYE ole)

U.S. Brand Names Chenodal™

Index Terms CDCA; Chenodeoxycholic Acid

Generic Availability (U.S.) No

Pharmacologic Category Bile Acid

Pregnancy Risk Factor X

Lactation Excretion in breast milk unknown/use caution

Use Oral dissolution of radiolucent cholesterol gallstones in selected patients as an alternative to surgery

Unlabeled/Investigational Use Cerebrotendinous xanthomatosis (CTX)

Available Dosage Forms

Tablet, oral:

Chenodal™: 250 mg

Dosing

Adult

Cerebrotendinous xanthomatosis (unlabeled use): Oral: 750 mg/day in 3 divided doses (Beringer, 1984)

Gallstone dissolution (monotherapy): Oral: Initial: 250 mg twice daily for the first 2 weeks and increasing by 250 mg/day each week thereafter until the recommended or maximum tolerated dose is achieved; maintenance: 13-16 mg/kg/day in 2 divided doses. **Note:** Dosages <10 mg/kg are usually ineffective and may increase the risk of cholecystectomy.

Gallstone dissolution (combination therapy; unlabeled dose): Oral: 5-7.5 mg/kg/day once daily at bedtime, in combination with ursodeoxycholic acid, with or without adjuvant lithotripsy (Jazrawi, 1992; Pereira, 1997; Petroni, 2001)

Pediatric Cerebrotendinous xanthomatosis (unlabeled use): Oral: 15 mg/kg/day in three divided doses (van Heijst, 1998)

Hepatic Impairment Use extreme caution; contraindicated for use in presence of known hepatocyte dysfunction or bile ductal abnormalities.

Monitoring and Teaching Issues

Laboratory Monitoring Serum aminotransferase levels (monthly for first 3 months, then every 3 months during therapy); serum cholesterol (every 6 months)

Patient Education Medication may need to be taken for 24 months before dissolution will occur. Blood studies and x-rays studies will be necessary during therapy. Report persistent diarrhea and gallstone attacks (abdominal pain, nausea and vomiting, yellowing of skin or eyes).

◆ **Cheratussin** *see* GuaiFENesin *on page 890*

◆ **Chickenpox Vaccine** *see* Varicella Virus Vaccine *on page 1850*

◆ **Children's Nasal Decongestant [OTC]** *see* Pseudoephedrine *on page 1529*

◆ **Chloditan** *see* Mitotane *on page 1242*

◆ **Chlodithane** *see* Mitotane *on page 1242*

◆ **Chloral** *see* Chloral Hydrate *on page 356*

Chloral Hydrate (KLOR al HYE drate)

U.S. Brand Names Somnote®

Index Terms Chloral; Hydrated Chloral; Trichloroacetaldehyde Monohydrate

Generic Availability (U.S.) Yes: Syrup and suppositories

Pharmacologic Category Hypnotic, Nonbenzodiazepine

Medication Safety Issues

High alert medication: The Institute for Safe Medication Practices (ISMP) includes this medication among its list of drugs which have a heightened risk of causing significant patient harm when used in error.

Pregnancy Risk Factor C

Lactation Enters breast milk/compatible

Use Short-term sedative and hypnotic (<2 weeks); sedative/hypnotic for diagnostic procedures; sedative prior to EEG evaluations

Controlled Substance C-IV

Available Dosage Forms

Capsule, oral:

Somnote®: 500 mg

Suppository, rectal: 500 mg (25s)

Syrup, oral: 500 mg/5 mL (5 mL, 473 mL, 480 mL)

Dosing

Adult

Sedation, anxiety: Oral, rectal: 250 mg 3 times/day

Hypnotic: Oral, rectal: 500-1000 mg at bedtime or 30 minutes prior to procedure, not to exceed 2 g/24 hours

Discontinuation: Withdraw gradually over 2 weeks if patient has been maintained on high doses for prolonged period of time. Do not stop drug abruptly; sudden withdrawal may result in delirium.

Geriatric Hypnotic: Initial: Oral: 250 mg at bedtime; adjust for renal impairment.

Pediatric

Sedation, anxiety: Oral, rectal: 5-15 mg/kg/dose every 8 hours, maximum: 500 mg/dose

Prior to EEG: Oral, rectal: 20-25 mg/kg/dose, 30-60 minutes prior to EEG; may repeat in 30 minutes to maximum of 100 mg/kg or 2 g total

Hypnotic: Oral, rectal: 20-40 mg/kg/dose up to a maximum of 50 mg/kg/24 hours or 1 g/dose or 2 g/24 hours

Conscious sedation: Oral: 50-75 mg/kg/dose 30-60 minutes prior to procedure; may repeat 30 minutes after initial dose if needed, to a total maximum dose of 120 mg/kg or 1 g total

Discontinuation: Withdraw gradually over 2 weeks if patient has been maintained on high doses for prolonged period of time. Do not stop drug abruptly; sudden withdrawal may result in delirium.

Renal Impairment

Cl_{cr} <50 mL/minute: Avoid use.

Hemodialysis effects: Supplemental dose is not necessary; dialyzable (50% to 100%).

Hepatic Impairment Avoid use in patients with severe hepatic impairment.

Administration

Oral Chilling the syrup may help to mask unpleasant taste. Do not crush capsule (contains drug in liquid form). Gastric irritation may be minimized by diluting dose in water or other oral liquid.

Monitoring and Teaching Issues

Physical Assessment For short-term use. Assess for history of addiction; long-term use can result in dependence, abuse, or tolerance. Monitor for excessive sedation. For inpatient use, institute safety measures to prevent falls.

Patient Education Drug may cause physical and/or psychological dependence. While using this medication, do not use alcohol. You may experience drowsiness, dizziness, blurred vision, nausea, vomiting, unpleasant taste, or diarrhea. Report skin rash, CNS changes (confusion, depression, increased sedation, excitation, headache, insomnia, or nightmares), unresolved GI distress, chest pain or palpitations, or ineffectiveness of medication.

Chlorambucil (klor AM byoo sil)

U.S. Brand Names Leukeran®

Index Terms CB-1348; Chlorambucilum; Chloraminophene; Chlorbutinum; WR-139013

Generic Availability (U.S.) No

Pharmacologic Category Antineoplastic Agent, Alkylating Agent

Medication Safety Issues

Sound-alike/look-alike issues:

Chlorambucil may be confused with Chloromycetin®

Leukeran® may be confused with Alkeran®, leucovorin, Leukine®, Myleran®

High alert medication: The Institute for Safe Medication Practices (ISMP) includes this medication among its list of drugs which have a heightened risk of causing significant patient harm when used in error.

Pregnancy Risk Factor D

Lactation Excretion in breast milk unknown/not recommended

Use Management of chronic lymphocytic leukemia (CLL), Hodgkin's lymphoma, non-Hodgkin's lymphoma (NHL)

Unlabeled/Investigational Use Treatment of nephrotic syndrome, Waldenström's macroglobulinemia

Available Dosage Forms

Tablet, oral:

Leukeran®: 2 mg

Dosing

Adult Refer to individual protocols.

CLL, NHL: Oral: 0.1 mg/kg/day for 3-6 weeks **or** 0.4 mg/kg (increased by 0.1mg/kg/dose until response/toxicity observed) biweekly **or** 0.4 mg/kg (increased by 0.1mg/kg/dose until response/toxicity observed) monthly **or** 0.03-0.1 mg/kg/day continuously

Hodgkin's lymphoma: Oral: 0.2 mg/kg/day for 3-6 weeks **or** 0.4 mg/kg (increased by 0.1 mg/kg/dose until response/toxicity observed) biweekly **or** 0.4 mg/kg (increased by 0.1mg/kg/dose until response/toxicity observed) monthly **or** 0.03-0.1 mg/kg/day continuously

Waldenström's macroglobulinemia (unlabeled use): Oral: 0.1 mg/kg/day (continuously) for at least 6 months **or** 0.3 mg/kg/day for 7 days every 6 weeks for at least 6 months

Geriatric Refer to adult dosing. Begin at the lower end of dosing range(s)

Pediatric Refer to individual protocols. Unlabeled uses:

General short courses: Oral: 0.1-0.2 mg/kg/day for 3-6 weeks **or** maintenance therapy: 0.03-0.1 mg/kg/day

Nephrotic syndrome: Oral: 0.1-0.2 mg/kg/day every day for ~8-12 weeks with low-dose prednisone

Chronic lymphocytic leukemia (CLL): Oral:

Biweekly regimen: Initial: 0.4 mg/kg/dose every 2 weeks; increase dose by 0.1 mg/kg every 2 weeks until a response occurs and/or myelosuppression occurs

Monthly regimen: Initial: 0.4 mg/kg, increase dose by 0.1 mg/kg every 4 weeks until a response occurs and/or myelosuppression occurs

Malignant lymphomas:

Non-Hodgkin's lymphoma: 0.1 mg/kg/day

Hodgkin's lymphoma: 0.2 mg/kg/day

Renal Impairment The FDA-approved labeling does not contain renal dosing adjustment guidelines. The following guidelines have been used by some clinicians (Aronoff, 2007): Adults:

Cl_{cr} 10-50 mL/minute: Administer 75% of dose

Cl_{cr} <10 mL/minute: Administer 50% of dose

Continuous ambulatory peritoneal dialysis (CAPD): Administer 50% of dose

Hepatic Impairment The FDA-approved labeling does not contain hepatic dosing adjustment guidelines. Chlorambucil is hepatically metabolized into active and inactive metabolites; dosage adjustment may be needed in patients with hepatic impairment.

Adjustment for Toxicity

Skin reactions: Discontinue treatment

Hematologic: Persistent neutropenia, thrombocytopenia, and/or lymphocytosis: Do not exceed 0.1 mg/kg/day

Concurrent or within 4 weeks of chemotherapy/radiotherapy: Initiate treatment cautiously; reduce dose; monitor closely. (May use the usual dose if radiation therapy is small doses of palliative radiation over isolated foci remote from bone marrow.)

Administration

Oral Usually administered as a single dose; preferably on an empty stomach.

Monitoring and Teaching Issues

Laboratory Monitoring Liver function tests, CBC with differential and platelets (weekly, with WBC monitored twice weekly during the first 3-6 weeks of treatment), serum uric acid

Physical Assessment Use caution in presence of seizure disorder or bone marrow suppression. Monitor for hematologic myelosuppression, hypersensitivity rash, drug fever, seizures, gastrointestinal upset, and hepatotoxicity. Teach sexually-active female patients necessity for contraception.

Patient Education Maintain adequate hydration, unless instructed to restrict fluid intake. Avoid alcohol and acidic, spicy, or hot foods. May cause menstrual irregularities and/or sterility. You will be more susceptible to infection. May cause nausea, vomiting, or mouth sores. Report CNS changes (agitation, confusion, hallucinations, seizures); easy bruising or bleeding; unusual rash; persistent nausea, vomiting, or mouth sores; yellowing of skin or dark urine; or respiratory difficulty.

◆ **Chlorambucilum** *see* Chlorambucil *on page 357*

◆ **Chloraminophene** *see* Chlorambucil *on page 357*

◆ **Chlorbutinum** *see* Chlorambucil *on page 357*

ChlordiazePOXIDE (klor dye az e POKS ide)

Index Terms Librium; Methaminodiazepoxide Hydrochloride

Generic Availability (U.S.) Yes

Pharmacologic Category Benzodiazepine

Medication Safety Issues

Sound-alike/look-alike issues:

ChlordiazePOXIDE may be confused with chlorproMAZINE

Librium may be confused with Librax®

Beers Criteria medication: This drug may be inappropriate for use in geriatric patients (high severity risk).

Lactation Enters breast milk

Use Management of anxiety disorder or for the short-term relief of symptoms of anxiety; withdrawal symptoms of acute alcoholism; preoperative apprehension and anxiety

Controlled Substance C-IV

Available Dosage Forms

Capsule, oral: 5 mg, 10 mg, 25 mg

Dosing

Adult

Anxiety:

Oral: 15-100 mg divided 3-4 times/day

I.M., I.V.: Initial: 50-100 mg followed by 25-50 mg 3-4 times/day as needed

Preoperative anxiety: I.M.: 50-100 mg prior to surgery

Ethanol withdrawal symptoms: Oral, I.V.: 50-100 mg to start, dose may be repeated in 2-4 hours as necessary to a maximum of 300 mg/24 hours

Note: Up to 300 mg may be given I.M. or I.V. during a 6-hour period, but not more than this in any 24-hour period.

Geriatric Anxiety: Oral: 5 mg 2-4 times/day; adjust for renal impairment. Avoid use if possible.

Pediatric Anxiety: Oral, I.M.:

<6 years: Not recommended

>6 years: 0.5 mg/kg/24 hours divided every 6-8 hours

Renal Impairment

Cl_{cr} <10 mL/minute: Administer 50% of dose.

Not dialyzable (0% to 5%)

Hepatic Impairment Avoid use.

Administration

I.M. Administer by deep I.M. injection slowly into the upper outer quadrant of the gluteus muscle. Use only the diluent provided for I.M. use. Solutions made with SWFI or NS cause pain with I.M. administration.

I.V. Administer slowly over at least 1 minute. Do not use the diluent provided for I.M. use. Air bubbles form during reconstitution.

Monitoring and Teaching Issues

Physical Assessment Assess for CNS depression. Assess for history of addiction; long-term use can result in dependence, abuse, or tolerance; periodically evaluate need for continued use. For inpatient use, institute safety measures. Taper dosage slowly when discontinuing. **I.V.:** Monitor vital signs frequently during infusion and observe safety precautions to prevent falls.

Patient Education Oral: Drug may cause physical and/or psychological dependence. Do not use alcohol. Maintain adequate hydration, unless instructed to restrict fluid intake. You may experience drowsiness, lightheadedness, impaired coordination, dizziness, blurred vision, dry mouth, constipation, or altered sexual drive or ability (reversible). Report persistent CNS effects (eg, euphoria, confusion, increased sedation, depression); chest pain, palpitations, or rapid heartbeat; muscle cramping, weakness, tremors, rigidity, or altered gait; or worsening of condition.

Related Information

Benzodiazepines *on page* 1988

◆ **Chlordiazepoxide and Clidinium** *see* Clidinium and Chlordiazepoxide *on page* 396

◆ **Chlormeprazine** *see* Prochlorperazine *on page* 1512

◆ **2-Chlorodeoxyadenosine** *see* Cladribine *on page* 389

◆ **Chloromag®** *see* Magnesium Chloride *on page* 1143

Chloroquine (KLOR oh kwin)

U.S. Brand Names Aralen®

Index Terms Chloroquine Phosphate

Generic Availability (U.S.) Yes

Pharmacologic Category Aminoquinoline (Antimalarial)

Medication Safety Issues

International issues:

Aralen [U.S., Mexico, and Philippines] may be confused with Paralen brand name for acetaminophen [Czech Republic]

Lactation Enters breast milk/not recommended (AAP considers "compatible"; AAP 2001 update pending)

Use Suppression/chemoprophylaxis or treatment of acute malaria due to susceptible *Plasmodium malariae, P. vivax, P. ovale, P. falciparum*; extraintestinal amebiasis

Unlabeled/Investigational Use Rheumatoid arthritis; discoid lupus erythematosus

Available Dosage Forms

Tablet, oral: 250 mg, 500 mg

Aralen®: 500 mg

Dosing

Adult & Geriatric

Malaria, suppression or prophylaxis: Oral: 500 mg/week (300 mg base) on the same day each week; begin 2 weeks prior to exposure; continue for 8 weeks after leaving endemic area; if suppressive therapy is not begun prior to exposure, double the initial loading dose to 1 g (600 mg base) and administer in 2 divided doses 6 hours apart, followed by the usual dosage regimen.

Malaria, acute attack: Oral: 1 g (600 mg base) on day 1, followed by 500 mg (300 mg base) 6 hours later, followed by 500 mg (300 mg base) on days 2 and 3.

Extraintestinal amebiasis: Oral: 1 g/day (600 mg base) for 2 days followed by 500 mg/day (300 mg base) for at least 2-3 weeks.

Rheumatoid arthritis, lupus erythematosus (unlabeled uses): Oral: 250 mg (150 mg base) once daily; reduce dosage following maximal response (taper to discontinue after response in lupus); generally requires 3-6 weeks. **Note:** Not considered first-line agent.

Pediatric

Malaria, suppression or prophylaxis of malaria: Oral: Administer 8.3 mg/kg/week (5 mg/kg base) on the same day each week (not to exceed 500 mg/dose [300 mg base/dose]); begin 1-2 weeks prior to exposure; continue for 4 weeks after leaving endemic area; if suppressive therapy is not begun prior to exposure, double the initial loading dose to 16.6 mg/kg (10 mg/kg base) (maximum: 1000 mg [600 mg base]) and administer in 2 divided doses 6 hours apart, followed by the usual dosage regimen

Malaria, acute attack: Oral: 16.6 mg/kg (10 mg/kg base) on day 1 (maximum: 1000 mg [600 mg base]), followed by 8.3 mg/kg (5 mg/kg base [300 mg base/dose]; maximum: 500 mg/dose [300 mg base/dose]) 6-, 24-, and 36 hours after first dose (CDC, 2009)

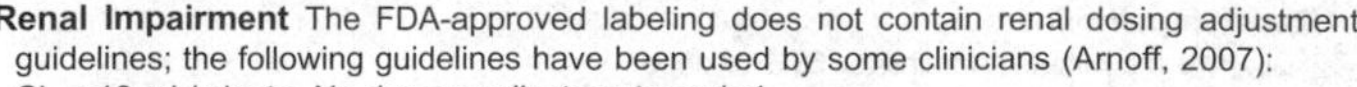

Renal Impairment The FDA-approved labeling does not contain renal dosing adjustment guidelines; the following guidelines have been used by some clinicians (Arnoff, 2007):

Cl_{cr} ≥10 mL/minute: No dosage adjustment needed.

Cl_{cr} <10 mL/minute: Administer 50% of dose.

Hemodialysis effects: Minimally removed by hemodialysis.

Hemodialysis, peritoneal dialysis: Administer 50% of dose.

Continuous renal replacement therapy (CRRT): Administer 100% of normal dose.

Administration

Oral May be taken with meals to decrease GI upset. Chloroquine phosphate tablets have also been mixed with chocolate syrup or enclosed in gelatin capsules to mask the bitter taste.

Monitoring and Teaching Issues

Laboratory Monitoring Periodic CBC in prolonged therapy.

Physical Assessment Assess results of CBC and monitor for retinopathy, hearing loss, or myopathy regularly. Teach patient to report anemia, muscle weakness, or visual or auditory changes.

Patient Education It is important to complete full course of therapy. May be taken with meals to decrease GI upset and bitter aftertaste. Avoid excessive alcohol when taking this medication. You should have regular ophthalmic exams (every 4-6 months) if using this medication over extended periods. May cause skin discoloration (blue/black), hair bleaching, or skin rash. If you have psoriasis, may cause exacerbation. May cause headache, nausea, vomiting, loss of appetite, or increased sensitivity to sunlight. Report vision changes, any change in hearing acuity or ringing in ears, rash or itching, persistent diarrhea or GI disturbances, chest pain or palpitations, CNS changes, unusual fatigue, or easy bruising or bleeding.

◆ **Chloroquine Phosphate** *see* Chloroquine *on page 359*

◆ **Chlorpheniramine and Dextromethorphan** *see* Dextromethorphan and Chlorpheniramine *on page 513*

◆ **Chlorpheniramine Maleate and Dextromethorphan Hydrobromide** *see* Dextromethorphan and Chlorpheniramine *on page 513*

ChlorproMAZINE (klor PROE ma zeen)

Index Terms Chlorpromazine Hydrochloride; CPZ; Thorazine

Generic Availability (U.S.) Yes

Pharmacologic Category Antimanic Agent; Antipsychotic Agent, Typical, Phenothiazine

Medication Safety Issues

Sound-alike/look-alike issues:

ChlorproMAZINE may be confused with chlordiazePOXIDE, chlorproPAMIDE, clomiPRAMINE, prochlorperazine, promethazine

Thorazine® may be confused with thiamine, thioridazine

Lactation Enters breast milk/not recommended (AAP rates "of concern"; AAP 2001 update pending)

Use Management of psychotic disorders (control of mania, treatment of schizophrenia); control of nausea and vomiting; relief of restlessness and apprehension before surgery; acute intermittent porphyria; adjunct in the treatment of tetanus; intractable hiccups; combativeness and/or explosive hyperexcitable behavior in children 1-12 years of age and in short-term treatment of hyperactive children

Unlabeled/Investigational Use Behavioral symptoms associated with dementia (elderly); psychosis/agitation related to Alzheimer's dementia

Available Dosage Forms

Injection, solution: 25 mg/mL (1 mL, 2 mL)

Tablet, oral: 10 mg, 25 mg, 50 mg, 100 mg, 200 mg

Dosing

Adult

Schizophrenia/psychoses:

Oral: Range: 30-800 mg/day in 1-4 divided doses, initiate at lower doses and titrate as needed; usual dose: 200-600 mg/day; some patients may require 1-2 g/day

I.M., I.V.: Initial: 25 mg, may repeat (25-50 mg) in 1-4 hours, gradually increase to a maximum of 400 mg/dose every 4-6 hours until patient is controlled; usual dose: 300-800 mg/day

Intractable hiccups:

Oral, I.M.: 25-50 mg 3-4 times/day

I.V. (refractory to oral or I.M. treatment): 25-50 mg via slow I.V. infusion

Nausea and vomiting:

Oral: 10-25 mg every 4-6 hours

I.M., I.V.: 25-50 mg every 4-6 hours

Geriatric

Behavioral symptoms associated with dementia (unlabeled use): Initial: 10-25 mg 1-2 times/day; increase at 4- to 7-day intervals by 10-25 mg/day. Increase dose intervals (eg, twice daily, 3 times/day) as necessary to control behavior response or side effects; maximum daily dose: 800 mg; gradual increases (titration) may prevent some side effects or decrease their severity.

Other indications: Refer to adult dosing.

Pediatric

Schizophrenia/psychoses: Children ≥6 months:

Oral: 0.5-1 mg/kg/dose every 4-6 hours; older children may require 200 mg/day or higher.

I.M., I.V.: 0.5-1 mg/kg/dose every 6-8 hours; maximum dose for <5 years (<22.7 kg): 40 mg/day; maximum for 5-12 years (22.7-45.5 kg): 75 mg/day

Nausea and vomiting: Children ≥6 months:

Oral: 0.5-1 mg/kg/dose every 4-6 hours as needed

I.M., I.V.: 0.5-1 mg/kg/dose every 6-8 hours; maximum dose for <5 years (<22.7 kg): 40 mg/day; maximum for 5-12 years (22.7-45.5 kg): 75 mg/day

Renal Impairment Not dialyzable (0% to 5%)

Hepatic Impairment Avoid use in severe hepatic dysfunction.

Administration

I.V. Do not administer SubQ (tissue damage and irritation may occur); for direct I.V. injection: Dilute with normal saline to a maximum concentration of 1 mg/mL, administer slow I.V. at a rate not to exceed 0.5 mg/minute in children and 1 mg/minute in adults. For treatment of intractable hiccups the manufacturer recommends diluting 25-50 mg of chlorpromazine in 500-1000 ml of normal saline. To reduce the risk of hypotension, patients receiving I.V. chlorpromazine must remain lying down during and for 30 minutes after the injection. **Note:** Avoid skin contact with solution; may cause contact dermatitis.

Monitoring and Teaching Issues

Laboratory Monitoring Lipid profile, fasting blood glucose/Hgb A_{1c}; BMI; CBC in patients with risk factors for leukopenia/neutropenia

Physical Assessment Review ophthalmic exam results. Monitor for suicide ideation and depression at beginning of therapy and periodically with long-term use. I.V./I.M.: Significant hypotension may occur. Initiate at lower doses and taper dosage slowly when discontinuing.

Patient Education Avoid alcohol. Maintain adequate hydration, unless instructed to restrict fluid intake. You may experience excess drowsiness, lightheadedness, dizziness, blurred vision, dry mouth, upset stomach, nausea, vomiting, anorexia, constipation, postural hypotension, urinary retention, ejaculatory dysfunction (reversible), decreased perspiration, or photosensitivity. Report persistent CNS effects (trembling fingers, altered gait or balance, excessive sedation, seizures, unusual movements, anxiety, suicide ideation, abnormal thoughts, confusion, personality changes); chest pain, palpitations, rapid heartbeat, or severe dizziness; unresolved urinary retention or changes in urinary pattern; altered menstrual pattern, change in libido, swelling or pain in breasts (male or female); vision changes, skin rash, irritation, or changes in color of skin (gray-blue); or worsening of condition.

Related Information

Antipsychotic Agents *on page 1986*

◆ **Chlorpromazine Hydrochloride** *see* ChlorproMAZINE *on page 360*

Chlorthalidone (klor THAL i done)

U.S. Brand Names Thalitone®

Index Terms Hygroton

Generic Availability (U.S.) Yes

Pharmacologic Category Diuretic, Thiazide

Pregnancy Risk Factor B

Lactation Enters breast milk/not recommended (AAP rates "compatible"; AAP 2001 update pending)

Use Management of mild-to-moderate hypertension when used alone or in combination with other agents; treatment of edema associated with heart failure or nephrotic syndrome. Recent studies have found chlorthalidone effective in the treatment of isolated systolic hypertension in the elderly.

Unlabeled/Investigational Use Pediatric hypertension

Available Dosage Forms

Tablet, oral: 25 mg, 50 mg

Thalitone®: 15 mg

Dosing

Adult

Hypertension: Oral: 25-100 mg/day or 100 mg 3 times/week; usual dosage range (JNC 7): 12.5-25 mg/day

Edema: Initial: 50-100 mg/day or 100 mg on alternate days; maximum dose: 200 mg/day

Heart failure-associated edema: 12.5-25 mg once daily; maximum daily dose: 100 mg (ACC/AHA 2009 Heart Failure Guidelines)

Geriatric Oral: Initial: 12.5-25 mg/day or every other day; there is little advantage to using doses >25 mg/day.

Pediatric Oral: Children (nonapproved): 2 mg/kg/dose 3 times/week or 1-2 mg/kg/day

Hypertension (unlabeled use): Initial: 0.3 mg/kg once daily, up to 2 mg/kg/day; maximum: 50 mg/day

Renal Impairment Cl_{cr} <10 mL/minute: Avoid use. Ineffective with low GFR (Aronoff, 2002)

Note: ACC/AHA 2009 Heart Failure Guidelines suggest that thiazides lose their efficacy when Cl_{cr} <40 mL/minute

Monitoring and Teaching Issues

Laboratory Monitoring Serum electrolytes, renal function

Physical Assessment Assess allergy history prior to beginning therapy. Monitor electrolyte balance and renal function on a regular basis throughout therapy. Assess blood pressure and fluid status regularly. Caution patients with diabetes to monitor glucose levels (may reduce effect of oral hypoglycemics).

Patient Education Take once-daily dose in morning or last of daily doses early in the day to avoid night-time disturbances. You may need to make dietary changes (eg, your prescriber may recommend a potassium supplement or foods high in potassium; do not increase your potassium intake unless recommended to do so). If using oral hypoglycemics, monitor glucose levels closely (this medication may reduce effect of oral hypoglycemics). May cause sensitivity to sunlight, anorexia, or GI distress. Report muscle twitching or cramps; nausea or vomiting; confusion; numbness of extremities; loss of appetite or GI distress; severe rash, redness, or itching of skin; chest pain or palpitations; respiratory difficulty; or unusual weight loss.

Related Information

Heart Failure (Systolic) *on page 2040*

◆ **Chlorthalidone and Atenolol** *see* Atenolol and Chlorthalidone *on page 164*

Chlorzoxazone (klor ZOKS a zone)

U.S. Brand Names Parafon Forte® DSC

Generic Availability (U.S.) Yes

Pharmacologic Category Skeletal Muscle Relaxant

Medication Safety Issues

Sound-alike/look-alike issues:

Parafon Forte® may be confused with Fam-Pren Forte

Beers Criteria medication: This drug may be inappropriate for use in geriatric patients (high severity risk).

Pregnancy Risk Factor C

Lactation Excretion in breast milk unknown/not recommended

Use Symptomatic treatment of muscle spasm and pain associated with acute musculoskeletal conditions

Mechanism of Action/Effect Acts on the spinal cord and subcortical levels by depressing polysynaptic reflexes

Contraindications Hypersensitivity to chlorzoxazone or any component of the formulation; impaired liver function

Warnings/Precautions This class of medication is poorly tolerated by the elderly due to anticholinergic effects, sedation, and weakness. Efficacy is questionable at dosages tolerated by elderly patients (Beers Criteria).

Drug Interactions

Metabolism/Transport Effects Substrate of CYP1A2 (minor), 2A6 (minor), 2D6 (minor), 2E1 (major), 3A4 (minor); **Inhibits** CYP2E1 (weak), 3A4 (weak)

Avoid Concomitant Use There are no known interactions where it is recommended to avoid concomitant use.

Decreased Effect

The levels/effects of Chlorzoxazone may be decreased by: Peginterferon Alfa-2b

Increased Effect/Toxicity

Chlorzoxazone may increase the levels/effects of: Alcohol (Ethyl); CNS Depressants; Methotrimeprazine

The levels/effects of Chlorzoxazone may be increased by: Conivaptan; Disulfiram; Droperidol; Isoniazid; Methotrimeprazine

Nutritional/Ethanol Interactions Ethanol: Avoid ethanol (may increase CNS depression).

Adverse Reactions Frequency not defined.

Central nervous system: Dizziness, drowsiness lightheadedness, paradoxical stimulation, malaise

Dermatologic: Rash, petechiae, ecchymoses (rare), angioneurotic edema

Gastrointestinal: Nausea, vomiting, stomach cramps

Genitourinary: Urine discoloration

Hepatic: Liver dysfunction

Miscellaneous: Anaphylaxis (very rare)

Pharmacodynamics/Kinetics

Onset of Action ~1 hour

Duration of Action 6-12 hours

Absorption Readily absorbed

Metabolism Extensively hepatic via glucuronidation

Excretion Urine (as conjugates)

Available Dosage Forms

Caplet, oral:

Parafon Forte® DSC: 500 mg

Tablet, oral: 500 mg

Dosing

Adult Muscle spasm: Oral: 250-500 mg 3-4 times/day up to 750 mg 3-4 times/day

Geriatric Oral: Initial: 250 mg 2-4 times/day; increase as necessary to 750 mg 3-4 times/day.

Pediatric Muscle spasm: Oral: 20 mg/kg/day or 600 mg/m^2/day in 3-4 divided doses

Monitoring and Teaching Issues

Laboratory Monitoring Periodic liver functions

Physical Assessment Do not discontinue abruptly if patient using chronically; taper dosage slowly.

Patient Education Take with food. Do not use alcohol. You may experience drowsiness, dizziness, lightheadedness, or postural hypotension. Report excessive drowsiness.

Geriatric Considerations No data available on the use of skeletal muscle relaxants in the elderly. Start dosing low and increase as necessary. The FDA recently approved a stronger warning about hepatotoxicity in the labeling of chlorzoxazone. Because it can cause unpredictable, fatal hepatic toxicity, the use of chlorzoxazone should be avoided.

This medication is considered to be potentially inappropriate in this patient population (Beers Criteria severity: High).

◆ **Cholera and Traveler's Diarrhea Vaccine** *see* Travelers' Diarrhea and Cholera Vaccine *on page 1806*

◆ **Cholera Vaccine** *see* Travelers' Diarrhea and Cholera Vaccine *on page 1806*

Cholestyramine Resin (koe LES teer a meen REZ in)

U.S. Brand Names Prevalite®; Questran®; Questran® Light

Generic Availability (U.S.) Yes

Pharmacologic Category Antilipemic Agent, Bile Acid Sequestrant

Pregnancy Risk Factor C

Lactation Does not enter breast milk/use caution

Use Adjunct in the management of primary hypercholesterolemia; pruritus associated with elevated levels of bile acids; diarrhea associated with excess fecal bile acids; binding toxicologic agents; pseudomembraneous colitis

Available Dosage Forms

Powder for suspension, oral: Cholestyramine resin 4 g/5 g of powder (210 g); Cholestyramine resin 4 g/5.7 g of powder (239.4 g); Cholestyramine resin 4 g/9 g of powder (378 g); Cholestyramine resin 4 g/5 g packet (60s); Cholestyramine resin 4 g/5.7 g packet (60s); Cholestyramine resin 4 g/9 g packet (60s)

Prevalite®: Cholestyramine resin 4 g/5.5 g of powder (231 g); Cholestyramine resin 4 g/5.5 g packet (42s, 60s)

Questran®: Cholestyramine resin 4 g/9 g of powder (378 g); Cholestyramine resin 4 g/9 g packet (60s)

Questran® Light: Cholestyramine resin 4 g/5 g of powder (210 g); Cholestyramine resin 4 g/5 g packet (60s)

Dosing

Adult & Geriatric Dyslipidemia: Oral (dosages are expressed in terms of anhydrous resin): 4 g 1-2 times/day to a maximum of 24 g/day (and a maximum of 6 times/day)

Pediatric Dyslipidemia: Oral (dosages are expressed in terms of anhydrous resin): Children: 240 mg/kg/day in 3 divided doses; need to titrate dose depending on indication

Renal Impairment Not removed by hemo- or peritoneal dialysis. Supplemental doses not necessary with dialysis or continuous arteriovenous or venovenous hemofiltration effects.

Administration

Oral Mix powder with water or other fluid prior to administration; not to be taken in dry form. Suspension should not be sipped or held in mouth for prolonged periods (may cause tooth discoloration or enamel decay).

Monitoring and Teaching Issues

Laboratory Monitoring Serum cholesterol and triglyceride levels before initiating treatment and periodically throughout treatment.

Patient Education Take once or twice a day as directed. Do not take the powder in its dry form; mix with fluid. Cholestyramine may lower absorption of many medications; check proper administration times. Ongoing medical follow-up and laboratory tests may be required. You may experience GI effects (these should resolve after continued use), nausea and vomiting, or constipation. Report unusual stomach cramping, pain or blood in stool, or unresolved nausea, vomiting, or constipation.

Related Information

Hyperlipidemia Management *on page 2046*

◆ **Choline Fenofibrate** *see* Fenofibric Acid *on page 742*

Choline Magnesium Trisalicylate (KOE leen mag NEE zhum trye sa LIS i late)

Index Terms Tricosal; Trilisate

Generic Availability (U.S.) Yes

Pharmacologic Category Salicylate

Pregnancy Risk Factor C/D (3rd trimester)

Lactation Enters breast milk/use caution

Use Management of osteoarthritis, rheumatoid arthritis, and other arthritis; acute painful shoulder

Available Dosage Forms

Liquid, oral: 500 mg/5 mL (240 mL)

Dosing

Adult Arthritis, pain: Oral (based on total salicylate content): 500 mg to 1.5 g 2-3 times/day **or** 3 g at bedtime; usual maintenance dose: 1-4.5 g/day

Geriatric Usual dose: 750 mg 3 times/day.

Pediatric Children: Oral (based on total salicylate content): <37 kg: 50 mg/kg/day given in 2 divided doses; 2250 mg/day for heavier children

Renal Impairment Avoid use in severe renal impairment.

Administration

Oral Liquid may be mixed with fruit juice just before drinking. Do not administer with antacids. Take with a full glass of water and remain in an upright position for 15-30 minutes after administration.

Monitoring and Teaching Issues

Laboratory Monitoring Serum magnesium with high-dose therapy or in patients with impaired renal function, serum salicylate levels, renal function

Physical Assessment Do not use for persons with allergic reaction to salicylates or other NSAIDs. Monitor for effectiveness of pain relief.

Patient Education Take with food or milk. While using this medication, do not use alcohol. You may experience nausea, vomiting, or gastric discomfort; GI bleeding, ulceration, or perforation can occur with or without pain. Report ringing in ears, persistent stomach pain, unresolved nausea or vomiting, respiratory difficulty or shortness of breath, unusual bruising or bleeding (mouth, urine, stool), or skin rash.

Related Information

Nonsalicylate / Nonsteroidal Anti-Inflammatory Agents *on page 2002*

◆ **Choriogonadotropin Alfa** *see* Chorionic Gonadotropin (Recombinant) *on page 365*

Chorionic Gonadotropin (Human) (kor ee ON ik goe NAD oh troe pin HYU man)

U.S. Brand Names Novarel®; Pregnyl®

Index Terms CG; hCG

Generic Availability (U.S.) Yes

Pharmacologic Category Gonadotropin; Ovulation Stimulator

Pregnancy Risk Factor X

Lactation Excretion in breast milk unknown/use caution

Use Induces ovulation and pregnancy in anovulatory, infertile females; treatment of hypogonadotropic hypogonadism, prepubertal cryptorchidism; spermatogenesis induction with follitropin alfa

Available Dosage Forms

Injection, powder for reconstitution: 10,000 units

Novarel®: 10,000 units

Pregnyl®: 10,000 units

Dosing

Adult & Geriatric

Induction of ovulation: Females: I.M.: 5000-10,000 units 1 day following last dose of menotropins

Spermatogenesis induction associated with hypogonadotropic hypogonadism: Males: Treatment regimens vary (range: 1000-2000 units 2-3 times a week). Administer hCG until serum testosterone levels are normal (may require 2-3 months of therapy), then may add follitropin alfa or menopausal gonadotropin if needed to induce spermatogenesis; continue hCG at the dose required to maintain testosterone levels.

Pediatric Various regimens:

Prepubertal cryptorchidism: I.M.:

4000 units 3 times/week for 3 weeks **or**

5000 units every second day for 4 injections **or**

500 units 3 times/week for 4-6 weeks **or**

15 injections of 500-1000 units given over 6 weeks

Hypogonadotropic hypogonadism: Males: I.M.:

500-1000 units 3 times/week for 3 weeks, followed by the same dose twice weekly for 3 weeks **or**

4000 units 3 times/week for 6-9 months, then reduce dosage to 2000 units 3 times/week for additional 3 months

Administration

I.M. I.M. administration only

Monitoring and Teaching Issues

Laboratory Monitoring

Male: Serum testosterone levels, semen analysis

Female: Serum progestin level (ovulation)

Physical Assessment If self-administered, teach patient appropriate injection technique and syringe/needle disposal.

Patient Education This medication can only be administered by injection. If self-administered, follow instruction for reconstitution, injection, and needle disposal. May cause headache, depression, irritability, or restlessness. Contact prescriber if symptoms are severe or do not resolve with use. Contact prescriber if breasts swell; if you experience swelling of legs or feet; or if there is pain, redness, or swelling at injection site.

Chorionic Gonadotropin (Recombinant)

(kor ee ON ik goe NAD oh troe pin ree KOM be nant)

U.S. Brand Names Ovidrel®

Index Terms Choriogonadotropin Alfa; r-hCG

Generic Availability (U.S.) No

Pharmacologic Category Gonadotropin; Ovulation Stimulator

Pregnancy Risk Factor X

Lactation Excretion in breast milk unknown/use caution

Use As part of an assisted reproductive technology (ART) program, induces ovulation in infertile females who have been pretreated with follicle stimulating hormones (FSH); induces ovulation and pregnancy in infertile females when the cause of infertility is functional

Mechanism of Action/Effect Luteinizing hormone analogue produced by recombinant DNA techniques; stimulates late follicular maturation and intitates rupture of the ovarian follicle once follicular development has occurred

Contraindications Hypersensitivity to hCG preparations or any component of the formulation; primary ovarian failure; uncontrolled thyroid or adrenal dysfunction; uncontrolled organic intracranial lesion (ie, pituitary tumor); abnormal uterine bleeding, ovarian cyst or enlargement of undetermined origin; sex hormone dependent tumors; pregnancy

Warnings/Precautions Ovarian enlargement may occur; may be accompanied by abdominal distention or abdominal pain and generally regresses without treatment within 2-3 weeks. If ovaries are abnormally enlarged on the last day of treatment, withhold hCG to reduce the risk of ovarian hyperstimulation syndrome (OHSS). OHSS is characterized by severe ovarian enlargement, abdominal pain/distention, nausea, vomiting, diarrhea, dyspnea, and oliguria, and may be accompanied by ascites, pleural effusion, hypovolemia, electrolyte imbalance, hemoperitoneum, and thromboembolic events. If severe hyperstimulation occurs, stop treatment and hospitalize patient. This syndrome develops rapidly with 24 hours to several days and generally occurs during the 7-10 days immediately following treatment.

Arterial thromboembolic events have been reported in association with and separate from OHSS. These medications should only be used by healthcare providers who are thoroughly familiar with infertility problems and their management. Multiple births may result from the use of these medications; advise patients of the potential risk of multiple births before starting the treatment. Safety and efficacy have not been established in the elderly or in children.

Drug Interactions

Avoid Concomitant Use There are no known interactions where it is recommended to avoid concomitant use.

Decreased Effect There are no known significant interactions involving a decrease in effect.

Increased Effect/Toxicity There are no known significant interactions involving an increase in effect.

Lab Interactions May interfere with interpretation of pregnancy tests; may cross-react with radioimmunoassay of luteinizing hormone and other gonadotropins

Adverse Reactions

2% to 10%:

Endocrine & metabolic: Ovarian cyst (3%), ovarian hyperstimulation (<2% to 3%)

Gastrointestinal: Abdominal pain (3% to 4%), nausea (3%), vomiting (3%)

Local: Injection site: Pain (8%), bruising (3% to 5%), reaction (<2% to 3%), inflammation (<2% to 2%)

Miscellaneous: Postoperative pain (5%)

<2%:

Cardiovascular: Cardiac arrhythmia, heart murmur

Central nervous system: Dizziness, emotional lability, fever, headache, insomnia, malaise

Dermatologic: Pruritus, rash

Endocrine & metabolic: Breast pain, hot flashes, hyperglycemia, intermenstrual bleeding, vaginal hemorrhage

Gastrointestinal: Abdominal enlargement, diarrhea, flatulence

Genitourinary: Cervical carcinoma, cervical lesion, dysuria, genital herpes, genital moniliasis, leukorrhea, urinary incontinence, urinary tract infection, vaginal discomfort, vaginal hemorrhage, vaginitis

Hematologic: Leukocytosis

Neuromuscular & skeletal: Back pain, paresthesia

Renal: Albuminuria

Respiratory: Cough, pharyngitis, upper respiratory tract infection

Miscellaneous: Ectopic pregnancy, hiccups

In addition, the following have been reported with menotropin therapy: Adnexal torsion, hemoperitoneum, mild-to-moderate ovarian enlargement, pulmonary and vascular complications. Ovarian neoplasms have also been reported (rare) with multiple drug regimens used for ovarian induction (relationship not established).

Pharmacodynamics/Kinetics

Bioavailability 40%

Time to Peak 12-24 hours

Half-Life Elimination Initial: 4 hours; Terminal: 29 hours

Excretion Urine (10% of dose)

Available Dosage Forms

Injection, solution:

Ovidrel®: 257.5 mcg/0.515 mL (0.515 mL)

Dosing

Adult Assisted reproductive technologies (ART) and ovulation induction in females: SubQ: 250 mcg given 1 day following the last dose of follicle stimulating agent. Use only after adequate follicular development has been determined. Hold treatment when there is an excessive ovarian response.

Geriatric Safety and efficacy have not been established.

Renal Impairment Safety and efficacy have not been established.

Hepatic Impairment Safety and efficacy have not been established.

Administration

Other For SubQ use only; inject into stomach area.

Stability

Storage Prefilled syringe: Prior to dispensing, store at 2°C to 8°C (36°F to 46°F). Patient may store at 25°C (77°F) for up to 30 days. Protect from light.

Monitoring and Teaching Issues

Laboratory Monitoring Ultrasound and/or estradiol levels to assess follicle development; ultrasound to assess number and size of follicles; ovulation (basal body temperature, serum progestin level, menstruation, sonography)

Physical Assessment If self-administered, teach patient proper storage, reconstitution, injection technique, and needle/syringe disposal.

Patient Education Note that there is a risk of multiple births associated with treatment. This drug must be administered exactly as scheduled (1 day following last dose of follicle stimulating agent); maintain a calendar of treatment days. Keep all ultrasound and laboratory appointments as instructed by prescriber. Avoid strenuous exercise, especially those with pelvic involvement. You may experience nausea, vomiting, GI upset, or hot flashes; if persistent consult prescriber. Report immediately any persistent abdominal pain, vomiting, or acute pelvic pain; chest pain or palpitations; or shortness of breath.

Pregnancy Considerations Intrauterine death and impaired birth were observed in animal studies. Ectopic pregnancy, premature labor, postpartum fever, and spontaneous abortion have been reported in clinical trials. Congenital abnormalities have also been observed, however, the incidence is similar during natural conception.

Additional Information Clinical studies have shown r-hCG to be clinically and statistically equivalent to urinary-derived hCG products.

◆ **CI-1008** *see* Pregabalin *on page 1504*

◆ **Cialis®** *see* Tadalafil *on page 1700*

Ciclesonide (Oral Inhalation) (sye KLES oh nide)

U.S. Brand Names Alvesco®

Generic Availability (U.S.) No

Pharmacologic Category Corticosteroid, Inhalant (Oral)

Pregnancy Risk Factor C

Lactation Excretion in breast milk unknown/use caution

Use Prophylactic management of bronchial asthma

Mechanism of Action/Effect Ciclesonide is a nonhalogenated, glucocorticoid prodrug that is hydrolyzed to the pharmacologically active metabolite des-ciclesonide following administration. Des-ciclesonide has a high affinity for the glucocorticoid receptor and exhibits anti-inflammatory activity. The mechanism of action for corticosteroids is believed to be a combination of three important properties – anti-inflammatory activity, immunosuppressive properties, and antiproliferative actions.

Contraindications Hypersensitivity to ciclesonide or any component of the formulation; primary treatment of acute asthma or status asthmaticus; moderate-to-severe bronchiectasis

Canadian labeling: Additional contraindications (not in U.S. labeling): Untreated fungal, bacterial, or tuberculosis infections of the respiratory tract; moderate-to-severe bronchiectasis

Warnings/Precautions May cause hypercorticism or suppression of hypothalamic-pituitary-adrenal (HPA) axis, particularly in younger children or in patients receiving high doses for prolonged periods. HPA axis suppression may lead to adrenal crisis. Withdrawal and discontinuation of a corticosteroid should be done slowly and carefully. Particular care is required when patients are transferred from systemic corticosteroids to inhaled products due to possible adrenal insufficiency or withdrawal from steroids, including an increase in allergic symptoms. Patients receiving >20 mg per day of prednisone (or equivalent) may be most susceptible. Fatalities have occurred due to adrenal insufficiency in asthmatic patients during and after transfer from systemic corticosteroids to aerosol steroids; aerosol steroids do **not** provide the systemic steroid needed to treat patients having trauma, surgery, or infections.

Bronchospasm may occur with wheezing after inhalation; if this occurs stop steroid and treat with a fast-acting bronchodilator. Supplemental steroids (oral or parenteral) may be needed during stress or severe asthma attacks. Not to be used in status asthmaticus or for the relief of acute bronchospasm. Oropharyngeal thrush due to candida albicans infection may occur with use. Prolonged use of corticosteroids may also increase the incidence of secondary infection, mask acute infection (including fungal infections), prolong or exacerbate viral infections, or limit response to vaccines. Exposure to chickenpox and measles should be avoided; corticosteroids should not be used to treat ocular herpes simplex. Close observation is required in patients with latent tuberculosis and/or TB reactivity; restrict use in active TB (only in conjunction with antituberculosis treatment). Use in patients with TB is contraindicated in the Canadian labeling. Prolonged treatment with corticosteroids has been associated with the development of Kaposi's sarcoma (case reports); if noted, discontinuation of therapy should be considered.

Use with caution in patients with thyroid disease, severe hepatic impairment, glaucoma, cataracts, patients at risk for osteoporosis, and patients at risk for seizures.

Orally inhaled corticosteroids may cause a reduction in growth velocity in pediatric patients (~1 cm per year [range: 0.3-1.8 cm per year] and related to dose and duration of exposure). To minimize the systemic effects of orally inhaled corticosteroids, each patient should be titrated to the lowest effective dose. Growth should be routinely monitored in pediatric patients.

Drug Interactions

Metabolism/Transport Effects Substrate of CYP3A4 (major), 2D6 (minor)

Avoid Concomitant Use

Avoid concomitant use of Ciclesonide (Oral Inhalation) with any of the following: Aldesleukin

Decreased Effect

Ciclesonide (Oral Inhalation) may decrease the levels/effects of: Aldesleukin; Corticorelin

Increased Effect/Toxicity

The levels/effects of Ciclesonide (Oral Inhalation) may be increased by: CYP3A4 Inhibitors (Moderate); Dasatinib

Adverse Reactions

>10%:

Central nervous system: Headache (≤11%)

Respiratory: Nasopharyngitis (≤11%)

1% to 10%:

Cardiovascular: Facial edema (≥3%)

Central nervous system: Dizziness (≥3%), fatigue (≥3%), dysphonia (1%)

Dermatologic: Urticaria (≥3%)

Gastrointestinal: Gastroenteritis (≥3%), oral candidiasis (≥3%)

Neuromuscular & skeletal: Arthralgia (≤4%), musculoskeletal chest pain (≥3%), back pain (≥3%), extremity pain (≥3%)

Ocular: Conjunctivitis (≥3%)

Otic: Ear pain (2%)

Respiratory: Upper respiratory infection (≤9%), epistaxis (≤8%), nasal congestion (≤6%), sinusitis (≤6%), pharyngolaryngeal pain (≤ 5%), hoarseness (≥3%), pneumonia (≥3%), paradoxical bronchospasm (2%)

Miscellaneous: Influenza (≥3%)

Pharmacodynamics/Kinetics

Absorption 52% (lung deposition)

Bioavailability >50% (active metabolite)

Time to Peak ~1 hour (active metabolite)

Protein Binding ≥99%

Half-Life Elimination ~5-7 hours

Metabolism Ciclesonide hydrolyzed to active metabolite, des-ciclesonide via esterases in nasal mucosa; further metabolism via hepatic CYP3A4 and 2D6

Excretion Feces (78%)

Available Dosage Forms

Aerosol, for oral inhalation:

Alvesco®: 80 mcg/inhalation (6.1 g); 160 mcg/inhalation (6.1 g)

Dosing

Adult & Geriatric Asthma: Oral inhalation (Alvesco®): **Note:** Titrate to the lowest effective dose once asthma stability is achieved:

U.S. labeling:

Prior therapy with bronchodilators alone: Initial: 80 mcg twice daily (maximum dose: 320 mcg/day)

Prior therapy with inhaled corticosteroids: Initial: 80 mcg twice daily (maximum dose: 640 mcg/day)

Prior therapy with oral corticosteroids: Initial: 320 mcg twice daily (maximum dose: 640 mcg/day)

Canadian labeling: Initial: 400 mcg once daily; maintenance: 100-800 mcg/day (1-2 puffs once or twice daily)

Conversion from oral to inhaled steroid: Initiation of oral inhalation therapy should begin in patients who have previously been stabilized on oral corticosteroids (OCS). A gradual dose reduction of OCS should begin ~7-10 days after starting inhaled therapy. U.S. labeling recommends reducing prednisone dose no more rapidly than ≤2.5 mg/day on a weekly basis. The Canadian labeling recommends decreasing the daily dose of prednisone by 1 mg (or equivalent of other OCS) every 7 days in closely monitored patients, and every 10 days in patients whom close monitoring is not possible. In the presence of withdrawal symptoms, resume previous OCS dose for 1 week before attempting further dose reductions.

Pediatric Asthma: Oral inhalation (Alvesco®): **Note:** Titrate to the lowest effective dose once asthma stability is achieved:

U.S. labeling: Children ≥12 years: Refer to adult dosing.

Canadian labeling:

Children 6-11 years: Initial: 100-200 mcg once daily; maintenance: 100-200 mcg/day (1-2 puffs once daily)

Children ≥12 years: Refer to adult dosing.

Administration

Inhalation Remove mouthpiece cover, place inhaler in mouth, close lips around mouthpiece, and inhale slowly and deeply. Press down on top of inhaler after slow inhalation has begun. Remove inhaler while holding breath for approximately 10 seconds. Breathe out slowly and replace mouthpiece on inhaler. Do not wash or place inhaler in water. Clean mouthpiece using a dry cloth or tissue once weekly. Discard after the "discard by" date or after labeled number of doses has been used, even if container is not completely empty.

Shaking is not necessary since drug is formulated as a solution aerosol. Prime inhaler prior to initial use or if not in use for ≥1 week by releasing 3 puffs into the air.

Stability

Storage Store at 15°C to 30°C (59°F to 86°F); do not freeze.

Monitoring and Teaching Issues

Physical Assessment Growth should be monitored periodically with long-term use in children. Do not discontinue abruptly after long-term use.

Patient Education Not intended for treatment of acute asthma attacks. You may be susceptible to infections. Avoid exposure to chickenpox or measles. Report persistent headache, nosebleeds, fungal infection in the mouth, bad taste, sore throat or tongue, worsening of condition, or lack of improvement.

Pregnancy Considerations Teratogenic effects were reported in some, but not all animal studies. There are no adequate and well-controlled studies in pregnant women. The extent of intranasal absorption of ciclesonide systemically is low but variable; use during pregnancy with caution. Hypoadrenalism may occur in infants born to mothers receiving corticosteroids during pregnancy.

Additional Information The incidence of oral candidiasis, as well as other localized oropharyngeal effects, observed with ciclesonide use has been reported to be approximately one-half of that seen with other commonly inhaled corticosteroids such as budesonide and fluticasone. Small particle size, minimal activation, and deposition in the oropharynx may explain this decreased incidence.

Ciclesonide (Nasal) (sye KLES oh nide)

U.S. Brand Names Omnaris™

Generic Availability (U.S.) No

Pharmacologic Category Corticosteroid, Nasal

Pregnancy Risk Factor C

Lactation Excretion in breast milk unknown/use caution

Use Management of seasonal and perennial allergic rhinitis

Available Dosage Forms

Suspension, intranasal:

Omnaris™: 50 mcg/inhalation (12.5 g)

Dosing

Adult & Geriatric

Perennial allergic rhinitis: 2 sprays (50 mcg/spray) per nostril once daily; maximum: 200 mcg/day

Seasonal allergic rhinitis: 2 sprays (50 mcg/spray) per nostril once daily; maximum: 200 mcg/day

Pediatric

Perennial allergic rhinitis: Children ≥12 years: Refer to adult dosing:

Seasonal allergic rhinitis:

U.S. labeling: Children ≥6 year: Refer to adult dosing.

Canadian labeling: Children ≥12 years: Refer to adult dosing.

Administration

Other Intranasal: Shake bottle gently before using. Prime pump prior to first use (press 8 times until fine mist appears) or if spray has not been used in 4 consecutive days (press 1 time or until a fine mist appears). Blow nose to clear nostrils. Insert applicator into nostril, keeping bottle upright, and close off the other nostril. Breathe in through nose. While inhaling, press pump to release spray. Avoid spraying directly onto the nasal septum. Nasal applicator may be removed and rinsed with warm water to clean. Discard after the "discard by" date or after labeled number of doses has been used, even if bottle is not completely empty.

Cidofovir (si DOF o veer)

U.S. Brand Names Vistide®

Generic Availability (U.S.) No

Pharmacologic Category Antiviral Agent

Pregnancy Risk Factor C

Lactation Excretion in breast milk unknown/contraindicated

Use Treatment of cytomegalovirus (CMV) retinitis in patients with acquired immunodeficiency syndrome (AIDS). **Note:** Should be administered with probenecid.

Mechanism of Action/Effect Nucleotide analog that selectively inhibits viral DNA polymerase, suppressing viral DNA synthesis

Contraindications Hypersensitivity to cidofovir; history of clinically-severe hypersensitivity to probenecid or other sulfa-containing medications; serum creatinine >1.5 mg/dL; Cl_{cr} <55 mL/minute; urine protein ≥100 mg/dL (≥2+ proteinuria); use with or within 7 days of nephrotoxic agents; direct intraocular injection

Warnings/Precautions Hazardous agent - use appropriate precautions for handling and disposal. **[U.S. Boxed Warning]: Dose-dependent nephrotoxicity requires dose adjustment or discontinuation if changes in renal function occur during therapy (eg, proteinuria, glycosuria, decreased serum phosphate, uric acid or bicarbonate, and elevated creatinine). Neutropenia has been reported;** monitor counts during therapy. Cases of ocular hypotony have also occurred; monitor intraocular pressure. Monitor for signs of metabolic acidosis. Safety and efficacy have not been established in children or the elderly. Administration must be accompanied by oral probenecid and intravenous saline prehydration. **[U.S. Boxed Warning]: Indicated only for CMV retinitis treatment in HIV patients; possibly carcinogenic and teratogenic based on animal data. May cause hypospermia.**

Drug Interactions

Avoid Concomitant Use There are no known interactions where it is recommended to avoid concomitant use.

Decreased Effect There are no known significant interactions involving a decrease in effect.

Increased Effect/Toxicity There are no known significant interactions involving an increase in effect.

Adverse Reactions

>10%:

- Central nervous system: Chills, fever, headache, pain
- Dermatologic: Alopecia, rash
- Gastrointestinal: Nausea, vomiting, diarrhea, anorexia
- Hematologic: Anemia, neutropenia
- Neuromuscular & skeletal: Weakness
- Ocular: Intraocular pressure decreased, iritis, ocular hypotony, uveitis
- Renal: Creatinine increased, proteinuria, renal toxicity
- Respiratory: Cough, dyspnea
- Miscellaneous: Infection, oral moniliasis, serum bicarbonate decreased

1% to 10%:

- Renal: Fanconi syndrome
- Respiratory: Pneumonia

Frequency not defined (limited to important or life-threatening reactions):

- Cardiovascular: Cardiomyopathy, cardiovascular disorder, CHF, edema, postural hypotension, shock, syncope, tachycardia
- Central nervous system: Agitation, amnesia, anxiety, confusion, convulsion, dizziness, hallucinations, insomnia, malaise, vertigo
- Dermatologic: Photosensitivity reaction, skin discoloration, urticaria
- Endocrine & metabolic: Adrenal cortex insufficiency
- Gastrointestinal: Abdominal pain, aphthous stomatitis, colitis, constipation, dysphagia, fecal incontinence, gastritis, GI hemorrhage, gingivitis, melena, proctitis, splenomegaly, stomatitis, tongue discoloration
- Genitourinary: Urinary incontinence
- Hematologic: Hypochromic anemia, leukocytosis, leukopenia, lymphadenopathy, lymphoma-like reaction, pancytopenia, thrombocytopenia, thrombocytopenic purpura
- Hepatic: Hepatomegaly, hepatosplenomegaly, jaundice, liver function tests abnormal, liver damage, liver necrosis
- Local: Injection site reaction
- Neuromuscular & skeletal: Tremor
- Ocular: Amblyopia, blindness, cataract, conjunctivitis, corneal lesion, diplopia, vision abnormal
- Otic: Hearing loss
- Miscellaneous: Allergic reaction, sepsis

Pharmacodynamics/Kinetics

Protein Binding <6%

Half-Life Elimination Plasma: ~2.6 hours

Metabolism Minimal; phosphorylation occurs intracellularly

Excretion Urine

Pharmacokinetic Note Data is based on a combination of cidofovir administered with probenecid.

Available Dosage Forms

Injection, solution [preservative free]:

Vistide®: 75 mg/mL (5 mL)

Dosing

Adult & Geriatric Treatment of cytomegalovirus (CMV) retinitis: I.V.:

Induction treatment: 5 mg/kg once weekly for 2 consecutive weeks

Maintenance treatment: 5 mg/kg administered once every 2 weeks

Note: Probenecid must be administered orally with each dose of cidofovir.

Probenecid dose: 2 g 3 hours prior to cidofovir dose, 1 g at 2 hours and 8 hours after completion of the infusion

Hydration: Patients should also receive 1 L of normal saline intravenously prior to each infusion of cidofovir; saline should be infused over 1-2 hours. A second liter may be administered over 1- to 3- hours at the start of cidofovir infusion or immediately following infusion, if tolerated.

Renal Impairment

Changes in renal function during therapy: If the creatinine increases by 0.3-0.4 mg/dL, reduce the cidofovir dose to 3 mg/kg; discontinue therapy for increases ≥0.5 mg/dL or development of ≥3+ proteinuria

Pre-existing renal impairment: Use is contraindicated with serum creatinine >1.5 mg/dL, Cl_{cr} <55 mL/minute, or urine protein ≥100 mg/dL (≥2+ proteinuria)

Administration

I.V. For I.V. infusion only. Infuse over 1 hour. Hydrate with 1 L of 0.9% NS I.V. prior to cidofovir infusion. A second liter may be administered over a 1- to 3-hour period immediately following infusion, if tolerated.

Stability

Reconstitution Dilute dose in NS 100 mL prior to infusion.

Storage Store at controlled room temperature 20°C to 25°C (68°F to 77°F). Store admixtures under refrigeration for ≤24 hours. Cidofovir infusion admixture should be administered within 24 hours of preparation at room temperature or refrigerated. Admixtures should be allowed to equilibrate to room temperature prior to use.

Monitoring and Teaching Issues

Laboratory Monitoring Serum creatinine, serum bicarbonate, acid-base status, urine protein, WBC should be monitored with each dose; monitor intraocular pressure frequently.

Physical Assessment Assess patient allergy history (sulfa) prior to beginning therapy. Administration must be accompanied by oral probenecid and intravenous saline prehydration. Infusion site should be monitored closely to avoid extravasation. Monitor for CNS changes, anemia, interocular pressure, renal damage, proteinuria, and elevated creatine regularly during therapy. For patients with diabetes, serum glucose should be monitored closely (may cause hyperglycemia). Instruct patient to report any changes in vision or eye pain.

Patient Education This drug can only be administered I.V. Report immediately any pain, stinging, or swelling at infusion site. You may be more susceptible to infection. May cause hair loss (reversible), headache, anxiety, confusion, diarrhea, nausea, heartburn, vomiting, constipation, or postural hypotension. Report severe unresolved vomiting, constipation, or diarrhea; chills, fever, signs of infection; respiratory difficulty or unusual coughing; palpitations, chest pain, or syncope; CNS changes (eg, hallucinations, depression, excessive sedation, amnesia, seizures, insomnia); or vision changes.

Geriatric Considerations Since elderly individuals frequently have reduced kidney function, particular attention should be paid to assessing renal function before and frequently during administration.

Breast-Feeding Considerations The CDC recommends **not** to breast-feed if diagnosed with HIV to avoid postnatal transmission of the virus.

Pregnancy Considerations [U.S. Boxed Warning]: Possibly carcinogenic and teratogenic based on animal data. May cause hypospermia. Cidofovir was shown to be teratogenic and embryotoxic in animal studies, some at doses which also produced maternal toxicity. Reduced testes weight and hypospermia were also noted in animal studies. There are no adequate and well-controlled studies in pregnant women; use during pregnancy only if the potential benefit to the mother outweighs the possible risk to the fetus. Women of childbearing potential should use effective contraception during therapy and for 1 month following treatment. Males should use a barrier contraceptive during therapy and for 3 months following treatment.

Cilostazol (sil OH sta zol)

U.S. Brand Names Pletal®

Index Terms OPC-13013

Generic Availability (U.S.) Yes

Pharmacologic Category Antiplatelet Agent; Phosphodiesterase Enzyme Inhibitor

Medication Safety Issues

Sound-alike/look-alike issues:

Pletal® may be confused with Plendil®

Pregnancy Risk Factor C

Lactation Excretion in breast milk unknown/not recommended

Use Symptomatic management of peripheral vascular disease, primarily intermittent claudication

Unlabeled/Investigational Use Adjunct with aspirin and clopidogrel for prevention of stent thrombosis and restenosis after coronary stent placement

Mechanism of Action/Effect Cilostazol and its metabolites are inhibitors of phosphodiesterase III. As a result, cyclic AMP is increased leading to reversible inhibition of platelet aggregation, vasodilation, and inhibition of vascular smooth muscle cell proliferation.

Contraindications Hypersensitivity to cilostazol or any component of the formulation; heart failure (HF) of any severity; hemostatic disorders or active bleeding

Warnings/Precautions [U.S. Boxed Warning]: The use of this drug is contraindicated in patients with heart failure. Use with caution in severe underlying heart disease. Use with caution in patients receiving other platelet aggregation inhibitors or in patients with thrombocytopenia. Discontinue therapy if thrombocytopenia or leukopenia occur; progression to agranulocytosis (reversible) has been reported when cilostazol was not immediately stopped. When cilostazol and clopidogrel are used concurrently, manufacturer recommends checking bleeding times. Withhold for at least 4-6 half-lives prior to elective surgical procedures. Use with caution in patients receiving CYP3A4 inhibitors (eg, ketoconazole or erythromycin) or CYP2C19 inhibitors (eg, omeprazole). If concurrent use is warranted, consider dosage adjustment of cilostazol. Use caution in moderate-to-severe hepatic impairment. Use cautiously in severe renal impairment (Cl_{cr} <25 mL/minute).

Drug Interactions

Metabolism/Transport Effects **Substrate** of CYP1A2 (minor), 2C19 (minor), 2D6 (minor), 3A4 (major)

Avoid Concomitant Use There are no known interactions where it is recommended to avoid concomitant use.

Decreased Effect

The levels/effects of Cilostazol may be decreased by: CYP3A4 Inducers (Strong); Deferasirox; Herbs (CYP3A4 Inducers); Nonsteroidal Anti-Inflammatory Agents; Peginterferon Alfa-2b

Increased Effect/Toxicity

Cilostazol may increase the levels/effects of: Anticoagulants; Antiplatelet Agents; Collagenase (Systemic); Drotrecogin Alfa; Ibritumomab; Salicylates; Thrombolytic Agents; Tositumomab and Iodine I 131 Tositumomab

The levels/effects of Cilostazol may be increased by: Antifungal Agents (Azole Derivatives, Systemic); Conivaptan; CYP2C19 Inhibitors (Moderate); CYP2C19 Inhibitors (Strong); CYP3A4 Inhibitors (Moderate); CYP3A4 Inhibitors (Strong); Dasatinib; Esomeprazole; Glucosamine; Herbs (Anticoagulant/Antiplatelet Properties); Macrolide Antibiotics; Nonsteroidal Anti-Inflammatory Agents; Omega-3-Acid Ethyl Esters; Omeprazole; Pentosan Polysulfate Sodium; Pentoxifylline; Prostacyclin Analogues

Nutritional/Ethanol Interactions

Food: Taking cilostazol with a high-fat meal may increase peak concentration by 90%. Avoid concurrent ingestion of grapefruit juice due to the potential to inhibit CYP3A4.

Herb/Nutraceutical: St John's wort may decrease the levels/effects of cilostazol. Avoid alfalfa, anise, bilberry, bladderwrack, bromelain, cat's claw, chamomile, coleus, cordyceps, dong quai, evening primrose oil, fenugreek, feverfew, garlic, ginger, ginkgo biloba, ginseng (American), ginseng (Panax), ginseng (Siberian), grape seed, green tea, guggul, horse chestnut seed, horseradish, licorice, prickly ash, red clover, reishi, SAMe (S-adenosylmethionine), sweet clover, turmeric, white willow (all have additional antiplatelet activity).

Adverse Reactions

>10%:

Central nervous system: Headache (27% to 34%)
Gastrointestinal: Abnormal stools (12% to 15%), diarrhea (12% to 19%)
Respiratory: Rhinitis (7% to 12%)
Miscellaneous: Infection (10% to 14%)

2% to 10%:

Cardiovascular: Peripheral edema (7% to 9%), palpitation (5% to 10%), tachycardia (4%)
Central nervous system: Dizziness (9% to 10%), vertigo (up to 3%)
Gastrointestinal: Dyspepsia (6%), nausea (6% to 7%), abdominal pain (4% to 5%), flatulence (2% to 3%)
Neuromuscular & skeletal: Back pain (6% to 7%), myalgia (2% to 3%)
Respiratory: Pharyngitis (7% to 10%), cough (3% to 4%)

Pharmacodynamics/Kinetics

Onset of Action 2-4 weeks; may require up to 12 weeks

Protein Binding Cilostazol 95% to 98%; active metabolites 66% to 97%

Half-Life Elimination 11-13 hours

Metabolism Hepatic via CYP3A4 (primarily), 1A2, 2C19, and 2D6; at least one metabolite has significant activity

Excretion Urine (74%) and feces (20%) as metabolites

Available Dosage Forms

Tablet, oral: 50 mg, 100 mg

Pletal®: 50 mg, 100 mg

Dosing

Adult & Geriatric Peripheral vascular disease: Oral: 100 mg twice daily

Dosage adjustment for cilostazol with concomitant medications:

CYP2C19 inhibitors (see Drug Interactions): Dosage of cilostazol should be reduced to 50 mg twice daily

CYP3A4 inhibitors (see Drug Interactions): Dosage of cilostazol should be reduced to 50 mg twice daily

Administration

Oral Administer cilostazol 30 minutes before or 2 hours after meals.

Stability

Storage Store at 25°C (77°F); excursions permitted to 15°C to 30°C (59°F to 86°F).

Monitoring and Teaching Issues

Patient Education Take on empty stomach (30 minutes before or 2 hours after meals). Inform prescribers and dentists that you are taking this medication prior to scheduling any surgery or dental procedure. You may experience nervousness, dizziness, fatigue, nausea, vomiting, flatulence, or postural hypotension. Report chest pain, palpitations, unusual heartbeat, swelling of extremities, unusual bleeding, unresolved GI upset or pain, dizziness, nervousness, sleeplessness, fatigue, muscle cramping or tremor, or unusual cough.

Dietary Considerations It is best to take cilostazol 30 minutes before or 2 hours after meals.

Geriatric Considerations Elderly must be evaluated for cardiac status. Since CHF is common, this disease cannot be overlooked.

Breast-Feeding Considerations It is not known whether cilostazol is excreted in human milk. Because of the potential risk to nursing infants, a decision to discontinue the drug or discontinue nursing should be made.

Pregnancy Considerations In animal studies, abnormalities of the skeletal, renal and cardiovascular system were increased. In addition, the incidence of stillbirth and decreased birth weights were increased.

◆ **Ciloxan®** *see* Ciprofloxacin (Ophthalmic) *on page* 379

Cimetidine (sye MET i deen)

U.S. Brand Names Tagamet HB 200® [OTC]

Generic Availability (U.S.) Yes

Pharmacologic Category Histamine H_2 Antagonist

Medication Safety Issues

Sound-alike/look-alike issues:

Cimetidine may be confused with simethicone

Beers Criteria medication: This drug may be inappropriate for use in geriatric patients (low severity risk).

Pregnancy Risk Factor B

Lactation Enters breast milk/not recommended (AAP rates "compatible"; AAP 2001 update pending)

Use Short-term treatment of active duodenal ulcers and benign gastric ulcers; maintenance therapy of duodenal ulcer; treatment of gastric hypersecretory states; treatment of gastroesophageal reflux disease (GERD)

OTC labeling: Prevention or relief of heartburn, acid indigestion, or sour stomach

Unlabeled/Investigational Use Part of a multidrug regimen for *H. pylori* eradication to reduce the risk of duodenal ulcer recurrence

Available Dosage Forms

Solution, oral: 300 mg/5 mL (237 mL, 240 mL, 250 mL, 473 mL, 480 mL)

Tablet, oral: 200 mg, 300 mg, 400 mg, 800 mg

Tagamet HB 200® [OTC]: 200 mg

Dosing

Adult & Geriatric

Short-term treatment of active ulcers: Oral: 300 mg 4 times/day or 800 mg at bedtime or 400 mg twice daily for up to 8 weeks

Note: Higher doses of 1600 mg at bedtime for 4 weeks may be beneficial for a subpopulation of patients with larger duodenal ulcers (>1 cm defined endoscopically) who are also heavy smokers (≥1 pack/day).

Duodenal ulcer prophylaxis: 400 mg at bedtime

Gastric hypersecretory conditions: 300-600 mg every 6 hours; dosage not to exceed 2.4 g/day

Gastroesophageal reflux disease: 400 mg 4 times/day or 800 mg twice daily for 12 weeks

Peptic ulcer disease eradication of *Helicobacter pylori* (unlabeled use): 400 mg twice daily; requires combination therapy with antibiotics

Heartburn, acid indigestion, sour stomach (OTC labeling): 200 mg up to twice daily; may take 30 minutes prior to eating foods or beverages expected to cause heartburn or indigestion

Pediatric

Oral: 20-40 mg/kg/day in divided doses every 6 hours

Heartburn, acid indigestion, sour stomach (OTC labeling): Children ≥12 years: Oral: Refer to adult dosing.

Renal Impairment

Cl_{cr} 10-50 mL/minute: Administer 50% of normal dose

Cl_{cr} <10 mL/minute: Administer 25% of normal dose

Slightly dialyzable (5% to 20%); administer after dialysis

Hepatic Impairment Usual dose is safe in mild liver disease but use with caution and in reduced dosage in severe liver disease. Increased risk of CNS toxicity in cirrhosis suggested by enhanced penetration of CNS.

Administration

Oral Administer with meals so that the drug's peak effect occurs at the proper time (peak inhibition of gastric acid secretion occurs at 1 and 3 hours after dosing in fasting subjects and approximately 2 hours in nonfasting subjects. This correlates well with the time food is no longer in the stomach offering a buffering effect). Stagger doses of antacids with cimetidine.

Monitoring and Teaching Issues

Laboratory Monitoring CBC, gastric pH, occult blood with GI bleeding; monitor renal function to correct dose.

Physical Assessment Use caution in presence of renal impairment. Monitor for CNS changes, agitation, and gastric bleeding regularly during therapy.

Patient Education Take with meals. Avoid excess alcohol. May cause headache, dizziness, agitation, nausea, vomiting, or diarrhea. Report chest pain or palpitations; CNS changes (confusion, agitation); persistent diarrhea, nausea, vomiting, or heartburn; black tarry stools or coffee ground-like emesis; rash; unusual bleeding or bruising; sore throat; or fever; or unexplained weight loss.

◆ **Cimzia®** *see* Certolizumab Pegol *on page 348*

Cinacalcet (sin a KAL cet)

U.S. Brand Names Sensipar®

Index Terms AMG 073; Cinacalcet Hydrochloride

Generic Availability (U.S.) No

Pharmacologic Category Calcimimetic

Pregnancy Risk Factor C

Lactation Excretion in breast milk unknown/not recommended

Use Treatment of secondary hyperparathyroidism in patients with chronic kidney disease (CKD) on dialysis; treatment of hypercalcemia in patients with parathyroid carcinoma; treatment of severe hypercalcemia in patients with primary hyperparathyroidism who are unable to undergo parathyroidectomy

Mechanism of Action/Effect Lowers parathyroid hormone (PTH) and serum calcium by increasing the sensitivity of the calcium-sensing receptor on the parathyroid gland, thereby preventing progressive bone disease

Contraindications Hypocalcemia (serum calcium lower than the lower limit of normal range)

Canadian labeling: Additional contraindications (not in U.S. labeling): Hypersensitivity to any component of the formulation

Warnings/Precautions Use is contraindicated in hypocalcemia. Monitor serum calcium and for symptoms of hypocalcemia (eg, cramps, myalgia, paresthesia, seizure, tetany); may require treatment interruption, dose reduction, or initiation (or dose increases) of calcium-based phosphate binder or vitamin D to raise serum calcium depending on calcium levels or symptoms of hypocalcemia. Use with caution in patients with a seizure disorder (seizure threshold is lowered by significant serum calcium reductions); monitor calcium levels closely. Adynamic bone disease may develop if intact parathyroid hormone (iPTH) levels are suppressed (<100 pg/mL).

Use caution in patients with moderate-to-severe hepatic impairment (Child-Pugh classes B and C); monitor serum calcium, serum phosphorus and iPTH closely. In the U.S., the long-term safety and efficacy of cinacalcet has not been evaluated in chronic kidney disease (CKD) patients with hyperparathyroidism not requiring dialysis. Not indicated for CKD patients not receiving dialysis. Although possibly related to lower baseline calcium levels, clinical studies have shown an increased incidence of hypocalcemia (<8.4 mg/dL) in patients not requiring dialysis. Monitor serum calcium and iPTH concentrations closely in patients on concurrent CYP3A4 inhibitors; dosage adjustment may be required. Cinacalcet is a strong inhibitor of CYP2D6; if on concurrent therapy with a CYP2D6 substrate, dosage adjustment of the CYP2D6 substrate may be necessary. May cause a decrease in testosterone levels (free and total); although below normal testosterone levels may occur in patients with end-stage renal disease, the clinical significance has not been determined. Use with caution in patients with cardiovascular disease; idiosyncratic hypotension, worsening of heart failure, and/or arrhythmia have been reported in patients with impaired cardiovascular function; may correlate with decreased serum calcium.

Drug Interactions

Metabolism/Transport Effects Substrate (minor) of CYP1A2, 2D6, 3A4; **Inhibits** CYP2D6 (major)

Avoid Concomitant Use

Avoid concomitant use of Cinacalcet with any of the following: Tamoxifen; Thioridazine

Decreased Effect

Cinacalcet may decrease the levels/effects of: Codeine; Tacrolimus; Tacrolimus (Systemic); TraMADol

The levels/effects of Cinacalcet may be decreased by: Peginterferon Alfa-2b

Increased Effect/Toxicity

Cinacalcet may increase the levels/effects of: Atomoxetine; CYP2D6 Substrates; Fesoterodine; Nebivolol; Tamoxifen; Tetrabenazine; Thioridazine; Tricyclic Antidepressants

The levels/effects of Cinacalcet may be increased by: Antifungal Agents (Azole Derivatives, Systemic); Conivaptan; CYP3A4 Inhibitors (Moderate); CYP3A4 Inhibitors (Strong); Dasatinib

Nutritional/Ethanol Interactions Food: Food increases bioavailability.

Adverse Reactions

>10%:

Central nervous system: Fatigue (12% to 21%), headache (≤21%), depression (10% to 18%)

Endocrine & metabolic: Hypocalcemia (≤66%), dehydration (≤24%), hypercalcemia (12% to 21%)

Gastrointestinal: Nausea (31% to 66%), vomiting (27% to 52%), diarrhea (≤21%), anorexia (6% to 21%), constipation (10% to 18%)

Hematologic: Anemia (6% to 17%)

Neuromuscular & skeletal: Parasthesia (14% to 29%), fracture (12% to 21%), weakness (7% to 17%), arthralgia (6% to 17%), myalgia (≤15%), limb pain (10% to 12%)

Respiratory: Upper respiratory infection (10% to 12%)

1% to 10%:

Cardiovascular: Hypertension (≤7%)

Central nervous system: Dizziness (≤10%), seizure (1%)

Endocrine & metabolic: Testosterone decreased

Neuromuscular & skeletal: Chest pain (noncardiac; ≤6%)

Pharmacodynamics/Kinetics

Time to Peak ~2-6 hours

Protein Binding ~93% to 97%

Half-Life Elimination Terminal: 30-40 hours; moderate hepatic impairment: 65 hours; severe hepatic impairment: 84 hours

Metabolism Hepatic (extensive) via CYP3A4, 2D6, 1A2; forms inactive metabolites

Excretion Urine ~80% (as metabolites); feces ~15%

Available Dosage Forms

Tablet, oral:

Sensipar®: 30 mg, 60 mg, 90 mg

Dosing

Adult Note: Do not titrate dose more frequently than every 2-4 weeks. Dosage adjustment may be required in patients on concurrent CYP3A4 inhibitors.

Secondary hyperparathyroidism: Oral: Initial: 30 mg once daily (maximum daily dose: 180 mg); increase dose incrementally (60 mg, 90 mg, 120 mg, 180 mg once daily) as necessary to maintain intact parathyroid hormone (iPTH) level between 150-300 pg/mL.

Parathyroid carcinoma, primary hyperparathyroidism: Oral: Initial: 30 mg twice daily (maximum daily dose: 360 mg daily as 90 mg 4 times/day); increase dose incrementally (60 mg twice daily, 90 mg twice daily, 90 mg 3-4 times/day) as necessary to normalize serum calcium levels.

Geriatric Refer to adult dosing. No adjustment required.

Renal Impairment No adjustment required.

Hepatic Impairment Patients with moderate-to-severe dysfunction (Child-Pugh classes B and C) have an increased exposure to cinacalcet and increased half-life. Dosage adjustments may be necessary based on serum calcium, serum phosphorus and/or iPTH.

Adjustment for Toxicity Dosage adjustment for hypocalcemia:

If serum calcium >7.5 mg/dL but <8.4 mg/dL **or** if hypocalcemia symptoms occur: Use calcium-containing phosphate binders and/or vitamin D to raise calcium levels.

If serum calcium <7.5 mg/dL **or** if hypocalcemia symptoms persist and the dose of vitamin D cannot be increased: Withhold cinacalcet until serum calcium ≥8 mg/dL and/or symptoms of hypocalcemia resolve. Reinitiate cinacalcet at the next lowest dose.

If iPTH <150-300 pg/mL: Reduce dose or discontinue cinacalcet and/or vitamin D.

Administration

Oral Administer with food or shortly after a meal. Do not break or divide tablet; should be taken whole.

Stability

Storage Store at 25°C (77°F); excursions permitted to 15°C to 30°C (59°F to 86°F).

Monitoring and Teaching Issues

Laboratory Monitoring

Secondary hyperparathyroidism: Serum calcium and phosphorus levels prior to initiation and within a week of initiation or dosage adjustment; iPTH should be measured 1-4 weeks after initiation or dosage adjustment. After the maintenance dose is established, monthly calcium and phosphorus levels and iPTH every 1-3 months are required. Wait at least 12 hours after dose before drawing iPTH levels.

Parathyroid carcinoma and primary hyperparathyroidism: Serum calcium levels prior to initiation and within a week of initiation or dosage adjustment; once maintenance dose is established, obtain serum calcium every 2 months.

Physical Assessment Use caution with history of seizure disorder; assess serum calcium levels closely prior to initiating therapy, after dose change, and regularly during maintenance therapy. Monitor for hypocalcemia (paresthesias, myalgia, cramping, tetany, seizures) at beginning of therapy and regularly thereafter.

Patient Education Take with food; do not break, chew, or crush tablet (swallow whole). You may experience dizziness, nausea, vomiting, loss of appetite, or diarrhea. Report any muscle cramping, twitches, tremors, or spasms; chest pain or palpitations; or unresolved gastrointestinal disturbance.

Dietary Considerations Take with food or shortly after a meal. May be taken with vitamin D and/or phosphate binders.

Breast-Feeding Considerations Due to the potential for serious adverse effects in the nursing infant, the manufacturer recommends discontinuing nursing or discontinuing cinacalcet.

Pregnancy Considerations In animal studies, there were no teratogenic effects observed, although decreased pup weights were noted. There are no adequate or well-controlled studies in pregnant women. Use in pregnancy only if potential benefit to mother justifies risk to the fetus. Women who become pregnant during cinacalcet treatment are encouraged to enroll in Amgen's Pregnancy Surveillance Program (1-800-772-6436).

◆ **Cinacalcet Hydrochloride** *see* Cinacalcet *on page* *373*

◆ **Cipro®** *see* Ciprofloxacin (Systemic) *on page* *375*

◆ **Ciprodex®** *see* Ciprofloxacin and Dexamethasone *on page* *380*

Ciprofloxacin (Systemic) (sip roe FLOKS a sin)

U.S. Brand Names Cipro®; Cipro® I.V.; Cipro® XR; Proquin® XR

Index Terms Ciprofloxacin Hydrochloride

Generic Availability (U.S.) Yes: Excludes suspension

Pharmacologic Category Antibiotic, Quinolone

Medication Safety Issues

Sound-alike/look-alike issues:

Ciprofloxacin may be confused with cephalexin

Cipro® may be confused with Ceftin®

Medication Guide Available Yes

Pregnancy Risk Factor C

Lactation Enters breast milk/not recommended (AAP rates "compatible"; AAP 2001 update pending)

Use

Children: Complicated urinary tract infections and pyelonephritis due to *E. coli*. **Note:** Although effective, ciprofloxacin is not the drug of first choice in children.

Children and Adults: To reduce incidence or progression of disease following exposure to aerolized *Bacillus anthracis*.

Adults: Treatment of the following infections when caused by susceptible bacteria: Urinary tract infections; acute uncomplicated cystitis in females; chronic bacterial prostatitis; lower respiratory tract infections (including acute exacerbations of chronic bronchitis); acute sinusitis; skin and skin structure infections; bone and joint infections; complicated intra-abdominal infections (in combination with metronidazole); infectious diarrhea; typhoid fever due to *Salmonella typhi* (eradication of chronic typhoid carrier state has not been proven); uncomplicated cervical and urethra gonorrhea (due to *N. gonorrhoeae*); nosocomial pneumonia; empirical therapy for febrile neutropenic patients (in combination with piperacillin)

Note: As of April 2007, the CDC no longer recommends the use of fluoroquinolones for the treatment of gonococcal disease.

Unlabeled/Investigational Use Acute pulmonary exacerbations in cystic fibrosis (children); cutaneous/gastrointestinal/oropharyngeal anthrax (treatment, children and adults); disseminated gonococcal infection (adults); chancroid (adults); prophylaxis to *Neisseria meningitidis* following close contact with an infected person; empirical therapy (oral) for febrile neutropenia in low-risk cancer patients; HACEK group endocarditis; infectious diarrhea (children)

Mechanism of Action/Effect Inhibits DNA-gyrase in susceptible organisms; inhibits relaxation of supercoiled DNA and promotes breakage of double-stranded DNA

Contraindications Hypersensitivity to ciprofloxacin, any component of the formulation, or other quinolones; concurrent administration of tizanidine

Warnings/Precautions [U.S. Boxed Warning]: There have been reports of tendon inflammation and/or rupture with quinolone antibiotics; risk may be increased with concurrent corticosteroids, organ transplant recipients, and in patients >60 years of age. Rupture of the Achilles tendon sometimes requiring surgical repair has been reported most frequently; but other tendon sites (eg, rotator cuff, biceps) have also been reported. Strenuous physical activity, rheumatoid arthritis, and renal impairment may be an independent risk factor for tendonitis. Discontinue at first sign of tendon inflammation or pain. May occur even after discontinuation of therapy. Use with caution in patients with rheumatoid arthritis; may increase risk of tendon rupture. CNS stimulation may occur (tremor, restlessness, confusion, and very rarely hallucinations or seizures). Use with caution in patients with known or suspected CNS disorder. Potential for seizures, although very rare, may be increased with concomitant NSAID therapy. Use with caution in individuals at risk of seizures. Fluoroquinolones may prolong QT_c interval; avoid use in patients with a history of QT_c prolongation, uncorrected hypokalemia, hypomagnesemia, or concurrent administration of other medications known to prolong the QT interval (including Class Ia and Class III antiarrhythmics, cisapride, erythromycin, antipsychotics, and tricyclic antidepressants). Prolonged use may result in fungal or bacterial superinfection, including *C. difficile*-associated diarrhea (CDAD) and pseudomembranous colitis; CDAD has been observed >2 months postantibiotic treatment. Rarely crystalluria has occurred; urine alkalinity may increase the risk. Ensure adequate hydration during therapy. Adverse effects, including those related to joints and/or surrounding tissues, are increased in pediatric patients and therefore, ciprofloxacin should not be considered as drug of choice in children (exception is anthrax treatment). Rare cases of peripheral neuropathy may occur.

Fluoroquinolones have been associated with the development of serious, and sometimes fatal, hypoglycemia, most often in elderly diabetics but also in patients without diabetes. This occurred most frequently with gatifloxacin (no longer available systemically), but may occur at a lower frequency with other quinolones.

Severe hypersensitivity reactions, including anaphylaxis, have occurred with quinolone therapy. Reactions may present as typical allergic symptoms after a single dose, or may manifest as severe idiosyncratic dermatologic, vascular, pulmonary, renal, hepatic, and/or hematologic events, usually after multiple doses. Prompt discontinuation of drug should occur if skin rash or other symptoms arise. **[U.S. Boxed Warning]: Quinolones may exacerbate myasthenia gravis; avoid use (rare, potentially life-threatening weakness of respiratory muscles may occur).** Use caution in renal impairment. Avoid excessive sunlight and take precautions to limit exposure (eg, loose fitting clothing, sunscreen); may cause moderate-to-severe phototoxicity reactions. Discontinue use if photosensitivity occurs. Since ciprofloxacin is ineffective in the treatment of syphilis and may mask symptoms, all patients should be tested for syphilis at the time of gonorrheal diagnosis and 3 months later. Hemolytic reactions may (rarely) occur with quinolone use in patients with latent or actual G6PD deficiency.

Ciprofloxacin is a potent inhibitor of CYP1A2. Coadministration of drugs which depend on this pathway may lead to substantial increases in serum concentrations and adverse effects.

Drug Interactions

Metabolism/Transport Effects Substrate of P-glycoprotein; **Inhibits** CYP1A2 (strong), 3A4 (weak)

Avoid Concomitant Use

Avoid concomitant use of Ciprofloxacin (Systemic) with any of the following: BCG; TiZANidine

Decreased Effect

Ciprofloxacin (Systemic) may decrease the levels/effects of: BCG; Mycophenolate; Phenytoin; Sulfonylureas; Typhoid Vaccine

The levels/effects of Ciprofloxacin (Systemic) may be decreased by: Antacids; Calcium Salts; Didanosine; Iron Salts; Magnesium Salts; P-Glycoprotein Inducers; Quinapril; Sevelamer; Sucralfate; Zinc Salts

Increased Effect/Toxicity

Ciprofloxacin (Systemic) may increase the levels/effects of: Bendamustine; Caffeine; Corticosteroids (Systemic); CYP1A2 Substrates; Erlotinib; Methotrexate; Pentoxifylline; QTc-Prolonging Agents; ROPINIRole; Ropivacaine; Sulfonylureas; Theophylline Derivatives; TiZANidine; Vitamin K Antagonists

The levels/effects of Ciprofloxacin (Systemic) may be increased by: Insulin; Nonsteroidal Anti-Inflammatory Agents; P-Glycoprotein Inhibitors; Probenecid

Nutritional/Ethanol Interactions

Food: Food decreases rate, but not extent, of absorption. Ciprofloxacin serum levels may be decreased if taken with dairy products or calcium-fortified juices. Ciprofloxacin may increase serum caffeine levels if taken with caffeine.

Enteral feedings may decrease plasma concentrations of ciprofloxacin probably by >30% inhibition of absorption. Ciprofloxacin should not be administered with enteral feedings. The feeding would need to be discontinued for 1-2 hours prior to and after ciprofloxacin administration. Nasogastric administration produces a greater loss of ciprofloxacin bioavailability than does nasoduodenal administration.

Herb/Nutraceutical: Avoid dong quai, St John's wort (may also cause photosensitization).

Lab Interactions Some quinolones may produce a false-positive urine screening result for opiates using commercially-available immunoassay kits. This has been demonstrated most consistently for levofloxacin and ofloxacin, but other quinolones have shown cross-reactivity in certain assay kits. Confirmation of positive opiate screens by more specific methods should be considered.

Adverse Reactions 1% to 10%:

Central nervous system: Neurologic events (children 2%, includes dizziness, insomnia, nervousness, somnolence); fever (children 2%); headache (I.V. administration); restlessness (I.V. administration)

Dermatologic: Rash (children 2%, adults 1%)

Gastrointestinal: Nausea (3%); diarrhea (children 5%, adults 2%); vomiting (children 5%, adults 1%); abdominal pain (children 3%, adults <1%); dyspepsia (children 3%)

Hepatic: ALT increased, AST increased (adults 1%)

Local: Injection site reactions (I.V. administration)

Respiratory: Rhinitis (children 3%)

Pharmacodynamics/Kinetics

Absorption Oral: Immediate release tablet: Rapid (~50% to 85%)

Time to Peak Oral:

Immediate release tablet: 0.5-2 hours

Extended release tablet: Cipro® XR: 1-2.5 hours; Proquin® XR: 3.5-8.7 hours

Protein Binding 20% to 40%

Half-Life Elimination Children: 2.5 hours; Adults: Normal renal function: 3-5 hours

Metabolism Partially hepatic; forms 4 metabolites (limited activity)

Excretion Urine (30% to 50% as unchanged drug); feces (15% to 43%)

Available Dosage Forms

Infusion, premixed in D_5W: 200 mg (100 mL); 400 mg (200 mL)

Cipro® I.V.: 200 mg (100 mL); 400 mg (200 mL)

Infusion, premixed in D_5W [preservative free]: 200 mg (100 mL); 400 mg (200 mL)

Injection, solution: 10 mg/mL (20 mL, 40 mL, 120 mL)

Injection, solution [preservative free]: 10 mg/mL (20 mL)

Microcapsules for suspension, oral:

Cipro®: 250 mg/5 mL (100 mL); 500 mg/5 mL (100 mL)

Tablet, oral: 100 mg, 250 mg, 500 mg, 750 mg

Cipro®: 250 mg, 500 mg

Tablet, extended release, oral: 500 mg, 1000 mg

Cipro® XR: 500 mg, 1000 mg

Proquin® XR: 500 mg

Dosing

Adult Note: Extended release tablets and immediate release formulations are not interchangeable. Unless otherwise specified, oral dosing reflects the use of immediate release formulations.

Anthrax:

Inhalational (postexposure prophylaxis):

Oral: 500 mg every 12 hours for 60 days

I.V.: 400 mg every 12 hours for 60 days

Cutaneous (treatment, CDC guidelines): Oral: Immediate release formulation: 500 mg every 12 hours for 60 days. **Note:** In the presence of systemic involvement, extensive edema, lesions on head/neck, refer to I.V. dosing for treatment of inhalational/gastrointestinal/oropharyngeal anthrax.

Inhalational/gastrointestinal/oropharyngeal (treatment, CDC guidelines): I.V.: 400 mg every 12 hours. **Note:** Initial treatment should include two or more agents predicted to be effective (per CDC recommendations). Continue combined therapy for 60 days.

Bone/joint infections:

Oral: 500-750 mg twice daily for 4-6 weeks

I.V.:

Mild/moderate: 400 mg every 12 hours for 4-6 weeks

Severe/complicated: 400 mg every 8 hours for 4-6 weeks

Chancroid (unlabeled use): Oral: 500 mg twice daily for 3 days (CDC, 2010)

Endocarditis due to HACEK organisms (AHA guidelines, unlabeled use): Note: Not first-line option; use only if intolerant of beta-lactam therapy:

Oral: 500 mg every 12 hours for 4 weeks

I.V.: 400 mg every 12 hours for 4 weeks

Febrile neutropenia: I.V.: 400 mg every 8 hours for 7-14 days (combination therapy generally recommended)

Gonococcal infections:

Urethral/cervical gonococcal infections: Oral: 250-500 mg as a single dose (CDC recommends concomitant doxycycline or azithromycin due to possible coinfection with *Chlamydia*; **Note:** As of April 2007, the CDC no longer recommends the use of fluoroquinolones for the treatment of uncomplicated gonococcal disease.

Disseminated gonococcal infection (CDC guidelines): Oral: 500 mg twice daily to complete 7 days of therapy (initial treatment with ceftriaxone 1 g I.M./I.V. daily for 24-48 hours after improvement begins); **Note:** As of April 2007, the CDC no longer recommends the use of fluoroquinolones for the treatment of more serious gonococcal disease, unless no other options exist and susceptibility can be confirmed via culture.

Granuloma inguinale (donovanosis) (unlabeled use): Oral: 750 mg twice daily for at least 3 weeks (and until lesions have healed) (CDC, 2010)

Infectious diarrhea: Oral:

Salmonella: 500 mg twice daily for 5-7 days

Shigella: 500 mg twice daily for 3 days

Traveler's diarrhea: Mild: 750 mg for one dose; Severe: 500 mg twice daily for 3 days

Vibrio cholerae: 1 g for one dose

Intra-abdominal, complicated, community-acquired (in combination with metronidazole): Note: Avoid using in settings where *E. coli* susceptibility to fluoroquinolones is <90%:

Oral: 500 mg every 12 hours for 7-14 days

I.V.: 400 mg every 12 hours for 7-14 days; **Note:** 2010 IDSA guidelines recommend treatment duration of 4-7 days (provided source controlled)

Lower respiratory tract, skin/skin structure infections:

Oral: 500-750 mg twice daily for 7-14 days

I.V.:

Mild/moderate: 400 mg every 12 hours for 7-14 days

Severe/complicated: 400 mg every 8 hours for 7-14 days

Nosocomial pneumonia: I.V.: 400 mg every 8 hours for 10-14 days

Prostatitis (chronic, bacterial): Oral: 500 mg every 12 hours for 28 days

Sinusitis (acute): Oral: 500 mg every 12 hours for 10 days

Typhoid fever: Oral: 500 mg every 12 hours for 10 days

Urinary tract infection:

Acute uncomplicated, cystitis:

Oral:

Immediate release formulation: 250 mg every 12 hours for 3 days

Extended release formulation (Cipro® XR, Proquin® XR): 500 mg every 24 hours for 3 days

I.V.: 200 mg every 12 hours for 7-14 days

Complicated (including pyelonephritis):

Oral:

Immediate release formulation: 500 mg every 12 hours for 7-14 days

Extended release formulation (Cipro® XR): 1000 mg every 24 hours for 7-14 days

I.V.: 400 mg every 12 hours for 7-14 days

Geriatric Refer to adult dosing. Adjust dose carefully based on renal function.

Pediatric See Warnings/Precautions. **Note:** Extended release tablets and immediate release formulations are not interchangeable. Unless otherwise specified, oral dosing reflects the use of immediate release formulations.

Anthrax:

Inhalational (postexposure prophylaxis):

Oral: 15 mg/kg/dose every 12 hours for 60 days; maximum: 500 mg/dose

I.V.: 10 mg/kg/dose every 12 hours for 60 days; do **not** exceed 400 mg/dose (800 mg/day)

Cutaneous (treatment, CDC guidelines): Oral: 10-15 mg/kg every 12 hours for 60 days (maximum: 1 g/day); amoxicillin 80 mg/kg/day divided every 8 hours is an option for completion of treatment after clinical improvement. **Note:** In the presence of systemic involvement, extensive edema, lesions on head/neck, refer to I.V. dosing for treatment of inhalational/gastrointestinal/oropharyngeal anthrax.

Inhalational/gastrointestinal/oropharyngeal (treatment, CDC guidelines): I.V.: Initial: 10-15 mg/kg every 12 hours for 60 days (maximum: 500 mg/dose); switch to oral therapy when clinically appropriate; refer to adult dosing for notes on combined therapy and duration

Cystic fibrosis (unlabeled use): Children 5-17 years:
Oral: 40 mg/kg/day divided every 12 hours administered following 1 week of I.V. therapy has been reported in a clinical trial; total duration of therapy: 10-21 days
I.V.: 30 mg/kg/day divided every 8 hours for 1 week, followed by oral therapy, has been reported in a clinical trial
Urinary tract infection (complicated) or pyelonephritis: Children 1-17 years:
Oral: 20-30 mg/kg/day in 2 divided doses (every 12 hours) for 10-21 days; maximum: 1.5 g/day
I.V.: 6-10 mg/kg every 8 hours for 10-21 days (maximum: 400 mg/dose)

Renal Impairment Adults:
Cl_{cr} 30-50 mL/minute: Oral: Administer 250-500 mg every 12 hours.
Cl_{cr} <30 mL/minute: Acute uncomplicated pyelonephritis or complicated UTI: Oral: Extended release formulation: 500 mg every 24 hours
Cl_{cr} 5-29 mL/minute:
Oral: Administer 250-500 mg every 18 hours.
I.V.: Administer 200-400 mg every 18-24 hours.
Dialysis: Only small amounts of ciprofloxacin are removed by hemo- or peritoneal dialysis (<10%); usual dose: Oral: 250-500 mg every 24 hours following dialysis.
Continuous renal replacement therapy (CRRT): I.V.:
CVVH: 200 mg every 12 hours
CVVHD or CVVHDF: 200-400 mg every 12 hours

Administration

Oral May administer with food to minimize GI upset; avoid antacid use; maintain proper hydration and urine output. Administer immediate release ciprofloxacin and Cipro® XR at least 2 hours before or 6 hours after, and Proquin® XR at least 4 hours before or 6 hours after antacids or other products containing calcium, iron, or zinc (including dairy products or calcium-fortified juices). Separate oral administration from drugs which may impair absorption (see Drug Interactions).
Oral suspension: Should not be administered through feeding tubes (suspension is oil-based and adheres to the feeding tube). Patients should avoid chewing on the microcapsules.
Nasogastric/orogastric tube: Crush immediate-release tablet and mix with water. Flush feeding tube before and after administration. Hold tube feedings at least 1 hour before and 2 hours after administration.
Tablet, extended release: Do not crush, split, or chew. May be administered with meals containing dairy products (calcium content <800 mg), but not with dairy products alone. Proquin® XR should be administered with a main meal of the day; evening meal is preferred.

I.V. Administer by slow I.V. infusion over 60 minutes into a large vein.

Stability

Reconstitution Injection, vial: May be diluted with NS, D_5W, SWFI, $D_{10}W$, $D_5{}^1/_4NS$, $D_5{}^1/_2NS$, LR.

Storage
Injection:
Premixed infusion: Store between 5°C to 25°C (41°F to 77°F); avoid freezing. Protect from light.
Vial: Store between 5°C to 30°C (41°F to 86°F); avoid freezing. Protect from light. Diluted solutions of 0.5-2 mg/mL are stable for up to 14 days refrigerated or at room temperature.
Microcapsules for oral suspension: Prior to reconstitution, store below 25°C (77°F). Protect from freezing. Following reconstitution, store below 30°C (86°F) for up to 14 days. Protect from freezing.
Tablet:
Immediate release: Store below 30°C (86°F).
Extended release: Store at room temperature of 15°C to 30°C (59°F to 86°F).

Monitoring and Teaching Issues

Laboratory Monitoring CBC, renal and hepatic function during prolonged therapy; culture and sensitivity specimen should be taken prior to initiating therapy

Physical Assessment Assess results of culture and sensitivity tests prior to beginning therapy. Use caution in patients with known or suspected CNS disorder, current or potential for QT prolongation, renal or hepatic impairment, or diabetes. I.V.: See Administration specifics. Monitor for hypersensitivity reactions (severe reactions, including anaphylaxis, have occurred with quinolone therapy), *C. difficile*-associated colitis (can occur post-treatment), and changes in CNS.

Patient Education Infusion: Report immediately any redness, swelling, or pain at infusion site; any swelling of mouth, lips, tongue, or throat; chest pain or tightness; respiratory difficulty; back pain; sudden itching; or skin rash. Oral: Take exactly according to specific instructions (eg, timing with meals, dairy products, antacids or products containing calcium, iron or zinc differs with each formulation). Do not crush, split, or chew extended release tablets or chew on microcapsules in oral suspension. Maintain adequate hydration, unless instructed to restrict fluid intake. You may experience nausea, vomiting, anorexia, or increased sensitivity to sunlight. If tendon inflammation or pain occurs or if you experience signs of an allergic reaction (eg, itching, skin rash, respiratory difficulty, facial edema or difficulty swallowing, loss of consciousness, tingling, chest pain, palpitations), discontinue use and contact prescriber immediately. Report persistent GI disturbances, CNS changes (eg, excessive sleepiness, agitation, tremors), vision changes, respiratory difficulty, signs of opportunistic infection (eg, sore throat, chills, fever, burning, itching on urination, vaginal discharge, white plaques in mouth), persistent diarrhea, or worsening of condition.

Dietary Considerations Food: Drug may cause GI upset; take without regard to meals (manufacturer prefers that immediate release tablet is taken 2 hours after meals). Extended release tablet may be taken with meals that contain dairy products (calcium content <800 mg), but not with dairy products alone.

Dairy products, calcium-fortified juices, oral multivitamins, and mineral supplements: Absorption of ciprofloxacin is decreased by divalent and trivalent cations. The manufacturer states that the usual dietary intake of calcium (including meals which include dairy products) has not been shown to interfere with ciprofloxacin absorption. Immediate release ciprofloxacin and Cipro® XR may be taken 2 hours before or 6 hours after, and Proquin® XR may be taken 4 hours before or 6 hours after, any of these products.

Caffeine: Patients consuming regular large quantities of caffeinated beverages may need to restrict caffeine intake if excessive cardiac or CNS stimulation occurs.

Geriatric Considerations See Warnings/Precautions regarding tendon rupture in patients >60 years of age. Ciprofloxacin should not be used as first-line therapy unless the culture and sensitivity findings show resistance to usual therapy. The interactions with caffeine and theophylline can result in serious toxicity in the elderly. Adjust dose for renal function.

Breast-Feeding Considerations Ciprofloxacin is excreted in breast milk. Breast-feeding is not recommended by the manufacturer. Due to the low concentrations in human milk, minimal toxicity would be expected in the nursing infant and infant serum levels were undetectable in one report. Nondose-related effects could include modification of bowel flora. There has been a single case report of perforated pseudomembranous colitis in a breast-feeding infant whose mother was taking ciprofloxacin.

Pregnancy Considerations Adverse events have been observed in some animal studies; therefore, the manufacturer classifies ciprofloxacin as pregnancy category C. Ciprofloxacin crosses the placenta and produces measurable concentrations in the amniotic fluid and cord serum. An increased risk of teratogenic effects has not been observed in animals or humans following ciprofloxacin use during pregnancy; however, because of concerns of cartilage damage in immature animals, ciprofloxacin should only be used during pregnancy if a safer option is not available. Ciprofloxacin is recommended for prophylaxis and treatment of pregnant women exposed to anthrax. Serum concentrations of ciprofloxacin may be lower during pregnancy than in nonpregnant patients.

Additional Information Although the systemic use of ciprofloxacin is only FDA-approved in children for the treatment of complicated UTI and postexposure treatment of inhalation anthrax, use of the fluoroquinolones in pediatric patients is increasing. Current recommendations by the American Academy of Pediatrics note that the systemic use of these agents in children should be restricted to infections caused by multidrug resistant pathogens with no safe or effective alternative, and when parenteral therapy is not feasible or other oral agents are not available.

Related Information

Antimicrobial Drugs of Choice *on page 2008*

Community-Acquired Pneumonia in Adults *on page 2021*

Compatibility of Drugs *on page 1994*

I.V. to Oral Conversion *on page 1956*

Prophylaxis for Patients Exposed to Common Communicable Diseases *on page 2073*

Ciprofloxacin (Ophthalmic) (sip roe FLOKS a sin)

U.S. Brand Names Ciloxan®

Index Terms Ciprofloxacin Hydrochloride

Generic Availability (U.S.) Yes: Excludes ointment

Pharmacologic Category Antibiotic, Ophthalmic; Antibiotic, Quinolone

Medication Safety Issues

Sound-alike/look-alike issues:

Ciprofloxacin may be confused with cephalexin

Ciloxan® may be confused with cinoxacin, Cytoxan

Pregnancy Risk Factor C

Lactation Use caution (AAP rates "compatible"; AAP 2001 update pending)

Use Treatment of superficial ocular infections (corneal ulcers, conjunctivitis) due to susceptible strains

Available Dosage Forms

Ointment, ophthalmic:

Ciloxan®: 3.33 mg/g (3.5 g)

Solution, ophthalmic: 3.5 mg/mL (2.5 mL, 5 mL, 10 mL)

Ciloxan®: 3.5 mg/mL (5 mL)

Dosing

Adult & Geriatric

Bacterial conjunctivitis:

Ophthalmic solution: Instill 1-2 drops in eye(s) every 2 hours while awake for 2 days and 1-2 drops every 4 hours while awake for the next 5 days

Ophthalmic ointment: Apply a 1/2" ribbon into the conjunctival sac 3 times/day for the first 2 days, followed by a 1/2" ribbon applied twice daily for the next 5 days

Corneal ulcer: *Ophthalmic solution:* Instill 2 drops into affected eye every 15 minutes for the first 6 hours, then 2 drops into the affected eye every 30 minutes for the remainder of the first day. On day 2, instill 2 drops into the affected eye hourly. On days 3-14, instill 2 drops into affected eye every 4 hours. Treatment may continue after day 14 if re-epithelialization has not occurred.

Pediatric

Bacterial conjunctivitis:

Ophthalmic solution: Children >1 year: Refer to adult dosing.

Ophthalmic ointment: Children >2 years: Refer to adult dosing.

Corneal ulcer: *Ophthalmic solution:* Children >1 year: Refer to adult dosing.

Administration

Other For topical ophthalmic use only; avoid touching tip of applicator to eye or other surfaces.

Monitoring and Teaching Issues

Patient Education Wash hands prior to instilling eye medication. Do not touch dropper to eye or any other surface. Do not wear contact lenses while using this medication (check with prescriber before using again). Tilt head back, look upward, and pull lower eyelid down to make a pouch. Drop prescribed number of drops directly into eye. Close eye, place one finger at corner of eye near nose, and apply gentle pressure. Do not blink or rub eye. If also using ointment, use drops before ointment. May cause temporary stinging or burning. Report persistent eye discomfort, itching, redness, unusual tearing, feeling as if something is in your eye, blurred vision, eye pain, worsening vision, a bad taste in your mouth, sensitivity to light, skin rash, difficulty breathing, or worsening of symptoms.

Ciprofloxacin (Otic) (sip roe FLOKS a sin)

U.S. Brand Names Cetraxal®

Index Terms Ciprofloxacin Hydrochloride

Generic Availability (U.S.) No

Pharmacologic Category Antibiotic, Otic; Antibiotic, Quinolone

Medication Safety Issues

Sound-alike/look-alike issues:

Cetraxal® may be confused with cefTRIAXone

Ciprofloxacin may be confused with cephalexin

Pregnancy Risk Factor C

Lactation Not recommended (AAP rates "compatible"; AAP 2001 update pending)

Use Treatment of acute otitis externa due to susceptible strains of *Pseudomonas aeruginosa* or *Staphylococcus aureus*

Available Dosage Forms

Solution, otic [preservative free]:

Cetraxal®: 0.5 mg/0.25 mL (14s)

Dosing

Adult & Geriatric Acute otitis externa: Otic solution: Instill 0.25 mL (contents of 1 single-dose container) into affected ear twice daily for 7 days

Pediatric Acute otitis externa: Otic solution: Children ≥1 year: Refer to adult dosing.

Administration

Other For otic use only. Prior to use, warm solution by holding container in hands for at least 1 minute. Patient should lie down with affected ear upward and medication instilled. Patients should remain in the position for at least 1 minute to allow penetration of solution.

Monitoring and Teaching Issues

Patient Education Store containers in foil pouch until immediately prior to use. Wash hands prior to instilling medication. Warm container by holding in hands for at least 1 minute before instilling (cold solution may cause dizziness). Lie with affected ear upward and then instill solution. Remain in this position for 1 minute. Repeat for opposite ear if necessary. Report increased pain, headache, rash, or if condition does not improve after one week.

Ciprofloxacin and Dexamethasone (sip roe FLOKS a sin & deks a METH a sone)

U.S. Brand Names Ciprodex®

Index Terms Ciprofloxacin Hydrochloride and Dexamethasone; Dexamethasone and Ciprofloxacin

Generic Availability (U.S.) No

Pharmacologic Category Antibiotic, Otic; Antibiotic/Corticosteroid, Otic; Corticosteroid, Otic

Pregnancy Risk Factor C

Lactation Excretion in breast milk unknown/not recommended

Use Treatment of acute otitis media in pediatric patients with tympanostomy tubes or acute otitis externa in children and adults

Available Dosage Forms

Suspension, otic:

Ciprodex®: Ciprofloxacin 0.3% and dexamethasone 0.1% (7.5 mL)

Dosing

Adult & Geriatric Acute otitis externa: Otic: Instill 4 drops into affected ear(s) twice daily for 7 days

Pediatric Acute otitis media in patients with tympanostomy tubes or acute otitis externa: Otic: Instill 4 drops into affected ear(s) twice daily for 7 days

Administration

Other Otic: Prior to instillation, bottle should be warmed in hands for 1-2 minutes. Shake suspension well immediately before using. Patient should lie with affected ear upward and remain in this position for 60 seconds following application. Drops should be instilled directly into tympanostomy tube (if present) and tragus should be pumped 5 times to facilitate penetration into the middle ear.

Monitoring and Teaching Issues

Physical Assessment See individual agents.

Patient Education See individual agents.

Related Information

Ciprofloxacin (Otic) *on page 380*

Ciprofloxacin and Hydrocortisone (sip roe FLOKS a sin & hye droe KOR ti sone)

U.S. Brand Names Cipro® HC

Index Terms Ciprofloxacin Hydrochloride and Hydrocortisone; Hydrocortisone and Ciprofloxacin

Generic Availability (U.S.) No

Pharmacologic Category Antibiotic/Corticosteroid, Otic

Pregnancy Risk Factor C

Use Treatment of acute otitis externa, sometimes known as "swimmer's ear"

Available Dosage Forms

Suspension, otic:

Cipro® HC: Ciprofloxacin 0.2% and hydrocortisone 1% (10 mL)

Dosing

Adult & Geriatric Otitis externa: Otic: The recommended dosage for all patients is three drops of the suspension in the affected ear twice daily for 7 days; twice-daily dosing schedule is more convenient for patients than that of existing treatments with hydrocortisone, which are typically administered 3 or 4 times a day; a twice-daily dosage schedule may be especially helpful for parents and caregivers of young children

Pediatric Children ≥1 year: Refer to adult dosing.

Monitoring and Teaching Issues

Physical Assessment See individual agents.

Patient Education See individual agents.

Related Information

Ciprofloxacin (Otic) *on page 380*

- **Ciprofloxacin Hydrochloride** *see* Ciprofloxacin (Ophthalmic) *on page 379*
- **Ciprofloxacin Hydrochloride** *see* Ciprofloxacin (Otic) *on page 380*
- **Ciprofloxacin Hydrochloride** *see* Ciprofloxacin (Systemic) *on page 375*
- **Ciprofloxacin Hydrochloride and Dexamethasone** *see* Ciprofloxacin and Dexamethasone *on page 380*
- **Ciprofloxacin Hydrochloride and Hydrocortisone** *see* Ciprofloxacin and Hydrocortisone *on page 381*
- **Cipro® HC** *see* Ciprofloxacin and Hydrocortisone *on page 381*
- **Cipro® I.V.** *see* Ciprofloxacin (Systemic) *on page 375*
- **Cipro® XR** *see* Ciprofloxacin (Systemic) *on page 375*

Cisapride (SIS a pride)

U.S. Brand Names Propulsid®

Generic Availability (U.S.) No

Pharmacologic Category Gastrointestinal Agent, Prokinetic

Medication Safety Issues

Sound-alike/look-alike issues:

Propulsid® may be confused with propranolol

Medication Guide Available Yes

Prescribing and Access Restrictions In U.S., available via limited-access protocol only. Call 877-795-4247 for more information.

Pregnancy Risk Factor C

Lactation Enters breast milk/use caution (AAP rates "compatible"; AAP 2001 update pending)

Use Treatment of nocturnal symptoms of gastroesophageal reflux disease (GERD); has demonstrated effectiveness for gastroparesis, refractory constipation, and nonulcer dyspepsia

Dosing

Adult & Geriatric GERD or gastrointestinal dysmotility: Oral: Initial: 5-10 mg 4 times/day at least 15 minutes before meals and at bedtime; in some patients the dosage will need to be increased to 20 mg to obtain a satisfactory result.

Pediatric Gastrointestinal dysmotility: Oral: Children: 0.15-0.3 mg/kg/dose 3-4 times/day; maximum: 10 mg/dose

Hepatic Impairment Initiate at 50% usual dose.

Monitoring and Teaching Issues

Laboratory Monitoring A 12-lead ECG should be performed prior to administration of cisapride. Treatment with cisapride should not be initiated if the QT_c value exceeds 450 milliseconds. Serum electrolytes (potassium, calcium, and magnesium) and creatinine should be assessed prior to administration of cisapride and whenever conditions develop that may affect electrolyte balance or renal function.

Physical Assessment Evaluate cardiac status thoroughly prior to therapy (12-lead ECG). Assess ECG and electrolyte balance. Monitor for tachycardia, fatigue, diarrhea, and other abdominal symptoms.

Patient Education Take before meals. Avoid alcohol and grapefruit juice. May cause increased sedation, headache, and anxiety. Immediately report rapid heartbeat, palpitations, chest pain, or tightness. Report severe abdominal pain, prolonged diarrhea, weight loss, and extreme fatigue.

Cisatracurium (sis a tra KYOO ree um)

U.S. Brand Names Nimbex®

Index Terms Cisatracurium Besylate

Generic Availability (U.S.) No

Pharmacologic Category Neuromuscular Blocker Agent, Nondepolarizing

Medication Safety Issues

Sound-alike/look-alike issues:

Nimbex® may be confused with Revex®

High alert medication: The Institute for Safe Medication Practices (ISMP) includes this medication among its list of drugs which have a heightened risk of causing significant patient harm when used in error.

United States Pharmacopeia (USP) 2006: The Interdisciplinary Safe Medication Use Expert Committee of the USP has recommended the following:

- Hospitals, clinics, and other practice sites should institute special safeguards in the storage, labeling, and use of these agents and should include these safeguards in staff orientation and competency training.
- Healthcare professionals should be on high alert (especially vigilant) whenever a neuromuscular-blocking agent (NMBA) is stocked, ordered, prepared, or administered.

Pregnancy Risk Factor B

Lactation Excretion in breast milk unknown/use caution

Use Adjunct to general anesthesia to facilitate endotracheal intubation and to relax skeletal muscles during surgery; to facilitate mechanical ventilation in ICU patients; does not relieve pain or produce sedation

Mechanism of Action/Effect Blocks neural transmission at the myoneural junction by binding with cholinergic receptor sites

Contraindications Hypersensitivity to cisatracurium besylate or any component of the formulation

Warnings/Precautions Maintenance of an adequate airway and respiratory support is critical; certain clinical conditions may result in potentiation or antagonism of neuromuscular blockade:

Potentiation: Electrolyte abnormalities, severe hyponatremia, severe hypocalcemia, severe hypokalemia, hypermagnesemia, neuromuscular diseases, acidosis, acute intermittent porphyria, renal failure, hepatic failure

Antagonism: Alkalosis, hypercalcemia, demyelinating lesions, peripheral neuropathies, diabetes mellitus

Increased sensitivity in patients with myasthenia gravis, Eaton-Lambert syndrome; resistance in burn patients (>30% of body) for period of 5-70 days postinjury; resistance in patients with muscle trauma, denervation, immobilization, infection. Cross-sensitivity with other neuromuscular-blocking agents may occur; use extreme caution in patients with previous anaphylactic reactions. Bradycardia may be more common with cisatracurium than with other neuromuscular blocking agents since it has no clinically significant effects on heart rate to counteract the bradycardia produced by anesthetics. Use caution in the elderly. Should be administered by adequately trained individuals familiar with its use. Some dosage forms may contain benzyl alcohol which has been associated with "gasping syndrome" in neonates.

Drug Interactions

Avoid Concomitant Use

Avoid concomitant use of Cisatracurium with any of the following: QuiNINE

Decreased Effect

The levels/effects of Cisatracurium may be decreased by: Acetylcholinesterase Inhibitors; Loop Diuretics

Increased Effect/Toxicity

Cisatracurium may increase the levels/effects of: Cardiac Glycosides; Corticosteroids (Systemic); OnabotulinumtoxinA; RimabotulinumtoxinB

The levels/effects of Cisatracurium may be increased by: AbobotulinumtoxinA; Aminoglycosides; Calcium Channel Blockers; Capreomycin; Colistimethate; Inhalational Anesthetics; Ketorolac; Ketorolac (Systemic); Lincosamide Antibiotics; Lithium; Loop Diuretics; Magnesium Salts; Polymyxin B; Procainamide; QuiNIDine; QuiNINE; Spironolactone; Tetracycline Derivatives; Vancomycin

Pharmacodynamics/Kinetics

Onset of Action I.V.: 2-3 minutes; Peak effect: 3-5 minutes

Duration of Action Recovery begins in 20-35 minutes when anesthesia is balanced; recovery is attained in 90% of patients in 25-93 minutes

Half-Life Elimination 22-29 minutes

Metabolism Undergoes rapid nonenzymatic degradation in the bloodstream (Hofmann elimination) to laudanosine and inactive metabolites; laudanosine may cause CNS stimulation (association not established in humans) and has less accumulation with prolonged use than atracurium due to lower requirements for clinical effect

Available Dosage Forms

Injection, solution:

Nimbex®: 2 mg/mL (5 mL, 10 mL); 10 mg/mL (20 mL)

Dosing

Adult & Geriatric Neuromuscular blockade: I.V. (not to be used I.M.):

Operating room administration:

Intubating doses: 0.15-0.2 mg/kg as components of propofol/nitrous oxide/oxygen induction-intubation technique. (**Note:** May produce generally good or excellent conditions for tracheal intubation in 1.5-2 minutes with clinically effective duration of action during propofol anesthesia of 55-61 minutes.) Initial dose after succinylcholine for intubation: 0.1 mg/kg; maintenance dose: 0.03 mg/kg 40-60 minutes after initial dose, then at ~20-minute intervals based on clinical criteria.

Continuous infusion: After an initial bolus, a diluted solution can be given by continuous infusion for maintenance of neuromuscular blockade during extended surgery; adjust the rate of administration according to the patient's response as determined by peripheral nerve stimulation. An initial infusion rate of 3 mcg/kg/minute may be required to rapidly counteract the spontaneous recovery of neuromuscular function; thereafter, a rate of 1-2 mcg/kg/minute should be adequate to maintain continuous neuromuscular block in the 89% to 99% range in most pediatric and adult patients. Consider reduction of the infusion rate by 30% to 40% when administering during stable isoflurane, enflurane, sevoflurane, or desflurane anesthesia. Spontaneous recovery from neuromuscular blockade following discontinuation of infusion of cisatracurium may be expected to proceed at a rate comparable to that following single bolus administration.

Intensive care unit administration: Follow the principles for infusion in the operating room. At initial signs of recovery from bolus dose, begin the infusion at a dose of 3 mcg/kg/minute and adjust rates accordingly; dosage ranges of 0.5-10 mcg/kg/minute have been reported. If patient is allowed to recover from neuromuscular blockade, readministration of a bolus dose may be necessary to quickly re-establish neuromuscular block prior to reinstituting the infusion. See table.

Cisatracurium Besylate Infusion Chart

Drug Delivery Rate (mcg/kg/min)	Infusion Rate (mL/kg/min) 0.1 mg/mL (10 mg/100 mL)	Infusion Rate (mL/kg/min) 0.4 mg/mL (40 mg/100 mL)
1	0.01	0.0025
1.5	0.015	0.00375
2	0.02	0.005
3	0.03	0.0075
5	0.05	0.0125

Pediatric Neuromuscular blockade: I.V. (not to be used I.M.):

Operating room administration:

Infants 1-23 months: *Intubating dose:* 0.15 mg/kg over 5-10 seconds during either halothane (not available in U.S.) or opioid anesthesia

Children 2-12 years: *Intubating doses:* 0.1-0.15 mg/kg over 5-15 seconds during either halothane (not available in U.S.) or opioid anesthesia. (**Note:** When given during stable opioid/nitrous oxide/oxygen anesthesia, 0.1 mg/kg produces maximum neuromuscular block in an average of 2.8 minutes and clinically effective block for 28 minutes.)

Children ≥2 years: *Continuous infusion:* Refer to adult dosing.

Intensive care unit administration: Refer to adult dosing.

Renal Impairment Because slower times to onset of complete neuromuscular block were observed in renal dysfunction patients, extending the interval between the administration of cisatracurium and intubation attempt may be required to achieve adequate intubation conditions.

Administration

I.M. Not for I.M. injection, too much tissue irritation.

I.V. Administer I.V. only. The use of a peripheral nerve stimulator will permit the most advantageous use of cisatracurium, minimize the possibility of overdosage or underdosage and assist in the evaluation of recovery.

Give undiluted as a bolus injection. Continuous administration requires the use of an infusion pump.

Stability

Storage Refrigerate intact vials at 2°C to 8°C (36°F to 46°F). Use vials within 21 days upon removal from the refrigerator to room temperature (25°C to 77°F). Per the manufacturer, dilutions of 0.1-0.2 mg/mL in 0.9% sodium chloride (NS) or dextrose 5% in water (D_5W) are stable for up to 24 hours at room temperature or under refrigeration and in D_5LR for up to 24 hours in the refrigerator. *Additional stability data:* Dilutions of 0.1, 2, and 5 mg/mL in D_5W or

NS are stable in the refrigerator for up to 30 days; at room temperature (23°C), dilutions of 0.1 and 2 mg/mL began exhibiting substantial drug loss between 7-14 days; dilutions of 5 mg/mL in D_5W or NS are stable for up to 30 days at room temperature (23°C) (Xu, 1998). Usual concentration: 0.1-0.4 mg/mL.

Monitoring and Teaching Issues

Physical Assessment Dosage and rate of administration should be individualized and titrated to the desired effect, according to relevant clinical factors, premedication, concomitant medications, age, and general condition of the patient. Ventilatory support must be instituted and maintained until adequate respiratory muscle function and/or airway protection are assured. This drug is not an anesthetic or analgesic; pain must be treated with other agents. Continuous monitoring of vital signs, cardiac status, respiratory status, and degree of neuromuscular block (objective assessment with peripheral external nerve stimulator) is mandatory during infusion and until full muscle tone has returned. Safety precautions must be maintained until full muscle tone has returned. **Note:** It may take longer for return of muscle tone in obese or elderly patients or patients with renal or hepatic disease, myasthenia gravis, myopathy, other neuromuscular disease, dehydration, electrolyte imbalance, or severe acid/base imbalance.

Long-term use: Monitor level of neuromuscular blockade, skeletal muscle movement, and respiratory effort. Reposition patient and provide appropriate skin care, mouth care, and care of patient's eyes every 2-3 hours while sedated. Provide appropriate emotional and sensory support (auditory and environmental).

Patient Education Patient will usually be unconscious prior to administration. Reassurance of constant monitoring and emotional support to reduce fear and anxiety should precede and follow administration. Following return of muscle tone, do not attempt to change position or rise from bed without assistance.

Additional Information Cisatracurium is classified as an intermediate-duration neuromuscular-blocking agent. It does not appear to have a cumulative effect on the duration of blockade. Neuromuscular-blocking potency is 3 times that of atracurium; maximum block is up to 2 minutes longer than for equipotent doses of atracurium.

Related Information

Compatibility of Drugs *on page* *1994*

◆ **Cisatracurium Besylate** *see* Cisatracurium *on page* *382*

CISplatin (SIS pla tin)

Index Terms CDDP; Platinol; Platinol-AQ

Generic Availability (U.S.) Yes

Pharmacologic Category Antineoplastic Agent, Alkylating Agent; Antineoplastic Agent, Platinum Analog

Medication Safety Issues

Sound-alike/look-alike issues:

CISplatin may be confused with CARBOplatin, oxaliplatin

High alert medication: This medication is in a class the Institute for Safe Medication Practices (ISMP) includes among its list of drugs which have a heightened risk of causing significant patient harm when used in error.

Doses >100 mg/m^2 once every 3-4 weeks are rarely used and should be verified with the prescriber.

Pregnancy Risk Factor D

Lactation Enters breast milk/not recommended

Use Treatment of advanced bladder cancer, metastatic testicular cancer, and metastatic ovarian cancer

Unlabeled/Investigational Use Treatment of head and neck cancer, breast cancer, gastric cancer, esophageal cancer, cervical cancer, prostate cancer, nonsmall cell lung cancer, small cell lung cancer; Hodgkin's and non-Hodgkin's lymphoma; neuroblastoma; sarcomas, myeloma, melanoma, mesothelioma, hepatoblastoma, and osteosarcoma

Mechanism of Action/Effect Inhibits DNA synthesis

Contraindications Hypersensitivity to cisplatin, other platinum-containing compounds, or any component of the formulation (anaphylactic-like reactions have been reported); pre-existing renal impairment; myelosuppression; hearing impairment

Warnings/Precautions Hazardous agent - use appropriate precautions for handling and disposal. **[U.S. Boxed Warning]: Doses >100 mg/m^2 once every 3-4 weeks are rarely used and should be verified with the prescriber.** Patients should receive adequate hydration, with or without diuretics, prior to and for 24 hours after cisplatin administration. Reduce dosage in renal impairment. **[U.S. Boxed Warning]: Cumulative renal toxicity may be severe.** Elderly patients may be more susceptible to nephrotoxicity and peripheral neuropathy; select dose cautiously and monitor closely. **[U.S. Boxed Warnings]: Dose-related toxicities include myelosuppression, nausea, and vomiting. Ototoxicity, especially pronounced in children, is manifested by tinnitus or loss of high frequency hearing and occasionally, deafness.** Severe and possibly irreversible neuropathies may occur with higher than recommended doses or more frequent regimen. Serum electrolytes, particularly magnesium and potassium, should be monitored and replaced as needed during and after cisplatin therapy. When administered as sequential infusions, taxane derivatives (docetaxel, paclitaxel) should be administered before platinum derivatives (carboplatin, cisplatin). **[U.S. Boxed Warnings]: Anaphylactic-like reactions have been reported; may be managed with epinephrine,**

corticosteroids, and/or antihistamines. Should be administered under the supervision of an experienced cancer chemotherapy physician.

Drug Interactions

Avoid Concomitant Use

Avoid concomitant use of CISplatin with any of the following: BCG; Natalizumab; Pimecrolimus; Roflumilast; Tacrolimus (Topical); Vaccines (Live)

Decreased Effect

CISplatin may decrease the levels/effects of: BCG; Phenytoin; Sipuleucel-T; Vaccines (Inactivated); Vaccines (Live)

The levels/effects of CISplatin may be decreased by: Echinacea

Increased Effect/Toxicity

CISplatin may increase the levels/effects of: Aminoglycosides; Leflunomide; Natalizumab; Taxane Derivatives; Topotecan; Vaccines (Live); Vinorelbine

The levels/effects of CISplatin may be increased by: Denosumab; Loop Diuretics; Pimecrolimus; Roflumilast; Tacrolimus (Topical); Trastuzumab

Nutritional/Ethanol Interactions Herb/Nutraceutical: Avoid black cohosh, dong quai in estrogen-dependent tumors.

Adverse Reactions

>10%:

Central nervous system: Neurotoxicity: Peripheral neuropathy is dose- and duration-dependent.

Gastrointestinal: Nausea and vomiting (76% to 100%)

Hematologic: Myelosuppression (25% to 30%; nadir: day 18-23; recovery: by day 39; mild with moderate doses, mild-to-moderate with high-dose therapy)

Hepatic: Liver enzymes increased

Renal: Nephrotoxicity (acute renal failure and chronic renal insufficiency)

Otic: Ototoxicity (10% to 30%; manifested as high frequency hearing loss; ototoxicity is especially pronounced in children)

1% to 10%: Local: Tissue irritation

Pharmacodynamics/Kinetics

Protein Binding >90%

Half-Life Elimination Initial: 20-30 minutes; Beta: 60 minutes; Terminal: ~24 hours; Secondary half-life: 44-73 hours

Metabolism Nonenzymatic; inactivated (in both cell and bloodstream) by sulfhydryl groups; covalently binds to glutathione and thiosulfate

Excretion Urine (>90%); feces (10%)

Available Dosage Forms

Injection, solution [preservative free]: 1 mg/mL (50 mL, 100 mL, 200 mL)

Dosing

Adult VERIFY ANY CISPLATIN DOSE EXCEEDING 100 mg/m^2 PER COURSE. Pretreatment hydration with 1-2 L of I.V. fluid is recommended. Details concerning dosing in combination regimens should also be consulted.

Advanced bladder cancer: I.V.: 50-70 mg/m^2 every 3-4 weeks

Metastatic ovarian cancer: I.V.: 75-100 mg/m^2 every 4 weeks (combination therapy) or 100 mg/m^2 every 4 weeks (as a single agent)

Metastatic testicular cancer: I.V.: 10-20 mg/m^2/day for 5 days repeated every 3 weeks (Saxman, 1998)

Head and neck cancer (unlabeled use): I.V.: 100 mg/m^2 every 3 weeks for 3 doses (as a single agent) (Bernier, 2004; Cooper, 2004)

Malignant pleural mesothelioma (unlabeled use): I.V.: 75 mg/m^2 on day 1 of each 21-day cycle (in combination with pemetrexed) (Vogelzang, 2003) **or** 100 mg/m^2 on day 1 of a 28-day cycle (in combination with gemcitabine) (Nowak, 2002) **or** 80 mg/m^2 on day 1 of a 21-day cycle (in combination with gemcitabine) (van Haarst, 2002)

Intraperitoneal: Ovarian cancer (unlabeled use): 100 mg/m^2 on day 2 of a 21-day treatment cycle (Armstrong, 2006)

Geriatric Refer to adult dosing. Select dose cautiously and monitor closely in the elderly; may be more susceptible to nephrotoxicity and peripheral neuropathy.

Pediatric VERIFY ANY CISPLATIN DOSE EXCEEDING 100 mg/m^2 PER COURSE. Pretreatment hydration is recommended. Details concerning dosing in combination regimens should also be consulted.

Hepatoblastoma (unlabeled use; combination chemotherapy): I.V.: 80 mg/m^2 continuous infusion over 24 hours on day 1 of a 21-day treatment cycle (Pritchard, 2000)

Medulloblastoma (unlabeled use; combination chemotherapy): I.V.: 75 mg/m^2 on either day 0 or day 1 of each chemotherapy cycle (Packer, 2006)

Osteosarcoma (unlabeled use; combination chemotherapy): I.V.: 60 mg/m^2/day for 2 days weeks 2, 7, 25, and 28 (neoadjuvant) or weeks 5, 10, 25, and 28 (adjuvant) (Goorin, 2003)

Bone marrow/stem cell transplant (unlabeled use): Continuous I.V. infusion: High dose: 55 mg/m^2/day for 72 hours; total dose = 165 mg/m^2

Renal Impairment Note: The manufacturer(s) recommend that repeat courses of cisplatin should not be given until serum creatinine is <1.5 mg/dL and/or BUN is <25 mg/dL. The FDA-approved labeling does not contain renal dosing adjustment guidelines. The following guidelines have been used by some clinicians:

Aronoff, 2007:

Cl_{cr} 10-50 mL/minute: Administer 75% of dose

Cl_{cr} <10 mL/minute: Administer 50% of dose

Hemodialysis: Partially cleared by hemodialysis.
Administer 50% of dose posthemodialysis
Continuous ambulatory peritoneal dialysis (CAPD): Administer 50% of dose
Continuous renal replacement therapy (CRRT): Administer 75% of dose

Kintzel, 1995:
Cl_{cr} 46-60 mL/minute: Administer 75% of dose
Cl_{cr} 31-45 mL/minute: Administer 50% of dose
Cl_{cr} <30 mL/minute: Consider use of alternative drug

Administration

I.V. Irritant. Perform pretreatment hydration (see Dosing).

I.V.: Rate of administration has varied from a 15- to 120-minute infusion, 1 mg/minute infusion, 6- to 8-hour infusion, 24-hour infusion, or per protocol.

Stability

Reconstitution The infusion solution should have a final sodium chloride concentration ≥0.2%.

Storage Store intact vials at room temperature 15°C to 25°C (59°F to 77°F). Protect from light. Do not refrigerate solution as a precipitate may form. Further dilution **stability is dependent on the chloride ion concentration** and should be mixed in solutions of NS (at least 0.3% NaCl). After initial entry into the vial, solution is stable for 28 days protected from light or for at least 7 days under fluorescent room light at room temperature.

Further dilutions in NS, D_5/0.45% NaCl or D_5/NS to a concentration of 0.05-2 mg/mL are stable for 72 hours at 4°C to 25°C. The infusion solution should have a final sodium chloride concentration ≥0.2%.

Monitoring and Teaching Issues

Laboratory Monitoring Renal function (serum creatinine, BUN, Cl_{cr}); electrolytes (particularly magnesium, calcium, potassium) before and within 48 hours after cisplatin therapy; liver function periodically, CBC with differential and platelet count, urinalysis

Physical Assessment Verify any dose exceeding 100 mg/m^2 per course. Assess other drugs patient may be taking for potential interactions (especially ototoxins or nephrotoxins). Patient should be vigorously hydrated prior to and for 24 hours following infusion. Assess auditory status prior to each treatment and regularly during therapy. Cisplatin is emetogenic; antiemetic should be administered prior to each treatment and as needed between infusions. Infusion site must be monitored closely to reduce potential for extravasation. Anaphylaxis-like reaction is possible; emergency medication should be readily available. Monitor for acute or chronic renal failure; peripheral neuropathy and ototoxicity may be irreversible. Teach patient importance of adequate hydration.

Patient Education This medication can only be administered by I.V. Report immediately any burning, pain, itching, or redness at infusion site; difficulty breathing or swallowing; swelling of mouth or throat; or chest pain or palpitations. It is important that you maintain adequate hydration, unless instructed to restrict fluid intake, and adequate nutrition. May cause severe nausea or vomiting that can be delayed for up to 48 hours after infusion and last for 1 week (consult prescriber for appropriate antiemetic medication). May cause mouth sores or loss of hair (reversible). You will be susceptible to infection. Report promptly any pain, tingling, loss of sensation, or cramping in extremities; ringing in ears or change in hearing; difficulty breathing or swallowing; fever or chills; unusual fatigue; or unusual bruising/bleeding.

Dietary Considerations Some products may contain sodium.

Pregnancy Considerations Animal studies have demonstrated teratogenicity and embryotoxicity. There are no adequate and well-controlled studies in pregnant women. Women of childbearing potential should be advised to avoid pregnancy. If used in pregnancy, or if patient becomes pregnant during treatment, the patient should be apprised of potential hazard to the fetus.

◆ **13-*cis*-Retinoic Acid** *see* Isotretinoin *on page 1030*

Citalopram (sye TAL oh pram)

U.S. Brand Names CeleXA®

Index Terms Citalopram Hydrobromide; Nitalapram

Generic Availability (U.S.) Yes

Pharmacologic Category Antidepressant, Selective Serotonin Reuptake Inhibitor

Medication Safety Issues

Sound-alike/look-alike issues:
CeleXA® may be confused with CeleBREX®, Cerebra®, Cerebyx®, Ranexa™, ZyPREXA®

Medication Guide Available Yes

Pregnancy Risk Factor C

Lactation Enters breast milk/consider risk:benefit

Use Treatment of depression

Unlabeled/Investigational Use Treatment of mild dementia-associated agitation in nonpsychotic patients; smoking cessation; ethanol abuse; obsessive-compulsive disorder (OCD) in children; diabetic neuropathy

Mechanism of Action/Effect A bicyclic phthalane derivative, citalopram selectively inhibits serotonin reuptake in the presynaptic neurons thus increasing serotonergic activity in the brain.

Contraindications Hypersensitivity to citalopram or any component of the formulation; concomitant use with MAO inhibitors or within 2 weeks of discontinuing MAO inhibitors; concomitant use with pimozide

Warnings/Precautions [U.S. Boxed Warning]: Antidepressants increase the risk of suicidal thinking and behavior in children, adolescents, and young adults (18-24 years of age) with major depressive disorder (MDD) and other psychiatric disorders; consider risk prior to prescribing. Short-term studies did not show an increased risk in patients >24 years of age and showed a decreased risk in patients ≥65 years. Closely monitor patients for clinical worsening, suicidality, or unusual changes in behavior, particularly during the initial 1-2 months of therapy or during periods of dosage adjustments (increases or decreases); the patient's family or caregiver should be instructed to closely observe the patient and communicate condition with healthcare provider. A medication guide concerning the use of antidepressants should be dispensed with each prescription. **Citalopram is not FDA approved for use in children.**

The possibility of a suicide attempt is inherent in major depression and may persist until remission occurs. Use caution in high-risk patients. Worsening depression and severe abrupt suicidality that are not part of the presenting symptoms may require discontinuation or modification of drug therapy. The patient's family or caregiver should be alerted to monitor patients for the emergence of suicidality and associated behaviors (such as agitation, irritability, hostility, impulsivity, and hypomania) and call healthcare provider.

May worsen psychosis in some patients or precipitate a shift to mania or hypomania in patients with bipolar disorder. Patients presenting with depressive symptoms should be screened for bipolar disorder. Monotherapy in patients with bipolar disorder should be avoided. **Citalopram is not FDA approved for the treatment of bipolar depression.**

Serotonin syndrome and neuroleptic malignant syndrome (NMS)-like reactions have occurred with serotonin/norepinephrine reuptake inhibitors (SNRIs) and selective serotonin reuptake inhibitors (SSRIs) when used alone, and particularly when used in combination with serotonergic agents (eg, triptans) or antidopaminergic agents (eg, antipsychotics). Concurrent use with MAO inhibitors is contraindicated. May increase the risks associated with electroconvulsive therapy. Has a low potential to impair cognitive or motor performance; caution operating hazardous machinery or driving.

Use with caution in patients with hepatic or renal dysfunction, in elderly patients, concomitant CNS depressants, and pregnancy (high doses of citalopram have been associated with teratogenicity in animals). Use caution with concomitant use of aspirin, NSAIDs, warfarin, or other drugs that affect coagulation; the risk of bleeding may be potentiated. May cause hyponatremia/SIADH (elderly at increased risk); volume depletion and diuretics may increase risk. May cause or exacerbate sexual dysfunction. Upon discontinuation of citalopram therapy, gradually taper dose. If intolerable symptoms occur following a decrease in dosage or upon discontinuation of therapy, then resuming the previous dose with a more gradual taper should be considered.

Drug Interactions

Metabolism/Transport Effects Substrate of CYP2C19 (major), 2D6 (minor), 3A4 (major); **Inhibits** CYP1A2 (weak), 2B6 (weak), 2C19 (weak), 2D6 (weak)

Avoid Concomitant Use

Avoid concomitant use of Citalopram with any of the following: Artemether; Dronedarone; Iobenguane I 123; Lumefantrine; MAO Inhibitors; Methylene Blue; Nilotinib; Pimozide; QuiNINE; Sibutramine; Tetrabenazine; Thioridazine; Toremifene; Tryptophan; Vandetanib; Ziprasidone

Decreased Effect

Citalopram may decrease the levels/effects of: Iobenguane I 123

The levels/effects of Citalopram may be decreased by: CarBAMazepine; CYP2C19 Inducers (Strong); CYP3A4 Inducers (Strong); Cyproheptadine; Deferasirox; Peginterferon Alfa-2b

Increased Effect/Toxicity

Citalopram may increase the levels/effects of: Alcohol (Ethyl); Alpha-/Beta-Blockers; Anticoagulants; Antidepressants (Serotonin Reuptake Inhibitor/Antagonist); Antiplatelet Agents; Aspirin; BusPIRone; CarBAMazepine; CloZAPine; CNS Depressants; Collagenase (Systemic); Desmopressin; Dextromethorphan; Dronedarone; Drotrecogin Alfa; Haloperidol; Ibritumomab; Lithium; Methadone; Methylene Blue; Mexiletine; NSAID (COX-2 Inhibitor); NSAID (Nonselective); Pimozide; QTc-Prolonging Agents; QuiNINE; RisperiDONE; Salicylates; Serotonin Modulators; Tetrabenazine; Thioridazine; Thrombolytic Agents; Toremifene; Tositumomab and Iodine I 131 Tositumomab; TraMADol; Tricyclic Antidepressants; Vandetanib; Vitamin K Antagonists; Ziprasidone

The levels/effects of Citalopram may be increased by: Alfuzosin; Analgesics (Opioid); Artemether; BusPIRone; Chloroquine; Cimetidine; Ciprofloxacin; Ciprofloxacin (Systemic); Conivaptan; CYP2C19 Inhibitors (Moderate); CYP2C19 Inhibitors (Strong); CYP3A4 Inhibitors (Moderate); CYP3A4 Inhibitors (Strong); Fluconazole; Gadobutrol; Glucosamine; Herbs (Anticoagulant/Antiplatelet Properties); Lumefantrine; Macrolide Antibiotics; MAO Inhibitors; Metoclopramide; Nilotinib; Omega-3-Acid Ethyl Esters; Pentosan Polysulfate Sodium; Pentoxifylline; Prostacyclin Analogues; QuiNINE; Sibutramine; TraMADol; Tryptophan

Nutritional/Ethanol Interactions

Ethanol: Avoid ethanol (may increase CNS depression).

Herb/Nutraceutical: Avoid valerian, St John's wort, SAMe, kava kava, and gotu kola (may increase CNS depression).

Adverse Reactions

>10%:

Central nervous system: Somnolence (18%; dose related), insomnia (15%; dose related)

Gastrointestinal: Nausea (21%), xerostomia (20%)

Miscellaneous: Diaphoresis (11%; dose related)

1% to 10%:

Cardiovascular: Heart rate decreased, postural hypotension, tachycardia

Central nervous system: Fatigue (5%; dose related), anorexia (4%), anxiety (4%), agitation (3%), fever (2%), yawning (2%; dose related), amnesia, apathy, concentration impaired, confusion, depression, migraine, suicide attempt

Dermatologic: Rash, pruritus

Endocrine & metabolic: Libido decreased (1% to 4%), dysmenorrhea (3%), amenorrhea, sexual dysfunction

Gastrointestinal: Diarrhea (8%), dyspepsia (5%), vomiting (4%), abdominal pain (3%), flatulence, salivation increased, taste perversion, weight gain/loss

Genitourinary: Ejaculation disorder (6%), impotence (3%; dose related), polyuria

Neuromuscular & skeletal: Tremor (8%), arthralgia (2%), myalgia (2%), paresthesia

Ocular: Abnormal accommodation

Respiratory: Rhinitis (5%), upper respiratory tract infection (5%), sinusitis (3%), cough

Pharmacodynamics/Kinetics

Onset of Action Depression: The onset of action is within a week; however, individual response varies greatly and full response may not be seen until 8-12 weeks after initiation of treatment.

Bioavailability 80%

Time to Peak Serum: 1-6 hours, average within 4 hours

Protein Binding Plasma: ~80%

Half-Life Elimination 24-48 hours (average: 35 hours); doubled with hepatic impairment

Metabolism Extensively hepatic, via CYP3A4 and 2C19 (major pathways), and 2D6 (minor pathway); forms metabolites, N-demethylcitalopram (DCT) and didemethylcitalopram (DDCT) which are at least eight times less potent than citalopram

Excretion Urine (Citalopram 10% and DCT 5%)

Note: Clearance was decreased, while AUC and half-life were significantly increased in elderly patients and in patients with hepatic impairment. Mild-to-moderate renal impairment may reduce clearance (17%) and prolong half-life of citalopram. No pharmacokinetic information is available concerning patients with severe renal impairment.

Available Dosage Forms

Solution, oral: 10 mg/5 mL (240 mL)

Tablet, oral: 10 mg, 20 mg, 40 mg

CeleXA®: 10 mg, 20 mg, 40 mg

Dosing

Adult Depression: Oral: Initial: 20 mg/day, generally with an increase to 40 mg/day; doses of more than 40 mg are not usually necessary. Should a dose increase be necessary, it should occur in 20 mg increments at intervals of no less than 1 week. Maximum dose: 60 mg/day.

Geriatric

Depression: Oral: Initial: 20 mg once daily; increase dose to 40 mg/day in nonresponsive patients

Alzheimer's dementia-related depression (unlabeled use): Oral: Initial: 5-10 mg/day; may increase at multi-week intervals to maximum of 40 mg/day

Pediatric Children and Adolescents: Obsessive-compulsive disorder (unlabeled use): Oral: 10-40 mg/day

Renal Impairment

Mild-to-moderate impairment: No dosage adjustment needed.

Severe impairment: Cl_{cr} <20 mL/minute: Use with caution.

Hepatic Impairment Oral: 20 mg once daily; increase dose to 40 mg/day in nonresponsive patients.

Administration

Oral May be administered without regard to food.

Stability

Storage Store at 25°C (77°F); excursions permitted to 15°C to 30°C (59°F to 86°F).

Monitoring and Teaching Issues

Laboratory Monitoring Liver function tests and CBC with continued therapy

Physical Assessment Assess mental status for depression, signs of clinical worsening, suicide ideation, anxiety, social functioning, mania, or panic attack. Teach patient hypotensive precautions. Taper dosage slowly when discontinuing.

Patient Education It may take up to 3 weeks to see therapeutic effects from this medication. May be taken with or without food. Avoid alcohol. You may experience sexual dysfunction (reversible). May cause dizziness, anxiety, blurred vision, nausea, or dry mouth. Report confusion or impaired concentration, suicide ideation, severe headache, palpitations, rash, insomnia or nightmares, changes in personality, muscle weakness or tremors, altered gait pattern, signs and symptoms of respiratory infection, or excessive perspiration.

Dietary Considerations May be taken without regard to food.

Geriatric Considerations In open-label and placebo-controlled studies, elderly patients with or without dementia have shown significant improvement in depressive symptoms, irritability, anxiety, behavior, and restlessness. Effects on intellectual function have not been consistent. Thus, it appears that citalopram has additional effects in stabilizing emotion. A seven- to eightfold variation in citalopram S(+) (active) and R(-) enantiomer concentrations have been reported in the elderly. The racemic citalopram concentration-to-dose ratio was 1.8 times greater in elderly patients compared to younger patients.

Clearance was decreased, while AUC and half-life were significantly increased in elderly patients and in patients with hepatic impairment. Mild-to-moderate renal impairment may reduce clearance of citalopram (17% reduction noted in trials). No pharmacokinetic information is available concerning patients with severe renal impairment. The elderly are more prone to SSRI/SNRI-induced hyponatremia.

Breast-Feeding Considerations Citalopram and its metabolites are excreted in human milk. According to the manufacturer, the decision to continue or discontinue breast-feeding during therapy should take into account the risk of exposure to the infant and the benefits of treatment to the mother. Excessive somnolence, decreased feeding, colic, irritability, restlessness, and weight loss have been reported in breast-fed infants. The long-term effects on development and behavior have not been studied; therefore, citalopram should be prescribed to a mother who is breast-feeding only when the benefits outweigh the potential risks.

Pregnancy Considerations Due to adverse effects observed in animal studies, citalopram is classified as pregnancy category C. Citalopram and its metabolites cross the human placenta. Nonteratogenic effects in the newborn following SSRI exposure late in the third trimester include respiratory distress, cyanosis, apnea, seizures, temperature instability, feeding difficulty, vomiting, hypoglycemia, hypo- or hypertonia, hyper-reflexia, jitteriness, irritability, constant crying, and tremor. An increased risk of low birth weight and lower Apgar scores have also been reported. Exposure to SSRIs after the twentieth week of gestation has been associated with persistent pulmonary hypertension of the newborn (PPHN). Adverse effects may be due to toxic effects of the SSRI or drug withdrawal without a taper. The long-term effects of *in utero* SSRI exposure on infant development and behavior are not known.

Due to pregnancy-induced physiologic changes, women who are pregnant may require increased doses of citalopram to achieve euthymia. Women treated for major depression and who are euthymic prior to pregnancy are more likely to experience a relapse when medication is discontinued as compared to pregnant women who continue taking antidepressant medications. The ACOG recommends that therapy with SSRIs or SNRIs during pregnancy be individualized; treatment of depression during pregnancy should incorporate the clinical expertise of the mental health clinician, obstetrician, primary healthcare provider, and pediatrician. If treatment during pregnancy is required, consider tapering therapy during the third trimester in order to prevent withdrawal symptoms in the infant. If this is done and the woman is considered to be at risk of relapse from her major depressive disorder, the medication can be restarted following delivery, although the dose should be readjusted to that required before pregnancy. Treatment algorithms have been developed by the ACOG and the APA for the management of depression in women prior to conception and during pregnancy (Yonkers, 2009).

Related Information

Antidepressant Agents *on page 1982*

- **Citalopram Hydrobromide** *see* Citalopram *on page 386*
- **Citric Acid and Sodium Citrate** *see* Sodium Citrate and Citric Acid *on page 1660*
- **Citrovorum Factor** *see* Leucovorin Calcium *on page 1080*
- **CL-118,532** *see* Triptorelin *on page 1824*
- **Cl-719** *see* Gemfibrozil *on page 859*
- **CL-232315** *see* Mitoxantrone *on page 1244*

Cladribine (KLA dri been)

U.S. Brand Names Leustatin®

Index Terms 2-CdA; 2-Chlorodeoxyadenosine; NSC-105014

Generic Availability (U.S.) Yes

Pharmacologic Category Antineoplastic Agent, Antimetabolite; Antineoplastic Agent, Antimetabolite (Purine Analog)

Medication Safety Issues

Sound-alike/look-alike issues:

Cladribine may be confused with clevidipine, clofarabine, fludarabine
Leustatin® may be confused with lovastatin

High alert medication: The Institute for Safe Medication Practices (ISMP) includes this medication among its list of drugs which have a heightened risk of causing significant patient harm when used in error.

Pregnancy Risk Factor D

Lactation Excretion in breast milk unknown/not recommended

Use Treatment of hairy cell leukemia

Unlabeled/Investigational Use Treatment of chronic lymphocytic leukemia (CLL), chronic myelogenous leukemia (CML), non-Hodgkin's lymphomas, progressive multiple sclerosis

Mechanism of Action/Effect A prodrug which incorporates DNA causing breakage of DNA strands and shutdown of DNA synthesis. Cladribine is cell-cycle nonspecific.

Contraindications Hypersensitivity to cladribine or any component of the formulation

Warnings/Precautions Hazardous agent - use appropriate precautions for handling and disposal. **[U.S. Boxed Warnings]: Dose-dependent, reversible myelosuppression will occur; use with caution in patients with pre-existing hematologic or immunologic abnormalities. Neurologic toxicity has been reported, usually with higher doses, but**

may occur at normal doses. Acute renal toxicity has been reported with high doses; use caution when administering with other nephrotoxic agents. Use caution with renal or hepatic impairment. Fever may occur, with or without neutropenia. Use caution in patients with high tumor burden; tumor lysis syndrome may occur. **[U.S. Boxed Warning]: Should be administered under the supervision of an experienced cancer chemotherapy physician.** Safety and efficacy in children have not been established.

Drug Interactions

Avoid Concomitant Use

Avoid concomitant use of Cladribine with any of the following: BCG; Natalizumab; Pimecrolimus; Roflumilast; Tacrolimus (Topical); Vaccines (Live)

Decreased Effect

Cladribine may decrease the levels/effects of: BCG; Sipuleucel-T; Vaccines (Inactivated); Vaccines (Live)

The levels/effects of Cladribine may be decreased by: Echinacea

Increased Effect/Toxicity

Cladribine may increase the levels/effects of: Leflunomide; Natalizumab; Vaccines (Live)

The levels/effects of Cladribine may be increased by: Denosumab; Pimecrolimus; Roflumilast; Tacrolimus (Topical); Trastuzumab

Nutritional/Ethanol Interactions Ethanol: Avoid ethanol (due to GI irritation).

Adverse Reactions

>10%:

Central nervous system: Fever (69%; ≥104°F: 11%), fatigue (11% to 45%), headache (7% to 22%)
Dermatologic: Rash (10% to 27%)
Gastrointestinal: Nausea (28%), appetite decreased (17%), vomiting (13%)
Hematologic: Myelosuppression, common, dose limiting (nadir: 5-10 days, recovery: 4-8 weeks); neutropenia (70%); anemia (37%); thrombocytopenia (12%)
Local: Injection site reactions (9% to 19%)
Respiratory: Abnormal breath sounds (11%)
Miscellaneous: Infection (28%)

1% to 10%:

Cardiovascular: Edema (6%), tachycardia (6%), thrombosis (2%)
Central nervous system: Dizziness (9%), chills (9%), insomnia (7%), malaise (5% to 7%), pain (6%)
Dermatologic: Purpura (10%), petechiae (8%), pruritus (6%), erythema (6%)
Gastrointestinal: Diarrhea (10%), constipation (9%), abdominal pain (6%)
Local: Phlebitis (2%)
Neuromuscular & skeletal: Weakness (9%), myalgia (7%), arthralgia (5%)
Respiratory: Cough (7% to 10%), abnormal chest sounds (9%), dyspnea (7%), epistaxis (5%)
Miscellaneous: Diaphoresis (9%)

Pharmacodynamics/Kinetics

Absorption Oral: 55%; SubQ: 100%; Rectal: 20%

Protein Binding 20%

Half-Life Elimination Biphasic: Alpha: 25 minutes; Beta: 6.7 hours; Terminal, mean: Normal renal function: 5.4 hours

Metabolism Hepatic; 5′-triphosphate moiety-active

Excretion Urine (18% to 44%); Clearance: Estimated systemic: 640 mL/hour/kg

Available Dosage Forms

Injection, solution [preservative free]: 1 mg/mL (10 mL)
Leustatin®: 1 mg/mL (10 mL)

Dosing

Adult & Geriatric Refer to individual protocols.

Hairy cell leukemia: I.V. Continuous infusion:
0.09 mg/kg/day days 1-7; may be repeated every 28-35 days **or**
3.4 mg/m^2/day SubQ days 1-7 (unlabeled dose)

Chronic lymphocytic leukemia (unlabeled use): I.V. Continuous infusion:
0.1 mg/kg/day days 1-7 **or**
0.028-0.14 mg/kg/day as a 2-hour infusion days 1-5

Chronic myelogenous leukemia (unlabeled use): I.V. 15 mg/m^2/day as a 1-hour infusion days 1-5; if no response, increase dose to 20 mg/m^2/day in the second course.

Pediatric Refer to individual protocols.

Acute leukemias (unlabeled use): 6.2-7.5 mg/m^2/day continuous infusion for days 1-5; maximum tolerated dose was 8.9 mg/m^2/day.

Renal Impairment The FDA-approved labeling recommends that caution should be used in patients with renal impairment; however, no specific dosage adjustment guidelines are available due to lack of data. The following guidelines have been used by some clinicians (Aronoff, 2007):

Children:
Cl_{cr} 10-50 mL/minute: Administer 50% of dose
Cl_{cr} <10 mL/minute: Administer 30% of dose
Hemodialysis: Administer 30% of dose
Continuous renal replacement therapy (CRRT): Administer 50% of dose

Adults:
Cl_{cr} 10-50 mL/minute: Administer 75% of dose
Cl_{cr} <10 mL/minute: Administer 50% of dose
Continuous ambulatory peritoneal dialysis (CAPD): Administer 50% of dose

Hepatic Impairment The FDA-approved labeling recommends that caution should be used in patients with hepatic impairment; however, no specific dosage adjustment guidelines are available due to lack of data.

Administration

I.V. Administer as a 1- to 2-hour infusion or by continuous infusion

Stability

Reconstitution Dilute in 500 mL; dilute to a total volume of 100 mL for 7-day infusion. Solutions for 7-day infusion should be prepared in bacteriostatic NS; the manufacturer recommends filtering with a 0.22 micron filter when preparing 7-day infusions.

Storage Store intact vials under refrigeration 2°C to 8°C (36°F to 46°F). Protect from light. Dilutions in 500 mL NS are stable for 72 hours. Stable in PVC containers for 24 hours at room temperature of 15°C to 30°C (59°F to 86°F) and 7 days in Pharmacia Deltec® cassettes.

Monitoring and Teaching Issues

Laboratory Monitoring Liver and renal function tests, CBC with differential, platelets, uric acid

Physical Assessment Monitor for myelosuppression, cardiac changes, and renal failure regularly during therapy and following therapy (patients should be considered immunosuppressed for up to 1 year after cladribine therapy).

Patient Education This drug can only be administered by infusion. It is important to maintain adequate nutrition and hydration during therapy. You will be more susceptible to infection during therapy and for up to 1 year following therapy. May cause nausea, vomiting, muscle weakness or pain, or mouth sores. Report immediately rash, unusual excessive fatigue, and/or signs of infection. Report rapid heartbeat or palpitations; unusual bruising or bleeding; persistent GI disturbances; diarrhea or constipation; yellowing of eyes or skin; change in color of urine or stool; swelling, warmth, or pain in extremities; or difficult respirations.

Breast-Feeding Considerations Due to the potential for serious adverse reactions in the nursing infant, breast-feeding is not recommended.

Pregnancy Considerations Teratogenic effects and fetal mortality were observed in animal studies. There are no adequate and well-controlled studies in pregnant women. Women of childbearing potential should avoid becoming pregnant.

- ◆ **Claforan®** *see* Cefotaxime *on page 322*
- ◆ **Claravis™** *see* Isotretinoin *on page 1030*
- ◆ **Clarinex®** *see* Desloratadine *on page 492*

Clarithromycin (kla RITH roe mye sin)

U.S. Brand Names Biaxin®; Biaxin® XL

Generic Availability (U.S.) Yes

Pharmacologic Category Antibiotic, Macrolide

Medication Safety Issues

Sound-alike/look-alike issues:

Clarithromycin may be confused with Claritin®, clindamycin, erythromycin

Pregnancy Risk Factor C

Lactation Excretion in breast milk unknown/use caution

Use

Children:

Acute otitis media (*H. influenzae, M. catarrhalis*, or *S. pneumoniae*)

Community-acquired pneumonia due to susceptible *Mycoplasma pneumoniae, S. pneumoniae*, or *Chlamydia pneumoniae* (TWAR)

Pharyngitis/tonsillitis due to susceptible *S. pyogenes*, acute maxillary sinusitis due to susceptible *H. influenzae, S. pneumoniae*, or *Moraxella catarrhalis*, uncomplicated skin/skin structure infections due to susceptible *S. aureus, S. pyogenes*, and mycobacterial infections

Prevention of disseminated mycobacterial infections due to MAC disease in patients with advanced HIV infection

Adults:

Pharyngitis/tonsillitis due to susceptible *S. pyogenes*

Acute maxillary sinusitis due to susceptible *H. influenzae, M. catarrhalis*, or *S. pneumoniae*

Acute exacerbation of chronic bronchitis due to susceptible *H. influenzae, H. parainfluenzae, M. catarrhalis*, or *S. pneumoniae*

Community-acquired pneumonia due to susceptible *H. influenzae, H. parainfluenzae, Mycoplasma pneumoniae, S. pneumoniae*, or *Chlamydia pneumoniae* (TWAR), *Moraxella catarrhalis*

Uncomplicated skin/skin structure infections due to susceptible *S. aureus, S. pyogenes*

Disseminated mycobacterial infections due to *M. avium* or *M. intracellulare*

Prevention of disseminated mycobacterial infections due to *M. avium* complex (MAC) disease (eg, patients with advanced HIV infection)

Duodenal ulcer disease due to *H. pylori* in regimens with other drugs including amoxicillin and lansoprazole or omeprazole, ranitidine bismuth citrate, bismuth subsalicylate, tetracycline, and/or an H_2 antagonist

Unlabeled/Investigational Use Pertussis (CDC guidelines); alternate antibiotic for prophylaxis of infective endocarditis in patients who are allergic to penicillin and undergoing surgical or dental procedures (ACC/AHA guidelines)

Mechanism of Action/Effect Exerts its antibacterial action by binding to 50S ribosomal subunit resulting in inhibition of protein synthesis. The 14-OH metabolite of clarithromycin is twice as active as the parent compound against some organisms.

Contraindications Hypersensitivity to clarithromycin, erythromycin, or any macrolide antibiotic; use with ergot derivatives, pimozide, cisapride

Warnings/Precautions Dosage adjustment required with severe renal impairment; decreased dosage or prolonged dosing interval may be appropriate. Use with caution in patients with myasthenia gravis. Colchicine toxicity (including fatalities) has been reported with concomitant use. Prolonged use may result in fungal or bacterial superinfection, including *C. difficile*-associated diarrhea (CDAD) and pseudomembranous colitis; CDAD has been observed >2 months postantibiotic treatment. Macrolides (including clarithromycin) have been associated with rare QT prolongation and ventricular arrhythmias, including torsade de pointes. Use caution in patients with coronary artery disease. Avoid use of extended release tablets (Biaxin® XL) in patients with known stricture/narrowing of the GI tract.

Drug Interactions

Metabolism/Transport Effects Substrate of CYP3A4 (major); **Inhibits** CYP1A2 (weak), CYP3A4 (strong), P-glycoprotein

Avoid Concomitant Use

Avoid concomitant use of Clarithromycin with any of the following: Alfuzosin; Artemether; BCG; Cisapride; Conivaptan; Dihydroergotamine; Disopyramide; Dronedarone; Eplerenone; Ergotamine; Everolimus; Halofantrine; Lumefantrine; Lurasidone; Nilotinib; Nisoldipine; Pimozide; QuiNINE; Ranolazine; Rivaroxaban; RomiDEPsin; Salmeterol; Silodosin; Tamsulosin; Tetrabenazine; Thioridazine; Tolvaptan; Topotecan; Toremifene; Vandetanib; Ziprasidone

Decreased Effect

Clarithromycin may decrease the levels/effects of: BCG; Clopidogrel; Prasugrel; Typhoid Vaccine; Zidovudine

The levels/effects of Clarithromycin may be decreased by: CYP3A4 Inducers (Strong); Deferasirox; Etravirine; Herbs (CYP3A4 Inducers); Protease Inhibitors

Increased Effect/Toxicity

Clarithromycin may increase the levels/effects of: Alfentanil; Alfuzosin; Almotriptan; Alosetron; Antifungal Agents (Azole Derivatives, Systemic); Antineoplastic Agents (Vinca Alkaloids); Benzodiazepines (metabolized by oxidation); Bortezomib; Brinzolamide; BusPIRone; Calcium Channel Blockers; CarBAMazepine; Cardiac Glycosides; Ciclesonide; Cilostazol; Cisapride; CloZAPine; Colchicine; Conivaptan; Corticosteroids (Orally Inhaled); Corticosteroids (Systemic); CycloSPORINE; CycloSPORINE (Systemic); CYP3A4 Substrates; Dabigatran Etexilate; Dienogest; Dihydroergotamine; Disopyramide; Dronedarone; Dutasteride; Eletriptan; Eplerenone; Ergot Derivatives; Ergotamine; Everolimus; FentaNYL; Fesoterodine; GlipiZIDE; GlyBURIDE; GuanFACINE; Halofantrine; HMG-CoA Reductase Inhibitors; Ixabepilone; Lumefantrine; Lurasidone; Maraviroc; MethylPREDNISolone; Nilotinib; Nisoldipine; Paricalcitol; Pazopanib; P-Glycoprotein Substrates; Phosphodiesterase 5 Inhibitors; Pimecrolimus; Pimozide; Protease Inhibitors; QTc-Prolonging Agents; QuiNIDine; QuiNINE; Ranolazine; Repaglinide; Rifamycin Derivatives; Rivaroxaban; RomiDEPsin; Salmeterol; Saxagliptin; Selective Serotonin Reuptake Inhibitors; Silodosin; Sirolimus; SORAfenib; Tacrolimus; Tacrolimus (Systemic); Tacrolimus (Topical); Tadalafil; Tamsulosin; Temsirolimus; Tetrabenazine; Theophylline Derivatives; Thioridazine; Tolvaptan; Topotecan; Toremifene; Vandetanib; Vilazodone; Vitamin K Antagonists; Zidovudine; Ziprasidone; Zopiclone

The levels/effects of Clarithromycin may be increased by: Alfuzosin; Antifungal Agents (Azole Derivatives, Systemic); Artemether; Chloroquine; Ciprofloxacin; Ciprofloxacin (Systemic); CYP3A4 Inhibitors (Moderate); CYP3A4 Inhibitors (Strong); Gadobutrol; Lumefantrine; Nilotinib; Protease Inhibitors; QuiNINE

Nutritional/Ethanol Interactions

Food: Immediate release: Food delays rate, but not extent of absorption; Extended release: Food increases clarithromycin AUC by ~30% relative to fasting conditions.

Herb/Nutraceutical: St John's wort may decrease clarithromycin levels.

Adverse Reactions 1% to 10%:

Central nervous system: Headache (adults and children 2%)

Dermatologic: Rash (children 3%)

Gastrointestinal: Abnormal taste (adults 3% to 7%), diarrhea (adults 3% to 6%; children 6%), vomiting (children 6%), nausea (adults 3%), abdominal pain (adults 2%; children 3%), dyspepsia (adults 2%)

Hepatic: Prothrombin time increased (adults 1%)

Renal: BUN increased (4%)

Pharmacodynamics/Kinetics

Absorption Immediate release: Rapid; food delays rate, but not extent of absorption

Bioavailability ~50%

Time to Peak Immediate release: 2-4 hours

Protein Binding 42% to 50%

Half-Life Elimination Immediate release: Clarithromycin: 3-7 hours; 14-OH-clarithromycin: 5-9 hours

Metabolism Partially hepatic via CYP3A4; converted to 14-OH clarithromycin (active metabolite)

Excretion Primarily urine (20% to 40% as unchanged drug; additional 10% to 15% as metabolite)

Clearance: Approximates normal GFR

Available Dosage Forms

Granules for suspension, oral: 125 mg/5 mL (50 mL, 100 mL); 250 mg/5 mL (50 mL, 100 mL)

Biaxin®: 125 mg/5 mL (50 mL, 100 mL); 250 mg/5 mL (50 mL, 100 mL)

Tablet, oral: 250 mg, 500 mg

Biaxin®: 250 mg, 500 mg

Tablet, extended release, oral: 500 mg
Biaxin® XL: 500 mg

Dosing

Adult & Geriatric

Usual dosage range: Oral: 250-500 mg every 12 hours **or** 1000 mg (two 500 mg extended release tablets) once daily for 7-14 days

Acute exacerbation of chronic bronchitis: Oral:

M. catarrhalis and *S. pneumoniae*: 250 mg every 12 hours for 7-14 days **or** 1000 mg (two 500 mg extended release tablets) once daily for 7 days

H. influenzae: 500 mg every 12 hours for 7-14 days **or** 1000 mg (two 500 mg extended release tablets) once daily for 7 days

H. parainfluenzae: 500 mg every 12 hours for 7 days **or** 1000 mg (two 500 mg extended release tablets) once daily for 7 days

Acute maxillary sinusitis: Oral: 500 mg every 12 hours **or** 1000 mg (two 500 mg extended release tablets) once daily for 14 days

Mycobacterial infection (prevention and treatment): Oral: 500 mg twice daily (use with other antimycobacterial drugs, eg, ethambutol or rifampin)

Peptic ulcer disease: Eradication of *Helicobacter pylori*: Dual or triple combination regimens with bismuth subsalicylate, amoxicillin, an H_2-receptor antagonist, or proton-pump inhibitor: 500 mg every 8-12 hours for 10-14 days

Pertussis (unlabeled use; CDC, 2005): Oral: 500 mg twice daily for 7 days

Pharyngitis, tonsillitis: Oral: 250 mg every 12 hours for 10 days

Pneumonia: Oral:

C. pneumoniae, *M. pneumoniae*, and *S. pneumoniae*: 250 mg every 12 hours for 7-14 days **or** 1000 mg (two 500 mg extended release tablets) once daily for 7 days

H. influenzae: 250 mg every 12 hours for 7 days **or** 1000 mg (two 500 mg extended release tablets) once daily for 7 days

H. parainfluenzae and *M. catarrhalis*: 1000 mg (two 500 mg extended release tablets) once daily for 7 days

Prophylaxis against infective endocarditis (unlabeled use): Oral: 500 mg 30-60 minutes prior to procedure. **Note:** American Heart Association (AHA) guidelines now recommend prophylaxis only in patients undergoing invasive procedures and in whom underlying cardiac conditions may predispose to a higher risk of adverse outcomes should infection occur. As of April 2007, routine prophylaxis for GI/GU procedures is no longer recommended by the AHA.

Skin and skin structure infection, uncomplicated: Oral: 250 mg every 12 hours for 7-14 days

Pediatric

Community-acquired pneumonia, sinusitis, bronchitis, skin infections: Oral: 15 mg/kg/day divided every 12 hours for 10 days

Mycobacterial infection (prevention and treatment): Oral:

Manufacturer's recommendation: 7.5 mg/kg/dose (maximum: 500 mg/dose) twice daily. **Note:** Safety of clarithromycin for MAC not studied in children <20 months.

HIV-exposed/-positive (unlabeled use; CDC, 2009):

Primary prophylaxis: 7.5 mg/kg/dose (maximum: 500 mg/dose) twice daily

Secondary prophylaxis: 7.5 mg/kg/dose (maximum: 500 mg/dose) twice daily, plus ethambutol, with or without rifabutin

Treatment: 7.5-15 mg/kg/dose (maximum: 500 mg/dose) twice daily plus ethambutol, plus rifabutin (for severe disease)

Pertussis (unlabeled use; CDC, 2005): Oral:

Children 1-5 months: 15 mg/kg/day divided every 12 hours for 7 days

Children ≥6 months: 15 mg/kg/day divided every 12 hours for 7 days (maximum: 1 g/day)

Prophylaxis against infective endocarditis (unlabeled use): Oral: 15 mg/kg 30-60 minutes before procedure (maximum: 500 mg). **Note:** American Heart Association (AHA) guidelines now recommend prophylaxis only in patients undergoing invasive procedures and in whom underlying cardiac conditions may predispose to a higher risk of adverse outcomes should infection occur. As of April 2007, routine prophylaxis for GI/GU procedures is no longer recommended by the AHA.

Renal Impairment

Cl_{cr} <30 mL/minute: Half the normal dose or double the dosing interval.
Hemodialysis: Administer after HD session is completed.

In combination with ritonavir:

Cl_{cr} 30-60 mL/minute: Reduce dose by 50%.
Cl_{cr} <30 mL/minute: Reduce dose by 75%.

Hepatic Impairment No dosing adjustment is needed as long as renal function is normal.

Administration

Oral Clarithromycin immediate release tablets and oral suspension may be administered with or without meals. Give every 12 hours rather than twice daily to avoid peak and trough variation. Shake suspension well before each use.

Extended release tablets: Should be given with food. Do not crush or chew extended release tablet.

Stability

Storage

Immediate release 250 mg tablets and granules for oral suspension: Store at controlled room temperature of 15°C to 30°C (59°F to 86°F). Reconstituted oral suspension should not be refrigerated because it might gel; microencapsulated particles of clarithromycin in suspension are stable for 14 days when stored at room temperature. Protect tablets from light.

Immediate release 500 mg tablets and Biaxin® XL: Store at controlled room temperature of 20°C to 25°C (68°F to 77°F); excursions permitted to 15°C to 30°C (59°F to 86°F).

Monitoring and Teaching Issues

Laboratory Monitoring CBC with differential, BUN, creatinine; perform culture and sensitivity studies prior to initiating drug therapy

Physical Assessment Assess results of culture and sensitivity tests and patient's allergy history prior to therapy. Use with caution in presence of severe renal impairment, myasthenia gravis, or coronary artery disease. Evaluate results of laboratory monitoring with long-term use.

Patient Education Tables and suspension may be taken with or without meals or milk. Extended release formulation (XL) should be taken with meals; do not break or chew extended release tablets. Maintain adequate hydration, unless instructed to restrict fluid intake. May cause nausea, heartburn, abnormal taste, diarrhea, headaches, or abdominal pain. Report rapid heartbeat or palpitations, persistent fever or chills, easy bruising or bleeding, joint pain, severe persistent diarrhea, skin rash, sores in mouth, or foul-smelling urine.

Dietary Considerations Clarithromycin immediate release tablets and oral suspension may be given with or without meals, and may be taken with milk. Extended release tablets should be taken with food.

Geriatric Considerations Considered one of the drugs of choice in the outpatient treatment of community-acquired pneumonia in elderly. After doses of 500 mg every 12 hours for 5 days, 12 healthy elderly subjects had significantly increased C_{max} and C_{min}, elimination half-lives of clarithromycin and 14-OH clarithromycin compared to 12 healthy young subjects. These changes were attributed to a significant decrease in renal clearance; at a dose of 1000 mg twice daily, 100% of 13 elderly subjects experienced an adverse event compared to only 10% taking 500 mg twice daily.

Breast-Feeding Considerations It is not known if clarithromycin is excreted in human breast milk. The manufacturer recommends that caution be exercised when administering clarithromycin to breast-feeding women.

Other macrolides are considered compatible with breast-feeding and clarithromycin is used therapeutically in infants. Nondose-related effects could include modification of bowel flora.

Pregnancy Considerations Adverse fetal effects have been documented in some animal studies; therefore, clarithromycin is classified as pregnancy category C. Clarithromycin crosses the placenta. The manufacturer recommends that clarithromycin not be used in a pregnant woman unless there are no alternative therapies. An increased risk of teratogenic events has not been observed following maternal use of clarithromycin.

Related Information

Antimicrobial Drugs of Choice *on page* 2008
Community-Acquired Pneumonia in Adults *on page* 2021
Helicobacter pylori Treatment *on page* 2045

◆ **Clarithromycin, Lansoprazole, and Amoxicillin** *see* Lansoprazole, Amoxicillin, and Clarithromycin *on page* 1064
◆ **Claritin® 24 Hour Allergy [OTC]** *see* Loratadine *on page* 1128
◆ **Claritin-D® 12 Hour Allergy & Congestion [OTC]** *see* Loratadine and Pseudoephedrine *on page* 1129
◆ **Claritin-D® 24 Hour Allergy & Congestion [OTC]** *see* Loratadine and Pseudoephedrine *on page* 1129
◆ **Claritin® Children's Allergy [OTC]** *see* Loratadine *on page* 1128
◆ **Claritin® Liqui-Gels® 24 Hour Allergy [OTC]** *see* Loratadine *on page* 1128
◆ **Claritin® RediTabs® 24 Hour Allergy [OTC]** *see* Loratadine *on page* 1128
◆ **Clavulanic Acid and Amoxicillin** *see* Amoxicillin and Clavulanate Potassium *on page* 113
◆ **Cleocin®** *see* Clindamycin (Topical) *on page* 400
◆ **Cleocin HCl®** *see* Clindamycin (Systemic) *on page* 397
◆ **Cleocin Pediatric®** *see* Clindamycin (Systemic) *on page* 397
◆ **Cleocin Phosphate®** *see* Clindamycin (Systemic) *on page* 397
◆ **Cleocin T®** *see* Clindamycin (Topical) *on page* 400
◆ **Cleocin® Vaginal Ovule** *see* Clindamycin (Topical) *on page* 400

Clevidipine (klev ID i peen)

U.S. Brand Names Cleviprex™

Index Terms Clevidipine Butyrate

Generic Availability (U.S.) No

Pharmacologic Category Calcium Channel Blocker; Calcium Channel Blocker, Dihydropyridine

Medication Safety Issues

Sound-alike/look-alike issues:

Clevidipine may be confused with cladribine, clofarabine, clomiPRAMINE
Cleviprex™ may be confused with Claravis™

Pregnancy Risk Factor C

Lactation Excretion in breast milk unknown/not recommended

Use Management of hypertension when oral treatment is not feasible or not desirable

Mechanism of Action/Effect Dihydropyridine calcium channel blocker with potent arterial vasodilating activity. Inhibits calcium ion influx in arterial smooth muscle, producing a decrease in mean arterial pressure (MAP) by reducing systemic vascular resistance.

Contraindications Hypersensitivity to clevidipine or any component of the formulation (soybeans, soy products, eggs, egg products); hypertriglyceridemia or complications of hypertriglyceridemia (eg, acute pancreatitis); lipoid nephrosis; severe aortic stenosis

Warnings/Precautions Symptomatic hypotension with or without syncope and reflex tachycardia may rarely occur. Blood pressure must be lowered at a rate appropriate for the patient's clinical condition; dosage reductions may be necessary. Treatment of clevidipine-induced tachycardia with beta-blockers is **not** recommended. After prolonged use, discontinuation may cause rebound hypertension; monitor closely for ≥8 hours after discontinuation. Use with caution in patients with heart failure (may worsen symptoms). Clevidipine is formulated within a 20% fat emulsion (0.2 g/mL); hypertriglyceridemia is an expected side effect with high-dose or extended treatment periods; median infusion duration in clinical trials was approximately 6.5 hours (Aronson, 2008). Patients who develop hypertriglyceridemia (eg, >500 mg/dL) are at risk of developing pancreatitis. A reduction in the quantity of concurrently administered lipids may be necessary. Use is contraindicated in patients with hypertriglyceridemia or complications associated with hypertriglyceridemia (eg, acute pancreatitis) and lipoid nephrosis. Withdrawal from concomitant beta-blocker therapy should be done gradually. Initiate therapy at the low end of the dosage range in the elderly, with careful upward titration if needed. Vials may support microbial growth; maintain aseptic technique while handling.

Drug Interactions

Avoid Concomitant Use There are no known interactions where it is recommended to avoid concomitant use.

Decreased Effect

Clevidipine may decrease the levels/effects of: QuiNIDine

The levels/effects of Clevidipine may be decreased by: Calcium Salts; Herbs (Hypertensive Properties); Methylphenidate; Yohimbine

Increased Effect/Toxicity

Clevidipine may increase the levels/effects of: Amifostine; Antihypertensives; Calcium Channel Blockers (Nondihydropyridine); Hypotensive Agents; Magnesium Salts; Neuromuscular-Blocking Agents (Nondepolarizing); Nitroprusside; RiTUXimab

The levels/effects of Clevidipine may be increased by: Alpha1-Blockers; Calcium Channel Blockers (Nondihydropyridine); Diazoxide; Herbs (Hypotensive Properties); Magnesium Salts; MAO Inhibitors; Pentoxifylline; Phosphodiesterase 5 Inhibitors; Prostacyclin Analogues

Nutritional/Ethanol Interactions Herb/Nutraceutical: Avoid bayberry, blue cohosh, cayenne, ephedra, ginger, ginseng (American), kola, licorice (may worsen hypertension). Avoid black cohosh, California poppy, coleus, golden seal, hawthorn, mistletoe, periwinkle, quinine, shepherd's purse (may have increased antihypertensive effect).

Adverse Reactions

>10%:

Central nervous system: Fever (19%), insomnia (12%)
Gastrointestinal: Nausea (5% to 21%)

1% to 10%:

Central nervous system: Headache (6%)
Gastrointestinal: Vomiting (3%)
Hematologic: Postprocedural hemorrhage (3%)
Renal: Acute renal failure (9%)
Respiratory: Pneumonia (3%), respiratory failure (3%)

Pharmacodynamics/Kinetics

Onset of Action 2-4 minutes after start of infusion

Duration of Action I.V.: 5-15 minutes

Protein Binding >99.5%

Half-Life Elimination Biphasic: Initial: 1 minute (predominant); Terminal: 15 minutes

Metabolism Rapid hydrolysis primarily by esterases in blood and extravascular tissues to an inactive carboxylic acid metabolite and formaldehyde

Excretion Urine (63% to 74% as metabolites); feces (7% to 22% as metabolites)

Available Dosage Forms

Injection, emulsion:

Cleviprex™: 0.5 mg/mL (50 mL, 100 mL)

Dosing

Adult Management of hypertension: I.V.: Initial: 1-2 mg/hour

Titration: Initial: dose may be doubled at 90-second intervals toward blood pressure goal. As blood pressure approaches goal, dose may be increased by less than double every 5-10 minutes. **Note:** For every 1-2 mg/hour increase in dose, an approximate reduction of 2-4 mm Hg in systolic blood pressure may occur.

Usual maintenance: 4-6 mg/hour; maximum: 21 mg/hour (1000 mL within a 24-hour period). There is limited short-term experience with doses up to 32 mg/hour. Data is limited beyond 72 hours.

Geriatric Refer to adult dosing. Initiate at the low end of the dosage range. Specific guidelines for adjustment of clevidipine are not available, but careful monitoring is warranted.

Renal Impairment No adjustment required with initial infusion rate.

Hepatic Impairment No adjustment required with initial infusion rate.

Administration

I.V. I.V.: Maintain aseptic technique. Do not use if contamination is suspected. Do not dilute. Invert vial gently several times to ensure uniformity of emulsion prior to administration. Administer as a slow continuous infusion via central or peripheral line, using infusion device allowing for calibrated infusion rates. Use within 4 hours of puncturing vial; discard any tubing and unused portion, including that currently being infused.

Stability

Storage Store in refrigerator at 2°C to 8°C (36°F to 46°F). Unopened vials are stable for 2 months at room temperature. Vials are stable for 4 hours once opened. Protect from light during storage. Do not freeze.

Monitoring and Teaching Issues

Physical Assessment Assess allergy history prior to treatment (soybeans or soy products, eggs or egg products). Use caution in presence of impaired lipid metabolism or heart failure. Assess cardiac status and blood pressure closely and titrate upward carefully, if needed. Patient should be monitored for a minimum of 8 hours after discontinuation (rebound hypertension may occur).

Patient Education This medication can only be administered by infusion. Report immediately any pain, burning, or swelling at infusion site or any signs of allergic reaction (eg, respiratory difficulty or swallowing, back pain, chest tightness, rash, hives, swelling of lips or mouth). Ask for assistance when rising or changing position until response to drug is known. Report chest pain or palpitations, headache, dizziness, nausea, vomiting, or difficulty breathing.

Dietary Considerations Clevidipine is formulated in an oil-in-water emulsion containing 200 mg/mL of lipid (2 kcal/mL). If on parenteral nutrition, may need to adjust the amount of lipid infused. Emulsion contains soybean oil, egg yolk phospholipids, and glycerin.

Geriatric Considerations No overall differences in safety or efficacy noted in the initial studies in elderly. Doses should be started at low end of dosage range and titrated slowly since elderly may experience a greater hypotensive response, reflecting their greater frequency of renal and cardiac disease with decreased function and concomitant drug therapy.

Pregnancy Considerations Adverse events were observed in animal reproduction studies. There are no adequate and well-controlled studies in pregnant women. Use only if potential benefit justifies potential risks.

Related Information

Calcium Channel Blockers *on page* 1993

Hyperlipidemia Management *on page* 2046

Hypertension *on page* 2052

◆ **Clevidipine Butyrate** *see* Clevidipine *on page* 394

◆ **Cleviprex™** *see* Clevidipine *on page* 394

Clidinium and Chlordiazepoxide (kli DI nee um & klor dye az e POKS ide)

U.S. Brand Names Librax® *[original formulation]*

Index Terms Chlordiazepoxide and Clidinium

Generic Availability (U.S.) Yes

Pharmacologic Category Antispasmodic Agent, Gastrointestinal; Benzodiazepine

Medication Safety Issues

Sound-alike/look-alike issues:

Librax® may be confused with Librium

Librax® formulation may be cause for confusion:

In November 2004, Valeant Pharmaceuticals licensed the Librax® trademark to Victory Pharmaceuticals. Subsequently, the product was reformulated to contain chlordiazepoxide and methscopolamine. In January 2006, Valeant Pharmaceuticals began redistributing the original formulation of Librax®, containing clidinium and chlordiazepoxide. Victory Pharmaceuticals has discontinued their product. **Note:** The formulation of Librax® distributed in Canada (Valeant Canada Ltd) always contained clidinium and chlordiazepoxide.

Beers Criteria medication: This drug may be inappropriate for use in geriatric patients (high severity risk).

Pregnancy Risk Factor D

Lactation Enters breast milk/contraindicated

Use Adjunct treatment of peptic ulcer; treatment of irritable bowel syndrome

Available Dosage Forms

Capsule: Clidinium 2.5 mg and chlordiazepoxide 5 mg

Librax® [original formulation]: Clidinium 2.5 mg and chlordiazepoxide 5 mg

Dosing

Adult & Geriatric Adjunct treatment of peptic ulcer; treatment of IBS: Oral: 1-2 capsules 3-4 times/day, before meals or food and at bedtime. **Caution:** Do not abruptly discontinue after prolonged use; taper dose gradually.

Administration

Oral Administer before meals. **Caution:** Do not abruptly discontinue after prolonged use; taper dose gradually.

Monitoring and Teaching Issues

Laboratory Monitoring CBC, liver function

Physical Assessment See individual agents.

Patient Education See individual agents.

Related Information

ChlordiazePOXIDE *on page 358*

- **Climara®** *see* Estradiol (Systemic) *on page 670*
- **Clindagel®** *see* Clindamycin (Topical) *on page 400*
- **ClindaMax®** *see* Clindamycin (Topical) *on page 400*

Clindamycin (Systemic) (klin da MYE sin)

U.S. Brand Names Cleocin HCl®; Cleocin Pediatric®; Cleocin Phosphate®

Index Terms Clindamycin Hydrochloride; Clindamycin Palmitate

Generic Availability (U.S.) Yes

Pharmacologic Category Antibiotic, Lincosamide

Medication Safety Issues

Sound-alike/look-alike issues:

Cleocin® may be confused with bleomycin, Clinoril®, Cubicin®, Lincocin®

Clindamycin may be confused with clarithromycin, Claritin®, vancomycin

Pregnancy Risk Factor B

Lactation Enters breast milk/not recommended (AAP rates "compatible"; AAP 2001 update pending)

Use Treatment of susceptible bacterial infections, mainly those caused by anaerobes, streptococci, pneumococci, and staphylococci; pelvic inflammatory disease (I.V.)

Unlabeled/Investigational Use May be useful in PCP; alternate treatment for toxoplasmosis; bacterial vaginosis (oral); alternate treatment for MRSA infections

Mechanism of Action/Effect Reversibly binds to 50S ribosomal subunits preventing peptide bond formation thus inhibiting bacterial protein synthesis; bacteriostatic or bactericidal depending on drug concentration, infection site, and organism

Contraindications Hypersensitivity to clindamycin, lincomycin, or any component of the formulation

Warnings/Precautions Dosage adjustment may be necessary in patients with severe hepatic dysfunction. **[U.S. Boxed Warning]: Can cause severe and possibly fatal colitis.** Prolonged use may result in fungal or bacterial superinfection, including *C. difficile*-associated diarrhea (CDAD) and pseudomembranous colitis; CDAD has been observed >2 months postantibiotic treatment. Use with caution in patients with a history of gastrointestinal disease. Discontinue drug if significant diarrhea, abdominal cramps, or passage of blood and mucus occurs. Some dosage forms contain benzyl alcohol or tartrazine. Use caution in atopic patients. Not appropriate for use in the treatment of meningitis due to inadequate penetration into the CSF.

Drug Interactions

Avoid Concomitant Use

Avoid concomitant use of Clindamycin (Systemic) with any of the following: BCG; Erythromycin; Erythromycin (Systemic)

Decreased Effect

Clindamycin (Systemic) may decrease the levels/effects of: BCG; Erythromycin (Systemic); Typhoid Vaccine

The levels/effects of Clindamycin (Systemic) may be decreased by: Erythromycin; Kaolin

Increased Effect/Toxicity

Clindamycin (Systemic) may increase the levels/effects of: Neuromuscular-Blocking Agents

Nutritional/Ethanol Interactions

Food: Peak concentrations may be delayed with food.

Herb/Nutraceutical: St John's wort may decrease clindamycin levels.

Adverse Reactions Frequency not defined.

Cardiovascular: Cardiac arrest (rare; I.V. administration), hypotension (rare; I.V. administration)

Dermatologic: Erythema multiforme (rare), exfoliative dermatitis (rare), pruritus, rash, Stevens-Johnson syndrome (rare), urticaria

Gastrointestinal: Abdominal pain, diarrhea, esophagitis, nausea, pseudomembranous colitis, vomiting

Genitourinary: Vaginitis

Hematologic: Agranulocytosis, eosinophilia (transient), neutropenia (transient), thrombocytopenia

Hepatic: Jaundice, liver function test abnormalities

Local: Induration/pain/sterile abscess (I.M.), thrombophlebitis (I.V.)

Neuromuscular & skeletal: Polyarthritis (rare)

Renal: Renal dysfunction (rare)

Miscellaneous: Anaphylactoid reactions (rare)

Pharmacodynamics/Kinetics

Absorption Oral, hydrochloride: Rapid (90%)

Time to Peak Serum: Oral: Within 60 minutes; I.M.: 1-3 hours

Half-Life Elimination Neonates: Premature: 8.7 hours; Full-term: 3.6 hours; Children: ~2 hours; Adults: ~2-3 hours; Elderly 4 hours (range 3.4-5.1 hours)

Metabolism Hepatic; forms metabolites (variable activity); Clindamycin phosphate is converted to clindamycin HCl (active)

Excretion Urine (10%) and feces (~4%) as active drug and metabolites

Available Dosage Forms

Capsule, oral: 75 mg, 150 mg, 300 mg

Cleocin HCl®: 75 mg, 150 mg, 300 mg

Granules for solution, oral: 75 mg/5 mL (100 mL)

Cleocin Pediatric®: 75 mg/5 mL (100 mL)

Infusion, premixed in D_5W:

Cleocin Phosphate®: 300 mg (50 mL); 600 mg (50 mL); 900 mg (50 mL)

Injection, solution: 150 mg/mL (2 mL, 4 mL, 6 mL, 60 mL)

Cleocin Phosphate®: 150 mg/mL (2 mL, 4 mL, 6 mL, 60 mL)

Dosing

Adult & Geriatric

Usual dose:

Oral: 150-450 mg/dose every 6-8 hours; maximum dose: 1.8 g/day

I.M., I.V.: 1.2-2.7 g/day in 2-4 divided doses; maximum dose: 4.8 g/day

Amnionitis: *I.V.:* 450-900 mg every 8 hours

Anthrax (unlabeled use): *I.V.:* 900 mg every 8 hours with ciprofloxacin or doxycycline

Babesiosis (unlabeled use):

Oral: 600 mg 3 times/day for 7-10 days with quinine (*Medical Letter*, 2007)

I.V.: 1.2 g twice daily for 7-10 days with quinine (*Medical Letter*, 2007)

Bacterial vaginosis (unlabeled use): *Oral:* 300 mg twice daily for 7 days (CDC, 2010)

Bite wounds (canine): *Oral:* 300 mg 4 times/day with a fluoroquinolone

Cellulitis due to MRSA (unlabeled use): Oral: 300-450 mg 3 times/day for 5-10 days (Liu, 2011)

Complicated skin/soft tissue infection due to MRSA (unlabeled use): I.V., Oral: 600 mg 3 times/day for 7-14 days (Liu, 2011)

Gangrenous pyomyositis: *I.V.:* 900 mg every 8 hours with penicillin G

Group B streptococcus (neonatal prophylaxis): *I.V.:* 900 mg every 8 hours until delivery

Orofacial/parapharyngeal space infections:

Oral: 150-450 mg every 6 hours for at least 7 days; maximum dose: 1.8 g/day

I.V.: 600-900 mg every 8 hours

Osteomyelitis due to MRSA (unlabeled use): *I.V., Oral:* 600 mg 3 times/day for a minimum of 8 weeks (some experts combine with rifampin) (Liu, 2011)

Pelvic inflammatory disease: *I.V.:* 900 mg every 8 hours with gentamicin (conventional or single daily dosing); 24 hours after clinical improvement may convert to oral doxycycline 100 mg twice daily **or** clindamycin 450 mg 4 times/day to complete 14 days of total therapy. Avoid doxycycline if tubo-ovarian abscess is present. (CDC, 2010)

***Pneumocystis jiroveci* pneumonia (unlabeled use):**

I.V.: 600-900 mg every 6-8 hours with primaquine for 21 days (CDC, 2009)

Oral: 300-450 mg every 6-8 hours with primaquine for 21 days (CDC,2009)

Pneumonia due to MRSA (unlabeled use): *I.V., Oral:* 600 mg 3 times/day for 7-21 days (Liu, 2011)

Prophylaxis against infective endocarditis (unlabeled use):

Oral: 600 mg 30-60 minutes before procedure with no follow-up dose needed (Wilson, 2007)

I.M., I.V.: 600 mg 30-60 minutes before procedure. Intramuscular injections should be avoided in patients who are receiving anticoagulant therapy. In these circumstances, orally administered regimens should be given whenever possible. Intravenously administered antibiotics should be used for patients who are unable to tolerate or absorb oral medications. (Wilson, 2007)

Note: American Heart Association (AHA) guidelines now recommend prophylaxis only in patients undergoing invasive procedures and in whom underlying cardiac conditions may predispose to a higher risk of adverse outcomes should infection occur. As of April 2007, routine prophylaxis for GI/GU procedures is no longer recommended by the AHA.

Prophylaxis in total joint replacement patients undergoing dental procedures which produce bacteremia (unlabeled use):

Oral: 600 mg 1 hour prior to procedure (ADA, 2003)

I.V.: 600 mg 1 hour prior to procedure (for patients unable to take oral medication) (ADA, 2003)

Septic arthritis due to MRSA (unlabeled use): *I.V., Oral:* 600 mg 3 times/day for 3-4 weeks (Liu, 2011)

Toxic shock syndrome: *I.V.:* 900 mg every 8 hours with penicillin G or ceftriaxone

Toxoplasmosis (HIV-exposed/positive; secondary prevention [unlabeled use]): *Oral:* 600 mg every 8 hours (with pyrimethamine and leucovorin calcium) (CDC, 2009)

Pediatric

Usual dose:

Oral: Infants and Children: 8-20 mg/kg/day as hydrochloride; 8-25 mg/kg/day as palmitate in 3-4 divided doses; minimum dose of palmitate: 37.5 mg 3 times/day

I.M., I.V.:

<1 month: 15-20 mg/kg/day in 3-4 divided doses

>1 month: 20-40 mg/kg/day in 3-4 divided doses

Anthrax (unlabeled use): *I.V.:* 7.5 mg/kg every 6 hours

Babesiosis (unlabeled use): *Oral:* 20-40 mg/kg divided every 8 hours for 7-10 days plus quinine (*Medical Letter*, 2007)

Cellulitis due to MRSA (unlabeled use): *Oral:* 10-13 mg/kg/dose every 6-8 hours for 5-10 days (maximum: 40 mg/kg/day) (Liu, 2011)

Complicated skin/soft tissue infection due to MRSA (unlabeled use): *I.V., Oral:* 10-13 mg/kg/dose every 6-8 hours for 7-14 days (maximum: 40 mg/kg/day) (Liu, 2011)

Orofacial infections:

Oral: 10-20 mg/kg/day in 3-4 equally divided doses

I.V.: 15-25 mg/kg/day in 3-4 equally divided doses

Osteomyelitis due to MRSA (unlabeled use): *I.V., Oral:* 10-13 mg/kg/dose every 6-8 hours for a minimum of 4-6 weeks (maximum: 40 mg/kg/day) (Liu, 2011)

Pneumonia due to MRSA (unlabeled use): *I.V., Oral:* 10-13 mg/kg/dose every 6-8 hours for 7-21 days (maximum: 40 mg/kg/day) (Liu, 2011)

Prophylaxis against infective endocarditis (unlabeled use):

Oral: 20 mg/kg 30-60 minutes before procedure (Wilson, 2007)

I.M., I.V.: 20 mg/kg 30-60 minutes before procedure. Intramuscular injections should be avoided in patients who are receiving anticoagulant therapy. In these circumstances, orally administered regimens should be given whenever possible. Intravenously administered antibiotics should be used for patients who are unable to tolerate or absorb oral medications. (Wilson, 2007).

Note: American Heart Association (AHA) guidelines now recommend prophylaxis only in patients undergoing invasive procedures and in whom underlying cardiac conditions may predispose to a higher risk of adverse outcomes should infection occur. As of April 2007, routine prophylaxis for GI/GU procedures is no longer recommended by the AHA.

Septic arthritis due to MRSA (unlabeled use): *I.V., Oral:* 10-13 mg/kg/dose every 6-8 hours for minimum of 3-4 weeks (maximum: 40 mg/kg/day) (Liu, 2011)

Toxoplasmosis (HIV-exposed/-positive; secondary prevention [unlabeled use]): *Oral:* 20-30 mg/kg/day divided every 6-8 hours (plus pyrimethamine and leucovorin calcium) (CDC, 2009)

Renal Impairment No adjustment required.

Hepatic Impairment Systemic use: No adjustment required. Use caution with severe hepatic impairment.

Administration

Oral Administer oral dosage form with a full glass of water to minimize esophageal ulceration. Give around-the-clock to promote less variation in peak and trough serum levels.

I.M. Deep I.M. sites, rotate sites. Do not exceed 600 mg in a single injection.

I.V. Never administer as bolus; administer by I.V. intermittent infusion over at least 10-60 minutes, at a rate **not** to exceed 30 mg/minute (do not exceed 1200 mg/hour). Final concentration for administration should not exceed 18 mg/mL.

Stability

Storage

Capsule: Store at room temperature of 20°C to 25°C (68°F to 77°F).

I.V.: Infusion solution in NS or D_5W solution is stable for 16 days at room temperature, 32 days refrigerated, or 8 weeks frozen. Prior to use, store vials and premixed bags at controlled room temperature 20°C to 25°C (68°F to 77°F). After initial use, discard any unused portion of vial after 24 hours.

Oral solution: Do not refrigerate reconstituted oral solution (it will thicken). Following reconstitution, oral solution is stable for 2 weeks at room temperature of 20°C to 25°C (68°F to 77°F).

Monitoring and Teaching Issues

Laboratory Monitoring CBC, liver and renal function periodically with prolonged therapy

Physical Assessment Evaluate patient's allergy history before initiating therapy. Cardiac status and blood pressure should be monitored and patient kept recumbent after infusion until blood pressure is stabilized.

Patient Education

I.M., I.V.: Report any burning, pain, swelling, or redness at infusion or injection site.

Oral: Take each dose with a full glass of water. You may experience nausea or vomiting. Report dizziness; persistent GI effects (pain, diarrhea, vomiting); skin redness, rash, or burning; fever; chills; unusual bruising or bleeding; signs of infection; excessive fatigue; yellowing of eyes or skin; change in color of urine or blackened stool; swelling, warmth, or pain in extremities; difficult respirations; bloody or fatty stool (do not take antidiarrheal without consulting prescriber); or lack of improvement or worsening of condition.

Dietary Considerations May be taken with food.

Geriatric Considerations Clindamycin has not been studied in the elderly; however, since it is eliminated principally by nonrenal mechanisms, major alteration in its pharmacokinetics are not expected. Elderly patients are often at a higher risk for developing serious colitis and require close monitoring.

Breast-Feeding Considerations Small amounts of clindamycin transfer to human milk. The manufacturer does not recommend the use of clindamycin during breast-feeding. Nondose-related effects could include modification of bowel flora. There has been one published case of bloody stools in a nursing infant, but a causal relationship was not proven.

Pregnancy Considerations Because adverse effects were not observed in animals, clindamycin is classified as pregnancy category B. Clindamycin crosses the placenta throughout pregnancy and at term, but use during pregnancy has not been shown to cause adverse fetal effects. Clindamycin pharmacokinetics are not affected by pregnancy. Clindamycin therapy is recommended in certain pregnant patients for prophylaxis of group B streptococcal disease in newborns, prophylaxis and treatment of *Toxoplasma gondii* encephalitis, or for the treatment of *Pneumocystis* pneumonia (PCP), bacterial vaginosis, or malaria.

Additional Information *In vitro* susceptibility rates to clindamycin are higher in community acquired versus hospital acquired MRSA, although this may vary by geographic region. The D-zone test is recommended for detection of inducible resistance to clindamycin in erythromycin-resistant but clindamycin-susceptible isolates (Liu, 2011).

Related Information

Antimicrobial Drugs of Choice *on page 2008*
Community-Acquired Pneumonia in Adults *on page 2021*
Compatibility of Drugs *on page 1994*
I.V. to Oral Conversion *on page 1956*

Clindamycin (Topical) (klin da MYE sin)

U.S. Brand Names Cleocin T®; Cleocin®; Cleocin® Vaginal Ovule; Clindagel®; ClindaMax®; ClindaReach®; Clindesse®; Evoclin®

Index Terms Clindamycin Phosphate

Generic Availability (U.S.) Yes: Excludes foam, vaginal suppositories

Pharmacologic Category Antibiotic, Lincosamide; Topical Skin Product, Acne

Medication Safety Issues

Sound-alike/look-alike issues:

Cleocin® may be confused with bleomycin, Clinoril®, Cubicin®, Lincocin®
Clindamycin may be confused with clarithromycin, Claritin®, vancomycin

Pregnancy Risk Factor B

Lactation Enters breast milk/not recommended (AAP rates "compatible"; AAP 2001 update pending)

Use Treatment of bacterial vaginosis (vaginal cream, vaginal suppository); topically in treatment of severe acne

Available Dosage Forms

Aerosol, topical: 1% (50 g, 100 g)
Evoclin®: 1% (50 g, 100 g)

Cream, vaginal: 2% (40 g)
Cleocin®: 2% (40 g)
Clindesse®: 2% (5 g)

Gel, topical: 1% (30 g, 60 g)
Cleocin T®: 1% (30 g, 60 g)
Clindagel®: 1% (40 mL, 75 mL)
ClindaMax®: 1% (30 g, 60 g)

Lotion, topical: 1% (60 mL)
Cleocin T®: 1% (60 mL)
ClindaMax®: 1% (60 mL)

Pledget, topical: 1% (60s, 69s)
Cleocin T®: 1% (60s)
ClindaReach®: 1% (120s)

Solution, topical: 1% (30 mL, 60 mL)
Cleocin T®: 1% (30 mL, 60 mL)

Suppository, vaginal:
Cleocin® Vaginal Ovule: 100 mg (3s)

Dosing

Adult & Geriatric

Acne: *Topical:*
Gel, pledget, lotion, solution: Apply a thin film twice daily
Foam (Evoclin®): Apply once daily

Bacterial vaginosis: *Intravaginal:*
Suppositories: Insert one ovule (100 mg clindamycin) daily into vagina at bedtime for 3 days
Cream:
Cleocin®: One full applicator inserted intravaginally once daily before bedtime for 3 or 7 consecutive days in nonpregnant patients or for 7 consecutive days in pregnant patients
Clindesse®: One full applicator inserted intravaginally as a single dose at anytime during the day in nonpregnant patients

Pediatric Acne: *Topical:* Children ≥12 years: Refer to adult dosing.

Administration

Topical Foam: Dispense directly into cap or onto a cool surface. Do not dispense directly into hands. Avoid contact with eyes.

Other Intravaginal:
Cream: Insertion should be as far as possible into the vagina without causing discomfort.
Ovule: The foil should be removed; if the applicator is used for insertion, it should be washed for additional use.

Monitoring and Teaching Issues

Patient Education

Topical, foam: Wash hands thoroughly or wear gloves. Do not dispense directly onto hands or face (foam will begin to melt on contact with warm skin). Dispense an amount that will cover the affected area directly into the cap or onto a cool surface. If can seems warm or foam seems runny, run can under cold water. Pick up small amounts of foam with fingertips and gently massage into affected areas until foam disappears. Wash hands thoroughly. Wait 30 minutes before shaving or applying make-up.

Topical gel, lotion, or solution: Wash hands thoroughly before applying or wear gloves. Apply thin film of gel, lotion, or solution to affected area. May apply porous dressing. Wash hands thoroughly. Wait 30 minutes before shaving or applying make-up. Report persistent burning, swelling, itching, excessive dryness, or worsening of condition.

Vaginal: Wash hands before using. At bedtime: If using applicator, gently insert full applicator into vagina and expel cream. Wash applicator with soap and water following use. If using suppository, insert high into vagina. Remain lying down for 30 minutes following administration. Avoid intercourse during therapy. Report dizziness, nausea, vomiting, stomach cramps, headache, or lack of improvement or worsening of condition.

Related Information

Antimicrobial Drugs of Choice *on page 2008*

Clindamycin and Benzoyl Peroxide (klin da MYE sin & BEN zoe il peer OKS ide)

U.S. Brand Names Acanya®; BenzaClin®; Duac® CS [DSC]

Index Terms Benzoyl Peroxide and Clindamycin; Clindamycin Phosphate and Benzoyl Peroxide

Generic Availability (U.S.) Yes

Pharmacologic Category Acne Products; Topical Skin Product; Topical Skin Product, Acne

Pregnancy Risk Factor C

Lactation Excretion in breast milk unknown/not recommended

Use Topical treatment of acne vulgaris

Available Dosage Forms

Gel, topical: Clindamycin 1% and benzoyl peroxide 5% (50 g)

Acanya®: Clindamycin 1.2% and benzoyl peroxide 2.5% (50 g)

BenzaClin®: Clindamycin 1% and benzoyl peroxide 5% (25 g, 35 g, 50 g)

Duac®: Clindamycin 1% and benzoyl peroxide 5% (45 g)

Dosing

Adult & Geriatric Apply to affected areas after skin has been cleansed and dried:

Acne: Topical:

Acanya®: Apply pea-sized amount once daily; use >12 weeks has not been studied.

BenzaClin®: Apply twice daily (morning and evening).

Inflammatory acne: Topical: *Duac® CS:* Apply once daily in the evening.

Pediatric Children ≥12 years: Refer to adult dosing.

Administration

Topical Skin should be clean and dry before applying. For external use only; avoid applying to inside nose, mouth, eyes, and mucous membranes.

Monitoring and Teaching Issues

Physical Assessment See individual agents.

Patient Education See individual agents.

Related Information

Clindamycin (Topical) *on page 400*

Clindamycin and Tretinoin (klin da MYE sin & TRET i noyn)

U.S. Brand Names Veltin™; Ziana™

Index Terms Clindamycin Phosphate and Tretinoin; Tretinoin and Clindamycin; Veltin™

Generic Availability (U.S.) No

Pharmacologic Category Acne Products; Retinoic Acid Derivative; Topical Skin Product; Topical Skin Product, Acne

Pregnancy Risk Factor C

Lactation Excretion in breast milk unknown/use caution

Use Treatment of acne vulgaris

Available Dosage Forms

Gel, topical:

Veltin™: Clindamycin phosphate 1.2% and tretinoin 0.025% (30 g, 60 g)

Ziana™: Clindamycin phosphate 1.2% and tretinoin 0.025% (30 g, 60 g)

Dosing

Adult Acne: Topical: Apply once daily

Pediatric Acne: Topical: Children ≥12 years: Refer to adult dosing.

Administration

Topical At bedtime, clean face with a mild soap and pat dry before applying medication. A pea-size amount should be applied to one fingertip and then dotted on chin, cheeks, nose, and forehead. Gently rub over entire face or entire affected area while avoiding eyes, mouth, angles of nose, and mucous membranes.

Monitoring and Teaching Issues

Physical Assessment See individual agents.

Patient Education See individual agents.

- **Clindamycin Hydrochloride** *see* Clindamycin (Systemic) *on page 397*
- **Clindamycin Palmitate** *see* Clindamycin (Systemic) *on page 397*
- **Clindamycin Phosphate** *see* Clindamycin (Topical) *on page 400*
- **Clindamycin Phosphate and Benzoyl Peroxide** *see* Clindamycin and Benzoyl Peroxide *on page 401*
- **Clindamycin Phosphate and Tretinoin** *see* Clindamycin and Tretinoin *on page 401*
- **ClindaReach®** *see* Clindamycin (Topical) *on page 400*

◆ **Clindesse®** *see* Clindamycin (Topical) *on page 400*

◆ **Clinoril®** *see* Sulindac *on page 1689*

◆ **Clomid®** *see* ClomiPHENE *on page 402*

ClomiPHENE (KLOE mi feen)

U.S. Brand Names Clomid®; Serophene®

Index Terms Clomiphene Citrate

Generic Availability (U.S.) Yes

Pharmacologic Category Ovulation Stimulator; Selective Estrogen Receptor Modulator (SERM)

Medication Safety Issues

Sound-alike/look-alike issues:

ClomiPHENE may be confused with clomiPRAMINE, clonidine

Clomid® may be confused with clonidine

Serophene® may be confused with Sarafem®

Pregnancy Risk Factor X

Lactation Excretion in breast milk unknown/use caution

Use Treatment of ovulatory failure in patients desiring pregnancy

Mechanism of Action/Effect Clomiphene is a racemic mixture consisting of zuclomiphene (~38%) and enclomiphene (~62%) each with distinct pharmacologic properties. Zuclomiphene is more potent in inducing ovulation. Ovulation occurs by stimulating the release of pituitary gonadotropins, causing growth of the ovarian follicle followed by follicular rupture.

Contraindications Hypersensitivity to clomiphene citrate or any of its components; liver disease; abnormal uterine bleeding; enlargement or development of ovarian cyst (not due to polycystic ovarian syndrome); uncontrolled thyroid or adrenal dysfunction; presence of an organic intracranial lesion such as pituitary tumor; pregnancy

Warnings/Precautions Ovarian enlargement may occur with use; may be accompanied by abdominal distention or abdominal pain and generally regresses without treatment within 2-3 weeks. Do not continue dosing until ovaries are of normal size. Ovarian hyperstimulation syndrome (OHSS) is characterized by severe ovarian enlargement, abdominal pain/distention, nausea, vomiting, diarrhea, dyspnea, and oliguria, and may be accompanied by ascites, pleural effusion, hypovolemia, electrolyte imbalance, hemoperitoneum, and thromboembolic events. If severe hyperstimulation occurs, stop treatment and hospitalize patient. This syndrome develops rapidly within 24 hours to several days and generally occurs during the 7-10 days immediately following treatment. Use with caution in patients unusually sensitive to pituitary gonadotropins (eg, PCOS). To minimize risks, use only at the lowest effective dose. Blurring or other visual symptoms can occur; patients with visual disturbances should discontinue therapy and have an eye exam. Multiple births may result from the use of these medications; advise patient of the potential risk of multiple births before starting the treatment.

Drug Interactions

Avoid Concomitant Use There are no known interactions where it is recommended to avoid concomitant use.

Decreased Effect There are no known significant interactions involving a decrease in effect.

Increased Effect/Toxicity There are no known significant interactions involving an increase in effect.

Lab Interactions Clomiphene may increase levels of serum thyroxine and thyroxine-binding globulin (TBG)

Adverse Reactions

>10%: Endocrine & metabolic: Ovarian enlargement (14%)

1% to 10%:

Central nervous system: Headache (1%)

Endocrine & metabolic: Hot flashes (10%), breast discomfort (2%), abnormal uterine bleeding (1%)

Gastrointestinal: Distention/bloating/discomfort (6%), nausea (2%), vomiting (2%)

Ocular: Visual symptoms (2%, includes blurring of vision, diplopia, floaters, lights, phosphenes, photophobia, scotomata, waves)

Pharmacodynamics/Kinetics

Onset of Action Ovulation: 5-10 days following course of treatment

Duration of Action Effects are cumulative; ovulation may occur in the cycle following the last treatment

Time to Peak ~6 hours

Half-Life Elimination 5-7 days

Metabolism Hepatic; undergoes enterohepatic recirculation

Excretion Primarily feces; urine (small amounts)

Available Dosage Forms

Tablet, oral: 50 mg

Clomid®: 50 mg

Serophene®: 50 mg

Dosing

Adult & Geriatric Ovulation induction: Oral: Females:

Initial course: 50 mg once daily for 5 days. Begin on or about the fifth day of cycle if progestin-induced bleeding is scheduled or spontaneous uterine bleeding occurs prior to therapy.

Dose adjustment: Subsequent doses may be increased to 100 mg once daily for 5 days only if ovulation does not occur at the initial dose. A low dose or duration of course is recommended in patients where unusual sensitivity to pituitary gonadotropin is suspected (eg, PCOS).

Repeat courses: If needed, the 5-day cycle may be repeated as early as 30 days after the previous one. Exclude the presence of pregnancy.

Maximum dose: 100 mg once daily for 5 days for 6 cycles. Discontinue if ovulation does not occur after 3 courses of treatment; or if 3 ovulatory responses occur but pregnancy is not achieved. Re-evaluate if menses does not occur following ovulatory response. Doses larger than 150 mg have been reported, however, pregnancy rates are low.

Administration

Oral The total daily dose should be taken at one time to maximize effectiveness.

Stability

Storage Store at room temperature of 15°C to 30°C (59°F to 86°F). Protect from light, heat, and excessive humidity.

Monitoring and Teaching Issues

Laboratory Monitoring Basal body temperature, serum progesterone, urinary luteinizing hormone; pregnancy test prior to repeat courses

Physical Assessment Teach patient proper use (eg, measuring basal body temperature and timing of intercourse).

Patient Education There may be a risk of multiple pregnancies with therapy. Follow recommended schedule of dosing exactly. May cause hot flashes. Report sudden abdominal discomfort, bloating or pain, nausea, or vomiting.

Breast-Feeding Considerations Clomiphene may decrease lactation.

Pregnancy Considerations Embryotoxic effects were observed in animal studies. The incidence of adverse fetal effects following maternal use of clomiphene for ovulation induction is similar to those seen in the general population. Clomiphene is not indicated for use in women who are already pregnant.

◆ **Clomiphene Citrate** *see* ClomiPHENE *on page 402*

ClomiPRAMINE (kloe MI pra meen)

U.S. Brand Names Anafranil®

Index Terms Clomipramine Hydrochloride

Generic Availability (U.S.) Yes

Pharmacologic Category Antidepressant, Tricyclic (Tertiary Amine)

Medication Safety Issues

Sound-alike/look-alike issues:

ClomiPRAMINE may be confused with chlorproMAZINE, clevidipine, clomiPHENE, desipramine, Norpramin®

Anafranil® may be confused with alfentanil, enalapril, nafarelin

Medication Guide Available Yes

Pregnancy Risk Factor C

Lactation Enters breast milk/not recommended (AAP rates "of concern"; AAP 2001 update pending)

Use Treatment of obsessive-compulsive disorder (OCD)

Unlabeled/Investigational Use Depression, panic attacks, chronic pain

Mechanism of Action/Effect Clomipramine appears to affect serotonin uptake while its active metabolite, desmethylclomipramine, affects norepinephrine uptake

Contraindications Hypersensitivity to clomipramine, other tricyclic agents, or any component of the formulation; use of MAO inhibitors within 14 days; use in a patient during the acute recovery phase of MI

Warnings/Precautions [U.S. Boxed Warning]: Antidepressants increase the risk of suicidal thinking and behavior in children, adolescents, and young adults (18-24 years of age) with major depressive disorder (MDD) and other psychiatric disorders; consider risk prior to prescribing. Short-term studies did not show an increased risk in patients >24 years of age and showed a decreased risk in patients ≥65 years. Closely monitor for clinical worsening, suicidality, or unusual changes in behavior; the patient's family or caregiver should be instructed to closely observe the patient and communicate condition with healthcare provider. A medication guide should be dispensed with each prescription. **Clomipramine is FDA approved for the treatment of OCD in children ≥10 years of age.**

The possibility of a suicide attempt is inherent in major depression and may persist until remission occurs. Monitor for worsening of depression or suicidality, especially during initiation of therapy (generally first 1-2 months) or with dose increases or decreases. Use caution in high-risk patients. Worsening depression and severe abrupt suicidality that are not part of the presenting symptoms may require discontinuation or modification of drug therapy. The patient's family or caregiver should be alerted to monitor patients for the emergence of suicidality and associated behaviors (such as agitation, irritability, hostility, impulsivity, and hypomania) and notify the healthcare provider.

May worsen psychosis in some patients or precipitate a shift to mania or hypomania in patients with bipolar disorder. Patients presenting with depressive symptoms should be screened for bipolar disorder. Monotherapy in patients with bipolar disorder should be avoided. **Clomipramine is not FDA approved for bipolar depression.**

TCAs may rarely cause bone marrow suppression; monitor for any signs of infection and obtain CBC if symptoms (eg, fever, sore throat) evident. May cause seizures (relationship to dose and/or duration of therapy) - do not exceed maximum doses. Use caution in patients with a previous seizure disorder or condition predisposing to seizures such as brain damage, alcoholism, or concurrent therapy with other drugs which lower the seizure threshold. May increase the risks associated with electroconvulsive therapy. Has been associated with a high incidence of sexual dysfunction. Weight gain may occur. Hyperpyrexia has been observed with TCAs in combination with anticholinergics and/or neuroleptics, particularly during hot weather.

The degree of sedation, anticholinergic effects, and conduction abnormalities are high relative to other antidepressants. Clomipramine often causes drowsiness/sedation, resulting in impaired performance of tasks requiring alertness (eg, operating machinery or driving). Sedative effects may be additive with other CNS depressants and/or ethanol. The risk of orthostasis is moderate to high relative to other antidepressants. Use with caution in patients with a history of cardiovascular disease (including previous MI, stroke, tachycardia, or conduction abnormalities). Use with caution in patients with urinary retention, benign prostatic hyperplasia, narrow-angle glaucoma, xerostomia, visual problems, constipation, or a history of bowel obstruction.

Consider discontinuing, when possible, prior to elective surgery. Therapy should not be abruptly discontinued in patients receiving high doses for prolonged periods. Use with caution in hyperthyroid patients or those receiving thyroid supplementation. Use with caution in patients with hepatic or renal dysfunction and in elderly patients.

Drug Interactions

Metabolism/Transport Effects Substrate of CYP1A2 (major), 2C19 (major), 2D6 (major), 3A4 (minor); **Inhibits** CYP2D6 (moderate)

Avoid Concomitant Use

Avoid concomitant use of ClomiPRAMINE with any of the following: Artemether; Dronedarone; Iobenguane I 123; Lumefantrine; MAO Inhibitors; Methylene Blue; Nilotinib; Pimozide; QuiNINE; Sibutramine; Tetrabenazine; Thioridazine; Toremifene; Vandetanib; Ziprasidone

Decreased Effect

ClomiPRAMINE may decrease the levels/effects of: Acetylcholinesterase Inhibitors (Central); Alpha2-Agonists; Codeine; Iobenguane I 123

The levels/effects of ClomiPRAMINE may be decreased by: Acetylcholinesterase Inhibitors (Central); Barbiturates; CYP1A2 Inducers (Strong); CYP2C19 Inducers (Strong); Peginterferon Alfa-2b; St Johns Wort

Increased Effect/Toxicity

ClomiPRAMINE may increase the levels/effects of: Alcohol (Ethyl); Alpha-/Beta-Agonists (Direct-Acting); Alpha1-Agonists; Amphetamines; Anticholinergics; Aspirin; Beta2-Agonists; CNS Depressants; CYP2D6 Substrates; Desmopressin; Dronedarone; Fesoterodine; Methylene Blue; Milnacipran; Nebivolol; NSAID (COX-2 Inhibitor); NSAID (Nonselective); Pimozide; QTc-Prolonging Agents; QuiNIDine; QuiNINE; Serotonin Modulators; Sulfonylureas; Tamoxifen; Tetrabenazine; Thioridazine; Toremifene; TraMADol; Vandetanib; Vitamin K Antagonists; Yohimbine; Ziprasidone

The levels/effects of ClomiPRAMINE may be increased by: Alfuzosin; Altretamine; Artemether; BuPROPion; CarBAMazepine; Chloroquine; Cimetidine; Cinacalcet; Ciprofloxacin; Ciprofloxacin (Systemic); Conivaptan; CYP1A2 Inhibitors (Moderate); CYP1A2 Inhibitors (Strong); CYP2C19 Inhibitors (Moderate); CYP2C19 Inhibitors (Strong); CYP2D6 Inhibitors (Moderate); CYP2D6 Inhibitors (Strong); Dexmethylphenidate; Divalproex; DULoxetine; Gadobutrol; Grapefruit Juice; Lithium; Lumefantrine; MAO Inhibitors; Methylphenidate; Metoclopramide; Nilotinib; Pramlintide; Propoxyphene; Protease Inhibitors; QuiNIDine; QuiNINE; Selective Serotonin Reuptake Inhibitors; Sibutramine; Terbinafine; Terbinafine (Systemic); Valproic Acid

Nutritional/Ethanol Interactions

Ethanol: Avoid ethanol (may increase CNS depression).
Food: Serum concentrations/toxicity may be increased by grapefruit juice.
Herb/Nutraceutical: Avoid valerian, St John's wort, SAMe, kava kava.

Lab Interactions Increased glucose; may interfere with urine detection of methadone (false-positive)

Adverse Reactions Data shown for children reflects both children and adolescents studied in clinical trials.

>10%:

Central nervous system: Dizziness (54%), somnolence (54%), drowsiness, headache (52%; children 28%), fatigue (39%), insomnia (25%; children 11%), malaise, nervousness (18%; children 4%)
Endocrine & metabolic: Libido changes (21%), hot flushes (5%)
Gastrointestinal: Xerostomia (84%, children 63%) constipation (47%; children 22%), nausea (33%; children 9%), dyspepsia (22%; children 13%), weight gain (18%; children 2%), diarrhea (13%; children 7%), anorexia (12%; children 22%), abdominal pain (11%), appetite increased (11%)
Genitourinary: Ejaculation failure (42%), impotence (20%), micturition disorder (14%; children 4%)
Neuromuscular & skeletal: Tremor (54%), myoclonus (13%; children 2%), myalgia (13%)
Ocular: Abnormal vision (18%; children 7%)
Respiratory: Pharyngitis (14%), rhinitis (12%)
Miscellaneous: Diaphoresis increased (29%; children 9%)

1% to 10%:

Cardiovascular: Flushing (8%), postural hypotension (6%), palpitation (4%), tachycardia (4%; children 2%), chest pain (4%), edema (2%)

Central nervous system: Anxiety (9%), memory impairment (9%), twitching (7%), depression (5%), concentration impaired (5%), fever (4%), hypertonia (4%), abnormal dreaming (3%), agitation (3%), confusion (3%), migraine (3%), pain (3%), psychosomatic disorder (3%), speech disorder (3%), yawning (3%), aggressiveness (children 2%), chills (2%), depersonalization (2%), emotional lability (2%), irritability (2%), panic reaction (1%)

Dermatologic: Rash (8%), pruritus (6%), purpura (3%), dermatitis (2%), acne (2%), dry skin (2%), urticaria (1%)

Endocrine & metabolic: Amenorrhea (1%), breast enlargement (2%), breast pain (1%), hot flashes (5%), lactation (nonpuerperal) (4%)

Gastrointestinal: Taste disturbance (8%), vomiting (7%), flatulence (6%), tooth disorder (5%), dysphagia (2%), esophagitis (1%)

Genitourinary: UTI (2% to 6%), micturition frequency (5%), dysuria (2%), leucorrhea (2%), vaginitis (2%), urinary retention (2%)

Neuromuscular & skeletal: Paresthesia (9%), back pain (6%), arthralgia (3%), paresis (children 2%), weakness (1%)

Ocular: Lacrimation abnormal (3%), mydriasis (2%), conjunctivitis (1%)

Otic: Tinnitus (6%)

Respiratory: Sinusitis (6%), coughing (6%), bronchospasm (2%; children 7%), epistaxis (2%)

Pharmacodynamics/Kinetics

Absorption Rapid

Time to Peak 2-6 hours

Protein Binding 97%, primarily to albumin

Half-Life Elimination Clomipramine: Mean: 32 hours (range: 19-37 hours); DMI: Mean: 69 hours (range: 54-77 hours)

Metabolism Hepatic to desmethylclomipramine (DMI; active); extensive first-pass effect

Excretion Urine and feces

Available Dosage Forms

Capsule, oral: 25 mg, 50 mg, 75 mg

Anafranil®: 25 mg, 50 mg, 75 mg

Dosing

Adult & Geriatric Treatment of OCD: Oral: Initial: 25 mg/day; may gradually increase as tolerated over the first 2 weeks to 100 mg/day in divided doses; Maintenance: May further increase to recommended maximum of 250 mg/day; may give as a single daily dose at bedtime once tolerated

Pediatric Treatment of OCD: Oral: Children >10 years: Initial: 25 mg/day and gradually increase, as tolerated, to a maximum of 3 mg/kg/day or 100 mg/day (whichever is less). Maintenance: May further increase to recommended maximum of 3 mg/kg/day or 200 mg/day (whichever is less); may give as a single daily dose at bedtime once tolerated. **Note:** The safety and efficacy of clomipramine in pediatric patients ≤10 years of age have not been established and, therefore, dosing recommendations cannot be made.

Administration

Oral During titration, may divide doses and administer with meals to decrease gastrointestinal side effects. After titration, may administer total daily dose at bedtime to decrease daytime sedation.

Monitoring and Teaching Issues

Laboratory Monitoring Monitor ECG in older adults and patients with cardiac disease

Physical Assessment Observe for clinical worsening, suicidality, or unusual behavior changes, especially during the initial few months of therapy or during dosage changes. If history of cardiac problems, monitor cardiac status closely. Be alert to the potential of new or increased seizure activity. Instruct family or caregiver to observe the patient's behavior closely and communicate any changes to prescriber. Taper dosage slowly when discontinuing.

Patient Education Take multiple dose medication with meals to reduce side effects. Take single daily dose at bedtime to reduce daytime sedation. The effect of this drug may take several weeks to appear. Do not use alcohol. May cause weight gain, dizziness, drowsiness, headache, seizures, dry mouth or unpleasant aftertaste, constipation, or orthostatic hypotension. Report unresolved constipation or GI upset, unusual muscle weakness, palpitations, or persistent CNS disturbances (hallucinations, suicidality, seizures, delirium, insomnia, or impaired gait).

Geriatric Considerations Not approved as an antidepressant, clomipramine's anticholinergic and hypotensive effects limit its use versus other preferred antidepressants. Elderly patients were found to have higher dose-normalized plasma concentrations as a result of decreased demethylation (decreased 50%) and hydroxylation (25%).

Breast-Feeding Considerations Based on information from three mother-infant pairs, following maternal use of clomipramine 75-150 mg/day, the estimated exposure to the breast-feeding infant would be 0.4% to 4% of the weight-adjusted maternal dose. Adverse events have not been reported in nursing infants (information from seven cases). Infants should be monitored for signs of adverse events; routine monitoring of infant serum concentrations is not recommended.

Pregnancy Considerations Adverse events were observed in some animal reproduction studies. Withdrawal symptoms (including jitteriness, tremor, and seizures) have been observed in neonates whose mothers took clomipramine up to delivery.

Related Information

Antidepressant Agents *on page 1982*

◆ **Clomipramine Hydrochloride** *see* ClomiPRAMINE *on page 403*

ClonazePAM (kloe NA ze pam)

U.S. Brand Names KlonoPIN®

Generic Availability (U.S.) Yes

Pharmacologic Category Benzodiazepine

Medication Safety Issues

Sound-alike/look-alike issues:

ClonazePAM may be confused with clofazimine, cloNIDine, clorazepate, cloZAPine, LORazepam

KlonoPIN® may be confused with clofazimine, cloNIDine, clorazepate, cloZAPine, LORazepam

Medication Guide Available Yes

Pregnancy Risk Factor D

Lactation Enters breast milk/not recommended

Use Alone or as an adjunct in the treatment of petit mal variant (Lennox-Gastaut), akinetic, and myoclonic seizures; petit mal (absence) seizures unresponsive to succimides; panic disorder with or without agoraphobia

Unlabeled/Investigational Use Restless legs syndrome; neuralgia; multifocal tic disorder; parkinsonian dysarthria; bipolar disorder; adjunct therapy for schizophrenia; burning mouth syndrome

Mechanism of Action/Effect The exact mechanism is unknown, but believed to be related to its ability to enhance the activity of GABA; suppresses the spike-and-wave discharge in absence seizures by depressing nerve transmission in the motor cortex

Contraindications Hypersensitivity to clonazepam or any component of the formulation (cross-sensitivity with other benzodiazepines may exist); significant liver disease; narrow-angle glaucoma; pregnancy

Warnings/Precautions Antiepileptics are associated with an increased risk of suicidal behavior/thoughts with use (regardless of indication); patients should be monitored for signs/symptoms of depression, suicidal tendencies, and other unusual behavior changes during therapy and instructed to inform their healthcare provider immediately if symptoms occur.

Use with caution in elderly or debilitated patients, patients with hepatic disease (including alcoholics), or renal impairment. Use with caution in patients with respiratory disease or impaired gag reflex or ability to protect the airway from secretions (salivation may be increased). Worsening of seizures may occur when added to patients with multiple seizure types. Concurrent use with valproic acid may result in absence status. Monitoring of CBC and liver function tests has been recommended during prolonged therapy.

Causes CNS depression (dose related) resulting in sedation, dizziness, confusion, or ataxia which may impair physical and mental capabilities. Patients must be cautioned about performing tasks which require mental alertness (eg, operating machinery or driving). Use with caution in patients receiving other CNS depressants or psychoactive agents. Effects with other sedative drugs or ethanol may be potentiated. Benzodiazepines have been associated with falls and traumatic injury and should be used with extreme caution in patients who are at risk of these events (especially the elderly).

Use caution in patients with depression, particularly if suicidal risk may be present. Use with caution in patients with a history of drug dependence. Benzodiazepines have been associated with dependence and acute withdrawal symptoms, including seizures, on discontinuation or reduction in dose. Acute withdrawal, including seizures, may be precipitated in patients after administration of flumazenil to patients receiving long-term benzodiazepine therapy.

Benzodiazepines have been associated with anterograde amnesia. Paradoxical reactions, including hyperactive or aggressive behavior, have been reported with benzodiazepines, particularly in adolescent/pediatric or psychiatric patients. Does not have analgesic, antidepressant, or antipsychotic properties.

Drug Interactions

Metabolism/Transport Effects Substrate of CYP3A4 (major)

Avoid Concomitant Use

Avoid concomitant use of ClonazePAM with any of the following: OLANZapine

Decreased Effect

The levels/effects of ClonazePAM may be decreased by: CarBAMazepine; CYP3A4 Inducers (Strong); Deferasirox; Rifamycin Derivatives; St Johns Wort; Theophylline Derivatives; Yohimbine

Increased Effect/Toxicity

ClonazePAM may increase the levels/effects of: Alcohol (Ethyl); CloZAPine; CNS Depressants; Methotrimeprazine; Phenytoin

The levels/effects of ClonazePAM may be increased by: Antifungal Agents (Azole Derivatives, Systemic); Aprepitant; Calcium Channel Blockers (Nondihydropyridine); Cimetidine; Conivaptan; Contraceptives (Estrogens); Contraceptives (Progestins); CYP3A4 Inhibitors (Moderate); CYP3A4 Inhibitors (Strong); Dasatinib; Droperidol; Fluconazole; Fosaprepitant; Grapefruit Juice; Isoniazid; Macrolide Antibiotics; Methotrimeprazine; Nefazodone; OLANZapine; Proton Pump Inhibitors; Selective Serotonin Reuptake Inhibitors

Nutritional/Ethanol Interactions

Ethanol: Avoid ethanol (may increase CNS depression).

Food: Clonazepam serum concentration is unlikely to be increased by grapefruit juice because of clonazepam's high oral bioavailability.

Herb/Nutraceutical: St John's wort may decrease clonazepam levels. Avoid valerian, St John's wort, kava kava, gotu kola (may increase CNS depression).

Adverse Reactions Reactions reported in patients with seizure and/or panic disorder. Frequency not defined.

Cardiovascular: Edema (ankle or facial), palpitation

Central nervous system: Amnesia, ataxia (seizure disorder ~30%; panic disorder 5%), behavior problems (seizure disorder ~25%), coma, confusion, depression, dizziness, drowsiness (seizure disorder ~50%), emotional lability, fatigue, fever, hallucinations, headache, hypotonia, hysteria, insomnia, intellectual ability reduced, memory disturbance, nervousness; paradoxical reactions (including aggressive behavior, agitation, anxiety, excitability, hostility, irritability, nervousness, nightmares, sleep disturbance, vivid dreams); psychosis, slurred speech, somnolence (panic disorder 37%), suicidal attempt, suicide ideation, vertigo

Dermatologic: Hair loss, hirsutism, skin rash

Endocrine & metabolic: Dysmenorrhea, libido increased/decreased

Gastrointestinal: Abdominal pain, anorexia, appetite increased/decreased, coated tongue, constipation, dehydration, diarrhea, gastritis, gum soreness, nausea, weight changes (loss/gain), xerostomia

Genitourinary: Colpitis, dysuria, ejaculation delayed, enuresis, impotence, micturition frequency, nocturia, urinary retention, urinary tract infection

Hematologic: Anemia, eosinophilia, leukopenia, thrombocytopenia

Hepatic: Alkaline phosphatase increased (transient), hepatomegaly, serum transaminases increased (transient)

Neuromuscular & skeletal: Choreiform movements, coordination abnormal, dysarthria, muscle pain, muscle weakness, myalgia, tremor

Ocular: Blurred vision, eye movements abnormal, diplopia, nystagmus

Respiratory: Chest congestion, cough, bronchitis, hypersecretions, pharyngitis, respiratory depression, respiratory tract infection, rhinitis, rhinorrhea, shortness of breath, sinusitis

Miscellaneous: Allergic reaction, aphonia, dysdiadochokinesis, encopresis, "glassy-eyed" appearance, hemiparesis, lymphadenopathy

Pharmacodynamics/Kinetics

Onset of Action 20-60 minutes

Duration of Action Infants and young children: 6-8 hours; Adults: ≤12 hours

Absorption Well absorbed

Time to Peak Serum: 1-3 hours; Steady-state: 5-7 days

Protein Binding 85%

Half-Life Elimination Children: 22-33 hours; Adults: 19-50 hours

Metabolism Extensively hepatic via glucuronide and sulfate conjugation

Excretion Urine (<2% as unchanged drug); metabolites excreted as glucuronide or sulfate conjugates

Controlled Substance C-IV

Available Dosage Forms

Tablet, oral: 0.5 mg, 1 mg, 2 mg

KlonoPIN®: 0.5 mg, 1 mg, 2 mg

Tablet, orally disintegrating, oral: 0.125 mg, 0.25 mg, 0.5 mg, 1 mg, 2 mg

Dosing

Adult

Burning mouth syndrome (unlabeled use): Oral: 0.25-3 mg/day in 2 divided doses, in morning and evening.

Seizure disorders: Oral:

Initial daily dose not to exceed 1.5 mg given in 3 divided doses; may increase by 0.5-1 mg every third day until seizures are controlled or adverse effects seen (maximum: 20 mg/day)

Usual maintenance dose: 0.05-0.2 mg/kg; do not exceed 20 mg/day

Panic disorder: Oral: 0.25 mg twice daily; increase in increments of 0.125-0.25 mg twice daily every 3 days; target dose: 1 mg/day (maximum: 4 mg/day)

Discontinuation of treatment: To discontinue, treatment should be withdrawn gradually. Decrease dose by 0.125 mg twice daily every 3 days until medication is completely withdrawn.

Geriatric Refer to adult dosing. Initiate with low doses and observe closely.

Pediatric

Seizure disorders (see Use): Oral:

Children <10 years or 30 kg:

Initial daily dose: 0.01-0.03 mg/kg/day (maximum: 0.05 mg/kg/day) given in 2-3 divided doses; increase by no more than 0.5 mg every third day until seizures are controlled or adverse effects seen.

Usual maintenance dose: 0.1-0.2 mg/kg/day divided 3 times/day; not to exceed 0.2 mg/kg/day.

Children >10 years or 30 kg: Refer to adult dosing.

Renal Impairment Hemodialysis: Supplemental dose is not necessary.

Administration

Oral Orally-disintegrating tablet: Open pouch and peel back foil on the blister; do not push tablet through foil. Use dry hands to remove tablet and place in mouth. May be swallowed with or without water. Use immediately after removing from package.

Monitoring and Teaching Issues

Laboratory Monitoring Renal function

Physical Assessment Assess for signs of CNS depression. Assess history of addiction; long-term use can result in dependence, abuse, or tolerance; periodically evaluate need for continued use. For inpatient use, institute safety measures to prevent falls. Taper dosage slowly when discontinuing. Teach patient seizure precautions (if administered for seizures).

Patient Education Drug may cause physical and/or psychological dependence. While using this medication, do not use alcohol. You may experience drowsiness, dizziness, blurred vision, nausea, vomiting, loss of appetite, dry mouth, or constipation. If medication is used to control seizures, wear identification that you are taking an antiepileptic medication. Report excessive drowsiness, dizziness, fatigue, or impaired coordination; CNS changes (confusion, depression, increased sedation, excitation, headache, agitation, insomnia, or nightmares) or changes in cognition; respiratory difficulty or shortness of breath; changes in urinary pattern; changes in sexual activity; muscle cramping, weakness, tremors, or rigidity; ringing in ears or visual disturbances; excessive perspiration; excessive GI symptoms (cramping, constipation, vomiting, anorexia); or worsening of seizure activity or loss of seizure control.

Geriatric Considerations Hepatic clearance may be decreased allowing accumulation of active drug. Also, metabolites of clonazepam are renally excreted and may accumulate in the elderly as renal function declines with age. Observe for signs of CNS and pulmonary toxicity.

Breast-Feeding Considerations Clonazepam enters breast milk. Drowsiness, lethargy, or weight loss in nursing infants have been observed in case reports following maternal use of some benzodiazepines.

Pregnancy Considerations Clonazepam was shown to be teratogenic in some animal studies. Clonazepam crosses the placenta. Teratogenic effects have been observed with some benzodiazepines; however, additional studies are needed. Epilepsy itself, the number of medications, genetic factors, or a combination of these probably influence the teratogenicity of anticonvulsant therapy. The incidence of premature birth and low birth weights may be increased following maternal use of benzodiazepines; hypoglycemia and respiratory problems in the neonate may occur following exposure late in pregnancy. Neonatal withdrawal symptoms may occur within days to weeks after birth and "floppy infant syndrome" (which also includes withdrawal symptoms) has been reported with some benzodiazepines, including clonazepam.

Patients exposed to clonazepam during pregnancy are encouraged to enroll themselves into the AED Pregnancy Registry by calling 1-888-233-2334. Additional information is available at www.aedpregnancyregistry.org.

Additional Information Ethosuximide or valproic acid may be preferred for treatment of absence (petit mal) seizures. Clonazepam-induced behavioral disturbances may be more frequent in mentally handicapped patients. Abrupt discontinuation after sustained use (generally >10 days) may cause withdrawal symptoms. Flumazenil, a competitive benzodiazepine antagonist at the CNS receptor site, reverses benzodiazepine-induced CNS depression.

Related Information

Anticonvulsant Drugs of Choice *on page 1981*
Benzodiazepines *on page 1988*

CloNIDine (KLON i deen)

U.S. Brand Names Catapres-TTS®-1; Catapres-TTS®-2; Catapres-TTS®-3; Catapres®; Duraclon®; Kapvay™; Nexiclon™ XR

Index Terms Clonidine Hydrochloride

Generic Availability (U.S.) Yes: Excludes extended release tablets, oral suspension

Pharmacologic Category Alpha$_2$-Adrenergic Agonist

Medication Safety Issues

Sound-alike/look-alike issues:

CloNIDine may be confused with Clomid®, clomiPHENE, clonazePAM, cloZAPine, KlonoPIN®, quiNIDine

Catapres® may be confused with Cataflam®, Cetapred®, Combipres

Dosing issues:

Use caution when interpreting dosing information. Pediatric dose for epidural infusion expressed as mcg/kg/**hour**.

High alert medication: The Institute for Safe Medication Practices (ISMP) includes this medication (epidural administration) among its list of drug classes which have a heightened risk of causing significant patient harm when used in error.

Beers Criteria medication: This drug may be inappropriate for use in geriatric patients (low severity risk).

Transdermal patch may contain conducting metal (eg, aluminum); remove patch prior to MRI.

Pregnancy Risk Factor C

Lactation Enters breast milk/not recommended

Use

Oral:

Immediate release: Management of hypertension (monotherapy or as adjunctive therapy)

Extended release:

Kapvay™: Treatment of attention-deficit/hyperactivity disorder (ADHD) (monotherapy or as adjunctive therapy)

Nexiclon™ XR: Management of hypertension (monotherapy or as adjunctive therapy)

Epidural (Duraclon®): For continuous epidural administration as adjunctive therapy with opioids for treatment of severe cancer pain in patients tolerant to or unresponsive to opioids alone; epidural clonidine is generally more effective for neuropathic pain and less effective (or possibly ineffective) for somatic or visceral pain

Transdermal patch: Management of hypertension (monotherapy or as adjunctive therapy)

Unlabeled/Investigational Use Heroin or nicotine withdrawal; severe pain; dysmenorrhea; vasomotor symptoms associated with menopause; ethanol dependence; prophylaxis of migraines; glaucoma; diabetes-associated diarrhea; impulse control disorder, clozapine-induced sialorrhea; aid in the diagnosis of growth hormone deficiency

Mechanism of Action/Effect Stimulates alpha$_2$-adrenoceptors in the brain stem, thus activating an inhibitory neuron, resulting in reduced sympathetic outflow from the CNS, producing a decrease in peripheral resistance, renal vascular resistance, heart rate, and blood pressure; epidural clonidine may produce pain relief at spinal presynaptic and postjunctional alpha$_2$-adrenoceptors by preventing pain signal transmission; pain relief occurs only for the body regions innervated by the spinal segments where analgesic concentrations of clonidine exist; in the treatment of ADHD, the mechanism of action is unknown.

Contraindications Hypersensitivity to clonidine hydrochloride or any component of the formulation

Epidural administration: Injection site infection; concurrent anticoagulant therapy; bleeding diathesis; administration above the C4 dermatome

Warnings/Precautions May cause CNS depression, which may impair physical or mental abilities; patients must be cautioned about performing tasks which require mental alertness (eg, operating machinery or driving). Sedating effects may be potentiated when used with other CNS-depressant drugs or ethanol. Use with caution in patients with severe coronary insufficiency; conduction disturbances; recent MI, CVA, or chronic renal insufficiency. May cause dose dependent reductions in heart rate; use with caution in patients with preexisting bradycardia or those predisposed to developing bradycardia. Caution in sinus node dysfunction. Use with caution in patients concurrently receiving agents known to reduce SA node function and/or AV nodal conduction (eg, digoxin, diltiazem, metoprolol, verapamil). May cause significant xerostomia. Clonidine may cause eye dryness in patients who wear contact lenses.

[U.S. Boxed Warning]: Must dilute concentrated epidural injectable (500 mcg/mL) solution prior to use. Epidural clonidine is not recommended for perioperative, obstetrical, or postpartum pain due to risk of hemodynamic instability. Clonidine injection should be administered via a continuous epidural infusion device. Monitor closely for catheter-related infection such as meningitis or epidural abscess. Epidural clonidine is not recommended for use in patients with severe cardiovascular disease or hemodynamic instability; may lead to cardiovascular instability (hypotension, bradycardia). Symptomatic hypotension may occur with use; in all patients, use epidural clonidine with caution due to the potential for severe hypotension especially in women and those of low body weight. Most hypotensive episodes occur within the first 4 days of initiation; however, episodes may occur throughout the duration of therapy.

Gradual withdrawal is needed (taper oral immediate release or epidural dose gradually over 2-4 days to avoid rebound hypertension) if drug needs to be stopped. Patients should be instructed about abrupt discontinuation (causes rapid increase in BP and symptoms of sympathetic overactivity). In patients on both a beta-blocker and clonidine where withdrawal of clonidine is necessary, withdraw the beta-blocker first and several days before clonidine withdrawal, then slowly decrease clonidine. In children and adolescents, extended release formulation (Kapvay™) should be tapered in decrements of no more than 0.1 mg every 3-7 days. Discontinue oral immediate release formulations within 4 hours of surgery then restart as soon as possible afterwards. Discontinue oral extended release formulations up to 28 hours prior to surgery, then restart the following day.

Oral formulations of clonidine (immediate release versus extended release) are not interchangeable on a mg:mg basis due to different pharmacokinetic profiles. This includes commercially available oral suspension (Nexiclon™ XR) which is an extended release preparation and should not be used interchangeably with any extemporaneously prepared clonidine oral suspension.

Transdermal patch may contain conducting metal (eg, aluminum); remove patch prior to MRI. Due to the potential for altered electrical conductivity, remove transdermal patch before cardioversion or defibrillation. Localized contact sensitization to the transdermal system has been reported; in these patients, allergic reactions (eg, generalized rash, urticaria, angioedema) have also occurred following subsequent substitution of oral therapy.

Clonidine may be inappropriate for use in the elderly due to CNS adverse events and orthostatic hypotension (Beers Criteria). In pediatric patients, epidural clonidine should be reserved for cancer patients with severe intractable pain, unresponsive to other analgesics or epidural or spinal opioids. Use oral formulations with caution in pediatric patients since children commonly have gastrointestinal illnesses with vomiting and are susceptible to hypertensive episodes due to abrupt inability to take oral medication.

Drug Interactions

Avoid Concomitant Use

Avoid concomitant use of CloNIDine with any of the following: Iobenguane I 123

Decreased Effect

CloNIDine may decrease the levels/effects of: Iobenguane I 123

The levels/effects of CloNIDine may be decreased by: Antidepressants (Alpha2-Antagonist); Herbs (Hypertensive Properties); Serotonin/Norepinephrine Reuptake Inhibitors; Tricyclic Antidepressants; Yohimbine

Increased Effect/Toxicity

CloNIDine may increase the levels/effects of: Amifostine; Antihypertensives; Hypotensive Agents; RiTUXimab

The levels/effects of CloNIDine may be increased by: Beta-Blockers; Diazoxide; Herbs (Hypotensive Properties); MAO Inhibitors; Methylphenidate; Pentoxifylline; Phosphodiesterase 5 Inhibitors; Prostacyclin Analogues

Nutritional/Ethanol Interactions

Ethanol: Avoid ethanol (may increase CNS depression). *In vitro* studies have shown high concentrations of alcohol may increase the rate of release of Nexiclon™ XR.

Herb/Nutraceutical: Avoid dong quai if using for hypertension (has estrogenic activity). Avoid ephedra, yohimbe, ginseng (may worsen hypertension). Avoid valerian, St John's wort, kava kava, gotu kola (may increase CNS depression).

Lab Interactions Positive Coombs' test

Adverse Reactions Frequency not always defined.

Oral, Transdermal: Incidence of adverse events may be less with transdermal compared to oral due to the lower peak/trough ratio.

Cardiovascular: Bradycardia (≤4%), palpitation (1%), tachycardia (1%), arrhythmia, atrioventricular block, chest pain, CHF, ECG abnormalities, flushing, orthostatic hypotension, pallor, Raynaud's phenomenon, syncope

Central nervous system: Drowsiness (12% to 38%), headache (1% to 29%), fatigue (4% to 16%), dizziness (2% to 16%), sedation (3% to 10%), insomnia (≤6%), lethargy (3%), nervousness (1% to 3%), mental depression (1%), aggression, agitation, anxiety, behavioral changes, CVA, delirium, delusional perception, fever, hallucinations (visual and auditory), irritability, malaise, nightmares, restlessness, vivid dreams

Dermatologic: Transient localized skin reactions characterized by pruritus and erythema (transdermal 15% to 50%), contact dermatitis (transdermal 8% to 34%), vesiculation (transdermal 7%), allergic contact sensitization (transdermal 5%), hyperpigmentation (transdermal 5%), burning (transdermal 3%), edema (3%), excoriation (transdermal 3%) blanching (transdermal 1%), generalized macular rash (1%), papules (transdermal 1%), throbbing (transdermal 1%), alopecia, angioedema, hives, localized hypopigmentation (transdermal), rash, urticaria

Endocrine & metabolic: Sexual dysfunction (3%), gynecomastia (1%), creatine phosphokinase increased (transient; oral), hyperglycemia (transient; oral), libido decreased

Gastrointestinal: Xerostomia (≤40%), constipation (2% to 10%), anorexia (1%), taste perversion (1%), weight gain (<1%), abdominal pain (oral), diarrhea, nausea, parotid gland pain (oral), parotitis (oral), pseudo-obstruction (oral), throat pain, vomiting

Genitourinary: Erectile dysfunction (2% to 3%), nocturia (1%), dysuria, enuresis, urinary retention

Hematologic: Thrombocytopenia (oral)

Hepatic: Liver function test (mild transient abnormalities; ≤1%), hepatitis

Neuromuscular & skeletal: Weakness (10%), arthralgia (1%), myalgia (1%), leg cramps (<1%), numbness (localized, transdermal), pain in extremities, paresthesia, tremor

Ocular: Accommodation disorder, blurred vision, burning eyes, dry eyes, lacrimation decreased, lacrimation increased

Otic: Ear pain, otitis media

Renal: Pollakiuria

Respiratory: Asthma, epistaxis, nasal congestion, nasal dryness, nasopharyngitis, respiratory tract infection, rhinorrhea

Miscellaneous: Withdrawal syndrome (1%), flu-like syndrome, thirst

Epidural: Note: The following adverse events occurred more often than placebo in cancer patients with intractable pain being treated with concurrent epidural morphine.

>10%:

Cardiovascular: Hypotension (45%), postural hypotension (32%)

Central nervous system: Confusion (13%), dizziness (13%)

Gastrointestinal: Xerostomia (13%)

1% to 10%:

Cardiovascular: Chest pain (5%)

Central nervous system: Hallucinations (5%)

Gastrointestinal: Nausea/vomiting (8%)

Otic: Tinnitus (5%)

Miscellaneous: Diaphoresis (5%)

Pharmacodynamics/Kinetics

Onset of Action Oral: 0.5-1 hour; Transdermal: Initial application: 2-3 days

Duration of Action 6-10 hours

Absorption Oral: Extended release tablets (Kapvay™) are not bioequivalent with immediate release formulations; peak plasma concentrations are 50% lower compared to immediate release formulations

Bioavailability Oral: Immediate release: 75% to 85%; Extended release (Kapvay™): 89% (relative to immediate release formulation)

Time to Peak Oral: Immediate release: 3-5 hours; Extended release: 7-8 hours

Protein Binding 20% to 40%

Half-Life Elimination Adults: Normal renal function: 12-16 hours; Renal impairment: Up to 41 hours

Epidural administration: CSF half-life elimination: 0.8-1.8 hours

Metabolism Extensively hepatic to inactive metabolites; undergoes enterohepatic recirculation

Excretion Urine (40% to 60%as unchanged drug)

Available Dosage Forms

Injection, solution [preservative free]: 100 mcg/mL (10 mL); 500 mcg/mL (10 mL)
Duraclon®: 100 mcg/mL (10 mL); 500 mcg/mL (10 mL)

Patch, transdermal: 0.1 mg/24 hours (4s); 0.2 mg/24 hours (4s); 0.3 mg/24 hours (4s)
Catapres-TTS®-1: 0.1 mg/24 hours (4s)
Catapres-TTS®-2: 0.2 mg/24 hours (4s)
Catapres-TTS®-3: 0.3 mg/24 hours (4s)

Suspension, extended release, oral:
Nexiclon™ XR: 0.09 mg/mL (118 mL)

Tablet, oral: 0.1 mg, 0.2 mg, 0.3 mg
Catapres®: 0.1 mg, 0.2 mg, 0.3 mg

Tablet, extended release, oral:
Kapvay™: 0.1 mg
Nexiclon™ XR: 0.17 mg

Dosing

Adult Note: Dosing is expressed as the salt (clonidine hydrochloride) unless otherwise noted. Formulations of clonidine (immediate release versus extended release) are not interchangeable on a mg:mg basis due to different pharmacokinetic profiles. This includes commercially available oral suspension (Nexiclon™ XR) which is an extended release preparation and should not be used interchangeably with any extemporaneously prepared clonidine oral suspension.

Hypertension:

Oral:

Immediate release: Initial dose: 0.1 mg twice daily (maximum recommended dose: 2.4 mg/day); usual dose range (JNC 7): 0.1-0.8 mg/day in 2 divided doses

Extended release (Nexiclon™ XR): Initial: 0.17 mg clonidine base once daily at bedtime; may increase increments of 0.09 mg/day every 7 days; maintenance: usual dose range: 0.17-0.52 mg clonidine base once daily; maximum: 0.52 mg/day clonidine base

Conversion between immediate release clonidine hydrochloride and extended release (Nexiclon™ XR) clonidine base:

Current dose immediate release tablets 0.05 mg twice daily: Convert to extended release tablet of 0.09 mg clonidine base once daily

Current dose immediate release tablets 0.1 mg twice daily: Convert to extended release tablet of 0.17 mg clonidine base once daily

Current dose immediate release tablets 0.2 mg twice daily: Convert to extended release tablet of 0.34 mg clonidine base once daily

Current dose immediate release tablets 0.3 mg twice daily: convert to extended release tablets of 0.52 mg clonidine base once daily

Transdermal: Initial: 0.1 mg/24 hour patch applied once every 7 days and increase by 0.1 mg at 1- to 2-week intervals (dosages >0.6 mg/24 hours do not improve efficacy); usual dose range (JNC 7): 0.1-0.3 mg/24 hour patch applied applied once every 7 days

Acute hypertension (urgency) (unlabeled use): Oral: Initial 0.1-0.2 mg; may be followed by additional doses of 0.1 mg every hour, if necessary, to a maximum total dose of 0.7 mg (Atkin, 1992; Jaker, 1989)

Unlabeled route of administration: Sublingual: Initial: 0.1-0.2 mg; followed by 0.05-0.1 mg every hour until blood pressure controlled or a cumulative dose of 0.7 mg is reached (Cunningham, 1994; Matuschka, 1999)

Nicotine withdrawal symptoms (unlabeled use; Fiore, 2008):

Oral: Initial: 0.1 mg twice daily; titreate by 0.1 mg/day every 7 days if needed; dosage range used in clinical trials: 0.15-0.75 mg/day; duration of therapy ranged from 3-10 weeks in clinical trials

Transdermal: Initial: 0.1 mg/24 hour patch applied once every 7 days and increase by 0.1 mg at 1-week intervals if necessary; dosage range used in clinical trials: 0.1-0.2 mg/24 hour patch applied once every 7 days; duration of therapy ranged from 3-10 weeks in clinical trials

Note: If transitioning from oral to transdermal therapy, overlap oral regimen for 1-2 days; transdermal route takes 2-3 days to achieve therapeutic effects.

Conversion from oral to transdermal:

Day 1: Place Catapres-TTS® 1; administer 100% of oral dose.
Day 2: Administer 50% of oral dose.
Day 3: Administer 25% of oral dose.
Day 4: Patch remains, no further oral supplement necessary.

Pain management: Epidural infusion: Reserved for cancer patients with severe intractable pain, unresponsive to other opioid analgesics: Starting dose: 30 mcg/hour; titrate as required for relief of pain or presence of side effects; experience with doses >40 mcg/hour is limited; should be considered an adjunct to opioid therapy

Geriatric Hypertension: Oral:

Immediate release: Initial: 0.1 mg once daily at bedtime, increase gradually as needed.

Extended release (Nexiclon™ XR): No specific recommendations are provided by the manufacturer although a lower initial dose is recommended.

Pediatric Note: Dosing is expressed as the salt (clonidine hydrochloride) unless otherwise noted. Formulations of clonidine (immediate release versus extended release) are not interchangeable on a mg:mg basis due to different pharmacokinetic profiles. This includes commercially available oral suspension (Nexiclon™ XR) which is an extended release preparation and should not be used interchangeably with any extemporaneously prepared clonidine oral suspension.

Hypertension (unlabeled use): Oral: Children ≥12 years: Immediate release: Initial: 0.2 mg/day in 2 divided doses; increase gradually, if needed, in 0.1 mg/day increments at weekly intervals; maximum: 2.4 mg/day (rarely required) (NHBPEP, Fourth Report)

Severe hypertension (unlabeled use): Oral: Children: Immediate release: 0.05-0.1 mg/dose; may repeat up to a maximum total dose of 0.8 mg (NHBPEP, Fourth Report)

Clonidine tolerance test (test of growth hormone release from pituitary) (unlabeled use): Oral:

0.15 mg/m^2 as a single dose (Lanes, 1982)

or

5 mcg/kg as a single dose; maximum dose: 250 mcg (Richmond, 2008)

ADHD: Oral: **Note:** May be used alone or as an adjunct to stimulants.

Immediate release (unlabeled indication; Pliszka, 2007):

Children ≤45 kg: Initial: 0.05 mg at bedtime; sequentially increase every 3-7 days by 0.05 mg increments as twice daily, then 3 times daily, then 4 times daily; maximum daily dose: 0.2 mg/day for patients weighing 27-40.5 kg; 0.3 mg/day for patients weighing 40.5-45 kg. When discontinuing therapy, taper gradually over 1-2 weeks.

Children >45 kg: Initial: 0.1 mg at bedtime; sequentially increase every 3-7 days by 0.1 mg increments as twice daily, then 3 times daily, then 4 times daily; maximum daily dose: 0.4 mg/day. When discontinuing therapy, taper gradually over 1-2 weeks.

Extended release (Kapvay™): Children ≥6 years: Initial: 0.1 mg at bedtime; increase in 0.1 mg/day increments every 7 days until desired response, doses should be administered twice daily (either split equally or with the higher split dosage given at bedtime); maximum: 0.4 mg/day. **Note:** Maintenance treatment for >5 weeks has not been evaluated. When discontinuing therapy, taper daily dose by ≤0.1 mg every 3-7 days.

Pain management: Epidural infusion: Reserved for cancer patients with severe intractable pain, unresponsive to other opioid analgesics: Initial: 0.5 mcg/kg/**hour**; adjust with caution, based on clinical effect

Renal Impairment Bradycardia, sedation, and hypotension may be more likely to occur in patients with renal failure; may consider using doses at the lower end of the dosing range and monitor closely.

Not dialyzable (0% to 5%) via hemodialysis; supplemental dose is not necessary; unclear how much is removed via peritoneal dialysis. Oral antihypertensive drugs given preferentially at night may reduce the nocturnal surge of blood pressure and minimize the intradialytic hypotension that may occur when taken the morning before a dialysis session (K/DOQI, 2005).

Oral: Extended release (Nexiclon™ XR):

Moderate-to-severe impairment (not on dialysis): No dosage adjustment recommended; titrate slowly

End-stage kidney disease (on maintenance dialysis): Initial: 0.09 mg clonidine base/day; titrate slowly

Administration

Oral May be taken with our without food. Do not discontinue clonidine abruptly. If needed, gradually reduce dose over 2-4 days to avoid rebound hypertension.

Extended release products:

Kapvay™: Swallow whole; do not crush, split, or chew.

Nexiclon™ XR: Tablets may be split. Shake suspension well before use.

Topical Transdermal patch: Patches should be applied weekly at a consistent time to a clean, hairless area of the upper outer arm or chest. Rotate patch sites weekly. Redness under patch may be reduced if a topical corticosteroid spray is applied to the area before placement of the patch.

Other Epidural: Specialized techniques are required for continuous epidural administration; administration via this route should only be performed by qualified individuals familiar with the techniques of epidural administration and patient management problems associated with this route. Familiarization of the epidural infusion device is essential. Do not discontinue clonidine abruptly; if needed, gradually reduce dose over 2-4 days to avoid withdrawal symptoms.

Stability

Reconstitution Epidural formulation: Prior to administration, the 500 mcg/mL concentration must be diluted in 0.9% sodium chloride for injection (preservative-free) to a final concentration of 100 mcg/mL.

Storage

Epidural formulation: Store at 25°C (77°F); excursions permitted to 15°C to 30°C (59°F to 86°F). **Preservative free;** discard unused portion.

Oral suspension, tablets: Store at 25°C (77°F); excursions permitted to 15°C to 30°C (59°F to 86°F). Protect from light.

Transdermal patches: Store below 30°C (86°F).

Monitoring and Teaching Issues

Laboratory Monitoring Clonidine tolerance test: Growth hormone concentrations, blood glucose (Huang, 2001)

Physical Assessment Use with caution and monitor closely in presence of pre-existing renal impairment, cardiovascular disease, hemodynamic instability, CNS disease or depression. Monitor blood pressure and mental status throughout. Advise patients using oral hypoglycemic agents or insulin to check glucose levels closely; clonidine may decrease the symptoms of hypoglycemia. When discontinuing, monitor blood pressure and taper dose gradually (over 1 week for oral, 2-4 days for epidural).

Patient Education Take at bedtime. If using patch, check daily for correct placement; rotate patch sites weekly. Remove patch while having MRI scan; can cause burns. Do not skip doses or discontinue without consulting prescriber (this drug must be discontinued on a specific schedule to prevent serious adverse effects). This medication may cause drowsiness, dizziness, fatigue, insomnia, decreased libido or sexual function (will resolve when drug is discontinued), postural hypotension, constipation, dry mouth, or nausea. Report chest pain, palpitations, or change in heartbeat; changes in urinary pattern; persistent nervousness, depression, lethargy, insomnia, or nightmares; sudden weight gain; unusual or persistent swelling of ankles, feet, or extremities; or skin reaction to transdermal patch.

Geriatric Considerations Because of its potential CNS adverse effects, clonidine may not be considered a drug of choice in the elderly. If the decision is to use clonidine, adjust dose based on response and adverse reactions.

This medication is considered to be potentially inappropriate in this patient population (Beers Criteria severity: Low).

Breast-Feeding Considerations Enters breast milk with concentrations approximately twice maternal serum concentrations

Pregnancy Considerations Adverse events have been observed in some animal reproduction studies. Clonidine crosses the placenta; concentrations in the umbilical cord plasma are similar to those in the maternal serum and concentrations in the amniotic fluid may be 4 times those in the maternal serum. **[U.S. Boxed Warning]: Epidural clonidine is not recommended for obstetrical or postpartum pain** due to risk of hemodynamic instability.

Additional Information Each 0.1 mg of clonidine hydrochloride (salt form) is equivalent to 0.087 mg of the free base.

Transdermal clonidine should only be used in patients unable to take oral medication. The transdermal product is much more expensive than oral clonidine and produces no better therapeutic effects.

When used for ADHD treatment, clonidine is recommended to be used as part of a comprehensive treatment program (eg, psychological, educational, and social) for attention-deficit disorder.

◆ **Clonidine Hydrochloride** *see* CloNIDine *on page 408*

Clopidogrel (kloh PID oh grel)

U.S. Brand Names Plavix®

Index Terms Clopidogrel Bisulfate

Generic Availability (U.S.) No

Pharmacologic Category Antiplatelet Agent; Antiplatelet Agent, Thienopyridine

Medication Safety Issues

Sound-alike/look-alike issues:

Plavix® may be confused with Elavil®, Paxil®

Medication Guide Available Yes

Pregnancy Risk Factor B

Lactation Excretion in breast milk unknown/not recommended

Use Reduces rate of atherothrombotic events (myocardial infarction, stroke, vascular deaths) in patients with recent MI or stroke, or established peripheral arterial disease; reduces rate of atherothrombotic events in patients with unstable angina (UA) or non-ST-segment elevation (NSTEMI) managed medically or with percutaneous coronary intervention (PCI) (with or without stent) or CABG; reduces rate of death and atherothrombotic events in patients with ST-segment elevation MI (STEMI) managed medically

Unlabeled/Investigational Use In aspirin-allergic patients, initial treatment of acute coronary syndromes (ACS) or prevention of coronary artery bypass graft closure (saphenous vein)

Mechanism of Action/Effect Irreversibly blocks platelet aggregation; platelets blocked by clopidogrel are affected for the remainder of their lifespan (~7-10 days).

Contraindications Hypersensitivity to clopidogrel or any component of the formulation; active pathological bleeding such as peptic ulcer or intracranial hemorrhage

Canadian labeling: Additional contraindications (not in U.S. labeling): Significant liver impairment or cholestatic jaundice

Warnings/Precautions [U.S. Boxed Warning]: Patients with one or more copies of the variant *CYP2C19*2* and/or *CYP2C19*3* alleles (and potentially other reduced-function variants) may have reduced conversion of clopidogrel to its active thiol metabolite. Lower active metabolite exposure may result in reduced platelet inhibition and, thus, a higher rate of cardiovascular events following MI or stent thrombosis following PCI. Although evidence is insufficient to recommend routine genetic testing, tests are available to determine CYP2C19 genotype and may be used to determine therapeutic strategy; alternative treatment or treatment strategies may be considered if patient is identified as a CYP2C19 poor metabolizer. Genetic testing may be considered prior to initiating clopidogrel in patients at moderate or high risk for poor outcomes (eg, PCI in patients with extensive and/or very complex disease). The optimal dose for CYP2C19 poor metabolizers has yet to be determined. After initiation of clopidogrel, functional testing (eg, VerifyNow® P2Y12 assay) may also be done to determine clopidogrel responsiveness (Holmes, 2010).

Use with caution in patients who may be at risk of increased bleeding, including patients with PUD, trauma, or surgery. In patients with coronary stents, premature interruption of therapy may result in stent thrombosis with subsequent fatal and nonfatal MI. Duration of therapy, in general, is determined by the type of stent placed (bare metal or drug eluting) and whether an ACS event was ongoing at the time of placement. Consider discontinuing 5 days before elective surgery (except in patients with cardiac stents that have not completed their full course of dual antiplatelet therapy; patient-specific situations need to be discussed with cardiologist; AHA/ACC/SCAI/ACS/ADA Science Advisory provides recommendations). Use caution in concurrent treatment with anticoagulants (eg, heparin, warfarin) or other antiplatelet drugs; bleeding risk is increased. Concurrent use with drugs known to inhibit CYP2C19 (eg, proton pump inhibitors) may reduce levels of active metabolite and subsequently reduce clinical efficacy and increase the risk of cardiovascular events; if possible, avoid concurrent use of moderate-to-strong CYP2C19 inhibitors. In patients requiring antacid therapy, consider use of an acid-reducing agent lacking (eg, ranitidine) or with less CYP2C19 inhibition. If a PPI is necessary, the use of pantoprazole, a weak CYP2C19 inhibitor, has been shown to have less of an effect on the pharmacologic activity of clopidogrel. Of the PPIs, lansoprazole exhibits the most potent CYP2C19 inhibitory effects (Li, 2004).Use with caution in patients with severe liver or renal disease (experience is limited). Cases of TTP (usually occurring within the first 2 weeks of therapy), resulting in some fatalities, have been reported; urgent plasmapheresis is required. Use in patients with severe hepatic impairment or cholestatic jaundice is contraindicated in the Canadian labeling. Cases of TTP (usually occurring within the first 2 weeks of therapy), resulting in some fatalities, have been reported; urgent plasmapheresis is required.

Drug Interactions

Metabolism/Transport Effects Substrate of CYP2C19, 3A4, 1A2 (minor); **Inhibits** CYP2B6 (moderate), 2C9 (weak)

Avoid Concomitant Use

Avoid concomitant use of Clopidogrel with any of the following: CYP2C19 Inhibitors (Moderate); CYP2C19 Inhibitors (Strong); Omeprazole

Decreased Effect

The levels/effects of Clopidogrel may be decreased by: Amiodarone; Calcium Channel Blockers; CYP2C19 Inhibitors (Moderate); CYP2C19 Inhibitors (Strong); Dexlansoprazole; Esomeprazole; Lansoprazole; Macrolide Antibiotics; Nonsteroidal Anti-Inflammatory Agents; Omeprazole; Pantoprazole; RABEprazole

Increased Effect/Toxicity

Clopidogrel may increase the levels/effects of: Anticoagulants; Antiplatelet Agents; Collagenase (Systemic); CYP2B6 Substrates; Drotrecogin Alfa; Ibritumomab; Salicylates; Thrombolytic Agents; Tositumomab and Iodine I 131 Tositumomab; Warfarin

The levels/effects of Clopidogrel may be increased by: Dasatinib; Glucosamine; Herbs (Anticoagulant/Antiplatelet Properties); Nonsteroidal Anti-Inflammatory Agents; Omega-3-Acid Ethyl Esters; Pentosan Polysulfate Sodium; Pentoxifylline; Prostacyclin Analogues; Rifamycin Derivatives

Nutritional/Ethanol Interactions Herb/Nutraceutical: Avoid alfalfa, anise, bilberry, bladderwrack, bromelain, cat's claw, chamomile, coleus, cordyceps, dong quai, evening primrose oil, fenugreek, feverfew, garlic, ginger, ginkgo biloba, ginseng (American), ginseng (Panax), ginseng (Siberian), grape seed, green tea, guggul, horse chestnut seed, horseradish, licorice, prickly ash, red clover, reishi, SAMe (S-adenosylmethionine), sweet clover, turmeric, white willow (all have additional antiplatelet activity).

Adverse Reactions As with all drugs which may affect hemostasis, bleeding is associated with clopidogrel. Hemorrhage may occur at virtually any site. Risk is dependent on multiple variables, including the concurrent use of multiple agents which alter hemostasis and patient susceptibility.

3% to 10%:
- Dermatologic: Rash (4%), pruritus (3%)
- Hematologic: Bleeding (major 4%; minor 5%), purpura/bruising (5%), epistaxis (3%)

1% to 3%:
- Gastrointestinal: GI hemorrhage (2%)
- Hematologic: Hematoma

Pharmacodynamics/Kinetics

Onset of Action

Onset of action: Inhibition of platelet aggregation (IPA): Dose-dependent:
- 300-600 mg loading dose: Detected within 2 hours
- 50-100 mg/day: Detected by the second day of treatment

Peak effect: Time to maximal IPA: Dose-dependent: **Note:** Degree of IPA based on adenosine diphosphate (ADP) concentration used during light aggregometry:
- 300-600 mg loading dose:
  - ADP 5 µmol/L: 20% to 30% IPA at 6 hours post administration (Montelescot, 2006)
  - ADP 20 µmol/L: 30% to 37% IPA at 6 hours post administration (Montelescot, 2006)
- 50-100 mg/day: ADP 5 µmol/L: 50% to 60% IPA at 5-7 days (Herbert, 1993)

Absorption Well absorbed

Time to Peak Serum: ~0.75 hours

Protein Binding Parent drug: 98%; Inactive metabolite: 94%

Half-Life Elimination Parent drug: ~6 hours; Active metabolite: ~30 minutes

Metabolism Extensively hepatic via esterase-mediated hydrolysis to a carboxylic acid derivative (inactive) and via CYP450-mediated (CYP2C19 primarily) oxidation to a thiol metabolite (active)

Excretion Urine (50%); feces (46%)

Available Dosage Forms

Tablet, oral:

Plavix®: 75 mg, 300 mg

Dosing

Adult & Geriatric

Recent MI, recent stroke, or established arterial disease: Oral: 75 mg once daily

Acute coronary syndrome:

Unstable angina, non-ST-segment elevation myocardial infarction (UA/NSTEMI): Initial: 300 mg loading dose, followed by 75 mg once daily (in combination with aspirin 81-325 mg once daily). **Note:** A loading dose of 600 mg given at least 2 hours (or 24 hours in patients unable to take aspirin) prior to PCI is recommended (*Chest* guidelines, 2008)

ST-segment elevation myocardial infarction (STEMI): 75 mg once daily (in combination with aspirin 162-325 mg initially followed by 81-162 mg/day). **Note:** CLARITY-TIMI 28 used a 300 mg loading dose (with thrombolysis) demonstrating an improvement in the patency rate of the infarct related artery and reduction in ischemic complications. The duration of therapy was <28 days (usually until hospital discharge) unless nonprimary percutaneous coronary intervention (PCI) was performed (Sabatine, 2005).

The American College of Chest Physicians (Goodman, 2008) recommends:

Patients ≤75 years: Initial: 300 mg loading dose, followed by 75 mg once daily for up to 28 days (in combination with aspirin)

Patients >75 years: 75 mg once daily for up to 28 days (with or without thrombolysis)

Percutaneous coronary intervention (PCI): Loading dose: 300-600 mg given as early as possible before or at the time of primary or nonprimary PCI followed by 75 mg once daily. **Note:** If an initial loading dose of 300 mg was given prior to PCI, a supplemental loading dose of 300 mg (total loading dose = 600 mg) may be administered (Kushner, 2009).

Note: *Coronary artery stents:* Premature interruption of therapy may result in stent thrombosis with subsequent fatal and nonfatal MI. The 2009 focused update of the ACCF/AHA/SCAI joint STEMI/PCI guidelines recommend clopidogrel for at least 12 months in patients receiving either a bare metal stent (BMS) or drug eluting stent (DES) during PCI for ACS; durations >15 months may be considered in patients with DES placement (Kushner, 2009). Patients who undergo PCI without ongoing ACS are not addressed in this focused update; however, the 2008 *Chest* guidelines recommend for patients receiving a BMS without ongoing ACS, clopidogrel may be continued for at least 1 month; patients receiving a DES should receive clopidogrel for at least 12 months (Becker, 2008).

CYP2C19 poor metabolizers (ie, *CYP2C19*2* or **3* carriers): An appropriate regimen for this patient population has not been established in clinical outcome trials; however, a higher dose regimen of 600 mg loading dose followed by 150 mg once daily has demonstrated an increase in antiplatelet response in this patient population.

Prevention of coronary artery bypass graft closure (saphenous vein): Aspirin-allergic patients (unlabeled use) [*Chest* guidelines, 2008]: Loading dose: 300 mg administered 6 hours following procedure; maintenance: 75 mg/day

Renal Impairment No adjustment is necessary.

Hepatic Impairment Use with caution; experience is limited. **Note:** Inhibition of ADP-induced platelet aggregation and mean bleeding time prolongation were similar in patients with severe hepatic impairment compared to healthy subjects after repeated doses of 75 mg once daily for 10 days.

Administration

Oral May be administered without regard to meals.

Stability

Storage Store at 25°C (77°F); excursions permitted to 15°C to 30°C (59°F to 86°F).

Monitoring and Teaching Issues

Laboratory Monitoring Hemoglobin and hematocrit periodically

Physical Assessment Monitor for unusual bleeding.

Patient Education May cause headache or dizziness. It may take longer than usual to stop bleeding. Inform prescribers and dentists that you are taking this medication prior to scheduling any surgery or dental procedure. Report immediately unusual or acute chest pain or respiratory difficulties; skin rash; unresolved bleeding, diarrhea, or GI distress; nosebleed; or acute headache.

Dietary Considerations May be taken without regard to meals.

Geriatric Considerations Plasma concentrations of the main metabolite of clopidogrel were significantly higher in the elderly (≥75 years). This was not associated with changes in bleeding time or platelet aggregation. No dosage adjustment is recommended.

Pregnancy Considerations Teratogenic effects were not observed in animal studies. Use during pregnancy only if clearly needed.

◆ **Clopidogrel Bisulfate** *see* Clopidogrel *on page 413*

Clorazepate (klor AZ e pate)

U.S. Brand Names Tranxene® T-Tab®

Index Terms Clorazepate Dipotassium; Tranxene T-Tab

Generic Availability (U.S.) Yes

Pharmacologic Category Benzodiazepine

Medication Safety Issues

Sound-alike/look-alike issues:

Clorazepate may be confused with clofibrate, clonazepam, KlonoPIN®

Beers Criteria medication: This drug may be inappropriate for use in geriatric patients (high severity risk).

Medication Guide Available Yes

Lactation Enters breast milk/not recommended

Use Treatment of generalized anxiety disorder; management of ethanol withdrawal; adjunct anticonvulsant in management of partial seizures

Controlled Substance C-IV

Available Dosage Forms

Tablet, oral: 3.75 mg, 7.5 mg, 15 mg
Tranxene® T-Tab®: 3.75 mg, 7.5 mg, 15 mg

Dosing

Adult

Anxiety: Oral: 7.5-15 mg 2-4 times/day

Ethanol withdrawal: Oral: Initial: 30 mg, then 15 mg 2-4 times/day on first day; maximum daily dose: 90 mg; gradually decrease dose over subsequent days.

Seizures (anticonvulsant): Oral: Initial: Up to 7.5 mg/dose 2-3 times/day; increase dose by 7.5 mg at weekly intervals; not to exceed 90 mg/day

Geriatric Oral: Anxiety: 7.5 mg 1-2 times/day; use is not recommended in the elderly.

Pediatric

Seizures (anticonvulsant): Oral:

Children 9-12 years: Initial: 3.75-7.5 mg/dose twice daily; increase dose by 3.75 mg at weekly intervals, not to exceed 60 mg/day in 2-3 divided doses.

Children >12 years: Refer to adult dosing.

Monitoring and Teaching Issues

Physical Assessment Assess for CNS depression and potential for suicide ideation. Assess history of addiction; long-term use can result in dependence, abuse, or tolerance; periodically evaluate need for continued use. For inpatient use, institute safety measures to prevent falls. Taper dosage slowly when discontinuing.

Patient Education Drug may cause physical and/or psychological dependence. Do not use alcohol. You may experience drowsiness, lightheadedness, impaired coordination, dizziness, blurred vision, nausea, vomiting, dry mouth, constipation, altered sexual drive or ability (reversible), or photosensitivity. Report persistent CNS effects (eg, confusion, depression, suicide ideation, increased sedation, excitation, headache, agitation, insomnia or nightmares, dizziness, fatigue, impaired coordination, changes in personality, or changes in cognition); changes in urinary pattern; muscle cramping, weakness, tremors, or rigidity; ringing in ears or visual disturbances; chest pain, palpitations, or rapid heartbeat; excessive perspiration; excessive GI symptoms (cramping, constipation, vomiting, anorexia); or worsening of condition.

Related Information

Benzodiazepines *on page 1988*

◆ **Clorazepate Dipotassium** *see* Clorazepate *on page 415*

Clotrimazole (Oral) (kloe TRIM a zole)

Index Terms Mycelex

Generic Availability (U.S.) Yes

Pharmacologic Category Antifungal Agent, Oral Nonabsorbed

Medication Safety Issues

Sound-alike/look-alike issues:

Clotrimazole may be confused with co-trimoxazole
Mycelex may be confused with Myoflex®

International issues:

Cloderm: Brand name for clotrimazole [Germany], but also brand name for alclomethasone [Indonesia]; clobetasol [China, India, Malaysia, Singapore, Thailand]; clocortolone [U.S., Canada]

Canesten: Brand name for clotrimazole [multiple international markets] may be confused with Canesten Bifonazol Comp brand name for bifonazole/urea [Austria]; Canesten Extra brand name for bifonazole [China, Germany]; Canesten Extra Nagelset brand name for bifonazole/urea [Denmark]; Canesten Fluconazole brand name for fluconazole [New Zealand]; Canesten Oasis brand name for sodium citrate [Great Britain]; Canesten Once Daily brand name for bifonazole [Australia]; Canesten Oral brand name for fluconazole [United Kingdom]; Cenestin® brand name for estrogens (conjugated A/synthetic) [U.S., Canada]

Mycelex: Brand name for clotrimazole [U.S.] may be confused with Mucolex brand name for carbocysteine [Ireland, Portugal, Thailand]; guaifenesin [China]

Pregnancy Risk Factor C

Lactation Excretion in breast milk unknown

Use Treatment of susceptible fungal infections, including oropharyngeal candidiasis; limited data suggest that clotrimazole troches may be effective for prophylaxis against oropharyngeal candidiasis in neutropenic patients

Available Dosage Forms

Troche, oral: 10 mg

Dosing

Adult & Geriatric Oropharyngeal candidiasis: Oral:

Prophylaxis: 10 mg troche dissolved 3 times/day for the duration of chemotherapy or until steroids are reduced to maintenance levels

Treatment: 10 mg troche dissolved slowly 5 times/day for 14 consecutive days

Pediatric Oropharyngeal candidiasis: Children >3 years: Refer to adult dosing.

Administration

Oral Troche: Allow to dissolve slowly over 15-30 minutes.

Monitoring and Teaching Issues

Laboratory Monitoring Periodic liver function during oral therapy with clotrimazole troche

Patient Education Do not swallow oral medication whole; allow to dissolve slowly in mouth. You may experience nausea or vomiting. Report signs of opportunistic infection (eg, white plaques in mouth, fever, chills, perianal itching, vaginal itching or discharge, fatigue, unhealed wounds or sores).

◆ **Clotrimazole and Betamethasone** *see* Betamethasone and Clotrimazole *on page* 208

Clozapine (KLOE za peen)

U.S. Brand Names Clozaril®; FazaClo®

Generic Availability (U.S.) Yes: Excludes orally-disintegrating tablet

Pharmacologic Category Antipsychotic Agent, Atypical

Medication Safety Issues

Sound-alike/look-alike issues:

CloZAPine may be confused with clonazePAM, cloNIDine, KlonoPIN®

Clozaril® may be confused with Clinoril®, Colazal®

Prescribing and Access Restrictions

U.S.: Clozaril® is deemed to have an approved REMS program. As a requirement of the REMS program, access to this medication is restricted. Patient-specific registration is required to dispense clozapine. Monitoring systems for individual clozapine manufacturers are independent. If a patient is switched from one brand/manufacturer of clozapine to another, the patient must be entered into a new registry (must be completed by the prescriber and delivered to the dispensing pharmacy). Healthcare providers, including pharmacists dispensing clozapine, should verify the patient's hematological status and qualification to receive clozapine with all existing registries. The manufacturer of Clozaril® requests that healthcare providers submit all WBC/ANC values following discontinuation of therapy to the Clozaril National Registry for all nonrechallengable patients until WBC is ≥3500/mm^3 and ANC is ≥2000/mm^3.

Canada: Distribution of clozapine is available only through the Clozaril Support and Assistance Network (CSAN). Details regarding CSAN are available to Canadian practitioners at (800-267-2726).

Pregnancy Risk Factor B

Lactation Enters breast milk/not recommended (AAP rates "of concern"; AAP 2001 update pending)

Use Treatment-refractory schizophrenia; to reduce risk of recurrent suicidal behavior in schizophrenia or schizoaffective disorder

Unlabeled/Investigational Use Schizoaffective disorder, bipolar disorder, childhood psychosis, severe obsessive-compulsive disorder; psychosis/agitation related to Alzheimer's dementia

Mechanism of Action/Effect Clozapine (dibenzodiazepine antipsychotic) exhibits weak antagonism of D_1, D_2, D_3, and D_5 dopamine receptor subtypes, but shows high affinity for D_4; in addition, it blocks the serotonin ($5HT_2$), alpha-adrenergic, histamine H_1, and cholinergic receptors

Contraindications Hypersensitivity to clozapine or any component of the formulation; history of agranulocytosis or severe granulocytopenia with clozapine; uncontrolled epilepsy, severe central nervous system depression or comatose state; paralytic ileus; myeloproliferative disorders or use with other agents which have a well-known risk of agranulocytosis or bone marrow suppression

Canadian labeling: Additional contraindications (not in U.S. labeling): Active hepatic disease associated with nausea, anorexia, or jaundice; progressive hepatic disease or hepatic failure; severe renal impairment; severe cardiac disease (eg, myocarditis); patients unable to undergo blood testing

Warnings/Precautions [U.S. Boxed Warning]: Elderly patients with dementia-related psychosis treated with antipsychotics are at an increased risk of death compared to placebo. Most deaths appeared to be either cardiovascular (eg, heart failure, sudden death) or infectious (eg, pneumonia) in nature. Clozapine is not approved for the treatment of dementia-related psychosis.

[U.S. Boxed Warning]: Significant risk of agranulocytosis, potentially life-threatening. Therapy should not be initiated in patients with WBC <3500 cells/mm^3 or ANC <2000 cells/mm^3 or history of myeloproliferative disorder. WBC testing should occur periodically on an on-going basis (see prescribing information for monitoring details) to ensure that acceptable WBC/ANC counts are maintained. Initial episodes of moderate leukopenia or granulopoietic suppression confer up to a 12-fold increased risk for subsequent episodes of agranulocytosis. WBCs must be monitored weekly for at least 4 weeks after therapy discontinuation or until WBC is ≥3500/mm^3 and ANC is ≥2000/mm^3. Use with caution in patients receiving other marrow suppressive agents. Eosinophilia has been reported to occur with clozapine. Interrupt therapy for eosinophil count >4000/mm^3. May resume therapy when eosinophil count <3000/mm^3.

(**Note:** The Canadian labeling recommends discontinuing therapy for eosinophil count >3000/mm^3; may resume therapy when eosinophil count <1000/mm^3). Due to the significant risk of agranulocytosis, it is strongly recommended that a patient must fail at least two trials of other primary medications for the treatment of schizophrenia (of adequate dose and duration) before initiating therapy with clozapine.

Cognitive and/or motor impairment (sedation) is common with clozapine, resulting in impaired performance of tasks requiring alertness (eg, operating machinery or driving); use caution in patients receiving general anesthesia. **[U.S. Boxed Warning]: Seizures have been associated with clozapine use in a dose-dependent manner;** use with caution in patients at risk of seizures, including those with a history of seizures, head trauma, brain damage, alcoholism, or concurrent therapy with medications which may lower seizure threshold. Benign transient temperature elevation (>100.4°F) may occur; peaking within the first 3 weeks of treatment. Rule out infection, agranulocytosis, and neuroleptic malignant syndrome (NMS) in patients presenting with fever. However, clozapine may also be associated with severe febrile reactions, including neuroleptic malignant syndrome (NMS). Clozapine's potential for extrapyramidal symptoms (including tardive dyskinesia) appears to be extremely low. Risk of dystonia (and probably other EPS) may be greater with increased doses, use of conventional antipsychotics, males, and younger patients.

Deep vein thrombosis, myocarditis, pericarditis, pericardial effusion, cardiomyopathy, and HF have also been associated with clozapine. **[U.S. Boxed Warning]: Fatalities due to myocarditis have been reported; highest risk in the first month of therapy, however, later cases also reported.** Myocarditis or cardiomyopathy should be considered in patients who present with signs/symptoms of heart failure (dyspnea, fatigue, orthopnea, paroxysmal nocturnal dyspnea, peripheral edema), chest pain, palpitations, new electrocardiographic abnormalities (arrhythmias, ST-T wave abnormalities), or unexplained fever. Patients with tachycardia during the first month of therapy should be closely monitored for other signs of myocarditis. Discontinue clozapine if myocarditis is suspected; do not rechallenge in patients with clozapine-related myocarditis. The reported rate of myocarditis in clozapine-treated patients appears to be 17-322 times greater than in the general population. Clozapine should be discontinued in patients with confirmed cardiomyopathy unless benefit clearly outweighs risk. Rare cases of thromboembolism, including pulmonary embolism and stroke resulting in fatalities, have been associated with clozapine.

An increased incidence of cerebrovascular effects (eg, transient ischemic attack, stroke), including fatalities, has been reported in placebo-controlled trials of atypical antipsychotics in elderly patients with dementia-related psychosis.

May cause anticholinergic effects; use with caution in patients with urinary retention, benign prostatic hyperplasia, narrow-angle glaucoma, xerostomia, visual problems, constipation, or history of bowel obstruction. May cause hyperglycemia; in some cases may be extreme and associated with ketoacidosis, hyperosmolar coma, or death. Use with caution in patients with diabetes or other disorders of glucose regulation; monitor for worsening of glucose control. Antipsychotic use has been associated with esophageal dysmotility and aspiration; use with caution in patients at risk of pneumonia (eg, Alzheimer's disease). Use with caution in patients with hepatic disease or impairment; monitor hepatic function regularly. Hepatitis has been reported as a consequence of therapy. Discontinuation of therapy may be necessary with significant elevations in liver function tests; may reinitiate with close monitoring and if values return to normal. Use with caution in patients with renal disease.

Use caution with cardiovascular or pulmonary disease; gradually increase dose. **[U.S. Boxed Warning]: May cause orthostatic hypotension (with or without syncope);** generally occurs more frequently with initial titration and in association with rapid dose increases; use with caution in patients at risk of hypotension or in patients where transient hypotensive episodes would be poorly tolerated (cardiovascular disease or cerebrovascular disease). Concurrent use with benzodiazepines may increase the risk of severe cardiopulmonary reactions. May cause tachycardia (including sustained); sustained tachycardia is not limited to a reflex response to orthostatic hypotension, and is present in all positions.

The possibility of a suicide attempt is inherent in psychotic illness or bipolar disorder; use caution in high-risk patients during initiation of therapy. Prescriptions should be written for the smallest quantity consistent with good patient care.

Medication should not be stopped abruptly; taper off over 1-2 weeks. If conditions warrant abrupt discontinuation (leukopenia, myocarditis, cardiomyopathy), monitor patient for psychosis and cholinergic rebound (headache, nausea, vomiting, diarrhea). Significant weight gain has been observed with antipsychotic therapy; incidence varies with product. Monitor waist circumference and BMI. Elderly patients are more susceptible to adverse effects (including agranulocytosis, cardiovascular, anticholinergic, and tardive dyskinesia). Clozapine levels may be lower in patients who smoke. Smoking cessation may cause toxicity in a patient stabilized on clozapine. Monitor change in smoking. FazaClo® oral disintegrating tablets contain phenylalanine.

Drug Interactions

Metabolism/Transport Effects Substrate of CYP1A2 (major), 2A6 (minor), 2C9 (minor), 2C19 (minor), 2D6 (minor), 3A4 (minor); **Inhibits** CYP1A2 (weak), 2C9 (weak), 2C19 (weak), 2D6 (moderate), 2E1 (weak), 3A4 (weak)

Avoid Concomitant Use

Avoid concomitant use of CloZAPine with any of the following: Metoclopramide; Thioridazine

Decreased Effect

CloZAPine may decrease the levels/effects of: Amphetamines; Anti-Parkinson's Agents (Dopamine Agonist); Codeine; Quinagolide; TraMADol

The levels/effects of CloZAPine may be decreased by: CarBAMazepine; CYP1A2 Inducers (Strong); Lithium formulations; Omeprazole; Peginterferon Alfa-2b; Phenytoin

Increased Effect/Toxicity

CloZAPine may increase the levels/effects of: Alcohol (Ethyl); Anticholinergics; CNS Depressants; CYP2D6 Substrates; Fesoterodine; Methotrimeprazine; Methylphenidate; Nebivolol; Tamoxifen; Thioridazine

The levels/effects of CloZAPine may be increased by: Acetylcholinesterase Inhibitors (Central); Benzodiazepines; Cimetidine; Conivaptan; CYP1A2 Inhibitors (Moderate); CYP1A2 Inhibitors (Strong); Droperidol; Lithium formulations; Macrolide Antibiotics; MAO Inhibitors; Methotrimeprazine; Methylphenidate; Metoclopramide; Nefazodone; Omeprazole; Pramlintide; Selective Serotonin Reuptake Inhibitors; Tetrabenazine

Nutritional/Ethanol Interactions

Ethanol: Avoid ethanol (may increase CNS depression).

Herb/Nutraceutical: St John's wort may decrease clozapine levels. Avoid kava kava, gotu kola, valerian, St John's wort (may increase CNS depression).

Adverse Reactions

>10%:

Cardiovascular: Tachycardia (25%)

Central nervous system: Drowsiness (39% to 46%), dizziness (19% to 27%), insomnia (2% to 20%)

Gastrointestinal: Sialorrhea (31% to 48%), weight gain (4% to 31%), constipation (14% to 25%), nausea/vomiting (3% to 17%)

1% to 10%:

Cardiovascular: Hypotension (9%), syncope (6%), hypertension (4%), angina (1%), ECG changes (1%)

Central nervous system: Headache (7%), agitation (4%), akinesia (4%), nightmares (4%), restlessness (4%), akathisia (3%), confusion (3%), seizure (3%), anxiety (1%), ataxia (1%), depression (1%), lethargy (1%), myoclonic jerks (1%), slurred speech (1%)

Dermatologic: Rash (2%)

Gastrointestinal: Abdominal discomfort/heartburn (4% to 14%), xerostomia (6%), diarrhea (2%), anorexia (1%), throat discomfort (1%)

Genitourinary: Urinary abnormalities (eg, abnormal ejaculation, retention, urgency, incontinence; 1% to 2%)

Hematologic: Agranulocytosis (1%), eosinophilia (1%), leukocytosis, leukopenia

Hepatic: Liver function tests abnormal (1%)

Neuromuscular & skeletal: Tremor (6%), hypokinesia (4%), rigidity (3%), hyperkinesia (1%), weakness (1%), pain (1%), spasm (1%)

Ocular: Visual disturbances (5%)

Respiratory: Dyspnea (1%), nasal congestion (1%)

Miscellaneous: Diaphoresis (6%), tongue numbness (1%)

Pharmacodynamics/Kinetics

Bioavailability 50% to 60% (not affected by food)

Time to Peak 2.5 hours (range: 1-6 hours)

Protein Binding 97% to serum proteins

Half-Life Elimination Steady state: 12 hours (range: 4-66 hours)

Metabolism Extensively hepatic; forms metabolites with limited or no activity

Excretion Urine (~50%) and feces (30%) with trace amounts of unchanged drug

Available Dosage Forms

Tablet, oral: 25 mg, 50 mg, 100 mg, 200 mg

Clozaril®: 25 mg, 100 mg

Tablet, orally disintegrating, oral:

FazaClo®: 12.5 mg, 25 mg, 100 mg, 150 mg, 200 mg

Dosing

Adult

Schizophrenia: Initial: 12.5 mg once or twice daily; increased, as tolerated, in increments of 25-50 mg/day to a target dose of 300-450 mg/day after 2 weeks; may further titrate in increments not exceeding 100 mg and no more frequently than once or twice weekly. May require doses as high as 600-900 mg/day (maximum dose: 900 mg/day). **Note:** In some efficacy studies, total daily dosage was administered in 3 divided doses.

Suicidal behavior in schizophrenia or schizoaffective disorder: Initial: 12.5 mg once or twice daily; increased, as tolerated, in increments of 25-50 mg/day to a target dose of 300-450 mg/day after 2 weeks; mean dose is ~300 mg/day (range: 12.5-900 mg); treatment duration 2 years then reassess need. **Note:** If no longer a suicide risk, may resume prior antipsychotic therapy after gradually tapering off clozapine over 1-2 weeks.

Termination of therapy: If dosing is interrupted for ≥48 hours, therapy must be reinitiated at 12.5-25 mg/day; may be increased more rapidly than with initial titration, unless cardiopulmonary arrest occurred during initial titration.

In the event of planned termination of clozapine, gradual reduction in dose over a 1- to 2-week period is recommended. If conditions warrant abrupt discontinuation (leukopenia), monitor patient for psychosis and cholinergic rebound (headache, nausea, vomiting, diarrhea).

Geriatric

Schizophrenia: Oral: Experience in the elderly is limited; initial dose should be 12.5-25 mg/day; increase as tolerated by 25 mg/day to desired response. Elderly may require slower titration and daily increases may not be tolerated.

Psychosis/agitation related to Alzheimer's dementia (unlabeled use): Oral: Initial: 12.5 mg/day; if necessary, gradually increase as tolerated not to exceed 75-100 mg/day (Rabins, 2007)

Pediatric Children and Adolescents: Childhood psychosis (unlabeled use): Oral: Initial: 12.5-25 mg/day; increase to a target dose of 25-400 mg/day (Kumra, 2008; Turetz, 1997)

Adjustment for Toxicity

Eosinophilia:

U.S. labeling: Interrupt therapy for eosinophil count >4000/mm^3; may resume therapy when eosinophil count <3000/mm^3

Canadian labeling: Interrupt therapy for eosinophil count >3000/mm^3; may resume therapy when eosinophil count <1000/ mm^3

Moderate leukopenia or granulocytopenia (WBC <3000/mm^3 and/or ANC <1500/mm^3): Discontinue therapy; may rechallenge patient when WBC is >3500/mm^3 and ANC is >2000/mm^3. **Note:** Patient is at greater risk for developing agranulocytosis.

Severe leukopenia or granulocytopenia (WBC <2000/mm^3 and/or ANC <1000/mm^3 [U.S. labeling] or ANC <1500/mm^3 [Canadian labeling]): Discontinue therapy and do not rechallenge patient.

Platelets <50,000/mm^3: Canadian labeling recommends discontinuing therapy

Administration

Oral May be taken without regard to food. Total daily dose may be divided into uneven doses with larger dose administered at bedtime.

Canadian labeling: Maintenance dosing ≤200 mg/day may be administered as single dose in the evening.

Orally-disintegrating tablet: Should be removed from foil blister by peeling apart (do not push tablet through the foil). Remove immediately prior to use. Place tablet in mouth and allow to dissolve; swallow with saliva. If dosing requires splitting tablet, throw unused portion away.

Stability

Storage Store at ≤30°C (86°F).

FazaClo®: Store at 25°C (77°F); excursions permitted to 15°C to 30°C (59°F to 86°F). Protect from moisture; do not remove from package until ready to use.

Monitoring and Teaching Issues

Laboratory Monitoring ECG; WBC (see below), fasting lipid profile and fasting blood glucose/Hgb A_{1c} (prior to treatment, at 3 months, then annually; liver function tests; BMI, personal/family history of obesity; waist circumference (weight should be assessed prior to treatment, at 4 weeks, 8 weeks, 12 weeks, and then at quarterly intervals

WBC and ANC should be obtained at baseline and at least weekly for the first 6 months (26 weeks) of continuous treatment. If counts remain acceptable (WBC ≥3500/mm^3, ANC ≥2000/mm^3) during this time period, then they may be monitored every other week for the next 6 months (26 weeks). If WBC/ANC continue to remain within these acceptable limits after the second 6 months (26 weeks) of therapy, monitoring can be decreased to every 4 weeks. If clozapine is discontinued, a weekly WBC should be conducted for an additional 4 weeks or until WBC is ≥3500/mm^3 and ANC is ≥2000/mm^3. If clozapine therapy is interrupted due to moderate leukopenia, weekly WBC/ANC monitoring is required for 12 months in patients restarted on clozapine treatment. (**Note:** When therapy is interrupted for >3 days, the Canadian labeling recommends weekly hematologic testing for an additional 6 weeks). If therapy is interrupted for reasons other than leukopenia/granulocytopenia, the 6-month time period for initiation of biweekly WBCs may need to be reset. **This determination depends upon the treatment duration, the length of the break in therapy, and whether or not an abnormal blood event occurred.**

Consult manufacturer prescribing information for determination of appropriate WBC/ANC monitoring interval.

Physical Assessment Initiate at lower doses and taper dosage slowly when discontinuing. Instruct patients with diabetes to monitor blood glucose levels closely; may cause hyperglycemia. Be alert to the potential for cardiac abnormalities. Monitor weight prior to treatment and at least monthly. Consider titrating to a different antipsychotic agent for a weight gain ≥5% of initial weight. Review ophthalmic exam periodically and assess results of weekly laboratory tests.

Patient Education Avoid alcohol. Maintain adequate hydration. If you have diabetes, monitor blood glucose levels frequently. You may experience headache, excess drowsiness, dizziness, or blurred vision; constipation; dry mouth, nausea, or vomiting; or postural hypotension. You may be prone to infections; report fever, sore throat, or other possible signs of infection. Report persistent CNS effects (insomnia, depression, altered consciousness); palpitations, rapid heartbeat, or severe dizziness; vision changes; hypersalivation, tearing, or sweating; seizures; chest pain or shortness of breath; excessive fatigue; or worsening of condition.

Dietary Considerations May be taken without regard to food. Some products may contain phenylalanine.

Geriatric Considerations Not recommended for use in nonpsychotic patients (eg, dimentia-related psychotic symptoms). Studies in subjects >65 years of age have not been done. Orthostatic hypotension and sustained tachycardia have been noted in up to 25% of patients taking clozapine; therefore, elderly with cardiovascular disease may be at risk. The anticholinergic effects of clozapine may be prominent in elderly (eg, constipation, confusion, urinary retention).

Breast-Feeding Considerations Clozapine was found to accumulate in breast milk in concentrations higher than the maternal plasma.

Pregnancy Considerations Teratogenic effects were not seen in animal studies. Clozapine crosses the placenta and can be detected in the fetal blood and amniotic fluid. Antipsychotic use during the third trimester of pregnancy has a risk for abnormal muscle movements (extrapyramidal symptoms [EPS]) and withdrawal symptoms in newborns following delivery. Symptoms in the newborn may include agitation, feeding disorder, hypertonia, hypotonia, respiratory distress, somnolence, and tremor; these effects may be self-limiting or require hospitalization. Healthcare providers are encouraged to enroll women 18-45 years of age exposed to clozapine during pregnancy in the Atypical Antipsychotics Pregnancy Registry (1-866-961-2388). Women with amenorrhea associated with use of other antipsychotic agents may return to normal menstruation when switching to clozapine therapy. Reliable contraceptive measures should be employed by women of childbearing potential switching to clozapine therapy.

Related Information

Antipsychotic Agents *on page 1986*

- ◆ **Clozaril®** *see* Clozapine *on page 417*
- ◆ **CMA-676** *see* Gemtuzumab Ozogamicin *on page 863*
- ◆ **CMV-IGIV** *see* Cytomegalovirus Immune Globulin (Intravenous-Human) *on page 451*
- ◆ **CNTO-148** *see* Golimumab *on page 883*
- ◆ **Coagulant Complex Inhibitor** *see* Anti-inhibitor Coagulant Complex *on page 136*
- ◆ **Coagulation Factor VIIa** *see* Factor VIIa (Recombinant) *on page 731*

Codeine (KOE deen)

Index Terms Codeine Phosphate; Codeine Sulfate; Methylmorphine

Generic Availability (U.S.) Yes

Pharmacologic Category Analgesic, Opioid; Antitussive

Medication Safety Issues

Sound-alike/look-alike issues:

Codeine may be confused with Cardene®, Cophene®, Cordran®, iodine, Lodine®

High alert medication: The Institute for Safe Medication Practices (ISMP) includes this medication among its list of drug classes which have a heightened risk of causing significant patient harm when used in error.

Pregnancy Risk Factor C

Lactation Enters breast milk/use caution (AAP rates "compatible"; AAP 2001 update pending)

Use Treatment of mild-to-moderate pain; antitussive in lower doses

Mechanism of Action/Effect Inhibits perception of and response to pain; causes cough supression; produces generalized CNS depression

Contraindications Hypersensitivity to codeine or any component of the formulation; pregnancy (prolonged use or high doses at term)

Warnings/Precautions Use with caution in patients with hypersensitivity reactions to other phenanthrene-derivative opioid agonists (morphine, hydrocodone, hydromorphone, levorphanol, oxycodone, oxymorphone); respiratory diseases including asthma, emphysema, COPD, adrenal insufficiency, biliary tract impairment, CNS depression/coma, head trauma, morbid obesity, prostatic hyperplasia, urinary stricture, thyroid dysfunction, or severe liver or renal insufficiency; some preparations contain sulfites which may cause allergic reactions; tolerance or drug dependence may result from extended use. May obscure diagnosis or clinical course of patients with acute abdominal conditions. May cause CNS depression, which may impair physical or mental abilities; patients must be cautioned about performing tasks which require mental alertness (eg, operating machinery or driving). May cause hypotension; use with caution in patients with hypovolemia, cardiovascular disease (including acute MI), or drugs which may exaggerate hypotensive effects (including phenothiazines or general anesthetics). Use caution in patients with two or more copies of the variant CYP2D6*2 allele; may have extensive conversion to morphine and thus increased opioid-mediated effects.

Not recommended for use for cough control in patients with a productive cough; not recommended as an antitussive for children <2 years of age; the elderly and debilitated patients may be particularly susceptible to adverse effects of narcotics

Not approved for I.V. administration (although this route has been used clinically). If given intravenously, must be given slowly and the patient should be lying down. Rapid intravenous administration of narcotics may increase the incidence of serious adverse effects, in part due to limited opportunity to assess response prior to administration of the full dose. Access to respiratory support should be immediately available.

Concurrent use of agonist/antagonist analgesics may precipitate withdrawal symptoms and/or reduced analgesic efficacy in patients following prolonged therapy with mu opioid agonists. Abrupt discontinuation following prolonged use may also lead to withdrawal symptoms.

Drug Interactions

Metabolism/Transport Effects Substrate of CYP2D6 (major), 3A4 (minor); **Inhibits** CYP2D6 (weak)

Avoid Concomitant Use There are no known interactions where it is recommended to avoid concomitant use.

Decreased Effect

Codeine may decrease the levels/effects of: Pegvisomant

The levels/effects of Codeine may be decreased by: Ammonium Chloride; CYP2D6 Inhibitors (Moderate); CYP2D6 Inhibitors (Strong); Mixed Agonist / Antagonist Opioids

Increased Effect/Toxicity

Codeine may increase the levels/effects of: Alcohol (Ethyl); Alvimopan; CNS Depressants; Desmopressin; Selective Serotonin Reuptake Inhibitors; Thiazide Diuretics

The levels/effects of Codeine may be increased by: Amphetamines; Antipsychotic Agents (Phenothiazines); Droperidol; Somatostatin Analogs; Succinylcholine

Nutritional/Ethanol Interactions

Ethanol: Avoid or limit ethanol (may increase CNS depression).

Herb/Nutraceutical: St John's wort may decrease codeine levels. Avoid valerian, St John's wort, kava kava, gotu kola (may increase CNS depression).

Lab Interactions Some quinolones may produce a false-positive urine screening result for opiates using commercially-available immunoassay kits. This has been demonstrated most consistently for levofloxacin and ofloxacin, but other quinolones have shown cross-reactivity in certain assay kits. Confirmation of positive opiate screens by more specific methods should be considered.

Adverse Reactions

Frequency not defined: ALT increased, AST increased

>10%:

- Central nervous system: Drowsiness
- Gastrointestinal: Constipation

1% to 10%:

- Cardiovascular: Hypotension, tachycardia or bradycardia
- Central nervous system: Confusion, dizziness, false feeling of well being, headache, lightheadedness, malaise, paradoxical CNS stimulation, restlessness
- Dermatologic: Rash, urticaria
- Gastrointestinal: Anorexia, nausea, vomiting, xerostomia
- Genitourinary: Ureteral spasm, urination decreased
- Hepatic: LFTs increased
- Local: Burning at injection site
- Neuromuscular & skeletal: Weakness
- Ocular: Blurred vision
- Respiratory: Dyspnea
- Miscellaneous: Histamine release

Pharmacodynamics/Kinetics

Onset of Action Oral: 0.5-1 hour; I.M.: 10-30 minutes; Peak effect: Oral: 1-1.5 hours; I.M.: 0.5-1 hour

Duration of Action 4-6 hours

Absorption Oral: Adequate

Protein Binding 7%

Half-Life Elimination 2.5-3.5 hours

Metabolism Hepatic to morphine (active)

Excretion Urine (3% to 16% as unchanged drug, norcodeine, and free and conjugated morphine)

Controlled Substance C-II

Available Dosage Forms

Powder, for prescription compounding: USP: 100% (10 g, 25 g)

Tablet, oral: 15 mg, 30 mg, 60 mg

Dosing

Adult & Geriatric Note: These are guidelines and do not represent the maximum doses that may be required in all patients. Doses should be titrated to pain relief/prevention. Doses >1.5 mg/kg body weight are not recommended.

Pain management (analgesic):

Oral, regular release: 30 mg every 4-6 hours as needed; patients with prior opiate exposure may require higher initial doses. Usual range: 15-120 mg every 4-6 hours as needed. **Note:** The American Pain Society recommends an initial dose of 30-60 mg for adults with moderate pain.

Oral, controlled release formulation (Codeine Contin®, not available in U.S.): 50-300 mg every 12 hours. **Note:** A patient's codeine requirement should be established using prompt release formulations; conversion to long acting products may be considered when chronic, continuous treatment is required. Higher dosages should be reserved for use only in opioid-tolerant patients.

I.M., SubQ: 30 mg every 4-6 hours as needed; patients with prior opiate exposure may require higher initial doses. Usual range: 15-120 mg every 4-6 hours as needed; more frequent dosing may be needed

Cough (antitussive): Oral (for nonproductive cough): 10-20 mg/dose every 4-6 hours as needed; maximum: 120 mg/day

Pediatric Note: These are guidelines and do not represent the maximum doses that may be required in all patients. Doses should be titrated to pain relief/prevention. Doses >1.5 mg/kg body weight are not recommended.

Analgesic: Oral, I.M., SubQ: Children: 0.5-1 mg/kg/dose every 4-6 hours as needed; maximum: 60 mg/dose

Antitussive: Oral (for nonproductive cough): Children: 1-1.5 mg/kg/day in divided doses every 4-6 hours as needed: Alternative dose according to age:

2-6 years: 2.5-5 mg every 4-6 hours as needed; maximum: 30 mg/day

6-12 years: 5-10 mg every 4-6 hours as needed; maximum: 60 mg/day

Renal Impairment

Cl_{cr} 10-50 mL/minute: Administer 75% of dose.

Cl_{cr} <10 mL/minute: Administer 50% of dose.

Hepatic Impairment Dosing adjustment is probably necessary in hepatic insufficiency.

Stability

Storage Store injection between 15°C to 30°C; avoid freezing. Do not use if injection is discolored or contains a precipitate. Protect injection from light.

Monitoring and Teaching Issues

Physical Assessment Monitor for effectiveness of pain relief and CNS status prior to treatment and periodically throughout. May cause physical and/or psychological dependence. For inpatients, implement safety measures to prevent falls. Assess patient's physical and/or psychological dependence. Discontinue slowly after prolonged use.

Patient Education May cause physical and/or psychological dependence. Do not use alcohol, sedatives, tranquilizers, antihistamines, or pain medications without consulting prescriber. Maintain adequate hydration, unless instructed to restrict fluid intake. May cause dizziness, drowsiness, confusion, agitation, impaired coordination, or blurred vision; nausea or vomiting; loss of appetite; or constipation (if unresolved, consult prescriber about use of stool softeners). Report confusion, insomnia, excessive nervousness, excessive sedation or drowsiness, or shakiness; acute GI upset; respiratory difficulty or shortness of breath; facial flushing, rapid heartbeat, or palpitations; urinary difficulty; unusual muscle weakness; or vision changes.

Geriatric Considerations The elderly may be particularly susceptible to CNS depression and confusion as well as the constipating effects of narcotics.

Breast-Feeding Considerations Codeine and its metabolite (morphine) are found in breast milk and can be detected in the serum of nursing infants. The relative dose to a nursing infant has been calculated to be ~1% of the weight-adjusted maternal dose. Higher levels of morphine may be found in the breast milk of lactating mothers who are "ultra-rapid metabolizers" of codeine; patients with two or more copies of the variant CYP2D6*2 allele may have extensive conversion to morphine and thus increased opioid-mediated effects. In one case, excessively high serum concentrations of morphine were reported in a breast-fed infant following maternal use of acetaminophen with codeine. The mother was later found to be an "ultra-rapid metabolizer" of codeine; symptoms in the infant included feeding difficulty and lethargy, followed by death. Caution should be used since most persons are not aware if they have the genotype resulting in "ultra-rapid metabolizer" status. When codeine is used in breast-feeding women, it is recommended to use the lowest dose for the shortest duration of time and observe the infant for increased sleepiness, difficulty in feeding or breathing, or limpness.

Pregnancy Considerations Animal reproduction studies have not been conducted. Neonatal abstinence syndrome (NAS) has been observed in the newborn following maternal use of codeine during pregnancy. Symptoms of opiate withdrawal may include excessive crying, diarrhea, fever, hyper-reflexia, irritability, tremors, or vomiting. Perinatal stroke has also been reported.

Related Information

Opioid Analgesics *on page 2003*

- **Codeine, Acetaminophen, Butalbital, and Caffeine** *see* Butalbital, Acetaminophen, Caffeine, and Codeine *on page 261*
- **Codeine and Acetaminophen** *see* Acetaminophen and Codeine *on page 41*
- **Codeine and Butalbital Compound** *see* Butalbital, Aspirin, Caffeine, and Codeine *on page 262*
- **Codeine and Guaifenesin** *see* Guaifenesin and Codeine *on page 891*
- **Codeine, Butalbital, Aspirin, and Caffeine** *see* Butalbital, Aspirin, Caffeine, and Codeine *on page 262*
- **Codeine Phosphate** *see* Codeine *on page 421*
- **Codeine Sulfate** *see* Codeine *on page 421*
- **Cogentin®** *see* Benztropine *on page 202*
- **ColBenemid** *see* Colchicine and Probenecid *on page 426*

Colchicine (KOL chi seen)

U.S. Brand Names Colcrys®

Generic Availability (U.S.) No

Pharmacologic Category Colchicine

Medication Safety Issues

Sound-alike/look-alike issues:

Colchicine may be confused with Cortrosyn®

Medication Guide Available Yes

Pregnancy Risk Factor C

Lactation Enters breast milk/use caution (AAP rates "compatible"; AAP 2001 update pending)

Use Prevention and treatment of acute gout flares; treatment of familial Mediterranean fever (FMF)

Unlabeled/Investigational Use Primary biliary cirrhosis; pericarditis

Mechanism of Action/Effect Reduces the deposition of urate crystals that perpetuates the inflammatory response

Contraindications Concomitant use of a P-glycoprotein (P-gp) or strong CYP3A4 inhibitor in presence of renal or hepatic impairment

Warnings/Precautions Hazardous agent - use appropriate precautions for handling and disposal. Myelosuppression (eg, thrombocytopenia, leukopenia, granulocytopenia, pancytopenia) and aplastic anemia have been reported in patients receiving therapeutic doses. Neuromuscular toxicity (including rhabdomyolysis) has been reported in patients receiving therapeutic doses; patients with renal dysfunction and elderly patients are at increased risk. Concomitant use of cyclosporine, diltiazem, verapamil, fibrates, and statins may increase the risk of myopathy. Clearance is decreased in renal or hepatic impairment; monitor closely for adverse effects/toxicity. Dosage adjustments may be required depending on degree of impairment or indication, and may be affected by the use of concurrent medication (CYP3A4 or P-gp inhibitors). Concurrent use of P-gp or strong CYP3A4 inhibitors is contraindicated in renal impairment; fatal toxicity has been reported. Colchicine does not have analgesic activity and should not be used to treat pain from other causes. Colchicine requires dosage adjustment when used concurrently with protease inhibitor regimens. Colchicine does not have analgesic activity and should not be used to treat pain from other causes.

Drug Interactions

Metabolism/Transport Effects Substrate of CYP3A4 (major), P-glycoprotein; **Induces** CYP2C8 (weak), 2C9 (weak), 2E1 (weak), 3A4 (weak)

Avoid Concomitant Use There are no known interactions where it is recommended to avoid concomitant use.

Decreased Effect

Colchicine may decrease the levels/effects of: Cyanocobalamin; Saxagliptin

The levels/effects of Colchicine may be decreased by: P-Glycoprotein Inducers

Increased Effect/Toxicity

Colchicine may increase the levels/effects of: HMG-CoA Reductase Inhibitors

The levels/effects of Colchicine may be increased by: CYP3A4 Inhibitors (Moderate); CYP3A4 Inhibitors (Strong); Dasatinib; Digoxin; Fibric Acid Derivatives; P-Glycoprotein Inhibitors

Nutritional/Ethanol Interactions

Ethanol: Avoid ethanol.

Food: Cyanocobalamin (vitamin B_{12}): Malabsorption of the substrate. May result in macrocytic anemia or neurologic dysfunction. Grapefruit juice may increase colchicine serum concentrations.

Herb/Nutraceutical: Vitamin B_{12} absorption may be decreased by colchicine.

Lab Interactions May cause false-positive results in urine tests for erythrocytes or hemoglobin

Adverse Reactions

>10%: Gastrointestinal: Gastrointestinal disorders including abdominal pain, cramping, nausea, vomiting (up to 26%), diarrhea (up to 23%)

1% to 10%: Respiratory: Pharyngolaryngeal pain (3%)

Pharmacodynamics/Kinetics

Onset of Action Oral: Pain relief: ~18-24 hours

Bioavailability ~45%

Time to Peak Serum: Oral: 0.5-3 hours

Protein Binding ~39%

Half-Life Elimination 27-31 hours (multiple oral doses; young, healthy volunteers)

Metabolism Hepatic via CYP3A4; 3 metabolites (2 primary, 1 minor)

Excretion Urine (40% to 65% as unchanged drug); enterohepatic recirculation and biliary excretion also possible

Available Dosage Forms

Tablet, oral: 0.6 mg

Colcrys®: 0.6 mg

Dosing

Adult

Familial Mediterranean fever (FMF): Oral: 1.2-2.4 mg/day in 1-2 divided doses; titration: Increase or decrease dose in 0.3 mg increments based on efficacy or adverse effects; maximum: 2.4 mg/day

Gout: Oral:

Flare treatment: Initial: 1.2 mg at the first sign of flare, followed in 1 hour with a single dose of 0.6 mg (maximum: 1.8 mg within 1 hour). Patients receiving prophylaxis therapy may receive treatment dosing; wait 12 hours before resuming prophylaxis dose. **Note:** Current FDA-approved dose for gout flare is substantially lower than what has been historically used clinically. Doses larger than the currently recommended dosage for gout flare have not been proven to be more effective.

Prophylaxis: 0.6 mg once or twice daily; maximum: 1.2 mg/day

Pericarditis (unlabeled use): Oral: 0.6 mg twice daily (Antman, 2004)

Primary biliary cirrhosis (unlabeled use): Oral: 0.6 mg twice daily (Kaplan, 2005); **Note:** Use reserved for patients refractory to ursodiol.

Dosage adjustment for concomitant therapy with CYP3A4 or P-glycoprotein (P-gp) inhibitors: *Dosage adjustment also required in patients receiving CYP3A4 or P-gp inhibitors up to 14 days prior to initiation of colchicine.* **Note:** Treatment of gout flare with colchicine is not recommended in patients receiving prophylactic colchicine and CYP3A4 inhibitors.

Coadministration of **strong** CYP3A4 inhibitor (eg, atazanavir, clarithromycin, darunavir, indinavir, itraconazole, ketoconazole, lopinavir/ritonavir, nefazodone, nelfinavir, ritonavir, saquinavir, telithromycin, tipranavir):

FMF: Maximum dose: 0.6 mg/day (0.3 mg twice daily)

Gout prophylaxis:

If original dose is 0.6 mg twice daily, adjust dose to 0.3 mg once daily

If original dose is 0.6 mg once daily, adjust dose to 0.3 mg every other day

Gout flare treatment: Initial: 0.6 mg, followed in 1 hour by a single dose of 0.3 mg; do not repeat for at least 3 days

Coadministration of **moderate** CYP3A4 inhibitor (eg, aprepitant, diltiazem, erythromycin, fluconazole, fosamprenavir, grapefruit juice, verapamil):

FMF: Maximum dose: 1.2 mg/day (0.6 mg twice daily)

Gout prophylaxis:

If original dose is 0.6 mg twice daily, adjust dose to 0.3 mg twice daily **or** 0.6 mg once daily

If original dose is 0.6 mg once daily, adjust dose to 0.3 mg once daily

Gout flare treatment: 1.2 mg as a single dose; do not repeat for at least 3 days

Coadministration of P-gp inhibitor (eg, cyclosporine, ranolazine):

FMF: Maximum dose: 0.6 mg/day (0.3 mg twice daily)

Gout prophylaxis:

If original dose is 0.6 mg twice daily, adjust dose to 0.3 mg once daily

If original dose is 0.6 mg once daily, adjust dose to 0.3 mg every other day

Gout flare treatment: Initial: 0.6 mg as a single dose; do not repeat for at least 3 days

Geriatric Use caution; reduce prophylactic daily dose by 50% in individuals >70 years (Terkeltaub, 2009)

Pediatric

Familial Mediterranean fever (FMF): Oral:

Children 4-6 years: 0.3-1.8 mg/day in 1-2 divided doses

Children 6-12 years: 0.9-1.8 mg/day in 1-2 divided doses

Children >12 years: Refer to adult dosing.

Gout prophylaxis/treatment: Oral: Children >16 years: Refer to adult dosing.

Renal Impairment Concurrent use of colchicine and P-gp or strong CYP3A4 inhibitors is **contraindicated** in renal impairment. Fatal toxicity has been reported. Treatment of gout flares is not recommended in patients with renal impairment receiving prophylactic colchicine.

FMF:

Cl_{cr} 30-80 mL/minute: Monitor closely for adverse effects; dose reduction may be necessary.

Cl_{cr} <30 mL/minute: Initial dose: 0.3 mg/day; use caution if dose titrated; monitor for adverse effects.

Dialysis: 0.3 mg as a single dose; use caution if dose titrated; dosing can be increased with close monitoring; monitor for adverse effects. Not removed by dialysis.

Gout prophylaxis:

Cl_{cr} 30-80 mL/minute: Dosage adjustment not required; monitor closely for adverse effects.

Cl_{cr} <30 mL/minute: Initial dose: 0.3 mg/day; use caution if dose titrated; monitor for adverse effects.

Dialysis: 0.3 mg twice weekly; monitor closely for adverse effects.

Gout flare treatment:

Cl_{cr} 30-80 mL/minute: Dosage adjustment not required; monitor closely for adverse effects.

Cl_{cr} <30 mL/minute: Dosage reduction not required but may be considered; treatment course should not be repeated more frequently than every 14 days.

Dialysis: 0.6 mg as a single dose; treatment course should not be repeated more frequently than every 14 days. Not removed by dialysis.

Hemodialysis: Avoid chronic use of colchicine.

Hepatic Impairment Concurrent use of colchicine and P-glycoprotein or strong CYP3A4 inhibitors is **contraindicated** in hepatic impairment. Fatal toxicity has been reported. Treatment of gout flare with colchicine is not recommended in patients with hepatic impairment receiving prophylactic colchicine.

FMF:

Mild-to-moderate impairment: Use caution; monitor closely for adverse effects.

Severe impairment: Consider dosage reduction.

Gout prophylaxis:

Mild-to-moderate impairment: Dosage adjustment not required; monitor closely for adverse effects.

Severe impairment: Dosage adjustment should be considered.

Gout flare treatment:

Mild-to-moderate impairment: Dosage adjustment not required; monitor closely for adverse effects.

Severe impairment: Dosage reduction not required but may be considered; treatment course should not be repeated more frequently than every 14 days.

Administration

Oral Administer orally with water and maintain adequate fluid intake. May be administered without regard to meals.

Stability

Storage Store at 20°C to 25°C (68°F to 77°F). Protect from light.

Monitoring and Teaching Issues

Laboratory Monitoring CBC, renal and hepatic function on a regular basis

Patient Education Consult prescriber about a low-purine diet. Maintain adequate hydration, unless instructed to restrict fluid intake. Avoid grapefruit and grapefruit juice. You may experience diarrhea, nausea, vomiting, anorexia, or hair loss (reversible). Stop medication and report to prescriber if severe vomiting, watery or bloody diarrhea, or abdominal pain occurs. Report muscle tremors or weakness, numbness or tingling in fingers or toes, fatigue, numbness or tingling in fingers or toes, easy bruising or bleeding, yellowing of eyes or skin, or pale stool or dark urine.

Dietary Considerations May be taken without regard to meals. May need to supplement with vitamin B_{12}. Avoid grapefruit juice.

Geriatric Considerations Colchicine appears to be more toxic in older adults, particularly in the presence of renal, gastrointestinal, or cardiac disease. The most predictable oral side effects are gastrointestinal (eg, vomiting, abdominal pain, and nausea). If colchicine is stopped at this point, other more severe adverse effects may be avoided, such as bone marrow suppression, peripheral neuritis, etc.

Breast-Feeding Considerations Colchicine enters breast milk; exclusively breast-fed infants are expected to receive <10% of the weight-adjusted maternal dose (limited data).

Pregnancy Considerations Adverse events were observed in animal reproduction studies. Colchicine crosses the human placenta. Use during pregnancy in the treatment of familial Mediterranean fever has not shown an increase in miscarriage, stillbirth, or teratogenic effects (limited data).

Additional Information Oral colchicine had been available as an unapproved medication without FDA-approved prescribing information. In August 2009, the FDA approved prescribing information for a brand name colchicine product. The currently approved prescribing information recommends a lower than historically used dosage for the treatment of acute gout. This recommendation is based on data from the AGREE trial. In this trial, low-dose colchicine (1.8 mg total) had similar efficacy to high dose colchicine (4.8 mg total). Additionally, the low dosage regimen was associated with a lower incidence (26% vs 77%) of GI adverse events. Parenteral formulation of colchicine is no longer available in the U.S.; serious life-threatening complications (eg, neutropenia, acute renal failure, thrombocytopenia, heart failure) associated with intravenous colchicine have occurred prior to market withdrawal. The risks associated with oral colchicine are believed to be lower compared to intravenous use.

Colchicine and Probenecid (KOL chi seen & proe BEN e sid)

Index Terms ColBenemid; Probenecid and Colchicine

Generic Availability (U.S.) Yes

Pharmacologic Category Anti-inflammatory Agent; Antigout Agent; Uricosuric Agent

Pregnancy Risk Factor C

Lactation

Colchicine: Compatible

Probenecid: Excretion in breast milk unknown

Use Treatment of chronic gouty arthritis when complicated by frequent, recurrent acute attacks of gout

Available Dosage Forms

Tablet: Colchicine 0.5 mg and probenecid 0.5 g

Dosing

Adult & Geriatric Gout: Oral: 1 tablet/day for 1 week, then 1 tablet twice daily thereafter

Renal Impairment Probenecid may not be effective in patients with chronic renal insufficiency particularly when Cl_{cr} is ≤30 mL/minute.

Administration

Oral Do not initiate therapy until acute attack has subsided.

Monitoring and Teaching Issues

Physical Assessment See individual agents.

Patient Education See individual agents.

Related Information

Colchicine *on page 423*

Probenecid *on page 1508*

◆ **Colcrys®** *see* Colchicine *on page 423*

Colesevelam (koh le SEV a lam)

U.S. Brand Names Welchol®

Generic Availability (U.S.) No

Pharmacologic Category Antilipemic Agent, Bile Acid Sequestrant

Pregnancy Risk Factor B

Lactation Excretion in breast milk unknown

Use Management of elevated LDL in primary hypercholesterolemia (Fredrickson type IIa) when used alone or in combination with an HMG-CoA reductase inhibitor; management of heterozygous familial hypercholesterolemia (heFH) in adolescent patients (males and postmenarchal females 10-17 years of age) when used alone or in combination with an HMG-CoA reductase inhibitor, in patients who after an adequate trial of dietary therapy have LDL-C ≥190 mg/dL or LDL-C ≥160 mg/dL with positive family history of premature cardiovascular disease (CVD) or with two or more CVD risk factors; improve glycemic control in type 2 diabetes mellitus (noninsulin dependent, NIDDM) in conjunction with diet, exercise, and insulin or oral antidiabetic agents

Mechanism of Action/Effect Colesevelam binds bile acids including glycocholic acid in the intestine, impeding their reabsorption. Increases the fecal loss of bile salt-bound LDL-C.

Contraindications History of bowel obstruction; serum triglyceride concentration >500 mg/dL; history of hypertriglyceridemia-induced pancreatitis

Warnings/Precautions Use with caution in treating patients with serum triglyceride concentrations >300 mg/dL (may cause increased concentrations) or in patients susceptible to fat-soluble vitamin deficiencies. Discontinue if triglyceride concentrations exceed 500 mg/dL or hypertriglyceridemia-induced pancreatitis occurs. Use in patients with gastroparesis, other severe GI motility disorders, or a history of major GI tract surgery is not recommended due to constipating effects of colesevelam. Patients with dysphagia or swallowing disorders should use the oral suspension form of colesevelam due to large tablet size and risk for esophageal obstruction.

Minimal effects are seen on HDL-C and triglyceride levels. Secondary causes of hypercholesterolemia should be excluded before initiation. Colesevelam has not been studied in Fredrickson Type I, III, IV, or V dyslipidemias. Colesevelam is not indicated for the management of type 1 diabetes, particularly in the acute management (eg, DKA). It is also not indicated in type 2 diabetes mellitus as monotherapy and must be used as an adjunct to diet, exercise, and glycemic control with insulin or oral antidiabetic agents. Combination with dipeptidyl peptidase 4 inhibitors or thiazolidinediones has not been studied extensively.

Some products may contain phenylalanine.

Drug Interactions

Avoid Concomitant Use There are no known interactions where it is recommended to avoid concomitant use.

Decreased Effect

Colesevelam may decrease the levels/effects of: Amiodarone; Antidiabetic Agents (Thiazolidinedione); Chenodiol; Contraceptives (Estrogens); Contraceptives (Progestins); Corticosteroids (Oral); Ethinyl Estradiol; Ezetimibe; GlyBURIDE; Leflunomide; Loop Diuretics; Methotrexate; Niacin; Nonsteroidal Anti-Inflammatory Agents; Norethindrone; Phenytoin; Pravastatin; Propranolol; Raloxifene; Tetracycline Derivatives; Thiazide Diuretics; Thyroid Products; Ursodiol; Vitamin D Analogs; Vitamin K Antagonists

Increased Effect/Toxicity There are no known significant interactions involving an increase in effect.

Adverse Reactions

>10%: Gastrointestinal: Constipation (11%)

2% to 10%:

Gastrointestinal: Dyspepsia (8%)

Neuromuscular & skeletal: Weakness (4%), myalgia (2%)

Respiratory: Pharyngitis (3%)

Incidence less than or equal to placebo: Infection, headache, pain, back pain, abdominal pain, flu syndrome, flatulence, diarrhea, nausea, sinusitis, rhinitis, cough

Pharmacodynamics/Kinetics

Onset of Action Peak effect: Therapeutic: ~2 weeks

Absorption Insignificant

Half-Life Elimination 0.05% was excreted in the urine after 1 month of chronic dosing

Excretion Urine (0.05%) after 1 month of chronic dosing

Available Dosage Forms

Granules for suspension, oral:

Welchol®: 3.75 g/packet (30s)

Tablet, oral:

Welchol®: 625 mg

Dosing

Adult & Geriatric

Dyslipidemia: Oral: 1.875 g (oral suspension or 3 tablets) twice daily **or** 3.75 g (oral suspension or 6 tablets) once daily

Type 2 diabetes: *Combination therapy with insulin or oral antidiabetic agents:* Oral: 1.875 g (oral suspension or 3 tablets) twice daily **or** 3.75 g (oral suspension or 6 tablets) once daily

Pediatric Dyslipidemia (heterozygous familial hypercholesterolemia): Children 10-17 years (males and postmenarchal females): Oral:

Once-daily dosing: 3.75 g (oral suspension or 6 tablets)

Twice-daily dosing: 1.875 g (oral suspension or 3 tablets)

Note: Due to large tablet size, oral suspension is recommended in pediatric patients.

Administration

Oral Educate the patient on dietary guidelines.

Tablets: Administer with meal(s) and a liquid. Due to tablet size, it is recommended that any patient who has trouble swallowing tablets should use the oral suspension form.

Granules for oral suspension: Administer with meal(s). Mix powder with water prior to administration; not to be taken in dry form (to avoid GI distress). One packet should be added to 1/2-1 cup (4-8 ounces) of water and mixed well.

Stability

Storage Store at room temperature. Protect from moisture.

Monitoring and Teaching Issues

Laboratory Monitoring Serum cholesterol, LDL, and triglyceride levels should be obtained before initiating treatment and periodically thereafter (in accordance with NCEP guidelines).

Patient Education Many other medications should be taken 1 hour before or 4 hours after colesevelam. You may experience constipation. Report persistent GI upset, skeletal or muscle pain or weakness, or respiratory difficulties.

Dietary Considerations Should be taken with meal(s) and a liquid. Follow dietary guidelines. Some products may contain phenylalanine.

Geriatric Considerations The definition of and, therefore, when to treat hyperlipidemia in elderly is a controversial issue. The National Cholesterol Education Program recommends that all adults maintain a plasma cholesterol <160 mg/dL. Elderly with one additional risk factor, goal LDL would be <130 mg/dL. It is the authors' belief that pharmacologic treatment be reserved for those who are unable to obtain a desirable plasma cholesterol concentration by diet alone and for whom the benefits of treatment are believed to outweigh the potential adverse effects, drug interactions, and cost of treatment.

Pregnancy Considerations There are no adequate and well-controlled studies in pregnant women; use only in pregnancy if clearly needed.

Related Information

Hyperlipidemia Management *on page 2046*

◆ **Colestid®** *see* Colestipol *on page 428*

◆ **Colestid® Flavored** *see* Colestipol *on page 428*

Colestipol (koe LES ti pole)

U.S. Brand Names Colestid®; Colestid® Flavored

Index Terms Colestipol Hydrochloride

Generic Availability (U.S.) Yes

Pharmacologic Category Antilipemic Agent, Bile Acid Sequestrant

Medication Safety Issues

Sound-alike/look-alike issues:

Colestipol may be confused with calcitriol

Pregnancy Risk Factor C

Lactation Not recommended

Use Adjunct in management of primary hypercholesterolemia; regression of arteriolosclerosis; relief of pruritus associated with elevated levels of bile acids; possibly used to decrease plasma half-life of digoxin in toxicity

Available Dosage Forms

Granules for suspension, oral: 5 g/scoop (500 g); 5 g/packet (30s, 90s)

Colestid®: 5 g/scoop (300 g, 500 g); 5 g/packet (30s, 90s)

Colestid® Flavored: 5 g/scoop (450 g); 5 g/packet (60s)

Tablet, oral: 1 g

Colestid®: 1 g

Dosing

Adult & Geriatric Dyslipidemia: Oral:

Granules: 5-30 g/day given once or in divided doses 2-4 times/day; initial dose: 5 g 1-2 times/day; increase by 5 g at 1- to 2-month intervals

Tablets: 2-16 g/day; initial dose: 2 g 1-2 times/day; increase by 2 g at 1- to 2-month intervals

Administration

Oral Dry powder should be added to at least 90 mL of liquid and stirred until completely mixed. Other drugs should be administered at least 1 hour before or 4 hours after colestipol.

Monitoring and Teaching Issues

Physical Assessment Monitor bowel function. Be alert to potential for constipation or hemorrhoid problems.

Patient Education Take granules with 3-4 oz of water or fruit juice. Rinse glass with small amount of water to ensure full dose is taken. Take tablets one at a time. Other medications should be taken 1 hour before or 4 hours after colestipol. You may experience constipation, drowsiness, or dizziness. Report acute gastric pain, tarry stools, or respiratory difficulty.

Related Information

Hyperlipidemia Management *on page 2046*

◆ **Colestipol Hydrochloride** *see* Colestipol *on page 428*

◆ **Colocort®** *see* Hydrocortisone (Topical) *on page 920*

◆ **Colyte®** *see* Polyethylene Glycol-Electrolyte Solution *on page 1474*

◆ **CombiPatch®** *see* Estradiol and Norethindrone *on page 674*

◆ **Combivent®** *see* Ipratropium and Albuterol *on page 1011*

◆ **Combivir®** *see* Zidovudine and Lamivudine *on page 1894*

◆ **Combunox™ [DSC]** *see* Oxycodone and Ibuprofen *on page 1384*

◆ **Commit® [OTC]** *see* Nicotine *on page 1312*

◆ **Compazine** *see* Prochlorperazine *on page 1512*

◆ **Compound F** *see* Hydrocortisone (Systemic) *on page 917*

◆ **Compound F** *see* Hydrocortisone (Topical) *on page 920*

◆ **Compound S** *see* Zidovudine *on page 1890*

- **Compound S, Abacavir, and Lamivudine** *see* Abacavir, Lamivudine, and Zidovudine *on page* 32
- **Compoz® [OTC]** *see* DiphenhydrAMINE (Systemic) *on page* 543
- **Compro®** *see* Prochlorperazine *on page* 1512
- **Comtan®** *see* Entacapone *on page* 627
- **Comvax®** *see* *Haemophilus* b Conjugate and Hepatitis B Vaccine *on page* 892
- **Concerta®** *see* Methylphenidate *on page* 1204
- **Conjugated Estrogen** *see* Estrogens (Conjugated/Equine, Systemic) *on page* 682
- **Conjugated Estrogen** *see* Estrogens (Conjugated/Equine, Topical) *on page* 686
- **Constulose** *see* Lactulose *on page* 1053
- **Copaxone®** *see* Glatiramer Acetate *on page* 869
- **Copegus®** *see* Ribavirin *on page* 1571
- **Copolymer-1** *see* Glatiramer Acetate *on page* 869
- **Cordarone®** *see* Amiodarone *on page* 98
- **Coreg®** *see* Carvedilol *on page* 304
- **Coreg CR®** *see* Carvedilol *on page* 304
- **Corgard®** *see* Nadolol *on page* 1278
- **Coricidin® HBP Cough & Cold [OTC]** *see* Dextromethorphan and Chlorpheniramine *on page* 513
- **Cortaid® Advanced [OTC]** *see* Hydrocortisone (Topical) *on page* 920
- **Cortaid® Intensive Therapy [OTC]** *see* Hydrocortisone (Topical) *on page* 920
- **Cortaid® Maximum Strength [OTC]** *see* Hydrocortisone (Topical) *on page* 920
- **Cortef®** *see* Hydrocortisone (Systemic) *on page* 917
- **Cortenema®** *see* Hydrocortisone (Topical) *on page* 920
- **CortiCool® [OTC]** *see* Hydrocortisone (Topical) *on page* 920
- **Cortifoam®** *see* Hydrocortisone (Topical) *on page* 920
- **Cortisol** *see* Hydrocortisone (Systemic) *on page* 917
- **Cortisol** *see* Hydrocortisone (Topical) *on page* 920
- **Cortizone-10® Hydratensive Healing [OTC]** *see* Hydrocortisone (Topical) *on page* 920
- **Cortizone-10® Hydratensive Soothing [OTC]** *see* Hydrocortisone (Topical) *on page* 920
- **Cortizone-10® Intensive Healing Eczema [OTC]** *see* Hydrocortisone (Topical) *on page* 920
- **Cortizone-10® Maximum Strength [OTC]** *see* Hydrocortisone (Topical) *on page* 920
- **Cortizone-10® Maximum Strength Cooling Relief [OTC]** *see* Hydrocortisone (Topical) *on page* 920
- **Cortizone-10® Maximum Strength Easy Relief [OTC]** *see* Hydrocortisone (Topical) *on page* 920
- **Cortizone-10® Maximum Strength Intensive Healing Formula [OTC]** *see* Hydrocortisone (Topical) *on page* 920
- **Cortizone-10® Plus Maximum Strength [OTC]** *see* Hydrocortisone (Topical) *on page* 920
- **Corvert®** *see* Ibutilide *on page* 943
- **Cosmegen®** *see* DACTINomycin *on page* 455
- **Co-Trimoxazole** *see* Sulfamethoxazole and Trimethoprim *on page* 1686
- **Coumadin®** *see* Warfarin *on page* 1877
- **Covera-HS®** *see* Verapamil *on page* 1858
- **Coviracil** *see* Emtricitabine *on page* 613
- **Cozaar®** *see* Losartan *on page* 1133
- **CP358774** *see* Erlotinib *on page* 652
- **CPM** *see* Cyclophosphamide *on page* 434
- **CPT-11** *see* Irinotecan *on page* 1015
- **CPZ** *see* ChlorproMAZINE *on page* 360
- **Creon®** *see* Pancrelipase *on page* 1400
- **Crestor®** *see* Rosuvastatin *on page* 1613
- **Crinone®** *see* Progesterone *on page* 1514
- **Critic-Aid® Clear AF [OTC]** *see* Miconazole (Topical) *on page* 1224
- **Crixivan®** *see* Indinavir *on page* 967
- **Cromoglycic Acid** *see* Cromolyn (Systemic, Oral Inhalation) *on page* 429

Cromolyn (Systemic, Oral Inhalation) (KROE moe lin)

U.S. Brand Names Gastrocrom®
Index Terms Cromoglycic Acid; Cromolyn Sodium; Disodium Cromoglycate; DSCG
Generic Availability (U.S.) No
Pharmacologic Category Mast Cell Stabilizer

Pregnancy Risk Factor B

Lactation Excretion in breast milk unknown/use caution

Use

Inhalation: May be used as an adjunct in the prophylaxis of allergic disorders, including asthma; prevention of exercise-induced bronchospasm

Oral: Systemic mastocytosis

Unlabeled/Investigational Use Oral: Food allergy, treatment of inflammatory bowel disease

Mechanism of Action/Effect Prevents the mast cell release of histamine, leukotrienes, and slow-reacting substance of anaphylaxis

Contraindications Hypersensitivity to cromolyn or any component of the formulation; acute asthma attacks

Warnings/Precautions Severe anaphylactic reactions may occur rarely; cromolyn is a prophylactic drug with no benefit for acute situations; caution should be used when withdrawing the drug or tapering the dose as symptoms may reoccur; use with caution in patients with a history of cardiac arrhythmias. Dosage of oral product should be decreased with hepatic or renal dysfunction.

Drug Interactions

Avoid Concomitant Use There are no known interactions where it is recommended to avoid concomitant use.

Decreased Effect There are no known significant interactions involving a decrease in effect.

Increased Effect/Toxicity There are no known significant interactions involving an increase in effect.

Adverse Reactions Frequency not defined.

Cardiovascular: Angioedema, chest pain, edema, flushing, palpitation, premature ventricular contractions, tachycardia

Central nervous system: Anxiety, behavior changes, convulsions, depression, dizziness, fatigue, hallucinations, headache, irritability, insomnia, lethargy, migraine, nervousness, hypoesthesia, postprandial lightheadedness, psychosis

Dermatologic: Erythema, photosensitivity, pruritus, purpura, rash, urticaria

Gastrointestinal: Abdominal pain, constipation, diarrhea, dyspepsia, dysphagia, esophagospasm, flatulence, glossitis, nausea, stomatitis, vomiting

Genitourinary: Dysuria, urinary frequency

Hematologic: Neutropenia, pancytopenia, polycythemia

Hepatic: Liver function test abnormal

Local: Burning

Neuromuscular & skeletal: Arthralgia, leg stiffness, leg weakness, myalgia, paresthesia

Otic: Tinnitus

Respiratory: Dyspnea, pharyngitis

Miscellaneous: Lupus erythematosus

Pharmacodynamics/Kinetics

Onset of Action Response to treatment: Oral: May occur within 2-6 weeks

Absorption

Inhalation: ~8% reaches lungs upon inhalation; well absorbed

Oral: <1% of dose absorbed

Time to Peak Serum: Inhalation: ~15 minutes

Half-Life Elimination 80-90 minutes

Excretion Urine and feces (equal amounts as unchanged drug); exhaled gases (small amounts)

Available Dosage Forms

Solution, for nebulization: 20 mg/2 mL (60s, 120s)

Solution, oral:

Gastrocrom®: 100 mg/5 mL (96s)

Dosing

Adult & Geriatric

Asthma: For chronic control of asthma, taper frequency to the lowest effective dose (ie, 4 times/day to 3 times/day to twice daily). **Note:** Not effective for immediate relief of symptoms in acute asthmatic attacks; must be used at regular intervals for 2-4 weeks to be effective.

Nebulization solution: Initial: 20 mg 4 times/day; usual dose: 20 mg 3-4 times/day

Prophylaxis of bronchospasm (allergen- or exercise-induced):

Note: Administer 10-15 minutes prior to exercise or allergen exposure but no longer than 1 hour before:

Nebulization solution: Single dose of 20 mg

Mastocytosis: Oral: 200 mg 4 times/day; given 1/2 hour prior to meals and at bedtime. If control of symptoms is not seen within 2-3 weeks, dose may be increased to a maximum 40 mg/kg/day

Food allergy (unlabeled use), inflammatory bowel disease (unlabeled use): Oral: Initial dose: 200 mg 4 times/day; may double the dose if effect is not satisfactory within 2-3 weeks; up to 400 mg 4 times/day

Pediatric

Asthma: inhalation: For chronic control of asthma, taper frequency to the lowest effective dose (ie, 4 times/day to 3 times/day to twice daily): **Note:** Not effective for immediate relief of symptoms in acute asthmatic attacks; must be used at regular intervals for 2-4 weeks to be effective.

Nebulization solution: Children >2 years: Initial: 20 mg 4 times/day; usual dose: 20 mg 3-4 times/day

Prevention of allergen- or exercise-induced bronchospasm: Note: Administer 10-15 minutes prior to exercise or allergen exposure but no longer than 1 hour before:
Nebulization solution: Children >2 years: Refer to adult dosing.

Systemic mastocytosis: Oral:
Children 2-12 years: 100 mg 4 times/day; not to exceed 40 mg/kg/day; given 1/2 hour prior to meals and at bedtime
Children >12 years: Refer to adult dosing.

Food allergy (unlabeled use), inflammatory bowel disease (unlabeled use): Oral:
Children <2 years: Not recommended
Children 2-12 years: Initial dose: 100 mg 4 times/day; may double the dose if effect is not satisfactory within 2-3 weeks; not to exceed 40 mg/kg/day
Children >12 years: Refer to adult dosing.
Note: Once desired effect is achieved, dose may be tapered to lowest effective dose

Renal Impairment Specific guidelines not available; consider lower dose of oral product.

Hepatic Impairment Specific guidelines not available; consider lower dose of oral product.

Administration

Oral Oral solution: Open ampul and squeeze contents into glass of water; stir well. Administer at least 30 minutes before meals and at bedtime.

Stability

Storage Store at room temperature of 15°C to 30°C (59°F to 86°F). Protect from light. Do not use oral solution if solution becomes discolored or forms a precipitate.

Monitoring and Teaching Issues

Laboratory Monitoring Periodic pulmonary function

Physical Assessment This is prophylactic therapy, not to be used for acute situations.

Patient Education

Oral: Take at least 30 minutes before meals. You may experience dizziness, nervousness, diarrhea, headache, or muscle pain. Report persistent insomnia; skin rash; abdominal pain or difficulty swallowing; unusual cough, bronchospasm, or respiratory difficulty; or if condition worsens or fails to improve.

Nebulizer: Prepare nebulizer according to package instructions. Clear as much mucus as possible before use. Rinse mouth following each use to reduce unpleasant aftertaste. Report if symptoms worsen or condition fails to improve.

Dietary Considerations Oral: Should be taken at least 30 minutes before meals.

Breast-Feeding Considerations No data available on whether cromolyn enters into breast milk or clinical effects on the infant. Use of cromolyn is not considered a contraindication to breast-feeding.

Pregnancy Considerations Adverse events were not observed in animal reproduction studies. No data available on whether cromolyn crosses the placenta or clinical effects on the fetus. Available evidence suggests safe use during pregnancy.

Related Information

Asthma *on page 2015*

- **Cromolyn Sodium** *see* Cromolyn (Systemic, Oral Inhalation) *on page 429*
- **Crystalline Penicillin** *see* Penicillin G (Parenteral/Aqueous) *on page 1433*
- **CS-747** *see* Prasugrel *on page 1493*
- **CsA** *see* CycloSPORINE (Ophthalmic) *on page 442*
- **CsA** *see* CycloSPORINE (Systemic) *on page 437*
- **CTLA-4Ig** *see* Abatacept *on page 33*
- **CTX** *see* Cyclophosphamide *on page 434*
- **Cutivate®** *see* Fluticasone (Topical) *on page 803*
- **Cuvposa™** *see* Glycopyrrolate *on page 881*
- **CyA** *see* CycloSPORINE (Ophthalmic) *on page 442*
- **CyA** *see* CycloSPORINE (Systemic) *on page 437*

Cyanocobalamin (sye an oh koe BAL a min)

U.S. Brand Names CaloMist™; Ener-B® [OTC]; Nascobal®; Twelve Resin-K [OTC]

Index Terms Vitamin B_{12}

Generic Availability (U.S.) Yes: Excludes nasal spray

Pharmacologic Category Vitamin, Water Soluble

Pregnancy Risk Factor A/C (dose exceeding RDA recommendation); C (intranasal)

Lactation Enters breast milk/compatible

Use Treatment of pernicious anemia; vitamin B_{12} deficiency due to dietary deficiencies or malabsorption diseases, inadequate secretion of intrinsic factor, and inadequate utilization of B_{12} (eg, during neoplastic treatment); increased B_{12} requirements due to pregnancy, thyrotoxicosis, hemorrhage, malignancy, liver or kidney disease

CaloMist™: Maintenance of vitamin B_{12} concentrations after initial correction in patients with B_{12} deficiency without CNS involvement

Available Dosage Forms

Injection, solution: 1000 mcg/mL (1 mL, 10 mL, 30 mL)
Lozenge, oral: 50 mcg (100s); 100 mcg (100s); 250 mcg (100s, 250s); 500 mcg (100s, 250s)
Lozenge, sublingual: 500 mcg (100s)

Solution, intranasal:
CaloMist™: 25 mcg/spray (10.7 mL)
Nascobal®: 500 mcg/spray (2.3 mL)
Tablet, for buccal application/oral/sublingual:
Twelve Resin-K [OTC]: 1000 mcg
Tablet, oral: 50 mcg, 100 mcg, 250 mcg, 500 mcg, 1000 mcg
Ener-B® [OTC]: 100 mcg, 500 mcg, 1000 mcg
Tablet, sublingual: 1000 mcg, 2500 mcg, 5000 mcg
Tablet, timed release, oral: 1000 mcg
Ener-B® [OTC]: 1500 mcg

Dosing

Adult & Geriatric

Recommended intake: 2.4 mcg/day
Pregnancy: 2.6 mcg/day
Lactation: 2.8 mcg/day

Vitamin B_{12} deficiency:
Intranasal:
Nascobal®: 500 mcg in one nostril once weekly
CaloMist™: Maintenance therapy (following correction of vitamin B_{12} deficiency): 25 mcg in each nostril daily (50 mcg/day). If inadequate response, 25 mcg in each nostril twice daily (100 mcg/day).
Oral: 250 mcg/day
I.M., deep SubQ: Initial: 30 mcg/day for 5-10 days; maintenance: 100-200 mcg/month

Pernicious anemia: I.M., deep SubQ (administer concomitantly with folic acid if needed, 1 mg/day for 1 month): 100 mcg/day for 6-7 days; if improvement, administer same dose on alternate days for 7 doses, then every 3-4 days for 2-3 weeks; once hematologic values have returned to normal, maintenance dosage: 100 mcg/month. **Note:** Alternative dosing of 1000 mcg/day for 5 days (followed by 500-1000 mcg/month) has been used.
Hematologic remission (without evidence of nervous system involvement):
Intranasal (Nascobal®): 500 mcg in one nostril once weekly
Oral: 1000-2000 mcg/day
I.M., SubQ: 100-1000 mcg/month

Schilling test: I.M.: 1000 mcg

Pediatric

Adequate intake:
Children:
0-6 months: 0.4 mcg/day
7-12 months: 0.5 mcg/day

Recommended intake:
Children:
1-3 years: 0.9 mcg/day
4-8 years: 1.2 mcg/day
9-13 years: 1.8 mcg/day
Children >14 years: Refer to adult dosing.

Vitamin B_{12} deficiency: I.M., deep SubQ: Dosage in children is not well established: 0.2 mcg/kg for 2 days, followed by 1000 mcg/day for 2-7 days, followed by 100 mcg/week for one month; for malabsorptive causes of B_{12} deficiency, monthly maintenance doses of 100 mcg have been recommended **or** as an alternative 100 mcg/day for 10-15 days, then once or twice weekly for several months

Pernicious anemia: I.M., deep SubQ (administer concomitantly with folic acid if needed, 1 mg/day for 1 month): 30-50 mcg/day for 2 or more weeks (to a total dose of 1000-5000 mcg), then follow with 100 mcg/month as maintenance dosage

Administration

Oral Not recommended due to variable absorption; however, oral therapy of 1000-2000 mcg/day has been effective for anemia if I.M./SubQ routes refused or not tolerated.

I.M. I.M. or deep SubQ are preferred routes of administration.

I.V. Not recommended

Other Intranasal: Nasal spray:
Nascobal®: Prior to initial dose, activate (prime) spray nozzle by pumping unit quickly and firmly until first appearance of spray, then prime twice more. The unit must be reprimed once immediately before each subsequent use. Administer 1 hour before or after ingestion of hot foods/liquids.
CaloMist™: Prime unit by spraying 7 times. If ≥5 days since use, reprime with 2 sprays. Separate from other intranasal medications by several hours.

Monitoring and Teaching Issues

Laboratory Monitoring Erythrocyte and reticulocyte count, hemoglobin, hematocrit; monitor potassium concentrations during early therapy

Physical Assessment Provide patient appropriate nutritional counseling.

Patient Education Pernicious anemia may require treatment for life. Report skin rash, muscle cramps, or weakness.

◆ **Cyanokit®** *see* Hydroxocobalamin *on page* 928

◆ **Cyclessa®** *see* Ethinyl Estradiol and Desogestrel *on page* 695

Cyclobenzaprine (sye kloe BEN za preen)

U.S. Brand Names Amrix®; Fexmid®; Flexeril®

Index Terms Cyclobenzaprine Hydrochloride

Generic Availability (U.S.) Yes: Excludes capsule

Pharmacologic Category Skeletal Muscle Relaxant

Medication Safety Issues

Sound-alike/look-alike issues:

Cyclobenzaprine may be confused with cycloSERINE, cyproheptadine

Flexeril® may be confused with Floxin®

International issues:

Flexin: Brand name for cyclobenzaprine [Chile], but also the brand name for diclofenac [Argentina] and orphenadrine [Israel]

Flexin [Chile] may be confused with Floxin brand name for flunarizine [Thailand], norfloxacin [South Africa], ofloxacin [U.S., Canada], and perfloxacin [Philippines]; Fluoxin brand name for fluoxetine [Czech Republic]

Beers Criteria medication: This drug may be inappropriate for use in geriatric patients (high severity risk).

Pregnancy Risk Factor B

Lactation Excretion in breast milk unknown/use caution

Use Treatment of muscle spasm associated with acute, painful musculoskeletal conditions

Unlabeled/Investigational Use Treatment of muscle spasm associated with acute temporomandibular joint pain (TMJ)

Mechanism of Action/Effect Centrally-acting skeletal muscle relaxant pharmacologically related to tricyclic antidepressants; reduces tonic somatic motor activity influencing both alpha and gamma motor neurons

Contraindications Hypersensitivity to cyclobenzaprine or any component of the formulation; during or within 14 days of MAO inhibitors; hyperthyroidism; congestive heart failure; arrhythmias; heart block or conduction disturbances; acute recovery phase of MI

Warnings/Precautions May cause CNS depression, which may impair physical or mental abilities; patients must be cautioned about performing tasks which require mental alertness (eg, operating machinery or driving). Cyclobenzaprine shares the toxic potentials of the tricyclic antidepressants (including arrhythmias, tachycardia, and conduction time prolongation) and the usual precautions of tricyclic antidepressant therapy should be observed; use with caution in patients with urinary hesitancy or retention, angle-closure glaucoma or increased intraocular pressure, hepatic impairment, or in the elderly. This class of medication is poorly tolerated by the elderly due to anticholinergic effects, sedation, and weakness; efficacy is questionable at dosages tolerated by elderly patients (Beers Criteria). Extended release capsules not recommended for use in mild-to-severe hepatic impairment or in the elderly. Do not use concomitantly or within 14 days after MAO inhibitors; combination may cause hypertensive crisis, severe convulsions. Effects may be potentiated when used with other CNS depressants or ethanol.

Drug Interactions

Metabolism/Transport Effects Substrate of CYP1A2 (major), 2D6 (minor), 3A4 (minor)

Avoid Concomitant Use

Avoid concomitant use of Cyclobenzaprine with any of the following: MAO Inhibitors

Decreased Effect

Cyclobenzaprine may decrease the levels/effects of: Acetylcholinesterase Inhibitors (Central)

The levels/effects of Cyclobenzaprine may be decreased by: Acetylcholinesterase Inhibitors (Central); Peginterferon Alfa-2b

Increased Effect/Toxicity

Cyclobenzaprine may increase the levels/effects of: Alcohol (Ethyl); Anticholinergics; CNS Depressants; MAO Inhibitors; Methotrimeprazine

The levels/effects of Cyclobenzaprine may be increased by: Conivaptan; CYP1A2 Inhibitors (Moderate); CYP1A2 Inhibitors (Strong); Methotrimeprazine; Pramlintide

Nutritional/Ethanol Interactions

Food: Food increases bioavailability (peak plasma concentrations increased by 35% and area under the curve by 20%) of the extended release capsule.

Ethanol: Avoid ethanol (may increase CNS depression).

Herb/Nutraceutical: Avoid valerian, kava kava, gotu kola (may increase CNS depression).

Lab Interactions May cause false-positive serum TCA screen.

Adverse Reactions

>10%:

Central nervous system: Drowsiness (29% to 39%), dizziness (1% to 11%)

Gastrointestinal: Xerostomia (21% to 32%)

1% to 10%:

Central nervous system: Fatigue (1% to 6%), headache (1% to 5%), confusion (1% to 3%), irritability (1% to 3%), mental acuity decreased (1% to 3%), nervousness (1% to 3%), somnolence (1% to 2%)

Gastrointestinal: Dyspepsia (≤4%), abdominal pain (1% to 3%), constipation (1% to 3%), diarrhea (1% to 3%), nausea (1% to 3%), unpleasant taste (1% to 3%)

Neuromuscular & skeletal: Weakness (1% to 3%)

Ocular: Blurred vision (1% to 3%)

Respiratory: Pharyngitis (1% to 3%), upper respiratory infection (1% to 3%)

Pharmacodynamics/Kinetics

Bioavailability 33% to 55%

Time to Peak Extended release capsule: 7-8 hours

Half-Life Elimination Range: 8-37 hours; Immediate release tablet: 18 hours; Extended release capsule: 32-33 hours

Metabolism Hepatic via CYP3A4, 1A2, and 2D6; may undergo enterohepatic recirculation

Excretion Urine (as inactive metabolites); feces (as unchanged drug)

Available Dosage Forms

Capsule, extended release, oral:

Amrix®: 15 mg, 30 mg

Tablet, oral: 5 mg, 10 mg

Fexmid®: 7.5 mg

Flexeril®: 5 mg, 10 mg

Dosing

Adult Muscle spasm: Oral: **Note:** Do not use longer than 2-3 weeks

Capsule, extended release: Usual: 15 mg once daily; some patients may require up to 30 mg once daily

Tablet, immediate release: Initial: 5 mg 3 times/day; may increase up to 10 mg 3 times/day if needed

Geriatric

Capsule, extended release: Use not recommended

Tablet, immediate release: Initial: 5 mg; titrate dose slowly and consider less frequent dosing

Pediatric Muscle spasm: Oral: Tablet, immediate release: Children ≥15 years: Refer to adult dosing.

Hepatic Impairment

Capsule, extended release: Mild-to-severe impairment: Use not recommended.

Tablet, immediate release:

Mild impairment: Initial: 5 mg; use with caution; titrate slowly and consider less frequent dosing

Moderate-to-severe impairment: Use not recommended

Administration

Oral Extended release capsules: Administer at the same time each day. Do not crush or chew.

Stability

Storage

Amrix®, Flexeril®: Store at 25°C (77°F); excursions permitted to 15°C to 30°C (59°F to 86°F).

Fexmid®: Store at 20°C to 25°C (68°F to 77°F).

Monitoring and Teaching Issues

Physical Assessment May cause significant CNS depression. Caution patients about sedation.

Patient Education Do not use alcohol. You may experience drowsiness, dizziness, lightheadedness, or urinary retention. Report excessive drowsiness or skin rash.

Geriatric Considerations High doses in the elderly caused drowsiness and dizziness; therefore, use the lowest dose possible. Because cyclobenzaprine causes anticholinergic effects, it may not be the skeletal muscle relaxant of choice in the elderly.

This medication is considered to be potentially inappropriate in this patient population (Beers Criteria severity: High).

Pregnancy Considerations Teratogenic effects were not observed in animal studies. There are no adequate and well-controlled studies in pregnant women. Use during pregnancy only if clearly needed.

◆ **Cyclobenzaprine Hydrochloride** *see* Cyclobenzaprine *on page* 432

Cyclophosphamide (sye kloe FOS fa mide)

Index Terms CPM; CTX; CYT; Cytoxan; Neosar

Generic Availability (U.S.) Yes

Pharmacologic Category Antineoplastic Agent, Alkylating Agent

Medication Safety Issues

Sound-alike/look-alike issues:

Cyclophosphamide may be confused with cycloSPORINE, ifosfamide

Cytoxan may be confused with cefOXitin, Centoxin®, Ciloxan®, cytarabine, CytoGam®, Cytosar®, Cytosar-U®, Cytotec®

High alert medication: This medication is in a class the Institute for Safe Medication Practices (ISMP) includes among its list of drugs which have a heightened risk of causing significant patient harm when used in error.

Pregnancy Risk Factor D

Lactation Enters breast milk/contraindicated

Use

Oncology-related uses: Treatment of Hodgkin's lymphoma, non-Hodgkin's lymphoma (including Burkitt's lymphoma), chronic lymphocytic leukemia (CLL), chronic myelocytic leukemia (CML), acute myelocytic leukemia (AML), acute lymphocytic leukemia (ALL), mycosis fungoides, multiple myeloma, neuroblastoma, retinoblastoma; breast cancer; ovarian adenocarcinoma

Nononcology uses: Treatment of refractory nephrotic syndrome in children

Unlabeled/Investigational Use

Oncology-related uses: Ewing's sarcoma, rhabdomyosarcoma, Wilms tumor, ovarian germ cell tumors, small cell lung cancer, testicular cancer, pheochromocytoma, bone marrow transplantation conditioning regimen

Nononcology uses: Severe rheumatoid disorders, Wegener's granulomatosis, myasthenia gravis, multiple sclerosis, systemic lupus erythematosus, lupus nephritis, autoimmune hemolytic anemia, idiopathic thrombocytic purpura (ITP), and antibody-induced pure red cell aplasia; juvenile idiopathic arthritis (JIA)

Mechanism of Action/Effect Interferes with the normal function of DNA by alkylation and cross-linking the strands of DNA, and by possible protein modification; cyclophosphamide also possesses potent immunosuppressive activity; note that cyclophosphamide must be metabolized to its active form in the liver

Contraindications Hypersensitivity to cyclophosphamide or any component of the formulation; severely depressed bone marrow function

Warnings/Precautions Hazardous agent - use appropriate precautions for handling and disposal. Dosage adjustment may be needed for renal or hepatic failure. Hemorrhagic cystitis may occur; increased hydration and frequent voiding is recommended. Immunosuppression may occur; monitor for infections. May cause cardiotoxicity (HF, usually with higher doses); may potentiate the cardiotoxicity of anthracyclines. May impair fertility; interferes with oogenesis and spermatogenesis. Secondary malignancies (usually delayed) have been reported

Drug Interactions

Metabolism/Transport Effects **Substrate** of CYP2A6 (minor), 2B6 (major), 2C9 (minor), 2C19 (minor), 3A4 (minor); **Inhibits** CYP3A4 (weak); **Induces** CYP2B6 (weak), 2C8 (weak), 2C9 (weak)

Avoid Concomitant Use

Avoid concomitant use of Cyclophosphamide with any of the following: BCG; Belimumab; Etanercept; Natalizumab; Pimecrolimus; Roflumilast; Tacrolimus (Topical); Vaccines (Live)

Decreased Effect

Cyclophosphamide may decrease the levels/effects of: BCG; Cardiac Glycosides; Sipuleucel-T; Vaccines (Inactivated); Vaccines (Live); Vitamin K Antagonists

The levels/effects of Cyclophosphamide may be decreased by: CYP2B6 Inducers (Strong); Echinacea

Increased Effect/Toxicity

Cyclophosphamide may increase the levels/effects of: Leflunomide; Natalizumab; Succinylcholine; Vaccines (Live); Vitamin K Antagonists

The levels/effects of Cyclophosphamide may be increased by: Allopurinol; Belimumab; Conivaptan; CYP2B6 Inhibitors (Moderate); CYP2B6 Inhibitors (Strong); Denosumab; Etanercept; Pentostatin; Pimecrolimus; Quazepam; Roflumilast; Tacrolimus (Topical); Trastuzumab

Nutritional/Ethanol Interactions Herb/Nutraceutical: Avoid black cohosh, dong quai in estrogen-dependent tumors.

Lab Interactions Increased uric acid in serum and urine; false-positive Pap test; suppression of some skin tests

Adverse Reactions

>10%:

Dermatologic: Alopecia (40% to 60%) but hair will usually regrow although it may be a different color and/or texture. Hair loss usually begins 3-6 weeks after the start of therapy.

Endocrine & metabolic: Fertility: May cause sterility; interferes with oogenesis and spermatogenesis; may be irreversible in some patients; gonadal suppression (amenorrhea)

Gastrointestinal: Nausea and vomiting, usually beginning 6-10 hours after administration; anorexia, diarrhea, mucositis, and stomatitis are also seen

Genitourinary: Severe, potentially fatal acute hemorrhagic cystitis (7% to 40%)

Hematologic: Thrombocytopenia and anemia are less common than leukopenia

Onset: 7 days

Nadir: 10-14 days

Recovery: 21 days

1% to 10%:

Cardiovascular: Facial flushing

Central nervous system: Headache

Dermatologic: Skin rash

Respiratory: Nasal congestion occurs when I.V. doses are administered too rapidly; patients experience runny eyes, rhinorrhea, sinus congestion, and sneezing during or immediately after the infusion.

Pharmacodynamics/Kinetics

Absorption Oral: Well absorbed

Bioavailability >75%

Time to Peak Serum: Oral: ~1 hour

Protein Binding 10% to 60%

Half-Life Elimination 3-12 hours

Metabolism Hepatic to active metabolites acrolein, 4-aldophosphamide, 4-hydroperoxycyclophosphamide, and nor-nitrogen mustard

Excretion Urine (<30% as unchanged drug, 85% to 90% as metabolites)

Available Dosage Forms

Injection, powder for reconstitution: 500 mg, 1 g, 2 g

Tablet, oral: 25 mg, 50 mg

Dosing

Adult Details concerns dosing in combination regimens should also be consulted.

Single I.V. doses: 400-1800 mg/m^2 (30-50 mg/kg) per treatment course (1-5 days) which can be repeated at 2-4 week intervals

Continuous I.V. daily doses: 60-120 mg/m^2 (1-2.5 mg/kg) per day

Malignancy: Oral: Usual range (in the manufacturer's labeling): 1-5 mg/kg/day (initial and maintenance dosing)

Breast cancer (unlabeled dosing; combination chemotherapy): Oral:

CEF: 75 mg/m^2/day days 1-14 every 28 days (Levine, 1998)

CMF: 100 mg/m^2/day days 1-14 every 28 days (Bonadonna, 1995; Levine, 1998)

Nephrotic syndrome (refractory; unlabeled use): Oral: 2.5-3 mg/kg/day every day for 60-90 days (when refractory or intolerant to corticosteroid treatment)

JIA/vasculitis (unlabeled use): I.V.: 10 mg/kg every 2 weeks

SLE (unlabeled use): I.V.: 500 mg/m^2 every month; may increase up to a maximum dose of 1 g/m^2 every month (Austin, 1986)

Autologous BMT (unlabeled use): IVPB: 50 mg/kg/dose x 4 days **or** 60 mg/kg/dose for 2 days; total dose is usually divided over 2-4 days

High-dose BMT (unlabeled use):

I.V.:

60 mg/kg/day for 2 days (total dose: 120 mg/kg)

50 mg/kg/day for 4 days (total dose: 200 mg/kg)

1.8 g/m^2/day for 4 days (total dose: 7.2 g/m^2)

Continuous I.V.:

1.5 g/m^2/24 hours for 96 hours (total dose: 6 g/m^2)

1875 mg/m^2/24 hours for 72 hours (total dose: 5625 mg/m^2)

Note: Duration of infusion is 1-24 hours; generally combined with other high-dose chemotherapeutic drugs, lymphocyte immune globulin, or total body irradiation (TBI).

Geriatric Details concerns dosing in combination regimens should also be consulted: Initial and maintenance for induction: 1-2 mg/kg/day; adjust for renal clearance.

Pediatric Details concerns dosing in combination regimens should also be consulted.

Chemotherapy: Refer to adult dosing.

Malignancy: Oral: Usual range (in the manufacturer's labeling): 1-5 mg/kg/day (initial and maintenance dosing)

Nephrotic syndrome: Oral: 2.5-3 mg/kg/day every day for 60-90 days (when refractory or intolerant to corticosteroid treatment)

JIA/vasculitis (unlabeled use): Refer to adult dosing.

SLE (unlabeled use): I.V.: 500 mg/m^2 every month; may increase up to a maximum dose of 1 g/m^2 every month (Austin, 1986)

Renal Impairment The FDA-approved labeling states there is insufficient evidence to recommend dosage adjustment and therefore, does not contain renal dosing adjustment guidelines. The following guidelines have been used by some clinicians (Aronoff, 2007): Children and Adults:

Cl_{cr} <10 mL/minute: Administer 75% of normal dose

Hemodialysis effects: Moderately dialyzable (20% to 50%)

Administer 50% of dose posthemodialysis

Continuous ambulatory peritoneal dialysis (CAPD): Administer 75% of normal dose

Continuous renal replacement therapy (CRRT): Administer 100% of normal dose

Hepatic Impairment The pharmacokinetics of cyclophosphamide are not significantly altered in the presence of hepatic insufficiency. The FDA-approved labeling does not contain hepatic dosing adjustment guidelines. The following guidelines have been used by some clinicians (Floyd, 2006):

Serum bilirubin 3.1-5 mg/dL or transaminases >3 times ULN: Administer 75% of dose

Serum bilirubin >5 mg/mL: Avoid use

Administration

Oral Tablets are not scored and should not be cut or crushed. To minimize the risk of bladder irritation, do not administer tablets at bedtime.

I.V. IVPB or continuous intravenous infusion; I.V. infusions may be administered over 1-24 hours. Doses >500 mg to approximately 2 g may be administered over 20-30 minutes.

To minimize bladder toxicity, increase normal fluid intake during and for 1-2 days after cyclophosphamide dose. Most adult patients will require a fluid intake of at least 2 L/day. High-dose regimens should be accompanied by vigorous hydration with or without mesna therapy.

Stability

Reconstitution Reconstitute vials with SWI, NS, or D_5W to a concentration of 20 mg/mL.

Storage Store intact vials of powder at room temperature of 15°C to 30°C (59°F to 86°F). Reconstituted solutions are stable for 24 hours at room temperature and 6 days under refrigeration 2°C to 8°C (36°F to 46°F). Further dilutions in D_5W or NS are stable for 24 hours at room temperature (25°C) and 6 days at refrigeration.

Monitoring and Teaching Issues

Laboratory Monitoring CBC with differential, platelet count, ESR, BUN, UA, serum electrolytes, serum creatinine

Physical Assessment Assess other drugs patient may be taking that may increase or prolong nephrotoxicity and cardiotoxicity. Note infusion specifics in Administration, including recommendations for pre- and posthydration. Infusion site must be monitored to prevent extravasation. Assess results of urinalysis, BUN, and serum creatinine (detect nephrotoxicity); CBC with differential and platelet count (detect myelosuppression). Monitor for hemorrhagic cystitis, leukopenia, and renal tubular necrosis prior to each infusion and regularly during therapy. Teach patient importance of adequate hydration.

Patient Education Take during or after meals; do not take at night. Maintain adequate hydration unless instructed to restrict fluid intake and void frequently to reduce incidence of bladder irritation. You will be more susceptible to infection. May cause loss of hair (reversible, although regrowth hair may be different color or texture), infertility or amenorrhea, nausea or vomiting, headache, nasal congestion or cold symptoms, or mouth sores. Report any difficulty or pain with urination; chest pain, rapid heartbeat, or palpitations; easy bruising or bleeding; unusual rash; persistent nausea or vomiting; swelling of extremities; respiratory difficulty; or unusual fatigue.

Dietary Considerations Tablets should be administered during or after meals.

Geriatric Considerations Toxicity to immunosuppressives is increased in the elderly. Start with lowest recommended adult doses. Signs of infection, such as fever and WBC rise, may not occur. Lethargy and confusion may be more prominent signs of infection; adjust dose for renal function.

Additional Information In patients with CYP2B6 G516T variant allele, cyclophosphamide metabolism is markedly increased; metabolism is not influenced by CYP2C9 and CYP2C19 isotypes.

◆ **Cycloset®** *see* Bromocriptine *on page 231*

◆ **Cycloset®** *see* Bromocriptine *on page 231*

◆ **Cyclosporin A** *see* CycloSPORINE (Ophthalmic) *on page 442*

◆ **Cyclosporin A** *see* CycloSPORINE (Systemic) *on page 437*

CycloSPORINE (Systemic) (SYE kloe spor een)

U.S. Brand Names Gengraf®; Neoral®; SandIMMUNE®

Index Terms CsA; CyA; Cyclosporin A

Generic Availability (U.S.) Yes

Pharmacologic Category Calcineurin Inhibitor; Immunosuppressant Agent

Medication Safety Issues

Sound-alike/look-alike issues:

CycloSPORINE may be confused with cyclophosphamide, Cyklokapron®, cycloSERINE

CycloSPORINE modified (Neoral®, Gengraf®) may be confused with cycloSPORINE non-modified (SandIMMUNE®)

Gengraf® may be confused with Prograf®

Neoral® may be confused with Neurontin®, Nizoral®

SandIMMUNE® may be confused with SandoSTATIN®

Pregnancy Risk Factor C

Lactation Enters breast milk/not recommended

Use Prophylaxis of organ rejection in kidney, liver, and heart transplants, has been used with azathioprine and/or corticosteroids; severe, active rheumatoid arthritis (RA) not responsive to methotrexate alone; severe, recalcitrant plaque psoriasis in nonimmunocompromised adults unresponsive to or unable to tolerate other systemic therapy

Unlabeled/Investigational Use Allogenic stem cell transplants for prevention and treatment of graft-versus-host disease; also used in some cases of severe autoimmune disease (eg, SLE) that are resistant to corticosteroids and other therapy; focal segmental glomerulosclerosis; severe ulcerative colitis

Mechanism of Action/Effect Inhibits T-lymphocytes and lymphokine production and release in a reversible manner.

Contraindications Hypersensitivity to cyclosporine or any component of the formulation. I.V. cyclosporine is contraindicated in hypersensitivity to polyoxyethylated castor oil (Cremophor® EL).

Rheumatoid arthritis and psoriasis: Abnormal renal function, uncontrolled hypertension, malignancies. Concomitant treatment with PUVA or UVB therapy, methotrexate, other immunosuppressive agents, coal tar, or radiation therapy are also contraindications for use in patients with psoriasis.

Warnings/Precautions Hazardous agent - use appropriate precautions for handling and disposal. **[U.S. Boxed Warning]: Renal impairment, including structural kidney damage has occurred (when used at high doses); monitor renal function closely.** Elevations in serum creatinine and BUN generally respond to dosage reductions. Use caution with other potentially nephrotoxic drugs (eg, acyclovir, aminoglycoside antibiotics, amphotericin B, ciprofloxacin). **[U.S. Boxed Warning]: Increased risk of lymphomas and other malignancies, particularly those of the skin;** risk is related to intensity/duration of therapy and the use of >1 immunosuppressive agent; all patients should avoid excessive sun/UV light exposure. **[U.S. Boxed Warning]: Increased risk of infection; fatal infections have been reported.** Latent viral infections may be activated (including BK virus which is associated with nephropathy) and result in serious adverse effects. **[U.S. Boxed Warning]: May cause hypertension.** Use caution when changing dosage forms. **[U.S. Boxed Warning]: Cyclosporine (modified) has increased bioavailability as compared to cyclosporine (non-modified) and cannot be used interchangeably without close monitoring.** Monitor cyclosporine concentrations closely following the addition, modification, or deletion of other medications; live, attenuated vaccines may be less effective; use should be avoided. Increased hepatic enzymes and bilirubin have occurred (when used at high doses); improvement usually seen with dosage reduction.

Transplant patients: To be used initially with corticosteroids. May cause significant hyperkalemia and hyperuricemia, seizures (particularly if used with high dose corticosteroids), and encephalopathy. Other neurotoxic events (eg, optic disc edema including papilledema and visual impairment) have been reported rarely. Make dose adjustments based on cyclosporine blood concentrations. **[U.S. Boxed Warning]: Adjustment of dose should only be made under the direct supervision of an experienced physician.** Anaphylaxis has been reported with I.V. use; reserve for patients who cannot take oral form. **[U.S. Boxed Warning]: Risk of skin cancer may be increased in transplant patients.** Due to the increased risk for nephrotoxicity in renal transplantation, avoid using standard doses of cyclosporine in combination with everolimus; reduced cyclosporine doses are recommended; monitor cyclosporine concentrations closely. Cyclosporine and everolimus combination therapy may increase the risk for proteinuria. Cyclosporine combined with either everolimus or sirolimus may increase the risk for thrombotic microangiopathy/thrombotic thrombocytopenic purpura/hemolytic uremic syndrome (TMA/TTP/HUS).

Psoriasis: Patients should avoid excessive sun exposure; safety and efficacy in children <18 years of age have not been established. **[U.S. Boxed Warning]: Risk of skin cancer may be increased with a history of PUVA and possibly methotrexate or other immunosuppressants, UVB, coal tar, or radiation.**

Rheumatoid arthritis: Safety and efficacy for use in juvenile idiopathic arthritis (JIA) have not been established. If receiving other immunosuppressive agents, radiation or UV therapy, concurrent use of cyclosporine is not recommended.

Products may contain corn oil, ethanol, or propylene glycol; injection also contains Cremophor® EL (polyoxyethylated castor oil), which has been associated with rare anaphylactic reactions.

Drug Interactions

Metabolism/Transport Effects Substrate of CYP3A4 (major), P-glycoprotein; **Inhibits** CYP2C9 (weak), CYP3A4 (moderate), P-glycoprotein

Avoid Concomitant Use

Avoid concomitant use of CycloSPORINE (Systemic) with any of the following: Aliskiren; BCG; Bosentan; Dronedarone; Natalizumab; Pimecrolimus; Pitavastatin; Roflumilast; Silodosin; Sitaxentan; Tacrolimus; Tacrolimus (Systemic); Tacrolimus (Topical); Tolvaptan; Topotecan; Vaccines (Live)

Decreased Effect

CycloSPORINE (Systemic) may decrease the levels/effects of: BCG; GlyBURIDE; Mycophenolate; Sipuleucel-T; Vaccines (Inactivated); Vaccines (Live)

The levels/effects of CycloSPORINE (Systemic) may be decreased by: Armodafinil; Ascorbic Acid; Barbiturates; Bosentan; CarBAMazepine; CYP3A4 Inducers (Strong); Deferasirox; Dexamethasone; Dexamethasone (Systemic); Echinacea; Efavirenz; Fibric Acid Derivatives; Griseofulvin; Imipenem; MethylPREDNISolone; Modafinil; Nafcillin; Orlistat; P-Glycoprotein Inducers; Phenytoin; PrednisoLONE; PrednisoLONE (Systemic); PredniSONE; Probucol; Rifamycin Derivatives; Somatostatin Analogs; St Johns Wort; Sulfinpyrazone [Off Market]; Sulfonamide Derivatives; Terbinafine; Vitamin E

Increased Effect/Toxicity

CycloSPORINE (Systemic) may increase the levels/effects of: Aliskiren; Ambrisentan; Bosentan; Calcium Channel Blockers (Dihydropyridine); Calcium Channel Blockers (Nondihydropyridine); Cardiac Glycosides; Caspofungin; Colchicine; CYP3A4 Substrates; Dabigatran Etexilate; Dexamethasone; Dexamethasone (Systemic); DOXOrubicin; Dronedarone; Eplerenone; Etoposide; Etoposide Phosphate; Everolimus; Ezetimibe; FentaNYL; Fibric Acid Derivatives; Halofantrine; HMG-CoA Reductase Inhibitors; Imipenem; Leflunomide; Lurasidone; Methotrexate; MethylPREDNISolone; Minoxidil; Minoxidil (Systemic); Minoxidil (Topical); Natalizumab; P-Glycoprotein Substrates; Pitavastatin; PrednisoLONE; PrednisoLONE (Systemic); PredniSONE; Protease Inhibitors; Ranolazine; Repaglinide; Rivaroxaban; Salmeterol; Saxagliptin; Silodosin; Sirolimus; Sitaxentan; Tacrolimus; Tacrolimus (Systemic); Tacrolimus (Topical); Tolvaptan; Topotecan; Vaccines (Live); Vilazodone

The levels/effects of CycloSPORINE (Systemic) may be increased by: ACE Inhibitors; Aminoglycosides; Amiodarone; Amphotericin B; Androgens; Antifungal Agents (Azole Derivatives, Systemic); Bromocriptine; Calcium Channel Blockers (Nondihydropyridine); Carvedilol; Conivaptan; CYP3A4 Inhibitors (Moderate); CYP3A4 Inhibitors (Strong); Dasatinib; Denosumab; Dexamethasone; Dexamethasone (Systemic); Ezetimibe; Fluconazole; GlyBURIDE; Grapefruit Juice; Imatinib; Imipenem; Macrolide Antibiotics; Melphalan; Methotrexate; MethylPREDNISolone; Metoclopramide; MetroNIDAZOLE; MetroNIDAZOLE (Systemic); Nonsteroidal Anti-Inflammatory Agents; Norfloxacin; Omeprazole; P-Glycoprotein Inhibitors; Pimecrolimus; PrednisoLONE; PrednisoLONE (Systemic); PredniSONE; Protease Inhibitors; Pyrazinamide; Quinupristin; Roflumilast; Sirolimus; Sulfonamide Derivatives; Tacrolimus; Tacrolimus (Systemic); Tacrolimus (Topical); Temsirolimus; Trastuzumab

Nutritional/Ethanol Interactions

Food: Grapefruit juice increases cyclosporine serum concentrations.

Herb/Nutraceutical: Avoid St John's wort; as an enzyme inducer, it may increase the metabolism of and decrease plasma levels of cyclosporine; organ rejection and graft loss have been reported. Avoid cat's claw, echinacea (have immunostimulant properties).

Lab Interactions Specific whole blood, HPLC assay for cyclosporine may be falsely elevated if sample is drawn from the same line through which dose was administered (even if flush has been administered and/or dose was given hours before).

Adverse Reactions Adverse reactions reported with systemic use, including rheumatoid arthritis, psoriasis, and transplantation (kidney, liver, and heart). Percentages noted include the highest frequency regardless of indication/dosage. Frequencies may vary for specific conditions or formulation.

>10%:

Cardiovascular: Hypertension (8% to 53%), edema (5% to 14%)
Central nervous system: Headache (2% to 25%)
Dermatologic: Hirsutism (21% to 45%), hypertrichosis (5% to 19%)
Endocrine & metabolic: Triglycerides increased (15%), female reproductive disorder (9% to 11%)
Gastrointestinal: Nausea (23%), diarrhea (3% to 13%), gum hyperplasia (2% to 16%), abdominal discomfort (<1% to 15%), dyspepsia (2% to 12%)
Neuromuscular & skeletal: Tremor (7% to 55%), paresthesia (1% to 11%), leg cramps/muscle contractions (2% to 12%)
Renal: Renal dysfunction/nephropathy (10% to 38%), creatinine increased (16% to ≥50%)
Respiratory: Upper respiratory infection (1% to 14%)
Miscellaneous: Infection (3% to 25%)

Kidney, liver, and heart transplant only (≤2% unless otherwise noted):

Cardiovascular: Flushes (<1% to 4%), MI
Central nervous system: Convulsions (1% to 5%), anxiety, confusion, fever, lethargy
Dermatologic: Acne (1% to 6%), brittle fingernails, hair breaking, pruritus
Endocrine & metabolic: Gynecomastia (<1% to 4%), hyperglycemia
Gastrointestinal: Nausea (2% to 10%), vomiting (2% to 10%), diarrhea (3% to 8%), abdominal discomfort (<1% to 7%), cramps (0% to 4%), anorexia, constipation, gastritis, mouth sores, pancreatitis, swallowing difficulty, upper GI bleed, weight loss
Hematologic: Leukopenia (<1% to 6%), anemia, thrombocytopenia
Hepatic: Hepatotoxicity (<1% to 7%)
Neuromuscular & skeletal: Paresthesia (1% to 3%), joint pain, muscle pain, tingling, weakness
Ocular: Conjunctivitis, visual disturbance
Otic: Hearing loss, tinnitus
Renal: Hematuria
Respiratory: Sinusitis (<1% to 7%)
Miscellaneous: Lymphoma (<1% to 6%), allergic reactions, hiccups, night sweats

Rheumatoid arthritis only (1% to <3% unless otherwise noted):

Cardiovascular: Hypertension (8%), edema (5%), chest pain (4%), arrhythmia (2%), abnormal heart sounds, cardiac failure, MI, peripheral ischemia
Central nervous system: Dizziness (8%), pain (6%), insomnia (4%), depression (3%), migraine (2%), anxiety, hypoesthesia, emotional lability, impaired concentration, malaise, nervousness, paranoia, somnolence, vertigo
Dermatologic: Purpura (3%), abnormal pigmentation, angioedema, cellulitis, dermatitis, dry skin, eczema, folliculitis, nail disorder, pruritus, skin disorder, urticaria
Endocrine & metabolic: Menstrual disorder (3%), breast fibroadenosis, breast pain, diabetes mellitus, goiter, hot flashes, hyperkalemia, hyperuricemia, hypoglycemia, libido increased/decreased
Gastrointestinal: Vomiting (9%), flatulence (5%), gingivitis (4%), gum hyperplasia (2%), constipation, dry mouth, dysphagia, enanthema, eructation, esophagitis, gastric ulcer, gastritis, gastroenteritis, gingival bleeding, glossitis, peptic ulcer, salivary gland enlargement, taste perversion, tongue disorder, tooth disorder, weight loss/gain
Genitourinary: Leukorrhea (1%), abnormal urine, micturition urgency, nocturia, polyuria, pyelonephritis, urinary incontinence, uterine hemorrhage
Hematologic: Anemia, leukopenia
Hepatic: Bilirubinemia
Neuromuscular & skeletal: Paresthesia (8%), tremor (8%), leg cramps/muscle contractions (2%), arthralgia, bone fracture, joint dislocation, myalgia, neuropathy, stiffness, synovial cyst, tendon disorder, weakness
Ocular: Abnormal vision, cataract, conjunctivitis, eye pain
Otic: Tinnitus, deafness, vestibular disorder
Renal: BUN increased, hematuria, renal abscess
Respiratory: Cough (5%), dyspnea (5%), sinusitis (4%), abnormal chest sounds, bronchospasm, epistaxis
Miscellaneous: Infection (9%), abscess, allergy, bacterial infection, carcinoma, fungal infection, herpes simplex, herpes zoster, lymphadenopathy, moniliasis, diaphoresis increased, tonsillitis, viral infection

Psoriasis only (1% to <3% unless otherwise noted):

Cardiovascular: Chest pain, flushes
Central nervous system: Psychiatric events (4% to 5%), pain (3% to 4%), dizziness, fever, insomnia, nervousness, vertigo
Dermatologic: Hypertrichosis (5% to 7%), acne, dry skin, folliculitis, keratosis, pruritus, rash, skin malignancies
Endocrine & metabolic: Hot flashes
Gastrointestinal: Nausea (5% to 6%), diarrhea (5% to 6%), gum hyperplasia (4% to 6%), abdominal discomfort (3% to 6%), dyspepsia (2% to 3%), abdominal distention, appetite increased, constipation, gingival bleeding
Genitourinary: Micturition increased
Hematologic: Bleeding disorder, clotting disorder, platelet disorder, red blood cell disorder
Hepatic: Hyperbilirubinemia

Neuromuscular & skeletal: Paresthesia (5% to 7%), arthralgia (1% to 6%)
Ocular: Abnormal vision
Respiratory: Bronchospasm (5%), cough (5%), dyspnea (5%), rhinitis (5%), respiratory infection
Miscellaneous: Flu-like syndrome (8% to 10%)

Pharmacodynamics/Kinetics

Absorption Oral:

Cyclosporine (non-modified): Erratic and incomplete; dependent on presence of food, bile acids, and GI motility; larger oral doses are needed in pediatrics due to shorter bowel length and limited intestinal absorption

Cyclosporine (modified): Erratic and incomplete; increased absorption, up to 30% when compared to cyclosporine (non-modified); less dependent on food, bile acids, or GI motility when compared to cyclosporine (non-modified)

Bioavailability Oral:

Cyclosporine (non-modified): Dependent on patient population and transplant type (<10% in adult liver transplant patients and as high as 89% in renal transplant patients); bioavailability of Sandimmune® capsules and oral solution are equivalent; bioavailability of oral solution is ~30% of the I.V. solution

Children: 28% (range: 17% to 42%); gut dysfunction common in BMT patients and oral bioavailability is further reduced

Cyclosporine (modified): Bioavailability of Neoral® capsules and oral solution are equivalent:

Children: 43% (range: 30% to 68%)

Adults: 23% greater than with cyclosporine (non-modified) in renal transplant patients; 50% greater in liver transplant patients

Time to Peak Serum: Oral:

Cyclosporine (non-modified): 2-6 hours; some patients have a second peak at 5-6 hours
Cyclosporine (modified): Renal transplant: 1.5-2 hours

Protein Binding 90% to 98% to lipoproteins

Half-Life Elimination Oral: May be prolonged with hepatic impairment and shorter in pediatric patients due to the higher metabolism rate

Cyclosporine (non-modified): Biphasic: Alpha: 1.4 hours; Terminal: 19 hours (range: 10-27 hours)

Cyclosporine (modified): Biphasic: Terminal: 8.4 hours (range: 5-18 hours)

Metabolism Extensively hepatic via CYP3A4; forms at least 25 metabolites; extensive first-pass effect following oral administration

Excretion Primarily feces; urine (6%, 0.1% as unchanged drug and metabolites)

Available Dosage Forms

Capsule, oral: 25 mg, 100 mg
Gengraf®: 25 mg, 100 mg

Capsule, softgel, oral: 25 mg, 50 mg, 100 mg
Neoral®: 25 mg, 100 mg
SandIMMUNE®: 25 mg, 100 mg

Injection, solution: 50 mg/mL (5 mL)
SandIMMUNE®: 50 mg/mL (5 mL)

Injection, solution [preservative free]: 50 mg/mL (5 mL)

Solution, oral: 100 mg/mL (50 mL)
Gengraf®: 100 mg/mL (50 mL)
Neoral®: 100 mg/mL (50 mL)
SandIMMUNE®: 100 mg/mL (50 mL)

Dosing

Adult Neoral®/Genraf® and Sandimmune® are not bioequivalent and cannot be used interchangeably.

Newly-transplanted patients: Adjunct therapy with corticosteroids is recommended. Initial dose should be given 4-12 hours prior to transplant or may be given postoperatively; adjust initial dose to achieve desired plasma concentration.

Oral: Dose is dependent upon type of transplant and formulation:

Cyclosporine (modified):

Renal: 9 ± 3 mg/kg/day, divided twice daily
Liver: 8 ± 4 mg/kg/day, divided twice daily
Heart: 7 ± 3 mg/kg/day, divided twice daily

Cyclosporine (non-modified): Initial doses of 10-14 mg/kg/day have been used for renal transplants (the manufacturer's labeling includes dosing from initial clinical trials of 15 mg/kg/day [range: 14-18 mg/kg/day]; however, this higher dosing level is rarely used any longer). Continue initial dose daily for 1-2 weeks; taper by 5% per week to a maintenance dose of 5-10 mg/kg/day; some renal transplant patients may be dosed as low as 3 mg/kg/day

Note: When using the non-modified formulation, cyclosporine levels may increase in liver transplant patients when the T-tube is closed; dose may need decreased

I.V.: Cyclosporine (non-modified): Manufacturer's labeling: Initial dose: 5-6 mg/kg/day or one-third of the oral dose as a single dose, infused over 2-6 hours; use should be limited to patients unable to take capsules or oral solution; patients should be switched to an oral dosage form as soon as possible

Note: Many transplant centers administer cyclosporine as "divided dose" infusions (in 2-3 doses/day) or as a continuous (24-hour) infusion; dosages range from 3-7.5 mg/kg/day. Specific institutional protocols should be consulted.

Note: Conversion to cyclosporine (modified) from cyclosporine (non-modified): Start with daily dose previously used and adjust to obtain preconversion cyclosporine trough concentration. Plasma concentrations should be monitored every 4-7 days and dose adjusted as necessary, until desired trough level is obtained. When transferring patients with previously poor absorption of cyclosporine (non-modified), monitor trough levels at least twice weekly (especially if initial dose exceeds 10 mg/kg/day); high plasma levels are likely to occur.

Rheumatoid arthritis: Oral: Cyclosporine (modified): Initial dose: 2.5 mg/kg/day, divided twice daily; salicylates, NSAIDs, and oral glucocorticoids may be continued (refer to Drug Interactions); dose may be increased by 0.5-0.75 mg/kg/day if insufficient response is seen after 8 weeks of treatment; additional dosage increases may be made again at 12 weeks (maximum dose: 4 mg/kg/day). Discontinue if no benefit is seen by 16 weeks of therapy.

Note: Increase the frequency of blood pressure monitoring after each alteration in dosage of cyclosporine. Cyclosporine dosage should be decreased by 25% to 50% in patients with no history of hypertension who develop sustained hypertension during therapy and, if hypertension persists, treatment with cyclosporine should be discontinued.

Psoriasis: Oral: Cyclosporine (modified): Initial dose: 2.5 mg/kg/day, divided twice daily; dose may be increased by 0.5 mg/kg/day if insufficient response is seen after 4 weeks of treatment; additional dosage increases may be made every 2 weeks if needed (maximum dose: 4 mg/kg/day). Discontinue if no benefit is seen by 6 weeks of therapy. Once patients are adequately controlled, the dose should be decreased to the lowest effective dose. Doses <2.5 mg/kg/day may be effective. Treatment longer than 1 year is not recommended.

Note: Increase the frequency of blood pressure monitoring after each alteration in dosage of cyclosporine. Cyclosporine dosage should be decreased by 25% to 50% in patients with no history of hypertension who develop sustained hypertension during therapy and, if hypertension persists, treatment with cyclosporine should be discontinued.

Focal segmental glomerulosclerosis (unlabeled use): Oral: Initial: 3.5-5 mg/kg/day divided every 12 hours (in combination with oral prednisone) (Braun, 2008; Cattran, 1999)

Lupus nephritis (unlabeled use): Oral: Initial: 4 mg/kg/day for 1 month (reduce dose if trough concentrations >200 ng/mL); reduce dose by 0.5 mg/kg every 2 weeks to a maintenance dose of 2.5-3 mg/kg/day (Moroni, 2006)

Severe ulcerative colitis (steroid-refractory) (unlabeled use):

I.V.: Cyclosporine (non-modified): 2-4 mg/kg/day, infused continuously over 24 hours. (Lichtiger, 1994; Van Assche, 2003). **Note:** Some studies suggest no therapeutic difference between low-dose (2 mg/kg) and high-dose (4 mg/kg) cyclosporine regimens (Van Assche, 2003).

Oral: Cyclosporine (modified): 2.3-3 mg/kg every 12 hours (Weber 2006; De Saussure 2005)

Note: Patients responsive to I.V. therapy should be switched to oral therapy when possible.

Geriatric Refer to adult dosing. **Sandimmune® and Neoral®/Genraf® are not bioequivalent and cannot be used interchangeably.**

Pediatric Transplant: Refer to adult dosing. Children may require, and are able to tolerate, larger doses than adults.

Renal Impairment For severe psoriasis:

Serum creatinine levels ≥25% above pretreatment levels: Take another sample within 2 weeks; if the level remains ≥25% above pretreatment levels, decrease dosage of cyclosporine (modified) by 25% to 50%. If two dosage adjustments do not reverse the increase in serum creatinine levels, treatment should be discontinued.

Serum creatinine levels ≥50% above pretreatment levels: Decrease cyclosporine dosage by 25% to 50%. If two dosage adjustments do not reverse the increase in serum creatinine levels, treatment should be discontinued.

Hemodialysis: Supplemental dose is not necessary.

Peritoneal dialysis: Supplemental dose is not necessary.

Hepatic Impairment Dosage adjustment is probably necessary; monitor levels closely

Administration

Oral Oral solution: Do not administer liquid from plastic or styrofoam cup. May dilute Neoral® oral solution with orange juice or apple juice. May dilute Sandimmune® oral solution with milk, chocolate milk, or orange juice. Avoid changing diluents frequently. Mix thoroughly and drink at once. Use syringe provided to measure dose. Mix in a glass container and rinse container with more diluent to ensure total dose is taken. Do not rinse syringe before or after use (may cause dose variation).

Combination therapy with renal transplantation:

Everolimus: Administer cyclosporine at the same time as everolimus

Sirolimus: Administer cyclosporine 4 hours prior to sirolimus

I.V. The manufacturer recommends that following dilution, intravenous admixture be administered over 2-6 hours. However, many transplant centers administer as divided doses (2-3 doses/day) or as a 24-hour continuous infusion. Patients should be under continuous observation for at least the first 30 minutes of the infusion, and should be monitored frequently thereafter. To minimize leaching of DEHP, non-PVC sets should be used for administration.

Stability

Reconstitution Injection: To minimize leaching of DEHP, non-PVC containers and sets should be used for preparation and administration.

Sandimmune® injection: Injection should be further diluted (1 mL [50 mg] of concentrate in 20-100 mL of D_5W or NS) for administration by intravenous infusion.

Storage

Capsule: Store at controlled room temperature.

Injection: Store at controlled room temperature; do not refrigerate. Ampuls and vials should be protected from light. Stability of injection of parenteral admixture at room temperature (25°C) is 6 hours in PVC; 12-24 hours in Excel®, PAB® containers, or glass.

Oral solution: Store at controlled room temperature; do not refrigerate. Use within 2 months after opening; should be mixed in glass containers.

Monitoring and Teaching Issues

Laboratory Monitoring Cyclosporine levels, serum electrolytes, renal function, hepatic function

Physical Assessment Monitor kidney and hepatic function closely. Monitor blood pressure and assess for signs of fluid retention periodically. I.V.: Monitor closely for first 30 minutes of infusion and frequently thereafter to assess for adverse reactions.

Patient Education Oral: Take dose at the same time each day. You will be susceptible to infection. Avoid excessive exposure to sun. Practice good oral hygiene to reduce gum inflammation; see a dentist regularly during treatment. Report severe headache; mouth sores or swollen gums; signs of infection; persistent nausea, vomiting, or diarrhea; or change in urination. Increase in blood pressure or damage to the kidney is possible. Your prescriber will need to monitor you closely. Do not change one brand of cyclosporine for another; any changes must be done by your prescriber. If you are taking this medication for psoriasis, your risk of cancer may be increased when taking additional medications.

Oral solution: Dilute Neoral® with orange juice or apple juice. Dilute Sandimmune® with milk, chocolate milk, or orange juice. Mix thoroughly and drink at once. Mix in a glass container (do not use plastic or styrofoam) and rinse container with more juice/milk to ensure total dose is taken.

Dietary Considerations Administer this medication consistently with relation to time of day and meals. Avoid grapefruit juice with oral cyclosporine use.

Geriatric Considerations Cyclosporine has not been specifically studied in the elderly. Cyclosporine is being used in combination therapy for the treatment of severe rheumatoid arthritis.

Pregnancy Considerations Adverse events were not observed following the use of oral cyclosporine in animal reproduction studies (using doses that were not maternally toxic). In humans, cyclosporine crosses the placenta; maternal concentrations do not correlate with those found in the umbilical cord. Cyclosporine may be detected in the serum of newborns for several days after birth. Based on clinical use, premature births and low birth weight were consistently observed in pregnant transplant patients (additional pregnancy complications also present).

A pregnancy registry has been established for pregnant women taking immunosuppressants following any solid organ transplant (National Transplantation Pregnancy Registry, Temple University, 877-955-6877).

Additional Information Cyclosporine (modified): Refers to the capsule dosage formulation of cyclosporine in an aqueous dispersion (previously referred to as "microemulsion"). Cyclosporine (modified) has increased bioavailability as compared to cyclosporine (non-modified) and cannot be used interchangeably without close monitoring.

Related Information

Peak and Trough Guidelines *on page 1958*

CycloSPORINE (Ophthalmic) (SYE kloe spor een)

U.S. Brand Names Restasis®

Index Terms CsA; CyA; Cyclosporin A

Generic Availability (U.S.) No

Pharmacologic Category Immunosuppressant Agent

Medication Safety Issues

Sound-alike/look-alike issues:

CycloSPORINE may be confused with cyclophosphamide, Cyklokapron®, cycloSERINE

Pregnancy Risk Factor C

Lactation Excretion unknown/use caution

Use Increase tear production when suppressed tear production is presumed to be due to keratoconjunctivitis sicca-associated ocular inflammation (in patients not already using topical anti-inflammatory drugs or punctal plugs)

Contraindications Hypersensitivity to cyclosporine or any component of the formulation. Ophthalmic emulsion is contraindicated in patients with active ocular infections.

Warnings/Precautions Ophthalmic emulsion: Safety and efficacy have not been established in patients <16 years of age.

Drug Interactions

Avoid Concomitant Use There are no known interactions where it is recommended to avoid concomitant use.

Decreased Effect There are no known significant interactions involving a decrease in effect.

Increased Effect/Toxicity There are no known significant interactions involving an increase in effect.

Adverse Reactions

>10%: Ocular: Burning (17%)

1% to 10%: Ocular: Hyperemia (conjunctival 5%), eye pain, pruritus, stinging

Available Dosage Forms

Emulsion, ophthalmic [preservative free]:

Restasis®: 0.05% (0.4 mL)

Dosing

Adult & Geriatric Keratoconjunctivitis sicca: Ophthalmic (Restasis®): Instill 1 drop in each eye every 12 hours

Pediatric Keratoconjunctivitis sicca: Ophthalmic: Children ≥16 years: Refer to adult dosing.

Administration

Other Prior to use, invert vial several times to obtain a uniform emulsion. Remove contact lenses prior to instillation of drops; may be reinserted 15 minutes after administration. May be used with artificial tears; allow 15 minute interval between products.

Stability

Storage Store at 15°C to 25°C (59°F to 77°F). Vials are single-use; discard immediately following administration.

Monitoring and Teaching Issues

Breast-Feeding Considerations Cyclosporine is found in breast milk following oral administration. Serum concentrations are below the limit of detection (<0.1 ng/mL) following ophthalmic use.

Pregnancy Considerations Adverse events were not observed following the use of oral cyclosporine in animal reproduction studies when using doses that were approximately 300,000 times greater than a human ophthalmic dose (assuming complete absorption).

◆ **Cymbalta®** *see* DULoxetine *on page 596*

Cyproheptadine (si proe HEP ta deen)

Index Terms Cyproheptadine Hydrochloride; Periactin

Generic Availability (U.S.) Yes

Pharmacologic Category Histamine H_1 Antagonist; Histamine H_1 Antagonist, First Generation; Piperidine Derivative

Medication Safety Issues

Sound-alike/look-alike issues:

Cyproheptadine may be confused with cyclobenzaprine

Periactin may be confused with Perative®, Percodan®, Persantine®

Beers Criteria medication: This drug may be inappropriate for use in geriatric patients (high severity risk).

Pregnancy Risk Factor B

Lactation Excretion in breast milk unknown/contraindicated

Use Perennial and seasonal allergic rhinitis and other allergic symptoms including urticaria

Unlabeled/Investigational Use Migraine headache prophylaxis, pruritus, spasticity associated with spinal cord damage

Available Dosage Forms

Syrup, oral: 2 mg/5 mL (473 mL, 480 mL)

Tablet, oral: 4 mg

Dosing

Adult

Allergic conditions: Oral: 4-20 mg/day divided every 8 hours (not to exceed 0.5 mg/kg/day); some patients may require up to 32 mg/day for adequate control of symptoms

Spasticity associated with spinal cord damage (unlabeled use): Oral: Initial: 2-4 mg every 8 hours; maximum: 8 mg every 8 hours (Barbeau, 1982; Wainberg, 1990)

Geriatric Initiate therapy at the lower end of the dosage range.

Pediatric

Allergic conditions: Oral: Children: 0.25 mg/kg/day or 8 mg/m^2/day in 2-3 divided doses **or**

2-6 years: 2 mg every 8-12 hours (not to exceed 12 mg/day)

7-14 years: 4 mg every 8-12 hours (not to exceed 16 mg/day)

Migraine headache prophylaxis (unlabeled use): Oral: 4 mg every 8-12 hours

Monitoring and Teaching Issues

Physical Assessment Monitor weight periodically. Monitor for excess anticholinergic effects at beginning of therapy and periodically throughout.

Patient Education Avoid use of alcohol. You may experience drowsiness, dizziness, dry mouth, nausea, or abdominal pain. Report persistent sedation, confusion, agitation, blurred vision, respiratory difficulty, or lack of improvement or worsening of condition.

◆ **Cyproheptadine Hydrochloride** *see* Cyproheptadine *on page 443*

Cyproterone (sye PROE ter one)

Index Terms Cyproterone Acetate

Generic Availability (U.S.) Yes

Pharmacologic Category Antiandrogen

Pregnancy Risk Factor Not indicated for use in women

Use Palliative treatment of advanced prostate carcinoma

Mechanism of Action/Effect Cyproterone is a steroidal compound with antiandrogenic, antigonadotropic, and progestin-like activity.

Contraindications Hypersensitivity to cyproterone or any component of the formulation; active liver disease or hepatic dysfunction; renal impairment

Warnings/Precautions Cyproterone has been associated with hepatic toxicity (jaundice, hepatitis, hepatic failure); typically this toxicity develops after several months of therapy. Monitor hepatic function and consider discontinuation of therapy in patients with evidence of hepatic injury.

Use caution in patients with a history of depression. Cyproterone has been associated with an increased incidence of depression, particularly early in the course of therapy (initial 6-8 weeks). Use with caution in patients with diabetes or impaired glucose tolerance, may cause alterations in glucose metabolism. Use with caution in conditions that may be aggravated by fluid retention, or cardiovascular disease. May increase the risk of thromboembolism and/or alter lipid profiles.

Drug Interactions

Avoid Concomitant Use There are no known interactions where it is recommended to avoid concomitant use.

Decreased Effect

The levels/effects of Cyproterone may be decreased by: Aminoglutethimide

Increased Effect/Toxicity

The levels/effects of Cyproterone may be increased by: Herbs (Progestogenic Properties)

Nutritional/Ethanol Interactions

Ethanol: May reduce the effect of cyproterone (not established in the treatment of prostatic carcinoma); avoid concurrent use.

Adverse Reactions Frequency not defined.

Cardiovascular: Heart failure, hemorrhage, hypotension, MI, stroke, shock, stroke, syncope, tachycardia, thrombosis (DVT, pulmonary embolism, retinal vein thrombosis)

Central nervous system: Depression, dizziness, encephalopathy, fatigue, headache, lassitude

Dermatologic: Dry skin (sebum reduction), eczema, erythema, exfoliative dermatitis, hirsutism, nodosum, patchy loss of body hair, photosensitivity, pruritus, rash, scleroderma, skin discoloration, urticaria

Endocrine & metabolic: Adrenal suppression (dose related), benign nodular breast hyperplasia, diabetes mellitus, galactorrhea, gynecomastia, hot flashes, hypercalcemia, hyperglycemia, impotence, inhibition of spermatogenesis, libido increased, negative nitrogen balance, weight gain/loss

Gastrointestinal: Anorexia, constipation, diarrhea, dyspepsia, glossitis, nausea, pancreatitis, vomiting

Genitourinary: Bladder carcinoma, hematuria, urinary frequency

Hematologic: Anemia, fibrinogen increased, hemolytic anemia, leukopenia, leukocytosis, PT decreased, thrombocytopenia

Hepatic: Ascites, cholestatic jaundice, cirrhosis, hepatic dysfunction (dose related), hepatic carcinoma, hepatic coma, hepatic failure, hepatic necrosis, hepatitis, hepatoma, hepatomegaly, transaminases increased

Local: Injection site reaction

Neuromuscular and skeletal: Myasthenia, osteoporosis, weakness

Ocular: Abnormal accommodation, abnormal vision, blindness, optic neuritis, optic atrophy, retinal disorder

Renal: Renal failure, serum creatinine increased

Respiratory: Asthma, bronchospasm, cough, dyspnea, pulmonary embolism, pulmonary fibrosis

Miscellaneous: Allergic reaction

Pharmacodynamics/Kinetics

Absorption Oral: Rapid and complete

Time to Peak Plasma: Oral: 3-4 hours; Depot injection: 3 days

Half-Life Elimination Oral: 38 hours; Depot injection: 4 days

Metabolism Hepatic, some metabolites have activity

Excretion Urine (35%, as metabolites); feces (60%)

Product Availability Not available in U.S.

Dosing

Adult & Geriatric Prostatic carcinoma (palliative treatment): Males:

Oral: 200-300 mg/day in 2-3 divided doses; following orchiectomy, reduce dose to 100-200 mg/day; should be taken with meals

I.M. (depot): 300 mg (3 mL) once weekly; reduce dose in orchiectomized patients to 300 mg every 2 weeks

Renal Impairment Use is contraindicated.

Hepatic Impairment Use is contraindicated with hepatic impairment or active liver disease.

Administration

Oral Administer at the same time each day, with meals.

Stability

Storage Store at controlled room temperature of 25°C (77°F).

Monitoring and Teaching Issues

Laboratory Monitoring Liver function tests should be performed at baseline and periodically thereafter, or whenever signs or symptoms suggestive of hepatotoxicity are noted. Adrenal function should be monitored periodically.

Dietary Considerations Take with meals.

Pregnancy Considerations In males, sperm count and volume of ejaculate will be reduced. After ~2 months of treatment, infertility may be noted.

◆ **Cyproterone Acetate** *see* Cyproterone *on page* *443*

◆ **CYT** *see* Cyclophosphamide *on page* *434*

Cytarabine (sye TARE a been)

Index Terms Ara-C; Arabinosylcytosine; Cytarabine (Conventional); Cytarabine Hydrochloride; Cytosar-U; Cytosine Arabinosine Hydrochloride

Generic Availability (U.S.) Yes

Pharmacologic Category Antineoplastic Agent, Antimetabolite; Antineoplastic Agent, Antimetabolite (Pyrimidine Analog)

Medication Safety Issues

Sound-alike/look-alike issues:

Cytarabine may be confused with Cytadren®, Cytosar®, Cytoxan, vidarabine

Cytarabine (conventional) may be confused with cytarabine liposomal

Cytosar-U may be confused with cytarabine, Cytovene®, Cytoxan, Neosar®

High alert medication: This medication is in a class the Institute for Safe Medication Practices (ISMP) includes among its list of drugs which have a heightened risk of causing significant patient harm when used in error.

Intrathecal medication safety: The American Society of Clinical Oncology (ASCO)/Oncology Nursing Society (ONS) chemotherapy administration safety standards (Jacobson, 2009) encourage the following safety measures for intrathecal chemotherapy:

- Intrathecal medication should not be prepared during the preparation of any other agents
- After preparation, store in an isolated location or container clearly marked with a label identifying as "intrathecal" use only
- Delivery to the patient should only be with other medications intended for administration into the central nervous system

Pregnancy Risk Factor D

Lactation Excretion in breast milk unknown/not recommended

Use Remission induction in acute myeloid leukemia (AML), treatment of acute lymphocytic leukemia (ALL) and chronic myelocytic leukemia (CML; blast phase); prophylaxis and treatment of meningeal leukemia

Unlabeled/Investigational Use Postinduction, postremission consolidation, and salvage treatment of AML; treatment of primary central nervous system (CNS) lymphoma; treatment of relapsed or refractory Hodgkin's lymphoma; treatment of non-Hodgkin's lymphomas (NHL)

Mechanism of Action/Effect Inhibition of DNA synthesis in S Phase of cell division; degree of its cytotoxicity correlates linearly with its incorporation into DNA, therefore, incorporation into the DNA is responsible for drug activity and toxicity

Contraindications Hypersensitivity to cytarabine or any component of the formulation

Warnings/Precautions Hazardous agent - use appropriate precautions for handling and disposal. **[U.S. Boxed Warning]: Potent myelosuppressive agent;** use with caution in patients with prior bone marrow suppression; monitor for signs of febrile neutropenia.

High-dose regimens are associated with CNS, gastrointestinal, ocular (prophylaxis with ophthalmic corticosteroid drops is recommended), pulmonary toxicities and cardiomyopathy. Neurotoxicity associated with high dose treatment may present as acute cerebellar toxicity, or may be severe with seizure and/or coma; may be delayed, occurring up to 3-8 days after treatment has begun. Risk factors for neurotoxicity include cumulative cytarabine dose, prior CNS disease and renal impairment. Tumor lysis syndrome and subsequent hyperuricemia may occur with high dose cytarabine; monitor, consider allopurinol and hydrate accordingly. There have been case reports of fatal cardiomyopathy when high dose cytarabine was used in combination with cyclophosphamide as a preparation regimen for transplantation.

Use with caution in patients with impaired renal and hepatic function; may be at higher risk for CNS toxicities; dosage adjustments may be necessary. Cytarabine syndrome is characterized by fever, myalgia, bone pain, chest pain, maculopapular rash, conjunctivitis, and malaise, and may occur 6-12 hours following administration; may be managed with corticosteroids. There have been reports of acute pancreatitis in patients receiving continuous infusion and in patients previously treated with L-asparaginase. **[U.S. Boxed Warning]: Should be administered under the supervision of an experienced cancer chemotherapy physician.** Some products may contain benzyl alcohol; do not use products containing benzyl alcohol or products reconstituted with bacteriostatic diluent intrathecally or for high-dose cytarabine regimens. When used for intrathecal administration, should not be prepared during the preparation of any other agents; after preparation, store intrathecal medications in an isolated location or container clearly marked with a label identifying as "intrathecal" use only; delivery of intrathecal medications to the patient should only be with other medications intended for administration into the central nervous system (Jacobson, 2009).

Drug Interactions

Avoid Concomitant Use

Avoid concomitant use of Cytarabine with any of the following: BCG; Natalizumab; Pimecrolimus; Roflumilast; Tacrolimus (Topical); Vaccines (Live)

Decreased Effect

Cytarabine may decrease the levels/effects of: BCG; Cardiac Glycosides; Flucytosine; Sipuleucel-T; Vaccines (Inactivated); Vaccines (Live)

The levels/effects of Cytarabine may be decreased by: Echinacea

Increased Effect/Toxicity

Cytarabine may increase the levels/effects of: Leflunomide; Natalizumab; Vaccines (Live)

The levels/effects of Cytarabine may be increased by: Denosumab; Pimecrolimus; Roflumilast; Tacrolimus (Topical); Trastuzumab

Adverse Reactions Note: Frequency not defined.

Frequent:

Central nervous system: Fever
Dermatologic: Rash
Gastrointestinal: Anal inflammation, anal ulceration, anorexia, diarrhea, mucositis, nausea, vomiting
Hematologic: Myelosuppression, neutropenia (onset: 1-7 days; nadir [biphasic]: 7-9 days and at 15-24 days; recovery [biphasic]: 9-12 and at 24-34 days), thrombocytopenia (onset: 5 days; nadir: 12-15 days; recovery 15-25 days), anemia, bleeding, leukopenia, megaloblastosis, reticulocytes decreased
Hepatic: Hepatic dysfunction, transaminases increased (acute)
Local: Thrombophlebitis

Less frequent:

Cardiovascular: Chest pain, pericarditis
Central nervous system: Dizziness, headache, neural toxicity, neuritis
Dermatologic: Alopecia, pruritus, skin freckling, skin ulceration, urticaria
Gastrointestinal: Abdominal pain, bowel necrosis, esophageal ulceration, esophagitis, pancreatitis, sore throat
Genitourinary: Urinary retention
Hepatic: Jaundice
Local: Injection site cellulitis
Ocular: Conjunctivitis
Renal: Renal dysfunction
Respiratory: Dyspnea
Miscellaneous: Allergic edema, anaphylaxis, sepsis

Infrequent and/or case reports: Amylase increased, aseptic meningitis, cardiopulmonary arrest (acute), cerebral dysfunction, cytarabine syndrome (bone pain, chest pain, conjunctivitis, fever, maculopapular rash, malaise, myalgia); exanthematous pustulosis, hyperuricemia, injection site inflammation (SubQ injection), injection site pain (SubQ injection), interstitial pneumonitis, lipase increased, paralysis (intrathecal and I.V. combination therapy), rhabdomyolysis, veno-occlusive liver disease

Adverse events associated with high-dose cytarabine (CNS, gastrointestinal, ocular, and pulmonary toxicities are more common with high-dose regimens):

Cardiovascular: Cardiomegaly, cardiomyopathy (in combination with cyclophosphamide)
Central nervous system: Coma, neurotoxicity (dose-related, cerebellar toxicity may occur in patients receiving high-dose cytarabine [>36-48 g/m^2/cycle]; incidence may up to 55% in patients with renal impairment), personality change, somnolence
Dermatologic: Alopecia (complete), desquamation, rash (severe)
Gastrointestinal: Gastrointestinal ulcer, peritonitis, pneumatosis cystoides intestinalis
Hepatic: Hyperbilirubinemia, liver abscess, liver damage, necrotizing colitis
Neuromuscular & skeletal: Peripheral neuropathy (motor and sensory)
Ocular: Corneal toxicity, hemorrhagic conjunctivitis
Respiratory: Pulmonary edema, syndrome of sudden respiratory distress
Miscellaneous: Sepsis

Adverse events associated with intrathecal cytarabine administration:

Central nervous system: Accessory nerve paralysis, fever, necrotizing leukoencephalopathy (with concurrent cranial irradiation, I.T. methotrexate, and I.T. hydrocortisone), neurotoxicity, paraplegia
Gastrointestinal: Dysphagia, nausea, vomiting
Ocular: Blindness (with concurrent systemic chemotherapy and cranial irradiation), diplopia
Respiratory: Cough, hoarseness
Miscellaneous: Aphonia

Pharmacodynamics/Kinetics

Time to Peak I.M., SubQ: 20-60 minutes

Half-Life Elimination I.V.: Initial: 7-20 minutes; Terminal: 1-3 hours; I.T.: 2-6 hours

Metabolism Primarily hepatic; metabolized by deoxycytidine kinase and other nucleotide kinases to aracytidine triphosphate (active); about 86% to 96% of dose is metabolized to inactive uracil arabinoside (ARA-U); intrathecal administration results in little conversion to ARA-U due to the low levels of deaminase in the cerebral spinal fluid

Excretion Urine (~80%; 90% as metabolite ARA-U) within 24 hours

Available Dosage Forms

Injection, powder for reconstitution: 100 mg, 500 mg, 1 g, 2 g
Injection, solution: 20 mg/mL (25 mL); 100 mg/mL (20 mL)
Injection, solution [preservative free]: 20 mg/mL (5 mL, 50 mL); 100 mg/mL (20 mL)

Dosing

Adult & Geriatric Details concerning dosing in combination regimens should also be consulted.

AML remission induction: I.V.: Standard-dose (provided in the FDA-approved labeling): 100 mg/m^2/day continuous infusion for 7 days or 100 mg/m^2/dose continuous infusion every 12 hours for 7 days

Remission maintenance (unlabeled use):
I.V.: 70-200 mg/m^2/day for 2-5 days at monthly intervals
SubQ: 1-1.5 mg/kg single dose for maintenance at 1- to 4-week intervals

High-dose therapies (unlabeled uses): I.V.:
Doses of 1-3 g/m^2 have been used for refractory or secondary leukemias or refractory non-Hodgkin's lymphoma.
Doses of 1-3 g/m^2 every 12 hours for up to 12 doses have been used for leukemia

Bone marrow transplant (unlabeled use): I.V.: 1.5 g/m^2 continuous infusion over 48 hours

Meningeal leukemia: I.T.: Dosing provided in the FDA-approved labeling: Usual dose 30 mg/m^2 every 4 days; range: 5-75 mg/m^2 once daily for 4 days or once every 4 days until CNS findings normalize, followed by 1 additional treatment. **Note:** Optimal intrathecal chemotherapy dosing should be based on age rather than on body surface area (BSA); CSF volume correlates with age and not to BSA (Bleyer, 1983; Kerr, 2001).

Unlabeled uses or doses for intrathecal therapy: I.T.:

CNS prophylaxis (ALL): 100 mg weekly for 8 doses, then every 2 weeks for 8 doses, then monthly for 6 doses (high-risk patients) **or** 100 mg on day 7 or 8 with each chemotherapy cycle for 4 doses (low risk patients) **or** 16 doses (high-risk patients) (Cortes, 1995)

or as part of ITT: 40 mg days 0 and 14 during induction, days 1, 4, 8, and 11 during CNS therapy phase, every 18 weeks during intensification and maintenance phases (Storring, 2009)

CNS prophylaxis (APL, as part of ITT): 50 mg per dose; administer 1 dose prior to consolidation and 2 doses during each of 2 consolidation phases (total of 5 doses) (Ades, 2006; Ades, 2008)

CNS leukemia treatment (ALL, as part of ITT): 40 mg twice weekly until CSF cleared (Storring, 2009)

CNS lymphoma treatment: 50 mg twice a week for 4 weeks, then weekly for 4-8 weeks, then every other week for 4 weeks, then every 4 weeks for 4 doses (Glantz, 1999)

Leptomeningeal metastases treatment: 50 mg twice a week for 4 weeks, then weekly for 4 weeks then monthly for 4 doses (NCCN CNS cancer guidelines v.1.2010) **or** 40-60 mg per dose (DeAngelis, 2005)

Pediatric Details concerning dosing in combination regimens should also be consulted.

AML remission induction: I.V.: Refer to adult dosing.

Remission maintenance, high-dose therapies (unlabeled uses): Refer to adult dosing.

Meningeal leukemia: I.T.: Dosing provided in the FDA-approved labeling: Usual dose 30 mg/m^2 every 4 days; range: 5-75 mg/m^2 once daily for 4 days or once every 4 days until CNS findings normalize, followed by 1 additional treatment. **Note:** Optimal intrathecal chemotherapy dosing should be based on age rather than on body surface area (BSA); CSF volume correlates with age and not to BSA (Bleyer, 1983; Kerr, 2001).

Age-based dosing (unlabeled dosing): I.T.:

CNS prophylaxis:

<1 year: 20 mg per dose
1-2 years: 30 mg per dose
2-3 years: 50 mg per dose
≥3 years: 70 mg per dose

ALL CNS prophylaxis, age-specific doses from literature:

Administer on day 0 of induction therapy (Gaynon, 1993):

1-2 years: 30 mg per dose
2-3 years: 50 mg per dose
≥3 years: 70 mg per dose

Administer as part of intrathecal triple therapy (ITT) on days 1 and 15 of induction therapy; days 1, 15, 50, and 64 (standard risk patients) or days 1, 15, 29, and 43 (high-risk patients) during consolidation therapy; day 1 of reinduction therapy, and during maintenance therapy (very high-risk patients receive on days 1, 22, 45, and 59 of induction, days 8, 22, 36, and 50 of consolidation therapy, days 8 and 38 of reinduction therapy, and during maintenance) (Lin, 2007):

<1 year: 18 mg per dose
1-2 years: 24 mg per dose
2-3 years: 30 mg per dose
≥3 years: 36 mg per dose

Administer on day 0 of induction therapy, then as part of ITT on days 7, 14, and 21 during consolidation therapy; as part of ITT on days 0, 28, and 35 for 2 cycles of delayed intensification therapy, and then maintenance treatment as part of ITT on day 0 every 12 weeks for 38 months (boys) or 26 months (girls) from initial induction treatment (Matloub, 2006):

<2 years: 16 mg per dose
2-3 years: 20 mg per dose
≥3 years: 24-30 mg per dose

Administer on day 15 of induction therapy, days 1 and 15 of reinduction phase; and day 1 of cycle 2 of maintenance 1A phase (Pieters, 2007):

<1 year: 15 mg per dose
≥1 year: 20 mg per dose

Treatment, CNS leukemia (ALL): I.T.: Administer as part of ITT weekly until CSF remission, then every 4 weeks throughout continuation treatment (Lin, 2007):

<1 year: 18 mg per dose
1-2 years: 24 mg per dose
2-3 years: 30 mg per dose
≥3 years: 36 mg per dose

Renal Impairment The FDA-approved labeling does not contain renal dosing adjustment guidelines; the following guidelines have been used by some clinicians:

Aronoff, 2007 (cytarabine 100-200 mg/m^2): Children and Adults: No adjustment necessary

Kintzel, 1995 (high-dose cytarabine 1-3 g/m^2):

Cl_{cr} 46-60 mL/minute: Administer 60% of dose
Cl_{cr} 31-45 mL/minute: Administer 50% of dose
Cl_{cr} <30 mL/minute: Consider use of alternative drug

Smith, 1997 (high-dose cytarabine ≥2 g/m^2/dose):

Serum creatinine 1.5-1.9 mg/dL or increase (from baseline) of 0.5-1.2 mg/dL: Reduce dose to 1 g/m^2/dose

Serum creatinine ≥2 mg/dL or increase (from baseline) of >1.2 mg/dL: Reduce dose to 0.1 g/m^2/day as a continuous infusion

Hepatic Impairment Dose may need to be adjusted in patients with liver failure since cytarabine is partially detoxified in the liver. The FDA-approved labeling does not contain hepatic dosing adjustment guidelines; the following guideline has been used by some clinicians:

Floyd, 2006: Transaminases (any elevation): Administer 50% of dose; may increase subsequent doses in the absence of toxicities

Koren, 1992 (dose level not specified): Bilirubin >2 mg/dL: Administer 50% of dose; may increase subsequent doses in the absence of toxicities

Administration

I.V. Infuse as a continuous infusion or infuse over 1-3 hours (infusion rate based on protocol). GI adverse effects may be more pronounced with divided I.V. bolus doses than with continuous infusion.

Other

I.T.: Intrathecal doses should be administered as soon as possible after preparation.

May also be administered SubQ.

Stability

Reconstitution Use appropriate precautions for handling and disposal. **Note:** Solutions containing bacteriostatic agents may be used for SubQ and standard-dose (100-200 mg/m^2) I.V. cytarabine preparations, but should not be used for the preparation of either intrathecal doses or high-dose I.V. therapies.

I.V.:

Powder for reconstitution: Reconstitute with bacteriostatic water for injection (for standard-dose).

For I.V. infusion: Further dilute in 250-1000 mL 0.9% NaCl or D_5W.

Intrathecal: Powder for reconstitution: Reconstitute with preservative free sodium chloride 0.9%; may further dilute to preferred final volume (volume generally based on institution or practitioner preference; may be up to 12 mL) with Elliott's B solution, sodium chloride 0.9% or lactated Ringer's. Intrathecal medications should not be prepared during the preparation of any other agents.

Intrathecal triple therapy (ITT): Cytarabine 30-50 mg with hydrocortisone sodium succinate 15-25 mg and methotrexate 12 mg; compatible together for up to 24 hours in a syringe; however, should be administered administer as soon as possible after preparation because intrathecal preparations are preservative free

Storage Store intact vials of powder for injection at room temperature of 20°C to 25°C (68°F to 77°F); store intact vials of solution at room temperature of 15°C to 30°C (59°F to 86°F).

I.V.:

Powder for reconstitution: Reconstituted solutions should be stored at room temperature and used within 48 hours.

For I.V. infusion: Solutions for I.V. infusion diluted in D_5W or NS are stable for 7 days at room temperature, although the manufacturer recommends administration as soon as possible after preparation.

Intrathecal: Administer as soon as possible after preparation. After preparation, store intrathecal medications in an isolated location or container clearly marked with a label identifying as "intrathecal" use only.

Monitoring and Teaching Issues

Laboratory Monitoring Liver function, CBC with differential and platelet count, serum creatinine, BUN, serum uric acid

Physical Assessment Use caution in presence of impaired renal or hepatic function, prior bone marrow suppression, or prior CNS disease; dosage adjustment may be necessary. Ocular pain and conjunctivitis reactions may be reduced with ophthalmic corticosteroid premedication. Patient should be monitored closely throughout treatment, especially with high-dose regimens, for adverse gastrointestinal and pulmonary response, CNS toxicities, and cardiomyopathy.

Patient Education This drug is administered by infusion or injection. Report immediately any redness, swelling, burning, or pain at injection/infusion site; sudden difficulty breathing or swallowing; chest pain; or chills. Maintain adequate hydration. You will be more susceptible to infection. May cause nausea, vomiting, loss of appetite, diarrhea, mouth sores, dizziness, headache, confusion, or brittle or dry hair or loss of hair (may reverse after treatment). Report immediately any signs of respiratory distress, chest pain or palpitations, CNS changes, change in gait, skin rash or ulceration, unusual bruising or bleeding, persistent GI upset, yellowing of eyes or skin, change in color of urine, pain on urination, blackened stool, pain passing stool, pain or numbness in joints or muscles, blurred vision, or change in visual acuity.

Breast-Feeding Considerations Due to the potential for serious adverse reactions in the nursing infant, breast-feeding is not recommended.

Pregnancy Considerations Cytarabine is teratogenic in animal studies. Limb and ear defects have been noted in case reports when cytarabine has been used during pregnancy. The following have also been noted in the neonate: Pancytopenia, WBC depression, electrolyte abnormalities, prematurity, low birth weight, decreased hematocrit or platelets. Risk to the fetus is decreased if therapy is avoided during the 1st trimester; however, women of childbearing potential should be advised of the potential risks.

Additional Information I.V. doses ≥1.5 g/m^2 may produce conjunctivitis which can be ameliorated with prophylactic use of corticosteroid (0.1% dexamethasone) eye drops. Dexamethasone eye drops should be administered at 1-2 drops every 6 hours during and for 2-7 days after cytarabine is done.

◆ **Cytarabine (Conventional)** *see* Cytarabine *on page* 445

◆ **Cytarabine Hydrochloride** *see* Cytarabine *on page* 445

Cytarabine (Liposomal) (sye TARE a been lip po SOE mal)

U.S. Brand Names DepoCyt®

Generic Availability (U.S.) No

Pharmacologic Category Antineoplastic Agent, Antimetabolite (Pyrimidine Antagonist)

Medication Safety Issues

Sound-alike/look-alike issues:

Cytarabine may be confused with Cytadren®, Cytosar®, Cytoxan, vidarabine

Cytarabine liposomal may be confused with conventional cytarabine

DepoCyt® may be confused with Depoject®

High alert medication: This medication is in a class the Institute for Safe Medication Practices (ISMP) includes among its list of drugs which have a heightened risk of causing significant patient harm when used in error.

Intrathecal medication safety: The American Society of Clinical Oncology (ASCO)/Oncology Nursing Society (ONS) chemotherapy administration safety standards (Jacobson, 2009) encourage the following safety measures for intrathecal chemotherapy:

- Intrathecal medication should not be prepared during the preparation of any other agents
- After preparation, store in an isolated location or container clearly marked with a label identifying as "intrathecal" use only
- Delivery to the patient should only be with other medications intended for administration into the central nervous system

Pregnancy Risk Factor D

Lactation Excretion in breast milk unknown/not recommended

Use Treatment of lymphomatous meningitis

Mechanism of Action/Effect This is a sustained-release formulation of the active ingredient cytarabine. Acts to inhibit DNA polymerase which decreases DNA synthesis and repair.

Contraindications Hypersensitivity to cytarabine or any component of the formulation; active meningeal infection

Warnings/Precautions Hazardous agent - use appropriate precautions for handling and disposal. **[U.S. Boxed Warning]: Chemical arachnoiditis (nausea, vomiting, headache, fever) occurs commonly; may be fatal if untreated. The incidence and severity of chemical arachnoiditis is reduced by coadministration with dexamethasone.** Hydrocephalus has been reported and may be precipitated by chemical arachnoiditis. May cause neurotoxicity (including myelopathy), which may lead to permanent neurologic deficit. Blockage to CSF flow may increase the risk of neurotoxicity. Peripheral neurotoxicity has also been reported. Monitor for neurotoxicity; reduce subsequent doses; discontinue with persistent neurotoxicity. The risk of adverse events, including neurotoxicity, is increased with concurrent radiation therapy or systemic chemotherapy. Infectious meningitis may be associated with intrathecal administration. **[U.S. Boxed Warning]: Should be administered under the supervision of an experienced cancer chemotherapy physician.** For intrathecal use only. Intrathecal medications should not be prepared during the preparation of any other agents; after preparation, store intrathecal medications in an isolated location or container clearly marked with a label identifying as "intrathecal" use only; delivery of intrathecal medications to the patient should only be with other medications intended for administration into the central nervous system (Jacobson, 2009). Safety and efficacy in pediatric patients have not been established.

Drug Interactions

Avoid Concomitant Use

Avoid concomitant use of Cytarabine (Liposomal) with any of the following: BCG; Natalizumab; Pimecrolimus; Roflumilast; Tacrolimus (Topical); Vaccines (Live)

Decreased Effect

Cytarabine (Liposomal) may decrease the levels/effects of: BCG; Sipuleucel-T; Vaccines (Inactivated); Vaccines (Live)

The levels/effects of Cytarabine (Liposomal) may be decreased by: Echinacea

Increased Effect/Toxicity

Cytarabine (Liposomal) may increase the levels/effects of: Leflunomide; Natalizumab; Vaccines (Live)

The levels/effects of Cytarabine (Liposomal) may be increased by: Denosumab; Pimecrolimus; Roflumilast; Tacrolimus (Topical); Trastuzumab

Lab Interactions Since cytarabine liposomes are similar in appearance to WBCs, care must be taken in interpreting CSF examinations in patients receiving cytarabine liposomal.

Adverse Reactions

>10%:

Cardiovascular: Peripheral edema (11%)

Central nervous system: Chemical arachnoiditis (without dexamethasone premedication: 100%; with dexamethasone premedication: 33% to 42%; grade 4: 19% to 30%; onset: ≤5 days); headache (56%), confusion (33%), fever (32%), fatigue (25%), seizure (20% to 22%), dizziness (18%), lethargy (16%), insomnia (14%), memory impairment (14%), pain (14%)

Endocrine & metabolic: Dehydration (13%)

Gastrointestinal: Nausea (46%), vomiting (44%), constipation (25%), diarrhea (12%), appetite decreased (11%)

Genitourinary: Urinary tract infection (14%)

Hematologic: Anemia (12%), thrombocytopenia (3% to 11%)

Neuromuscular & skeletal: Weakness (40%), back pain (24%), abnormal gait (23%), limb pain (15%), neck pain (14%), arthralgia (11%), neck stiffness (11%)

Ocular: Blurred vision (11%)

1% to 10%:

Cardiovascular: Tachycardia (9%), hypotension (8%), hypertension (6%), syncope (3%), edema (2%)

Central nervous system: Agitation (10%), hypoesthesia (10%), depression (8%), anxiety (7%), sensory neuropathy (3%)

Dermatologic: Pruritus (2%)

Endocrine & metabolic: Hypokalemia (7%), hyponatremia (7%), hyperglycemia (6%)

Gastrointestinal: Abdominal pain (9%), dysphagia (8%), anorexia (5%), hemorrhoids (3%), mucosal inflammation (3%)

Genitourinary: Incontinence (7%), urinary retention (5%)

Hematologic: Neutropenia (10%), contusion (2%)

Neuromuscular & skeletal: Muscle weakness (10%), tremor (9%), peripheral neuropathy (4%), abnormal reflexes (3%)

Otic: Hypoacusis (6%)

Respiratory: Dyspnea (10%), cough (7%), pneumonia (6%)

Miscellaneous: Diaphoresis (2%)

Pharmacodynamics/Kinetics

Absorption Systemic exposure following intrathecal administration is negligible since transfer rate from CSF to plasma is slow

Time to Peak CSF: Intrathecal: <1 hour

Half-Life Elimination CSF: 6-82 hours

Available Dosage Forms

Injection, suspension, intrathecal [preservative free]:

DepoCyt®: 10 mg/mL (5 mL)

Dosing

Adult & Geriatric Note: Patients should be started on dexamethasone 4 mg twice daily (oral or I.V.) for 5 days, beginning on the day of cytarabine liposomal injection

Lymphomatous meningitis: I.T.:

Induction: 50 mg every 14 days for a total of 2 doses (weeks 1 and 3)

Consolidation: 50 mg every 14 days for 3 doses (weeks 5, 7, and 9), followed by an additional dose at week 13

Maintenance: 50 mg every 28 days for 4 doses (weeks 17, 21, 25, and 29)

Adjustment for Toxicity If drug-related neurotoxicity develops, reduce dose to 25 mg. If toxicity persists, discontinue treatment.

Administration

Other For intrathecal use only. Dose should be removed from vial immediately before administration (must be administered within 4 hours of removal). An in-line filter should **not** be used. Administer directly into the CSF via an intraventricular reservoir or by direct injection into the lumbar sac. Injection should be made slowly (over 1-5 minutes). Patients should lie flat for 1 hour after lumbar puncture.

Stability

Reconstitution Use appropriate precautions for handling and disposal. Allow vial to warm to room temperature prior to withdrawal from vial. Particles may settle in diluent over time, and may be resuspended by gentle agitation or inversion of the vial. Further reconstitution or dilution is not required. Intrathecal medications should not be prepared during the preparation of any other agents.

Storage Store under refrigeration at 2°C to 8°C (36°F to 46°F); protect from freezing. Avoid aggressive agitation. Solutions should be used within 4 hours of withdrawal from the vial.

After preparation, store intrathecal medications in an isolated location or container clearly marked with a label identifying as "intrathecal" use only.

Monitoring and Teaching Issues

Laboratory Monitoring Since cytarabine liposomes are similar in appearance to WBCs, care must be taken in interpreting CSF examinations in patients receiving cytarabine liposomal.

Physical Assessment This medication is only for intrathecal administration. Patient must be monitored continuously for adverse reactions that can be immediate (eg, neurotoxicity [myelopathy, ataxia, confusion, coma] and chemical arachnoiditis [neck pain, neck rigidity, headache, fever, nausea, vomiting, back pain]); potential for adverse reactions increased with concurrent radiation therapy or systemic chemotherapy. Incidence and severity of chemical arachnoiditis is reduced by coadministration with dexamethasone. Provide patient teaching according to patient condition.

Patient Education This medication can only be given by infusion into the spinal cord. You will be monitored closely during and after each infusion. Report immediately any neck pain or rigidity, headache, fever, nausea, or vomiting. Report any swelling of extremities, acute weakness, unusual gait pattern, or CNS changes (confusion, speech difficulty).

Breast-Feeding Considerations Although the systemic exposure following intrathecal administration of cytarabine liposomal is negligible, breast-feeding is not recommended due to the potential for serious adverse reactions in the nursing infant.

Pregnancy Considerations Reproductive studies have not been conducted with cytarabine liposomal. Cytarabine, the active component, has been associated with fetal malformations when given as a component of combination chemotherapy during the first trimester. Systemic exposure following intrathecal administration of cytarabine liposomal is negligible. There are no adequate and well-controlled studies in pregnant women. Women of childbearing potential should avoid becoming pregnant during treatment.

◆ **CytoGam®** *see* Cytomegalovirus Immune Globulin (Intravenous-Human) *on page* 451

Cytomegalovirus Immune Globulin (Intravenous-Human)

(sye toe meg a low VYE rus i MYUN GLOB yoo lin in tra VEE nus HYU man)

U.S. Brand Names CytoGam®

Index Terms CMV-IGIV

Generic Availability (U.S.) No

Pharmacologic Category Blood Product Derivative; Immune Globulin

Medication Safety Issues

Sound-alike/look-alike issues:

CytoGam® may be confused with Cytoxan, Gamimune® N

Pregnancy Risk Factor C

Lactation Excretion in breast milk unknown

Use Prophylaxis of cytomegalovirus (CMV) disease associated with kidney, lung, liver, pancreas, and heart transplants; concomitant use with ganciclovir should be considered in organ transplants (other than kidney) from CMV seropositive donors to CMV seronegative recipients

Unlabeled/Investigational Use Adjunct therapy in the treatment of CMV disease in immunocompromised patients

Available Dosage Forms

Injection, solution [preservative free]:

CytoGam®: 50 mg ± 10 mg/mL (50 mL)

Dosing

Adult

Kidney transplant: I.V.:

Initial dose (within 72 hours of transplant): 150 mg/kg/dose

2, 4, 6, and 8 weeks after transplant: 100 mg/kg/dose

12 and 16 weeks after transplant: 50 mg/kg/dose

Liver, lung, pancreas, or heart transplant: I.V.:

Initial dose (within 72 hours of transplant): 150 mg/kg/dose

2, 4, 6, and 8 weeks after transplant: 150 mg/kg/dose

12 and 16 weeks after transplant: 100 mg/kg/dose

Severe CMV pneumonia: I.V.: Various regimens have been used, including 400 mg/kg CMV-IGIV in combination with ganciclovir on days 1, 2, 7, or 8, followed by 200 mg/kg CMV-IGIV on days 14 and 21

Geriatric Use with caution in patients >65 years of age; elderly may be at increased risk of renal insufficiency.

Renal Impairment Use with caution; specific dosing adjustments are not available. Infusion rate should be the minimum practical; do not exceed 180 mg/kg/hour.

Administration

I.V. For I.V. use only. Administer as separate infusion. Infuse beginning at 15 mg/kg/hour, then increase to 30 mg/kg/hour after 30 minutes if no untoward reactions. May titrate up to 60 mg/kg/hour. Do not administer faster than 75 mL/hour. Begin infusion within 6 hours of entering vial, complete infusion within 12 hours.

Monitoring and Teaching Issues

Physical Assessment Assess for history of previous allergic reactions. Monitor vital signs during infusion and observe for adverse or allergic reactions.

Patient Education This medication can only be administered by infusion. You will be monitored closely during the infusion. You may experience nausea. Do not have any vaccinations for the next 3 months without consulting prescriber. Immediately report chills, muscle cramping, low back pain, chest pain or tightness, or respiratory difficulty.

◆ **Cytosar-U** *see* Cytarabine *on page* 445

◆ **Cytosine Arabinosine Hydrochloride** *see* Cytarabine *on page* 445

◆ **Cytostasan** *see* Bendamustine *on page* 198

◆ **Cytotec®** *see* Misoprostol *on page* 1242

◆ **Cytovene®-IV** *see* Ganciclovir (Systemic) *on page* 849

◆ **Cytoxan** *see* Cyclophosphamide *on page* 434

◆ **Cytra-2** *see* Sodium Citrate and Citric Acid *on page* 1660

◆ **D2** *see* Ergocalciferol *on page* 650

◆ **D2E7** *see* Adalimumab *on page* 48

◆ **d4T** *see* Stavudine *on page 1680*

◆ **DAB_{389}IL-2** *see* Denileukin Diftitox *on page 484*

◆ **DAB389 Interleukin-2** *see* Denileukin Diftitox *on page 484*

◆ **DABIL2** *see* Denileukin Diftitox *on page 484*

Dacarbazine (da KAR ba zeen)

Index Terms DIC; Dimethyl Triazeno Imidazole Carboxamide; DTIC; DTIC-Dome; Imidazole Carboxamide; Imidazole Carboxamide Dimethyltriazene; WR-139007

Generic Availability (U.S.) Yes

Pharmacologic Category Antineoplastic Agent, Alkylating Agent (Triazene)

Medication Safety Issues

Sound-alike/look-alike issues:

Dacarbazine may be confused with Dicarbosil®, procarbazine

High alert medication: This medication is in a class the Institute for Safe Medication Practices (ISMP) includes among its list of drugs which have a heightened risk of causing significant patient harm when used in error.

Pregnancy Risk Factor C

Lactation Excretion in breast milk unknown/not recommended

Use Treatment of malignant melanoma, Hodgkin's disease

Unlabeled/Investigational Use Treatment of soft-tissue sarcomas, islet cell tumors, pheochromocytoma, medullary carcinoma of the thyroid

Mechanism of Action/Effect Dacarbazine is an alkylating agent. It is converted to the active alkylating metabolite MTIC. The cytotoxic effects of MTIC are manifested through alkylation of DNA and appears to attack cross-links strands of DNA resulting in the inhibition of DNA, RNA, and protein synthesis.

Contraindications Hypersensitivity to dacarbazine or any component of the formulation

Warnings/Precautions Hazardous agent - use appropriate precautions for handling and disposal. **[U.S. Boxed Warnings]: Bone marrow suppression is a common toxicity;** leukopenia and thrombocytopenia may be severe; may result in treatment delays or discontinuation; monitor closely. **Hepatotoxicity with hepatocellular necrosis and hepatic vein thrombosis has been reported (rare),** usually with combination chemotherapy, but may occur with dacarbazine alone. The half-life is increased in patients with renal and/or hepatic impairment; use caution, monitor for toxicity and consider dosage reduction. Anaphylaxis may occur following dacarbazine administration. Extravasation may result in tissue damage and severe pain. **[U.S. Boxed Warnings]: May be carcinogenic and/or teratogenic. Should be administered under the supervision of an experienced cancer chemotherapy physician.** Carefully evaluate the potential benefits of therapy against the risk for toxicity.

Drug Interactions

Metabolism/Transport Effects Substrate (major) of CYP1A2, 2E1

Avoid Concomitant Use

Avoid concomitant use of Dacarbazine with any of the following: BCG; Natalizumab; Pimecrolimus; Roflumilast; Tacrolimus (Topical); Vaccines (Live)

Decreased Effect

Dacarbazine may decrease the levels/effects of: BCG; Sipuleucel-T; Vaccines (Inactivated); Vaccines (Live)

The levels/effects of Dacarbazine may be decreased by: CYP1A2 Inducers (Strong); Echinacea; SORAfenib

Increased Effect/Toxicity

Dacarbazine may increase the levels/effects of: Leflunomide; Natalizumab; Vaccines (Live)

The levels/effects of Dacarbazine may be increased by: CYP1A2 Inhibitors (Moderate); CYP1A2 Inhibitors (Strong); CYP2E1 Inhibitors (Moderate); CYP2E1 Inhibitors (Strong); Denosumab; MAO Inhibitors; Pimecrolimus; Roflumilast; Tacrolimus (Topical); Trastuzumab

Nutritional/Ethanol Interactions

Ethanol: Avoid ethanol (due to GI irritation).

Herb/Nutraceutical: Avoid dong quai, St John's wort (may also cause photosensitization).

Adverse Reactions Frequency not always defined.

Dermatologic: Alopecia

Gastrointestinal: Nausea and vomiting (>90%), anorexia

Hematologic: Myelosuppression (onset: 5-7 days; nadir: 7-10 days; recovery: 21-28 days), leukopenia, thrombocytopenia

Local: Pain on infusion

Pharmacodynamics/Kinetics

Protein Binding ~5%

Half-Life Elimination Biphasic: Initial: 20-40 minutes, Terminal: 5 hours; Patients with renal and hepatic dysfunction: Initial: 55 minutes, Terminal: 7.2 hours

Metabolism Extensively hepatic to the active metabolite MTIC [(methyl-triazene-1-yl)-imidazole-4-carboxamide]

Excretion Urine (~40% as unchanged drug)

Available Dosage Forms

Injection, powder for reconstitution: 100 mg, 200 mg

Dosing

Adult & Geriatric Details concerning dosing in combination regimens should also be consulted.

Hodgkin's disease (combination chemotherapy): I.V.: 375 mg/m^2/dose days 1 and 15 every 4 weeks (ABVD regimen)

Metastatic melanoma: I.V.: 250 mg/m^2/dose days 1-5 every 3 weeks

Metastatic melanoma (unlabeled dosing; in combination with cisplatin and vinblastine): I.V:. 800 mg/m^2 on day 1 every 3 weeks (Atkins, 2008; Eton, 2002)

Soft tissue sarcoma (unlabeled use; MAID regimen): I.V.: 250 mg/m^2/day continuous infusion for 4 days every 3 weeks (total of 1000 mg/m^2/cycle) (Antman, 1993; Antman, 1998)

Pediatric Details concerning dosing in combination regimens should also be consulted.

Hodgkin's disease (combination chemotherapy): I.V.: 375 mg/m^2/dose days 1 and 15 every 4 weeks (ABVD regimen; Hutchinson, 1998)

Renal Impairment The FDA-approved labeling does not contain dosage adjustment guidelines. The following guidelines have been used by some clinicians (Kintzel, 1995):

Cl_{cr} 46-60 mL/minute: Administer 80% of dose
Cl_{cr} 31-45 mL/minute: Administer 75% of dose
Cl_{cr} <30 mL/minute: Administer 70% of dose

Hepatic Impairment The FDA-approved labeling does not contain adjustment guidelines. May cause hepatotoxicity; monitor closely for signs of toxicity.

Administration

I.V. Irritant. Infuse over 30-60 minutes; may also be administered as a continuous infusion (unlabeled administration rate) depending on the protocol

Stability

Reconstitution Use appropriate precautions for handling and disposal. The manufacturer recommends reconstituting 100 mg and 200 mg vials with 9.9 mL and 19.7 mL SWFI, respectively, to a concentration of 10 mg/mL; some institutions use different standard dilutions (eg, 20 mg/mL).

Standard I.V. dilution: Dilute in 250-1000 mL D_5W or NS.

Storage Store intact vials under refrigeration (2°C to 8°C). Protect from light. The following stability information has also been reported: Intact vials are stable for 3 months at room temperature (Cohen, 2007). Reconstituted solution is stable for 24 hours at room temperature (20°C) and 96 hours under refrigeration (4°C) when protected from light, although the manufacturer recommends use within 72 hours if refrigerated and 8 hours at room temperature. Solutions for infusion (in D_5W or NS) are stable for 24 hours at room temperature if protected from light. Decomposed drug turns pink.

Monitoring and Teaching Issues

Laboratory Monitoring CBC with differential, liver function

Physical Assessment To be administered under the supervision of an experienced cancer chemotherapy physician. Use with caution and monitor for toxicity in presence of renal and/or hepatic impairment. Premedicate with antiemetic (emetic potential is moderately high). Patient must be monitored closely for anaphylactic reaction; emergency treatment should be available. Infusion site must be closely monitored; extravasation can cause severe cellulitis or tissue necrosis. Assess results of CBC with differential and LFTs prior to each treatment and throughout therapy.

Patient Education This drug can only be given by infusion. Report immediately any pain, burning, or swelling at infusion site; chest pain; or difficulty breathing or swallowing. Limit oral intake for 4-6 hours before infusion. Maintain adequate nutrition and hydration, unless instructed to restrict fluid intake. You will be more susceptible to infection. May cause nausea, vomiting, loss of appetite, hair loss (reversible), headache, fever, sinus congestion, or muscle aches. Report immediately any numbness in extremities or change in gait, respiratory distress or respiratory difficulty, change in urinary pattern, rash, easy bruising or bleeding, yellowing of eyes or skin, change in color of urine, or blackened stool.

Breast-Feeding Considerations Due to the potential for serious adverse reactions in the nursing infant, breast-feeding is not recommended.

Pregnancy Considerations [U.S. Boxed Warning]: This agent is carcinogenic and/or teratogenic when used in animals; adverse effects have been observed in animal studies. There are no adequate and well-controlled trials in pregnant women; use in pregnancy only if the potential benefit outweighs the potential risk to the fetus.

◆ **Dacliximab** *see* Daclizumab *on page 453*

Daclizumab (dac KLYE zue mab)

U.S. Brand Names Zenapax® [DSC]

Index Terms anti-Tac Monoclonal antibody; Dacliximab; MOAB anti-Tac

Generic Availability (U.S.) No

Pharmacologic Category Immunosuppressant Agent; Monoclonal Antibody

Pregnancy Risk Factor C

Lactation Excretion in breast milk unknown/not recommended

Use Prophylaxis of acute rejection in renal transplantation (in combination with cyclosporine and corticosteroids)

Unlabeled/Investigational Use Treatment of refractory acute graft-versus-host disease; prevention of cardiac transplant rejection

Mechanism of Action/Effect Daclizumab is a chimeric (90% human, 10% murine) monoclonal IgG antibody produced by recombinant DNA technology. Daclizumab inhibits immune reactions by binding and blocking the alpha-chain of the Tac subunit of the interleukin-2 receptor (CD25) complex located on the surface of activated lymphocytes.

Contraindications Hypersensitivity to daclizumab or any component of the formulation

Warnings/Precautions Severe acute hypersensitivity reactions, including anaphylaxis, have been observed on initial exposure and following re-exposure; medications for the management of severe allergic reaction should be available for immediate use. Hypersensitivity reactions may include bronchospasm, cyanosis, hypoxia, laryngeal edema, pulmonary edema, respiratory arrest, wheezing, hypotension, peripheral edema, diaphoresis, fever, loss of consciousness, rash, pruritus, urticaria, and/or injection site reactions. Permanently discontinue for severe hypersensitivity reaction. The risks of subsequent treatment courses are unknown and should be undertaken with caution.

An immunosuppressive regimen in cardiac transplant recipients which included daclizumab, cyclosporine, mycophenolate, and corticosteroids is associated with an increased in mortality (related to an increased incidence of severe infections), when compared to cyclosporine, mycophenolate, and corticosteroids plus placebo; higher mortality is also associated with concomitant use of antilymphocyte globulin. Patients on immunosuppressive therapy are at increased risk for infectious complications and secondary malignancies; long-term effects on immune function are unknown. Anti-idiotype antibodies have been measured in patients who have received daclizumab (adults 14%; children 34%); detection of antibodies may be influenced by multiple factors and may, therefore, be misleading. **[U.S. Boxed Warning]: Should be administered under the supervision of a physician experienced in immunosuppressive therapy and organ transplant management.**

Drug Interactions

Avoid Concomitant Use

Avoid concomitant use of Daclizumab with any of the following: BCG; Natalizumab; Pimecrolimus; Roflumilast; Tacrolimus (Topical); Vaccines (Live)

Decreased Effect

Daclizumab may decrease the levels/effects of: BCG; Sipuleucel-T; Vaccines (Inactivated); Vaccines (Live)

The levels/effects of Daclizumab may be decreased by: Echinacea

Increased Effect/Toxicity

Daclizumab may increase the levels/effects of: Leflunomide; Natalizumab; Vaccines (Live)

The levels/effects of Daclizumab may be increased by: Denosumab; Pimecrolimus; Roflumilast; Tacrolimus (Topical); Trastuzumab

Adverse Reactions Adverse effects reported during clinical trial use of daclizumab may be related to the patient population, transplant procedure, and concurrent transplant medications; incidences reported with daclizumab were similar to those reported with placebo. Diarrhea, fever, postoperative pain, pruritus, respiratory tract infection, urinary tract infection, hypertension (aggravated), and vomiting occurred more often in children than adults.

≥5%:

- Cardiovascular: Chest pain, edema (including peripheral), hyper-/hypotension, tachycardia, thrombosis
- Central nervous system: Dizziness, fatigue, fever, headache, insomnia, pain, post-traumatic pain
- Dermatologic: Acne, cellulitis, wound healing impaired
- Endocrine & metabolic: Hyperglycemia (32%)
- Gastrointestinal: Abdominal distention, abdominal pain, constipation, diarrhea, dyspepsia, epigastric pain, nausea, pyrosis, vomiting
- Genitourinary: Dysuria
- Hematologic: Bleeding
- Neuromuscular & skeletal: Back pain, musculoskeletal pain, tremor
- Renal: Oliguria, renal tubular necrosis
- Respiratory: Cough, dyspnea, pulmonary edema
- Miscellaneous: Anti-daclizumab antibody formation (children 34%; adults 14%), malignancy (2% to 6%), lymphocele, wound infection

≥2% to <5%:

- Central nervous system: Anxiety, depression, shivering
- Dermatologic: Hirsutism, pruritus, rash
- Endocrine & metabolic: Dehydration, diabetes mellitus, fluid overload
- Gastrointestinal: Flatulence, gastritis, hemorrhoids
- Genitourinary: Urinary retention, urinary tract bleeding
- Local: Injection site reaction
- Neuromuscular & skeletal: Arthralgia, leg cramps, myalgia, neuropathy, weakness
- Ocular: Vision blurred
- Renal: Hydronephrosis, renal damage, renal insufficiency
- Respiratory: Abnormal breath sounds, atelectasis, congestion, hypoxia, pharyngitis, pleural effusion, rales, rhinitis
- Miscellaneous: Diaphoresis, night sweats

Pharmacodynamics/Kinetics

Half-Life Elimination Estimated: Adults: Terminal: ~20 days (range 11-38 days); Children: ~13 days

Product Availability Zenapax®: Due to diminishing market demand, the manufacturer of daclizumab has discontinued production; it is anticipated that available supplies will be depleted in January 2010; all remaining lots will expire in 2011.

Dosing

Adult

Prophylaxis of acute renal transplant rejection: I.V.: 1 mg/kg within 24 hours before transplantation (day 0), then every 14 days for 4 additional doses (total of 5 doses). **Note:** Daclizumab is used adjunctively with other immunosuppressants (cyclosporine and corticosteroids).

Prevention of cardiac transplant rejection (unlabeled use): I.V.: 1 mg/kg (maximum dose: 100 mg); administer within 12 hours after heart transplant and on days 8, 22, 36, and 50 post-transplant (Hershberger, 2005)

Treatment of refractory acute graft-versus-host disease (unlabeled use): I.V.: 1 mg/kg on days 1, 4, 8, 15, and 22 (Bordigoni, 2006; Srinivasan, 2004) **or** 1 mg/kg (maximum dose: 100 mg); on days 1, 4, 8, 15, and 22 (Prezpiorka, 2000)

Geriatric Refer to adult dosing. Use with caution.

Pediatric

Prophylaxis of acute renal transplant rejection: I.V.: 1 mg/kg within 24 hours before transplantation (day 0), then every 14 days for 4 additional doses (total of 5 doses). **Note:** Daclizumab is used adjunctively with other immunosuppressants (cyclosporine and corticosteroids).

Treatment of refractory acute graft-versus-host disease (unlabeled use): I.V.: 1 mg/kg on days 1, 4, 8, 15, and 22 (Perales, 2007; Prezpiorka, 2000)

Renal Impairment No dosage adjustment needed.

Hepatic Impairment No data available for patients with severe impairment.

Administration

I.V. For I.V. administration following dilution. Administer within 4 hours of preparation if stored at room temperature; infuse over a 15-minute period via a peripheral or central vein.

Stability

Reconstitution Dilute in 50 mL 0.9% sodium chloride prior to administration; mix by gently inverting bag to avoid foaming; do not shake. Do not use if solution is discolored or particulate matter is present. Do not mix with other medications or infuse other medications through same I.V. line.

Storage Refrigerate intact vials at 2°C to 8°C (36°F to 46°F); do not freeze. Do not shake. Protect undiluted solution from direct light. Do not use if solution is discolored or particulate matter is present. Solutions diluted for infusion in 0.9% sodium chloride are stable for 24 hours at 4°C or for 4 hours at room temperature.

Monitoring and Teaching Issues

Laboratory Monitoring Serum glucose

Physical Assessment Assess cardiorespiratory and renal function (fluid overload) during infusion and periodically between infusions. May cause hyperglycemia. Be alert to the possibility of the development of infection. Malignancies may occur with long-term use. Hypersensitivity reactions can occur. Treatment for severe allergic reactions should be available for immediate use.

Patient Education This medication, which may help to reduce transplant rejection, can only be administered by infusion. You will be monitored closely during infusion. Report immediately any respiratory or swallowing difficulty; tightness in jaw or throat; chest pain; or rash or pain at infusion site. You will be more susceptible to infection. Maintain adequate nutrition and hydration, unless instructed to restrict fluid intake. May cause elevated blood sugar, headache, dizziness, fatigue, back pain, leg cramps, musculoskeletal pain, nausea, or vomiting. Report chest pain or palpitations, persistent dizziness, respiratory difficulty, rash, infection (fever or chills), thirst, excessive urination, or weight loss.

Pregnancy Considerations An increased risk of fetal loss was observed in animal reproduction studies. Generally, IgG molecules cross the placenta. Use during pregnancy only if the potential benefit to the mother outweighs the possible risk to the fetus. Women of childbearing potential should use effective contraception before, during, and for 4 months following daclizumab treatment.

◆ **Dacogen™** *see* Decitabine *on page 476*

◆ **DACT** *see* DACTINomycin *on page 455*

DACTINomycin (dak ti noe MYE sin)

U.S. Brand Names Cosmegen®

Index Terms ACT-D; Actinomycin; Actinomycin Cl; Actinomycin D; DACT

Generic Availability (U.S.) Yes

Pharmacologic Category Antineoplastic Agent, Antibiotic

Medication Safety Issues

Sound-alike/look-alike issues:

DACTINomycin may be confused with DAPTOmycin, DAUNOrubicin

Actinomycin may be confused with achromycin

High alert medication: The Institute for Safe Medication Practices (ISMP) includes this medication among its list of drug classes which have a heightened risk of causing significant patient harm when used in error.

Pregnancy Risk Factor D

Lactation Excretion in breast milk unknown/not recommended

Use Treatment of Wilms' tumor, childhood rhabdomyosarcoma, Ewing's sarcoma, metastatic testicular tumors (nonseminomatous), gestational trophoblastic neoplasm; regional perfusion (palliative or adjunctive) of locally recurrent or locoregional solid tumors (sarcomas, carcinomas and adenocarcinomas)

Unlabeled/Investigational Use Treatment of ovarian cancer (germ cell or stromal tumors), osteosarcoma, soft tissue sarcoma (other than rhabdomyosarcoma)

Mechanism of Action/Effect Causes cell death by binding to DNA inhibiting messenger RNA

Contraindications Hypersensitivity to dactinomycin or any component of the formulation; patients with concurrent or recent chickenpox or herpes zoster

Warnings/Precautions [U.S. Boxed Warnings]: Hazardous agent - use appropriate precautions for handling and disposal. Dactinomycin is extremely irritating to tissues; if extravasation occurs during I.V. use, severe damage to soft tissues will occur; has led to contracture of the arm (rare). Avoid inhalation of vapors or contact with skin, mucous membrane, or eyes; avoid exposure during pregnancy. Recommended for I.V.administration only. The manufacturer recommends intermittent ice (15 minutes 4 times/day) for suspected extravasation.

May cause veno-occlusive liver disease (VOD); use with caution in hepatobiliary dysfunction. Monitor for signs or symptoms of hepatic VOD, including bilirubin >1.4 mg/dL, unexplained weight gain, ascites, hepatomegaly, or unexplained right upper quadrant pain (Arndt, 2004). The risk of fatal VOD is increased in children <4 years of age.

Dactinomycin potentiates the effects of radiation therapy; use with caution in patients who have received radiation therapy; reduce dosages in patients who are receiving dactinomycin and radiation therapy simultaneously; combination with radiation therapy may result in increased GI toxicity and myelosuppression. Avoid dactinomycin use within 2 months of radiation treatment for right-sided Wilms' tumor, may increase the risk of hepatotoxicity.

Toxic effects may be delayed in onset (2-4 days following a course of treatment) and may require 1-2 weeks to reach maximum severity. Long-term observation of cancer survivors is recommended due to the increased risk of second primary tumors following treatment with radiation and antineoplastic agents. Regional perfusion therapy may result in local limb edema, soft tissue damage, and possible venous thrombosis; leakage of dactinomycin into systemic circulation may result in hematologic toxicity, infection, impaired wound healing, and mucositis. Dosage is usually expressed in **MICRO**grams and should be calculated on the basis of body surface area (BSA) in obese or edematous adult patients (to relate dose to lean body mass). Avoid administration of live vaccines during dactinomycin treatment. Avoid use in infants <6 months of age (toxic effects may occur more frequently). May be associated with an increased risk of myelosuppression in the elderly; use with caution. **[U.S. Boxed Warning]: Should be administered under the supervision of an experienced cancer chemotherapy physician.**

Drug Interactions

Avoid Concomitant Use

Avoid concomitant use of DACTINomycin with any of the following: BCG; Natalizumab; Pimecrolimus; Roflumilast; Tacrolimus (Topical); Vaccines (Live)

Decreased Effect

DACTINomycin may decrease the levels/effects of: BCG; Sipuleucel-T; Vaccines (Inactivated); Vaccines (Live)

The levels/effects of DACTINomycin may be decreased by: Echinacea

Increased Effect/Toxicity

DACTINomycin may increase the levels/effects of: Leflunomide; Natalizumab; Vaccines (Live)

The levels/effects of DACTINomycin may be increased by: Denosumab; Pimecrolimus; Roflumilast; Tacrolimus (Topical); Trastuzumab

Lab Interactions May interfere with bioassays of antibacterial drug levels

Adverse Reactions Frequency not defined.

Central nervous system: Fatigue, fever, lethargy, malaise

Dermatologic: Acne, alopecia (reversible), cheilitis; increased pigmentation, sloughing, or erythema of previously irradiated skin; skin eruptions

Endocrine & metabolic: Growth retardation, hyperuricemia, hypocalcemia

Gastrointestinal: Abdominal pain, anorexia, diarrhea, dysphagia, esophagitis, GI ulceration, mucositis, nausea, pharyngitis, proctitis, stomatitis, vomiting

Hematologic: Agranulocytosis, anemia, aplastic anemia, febrile neutropenia, leukopenia, neutropenia, pancytopenia, reticulocytopenia, thrombocytopenia, myelosuppression (onset: 7 days, nadir: 14-21 days, recovery: 21-28 days)

Hepatic: Ascites, bilirubin increased, hepatic failure, hepatitis, hepatomegaly, hepatopathy thrombocytopenia syndrome, hepatotoxicity, liver function test abnormality, veno-occlusive disease

Local: Erythema, edema, epidermolysis, pain, tissue necrosis, and ulceration (following extravasation)

Neuromuscular & skeletal: Myalgia

Renal: Renal function abnormality

Respiratory: Pneumonitis

Miscellaneous: Anaphylactoid reaction, infection

Pharmacodynamics/Kinetics

Half-Life Elimination ~36 hours; Children: Range: 14-43 hours

Metabolism Minimal

Excretion Urine and feces

Available Dosage Forms

Injection, powder for reconstitution: 0.5 mg

Cosmegen®: 0.5 mg

Dosing

Adult Details concerning dosing in combination regimens should also be consulted.

Note: Medication orders for dactinomycin are commonly written in MICROgrams (eg, 150 mcg) although many regimens list the dose in MILLIgrams (eg, mg/kg or mg/m^2). One-time doses for >1000 mcg, or multiple-day doses for >500 mcg/day are not common. The dose intensity per 2-week cycle should not exceed 15 mcg/kg/day for 5 days or 400-600 mcg/m^2/day for 5 days. Some practitioners recommend calculation of the dosage for obese or edematous adult patients on the basis of body surface area in an effort to relate dosage to lean body mass.

Usual doses:

I.V.: 15 mcg/kg/day for 5 days every 3-6 weeks **or** 400-600 mcg/m^2/day for 5 days every 3-6 weeks **or** 1000 mcg/m^2 on day 1 or 12 mcg/kg/day for 5 days (monotherapy) **or** 500 mcg/dose days 1 and 2 (as part of a combination chemotherapy regimen)

Regional perfusion (dosages and techniques may vary by institution; obese patients and patients with prior chemotherapy or radiation therapy may require lower doses): Lower extremity or pelvis: 50 mcg/kg; Upper extremity: 35 mcg/kg

Indication-specific dosing:

Testicular cancer: I.V.: 1000 mcg/m^2 on day 1 (as part of a combination chemotherapy regimen)

Gestational trophoblastic neoplasm: I.V.: 12 mcg/kg/day for 5 days (monotherapy) **or** 500 mcg/dose days 1 and 2 (as part of a combination chemotherapy regimen)

Wilms' tumor, Ewing's sarcoma, rhabdomyosarcoma: I.V.: 15 mcg/kg/day for 5 days (in various combination regimens and schedules)

Osteosarcoma (unlabeled use): I.V.: 600 mcg/m^2/dose days 1, 2, and 3 as part of a combination chemotherapy regimen (Goorin, 2003)

Ovarian (germ cell) tumor (unlabeled use): I.V.: 500 mcg/day for 5 days every 4 weeks (Gershenson, 1985) **or** 300 mcg/m^2/day for 5 days every 4 weeks (Slayton,1985)

Geriatric Refer to adult dosing. Elderly patients are at increased risk of myelosuppression; dosing should begin at the low end of the dosing range.

Pediatric Details concerning dosing in combination regimens should also be consulted.

Note: Medication orders for dactinomycin are commonly written in MICROgrams (eg, 150 mcg) although many regimens list the dose in MILLIgrams (eg, mg/kg or mg/m^2). One-time doses for >1000 mcg, or multiple-day doses for >500 mcg/day are not common. The dose intensity per 2-week cycle should not exceed 15 mcg/kg/day for 5 days or 400-600 mcg/m^2/day for 5 days.

Usual dose: I.V.: Children >6 months: 15 mcg/kg/day for 5 days every 3-6 weeks **or** 400-600 mcg/m^2/day for 5 days every 3-6 weeks

Wilms' tumor, rhabdomyosarcoma, Ewing's sarcoma: 15 mcg/kg/day for 5 days (in various combination regimens and schedules)

Osteosarcoma (unlabeled use): 600 mcg/m^2/dose days 1, 2, and 3 as part of a combination chemotherapy regimen (Goorin, 2003)

Renal Impairment No adjustment is necessary.

Administration

I.V. Slow I.V. push or infuse over 10-15 minutes. Avoid extravasation. Do not filter with cellulose ester membrane filters. Do not administer I.M. or SubQ.

Stability

Reconstitution Use appropriate precautions for handling and disposal. Dilute with 1.1 mL of preservative-free SWFI to yield a final concentration of 500 mcg/mL (diluent containing preservatives will cause precipitation). May further dilute in D_5W or NS. Cellulose ester membrane filters may partially remove dactinomycin from solution and should not be used during preparation or administration.

Storage Store at controlled room temperature of 15°C to 30°C (59°F to 86°F). Protect from light and humidity. Reconstituted solutions retain potency for 24 hours at room temperature or refrigerated. Solutions in 50 mL D_5W are stable for 24 hours at room temperature.

Monitoring and Teaching Issues

Laboratory Monitoring CBC with differential and platelet count, liver and renal function

Physical Assessment Use caution to prevent inadvertent exposure to this medication. Infusion site must be closely monitored; extravasation can cause severe cellulitis or tissue necrosis. Assess results of hematology, renal, and hepatic function tests on a regular basis throughout therapy (toxic effects may be delayed 2-4 days following a course of treatment and may take 1-2 weeks to reach maximum severity).

Patient Education This drug is given by infusion and you will be closely monitored. Report immediately any pain, burning, or swelling at infusion site; sudden chest pain, difficulty breathing or swallowing, or chills. Between infusions, maintain adequate nutrition and hydration. You will be more susceptible to infection. May cause fatigue or malaise, nausea, vomiting, loss of appetite, diarrhea, or hair loss (reversible). Report unresolved nausea, vomiting, diarrhea, or abdominal pain; difficulty swallowing; or rash.

Breast-Feeding Considerations It is not known if dactinomycin is excreted in human breast milk. Due to the potential for serious adverse reactions in the nursing infant, breast-feeding is not recommended.

Pregnancy Considerations Animal studies have demonstrated teratogenic effects and fetal loss. There are no adequate and well-controlled studies in pregnant women. Women of childbearing potential are advised not to become pregnant. Use only when potential benefit justifies potential risk to the fetus. **[U.S. Boxed Warning]: Avoid exposure during pregnancy.**

Dalfampridine (dal FAM pri deen)

U.S. Brand Names Ampyra™

Index Terms 4-aminopyridine; 4-AP; EL-970; Fampridine-SR

Pharmacologic Category Potassium Channel Blocker

Medication Safety Issues

Sound-alike/look-alike issues:

Ampyra™ may be confused with anakinra

Dalfampridine may be confused with delavirdine, desipramine

Medication Guide Available Yes

Pregnancy Risk Factor C

Lactation Excretion in breast milk unknown/not recommended

Use Treatment to improve walking in multiple sclerosis (MS) patients

Mechanism of Action/Effect Enhances nerve conduction leading to improvements in muscle contraction.

Contraindications History of seizure; moderate or severe renal impairment (Cl_{cr} ≤50 mL/minute)

Warnings/Precautions Dalfampridine administration is associated with a dose-dependent risk of seizure; discontinue use and do not reinitiate therapy if seizure occurs during treatment. Use is contraindicated in patients with a history of seizures. Use with caution in patients with mild renal impairment. No specific dosage adjustment is recommended by the manufacturer; however, risk of seizure may be increased secondary to reduced clearance in these patients. Use is contraindicated in moderate-to-severe renal impairment (Cl_{cr} ≤50 mL/minute). To avoid adverse reactions, dalfampridine should not be administered with other 4-aminopyridine formulations (eg, compounded immediate release fampridine)

Drug Interactions

Avoid Concomitant Use There are no known interactions where it is recommended to avoid concomitant use.

Decreased Effect There are no known significant interactions involving a decrease in effect.

Increased Effect/Toxicity There are no known significant interactions involving an increase in effect.

Adverse Reactions

>10%: Genitourinary: Urinary tract infection (12%)

1% to 10%:

Central nervous system: Insomnia (9%), dizziness (7%), headache (7%), multiple sclerosis relapse (4%), seizures (up to 4%; dose-dependent)

Gastrointestinal: Nausea (7%), constipation (3%), dyspepsia (2%)

Neuromuscular & skeletal: Weakness (7%), back pain (5%), balance disorder (5%), paresthesia (4%)

Respiratory: Nasopharyngitis (4%), pharyngolaryngeal pain (2%)

Pharmacodynamics/Kinetics

Absorption Rapid and complete

Bioavailability 96% (relative to aqueous solution)

Protein Binding Negligible

Half-Life Elimination 5-7 hours; prolonged in severe renal impairment (~3 times longer)

Metabolism No active metabolites detected

Excretion Urine (96%; 90% of total dose as unchanged drug); feces (0.5%)

Available Dosage Forms

Tablet, extended release, oral:

Ampyra™: 10 mg

Dosing

Adult & Geriatric Multiple sclerosis: Oral: 10 mg every 12 hours (maximum daily dose: 20 mg); no additional benefit seen with doses >20 mg/day

Renal Impairment

Mild renal impairment (Cl_{cr} 51-80 mL/minute): No specific adjustment recommended by the manufacturer; however, risk of seizure may be increased secondary to reduced clearance.

Moderate-to-severe renal impairment (Cl_{cr} ≤50 mL/minute): Contraindicated.

Administration

Oral May be administered with or without food. Do not chew, crush, dissolve, or divide tablet.

Stability

Storage Store at 25°C (77°F); excursions permitted to 15°C to 30°C (59°F to 86°F).

Monitoring and Teaching Issues

Laboratory Monitoring Renal function; EEG

Physical Assessment Assess carefully for renal impairment or history of seizures. If seizures occur, discontinue medication.

Patient Education Take with or without food. Discontinue and consult prescriber if you experience a seizure. You may experience dizziness or headache. Report any sign of urinary tract infection (change in urinary pattern or pain on urination), relapse of multiple sclerosis, persistent headache or dizziness, unusual muscle weakness, or difficulty with balance.

Dietary Considerations May be taken with or without food.

Geriatric Considerations Dalfampridine is contraindicated in patients with a Cl_{cr} ≤50 mL/minute. Because many older patients have impaired renal function, this medication should be used with caution and only when the renal function is known to be Cl_{cr} >50 mL/minute.

Breast-Feeding Considerations Due to the potential for serious adverse reactions in the nursing infant, breast-feeding is not recommended.

Pregnancy Considerations Adverse events have been observed in animal studies, including decreased growth and death. There are no adequate and well-controlled studies in pregnant women.

◆ **Dalfopristin and Quinupristin** *see* Quinupristin and Dalfopristin *on page* 1543

◆ **Daliresp™** *see* Roflumilast *on page* 1605

Dalteparin (dal TE pa rin)

U.S. Brand Names Fragmin®

Index Terms Dalteparin Sodium; NSC-714371

Generic Availability (U.S.) No

Pharmacologic Category Low Molecular Weight Heparin

Medication Safety Issues

High alert medication: The Institute for Safe Medication Practices (ISMP) includes this medication among its list of drugs which have a heightened risk of causing significant patient harm when used in error.

2009 National Patient Safety Goals: The Joint Commission (TJC) requires healthcare organizations that provide anticoagulant therapy to have a process in place to reduce the risk of anticoagulant-associated patient harm. Patients receiving anticoagulants should receive individualized care through a defined process that includes standardized ordering, dispensing, administration, monitoring and education. This does not apply to routine short-term use of anticoagulants for prevention of venous thromboembolism when the expectation is that the patient's laboratory values will remain within or close to normal values (NPSG.03.05.01).

Pregnancy Risk Factor B

Lactation Enters breast milk/use caution

Use Prevention of deep vein thrombosis which may lead to pulmonary embolism, in patients requiring abdominal surgery who are at risk for thromboembolism complications (eg, patients >40 years of age, obesity, patients with malignancy, history of deep vein thrombosis or pulmonary embolism, and surgical procedures requiring general anesthesia and lasting >30 minutes); prevention of DVT in patients undergoing hip-replacement surgery; patients immobile during an acute illness; acute treatment of unstable angina or non-Q-wave myocardial infarction; prevention of ischemic complications in patients on concurrent aspirin therapy; in patients with cancer, extended treatment (6 months) of acute symptomatic venous thromboembolism (DVT and/or PE) to reduce the recurrence of venous thromboembolism

Unlabeled/Investigational Use Active treatment of deep vein thrombosis (noncancer patients)

Mechanism of Action/Effect Low molecular weight heparin analog; the commercial product contains 3% to 15% heparin; has been shown to inhibit both factor Xa and factor IIa (thrombin), however, the antithrombotic effect of dalteparin is characterized by a higher ratio of antifactor Xa to antifactor IIa activity (ratio = 4)

Contraindications Hypersensitivity to dalteparin or any component of the formulation; thrombocytopenia associated with a positive *in vitro* test for antiplatelet antibodies in the presence of dalteparin; hypersensitivity to heparin or pork products; patients with active major bleeding; patients with unstable angina, non-Q-wave MI, or acute venous thromboembolism undergoing regional anesthesia; not for I.M. or I.V. use

Warnings/Precautions **[U.S. Boxed Warning]: Spinal or epidural hematomas, including subsequent paralysis, may occur with recent or anticipated neuraxial anesthesia (epidural or spinal) or spinal puncture in patients anticoagulated with LMWH or heparinoids.** Consider risk versus benefit prior to spinal procedures; risk is increased by the use of concomitant agents which may alter hemostasis, the use of indwelling epidural catheters for analgesia, a history of spinal deformity or spinal surgery, as well as traumatic or repeated epidural or spinal punctures. Patient should be observed closely for bleeding if enoxaparin is administered during or immediately following diagnostic lumbar puncture, epidural anesthesia, or spinal anesthesia.

Use with caution in patients with pre-existing thrombocytopenia, recent childbirth, subacute bacterial endocarditis, peptic ulcer disease, pericarditis or pericardial effusion, liver or renal function impairment, recent lumbar puncture, vasculitis, concurrent use of aspirin (increased bleeding risk), previous hypersensitivity to heparin, heparin-associated thrombocytopenia. Monitor platelet count closely. Rare thrombocytopenia may occur. Consider discontinuation of dalteparin in any patient developing significant thrombocytopenia related to initiation of dalteparin. Rare cases of thrombocytopenia with thrombosis have occurred. Use caution in patients with congenital or drug-induced thrombocytopenia or platelet defects. Cancer patients with thrombocytopenia may require dose adjustments for treatment of acute venous thromboembolism.

Use with caution in patients with known hypersensitivity to methylparaben or propylparaben. Monitor patient closely for signs or symptoms of bleeding. Certain patients are at increased risk of bleeding. Risk factors include bacterial endocarditis; congenital or acquired bleeding disorders; active ulcerative or angiodysplastic GI diseases; severe uncontrolled hypertension; hemorrhagic stroke; or use shortly after brain, spinal, or ophthalmology surgery; in patient treated concomitantly with platelet inhibitors; recent GI bleeding; thrombocytopenia or platelet defects; severe liver disease; hypertensive or diabetic retinopathy; or in patients undergoing invasive procedures.

Use with caution in patients with severe renal failure (has not been studied). Safety and efficacy in pediatric patients have not been established. Rare cases of thrombocytopenia with thrombosis have occurred. Multidose vials contain benzyl alcohol and should not be used in pregnant women. In neonates, large amounts of benzyl alcohol (>100 mg/kg/day) have been associated with fatal toxicity (gasping syndrome). Heparin can cause hyperkalemia by affecting aldosterone. Similar reactions could occur with dalteparin. Monitor for hyperkalemia. Do **not** administer intramuscularly. Not to be used interchangeably (unit for unit) with heparin or any other low molecular weight heparins.

There is no consensus for adjusting/correcting the weight-based dosage of LMWH for patients who are morbidly obese (BMI ≥40 kg/m^2). For patients undergoing inpatient bariatric surgery, the American College of Chest Physicians Practice Guidelines suggest using a higher thromboprophylaxis dose of LMWH for obese patients (Geerts, 2008).

Drug Interactions

Avoid Concomitant Use There are no known interactions where it is recommended to avoid concomitant use.

Decreased Effect There are no known significant interactions involving a decrease in effect.

Increased Effect/Toxicity

Dalteparin may increase the levels/effects of: Anticoagulants; Collagenase (Systemic); Drotrecogin Alfa; Ibritumomab; Tositumomab and Iodine I 131 Tositumomab

The levels/effects of Dalteparin may be increased by: 5-ASA Derivatives; Antiplatelet Agents; Dasatinib; Herbs (Anticoagulant/Antiplatelet Properties); Nonsteroidal Anti-Inflammatory Agents; Pentosan Polysulfate Sodium; Pentoxifylline; Prostacyclin Analogues; Salicylates; Thrombolytic Agents

Nutritional/Ethanol Interactions Herb/Nutraceutical: Alfalfa, anise, bilberry, bladderwrack, bromelain, cat's claw, celery, chamomile, coleus, cordyceps, dong quai, evening primrose oil, fenugreek, feverfew, garlic, ginger, ginkgo biloba, ginseng (American), ginseng (panax), ginseng (Siberian), grapeseed, green tea, guggul, horse chestnut seed, horseradish, licorice, prickly ash, red clover, reishi, SAMe (s-adenosylmethionine), sweet clover, turmeric, white willow (all have additional antiplatelet/anticoagulant activity)

Lab Interactions Increased AST, ALT levels

Adverse Reactions Note: As with all anticoagulants, bleeding is the major adverse effect of dalteparin. Hemorrhage may occur at virtually any site. Risk is dependent on multiple variables.

>10%:

Hematologic: Bleeding (3% to 14%)

1% to 10%:

Hematologic: Wound hematoma (up to 3%)

Hepatic: AST >3 times upper limit of normal (5% to 9%), ALT >3 times upper limit of normal (4% to 10%)

Local: Pain at injection site (up to 12%), injection site hematoma (up to 7%)

Pharmacodynamics/Kinetics

Onset of Action 1-2 hours

Duration of Action >12 hours

Bioavailability SubQ: 81% to 93%

Time to Peak Serum: 4 hours

Half-Life Elimination Route dependent: 2-5 hours

Available Dosage Forms

Injection, solution:

Fragmin®: 25,000 anti-Xa int. units/mL (3.8 mL)

Injection, solution [preservative free]:

Fragmin®: 10,000 anti-Xa int. units/mL (1 mL); 2500 anti-Xa int. units/0.2 mL (0.2 mL); 5000 anti-Xa int. units/0.2 mL (0.2 mL); 7500 anti-Xa int. units/0.3 mL (0.3 mL); 12,500 anti-Xa int. units/0.5 mL (0.5 mL); 15,000 anti-Xa int. units/0.6 mL (0.6 mL); 18,000 anti-Xa int. units/0.72 mL (0.72 mL)

Dosing

Adult & Geriatric

Abdominal surgery (DVT prophylaxis):

Low-to-moderate DVT risk: SubQ: 2500 int. units 1-2 hours prior to surgery, then once daily for 5-10 days postoperatively

High DVT risk: SubQ: 5000 int. units the evening prior to surgery and then once daily for 5-10 days postoperatively. Alternatively in patients with malignancy: 2500 int. units 1-2 hours prior to surgery, 2500 int. units 12 hours later, then 5000 int. units once daily for 5-10 days postoperatively.

Total hip surgery (DVT prophylaxis): SubQ: **Note:** Three treatment options are currently available. Dose is given for 5-10 days, although up to 14 days of treatment have been tolerated in clinical trials:

Postoperative start:

Initial: 2500 int. units 4-8 hours* after surgery

Maintenance: 5000 int. units once daily; start at least 6 hours after postsurgical dose

Preoperative (starting day of surgery):

Initial: 2500 int. units within 2 hours before surgery

Adjustment: 2500 int. units 4-8 hours* after surgery

Maintenance: 5000 int. units once daily; start at least 6 hours after postsurgical dose

Preoperative (starting evening prior to surgery):

Initial: 5000 int. units 10-14 hours before surgery

Adjustment: 5000 int. units 4-8 hours* after surgery

Maintenance: 5000 int. units once daily, allowing 24 hours between doses.

***Note:** Dose may be delayed if hemostasis is not yet achieved.

Unstable angina or non-Q-wave myocardial infarction: SubQ: 120 int. units/kg body weight (maximum dose: 10,000 int. units) every 12 hours for 5-8 days with concurrent aspirin therapy. Discontinue dalteparin once patient is clinically stable.

Venous thromboembolism: SubQ: Cancer patients:

Initial (month 1): 200 int. units/kg (maximum dose: 18,000 int. units) once daily for 30 days

Maintenance (months 2-6): ~150 int. units/kg (maximum dose: 18,000 int. units) once daily. If platelet count between 50,000-100,000/mm^3, reduce dose by 2,500 int. units until platelet count recovers to ≥100,000/mm^3. If platelet count <50,000/mm^3, discontinue dalteparin until platelet count recover to >50,000/mm^3.

Immobility/acute illness (DVT prophylaxis): 5000 int. units once daily

Renal Impairment In cancer patients, receiving treatment for venous thromboembolism, if Cl_{cr} <30 mL/minute, manufacturer recommends monitoring anti-Xa levels to determine appropriate dose.

Hepatic Impairment Use with caution in patients with hepatic insufficiency; specific dosage adjustments have not been recommended.

Administration

I.M. Do **not** administer I.M.

Other For deep SubQ injection only. May be injected in a U-shape to the area surrounding the navel, the upper outer side of the thigh, or the upper outer quadrangle of the buttock. Use thumb and forefinger to lift a fold of skin when injecting dalteparin to the navel area or thigh. Insert needle at a 45- to 90-degree angle. The entire length of needle should be inserted. Do not expel air bubble from fixed-dose syringe prior to injection. Air bubble (and extra solution, if applicable) may be expelled from graduated syringes. In order to minimize bruising, do not rub injection site.

To convert from I.V. unfractionated heparin (UFH) infusion to SubQ dalteparin (Nutescu, 2007): Calculate specific dose for dalteparin based on indication, discontinue UFH and begin dalteparin within 1 hour

To convert from SubQ dalteparin to I.V. UFH infusion (Nutescu, 2007): Discontinue dalteparin; calculate specific dose for I.V. UFH infusion based on indication; omit heparin bolus/ loading dose

Converting from SubQ dalteparin dosed every 12 hours: Start I.V. UFH infusion 10-11 hours after last dose of dalteparin

Converting from SubQ dalteparin dosed every 24 hours: Start I.V. UFH infusion 22-23 hours after last dose of dalteparin

Stability

Storage Store at temperatures of 20°C to 25°C (68°F to 77°F). Multidose vials may be stored for up to 2 weeks at room temperature after entering.

Monitoring and Teaching Issues

Laboratory Monitoring Periodic CBC including platelet count; stool occult blood tests; monitoring of PT and PTT is not necessary. Once patient has received 3-4 doses, anti-Xa levels, drawn 4-6 hours after dalteparin administration, may be used to monitor effect in patients with severe renal dysfunction or if abnormal coagulation parameters or bleeding should occur.

Physical Assessment Evaluate for increased bleeding risk prior to beginning treatment. Bleeding precautions should be observed during treatment. Teach patient about bleeding precautions.

Patient Education This drug can only be administered by injection. You may have a tendency to bleed easily while taking this drug. Report unusual fever; unusual bleeding or bruising (bleeding gums, nosebleed, blood in urine, dark stool); pain in joints or back; severe headache or confusion; skin rash; redness, swelling, or pain at injection site; or severe dizziness.

Geriatric Considerations No specific recommendations are necessary for the elderly.

Breast-Feeding Considerations In lactating women receiving prophylactic doses of dalteparin, small amounts of anti-xa activity was noted in breast milk. The milk/plasma ratio was <0.025 to 0.224. Oral absorption of low molecular weight heparin is extremely low.

Pregnancy Considerations Multiple-dose vials contain benzyl alcohol (avoid in pregnant women due to association with gasping syndrome in premature infants). Adverse effects were not observed in animal studies. There are no adequate and well-controlled studies in pregnant women. Use during pregnancy only if clearly needed.

Additional Information

Multidose vial contains 14 mg/mL benzyl alcohol.

◆ **Dalteparin Sodium** *see* Dalteparin *on page 459*

Danazol (DA na zole)

Index Terms Danocrine
Generic Availability (U.S.) Yes
Pharmacologic Category Androgen
Medication Safety Issues
Sound-alike/look-alike issues:
Danazol may be confused with Dantrium®
Danocrine may be confused with Dacriose®
Pregnancy Risk Factor X
Lactation Enters breast milk/contraindicated
Use Treatment of endometriosis, fibrocystic breast disease, and hereditary angioedema
Available Dosage Forms
Capsule, oral: 50 mg, 100 mg, 200 mg
Dosing
Adult & Geriatric
Endometriosis (females): Oral: Initial: 200-400 mg/day in 2 divided doses for mild disease; individualize dosage. Usual maintenance dose: 800 mg/day in 2 divided doses to achieve amenorrhea and rapid response to painful symptoms. Continue therapy uninterrupted for 3-6 months (up to 9 months).
Fibrocystic breast disease (females): Oral: Range: 100-400 mg/day in 2 divided doses
Hereditary angioedema (males/females): Oral: Initial: 200 mg 2-3 times/day; after favorable response, decrease the dosage by 50% or less at intervals of 1-3 months or longer if the frequency of attacks dictates. If an attack occurs, increase the dosage by up to 200 mg/day.
Monitoring and Teaching Issues
Laboratory Monitoring Liver and renal function
Physical Assessment Assess anticoagulants and hypoglycemic agents patient may be taking for potential interactions. Monitor for hypertension, increased LDL, CNS changes, jaundice, and hematuria. Caution patients with diabetes to monitor glucose levels closely; may enhance the glucose-lowering effect of hypoglycemic agents. Teach patient good self-breast-exam technique.
Patient Education Therapy may take up to several months depending on purpose for therapy. If you have diabetes, monitor serum glucose closely and notify prescriber of changes; this medication can alter hypoglycemic requirements. Consult prescriber for appropriate self-breast-exam technique. May cause headache, sleeplessness, anxiety, acne, growth of body hair, deepening of voice, loss of libido, impotence, or menstrual irregularity (usually reversible). Report changes in menstrual pattern, deepening of voice or unusual growth of body hair, persistent penile erections, fluid retention (eg, swelling of ankles, feet, or hands, respiratory difficulty, or sudden weight gain), change in color of urine or stool, yellowing of eyes or skin, or unusual bruising or bleeding.

◆ **Danocrine** *see* Danazol *on page* 462

◆ **Dantrium®** *see* Dantrolene *on page* 462

Dantrolene (DAN troe leen)

U.S. Brand Names Dantrium®; Revonto™
Index Terms Dantrolene Sodium
Generic Availability (U.S.) Yes: Capsule
Pharmacologic Category Skeletal Muscle Relaxant
Medication Safety Issues
Sound-alike/look-alike issues:
Dantrium® may be confused with danazol, Daraprim®
Revonto™ may be confused with Revatio®
Pregnancy Risk Factor C
Lactation Enters breast milk/not recommended
Use Treatment of spasticity associated with upper motor neuron disorders (eg, spinal cord injury, stroke, cerebral palsy, or multiple sclerosis); management of malignant hyperthermia; prevention of malignant hyperthermia in susceptible individuals (preoperative/postoperative administration)
Unlabeled/Investigational Use Neuroleptic malignant syndrome (NMS)
Available Dosage Forms
Capsule, oral: 25 mg, 50 mg, 100 mg
Dantrium®: 25 mg, 50 mg, 100 mg
Injection, powder for reconstitution:
Dantrium®: 20 mg
Revonto™: 20 mg
Dosing
Adult & Geriatric
Spasticity: Oral: Initial: 25 mg once daily for 7 days; increase to 25 mg 3 times/day for 7 days, increase to 50 mg 3 times/day for 7 days, and then increase to 100 mg 3 times/day; not to exceed 400 mg/day

Malignant hyperthermia:

Preoperative prophylaxis:

Oral: 4-8 mg/kg/day in 4 divided doses, begin 1-2 days prior to surgery with last dose 3-4 hours prior to surgery

I.V.: 2.5 mg/kg ~1¼ hours prior to anesthesia and infused over 1 hour with additional doses as needed and individualized

Crisis: I.V.: 2.5 mg/kg; continuously repeat dose until symptoms subside or a cumulative dose of 10 mg/kg is reached; if physiologic and metabolic abnormalities reappear, repeat regimen (**Note:** Manufacturer's labeling suggests an initial dose of 1 mg/kg; however, guidelines recommend 2.5 mg/kg initially [www.mhaus.org]).

Postcrisis follow-up: Oral: 4-8 mg/kg/day in 4 divided doses for 1-3 days; I.V. dantrolene may be used when oral therapy is not practical; individualize dosage beginning with 1 mg/kg or more as the clinical situation dictates

Neuroleptic malignant syndrome (unlabeled use): I.V.: 1-2.5 mg/kg, may repeat dose up to maximum cumulative dose of 10 mg/kg/day, then switch to oral dosage (Strawn, 2007; Susman, 2001)

Pediatric

Spasticity: Oral: Initial: 0.5 mg/kg/dose once daily for 7 days; increase to 0.5 mg/kg/dose 3 times/day for 7 days, increase to 1 mg/kg/dose 3 times/day for 7 days, and then increase to 2 mg/kg/dose 3 times/day; not to exceed 400 mg/day

Malignant hyperthermia: Refer to adult dosing.

Administration

I.V. Therapeutic or emergency dose can be administered with rapid continuous I.V. push. Follow-up doses should be administered over 2-3 minutes.

Monitoring and Teaching Issues

Laboratory Monitoring Liver function for potential hepatotoxicity

Physical Assessment I.V.: Monitor vital signs, cardiac function, respiratory status, and I.V. site (extravasation very irritating to tissues).

Patient Education Do not use alcohol. You may experience drowsiness, dizziness, lightheadedness, nausea, vomiting, or diarrhea.

◆ **Dantrolene Sodium** *see* Dantrolene *on page 462*

◆ **Daptacel®** *see* Diphtheria and Tetanus Toxoids, and Acellular Pertussis Vaccine *on page 552*

Darbepoetin Alfa (dar be POE e tin AL fa)

U.S. Brand Names Aranesp®; Aranesp® SingleJect®

Index Terms Erythropoiesis-Stimulating Agent (ESA); Erythropoiesis-Stimulating Protein; NESP; Novel Erythropoiesis-Stimulating Protein

Generic Availability (U.S.) No

Pharmacologic Category Colony Stimulating Factor; Growth Factor; Recombinant Human Erythropoietin

Medication Safety Issues

Sound-alike/look-alike issues:

Aranesp® may be confused with Aralast, Aricept®

Darbepoetin alfa may be confused with dalteparin, epoetin alfa, epoetin beta

Medication Guide Available Yes

Prescribing and Access Restrictions As a requirement of the REMS program, access to this medication is restricted. Healthcare providers and hospitals must be enrolled in the ESA APPRISE (Assisting Providers and Cancer Patients with Risk Information for the Safe use of ESAs) Oncology Program (866-284-8089; http://www.esa-apprise.com) to prescribe or dispense ESAs (ie, darbepoetin alfa, epoetin alfa) to patients with cancer.

Pregnancy Risk Factor C

Lactation Excretion in breast milk unknown/use caution

Use Treatment of anemia (elevate or maintain red blood cell level and decrease the need for transfusions) associated with chronic renal failure (including patients on dialysis and not on dialysis); treatment of anemia due to concurrent chemotherapy in patients with metastatic cancer (nonmyeloid malignancies)

Note: Darbepoetin is **not** indicated for use in cancer patients under the following conditions:

- receiving hormonal therapy, therapeutic biologic products, or radiation therapy unless also receiving concurrent myelosuppressive chemotherapy
- receiving myelosuppressive therapy when the expected outcome is curative

Unlabeled/Investigational Use Treatment of symptomatic anemia in myelodysplastic syndrome (MDS)

Mechanism of Action/Effect Stimulates production of red blood cells within the bone marrow. There is a dose response relationship with this effect. This results in an increase in red blood cell counts followed by a rise in hematocrit and hemoglobin levels. When administered SubQ or I.V., darbepoetin's half-life is ~3 times that of epoetin alfa.

Contraindications Hypersensitivity to darbepoetin or any component of the formulation; uncontrolled hypertension

Warnings/Precautions [U.S. Boxed Warning]: Erythropoiesis-stimulating agents (ESAs) increased the risk of serious cardiovascular events, thromboembolic events, stroke, and/or tumor progression in clinical studies; a rapid rise in hemoglobin (>1 g/dL over 2 weeks) or maintaining higher hemoglobin levels may contribute to these risks. **[U.S. Boxed Warning]: A shortened overall survival and/or increased risk of tumor progression or recurrence has been reported in studies with breast, cervical, head and neck, lymphoid,**

and non small cell lung cancer patients. It is of note that in these studies, patients received ESAs to a target hemoglobin of ≥12 g/dL; although risk has not been excluded when dosed to achieve a target hemoglobin of <12 g/dL. **[U.S. Boxed Warnings]: To decrease these risks, and risk of cardio- and thrombovascular events, use ESAs in cancer patients only for the treatment of anemia related to concurrent chemotherapy and use the lowest dose needed to avoid red blood cell transfusions. Discontinue ESA following completion of the chemotherapy course. ESAs are not indicated for patients receiving myelosuppressive therapy when the anticipated outcome is curative.** Use of ESAs has been associated with an increased risk of venous thromboembolism (VTE) without a reduction in transfusions in patients >65 years of age with cancer (Hershman, 2009). Improved anemia symptoms, quality of life, fatigue or well-being has not been demonstrated in controlled clinical trials. **[U.S. Boxed Warning]: Because of the risks of decreased survival and increased risk of tumor growth or progression, all healthcare providers and hospitals are required to enroll and comply with the ESA APPRISE (Assisting Providers and Cancer Patients with Risk Information for the Safe use of ESAs) Oncology Program prior to prescribing or dispensing ESAs to cancer patients.** Prescribers and patients will have to provide written documentation of discussed risks.

[U.S. Boxed Warning]: An increased risk of death, serious cardiovascular events, and stroke was reported in patients administered ESAs to target hemoglobin levels ≥13 g/dL; dosing should be individualized to achieve and maintain hemoglobin levels within 10-12 g/dL range. Hemoglobin rising >1 g/dL in a 2-week period may contribute to the risk. CRF patients who exhibit an inadequate hemoglobin response to ESA therapy may be at a higher risk for cardiovascular events and mortality compared to other patients. ESA therapy may reduce dialysis efficacy (due to increase in red blood cells and decrease in plasma volume); adjustments in dialysis parameters may be needed. CRF patients not requiring dialysis may have a better response to darbepoetin and may require lower doses. An increased risk of DVT has been observed in patients treated with epoetin undergoing surgical orthopedic procedures. Darbepoetin is **not** approved for reduction in allogeneic red blood cell transfusions in patients scheduled for surgical procedures. During therapy in any patient, hemoglobin levels should not exceed a target range of 10-12 g/dL and should not rise >1 g/dL per 2-week time period.

Use with caution in patients with hypertension or with a history of seizures; hypertensive encephalopathy and seizures have been reported. Use is contraindicated in patients with uncontrolled hypertension. If hypertension is difficult to control, reduce or hold darbepoetin alfa. Due to the delayed onset of erythropoiesis, darbepoetin alfa is **not** recommended for acute correction of severe anemia or as a substitute for emergency transfusion. Consider discontinuing in patients who receive a renal transplant.

Prior to treatment, correct or exclude deficiencies of iron, vitamin B_{12}, and/or folate, as well as other factors which may impair erythropoiesis (aluminum toxicity, inflammatory conditions, infections). Prior to and during therapy, iron stores must be evaluated. Supplemental iron is recommended if serum ferritin <100 mcg/L or serum transferrin saturation <20%. Poor response should prompt evaluation of these potential factors, as well as possible malignant processes, occult blood loss, hemolysis, and/or bone marrow fibrosis. Severe anemia and pure red cell aplasia (PRCA) with associated neutralizing antibodies to erythropoietin has been reported, predominantly in patients with CRF receiving SubQ darbepoetin (the I.V. route is preferred for hemodialysis patients). Cases have also been reported in patients with hepatitis C who were receiving ESAs, interferon, and ribavirin. Patients with a sudden loss of response to darbepoetin (with severe anemia and a low reticulocyte count) should be evaluated for PRCA with associated neutralizing antibodies to erythropoietin; discontinue treatment in patients with PRCA secondary to neutralizing antibodies to erythropoietin. Antibodies may cross-react; do not switch to another ESA in patients who develop antibody-mediated anemia.

Safety and efficacy in patients with underlying hematologic diseases (eg, porphyria, thalassemia, hemolytic anemia, and sickle cell disease) have not been established. Potentially serious allergic reactions have been reported (rarely). Discontinue immediately (and permanently) in patients who experience serious allergic/anaphylactic reactions. Some products may contain albumin and the packaging of some formulations may contain latex. Safety and efficacy in children with cancer have not been established; children >1 year of age with CRF have been converted from epoetin alfa to darbepoetin.

Drug Interactions

Avoid Concomitant Use There are no known interactions where it is recommended to avoid concomitant use.

Decreased Effect There are no known significant interactions involving a decrease in effect.

Increased Effect/Toxicity There are no known significant interactions involving an increase in effect.

Nutritional/Ethanol Interactions Ethanol: Should be avoided due to adverse effects on erythropoiesis.

Adverse Reactions

>10%:

Cardiovascular: Edema (21%), hypertension (4% to 20%), hypotension (20%)

Central nervous system: Fatigue (9% to 33%), fever (4% to 19%), headache (12% to 15%), dizziness (7% to 14%)

Gastrointestinal: Diarrhea (14% to 22%), constipation (5% to 18%), vomiting (2% to 14%), nausea (11%)

Neuromuscular & skeletal: Muscle spasm (17%), arthralgia (9% to 13%)

Respiratory: Upper respiratory infection (15%)

Miscellaneous: Infection (24%)

1% to 10%:

Cardiovascular: Peripheral edema (10%), arrhythmia/arrest (8%), angina/chest pain (7% to 8%), fluid overload (6%), thrombosis (6%), CHF (5%), MI (2%)

Central nervous system: Stroke (2% to 5%), seizure (≤1%), TIA (≤1%)

Dermatologic: Rash (7%), pruritus (6%)

Endocrine & metabolic: Dehydration (3% to 5%)

Gastrointestinal: Abdominal pain (10%)

Local: Vascular access hemorrhage (7%), injection site pain (6%), vascular access infection (6%), vascular access thrombosis (6%)

Neuromuscular & skeletal: Limb pain (8%), myalgia (8%), back pain (7%), weakness (5%)

Respiratory: Dyspnea (2% to 10%), cough (9%), bronchitis (5%), pneumonia (3%), pulmonary embolism (1%)

Miscellaneous: Flu-like syndrome (6%)

Pharmacodynamics/Kinetics

Onset of Action Increased hemoglobin levels not generally observed until 2-6 weeks after initiating treatment

Absorption SubQ: Slow

Bioavailability CRF: SubQ: Adults: ~37% (range: 30% to 50%); Children: 54% (range: 32% to 70%)

Time to Peak SubQ:

CRF: Adults: 48 hours (range: 12-72 hours; independent of dialysis); Children: 36 hours (range: 10-58 hours)

Cancer: Adults: 71-90 hours (range: 28-123 hours); Children: 71 hours (range: 21-143 hours)

Half-Life Elimination Note: Darbepoetin half-life is approximately threefold longer than epoetin alfa following I.V. administration

CRF: Adults:

I.V.: 21 hours

SubQ: Nondialysis patients: 70 hours (range: 35-139 hours); Dialysis patients: 46 hours (range: 12-89 hours)

Cancer: Adults: SubQ: 74 hours (range: 24-144 hours); Children: 49 hours

Available Dosage Forms

Injection, solution [preservative free]:

Aranesp®: 25 mcg/mL (1 mL); 40 mcg/mL (1 mL); 60 mcg/mL (1 mL); 100 mcg/mL (1 mL); 150 mcg/0.75 mL (0.75 mL); 200 mcg/mL (1 mL); 300 mcg/mL (1 mL)

Aranesp® SingleJect®: 25 mcg/0.42 mL (0.42 mL); 40 mcg/0.4 mL (0.4 mL); 60 mcg/0.3 mL (0.3 mL); 100 mcg/0.5 mL (0.5 mL); 150 mcg/0.3 mL (0.3 mL); 200 mcg/0.4 mL (0.4 mL); 300 mcg/0.6 mL (0.6 mL); 500 mcg/mL (1 mL)

Dosing

Adult & Geriatric Note: Hemoglobin levels should not exceed 12 g/dL and should not rise >1 g/dL per 2-week time period during therapy in any patient.

Anemia associated with CRF: Individualize dosing to achieve and maintain hemoglobin levels to a target range of 10-12 g/dL. Hemoglobin levels should not exceed 12 g/dL.

I.V., SubQ: Initial: 0.45 mcg/kg once weekly; alternative dose for nondialysis patients: 0.75 mcg/kg once every 2 weeks; Maintenance: titrate to maintain hemoglobin levels between 10-12 g/dL as described below (may be administered once weekly or every 2 weeks; nondialysis patients may require lower maintenance doses) **Note:** I.V. route is preferred in hemodialysis patients.

Dosage adjustment:

Decrease dose by ~25%: If hemoglobin approaches 12 g/dL **or** hemoglobin increases >1 g/dL in any 2-week period. If hemoglobin continues to increase, temporarily discontinue therapy until hemoglobin begins to decrease, then resume therapy with a ~25% reduction from previous dose.

Increase dose by ~25%: If hemoglobin does not increase by 1 g/dL after 4 weeks of therapy (with adequate iron stores). Do not increase dose more frequently than at 4-week intervals.

Inadequate or lack of response: If patient does not attain target hemoglobin range of 10-12 g/dL after appropriate dose titrations over 12 weeks:

Do not continue to increase dose and use the minimum effective dose that will maintain a hemoglobin level sufficient to avoid red blood cell transfusions **and** evaluate patient for other causes of anemia.

Monitor hemoglobin closely thereafter and if responsiveness improves, may resume making dosage adjustments as recommended above. If responsiveness does not improve and recurrent red blood cell transfusions continue to be needed, discontinue therapy.

Maintenance dose: Individualize to target hemoglobin range of 10-12 g/dL; limit additional dosage increase to every 4 weeks or longer. Patients generally require lower maintenance doses than initial doses to maintain target range.

Conversion from epoetin alfa: I.V., SubQ: Initial dose: Epoetin alfa doses may be converted to doses ranging from 6.25-200 mcg darbepoetin alfa per week (see conversion table on next page).

Anemia associated with chemotherapy: Titrate dosage to use the minimum effective dose that will maintain a hemoglobin level sufficient to avoid red blood cell transfusions. Do not initiate therapy if hemoglobin ≥10 g/dL. Discontinue darbepoetin following completion of chemotherapy.

SubQ: Initial: 2.25 mcg/kg once weekly **or** 500 mcg once every 3 weeks

Dosage adjustment:

Increase dose: If hemoglobin does not increase by 1 g/dL after 6 weeks of therapy (for patients receiving weekly therapy), the dose should be increased up to 4.5 mcg/kg once weekly

Decrease dose by 40%: If hemoglobin increases >1g/dL in any 2-week period **or** hemoglobin reaches a level sufficient to avoid red blood cell transfusion.

Withhold dose: If hemoglobin exceeds a level needed to avoid red blood cell transfusion. Resume treatment with a dose 40% below the previous dose when hemoglobin approaches a level where transfusions may be required.

Discontinue: On completion of chemotherapy or if after 8 weeks of therapy there is no hemoglobin response or transfusions still required

Symptomatic anemia associated with MDS (unlabeled use): Adults: SubQ: 150-300 mcg once weekly (NCCN MDS guidelines v.2.2010)

Conversion from epoetin alfa to darbepoetin alfa: See table.

Conversion From Epoetin Alfa to Darbepoetin Alfa (Initial Dose)

Previous Dosage of Epoetin Alfa (units/week)	Children Darbepoetin Alfa Dosage (mcg/week)	Adults Darbepoetin Alfa Dosage (mcg/week)
<1500	Not established	6.25
1500-2499	6.25	6.25
2500-4999	10	12.5
5000-10,999	20	25
11,000-17,999	40	40
18,000-33,999	60	60
34,000-89,999	100	100
≥90,000	200	200

Note: In patients receiving epoetin alfa 2-3 times per week, darbepoetin alfa is administered once weekly. In patients receiving epoetin alfa once weekly, darbepoetin alfa is administered once every 2 weeks. The darbepoetin dose to be administered every 2 weeks is derived by adding together 2 weekly epoetin alfa doses and then converting to the appropriate darbepoetin dose. Titrate dose to hemoglobin response thereafter (see Renal Impairment).

Pediatric Note: Hemoglobin levels should not exceed 12 g/dL and should not rise >1 g/dL per 2-week time period during therapy in any patient.

Anemia associated with CRF: I.V. (preferred for hemodialysis patients), SubQ:

Children ≥1 year: Conversion from epoetin alfa: Initial dose: Epoetin alfa doses of 1500 to ≥90,000 units per week may be converted to doses ranging from 6.25-200 mcg darbepoetin alfa per week (see pediatric column in conversion table below).

Children 11-18 years: Initial treatment (unlabeled use): Initial dose: 0.45 mcg/kg once weekly; titrate to hemoglobin response

Anemia associated with chemotherapy: SubQ: Children (unlabeled use): 2.25 mcg/kg once weekly (discontinue following completion of chemotherapy course)

Dosage adjustment: Refer to adult dosing.

Renal Impairment Dosage requirements for patients with chronic renal failure who do not require dialysis may be lower than in dialysis patients. Monitor patients closely during the time period in which a dialysis regimen is initiated, dosage requirement may increase. The National Kidney Foundation Clinical Practice Guidelines for Anemia in Chronic Kidney Disease: 2007 Update of Hemoglobin Target (September, 2007) recommend hemoglobin levels in the range of 11-12 g/dL for dialysis and nondialysis patients receiving ESAs; hemoglobin levels should not be maintained >13 g/dL.

Hemodialysis: I.V. route is preferred in hemodialysis patients.

Administration

I.V. May be administered by I.V. injection. The I.V. route is recommended in hemodialysis patients. Do not shake; vigorous shaking may denature darbepoetin alfa, rendering it biologically inactive. Do not dilute or administer in conjunction with other drug solutions. Discard any unused portion of the vial; do not pool unused portions.

Other May be administered SubQ.

Stability

Storage Store at 2°C to 8°C (36°F to 46°F); do not freeze. Do not shake. Protect from light. The following stability information has also been reported: May be stored at room temperature for up to 7 days (Cohen, 2007).

Monitoring and Teaching Issues

Laboratory Monitoring Hemoglobin (at least once per week until maintenance dose established and after dosage changes; monitor at regular intervals at least once per month once hemoglobin is stabilized); iron stores (transferrin saturation and ferritin) prior to and during therapy; serum chemistry (CRF patients)

Physical Assessment Evaluate history of hypertension or seizures and potential risk for thromboembolism prior to beginning therapy. Blood pressure should be monitored closely and controlled during therapy. If administered by intravenous infusion, lines should be monitored closely for possible clotting. Assess blood chemistries, hemoglobin/hematocrit, serum ferritin, and transferrin saturation prior to and on a regular basis during therapy. Monitor for hyper-/hypotension, edema, thrombosis, stroke, TIA, and anemia. Teach patient proper SubQ injection technique and syringe/needle disposal.

Patient Education If self-administered, follow exact directions for injection and needle disposal. You will require frequent blood tests to determine appropriate dosage and reduce potential for severe adverse effects; maintaining laboratory testing schedule is vital. You may experience fever, headache, trouble sleeping, itching, skin pain, nausea, vomiting, diarrhea, heartburn, or upper respiratory congestion. Report onset of severe headache, unusual dizziness, or blurred vision; chest pain or irregular heartbeat; leg pain and tenderness; muscular tremors or seizure activity; or difficulty breathing.

Dietary Considerations Supplemental iron intake may be required in patients with low iron stores.

Pregnancy Considerations There are no adequate and well-controlled studies in pregnant women. Darbepoetin alfa should be used in a pregnant woman only if potential benefit justifies the potential risk to the fetus.

Additional Information Oncology Comment: The American Society of Hematology (ASH) and American Society of Clinical Oncology (ASCO) 2007 updates to the clinical practice guidelines for the use of erythropoiesis-stimulating agents (ESAs) indicate that ESAs are most appropriate when used according to the dosage parameters within the Food and Drug Administration (FDA) approved labeling for epoetin and darbepoetin (Rizzo, 2008). While the previous guidelines addressed only the use of epoetin, the 2007 guidelines also address the use of darbepoetin, which is assessed as being equivalent to epoetin with respect to safety and efficacy. When used as an option for the treatment of chemotherapy-associated anemia (to increase hemoglobin and decrease red blood cell transfusions), therapy with ESAs should begin as the hemoglobin level approaches or falls below 10 g/dL. The ASH/ASCO guidelines recommend following the FDA approved dosing (and dosing adjustment) guidelines and target hemoglobin ranges as alternate dosing and schedules have not demonstrated consistent differences in effectiveness with regard to hemoglobin response. In patients who do not have a response within 6-8 weeks (hemoglobin rise <1-2 g/dL or no reduction in transfusions) ESA therapy should be discontinued.

The guidelines note that patients with an increased risk of thromboembolism (generally includes previous history of thrombosis, surgery, and/or prolonged periods of immobilization) and patients receiving concomitant medications that may increase thromboembolic risk, should begin ESA therapy only after careful consideration. With the exception of low-risk myelodysplasia-associated anemia (which has evidence supporting the use of ESAs without concurrent chemotherapy), the guidelines do not support the use of ESAs in the absence of concurrent chemotherapy.

Darifenacin (dar i FEN a sin)

U.S. Brand Names Enablex®

Index Terms Darifenacin Hydrobromide; UK-88,525

Generic Availability (U.S.) No

Pharmacologic Category Anticholinergic Agent

Pregnancy Risk Factor C

Lactation Excretion in breast milk unknown/use caution

Use Management of symptoms of bladder overactivity (urge incontinence, urgency, and frequency)

Mechanism of Action/Effect Blocks muscarinic/cholinergic receptors (M3 subtype) on the smooth muscle of the urinary bladder to limit bladder contractions, reducing the symptoms of bladder irritability/overactivity (urge incontinence, urgency and frequency).

Contraindications Hypersensitivity to darifenacin or any component of the formulation; uncontrolled narrow-angle glaucoma; urinary retention, paralytic ileus, GI or GU obstruction

Warnings/Precautions May cause drowsiness and/or blurred vision, which may impair physical or mental abilities; patients must be cautioned about performing tasks which require mental alertness (eg, operating machinery or driving). May occur in the presence of increased environmental temperature; use caution in hot weather and/or exercise. Use with caution with hepatic impairment; dosage limitation is required in moderate hepatic impairment (Child-Pugh class B). Not recommended for use in severe hepatic impairment (Child-Pugh class C). Use with caution in patients with clinically-significant bladder outlet obstruction or prostatic hyperplasia (nonobstructive). Use caution in patients with decreased GI motility, constipation, hiatal hernia, reflux esophagitis, and ulcerative colitis. Use caution in patients with myasthenia gravis. In patients with controlled narrow-angle glaucoma, darifenacin should be used with extreme caution and only when the potential benefit outweighs risks of treatment. Use with caution in patients taking strong CYP3A4 inhibitors (see Drug Interactions); dosage limitation of darifenacin is required.

Drug Interactions

Metabolism/Transport Effects Substrate of CYP2D6 (minor), CYP3A4 (major); **Inhibits** CYP2D6 (moderate), 3A4 (weak)

Avoid Concomitant Use

Avoid concomitant use of Darifenacin with any of the following: Thioridazine

Decreased Effect

Darifenacin may decrease the levels/effects of: Acetylcholinesterase Inhibitors (Central); Codeine; Secretin; TraMADol

The levels/effects of Darifenacin may be decreased by: Acetylcholinesterase Inhibitors (Central); CYP3A4 Inducers (Strong); Deferasirox; Herbs (CYP3A4 Inducers); Peginterferon Alfa-2b

Increased Effect/Toxicity

Darifenacin may increase the levels/effects of: AbobotulinumtoxinA; Anticholinergics; Cannabinoids; CYP2D6 Substrates; Fesoterodine; Nebivolol; OnabotulinumtoxinA; Potassium Chloride; RimabotulinumtoxinB; Tamoxifen; Thioridazine

The levels/effects of Darifenacin may be increased by: Conivaptan; CYP3A4 Inhibitors (Moderate); CYP3A4 Inhibitors (Strong); Dasatinib; Pramlintide

Nutritional/Ethanol Interactions Herb/Nutraceutical: Darifenacin serum concentration may be decreased by St John's wort (avoid concurrent use.)

Adverse Reactions

>10%: Gastrointestinal: Xerostomia (19% to 35%), constipation (15% to 21%)

1% to 10%:

Cardiovascular: Hypertension (≥1%), peripheral edema (≥1%)

Central nervous system: Headache (7%), dizziness (<2%), pain (≥1%)

Dermatological: Dry skin (≥1%), pruritus (≥1%), rash (≥1%)

Gastrointestinal: Dyspepsia (3% to 8%), abdominal pain (2% to 4%), nausea (2% to 4%), vomiting (≥1%), weight gain (≥1%)

Genitourinary: Urinary tract infection (4% to 5%), vaginitis (≥1%), urinary retention (acute)

Neuromuscular & skeletal: Weakness (<3%), arthralgia (≥1%), back pain (≥1%)

Ocular: Dry eyes (2%), abnormal vision (≥1%)

Respiratory: Bronchitis (≥1%), pharyngitis (≥1%), rhinitis (≥1%), sinusitis (≥1%)

Miscellaneous: Flu-like syndrome (1% to 3%)

Pharmacodynamics/Kinetics

Bioavailability 15% to 19%

Time to Peak Plasma: ~7 hours

Protein Binding ~98% (primarily alpha$_1$-acid glycoprotein)

Half-Life Elimination ~13-19 hours

Metabolism Hepatic, via CYP3A4 (major) and CYP2D6 (minor)

Excretion Urine (60%), feces (40%); as metabolites (inactive)

Available Dosage Forms

Tablet, extended release, oral:

Enablex®: 7.5 mg, 15 mg

Dosing

Adult & Geriatric

Symptoms of bladder overactivity: Oral: Initial: 7.5 mg once daily. If response is not adequate after a minimum of 2 weeks, dosage may be increased to 15 mg once daily.

Dosage adjustment with concomitant potent CYP3A4 inhibitors (eg, azole antifungals, erythromycin, isoniazid, protease inhibitors): Daily dosage should not exceed 7.5 mg/day

Renal Impairment No adjustment required.

Hepatic Impairment

Moderate impairment (Child-Pugh class B): Daily dosage should not exceed 7.5 mg/day

Severe impairment (Child-Pugh class C): Has not been evaluated; use is not recommended

Administration

Oral Tablet should be taken with liquid and swallowed whole; do not chew, crush, or split tablet. May be taken without regard to food.

Stability

Storage Store at 25°C (77°F); excursions permitted to 15°C to 30°C (59°F to 86°F). Protect from light.

Monitoring and Teaching Issues

Patient Education Swallow tablet whole. May cause headache, dizziness, nervousness, sleepiness, abdominal discomfort, diarrhea, constipation, dry mouth, nausea, or vomiting. Report back pain, muscle spasms, alteration in gait, or numbness of extremities; unresolved or persistent constipation, diarrhea, or vomiting; symptoms of upper respiratory infection or flu; or difficulty urinating, pain on urination, or abdominal pain.

Dietary Considerations May be taken without regard to meals, with or without food.

Geriatric Considerations There is a trend for decreased clearance with age, though no change in dose is recommended. The selectivity of darifenacin for the M3 receptor on the bladder may offer an advantage (less CNS and cardiovascular effects) over other anticholinergic agents used in the treatment of overactive bladder.

Breast-Feeding Considerations Although human data are not available, darifenacin is excreted in the breast milk in animals.

Pregnancy Considerations Teratogenic effects and developmental delay were observed in some animal studies. There are no adequate and well-controlled studies in pregnant women; should be used only if potential benefit outweighs possible risk to the fetus.

Related Information

Pharmacotherapy of Urinary Incontinence *on page* 2071

◆ **Darifenacin Hydrobromide** *see* Darifenacin *on page* 467

Darunavir (dar OO na veer)

U.S. Brand Names Prezista®

Index Terms Darunavir Ethanolate; TMC-114

Generic Availability (U.S.) No

Pharmacologic Category Antiretroviral Agent, Protease Inhibitor

Pregnancy Risk Factor C

Lactation Excretion in breast milk unknown/not recommended

Use Treatment of HIV-1 infections in combination with ritonavir and other antiretroviral agents

Mechanism of Action/Effect Blocks the site of HIV-1 protease activity, resulting in the formation of immature, noninfectious viral particles.

Contraindications Coadministration with medications highly dependent upon CYP3A4 for clearance and for which increased levels are associated with serious and/or life-threatening events (includes alfuzosin, cisapride, ergot alkaloids [eg, dihydroergotamine, ergonovine, ergotamine, methylergonovine], lovastatin, midazolam [oral], pimozide, rifampin, sildenafil (when used for pulmonary artery hypertension [eg, Revatio®]), simvastatin, St John's wort, triazolam

Canadian labeling: Additional contraindications: Hypersensitivity to darunavir or any component of the formulation; coadministration with amiodarone, lidocaine (systemic), quinidine; severe (Child-Pugh class C) hepatic impairment

Warnings/Precautions Coadministration with ritonavir is required (DHHS, 2011). Use with caution in patients taking strong CYP3A4 inhibitors, moderate or strong CYP3A4 inducers and major CYP3A4 substrates (see Drug Interactions); consider alternative agents that avoid or lessen the potential for CYP-mediated interactions. Do not coadminister colchicine in patient with renal or hepatic impairment; avoid concurrent use with salmeterol.

Use with caution in patients with hepatic impairment, including active chronic hepatitis; consider interruption or discontinuation with worsening hepatic function. Not recommended in severe hepatic impairment (contraindicated in Canadian labeling). Infrequent cases of drug-induced hepatitis (including acute and cytolytic) have been reported. Liver injury has been reported with use (including some fatalities), though generally in patients on multiple medications, with advanced HIV disease, hepatitis B/C coinfection, and/or immune reconstitution syndrome. Monitor patients closely; consider interrupting or discontinuing therapy if signs/symptoms of liver impairment occur.

May cause fat redistribution (buffalo hump, increased abdominal girth, breast engorgement, facial atrophy). Immune reconstitution syndrome, including inflammatory responses to indolent infections, has been associated with antiretroviral therapy; additional evaluation and treatment may be required. May increase cholesterol and/or triglycerides. Pancreatitis has been observed with use. Risk for pancreatitis may be increased in patients with elevated triglycerides, advanced HIV disease, or history of pancreatitis. Protease inhibitors have been associated with glucose dysregulation; use caution in patients with diabetes. Use with caution in patients with sulfonamide allergy (contains sulfa moiety) or hemophilia. Protease inhibitors have been associated with a variety of hypersensitivity events (some severe), including rash, anaphylaxis (rare), angioedema, bronchospasm, erythema multiforme, Stevens-Johnson syndrome (rare), and/or toxic epidermal necrolysis. Discontinue treatment if severe skin reactions develop. Severe skin reactions may be accompanied by fever, malaise, fatigue, arthralgias, hepatitis, oral lesion, blisters, conjunctivitis, and/or eosinophilia. Mild-to-moderate rash may occur early in treatment and resolve with continued therapy. Treatment history and resistance data should guide use of darunavir with ritonavir.

Drug Interactions

Metabolism/Transport Effects Substrate of CYP3A4 (major); **Inhibits** P-glycoprotein

Avoid Concomitant Use

Avoid concomitant use of Darunavir with any of the following: Alfuzosin; Amiodarone; Cisapride; Conivaptan; Dronedarone; Eplerenone; Ergot Derivatives; Everolimus; Halofantrine; Lopinavir; Lovastatin; Lurasidone; Midazolam; Nilotinib; Nisoldipine; PHENobarbital; Phenytoin; Pimozide; QuiNIDine; Ranolazine; Rifampin; Rivaroxaban; RomiDEPsin; Salmeterol; Saquinavir; Silodosin; Simvastatin; St Johns Wort; Tamsulosin; Tolvaptan; Topotecan; Toremifene; Triazolam; Voriconazole

Decreased Effect

Darunavir may decrease the levels/effects of: Abacavir; Clarithromycin; Contraceptives (Estrogens); Delavirdine; Didanosine; Divalproex; Etravirine; Meperidine; Methadone; Norethindrone; PARoxetine; Prasugrel; Sertraline; Theophylline Derivatives; Valproic Acid; Voriconazole; Warfarin; Zidovudine

The levels/effects of Darunavir may be decreased by: CarBAMazepine; Contraceptives (Estrogens); CYP3A4 Inducers (Strong); Deferasirox; Efavirenz; Garlic; Lopinavir; PHENobarbital; Phenytoin; Rifampin; Saquinavir; St Johns Wort; Tenofovir

Increased Effect/Toxicity

Darunavir may increase the levels/effects of: Alfuzosin; Almotriptan; Alosetron; ALPRAZolam; Amiodarone; Antifungal Agents (Azole Derivatives, Systemic); Bortezomib; Brinzolamide; Calcium Channel Blockers (Dihydropyridine); Calcium Channel Blockers (Nondihydropyridine); CarBAMazepine; Ciclesonide; Cisapride; Clarithromycin; Colchicine; Conivaptan; Corticosteroids (Orally Inhaled); CycloSPORINE; CycloSPORINE (Systemic); CYP2D6 Substrates; CYP3A4 Substrates; Dabigatran Etexilate; Dienogest; Digoxin; Dronedarone; Dutasteride; Efavirenz; Enfuvirtide; Eplerenone; Ergot Derivatives; Everolimus; FentaNYL; Fesoterodine; Fusidic Acid; GuanFACINE; Halofantrine; HMG-CoA Reductase Inhibitors;

Ixabepilone; Lidocaine; Lidocaine (Systemic); Lidocaine (Topical); Lovastatin; Lumefantrine; Lurasidone; Maraviroc; Meperidine; MethylPREDNISolone; Midazolam; Nefazodone; Nilotinib; Nisoldipine; Paricalcitol; Pazopanib; P-Glycoprotein Substrates; Pimecrolimus; Pimozide; Protease Inhibitors; QuiNIDine; Ranolazine; Rifabutin; Rivaroxaban; RomiDEPsin; Salmeterol; Saxagliptin; Sildenafil; Silodosin; Simvastatin; Sirolimus; SORAfenib; Tacrolimus; Tacrolimus (Systemic); Tacrolimus (Topical); Tadalafil; Tamsulosin; Temsirolimus; Tenofovir; Tolvaptan; Topotecan; Toremifene; TraZODone; Triazolam; Tricyclic Antidepressants; Vardenafil; Vilazodone

The levels/effects of Darunavir may be increased by: Antifungal Agents (Azole Derivatives, Systemic); Clarithromycin; CycloSPORINE; CycloSPORINE (Systemic); CYP3A4 Inhibitors (Moderate); CYP3A4 Inhibitors (Strong); Dasatinib; Delavirdine; Efavirenz; Enfuvirtide; Etravirine; Fusidic Acid; Rifabutin

Nutritional/Ethanol Interactions

Food: Bioavailability is increased when administered with food.

Herb/nutraceutical: St John's wort may decrease the plasma levels of darunavir; concomitant use is contraindicated.

Adverse Reactions As a class, protease inhibitors potentially cause dyslipidemias which includes elevated cholesterol and triglycerides and a redistribution of body fat centrally to cause increased abdominal girth, buffalo hump, facial atrophy, and breast enlargement. These agents also cause hyperglycemia. Frequency of adverse events is reported for darunavir/ritonavir. See also Ritonavir monograph.

>10%:

Endocrine & metabolic: Hypercholesterolemia (grade 2: 16% to 25%; grade 3: 1% to 10%), LDL increased (grade 2: 14%; grade 3: 5% to 8%)

Gastrointestinal: Vomiting (children 13%; adults 2% to 5%), diarrhea (8% to 14%)

2% to 10%:

Central nervous system: Headache (children 9%; adults 3% to 6%), fatigue (children 3%; adults ≤2%)

Dermatologic: Rash (5% to 10%)

Endocrine & metabolic: Hyperglycemia (grade 2: 7% to 10%; grade 3: ≤1%; grade 4: <1%), triglycerides increased (grade 2: 3% to 10%; grade 3: 1% to 7%; grade 4: ≤3%), diabetes mellitus (2%)

Gastrointestinal: Abdominal pain (children 10%; adults 5% to 6%), nausea (3% to 7%), amylase increased (grade 2: 5% to 6%; grade 3: 3% to 7%), lipase increased (grade 2: 2% to 3%; grade 3: ≤2%; grade 4: <1%), abdominal distention (2%), anorexia (2%), dyspepsia (2%)

Hepatic: ALT increased (grade 2: 7%, grade 3: 2% to 3%; grade 4: ≤1%), AST increased (grade 2: 6%; grade 3: 2% to 4%; grade 4: <1%), alkaline phosphatase (grade 2: ≤2%; grade 3: <1%)

Neuromuscular & skeletal: Weakness (≤3%)

Pharmacodynamics/Kinetics

Absorption Increased 30% with food

Bioavailability 82%

Protein Binding ~95%; primarily to alpha$_1$ acid glycoprotein (AAG)

Half-Life Elimination ~15 hours

Metabolism Hepatic, via CYP3A4 to minimally-active metabolites

Excretion Feces (~80%, 41% as unchanged drug); urine (~14%, 8% as unchanged drug)

Available Dosage Forms

Tablet, oral:

Prezista®: 75 mg, 150 mg, 400 mg, 600 mg

Dosing

Adult & Geriatric Treatment of HIV infection: Oral:

Therapy-naive: 800 mg once daily; coadministration with ritonavir 100 mg once daily is required. **Note:** Recommended (with ritonavir) as a first-line therapy with tenofovir/emtricitabine in antiretroviral naïve patients (DHHS, 2011).

Therapy-experienced: **Note:** If genotypic testing is not possible, 600 mg twice daily, coadministered with ritonavir 100 mg twice daily, is recommended.

With no resistance-associated substitutions: 800 mg once daily; coadministration with ritonavir 100 mg once daily is required

With ≥1 resistance-associated substitution: 600 mg twice daily; coadministration with ritonavir 100 mg twice daily is required

Dosage adjustments for concomitant therapy: Oral:

Coadministration with bosentan:

Coadministration of bosentan in patients currently receiving darunavir/ritonavir: For patients receiving ritonavir for at least 10 days, begin with bosentan 62.5 mg once daily or every other day based on tolerability

Coadministration of darunavir/ritonavir in patients currently receiving bosentan: Discontinue bosentan 36 hours prior to the initiation of ritonavir. After at least 10 days of ritonavir, resume bosentan 62.5 mg once daily or every other day based on tolerability.

Coadministration with colchicine:

Familial Mediterranean fever (FMF): Maximum colchicine dose: 0.6 mg/day (0.3 mg twice daily)

Gout prophylaxis:
If original colchicine dose is 0.6 mg twice daily, adjust dose to 0.3 mg once daily
If original colchicine dose is 0.6 mg once daily, adjust dose to 0.3 mg every other day
Gout flare treatment: Initial: Colchicine 0.6 mg, followed in 1 hour by a single dose of 0.3 mg; do not repeat for at least 3 days

Coadministration with phosphodiesterase-5 enzyme (PDE-5) inhibitor:
Pulmonary arterial hypertension: Darunavir/ritonavir coadministered with tadalafil:
Patient receiving darunavir with ritonavir for at least 1 week: Initiate tadalafil at 20 mg once daily; increase to 40 mg once daily based on individual tolerability
Patient receiving tadalafil when initiating darunavir/ritonavir: Discontinue tadalafil at least 24 hours prior to starting darunavir/ritonavir. After at least 1 week following the initiation of ritonavir, resume tadalafil at 20 mg once daily; increase to 40 mg once daily based on individual tolerability.
Erectile dysfunction: Darunavir/ritonavir coadministered with:
Sildenafil (Viagra®): Maximum sildenafil dose: 25 mg in a 48-hour period
Tadalafil (Cialis®): Maximum tadalafil dose: 10 mg in a 72-hour period
Vardenafil: Maximum vardenafil dose: 2.5 mg in a 72-hour period

Pediatric Treatment of HIV infection: Oral: **Note:** Do not use once-daily dosing in pediatric patients; maximum dose: 600 mg darunavir/100 mg ritonavir twice daily.
Children ≥6 years:
≥20 kg to <30 kg: 375 mg twice daily; coadministration with ritonavir 50 mg twice daily is required
≥30 kg to <40 kg: 450 mg twice daily; coadministration with ritonavir 60 mg twice daily is required
≥40 kg: 600 mg twice daily; coadministration with ritonavir 100 mg twice daily is required

Renal Impairment No adjustment required for mild-to-moderate impairment. No data available for use in severe renal failure or end-stage renal disease.

Hepatic Impairment No adjustment for mild-to-moderate impairment (Child-Pugh classes A and B). Not recommended for patients with severe impairment (contraindicated in Canadian labeling).

Adjustment for Toxicity
Severe rash: Discontinue treatment.
New or worsening liver dysfunction: Consider interrupting or discontinuing treatment.

Administration

Oral Coadministration with ritonavir and food is required (bioavailability is increased).

Stability

Storage Store at 25°C (77°F); excursions permitted to 15°C to 30°C (59°F to 86°F).

Monitoring and Teaching Issues

Laboratory Monitoring Viral load, CD4, serum glucose; transaminase levels prior to and during therapy (increase monitoring in patients at risk for liver impairment), cholesterol, triglycerides

Physical Assessment Evaluate CD4 count, viral load, transaminase levels, serum glucose, and lipid levels prior to and at regular intervals during therapy. Monitor for hypersensitivity reaction, gastrointestinal disturbances that can lead to dehydration and weight loss, and hyperlipidemia regularly during therapy. Caution patients with diabetes to monitor glucose levels closely; protease inhibitors may cause alterations in glucose regulation. Teach patient proper timing of multiple medications.

Patient Education This drug will not cure HIV, nor has it been found to reduce transmission of HIV; use appropriate precautions to prevent spread to other persons. This drug is prescribed as one part of a multidrug combination; take exactly as directed for full course of therapy. Take with food. Maintain adequate nutrition and hydration, unless instructed to restrict fluid intake. Frequent blood tests may be required. You may be advised to check your glucose levels; this drug can cause hyperglycemia. May cause body changes due to redistribution of body fat, facial atrophy, or breast enlargement (normal effects of drug); nausea or vomiting; diarrhea; or headache. Inform prescriber if you experience signs of hypersensitivity (rash, difficulty swallowing or breathing, swelling of mouth or tongue); unresolved persistent vomiting, diarrhea, or abdominal pain; respiratory difficulty or chest pain; unusual bleeding or bruising; or dark-colored urine or light stool.

Dietary Considerations Absorption increased with food. Take with meals.

Breast-Feeding Considerations In infants born to mothers who are HIV positive, HAART while breast-feeding may decrease postnatal infection. However, maternal or infant antiretroviral therapy does not completely eliminate the risk of postnatal HIV transmission. In addition, multiclass-resistant virus has been detected in breast-feeding infants despite maternal therapy.

In the United States where formula is accessible, affordable, safe, and sustainable, complete avoidance of breast-feeding by HIV-infected women is recommended to decrease potential transmission of HIV.

Pregnancy Considerations It is not known if darunavir crosses the human placenta. Teratogenic effects have not been observed in animal reproduction studies. However, there are no adequate and well-controlled studies in pregnant women. Pregnancy and protease inhibitors are both associated with an increased risk of hyperglycemia. Glucose levels should be closely monitored. The Perinatal HIV Guidelines Working Group notes there is insufficient data to recommend use during pregnancy; however, if used, darunavir must be given with low-dose ritonavir boosting. Healthcare providers are encouraged to enroll pregnant women exposed to antiretroviral medications in the Antiretroviral Pregnancy Registry (1-800-258-4263 or www.APRegistry.com). Healthcare providers caring for HIV-infected women and their infants may contact the National Perinatal HIV Hotline (888-448-8765) for clinical consultation.

Women receiving estrogen (as hormonal contraception or replacement therapy) have an increased incidence of rash. Alternative forms of contraception may be needed.

- **Darunavir Ethanolate** *see* Darunavir *on page 469*
- **Darvon® [DSC]** *see* Propoxyphene *on page 1522*
- **Darvon-N® [DSC]** *see* Propoxyphene *on page 1522*
- **Daunomycin** *see* DAUNOrubicin Hydrochloride *on page 474*

DAUNOrubicin Citrate (Liposomal) (daw noe ROO bi sin SI trate lip po SOE mal)

U.S. Brand Names DaunoXome®

Index Terms DAUNOrubicin Liposomal; Liposomal DAUNOrubicin; NSC-697732

Generic Availability (U.S.) No

Pharmacologic Category Antineoplastic Agent, Anthracycline

Medication Safety Issues

Sound-alike/look-alike issues:

DAUNOrubicin liposomal may be confused with DACTINomycin, DOXOrubicin, DOXOrubicin liposomal, epirubicin, IDArubicin, valrubicin

Liposomal formulation (DaunoXome®) may be confused with the conventional formulation (Cerubidine®, Rubex®)

High alert medication: The Institute for Safe Medication Practices (ISMP) includes this medication among its list of drug classes which have a heightened risk of causing significant patient harm when used in error.

Pregnancy Risk Factor D

Lactation Excretion in breast milk unknown/not recommended

Use First-line treatment of advanced HIV-associated Kaposi's sarcoma (KS)

Mechanism of Action/Effect Binds to DNA and inhibits DNA synthesis causing cell death

Contraindications Hypersensitivity to daunorubicin citrate (liposomal), daunorubicin, or any component of the formulation

Warnings/Precautions Hazardous agent - use appropriate precautions for handling and disposal. **[U.S. Boxed Warning]: Monitor cardiac function regularly; especially in patients with previous therapy with high cumulative doses of anthracyclines, cyclophosphamide, or thoracic radiation, or who have pre-existing cardiac disease.** Although the risk increases with cumulative dose, irreversible cardiotoxicity may occur with anthracycline treatment at any dose level. Patients with pre-existing heart disease, hypertension, concurrent administration of other antineoplastic agents, prior or concurrent chest irradiation, and advanced age are at increased risk. Evaluate left ventricular ejection fraction (LVEF) prior to treatment and periodically during treatment.

[U.S. Boxed Warning]: May cause bone marrow suppression, particularly neutropenia; monitor closely for infections. **[U.S. Boxed Warning]: Use caution with hepatic impairment;** dosage reduction is recommended. Use caution with renal impairment; may require dose adjustment. **[U.S. Boxed Warning]: The lipid component is associated with infusion-related reactions (back pain, flushing, chest tightness) usually within the first 5 minutes of infusion;** monitor, interrupt infusion, and resume at reduced infusion rate. Safety and efficacy in children and the elderly have not been established. **[U.S. Boxed Warning]: Should be administered under the supervision of an experienced cancer chemotherapy physician.**

Drug Interactions

Metabolism/Transport Effects Substrate of P-glycoprotein

Avoid Concomitant Use

Avoid concomitant use of DAUNOrubicin Citrate (Liposomal) with any of the following: BCG; Natalizumab; Pimecrolimus; Roflumilast; Tacrolimus (Topical); Vaccines (Live)

Decreased Effect

DAUNOrubicin Citrate (Liposomal) may decrease the levels/effects of: BCG; Cardiac Glycosides; Sipuleucel-T; Vaccines (Inactivated); Vaccines (Live)

The levels/effects of DAUNOrubicin Citrate (Liposomal) may be decreased by: Cardiac Glycosides; Echinacea; P-Glycoprotein Inducers

Increased Effect/Toxicity

DAUNOrubicin Citrate (Liposomal) may increase the levels/effects of: Leflunomide; Natalizumab; Vaccines (Live)

The levels/effects of DAUNOrubicin Citrate (Liposomal) may be increased by: Bevacizumab; Denosumab; P-Glycoprotein Inhibitors; Pimecrolimus; Roflumilast; Tacrolimus (Topical); Taxane Derivatives; Trastuzumab

Adverse Reactions

>10%:

Cardiovascular: Edema (11%)

Central nervous system: Fatigue (49%), fever (47%), headache (25%), neutropenic fever (17%)

Gastrointestinal: Nausea (54%), diarrhea (38%), abdominal pain (23%), anorexia (23%), vomiting (23%)

Hematologic: Myelosuppression (onset: 7 days; nadir: 14 days; recovery 21 days), neutropenia (up to 55%; grade 4: 15%), anemia (up to 55%; grade 4: 2%), thrombocytopenia (up to 12%; grade 4: 1%)
Neuromuscular & skeletal: Rigors (19%), back pain (16%), neuropathy (13%)
Respiratory: Cough (28%), dyspnea (26%), rhinitis (12%)
Miscellaneous: Opportunistic infections (40%), allergic reactions (24%), diaphoresis (14%), infusion-related reactions (14%; includes back pain, flushing, chest tightness)

1% to 10%:

Cardiovascular: Chest pain (10%), hypertension (≤5%), palpitation (≤5%), syncope (≤5%), tachycardia (≤5%), LVEF decreased (3%), CHF/cardiomyopathy
Central nervous system: Depression (10%), malaise (10%), dizziness (8%), insomnia (6%), abnormal thinking (≤5%), amnesia (≤5%), anxiety (≤5%), ataxia (≤5%), confusion (≤5%), emotional lability (≤5%), hallucination (≤5%), meningitis (≤5%), seizure (≤5%), somnolence (≤5%)
Dermatologic: Alopecia (8%), pruritus (7%), dry skin (≤5%), folliculitis (≤5%), seborrhea (≤5%)
Endocrine & metabolic: Dehydration (≤5%), hot flashes (≤5%)
Gastrointestinal: Stomatitis (10%), constipation (7%), tenesmus (5%), appetite increased (≤5%), dental caries (≤5%), dysphagia (≤5%), gastrointestinal hemorrhage (≤5%), gastritis (≤5%), gingival bleeding (≤5%), hemorrhoids (≤5%), melena (≤5%), splenomegaly (≤5%), taste perversion (≤5%), xerostomia (≤5%)
Genitourinary: Dysuria (≤5%), nocturia (≤5%), polyuria (≤5%)
Hepatic: Hepatomegaly (≤5%)
Local: Injection site inflammation (≤5%)
Neuromuscular & skeletal: Arthralgia (7%), myalgia (7%), gait abnormal (≤5%), hyperkinesia (≤5%), hypertonia (≤5%), tremor (≤5%)
Ocular: Abnormal vision (5%) conjunctivitis (≤5%), eye pain (≤5%)
Otic: Deafness (≤5%), earache (≤5%), tinnitus (≤5%)
Respiratory: Sinusitis (8%), hemoptysis (≤5%), pulmonary infiltrate (≤5%), sputum increased (≤5%)
Miscellaneous: Flu-like syndrome (5%), hiccups (≤5%), lymphadenopathy (≤5%), thirst (≤5%)

Pharmacodynamics/Kinetics

Half-Life Elimination Distribution: 4.4 hours; Terminal: 3-5 hours

Metabolism Similar to daunorubicin, but metabolite plasma levels are low

Excretion Primarily feces; some urine

Clearance, plasma: 17.3 mL/minute

Available Dosage Forms

Injection, solution [preservative free]:
DaunoXome®: 2 mg/mL (25 mL)

Dosing

Adult Refer to individual protocols.

Advanced HIV-associated Kaposi's sarcoma: I.V.: 40 mg/m^2 every 2 weeks

Geriatric Refer to adult dosing. Use with caution.

Renal Impairment

S_{cr} 1.2-3 mg/dL: Reduce dose to 75% of normal.
S_{cr} >3 mg/dL: Reduce dose to 50% of normal.

Hepatic Impairment

Serum bilirubin 1.2-3 mg/dL: Reduce to 75% of normal dose.
Serum bilirubin >3 mg/dL: Reduce to 50% of normal dose.

Adjustment for Toxicity Withhold treatment for ANC <750/mm^3

Administration

I.V. Infuse over 1 hour; do not mix with other drugs. Avoid extravasation.

Stability

Reconstitution Only fluid which may be mixed with DaunoXome® is D_5W. Dilute to a 1:1 solution (1 mg daunorubicin liposomal/mL D_5W). Must **not** be mixed with saline, bacteriostatic agents (such as benzyl alcohol), or any other solution.

Storage Store intact vials of solution under refrigeration at 2°C to 8°C (36°F to 46°F); do not freeze. Protect from light. Diluted daunorubicin liposomal for infusion may be refrigerated at 2°C to 8°C (36°F to 46°F) for a maximum of 6 hours. Do not use with in-line filters.

Monitoring and Teaching Issues

Laboratory Monitoring CBC with differential and platelets (prior to each dose), liver function tests, renal function tests; evaluate cardiac function (baseline left ventricular ejection fraction [LVEF] prior to treatment initiation; repeat LVEF at total cumulative doses of 320 mg/m^2, and every 160 mg/m^2 thereafter; patients with pre-existing cardiac disease, history of prior chest irradiation, or history of prior anthracycline treatment should have baseline LVEF and every 160 mg/m^2 thereafter)

Physical Assessment Evaluate patient for use cautions prior to beginning therapy (eg, pre-existing bone marrow depressions, impaired hepatic or renal function, or cardiac disease). Infusion site should be closely monitored to avoid extravasation. Patient must be monitored closely during infusions for infusion-related reaction (back pain, flushing, chest tightness). If infusion reaction occurs, interrupt infusion and restart at reduced rate.

Patient Education This medication can only be administered by infusion. You will be monitored closely. Report immediately any swelling, pain, burning, or redness at infusion site; chest pain or tightness; or difficulty breathing or swallowing. It is important that you maintain adequate nutrition between treatments and adequate hydration, unless instructed to restrict fluid intake. You will be more susceptible to infection. May cause nausea or vomiting, diarrhea, loss of hair (reversible), or red-pink urine (normal). Report immediately chest pain, palpitations, rapid heartbeat, swelling of extremities, or difficulty breathing. Report unresolved nausea, vomiting, or diarrhea; alterations in urinary pattern (increased or decreased); opportunistic infection (eg, fever, chills, unusual bruising or bleeding, fatigue, purulent vaginal discharge, unhealed mouth sores); CNS changes (depression, insomnia, abnormal thinking, confusion, seizures); abdominal pain or blood in stools; excessive fatigue; or yellowing of eyes or skin.

Pregnancy Considerations Teratogenic effects and embryotoxicity were noted in animal studies. There are no adequate and well-controlled studies in pregnant women. Women of childbearing potential should avoid becoming pregnant while receiving treatment.

DAUNOrubicin Hydrochloride (daw noe ROO bi sin hye droe KLOR ide)

U.S. Brand Names Cerubidine®

Index Terms Daunomycin; Rubidomycin Hydrochloride

Generic Availability (U.S.) Yes

Pharmacologic Category Antineoplastic Agent, Anthracycline

Medication Safety Issues

Sound-alike/look-alike issues:

DAUNOrubicin may be confused with DACTINomycin, DOXOrubicin, DOXOrubicin liposomal, epirubicin, IDArubicin, valrubicin

Conventional formulation (Cerubidine®, DAUNOrubicin hydrochloride) may be confused with the liposomal formulation (DaunoXome®)

High alert medication: The Institute for Safe Medication Practices (ISMP) includes this medication among its list of drug classes which have a heightened risk of causing significant patient harm when used in error.

Pregnancy Risk Factor D

Lactation Excretion in breast milk unknown/not recommended

Use Treatment of acute lymphocytic leukemia (ALL) and acute myeloid leukemia (AML)

Mechanism of Action/Effect Inhibition of DNA and RNA synthesis by intercalation between DNA base pairs and by steric obstruction. Daunomycin intercalates at points of local uncoiling of the double helix. Although the exact mechanism is unclear, it appears that direct binding to DNA (intercalation) and inhibition of DNA repair (topoisomerase II inhibition) result in blockade of DNA and RNA synthesis and fragmentation of DNA.

Contraindications Hypersensitivity to daunorubicin or any component of the formulation

Warnings/Precautions Hazardous agent - use appropriate precautions for handling and disposal. Use with caution in patients who have received radiation therapy; reduce dosage in patients who are receiving radiation therapy simultaneously. **[U.S. Boxed Warnings]: Use caution with renal impairment or in the presence of hepatic dysfunction; dosage reduction is recommended. Potent vesicant; if extravasation occurs, severe local tissue damage leading to ulceration and necrosis, and pain may occur. For I.V. administration only. Severe bone marrow suppression may occur.**

[U.S. Boxed Warning]: May cause cumulative, dose-related myocardial toxicity (concurrent or delayed). Total cumulative dose should take into account previous or concomitant treatment with cardiotoxic agents or irradiation of chest. The incidence of irreversible myocardial toxicity increases as the total cumulative (lifetime) dosages approach:

550 mg/m^2 in adults
400 mg/m^2 in adults receiving chest radiation
300 mg/m^2 in children >2 years of age
10 mg/kg in children <2 years of age

Although the risk increases with cumulative dose, irreversible cardiotoxicity may occur at any dose level. Patients with pre-existing heart disease, hypertension, concurrent administration of other antineoplastic agents, prior or concurrent chest irradiation, advanced age; and infants and children are at increased risk. Monitor left ventricular (LV) function (baseline and periodic) with ECHO or MUGA scan; monitor ECG.

Secondary leukemias may occur when used with combination chemotherapy or radiation therapy. **[U.S. Boxed Warning]: Should be administered under the supervision of an experienced cancer chemotherapy physician.**

Drug Interactions

Metabolism/Transport Effects Substrate of P-glycoprotein

Avoid Concomitant Use

Avoid concomitant use of DAUNOrubicin Hydrochloride with any of the following: BCG; Natalizumab; Pimecrolimus; Roflumilast; Tacrolimus (Topical); Vaccines (Live)

Decreased Effect

DAUNOrubicin Hydrochloride may decrease the levels/effects of: BCG; Cardiac Glycosides; Sipuleucel-T; Vaccines (Inactivated); Vaccines (Live)

The levels/effects of DAUNOrubicin Hydrochloride may be decreased by: Cardiac Glycosides; Echinacea; P-Glycoprotein Inducers

Increased Effect/Toxicity

DAUNOrubicin Hydrochloride may increase the levels/effects of: Leflunomide; Natalizumab; Vaccines (Live)

The levels/effects of DAUNOrubicin Hydrochloride may be increased by: Bevacizumab; Denosumab; P-Glycoprotein Inhibitors; Pimecrolimus; Roflumilast; Tacrolimus (Topical); Taxane Derivatives; Trastuzumab

Nutritional/Ethanol Interactions Ethanol: Avoid ethanol (due to GI irritation).

Lab Interactions Increased potassium (S)

Adverse Reactions

>10%:

Cardiovascular: Transient ECG abnormalities (supraventricular tachycardia, S-T wave changes, atrial or ventricular extrasystoles); generally asymptomatic and self-limiting. CHF, dose related, may be delayed for 7-8 years after treatment.

Dermatologic: Alopecia(reversible), radiation recall

Gastrointestinal: Mild nausea or vomiting, stomatitis

Genitourinary: Discoloration of urine (red)

Hematologic: Myelosuppression (onset: 7 days; nadir: 10-14 days; recovery: 21-28 days), primarily leukopenia; thrombocytopenia and anemia

1% to 10%:

Dermatologic: Skin "flare" at injection site; discoloration of saliva, sweat, or tears

Endocrine & metabolic: Hyperuricemia

Gastrointestinal: Abdominal pain, GI ulceration, diarrhea

Pharmacodynamics/Kinetics

Half-Life Elimination Distribution: 2 minutes; Elimination: 14-20 hours; Terminal: 18.5 hours; Daunorubicinol plasma half-life: 24-48 hours

Metabolism Primarily hepatic to daunorubicinol (active), then to inactive aglycones, conjugated sulfates, and glucuronides

Excretion Feces (40%); urine (~25% as unchanged drug and metabolites)

Available Dosage Forms

Injection, powder for reconstitution: 20 mg

Cerubidine®: 20 mg

Injection, solution [preservative free]: 5 mg/mL (4 mL, 10 mL)

Dosing

Adult Refer to individual protocols. **Note:** Cumulative dose should not exceed 550 mg/m^2 in adults without risk factors for cardiotoxicity and should not exceed 400 mg/m^2 in adults receiving chest irradiation.

Range: I.V.: 30-60 mg/m^2/day for 3 days, repeat dose in 3-4 weeks

ALL combination therapy: I.V.: 45 mg/m^2/day for 3 days

AML combination therapy (induction): I.V.: Adults <60 years: Induction: 45 mg/m^2/day for 3 days of the first course of induction therapy; subsequent courses: 45 mg/m^2/day for 2 days

Geriatric

ALL combination therapy: I.V.: 45 mg/m^2/day for 3 days

AML combination therapy (induction): Elderly ≥60 years: Induction: 30 mg/m^2/day for 3 days of the first course of induction therapy; subsequent courses: 30 mg/m^2/day for 2 days

Pediatric Refer to individual protocols. **Note:** Cumulative dose should not exceed 300 mg/m^2 in children >2 years or 10 mg/kg in children <2 years of age; maximum cumulative doses for younger children are unknown.

ALL combination therapy: I.V.:

Children <2 years or BSA <0.5 m^2: 1 mg/kg/dose per protocol, with frequency dependent on regimen employed

Children ≥2 years and BSA ≥0.5 m^2: Remission induction: 25 mg/m^2 on day 1 every week for up to 4-6 cycles

AML combination therapy (induction): Children ≥2 years and BSA ≥0.5 m^2: I.V. continuous infusion: 30-60 mg/m^2/day on days 1-3 of cycle

Renal Impairment

The FDA-approved labeling recommends the following adjustment: S_{cr} >3 mg/dL: Administer 50% of normal dose.

The following guidelines have been used by some clinicians (Aronoff, 2007):

Children:

Cl_{cr} <30 mL/minute: Administer 50% of dose.

Hemodialysis/continuous ambulatory peritoneal dialysis (CAPD): Administer 50% of dose.

Adults: No adjustment recommended.

Hepatic Impairment

The FDA-approved labeling recommends the following adjustments:

Serum bilirubin 1.2-3 mg/dL: Administer 75% of dose.

Serum bilirubin >3 mg/dL: Administer 50% of dose.

The following guidelines have been used by some clinicians (Floyd, 2006):

Serum bilirubin 1.2-3 mg/dL: Administer 75% of dose

Serum bilirubin 3.1-5 mg/dL: Administer 50% of dose

Serum bilirubin >5 mg/dL: Avoid use

Administration

I.V. Vesicant. **Never** administer I.M. or SubQ. Administer as slow I.V. push over 1-5 minutes into the tubing of a rapidly infusing I.V. solution of D_5W or NS or dilute in 100 mL of D_5W or NS and infuse over 15-30 minutes.

Stability

Reconstitution Dilute vials of powder for injection with 4 mL SWFI for a final concentration of 5 mg/mL. May further dilute in 100 mL D_5W or NS.

Storage Store intact vials of powder for injection at room temperature of 15°C to 30°C (59°F to 86°F); intact vials of solution for injection should be refrigerated at 2°C to 8°C (36°F to 46°F). Protect from light. Reconstituted solution is stable for 4 days at 15°C to 25°C. Further dilution in D_5W, LR, or NS is stable at room temperature (25°C) for up to 4 weeks if protected from light.

Monitoring and Teaching Issues

Laboratory Monitoring CBC with differential and platelet count, liver function test, ECG, left ventricular ejection function (echocardiography [ECHO] or multigated radionuclide angiography [MUGA] scan), renal function test

Physical Assessment Use with caution in presence of pre-existing bone marrow suppression, impaired hepatic or renal function, or cardiac disease. Infusion site must be closely monitored; extravasation can cause severe cellulitis or tissue necrosis. Monitor for tachycardia, cough, dyspnea, and gastrointestinal upset prior to each infusion and throughout therapy.

Patient Education This medication can only be administered I.V. Report immediately any swelling, pain, burning, or redness at infusion site. Avoid alcohol. It is important to maintain adequate nutrition and hydration, unless instructed to restrict fluid intake. You will be more susceptible to infection. May cause nausea or vomiting, diarrhea, loss of hair (reversible), or red-pink urine (normal). Report immediately chest pain, swelling of extremities, respiratory difficulty, palpitations, or rapid heartbeat. Report unresolved nausea, vomiting, or diarrhea; alterations in urinary pattern (increased or decreased); opportunistic infection (eg, fever, chills, unusual bruising or bleeding fatigue, purulent vaginal discharge, unhealed mouth sores); abdominal pain or blood in stools; excessive fatigue; or yellowing of eyes or skin.

Pregnancy Considerations May cause fetal harm when administered to a pregnant woman. Animal studies have shown an increased incidence of fetal abnormalities.

- **DAUNOrubicin Liposomal** *see* DAUNOrubicin Citrate (Liposomal) *on page 472*
- **DaunoXome®** *see* DAUNOrubicin Citrate (Liposomal) *on page 472*
- **1-Day™ [OTC]** *see* Tioconazole *on page 1769*
- **Daypro®** *see* Oxaprozin *on page 1374*
- **Daytrana™** *see* Methylphenidate *on page 1204*
- **DDAVP®** *see* Desmopressin *on page 493*
- **ddI** *see* Didanosine *on page 524*
- **1-Deamino-8-D-Arginine Vasopressin** *see* Desmopressin *on page 493*
- **Decadron** *see* Dexamethasone (Systemic) *on page 499*

Decitabine (de SYE ta been)

U.S. Brand Names Dacogen™

Index Terms 5-Aza-2'-deoxycytidine; 5-Aza-dCyd; Deoxyazacytidine; Dezocitidine

Generic Availability (U.S.) No

Pharmacologic Category Antineoplastic Agent, DNA Methylation Inhibitor

Medication Safety Issues

High alert medication: This medication is in a class the Institute for Safe Medication Practices (ISMP) includes among its list of drug classes which have a heightened risk of causing significant patient harm when used in error.

Pregnancy Risk Factor D

Lactation Excretion in breast milk unknown/not recommended

Use Treatment of myelodysplastic syndrome (MDS)

Unlabeled/Investigational Use Treatment of acute myelogenous leukemia (AML), sickle cell anemia

Mechanism of Action/Effect Hypomethylating agent

Contraindications There are no contraindications listed within the manufacturer's labeling.

Warnings/Precautions Hazardous agent - use appropriate precautions for handling and disposal. The dose-limiting toxicity is bone marrow suppression; worsening neutropenia is common in first two treatment cycles and may not correlate with progression of underlying MDS; may require dosage adjustment (after the first cycle), growth factor support and/or antimicrobial agents; monitor for infection. Not studied in hepatic and renal disease; use caution.

Drug Interactions

Avoid Concomitant Use There are no known interactions where it is recommended to avoid concomitant use.

Decreased Effect There are no known significant interactions involving a decrease in effect.

Increased Effect/Toxicity There are no known significant interactions involving an increase in effect.

Adverse Reactions

>10%:

Cardiovascular: Peripheral edema (25% to 27%), pallor (23%), edema (5% to 18%), cardiac murmur (16%), hypotension (6% to 11%)

Central nervous system: Fever (6% to 53%), fatigue (46%), headache (23% to 28%), insomnia (14% to 28%), dizziness (18% to 21%), chills (16%), pain (5% to 13%), confusion (8% to 12%), lethargy (12%), anxiety (9% to 11%), hypoesthesia (11%)

Dermatologic: Petechiae (12% to 39%), bruising (9% to 22%), rash (11% to 19%), erythema (5% to 14%), cellulitis (9% to 12%), lesions (5% to 11%), pruritus (9% to 11%)

Endocrine & metabolic: Hyperglycemia (6% to 33%), hypoalbuminemia (7% to 24%), hypomagnesemia (5% to 24%), hypokalemia (12% to 22%), hyperkalemia (13%), hyponatremia (19%)

Gastrointestinal: Nausea (40% to 42%), constipation (30% to 35%), diarrhea (28% to 34%), vomiting (16% to 25%), anorexia/appetite decreased (8% to 23%), abdominal pain (5% to 14%), oral mucosal petechiae (13%), stomatitis (11% to 12%), dyspepsia (10% to 12%)

Hematologic: Neutropenia (38% to 90%; grades 3/4: 37% to 87%; recovery 28-50 days), thrombocytopenia (27% to 89%; grades 3/4: 24% to 85%), anemia (31% to 82%; grades 3/4: 22%), febrile neutropenia (20% to 29%; grades 3/4: 23%), leukopenia (6% to 28%; grades 3/4: 22%), lymphadenopathy (12%)
Hepatic: Hyperbilirubinemia (6% to 14%), alkaline phosphatase increased (11%)
Local: Tenderness (11%)
Neuromuscular & skeletal: Rigors (22%), arthralgia (17% to 20%), limb pain (18% to 19%), back pain (17% to 18%), weakness (15%)
Respiratory: Cough (27% to 40%), dyspnea (29%), pneumonia (20% to 22%), pharyngitis (16%), lung crackles (14%), epistaxis (13%)

5% to 10%:
Cardiovascular: Tachycardia (8%), chest pain/discomfort (6% to 7%), facial edema (6%), hypertension (6%), heart failure (5%)
Central nervous system: Depression (9%), malaise (5%)
Dermatologic: Alopecia (8%), dry skin (8%), urticaria (6%)
Endocrine & metabolic: Hyperuricemia (10%), LDH increased (8%), bicarbonate increased (6%), dehydration (6% to 8%), hypochloremia (6%), bicarbonate decreased (5%), hypoproteinemia (5%)
Gastrointestinal: Mucosal inflammation (9%), weight loss (9%), gingival bleeding (8%), hemorrhoids (8%), loose stools (7%), tongue ulceration (7%), dysphagia (5% to 6%), oral candidiasis (6%), toothache (6%), abdominal distension (5%), gastroesophageal reflux (5%), glossodynia (5%), lip ulceration (5%), oral pain (5%), tooth abscess (5%)
Genitourinary: Urinary tract infection (7%), dysuria (6%), polyuria (5%)
Hematologic: Bacteremia (5% to 8%), hematoma (5%), pancytopenia (5%), thrombocythemia (5%)
Hepatic: Ascites (10%), AST increased (10%), hypobilirubinemia (5%)
Local: Catheter infection (8%), catheter site erythema (5%), catheter site pain (5%), injection site swelling (5%)
Neuromuscular & skeletal: Myalgia (5% to 9%), falling (8%), chest wall pain (7%), muscle spasm (7%), bone pain (6%), musculoskeletal pain/discomfort (5% to 6%), crepitation (5%)
Ocular: Blurred vision (6%)
Otic: Ear pain (6%)
Respiratory: Breath sounds abnormal (5% to 10%), hypoxia (10%), upper respiratory tract infection (10%), pharyngolaryngeal pain (8%), rales (8%), pulmonary edema (6%), sinusitis (5% to 6%), pleural effusion (5%), postnasal drip (5%), sinus congestion (5%)
Miscellaneous: Candidal infection (10%), staphylococcal infection (7%), transfusion reaction (7%), night sweats (5%)

Pharmacodynamics/Kinetics

Time to Peak At end of infusion

Protein Binding <1%

Half-Life Elimination ~30-35 minutes

Metabolism Possibly via deamination by cytidine deaminase

Available Dosage Forms

Injection, powder for reconstitution:
Dacogen™: 50 mg

Dosing

Adult & Geriatric

MDS: I.V.:
15 mg/m^2 over 3 hours every 8 hours (45 mg/m^2/day) for 3 days (135 mg/m^2/cycle) every 6 weeks (treatment is recommended for at least 4 cycles and may continue until the patient no longer continues to benefit)
Adjustment for prolonged hematologic toxicity (ANC <1000/mm^3 and platelets <50,000/mm^3):
>6 weeks but <8 weeks: Delay dose for up to 2 weeks and temporarily reduce dose to 11 mg/m^2 every 8 hours (33 mg/m^2/day) for 3 days
>8 weeks but <10 weeks: Assess for disease progression; if no disease progression, delay dose for up to 2 weeks and reduce dose to 11 mg/m^2 every 8 hours (33 mg/m^2/day) for 3 days; maintain or increase dose with subsequent cycles if clinically indicated

or

20 mg/m^2 over 1 hour daily for 5 days every 28 days (delay subsequent treatment cycles until hematologic recovery (ANC ≥1000/mm^3 and platelets ≥50,000/mm^3)

AML (unlabeled use): I.V.: 20 mg/m^2 over 1 hour daily for 5 days every 28 days (Cashen, 2010)

Adjustment for Toxicity

Hematologic toxicity (ANC <1000/mm^3 and platelets <50,000/mm^3): Delay and/or reduce dose; refer to adult dosing for recommendations specific to each MDS dosing regimen
Nonhematologic toxicity: Temporarily hold treatment until resolution for any of the following toxicities:
Serum creatinine ≥2 mg/dL
ALT, bilirubin ≥2 times ULN
Active or uncontrolled infection

Administration

I.V. Infuse over 1-3 hours. Premedication with antiemetics is recommended.

Stability

Reconstitution Vials should be reconstituted with 10 mL SWFI to a concentration of 5 mg/mL. Immediately further dilute with 50-250 mL NS, D_5W, or lactated Ringer's to a final concentration of 0.1-1 mg/mL. Use appropriate precautions for handling and disposal. Solutions not administered within 15 minutes of preparation should be prepared with cold (2°C to 8°C [36°F to 46°F]) infusion solutions.

Storage Store vials at 25°C (77°F); excursions permitted to 15°C to 30°C (59°F to 86°F). Solutions diluted for infusion may be stored for up to 7 hours under refrigeration at 2°C to 8°C (36°F to 46°F) if prepared with cold infusion fluids.

Monitoring and Teaching Issues

Laboratory Monitoring CBC with differential and platelets with each cycle, more frequently if needed; liver enzymes; serum creatinine

Physical Assessment Use caution in presence of hepatic impairment. Premedication with antiemetic is recommended. Monitor for worsening neutropenia, thrombocytopenia, anemia, pulmonary edema, gastrointestinal disturbance, CNS changes, hyperglycemia, and infection prior to each cycle and periodically as indicated during therapy. Advise patients with diabetes to monitor serum glucose closely (may cause hyperglycemia).

Patient Education This medication can only be administered by intravenous infusion. Report immediately any redness, swelling, pain, or burning at infusion site, or any adverse response during infusion (eg, respiratory difficulty, facial edema, pain, restlessness, tremor, wheezing). Maintain adequate nutrition and hydration, unless instructed to restrict fluid intake. You may be more susceptible to infection. If you have diabetes, you should monitor serum glucose closely; may cause hyperglycemia. May cause lethargy, dizziness, visual changes, confusion, anxiety, nausea, vomiting, loss of appetite, dry mouth, mouth sores, loss of hair (may grow back when treatment is discontinued), diarrhea, or constipation. Report respiratory difficulty; chest pain or palpitations; unusual bleeding, bruising, or rash; or any sign of urinary tract infection (itching or burning) or opportunistic infection (eg, sore throat, fever, chills, fatigue, thrush, vaginal discharge, diarrhea).

Breast-Feeding Considerations Due to the potential for serious adverse reactions in the nursing infant, breast-feeding is not recommended.

Pregnancy Considerations Teratogenic effects, decreased fetal weight, and increased fetal deaths were observed in animal studies. There are no adequate and well-controlled studies in pregnant women. Women of childbearing potential should be advised to avoid pregnancy during treatment and for 1 month after treatment. In addition, males should be advised to avoid fathering a child while on decitabine therapy and for 2 months after treatment.

◆ **Declomycin** *see* Demeclocycline *on page* 484

Deferoxamine (de fer OKS a meen)

U.S. Brand Names Desferal®

Index Terms Deferoxamine Mesylate; Desferrioxamine

Generic Availability (U.S.) Yes

Pharmacologic Category Antidote; Chelating Agent

Medication Safety Issues

Sound-alike/look-alike issues:

Deferoxamine may be confused with cefuroxime, deferasirox

Desferal® may be confused with desflurane, Dexferrum®, Disophrol®

International issues:

Desferal [U.S., Canada, and multiple international markets] may be confused with Deseril brand name for methysergide [Australia, Belgium, Great Britain, Netherlands]

Pregnancy Risk Factor C

Lactation Excretion in breast milk unknown/use caution

Use Adjunct in the treatment of acute iron intoxication; treatment of chronic iron overload secondary to multiple transfusions

Canadian labeling (unlabeled use in the U.S.): Diagnosis of aluminum overload; treatment of chronic aluminum overload in patients with end-stage renal failure undergoing maintenance dialysis

Unlabeled/Investigational Use Diagnosis or treatment of aluminum induced toxicity associated with chronic kidney disease (CKD)

Available Dosage Forms

Injection, powder for reconstitution: 500 mg, 2 g

Desferal®: 500 mg, 2 g

Dosing

Adult

Acute iron toxicity: Note: The I.V. route should be used for patients in a state of cardiovascular collapse.

I.M., I.V.: Initial: 1000 mg, may be followed by 500 mg every 4 hours for 2 doses; subsequent doses of 500 mg have been administered every 4-12 hours based on clinical response (maximum recommended dose: 6 g/day [per manufacturer])

Canadian labeling:

I.M.: Initial: 90 mg/kg/dose (maximum/dose: 2 g) followed by 45 mg/kg every 4-12 hours as needed (maximum: 6 g/24 hours)

I.V.: 15 mg/kg/hour up to a maximum of 80 mg/kg/dose or maximum of 6 g/24 hours

Chronic iron overload:

I.M., I.V.: Initial: I.M.: 500-1000 mg/day; in addition, 2000 mg should be given I.V. with each unit of blood transfused (administer separately from blood); maximum: 1 g/day in absence of transfusions; 6 g/day if patient received transfusions

SubQ: 1-2 g every day or 20-40 mg/kg/day over 8-24 hours

Unlabeled dosing: I.V., SubQ: 25-50 mg/kg over 8-10 hours 5-7 days/week (Brittenham, 2011)

Canadian labeling: I.V., SubQ: 1-4 g (20-60 mg/kg) over ~12 hours (may further increase iron excretion with infusion over 24 hours)

Diagnosis of aluminum-induced toxicity with CKD (unlabeled use; K/DOQI guidelines, 2003): I.V.: Test dose: 5 mg/kg during the last hour of dialysis if serum aluminum levels are 60-200 mcg/L, or clinical signs/symptoms of toxicity, or aluminum exposure prior to parathyroid surgery. Measure aluminum just prior to deferoxamine; remeasure 2 days later (test is positive if serum aluminum is ≥50 mcg/L). Do not use if aluminum serum levels are >200 mcg/L.

Canadian labeling: **Note:** Measure serum aluminum levels prior to and after administration of deferoxamine. I.V.: Test dose: 5 mg/kg/dose (infusion rate not to exceed 15 mg/kg/hour) following hemodialysis (preferred) or during the last hour of dialysis if serum aluminum levels are >60 mcg/L in association with serum ferritin levels >100 mcg/L; continuous rise in serum aluminum over the next 24-48 hours suggests overload. Remeasure serum aluminum levels prior to next hemodialysis, test is considered positive if serum aluminum levels increase >150 mcg/L above baseline.

Treatment of aluminum toxicity with CKD (unlabeled use; K/DOQI guidelines, 2003): I.V.: Administer after diagnostic deferoxamine test dose. **Note:** The risk for deferoxamine-associated neurotoxicity is increased if aluminum serum levels are >200 mcg/L; withhold deferoxamine and administer intensive dialysis until <200 mcg/L.

Aluminum rise ≥300 mcg/L: 5 mg/kg once a week 5 hours before dialysis for 4 months

Aluminum rise <300 mcg/L: 5 mg/kg once a week during the last hour of dialysis for 2 months

Canadian labeling: Treatment should be considered for symptomatic patients with serum aluminum levels >60 mcg/L and a positive deferoxamine test dose.

Hemodialysis: I.V.: 5 mg/kg/dose (infusion rate not to exceed 15 mg/kg/hour) once weekly for 3 months following hemodialysis (preferred) or during the last hour of dialysis administered. Withhold treatment for 1 month then perform deferoxamine test. Further treatment is not recommended if 2 consecutive tests (performed 1 month apart) yield an increase in serum aluminum levels <75 mcg/mL.

Continuous ambulatory or cyclic peritoneal dialysis: Intraperitoneal (preferred), I.M., SubQ infusion (slow), or I.V. infusion (slow): 5 mg/kg/dose once weekly prior to final daily exchange

Geriatric Refer to adult dosing. May initiate at the lower end of the dosing range.

Pediatric

Acute iron toxicity: Children ≥3 years: Refer to "Note" in adult dosing.

I.M.: 90 mg/kg/dose every 8 hours (maximum: 6 g/24 hours)

I.V.: 15 mg/kg/hour (maximum: 6 g/24 hours)

Canadian labeling:

I.M.: 90 mg/kg/dose (maximum/dose: 1 g) followed by 45 mg/kg every 4-12 hours as needed (maximum: 6 g/24 hours)

I.V.: 15 mg/kg/hour up to a maximum of 80 mg/kg/dose or maximum of 6 g/24 hours

Chronic iron overload: Children ≥3 years:

I.V.: 15 mg/kg/hour (maximum: 6 g/24 hours)

SubQ: 20-40 mg/kg/day over 8-12 hours (maximum: 1000-2000 mg/day)

Unlabeled dosing: I.V., SubQ: 25-30 mg/kg over 8-10 hours 5-7 days/week (Brittenham, 2011)

Diagnosis of aluminum induced toxicity with CKD (unlabeled use; K/DOQI guidelines, 2003): Children: I.V.: Test dose: 5 mg/kg during the last hour of dialysis if serum aluminum levels are 60-200 mcg/L, or clinical signs/symptoms of toxicity, or aluminum exposure prior to parathyroid surgery. Measure aluminum just prior to deferoxamine; remeasure 2 days later (test is positive if serum aluminum is ≥50 mcg/L). Do not use if aluminum serum levels are >200 mcg/L.

Treatment of aluminum toxicity with CKD (unlabeled use; K/DOQI guidelines, 2003): Children: I.V.: Administer after diagnostic deferoxamine test dose. **Note:** The risk for deferoxamine-associated neurotoxicity is increased if aluminum serum levels are >200 mcg/L; withhold deferoxamine and administer intensive dialysis until <200 mcg/L.

Aluminum rise ≥300 mcg/L: 5 mg/kg once a week 5 hours before dialysis for 4 months

Aluminum rise <300 mcg/L: 5 mg/kg once a week during the last hour of dialysis for 2 months

Renal Impairment Severe renal disease or anuria: Use is contraindicated in the FDA-approved labeling.

The following adjustments have been used by some clinicians (Aronoff, 2007): Adults:

Cl_{cr} >50 mL/minute: No adjustment required

Cl_{cr} 10-50 mL/minute, CRRT: Administer 25% to 50% of normal dose

Cl_{cr}<10 mL/minute, hemodialysis, peritoneal dialysis: Avoid use

Administration

I.V. Urticaria, flushing of the skin, hypotension, and shock have occurred following rapid I.V. administration; limiting infusion rate to 15mg/kg/hour may help avoid infusion-related adverse effects.

Acute iron toxicity: The manufacturer states that the I.M. route is preferred; however, the I.V. route is generally preferred in patients with severe toxicity (ie, patients in shock). For the first 1000 mg, infuse at 15 mg/kg/hour. Subsequent doses may be given over 4-12 hours at a rate not to exceed 125 mg/hour.

Chronic iron overload: Longer infusion times (24 hours) and I.V. administration may be required in patients with severe cardiac iron deposition (Brittenham, 2011).

Diagnosis or treatment of aluminum-induced toxicity with CKD: Administer dose over 1 hour during the last hour of dialysis (K/DOQI guidelines, 2003).

Other SubQ: When administered for chronic iron overload, daily dose is usually given over 8-12 hours using portable infusion pump. Topical anesthetic or glucocorticoid creams may be used for induration or erythema (Brittenham, 2011).

Monitoring and Teaching Issues

Laboratory Monitoring Serum iron, total iron-binding capacity, ferritin, CBC with differential, serum creatinine, liver function tests, serum chemistries, serum aluminum (yearly; every 3 months in patients on aluminum-containing medications)

Physical Assessment Infuse slowly and monitor infusion site. Monitor for acute reactions; urticaria, hypotension, and shock can occur following rapid I.V. administration. With chronic therapy, perform ophthalmologic exam (fundoscopy, slit-lamp exam) and audiometry. Teach patient proper injection technique and syringe/needle disposal. Monitor for adverse cardiac, respiratory, or CNS symptoms and teach patient importance of reporting adverse symptoms.

Patient Education You will be monitored closely for effects of this medication and frequent blood or urine tests may be necessary. Your urine may show a reddish discoloration. Report chest pain; rapid heartbeat; headache; pain, swelling, or irritation at infusion site; skin rash; changes or loss of hearing or vision; or acute abdominal or leg cramps.

◆ **Deferoxamine Mesylate** *see* Deferoxamine *on page 478*

Degarelix (deg a REL ix)

U.S. Brand Names Firmagon®

Index Terms Degarelix Acetate; FE200486

Generic Availability (U.S.) No

Pharmacologic Category Antineoplastic Agent, Gonadotropin-Releasing Hormone Antagonist; Gonadotropin Releasing Hormone Antagonist

Medication Safety Issues

Sound-alike/look-alike issues:

Degarelix may be confused with cetrorelix, ganirelix

Pregnancy Risk Factor X

Lactation Excretion in breast milk unknown/not recommended

Use Treatment of advanced prostate cancer

Mechanism of Action/Effect Binds to and blocks gonadotropin-releasing hormone (GnRH) receptors in the anterior pituitary gland, decreasing secretion of luteinizing hormone (LH) and follicle stimulation hormone (FSH), resulting in rapid androgen deprivation by decreasing testosterone levels (without an initial surge in testosterone levels).

Contraindications Hypersensitivity to degarelix or any component of the formulation; pregnancy (or potential to become pregnant)

Warnings/Precautions Hazardous agent - use appropriate precautions for handling and disposal. Long-term androgen deprivation therapy may prolong the QT interval; use with caution in patients with a known history of QT prolongation or other risk factors for QT prolongation (eg, concomitant use of medications known to prolong QT interval, heart failure, and/or electrolyte abnormalities). Androgen-deprivation therapy may increase the risk for cardiovascular disease (Levine, 2010) and decreased bone mineral density. Androgen deprivation therapy may cause obesity and insulin resistance; the risk for diabetes is increased.

Degarelix exposure is decreased in patients with hepatic impairment, dosage adjustment is not recommended in patients with mild-to-moderate hepatic impairment, although testosterone levels should be monitored. Has not been studied in patients with severe hepatic impairment; use with caution. Data for use in patients with moderate-to-severe renal impairment (Cl_{cr} <50 mL/minute) is limited; use with caution.

Drug Interactions

Avoid Concomitant Use

Avoid concomitant use of Degarelix with any of the following: Artemether; Dronedarone; Lumefantrine; Nilotinib; Pimozide; QuiNINE; Tetrabenazine; Thioridazine; Toremifene; Vandetanib; Ziprasidone

Decreased Effect There are no known significant interactions involving a decrease in effect.

Increased Effect/Toxicity

Degarelix may increase the levels/effects of: Dronedarone; Pimozide; QTc-Prolonging Agents; QuiNINE; Tetrabenazine; Thioridazine; Toremifene; Vandetanib; Ziprasidone

The levels/effects of Degarelix may be increased by: Alfuzosin; Artemether; Chloroquine; Ciprofloxacin; Ciprofloxacin (Systemic); Gadobutrol; Lumefantrine; Nilotinib; QuiNINE

Lab Interactions Suppression of pituitary-gonadal function may affect diagnostic tests of pituitary gonadotropic and gonadal functions.

Adverse Reactions

>10%:

Endocrine & metabolic: Hot flashes (26%)

Local: Injections site reactions (35%, grade 3: ≤2%; pain 28%, erythema 17%, swelling 6%, induration 4%, nodule 3%)

1% to 10%:

Cardiovascular: Hypertension (6%)

Central nervous system: Chills (5%), dizziness (1% to 5%), fever (1% to 5%), headache (1% to 5%), insomnia (1% to 5%), fatigue (3%)

Dermatologic: Hyperhydrosis

Endocrine & metabolic: Hypercholesterolemia (3%), gynecomastia, testicular atrophy

Gastrointestinal: Weight gain (9%), constipation (5%), nausea (1% to 5%), diarrhea

Genitourinary: Urinary tract infection (5%), erectile dysfunction

Hepatic: ALT increased (10%; grade 3: <1%), AST increased (5%; grade 3: <1%), GGT increased

Neuromuscular & skeletal: Back pain (6%), arthralgia (5%), weakness (1% to 5%)

Miscellaneous: Antidegarelix antibody formation (10%), night sweats (1% to 5%)

Pharmacodynamics/Kinetics

Onset of Action Rapid; ~96% of patients had testosterone levels ≤50 ng/dL within 3 days (Klotz, 2008)

Bioavailability Biphasic release: Rapid release initially, then slow release from depot formed after subcutaneous injection administration (Tornoe, 2007)

Time to Peak Plasma: Loading dose: SubQ: Within 2 days

Protein Binding ~90%

Half-Life Elimination Loading dose: SubQ: ~53 days

Metabolism Hepatobiliary, via peptide hydrolysis

Excretion Feces (~70% to 80%, primarily as peptide fragments); urine (~20% to 30%)

Available Dosage Forms

Injection, powder for reconstitution:

Firmagon®: 80 mg, 120 mg

Dosing

Adult & Geriatric Prostate cancer: SubQ:

Loading dose: 240 mg administered as two 120 mg (3 mL) injections

Maintenance dose: 80 mg every 28 days (beginning 28 days after initial loading dose)

Renal Impairment Cl_{cr} <50 mL/minute: Use with caution.

Hepatic Impairment

Mild-to-moderate hepatic impairment: No adjustment required; monitor serum testosterone levels.

Severe hepatic impairment: Has not been studied; use with caution.

Administration

I.V. Not for I.V. use.

Other Not for I.V. use. Administer SubQ in the abdominal area by grasping skin and elevating SubQ tissue; insert the needle deeply at an angle not ≤45 degrees. Avoid pressure exposed areas (eg, waistband, belt, or near ribs); rotate injection site. Inject loading dose as two 3 mL injections (40 mg/mL); maintenance dose should be administered as a single 4 mL injection (20 mg/mL); begin maintenance dose 28 days after initial loading dose.

Stability

Reconstitution Use appropriate precautions (wear gloves for preparation and administration) for handling and disposal. Reconstitute with preservative free sterile water for injection (reconstitute each 120 mg vial with 3 mL; reconstitute the 80 mg vial with 4.2 mL). Swirl gently; do not shake (to prevent foaming). Dissolution may take up to 15 minutes. Keep vial upright at all times. Tilt vial slightly, keeping needle in lowest section of vial to withdraw for administration. Administer within 1 hour of reconstitution.

Storage Store at 25°C (77°F); excursions permitted to 15°C to 30°C (59°F to 86°F).

Monitoring and Teaching Issues

Laboratory Monitoring Prostate-specific antigen (PSA) periodically, serum testosterone levels (if PSA increases; in patients with hepatic impairment: monitor testosterone levels monthly until achieve castration levels, then consider monitoring every other month), liver function tests (at baseline), serum electrolytes (calcium, magnesium, potassium, sodium); bone mineral density

Physical Assessment Use with caution in presence or history of cardiovascular disease; minimize cardiovascular risk factors. Evaluate PSA and serum testosterone levels, LFTs, electrolytes, and bone density on a regular basis during therapy. Supplemental calcium and vitamin D may reduce risk of osteoporosis due to androgen deprivation.

Patient Education This drug can only be administered by injection in abdominal area at regularly scheduled intervals. It is important that you maintain adequate nutrition and fluid intake; dietary supplements of calcium or vitamins may be recommended. You may experience hot flashes, dizziness, headache, insomnia, fatigue, nausea, diarrhea, or constipation. Report any injection site reaction (pain, redness, swelling), acute headache, signs of urinary tract infection (pain, itching, change in urinary pattern), or persistent back or muscle pain or weakness.

Dietary Considerations Supplementation with 500 mg calcium and 400 int. units of vitamin D is recommended (due to the increased risk for osteoporosis with androgen deprivation therapy).

Geriatric Considerations No dosage adjustments are necessary in elderly. Monitor serum lipids and for hypertension.

Pregnancy Considerations Animal studies have demonstrated embryo and fetal loss. Use is contraindicated in women who are or may become pregnant.

- **Degarelix Acetate** *see* Degarelix *on page 480*
- **Dehydrobenzperidol** *see* Droperidol *on page 593*
- **Delatestryl®** *see* Testosterone *on page 1739*

Delavirdine (de la VIR deen)

U.S. Brand Names Rescriptor®

Index Terms U-90152S

Generic Availability (U.S.) No

Pharmacologic Category Antiretroviral Agent, Reverse Transcriptase Inhibitor (Non-nucleoside)

Medication Safety Issues

Sound-alike/look-alike issues:

Delavirdine may be confused with dalfampridine

Pregnancy Risk Factor C

Lactation Excretion in breast milk unknown/contraindicated

Use Treatment of HIV-1 infection in combination with at least two additional antiretroviral agents

Mechanism of Action/Effect Delavirdine binds directly to reverse transcriptase, blocking RNA-dependent and DNA-dependent DNA polymerase activities

Contraindications Hypersensitivity to delavirdine or any component of the formulation; concurrent use of alprazolam, astemizole, cisapride, ergot alkaloids, midazolam, pimozide, rifampin, terfenadine, or triazolam

Warnings/Precautions Use with caution in patients with hepatic or renal dysfunction; due to rapid emergence of resistance, delavirdine should not be used as monotherapy or as a component of an initial antiretroviral regimen; cross-resistance may be conferred to other non-nucleoside reverse transcriptase inhibitors, although potential for cross-resistance with protease inhibitors is low. Long-term effects of delavirdine are not known. May cause redistribution of fat (eg, buffalo hump, peripheral wasting with increased abdominal girth, cushingoid appearance). Immune reconstitution syndrome may develop resulting in the occurrence of an inflammatory response to an indolent or residual opportunistic infection; further evaluation and treatment may be required. Safety and efficacy have not been established in children. Rash, which occurs frequently, may require discontinuation of therapy; usually occurs within 1-3 weeks and lasts <2 weeks. Most patients may resume therapy following a treatment interruption. Use with caution in patients taking strong CYP3A4 inhibitors, moderate or strong CYP3A4 inducers and major CYP3A4 substrates (see Drug Interactions); consider alternative agents that avoid or lessen the potential for CYP-mediated interactions.

Drug Interactions

Metabolism/Transport Effects Substrate of CYP2D6 (minor), 3A4 (major); **Inhibits** CYP1A2 (weak), 2C9 (strong), 2C19 (strong), 2D6 (strong), 3A4 (strong)

Avoid Concomitant Use

Avoid concomitant use of Delavirdine with any of the following: Alfuzosin; Clopidogrel; Conivaptan; Dronedarone; Eplerenone; Etravirine; Everolimus; Fosamprenavir; H2-Antagonists; Halofantrine; Lurasidone; Nilotinib; Nisoldipine; Proton Pump Inhibitors; Ranolazine; Rivaroxaban; RomiDEPsin; Salmeterol; Silodosin; St Johns Wort; Tamoxifen; Tamsulosin; Thioridazine; Tolvaptan; Toremifene

Decreased Effect

Delavirdine may decrease the levels/effects of: Clopidogrel; Codeine; Etravirine; Prasugrel; TraMADol

The levels/effects of Delavirdine may be decreased by: Antacids; CYP3A4 Inducers (Strong); Deferasirox; Fosamprenavir; H2-Antagonists; Peginterferon Alfa-2b; Protease Inhibitors; Proton Pump Inhibitors; Rifamycin Derivatives; St Johns Wort

Increased Effect/Toxicity

Delavirdine may increase the levels/effects of: Alfuzosin; Almotriptan; Alosetron; Atomoxetine; Bortezomib; Brinzolamide; Carvedilol; Ciclesonide; Colchicine; Conivaptan; Corticosteroids (Orally Inhaled); CYP2C19 Substrates; CYP2C9 Substrates (High risk); CYP2D6 Substrates; CYP3A4 Substrates; Dienogest; Dronedarone; Dutasteride; Eplerenone; Etravirine; Everolimus; FentaNYL; Fesoterodine; Fosamprenavir; GuanFACINE; Halofantrine; Ixabepilone; Lumefantrine; Lurasidone; Maraviroc; MethylPREDNISolone; Nebivolol; Nilotinib; Nisoldipine; PACLitaxel; Paricalcitol; Pazopanib; Pimecrolimus; Protease Inhibitors; Ranolazine; Rifamycin Derivatives; Rivaroxaban; RomiDEPsin; Salmeterol; Saxagliptin; Silodosin; SORAfenib; Tadalafil; Tamoxifen; Tamsulosin; Tetrabenazine; Thioridazine; Tolvaptan; Toremifene; Vilazodone

Nutritional/Ethanol Interactions Herb/Nutraceutical: Delavirdine serum concentration may be decreased by St John's wort; avoid concurrent use.

Adverse Reactions

Frequency of adverse reactions reported from occurrence in clinical trials with delavirdine when used as part of combination antiretroviral therapy.

>10%:

Central nervous system: Headache (19% to 20%), depressive symptoms (10% to 15%), fever (4% to 12%)

Dermatologic: Rash (16% to 32%)

Gastrointestinal: Nausea (20% to 25%), vomiting (3% to 11%)

1% to 10%:

Central nervous system: Anxiety (6% to 8%)

Endocrine & metabolic: Transaminases increased (2% to 5%), amylase increased (3%), bilirubin increased (2%)

Gastrointestinal: Diarrhea, vomiting, abdominal pain (4% to 6%)

Hematologic: Prothrombin time increased (2%), hemoglobin decreased (1% to 3%)

Respiratory: Bronchitis (6% to 8%)

Frequency not defined (limited to important or life threatening): Abscess, adenopathy, alkaline phosphatase increased, allergic reaction, angioedema, anorexia, arrhythmia, bloody stool, bone pain, bruising, cardiac insufficiency, cardiac rate abnormal, cardiomyopathy, chest congestion, cognitive impairment, colitis, confusion, conjunctivitis, dermal leukocytoclastic vasculitis, desquamation, diverticulitis, dyspnea, emotional lability, eosinophilia, erythema multiforme, fecal incontinence, fungal dermatitis, gamma glutamyl transpeptidase increased, gastroenteritis, gastrointestinal bleeding, granulocytosis, gum hemorrhage, hallucination, hematuria, hepatomegaly, hyperglycemia, hyperkalemia, hypertension, hypertriglyceridemia, hyperuricemia, hypocalcemia, hyponatremia, hypophosphatemia, infection, jaundice, kidney pain, leukopenia, lipase increased, menstrual irregularities, moniliasis (oral/vaginal), pancreatitis, pancytopenia, paralysis, peripheral vascular disorder, pneumonia, postural hypotension, purpura, redistribution of body fat, renal calculi, serum creatinine increased, spleen disorder, Stevens-Johnson syndrome, tetany, thrombocytopenia, urinary tract infection, vertigo

Pharmacodynamics/Kinetics

Absorption Rapid

Bioavailability Tablet: 85% as tablet; ~100% as oral slurry

Time to Peak Plasma: 1 hour

Protein Binding ~98%, primarily to albumin

Half-Life Elimination 5.8 hours (range: 2-11 hours)

Metabolism Hepatic via CYP3A4 and 2D6 (**Note:** May reduce CYP3A activity and inhibit its own metabolism.)

Excretion Urine (51%, <5% as unchanged drug); feces (44%); nonlinear kinetics exhibited

Available Dosage Forms

Tablet, oral:

Rescriptor®: 100 mg, 200 mg

Dosing

Adult & Geriatric HIV-1 infection (part of combination): Oral: 400 mg 3 times/day

Note: Only a single delavirdine mutation causes resistance; use is not recommended in initial antiretroviral regimens (DHHS, 2011).

Pediatric HIV-1 infection (part of combination): Adolescents ≥16 years: Refer to adult dosing.

Administration

Oral Patients with achlorhydria should take the drug with an acidic beverage. Antacids and delavirdine should be separated by 1 hour. A dispersion of delavirdine may be prepared by adding four 100 mg tablets to at least 3 oz of water. Allow to stand for a few minutes and stir until uniform dispersion. Drink immediately. Rinse glass and mouth, then swallow the rinse to ensure total dose administered. The 200 mg tablets should be taken intact.

Stability

Storage Store at 20°C to 25°C (68°F to 77°F). Protect from humidity.

Monitoring and Teaching Issues

Laboratory Monitoring Liver function tests if administered with saquinavir; viral load

Physical Assessment Assess decrease in infections and progress of disease, viral load, and CD4 count periodically during therapy. Monitor for rash and gastrointestinal upset. Teach patient proper timing of multiple medications.

Patient Education You will be provided with a list of specific medications that should not be used during therapy. This drug will not cure HIV, nor has it been found to reduce transmission of HIV; use appropriate precautions to prevent spread to other persons. This drug is prescribed as one part of a multidrug combination; take exactly as directed for full course of therapy. May be taken with or without food. Take 200 mg tablets intact (do not chew or dissolve). You may mix four 100 mg tablets in 3-5 oz of water; allow to stand a few minutes and stir; drink immediately; rinse glass and mouth (swallow rinse solution) following ingestion to ensure total dose administered. Maintain adequate hydration, unless instructed to restrict fluid intake. Frequent blood tests may be required. May cause nausea or vomiting; consult prescriber if symptoms persist. Report skin rash, muscle weakness, persistent headache, depression, fatigue, or gastrointestinal upset.

Dietary Considerations May be taken without regard to meals.

Breast-Feeding Considerations In infants born to mothers who are HIV positive, HAART while breast-feeding may decrease postnatal infection. However, maternal or infant antiretroviral therapy does not completely eliminate the risk of postnatal HIV transmission. In addition, multiclass-resistant virus has been detected in breast-feeding infants despite maternal therapy.

In the United States where formula is accessible, affordable, safe, and sustainable, complete avoidance of breast-feeding by HIV-infected women is recommended to decrease potential transmission of HIV.

Pregnancy Considerations It is not known if delavirdine crosses the human placenta. Delavirdine was shown to be teratogenic in some animal studies. There are no adequate and well-controlled studies in pregnant women and use during pregnancy is not recommended unless other alternatives are not available. Healthcare providers are encouraged to enroll pregnant women exposed to antiretroviral medications in the Antiretroviral Pregnancy

Registry (1-800-258-4263 or www.APRegistry.com). Healthcare providers caring for HIV-infected women and their infants may contact the National Perinatal HIV Hotline (888-448-8765) for clinical consultation.

Additional Information Potential compliance problems, frequency of administration, and adverse effects should be discussed with patients before initiating therapy to help prevent the emergence of resistance.

- ◆ **Delestrogen®** *see* Estradiol (Systemic) *on page 670*
- ◆ **Delta-9-tetrahydro-cannabinol** *see* Dronabinol *on page 590*
- ◆ **Delta-9 THC** *see* Dronabinol *on page 590*
- ◆ **Deltacortisone** *see* PredniSONE *on page 1500*
- ◆ **Deltadehydrocortisone** *see* PredniSONE *on page 1500*
- ◆ **Demadex®** *see* Torsemide *on page 1795*

Demeclocycline (dem e kloe SYE kleen)

Index Terms Declomycin; Demeclocycline Hydrochloride; Demethylchlortetracycline

Generic Availability (U.S.) Yes

Pharmacologic Category Antibiotic, Tetracycline Derivative

Pregnancy Risk Factor D

Lactation Enters breast milk/not recommended

Use Treatment of susceptible bacterial infections (acne, gonorrhea, pertussis, and urinary tract infections) caused by both gram-negative and gram-positive organisms

Unlabeled/Investigational Use Treatment of chronic syndrome of inappropriate secretion of antidiuretic hormone (SIADH)

Available Dosage Forms

Tablet, oral: 150 mg, 300 mg

Dosing

Adult & Geriatric

Susceptible infections: Oral: 150 mg 4 times/day or 300 mg twice daily

SIADH (unlabeled use): Oral: 900-1200 mg/day or 13-15 mg/kg/day divided every 6-8 hours initially, then decrease to 600-900 mg/day

Pediatric Susceptible infections: Oral: ≥8 years: 8-12 mg/kg/day divided every 6-12 hours

Renal Impairment Should be avoided in patients with renal dysfunction.

Hepatic Impairment Should be avoided in patients with hepatic dysfunction.

Administration

Oral Administer 1 hour before or 2 hours after food or milk with plenty of fluid.

Monitoring and Teaching Issues

Laboratory Monitoring CBC, renal and hepatic function; perform culture and sensitivity studies prior to initiating therapy

Physical Assessment Assess results of culture and sensitivity tests and patient's allergy history prior to beginning therapy. Monitor for rash, anaphylactic reactions, anemia, and CNS changes. Advise patients with diabetes about use of Clinitest®.

Patient Education Take on an empty stomach (1 hour before or 2 hours after meals with plenty of fluid). Take at regularly scheduled intervals around-the-clock. Avoid antacids, iron, and dairy products within 2 hours of taking demeclocycline. May cause photosensitivity, dizziness, lightheadedness, nausea, vomiting, or diarrhea. Report rash or intense itching, yellowing of skin or eyes, change in color of urine or stools, fever or chills, dark urine or pale stools, vaginal itching or discharge, foul-smelling stools, excessive thirst or urination, acute headache, unresolved or persistent diarrhea, or respiratory difficulty.

- ◆ **Demeclocycline Hydrochloride** *see* Demeclocycline *on page 484*
- ◆ **Demerol®** *see* Meperidine *on page 1172*
- ◆ **4-Demethoxydaunorubicin** *see* IDArubicin *on page 945*
- ◆ **Demethylchlortetracycline** *see* Demeclocycline *on page 484*

Denileukin Diftitox (de ni LOO kin DIF ti toks)

U.S. Brand Names ONTAK®

Index Terms DAB389 Interleukin-2; DAB_{389}IL-2; DABIL2

Generic Availability (U.S.) No

Pharmacologic Category Antineoplastic Agent, Miscellaneous

Medication Safety Issues

High alert medication: The Institute for Safe Medication Practices (ISMP) includes this medication among its list of drug classes which have a heightened risk of causing significant patient harm when used in error.

Lactation Excretion in breast milk unknown/not recommended

Use Treatment of persistent or recurrent cutaneous T-cell lymphoma (CTCL) whose malignant cells express the CD25 component of the IL-2 receptor

Unlabeled/Investigational Use Treatment of CTCL types mycosis fungoides (MF) and Sézary syndrome (SS); peripheral T-cell lymphoma (second-line treatment)

Mechanism of Action/Effect Interacts with receptors on surface of malignant cells to inhibit intracellular protein synthesis rapidly leading to cell death.

Contraindications There are no contraindications listed within the manufacturer's labeling.

Warnings/Precautions Hazardous agent - use appropriate precautions for handling and disposal. **[U.S. Boxed Warning]: Has been associated with a potentially severe, including life-threatening, capillary leak syndrome; monitor weight, edema, blood pressure, and serum albumin prior to and during treatment.** Symptoms of capillary leak syndrome (hypotension, edema, hypoalbuminemia) may be delayed, occurring up to 2 weeks post infusion; symptoms may persist or worsen after cessation of denileukin diftitox. Withhold treatment if serum albumin <3 g/dL; pre-existing low serum albumin levels may correlate with capillary leak syndrome. **[U.S. Boxed Warning]: Serious and fatal infusion reactions have occurred. Administer in a facility appropriate for cardiopulmonary resuscitation. Discontinue immediately and permanently with serious infusion reaction.** Infusion reaction symptoms usually occur within 24 hours of infusion and resolve within 48 hours of last infusion of cycle. Incidence of infusion reaction has been reported to be lower in cycles 3 and 4 (compared to cycles 1 and 2). The manufacturer recommends premedicating with an antihistamine and acetaminophen; corticosteroid (eg, dexamethasone) premedication may help to reduce the incidence of hypersensitivity and edema (Foss, 2001). **[U.S. Boxed Warning]: Loss of visual acuity, usually associated with loss of color vision (with or without retinal pigment mottling) has been reported;** most patients have persistent visual impairment.

Confirm CD25 expression on malignant cells prior to treatment. May develop immunogenicity; patients with antibodies have a two- to threefold increase in clearance; the presence of antibodies does not correlate with risk for hypersensitivity/infusion related reactions. Monitor closely for infection; may impair immune function. Use with caution in patients >65 years of age; adverse events (anemia, anorexia, confusion, hypotension, rash, nausea/vomiting) may occur more frequently. Safety and efficacy in children have not been established. Should be administered under the supervision of an experienced cancer chemotherapy physician.

Drug Interactions

Avoid Concomitant Use

Avoid concomitant use of Denileukin Diftitox with any of the following: BCG; Belimumab; Natalizumab; Pimecrolimus; Roflumilast; Tacrolimus (Topical); Vaccines (Live)

Decreased Effect

Denileukin Diftitox may decrease the levels/effects of: BCG; Sipuleucel-T; Vaccines (Inactivated); Vaccines (Live)

The levels/effects of Denileukin Diftitox may be decreased by: Echinacea

Increased Effect/Toxicity

Denileukin Diftitox may increase the levels/effects of: Belimumab; Leflunomide; Natalizumab; Vaccines (Live)

The levels/effects of Denileukin Diftitox may be increased by: Denosumab; Pimecrolimus; Roflumilast; Tacrolimus (Topical); Trastuzumab

Adverse Reactions

>10%:

Cardiovascular: Capillary leak syndrome (33%; serious: 11%), peripheral edema (20% to 26%), vasodilation (22%), hypotension (7% to 16%), chest pain (4% to 13%), tachycardia (12%), thrombosis-related events (7% to 11%)

Central nervous system: Fever (49% to 64%), fatigue (44% to 47%), headache (26% to 29%), dizziness (11% to 13%), pain (11% to 13%)

Dermatologic: Rash (20% to 24%), pruritus (16% to 18%)

Endocrine & metabolic: Hypoalbuminemia (14% to 17%)

Gastrointestinal: Nausea (47% to 60%), vomiting (13% to 35%), diarrhea (22%), anorexia (9% to 20%), taste disturbance (11% to 13%)

Hematologic: Lymphopenia (70%; 24% had lymphopenia at baseline)

Hepatic: ALT increased (84%), AST increased (84%)

Neuromuscular & skeletal: Rigors (42% to 47%), myalgia (18% to 20%), weakness (18%), back pain (16% to 18%), arthralgia (13% to 16%)

Respiratory: Cough (18% to 20%), upper respiratory infection (13%), dyspnea (11% to 13%)

Miscellaneous: Antibody formation (76% to 100%) neutralizing antibodies (45% to 97%), flu-like syndrome (≤85%), infusion reaction (71%; serious: 8%), infection (48%)

1% to 10%:

Cardiovascular: Arrhythmia (6%), hypertension (6%)

Hematologic: Leukopenia (grades 3/4: 3% to 6%), neutropenia (grades 3/4: 3%), thrombocytopenia (grades 3/4: 3%)

Local: Injection site reaction (8%)

Ocular: Visual changes (serious: 4%; includes loss of visual acuity)

Renal: Serum creatinine increased (3% to 10%), proteinuria/casts/hematuria (6%)

Pharmacodynamics/Kinetics

Half-Life Elimination Distribution: 2-5 minutes; Terminal: 70-80 minutes

Metabolism Hepatic via proteolytic degradation (animal studies)

Available Dosage Forms

Injection, solution:

ONTAK®: 150 mcg/mL (2 mL)

Dosing

Adult & Geriatric Note: Premedicate with an antihistamine and acetaminophen prior to each infusion; corticosteroid premedication (eg, dexamethasone) may reduce the incidence of hypersensitivity and edema (Foss, 2001). Withhold treatment if serum albumin <3 g/dL.

Persistent or recurrent cutaneous T-cell lymphoma: I.V.: 9 or 18 mcg/kg/day days 1 through 5 every 21 days for 8 cycles.

Adjustment for Toxicity

Serum albumin <3 g/dL: Withhold treatment

Severe infusion reaction: Permanently discontinue treatment

Administration

I.V. For I.V. use only. Infuse over 30-60 minutes. Should **not** be given as a rapid I.V. bolus. Discontinue or reduce infusion rate for infusion related reactions; discontinue for severe infusion reaction. Do not administer through an in-line filter. Premedicate with an antihistamine and acetaminophen; consider corticosteroid premedication.

Stability

Reconstitution Must be brought to room temperature (25°C or 77°F) before preparing the dose. Do **not** heat vials. Thaw in refrigerator for not more than 24 hours or at room temperature for 1-2 hours. Solution may be mixed by gentle swirling; avoid vigorous agitation. Dilute with NS to a concentration of ≥15 mcg/mL; the concentration must be ≥15 mcg/mL during all steps of preparation. Add drug to the empty sterile I.V. bag first, then add NS. Do not prepare with glass syringes or in glass containers.

Storage Store intact vials frozen at or below -10°C (14°F); do not refreeze after thawing. Solutions ≥15 mcg/mL in NS should be used within 6 hours.

Monitoring and Teaching Issues

Laboratory Monitoring Baseline CD25 expression (on malignant cells); serum albumin level (prior to each treatment), CBC, blood chemistry panel, renal and hepatic function tests (prior to initiation of therapy and weekly during therapy). Information on assay for malignant cell CD25 expression is available at 1-877-873-4724.

Physical Assessment Premedicate with antihistamine and acetaminophen prior to each infusion. Patient must be monitored closely for acute hypersensitivity reaction during and for 24-48 hours following infusion (resuscitation equipment should be immediately available during infusion). Discontinue permanently if serious infusion reaction occurs. Following infusion, patient should be monitored or taught to monitor for delayed vascular leak syndrome, gastrointestinal effects, fever, pain, or respiratory infection. Teach patient to report signs of infection.

Patient Education This medication can only be administered via intravenous infusion. During infusion, report immediately any chills; chest pain, respiratory difficulty, or tightness in throat; or redness, swelling, pain, or burning at infusion site. Maintain adequate hydration, unless instructed to restrict fluids. You may be more susceptible to infection. May cause nausea, vomiting, anorexia, flatulence, constipation, diarrhea, headache, back or muscle pain, dizziness, weakness, or confusion. Report unresolved GI effects; headache or back or muscle pain; skin dryness, rash, or sores; altered urinary patterns; flu syndrome or infection (eg, weakness, fatigue, white plaques or sores in mouth, vaginal discharge, chills, fever); CNS disturbances (insomnia, dizziness, agitation, confusion, depression); unusual bleeding or bruising; blood in urine or stool; or swelling of extremities.

Breast-Feeding Considerations The excretion of denileukin diftitox in breast milk is unknown, however, it is recommended that a breast-feeding woman who is treated with denileukin diftitox should discontinue nursing.

Pregnancy Considerations Animal reproduction studies have not been conducted. There are no adequate and well-controlled studies in pregnant women. Should be given to a pregnant woman only if clearly needed

Additional Information Oncology Comment: The National Comprehensive Cancer Network® (NCCN) Non-Hodgkin's Lymphoma Guidelines (v.2.2009) list denileukin diftitox as a second-line treatment option for systemic therapy of peripheral (cutaneous) T-cell lymphoma in patients who are not candidates for high dose therapy or autologous stem cell rescue. In mycosis fungoides (MF) and Sézary syndrome (SS), denileukin diftitox is a therapy option, either as monotherapy or in combination with bexarotene (Foss, 2005). Participation in a clinical trial is encouraged for this patient population.

Corticosteroids may be considered for prevention of hypersensitivity reaction. In a small study (Foss, 2001) reviewing denileukin diftitox and premedication with either prednisone 20 mg orally or dexamethasone 8 mg I.V. on day 1 followed by dexamethasone 8 mg I.V. on days 2-5, a reduction in adverse events was observed when compared to a previous (Olsen, 2001) phase III study. A statistically significant reduction in the incidence of edema was demonstrated. Improved response rates (compared to the phase III study) were noted, likely due to in increase in tolerability due to corticosteroid premedication. While some studies did not allow premedication with corticosteroids (Kuzel, 2007; Olsen, 2001) as part of the trial design, dexamethasone premedication has been utilized in other studies and case reports (Foss, 2005; Frankel, 2006; Gerena-Lewis, 2009; Talpur, 2002) with denileukin diftitox use for cutaneous T-cell lymphoma as well as other (unlabeled) uses.

Denosumab (den OH sue mab)

U.S. Brand Names Prolia™; Xgeva™

Index Terms AMG-162

Generic Availability (U.S.) No

Pharmacologic Category Monoclonal Antibody

Medication Guide Available Yes

Pregnancy Risk Factor C

Lactation Excretion unknown/not recommended

Use Treatment of osteoporosis in postmenopausal women at high risk for fracture; prevention of skeletal-related events (eg, fracture, spinal cord compression, bone pain requiring radiation therapy) in patients with bone metastases from solid tumors

Unlabeled/Investigational Use Prevention of bone loss due to androgen deprivation therapy in nonmetastatic prostate cancer; prevention of bone loss due to aromatase inhibitor therapy in breast cancer; treatment of bone destruction caused by rheumatoid arthritis

Mechanism of Action/Effect Denosumab is a monoclonal antibody which causes decreased bone resorption and increased bone mass.

Contraindications

Prolia™: Hypocalcemia

Xgeva™: There are no contraindications listed in the manufacturer's labeling.

Warnings/Precautions Denosumab may cause or exacerbate hypocalcemia. Monitor calcium levels; correct pre-existing hypocalcemia prior to therapy. Use caution in patients with a history of hypoparathyroidism, thyroid surgery, parathyroid surgery, malabsorption syndromes, excision of small intestine, severe renal impairment or other conditions which would predispose the patient to hypocalcemia; monitor closely during therapy. Ensure adequate calcium and vitamin D intake; supplement with calcium and vitamin D; magnesium supplementation may also be necessary. Incidence of infections may be increased, including serious skin infections, abdominal, urinary, ear, or periodontal infections. Endocarditis has also been reported following use. Patients should be advised to contact healthcare provider if signs or symptoms of severe infection or cellulitis develop. Use with caution in patients with impaired immune systems or using concomitant immunosuppressive therapy; may be at increased risk for serious infections. Evaluate the need for continued treatment with serious infection. Osteonecrosis of the jaw (ONJ) has been reported in patients receiving denosumab. Risk factors include invasive dental procedures (eg, tooth extraction, dental implants, boney surgery); a diagnosis of cancer, concomitant chemotherapy or corticosteroids, poor oral hygiene, ill-fitting dentures; and comorbid disorders (anemia, coagulopathy, infection, pre-existing dental disease). Patients should maintain good oral hygiene during treatment. A dental exam and preventative dentistry should be performed prior to therapy. The benefit/risk must be assessed by the treating physician and/or dentist/surgeon prior to any invasive dental procedure; avoid invasive procedures in patients with bone metastases receiving therapy for prevention of skeletal-related events. Patients developing ONJ while on denosumab therapy should receive care by a dentist or oral surgeon; extensive dental surgery to treat ONJ may exacerbate ONJ.

Postmenopausal osteoporosis: For use in women at high risk for fracture which is defined as a history of osteoporotic fracture or multiple risk factors for fracture. May also be used in women who failed or did not tolerate other therapies.

Bone metastases: Denosumab is not indicated for the prevention of skeletal-related events in patients with multiple myeloma. In trials of with multiple myeloma patients, denosumab was noninferior to zoledronic acid in delaying time to first skeletal-related event and mortality was increased in a subset of the denosumab-treated group.

Denosumab therapy results in significant suppression of bone turnover; the long term effects of treatment are not known but may contribute to adverse outcomes such as ONJ, atypical fractures, or delayed fracture healing; monitor. Use with caution in patients with renal impairment (Cl_{cr} <30 mL/minute) or patients on dialysis; risk of hypocalcemia is increased. Dose adjustment is not needed. Dermatitis, eczema, and rash (which are not necessarily specific to the injection site) have been reported. Consider discontinuing use if symptoms occur. Packaging may contain natural latex rubber. Safety and efficacy have not been established in children; use may impair bone growth in children with open growth plates or inhibit eruption of dentition.

Drug Interactions

Avoid Concomitant Use There are no known interactions where it is recommended to avoid concomitant use.

Decreased Effect There are no known significant interactions involving a decrease in effect.

Increased Effect/Toxicity

Denosumab may increase the levels/effects of: Immunosuppressants

Nutritional/Ethanol Interactions Ethanol: Avoid ethanol (may increase risk of osteoporosis).

Adverse Reactions A postmarketing safety program for Prolia™ is available to collect information on adverse events; more information is available at http://www.proliasafety.com. To report adverse events for either Prolia™ or Xgeva™, prescribers may also call Amgen at 800-772-6436 or FDA at 800-332-1088. **Note:** Adverse events and frequencies occurred in patients with osteoporosis unless otherwise noted as occurring in patients with cancer.

>10%:

- Central nervous system: Fatigue (cancer patients: 45%), headache (cancer patients: 13%)
- Dermatologic: Dermatitis (11%), eczema (11%), rash (3% to 11%)
- Endocrine & metabolic: Hypophosphatemia (cancer patients: 32%; grade 3: 15%), hypocalcemia (2%; cancer patients: 18%; grade 3: 3%)
- Gastrointestinal: Nausea (cancer patients: 31%), diarrhea (cancer patients: 20%)
- Neuromuscular & skeletal: Limb pain (12%), weakness (cancer patients: 45%; osteoporosis: 2%)
- Respiratory: Dyspnea (cancer patients: 21%), cough (cancer patients: 15%)

1% to 10%:

- Cardiovascular: Peripheral edema (5%), angina (3%)
- Endocrine & metabolic: Hypercholesterolemia (7%)
- Gastrointestinal: Flatulence (2%)
- Neuromuscular & skeletal: Sciatica (5%), bone pain (4%), myalgia (3%), osteonecrosis of the jaw ([ONJ] cancer patients: 2%)
- Respiratory: Upper respiratory tract infection (5%)
- Miscellaneous: New malignancies (5%), infections (nonfatal, serious; 4%)

Pharmacodynamics/Kinetics

Onset of Action Decreases markers of bone resorption by ~85% within 3 days; maximal reductions observed within 1 month

Duration of Action Markers of bone resorption return to baseline within 12 months of discontinuing therapy

Bioavailability SubQ: 62%

Time to Peak Serum: 10 days (range 3-21 days)

Half-Life Elimination ~25-28 days

Available Dosage Forms

Injection, solution [preservative free]:

Prolia™: 60 mg/mL (1 mL)

Xgeva™: 70 mg/mL (1.7 mL)

Dosing

Adult & Geriatric

Prevention of skeletal-related events in bone metastases from solid tumors (Xgeva™): SubQ: 120 mg every 4 weeks

Treatment of osteoporosis in postmenopausal females (Prolia™): SubQ: 60 mg as a single dose, once every 6 months

Prevention of androgen-induced bone loss in nonmetastatic prostate cancer (unlabeled use): SubQ: 60 mg as a single dose, once every 6 months (Smith, 2009)

Prevention of aromatase inhibitor-induced bone loss in breast cancer (unlabeled use): SubQ: 60 mg as a single dose, once every 6 months for 4 doses (Ellis, 2008)

Renal Impairment Dose adjustment is not needed; monitor patients with severe impairment (Cl_{cr} <30 mL/minute or on dialysis) due to increased risk of hypocalcemia.

Administration

Other SubQ: Prior to administration, bring to room temperature in original container (allow to stand ~15-30 minutes); do not warm by any other method. Solution may contain trace amounts of translucent to white protein particles; do not use if cloudy, discolored (normal solution should be clear and colorless to pale yellow), or contains excessive particles or foreign matter. Avoid vigorous shaking. Administer via SubQ injection in the upper arm, upper thigh, or abdomen.

Osteoporosis: If a dose is missed, administer as soon as possible, then continue dosing every 6 months from the date of the last injection.

Stability

Storage Prior to use, store in original carton under refrigeration, 2°C to 8°C (36°F to 46°F). Do not freeze. Prior to use, bring to room temperature of 25°C (77°F) in original container (usually takes 15-30 minutes). Use within 14 days once at room temperature. Protect from direct heat and light; do not expose to temperatures >25°C (77°F).

Monitoring and Teaching Issues

Laboratory Monitoring Serum calcium, phosphorus and magnesium, especially in patients predisposed to hypocalcemia (severe renal impairment, malabsorption syndromes, hypoparathyroidism).

Osteoporosis: Bone mineral density as measured by central dual-energy x-ray absorptiometry (DXA) of the hip or spine (prior to initiation of therapy and at least every 2 years; serum calcium and 25(OH)D; may consider monitoring biochemical markers of bone turnover (National Osteoporosis Foundation Guidelines, 2010)

Physical Assessment Use with caution if impaired immune system. Correct pre-existing hypocalcemia prior to beginning therapy and monitor closely for hypocalcemia, especially in patients with abdominal or parathyroid surgery, renal impairment, malabsorption syndrome, or hypoparathyroidism. For patients at risk for osteonecrosis of the jaw, including those who have received chemotherapy or corticosteroids or who have had poor oral care or oral surgery, dental exams and preventive dentistry are necessary before beginning treatment. Teach patient importance of adequate dietary calcium and vitamin D.

Patient Education This medication can only be administered by injection; report immediately any irritation or pain at injection site. Your diet should include adequate calcium and vitamin D; consult prescriber about appropriate dietary intake. Advise prescriber of any dental problems you may have; you may be instructed to have dental evaluation prior to therapy. You may experience increased fatigue, skin irritation, or decreased calcium or phosphate levels. Report immediately any signs or symptoms of unusual or persistent infection (fever or chills, cough, sore throat, abdominal pain, pain or difficulty when passing urine, or skin rash.

Dietary Considerations Ensure adequate calcium and vitamin D intake. Calcium 1000 mg/day and vitamin D ≥400 units/day is recommended in product labeling (Prolia™).

Women and men >50 years of age should consume elemental calcium 1200-1500 mg/day and vitamin D 800-1000 int. units/day (National Osteoporosis Foundation Guidelines, 2010).

Breast-Feeding Considerations According to the manufacturer, the decision to continue or discontinue breast-feeding during therapy should take into account the risk of exposure to the infant and the benefits of treatment to the mother. In animal studies, mammary gland development was impaired following exposure to denosumab during pregnancy, resulting in impaired lactation postpartum.

Pregnancy Considerations Adverse fetal events were observed in studies of genetically engineered mice developed to be missing RANKL (the target of denosumab). In studies of monkeys where denosumab was administered during the 1st trimester of pregnancy only, adverse fetal events were not observed. However, fetal exposure to monoclonal antibodies is expected to increase as pregnancy progresses. If a pregnant woman is inadvertently exposed, patients or their prescribers may contact the Amgen Pregnancy Surveillance Program (800-772-6436).

Related Information

Osteoporosis Management *on page 2067*

◆ **Deodorized Tincture of Opium (error-prone synonym)** *see* Opium Tincture *on page 1363*

◆ **Deoxyazacytidine** *see* Decitabine *on page 476*

◆ **Depacon®** *see* Valproic Acid *on page 1832*

◆ **Depakene®** *see* Valproic Acid *on page 1832*

◆ **Depakote®** *see* Divalproex *on page 557*

◆ **Depakote® ER** *see* Divalproex *on page 557*

◆ **Depakote® Sprinkle** *see* Divalproex *on page 557*

◆ **DepoCyt®** *see* Cytarabine (Liposomal) *on page 449*

◆ **Depo®-Estradiol** *see* Estradiol (Systemic) *on page 670*

◆ **Depo-Medrol®** *see* MethylPREDNISolone *on page 1208*

◆ **Depo-Provera®** *see* MedroxyPROGESTERone *on page 1154*

◆ **Depo-Provera® Contraceptive** *see* MedroxyPROGESTERone *on page 1154*

◆ **depo-subQ provera 104®** *see* MedroxyPROGESTERone *on page 1154*

◆ **Depo®-Testosterone** *see* Testosterone *on page 1739*

◆ **Deprenyl** *see* Selegiline *on page 1630*

◆ **DermaFungal [OTC]** *see* Miconazole (Topical) *on page 1224*

◆ **Dermagran® AF [OTC]** *see* Miconazole (Topical) *on page 1224*

◆ **Dermamycin® [OTC]** *see* DiphenhydrAMINE (Topical) *on page 546*

◆ **Dermarest® Eczema Medicated [OTC]** *see* Hydrocortisone (Topical) *on page 920*

◆ **Derma-Smoothe/FS®** *see* Fluocinolone (Topical) *on page 785*

◆ **DermOtic®** *see* Fluocinolone (Otic) *on page 785*

◆ **Desferal®** *see* Deferoxamine *on page 478*

◆ **Desferrioxamine** *see* Deferoxamine *on page 478*

◆ **Desiccated Thyroid** *see* Thyroid, Desiccated *on page 1757*

Desipramine (des IP ra meen)

U.S. Brand Names Norpramin®

Index Terms Desipramine Hydrochloride; Desmethylimipramine Hydrochloride

Generic Availability (U.S.) Yes

Pharmacologic Category Antidepressant, Tricyclic (Secondary Amine)

Medication Safety Issues

Sound-alike/look-alike issues:

Desipramine may be confused with clomiPRAMINE, dalfampridine, deserpidine, diphenhydrAMINE, disopyramide, imipramine, nortriptyline

Norpramin® may be confused with clomiPRAMINE, imipramine, Normodyne®, Norpace®, nortriptyline, Tenormin®

International issues:

Norpramin: Brand name for desipramine [U.S., Canada], but also the brand name for enalapril/hydrochlorothiazide [Portugal]; omeprazole [Spain]

Medication Guide Available Yes

Lactation Enters breast milk (AAP rates "of concern"; AAP 2001 update pending)

Use Treatment of depression

Unlabeled/Investigational Use Analgesic adjunct in chronic pain; peripheral neuropathies; substance-related disorders (eg, cocaine withdrawal); attention-deficit/hyperactivity disorder (ADHD); depression in children ≤12 years of age

Available Dosage Forms

Tablet, oral: 10 mg, 25 mg, 50 mg, 75 mg, 100 mg, 150 mg

Norpramin®: 10 mg, 25 mg, 50 mg, 75 mg, 100 mg, 150 mg

Dosing

Adult

Depression: Oral: Initial: 75 mg/day in divided doses; increase gradually to 150-200 mg/day in divided or single dose; maximum: 300 mg/day

Cocaine withdrawal (unlabeled use): 50-200 mg/day in divided or single dose

Neuropathic pain (unlabeled use): Oral: Initial: 10-25 mg/day; increase dose every 3 days as necessary until the desired effect is obtained; usual effective dose: 50-150 mg/day (maximum dose: 150 mg/day)

Geriatric Oral: Initial: 10-25 mg/day; increase by 10-25 mg every 3 days for inpatients and every week for outpatients if tolerated; usual maintenance dose: 75-100 mg/day, but doses up to 150 mg/day may be necessary.

Pediatric Depression: Oral:

Children 6-12 years (unlabeled use): 10-30 mg/day or 1-3 mg/kg/day in divided doses; do not exceed 5 mg/kg/day

Adolescents: Initial: 25-50 mg/day; gradually increase to 100 mg/day in single or divided doses; maximum: 150 mg/day

Renal Impairment Hemodialysis/peritoneal dialysis effects: Supplemental dose is not necessary.

Monitoring and Teaching Issues

Physical Assessment Monitor CNS status. Assess cardiac and seizure history prior to initiating therapy. Assess for suicidal tendencies before beginning therapy, during initiation of therapy, or following an increase or decrease of dosage. Caution patients with diabetes to monitor glucose levels closely; may increase or decrease serum glucose levels. Taper dose slowly when discontinuing.

Patient Education It may take 2-3 weeks to achieve desired results. Avoid alcohol. Maintain adequate hydration, unless instructed to restrict fluid intake. May cause drowsiness, lightheadedness, impaired coordination, dizziness, blurred vision, loss of appetite or disturbed taste, constipation, urinary retention, postural hypotension, altered sexual drive or ability (reversible), or photosensitivity. Report chest pain, palpitations, or rapid heartbeat; persistent adverse CNS effects (eg, suicide ideation, nervousness, restlessness, insomnia, anxiety, excitation, headache, agitation, impaired coordination, changes in cognition); muscle cramping, weakness, tremors, or rigidity; seizures; blurred vision or eye pain; breast enlargement or swelling; yellowing of skin or eyes; or worsening of condition.

Related Information

Antidepressant Agents *on page* 1982

Peak and Trough Guidelines *on page* 1958

Pharmacotherapy of Urinary Incontinence *on page* 2071

◆ **Desipramine Hydrochloride** *see* Desipramine *on page* 489

Desirudin (des i ROO din)

U.S. Brand Names Iprivask®

Index Terms CGP-39393; Desulfato-Hirudin; Desulfatohirudin; Desulphatohirudin; r-Hirudin; Recombinant Desulfatohirudin; Recombinant Hirudin

Generic Availability (U.S.) No

Pharmacologic Category Anticoagulant, Thrombin Inhibitor

Medication Safety Issues

High alert medication: The Institute for Safe Medication Practices (ISMP) includes this medication among its list of drugs which have a heightened risk of causing significant patient harm when used in error.

Pregnancy Risk Factor C

Lactation Excretion in breast milk unknown/use caution

Use Prophylaxis of deep vein thrombosis (DVT) in patients undergoing surgery for hip replacement

Mechanism of Action/Effect Desirudin is a direct, highly selective thrombin inhibitor. Reversibly binds to the active thrombin site of free and clot-associated thrombin. Inhibits fibrin formation, activation of coagulation factors V, VII, and XIII, and thrombin-induced platelet aggregation resulting in a dose-dependent prolongation of the activated partial thromboplastin time (aPTT).

Contraindications Hypersensitivity to natural or recombinant hirudins; active bleeding and/or irreversible coagulation disorders

Warnings/Precautions [U.S. Boxed Warning]: Patients with recent or anticipated neuraxial anesthesia (epidural or spinal anesthesia) are at risk of epidural or spinal hematoma and subsequent paralysis. Consider risk versus benefit prior to neuraxial anesthesia; risk is increased by concomitant agents which may alter hemostasis, as well as traumatic or repeated epidural or spinal puncture. Patient should be observed closely for bleeding and signs and symptoms of neurological impairment if therapy is administered during or immediately following diagnostic lumbar puncture, epidural anesthesia, or spinal anesthesia.

Allergic and hypersensitivity reactions, including anaphylaxis and fatal anaphylactoid reactions have been reported with other hirudin derivatives. Exercise caution when re-exposing patients (anaphylaxis has been reported). Monitor patient closely for signs or symptoms of bleeding. Certain patients are at increased risk of bleeding. Risk factors include bacterial endocarditis; congenital or acquired bleeding disorders; active ulcerative or angiodysplastic GI diseases; severe uncontrolled hypertension; history of hemorrhagic stroke; use shortly after brain, spinal, or ophthalmology surgery; patients treated concomitantly with platelet inhibitors; recent GI bleeding; thrombocytopenia or platelet defects; renal impairment; hepatic impairment; hypertensive or diabetic retinopathy; or in patients undergoing invasive procedures. Do not administer with other agents that increase the risk of hemorrhage unless coadministration cannot be avoided. Discontinue if bleeding occurs. Contraindicated with active bleeding and/or irreversible coagulation disorders.

Do **not** administer intramuscularly (I.M.). Do not use interchangeably (unit-for-unit) with other hirudins. Use with caution in patients with moderate-to-severe renal dysfunction (Cl_{cr} <60 mL/minute/1.73 m^2); dosage reduction is necessary; monitor aPTT and renal function daily. The American College of Chest Physicians recommends against the use of desirudin in patients with Cl_{cr} <30 mL/minute (Hirsh, 2008). Use with caution in the elderly; elimination half-life prolonged in patients >75 years of age.

Drug Interactions

Avoid Concomitant Use There are no known interactions where it is recommended to avoid concomitant use.

Decreased Effect There are no known significant interactions involving a decrease in effect.

Increased Effect/Toxicity

Desirudin may increase the levels/effects of: Anticoagulants; Collagenase (Systemic); Ibritumomab; Tositumomab and Iodine I 131 Tositumomab

The levels/effects of Desirudin may be increased by: Antiplatelet Agents; Dasatinib; Herbs (Anticoagulant/Antiplatelet Properties); Nonsteroidal Anti-Inflammatory Agents; Pentosan Polysulfate Sodium; Prostacyclin Analogues; Salicylates; Thrombolytic Agents

Nutritional/Ethanol Interactions Herb/Nutraceutical: Avoid alfalfa, anise, bilberry, bladderwrack, bromelain, cat's claw, celery, coleus, cordyceps, dong quai, evening primrose oil, fenugreek, feverfew, garlic, ginger, ginkgo biloba, ginseng (American/Panax/Siberian), grapeseed, green tea, guggul, horse chestnut seed, horseradish, licorice, prickly ash, red clover, reishi, sweet clover, turmeric, white willow (all possess anticoagulant or antiplatelet activity and as such, may enhance the anticoagulant effects of desirudin).

Adverse Reactions As with all anticoagulants, bleeding is the major adverse effect. Hemorrhage may occur at any site.

2% to 10%:

Gastrointestinal: Nausea (2%)

Hematologic: Hematoma (6%), hemorrhage (major, <1% to 3%; may include cases of intracranial, retroperitoneal, intraocular, intraspinal, or prosthetic joint hemorrhage), anemia (3%)

Local: Injection site mass (4%), deep thrombophlebitis (2%)

Miscellaneous: Wound secretion (4%)

Pharmacodynamics/Kinetics

Absorption Subcutaneous: Complete

Time to Peak Plasma: 1-3 hours

Half-Life Elimination ~2 hours; Prolonged with renal impairment (Cl_{cr} <31 mL/minute/1.73 m^2: Up to 12 hours)

Excretion Urine (40% to 50% as unchanged drug)

Available Dosage Forms

Injection, powder for reconstitution [preservative free]:

Iprivask®: 15 mg

Dosing

Adult & Geriatric DVT prophylaxis: SubQ: 15 mg every 12 hours; initial dose may be given up to 5-15 minutes prior to surgery (after induction of regional anesthesia, if used); has been administered for up to 12 days (average: 9-12 days) in clinical trials

Renal Impairment

Moderate renal impairment (Cl_{cr} ≥31-60 mL/minute/1.73 m^2): 5 mg every 12 hours

Severe renal impairment (Cl_{cr} <31 mL/minute/1.73 m^2): 1.7 mg every 12 hours; **Note:** The American College of Chest Physicians recommends against the use of desirudin in patients with Cl_{cr} <30 mL/minute (Hirsh, 2008).

Administration

I.M. Do **not** administer I.M.

Other For SubQ administration only. Administration should be alternated between the left and right anterolateral and left and right posterolateral thigh or abdominal wall. Insert needle into a skin fold held between the thumb and forefinger; the skin fold should be held throughout the injection. Do not rub injection site. Do not mix with other injections or infusions. Administer according to recommended regimen.

Stability

Reconstitution Attach enclosed vial adapter to vial containing desirudin. Remove syringe cap and attach provided syringe containing diluent to adapter on vial. Slowly push plunger down to transfer entire contents of syringe into vial. Do not remove syringe from vial adapter. Gently swirl solution; round tablet in vial will dissolve within 10 seconds. Resultant solution concentration is 31.5 mg/mL (15.75 mg/0.5 mL provides a 15 mg dose). Turn vial upside down; withdraw appropriate dose amount back into syringe. Remove syringe from vial. Attach enclosed Eclipse™ needle (or any needle appropriate for subcutaneous administration); pull pink lever down and uncap needle; ready for injection. After injection, flip up pink lever to cover needle until it snaps into place; dispose of syringe appropriately.

Storage Store at 25°C (77°F); excursions permitted to 15°C to 30°C (59°F to 86°F). Protect from light. Following reconstitution, solution may be stored at room temperature for up to 24 hours. Discard unused solution after 24 hours.

Monitoring and Teaching Issues

Laboratory Monitoring Monitor aPTT, serum creatinine/creatinine clearance, CBC; stool occult blood tests. Serum creatinine and aPTT should be monitored daily in patients with moderate-to-severe renal insufficiency. Interrupt therapy if aPTT exceeds 2 times normal; resume at a reduced dose when aPTT is <2 times control.

Physical Assessment Evaluate any previous exposure to other hirudin derivatives. Use caution in presence of renal impairment and increased risk of bleeding. Patient must be monitored closely for anaphylactic reaction; treatment for anaphylactic reactions should be available. Bleeding precautions should be observed and patient monitored for signs or symptoms of bleeding (discontinue if bleeding occurs). Monitor for hypersensitivity reaction and bleeding regularly during therapy. Teach patient bleeding precautions.

Patient Education This drug can only be administered by SubQ injection. Report immediately any pain, swelling, burning, or bleeding at injection site; chest pain or difficulty breathing; or swelling of mouth or throat. You may have a tendency to bleed easily; brush teeth with soft brush, floss with waxed floss, use electric razor, avoid scissors or anything sharp, and use caution to prevent falls or injury.

Geriatric Considerations Serious adverse drug events are more common in persons ≥75 years of age. Dosage adjustment may be necessary based on kidney function.

Pregnancy Considerations Teratogenic effects were observed in some animal reproductive studies. There are no adequate and well-controlled studies in pregnant women. Desirudin should be used in pregnant women only if clinical benefit outweighs risks of therapy.

Desloratadine (des lor AT a deen)

U.S. Brand Names Clarinex®

Generic Availability (U.S.) No

Pharmacologic Category Histamine H_1 Antagonist; Histamine H_1 Antagonist, Second Generation; Piperidine Derivative

Medication Safety Issues

Sound-alike/look-alike issues:

Clarinex® may be confused with Celebrex®

Pregnancy Risk Factor C

Lactation Enters breast milk/not recommended

Use Relief of nasal and non-nasal symptoms of seasonal allergic rhinitis (SAR) and perennial allergic rhinitis (PAR); treatment of chronic idiopathic urticaria (CIU)

Mechanism of Action/Effect Desloratadine is a long-acting antihistamine with selective H_1 receptor antagonistic activity.

Contraindications Hypersensitivity to desloratadine, loratadine, or any component of the formulation

Warnings/Precautions Dose should be adjusted in patients with liver or renal impairment. Use with caution in patients known to be slow metabolizers of desloratadine (incidence of side effects may be increased). Some products may contain phenylalanine. Safety and efficacy have not been established for children <6 months of age.

Drug Interactions

Metabolism/Transport Effects Substrate of P-glycoprotein

Avoid Concomitant Use There are no known interactions where it is recommended to avoid concomitant use.

Decreased Effect

Desloratadine may decrease the levels/effects of: Acetylcholinesterase Inhibitors (Central); Benzylpenicilloyl Polylysine; Betahistine

The levels/effects of Desloratadine may be decreased by: Acetylcholinesterase Inhibitors (Central); Amphetamines; P-Glycoprotein Inducers

Increased Effect/Toxicity

Desloratadine may increase the levels/effects of: Alcohol (Ethyl); Anticholinergics; CNS Depressants

The levels/effects of Desloratadine may be increased by: Droperidol; P-Glycoprotein Inhibitors; Pramlintide

Nutritional/Ethanol Interactions

Ethanol: Avoid ethanol (may increase risk of sedation).

Food: Does not affect bioavailability.

Adverse Reactions

>10%: Central nervous system: Headache (14%)

1% to 10%:

Central nervous system: Fatigue (2% to 5%), somnolence (2%), dizziness (4%)
Endocrine & metabolic: Dysmenorrhea (2%)
Gastrointestinal: Xerostomia (3%), nausea (5%), dyspepsia (3%)
Neuromuscular & skeletal: Myalgia (2% to 3%)
Respiratory: Pharyngitis (3% to 4%)

Pharmacodynamics/Kinetics

Time to Peak 3 hours

Protein Binding Desloratadine: 82% to 87%; 3-hydroxydesloratadine: 85% to 89%

Half-Life Elimination 27 hours

Metabolism Hepatic to active metabolite, 3-hydroxydesloratadine (specific enzymes not identified); undergoes glucuronidation. Decreased in slow metabolizers of desloratadine. Not expected to affect or be affected by medications metabolized by CYP with normal doses.

Excretion Urine and feces (as metabolites)

Available Dosage Forms

Syrup, oral:

Clarinex®: 0.5 mg/mL (480 mL)

Tablet, oral:

Clarinex®: 5 mg

Tablet, orally disintegrating, oral:

Clarinex®: 2.5 mg, 5 mg

Dosing

Adult & Geriatric Seasonal or perennial allergic rhinitis, chronic idiopathic urticaria: Oral: 5 mg once daily

Pediatric Seasonal or perennial allergic rhinitis, chronic idiopathic urticaria: Oral:

Children:

6-11 months: 1 mg once daily

12 months to 5 years: 1.25 mg once daily

6-11 years: 2.5 mg once daily

Children ≥12 years: Refer to adult dosing.

Renal Impairment

Children: Not established

Adults: 5 mg every other day

Hepatic Impairment 5 mg every other day

Administration

Oral May be taken with or without food.

RediTabs® should be placed on the tongue; tablet will disintegrate immediately. May be taken with or without water.

Syrup: A commercially-available measuring dropper or syringe calibrated to deliver 2 mL or 2.5 mL should be used to administer age-appropriate doses in children.

Stability

Storage Syrup, tablet, orally-disintegrating tablet: Store at 25°C (77°F); excursions permitted between 15°C to 30°C (59°F to 86°F). Protect from moisture and excessive heat (85°F). Use orally-disintegrating tablet immediately after opening blister package. Syrup should be protected from light.

Monitoring and Teaching Issues

Patient Education Avoid use of alcohol. You may experience headache, drowsiness, dizziness, dry mouth, dry throat, or nausea. Report rapid heartbeat, shortness of breath, or skin rash.

Dietary Considerations May be taken with or without food. Some products may contain phenylalanine.

Pregnancy Considerations There are no adequate and well-controlled studies in pregnant women. Use during pregnancy only if clearly needed.

◆ **Desmethylimipramine Hydrochloride** *see* Desipramine *on page 489*

Desmopressin (des moe PRES in)

U.S. Brand Names DDAVP®; Stimate®

Index Terms 1-Deamino-8-D-Arginine Vasopressin; Desmopressin Acetate

Generic Availability (U.S.) Yes

Pharmacologic Category Antihemophilic Agent; Hemostatic Agent; Vasopressin Analog, Synthetic

Pregnancy Risk Factor B

Lactation Excretion in breast milk unknown/use caution

Use

Injection: Treatment of diabetes insipidus; maintenance of hemostasis and control of bleeding in hemophilia A with factor VIII coagulant activity levels >5% and mild-to-moderate classic von Willebrand's disease (type 1) with factor VIII coagulant activity levels >5%

Nasal solutions (DDAVP® Nasal Spray and DDAVP® Rhinal Tube): Treatment of central diabetes insipidus

Nasal spray (Stimate®): Maintenance of hemostasis and control of bleeding in hemophilia A with factor VIII coagulant activity levels >5% and mild-to-moderate classic von Willebrand's disease (type 1) with factor VIII coagulant activity levels >5%

Tablet: Treatment of central diabetes insipidus, temporary polyuria and polydipsia following pituitary surgery or head trauma, primary nocturnal enuresis

Unlabeled/Investigational Use Uremic bleeding associated with acute or chronic renal failure; prevention of surgical bleeding in patients with uremia

Mechanism of Action/Effect Enhances reabsorption of water in the kidneys by increasing permeability of the collecting ducts; raises plasma levels of von Willebrand factor and factor VIII

Contraindications Hypersensitivity to desmopressin or any component of the formulation; hyponatremia or a history of hyponatremia; moderate-to-severe renal impairment (Cl_{cr}<50 mL/minute)

Canadian labeling: Additional contraindications (not in U.S. labeling): Type 2B or platelet-type (pseudo) von Willebrand's disease (injection, intranasal, oral, sublingual); known hyponatremia, habitual or psychogenic polydipsia, cardiac insufficiency or other conditions requiring diuretic therapy (intranasal, sublingual); nephrosis, severe hepatic dysfunction (sublingual); primary nocturnal enuresis (intranasal)

Warnings/Precautions Allergic reactions and anaphylaxis have been reported rarely with both the I.V. and intranasal formulations. Fluid intake should be adjusted downward in the elderly and very young patients to decrease the possibility of water intoxication and hyponatremia. Use may rarely lead to extreme decreases in plasma osmolality, resulting in seizures, coma, and death. Use caution with cystic fibrosis, heart failure, renal dysfunction, polydipsia (habitual or psychogenic [contraindicated in Canadian labeling]), or other conditions associated with fluid and electrolyte imbalance due to potential hyponatremia. Use caution with coronary artery insufficiency or hypertensive cardiovascular disease; may increase or decrease blood pressure leading to changes in heart rate. Consider switching from nasal to intravenous solution if changes in the nasal mucosa (scarring, edema) occur leading to unreliable absorption. Use caution in patients predisposed to thrombus formation; thrombotic events (acute cerebrovascular thrombosis, acute myocardial infarction) have occurred (rare).

Desmopressin (intranasal and I.V.), when used for hemostasis in hemophilia, is not for use in hemophilia B, type 2B von Willebrand disease, severe classic von Willebrand disease (type 1), or in patients with factor VIII antibodies. In general, desmopressin is also not recommended for use in patients with ≤5% factor VIII activity level, although it may be considered in selected patients with activity levels between 2% and 5%.

Consider switching from nasal to intravenous administration if changes in the nasal mucosa (scarring, edema) occur leading to unreliable absorption. Consider alternative rout of administration (I.V. or intranasal) with inadequate therapeutic response at maximum recommended oral doses. Therapy should be interrupted if patient experiences an acute illness (eg, fever, recurrent vomiting or diarrhea), vigorous exercise, or any condition associated with an increase in water consumption. Some patients may demonstrate a change in response after long-term therapy (>6 months) characterized as decreased response or a shorter duration of response.

Drug Interactions

Avoid Concomitant Use There are no known interactions where it is recommended to avoid concomitant use.

Decreased Effect

The levels/effects of Desmopressin may be decreased by: Demeclocycline; Lithium

Increased Effect/Toxicity

Desmopressin may increase the levels/effects of: Lithium

The levels/effects of Desmopressin may be increased by: Analgesics (Opioid); CarBAMazepine; ChlorproMAZINE; LamoTRIgine; Nonsteroidal Anti-Inflammatory Agents; Selective Serotonin Reuptake Inhibitors; Tricyclic Antidepressants

Nutritional/Ethanol Interactions Ethanol: Avoid ethanol (may decrease antidiuretic effect).

Adverse Reactions Frequency may not be defined (may be dose or route related).

Cardiovascular: Blood pressure increased/decreased (I.V.), facial flushing

Central nervous system: Headache (2% to 5%), dizziness (intranasal; ≤3%), chills (intranasal; 2%)

Dermatologic: Rash

Endocrine & metabolic: Hyponatremia, water intoxication

Gastrointestinal: Abdominal pain (intranasal; 2%), gastrointestinal disorder (intranasal; ≤2%), nausea (intranasal; ≤2%), abdominal cramps, sore throat

Hepatic: Transient increases in liver transaminases (associated primarily with tablets)

Local: Injection: Burning pain, erythema, and swelling at the injection site

Neuromuscular & Skeletal: Weakness (intranasal; ≤2%)

Ocular: Conjunctivitis (intranasal; ≤2%), eye edema (intranasal; ≤2%), lacrimation disorder (intranasal; ≤2%)

Respiratory: Rhinitis (intranasal; 3% to 8%), epistaxis (intranasal; ≤3%), nostril pain (intranasal; ≤2%), cough, nasal congestion, upper respiratory infection

Pharmacodynamics/Kinetics

Onset of Action

Intranasal: Antidiuretic: 15-30 minutes; Increased factor VIII and von Willebrand factor (vWF) activity (dose related): 30 minutes

Peak effect: Antidiuretic: 1 hour; Increased factor VIII and vWF activity: 1.5 hours

I.V. infusion: Increased factor VIII and vWF activity: 30 minutes (dose related)

Peak effect: 1.5-2 hours

Oral tablet: Antidiuretic: ~1 hour

Peak effect: 4-7 hours

Duration of Action Intranasal, I.V. infusion, Oral tablet: ~6-14 hours

Absorption Sublingual: Rapid

Bioavailability

Intranasal: ~3.5%

Oral tablet: 5% compared to intranasal, 0.16% compared to I.V.

Half-Life Elimination Intranasal: ~3.5 hours; I.V. infusion: 3 hours; Oral tablet: 2-3 hours

Renal impairment: ≤9 hours

Metabolism Unknown

Excretion Urine

Available Dosage Forms

Injection, solution: 4 mcg/mL (1 mL, 10 mL)

DDAVP®: 4 mcg/mL (1 mL, 10 mL)

Solution, intranasal: 0.1 mg/mL (2.5 mL, 5 mL)

DDAVP®: 0.1 mg/mL (2.5 mL, 5 mL)

Stimate®: 1.5 mg/mL (2.5 mL)

Tablet, oral: 0.1 mg, 0.2 mg

DDAVP®: 0.1 mg, 0.2 mg

Dosing

Adult & Geriatric

Diabetes insipidus:

I.V., SubQ: U.S. labeling: 2-4 mcg/day (0.5-1 mL) in 2 divided doses or 1/10 of the maintenance intranasal dose. Fluid restriction should be observed.

I.M., I.V., SubQ: Canadian labeling (not in U.S. labeling): 1-4 mcg (0.25-1 mL) once daily or 1/10 of the maintenance intranasal dose. Fluid restriction should be observed.

Intranasal (100 mcg/mL nasal solution): 10-40 mcg/day (0.1-0.4 mL) divided 1-3 times/day; adjust morning and evening doses separately for an adequate diurnal rhythm of water turnover. **Note:** The nasal spray pump can only deliver doses of 10 mcg (0.1 mL) or multiples of 10 mcg (0.1 mL); if doses other than this are needed, the rhinal tube delivery system is preferred. Fluid restriction should be observed.

Oral:

U.S. labeling: Initial: 0.05 mg twice daily; total daily dose should be increased or decreased as needed to obtain adequate antidiuresis (range: 0.1-1.2 mg divided 2-3 times/day). Fluid restriction should be observed.

Canadian labeling (not in U.S. labeling): Initial: 0.1 mg 3 times/day; total daily dose should be increased or decreased as needed to obtain adequate antidiuresis (range: 0.3-1.2 mg divided 3 times/day). Fluid restriction should be observed.

Sublingual formulation: Canadian labeling (not in U.S. labeling): Initial: 60 mcg 3 times/day; total daily dose should be increased or decreased as needed to obtain adequate antidiuresis. Usual maintenance: 60-120 mcg 3 times/day (range: 120-720 mcg divided 2-3 times/day). Fluid restriction should be observed.

Nocturnal enuresis: *Oral:* 0.2 mg at bedtime; dose may be titrated up to 0.6 mg to achieve desired response.

Hemophilia A and mild-to-moderate von Willebrand disease (type 1):

I.V.: 0.3 mcg/kg by slow infusion; if used preoperatively, administer 30 minutes before procedure

Canadian labeling (not in U.S. labeling): Maximum I.V. dose: 20 mcg

Intranasal (using high concentration spray [1.5 mg/mL]): <50 kg: 150 mcg (1 spray); >50 kg: 300 mcg (1 spray each nostril); repeat use is determined by the patient's clinical condition and laboratory work. If using preoperatively, administer 2 hours before surgery.

Uremic bleeding associated with acute or chronic renal failure (unlabeled use) (Watson, 1984): I.V.: 0.4 mcg/kg over 10 minutes

Prevention of surgical bleeding in patients with uremia (unlabeled use) (Mannucci, 1983): I.V.: 0.3 mcg/kg over 30 minutes

Pediatric

Diabetes insipidus:

I.M., I.V., SubQ: Canadian labeling (not in U.S. labeling): ≥3 months: 0.4 mcg (0.1 mL) once daily or 1/10 of the maintenance intranasal dose. Fluid restriction should be observed.

I.V., SubQ:

Children <12 years: No definitive dosing available. Adult dosing should **not** be used in this age group; adverse events such as hyponatremia-induced seizures may occur. Dose should be reduced. Some have suggested an initial dosage range of 0.1-1 mcg in 1 or 2 divided doses (Cheetham, 2002). Initiate at low dose and increase as necessary. Closely monitor serum sodium levels and urine output; fluid restriction is recommended.

Children ≥12 years: Refer to adult dosing.

Intranasal (using 100 mcg/mL nasal solution):

3 months to 12 years: Initial: 5 mcg/day (0.05 mL/day) divided 1-2 times/day; range: 5-30 mcg/day (0.05-0.3 mL/day) divided 1-2 times/day; adjust morning and evening doses separately for an adequate diurnal rhythm of water turnover. **Note:** The nasal spray pump can only deliver doses of 10 mcg (0.1 mL) or multiples of 10 mcg (0.1 mL); if doses other than this are needed, the rhinal tube delivery system is preferred. Fluid restriction should be observed.

Children ≥12 years: Refer to adult dosing.

Oral:

U.S. labeling: ≥4 years: Initial: 0.05 mg twice daily; total daily dose should be increased or decreased as needed to obtain adequate antidiuresis (range: 0.1-1.2 mg divided 2-3 times/day). Fluid restriction should be observed.

Canadian labeling (not in U.S. labeling): ≥5 years: Initial: 0.1 mg 3 times/day; total daily dose should be increased or decreased as needed to obtain adequate antidiuresis (range: 0.3-1.2 mg divided 3 times/day). Divide daily doses so that the evening dose is 2 times higher than the morning or afternoon dose to ensure adequate antidiuresis during the night. Fluid restriction should be observed.

Sublingual formulation: Canadian labeling (not in U.S. labeling): ≥3 months: Initial: 60 mcg 3 times/day; total daily dose should be increased or decreased as needed to obtain adequate antidiuresis. Usual maintenance: 60-120 mcg 3 times/day (range: 120-720 mcg divided 2-3 times/day); divide daily doses so that the evening dose is 2 times higher than the morning or afternoon dose to ensure adequate antidiuresis during the night. Fluid restriction should be observed.

Hemophilia A and von Willebrand disease (type 1):

I.V.: ≥3 months: 0.3 mcg/kg by slow infusion; may repeat dose if needed; if used preoperatively, administer 30 minutes before procedure

Canadian labeling (not in U.S. labeling): Maximum I.V. dose: 20 mcg

Note: Adverse events such as hyponatremia-induced seizures have been reported especially in young children using this dosing regimen (Das, 2005; Molnar, 2005; Smith, 1989; Thumfart, 2005; Weinstein, 1989). Fluid restriction and careful monitoring of serum sodium levels and urine output are necessary.

Intranasal (using high concentration spray [1.5 mg/mL]): ≥11 months: Refer to adult dosing.

Nocturnal enuresis:

Oral:

Children ≥6 years: 0.2 mg at bedtime. Dose may be titrated up to 0.6 mg to achieve desired response. Fluid intake should be limited 1 hour prior to dose until the next morning, or at least 8 hours after administration. **Note:** In the Canadian labeling, use is approved for patients ≥5 years.

Children >12 years: Refer to adult dosing.

Sublingual: Canadian labeling (not in U.S. labeling): ≥5 years: Initial: 120 mcg at bedtime; dose may be titrated up to 360 mcg to achieve desired response. Fluid intake should be limited 1 hour prior to dose until the next morning, or at least 8 hours after administration.

Renal Impairment Cl_{cr} <50 mL/minute: Use is contraindicated according to the manufacturer; however, has been used in acute and chronic renal failure patients experiencing uremic bleeding or for prevention of surgical bleeding (unlabeled uses; Mannuccio, 1983; Watson, 1984).

Administration

I.M. Central diabetes insipidus: Withdraw dose from ampul into appropriate syringe size (eg, insulin syringe). Further dilution is not required. Administer as direct injection.

I.V.

I.V. push: Central diabetes insipidus: Withdraw dose from ampul into appropriate syringe size (eg, insulin syringe). Further dilution is not required. Administer as direct injection.

I.V. infusion:

Hemophilia A, von Willebrand disease (type 1), and prevention of surgical bleeding in patients with uremia (unlabeled; Mannucci, 1983): Infuse over 15-30 minutes

Acute uremic bleeding (unlabeled; Watson, 1984): May infuse over 10 minutes

Other

Intranasal:

DDAVP®: Nasal pump spray: Delivers 0.1 mL (10 mcg); for doses <10 mcg or for other doses which are not multiples, use rhinal tube. DDAVP® Nasal spray delivers fifty 10 mcg doses. For 10 mcg dose, administer in one nostril. Any solution remaining after 50 doses should be discarded. Pump must be primed prior to first use.

DDAVP® Rhinal tube: Insert top of dropper into tube (arrow marked end) in downward position. Squeeze dropper until solution reaches desired calibration mark. Disconnect dropper. Grasp the tube 3/4 inch from the end and insert tube into nostril until the fingertips reach the nostril. Place opposite end of tube into the mouth (holding breath). Tilt head back and blow with a strong, short puff into the nostril (for very young patients, an adult should blow solution into the child's nose). Reseal dropper after use.

SubQ: Central diabetes insipidus: Withdraw dose from ampul into appropriate syringe size (eg, insulin syringe). Further dilution is not required. Administer as direct injection.

Stability

Reconstitution DDAVP®: Dilute solution for injection in 10-50 mL NS for I.V. infusion (10 mL for children ≤10 kg: 50 mL for adults and children >10 kg).

Storage

DDAVP®:

Nasal spray: Store at controlled room temperature of 20°C to 25°C (68°F to 77°F). Keep nasal spray in upright position.

Rhinal Tube solution: Store refrigerated at 2°C to 8°C (36°F to 46°F). May store at controlled room temperature of 20°C to 25°C (68°F to 77°F) for up to 3 weeks.

Solution for injection: Store refrigerated at 2°C to 8°C (36°F to 46°F).

Tablet: Store at controlled room temperature of 20°C to 25°C (68°F to 77°F).

DDAVP® Melt (CAN; not available in U.S.): Store at 15°C to 25°C (59°F to 77°F) in original container. Protect from moisture.

Stimate® nasal spray: Store refrigerated at 2°C to 8°C (36°F to 46°F). May store at controlled room temperature of 22°C (72°F) for up to 3 weeks.

Monitoring and Teaching Issues

Laboratory Monitoring For all indications, fluid intake, urine volume, and signs and symptoms of hyponatremia should be closely monitored especially in high-risk patient subgroups (eg, young children, elderly, patients with heart failure).

Diabetes insipidus: Urine specific gravity, plasma and urine osmolality, serum electrolytes

Hemophilia A: Factor VIII coagulant activity, factor VIII ristocetin cofactor activity, and factor VIII antigen levels, aPTT

von Willebrand disease: Factor VIII coagulant activity, factor VIII ristocetin cofactor activity, and factor VIII von Willebrand antigen levels, bleeding time

Nocturnal enuresis: Serum electrolytes if used for >7 days

Physical Assessment Evaluate for any history of or potential for hyponatremia or renal impairment prior to beginning therapy. Monitor for thromboembolism, hyponatremia, and water intoxication regularly throughout therapy.

Patient Education Avoid alcohol; may decrease effect of medication. Avoid overhydration; follow prescriber instructions for fluid intake. Report increased weight or swelling of extremities; excessive thirst; unresolved headache; chest pain or palpitation; respiratory difficulty; acute heartburn, nausea, vomiting, or abdominal cramping; CNS changes (agitation, chills, coma, dizziness, insomnia, confusion); or rash. If using intranasal product, inspect nasal membranes regularly and report swelling, redness, irritation, or increased nasal congestion.

Geriatric Considerations Elderly patients should be cautioned not to increase their fluid intake beyond that sufficient to satisfy their thirst in order to avoid water intoxication and hyponatremia. Under experimental conditions, elderly have been shown to have a decreased responsiveness to vasopressin with respect to its effects on water homeostasis.

Pregnancy Considerations Adverse events were not observed in animal reproductive studies. There are no adequate and well-controlled studies in pregnant women. Anecdotal reports suggest congenital anomalies and low birth weight. However, causal relationship has not been established. Desmopressin has been used safely during pregnancy.

Additional Information 10 mcg of desmopressin acetate is equivalent to 40 int. units

- **Desmopressin Acetate** *see* Desmopressin *on page 493*
- **Desogen®** *see* Ethinyl Estradiol and Desogestrel *on page 695*
- **Desogestrel and Ethinyl Estradiol** *see* Ethinyl Estradiol and Desogestrel *on page 695*
- **Desoxyephedrine Hydrochloride** *see* Methamphetamine *on page 1190*
- **Desoxyn®** *see* Methamphetamine *on page 1190*

◆ **Desoxyphenobarbital** *see* Primidone *on page 1507*

◆ **Desulfato-Hirudin** *see* Desirudin *on page 490*

◆ **Desulphatohirudin** *see* Desirudin *on page 490*

Desvenlafaxine (des ven la FAX een)

U.S. Brand Names Pristiq®

Index Terms O-desmethylvenlafaxine; ODV

Generic Availability (U.S.) No

Pharmacologic Category Antidepressant, Serotonin/Norepinephrine Reuptake Inhibitor

Medication Guide Available Yes

Pregnancy Risk Factor C

Lactation Enters breast milk/not recommended

Use Treatment of major depressive disorder

Mechanism of Action/Effect Desvenlafaxine is a serotonin and norepinephrine reuptake inhibitor.

Contraindications Hypersensitivity to desvenlafaxine, venlafaxine or any component of the formulation; use of MAO inhibitors within 14 days; should not initiate MAO inhibitor within 7 days of discontinuing desvenlafaxine

Warnings/Precautions [U.S. Boxed Warning]: Antidepressants increase the risk of suicidal thinking and behavior in children, adolescents, and young adults (18-24 years of age) with major depressive disorder (MDD) and other psychiatric disorders; consider risk prior to prescribing. Short-term studies did not show an increased risk in patients >24 years of age and showed a decreased risk in patients ≥65 years. Closely monitor for clinical worsening, suicidality, or unusual changes in behavior; the patient's family or caregiver should be instructed to closely observe the patient and communicate condition with healthcare provider. A medication guide should be dispensed with each prescription. **Desvenlafaxine is not FDA approved for use in children.**

The possibility of a suicide attempt is inherent in major depression and may persist until remission occurs. Monitor for worsening of depression or suicidality, especially during initiation of therapy (generally first 1-2 months) or with dose increases or decreases. Use caution in high-risk patients. Worsening depression and severe abrupt suicidality that are not part of the presenting symptoms may require discontinuation or modification of drug therapy. The patient's family or caregiver should be alerted to monitor patients for the emergence of suicidality and associated behaviors (such as agitation, irritability, hostility, impulsivity, and hypomania) and call healthcare provider.

May worsen psychosis in some patients or precipitate a shift to mania or hypomania in patients with bipolar disorder. Patients presenting with depressive symptoms should be screened for bipolar disorder. Monotherapy in patients with bipolar disorder should be avoided. **Desvenlafaxine is not FDA approved for the treatment of bipolar depression.**

Serotonin syndrome and neuroleptic malignant syndrome (NMS)-like reactions have occurred with serotonin/norepinephrine reuptake inhibitors (SNRIs) and selective serotonin reuptake inhibitors (SSRIs) when used alone, and particularly when used in combination with serotonergic agents (eg, triptans) or antidopaminergic agents (eg, antipsychotics). Concurrent use with MAO inhibitors is contraindicated. Do not begin desvenlafaxine within 14 days of terminating MAO-I therapy; do not initiate MAO-I treatment within 7 days of discontinuing desvenlafaxine. May cause sustained increase in blood pressure or heart rate; dose related. Control pre-existing hypertension prior to initiation of desvenlafaxine. Use caution in patients with recent history of MI, unstable heart disease, or cerebrovascular disease; may cause increases in serum lipids (cholesterol, LDL, triglycerides). Use caution in patients with renal impairment; dose reduction required in severe renal impairment. Use caution in patients with hepatic impairment; clearance is decreased and average AUC is increased; dosage adjustment is recommended. May cause hyponatremia/SIADH (elderly at increased risk); volume depletion (diuretics may increase risk).

Interstitial lung disease and eosinophilic pneumonia have been rarely reported with venlafaxine (the parent drug of desvenlafaxine); may present as progressive dyspnea, cough, and/or chest pain. Prompt evaluation and possible discontinuation of therapy may be necessary. Use cautiously in patients with a history of seizures. The risks of cognitive or motor impairment are low. May cause or exacerbate sexual dysfunction. May impair platelet aggregation, resulting in bleeding.

Abrupt discontinuation or dosage reduction after extended (≥6 weeks) therapy may lead to agitation, dysphoria, nervousness, anxiety, and other symptoms; discontinuation symptoms may also occur when switching from another antidepressant. When discontinuing therapy or switching antidepressants, dosage should be tapered gradually over at least a 2-week period. If intolerable symptoms occur following a decrease in dosage or upon discontinuation of therapy, then resuming the previous dose with a more gradual taper should be considered. Use caution in patients with increased intraocular pressure or at risk of acute narrow-angle glaucoma.

Drug Interactions

Metabolism/Transport Effects Substrate of 3A4 (minor); **Inhibits** 3A4 (weak)

Avoid Concomitant Use

Avoid concomitant use of Desvenlafaxine with any of the following: Iobenguane I 123; MAO Inhibitors; Methylene Blue; Sibutramine

Decreased Effect

Desvenlafaxine may decrease the levels/effects of: Alpha2-Agonists; Iobenguane I 123

Increased Effect/Toxicity

Desvenlafaxine may increase the levels/effects of: Alcohol (Ethyl); Alpha-/Beta-Agonists; Aspirin; CNS Depressants; Methotrimeprazine; Methylene Blue; NSAID (Nonselective); Serotonin Modulators; Vitamin K Antagonists

The levels/effects of Desvenlafaxine may be increased by: Droperidol; MAO Inhibitors; Methotrimeprazine; Sibutramine

Nutritional/Ethanol Interactions

Ethanol: Avoid ethanol (may increase CNS effects).

Herb/Nutraceutical: Avoid St John's wort (may increase risk of serotonin syndrome and/or excessive sedation).

Adverse Reactions Reported for 50-100 mg/day.

>10%:

Central nervous system: Dizziness (10% to 13%), insomnia (9% to 12%)

Gastrointestinal: Nausea (22% to 26%), xerostomia (11% to 17%), diarrhea (9% to 11%)

Miscellaneous: Diaphoresis (10% to 11%)

1% to 10%:

Cardiovascular: Palpitation (≤3%), orthostatic hypotension (<2%; elderly 8%), syncope (<2%), hypertension (dose related; ≤1% of patients taking 50-100 mg daily had sustained diastolic BP ≥90 mm Hg)

Central nervous system: Somnolence (≤9%), fatigue (7%), anxiety (3% to 5%), abnormal dreams (2% to 3%), irritability (2%), vertigo (1% to 2%), feeling jittery (≤2%), depersonalization (<2%), extrapyramidal symptoms (<2%), hypomania (<2%), seizures (<2%), concentration decreased (≤1%)

Dermatologic: Rash (1%)

Endocrine & metabolic: Libido decreased (males 4% to 5%), cholesterol (increased by ≥50 mg/dL and ≥261 mg/dL: 3% to 4%), anorgasmia (females 1%; males ≤3%), hot flushes (1%), low density lipoprotein cholesterol (increased by ≥50 mg/dL and ≥190 mg/dL: ≤1%), sexual dysfunction (males ≤1%)

Gastrointestinal: Constipation (9%), anorexia (5% to 8%), vomiting (≤4%), weight loss (≤2%), weight gain (<2%)

Genitourinary: Urinary hesitancy (≤1%)

Hepatic: Liver function tests abnormal (<2%)

Neuromuscular & skeletal: Tremor (≤3%), paresthesia (2%), weakness (≤2%), stiffness (<2%)

Ocular: Blurred vision (3% to 4%), mydriasis (2%)

Otic: Tinnitus (≤2%)

Renal: Proteinuria (6% to 8%)

Respiratory: Epistaxis (<2%)

Miscellaneous: Ejaculation retarded (1% to 5%), erectile dysfunction (3% to 6%), hypersensitivity reaction (<2%), yawning (1%), ejaculation failure (≤1%)

Class-wide adverse effects: Gastrointestinal hemorrhage, hallucinations, photosensitivity

Pharmacodynamics/Kinetics

Bioavailability ~80%

Time to Peak Serum: ~7.5 hours

Protein Binding 30%

Half-Life Elimination ~11 hours; prolonged in renal failure

Metabolism Hepatic via conjugation, and oxidation via CYP3A4 (minor pathway)

Excretion Urine (45% as unchanged drug; ~24% as metabolites)

Available Dosage Forms

Tablet, extended release, oral:

Pristiq®: 50 mg, 100 mg

Dosing

Adult & Geriatric Depression: Oral: 50 mg once daily; doses up to 400 mg once daily have been studied; however, the manufacturer states there is no evidence that doses >50 mg/day confer any additional benefit. A flat dose response curve for efficacy between 50-400 mg/day has been noted as well as an increase in adverse events.

Note: Gradually taper dose (by increasing dosing interval) if discontinuing.

Renal Impairment

Cl_{cr} >50 mL/minute: No dosage adjustment required

Cl_{cr} 30-50 mL/minute: 50 mg once daily (maximum)

Cl_{cr} <30 mL/minute: 50 mg every other day (maximum)

Hemodialysis: 50 mg every other day (maximum). Supplemental doses not required after HD.

Hepatic Impairment 50 mg once daily; maximum dose: 100 mg/day

Administration

Oral May be taken with or without food. Swallow tablet whole; do not crush, chew, break, or dissolve. When discontinuing therapy, extend dosing interval to taper.

Monitoring and Teaching Issues

Laboratory Monitoring Lipid panel

Physical Assessment Observe for clinical worsening, suicidality, or unusual behavior changes; especially during the initial few months of therapy or during dosage changes. Monitor vital signs at the beginning and periodically throughout therapy. Taper dosage slowly when discontinuing.

Patient Education It may take 2-3 weeks to achieve desired results. Extended release capsules should be swallowed whole; do not crush or chew. Avoid alcohol. Maintain adequate hydration, unless instructed to restrict fluid intake. You may experience excess drowsiness or insomnia, lightheadedness, dizziness, blurred vision, headache, nausea, vomiting, anorexia, dry mouth, constipation, diarrhea, postural hypotension, urinary retention, or sexual dysfunction (reversible). Report persistent CNS effects (eg, insomnia, restlessness, fatigue, anxiety, abnormal thoughts, suicide ideation, confusion, personality changes, impaired cognitive function), muscle cramping or tremors, chest pain, palpitations, rapid heartbeat, unusual bleeding or bruising, or worsening of condition.

Dietary Considerations May be taken with or without food.

Geriatric Considerations No dose adjustment is necessary for age alone; adjust dose for renal function in the elderly. According to desvenlafaxine's manufacturer, 5% of the 3292 patients in clinical trials were 65 years of age or older. No differences in safety or efficacy were reported between younger and older adults. The elderly are more prone to SSRI/SNRI-induced hyponatremia.

Breast-Feeding Considerations Desvenlafaxine is found in human milk. The manufacturer recommends breast-feeding during therapy only if the expected benefits to the mother outweigh any potential risk to the infant.

Pregnancy Considerations Desvenlafaxine is classified as pregnancy category C due to adverse effects observed in animal studies. Nonteratogenic effects in the newborn following SSRI/SNRI exposure late in the third trimester include respiratory distress, cyanosis, apnea, seizures, temperature instability, feeding difficulty, vomiting, hypoglycemia, hyper- or hypotonia, hyper-reflexia, jitteriness, irritability, constant crying, and tremor. The long-term effects on neurobehavior have not been studied.

Women treated for major depression and who are euthymic prior to pregnancy are more likely to experience a relapse when medication is discontinued as compared to pregnant women who continue taking antidepressant medications. The ACOG recommends that therapy with SSRIs or SNRIs during pregnancy be individualized; treatment of depression during pregnancy should incorporate the clinical expertise of the mental health clinician, obstetrician, primary healthcare provider, and pediatrician. If treatment during pregnancy is required, consider tapering therapy during the third trimester in order to prevent withdrawal symptoms in the infant. If this is done and the woman is considered to be at risk from her major depressive disorder, the medication can be restarted following delivery, although the dose should be readjusted to that required before pregnancy. Treatment algorithms have been developed by the ACOG and the APA for the management of depression in women prior to conception and during pregnancy (Yonkers, 2009).

Desvenlafaxine is the major active metabolite of venlafaxine; also refer to the Venlafaxine monograph.

Related Information

Antidepressant Agents *on page 1982*

◆ **Desyrel** *see* TraZODone *on page 1808*

◆ **Detemir Insulin** *see* Insulin Detemir *on page 984*

◆ **Detrol®** *see* Tolterodine *on page 1783*

◆ **Detrol® LA** *see* Tolterodine *on page 1783*

◆ **Detryptoreline** *see* Triptorelin *on page 1824*

Dexamethasone (Systemic) (deks a METH a sone)

U.S. Brand Names Baycadron™; Dexamethasone Intensol™; DexPak® 10 Day TaperPak®; DexPak® 13 Day TaperPak®; DexPak® 6 Day TaperPak®

Index Terms Decadron; Dexamethasone Sodium Phosphate

Generic Availability (U.S.) Yes

Pharmacologic Category Anti-inflammatory Agent; Antiemetic; Corticosteroid, Systemic

Medication Safety Issues

Sound-alike/look-alike issues:

Dexamethasone may be confused with desoximetasone, dextroamphetamine

Decadron® may be confused with Percodan®

Pregnancy Risk Factor C

Lactation Excretion in breast milk unknown/use caution

Use Primarily as an anti-inflammatory or immunosuppressant agent in the treatment of a variety of diseases including those of allergic, dermatologic, endocrine, hematologic, inflammatory, neoplastic, nervous system, renal, respiratory, rheumatic, and autoimmune origin; may be used in management of cerebral edema, chronic swelling, as a diagnostic agent, diagnosis of Cushing's syndrome, antiemetic

Unlabeled/Investigational Use

Dexamethasone suppression test: General indicator consistent with depression and/or suicide

Accelerate fetal lung maturation in patients with preterm labor

Mechanism of Action/Effect Decreases inflammation by suppression of neutrophil migration, decreased production of inflammatory mediators, and reversal of increased capillary permeability; suppresses normal immune response. Dexamethasone's mechanism of antiemetic activity is unknown.

Contraindications Hypersensitivity to dexamethasone or any component of the formulation; systemic fungal infections, cerebral malaria

Warnings/Precautions Use with caution in patients with thyroid disease, hepatic impairment, renal impairment, cardiovascular disease, diabetes, glaucoma, cataracts, myasthenia gravis, patients at risk for osteoporosis, patients at risk for seizures, or GI diseases (diverticulitis, peptic ulcer, ulcerative colitis) due to perforation risk. Use caution following acute MI (corticosteroids have been associated with myocardial rupture). Because of the risk of adverse effects, systemic corticosteroids should be used cautiously in the elderly in the smallest possible effective dose for the shortest duration. May affect growth velocity; growth should be routinely monitored in pediatric patients. Withdraw therapy with gradual tapering of dose.

May cause hypercorticism or suppression of hypothalamic-pituitary-adrenal (HPA) axis, particularly in younger children or in patients receiving high doses for prolonged periods. HPA axis suppression may lead to adrenal crisis. Withdrawal and discontinuation of a corticosteroid should be done slowly and carefully. Particular care is required when patients are transferred from systemic corticosteroids to inhaled products due to possible adrenal insufficiency or withdrawal from steroids, including an increase in allergic symptoms. Patients receiving >20 mg per day of prednisone (or equivalent) may be most susceptible. Fatalities have occurred due to adrenal insufficiency in asthmatic patients during and after transfer from systemic corticosteroids to aerosol steroids; aerosol steroids do not provide the systemic steroid needed to treat patients having trauma, surgery, or infections. Dexamethasone does not provide adequate mineralocorticoid activity in adrenal insufficiency (may be employed as a single dose while cortisol assays are performed). The lowest possible dose should be used during treatment; discontinuation and/or dose reductions should be gradual.

Acute myopathy has been reported with high dose corticosteroids, usually in patients with neuromuscular transmission disorders; may involve ocular and/or respiratory muscles; monitor creatine kinase; recovery may be delayed. Corticosteroid use may cause psychiatric disturbances, including depression, euphoria, insomnia, mood swings, and personality changes. Pre-existing psychiatric conditions may be exacerbated by corticosteroid use. Prolonged use of corticosteroids may also increase the incidence of secondary infection, mask acute infection (including fungal infections), prolong or exacerbate viral infections, or limit response to vaccines. Exposure to chickenpox should be avoided; corticosteroids should not be used to treat ocular herpes simplex. Corticosteroids should not be used for cerebral malaria or viral hepatitis. Close observation is required in patients with latent tuberculosis and/or TB reactivity; restrict use in active TB (only in conjunction with antituberculosis treatment). Prolonged treatment with corticosteroids has been associated with the development of Kaposi's sarcoma (case reports); if noted, discontinuation of therapy should be considered. High-dose corticosteroids should not be used to manage acute head injury.

Drug Interactions

Metabolism/Transport Effects Substrate of CYP3A4 (major), P-glycoprotein; **Induces** CYP2A6 (weak), CYP2B6 (weak), CYP2C8 (weak), CYP2C9 (weak), CYP3A4 (strong), P-glycoprotein

Avoid Concomitant Use

Avoid concomitant use of Dexamethasone (Systemic) with any of the following: Aldesleukin; BCG; Dabigatran Etexilate; Dronedarone; Everolimus; Lurasidone; Natalizumab; Nilotinib; Nisoldipine; Pazopanib; Pimecrolimus; Praziquantel; Ranolazine; Roflumilast; RomiDEPsin; Tacrolimus (Topical); Tolvaptan; Vandetanib

Decreased Effect

Dexamethasone (Systemic) may decrease the levels/effects of: Aldesleukin; Antidiabetic Agents; BCG; Calcitriol; Caspofungin; Corticorelin; CycloSPORINE; CycloSPORINE (Systemic); CYP3A4 Substrates; Dabigatran Etexilate; Dronedarone; Everolimus; Exemestane; Gefitinib; GuanFACINE; Imatinib; Isoniazid; Ixabepilone; Lurasidone; Maraviroc; NIFEdipine; Nilotinib; Nisoldipine; Pazopanib; P-Glycoprotein Substrates; Praziquantel; Ranolazine; RomiDEPsin; Salicylates; Sipuleucel-T; SORAfenib; Tadalafil; Tolvaptan; Ulipristal; Vaccines (Inactivated); Vandetanib

The levels/effects of Dexamethasone (Systemic) may be decreased by: Aminoglutethimide; Antacids; Barbiturates; Bile Acid Sequestrants; CYP3A4 Inducers (Strong); Deferasirox; Echinacea; Herbs (CYP3A4 Inducers); Mitotane; P-Glycoprotein Inducers; Primidone; Rifamycin Derivatives

Increased Effect/Toxicity

Dexamethasone (Systemic) may increase the levels/effects of: Acetylcholinesterase Inhibitors; Amphotericin B; CycloSPORINE; CycloSPORINE (Systemic); Leflunomide; Lenalidomide; Loop Diuretics; Natalizumab; NSAID (COX-2 Inhibitor); NSAID (Nonselective); Thalidomide; Thiazide Diuretics; Vaccines (Live); Warfarin

The levels/effects of Dexamethasone (Systemic) may be increased by: Antifungal Agents (Azole Derivatives, Systemic); Aprepitant; Asparaginase; Calcium Channel Blockers (Nondihydropyridine); Conivaptan; CycloSPORINE; CycloSPORINE (Systemic); CYP3A4 Inhibitors (Moderate); CYP3A4 Inhibitors (Strong); Dasatinib; Denosumab; Estrogen Derivatives; Fluconazole; Fosaprepitant; Macrolide Antibiotics; Neuromuscular-Blocking Agents (Nondepolarizing); P-Glycoprotein Inhibitors; Pimecrolimus; Quinolone Antibiotics; Roflumilast; Salicylates; Tacrolimus (Topical); Trastuzumab

Nutritional/Ethanol Interactions

Ethanol: Avoid ethanol (may enhance gastric mucosal irritation).
Food: Dexamethasone interferes with calcium absorption. Limit caffeine.
Herb/Nutraceutical: Avoid cat's claw, echinacea (have immunostimulant properties).

Adverse Reactions Frequency not defined.

Cardiovascular: Arrhythmia, bradycardia, cardiac arrest, cardiomyopathy, CHF, circulatory collapse, edema, hypertension, myocardial rupture (post-MI), syncope, thromboembolism, vasculitis

Central nervous system: Depression, emotional instability, euphoria, headache, intracranial pressure increased, insomnia, malaise, mood swings, neuritis, personality changes, pseudotumor cerebri (usually following discontinuation), psychic disorders, seizure, vertigo

Dermatologic: Acne, allergic dermatitis, alopecia, angioedema, bruising, dry skin, erythema, fragile skin, hirsutism, hyper-/hypopigmentation, hypertrichosis, perianal pruritus (following I.V. injection), petechiae, rash, skin atrophy, skin test reaction impaired, striae, urticaria, wound healing impaired

Endocrine & metabolic: Adrenal suppression, carbohydrate tolerance decreased, Cushing's syndrome, diabetes mellitus, glucose intolerance decreased, growth suppression (children), hyperglycemia, hypokalemic alkalosis, menstrual irregularities, negative nitrogen balance, pituitary-adrenal axis suppression, protein catabolism, sodium retention

Gastrointestinal: Abdominal distention, appetite increased, gastrointestinal hemorrhage, gastrointestinal perforation, nausea, pancreatitis, peptic ulcer, ulcerative esophagitis, weight gain

Genitourinary: Altered (increased or decreased) spermatogenesis

Hepatic: Hepatomegaly, transaminases increased

Local: Postinjection flare (intra-articular use), thrombophlebitis

Neuromuscular & skeletal: Arthropathy, aseptic necrosis (femoral and humoral heads), fractures, muscle mass loss, myopathy (particularly in conjunction with neuromuscular disease or neuromuscular-blocking agents), neuropathy, osteoporosis, parasthesia, tendon rupture, vertebral compression fractures, weakness

Ocular: Cataracts, exophthalmos, glaucoma, intraocular pressure increased

Renal: Glucosuria

Respiratory: Pulmonary edema

Miscellaneous: Abnormal fat deposition, anaphylactoid reaction, anaphylaxis, avascular necrosis, diaphoresis, hiccups, hypersensitivity, impaired wound healing, infections, Kaposi's sarcoma, moon face, secondary malignancy

Pharmacodynamics/Kinetics

Onset of Action Acetate: Prompt

Duration of Action Metabolic effect: 72 hours; acetate is a long-acting repository preparation

Time to Peak Serum: Oral: 1-2 hours; I.M.: ~8 hours

Half-Life Elimination Normal renal function: 1.8-3.5 hours; Biological half-life: 36-54 hours

Metabolism Hepatic

Excretion Urine and feces

Available Dosage Forms

Elixir, oral: 0.5 mg/5 mL (237 mL)
Baycadron™: 0.5 mg/5 mL (237 mL)

Injection, solution: 4 mg/mL (1 mL, 5 mL, 30 mL); 10 mg/mL (1 mL, 10 mL)

Injection, solution [preservative free]: 10 mg/mL (1 mL)

Solution, oral: 0.5 mg/5 mL (240 mL, 500 mL)
Dexamethasone Intensol™: 1 mg/mL (30 mL)

Tablet, oral: 0.5 mg, 0.75 mg, 1 mg, 1.5 mg, 2 mg, 4 mg, 6 mg
DexPak® 6 Day TaperPak®: 1.5 mg
DexPak® 10 Day TaperPak®: 1.5 mg
DexPak® 13 Day TaperPak®: 1.5 mg

Dosing

Adult

Anti-inflammatory:
Oral, I.M., I.V.: 0.75-9 mg/day in divided doses every 6-12 hours
Intra-articular, intralesional, or soft tissue: 0.4-6 mg/day

Extubation or airway edema: Oral, I.M., I.V.: 0.5-2 mg/kg/day in divided doses every 6 hours beginning 24 hours prior to extubation and continuing for 4-6 doses afterwards

Antiemetic:
Prophylaxis: Oral, I.V.: 10-20 mg 15-30 minutes before treatment on each treatment day
Continuous infusion regimen: Oral or I.V.: 10 mg every 12 hours on each treatment day
Mildly emetogenic therapy: Oral, I.M., I.V.: 4 mg every 4-6 hours
Delayed nausea/vomiting: Oral: 4-10 mg 1-2 times/day for 2-4 days **or**
8 mg every 12 hours for 2 days; then
4 mg every 12 hours for 2 days **or**
20 mg 1 hour before chemotherapy; then
10 mg 12 hours after chemotherapy; then
8 mg every 12 hours for 4 doses; then
4 mg every 12 hours for 4 doses

Multiple myeloma: Oral, I.V.: 40 mg/day, days 1 to 4, 9 to 12, and 17 to 20, repeated every 4 weeks (alone or as part of a regimen)

Cerebral edema: I.V. 10 mg stat, 4 mg I.M./I.V. (should be given as sodium phosphate) every 6 hours until response is maximized, then switch to oral regimen, then taper off if appropriate; dosage may be reduced after 2-4 days and gradually discontinued over 5-7 days

Dexamethasone suppression test (depression/suicide indicator) (unlabeled use): Oral: 1 mg at 11 PM, draw blood at 8 AM the following day for plasma cortisol determination

Cushing's syndrome, diagnostic: Oral: 1 mg at 11 PM, draw blood at 8 AM; greater accuracy for Cushing's syndrome may be achieved by the following:
Dexamethasone 0.5 mg by mouth every 6 hours for 48 hours (with 24-hour urine collection for 17-hydroxycorticosteroid excretion)
Differentiation of Cushing's syndrome due to ACTH excess from Cushing's due to other causes: Oral: Dexamethasone 2 mg every 6 hours for 48 hours (with 24-hour urine collection for 17-hydroxycorticosteroid excretion)
Multiple sclerosis (acute exacerbation): Oral: 30 mg/day for 1 week, followed by 4-12 mg/day for 1 month
Treatment of shock:
Addisonian crisis/shock (eg, adrenal insufficiency/responsive to steroid therapy): I.V.: 4-10 mg as a single dose, which may be repeated if necessary
Unresponsive shock (eg, unresponsive to steroid therapy): I.V.: 1-6 mg/kg as a single I.V. dose or up to 40 mg initially followed by repeat doses every 2-6 hours while shock persists
Physiological replacement: Oral, I.M., I.V. (should be given as sodium phosphate): 0.03-0.15 mg/kg/day **or** 0.6-0.75 mg/m^2/day in divided doses every 6-12 hours

Geriatric Refer to adult dosing. Use cautiously in the elderly in the smallest possible dose.

Pediatric

Antiemetic (prior to chemotherapy): Refer to individual protocols and emetogenic potential: I.V.: 10 mg/m^2/dose every 12-24 hours on days of chemotherapy for severely emetogenic chemotherapy courses
Anti-inflammatory and/or immunosuppressant: Oral, I.M., I.V.: 0.08-0.3 mg/kg/day **or** 2.5-10 mg/m^2/day in divided doses every 6-12 hours
Extubation or airway edema: Oral, I.M., I.V.: 0.5-2 mg/kg/day in divided doses every 6 hours beginning 24 hours prior to extubation and continuing for 4-6 doses afterwards
Cerebral edema: I.V.: Loading dose: 1-2 mg/kg/dose as a single dose; maintenance: 1-1.5 mg/kg/day (maximum: 16 mg/day) in divided doses every 4-6 hours, taper off over 1-6 weeks
Bacterial meningitis: Infants and Children >6 weeks: I.V.: 0.15 mg/kg/dose every 6 hours for the first 2-4 days of antibiotic treatment; start dexamethasone 10-20 minutes before or with the first dose of antibiotic
Physiologic replacement: Oral, I.M., I.V.: 0.03-0.15 mg/kg/day or 0.6-0.75 mg/m^2/day in divided doses every 6-12 hours

Renal Impairment Hemodialysis or peritoneal dialysis: Supplemental dose is not necessary.

Administration

Oral Administer oral formulation with meals to decrease GI upset.

I.V. Administer as a 5-10 minute bolus; rapid injection is associated with a high incidence of perineal discomfort.

Topical Topical formulation is for external use. Do not use on open wounds.

Stability

Reconstitution Injection should be diluted in 50-100 mL NS or D_5W.

Storage Injection solution: Store at room temperature; protect from light and freezing.
Stability of injection of parenteral admixture at room temperature (25°C): 24 hours.
Stability of injection of parenteral admixture at refrigeration temperature (4°C): 2 days; protect from light and freezing.

Monitoring and Teaching Issues

Laboratory Monitoring Hemoglobin, occult blood loss, serum potassium, glucose
Dexamethasone suppression test, overnight: 8 AM cortisol <6 mg/100 mL (dexamethasone 1 mg). Plasma cortisol determination should be made on the day after giving dose.

Physical Assessment Caution patients with diabetes to monitor glucose levels closely (corticosteroids may alter glucose levels).

Patient Education Oral: Take with or after meals. Avoid alcohol and limit intake of caffeine or stimulants. Prescriber may recommend increased dietary vitamins, minerals, or iron. If you have diabetes, monitor glucose levels closely (antidiabetic medication may need to be adjusted). Inform prescriber if you are experiencing greater-than-normal levels of stress (medication may need adjustment). You may be more susceptible to infection. Some forms of this medication may cause GI upset. Report promptly excessive nervousness or sleep disturbances, signs of infection (eg, sore throat, unhealed injuries), excessive growth of body hair or loss of skin color, vision changes, weight gain, swelling of face or extremities, respiratory difficulty, muscle weakness, tarry stool, persistent abdominal pain, or worsening of condition or failure to improve.

Dietary Considerations May be taken with meals to decrease GI upset. May need diet with increased potassium, pyridoxine, vitamin C, vitamin D, folate, calcium, and phosphorus.

Geriatric Considerations Because of the risk of adverse effects, systemic corticosteroids should be used cautiously in the elderly in the smallest possible dose, and for the shortest possible time.

Breast-Feeding Considerations Corticosteroids are excreted in human milk; information specific to dexamethasone has not been located.

Pregnancy Considerations Adverse events have been observed with corticosteroids in animal reproduction studies. Dexamethasone crosses the placenta; and is partially metabolized to an inactive metabolite by placental enzymes. Due to its positive effect on stimulating fetal lung maturation, the injection is often used in patients with premature labor (24-34 weeks gestation). Some studies have shown an association between first trimester systemic corticosteroid use and oral clefts; adverse events in the fetus/neonate have been noted in case reports following large doses of systemic corticosteroids during pregnancy. Women exposed to dexamethasone during pregnancy for the treatment of an autoimmune disease may contact the OTIS Autoimmune Diseases Study at 877-311-8972.

Additional Information Effects of inhaled/intranasal steroids on growth have been observed in the absence of laboratory evidence of HPA axis suppression, suggesting that growth velocity is a more sensitive indicator of systemic corticosteroid exposure in pediatric patients than some commonly used tests of HPA axis function. The long-term effects of this reduction in growth velocity associated with orally-inhaled and intranasal corticosteroids, including the impact on final adult height, are unknown. The potential for "catch up" growth following discontinuation of treatment with inhaled corticosteroids has not been adequately studied.

Withdrawal/tapering of therapy: Corticosteroid tapering following short-term use is limited primarily by the need to control the underlying disease state; tapering may be accomplished over a period of days. Following longer-term use, tapering over weeks to months may be necessary to avoid signs and symptoms of adrenal insufficiency and to allow recovery of the HPA axis. Testing of HPA axis responsiveness may be of value in selected patients. Subtle deficits in HPA response may persist for months after discontinuation of therapy, and may require supplemental dosing during periods of acute illness or surgical stress.

Related Information

Corticosteroids *on page 1996*

Dexamethasone (Ophthalmic) (deks a METH a sone)

U.S. Brand Names Maxidex®; Ozurdex®

Index Terms Dexamethasone Sodium Phosphate

Generic Availability (U.S.) Yes: Ophthalmic solution

Pharmacologic Category Anti-inflammatory Agent, Ophthalmic; Corticosteroid, Ophthalmic

Medication Safety Issues

Sound-alike/look-alike issues:

Dexamethasone may be confused with desoximetasone, dextroamphetamine

Maxidex® may be confused with Maxzide®

Pregnancy Risk Factor C

Lactation Excretion in breast milk unknown/use caution

Use Management of steroid responsive inflammatory conditions such as allergic conjunctivitis, iritis, or cyclitis; symptomatic treatment of corneal injury from chemical, radiation, or thermal burns, or penetration of foreign bodies

Ophthalmic intravitreal implant (Ozurdex®): Treatment of macular edema following branch retinal vein occlusion (BRVO) or central retinal vein occlusion (CRVO); treatment of non-infective uveitis

Available Dosage Forms

Implant, intravitreal:

Ozurdex®: 0.7 mg (1s)

Solution, ophthalmic: 0.1% (5 mL)

Suspension, ophthalmic:

Maxidex®: 0.1% (5 mL)

Dosing

Adult

Anti-inflammatory:

Ophthalmic solution: Instill 1-2 drops into conjunctival sac every hour during the day and every other hour during the night; gradually reduce dose to every 3-4 hours, then to 3-4 times/day.

Ophthalmic suspension: Instill 1-2 drops into conjunctival sac up to 4-6 times/day; may use hourly in severe disease; taper prior to discontinuation.

Macular edema (following BRVO or CRVO): *Ophthalmic injection:* Ocular implant (Ozurdex®): Intravitreal: 0.7 mg implant injected in affected eye

Noninfective uveitis: *Ophthalmic injection:* Ocular implant (Ozurdex®): Intravitreal: 0.7 mg implant injected in affected eye

Geriatric Refer to adult dosing. Solution/suspension: Use cautiously in the elderly in the smallest possible dose.

Pediatric Ophthalmic anti-inflammatory: *Solution, suspension:* Instill 1-2 drops every hour during the day and every other hour during the night; gradually reduce dose to every 3-4 hours, then to 3-4 times/day; others have used 2-4 times/day dosing (Cassidy, 2001)

Administration

Other

Ophthalmic solution, suspension: Remove soft contact lenses prior to using solutions containing benzalkonium chloride. Do not touch tip of container to eye.

Ophthalmic implant (intravitreal injection): Ozurdex®: Administer under controlled aseptic conditions (eg, sterile gloves, sterile drape, sterile eyelid speculum). Adequate anesthesia and a broad-spectrum bactericidal agent should be administered prior to injection. In the sterile field, open foil pouch, remove applicator, and pull the safety tab straight off of the applicator (do not twist or flex the tab). If administration is required in the second eye, a new applicator should be used and the sterile field, syringe, gloves, drapes, and eyelid speculum should be changed.

Monitoring and Teaching Issues

Physical Assessment Monitor intraocular pressure if used >10 days.

Patient Education For use in eyes only. Wash hands before using. Lie down or tilt your head back and look upward. Put drops of suspension or solution inside lower eyelid. Close eye and roll eyeball in all directions. Do not blink for 1/2 minute. Apply gentle pressure to inner corner of eye for 30 seconds. Do not use any other eye preparation for at least 10 minutes. Do not let tip of applicator touch eye; do not contaminate tip of applicator (may cause eye infection, eye damage, or vision loss). You may be more sensitive to bright light. Inform prescriber if condition worsens, fails to improve, or if you experience eye pain or disturbances of vision.

◆ **Dexamethasone and Ciprofloxacin** *see* Ciprofloxacin and Dexamethasone *on page* 380

◆ **Dexamethasone Intensol™** *see* Dexamethasone (Systemic) *on page* 499

◆ **Dexamethasone Sodium Phosphate** *see* Dexamethasone (Ophthalmic) *on page* 503

◆ **Dexamethasone Sodium Phosphate** *see* Dexamethasone (Systemic) *on page* 499

Dexchlorpheniramine (deks klor fen EER a meen)

Index Terms Dexchlorpheniramine Maleate

Generic Availability (U.S.) Yes

Pharmacologic Category Alkylamine Derivative; Histamine H_1 Antagonist; Histamine H_1 Antagonist, First Generation

Medication Safety Issues

Beers Criteria medication: This drug may be inappropriate for use in geriatric patients (high severity risk).

Pregnancy Risk Factor B

Lactation Excretion in breast milk unknown/not recommended

Use Perennial and seasonal allergic rhinitis and other allergic symptoms including urticaria

Available Dosage Forms

Syrup, oral: 2 mg/5 mL (473 mL)

Dosing

Adult & Geriatric Allergy symptoms: Oral: 2 mg every 4-6 hours or 4-6 mg timed release at bedtime or every 8-10 hours

Pediatric Allergy symptoms: Oral:

2-5 years: 0.5 mg every 4-6 hours (do not use timed release)

6-11 years: 1 mg every 4-6 hours or 4 mg timed release at bedtime

Administration

Oral May be administered without regard to meals.

Monitoring and Teaching Issues

Patient Education Avoid use of alcohol. You may experience drowsiness, dizziness, dry mouth, nausea, or abdominal pain. Report persistent sedation, confusion, agitation, blurred vision, respiratory difficulty, lack of improvement, or worsening of condition.

◆ **Dexchlorpheniramine Maleate** *see* Dexchlorpheniramine *on page* 504

◆ **Dexedrine® Spansule®** *see* Dextroamphetamine *on page* 509

◆ **Dexferrum®** *see* Iron Dextran Complex *on page* 1021

◆ **Dexilant™** *see* Dexlansoprazole *on page* 504

Dexlansoprazole (deks lan SOE pra zole)

U.S. Brand Names Dexilant™; Kapidex™ [DSC]

Index Terms Kapidex; TAK-390MR

Generic Availability (U.S.) No

Pharmacologic Category Proton Pump Inhibitor; Substituted Benzimidazole

Medication Safety Issues

Sound-alike/look-alike issues:

Dexlansoprazole may be confused with aripiprazole, lansoprazole

Kapidex™ [DSC] may be confused with Casodex®, Kadian®

International issues:

Kapidex™ [DSC] may be confused with Capadex which is a brand name for propoxyphene/acetaminophen combination product in Australia and New Zealand

Pregnancy Risk Factor B

Lactation Excretion in breast milk unknown/not recommended

Use Short-term (4 weeks) treatment of heartburn associated with nonerosive GERD; short-term (up to 8 weeks) treatment of all grades of erosive esophagitis; to maintain healing of erosive esophagitis for up to 6 months

Mechanism of Action/Effect A proton pump inhibitor which decreases acid secretion in gastric parietal cells

Contraindications Hypersensitivity to dexlansoprazole or any component of the formulation

Warnings/Precautions Use of proton pump inhibitors may increase the risk of gastrointestinal infections (eg, *Salmonella, Campylobacter*). Relief of symptoms does not preclude the presence of a gastric malignancy. Atrophic gastritis (by biopsy) has been noted with long-term omeprazole therapy; this may also occur with dexlansoprazole. No occurrences of enterochromaffin-like (ECL) cell carcinoids, dysplasia, or neoplasia, such as those seen in rodent studies, have been reported in humans. Patients with moderate hepatic impairment (Child-Pugh class B) may require dosage reductions; no studies have been conducted in patients with severe hepatic impairment. Proton pump inhibitors may diminish the therapeutic effect of clopidogrel, thought to be due to reduced formation of the active metabolite of clopidogrel; an increase in the risk of cardiovascular events may occur. The manufacturer of clopidogrel recommends avoidance of concomitant administration of another PPI (ie, omeprazole); given the potency of CYP2C19 inhibitory activity, similar recommendations with dexlansoprazole would appear prudent.

Increased incidence of osteoporosis-related bone fractures of the hip, spine, or wrist may occur with proton pump inhibitor therapy. Patients on high-dose (multiple daily doses) or long-term therapy (≥1 year) should be monitored. Use the lowest effective dose for the shortest duration of time, use vitamin D and calcium supplementation, and follow appropriate guidelines to reduce risk of fractures in patients at risk.

Drug Interactions

Metabolism/Transport Effects Substrate of CYP2C9 (minor), 2C19 (major), 3A4 (major); **Inhibits** CYP2C9 (weak), 2C19 (moderate), 2D6 (weak), 3A4 (weak); **Induces** CYP1A2 (weak)

Avoid Concomitant Use

Avoid concomitant use of Dexlansoprazole with any of the following: Delavirdine; Erlotinib; Nelfinavir; Posaconazole

Decreased Effect

Dexlansoprazole may decrease the levels/effects of: Atazanavir; Bisphosphonate Derivatives; Cefditoren; Clopidogrel; Dabigatran Etexilate; Dasatinib; Delavirdine; Erlotinib; Gefitinib; Indinavir; Iron Salts; Itraconazole; Ketoconazole; Ketoconazole (Systemic); Mesalamine; Mycophenolate; Nelfinavir; Posaconazole

The levels/effects of Dexlansoprazole may be decreased by: Tipranavir

Increased Effect/Toxicity

Dexlansoprazole may increase the levels/effects of: Amphetamines; Benzodiazepines (metabolized by oxidation); Dexmethylphenidate; Methotrexate; Methylphenidate; Phenytoin; Raltegravir; Saquinavir; Tacrolimus; Tacrolimus (Systemic); Voriconazole

The levels/effects of Dexlansoprazole may be increased by: Fluconazole; Ketoconazole; Ketoconazole (Systemic)

Nutritional/Ethanol Interactions Ethanol: Avoid ethanol (may cause gastric mucosal irritation).

Adverse Reactions 2% to 10%:

Gastrointestinal: Diarrhea (5%), abdominal pain (4%), nausea (3%), flatulence (1% to 3%), vomiting (1% to 2%)

Respiratory: Upper respiratory tract infection (2% to 3%)

Pharmacodynamics/Kinetics

Bioavailability May be increased when administered with food

Time to Peak Serum: **Note:** Two distinct peaks secondary to dual release formulation:

Peak 1: 1-2 hours

Peak 2: 4-5 hours

Protein Binding ~96% to 99%

Half-Life Elimination ~1-2 hours

Metabolism Hepatic via CYP2C19-mediated hydroxylation and CYP3A4-mediated oxidation; followed by reduction to sulfate, glucuronide, and glutathione conjugates (inactive)

Excretion Urine (~51% as metabolites); feces (~48% as metabolites)

Available Dosage Forms

Capsule, delayed release, oral:

Dexilant™: 30 mg, 60 mg

Dosing

Adult & Geriatric

Erosive esophagitis: Oral: Short-term treatment: 60 mg once daily for up to 8 weeks; maintenance therapy: 30 mg once daily for up to 6 months

Symptomatic GERD: Oral: Short-term treatment: 30 mg once daily for 4 weeks

Renal Impairment No dosage adjustment is needed.

Hepatic Impairment

Mild hepatic impairment (Child-Pugh class A): No dosage adjustment is needed.

Moderate hepatic impairment (Child-Pugh class B): Consider a maximum dose of 30 mg/day.

Severe hepatic impairment (Child-Pugh class C): Use has not been studied in patients with severe hepatic impairment.

Administration

Oral May be administered without regard to meals; some patients may benefit from premeal administration if symptoms do not adequately respond to post-meal dosing. Capsules should be swallowed whole; alternatively, patients who are unable to swallow capsules may open the capsule, sprinkle the intact granules onto 1 tablespoon of applesauce, and swallow intact granules immediately.

Stability

Storage Store at 25°C (77°F); excursions permitted to 15°C to 30°C (59°F to 86°F).

Monitoring and Teaching Issues

Patient Education Do not crush or chew capsules. Capsule may be opened and contents added to applesauce. Avoid alcohol. You may experience stomach pain, diarrhea, nausea and/or vomiting, or gas. Report persistent abdominal pain, unresolved severe diarrhea, or persistent vomiting.

Dietary Considerations May be taken without regard to meals; some patients may benefit from premeal administration if symptoms do not adequately respond to post-meal dosing.

Geriatric Considerations No dose adjustment is recommended based on age or renal function. An increased half-life (2.23 vs 1.5 hours) and greater AUC (34.5%) in elderly compared to younger subjects are not considered to be clinically significant.

An increased risk of fractures of the hip, spine, or wrist has been observed in epidemiologic studies with proton pump inhibitor (PPI) use, primarily in older adults ≥50 years of age. The greatest risk was seen in patients receiving high doses or on long-term therapy (≥1 year). Calcium and vitamin D supplementation and close monitoring are recommended to reduce the risk of fracture in high-risk patients.

Pregnancy Considerations Animal studies have not shown teratogenic effects to the fetus. However, there are no adequate and well-controlled studies in pregnant women; use during pregnancy only if clearly needed.

Dexmethylphenidate (dex meth il FEN i date)

U.S. Brand Names Focalin®; Focalin® XR

Index Terms Dexmethylphenidate Hydrochloride

Generic Availability (U.S.) Yes: Tablet

Pharmacologic Category Central Nervous System Stimulant

Medication Safety Issues

Sound-alike/look-alike issues:

Dexmethylphenidate may be confused with methadone

Focalin® may be confused with Folotyn®

Medication Guide Available Yes

Pregnancy Risk Factor C

Lactation Excretion in breast milk unknown/use caution

Use Treatment of attention-deficit/hyperactivity disorder (ADHD)

Mechanism of Action/Effect CNS stimulant

Contraindications Hypersensitivity to dexmethylphenidate, methylphenidate, or any component of the formulation; marked anxiety, tension, and agitation; glaucoma; motor tics, family history or diagnosis of Tourette's syndrome; use with or within 14 days following MAO inhibitor therapy

Warnings/Precautions CNS stimulant use has been associated with serious cardiovascular events including sudden death in patients with pre-existing structural cardiac abnormalities or other serious heart problems (sudden death in children and adolescents; sudden death, stroke, and MI in adults). These products should be avoided in patients with known serious structural cardiac abnormalities, cardiomyopathy, serious heart rhythm abnormalities, or other serious cardiac problems that could increase the risk of sudden death that these conditions alone carry. Patients should be carefully evaluated for cardiac disease prior to initiation of therapy. Use of stimulants can cause an increase in blood pressure (average 2-4 mm Hg) and increases in heart rate (average 3-6 bpm), although some patients may have larger than average increases. Use caution with hypertension, hyperthyroidism, or other cardiovascular conditions that might be exacerbated by increases in blood pressure or heart rate.

Has demonstrated value as part of a comprehensive treatment program for ADHD. Use with caution in patients with bipolar disorder (may induce mixed/manic episode). May exacerbate symptoms of behavior and thought disorder in psychotic patients; new onset psychosis or mania may occur with stimulant use; observe for symptoms of aggression and/or hostility. Use caution with seizure disorders (may reduce seizure threshold). Use caution in patients with history of ethanol or drug abuse. May exacerbate symptoms of behavior and thought disorder in psychotic patients. **[U.S. Boxed Warning]: Potential for drug dependency exists - avoid abrupt discontinuation in patients who have received for prolonged periods.** Visual disturbances have been reported (rare). Stimulant use has been associated with growth suppression. Growth should be monitored during treatment.

Drug Interactions

Avoid Concomitant Use

Avoid concomitant use of Dexmethylphenidate with any of the following: Iobenguane I 123; MAO Inhibitors

Decreased Effect

Dexmethylphenidate may decrease the levels/effects of: Iobenguane I 123

Increased Effect/Toxicity

Dexmethylphenidate may increase the levels/effects of: PHENobarbital; Phenytoin; Primidone; Sympathomimetics; Tricyclic Antidepressants; Vitamin K Antagonists

The levels/effects of Dexmethylphenidate may be increased by: Antacids; Atomoxetine; Cannabinoids; H2-Antagonists; MAO Inhibitors; Proton Pump Inhibitors

Nutritional/Ethanol Interactions

Ethanol: Avoid ethanol (may cause CNS depression).

Food: High-fat meal may increase time to peak concentration.

Herb/Nutraceutical: Avoid ephedra (may cause hypertension or arrhythmias) and yohimbe (also has CNS stimulatory activity).

Adverse Reactions Actual frequency may be dependent upon dose and/or formulation.

>10%:

Central nervous system: Headache (25% to 39%), insomnia (children 5% to 17%), restlessness (adults 12%), anxiety (5% to 11%)

Gastrointestinal: Appetite decreased (children 30%), xerostomia (adults 7% to 20%), abdominal pain (children 15%)

1% to 10%:

Central nervous system: Dizziness (adults 6%), fever (children 5%), irritability (children ≤5%), depression (children ≤3%), mood swings (children ≤3%)

Dermatologic: Pruritus (children ≤3%)

Gastrointestinal: Nausea (children 9%), dyspepsia (5% to 9%), vomiting (children 2% to 9%), anorexia (children 5% to 7%), pharyngolaryngeal pain (adults 4% to 7%)

Respiratory: Nasal congestion (children ≤5%)

Frequency not defined: Ocular: Accommodation difficulties, blurred vision

Also refer to Methylphenidate for adverse effects seen with other methylphenidate products.

Pharmacodynamics/Kinetics

Onset of Action Extended release: ≥0.5 hours

Duration of Action Extended release: 12 hours

Absorption Immediate release: Rapid; Extended release: Bimodal

Bioavailability 22% to 25%

Time to Peak Fasting:

Immediate release: 1-1.5 hours

Extended release: First peak: 1.5 hours (range: 1-4 hours); Second peak: 6.5 hours (range: 4.5-7 hours)

Protein Binding 12% to 15%

Half-Life Elimination Immediate release: Adults: 2-4.5 hours; children: 2-3 hours

Metabolism Via de-esterification to inactive metabolite, *d*-α-phenyl-piperidine acetate (*d*-ritalinic acid)

Excretion Urine (90%, primarily as inactive metabolite)

Controlled Substance C-II

Available Dosage Forms

Capsule, extended release, oral:

Focalin® XR: 5 mg, 10 mg, 15 mg, 20 mg, 30 mg

Tablet, oral: 2.5 mg, 5 mg, 10 mg

Focalin®: 2.5 mg, 5 mg, 10 mg

Dosing

Adult & Geriatric

Treatment of ADHD: Patients not currently taking methylphenidate: Oral:

Immediate release: Initial: 2.5 mg twice daily; dosage may be adjusted in increments of 2.5-5 mg at weekly intervals (maximum dose: 20 mg/day); doses should be taken at least 4 hours apart

Extended release: Initial: 10 mg once daily; dosage may be adjusted in increments of 10 mg/day at weekly intervals (maximum dose: 40 mg/day)

Conversion to dexmethylphenidate from methylphenidate:

Immediate release: Initial: Half the total daily dose of racemic methylphenidate (maximum dexmethylphenidate dose: 20 mg/day)

Extended release: Initial: Half the total daily dose of racemic methylphenidate (maximum dexmethylphenidate dose: 40 mg/day)

Conversion from dexmethylphenidate immediate release to dexmethylphenidate extended release: When changing from Focalin® tablets to Focalin® XR capsules, patients may be switched to the same daily dose using Focalin® XR (maximum dose: 40 mg/day)

Dose reductions and discontinuation: Reduce dose or discontinue in patients with paradoxical aggravation of symptoms. Discontinue if no improvement is seen after one month of treatment.

Pediatric

Treatment of ADHD: Children ≥6 years: Patients not currently taking methylphenidate: Oral:

Immediate release: Initial: 2.5 mg twice daily; dosage may be adjusted in increments of 2.5-5 mg at weekly intervals (maximum dose: 20 mg/day); doses should be taken at least 4 hours apart

Extended release: Initial: 5 mg once daily; dosage may be adjusted in increments of 5 mg/day at weekly intervals (maximum dose: 30 mg/day)

Conversion to dexmethylphenidate from methylphenidate:

Immediate release: Initial: Half the total daily dose of racemic methylphenidate (maximum dexmethylphenidate dose: 20 mg/day)

Extended release: Initial: Half the total daily dose of racemic methylphenidate (maximum dexmethylphenidate dose: 30 mg/day)

Conversion from dexmethylphenidate immediate release to dexmethylphenidate extended release: When changing from Focalin® tablets to Focalin® XR capsules, patients may be switched to the same daily dose using Focalin® XR (maximum dose: 30 mg/day)

Dose reductions and discontinuation: Refer to adult dosing.

Renal Impairment No data available. However, considering extensive metabolism to inactive compounds, renal insufficiency expected to have minimal effect on kinetics of dexmethylphenidate.

Hepatic Impairment No data available.

Administration

Oral

Capsule: Should be administered once daily in the morning; do not crush or chew. Capsules may be opened and contents sprinkled over a spoonful of applesauce; consume immediately; do not store for future use.

Tablet: Should be administered at least 4 hours apart; may be taken with or without food.

Stability

Storage Store at 25°C (77°F); excursions permitted to 15°C to 30°C (59°F to 86°F). Protect from light and moisture.

Monitoring and Teaching Issues

Laboratory Monitoring CBC with differential, ECG, platelet count

Physical Assessment This drug should be used as part of a comprehensive treatment program for ADHD. Perform careful cardiovascular assessment prior to initiating therapy. Monitor vital signs at beginning of therapy and periodically throughout. In children, monitor growth pattern. If growth/weight gain is not as expected, may need to discontinue medication. Taper dosage when discontinuing from long-term therapy.

Patient Education Response may take some time. You may experience decreased appetite or weight loss, restlessness, impaired judgment, headache, dry mouth, or dizziness. Report unresolved rapid heartbeat, chest pain, difficulty breathing, excessive agitation, nervousness, insomnia, tremors, dizziness, or skin rash.

Dietary Considerations May be taken without regard to meals.

Breast-Feeding Considerations It is not known if dexmethylphenidate is excreted into breast milk. Dexmethylphenidate is the more active *d-threo*-enantiomer of racemic methylphenidate, and methylphenidate is excreted into breast milk. Refer to Methylphenidate monograph for additional information.

Pregnancy Considerations Teratogenic effects were noted in animal studies. There are no adequate and well-controlled studies in pregnant women. Use only if the potential benefit to the mother outweighs the possible risks to the fetus.

Additional Information Focalin® XR capsules use a bimodal release where 1/2 the dose is provided in immediate release beads and 1/2 the dose is in delayed release beads. A single, once-daily dose of a capsule provides the same amount of dexmethylphenidate as two tablets given 4 hours apart.

◆ **Dexmethylphenidate Hydrochloride** *see* Dexmethylphenidate *on page 506*

◆ **DexPak® 6 Day TaperPak®** *see* Dexamethasone (Systemic) *on page 499*

◆ **DexPak® 10 Day TaperPak®** *see* Dexamethasone (Systemic) *on page 499*

◆ **DexPak® 13 Day TaperPak®** *see* Dexamethasone (Systemic) *on page 499*

Dexrazoxane (deks ray ZOKS ane)

U.S. Brand Names Totect®; Zinecard®

Index Terms ICRF-187

Generic Availability (U.S.) Yes

Pharmacologic Category Antidote; Cardioprotectant

Medication Safety Issues

Sound-alike/look-alike issues:

Zinecard® may be confused with Gemzar®

Pregnancy Risk Factor C (Zinecard®) / D (Totect®)

Lactation Excretion in breast milk unknown/not recommended

Use

Zinecard®: Reduction of the incidence and severity of cardiomyopathy associated with doxorubicin administration in women with metastatic breast cancer who have received a cumulative doxorubicin dose of 300 mg/m^2 and who would benefit from continuing therapy with doxorubicin. (Not recommended for use with initial doxorubicin therapy.)

Totect®: Treatment of anthracycline-induced extravasation.

Unlabeled/Investigational Use Reduction of the incidence and severity of cardiomyopathy associated with doxorubicin administration (cumulative doses >300 mg/m^2) in patients with malignancies other than metastatic breast cancer who would benefit from continuing therapy with doxorubicin; reduction of the incidence and severity of cardiomyopathy associated with continued epirubicin administration for advanced breast cancer

Available Dosage Forms

Injection, powder for reconstitution: 250 mg, 500 mg

Totect®: 500 mg

Zinecard®: 250 mg, 500 mg

Dosing

Adult & Geriatric

Prevention of doxorubicin cardiomyopathy: I.V.: A 10:1 ratio of dexrazoxane:doxorubicin (500 mg/m^2 dexrazoxane: 50 mg/m^2 doxorubicin). **Note:** Cardiac monitoring should continue during dexrazoxane therapy; doxorubicin/dexrazoxane should be discontinued in patients who develop a decline in LVEF or clinical CHF.

Treatment of anthracycline extravasation: I.V.: 1000 mg/m^2 on days 1 and 2 (maximum dose: 2000 mg), followed by 500 mg/m^2 on day 3 (maximum dose: 1000 mg); begin treatment as soon as possible, within 6 hours of extravasation

Pediatric Prevention of doxorubicin cardiomyopathy (unlabeled use): I.V.: A 10:1 ratio of dexrazoxane:doxorubicin (eg, 300 mg/m^2 dexrazoxane: 30 mg/m^2 doxorubicin) was used in patients with high-risk acute lymphoblastic leukemia (Moghrabi, 2007)

Renal Impairment Moderate-to-severe (Cl_{cr}<40 mL/minute):

Prevention of cardiomyopathy: Reduce dose by 50%, using a 5:1 dexrazoxane:doxorubicin ratio (250 mg/m^2 dexrazoxane: 50 mg/m^2 doxorubicin)

Anthracycline-induced extravasation: Reduce dose by 50%

Hepatic Impairment

Prevention of cardiomyopathy: Since doxorubicin dosage is reduced in hyperbilirubinemia, a proportional reduction in dexrazoxane dosage is recommended (maintain a 10:1 ratio of dexrazoxane:doxorubicin)

Anthracycline-induced extravasation: Use has not been evaluated in patients with hepatic dysfunction

Administration

I.V.

Prevention of doxorubicin cardiomyopathy: Administer by slow I.V. push or rapid (5-15 minutes) I.V. infusion. Administer doxorubicin within 30 minutes after beginning the infusion with dexrazoxane.

Treatment of anthracycline extravasation: Administer I.V. over 1-2 hours; begin infusion as soon as possible, within 6 hours of extravasation. Infusion solution should be at room temperature prior to administration. Infuse in a large vein in an area remote from the extravasation. If extravasation is also being managed with cooling, withhold cooling beginning 15 minutes before dexrazoxane infusion; continue withholding cooling until 15 minutes after infusion is completed. Day 2 and 3 doses should be administered at approximately the same time (± 3 hours) as the dose on day 1. For I.V. administration; **not** for local infiltration into extravasation

Monitoring and Teaching Issues

Laboratory Monitoring Frequent complete blood counts are recommended; liver function; serum creatinine

Physical Assessment Monitor cardiac function closely. Assess infusion site frequently. Avoid extravasation.

Patient Education This I.V. medication is given to reduce incidence of cardiac complications with doxorubicin. Report promptly any pain at infusion site. You will be more susceptible to infections. Report shortness of breath, chest discomfort, unusual bleeding, fever, or swelling of extremities.

Dextroamphetamine (deks troe am FET a meen)

U.S. Brand Names Dexedrine® Spansule®; ProCentra®

Index Terms Dextroamphetamine Sulfate

Generic Availability (U.S.) Yes: Excludes capsule (sustained release), oral solution

Pharmacologic Category Stimulant

Medication Safety Issues

Sound-alike/look-alike issues:

Dexedrine® may be confused with dextran, Excedrin®

Dextroamphetamine may be confused with dexamethasone

Beers Criteria medication: This drug may be inappropriate for use in geriatric patients (high severity risk).

Medication Guide Available Yes

Pregnancy Risk Factor C

Lactation Enters breast milk/not recommended

Use Narcolepsy; attention-deficit/hyperactivity disorder (ADHD)

Unlabeled/Investigational Use Depression

Controlled Substance C-II

Available Dosage Forms

Capsule, extended release, oral: 5 mg, 10 mg, 15 mg

Capsule, sustained release, oral:

Dexedrine® Spansule®: 5 mg, 10 mg, 15 mg

Solution, oral:

ProCentra®: 5 mg/5 mL (480 mL)

Tablet, oral: 5 mg, 10 mg

Dosing

Adult Narcolepsy: Oral: Initial: 10 mg/day, may increase at 10 mg/day increments in weekly intervals until side effects appear (maximum dose: 60 mg/day)

Geriatric Refer to adult dosing; start at lowest dose. Use with caution.

Pediatric

Narcolepsy: Oral: Children 6-12 years: Initial: 5 mg/day, may increase at 5 mg/day increments in weekly intervals until side effects appear (maximum dose: 60 mg/day)

Attention-deficit/hyperactivity disorder (ADHD): Oral:

Children 3-5 years: Immediate release tablets or oral solution: Initial: 2.5 mg/day; may increase at 2.5 mg/day increments in weekly intervals until optimal response is obtained, usual range: 0.1-0.5 mg/kg/dose (maximum dose: 40 mg/day)

Children ≥6 years: Initial: 5 mg once or twice daily; may increase at 5 mg/day increments in weekly intervals until optimal response is reached, usual range: 0.1-0.5 mg/kg/dose (5-20 mg/day) (maximum dose: 40 mg/day)

Administration

Oral Administer initial dose upon awakening; do not administer doses late in the evening due to potential for insomnia.

Immediate release tablets and oral solution: If needed, 1-2 additional doses may be administered at intervals of 4-6 hours.

Extended release or sustained release capsules: Do not crush sustained release drug products. Formulations may be used for once-daily administration, if appropriate.

Monitoring and Teaching Issues

Physical Assessment Assess for history of suicidal tendencies. Perform careful cardiovascular assessment prior to initiating therapy. Periodically evaluate the need for continued use. Monitor vital signs at start of therapy, when changing dosage, and at regular intervals throughout. Monitor serum glucose closely in patients with diabetes (amphetamines may alter doses of diabetic medications). Monitor weight; may see weight loss. Taper dosage slowly when discontinuing.

Patient Education Take early in day to avoid sleep disturbance, 30 minutes before meals. Avoid alcohol or caffeine. You may experience restlessness, impaired judgment, dry mouth, nausea or vomiting, constipation, or diarrhea. Patients with diabetes need to monitor serum glucose closely. Report chest pain, palpitations, difficulty breathing, fainting, extreme fatigue or depression, CNS changes (aggressiveness, restlessness, euphoria, sleep disturbances), or weight loss.

Dextroamphetamine and Amphetamine

(deks troe am FET a meen & am FET a meen)

U.S. Brand Names Adderall XR®; Adderall®

Index Terms Amphetamine and Dextroamphetamine

Generic Availability (U.S.) Yes

Pharmacologic Category Stimulant

Medication Safety Issues

Sound-alike/look-alike issues:

Adderall® may be confused with Inderal®

Beers Criteria medication: This drug may be inappropriate for use in geriatric patients (high severity risk).

Medication Guide Available Yes

Pregnancy Risk Factor C

Lactation Enters breast milk/contraindicated

Use Attention-deficit/hyperactivity disorder (ADHD); narcolepsy

Mechanism of Action/Effect Amphetamines release catecholamines from storage sites in the nerve terminals.

Contraindications Hypersensitivity to dextroamphetamine, amphetamine, or any component of the formulation; advanced arteriosclerosis; symptomatic cardiovascular disease; moderate-to-severe hypertension; hyperthyroidism; hypersensitivity or idiosyncrasy to the sympathomimetic amines; glaucoma; agitated states; patients with a history of drug abuse; with or within 14 days following MAO inhibitor (hypertensive crisis)

Warnings/Precautions [U.S. Boxed Warning]: Use has been associated with serious cardiovascular events including sudden death in patients with pre-existing structural cardiac abnormalities or other serious heart problems (sudden death in children and adolescents; sudden death, stroke and MI in adults. These products should be avoided in the patients with known serious structural cardiac abnormalities, cardiomyopathy, serious heart rhythm abnormalities, or other serious cardiac problems that could increase the risk of sudden death that these conditions alone carry. Patients should be carefully evaluated for cardiac disease prior to initiation of therapy. Use with caution in patients with hypertension and other cardiovascular conditions that might be exacerbated by increases in blood pressure or heart rate. Amphetamines may impair the ability to engage in potentially hazardous activities. May cause visual disturbances.

Use with caution in patients with psychiatric or seizure disorders. May exacerbate symptoms of behavior and thought disorder in psychotic patients. Stimulants may unmask tics in individuals with coexisting Tourette's syndrome. **[U.S. Boxed Warning]: Potential for drug dependency exists; prolonged use may lead to drug dependency.** Use is contraindicated in patients with history of ethanol or drug abuse. Prescriptions should be written for the smallest quantity consistent with good patient care to minimize possibility of overdose. Abrupt discontinuation following high doses or for prolonged periods may result in symptoms for withdrawal.

May be inappropriate for use in the elderly due to CNS stimulant adverse effects (Beers Criteria). Safety and efficacy have not been established in children <3 years of age. Appetite suppression may occur; monitor weight during therapy, particularly in children. Use of stimulants has been associated with suppression of growth; monitor growth rate during treatment.

Drug Interactions

Metabolism/Transport Effects Amphetamine: **Inhibits** CYP2D6 (weak)

Avoid Concomitant Use

Avoid concomitant use of Dextroamphetamine and Amphetamine with any of the following: Iobenguane I 123; MAO Inhibitors

Decreased Effect

Dextroamphetamine and Amphetamine may decrease the levels/effects of: Antihistamines; Ethosuximide; Iobenguane I 123; PHENobarbital; Phenytoin

The levels/effects of Dextroamphetamine and Amphetamine may be decreased by: Ammonium Chloride; Antipsychotics; Gastrointestinal Acidifying Agents; Lithium; Methenamine; Peginterferon Alfa-2b

Increased Effect/Toxicity

Dextroamphetamine and Amphetamine may increase the levels/effects of: Analgesics (Opioid); Sympathomimetics

The levels/effects of Dextroamphetamine and Amphetamine may be increased by: Alkalinizing Agents; Antacids; Atomoxetine; Cannabinoids; Carbonic Anhydrase Inhibitors; MAO Inhibitors; Proton Pump Inhibitors; Tricyclic Antidepressants

Nutritional/Ethanol Interactions

Ethanol: Avoid ethanol (may increase CNS depression).

Food: Dextroamphetamine serum levels may be altered if taken with acidic food, juices, or vitamin C. Avoid caffeine.

Herb/Nutraceutical: Avoid ephedra (may cause hypertension or arrhythmias).

Lab Interactions Increased corticosteroid levels (greatest in evening); may interfere with urinary steroid testing

Adverse Reactions

As reported with Adderall XR®:

>10%:

Central nervous system: Insomnia (12% to 27%), headache (up to 26% in adults)

Gastrointestinal: Appetite decreased (22% to 36%), abdominal pain (11% to 14%), dry mouth (2% to 35%), weight loss (4% to 11%)

1% to 10%:

Cardiovascular: Tachycardia (up to 6% in adults), palpitation (2% to 4%)

Central nervous system: Emotional lability (2% to 9%), agitation (up to 8% in adults), anxiety (8%), dizziness (2% to 7%), nervousness (6%), fever (5%), somnolence (2% to 4%)

Dermatologic: Photosensitization (2% to 4%)

Endocrine & metabolic: Dysmenorrhea (2% to 4%), impotence (2% to 4%), libido decreased (2% to 4%)

Gastrointestinal: Nausea (2% to 8%), vomiting (2% to 7%), diarrhea (2% to 6%), constipation (2% to 4%), dyspepsia (2% to 4%), tooth disorder (2% to 4%)

Genitourinary: Urinary tract infection (5%)

Neuromuscular & skeletal: Twitching (2% to 4%), weakness (2% to 6%)

Respiratory: Dyspnea (2% to 4%)

Miscellaneous: Diaphoresis (2% to 4%), infection (2% to 4%), speech disorder (2% to 4%)

Adverse reactions reported with other amphetamines include: Adverse reactions reported with other amphetamines include: Anaphylaxis, angioedema, anorexia, cardiomyopathy, depression, dyskinesia, dysphoria, euphoria, exacerbation of motor and phonic tics, exacerbation of Tourette's syndrome, hypertension, MI, overstimulation, psychosis, rash, restlessness, seizure, stroke, taste disturbance, tremor, urticaria

Pharmacodynamics/Kinetics

Onset of Action 30-60 minutes

Duration of Action 4-6 hours

Absorption Well-absorbed

Time to Peak T_{max}: Adderall®: 3 hours; Adderall XR®: 7 hours

Half-Life Elimination

Children 6-12 years: d-amphetamine: 9 hours; l-amphetamine: 11 hours

Adolescents 13-17 years: d-amphetamine: 11 hours; l-amphetamine: 13-14 hours

Adults: d-amphetamine: 10 hours; l-amphetamine: 13 hours

Metabolism Hepatic via cytochrome P450 monooxygenase and glucuronidation

Excretion Urine (highly dependent on urinary pH); 70% of a single dose is eliminated within 24 hours; excreted as unchanged amphetamine (30%, may range from ~1% in alkaline urine to ~75% in acidic urine), benzoic acid, hydroxyamphetamine, hippuric acid, norephedrine, and *p*-hydroxynorephedrine

Pharmacokinetic Note See Dextroamphetamine monograph.

Controlled Substance C-II

Available Dosage Forms

Capsule, extended release:

5 mg [dextroamphetamine sulfate 1.25 mg, dextroamphetamine saccharate 1.25 mg, amphetamine aspartate monohydrate 1.25 mg, amphetamine sulfate 1.25 mg]

10 mg [dextroamphetamine sulfate 2.5 mg, dextroamphetamine saccharate 2.5 mg, amphetamine aspartate monohydrate 2.5 mg, amphetamine sulfate 2.5 mg]

15 mg [dextroamphetamine sulfate 3.75 mg, dextroamphetamine saccharate 3.75 mg, amphetamine aspartate monohydrate 3.75 mg, amphetamine sulfate 3.75 mg]

20 mg [dextroamphetamine sulfate 5 mg, dextroamphetamine saccharate 5 mg, amphetamine aspartate monohydrate 5 mg, amphetamine sulfate 5 mg]

25 mg [dextroamphetamine sulfate 6.25 mg, dextroamphetamine saccharate 6.25 mg, amphetamine aspartate monohydrate 6.25 mg, amphetamine sulfate 6.25 mg]

30 mg [dextroamphetamine sulfate 7.5 mg, dextroamphetamine saccharate 7.5 mg, amphetamine aspartate monohydrate 7.5 mg, amphetamine sulfate 7.5 mg]

Adderall XR®:

5 mg [dextroamphetamine 1.25 mg, dextroamphetamine saccharate 1.25 mg, amphetamine aspartate monohydrate 1.25 mg, amphetamine sulfate 1.25 mg]

10 mg [dextroamphetamine sulfate 2.5 mg, dextroamphetamine saccharate 2.5 mg, amphetamine aspartate monohydrate 2.5 mg, amphetamine sulfate 2.5 mg]

15 mg [dextroamphetamine sulfate 3.75 mg, dextroamphetamine saccharate 3.75 mg, amphetamine aspartate monohydrate 3.75 mg, amphetamine sulfate 3.75 mg]

20 mg [dextroamphetamine sulfate 5 mg, dextroamphetamine saccharate 5 mg, amphetamine aspartate monohydrate 5 mg, amphetamine sulfate 5 mg]

25 mg [dextroamphetamine sulfate 6.25 mg, dextroamphetamine saccharate 6.25 mg, amphetamine aspartate monohydrate 6.25 mg, amphetamine sulfate 6.25 mg]
30 mg [dextroamphetamine sulfate 7.5 mg, dextroamphetamine saccharate 7.5 mg, amphetamine aspartate monohydrate 7.5 mg, amphetamine sulfate 7.5 mg]

Tablet: 5 mg, 7.5 mg, 10 mg, 12.5 mg, 15 mg, 20 mg, 30 mg

5 mg [dextroamphetamine sulfate 1.25 mg, dextroamphetamine saccharate 1.25 mg, amphetamine aspartate monohydrate 1.25 mg, amphetamine sulfate 1.25 mg]
7.5 mg [dextroamphetamine sulfate 1.875 mg, dextroamphetamine saccharate 1.875 mg, amphetamine aspartate monohydrate 1.875 mg, amphetamine sulfate 1.875 mg]
10 mg [dextroamphetamine sulfate 2.5 mg, dextroamphetamine saccharate 2.5 mg, amphetamine aspartate monohydrate 2.5 mg, amphetamine sulfate 2.5 mg]
12.5 mg [dextroamphetamine sulfate 3.125 mg, dextroamphetamine saccharate 3.125 mg, amphetamine aspartate monohydrate 3.125 mg, amphetamine sulfate 3.125 mg]
15 mg [dextroamphetamine sulfate 3.75 mg, dextroamphetamine saccharate 3.75 mg, amphetamine aspartate monohydrate 3.75 mg, amphetamine sulfate 3.75 mg]
20 mg [dextroamphetamine sulfate 5 mg, dextroamphetamine saccharate 5 mg, amphetamine aspartate monohydrate 5 mg, amphetamine sulfate 5 mg]
30 mg [dextroamphetamine sulfate 7.5 mg, dextroamphetamine saccharate 7.5 mg, amphetamine aspartate monohydrate 7.5 mg, amphetamine sulfate 7.5 mg]

Adderall®:

5 mg [dextroamphetamine sulfate 1.25 mg, dextroamphetamine saccharate 1.25 mg, amphetamine aspartate monohydrate 1.25 mg, amphetamine sulfate 1.25 mg]
7.5 mg [dextroamphetamine 1.875 mg, dextroamphetamine saccharate 1.875 mg, amphetamine aspartate monohydrate 1.875 mg, amphetamine sulfate 1.875 mg]
10 mg [dextroamphetamine sulfate 2.5 mg, dextroamphetamine saccharate 2.5 mg, amphetamine aspartate monohydrate 2.5 mg, amphetamine sulfate 2.5 mg]
12.5 mg [dextroamphetamine sulfate 3.125 mg, dextroamphetamine saccharate 3.125 mg, amphetamine aspartate monohydrate 3.125 mg, amphetamine sulfate 3.125 mg]
15 mg [dextroamphetamine sulfate 3.75 mg, dextroamphetamine saccharate 3.75 mg, amphetamine aspartate monohydrate 3.75 mg, amphetamine sulfate 3.75 mg]
20 mg [dextroamphetamine sulfate 5 mg, dextroamphetamine saccharate 5 mg, amphetamine aspartate monohydrate 5 mg, amphetamine sulfate 5 mg]
30 mg [dextroamphetamine sulfate 7.5 mg, dextroamphetamine saccharate 7.5 mg, amphetamine aspartate monohydrate 7.5 mg, amphetamine sulfate 7.5 mg]

Dosing

Adult & Geriatric Note: Use lowest effective individualized dose; administer first dose as soon as awake; use intervals of 4-6 hours between additional doses.

ADHD: Oral:

Adderall®: Initial: 5 mg once or twice daily; increase daily dose in 5 mg increments at weekly intervals until optimal response is obtained; usual maximum dose: 40 mg/day given in 1-3 divided doses per day.

Adderall XR®: Initial: 20 mg once daily in the morning; higher doses (up to 60 mg once daily) have been evaluated; however, there is not adequate evidence that higher doses afforded additional benefit

Narcolepsy: *Adderall®*: Oral: Initial: 10 mg/day; increase daily dose in 10 mg increments at weekly intervals until optimal response is obtained; maximum dose: 60 mg/day given in 1-3 divided doses per day with intervals of 4-6 hours between doses.

Pediatric

Note: Use lowest effective individualized dose; administer first dose as soon as awake

ADHD: Oral:

Children: <3 years: Not recommended.

Children: 3-5 years (Adderall®): Initial 2.5 mg/day given every morning; increase daily dose in 2.5 mg increments at weekly intervals until optimal response is obtained; maximum dose: 40 mg/day given in 1-3 divided doses per day. Use intervals of 4-6 hours between additional doses.

Children: ≥6 years:

Adderall®: Initial: 5 mg once or twice daily; increase daily dose in 5 mg increments at weekly intervals until optimal response is obtained; usual maximum dose: 40 mg/day given in 1-3 divided doses per day. Use intervals of 4-6 hours between additional doses.

Adderall XR®: 5-10 mg once daily in the morning; if needed, may increase daily dose in 5-10 mg increments at weekly intervals (maximum dose: 30 mg/day)

Adolescents 13-17 years (Adderall XR®): 10 mg once daily in the morning; maybe increased to 20 mg/day after 1 week if symptoms are not controlled; higher doses (up to 60 mg)/day have been evaluated; however, there is not adequate evidence that higher doses afforded additional benefit.

Narcolepsy: *Adderall®*: Oral:

Children: 6-12 years: Initial: 5 mg/day; increase daily dose in 5 mg increments at weekly intervals until optimal response is obtained; maximum dose: 60 mg/day given in 1-3 divided doses per day with intervals of 4-6 hours between doses.

Children >12 years: Refer to adult dosing.

Administration

Oral

Adderall®: To avoid insomnia, last daily dose should be administered no less than 6 hours before retiring.

Adderall XR®: Should be given by noon. Capsule may be swallowed whole or it may be opened and the contents sprinkled on applesauce. Applesauce should be consumed immediately without chewing. Do not divide the contents of the capsule.

Stability

Storage Store at controlled room temperature of 15°C to 30°C (59°F to 86°F). Protect from light.

Monitoring and Teaching Issues

Physical Assessment See individual agents.

Patient Education See individual agents.

Geriatric Considerations This medication is considered to be potentially inappropriate in this patient population (Beers Criteria severity: High).

Pregnancy Considerations Use during pregnancy may lead to increased risk of premature delivery and low birth weight. Infants may experience symptoms of withdrawal. Teratogenic effects were reported when taken during the 1st trimester.

Additional Information Treatment of ADHD may include "drug holidays" or periodic discontinuation of medication in order to assess the patient's requirements, decrease tolerance, and limit suppression of linear growth and weight; the combination of equal parts of *d, l*-amphetamine aspartate, *d, l*-amphetamine sulfate, dextroamphetamine saccharate and dextroamphetamine sulfate results in a 75:25 ratio of the dextro and levo isomers of amphetamine.

The duration of action of Adderall® is longer than methylphenidate; behavioral effects of a single morning dose of Adderall® may last throughout the school day; a single morning dose of Adderall® has been shown in several studies to be as effective as twice daily dosing of methylphenidate for the treatment of ADHD (see Pelham et al, *Pediatrics*, 1999, 104(6):1300-11; Manos, 1999; Pliszka, 2000).

Related Information

Dextroamphetamine *on page 509*

◆ **Dextroamphetamine Sulfate** *see* Dextroamphetamine *on page 509*

Dextromethorphan and Chlorpheniramine

(deks troe meth OR fan & klor fen IR a meen)

U.S. Brand Names Coricidin® HBP Cough & Cold [OTC]; Dimetapp® Children's Long Acting Cough Plus Cold [OTC]; Robitussin® Children's Cough & Cold Long-Acting [OTC]; Robitussin® Cough & Cold Long-Acting [OTC]; Scot-Tussin® DM Maximum Strength [OTC]; Triaminic® Children's Softchews® Cough & Runny Nose [OTC]

Index Terms Chlorpheniramine and Dextromethorphan; Chlorpheniramine Maleate and Dextromethorphan Hydrobromide; Dextromethorphan Hydrobromide and Chlorpheniramine Maleate

Generic Availability (U.S.) No

Pharmacologic Category Alkylamine Derivative; Antitussive; Histamine H_1 Antagonist; Histamine H_1 Antagonist, First Generation

Use Symptomatic relief of runny nose, sneezing, itchy/watery eyes, cough, and other upper respiratory symptoms associated with hay fever, common cold, or upper respiratory allergies

Available Dosage Forms

Syrup:

Dimetapp® Children's Long Acting Cough Plus Cold [OTC]: Dextromethorphan 7.5 mg and chlorpheniramine 1 mg per 5 mL (118 mL)

Robitussin® Children's Cough and Cold Long-Acting [OTC]: Dextromethorphan 15 mg and chlorpheniramine 2 mg per 5 mL (118 mL)

Robitussin® Cough and Cold Long-Acting [OTC]: Dextromethorphan 15 mg and chlorpheniramine 2 mg per 5 mL (118 mL)

Scot-Tussin® DM Maximum Strength [OTC]: Dextromethorphan 15 mg and chlorpheniramine 2 mg per 5 mL (118 mL)

Tablet:

Coricidin® HBP Cough and Cold [OTC]: Dextromethorphan 30 mg and chlorpheniramine 4 mg

Tablet, softchew:

Triaminic® Children's Softchews® Cough & Runny Nose [OTC]: Dextromethorphan 5 mg and chlorpheniramine 1 mg

Dosing

Adult & Geriatric General dosing guidelines; consult specific product labeling.

Cough, cold symptoms: Oral: Dextromethorphan 30 mg and chlorpheniramine 4 mg every 6 hours as needed (maximum: 120 mg dextromethorphan and 16 mg chlorpheniramine/24 hours)

Pediatric General dosing guidelines; consult specific product labeling.

Cough, cold symptoms: Oral:

Children 6-11 years:

Liquid: Dextromethorphan 15 mg and chlorpheniramine 2 mg every 6 hours as needed (maximum: 60 mg dextromethorphan and 8 mg chlorpheniramine/24 hours)

Chewable tablet: Dextromethorphan 10 mg and chlorpheniramine 2 mg every 4-6 hours as needed (maximum: 50 mg dextromethorphan and 10 mg chlorpheniramine/24 hours)

Children ≥12 years: Refer to adult dosing.

Administration

Oral Triaminic® Children's Softchews® Cough & Runny Nose: Dissolve in mouth or chew prior to swallowing.

Dextromethorphan and Quinidine (deks troe meth OR fan & KWIN i deen)

U.S. Brand Names Nuedexta™

Index Terms Dextromethorphan Hydrobromide and Quinidine Sulfate; Quinidine and Dextromethorphan

Pharmacologic Category Antiarrhythmic Agent, Class Ia; N-Methyl-D-Aspartate Receptor Antagonist

Pregnancy Risk Factor C

Lactation Use caution

Use Treatment of pseudobulbar affect (PBA)

Available Dosage Forms

Capsule, oral:

Nuedexta™: Dextromethorphan hydrobromide 20 mg and quinidine sulfate 10 mg

Dosing

Adult Pseudobulbar affect: Oral: One capsule once daily for 7 days, then increase to 1 capsule twice daily; reassess patient periodically to determine if continued use is necessary

Renal Impairment Dose adjustment not required for mild or moderate renal impairment; not studied with severe impairment.

Hepatic Impairment Dose adjustment not required for mild or moderate hepatic impairment; however, an increase in adverse reactions is observed with moderate hepatic dysfunction; not studied with severe impairment.

Administration

Oral May be administered with or without food. Administer twice-daily doses every 12 hours.

Monitoring and Teaching Issues

Laboratory Monitoring Potassium and magnesium prior to and during therapy; CBC, liver and renal function tests

- ◆ **Dextromethorphan Hydrobromide and Chlorpheniramine Maleate** *see* Dextromethorphan and Chlorpheniramine *on page 513*
- ◆ **Dextromethorphan Hydrobromide and Quinidine Sulfate** *see* Dextromethorphan and Quinidine *on page 514*
- ◆ **Dextropropoxyphene** *see* Propoxyphene *on page 1522*
- ◆ **Dex-Tuss** *see* Guaifenesin and Codeine *on page 891*
- ◆ **Dezocitidine** *see* Decitabine *on page 476*
- ◆ **dFdC** *see* Gemcitabine *on page 855*
- ◆ **dFdCyd** *see* Gemcitabine *on page 855*
- ◆ **DHAD** *see* Mitoxantrone *on page 1244*
- ◆ **DHAQ** *see* Mitoxantrone *on page 1244*
- ◆ **DHE** *see* Dihydroergotamine *on page 535*
- ◆ **D.H.E. 45®** *see* Dihydroergotamine *on page 535*
- ◆ **DHPG Sodium** *see* Ganciclovir (Systemic) *on page 849*
- ◆ **Diabeta** *see* GlyBURIDE *on page 877*
- ◆ **DiaBeta®** *see* GlyBURIDE *on page 877*
- ◆ **DiabetAid® Antifungal Foot Bath [OTC]** *see* Miconazole (Topical) *on page 1224*
- ◆ **Diabetic Siltussin DAS-Na [OTC]** *see* GuaiFENesin *on page 890*
- ◆ **Diabetic Tussin® EX [OTC]** *see* GuaiFENesin *on page 890*
- ◆ **Diaminocyclohexane Oxalatoplatinum** *see* Oxaliplatin *on page 1370*
- ◆ **Diamode [OTC]** *see* Loperamide *on page 1126*
- ◆ **Diamox® Sequels®** *see* AcetaZOLAMIDE *on page 42*
- ◆ **Diastat®** *see* Diazepam *on page 514*
- ◆ **Diastat® AcuDial™** *see* Diazepam *on page 514*

Diazepam (dye AZ e pam)

U.S. Brand Names Diastat®; Diastat® AcuDial™; Diazepam Intensol™; Valium®

Generic Availability (U.S.) Yes

Pharmacologic Category Benzodiazepine

Medication Safety Issues

Sound-alike/look-alike issues:

Diazepam may be confused with diazoxide, diltiazem, Ditropan, LORazepam
Valium® may be confused with Valcyte®

Beers Criteria medication: This drug may be inappropriate for use in geriatric patients (high severity risk).

Pregnancy Risk Factor D

Lactation Enters breast milk/not recommended (AAP rates "of concern"; AAP 2001 update pending)

Use Management of anxiety disorders, ethanol withdrawal symptoms; skeletal muscle relaxant; treatment of convulsive disorders; preoperative or preprocedural sedation and amnesia

Rectal gel: Management of selected, refractory epilepsy patients on stable regimens of antiepileptic drugs requiring intermittent use of diazepam to control episodes of increased seizure activity

Unlabeled/Investigational Use Panic disorders; short-term treatment of spasticity in children with cerebral palsy

Mechanism of Action/Effect Binds to stereospecific benzodiazepine receptors on the postsynaptic GABA neuron at several sites within the central nervous system, including the limbic system, reticular formation. Enhancement of the inhibitory effect of GABA on neuronal excitability results by increased neuronal membrane permeability to chloride ions. This shift in chloride ions results in hyperpolarization (a less excitable state) and stabilization.

Contraindications Hypersensitivity to diazepam or any component of the formulation (cross-sensitivity with other benzodiazepines may exist); myasthenia gravis; severe respiratory insufficiency; severe hepatic insufficiency; sleep apnea syndrome; acute narrow-angle glaucoma; not for use in children <6 months of age (oral)

Warnings/Precautions Withdrawal has also been associated with an increase in the seizure frequency. Use with caution with drugs which may decrease diazepam metabolism. Use with caution in debilitated patients, obese patients, patients with hepatic disease (including alcoholics), or renal impairment. Active metabolites with extended half-lives may lead to delayed accumulation and adverse effects. Use with caution in patients with respiratory disease or impaired gag reflex.

Acute hypotension, muscle weakness, apnea, and cardiac arrest have occurred with parenteral administration. Acute effects may be more prevalent in patients receiving concurrent barbiturates, narcotics, or ethanol. Appropriate resuscitative equipment and qualified personnel should be available during administration and monitoring. Avoid use of the injection in patients with shock, coma, or acute ethanol intoxication. Intra-arterial injection or extravasation of the parenteral formulation should be avoided. Parenteral formulation contains propylene glycol, which has been associated with toxicity when administered in high dosages. Administration of rectal gel should only be performed by individuals trained to recognize characteristic seizure activity and monitor response.

Causes CNS depression (dose-related) resulting in sedation, dizziness, confusion, or ataxia which may impair physical and mental capabilities. Patients must be cautioned about performing tasks which require mental alertness (eg, operating machinery or driving). Use with caution in patients receiving other CNS depressants or psychoactive agents. Effects with other sedative drugs or ethanol may be potentiated. The dosage of narcotics should be reduced by approximately 1/3 when diazepam is added. Benzodiazepines have been associated with falls and traumatic injury and should be used with extreme caution in patients who are at risk of these events (especially the elderly). Benzodiazepines with long half-lives may produce prolonged sedation and increase the risk of falls and fracture. Short- or intermediate-acting benzodiazepines are preferred in elderly patients (Beers Criteria).

Use with caution in patients taking strong CYP3A4 inhibitors, moderate or strong CYP3A4 and CYP2C19 inducers and major CYP3A4 substrates.

Use caution in patients with depression or anxiety associated with depression, particularly if suicidal risk may be present. Use with caution in patients with a history of drug dependence. Benzodiazepines have been associated with dependence and acute withdrawal symptoms on discontinuation or reduction in dose. Acute withdrawal, including seizures, may be precipitated in patients after administration of flumazenil to patients receiving long-term benzodiazepine therapy.

Diazepam has been associated with anterograde amnesia. Psychiatric and paradoxical reactions, including hyperactive or aggressive behavior, have been reported with benzodiazepines, particularly in adolescent/pediatric or elderly patients. Does not have analgesic, antidepressant, or antipsychotic properties.

Rectal gel: Safety and efficacy have not been established in children <2 years of age.

Oral: Safety and efficacy have not been established in children <6 months of age.

Injection: Safety and efficacy have not been established in children <30 days of age. Solution for injection may contain sodium benzoate, benzyl alcohol, or benzoic acid. Large amounts have been associated with "gasping syndrome" in neonates.

Drug Interactions

Metabolism/Transport Effects Substrate of CYP1A2 (minor), 2B6 (minor), 2C9 (minor), 2C19 (major), 3A4 (major); **Inhibits** CYP2C19 (weak), 3A4 (weak)

Avoid Concomitant Use

Avoid concomitant use of Diazepam with any of the following: OLANZapine

Decreased Effect

The levels/effects of Diazepam may be decreased by: CarBAMazepine; CYP2C19 Inducers (Strong); CYP3A4 Inducers (Strong); Deferasirox; Rifamycin Derivatives; St Johns Wort; Theophylline Derivatives; Yohimbine

Increased Effect/Toxicity

Diazepam may increase the levels/effects of: Alcohol (Ethyl); CloZAPine; CNS Depressants; Methotrimeprazine; Phenytoin

The levels/effects of Diazepam may be increased by: Antifungal Agents (Azole Derivatives, Systemic); Aprepitant; Calcium Channel Blockers (Nondihydropyridine); Cimetidine; Conivaptan; Contraceptives (Estrogens); Contraceptives (Progestins); CYP2C19 Inhibitors (Moderate); CYP2C19 Inhibitors (Strong); CYP3A4 Inhibitors (Moderate); CYP3A4 Inhibitors

(Strong); Dasatinib; Disulfiram; Droperidol; Fluconazole; Fosamprenavir; Fosaprepitant; Grapefruit Juice; Isoniazid; Macrolide Antibiotics; Methotrimeprazine; Nefazodone; OLANZapine; Proton Pump Inhibitors; Ritonavir; Saquinavir; Selective Serotonin Reuptake Inhibitors

Nutritional/Ethanol Interactions

Ethanol: Avoid ethanol (may increase CNS depression).

Food: Diazepam serum concentrations may be increased if taken with food. Grapefruit juice may increase diazepam serum concentrations; avoid concurrent use.

Herb/Nutraceutical: St John's wort may decrease diazepam levels. Avoid valerian, St John's wort, kava kava, gotu kola (may increase CNS depression).

Lab Interactions False-negative urinary glucose determinations when using Clinistix® or Diastix®

Adverse Reactions Frequency not defined. Adverse reactions may vary by route of administration.

Cardiovascular: Hypotension, vasodilatation

Central nervous system: Amnesia, ataxia, confusion, depression, drowsiness, fatigue, headache, slurred speech, paradoxical reactions (eg, aggressiveness, agitation, anxiety, delusions, hallucinations, inappropriate behavior, increased muscle spasms, insomnia, irritability, psychoses, rage, restlessness, sleep disturbances, stimulation), vertigo

Dermatologic: Rash

Endocrine & metabolic: Libido changes

Gastrointestinal: Constipation, diarrhea, nausea, salivation changes (dry mouth or hypersalivation)

Genitourinary: Incontinence, urinary retention

Hepatic: Jaundice

Local: Phlebitis, pain with injection

Neuromuscular & skeletal: Dysarthria, tremor, weakness

Ocular: Blurred vision, diplopia

Respiratory: Apnea, asthma, respiratory rate decreased

Pharmacodynamics/Kinetics

Onset of Action I.V.: Status epilepticus: Almost immediate

Duration of Action I.V.: Status epilepticus: 20-30 minutes

Absorption Oral: 85% to 100%, more reliable than I.M.

Protein Binding 98%

Half-Life Elimination Parent drug: Adults: 20-50 hours; increased half-life in neonates, elderly, and those with severe hepatic disorders; Active major metabolite (desmethyldiazepam): 50-100 hours; may be prolonged in neonates

Metabolism Hepatic

Controlled Substance C-IV

Available Dosage Forms

Gel, rectal: 10 mg (2 mL); 20 mg (4 mL); 5 mg/mL (0.5 mL)

Diastat®: 5 mg/mL (0.5 mL)

Diastat® AcuDial™: 10 mg (2 mL); 20 mg (4 mL)

Injection, solution: 5 mg/mL (2 mL, 10 mL)

Solution, oral: 5 mg/5 mL (5 mL, 500 mL)

Diazepam Intensol™: 5 mg/mL (30 mL)

Tablet, oral: 2 mg, 5 mg, 10 mg

Valium®: 2 mg, 5 mg, 10 mg

Dosing

Adult Note: Oral absorption is more reliable than I.M.

Acute ethanol withdrawal: *Oral:* 10 mg 3-4 times during first 24 hours, then decrease to 5 mg 3-4 times/day as needed

Anticonvulsant (acute treatment): *Rectal gel:* 0.2 mg/kg. **Note:** Dosage should be rounded upward to the next available dose, 2.5, 5, 7.5, 10, 12.5, 15, 17.5, and 20 mg/dose; dose may be repeated in 4-12 hours if needed; do not use for more than 5 episodes per month or more than one episode every 5 days.

Anxiety (symptoms/disorders):

Oral: 2-10 mg 2-4 times/day

I.M., I.V.: 2-10 mg, may repeat in 3-4 hours if needed

Muscle spasm: *I.V., I.M.:* Initial: 5-10 mg; then 5-10 mg in 3-4 hours, if necessary. Larger doses may be required if associated with tetanus.

Sedation in the ICU patient: *I.V.:* 0.03-0.1 mg/kg every 30 minutes to 6 hours

Skeletal muscle relaxant (adjunct therapy): *Oral:* 2-10 mg 3-4 times/day

Status epilepticus:

I.V.: 5-10 mg every 5-10 minutes given over ≤5 mg/minute (maximum dose: 30 mg)

Rectal gel: Premonitory/out-of-hospital treatment: 10 mg once; may repeat once if necessary

Rapid tranquilization of agitated patient (administer every 30-60 minutes): *Oral:* 5-10 mg; average total dose for tranquilization: 20-60 mg

Geriatric Oral absorption is more reliable than I.M.. Elderly and/or debilitated patients:

Oral: 2-2.5 mg 1-2 times/day initially; increase gradually as needed and tolerated.

Rectal gel: Due to the increased half-life in elderly and debilitated patients, consider reducing dose.

Pediatric

Anticonvulsant (acute treatment): *Rectal gel:*

Children <2 years: Safety and efficacy have not been studied

Children 2-5 years: 0.5 mg/kg

Children 6-11 years: 0.3 mg/kg

Children ≥12 years: Refer to adult dosing.

Note: Dosage should be rounded upward to the next available dose, 2.5, 5, 7.5, 10, 12.5, 15, 17.5, and 20 mg/dose; dose may be repeated in 4-12 hours if needed; do not use for more than 5 episodes per month or more than one episode every 5 days.

Conscious sedation for procedures:

Oral:

Children: 0.2-0.3 mg/kg (maximum dose: 10 mg) 45-60 minutes prior to procedure

Adolescents: 10 mg

I.V.: Adolescents: 5 mg; may repeat with 2.5 mg if needed

Febrile seizure prophylaxis: *Oral:* Children: 1 mg/kg/day divided every 8 hours; initiate therapy at first sign of fever and continue for 24 hours after fever is gone

Muscle spasm associated with tetanus: *I.V., I.M.:*

Infants >30 days: 1-2 mg/dose every 3-4 hours as needed

Children ≥5 years: 5-10 mg/dose every 3-4 hours as needed

Sedation or muscle relaxation or anxiety:

Oral: Children: 0.12-0.8 mg/kg/day in divided doses every 6-8 hours

I.M., I.V.: Children: 0.04-0.3 mg/kg/dose every 2-4 hours to a maximum of 0.6 mg/kg within an 8-hour period if needed

Spasticity in cerebral palsy (unlabeled use): *Oral:* Dose should be individualized:

Children ≤5 years: <8.5 kg: 0.5-1 mg at bedtime; 8.5-15 kg: 1-2 mg at bedtime (Mathew, 2005)

Children 5-16 years: 1.25 mg 3 times daily to 5 mg 4 times daily (Engle, 1966)

Status epilepticus:

I.V.: Infants >30 days and Children: 0.1-0.3 mg/kg given over ≤5 mg/minute; may repeat dose after 5-10 minutes; maximum: 10 mg/dose (Hegenbarth, 2008)

Rectal: 0.5 mg/kg/dose then 0.25 mg/kg/dose in 10 minutes if needed (prepare dose using parenteral formulation)

Renal Impairment No dose adjustment recommended; decrease dose if administered for prolonged periods.

I.V.: Risk of propylene glycol toxicity; monitor closely if using for prolonged periods or at high doses.

Hemodialysis: Not dialyzable (0% to 5%); supplemental dose is not necessary.

Hepatic Impairment Use caution.

Administration

Oral Intensol™ should be diluted before use.

I.V. Continuous infusion is not recommended because of precipitation in I.V. fluids and absorption of drug into infusion bags and tubing. In children, do not exceed 1-2 mg/minute IVP; in adults 5 mg/minute.

Other Rectal gel: Prior to administration, confirm that prescribed dose is visible and correct, and that the green "ready" band is visible. Patient should be positioned on side (facing person responsible for monitoring), with top leg bent forward. Insert rectal tip (lubricated) into rectum and push in plunger gently over 3 seconds. Remove tip of rectal syringe after 3 additional seconds. Buttocks should be held together for 3 seconds after removal. Dispose of syringe appropriately.

Stability

Reconstitution Per manufacturer, do not mix I.V. product with other medications.

Storage

Injection: Store at 20° to 25°C (68° to 77°F); excursions permitted to 15°C to 30°C (59°F to 86°F). Protect from light. Potency is retained for up to 3 months when kept at room temperature. Most stable at pH 4-8; hydrolysis occurs at pH <3.

Rectal gel: Store at 25°C (77°F); excursion permitted to 15°C to 30°C (59°F to 86°F).

Tablet: Store at 15°C to 30°C (59°F to 86°F).

Monitoring and Teaching Issues

Physical Assessment Assess for history of addiction; long-term use can result in dependence, abuse, or tolerance; periodically evaluate need for continued use. Monitor blood pressure and CNS status. For inpatient use, institute safety measures to prevent falls. Taper dosage slowly when discontinuing. Teach patient seizure precautions (if administered for seizures).

Patient Education Drug may cause physical and/or psychological dependence. While using this medication, do not use alcohol. Maintain adequate hydration, unless instructed to restrict fluid intake. You may experience drowsiness, dizziness, blurred vision, nausea, vomiting, loss of appetite, dry mouth, or constipation. If medication is used to control seizures, wear identification that you are taking an antiepileptic medication. Report CNS changes (confusion, depression, excitation, insomnia, dizziness, fatigue, or impaired coordination) or changes in cognition, respiratory difficulty, or worsening of seizure activity or loss of seizure control.

Geriatric Considerations Due to its long-acting metabolite, diazepam is not considered a drug of choice in the elderly. Long-acting benzodiazepines have been associated with falls in the elderly. Interpretive guidelines from the Centers for Medicare and Medicaid Services (CMS) strongly discourage the use of this agent in residents of long-term care facilities.

This medication is considered to be potentially inappropriate in this patient population (Beers Criteria severity: High).

Breast-Feeding Considerations Diazepam and N-desmethyldiazepam can be found in breast milk; the oxazepam metabolite has also been detected in the urine of a nursing infant. Drowsiness, lethargy, or weight loss in nursing infants have been observed in case reports following maternal use of some benzodiazepines, including diazepam.

Pregnancy Considerations Teratogenic effects have been reported in animal studies. In humans, diazepam and its metabolites (N-desmethyldiazepam, temazepam, and oxazepam) cross the placenta. Teratogenic effects have been observed with diazepam; however, additional studies are needed. The incidence of premature birth and low birth weights may be increased following maternal use of benzodiazepines; hypoglycemia and respiratory problems in the neonate may occur following exposure late in pregnancy. Neonatal withdrawal symptoms may occur within days to weeks after birth and "floppy infant syndrome" (which also includes withdrawal symptoms) has been reported with some benzodiazepines (including diazepam).

Additional Information Diazepam does not have any analgesic effects.

Diastat® AcuDial™: When dispensing, consult package information for directions on setting patient's dose; confirm green "ready" band is visible prior to dispensing product.

Related Information

Benzodiazepines *on page 1988*

◆ **Diazepam Intensol™** *see* Diazepam *on page 514*

◆ **DIC** *see* Dacarbazine *on page 452*

Diclofenac (Systemic) (dye KLOE fen ak)

U.S. Brand Names Cambia™; Cataflam®; Voltaren®-XR; Zipsor™

Index Terms Diclofenac Potassium; Diclofenac Sodium

Generic Availability (U.S.) Yes: Excludes capsule, oral solution

Pharmacologic Category Nonsteroidal Anti-inflammatory Drug (NSAID); Nonsteroidal Anti-inflammatory Drug (NSAID), Oral

Medication Safety Issues

Sound-alike/look-alike issues:

Diclofenac may be confused with Diflucan®, Duphalac®

Cataflam® may be confused with Catapres®

Voltaren® may be confused with traMADol, Ultram®, Verelan®

International issues:

Flexin: Brand name for diclofenac [Argentina], but also the brand name for cyclobenzaprine [Chile] and orphenadirine [Israel]

Flexin [Argentina] may be confused with Floxin brand name for flunarizine [Thailand], norfloxacin [South Africa], ofloxacin [U.S., Canada], and perfloxacin [Philippines]; Fluoxin brand name for fluoxetine [Czech Republic]

Medication Guide Available Yes

Pregnancy Risk Factor C (oral)/D (≥30 weeks gestation [oral])

Lactation Excreted in breast milk/not recommended

Use

Capsule: Relief of mild-to-moderate acute pain

Immediate-release tablet: Ankylosing spondylitis; primary dysmenorrhea; acute and chronic treatment of rheumatoid arthritis, osteoarthritis

Delayed-release tablet: Acute and chronic treatment of rheumatoid arthritis, osteoarthritis, ankylosing spondylitis

Extended-release tablet: Chronic treatment of osteoarthritis, rheumatoid arthritis

Oral solution: Treatment of acute migraine with or without aura

Suppository (CAN; not available in U.S.): Symptomatic treatment of rheumatoid arthritis and osteoarthritis (including degenerative joint disease of hip)

Unlabeled/Investigational Use Juvenile idiopathic arthritis (JIA)

Mechanism of Action/Effect Reversibly inhibits cyclooxygenase-1 and 2 (COX-1 and 2) enzymes, which results in decreased formation of prostaglandin precursors; has antipyretic, analgesic, and anti-inflammatory properties

Contraindications Hypersensitivity to diclofenac or any component of the formulation; hypersensitivity to bovine protein (capsule formulation only); patients who exhibit asthma, urticaria, or other allergic-type reactions after taking aspirin or other NSAIDs; perioperative pain in the setting of coronary artery bypass graft (CABG) surgery

Canadian labeling: Additional contraindications (not in U.S. labeling): Uncontrolled heart failure, active gastric/duodenal/peptic ulcer; active GI bleed or perforation; regional ulcer, gastritis, or ulcerative colitis; cerebrovascular bleeding or other bleeding disorders; inflammatory bowel disease; severe hepatic impairment; active hepatic disease; severe renal impairment (Cl_{cr} <30 mL/minute) or deteriorating renal disease; known hyperkalemia; patients <16 years of age; breast-feeding; pregnancy (third trimester); use of diclofenac suppository if recent history of bleeding or inflammatory lesions of rectum/anus

Warnings/Precautions [U.S. Boxed Warning]: NSAIDs are associated with an increased risk of adverse cardiovascular thrombotic events, including MI and stroke. Risk may be increased with duration of use or pre-existing cardiovascular risk factors or disease. Carefully evaluate individual cardiovascular risk profiles prior to prescribing. May cause new-onset hypertension or worsening of existing hypertension. Monitor blood pressure closely. Use caution with fluid retention. Avoid use in heart failure. Concurrent administration of ibuprofen, and potentially other nonselective NSAIDs, may interfere with aspirin's cardioprotective effect. **[U.S. Boxed Warning]: Use is contraindicated for treatment of perioperative pain in the setting of coronary artery bypass graft (CABG) surgery.** Risk of MI and stroke may be increased with use following CABG surgery.

NSAID use may compromise existing renal function; dose-dependent decreases in prostaglandin synthesis may result from NSAID use, reducing renal blood flow which may cause renal decompensation. NSAID use may increase the risk for hyperkalemia. Patients with impaired renal function, dehydration, heart failure, liver dysfunction, those taking diuretics and ACEI, and the elderly are at greater risk of renal toxicity and hyperkalemia. Rehydrate patient before starting therapy; monitor renal function closely. Not recommended for use in patients with advanced renal disease. Long-term NSAID use may result in renal papillary necrosis while persistent urinary symptoms (eg, dysuria, bladder pain), cystitis, or hematuria may occur anytime after initiating NSAID therapy. Discontinue therapy with symptom onset and evaluate for origin.

[U.S. Boxed Warning]: NSAIDs may increase risk of gastrointestinal irritation, inflammation, ulceration, bleeding, and perforation. These events may occur at any time during therapy and without warning. Use caution with a history of GI disease (bleeding or ulcers), concurrent therapy with aspirin, anticoagulants and/or corticosteroids, smoking, use of alcohol, the elderly or debilitated patients. When used concomitantly with ≤325 mg of aspirin, a substantial increase in the risk of gastrointestinal complications (eg, ulcer) occurs; concomitant gastroprotective therapy (eg, proton pump inhibitors) is recommended (Bhatt, 2008).

Use the lowest effective dose for the shortest duration of time, consistent with individual patient goals, to reduce risk of cardiovascular or GI adverse events. Alternate therapies should be considered for patients at high risk.

NSAIDs may cause photosensitivity or serious skin adverse events including exfoliative dermatitis, Stevens-Johnson syndrome (SJS), and toxic epidermal necrolysis (TEN); discontinue use at first sign of skin rash or hypersensitivity. Anaphylactoid reactions may occur, even without prior exposure; patients with "aspirin triad" (bronchial asthma, aspirin intolerance, rhinitis) may be at increased risk. Do not use in patients who experience bronchospasm, asthma, rhinitis, or urticaria with NSAID or aspirin therapy. Use caution in other forms of asthma. Platelet adhesion and aggregation may be decreased; may prolong bleeding time; patients with coagulation disorders or who are receiving anticoagulants should be monitored closely. Anemia may occur; patients on long-term NSAID therapy should be monitored for anemia. Rarely, NSAID use may cause severe blood dyscrasias (eg, agranulocytosis, aplastic anemia, thrombocytopenia).

Use with caution in patients with impaired hepatic function. Closely monitor patients with any abnormal LFT. Diclofenac can cause transaminase elevations; initiate monitoring 4-8 weeks into therapy. Rarely, severe hepatic reactions (eg, fulminant hepatitis, liver failure) have occurred; discontinue all formulations if signs or symptoms of liver disease develop, or if systemic manifestations occur. Use with caution in hepatic porphyria (may trigger attack).

NSAIDS may cause drowsiness, dizziness, blurred vision, and other neurologic effects which may impair physical or mental abilities; patients must be cautioned about performing tasks which require mental alertness (eg, operating machinery or driving). Discontinue use with blurred or diminished vision and perform ophthalmologic exam. Monitor vision with long-term therapy. The elderly are at increased risk for adverse effects (especially peptic ulceration, CNS effects, and renal toxicity) from NSAIDs even at low doses. May increase the risk of aseptic meningitis, especially in patients with systemic lupus erythematosus (SLE) and mixed connective tissue disorders.

Withhold for at least 4-6 half-lives prior to surgical or dental procedures. Safety and efficacy have not been established in children.

Capsule: Contains gelatin; use is contraindicated in patients with history of hypersensitivity to bovine protein.

Oral solution: Only indicated for the acute treatment of migraine; not indicated for migraine prophylaxis or cluster headache. Not bioequivalent to other forms of diclofenac (even same dose); do not interchange products. Contains phenylalanine.

Drug Interactions

Metabolism/Transport Effects Substrate (minor) of CYP1A2, 2B6, 2C8, 2C9, 2C19, 2D6, 3A4; **Inhibits** CYP1A2 (moderate), 2C9 (weak), 2E1 (weak), 3A4 (weak)

Avoid Concomitant Use

Avoid concomitant use of Diclofenac (Systemic) with any of the following: Ketorolac; Ketorolac (Systemic)

Decreased Effect

Diclofenac (Systemic) may decrease the levels/effects of: ACE Inhibitors; Angiotensin II Receptor Blockers; Antiplatelet Agents; Beta-Blockers; Eplerenone; HydrALAZINE; Loop Diuretics; Potassium-Sparing Diuretics; Salicylates; Thiazide Diuretics

The levels/effects of Diclofenac (Systemic) may be decreased by: Bile Acid Sequestrants; Nonsteroidal Anti-Inflammatory Agents; Peginterferon Alfa-2b; Salicylates

Increased Effect/Toxicity

Diclofenac (Systemic) may increase the levels/effects of: Aminoglycosides; Anticoagulants; Antiplatelet Agents; Bisphosphonate Derivatives; Collagenase (Systemic); CycloSPORINE; CycloSPORINE (Systemic); CYP1A2 Substrates; Desmopressin; Digoxin; Drotrecogin Alfa; Eplerenone; Haloperidol; Ibritumomab; Lithium; Methotrexate; Nonsteroidal Anti-Inflammatory Agents; PEMEtrexed; Potassium-Sparing Diuretics; PRALAtrexate; Quinolone Antibiotics; Salicylates; Thrombolytic Agents; Tositumomab and Iodine I 131 Tositumomab; Vancomycin; Vitamin K Antagonists

The levels/effects of Diclofenac (Systemic) may be increased by: Antidepressants (Tricyclic, Tertiary Amine); Conivaptan; Corticosteroids (Systemic); Dasatinib; Glucosamine; Herbs (Anticoagulant/Antiplatelet Properties); Ketorolac; Ketorolac (Systemic); Nonsteroidal Anti-Inflammatory Agents; Omega-3-Acid Ethyl Esters; Pentosan Polysulfate Sodium; Pentoxifylline; Probenecid; Prostacyclin Analogues; Selective Serotonin Reuptake Inhibitors; Serotonin/Norepinephrine Reuptake Inhibitors; Treprostinil; Voriconazole

Nutritional/Ethanol Interactions

Ethanol: Avoid ethanol (may enhance gastric mucosal irritation).

Herb/Nutraceutical: Avoid alfalfa, anise, bilberry, bladderwrack, bromelain, cat's claw, celery, chamomile, coleus, cordyceps, dong quai, evening primrose, fenugreek, feverfew, garlic, ginger, ginkgo biloba, grapeseed, green tea, ginseng (Siberian), guggul, horse chestnut, horseradish, licorice, prickly ash, red clover, reishi, SAMe (s-adenosylmethionine), sweet clover, turmeric, white willow (all have additional antiplatelet activity).

Adverse Reactions

Oral:

1% to 10%:

Cardiovascular: Edema
Central nervous system: Dizziness, headache
Dermatologic: Pruritus, rash
Endocrine & metabolic: Fluid retention
Gastrointestinal: Abdominal distension, abdominal pain, constipation, diarrhea, dyspepsia, flatulence, GI perforation, heartburn, nausea, peptic ulcer/GI bleed, vomiting
Hematologic: Anemia, bleeding time increased
Hepatic: Liver enzyme abnormalities (>3 x ULN; ≤4%)
Otic: Tinnitus
Renal: Renal function abnormal
Miscellaneous: Diaphoresis increased

Rectal suppository (CAN; not available in U.S.): Also refer to adverse reactions associated with oral formulations.

Pharmacodynamics/Kinetics

Onset of Action

Cataflam® is more rapid than sodium salt (Voltaren®) because it dissolves in the stomach instead of the duodenum

Suppository: more rapid onset, but slower rate of absorption when compared to enteric coated tablet

Bioavailability 55%

Time to Peak Serum: Cambia™: ~0.25 hours; Cataflam®: ~1 hour; Voltaren®: ~2 hours; Voltaren® XR ~5 hours; Zipsor™: ~0.5 hour; Suppository: ≤1 hour. **Note:** Suppository: C_{max}: Approximately two-thirds of that observed with enteric coated tablet (equivalent 50 mg dose).

Protein Binding >99%, primarily to albumin

Half-Life Elimination ~2 hours

Metabolism Hepatic; undergoes first-pass metabolism; forms several metabolites (1 with weak activity)

Excretion Urine (~65%); feces (~35%)

Available Dosage Forms

Capsule, liquid filled, oral:
Zipsor™: 25 mg

Powder for solution, oral:
Cambia™: 50 mg/packet (1s)

Tablet, oral: 50 mg
Cataflam®: 50 mg

Tablet, delayed release, enteric coated, oral: 25 mg, 50 mg, 75 mg

Tablet, extended release, oral: 100 mg
Voltaren®-XR: 100 mg

Dosing

Adult

Analgesia: Oral:

Immediate release tablet: Starting dose: 50 mg 3 times/day (maximum dose: 150 mg/day); may administer 100 mg loading dose, followed by 50 mg every 8 hours (maximum dose day 1: 200 mg/day; maximum dose day 2 and thereafter: 150 mg/day)

Immediate release capsule: 25 mg 4 times/day

Primary dysmenorrhea: Oral: Immediate release tablet: Starting dose: 50 mg 3 times/day (maximum dose: 150 mg/day); may administer 100 mg loading dose, followed by 50 mg every 8 hours (maximum dose day 1: 200 mg/day; maximum dose day 2 and thereafter: 150 mg/day)

Rheumatoid arthritis:

Oral: Immediate or delayed release tablet: 150-200 mg/day in 2-4 divided doses; Extended release tablet: 100-200 mg/day

Canadian labeling: 150 mg/day in 3 divided doses (75-150 mg/day of slow release tablet)

Rectal suppository (not available in U.S.): *Canadian labeling:* Insert 50 mg or 100 mg rectally as single dose to substitute for final (third) oral daily dose (maximum combined dose [rectal and oral]: 150 mg/day

Osteoarthritis:

Oral: Immediate or delayed release tablet: 100-150 mg/day in 2-3 divided doses; Extended release tablet: 100 mg/day

Canadian labeling: 150 mg/day in 3 divided doses (75-150 mg/day of slow release tablet)

Rectal suppository (not available in U.S.): *Canadian labeling:* Insert 50 mg or 100 mg rectally as single dose to substitute for final (third) oral daily dose (maximum combined dose [rectal and oral]: 150 mg/day

Ankylosing spondylitis: Oral: Delayed release tablet: 100-125 mg/day in 4-5 divided doses

Migraine: Oral: Oral solution: 50 mg (one packet) as a single dose at the time of migraine onset; safety and efficacy of a second dose have not been established.

Geriatric Refer to adult dosing. No specific dosing recommendations; elderly may demonstrate adverse effects at lower doses than younger adults, and >60% may develop asymptomatic peptic ulceration with or without hemorrhage; monitor renal function.

Renal Impairment Not recommended in patients with advanced renal disease or significant renal impairment.

Hepatic Impairment May require dosage adjustment; use oral solution only if benefits outweigh risks.

Administration

Oral Do not crush tablets. Administer with food or milk to avoid gastric distress. Take with full glass of water to enhance absorption.

Oral solution: Empty contents of packet into 1-2 ounces (30-60 mL) of water (do not use other liquids), mix well and administer immediately; food may reduce effectiveness.

Other Rectal suppository: Remove entire plastic wrapping prior to inserting rectally.

Stability

Storage

Capsule, oral solution: Store at 25°C (77°F); excursions permitted to 15°C to 30°C (59°F to 86°F). Protect from moisture.

Suppository (CAN; not available in U.S.): Store at 15°C to 30°C (59°F to 86°F); protect from heat.

Tablet: Store below 30°C (86°F). Protect from moisture; store in tight container.

Monitoring and Teaching Issues

Laboratory Monitoring CBC, liver enzymes (periodically during chronic therapy starting 4-8 weeks after initiation); urine output and BUN/serum creatinine, occult blood loss

Physical Assessment Evaluate cardiac risk and potential for GI bleeding prior to prescribing this medication. Monitor blood pressure at the beginning of therapy and periodically during use. Schedule ophthalmic evaluations for patients who develop eye complaints during long-term NSAID therapy.

Patient Education Do not crush or chew tablets. Take with 8 oz of water, along with food or milk products to reduce GI distress. Avoid alcohol. You may experience dizziness, nervousness, headache, nausea, vomiting, dry mouth, heartburn, or constipation; GI bleeding, ulceration, or perforation can occur with or without pain; discontinue medication and contact prescriber if persistent abdominal pain or cramping or blood in stool occurs. Report chest pain or palpitations; respiratory difficulty; bruising/bleeding or blood in urine, stool, mouth, or vomitus; unusual fatigue; skin rash or itching; jaundice, unusual weight gain, or swelling of extremities; change in vision or ringing in ears.

Dietary Considerations Oral formulations may be taken with food to decrease GI distress. Food may reduce effectiveness of oral solution. Some products may contain phenylalanine. Diclofenac potassium = Cataflam®; potassium content: 5.8 mg (0.15 mEq) per 50 mg tablet

Geriatric Considerations Elderly are a high-risk population for adverse effects from nonsteroidal anti-inflammatory agents. As much as 60% of the elderly can develop peptic ulceration and/or hemorrhage asymptomatically. The concomitant use of H_2 blockers and sucralfate is not effective as prophylaxis with the exception of NSAID-induced duodenal ulcers which may be prevented by the use of ranitidine. Misoprostol and proton pump inhibitors are the only agents proven to help prevent the development of NSAID-induced ulcers. Also, concomitant disease and drug use contribute to the risk for GI adverse effects. Use lowest effective dose for shortest period possible. Consider renal function decline with age. Use of NSAIDs can compromise existing renal function especially when Cl_{cr} is ≤30 mL/minute. CNS adverse effects such as confusion, agitation, and hallucination are generally seen in overdose or high dose situations, but elderly may demonstrate these adverse effects at lower doses than younger adults.

Breast-Feeding Considerations Low concentrations of diclofenac can be found in breast milk. Breast-feeding is not recommended by the manufacturer. Use while breast-feeding is contraindicated in Canadian labeling.

Pregnancy Considerations Adverse events were not observed in the initial animal reproduction studies; therefore, manufacturers classify most dosage forms of diclofenac as pregnancy category C (oral: category D ≥30 weeks gestation). Diclofenac crosses the placenta and can be detected in fetal tissue and amniotic fluid. NSAID exposure during the first trimester is not strongly associated with congenital malformations; however, cardiovascular anomalies and cleft palate have been observed following NSAID exposure in some studies. The use of a NSAID close to conception may be associated with an increased risk of miscarriage. Nonteratogenic effects have been observed following NSAID administration during the third trimester including: Myocardial degenerative changes, prenatal constriction of the ductus arteriosus, fetal tricuspid regurgitation, failure of the ductus arteriosus to close postnatally; renal dysfunction or failure, oligohydramnios; gastrointestinal bleeding or perforation, increased risk of necrotizing enterocolitis; intracranial bleeding (including intraventricular hemorrhage), platelet dysfunction with resultant bleeding; pulmonary hypertension. Because they may cause premature closure of the ductus arteriosus, use of NSAIDs late in pregnancy should be avoided (use after 31 or 32 weeks gestation is not recommended by some clinicians). Product labeling for Zipsor™ specifically notes that use at ≥30 weeks gestation should be avoided and, therefore, classifies diclofenac as pregnancy category D at this time. Use in the third trimester is contraindicated in the Canadian labeling. The chronic use of NSAIDs in women of reproductive age may be associated with infertility that is reversible upon discontinuation of the medication. A registry is available for pregnant women exposed to autoimmune medications including diclofenac. For additional information contact the Organization of Teratology Information Specialists, OTIS Autoimmune Diseases Study, at 877-311-8972

Related Information

Nonsalicylate / Nonsteroidal Anti-Inflammatory Agents *on page* 2002

Diclofenac (Topical) (dye KLOE fen ak)

U.S. Brand Names Flector®; Pennsaid®; Solaraze®; Voltaren® Gel

Index Terms Diclofenac Diethylamine [CAN]; Diclofenac Epolamine; Diclofenac Sodium

Generic Availability (U.S.) No

Pharmacologic Category Nonsteroidal Anti-inflammatory Drug (NSAID); Nonsteroidal Anti-inflammatory Drug (NSAID), Topical

Medication Safety Issues

Sound-alike/look-alike issues:

Diclofenac may be confused with Diflucan®, Duphalac®

Voltaren® may be confused with traMADol, Ultram®, Verelan®

International issues:

Flexin: Brand name for diclofenac [Argentina], but also the brand name for cyclobenzaprine [Chile] and orphenadirine [Israel]

Flexin [Argentina] may be confused with Floxin brand name for flunarizine [Thailand], norfloxacin [South Africa], ofloxacin [U.S., Canada], and perfloxacin [Philippines]; Fluoxin brand name for fluoxetine [Czech Republic]

Transdermal patch (Flector®) contains conducting metal (eg, aluminum); remove patch prior to MRI.

Medication Guide Available Yes

Pregnancy Risk Factor B (topical gel 3%); C (topical gel 1%, topical solution, topical patch) D (topical solution ≥30 weeks gestation)

Lactation Not recommended

Use

Topical gel 1%: Relief of osteoarthritis pain in joints amenable to topical therapy (eg, ankle, elbow, foot, hand, knee, wrist)

Canadian labeling (not in U.S. labeling): Relief of pain associated with acute, localized joint/ muscle injuries (eg, sports injuries, strains) in patients ≥16 years of age

Topical gel 3%: Actinic keratosis (AK) in conjunction with sun avoidance

Topical patch: Acute pain due to minor strains, sprains, and contusions

Topical solution: Relief of osteoarthritis pain of the knee

Available Dosage Forms

Gel, topical:

Solaraze®: 3% (100 g)

Voltaren® Gel: 1% (100 g)

Patch, transdermal:

Flector®: 1.3% (30s)

Solution, topical:

Pennsaid®: 1.5% (150 mL)

Dosing

Adult

Osteoarthritis:

Topical gel (Voltaren®): **Note:** Maximum total body dose of 1% gel should not exceed 32 g per day

Lower extremities: Apply 4 g of 1% gel to affected area 4 times daily (maximum: 16 g per joint per day)

Upper extremities: Apply 2 g of 1% gel to affected area 4 times daily (maximum: 8 g per joint per day)

Topical solution: Apply 40 drops to each affected knee(s) 4 times daily

Actinic keratosis (AK): Topical (Solaraze® Gel): Apply 3% gel to lesion area twice daily for 60-90 days

Acute pain (strains, sprains, contusions): Topical:

Patch: Apply 1 patch twice daily to most painful area of skin

Gel (Voltaren® Emulgel™ [CAN; not available in U.S.]): Apply to affected area(s) of skin 3 or 4 times daily for up to 7 days

Geriatric Refer to adult dosing. No specific dosing recommendations; elderly may demonstrate adverse effects at lower doses than younger adults, and >60% may develop asymptomatic peptic ulceration with or without hemorrhage; monitor renal function.

Administration

Topical

Topical gel: Do not cover with occlusive dressings or apply sunscreens, cosmetics, lotions, moisturizers, insect repellents or other topical medications to affected area. Do not wash area for 1 hour following application. Wash hands immediately after application (unless hands are treated joint). Avoid sunlight to exposure areas.

1% formulation: Apply gel to affected area or joint and rub into skin gently, making sure to apply to entire affected area or joint.

3% formulation: Apply to lesion with gel and smooth into skin gently.

Topical solution: Apply to clean, dry, intact skin; do not apply to eyes, mucous membranes, or open wounds. Wash hands before and after use. Apply 10 drops at a time directly onto knee or into hand then onto knee (helps avoid spillage). Spread evenly around knee (front, back, sides). Allow knee to dry before applying clothing. Do not shower or bathe for at least 30 minutes after applying. Do not apply heat or occlusive dressing to treated knee; protect treated knee from sunlight. Cosmetics, insect repellant, lotion, moisturizer, sunscreens, or other topical medication may be applied to treated knee once solution has dried.

Transdermal patch: Apply to intact, nondamaged skin. Remove transparent liner prior to applying to skin. Wash hands after applying as well as after removal of patch. May tape down edges of patch, if peeling occurs. Should not be worn while bathing or showering. Fold used patches so the adhesive side sticks to itself; dispose of used patches out of reach of children and pets.

Monitoring and Teaching Issues

Laboratory Monitoring CBC, liver enzymes (periodically during chronic therapy starting 4-8 weeks after initiation), BUN/serum creatinine; monitor urine output; occult blood loss

Patient Education

Gel: This preparation is for topical use only. Use at regular intervals. Wash hands before and after use. Gently apply enough of the gel to cover the lesion. Do not wrap skin where applied in airtight or occlusive dressing. Advise prescriber if you are using any other skin preparations. Avoid direct sunlight and sunlamps while using this medication. You may experience dry skin, itching, peeling, swelling, or tingling at site of application. If severe skin reaction develops, stop applications and notify your prescriber at once.

Transdermal patch: Remove patch prior to MRI. Do not wear during bathing or showering. Apply to clear, healthy skin, avoiding eyes and mucous membranes.

Diclofenac and Misoprostol (dye KLOE fen ak & mye soe PROST ole)

U.S. Brand Names Arthrotec®

Index Terms Misoprostol and Diclofenac

Generic Availability (U.S.) No

Pharmacologic Category Nonsteroidal Anti-inflammatory Drug (NSAID), Oral; Prostaglandin

Medication Guide Available Yes

Pregnancy Risk Factor X

Lactation Enters breast milk/use caution

Use Treatment of osteoarthritis and rheumatoid arthritis in patients at high risk for NSAID-induced gastric and duodenal ulceration

Available Dosage Forms

Tablet:

Arthrotec® 50: Diclofenac 50 mg and misoprostol 200 mcg

Arthrotec® 75: Diclofenac 75 mg and misoprostol 200 mcg

Dosing

Adult & Geriatric

Osteoarthritis: Oral: Arthotec® 50: 1 tablet 3 times/day

Rheumatoid arthritis: Oral: Arthotec® 50: 1 tablet 3 or 4 times/day

Note: For both indications, may administer Arthrotec® 50 or Arthrotec® 75 one tablet twice daily if recommended dose is not tolerated; however, these options are less effective in preventing GI ulceration. May adjust dose using individual agents in combination with Arthrotec®. The maximum daily dose of misoprostal is 800 mcg and the maximum single dose of misoprostal is 200 mcg. The maximum daily dose of diclofenac is 150 mg/day (osteoarthritis) or 225 mg/day (rheumatoid arthritis).

Renal Impairment Not recommended for use in patients with advanced renal disease. In renal insufficiency, diclofenac should be used with caution due to potential detrimental effects on renal function, and misoprostol dosage reduction may be required if adverse effects occur (misoprostol is renally eliminated).

Hepatic Impairment May require dosage adjustment.

Administration

Oral Incidence of diarrhea may be lessened by having patient take dose right after meals and avoiding magnesium containing antacids. Tablets should not be crushed or chewed. Therapy is usually begun on the second or third day of the next normal menstrual period in women of child bearing potential.

Monitoring and Teaching Issues

Laboratory Monitoring CBC, liver enzymes (periodically during chronic therapy starting 4-8 weeks after initiation), urine output and BUN/serum creatinine in patients receiving diuretics, occult blood loss

Physical Assessment See individual agents.

Patient Education See individual agents.

Related Information

Diclofenac (Systemic) *on page 518*

Misoprostol *on page 1242*

◆ **Diclofenac Diethylamine [CAN]** *see* Diclofenac (Topical) *on page 522*

◆ **Diclofenac Epolamine** *see* Diclofenac (Topical) *on page 522*

◆ **Diclofenac Potassium** *see* Diclofenac (Systemic) *on page 518*

◆ **Diclofenac Sodium** *see* Diclofenac (Systemic) *on page 518*

◆ **Diclofenac Sodium** *see* Diclofenac (Topical) *on page 522*

Dicloxacillin (dye kloks a SIL in)

Index Terms Dicloxacillin Sodium
Generic Availability (U.S.) Yes
Pharmacologic Category Antibiotic, Penicillin
Pregnancy Risk Factor B
Lactation Excretion in breast milk unknown/use caution
Use Treatment of systemic infections such as pneumonia, skin and soft tissue infections, and osteomyelitis caused by penicillinase-producing staphylococci
Available Dosage Forms
Capsule, oral: 250 mg, 500 mg
Dosing
Adult & Geriatric
Susceptible infections: Oral: 125-500 mg every 6 hours
Erysipelas, furunculosis, mastitis, otitis externa, septic bursitis, skin abscess: Oral: 500 mg every 6 hours
Impetigo: 250 mg every 6 hours
Prosthetic joint (long-term suppression therapy): Oral: 250 mg twice daily
Staphylococcus aureus**, methicillin susceptible infection if no I.V. access:** Oral: 500-1000 mg every 6-8 hours
Pediatric Use in newborns is not recommended.
Susceptible infections: Oral:
Children <40 kg: 12.5-25 mg/kg/day divided every 6 hours; doses of 50-100 mg/kg/day in divided doses every 6 hours have been used for therapy of osteomyelitis
Children >40 kg: 125-250 mg every 6 hours
Furunculosis: Oral: 25-50 mg/kg/day divided every 6 hours
Osteomyelitis: Oral: 50-100 mg/kg/day in divided doses every 6 hours
Renal Impairment
Dosage adjustment is not necessary.
Not dialyzable (0% to 5%); supplemental dose is not necessary.
Peritoneal dialysis effects: Supplemental dose is not necessary.
Continuous arteriovenous or venovenous hemofiltration: Supplemental dose is not necessary.
Administration
Oral Administer 1 hour before or 2 hours after meals. Administer around-the-clock to promote less variation in peak and trough serum levels.
Monitoring and Teaching Issues
Laboratory Monitoring Perform culture and sensitivity studies prior to initiating therapy.
Physical Assessment Assess allergy history prior to beginning therapy.
Patient Education Take medication with a large glass of water 1 hour before or 2 hours after meals. Take at regular intervals around-the-clock. May cause some gastric distress and diarrhea. Report fever, vaginal itching, persistent diarrhea, sores in the mouth, loose foul-smelling stools, yellowing of skin or eyes, or change in color of urine or stool.

◆ **Dicloxacillin Sodium** *see* Dicloxacillin *on page 524*

Didanosine (dye DAN oh seen)

U.S. Brand Names Videx®; Videx® EC
Index Terms ddI; Dideoxyinosine
Generic Availability (U.S.) Yes: Delayed release capsule
Pharmacologic Category Antiretroviral Agent, Reverse Transcriptase Inhibitor (Nucleoside)
Medication Safety Issues
Sound-alike/look-alike issues:
Videx® may be confused with Lidex®
Medication Guide Available Yes
Pregnancy Risk Factor B
Lactation Excretion in breast milk unknown/contraindicated
Use Treatment of HIV infection; always to be used in combination with at least two other antiretroviral agents
Mechanism of Action/Effect Didanosine, a purine nucleoside (adenosine) analog and the deamination product of dideoxyadenosine (ddA), inhibits HIV replication *in vitro* in both T cells and monocytes. Didanosine is converted within the cell to the mono-, di-, and triphosphates of ddA. These ddA triphosphates act as substrate and inhibitor of HIV reverse transcriptase substrate and inhibitor of HIV reverse transcriptase thereby blocking viral DNA synthesis and suppressing HIV replication.
Contraindications Concurrent administration with allopurinol or ribavirin
Warnings/Precautions [U.S. Boxed Warning]: Pancreatitis (sometimes fatal) has been reported; incidence is dose related. Risk factors for developing pancreatitis may include a previous history of the condition, concurrent cytomegalovirus or *Mycobacterium avium-intracellulare* infection, renal impairment, advanced age, and concomitant use of stavudine,

pentamidine, or hydroxyurea. Discontinue didanosine if clinical signs of pancreatitis occur. **[U.S. Boxed Warning]: Lactic acidosis, symptomatic hyperlactatemia, and severe hepatomegaly with steatosis (sometimes fatal) have occurred with antiretroviral nucleoside analogues, including didanosine.** Hepatotoxicity may occur even in the absence of marked transaminase elevations; suspend therapy in any patient developing clinical/laboratory findings which suggest hepatotoxicity. Hepatotoxicity and hepatic failure (including fatal cases) have been reported in HIV patients receiving combination drug therapy with didanosine and stavudine or hydroxyurea, or didanosine, stavudine, and hydroxyurea; avoid these combinations. Not currently recommended in combination with tenofovir due to failure and resistance. Noncirrhotic portal hypertension may develop within months to years of starting didanosine therapy. Signs may include elevated liver enzymes, esophageal varices, hematemesis, ascites, and splenomegaly. Noncirrhotic portal hypertension may lead to liver failure and/or death. Discontinue use in patients with evidence of this condition. Pregnant women may be at increased risk of lactic acidosis and liver damage. Use with caution in patients with hepatic impairment; safety and efficacy have not been established in patients with significant hepatic disease. Patients on combination antiretroviral therapy with hepatic impairment may be at increased risk of potentially severe and fatal hepatic toxicity; consider interruption or discontinuation of therapy if hepatic impairment worsens.

Peripheral neuropathy occurs in ~20% of patients receiving the drug. If symptomatic, discontinue therapy; after resolution of symptoms, reinitiation of therapy at a reduced dose may be tolerated. Permanently discontinue if neuropathy recurs. Retinal changes (including retinal depigmentation) and optic neuritis have been reported in adults and children using didanosine. Patients should undergo retinal examination every 6-12 months. Use caution in renal impairment; dose reduction recommended for Cl_{cr} <60 mL/minute. May cause redistribution of fat (eg, buffalo hump, peripheral wasting with increased abdominal girth, cushingoid appearance). Patients may develop immune reconstitution syndrome resulting in the occurrence of an inflammatory response to an indolent or residual opportunistic infection; further evaluation and treatment may be required. Didanosine delayed release capsules are indicated for once-daily use.

Drug Interactions

Avoid Concomitant Use

Avoid concomitant use of Didanosine with any of the following: Alcohol (Ethyl); Allopurinol; Febuxostat; Hydroxyurea; Ribavirin; Tenofovir

Decreased Effect

Didanosine may decrease the levels/effects of: Antifungal Agents (Azole Derivatives, Systemic); Atazanavir; Indinavir; Quinolone Antibiotics

The levels/effects of Didanosine may be decreased by: Atazanavir; Darunavir; Lopinavir; Methadone; Tenofovir; Tipranavir

Increased Effect/Toxicity

Didanosine may increase the levels/effects of: Hydroxyurea

The levels/effects of Didanosine may be increased by: Alcohol (Ethyl); Allopurinol; Febuxostat; Ganciclovir-Valganciclovir; Hydroxyurea; Ribavirin; Stavudine; Tenofovir

Nutritional/Ethanol Interactions

Ethanol: Avoid ethanol (increases risk of pancreatitis).

Food: Decreases AUC and C_{max}. Didanosine serum levels may be decreased by 55% if taken with food.

Adverse Reactions As reported in monotherapy studies; risk of toxicity may increase when combined with other agents.

>10%:

Gastrointestinal: Diarrhea (19% to 28%), amylase increased (15% to 17%), abdominal pain (7% to 13%)

Neuromuscular & skeletal: Peripheral neuropathy (17% to 20%)

1% to 10%:

Dermatologic: Rash/pruritus (7% to 9%)

Endocrine & metabolic: Uric acid increased (2% to 3%)

Gastrointestinal: Pancreatitis (1% to 7% dose dependent); patients >65 years of age had a higher frequency of pancreatitis than younger patients patients (10% vs 5% in younger patients)

Hepatic: AST increased (7% to 9%), ALT increased (6% to 9%), alkaline phosphatase increased (1% to 4%)

Pharmacodynamics/Kinetics

Absorption Subject to degradation by acidic pH of stomach; some formulations are buffered to resist acidic pH; ≤55% reduction in peak plasma concentration is observed in presence of food. Delayed release capsules contain enteric-coated beadlets which dissolve in the small intestine.

Bioavailability Children: 25%; Adults: 42%

Time to Peak Delayed release capsules: 2 hours; Powder for suspension: 0.25-1.5 hours

Protein Binding <5%

Half-Life Elimination

Children and Adolescents: 0.8 hour

Adults: Normal renal function: 1.5 hours; however, active metabolite, ddATP, has an intracellular half-life >12 hours *in vitro*; Renal impairment: 2.5-5 hours

Metabolism Has not been evaluated in humans; studies conducted in dogs, show extensive metabolism with allantoin, hypoxanthine, xanthine, and uric acid being the major metabolites found in urine

Excretion Urine (~55% as unchanged drug)
Clearance: Total body: Averages 800 mL/minute

Available Dosage Forms

Capsule, delayed release, enteric coated beadlets, oral: 125 mg, 200 mg, 250 mg, 400 mg
Videx® EC: 125 mg, 200 mg, 250 mg, 400 mg

Capsule, delayed release, enteric coated pellets, oral: 200 mg, 250 mg, 400 mg

Powder for solution, oral:
Videx®: 2 g/bottle, 4 g/bottle

Dosing

Adult Treatment of HIV infection: Oral:
Dosing based on patient weight:
Pediatric powder for oral solution (Videx®):
<60 kg: 125 mg twice daily (preferred) or 250 mg once daily
≥60 kg: 200 mg twice daily (preferred) or 400 mg once daily
Delayed release capsule (Videx® EC):
25 kg to <60 kg: 250 mg once daily
≥60 kg: 400 mg once daily

When taken with tenofovir:
<60 kg and Cl_{cr} ≥60 mL/minute: 200 mg once daily
≥60 kg and Cl_{cr} ≥60 mL/minute: 250 mg once daily
Note: Combined use of tenofovir with didanosine is no longer recommended (DHHS, 2011).

Geriatric Refer to adult dosing. Elderly patients have a higher frequency of pancreatitis (10% versus 5% in younger patients); monitor renal function and dose accordingly.

Pediatric Treatment of HIV infection: Oral:
Pediatric powder for oral solution (Videx®): **Note:** Once-daily dosing of the oral solution is not FDA approved in children.
Infants: 2 weeks to 8 months: 100 mg/m^2 twice daily is recommended by the manufacturer; 50 mg/m^2 may be considered in infants 2 weeks to <3 months (AIDS*info* guidelines)
Infants and Children >8 months: 120 mg/m^2 twice daily, not to exceed adult dose, is recommended by the manufacturer. **Note:** AIDS*info* guidelines suggest a range of 90-150 mg/m^2 twice daily
Adolescents: Dosing based on patient weight: Refer to adult dosing.
Children 3-21 years (unlabeled dose): Treatment-naive: 240 mg/m^2/dose once daily (maximum: 400 mg/dose) (AIDS*info* guidelines)
Delayed release capsule (Videx® EC):
Children ≥6 years:
20 kg to <25 kg: 200 mg once daily
25 kg to <60 kg: 250 mg once daily
≥60 kg: 400 mg once daily
Children 3-21 years (unlabeled dose): Treatment-naive: 240 mg/m^2/dose once daily (maximum: 400 mg/dose) (AIDS*info* guidelines)

Renal Impairment
Children: No specific guidelines available; consider dosage reduction using adjustments for adults.
Adults: Dosing based on patient weight, creatinine clearance, and dosage form: See table.

Recommended Dose (mg) of Didanosine by Body Weight – Adults

Creatinine Clearance (mL/min)	≥60 kg		<60 kg	
	Powder for Oral Solution	Delayed Release Capsule	Powder for Oral Solution	Delayed Release Capsule
≥60	400 mg daily or 200 mg twice daily	400 mg daily	250 mg daily or 125 mg twice daily	250 mg daily
30-59	200 mg daily or 100 mg twice daily	200 mg daily	150 mg daily or 75 mg twice daily	125 mg daily
10-29	150 mg daily	125 mg daily	100 mg daily	125 mg daily
<10	100 mg daily	125 mg daily	75 mg daily	See Note.

Note: Per manufacturer, not suitable for use in patients <60 kg with Cl_{cr} <10 mL/minute; use alternate formulation.

Patients requiring hemodialysis or CAPD: Dose per Cl_{cr} <10 mL/minute. Didanosine is not removed via CAPD and minimal amount of dose (≤7%) is removed by hemodialysis; no supplemental dosing necessary.

Hepatic Impairment No dosage adjustment needed.

Administration

Oral Pediatric powder for oral solution: Administer on an empty stomach at least 30 minutes before or 2 hours after eating. Prior to dispensing, the powder should be mixed with purified water USP to an initial concentration of 20 mg/mL and then further diluted with an appropriate antacid suspension to a final mixture of 10 mg/mL. Shake well prior to use.
Videx® EC: Administer on an empty stomach at least 1 hour before or 2 hours after eating; swallow capsule whole.

Stability

Reconstitution Videx® pediatric powder: Add 100 mL or 200 mL purified water, USP to the 2 g or 4 g container, respectively, to achieve a 20 mg/mL solution. Immediately mix the resulting solution with an equal volume of Mylanta® Maximum Strength (or equivalent) to achieve a final concentration of 10 mg/mL.

Storage Delayed release capsules should be stored in tightly closed bottles at controlled room temperature of 25°C (77°F). Unreconstituted powder should be stored at 15°C to 30°C (59°F to 86°F). Reconstituted pediatric solution is stable for 30 days if refrigerated.

Monitoring and Teaching Issues

Laboratory Monitoring Serum potassium, uric acid, creatinine, hemoglobin, CBC with neutrophil, platelet count, CD4 cells, liver function, serum bilirubin, albumin, INR, amylase; viral load

Physical Assessment Use caution in presence of or at risk for hepatotoxicity. Monitor for hepatotoxicity, peripheral neuropathy, gastrointestinal pain, and vision changes regularly during therapy. Teach patient proper timing of multiple medications.

Patient Education This drug will not cure HIV, nor has it been found to reduce transmission of HIV; use appropriate precautions to prevent spread to other persons. This drug is prescribed as one part of a multidrug combination; take exactly as directed for full course of therapy. Do not break or chew delayed release capsules. Maintain adequate hydration, unless instructed to restrict fluid intake. Frequent blood tests may be required. You may be advised to have a retinal exam periodically. May cause nausea, vomiting, diarrhea, or changes in body fat (increased in upper back, neck, breast, and around trunk; decreased in legs, arms, and face). Report immediately any loss of sensation, numbness, or tingling in fingers, toes, or feet; persistent unresolved abdominal distress (pain, nausea, vomiting, diarrhea); changes in vision; or signs of infection (burning on urination, perineal itching, white plaques in mouth, unhealed sores, persistent sore throat, cough).

Dietary Considerations Take on an empty stomach; administer at least 30 minutes before or 2 hours after eating

Geriatric Considerations Since the elderly often have a creatinine clearance <60 mL/minute, monitor closely for adverse reactions and adjust dose accordingly to maintain efficacy (CD4 counts).

Breast-Feeding Considerations In infants born to mothers who are HIV positive, HAART while breast-feeding may decrease postnatal infection. However, maternal or infant antiretroviral therapy does not completely eliminate the risk of postnatal HIV transmission. In addition, multiclass-resistant virus has been detected in breast-feeding infants despite maternal therapy.

In the United States where formula is accessible, affordable, safe, and sustainable, complete avoidance of breast-feeding by HIV-infected women is recommended to decrease potential transmission of HIV.

Pregnancy Considerations Adverse events have not been observed in animal reproduction studies. Didanosine has been shown to cross the placenta. Based on data from the Antiretroviral Pregnancy Registry, birth defects have been observed in 4.6% of offspring with first trimester exposure (in comparison to 2.7% observed in U.S. population); no pattern of defects has been observed. Cases of lactic acidosis/hepatic steatosis syndrome related to mitochondrial toxicity have been reported in pregnant women receiving nucleoside analogues. It is not known if pregnancy itself potentiates this known side effect; however, women may be at increased risk of lactic acidosis and liver damage. In addition, these adverse events are similar to other rare but life-threatening syndromes which occur during pregnancy (eg, HELLP syndrome). Hepatic enzymes and electrolytes should be monitored frequently during the third trimester of pregnancy and clinicians should watch for early signs of the syndrome. Combination treatment with stavudine may also contribute to the risk of lactic acidosis, and should be considered only if benefit outweighs risk. Pharmacokinetics are not significantly altered during pregnancy; dose adjustments are not needed. The Perinatal HIV Guidelines Working Group considers didanosine to be an alternative NRTI in dual nucleoside combination regimens; use with stavudine only if no other alternatives are available. Healthcare providers are encouraged to enroll pregnant women exposed to antiretroviral medications in the Antiretroviral Pregnancy Registry (1-800-258-4263 or www.APRegistry.com). Healthcare providers caring for HIV-infected women and their infants may contact the National Perinatal HIV Hotline (888-448-8765) for clinical consultation.

Additional Information A high rate of early virologic nonresponse was observed was observed when the combination of didanosine, lamivudine, and tenofovir or the triple NRTI combination of didanosine, tenofovir and emtricitabine were used as the initial regimen in treatment-naive patients. Use of either of these combinations is not recommended; patients currently on these regimens should be closely monitored for modification of therapy. Early virologic failure and increased toxicity was also observed with tenofovir and didanosine delayed release capsules, plus either efavirenz or nevirapine; use is not recommended. In addition, preliminary data show inferior virologic response with the combination of atazanavir, didanosine and emtricitabine; use should be avoided (DHHS, 2011).

◆ **Dideoxyinosine** *see* Didanosine *on page 524*

◆ **Dienogest and Estradiol** *see* Estradiol and Dienogest *on page 673*

Diethylpropion (dye eth il PROE pee on)

Index Terms Amfepramone; Diethylpropion Hydrochloride

Generic Availability (U.S.) Yes

Pharmacologic Category Anorexiant; Sympathomimetic

Medication Safety Issues

Beers Criteria medication: This drug may be inappropriate for use in geriatric patients (high severity risk).

Pregnancy Risk Factor B

Lactation Enters breast milk/use caution

Use Short-term (few weeks) adjunct in the management of exogenous obesity

Pharmacotherapy for weight loss is recommended only for obese patients with a body mass index ≥30 kg/m^2, or ≥27 kg/m^2 in the presence of other risk factors such as hypertension, diabetes, and/or dyslipidemia or a high waist circumference; therapy should be used in conjunction with a comprehensive weight management program.

Controlled Substance C-IV

Available Dosage Forms

Tablet, oral: 25 mg

Tablet, controlled release, oral: 75 mg

Dosing

Adult & Geriatric Obesity (short-term adjunct): Oral:

Tablet: 25 mg 3 times/day before meals or food

Tablet, controlled release: 75 mg at midmorning

Pediatric Children >16 years: Refer to adult dosing.

Administration

Oral Dose should not be administered in evening or at bedtime.

Tablet: Administer 1 hour before meals.

Tablet, controlled release: Do not crush tablet; administer at midmorning.

Monitoring and Teaching Issues

Physical Assessment Assess for history of psychopathology, homicidal or suicidal tendencies, or addiction; long-term use can result in dependence, abuse, or tolerance. Periodically evaluate the need for continued use. Monitor serum glucose closely in patients with diabetes (amphetamines may alter antidiabetic requirements). Taper dosage slowly when discontinuing.

Patient Education Drug may cause physical and/or psychological dependence. Do not crush or chew extended release tablets. Take early in day to avoid sleep disturbance, 1 hour before meals. Avoid alcohol, caffeine, or OTC medications that act as stimulants. You may experience restlessness, euphoria, or impaired judgment; dry mouth; nausea or vomiting; constipation; diarrhea; or altered libido (reversible). Patients with diabetes need to monitor serum glucose closely (may alter antidiabetic medication requirements). Report chest pain, palpitations, or irregular heartbeat; muscle weakness or tremors; extreme fatigue or depression; CNS changes (aggressiveness, restlessness, euphoria, sleep disturbances); severe abdominal distress or cramping; changes in sexual activity; changes in urinary pattern; or blurred vision.

Related Information

Obesity Treatment Guidelines *on page 2064*

◆ **Diethylpropion Hydrochloride** *see* Diethylpropion *on page 527*

Difenoxin and Atropine (dye fen OKS in & A troe peen)

U.S. Brand Names Motofen®

Index Terms Atropine and Difenoxin

Generic Availability (U.S.) No

Pharmacologic Category Antidiarrheal

Pregnancy Risk Factor C

Lactation Enters breast milk/contraindicated

Use Treatment of diarrhea

Controlled Substance C-IV

Available Dosage Forms

Tablet, oral:

Motofen®: Difenoxin 1 mg and atropine 0.025 mg

Dosing

Adult Diarrhea: Oral: Initial: 2 tablets (each tablet contains difenoxin hydrochloride 1 mg and atropine sulfate 0.025 mg), then 1 tablet after each loose stool; 1 tablet every 3-4 hours, up to 8 tablets in a 24-hour period; if no improvement after 48 hours, continued administration is not indicated

Geriatric Refer to adult dosing; use with caution.

Monitoring and Teaching Issues

Physical Assessment See individual agents.

Patient Education See individual agents.

Related Information

Atropine *on page 172*

◆ **Differin®** *see* Adapalene *on page 51*

◆ **Diflucan®** *see* Fluconazole *on page 772*

◆ **Difluorodeoxycytidine Hydrochlorothiazide** *see* Gemcitabine *on page 855*

Difluprednate (dye floo PRED nate)

U.S. Brand Names Durezol®

Generic Availability (U.S.) No

Pharmacologic Category Corticosteroid, Ophthalmic

Medication Safety Issues

Sound-alike/look-alike issues:

Durezol™ may be confused with Durasal

Pregnancy Risk Factor C

Lactation Excretion in breast milk unknown/use caution

Use Treatment of inflammation and pain following ocular surgery

Available Dosage Forms

Emulsion, ophthalmic:

Durezol®: 0.05% (5 mL)

Dosing

Adult & Geriatric Anti-inflammatory: Ophthalmic: Adults: Instill 1 drop in conjunctival sac of the affected eye(s) 4 times/day beginning 24 hours after surgery, continue for 2 weeks, then decrease to 2 times/day for 1 week, then taper based on response

Monitoring and Teaching Issues

Patient Education Do not allow dropper to touch any surface of the eye to avoid contamination. If pain in eye, redness, or itching becomes aggravated, contact prescriber. Do not wear contact lens while using this medication.

◆ **Digibind® [DSC]** *see* Digoxin Immune Fab *on page 533*

◆ **DigiFab®** *see* Digoxin Immune Fab *on page 533*

◆ **Digitalis** *see* Digoxin *on page 529*

Digoxin (di JOKS in)

U.S. Brand Names Lanoxin®

Index Terms Digitalis

Generic Availability (U.S.) Yes

Pharmacologic Category Antiarrhythmic Agent, Miscellaneous; Cardiac Glycoside

Medication Safety Issues

Sound-alike/look-alike issues:

Digoxin may be confused with Desoxyn®, doxepin

Lanoxin® may be confused with Lasix®, levothyroxine, Levoxyl®, Levsinex®, Lomotil®, Lonox®, Mefoxin®, naloxone, Xanax®

High alert medication: The Institute for Safe Medication Practices (ISMP) includes this medication among its list of drugs which have a heightened risk of causing significant patient harm when used in error.

Beers Criteria medication: This drug may be inappropriate for use in geriatric patients (low severity risk).

International issues:

Lanoxin [U.S., Canada, and multiple international markets] may be confused with Limoxin brand name for ambroxol [Indonesia] and amoxicillin [Mexico]

Pregnancy Risk Factor C

Lactation Enters breast milk/use caution (AAP rates "compatible"; AAP 2001 update pending)

Use Treatment of mild-to-moderate (or stage C as recommended by the ACCF/AHA) heart failure (HF); atrial fibrillation (rate-control)

Note: In treatment of atrial fibrillation (AF), use is not considered first-line unless AF coexistent with heart failure or in sedentary patients (Fuster, 2006).

Unlabeled/Investigational Use Fetal tachycardia with or without hydrops; to slow ventricular rate in supraventricular tachyarrhythmias such as supraventricular tachycardia (SVT) excluding atrioventricular reciprocating tachycardia (AVRT)

Mechanism of Action/Effect

Heart failure: Inhibition of the sodium/potassium ATPase pump in myocardial cells results in a transient increase of intracellular sodium, which in turn promotes calcium influx via the sodium-calcium exchange pump leading to increased contractility.

Supraventricular arrhythmias: Direct suppression of the AV node conduction to increase effective refractory period and decrease conduction velocity - positive inotropic effect, enhanced vagal tone, and decreased ventricular rate to fast atrial arrhythmias. Atrial fibrillation may decrease sensitivity and increase tolerance to higher serum digoxin concentrations.

Contraindications Hypersensitivity to digoxin (rare) or other forms of digitalis, or any component of the formulation; ventricular fibrillation

Warnings/Precautions Watch for proarrhythmic effects (especially with digoxin toxicity). Withdrawal in clinically stable patients with HF may lead to recurrence of HF symptoms. During an episode of atrial fibrillation or flutter in patients with an accessory bypass tract (eg, Wolff-Parkinson-White syndrome), use has been associated with increased anterograde conduction down the accessory pathway leading to ventricular fibrillation; avoid use in such patients. Avoid use in patients with second- or third-degree heart block (except in patients with a functioning artificial pacemaker); incomplete AV block (eg, Stokes-Adams attack) may progress to complete block with digoxin administration. HF patients with preserved left ventricular function including patients with restrictive cardiomyopathy, constrictive pericarditis, and amyloid heart disease may be susceptible to digoxin toxicity; avoid use unless used to control ventricular response with atrial fibrillation. Digoxin should not be used in patients with low EF, sinus rhythm, and no HF symptoms since the risk of harm may be greater than clinical benefit. Avoid use in patients with hypertrophic cardiomyopathy (HCM) and outflow tract obstruction unless used to control ventricular response with atrial fibrillation; outflow obstruction may worsen due to the positive inotropic effects of digoxin.

Use with caution in patients with hyperthyroidism, hypothyroidism, recent acute MI (within 6 months), sinus nodal disease (eg, sick sinus syndrome). Reduce dose with renal impairment and when amiodarone, propafenone, quinidine, or verapamil are added to a patient on digoxin; use with caution in patients taking strong inducers or inhibitors of P-glycoprotein (eg, cyclosporine). Avoid rapid I.V. administration of calcium in digitalized patients; may produce serious arrhythmias.

Atrial arrhythmias associated with hypermetabolic states are very difficult to treat; treat underlying condition first; if digoxin is used, ensure digoxin toxicity does not occur. Patients with beri beri heart disease may fail to adequately respond to digoxin therapy; treat underlying thiamine deficiency concomitantly. Correct electrolyte disturbances, especially hypokalemia or hypomagnesemia, prior to use and throughout therapy; toxicity may occur despite therapeutic digoxin concentrations. Hypercalcemia may increase the risk of digoxin toxicity; maintain normocalcemia. It is not necessary to routinely reduce or hold digoxin therapy prior to elective electrical cardioversion for atrial fibrillation; however, exclusion of digoxin toxicity (eg, clinical and ECG signs) is necessary prior to cardioversion. If signs of digoxin excess exist, withhold digoxin and delay cardioversion until toxicity subsides; usually >24 hours. Use with caution in the elderly; may develop exaggerated serum/tissue concentrations due to age-related alterations in clearance and pharmacodynamics differences; dosage reduction may be necessary; in general, avoid doses >0.125 mg/day (Beers Criteria).

Drug Interactions

Metabolism/Transport Effects Substrate of CYP3A4 (minor), P-glycoprotein

Avoid Concomitant Use There are no known interactions where it is recommended to avoid concomitant use.

Decreased Effect

Digoxin may decrease the levels/effects of: Antineoplastic Agents (Anthracycline)

The levels/effects of Digoxin may be decreased by: 5-ASA Derivatives; Acarbose; Aminoglycosides; Antineoplastic Agents; Antineoplastic Agents (Anthracycline); Bile Acid Sequestrants; Kaolin; Penicillamine; P-Glycoprotein Inducers; Potassium-Sparing Diuretics; St Johns Wort; Sucralfate

Increased Effect/Toxicity

Digoxin may increase the levels/effects of: Adenosine; Colchicine; Dronedarone; Midodrine

The levels/effects of Digoxin may be increased by: Aminoquinolines (Antimalarial); Amiodarone; Atorvastatin; Beta-Blockers; Calcium Channel Blockers (Nondihydropyridine); Calcium Polystyrene Sulfonate; Carvedilol; Conivaptan; CycloSPORINE; CycloSPORINE (Systemic); Dronedarone; Etravirine; Glycopyrrolate; Itraconazole; Macrolide Antibiotics; Milnacipran; Nefazodone; Neuromuscular-Blocking Agents; Nonsteroidal Anti-Inflammatory Agents; Paricalcitol; P-Glycoprotein Inhibitors; Posaconazole; Potassium-Sparing Diuretics; Propafenone; Protease Inhibitors; QuiNIDine; QuiNINE; Ranolazine; Reserpine; SitaGLIPtin; Sodium Polystyrene Sulfonate; Spironolactone; Telmisartan; Tolvaptan; Vitamin D Analogs

Nutritional/Ethanol Interactions

Food: Digoxin peak serum concentrations may be decreased if taken with food. Meals containing increased fiber (bran) or foods high in pectin may decrease oral absorption of digoxin.

Herb/Nutraceutical: Avoid ephedra (risk of cardiac stimulation). Avoid natural licorice (causes sodium and water retention and increases potassium loss).

Lab Interactions Spironolactone may interfere with digoxin radioimmunoassay.

Adverse Reactions Incidence not always reported.

Cardiovascular: Accelerated junctional rhythm, asystole, atrial tachycardia with or without block, AV dissociation, first-, second- (Wenckebach), or third-degree heart block, facial edema, PR prolongation, PVCs (especially bigeminy or trigeminy), ST segment depression, ventricular tachycardia or ventricular fibrillation

Central nervous system: Dizziness (6%), mental disturbances (5%), headache (4%), apathy, anxiety, confusion, delirium, depression, fever, hallucinations

Dermatologic: Rash (erythematous, maculopapular [most common], papular, scarlatiniform, vesicular or bullous), pruritus, urticaria, angioneurotic edema

Gastrointestinal: Nausea (4%), vomiting (2%), diarrhea (4%), abdominal pain, anorexia

Neuromuscular & skeletal: Weakness

Ocular: Visual disturbances (blurred or yellow vision)

Respiratory: Laryngeal edema

Children are more likely to experience cardiac arrhythmia as a sign of excessive dosing. The most common are conduction disturbances or tachyarrhythmia (atrial tachycardia with or without block) and junctional tachycardia. Ventricular tachyarrhythmias are less common. In infants, sinus bradycardia may be a sign of digoxin toxicity. Any arrhythmia seen in a child on digoxin should be considered as digoxin toxicity. The gastrointestinal and central nervous system symptoms are not frequently seen in children.

Pharmacodynamics/Kinetics

Onset of Action

Heart rate control: Oral: 1-2 hours; I.V.: 5-60 minutes

Peak effect: Heart rate control: Oral: 2-8 hours; I.V.: 1-6 hours; **Note:** In patients with atrial fibrillation, median time to ventricular rate control in one study was 6 hours (range: 3-15 hours) (Siu, 2009)

Duration of Action Adults: 3-4 days

Absorption By passive nonsaturable diffusion in the upper small intestine; food may delay, but does not affect extent of absorption

Bioavailability Oral (formulation dependent): Elixir: 70% to 85%; Tablet: 60% to 80%

Time to Peak Serum: Oral: 1-3 hours

Protein Binding ~25%; in uremic patients, digoxin is displaced from plasma protein binding sites

Half-Life Elimination

Age, renal and cardiac function dependent:

- Neonates: Premature: 61-170 hours; Full-term: 35-45 hours
- Infants: 18-25 hours
- Children: 18-36 hours
- Adults: 36-48 hours
- Adults, anephric: 3.5-5 days

Parent drug: 38 hours; Metabolites: Digoxigenin: 4 hours; Monodigitoxoside: 3-12 hours

Metabolism Via sequential sugar hydrolysis in the stomach or by reduction of lactone ring by intestinal bacteria (in ~10% of population, gut bacteria may metabolize up to 40% of digoxin dose); once absorbed, only ~16% is metabolized to 3-beta-digoxigenin, 3-keto-digoxigenin, and glucuronide and sulfate conjugates; metabolites may contribute to therapeutic and toxic effects of digoxin; metabolism is reduced with decompensated HF

Excretion Urine (50% to 70% as unchanged drug)

Available Dosage Forms

Injection, solution: 250 mcg/mL (1 mL, 2 mL)

Lanoxin®: 100 mcg/mL (1 mL); 250 mcg/mL (2 mL)

Solution, oral: 50 mcg/mL (2.5 mL, 5 mL, 60 mL)

Tablet, oral: 125 mcg, 250 mcg

Lanoxin®: 125 mcg, 250 mcg

Dosing

Adult Note: When changing from oral (tablets or liquid) or I.M. to I.V. therapy, dosage should be reduced by 20% to 25%.

Atrial fibrillation (rate control) in patients with heart failure: Loading dose: I.V.: 0.25 mg every 2 hours, up to 1.5 mg within 24 hours; for nonacute situations, may administer 0.5 mg orally once daily for 2 days followed by oral maintenance dose. Maintenance dose: I.V., Oral: 0.125-0.375 mg once daily (Fuster, 2006)

Heart failure: Daily maintenance dose (**Note:** Loading dose not recommended): Oral: 0.125-0.25 mg once daily; higher daily doses (up to 0.5 mg/day) are rarely necessary. If patient is >70 years of age, has impaired renal function, or has a low lean body mass, low doses (eg, 0.125 mg daily or every other day) should be used (Hunt, 2009).

Supraventricular tachyarrhythmias (rate control):

Initial: Total digitalizing dose:

Oral: 0.75-1.5 mg

I.V., I.M.: 0.5-1 mg (**Note:** I.M. not preferred due to severe injection site pain.)

Give 1/2 (one-half) of the total digitalizing dose (TDD) as the initial dose, then give 1/4 (one-quarter) of the TDD in each of 2 subsequent doses at 6- to 8-hour intervals. Obtain ECG 6 hours after each dose to assess potential toxicity.

Daily maintenance dose:

Oral: 0.125-0.5 mg once daily

I.V., I.M.: 0.1-0.4 mg once daily (**Note:** I.M. not preferred due to severe injection site pain.)

Geriatric Dose is based on lean body weight and normal renal function for age. Decrease dose in patients with decreased renal function (see Renal Impairment).

Heart failure: If patient is >70 years of age, low doses (eg, 0.125 mg daily or every other day) should be used (Hunt, 2009).

Pediatric Atrial dysrhythmias (rate control), HF: When changing from oral (tablets or liquid) or I.M. to I.V. therapy, dosage should be reduced by 20% to 25%. See table.

Dosage Recommendations for Digoxin[1]

Age	Total Digitalizing Dose[2,3] (mcg/kg)		Daily Maintenance Dose[3,4] (mcg/kg)	
	Oral	I.V. or I.M.[5]	Oral	I.V. or I.M.[5]
Preterm infant	20-30	15-25	5-7.5	4-6
Full-term infant	25-35	20-30	6-10	5-8
1 mo - 2 y	35-60	30-50	10-15	7.5-12
2-5 y	30-40	25-35	7.5-10	6-9
5-10 y	20-35	15-30	5-10	4-8
>10 y	10-15	8-12	2.5-5	2-3

[1] **Heart failure:** A lower serum digoxin concentration may be adequate to treat heart failure (compared to cardiac arrhythmias); consider doses at the lower end of the recommended range for treatment of heart failure; a digitalizing dose (loading dose) may not be necessary when treating heart failure (Ross, 2001).

[2] **Do not give full total digitalizing dose (TDD) at once.** Give one-half of the total digitalizing dose (TDD) in the initial dose, then give one-quarter of the TDD in each of two subsequent doses at 6- to 8-hour intervals. Obtain ECG 6 hours after each dose to assess potential toxicity.

[3]Based on lean body weight and normal renal function for age. Decrease dose in patients with decreased renal function; digitalizing dose often not recommended in infants and children.

[4]Divided every 12 hours in infants and children <10 years of age. Given once daily to children >10 years of age and adults.

[5]I.M. not preferred due to severe injection site pain. If I.M. route is necessary, administer as deep injection followed by massage of injection site.

Renal Impairment

Loading dose: If loading dose necessary, reduce dose by 50% in ESRD.

Maintenance dose:

Cl_{cr} 10-50 mL/minute: Administer 25% to 75% of dose or every 36 hours.

Cl_{cr} <10 mL/minute: Administer 10% to 25% of dose or every 48 hours.

Not dialyzable (0% to 5%)

Administration

I.M. I.V. route preferred. If I.M. injection necessary, administer by deep injection followed by massage at the injection site. Inject no more than 2 mL per injection site. May cause intense pain.

I.V. May be administered undiluted or diluted fourfold in D_5W, NS, or SWFI for direct injection. Less than fourfold dilution may lead to drug precipitation. Inject slowly over ≥5 minutes

Stability

Storage Store at 25°C (77°F); excursions permitted to 15°C to 30°C (59°F to 86°F). Protect elixir, injection, and tablets from light.

Monitoring and Teaching Issues

Laboratory Monitoring

When to draw serum digoxin concentrations: Digoxin serum concentrations should be drawn **at least 6-8 hours after last dose, regardless of route of administration (optimally 12-24 hours after a dose). Note:** Serum digoxin concentrations may decrease in response to exercise due to increased skeletal muscle uptake; a period of rest (eg, ~2 hours) after exercise may be necessary prior to drawing serum digoxin concentrations.

Initiation of therapy:

If a loading dose is given: Digoxin serum concentration may be drawn within 12-24 hours after the initial loading dose administration. Concentrations drawn this early may confirm the relationship of digoxin plasma concentrations and response but are of little value in determining maintenance doses.

If a loading dose is not given: Digoxin serum concentration should be obtained after 3-5 days of therapy.

Maintenance therapy:

Trough concentrations should be followed just prior to the next dose or at a minimum of 6-8 hours after last dose.

Digoxin serum concentrations should be obtained within 5-7 days (approximate time to steady-state) after any dosage changes. Continue to obtain digoxin serum concentrations 7-14 days after any change in maintenance dose. **Note:** In patients with end-stage renal disease, it may take 15-20 days to reach steady-state.

Patients who are receiving electrolyte-depleting medications such as diuretics, serum potassium, magnesium, and calcium should be monitored closely.

Digoxin serum concentrations should be obtained whenever any of the following conditions occur:

Questionable patient compliance or to evaluate clinical deterioration following an initial good response

Changing renal function

Suspected digoxin toxicity

Initiation or discontinuation of therapy with drugs (eg, amiodarone, quinidine, verapamil) which potentially interact with digoxin.

Any disease changes (eg, thyroid disease)

Physical Assessment Assess results of laboratory tests when beginning or changing dosage, especially with I.V. administration. Monitor for signs of digoxin toxicity. I.V.: Monitor ECG continuously. Oral: Monitor apical pulse before administering any dose.

Patient Education Maintain adequate dietary intake of potassium (do not increase without consulting prescriber). Adequate dietary potassium will reduce risk of digoxin toxicity. Take pulse at the same time each day; hold medication as directed by prescriber. Notify prescriber of acute changes in pulse. Report loss of appetite, nausea, vomiting, persistent diarrhea, swelling of extremities, palpitations, "yellowing" or blurred vision, mental confusion or depression, or unusual fatigue.

Dietary Considerations Maintain adequate amounts of potassium in diet to decrease risk of hypokalemia (hypokalemia may increase risk of digoxin toxicity).

Geriatric Considerations Digitalis preparations (primarily digoxin) are frequently used to treat common cardiac diseases in the elderly (heart failure, atrial fibrillation). Elderly are at risk for toxicity due to age-related changes; volume of distribution is diminished significantly; half-life is increased as a result of decreased total body clearance. Additionally, elderly frequently have concomitant diseases which affect the pharmacokinetics in digitalis glycosides; hypo- and hyperthyroidism and renal function decline will affect clearance of digoxin. Exercise in elderly will reduce serum concentrations of digoxin due to increased skeletal muscle uptake. Therefore, a knowledge of the physical activity of elderly helps interpret serum assays. Must be observant for noncardiac signs of toxicity in elderly such as anorexia, vision changes (blurred), confusion, and depression. Changes in dose may be necessary with declining renal function with age; monitor closely.

This medication is considered to be potentially inappropriate in this patient population (Beers Criteria severity: Low).

Breast-Feeding Considerations Digoxin is excreted into breast milk and similar concentrations are found within mother's serum and milk. The manufacturer recommends that caution be used in nursing women.

Pregnancy Considerations Animal reproduction studies have not been conducted. Digoxin crosses the placenta and can be detected in the fetus. Digoxin is recommended as first-line in the treatment of fetal tachycardia determined to be SVT. In pregnant women with atrial fibrillation or SVT, use of digoxin is recommended (Class I recommendation; Blomström-Lundqvist, 2003; Fuster, 2006).

Related Information

Antiarrhythmic Drugs *on page 1978*

Heart Failure (Systolic) *on page 2040*

Peak and Trough Guidelines *on page 1958*

Digoxin Immune Fab (di JOKS in i MYUN fab)

U.S. Brand Names Digibind® [DSC]; DigiFab®

Index Terms Antidigoxin Fab Fragments, Ovine

Generic Availability (U.S.) No

Pharmacologic Category Antidote

Pregnancy Risk Factor C

Lactation Excretion in breast milk unknown/use caution

Use Treatment of life-threatening or potentially life-threatening digoxin intoxication, including:

- acute digoxin ingestion (ie, >10 mg in adults or >4 mg in children)
- chronic ingestions leading to steady-state digoxin concentrations >6 ng/mL in adults or >4 ng/mL in children
- manifestations of digoxin toxicity due to overdose (life-threatening ventricular arrhythmias, progressive bradycardia, second- or third-degree heart block not responsive to atropine, serum potassium >5 mEq/L in adults or >6 mEq in children)

Available Dosage Forms

Injection, powder for reconstitution:

DigiFab®: 40 mg

Dosing

Adult & Geriatric Each vial of Digibind® 38 mg or DigiFab™ 40 mg will bind ~0.5 mg of digoxin or digitoxin.

Note: Estimation of the dose is based on the body burden of digitalis. This may be calculated if the amount ingested is known or the postdistribution serum drug level is known (round dose to the nearest whole vial). If the amount of ingestion is unknown, general dosing guidelines should be used.

Acute ingestion of unknown amount: I.V.: 20 vials is adequate to treat most life-threatening ingestions. May give as a single dose or give 10 vials, observe response, and give a second 10 vial dose if indicated.

Acute ingestion of known amount: I.V.:

Based on number of tablets/capsules ingested:

Step 1:

Total body load (mg) = Amount (mg) digoxin capsules/digitoxin ingested

Step 2:

Dose (vials) = Total body load (mg) / (0.5 mg digitalis bound/vial)

Alternatively, the following table gives an estimation of the number of vials needed based on the number of digoxin tablets or capsules ingested.

Number of Digoxin Tablets or Capsules Ingested[1]	Dose of Digoxin Immune Fab (# of Vials)
25	10
50	20
75	30
100	40
150	60
200	80

[1]250 mcg tablets with 80% bioavailability or 200 mcg Lanoxicaps® capsules with 100% bioavailability.

Based on steady-state serum digoxin concentration: Adults:

Step 1:

Dose (vials) = (serum digoxin concentration [ng/mL] x weight [kg]) / 100

Alternatively, the following table gives an estimation of the number of vials needed based on the steady-state serum digoxin concentration.

Adult Dose Estimates of Digibind® (in # of Vials) From Steady-State Serum Digoxin Concentration

Patient Weight (kg)	Serum Digoxin Concentration (ng/mL)						
	1	2	4	8	12	16	20
40	0.5 v	1 v	2 v	3 v	5 v	7 v	8 v
60	0.5 v	1 v	3 v	5 v	7 v	10 v	12 v
70	1 v	2 v	3 v	6 v	9 v	11 v	14 v
80	1 v	2 v	3 v	7 v	10 v	13 v	16 v
100	1 v	2 v	4 v	8 v	12 v	16 v	20 v

v = vials.

Based on steady-state serum digitoxin concentration: Children and Adults: If the calculated dose based on the digitoxin concentration is different than that for the digoxin concentration, use the higher dose.

Step 1:

Dose (vials) = [serum **digitoxin** concentration (ng/mL) x weight (kg)] / 1000

Chronic toxicity (serum digoxin concentration unavailable): I.V.: Adults: 6 vials is adequate to reverse most cases of toxicity

Pediatric Each vial of Digibind® 38 mg or DigiFab™ 40 mg will bind ~0.5 mg of digoxin or digitoxin.

Note: Estimation of the dose is based on the body burden of digitalis. This may be calculated if the amount ingested is known or the postdistribution serum drug level is known (round dose to the nearest whole vial). If the amount of ingestion is unknown, general dosing guidelines should be used.

Acute ingestion of unknown amount: I.V.: Refer to adult dosing.

Acute ingestion of known amount: I.V.: Refer to adult dosing.

Based on steady-state serum digoxin concentration: Infants and Children ≤20 kg: May require smaller doses; calculate dose in milligrams, reconstitute with NS, and administer dose via tuberculin syringe

Step 1:

Dose (mg) = [(serum digoxin concentration [ng/mL] x weight [kg]) / 100] x (mg/vial)

Note: Digibind® 38 mg/vial or DigiFab™ 40 mg/vial

Alternatively, the following table gives an estimation of the amount of **Digibind®** needed based on the steady-state serum digoxin concentration.

Infants and Small Children Dose Estimates of Digibind® (in mg) From Steady-State Serum Digoxin Concentration

Patient Weight (kg)	Serum Digoxin Concentration (ng/mL)						
	1	2	4	8	12	16	20
1	0.4 mg[1]	1 mg[1]	1.5 mg[1]	3 mg[1]	5 mg	6 mg	8 mg
3	1 mg[1]	2 mg[1]	5 mg	9 mg	14 mg	18 mg	23 mg
5	2 mg[1]	4 mg	8 mg	15 mg	23 mg	30 mg	38 mg
10	4 mg	8 mg	15 mg	30 mg	46 mg	61 mg	76 mg
20	8 mg	15 mg	30 mg	61 mg	91 mg	122 mg	152 mg

[1]Dilution of reconstituted vial to 1 mg/mL may be desirable.

Alternatively, the following table gives an estimation of the amount of **DigiFab™** needed based on the steady-state serum digoxin concentration.

Infants and Small Children Dose Estimates of DigiFab™ (in mg) From Steady-State Serum Digoxin Concentration

Patient Weight (kg)	Serum Digoxin Concentration (ng/mL)						
	1	2	4	8	12	16	20
1	0.4 mg[1]	1 mg[1]	1.5 mg[1]	3 mg[1]	5 mg	6.5 mg	8 mg
3	1 mg[1]	2.5 mg[1]	5 mg	10 mg	14 mg	19 mg	24 mg
5	2 mg[1]	4 mg	8 mg	16 mg	24 mg	32 mg	40 mg
10	4 mg	8 mg	16 mg	32 mg	48 mg	64 mg	80 mg
20	8 mg	16 mg	32 mg	64 mg	96 mg	128 mg	160 mg

[1]Dilution of reconstituted vial to 1 mg/mL may be desirable.

Based on steady-state digitoxin concentration: Refer to adult dosing.

Chronic toxicity (serum digoxin concentration unavailable): I.V.: Infants and Children ≤20 kg: 1 vial is adequate to reverse most cases of toxicity

Renal Impairment Renal elimination of complexed digoxin may be decreased in renal failure. Potential "rebound" may occur when immune fragments are hepatically metabolized, leaving unbound digoxin.

Administration

I.V. Continuous I.V. infusion over ≥30 minutes is preferred. May give by bolus injection if cardiac arrest is imminent. Small doses (infants/small children) may be administered using tuberculin syringe.

Monitoring and Teaching Issues

Laboratory Monitoring Serum potassium, serum digoxin concentration prior to first dose of digoxin immune Fab; **digoxin levels will greatly increase with digoxin immune Fab use and are not an accurate determination of body stores** (has no clinical meaning; avoid monitoring serum concentrations); standard digoxin concentration measurements may be misleading until Fab fragments are eliminated from the body.

Patients with renal failure should be monitored for a prolonged period for reintoxication with digoxin following the rerelease of bound digoxin into the blood.

Physical Assessment Assess allergy history prior to administration. Assess cardiac status, vital signs, and blood pressure during and following infusion. Monitor for signs of reoccurrence of cardiac toxicity.

Patient Education Immediately report dizziness, palpitations, cramping, respiratory difficulty, rash, or itching.

Dihydrocodeine, Aspirin, and Caffeine

(dye hye droe KOE deen, AS pir in, & KAF een)

U.S. Brand Names Synalgos®-DC

Index Terms Dihydrocodeine Compound

Generic Availability (U.S.) No

Pharmacologic Category Analgesic, Opioid

Medication Safety Issues

Sound-alike/look-alike issues:

Synalgos®-DC may be confused with Synagis®

High alert medication: The Institute for Safe Medication Practices (ISMP) includes this medication among its list of drug classes which have a heightened risk of causing significant patient harm when used in error.

Pregnancy Risk Factor B/D (prolonged use or high doses at term)

Lactation Excretion in breast milk unknown/use caution

Use Management of mild-to-moderate pain that requires relaxation

Controlled Substance C-III

Available Dosage Forms

Capsule, oral:

Synalgos®-DC: Dihydrocodeine 16 mg, aspirin 356.4 mg, and caffeine 30 mg

Dosing

Adult Pain: Oral: 1-2 capsules every 4-6 hours as needed

Geriatric Initial dosing should be cautious (low end of adult dosing range).

Monitoring and Teaching Issues

Physical Assessment See individual agents.

Patient Education See individual agents.

Related Information

Aspirin *on page 155*

◆ **Dihydrocodeine Compound** *see* Dihydrocodeine, Aspirin, and Caffeine *on page 535*

Dihydroergotamine (dye hye droe er GOT a meen)

U.S. Brand Names D.H.E. 45®; Migranal®

Index Terms DHE; Dihydroergotamine Mesylate

Generic Availability (U.S.) Yes: Injection

Pharmacologic Category Antimigraine Agent; Ergot Derivative

Pregnancy Risk Factor X

Lactation Enters breast milk/contraindicated

Use Treatment of migraine headache with or without aura; injection also indicated for treatment of cluster headaches

Unlabeled/Investigational Use Adjunct for DVT prophylaxis for hip surgery, for orthostatic hypotension, xerostomia secondary to antidepressant use, and pelvic congestion with pain

Available Dosage Forms

Injection, solution: 1 mg/mL (1 mL)

D.H.E. 45®: 1 mg/mL (1 mL)

Solution, intranasal:

Migranal®: 4 mg/mL (1 mL)

Dosing

Adult

Migraine, cluster headache:

I.M., SubQ: 1 mg at first sign of headache; repeat hourly to a maximum dose of 3 mg/day; maximum dose: 6 mg/week

I.V.: 1 mg at first sign of headache; repeat hourly up to a maximum dose of 2 mg/day; maximum dose: 6 mg/week

Intranasal: 1 spray (0.5 mg) of nasal spray should be administered into each nostril; if needed, repeat after 15 minutes, up to a total of 4 sprays (2 mg). **Note:** Do not exceed 6 sprays (3 mg) in a 24-hour period and no more than 8 sprays (4 mg) in a week.

Intractable migraine (status migrainosus; >72 hours): *I.V.:* Raskin protocol (unlabeled dosing): Initial test dose: 0.5 mg (following premedication with metoclopramide); subsequent dosing is titrated (range: 0.2-1 mg) every 8 hours for 2-3 days and administered with or without metoclopramide based on response and tolerance (Raskin, 1986; Raskin, 1990). **Note:** Some clinicians use modified versions of this protocol, with additional adjunctive medications and/or alternate antiemetic agents.

Geriatric Refer to adult dosing. Patients >65 years of age were not included in controlled clinical studies.

Renal Impairment Contraindicated in severe renal impairment

Hepatic Impairment Dosage reductions are probably necessary but specific guidelines are not available; contraindicated in severe hepatic dysfunction.

Administration

I.M. May administer by intramuscular injection.

I.V. Administer slowly over 2-3 minutes (Raskin protocol)

Other

Intranasal: Prior to administration of nasal spray, the nasal spray applicator must be primed (pumped 4 times); in order to let the drug be absorbed through the skin in the nose, patients should not inhale deeply through the nose while spraying or immediately after spraying; for best results, treatment should be initiated at the first symptom or sign of an attack; however, nasal spray can be used at any stage of a migraine attack

SubQ: May administer by subcutaneous injection.

Monitoring and Teaching Issues

Physical Assessment Cardiovascular status should be evaluated prior to initiating medication and periodically thereafter. Teach patient proper storage, administration, injection technique, and syringe/needle disposal.

Patient Education Take this drug as rapidly as possible when first headache symptoms occur. May cause drowsiness or feelings of numbness or tingling of fingers, toes, or face. Report heart palpitations, severe nausea or vomiting, and severe numbness of fingers or toes.

- **Dihydroergotamine Mesylate** *see* Dihydroergotamine *on page* *535*
- **Dihydrohydroxycodeinone** *see* OxyCODONE *on page* *1380*
- **Dihydromorphinone** *see* HYDROmorphone *on page* *922*
- **Dihydroxyanthracenedione** *see* Mitoxantrone *on page* *1244*
- **Dihydroxyanthracenedione Dihydrochloride** *see* Mitoxantrone *on page* *1244*
- **1,25 Dihydroxycholecalciferol** *see* Calcitriol *on page* *271*
- **Dihydroxydeoxynorvinkaleukoblastine** *see* Vinorelbine *on page* *1868*
- **Dilacor XR®** *see* Diltiazem *on page* *536*
- **Dilantin®** *see* Phenytoin *on page* *1453*
- **Dilantin-125®** *see* Phenytoin *on page* *1453*
- **Dilatrate®-SR** *see* Isosorbide Dinitrate *on page* *1028*
- **Dilaudid®** *see* HYDROmorphone *on page* *922*
- **Dilaudid-HP®** *see* HYDROmorphone *on page* *922*
- **Dilt-CD** *see* Diltiazem *on page* *536*
- **Diltia XT®** *see* Diltiazem *on page* *536*

Diltiazem (dil TYE a zem)

U.S. Brand Names Cardizem®; Cardizem® CD; Cardizem® LA; Cartia XT®; Dilacor XR®; Dilt-CD; Dilt-XR; Diltia XT®; Diltzac; Matzim™ LA; Taztia XT®; Tiazac®

Index Terms Diltiazem Hydrochloride

Generic Availability (U.S.) Yes

Pharmacologic Category Antiarrhythmic Agent, Class IV; Calcium Channel Blocker; Calcium Channel Blocker, Nondihydropyridine

Medication Safety Issues

Sound-alike/look-alike issues:

Cardizem® may be confused with Cardene®, Cardene SR®, Cardizem CD®, Cardizem SR®, cardiem, cortisone

Cartia XT® may be confused with Procardia XL®

Diltiazem may be confused with Calan®, diazepam, Dilantin®

Tiazac® may be confused with Tigan®, Tiazac® XC [CAN], Ziac®

High alert medication: The Institute for Safe Medication Practices (ISMP) includes this medication (I.V. formulation) among its list of drug classes which have a heightened risk of causing significant patient harm when used in error.

Significant differences exist between oral and I.V. dosing. Use caution when converting from one route of administration to another.

International issues:

Cardizem [U.S., Canada, and multiple international markets] may be confused with Cardem brand name for celiprolol [Spain]

Cartia XT [U.S.] may be confused with Cartia brand name for aspirin [multiple international markets]

Dilacor XR [U.S.] may be confused with Dilacor brand name for verapamil [Brazil]

Dipen [Greece] may be confused with Depen brand name for penicillamine [U.S.]; Depin brand name for nifedipine [India]; Depon brand name for acetaminophen [Greece]

Tiazac: Brand name for diltiazem [U.S, Canada], but also the brand name for pioglitazone [Chile]

Pregnancy Risk Factor C

Lactation Enters breast milk/not recommended (AAP considers "compatible"; AAP 2001 update pending)

Use

Oral: Essential hypertension; chronic stable angina or angina from coronary artery spasm

Injection: Control of rapid ventricular rate in patients with atrial fibrillation or atrial flutter; conversion of paroxysmal supraventricular tachycardia (PSVT)

Unlabeled/Investigational Use

ACLS guidelines: Injection: Stable narrow-complex tachycardia uncontrolled or unconverted by adenosine or vagal maneuvers or if SVT is recurrent

Pediatric hypertension

Mechanism of Action/Effect Nondihydropyridine calcium channel blocker which inhibits calcium ion from entering the "slow channels" or select voltage-sensitive areas of vascular smooth muscle and myocardium during depolarization, producing a relaxation of coronary vascular smooth muscle and coronary vasodilation; increases myocardial oxygen delivery in patients with vasospastic angina

Contraindications

Oral: Hypersensitivity to diltiazem or any component of the formulation; sick sinus syndrome (except in patients with a functioning artificial pacemaker); second- or third-degree AV block (except in patients with a functioning artificial pacemaker); severe hypotension (systolic <90 mm Hg); acute MI and pulmonary congestion

Intravenous (I.V.): Hypersensitivity to diltiazem or any component of the formulation; sick sinus syndrome (except in patients with a functioning artificial pacemaker); second- or third-degree AV block (except in patients with a functioning artificial pacemaker); severe hypotension (systolic <90 mm Hg); cardiogenic shock; administration concomitantly or within a few hours of the administration of I.V. beta-blockers; atrial fibrillation or flutter associated with accessory bypass tract (eg, Wolff-Parkinson-White syndrome); ventricular tachycardia (with wide-complex tachycardia, must determine whether origin is supraventricular or ventricular)

Canadian labeling: Additional contraindications (not in U.S. labeling): I.V. and Oral: Pregnancy; use in women of childbearing potential

Warnings/Precautions Can cause first-, second-, and third-degree AV block or sinus bradycardia and risk increases with agents known to slow cardiac conduction. The most common side effect is peripheral edema; occurs within 2-3 weeks of starting therapy. Symptomatic hypotension with or without syncope can rarely occur; blood pressure must be lowered at a rate appropriate for the patient's clinical condition. Use caution when using diltiazem together with a beta-blocker; may result in conduction disturbances, hypotension, and worsened LV function. Simultaneous administration of I.V. diltiazem and an I.V. beta-blocker or administration within a few hours of each other may result in asystole and is contraindicated. Use with other agents known to either reduce SA node function and/or AV nodal conduction (eg, digoxin) or reduce sympathetic outflow (eg, clonidine) may increase the risk of serious bradycardia. Use caution in left ventricular dysfunction (may exacerbate condition). Avoid use of diltiazem in patients with heart failure and reduced ejection fraction (Hunt, 2009). Use with caution with hypertrophic obstructive cardiomyopathy; routine use is currently not recommended due to insufficient evidence (Maron, 2003). Use with caution in hepatic or renal dysfunction. Transient dermatologic reactions have been observed with use; if reaction persists, discontinue. May (rarely) progress to erythema multiforme or exfoliative dermatitis.

Drug Interactions

Metabolism/Transport Effects **Substrate** of CYP2C9 (minor), 2D6 (minor), 3A4 (major), P-glycoprotein; **Inhibits** CYP2C9 (weak), 2D6 (weak), 3A4 (moderate)

Avoid Concomitant Use

Avoid concomitant use of Diltiazem with any of the following: Tolvaptan

Decreased Effect

Diltiazem may decrease the levels/effects of: Clopidogrel

The levels/effects of Diltiazem may be decreased by: Barbiturates; Calcium Salts; CarBAMazepine; Colestipol; CYP3A4 Inducers (Strong); Deferasirox; Herbs (CYP3A4 Inducers); Herbs (Hypertensive Properties); Methylphenidate; Nafcillin; Peginterferon Alfa-2b; P-Glycoprotein Inducers; Rifamycin Derivatives; Yohimbine

Increased Effect/Toxicity

Diltiazem may increase the levels/effects of: Alfentanil; Amifostine; Amiodarone; Antihypertensives; Aprepitant; Atorvastatin; Benzodiazepines (metabolized by oxidation); Beta-Blockers; BusPIRone; Calcium Channel Blockers (Dihydropyridine); CarBAMazepine; Cardiac Glycosides; Colchicine; Corticosteroids (Systemic); CycloSPORINE; CycloSPORINE (Systemic); CYP3A4 Substrates; Dronedarone; Eletriptan; Eplerenone; Everolimus; Fingolimod; Fosaprepitant; Halofantrine; Hypotensive Agents; Lithium; Lovastatin; Lurasidone; Magnesium Salts; Midodrine; Neuromuscular-Blocking Agents (Nondepolarizing); Nitroprusside; Phenytoin; Pimecrolimus; QuiNIDine; Ranolazine; Red Yeast Rice; RiTUXimab; Salicylates; Salmeterol; Saxagliptin; Simvastatin; Tacrolimus; Tacrolimus (Systemic); Tacrolimus (Topical); Tolvaptan; Vilazodone

The levels/effects of Diltiazem may be increased by: Alpha1-Blockers; Anilidopiperidine Opioids; Antifungal Agents (Azole Derivatives, Systemic); Aprepitant; Atorvastatin; Calcium Channel Blockers (Dihydropyridine); Cimetidine; Conivaptan; CycloSPORINE; CycloSPORINE (Systemic); CYP3A4 Inhibitors (Moderate); CYP3A4 Inhibitors (Strong); Dasatinib; Diazoxide; Dronedarone; Fluconazole; Fosaprepitant; Grapefruit Juice; Herbs (Hypotensive Properties); Lovastatin; Macrolide Antibiotics; Magnesium Salts; MAO Inhibitors; Pentoxifylline; P-Glycoprotein Inhibitors; Phosphodiesterase 5 Inhibitors; Prostacyclin Analogues; Protease Inhibitors; Simvastatin

Nutritional/Ethanol Interactions

Ethanol: Avoid ethanol (may increase risk of hypotension or vasodilation).

Food: Diltiazem serum levels may be elevated if taken with food. Serum concentrations were not altered by grapefruit juice in small clinical trials.

Herb/Nutraceutical: St John's wort may decrease diltiazem levels. Avoid bayberry, blue cohosh, cayenne, ephedra, ginger, ginseng (American), kola, licorice, yohimbe (may worsen hypertension). Avoid black cohosh, California poppy, coleus, garlic, golden seal, hawthorn, mistletoe, periwinkle, quinine, shepherd's purse (may have increased antihypertensive effect).

Adverse Reactions Note: Frequencies represent ranges for various dosage forms. Patients with impaired ventricular function and/or conduction abnormalities may have higher incidence of adverse reactions.

>10%:

Cardiovascular: Edema (2% to 15%)

Central nervous system: Headache (5% to 12%)

2% to 10%:

Cardiovascular: AV block (first degree 2% to 8%), edema (lower limb 2% to 8%), pain (6%), bradycardia (2% to 6%), hypotension (<2% to 4%), vasodilation (2% to 3%), extrasystoles (2%), flushing (1% to 2%), palpitation (1% to 2%)

Central nervous system: Dizziness (3% to 10%), nervousness (2%)

Dermatologic: Rash (1% to 4%)

Endocrine & metabolic: Gout (1% to 2%)

Gastrointestinal: Dyspepsia (1% to 6%), constipation (<2% to 4%), vomiting (2%), diarrhea (1% to 2%)

Local: Injection site reactions: Burning, itching (4%)

Neuromuscular & skeletal: Weakness (1% to 4%), myalgia (2%)

Respiratory: Rhinitis (<2% to 10%), pharyngitis (2% to 6%), dyspnea (1% to 6%), bronchitis (1% to 4%), cough (≤3), sinus congestion (1% to 2%)

Pharmacodynamics/Kinetics

Onset of Action Oral: Immediate release tablet: 30-60 minutes; I.V.: 3 minutes

Duration of Action I.V.: Bolus: 1-3 hours; Continuous infusion (after discontinuation): 0.5-10 hours

Absorption Immediate release tablet: >90%; Extended release capsule: ~93%

Bioavailability Oral: ~40% (undergoes extensive first-pass metabolism)

Time to Peak Serum: Immediate release tablet: 2-4 hours; Extended release tablet: 11-18 hours; Extended release capsule: 10-14 hours

Protein Binding 70% to 80%

Half-Life Elimination Immediate release tablet: 3-4.5 hours, may be prolonged with renal impairment; Extended release tablet: 6-9 hours; Extended release capsules: 5-10 hours; I.V.: single dose: ~3.4 hours; continuous infusion: 4-5 hours

Metabolism Hepatic (extensive first-pass effect); following single I.V. injection, plasma concentrations of N-monodesmethyldiltiazem and desacetyldiltiazem are typically undetectable; however, these metabolites accumulate to detectable concentrations following 24-hour constant rate infusion. N-monodesmethyldiltiazem appears to have 20% of the potency of diltiazem; desacetyldiltiazem is about 25% to 50% as potent as the parent compound.

Excretion Urine (2% to 4% as unchanged drug; 6% to 7% as metabolites); feces

Available Dosage Forms

Capsule, extended release, oral: 60 mg, 90 mg, 120 mg, 180 mg, 240 mg, 300 mg, 360 mg, 420 mg
Cardizem® CD: 120 mg, 180 mg, 240 mg, 300 mg, 360 mg
Cartia XT®: 120 mg, 180 mg, 240 mg, 300 mg
Dilacor XR®: 240 mg
Dilt-CD: 120 mg, 180 mg, 240 mg, 300 mg
Dilt-XR: 120 mg, 180 mg, 240 mg
Diltia XT®: 120 mg, 180 mg, 240 mg
Diltzac: 120 mg, 180 mg, 240 mg, 300 mg, 360 mg
Taztia XT®: 120 mg, 180 mg, 240 mg, 300 mg, 360 mg
Tiazac®: 120 mg, 180 mg, 240 mg, 300 mg, 360 mg, 420 mg

Injection, powder for reconstitution: 100 mg

Injection, solution: 5 mg/mL (5 mL, 10 mL, 25 mL)

Tablet, oral: 30 mg, 60 mg, 90 mg, 120 mg
Cardizem®: 30 mg, 60 mg, 90 mg, 120 mg

Tablet, extended release, oral: 240 mg
Cardizem® LA: 120 mg, 180 mg, 240 mg, 300 mg, 360 mg, 420 mg
Matzim™ LA: 180 mg, 240 mg, 300 mg, 360 mg, 420 mg

Dosing

Adult

Angina: Oral:

Capsule, extended release:

Dilacor XR®, Dilt-XR, Diltia XT®: Initial: 120 mg once daily; titrate over 7-14 days; usual dose range: 120-320 mg/day: maximum: 480 mg/day

Cardizem® CD, Cartia XT®, Dilt-CD: Initial: 120-180 mg once daily; titrate over 7-14 days; usual dose range: 120-320 mg/day; maximum: 480 mg/day

Tiazac®, Taztia XT®: Initial: 120-180 mg once daily; titrate over 7-14 days; usual dose range: 120-320 mg/day; maximum: 540 mg/day

Tablet, extended release (Cardizem® LA, Tiazac® XC [CAN; not available in U.S.]): 180 mg once daily; may increase at 7- to 14-day intervals; usual dose range: 120-320 mg/day; maximum: 360 mg/day

Tablet, immediate release (Cardizem®): Usual starting dose: 30 mg 4 times/day; titrate dose gradually at 1- to 2-day intervals; usual dose range: 120-320 mg/day

Hypertension: Oral:

Capsule, extended release (once-daily dosing):

Cardizem® CD, Cartia XT®, Dilt-CD: Initial: 180-240 mg once daily; dose adjustment may be made after 14 days; usual dose range (JNC 7): 180-420 mg/day; maximum: 480 mg/day

Dilacor® XR, Diltia XT®, Dilt-XR: Initial: 180-240 mg once daily; dose adjustment may be made after 14 days; usual dose range (JNC 7): 180-420 mg/day; maximum: 540 mg/day

Tiazac®, Taztia XT®: Initial: 120-240 mg once daily; dose adjustment may be made after 14 days; usual dose range (JNC 7): 180-420 mg/day; maximum: 540 mg/day

Capsule, extended release (twice-daily dosing): Initial: 60-120 mg twice daily; dose adjustment may be made after 14 days; usual range: 240-360 mg/day

Note: Diltiazem is available as a generic intended for either once- or twice-daily dosing, depending on the formulation; verify appropriate extended release capsule formulation is administered.

Tablet, extended release (Cardizem® LA, Tiazac® XC [CAN; not available in U.S.]): Initial: 180-240 mg once daily; dose adjustment may be made after 14 days; usual dose range (JNC 7): 120-540 mg/day

Atrial fibrillation, atrial flutter, PSVT: I.V.:

Initial bolus dose: 0.25 mg/kg actual body weight over 2 minutes (average adult dose: 20 mg); ACLS guideline recommends 15-20 mg

Repeat bolus dose (may be administered after 15 minutes if the response is inadequate): 0.35 mg/kg actual body weight over 2 minutes (average adult dose: 25 mg); ACLS guideline recommends 20-25 mg

Continuous infusion (infusions >24 hours or infusion rates >15 mg/hour are not recommended): Initial infusion rate of 10 mg/hour; rate may be increased in 5 mg/hour increments up to 15 mg/hour as needed; some patients may respond to an initial rate of 5 mg/hour.

If diltiazem injection is administered by continuous infusion for >24 hours, the possibility of decreased diltiazem clearance, prolonged elimination half-life, and increased diltiazem and/or diltiazem metabolite plasma concentrations should be considered.

Conversion from I.V. diltiazem to oral diltiazem:

Oral dose (mg/day) is approximately equal to [rate (mg/hour) x 3 + 3] x 10.

3 mg/hour = 120 mg/day
5 mg/hour = 180 mg/day
7 mg/hour = 240 mg/day
11 mg/hour = 360 mg/day

Geriatric Refer to adult dosing. **Note:** Patients ≥60 years may respond to a lower initial dose (eg, 120 mg once daily using extended release capsule)

Pediatric

Children: Minimal information available; some centers use the following:

Hypertension (unlabeled use): Oral: Initial: 1.5-2 mg/kg/day in 3 divided doses (maximum: 6 mg/kg/day, up to 360 mg/day) (Flynn, 2000)

Adolescents: Refer to adult dosing.

Renal Impairment Use with caution; no dosing adjustments recommended.

Dialysis: Not removed by hemo- or peritoneal dialysis; supplemental dose is not necessary.

Hepatic Impairment Use with caution; no specific dosing recommendations available; extensively metabolized by the liver; half-life is increased in patients with cirrhosis.

Administration

Oral

Immediate release tablet (Cardizem®): Administer before meals and at bedtime.

Long acting dosage forms: Do not open, chew, or crush; swallow whole.

Cardizem® CD, Cardizem® LA, Cartia XT®, Dilt-CD: May be administered without regards to meals.

Dilacor XR®, Dilt-XR, Diltia XT®: Administer on an empty stomach.

Taztia XT™, Tiazac®: Capsules may be opened and sprinkled on a spoonful of applesauce. Applesauce should not be hot and should be swallowed without chewing, followed by drinking a glass of water.

Tiazac® XC [CAN; not available in U.S.]: Administer at bedtime

I.V. Bolus doses given over 2 minutes with continuous ECG and blood pressure monitoring. Continuous infusion should be via infusion pump.

Stability

Storage

Capsule, tablet: Store at room temperature. Protect from light.

Solution for injection: Store in refrigerator at 2°C to 8°C (36°F to 46°F); do not freeze. May be stored at room temperature for up to 1 month. Following dilution to ≤1 mg/mL with $D_5$1/2NS, D_5W, or NS, solution is stable for 24 hours at room temperature or under refrigeration.

Monitoring and Teaching Issues

Laboratory Monitoring Liver function tests

Physical Assessment Evaluate for use-related precautions prior to beginning therapy. Assess potential for interactions with other agents that may cause increased risk of bradycardia, conduction delays, or decreased cardiac output. I.V. requires use of infusion pump and continuous cardiac and hemodynamic monitoring. Assess therapeutic effectiveness according to use (hypertension, angina, atrial fib/flutter, or PSVT).

Patient Education Oral: Do not crush or chew extended release form. Avoid or limit alcohol and caffeine. May cause dizziness or lightheadedness, nausea, vomiting, or constipation. Report chest pain, palpitations, or irregular heartbeat; persistent diarrhea; unusual cough or respiratory difficulty; swelling of extremities; muscle tremors or weakness; confusion or acute lethargy; or skin rash.

Geriatric Considerations Elderly may experience a greater hypotensive response; constipation may be encountered more often in elderly. Calcium channel blockers are no more effective in elderly than other therapies; however, they do not cause significant CNS effects which is an advantage over other antihypertensive agents (eg, beta-blockers, clonidine).

Breast-Feeding Considerations Diltiazem is excreted into breastmilk in concentrations similar to those in the maternal plasma.

Pregnancy Considerations Teratogenic and embryotoxic effects have been demonstrated in animal reproduction studies.

Related Information

Antiarrhythmic Drugs *on page 1978*

Calcium Channel Blockers *on page 1993*

◆ **Diltiazem Hydrochloride** *see* Diltiazem *on page 536*

◆ **Dilt-XR** *see* Diltiazem *on page 536*

◆ **Diltzac** *see* Diltiazem *on page 536*

◆ **Dimetapp® Children's Long Acting Cough Plus Cold [OTC]** *see* Dextromethorphan and Chlorpheniramine *on page 513*

◆ **Dimetapp® Children's Nighttime Cold & Congestion [OTC]** *see* Diphenhydramine and Phenylephrine *on page 546*

◆ **Dimethyl Triazeno Imidazole Carboxamide** *see* Dacarbazine *on page 452*

Dinoprostone (dye noe PROST one)

U.S. Brand Names Cervidil®; Prepidil®; Prostin E2®

Index Terms PGE_2; Prostaglandin E_2

Generic Availability (U.S.) No

Pharmacologic Category Abortifacient; Prostaglandin

Medication Safety Issues

Sound-alike/look-alike issues:

Prepidil® may be confused with Bepridil®

International issues:

Cervidil®: Brand name for gemeprost in Italy

Pregnancy Risk Factor C

Lactation Excretion in breast milk unknown

Use

Endocervical gel: Promote cervical ripening in patients at or near term in whom there is a medical or obstetrical indication for the induction of labor

Suppositories: Terminate pregnancy from 12th through 20th week of gestation; evacuate uterus in cases of missed abortion or intrauterine fetal death up to 28 weeks of gestation; manage benign hydatidiform mole (nonmetastatic gestational trophoblastic disease)

Vaginal insert: Initiation and/or continuation of cervical ripening in patients at or near term in whom there is a medical or obstetrical indication for the induction of labor

Mechanism of Action/Effect A synthetic prostaglandin E_2 abortifacient that stimulates uterine contractions similar to those seen during natural labor. Prostaglandin E_2 plays a role in cervical ripening, which allows the fetus to pass through the birth canal.

Contraindications Hypersensitivity to prostaglandins or any component of the formulation

Endocervical gel *and* vaginal insert: Patients in whom oxytocic drugs are contraindicated; history of cesarean section or major uterine surgery; presence of cephalopelvic disproportion; fetal distress when delivery is not imminent; unexplained vaginal bleeding during this pregnancy. In addition:

Endocervical gel: History of difficult labor and/or traumatic delivery, ≥6 previous term pregnancies with nonvertex presentation, hyperactive or hypertonic uterine patterns, obstetric emergencies when surgical intervention would be favorable, placenta previa, when vaginal delivery is not indicated (eg, vasa previa, active herpes genitalia)

Vaginal insert: Patients already receiving I.V. oxytocic drugs, ≥6 previous term pregnancies

Suppository: Acute pelvic inflammatory disease; active cardiac, pulmonary, renal, or hepatic disease

Warnings/Precautions [U.S. Boxed Warning]: Dinoprostone should be used only by medically-trained personnel in a hospital.

Postpartum DIC has been reported following dinoprostone for labor induction. Risk may be increased in women ≥30 years of age, gestation age >40 weeks, or women with pregnancy complications. Use caution in patients with hepatic or renal impairment.

Endocervical gel: Use caution with ruptured membranes, glaucoma, or a history of asthma. Intracervical placement of gel may lead to anaphylactoid syndrome of pregnancy (rare).

Vaginal insert: Use caution with ruptured membranes; nonvertex or nonsingleton pregnancy; previous uterine hypertony; history of asthma or glaucoma. Must be removed prior to administration of oxytocin, in case of hyperstimulation or if labor begins, fetal or maternal distress, and prior to amniotomy. Intravaginal placement of insert may lead to anaphylactoid syndrome of pregnancy (rare).

Suppository: Transient pyrexia and decreased blood pressure may be observed with treatment. Use caution with history of asthma; hypotension or hypertension; cardiovascular disease; anemia; jaundice; diabetes; epilepsy; compromised uteri; cervicitis, endocervical infections or acute vaginitis. Measures should be taken to ensure complete abortion. Commercially available suppositories should not be used for extemporaneous preparation of any other dosage form of drug. Do not use for cervical ripening or other indications in patients with term pregnancy.

Drug Interactions

Avoid Concomitant Use

Avoid concomitant use of Dinoprostone with any of the following: Carbetocin

Decreased Effect There are no known significant interactions involving a decrease in effect.

Increased Effect/Toxicity

Dinoprostone may increase the levels/effects of: Carbetocin; Oxytocin

Adverse Reactions

Endocervical gel: 1% to 10%:

Central nervous system: Fever (1%)
Gastrointestinal: GI upset (6%)
Genitourinary: Abnormal uterine contractions (7%), warm feeling in vagina (2%)
Neuromuscular & skeletal: Back pain (3%)

Suppository: Frequency not defined:

Cardiovascular: Arrhythmia, chest pain, chest tightness, hypotension, syncope
Central nervous system: Chills, dizziness, fever, headache, shivering, tension
Dermatologic: Rash, skin discoloration
Endocrine & metabolic: Breast tenderness, endometritis, hot flashes
Gastrointestinal: Dehydration, diarrhea, nausea, vomiting
Genitourinary: uterine rupture, urinary retention, vaginal pain, vaginismus, vaginitis, vulvitis
Neuromuscular & skeletal: Arthralgia, backache, joint inflammation/pain (new or exacerbated), leg cramps (nocturnal), muscle cramp/pain, myalgia, paresthesia, stiff neck, tremor, weakness
Ocular: Blurred vision, eye pain
Otic: Hearing impairment
Respiratory: Cough, dyspnea, laryngitis, pharyngitis, wheezing
Miscellaneous: Diaphoresis

Vaginal insert: 1% to 10%: Genitourinary: Uterine hyperstimulation *without* fetal distress (2% to 5%), uterine hyperstimulation *with* fetal distress (3%)

Pharmacodynamics/Kinetics

Onset of Action Uterine contractions: Vaginal suppository: Within 10 minutes

Duration of Action Vaginal insert: 0.3 mg/hour over 12 hours; Vaginal suppository: Up to 2-3 hours

Absorption Vaginal suppository: Slow

Time to Peak Endocervical gel: 30-45 minutes

Half-Life Elimination 2.5-5 minutes

Metabolism Metabolized in the lungs; forms metabolites which are further metabolized in the liver and kidney

Excretion Primarily urine; feces (small amounts)

Available Dosage Forms

Gel, endocervical:

Prepidil®: 0.5 mg/3 g (3 g)

Insert, vaginal:

Cervidil®: 10 mg (1s)

Suppository, vaginal:

Prostin E2®: 20 mg (5s)

Dosing

Adult & Geriatric

Abortifacient: *Vaginal suppository:* Insert 20 mg (1 suppository) high in vagina, repeat at 3- to 5-hour intervals until abortion occurs; continued administration for longer than 2 days is not advisable

Cervical ripening:

Endocervical gel: Using catheter supplied with gel, insert 0.5 mg into the cervical canal. May repeat every 6 hours if needed. Maximum cumulative dose: 1.5 mg/24 hours

Vaginal insert: Insert 10 mg transversely into the posterior fornix of the vagina (to be removed at the onset of active labor or after 12 hours)

Pediatric Females of reproductive age: Refer to adult dosing.

Administration

Other

Endocervical gel: Bring to room temperature just prior to use. Do not force the warming process (eg, water bath, microwave). Avoid contact with skin while handling; wash hands thoroughly with soap and water after administration. For cervical ripening, patient should be supine in the dorsal position. The appropriate catheter length should be based on degree of effacement; 20 mm for no effacement; 10 mm if 50% effaced. Patient should remain supine for 15-30 minutes following administration. The manufacturer recommends waiting 6-12 hours after dinoprostone gel administration before initiating oxytocin.

Vaginal insert: One vaginal insert is placed transversely in the posterior fornix of the vagina immediately after removal from its foil package. Patients should remain in the recumbent position for 2 hours after insertion, but thereafter may be ambulatory. Do not use without retrieval system. Product does not need warmed prior to use. A water miscible lubricant may be used to facilitate insertion (avoid excessive use of lubricant). Ensure complete removal of system at completion of therapy. The manufacturer recommends waiting ≥30 minutes after removing the dinoprostone vaginal insert before initiating oxytocin.

Vaginal suppository: Insert high into vagina after removal from its foil package. Bring to room temperature just prior to use. Patient should remain supine for 10 minutes following insertion.

Stability

Storage

Endocervical gel should be stored under refrigeration at 2°C to 8°C (36°F to 46°F).

Suppositories must be kept frozen; store in freezer not above -20°C (-4°F).

Vaginal insert should be stored in freezer between -20°C and -10°C (-4°F and 14°F).

Monitoring and Teaching Issues

Physical Assessment Monitor temperature, uterine tone, and vaginal discharge closely throughout procedure and postprocedure. Monitor abortion for completeness (other measures may be necessary if incomplete).

Patient Education Nausea and vomiting, cramping or uterine pain, or fever may occur. Report acute pain, respiratory difficulty, or skin rash. Closely monitor for vaginal discharge for several days. Report heavy vaginal bleeding, itching, malodorous or bloody discharge, or severe cramping.

Breast-Feeding Considerations Endogenous PGE_2 can be detected in breast milk. High levels have been associated with diarrhea in nursing infants.

Pregnancy Considerations Skeletal anomalies and embryotoxicity have been observed in animal studies. Although these effects would not be expected in humans when administered after the period of organogenesis, a sustained increase in uterine tone may have increased risks of adverse events to the fetus.

Fetal distress without corresponding maternal uterine hyperstimulation was observed in 3% to 4% of infants exposed to Cervidil® *in utero.* No adverse effects on physical or psychomotor function were observed in a 3 year follow-up study of exposed infants. Abnormal fetal heart rates were observed in 17% of infants exposed to Prepidil® gel *in utero.* Deceleration, intrauterine fetal sepsis, fetal depression and fetal acidosis have also been reported with administration of the gel.

When used for termination of pregnancy, dinoprostone is not considered feticidal, but is used to terminate pregnancy due to its ability to stimulate uterine contractions; do not use if fetus has reached the stage of viability.

- **Diotame [OTC]** *see* Bismuth *on page* *221*
- **Diovan®** *see* Valsartan *on page* *1838*
- **Diovan HCT®** *see* Valsartan and Hydrochlorothiazide *on page* *1840*
- **Dipentum®** *see* Olsalazine *on page* *1353*
- **Diphen [OTC]** *see* DiphenhydrAMINE (Systemic) *on page* *543*
- **Diphenhist® [OTC]** *see* DiphenhydrAMINE (Systemic) *on page* *543*
- **Diphenhist® [OTC]** *see* DiphenhydrAMINE (Topical) *on page* *546*

DiphenhydrAMINE (Systemic) (dye fen HYE dra meen)

U.S. Brand Names Aler-Cap [OTC]; Aler-Dryl [OTC]; Aler-Tab [OTC]; AllerMax® [OTC]; Altaryl [OTC]; Anti-Hist [OTC]; Banophen™ [OTC]; Benadryl® Allergy Quick Dissolve [OTC]; Benadryl® Allergy [OTC]; Benadryl® Children's Allergy FastMelt® [OTC]; Benadryl® Children's Allergy Perfect Measure™ [OTC]; Benadryl® Children's Allergy [OTC]; Benadryl® Children's Dye Free Allergy [OTC]; Benadryl® Dye-Free Allergy [OTC]; Compoz® [OTC]; Diphen [OTC]; Diphenhist® [OTC]; Genahist™ [OTC] [DSC]; Histaprin [OTC]; Nytol® Quick Caps [OTC]; Nytol® Quick Gels [OTC]; PediaCare® Children's Allergy [OTC]; PediaCare® Children's NightTime Cough [OTC]; Siladryl Allergy [OTC]; Silphen [OTC]; Simply Sleep® [OTC]; Sleep-ettes D [OTC]; Sleep-Tabs [OTC]; Sleepinal® [OTC]; Sominex® Maximum Strength [OTC]; Sominex® [OTC]; Theraflu® Thin Strips® Multi Symptom [OTC]; Triaminic Thin Strips® Children's Cough & Runny Nose [OTC]; Twilite® [OTC]; Unisom® SleepGels® Maximum Strength [OTC]; Unisom® SleepMelts™ [OTC]

Index Terms Diphenhydramine Citrate; Diphenhydramine Hydrochloride; Diphenhydramine Tannate

Generic Availability (U.S.) Yes: Excludes orally-disintegrating tablet, strip

Pharmacologic Category Ethanolamine Derivative; Histamine H_1 Antagonist; Histamine H_1 Antagonist, First Generation

Medication Safety Issues

Sound-alike/look-alike issues:

DiphenhydrAMINE may be confused with desipramine, dicyclomine, dimenhyDRINATE

Benadryl® may be confused with benazepril, Bentyl®, Benylin®, Caladryl®

Beers Criteria medication: This drug may be inappropriate for use in geriatric patients (high severity risk).

International issues:

Sominex®: Brand name for promethazine in Great Britain

Pregnancy Risk Factor B

Lactation Enters breast milk/contraindicated

Use Symptomatic relief of allergic symptoms caused by histamine release including nasal allergies and allergic dermatosis; adjunct to epinephrine in the treatment of anaphylaxis; nighttime sleep aid; prevention or treatment of motion sickness; antitussive; management of Parkinsonian syndrome including drug-induced extrapyramidal symptoms

Mechanism of Action/Effect Competes with histamine for H_1-receptor sites on effector cells in the gastrointestinal tract, blood vessels, and respiratory tract; anticholinergic and sedative effects are also seen

Contraindications Hypersensitivity to diphenhydramine or any component of the formulation; acute asthma; neonates or premature infants; breast-feeding; use as a local anesthetic (injection)

Warnings/Precautions Causes sedation, caution must be used in performing tasks which require alertness (eg, operating machinery or driving). Sedative effects of CNS depressants or ethanol are potentiated. Should not be used as a hypnotic in the elderly; may cause excessive sedation and confusion; may be inappropriate in this age group when used as an antihistamine due to potent anticholinergic effects (nonanticholinergic antihistamines preferred); when used for emergency allergic reactions, use the smallest effective dose (Beers Criteria). Antihistamines may cause excitation in young children. Use with caution in patients with angle-closure glaucoma, pyloroduodenal obstruction (including stenotic peptic ulcer), urinary tract obstruction (including bladder neck obstruction and symptomatic prostatic hyperplasia), asthma, hyperthyroidism, increased intraocular pressure, and cardiovascular disease (including hypertension and tachycardia). Some preparations contain soy protein; avoid use in patients with soy protein or peanut allergies. Some products may contain phenylalanine.

Self-medication (OTC use): Do not use with other products containing diphenhydramine, even ones used on the skin. Oral products are not for OTC use in children <6 years of age.

Drug Interactions

Metabolism/Transport Effects Inhibits CYP2D6 (moderate)

Avoid Concomitant Use There are no known interactions where it is recommended to avoid concomitant use.

Decreased Effect

DiphenhydrAMINE (Systemic) may decrease the levels/effects of: Acetylcholinesterase Inhibitors (Central); Benzylpenicilloyl Polylysine; Betahistine; Codeine; TraMADol

The levels/effects of DiphenhydrAMINE (Systemic) may be decreased by: Acetylcholinesterase Inhibitors (Central); Amphetamines

Increased Effect/Toxicity

DiphenhydrAMINE (Systemic) may increase the levels/effects of: Alcohol (Ethyl); Anticholinergics; CNS Depressants; CYP2D6 Substrates; Fesoterodine; Nebivolol; Tamoxifen

The levels/effects of DiphenhydrAMINE (Systemic) may be increased by: Droperidol; Pramlintide

Nutritional/Ethanol Interactions

Ethanol: Avoid ethanol (may increase CNS depression).

Herb/Nutraceutical: Avoid valerian, St John's wort, kava kava, gotu kola (may increase CNS depression).

Lab Interactions May interfere with urine detection of methadone and PCP (false-positives); may cause false-positive serum TCA screen; may suppress the wheal and flare reactions to skin test antigens

Adverse Reactions Frequency not defined.

Cardiovascular: Chest tightness, extrasystoles, hypotension, palpitation, tachycardia

Central nervous system: Chills, confusion, convulsion, disturbed coordination, dizziness, euphoria, excitation, fatigue, headache, insomnia, irritability, nervousness, paradoxical excitement, restlessness, sedation, sleepiness, vertigo

Endocrine & metabolic: Menstrual irregularities (early menses)

Gastrointestinal: Anorexia, constipation, diarrhea, dry mucous membranes, epigastric distress, nausea, throat tightness, vomiting, xerostomia

Genitourinary: Difficult urination, urinary frequency, urinary retention

Hematologic: Agranulocytosis, hemolytic anemia, thrombocytopenia

Neuromuscular & skeletal: Neuritis, paresthesia, tremor

Ocular: Blurred vision, diplopia

Otic: Labyrinthitis (acute), tinnitus

Respiratory: Nasal stuffiness, thickening of bronchial secretions, wheezing

Miscellaneous: Anaphylactic shock, diaphoresis

Pharmacodynamics/Kinetics

Onset of Action Maximum sedative effect: 1-3 hours

Duration of Action 4-7 hours

Bioavailability Oral: ~40% to 70%

Time to Peak Serum: 2-4 hours

Protein Binding 78%

Half-Life Elimination 2-10 hours; Elderly: 13.5 hours

Metabolism Extensively hepatic n-demethylation via CYP2D6; minor demethylation via CYP1A2, 2C9 and 2C19; smaller degrees in pulmonary and renal systems; significant first-pass effect

Excretion Urine (as unchanged drug)

Available Dosage Forms

Caplet, oral:
- Aler-Dryl [OTC]: 50 mg
- AllerMax® [OTC]: 50 mg
- Anti-Hist [OTC]: 25 mg
- Compoz® [OTC]: 50 mg
- Histaprin [OTC]: 25 mg
- Nytol® Quick Caps [OTC]: 25 mg
- Simply Sleep® [OTC]: 25 mg
- Sleep-ettes D [OTC]: 50 mg
- Sominex® Maximum Strength [OTC]: 50 mg
- Twilite® [OTC]: 50 mg

Capsule, oral: 25 mg, 50 mg
- Aler-Cap [OTC]: 25 mg
- Banophen™ [OTC]: 25 mg
- Benadryl® Allergy [OTC]: 25 mg
- Diphen [OTC]: 25 mg
- Diphenhist® [OTC]: 25 mg
- Sleepinal® [OTC]: 50 mg

Capsule, softgel, oral:
- Benadryl® Dye-Free Allergy [OTC]: 25 mg
- Compoz® [OTC]: 50 mg
- Nytol® Quick Gels [OTC]: 50 mg
- Unisom® SleepGels® Maximum Strength [OTC]: 50 mg

Captab, oral:
- Diphenhist® [OTC]: 25 mg

Elixir, oral:
- Altaryl [OTC]: 12.5 mg/5 mL (120 mL, 480 mL, 3840 mL)
- Banophen™ [OTC]: 12.5 mg/5 mL (120 mL, 480 mL)

Injection, solution: 50 mg/mL (1 mL, 10 mL)

Injection, solution [preservative free]: 50 mg/mL (1 mL)

Liquid, oral:
- AllerMax® [OTC]: 12.5 mg/5 mL (120 mL)
- Benadryl® Children's Allergy [OTC]: 12.5 mg/5 mL (118 mL, 236 mL)
- Benadryl® Children's Allergy Perfect Measure™ [OTC]: 12.5 mg/5 mL (5 mL)
- Benadryl® Children's Dye Free Allergy [OTC]: 12.5 mg/5 mL (118 mL)
- Siladryl Allergy [OTC]: 12.5 mg/5 mL (118 mL, 237 mL, 473 mL)

Solution, oral: 12.5 mg/5 mL (5 mL, 10 mL, 20 mL)
- Diphenhist® [OTC]: 12.5 mg/5 mL (120 mL, 480 mL)

Strip, orally disintegrating, oral:
- Benadryl® Allergy Quick Dissolve [OTC]: 25 mg (10s)
- Theraflu® Thin Strips® Multi Symptom [OTC]: 25 mg (12s, 24s)
- Triaminic Thin Strips® Children's Cough & Runny Nose [OTC]: 12.5 mg (14s)

Syrup, oral:
- PediaCare® Children's Allergy [OTC]: 12.5 mg/5 mL (118 mL)
- PediaCare® Children's NightTime Cough [OTC]: 12.5 mg/5 mL (118 mL)
- Silphen [OTC]: 12.5 mg/5 mL (118 mL, 237 mL, 473 mL)

Tablet, oral: 25 mg, 50 mg

Aler-Tab [OTC]: 25 mg

Banophen™ [OTC]: 25 mg

Benadryl® Allergy [OTC]: 25 mg

Sleep-Tabs [OTC]: 25 mg

Sominex® [OTC]: 25 mg

Tablet, orally dissolving, oral:

Benadryl® Children's Allergy FastMelt® [OTC]: 12.5 mg

Unisom® SleepMelts™ [OTC]: 25 mg

Dosing

Adult Note: Dosages are expressed as the hydrochloride salt.

Allergic reactions or motion sickness:

Oral: 25-50 mg every 6-8 hours

I.M., I.V.: 10-50 mg per dose; single doses up to 100 mg may be used if needed; not to exceed 400 mg/day

Antitussive: Oral: 25 mg every 4 hours; maximum: 150 mg/24 hours

Night-time sleep aid: Oral: 50 mg at bedtime

Dystonic reaction: I.M., I.V.: 50 mg in a single dose; may repeat in 20-30 minutes if necessary

Geriatric Initial: 25 mg 2-3 times/day increasing as needed

Pediatric Note: Dosages are expressed as the hydrochloride salt.

Allergic reactions or motion sickness: Oral, I.M., I.V.: 5 mg/kg/day or 150 mg/m^2/day in divided doses every 6-8 hours, not to exceed 300 mg/day

Alternate dosing by age: Oral:

2 to <6 years: 6.25 mg every 4-6 hours; maximum: 37.5 mg/day

6 to <12 years: 12.5-25 mg every 4-6 hours; maximum: 150 mg/day

≥12 years: 25-50 mg every 4-6 hours; maximum: 300 mg/day

Night-time sleep aid: Oral: Children ≥12 years: 50 mg at bedtime

Antitussive: Oral:

2 to <6 years: 6.25 mg every 4 hours; maximum: 37.5 mg/day

6 to <12 years: 12.5 mg every 4 hours; maximum: 75 mg/day

≥12 years: 25 mg every 4 hours; maximum: 150 mg/day

Treatment of dystonic reactions: I.M., I.V.: 0.5-1 mg/kg/dose

Administration

Oral When used to prevent motion sickness, first dose should be given 30 minutes prior to exposure.

I.V. Injection solution: For I.V. or I.M. administration only. Local necrosis may result with SubQ or intradermal use. For I.V. administration, inject at a rate ≤25 mg/minute.

Stability

Storage Injection: Store at room temperature of 15°C to 30°C (59°F to 86°F); protect from freezing. Protect from light.

Monitoring and Teaching Issues

Patient Education Avoid use of alcohol. You may experience drowsiness, dizziness, dry mouth, nausea, or vomiting. Report persistent sedation, confusion, agitation, blurred vision, respiratory difficulty, lack of improvement, or worsening of condition.

Dietary Considerations

Benadryl® Allergy strips contain sodium 4 mg per 25 mg strip.

Benadryl® Children's Allergy chewable tablets contain phenylalanine 4.2 mg, magnesium 15 mg, and sodium 2 mg per 12.5 mg tablet.

Benadryl® Children's Allergy Fastmelt® contains phenylalanine 4.5 mg/tablet and soy protein isolate (contraindicated in patients with soy protein allergies; use caution in peanut allergic individuals, ~10% are estimated to also have soy protein allergies).

Geriatric Considerations Diphenhydramine has high sedative and anticholinergic properties, so it may not be considered the antihistamine of choice for prolonged use in the elderly. Its use as a sleep aid is discouraged due to its anticholinergic effects; interpretive guidelines from the Centers for Medicare and Medicaid Services (CMS) discourage the use of diphenhydramine as a sedative or anxiolytic in long-term care facilities.

This medication is considered to be potentially inappropriate in this patient population (Beers Criteria severity: High).

Breast-Feeding Considerations Infants may be more sensitive to the effects of antihistamines. Use while breast-feeding is contraindicated by the manufacturer.

Pregnancy Considerations Teratogenic effects were not observed in animal studies. Diphenhydramine crosses the human placenta. One retrospective study showed an increased risk of cleft palate formation following maternal use of diphenhydramine during the 1st trimester of pregnancy; however, later studies have not confirmed this finding. Signs of toxicity and symptoms of withdrawal have been reported in infants following high doses or chronic maternal use close to term. Diphenhydramine has been evaluated for the treatment of hyperemesis gravidarum. It is generally not considered the antihistamine of choice for treating allergic rhinitis or nausea and vomiting during pregnancy.

Additional Information Diphenhydramine citrate 19 mg is equivalent to diphenhydramine hydrochloride 12.5 mg

DiphenhydrAMINE (Topical) (dye fen HYE dra meen)

U.S. Brand Names Banophen™ Anti-Itch [OTC]; Benadryl® Extra Strength Itch Stopping [OTC]; Benadryl® Itch Relief Extra Strength [OTC]; Benadryl® Itch Stopping Extra Strength [OTC]; Benadryl® Itch Stopping [OTC]; Dermamycin® [OTC]; Diphenhist® [OTC]

Index Terms Diphenhydramine Hydrochloride

Generic Availability (U.S.) Yes: Excludes gel, liquid stick, spray

Pharmacologic Category Ethanolamine Derivative; Histamine H_1 Antagonist; Histamine H_1 Antagonist, First Generation; Topical Skin Product

Medication Safety Issues

Institute for Safe Medication Practices (ISMP) has reported cases of patients mistakenly *swallowing* Benadryl® Itch Stopping [OTC] gel intended for topical application. Unclear labeling and similar packaging of the topical gel in containers resembling an oral liquid are factors believed to be contributing to the administration errors. The topical gel contains camphor which can be toxic if swallowed. ISMP has requested the manufacturer to make the necessary changes to prevent further confusion.

Sound-alike/look-alike issues:

DiphenhydrAMINE may be confused with desipramine, dicyclomine, dimenhyDRINATE

Benadryl® may be confused with benazepril, Bentyl®, Benylin®, Caladryl®

Use Topically for relief of pain and itching associated with insect bites, minor cuts and burns, or rashes due to poison ivy, poison oak, and poison sumac

Available Dosage Forms

Cream, topical: 2% (30 g)

Banophen™ Anti-Itch [OTC]: 2% (28.4 g)

Benadryl® Itch Stopping [OTC]: 1% (14.2 g, 28.3 g)

Benadryl® Itch Stopping Extra Strength [OTC]: 2% (14.2 g, 28.3 g)

Dermamycin® [OTC]: 2% (28 g)

Diphenhist® [OTC]: 2% (28.4 g)

Gel, topical:

Benadryl® Extra Strength Itch Stopping [OTC]: 2% (120 mL)

Liquid, topical:

Benadryl® Itch Relief Extra Strength [OTC]: 2% (14 mL)

Benadryl® Itch Stopping Extra Strength [OTC]: 2% (59 mL)

Dermamycin® [OTC]: 2% (60 mL)

Dosing

Adult Relief of pain and itching: Topical: Apply 1% or 2% to affected area up to 3-4 times/day

Pediatric Relief of pain and itching: Topical: Children ≥2 years: Apply 1% or 2% to affected area up to 3-4 times/day

◆ **Diphenhydramine and ASA** *see* Aspirin and Diphenhydramine *on page 159*

◆ **Diphenhydramine and Aspirin** *see* Aspirin and Diphenhydramine *on page 159*

Diphenhydramine and Phenylephrine (dye fen HYE dra meen & fen il EF rin)

U.S. Brand Names Aldex® CT; Benadryl-D® Allergy & Sinus [OTC]; Benadryl-D® Children's Allergy & Sinus [OTC]; Dimetapp® Children's Nighttime Cold & Congestion [OTC]; Robitussin® Night Time Cough & Cold [OTC]; Triaminic® Children's Night Time Cold & Cough [OTC]; Triaminic® Children's Thin Strips® Night Time Cold & Cough [OTC]

Index Terms Diphenhydramine Hydrochloride and Phenylephrine Hydrochloride; Diphenhydramine Tannate and Phenylephrine Tannate; Phenylephrine and Diphenhydramine; Phenylephrine Hydrochloride and Diphenhydramine Hydrochloride; Phenylephrine Tannate and Diphenhydramine Tannate

Generic Availability (U.S.) No

Pharmacologic Category Alpha/Beta Agonist; Decongestant; Ethanolamine Derivative; Histamine H_1 Antagonist; Histamine H_1 Antagonist, First Generation

Pregnancy Risk Factor C

Lactation Excretion in breast milk unknown/contraindicated

Use Temporary relief of symptoms of allergic rhinitis, sinusitis, and other upper respiratory conditions, including sinus/nasal congestion, sneezing, stuffy/runny nose, itchy/watery eyes, and cough

Available Dosage Forms

Liquid, oral:

Benadryl-D® Children's Allergy & Sinus [OTC]: Diphenhydramine 12.5 mg and phenylephrine 5 mg per 5 mL (118 mL)

Strip, orally disintegrating:

Triaminic® Children's Thin Strips® Night Time Cold & Cough [OTC]: Diphenhydramine 12.5 mg and phenylephrine 5 mg

Syrup, oral:

Dimetapp® Children's Nighttime Cold and Congestion [OTC]: Diphenhydramine 6.25 mg and phenylephrine 2.5 mg per 5 mL (120 mL)

Robitussin® Night Time Cough & Cold [OTC]: Diphenhydramine 6.25 mg and phenylephrine 2.5 mg per 5 mL (120 mL)

Triaminic® Children's Night Time Cold & Cough [OTC]: Diphenhydramine 6.25 mg and phenylephrine 2.5 mg per 5 mL (118 mL)

Tablet, oral:

Benadryl-D® Allergy & Sinus [OTC]: Diphenhydramine 25 mg and phenylephrine 10 mg

Tablet, chewable, oral:

Aldex® CT: Diphenhydramine 12.5 mg and phenylephrine 5 mg

Dosing

Adult Allergic symptoms, nasal congestion: Oral:

Aldex® CT: 1-2 tablets every 6 hours

OTC labeling: **Note:** General dosing guidelines; refer to specific product labeling:

10-20 mL every 4 hours as needed (maximum: 6 doses/24 hours) **or** 1 tablet every 4 hours as needed (maximum: 6 doses/24 hours)

Geriatric Refer to adult dosing.

Pediatric Allergic symptoms, nasal congestion: Oral:

Aldex® CT:

Children 6-11 years: One-half to 1 tablet every 6 hours

Children ≥12 years: Refer to adult dosing.

OTC labeling:

Children <6 years: Use not recommended

Children 6-11 years:

Benadryl-D® Children's Allergy & Sinus: 5 mL every 4 hours as needed (maximum: 6 doses/24 hours)

Dimetapp® Children's Nighttime Cold and Congestion, Triaminic® Children's Night Time Cold & Cough: 10 mL every 4 hours as needed (maximum: 6 doses/24 hours)

Triaminic® Children's Thin Strips® Night Time Cold & Cough: One strip every 4 hours as needed (maximum: 6 doses/24 hours)

Children ≥12 years: Refer to adult dosing.

Monitoring and Teaching Issues

Physical Assessment See individual agents.

Patient Education See individual agents.

- ◆ **Diphenhydramine Citrate** *see* DiphenhydrAMINE (Systemic) *on page 543*
- ◆ **Diphenhydramine Citrate and Aspirin** *see* Aspirin and Diphenhydramine *on page 159*
- ◆ **Diphenhydramine Hydrochloride** *see* DiphenhydrAMINE (Systemic) *on page 543*
- ◆ **Diphenhydramine Hydrochloride** *see* DiphenhydrAMINE (Topical) *on page 546*
- ◆ **Diphenhydramine Hydrochloride and Phenylephrine Hydrochloride** *see* Diphenhydramine and Phenylephrine *on page 546*
- ◆ **Diphenhydramine Tannate** *see* DiphenhydrAMINE (Systemic) *on page 543*
- ◆ **Diphenhydramine Tannate and Phenylephrine Tannate** *see* Diphenhydramine and Phenylephrine *on page 546*

Diphenoxylate and Atropine (dye fen OKS i late & A troe peen)

U.S. Brand Names Lomotil®

Index Terms Atropine and Diphenoxylate

Generic Availability (U.S.) Yes

Pharmacologic Category Antidiarrheal

Medication Safety Issues

Sound-alike/look-alike issues:

Lomotil® may be confused with LaMICtal®, LamISIL®, lamoTRIgine, Lanoxin®, Lasix®, ludiomil

Lonox® may be confused with Lanoxin®, Loprox®

Pregnancy Risk Factor C

Lactation Enters breast milk/use caution

Use Treatment of diarrhea

Controlled Substance C-V

Available Dosage Forms

Solution, oral: Diphenoxylate 2.5 mg and atropine 0.025 mg per 5 mL

Tablet: Diphenoxylate 2.5 mg and atropine 0.025 mg

Dosing

Adult & Geriatric Diarrhea: Oral: Diphenoxylate 5 mg 4 times/day until control achieved (maximum: 20 mg/day), then reduce dose as needed; some patients may be controlled on doses of 5 mg/day

Pediatric Diarrhea: Oral: Children 2-12 years (use with caution in young children due to variable responses): Liquid: Diphenoxylate 0.3-0.4 mg/kg/day in 4 divided doses until control achieved (maximum: 10 mg/day), then reduce dose as needed; some patients may be controlled on doses as low as 25% of the initial daily dose

Administration

Oral If there is no response within 48 hours of continuous therapy, this medication is unlikely to be effective and should be discontinued; if chronic diarrhea is not improved symptomatically within 10 days at maximum dosage, control is unlikely with further use. Use of the liquid preparation is recommended in children <13 years of age; use plastic dropper provided when measuring liquid.

Monitoring and Teaching Issues

Physical Assessment See individual agents.

Patient Education See individual agents.

Related Information

Atropine *on page 172*

◆ **Diphenylhydantoin** *see* Phenytoin *on page 1453*

Diphtheria and Tetanus Toxoids, Acellular Pertussis and *Haemophilus influenzae* b Conjugate Vaccine

(dif THEER ee a & TET a nus TOKS oyds, ay CEL yoo lar per TUS sis & hem OF fi lus in floo EN za bee KON joo gate vak SEEN)

U.S. Brand Names TriHIBit® [DSC]

Index Terms *Haemophilus influenzae* b Conjugate Vaccine and Diphtheria, Tetanus Toxoids, and Acellular Pertussis Vaccine; DTaP/Hib

Generic Availability (U.S.) No

Pharmacologic Category Vaccine, Inactivated (Bacterial)

Pregnancy Risk Factor C

Use Active immunization of children 15-18 months of age for prevention of diphtheria, tetanus, pertussis, and invasive disease caused by *H. influenzae* type b

The Advisory Committee on Immunization Practices (ACIP) recommends the use of TriHIBit® for the fourth dose of the diphtheria, tetanus, pertussis, and *Haemophilus* vaccine series. Whenever feasible, the same manufacturer should be used to provide the pertussis component; however, vaccination should not be deferred if a specific brand is not known or is not available.

Available Dosage Forms

Injection, suspension [preservative free]:

TriHIBit®: Diphtheria 6.7 Lf units, tetanus 5 Lf units, acellular pertussis antigens [inactivated pertussis toxin 23.4 mcg, filamentous hemagglutinin 23.4 mcg], and *Haemophilus* b capsular polysaccharide 10 mcg [bound to tetanus toxoid 24 mcg] per 0.5 mL (0.5 mL) [Tripedia® vaccine used to reconstitute ActHIB® forms TriHIBit®]

Dosing

Pediatric Immunization: Children 15-18 months: I.M.: 0.5 mL: **Note:** For use as the fourth dose of the DTaP and Hib series (see individual vaccines).

Administration

I.M. For I.M use only; do not administer I.V. or SubQ. Administer in the anterolateral aspects of the thigh or the deltoid muscle of the upper arm. Do not inject in the gluteal area or where there may be a major nerve trunk. Do not administer additional vaccines or immunoglobulins at the same site or using the same syringe.

For patients at risk of hemorrhage following intramuscular injection, the ACIP recommends "it should be administered intramuscularly if, in the opinion of the physician familiar with the patients bleeding risk, the vaccine can be administered by this route with reasonable safety. If the patient receives antihemophilia or other similar therapy, intramuscular vaccination can be scheduled shortly after such therapy is administered. A fine needle (23 gauge or smaller) can be used for the vaccination and firm pressure applied to the site (without rubbing) for at least 2 minutes. The patient should be instructed concerning the risk of hematoma from the injection." Patients on anticoagulant therapy should be considered to have the same bleeding risks and treated as those with clotting factor disorders (CDC, 2011).

Simultaneous administration of vaccines helps ensure the patients will be fully vaccinated by the appropriate age. Simultaneous administration of vaccines is defined as administering >1 vaccine on the same day at different anatomic sites. The use of licensed combination vaccines is generally preferred over separate injections of the equivalent components. Separate vaccines should not be combined in the same syringe unless indicated by product specific labeling. Separate needles and syringes should be used for each injection. The ACIP prefers each dose of a specific vaccine in a series come from the same manufacturer when possible. Adolescents and adults should be vaccinated while seated or lying down. In general, preterm infants should be vaccinated at the same chronological age as full-term infants (CDC. 2011).

Antipyretics have not been shown to prevent febrile seizures. Antipyretics may be used to treat fever or discomfort following vaccination (CDC, 2011). One study reported that routine prophylactic administration of acetaminophen to prevent fever prior to vaccination decreased the immune response of some vaccines; the clinical significance of this reduction in immune response has not been established (Prymula, 2009).

Monitoring and Teaching Issues

Physical Assessment Federal law requires entry into the patient's medical record.

Related Information

Immunization Recommendations *on page 1941*

Diphtheria and Tetanus Toxoids, Acellular Pertussis, and Poliovirus Vaccine

(dif THEER ee a & TET a nus TOKS oyds, ay CEL yoo lar per TUS sis & POE lee oh VYE rus vak SEEN)

U.S. Brand Names Kinrix®

Index Terms Diphtheria and Tetanus Toxoids and Acellular Pertussis Adsorbed, and Inactivated Poliovirus Vaccine Combined; Diphtheria, Tetanus Toxoids, Acellular Pertussis (DTaP); DTaP-IPV; Poliovirus, Inactivated (IPV)

Generic Availability (U.S.) No

Pharmacologic Category Vaccine, Inactivated (Bacterial); Vaccine, Inactivated (Viral)

Pregnancy Risk Factor C

Use Active immunization against diphtheria, tetanus, pertussis, and poliomyelitis, used as the 5th dose in the DTaP series and the 4th dose in the IPV series

The Advisory Committee on Immunization Practices (ACIP) recommends routine vaccination for use as the fifth dose in the DTaP series and the fourth dose in the IPV series in children who received DTaP (Infanrix®) and/or DTaP-Hepatitis B-IPV (Pediarix®) as the first 3 doses and DTaP (Infanrix®) as the fourth dose. Whenever feasible, the same manufacturer should be used to provide the pertussis component; however, vaccination should not be deferred if a specific brand is not known or is not available.

Available Dosage Forms

Injection, suspension [preservative free]:

Kinrix®: Diphtheria toxoid 25 Lf, tetanus toxoid 10 Lf, acellular pertussis antigens [inactivated pertussis toxin 25 mcg, filamentous hemagglutinin 25 mcg, pertactin 8 mcg], type 1 poliovirus 40 D-antigen units, type 2 poliovirus 8 D-antigen units, and type 3 poliovirus 32 D-antigen units per 0.5 mL (0.5 mL)

Dosing

Pediatric Immunization: I.M.: Children 4-6 years: 0.5 mL; **Note:** For use as the 5th dose in the DTaP series and the 4th dose in the IPV series

Administration

I.M. For I.M. use only; do not administer intradermally, I.V., or SubQ. Shake well prior to use; do not use unless a homogeneous, turbid, white suspension forms. Discard if the suspension is discolored or if there are cracks in the vial or syringe. Administer in the deltoid muscle of the upper arm. Do not administer additional vaccines or immunoglobulins at the same site, or using the same syringe.

For patients at risk of hemorrhage following intramuscular injection, the ACIP recommends "it should be administered intramuscularly if, in the opinion of the physician familiar with the patients bleeding risk, the vaccine can be administered by this route with reasonable safety. If the patient receives antihemophilia or other similar therapy, intramuscular vaccination can be scheduled shortly after such therapy is administered. A fine needle (23 gauge or smaller) can be used for the vaccination and firm pressure applied to the site (without rubbing) for at least 2 minutes. The patient should be instructed concerning the risk of hematoma from the injection." Patients on anticoagulant therapy should be considered to have the same bleeding risks and treated as those with clotting factor disorders (CDC, 2011).

Simultaneous administration of vaccines helps ensure the patients will be fully vaccinated by the appropriate age. Simultaneous administration of vaccines is defined as administering >1 vaccine on the same day at different anatomic sites. The use of licensed combination vaccines is generally preferred over separate injections of the equivalent components. Separate vaccines should not be combined in the same syringe unless indicated by product specific labeling. Separate needles and syringes should be used for each injection. The ACIP prefers each dose of a specific vaccine in a series come from the same manufacturer when possible. Adolescents and adults should be vaccinated while seated or lying down. In general, preterm infants should be vaccinated at the same chronological age as full-term infants (CDC, 2011).

Antipyretics have not been shown to prevent febrile seizures. Antipyretics may be used to treat fever or discomfort following vaccination (CDC, 2011). One study reported that routine prophylactic administration of acetaminophen to prevent fever prior to vaccination decreased the immune response of some vaccines; the clinical significance of this reduction in immune response has not been established (Prymula, 2009).

Monitoring and Teaching Issues

Physical Assessment Evaluate patient's prior immunization history, current state of health, and appropriateness for vaccination prior to therapy. Defer treatment in presence of acute illness or fever. Treatment for anaphylactic reactions should be immediately available. For I.M. use only. Federal law requires entry into the patient's medical record.

Patient Education Notify prescriber immediately of any acute reaction to vaccination (eg, difficulty breathing or swallowing, chest pain or palpitations, acute headache, rash, seizures, high fever). Follow directions for care of injection site; report persistent redness, swelling, or signs of infection at injection site. May cause drowsiness or loss of appetite; if these persist beyond 1-2 days or become severe, consult prescriber.

Related Information

Immunization Recommendations *on page* 1941

Diphtheria and Tetanus Toxoids, Acellular Pertussis, Hepatitis B (Recombinant), Poliovirus (Inactivated), and *Haemophilus influenzae* B Conjugate (Adsorbed) Vaccine

(dif THEER ee a & TET a nus TOKS oyds, ay CEL yoo lar per TUS sis, hep a TYE tis bee ree KOM be nant, POE lee oh VYE rus in ak ti VAY ted, & hem OF fi lus in floo EN za bee KON joo gate ad SORBED vak SEEN)

Index Terms Diphtheria and Tetanus Toxoids and Acellular Pertussis, Hepatitis B (Recombinant), Inactivated Poliovirus Vaccine, and *Haemophilus influenzae* Type B Combined; DTaP-HepB-IPV-Hib

Generic Availability (U.S.) No

Pharmacologic Category Vaccine, Inactivated (Bacterial, Viral)

Medication Safety Issues

Sound-alike/look-alike issues:

Infanrix Hexa™ may be confused with Infanrix®

Use Active primary immunization against diphtheria, tetanus, pertussis, hepatitis B, poliomyelitis and disease caused by *Haemophilus influenzae* type b in infants and children 6 weeks to 2 years of age; booster immunization (at 18 months) in infants who previously received a full primary vaccination course of each component of the vaccine

Product Availability Not available in U.S.

Dosing

Pediatric Note: Vaccinate preterm infants according to their chronological age from birth.

Children 6 weeks to 2 years:

Primary immunization: I.M.: 0.5 mL; repeat in 8-week intervals for a total of 3 doses. Vaccination usually begins at 2 months, but may be started at 6 weeks of age. Do not administer to infants <6 weeks of age.

Use in children previously vaccinated with one or more doses of hepatitis B vaccine: Children who received 1 dose of hepatitis B vaccine at birth may receive a 3 dose series of Infanrix Hexa™ beginning no earlier than at 6 weeks of age. Use in infants who received more than 1 dose of hepatitis B vaccine has not been studied.

Where immunization against poliovirus is desired, Infanrix Hexa™ may be administered instead to infants scheduled to receive concurrent Infanrix™ (diphtheria, tetanus and acellular pertussis vaccine) and hepatitis B vaccine.

Booster immunization: I.M.: 0.5 mL administered at 18 months (in infants who have received a full primary vaccination course of each component of Infanrix Hexa™)

Note: Dosing delays should not interfere with the final immunity achieved with Infanrix Hexa™. Regardless of the time that elapses between doses, it is not necessary to restart the vaccination series.

Administration

I.M. Administer by I.M. injection only, preferably in the anterolateral aspects of the thigh or the deltoid muscle of the upper arm. Do not administer intravenously or subcutaneously. Do not inject into the gluteal area (suboptimal hepatitis B immune response) or areas where major nerve trunks may be located. Fractional dosing (use of reduced volume) is not recommended. If more than one vaccine is to be given by IM injection use separate limbs. Rotate injection sites when completing vaccination series.

Acetaminophen may be used when needed to provide comfort; however, routine prophylactic administration of acetaminophen to prevent fever due to vaccine use is not recommended. There is evidence of a decreased immune response to some vaccines associated with acetaminophen administration; the clinical significance of this reduction in immune response has not been established.

Diphtheria and Tetanus Toxoids, Acellular Pertussis, Poliovirus and *Haemophilus* b Conjugate Vaccine

(dif THEER ee a & TET a nus TOKS oyds ay CEL yoo lar per TUS sis POE lee oh VYE rus & hem OF fi lus in floo EN za bee KON joo gate vak SEEN)

U.S. Brand Names Pentacel®

Index Terms *Haemophilus* B Conjugate (Hib); *Haemophilus* B Polysaccharide; Diphtheria Toxoid; Diphtheria, Tetanus Toxoids, Acellular Pertussis (DTaP); DTaP-IPV/Hib; Pertussis, Acellular (Adsorbed); Poliovirus, Inactivated (IPV); Tetanus Toxoid

Generic Availability (U.S.) No

Pharmacologic Category Vaccine, Inactivated (Bacterial); Vaccine, Inactivated (Viral)

Medication Safety Issues

Pentacel® is supplied in two vials, one containing DTaP-IPV liquid and one containing Hib powder, which must be mixed together in order to administer the recommended vaccine components.

Pregnancy Risk Factor C

Use Active immunization against diphtheria, tetanus, pertussis, poliomyelitis, and invasive disease caused by *H. influenzae* type b in children 6 weeks through 4 years of age

Advisory Committee on Immunization Practices (ACIP) recommends that Pentacel® (DTaP-IPV/Hib) may be used to provide the recommended DTaP, IPV, and Hib immunization in children <5 years of age. Whenever feasible, the same manufacturer should be used to provide the pertussis component; however, vaccination should not be deferred if a specific brand is not known or is not available. The Hib component in Pentacel® contains a tetanus toxoid conjugate. A Hib vaccine containing the PRP-OMP conjugate (PedvaxHIB®) may provide a more rapid seroconversion following the first dose and may be preferable to use in certain populations (eg, American Indian or Alaska Native children).

Available Dosage Forms

Injection, suspension:

Pentacel®: Diphtheria toxoid 15 Lf, tetanus toxoid 5 Lf, acellular pertussis antigens, poliovirus, and *Haemophilus* b capsular polysaccharide 10 mcg per 0.5 mL (0.5 mL)

Dosing

Pediatric Primary immunization: Children 6 weeks to ≤4 years: I.M.: 0.5 mL per dose administered at 2, 4, 6 and 15-18 months of age (total of 4 doses). The first dose may be administered as early as 6 weeks of age. Following completion of the 4-dose series, children should receive a dose of DTaP vaccine at 4-6 years of age (Daptacel® recommended due to same pertussis antigen used in both products).

Note: Per the ACIP, polio vaccine should not be administered more frequently than 4 weeks apart. Use of the minimum age and minimum intervals during the first 6 months of life should only be done when the vaccine recipient is at risk for imminent exposure to circulating poliovirus (shorter intervals and earlier start dates may lead to lower seroconversion. Pentacel® is not indicated for the polio booster dose given at 4-6 years of age; Kinrix® or IPV should be used.

Children previously vaccinated with ≥1 dose of Daptacel® or IPV vaccines: Pentacel® may be used to complete the first 4 doses of the DTaP or IPV series in children scheduled to receive the other components in the vaccine.

Children previously vaccinated with ≥1 dose of *Haemophilus* b Conjugate vaccine: Pentacel® may be used to complete the series in children scheduled to receive the other components in the vaccine; however, if different brands of *Haemophilus* b Conjugate vaccine are administered to complete the series, 3 primary immunizing doses are needed, followed by a booster dose.

Note: Completion of 3 doses of Pentacel® provides primary immunization against diphtheria, tetanus, *H. influenzae* type B, and poliomyelitis. Completion of the 4-dose series with Pentacel® provides primary immunization against pertussis. It also provides a booster vaccination against diphtheria, tetanus, *H. influenzae* type B, and poliomyelitis.

Administration

I.M. For I.M. administration only. Do not administer I.V. or SubQ. Administer in the anterolateral aspect of thigh in children <1 year of age or deltoid muscle of upper arm in older children. Do not administer to gluteal area or areas near a major nerve trunk. Do not administer additional vaccines or immunoglobulins at the same site or using the same syringe.

For patients at risk of hemorrhage following intramuscular injection, the ACIP recommends: "It should be administered intramuscularly if, in the opinion of the physician familiar with the patient's bleeding risk, the vaccine can be administered by this route with reasonable safety. If the patient receives antihemophilia or other similar therapy, intramuscular vaccination can be scheduled shortly after such therapy is administered. A fine needle (23-gauge or smaller) can be used for the vaccination and firm pressure applied to the site (without rubbing) for at least 2 minutes. The patient should be instructed concerning the risk of hematoma from the injection." Patients on anticoagulant therapy should be considered to have the same bleeding risks and treated as those with clotting factor disorders (CDC, 2011).

Simultaneous administration of vaccines helps ensure the patients will be fully vaccinated by the appropriate age. Simultaneous administration of vaccines is defined as administering >1 vaccine on the same day at different anatomic sites. The use of licensed combination vaccines is generally preferred over separate injections of the equivalent components. Separate vaccines should not be combined in the same syringe unless indicated by product specific labeling. Separate needles and syringes should be used for each injection. The ACIP prefers each dose of a specific vaccine in a series come from the same manufacturer when possible. Adolescents and adults should be vaccinated while seated or lying down. In general, preterm infants should be vaccinated at the same chronological age as full-term infants (CDC, 2011).

Antipyretics have not been shown to prevent febrile seizures. Antipyretics may be used to treat fever or discomfort following vaccination (CDC, 2011). One study reported that routine prophylactic administration of acetaminophen to prevent fever prior to vaccination decreased the immune response of some vaccines; the clinical significance of this reduction in immune response has not been established (Prymula, 2009).

Monitoring and Teaching Issues

Physical Assessment Federal law requires entry into the patient's medical record.

Related Information

Immunization Recommendations *on page 1941*

◆ **Diphtheria and Tetanus Toxoids and Acellular Pertussis Adsorbed, and Inactivated Poliovirus Vaccine Combined** *see* Diphtheria and Tetanus Toxoids, Acellular Pertussis, and Poliovirus Vaccine *on page 548*

◆ **Diphtheria and Tetanus Toxoids and Acellular Pertussis Adsorbed, Hepatitis B (Recombinant) and Inactivated Poliovirus Vaccine Combined** *see* Diphtheria, Tetanus Toxoids, Acellular Pertussis, Hepatitis B (Recombinant), and Poliovirus Vaccine *on page 555*

◆ **Diphtheria and Tetanus Toxoids and Acellular Pertussis, Hepatitis B (Recombinant), Inactivated Poliovirus Vaccine, and *Haemophilus influenzae* Type B Combined** *see* Diphtheria and Tetanus Toxoids, Acellular Pertussis, Hepatitis B (Recombinant), Poliovirus (Inactivated), and *Haemophilus influenzae* B Conjugate (Adsorbed) Vaccine *on page 550*

Diphtheria and Tetanus Toxoids, and Acellular Pertussis Vaccine

(dif THEER ee a & TET a nus TOKS oyds & ay CEL yoo lar per TUS sis vak SEEN)

U.S. Brand Names Adacel®; Boostrix®; Daptacel®; Infanrix®; Tripedia® [DSC]

Index Terms DTaP; Tdap; Tetanus Toxoid, Reduced Diphtheria Toxoid, and Acellular Pertussis, Adsorbed

Generic Availability (U.S.) No

Pharmacologic Category Vaccine, Inactivated (Bacterial)

Medication Safety Issues

Sound-alike/look-alike issues:

Adacel® (Tdap) may be confused with Daptacel® (DTaP)

Tdap (Adacel®, Boostrix®) may be confused with DTaP (Daptacel®, Infanrix®, Tripedia®)

Carefully review product labeling to prevent inadvertent administration of Tdap when DTaP is indicated. Tdap contains lower amounts of diphtheria toxoid and some pertussis antigens than DTaP.

Tdap is not indicated for use in children <10 years of age

DTaP is not indicated for use in persons ≥7 years of age

Guidelines are available in case of inadvertent administration of these products; refer to ACIP recommendations, February 2006 available at http://www.cdc.gov/mmwr/preview/mmwrhtml/rr55e223a1.htm

Note:

DTaP: Diphtheria and tetanus toxoids and acellular pertussis vaccine

DTP: Diphtheria and tetanus toxoids and pertussis vaccine (unspecified pertussis antigens)

DTwP: Diphtheria and tetanus toxoids and whole-cell pertussis vaccine (no longer available on U.S. market)

Tdap: Tetanus toxoid, reduced diphtheria toxoid, and acellular pertussis vaccine

Pregnancy Risk Factor C

Lactation Excretion in breast milk unknown/use caution

Use

Daptacel®, Infanrix®, Tripedia® (DTaP): Active immunization against diphtheria, tetanus, and pertussis from age 6 weeks through 6 years of age (prior to seventh birthday)

Adacel®, Boostrix® (Tdap): Active booster immunization against diphtheria, tetanus, and pertussis

The Advisory Committee on Immunization Practices (ACIP) recommends routine vaccination for the following:

Children 6 weeks to <7 years (DTaP):

- For primary immunization against diphtheria, tetanus and pertussis
- Pediatric patients who are wounded in bombings or similar mass casualty events and who have penetrating injuries or nonintact skin exposure, and have an uncertain vaccination history should receive a tetanus booster with DTaP (if no contraindications exist) (CDC, 57 [RR6], 2008)

Children 7-10 years (Tdap):

- Children not fully vaccinated against pertussis should receive a single dose of Tdap (if no contraindications exist) (CDC, 60[1], 2011)
- Children never vaccinated against diphtheria, tetanus, or pertussis, or whose vaccination status is not known should receive a series of three vaccinations containing tetanus and diphtheria toxoids and the first dose should be with Tdap (CDC, 60[1], 2011)

Adolescents 11-18 years (Tdap):

- A single dose of Tdap as a booster dose in adolescents who have completed the recommended childhood DTaP vaccination series (preferred age of administration is 11-12 years) (CDC, 60[1], 2011)

Adolescents ≥11 years and Adults (Tdap):

- Persons wounded in bombings or similar mass casualty events and who cannot confirm receipt of a tetanus booster within the previous 5 years and who have penetrating injuries or nonintact skin exposure should receive a single dose of Tdap (CDC, 57 [RR6] 2008)

Adults 19-64 years (Tdap): A single dose of Tdap should be given to replace a single dose of the 10-year Td booster in patients who have not previously received Tdap or for whom vaccine status is not known, and as soon as feasible to all:

- Postpartum women (CDC, 57[RR4], 2008; CDC, 60[4], 2011)
- Close contacts of children <12 months of age; Tdap should ideally be administered at least 2 weeks prior to beginning close contact (CDC, 60[4], 2011; CDC, 55[RR17], 2006)
- Healthcare providers with direct patient contact (CDC, 60[4], 2011; CDC, 55[RR17], 2006)

Adults ≥65 years who have not previously received Tdap:

- All adults ≥65 years may receive a single dose of Tdap in place of a dose of Td (CDC, 60 [1], 2011)
- Adults ≥65 years who anticipate close contact with children <12 months of age should receive a single dose of Tdap in place a of a dose of Td (CDC, 60[1], 2011)

Note: Tdap is currently recommended for a single dose only (all age groups) (CDC, 60[1], 2011)

Available Dosage Forms

Injection, suspension [Tdap, booster formulation]:

Adacel®: Diphtheria 2 Lf units, tetanus 5 Lf units, and acellular pertussis antigens per 0.5 mL (0.5 mL)

Boostrix®: Diphtheria 2.5 Lf units, tetanus 5 Lf units, and acellular pertussis antigens per 0.5 mL (0.5 mL)

Injection, suspension [DTaP, active immunization formulation]:

Daptacel®: Diphtheria 15 Lf units, tetanus 5 Lf units, and acellular pertussis antigens per 0.5 mL (0.5 mL)

Infanrix®: Diphtheria 25 Lf units, tetanus 10 Lf units, and acellular pertussis antigens per 0.5 mL (0.5 mL) [preservative free]

Tripedia®: Diphtheria 6.7 Lf units, tetanus 5 Lf units, and acellular pertussis antigens per 0.5 mL (0.5 mL)

Note: Tripedia® vaccine is also used to reconstitute ActHIB® to prepare TriHIBit® vaccine (diphtheria, tetanus toxoids, and acellular pertussis and *Haemophilus influenzae* b conjugate vaccine combination)

Dosing

Adult & Geriatric Note: Tdap can be administered regardless of the interval between the last tetanus or diphtheria toxoid containing vaccine. Tdap is currently recommended for a single dose only (CDC, 60[1], 2011)

Booster Immunization: ACIP recommendations: I.M.:

Adults 19-64 years: 0.5 mL per dose. A single dose of Tdap should be given to replace a single dose of the 10 year Td booster in patients who have not previously received Tdap or for whom vaccine status is not known. A single dose of Tdap is recommended for health care personnel who have not previously received Tdap and who have direct patient contact (CDC, 55[17], 2006; CDC, 60[4], 2011).

Adults ≥65 years: 0.5 mL per dose. A single dose of Tdap may be given to older adults who have not previously received Tdap (CDC, 60[1], 2011)

Booster Immunization: Manufacturer's recommendations: I.M.: Adults ≤64 years (Adacel®, Boostrix®): 0.5 mL as a single dose, administered 5 years after last dose of tetanus toxoid, diphtheria toxoid, and/or pertussis-containing vaccine

Wound management: I.M.: Adacel® or Boostrix® may be used as an alternative to Td vaccine when a tetanus toxoid-containing vaccine is needed for wound management, and in whom the pertussis component is also indicated. Tetanus prophylaxis in patients with wounds should consider if the wound is clean or contaminated, the immunization status of the patient, proper use of tetanus toxoid and/or tetanus immune globulin (TIG), wound cleaning, and (if required) surgical debridement and the proper use of antibiotics. Patients with an uncertain or incomplete tetanus immunization status should have additional follow up to ensure a series is completed. Patients with a history of Arthus reaction following a previous dose of a tetanus toxoid-containing vaccine should not receive a tetanus toxoid-containing vaccine until >10 years after the most recent dose even if they have a wound that is neither clean nor minor. See table.

Tetanus Prophylaxis in Wound Management

History of Tetanus Immunization Doses	Clean, Minor Wounds		All Other Wounds[1]	
	Tetanus Toxoid[2]	TIG	Tetanus Toxoid[2]	TIG
Uncertain or <3 doses	Yes	No	Yes	Yes
3 or more doses	No[3]	No	No[4]	No

[1]Such as, but not limited to, wounds contaminated with dirt, feces, soil, and saliva; puncture wounds; wounds from crushing, tears, burns, and frostbite.

[2]Tetanus toxoid in this chart refers to a tetanus toxoid-containing vaccine. For children <7 years of age, DTaP (DT, if pertussis vaccine contraindicated) is preferred to tetanus toxoid alone. For children ≥7 years and Adults, Td preferred to tetanus toxoid alone; Tdap may be preferred if the patient has not previously been vaccinated with Tdap.

[3]Yes, if ≥10 years since last dose.

[4]Yes, if ≥5 years since last dose.

Adapted from CDC "Yellow Book" (*Health Information for International Travel 2010*), "Routine Vaccine-Preventable Diseases, Tetanus" (available at http://www.cdc.gov/yellowbook) and *MMWR* 2006, 55(RR-17).

Abbreviations: **DT** = Diphtheria and Tetanus Toxoids (formulation for age ≤6 years); **DTaP** = Diphtheria and Tetanus Toxoids, and Acellular Pertussis (formulation for age ≤6 years; Daptacel®, Infanrix®, Tripedia®); **Td** = Diphtheria and Tetanus Toxoids (formulation for age ≥7 years; Decavac®); **TT**= Tetanus toxoid (adsorbed [formulation for age ≥7 years]); **Tdap** = Diphtheria and Tetanus Toxoids, and Acellular Pertussis (Adacel® or Boostrix® [formulations for age ≥7 years]); **TIG** = Tetanus Immune Globulin

Pediatric Note: Tdap can be administered regardless of the interval between the last tetanus or diphtheria toxoid containing vaccine. Tdap is currently recommended for a single dose only (CDC, 60[1], 2011)

Primary immunization: I.M.:

Children 6 weeks to <7 years: **Note:** Whenever possible, the same product should be used for all doses. Interruption of recommended schedule does not require starting the series over; a delay between doses should not interfere with final immunity.

Daptacel®, Infanrix®, Tripedia®: 0.5 mL per dose, total of 5 doses administered as follows:

Three doses, usually given at 2-, 4-, and 6 months of age; may be given as early as 6 weeks of age and repeated every 4-8 weeks

Fourth dose: Given at ~15-20 months of age, but at least 6 months after third dose. The fourth dose may be given as early as 12 months of age, but at least 6 months must have elapsed between the third dose and the fourth dose.

Fifth dose: Given at 4-6 years of age, prior to starting school or kindergarten; if the fourth dose is given at ≥4 years of age, the fifth dose may be omitted

For children who start primary immunization series ≥4 months of age, refer to current ACIP "Catch-up Immunization Schedule".

Children 7-10 years: Not fully vaccinated against pertussis, or never vaccinated against diphtheria, tetanus, or pertussis, or whose vaccination status is not known: Administer a series of 3 vaccinations containing tetanus and diphtheria toxoids; the first dose should be with Tdap (CDC, 60[1], 2011).

Booster Immunization: ACIP recommendations: I.M.: Adolescents 11-18 years: 0.5 mL per dose. Tdap should be given as a single booster dose at age 11 or 12 years in adolescents who have completed a childhood vaccination series, followed by booster doses of Td every 10 years. Adolescents who have not received Tdap at age 11 or 12 should receive a single dose of Tdap in place of a single Td booster dose (CDC, 55[3], 2006; CDC, 60[1], 2011).

Booster Immunization: Manufacturer's recommendations: I.M.:

Children ≥10 years (Boostrix®): 0.5 mL as a single dose, administered 5 years after last dose of tetanus toxoid, diphtheria toxoid, and/or pertussis-containing vaccine

Children ≥11 years (Adacel®): 0.5 mL as a single dose, administered 5 years after last dose of tetanus toxoid, diphtheria toxoid and/or pertussis-containing vaccine

Wound management: Refer to adult dosing.

Administration

I.M. Shake suspension well.

Adacel®, Boostrix®: Administer only I.M. in deltoid muscle of upper arm.

Daptacel®, Infanrix®, Tripedia®: Administer only I.M. in anterolateral aspect of thigh or deltoid muscle of upper arm.

If feasible, the same brand of DTaP should be used for all doses in the series (CDC, 60 [2], 2011).

For patients at risk of hemorrhage following intramuscular injection, the ACIP recommends "it should be administered intramuscularly if, in the opinion of the physician familiar with the patients bleeding risk, the vaccine can be administered by this route with reasonable safety. If the patient receives antihemophilia or other similar therapy, intramuscular vaccination can be scheduled shortly after such therapy is administered. A fine needle (23 gauge or smaller) can be used for the vaccination and firm pressure applied to the site (without rubbing) for at least 2 minutes. The patient should be instructed concerning the risk of hematoma from the injection." Patients on anticoagulant therapy should be considered to have the same bleeding risks and treated as those with clotting factor disorders (CDC, 60[2], 2011).

Simultaneous administration of vaccines helps ensure the patients will be fully vaccinated by the appropriate age. Simultaneous administration of vaccines is defined as administering >1 vaccine on the same day at different anatomic sites. The use of licensed combination vaccines is generally preferred over separate injections of the equivalent components. Separate vaccines should not be combined in the same syringe unless indicated by product specific labeling. Separate needles and syringes should be used for each injection. The ACIP prefers each dose of a specific vaccine in a series come from the same manufacturer when possible. Adolescents and adults should be vaccinated while seated or lying down. In general, preterm infants should be vaccinated at the same chronological age as full-term infants (CDC, 60[2], 2011).

Antipyretics have not been shown to prevent febrile seizures. Antipyretics may be used to treat fever or discomfort following vaccination (CDC, 2011). One study reported that routine prophylactic administration of acetaminophen to prevent fever prior to vaccination decreased the immune response of some vaccines; the clinical significance of this reduction in immune response has not been established (Prymula, 2009).

Monitoring and Teaching Issues

Physical Assessment Federal law requires entry into the patient's medical record.

Related Information

Immunization Recommendations *on page 1941*

Prophylaxis for Patients Exposed to Common Communicable Diseases *on page 2073*

◆ **Diphtheria CRM$_{197}$ Protein** *see* Pneumococcal Conjugate Vaccine (7-Valent) *on page 1469*

◆ **Diphtheria CRM$_{197}$ Protein** *see* Pneumococcal Conjugate Vaccine (13-Valent) *on page 1470*

◆ **Diphtheria, Tetanus Toxoids, Acellular Pertussis (DTaP)** *see* Diphtheria and Tetanus Toxoids, Acellular Pertussis, and Poliovirus Vaccine *on page 548*

◆ **Diphtheria, Tetanus Toxoids, Acellular Pertussis (DTaP)** *see* Diphtheria and Tetanus Toxoids, Acellular Pertussis, Poliovirus and *Haemophilus* b Conjugate Vaccine *on page 550*

Diphtheria, Tetanus Toxoids, Acellular Pertussis, Hepatitis B (Recombinant), and Poliovirus Vaccine

(dif THEER ee a, TET a nus TOKS oyds, ay CEL yoo lar per TUS sis, hep a TYE tis bee ree KOM be nant, & POE lee oh VYE rus vak SEEN)

U.S. Brand Names Pediarix®

Index Terms Diphtheria and Tetanus Toxoids and Acellular Pertussis Adsorbed, Hepatitis B (Recombinant) and Inactivated Poliovirus Vaccine Combined; DTaP-HepB-IPV

Generic Availability (U.S.) No

Pharmacologic Category Vaccine, Inactivated (Bacterial); Vaccine, Inactivated (Viral)

Pregnancy Risk Factor C

Use Combination vaccine for the active immunization against diphtheria, tetanus, pertussis, hepatitis B virus (all known subtypes), and poliomyelitis (caused by poliovirus types 1, 2, and 3)

The Advisory Committee on Immunization Practices (ACIP) recommends Pediarix® for the following:

- Primary vaccination for DTaP, Hep B, and IPV in children at 2, 4, and 6 months of age.
- To complete the primary vaccination series in children who have received DTaP (Infanrix®) and who are scheduled to receive the other components of the vaccine. Whenever feasible, the same manufacturer should be used to provide the pertussis component; however, vaccination should not be deferred if a specific brand is not known or is not available. HepB and IPV from different manufacturers are interchangeable.

Available Dosage Forms

Injection, suspension [preservative free]:

Pediarix®: Diphtheria toxoid 25 Lf, tetanus toxoid 10 Lf, acellular pertussis antigens per 0.5 mL (0.5 mL)

Dosing

Pediatric

Primary immunization: Children 6 weeks to <7 years: I.M.: 0.5 mL/dose; administer as a 3-dose series at 2-, 4-, and 6 months of age in 6- to 8-week intervals (preferably 8-week intervals). Vaccination usually begins at 2 months, but may be started as early as 6 weeks of age.

Note: Pediarix® is approved for the first 3 doses of polio vaccine. Per the ACIP, polio vaccine is given at 2, 4 and 6 months of age and should not be administered more frequently than 4 weeks apart. Use of the minimum age and minimum intervals during the first 6 months of life should only be done when the vaccine recipient is at risk for imminent exposure to circulating poliovirus (shorter intervals and earlier start dates may lead to lower seroconversion).

Use in children previously vaccinated with one or more component, and who are also scheduled to receive all vaccine components:

Hepatitis B vaccine: Infants previously vaccinated with 1 or 2 doses of another hepatitis B vaccine may use Pediarix® to complete the 3-dose series. Not for use as birth dose of hepatitis B vaccine. Infants born to HB_sAg-positive women should begin dosing with DTaP-HepB-IPV by age 6-8 weeks after receiving the single antigen hepatitis B vaccine at birth.

Diphtheria and tetanus toxoids, and acellular pertussis vaccine (DTaP): Infants previously vaccinated with 1 or 2 doses of Infanrix® may use Pediarix® to complete the first 3 doses of the series; use of Pediarix® to complete DTaP vaccination started with products other than Infanrix® is not recommended.

Inactivated polio vaccine (IPV): Infants previously vaccinated with 1 or 2 doses of IPV may use Pediarix® to complete the first 3 doses of the series.

Administration

I.M. For I.M. use only; do not administer I.V., SubQ, or intradermally. Shake well prior to use; do not use unless a homogeneous, turbid, white suspension forms. Administer in the anterolateral aspects of the thigh or the deltoid muscle of the upper arm. Do not inject in the gluteal area (suboptimal hepatitis B immune response) or where there may be a major nerve trunk. Do not administer additional vaccines or immunoglobulins at the same site, or using the same syringe.

For patients at risk of hemorrhage following intramuscular injection, the ACIP recommends "it should be administered intramuscularly if, in the opinion of the physician familiar with the patients bleeding risk, the vaccine can be administered by this route with reasonable safety. If the patient receives antihemophilia or other similar therapy, intramuscular vaccination can be scheduled shortly after such therapy is administered. A fine needle (23 gauge or smaller) can be used for the vaccination and firm pressure applied to the site (without rubbing) for at least 2 minutes. The patient should be instructed concerning the risk of hematoma from the injection." Patients on anticoagulant therapy should be considered to have the same bleeding risks and treated as those with clotting factor disorders (CDC, 2011).

Simultaneous administration of vaccines helps ensure the patients will be fully vaccinated by the appropriate age. Simultaneous administration of vaccines is defined as administering >1 vaccine on the same day at different anatomic sites. The use of licensed combination vaccines is generally preferred over separate injections of the equivalent components. Separate vaccines should not be combined in the same syringe unless indicated by product specific labeling. Separate needles and syringes should be used for each injection. The ACIP prefers each dose of a specific vaccine in a series come from the same manufacturer when possible. Adolescents and adults should be vaccinated while seated or lying down. In general, preterm infants should be vaccinated at the same chronological age as full-term infants (CDC, 2011).

Antipyretics have not been shown to prevent febrile seizures. Antipyretics may be used to treat fever or discomfort following vaccination (CDC, 2011). One study reported that routine prophylactic administration of acetaminophen to prevent fever prior to vaccination decreased the immune response of some vaccines; the clinical significance of this reduction in immune response has not been established (Prymula, 2009).

Monitoring and Teaching Issues

Physical Assessment Children who are moderately-to-severely ill should not get this vaccination until they have recovered. Assess any hypersensitivity history prior to administering. Treatment for anaphylactic/anaphylactoid reaction should be available. Antipyretics should be administered at time of and for 24 hours following vaccination to patients at high-risk for seizures. Federal law requires entry into the patient's medical record.

Patient Education Inform prescriber of all previous allergic reactions. Three doses will be required for effective immunity; consult prescriber for appropriate schedule of vaccinations. May cause increased sleeping, restlessness, fussiness, decreased appetite, or fever. Use antipyretic if directed by prescriber. May cause some redness, pain, or swelling at injection site; consult prescriber if excessive or persistent. Notify prescriber immediately of any severe reactions (eg, fever >105°F within 48 hours, inconsolable crying that occurs within 48 hours and lasts 3 hours, seizures that occur within 3 days).

Related Information

Immunization Recommendations *on page* 1941

◆ **Diphtheria Toxoid** *see* Diphtheria and Tetanus Toxoids, Acellular Pertussis, Poliovirus and *Haemophilus* b Conjugate Vaccine *on page* 550

◆ **Diphtheria Toxoid Conjugate** *see Haemophilus* b Conjugate Vaccine *on page* 893

◆ **Diprolene®** *see* Betamethasone *on page* 205

◆ **Diprolene® AF** *see* Betamethasone *on page* 205

◆ **Dipropylacetic Acid** *see* Valproic Acid *on page* 1832

Dipyridamole (dye peer ID a mole)

U.S. Brand Names Persantine®

Generic Availability (U.S.) Yes

Pharmacologic Category Antiplatelet Agent; Vasodilator

Medication Safety Issues

Sound-alike/look-alike issues:

Dipyridamole may be confused with disopyramide

Persantine® may be confused with Periactin®, Permitil®

Beers Criteria medication: This drug may be inappropriate for use in geriatric patients (low severity risk).

Pregnancy Risk Factor B

Lactation Enters breast milk/use caution

Use

Oral: Used with warfarin to decrease thrombosis in patients after artificial heart valve replacement

I.V.: Diagnostic agent in CAD

Unlabeled/Investigational Use Stroke prevention (in combination with aspirin)

Available Dosage Forms

Injection, solution: 5 mg/mL (2 mL, 10 mL)

Tablet, oral: 25 mg, 50 mg, 75 mg

Persantine®: 25 mg, 50 mg, 75 mg

Dosing

Adult & Geriatric

Adjunctive therapy for prophylaxis of thromboembolism with cardiac valve replacement: Oral: 75-100 mg 4 times/day

Evaluation of coronary artery disease: I.V.: 0.14 mg/kg/minute for 4 minutes; maximum dose: 60 mg

Following dipyridamole infusion, inject thallium-201 within 5 minutes. **Note:** Aminophylline should be available for urgent/emergent use; dosing of 50-100 mg (range: 50-250 mg) I.V. push over 30-60 seconds.

Pediatric

Adjunctive therapy for prophylaxis of thromboembolism with cardiac valve replacement: Oral: Children ≥12 years: Refer to adult dosing.

Administration

Oral Administer with water 1 hour before meals.

I.V. I.V.: Infuse diluted solution over 4 minutes.

Monitoring and Teaching Issues

Physical Assessment Observe bleeding precautions. Oral: Monitor blood pressure on a regular basis. I.V.: Continuous ECG and blood pressure monitoring necessary during infusion.

Patient Education Take tablet with water 1 hour before meals. Inform prescribers and dentists that you are taking this medication prior to scheduling any surgery or dental procedure. You may experience mild headache, transient diarrhea, or temporary dizziness. You may have a tendency to bleed easily. Report chest pain, redness around mouth, acute abdominal cramping or severe diarrhea, acute and persistent headache or dizziness, rash, respiratory difficulty, or swelling of extremities.

◆ **Dipyridamole and Aspirin** *see* Aspirin and Dipyridamole *on page 160*
◆ **Disodium Cromoglycate** *see* Cromolyn (Systemic, Oral Inhalation) *on page 429*
◆ ***d*-Isoephedrine Hydrochloride** *see* Pseudoephedrine *on page 1529*

Disulfiram (dye SUL fi ram)

U.S. Brand Names Antabuse®
Generic Availability (U.S.) Yes
Pharmacologic Category Aldehyde Dehydrogenase Inhibitor
Medication Safety Issues
Sound-alike/look-alike issues:
Disulfiram may be confused with Diflucan®
Antabuse® may be confused with Anturane®
Pregnancy Risk Factor C
Lactation Excretion in breast milk unknown
Use Management of chronic alcoholism
Available Dosage Forms
Tablet, oral: 250 mg
Antabuse®: 250 mg, 500 mg
Dosing
Adult & Geriatric Note: Do not administer until the patient has abstained from ethanol for at least 12 hours.

Alcoholism: Oral: Initial: 500 mg/day as a single dose for 1-2 weeks; maximum daily dose is 500 mg. Average maintenance dose: 250 mg/day; range: 125-500 mg; duration of therapy is to continue until the patient is fully recovered socially and a basis for permanent self control has been established. Maintenance therapy may be required for months or even years.

Administration
Oral Administration of any medications containing alcohol, including topicals, is contraindicated. Do not administer disulfiram if ethanol has been consumed within the prior 12 hours.
Monitoring and Teaching Issues
Laboratory Monitoring Monitor liver function before and 10-14 days after beginning therapy.
Physical Assessment Do not administer until the patient has abstained from ethanol for 12 hours. Assess results of laboratory tests and for CNS changes prior to treatment and periodically. Advise patient about disulfiram reaction if alcohol is ingested.
Patient Education Tablets can be crushed or mixed with water or juice. Metallic aftertaste may occur; this will go away. Do not drink any alcohol, including products containing alcohol (such as cough and cold syrups or some mouthwashes), or use alcohol-containing skin products while taking this medication and for at least 3 days (preferably 14 days) after stopping this medication. Drowsiness, tiredness, or visual changes may occur. Notify prescriber of any weakness, nausea, vomiting, decreased appetite, yellowing of skin or eyes, dark-colored urine, or numbness of fingers or feet.

◆ **Ditropan** *see* Oxybutynin *on page 1378*
◆ **Ditropan XL®** *see* Oxybutynin *on page 1378*

Divalproex (dye VAL proe ex)

U.S. Brand Names Depakote®; Depakote® ER; Depakote® Sprinkle
Index Terms Divalproex Sodium; Valproate Semisodium; Valproic Acid Derivative
Generic Availability (U.S.) Yes
Pharmacologic Category Anticonvulsant, Miscellaneous; Antimanic Agent; Histone Deacetylase Inhibitor
Medication Safety Issues
Sound-alike/look-alike issues:
Depakote® may be confused with Depakene®, Depakote® ER, Senokot®
Depakote® ER may be confused with Depakote®, divalproex enteric coated
Pregnancy Risk Factor D
Lactation Enters breast milk/not recommended (AAP considers "compatible"; AAP 2001 update pending)
Use Monotherapy and adjunctive therapy in the treatment of patients with complex partial seizures; monotherapy and adjunctive therapy of simple and complex absence seizures; adjunctive therapy in patients with multiple seizure types that include absence seizures
Depakote®, Depakote® ER: Mania associated with bipolar disorder; migraine prophylaxis
Mechanism of Action/Effect Causes increased availability of gamma-aminobutyric acid (GABA), an inhibitory neurotransmitter, to brain neurons or may enhance the action of GABA or mimic its action at postsynaptic receptor sites
Contraindications Hypersensitivity to divalproex, derivatives, or any component of the formulation; hepatic disease or significant impairment; urea cycle disorders
Warnings/Precautions
[U.S. Boxed Warning]: Hepatic failure resulting in fatalities has occurred in patients; children <2 years of age are at considerable risk. Other risk factors include organic brain disease, mental retardation with severe seizure disorders, congenital metabolic disorders, and patients on multiple anticonvulsants. Hepatotoxicity has usually been reported within 6 months

of therapy initiation. Monitor patients closely for appearance of malaise, weakness, facial edema, anorexia, jaundice, and vomiting; discontinue immediately with signs/symptom of significant or suspected impairment. Liver function tests should be performed at baseline and at regular intervals after initiation of therapy, especially within the first 6 months. Hepatic dysfunction may progress despite discontinuing treatment. Should only be used as monotherapy in children <2 years of age and patients at high risk for hepatotoxicity. Contraindicated with severe impairment.

[U.S. Boxed Warning]: Cases of life-threatening pancreatitis, occurring at the start of therapy or following years of use, have been reported in adults and children. Some cases have been hemorrhagic with rapid progression of initial symptoms to death. Promptly evaluate symptoms of abdominal pain, nausea, vomiting, and/or anorexia; should generally be discontinued if pancreatitis is diagnosed.

[U.S. Boxed Warning]: May cause teratogenic effects such as neural tube defects (eg, spina bifida). Use in women of childbearing potential requires that benefits of use in mother be weighed against the potential risk to fetus, especially when used for conditions not associated with permanent injury or risk of death (eg, migraine).

May cause severe thrombocytopenia, inhibition of platelet aggregation, and bleeding. Tremors may indicate overdosage; use with caution in patients receiving other anticonvulsants. Hypersensitivity reactions affecting multiple organs have been reported in association with divalproex use; may include dermatologic and/or hematologic changes (eosinophilia, neutropenia, thrombocytopenia) or symptoms of organ dysfunction.

Hyperammonemia and/or encephalopathy, sometimes fatal, have been reported following the initiation of divalproex therapy and may be present with normal transaminase levels. Ammonia levels should be measured in patients who develop unexplained lethargy and vomiting, changes in mental status, or in patients who present with hypothermia (unintentional drop in core body temperature to <35°C/95°F). Discontinue therapy if ammonia levels are increased and evaluate for possible urea cycle disorder (UCD); contraindicated in patients with UCD. Evaluation of UCD should be considered for the following patients prior to the start of therapy: History of unexplained encephalopathy or coma; encephalopathy associated with protein load; pregnancy or postpartum encephalopathy; unexplained mental retardation; history of elevated plasma ammonia or glutamine; history of cyclical vomiting and lethargy; episodic extreme irritability, ataxia; low BUN or protein avoidance; family history of UCD or unexplained infant deaths (particularly male); or signs or symptoms of UCD (hyperammonemia, encephalopathy, respiratory alkalosis). Hypothermia has been reported with divalproex therapy; may or may not be associated with hyperammonemia; may also occur with concomitant topiramate therapy.

In vitro studies have suggested divalproex stimulates the replication of HIV and CMV viruses under experimental conditions. The clinical consequence of this is unknown, but should be considered when monitoring affected patients.

Antiepileptics are associated with an increased risk of suicidal behavior/thoughts with use (regardless of indication); patients should be monitored for signs/symptoms of depression, suicidal tendencies, and other unusual behavior changes during therapy and instructed to inform their healthcare provider immediately if symptoms occur.

Anticonvulsants should not be discontinued abruptly because of the possibility of increasing seizure frequency; divalproex should be withdrawn gradually to minimize the potential of increased seizure frequency, unless safety concerns require a more rapid withdrawal. Concomitant use with carbapenem antibiotics may reduce valproic acid levels to subtherapeutic levels; monitor levels frequently and consider alternate therapy if levels drop significantly or lack of seizure control occurs. Concomitant use with clonazepam may induce absence status. Patients treated for bipolar disorder should be monitored closely for clinical worsening or suicidality; prescriptions should be written for the smallest quantity consistent with good patient care.

CNS depression may occur with divalproex use. Patients must be cautioned about performing tasks which require mental alertness (operating machinery or driving). Effects with other sedative drugs or ethanol may be potentiated. Use with caution in the elderly.

Drug Interactions

Metabolism/Transport Effects For divalproex: **Substrate** (minor) of CYP2A6, 2B6, 2C9, 2C19, 2E1; **Inhibits** CYP2C9 (weak), 2C19 (weak), 2D6 (weak), 3A4 (weak); **Induces** CYP2A6 (weak)

Avoid Concomitant Use There are no known interactions where it is recommended to avoid concomitant use.

Decreased Effect

Divalproex may decrease the levels/effects of: CarBAMazepine; OXcarbazepine; Phenytoin

The levels/effects of Divalproex may be decreased by: Barbiturates; CarBAMazepine; Carbapenems; Ethosuximide; Methylfolate; Phenytoin; Primidone; Protease Inhibitors; Rifampin

Increased Effect/Toxicity

Divalproex may increase the levels/effects of: Barbiturates; Ethosuximide; LamoTRIgine; LORazepam; Paliperidone; Primidone; RisperiDONE; Rufinamide; Temozolomide; Tricyclic Antidepressants; Vorinostat; Zidovudine

The levels/effects of Divalproex may be increased by: ChlorproMAZINE; Felbamate; GuanFACINE; Salicylates; Topiramate

Nutritional/Ethanol Interactions

Ethanol: Avoid ethanol (may increase CNS depression).

Food: Food may delay but does not affect the extent of absorption. Valproic acid serum concentrations may be decreased if taken with food. Milk has no effect on absorption.

Herb/Nutraceutical: Avoid evening primrose (seizure threshold decreased).

Lab Interactions Divalproex may cause abnormalities in liver function tests; false-positive result for urine ketones

Adverse Reactions

>10%:

Central nervous system: Headache (≤31%), somnolence (≤30%), dizziness (12% to 25%), insomnia (>1% to 15%), nervousness (>1% to 11%), pain (1% to 11%)

Dermatologic: Alopecia (>1% to 24%)

Gastrointestinal: Nausea (15% to 48%), vomiting (7% to 27%), diarrhea (7% to 23%), abdominal pain (7% to 23%), dyspepsia (7% to 23%), anorexia (>1% to 12%)

Hematologic: Thrombocytopenia (1% to 24%; dose related)

Neuromuscular & skeletal: Tremor (≤57%), weakness (6% to 27%)

Ocular: Diplopia (>1% to 16%), amblyopia/blurred vision (≤12%)

Miscellaneous: Infection (≤20%), flu-like syndrome (12%)

1% to 10%:

Cardiovascular: Peripheral edema (>1% to 8%), chest pain (>1% to <5%), edema (>1% to <5%), facial edema (>1% to <5%), hypertension (>1% to <5%), hypotension (>1% to <5%), palpitation (>1% to <5%), postural hypotension (>1% to <5%), tachycardia (>1% to <5%), vasodilation(>1% to <5%), arrhythmia

Central nervous system: Ataxia (>1% to 8%), amnesia (>1% to 7%), emotional lability (>1% to 6%), fever (>1% to 6%), abnormal thinking (≤6%), depression (>1% to 5%), abnormal dreams (>1% to <5%), agitation (>1% to <5%), anxiety (>1% to <5%), catatonia (>1% to <5%), chills (>1% to <5%), confusion (>1% to <5%), coordination abnormal (>1% to <5%), hallucination (>1% to <5%), malaise (>1% to <5%), personality disorder (>1% to <5%), speech disorder (>1% to <5%), tardive dyskinesia (>1% to <5%), vertigo (>1% to <5%), euphoria (1%), hypoesthesia (1%)

Dermatologic: Rash (>1% to 6%), bruising (>1% to 5%), discoid lupus erythematosus (>1% to <5%), dry skin (>1% to <5%), furunculosis (>1% to <5%), petechia (>1% to <5%), pruritus (>1% to <5), seborrhea (>1% to <5%)

Endocrine & metabolic: Amenorrhea (>1% to <5%), dysmenorrhea (>1% to <5%), metrorrhagia (>1% to <5%), hypoproteinemia

Gastrointestinal: Weight gain (4% to 9%), weight loss (6%), appetite increased (≤6%), constipation (>1% to 5%), xerostomia (>1% to 5%), eructation (>1% to <5%), fecal incontinence (>1% to <5%), flatulence (>1% to <5%), gastroenteritis (>1% to <5%), glossitis (>1% to <5%), hematemesis (>1% to <5%), pancreatitis (>1% to <5%), periodontal abscess (>1% to <5%), stomatitis (>1% to <5%), taste perversion (>1% to <5%), dysphagia, gum hemorrhage, mouth ulceration

Genitourinary: Cystitis (>1% to 5%), dysuria (>1% to 5%), urinary frequency (>1% to <5%), urinary incontinence (>1% to <5%), vaginal hemorrhage (>1% to 5%), vaginitis (>1% to <5%)

Hepatic: ALT increased (>1% to <5%), AST increased (>1% to <5%)

Local: Injection site pain (3%), injection site reaction (2%), injection site inflammation (1%)

Neuromuscular & skeletal: Back pain (≤8%), abnormal gait (>1% to <5%), arthralgia (>1% to <5%), arthrosis (>1% to <5%), dysarthria (>1% to <5%), hypertonia (>1% to <5%), hypokinesia (>1% to <5%), leg cramps (>1% to <5%), myalgia (>1% to <5%), myasthenia (>1% to <5%), neck pain (>1% to <5%), neck rigidity (>1% to <5%), paresthesia (>1% to <5%), reflex increased (>1% to <5%), twitching (>1% to <5%)

Ocular: Nystagmus (1% to 8%), dry eyes (>1% to 5%), eye pain (>1% to 5%), abnormal vision (>1% to <5%), conjunctivitis (>1% to <5%)

Otic: Tinnitus (1% to 7%), ear pain (>1% to 5%), deafness (>1% to <5%), otitis media (>1% to <5%)

Respiratory: Pharyngitis (2% to 8%), bronchitis (5%), rhinitis (>1% to 5%), dyspnea (1% to 5%), cough (>1% to <5%), epistaxis (>1% to <5%), pneumonia (>1% to <5%), sinusitis (>1% to <5%)

Miscellaneous: Diaphoresis (1%), hiccups

Pharmacodynamics/Kinetics

Bioavailability Depakote® ER: ~90% relative to I.V. dose and ~89% relative to delayed release formulation

Time to Peak Serum: Depakote® tablet: ~4 hours; Depakote® ER: 4-17 hours

Protein Binding Dose dependent: 80% to 90%; decreased in the elderly and with hepatic or renal dysfunction

Half-Life Elimination Increased in neonates and with liver disease; Children >2 months: 7-13 hours; Adults: 9-16 hours

Metabolism Extensively hepatic via glucuronide conjugation and mitochondrial beta-oxidation. The relationship between dose and total valproate concentration is nonlinear; concentration does not increase proportionally with the dose, but increases to a lesser extent due to saturable plasma protein binding. The kinetics of unbound drug are linear.

Excretion Urine (30% to 50% as glucuronide conjugate, 3% as unchanged drug)

Available Dosage Forms

Capsule, sprinkle, oral: 125 mg

Depakote® Sprinkle: 125 mg

Tablet, delayed release, oral: 125 mg, 250 mg, 500 mg

Depakote®: 125 mg, 250 mg, 500 mg

Tablet, extended release, oral: 250 mg, 500 mg

Depakote® ER: 250 mg, 500 mg

Dosing

Adult Equivalent oral dosages of divalproex and valproic acid deliver the same quantities of valproate ion.

Seizures: Oral: Administer doses >250 mg/day in divided doses.

Simple and complex absence seizure: Initial: 15 mg/kg/day; increase by 5-10 mg/kg/day at weekly intervals until therapeutic levels are achieved; maximum: 60 mg/kg/day.

Complex partial seizure: Initial: 10-15 mg/kg/day; increase by 5-10 mg/kg/day at weekly intervals until therapeutic levels are achieved; maximum: 60 mg/kg/day.

Note: Regular release and delayed release formulations are usually given in 2-4 divided doses/day; extended release formulation (Depakote® ER) is usually given once daily. Conversion to Depakote® ER from a stable dose of Depakote® may require an increase in the total daily dose between 8% and 20% to maintain similar serum concentrations.

Mania: Oral:

Depakote® tablet: Initial: 750 mg/day in divided doses; dose should be adjusted as rapidly as possible to desired clinical effect; maximum recommended dosage: 60 mg/kg/day

Depakote® ER: Initial: 25 mg/kg/day given once daily; dose should be adjusted as rapidly as possible to desired clinical effect; maximum recommended dose: 60 mg/kg/day.

Migraine prophylaxis: Oral:

Depakote® tablet: 250 mg twice daily; adjust dose based on patient response, up to 1000 mg/day

Depakote® ER: 500 mg once daily for 7 days, then increase to 1000 mg once daily; adjust dose based on patient response; usual dosage range: 500-1000 mg/day

Geriatric Initiate at lower doses; dose escalation should be managed more slowly (in persons of advanced age). Refer to adult dosing.

Pediatric Equivalent oral dosages of divalproex and valproic acid deliver the same quantities of valproate ion.

Seizures: Oral:

Simple and complex absence seizures: Refer to adult dosing. Larger maintenance doses may be required in younger children.

Complex partial seizures: Children ≥10 years: Refer to adult dosing. Larger maintenance doses may be required in younger children.

Note: Depakote® ER is not recommended for use in children <10 years of age.

Migraine prophylaxis: Oral: Children ≥12 years: Refer to adult dosing.

Renal Impairment A 27% reduction in clearance of unbound valproate is seen in patients with Cl_{cr} <10 mL/minute. Hemodialysis reduces valproate concentrations by 20%, therefore, no dose adjustment is needed in patients with renal failure. Protein binding is reduced, monitoring only total valproate concentrations may be misleading.

Hepatic Impairment Dosage reduction is required. Clearance is decreased with liver impairment. Hepatic disease is also associated with decreased albumin concentrations and 2- to 2.6-fold increase in the unbound fraction. Free concentrations of valproate may be elevated while total concentrations appear normal. Use is contraindicated in severe impairment.

Administration

Oral

Depakote® ER: Swallow whole; do not crush or chew. Patients who need dose adjustments smaller than 500 mg/day for migraine prophylaxis should be changed to Depakote® delayed release tablets.

Depakote® Sprinkle capsules may be swallowed whole or open capsule and sprinkle on small amount (1 teaspoonful) of soft food and use immediately (do not store or chew).

Stability

Storage

Depakote® tablet: Store below 30°C (86°F).

Depakote® Sprinkles: Store below 25°C (77°F).

Depakote® ER: Store at controlled room temperature of 25°C (77°F).

Monitoring and Teaching Issues

Laboratory Monitoring Liver enzymes (at baseline and during therapy), CBC with platelets (baseline and periodic intervals), PT/PTT (especially prior to surgery), serum ammonia (with symptoms of lethargy, mental status change), serum valproate levels

Physical Assessment Do not discontinue abruptly; wean patient off of medication. Teach patient safety and seizure precautions.

Patient Education Oral: Do not crush or chew capsule or enteric-coated pill. While using this medication, do not use alcohol. Maintain adequate hydration, unless instructed to restrict fluid intake. You may experience nervousness, decreased appetite, insomnia, headache, sleepiness, dizziness, visual changes, and hair loss. Report suicide ideation or depression; alterations in menstrual cycle; abdominal cramps, unresolved diarrhea, vomiting, or constipation; skin rash; tremors; unusual bruising or bleeding; blood in urine, stool, or vomitus; malaise; weakness; facial swelling; yellowing of skin or eyes; persistent abdominal pain; excessive sedation; change in mental status; extreme lethargy; or restlessness.

Dietary Considerations Divalproex may cause GI upset; take with large amount of water or food to decrease GI upset. May need to split doses to avoid GI upset.

Depakote® Sprinkle capsule contents may be mixed with semisolid food (eg, applesauce or pudding) in patients having difficulty swallowing; particles should be swallowed and not chewed.

Geriatric Considerations Although there is little data in elderly for the use of divalproex in the treatment of seizures, there are a number of studies which demonstrate its benefit in the treatment of agitation and dementia and other psychiatric disorders. It is important that the clinician understand that serum concentrations do not correlate with behavior response; likewise, it is imperative to monitor LFTs and CBC during the first 6 months of therapy. See Warnings/Precautions, Laboratory Monitoring, and Additional Information.

Elimination is decreased in elderly. Studies of older adults with dementia show a high incidence of somnolence (which is usually transient); cognitive side effects generally minimal. In some patients, this was associated with weight loss. Starting doses should be lower and increased slowly, with careful monitoring of nutritional intake and dehydration. Safety and efficacy for use in patients >65 years of age have not been studied for migraine prophylaxis.

Breast-Feeding Considerations Breast milk concentrations of valproic acid have been reported as 1% to 10% of maternal concentration. The weight-adjusted dose to the infant has been calculated to be ~4%.

Pregnancy Considerations [U.S. Boxed Warning]: May cause teratogenic effects such as neural tube defects (eg, spina bifida). Teratogenic effects have been reported in animals and humans. Valproic acid crosses the placenta. Neural tube, cardiac, facial (characteristic pattern of dysmorphic facial features), skeletal, multiple other defects reported. Epilepsy itself, number of medications, genetic factors, or a combination of these probably influence the teratogenicity of anticonvulsant therapy. Information from the North American Antiepileptic Drug Pregnancy Registry notes a fourfold increase in congenital malformations with exposure to valproic acid monotherapy during the 1st trimester of pregnancy when compared to monotherapy with other antiepileptic drugs (AED). The risk of neural tube defects is ~1% to 2% (general population risk estimated to be 0.14% to 0.2%). The effect of folic acid supplementation to decrease this risk is unknown, however, folic acid supplementation is recommended for all women contemplating pregnancy. An information sheet describing the teratogenic potential is available from the manufacturer.

Nonteratogenic effects have also been reported. Afibrinogenemia leading to fatal hemorrhage and hepatotoxicity have been noted in case reports of infants following *in utero* exposure to valproic acid. Developmental delay, autism and/or autism spectrum disorder have also been reported. Use in women of childbearing potential requires that benefits of use in mother be weighed against the potential risk to fetus, especially when used for conditions not associated with permanent injury or risk of death (eg, migraine).

Patients exposed to valproic acid during pregnancy are encouraged to enroll themselves into the AED Pregnancy Registry by calling 1-888-233-2334. Additional information is available at www.aedpregnancyregistry.org.

Additional Information Divalproex sodium is a compound of sodium valproate and valproic acid; divalproex dissociates to valproate in the GI tract.

Extended release tablets have 10% to 20% less fluctuation in serum concentration than delayed release tablets. Extended release tablets are not bioequivalent to delayed release tablets.

Related Information

Anticonvulsant Drugs of Choice *on page 1981*

◆ **Divalproex Sodium** *see* Divalproex *on page 557*

◆ **Divigel®** *see* Estradiol (Systemic) *on page 670*

◆ **5071-1DL(6)** *see* Megestrol *on page 1158*

◆ ***D*-Mannitol** *see* Mannitol *on page 1146*

◆ **4-DMDR** *see* IDArubicin *on page 945*

DOBUTamine (doe BYOO ta meen)

Index Terms Dobutamine Hydrochloride

Generic Availability (U.S.) Yes

Pharmacologic Category Adrenergic Agonist Agent

Medication Safety Issues

Sound-alike/look-alike issues:

DOBUTamine may be confused with DOPamine

High alert medication: The Institute for Safe Medication Practices (ISMP) includes this medication among its list of drugs which have a heightened risk of causing significant patient harm when used in error.

Pregnancy Risk Factor B

Lactation Excretion in breast milk unknown

Use Short-term management of patients with cardiac decompensation

Unlabeled/Investigational Use Positive inotropic agent for use in myocardial dysfunction related to sepsis; stress echocardiography

Mechanism of Action/Effect Stimulates $beta_1$-adrenergic receptors, causing increased contractility and heart rate, with little effect on $beta_2$- or alpha-receptors

Contraindications Hypersensitivity to dobutamine or sulfites (some contain sodium metabisulfate), or any component of the formulation; idiopathic hypertrophic subaortic stenosis (IHSS)

Warnings/Precautions May increase heart rate. Patients with atrial fibrillation may experience an increase in ventricular response. An increase in blood pressure is more common, but occasionally a patient may become hypotensive. May exacerbate ventricular ectopy. If needed, correct hypovolemia first to optimize hemodynamics. Ineffective therapeutically in the presence of mechanical obstruction such as severe aortic stenosis. Use caution post-MI (can increase myocardial oxygen demand). Use cautiously in the elderly starting at lower end of the dosage range. Use with extreme caution in patients taking MAO inhibitors. Dobutamine in combination with stress echo may be used diagnostically. Product may contain sodium sulfite.

Drug Interactions

Avoid Concomitant Use

Avoid concomitant use of DOBUTamine with any of the following: Iobenguane I 123

Decreased Effect

DOBUTamine may decrease the levels/effects of: Iobenguane I 123

The levels/effects of DOBUTamine may be decreased by: Calcium Salts

Increased Effect/Toxicity

DOBUTamine may increase the levels/effects of: Sympathomimetics

The levels/effects of DOBUTamine may be increased by: Atomoxetine; Cannabinoids; COMT Inhibitors

Lab Interactions May affect serum assay of chloramphenicol.

Adverse Reactions Incidence of adverse events is not always reported.

Cardiovascular: Increased heart rate, increased blood pressure, increased ventricular ectopic activity, hypotension, premature ventricular beats (5%, dose related), anginal pain (1% to 3%), nonspecific chest pain (1% to 3%), palpitation (1% to 3%)

Central nervous system: Fever (1% to 3%), headache (1% to 3%), paresthesia

Endocrine & metabolic: Slight decrease in serum potassium

Gastrointestinal: Nausea (1% to 3%)

Hematologic: Thrombocytopenia (isolated cases)

Local: Phlebitis, local inflammatory changes and pain from infiltration, cutaneous necrosis (isolated cases)

Neuromuscular & skeletal: Mild leg cramps

Respiratory: Dyspnea (1% to 3%)

Pharmacodynamics/Kinetics

Onset of Action I.V.: 1-10 minutes; Peak effect: 10-20 minutes

Half-Life Elimination 2 minutes

Metabolism In tissues and hepatically to inactive metabolites

Excretion Urine (as metabolites)

Available Dosage Forms

Infusion, premixed in D_5W: 1 mg/mL (250 mL, 500 mL); 2 mg/mL (250 mL); 4 mg/mL (250 mL)

Injection, solution: 12.5 mg/mL (20 mL, 40 mL, 100 mL)

Dosing

Adult & Geriatric Cardiac decompensation: I.V. infusion: 2.5-20 mcg/kg/minute; maximum: 40 mcg/kg/minute, titrate to desired response; see table.

Infusion Rates of Various Dilutions of Dobutamine

Desired Delivery Rate (mcg/kg/min)	Infusion Rate (mL/kg/min)	
	500 mcg/mL	1000 mcg/mL
2.5	0.005	0.0025
5	0.01	0.005
7.5	0.015	0.0075
10	0.02	0.01
12.5	0.025	0.0125
15	0.03	0.015

Pediatric Cardiac decompensation: Refer to adult dosing.

Administration

I.V. Always administer via infusion device; administer into large vein.

Stability

Reconstitution Remix solution every 24 hours. Pink discoloration of solution indicates slight oxidation but **no** significant loss of potency.

Standard adult diluent: 250 mg/500 mL D_5W; 500 mg/500 mL D_5W.

Storage Store reconstituted solution under refrigeration for 48 hours or 6 hours at room temperature. Stability of parenteral admixture at room temperature (25°C) is 48 hours; at refrigeration (4°C) stability is 7 days.

Monitoring and Teaching Issues

Laboratory Monitoring Serum glucose, renal function

Physical Assessment Infusion pump and frequent cardiac monitoring are required.

Patient Education When administered in emergencies, patient education should be appropriate to the situation. If patient is aware, instruct to promptly report chest pain, palpitations, rapid heartbeat, headache, nervousness or restlessness, nausea or vomiting, or respiratory difficulty.

Geriatric Considerations A recent study demonstrated beneficial hemodynamic effects in elderly patients; monitor closely.

Additional Information Dobutamine lowers central venous pressure and wedge pressure but has little effect on pulmonary vascular resistance.

Dobutamine therapy should be avoided in patients with stable heart failure due to an increase in mortality. In patients with intractable heart failure, dobutamine may be used as a short-term infusion to provide symptomatic benefit. It is not known whether short-term dobutamine therapy in end-stage heart failure has any outcome benefit.

Dobutamine infusion during echocardiography is used as a cardiovascular stress. Wall motion abnormalities developing with increasing doses of dobutamine may help to identify ischemic and/or hibernating myocardium.

Related Information

Compatibility of Drugs *on page 1994*

◆ **Dobutamine Hydrochloride** *see* DOBUTamine *on page 561*

Docetaxel (doe se TAKS el)

U.S. Brand Names Taxotere®

Index Terms RP-6976

Generic Availability (U.S.) Yes: Excludes injection solution concentrate

Pharmacologic Category Antineoplastic Agent, Antimicrotubular; Antineoplastic Agent, Natural Source (Plant) Derivative; Antineoplastic Agent, Taxane Derivative

Medication Safety Issues

Sound-alike/look-alike issues:

DOCEtaxel may confused with PACLitaxel

Taxotere® may be confused with Taxol®

Docetaxel is available as a one-vial formulation at concentrations of 10 mg/mL (generic formulation) and 20 mg/mL (concentrate; Taxotere®). Docetaxel was previously available as a two-vial formulation which included two vials (a concentrated docetaxel vial and a diluent vial), resulting in a reconstituted concentration of 10 mg/mL. The two-vial formulation has been discontinued by the manufacturer. Admixture errors have occurred due to the availability of two concentrations (10 mg/mL and 20 mg/mL).

High alert medication: This medication is in a class the Institute for Safe Medication Practices (ISMP) includes among its list of drug classes which have a heightened risk of causing significant patient harm when used in error.

Pregnancy Risk Factor D

Lactation Excretion in breast milk unknown/not recommended

Use Treatment of breast cancer (locally advanced/metastatic or adjuvant treatment of operable node-positive); locally-advanced or metastatic nonsmall cell lung cancer (NSCLC); hormone refractory, metastatic prostate cancer; advanced gastric adenocarcinoma; locally-advanced squamous cell head and neck cancer

Unlabeled/Investigational Use Treatment of bladder cancer (metastatic), ovarian cancer, cervical cancer (relapsed), esophageal cancer, small cell lung cancer (relapsed), soft tissue sarcoma, Ewing's sarcoma, osteosarcoma, and unknown-primary adenocarcinoma

Available Dosage Forms

Injection, solution: 10 mg/mL (2 mL, 8 mL, 16 mL)

Taxotere®: 20 mg/mL (1 mL, 4 mL)

Dosing

Adult & Geriatric Note: Premedicate with corticosteroids, beginning the day before docetaxel administration, (administer corticosteroids for 3 days) to reduce the severity of hypersensitivity reactions and fluid retention. Details concerning dosing in combination regimens should also be consulted.

Breast cancer: I.V.:

Locally-advanced or metastatic: 60-100 mg/m^2 every 3 weeks (as a single agent)

Operable, node-positive (adjuvant treatment): 75 mg/m^2 every 3 weeks for 6 courses (in combination with doxorubicin and cyclophosphamide)

Weekly administration (unlabeled dosing): 40 mg/m^2/dose once a week (as a single agent) for 6 weeks followed by a 2-week rest, repeat until disease progression or unacceptable toxicity (Burstein, 2000) **or** 35 mg/m^2/dose once a week (in combination with trastuzumab) for 3 weeks followed by a 1-week rest; repeat until disease progression or unacceptable toxicity (Esteva, 2002)

Nonsmall cell lung cancer: I.V.: 75 mg/m^2 every 3 weeks (as monotherapy or in combination with cisplatin)

Prostate cancer: I.V.: 75 mg/m^2 every 3 weeks (in combination with prednisone)

Gastric adenocarcinoma: I.V.: 75 mg/m^2 every 3 weeks (in combination with cisplatin and fluorouracil)

Head and neck cancer: I.V.: 75 mg/m^2 every 3 weeks (in combination with cisplatin and fluorouracil) for 3 or 4 cycles, followed by radiation therapy

Bladder cancer, metastatic (unlabeled use): I.V.: 100 mg/m^2 every 3 weeks (as a single agent) (McCaffrey, 1997)

Esophageal cancer (unlabeled use): I.V.: 75 mg/m^2 every 3 weeks (in combination with cisplatin and fluorouracil) (Ajani, 2007; Van Cutsem, 2006)

Ovarian cancer (unlabeled use): I.V.: 60 mg/m^2 every 3 weeks (in combination with carboplatin) (Markman, 2001) **or** 75 mg/m^2 every 3 weeks (in combination with carboplatin) (Vasey, 2004) **or** 35 mg/m^2 (maximum dose: 70 mg) weekly for 3 weeks followed by a 1-week rest (in combination with carboplatin) (Kushner, 2007)

Soft tissue sarcoma (unlabeled use): I.V.: 100 mg/m^2 on day 8 of a 3-week treatment cycle (in combination with gemcitabine and filgrastim or pegfilgrastim) (Leu, 2004; Maki, 2007)

Unknown-primary, adenocarcinoma (unlabeled use): I.V.: 65 mg/m^2 every 3 weeks (in combination with carboplatin) (Greco, 2000) **or** 75 mg/m^2 on day 8 of a 3-week treatment cycle (in combination with gemcitabine) (Pouessel, 2004)

Renal Impairment Renal excretion is minimal (<5%), therefore, the need for dosage adjustments for renal dysfunction is unlikely (Li, 2007). Not removed by hemodialysis, may be administered before or after hemodialysis (Janus, 2010).

Hepatic Impairment

The FDA-approved labeling recommends the following adjustments:

Total bilirubin greater than the ULN, or AST and/or ALT >1.5 times ULN concomitant with alkaline phosphatase >2.5 times ULN: Use is not recommended.

Hepatic impairment dosing adjustment specific for gastric adenocarcinoma:

AST/ALT >2.5 to ≤5 times ULN and alkaline phosphatase ≤2.5 times ULN: Administer 80% of dose

AST/ALT >1.5 to ≤5 times ULN and alkaline phosphatase >2.5 to ≤5 times ULN: Administer 80% of dose

AST/ALT >5 times ULN and /or alkaline phosphatase >5 times ULN: Discontinue docetaxel

The following guidelines have been used by some clinicians (Floyd, 2006):

Transaminases 1.6-6 times ULN: Administer 75% of dose

Transaminases >6 times ULN: Use clinical judgment

Adjustment for Toxicity Note: Toxicity includes febrile neutropenia, neutrophils ≤500/mm^3 for >1 week, severe or cumulative cutaneous reactions; in nonsmall cell lung cancer, this may also include platelets <25,000/mm^3 and other grade 3/4 nonhematologic toxicities.

Breast cancer (single agent): Patients dosed initially at 100 mg/m^2; reduce dose to 75 mg/m^2; **Note:** If the patient continues to experience these adverse reactions, the dosage should be reduced to 55 mg/m^2 or therapy should be discontinued; discontinue for peripheral neuropathy ≥ grade 3. Patients initiated at 60 mg/m^2 who do not develop toxicity may tolerate higher doses.

Breast cancer, adjuvant treatment (combination chemotherapy): TAC regimen should be administered when neutrophils are ≥1500 cells/mm^3. Patients experiencing febrile neutropenia should receive G-CSF in all subsequent cycles. Patients with persistent febrile neutropenia (while on G-CSF), patients experiencing severe/cumulative cutaneous reactions, moderate neurosensory effects (signs/symptoms) or grade 3 or 4 stomatitis should receive a reduced dose (60 mg/m^2) of docetaxel. Discontinue therapy with persistent toxicities after dosage reduction.

Nonsmall cell lung cancer:

Monotherapy: Patients dosed initially at 75 mg/m^2 should have dose held until toxicity is resolved, then resume at 55 mg/m^2; discontinue for peripheral neuropathy ≥ grade 3.

Combination therapy (with cisplatin): Patients dosed initially at 75 mg/m^2 should have the docetaxel dosage reduced to 65 mg/m^2 in subsequent cycles; if further adjustment is required, dosage may be reduced to 50 mg/m^2

Prostate cancer: Reduce dose to 60 mg/m^2; discontinue therapy if toxicities persist at lower dose.

Gastric cancer, head and neck cancer: **Note:** Cisplatin may require dose reductions/therapy delays for peripheral neuropathy, ototoxicity, and /or nephrotoxicity. Patients experiencing febrile neutropenia, documented infection with neutropenia or neutropenia >7 days should receive G-CSF in all subsequent cycles. For neutropenic complications despite G-CSF use, further reduce dose to 60 mg/m^2. Neutropenic complications in subsequent cycles should be further dose reduced to 45 mg/m^2. Patients who experience grade 4 thrombocytopenia should receive a dose reduction from 75 mg/m^2 to 60 mg/m^2. Discontinue therapy for persistent toxicities.

Gastrointestinal toxicity for docetaxel in combination with cisplatin and fluorouracil for treatment of gastric cancer or head and neck cancer:

Diarrhea, grade 3:
- First episode: Reduce fluorouracil dose by 20%
- Second episode: Reduce docetaxel dose by 20%

Diarrhea, grade 4:
- First episode: Reduce fluorouracil and docetaxel doses by 20%
- Second episode: Discontinue treatment

Stomatitis, grade 3:
- First episode: Reduce fluorouracil dose by 20%
- Second episode: Discontinue fluorouracil for all subsequent cycles
- Third episode: Reduce docetaxel dose by 20%

Stomatitis, grade 4:
- First episode: Discontinue fluorouracil for all subsequent cycles
- Second episode: Reduce docetaxel dose by 20%

Administration

I.V. Administer I.V. infusion over 1-hour through nonsorbing polyethylene lined (non-DEHP) tubing; in-line filter is not necessary (the use of a filter during administration is not recommended by the manufacturer). Infusion should be completed within 4 hours of final preparation. **Note:** Premedication with corticosteroids for 3 days, beginning the day before docetaxel administration, is recommended to prevent hypersensitivity reactions and fluid retention.

Monitoring and Teaching Issues

Laboratory Monitoring CBC with differential, liver function tests, bilirubin, alkaline phosphatase, renal function

Physical Assessment Severe hypersensitivity reactions have been reported; premedication with dexamethasone may be advisable. Patient should be monitored continuously during infusion; dosing adjustment may be necessary. Monitor for neutropenia, severe fluid retention, pleural effusion, opportunistic infections, and anemia prior to each infusion and on a regular basis.

Patient Education This medication can only be administered by infusion; report immediately any pain, burning, swelling, or redness at infusion site, difficulty breathing or swallowing, chest pain, or sudden chills. It is important to maintain adequate nutrition and hydration, unless instructed to restrict fluid intake. You will be more susceptible to infection. May cause nausea or vomiting, loss of hair (reversible), or diarrhea. Report immediately swelling of extremities, respiratory difficulty, unusual weight gain, abdominal distention, chest pain, palpitations, fever, chills, unusual bruising or bleeding, signs of infection, excessive fatigue, or rash.

Dofetilide (doe FET il ide)

U.S. Brand Names Tikosyn®

Generic Availability (U.S.) No

Pharmacologic Category Antiarrhythmic Agent, Class III

Prescribing and Access Restrictions Tikosyn® is deemed to have an approved REMS program. As a requirement of the REMS program, access to this medication is restricted. Tikosyn® is only available to prescribers and hospitals that have confirmed their participation in a designated Tikosyn® Education Program. The program provides comprehensive education about the importance of in-hospital treatment initiation and individualized dosing.

T.I.P.S. is the Tikosyn® In Pharmacy System designated to allow retail pharmacies to stock and dispense Tikosyn® once they have been enrolled. A participating pharmacy must confirm receipt of the T.I.P.S. program materials and educate its pharmacy staff about the procedures required to fill an outpatient prescription for Tikosyn®. The T.I.P.S. enrollment form is available at www.tikosyn.com. Tikosyn® is only available from a special mail order pharmacy, and enrolled retail pharmacies. Pharmacists must verify that the hospital/prescriber is a confirmed participant before Tikosyn® is provided. For participant verification, the pharmacist may call 1-800-788-7353 or use the web site located at www.tikosynlist.com. Further details and directions on the program are provided at www.tikosyn.com.

Dofetilide therapy must be initiated/adjusted in a hospital setting with proper monitoring under the guidance of experienced personnel.

Pregnancy Risk Factor C

Lactation Excretion in breast milk unknown/not recommended

Use Maintenance of normal sinus rhythm in patients with chronic atrial fibrillation/atrial flutter of longer than 1-week duration who have been converted to normal sinus rhythm; conversion of atrial fibrillation and atrial flutter to normal sinus rhythm

Mechanism of Action/Effect Blocks cardiac potassium ion channels and increases action potential duration due to delayed repolarization

Contraindications Hypersensitivity to dofetilide or any component of the formulation; patients with congenital or acquired long QT syndromes, do not use if a baseline QT interval or QT_c is >440 msec (500 msec in patients with ventricular conduction abnormalities); severe renal impairment (estimated Cl_{cr} <20 mL/minute); concurrent use with verapamil, cimetidine, hydrochlorothiazide (alone or in combinations), trimethoprim (alone or in combination with sulfamethoxazole), itraconazole, ketoconazole, prochlorperazine, or megestrol; baseline heart rate <50 beats/minute; other drugs that prolong QT intervals (phenothiazines, cisapride, bepridil, tricyclic antidepressants, moxifloxacin; hypokalemia or hypomagnesemia; concurrent amiodarone, clarithromycin, or erythromycin

Warnings/Precautions [U.S. Boxed Warning]: Must be initiated (or reinitiated) in a setting with continuous monitoring and staff familiar with the recognition and treatment of life-threatening arrhythmias. Patients must be monitored with continuous ECG for a minimum of 3 days, or for a minimum of 12 hours after electrical or pharmacological cardioversion to normal sinus rhythm, whichever is greater. Patients should be readmitted for continuous monitoring if dosage is later increased.

Reserve for patients who are highly symptomatic with atrial fibrillation/atrial flutter; torsade de pointes significantly increases with doses >500 mcg twice daily; hold Class Ia or Class III antiarrhythmics for at least three half-lives prior to starting dofetilide; use in patients on amiodarone therapy only if serum amiodarone level is <0.3 mg/L or if amiodarone was stopped for >3 months previously; correct hypokalemia or hypomagnesemia before initiating dofetilide and maintain within normal limits during treatment. Risk of hypokalemia and/or hypomagnesemia may be increased by potassium-depleting diuretics, increasing the risk of torsade de pointes. Concurrent use with other drugs known to prolong QT_c interval is not recommended.

Patients with sick sinus syndrome or with second or third-degree heart block should not receive dofetilide unless a functional pacemaker is in place. Defibrillation threshold is reduced in patients with ventricular tachycardia or ventricular fibrillation undergoing implantation of a cardioverter-defibrillator device. Use with caution in renal impairment; not recommended in patients receiving drugs which may compete for renal secretion via cationic transport. Use with caution in patients with severe hepatic impairment.

In the Cardiac Arrhythmia Suppression Trial (CAST), recent (>6 days but <2 years ago) myocardial infarction patients with asymptomatic, non-life-threatening ventricular arrhythmias did not benefit and may have been harmed by attempts to suppress the arrhythmia with flecainide or encainide. An increased mortality or nonfatal cardiac arrest rate (7.7%) was seen in the active treatment group compared with patients in the placebo group (3%). The applicability of the CAST results to other populations is unknown. Antiarrhythmic agents should be reserved for patients with life-threatening ventricular arrhythmias.

Drug Interactions

Metabolism/Transport Effects Substrate of CYP3A4 (minor)

Avoid Concomitant Use

Avoid concomitant use of Dofetilide with any of the following: Antifungal Agents (Azole Derivatives, Systemic); Artemether; Cimetidine; Dronedarone; Lumefantrine; Megestrol; Nilotinib; Pimozide; Prochlorperazine; QuiNINE; Saquinavir; Tetrabenazine; Thiazide Diuretics; Thioridazine; Toremifene; Trimethoprim; Vandetanib; Verapamil; Ziprasidone

Decreased Effect There are no known significant interactions involving a decrease in effect.

Increased Effect/Toxicity

Dofetilide may increase the levels/effects of: Dronedarone; Pimozide; QTc-Prolonging Agents; QuiNINE; Tetrabenazine; Thioridazine; Toremifene; Vandetanib; Ziprasidone

The levels/effects of Dofetilide may be increased by: Alfuzosin; Antifungal Agents (Azole Derivatives, Systemic); Artemether; Chloroquine; Cimetidine; Ciprofloxacin; Ciprofloxacin (Systemic); Conivaptan; Eribulin; Fingolimod; Gadobutrol; Loop Diuretics; Lumefantrine; Megestrol; Nilotinib; Prochlorperazine; QuiNINE; Saquinavir; Thiazide Diuretics; Trimethoprim; Verapamil

Nutritional/Ethanol Interactions Herb/Nutraceutical: St John's wort may decrease dofetilide levels. Avoid ephedra (may worsen arrhythmia).

Adverse Reactions

Supraventricular arrhythmia patients (incidence > placebo)

>10%: Central nervous system: Headache (11%)

2% to 10%:

Central nervous system: Dizziness (8%), insomnia (4%)

Cardiovascular: Ventricular tachycardia (2.6% to 3.7%), chest pain (10%), torsade de pointes (3.3% in CHF patients and 0.9% in patients with a recent MI; up to 10.5% in patients receiving doses in excess of those recommended). Torsade de pointes occurs most frequently within the first 3 days of therapy.

Dermatologic: Rash (3%)

Gastrointestinal: Nausea (5%), diarrhea (3%), abdominal pain (3%)

Neuromuscular & skeletal: Back pain (3%)

Respiratory: Respiratory tract infection (7%), dyspnea (6%)

Miscellaneous: Flu syndrome (4%)

<2%:

Central nervous system: CVA, facial paralysis, flaccid paralysis, migraine, paralysis

Cardiovascular: AV block (0.4% to 1.5%), ventricular fibrillation (0% to 0.4%), bundle branch block, heart block, edema, heart arrest, myocardial infarct, sudden death, syncope

Dermatologic: Angioedema

Gastrointestinal: Liver damage

Neuromuscular & skeletal: Paresthesia

Respiratory: Cough

>2% (incidence ≤ placebo): Anxiety, pain, angina, atrial fibrillation, hypertension, palpitation, supraventricular tachycardia, peripheral edema, urinary tract infection, weakness, arthralgia, diaphoresis

Pharmacodynamics/Kinetics

Absorption Well absorbed

Bioavailability >90%

Time to Peak Serum: Fasting: 2-3 hours

Protein Binding 60% to 70%

Half-Life Elimination 10 hours

Metabolism Hepatic via CYP3A4, but low affinity for it; metabolites formed by N-dealkylation and N-oxidation

Excretion Urine (80%; 80% as unchanged drug, 20% as inactive or minimally active metabolites); renal elimination consists of glomerular filtration and active tubular secretion via cationic transport system

Available Dosage Forms

Capsule, oral:

Tikosyn®: 125 mcg, 250 mcg, 500 mcg

Dosing

Adult Note: QT_c must be determined prior to first dose

Antiarrhythmic: Oral:

Initial: 500 mcg orally twice daily. Initial dosage must be adjusted in patients with estimated Cl_{cr} <60 mL/minute. Dofetilide may be initiated at lower doses than recommended based on physician discretion.

Modification of dosage in response to initial dose: QT_c interval should be measured 2-3 hours after the initial dose. If the QT_c >15% of baseline, or if the QT_c is >500 msec (550 msec in patients with ventricular conduction abnormalities), dofetilide should be adjusted. If the starting dose is 500 mcg twice daily, then adjust to 250 mcg twice daily. If the starting dose was 250 mcg twice daily, then adjust to 125 mcg twice daily. If the starting dose was 125 mcg twice daily, then adjust to 125 mcg every day.

Continued monitoring for doses 2-5: QT_c interval must be determined 2-3 hours after each subsequent dose of dofetilide for in-hospital doses 2-5. If the measured QT_c is >500 msec (550 msec in patients with ventricular conduction abnormalities) dofetilide should be stopped.

Geriatric Refer to adult dosing. No specific dosage adjustments are recommended based on age; however, careful assessment of renal function is particularly important in this population.

Renal Impairment Note: The manufacturer recommends using actual body weight when using the Cockcroft-Gault equation to calculate creatinine clearance.

Cl_{cr} >60 mL/minute: Administer 500 mcg twice daily.
Cl_{cr} 40-60 mL/minute: Administer 250 mcg twice daily.
Cl_{cr} 20-39 mL/minute: Administer 125 mcg twice daily.
Cl_{cr} <20 mL/minute: Contraindicated in this group

Hepatic Impairment No dosage adjustments required in Child-Pugh class A and B; patients with severe hepatic impairment were not studied.

Administration

Oral Do not open capsules.

Monitoring and Teaching Issues

Laboratory Monitoring Serum creatinine; check serum potassium and magnesium levels if on medications where these electrolyte disturbances can occur, or if patient has a history of hypokalemia or hypomagnesemia.

Physical Assessment Must be initiated or reinitiated by a cardiologist in a setting with continuous ECG monitoring for a period of time at beginning or adjustment of therapy. Monitor for signs of electrolyte imbalance.

Patient Education Do not open capsules. If you miss a dose, take your normal amount at the next scheduled time. You will need regular cardiac checkups and blood tests when taking this medication. You may experience headache, dizziness, difficulty sleeping, abdominal pain, diarrhea, or nausea. Inform prescriber immediately if you experience fainting, severe GI discomfort or diarrhea, chest palpitations, irregular heartbeat, chest pain, increased thirst, respiratory difficulty, skin rash, back pain, or alteration in muscle strength or gait.

Geriatric Considerations No specific dosage adjustments are recommended based on age; however, evaluation for use of this drug in the elderly is imperative. A complete review of medications, to assure there is no inadvertent use of contraindicated medications and those with potential drug interactions, can be re-evaluated for continued need. Laboratory values must be assessed prior to initiating medication; careful assessment of renal function is particularly important in the elderly population.

Pregnancy Considerations Dofetilide has been shown to adversely affect *in utero* growth, organogenesis, and survival of rats and mice. There are no adequate and well-controlled studies in pregnant women. Dofetilide should be used with extreme caution in pregnant women and in women of childbearing age only when the benefit to the patient unequivocally justifies the potential risk to the fetus.

Related Information

Antiarrhythmic Drugs *on page 1978*

Dolasetron (dol A se tron)

U.S. Brand Names Anzemet®

Index Terms Dolasetron Mesylate; MDL 73,147EF

Generic Availability (U.S.) No

Pharmacologic Category Antiemetic; Selective 5-HT_3 Receptor Antagonist

Medication Safety Issues

Sound-alike/look-alike issues:

Anzemet® may be confused with Aldomet®, Antivert®, Avandamet®
Dolasetron may be confused with granisetron, ondansetron, palonosetron

Pregnancy Risk Factor B

Lactation Excretion in breast milk unknown/use caution

Use

U.S. labeling:

Injection: Prevention and treatment of postoperative nausea and vomiting
Oral: Prevention of nausea and vomiting associated with emetogenic cancer chemotherapy (initial and repeat courses); prevention of postoperative nausea and vomiting

Canadian labeling: Injection, oral: Prevention of nausea and vomiting associated with emetogenic cancer chemotherapy (initial and repeat courses)

Mechanism of Action/Effect Selective 5-HT_3 receptor antagonist, blocking serotonin, both peripherally on vagal nerve terminals and centrally in the chemoreceptor trigger zone

Contraindications

U.S. labeling:

Injection: Hypersensitivity to dolasetron or any component of the formulation; use for the prevention of chemotherapy-induced nausea and vomiting
Tablet: Hypersensitivity to dolasetron or any component of the formulation

Canadian labeling: Injection, tablet: Hypersensitivity to dolasetron or any component of the formulation; use in children and adolescents <18 years of age; use for the prevention or treatment of postoperative nausea and vomiting

Warnings/Precautions Dolasetron is associated with a number of dose-dependent increases in ECG intervals (eg, PR, QRS duration, QT/QT_c, JT), usually occurring 1-2 hours after I.V. administration and usually lasting 6-8 hours; however, may last ≥24 hours and rarely lead to heart block or arrhythmia. Clinically relevant QT-interval prolongation may occur resulting in torsade de pointes, when used in conjunction with other agents that prolong the QT interval (eg, Class I and III antiarrhythmics). Avoid use in patients at greater risk for QT prolongation (eg, patients with congenital long QT syndrome, medications known to prolong QT interval, electrolyte abnormalities, and cumulative high-dose anthracycline therapy) and/or ventricular arrhythmia. Correct potassium or magnesium abnormalities prior to initiating therapy. I.V. formulations of 5-HT_3 antagonists have more association with ECG interval changes, compared to oral formulations. Reduction in heart rate may also occur with the 5-HT_3 antagonists. Use with caution in children and adolescents who have or may develop QT_c prolongation; rare cases of supraventricular and ventricular arrhythmias, cardiac arrest, and MI have been reported in this population.

Use with caution in patients allergic to other 5-HT_3 receptor antagonists; cross-reactivity has been reported with other 5-HT_3 receptor antagonists. **For chemotherapy-associated nausea and vomiting, should be used on a scheduled basis, not on an "as needed" (PRN) basis,** since data support the use of this drug only in the prevention of nausea and vomiting (due to antineoplastic therapy) and not in the rescue of nausea and vomiting. Not intended for treatment of nausea and vomiting or for chronic continuous therapy.

Drug Interactions

Metabolism/Transport Effects Substrate (minor) of CYP2C9, 3A4; **Inhibits** CYP2D6 (weak)

Avoid Concomitant Use

Avoid concomitant use of Dolasetron with any of the following: Apomorphine; Artemether; Dronedarone; Lumefantrine; Nilotinib; Pimozide; QuiNINE; Tetrabenazine; Thioridazine; Toremifene; Vandetanib; Ziprasidone

Decreased Effect There are no known significant interactions involving a decrease in effect.

Increased Effect/Toxicity

Dolasetron may increase the levels/effects of: Apomorphine; Dronedarone; Pimozide; QTc-Prolonging Agents; QuiNINE; Tetrabenazine; Thioridazine; Toremifene; Vandetanib; Ziprasidone

The levels/effects of Dolasetron may be increased by: Alfuzosin; Artemether; Chloroquine; Ciprofloxacin; Ciprofloxacin (Systemic); Conivaptan; Gadobutrol; Lumefantrine; Nilotinib; QuiNINE

Nutritional/Ethanol Interactions Food: Food does not affect the bioavailability of oral doses.

Adverse Reactions Adverse events may vary according to indication

>10%:

Central nervous system: Headache (7% to 24%)

Gastrointestinal: Diarrhea (2% to 12%)

1% to 10%:

Cardiovascular: Bradycardia (4% to 5%), hypertension (≤3%), tachycardia (2% to 3%)

Central nervous system: Dizziness (1% to 6%), fatigue (3% to 6%), fever (4%), pain (≤2%), chills/shivering (1% to 2%)

Gastrointestinal: Dyspepsia (≤3%), abdominal pain (≤3%)

Hepatic: Abnormal hepatic function (4%)

Renal: Oliguria (3%)

Pharmacodynamics/Kinetics

Absorption Oral: Rapid and complete

Bioavailability Oral: ~75% (not affected by food)

Time to Peak Hydrodolasetron: I.V.: 0.6 hours; Oral: ~1 hour

Protein Binding Hydrodolasetron: 69% to 77% (50% bound to $alpha_1$-acid glycoprotein)

Half-Life Elimination Dolasetron: ≤10 minutes; hydrodolasetron: Adults: 6-8 hours; Children: 4-6 hours; Severe renal impairment: 11 hours; Severe hepatic impairment: 11 hours

Metabolism Hepatic; rapid reduction by carbonyl reductase to hydrodolasetron (active metabolite); further metabolized by CYP2D6, CYP3A, and flavin monooxygenase

Excretion Urine ~67% (53% to 61% of the total dose as active metabolite hydrodolasetron); feces ~33%

Available Dosage Forms

Injection, solution:

Anzemet®: 20 mg/mL (0.625 mL, 5 mL, 25 mL)

Tablet, oral:

Anzemet®: 50 mg, 100 mg

Dosing

Adult & Geriatric Note: In the U.S., use of dolasetron injection is contraindicated for the prevention of chemotherapy induced nausea and vomiting. In Canada, use of dolasetron is contraindicated in the prevention and treatment of postoperative nausea and vomiting in adults.

Prevention of chemotherapy-associated nausea and vomiting (including initial and repeat courses):

U.S. labeling: Oral: 100 mg within 1 hour before chemotherapy

Canadian labeling:

Oral: 100 mg within 1 hour before chemotherapy

I.V.: 100 mg or in patients <56 kg or >90 kg: 1.8 mg/kg ~30 minutes before chemotherapy

Postoperative nausea and vomiting: *U.S. labeling:*

Prevention:

Oral: 100 mg within 2 hours before surgery

I.V.: 12.5 mg ~15 minutes before cessation of anesthesia

Treatment: I.V.: 12.5 mg as soon as nausea or vomiting present

Pediatric Note: In Canada, use of dolasetron is contraindicated in children and adolescents <18 years of age.

Prevention of chemotherapy-associated nausea and vomiting (including initial and repeat courses): Children 2-16 years: Oral: 1.8 mg/kg within 1 hour before chemotherapy; maximum: 100 mg/dose

Postoperative nausea and vomiting: Children 2-16 years:

Prevention:

Oral: 1.2 mg/kg within 2 hours before surgery; maximum: 100 mg/dose

I.V.: 0.35 mg/kg ~15 minutes before cessation of anesthesia; maximum: 12.5 mg

Treatment: I.V.: 0.35 mg/kg as soon as nausea or vomiting present; maximum: 12.5 mg/dose

Renal Impairment No dosage adjustment necessary.

Hepatic Impairment No dosage adjustment necessary.

Administration

Oral When unable to administer in tablet form, dolasetron injection may be diluted in apple or apple-grape juice and taken orally; this dilution is stable for 2 hours at room temperature.

I.V. I.V. injection may be given either undiluted IVP over 30 seconds or diluted in 50 mL of compatible fluid and infused over 15 minutes. Flush line before and after dolasetron administration.

Stability

Reconstitution Dilute in 50 mL of a compatible solution (ie, 0.9% NS, D_5W, $D_5{}^1/_2NS$, D_5LR, LR, and 10% mannitol injection).

Storage Store intact vials and tablets at room temperature of 20°C to 25°C (68°F to 77°F). Protect from light. Solutions diluted for infusion are stable under normal lighting conditions at room temperature for 24 hours or under refrigeration for 48 hours.

Monitoring and Teaching Issues

Laboratory Monitoring Potassium, magnesium

Physical Assessment Assess allergy history (selective 5-HT_3 receptor antagonists) prior to administering. Use with caution in presence of or risk for cardiac conduction abnormalities (eg, QT prolongation, medication known to prolong QT interval, electrolyte abnormalities). Oral and I.V. doses have different schedules and should not be administered on "PRN" basis.

Patient Education This drug is given to reduce the incidence of nausea and vomiting. If this medication is given by intravenous infusion you will be monitored during infusion. Report immediately any chest pain, respiratory difficulty, or pain or itching at infusion site. You may experience headache, drowsiness, or dizziness. Report chest pain or palpitations, persistent headache, excessive drowsiness, fever, constipation, or diarrhea.

Dietary Considerations May be taken without regard to meals.

Geriatric Considerations In controlled trials, no difference in overall safety and efficacy were observed between elderly and younger adults. Pharmacokinetics are similar in younger adults and elderly. No dosage adjustment necessary.

Pregnancy Considerations Teratogenic effects were not observed in animal studies. There are no adequate and well-controlled studies in pregnant women.

Additional Information Efficacy of dolasetron, for chemotherapy treatment, is enhanced with concomitant administration of dexamethasone 20 mg (increases complete response by 10% to 20%). Oral administration of the intravenous solution is equivalent to tablets.

◆ **Dolasetron Mesylate** *see* Dolasetron *on page 567*

◆ **Dolgic® Plus** *see* Butalbital, Acetaminophen, and Caffeine *on page 260*

◆ **Dolophine®** *see* Methadone *on page 1186*

Donepezil (doh NEP e zil)

U.S. Brand Names Aricept®; Aricept® ODT

Index Terms E2020

Generic Availability (U.S.) Yes

Pharmacologic Category Acetylcholinesterase Inhibitor (Central)

Medication Safety Issues

Sound-alike/look-alike issues:

Aricept® may be confused with AcipHex®, Ascriptin®, and Azilect®

Pregnancy Risk Factor C

Lactation Excretion in breast milk unknown/not recommended

Use Treatment of mild, moderate, or severe dementia of the Alzheimer's type

Unlabeled/Investigational Use Behavioral syndromes in dementia; mild-to-moderate dementia associated with Parkinson's disease; Lewy body dementia

Mechanism of Action/Effect Alzheimer's disease is characterized by cholinergic deficiency in the cortex and basal forebrain, which contributes to cognitive deficits. Donepezil reversibly and noncompetitively inhibits centrally-active acetylcholinesterase, the enzyme responsible for hydrolysis of acetylcholine. This appears to result in increased concentrations of acetylcholine available for synaptic transmission in the central nervous system.

Contraindications Hypersensitivity to donepezil, piperidine derivatives, or any component of the formulation

Warnings/Precautions Cholinesterase inhibitors may have vagotonic effects which may cause bradycardia and/or heart block with or without a history of cardiac disease; syncopal episodes have been associated with donepezil. Alzheimer's treatment guidelines consider bradycardia to be a relative contraindication for use of centrally-active cholinesterase inhibitors. Use with caution with sick sinus syndrome or other supraventricular cardiac conduction abnormalities, COPD, or asthma. Use with caution in patients with a history of seizure disorder; cholinomimetics may potentially cause generalized seizures, although seizure activity may also result from Alzheimer's disease. Use with caution in patients at risk of ulcer disease (eg, previous history or NSAID use), or in patients with bladder outlet obstruction. May cause dose-related diarrhea, nausea, and/or vomiting, which usually resolves in 1-3 weeks. May cause anorexia and/or weight loss (dose-related). May exaggerate neuromuscular blockade effects of depolarizing neuromuscular-blocking agents (eg, succinylcholine).

Drug Interactions

Metabolism/Transport Effects Substrate (minor) of CYP2D6, 3A4

Avoid Concomitant Use There are no known interactions where it is recommended to avoid concomitant use.

Decreased Effect

Donepezil may decrease the levels/effects of: Anticholinergics; Neuromuscular-Blocking Agents (Nondepolarizing)

The levels/effects of Donepezil may be decreased by: Anticholinergics; Peginterferon Alfa-2b

Increased Effect/Toxicity

Donepezil may increase the levels/effects of: Antipsychotics; Beta-Blockers; Cholinergic Agonists; Succinylcholine

The levels/effects of Donepezil may be increased by: Conivaptan; Corticosteroids (Systemic)

Nutritional/Ethanol Interactions Herb/Nutraceutical: St John's wort may decrease donepezil levels. Ginkgo biloba may increase adverse effects/toxicity of acetylcholinesterase inhibitors.

Adverse Reactions

>10%:

Central nervous system: Insomnia (2% to 14%)

Gastrointestinal: Nausea (3% to 19%; dose related), diarrhea (5% to 15%; dose related)

Miscellaneous: Accident (7% to 13%), infection (11%)

1% to 10%:

Cardiovascular: Hypertension (3%), chest pain (2%), hemorrhage (2%), syncope (2%), hypotension, atrial fibrillation, bradycardia, ECG abnormal, edema, heart failure, hot flashes, peripheral edema, vasodilation

Central nervous system: Headache (3% to 10%), pain (3% to 9%), fatigue (1% to 8%), dizziness (2% to 8%), abnormal dreams (3%), hostility (3%), nervousness (1% to 3%), hallucinations (3%), depression (2% to 3%), confusion (2%), emotional lability (2%), personality disorder (2%), fever (2%), somnolence (2%), abnormal crying, aggression, agitation, anxiety, aphasia, delusions, irritability, restlessness, seizure, vertigo

Dermatologic: Bruising (4% to 5%), eczema (3%), pruritus, rash, skin ulcer, urticaria

Endocrine & metabolic: Dehydration (1% to 2%), hyperlipemia (2%), libido increased

Gastrointestinal: Anorexia (2% to 8%), vomiting (3% to 9%; dose related), weight loss (3% to 5%; dose related), abdominal pain, bloating, constipation, dyspepsia, epigastric pain, fecal incontinence, gastroenteritis, GI bleeding, toothache

Genitourinary: Urinary frequency (2%), urinary incontinence (1% to 3%), cystitis, hematuria, glycosuria, nocturia, UTI

Hematologic: Contusion (≤2%), anemia

Hepatic: Alkaline phosphatase increased

Neuromuscular & skeletal: Muscle cramps (3% to 8%), back pain (3%), CPK increased (3%), arthritis (1% to 2%), ataxia, bone fracture, gait abnormal, lactate dehydrogenase increased, paresthesia, tremor, weakness (1% to 2%)

Ocular: Blurred vision, cataract, eye irritation

Respiratory: Bronchitis, cough increased, dyspnea, pharyngitis, pneumonia, sore throat

Miscellaneous: Diaphoresis, fungal infection, flu symptoms, wandering

Pharmacodynamics/Kinetics

Absorption Well absorbed

Bioavailability 100%

Time to Peak Plasma: Tablet, 10 mg: 3 hours; Tablet, 23 mg: ~8 hours; **Note:** Peak plasma concentrations almost twofold higher for the 23 mg tablet compared to the 10 mg tablet

Protein Binding 96%, primarily to albumin (75%) and α_1-acid glycoprotein (21%)

Half-Life Elimination 70 hours; time to steady-state: 15 days

Metabolism Extensively to four major metabolites (two are active) via CYP2D6 and 3A4; undergoes glucuronidation

Excretion Urine 57% (17% as unchanged drug); feces 15%

Available Dosage Forms

Tablet, oral: 5 mg, 10 mg

Aricept®: 5 mg, 10 mg, 23 mg

Tablet, orally disintegrating, oral: 5 mg, 10 mg

Aricept® ODT: 5 mg, 10 mg

Dosing

Adult Alzheimer's dementia: Oral:

Mild-to-moderate: Initial: 5 mg once daily; may increase to 10 mg once daily after 4-6 weeks; effective dosage range in clinical studies: 5-10 mg/day

Moderate-to-severe: Initial: 5 mg once daily; may increase to 10 mg once daily after 4-6 weeks; may increase further to 23 mg once daily after ≥3 months; effective dosage range in clinical studies: 10-23 mg/day

Geriatric Refer to adult dosing. **Note:** The Canadian labeling recommends a maximum dose of 5 mg once daily in elderly women of low body weight.

Administration

Oral Administer at bedtime without regard to food.

Aricept® 5 mg or 10 mg tablet: Swallow whole with water; do not split or crush per manufacturer's labeling. However, data available from the manufacturer showed that bioavailability was not affected by disintegration or dissolution when administered as a solution compared to a tablet during a bioequivalence study (data on file, Eisai Inc).

Aricept® 23 mg tablet: Swallow whole with water; do **NOT** crush or chew due to an increased rate of absorption. The 23 mg strength is provided in a unique film-coated formulation different from the 5 mg or 10 mg tablet strengths, which results in an altered pharmacokinetic profile.

Aricept® ODT: Allow tablet to dissolve completely on tongue and follow with water.

Stability

Storage Store at 15°C to 30°C (59°F to 86°F).

Monitoring and Teaching Issues

Physical Assessment Assess bladder adequacy prior to treatment. Assess for cholinergic crisis. Monitor pulse.

Patient Education This medication will not cure the disease, but may help reduce symptoms. May cause dizziness, sedation, or hypotension; vomiting or loss of appetite; or diarrhea. Report persistent abdominal discomfort; significantly increased salivation, sweating, tearing, or urination; flushed skin; chest pain or palpitations; acute headache; unresolved diarrhea; excessive fatigue, insomnia, dizziness, or depression; increased muscle, joint, or body pain; vision changes or blurred vision; or shortness of breath or wheezing.

Dietary Considerations May take with or without food.

Pregnancy Considerations Teratogenic effects were not observed in animal studies. There are no adequate and well-controlled studies in pregnant women.

DOPamine (DOE pa meen)

Index Terms Dopamine Hydrochloride; Intropin

Generic Availability (U.S.) Yes

Pharmacologic Category Adrenergic Agonist Agent

Medication Safety Issues

Sound-alike/look-alike issues:

DOPamine may be confused with DOBUTamine, Dopram®

High alert medication: The Institute for Safe Medication Practices (ISMP) includes this medication among its list of drugs which have a heightened risk of causing significant patient harm when used in error.

Pregnancy Risk Factor C

Lactation Excretion in breast milk unknown

Use Adjunct in the treatment of shock (eg, MI, open heart surgery, renal failure, cardiac decompensation) which persists after adequate fluid volume replacement

Unlabeled/Investigational Use Symptomatic bradycardia or heart block unresponsive to atropine or pacing

Mechanism of Action/Effect Stimulates both adrenergic and dopaminergic receptors, lower doses are mainly dopaminergic stimulating and produce renal and mesenteric vasodilation, higher doses also are both dopaminergic and $beta_1$-adrenergic stimulating and produce cardiac stimulation and renal vasodilation; large doses stimulate alpha-adrenergic receptors

Contraindications Hypersensitivity to sulfites (commercial preparation contains sodium bisulfite); pheochromocytoma; ventricular fibrillation

Warnings/Precautions Use with caution in patients with cardiovascular disease or cardiac arrhythmias or patients with occlusive vascular disease. Correct hypovolemia and electrolytes when used in hemodynamic support. May cause increases in HR and arrhythmia. Use with caution in post-MI patients. Use with extreme caution in patients taking MAO inhibitors. Avoid extravasation; infuse into a large vein if possible. Avoid infusion into leg veins. Watch I.V. site closely. **[U.S. Boxed Warning]: If extravasation occurs, infiltrate the area with diluted phentolamine (5-10 mg in 10-15 mL of saline) with a fine hypodermic needle. Phentolamine should be administered as soon as possible after extravasation is noted.** Product may contain sodium metabisulfite.

Drug Interactions

Avoid Concomitant Use

Avoid concomitant use of DOPamine with any of the following: Inhalational Anesthetics; Iobenguane I 123; Lurasidone

Decreased Effect

DOPamine may decrease the levels/effects of: Iobenguane I 123

Increased Effect/Toxicity

DOPamine may increase the levels/effects of: Lurasidone; Sympathomimetics

The levels/effects of DOPamine may be increased by: Atomoxetine; Cannabinoids; COMT Inhibitors; Inhalational Anesthetics

Adverse Reactions Frequency not defined.

Cardiovascular: Ectopic beats, tachycardia, anginal pain, palpitation, hypotension, vasoconstriction

Central nervous system: Headache

Gastrointestinal: Nausea and vomiting

Respiratory: Dyspnea

Pharmacodynamics/Kinetics

Onset of Action Adults: 5 minutes

Duration of Action Adults: <10 minutes

Half-Life Elimination 2 minutes

Metabolism Renal, hepatic, plasma; 75% to inactive metabolites by monoamine oxidase and 25% to norepinephrine

Excretion Urine (as metabolites)

Clearance: Neonates: Varies and appears to be age related; prolonged clearance with combined hepatic and renal impairment

Pharmacokinetic Note Dopamine has exhibited nonlinear kinetics in children; with medication changes, may not achieve steady-state for ~1 hour rather than 20 minutes.

Available Dosage Forms

Infusion, premixed in D_5W: 0.8 mg/mL (250 mL, 500 mL); 1.6 mg/mL (250 mL, 500 mL); 3.2 mg/mL (250 mL)

Injection, solution: 40 mg/mL (5 mL, 10 mL); 80 mg/mL (5 mL, 10 mL); 160 mg/mL (5 mL)

Dosing

Adult & Geriatric

Hemodynamic support: I.V. infusion: 1-5 mcg/kg/minute up to 50 mcg/kg/minute, titrate to desired response; infusion may be increased by 1-4 mcg/kg/minute at 10- to 30-minute intervals until optimal response is obtained

Note: If dosages >20-30 mcg/kg/minute are needed, a more direct-acting vasopressor may be more beneficial (ie, epinephrine, norepinephrine).

Hemodynamic effects of dopamine are dose dependent:

Low-dose: 1-5 mcg/kg/minute, increased renal blood flow and urine output

Intermediate-dose: 5-15 mcg/kg/minute, increased renal blood flow, heart rate, cardiac contractility, and cardiac output

High-dose: >15 mcg/kg/minute, alpha-adrenergic effects begin to predominate, vasoconstriction, increased blood pressure

Pediatric Hemodynamic support: I.V. infusion:

Children: 1-20 mcg/kg/minute, maximum: 50 mcg/kg/minute continuous infusion, titrate to desired response.

Administration

I.V. Vesicant. **Must be diluted prior to use.** Do not discontinue suddenly - sudden discontinuation may lead to marked hypotension.

Stability

Storage Protect from light. Solutions that are darker than slightly yellow should not be used.

Monitoring and Teaching Issues

Laboratory Monitoring Serum glucose, renal function

Physical Assessment Infusion pump, continuous cardiac and hemodynamic monitoring, and frequent assessment of I.V. site is required for inpatient therapy.

Patient Education When administered in emergencies, patient education should be appropriate to the situation. If patient is aware, instruct to promptly report chest pain, palpitations, rapid heartbeat, headache, nervousness or restlessness, nausea or vomiting, or respiratory difficulty.

Geriatric Considerations Has not been specifically studied in the elderly; monitor closely, especially due to increase in cardiovascular disease with age.

Additional Information Dopamine is most frequently used for treatment of hypotension because of its peripheral vasoconstrictor action. In this regard, dopamine is often used together with dobutamine and minimizes hypotension secondary to dobutamine-induced vasodilation. Thus, pressure is maintained by increased cardiac output (from dobutamine) and vasoconstriction (by dopamine). It is critical neither dopamine nor dobutamine be used in patients in the absence of correcting any hypovolemia as a cause of hypotension.

Low-dose dopamine is often used in the intensive care setting for presumed beneficial effects on renal function. However, there is no clear evidence that low-dose dopamine confers any renal or other benefit. Indeed, dopamine may act on dopamine receptors in the carotid bodies causing chemoreflex suppression. In patients with heart failure, dopamine may inhibit breathing and cause pulmonary shunting. Both these mechanisms would act to decrease minute ventilation and oxygen saturation. This could potentially be deleterious in patients with respiratory compromise and patients being weaned from ventilators.

Related Information

Compatibility of Drugs *on page* 1994

◆ **Dopamine Hydrochloride** *see* DOPamine *on page* 571

◆ **Doribax®** *see* Doripenem *on page* 573

Doripenem (dore i PEN em)

U.S. Brand Names Doribax®

Index Terms S-4661

Generic Availability (U.S.) No

Pharmacologic Category Antibiotic, Carbapenem

Medication Safety Issues

Sound-alike/look-alike issues:

Doribax® may be confused with Zovirax®

Pregnancy Risk Factor B

Lactation Excretion in breast milk unknown/use caution

Use Treatment of complicated intra-abdominal infections and complicated urinary tract infections (including pyelonephritis) due to susceptible gram-positive, gram-negative (including *Pseudomonas aeruginosa*), and anaerobic bacteria

Unlabeled/Investigational Use Treatment of nosocomial pneumonia

Mechanism of Action/Effect Inhibits cell wall synthesis in susceptible bacteria

Contraindications Known serious hypersensitivity to doripenem or other carbapenems (eg, imipenem, ertapenem, meropenem); anaphylactic reactions to beta-lactam antibiotics

Warnings/Precautions Serious hypersensitivity reactions, including anaphylaxis, and skin reactions have been reported in patients receiving beta-lactams. Prolonged use may result in fungal or bacterial superinfection, including *C. difficile*-associated diarrhea (CDAD) and pseudomembranous colitis; CDAD has been observed >2 months postantibiotic treatment. Use with caution in patients with renal impairment; dosage adjustment required in patients with moderate-to-severe renal dysfunction. May decrease divalproex sodium/valproic acid concentrations leading to breakthrough seizures; concomitant use not recommended. Administer via intravenous infusion only. Per manufacturer's labeling, investigational experience of doripenem via inhalation resulted in pneumonitis.

Drug Interactions

Avoid Concomitant Use

Avoid concomitant use of Doripenem with any of the following: BCG; Probenecid

Decreased Effect

Doripenem may decrease the levels/effects of: BCG; Divalproex; Typhoid Vaccine; Valproic Acid

Increased Effect/Toxicity

The levels/effects of Doripenem may be increased by: Probenecid

Adverse Reactions

>10%:

Central nervous system: Headache (4% to 16%)

Gastrointestinal: Nausea (4% to 12%), diarrhea (6% to 11%)

1% to 10%:

Dermatologic: Rash (1% to 5%; includes allergic/bullous dermatitis, erythema, macular/papular eruptions, urticaria, and erythema multiforme), pruritus (≤3%)

Gastrointestinal: Oral candidiasis (1%)

Hematologic: Anemia (2% to 10%)

Hepatic: Transaminases increased (1% to 2%)

Local: Phlebitis (4% to 8%)

Renal: Renal impairment/failure (≤1%)

Miscellaneous: Vulvomycotic infection (1% to 2%)

Pharmacodynamics/Kinetics

Protein Binding 8% to 9%

Half-Life Elimination ~1 hour

Metabolism Non-CYP-mediated metabolism via dehydropeptidase-I to doripenem-M1 (inactive metabolite)

Excretion Urine (70% as unchanged drug; 15% as doripenem-M1 metabolite); feces (<1%)

Available Dosage Forms

Injection, powder for reconstitution:

Doribax®: 250 mg, 500 mg

Dosing

Adult & Geriatric

Intra-abdominal infection, complicated, severe: 500 mg every 8 hours for 5-14 days. **Note:** 2010 IDSA guidelines recommend treatment duration of 4-7 days (provided source controlled). Not recommended for mild-to-moderate, community-acquired intra-abdominal infections due to risk of toxicity and the development of resistant organisms (Solomkin, 2010).

Urinary tract infection (complicated) or pyelonephritis: I.V.: 500 mg every 8 hours for 10-14 days

Renal Impairment

Cl_{cr} 30-50 mL/minute: 250 mg every 8 hours

Cl_{cr} 11-29 mL/minute: 250 mg every 12 hours

Hemodialysis: Dialyzable (~52% of dose removed during 4-hour session in ESRD patients)

Administration

I.V. Infuse over 1 hour

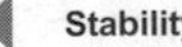

Stability

Reconstitution Reconstitute 250 mg vial with 10 mL of SWFI or NS; further dilute for infusion with 50 mL or 100 mL of NS or D_5W. Shake gently until clear. Reconstitute 500 mg vial with 10 mL of SWFI or NS; further dilute for infusion with 100 mL of NS or D_5W. Shake gently until clear. Reconstituted vial may be stored for up to 1 hour prior to preparation of infusion solution. To prepare a 250 mg dose using a 500 mg vial, reconstitute the 500 mg vial with 10 mL of SWFI or NS and further dilute with 100 mL of compatible solution as above, but remove and discard 55 mL from the infusion bag to leave the remaining solution containing the 250 mg dose.

Storage Store dry powder vials at 15°C to 30°C (59°F to 86°F). Stability of solution when diluted in NS is 12 hours at room temperature or 72 hours under refrigeration; stability in D_5W is 4 hours at room temperature and 24 hours under refrigeration.

Monitoring and Teaching Issues

Laboratory Monitoring Periodic renal assessment; consider hematologic monitoring during prolonged therapy

Physical Assessment Assess results of culture and sensitivity tests and patient history of previous allergies or adverse drug reactions. Use caution in presence of renal impairment. Patient must be monitored closely for adverse reactions, especially anaphylaxis or skin reactions.

Patient Education This medication can only be administered intravenously. Report warmth, swelling, or irritation at infusion site; difficulty breathing; facial swelling; or acute anxiety. Maintain adequate nutrition and hydration, unless instructed to restrict fluid intake. Report prolonged GI effects (diarrhea, nausea), skin rash, or excessive or persistent fatigue or weakness.

Geriatric Considerations Careful attention to dose adjustment based on renal function, as well as monitoring renal function during treatment is recommended. According to the manufacturer, 28% of clinical trial patients were ≥65 years and 12% were ≥75 years, with no differences in overall age-related safety findings.

Breast-Feeding Considerations It is not known if doripenem is excreted into breast milk. The manufacturer recommends that caution be exercised when administering doripenem to nursing women.

Pregnancy Considerations Adverse events have not been observed in animal studies; therefore, the manufacturer classifies doripenem as pregnancy category B. There are no adequate and well-controlled studies completed in pregnant women.

Dornase Alfa (DOOR nase AL fa)

U.S. Brand Names Pulmozyme®

Index Terms Recombinant Human Deoxyribonuclease; rhDNase

Generic Availability (U.S.) No

Pharmacologic Category Enzyme

Pregnancy Risk Factor B

Lactation Excretion in breast milk unknown/use caution

Use Management of cystic fibrosis patients to reduce the frequency of respiratory infections that require parenteral antibiotics in patients with FVC ≥40% of predicted; in conjunction with standard therapies, to improve pulmonary function in patients with cystic fibrosis

Available Dosage Forms

Solution, for nebulization [preservative free]:

Pulmozyme®: 2.5 mg/2.5 mL (30s)

Dosing

Adult & Geriatric Mucolytic: Inhalation: 2.5 mg once daily through selected nebulizers

Pediatric

Mucolytic (cystic fibrosis): Inhalation:

Children ≥3 months: 2.5 mg once daily through selected nebulizers; experience in children <5 years is limited

Note: Patients unable to inhale or exhale orally throughout the entire treatment period may use Pari-Baby™ nebulizer. Some patients may benefit from twice daily administration.

Monitoring and Teaching Issues

Physical Assessment Teach patient appropriate use of nebulizer.

Patient Education Inform prescriber of any allergies you have. Report skin rash, respiratory difficulty, wheezing, or cough. Self-administered nebulizer: Do not combine with any other medications in the nebulizer. Wash hands before and after treatment. Wash and dry nebulizer after each treatment. Twist open the top of one unit dose vial and squeeze contents into nebulizer reservoir. Connect nebulizer reservoir to the mouthpiece or face mask. Connect nebulizer to compressor. Sit in comfortable, upright position. Put on face mask and turn on compressor. Avoid leakage around the mask to avoid mist getting into eyes. Breathe calmly and deeply until no more mist is formed in nebulizer (about 5 minutes).

◆ **Doryx®** *see* Doxycycline *on page* 586

Dorzolamide (dor ZOLE a mide)

U.S. Brand Names Trusopt®

Index Terms Dorzolamide Hydrochloride

Generic Availability (U.S.) Yes

Pharmacologic Category Carbonic Anhydrase Inhibitor; Ophthalmic Agent, Antiglaucoma

Pregnancy Risk Factor C

Lactation Excretion in breast milk unknown/not recommended

Use Treatment of elevated intraocular pressure in patients with ocular hypertension or open-angle glaucoma

Available Dosage Forms

Solution, ophthalmic: 2% (10 mL)

Trusopt®: 2% (10 mL)

Dosing

Adult & Geriatric Reduction of intraocular pressure: Ophthalmic: Instill 1 drop in the affected eye(s) 3 times/day

Pediatric Refer to adult dosing.

Administration

Other If more than one topical ophthalmic drug is being used, administer the drugs at least 10 minutes apart. Remove contact lens prior to administration and wait 15 minutes before reinserting. Instruct patients to avoid allowing the tip of the dispensing container to contact the eye or surrounding structures. Ocular solutions can become contaminated by common bacteria known to cause ocular infections. Serious damage to the eye and subsequent loss of vision may occur from using contaminated solutions.

Monitoring and Teaching Issues

Patient Education For use in eyes only. If serious or unusual reactions or signs of hypersensitivity occur, contact ophthalmologist. If any ocular reactions occur, particularly conjunctivitis and lid reactions, notify prescriber. Avoid allowing the tip of the dispensing container to contact the eye or surrounding structures. Take out contact lenses before using medicine. Lenses can be replaced 15 minutes after medicine is given.

◆ **Dorzolamide Hydrochloride** *see* Dorzolamide *on page* 574

◆ **Dovonex®** *see* Calcipotriene *on page* 268

Doxazosin (doks AY zoe sin)

U.S. Brand Names Cardura®; Cardura® XL

Index Terms Doxazosin Mesylate

Generic Availability (U.S.) Yes: Excludes extended release tablet

Pharmacologic Category Alpha$_1$ Blocker

Medication Safety Issues

Sound-alike/look-alike issues:

Doxazosin may be confused with doxapram, doxepin, DOXOrubicin

Cardura® may be confused with Cardene®, Cordarone®, Cordran®, Coumadin®, K-Dur®, Ridaura®

Beers Criteria medication: This drug may be inappropriate for use in geriatric patients (low severity risk).

Pregnancy Risk Factor C

Lactation Excretion in breast milk unknown/use caution

Use

Immediate release formulation: Treatment of hypertension as monotherapy or in conjunction with diuretics, ACE inhibitors, beta-blockers, or calcium antagonists

Immediate release and extended release formulations: Treatment of urinary outflow obstruction and/or obstructive and irritative symptoms associated with benign prostatic hyperplasia (BPH)

Unlabeled/Investigational Use Pediatric hypertension

Mechanism of Action/Effect

Hypertension: Competitively inhibits postsynaptic alpha$_1$-adrenergic receptors which results in vasodilation of veins and arterioles and a decrease in total peripheral resistance and blood pressure; ~50% as potent on a weight by weight basis as prazosin.

BPH: Competitively inhibits postsynaptic alpha$_1$-adrenergic receptors in prostatic stromal and bladder neck tissues. This reduces the sympathetic tone-induced urethral stricture causing BPH symptoms.

Contraindications Hypersensitivity to quinazolines (prazosin, terazosin), doxazosin, or any component of the formulation

Warnings/Precautions Can cause significant orthostatic hypotension and syncope, especially with first dose; anticipate a similar effect if therapy is interrupted for a few days, if dosage is rapidly increased, or if another antihypertensive drug (particularly vasodilators) or a PDE-5 inhibitor is introduced. Discontinue if symptoms of angina occur or worsen. Patients should be cautioned about performing hazardous tasks when starting new therapy or adjusting dosage upward. Prostate cancer should be ruled out before starting for BPH. Use with caution in mild-to-moderate hepatic impairment; not recommended in severe dysfunction. Intraoperative floppy iris syndrome has been observed in cataract surgery patients who were on or were previously treated with alpha$_1$-blockers. Causality has not been established and there appears to be no benefit in discontinuing alpha-blocker therapy prior to surgery. May be inappropriate in the elderly due to potential for dry mouth, hypotension, and urinary problems (Beers Criteria).

The extended release formulation consists of drug within a nondeformable matrix; following drug release/absorption, the matrix/shell is expelled in the stool. The use of nondeformable products in patients with known stricture/narrowing of the GI tract has been associated with symptoms of obstruction. Use caution in patients with increased GI retention (eg, chronic

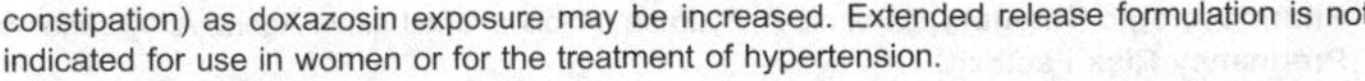

constipation) as doxazosin exposure may be increased. Extended release formulation is not indicated for use in women or for the treatment of hypertension.

Drug Interactions

Avoid Concomitant Use

Avoid concomitant use of Doxazosin with any of the following: Alpha1-Blockers

Decreased Effect

The levels/effects of Doxazosin may be decreased by: Herbs (Hypertensive Properties); Methylphenidate; Yohimbine

Increased Effect/Toxicity

Doxazosin may increase the levels/effects of: Alpha1-Blockers; Amifostine; Antihypertensives; Calcium Channel Blockers; Hypotensive Agents; RiTUXimab

The levels/effects of Doxazosin may be increased by: Beta-Blockers; Diazoxide; Herbs (Hypotensive Properties); MAO Inhibitors; Pentoxifylline; Phosphodiesterase 5 Inhibitors; Prostacyclin Analogues

Nutritional/Ethanol Interactions Herb/Nutraceutical: Avoid dong quai if using for hypertension (has estrogenic activity). Avoid ephedra, yohimbe, ginseng (may worsen hypertension). Avoid saw palmetto when used for BPH (due to limited experience with this combination). Avoid garlic (may have increased antihypertensive effect).

Adverse Reactions Note: Type and frequency of adverse reactions reflect combined data from BPH and hypertension trials and immediate release and extended release products.

>10%: Central nervous system: Dizziness (5% to 19%), headache (5% to 14%)

1% to 10%:

- Cardiovascular: Orthostatic hypotension (dose related; 0.3% up to 2%), edema (3% to 4%), hypotension (1% to 2%), palpitation (1% to 2%), chest pain (1% to 2%), arrhythmia (1%), syncope (2%), flushing (1%)
- Central nervous system: Fatigue (8% to 12%), somnolence (1% to 5%), nervousness (2%), pain (2%), vertigo (2% to 4%), insomnia (1%), anxiety (1%), paresthesia (1%), movement disorder (1%), ataxia (1%), hypertonia (1%), depression (1%)
- Dermatologic: Rash (1%), pruritus (1%)
- Endocrine & metabolic: Sexual dysfunction (2%)
- Gastrointestinal: Abdominal pain (2%), diarrhea (2%), dyspepsia (1% to 2%), nausea (1% to 3%), xerostomia (1% to 2%), constipation (1%), flatulence (1%)
- Genitourinary: Urinary tract infection (1%), impotence (1%), polyuria (2%), incontinence (1%)
- Neuromuscular & skeletal: Back pain (2% to 3%), weakness (1% to 7%), arthritis (1%), muscle weakness (1%), myalgia (≤1%), muscle cramps (1%)
- Ocular: Abnormal vision (1% to 2%), conjunctivitis (1%)
- Otic: Tinnitus (1%)
- Respiratory: Respiratory tract infection (5%), rhinitis (3%), dyspnea (1% to 3%), respiratory disorder (1%), epistaxis (1%)
- Miscellaneous: Diaphoresis increased (1%), flu-like syndrome (1%)

Pharmacodynamics/Kinetics

Duration of Action >24 hours

Bioavailability Immediate release: ~65%; Extended release relative to immediate release: 54% to 59%

Time to Peak Serum: Immediate release: 2-3 hours; Extended release: 8-9 hours

Protein Binding ~98%

Half-Life Elimination Immediate release: ~22 hours; Extended release: 15-19 hours

Metabolism Extensively hepatic to active metabolites; primarily via CYP3A4; secondary pathways involve CYP2D6 and 2C19

Excretion Feces (63%, primarily as metabolites); urine (9%, primarily as metabolites)

Pharmacokinetic Note Not significantly affected by increased age.

Available Dosage Forms

Tablet, oral: 1 mg, 2 mg, 4 mg, 8 mg

Cardura®: 1 mg, 2 mg, 4 mg, 8 mg

Tablet, extended release, oral:

Cardura® XL: 4 mg, 8 mg

Dosing

Adult

BPH: Oral:

Immediate release: 1 mg once daily in morning or evening; may be increased to 2 mg once daily. Thereafter titrate upwards, if needed, over several weeks, balancing therapeutic benefit with doxazosin-induced postural hypotension. Goal: 4-8 mg/day; maximum dose: 8 mg/day

Reinitiation of therapy: If therapy is discontinued for several days, restart at 1 mg dose and titrate as before

Extended release: 4 mg once daily with breakfast; titrate based on response and tolerability every 3-4 weeks to maximum recommended dose of 8 mg/day

Reinitiation of therapy: If therapy is discontinued for several days, restart at 4 mg dose and titrate as before

Note: Conversion to extended release from immediate release: Omit final evening dose of immediate release prior to starting morning dosing with extended release product; initiate extended release product using 4 mg once daily

Hypertension: Oral: *Immediate release:* 1 mg once daily in morning or evening; may be increased to 2 mg once daily. Thereafter titrate upwards, if needed, over several weeks, balancing therapeutic benefit with doxazosin-induced postural hypotension. Maximum dose: 16 mg/day

Reinitiation of therapy: If therapy is discontinued for several days, restart at 1 mg dose and titrate as before

Geriatric Immediate release: Oral: Initial: 0.5 mg once daily

Pediatric Hypertension (unlabeled use): Oral: Immediate release: Initial: 1 mg once daily; maximum: 4 mg/day

Hepatic Impairment Use with caution in mild-to-moderate hepatic dysfunction. Do not use with severe impairment.

Administration

Oral Cardura® XL: Tablets should be swallowed whole; do not crush, chew, or divide. Administer with morning meal.

Stability

Storage Store at 25°C (77°F); excursions permitted to 15°C to 30°C (59°F to 86°F).

Monitoring and Teaching Issues

Physical Assessment Assess blood pressure and monitor for hypotension, CNS changes, and urinary retention prior to treatment and on a regular basis. When discontinuing, blood pressure should be closely monitored and dose tapered slowly over 1 week or more.

Patient Education Do not crush or chew extended release forms, swallow whole. Tablet shell may be visible in the stool. Follow recommended diet and exercise program. May cause drowsiness, dizziness, postural hypotension, or nausea. Report increased nervousness or depression; sudden weight gain; unusual or persistent swelling of ankles, feet, or extremities; palpitations or rapid heartbeat; or muscle weakness, fatigue, or pain.

Dietary Considerations Cardura® XL: Take with morning meal.

Geriatric Considerations Adverse reactions such as dry mouth and urinary problems can be particularly bothersome in the elderly. In studies of the extended-release tablets, the incidence of hypotension was higher in the elderly compared to younger patients.

This medication is considered to be potentially inappropriate in this patient population (Beers Criteria severity: Low).

Breast-Feeding Considerations The extended release formulation is not indicated for use in women.

Pregnancy Considerations Adverse events were observed in some animal reproduction studies. Delayed postnatal development was also noted. There are no adequate and well-controlled studies in pregnant women.

Additional Information First-dose hypotension occurs less frequently with doxazosin as compared to prazosin; this may be due to its slower onset of action.

Related Information

Pharmacotherapy of Urinary Incontinence *on page 2071*

◆ **Doxazosin Mesylate** *see* Doxazosin *on page 575*

Doxepin (Systemic) (DOKS e pin)

U.S. Brand Names Silenor®

Index Terms Doxepin Hydrochloride

Generic Availability (U.S.) Yes: Excludes tablet

Pharmacologic Category Antidepressant, Tricyclic (Tertiary Amine)

Medication Safety Issues

Sound-alike/look-alike issues:

Doxepin may be confused with digoxin, doxapram, doxazosin, Doxidan®, doxycycline

SINEquan® may be confused with saquinavir, Serentil®, SEROquel®, Singulair®, Zonegran®

Beers Criteria medication: This drug may be inappropriate for use in geriatric patients (high severity risk).

International issues:

Doxal® [Finland] may be confused with Doxil® which is a brand name for doxorubicin in the U.S.

Doxal® [Finland]: Brand name for doxycycline in Austria; brand name for pyridoxine/thiamine in Brazil

Medication Guide Available Yes

Pregnancy Risk Factor C

Lactation Enters breast milk/use caution (AAP rates "of concern"; AAP 2001 update pending)

Use Depression; treatment of insomnia (with difficulty of sleep maintenance)

Unlabeled/Investigational Use Analgesic for certain chronic and neuropathic pain; anxiety

Available Dosage Forms

Capsule, oral: 10 mg, 25 mg, 50 mg, 75 mg, 100 mg, 150 mg

Solution, oral: 10 mg/mL (118 mL, 120 mL)

Tablet, oral:

Silenor®: 3 mg, 6 mg

Dosing

Adult

Depression and/or anxiety: Oral: Initial: 25-150 mg/day at bedtime or in 2-3 divided doses; may gradually increase up to 300 mg/day; single dose should not exceed 150 mg; select patients may respond to 25-50 mg/day.

Insomnia (Silenor®): Oral: 3-6 mg once daily 30 minutes prior to bedtime; maximum dose: 6 mg/day

Geriatric

Depression and/or anxiety: Oral: Initial: 10-25 mg at bedtime; increase by 10-25 mg every 3 days for inpatients and weekly for outpatients if tolerated. Rarely does the maximum dose required exceed 75 mg/day; a single bedtime dose is recommended.

Insomnia: Oral: 3 mg once daily 30 minutes prior to bedtime; increase to 6 mg once daily if clinically needed

Hepatic Impairment Use a lower dose and adjust gradually.

Silenor®: Initial: 3 mg once daily

Administration

Oral Do not mix oral concentrate with carbonated beverages (physically incompatible).

Silenor®: Administer within 30 minutes prior to bedtime; do not take within 3 hours of food

Monitoring and Teaching Issues

Physical Assessment Monitor CNS status. Be alert for signs of clinical worsening, suicidal ideation, or other changes in behavior. Taper dosage slowly when discontinuing.

Patient Education It may take several weeks to achieve desired results. Avoid alcohol. Maintain adequate hydration, unless instructed to restrict fluid intake. You may experience drowsiness, lightheadedness, impaired coordination, dizziness, blurred vision, constipation, urinary retention, postural hypotension, altered sexual drive or ability (reversible), or photosensitivity. Report persistent CNS effects (eg, nervousness, restlessness, insomnia, anxiety, excitation, suicide ideation, headache, agitation, impaired coordination, changes in cognition); muscle cramping, weakness, tremors, or rigidity; chest pain, palpitations, or irregular heartbeat; blurred vision or eye pain; yellowing of skin or eyes; or worsening of condition.

Related Information

Antidepressant Agents *on page* 1982

Doxepin (Topical) (DOKS e pin)

U.S. Brand Names Prudoxin™; Zonalon®

Index Terms Doxepin Hydrochloride

Generic Availability (U.S.) No

Pharmacologic Category Topical Skin Product

Medication Safety Issues

Sound-alike/look-alike issues:

Doxepin may be confused with digoxin, doxapram, doxazosin, Doxidan®, doxycycline

Zonalon® may be confused with Zone-A Forte®

International issues:

Doxal® [Finland] may be confused with Doxil® which is a brand name for doxorubicin in the U.S.

Doxal® [Finland]: Brand name for doxycycline in Austria; brand name for pyridoxine/thiamine in Brazil

Pregnancy Risk Factor B

Lactation Enters breast milk/not recommended (AAP rates "of concern"; AAP 2001 update pending)

Use Short-term (<8 days) management of moderate pruritus in adults with atopic dermatitis or lichen simplex chronicus

Unlabeled/Investigational Use Cream: Treatment of burning mouth syndrome and neuropathic pain

Available Dosage Forms

Cream, topical:

Prudoxin™: 5% (45 g)

Zonalon®: 5% (30 g, 45 g)

Dosing

Adult

Burning mouth syndrome (unlabeled use): Oral topical: Cream: Apply 3-4 times daily.

Pruritus: Topical: Apply a thin film 4 times/day with at least 3- to 4-hour interval between applications; not recommended for use >8 days. (Oral administration of doxepin 25-50 mg has also been used, but systemic adverse effects are increased.)

Geriatric Pruritus: Topical: Refer to adult dosing.

Administration

Topical Apply thin film to affected area; use of occlusive dressings is not recommended.

Monitoring and Teaching Issues

Patient Education Apply in thin layer; do not overuse. Report increased skin irritation, worsening of condition, or lack of improvement.

◆ **Doxepin Hydrochloride** *see* Doxepin (Systemic) *on page* 577

◆ **Doxepin Hydrochloride** *see* Doxepin (Topical) *on page* 578

Doxercalciferol (doks er kal si fe FEER ole)

U.S. Brand Names Hectorol®
Index Terms 1α-Hydroxyergocalciferol
Generic Availability (U.S.) No
Pharmacologic Category Vitamin D Analog
Pregnancy Risk Factor B
Lactation Excretion in breast milk unknown/not recommended
Use Treatment of secondary hyperparathyroidism in patients with chronic kidney disease
Available Dosage Forms
Capsule, softgel, oral:
Hectorol®: 0.5 mcg, 1 mcg, 2.5 mcg
Injection, solution:
Hectorol®: 2 mcg/mL (1 mL, 2 mL)
Dosing
Adult & Geriatric Secondary hyperparathyroidism:
Oral:
Dialysis patients: Dose should be titrated to lower iPTH to 150-300 pg/mL; dose is adjusted at 8-week intervals (maximum dose: 20 mcg 3 times/week)
Initial dose: iPTH >400 pg/mL: 10 mcg 3 times/week at dialysis
Dose titration:
iPTH level decreased by 50% and >300 pg/mL: Dose can be increased to 12.5 mcg 3 times/week for 8 more weeks; this titration process can continue at 8-week intervals; each increase should be by 2.5 mcg/dose
iPTH level 150-300 pg/mL: Maintain current dose
iPTH level <100 pg/mL: Suspend doxercalciferol for 1 week; resume at a reduced dose; decrease each dose (not weekly dose) by at least 2.5 mcg
Predialysis patients: Dose should be titrated to lower iPTH to 35-70 pg/mL with stage 3 disease or to 70-110 pg/mL with stage 4 disease: Dose may be adjusted at 2-week intervals (maximum dose: 3.5 mcg/day)
Initial dose: 1 mcg/day
Dose titration:
iPTH level >70 pg/mL with stage 3 disease or >110 pg/mL with stage 4 disease: Increase dose by 0.5 mcg every 2 weeks as necessary
iPTH level 35-70 pg/mL with stage 3 disease or 70-110 pg/mL with stage 4 disease: Maintain current dose
iPTH level is <35 pg/mL with stage 3 disease or <70 pg/mL with stage 4 disease: Suspend doxercalciferol for 1 week, then resume at a reduced dose (at least 0.5 mcg lower)
I.V.:
Dialysis patients: Dose should be titrated to lower iPTH to 150-300 pg/mL; dose is adjusted at 8-week intervals (maximum dose: 18 mcg/week)
Initial dose: iPTH level >400 pg/mL: 4 mcg 3 times/week after dialysis, administered as a bolus dose
Dose titration:
iPTH level decreased by <50% and >300 pg/mL: Dose can be increased by 1-2 mcg at 8-week intervals, as necessary
iPTH level decreased by >50% and >300 pg/mL: Maintain current dose
iPTH level 150-300 pg/mL: Maintain current dose
iPTH level <100 pg/mL: Suspend doxercalciferol for 1 week; resume at a reduced dose (at least 1 mcg lower)
Hypercalcemia, hyperphosphatemia, or serum calcium times phosphorus product >55 mg^2/dL^2: Decrease or suspend dose and/or adjust dose of phosphate binders; if dose is suspended, resume at a reduced dose (at least 1 mcg lower)
Renal Impairment No adjustment is required.
Hepatic Impairment Use with caution; no guidelines for dosage adjustment.
Monitoring and Teaching Issues
Laboratory Monitoring
Dialysis patients: Before initiating, check iPTH, serum calcium, and phosphorus. Check weekly for first 12 weeks of therapy. Thereafter, serum iPTH, calcium, phosphorus, and alkaline phosphatase should be periodically monitored.
Predialysis patients: iPTH, serum calcium and phosphorus every 2 weeks for 3 months following initiation and dose adjustments, then monthly for 3 months, then every 3 months.
Physical Assessment Provide appropriate nutritional counseling.
Patient Education Stop other vitamin D products. Report headache, dizziness, weakness, sleepiness, severe nausea, vomiting, dry mouth, loss of appetite, constipation, metallic taste, muscle and/or bone pain, malaise, and difficulty thinking or concentrating. Follow diet and calcium supplements as directed by prescriber.

◆ **Doxil®** *see* DOXOrubicin (Liposomal) *on page* 582

DOXOrubicin (doks oh ROO bi sin)

U.S. Brand Names Adriamycin®
Index Terms ADR (error-prone abbreviation); Adria; Doxorubicin Hydrochloride; Hydroxydaunomycin Hydrochloride; Hydroxyldaunorubicin Hydrochloride
Generic Availability (U.S.) Yes

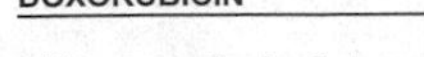

Pharmacologic Category Antineoplastic Agent, Anthracycline

Medication Safety Issues

Sound-alike/look-alike issues:

DOXOrubicin may be confused with DACTINomycin, DAUNOrubicin, DAUNOrubicin liposomal, doxacurium, doxapram, doxazosin, DOXOrubicin liposomal, epirubicin, IDArubicin, valrubicin

Adriamycin PFS® may be confused with achromycin, Aredia®, Idamycin®

Conventional formulation (Adriamycin PFS®, Adriamycin RDF®) may be confused with the liposomal formulation (Doxil®)

Use caution when selecting product for preparation and dispensing; indications, dosages and adverse event profiles differ between conventional DOXOrubicin hydrochloride solution and DOXOrubicin liposomal. Both formulations are the same concentration. As a result, serious errors have occurred.

High alert medication: The Institute for Safe Medication Practices (ISMP) includes this medication among its list of drug classes which have a heightened risk of causing significant patient harm when used in error.

ADR is an error-prone abbreviation

International issues:

Doxil® may be confused with Doxal® which is a brand name for doxepin in Finland, a brand name for doxycycline in Austria, and a brand name for pyridoxine/thiamine combination in Brazil

Rubex, a discontinued brand name for DOXOrubicin in the U.S, is a brand name for ascorbic acid in Ireland

Pregnancy Risk Factor D

Lactation Enters breast milk/not recommended

Use Treatment of acute lymphocytic leukemia (ALL), acute myeloid leukemia (AML), Hodgkin's disease, malignant lymphoma, soft tissue and bone sarcomas, thyroid cancer, small cell lung cancer, breast cancer, gastric cancer, ovarian cancer, bladder cancer, neuroblastoma, and Wilms' tumor

Unlabeled/Investigational Use Treatment of multiple myeloma, endometrial carcinoma, uterine sarcoma, head and neck cancer, liver cancer, kidney cancer

Mechanism of Action/Effect Inhibits DNA and RNA synthesis, active throughout cell cycle, results in cell death.

Contraindications Hypersensitivity to doxorubicin, any component of the formulation, or to other anthracyclines or anthracenediones; recent MI, severe myocardial insufficiency, severe arrhythmia; previous therapy with high cumulative doses of doxorubicin, daunorubicin, idarubicin, or other anthracycline and anthracenediones; baseline neutrophil count $<1500/mm^3$; severe hepatic impairment

Warnings/Precautions Hazardous agent - use appropriate precautions for handling and disposal. **[U.S. Boxed Warning]: May cause cumulative, dose-related, myocardial toxicity (early or delayed).** Cardiotoxicity is dose-limiting. Total cumulative dose should take into account previous or concomitant treatment with cardiotoxic agents or irradiation of chest. The incidence of irreversible myocardial toxicity increases as the total cumulative (lifetime) dosages approach 450-500 mg/m^2. Although the risk increases with cumulative dose, irreversible cardiotoxicity may occur at any dose level. Patients with pre-existing heart disease, hypertension, concurrent administration of other antineoplastic agents, prior or concurrent chest irradiation, advanced age; and infants and children are at increased risk. Alternative administration schedules (weekly or continuous infusions) have are associated with less cardiotoxicity Baseline and periodic monitoring of ECG and LVEF (with either ECHO or MUGA scan) is recommended. **[U.S. Boxed Warnings]: Reduce dose in patients with impaired hepatic function; dose-limiting severe myelosuppression (primarily leukopenia and neutropenia) may occur. Secondary acute myelogenous leukemia and myelodysplastic syndrome have been reported following treatment.** May cause tumor lysis syndrome and hyperuricemia (in patients with rapidly growing tumors).

Children are at increased risk for developing delayed cardiotoxicity; follow-up cardiac function monitoring is recommended. Doxorubicin may contribute to prepubertal growth failure in children; may also contribute to gonadal impairment (usually temporary). Radiation recall pneumonitis has been reported in children receiving concomitant dactinomycin and doxorubicin. **[U.S. Boxed Warnings]: For I.V. administration only. Potent vesicant; if extravasation occurs, severe local tissue damage leading to ulceration, necrosis, and pain may occur. Should be administered under the supervision of an experienced cancer chemotherapy physician.**

Drug Interactions

Metabolism/Transport Effects Substrate of CYP2D6 (major), CYP3A4 (major), P-glycoprotein; **Inhibits** CYP2B6 (moderate), 2D6 (weak), 3A4 (weak); **Induces** P-glycoprotein

Avoid Concomitant Use

Avoid concomitant use of DOXOrubicin with any of the following: BCG; Dabigatran Etexilate; Natalizumab; Pimecrolimus; Roflumilast; Tacrolimus (Topical); Vaccines (Live)

Decreased Effect

DOXOrubicin may decrease the levels/effects of: BCG; Cardiac Glycosides; Dabigatran Etexilate; P-Glycoprotein Substrates; Sipuleucel-T; Stavudine; Vaccines (Inactivated); Vaccines (Live); Vitamin K Antagonists; Zidovudine

The levels/effects of DOXOrubicin may be decreased by: Cardiac Glycosides; CYP3A4 Inducers (Strong); Deferasirox; Echinacea; Herbs (CYP3A4 Inducers); Peginterferon Alfa-2b; P-Glycoprotein Inducers

Increased Effect/Toxicity

DOXOrubicin may increase the levels/effects of: CYP2B6 Substrates; Leflunomide; Natalizumab; Vaccines (Live); Vitamin K Antagonists; Zidovudine

The levels/effects of DOXOrubicin may be increased by: Bevacizumab; Conivaptan; CycloSPORINE; CycloSPORINE (Systemic); CYP2D6 Inhibitors (Moderate); CYP2D6 Inhibitors (Strong); CYP3A4 Inhibitors (Moderate); CYP3A4 Inhibitors (Strong); Darunavir; Dasatinib; Denosumab; P-Glycoprotein Inhibitors; Pimecrolimus; Roflumilast; SORAfenib; Tacrolimus (Topical); Taxane Derivatives; Trastuzumab

Nutritional/Ethanol Interactions Herb/Nutraceutical: Avoid St John's wort (may decrease doxorubicin levels). Avoid black cohosh, dong quai in estrogen-dependent tumors.

Adverse Reactions Frequency not defined.

Cardiovascular:

Acute cardiotoxicity: Atrioventricular block, bradycardia, bundle branch block, ECG abnormalities, extrasystoles (atrial or ventricular), sinus tachycardia, ST-T wave changes, supraventricular tachycardia, tachyarrhythmia, ventricular tachycardia

Delayed cardiotoxicity: LVEF decreased, CHF (manifestations include ascites, cardiomegaly, dyspnea, edema, gallop rhythm, hepatomegaly, oliguria, pleural effusion, pulmonary edema, tachycardia); myocarditis, pericarditis

Central nervous system: Malaise

Dermatologic: Alopecia, itching, photosensitivity, radiation recall, rash; discoloration of saliva, sweat, or tears

Endocrine & metabolic: Amenorrhea, dehydration, infertility (may be temporary), hyperuricemia

Gastrointestinal: Abdominal pain, anorexia, colon necrosis, diarrhea, GI ulceration, mucositis, nausea, vomiting

Genitourinary: Discoloration of urine

Hematologic: Leukopenia/neutropenia (75%; nadir: 10-14 days; recovery: by day 21); thrombocytopenia and anemia

Local: Skin "flare" at injection site, urticaria

Neuromuscular & skeletal: Weakness

Pharmacodynamics/Kinetics

Absorption Oral: Poor (<50%)

Protein Binding Plasma: 70% to 76%

Half-Life Elimination

Distribution: 5-10 minutes

Elimination: Doxorubicin: 1-3 hours; Metabolites: 3-3.5 hours

Terminal: 17-48 hours

Male: 54 hours; Female: 35 hours

Metabolism Primarily hepatic to doxorubicinol (active), then to inactive aglycones, conjugated sulfates, and glucuronides

Excretion Feces (~40% to 50% as unchanged drug); urine (~5% to 12% as unchanged drug and metabolites)

Clearance: Male: 113 L/hour; Female: 44 L/hour

Available Dosage Forms

Injection, powder for reconstitution:

Adriamycin®: 10 mg, 20 mg, 50 mg

Injection, solution [preservative free]: 2 mg/mL (5 mL, 10 mL, 25 mL, 37.5 mL, 75 mL, 100 mL)

Adriamycin®: 2 mg/mL (5 mL, 10 mL, 25 mL, 100 mL)

Dosing

Adult & Geriatric Refer to individual protocols. **Note:** Lower dosage should be considered for patients with inadequate marrow reserve (due to old age, prior treatment or neoplastic marrow infiltration).

Usual or typical dosages: I.V.: 60-75 mg/m^2/dose every 21 days **or**
60 mg/m^2/dose every 2 weeks (dose dense) **or**
40-60 mg/m^2/dose every 3-4 weeks **or**
20-30 mg/m^2/day for 2-3 days every 4 weeks **or**
20 mg/m^2/dose once weekly

Pediatric Refer to individual protocols. **Note:** Lower dosage should be considered for patients with inadequate marrow reserve (due to prior treatment or neoplastic marrow infiltration).

Usual/typical dosages: Children: I.V.:
35-75 mg/m^2/dose every 21 days **or**
20-30 mg/m^2/dose once weekly **or**
60-90 mg/m^2 given as a continuous infusion over 96 hours every 3-4 weeks

Renal Impairment

Adjustments are not required.

Hemodialysis: Supplemental dose is not necessary.

Hepatic Impairment

The FDA-approved labeling recommends the following adjustments:

Serum bilirubin 1.2-3 mg/dL: Administer 50% of dose

Serum bilirubin 3.1-5 mg/dL: Administer 25% of dose

Severe hepatic impairment: Use is contraindicated

The following guidelines have been used by some clinicians: Floyd, 2006:

Transaminases 2-3 times ULN: Administer 75% of dose

Transaminases >3 times ULN or serum bilirubin 1.2-3 mg/dL: Administer 50% of dose

Serum bilirubin 3.1-5 mg/dL: Administer 25% of dose

Serum bilirubin >5 mg/dL: Do not administer

Adjustment for Toxicity The following delays and/or dose reductions have been used:

Neutropenic fever/infection: Consider reducing to 75% of dose in subsequent cycles

ANC <1000/mm^3: Delay treatment until ANC recovers to ≥1000/mm^3

Platelets <100,000/mm^3: Delay treatment until platelets recover to ≥100,000/mm^3

Administration

I.V. Vesicant. I.V. push over at least 3-5 minutes or IVPB over 15-60 minutes. Infusion via central venous line recommended.

Stability

Reconstitution Reconstitute lyophilized powder with NS to a final concentration of 2 mg/mL (may further dilute in 50-1000 mL D_5W or NS for infusion). Unstable in solutions with a pH <3 or >7.

Storage Store intact vials of solution under refrigeration at 2°C to 8°C. Protected from light. Store intact vials of lyophilized powder at room temperature (15°C to 30°C). Reconstituted vials are stable for 7 days at room temperature (25°C) and 15 days under refrigeration (5°C) when protected from light. Infusions are stable for 48 hours at room temperature (25°C) when protected from light. Solutions diluted in 50-1000 mL D_5W or NS are stable for 48 hours at room temperature (25°C) when protected from light.

Monitoring and Teaching Issues

Laboratory Monitoring CBC with differential and platelet count; liver function tests (bilirubin, ALT/AST, alkaline phosphatase); serum uric acid, calcium, potassium, phosphate and creatinine; cardiac function (baseline, periodic, and followup): ECG, left ventricular ejection fraction (echocardiography [ECHO] or multigated radionuclide angiography [MUGA])

Physical Assessment Premedication with antiemetic is recommended (especially with larger doses). Infusion site must be closely monitored; extravasation can cause sloughing or tissue necrosis (do not apply heat or sodium bicarbonate). Teach patient importance of adequate hydration.

Patient Education This medication can only be administered intravenously. Report immediately any swelling, pain, burning, or redness at infusion site. Maintain adequate nutrition. You will be more susceptible to infection. May cause nausea or vomiting, diarrhea, loss of hair (reversible), or darker yellow urine (normal). Report immediately chest pain, swelling of extremities, respiratory difficulty, palpitations, or rapid heartbeat. Report unresolved nausea, vomiting, or diarrhea; alterations in urinary pattern (increased or decreased); opportunistic infection (fever, chills, unusual bruising or bleeding fatigue, purulent vaginal discharge, unhealed mouth sores); abdominal pain or blood in stools; excessive fatigue; or yellowing of eyes or skin.

Breast-Feeding Considerations Doxorubicin and its metabolites are found in breast milk. Due to the potential for serious adverse reactions in the nursing infant, breast-feeding should be discontinued during treatment.

Pregnancy Considerations Teratogenicity and embryotoxicity were observed in animal studies. There are no adequate and well-controlled studies in pregnant women. Advise patients to avoid becoming pregnant (females) and to avoid causing pregnancy (males) during treatment. According to the National Comprehensive Cancer Network (NCCN) breast cancer guidelines, doxorubicin, if indicated, may be administered to pregnant women with breast cancer as part of a combination chemotherapy regimen, although chemotherapy should not be administered during the first trimester or after 35 weeks gestation.

◆ **Doxorubicin Hydrochloride** *see* DOXOrubicin *on page* 579

◆ **DOXOrubicin Hydrochloride (Liposomal)** *see* DOXOrubicin (Liposomal) *on page* 582

◆ **DOXOrubicin Hydrochloride Liposome** *see* DOXOrubicin (Liposomal) *on page* 582

DOXOrubicin (Liposomal) (doks oh ROO bi sin lip pah SOW mal)

U.S. Brand Names Doxil®

Index Terms DOXOrubicin Hydrochloride (Liposomal); DOXOrubicin Hydrochloride Liposome; Liposomal DOXOrubicin; Pegylated DOXOrubicin Liposomal; Pegylated Liposomal DOXOrubicin

Generic Availability (U.S.) No

Pharmacologic Category Antineoplastic Agent, Anthracycline

Medication Safety Issues

Sound-alike/look-alike issues:

DOXOrubicin liposomal may be confused with DACTINomycin, DAUNOrubicin, DAUNOrubicin liposomal, doxacurium, doxapram, doxazosin, DOXOrubicin, epirubicin, IDArubicin, valrucibin

DOXOrubicin liposomal may be confused with DAUNOrubicin liposomal

Doxil® may be confused with Doxy®, Paxil®

Liposomal formulation (Doxil®) may be confused with the conventional formulation (Adriamycin PFS®, Adriamycin RDF®)

International issues:

Doxil [U.S., Israel] may be confused with Doxal brand name for doxepin [Finland} and pyridoxine/thiamine [Brazil]

High alert medication: The Institute for Safe Medication Practices (ISMP) includes this medication among its list of drug classes which have a heightened risk of causing significant patient harm when used in error.

Use caution when selecting product for preparation and dispensing; indications, dosages and adverse event profiles differ between conventional DOXOrubicin hydrochloride solution and DOXOrubicin liposomal. Both formulations are the same concentration. As a result, serious errors have occurred. Liposomal formulation of doxorubicin should NOT be substituted for doxorubicin hydrochloride on a mg-per-mg basis.

Pregnancy Risk Factor D

Lactation Excretion in breast milk unknown/contraindicated

Use Treatment of ovarian cancer, multiple myeloma, and AIDS-related Kaposi's sarcoma

Unlabeled/Investigational Use Treatment of metastatic breast cancer, Hodgkin's lymphoma, cutaneous T-cell lymphomas (mycosis fungoides and Sézary syndrome), advanced soft tissue sarcomas; recurrent or metastatic cervical cancer, advanced or metastatic uterine sarcoma

Mechanism of Action/Effect Inhibits DNA and RNA synthesis of susceptible bacteria, active throughout cell cycle, results in cell death

Contraindications Hypersensitivity to doxorubicin liposomal, conventional doxorubicin, or any component of the formulation; breast-feeding

Warnings/Precautions Hazardous agent - use appropriate precautions for handling and disposal.

[U.S. Boxed Warning]: Doxorubicin may cause cumulative, dose-related myocardial toxicity (concurrent or delayed). Doxorubicin liposomal should be used with caution in patients with high cumulative doses of any anthracycline. Total cumulative dose should also account for previous or concomitant treatment with other cardiotoxic agents or irradiation of chest. The incidence of irreversible myocardial toxicity increases as the total cumulative (lifetime) dosages approach 450-550 mg/m^2; or 400 mg/m^2 in patients who have received prior mediastinal radiation therapy or concurrent therapy with other cardiotoxic agents (eg, cyclophosphamide). Although the risk increases with cumulative dose, irreversible cardiotoxicity may occur with anthracycline treatment at any dose level. Patients with pre-existing heart disease, hypertension, concurrent administration of other antineoplastic agents, prior or concurrent chest irradiation, and advanced age are at increased risk. Evaluate left ventricular ejection fraction (LVEF) prior to treatment and periodically during treatment. The onset of symptoms of anthracycline-induced HF and/or cardiomyopathy may be delayed.

[U.S. Boxed Warning]: Acute infusion reactions may occur, some may be serious/life-threatening, including fatal allergic/anaphylactoid-like reactions. Infusion reactions typically occur with the first infusion and may include flushing, dyspnea, facial swelling, headache, chills, back pain, hypotension, and/or tightness of chest/throat. Reactions usually resolve with termination of infusion, or in some cases, slowing the infusion rate. Medication for the treatment of reactions should be readily available in the event of severe reactions. Infuse doxorubicin liposomal at 1 mg/minute initially to minimize risk of infusion reaction.

[U.S. Boxed Warning]: Use with caution in patients with hepatic impairment; dosage reduction is recommended. Use in patients with hepatic impairment has not been adequately studied; dosing adjustment recommendations in multiple myeloma patients with hepatic impairment is not available. **[U.S. Boxed Warning]: Severe myelosuppression may occur.** Palmar-plantar erythrodysesthesia (hand-foot syndrome) has been reported in up to 51% of patients with ovarian cancer, 19% of patients with multiple myeloma, and ~3% in patients with Kaposi's sarcoma. May occur early in treatment, but is usually seen after 2-3 treatment cycles. Dosage modification may be required. In severe cases, treatment discontinuation may be required. **[U.S. Boxed Warning]: Liposomal formulations of doxorubicin should NOT be substituted for conventional doxorubicin hydrochloride on a mg-per-mg basis.**

Doxorubicin may potentiate the toxicity of cyclophosphamide (hemorrhagic cystitis) and mercaptopurine (hepatotoxicity). Radiation recall reaction has been reported with doxorubicin liposomal treatment after radiation therapy. Radiation-induced toxicity (to the myocardium, mucosa, skin, and liver) may be increased by doxorubicin. Safety and efficacy in children have not been established.

Drug Interactions

Metabolism/Transport Effects Substrate of CYP2D6 (major), CYP3A4 (major), P-glycoprotein; **Inhibits** CYP2B6 (moderate), 2D6 (weak), 3A4 (weak); **Induces** P-glycoprotein

Avoid Concomitant Use

Avoid concomitant use of DOXOrubicin (Liposomal) with any of the following: BCG; Natalizumab; Pimecrolimus; Roflumilast; Tacrolimus (Topical); Vaccines (Live)

Decreased Effect

DOXOrubicin (Liposomal) may decrease the levels/effects of: BCG; Cardiac Glycosides; Sipuleucel-T; Stavudine; Vaccines (Inactivated); Vaccines (Live); Zidovudine

The levels/effects of DOXOrubicin (Liposomal) may be decreased by: Cardiac Glycosides; CYP3A4 Inducers (Strong); Deferasirox; Echinacea; Herbs (CYP3A4 Inducers); Peginterferon Alfa-2b

Increased Effect/Toxicity

DOXOrubicin (Liposomal) may increase the levels/effects of: CYP2B6 Substrates; Leflunomide; Natalizumab; Vaccines (Live); Zidovudine

The levels/effects of DOXOrubicin (Liposomal) may be increased by: Bevacizumab; Conivaptan; CYP2D6 Inhibitors (Moderate); CYP2D6 Inhibitors (Strong); CYP3A4 Inhibitors (Moderate); CYP3A4 Inhibitors (Strong); Darunavir; Dasatinib; Denosumab; Pimecrolimus; Roflumilast; Tacrolimus (Topical); Taxane Derivatives; Trastuzumab

Nutritional/Ethanol Interactions

Ethanol: Avoid ethanol (due to GI irritation).

Herb/Nutraceutical: St John's wort may decrease doxorubicin levels.

Adverse Reactions

>10%:

Cardiovascular: Peripheral edema (≤11%)

Central nervous system: Fever (8% to 21%), headache (≤11%), pain (≤21%)

Dermatologic: Palmar-plantar erythrodysesthesia/hand-foot syndrome (≤51% in ovarian cancer [grades 3/4: 24%]; 3% in Kaposi's sarcoma), rash (≤29% in ovarian cancer, ≤5% in Kaposi's sarcoma), alopecia (9% to 19%)

Gastrointestinal: Nausea (17% to 46%), stomatitis (5% to 41%), vomiting (8% to 33%), constipation (≤30%), diarrhea (5% to 21%), anorexia (≤20%), mucositis (≤14%), dyspepsia (≤12%), intestinal obstruction (≤11%)

Hematologic: Myelosuppression (onset: 7 days; nadir: 10-14 days; recovery: 21-28 days), thrombocytopenia (13% to 65%; grades 3/4: 1%), neutropenia (12% to 62%; grade 4: 4%), leukopenia (36%), anemia (6% to 74%; grade 4: <1%)

Neuromuscular & skeletal: Weakness (7% to 40%), back pain (≤12%)

Respiratory: Pharyngitis (≤16%), dyspnea (≤15%)

Miscellaneous: Infection (≤12%)

1% to 10%:

Cardiovascular: Cardiac arrest, chest pain, deep thrombophlebitis, edema, hypotension, pallor, tachycardia, vasodilation

Central nervous system: Agitation, anxiety, chills, confusion, depression, dizziness, emotional lability, insomnia, somnolence, vertigo

Dermatologic: Acne, bruising, dry skin (6%), exfoliative dermatitis, fungal dermatitis, furunculosis, maculopapular rash, pruritus, skin discoloration, vesiculobullous rash

Endocrine & metabolic: Dehydration, hypercalcemia, hyperglycemia, hypokalemia, hyponatremia

Gastrointestinal: Abdomen enlarged, anorexia, ascites, cachexia, dyspepsia, dysphagia, esophagitis, flatulence, gingivitis, glossitis, ileus, mouth ulceration, oral moniliasis, rectal bleeding, taste perversion, weight loss, xerostomia

Genitourinary: Cystitis, dysuria, leukorrhea, pelvic pain, polyuria, urinary incontinence, urinary tract infection, urinary urgency, vaginal bleeding, vaginal moniliasis

Hematologic: Hemolysis, prothrombin time increased

Hepatic: ALT increased, alkaline phosphatase increased, hyperbilirubinemia

Local: Thrombophlebitis

Neuromuscular & skeletal: Arthralgia, hypertonia, myalgia, neuralgia, neuritis (peripheral), neuropathy, paresthesia (≤10%), pathological fracture

Ocular: Conjunctivitis, dry eyes, retinitis

Otic: Ear pain

Renal: Albuminuria, hematuria

Respiratory: Apnea, cough (≤10%), epistaxis, pleural effusion, pneumonia, rhinitis, sinusitis

Miscellaneous: Allergic reaction; infusion-related reactions (7%; includes bronchospasm, chest tightness, chills, dyspnea, facial edema, flushing, headache, herpes simplex/zoster, hypotension, pruritus); moniliasis, diaphoresis

Pharmacodynamics/Kinetics

Protein Binding Unknown; nonliposomal (conventional) doxorubicin: 70%

Half-Life Elimination Terminal: Distribution: 4.7-5.2 hours, Elimination: 44-55 hours

Metabolism Hepatic and in plasma to doxorubicinol and the sulfate and glucuronide conjugates of 4-demethyl,7-deoxyaglycones

Excretion Urine (5% as doxorubicin or doxorubicinol)

Available Dosage Forms

Injection, solution:

Doxil®: 2 mg/mL (10 mL, 25 mL)

Dosing

Adult & Geriatric Details concerning dosing in combination regimens should also be consulted. **Liposomal formulations of doxorubicin should NOT be substituted for conventional doxorubicin hydrochloride on a mg-per-mg basis.**

AIDS-related Kaposi's sarcoma: I.V.: 20 mg/m^2/dose once every 3 weeks

Multiple myeloma: I.V.: 30 mg/m^2/dose every 3 weeks (in combination with bortezomib) **or**

Unlabeled dosing: I.V.: 40 mg/m^2/dose every 4 weeks (in combination with vincristine and dexamethasone) (Rifkin, 2006)

Ovarian cancer: I.V.: 50 mg/m^2/dose every 4 weeks (minimum of 4 cycles is recommended)

Breast cancer (unlabeled use): I.V.: 50 mg/m^2/dose every 4 weeks (Keller, 2004)

Uterine sarcoma (unlabeled use): I.V.: 50 mg/m^2/dose every 4 weeks (Sutton, 2005)

Hepatic Impairment Note: Dosage adjustment information is not available in patients with multiple myeloma.

Bilirubin 1.2-3 mg/dL: Administer 50% of dose

Bilirubin >3 mg/dL: Administer 25% of dose

Adjustment for Toxicity

Recommended Dose Modification Guidelines

Toxicity Grade	Dose Adjustment
HAND FOOT SYNDROME (HFS)	
1 (Mild erythema, swelling, or desquamation not interfering with daily activities)	Redose unless patient has experienced previous Grade 3 or 4 HFS toxicity. If so, delay up to 2 weeks and decrease dose by 25%; return to original dosing interval.
2 (Erythema, desquamation, or swelling interfering with, but not precluding, normal physical activities; small blisters or ulcerations <2 cm in diameter)	Delay dosing up to 2 weeks or until resolved to Grade 0-1. If after 2 weeks there is no resolution, discontinue liposomal doxorubicin. Otherwise, if no prior Grade 3-4 HFS, continue treatment at previous dose and dosage interval. If a prior Grade 3-4 HFS has occurred, continue prior dosage interval, but decrease dose by 25%.
3 (Blistering, ulceration, or swelling interfering with walking or normal daily activities; cannot wear regular clothing)	Delay dosing up to 2 weeks or until resolved to Grade 0-1. Decrease dose by 25% and return to original dosing interval; if after 2 weeks there is no resolution, discontinue liposomal doxorubicin.
4 (Diffuse or local process causing infectious complications, or a bedridden state or hospitalization)	Delay dosing up to 2 weeks or until resolved to Grade 0-1. Decrease dose by 25% and return to original dosing interval. If after 2 weeks there is no resolution, discontinue liposomal doxorubicin.
STOMATITIS	
1 (Painless ulcers, erythema, or mild soreness)	Redose unless patient has experienced previous Grade 3 or 4 toxicity. If so, delay up to 2 weeks and decrease by 25%. Return to original dosing interval.
2 (Painful erythema, edema, or ulcers, but can eat)	Delay dosing up to 2 weeks or until resolved to Grade 0-1. If after 2 weeks there is no resolution, discontinue liposomal doxorubicin. Otherwise, if not prior Grade 3-4 stomatitis, continue treatment at previous dose and dosage interval. If prior Grade 3-4 toxicity, continue treatment with previous dosage interval, but decrease dose by 25%.
3 (Painful erythema, edema, or ulcers, and cannot eat)	Delay dosing up to 2 weeks or until resolved to Grade 0-1. Decrease dose by 25% and return to original dosing interval. If after 2 weeks there is no resolution, discontinue liposomal doxorubicin.
4 (Requires parenteral or enteral support)	Delay dosing up to 2 weeks or until resolved to Grade 0-1. Decrease dose by 25% and return to original dosing interval. If after 2 weeks there is no resolution, discontinue liposomal doxorubicin.

Hematological Toxicity (see below for multiple myeloma)

Grade	ANC	Platelets	Modification
1	1500-1900	75,000-150,000	Resume treatment with no dose reduction.
2	1000-<1500	50,000-<75,000	Wait until ANC ≥1500 and platelets ≥75,000; redose with no dose reduction.
3	500-999	25,000-<50,000	Wait until ANC ≥1500 and platelets ≥75,000; redose with no dose reduction.
4	<500	<25,000	Wait until ANC ≥1500 and platelets ≥75,000; redose at 25% dose reduction or continue full dose with cytokine support.

Dosing Adjustment for Toxicity in Treatment with Bortezomib (for Multiple Myeloma) (see Bortezomib monograph for bortezomib dosage reduction with toxicity guidelines):

Fever ≥38°C and ANC <1000/mm³: If prior to doxorubicin liposomal treatment (day 4), do not administer; if after doxorubicin liposomal administered, reduce dose by 25% in next cycle.

ANC <500/mm³, platelets <25,000/mm³, hemoglobin <8 g/dL: If prior to doxorubicin liposomal treatment (day 4); do not administer; if after doxorubicin liposomal administered, reduce dose by 25% in next cycle if bortezomib dose reduction occurred for hematologic toxicity.

Grade 3 or 4 nonhematologic toxicity: Delay dose until resolved to grade <2; reduce dose by 25% for all subsequent doses.

Neuropathic pain or peripheral neuropathy: No dose reductions needed for doxorubicin liposomal, refer to Bortezomib monograph for bortezomib dosing adjustment.

Administration

I.V. Irritant; avoid extravasation. Administer IVPB over 60 minutes; manufacturer recommends administering at initial rate of 1 mg/minute to minimize risk of infusion reactions until the absence of a reaction has been established, then increase the infusion rate for completion over 1 hour. **Do not administer intramuscular or subcutaneous. Do not infuse with in-line filters.**

Stability

Reconstitution Doses of doxorubicin liposomal ≤90 mg must be diluted in 250 mL of D_5W prior to administration. Doses >90 mg should be diluted in 500 mL D_5W. Solution is not a clear, but has a red, translucent appearance due to the liposomal dispersion. Use appropriate precautions for handling and disposal.

Storage Store intact vials of solution under refrigeration at 2°C to 8°C (36°F to 46°F); avoid freezing. Prolonged freezing may adversely affect liposomal drug products, however, short-term freezing (<1 month) does not appear to have a deleterious effect. Diluted doxorubicin hydrochloride liposome injection may be refrigerated at 2°C to 8°C (36°F to 46°F); administer within 24 hours. **Do not infuse with in-line filters.**

Monitoring and Teaching Issues

Laboratory Monitoring CBC with differential, platelet count, echocardiogram, liver function tests (ALT/AST, bilirubin, alkaline phosphatase)

Physical Assessment Use caution in presence of hepatic impairment, heart disease, or high cumulative doses of any anthracycline; dosage adjustment may be necessary. Premedication with antiemetic is recommended, especially with larger doses. Infusion site must be closely monitored to prevent extravasation. Patient must be monitored for infusion reactions continuously during and following infusion (acute allergic/anaphylactic reactions may be fatal); medication/equipment for treating reactions should be readily available. Teach patient importance of adequate nutrition and hydration.

Patient Education This medication can only be administered by infusion. Report immediately any swelling, pain, burning, or redness at infusion site; back pain; difficulty breathing; rapid heartbeat; or chills. Avoid alcohol; may cause gastrointestinal irritation. It is important to maintain adequate nutrition and hydration, unless instructed to restrict fluid intake. You will be more susceptible to infection. You may experience weakness, tiredness, or fatigue. May cause nausea or vomiting, sore mouth or gums, diarrhea, loss of hair (reversible), or red-pink urine (normal). Seek immediate emergency care if you experience chest pain or rapid or irregular heart beat. Report any swelling of extremities; respiratory difficulty; unresolved nausea, vomiting, abdominal pain, diarrhea, or blood in stool; alterations in urinary pattern; opportunistic infection (fever, chills, unusual bruising or bleeding, fatigue, purulent vaginal discharge, unhealed mouth sores); excessive fatigue; redness, swelling, pain, or blisters on the palms of the hands and/or the soles of the feet; or yellowing of eyes or skin.

Breast-Feeding Considerations Due to the potential for serious adverse reactions in the nursing infant, breast-feeding is contraindicated.

Pregnancy Considerations May cause fetal harm if administered during pregnancy. There are no adequate and well-controlled studies in pregnant women. Women of childbearing potential should avoid becoming pregnant during treatment.

Additional Information Oncology Comment: Doxorubicin liposomal is listed within National Comprehensive Cancer Network® (NCCN) guidelines for the treatment of the following types of malignancies:

Breast cancer: As a preferred single-agent therapy for recurrent or metastatic breast cancer

Cervical cancer: As second-line treatment for recurrent or metastatic cervical cancer

Hodgkin's lymphoma: As second-line chemotherapy (in combination with gemcitabine and vinorelbine)

Non-Hodgkin's lymphomas: As a first-line systemic treatment for cutaneous T-cell lymphomas, mycosis fungoides, and Sezary syndrome, in patients with generalized tumor disease or tumor disease with blood involvement

Ovarian cancer: As a preferred agent for recurrent ovarian cancer

Multiple myeloma: As primary induction therapy for both transplant candidates and nontransplant candidates (in combination with vincristine and dexamethasone), and as salvage therapy (in combination with bortezomib)

Soft tissue sarcoma: As a systemic single-agent treatment for metastatic disease for extremity, retroperitoneal, or intra-abdominal (other than GIST) soft tissue sarcomas

Uterine cancer: As a single-agent treatment for advanced or metastatic uterine sarcoma

◆ **Doxy 100™** *see* Doxycycline *on page* 586

Doxycycline (doks i SYE kleen)

U.S. Brand Names Adoxa®; Adoxa® Pak™ 1/150; Adoxa® Pak™ 1/75; Alodox™; Doryx®; Doxy 100™; Monodox®; Oracea®; Oraxyl™; Periostat®; Vibramycin®

Index Terms Doxycycline Calcium; Doxycycline Hyclate; Doxycycline Monohydrate

Generic Availability (U.S.) Yes: Excludes capsule (variable release), syrup

Pharmacologic Category Antibiotic, Tetracycline Derivative

Medication Safety Issues

Sound-alike/look-alike issues:

Doxycycline may be confused with dicyclomine, doxepin, doxylamine

Doxy100™ may be confused with Doxil®

Monodox® may be confused with Maalox®

Oracea® may be confused with Orencia®

Vibramycin® may be confused with vancomycin, Vibativ™

Pregnancy Risk Factor D

Lactation Enters breast milk/not recommended

Use Principally in the treatment of infections caused by susceptible *Rickettsia*, *Chlamydia*, and *Mycoplasma*; alternative to mefloquine for malaria prophylaxis; treatment for syphilis, uncomplicated *Neisseria gonorrhoeae*, *Listeria*, *Actinomyces israelii*, and *Clostridium* infections in penicillin-allergic patients; used for community-acquired pneumonia and other common infections due to susceptible organisms; anthrax due to *Bacillus anthracis,* including inhalational anthrax (postexposure); treatment of infections caused by uncommon susceptible gram-negative and gram-positive organisms including *Borrelia recurrentis*, *Ureaplasma urealyticum*, *Haemophilus ducreyi*, *Yersinia pestis*, *Francisella tularensis*, *Vibrio cholerae*, *Campylobacter fetus*, *Brucella* spp, *Bartonella bacilliformis*, and *Klebsiella granulomatis,* Q fever, Lyme disease; treatment of inflammatory lesions associated with rosacea; intestinal amebiasis; severe acne

Unlabeled/Investigational Use Sclerosing agent for pleural effusion injection; vancomycin-resistant enterococci (VRE); alternate treatment for MRSA infections

Mechanism of Action/Effect Inhibits protein synthesis by binding with the 30S and possibly the 50S ribosomal subunit(s) of susceptible bacteria; may also cause alterations in the cytoplasmic membrane

Doxycycline inhibits collagenase *in vitro* and has been shown to inhibit collagenase in the gingival crevicular fluid in adults with periodontitis

Contraindications Hypersensitivity to doxycycline, tetracycline or any component of the formulation

Warnings/Precautions Photosensitivity reaction may occur with this drug; avoid prolonged exposure to sunlight or tanning equipment. Antianabolic effects of tetracyclines can increase BUN (dose-related). Autoimmune syndromes have been reported. Hepatotoxicity rarely occurs; if symptomatic, conduct LFT and discontinue drug. Pseudotumor cerebri has been (rarely) reported with tetracycline use; usually resolves with discontinuation. Prolonged use may result in fungal or bacterial superinfection, including *C. difficile*-associated diarrhea (CDAD) and pseudomembranous colitis; CDAD has been observed >2 months postantibiotic treatment. May cause tissue hyperpigmentation, enamel hypoplasia, or permanent tooth discoloration; use of tetracyclines should be avoided during tooth development (children ≤8 years of age) unless other drugs are not likely to be effective or are contraindicated. However, recommended in treatment of anthrax exposure and tickborne rickettsial diseases. Do not use during pregnancy. In addition to affecting tooth development, tetracycline use has been associated with retardation of skeletal development and reduced bone growth.

Additional specific warnings: Oracea®: Should not be used for the treatment or prophylaxis of bacterial infections, since the lower dose of drug per capsule may be subefficacious and promote resistance. Syrup contains sodium metabisulfite. Effectiveness of products intended for use in periodontitis has not been established in patients with coexistent oral candidiasis; use with caution in patients with a history or predisposition to oral candidiasis.

Drug Interactions

Metabolism/Transport Effects Inhibits CYP3A4 (moderate)

Avoid Concomitant Use

Avoid concomitant use of Doxycycline with any of the following: BCG; Retinoic Acid Derivatives

Decreased Effect

Doxycycline may decrease the levels/effects of: BCG; Penicillins; Typhoid Vaccine

The levels/effects of Doxycycline may be decreased by: Antacids; Barbiturates; Bile Acid Sequestrants; Bismuth; Bismuth Subsalicylate; CarBAMazepine; Iron Salts; Magnesium Salts; Phenytoin; Quinapril; Sucralfate

Increased Effect/Toxicity

Doxycycline may increase the levels/effects of: Neuromuscular-Blocking Agents; Retinoic Acid Derivatives; Vitamin K Antagonists

Nutritional/Ethanol Interactions

Ethanol: Chronic ethanol ingestion may reduce the serum concentration of doxycycline.

Food: Doxycycline serum levels may be slightly decreased if taken with food or milk. Administration with iron or calcium may decrease doxycycline absorption. May decrease absorption of calcium, iron, magnesium, zinc, and amino acids.

Herb/Nutraceutical: St John's wort may decrease doxycycline levels. Avoid dong quai, St John's wort (may also cause photosensitization).

Lab Interactions False-negative urine glucose using Clinistix®

Adverse Reactions Frequency not defined.

Cardiovascular: Intracranial hypertension, pericarditis

Dermatologic: Angioneurotic edema, erythema multiforme, exfoliative dermatitis (rare), photosensitivity, rash, skin hyperpigmentation, Stevens-Johnson syndrome, toxic epidermal necrolysis, urticaria

Endocrine & metabolic: Brown/black discoloration of thyroid gland (no dysfunction reported), hypoglycemia

Gastrointestinal: Anorexia, diarrhea, dysphagia, enterocolitis, esophagitis (rare), esophageal ulcerations (rare), glossitis, inflammatory lesions in anogenital region, nausea, oral (mucosal) pigmentation, pseudomembranous colitis, tooth discoloration (children), vomiting

Hematologic: Eosinophilia, hemolytic anemia, neutropenia, thrombocytopenia

Hepatic: Hepatotoxicity (rare)

Renal: BUN increased (dose related)

Miscellaneous: Anaphylactoid purpura, anaphylaxis, bulging fontanels (infants), serum sickness, SLE exacerbation

Note: Adverse effects in clinical trials occurring at a frequency more than 1% greater than placebo:

Periostat®: Diarrhea, dyspepsia, joint pain, menstrual cramp, nausea, dyspepsia, pain

Oracea®: Abdominal distention, abdominal pain, anxiety, AST increased, back pain, fungal infection, hyperglycemia, influenza, LDH increased, nasal congestion, nasopharyngitis, pain, sinus headache, sinusitis, xerostomia

Pharmacodynamics/Kinetics

Absorption Oral: Almost complete

Bioavailability Reduced at high pH; may be clinically significant in patients with gastrectomy, gastric bypass surgery, or who are otherwise deemed achlorhydric

Time to Peak Serum: 1.5-4 hours

Protein Binding 90%

Half-Life Elimination 12-15 hours (usually increases to 22-24 hours with multiple doses); End-stage renal disease: 18-25 hours; Oracea®: 21 hours

Metabolism Not hepatic; partially inactivated in GI tract by chelate formation

Excretion Feces (30%); urine (23%)

Available Dosage Forms

Capsule, oral: 50 mg, 100 mg
Adoxa®: 150 mg
Monodox®: 50 mg, 75 mg, 100 mg
Oraxyl™: 20 mg
Vibramycin®: 100 mg

Capsule, variable release, oral:
Oracea®: 40 mg [30 mg (immediate release) and 10 mg (delayed release)]

Injection, powder for reconstitution: 100 mg
Doxy 100™: 100 mg

Powder for suspension, oral:
Vibramycin®: 25 mg/5 mL (60 mL)

Syrup, oral:
Vibramycin®: 50 mg/5 mL (473 mL)

Tablet, oral: 20 mg, 50 mg, 75 mg, 100 mg, 150 mg
Adoxa®: 50 mg
Adoxa® Pak™ 1/150: 150 mg
Adoxa® Pak™ 1/75: 75 mg
Alodox™: 20 mg
Periostat®: 20 mg

Tablet, delayed release coated beads, oral: 75 mg, 100 mg

Tablet, delayed release coated pellets, oral:
Doryx®: 75 mg, 100 mg, 150 mg

Dosing

Adult & Geriatric

Usual dosage range: Oral, I.V.: 100-200 mg/day in 1-2 divided doses

Anthrax:

Inhalational (postexposure prophylaxis): Oral, I.V. (use oral route when possible): 100 mg every 12 hours for 60 days (ACIP, 2010)

Cutaneous (treatment): Oral: 100 mg every 12 hours for 60 days. **Note:** In the presence of systemic involvement, extensive edema, lesions on head/neck, refer to I.V. dosing for treatment of inhalational/gastrointestinal/oropharyngeal anthrax

Inhalational/gastrointestinal/oropharyngeal (treatment): I.V.: Initial: 100 mg every 12 hours; switch to oral therapy when clinically appropriate; some recommend initial loading dose of 200 mg, followed by 100 mg every 8-12 hours (Franz, 1997). **Note:** Initial treatment should include two or more agents predicted to be effective (CDC, 2001). Agents suggested for use in conjunction with doxycycline or ciprofloxacin include rifampin, vancomycin, imipenem, penicillin, ampicillin, chloramphenicol, clindamycin, and clarithromycin. May switch to oral antimicrobial therapy when clinically appropriate. Continue combined therapy for 60 days

Brucellosis: Oral: 100 mg twice daily for 6 weeks with rifampin or streptomycin

Cellulitis (purulent) due to community-acquired MRSA (unlabeled use): Oral: 100 mg twice daily for 5-10 days (Liu, 2011)

Chlamydial infections, uncomplicated: Oral: 100 mg twice daily for ≥7 days

Community-acquired pneumonia, bronchitis: Oral, I.V.: 100 mg twice daily (Ailani, 1999; Mandell, 2007)

Epididymitis: Oral: 100 mg twice daily for 10 days (in combination with ceftriaxone) (CDC, 2010)

Gonococcal infection, uncomplicated (cervix, pharynx, rectum, urethra): Oral: 100 mg twice daily for 7 days (in combination with a cephalosporin) (CDC, 2010)

Alternatively, the manufacturer recommends a single-visit dose in nonanorectal infections in men: 300 mg initially, repeat dose in 1 hour (total dose: 600 mg)

Granuloma inguinale (donovanosis): Oral: 100 mg twice daily for at least 3 weeks (and until lesions have healed) (CDC, 2010)

Lyme disease: Oral (Halperin, 2007; Wormser, 2006):

Prevention: Initiate within 72 hours of tick removal: 200 mg administered as a single dose

Treatment (early lyme disease without neurologic manifestations): 100 mg twice daily for 10-21 days

Treatment (meningitis or other early neurologic manifestations): 100-200 mg twice daily for 14 days (range: 10-28 days)

Lymphogranuloma venereum: Oral: 100 mg twice daily for 21 days (CDC, 2010)

Malaria prophylaxis: 100 mg/day. Start 1-2 days prior to travel to endemic area; continue daily during travel and for 4 weeks after leaving endemic area

Nongonococcal urethritis: Oral: 100 mg twice daily for 7 days (CDC, 2010)

Pelvic inflammatory disease:

Treatment, inpatient: Oral, I.V.: 100 mg twice daily (in combination with cefoxitin or cefotetan); may transition to oral doxycycline (add clindamycin or metronidazole if tubo-ovarian abscess present) to complete 14 days of treatment (CDC, 2010)

Treatment, outpatient: Oral: 100 mg twice daily for 14 days (with or without metronidazole); preceded by a single I.M. dose of cefoxitin (plus oral probenecid) or ceftriaxone (CDC, 2010)

Periodontitis: Oral: 20 mg twice daily as an adjunct following scaling and root planing; may be administered for up to 9 months. Safety beyond 12 months of treatment and efficacy beyond 9 months of treatment have not been established.

Proctitis: Oral: 100 mg twice daily for 7 days (in combination with ceftriaxone) (CDC, 2010)

Q fever: Oral: 100 mg every 12 hours for 15-21days (CDC, 2009)

Rosacea (Oracea®): Oral: 40 mg once daily in the morning

Sclerosing agent for pleural effusion (unlabeled use): Intrapleural: 500 mg as a single dose in 100 mL NS (Porcel, 2006); may require a repeat dose (Kvale, 2007)

Syphilis:

Primary/secondary syphilis: Oral: 100 mg twice daily for 14 days (CDC, 2010)

Latent syphilis: Oral: 100 mg twice daily for 28 days (CDC, 2010)

Tickborne rickettsial disease: Oral, I.V.: 100 mg twice daily for 5-7 days; severe or complicated disease may require longer treatment; human granulocytotropic anaplasmosis (HGA) should be treated for 10-14 days.

Tularemia: I.V. (may transition to oral if clinically appropriate): Initial: 100 mg every 12 hours for 14-21 days (Dennis, 2001)

Vibrio cholerae: Oral: 300 mg as a single dose (WHO, 2004)

***Yersinia pestis* (plague):** Oral, I.V.: 200 mg initially then 100 mg twice daily **or** 200 mg once daily for 10 days (Daya, 2005; Inglesby, 2000)

Pediatric

Usual dosage range:

Children >8 years (≤45 kg): Oral, I.V.: 2-5 mg/kg/day in 1-2 divided doses, not to exceed 200 mg/day

Children >8 years (>45 kg): Oral, I.V.: Refer to adult dosing.

Anthrax:

Inhalational (postexposure prophylaxis) (ACIP, 2010): Oral, I.V. (use oral route when possible):

≤8 years: 2.2 mg/kg every 12 hours for 60 days

>8 years and ≤45 kg: 2.2 mg/kg every 12 hours for 60 days

>8 years and >45 kg: 100 mg every 12 hours for 60 days

Cutaneous (treatment): Oral: See Dosing for "Inhalational (postexposure prophylaxis)"

Note: In the presence of systemic involvement, extensive edema, and/or lesions on head/neck, doxycycline should initially be administered I.V.

Inhalational/gastrointestinal/oropharyngeal (treatment): I.V.: Refer to dosing for inhalational anthrax (postexposure prophylaxis); switch to oral therapy when clinically appropriate.

Note: Initial treatment should include two or more agents predicted to be effective (CDC, 2001). Agents suggested for use in conjunction with doxycycline or ciprofloxacin include rifampin, vancomycin, imipenem, penicillin, ampicillin, chloramphenicol, clindamycin, and clarithromycin. May switch to oral antimicrobial therapy when clinically appropriate. Continue combined therapy for 60 days

Cellulitis (purulent) due to community-acquired MRSA (unlabeled use): Oral: Children >8 years and ≤45 kg: 2 mg/kg/dose every 12 hours for 5-10 days; >45 kg: Refer to adult dosing (Liu, 2011)

Chlamydial infections, uncomplicated: Children >8 years and >45 kg: Oral: 100 mg twice daily for 7 days

Lyme disease: Children ≥8 years: Oral (Halperin, 2007; Wormser, 2006):

Prevention: 4 mg/kg (maximum: 200 mg) administered as a single dose; **Note:** Initiate within 72 hours of tick removal

Treatment (early lyme disease without neurologic manifestations): 1-2 mg/kg twice daily for 10-21 days (maximum: 100 mg/dose)

Treatment (meningitis and other early neurologic manifestations): 4-8 mg/kg/day in 2 divided doses for 10-28 days (maximum: 200 mg/dose)

Malaria prophylaxis: Children ≥8 years: Oral: 2 mg/kg/day (maximum: 100 mg/day). Start 1-2 days prior to travel to endemic area; continue daily during travel and for 4 weeks after leaving endemic area

Q fever: Oral: 2.2 mg/kg twice/day for 15-21 days. Some clinicians may recommend trimethoprim/sulfamethoxazole for children <8 years of age (Hartzell, 2008). **Note:** Use of tetracyclines should be avoided during tooth development (children ≤8 years of age) unless other drugs are unlikely to be effective or are contraindicated.

Tickborne rickettsial disease: Note: The American Academy of Pediatrics Committee on Infectious Diseases identifies doxycycline as the drug of choice in children of any age.

Children ≤8 years: Oral, I.V.: 2.2 mg/kg (maximum dose: 100 mg) every 12 hours for 5-7 days

Children >8 years and >45 kg: Oral, I.V.: 100 mg twice daily for 5-7days; severe or complicated disease may require longer treatment; human granulocytotropic anaplasmosis (HGA) should be treated for 10-14 days

Tularemia: I.V. (may transition to oral if clinically indicated) (Dennis, 2001):

Children <45 kg: 2.2 mg/kg every 12 hours for 14-21 days

Children ≥45 kg: 100 mg every 12 hours for 14-21 days

Renal Impairment No adjustment necessary.

Not dialyzable; 0% to 5% by hemo- and peritoneal methods or by continuous arteriovenous or venovenous hemofiltration; supplemental dose is not necessary.

Administration

Oral Oral administration is preferable unless patient has significant nausea and vomiting; I.V. and oral routes are bioequivalent. May give with meals to decrease GI upset. Capsule and tablet: Administer with at least 8 ounces of water and have patient sit up for at least 30 minutes after taking to reduce the risk of esophageal irritation and ulceration.

Oracea®: Take on an empty stomach 1 hour before or 2 hours after meals.

Doryx®: May be administered by carefully breaking up the tablet and sprinkling tablet contents on a spoonful of cold applesauce. The delayed release pellets must not be crushed or damaged when breaking up tablet. Should be administered immediately after preparation and without chewing.

I.V. Infuse slowly, usually over 1-4 hours. Avoid extravasation. Oral administration is preferable unless patient has significant nausea and vomiting; I.V. and oral routes are bioequivalent.

Other Intrapleural (unlabeled route): Add to 100 mL NS and instill into chest tube (Porcel, 2006)

Stability

Reconstitution I.V. infusion: Following reconstitution with sterile water for injection, dilute to a final concentration of 0.1-1 mg/mL using a compatible solution.

Storage

Capsule, tablet: Store at controlled room temperature of 25°C (77°F); excursions permitted to 15°C to 30°C (59°F to 86°F). Protect from light.

I.V. infusion: Protect from light. Stability varies based on solution.

Monitoring and Teaching Issues

Laboratory Monitoring Perform culture and sensitivity testing prior to initiating therapy. CBC, renal and liver function tests periodically with prolonged therapy.

Physical Assessment Assess results of culture and sensitivity test and patient's allergy history prior to beginning therapy. I.V.: Infusion site must be closely monitored; extravasation can be very irritating to veins (use of central line is preferable). Teach patient importance of adequate hydration and photosensitivity precautions.

Patient Education If administered by infusion, report immediately any acute back pain, difficulty breathing or swallowing, chest tightness, pain, redness, or swelling at infusion site. Oral: Medication may be taken with food if gastric irritation occurs. Avoid alcohol and maintain adequate hydration, unless instructed to restrict fluid intake. You may be sensitive to sunlight. May cause nausea, vomiting, or diarrhea. Report skin rash or itching; easy bruising or bleeding; yellowing of skin or eyes; pale stool or dark urine; unhealed mouth sores; vaginal itching or discharge; persistent diarrhea; and fever, chills, or unusual cough.

Dietary Considerations

Tetracyclines (in general): Take with food if gastric irritation occurs. While administration with food may decrease GI absorption of doxycycline by up to 20%, administration on an empty stomach is not recommended due to GI intolerance. Of currently available tetracyclines, doxycycline has the least affinity for calcium.

Oracea®: Take on an empty stomach 1 hour before or 2 hours after meals.

Some products may contain sodium.

Geriatric Considerations Dose adjustment for renal function is not necessary.

Breast-Feeding Considerations Tetracyclines, including doxycycline, are excreted in breast milk and therefore, breast-feeding is not recommended by the manufacturer.

Doxycycline is less bound to the calcium in maternal milk which may lead to increased absorption compared to other tetracyclines. Only minimal amounts of doxycycline are excreted in human milk and the relative amount of tooth staining has been reported to be lower when compared to other tetracycline analogs. Nondose-related effects could include modification of bowel flora.

Pregnancy Considerations Because use during pregnancy may cause fetal harm, doxycycline is classified as pregnancy category D. Exposure to tetracyclines during the second or third trimester may cause permanent discoloration of the teeth. Most reports do not show an increase risk for teratogenicity with the exception of a potential small increased risk for cleft palate or esophageal atresia/stenosis. When considering treatment for life-threatening infection and/or prolonged duration of therapy (such as in anthrax), the potential risk to the fetus must be balanced against the severity of the potential illness.

Additional Information Oracea® capsules are not bioequivalent to other doxycycline products.

Related Information

Antimicrobial Drugs of Choice *on page 2008*

Community-Acquired Pneumonia in Adults *on page 2021*

I.V. to Oral Conversion *on page 1956*

Prophylaxis for Patients Exposed to Common Communicable Diseases *on page 2073*

◆ **Doxycycline Calcium** *see* Doxycycline *on page 586*

◆ **Doxycycline Hyclate** *see* Doxycycline *on page 586*

◆ **Doxycycline Monohydrate** *see* Doxycycline *on page 586*

◆ **DPA** *see* Valproic Acid *on page 1832*

◆ **DPH** *see* Phenytoin *on page 1453*

◆ **Dramamine® Less Drowsy Formula [OTC]** *see* Meclizine *on page 1153*

◆ **Drisdol®** *see* Ergocalciferol *on page 650*

Dronabinol (droe NAB i nol)

U.S. Brand Names Marinol®

Index Terms Delta-9 THC; Delta-9-tetrahydro-cannabinol; Tetrahydrocannabinol; THC

Generic Availability (U.S.) Yes

Pharmacologic Category Antiemetic; Appetite Stimulant

Medication Safety Issues

Sound-alike/look-alike issues:

Dronabinol may be confused with droperidol

Pregnancy Risk Factor C

Lactation Enters breast milk/contraindicated

Use Chemotherapy-associated nausea and vomiting refractory to other antiemetic(s); AIDS-related anorexia

Unlabeled/Investigational Use Cancer-related anorexia

Controlled Substance C-III

Available Dosage Forms

Capsule, soft gelatin, oral: 2.5 mg, 5 mg, 10 mg

Marinol®: 2.5 mg, 5 mg, 10 mg

Dosing

Adult & Geriatric

Antiemetic: Oral: 5 mg/m^2 1-3 hours before chemotherapy, then give 5 mg/m^2/dose every 2-4 hours after chemotherapy for a total of 4-6 doses/day; dose may be increased up to a maximum of 15 mg/m^2/dose if needed (dosage may be increased by 2.5 mg/m^2 increments).

Appetite stimulant (AIDS-related): Oral: Initial: 2.5 mg twice daily (before lunch and dinner); titrate up to a maximum of 20 mg/day.

Pediatric Antiemetic: Oral: Refer to adult dosing.

Hepatic Impairment Usual dose should be reduced in patients with severe liver failure.

Monitoring and Teaching Issues

Physical Assessment Use caution in the presence of heart disease, hepatic disease, or seizure disorders. Monitor closely for adverse psychotic reactions; this drug is the psychoactive substance in marijuana.

Patient Education Avoid alcohol. May cause psychotic reaction, impaired coordination or judgment, faintness, dizziness, drowsiness, clumsiness, unsteadiness, or muscular weakness. Report excessive or persistent CNS changes (euphoria, anxiety, depression, memory lapse, bizarre thought patterns, excitability, inability to control thoughts or behavior, fainting), respiratory difficulties, and rapid heartbeat.

Dronedarone (droe NE da rone)

U.S. Brand Names Multaq®

Index Terms Dronedarone Hydrochloride; SR33589

Generic Availability (U.S.) No

Pharmacologic Category Antiarrhythmic Agent, Class III

Medication Guide Available Yes

Pregnancy Risk Factor X

Lactation Excretion in breast milk unknown/contraindicated

Use To reduce the risk of hospitalization related to paroxysmal or persistent atrial fibrillation (AF) or atrial flutter (AFL) in patients with a recent episode of AF/AFL and associated cardiovascular risk factors (eg, age >70 years, hypertension, diabetes, prior cerebrovascular accident, left atrial diameter ≥50 mm or left ventricular ejection fraction <40%), who are in normal sinus rhythm or will be cardioverted

Mechanism of Action/Effect A noniodinated antiarrhythmic agent structurally related to amiodarone exhibiting properties of all 4 antiarrhythmic classes. Dronedarone prolongs the action potential and refractory period in myocardial tissue, and slows heart rate through inhibition of calcium channels and $beta_1$-receptors.

Contraindications NYHA Class IV heart failure (HF); NYHA Class II-III HF with recent decompensation requiring hospitalization or referral to a specialized HF clinic; second- or third-degree heart block or sick sinus syndrome (except in patients with a functioning artificial pacemaker); bradycardia <50 bpm; concomitant use of strong CYP3A4 inhibitors (eg, ketoconazole, itraconazole, voriconazole, cyclosporine, telithromycin, clarithromycin, nefazodone, or ritonavir); concomitant use of drugs or herbal products known to prolong the QT interval increasing the risk for torsade de pointes (eg, phenothiazine antipsychotics, tricyclic antidepressants, certain oral macrolide antibiotics, or class I and III antiarrhythmics); QT_c (Bazett) interval ≥500 msec or PR interval >280 msec; severe hepatic impairment; pregnancy; breastfeeding

Warnings/Precautions [U.S. Boxed Warning]: In patients with severe HF requiring recent hospitalization or referral to a specialized HF clinic for worsening symptoms, patients receiving dronedarone had a greater than twofold increase in mortality; use is contraindicated in patients with NYHA Class IV HF or NYHA Class II-III HF with recent decompensation requiring hospitalization or referral to a specialized HF clinic. If patients develop new or worsening HF symptoms (eg, weight gain, dependent edema, or increasing shortness of breath) while on therapy, consider suspension or discontinuation of dronedarone.

Dronedarone induces a moderate prolongation of the QT interval (average ~10 msec); much greater effects have been observed. Use in patients with QT_c (Bazett) interval ≥500 msec is contraindicated; discontinue use of dronedarone if this occurs during therapy. Following initiation, dronedarone may produce a slight increase in serum creatinine (~0.1 mg/dL) due to inhibition of tubular secretion; glomerular filtration rate is not affected; effect is reversible upon discontinuation.

Severe liver injury, including acute liver failure leading to liver transplant, has been rarely reported. If liver injury is suspected, discontinue therapy and evaluate liver enzymes/bilirubin. Appropriate treatment should be started and therapy should not be reinitiated if liver injury is confirmed. Advise patients to report any signs or symptoms of hepatic injury (unusual fatigue, jaundice, nausea, vomiting, abdominal pain, and/or fever). Consider periodic monitoring of serum liver enzymes and bilirubin, especially during the first 6 months of therapy. Use with caution in patients with mild-to-moderate hepatic impairment; use is contraindicated in severe hepatic impairment.

Chronic administration of antiarrhythmic drugs may affect defibrillation or pacing thresholds; assess when initiating dronedarone and during therapy. Correct electrolyte disturbances, especially hypokalemia or hypomagnesemia, prior to use and throughout therapy. Dronedarone is a moderate inhibitor of CYP3A4 and CYP2D6 enzymes and has potential to inhibit p-glycoprotein, which may lead to increased serum concentrations/toxicity of a number of medications. Use caution when initiating dronedarone in patients on warfarin. Cases of increased INR with or without bleeding have occurred in patients treated with warfarin; monitor INR closely after initiating dronedarone in these patients. Women of childbearing potential should use effective contraceptive methods during treatment.

Drug Interactions

Metabolism/Transport Effects Inhibits P-glycoprotein

Avoid Concomitant Use

Avoid concomitant use of Dronedarone with any of the following: Artemether; CycloSPORINE; CycloSPORINE (Systemic); CYP3A4 Inducers (Strong); CYP3A4 Inhibitors (Strong); Grapefruit Juice; Lumefantrine; Nilotinib; Pimozide; QTc-Prolonging Agents; QuiNINE; Silodosin; St Johns Wort; Tetrabenazine; Thioridazine; Tolvaptan; Topotecan; Toremifene; Vandetanib; Ziprasidone

Decreased Effect

Dronedarone may decrease the levels/effects of: Codeine; TraMADol

The levels/effects of Dronedarone may be decreased by: CYP3A4 Inducers (Strong); Deferasirox; St Johns Wort

Increased Effect/Toxicity

Dronedarone may increase the levels/effects of: Atorvastatin; Beta-Blockers; Calcium Channel Blockers (Nondihydropyridine); Colchicine; CYP2D6 Substrates; CYP3A4 Substrates; Dabigatran Etexilate; Digoxin; Eplerenone; Everolimus; FentaNYL; Fesoterodine; Lovastatin; Lurasidone; P-Glycoprotein Substrates; Pimecrolimus; Pimozide; QTc-Prolonging Agents; QuiNINE; Red Yeast Rice; Rivaroxaban; Salmeterol; Saxagliptin; Silodosin; Simvastatin; Tamoxifen; Tetrabenazine; Thioridazine; Tolvaptan; Topotecan; Toremifene; Vandetanib; Vilazodone; Vitamin K Antagonists; Ziprasidone

The levels/effects of Dronedarone may be increased by: Alfuzosin; Artemether; Calcium Channel Blockers (Nondihydropyridine); Chloroquine; Ciprofloxacin; Ciprofloxacin (Systemic); CycloSPORINE; CycloSPORINE (Systemic); CYP3A4 Inhibitors (Moderate); CYP3A4 Inhibitors (Strong); Digoxin; Eribulin; Fingolimod; Gadobutrol; Grapefruit Juice; Lumefantrine; Nilotinib; QTc-Prolonging Agents; QuiNINE

Nutritional/Ethanol Interactions

Food: Increases the rate and extent of absorption of dronedarone. Grapefruit juice increases bioavailability of dronedarone threefold; altered effects are possible; use should be avoided during therapy.

Herb/Nutraceutical: St John's wort may decrease dronedarone levels. Avoid ephedra (may worsen arrhythmia). Avoid dong quai.

Adverse Reactions

>10%:

- Cardiovascular: QT_c (Bazett) prolongation (28% [placebo: 19%]; defined as >450 msec in males or >470 msec in females)
- Renal: Serum creatinine increased ≥10% (51%; occurred 5 days after initiation)

1% to 10%:

- Cardiovascular: Bradycardia (3%)
- Dermatologic: Allergic dermatitis (≤5%), dermatitis (≤5%), eczema (≤5%), pruritus (≤5%), rash (≤5%; described as generalized, macular, maculopapular, erythematous)
- Gastrointestinal: Diarrhea (9%), nausea (5%), abdominal pain (4%), dyspepsia (2%), vomiting (2%)
- Neuromuscular & skeletal: Weakness (7%)

Pharmacodynamics/Kinetics

Bioavailability Oral: Without food: 4%; With high-fat meal: 15%

Time to Peak Plasma: 3-6 hours

Protein Binding >98%

Half-Life Elimination 13-19 hours

Metabolism Hepatic via CYP3A4 to active N-debutyl metabolite (1/10 to 1/3 as potent as dronedarone) and other inactive metabolites

Excretion Feces (84% mainly as metabolites); urine (~6% mainly as metabolites)

Available Dosage Forms

Tablet, oral:

Multaq®: 400 mg

Dosing

Adult & Geriatric Atrial fibrillation/atrial flutter: Oral: 400 mg twice daily

Renal Impairment No dosage adjustment necessary.

Hepatic Impairment No dosage adjustment necessary for moderate hepatic impairment. Contraindicated with severe hepatic impairment.

Administration

Oral Administer with morning and evening meal.

Stability

Storage Store at 25°C (77°F); excursions permitted to 15°C to 30°C (59°F to 86°F).

Monitoring and Teaching Issues

Laboratory Monitoring Serum electrolytes (potassium, magnesium); serum liver enzymes and bilirubin (periodically, especially during the first 6 months of therapy)

Patient Education Take with food. Avoid grapefruit juice. You may experience diarrhea, nausea, or weakness. Report weight gain, swelling of extremities, or shortness of breath.

Dietary Considerations Take with a meal. Grapefruit juice is not recommended.

Geriatric Considerations Clinical studies, involving over 2000 patients 75 years of age and older, did not demonstrate any difference in safety and efficacy between younger adults and elderly. No dosage adjustments necessary for age.

Breast-Feeding Considerations It is not known whether dronedarone is secreted in human milk. Because the potential for serious adverse reactions exists, a decision should be made whether to discontinue nursing or discontinue the drug, taking into account the importance of the drug to the mother.

Pregnancy Considerations Teratogenic effects were observed in animal studies. May cause fetal harm when administered to a pregnant woman, use is contraindicated.

◆ **Dronedarone Hydrochloride** *see* Dronedarone *on page 591*

Droperidol (droe PER i dole)

Index Terms Dehydrobenzperidol

Generic Availability (U.S.) Yes

Pharmacologic Category Antiemetic; Antipsychotic Agent, Typical

Medication Safety Issues

Sound-alike/look-alike issues:

Droperidol may be confused with dronabinol

Inapsine® may be confused with asenapine, Nebcin®

Pregnancy Risk Factor C

Lactation Excretion in breast milk unknown/use caution

Use Prevention and/or treatment of nausea and vomiting from surgical and diagnostic procedures

Available Dosage Forms

Injection, solution: 2.5 mg/mL (2 mL)

Injection, solution [preservative free]: 2.5 mg/mL (2 mL)

Dosing

Adult & Geriatric Note: Titrate carefully to desired effect

Prevention of PONV: I.M., I.V.:

Manufacturer labeling: Maximum initial dose: 2.5 mg; additional doses of 1.25 mg may be administered with caution to achieve desired effect

Consensus guideline recommendations: 0.625-1.25 mg I.V. administered after surgery (Gan, 2007)

Canadian labeling:

Prevention and treatment of PONV: I.V.: 0.625-1.25 mg 30 minutes prior to anticipated end of surgery, and then every 6 hours as needed for breakthrough PONV

Pediatric Note: Titrate carefully to desired effect

Prevention of postoperative nausea and vomiting (PONV): I.M., I.V.: Children 2-12 years:

Manufacturer labeling: Maximum dose: 0.1 mg/kg; additional doses may be repeated with caution to achieve desired effect

Consensus guideline recommendations: 0.01-0.015 mg/kg (maximum: 1.25 mg) I.V. administered after surgery (Gan, 2007)

Canadian labeling:

Prevention and treatment of PONV: I.V.: Children >2 years and Adolescents: 0.02-0.05 mg/kg (maximum dose: 1.25 mg) 30 minutes prior to anticipated end of surgery, and then every 6 hours as needed for breakthrough PONV

Renal Impairment

U.S. labeling: Specific dosing recommendations are not provided; use with caution.

Canadian labeling: I.V.: 0.625 mg; additional dosing should be administered with caution.

Hepatic Impairment

U.S. labeling: Specific dosing recommendations are not provided; use with caution.

Canadian labeling: I.V.: 0.625 mg; additional dosing should be administered with caution.

Administration

I.V. According to the manufacturer, I.V. push administration should be slow. For I.V. infusion, dilute in 50-100 mL NS or D_5W.

Monitoring and Teaching Issues

Laboratory Monitoring Serum magnesium and potassium

Physical Assessment Monitor vital signs and cardiac and respiratory status on a frequent basis and especially immediately following administration and for several hours afterward. Monitor for extrapyramidal symptoms for 24-48 hours after therapy. Teach and use safety precautions until the patient is stable.

Patient Education This drug may cause you to feel very sleepy; do not attempt to get up without assistance. May cause dizziness or constipation. Immediately report any respiratory difficulty, confusion, or palpitations.

Drospirenone and Estradiol (droh SPYE re none & es tra DYE ole)

U.S. Brand Names Angeliq®

Index Terms E2 and DRSP; Estradiol and Drospirenone

Generic Availability (U.S.) No

Pharmacologic Category Estrogen and Progestin Combination

Lactation Enters breast milk/not recommended

Use Treatment of moderate-to-severe vasomotor symptoms associated with menopause; treatment of vulvar and vaginal atrophy associated with menopause

Available Dosage Forms

Tablet:

Angeliq®: Drospirenone 0.5 mg and estradiol 1 mg

Dosing

Adult & Geriatric

Moderate-to-severe vasomotor symptoms associated with menopause: Oral: One tablet daily; re-evaluate patients at 3- and 6-month intervals to determine if treatment is still necessary.

Atrophic vaginitis in females with an intact uterus: Oral: One tablet daily; re-evaluate patients at 3- and 6-month intervals to determine if treatment is still necessary.

Note: The lowest dose of estrogen/progestin that will control symptoms should be used; medication should be discontinued as soon as possible.

Renal Impairment Use in contraindicated.

Hepatic Impairment Use in contraindicated.

Monitoring and Teaching Issues

Laboratory Monitoring Glycemic control in patients with diabetes; lipid profiles in patients being treated for hyperlipidemias; thyroid function in patients on thyroid hormone replacement therapy

Physical Assessment See individual agents.

Patient Education See individual agents.

◆ **Drospirenone and Ethinyl Estradiol** *see* Ethinyl Estradiol and Drospirenone *on page 696*

◆ **Drospirenone, Ethinyl Estradiol, and Levomefolate Calcium** *see* Ethinyl Estradiol, Drospirenone, and Levomefolate *on page 706*

Drotrecogin Alfa (dro TRE coe jin AL fa)

U.S. Brand Names Xigris®

Index Terms Activated Protein C, Human, Recombinant; Drotrecogin Alfa, Activated; Protein C (Activated), Human, Recombinant; rhAPC

Generic Availability (U.S.) No

Pharmacologic Category Protein C (Activated)

Medication Safety Issues

Dosing issues:

Use caution when interpreting dosing information. Maintenance dose expressed as mcg/kg/**hour**.

Pregnancy Risk Factor C

Lactation Excretion in breast milk unknown/not recommended

Use Reduction of mortality from severe sepsis (associated with organ dysfunction) in adults at high risk of death (eg, APACHE II score ≥25)

Unlabeled/Investigational Use Purpura fulminans

Mechanism of Action/Effect Decreases mortality from severe sepsis by blocking thrombotic activity. Blocks factor Va and VIIIa. In addition, may have other anti-inflammatory effects.

Contraindications Hypersensitivity to drotrecogin alfa or any component of the formulation; active internal bleeding; recent hemorrhagic stroke (within 3 months); severe head trauma (within 2 months); recent intracranial or intraspinal surgery (within 2 months); intracranial neoplasm or mass lesion; evidence of cerebral herniation; presence of an epidural catheter; trauma with an increased risk of life-threatening bleeding

Warnings/Precautions Increases risk of bleeding; careful evaluation of risks and benefit is required prior to initiation. Bleeding risk is increased in patients receiving concurrent therapeutic heparin, oral anticoagulants, glycoprotein IIb/IIIa antagonists, platelet aggregation inhibitors, or aspirin at a dosage of >650 mg/day (within 7 days). In addition, an increased bleeding risk is associated with prolonged INR (>3), gastrointestinal bleeding (within 6 weeks), decreased platelet count (<30,000/mm^3), thrombolytic therapy (within 3 days), recent ischemic stroke (within 3 months), intracranial AV malformation or aneurysm, known bleeding diathesis, severe hepatic disease (chronic), or other condition where bleeding is a significant hazard or difficult to manage due to its location. Discontinue if significant bleeding occurs (may consider continued use after stabilization). Treatment interruption required for invasive procedures. During treatment, aPTT cannot be used to assess coagulopathy (PT/INR not affected).

Efficacy not established in adult patients at a low risk of death. Patients with pre-existing nonsepsis-related medical conditions with a poor prognosis (anticipated survival <28 days), patients with acute pancreatitis (no established source of infection), HIV-infected patients with a CD4 count ≤50 cells/mm^3, chronic dialysis patients, pre-existing hypercoagulable conditions, and patients who had received bone marrow, liver, lung, pancreas, or small bowel transplants were excluded from the clinical trial which established benefit. In addition, patients weighing

>135 kg were not evaluated. Safety and efficacy have not been established in pediatric patients.

Drug Interactions

Avoid Concomitant Use There are no known interactions where it is recommended to avoid concomitant use.

Decreased Effect There are no known significant interactions involving a decrease in effect.

Increased Effect/Toxicity

Drotrecogin Alfa may increase the levels/effects of: Anticoagulants; Collagenase (Systemic); Fondaparinux; Ibritumomab; Tositumomab and Iodine I 131 Tositumomab

The levels/effects of Drotrecogin Alfa may be increased by: Antiplatelet Agents; Antithrombin; Danaparoid; Dasatinib; Heparin; Heparin (Low Molecular Weight); Herbs (Anticoagulant/Antiplatelet Properties); Nonsteroidal Anti-Inflammatory Agents; Pentosan Polysulfate Sodium; Prostacyclin Analogues; Salicylates; Thrombolytic Agents; Vitamin K Antagonists

Nutritional/Ethanol Interactions Herb/Nutraceutical: Recent use/intake of herbs with anti-coagulant or antiplatelet activity (including cat's claw, feverfew, garlic, ginkgo, ginseng, and horse chestnut seed) may increase the risk of bleeding.

Lab Interactions May interfere with one-stage coagulation assays based on the aPTT (such as factor VIII, IX, and XI assays).

Adverse Reactions As with all drugs which may affect hemostasis, bleeding is the major adverse effect associated with drotrecogin alfa. Hemorrhage may occur at virtually any site. Risk is dependent on multiple variables, including the dosage administered, concurrent use of multiple agents which alter hemostasis, and patient predisposition.

>10%:

Dermatologic: Bruising

Gastrointestinal: Gastrointestinal bleeding

1% to 10%: Hematologic: Bleeding (serious 2.4% during infusion vs 3.5% during 28-day study period; individual events listed as <1%)

Pharmacodynamics/Kinetics

Duration of Action Plasma nondetectable within 2 hours of discontinuation

Half-Life Elimination 1.6 hours

Metabolism Inactivated by endogenous plasma protease inhibitors; mean clearance: 40 L/hour; increased with severe sepsis (~50%)

Available Dosage Forms

Injection, powder for reconstitution [preservative free]:

Xigris®: 5 mg, 20 mg

Dosing

Adult & Geriatric

Purpura fulminans (unlabeled use): 24 mcg/kg/**hour**

Severe sepsis: I.V.: 24 mcg/kg/**hour** for a total of 96 hours; stop infusion **immediately** if clinically-important bleeding is identified. **Note:** Use actual body weight for dosing.

For patient eligibility, may utilize the APACHE II scoring system (http://www.sfar.org/scores2/apache22.html).

Pediatric Purpura fulminans (unlabeled use): Refer to adult dosing.

Renal Impairment No specific adjustment recommended.

Administration

I.V. Administer via infusion pump. Administration must be completed within 12 hours of solution preparation. Suspend administration for 2 hours prior to invasive procedures or other procedure with significant bleeding risk; may continue treatment immediately following uncomplicated, minimally-invasive procedures, but delay for 12 hours after major invasive procedures/surgery.

Stability

Reconstitution Reconstitute 5 mg vials with 2.5 mL and 20 mg vials with 10 mL sterile water for injection (resultant solution ~2 mg/mL). Must be further diluted (within 3 hours of reconstitution) in 0.9% sodium chloride, typically to a concentration between 100 mcg/mL and 200 mcg/mL when using infusion pump and between 100 mcg/mL and 1000 mcg/mL when infused via syringe pump. Although product information states administration must be completed within 12 hours of preparation, additional studies (data on file, Lilly Research Laboratories) show that the final solution is stable for 14 hours at 15°C to 30°C (59°F to 86°F). If not used immediately, a prepared solution may be stored in the refrigerator for up to 12 hours. The total expiration time (refrigeration and administration) should be ≤24 hours from time of preparation.

Storage Store vials under refrigeration at 2°C to 8°C (36°F to 46°F); do not freeze. Protect from light.

Monitoring and Teaching Issues

Laboratory Monitoring Hemoglobin/hematocrit, PT/INR, platelet count

Physical Assessment Patient must be monitored very closely for bleeding during and following infusion. If significant bleeding occurs, infusion should be stopped and prescriber notified immediately. Bleeding precautions must be observed.

Patient Education This medication can only be administered by infusion. You will be monitored closely.

Additional Information Prepared by recombinant DNA technology in human cell line

Related Information

Compatibility of Drugs *on page 1994*

◆ **Drotrecogin Alfa, Activated** *see* Drotrecogin Alfa *on page 594*

- ◆ **Droxia®** *see* Hydroxyurea *on page* *931*
- ◆ **DSCG** *see* Cromolyn (Systemic, Oral Inhalation) *on page* *429*
- ◆ **DTaP** *see* Diphtheria and Tetanus Toxoids, and Acellular Pertussis Vaccine *on page* *552*
- ◆ **DTaP-HepB-IPV** *see* Diphtheria, Tetanus Toxoids, Acellular Pertussis, Hepatitis B (Recombinant), and Poliovirus Vaccine *on page* *555*
- ◆ **DTaP-HepB-IPV-Hib** *see* Diphtheria and Tetanus Toxoids, Acellular Pertussis, Hepatitis B (Recombinant), Poliovirus (Inactivated), and *Haemophilus influenzae* B Conjugate (Adsorbed) Vaccine *on page* *550*
- ◆ **DTaP/Hib** *see* Diphtheria and Tetanus Toxoids, Acellular Pertussis and *Haemophilus influenzae* b Conjugate Vaccine *on page* *548*
- ◆ **DTaP-IPV** *see* Diphtheria and Tetanus Toxoids, Acellular Pertussis, and Poliovirus Vaccine *on page* *548*
- ◆ **DTaP-IPV/Hib** *see* Diphtheria and Tetanus Toxoids, Acellular Pertussis, Poliovirus and *Haemophilus* b Conjugate Vaccine *on page* *550*
- ◆ **DTIC** *see* Dacarbazine *on page* *452*
- ◆ **DTIC-Dome** *see* Dacarbazine *on page* *452*
- ◆ **DTO (error-prone abbreviation)** *see* Opium Tincture *on page* *1363*
- ◆ **D-Trp(6)-LHRH** *see* Triptorelin *on page* *1824*
- ◆ **Duac® CS [DSC]** *see* Clindamycin and Benzoyl Peroxide *on page* *401*
- ◆ **Duetact™** *see* Pioglitazone and Glimepiride *on page* *1462*

DULoxetine (doo LOX e teen)

U.S. Brand Names Cymbalta®

Index Terms (+)-(*S*)-*N*-Methyl-γ-(1-naphthyloxy)-2-thiophenepropylamine Hydrochloride; Duloxetine Hydrochloride; LY248686

Generic Availability (U.S.) No

Pharmacologic Category Antidepressant, Serotonin/Norepinephrine Reuptake Inhibitor

Medication Safety Issues

Sound-alike/look-alike issues:

Cymbalta® may be confused with Symbyax®

DULoxetine may be confused with FLUoxetine

Medication Guide Available Yes

Pregnancy Risk Factor C

Lactation Enters breast milk/not recommended

Use Acute and maintenance treatment of major depressive disorder (MDD); treatment of generalized anxiety disorder (GAD); management of pain associated with diabetic neuropathy; management of fibromyalgia; chronic musculoskeletal pain

Unlabeled/Investigational Use Treatment of stress incontinence

Mechanism of Action/Effect Inhibits reuptake of both norepinephrine and serotonin (SNRI); improves symptoms of depression and chronic pain

Contraindications Concomitant use or within 2 weeks of MAO inhibitors; uncontrolled narrow-angle glaucoma

Canadian labeling: Additional contraindications (not in U.S. labeling): Hypersensitivity to duloxetine or any component of the formulation; hepatic impairment; severe renal impairment (eg, Cl_{cr} <30 mL/minute) or end-stage renal disease (ESRD); concomitant use with thioridazine or with CYP1A2 inhibitors

Warnings/Precautions [U.S. Boxed Warning]: Antidepressants increase the risk of suicidal thinking and behavior in children, adolescents, and young adults (18-24 years of age) with major depressive disorder (MDD) and other psychiatric disorders; consider risk prior to prescribing. Short-term studies did not show an increased risk in patients >24 years of age and showed a decreased risk in patients ≥65 years. Closely monitor for clinical worsening, suicidality, or unusual changes in behavior; the patient's family or caregiver should be instructed to closely observe the patient and communicate condition with healthcare provider. A medication guide concerning the use of antidepressants in children and teenagers should be dispensed with each prescription. **Duloxetine is not FDA approved for use in children.**

The possibility of a suicide attempt is inherent in major depression and may persist until remission occurs. Patients treated with antidepressants should be observed for clinical worsening and suicidality, especially during the initial (generally first 1-2 months) few months of a course of drug therapy, or at times of dose changes, either increases or decreases. Use caution in high-risk patients. Worsening depression and severe abrupt suicidality that are not part of the presenting symptoms may require discontinuation or modification of drug therapy. The patient's family or caregiver should be alerted to monitor patients for the emergence of suicidality and associated behaviors (such as agitation, irritability, hostility, impulsivity, and hypomania) and call healthcare provider.

May worsen psychosis in some patients or precipitate a shift to mania or hypomania in patients with bipolar disorder. Patients presenting with depressive symptoms should be screened for bipolar disorder. Monotherapy in patients with bipolar disorder should be avoided. **Duloxetine is not FDA approved for the treatment of bipolar depression.**

May cause orthostatic hypotension/syncope at therapeutic doses especially within the first week of therapy and after dose increases. Monitor blood pressure with initiation of therapy, dose increases (especially in patients receiving >60 mg/day), or with concomitant use of vasodilators or CYP1A2 inhibitors. Use caution in patients with hypertension. May increase blood pressure. Rare cases of hypertensive crisis have been reported in patients with pre-existing hypertension; evaluate blood pressure prior to initiating therapy and periodically thereafter; consider dose reduction or gradual discontinuation of therapy in individuals with sustained hypertension during therapy.

Modest increases in serum glucose and hemoglobin A_{1c} (Hb A_{1c}) levels have been observed in some diabetic patients receiving duloxetine therapy for diabetic peripheral neuropathy (DPN). Duloxetine may cause increased urinary resistance; advise patient to report symptoms of urinary hesitation/difficulty. Has a low potential to impair cognitive or motor performance. Use caution with a previous seizure disorder or condition predisposing to seizures such as brain damage or alcoholism. Avoid use in patients with substantial ethanol intake, evidence of chronic liver disease, or hepatic impairment (contraindicated in Canadian labeling). Rare cases of hepatic failure (including fatalities) have been reported with use. Hepatitis with abdominal pain, hepatomegaly, elevated transaminase levels >20 times the upper limit of normal (ULN) with and without jaundice have all been observed. Discontinue therapy with the presentation of jaundice or other signs of hepatic dysfunction and do not reinitiate therapy unless another source or cause is identified.

May cause hyponatremia/SIADH (elderly at increased risk); volume depletion (diuretics may increase risk). Use with caution in patients with controlled narrow angle glaucoma. May cause or exacerbate sexual dysfunction. Use caution with renal impairment (contraindicated in Canadian labeling for severe renal impairment or ESRD). Use caution with concomitant CNS depressants. May impair platelet aggregation; use caution with concomitant use of NSAIDs, ASA, or other drugs that affect coagulation; the risk of bleeding may be potentiated.

Serotonin syndrome and neuroleptic malignant syndrome (NMS)-like reactions have occurred with serotonin/norepinephrine reuptake inhibitors (SNRIs) and selective serotonin reuptake inhibitors (SSRIs) when used alone, and particularly when used in combination with serotonergic agents (eg, triptans) or antidopaminergic agents (eg, antipsychotics). Concurrent use with MAO inhibitors is contraindicated. Use caution during concurrent therapy with triptans and drugs which lower the seizure threshold; concurrent use of serotonin precursors (eg, tryptophan) is not recommended. To discontinue therapy with duloxetine, gradually taper dose. If intolerable symptoms occur following a decrease in dosage or upon discontinuation of therapy, then resuming the previous dose with a more gradual taper should be considered. May increase the risks associated with electroconvulsive therapy. Consider discontinuing, when possible, prior to elective surgery. Formulation contains sucrose; patients with fructose intolerance, glucose-galactose malabsorption, or sucrose-isomaltase deficiency should avoid use.

Drug Interactions

Metabolism/Transport Effects **Substrate** (major) of CYP1A2, 2D6; **inhibits** CYP2D6 (moderate)

Avoid Concomitant Use

Avoid concomitant use of DULoxetine with any of the following: Iobenguane I 123; MAO Inhibitors; Methylene Blue; Sibutramine; Thioridazine

Decreased Effect

DULoxetine may decrease the levels/effects of: Alpha2-Agonists; Codeine; Iobenguane I 123

The levels/effects of DULoxetine may be decreased by: CYP1A2 Inducers (Strong); Peginterferon Alfa-2b

Increased Effect/Toxicity

DULoxetine may increase the levels/effects of: Alcohol (Ethyl); Alpha-/Beta-Agonists; Aspirin; CNS Depressants; CYP2D6 Substrates; Fesoterodine; Methotrimeprazine; Methylene Blue; Nebivolol; NSAID (Nonselective); Serotonin Modulators; Tamoxifen; Thioridazine; Tricyclic Antidepressants

The levels/effects of DULoxetine may be increased by: CYP1A2 Inhibitors (Moderate); CYP1A2 Inhibitors (Strong); CYP2D6 Inhibitors (Moderate); CYP2D6 Inhibitors (Strong); Darunavir; Droperidol; FluvoxaMINE; MAO Inhibitors; Methotrimeprazine; PARoxetine; Sibutramine

Nutritional/Ethanol Interactions

Ethanol: Avoid ethanol (may increase CNS depression and/or hepatotoxic potential of duloxetine).

Herb/Nutraceutical: Avoid valerian, St John's wort, SAMe, kava kava, and gotu kola (may increase CNS depression).

Adverse Reactions

>10%:

Central nervous system: Headache (13% to 14%), somnolence (10% to 12%; dose related), fatigue (10 to 11%), dizziness (10%), insomnia (10%; dose related)

Gastrointestinal: Nausea (23% to 25%), xerostomia (11% to 15%; dose related), constipation (10%; dose related), diarrhea (9% to 10%), appetite decreased (7% to 9%; dose related)

1% to 10%:

Cardiovascular: Palpitation (1% to 2%)

Central nervous system: Agitation (3% to 5%), anxiety (3%), dreams abnormal (1% to 2%), yawning (1% to 2%), hypoesthesia (≥1%), lethargy (≥1%), vertigo (≥1%), chills (1%), sleep disorder (1%)

Dermatologic: Hyperhydrosis (6% to 7%)

Endocrine & metabolic: Libido decreased (2% to 4%), hot flushes (1% to 3%), orgasm abnormality (1% to 3%)
Gastrointestinal: Abdominal pain (4% to 6%), vomiting (3% to 5%), dyspepsia (2%), weight loss (2%), flatulence (≥1%), taste abnormal (≥1%), weight gain (≥1%)
Genitourinary: Erectile dysfunction (4% to 5%), ejaculation delayed (3%; dose related), ejaculatory dysfunction (2%)
Hepatic: ALT >3x ULN (1%)
Neuromuscular & skeletal: Muscle spasms (3%), tremor (2% to 3%; dose related), musculoskeletal pain (≥1%), paresthesia (≥1%), rigors (≥1%)
Ocular: Blurred vision (1% to 3%)
Respiratory: Nasopharyngitis (5%), cough (3%)
Miscellaneous: Influenza (3%)

Pharmacodynamics/Kinetics

Absorption Well absorbed, 2-hour delay in absorption after ingestion; food decreases extent of absorption ~10% (no effect on C_{max})

Time to Peak 6 hours; 10 hours when ingested with food

Protein Binding >90%; primarily to albumin and α_1-acid glycoprotein

Half-Life Elimination 12 hours (range 8-17 hours)

Metabolism Hepatic, via CYP1A2 and CYP2D6; forms multiple metabolites (inactive)

Excretion Urine (~70%; <1% of total dose as unchanged drug); feces (~20%)

Available Dosage Forms

Capsule, delayed release, enteric coated pellets, oral:
Cymbalta®: 20 mg, 30 mg, 60 mg

Dosing

Adult

Major depressive disorder: Oral: Initial: 40-60 mg/day; dose may be divided (ie, 20 or 30 mg twice daily) or given as a single daily dose of 60 mg; maintenance: 60 mg once daily; for doses >60 mg/day, titrate dose in increments of 30 mg/day over 1 week as tolerated to a maximum dose: 120 mg/day. **Note:** Doses >60 mg/day have not been demonstrated to be more effective.

Diabetic neuropathy: Oral: 60 mg once daily; lower initial doses may be considered in patients where tolerability is a concern and/or renal impairment is present. **Note:** Doses up to 120 mg/day administered in clinical trials offered no additional benefit and were less well tolerated than dose of 60 mg/day.

Fibromyalgia: Oral: 30 mg once daily for 1 week, then increase to 60 mg once daily as tolerated. **Note:** Doses up to 120 mg/day administered in clinical trials offered no additional benefit and were less well tolerated than dose of 60 mg/day.

Generalized anxiety disorder: Oral: Initial: 30-60 mg/day as a single daily dose; patients initiated at 30 mg/day should be titrated to 60 mg/day after 1 week; maximum dose: 120 mg/day. **Note:** Doses >60 mg/day have not been demonstrated to be more effective than 60 mg/day.

Chronic musculoskeletal pain: Oral: 30 mg once daily for 1 week, then increase to 60 mg once daily as tolerated

Stress incontinence (unlabeled use): Oral: 40 mg twice daily

Geriatric

Major depressive disorder: Oral: Manufacturer does not recommend specific dosage adjustment. Conservatively, may initiate at a dose of 20 mg 1-2 times/day; increase to 40-60 mg/day as a single daily dose or in divided doses **or** initiate therapy at 30 mg/day for 1 week then increase to 60 mg/day as tolerated.

Other indications: Refer to adult dosing.

Renal Impairment Not recommended for use in Cl_{cr} <30 mL/minute or ESRD (contraindicated in Canadian labeling). In mild-moderate impairment, lower initial doses may be considered with titration guided by response and tolerability.

Hepatic Impairment Not recommended for use in hepatic impairment (contraindicated in Canadian labeling).

Administration

Oral Capsule should be swallowed whole; do not crush. Although the manufacturer does not recommend opening the capsule to facilitate administration; the contents of capsule may be sprinkled on applesauce or in apple juice and swallowed (without chewing) immediately. Do not sprinkle contents on chocolate pudding (Wells, 2008). Administer without regard to meals.

Stability

Storage Store at 25°C (77°F); excursions permitted to 15°C to 30°C (59°F to 86°F)

Monitoring and Teaching Issues

Laboratory Monitoring Glucose levels and Hb A_{1c} levels in diabetic patients, creatinine, BUN, transaminases

Physical Assessment Monitor blood pressure (can cause elevation or orthostatic hypotension) at the beginning of treatment and periodically throughout. Monitor for worsening of depression and suicide ideation. Taper dosage slowly when discontinuing. Do not discontinue abruptly.

Patient Education Swallow capsule whole; do not open or crush. It may take 2-3 weeks to achieve desired results. Maintain adequate hydration, unless instructed to restrict fluid intake. Avoid alcohol use. If you have diabetes, monitor blood glucose levels closely. May cause increase in glycemic levels. Can cause drowsiness, dizziness, fatigue, or insomnia. You may experience headache, nausea, diarrhea, constipation, appetite decrease, or xerostomia. Report persistent insomnia, dizziness, headache, suicide ideation, worsening of anxiety, panic attacks, agitation, irritability, akathisia, hostility, hypomania, and mania.

Dietary Considerations May be taken without regard to meals.

Geriatric Considerations In an 8-week study of elderly patients with a history of recurrent major depressive disorder, improvements in verbal learning and memory, and depression response and remission rates were significantly greater in subjects randomized to duloxetine 60 mg per day compared to placebo. Duloxetine was well tolerated. No dose adjustment is necessary for age alone; adjust dose for renal function in the elderly. Higher doses are generally required for treatment of general anxiety disorder, neuropathic pain and stress urinary incontinence (unlabeled use). The elderly are more prone to SSRI/SNRI-induced hyponatremia.

Breast-Feeding Considerations Duloxetine is excreted in human milk. The average relative dose to the infant was calculated to be ~0.14% (maximum: 0.25%) of the weight-adjusted maternal dose. Duloxetine is not stable at an acidic pH; therefore, any drug which reaches the stomach of the breast-feeding infant may degrade, thus decreasing the amount reaching the systemic circulation. Breast-feeding is not recommended by the manufacturer. The long term effects on neurobehavior have not been studied, thus one should prescribe duloxetine to a mother who is breast-feeding only when the benefits outweigh the potential risks.

Pregnancy Considerations Duloxetine is classified as pregnancy category C due to adverse effects observed in animal studies. Nonteratogenic effects in the newborn following SSRI/SNRI exposure late in the third trimester include respiratory distress, cyanosis, apnea, seizures, temperature instability, feeding difficulty, vomiting, hypoglycemia, hyper- or hypotonia, hyper-reflexia, jitteriness, irritability, constant crying, and tremor. The long-term effects on neurobehavior have not been studied.

Women treated for major depression and who are euthymic prior to pregnancy are more likely to experience a relapse when medication is discontinued as compared to pregnant women who continue taking antidepressant medications. The ACOG recommends that therapy with SSRIs or SNRIs during pregnancy be individualized; treatment of depression during pregnancy should incorporate the clinical expertise of the mental health clinician, obstetrician, primary healthcare provider, and pediatrician. If treatment during pregnancy is required, consider tapering therapy during the third trimester in order to prevent withdrawal symptoms in the infant. If this is done and the woman is considered to be at risk of relapse from her major depressive disorder, the medication can be restarted following delivery, although the dose should be readjusted to that required before pregnancy. Treatment algorithms have been developed by the ACOG and the APA for the management of depression in women prior to conception and during pregnancy (Yonkers, 2009).

Related Information

Antidepressant Agents *on page 1982*

◆ **Duloxetine Hydrochloride** *see* DULoxetine *on page 596*

◆ **DuoNeb®** *see* Ipratropium and Albuterol *on page 1011*

◆ **DuP 753** *see* Losartan *on page 1133*

◆ **Duraclon®** *see* CloNIDine *on page 408*

◆ **Duragesic®** *see* FentaNYL *on page 744*

◆ **Duramorph** *see* Morphine (Systemic) *on page 1258*

◆ **Durezol®** *see* Difluprednate *on page 529*

◆ **Duricef** *see* Cefadroxil *on page 311*

Dutasteride (doo TAS teer ide)

U.S. Brand Names Avodart®

Generic Availability (U.S.) No

Pharmacologic Category 5 Alpha-Reductase Inhibitor

Pregnancy Risk Factor X

Lactation Excretion in breast milk unknown/contraindicated in women of childbearing potential

Use Treatment of symptomatic benign prostatic hyperplasia (BPH) as monotherapy or combination therapy with tamsulosin

Unlabeled/Investigational Use Treatment of male patterned baldness; prostate cancer prevention (to reduce the incidence)

Mechanism of Action/Effect Inhibits the conversion of testosterone to dihydrotestosterone (DHT) via 5α-reductase DHT stimulates prostatic cell hyperplasia.

Contraindications Hypersensitivity to dutasteride, other 5α-reductase inhibitors (eg, finasteride), or any component of the formulation; children; women of childbearing potential; pregnancy

Warnings/Precautions Hazardous agent - use appropriate precautions for handling and disposal. Pregnant women or women trying to conceive should not handle the product; active ingredient can be absorbed through the skin and may negatively impact fetal development. Urological diseases, including prostate cancer, and/or obstructive uropathy should be ruled out before initiating. Urological diseases including cancer and/or obstructive uropathy should be ruled out before initiating. Avoid donating blood during or for 6 months following treatment due to risk of administration to a pregnant female transfusion recipient. Use caution in hepatic impairment and with concurrent use of potent, chronic CYP3A4 inhibitors. Reduces prostate specific antigen (PSA); re-establish a new baseline after 3-6 months of use. When compared to placebo, 5-alpha-reductase inhibitors (5-ARI) have been shown to reduce the incidence of prostate cancer, although an increase in the incidence of high-grade prostate cancers has been observed with another 5-ARI, finasteride (Kramer, 2009; Thompson, 2003).

Drug Interactions

Metabolism/Transport Effects Substrate of CYP3A4 (minor)

Avoid Concomitant Use There are no known interactions where it is recommended to avoid concomitant use.

Decreased Effect There are no known significant interactions involving a decrease in effect.

Increased Effect/Toxicity

The levels/effects of Dutasteride may be increased by: CYP3A4 Inhibitors (Strong)

Nutritional/Ethanol Interactions

Ethanol: No effect or interaction noted.

Food: Maximum serum concentrations reduced by 10% to 15% when taken with food; not clinically significant.

Herb/Nutraceutical: St John's wort may decrease dutasteride levels. Avoid saw palmetto (concurrent use has not been adequately studied).

Lab Interactions PSA levels decrease in treated patients. After 6 months of therapy, PSA levels stabilize to a new baseline that is ~50% of pretreatment values. If following serial PSAs in a patient, re-establish a new baseline after 3-6 months of use. If interpreting an isolated PSA value in a patient treated for 6 months, then double the PSA value for comparison.

Adverse Reactions

>10%: Endocrine & metabolic: Serum testosterone increased, thyroid-stimulating hormone increased

1% to 10%: Endocrine & metabolic: Impotence (1% to 5%), libido decreased (≤3%), ejaculation disorders (≤1%), gynecomastia (including breast tenderness, breast enlargement) (≤1%)

Note: Frequency of adverse events (except gynecomastia) tends to decrease with continued use (>6 months).

Pharmacodynamics/Kinetics

Absorption Absorbed via skin when handling capsules

Bioavailability ~60% (range: 40% to 94%)

Time to Peak 2-3 hours

Protein Binding 99% to albumin; ~97% to α_1-acid glycoprotein; >96% to semen protein

Half-Life Elimination Terminal: ~5 weeks

Metabolism Hepatic via CYP3A4 isoenzyme; forms metabolites: 6-hydroxydutasteride has activity similar to parent compound, 4'-hydroxydutasteride and 1,2-dihydrodutasteride are much less potent than parent *in vitro*

Excretion Feces (40% as metabolites, ~5% as unchanged drug); urine (<1% as unchanged drug); ~55% of dose unaccounted for

Available Dosage Forms

Capsule, softgel, oral:

Avodart®: 0.5 mg

Dosing

Adult & Geriatric Males:

Benign prostatic hyperplasia (BPH): Oral: 0.5 mg once daily alone or in combination with tamsulosin

Prostate cancer prevention (unlabeled use): Oral: 0.5 mg once daily; planned duration of treatment was 4 years (Andriole, 2004; Kramer, 2009)

Renal Impairment No adjustment is required.

Hepatic Impairment Use caution; no specific adjustments recommended.

Administration

Oral May be administered without regard to meals. Capsule should be swallowed whole; do not chew or open; contact with opened capsule can cause oropharyngeal irritation. Should not be touched or handled by women who are pregnant or are of childbearing age.

Stability

Storage Store at controlled room temperature of 25°C (77°F); excursions permitted to 15°C to 30°C (59°F to 86°F).

Monitoring and Teaching Issues

Laboratory Monitoring New baseline PSA level after 3-6 months of therapy

Dietary Considerations May be taken without regard to meals.

Pregnancy Considerations Preclinical data (animal studies) suggests that the suppression of circulating levels of dihydrotestosterone may inhibit the development of the external genital organs and lead to feminization of a male fetus carried by a woman exposed to dutasteride. Pregnant woman and those who may become pregnant should not handle the capsules because dutasteride is absorbed through the skin. It is distributed into the semen.

Dutasteride and Tamsulosin (doo TAS teer ide & tam SOO loe sin)

U.S. Brand Names Jalyn™

Index Terms Tamsulosin and Dutasteride; Tamsulosin Hydrochloride and Dutasteride

Generic Availability (U.S.) No

Pharmacologic Category 5 Alpha-Reductase Inhibitor; $Alpha_1$ Blocker

Pregnancy Risk Factor X

Lactation Excretion in breast milk unknown/not indicated for use in women

Use Treatment of symptomatic benign prostatic hyperplasia (BPH)

Available Dosage Forms

Capsule, oral:

Jalyn™: Dutasteride 0.5 mg and tamsulosin hydrochloride 0.4 mg

Dosing

Adult & Geriatric Males:

Benign prostatic hyperplasia (BPH): Oral: One capsule (0.5 mg dutasteride/0.4 mg tamsulosin) once daily ~30 minutes after the same meal each day

Renal Impairment

Cl_{cr} 10-30 mL/minute/1.73 m^2: No adjustment needed

Cl_{cr} <10 mL/minute/1.73 m^2: Not studied

Hepatic Impairment Use caution; no specific adjustments recommended

Administration

Oral Administer 30 minutes after the same meal each day. Capsules should be swallowed whole; do not crush, chew, or open. Oropharyngeal contact with capsule contents may result in irritation of the mucosa.

Monitoring and Teaching Issues

Laboratory Monitoring New baseline PSA level after 3-6 months of therapy

Physical Assessment See individual agents.

Patient Education See individual agents.

- **DW286** *see* Gemifloxacin *on page* 861
- **Dyazide®** *see* Hydrochlorothiazide and Triamterene *on page* 914
- **Dynacin®** *see* Minocycline *on page* 1236
- **DynaCirc CR®** *see* Isradipine *on page* 1033
- **E2 and DRSP** *see* Drospirenone and Estradiol *on page* 594
- **E2020** *see* Donepezil *on page* 569
- **E 2080** *see* Rufinamide *on page* 1617
- **E7389** *see* Eribulin *on page* 652
- **Easprin®** *see* Aspirin *on page* 155
- **EC-Naprosyn®** *see* Naproxen *on page* 1289
- ***E. coli* Asparaginase** *see* Asparaginase *on page* 152
- **Ecotrin® [OTC]** *see* Aspirin *on page* 155
- **Ecotrin® Arthritis Strength [OTC]** *see* Aspirin *on page* 155
- **Ecotrin® Low Strength [OTC]** *see* Aspirin *on page* 155

Eculizumab (e kue LIZ oo mab)

U.S. Brand Names Soliris®

Generic Availability (U.S.) No

Pharmacologic Category Monoclonal Antibody; Monoclonal Antibody, Complement Inhibitor

Medication Safety Issues

Sound-alike/look-alike issues:

Eculizumab may be confused with efalizumab

Medication Guide Available Yes

Prescribing and Access Restrictions Patients and providers must enroll with Soliris® OneSource™ (1-888-765-4747) program prior to treatment initiation.

Pregnancy Risk Factor C

Lactation Excretion in breast milk unknown/use caution

Use Treatment of paroxysmal nocturnal hemoglobinuria (PNH) to reduce hemolysis

Mechanism of Action/Effect Complement-mediated intravascular hemolysis is a key clinical feature of paroxysmal nocturnal hemoglobinuria. Eculizumab is a humanized monoclonal IgG antibody that blocks the formation of a key component of the complement cascade (C5b). Without this factor, the subsequent formation of the membrane attack complex (MAC) by the final group of complement proteins (C5b-9) cannot occur. This results in stabilization of hemoglobin levels and a reduction in the need for RBC transfusions.

Contraindications Unresolved serious *Neisseria meningitidis* infection; patients not currently vaccinated against *Neisseria meningitidis*

Warnings/Precautions **[U.S. Boxed Warning]: The risk for meningococcal *(Neisseria meningitides)* infections (septicemia and/or meningitis) is increased with PNH and may be further increased in patients receiving eculizumab; vaccinate with meningococcal vaccine at least 2 weeks prior to initiation of treatment;** revaccinate according to current guidelines. Quadrivalent, conjugated meningococcal vaccines are recommended. Meningococcal infections developed in some patients despite vaccination. **[U.S. Boxed Warning]: Monitor for early signs of meningococcal infections; evaluate and treat promptly.** Consider withholding eculizumab during the treatment of serious meningococcal infections. In addition to meningitis, the risk of other infections, especially encapsulated bacteria (eg, *Streptococcus pneumoniae, H. influenzae*) is increased with eculizumab treatment. Use caution in patients with concurrent systemic infection. Patients should be up to date with all immunizations before initiating therapy.

Infusion reactions, including anaphylaxis or hypersensitivity, may occur; interrupt infusion for severe reaction. Continue monitoring for 1 hour after completion of infusion. Patients with PNH who discontinue treatment may be at increased risk for serious hemolysis; monitor closely for at least 8 weeks after treatment discontinuation. Consider RBC transfusion, exchange transfusion, anticoagulation, corticoids or reinitiation of eculizumab for serious hemolysis after discontinuation. In clinical trials, anticoagulant therapy was continued in patients who were receiving these

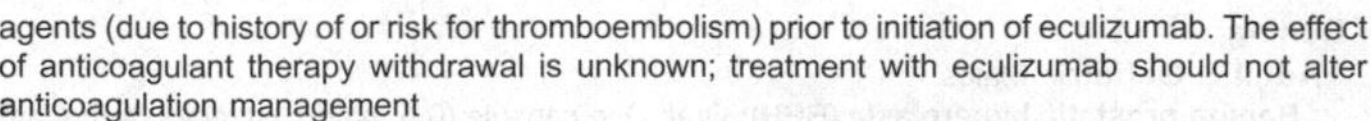

agents (due to history of or risk for thromboembolism) prior to initiation of eculizumab. The effect of anticoagulant therapy withdrawal is unknown; treatment with eculizumab should not alter anticoagulation management

Drug Interactions

Avoid Concomitant Use

Avoid concomitant use of Eculizumab with any of the following: BCG; Natalizumab; Pimecrolimus; Roflumilast; Tacrolimus (Topical); Vaccines (Live)

Decreased Effect

Eculizumab may decrease the levels/effects of: BCG; Sipuleucel-T; Vaccines (Inactivated); Vaccines (Live)

The levels/effects of Eculizumab may be decreased by: Echinacea

Increased Effect/Toxicity

Eculizumab may increase the levels/effects of: Leflunomide; Natalizumab; Vaccines (Live)

The levels/effects of Eculizumab may be increased by: Denosumab; Pimecrolimus; Roflumilast; Tacrolimus (Topical); Trastuzumab

Adverse Reactions

>10%:

Central nervous system: Headache (44%; serious: 2%; usually occurs within 48 hours of each of the first 2 induction doses), fatigue (12%)
Gastrointestinal: Nausea (16%). abdominal pain, diarrhea, vomiting
Genitourinary: Urinary tract infection
Neuromuscular & skeletal: Back pain (19%), arthralgia
Respiratory: Nasopharyngitis (23%), cough (12%)

1% to 10%:

Central nervous system: Fever (serious: 2%)
Gastrointestinal: Constipation (7%)
Hematologic: Anemia (serious: 2%)
Neuromuscular & skeletal: Limb pain (7%), myalgia (7%)
Respiratory: Respiratory tract infection (7%), sinusitis (7%)
Miscellaneous: Herpes infections (7%), flu-like syndrome (5%), viral infection (serious: 2%), meningococcal infection (1%)

Pharmacodynamics/Kinetics

Onset of Action PNH: Reduced hemolysis: ≤1 week

Half-Life Elimination ~11 days (range: ~8-15 days)

Available Dosage Forms

Injection, solution [preservative free]:
Soliris®: 10 mg/mL (30 mL)

Dosing

Adult & Geriatric Note: Patients must receive meningococcal vaccine at least 2 weeks prior to treatment initiation; revaccinate according to current guidelines. Treatment should be administered at the recommended time interval although administration may be varied by ±2 days.

PNH: I.V.: 600 mg every 7 days for the first 4 weeks, followed by 900 mg 7 days later; then maintenance: 900 mg every 14 days thereafter

Renal Impairment Not studied in renal dysfunction.

Hepatic Impairment Not studied in hepatic dysfunction.

Administration

I.V. Allow to warm to room temperature prior to administration. Infuse over 35 minutes. Decrease infusion rate or discontinue for infusion reactions; do not exceed a maximum 2-hour duration of infusion. Monitor for at least 1 hour following completion of infusion (for signs/symptoms of infusion reaction).

Stability

Reconstitution Dilute with an equal volume of D_5W, sodium chloride 0.9%, sodium chloride 0.45%, or Ringer's injection to a final concentration of 5 mg/mL (eg, 600 mg in a total volume of 120 mL or 900 mg in a total volume of 180 mL). Gently invert bag to mix.

Storage Prior to dilution, store vials at 2°C to 8°C (36°F to 46°F); do not freeze. Protect from light; do not shake. Following dilution, store at room temperature or refrigerate; protect from light; use within 24 hours.

Monitoring and Teaching Issues

Laboratory Monitoring CBC with differential, lactic dehydrogenase (LDH), AST, urinalysis
After discontinuation: Serum LDH, hemoglobin, serum creatinine (monitor for at least 8 weeks after discontinuation)

Serum LDH levels greater than pretreatment level along with: >25% decrease in PNH clone size in ≤1 week, or hemoglobin level <5 g/dL, or a hemoglobin decrease of >4 g/dL in ≤1 week, or 50% increase in serum creatinine, or angina, mental status change, or thrombosis is indicative of serious hemolysis

Physical Assessment Patient should receive the meningococcal vaccine at least 2 weeks prior to starting therapy and be up to date on all vaccinations. Monitor closely during infusion and for 1 hour after infusion.

Patient Education You may experience headache within 2 days of the first 2 doses. Other side effects include nausea, back pain, sore throat, or cough. Monitor for infections. Meningococcal vaccination is recommended at least 2 weeks prior to starting therapy. Report immediately a severe headache with nausea or vomiting, high fever, stiff neck or back, rash, confusion, severe muscle aches with flu-like symptoms, or eyes sensitive to light.

Breast-Feeding Considerations It is not known if eculizumab is excreted in human milk. However, human IgG is excreted in breast milk, and therefore, eculizumab may also be excreted in milk. The risks to the infant from gastrointestinal or limited systemic exposure are unknown.

Pregnancy Considerations Animal studies have demonstrated fetal abnormalities. Eculizumab is a recombinant IgG molecule with IgG2 and IgG4 sequences; human IgG is known to cross the placenta, however IgG2 may have reduced placental transfer compared to other IgG subclasses. There are no adequate and well-controlled studies in pregnant women. Pregnant women with PNH and their fetuses have high rates of morbidity and mortality during pregnancy and the postpartum period. Limited information is available related to use during pregnancy. Use during pregnancy only if clearly needed.

- **Edecrin®** *see* Ethacrynic Acid *on page 692*
- **Edex®** *see* Alprostadil *on page 83*
- **Edluar™** *see* Zolpidem *on page 1905*

Edrophonium (ed roe FOE nee um)

U.S. Brand Names Enlon®

Index Terms Edrophonium Chloride

Generic Availability (U.S.) No

Pharmacologic Category Acetylcholinesterase Inhibitor; Antidote; Diagnostic Agent

Pregnancy Risk Factor C

Lactation Excretion in breast milk unknown

Use Diagnosis of myasthenia gravis; differentiation of cholinergic crises from myasthenia crises; reversal of nondepolarizing neuromuscular blockers

Available Dosage Forms

Injection, solution:

Enlon®: 10 mg/mL (15 mL)

Dosing

Adult & Geriatric Usually administered I.V., however, if not possible, I.M. or SubQ may be used.

Diagnosis of Myasthenia gravis:

I.V.: 2 mg test dose administered over 15-30 seconds; 8 mg given 45 seconds later if no response is seen. Test dose may be repeated after 30 minutes.

I.M.: Initial: 10 mg; if no cholinergic reaction occurs, give 2 mg 30 minutes later to rule out false-negative reaction.

Titration of oral anticholinesterase therapy: 1-2 mg given 1 hour after oral dose of anticholinesterase; if strength improves, an increase in neostigmine or pyridostigmine dose is indicated.

Differentiation of cholinergic from myasthenic crisis: I.V.: 1 mg; may repeat after 1 minute. **Note:** Intubation and controlled ventilation may be required if patient has cholinergic crisis.

Reversal of nondepolarizing neuromuscular blocking agents (neostigmine with atropine usually preferred): I.V.: 10 mg over 30-45 seconds; may repeat every 5-10 minutes up to 40 mg.

Termination of paroxysmal atrial tachycardia: I.V. rapid injection: 5-10 mg

Pediatric Usually administered I.V., however, if not possible, I.M. or SubQ may be used:

Infants:

I.M.: 0.5-1 mg

I.V.: Initial: 0.1 mg, followed by 0.4 mg if no response; total dose = 0.5 mg

Children:

Diagnosis: Initial: 0.04 mg/kg over 1 minute followed by 0.16 mg/kg if no response, to a maximum total dose of 5 mg for children <34 kg, or 10 mg for children >34 kg **or**

Alternative dosing (manufacturer's recommendation):

≤34 kg: 1 mg; if no response after 45 seconds, repeat dosage in 1 mg increments every 30-45 seconds, up to a total of 5 mg

>34 kg: 2 mg; if no response after 45 seconds, repeat dosage in 1 mg increments every 30-45 seconds, up to a total of 10 mg

I.M.:

<34 kg: 1 mg

>34 kg: 5 mg

Titration of oral anticholinesterase therapy: 0.04 mg/kg once given 1 hour after oral intake of the drug being used in treatment. If strength improves, an increase in neostigmine or pyridostigmine dose is indicated.

Renal Impairment Dose may need to be reduced in patients with chronic renal failure.

Monitoring and Teaching Issues

Physical Assessment Administration of edrophonium for MG diagnosis is supervised by a neurologist and use as a neuromuscular blocking agent is supervised by an anesthesiologist. Patient must be monitored closely during and following procedure for cholinergic crisis; keep atropine at hand for antidote. Patients receiving the medication for MG testing will have been advised by their neurologist about drug effects. Those patients receiving medication for neuromuscular block will be unaware of drug effects. Patient should never be left alone until all drug effects and the possibility of cholinergic crisis have passed.

- **Edrophonium Chloride** *see* Edrophonium *on page 603*

◆ **E.E.S.®** *see* Erythromycin (Systemic) *on page* 658

Efavirenz (e FAV e renz)

U.S. Brand Names Sustiva®

Generic Availability (U.S.) No

Pharmacologic Category Antiretroviral Agent, Reverse Transcriptase Inhibitor (Non-nucleoside)

Prescribing and Access Restrictions Efavirenz oral solution is available only through an expanded access (compassionate use) program. Enrollment information may be obtained by calling 877-372-7097.

Pregnancy Risk Factor D

Lactation Enters breast milk/contraindicated

Use Treatment of HIV-1 infections in combination with at least two other antiretroviral agents

Mechanism of Action/Effect As a non-nucleoside reverse transcriptase inhibitor, efavirenz has activity against HIV-1 by binding to reverse transcriptase. It consequently blocks the RNA-dependent and DNA-dependent DNA polymerase activities including HIV-1 replication. It does not require intracellular phosphorylation for antiviral activity.

Contraindications Hypersensitivity to efavirenz or any component of the formulation; concurrent use of bepridil, cisapride, midazolam, pimozide, triazolam, voriconazole (with standard [eg, unadjusted] voriconazole and efavirenz doses), or ergot alkaloids (includes dihydroergotamine, ergotamine, ergonovine, methylergonovine)

Warnings/Precautions Do not use as single-agent therapy; avoid pregnancy; women of childbearing potential should undergo pregnancy testing prior to initiation of therapy; use caution with other agents metabolized by cytochrome P450 isoenzyme 3A4 (see Contraindications); use caution with history of mental illness/drug abuse (predisposition to psychological reactions); may cause CNS and psychiatric symptoms, which include impaired concentration, dizziness or drowsiness (avoid potentially hazardous tasks such as driving or operating machinery if these effects are noted); CNS effects may be potentiated when used with other sedative drugs or ethanol. Serious psychiatric side effects have been associated with efavirenz, including severe depression, suicide, paranoia, and mania. May cause mild-to-moderate maculopapular rash; usually occurs within 2 weeks of starting therapy; discontinue if severe rash (involving blistering, desquamation, mucosal involvement, or fever) develops. Children are more susceptible.

Caution in patients with known or suspected hepatitis B or C infection (monitoring of liver function is recommended) or Child-Pugh class A hepatic impairment; not recommended in Child-Pugh class B or C hepatic impairment. Persistent elevations of serum transaminases >5 times the upper limit of normal should prompt evaluation - benefit of continued therapy should be weighed against possible risk of hepatotoxicity. Increases in total cholesterol and triglycerides have been reported; screening should be done prior to therapy and periodically throughout treatment. May cause redistribution of fat (eg, buffalo hump, peripheral wasting with increased abdominal girth, cushingoid appearance). Patients may develop immune reconstitution syndrome resulting in the occurrence of an inflammatory response to an indolent or residual opportunistic infection; further evaluation and treatment may be required. Use with caution in patients with a history of seizure disorder; seizures have been associated with use.

Drug Interactions

Metabolism/Transport Effects **Substrate** (major) of CYP2B6, 3A4; **Inhibits** CYP2C9 (moderate), 2C19 (moderate), 3A4 (moderate); **Induces** CYP2B6 (weak), 3A4 (strong)

Avoid Concomitant Use

Avoid concomitant use of Efavirenz with any of the following: Bepridil [Off Market]; Cisapride; Clopidogrel; Dienogest; Dronedarone; Ergot Derivatives; Etravirine; Lurasidone; Midazolam; Nevirapine; Nilotinib; Nisoldipine; Pazopanib; Pimozide; Posaconazole; Praziquantel; Ranolazine; Roflumilast; RomiDEPsin; St Johns Wort; Tolvaptan; Triazolam; Vandetanib

Decreased Effect

Efavirenz may decrease the levels/effects of: Atazanavir; Atorvastatin; Buprenorphine; Caspofungin; Clopidogrel; CycloSPORINE; CycloSPORINE (Systemic); CYP3A4 Substrates; Darunavir; Dienogest; Dronedarone; Etonogestrel; Etravirine; Everolimus; Exemestane; Gefitinib; GuanFACINE; Imatinib; Itraconazole; Ixabepilone; Lopinavir; Lovastatin; Lurasidone; Maraviroc; Methadone; NIFEdipine; Nilotinib; Nisoldipine; Norgestimate; Pazopanib; Posaconazole; Pravastatin; Praziquantel; Protease Inhibitors; Raltegravir; Ranolazine; Rifabutin; Roflumilast; RomiDEPsin; Saxagliptin; Sertraline; Simvastatin; Sirolimus; SORAfenib; Tacrolimus; Tacrolimus (Systemic); Tadalafil; Tolvaptan; Ulipristal; Vandetanib; Vitamin K Antagonists; Voriconazole

The levels/effects of Efavirenz may be decreased by: CYP2B6 Inducers (Strong); CYP3A4 Inducers (Strong); Deferasirox; Nevirapine; Phenytoin; Rifabutin; Rifampin; St Johns Wort

Increased Effect/Toxicity

Efavirenz may increase the levels/effects of: Alcohol (Ethyl); Bepridil [Off Market]; Carvedilol; Cisapride; CNS Depressants; Colchicine; CYP2C19 Substrates; CYP2C9 Substrates (High risk); CYP3A4 Substrates; Eplerenone; Ergot Derivatives; Etravirine; FentaNYL; Halofantrine; Lurasidone; Methotrimeprazine; Midazolam; Nevirapine; PACLitaxel; Phenytoin; Pimecrolimus; Pimozide; Protease Inhibitors; Ranolazine; Salmeterol; Saxagliptin; Tolvaptan; Triazolam; Vilazodone; Vitamin K Antagonists

The levels/effects of Efavirenz may be increased by: Conivaptan; CYP2B6 Inhibitors (Moderate); CYP2B6 Inhibitors (Strong); Darunavir; Droperidol; Methotrimeprazine; Nevirapine; Quazepam; Voriconazole

Nutritional/Ethanol Interactions

Ethanol: Avoid ethanol (hepatic and CNS adverse effects).

Food: Avoid high-fat meals (increase the absorption of efavirenz).

Herb/Nutraceutical: St John's wort may decrease efavirenz serum levels. Avoid concurrent use.

Lab Interactions False-positive tests for cannabinoids have been reported when the CEDIA DAU Multilevel THC assay is used. False-positive results with other assays for cannabinoids have not been observed. False-positive tests for benzodiazepines have been reported and are likely due to the 8-hydroxy-efavirenz major metabolite.

Adverse Reactions Unless otherwise noted, frequency of adverse events is as reported in adults receiving combination antiretroviral therapy.

>10%:

Central nervous system: Dizziness (2% to 28%; children 16%), fever (children 21%), depression (up to 19%; severe: 1% to 2%), insomnia (up to 16%), anxiety (2% to 13%), pain (1% to 13%; children 14%), headache (2% to 8%; children 11%)

Dermatologic: Rash (5% to 26%, grade 3/4: <1%; children up to 46%, grade 3/4: 2% to 4%)

Endocrine & metabolic: HDL increased (25% to 35%), total cholesterol increased (20% to 40%), triglycerides increased (≥751 mg/dL: 6% to 11%)

Gastrointestinal: Diarrhea (3% to 14%; children: up to 39%), nausea (2% to 12%; children 12%), vomiting (3% to 6%; children 12%)

Respiratory: Cough (children 16%)

1% to 10%:

Central nervous system: Impaired concentration (up to 8%), somnolence (up to 7%), fatigue (up to 8%), abnormal dreams (1% to 6%), nervousness (2% to 7%), hallucinations (1%)

Dermatologic: Pruritus (up to 9%)

Endocrine & metabolic: Hyperglycemia (>250 mg/dL: 2% to 5%)

Gastrointestinal: Dyspepsia (up to 4%), abdominal pain (2% to 3%), anorexia (up to 2%), amylase increased (grade 3/4: up to 6%)

Hematologic: Neutropenia (grade 3/4: 2% to 10%)

Hepatic: Transaminases increased (grade 3/4: 2% to 8%, incidence higher with hepatitis B and/or C coinfection)

Pharmacodynamics/Kinetics

Absorption Increased by fatty meals

Time to Peak 3-5 hours

Protein Binding >99%, primarily to albumin

Half-Life Elimination Single dose: 52-76 hours; Multiple doses: 40-55 hours

Metabolism Hepatic via CYP3A4 and 2B6 to inactive hydroxylated metabolites; may induce its own metabolism

Excretion Feces (16% to 61% primarily as unchanged drug); urine (14% to 34% as metabolites)

Available Dosage Forms

Capsule, oral:

Sustiva®: 50 mg, 200 mg

Tablet, oral:

Sustiva®: 600 mg

Dosing

Adult & Geriatric

HIV infection (as part of combination; a preferred regimen for therapy-naive patients with tenofovir and emtricitabine [DHHS, 2011]): Oral: 600 mg once daily

Dosage adjustment for concomitant voriconazole: Reduce efavirenz dose to 300 mg once daily and increase voriconazole to 400 mg every 12 hours

Pediatric Dosage is based on body weight.

HIV infection (as part of combination therapy): Oral: Children ≥3 years:

10 kg to <15 kg: 200 mg once daily
15 kg to <20 kg: 250 mg once daily
20 kg to <25 kg: 300 mg once daily
25 kg to <32.5 kg: 350 mg once daily
32.5 kg to <40 kg: 400 mg once daily
≥40 kg: 600 mg once daily

Renal Impairment No adjustment is necessary.

Hepatic Impairment

Mild impairment (Child-Pugh class A): No dosage adjustment recommended; use with caution.

Moderate-to-severe impairment (Child-Pugh class B or C): Use not recommended.

Administration

Oral Administer on an empty stomach. Dosing at or before bedtime is recommended to limit central nervous system effects (DHHS, 2011). Tablets should not be broken. Some clinicians recommend opening capsules and adding to liquid or food for patients that cannot swallow capsules; however, no pharmacokinetic data are available and this is not recommended (DHHS [pediatric], 2010).

Stability

Storage Store at controlled room temperature of 25°C (77°F); excursion permitted to 15°C to 30°C (59°F to 86°F).

Monitoring and Teaching Issues

Laboratory Monitoring Monitor serum transaminases (discontinuation of treatment should be considered for persistent elevations greater than five times the upper limit of normal), cholesterol, and triglycerides.

Physical Assessment Use caution in presence of or history of hepatic impairment or mental illness/drug abuse (increased risk of serious psychiatric side effects). Assess decrease in infections and progression of disease, viral load, and CD4 count. Monitor for CNS effects, redistribution of body fat, hyperglycemia, hyperlipidemia, and cushingoid appearance periodically during therapy. Teach patient proper timing of multiple medications.

Patient Education This drug will not cure HIV, nor has it been found to reduce transmission of HIV; use appropriate precautions to prevent spread to other persons. This medication will be prescribed with a combination of other medications; time these medications as directed by prescriber. Take on an empty stomach. Maintain adequate hydration, unless instructed to restrict fluid intake. Frequent blood tests may be required. You may be advised to check your glucose levels; this drug can cause hyperglycemia. May cause dizziness, insomnia, impaired concentration, nausea, vomiting, abdominal pain, or diarrhea. May cause changes in body fat, increased fat in upper back and neck and around trunk, and loss of fat from extremities and face. Report immediately any CNS changes (depression, anxiety, suicide ideation, abnormal dreams, hallucinations, nervousness, impaired concentration), rash, or persistent gastrointestinal upset.

Dietary Considerations Should be taken on an empty stomach.

Breast-Feeding Considerations Pharmacokinetic data from a small study indicates that peak serum concentrations may be significantly increased in lactating women.

In infants born to mothers who are HIV positive, HAART while breast-feeding may decrease postnatal infection. However, maternal or infant antiretroviral therapy does not completely eliminate the risk of postnatal HIV transmission. In addition, multiclass-resistant virus has been detected in breast-feeding infants despite maternal therapy.

In the United States where formula is accessible, affordable, safe, and sustainable, complete avoidance of breast-feeding by HIV-infected women is recommended to decrease potential transmission of HIV. Although breast-feeding is not recommended, plasma concentrations of efavirenz in nursing infants have been reported as ~13% of maternal plasma concentrations.

Pregnancy Considerations Teratogenic effects have been observed in primates receiving efavirenz. Based on data from the Antiretroviral Pregnancy Registry, birth defects have been observed in 2.8% of offspring with first trimester exposure (in comparison to 2.7% observed in U.S. population) and a pattern of severe CNS defects have been reported. Pregnancy should be avoided and alternate therapy should be considered in women of childbearing potential. Women of childbearing potential should undergo pregnancy testing prior to initiation of efavirenz. Barrier contraception should be used in combination with other (hormonal) methods of contraception and for 12 weeks after efavirenz is discontinued. If therapy with efavirenz is administered during pregnancy, avoid use during the first trimester (DHHS, 2011); use in the second and third trimesters only after considering other alternatives. Pharmacokinetic data from small study indicates that peak serum levels in the third trimester may be significantly increased. Healthcare providers are encouraged to enroll pregnant women exposed to antiretroviral medications in the Antiretroviral Pregnancy Registry (1-800-258-4263 or www.APRegistry.com). Healthcare providers caring for HIV-infected women and their infants may contact the National Perinatal HIV Hotline (888-448-8765) for clinical consultation.

Additional Information Early virologic failure was observed with tenofovir and didanosine delayed release capsules, plus either efavirenz or nevirapine; use caution in treatment-naive patients with high baseline viral loads.

Efavirenz, Emtricitabine, and Tenofovir

(e FAV e renz, em trye SYE ta been, & te NOE fo veer)

U.S. Brand Names Atripla®

Index Terms Emtricitabine, Efavirenz, and Tenofovir; FTC, TDF, and EFV; Tenofovir Disoproxil Fumarate, Efavirenz, and Emtricitabine

Generic Availability (U.S.) No

Pharmacologic Category Antiretroviral Agent, Reverse Transcriptase Inhibitor (Non-nucleoside); Antiretroviral Agent, Reverse Transcriptase Inhibitor (Nucleoside); Antiretroviral Agent, Reverse Transcriptase Inhibitor (Nucleotide)

Pregnancy Risk Factor D

Lactation See individual agents.

Use Treatment of HIV infection

Mechanism of Action/Effect See individual agents.

Contraindications History of clinically-significant hypersensitivity (eg, Stevens-Johnson syndrome, erythema multiforme, or toxic skin reactions) to efavirenz, concurrent use of bepridil, cisapride, midazolam, triazolam, voriconazole, ergot alkaloids (includes dihydroergotamine, ergotamine, ergonovine, methylergonovine), St John's wort, pimozide

Warnings/Precautions **[U.S. Boxed Warning]: Lactic acidosis and severe hepatomegaly with steatosis have been reported with nucleoside analogues, including fatal cases.** Use caution in hepatic impairment. Use with caution in patients with risk factors for liver disease (risk may be increased in obese patients or prolonged exposure) and suspend treatment in any patient who develops clinical or laboratory findings suggestive of lactic acidosis or hepatotoxicity (transaminase elevation may/may not accompany hepatomegaly and steatosis). Persistent elevations of serum transaminases >5 times the upper limit of normal should prompt evaluation - benefit of continued therapy should be weighed against possible risk of hepatotoxicity. May cause redistribution of fat (eg, buffalo hump, peripheral wasting with increased abdominal girth, cushingoid appearance).

[U.S. Boxed Warning]: Safety and efficacy during coinfection of HIV and HBV have not been established; acute, severe exacerbations of HBV have been reported following discontinuation of antiretroviral therapy. All patients with HIV should be tested for HBV prior to initiation of treatment. Caution in patients with known or suspected hepatitis B or C infection (monitoring of liver function is recommended). In HBV coinfected patients, monitor hepatic function closely for several months following discontinuation.

Avoid pregnancy; women of childbearing potential should undergo pregnancy testing prior to initiation of therapy. Use with caution in patients taking strong CYP3A4 inhibitors, moderate or strong CYP3A4 inducers and major CYP3A4 substrates (see Drug Interactions); consider alternative agents that avoid or lessen the potential for CYP-mediated interactions. Immune reconstitution syndrome may develop resulting in the occurrence of an inflammatory response to an indolent or residual opportunistic infection; further evaluation and treatment may be required. Discontinue if severe rash (involving blistering, desquamation, mucosal involvement or fever) develops. Do not use concurrently with adefovir or lamivudine (or lamivudine-combination products). To avoid duplicate therapy, do not use concurrently with efavirenz emtricitabine, tenofovir, or any combination of these drugs.

Use caution with history of mental illness/drug abuse (predisposition to psychological reactions); may cause CNS and psychiatric symptoms, which include impaired concentration, dizziness or drowsiness (avoid potentially hazardous tasks such as driving or operating machinery if these effects are noted); serious psychiatric side effects have been associated with efavirenz, including severe depression, suicidal ideation, paranoia, and mania. Seizures have been associated with efavirenz use; use caution in patients with a history of seizure disorder.

May cause osteomalacia (which may contribute to fractures) and/or renal toxicity (acute renal failure and/or Fanconi syndrome); avoid use with concurrent or recent nephrotoxic therapy; monitor renal function and possible bone abnormalities during therapy. Product is a fixed-dose combination and is not appropriate for use in renal impairment (Cl_{cr} <50 mL/minute).

Use has been associated with decreases in bone mineral density. Consider monitoring of bone density in patients at risk for osteopenia or with a history of pathologic fractures; consider calcium and vitamin D supplementation. Fixed dose combination product; safety and efficacy have not been established in pediatric patients <18 years of age. In children <40 kg, the dose of efavirenz would be excessive.

Drug Interactions

Metabolism/Transport Effects

Efavirenz: **Substrate** (major) of CYP2B6, 3A4; **Inhibits** CYP2C9 (moderate), 2C19 (moderate), 3A4 (moderate); **Induces** CYP2B6 (weak), 3A4 (strong)

Tenofovir: **Inhibits** CYP1A2 (weak)

Avoid Concomitant Use

Avoid concomitant use of Efavirenz, Emtricitabine, and Tenofovir with any of the following: Bepridil [Off Market]; Cisapride; Clopidogrel; Didanosine; Dienogest; Dronedarone; Ergot Derivatives; Etravirine; LamiVUDine; Lurasidone; Midazolam; Nevirapine; Nilotinib; Nisoldipine; Pazopanib; Pimozide; Posaconazole; Praziquantel; Ranolazine; Roflumilast; RomiDEPsin; St Johns Wort; Tolvaptan; Triazolam; Vandetanib

Decreased Effect

Efavirenz, Emtricitabine, and Tenofovir may decrease the levels/effects of: Atazanavir; Atorvastatin; Buprenorphine; Caspofungin; Clopidogrel; CycloSPORINE; CycloSPORINE (Systemic); CYP3A4 Substrates; Darunavir; Didanosine; Dienogest; Dronedarone; Etonogestrel; Etravirine; Everolimus; Exemestane; Gefitinib; GuanFACINE; Imatinib; Itraconazole; Ixabepilone; Lopinavir; Lovastatin; Lurasidone; Maraviroc; Methadone; NIFEdipine; Nilotinib; Nisoldipine; Norgestimate; Pazopanib; Posaconazole; Pravastatin; Praziquantel; Protease Inhibitors; Raltegravir; Ranolazine; Rifabutin; Roflumilast; RomiDEPsin; Saxagliptin; Sertraline; Simvastatin; Sirolimus; SORAfenib; Tacrolimus; Tacrolimus (Systemic); Tadalafil; Tolvaptan; Ulipristal; Vandetanib; Vitamin K Antagonists; Voriconazole

The levels/effects of Efavirenz, Emtricitabine, and Tenofovir may be decreased by: Adefovir; CYP2B6 Inducers (Strong); CYP3A4 Inducers (Strong); Deferasirox; Nevirapine; Phenytoin; Rifabutin; Rifampin; St Johns Wort

Increased Effect/Toxicity

Efavirenz, Emtricitabine, and Tenofovir may increase the levels/effects of: Adefovir; Alcohol (Ethyl); Bepridil [Off Market]; Carvedilol; Cisapride; CNS Depressants; Colchicine; CYP2C19 Substrates; CYP2C9 Substrates (High risk); CYP3A4 Substrates; Didanosine; Eplerenone; Ergot Derivatives; Etravirine; FentaNYL; Ganciclovir-Valganciclovir; Halofantrine; Lurasidone; Methotrimeprazine; Midazolam; Nevirapine; PACLitaxel; Phenytoin; Pimecrolimus; Pimozide; Protease Inhibitors; Ranolazine; Salmeterol; Saxagliptin; Tolvaptan; Triazolam; Vilazodone; Vitamin K Antagonists

The levels/effects of Efavirenz, Emtricitabine, and Tenofovir may be increased by: Acyclovir-Valacyclovir; Atazanavir; Conivaptan; CYP2B6 Inhibitors (Moderate); CYP2B6 Inhibitors (Strong); Darunavir; Droperidol; Ganciclovir-Valganciclovir; LamiVUDine; Lopinavir; Methotrimeprazine; Nevirapine; Protease Inhibitors; Quazepam; Ribavirin; Voriconazole

Nutritional/Ethanol Interactions

Ethanol: Avoid ethanol (hepatic and CNS adverse effects).

Food: Avoid high-fat meals (increase the absorption of efavirenz). Food decreases peak plasma concentrations of emtricitabine, but does not alter the extent of absorption or overall systemic exposure. Fatty meals may increase the bioavailability of tenofovir.

Herb/Nutraceutical: St John's wort may decrease efavirenz serum levels. Concurrent use is contraindicated.

Lab Interactions False-positive test for cannabinoids have been reported when the CEDIA DAU Multilevel THC assay is used in patients receiving efavirenz. False-positive results with other assays for cannabinoids have not been observed.

Adverse Reactions The complete adverse reaction profile of combination therapy has not been established. **See individual agents.** The following adverse effects were noted in clinical trials with combination therapy:

>10%: Endocrine & metabolic: Hypercholesterolemia (22%)

1% to 10%:

Central nervous system: Depression (9%), fatigue (9%), dizziness (8%), headache (6%), anxiety (5%), insomnia (5%), somnolence (4%), abnormal dreams

Dermatologic: Rash (7%)

Endocrine & metabolic: Triglycerides increased (4%), hyperglycemia (2%)

Gastrointestinal: Nausea (9%), diarrhea (9%), serum amylase increased (8%), vomiting (2%)

Hematologic: Neutropenia (3%)

Hepatic: AST increased (3%), ALT increased (2%), alkaline phosphatase increased (1%)

Neuromuscular & skeletal: Creatine increased (9%)

Renal: Hematuria (3%)

Respiratory: Sinusitis (8%), upper respiratory infection (8%), nasopharyngitis (5%)

Pharmacodynamics/Kinetics

Pharmacokinetic Note See individual agents.

Available Dosage Forms

Tablet:

Atripla®: Efavirenz 600 mg, emtricitabine 200 mg, and tenofovir disoproxil fumarate 300 mg

Dosing

Adult & Geriatric HIV infection: Oral: One tablet once daily

Renal Impairment Moderate-to-severe renal impairment (Cl_{cr} <50 mL/minute): Use not recommended.

Administration

Oral Should be taken on an empty stomach, normally at bedtime to increase gastrointestinal tolerance and decrease nervous system manifestations.

Stability

Storage Store at 25°C (77°F); excursions permitted between 15°C to 30°C (59°F to 86°F). Dispense only in original container.

Monitoring and Teaching Issues

Laboratory Monitoring Testing for HBV is recommended prior to the initiation of antiretroviral therapy. Monitor CBC with differential, reticulocyte count, serum creatine kinase, CD4 count, HIV RNA plasma levels, renal and hepatic function tests, cholesterol, triglycerides, bone density (long-term), serum phosphorus. Serum transaminases (discontinuation of treatment should be considered for persistent elevations >5 times ULN).

Patients with HIV and HBV coinfection should have hepatic function monitored for several months following discontinuation.

Physical Assessment See individual agents.

Patient Education See individual agents.

Dietary Considerations Should be taken on an empty stomach. In patients with history of bone fracture or osteopenia, consider calcium and vitamin D supplementation.

Breast-Feeding Considerations See individual agents.

Pregnancy Considerations See individual agents.

- ◆ **Effer-K®** *see* Potassium Bicarbonate and Potassium Citrate *on page* 1479
- ◆ **Effexor®** *see* Venlafaxine *on page* 1855
- ◆ **Effexor XR®** *see* Venlafaxine *on page* 1855
- ◆ **Effient®** *see* Prasugrel *on page* 1493
- ◆ **Eformoterol and Budesonide** *see* Budesonide and Formoterol *on page* 239
- ◆ **Egrifta™** *see* Tesamorelin *on page* 1737
- ◆ **EL-970** *see* Dalfampridine *on page* 458
- ◆ **Elavil** *see* Amitriptyline *on page* 103
- ◆ **Eldepryl®** *see* Selegiline *on page* 1630
- ◆ **Eldopaque® [OTC]** *see* Hydroquinone *on page* 927
- ◆ **Eldopaque Forte®** *see* Hydroquinone *on page* 927
- ◆ **Eldoquin® [OTC]** *see* Hydroquinone *on page* 927
- ◆ **Eldoquin Forte®** *see* Hydroquinone *on page* 927
- ◆ **Electrolyte Lavage Solution** *see* Polyethylene Glycol-Electrolyte Solution *on page* 1474
- ◆ **Electrolyte Lavage Solution** *see* Polyethylene Glycol-Electrolyte Solution and Bisacodyl *on page* 1475
- ◆ **Elestat®** *see* Epinastine *on page* 628
- ◆ **Elestrin®** *see* Estradiol (Systemic) *on page* 670

Eletriptan (el e TRIP tan)

U.S. Brand Names Relpax®

Index Terms Eletriptan Hydrobromide

Generic Availability (U.S.) No

Pharmacologic Category Antimigraine Agent; Serotonin 5-$HT_{1B, 1D}$ Receptor Agonist

Pregnancy Risk Factor C

Lactation Enters breast milk/use caution

Use Acute treatment of migraine, with or without aura

Mechanism of Action/Effect Selective agonist for serotonin receptor in cranial arteries; causes vasoconstriction and relief of migraine

Contraindications Hypersensitivity to eletriptan or any component of the formulation; ischemic heart disease (angina pectoris, history of myocardial infarction, or proven silent ischemia) or in patients with symptoms consistent with ischemic heart disease, coronary artery vasospasm, or Prinzmetal's angina; cerebrovascular syndromes (including strokes, transient ischemic attacks); peripheral vascular syndromes (including ischemic bowel disease); uncontrolled hypertension; use within 24 hours of ergotamine derivatives; use within 24 hours of another 5-HT_1 agonist; management of hemiplegic or basilar migraine; severe hepatic impairment

Warnings/Precautions Only indicated for treatment of acute migraine; not indicated for migraine prophylaxis, or for the treatment of cluster headache, hemiplegic or basilar migraine. If a patient does not respond to the first dose, the diagnosis of migraine should be reconsidered. Do not give to patients with risk factors for CAD until a cardiovascular evaluation has been performed; if evaluation is satisfactory, the healthcare provider should administer the first dose and cardiovascular status should be periodically evaluated. Cardiac events (coronary artery vasospasm, transient ischemia, MI, ventricular tachycardia/fibrillation, cardiac arrest, and death), cerebral/subarachnoid hemorrhage, stroke, peripheral vascular ischemia, and colonic ischemia have been reported with 5-HT_1 agonist administration. Significant elevation in blood pressure, including hypertensive crisis, has also been reported on rare occasions in patients with and without a history of hypertension. Use with caution with mild-to-moderate hepatic impairment. Symptoms of agitation, confusion, hallucinations, hyper-reflexia, myoclonus, shivering, and tachycardia (serotonin syndrome) may occur with concomitant proserotonergic drugs (ie, SSRIs/SNRIs or triptans) or agents which reduce eletriptan's metabolism. Concurrent use of serotonin precursors (eg, tryptophan) is not recommended. Use not recommended within 72 hours in patients taking strong CYP3A4 inhibitors.

Drug Interactions

Metabolism/Transport Effects Substrate of CYP3A4 (major)

Avoid Concomitant Use

Avoid concomitant use of Eletriptan with any of the following: Ergot Derivatives; Sibutramine

Decreased Effect There are no known significant interactions involving a decrease in effect.

Increased Effect/Toxicity

Eletriptan may increase the levels/effects of: Ergot Derivatives; Serotonin Modulators

The levels/effects of Eletriptan may be increased by: Antifungal Agents (Azole Derivatives, Systemic); Calcium Channel Blockers (Nondihydropyridine); Conivaptan; CYP3A4 Inhibitors (Moderate); CYP3A4 Inhibitors (Strong); Dasatinib; Ergot Derivatives; Fluconazole; Macrolide Antibiotics; Sibutramine

Nutritional/Ethanol Interactions Food: High-fat meal increases bioavailability.

Adverse Reactions 1% to 10%:

Cardiovascular: Chest pain/tightness (1% to 4%; placebo 1%), palpitation

Central nervous system: Dizziness (3% to 7%; placebo 3%), somnolence (3% to 7%; placebo 4%), headache (3% to 4%; placebo 3%), chills, pain, vertigo

Gastrointestinal: Nausea (4% to 8%; placebo 5%), xerostomia (2% to 4%, placebo 2%), dysphagia (1% to 2%), abdominal pain/discomfort (1% to 2%; placebo 1%), dyspepsia (1% to 2%; placebo 1%)

Neuromuscular & skeletal: Weakness (4% to 10%), paresthesia (3% to 4%), back pain, hypertonia, hypoesthesia

Respiratory: Pharyngitis

Miscellaneous: Diaphoresis

Pharmacodynamics/Kinetics

Absorption Well absorbed

Bioavailability ~50%, increased with high-fat meal

Time to Peak Plasma: 1.5-2 hours

Protein Binding ~85%

Half-Life Elimination ~4 hours (Elderly: 4.4-5.7 hours); Metabolite: ~13 hours

Metabolism Hepatic via CYP3A4; forms one metabolite (active)

Available Dosage Forms

Tablet, oral:

Relpax®: 20 mg, 40 mg

Dosing

Adult & Geriatric Acute migraine: Oral: Initial: 20-40 mg (maximum: 40 mg/dose); if the headache improves but returns, dose may be repeated after 2 hours have elapsed since first dose (maximum: 80 mg/day)

Note: If the first dose is ineffective, diagnosis needs to be re-evaluated. Safety of treating >3 headaches/month has not been established.

Renal Impairment No dosing adjustment needed; monitor for increased blood pressure.

Hepatic Impairment

Mild-to-moderate impairment: No adjustment necessary.

Severe impairment: Use is contraindicated.

Stability

Storage Store at 25°C (77°F); excursions permitted to 15°C to 30°C (59°F to 86°F).

Monitoring and Teaching Issues

Physical Assessment For use with clear diagnosis of migraine. Cardiovascular status should be evaluated prior to initiating medication and periodically thereafter. Monitor for hypertension and cardiac events.

Patient Education This drug is to be used to reduce your migraine, not to prevent the number of attacks. Do not crush, break, or chew tablet. If headache improves but returns, dose may be repeated after 2 hours. Do not exceed two doses in 24 hours. May cause dizziness, drowsiness, nausea, vomiting, or abdominal pain. Report immediately any chest pain, tightness, or palpitations; muscle weakness or tremors; back pain; respiratory difficulty; changes in CNS (abnormal thought processes, depression, insomnia, confusion, agitation); swelling of eyelids, face, lips, or throat; rash; or hives.

Geriatric Considerations Since elderly often have cardiovascular disease, careful evaluation of the use of 5-HT agonists is needed to avoid complications with the use of these agents. Safety and efficacy in elderly >65 years of age have not been established, however, pharmacokinetic disposition is similar to that in younger adults. Use lowest recommended doses initially.

Breast-Feeding Considerations Eight women were given a single dose of eletriptan 80 mg. The amount of drug detected in breast milk over 24 hours was ~0.02% of the maternal dose and the milk-to-plasma ratio was variable. The presence of the active metabolite was not measured.

Pregnancy Considerations Teratogenic effects were observed in animal studies.

Related Information

Antimigraine Drugs: 5-HT_1 Receptor Agonists *on page 1985*

- **Eletriptan Hydrobromide** *see* Eletriptan *on page 608*
- **Eligard®** *see* Leuprolide *on page 1082*
- **Elitek™** *see* Rasburicase *on page 1562*
- **Elixophyllin® Elixir** *see* Theophylline *on page 1748*
- **ella®** *see* Ulipristal *on page 1826*
- **Ellence®** *see* Epirubicin *on page 633*
- **Elmiron®** *see* Pentosan Polysulfate Sodium *on page 1440*
- **Elocon®** *see* Mometasone (Topical) *on page 1255*
- **Eloxatin®** *see* Oxaliplatin *on page 1370*
- **Elspar®** *see* Asparaginase *on page 152*

Eltrombopag (el TROM boe pag)

U.S. Brand Names Promacta®

Index Terms Eltrombopag Olamine; Revolade®; SB-497115; SB-497115-GR

Generic Availability (U.S.) No

Pharmacologic Category Colony Stimulating Factor; Thrombopoietic Agent

Medication Guide Available Yes

Prescribing and Access Restrictions As a requirement of the REMS program, access to this medication is restricted. Eltrombopag is approved for marketing under a Food and Drug Administration (FDA) approved, risk management, and restricted distribution program called Promacta® Cares™ (1-877-977-6622). Patients, prescribers, and pharmacies must be enrolled in the program.

Pregnancy Risk Factor C

Lactation Excretion in breast milk unknown/not recommended

Use Treatment of thrombocytopenia in patients with chronic immune (idiopathic) thrombocytopenic purpura (ITP) at risk for bleeding who have had insufficient response to corticosteroids, immune globulin, or splenectomy

Mechanism of Action/Effect Thrombopoietin (TPO) nonpeptide agonist which increases platelet counts by binding to and activating the human TPO receptor.

Contraindications There are no contraindications listed within the manufacturer's labeling.

Warnings/Precautions [U.S. Boxed Warning]: May cause hepatotoxicity; obtain ALT, AST, and bilirubin prior to treatment initiation, every 2 weeks during adjustment phase, then monthly (after stable dose established); obtain fractionation for elevated bilirubin levels. Repeat abnormal liver function tests within 3-5 days; if confirmed abnormal, monitor weekly until resolves, stabilizes, or returns to baseline. Discontinue treatment for ALT levels ≥3 times the upper limit of normal (ULN) and which are progressive, or persistent (≥4 weeks), or accompanied by increased direct bilirubin, or accompanied by clinical signs of liver injury or evidence of hepatic decompensation. Reinitiation is not recommended; hepatotoxicity usually recurred with retreatment after therapy interruption; however, if the benefit of treatment outweighs the hepatotoxicity risk, initiate carefully, and monitor liver function tests weekly during the dose adjustment phase; permanently discontinue if hepatotoxicity recurs with rechallenge. Use with caution in patients with pre-existing hepatic impairment (clearance may be reduced); dosage reductions are recommended in patients with hepatic dysfunction; monitor closely.

[U.S. Boxed Warning]: Eltrombopag is available through a restricted access program called Promacta® Cares™; prescribers, pharmacies, and patients must be registered with the program. The program maintains a patient registry and requires prescribers to monitor and report baseline and periodic safety information related to hepatotoxicity, thromboembolic events, bone marrow reticulin events, rebound thrombocytopenia (after cessation), and malignancies. May increase the risk for bone marrow reticulin formation or progression; collagen fibrosis (not associated with cytopenias) was observed in clinical trials. In an extension study, myelofibrosis (≤grade 1) was observed in a majority of bone marrow biopsies performed after 1 year of treatment. Monitor peripheral blood smear for cellular morphologic abnormalities; analyze CBC monthly; discontinue treatment with onset of new or worsening abnormalities (eg, teardrop and nucleated RBC, immature WBC) or cytopenias and consider bone marrow biopsy (with staining for fibrosis). Upon discontinuation of therapy, thrombocytopenia may worsen; severity may be greater than pretreatment level. Risk of bleeding is increased during rebound thrombocytopenia, particularly in patients receiving anticoagulants or antiplatelet agents; monitor closely; monitor for at least 4 weeks after treatment discontinuation.

Thromboembolism may occur with excess increases in platelet levels. Use with caution in patients with known risk factors for thromboembolism (eg, Factor V Leiden, ATIII deficiency, antiphospholipid syndrome, chronic liver disease). Portal venous thrombosis was reported in a study of non-ITP patients with chronic liver disease (not an FDA-approved indication) receiving eltrombopag 75 mg once daily for 14 days as a preparative regimen prior to invasive procedures to reduce platelet transfusions. Stimulation of cell surface thrombopoietin (TPO) receptors may increase the risk for hematologic malignancies.

Cataract formation or worsening was observed in clinical trials. Monitor regularly for signs and symptoms of cataracts; obtain ophthalmic exam at baseline and during therapy. Use with caution in patients at risk for cataracts (eg, advanced age, long-term glucocorticoid use). Allow at least 4 hours between dosing of eltrombopag and antacids, minerals (eg, iron, calcium, aluminum, magnesium, selenium, zinc), or foods high in calcium; may reduce eltrombopag levels. Patients of East-Asian ethnicity (eg, Chinese, Japanese, Korean, Taiwanese) may have greater drug exposure (compared to non-east Asians); therapy should be initiated with lower starting doses.

Indicated only when the degree of thrombocytopenia and clinical conditions increase the risk for bleeding; use the lowest dose necessary to achieve and maintain platelet count ≥50,000/mm^3. Do not use to normalize platelet counts. Discontinue if platelet count does not respond to a level to avoid clinically important bleeding after 4 weeks at the maximum recommended dose.

Drug Interactions

Metabolism/Transport Effects

Substrate of CYP1A2 (minor), CYP2C8 (minor), UGT1A1, UGT1A3; **Inhibits** CYP2C8 inhibitor (moderate), SLCO1B1, UGT1A1, UGT1A3, UGT1A4, UGT1A6, UGT1A9, UGT2B7, and UGT2B15

Avoid Concomitant Use There are no known interactions where it is recommended to avoid concomitant use.

Decreased Effect

The levels/effects of Eltrombopag may be decreased by: Aluminum Hydroxide; Calcium Salts; Iron Salts; Magnesium Salts; Selenium; Sucralfate; Zinc Salts

Increased Effect/Toxicity

Eltrombopag may increase the levels/effects of: CYP2C8 Substrates (High risk); OATP1B1/SLCO1B1 Substrates; Rosuvastatin

Nutritional/Ethanol Interactions Food: Food, especially dairy products, may decrease the absorption of eltrombopag; allow at least 4 hours between dosing of eltrombopag and polyvalent cation intake (eg, dairy products, calcium-rich foods, multivitamins with minerals).

Adverse Reactions

>10%: Hepatic: Liver function tests abnormal (11%)

1% to 10%:

Central nervous system: Headache (10%), fatigue (4%)

Dermatologic: Rash (3%), alopecia (2%)

Gastrointestinal: Diarrhea (9%), nausea (4% to 9%), vomiting (6%), xerostomia (2%)

Genitourinary: Urinary tract infection (5%)

Hematologic: Myelofibrosis (Extension study: Grade ≤1: 93%; grade 2: 7%), rebound thrombocytopenia (8%)

Hepatic: Hyperbilirubinemia (6%), ALT increased (5% to 6%), AST increased (4%), alkaline phosphatase increased (2%)

Neuromuscular & skeletal: Myalgia (5%), back pain (3%), paresthesia (3%)

Ocular: Cataract (4% to 7%)

Respiratory: Upper respiratory infection (7%), oropharyngeal pain (4%), pharyngitis (4%)

Miscellaneous: Influenza (3%)

Pharmacodynamics/Kinetics

Onset of Action Platelet count increase: Within 1-2 weeks; Peak platelet count increase: 14-16 days

Duration of Action Platelets return to baseline: 1-2 weeks after last dose

Bioavailability ~52%

Time to Peak 2-6 hours

Protein Binding >99%

Half-Life Elimination ~21-32 hours in healthy individuals; ~26-35 hours in patients with ITP

Metabolism Extensive hepatic metabolism; via CYP 1A2, 2C8 oxidation and UGT 1A1, 1A3 glucuronidation

Excretion Feces (~59%, 20% as unchanged drug, 21% glutathione-related conjugates); urine (31%, 20% glucuronide of the phenypyrazole moiety)

Available Dosage Forms

Tablet, oral:

Promacta®: 25 mg, 50 mg, 75 mg

Dosing

Adult & Geriatric Note: Use the lowest dose to achieve and maintain platelet count ≥50,000/mm^3 as needed to reduce the risk of bleeding. Adjust dose based on platelet count response; initial platelet response generally occurs within 1-2 weeks. Discontinue if platelet count does not respond to a level that avoids clinically important bleeding after 4 weeks at the maximum daily dose of 75 mg.

Immune (idiopathic) thrombocytopenic purpura (ITP): Oral: Initial: 50 mg once daily; adjust dose to achieve and maintain platelet count ≥50,000/mm^3 to reduce the risk of bleeding; maximum dose: 75 mg once daily

Initial dosage for patients of East-Asian ethnicity (eg, Chinese, Japanese, Korean, Taiwanese): Oral: 25 mg once daily

Dosage adjustment recommendations (based on platelet response):

Platelet count <50,000/mm^3 (after at least 2 weeks): Increase daily dose by 25 mg (if taking 25 mg every other day, increase dose to 25 mg once daily prior to increasing the dose amount by 25 mg/day); maximum dose: 75 mg/day

Platelet count ≥200,000/mm^3 and ≤400,000/mm^3 (at any time): Reduce daily dose by 25 mg; reassess in 2 weeks

Platelet count >400,000/mm^3: Withhold dose; assess platelet count twice weekly; when platelet count <150,000/mm^3, resume with the daily dose reduced by 25 mg

Platelet count >400,000/mm^3 after 2 weeks at the lowest dose: Discontinue treatment

Renal Impairment Initial dose: Adjustment not required; monitor closely

Hepatic Impairment

Adjustment for hepatic impairment prior to initiating treatment:

Mild, moderate, or severe impairment (Child-Pugh classes A, B, or C): Initial dose: 25 mg once daily

Patients of East-Asian ethnicity with hepatic impairment (Child-Pugh classes A, B, or C): Initial dose: 25 mg once every other day

Adjustment for hepatic impairment during treatment:

Hepatic impairment (Child-Pugh classes A, B, or C) after treatment initiation or after dose increases: Wait 3 weeks (instead of 2 weeks) prior to increasing dose for platelet count <50,000/mm^3

ALT levels ≥3 times the upper limit of normal (ULN) **and** which are progressive, persistent (≥4 weeks), accompanied by increased direct bilirubin, or accompanied by clinical signs of liver injury or evidence of hepatic decompensation: Discontinue treatment.

Adjustment for Toxicity

Excessive platelet response (platelets >400,000/mm^3 after 2 weeks at the lowest dose): Discontinue treatment.

New or worsening cellular abnormalities or cytopenias: Discontinue treatment.

Administration

Oral Administer on an empty stomach, 1 hour before or 2 hours after a meal. Do not administer concurrently with antacids, foods high in calcium, or minerals (eg, iron, calcium, aluminum, magnesium, selenium, zinc); separate by at least 4 hours. Do not administer more than one dose within 24 hours.

Stability

Storage Store at room temperature of 25°C (77°F); excursions permitted to 15°C to 30°C (59°F to 86°F).

Monitoring and Teaching Issues

Laboratory Monitoring Liver tests, including ALT, AST, and bilirubin (baseline, every 2 weeks during dosage titration, then monthly; evaluate abnormal liver function tests within 3-5 days; monitor weekly if retreating [not recommended] after therapy interruption for hepatotoxicity); bilirubin fractionation (for elevated bilirubin); CBC with differential and platelet count (weekly at initiation and during dosage titration, then monthly when stable; continue monitoring for ≥4 weeks after cessation); peripheral blood smear (baseline and monthly when stable)

Physical Assessment Patient and provider must be registered with the Promacta® Cares™ program. Dosage adjustments may be necessary in patients with hepatic impairment.

Patient Education Take on an empty stomach, 1 hour before or 2 hours after a meal and at least 4 hours before or after any dairy products or multivitamins with minerals. You will require frequent blood tests to determine appropriate dosage and to reduce potential for severe adverse effects; maintaining laboratory testing schedule is vital. May cause nausea; vomiting; loss of appetite; or muscle, joint, back, or limb pain. Report new or persistent fatigue, yellowing of skin or eyes, unusual or increased bruising or bleeding, or change in vision.

Dietary Considerations Take on an empty stomach (1 hour before or 2 hours after a meal). Food, especially dairy products, may decrease the absorption of eltrombopag; allow at least 4 hours between dosing of eltrombopag and polyvalent cation intake (eg, dairy products, calcium-rich foods, multivitamins with minerals).

Breast-Feeding Considerations Due to the potential for serious adverse effects in the nursing infant, breast-feeding is not recommended.

Pregnancy Considerations Adverse effects were observed in animal studies. There are no adequate and well-controlled studies in pregnant women. Use during pregnancy only if the potential benefit to the mother outweighs the potential risk to the fetus. A Promacta® pregnancy registry has been established to monitor outcomes of women exposed to eltrombopag during pregnancy (1-888-825-5249).

- ◆ **Eltrombopag Olamine** *see* Eltrombopag *on page 610*
- ◆ **Embeda™** *see* Morphine and Naltrexone *on page 1263*
- ◆ **Emcyt®** *see* Estramustine *on page 675*
- ◆ **Emend®** *see* Aprepitant *on page 139*
- ◆ **Emend® for Injection** *see* Fosaprepitant *on page 826*
- ◆ **Emsam®** *see* Selegiline *on page 1630*

Emtricitabine (em trye SYE ta been)

U.S. Brand Names Emtriva®

Index Terms BW524W91; Coviracil; FTC

Generic Availability (U.S.) No

Pharmacologic Category Antiretroviral Agent, Reverse Transcriptase Inhibitor (Nucleoside)

Pregnancy Risk Factor B

Lactation Excretion in breast milk unknown/contraindicated

Use Treatment of HIV infection in combination with at least two other antiretroviral agents

Mechanism of Action/Effect Nucleoside reverse transcriptase inhibitor which interferes with viral RNA-dependent DNA synthesis, resulting in inhibition of viral replication.

Contraindications Hypersensitivity to emtricitabine or any component of the formulation

Warnings/Precautions [U.S. Boxed Warning]: Lactic acidosis, severe hepatomegaly with steatosis, and hepatic failure have occurred rarely with emtricitabine (similar to other nucleoside analogues). Some cases have been fatal; stop treatment if lactic acidosis or hepatotoxicity occur. Prior liver disease, obesity, extended duration of therapy, and female gender may represent risk factors for severe hepatic reactions. Testing for hepatitis B is recommended prior to the initiation of therapy; **[U.S. Boxed Warnings]: Hepatitis B may be exacerbated following discontinuation of emtricitabine; not indicated for treatment of chronic hepatitis B; safety and efficacy in HIV/HBV coinfected patients not established.** May be associated with fat redistribution (buffalo hump, increased abdominal girth, breast engorgement, facial atrophy, and dyslipidemia). Immune reconstitution syndrome may develop resulting in the occurrence of an inflammatory response to an indolent or residual opportunistic infection; further evaluation and treatment may be required. Use caution in patients with renal impairment (dosage adjustment required).

Drug Interactions

Avoid Concomitant Use

Avoid concomitant use of Emtricitabine with any of the following: LamiVUDine

Decreased Effect There are no known significant interactions involving a decrease in effect.

Increased Effect/Toxicity

The levels/effects of Emtricitabine may be increased by: Ganciclovir-Valganciclovir; LamiVUDine; Ribavirin

Nutritional/Ethanol Interactions Food: Food decreases peak plasma concentrations, but does not alter the extent of absorption or overall systemic exposure.

Adverse Reactions Clinical trials were conducted in patients receiving other antiretroviral agents, and it is not possible to correlate frequency of adverse events with emtricitabine alone. The range of frequencies of adverse events is generally comparable to comparator groups, with the exception of hyperpigmentation, which occurred more frequently in patients receiving emtricitabine. Unless otherwise noted, percentages are as reported in adults.

>10%:

Central nervous system: Dizziness (4% to 25%), headache (6% to 22%), fever (children 18%), insomnia (5% to 16%), abnormal dreams (2% to 11%)

Dermatologic: Hyperpigmentation (children 32%; adults 2% to 4%; primarily of palms and/or soles but may include tongue, arms, lip and nails; generally mild and nonprogressive without associated local reactions such as pruritus or rash); rash (17% to 30%; includes pruritus, maculopapular rash, vesiculobullous rash, pustular rash, and allergic reaction)

Gastrointestinal: Diarrhea (children 20%; adults 9% to 23%), vomiting (children 23%; adults 9%), nausea (13% to 18%), abdominal pain (8% to 14%), gastroenteritis (children 11%)

Neuromuscular & skeletal: Weakness (12% to 16%), CPK increased (grades 3/4: 11% to 12%)

Otic: Otitis media (children 23%)

Respiratory: Cough (children 28%; adults 14%), rhinitis (children 20%; adults 12% to 18%), pneumonia (children 15%)

Miscellaneous: Infection (children 44%)

1% to 10%:

Central nervous system: Depression (6% to 9%), neuropathy/neuritis (4%)

Endocrine & metabolic: Serum triglycerides increased (grades 3/4: 4% to 10%), disordered glucose homeostasis (grades 3/4: 2% to 3%), serum amylase increased (grades 3/4: children 9%; adults 2% to 5%), serum lipase increased (grades 3/4: ≤1%)

Gastrointestinal: Dyspepsia (4% to 8%), serum amylase increased (grades 3/4: 8%)

Genitourinary: Hematuria (grades 3/4: 3%)

Hematologic: Anemia (children: 7%), neutropenia (grades 3/4: children 2%; adults 5%)

Hepatic: Transaminases increased (grades 3/4: 2% to 6%), alkaline phosphatase increased (>550 units/L: 1%), bilirubin increased (grades 3/4: 1%)

Neuromuscular & skeletal: Creatinine kinase increased (grades 3/4: 9%), myalgia (4% to 6%), paresthesia (5% to 6%), arthralgia (3% to 5%)

Respiratory: Upper respiratory tract infection (8%), sinusitis (8%), pharyngitis (5%)

Pharmacodynamics/Kinetics

Absorption Rapid, extensive

Bioavailability Capsule: 93%; solution: 75%

Time to Peak Plasma: 1-2 hours

Protein Binding <4%

Half-Life Elimination Normal renal function: Adults: 10 hours; children: 5-18 hours

Metabolism Limited, via oxidation and conjugation (not via CYP isoenzymes)

Excretion Urine (86% primarily as unchanged drug, 13% as metabolites); feces (14%)

Available Dosage Forms

Capsule, oral:

Emtriva®: 200 mg

Solution, oral:

Emtriva®: 10 mg/mL (170 mL)

Dosing

Adult & Geriatric HIV infection: Oral:

Capsule: 200 mg once daily

Solution: 240 mg once daily

Note: Emtricitabine in combination with tenofovir is recommended as a component of first line regimens (with atazanavir/ritonavir, with darunavir/ritonavir, with efavirenz, or with raltegravir) in treatment-naive patients (DHHS,2011).

Pediatric HIV infection: Oral:

Children: 0-3 months: Solution: 3 mg/kg/day

Children: 3 months to 17 years:

Capsule: Children >33 kg: 200 mg once daily

Solution: 6 mg/kg once daily; maximum: 240 mg/day

Renal Impairment Adults (consider similar adjustments in children):

Cl_{cr} 30-49 mL/minute: Capsule: 200 mg every 48 hours; solution: 120 mg every 24 hours

Cl_{cr} 15-29 mL/minute: Capsule: 200 mg every 72 hours; solution: 80 mg every 24 hours

Cl_{cr} <15 mL/minute (including hemodialysis patients): Capsule: 200 mg every 96 hours; solution: 60 mg every 24 hours; administer after dialysis

Hepatic Impairment No adjustment required.

Administration

Oral May be administered with or without food.

Stability

Storage Store capsules at 15°C to 30°C (59°F to 86°F). Solution should be stored under refrigeration at 2°C to 8°C (36°F to 46°F). Once dispensed, may be stored at 15°C to 30°C (59°F to 86°F) if used within 3 months.

Monitoring and Teaching Issues

Laboratory Monitoring Viral load, CD4, liver function tests; hepatitis B testing is recommended prior to initiation of therapy

Physical Assessment Assess viral load and CD4 count. Monitor for lactic acidosis periodically during therapy. Teach patient proper timing of multiple medications.

Patient Education This drug will not cure HIV, nor has it been found to reduce transmission of HIV. Use appropriate precautions to prevent spread to other people. This drug is prescribed as one part of a multi-drug combination; time multiple medications exactly as directed for full course of therapy. Take with or without food. Maintain adequate hydration, unless instructed to restrict fluid intake. Frequent blood tests may be required. May cause hyperpigmentation of hands, soles, or lips (normal). May cause headache, dizziness, insomnia, nausea, vomiting, abdominal pain, and diarrhea. Report persistent fast or rapid heartbeat, weakness or tiredness, muscle pain, respiratory difficulty, gastrointestinal upset, rash, diarrhea, signs of infection (burning on urination, perineal itching, white plaques in mouth, unhealed sores, persistent sore throat, or cough), yellowing of skin or eyes, dark urine, or light stool.

Dietary Considerations May be taken with or without food.

Breast-Feeding Considerations In infants born to mothers who are HIV positive, HAART while breast-feeding may decrease postnatal infection. However, maternal or infant antiretroviral therapy does not completely eliminate the risk of postnatal HIV transmission. In addition, multiclass-resistant virus has been detected in breast-feeding infants despite maternal therapy.

In the United States where formula is accessible, affordable, safe, and sustainable, complete avoidance of breast-feeding by HIV-infected women is recommended to decrease potential transmission of HIV.

Pregnancy Considerations Adverse events were not observed in animal studies. Emtricitabine crosses the placenta; no increased risk of overall birth defects has been observed according to data collected by the antiretroviral pregnancy registry. Cases of lactic acidosis/hepatic steatosis syndrome related to mitochondrial toxicity have been reported in pregnant women receiving nucleoside analogues. It is not known if pregnancy itself potentiates this known side effect; however, women may be at increased risk of lactic acidosis and liver damage. In addition, these adverse events are similar to other rare but life-threatening syndromes which occur during pregnancy (eg, HELLP syndrome). Hepatic enzymes and electrolytes should be monitored frequently during the third trimester of pregnancy and clinicians should watch for early signs of the syndrome. A pharmacokinetic study shows a slight decrease in emtricitabine serum levels during the third trimester; however, there is no clear need to adjust the dose. The Perinatal HIV Guidelines Working Group considers emtricitabine to be an alternative NRTI in dual nucleoside combination regimens. Healthcare providers are encouraged to enroll pregnant women exposed to antiretroviral medications in the Antiretroviral Pregnancy Registry (1-800-258-4263 or www.APRegistry.com). Healthcare providers caring for HIV-infected women and their infants may contact the National Perinatal HIV Hotline (888-448-8765) for clinical consultation.

Additional Information Data suggest that the combination of atazanavir/didanosine and emtricitabine is associated with inferior virologic responses; use is not recommended (DHHS, 2011). If a patient is coinfected with HIV/HBV, use of a single agent active against HBV may lead to HBV resistance; always use emtricitabine with tenofovir in these patients (DHHS, 2011).

Emtricitabine and Tenofovir (em trye SYE ta been & te NOE fo veer)

U.S. Brand Names Truvada®

Index Terms Tenofovir and Emtricitabine

Generic Availability (U.S.) No

Pharmacologic Category Antiretroviral Agent, Reverse Transcriptase Inhibitor (Nucleoside); Antiretroviral Agent, Reverse Transcriptase Inhibitor (Nucleotide)

Pregnancy Risk Factor B

Lactation See individual agents.

Use Treatment of HIV infection in combination with other antiretroviral agents

Unlabeled/Investigational Use Treatment of hepatitis B in patients with antiviral-resistant HBV or coinfection with HIV; pre-exposure prophylaxis (PrEP) for prevention of HIV infection in men who have sex with men who are at high risk for acquiring HIV

Mechanism of Action/Effect Inhibits the production of new HIV virus by blocking the viral enzyme responsible for making DNA from viral RNA.

Contraindications There are no contraindications listed within the FDA-approved labeling.

Warnings/Precautions Not recommended as a component of a triple nucleoside regimen.

[U.S. Boxed Warning]: Lactic acidosis and severe hepatomegaly with steatosis have been reported with nucleoside and nucleotide analogues (eg, tenofovir), including fatal cases. Use with caution in patients with risk factors for liver disease (risk may be increased in obese patients or prolonged exposure) and suspend treatment in any patient who develops clinical or laboratory findings suggestive of lactic acidosis (transaminase elevation may/may not accompany hepatomegaly and steatosis). Use caution in hepatic impairment; no dosage adjustment is required; limited studies indicate the pharmacokinetics of tenofovir are not altered in hepatic dysfunction.

Use caution in moderate renal impairment (Cl_{cr} <50 mL/minute); dosage adjustment required. Calculate creatinine clearance prior to initiation in all patients; monitor renal function during therapy (including recalculation of creatinine clearance and serum phosphorus) in patients at risk for renal impairment, including those with previous renal decline on adefovir. May cause osteomalacia and/or renal toxicity; avoid use in patients with Cl_{cr} <30 mL/minute or concurrent therapy with other nephrotoxic drugs; monitor for possible bone abnormalities during therapy. All patients with HIV should be tested for HBV prior to initiation of treatment.

[U.S. Boxed Warning]: Safety and efficacy during coinfection of HIV and HBV have not been established; acute, severe exacerbations of HBV have been reported following discontinuation of antiretroviral therapy. In HBV coinfected patients, monitor hepatic function closely for several months following discontinuation. May cause redistribution of fat (eg, buffalo hump, peripheral wasting with increased abdominal girth, cushingoid appearance). Immune reconstitution syndrome may develop resulting in the occurrence of an inflammatory response to an indolent or residual opportunistic infection; further evaluation and treatment may be required. Do not use concurrently with adefovir, emtricitabine, tenofovir, lamivudine, or lamivudine-combination products. Safety and efficacy have not been established in pediatric patients.

Drug Interactions

Avoid Concomitant Use

Avoid concomitant use of Emtricitabine and Tenofovir with any of the following: Didanosine; LamiVUDine

Decreased Effect

Emtricitabine and Tenofovir may decrease the levels/effects of: Atazanavir; Didanosine; Protease Inhibitors

The levels/effects of Emtricitabine and Tenofovir may be decreased by: Adefovir

Increased Effect/Toxicity

Emtricitabine and Tenofovir may increase the levels/effects of: Adefovir; Didanosine; Ganciclovir-Valganciclovir

The levels/effects of Emtricitabine and Tenofovir may be increased by: Acyclovir-Valacyclovir; Atazanavir; Ganciclovir-Valganciclovir; LamiVUDine; Lopinavir; Protease Inhibitors; Ribavirin

Nutritional/Ethanol Interactions Food: Food decreases peak plasma concentrations, but does not alter the extent of absorption or overall systemic exposure.

Adverse Reactions The adverse reaction profile of combination therapy has not been established. See individual agents.

Available Dosage Forms

Tablet:

Truvada®: Emtricitabine 200 mg and tenofovir 300 mg

Dosing

Adult & Geriatric Note: Concurrent use with adefovir, emtricitabine, lamivudine, and/or tenofovir alone or as a combination product should be avoided.

HIV: Oral: One tablet (emtricitabine 200 mg and tenofovir 300 mg) once daily

Treatment of hepatitis B in patients with antiviral-resistant HBV or coinfection with HIV (unlabeled use): Oral: One tablet (emtricitabine 200 mg and tenofovir 300 mg) once daily (Lok, 2009)

Pre-exposure prophylaxis (PrEP) for prevention of HIV infection in high-risk men who have sex with men (unlabeled use): Oral: One tablet (emtricitabine 200 mg and tenofovir 300 mg) once daily; in Cl_{cr} <60 mL/minute, use is not recommended (CDC interim guidance, 2011)

Renal Impairment

Cl_{cr} ≥50 mL/minute: No adjustment necessary.

Cl_{cr} 30-49 mL/minute: Increase interval to every 48 hours.

Cl_{cr} <30 mL/minute or hemodialysis: Not recommended.

Hepatic Impairment No dosing adjustment necessary for tenofovir in moderate-to-severe hepatic compromise; no specific data available on emtricitabine in hepatic impairment, but given limited hepatic metabolism, dose adjustments are unlikely.

Administration

Oral May be administered with or without food. If used with didanosine, refer to didanosine monograph for additional information.

Stability

Storage Store tablets at 25°C (77°F); excursions permitted to 15°C to 30°C (59°F to 86°F).

Monitoring and Teaching Issues

Laboratory Monitoring CBC with differential, reticulocyte count, serum creatine kinase, CD4 count, HIV RNA plasma levels, renal and hepatic function tests, serum phosphorus; testing for HBV is recommended prior to the initiation of antiretroviral therapy

High-risk males using therapy for the unlabeled indication of HIV pre-exposure prophylaxis (CDC interim guidance, 2011): Documented negative HIV test (immediately prior to use, then every 2-3 months during therapy), BUN and serum creatinine (prior to initiation, 3 months after initiation, then annually); testing for HBV (prior to initiation) and sexually-transmitted infections (STIs) (prior to initiation, then every 6 months, even if asymptomatic) are also recommended

Physical Assessment See individual agents.

Patient Education See individual agents.

Dietary Considerations May be taken without regard to meals. Consider calcium and vitamin D supplementation in patients with history of bone fracture or osteopenia.

Breast-Feeding Considerations See individual agents.

Pregnancy Considerations See individual agents.

Additional Information When emtricitabine/tenofovir was studied in a large, multinational, randomized, double-blind, placebo-controlled clinical trial for pre-exposure prophylaxis (PrEP) for HIV prevention in men who have sex with men, a 44% reduction in the incidence of HIV acquisition was observed (Grant, 2010). PrEP should be accompanied by a comprehensive HIV prevention program (eg, risk reduction counseling, access to condoms), with particular emphasis on medication adherence. In addition, regular monitoring (eg, HIV status, risk behavior, adherence, adverse effects) is highly recommended. At present, the long-term effects of emtricitabine and tenofovir use in HIV-uninfected men or men who become HIV-infected while on prophylaxis therapy is unknown. (CDC interim guidance, 2011).

- ◆ **Emtricitabine, Efavirenz, and Tenofovir** *see* Efavirenz, Emtricitabine, and Tenofovir *on page 606*
- ◆ **Emtriva®** *see* Emtricitabine *on page 613*
- ◆ **ENA 713** *see* Rivastigmine *on page 1601*
- ◆ **Enablex®** *see* Darifenacin *on page 467*

Enalapril (e NAL a pril)

U.S. Brand Names Vasotec®

Index Terms Enalapril Maleate; Enalaprilat

Generic Availability (U.S.) Yes

Pharmacologic Category Angiotensin-Converting Enzyme (ACE) Inhibitor

Medication Safety Issues

Sound-alike/look-alike issues:

Enalapril may be confused with Anafranil®, Elavil®, Eldepryl®, ramipril

Significant differences exist between oral and I.V. dosing. Use caution when converting from one route of administration to another.

International issues:

Acepril [Hungary, Switzerland] may be confused with Accupril which is a brand name for quinapril [U.S.]

Acepril: Brand name for enalapril [Hungary, Switzerland], but also brand name for captopril [Great Britain]; lisinopril [Malaysia]

Pregnancy Risk Factor C (1st trimester); D (2nd and 3rd trimesters)

Lactation Enters breast milk/not recommended (AAP rates "compatible"; AAP 2001 update pending)

Use Treatment of hypertension; treatment of symptomatic heart failure; treatment of asymptomatic left ventricular dysfunction

Unlabeled/Investigational Use

Unlabeled: To delay the progression of nephropathy and reduce risks of cardiovascular events in hypertensive patients with type 1 or 2 diabetes mellitus; hypertensive crisis, diabetic nephropathy, hypertension secondary to scleroderma renal crisis, diagnosis of aldosteronism, idiopathic edema, Bartter's syndrome, postmyocardial infarction for prevention of ventricular failure

Investigational: Severe congestive heart failure in infants, neonatal hypertension, acute cardiogenic pulmonary edema (enalaprilat)

Mechanism of Action/Effect Competitive inhibitor of angiotensin-converting enzyme (ACE); prevents conversion of angiotensin I to angiotensin II, a potent vasoconstrictor; results in lower levels of angiotensin II which causes an increase in plasma renin activity and a reduction in aldosterone secretion

Contraindications Hypersensitivity to enalapril or enalaprilat; angioedema related to previous treatment with an ACE inhibitor; patients with idiopathic or hereditary angioedema

Warnings/Precautions Anaphylactic reactions may occur rarely with ACE inhibitors. At any time during treatment (especially following first dose) angioedema may occur rarely with ACE inhibitors; it may involve the head and neck (potentially compromising airway) or the intestine (presenting with abdominal pain). African-Americans may be at an increased risk. Prolonged frequent monitoring may be required especially if tongue, glottis, or larynx are involved as they are associated with airway obstruction. Patients with a history of airway surgery may have a higher risk of airway obstruction. Aggressive early and appropriate management is critical. Use in patients with idiopathic or hereditary angioedema or previous angioedema associated with ACE inhibitor therapy is contraindicated. Severe anaphylactoid reactions may be seen during hemodialysis (eg, CVVHD) with high-flux dialysis membranes (eg, AN69), and rarely, during low density lipoprotein apheresis with dextran sulfate cellulose. Rare cases of anaphylactoid reactions have been reported in patients undergoing sensitization treatment with hymenoptera (bee, wasp) venom while receiving ACE inhibitors.

Symptomatic hypotension with or without syncope can occur with ACE inhibitors (usually with the first several doses); effects are most often observed in volume depleted patients; correct volume depletion prior to initiation; close monitoring of patient is required especially with initial dosing and dosing increases; blood pressure must be lowered at a rate appropriate for the patient's clinical condition. Initiation of therapy in patients with ischemic heart disease or cerebrovascular disease warrants close observation due to the potential consequences posed by falling blood pressure (eg, MI, stroke). Use with caution in hypertrophic cardiomyopathy with outflow tract obstruction, severe aortic stenosis, or before, during, or immediately after major surgery. **[U.S. Boxed Warning]: Based on human data, ACEIs can cause injury and death to the developing fetus when used in the second and third trimesters. ACEIs should be discontinued as soon as possible once pregnancy is detected.** Injection contains benzyl alcohol which has been associated with "gasping syndrome" in neonates.

Hyperkalemia may occur with ACE inhibitors; risk factors include renal dysfunction, diabetes mellitus, concomitant use of potassium-sparing diuretics, potassium supplements, and/or potassium-containing salts. Use cautiously, if at all, with these agents and monitor potassium closely. Cough may occur with ACE inhibitors. Other causes of cough should be considered (eg, pulmonary congestion in patients with heart failure) and excluded prior to discontinuation.

May be associated with deterioration of renal function and/or increases in serum creatinine, particularly in patients with low renal blood flow (eg, renal artery stenosis, heart failure) whose glomerular filtration rate (GFR) is dependent on efferent arteriolar vasoconstriction by angiotensin II; deterioration may result in oliguria, acute renal failure, and progressive azotemia. Small increases in serum creatinine may occur following initiation; consider discontinuation only in patients with progressive and/or significant deterioration in renal function. Use with caution in patients with unstented unilateral/bilateral renal artery stenosis. When unstented bilateral renal artery stenosis is present, use is generally avoided due to the elevated risk of deterioration in renal function unless possible benefits outweigh risks. Concurrent use of angiotensin receptor blockers may increase the risk of clinically-significant adverse events (eg, renal dysfunction, hyperkalemia).

Rare toxicities associated with ACE inhibitors include cholestatic jaundice (which may progress to fulminant hepatic necrosis), agranulocytosis, neutropenia or leukopenia with myeloid hypoplasia. Patients with collagen vascular diseases (especially with concomitant renal impairment) or renal impairment alone may be at increased risk for hematologic toxicity; periodically monitor CBC with differential in these patients.

Drug Interactions

Metabolism/Transport Effects Substrate of CYP3A4 (minor)

Avoid Concomitant Use There are no known interactions where it is recommended to avoid concomitant use.

Decreased Effect

The levels/effects of Enalapril may be decreased by: Antacids; Aprotinin; CYP3A4 Inducers (Strong); Deferasirox; Herbs (CYP3A4 Inducers); Herbs (Hypertensive Properties); Methylphenidate; Nonsteroidal Anti-Inflammatory Agents; Salicylates; Yohimbine

Increased Effect/Toxicity

Enalapril may increase the levels/effects of: Allopurinol; Amifostine; Antihypertensives; AzaTHIOprine; CycloSPORINE; CycloSPORINE (Systemic); Ferric Gluconate; Gold Sodium Thiomalate; Hypotensive Agents; Iron Dextran Complex; Lithium; RiTUXimab

The levels/effects of Enalapril may be increased by: Angiotensin II Receptor Blockers; Conivaptan; Diazoxide; DPP-IV Inhibitors; Eplerenone; Everolimus; Herbs (Hypotensive Properties); Loop Diuretics; MAO Inhibitors; Pentoxifylline; Phosphodiesterase 5 Inhibitors;

Potassium Salts; Potassium-Sparing Diuretics; Prostacyclin Analogues; Sirolimus; Temsirolimus; Thiazide Diuretics; TiZANidine; Tolvaptan; Trimethoprim

Nutritional/Ethanol Interactions Herb/Nutraceutical: Avoid bayberry, blue cohosh, cayenne, ephedra, ginger, ginseng (American), kola, licorice (may worsen hypertension). Avoid black cohosh, california poppy, coleus, golden seal, hawthorn, mistletoe, periwinkle, quinine, shepherd's purse (may have increased antihypertensive effect).

Lab Interactions Positive Coombs' [direct]; may cause false-positive results in urine acetone determinations using sodium nitroprusside reagent

Adverse Reactions Note: Frequency ranges include data from hypertension and heart failure trials. Higher rates of adverse reactions have generally been noted in patients with CHF. However, the frequency of adverse effects associated with placebo is also increased in this population.

1% to 10%:

Cardiovascular: Hypotension (0.9% to 7%), chest pain (2%), syncope (0.5% to 2%), orthostasis (2%), orthostatic hypotension (2%)

Central nervous system: Headache (2% to 5%), dizziness (4% to 8%), fatigue (2% to 3%)

Dermatologic: Rash (2%)

Gastrointestinal: Abnormal taste, abdominal pain, vomiting, nausea, diarrhea, anorexia, constipation

Neuromuscular & skeletal: Weakness

Renal: Serum creatinine increased (0.2% to 20%), worsening of renal function (in patients with bilateral renal artery stenosis or hypovolemia)

Respiratory (1% to 2%): Bronchitis, cough, dyspnea

Pharmacodynamics/Kinetics

Onset of Action Oral: ~1 hour, I.V.: ≤15 minutes; Peak effect: Oral: 4-6 hours, I.V.: 1-4 hours

Duration of Action Oral: 12-24 hours; I.V.: ~6 hours

Absorption Oral: 55% to 75%

Time to Peak Serum: Oral: Enalapril: 0.5-1.5 hours; Enalaprilat (active): 3-4.5 hours

Protein Binding 50% to 60%

Half-Life Elimination

Enalapril: Adults: Healthy: 2 hours; Congestive heart failure: 3.4-5.8 hours

Enalaprilat: Infants 6 weeks to 8 months of age: 6-10 hours; Adults: 35-38 hours

Metabolism Prodrug, undergoes hepatic biotransformation to enalaprilat

Excretion Urine (60% to 80%); some feces

Available Dosage Forms

Injection, solution: 1.25 mg/mL (1 mL, 2 mL)

Tablet, oral: 2.5 mg, 5 mg, 10 mg, 20 mg

Vasotec®: 2.5 mg, 5 mg, 10 mg, 20 mg

Dosing

Adult & Geriatric Use lower listed initial dose in patients with hyponatremia, hypovolemia, severe congestive heart failure, decreased renal function, or in those receiving diuretics.

Asymptomatic left ventricular dysfunction: Oral: 2.5 mg twice daily, titrated as tolerated to 20 mg/day

Heart failure:

Oral: Initial: 2.5 mg once or twice daily (usual range: 5-40 mg/day in 2 divided doses). Titrate slowly at 1- to 2-week intervals. Target dose: 10-20 mg twice daily (ACC/AHA 2009 Heart Failure Guidelines)

I.V.: Avoid I.V. administration in patients with unstable heart failure or those suffering acute myocardial infarction.

Hypertension:

Oral: 2.5-5 mg/day then increase as required, usually at 1- to 2-week intervals; usual dose range (JNC 7): 2.5-40 mg/day in 1-2 divided doses. **Note:** Initiate with 2.5 mg if patient is taking a diuretic which cannot be discontinued. May add a diuretic if blood pressure cannot be controlled with enalapril alone.

I.V. (Enalaprilat): 1.25 mg/dose, given over 5 minutes every 6 hours; doses as high as 5 mg/dose every 6 hours have been tolerated for up to 36 hours. **Note:** If patients are concomitantly receiving diuretic therapy, begin with 0.625 mg I.V. over 5 minutes; if the effect is not adequate after 1 hour, repeat the dose and administer 1.25 mg at 6-hour intervals thereafter; if adequate, administer 0.625 mg I.V. every 6 hours.

Conversion from I.V. to oral therapy if not concurrently on diuretics: 5 mg once daily; subsequent titration as needed; if concurrently receiving diuretics and responding to 0.625 mg I.V. every 6 hours, initiate with 2.5 mg/day.

Pediatric

Hypertension: Oral: Children 1 month to 17 years: Initial: 0.08 mg/kg/day (up to 5 mg) in 1-2 divided doses; adjust dosage based on patient response; doses >0.58 mg/kg (40 mg) have not been evaluated in pediatric patients

Heart failure (non-FDA approved):

Infants and Children:

Oral (Enalapril): Initial: 0.1 mg/kg/day in 1-2 divided doses; increase as required over 2 weeks to maximum of 0.5 mg/kg/day; mean dose required for CHF improvement in 39 children (9 days to 17 years) was 0.36 mg/kg/day; investigationally, select individuals have been treated with doses up to 0.94 mg/kg/day

I.V. (Enalaprilat): 5-10 mcg/kg/dose administered every 8-24 hours (as determined by blood pressure readings); monitor patients carefully; select patients may require higher doses

Adolescents: Refer to adult dosing.

Renal Impairment

Oral: Enalapril: Hypertension:

Cl_{cr} 30-80 mL/minute: Administer 5 mg/day titrated upwards to maximum of 40 mg.

Cl_{cr} <30 mL/minute: Administer 2.5 mg day titrated upward until blood pressure is controlled up to a maximum of 40 mg.

For heart failure patients with sodium <130 mEq/L or serum creatinine >1.6 mg/dL, initiate dosage with 2.5 mg/day, increasing to twice daily as needed; increase further in increments of 2.5 mg/dose at >4-day intervals to a maximum daily dose of 40 mg.

I.V.: Enalaprilat:

Cl_{cr} >30 mL/minute: Initiate with 1.25 mg every 6 hours and increase dose based on response.

Cl_{cr} <30 mL/minute: Initiate with 0.625 mg every 6 hours and increase dose based on response.

Moderately dialyzable (20% to 50%)

Administer dose postdialysis (eg, 0.625 mg I.V. every 6 hours) or administer 20% to 25% supplemental dose following dialysis; Clearance: 62 mL/minute

Peritoneal dialysis effects: Supplemental dose is not necessary, although some removal of drug occurs.

Hepatic Impairment Hydrolysis of enalapril to enalaprilat may be delayed and/or impaired in patients with severe hepatic impairment, but the pharmacodynamic effects of the drug do not appear to be significantly altered. No dosage adjustment is necessary.

Administration

I.V. Injection solution: Administer direct IVP over at least 5 minutes or dilute up to 50 mL and infuse.

Stability

Storage Enalaprilat: Clear, colorless solution which should be stored at <30°C. I.V. is stable for 24 hours at room temperature in D_5W or NS.

Monitoring and Teaching Issues

Laboratory Monitoring Serum creatinine and potassium; if patient has collagen vascular disease and/or renal impairment, periodically monitor CBC with differential

Physical Assessment Assess potential for interactions with other pharmacological agents or herbal products that may impact fluid balance or cardiac status. Blood pressure should be closely monitored with first dose or change in dose. Assess results of laboratory tests closely during first 3 months of therapy and regularly thereafter. Monitor for anaphylactic reaction, hypovolemia, angioedema, and postural hypotension.

Patient Education Do not use potassium supplement or salt substitutes without consulting prescriber. Take first dose at bedtime. This drug does not eliminate need for diet or exercise regimen as recommended by prescriber. May cause dizziness, fainting, lightheadedness, postural hypotension, nausea, vomiting, abdominal pain, dry mouth, or transient loss of appetite. Report persistent nausea and vomiting; chest pain or palpitations; mouth sores; fever or chills; swelling of extremities, face, mouth, or tongue; skin rash; numbness, tingling, or pain in muscles; or respiratory difficulty or unusual cough.

Dietary Considerations Limit salt substitutes or potassium-rich diet.

Geriatric Considerations Due to frequent decreases in glomerular filtration (also creatinine clearance) with aging, elderly patients may have exaggerated responses to ACE inhibitors; differences in clinical response due to hepatic changes are not observed. ACE inhibitors may be preferred agents in elderly patients with congestive heart failure and diabetes mellitus. Diabetic proteinuria is reduced and insulin sensitivity is enhanced. In general, the side effect profile is favorable in the elderly and causes little or no CNS confusion; use lowest dose recommendations initially; adjust dose for renal function in the elderly. Many elderly may be volume depleted due to diuretic use and/or blunted thirst reflex resulting in inadequate fluid intake.

Breast-Feeding Considerations Enalapril and enalaprilat are excreted in breast milk. Breast-feeding is not recommended by the manufacturer.

Pregnancy Considerations Due to adverse events observed in some animal studies, enalapril is considered pregnancy category C during the first trimester. Based on human data, enalapril is considered pregnancy category D if used during the second and third trimesters (per the manufacturer; however, one study suggests that fetal injury may occur at anytime during pregnancy). Enalaprilat, the active metabolite of enalapril, crosses the placenta. First trimester exposure to ACE inhibitors may cause major congenital malformations. An increased risk of cardiovascular and/or central nervous system malformations was observed in one study; however, an increased risk of teratogenic events was not observed in other studies. Second and third trimester use of an ACE inhibitor is associated with oligohydramnios. Oligohydramnios due to decreased fetal renal function may lead to fetal limb contractures, craniofacial deformation, and hypoplastic lung development. The use of ACE inhibitors during the second and third trimesters is also associated with anuria, hypotension, renal failure (reversible or irreversible), skull hypoplasia, and death in the fetus/neonate. Chronic maternal hypertension itself is also associated with adverse events in the fetus/infant. ACE inhibitors are not recommended during pregnancy to treat maternal hypertension or heart failure. Those who are planning a pregnancy should be considered for other medication options if an ACE inhibitor is currently prescribed or the ACE inhibitor should be discontinued as soon as possible once pregnancy is detected. The exposed fetus should be monitored for fetal growth, amniotic fluid volume, and organ formation. Infants exposed to an ACE inhibitor *in utero*, especially during the second and third trimester, should be monitored for hyperkalemia, hypotension, and oliguria.

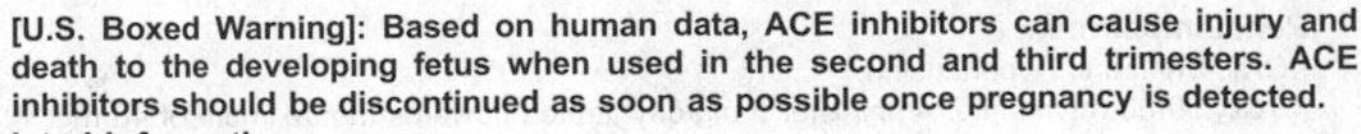

[U.S. Boxed Warning]: Based on human data, ACE inhibitors can cause injury and death to the developing fetus when used in the second and third trimesters. ACE inhibitors should be discontinued as soon as possible once pregnancy is detected.

Related Information

Angiotensin Agents *on page 1974*
Heart Failure (Systolic) *on page 2040*

Enalapril and Felodipine (e NAL a pril & fe LOE di peen)

U.S. Brand Names Lexxel® [DSC]

Index Terms Enalapril Maleate and Felodipine; Felodipine and Enalapril

Generic Availability (U.S.) No

Pharmacologic Category Angiotensin-Converting Enzyme (ACE) Inhibitor; Calcium Channel Blocker; Calcium Channel Blocker, Dihydropyridine

Pregnancy Risk Factor C/D (2nd and 3rd trimesters)

Lactation Enters breast milk/use caution

Use Treatment of hypertension, however, not indicated for initial treatment of hypertension; replacement therapy in patients receiving separate dosage forms (for patient convenience); when monotherapy with one component fails to achieve desired antihypertensive effect, or when dose-limiting adverse effects limit upward titration of monotherapy

Dosing

Adult Hypertension: Oral: Enalapril 5-20 mg and felodipine 2.5-10 mg once daily

Geriatric Recommended initial dose of felodipine is 2.5 mg daily. Titration of individual components is preferred.

Renal Impairment Cl_{cr} <30 mL/minute: Recommended initial dose of enalapril is 2.5 mg/day. Titration of individual components is preferred.

Hepatic Impairment Recommended initial dose of felodipine is 2.5 mg daily. Titration of individual components is preferred.

Monitoring and Teaching Issues

Laboratory Monitoring Serum creatinine and potassium; if patient has collagen vascular disease and/or renal impairment, periodically monitor CBC with differential

Physical Assessment See individual agents.

Patient Education See individual agents.

Related Information

Enalapril *on page 616*
Felodipine *on page 738*

Enalapril and Hydrochlorothiazide (e NAL a pril & hye droe klor oh THYE a zide)

U.S. Brand Names Vaseretic®

Index Terms Enalapril Maleate and Hydrochlorothiazide; Hydrochlorothiazide and Enalapril

Generic Availability (U.S.) Yes

Pharmacologic Category Angiotensin-Converting Enzyme (ACE) Inhibitor; Diuretic, Thiazide

Medication Safety Issues

International issues:

Norpramin: Brand name for enalapril/hydrochlorothiazide [Portugal], but also the brand name for desipramine [U.S., Canada]; omeprazole [Spain]

Pregnancy Risk Factor C/D (2nd and 3rd trimesters)

Lactation Enters breast milk (both ingredients)/compatible

Use Treatment of hypertension

Available Dosage Forms

Tablet: 5/12.5: Enalapril 5 mg and hydrochlorothiazide 12.5 mg; 10/25: Enalapril 10 mg and hydrochlorothiazide 25 mg

Vaseretic®: 10/25: enalapril 10 mg and hydrochlorothiazide 25 mg

Dosing

Adult Hypertension: Oral: Enalapril 5-10 mg and hydrochlorothiazide 12.5-25 mg once daily (maximum: 40 mg/day [enalapril]; 50 mg/day [hydrochlorothiazide])

Geriatric Refer to dosing in individual monographs; adjust for renal impairment.

Renal Impairment

Cl_{cr} >30 mL/minute: Administer usual dose.

Severe renal failure: Avoid; loop diuretics are recommended.

Monitoring and Teaching Issues

Laboratory Monitoring BUN, serum creatinine, and electrolytes; if patient has collagen vascular disease and/or renal impairment, periodically monitor CBC with differential

Physical Assessment See individual agents.

Patient Education See individual agents.

Related Information

Enalapril *on page 616*
Hydrochlorothiazide *on page 912*

◆ **Enalaprilat** *see* Enalapril *on page 616*
◆ **Enalapril Maleate** *see* Enalapril *on page 616*
◆ **Enalapril Maleate and Felodipine** *see* Enalapril and Felodipine *on page 620*

◆ **Enalapril Maleate and Hydrochlorothiazide** *see* Enalapril and Hydrochlorothiazide *on page 620*
◆ **Enbrel®** *see* Etanercept *on page 690*
◆ **Enbrel® SureClick®** *see* Etanercept *on page 690*
◆ **Endocet®** *see* Oxycodone and Acetaminophen *on page 1383*
◆ **Endometrin®** *see* Progesterone *on page 1514*
◆ **Ener-B® [OTC]** *see* Cyanocobalamin *on page 431*
◆ **Enerjets [OTC]** *see* Caffeine *on page 267*

Enfuvirtide (en FYOO vir tide)

U.S. Brand Names Fuzeon®

Index Terms T-20

Generic Availability (U.S.) No

Pharmacologic Category Antiretroviral Agent, Fusion Protein Inhibitor

Pregnancy Risk Factor B

Lactation Excretion in breast milk unknown/contraindicated

Use Treatment of HIV-1 infection in combination with other antiretroviral agents in treatment-experienced patients with evidence of HIV-1 replication despite ongoing antiretroviral therapy

Mechanism of Action/Effect Inhibits the fusion of HIV-1 virus with CD4 cells

Contraindications Hypersensitivity to enfuvirtide or any component of the formulation

Warnings/Precautions Monitor closely for signs/symptoms of pneumonia; associated with an increased incidence during clinical trials, particularly in patients with a low CD4 cell count, high initial viral load, I.V. drug use, smoking, or a history of lung disease. May cause hypersensitivity reactions (symptoms may include rash, fever, nausea, vomiting, hypotension, and elevated transaminases). In addition, local injection site reactions are common. An inflammatory response to indolent or residual opportunistic infections (immune reconstitution syndrome) has occurred with antiretroviral therapy; further investigation is warranted. Administration using a needle-free device has been associated with nerve pain (including neuralgia and/or paresthesia lasting up to 6 months), bruising, and hematomas when administered at sites where large nerves are close to the skin; only administer medication in recommended sites and use caution in patients with coagulation disorders (eg, hemophilia) or receiving anticoagulants. Safety and efficacy have not been established in children <6 years of age.

Drug Interactions

Avoid Concomitant Use There are no known interactions where it is recommended to avoid concomitant use.

Decreased Effect There are no known significant interactions involving a decrease in effect.

Increased Effect/Toxicity

Enfuvirtide may increase the levels/effects of: Protease Inhibitors

The levels/effects of Enfuvirtide may be increased by: Protease Inhibitors

Adverse Reactions

>10%:

Gastrointestinal: Diarrhea (32%), nausea (23%)

Local: Injection site infection (children 11%), injection site reactions (98%; may include pain, erythema, induration, pruritus, ecchymosis, nodule or cyst formation)

1% to 10%:

Dermatologic: Folliculitis (2%)

Gastrointestinal: Weight loss (7%), abdominal pain (4%), appetite decreased (3%), pancreatitis (3%), anorexia (2%), xerostomia (2%)

Hematologic: Eosinophilia (2% to 9%)

Hepatic: Transaminases increased (4%, grade 4: 1%)

Local: Injection site infection (adults 2%)

Neuromuscular & skeletal: CPK increased (3% to 7%), limb pain (3%), myalgia (3%)

Ocular: Conjunctivitis (2%)

Respiratory: Sinusitis (6%), cough (4%), pneumonia (3%)

Miscellaneous: Infections (4% to 6%), herpes simplex (4%), flu-like syndrome (2%)

Pharmacodynamics/Kinetics

Bioavailability 84 ± 16%

Time to Peak 4-8 hours

Protein Binding 92%

Half-Life Elimination 3.8 hours

Metabolism Proteolytic hydrolysis (CYP isoenzymes do not appear to contribute to metabolism)

Clearance: Adults: 24.8 mL/hour/kg

Available Dosage Forms

Injection, powder for reconstitution [preservative free]:

Fuzeon®: 108 mg

Dosing

Adult & Geriatric HIV treatment: SubQ: 90 mg twice daily

Pediatric HIV treatment: SubQ:

Children 6-16 years: 2 mg/kg twice daily (maximum dose: 90 mg twice daily)

Adolescents ≥16 years: Refer to adult dosing.

Renal Impairment

Cl_{cr} >35 mL/minute: Clearance not affected; no dosage adjustment required.

Cl_{cr} ≤35 mL/minute: Limited data showed decreased clearance; however, no dosage adjustment recommended.

End-stage renal disease (on dialysis): Limited data showed decreased clearance; however, no dosage adjustment recommended.

Hepatic Impairment No dosage adjustment required.

Administration

Other Inject subcutaneously into upper arm, abdomen, or anterior thigh. Do not inject into moles, the navel, over a blood vessel or skin abnormalities such as scar tissue, surgical scars, bruises, or tattoos. In addition, do not inject in or near sites where large nerves are close to the skin including the elbow, knee, groin, or buttocks. Rotate injection site, give injections at a site different from the preceding injection site; do not inject into any site where an injection site reaction is evident. Bioequivalence was found to be similar in a study comparing standard administration using a needle versus a needle-free device.

Stability

Reconstitution Reconstitute with 1.1 mL SWFI; tap vial for 10 seconds and roll gently to ensure contact with diluent; then allow to stand until solution is completed; may require up to 45 minutes to form solution (108 mg/1.2 mL).

Storage Store powder at 15°C to 30°C (59°F to 86°F). Reconstituted solutions should be refrigerated and must be used within 24 hours.

Monitoring and Teaching Issues

Physical Assessment Use caution and monitor closely for symptoms of pneumonia with history of I.V. drug use, smoking, or lung disease. Assess CD4 level and viral load. Monitor for pneumonia, neuropathy, and CNS changes on a regular basis throughout therapy. Teach patient or caregiver proper use (eg, reconstitution, injection procedure, needle/syringe disposal, and proper timing of medications). Teach patient report hypersensitivity reactions and injection site infection.

Patient Education This drug will not cure HIV, nor has it been found to reduce transmission of HIV; use appropriate precautions to prevent spread to other persons. This drug is prescribed as one part of a multidrug combination; take exactly as directed for full course of therapy. This drug can only be administered by injection; follow exact injection instructions that come with your medication. Do not mix any other medications in the same syringe. Inject into the upper arm, abdomen, or anterior thigh; do not inject in the same area you did the time before and do not inject around the naval, into scar tissues, a bruise, a mole, or where there is an injection site reaction. Make sure you have an adequate supply of medications on hand; do not allow supply to run out. Do not miss or skip a dose; if you miss a dose, take the missed dose as soon as you can and take the next dose as scheduled. If it is close to the time for the next dose, wait and take the next dose as regularly scheduled. Do not take two doses at the same time. May cause injection site reactions, such as itching, swelling, redness, pain, hardened skin, or bumps. May cause insomnia, anorexia, or constipation. Notify prescriber immediately if you experience a hypersensitivity reaction (rash, fever, nausea, vomiting, hypotension, blood in urine) or injection site becomes infected (red, painful, swollen, drainage). Report CNS disturbances (depression, anxiety), weakness, loss of feeling, muscle pain, respiratory infections, difficulty breathing, flu-like symptoms, unusual cough, fever, alteration in urinary pattern, or swelling of legs or feet.

Breast-Feeding Considerations In infants born to mothers who are HIV positive, HAART while breast-feeding may decrease postnatal infection. However, maternal or infant antiretroviral therapy does not completely eliminate the risk of postnatal HIV transmission. In addition, multiclass-resistant virus has been detected in breast-feeding infants despite maternal therapy.

In the United States where formula is accessible, affordable, safe, and sustainable, complete avoidance of breast-feeding by HIV-infected women is recommended to decrease potential transmission of HIV.

Pregnancy Considerations Teratogenic effects were not observed in animal studies; however, there are no adequate and well-controlled studies in pregnant women, and data is insufficient to recommend use during pregnancy. Limited data suggests that enfuvirtide does not cross the placenta. Healthcare providers are encouraged to enroll pregnant women exposed to antiretroviral medications in the Antiretroviral Pregnancy Registry (1-800-258-4263 or www.APRegistry.com). Healthcare providers caring for HIV-infected women and their infants may contact the National Perinatal HIV Hotline (888-448-8765) for clinical consultation.

- **ENG** *see* Etonogestrel *on page 710*
- **Engerix-B®** *see* Hepatitis B Vaccine (Recombinant) *on page 905*
- **Engerix-B® and Havrix®** *see* Hepatitis A and Hepatitis B Recombinant Vaccine *on page 903*
- **Enhanced-potency Inactivated Poliovirus Vaccine** *see* Poliovirus Vaccine (Inactivated) *on page 1473*
- **Enjuvia™** *see* Estrogens (Conjugated B/Synthetic) *on page 679*
- **Enlon®** *see* Edrophonium *on page 603*

Enoxaparin (ee noks a PA rin)

U.S. Brand Names Lovenox®

Index Terms Enoxaparin Sodium

Generic Availability (U.S.) Yes: Injection solution (preservative free)

Pharmacologic Category Low Molecular Weight Heparin

Medication Safety Issues

Sound-alike/look-alike issues:

Lovenox® may be confused with Lasix®, Levaquin®, Lotronex®, Protonix®

High alert medication: The Institute for Safe Medication Practices (ISMP) includes this medication among its list of drugs which have a heightened risk of causing significant patient harm when used in error.

2009 National Patient Safety Goals: The Joint Commission (TJC) requires healthcare organizations that provide anticoagulant therapy to have a process in place to reduce the risk of anticoagulant-associated patient harm. Patients receiving anticoagulants should receive individualized care through a defined process that includes standardized ordering, dispensing, administration, monitoring and education. This does not apply to routine short-term use of anticoagulants for prevention of venous thromboembolism when the expectation is that the patient's laboratory values will remain within or close to normal values (NPSG.03.05.01).

Pregnancy Risk Factor B

Lactation Excretion in breast milk unknown/use caution

Use

Acute coronary syndromes: Unstable angina (UA), non-ST-elevation (NSTEMI), and ST-elevation myocardial infarction (STEMI)

DVT prophylaxis: Following hip or knee replacement surgery, abdominal surgery, or in medical patients with severely-restricted mobility during acute illness who are at risk for thromboembolic complications

DVT treatment (acute): Inpatient treatment (patients with and without pulmonary embolism) and outpatient treatment (patients without pulmonary embolism)

Note: High-risk patients include those with one or more of the following risk factors: >40 years of age, obesity, general anesthesia lasting >30 minutes, malignancy, history of deep vein thrombosis or pulmonary embolism

Unlabeled/Investigational Use Prophylaxis and treatment of thromboembolism in children; anticoagulant bridge therapy during temporary interruption of vitamin K antagonist therapy in patients at high risk for thromboembolism; DVT prophylaxis following moderate-risk general surgery, major gynecologic surgery and following higher-risk general surgery for cancer; management of venous thromboembolism (VTE) during pregnancy (Hirsh, 2008)

Mechanism of Action/Effect Low molecular weight heparin that blocks factor Xa and IIa to prevent thrombus and clot formation

Contraindications Hypersensitivity to enoxaparin, heparin, or any component of the formulation; thrombocytopenia associated with a positive *in vitro* test for antiplatelet antibodies in the presence of enoxaparin; hypersensitivity to pork products; active major bleeding; not for I.M. use

Warnings/Precautions **[U.S. Boxed Warning]: Spinal or epidural hematomas, including subsequent paralysis, may occur with recent or anticipated neuraxial anesthesia (epidural or spinal anesthesia) or spinal puncture in patients anticoagulated with LMWH or heparinoids.** Consider risk versus benefit prior to spinal procedures; risk is increased by the use of concomitant agents which may alter hemostasis, the use of indwelling epidural catheters for analgesia, a history of spinal deformity or spinal surgery, as well as a history of traumatic or repeated epidural or spinal punctures. Patient should be observed closely for bleeding and signs and symptoms of neurological impairment if therapy is administered during or immediately following diagnostic lumbar puncture, epidural anesthesia, or spinal anesthesia.

Do not administer intramuscularly. Not recommended for thromboprophylaxis in patients with prosthetic heart valves (especially pregnant women). Not to be used interchangeably (unit for unit) with heparin or any other low molecular weight heparins. Use caution in patients with history of heparin-induced thrombocytopenia. Monitor patient closely for signs or symptoms of bleeding. Certain patients are at increased risk of bleeding. Risk factors include bacterial endocarditis; congenital or acquired bleeding disorders; active ulcerative or angiodysplastic GI diseases; severe uncontrolled hypertension; history of hemorrhagic stroke; use shortly after brain, spinal, or ophthalmic surgery; patients treated concomitantly with platelet inhibitors; recent GI bleeding; thrombocytopenia or platelet defects; severe liver disease; hypertensive or diabetic retinopathy; or in patients undergoing invasive procedures. Monitor platelet count closely. Rare cases of thrombocytopenia have occurred. Discontinue therapy and consider alternative treatment if platelets are <100,000/mm^3 and/or thrombosis develops. Rare cases of thrombocytopenia with thrombosis have occurred. Use caution in patients with congenital or drug-induced thrombocytopenia or platelet defects. Risk of bleeding may be increased in women <45 kg and in men <57 kg. Use caution in patients with renal failure; dosage adjustment needed if Cl_{cr} <30 mL/minute. Use with caution in the elderly (delayed elimination may occur); dosage alteration/adjustment may be required (eg, omission of I.V. bolus in acute STEMI in patients ≥75 years of age). Monitor for hyperkalemia; can cause hyperkalemia possibly by suppressing aldosterone production. Multiple-dose vials contain benzyl alcohol (use caution in pregnant women). In neonates, large amounts of benzyl alcohol (>100 mg/kg/day) have been associated with fatal toxicity (gasping syndrome).

There is no consensus for adjusting/correcting the weight-based dosage of LMWH for patients who are morbidly obese (BMI ≥40 kg/m^2). For patients undergoing inpatient bariatric surgery, the American College of Chest Physicians Practice Guidelines suggest using a higher thromboprophylaxis dose of LMWH for obese patients (Geerts, 2008).

Drug Interactions

Avoid Concomitant Use There are no known interactions where it is recommended to avoid concomitant use.

Decreased Effect There are no known significant interactions involving a decrease in effect.

Increased Effect/Toxicity

Enoxaparin may increase the levels/effects of: Anticoagulants; Collagenase (Systemic); Drotrecogin Alfa; Ibritumomab; Tositumomab and Iodine I 131 Tositumomab

The levels/effects of Enoxaparin may be increased by: 5-ASA Derivatives; Antiplatelet Agents; Dasatinib; Herbs (Anticoagulant/Antiplatelet Properties); Nonsteroidal Anti-Inflammatory Agents; Pentosan Polysulfate Sodium; Pentoxifylline; Prostacyclin Analogues; Salicylates; Thrombolytic Agents

Nutritional/Ethanol Interactions Herb/Nutraceutical: Avoid cat's claw, dong quai, evening primrose, feverfew, garlic, ginger, ginkgo, red clover, horse chestnut, green tea, ginseng (all have additional antiplatelet activity).

Lab Interactions Increased AST, ALT levels

Adverse Reactions As with all anticoagulants, bleeding is the major adverse effect of enoxaparin. Hemorrhage may occur at virtually any site. Risk is dependent on multiple variables. At the recommended doses, single injections of enoxaparin do not significantly influence platelet aggregation or affect global clotting time (ie, PT or aPTT).

1% to 10%:

Central nervous system: Fever (5% to 8%), confusion, pain
Dermatologic: Erythema, bruising
Gastrointestinal: Nausea (3%), diarrhea
Hematologic: Hemorrhage (major, <1% to 4%; includes cases of intracranial, retroperitoneal, or intraocular hemorrhage; incidence varies with indication/population), thrombocytopenia (moderate 1%; severe 0.1% - see **"Note"** below), anemia (<2%)
Hepatic: ALT increased, AST increased
Local: Injection site hematoma (9%), local reactions (irritation, pain, ecchymosis, erythema)
Renal: Hematuria (<2%)

Note: Thrombocytopenia with thrombosis: Cases of heparin-induced thrombocytopenia (some complicated by organ infarction, limb ischemia, or death) have been reported.

Pharmacodynamics/Kinetics

Onset of Action Peak effect: SubQ: Antifactor Xa and antithrombin (antifactor IIa): 3-5 hours

Duration of Action 40 mg dose: Antifactor Xa activity: ~12 hours

Protein Binding Does not bind to heparin binding proteins

Half-Life Elimination Plasma: 2-4 times longer than standard heparin, independent of dose; based on anti-Xa activity: 4.5-7 hours

Metabolism Hepatic, to lower molecular weight fragments (little activity)

Excretion Urine (40% of dose; 10% as active fragments)

Available Dosage Forms

Injection, solution:
Lovenox®: 100 mg/mL (3 mL)

Injection, solution [preservative free]: 30 mg/0.3 mL (0.3 mL); 40 mg/0.4 mL (0.4 mL); 60 mg/0.6 mL (0.6 mL); 80 mg/0.8 mL (0.8 mL); 100 mg/mL (1 mL); 120 mg/0.8 mL (0.8 mL); 150 mg/mL (1 mL)
Lovenox®: 30 mg/0.3 mL (0.3 mL); 40 mg/0.4 mL (0.4 mL); 60 mg/0.6 mL (0.6 mL); 80 mg/0.8 mL (0.8 mL); 100 mg/mL (1 mL); 120 mg/0.8 mL (0.8 mL); 150 mg/mL (1 mL)

Dosing

Adult One mg of enoxaparin is equal to 100 int. units of anti-Xa activity (World Health Organization First International Low Molecular Weight Heparin Reference Standard).

DVT prophylaxis: SubQ:

Hip replacement surgery:

Twice-daily dosing: 30 mg every 12 hours, with initial dose within 12-24 hours after surgery, and every 12 hours for at least 10 days or until risk of DVT has diminished or the patient is adequately anticoagulated on warfarin.

Once-daily dosing: 40 mg once daily, with initial dose within 9-15 hours before surgery, and daily for at least 10 days (or up to 35 days postoperatively) or until risk of DVT has diminished or the patient is adequately anticoagulated on warfarin.

Knee replacement surgery: 30 mg every 12 hours, with initial dose within 12-24 hours after surgery, and every 12 hours for at least 10 days or until risk of DVT has diminished or the patient is adequately anticoagulated on warfarin.

Abdominal surgery: 40 mg once daily, with initial dose given 2 hours prior to surgery; continue until risk of DVT has diminished (usually 7-10 days).

Bariatric surgery: Roux-en-Y gastric bypass: Appropriate dosing strategies have not been clearly defined (Borkgren-Okonek, 2008; Scholten, 2002):

BMI ≤50 kg/m^2: 40 mg every 12 hours
BMI >50 kg/m^2: 60 mg every 12 hours

Note: Bariatric surgery guidelines suggest initiation 30-120 minutes before surgery and postoperatively until patient is fully mobile (Mechanick, 2009). Alternatively, limiting administration to the postoperative period may reduce perioperative bleeding.

Medical patients with severely-restricted mobility during acute illness: 40 mg once daily; continue until risk of DVT has diminished (usually 6-11 days).

DVT treatment (acute): SubQ: **Note:** Start warfarin on the first treatment day and continue enoxaparin until INR is between 2 and 3 (usually 5-7 days).

Inpatient treatment (with or without pulmonary embolism): 1 mg/kg/dose every 12 hours or 1.5 mg/kg once daily.

Outpatient treatment (without pulmonary embolism): 1 mg/kg/dose every 12 hours.

Percutaneous coronary intervention (PCI), adjunctive therapy: In enoxaparin-treated patients undergoing PCI, if balloon inflation occurs ≤8 hours after the last SubQ enoxaparin dose, no additional dosing is needed. If balloon inflation occurs 8-12 hours after the last SubQ enoxaparin dose, a single I.V. dose of 0.3 mg/kg should be administered (Hirsh, 2008; King, 2007)

ST-elevation MI (STEMI):

Patients <75 years of age: Initial: 30 mg I.V. single bolus plus 1 mg/kg (maximum 100 mg for the first 2 doses only) SubQ every 12 hours. The first SubQ dose should be administered with the I.V. bolus. Maintenance: After first 2 doses, administer 1 mg/kg SubQ every 12 hours.

Patients ≥75 years of age: Initial: SubQ: 0.75 mg/kg every 12 hours (**Note:** No I.V. bolus is administered in this population); a maximum dose of 75 mg is recommended for the first 2 doses. Maintenance: After first 2 doses, administer 0.75 mg/kg SubQ every 12 hours

Obesity: Use weight-based dosing; a maximum dose of 100 mg is recommended for the first 2 doses (Nutescu, 2009)

Additional notes on STEMI treatment: Therapy was continued for 8 days or until hospital discharge; optimal duration not defined. Unless contraindicated, all patients received aspirin (75-325 mg daily) in clinical trials. In patients with STEMI receiving thrombolytics, initiate enoxaparin dosing between 15 minutes before and 30 minutes after fibrinolytic therapy. In patients undergoing PCI, if balloon inflation occurs ≤8 hours after the last SubQ enoxaparin dose, no additional dosing is needed. If balloon inflation occurs 8-12 hours after last SubQ enoxaparin dose, a single I.V. dose of 0.3 mg/kg should be administered (Hirsh, 2008; King, 2007).

Unstable angina or non-ST-elevation MI (NSTEMI): 1 mg/kg every 12 hours in conjunction with oral aspirin therapy (100-325 mg once daily); continue until clinical stabilization (a minimum of at least 2 days)

Geriatric SubQ: Refer to adult dosing. Increased incidence of bleeding with doses of 1.5 mg/kg/day or 1 mg/kg every 12 hours; injection-associated bleeding and serious adverse reactions are also increased in the elderly. Careful attention should be paid to elderly patients, particularly those <45 kg. **Note:** Dosage alteration/adjustment may be required.

Pediatric One mg of enoxaparin is equal to 100 int. units of anti-Xa activity (World Health Organization First International Low Molecular Weight Heparin Reference Standard).

Thromboembolism (unlabeled use; Monagle, 2008): SubQ:

Infants <2 months: Initial:

Prophylaxis: 0.75 mg/kg every 12 hours

Treatment: 1.5 mg/kg every 12 hours

Infants >2 months and Children ≤18 years: Initial:

Prophylaxis: 0.5 mg/kg every 12 hours

Treatment: 1 mg/kg every 12 hours

Maintenance: See **Dosage Titration** table:

Enoxaparin Pediatric Dosage Titration

Antifactor Xa	Dose Titration	Time to Repeat Antifactor Xa Level
<0.35 units/mL	Increase dose by 25%	4 h after next dose
0.35-0.49 units/mL	Increase dose by 10%	4 h after next dose
0.5-1 unit/mL	Keep same dosage	Next day, then 1 wk later, then monthly (4 h after dose)
1.1-1.5 units/mL	Decrease dose by 20%	Before next dose
1.6-2 units/mL	Hold dose for 3 h and decrease dose by 30%	Before next dose, then 4 h after next dose
>2 units/mL	Hold all doses until antifactor Xa is 0.5 units/mL, then decrease dose by 40%	Before next dose and every 12 h until antifactor Xa <0.5 units/mL

Modified from Monagle P, Michelson AD, Bovill E, et al, "Antithrombotic Therapy in Children," *Chest*, 2001, 119:344S-70S.

Renal Impairment

Cl_{cr} ≥30 mL/minute: No specific adjustment recommended (per manufacturer); monitor closely for bleeding.

Cl_{cr} <30 mL/minute:

DVT prophylaxis in abdominal surgery, hip replacement, knee replacement, or in medical patients during acute illness: SubQ: 30 mg once daily

DVT treatment (inpatient or outpatient treatment in conjunction with warfarin): SubQ: 1 mg/kg once daily

STEMI:

<75 years: Initial: I.V.: 30 mg as a single dose with the first dose of the SubQ maintenance regimen administered at the same time as the I.V. bolus; Maintenance: SubQ: 1 mg/kg every 24 hours

≥75 years of age: Omit I.V. bolus; Maintenance: SubQ: 1 mg/kg every 24 hours

Unstable angina, NSTEMI: SubQ: 1 mg/kg once daily

Dialysis: Enoxaparin has not been FDA approved for use in dialysis patients. It's elimination is primarily via the renal route. Serious bleeding complications have been reported with use in patients who are dialysis dependent or have severe renal failure. LMWH administration at fixed doses without monitoring has greater unpredictable anticoagulant effects in patients with chronic kidney disease. If used, dosages should be reduced and anti-Xa levels frequently monitored, as accumulation may occur with repeated doses. Many clinicians would not use enoxaparin in this population especially without timely anti-Xa levels.

Hemodialysis: Supplemental dose is not necessary.

Peritoneal dialysis: Significant drug removal is unlikely based on physiochemical characteristics.

Administration

I.M. Do **not** administer I.M.

I.V. May be administered I.V. as part of treatment for ST-elevation myocardial infarction (STEMI) only in patients <75 years of age or during PCI. The manufacturer recommends using the multiple-dose vial to prepare I.V. doses. Do not mix or coadminister with other medications.

Other Should be administered by deep SubQ injection to the left or right anterolateral and left or right posterolateral abdominal wall. To avoid loss of drug from the 30 mg and 40 mg syringes, do not expel the air bubble from the syringe prior to injection. In order to minimize bruising, do not rub injection site. An automatic injector (Lovenox EasyInjector™) is available with the 30 mg and 40 mg syringes to aid the patient with self-injections. **Note:** Enoxaparin is available in 100 mg/mL and 150 mg/mL concentrations.

To convert from I.V. unfractionated heparin (UFH) infusion to SubQ enoxaparin (Nutescu, 2007): Calculate specific dose for enoxaparin based on indication, discontinue UFH and begin enoxaparin within 1 hour.

To convert from SubQ enoxaparin to I.V. UFH infusion (Nutescu, 2007): Discontinue enoxaparin, calculate specific dose for I.V. UFH infusion based on indication, omit heparin bolus/loading dose:

Converting from SubQ enoxaparin dosed every 12 hours: Start I.V. UFH infusion 10-11 hours after last dose of enoxaparin

Converting from SubQ enoxaparin dosed every 24 hours: Start I.V. UFH infusion 22-23 hours after last dose of enoxaparin

Stability

Storage Store at 25°C (77°F); excursions permitted to 15°C to 30°C (59°F to 86°F); do not freeze.

Monitoring and Teaching Issues

Laboratory Monitoring Platelets, occult blood, anti-Xa levels, serum creatinine; monitoring of PT and/or aPTT is not necessary. Routine monitoring of anti-Xa levels is not required, but has been utilized in patients with obesity and/or renal insufficiency. Monitoring anti-Xa levels is recommended in pregnant women receiving therapeutic doses of enoxaparin (Hirsh, 2008).

Physical Assessment Use caution in presence or history of conditions that increase risk of bleeding. Monitor for bleeding.

Patient Education This drug can only be administered by injection. If self-administered, follow exact directions for injection and needle disposal. You may have a tendency to bleed easily while taking this drug. Report unusual bleeding or bruising (bleeding gums, nosebleed, blood in urine, dark stool); pain in joints or back; redness, swelling, burning, or pain at injection site; severe headache or confusion; or any rash.

Geriatric Considerations No specific dosage adjustment recommendations for most indications, however, total clearance is lower and elimination is delayed in patients with renal failure. Adjustment may be necessary if renal impairment is present. In the treatment of STEMI, a lower dosage (0.75 mg/kg every 12 hours) and omission of the I.V. bolus, are recommended in patients ≥75 years of age.

Over 2800 patients, ≥65 years of age, have received enoxaparin sodium in pivotal clinical trials. The efficacy of enoxaparin injection in elderly (≥65 years) was similar to that seen in younger patients (<65 years). The incidence of bleeding complications was similar between elderly and younger patients when 30 mg every 12 hours or 40 mg once daily doses of enoxaparin injection was administered at doses of 1.5 mg/kg/day or 1 mg/kg every 12 hours. The risk of enoxaparin injection associated bleeding increased with age. Serious adverse events increased with age for patients receiving enoxaparin injections. Other clinical experience (including postmarketing surveillance and literature reports) has not revealed additional differences in the safety of enoxaparin injection between elderly and younger patients. Careful attention to dosing intervals and concomitant medications (especially antiplatelet medications) is advised. Monitoring of elderly patients with low body weight (<45 kg) and those predisposed to decreased renal function should be considered.

Breast-Feeding Considerations This drug has a high molecular weight that would minimize excretion in breast milk and is inactivated by the GI tract which further reduces the risk to the infant.

Pregnancy Considerations Animal studies have not shown teratogenic or fetotoxic effects. Pregnancy itself increases the risk of thromboembolism. Pregnant women with a history of thromboembolic disease are at increased risk of maternal and fetal complications. Enoxaparin does not cross the placenta. Use may be recommended in pregnant women for the management of VTE. Monitoring antifactor Xa levels is recommended. Risk of adverse events may be increased in pregnant women with mechanical heart valves; use is controversial and has not been adequately studied. Postmarketing reports include congenital abnormalities (cause and effect not established) and also fetal death when used in pregnant women. Multiple-dose vials contain benzyl alcohol; use caution in pregnant women.

◆ **Enoxaparin Sodium** *see* Enoxaparin *on page 622*
◆ **Enpresse®** *see* Ethinyl Estradiol and Levonorgestrel *on page 699*

Entacapone (en TA ka pone)

U.S. Brand Names Comtan®

Generic Availability (U.S.) No

Pharmacologic Category Anti-Parkinson's Agent, COMT Inhibitor

Pregnancy Risk Factor C

Lactation Excretion in breast milk unknown/use caution

Use Adjunct to levodopa/carbidopa therapy in patients with idiopathic Parkinson's disease who experience "wearing-off" symptoms at the end of a dosing interval

Mechanism of Action/Effect Entacapone inhibits COMT peripherally and alters the pharmacokinetics of levodopa so serum levels of levodopa become more sustained when used with levodopa/carbidopa combinations.

Contraindications Hypersensitivity to entacapone or any of component of the formulation

Warnings/Precautions May cause orthostatic hypotension and syncope; Parkinson's disease patients appear to have an impaired capacity to respond to a postural challenge; use with caution in patients at risk of hypotension (such as those receiving antihypertensive drugs) or where transient hypotensive episodes would be poorly tolerated (cardiovascular disease or cerebrovascular disease). Parkinson's patients being treated with dopaminergic agonists ordinarily require careful monitoring for signs and symptoms of postural hypotension, especially during dose escalation, and should be informed of this risk. May cause hallucinations, which may improve with reduction in levodopa therapy. Use with caution in patients with pre-existing dyskinesias; exacerbation of pre-existing dyskinesia and severe rhabdomyolysis has been reported. Levodopa dosage reduction may be required, particularly in patients with levodopa dosages >600 mg daily or with moderate-to-severe dyskinesia prior to initiation. Entacapone, in conjunction with other drug therapy that alters brain biogenic amine concentrations (eg, MAO inhibitors, SSRIs), has been associated with a syndrome resembling neuroleptic malignant syndrome (hyperpyrexia and confusion - some fatal) on abrupt withdrawal or dosage reduction. Concomitant use of entacapone and nonselective MAO inhibitors should be avoided. Selegiline is a selective MAO type B inhibitor (when given orally at ≤10 mg/day) and can be taken with entacapone.

Dopaminergic agents have been associated with compulsive behaviors and/or loss of impulse control, which has manifested as pathological gambling, libido increases (hypersexuality), and/or binge eating. Causality has not been established, and controversy exists as to whether this phenomenon is related to the underlying disease, prior behaviors/addictions and/or drug therapy. Dose reduction or discontinuation of therapy has been reported to reverse these behaviors in some, but not all cases. Risk for melanoma development is increased in Parkinson's disease patients; drug causation or factors contributing to risk have not been established. Patients should be monitored closely and periodic skin examinations should be performed. Dopaminergic agents from the ergot class have also been associated with fibrotic complications, such as retroperitoneal fibrosis, pulmonary infiltrates or effusion and pleural thickening. It is unknown whether non-ergot, pro-dopaminergic agents like entacapone confer this risk. Use caution in patients with hepatic impairment or severe renal impairment. Do not withdraw therapy abruptly. Discoloration of urine, saliva, or sweat to dark colors (red, brown, black) may be observed during therapy. Use with caution in patients with lower gastrointestinal disease or an increased risk of dehydration; has been associated with delayed development of diarrhea (usual onset after 4-12 weeks). Diarrhea may be a sign of drug-induced colitis. Discontinue use with prolonged diarrhea.

Drug Interactions

Metabolism/Transport Effects Inhibits CYP1A2 (weak), 2A6 (weak), 2C9 (weak), 2C19 (weak), 2D6 (weak), 2E1 (weak), 3A4 (weak)

Avoid Concomitant Use There are no known interactions where it is recommended to avoid concomitant use.

Decreased Effect There are no known significant interactions involving a decrease in effect.

Increased Effect/Toxicity

Entacapone may increase the levels/effects of: Alcohol (Ethyl); CNS Depressants; COMT Substrates; MAO Inhibitors; Methotrimeprazine

The levels/effects of Entacapone may be increased by: Droperidol; Methotrimeprazine

Nutritional/Ethanol Interactions

Ethanol: Avoid ethanol (may increase CNS adverse effects).

Food: Entacapone has been reported to chelate iron and decreasing serum iron levels were noted in clinical trials; however, clinically significant anemia has not been observed.

Adverse Reactions

>10%:

Gastrointestinal: Nausea (14%)
Neuromuscular & skeletal: Dyskinesia (25%), placebo (15%)

1% to 10%:

Cardiovascular: Orthostatic hypotension (4%), syncope (1%)
Central nervous system: Dizziness (8%), fatigue (6%), hallucinations (4%), anxiety (2%), somnolence (2%), agitation (1%)
Dermatologic: Purpura (2%)

Gastrointestinal: Diarrhea (10%), abdominal pain (8%), constipation (6%), vomiting (4%), dry mouth (3%), dyspepsia (2%), flatulence (2%), gastritis (1%), taste perversion (1%)

Genitourinary: Brown-orange urine discoloration (10%)

Neuromuscular & skeletal: Hyperkinesia (10%), hypokinesia (9%), back pain (4%), weakness (2%)

Respiratory: Dyspnea (3%)

Miscellaneous: Diaphoresis increased (2%), bacterial infection (1%)

Pharmacodynamics/Kinetics

Onset of Action Rapid; Peak effect: 1 hour

Absorption Rapid

Bioavailability 35%

Time to Peak Serum: 1 hour

Protein Binding 98%, primarily to albumin

Half-Life Elimination B phase: 0.4-0.7 hours; Y phase: 2.4 hours

Metabolism Isomerization to the *cis*-isomer, followed by direct glucuronidation of the parent and *cis*-isomer

Excretion Feces (90%); urine (10%)

Available Dosage Forms

Tablet, oral:

Comtan®: 200 mg

Dosing

Adult & Geriatric Parkinson's disease: Oral: 200 mg with each dose of levodopa/carbidopa, up to a maximum of 8 times/day (maximum daily dose: 1600 mg/day). To optimize therapy, the dosage of levodopa may need reduced or the dosing interval may need extended. Patients taking levodopa ≥800 mg/day or who had moderate-to-severe dyskinesias prior to therapy required an average decrease of 25% in the daily levodopa dose.

Renal Impairment No adjustment is required; dialysis patients were not studied.

Hepatic Impairment Dosage adjustment in chronic therapy with standard treatment has not been studied.

Administration

Oral Always administer in association with levodopa/carbidopa; can be combined with both the immediate and sustained release formulations of levodopa/carbidopa. May be administered without regard to meals. Should not be abruptly withdrawn from patient's therapy due to significant worsening of symptoms.

Monitoring and Teaching Issues

Laboratory Monitoring Liver function tests, serum iron (if signs of anemia)

Physical Assessment Monitor for postural hypotension, increased dyskinesias, and CNS changes (hallucinations, compulsive behaviors). Periodic skin examinations should be performed; risk for melanoma is increased in Parkinson's disease. Taper dose when discontinuing. Teach patient proper timing of multiple medications.

Patient Education This drug is prescribed as one part of a multidrug combination; take exactly as directed for full course of therapy. Avoid alcohol. Periodic laboratory tests and skin exams may be required. May cause dizziness, fatigue, sleepiness, postural hypotension, unusual taste, nausea, vomiting, flatulence, upset stomach, or brown- or orange-colored urine (normal). Report any CNS changes (unusual compulsiveness, increased libido, binge eating), any new or increased abnormal skeletal movements or weakness, persistent gastrointestinal problems, hallucinations, changes in the appearance of skin moles, or other unusual skin changes.

Dietary Considerations May be taken without regard to meals.

Geriatric Considerations No difference in adverse effects was noted in the elderly. Monitor levodopa dose.

Pregnancy Considerations Not recommended

◆ **Entacapone, Carbidopa, and Levodopa** *see* Levodopa, Carbidopa, and Entacapone *on page* 1091

◆ **Entereg®** *see* Alvimopan *on page* 90

◆ **Enterotoxigenic *Escherichia coli* and *Vibrio cholera* Vaccine** *see* Travelers' Diarrhea and Cholera Vaccine *on page* 1806

◆ **Entocort® EC** *see* Budesonide (Systemic, Oral Inhalation) *on page* 235

◆ **Enulose** *see* Lactulose *on page* 1053

◆ **EPEG** *see* Etoposide *on page* 712

◆ **Epidoxorubicin** *see* Epirubicin *on page* 633

◆ **Epiduo®** *see* Adapalene and Benzoyl Peroxide *on page* 52

◆ **Epiklor™** *see* Potassium Chloride *on page* 1480

◆ **Epiklor™/25** *see* Potassium Chloride *on page* 1480

Epinastine (ep i NAS teen)

U.S. Brand Names Elestat®

Index Terms Epinastine Hydrochloride

Generic Availability (U.S.) No

Pharmacologic Category Histamine H_1 Antagonist; Histamine H_1 Antagonist, Second Generation

Pregnancy Risk Factor C

Lactation Excretion in breast milk unknown/use caution

Use Treatment of allergic conjunctivitis

Available Dosage Forms

Solution, ophthalmic:

Elestat®: 0.05% (5 mL)

Dosing

Adult & Geriatric Allergic conjunctivitis: Ophthalmic: Instill 1 drop into each eye twice daily. Continue throughout period of exposure, even in the absence of symptoms.

Pediatric Allergic conjunctivitis: Ophthalmic: Children ≥3 years: Refer to adult dosing.

Administration

Other For ophthalmic use only; avoid touching tip of applicator to eye or other surfaces. Contact lenses should be removed prior to application, may be reinserted after 10 minutes. Do not wear contact lenses if eyes are red.

Monitoring and Teaching Issues

Physical Assessment For ophthalmic use only.

Patient Education For ophthalmic use only. Do not wear contact lenses if eyes are red. May cause headache. Wash hands before using. Remove contact lenses before application (may be reinserted after 10 minutes). Gently pull lower eyelid forward and instill prescribed amount in lower eyelid. Avoid touching tip of dropper to eye. Close eye and roll eyeball in all directions. May cause blurred vision, temporary stinging, or burning sensation.

◆ **Epinastine Hydrochloride** *see* Epinastine *on page 628*

EPINEPHrine (Systemic, Oral Inhalation) (ep i NEF rin)

U.S. Brand Names Adrenaclick™ [DSC]; Adrenalin®; EpiPen 2-Pak®; EpiPen Jr 2-Pak®; EpiPen®; EpiPen® Jr.; Primatene® Mist [OTC]; S2® [OTC]; Twinject®

Index Terms Adrenaline; Epinephrine Bitartrate; Epinephrine Hydrochloride; Racemic Epinephrine; Racepinephrine

Generic Availability (U.S.) Yes: Solution for injection

Pharmacologic Category Alpha/Beta Agonist

Medication Safety Issues

Sound-alike/look-alike issues:

EPINEPHrine may be confused with ePHEDrine

Epifrin® may be confused with ephedrine, EpiPen®

EpiPen® may be confused with Epifrin®

High alert medication: The Institute for Safe Medication Practices (ISMP) includes this medication among its list of drugs which have a heightened risk of causing significant patient harm when used in error.

Medication errors have occurred due to confusion with epinephrine products expressed as ratio strengths (eg, 1:1000 vs 1:10,000).

Epinephrine 1:1000 = 1 mg/mL and is most commonly used I.M.

Epinephrine 1:10,000 = 0.1 mg/mL and is used I.V.

Medication errors have occurred when topical epinephrine 1 mg/mL (1:1000) has been inadvertently injected. Vials of injectable and topical epinephrine look very similar. Epinephrine should always be appropriately labeled with the intended administration.

International issues:

EpiPen [U.S., Canada, and multiple international markets] may be confused with Epigen brand name for glycyrrhizinic acid [Argentina, Mexico, Russia] and Epopen brand name for epoetin alfa [Spain]

Pregnancy Risk Factor C

Lactation Excretion in breast milk unknown

Use Treatment of bronchospasms, bronchial asthma, viral croup, anaphylactic reactions, cardiac arrest; added to local anesthetics to decrease systemic absorption of intraspinal and local anesthetics and increase duration of action; decrease superficial hemorrhage

Unlabeled/Investigational Use ACLS guidelines: Ventricular fibrillation (VF) or pulseless ventricular tachycardia (VT) unresponsive to initial defibrillatory shocks; pulseless electrical activity; asystole; hypotension/shock unresponsive to volume resuscitation; symptomatic bradycardia unresponsive to atropine or pacing; inotropic support

Mechanism of Action/Effect Stimulates alpha-, beta$_1$-, and beta$_2$-adrenergic receptors resulting in relaxation of smooth muscle of the bronchial tree, cardiac stimulation (increasing myocardial oxygen consumption), and dilation of skeletal muscle vasculature; small doses can cause vasodilation via beta$_2$-vascular receptors; large doses may produce constriction of skeletal and vascular smooth muscle

Contraindications There are no absolute contraindications to the use of injectable epinephrine (including EpiPen®, EpiPen® Jr, and Twinject®) in a life-threatening situation.

Oral inhalation: Concurrent use or within 2 weeks of MAO inhibitors

Injectable solution: Per the manufacturer, contraindicated in narrow-angle glaucoma; shock; during general anesthesia with halogenated hydrocarbons or cyclopropane (currently not available in U.S.); individuals with organic brain damage; with local anesthesia of the digits; during labor; heart failure; coronary insufficiency

Warnings/Precautions Use with caution in elderly patients, patients with diabetes mellitus, cardiovascular diseases (eg, coronary artery disease, hypertension), thyroid disease, cerebrovascular disease, Parkinson's disease, or patients taking tricyclic antidepressants. Some products contain sulfites as preservatives; the presence of sulfites in some products (eg, EpiPen® and Twinject®) should not deter administration during a serious allergic or other emergency situation even if the patient is sulfite-sensitive. Accidental injection into digits, hands, or feet may result in local reactions, including injection site pallor, coldness and hypoesthesia or injury, resulting in bruising, bleeding, discoloration, erythema or skeletal injury; patient should seek immediate medical attention if this occurs. Rapid I.V. administration may cause death from cerebrovascular hemorrhage or cardiac arrhythmias; however, rapid I.V. administration during pulseless arrest is necessary.

Oral inhalation: Use with caution in patients with prostate enlargement or urinary retention; may cause temporary worsening of symptoms.

Self medication (OTC use): Oral inhalation: Prior to self-medication, patients should contact healthcare provider. The product should only be used in persons with a diagnosis of asthma. If symptoms are not relieved in 20 minutes or become worse do not continue to use the product - seek immediate medical assistance. The product should not be used more frequently or at higher doses than recommended unless directed by a healthcare provider. This product should not be used in patients who have required hospitalization for asthma or if a patient is taking prescription medication for asthma. Do not use if you have taken a MAO inhibitor (certain drugs used for depression, Parkinson's disease, or other conditions) within 2 weeks.

Drug Interactions

Avoid Concomitant Use

Avoid concomitant use of EPINEPHrine (Systemic, Oral Inhalation) with any of the following: Iobenguane I 123; Lurasidone

Decreased Effect

EPINEPHrine (Systemic, Oral Inhalation) may decrease the levels/effects of: Benzylpenicilloyl Polylysine; Iobenguane I 123

The levels/effects of EPINEPHrine (Systemic, Oral Inhalation) may be decreased by: Spironolactone

Increased Effect/Toxicity

EPINEPHrine (Systemic, Oral Inhalation) may increase the levels/effects of: Bromocriptine; Lurasidone; Sympathomimetics

The levels/effects of EPINEPHrine (Systemic, Oral Inhalation) may be increased by: Antacids; Atomoxetine; Beta-Blockers; Cannabinoids; Carbonic Anhydrase Inhibitors; COMT Inhibitors; Inhalational Anesthetics; MAO Inhibitors; Serotonin/Norepinephrine Reuptake Inhibitors; Tricyclic Antidepressants

Nutritional/Ethanol Interactions Herb/Nutraceutical: Avoid ephedra, yohimbe (may cause CNS stimulation).

Adverse Reactions Frequency not defined.

Cardiovascular: Angina, cardiac arrhythmia, chest pain, flushing, hypertension, pallor, palpitation, sudden death, tachycardia (parenteral), vasoconstriction, ventricular ectopy

Central nervous system: Anxiety (transient), apprehensiveness, cerebral hemorrhage, dizziness, headache, insomnia, lightheadedness, nervousness, restlessness

Gastrointestinal: Dry throat, loss of appetite, nausea, vomiting, xerostomia

Genitourinary: Acute urinary retention in patients with bladder outflow obstruction

Neuromuscular & skeletal: Tremor, weakness

Ocular: Allergic lid reaction, burning, eye pain, ocular irritation, precipitation of or exacerbation of narrow-angle glaucoma, transient stinging

Respiratory: Dyspnea, pulmonary edema

Miscellaneous: Diaphoresis

Pharmacodynamics/Kinetics

Onset of Action Bronchodilation: SubQ: ~5-10 minutes; Inhalation: ~1 minute

Metabolism Taken up into the adrenergic neuron and metabolized by monoamine oxidase and catechol-o-methyltransferase; circulating drug hepatically metabolized

Excretion Urine (as inactive metabolites, metanephrine, and sulfate and hydroxy derivatives of mandelic acid; small amounts as unchanged drug)

Available Dosage Forms

Aerosol, for oral inhalation:

Primatene® Mist [OTC]: 0.22 mg/inhalation (15 mL)

Injection, solution: 0.1 mg/mL (10 mL); 0.15 mg/0.15 mL (1.1 mL); 0.3 mg/0.3 mL (1.1 mL); 1 mg/mL (1 mL, 30 mL)

Adrenalin®: 1 mg/mL (1 mL, 30 mL)

EpiPen 2-Pak®: 0.3 mg/0.3 mL (2 mL)

EpiPen Jr 2-Pak®: 0.15 mg/0.3 mL (2 mL)

EpiPen®: 0.3 mg/0.3 mL (2 mL)

EpiPen® Jr.: 0.15 mg/0.3 mL (2 mL)

Twinject®: 0.15 mg/0.15 mL (1.1 mL); 0.3 mg/0.3 mL (1.1 mL)

Injection, solution [preservative free]: 1 mg/mL (1 mL)

Solution, for oral inhalation [preservative free]:

S2® [OTC]: 2.25% (0.5 mL)

Dosing

Adult & Geriatric

Asystole/pulseless arrest, pulseless VT/VF (ACLS, 2010):

I.V., I.O.: 1 mg every 3-5 minutes until return of spontaneous circulation; if this approach fails, higher doses of epinephrine (up to 0.2 mg/kg) have been used for treatment of specific problems (eg, beta-blocker or calcium channel blocker overdose)

Intratracheal: 2-2.5 mg every 3-5 minutes until I.V./I.O access established or return of spontaneous circulation; dilute in 5-10 mL NS or sterile water. **Note:** Absorption may be greater with sterile water (Naganobu, 2000).

Bradycardia (symptomatic; unresponsive to atropine or pacing): *I.V. infusion:* 2-10 mcg/minute **or** 0.1-0.5 mcg/kg/minute (7-35 mcg/minute in a 70 kg patient); titrate to desired effect (ACLS, 2010)

Bronchodilator:

SubQ: 0.3-0.5 mg (**1:1000** solution) every 20 minutes for 3 doses

Nebulization: S2® (racepinephrine, OTC labeling):

Hand-bulb nebulizer: Add 0.5 mL (~10 drops) to nebulizer; 1-3 inhalations up to every 3 hours if needed

Jet nebulizer: Add 0.5 mL (~10 drops) to nebulizer and dilute with 3 mL of NS; administer over ~15 minutes every 3-4 hours as needed

Inhalation: Primatene® Mist (OTC labeling): One inhalation, wait at least 1 minute; if not relieved, may use once more. Do not use again for at least 3 hours.

Hypersensitivity reaction: Note: SubQ administration results in slower absorption and is less reliable. I.M. administration in the anterolateral aspect of the middle third of the thigh is preferred in the setting of anaphylaxis (ACLS guidelines, 2010; Kemp, 2008).

I.M., SubQ: 0.2-0.5 mg (**1:1000** solution) every 5-15 minutes in the absence of clinical improvement (ACLS 2010; Kemp, 2008; Lieberman, 2010). If clinician deems appropriate, the 5-minute interval between injections may be shortened to allow for more frequent administration (Lieberman, 2010).

I.V.: 0.1 mg (**1:10,000** solution) over 5 minutes; may infuse at 1-4 mcg/minute to prevent the need to repeat injections frequently **or** may initiate with an infusion at 5-15 mcg/minute (with crystalloid administration) (ACLS, 2010; Brown, 2004). In general, I.V. administration should only be done in patients who are profoundly hypotensive or are in cardiopulmonary arrest refractory to volume resuscitation and several epinephrine injections (Lieberman, 2010).

Self-administration following severe allergic reactions (eg, insect stings, food): **Note:** The World Health Organization (WHO) and Anaphylaxis Canada recommend the availability of one dose for every 10-20 minutes of travel time to a medical emergency facility. More than 2 doses should only be administered under direct medical supervision.

Twinject®: I.M., SubQ: 0.3 mg; if anaphylactic symptoms persist, dose may be repeated in 5-15 minutes using the same device after partial disassembly

EpiPen®: I.M., SubQ: 0.3 mg; if anaphylactic symptoms persist, dose may be repeated in 5-15 minutes using an additional EpiPen®

Hypotension/shock, severe and fluid resistant (unlabeled use): *I.V. infusion:* Initial: 0.1-0.5 mcg/kg/minute (7-35 mcg/minute in a 70 kg patient); titrate to desired response (ACLS, 2010)

Pediatric

Cardiac arrest: Neonates (Neonatal resuscitation guidelines, 2010):

I.V.: 0.01-0.03 mg/kg (0.1-0.3 mL/kg of **1:10,000** solution) every 3-5 minutes until return of spontaneous circulation

Intratracheal: Although I.V. route is preferred, may administer 0.05-0.1 mg/kg (0.5-1 mL/kg of **1:10,000** solution) every 3-5 minutes until I.V. access established or return of spontaneous circulation

Asystole/pulseless arrest, pulseless VT/VF (after failed defibrillation attempts) (PALS, 2010): Infants and Children:

I.V., I.O.: 0.01 mg/kg (0.1 mL/kg of **1:10,000** solution) (maximum single dose: 1 mg) every 3-5 minutes until return of spontaneous circulation

Intratracheal: 0.1 mg/kg (0.1 mL/kg of **1:1000** solution) (maximum single dose: 2.5 mg) every 3-5 minutes until I.V./I.O access established or return of spontaneous circulation

Postresuscitation infusion to maintain cardiac output or stabilize: I.V., I.O.: 0.1-1 mcg/kg/minute; doses <0.3 mcg/kg/minute generally produce beta-adrenergic effects and higher doses (>0.3 mcg/kg/minute) generally produce alpha-adrenergic vasoconstriction; titrate dosage to desired effect

Bradycardia (symptomatic; unresponsive to atropine or pacing): Infants and Children:

I.V., I.O.: 0.01 mg/kg (0.1 mL/kg of **1:10,000** solution) (maximum single dose: 1 mg) every 3-5 minutes as needed

Intratracheal: 0.1 mg/kg or (0.1 mL/kg of **1:1000** solution) (maximum single dose: 2.5 mg) every 3-5 minutes as needed until I.V./I.O. access established

Continuous infusion: I.V., I.O.: 0.1-1 mcg/kg/minute; doses <0.3 mcg/kg/minute generally produce beta-adrenergic effects and higher doses (>0.3 mcg/kg/minute) generally produce alpha-adrenergic vasoconstriction; titrate dosage to desired effect

Bronchodilator:

SubQ: Infants and Children: 0.01 mg/kg (0.01 mL/kg of **1:1000** solution) (maximum single dose: 0.5 mg) every 20 minutes for 3 doses

Nebulization: S2® (racepinephrine, OTC labeling):

Children <4 years: Jet nebulizer: Croup: 0.05 mL/kg (maximum dose: 0.5 mL); dilute in 3 mL of NS. Administer over ~15 minutes; do not administer more frequently than every 2 hours

Children ≥4 years: Refer to adult dosing.

Inhalation: Children ≥4 years: Primatene® Mist: Refer to adult dosing.

Hypersensitivity reaction: Infants and Children: **Note:** SubQ administration results in slower absorption and is less reliable. I.M. administration in the anterolateral aspect of the middle third of the thigh is preferred in the setting of anaphylaxis (ACLS guidelines, 2010; Kemp, 2008).

I.M., SubQ: 0.01 mg/kg (0.01 mL/kg of **1:1000** solution) (maximum single dose: 0.3 mg) every 5-15 minutes; larger I.M. or SubQ doses, use of I.V. route, or continuous infusion may be needed for severe anaphylactic reactions (Kemp, 2008; Lieberman, 2010). If clinician deems appropriate, the 5-minute interval between injections may be shortened to allow for more frequent administration (Lieberman, 2010).

Self-administration following severe allergic reactions (eg, insect stings, food): **Note:** World Health Organization (WHO) and Anaphylaxis Canada recommend the availability of 1 dose for every 10-20 minutes of travel time to a medical emergency facility:

EpiPen® Jr: I.M., SubQ: Children 15-29 kg: 0.15 mg; if anaphylactic symptoms persist, dose may be repeated in 5-15 minutes using an additional EpiPen® Jr

EpiPen®: I.M., SubQ: Children ≥30 kg: 0.3 mg; if anaphylactic symptoms persist, dose may be repeated in 5-15 minutes using an additional EpiPen®

Twinject®: I.M., SubQ:

Children 15-29 kg: 0.15 mg; if anaphylactic symptoms persist, dose may be repeated in 5-15 minutes using the same device after partial disassembly

Children ≥30 kg: 0.3 mg; if anaphylactic symptoms persist, dose may be repeated in 5-15 minutes using the same device after partial disassembly

Alternate auto-injector dose: I.M. (Sicherer, 2007):

Children 10-25 kg: 0.15 mg

Children >25 kg: 0.3 mg

Hypotension/shock, fluid-resistant (unlabeled use): Continuous I.V. infusion: 0.1-1 mcg/kg/minute; doses up to 5 mcg/kg/minute may rarely be necessary (Hegenbarth, 2008)

Administration

I.M. I.M. administration into the buttocks should be avoided. I.M. administration in the anterolateral aspect of the middle third of the thigh is preferred in the setting of anaphylaxis (ACLS guidelines, 2010; Kemp, 2008). EpiPen®, EpiPen® Jr, and Twinject® Auto-Injectors should only be injected into the anterolateral aspect of the thigh, through clothing if necessary.

Note: EpiPen® and EpiPen® Jr Auto-Injectors contain a single, fixed-dose of epinephrine. Twinject® Auto-Injectors contain two doses; the first fixed-dose is available for auto-injection; the second dose is available for manual injection following partial disassembly of device.

I.V. When administering as a continuous infusion, central line administration is preferred. I.V. infusions require an infusion pump.

Inhalation S2®: If using jet nebulizer: Administer over ~15 minutes; must be diluted. If using hand-held rubber bulb nebulizer, dilution is not required.

Other

Intratracheal: Dilute in NS or sterile water. Absorption may be greater with sterile water (Naganobu, 2000). Pass catheter beyond tip of tracheal tube, stop compressions, spray drug quickly down tube. Follow immediately with several quick insufflations and continue chest compressions.

Subcutaneous: SubQ administration results in slower absorption and is less reliable. I.M. administration into the buttocks should be avoided. I.M. administration in the anterolateral aspect of the middle third of the thigh is preferred in the setting of anaphylaxis (ACLS guidelines, 2010; Kemp, 2008). EpiPen®, EpiPen® Jr, and Twinject® Auto-Injectors should only be injected into the anterolateral aspect of the thigh, through clothing if necessary.

Note: EpiPen® and EpiPen® Jr Auto-Injectors contain a single, fixed-dose of epinephrine. Twinject® Auto-Injectors contain two doses; the first fixed-dose is available for auto-injection; the second dose is available for manual injection following partial disassembly of device.

Stability

Reconstitution

S2®: Dilution not required when administered via hand-bulb nebulizer; dilute with NS 3-5 mL if using jet nebulizer.

Standard I.V. diluent: 1 mg/250 mL NS.

Preparation of adult I.V. infusion: Dilute 1 mg in 250 mL of D_5W or NS (4 mcg/mL).

Storage Epinephrine is sensitive to light and air. Protection from light is recommended. Oxidation turns drug pink, then a brown color. **Solutions should not be used if they are discolored or contain a precipitate.**

Adrenalin®: Store between 15°C to 25°C (59°F to 77°F); do not freeze. Protect from light. The 1:1000 solution should be discarded 30 days after initial use.

EpiPen® and EpiPen® Jr: Store at 25°C (77°F); excursions permitted to 15°C to 30°C (59°F to 86°F); do not freeze or refrigerate. Protect from light by storing in carrier tube provided.

Twinject®: Store between 20°C to 25°C (68°F to 77°F); excursions permitted to 15°C to 30°C (59°F to 86°F); do not freeze or refrigerate. Protect from light.

Primatene® Mist: Store between 20°C to 25°C (68°F to 77°F).

S2®: Store between 2°C to 20°C (36°F to 68°F). Protect from light.

Stability of injection of parenteral admixture at room temperature (25°C) or refrigeration (4°C) is 24 hours.

Monitoring and Teaching Issues

Physical Assessment Monitor vital signs. I.V. central line with infusion pump and continuous cardiac/hemodynamic monitoring is necessary.

Patient Education Avoid other stimulants to avoid serious overdose reactions. You may experience dizziness, blurred vision, restlessness, or difficulty urinating. Report excessive nervousness or excitation, inability to sleep, facial flushing, pounding heartbeat, muscle tremors or weakness, chest pain or palpitations, or increased sweating.

Aerosol: Use aerosol or nebulizer as per instructions. Clear as much mucus as possible before use. Rinse mouth following each use. If more than one inhalation is necessary, wait 1 minute between inhalations. May cause restlessness or nervousness. Report persistent nervousness, restlessness, sleeplessness, palpitations, tachycardia, chest pain, muscle tremors, dizziness, flushing, or if breathing difficulty persists.

Geriatric Considerations The use of epinephrine in the treatment of acute exacerbations of asthma was studied in the elderly. A dose of 0.3 mg SubQ every 20 minutes for three doses was well tolerated in elderly patients with no history of angina or recent myocardial infarction. There was no significant difference in the incidence of ventricular arrhythmias in elderly versus younger adults.

Pregnancy Considerations Teratogenic effects have been observed in animal reproduction studies. Epinephrine crosses the placenta and may cause fetal anoxia. Use during pregnancy when the potential benefit to the mother outweighs the possible risk to the fetus.

Additional Information Twinject® and EpiPen® are not interchangeable due to packaging considerations.

EPINEPHrine (Nasal) (ep i NEF rin)

U.S. Brand Names Adrenalin®

Index Terms Adrenaline; Epinephrine Hydrochloride

Generic Availability (U.S.) No

Pharmacologic Category Alpha/Beta Agonist

Medication Safety Issues

Sound-alike/look-alike issues:

EPINEPHrine may be confused with ePHEDrine

Use Treatment of nasal congestion

Available Dosage Forms

Solution, intranasal:

Adrenalin®: 1 mg/mL (30 mL)

Dosing

Adult & Geriatric Decongestant: *Intranasal:* Apply **1:1000** solution locally as drops or spray or with sterile swab

Pediatric Decongestant: Children ≥6 years: Refer to adult dosing

Monitoring and Teaching Issues

Physical Assessment Monitor vital signs.

Patient Education Avoid other stimulants to avoid serious overdose reactions. You may experience dizziness, blurred vision, restlessness, or difficulty urinating. Report excessive nervousness or excitation, inability to sleep, facial flushing, pounding heartbeat, muscle tremors or weakness, chest pain or palpitations, or increased sweating.

- ◆ **Epinephrine and Lidocaine** *see* Lidocaine and Epinephrine *on page 1109*
- ◆ **Epinephrine Bitartrate** *see* EPINEPHrine (Systemic, Oral Inhalation) *on page 629*
- ◆ **Epinephrine Hydrochloride** *see* EPINEPHrine (Nasal) *on page 633*
- ◆ **Epinephrine Hydrochloride** *see* EPINEPHrine (Systemic, Oral Inhalation) *on page 629*
- ◆ **EpiPen®** *see* EPINEPHrine (Systemic, Oral Inhalation) *on page 629*
- ◆ **EpiPen 2-Pak®** *see* EPINEPHrine (Systemic, Oral Inhalation) *on page 629*
- ◆ **EpiPen® Jr.** *see* EPINEPHrine (Systemic, Oral Inhalation) *on page 629*
- ◆ **EpiPen Jr 2-Pak®** *see* EPINEPHrine (Systemic, Oral Inhalation) *on page 629*
- ◆ **Epipodophyllotoxin** *see* Etoposide *on page 712*
- ◆ **Epipodophyllotoxin** *see* Etoposide Phosphate *on page 715*
- ◆ **EpiQuin® Micro** *see* Hydroquinone *on page 927*

Epirubicin (ep i ROO bi sin)

U.S. Brand Names Ellence®

Index Terms Epidoxorubicin; Epirubicin Hydrochloride; Pidorubicin; Pidorubicin Hydrochloride

Generic Availability (U.S.) Yes

Pharmacologic Category Antineoplastic Agent, Anthracycline

Medication Safety Issues

Sound-alike/look-alike issues:

Epirubicin may be confused with DOXOrubicin, DAUNOrubicin, eribulin, idarubicin

Ellence® may be confused with Elase®

High alert medication: This drug is in a class the Institute for Safe Medication Practices (ISMP) includes among its list of drug classes which have a heightened risk of causing significant patient harm when used in error.

Pregnancy Risk Factor D

Lactation Excretion in breast milk unknown/not recommended

Use Adjuvant therapy for primary breast cancer

Unlabeled/Investigational Use Treatment of esophageal cancer, gastric cancer, soft tissue sarcoma, uterine sarcoma

Mechanism of Action/Effect Epirubicin is an anthracycline agent which inhibits DNA and RNA synthesis throughout the cell cycle.

Contraindications Hypersensitivity to epirubicin or any component of the formulation, other anthracyclines, or anthracenediones; previous anthracycline treatment up to maximum cumulative dose; severe myocardial insufficiency, severe arrhythmias; recent myocardial infarction; severe hepatic dysfunction; baseline neutrophil count <1500/mm^3

Warnings/Precautions Hazardous agent - use appropriate precautions for handling and disposal.

[U.S. Boxed Warning]: Myocardial toxicity, including heart failure (HF) may occur, particularly in patients who have received prior anthracyclines, prior or concomitant radiotherapy to the mediastinal/pericardial area, or who have pre-existing cardiac disease. **May be concurrent or delayed.** Acute toxicity, primarily arrhythmia, and delayed toxicity, including decreased left ventricular ejection fraction (LVEF) and HF, have been described. Delayed toxicity usually develops late in the course of therapy or within 2-3 months after completion, however, events with an onset of several months to years after termination of treatment have been described. The risk HF of delayed cardiotoxicity increases more steeply with cumulative doses >900 mg/m^2, and this dose should be exceeded only with extreme caution. The risk of HF is ~0.9% at a cumulative dose of 550 mg/m^2, ~1.6% at a cumulative dose of 700 mg/m^2, and ~3.3% at a cumulative dose of 900 mg/m^2. Cardiotoxicity may also occur at lower cumulative doses or without risk factors. Toxicity may be additive with other anthracyclines or anthracenediones, and may be increased in pediatric patients. Regular monitoring of LVEF and discontinuation at the first sign of impairment is recommended especially in patients with cardiac risk factors or impaired cardiac function.

[U.S. Boxed Warning]: May cause severe myelosuppression; neutropenia is the dose-limiting toxicity; severe thrombocytopenia or anemia may occur. Patients should recover from myelosuppression due to prior chemotherapy treatment before beginning treatments. Thrombophlebitis and thromboembolic phenomena (including pulmonary embolism) have occurred.

[U.S. Boxed Warning]: Reduce dosage in patients with mild-to-moderate hepatic impairment (contraindicated in severe hepatic impairment) and in patients with serum creatinine >5 mg/dL (has not been studied in patients on dialysis); monitor hepatic and renal function at baseline and during treatment. May cause tumor lysis syndrome. Radiation recall has been reported; epirubicin may have radiosensitizing activity. **[U.S. Boxed Warnings]: Treatment with anthracyclines may increase the risk of secondary acute myelogenous leukemia (AML).** AML is more common when given in combination with other antineoplastic agents, after multiple courses of prior chemotherapy, or with escalated cumulative anthracycline doses (>720 mg/m^2 for epirubicin). The risk for treatment-related AML or myelodysplastic syndrome (MDS) is estimated at 0.3% at 3 years, 0.5% at 5 years, 0.6% at 8 years after treatment. **For I.V. administration only, severe local tissue damage and necrosis will result if extravasation occurs (vesicant); not for I.M. or SubQ use.** Women ≥70 years of age should be closely monitored for toxicity. **[U.S. Boxed Warning]: Should be administered under the supervision of an experienced cancer chemotherapy physician.**

Drug Interactions

Avoid Concomitant Use

Avoid concomitant use of Epirubicin with any of the following: BCG; Cimetidine; Natalizumab; Pimecrolimus; Roflumilast; Tacrolimus (Topical); Vaccines (Live)

Decreased Effect

Epirubicin may decrease the levels/effects of: BCG; Cardiac Glycosides; Sipuleucel-T; Vaccines (Inactivated); Vaccines (Live)

The levels/effects of Epirubicin may be decreased by: Cardiac Glycosides; Echinacea

Increased Effect/Toxicity

Epirubicin may increase the levels/effects of: Leflunomide; Natalizumab; Vaccines (Live)

The levels/effects of Epirubicin may be increased by: Bevacizumab; Cimetidine; Denosumab; Pimecrolimus; Roflumilast; Tacrolimus (Topical); Taxane Derivatives; Trastuzumab

Nutritional/Ethanol Interactions

Ethanol: Avoid ethanol (due to GI irritation).

Herb/Nutraceutical: Avoid black cohosh, dong quai in estrogen-dependent tumors.

Adverse Reactions Percentages reported as part of combination chemotherapy regimens.

>10%:

Central nervous system: Lethargy (1% to 46%)

Dermatologic: Alopecia (69% to 96%)

Endocrine & metabolic: Amenorrhea (69% to 72%), hot flashes (5% to 39%)

Gastrointestinal: Nausea/vomiting (83% to 92%; grades 3/4: 22% to 25%), mucositis (9% to 59%; grades 3/4: ≤9%), diarrhea (7% to 25%)

Hematologic: Leukopenia (50% to 80%; grades 3/4: 2% to 59%), neutropenia (54% to 80%; grades 3/4: 11% to 67%; nadir: 10-14 days; recovery: 21 days), anemia (13% to 72%; grades 3/4: ≤6%), thrombocytopenia (5% to 49%; grades 3/4: ≤5%)

Local: Injection site reactions (3% to 20%; grades 3/4: <1%)

Ocular: Conjunctivitis (1% to 15%)

Miscellaneous: Infection (15% to 22%; grades 3/4: ≤2%)

1% to 10%:

Cardiovascular: LVEF decreased (asymptomatic; delayed: 1% to 2%), HF (0.4% to 1.5%)

Central nervous system: Fever (1% to 5%)

Dermatologic: Rash (1% to 9%), skin changes (1% to 5%)
Gastrointestinal: Anorexia (2% to 3%)
Hematologic: Neutropenic fever (grades 3/4: ≤6%)

Pharmacodynamics/Kinetics

Protein Binding ~77% to albumin

Half-Life Elimination Triphasic; Mean terminal: 33 hours

Metabolism Extensive via hepatic and extrahepatic (including RBCs) routes

Excretion Feces (34% to 35%); urine (20% to 27%)

Available Dosage Forms

Injection, powder for reconstitution: 50 mg

Injection, solution [preservative free]: 2 mg/mL (25 mL, 100 mL)
Ellence®: 2 mg/mL (25 mL, 100 mL)

Dosing

Adult Note: Patients receiving 120 mg/m^2/cycle as part of combination therapy should also receive prophylactic therapy with sulfamethoxazole/trimethoprim or a fluoroquinolone. Details concerning dosing in combination regimens should also be consulted. Lower starting doses may be necessary for heavily pretreated patients, patients with pre-existing myelosuppression, or with bone marrow involvement.

Breast cancer, adjuvant treatment: I.V.: Usual dose: 100-120 mg/m^2 per 3- or 4-week treatment cycle as follows:
60 mg/m^2 on days 1 and 8 every 28 days for 6 cycles in combination with cyclophosphamide and fluorouracil (CEF-120 regimen; Levine, 2005) **or**
100 mg/m^2 on day 1 every 21 days for 6 cycles in combination with cyclophosphamide and fluorouracil (FEC-100 regimen; Bonneterre, 2005) **or**

Breast cancer (unlabeled regimens; as a part of combination chemotherapy): I.V.:
60 mg/m^2 on day 1 every 21 days for 8 cycles (EC regimen; Piccart, 2001) **or**
75 mg/m^2 on day 1 every 21 days for 4 cycles (FEC regimen; Buzdar, 2005) **or**
75 mg/m^2 on day 1 every 21 days for 6 cycles (EP and EC regimens; Langley, 2005) **or**
90 mg/m^2 on day 1 every 21 days for 4 or 6 cycles (FEC regimen ± paclitaxel; Martin, 2008) **or**
50 mg/m^2 on days 1 and 8 every 21-28 days for 6-9 cycles (CEF regimen; Ackland, 2001)

Esophageal cancer (unlabeled use; as part of combination chemotherapy): I.V.:
50 mg/m^2 on day 1 every 21 days for up to 8 cycles (ECF, ECX, EOF, and EOX regimens; Cunningham, 2008) **or**
50 mg/m^2 on day 1 every 21 days for 3 preoperative and 3 postoperative cycles (ECF regimen; Cunningham, 2006)

Gastric cancer (unlabeled use; as part of combination chemotherapy): I.V.:
50 mg/m^2 on day 1 every 21 days for up to 8 cycles (ECF, ECX, EOF, and EOX regimens [Cunningham, 2008]; ECF regimen [Waters, 1999]) **or**
50 mg/m^2 on day 1 every 21 days for 3 preoperative and 3 postoperative cycles (ECF regimen; Cunningham, 2006)

Dosage modifications:
Delay day 1 dose until platelets are ≥100,000/mm^3, ANC ≥1500/mm^3, and nonhematologic toxicities have recovered to ≤grade 1
Reduce day 1 dose in subsequent cycles to 75% of previous day 1 dose if patient experiences nadir platelet counts <50,000/mm^3, ANC <250/mm^3, neutropenic fever, or grade 3/4 nonhematologic toxicity during the previous cycle
For divided doses (day 1 and day 8), reduce day 8 dose to 75% of day 1 dose if platelet counts are 75,000-100,000/mm^3 and ANC is 1000-1499/mm^3; omit day 8 dose if platelets are <75,000/mm^3, ANC <1000/mm^3, or grade 3/4 nonhematologic toxicity

Dosage adjustment in bone marrow dysfunction: Heavily-treated patients, patients with pre-existing bone marrow depression or neoplastic bone marrow infiltration: Lower starting doses (75-90 mg/m^2) should be considered.

Geriatric Plasma clearance of epirubicin in elderly female patients was noted to be reduced by 35%. Although no initial dosage reduction is specifically recommended, particular care should be exercised in monitoring toxicity and adjusting subsequent dosage in elderly patients (particularly females >70 years of age).

Renal Impairment The FDA-approved labeling recommends that in patients with severe renal impairment (serum creatinine >5 mg/dL), lower doses should be considered. Aronoff (2007) recommends no dosage adjustment needed for Cl_{cr} <50 mL/minute.

Hepatic Impairment The FDA-approved labeling recommends the following guidelines (based on clinical trial information):
Bilirubin 1.2-3 mg/dL or AST 2-4 times the upper limit of normal: Administer 50% of recommended starting dose.
Bilirubin >3 mg/dL or AST >4 times the upper limit of normal: Administer 25% of recommended starting dose.
Severe hepatic impairment: Use is contraindicated.

Administration

I.V. Infuse over 15-20 minutes or slow I.V. push (for lower doses [due to dose modification or organ dysfunction]) over 3-10 minutes into a free-flowing I.V. solution. Avoid the use of veins over joints or in extremities with compromised venous or lymphatic drainage. Monitor infusion site; avoid extravasation.

Stability

Reconstitution Use appropriate precautions for handling and disposal. Reconstitute lyophilized powder with SWFI (25 mL for the 50 mg vial or 100 mL for the 200 mg vial) to a final concentration of 2 mg/mL.

Storage Store intact vials of solution under refrigeration at 2°C to 8°C (36°F to 46°F). Store intact vials of lyophilized powder at room temperature of 25°C (77°F); excursions permitted to 15°C to 30°C (59°F to 86°F). Protect from light. Reconstituted solutions are stable for 24 hours when stored at 2°C to 8°C (36°F to 46°F) or at room temperature. Discard unused solution from single dose vials within 24 hours of entry.

Monitoring and Teaching Issues

Laboratory Monitoring Baseline and repeated measurements of CBC with differential and platelet count, liver function tests, renal function, ECG, and LVEF. The method used for assessment of LVEF (echocardiogram or MUGA) should be consistent during routine monitoring.

Physical Assessment Use caution in presence of hepatic or renal impairment; evaluate at baseline and during treatment. Note specific infusion directions. Premedication with an antiemetic may be useful (emetogenic). Infusion site must be monitored closely to prevent extravasation; severe local tissue necrosis will result if extravasation occurs. Monitor for acute nausea and vomiting, anemia, infection, bleeding, and cardiotoxicity; cardiotoxicity may occur 1 to several months after termination of treatment. Teach patient importance of adequate hydration.

Patient Education This medication can only be administered by infusion. Report immediately any swelling, pain, burning, or redness at infusion site, sudden difficulty breathing or swallowing, chest pain, or chills. Maintain adequate nutrition and hydration, unless instructed to restrict fluid intake. You will be more susceptible to infection. May cause nausea or vomiting; if severe, contact prescriber for antiemetic. May cause diarrhea, loss of hair (reversible), hyperpigmentation of skin or nails, mouth sores, or changes in menstrual cycle (consult prescriber). Report chest pain, swelling of extremities, palpitations, or rapid heartbeat; respiratory difficulty or unusual cough; pain, redness, unusual warmth in extremities; unresolved nausea, vomiting, or diarrhea; alterations in urinary pattern (increased or decreased); opportunistic infection (fever, chills, unusual bruising or bleeding, fatigue, purulent vaginal discharge, unhealed mouth sores); skin rash; abdominal pain; or blood in urine or stool.

Breast-Feeding Considerations Excretion in human breast milk is unknown, however, other anthracyclines are excreted. Due to the potential for serious adverse reactions in the nursing infant, breast-feeding is not recommended.

Pregnancy Considerations Teratogenic effects and embryotoxicity were noted in animal studies. There are no adequate and well-controlled studies in pregnant women. If a pregnant woman is treated with epirubicin, or if a woman becomes pregnant while receiving this drug, she should be informed of the potential hazard to the fetus. Women of childbearing potential should be advised to avoid becoming pregnant. Men undergoing treatment should use effective contraception. Epirubicin may cause irreversible amenorrhea in premenopausal women.

◆ **Epirubicin Hydrochloride** *see* Epirubicin *on page* 633

◆ **Epitol®** *see* CarBAMazepine *on page* 287

◆ **Epivir®** *see* LamiVUDine *on page* 1054

◆ **Epivir-HBV®** *see* LamiVUDine *on page* 1054

Eplerenone (e PLER en one)

U.S. Brand Names Inspra™

Generic Availability (U.S.) Yes

Pharmacologic Category Diuretic, Potassium-Sparing; Selective Aldosterone Blocker

Medication Safety Issues

Sound-alike/look-alike issues:

Inspra™ may be confused with Spiriva®

Pregnancy Risk Factor B

Lactation Excretion in breast milk unknown/not recommended

Use Treatment of hypertension (may be used alone or in combination with other antihypertensive agents); treatment of heart failure (HF) following acute MI

Mechanism of Action/Effect Aldosterone increases blood pressure primarily by inducing sodium reabsorption. Eplerenone reduces blood pressure by blocking aldosterone binding at mineralocorticoid receptors found in the kidney, heart, blood vessels and brain.

Contraindications Serum potassium >5.5 mEq/L at initiation; Cl_{cr} ≤30 mL/minute; concomitant use of strong CYP3A4 inhibitors (see Drug Interactions for details)

The following additional contraindications apply to patients with hypertension: Type 2 diabetes mellitus (noninsulin dependent, NIDDM) with microalbuminuria; serum creatinine >2.0 mg/dL in males or >1.8 mg/dL in females; Cl_{cr} <50 mL/minute; concomitant use with potassium supplements or potassium-sparing diuretics

Warnings/Precautions Dosage adjustment needed for patients on moderate CYP3A4 inhibitors. Monitor closely for hyperkalemia; increases in serum potassium were dose related during clinical trials and rates of hyperkalemia also increased with declining renal function. Safety and efficacy have not been established in patients with severe hepatic impairment. Use with caution in HF patients post-MI with diabetes (especially if patient has proteinuria); risk of hyperkalemia is increased. Risk of hyperkalemia is increased with declining renal function. Use with caution in patients with mild renal impairment; contraindicated with moderate-severe impairment (HTN: Cl_{cr} <50 mL/minute; other indications: Cl_{cr} ≤30 mL/minute).

Drug Interactions

Metabolism/Transport Effects Substrate of CYP3A4 (major)

Avoid Concomitant Use

Avoid concomitant use of Eplerenone with any of the following: CYP3A4 Inhibitors (Strong); Itraconazole; Ketoconazole; Ketoconazole (Systemic); Posaconazole; Tacrolimus; Voriconazole

Decreased Effect

The levels/effects of Eplerenone may be decreased by: CYP3A4 Inducers (Strong); Deferasirox; Herbs (CYP3A4 Inducers); Herbs (Hypertensive Properties); Methylphenidate; Nonsteroidal Anti-Inflammatory Agents; Yohimbine

Increased Effect/Toxicity

Eplerenone may increase the levels/effects of: ACE Inhibitors; Amifostine; Angiotensin II Receptor Blockers; Antihypertensives; Hypotensive Agents; Potassium Salts; Potassium-Sparing Diuretics; RiTUXimab; Tacrolimus

The levels/effects of Eplerenone may be increased by: Calcium Channel Blockers (Nondihydropyridine); CYP3A4 Inhibitors (Moderate); CYP3A4 Inhibitors (Strong); Dasatinib; Diazoxide; Fluconazole; Herbs (Hypotensive Properties); Itraconazole; Ketoconazole; Ketoconazole (Systemic); Macrolide Antibiotics; MAO Inhibitors; Nonsteroidal Anti-Inflammatory Agents; Pentoxifylline; Phosphodiesterase 5 Inhibitors; Posaconazole; Prostacyclin Analogues; Protease Inhibitors; Voriconazole

Nutritional/Ethanol Interactions

Food: Grapefruit juice increases eplerenone AUC ~25%.

Herb/Nutraceutical: St John's wort may decrease levels of eplerenone. Avoid black cohosh, California poppy, coleus, golden seal, hawthorn, mistletoe, periwinkle, quinine, shepherd's purse (may have increased antihypertensive effect). Avoid bayberry, blue cohosh, cayenne, ephedra, ginger, ginseng (American), kola, licorice (may diminish the antihypertensive effect).

Adverse Reactions

>10%: Endocrine & metabolic: Hyperkalemia ([HF post-MI: K >5.5 mEq/L: 16%; K ≥6 mEq/L: 6%] [HTN: K >5.5 mEq/L at doses ≤100 mg: ≤1%; doses >100 mg: 9%]), hypertriglyceridemia (1% to 15%, dose related)

1% to 10%:

Central nervous system: Dizziness (3%), fatigue (2%)

Endocrine & metabolic: Hyponatremia (2%, dose related), breast pain (males <1% to 1%), gynecomastia (males <1% to 1%), hypercholesterolemia (<1% to 1%)

Gastrointestinal: Diarrhea (2%), abdominal pain (1%)

Genitourinary: Abnormal vaginal bleeding (<1% to 2%)

Renal: Creatinine increased (HF post-MI: 6%), albuminuria (1%)

Respiratory: Cough (2%)

Miscellaneous: Flu-like syndrome (2%)

Pharmacodynamics/Kinetics

Bioavailability 69%

Time to Peak Plasma: ~1.5 hours; may take up to 4 weeks for full antihypertensive effect

Protein Binding ~50%; primarily to alpha$_1$-acid glycoproteins

Half-Life Elimination 4-6 hours

Metabolism Primarily hepatic via CYP3A4; metabolites inactive

Excretion Urine (~67%); feces (32%); <5% as unchanged drug in urine and feces

Available Dosage Forms

Tablet, oral: 25 mg, 50 mg

Inspra™: 25 mg, 50 mg

Dosing

Adult & Geriatric

Hypertension: Oral: Initial: 50 mg once daily; may increase to 50 mg twice daily if response is not adequate; may take up to 4 weeks for full therapeutic response. Doses >100 mg/day are associated with increased risk of hyperkalemia and no greater therapeutic effect.

Dose modification during concurrent use with moderate CYP3A4 inhibitors: Initial: 25 mg once daily

Heart failure (post-MI): Oral: Initial: 25 mg once daily; dosage goal: Titrate to 50 mg once daily within 4 weeks, as tolerated

Dosage adjustment per serum potassium concentrations for HF (post-MI):

<5.0 mEq/L:

Increase dose from 25 mg every other day to 25 mg daily **or**

Increase dose from 25 mg daily to 50 mg daily

5.0-5.4 mEq/L: No adjustment needed

5.5-5.9 mEq/L:

Decrease dose from 50 mg daily to 25 mg daily **or**

Decrease dose from 25 mg daily to 25 mg every other day **or**

Decrease dose from 25 mg every other day to withhold medication

≥6.0 mEq/L: Withhold medication until potassium <5.5 mEq/L, then restart at 25 mg every other day

Renal Impairment

Hypertension: Cl_{cr} <50 mL/minute or serum creatinine >2.0 mg/dL in males or >1.8 mg/dL in females: Use is contraindicated; risk of hyperkalemia increases with declining renal function

All other indications: Cl_{cr} ≤30 mL/minute: Use is contraindicated.

Hepatic Impairment No dosage adjustment needed for mild-to-moderate impairment. Safety and efficacy not established for severe impairment.

Administration

Oral May be administered with or without food.

Stability

Storage Store at controlled room temperature of 25°C (77°F).

Monitoring and Teaching Issues

Laboratory Monitoring Serum potassium (levels monitored prior to therapy, within the first week, and at 1 month after start of treatment or dose adjustment, then periodically [monthly in clinical trials]); renal function

Physical Assessment Assess potassium levels, blood pressure, and renal function prior to and periodically during therapy. Monitor for hypotension and hyperkalemia at beginning of and at regular intervals during therapy.

Patient Education Take at the same time of day, without regard for meals. It may take up to 4 weeks to achieve desired results. Do not use potassium supplement or salt substitutes without consulting prescriber. This drug does not eliminate need for diet or exercise regimen as recommended by prescriber. May cause dizziness, high triglyceride levels, and increased potassium levels. Report muscle weakness, diarrhea, and abdominal pain.

Dietary Considerations May be taken with or without food. Do not use salt substitutes containing potassium.

Geriatric Considerations Since this medication is contraindicated in the treatment of hypertension in patients with a Cl_{cr} <50 mL/minute, it will have limited use in the elderly. Due to physiologic changes, elderly may be at increased risk of hyperkalemia when using this medication.

Pregnancy Considerations No teratogenic effects were seen in animal studies, however, there are no adequate and well-controlled studies in pregnant women. Use during pregnancy only if the potential benefit to the mother outweighs the possible risk to the fetus.

◆ **EPO** *see* Epoetin Alfa *on page* 638

Epoetin Alfa (e POE e tin AL fa)

U.S. Brand Names Epogen®; Procrit®

Index Terms *r*HuEPO-α; EPO; Erythropoiesis-Stimulating Agent (ESA); Erythropoietin

Generic Availability (U.S.) No

Pharmacologic Category Colony Stimulating Factor

Medication Safety Issues

Sound-alike/look-alike issues:

Epoetin alfa may be confused with darbepoetin alfa, epoetin beta

Epogen® may be confused with Neupogen®

International issues:

Epopen [Spain] may be confused with EpiPen brand name for epinephrine [U.S., Canada, and multiple international markets]

Medication Guide Available Yes

Prescribing and Access Restrictions As a requirement of the REMS program, access to this medication is restricted. Healthcare providers and hospitals must be enrolled in the ESA APPRISE (Assisting Providers and Cancer Patients with Risk Information for the Safe use of ESAs) Oncology Program (866-284-8089; http://www.esa-apprise.com) to prescribe or dispense ESAs (ie, epoetin alfa, darbepoetin alfa) to patients with cancer.

Pregnancy Risk Factor C

Lactation Excretion in breast milk unknown/use caution

Use Treatment of anemia (elevate or maintain red blood cell level and decrease the need for transfusions) associated with HIV (zidovudine) therapy, chronic renal failure (including patients on dialysis and not on dialysis); reduction of allogeneic blood transfusion for elective, noncardiac, nonvascular surgery; treatment of anemia due to concurrent chemotherapy in patients with metastatic cancer (nonmyeloid malignancies) receiving chemotherapy for a minimum of 2 months

Note: Erythropoietin is **not** indicated for use in cancer patients under the following conditions:

- receiving hormonal therapy, therapeutic biologic products, or radiation therapy unless also receiving concurrent myelosuppressive chemotherapy
- receiving myelosuppressive therapy when the expected outcome is curative
- anemia due to other factors (eg, iron deficiency, folate deficiency, or gastrointestinal bleed)

Not intended for patients who require immediate correction of severe anemia or as a substitute for emergency transfusion.

Unlabeled/Investigational Use Treatment of anemia associated with critical illness; anemia of prematurity; symptomatic anemia in myelodysplastic syndrome (MDS)

Mechanism of Action/Effect Induces red blood cell production in the bone marrow to be released into the blood stream where they mature to erythrocytes; results in rise in hematocrit and hemoglobin levels

Contraindications Hypersensitivity to albumin (human) or mammalian cell-derived products; uncontrolled hypertension

Warnings/Precautions [U.S. Boxed Warning]: Erythropoiesis-stimulating agents (ESAs) increased the risk of serious cardiovascular events, thromboembolic events, stroke, mortality, and/or tumor progression in clinical studies; a rapid rise in hemoglobin (>1 g/dL over 2 weeks) or maintaining higher hemoglobin levels may contribute to these risks.**[U.S. Boxed Warning]: A shortened overall survival and/or increased risk of tumor progression or recurrence has been reported in studies with breast, cervical, head and neck, lymphoid, and non small cell lung cancer patients.** It is of note that in these studies, patients received ESAs to a target hemoglobin of ≥12 g/dL; although risk has not been excluded when dosed to achieve a target hemoglobin of <12 g/dL. **[U.S. Boxed Warnings]: To decrease these risks, and risk of cardio- and thrombovascular events, use the lowest dose needed to avoid red blood cell transfusions. Use ESAs in cancer patients only for the treatment of anemia related to concurrent chemotherapy; discontinue ESA following completion of the chemotherapy course. ESAs are not indicated for patients receiving myelosuppressive therapy when the anticipated outcome is curative.** Use of ESAs has been associated with an increased risk of venous thromboembolism (VTE) without a reduction in transfusions in patients with cancer (Hershman, 2009). Improved anemia symptoms, quality of life, fatigue or well-being has not been demonstrated in controlled clinical trials. **[U.S. Boxed Warning]: Because of the risks of decreased survival and increased risk of tumor growth or progression, all healthcare providers and hospitals are required to enroll and comply with the ESA APPRISE (Assisting Providers and Cancer Patients with Risk Information for the Safe use of ESAs) Oncology Program prior to prescribing or dispensing ESAs to cancer patients.** Prescribers and patients will have to provide written documentation of discussed risks.

[U.S. Boxed Warning]: An increased risk of death, serious cardiovascular events, and stroke was reported in chronic renal failure patients administered ESAs to target hemoglobin levels ≥13 g/dL; dosing should be individualized to achieve and maintain hemoglobin levels within 10-12 g/dL range. Hemoglobin rising >1 g/dL in a 2-week period may contribute to the risk. Chronic renal failure patients who exhibit an inadequate hemoglobin response to ESA therapy may be at a higher risk for cardiovascular events and mortality compared to other patients. ESA therapy may reduce dialysis efficacy (due to increase in red blood cells and decrease in plasma volume); adjustments in dialysis parameters may be needed. Patients treated with epoetin may require increased heparinization during dialysis to prevent clotting of the artificial kidney. **[U.S. Boxed Warning]: Epoetin alfa increased the rate of DVT in perisurgery patients not receiving anticoagulant prophylaxis; consider DVT prophylaxis.** Increased mortality was also observed in patients undergoing coronary artery bypass surgery who received epoetin alfa; these deaths were associated with thrombotic events. Epoetin is not approved for reduction of red blood cell transfusion in patients undergoing cardiac or vascular surgery and is not indicated for anemic patients willing to donate autologous blood. During therapy in any patient, hemoglobin levels should not exceed a target range of 10-12 g/dL and should not rise >1 g/dL per 2-week time period.

Use with caution in patients with hypertension or with a history of seizures; hypertensive encephalopathy and seizures have been reported. If hypertension is difficult to control, reduce or hold epoetin alfa. An excessive rate of rise of hemoglobin is associated with hypertension or exacerbation of hypertension; decrease the epoetin dose if the hemoglobin increase exceeds 1 g/dL in any 2-week period. Blood pressure should be controlled prior to start of therapy and monitored closely throughout treatment. Due to the delayed onset of erythropoiesis, epoetin alfa is **not** recommended for acute correction of severe anemia or as a substitute for emergency transfusion.

Prior to treatment, correct or exclude deficiencies of iron, vitamin B_{12}, and/or folate, as well as other factors which may impair erythropoiesis (aluminum toxicity, inflammatory conditions, infections). Prior to and periodically during therapy, iron stores must be evaluated. Supplemental iron is recommended if serum ferritin <100 mcg/L or serum transferrin saturation <20%. Poor response should prompt evaluation of these potential factors, as well as possible malignant processes, occult blood loss, hemolysis, and/or bone marrow fibrosis. Severe anemia and pure red cell aplasia (PRCA) with associated neutralizing antibodies to erythropoietin has been reported, predominantly in patients with CRF receiving SubQ epoetin (the I.V. route is preferred for hemodialysis patients). Cases have also been reported in patients with hepatitis C who were receiving ESAs, interferon, and ribavirin. Patients with a sudden loss of response to epoetin alfa (with severe anemia and a low reticulocyte count) should be evaluated for PRCA with associated neutralizing antibodies to erythropoietin; discontinue treatment in patients with PRCA secondary to neutralizing antibodies to epoetin.

Safety and efficacy in patients with underlying hematologic diseases have not been established, including hypercoagulation disorders and sickle cell disease. Potentially serious allergic reactions have been reported (rarely). Discontinue immediately (and permanently) in patients who experience serious allergic/anaphylactic reactions. Use caution with porphyria, exacerbation of porphyria has been reported (rarely) in patients with chronic renal failure. Some products may contain albumin. Multidose vials contain benzyl alcohol; do not use in premature infants.

Drug Interactions

Avoid Concomitant Use There are no known interactions where it is recommended to avoid concomitant use.

Decreased Effect There are no known significant interactions involving a decrease in effect.

Increased Effect/Toxicity There are no known significant interactions involving an increase in effect.

Adverse Reactions

>10%:

Cardiovascular: Hypertension (5% to 24%), thrombotic/vascular events (coronary artery bypass graft surgery: 23%), edema (6% to 17%), deep vein thrombosis (≤11%)

Central nervous system: Fever (29% to 51%), dizziness (5% to 21%), insomnia (13% to 21%), headache (10% to 19%)

Dermatologic: Pruritus (14% to 22%), skin pain (4% to 18%), rash (≤16%)

Gastrointestinal: Nausea (11% to 58%), constipation (42% to 53%), vomiting (8% to 29%), diarrhea (6% to 21%), dyspepsia (7% to 11%)

Genitourinary: Urinary tract infection (3% to 12%)

Local: Injection site reaction (<10% to 29%)
Neuromuscular & skeletal: Arthralgia (≤11%), paresthesia (≤11%)
Respiratory: Cough (≤18%), congestion (≤15%), dyspnea (13% to 14%), upper respiratory infection (≤11%)

1% to 10%:

Central nervous system: Seizure (1% to 3%)
Local: Clotted vascular access (7%)

Pharmacodynamics/Kinetics

Onset of Action Several days; Peak effect: Hemoglobin level: 2-6 weeks

Bioavailability SubQ: ~21% to 31%; Intraperitoneal epoetin: 3% (Macdougall, 1989)

Time to Peak Serum: Chronic renal failure: SubQ: 5-24 hours

Half-Life Elimination Cancer: SubQ: 16-67 hours; Chronic renal failure: I.V.: 4-13 hours

Metabolism Some degradation does occur

Excretion Feces (majority); urine (small amounts, 10% unchanged in normal volunteers)

Available Dosage Forms

Injection, solution:

Epogen®: 10,000 units/mL (2 mL); 20,000 units/mL (1 mL)
Procrit®: 10,000 units/mL (2 mL); 20,000 units/mL (1 mL)

Injection, solution [preservative free]:

Epogen®: 2000 units/mL (1 mL); 3000 units/mL (1 mL); 4000 units/mL (1 mL); 10,000 units/mL (1 mL)
Procrit®: 2000 units/mL (1 mL); 3000 units/mL (1 mL); 4000 units/mL (1 mL); 10,000 units/mL (1 mL); 40,000 units/mL (1 mL)

Dosing

Adult & Geriatric Individuals with anemia due to iron deficiency, sickle cell disease, autoimmune hemolytic anemia, and bleeding, generally have appropriate endogenous EPO levels to drive erythropoiesis and would not ordinarily be candidates for EPO therapy. **Note:** Hemoglobin levels should not exceed 12 g/dL and should not rise >1 g/dL per 2-week time period during therapy in any patient.

Chronic renal failure patients: I.V. (preferred for hemodialysis patients), SubQ: Initial dose: 50-100 units/kg 3 times/week. Individualize dosing to achieve and maintain hemoglobin levels between 10-12 g/dL. Hemoglobin levels should not exceed a target range of 10-12 g/dL.

Dosage adjustment:

Decrease dose by 25%: If hemoglobin approaches 12 g/dL **or** hemoglobin increases >1 g/dL in any 2-week period. If hemoglobin continues to increase, temporarily discontinue therapy until hemoglobin begins to decrease, then resume therapy with a ~25% reduction from previous dose.

Increase dose by 25%: If hemoglobin <10 g/dL and does not increase by 1 g/dL after 4 weeks of therapy (with adequate iron stores) **or** hemoglobin decreases below 10 g/dL. If transferrin saturation >20%, may increase epoetin dose. Do not increase dose more frequently than at 4-week intervals, unless clinically indicated (hemoglobin response time for dose increases may be 2-6 weeks).

Inadequate or lack of response: If patient does not attain target hemoglobin range of 10-12 g/dL after appropriate dose titrations over 12 weeks:

Do not continue to increase dose and use the minimum effective dose that will maintain a hemoglobin level sufficient to avoid red blood cell transfusions **and** evaluate patient for other causes of anemia.

Monitor hemoglobin closely thereafter, and if responsiveness improves, may resume making dosage adjustments as recommended above. If responsiveness does not improve and recurrent red blood cell transfusions continue to be needed, discontinue therapy.

Maintenance dose: Individualize to target hemoglobin range of 10-12 g/dL; limit additional dosage increases to every 4 weeks (or longer)

Dialysis patients: Median dose: 75 units/kg 3 times/week
Nondialysis patients: Dosing range: 75-150 units/kg/week

Zidovudine-treated, HIV-infected patients (with serum erythropoietin levels ≤500 mU/mL and zidovudine doses ≤4200 mg/week; patient with erythropoietin levels >500 mU/mL is unlikely to respond). Titrate dosage to use the minimum effective dose that will maintain a hemoglobin level sufficient to avoid red blood cell transfusions. Hemoglobin levels should not exceed 12 g/dL

I.V.: 100 units/kg 3 times/week for 8 weeks

Dosage adjustment:

Increase dose in increments of 50-100 units/kg administered 3 times/week: If response is not satisfactory in terms of reducing transfusion requirements or increasing hemoglobin after 8 weeks of therapy. Evaluate response every 4-8 weeks thereafter and adjust the dose accordingly by 50-100 units/kg increments administered 3 times/week. If patient has not responded satisfactorily to 300 unit/kg dose 3 times/week, a response to higher doses is unlikely.

Withhold dose: If hemoglobin exceeds 12 g/dL and resume treatment at a 25% dose reduction when hemoglobin drops below 11g/dL.

Cancer patient on chemotherapy: Treatment of patients with erythropoietin levels >200 mU/mL is **not recommended by the manufacturer.** Titrate dosage to use the minimum effective dose that will maintain a hemoglobin level sufficient to avoid red blood cell transfusions. Do not initiate therapy if hemoglobin ≥10 g/dL. Discontinue erythropoietin following completion of chemotherapy.

SubQ: Initial dose: 150 units/kg 3 times/week or 40,000 units once weekly; commonly used doses range from 10,000 units 3 times/week to 40,000-60,000 units once weekly.

Dosage adjustment:

Increase dose: If response is not satisfactory after a sufficient period of evaluation (no reduction in transfusion requirements or increase in hemoglobin after 4 weeks of 3 times/week therapy) **or** (no increase in hemoglobin by ≥1 g/dL after 4 weeks of once-weekly therapy, in the absence of RBC transfusion), the dose may be increased every 4 weeks (or longer) to 300 units/kg 3 times/week, **or** when dosed weekly, increased all at once to 60,000 units weekly. If patient does not respond, a response to higher doses is unlikely.

Withhold dose: If hemoglobin exceeds a level needed to avoid red blood cell transfusion. Resume treatment with a 25% dose reduction when hemoglobin approaches a level where transfusions may be required.

Reduce dose by 25%: If hemoglobin increases >1 g/dL in any 2-week period **or** hemoglobin reaches a level sufficient to avoid red blood cell transfusion.

Discontinue: If after 8 weeks of therapy there is no response (ie, increased hemoglobin levels) or transfusions still required.

Surgery patients: Prior to initiating treatment, measure hemoglobin to establish that it is >10 g/dL and ≤13 g/dL: SubQ: Initial dose: 300 units/kg/day for 10 days before surgery, on the day of surgery, and for 4 days after surgery

Alternative dose: 600 units/kg in once weekly doses (21, 14, and 7 days before surgery) plus a fourth dose on the day of surgery

Anemia of critical illness (unlabeled use): SubQ: 40,000 units once weekly

Symptomatic anemia associated with MDS (unlabeled use): SubQ: 40,000-60,000 units 1-3 times/week (NCCN MDS guidelines v.2.2010)

Pediatric Note: Hemoglobin levels should not exceed 12 g/dL and should not rise >1 g/dL per 2-week time period during therapy in any patient.

Anemia of prematurity (unlabeled use): Infants: I.V., SubQ: Dosing range: 500-1250 units/kg/week; commonly used dose: 250 units/kg 3 times/week; supplement with oral iron therapy 3-8 mg/kg/day

Chronic renal failure patients: I.V. (preferred for hemodialysis patients), SubQ: Initial dose: 50 units/kg 3 times/week. Individualize dosing to achieve and maintain hemoglobin levels between 10-12 g/dL. Hemoglobin levels should not exceed 12 g/dL.

Dosage adjustment:

Decrease dose by 25%: If hemoglobin approaches 12 g/dL **or** hemoglobin increases >1 g/dL in any 2-week period. If hemoglobin continues to increase, temporarily discontinue therapy until hemoglobin begins to decrease, then resume therapy with a ~25% reduction from previous dose.

Increase dose by 25%: If hemoglobin <10 g/dL and does not increase by 1 g/dL after 4 weeks of therapy (with adequate iron stores) **or** hemoglobin decreases below 10 g/dL. If transferrin saturation >20%, may increase epoetin dose. Do not increase dose more frequently than at 4-week intervals, unless clinically indicated (hemoglobin response time for dose increases may be 2-6 weeks).

Inadequate or lack of response: If patient does not attain target hemoglobin range of 10-12 g/dL after appropriate dose titrations over 12 weeks:

Do not continue to increase dose and use the minimum effective dose that will maintain a hemoglobin level sufficient to avoid red blood cell transfusions **and** evaluate patient for other causes of anemia.

Monitor hemoglobin closely thereafter, and if responsiveness improves, may resume making dosage adjustments as recommended above. If responsiveness does not improve and recurrent red blood cell transfusions continue to be needed, discontinue therapy.

Maintenance dose: Individualize to target hemoglobin range of 10-12 g/dL; limit additional dosage increases to every 4 weeks (or longer)

Dialysis patients: 167 units/kg/week (hemodialysis) **or** 76 units/kg/week (peritoneal dialysis), in 2-3 divided doses per week

Nondialysis patients: Dosing range: 50-250 units/kg 1-3 times/week

Zidovudine-treated, HIV-infected patients (patient with erythropoietin levels >500 mU/mL is unlikely to respond): I.V., SubQ: Limited data available; reported dosing range: 50-400 units/kg 2-3 times/week.

Note: Titrate dosage to use the minimum effective dose that will maintain a hemoglobin level sufficient to avoid red blood cell transfusions. Hemoglobin levels should not exceed 12 g/dL.

Cancer patients on chemotherapy: I.V.: 600 units/kg once weekly (maximum: 40,000 units). Treatment of patients with erythropoietin levels >200 mU/mL is **not recommended by the manufacturer.** Titrate dosage to use the minimum effective dose that will maintain a hemoglobin level sufficient to avoid red blood cell transfusions. Do not initiate therapy if hemoglobin ≥10 g/dL. Discontinue erythropoietin following completion of chemotherapy.

Dosage adjustment:

Increase dose: If response is not satisfactory after a sufficient period of evaluation (no increase in hemoglobin by ≥1 g/dL after 4 weeks of once-weekly therapy, in the absence of RBC transfusion), the dose may be increased every 4 weeks (or longer) to 900 units/kg/week; maximum 60,000 units. If patient does not respond, a response to higher doses is unlikely.

Withhold dose: If hemoglobin exceeds a level needed to avoid red blood cell transfusion. Resume treatment with a 25% dose reduction when hemoglobin approaches a level where transfusions may be required.

Reduce dose by 25%: If hemoglobin increases >1 g/dL in any 2-week period **or** hemoglobin reaches a level sufficient to avoid red blood cell transfusion.

Discontinue: If after 8 weeks of therapy there is no response (ie, increased hemoglobin levels) or transfusions still required.

Renal Impairment The National Kidney Foundation Clinical Practice Guideline for Anemia in Chronic Kidney Disease: 2007 Update of Hemoglobin Target (September, 2007) recommend hemoglobin levels in the range of 11-12 g/dL for dialysis and nondialysis patients receiving ESAs; hemoglobin levels should not be >13 g/dL.

Hemodialysis: Supplemental dose is not necessary. I.V. route is preferred for hemodialysis patients.

Peritoneal dialysis: Supplemental dose is not necessary.

Administration

I.V. Patients with CRF on hemodialysis: I.V. route preferred; it may be administered into the venous line at the end of the dialysis procedure

Note: SubQ administration is the preferred route in other patient populations.

Other SubQ: SubQ is the preferred route of administration **except** in hemodialysis patients; 1:1 dilution with bacteriostatic NS (containing benzyl alcohol) acts as a local anesthetic to reduce pain at the injection site.

Stability

Reconstitution Prior to SubQ administration, preservative free solutions may be mixed with bacteriostatic NS containing benzyl alcohol 0.9% in a 1:1 ratio.

Storage Vials should be stored at 2°C to 8°C (36°F to 46°F); **do not freeze or shake**. Protect from light.

Single-dose 1 mL vial contains no preservative: Use one dose per vial. Do not re-enter vial; discard unused portions.

Single-dose vials (except 40,000 units/mL vial) are stable for 2 weeks at room temperature (Cohen, 2007). Single-dose 40,000 units/mL vial is stable for 1 week at room temperature.

Multidose 1 mL or 2 mL vial contains preservative. Store at 2°C to 8°C after initial entry and between doses. Discard 21 days after initial entry.

Multidose vials (with preservative) are stable for 1 week at room temperature (Cohen, 2007).

Prefilled syringes containing the 20,000 units/mL formulation with preservative are stable for 6 weeks refrigerated (2°C to 8°C) (Naughton, 2003).

Dilutions of 1:10 and 1:20 (1 part epoetin:19 parts sodium chloride) are stable for 18 hours at room temperature (Ohls, 1996).

Prior to SubQ administration, preservative free solutions may be mixed with bacteriostatic NS containing benzyl alcohol 0.9% in a 1:1 ratio (Corbo, 1992).

Dilutions of 1:10 in $D_{10}W$ with human albumin 0.05% or 0.1% are stable for 24 hours.

Monitoring and Teaching Issues

Laboratory Monitoring See table.

Test	Initial Phase Frequency	Maintenance Phase Frequency
Hemoglobin	1-2 x/week	2-4 x/month
Blood pressure	3 x/week	3 x/week
Serum ferritin	Monthly	Quarterly
Transferrin saturation	Monthly	Quarterly
Serum chemistries including CBC with differential, creatinine, blood urea nitrogen, potassium, phosphorous	Regularly per routine	Regularly per routine

Physical Assessment Evaluate history of hypertension or seizures and potential risk for thromboembolism prior to beginning therapy. Blood pressure should be monitored closely and controlled during therapy. If administered by intravenous infusion, lines should be monitored closely for possible clotting. Assess blood chemistries, hemoglobin/hematocrit, serum ferritin, and transferrin saturation prior to and on a regular basis during therapy; dosage adjustment and iron supplements may be necessary. Monitor for hypertension, thrombotic events, edema, and anemia. Serious allergic or anaphylactic reactions may require discontinuation of treatment. Teach patient proper SubQ injection technique and syringe/needle disposal.

Patient Education If self-administered, follow exact directions for injection and needle disposal. You will require frequent blood tests to determine appropriate dosage and reduce potential for severe adverse effects; maintaining laboratory testing schedule is vital. Report skin rash; difficulty swallowing; onset of severe headache, unusual dizziness, or blurred vision; chest pain; muscular tremors or seizure activity; or difficulty breathing.

Geriatric Considerations There is limited information about the use of epoetin alfa in the elderly. Endogenous erythropoietin secretion has been reported to be decreased in elderly with normocytic or iron deficiency anemias or those with a serum hemoglobin concentration <12 g/dL; one study did not find such a relationship in the elderly with chronic anemia. A blunted erythropoietin response to anemia has been reported in patients with cancer, rheumatoid arthritis, and AIDS.

Breast-Feeding Considerations When administered enterally to neonates (mixed with human milk or infant formula), *r*HuEPO-α did not significantly increase serum EPO concentrations. If passage via breast milk does occur, risk to a nursing infant appears low.

Pregnancy Considerations Epoetin alfa has been shown to have adverse effects (decreased weight gain, delayed development, delayed ossification) in animal studies. Studies suggest that *r*HuEPO-α does not cross the human placenta. Based on case reports, treatment with *r*HuEPO-α may be an option in pregnant women with ESRD on dialysis. Amenorrheic premenopausal women should be cautioned that menstruation may resume following treatment with *r*HuEPO-α and contraception should be considered if pregnancy is to be avoided.

Additional Information Factors limiting response to epoetin alfa: Delayed onset of erythropoiesis (2-6 weeks to increase hemoglobin), iron deficiency (most patients require iron supplementation); underlying infection, inflammatory or malignant process; blood loss (occult), underlying hematologic disease (thalassemia, refractory anemia, MDS); vitamin deficiency (folic acid or cyanocobalamin), hemolysis, aluminum overload, osteitis fibrosa cystica, and PRCA

Oncology Comment: The American Society of Hematology (ASH) and American Society of Clinical Oncology (ASCO) 2007 updates to the clinical practice guidelines for the use of erythropoiesis-stimulating agents (ESAs) indicate that ESAs are most appropriate when used according to the dosage parameters within the Food and Drug Administration (FDA) approved labeling for epoetin and darbepoetin (Rizzo, 2008). While the previous guidelines addressed only the use of epoetin, the 2007 guidelines also address the use of darbepoetin, which is assessed as being equivalent to epoetin with respect to safety and efficacy. When used as an option for the treatment of chemotherapy-associated anemia (to increase hemoglobin and decrease red blood cell transfusions), therapy with ESAs should begin as the hemoglobin level approaches or falls below 10 g/dL. The ASH/ASCO guidelines recommend following the FDA approved dosing (and dosing adjustment) guidelines and target hemoglobin ranges as alternate dosing and schedules have not demonstrated consistent differences in effectiveness with regard to hemoglobin response. In patients who do not have a response within 6-8 weeks (hemoglobin rise <1-2 g/dL or no reduction in transfusions) ESA therapy should be discontinued.

The guidelines note that patients with an increased risk of thromboembolism (generally includes previous history of thrombosis, surgery, and/or prolonged periods of immobilization) and patients receiving concomitant medications that may increase thromboembolic risk, should begin ESA therapy only after careful consideration. With the exception of low-risk myelodysplasia-associated anemia (which has evidence supporting the use of ESAs without concurrent chemotherapy), the guidelines do not support the use of ESAs in the absence of concurrent chemotherapy.

◆ **Epogen®** *see* Epoetin Alfa *on page 638*

Epoprostenol (e poe PROST en ole)

U.S. Brand Names Flolan®; Veletri®

Index Terms Epoprostenol Sodium; PGI_2; PGX; Prostacyclin

Generic Availability (U.S.) Yes

Pharmacologic Category Prostacyclin; Prostaglandin; Vasodilator

Medication Safety Issues

High alert medication: The Institute for Safe Medication Practices (ISMP) includes this medication among its list of drugs which have a heightened risk of causing significant patient harm when used in error.

Prescribing and Access Restrictions Orders for epoprostenol are distributed by two sources in the United States. Information on orders or reimbursement assistance may be obtained from either Accredo Health, Inc (1-800-935-6526) or TheraCom, Inc (1-877-356-5264).

Pregnancy Risk Factor B

Lactation Excretion in breast milk unknown/use caution

Use Treatment of idiopathic pulmonary arterial hypertension (IPAH); pulmonary hypertension associated with the scleroderma spectrum of disease (SSD) in NYHA Class III and Class IV patients who do not respond adequately to conventional therapy

Unlabeled/Investigational Use Acute vasodilator testing in pulmonary arterial hypertension (PAH)

Inhalation: Intraoperative treatment of pulmonary hypertension in patients undergoing cardiac surgery with cardiopulmonary bypass; post-cardiothoracic surgery pulmonary hypertension, right ventricular dysfunction, or refractory hypoxemia

Mechanism of Action/Effect Naturally occurring prostacyclin (PGI_2) which acts as a strong vasodilator in all vascular beds; inhibits platelet aggregation

Contraindications Hypersensitivity to epoprostenol or to structurally-related compounds; chronic use in patients with heart failure due to severe left ventricular systolic dysfunction; patients who develop pulmonary edema during dose initiation

Warnings/Precautions Initiation or transition to epoprostenol requires specialized cardiopulmonary monitoring in a critical care setting where clinicians are experienced in advanced management of pulmonary arterial hypertension. Abrupt interruptions or large sudden reductions in dosage may result in rebound pulmonary hypertension; some patients with PAH have developed pulmonary edema during dosing adjustment and acute vasodilator testing (not an approved use), which may be associated with concomitant heart failure (LV systolic dysfunction with significantly elevated left heart filling pressures) or pulmonary veno-occlusive disease/pulmonary capillary hemangiomatosis. During chronic use, unless contraindicated, anticoagulants should be coadministered to reduce the risk of thromboembolism. Use cautiously in patients who have conditions that increase bleeding risk (inhibits platelet aggregation). Use with caution in patients receiving anticoagulants and antiplatelet agents. Chronic continuous I.V. infusion of epoprostenol via a chronic indwelling central venous catheter (CVC) has been associated with local infections and serious blood stream infections. Clinical studies of epoprostenol in pulmonary hypertension did not include sufficient numbers of patients ≥65 years of age to substantiate its safety and efficacy in the geriatric population. As a result, in general, dose selection for an elderly patient should be cautious usually starting at the low end of the dosing range.

Drug Interactions

Avoid Concomitant Use There are no known interactions where it is recommended to avoid concomitant use.

Decreased Effect There are no known significant interactions involving a decrease in effect.

Increased Effect/Toxicity

Epoprostenol may increase the levels/effects of: Anticoagulants; Antihypertensives; Antiplatelet Agents

Adverse Reactions

Note: Adverse events reported during dose initiation and escalation include flushing (58%), headache (49%), nausea/vomiting (32%), hypotension (16%), anxiety/nervousness/agitation (11%), chest pain (11%), dizziness, abdominal pain, bradycardia, musculoskeletal pain, dyspnea, back pain, diaphoresis, dyspepsia, hypoesthesia/paresthesia, and tachycardia are also reported. The following adverse events have been reported during chronic administration for IPAH. Although some may be related to the underlying disease state, anxiety, diarrhea, flu-like syndrome, flushing, headache, jaw pain, nausea, nervousness, and vomiting are clearly contributed to epoprostenol.

>10%:

Cardiovascular: Chest pain (52% to 67%), palpitation (63%), tachycardia (35% to 43%), flushing (23% to 42%), arrhythmia (27%), bradycardia (15%), hypotension (13%)

Central nervous system: Dizziness (83%), headache (46% to 83%), chills/fever/sepsis/flu-like syndrome (13% to 25%), anxiety/nervousness/tremor (7% to 21%), depression/depression psychotic (13%)

Dermatologic: Skin ulcer (39%), eczema/rash/urticaria (25%)

Gastrointestinal: Nausea/vomiting (41% to 67%), anorexia (66%), diarrhea (37% to 50%), weight loss (27%)

Hematologic: Hemorrhage (11% to 19%)

Hepatic: Ascites (23%)

Local: Injection site reactions: Infection (21%), pain (13%)

Neuromuscular & skeletal: Weakness (87% to 100%), pain/neck pain/arthralgia (84%), jaw pain (54% to 75%), arthritis (52%), myalgia (44%), musculoskeletal pain (35%; predominantly involving legs and feet), back pain (13%), hypoesthesia/hyperparesthesia/paresthesia (5% to 12%)

Respiratory: Dyspnea (90%)

Miscellaneous: Diaphoresis (41%)

1% to 10%:

Cardiovascular: Supraventricular tachycardia (8%), cerebrovascular accident (4%), MI (4%)

Central nervous system: Insomnia (9%), seizure (4%), somnolence (4%)

Dermatologic: Rash (10%), pruritus (4%)

Endocrine & metabolic: Hypokalemia (6%), hyperkalemia (4%)

Gastrointestinal: Abdominal pain (14%), constipation (4% to 6%), weight gain (6%), flatulence (5%), abdominal enlargement (4%)

Genitourinary: Urinary tract infection (7%)

Hematologic: Thrombocytopenia (4%)

Ocular: Amblyopia (8%), vision abnormality (4%)

Renal: Hematuria (5%)

Respiratory: Epistaxis (4% to 9%), pleural effusion (4% to 7%), pharyngitis (5%), pneumonia (5%), pneumothorax (4%), pulmonary edema (4%)

Pharmacodynamics/Kinetics

Half-Life Elimination 6 minutes

Metabolism Rapidly hydrolyzed; subject to some enzymatic degradation; forms one active metabolite (6-keto-prostaglandin $F_{1}\alpha$) with minimal activity and 13 inactive metabolites

Excretion Urine (84%); feces (4%)

Available Dosage Forms

Injection, powder for reconstitution: 0.5 mg, 1.5 mg

Flolan®: 0.5 mg, 1.5 mg

Veletri®: 1.5 mg

Dosing

Adult & Geriatric

Pulmonary arterial hypertension (PAH): I.V.: Initial: 1-2 ng/kg/minute, increase dose in increments of 1-2 ng/kg/minute every 15 minutes or longer until dose-limiting side effects effects (eg, flushing, jaw pain, headache, or nausea) are noted or response to epoprostenol plateaus. Usual optimal dose (monotherapy): 25-40 ng/kg/minute (McLaughlin, 2009); significant patient variability in optimal dose exists. Maximum dose with chronic therapy has not been defined; however, doses as high as 195 ng/kg/minute have been described in children (Rosenzweig, 1999).

Dose adjustment during chronic phase of treatment:

If symptoms persist or recur following improvement, increase dose in 1-2 ng/kg/minute increments at intervals of at least 15 minutes. May also increase dose at intervals of 24-48 hours or longer (eg, every 1-2 weeks). **Note:** The need for increased doses should be expected with chronic use; incremental increases occur more frequently during the first few months after the drug is initiated.

In case of dose-limiting pharmacologic events (eg, hypotension, severe nausea, vomiting), decrease dose in 2 ng/kg/minute decrements at intervals of at least 15 minutes. Avoid abrupt withdrawal or sudden large dose reductions. **Note:** Adverse event may resolve without dosage adjustment.

Lung transplant: In patients receiving lung transplants, epoprostenol may be tapered after the initiation of cardiopulmonary bypass.

Acute vasodilator testing in patients with PAH (unlabeled use; McLaughlin, 2009): Note: Acute vasodilator testing should only be done in patients who might be considered candidates for calcium channel blocker therapy.

I.V.: Initial: 2 ng/kg/minute; increase dose in increments of 2 ng/kg/minute every 10-15 minutes; dosing range during testing: 2-10 ng/kg/minute

Intraoperative pulmonary hypertension during cardiac surgery with cardiopulmonary bypass (CPB) (unlabeled use): Inhalation (unlabeled route): **Note:** Institution-specific protocols vary.

Administration after induction of anesthesia before incision: 60 mcg (4 mL of 15,000 ng/mL concentration) via jet nebulizer; effect persists for ~25 minutes (Hache, 2003)

or

Intraoperative administration: *Nebulization via ventilator circuit:* Using a 15,000 ng/mL concentration and an oxygen flow of 8 L/minute, begin administration via jet nebulizer 5 minutes prior to weaning from CPB; discontinue at least 60 minutes after CPB weaned (Fattouch, 2006)

Post-cardiothoracic surgery pulmonary hypertension, right ventricular dysfunction, or refractory hypoxemia (unlabeled use) (DeWet, 2004): Inhalation (unlabeled route): **Note:** May need to change ventilator filter every 2 hours due to glycine buffer diluent; may cause ventilator valve malfunction. Tidal volume delivered by ventilator may require adjustment.

Nebulization via ventilator circuit: Using a 20,000 ng/mL concentration, prime nebulizer chamber with 15 mL; administer remainder at a constant rate of 8 mL/hour; delivers ~38 ng/kg/minute (based on a 70 kg patient); set oxygen flow at 2-3 L/minute; wean as tolerated.**Note:** Although not achieved with this regimen, in general, doses >50 ng/kg/minute do not provide additional benefit and may increase the risk of hypotension.

or

Nebulization via facemask with Venturi attachment: Using a 20,000 ng/mL concentration, prime nebulizer chamber with 15 mL; set oxygen flow at 2-3 L/minute; 8 mL/hour will be nebulized; wean as tolerated.

Weaning procedure: Reduce dose by 50% every 2-4 hours (ie, 20,000 ng/mL to 10,000 ng/mL to 5000 ng/mL) until a concentration of 2500 ng/mL is reached; carefully discontinue once patient remains stable on this concentration for at least 4 hours.

Pediatric Pulmonary arterial hypertension (PAH): Unlabeled use; refer to adult dosing.

Administration

I.V. The ambulatory infusion pump should be small and lightweight, be able to adjust infusion rates in 2 ng/kg/minute increments, have occlusion, end of infusion, and low battery alarms, have ± 6% accuracy of the programmed rate, and have positive continuous or pulsatile pressure with intervals ≤3 minutes between pulses. The reservoir should be made of polyvinyl chloride, polypropylene, or glass. Immediate access to back up pump, infusion sets and medication is essential to prevent treatment interruptions.

Inhalation Inhalation is an unlabeled route of administration.

Intraoperative administration: Administer via jet nebulizer connected to the inspiratory limb of the ventilator near the endotracheal tube with a bypass oxygen flow of 8 L/minute to achieve administration of a high proportion of small particles (Fattouch, 2006; Hache, 2003).

Post-cardiothoracic surgery: May also be administered via jet nebulizer connected to the inspiratory limb of the ventilator near the endotracheal tube or via face mask with a Venturi attachment for aerosolization with a bypass oxygen flow of 2-3 L/minute (De Wet, 2004). **Note:** Glycine buffer diluent may cause ventilator valve malfunction; it has been recommended that filters be changed on the ventilator every 2 hours; may also use a ventilator heating coil (De Wet, 2004).

Stability

Reconstitution

Preparation of Epoprostenol Infusion

To make solution with concentration:	Flolan® Instructions	Veletri® Instructions
	Note: Flolan® may only be prepared with sterile diluent provided.	**Note:** Veletri® may only be prepared with sterile water for injection (SWFI) or NS.
3000 ng/mL	Dissolve one 0.5 mg vial with 5 mL supplied diluent, withdraw 3 mL, and add to a sufficient volume of supplied diluent to make a total of 100 mL.	
5000 ng/mL	Dissolve one 0.5 mg vial with 5 mL supplied diluent, withdraw entire vial contents, and add to a sufficient volume of supplied diluent to make a total of 100 mL.	
10,000 ng/mL	Dissolve two 0.5 mg vials each with 5 mL supplied diluent, withdraw entire vial contents, and add to a sufficient volume of supplied diluent to make a total of 100 mL.	
15,000 ng/mL	Dissolve one 1.5 mg vial with 5 mL supplied diluent, withdraw entire vial contents, and add to a sufficient volume of supplied diluent to make a total of 100 mL.	Dissolve one 1.5 mg vial with 5 mL of SWFI or NS, withdraw entire vial contents, and add to a sufficient volume of the identical diluent to make a total of 100 mL.
20,000 ng/mL	Dissolve two 0.5 mg vials each with 5 mL supplied diluent, withdraw entire vial contents, and add to a sufficient volume of supplied diluent to make a total of **50 mL** (DeWet, 2004).	
30,000 ng/mL		Dissolve two 1.5 mg vials each with 5 mL of SWFI or NS, withdraw entire vial contents, and add to a sufficient volume of the identical diluent to make a total of 100 mL.

Storage Injection for reconstitution:

Flolan®: Prior to use, store vials at 15°C to 25°C (59°F to 77°F); do not freeze. Protect from light. Following reconstitution, solution must be stored under refrigeration at 2°C to 8°C (36°F to 46°F) if not used immediately; do not freeze. Protect from light. Discard if refrigerated for >48 hours. During use, a single reservoir of solution may be used at room temperature for a total duration of 8 hours, or used with a cold pouch for administration up to 24 hours. Cold packs should be changed every 12 hours.

Veletri®: Prior to use, store vials at 20°C to 25°C (68°F to 77°F); do not freeze. Protect from light. Following reconstitution, solution may be stored under refrigeration at 2°C to 8°C (36°F to 46°F) up to 5 days or at room temperature of 25°C (77°F) up to 48 hours if not used immediately; do not freeze. Protect from light. Discard if refrigerated for >5 days or if at room temperature for >48 hours. During use, a single reservoir of solution may be used at room temperature for up to 24 hours. If lower concentrations are used, pump reservoirs should be changed every 12 hours when administered at room temperature.

Monitoring and Teaching Issues

Physical Assessment Assess patient's or caregiver's ability to manage a central venous catheter in the home setting. Clinicians should routinely review with patient the importance of infection control practices for the management of a central venous catheter. **Institutional:** Continuous pulmonary and hemodynamic arterial monitoring, INR. **Home therapy:** Avoid sudden rate reduction or abrupt withdrawal or interruption of therapy. Monitor for improved pulmonary function and quality of life.

Patient Education Therapy on this drug will probably be long-term. You may experience mild headache, nausea, vomiting, diarrhea, weight loss, nervousness, dizziness, or muscular pains. Report immediately any signs or symptoms of acute or severe headache; back pain; increased difficult breathing; flushing; fever or chills; any unusual bleeding or bruising; chest pain; palpitations; difficulty breathing; increased pain, irritation, or pus formed at I.V. site; or any onset of unresolved diarrhea.

Pregnancy Considerations Teratogenic effects were not reported in animal studies. There are no adequate and well-controlled studies in pregnant women. Women with IPAH are encouraged to avoid pregnancy.

◆ **Epoprostenol Sodium** *see* Epoprostenol *on page 643*

Eprosartan (ep roe SAR tan)

U.S. Brand Names Teveten®

Generic Availability (U.S.) No

Pharmacologic Category Angiotensin II Receptor Blocker

Pregnancy Risk Factor C (1st trimester); D (2nd and 3rd trimesters)

Lactation Not recommended

Use Treatment of hypertension; may be used alone or in combination with other antihypertensives

Mechanism of Action/Effect Eprosartan is an angiotensin receptor antagonist which blocks the vasoconstriction and aldosterone-secreting effects of angiotensin II.

Contraindications Hypersensitivity to eprosartan or any component of the formulation

Warnings/Precautions [U.S. Boxed Warning]: Based on human data, drugs that act on the angiotensin system can cause injury and death to the developing fetus when used in the second and third trimesters. Angiotensin receptor blockers should be discontinued as soon as possible once pregnancy is detected. May cause hyperkalemia; avoid potassium supplementation unless specifically required by healthcare provider. Avoid use or use a smaller dose in patients who are volume depleted; correct depletion first. May be associated with deterioration of renal function and/or increases in serum creatinine, particularly in patients with low renal blood flow (eg, renal artery stenosis, heart failure) whose glomerular filtration rate (GFR) is dependent on efferent arteriolar vasoconstriction by angiotensin II. Use with caution in unstented unilateral/bilateral renal artery stenosis. When unstented bilateral renal artery stenosis is present, use is generally avoided due to the elevated risk of deterioration in renal function unless possible benefits outweigh risks. Use with caution in pre-existing renal insufficiency; significant aortic/mitral stenosis. Concurrent use of ACE inhibitors may increase the risk of clinically-significant adverse events (eg, renal dysfunction, hyperkalemia).

Drug Interactions

Metabolism/Transport Effects Inhibits CYP2C9 (weak)

Avoid Concomitant Use There are no known interactions where it is recommended to avoid concomitant use.

Decreased Effect

The levels/effects of Eprosartan may be decreased by: Herbs (Hypertensive Properties); Methylphenidate; Nonsteroidal Anti-Inflammatory Agents; Yohimbine

Increased Effect/Toxicity

Eprosartan may increase the levels/effects of: ACE Inhibitors; Amifostine; Antihypertensives; Hypotensive Agents; Lithium; Potassium-Sparing Diuretics; RiTUXimab

The levels/effects of Eprosartan may be increased by: Diazoxide; Eplerenone; Herbs (Hypotensive Properties); MAO Inhibitors; Pentoxifylline; Phosphodiesterase 5 Inhibitors; Potassium Salts; Prostacyclin Analogues; Tolvaptan; Trimethoprim

Nutritional/Ethanol Interactions Herb/Nutraceutical: Avoid dong quai if using for hypertension (has estrogenic activity). Avoid ephedra, yohimbe, ginseng (may worsen hypertension). Avoid garlic (may have increased antihypertensive effect).

Adverse Reactions 1% to 10%:

Central nervous system: Fatigue (2%), depression (1%)
Endocrine & metabolic: Hypertriglyceridemia (1%)
Gastrointestinal: Abdominal pain (2%)
Genitourinary: Urinary tract infection (1%)
Respiratory: Upper respiratory tract infection (8%), rhinitis (4%), pharyngitis (4%), cough (4%)
Miscellaneous: Viral infection (2%), injury (2%)

Pharmacodynamics/Kinetics

Bioavailability 300 mg dose: 13%

Time to Peak Serum: Fasting: 1-2 hours

Protein Binding 98%

Half-Life Elimination Terminal: 5-9 hours

Metabolism Minimally hepatic

Excretion Feces (90%); urine (7% primarily as unchanged drug)
Clearance: 7.9 L/hour

Available Dosage Forms

Tablet, oral:
Teveten®: 400 mg, 600 mg

Dosing

Adult & Geriatric Hypertension: Oral: Dosage must be individualized. Can administer once or twice daily with total daily doses of 400-800 mg. Usual starting dose is 600 mg once daily as monotherapy in patients who are euvolemic. Limited clinical experience with doses >800 mg.

Renal Impairment No starting dosage adjustment is necessary; however, carefully monitor the patient.

Hepatic Impairment No starting dosage adjustment is necessary; however, carefully monitor the patient.

Monitoring and Teaching Issues

Laboratory Monitoring Electrolytes, serum creatinine, BUN, urinalysis

Physical Assessment Use caution in presence of renal impairment. Assess potential for interactions with other pharmacological agents or herbal products that may impact blood pressure. Monitor for hypotension on a regular basis during therapy.

Patient Education This drug does not eliminate need for diet or exercise regimen as recommended by prescriber. May cause dizziness, fainting, lightheadedness, or postural hypotension. Report chest pain or palpitations; respiratory infection or cold symptoms; unusual cough; swelling of face, tongue, lips, or extremities; changes in urinary pattern; or extreme fatigue.

Geriatric Considerations No specific dose adjustments are necessary in the elderly due to the drug's major route of elimination. However, since many elderly may be volume depleted due to their "blunted thirst reflex" and use of diuretics, care and monitoring of blood pressure and volume status are necessary upon initiation.

Pregnancy Considerations Medications which act on the renin-angiotensin system are reported to have the following fetal/neonatal effects: Hypotension, neonatal skull hypoplasia, anuria, renal failure, and death; oligohydramnios is also reported. These effects are reported to occur with exposure during the second and third trimesters. There are no adequate and well-controlled studies in pregnant women. **[U.S. Boxed Warning]: Based on human data, drugs that act on the angiotensin system can cause injury and death to the developing fetus when used in the second and third trimesters. Angiotensin receptor blockers should be discontinued as soon as possible once pregnancy is detected.**

Related Information

Angiotensin Agents *on page* 1974

Eprosartan and Hydrochlorothiazide

(ep roe SAR tan & hye droe klor oh THYE a zide)

U.S. Brand Names Teveten® HCT

Index Terms Eprosartan Mesylate and Hydrochlorothiazide; Hydrochlorothiazide and Eprosartan

Generic Availability (U.S.) No

Pharmacologic Category Angiotensin II Receptor Blocker; Diuretic, Thiazide

Pregnancy Risk Factor C/D (2nd and 3rd trimesters)

Lactation Enters breast milk/not recommended

Use Treatment of hypertension (not indicated for initial treatment)

Available Dosage Forms

Tablet:

Teveten® HCT: 600 mg/12.5 mg: Eprosartan 600 mg and hydrochlorothiazide 12.5 mg; 600 mg/25 mg: Eprosartan 600 mg and hydrochlorothiazide 25 mg

Dosing

Adult & Geriatric Hypertension: Oral: Dose is individualized (combination substituted for individual components)

Usual recommended dose: Eprosartan 600 mg/hydrochlorothiazide 12.5 mg once daily (maximum dose: Eprosartan 600 mg/hydrochlorothiazide 25 mg once daily)

Renal Impairment Initial dose adjustments not recommended by manufacturer; carefully monitor patient. Hydrochlorothiazide is ineffective in patients with Cl_{cr} <30 mL/minute.

Hepatic Impairment Initial dose adjustments not recommended by manufacturer; carefully monitor patient.

Administration

Oral May be administered without regard to meals.

Monitoring and Teaching Issues

Laboratory Monitoring Serum electrolytes, BUN, creatinine

Physical Assessment See individual agents.

Patient Education See individual agents.

Related Information

Eprosartan *on page* 646

Hydrochlorothiazide *on page* 912

- **Eprosartan Mesylate and Hydrochlorothiazide** *see* Eprosartan and Hydrochlorothiazide *on page* 648
- **Epsom Salts** *see* Magnesium Sulfate *on page* 1144
- **EPT** *see* Teniposide *on page* 1728
- **Eptacog Alfa (Activated)** *see* Factor VIIa (Recombinant) *on page* 731

Eptifibatide (ep TIF i ba tide)

U.S. Brand Names Integrilin®

Index Terms Intrifiban

Generic Availability (U.S.) No

Pharmacologic Category Antiplatelet Agent, Glycoprotein IIb/IIIa Inhibitor

Medication Safety Issues

High alert medication: The Institute for Safe Medication Practices (ISMP) includes this medication among its list of drugs which have a heightened risk of causing significant patient harm when used in error.

Pregnancy Risk Factor B

Lactation Excretion in breast milk unknown/use caution

Use Treatment of patients with acute coronary syndrome (unstable angina/non-Q wave myocardial infarction [UA/NQMI]), including patients who are to be managed medically and those undergoing percutaneous coronary intervention (PCI including angioplasty, intracoronary stenting)

Unlabeled/Investigational Use To support PCI during ST-elevation myocardial infarction (administered at the time of primary PCI)

Mechanism of Action/Effect Eptifibatide is a glycoprotein IIb/IIIa receptor antagonist that reversibly blocks platelet aggregation and prevents thrombosis.

Contraindications Hypersensitivity to eptifibatide or any component of the product; active abnormal bleeding within the previous 30 days or a history of bleeding diathesis; history of stroke within 30 days or a history of hemorrhagic stroke; severe hypertension (systolic blood pressure >200 mm Hg or diastolic blood pressure >110 mm Hg) not adequately controlled on antihypertensive therapy; major surgery within the preceding 6 weeks; current or planned administration of another parenteral GP IIb/IIIa inhibitor; dependency on hemodialysis

Canadian labeling: Additional contraindications (not in U.S. labeling): PT >1.2 times control or INR ≥2.0; known history of intracranial disease (eg, neoplasm, arteriovenous malformation, aneurysm); severe renal impairment (Cl_{cr} <30 mL/minute); thrombocytopenia (<100,000 cells/mm^3); clinically significant liver disease

Warnings/Precautions Bleeding is the most common complication. Most major bleeding occurs at the arterial access site where the cardiac catheterization was done. When bleeding can not be controlled with pressure, discontinue infusion and heparin. Patients <70 kg may be at greater risk for major and minor bleeding. Use caution in patients with hemorrhagic retinopathy or with other drugs that affect hemostasis. Use with extreme caution in patients with platelet counts <100,000/mm^3 (contraindicated in the Canadian labeling). If platelet count decreases to <100,000/mm^3 during therapy, discontinue eptifibatide and heparin if administered concurrently.

Concurrent use with thrombolytics has not been established as safe and is generally not recommended (Goodman, 2008). Minimize invasive procedures, including arterial and venous punctures, I.M. injections, and nasogastric tube insertion. Prior to sheath removal, the aPTT or ACT should be checked (do not remove unless aPTT is <45 seconds or the ACT <150 seconds). Use caution in renal dysfunction (estimated Cl_{cr} <50 mL/minute, using Cockcroft-Gault equation); dosage adjustment required. Use is contraindicated in patients dependent upon hemodialysis.

Drug Interactions

Avoid Concomitant Use There are no known interactions where it is recommended to avoid concomitant use.

Decreased Effect

The levels/effects of Eptifibatide may be decreased by: Nonsteroidal Anti-Inflammatory Agents

Increased Effect/Toxicity

Eptifibatide may increase the levels/effects of: Anticoagulants; Antiplatelet Agents; Collagenase (Systemic); Drotrecogin Alfa; Ibritumomab; Salicylates; Thrombolytic Agents; Tositumomab and Iodine I 131 Tositumomab

The levels/effects of Eptifibatide may be increased by: Dasatinib; Glucosamine; Herbs (Anticoagulant/Antiplatelet Properties); Nonsteroidal Anti-Inflammatory Agents; Omega-3-Acid Ethyl Esters; Pentosan Polysulfate Sodium; Pentoxifylline; Prostacyclin Analogues

Nutritional/Ethanol Interactions Herb/Nutraceutical: Avoid alfalfa, anise, bilberry, bladderwrack, bromelain, cat's claw, celery, coleus, cordyceps, dong quai, evening primrose oil, fenugreek, feverfew, garlic, ginger, ginkgo biloba, ginseng (American), ginseng (Panax), ginseng (Siberian), grapeseed, green tea, guggul, horse chestnut seed, horseradish, licorice, prickly ash, red clover, reishi, same (s-adenosylmethionine), sweet clover, turmeric, and white willow (all have additional antiplatelet activity).

Adverse Reactions Bleeding is the major drug-related adverse effect. Access site is often primary source of bleeding complications. Incidence of bleeding is also related to heparin intensity. Patients weighing <70 kg may have an increased risk of major bleeding.

>10%: Hematologic: Bleeding (major: 1% to 11%; minor: 3% to 14%; transfusion required: 2% to 13%)

1% to 10%:

Cardiovascular: Hypotension (up to 7%)

Hematologic: Thrombocytopenia (1% to 3%)

Local: Injection site reaction

Pharmacodynamics/Kinetics

Onset of Action Within 1 hour

Duration of Action Platelet function restored ~4 hours following discontinuation

Protein Binding ~25%

Half-Life Elimination 2.5 hours

Excretion Primarily urine (as eptifibatide and metabolites); significant renal impairment may alter disposition of this compound

Clearance: Total body: 55-58 mL/kg/hour; Renal: ~50% of total in healthy subjects

Available Dosage Forms

Injection, solution:

Integrilin®: 0.75 mg/mL (100 mL); 2 mg/mL (10 mL, 100 mL)

Dosing

Adult

Acute coronary syndrome: I.V.: Bolus of 180 mcg/kg (maximum: 22.6 mg) over 1-2 minutes, begun as soon as possible following diagnosis, followed by a continuous infusion of 2 mcg/kg/minute (maximum: 15 mg/hour) until hospital discharge or initiation of CABG surgery, up to 72 hours. Concurrent aspirin and heparin therapy (target aPTT 50-70 seconds) are recommended. **Note:** If ST-elevation myocardial infarction (STEMI), the 2009 ACCF/AHA/SCAI guidelines suggest administration at the time of primary PCI (Kushner, 2009).

Percutaneous coronary intervention (PCI) with or without stenting: I.V.: Bolus of 180 mcg/kg (maximum: 22.6 mg) administered immediately before the initiation of PCI, followed by a continuous infusion of 2 mcg/kg/minute (maximum: 15 mg/hour). A second 180 mcg/kg bolus (maximum: 22.6 mg) should be administered 10 minutes after the first bolus. Infusion should be continued until hospital discharge or for up to 18-24 hours, whichever comes first; shorter infusion durations (ie, <2 hours) may be considered for nonemergent uncomplicated PCI in patients adequately pretreated with clopidogrel (Fung, 2007). Concurrent aspirin (162-325 mg 1-24 hours before PCI and daily thereafter) and heparin therapy (ACT 200-250 seconds during PCI) are recommended. Heparin infusion after PCI is discouraged. In patients who undergo coronary artery bypass graft surgery, discontinue infusion prior to surgery.

Geriatric Refer to adult dosing. No dosing adjustment for the elderly appears to be necessary; adjust carefully to renal function.

Renal Impairment Dialysis is a contraindication to use.

Note: The Cockcroft-Gault equation using actual body weight should be used to estimate renal function.

Acute coronary syndrome: Cl_{cr} <50 mL/minute: Use 180 mcg/kg bolus (maximum: 22.6 mg) and 1 mcg/kg/minute infusion (maximum: 7.5 mg/hour)

Percutaneous coronary intervention (PCI) with or without stenting: Cl_{cr} <50 mL/minute: Use 180 mcg/kg bolus (maximum: 22.6 mg) administered immediately before the initiation of PCI and followed by a continuous infusion of 1 mcg/kg/minute (maximum: 7.5 mg/hour). A second 180 mcg/kg (maximum: 22.6 mg) bolus should be administered 10 minutes after the first bolus.

Administration

I.V. Do not shake vial. Administer bolus doses by I.V. push over 1-2 minutes. Begin continuous infusion immediately following bolus administration; administer directly from the 100 mL vial.

Stability

Storage Vials should be stored refrigerated at 2°C to 8°C (36°F to 46°F). Vials can be kept at room temperature for 2 months, after which they must be discarded. Protect from light until administration. Do not use beyond the expiration date. Discard any unused portion left in the vial.

Monitoring and Teaching Issues

Laboratory Monitoring Laboratory tests at baseline and monitoring during therapy: Hematocrit and hemoglobin, platelet count, serum creatinine, PT/aPTT (maintain aPTT between 50-70 seconds unless PCI is to be performed), and ACT with PCI (maintain ACT between 200-300 seconds during PCI). Prior to sheath removal, the aPTT or ACT should be checked (do not remove unless aPTT is <45 seconds or the ACT <150 seconds).

Physical Assessment Monitor vital signs prior to, during, and after therapy. Monitor closely for signs of excessive/unusual bleeding. Observe and teach patient bleeding precautions.

Patient Education This medication can only be administered intravenously. You will have a tendency to bleed easily while medication is being administered. Report unusual bruising or bleeding (eg, blood in urine, stool, or vomitus; bleeding gums), dizziness or vision changes, or back pain.

Pregnancy Considerations Teratogenic effects were not observed in animal studies.

- ◆ **Epzicom®** *see* Abacavir and Lamivudine *on page* *32*
- ◆ **Equetro®** *see* CarBAMazepine *on page* *287*
- ◆ **ER-086526** *see* Eribulin *on page* *652*
- ◆ **Eraxis™** *see* Anidulafungin *on page* *130*
- ◆ **Erbitux®** *see* Cetuximab *on page* *352*

Ergocalciferol (er goe kal SIF e role)

U.S. Brand Names Calciferol™ [OTC]; Drisdol®; Drisdol® [OTC]

Index Terms Activated Ergosterol; D2; Viosterol; Vitamin D2

Generic Availability (U.S.) Yes: Capsule (softgel), tablet

Pharmacologic Category Vitamin D Analog

Medication Safety Issues

Sound-alike/look-alike issues:

Calciferol™ may be confused with calcitriol

Drisdol® may be confused with Drysol™

Ergocalciferol may be confused with alfacalcidol, cholecalciferol

Potential for medication errors: Liquid vitamin D preparations have the potential for dosing errors when administered to infants. Droppers should be clearly marked to easily provide 400 international units. For products intended for infants, the FDA recommends that accompanying droppers deliver no more than 400 international units per dose.

Pregnancy Risk Factor C (manufacturer); A/C (dose exceeding RDA recommendation; per expert analysis)

Lactation Enters breast milk/use caution

Use Treatment of refractory rickets, hypophosphatemia, hypoparathyroidism; dietary supplement

Unlabeled/Investigational Use Prevention and treatment of vitamin D deficiency in patients with chronic kidney disease (CKD)

Available Dosage Forms

Capsule, oral: 50,000 int. units

Drisdol®: 50,000 int. units

Capsule, softgel, oral: 50,000 int. units, 50,000 units

Solution, oral: 8000 int. units/mL (60 mL)

Calciferol™ [OTC]: 8000 int. units/mL (60 mL)

Drisdol® [OTC]: 8000 int. units/mL (60 mL)

Tablet, oral: 400 int. units

Dosing

Adult & Geriatric Note: 1 mcg = 40 int. units

Dietary Intake Reference ([DIR] 1997): Note: DIR is currently being reviewed (March 2009): Oral:

18-50 years: 5 mcg/day (200 int. units/day)

51-70 years: 10 mcg/day (400 int. units/day)

Osteoporosis prevention and treatment: Adults ≥50 years: 10 mcg/day (800-1000 int. units/day)

Vitamin D deficiency/insufficiency in patients with CKD stages 3-4 (K/DOQI guidelines): **Note:** Dose is based on 25-hydroxyvitamin D serum level (25[OH]D): Oral (treatment duration should be a total of 6 months):

Serum 25(OH)D <5 ng/mL:

50,000 int. units/week for 12 weeks, then 50,000 int. units/month

Serum 25(OH)D 5-15 ng/mL:

50,000 int. units/week for 4 weeks, then 50,000 int. units/month

Serum 25(OH)D 16-30 ng/mL:

50,000 int. units/month

Hypoparathyroidism: Oral: 625 mcg to 5 mg/day (25,000-200,000 int. units) and calcium supplements

Nutritional rickets and osteomalacia: Oral:

Adults with normal absorption: 25-125 mcg/day (1000-5000 int. units)

Adults with malabsorption: 250-7500 mcg (10,000-300,000 int. units)

Vitamin D *-dependent* rickets: Oral: 250 mcg to 1.5 mg/day (10,000-60,000 int. units)

Vitamin D *-resistant* rickets: Oral: 12,000-500,000 int. units/day

Familial hypophosphatemia: Oral: 10,000-60,000 int. units plus phosphate supplements

Pediatric Note: 1 mcg = 40 int. units

Adequate intake:

Infants and Children: Dietary Intake Reference ([DIR] 1997): Oral: 5 mcg (200 int. units)/day; **Note:** DIR is currently being reviewed (March 2009)

Infants and Children (Wagner, 2008): Oral: 10 mcg/day (400 int. units/day)

Breast-fed (fully or partially) Infants: Oral: 10 mcg/day (400 int. units/day) beginning in the first few days of life; continue supplementation until infant is weaned to ≥1 L/day or 1 quart/day of vitamin D-fortified formula or whole milk (after 12 months of age)

Nonbreast-fed Infants, Older Children ingesting <1000 mL of vitamin D-fortified formula or milk: Oral: 10 mcg/day (400 int. units/day)

Adolescents without adequate intake: Oral: 10 mcg/day (400 int. units/day)

Children with increased risk of vitamin D deficiency (chronic fat malabsorption, maintained on chronic antiseizure medications): Oral: Higher doses may be required; use laboratory testing (25 [OH]D, PTH, bone mineral status) to evaluate

Vitamin D deficiency/insufficiency in patients with CKD stages 3-4 (K/DOQI guidelines): **Note:** Dose is based on 25-hydroxyvitamin D serum level (25[OH]D): Oral (treatment duration should be a total of 3 months):

Serum 25(OH)D <5 ng/mL:

8000 int. units/day for 4 weeks, then 4000 int. units/day for 2 months **or**

50,000 int. units/week for 4 weeks, then 50,000 int. units twice a month for 2 months

Serum 25(OH)D 5-15 ng/mL:

4000 int units/day **or**

50,000 int units every other week

Serum 25(OH)D 16-30 ng/mL:

2000 int. units/day **or**

50,000 int. units every 4 weeks

Hypoparathyroidism: Oral: 1.25-5 mg/day (50,000-200,000 int. units) and calcium supplements

Nutritional rickets and osteomalacia: Oral:

Children with normal absorption: 25-125 mcg/day (1000-5000 int. units)

Children with malabsorption: 250-625 mcg/day (10,000-25,000 int. units)

Vitamin D *-dependent* rickets: Oral: 75-125 mcg/day (3000-5000 int. units); maximum: 1500 mcg/day

Vitamin D *-resistant* rickets: Oral: 12,000-500,000 int. units/day

Familial hypophosphatemia: Oral: 40,000-80,000 int. units plus phosphate supplements; dose may be reduced once growth is complete

Monitoring and Teaching Issues

Laboratory Monitoring Serum calcium, creatinine, BUN, phosphorus every 1-2 weeks

Children at increased risk of vitamin D deficiency (chronic fat malabsorption, chronic antiseizure medication use) require serum 25(OH)D, PTH, and bone mineral status to evaluate. If vitamin D supplement required, then 25(OH)D levels should be repeated at 3-month intervals until normal. PTH and bone mineral status should be monitored every 6 months until normal.

Vitamin D deficiency/insufficiency in patients with CKD stages 3-4: measure serum 25(OH)D levels after 3 months of treatment in children or after 6 months in adults. Discontinue ergocalciferol (or any vitamin D supplements) if the corrected total serum calcium level is >10.2 mg/dL.

Physical Assessment Provide patient appropriate nutritional counseling.

Patient Education Your prescriber may recommend a special diet. You may experience nausea, vomiting, or metallic taste. Report weakness, unresolved nausea or vomiting, or CNS irritability.

Eribulin (er i BUE lin)

U.S. Brand Names Halaven™

Index Terms B1939; E7389; ER-086526; Eribulin Mesylate; Halichondrin B Analog

Generic Availability (U.S.) No

Pharmacologic Category Antineoplastic Agent, Antimicrotubular

Medication Safety Issues

Sound-alike/look-alike issues:

Eribulin may be confused with epirubicin, erlotinib

High alert medication: This medication is in a class the Institute for Safe Medication Practices (ISMP) includes among its list of drug classes which have a heightened risk of causing significant patient harm when used in error.

Pregnancy Risk Factor D

Lactation Excretion in breast milk unknown/not recommended

Use Treatment of metastatic breast cancer in patients who have received at least 2 prior chemotherapy regimens

Available Dosage Forms

Injection, solution:

Halaven™: 0.5 mg/mL (2 mL)

Dosing

Adult & Geriatric Breast cancer, metastatic: I.V.: 1.4 mg/m^2/dose on days 1 and 8 of a 21-day treatment cycle

Renal Impairment

Cl_{cr} >50 mL/minute: No adjustment required.

Cl_{cr} 30-50 mL/minute: Reduce to 1.1 mg/m^2/dose.

Cl_{cr} <30 mL/minute: Use has not been studied.

Hepatic Impairment

Mild hepatic impairment (Child-Pugh class A): Reduce to 1.1 mg/m^2/dose.

Moderate hepatic impairment (Child-Pugh class B): Reduce to 0.7 mg/m^2/dose.

Severe hepatic impairment (Child-Pugh class C): Use has not been studied.

Adjustment for Toxicity

ANC <1000/mm^3 or platelets <75,000/mm^3 or grade 3 or 4 nonhematologic toxicity on day 1 or 8: Withhold dose; may delay day 8 dose up to 1 week. If toxicity resolves to ≤grade 2 by day 15 administer a reduced dose and wait at least 2 weeks before beginning the next cycle. Omit dose if not resolved to ≤grade 2 by day 15. Do not re-escalate dose after reduction.

Permanently reduce dose from 1.4 mg/m^2 to 1.1 mg/m^2 for the following:

ANC <500/mm^3 for >7 days

ANC <1000/mm^3 with fever or infection

Platelets <25,000/mm^3

Platelets <50,000/mm^3 requiring transfusion

Nonhematologic toxicity of grade 3 or 4

Dose omission or delay due to toxicity on day 8 of prior cycle

Permanently reduce dose from 1.1 mg/m^2 to 0.7 mg/m^2 for occurrence of any of the above events; discontinue treatment if the above toxicities occur at the 0.7 mg/m^2 dose level.

Administration

I.V. Infuse over 2-5 minutes. May be administered undiluted or diluted in 100 mL normal saline.

Monitoring and Teaching Issues

Laboratory Monitoring CBC with differential prior to each dose; renal and liver function tests; serum electrolytes, including potassium and magnesium

◆ **Eribulin Mesylate** *see* Eribulin *on page* 652

Erlotinib (er LOE tye nib)

U.S. Brand Names Tarceva®

Index Terms CP358774; Erlotinib Hydrochloride; OSI-774

Generic Availability (U.S.) No

Pharmacologic Category Antineoplastic Agent, Tyrosine Kinase Inhibitor; Epidermal Growth Factor Receptor (EGFR) Inhibitor

Medication Safety Issues

Sound-alike/look-alike issues:

Erlotinib may be confused with eribulin, gefitinib, imatinib, SUNItinib, vandetanib

High alert medication: This medication is in a class the Institute for Safe Medication Practices (ISMP) includes among its list of drug classes which have a heightened risk of causing significant patient harm when used in error.

Pregnancy Risk Factor D

Lactation Excretion in breast milk unknown/not recommended

Use Treatment of locally advanced or metastatic nonsmall cell lung cancer (NSCLC) refractory to at least 1 prior chemotherapy regimen (as monotherapy); maintenance treatment of locally advanced or metastatic NCSLC which has not progressed after 4-6 cycles of first line platinum-based chemotherapy; locally advanced, unresectable or metastatic pancreatic cancer (first-line therapy in combination with gemcitabine)

Unlabeled/Investigational Use First-line treatment of NSCLC with known EGFR mutation; treatment of head and neck cancer

Mechanism of Action/Effect Inhibits the intracellular phosphorylation of tyrosine kinase associated with epidermal growth factor receptor (EGFR) which is located on both normal and cancer cells causing cell death.

Contraindications There are no contraindications listed within the FDA-approved manufacturer's labeling.

Canadian labeling: Hypersensitivity to erlotinib or any component of the formulation

Warnings/Precautions Hazardous agent - use appropriate precautions for handling and disposal. Rare, sometimes fatal, pulmonary toxicity, including interstitial lung disease (acute respiratory distress syndrome, interstitial pneumonia, obliterative bronchiolitis, pneumonitis, pulmonary fibrosis, and pulmonary infiltrates) has occurred; symptoms may begin within 5 days to more than 9 months after treatment initiation (median: 39 days). Interrupt therapy for unexplained pulmonary symptoms (dyspnea, cough, and fever); discontinue for confirmed ILD.

Liver enzyme elevations have been reported. Hepatic failure and hepatorenal syndrome have also been reported, particularly in patients with baseline hepatic impairment. Monitor liver function; patients with any hepatic impairment (total bilirubin >ULN; Child-Pugh class A, B, or C) should be closely monitored, including those with hepatic disease due to tumor burden; use with extreme caution in patients with total bilirubin >3 times ULN. Dosage reduction, interruption or discontinuation may be recommended for changes in hepatic function. Acute renal failure and renal insufficiency (with/without hypokalemia) have been reported; use with caution in patients with or at risk for renal impairment. Monitor closely for dehydration; monitor renal function and electrolytes in patients at risk for dehydration. Gastrointestinal perforation has been reported with use; risk for perforation is increased with concurrent anti-angiogenic agents, corticosteroids, NSAIDs, and/or taxane based-therapy, and patients with history of peptic ulcers or diverticular disease; permanently discontinue in patients who develop perforation.

Bullous, blistering, or exfoliating skin conditions, some suggestive of Stevens-Johnson or toxic epidermal necrolysis (TEN) have been reported with use. Generalized or severe acneiform, erythematous or maculopapular rash may occur. Skin rash may correlate with treatment response and prolonged survival (Saif, 2008); management of skin rashes that are not serious should include alcohol-free lotions, topical antibiotics, or topical corticosteroids, or if necessary, oral antibiotics and systemic corticosteroids; avoid sunlight. Reduce dose or temporarily interrupt treatment for severe skin reactions; interrupt or discontinue treatment for bullous, blistering or exfoliative skin toxicity. Corneal perforation and ulceration have been reported with use; abnormal eyelash growth, keratoconjunctivitis sicca, or keratitis have also been reported and are known risk factors for corneal ulceration/perforation. Interrupt or discontinue treatment in patients presenting with eye pain or other acute or worsening ocular symptoms.

Use caution with cardiovascular disease; MI, CVA, and microangiopathic hemolytic anemia with thrombocytopenia have been noted in patients receiving concomitant erlotinib and gemcitabine. Elevated INR and bleeding events have been reported; use caution with concomitant anticoagulant therapy. Erlotinib levels may be lower in patients who smoke; advise patients to stop smoking. Smokers treated with 300 mg/day exhibited steady-state erlotinib levels comparable to former- and never-smokers receiving 150 mg/day (Hughes, 2009). Concurrent use with CYP3A4 inhibitors and moderate or strong CYP3A4 inducers may affect erlotinib levels; consider alternative agents to CYP3A4 inducers to avoid the potential for CYP-mediated interactions; use with caution in patients taking strong CYP3A4 inhibitors. Consider erlotinib dosage modification if concurrent use with CYP3A4 inhibitors/inducers cannot be avoided. In patients with NSCLC, EGFR mutations, specifically exon 19 deletions and exon 21 mutation (L858R), are associated with better response to erlotinib (Riely, 2006); erlotinib treatment is not recommended in patients with *K-ras* mutations; they are not likely to benefit from erlotinib treatment (Eberhard, 2005; Miller, 2008). Concurrent erlotinib plus platinum-based chemotherapy is not recommended for first line treatment of locally advanced or metastatic NSCLC due to a lack of clinical benefit. Product may contain lactose; avoid use in patients with Lapp lactase deficiency, glucose-galactose malabsorption, or glucose intolerance. Safety and efficacy have not been established in children.

Drug Interactions

Metabolism/Transport Effects Substrate of CYP1A2 (minor), 3A4 (major)

Avoid Concomitant Use

Avoid concomitant use of Erlotinib with any of the following: BCG; H2-Antagonists; Natalizumab; Pimecrolimus; Proton Pump Inhibitors; Roflumilast; Tacrolimus (Topical); Vaccines (Live)

Decreased Effect

Erlotinib may decrease the levels/effects of: BCG; Cardiac Glycosides; Sipuleucel-T; Vaccines (Inactivated); Vaccines (Live); Vitamin K Antagonists

The levels/effects of Erlotinib may be decreased by: Antacids; CYP3A4 Inducers (Strong); Deferasirox; Echinacea; H2-Antagonists; Herbs (CYP3A4 Inducers); Proton Pump Inhibitors; Rifampin

Increased Effect/Toxicity

Erlotinib may increase the levels/effects of: Leflunomide; Natalizumab; Vaccines (Live); Vitamin K Antagonists

The levels/effects of Erlotinib may be increased by: Antifungal Agents (Azole Derivatives, Systemic); Ciprofloxacin; Ciprofloxacin (Systemic); Conivaptan; CYP3A4 Inhibitors (Moderate); CYP3A4 Inhibitors (Strong); Dasatinib; Denosumab; FluvoxaMINE; Pimecrolimus; Roflumilast; Tacrolimus (Topical); Trastuzumab

Nutritional/Ethanol Interactions

Food: Erlotinib bioavailability is increased with food. Avoid grapefruit or grapefruit juice (may decrease the metabolism and increase erlotinib plasma concentrations).

Herb/Nutraceutical: Avoid St John's wort (may increase metabolism and decrease erlotinib concentrations).

Adverse Reactions

Adverse reactions reported with monotherapy:

>10%:

- Central nervous system: Fatigue (9% to 52%)
- Dermatologic: Rash (49% to 75%; grade 3: 6% to 8%; grade 4: <1%; median onset: 8 days), pruritus (7% to 13%), dry skin (4% to 12%)
- Gastrointestinal: Diarrhea (20% to 54%; grade 3: 2% to 6%; grade 4: <1%; median onset: 12 days), anorexia (9% to 52%), nausea (33%), vomiting (23%), stomatitis (17%), abdominal pain (11%)
- Ocular: Conjunctivitis (12%), keratoconjunctivitis sicca (12%)
- Respiratory: Dyspnea (41%), cough (33%)
- Miscellaneous: Infection (24%)

1% to 10%:

- Dermatologic: Acne (6%), dermatitis acneiform (5%), paronychia (4%)
- Gastrointestinal: Weight loss (4%)
- Hepatic: ALT increased (grade 2: 2% to 4%; grade 3: 1%), hyperbilirubinemia (grade 2: 4%; grade 3: <1%)
- Respiratory: Pneumonitis/pulmonary infiltrate (3%), pulmonary fibrosis (3%)

Adverse reactions reported with combination (erlotinib plus gemcitabine) therapy:

- Cardiovascular: Edema (37%), thrombotic events (grades 3/4: 11%), deep venous thrombosis (4%), cerebrovascular accident (2%; including cerebral hemorrhage), MI/myocardial ischemia (2%), arrhythmia, syncope
- Central nervous system: Fatigue (79%), fever (36%), depression (19%), dizziness (15%), headache (15%), anxiety (13%)
- Dermatologic: Rash (69%), alopecia (14%)
- Gastrointestinal: Nausea (60%), anorexia (52%), diarrhea (48%), abdominal pain (46%), vomiting (42%), weight loss (39%), stomatitis (22%), dyspepsia (17%), flatulence (13%), ileus, pancreatitis
- Hematologic: Hemolytic anemia, microangiopathic hemolytic anemia with thrombocytopenia (1%)
- Hepatic: ALT increased (grade 2: 31%, grade 3: 13%, grade 4: <1%), AST increased (grade 2: 24%, grade 3: 10%, grade 4 <1%), hyperbilirubinemia (grade 2: 17%, grade 3: 10%, grade 4: <1%)
- Neuromuscular & skeletal: Bone pain (25%), myalgia (21%), neuropathy (13%), rigors (12%)
- Renal: Renal insufficiency
- Respiratory: Dyspnea (24%), cough (16%), interstitial lung disease (ILD)-like events (3%)
- Miscellaneous: Infection (39%)

Pharmacodynamics/Kinetics

Absorption Oral: 60% on an empty stomach; almost 100% on a full stomach

Bioavailability Almost 100% when given with food; 60% without food

Time to Peak Plasma: 1-7 hours

Protein Binding 92% to 95% to albumin and α_1-acid glycoprotein

Half-Life Elimination 24-36 hours

Metabolism Hepatic, via CYP3A4 (major), CYP1A1 (minor), CYP1A2 (minor), and CYP1C (minor)

Excretion Primarily as metabolites: Feces (83%; 1% as unchanged drug); urine (8%)

Available Dosage Forms

Tablet, oral:

Tarceva®: 25 mg, 100 mg, 150 mg

Dosing

Adult & Geriatric Note: Details concerning dosing in combination regimens should also be consulted. Continue treatment until disease progression or unacceptable toxicity. Dose adjustments are likely to be needed when erlotinib is administered concomitantly with strong CYP3A4 inducers or inhibitors, or with continued smoking.

NSCLC, refractory: Oral: 150 mg once daily

NSCLC, maintenance therapy: Oral: 150 mg once daily

Pancreatic cancer: Oral: 100 mg once daily in combination with gemcitabine

NSCLC, first-line therapy in patients with EGFR mutations (unlabeled use): Oral: 150 mg once daily (Rosell, 2009)

Dosage adjustment for concomitant CYP3A4 inhibitors/inducers:

CYP3A4 inhibitors: Consider dose reductions for severe adverse reactions when erlotinib is administered concomitantly with strong CYP3A4 inhibitors (eg, azole antifungals, clarithromycin, erythromycin, nefazodone, protease inhibitors, telithromycin). Dose reduction (if required) should be done in decrements of 50 mg.

Concomitant CYP3A4 and CYP1A2 inhibitor (eg, ciprofloxacin): Consider dose reductions if severe adverse reactions occur.

CYP3A4 inducers: Alternatives to the enzyme-inducing agent should be utilized first. Concomitant administration with CYP3A4 inducers (eg, carbamazepine, phenobarbital, phenytoin, rifamycins, and St John's wort) may require erlotinib increased doses (increase as tolerated at 2-week intervals); doses >150 mg/day should be considered with rifampin (the maximum erlotinib dose studied in combination with rifampin was 450 mg). Immediately reduce erlotinib dose to recommended starting dose when CYP3A4 inducer is discontinued.

Dosage adjustment for concomitant smoking: A dose increase to a maximum dose of 300 mg (with careful monitoring) may be required in patients who continue to smoke; immediately reduce erlotinib dose to recommended starting dose upon smoking cessation.

Renal Impairment Interrupt treatment for risk of renal disease due to dehydration; may resume after euvolemia re-established.

Hepatic Impairment

The manufacturer recommends the following guidelines:

Patients with normal hepatic function at baseline: Total bilirubin >3 times ULN and/or transaminases >5 times ULN: Interrupt or discontinue treatment

Patients with baseline hepatic impairment:

Total bilirubin >3 times ULN: Use extreme caution

Worsening liver function (not yet severe): Interrupt treatment and/or reduce dose

Severe changes in liver function (eg, doubling of total bilirubin and/or tripling of transaminases): Interrupt or discontinue treatment

A reduced starting dose (75 mg once daily) has been recommended in patients with hepatic dysfunction (AST ≥3 times ULN or direct bilirubin 1-7 mg/dL), with individualized dosage escalation if tolerated (Miller, 2007).

Adjustment for Toxicity Dose reductions should be made in 50 mg decrements.

Diarrhea: Manage with loperamide; in severe diarrhea (unresponsive to loperamide) or dehydration due to diarrhea, reduce dose or temporarily interrupt treatment

Pulmonary symptoms: Acute onset (or worsening) of pulmonary symptoms (eg, dyspnea, cough, fever): Interrupt treatment and evaluate for drug-induced interstitial lung disease; discontinue permanently with development of interstitial lung disease

Severe skin reaction: Reduce dose or temporarily interrupt treatment

Bullous, blistering or exfoliative skin toxicity, acute or worsening ocular toxicities, or dehydration with risk for renal failure: Interrupt or discontinue treatment

Gastrointestinal perforation, hepatic failure: Discontinue treatment

Administration

Oral The manufacturer recommends administration on an empty stomach (at least 1 hour before or 2 hours after the ingestion of food).

For patients unable to swallow whole, tablets may be dissolved in 100 mL water and administered orally or via feeding tube (silicone-based); to ensure full dose is received, rinse container with 40 mL water, administer residue and repeat rinse (data on file, Genentech; Siu, 2007; Soulieres, 2004).

Stability

Storage Store at room temperature of 25°C (77°F); excursions permitted to 15°C and 30°C (59°F and 86°F).

Monitoring and Teaching Issues

Laboratory Monitoring Periodic liver function tests (transaminases, bilirubin, and alkaline phosphatase); renal function, electrolytes (in patients at risk for dehydration)

Physical Assessment Use with caution in presence or risk of cardiovascular disease, renal impairment, or hepatic impairment. Assess LFTs. Monitor for gastrointestinal perforation, diarrhea, ocular reactions, severe skin reactions, and interstitial lung disease; dose adjustments or discontinuation may be necessary.

Patient Education Take 1 hour before or 2 hours after food, and avoid grapefruit or grapefruit juice. If unable to swallow whole, tablets may be dissolved in 100 mL of water; rinse residue in container with 40 mL of water to assure full dose. If you are a smoker, inform prescriber if you stop smoking. Maintain adequate nutrition and hydration, unless instructed to restrict fluid intake. May cause fatigue, rash or dry skin, loss of hair (may grow back when treatment is completed), nausea, or anorexia. Report any persistent skin rash, blisters, or skin eruptions; persistent or severe gastrointestinal changes, including diarrhea, abdominal pain, nausea, or vomiting; eye pain or visual changes; difficulty breathing or unusual cough or fever; or signs of infection.

Dietary Considerations Take this medicine an empty stomach, 1 hour before or 2 hours after a meal. Avoid grapefruit juice.

Geriatric Considerations In clinical trials, there was no significant difference between older and younger adults in survival benefit, safety, or pharmacokinetics. No dosage adjustment necessary in elderly patients.

Pregnancy Considerations Animal studies have demonstrated fetal harm and abortion. There are no well-controlled studies in pregnant women. Women of childbearing potential should be advised to avoid pregnancy; adequate contraception is recommended during treatment and for 2 weeks after treatment has been completed.

Additional Information Oncology Comment: According to the National Comprehensive Cancer Network® (NCCN) pancreatic adenocarcinoma guidelines, gemcitabine combination therapy (including gemcitabine plus erlotinib) is an option for patients with good performance status in the treatment of locally-advanced or metastatic pancreatic cancer.

The NCCN guidelines for NSCLC recommend erlotinib as single agent treatment for disease progression after failure of first- or second-line treatment in patients with a performance status of 0-2. Erlotinib is considered a first-line single-agent therapy in patients with advanced or metastatic NSCLC who have a known active EGFR mutation or gene amplification. Erlotinib may also be used as maintenance treatment of recurrent or metastatic NCSLC which has not progressed after 4-6 cycles of first-line platinum-based chemotherapy.

Factors (in patients with NSCLC) which correlate positively with response to EGFR-tyrosine kinase inhibitor (TKI) therapy include skin rash (due to EGFR-TKI therapy), patients who have never smoked, EGFR mutation, and patients of Asian origin. EGFR mutations, specifically exon 19 deletions and exon 21 mutation (L858R) correlate with response to tyrosine kinase inhibitors (NCCN NSCLC guidelines v.2.2010; Riely, 2006). *K-ras* mutations correlated with poorer outcome with EGFR-TKI therapy in patients with NSCLC. (Cooley, 2008; Jackman, 2008; Masarelli, 2007; Shepherd, 2005).

◆ **Erlotinib Hydrochloride** *see* Erlotinib *on page* 652

◆ **Errin®** *see* Norethindrone *on page* 1334

Ertapenem (er ta PEN em)

U.S. Brand Names INVanz®

Index Terms Ertapenem Sodium; L-749,345; MK0826

Generic Availability (U.S.) No

Pharmacologic Category Antibiotic, Carbapenem

Medication Safety Issues

Sound-alike/look-alike issues:

Ertapenem may be confused with imipenem, meropenem

INVanz® may be confused with AVINza™, I.V. vancomycin

Pregnancy Risk Factor B

Lactation Enters breast milk/use caution

Use Treatment of the following moderate-severe infections: Complicated intra-abdominal infections, complicated skin and skin structure infections (including diabetic foot infections without osteomyelitis), complicated UTI (including pyelonephritis), acute pelvic infections (including postpartum endomyometritis, septic abortion, post surgical gynecologic infections), and community-acquired pneumonia. Prophylaxis of surgical site infection following elective colorectal surgery. Antibacterial coverage includes aerobic gram-positive organisms, aerobic gram-negative organisms, anaerobic organisms.

Note: Methicillin-resistant *Staphylococcus*, *Enterococcus* spp, penicillin-resistant strains of *Streptococcus pneumoniae*, beta-lactamase-positive strains of *Haemophilus influenzae* are **resistant** to ertapenem, as are most *Pseudomonas aeruginosa*.

Mechanism of Action/Effect Inhibits cell wall biosynthesis; cell wall assembly is arrested and the bacteria eventually lyse.

Contraindications Hypersensitivity to ertapenem, other carbapenems, or any component of the formulation; anaphylactic reactions to beta-lactam antibiotics. If using intramuscularly, known hypersensitivity to local anesthetics of the amide type (lidocaine is the diluent).

Warnings/Precautions Use caution with renal impairment. Dosage adjustment required in patients with moderate-to-severe renal dysfunction; elderly patients often require lower doses (based upon renal function). Prolonged use may result in superinfection, including pseudomembranous colitis. Has been associated with CNS adverse effects, including confusional states and seizures; use caution with CNS disorders (eg, brain lesions, history of seizures, or renal impairment). Serious hypersensitivity reactions, including anaphylaxis, have been reported (some without a history of previous allergic reactions to beta-lactams). Doses for I.M. administration are mixed with lidocaine; consult Lidocaine on page 1104 information for associated Warnings/Precautions. Safety and efficacy have not been established in children <3 months of age.

Drug Interactions

Avoid Concomitant Use

Avoid concomitant use of Ertapenem with any of the following: BCG

Decreased Effect

Ertapenem may decrease the levels/effects of: BCG; Divalproex; Typhoid Vaccine; Valproic Acid

Increased Effect/Toxicity

The levels/effects of Ertapenem may be increased by: Probenecid

Adverse Reactions Note: Percentages reported in adults.

1% to 10%:

Cardiovascular: Edema (3%), chest pain (1% to 2%), hypertension (1% to 2%), hypotension (1% to 2%), tachycardia (1% to 2%)

Central nervous system: Headache (6% to 7%); altered mental status (eg, agitation, confusion, disorientation, decreased mental acuity, changed mental status, somnolence, stupor) (3% to 5%); fever (2% to 5%), insomnia (3%), dizziness (2%), fatigue (1%), anxiety (1%)

Dermatologic: Rash (2% to 3%), pruritus (1% to 2%), erythema (1% to 2%)

Endocrine & metabolic: Hypokalemia (2%), hyperglycemia (1% to 2%), hyperkalemia (≤1%)

Gastrointestinal: Diarrhea (9% to 10%), nausea (6% to 9%), abdominal pain (4%), vomiting (4%), constipation (3% to 4%), acid regurgitation (1% to 2%), dyspepsia (1%), oral candidiasis (≤1%)

Genitourinary: Urine WBCs increased (2% to 3%), urine RBCs increased (1% to 3%), vaginitis (1% to 3%)

Hematologic: Thrombocytosis (4% to 7%), hematocrit/hemoglobin decreased (3% to 5%), eosinophils increased (1% to 2%), leukopenia (1% to 2%), neutrophils decreased (1% to 2%), thrombocytopenia (1%), prothrombin time increased (≤1%)

Hepatic: Hepatic enzyme increased (7% to 9%), alkaline phosphatase increase (4% to 7%), albumin decreased (1% to 2%), bilirubin (total) increased (1% to 2%)

Local: Infused vein complications (5% to 7%), phlebitis/thrombophlebitis (2%), extravasation (1% to 2%)

Neuromuscular & skeletal: Weakness (1%), leg pain (≤1%)

Renal: Serum creatinine increased (1%)

Respiratory: Dyspnea (1% to 3%), cough (1% to 2%), pharyngitis (1%), rales/rhonchi (1%), respiratory distress (≤1%)

Pharmacodynamics/Kinetics

Absorption I.M.: Almost complete

Bioavailability I.M.: ~90%

Time to Peak I.M.: ~2.3 hours

Protein Binding Concentration dependent, primarily to albumin: 85% at 300 mcg/mL, 95% at <100 mcg/mL

Half-Life Elimination

Children 3 months to 12 years: ~2.5 hours

Children ≥13 years and Adults: ~4 hours

Metabolism Non-CYP-mediated hydrolysis to inactive metabolite

Excretion Urine (~80% as unchanged drug and metabolite); feces (~10%)

Available Dosage Forms

Injection, powder for reconstitution:

INVanz®: 1 g

Dosing

Adult & Geriatric Note: I.V. therapy may be administered for up to 14 days; I.M. for up to 7 days

Community-acquired pneumonia and complicated urinary tract infections (including pyelonephritis): I.M., I.V.: 1 g/day; duration of total antibiotic treatment: 10-14 days (**Note:** Duration includes possible switch to appropriate oral therapy after at least 3 days of parenteral treatment, once clinical improvement demonstrated.)

Intra-abdominal infection: I.M., I.V.: 1 g/day for 5-14 days; **Note:** 2010 IDSA guidelines recommend a treatment duration of 4-7 days (provided source controlled) for community-acquired, mild-to-moderate IAI

Pelvic infections (acute): I.M., I.V.: 1 g/day for 3-10 days

Prophylaxis of surgical site following colorectal surgery: I.V.: 1 g given 1 hour preoperatively

Skin and skin structure infections (including diabetic foot infections): I.M., I.V.: 1 g/day for 7-14 days

Pediatric Note: I.V. therapy may be administered for up to 14 days; I.M. therapy for up to 7 days

Children 3 months to 12 years:

Community-acquired pneumonia and complicated urinary tract infections (including pyelonephritis): I.M., I.V.: 15 mg/kg twice daily (maximum: 1 g/day); duration of total antibiotic treatment: 10-14 days (**Note:** Duration includes possible switch to appropriate oral therapy after at least 3 days of parenteral treatment, once clinical improvement demonstrated.)

Intra-abdominal infection: I.M., I.V.: 15 mg/kg twice daily (maximum: 1 g/day) for 5-14 days

Pelvic infections (acute): I.M., I.V.: 15 mg/kg twice daily (maximum: 1 g/day) for 3-10 days

Skin and skin structure infections: I.M., I.V.: 15 mg/kg twice daily (maximum: 1 g/day) for 7-14 days

Children ≥13 years: Refer to adult dosing.

Renal Impairment

Children: No data available for pediatric patients with renal insufficiency.

Adults:

Cl_{cr} >30 mL/minute/1.73 m^2: No adjustment required

Cl_{cr} ≤30 mL/minute/1.73 m^2 and ESRD: 500 mg/day

Hemodialysis: When the daily dose is given within 6 hours prior to hemodialysis, a supplementary dose of 150 mg is required following hemodialysis.

Hepatic Impairment Adjustments cannot be recommended (lack of experience and research in this patient population).

Administration

I.M. Avoid injection into a blood vessel. Make sure patient does not have an allergy to lidocaine or another anesthetic of the amide type. Administer by deep I.M. injection into a large muscle mass (eg, gluteal muscle or lateral part of the thigh). Do not administer I.M. preparation or drug reconstituted for I.M. administration intravenously.

I.V. Infuse over 30 minutes

Stability

Reconstitution

I.M.: Reconstitute 1 g vial with 3.2 mL of 1% lidocaine HCl injection (without epinephrine). Shake well.

I.V.: Reconstitute 1 g vial with 10 mL of water for injection, 0.9% sodium chloride injection, or bacteriostatic water for injection. Shake well. For adults, transfer dose to 50 mL of 0.9% sodium chloride injection; for children, dilute dose with NS to a final concentration ≤20 mg/mL.

Storage Before reconstitution store at ≤25°C (77°F).

I.M.: Use within 1 hour after preparation.

I.V.: Reconstituted I.V. solution may be stored at room temperature and must be used within 6 hours **or** refrigerated, stored for up to 24 hours and used within 4 hours after removal from refrigerator. Do not freeze.

Monitoring and Teaching Issues

Physical Assessment Assess results of culture and sensitivity tests and patient history of previous allergies or adverse drug reactions. Use caution in presence of impaired renal function or CNS disorder. Patient must be monitored closely for adverse reactions, especially CNS adverse effects (history of seizures, head injuries, or other CNS events increases risk).

Patient Education This medication can only be administered intravenously or by intramuscular injections; report warmth, swelling, or irritation at infusion or injection site. Maintain adequate hydration, unless instructed to restrict fluid intake, and nutrition. Report unresolved nausea or vomiting. Report immediately any CNS changes (eg, dizziness, disorientation, headaches, confusion, or seizures). Report prolonged GI effects, persistent diarrhea, vomiting, or abdominal pain; change in respirations or respiratory difficulty; chest pain or palpitations; skin rash; foul-smelling vaginal discharge; or white plaques in mouth.

Dietary Considerations Some products may contain sodium.

Geriatric Considerations According to the package insert, the total and unbound AUCs were increased 37% and 67%, respectively, in healthy men and women ≥65 years of age compared to younger adults. No dose adjustment is required for patients with normal age-adjusted renal function.

Breast-Feeding Considerations Ertapenem is excreted in breast milk. The low concentrations in milk and low oral bioavailability suggest minimal exposure risk to the infant. Although the manufacturer recommends that caution be exercised when administering ertapenem to nursing women, most penicillins and carbapenems are safe for use in breast-feeding. Nondose-related effects could include modification of bowel flora.

Pregnancy Considerations With the exception of slightly decreased fetal weights in mice, teratogenic effects and fetal harm have not been shown in animal studies. Adequate and well-controlled studies have not been conducted in pregnant women and it is not known whether ertapenem can cause fetal harm.

Related Information

Antimicrobial Drugs of Choice *on page 2008*

Community-Acquired Pneumonia in Adults *on page 2021*

◆ **Ertapenem Sodium** *see* Ertapenem *on page 656*

◆ ***Erwinia* Asparaginase** *see* Asparaginase *on page 152*

◆ **Ery** *see* Erythromycin (Topical) *on page 661*

◆ **EryPed®** *see* Erythromycin (Systemic) *on page 658*

◆ **Ery-Tab®** *see* Erythromycin (Systemic) *on page 658*

◆ **Erythrocin®** *see* Erythromycin (Systemic) *on page 658*

◆ **Erythrocin® Lactobionate-I.V.** *see* Erythromycin (Systemic) *on page 658*

Erythromycin (Systemic) (er ith roe MYE sin)

U.S. Brand Names E.E.S.®; Ery-Tab®; EryPed®; Erythro-RX; Erythrocin®; Erythrocin® Lactobionate-I.V.; PCE®

Index Terms Erythromycin Base; Erythromycin Ethylsuccinate; Erythromycin Lactobionate; Erythromycin Stearate

Generic Availability (U.S.) Yes: Capsule, tablet (as base, ethylsuccinate, and stearate)

Pharmacologic Category Antibiotic, Macrolide

Medication Safety Issues

Sound-alike/look-alike issues:

Erythromycin may be confused with azithromycin, clarithromycin, Ethmozine®

Akne-Mycin® may be confused with AK-Mycin®

E.E.S.® may be confused with DES®

Eryc® may be confused with Emcyt®, Ery-Tab®

Ery-Tab® may be confused with Eryc®

Erythrocin® may be confused with Ethmozine®

Pregnancy Risk Factor B

Lactation Enters breast milk/use caution (AAP considers "compatible"; AAP 2001 update pending)

Use Treatment of susceptible bacterial infections including *S. pyogenes*, some *S. pneumoniae*, some *S. aureus*, *M. pneumoniae*, *Legionella pneumophila*, diphtheria, pertussis, *Chlamydia*, erythrasma, *N. gonorrhoeae*, *E. histolytica*, syphilis and nongonococcal urethritis, and *Campylobacter* gastroenteritis; used in conjunction with neomycin for decontaminating the bowel

Unlabeled/Investigational Use Treatment of gastroparesis, chancroid; preoperative gut sterilization

Mechanism of Action/Effect Inhibits RNA-dependent protein synthesis

Contraindications Hypersensitivity to erythromycin, any macrolide antibiotics, or any component of the formulation

Concomitant use with pimozide or cisapride

Warnings/Precautions Use caution with hepatic impairment with or without jaundice has occurred, it may be accompanied by malaise, nausea, vomiting, abdominal colic, and fever; discontinue use if these occur. Use caution with other medication relying on CYP3A4 metabolism; high potential for drug interactions exists. Prolonged use may result in fungal or bacterial superinfection, including *C. difficile*-associated diarrhea (CDAD) and pseudomembranous colitis; CDAD has been observed >2 months postantibiotic treatment. Use in infants has been associated with infantile hypertrophic pyloric stenosis (IHPS). Macrolides have been associated with rare QT_c prolongation and ventricular arrhythmias, including torsade de pointes. Use caution in elderly patients, as risk of adverse events may be increased. Use caution in myasthenia gravis patients; erythromycin may aggravate muscular weakness.

Drug Interactions

Metabolism/Transport Effects Substrate of CYP2B6 (minor), CYP3A4 (major), P-glycoprotein; **Inhibits** CYP1A2 (weak), CYP3A4 (moderate), P-glycoprotein

Avoid Concomitant Use

Avoid concomitant use of Erythromycin (Systemic) with any of the following: Artemether; BCG; Cisapride; Disopyramide; Dronedarone; Lincosamide Antibiotics; Lumefantrine; Nilotinib; Pimozide; QuiNINE; Silodosin; Tetrabenazine; Thioridazine; Tolvaptan; Topotecan; Toremifene; Vandetanib; Ziprasidone

Decreased Effect

Erythromycin (Systemic) may decrease the levels/effects of: BCG; Clopidogrel; Typhoid Vaccine; Zafirlukast

The levels/effects of Erythromycin (Systemic) may be decreased by: CYP3A4 Inducers (Strong); Deferasirox; Etravirine; Herbs (CYP3A4 Inducers); Lincosamide Antibiotics; P-Glycoprotein Inducers

Increased Effect/Toxicity

Erythromycin (Systemic) may increase the levels/effects of: Alfentanil; Antifungal Agents (Azole Derivatives, Systemic); Antineoplastic Agents (Vinca Alkaloids); Benzodiazepines (metabolized by oxidation); BusPIRone; Calcium Channel Blockers; CarBAMazepine; Cardiac Glycosides; Cilostazol; Cisapride; CloZAPine; Colchicine; Corticosteroids (Systemic); CycloSPORINE; CycloSPORINE (Systemic); CYP3A4 Substrates; Dabigatran Etexilate; Disopyramide; Dronedarone; Eletriptan; Eplerenone; Ergot Derivatives; Everolimus; FentaNYL; Fexofenadine; HMG-CoA Reductase Inhibitors; Lurasidone; P-Glycoprotein Substrates; Phosphodiesterase 5 Inhibitors; Pimecrolimus; Pimozide; QTc-Prolonging Agents; QuiNIDine; QuiNINE; Repaglinide; Rifamycin Derivatives; Rivaroxaban; Salmeterol; Saxagliptin; Selective Serotonin Reuptake Inhibitors; Silodosin; Sirolimus; Tacrolimus; Tacrolimus (Systemic); Tacrolimus (Topical); Temsirolimus; Tetrabenazine; Theophylline Derivatives; Thioridazine; Tolvaptan; Topotecan; Toremifene; Vandetanib; Vitamin K Antagonists; Ziprasidone; Zopiclone

The levels/effects of Erythromycin (Systemic) may be increased by: Alfuzosin; Antifungal Agents (Azole Derivatives, Systemic); Artemether; Chloroquine; Ciprofloxacin; Ciprofloxacin (Systemic); Conivaptan; CYP3A4 Inhibitors (Moderate); CYP3A4 Inhibitors (Strong); Gadobutrol; Lumefantrine; Nilotinib; P-Glycoprotein Inhibitors; QuiNINE

Nutritional/Ethanol Interactions

Ethanol: Avoid ethanol (may decrease absorption of erythromycin or enhance ethanol effects).
Food: Erythromycin serum levels may be altered if taken with food (formulation-dependent).
Herb/Nutraceutical: St John's wort may decrease erythromycin levels.

Lab Interactions False-positive urinary catecholamines

Adverse Reactions Frequency not defined. Incidence may vary with formulation.

Cardiovascular: QT_c prolongation, torsade de pointes, ventricular arrhythmia, ventricular tachycardia
Central nervous system: Seizure
Dermatitis: Pruritus, rash
Gastrointestinal: Abdominal pain, anorexia, diarrhea, infantile hypertrophic pyloric stenosis, nausea, oral candidiasis, pancreatitis, pseudomembranous colitis, vomiting
Hepatic: Cholestatic jaundice (most common with estolate), hepatitis, liver function tests abnormal
Local: Phlebitis at the injection site, thrombophlebitis
Neuromuscular & skeletal: Weakness
Otic: Hearing loss
Miscellaneous: Allergic reactions, anaphylaxis, hypersensitivity reactions, urticaria

Pharmacodynamics/Kinetics

Absorption Oral: Variable but better with salt forms than with base form; 18% to 45%; ethylsuccinate may be better absorbed with food

Time to Peak Serum: Base: 4 hours; Ethylsuccinate: 0.5-2.5 hours; delayed with food due to differences in absorption

Protein Binding Base: 73% to 81%

Half-Life Elimination Peak: 1.5-2 hours; End-stage renal disease: 5-6 hours

Metabolism Demethylation primarily via hepatic CYP3A4

Excretion Primarily feces; urine (2% to 15% as unchanged drug)

Available Dosage Forms

Capsule, delayed release, enteric coated pellets, oral: 250 mg

Granules for suspension, oral:
E.E.S.®: 200 mg/5 mL (100 mL, 200 mL)

Injection, powder for reconstitution:
Erythrocin® Lactobionate-I.V.: 500 mg

Powder, for prescription compounding:
Erythro-RX: USP: 100% (50 g)

Powder for suspension, oral:
EryPed®: 200 mg/5 mL (100 mL); 400 mg/5 mL (100 mL)

Tablet, oral: 250 mg, 400 mg, 500 mg
E.E.S.®: 400 mg
Erythrocin®: 250 mg, 500 mg

Tablet, delayed release, enteric coated, oral:
Ery-Tab®: 250 mg, 333 mg, 500 mg

Tablet, polymer coated particles, oral:
PCE®: 333 mg, 500 mg

Dosing

Adult & Geriatric Note: Due to differences in absorption, 400 mg erythromycin ethylsuccinate produces the same serum levels as 250 mg erythromycin base or stearate.

Usual dosage range:

Oral:
- Base: 250-500 mg every 6-12 hours
- Ethylsuccinate: 400-800 mg every 6-12 hours

I.V.: Lactobionate: 15-20 mg/kg/day divided every 6 hours or 500 mg to 1 g every 6 hours, or given as a continuous infusion over 24 hours (maximum: 4 g/24 hours)

Indication-specific dosing:

***Bartonella sp* infections (bacillary angiomatosis [BA], peliosis hepatis [PH]) (unlabeled use):** Oral: 500 mg (base) 4 times/day for 3 months (BA) or 4 months (PH)

Chancroid (unlabeled use): Oral: 500 mg (base) 3 times/day for 7 days; **Note:** Not a preferred agent; isolates with intermediate resistance have been documented (CDC, 2010)

Gastrointestinal prokinetic (unlabeled use): I.V.: 200 mg initially followed by 250 mg (base) orally 3 times/day 30 minutes before meals. Lower dosages have been used in some trials.

Granuloma inguinale (donovanosis) (unlabeled use): Oral: 500 mg (base) 4 times/day for 21 days (CDC, 2010)

Legionnaires' disease: Oral: 1.6-4 g (ethylsuccinate)/day or 1-4 g (base)/day in divided doses for 21 days. **Note:** No longer preferred therapy and only used in nonhospitalized patients.

Lymphogranuloma venereum: Oral: 500 mg (base) 4 times/day for 21 days; **Note:** Preferred therapy for pregnant or lactating women (CDC, 2010)

Nongonococcal urethritis (including coinfection with *C. trachomatis*): Oral: 500 mg (base) 4 times/day for 7 days or 800 mg (ethylsuccinate) 4 times/day for 7 days. **Note:** May use 250 mg (base) or 400 mg (ethylsuccinate) 4 times/day for 14 days if gastrointestinal intolerance.

Pertussis: Oral: 500 mg (base) every 6 hours for 14 days

Preop bowel preparation: Oral: 1 g erythromycin base at 1, 2, and 11 PM on the day before surgery combined with mechanical cleansing of the large intestine and oral neomycin

Pediatric Note: Due to differences in absorption, 400 mg erythromycin ethylsuccinate produces the same serum levels as 250 mg erythromycin base or stearate.

Usual dosage range: Infants and Children:

Oral:
- Base: 30-50 mg/kg/day in 2-4 divided doses; maximum: 2 g/day
- Ethylsuccinate: 30-50 mg/kg/day in 2-4 divided doses; maximum: 3.2 g/day
- Stearate: 30-50 mg/kg/day in 2-4 divided doses; maximum: 2 g/day

I.V.: Lactobionate: 15-50 mg/kg/day divided every 6 hours, not to exceed 4 g/day

Indication-specific dosing:

***Bartonella sp* infections (bacillary angiomatosis [BA], peliosis hepatis [PH]) (unlabeled use):** Oral: 40 mg/kg/day (ethylsuccinate) in 4 divided doses (maximum: 2 g/day) for 3 months (BA) or 4 months (PH)

Chlamydial infection *(C. trachomatis)*: Children <45 kg: Oral: 50 mg/kg/day (base or ethylsuccinate) in 4 divided doses for 14 days (CDC, 2010)

Conjunctivitis, neonatal *(C. trachomatis)*: Oral: 50 mg/kg/day (base or ethylsuccinate) in 4 divided doses for 14 days

Mild/moderate infection: Oral: 30-50 mg/kg/day in divided doses every 6-12 hours

Pertussis: Oral: 40-50 mg/kg/day in 4 divided doses for 14 days; maximum 2 g/day (not preferred agent for infants <1 month due to IHPS)

Pharyngitis, tonsillitis (streptococcal): Oral: 20 mg (base)/kg/day or 40 mg (ethylsuccinate)/kg/day in 2 divided doses for 10 days. **Note:** No longer preferred therapy due to increased organism resistance.

Pneumonia *(C. trachomatis)*: Infants: Oral: 50 mg/kg/day (base or ethylsuccinate) in 4 divided doses for 14 days (CDC, 2010)

Preop bowel preparation: Oral: 20 mg (base)/kg at 1, 2, and 11 PM on the day before surgery combined with mechanical cleansing of the large intestine and oral neomycin

Severe infection: I.V.: 15-50 mg/kg/day; maximum: 4 g/day

Renal Impairment Slightly dialyzable (5% to 20%); supplemental dose is not necessary in hemo- or peritoneal dialysis or in continuous arteriovenous or venovenous hemofiltration.

Administration

Oral Do not crush enteric coated drug product. GI upset, including diarrhea, is common. May be administered with food to decrease GI upset. Do not give with milk or acidic beverages.

I.V. Infuse 1 g over 20-60 minutes.

Stability

Reconstitution Erythromycin lactobionate should be reconstituted with sterile water for injection without preservatives to avoid gel formation. I.V. form has the longest stability in NS and should be prepared in this base solution whenever possible. Do not use D_5W as a diluent unless sodium bicarbonate is added to solution. If I.V. must be prepared in D_5W, 0.5 mL of the 8.4% sodium bicarbonate solution should be added per each 100 mL of D_5W.

Standard diluent: 500 mg/250 mL D_5W/NS; 750 mg/250 mL D_5W/NS; 1 g/250 mL D_5W/NS.

Storage

Injection: Store unreconstituted vials at 15°C to 30°C (59°F to 86°F). Reconstituted solution is stable for 2 weeks when refrigerated or for 8 hours at room temperature. Erythromycin I.V. infusion solution is stable at pH 6-8; stability of lactobionate is pH dependent; I.V. form has longest stability in NS. Stability of parenteral admixture at room temperature (25°C) and at refrigeration temperature (4°C) is 24 hours.

Oral suspension:

Granules: After mixing, store under refrigeration and use within 10 days.

Powder: Erythromycin ethylsuccinate may be stored at room temperature if used within 14 days. Refrigerate to preserve taste.

Tablet and capsule formulations: Store at <30°C (<86°F).

Monitoring and Teaching Issues

Laboratory Monitoring Perform culture and sensitivity studies prior to initiating drug therapy.

Physical Assessment Assess results of culture and sensitivity tests and patient's previous allergy history prior to therapy.

Patient Education Tablets/capsules: Take around-the-clock, with a full glass of water (not juice or milk); may take with food to reduce GI upset. Do not chew or crush extended release capsules or tablets. Avoid alcohol (may cause adverse response). May cause nausea, vomiting, or mouth sores. Report immediately any unusual malaise, nausea, vomiting, abdominal colic, or fever; skin rash or itching; easy bruising or bleeding; vaginal itching or discharge; watery or bloody diarrhea; yellowing of skin or eyes, pale stool or dark urine; persistent diarrhea; white plaques, sores, or fuzziness in mouth; or any change in hearing.

Dietary Considerations Drug may cause GI upset; may take with food. Some products may contain sodium.

Geriatric Considerations Dose does not need to be adjusted unless there is severe renal or hepatic impairment. Elderly may be at an increased risk for torsade de pointes, ototoxicity (particularly when dose is ≥4 g/day in conjunction with renal or hepatic impairment).

Breast-Feeding Considerations Erythromycin is excreted in breast milk; therefore, the manufacturer recommends that caution be exercised when administering erythromycin to breast-feeding women.

Due to the low concentrations in human milk, minimal toxicity would be expected in the nursing infant. One case report and a cohort study raise the possibility for a connection with pyloric stenosis in neonates exposed to erythromycin via breast milk and an alternative antibiotic may be preferred for breast-feeding mothers of infants in this age group. Nondose-related effects could include modification of bowel flora.

Pregnancy Considerations Adverse events were not observed in animal studies; therefore, erythromycin is classified as pregnancy category B. Erythromycin crosses the placenta and low concentrations are found in the fetal serum. No increased risk for congenital abnormalities has been documented, with the exception of a possible slight increase in risk for cardiovascular anomalies. Most studies do not support a link between prenatal exposure to erythromycin and pyloric stenosis in the neonate. In general, serum concentrations of erythromycin are lower in pregnant women. Erythromycin therapy in patients with preterm, premature rupture of membranes is associated with a range of health benefits to the neonate and long-term adverse events to the child have not been observed. However, maternal use of erythromycin in women with preterm labor, intact membranes, and no documented infection does not improve neonatal health and may have adverse effects in childhood (use is not recommended). Erythromycin is the antibiotic of choice for preterm premature rupture of membranes (with membrane rupture prior to 34 weeks gestation), the treatment of granuloma inguinale and lymphogranuloma venereum in pregnancy, and the treatment of or long-term suppression of *Bartonella* infection in HIV-infected pregnant patients. Erythromycin may be appropriate as an alternative agent for the prevention of group B streptococcal disease or the treatment of chlamydial infections in pregnant women (consult current guidelines).

Related Information

Antimicrobial Drugs of Choice *on page 2008*

Community-Acquired Pneumonia in Adults *on page 2021*

I.V. to Oral Conversion *on page 1956*

Prophylaxis for Patients Exposed to Common Communicable Diseases *on page 2073*

Erythromycin (Topical) (er ith roe MYE sin)

U.S. Brand Names Akne-mycin®; Ery

Generic Availability (U.S.) Yes: Gel, solution

Pharmacologic Category Acne Products; Antibiotic, Macrolide; Antibiotic, Topical; Topical Skin Product; Topical Skin Product, Acne

Medication Safety Issues

Sound-alike/look-alike issues:

Erythromycin may be confused with azithromycin, clarithromycin, Ethmozine®

Akne-Mycin® may be confused with AK-Mycin®

Pregnancy Risk Factor B

Lactation Use caution (AAP considers "compatible"; AAP 2001 update pending)

Use Treatment of acne vulgaris

Available Dosage Forms

Gel, topical: 2% (30 g, 60 g)

Ointment, topical:

Akne-mycin®: 2% (25 g)

Pledget, topical: 2%

Ery: 2%

Solution, topical: 2% (60 mL)

Dosing

Adult & Geriatric Acne: Topical: Usual dosage range: Apply over the affected area twice daily after the skin has been thoroughly washed and patted dry

Pediatric Topical: Refer to adult dosing.

Monitoring and Teaching Issues

Patient Education Apply as directed after skin has been cleansed and gently dried.

- **Erythromycin Base** *see* Erythromycin (Systemic) *on page 658*
- **Erythromycin Ethylsuccinate** *see* Erythromycin (Systemic) *on page 658*
- **Erythromycin Lactobionate** *see* Erythromycin (Systemic) *on page 658*
- **Erythromycin Stearate** *see* Erythromycin (Systemic) *on page 658*
- **Erythropoiesis-Stimulating Agent (ESA)** *see* Darbepoetin Alfa *on page 463*
- **Erythropoiesis-Stimulating Agent (ESA)** *see* Epoetin Alfa *on page 638*
- **Erythropoiesis-Stimulating Protein** *see* Darbepoetin Alfa *on page 463*
- **Erythropoietin** *see* Epoetin Alfa *on page 638*
- **Erythro-RX** *see* Erythromycin (Systemic) *on page 658*

Escitalopram (es sye TAL oh pram)

U.S. Brand Names Lexapro®

Index Terms Escitalopram Oxalate; Lu-26-054; S-Citalopram

Generic Availability (U.S.) No

Pharmacologic Category Antidepressant, Selective Serotonin Reuptake Inhibitor

Medication Safety Issues

Sound-alike/look-alike issues:

Lexapro® may be confused with Loxitane®

International issues:

Zavesca: Brand name for escitalopram [in multiple international markets; ISMP April 21, 2010], but also brand name for miglustat [Canada, U.S., and multiple international markets]

Medication Guide Available Yes

Pregnancy Risk Factor C

Lactation Enters breast milk/consider risk:benefit

Use Treatment of major depressive disorder; generalized anxiety disorders (GAD)

Unlabeled/Investigational Use Treatment of mild dementia-associated agitation in nonpsychotic patients

Mechanism of Action/Effect Escitalopram is the S-enantiomer of the racemic derivative citalopram, which selectively inhibits the reuptake of serotonin with little to no effect on norepinephrine or dopamine reuptake. It has no or very low affinity for 5-HT_{1-7}, alpha- and beta-adrenergic, D_{1-5}, H_{1-3}, M_{1-5}, and benzodiazepine receptors. Escitalopram does not bind to or has low affinity for Na^+, K^+, Cl^-, and Ca^{++} ion channels.

Contraindications Hypersensitivity to escitalopram, citalopram, or any component of the formulation; concomitant use with pimozide; concomitant use or within 2 weeks of MAO inhibitors

Warnings/Precautions [U.S. Boxed Warning]: Antidepressants increase the risk of suicidal thinking and behavior in children, adolescents, and young adults (18-24 years of age) with major depressive disorder (MDD) and other psychiatric disorders; consider risk prior to prescribing. Short-term studies did not show an increased risk in patients >24 years of age and showed a decreased risk in patients ≥65 years. Closely monitor patients for clinical worsening, suicidality, or unusual changes in behavior, particularly during the initial 1-2 months of therapy or during periods of dosage adjustments (increases or decreases); the patient's family or caregiver should be instructed to closely observe the patient and communicate condition with healthcare provider. A medication guide concerning the use of antidepressants should be dispensed with each prescription. **Escitalopram is not FDA approved for use in children <12 years of age.**

The possibility of a suicide attempt is inherent in major depression and may persist until remission occurs. Use caution in high-risk patients. Worsening depression and severe abrupt suicidality that are not part of the presenting symptoms may require discontinuation or modification of drug therapy. The patient's family or caregiver should be alerted to monitor patients for the emergence of suicidality and associated behaviors (such as agitation, irritability, hostility, impulsivity, and hypomania) and call healthcare provider.

May worsen psychosis in some patients or precipitate a shift to mania or hypomania in patients with bipolar disorder. Patients presenting with depressive symptoms should be screened for bipolar disorder. Monotherapy in patients with bipolar disorder should be avoided. Escitalopram is not FDA approved for the treatment of bipolar depression. Escitalopram is not FDA approved for the treatment of bipolar depression.

Serotonin syndrome and neuroleptic malignant syndrome (NMS)-like reactions have occurred with serotonin/norepinephrine reuptake inhibitors (SNRIs) and selective serotonin reuptake inhibitors (SSRIs) when used alone, and particularly when used in combination with serotonergic agents (eg, triptans) or antidopaminergic agents (eg, antipsychotics). Concurrent use or within 2 weeks of an MAO inhibitor is contraindicated. May increase the risks associated with electroconvulsive therapy. Has a low potential to impair cognitive or motor performance; caution operating hazardous machinery or driving.

Use caution with a previous seizure disorder or condition predisposing to seizures such as brain damage, alcoholism, or concurrent therapy with other drugs which lower the seizure threshold. May cause hyponatremia/SIADH (elderly at increased risk); volume depletion (diuretics may increase risk) may occur. May cause or exacerbate sexual dysfunction. Use caution with severe renal impairment or liver impairment; concomitant CNS depressants; pregnancy (high doses of citalopram have been associated with teratogenicity in animals). Use caution with concomitant use of aspirin, NSAIDs, warfarin, or other drugs that affect coagulation; the risk of bleeding may be potentiated.

Upon discontinuation of escitalopram therapy, gradually taper dose. If intolerable symptoms occur following a decrease in dosage or upon discontinuation of therapy, then resuming the previous dose with a more gradual taper should be considered.

Safety and efficacy have not been established in children <12 years of age with major depressive disorder or in children <18 years with generalized anxiety disorder.

Drug Interactions

Metabolism/Transport Effects Substrate (major) of CYP2C19, 3A4; **Inhibits** CYP2D6 (weak)

Avoid Concomitant Use

Avoid concomitant use of Escitalopram with any of the following: Artemether; Dronedarone; Iobenguane I 123; Lumefantrine; MAO Inhibitors; Methylene Blue; Nilotinib; Pimozide; QuiNINE; Sibutramine; Tetrabenazine; Thioridazine; Toremifene; Tryptophan; Vandetanib; Ziprasidone

Decreased Effect

Escitalopram may decrease the levels/effects of: Iobenguane I 123

The levels/effects of Escitalopram may be decreased by: CarBAMazepine; CYP2C19 Inducers (Strong); CYP3A4 Inducers (Strong); Cyproheptadine; Deferasirox

Increased Effect/Toxicity

Escitalopram may increase the levels/effects of: Alcohol (Ethyl); Alpha-/Beta-Blockers; Anticoagulants; Antidepressants (Serotonin Reuptake Inhibitor/Antagonist); Antiplatelet Agents; Aspirin; BusPIRone; CarBAMazepine; CloZAPine; CNS Depressants; Collagenase (Systemic); Desmopressin; Dextromethorphan; Dronedarone; Drotrecogin Alfa; Haloperidol; Ibritumomab; Lithium; Methadone; Methylene Blue; Mexiletine; NSAID (COX-2 Inhibitor); NSAID (Nonselective); Pimozide; QTc-Prolonging Agents; QuiNINE; RisperiDONE; Salicylates; Serotonin Modulators; Tetrabenazine; Thioridazine; Thrombolytic Agents; Toremifene; Tositumomab and Iodine I 131 Tositumomab; TraMADol; Tricyclic Antidepressants; Vandetanib; Vitamin K Antagonists; Ziprasidone

The levels/effects of Escitalopram may be increased by: Alfuzosin; Analgesics (Opioid); Artemether; BusPIRone; Chloroquine; Cimetidine; Ciprofloxacin; Ciprofloxacin (Systemic); Conivaptan; CYP2C19 Inhibitors (Moderate); CYP2C19 Inhibitors (Strong); CYP3A4 Inhibitors (Moderate); CYP3A4 Inhibitors (Strong); Gadobutrol; Glucosamine; Herbs (Anticoagulant/Antiplatelet Properties); Lumefantrine; Macrolide Antibiotics; MAO Inhibitors; Metoclopramide; Nilotinib; Omega-3-Acid Ethyl Esters; Pentosan Polysulfate Sodium; Pentoxifylline; Prostacyclin Analogues; QuiNINE; Sibutramine; TraMADol; Tryptophan

Nutritional/Ethanol Interactions

Ethanol: Avoid ethanol (may increase CNS depression).

Herb/Nutraceutical: Avoid valerian, St John's wort, SAMe, kava kava, and gotu kola (may increase CNS depression).

Adverse Reactions

>10%:

Central nervous system: Headache (24%), somnolence (6% to 13%), insomnia (9% to 12%)

Gastrointestinal: Nausea (15% to 18%)

Genitourinary: Ejaculation disorder (9% to 14%)

1% to 10%:

Central nervous system: Fatigue (5% to 8%), dizziness (5%), abnormal dreaming (3%), lethargy (3%), yawning (2%)

Endocrine & metabolic: Libido decreased (3% to 7%), anorgasmia (2% to 6%), menstrual disorder (2%)

Gastrointestinal: Xerostomia (6% to 9%), diarrhea (8%), constipation (3% to 5%), appetite decreased (3%), indigestion (3%), vomiting (3%), abdominal pain (2%), flatulence (2%), toothache (2%)

Genitourinary: Impotence (2% to 3%)

Neuromuscular & skeletal: Neck/shoulder pain (3%), paresthesia (2%)
Respiratory: Rhinitis (5%), sinusitis (3%)
Miscellaneous: Diaphoresis (4% to 5%), flu-like syndrome (5%)

Pharmacodynamics/Kinetics

Onset of Action Depression: The onset of action is within a week; however, individual response varies greatly and full response may not be seen until 8-12 weeks after initiation of treatment.

Time to Peak Escitalopram: ~5 hours; S-DCT: 14 hours

Protein Binding ~56% to plasma proteins

Half-Life Elimination Escitalopram: 27-32 hours; S-DCT: 59 hours

Metabolism Hepatic via CYP2C19 and 3A4 to an active metabolite, S-desmethylcitalopram (S-DCT; 1/7 the activity of escitalopram); S-DCT is metabolized to S-didesmethylcitalopram (S-DDCT; active; 1/27 the activity of escitalopram) via CYP2D6

Excretion Urine (Escitalopram: 8%; S-DCT: 10%)

Available Dosage Forms

Solution, oral:
Lexapro®: 1 mg/mL (240 mL)

Tablet, oral:
Lexapro®: 5 mg, 10 mg, 20 mg

Dosing

Adult Major depressive disorder, generalized anxiety disorder: Oral: Initial: 10 mg once daily; dose may be increased to 20 mg once daily after at least 1 week

Geriatric Major depressive disorder, generalized anxiety disorder: Oral: 10 mg once daily

Pediatric Major depressive disorder: Oral: Children ≥12 years: Initial: 10 mg once daily; dose may be increased to 20 mg once daily after at least 3 weeks

Renal Impairment
Mild-to-moderate impairment: No dosage adjustment needed.
Severe impairment: Cl_{cr} <20 mL/minute: Use with caution.

Hepatic Impairment 10 mg once daily

Administration

Oral Administer once daily (morning or evening), with or without food.

Stability

Storage Store at 25°C (77°F); excursions permitted to 15°C to 30°C (59°F to 86°F).

Monitoring and Teaching Issues

Physical Assessment Monitor for signs of clinical worsening, suicide ideation, mania, hypomania, anxiety, or panic attacks. Taper dosage slowly when discontinuing.

Patient Education Avoid alcohol. May cause fatigue, dizziness, lightheadedness, insomnia, impaired concentration, headache, nausea, vomiting, loss of appetite, diarrhea, sexual dysfunction (reversible when drug is discontinued), muscle pain, dry mouth, or tremor. Report immediately any CNS changes, such as increased depression, confusion, impaired concentration, severe headache, insomnia, nightmares, irritability, acute anxiety, panic attacks, suicide ideation, persistent GI changes, chest pain or palpitations, blurred vision or vision changes, or unusual bleeding (eg, blood in stool, urine, or vomitus; unusual bruising or nosebleeds).

Dietary Considerations May be taken with or without food.

Geriatric Considerations Bioavailability and half-life are increased by 50% in the elderly. The elderly are more prone to SSRI/SNRI-induced hyponatremia.

Breast-Feeding Considerations Escitalopram and its metabolite are excreted into breast milk. Limited data is available concerning the effects escitalopram may have in the nursing infant and the long-term effects on development and behavior have not been studied. According to the manufacturer, the decision to continue or discontinue breast-feeding during therapy should take into account the risk of exposure to the infant and the benefits of treatment to the mother. Escitalopram is the S-enantiomer of the racemic derivative citalopram; also refer to the Citalopram monograph.

Pregnancy Considerations Due to adverse effects observed in animal studies, escitalopram is classified as pregnancy category C. Escitalopram is distributed into the amniotic fluid. Limited data is available concerning the use of escitalopram during pregnancy. Nonteratogenic effects in the newborn following SSRI exposure late in the third trimester include respiratory distress, cyanosis, apnea, seizures, temperature instability, feeding difficulty, vomiting, hypoglycemia, hypo- or hypertonia, hyper-reflexia, jitteriness, irritability, constant crying, and tremor. An increased risk of low birth weight and lower Apgar scores have also been reported. Exposure to SSRIs after the twentieth week of gestation has been associated with persistent pulmonary hypertension of the newborn (PPHN). Adverse effects may be due to toxic effects of the SSRI or drug withdrawal without a taper. The long-term effects of *in utero* SSRI exposure on infant development and behavior are not known. Escitalopram is the S-enantiomer of the racemic derivative citalopram; also refer to the Citalopram monograph.

Women treated for major depression and who are euthymic prior to pregnancy are more likely to experience a relapse when medication is discontinued as compared to pregnant women who continue taking antidepressant medications. The ACOG recommends that therapy with SSRIs or SNRIs during pregnancy be individualized; treatment of depression during pregnancy should incorporate the clinical expertise of the mental health clinician, obstetrician, primary healthcare provider, and pediatrician. If treatment during pregnancy is required, consider tapering therapy during the third trimester in order to prevent withdrawal symptoms in the infant. If this is done and the woman is considered to be at risk of relapse from her major depressive disorder, the medication can be restarted following delivery, although the dose should be readjusted to that required before pregnancy. Treatment algorithms have been developed by the ACOG and the APA for the management of depression in women prior to conception and during pregnancy (Yonkers, 2009).

Additional Information The tablet and oral solution dosage forms are bioequivalent. Clinically, escitalopram 20 mg is equipotent to citalopram 40 mg. Do not coadminister with citalopram.

Related Information

Antidepressant Agents *on page 1982*

- **Escitalopram Oxalate** *see* Escitalopram *on page 662*
- **Esgic®** *see* Butalbital, Acetaminophen, and Caffeine *on page 260*
- **Esgic-Plus™** *see* Butalbital, Acetaminophen, and Caffeine *on page 260*
- **Eskalith** *see* Lithium *on page 1123*

Esmolol (ES moe lol)

U.S. Brand Names Brevibloc

Index Terms Esmolol Hydrochloride

Generic Availability (U.S.) Yes: Excludes infusion

Pharmacologic Category Antiarrhythmic Agent, Class II; Beta Blocker, Beta-1 Selective

Medication Safety Issues

Sound-alike/look-alike issues:

Esmolol may be confused with Osmitrol®

Brevibloc® may be confused with Brevital®, Bumex®, Buprenex®

High alert medication: The Institute for Safe Medication Practices (ISMP) includes this medication among its list of drugs which have a heightened risk of causing significant patient harm when used in error.

Pregnancy Risk Factor C

Lactation Excretion in breast milk unknown/use with caution

Use Treatment of supraventricular tachycardia (SVT) and atrial fibrillation/flutter (control ventricular rate); treatment of intraoperative and postoperative tachycardia and/or hypertension; treatment of noncompensatory sinus tachycardia

Unlabeled/Investigational Use In children, for SVT and postoperative hypertension

Mechanism of Action/Effect Class II antiarrhythmic: Beta$_1$-adrenergic receptor blocking agent that competes with beta$_1$-adrenergic agonists for available beta-receptor sites; it is a selective beta$_1$-antagonist with a very short duration of action; has little if any intrinsic sympathomimetic activity; and lacks membrane stabilizing action; it is administered intravenously and is used when beta-blockade of short duration is desired or in critically-ill patients in whom adverse effects of bradycardia, heart failure, or hypotension may necessitate rapid withdrawal of the drug

Contraindications Sinus bradycardia; heart block greater than first degree (except in patients with a functioning artificial pacemaker); cardiogenic shock; uncompensated cardiac failure

Warnings/Precautions Consider pre-existing conditions such as sick sinus syndrome before initiating. Hypotension is common; patients need close blood pressure monitoring. Administer cautiously in compensated heart failure and monitor for a worsening of the condition. Use caution in patients with PVD (can aggravate arterial insufficiency). Use caution with concurrent use of beta-blockers and either verapamil or diltiazem; bradycardia or heart block can occur. Use beta-blockers cautiously in patients with bronchospastic disease; monitor pulmonary status closely. Use cautiously in patients with diabetes because it can mask prominent hypoglycemic symptoms. Use with caution in patients with myasthenia gravis. Use caution in patients with renal dysfunction (active metabolite retained). Adequate alpha-blockade is required prior to use of any beta-blocker for patients with untreated pheochromocytoma. Use caution with history of severe anaphylaxis to allergens; patients taking beta-blockers may become more sensitive to repeated challenges. Treatment of anaphylaxis (eg, epinephrine) in patients taking beta-blockers may be ineffective or promote undesirable effects. Beta-blocker therapy should not be withdrawn abruptly (particularly in patients with CAD), but gradually tapered to avoid acute tachycardia, hypertension, and/or ischemia. Do not use in the treatment of hypertension associated with vasoconstriction related to hypothermia. Extravasation can lead to skin necrosis and sloughing.

Drug Interactions

Avoid Concomitant Use

Avoid concomitant use of Esmolol with any of the following: Methacholine

Decreased Effect

Esmolol may decrease the levels/effects of: Beta2-Agonists; Theophylline Derivatives

The levels/effects of Esmolol may be decreased by: Barbiturates; Herbs (Hypertensive Properties); Methylphenidate; Nonsteroidal Anti-Inflammatory Agents; Rifamycin Derivatives; Yohimbine

Increased Effect/Toxicity

Esmolol may increase the levels/effects of: Alpha-/Beta-Agonists (Direct-Acting); Alpha1-Blockers; Alpha2-Agonists; Amifostine; Antihypertensives; Antipsychotic Agents (Phenothiazines); Bupivacaine; Cardiac Glycosides; Fingolimod; Hypotensive Agents; Insulin; Lidocaine; Lidocaine (Systemic); Lidocaine (Topical); Mepivacaine; Methacholine; Midodrine; RiTUXimab; Sulfonylureas

The levels/effects of Esmolol may be increased by: Acetylcholinesterase Inhibitors; Aminoquinolines (Antimalarial); Amiodarone; Anilidopiperidine Opioids; Antipsychotic Agents (Phenothiazines); Calcium Channel Blockers (Nondihydropyridine); Diazoxide; Dipyridamole; Disopyramide; Dronedarone; Herbs (Hypotensive Properties); MAO Inhibitors; Pentoxifylline; Phosphodiesterase 5 Inhibitors; Propafenone; Propoxyphene; Prostacyclin Analogues; QuiNIDine; Reserpine

Adverse Reactions

>10%:

Cardiovascular: Asymptomatic hypotension (dose related: 25% to 38%), symptomatic hypotension (dose related: 12%)

Miscellaneous: Diaphoresis (10%)

1% to 10%:

Cardiovascular: Peripheral ischemia (1%)

Central nervous system: Dizziness (3%), somnolence (3%), confusion (2%), headache (2%), agitation (2%), fatigue (1%)

Gastrointestinal: Nausea (7%), vomiting (1%)

Local: Pain on injection (8%), infusion site reaction

Pharmacodynamics/Kinetics

Onset of Action Beta-blockade: I.V.: 2-10 minutes (quickest when loading doses are administered)

Duration of Action Hemodynamic effects: 10-30 minutes; prolonged following higher cumulative doses, extended duration of use

Protein Binding Esmolol: 55%; Acid metabolite: 10%

Half-Life Elimination Adults: Esmolol: 9 minutes; Acid metabolite: 3.7 hours; elimination of metabolite decreases with end-stage renal disease

Metabolism In blood by red blood cell esterases; forms acid metabolite (negligible activity; produces no clinically important effects) and methanol (does not achieve concentrations associated with methanol toxicity)

Excretion Urine (~73% to 88% as acid metabolite, <2% unchanged drug)

Available Dosage Forms

Infusion, premixed in NS [preservative free]:

Brevibloc: 2000 mg (100 mL); 2500 mg (250 mL)

Injection, solution [preservative free]: 10 mg/mL (10 mL)

Brevibloc: 10 mg/mL (10 mL)

Dosing

Adult & Geriatric Infusion requires an infusion pump (must be adjusted to individual response and tolerance):

Intraoperative tachycardia and/or hypertension (immediate control): I.V.: Initial bolus: 80 mg (1 mg/kg) over 30 seconds, followed by a 150 mcg/kg/minute infusion, if necessary. Adjust infusion rate as needed to maintain desired heart rate and/or blood pressure, up to 300 mcg/kg/minute.

For control of postoperative hypertension, as many as one-third of patients may require higher doses (250-300 mcg/kg/minute) to control blood pressure; the safety of doses >300 mcg/kg/minute has not been studied.

Supraventricular tachycardia (SVT) or gradual control of postoperative tachycardia/hypertension: I.V.: Loading dose: 500 mcg/kg over 1 minute; follow with a 50 mcg/kg/minute infusion for 4 minutes; response to this initial infusion rate may be a rough indication of the responsiveness of the ventricular rate.

Infusion may be continued at 50 mcg/kg/minute or, if the response is inadequate, titrated upward in 50 mcg/kg/minute increments (increased no more frequently than every 4 minutes) to a maximum of 200 mcg/kg/minute.

Note: To achieve more rapid response, following the initial loading dose and 50 mcg/kg/minute infusion, rebolus with a second 500 mcg/kg loading dose over 1 minute, and increase the maintenance infusion to 100 mcg/kg/minute for 4 minutes. If necessary, a third (and final) 500 mcg/kg loading dose may be administered, prior to increasing to an infusion rate of 150 mcg/kg/minute. After 4 minutes of the 150 mcg/kg/minute infusion, the infusion rate may be increased to a maximum rate of 200 mcg/kg/minute (without a bolus dose).

Guidelines for transfer to oral therapy (beta-blocker, calcium channel blocker):

Infusion should be reduced by 50% 30 minutes following the first dose of the alternative agent

Manufacturer suggests following the second dose of the alternative drug, patient's response should be monitored and if control is adequate for the first hour, esmolol may be discontinued.

Pediatric

Supraventricular tachycardias (SVT) (unlabeled use): I.V.: A limited amount of information regarding esmolol use in pediatric patients is currently available. Some centers have utilized doses of 100-500 mcg/kg given over 1 minute for control of supraventricular tachycardias.

Postoperative hypertension (unlabeled use): I.V.: Loading doses of 500 mcg/kg/minute over 1 minute with maximal doses of 50-250 mcg/kg/minute (mean: 173 mcg/kg/minute) have been used in addition to nitroprusside to treat postoperative hypertension after coarctation of aorta repair.

Renal Impairment Not removed by hemo- or peritoneal dialysis. Supplemental dose is not necessary.

Administration

I.V. Infusion into small veins or through a butterfly catheter should be avoided (can cause thrombophlebitis). Medication port of premixed bags should be used to withdraw only the initial bolus, if necessary (not to be used for withdrawal of additional bolus doses).

Stability

Storage Clear, colorless to light yellow solution which should be stored at 25°C (77°F); excursions permitted to 15°C to 30°C (59°F to 86°F); do not freeze. Protect from excessive heat.

Monitoring and Teaching Issues

Physical Assessment Requires continuous cardiac, hemodynamic, and infusion site monitoring (to prevent extravasation). Taper dosage slowly when discontinuing. Advise patients with diabetes to monitor glucose levels closely; beta-blockers may alter glucose tolerance.

Patient Education Esmolol is administered in emergencies; patient education should be appropriate to the situation.

Geriatric Considerations Due to alterations in the beta-adrenergic autonomic nervous system, beta-adrenergic blockade may result in less hemodynamic response than seen in younger adults. Studies indicate that despite decreased sensitivity to the chronotropic effects of beta-blockade with age, there appears to be an increased myocardial sensitivity to the negative inotropic effect during stress (ie, exercise). Controlled trials have shown the overall response rate for propranolol to be only 20% to 50% in elderly populations. Therefore, all beta-adrenergic blocking drugs may result in a decreased response as compared to younger adults.

Breast-Feeding Considerations It is not known if esmolol is excreted into breast milk. The manufacturer recommends that caution be exercised when administering esmolol to nursing women. The short half-life and the fact that it is not intended for chronic use should limit any exposure to the nursing infant.

Pregnancy Considerations Adverse events were not observed in animal reproduction studies; therefore, esmolol is classified as pregnancy category C. In a cohort study, an increased risk of cardiovascular defects was observed following maternal use of beta-blockers during pregnancy. Intrauterine growth restriction (IUGR), small placentas, as well as fetal/neonatal bradycardia, hypoglycemia, and/or respiratory depression have been observed following *in utero* exposure to beta-blockers as a class. Adequate facilities for monitoring infants at birth should be available. Untreated chronic maternal hypertension and pre-eclampsia are also associated with adverse events in the fetus, infant, and mother. Esmolol is a short-acting beta-blocker and not intended for the chronic treatment of hypertension in pregnancy. Esmolol has been evaluated for use during intubation as an agent to offset the exaggerated pressor response observed in pregnant women with hypertension undergoing surgery.

Related Information

Antiarrhythmic Drugs *on page 1978*

Beta-Blockers *on page 1990*

Hyperlipidemia Management *on page 2046*

◆ **Esmolol Hydrochloride** *see* Esmolol *on page 665*

Esmolol / Esomeprazole

Esomeprazole (es oh ME pray zol)

U.S. Brand Names NexIUM®; NexIUM® I.V.

Index Terms Esomeprazole Magnesium; Esomeprazole Sodium

Generic Availability (U.S.) No

Pharmacologic Category Proton Pump Inhibitor; Substituted Benzimidazole

Medication Safety Issues

Sound-alike/look-alike issues:

Esomeprazole may be confused with ARIPiprazole

NexIUM® may be confused with NexAVAR®

Pregnancy Risk Factor B

Lactation Excretion in breast milk unknown/not recommended

Use

Oral: Short-term (4-8 weeks) treatment of erosive esophagitis; maintaining symptom resolution and healing of erosive esophagitis; treatment of symptomatic gastroesophageal reflux disease (GERD); as part of a multidrug regimen for *Helicobacter pylori* eradication in patients with duodenal ulcer disease (active or history of within the past 5 years); prevention of gastric ulcers in patients at risk (age ≥60 years and/or history of gastric ulcer) associated with continuous NSAID therapy; long-term treatment of pathological hypersecretory conditions including Zollinger-Ellison syndrome

Canadian labeling: Additional use (not in U.S. labeling): Oral: Treatment of nonerosive reflux disease (NERD)

I.V.: Short-term (≤10 days) treatment of gastroesophageal reflux disease (GERD) when oral therapy is not possible or appropriate

Unlabeled/Investigational Use I.V.: Prevention of recurrent peptic ulcer bleeding postendoscopy

Mechanism of Action/Effect Prevents gastric acid secretion

Contraindications Hypersensitivity to esomeprazole, substituted benzimidazoles (eg, omeprazole, lansoprazole), or any component of the formulation

Warnings/Precautions Use of proton pump inhibitors may increase the risk of gastrointestinal infections (eg, *Salmonella, Campylobacter*). Relief of symptoms does not preclude the presence of a gastric malignancy. Atrophic gastritis (by biopsy) has been noted with long-term omeprazole therapy; this may also occur with esomeprazole. No reports of enterochromaffin-like (ECL) cell carcinoids, dysplasia, or neoplasia have occurred. Severe liver dysfunction may require dosage reductions. Safety and efficacy of I.V. therapy >10 days have not been established; transition from I.V. to oral therapy as soon possible. Bioavailability may be increased in Asian populations, the elderly, and patients with hepatic dysfunction. Decreased *H. pylori* eradication rates have been observed with short-term (≤7 days) combination therapy. The American College of Gastroenterology recommends 10-14 days of therapy (triple or quadruple) for eradication of *H. pylori* (Chey, 2007). Proton pump inhibitors may diminish the therapeutic effect of clopidogrel, thought to be due to reduced formation of the active metabolite of clopidogrel; an increase in the risk of cardiovascular events may occur. The manufacturer of clopidogrel recommends avoidance of concomitant administration of another PPI (ie, omeprazole); similar recommendations with esomeprazole would appear prudent.

Increased incidence of osteoporosis-related bone fractures of the hip, spine, or wrist may occur with proton pump inhibitor therapy. Patients on high-dose or long-term therapy should be monitored. Use the lowest effective dose for the shortest duration of time, use vitamin D and calcium supplementation, and follow appropriate guidelines to reduce risk of fractures in patients at risk.

Drug Interactions

Metabolism/Transport Effects Substrate of CYP2C19 (major), 3A4 (major); **Inhibits** CYP2C19 (moderate)

Avoid Concomitant Use

Avoid concomitant use of Esomeprazole with any of the following: Delavirdine; Erlotinib; Nelfinavir; Posaconazole

Decreased Effect

Esomeprazole may decrease the levels/effects of: Atazanavir; Bisphosphonate Derivatives; Cefditoren; Clopidogrel; Dabigatran Etexilate; Dasatinib; Delavirdine; Erlotinib; Gefitinib; Indinavir; Iron Salts; Itraconazole; Ketoconazole; Ketoconazole (Systemic); Mesalamine; Mycophenolate; Nelfinavir; Posaconazole

The levels/effects of Esomeprazole may be decreased by: CYP2C19 Inducers (Strong); Tipranavir

Increased Effect/Toxicity

Esomeprazole may increase the levels/effects of: Amphetamines; Benzodiazepines (metabolized by oxidation); Cilostazol; CYP2C19 Substrates; Dexmethylphenidate; Methotrexate; Methylphenidate; Raltegravir; Saquinavir; Tacrolimus; Tacrolimus (Systemic); Vitamin K Antagonists; Voriconazole

The levels/effects of Esomeprazole may be increased by: Conivaptan; Fluconazole; Ketoconazole; Ketoconazole (Systemic)

Nutritional/Ethanol Interactions Food: Absorption is decreased by 43% to 53% when taken with food.

Adverse Reactions Unless otherwise specified, percentages represent adverse reactions identified in clinical trials evaluating the oral formulation.

>10%: Central nervous system: Headache (I.V. 11%; oral ≤8%)

1% to 10%:

Cardiovascular: Hypertension (≤3%), chest pain (>1%)

Central nervous system: Pain (4%), dizziness (oral >1%; I.V. 3%), anxiety (2%), insomnia (2%), pyrexia (2%), fatigue (>1%)

Dermatologic: Rash (>1%), pruritus (I.V. ≤1%)

Endocrine & metabolic: Hypercholesterolemia (2%)

Gastrointestinal: Flatulence (oral ≤5%; I.V. 10%), diarrhea (oral ≤7%; I.V. 4%), abdominal pain (oral ≤6%; I.V. 6%), nausea (oral 5%; I.V. 6%), dyspepsia (oral >1%; I.V. 6%), gastritis (≤6%), constipation (oral 2%; I.V. 3%), vomiting (≤3%), benign GI neoplasm (>1%), dyspepsia (>1%), duodenitis (>1%), epigastric pain (>1%), esophageal disorder (>1%), gastroenteritis (>1%), GI mucosal discoloration (>1%), serum gastrin increased (>1%), tooth disorder (>1%), xerostomia (1%)

Genitourinary: Urinary tract infection (4%)

Hematologic: Anemia (>1%)

Hepatic: Transaminases increased (>1%)

Local: Injection site reaction (I.V. 2%)

Neuromuscular & skeletal: Arthralgia (3%), back pain (>1%), fracture (>1%), arthropathy (1%), myalgia (1%)

Respiratory: Respiratory infection (oral ≤9%; I.V. 1%), bronchitis (4%), sinusitis (oral ≤4%; I.V. 2%), coughing (>1%), rhinitis (>1%), dyspnea (1%)

Miscellaneous: Accident/injury (≤8%), viral infection (4%), allergy (2%), ear infection (2%), hernia (>1%), flu-like syndrome (1%)

Pharmacodynamics/Kinetics

Bioavailability Oral: 90% with repeat dosing

Time to Peak Oral: 1.5-2 hours

Protein Binding 97%

Half-Life Elimination ~1-1.5 hours

Metabolism Hepatic via CYP2C19 primarily and (to a lesser extent) via 3A4 to hydroxy, desmethyl, and sulfone metabolites (all inactive)

Excretion Urine (80%, primarily as inactive metabolites; <1% as active drug); feces (20%)

Available Dosage Forms

Capsule, delayed release, oral:

NexIUM®: 20 mg, 40 mg

Granules for suspension, delayed release, oral:

NexIUM®: 10 mg/packet (30s); 20 mg/packet (30s); 40 mg/packet (30s)

Injection, powder for reconstitution:
NexIUM® I.V.: 20 mg, 40 mg

Dosing

Adult

Erosive esophagitis (healing): Oral: Initial: 20-40 mg once daily for 4-8 weeks; if incomplete healing, may continue for an additional 4-8 weeks; maintenance: 20 mg once daily (controlled studies did not extend beyond 6 months)

Nonerosive reflux disease (NERD) (Canadian labeling): Initial: 20 mg once daily for 2-4 weeks; lack of symptom control after 4 weeks warrants further evaluation; maintenance (in patients with successful initial therapy): 20 mg once daily as needed

Symptomatic gastroesophageal reflux: Oral: 20 mg once daily for 4 weeks; may consider an additional 4 weeks of treatment if symptoms do not resolve

Treatment of GERD (short-term): I.V.: 20 mg or 40 mg once daily for ≤10 days; change to oral therapy as soon as appropriate

Prevention of recurrent peptic ulcer bleeding postendoscopy (unlabeled use; Sung, 2009): I.V. 80 mg over 30 minutes, followed by 8 mg/hour infusion for 72 hours, then 40 mg *orally* once daily for 27 additional days

***Helicobacter pylori* eradication:** Oral:

Manufacturer labeling: 40 mg once daily administered with amoxicillin 1000 mg *and* clarithromycin 500 mg twice daily for 10 days

American College of Gastroenterology guidelines (Chey, 2007):

Nonpenicillin allergy: 40 mg once daily administered with amoxicillin 1000 mg *and* clarithromycin 500 mg twice daily for 10-14 days

Penicillin allergy: 40 mg once daily administered with clarithromycin 500 mg *and* metronidazole 500 mg twice daily for 10-14 days **or** 40 mg once daily administered with bismuth subsalicylate 525 mg *and* metronidazole 250 mg *plus* tetracycline 500 mg 4 times/day for 10-14 days

Canadian labeling: 20 mg twice daily for 7 days; requires combination therapy

Prevention of NSAID-induced gastric ulcers: 20-40 mg once daily for up to 6 months

Treatment of NSAID-induced gastric ulcers (Canadian labeling): 20 mg once daily for 4-8 weeks.

Pathological hypersecretory conditions (Zollinger-Ellison syndrome): 40 mg twice daily; adjust regimen to individual patient needs; doses up to 240 mg/day have been administered

Geriatric Refer to adult dosing. No dosage adjustment needed.

Pediatric

Children 1-11 years: Oral: **Note:** Safety and efficacy of doses >1 mg/kg/day and/or therapy beyond 8 weeks have not been established.

Symptomatic GERD: 10 mg once daily for up to 8 weeks

Erosive esophagitis (healing):

<20 kg: 10 mg once daily for 8 weeks

≥20 kg: 10-20 mg once daily for 8 weeks

Nonerosive reflux disease (NERD) (Canadian labeling): 10 mg once daily for up to 8 weeks

Adolescents 12-17 years: Oral:

Symptomatic GERD: 20-40 mg once daily for up to 8 weeks

NERD (Canadian labeling): 20 mg once daily for 2-4 weeks

Renal Impairment No adjustment is necessary.

Hepatic Impairment Safety and efficacy not established in children with hepatic impairment.

Mild-to-moderate hepatic impairment (Child-Pugh class A or B): No dosage adjustment needed.

Severe hepatic impairment (Child-Pugh class C): Dose should not exceed 20 mg/day.

Administration

Oral

Capsule: Should be swallowed whole and taken at least 1 hour before eating (best if taken before breakfast). Capsule can be opened and contents mixed with 1 tablespoon of applesauce. Swallow immediately; mixture should not be chewed or warmed. For patients with difficulty swallowing, use of granules may be more appropriate.

Granules: Empty into container with 1 tablespoon of water and stir; leave 2-3 minutes to thicken. Stir and drink within 30 minutes. If any medicine remains after drinking, add more water, stir and drink immediately.

Tablet (Canadian formulation, not available in U.S.): Swallow whole or may be dispersed in a half a glass of noncarbonated water. Stir until tablets disintegrate, leaving a liquid containing pellets. Drink contents within 30 minutes. Do not chew or crush pellets. After drinking, rinse glass with water and drink.

I.V. May be administered by injection (≥3 minutes), intermittent infusion (10-30 minutes), or continuous infusion for up to 72 hours (Sung, 2009). Flush line prior to and after administration with NS, LR, or D_5W.

Other Nasogastric tube:

Capsule: Open capsule and place intact granules into a 60 mL catheter-tip syringe; mix with 50 mL of water. Replace plunger and shake vigorously for 15 seconds. Ensure that no granules remain in syringe tip. Do not administer if pellets dissolve or disintegrate. Use immediately after preparation. After administration, flush nasogastric tube with additional water.

Granules: Delayed release oral suspension granules can also be given by nasogastric or gastric tube. Add 15 mL of water to a catheter-tip syringe, add granules from packet. Shake the syringe, leave 2-3 minutes to thicken. Shake the syringe and administer through nasogastric or gastric tube (size 6 French or greater) within 30 minutes. Refill the syringe with 15 mL of water, shake and flush nasogastric/gastric tube.

Tablet (Canadian formulation, not available in U.S.): Disperse tablets in 50 mL of non-carbonated water. Stir until tablets disintegrate leaving a liquid containing pellets. After administration, flush with additional 25-50 mL of water to clear the syringe and tube.

Stability

Reconstitution Powder for injection:

For I.V. injection: Reconstitute powder with 5 mL NS.

For I.V. infusion: Initially reconstitute powder with 5 mL of NS, LR, or D_5W, then further dilute to a final volume of 50 mL.

Storage

Capsule, granules: Store at 15°C to 30°C (59°F to 86°F). Keep container tightly closed.

Powder for injection: Store at 25°C (77°F); excursions permitted to 15°C to 30°C (59°F to 86°F). Protect from light. Per the manufacturer, following reconstitution, solution for injection prepared in NS, and solution for infusion prepared in NS or LR should be used within 12 hours. Following reconstitution, solution for infusion prepared in D_5W should be used within 6 hours. Refrigeration is not required following reconstitution.

Additional stability data: Following reconstitution, solutions for infusion prepared in D_5W, NS, or LR in PVC bags are chemically and physically stable for 48 hours at room temperature (25°C) and for at least 120 hours under refrigeration (4°C) (Kupiec, 2008).

Monitoring and Teaching Issues

Laboratory Monitoring Susceptibility testing is recommended in patients who fail *H. pylori* eradication regimen.

Physical Assessment Assess effectiveness and interactions of other medications patient may be taking that are dependent on cytochrome P450 metabolism or on an acid environment for absorption.

Patient Education Take as directed, 1 hour before eating at same time each day. Swallow capsule whole; do not crush or chew. If you cannot swallow capsule whole, open capsule, mix contents with 1 tablespoon of applesauce, and swallow immediately; do not chew mixture. Do not store for future use. You may experience headache, constipation, diarrhea, or abdominal pain. Report persistent headache, diarrhea, abdominal pain, gas, changes in urination or pain on urination, or persistent muscular aches or pain.

Dietary Considerations Take at least 1 hour before meals; best if taken before breakfast. The contents of the capsule may be mixed in applesauce or water; pellets also remain intact when exposed to orange juice, apple juice, and yogurt.

Geriatric Considerations Dose adjustment is not necessary.

An increased risk of fractures of the hip, spine, or wrist has been observed in epidemiologic studies with proton pump inhibitor (PPI) use, primarily in older adults ≥50 years of age. The greatest risk was seen in patients receiving high doses or on long-term therapy (≥1 year). Calcium and vitamin D supplementation and close monitoring are recommended to reduce the risk of fracture in high-risk patients.

Breast-Feeding Considerations Esomeprazole excretion into breast milk has not been studied. However, omeprazole is excreted in breast milk, and therefore considered likely that esomeprazole is similarly excreted; breast-feeding is not recommended.

Pregnancy Considerations Teratogenic effects were not observed in animal studies. However, there are no adequate and well-controlled studies in pregnant women. Congenital abnormalities have been reported sporadically following omeprazole use during pregnancy.

Related Information

Helicobacter pylori Treatment *on page 2045*

- **Esomeprazole and Naproxen** *see* Naproxen and Esomeprazole *on page 1290*
- **Esomeprazole Magnesium** *see* Esomeprazole *on page 667*
- **Esomeprazole Sodium** *see* Esomeprazole *on page 667*
- **Esoterica® Daytime [OTC]** *see* Hydroquinone *on page 927*
- **Esoterica® Nighttime [OTC]** *see* Hydroquinone *on page 927*
- **Esterified Estrogens** *see* Estrogens (Esterified) *on page 687*
- **Estrace®** *see* Estradiol (Systemic) *on page 670*
- **Estraderm®** *see* Estradiol (Systemic) *on page 670*
- **Estradiol** *see* Estradiol (Systemic) *on page 670*

Estradiol (Systemic) (es tra DYE ole)

U.S. Brand Names Alora®; Climara®; Delestrogen®; Depo®-Estradiol; Divigel®; Elestrin®; Estrace®; Estraderm®; Estrasorb®; EstroGel®; Evamist™; Femring®; Femtrace®; Menostar®; Vivelle-Dot®

Index Terms Estradiol; Estradiol Acetate; Estradiol Transdermal; Estradiol Valerate

Generic Availability (U.S.) Yes: Oral tablet, patch, valerate oil for injection

Pharmacologic Category Estrogen Derivative

Medication Safety Issues

Sound-alike/look-alike issues:

Alora® may be confused with Aldara®

Elestrin™ may be confused with alosetron

Estraderm® may be confused with Testoderm®

Transdermal patch may contain conducting metal (eg, aluminum); remove patch prior to MRI.

Beers Criteria medication: This drug may be inappropriate for use in geriatric patients (low severity risk).

International issues:

Vivelle®: Brand name for ethinyl estradiol and norgestimate in Austria

Pregnancy Risk Factor X

Lactation Enters breast milk/use caution

Use Treatment of moderate-to-severe vasomotor symptoms associated with menopause; treatment of moderate-to-severe vulvar and vaginal atrophy associated with menopause; hypoestrogenism (due to hypogonadism, castration, or primary ovarian failure); advanced prostatic cancer (palliation); metastatic breast cancer (palliation) in men and postmenopausal women; postmenopausal osteoporosis (prophylaxis)

Available Dosage Forms

Emulsion, topical:

Estrasorb®: 2.5 mg/g (56s)

Gel, topical:

Divigel®: 0.1% (30s)

Elestrin®: 0.06% (144 g)

EstroGel®: 0.06% (50 g)

Injection, oil: 20 mg/mL (5 mL); 40 mg/mL (5 mL)

Delestrogen®: 10 mg/mL (5 mL); 20 mg/mL (5 mL); 40 mg/mL (5 mL)

Depo®-Estradiol: 5 mg/mL (5 mL)

Patch, transdermal: 0.025 mg/24 hours (4s); 0.0375 mg/24 hours (4s); 0.05 mg/24 hours (4s); 0.06 mg/24 hours (4s); 0.075 mg/24 hours (4s); 0.1 mg/24 hours (4s)

Alora®: 0.025 mg/24 hours (8s); 0.05 mg/24 hours (8s); 0.075 mg/24 hours (8s); 0.1 mg/24 hours (8s)

Climara®: 0.025 mg/24 hours (4s); 0.0375 mg/24 hours (4s); 0.05 mg/24 hours (4s); 0.06 mg/24 hours (4s); 0.075 mg/24 hours (4s); 0.1 mg/24 hours (4s)

Estraderm®: 0.05 mg/24 hours (8s); 0.1 mg/24 hours (8s)

Menostar®: 0.014 mg/24 hours (4s)

Vivelle-Dot®: 0.025 mg/24 hours (24s); 0.0375 mg/24 hours (24s); 0.05 mg/24 hours (24s); 0.075 mg/24 hours (24s); 0.1 mg/24 hours (24s)

Ring, vaginal:

Femring®: 0.05 mg/24 hours (1s); 0.1 mg/24 hours (1s)

Solution, topical:

Evamist™: 1.53 mg/spray (8.1 mL)

Tablet, oral: 0.5 mg, 1 mg, 2 mg

Estrace®: 0.5 mg, 1 mg, 2 mg

Femtrace®: 0.45 mg, 0.9 mg, 1.8 mg

Dosing

Adult & Geriatric All dosage needs to be adjusted based upon the patient's response:

Vulvar and vaginal atrophy associated with menopause:

I.M.: Valerate (Delestrogen®): 10-20 mg every 4 weeks

Intravaginal: Vaginal ring (Femring®): 0.05 mg intravaginally; following insertion, ring should remain in place for 3 months; dose may be increased to 0.1 mg if needed

Oral (Estrace®): 1-2 mg/day; administration should be cyclic (3 weeks on, 1 week off)

Topical gel (EstroGel®): 1.25 g/day applied at the same time each day

Transdermal (Alora®, Climara®, Estraderm®, Vivelle-Dot®): Refer to product-specific dosing.

Breast cancer, metastatic (appropriately selected patients): Oral (Estrace®): Males and postmenopausal females: 10 mg 3 times/day **or** (unlabeled dosing) postmenopausal women: 2 mg 3 times/day (Ellis, 2009)

Hypoestrogenism (female) due to hypogonadism, castration, or primary ovarian failure:

Oral (Estrace®): 1-2 mg/day; titrate as necessary to control symptoms using minimal effective dose for maintenance therapy

I.M: Valerate (Delestrogen®): 10-20 mg every 4 weeks

Transdermal (Alora®, Climara®, Estraderm®, Vivelle-Dot®): Refer to product-specific dosing.

Hypoestrogenism (female) due to hypogonadism: *I.M: Cypionate* (Depo®- Estradiol): 1.5-2 mg monthly

Osteoporosis prevention (females):

Oral (Estrace®): Lowest effective dose has not been determined; doses of 0.5 mg/day in a cyclic regimen for 23 days of a 28-week cycle were used in clinical studies

Transdermal (Alora®, Climara®, Estraderm®, Menostar®, Vivelle-Dot®): Refer to product-specific dosing (below)

Prostate cancer, advanced (androgen-dependent):

I.M.: Valerate (Delestrogen®): 30 mg or more every 1-2 weeks

Oral (Estrace®): 1-2 mg 3 times/day

Vasomotor symptoms associated with menopause:

Oral:

Estrace®: 1-2 mg daily, adjusted as necessary to limit symptoms; administration should be cyclic (3 weeks on, 1 week off)

Femtrace®: Initial dose: 0.45 mg/day; dosage range 0.45-1.8 mg/day

I.M. Cypionate (Depo®-Estradiol): 1-5 mg every 3-4 weeks

I.M. Valerate (Delestrogen®): 10-20 mg every 4 weeks

Topical emulsion (Estrasorb®): 3.48 g applied once daily in the morning

Topical gel:

Divigel®: 0.25 g/day; adjust dose based on patient response. Dosing range: 0.25-1 g/day

Elestrin®: 0.87 g/day applied at the same time each day

EstroGel®: 1.25 g/day applied at the same time each day

Topical spray (Evamist™): Initial: One spray (1.53 mg) per day. Adjust dose based on patient response. Dosing range: 1-3 sprays per day.

Transdermal (Alora®, Climara®, Estraderm®, Vivelle-Dot®): See product-specific dosing (below)

Vaginal ring (Femring®): Initial: 0.05 mg intravaginally; following insertion, ring should remain in place for 3 months; dose may be increased to 0.1 mg if needed

Transdermal product-specific dosing:

Note: Indicated dose may be used continuously in patients without an intact uterus. May be given continuously or cyclically (3 weeks on, 1 week off) in patients with an intact uterus **(exception - Menostar®, see specific dosing instructions).** When changing patients from oral to transdermal therapy, start transdermal patch 1 week after discontinuing oral hormone (may begin sooner if symptoms reappear within 1 week):

Transdermal once-weekly patch:

Vasomotor symptoms associated with menopause, vulvar and vaginal atrophy associated with menopause, female hypoestrogenism (due to hypogonadism, castration, or primary ovarian failure):

Climara®: Initial: Apply 0.025 mg/day patch once weekly. Adjust dose as necessary to control symptoms.

Prevention of osteoporosis in postmenopausal women:

Climara®: Apply patch once weekly; minimum effective dose 0.025 mg/day; adjust dosage based on response to therapy as indicated by biological markers and bone mineral density.

Menostar®: Apply patch once weekly (0.014 mg/day). In women with a uterus, also administer a progestin for 14 days every 6-12 months.

Transdermal twice-weekly patch:

Vasomotor symptoms associated with menopause, vulvar and vaginal atrophy associated with menopause, female hypoestrogenism (due to hypogonadism, castration, or primary ovarian failure): Titrate to lowest dose possible to control symptoms, adjusting initial dose after the first month of therapy:

Alora®, Estraderm®: Apply 0.05 mg patch twice weekly

Vivelle-Dot®: Apply 0.0375 mg patch twice weekly

Prevention of osteoporosis in postmenopausal women:

Alora®, Vivelle-Dot®: Apply 0.025 mg patch twice weekly; increase dose as necessary

Estraderm®: Apply 0.05 mg patch twice weekly; increase dose as necessary

Administration

I.M. The use of a progestin should be considered when administering estrogens to postmenopausal women with an intact uterus.

Injection for intramuscular administration only. Estradiol valerate should be injected into the upper outer quadrant of the gluteal muscle; administer with a dry needle (solution may become cloudy with wet needle).

Topical The use of a progestin should be considered when administering estrogens to postmenopausal women with an intact uterus.

Emulsion (Estrasorb®): Apply to clean, dry skin while in a sitting position. Contents of two pouches (total 3.48 g) are to be applied individually, once daily in the morning. Apply contents of first pouch to left thigh; massage into skin of left thigh and calf until thoroughly absorbed (~3 minutes). Apply excess from both hands to the buttocks. Apply contents of second pouch to the right thigh; massage into skin of right thigh and calf until thoroughly absorbed (~3 minutes). Apply excess from both hands to buttocks. Wash hands with soap and water. Allow skin to dry before covering legs with clothing. Do not apply to other areas of body. Do not apply to red or irritated skin.

Gel: Apply to clean, dry, unbroken skin at the same time each day. Allow to dry for 5 minutes prior to dressing. Gel is flammable; avoid fire or flame until dry. After application, wash hands with soap and water. Prior to the first use, pump must be primed. Do not apply gel to breast.

Divigel®: Apply entire contents of packet to right or left upper thigh each day (alternate sites). Do not apply to face, breasts, vaginal area or irritated skin. Apply over an area ~5x7 inches. Do not wash application site for 1 hour. Allow gel to dry before dressing

Elestrin®: Apply to upper arm and shoulder area using two fingers to spread gel. Apply after bath or shower; allow at least 2 hours between applying gel and going swimming. Wait at least 25 minutes before applying sunscreen to application area. Do not apply sunscreen to application area for ≥7 days (may increase absorption of gel).

EstroGel®: Apply gel to the arm, from the wrist to the shoulder. Spread gel as thinly as possible over one arm.

Spray: Evamist™: Prior to first use, prime pump by spraying 3 sprays with the cover on. To administer dose, hold container upright and vertical and rest the plastic cone flat against the skin while spraying. Spray to the inner surface of the forearm, starting near the elbow. If more than one spray is needed, apply to adjacent but not overlapping areas. Apply at the same time each day. Allow spray to dry for ~2 minutes. Do not wash application site for 30 minutes. Apply to clean, dry, unbroken skin. Do not apply to skin other than that of the forearm. Solution contained in the spray is flammable; avoid fire, flame, or smoking until spray has dried. If needed, sunscreen should be applied ~1 hour prior to application of Evamist™.

Transdermal patch: Do not apply transdermal system to breasts, but place on trunk of body (preferably abdomen). Rotate application sites allowing a 1-week interval between applications at a particular site. Do not apply to oily, damaged or irritated skin; avoid waistline or other areas where tight clothing may rub the patch off. Apply patch immediately after removing from protective pouch. In general, if patch falls off, the same patch may be reapplied or a new system may be used for the remainder of the dosing interval (not recommended with all products) When replacing patch, reapply to a new site. Swimming, bathing or showering are not expected to affect use of the patch. Note the following exceptions:

Estraderm®: Do not apply to an area exposed to direct sunlight.

Climara®, Menostar®: Swimming, bathing, or wearing patch while in a sauna have not been studied; adhesion of patch may be decreased or delivery of estradiol may be affected. Remove patch slowly after use to avoid skin irritation. If any adhesive remains on the skin after removal, first allow skin to dry for 15 minutes, then gently rub area with an oil-based cream or lotion. If patch falls off, a new patch should be applied for the remainder of the dosing interval.

Other Vaginal ring: Exact positioning is not critical for efficacy; however, patient should not feel anything once inserted. In case of discomfort, ring should be pushed further into vagina. If ring is expelled prior to 90 days, it may be rinsed off and reinserted. Ensure proper vaginal placement of the ring to avoid inadvertent urinary bladder insertion. If vaginal infection develops, Femring® may remain in place during local treatment of a vaginal infection.

Monitoring and Teaching Issues

Laboratory Monitoring Routine Papanicolaou smear, mammogram. Adequate diagnostic measures, including endometrial sampling, if indicated, should be performed to rule out malignancy in all cases of undiagnosed abnormal vaginal bleeding.

Physical Assessment Assess results of annual gynecological exam. Monitor for thromboembolism, hypertension, edema, and CNS changes on a regular basis during therapy. Before prescribing estrogen therapy to postmenopausal women, the risks and benefits must be weighed for each patient. Women should be informed of these risks and benefits, as well as possible effects of progestin when added to estrogen therapy. Estrogens with or without progestin should be used for shortest duration possible consistent with treatment goals and periodic assessment of risk:benefit should be made. Caution patients with diabetes to monitor glucose levels closely (may impair glucose tolerance). Remind patient about the importance of frequent self-breast exams and the need for annual gynecological exam.

Patient Education Follow directions for timing and application of your prescription. Annual gynecologic and regular self-breast exams are important. If you have diabetes, monitor glucose levels closely (may impair glucose tolerance). You may experience nausea, vomiting, abdominal pain, dizziness or mental depression, rash, headache, breast pain, or enlargement/ tenderness of breasts. Report unusual swelling of extremities; sudden acute pain in legs or calves, chest, or abdomen; shortness of breath; severe headache; sudden blindness or change in visual acuity; weakness or numbness of arm or leg; unusual vaginal bleeding; yellowing of skin or eyes; unusual bruising or bleeding; or skin rash. You may become intolerant to wearing contact lenses; notify prescriber if this occurs.

◆ **Estradiol Acetate** *see* Estradiol (Systemic) *on page* 670

Estradiol and Dienogest (es tra DYE ole & dye EN oh jest)

U.S. Brand Names Natazia™

Index Terms Dienogest and Estradiol; Estradiol Valerate and Dienogest

Generic Availability (U.S.) No

Pharmacologic Category Contraceptive; Estrogen and Progestin Combination

Pregnancy Risk Factor X

Lactation Enters breast milk/not recommended

Use Prevention of pregnancy

Unlabeled/Investigational Use Treatment of hypermenorrhea (menorrhagia); pain associated with endometriosis; dysmenorrhea; dysfunctional uterine bleeding

Available Dosage Forms

Tablet, oral [four-phasic formulation]:

Natazia™:

Days 1-2: Estradiol valerate 3 mg [2 dark yellow tablets]

Days 3-7: Estradiol valerate 2 mg and dienogest 2 mg [5 medium red tablets]

Days 8-24: Estradiol valerate 2 mg and dienogest 3 mg [17 light yellow tablets]

Days 25-26: Estradiol valerate 1 mg [2 dark red tablets]

Days 27-28: 2 white inactive tablets (28s)

Dosing

Adult Contraception: Female: Oral: Take 1 tablet daily in the order presented in the blister pack

Initial dosing: Start on day 1 of menstrual period (first day of bleeding). A nonhormonal contraceptive should be used for the first 9 days.

Switching from another combination oral contraceptive tablet: Take the first dark yellow tablet on the first day of withdrawal bleeding; do not continue taking tablets from previous contraceptive pack. If withdrawal bleeding does not occur, rule-out pregnancy before starting therapy. A nonhormonal contraceptive should be used for the first 9 days.

Switching from a vaginal ring or patch: Take the first dark yellow tablet on the day the ring or patch is removed. A nonhormonal contraceptive should be used for the first 9 days.

Switching from a progestin-only contraceptive: Take the first dark yellow tablet on the day of the next progestin-only tablet would have been given, or the day the progestin implant or IUD is removed, or on the day the next injection would have been given. A nonhormonal contraceptive should be used for the first 9 days.

Missed doses: If ≤12 hours late, take tablet as soon as remembering and take the next tablet at the usual time. If >12 hours late, instructions vary by day of cycle and number of tablets missed:

If missed ONE dose:

Days 1-17: Take missed tablet immediately; take next tablet at usual time; use back-up (nonhormonal) contraception for the next 9 days; continue taking 1 tablet each day for the rest of the cycle

Days 18-24: Do not continue using current blister pack (throw away); take day 1 of new blister pack; use back-up (nonhormonal) contraception for the next 9 days; continue taking 1 tablet each day for the rest of the cycle

Days 25-28: Take missed tablet immediately; take next tablet at usual time; continue taking 1 tablet each day for the rest of the cycle; no backup method of contraception is needed.

If missed TWO doses in a row:

Days 1-17: Do not take missed tablets; start by taking the tablet for the day it was first noticed that the tablet was missed; use back-up (nonhormonal) contraception for the next 9 days; continue taking 1 tablet each day for the rest of the cycle. If tablets were missed on days 17 and 18, follow directions for missed tablets on days 17-25.

Days 17-25: Do not continue using current blister pack (throw away); take day 3 of new blister pack; use back-up (nonhormonal) contraception for the next 9 days; continue taking 1 tablet each day for the rest of the cycle. If tablets were missed on days 25 and 26, follow directions for missed tablets on days 25-28.

Days 25-28: Do not continue using current blister pack (throw away); start a new pack on the same day, or start a new pack the day it would normally be started; continue taking 1 tablet each day for the rest of the cycle; no backup method of contraception is needed.

Pediatric

Contraception: Oral: Refer to adult dosing. Not to be used prior to menarche.

Renal Impairment Safety and efficacy have not been evaluated; dose adjustment not expected to be required.

Hepatic Impairment Discontinue if hepatic dysfunction occurs.

Administration

Oral Tablets should be taken at the same time each day in the order presented in the blister pack. Do not delay administration by >12 hours. In case of vomiting or diarrhea within 3-4 hours of taking a colored tablet, treat as if the dose was missed (or can take another tablet of the same color from an extra blister pack). Patients should be instructed not to take more than 2 tablets in any one day. A nonhormonal contraceptive (eg, condom or spermicide) should be used for the first 9 days of therapy. If patient is unsure of number of tablets missed, they should continue taking one tablet each day and use a back-up form of contraception.

◆ **Estradiol and Drospirenone** *see* Drospirenone and Estradiol *on page* 594

Estradiol and Norethindrone (es tra DYE ole & nor eth IN drone)

U.S. Brand Names Activella®; CombiPatch®; Mimvey™

Index Terms Norethindrone and Estradiol

Generic Availability (U.S.) Yes: Tablet

Pharmacologic Category Estrogen and Progestin Combination

Lactation Enters breast milk/use caution

Use Women with an intact uterus:

Tablet: Treatment of moderate-to-severe vasomotor symptoms associated with menopause; treatment of vulvar and vaginal atrophy; prophylaxis for postmenopausal osteoporosis

Transdermal patch: Treatment of moderate-to-severe vasomotor symptoms associated with menopause; treatment of vulvar and vaginal atrophy; treatment of hypoestrogenism due to hypogonadism, castration, or primary ovarian failure

Available Dosage Forms

Patch, transdermal:

CombiPatch®:

0.05/0.14: Estradiol 0.05 mg and norethindrone 0.14 mg per day (8s) [9 sq cm]

0.05/0.25: Estradiol 0.05 mg and norethindrone 0.25 mg per day (8s) [16 sq cm]

Tablet, oral: Estradiol 1 mg and norethindrone acetate 0.5 mg (28s)

Activella® 0.5/0.1: Estradiol 0.5 mg and norethindrone acetate 0.1 mg (28s)

Activella® 1/0.5, Mimvey™: Estradiol 1 mg and norethindrone acetate 0.5 mg (28s)

Dosing

Adult & Geriatric Note: Patients should be treated with the lowest effective dose and for the shortest duration, consistent with treatment goals.

Hypoestrogenism: Transdermal (patch):

Continuous combined regimen: Apply one patch twice weekly

Continuous sequential regimen: Apply estradiol-only patch for first 14 days of cycle, followed by one CombiPatch® applied twice weekly for the remaining 14 days of a 28-day cycle.

Osteoporosis, prevention in postmenopausal females (Activella®): Oral: 1 tablet daily

Menopause (moderate-to-severe vasomotor symptoms); vulvar and vaginal atrophy:

Oral (Activella®): 1 tablet daily

Transdermal (patch):

Continuous combined regimen: Apply one patch twice weekly

Continuous sequential regimen: Apply estradiol-only patch for first 14 days of cycle, followed by one CombiPatch® applied twice weekly for the remaining 14 days of a 28-day cycle.

Transdermal patch, combination pack (product-specific dosing for Canadian formulation):

Estalis®: Continuous combined regimen: Apply a new patch twice weekly during a 28-day cycle

Estalis-Sequi®: Continuous sequential regimen: Apply estradiol-only patch (Vivelle®) for first 14 days, followed by one Estalis® patch applied twice weekly during the last 14 days of a 28-day cycle

Note: In women previously receiving oral estrogens, initiate upon reappearance of menopausal symptoms following discontinuation of oral therapy.

Administration

Other Transdermal patch: Apply to clean dry skin. Do not apply transdermal patch to breasts; apply to lower abdomen, avoiding waistline. Rotate application sites.

Monitoring and Teaching Issues

Physical Assessment See individual agents.

Patient Education See individual agents.

Related Information

Estradiol (Systemic) *on page 670*

Norethindrone *on page 1334*

◆ **Estradiol Transdermal** *see* Estradiol (Systemic) *on page 670*

◆ **Estradiol Valerate** *see* Estradiol (Systemic) *on page 670*

◆ **Estradiol Valerate and Dienogest** *see* Estradiol and Dienogest *on page 673*

Estramustine (es tra MUS teen)

U.S. Brand Names Emcyt®

Index Terms Estramustine Phosphate; Estramustine Phosphate Sodium; NSC-89199

Generic Availability (U.S.) No

Pharmacologic Category Antineoplastic Agent, Alkylating Agent; Antineoplastic Agent, Hormone; Antineoplastic Agent, Hormone (Estrogen/Nitrogen Mustard)

Medication Safety Issues

Sound-alike/look-alike issues:

Emcyt® may be confused with Eryc®

Estramustine may be confused with exemestane.

High alert medication: The Institute for Safe Medication Practices (ISMP) includes this medication among its list of drug classes which have a heightened risk of causing significant patient harm when used in error.

Use Palliative treatment of progressive or metastatic prostate cancer

Mechanism of Action/Effect Combines the effects of estradiol and nitrogen mustard. It appears to bind to microtubule proteins, preventing normal tubulin function. The antitumor effect may be due solely to an estrogenic effect. Estramustine causes a marked decrease in plasma testosterone and an increase in estrogen levels.

Contraindications Hypersensitivity to estramustine, estradiol, nitrogen mustard, or any component of the formulation; active thrombophlebitis or thromboembolic disorders (except where tumor mass is the cause of thromboembolic disorder and the benefit may outweigh the risk)

Canadian labeling: Additional contraindications (not in the U.S. labeling): Severe hepatic or cardiac disease

Warnings/Precautions Hazardous agent - use appropriate precautions for handling and disposal. Glucose tolerance may be decreased; use with caution in patients with diabetes. Elevated blood pressure, peripheral edema (new-onset or exacerbation), or congestive heart disease may occur; use with caution in patients where fluid accumulation may be poorly tolerated, including cardiovascular disease (HF or hypertension), migraine, seizure disorder or renal dysfunction. Estrogen treatment for prostate cancer is associated with an increased risk of thrombosis and MI; use caution with history of cardiovascular disease (eg, thrombophlebitis, thrombosis, or thromboembolic disease) and cerebrovascular or coronary artery disease. Use with caution in patients with hepatic impairment (may be metabolized poorly) or with metabolic bone diseases. Allergic reactions and angioedema, including airway involvement, have been reported with use. Patients with prostate cancer and osteoblastic metastases should have their calcium monitored regularly. Estrogen use may cause gynecomastia and/or impotence. Avoid vaccination with live vaccines during treatment (risk of infection may be increased due to immunosuppression). Although the response to vaccines may be diminished, inactivated vaccines may be administered during treatment.

Drug Interactions

Avoid Concomitant Use

Avoid concomitant use of Estramustine with any of the following: BCG; Natalizumab; Pimecrolimus; Roflumilast; Tacrolimus (Topical); Vaccines (Live)

Decreased Effect

Estramustine may decrease the levels/effects of: BCG; Sipuleucel-T; Vaccines (Inactivated); Vaccines (Live)

The levels/effects of Estramustine may be decreased by: Calcium Salts; Echinacea

Increased Effect/Toxicity

Estramustine may increase the levels/effects of: Leflunomide; Natalizumab; Vaccines (Live)

The levels/effects of Estramustine may be increased by: Clodronate; Denosumab; Pimecrolimus; Roflumilast; Tacrolimus (Topical); Trastuzumab

Nutritional/Ethanol Interactions Food: Estramustine serum levels may be decreased if taken with milk and other dairy products, calcium supplements, and vitamins containing calcium.

Adverse Reactions

>10%:

- Cardiovascular: Edema (20%)
- Endocrine & metabolic: Gynecomastia (75%), breast tenderness (71%), libido decreased
- Gastrointestinal: Nausea (16%), diarrhea (13%), gastrointestinal upset (12%)
- Hepatic: LDH increased (2% to 33%), AST increased (2% to 33%)
- Respiratory: Dyspnea (12%)

1% to 10%:

- Cardiovascular: CHF (3%), MI (3%), cerebrovascular accident (2%), chest pain (1%), flushing (1%)
- Central nervous system: Lethargy (4%), insomnia (3%), emotional lability (2%), anxiety (1%), headache (1%)
- Dermatologic: Bruising (3%), dry skin (2%), pruritus (2%), hair thinning (1%), rash (1%), skin peeling (1%)
- Gastrointestinal: Anorexia (4%), flatulence (2%), burning throat (1%), gastrointestinal bleeding (1%), thirst (1%), vomiting (1%)
- Hematologic: Leukopenia (4%), thrombocytopenia (1%)
- Hepatic: Bilirubin increased (1% to 2%)
- Local: Thrombophlebitis (3%)
- Neuromuscular & skeletal: Leg cramps (9%)
- Ocular: Tearing (1%)
- Respiratory: Pulmonary embolism (2%), upper respiratory discharge (1%), hoarseness (1%)

Pharmacodynamics/Kinetics

Absorption Oral: 75%

Time to Peak Serum: 2-3 hours

Half-Life Elimination Terminal: 15-24 hours

Metabolism GI tract: Initial dephosphorylation; Hepatic: Oxidation and hydrolysis; metabolites include estramustine, estrone analog, estrone, and estradiol

Excretion Feces (2.9% to 4.8% as unchanged drug)

Available Dosage Forms

Capsule, oral:

Emcyt®: 140 mg

Dosing

Adult & Geriatric Details concerning dosing in combination regimens should also be consulted.

Prostate cancer: Oral: Males: 14 mg/kg/day (range: 10-16 mg/kg/day) in 3 or 4 divided doses

Combination therapy with docetaxel (unlabeled dose): 280 mg 3 times/day for 5 days (days 1 through 5) of a 21-day treatment cycle for up to 12 cycles (Petrylak, 2004)

Administration

Oral Administer on an empty stomach, at least 1 hour before or 2 hours after eating.

Stability

Storage Refrigerate at 2°C to 8°C (36°F to 46°F).

Monitoring and Teaching Issues

Laboratory Monitoring Serum calcium, liver function tests

Physical Assessment Use caution in presence of renal or hepatic impairment, metabolic disease, seizure disorders, or migraine history. Assess serum calcium levels and LFTs. Monitor for hypertension, CNS changes, and thromboembolism on a regular basis. Caution patients with diabetes to monitor glucose carefully; glucose tolerance may be decreased.

Patient Education It may take several weeks to manifest effects of this medication. Take on empty stomach, 1 hour before or 2 hours after meals or any supplements containing calcium; do not take with milk or milk products. Patients with diabetes should use caution and monitor glucose carefully; glucose tolerance may be decreased. May cause nausea, vomiting, flatulence, diarrhea, decreased libido (reversible), or breast tenderness or enlargement. Report sudden acute pain or cramping in legs or calves, unusual swelling in legs or feet, chest pain, shortness of breath, weakness or numbness of arms or legs, or respiratory difficulty.

Dietary Considerations Should be taken at least 1 hour before or 2 hours after eating. Milk products and calcium-rich foods or supplements may impair the oral absorption of estramustine phosphate sodium.

Breast-Feeding Considerations Estramustine is not indicated for use in women.

Pregnancy Considerations Estramustine is not indicated for use in women. Men who were impotent on estrogen therapy have regained potency while taking estramustine; effective contraception should be used for male patients with partners of childbearing potential.

- **Estramustine Phosphate** *see* Estramustine *on page 675*
- **Estramustine Phosphate Sodium** *see* Estramustine *on page 675*
- **Estrasorb®** *see* Estradiol (Systemic) *on page 670*
- **EstroGel®** *see* Estradiol (Systemic) *on page 670*
- **Estrogenic Substances, Conjugated** *see* Estrogens (Conjugated/Equine, Systemic) *on page 682*
- **Estrogenic Substances, Conjugated** *see* Estrogens (Conjugated/Equine, Topical) *on page 686*

Estrogens (Conjugated A/Synthetic)

(ES troe jenz KON joo gate ed aye sin THET ik)

U.S. Brand Names Cenestin®

Generic Availability (U.S.) No

Pharmacologic Category Estrogen Derivative

Medication Safety Issues

Sound-alike/look-alike issues:

Cenestin® may be confused with Senexon®

Beers Criteria medication: This drug may be inappropriate for use in geriatric patients (low severity risk).

International issues:

Cenestin [U.S., Canada] may be confused with Canesten which is a brand name for clotrimazole [multiple international markets] and a brand name for fluconazole [Great Britain]

Lactation Enters breast milk/use caution

Use Treatment of moderate-to-severe vasomotor symptoms of menopause; treatment of vulvar and vaginal atrophy

Mechanism of Action/Effect Estrogens modulate the pituitary secretion of gonadotropins, luteinizing hormone, and follicle-stimulating hormone through a negative feedback system; estrogen replacement reduces elevated levels of these hormones in postmenopausal women

Contraindications Hypersensitivity to estrogens or any component of the formulation; undiagnosed abnormal vaginal bleeding; history of or current thrombophlebitis or venous thromboembolic disorders (including DVT, PE); active or recent (within 1 year) arterial thromboembolic disease (eg, stroke, MI); carcinoma of the breast; estrogen-dependent tumor; hepatic dysfunction or disease; pregnancy

Warnings/Precautions

Cardiovascular-related considerations: **[U.S. Boxed Warning]: Estrogens with or without progestin should not be used to prevent coronary heart disease.** Use caution with cardiovascular disease or dysfunction. May increase the risks of hypertension, myocardial infarction (MI), stroke, pulmonary emboli (PE), and deep vein thrombosis; incidence of these effects was shown to be significantly increased in postmenopausal women using conjugated equine estrogens (CEE) in combination with medroxyprogesterone acetate (MPA). Nonfatal MI, PE, and thrombophlebitis have also been reported in males taking high doses of CEE (eg, for prostate cancer). Estrogen compounds are generally associated with lipid effects such as increased HDL-cholesterol and decreased LDL-cholesterol. Triglycerides may also be increased; use with caution in patients with familial defects of lipoprotein metabolism. Whenever possible, estrogens should be discontinued at least 4 weeks prior to and for 2 weeks following elective surgery associated with an increased risk of thromboembolism or during periods of prolonged immobilization.

Neurological considerations: **[U.S. Boxed Warning]: The risk of dementia may be increased in postmenopausal women;** increased incidence was observed in women ≥65 years of age taking CEE alone or in combination with MPA.

Cancer-related considerations: **[U.S. Boxed Warning]: Unopposed estrogens may increase the risk of endometrial carcinoma in postmenopausal women.** Estrogens may exacerbate endometriosis. Malignant transformation of residual endometrial implants has been reported posthysterectomy with estrogen only therapy. Consider adding a progestin in women with residual endometriosis posthysterectomy. Estrogens may increase the risk of breast cancer. An increased risk of invasive breast cancer was observed in postmenopausal women using CEE in combination with MPA; a smaller increase in risk was seen with estrogen therapy alone in observational studies. An increase in abnormal mammograms has also been reported with estrogen and progestin therapy. Estrogen use may lead to severe hypercalcemia in patients with breast cancer and bone metastases; discontinue estrogen if hypercalcemia occurs. Postmenopausal estrogen therapy and combined estrogen/progesterone therapy may increase the risk of ovarian cancer; however, the absolute risk to an individual woman is small. Although results from various studies are not consistent, risk does not appear to be significantly associated with the duration, route, or dose of therapy. In one study, the risk decreased after 2 years following discontinuation of therapy.

Estrogens may cause retinal vascular thrombosis; discontinue permanently if papilledema or retinal vascular lesions are observed on examination. Use with caution in patients with diseases which may be exacerbated by fluid retention, including asthma, epilepsy, migraine, diabetes or renal dysfunction. Use with caution in patients with a history of severe hypocalcemia, SLE, hepatic hemangiomas, porphyria, endometriosis, and gallbladder disease. Use caution with history of cholestatic jaundice associated with past estrogen use or pregnancy. May be inappropriate for use in the elderly due to potential of increased risk of breast and endometrial cancers and lack of proven cardioprotection (Beers Criteria). Safety and efficacy in pediatric patients have not been established. Prior to puberty, estrogens may cause premature closure of the epiphyses, premature breast development in girls or gynecomastia in boys. Vaginal bleeding and vaginal cornification may also be induced in girls.

Before prescribing estrogen therapy to postmenopausal women, the risks and benefits must be weighed for each patient. Women should be informed of these risks and benefits, as well as possible effects of progestin when added to estrogen therapy. Estrogens with or without progestin should be used for shortest duration possible consistent with treatment goals. Conduct periodic risk:benefit assessments.

When used solely for prevention of osteoporosis in women at significant risk, nonestrogen treatment options should be considered. When used solely for the treatment of vulvar and vaginal atrophy, topical vaginal products should be considered.

Drug Interactions

Metabolism/Transport Effects Based on estradiol and estrone: **Substrate** of CYP1A2 (major), 2A6 (minor), 2B6 (minor), 2C9 (minor), 2C19 (minor), 2D6 (minor), 2E1 (minor), 3A4 (major); **Inhibits** CYP1A2 (weak); **Induces** CYP3A4 (weak)

Avoid Concomitant Use

Avoid concomitant use of Estrogens (Conjugated A/Synthetic) with any of the following: Anastrozole

Decreased Effect

Estrogens (Conjugated A/Synthetic) may decrease the levels/effects of: Anastrozole; Chenodiol; Saxagliptin; Somatropin; Thyroid Products; Ursodiol

The levels/effects of Estrogens (Conjugated A/Synthetic) may be decreased by: CYP1A2 Inducers (Strong); CYP3A4 Inducers (Strong); Deferasirox; Herbs (CYP3A4 Inducers); Peginterferon Alfa-2b; Tipranavir

Increased Effect/Toxicity

Estrogens (Conjugated A/Synthetic) may increase the levels/effects of: Corticosteroids (Systemic); ROPINIRole; Tipranavir

The levels/effects of Estrogens (Conjugated A/Synthetic) may be increased by: Ascorbic Acid; Conivaptan; Herbs (Estrogenic Properties)

Nutritional/Ethanol Interactions

Ethanol: Avoid ethanol (routine use increases estrogen plasma concentrations and risk of breast cancer).

Food: Grapefruit juice may increase estrogen plasma concentrations, leading to increased adverse effects.

Herb/Nutraceutical: St John's wort may decrease levels. Herbs with estrogenic properties may enhance the adverse/toxic effect of estrogen derivatives; examples include alfalfa, black cohosh, bloodroot, hops, kudzu, licorice, red clover, saw palmetto, soybean, thyme, wild yam, yucca.

Lab Interactions Pathologist should be advised of estrogen/progesterone therapy when specimens are submitted. Reduced response to metyrapone test observed with conjugated estrogens (equine).

Adverse Reactions

>10%:

Central nervous system: Headache (11% to 68%), dizziness (11%), pain (11%)
Endocrine & metabolic: Breast pain (29%), endometrial thickening (19%), metrorrhagia (14%)
Gastrointestinal: Abdominal pain (9% to 28%), nausea (9% to 18%)
Neuromuscular & skeletal: Paresthesia (8% to 33%), back pain (14%)
Respiratory: Upper respiratory tract infection (13%)
Miscellaneous: Infection (2% to 14%)

1% to 10%:

Central nervous system: Anxiety (6%), fever (1%)
Gastrointestinal: Dyspepsia (10%), vomiting (7%), constipation (6%), diarrhea (6%), weight gain (6%)
Genitourinary: Vaginitis (8%)
Neuromuscular & skeletal: Leg cramps (10%), hypertonia (6%)
Respiratory: Rhinitis (6% to 8%), cough (6%)

In addition, the following have been reported with estrogen and/or progestin therapy:

Cardiovascular: Edema, hypertension, MI, stroke, venous thromboembolism

Central nervous system: Epilepsy exacerbation, irritability, mental depression, migraine, mood disturbances, nervousness

Dermatologic: Angioedema, chloasma, erythema multiforme, erythema nodosum, hemorrhagic eruption, hirsutism, melasma, pruritus, rash, scalp hair loss, urticaria

Endocrine & metabolic: Breast cancer, breast enlargement, breast tenderness, glucose tolerance impaired, HDL-cholesterol increased, hyper-/hypocalcemia, LDL-cholesterol decreased, libido changes, serum triglycerides/phospholipids increased, thyroid-binding globulin increased, total thyroid hormone (T_4) increased

Gastrointestinal: Abdominal cramps, bloating, cholecystitis, cholelithiasis, gallbladder disease, pancreatitis, weight gain/loss

Genitourinary: Alterations in frequency and flow of menses, cervical secretion changes, endometrial cancer, endometrial hyperplasia, uterine leiomyomata size increased, vaginal candidiasis

Hematologic: Aggravation of porphyria, antithrombin III and antifactor Xa decreased, fibrinogen levels increased, platelet aggregability and platelet count increased; prothrombin and factors VII, VIII, IX, X increased

Hepatic: Cholestatic jaundice, hepatic hemangiomas enlarged
Neuromuscular & skeletal: Arthralgias, chorea, leg cramps
Local: Thrombophlebitis
Ocular: Contact lens intolerance, retinal vascular thrombosis, corneal curvature steepening
Respiratory: Asthma exacerbation, pulmonary thromboembolism
Miscellaneous: Anaphylactoid/anaphylactic reactions, carbohydrate intolerance

Pharmacodynamics/Kinetics

Absorption Well absorbed over a period of several hours

Protein Binding Sex hormone-binding globulin (SHBG) and albumin

Metabolism Hepatic via CYP3A4; estradiol is converted to estrone and estriol; also undergoes enterohepatic recirculation; estrone sulfate is the main metabolite in postmenopausal women

Excretion Urine (primarily estriol, also as estradiol, estrone, and conjugates)

Available Dosage Forms

Tablet, oral:
Cenestin®: 0.3 mg, 0.45 mg, 0.625 mg, 0.9 mg, 1.25 mg

Dosing

Adult The lowest dose that will control symptoms should be used. Medication should be discontinued as soon as possible.

Menopause, moderate-to-severe vasomotor symptoms: Oral: 0.45 mg/day; may be titrated up to 1.25 mg/day; attempts to discontinue medication should be made at 3- to 6-month intervals

Vulvar and vaginal atrophy: Oral: 0.3 mg/day

Geriatric Refer to adult dosing. A higher incidence of stroke and invasive breast cancer were observed in women >75 years in a WHI substudy using conjugated equine estrogen.

Stability

Storage Store at room temperature of 25°C (77°F).

Monitoring and Teaching Issues

Laboratory Monitoring Yearly Papanicolaou smear, mammogram. Adequate diagnostic measures, including endometrial sampling, if indicated, should be performed to rule out malignancy in all cases of undiagnosed abnormal vaginal bleeding.

Physical Assessment Assess results of annual gynecological exam. Monitor for thromboembolism, hypertension, edema, and CNS changes on a regular basis during therapy. Before prescribing estrogen therapy to postmenopausal women, the risks and benefits must be weighed for each patient. Women should be informed of these risks and benefits, as well as possible effects of progestin when added to estrogen therapy. Estrogens with or without progestin should be used for shortest duration possible consistent with treatment goals and periodic assessment of risk:benefit should be made. Caution patients with diabetes to monitor glucose levels closely (may impair glucose tolerance). Remind patient about the importance of frequent self-breast exams and the need for annual gynecological exam.

Patient Education Annual gynecologic and regular self-breast exams are important. If you have diabetes, monitor glucose levels closely (may impair glucose tolerance). You may experience nausea, vomiting, abdominal pain, dizziness, mental depression, rash, headache, breast pain, or enlargement/tenderness of breasts. Report significant swelling of extremities; sudden acute pain in legs or calves, chest, or abdomen; shortness of breath; severe headache; sudden blindness; weakness or numbness of arm or leg; unusual vaginal bleeding; yellowing of skin or eyes; or unusual bruising or bleeding. You may become intolerant to wearing contact lenses; notify prescriber if this occurs.

Geriatric Considerations Before prescribing estrogen therapy to postmenopausal women, the risks and benefits must be weighed for each patient. Women should be informed of these risks and benefits, as well as possible side effects and the return of menstrual bleeding (when cycled with a progestin), and be involved in the decision to prescribe. A higher incidence of stroke and invasive breast cancer were observed in women >75 years in a WHI substudy using conjugated equine estrogen. Oral therapy may be more convenient for vaginal atrophy and urinary incontinence.

This medication is considered to be potentially inappropriate in this patient population (Beers Criteria severity: Low).

Breast-Feeding Considerations Estrogen has been shown to decrease the quantity and quality of human milk. Use only if clearly needed. Monitor the growth of the infant closely.

Pregnancy Considerations Use during pregnancy is contraindicated.

Additional Information Not biologically equivalent to conjugated estrogens from equine source. Contains 9 unique estrogenic compounds (equine source contains at least 10 active estrogenic compounds).

Related Information

Pharmacotherapy of Urinary Incontinence *on page 2071*

Estrogens (Conjugated B/Synthetic)

(ES troe jenz KON joo gate ed bee sin THET ik)

U.S. Brand Names Enjuvia™

Generic Availability (U.S.) No

Pharmacologic Category Estrogen Derivative

Medication Safety Issues

Sound-alike/look-alike issues:
Enjuvia™ may be confused with Januvia®

Beers Criteria medication: This drug may be inappropriate for use in geriatric patients (low severity risk).

Lactation Enters breast milk/use caution

Use Treatment of moderate-to-severe vasomotor symptoms of menopause; treatment of vulvar and vaginal atrophy associated with menopause; treatment of moderate-to-severe vaginal dryness and pain with intercourse associated with menopause

Mechanism of Action/Effect Estrogens modulate the pituitary secretion of gonadotropins, luteinizing hormone, and follicle-stimulating hormone through a negative feedback system; estrogen replacement reduces elevated levels of these hormones in postmenopausal women

Contraindications Hypersensitivity to estrogens or any component of the formulation; undiagnosed abnormal vaginal bleeding; history of or current thrombophlebitis or venous thromboembolic disorders (including DVT, PE); active or recent (within 1 year) arterial thromboembolic disease (eg, stroke, MI); carcinoma of the breast; estrogen-dependent tumor; hepatic dysfunction or disease; pregnancy

Warnings/Precautions

Cardiovascular-related considerations: **[U.S. Boxed Warning]: Estrogens with or without progestin should not be used to prevent coronary heart disease.** Use caution with cardiovascular disease or dysfunction. May increase the risks of hypertension, myocardial infarction (MI), stroke, pulmonary emboli (PE), and deep vein thrombosis; incidence of these effects was shown to be significantly increased in postmenopausal women using conjugated equine estrogens (CEE) in combination with medroxyprogesterone acetate (MPA). Nonfatal MI, PE, and thrombophlebitis have also been reported in males taking high doses of CEE (eg, for prostate cancer). Estrogen compounds are generally associated with lipid effects such as increased HDL-cholesterol and decreased LDL-cholesterol. Triglycerides may also be increased; use with caution in patients with familial defects of lipoprotein metabolism. Whenever possible, estrogens should be discontinued at least 4 weeks prior to and for 2 weeks following elective surgery associated with an increased risk of thromboembolism or during periods of prolonged immobilization.

Neurological considerations: **[U.S. Boxed Warning]: The risk of dementia may be increased in postmenopausal women;** increased incidence was observed in women ≥65 years of age taking CEE alone or in combination with MPA.

Cancer-related considerations: **[U.S. Boxed Warning]: Unopposed estrogens may increase the risk of endometrial carcinoma in postmenopausal women.** Estrogens may exacerbate endometriosis. Malignant transformation of residual endometrial implants has been reported posthysterectomy with estrogen only therapy. Consider adding a progestin in women with residual endometriosis posthysterectomy. Estrogens may increase the risk of breast cancer. An increased risk of invasive breast cancer was observed in postmenopausal women using CEE in combination with MPA; a smaller increase in risk was seen with estrogen therapy alone in observational studies. An increase in abnormal mammograms has also been reported with estrogen and progestin therapy. Estrogen use may lead to severe hypercalcemia in patients with breast cancer and bone metastases; discontinue estrogen if hypercalcemia occurs. Postmenopausal estrogen therapy and combined estrogen/progesterone therapy may increase the risk of ovarian cancer; however, the absolute risk to an individual woman is small. Although results from various studies are not consistent, risk does not appear to be significantly associated with the duration, route, or dose of therapy. In one study, the risk decreased after 2 years following discontinuation of therapy.

Estrogens may cause retinal vascular thrombosis; discontinue permanently if papilledema or retinal vascular lesions are observed on examination. Use with caution in patients with diseases which may be exacerbated by fluid retention, including asthma, epilepsy, migraine, diabetes or renal dysfunction. Use with caution in patients with a history of severe hypocalcemia, SLE, hepatic hemangiomas, porphyria, endometriosis, and gallbladder disease. Use caution with history of cholestatic jaundice associated with past estrogen use or pregnancy. May be inappropriate for use in the elderly due to potential of increased risk of breast and endometrial cancers and lack of proven cardioprotection (Beers Criteria). Safety and efficacy in pediatric patients have not been established. Prior to puberty, estrogens may cause premature closure of the epiphyses, premature breast development in girls or gynecomastia in boys. Vaginal bleeding and vaginal cornification may also be induced in girls.

Before prescribing estrogen therapy to postmenopausal women, the risks and benefits must be weighed for each patient. Women should be informed of these risks and benefits, as well as possible effects of progestin when added to estrogen therapy. Estrogens with or without progestin should be used for shortest duration possible consistent with treatment goals. Conduct periodic risk:benefit assessments. When used solely for the treatment of vaginal dryness and pain with intercourse, or vulvar and vaginal atrophy, topical vaginal products should be considered.

Drug Interactions

Metabolism/Transport Effects Based on estradiol and estrone: **Substrate** of CYP1A2 (major), 2A6 (minor), 2B6 (minor), 2C9 (minor), 2C19 (minor), 2D6 (minor), 2E1 (minor), 3A4 (major); **Inhibits** CYP1A2 (weak); **Induces** CYP3A4 (weak)

Avoid Concomitant Use

Avoid concomitant use of Estrogens (Conjugated B/Synthetic) with any of the following: Anastrozole

Decreased Effect

Estrogens (Conjugated B/Synthetic) may decrease the levels/effects of: Anastrozole; Chenodiol; Somatropin; Thyroid Products; Ursodiol

The levels/effects of Estrogens (Conjugated B/Synthetic) may be decreased by: CYP3A4 Inducers (Strong); Deferasirox; Herbs (CYP3A4 Inducers); Tipranavir

Increased Effect/Toxicity

Estrogens (Conjugated B/Synthetic) may increase the levels/effects of: Corticosteroids (Systemic); ROPINIRole; Tipranavir

The levels/effects of Estrogens (Conjugated B/Synthetic) may be increased by: Ascorbic Acid; Conivaptan; Herbs (Estrogenic Properties)

Nutritional/Ethanol Interactions

Ethanol: Avoid ethanol (routine use increases estrogen plasma concentrations and risk of breast cancer).

Food: Grapefruit juice may increase estrogen plasma concentrations, leading to increased adverse effects.

Herb/Nutraceutical: St John's wort may decrease levels. Herbs with estrogenic properties may enhance the adverse/toxic effect of estrogen derivatives; examples include alfalfa, black cohosh, bloodroot, hops, kudzu, licorice, red clover, saw palmetto, soybean, thyme, wild yam, and yucca.

Lab Interactions Pathologist should be advised of estrogen/progesterone therapy when specimens are submitted. Reduced response to metyrapone test observed with conjugated estrogens (equine).

Adverse Reactions

>10%:
- Central nervous system: Headache (15% to 25%), pain (10% to 19%)
- Endocrine & metabolic: Breast pain (up to 14%)
- Gastrointestinal: Abdominal pain (4% to 15%), nausea (7% to 12%)

1% to 10%:
- Central nervous system: Dizziness (1% to 7%)
- Endocrine & metabolic: Dysmenorrhea (1% to 8%)
- Gastrointestinal: Flatulence (4% to 7%)
- Genitourinary: Vaginitis (2% to 7%)
- Neuromuscular & skeletal: Paresthesia (up to 6%)
- Respiratory: Bronchitis (up to 7%), rhinitis (4% to 7%), sinusitis (3% to 7%)
- Miscellaneous: Flu-like syndrome (4% to 7%)

In addition, the following have been reported with estrogen and/or progestin therapy:
- Cardiovascular: Edema, hypertension, MI, stroke, venous thromboembolism
- Central nervous system: Epilepsy exacerbation, irritability, mental depression, migraine, mood disturbances, nervousness
- Dermatologic: Angioedema, chloasma, erythema multiforme, erythema nodosum, hemorrhagic eruption, hirsutism, loss of scalp hair, melasma, pruritus, rash, urticaria
- Endocrine & metabolic: Breast cancer, breast enlargement, breast tenderness, HDL-cholesterol increased, hyper-/hypocalcemia, impaired glucose tolerance, LDL-cholesterol decreased, libido (changes in), serum triglycerides/phospholipids increased, thyroid-binding globulin increased, total thyroid hormone (T_4) increased
- Gastrointestinal: Abdominal cramps, bloating, cholecystitis, cholelithiasis, gallbladder disease, pancreatitis, weight gain/loss
- Genitourinary: Alterations in frequency and flow of menses, changes in cervical secretions, endometrial cancer, endometrial hyperplasia, increased size of uterine leiomyomata, vaginal candidiasis
- Hematologic: Aggravation of porphyria; antithrombin III and antifactor Xa decreased; fibrinogen levels increased; platelet aggregability and platelet count increased; prothrombin and factors VII, VIII, IX, X increased
- Hepatic: Cholestatic jaundice, hepatic hemangiomas enlarged
- Local: Thrombophlebitis
- Neuromuscular & skeletal: Arthralgias, chorea, leg cramps
- Ocular: Contact lens intolerance, corneal curvature steepening, retinal vascular thrombosis
- Respiratory: Asthma exacerbation, pulmonary thromboembolism
- Miscellaneous: Anaphylactoid/anaphylactic reactions, carbohydrate intolerance

Pharmacodynamics/Kinetics

Absorption Well absorbed over a period of several hours

Protein Binding Sex hormone-binding globulin (SHBG) and albumin

Half-Life Elimination Conjugated estrone: 8-20 hours; conjugated equilin: 5-17 hours

Metabolism Hepatic via CYP3A4; estradiol is converted to estrone and estriol; also undergoes enterohepatic recirculation; estrone sulfate is the main metabolite in postmenopausal women

Excretion Urine (primarily estriol, also as estradiol, estrone, and conjugates)

Available Dosage Forms

Tablet, oral:

Enjuvia™: 0.3 mg, 0.45 mg, 0.625 mg, 0.9 mg, 1.25 mg

Dosing

Adult The lowest dose that will control symptoms should be used. Medication should be discontinued as soon as possible.

Menopause, moderate-to-severe vasomotor symptoms: Oral: 0.3 mg/day; may be titrated up to 1.25 mg/day. Attempts to discontinue medication should be made at 3- to 6-month intervals.

Vaginal dryness/vulvar and vaginal atrophy associated with menopause: Oral: 0.3 mg/day. Attempts to discontinue medication should be made at 3- to 6-month intervals.

Geriatric Refer to adult dosing. A higher incidence of stroke and invasive breast cancer were observed in women >75 years in a WHI substudy using conjugated equine estrogen.

Stability

Storage Store at room temperature of 25°C (77°F).

Monitoring and Teaching Issues

Laboratory Monitoring Papanicolaou smear, mammogram. Adequate diagnostic measures, including endometrial sampling, if indicated, should be performed to rule out malignancy in all cases of undiagnosed abnormal vaginal bleeding.

Physical Assessment Assess results of annual gynecological exam. Monitor for thromboembolism, hypertension, edema, and CNS changes on a regular basis during therapy. Before prescribing estrogen therapy to postmenopausal women, the risks and benefits must be weighed for each patient. Women should be informed of these risks and benefits, as well as possible effects of progestin when added to estrogen therapy. Estrogens with or without progestin should be used for shortest duration possible consistent with treatment goals and periodic assessment of risk:benefit should be made. Caution patients with diabetes to monitor glucose levels closely (may impair glucose tolerance). Remind patient about the importance of frequent self-breast exams and the need for annual gynecological exam.

Patient Education Annual gynecologic and regular self-breast exams are important. If you have diabetes, monitor glucose levels closely (may impair glucose tolerance). You may experience nausea, vomiting, abdominal pain, dizziness, depression, rash, headache, breast pain, or enlargement/tenderness of breasts. Report significant swelling of extremities; sudden acute pain in legs or calves, chest, or abdomen; shortness of breath; severe headache; sudden blindness; weakness or numbness of arm or leg; unusual vaginal bleeding; yellowing of skin or eyes; or unusual bruising or bleeding. You may become intolerant to wearing contact lenses; notify prescriber if this occurs.

Geriatric Considerations Enjuvia™ has not been studied in an elderly population. Before prescribing estrogen therapy to postmenopausal women, the risks and benefits must be weighed for each patient. Women should be informed of these risks and benefits, as well as possible side effects and the return of menstrual bleeding (when cycled with a progestin), and be involved in the decision to prescribe. A higher incidence of stroke and invasive breast cancer was observed in women >75 years of age in a WHI substudy. Oral therapy may be more convenient for vaginal atrophy and urinary incontinence.

This medication is considered to be potentially inappropriate in this patient population (Beers Criteria severity: Low).

Breast-Feeding Considerations Estrogen has been shown to decrease the quantity and quality of human milk. Use only if clearly needed. Monitor the growth of the infant closely.

Pregnancy Considerations Use during pregnancy is contraindicated.

Additional Information Not biologically equivalent to conjugated estrogens from equine source. Contains 10 unique estrogenic compounds (equine source contains at least 10 active estrogenic compounds).

Estrogens (Conjugated/Equine, Systemic)

(ES troe jenz KON joo gate ed, EE kwine)

U.S. Brand Names Premarin®

Index Terms C.E.S.; CE; CEE; Conjugated Estrogen; Estrogenic Substances, Conjugated

Generic Availability (U.S.) No

Pharmacologic Category Estrogen Derivative

Medication Safety Issues

Sound-alike/look-alike issues:

Premarin® may be confused with Primaxin®, Provera®, Remeron®

Beers Criteria medication: This drug may be inappropriate for use in geriatric patients (low severity risk).

Lactation Enters breast milk/use caution

Use Treatment of moderate-to-severe vasomotor symptoms associated with menopause; treatment of vulvar and vaginal atrophy; hypoestrogenism (due to hypogonadism, castration, or primary ovarian failure); prostatic cancer (palliation); breast cancer (palliation); osteoporosis (prophylaxis, postmenopausal women at significant risk only); abnormal uterine bleeding; moderate-to-severe dyspareunia (pain during intercourse) due to vaginal/vulvar atrophy of menopause

Unlabeled/Investigational Use Uremic bleeding

Mechanism of Action/Effect Estrogens modulate the pituitary secretion of gonadotropins, luteinizing hormone, and follicle-stimulating hormone through a negative feedback system; estrogen replacement reduces elevated levels of these hormones in postmenopausal women

Contraindications Hypersensitivity to estrogens or any component of the formulation; undiagnosed abnormal vaginal bleeding; history of or current thrombophlebitis or venous thromboembolic disorders (including DVT, PE); active or recent (within 1 year) arterial thromboembolic disease (eg, stroke, MI); carcinoma of the breast (except in appropriately selected patients being treated for metastatic disease); estrogen-dependent tumor; hepatic dysfunction or disease; pregnancy

Warnings/Precautions

Cardiovascular-related considerations: **[U.S. Boxed Warning]: Estrogens with or without progestin should not be used to prevent cardiovascular disease.** Use caution with cardiovascular disease or dysfunction. May increase the risks of hypertension, myocardial infarction (MI), stroke, pulmonary emboli (PE), and deep vein thrombosis; incidence of these effects was shown to be significantly increased in postmenopausal women using conjugated estrogens (CE) alone or in combination with medroxyprogesterone acetate (MPA). Nonfatal MI, PE, and thrombophlebitis have also been reported in males taking high doses of CE (eg, for prostate cancer). Estrogen compounds are generally associated with lipid effects such as increased HDL-cholesterol and decreased LDL-cholesterol. Triglycerides may also be increased; use with caution in patients with familial defects of lipoprotein metabolism. Whenever possible, estrogens should be discontinued at least 4 weeks prior to and for 2 weeks following elective surgery associated with an increased risk of thromboembolism or during periods of prolonged immobilization.

Neurological considerations: **[U.S. Boxed Warning]: The risk of dementia may be increased in postmenopausal women;** increased incidence was observed in women ≥65 years of age taking CE alone or in combination with MPA.

Cancer-related considerations: **[U.S. Boxed Warning]: Adequate diagnostic measures, including endometrial sampling, if indicated, should be performed to rule out malignancy in all cases of undiagnosed abnormal vaginal bleeding. Unopposed estrogens may increase the risk of endometrial carcinoma in postmenopausal women with an intact uterus.** Risk appears to be associated with long-term use The use of a progestin should be considered when administering estrogens to postmenopausal women with an intact uterus. Estrogens may exacerbate endometriosis. Malignant transformation of residual endometrial implants has been reported posthysterectomy with estrogen only therapy. Consider adding a progestin in women with residual endometriosis posthysterectomy. Presentation of irregular, unresolving vaginal bleeding warrants further evaluation including endometrial sampling, if indicated, to rule out malignancy. Estrogens may increase the risk of breast cancer. An increased risk of invasive breast cancer was observed in postmenopausal women using CE in combination with MPA; a smaller increase in risk was seen with estrogen therapy alone in observational studies. An increase in abnormal mammograms has also been reported with estrogen and progestin therapy. Estrogen use may lead to severe hypercalcemia in patients with breast cancer and bone metastases; discontinue estrogen if hypercalcemia occurs.

Estrogens may cause retinal vascular thrombosis; discontinue permanently if papilledema or retinal vascular lesions are observed on examination. Use with caution in patients with diseases which may be exacerbated by fluid retention, including asthma, epilepsy, migraine, diabetes, heart failure, or renal dysfunction. Use with caution in patients with a history of severe hypocalcemia, SLE, hepatic hemangiomas, porphyria, endometriosis, and gallbladder disease. Use caution with history of cholestatic jaundice associated with past estrogen use or pregnancy. May be inappropriate for use in the elderly due to potential of increased risk of breast and endometrial cancers and lack of proven cardioprotection (Beers Criteria). Prior to puberty, estrogens may cause premature closure of the epiphyses, premature breast development in girls or gynecomastia in boys. Vaginal bleeding and vaginal cornification may also be induced in girls.

[U.S. Boxed Warning]: Estrogens with or without progestin should be used for shortest duration possible at the lowest effective dose consistent with treatment goals. Before prescribing estrogen therapy to postmenopausal women, the risks and benefits must be weighed for each patient. Women should be informed of these risks and benefits, as well as possible effects of progestin when added to estrogen therapy. Estrogens with or without progestin should be used for shortest duration possible consistent with treatment goals. Conduct periodic risk:benefit assessments.

Drug Interactions

Metabolism/Transport Effects

Based on estradiol and estrone: **Substrate** of CYP1A2 (major), 2A6 (minor), 2B6 (minor), 2C9 (minor), 2C19 (minor), 2D6 (minor), 2E1 (minor), 3A4 (major); Inhibits CYP1A2 (weak), 2C8 (weak); Induces CYP3A4 (weak)

Avoid Concomitant Use

Avoid concomitant use of Estrogens (Conjugated/Equine, Systemic) with any of the following: Anastrozole

Decreased Effect

Estrogens (Conjugated/Equine, Systemic) may decrease the levels/effects of: Anastrozole; Chenodiol; Saxagliptin; Somatropin; Thyroid Products; Ursodiol

The levels/effects of Estrogens (Conjugated/Equine, Systemic) may be decreased by: CYP1A2 Inducers (Strong); CYP3A4 Inducers (Strong); Deferasirox; Herbs (CYP3A4 Inducers); Peginterferon Alfa-2b; Tipranavir

Increased Effect/Toxicity

Estrogens (Conjugated/Equine, Systemic) may increase the levels/effects of: Corticosteroids (Systemic); ROPINIRole; Tipranavir

The levels/effects of Estrogens (Conjugated/Equine, Systemic) may be increased by: Ascorbic Acid; Conivaptan; Herbs (Estrogenic Properties)

Nutritional/Ethanol Interactions

Ethanol: Avoid ethanol (routine use increases estrogen plasma concentrations and risk of breast cancer). Ethanol may also increase the risk of osteoporosis.

Food: Folic acid absorption may be decreased.

Herb/Nutraceutical: St John's wort may decrease levels. Herbs with estrogenic properties may enhance the adverse/toxic effect of estrogen derivatives; examples include alfalfa, black cohosh, bloodroot, hops, kudzu, licorice, red clover, saw palmetto, soybean, thyme, wild yam, yucca.

Lab Interactions Pathologist should be advised of estrogen/progesterone therapy when specimens are submitted. Reduced response to metyrapone test.

Adverse Reactions

Note: Percentages reported in postmenopausal women following oral use.

>10%:

Central nervous system: Headache (26% to 32%; placebo 28%)
Endocrine & metabolic: Breast pain (7% to 12%; placebo 9%)
Gastrointestinal: Abdominal pain (15% to 17%)
Genitourinary: Vaginal hemorrhage (2% to 14%)
Neuromuscular & skeletal: Back pain (13% to 14%)

1% to 10%:

Central nervous system: Nervousness (2% to 5%)
Dermatologic: Pruritus (4% to 5%)
Gastrointestinal: Flatulence (6% to 7%)
Genitourinary: Vaginitis (5% to 7%), leukorrhea (4% to 7%), vaginal moniliasis (5% to 6%)
Neuromuscular & skeletal: Weakness (7% to 8%), leg cramps (3% to 7%)

Additional adverse reactions reported with injection or vaginal cream; frequency not defined:

Genitourinary: Cystis-like syndrome, genital pruritus, vulvovaginal discomfort
Local: injection site: Edema, pain, phlebitis

In addition, the following have been reported with estrogen and/or progestin therapy:

Cardiovascular: DVT, edema, hypertension, MI, stroke, superficial venous thrombosis

Central nervous system: Dementia, dizziness, epilepsy exacerbation, headache, irritability, mental depression, migraine, mood disturbances, nervousness

Dermatologic: Angioedema, chloasma, erythema multiforme, erythema nodosum, hemorrhagic eruption, hirsutism, loss of scalp hair, melasma, pruritus, rash, urticaria

Endocrine & metabolic: Breast cancer, breast discharge, breast enlargement, breast tenderness, dysmenorrhea, fibrocystic breast changes, galactorrhea, glucose intolerance, HDL-cholesterol increased, hyper-/hypocalcemia, LDL-cholesterol decreased, libido (changes in), ovarian cancer, serum triglycerides/phospholipids increased, thyroid-binding globulin increased, total thyroid hormone (T_4) increased

Gastrointestinal: Abdominal cramps, bloating, cholecystitis, cholelithiasis, gallbladder disease, ischemic colitis, nausea, pancreatitis, vomiting, weight gain/loss

Genitourinary: Abnormal uterine bleeding/spotting, changes in cervical ectropion, changes in cervical secretions, endometrial cancer, endometrial hyperplasia, increased size of uterine leiomyomata, vaginal candidiasis

Hematologic: Aggravation of porphyria, antithrombin III and antifactor Xa decreased; factors II, II-VII-X complex, VII, VIII, VII-X complex, IX, X, and XII increased; increased beta-thromboglobulin, fibrinogen levels, plasminogen/plasminogen activity, platelet aggregability, platelet count, and prothrombin

Hepatic: Cholestatic jaundice, hepatic hemangiomas enlarged

Neuromuscular & skeletal: Arthralgias, chorea, leg cramps

Local: Thrombophlebitis

Ocular: Contact lens intolerance, corneal curvature steepening, retinal vascular thrombosis

Respiratory: Asthma exacerbation, pulmonary thromboembolism

Miscellaneous: Anaphylactoid/anaphylactic reactions, benign meningioma growth potentiation

Pharmacodynamics/Kinetics

Absorption Well absorbed

Time to Peak Total estrone: 7 hours

Protein Binding Binds to sex-hormone-binding globulin and albumin

Half-Life Elimination Total estrone: 27 hours

Metabolism Hepatic via CYP3A4; estradiol is converted to estrone and estriol; also undergoes enterohepatic recirculation (avoided with vaginal administration); estrone sulfate is the main metabolite in postmenopausal women

Excretion Urine (primarily estriol, also as estradiol, estrone, and conjugates)

Available Dosage Forms

Injection, powder for reconstitution:

Premarin®: 25 mg

Tablet, oral:

Premarin®: 0.3 mg, 0.45 mg, 0.625 mg, 0.9 mg, 1.25 mg

Dosing

Adult

Breast cancer palliation, metastatic disease in selected patients (male and female): Oral: 10 mg 3 times/day for at least 3 months

Uremic bleeding (unlabeled use): I.V.: 0.6 mg/kg/day for 5 days

Androgen-dependent prostate cancer palliation (males): Oral: 1.25-2.5 mg 3 times/day

Prevention of postmenopausal osteoporosis: Oral: Initial: 0.3 mg/day, cyclically* or daily, depending on medical assessment of patient. Dose may be adjusted based on bone mineral density and clinical response. The lowest effective dose should be used.

Menopause (moderate-to-severe vasomotor symptoms): Oral: Initial: 0.3 mg/day. May be given cyclically* or daily, depending on medical assessment of patient. The lowest dose that will control symptoms should be used. Medication should be discontinued as soon as possible.

Vulvar and vaginal atrophy: Oral: Initial: 0.3 mg/day. The lowest dose that will control symptoms should be used. May be given cyclically* or daily, depending on medical assessment of patient. Medication should be discontinued as soon as possible.

Female hypogonadism: Oral: 0.3-0.625 mg/day given cyclically*; dose may be titrated in 6- to 12-month intervals; progestin treatment should be added to maintain bone mineral density once skeletal maturity is achieved.

Female castration, primary ovarian failure: Oral: 1.25 mg/day given cyclically*; adjust according to severity of symptoms and patient response. For maintenance, adjust to the lowest effective dose.

Abnormal uterine bleeding:

Acute/heavy bleeding:

Oral (unlabeled route): 1.25 mg, may repeat every 4 hours for 24 hours, followed by 1.25 mg once daily for 7-10 days

I.M., I.V.: 25 mg, may repeat in 6-12 hours if needed

Note: Treatment should be followed by a low-dose oral contraceptive; medroxyprogesterone acetate along with or following estrogen therapy can also be given

Nonacute/lesser bleeding: Oral (unlabeled route): 1.25 mg once daily for 7-10 days

***Cyclic administration:** Either 3 weeks on, 1 week off **or** 25 days on, 5 days off

Geriatric Refer to adult dosing. A higher incidence of stroke and breast cancer was observed in women >75 years in a WHI substudy.

Pediatric Adolescents: Refer to adult dosing.

Hepatic Impairment

Mild-to-moderate liver impairment: Dosage reduction of estrogens is recommended.

Severe liver impairment: **Not recommended.**

Administration

Oral Administer at bedtime to minimize adverse effects. May be administered without regard to meals.

I.M. May be administered intramuscularly.

I.V. Administer I.V. doses slowly to avoid a flushing reaction.

Stability

Reconstitution Injection: Reconstitute with sterile water for injection; slowly inject diluent against side wall of the vial. Agitate gently; do not shake violently.

Storage

Injection: Refrigerate at 2°C to 8°C (36°F to 46°F) prior to reconstitution. Use immediately following reconstitution.

Tablets: Store at room temperature 20°C to 25°C (68°F to 77°F).

Monitoring and Teaching Issues

Laboratory Monitoring Routine physical examination that includes blood pressure and Papanicolaou smear. Adequate diagnostic measures, including endometrial sampling, if indicated, should be performed to rule out malignancy in all cases of undiagnosed abnormal vaginal bleeding.

Uremic bleeding: Bleeding time

Physical Assessment Assess results of annual gynecological exam. Monitor for thromboembolism, hypertension, edema, and CNS changes on a regular basis during therapy. Before prescribing estrogen therapy to postmenopausal women, the risks and benefits must be weighed for each patient. Women should be informed of these risks and benefits, as well as possible effects of progestin when added to estrogen therapy. Estrogens with or without progestin should be used for shortest duration possible consistent with treatment goals and periodic assessment of risk:benefit should be made. Caution patients with diabetes to monitor glucose levels closely (may impair glucose tolerance). Remind patient about the importance of frequent self-breast exams and the need for annual gynecological exam. Determine that patient is not pregnant before starting therapy. Do not give to females of childbearing age unless patient is capable of complying with contraceptive use. Advise patient about appropriate contraceptive measures as appropriate.

Patient Education Annual gynecologic exams and regular self-breast exams are important. If you have diabetes, monitor glucose levels closely (may impair glucose tolerance). You may experience nausea, vomiting, bloating, abdominal pain, dizziness, depression, rash, headache, breast pain, or enlargement/tenderness of breasts. Report significant swelling of extremities; sudden acute pain in legs, chest, or abdomen; shortness of breath; severe headache; CNS changes (dementia, mood disturbances, irritability, nervousness); sudden blindness; weakness or numbness of arm or leg; unusual vaginal bleeding; yellowing of skin or eyes; or unusual bruising or bleeding. You may become intolerant to wearing contact lenses; notify prescriber if this occurs.

Dietary Considerations Ensure adequate calcium and vitamin D intake when used for the prevention of osteoporosis. Powder for reconstitution for injection (25 mg) contains lactose 200 mg.

Geriatric Considerations Before prescribing estrogen therapy to postmenopausal women, the risks and benefits must be weighed for each patient. Women should be informed of these risks and benefits, as well as possible side effects and the return of menstrual bleeding (when cycled with a progestin), and be involved in the decision to prescribe. A higher incidence of stroke and invasive breast cancer was observed in women >75 years in a WHI substudy.

This medication is considered to be potentially inappropriate in this patient population (Beers Criteria severity: Low).

Breast-Feeding Considerations Estrogen has been shown to decrease the quantity and quality of human milk. Use only if clearly needed. Monitor the growth of the infant closely.

Pregnancy Considerations Estrogens are not indicated for use during pregnancy or immediately postpartum. In general, the use of estrogen and progestin as in combination hormonal contraceptives have not been associated with teratogenic effects when inadvertently taken early in pregnancy. These products are contraindicated for use during pregnancy.

Related Information

Depression *on page 2025*

Estrogens (Conjugated/Equine, Topical)

(ES troe jenz KON joo gate ed, EE kwine)

U.S. Brand Names Premarin®

Index Terms C.E.S.; CE; CEE; Conjugated Estrogen; Estrogenic Substances, Conjugated

Generic Availability (U.S.) No

Pharmacologic Category Estrogen Derivative

Medication Safety Issues

Sound-alike/look-alike issues:

Premarin® may be confused with Primaxin®, Provera®, Remeron®

Lactation Enters breast milk/use caution

Use Treatment of vulvar and vaginal atrophy; moderate-to-severe dyspareunia (pain during intercourse) due to vaginal/vulvar atrophy of menopause

Available Dosage Forms

Cream, vaginal:

Premarin®: 0.625 mg/g (42.5 g)

Dosing

Adult

Moderate-to-severe dyspareunia: Intravaginal: 0.5 g twice weekly (eg, Monday and Thursday) **or** once daily cyclically*

Vulvar and vaginal atrophy: Intravaginal: 0.5-2 g/day given cyclically*

***Cyclic administration:** Either 3 weeks on, 1 week off **or** 25 days on, 5 days off

Geriatric Refer to adult dosing. A higher incidence of stroke and breast cancer was observed in women >75 years in a WHI substudy.

Administration

Other Administer at bedtime to minimize adverse effects. Applicator calibrated in 0.5 g increments up to 2 g. To clean applicator, remove plunger from barrel. Wash with mild soap and warm water; do not boil or use hot water.

Monitoring and Teaching Issues

Laboratory Monitoring Routine physical examination that includes blood pressure and Papanicolaou smear. Adequate diagnostic measures, including endometrial sampling, if indicated, should be performed to rule out malignancy in all cases of undiagnosed abnormal vaginal bleeding.

Physical Assessment Assess results of annual gynecological exam. Monitor for thromboembolism, hypertension, edema, and CNS changes on a regular basis during therapy. Before prescribing estrogen therapy to postmenopausal women, the risks and benefits must be weighed for each patient. Women should be informed of these risks and benefits, as well as possible effects of progestin when added to estrogen therapy. Estrogens with or without progestin should be used for shortest duration possible consistent with treatment goals and periodic assessment of risk:benefit should be made. Caution patients with diabetes to monitor glucose levels closely (may impair glucose tolerance). Remind patient about the importance of frequent self-breast exams and the need for annual gynecological exam. Determine that patient is not pregnant before starting therapy.

Patient Education Annual gynecologic exams and regular self-breast exams are important. If you have diabetes, monitor glucose levels closely (may impair glucose tolerance). You may experience nausea, vomiting, bloating, abdominal pain, dizziness, depression, rash, headache, breast pain, or enlargement/tenderness of breasts. Report significant swelling of extremities; sudden acute pain in legs, chest, or abdomen; shortness of breath; severe headache; CNS changes (dementia, mood disturbances, irritability, nervousness); sudden blindness; weakness or numbness of arm or leg; unusual vaginal bleeding; yellowing of skin or eyes; or unusual bruising or bleeding. You may become intolerant to wearing contact lenses; notify prescriber if this occurs.

Related Information

Pharmacotherapy of Urinary Incontinence *on page 2071*

Estrogens (Conjugated/Equine) and Medroxyprogesterone

(ES troe jenz KON joo gate ed/EE kwine & me DROKS ee proe JES te rone)

U.S. Brand Names Premphase®; Prempro®

Index Terms Medroxyprogesterone and Estrogens (Conjugated); MPA and Estrogens (Conjugated)

Generic Availability (U.S.) No

Pharmacologic Category Estrogen and Progestin Combination

Medication Safety Issues

Sound-alike/look-alike issues:

Premphase® may be confused with Prempro®

Prempro® may be confused with Premphase®

Lactation Enters breast milk/use caution

Use Women with an intact uterus: Treatment of moderate-to-severe vasomotor symptoms associated with menopause; treatment of moderate-to-severe vulvar and vaginal atrophy due to menopause; postmenopausal osteoporosis (prophylaxis)

Available Dosage Forms

Tablet:

Premphase® [therapy pack contains two separate tablet formulations]: Conjugated estrogens 0.625 mg [14 maroon tablets] and conjugated estrogen 0.625 mg/medroxyprogesterone 5 mg [14 light blue tablets] (28s)

Prempro®:

0.3/1.5: Conjugated estrogens 0.3 mg and medroxyprogesterone 1.5 mg (28s)

0.45/1.5: Conjugated estrogens 0.45 mg and medroxyprogesterone 1.5 mg (28s)

0.625/2.5: Conjugated estrogens 0.625 mg and medroxyprogesterone 2.5 mg (28s)

0.625/5: Conjugated estrogens 0.625 mg and medroxyprogesterone 5 mg (28s)

Dosing

Adult

Treatment of moderate-to-severe vasomotor symptoms associated with menopause; treatment of vulvar and vaginal atrophy due to menopause in women with a uterus; osteoporosis prophylaxis in females with an intact uterus (**Note:** The lowest dose that will control symptoms should be used; medication should be discontinued as soon as possible):

Premphase®: Oral: One maroon conjugated estrogen 0.625 mg tablet daily on days 1 through 14 and 1 light blue conjugated estrogen 0.625 mg/mPA 5 mg tablet daily on days 15 through 28

Prempro®: Oral: One conjugated estrogen/MPA tablet once daily; maximum dose: 1 conjugated estrogen 0.625 mg/mPA 5 mg tablet daily

Geriatric Refer to adult dosing. A higher incidence of stroke and breast cancer was observed in women >75 years in a WHI substudy.

Monitoring and Teaching Issues

Laboratory Monitoring Serum cholesterol, HDL, LDL triglycerides

Physical Assessment See individual agents.

Patient Education See individual agents.

Related Information

Estrogens (Conjugated/Equine, Systemic) *on page 682*

MedroxyPROGESTERone *on page 1154*

Estrogens (Esterified) (ES troe jenz es TER i fied)

U.S. Brand Names Menest®

Index Terms Esterified Estrogens

Generic Availability (U.S.) No

Pharmacologic Category Estrogen Derivative

Medication Safety Issues

Sound-alike/look-alike issues:

Estratab® may be confused with Estratest®, Estratest® H.S.

Beers Criteria medication: This drug may be inappropriate for use in geriatric patients (low severity risk).

Lactation Enters breast milk/use caution

Use Treatment of moderate-to-severe vasomotor symptoms associated with menopause; treatment of moderate-to-severe vulvar and vaginal atrophy associated with menopause; hypoestrogenism (due to hypogonadism, castration, or primary ovarian failure); advanced prostatic cancer (palliation), metastatic breast cancer (palliation) in men and postmenopausal women

Available Dosage Forms

Tablet, oral:

Menest®: 0.3 mg, 0.625 mg, 1.25 mg, 2.5 mg

Dosing

Adult & Geriatric

Prostate cancer, advanced: Oral: 1.25-2.5 mg 3 times/day

Female hypoestrogenism due to hypogonadism: Oral: 2.5-7.5 mg/day in divided doses for 20 days followed by a 10-day rest period. Administer cyclically (3 weeks on and 1 week off). If bleeding does not occur by the end of the 10-day period, repeat the same dosing schedule; the number of courses dependent upon the responsiveness of the endometrium. If bleeding occurs before the end of the 10-day period, begin an estrogen-progestin cyclic regimen of 2.5-7.5 mg/day in divided doses for 20 days; during the last 5 days of estrogen therapy, give an oral progestin. If bleeding occurs before regimen is concluded, discontinue therapy and resume on the fifth day of bleeding.

Female hypoestrogenism due to castration and primary ovarian failure: Oral: 1.25 mg/day, cyclically. Adjust dosage upward or downward, according to the severity of symptoms and patient response. For maintenance, adjust dosage to lowest level that will provide effective control.

Vasomotor symptoms associated with menopause: Oral: 1.25 mg/day administered cyclically (3 weeks on and 1 week off). If patient has not menstruated within the last 2 months or more, cyclic administration is started arbitrary. If the patient is menstruating, cyclical administration is started on day 5 of the bleeding. For short-term use only and should be discontinued as soon as possible. Re-evaluate at 3- to 6-month intervals for tapering or discontinuation of therapy.

Vulvar and vaginal atrophy associated with menopause: Oral: 0.3 to ≥1.25 mg/day, depending on the tissue response of the individual patient. Administer cyclically. For short-term use only and should be discontinued as soon as possible. Re-evaluate at 3- to 6-month intervals for tapering or discontinuation of therapy.

Breast cancer, metastatic (appropriately selected patients): Males and postmenopausal females: Oral: 10 mg 3 times/day for at least 3 months

Administration

Oral Administer with food at same time each day.

Monitoring and Teaching Issues

Laboratory Monitoring Routine Papanicolaou smear, mammogram. Adequate diagnostic measures, including endometrial sampling, if indicated, should be performed to rule out malignancy in all cases of undiagnosed abnormal vaginal bleeding.

Physical Assessment Assess results of annual gynecological exam. Monitor for thromboembolism, hypertension, edema, and CNS changes on a regular basis during therapy. Before prescribing estrogen therapy to postmenopausal women, the risks and benefits must be weighed for each patient. Women should be informed of these risks and benefits, as well as possible effects of progestin when added to estrogen therapy. Estrogens with or without progestin should be used for shortest duration possible consistent with treatment goals and periodic assessment of risk:benefit should be made. Caution patients with diabetes to monitor glucose levels closely (may impair glucose tolerance). Remind patient about the importance of frequent self-breast exams and the need for annual gynecological exam.

Patient Education Annual gynecologic and regular self-breast exams are important. If you have diabetes, monitor glucose levels closely (may impair glucose tolerance). You may experience nausea, vomiting, abdominal pain, dizziness, mental depression, rash, hair loss, headache, breast pain, increased/decreased libido, enlargement/tenderness of breasts, or difficult/painful menstrual cycles. Report significant swelling of extremities; sudden acute pain in legs or calves, chest, or abdomen; shortness of breath; severe headache; sudden blindness; weakness or numbness of arm or leg; unusual vaginal bleeding; yellowing of skin or eyes; or unusual bruising or bleeding. You may become intolerant to wearing contact lenses; notify prescriber if this occurs.

◆ **Estrostep® Fe** *see* Ethinyl Estradiol and Norethindrone *on page* 701

Eszopiclone (es zoe PIK lone)

U.S. Brand Names Lunesta®

Generic Availability (U.S.) No

Pharmacologic Category Hypnotic, Nonbenzodiazepine

Medication Safety Issues

Sound-alike/look-alike issues:

Lunesta® may be confused with Neulasta®

Medication Guide Available Yes

Pregnancy Risk Factor C

Lactation Excretion in breast milk unknown/use caution

Use Treatment of insomnia

Mechanism of Action/Effect Interact with the GABA-receptor complex to promote sleep.

Contraindications There are no contraindications listed within the manufacturer's labeling.

Warnings/Precautions Symptomatic treatment of insomnia should be initiated only after careful evaluation of potential causes of sleep disturbance. Tolerance did not develop over 6 months of use. Use with caution in patients with depression or a history of drug dependence. Abrupt discontinuance may lead to withdrawal symptoms. Use with caution in patients receiving other CNS depressants or psychoactive medications. Hypnotics/sedatives have been associated with abnormal thinking and behavior changes including decreased inhibition, aggression, bizarre behavior, agitation, hallucinations, and depersonalization. These changes may occur unpredictably and may indicate previously unrecognized psychiatric disorders; evaluate appropriately. Amnesia may occur. May impair physical and mental capabilities. Postmarketing studies have indicated that the use of hypnotic/sedative agents for sleep has been associated with hypersensitivity reactions including anaphylaxis as well as angioedema. An increased risk for hazardous sleep-related activities such as sleep-driving (as well as cooking and eating food and making phone calls while asleep) has also been noted. Use caution in patients with respiratory compromise, hepatic dysfunction, elderly or those taking strong CYP3A4 inhibitors. Because of the rapid onset of action, administer immediately prior to bedtime or after the patient has gone to bed and is having difficulty falling asleep.

Drug Interactions

Metabolism/Transport Effects Substrate of CYP2E1 (minor), 3A4 (major)

Avoid Concomitant Use There are no known interactions where it is recommended to avoid concomitant use.

Decreased Effect

The levels/effects of Eszopiclone may be decreased by: CYP3A4 Inducers (Strong); Deferasirox; Flumazenil; Herbs (CYP3A4 Inducers)

Increased Effect/Toxicity

Eszopiclone may increase the levels/effects of: Alcohol (Ethyl); CNS Depressants; Methotrimeprazine

The levels/effects of Eszopiclone may be increased by: Antifungal Agents (Azole Derivatives, Systemic); Conivaptan; CYP3A4 Inhibitors (Moderate); CYP3A4 Inhibitors (Strong); Dasatinib; Droperidol; Methotrimeprazine

Nutritional/Ethanol Interactions

Ethanol: Use caution with concurrent use. Effects are additive and may decrease psychomotor function.

Food: Onset of action may be reduced if taken with or immediately after a heavy meal.

Herb/Nutraceutical: Avoid valerian, St John's wort, kava kava, gotu kola (may increase CNS depression).

Adverse Reactions

>10%:

Central nervous system: Headache (15% to 21%)

Gastrointestinal: Unpleasant taste (8% to 34%)

1% to 10%:

Cardiovascular: Chest pain, peripheral edema

Central nervous system: Somnolence (8% to 10%), dizziness (5% to 7%), pain (4% to 5%), nervousness (up to 5%), depression (1% to 4%), confusion (up to 3%), hallucinations (1% to 3%), anxiety (1% to 3%), abnormal dreams (1% to 3%), migraine

Dermatologic: Rash (3% to 4%), pruritus (1% to 4%)

Endocrine & metabolic: Libido decreased (up to 3%), dysmenorrhea (up to 3%), gynecomastia (males up to 3%)

Gastrointestinal: Xerostomia (3% to 7%), dyspepsia (2% to 6%), nausea (4% to 5%), diarrhea (2% to 4%), vomiting (up to 3%)

Genitourinary: Urinary tract infection (up to 3%)

Neuromuscular & skeletal: Neuralgia (up to 3%)

Miscellaneous: Infection (5% to 10%), viral infection (3%), accidental injury (up to 3%)

Pharmacodynamics/Kinetics

Absorption Rapid; high-fat/heavy meal may delay absorption

Time to Peak ~1 hour

Protein Binding 52% to 59%

Half-Life Elimination ~6 hours; Elderly (≥65 years): ~9 hours

Metabolism Hepatic via oxidation and demethylation (CYP2E1, 3A4); 2 primary metabolites; one with activity less than parent

Excretion Urine (up to 75%, primarily as metabolites; <10% as parent drug)

Controlled Substance C-IV

Available Dosage Forms

Tablet, oral:

Lunesta®: 1 mg, 2 mg, 3 mg

Dosing

Adult

Insomnia: Oral: Initial: 2 mg immediately before bedtime (maximum dose: 3 mg)

Concurrent use with strong CYP3A4 inhibitor: 1 mg immediately before bedtime; if needed, dose may be increased to 2 mg

Geriatric

Difficulty **falling** asleep: Initial: 1 mg before immediately bedtime; maximum dose: 2 mg.

Difficulty **staying** asleep: 2 mg immediately before bedtime.

Renal Impairment No adjustment required.

Hepatic Impairment

Mild-to-moderate: Use with caution; dosage adjustment unnecessary

Severe: Initial dose: 1 mg; maximum dose: 2 mg

Administration

Oral Because of the rapid onset of action, eszopiclone should be administered immediately prior to bedtime or after the patient has gone to bed and is having difficulty falling asleep. Do not take with, or immediately following, a high-fat meal. Do not crush or break tablet.

Stability

Storage Store at controlled room temperature of 25°C (77°F).

Monitoring and Teaching Issues

Physical Assessment Evaluate potential causes of insomnia prior to initiating medication. Assess for history of addiction; long-term use can result in dependence, abuse, or tolerance. Monitor for excessive CNS depression, abnormal thinking, and behavior changes. For inpatient use, institute safety measures to prevent falls.

Patient Education Drug may cause physical and/or psychological dependence. While using this medication, do not use alcohol. Take immediately prior to bedtime (quick onset) or when having difficulty falling asleep. Do not use unless you are able to get 8 or more hours of sleep before you must be active again. Swallow whole; do not crush or break tablet. You may experience drowsiness, dizziness, lightheadedness, difficulty with coordination, headache, or unpleasant taste. Report CNS changes (confusion, depression, increased sedation, excitation, severe headache, abnormal thinking, insomnia, or nightmares); respiratory difficulty; or unusual swelling, especially on face or neck.

Dietary Considerations Avoid taking after a heavy meal; may delay onset.

Geriatric Considerations In subjects >65 years of age, the AUC was increased by 41%. The manufacturer reports that in studies, the pattern of adverse reactions in elderly subjects was not different from that seen in younger adults.

Pregnancy Considerations No evidence of teratogenicity in animal models (high dose). There are no adequate or well-controlled studies in pregnant women; use only if clearly needed.

Etanercept (et a NER sept)

U.S. Brand Names Enbrel®; Enbrel® SureClick®

Generic Availability (U.S.) No

Pharmacologic Category Antirheumatic, Disease Modifying; Tumor Necrosis Factor (TNF) Blocking Agent

Medication Safety Issues

Sound-alike/look-alike issues:

Enbrel® may be confused with Levbid®

Medication Guide Available Yes

Pregnancy Risk Factor B

Lactation Excretion in breast milk unknown/not recommended

Use Treatment of moderately- to severely-active rheumatoid arthritis (RA); moderately- to severely-active polyarticular juvenile idiopathic arthritis (JIA); psoriatic arthritis; active ankylosing spondylitis (AS); moderate-to-severe chronic plaque psoriasis

Mechanism of Action/Effect Etanercept is a recombinant DNA-derived protein composed of tumor necrosis factor receptor (TNFR) linked to the Fc portion of human IgG1. Etanercept binds tumor necrosis factor (TNF) and blocks its interaction with cell surface receptors. TNF plays an important role in the inflammatory processes and the resulting joint pathology of rheumatoid arthritis (RA), polyarticular-course juvenile idiopathic arthritis (JIA), ankylosing spondylitis (AS), and plaque psoriasis.

Contraindications Hypersensitivity to etanercept or any component of the formulation; patients with sepsis (mortality may be increased)

Warnings/Precautions **[U.S. Boxed Warning]: Serious and potentially fatal infections have been reported including bacterial, mycobacterial, viral, and invasive fungal infections;** usually in patients taking concomitant immunosuppressive medication; infection may be disseminated, rather than localized, upon presentation. Cases of unrecognized invasive fungal infections (eg, histoplasmosis, blastomycosis, coccidioidomycosis, listeriosis, candidiasis, aspergillosis, pneumocystosis) have also been reported with anti-TNF agent use. Discontinue administration if patient develops a serious infection or sepsis. Caution should be exercised when considering the use in patients with chronic infection, history of recurrent infection, or predisposition to infection (eg, poorly-controlled diabetes or residence/travel from areas of endemic mycoses). Do not give to patients with an active chronic or localized infection. Patients should be educated about the symptoms of infection and closely monitored for signs and symptoms while undergoing treatment. **[U.S. Boxed Warning]: Tuberculosis (disseminated or extrapulmonary) has been reported in patients receiving etanercept; both reactivation of latent infection and new infections have been reported.** Patients should be evaluated for tuberculosis risk factors and for latent tuberculosis infection with a tuberculin skin test prior to starting therapy. Treatment of latent tuberculosis should be initiated before etanercept therapy; consider antituberculosis treatment if adequate course of treatment cannot be confirmed in patients with a history of latent or active tuberculosis or with risk factors despite negative skin test. Some patients who tested negative prior to therapy have developed active infection; monitor for signs and symptoms of tuberculosis in all patients. Rare reactivation of hepatitis B has occurred in chronic carriers of the virus; evaluate prior to initiation and during treatment in patients at risk for hepatitis B infection. Patients should be brought up to date with all immunizations before initiating therapy. Live vaccines should not be given concurrently with etanercept. Patients with a significant exposure to varicella virus should temporarily discontinue etanercept. Treatment with varicella zoster immune globulin should be considered.

[U.S. Boxed Warning]: Lymphoma and other malignancies have been reported in children and adolescent patients receiving TNF-blocking agents, including etanercept. Half of the malignancies reported in children were lymphomas (Hodgkin's and non-Hodgkin's) while other cases varied and included malignancies not typically observed in this population. The impact of etanercept on the development and course of malignancy is not fully defined. Compared to the general population, an increased risk of lymphoma has been noted in clinical trials; however, rheumatoid arthritis alone has been previously associated with an increased rate of lymphoma. Lymphomas and other malignancies were also observed (at rates higher than expected for the general population) in adult patients receiving etanercept. Etanercept is not recommended for use in patients with Wegener's granulomatosis who are receiving immunosuppressive therapy. Treatment may result in the formation of autoimmune antibodies; cases of autoimmune disease have not been described. Non-neutralizing antibodies to etanercept may also be formed. Rarely, a reversible lupus-like syndrome has occurred.

Allergic reactions may occur; if an anaphylactic reaction or other serious allergic reaction occurs, administration should be discontinued immediately and appropriate therapy initiated. Use with caution in patients with pre-existing or recent onset CNS demyelinating disorders; rare cases of new onset or exacerbation of CNS demyelinating disorders have occurred; may present with mental status changes and some may be associated with permanent disability. Optic neuritis, transverse myelitis, multiple sclerosis, and new onset or exacerbation of seizures have been reported. Use with caution in patients with heart failure or decreased left ventricular function; worsening and new-onset heart failure has been reported. Use caution in patients with a history of significant hematologic abnormalities; has been associated with pancytopenia and aplastic anemia (rare). Discontinue if significant hematologic abnormalities are confirmed. Use with caution in patients with moderate to severe alcoholic hepatitis. Compared to placebo, the mortality rate in patients treated with etanercept was similar at one month but significantly higher after 6 months

Due to a higher incidence of serious infections, concomitant use with anakinra is not recommended. Some dosage forms may contain dry natural rubber (latex). Some dosage forms may contain benzyl alcohol which has been associated with "gasping syndrome" in neonates.

Drug Interactions

Avoid Concomitant Use

Avoid concomitant use of Etanercept with any of the following: Abatacept; Anakinra; BCG; Belimumab; Canakinumab; Certolizumab Pegol; Cyclophosphamide; Natalizumab; Pimecrolimus; Rilonacept; Roflumilast; Tacrolimus (Topical); Vaccines (Live)

Decreased Effect

Etanercept may decrease the levels/effects of: BCG; Sipuleucel-T; Vaccines (Inactivated); Vaccines (Live)

The levels/effects of Etanercept may be decreased by: Echinacea

Increased Effect/Toxicity

Etanercept may increase the levels/effects of: Abatacept; Anakinra; Belimumab; Canakinumab; Certolizumab Pegol; Cyclophosphamide; Leflunomide; Natalizumab; Rilonacept; Vaccines (Live)

The levels/effects of Etanercept may be increased by: Denosumab; Pimecrolimus; Roflumilast; Tacrolimus (Topical); Trastuzumab

Nutritional/Ethanol Interactions Herb/Nutraceutical: Echinacea may decrease the therapeutic effects of etanercept (avoid concurrent use).

Adverse Reactions Percentages reported for adults except where specified.

>10%:

Central nervous system: Headache (17%; children 19%)
Gastrointestinal: Abdominal pain (5%; children 19%), vomiting (3%; children 13%)
Local: Injection site reaction (14% to 37%; erythema, itching, pain or swelling)
Respiratory: Respiratory tract infection (upper; 12% to 29%), rhinitis (12%)
Miscellaneous: Infection (35%; children 62%), positive ANA (11%), positive antidouble-stranded DNA antibodies (15% by RIA, 3% by *Crithidia luciliae* assay)

≥3% to 10%:

Central nervous system: Dizziness (7%)
Dermatologic: Rash (5%)
Gastrointestinal: Nausea (children 9%), dyspepsia (4%)
Neuromuscular & skeletal: Weakness (5%)
Respiratory: Pharyngitis (7%), cough (6%), respiratory disorder (5%), sinusitis (3%)

Pharmacodynamics/Kinetics

Onset of Action ~2-3 weeks; RA: 1-2 weeks

Time to Peak RA: SubQ: 35-103 hours

Half-Life Elimination RA: SubQ: 72-132 hour

Available Dosage Forms

Injection, powder for reconstitution:
Enbrel®: 25 mg

Injection, solution [preservative free]:
Enbrel®: 50 mg/mL (0.51 mL, 0.98 mL)
Enbrel® SureClick®: 50 mg/mL (0.98 mL)

Dosing

Adult

Rheumatoid arthritis, psoriatic arthritis, ankylosing spondylitis: SubQ:
Once-weekly dosing: 50 mg once weekly
Twice-weekly dosing: 25 mg given twice weekly (individual doses should be separated by 72-96 hours)

Plaque psoriasis: SubQ:
Initial: 50 mg twice weekly, 72-96 hours apart; maintain initial dose for 3 months (starting doses of 25 or 50 mg once weekly have also been used successfully)
Maintenance dose: 50 mg once weekly

Geriatric SubQ: Refer to adult dosing. Although greater sensitivity of some elderly patients cannot be ruled out, no overall differences in safety or effectiveness were observed.

Pediatric Juvenile idiopathic arthritis: Children 2-17 years: SubQ:
Once-weekly dosing: 0.8 mg/kg (maximum: 50 mg/dose) once weekly
Twice-weekly dosing: 0.4 mg/kg (maximum: 25 mg/dose) twice weekly (individual doses should be separated by 72-96 hours)

Administration

Other Administer subcutaneously. Rotate injection sites. New injections should be given at least one inch from an old site and never into areas where the skin is tender, bruised, red, or hard. **Note:** If the physician determines that it is appropriate, patients may self-inject after proper training in injection technique.
Powder for reconstitution: Follow package instructions carefully for reconstitution. The maximum amount injected at any single site should not exceed 25 mg.
Solution for injection: May be allowed to reach room temperature prior to injection.

Stability

Reconstitution Reconstitute lyophilized powder aseptically with 1 mL sterile bacteriostatic water for injection, USP (supplied); swirl gently, do not shake. Do not filter reconstituted solution during preparation or administration.

Storage

Prefilled syringes, autoinjectors: Store prefilled syringes and autoinjectors 2°C to 8°C (36°F to 46°F); do not freeze. Protect from light; do not shake. The following stability information has also been reported: May be stored at room temperature for up to 4 days (Cohen, 2007).

Powder for reconstitution: Must be refrigerated at 2°C to 8°C (36°F to 46°F); do not freeze. The following stability information has also been reported: May be stored at room temperature for up to 7 days (Cohen, 2007).

Monitoring and Teaching Issues

Laboratory Monitoring Latent TB screening prior to therapy initiation

Physical Assessment Monitor for signs and symptoms of infection, especially respiratory infections. Perform tuberculin skin test prior to initiating therapy; monitor for signs of tuberculosis throughout therapy. Assess for liver dysfunction. Monitor effectiveness of therapy (eg, pain, range of motion, mobility, ADL function, inflammation). If self-administered, teach patient appropriate injection technique and needle disposal.

Patient Education If self-injecting, follow instructions for injection and disposal of needles exactly. If redness, swelling, or irritation appears at the injection site, contact prescriber. You may experience headache or dizziness. If stomach pain or cramping; unusual bleeding or bruising; difficulty breathing; persistent fever; paleness; or blood in vomitus, stool, or urine occurs, stop medication and contact prescriber immediately. Also immediately report skin rash, unusual muscle or bone weakness, or signs of respiratory flu or other infection (eg, chills, fever, sore throat, easy bruising or bleeding, mouth sores, unhealed sores).

Geriatric Considerations Clinical trials including those ≥65 years of age with rheumatoid arthritis have not demonstrated any differences in safety and efficacy between elderly and younger adults to date. Since elderly have a higher incidence of infections in general, caution should be used, with close monitoring and patient education.

Breast-Feeding Considerations It is not known whether etanercept is excreted in human milk. Because many drugs and immunoglobulins are excreted in human milk and the potential for serious adverse reactions exists, a decision should be made whether to discontinue nursing or to discontinue the drug, taking into account the importance of the drug to the mother.

Pregnancy Considerations Developmental toxicity studies performed in animals have revealed no evidence of harm to the fetus. There are no studies in pregnant women; this drug should be used during pregnancy only if clearly needed. A pregnancy registry has been established to monitor outcomes of women exposed to etanercept during pregnancy (877-311-8972).

◆ **Ethacrynate Sodium** *see* Ethacrynic Acid *on page 692*

Ethacrynic Acid (eth a KRIN ik AS id)

U.S. Brand Names Edecrin®; Sodium Edecrin®

Index Terms Ethacrynate Sodium

Generic Availability (U.S.) No

Pharmacologic Category Diuretic, Loop

Medication Safety Issues

Sound-alike/look-alike issues:

Edecrin® may be confused with Eulexin, Ecotrin®

Beers Criteria medication: This drug may be inappropriate for use in geriatric patients (low severity risk).

Pregnancy Risk Factor B

Lactation Contraindicated

Use Management of edema associated with congestive heart failure; hepatic cirrhosis or renal disease; short-term management of ascites due to malignancy, idiopathic edema, and lymphedema

Available Dosage Forms

Injection, powder for reconstitution:

Sodium Edecrin®: 50 mg

Tablet, oral:

Edecrin®: 25 mg

Dosing

Adult I.V. formulation should be diluted in D_5W or NS (1 mg/mL) and infused over several minutes.

Edema:

Oral: 50-200 mg/day in 1-2 divided doses; may increase in increments of 25-50 mg at intervals of several days to a maximum of 400 mg/24 hours.

I.V.: 0.5-1 mg/kg/dose (maximum: 100 mg/dose); repeat doses not routinely recommended; however, if indicated, repeat doses every 8-12 hours.

Geriatric Oral: Initial: 25-50 mg/day

Pediatric

Edema: Oral: Children: 1 mg/kg/dose once daily; increase at intervals of 2-3 days as needed, to a maximum of 3 mg/kg/day.

Renal Impairment

Cl_{cr} <10 mL/minute: Avoid use.

Not removed by hemo- or peritoneal dialysis; supplemental dose is not necessary.

Administration

I.V. Injection should **not** be given SubQ or I.M. due to local pain and irritation. Single I.V. doses should not exceed 100 mg. Administer each 10 mg over a minute.

Monitoring and Teaching Issues

Laboratory Monitoring Renal function, serum electrolytes

Physical Assessment Monitor for dehydration and electrolyte imbalance on a regular basis.

Patient Education Take prescribed dose with food early in day. Include potassium-rich foods in your diet, but do not take potassium supplements without consulting prescriber. May cause dizziness, drowsiness, or diarrhea. Report hearing changes (ringing in ears); persistent headache; unusual confusion or nervousness; abdominal pain; palpitations or chest pain; flu-like symptoms; skin rash; blurred vision; swelling of ankles or feet; weight changes; increased fatigue; or joint/muscle swelling, pain, cramping, or trembling.

Ethambutol (e THAM byoo tole)

U.S. Brand Names Myambutol®

Index Terms Ethambutol Hydrochloride

Generic Availability (U.S.) Yes

Pharmacologic Category Antitubercular Agent

Medication Safety Issues

Sound-alike/look-alike issues:

Myambutol® may be confused with Nembutal®

Pregnancy Risk Factor C

Lactation Enters breast milk/use caution (AAP considers "compatible"; AAP 2001 update pending)

Use Treatment of pulmonary tuberculosis in conjunction with other antituberculosis agents

Unlabeled/Investigational Use Other mycobacterial diseases in conjunction with other antimycobacterial agents

Mechanism of Action/Effect Inhibits arabinosyl transferase resulting in impaired mycobacterial cell wall synthesis

Contraindications Hypersensitivity to ethambutol or any component of the formulation; optic neuritis (risk vs benefit decision); use in young children, unconscious patients, or any other patient who may be unable to discern and report visual changes

Warnings/Precautions May cause optic neuritis (unilateral or bilateral), resulting in decreased visual acuity or other vision changes. Discontinue promptly in patients with changes in vision, color blindness, or visual defects (effects normally reversible, but reversal may require up to a year). Irreversible blindness has been reported. Monitor visual acuity prior to and during therapy. Evaluation of visual acuity changes may be more difficult in patients with cataracts, optic neuritis, diabetic retinopathy, and inflammatory conditions of the eye; consideration should be given to whether or not visual changes are related to disease progression or effects of therapy. Use only in children whose visual acuity can accurately be determined and monitored (not recommended for use in children <13 years of age unless the benefit outweighs the risk). Dosage modification is required in patients with renal insufficiency; monitor renal function prior to and during treatment. Hepatic toxicity has been reported, possibly due to concurrent therapy; monitor liver function prior to and during treatment.

Drug Interactions

Avoid Concomitant Use There are no known interactions where it is recommended to avoid concomitant use.

Decreased Effect

The levels/effects of Ethambutol may be decreased by: Aluminum Hydroxide

Increased Effect/Toxicity There are no known significant interactions involving an increase in effect.

Lab Interactions Increased uric acid (S)

Adverse Reactions Frequency not defined.

Cardiovascular: Myocarditis, pericarditis

Central nervous system: Confusion, disorientation, dizziness, fever, hallucinations, headache, malaise

Dermatologic: Dermatitis, erythema multiforme, exfoliative dermatitis, pruritus, rash

Endocrine & metabolic: Acute gout or hyperuricemia

Gastrointestinal: Abdominal pain, anorexia, GI upset, nausea, vomiting

Hematologic: Eosinophilia, leukopenia, lymphadenopathy, neutropenia, thrombocytopenia

Hepatic: Hepatitis, hepatotoxicity (possibly related to concurrent therapy), LFTs abnormal

Neuromuscular & skeletal: Arthralgia, peripheral neuritis

Ocular: Optic neuritis; symptoms may include decreased acuity, scotoma, color blindness, or visual defects (usually reversible with discontinuation, irreversible blindness has been described)

Renal: Nephritis

Respiratory: Infiltrates (with or without eosinophilia), pneumonitis

Miscellaneous: Anaphylaxis, anaphylactoid reaction; hypersensitivity syndrome (cutaneous reactions, eosinophilia, and organ-specific inflammation)

Pharmacodynamics/Kinetics

Absorption ~80%

Time to Peak Serum: 2-4 hours

Protein Binding 20% to 30%

Half-Life Elimination 2.5-3.6 hours; End-stage renal disease: 7-15 hours

Metabolism Hepatic (20%) to inactive metabolite

Excretion Urine (~50% as unchanged drug, 8% to 15% as metabolites); feces (~20% as unchanged drug)

Available Dosage Forms

Tablet, oral: 100 mg, 400 mg

Myambutol®: 100 mg, 400 mg

Dosing

Adult & Geriatric

Disseminated *Mycobacterium avium* (MAC) treatment in patients with advanced HIV infection (unlabeled use; ATS/IDSA guidelines, 2007): Oral: 15 mg/kg ethambutol in combination with clarithromycin or azithromycin with/without rifabutin

Tuberculosis, active: Oral: FDA-approved labeling: Adolescents ≥13 years and Adults: Initial: 15 mg/kg once daily (maximum dose: 1.5 g); Retreatment (previous antituberculosis therapy): 25 mg/kg once daily (maximum dose: 2.5 g) for 60 days or until bacteriologic smears and cultures become negative, followed by 15 mg/kg daily.

Suggested doses by lean body weight (CDC, 2003):

Daily therapy: 15-25 mg/kg (maximum dose: 1.6 g)

40-55 kg: 800 mg

56-75 kg: 1200 mg

76-90 kg: 1600 mg

Twice weekly directly observed therapy (DOT): 50 mg/kg (maximum dose: 4 g)

40-55 kg: 2000 mg

56-75 kg: 2800 mg

76-90 kg: 4000 mg

Three times/week DOT: 25-30 mg/kg (maximum dose: 2.4 g)

40-55 kg: 1200 mg

56-75 kg: 2000 mg

76-90 kg: 2400 mg

Note: Used as part of a multidrug regimen. Treatment regimens consist of an initial 2 month phase, followed by a continuation phase of 4 or 7 additional months; frequency of dosing may differ depending on phase of therapy.

Nontuberculous mycobacterium *(M. kansasii)* (unlabeled use; ATS/IDSA guidelines, 2007): Oral: 15 mg/kg/day ethambutol for duration to include 12 months of culture-negative sputum; typically used in combination with rifampin and isoniazid; **Note:** Previous recommendations stated to use 25 mg/kg/day for the initial 2 months of therapy; however, IDSA guidelines state this may be unnecessary given the success of rifampin-based regimens with ethambutol 15 mg/kg/day or omitted altogether.

Pediatric

***Mycobacterium avium* (MAC), secondary prophylaxis or treatment: HIV-exposed/-infected:** Oral: Infants and Children: 15-25 mg/kg/day once daily (maximum: 2.5 g/day) with clarithromycin (or azithromycin) with or without rifabutin (CDC, 2009)

Tuberculosis, active: Oral: **Note:** Used as part of a multidrug regimen; treatment regimens consist of an initial 2-month phase, followed by a continuation phase of 4 or 7 additional months; frequency of dosing may differ depending on phase of therapy.

Children:

HIV negative: Daily therapy: 15-20 mg/kg/day (maximum: 1 g/day); Twice weekly directly observed therapy (DOT): 50 mg/kg (maximum: 2.5 g/dose) (*MMWR*, 2003)

HIV-exposed/-infected: Daily therapy: 15-25 mg/kg/day (maximum: 2.5 g/day) (CDC, 2009)

Adolescents ≥13 years: Refer to adult dosing.

Renal Impairment

MMWR, 2003: Cl_{cr} <30 mL/minute and hemodialysis: 15-25 mg/kg/dose 3 times weekly

Aronoff, 2007

Cl_{cr} 10-50 mL/minute: Administer every 24-36 hours

Cl_{cr} <10 mL/minute: Administer every 48 hours

Hemodialysis: Slightly dialyzable (5% to 20%); Administer dose postdialysis

Peritoneal dialysis: Dose for Cl_{cr} <10 mL/minute: Administer every 48 hours

Continuous arteriovenous or venovenous hemofiltration: Dose for Cl_{cr} 10-50 mL/minute: Administer every 24-36 hours

Stability

Storage Store at controlled room temperature of 20°C to 25°C (68°F to 77°F).

Monitoring and Teaching Issues

Laboratory Monitoring Baseline and periodic (monthly) visual testing (each eye individually, as well as both eyes tested together) in patients receiving >15 mg/kg/day; baseline and periodic renal, hepatic, and hematopoietic tests

Physical Assessment Use caution in presence of renal insufficiency. Assess results of visual tests at baseline and periodically throughout therapy. Monitor for CNS changes, neuritis, and ocular changes on a regular basis during therapy. Teach patient need to adhere to dosing program and importance of regular laboratory tests and ophthalmic evaluations.

Patient Education Take with meals. May cause GI distress, dizziness, disorientation, and drowsiness. You will need to have frequent ophthalmic exams and periodic medical check-ups to evaluate drug effects. Report vision changes, numbness or tingling of extremities, or persistent loss of appetite.

Dietary Considerations May be taken with food as absorption is not affected, may cause gastric irritation.

Geriatric Considerations Since most elderly patients acquired their tuberculosis before current antituberculin regimens were available, ethambutol is only indicated when patients are from areas where drug resistant *M. tuberculosis* is endemic, in HIV-infected elderly patients, and when drug resistant *M. tuberculosis* is suspected (see Renal Impairment).

Breast-Feeding Considerations The manufacturer suggests use during breast-feeding only if benefits to the mother outweigh the possible risk to the infant. Some references suggest that exposure to the infant is low and does not produce toxicity, and breast-feeding should not be discouraged. Other references recommend if breast-feeding, monitor the infant for rash, malaise, nausea, or vomiting.

Pregnancy Considerations Teratogenic effects have been seen in animals. There are no adequate and well-controlled studies in pregnant women; there have been reports of ophthalmic abnormalities in infants born to women receiving ethambutol as a component of antituberculous therapy. Use only during pregnancy if benefits outweigh risks.

- **Ethambutol Hydrochloride** *see* Ethambutol *on page* 693

Ethinyl Estradiol and Desogestrel (ETH in il es tra DYE ole & des oh JES trel)

U.S. Brand Names Apri®; Azurette™; Caziant®; Cesia® [DSC]; Cyclessa®; Desogen®; Kariva®; Mircette®; Ortho-Cept®; Reclipsen®; Solia® [DSC]; Velivet™

Index Terms Desogestrel and Ethinyl Estradiol; Ortho Cept

Generic Availability (U.S.) Yes

Pharmacologic Category Contraceptive; Estrogen and Progestin Combination

Medication Safety Issues

Sound-alike/look-alike issues:

Apri® may be confused with Apriso™

Ortho-Cept® may be confused with Ortho-Cyclen®

Pregnancy Risk Factor X

Lactation Enters breast milk/not recommended

Use Prevention of pregnancy

Unlabeled/Investigational Use Treatment of hypermenorrhea (menorrhagia); pain associated with endometriosis; dysmenorrhea; dysfunctional uterine bleeding

Available Dosage Forms

Tablet, low-dose formulations:

Azurette™:

Day 1-21: Ethinyl estradiol 0.02 mg and desogestrel 0.15 mg [21 white tablets]

Day 22-23: 2 inactive green tablets

Day 24-28: Ethinyl estradiol 0.01 mg [5 blue tablets] (28s)

Kariva®:

Day 1-21: Ethinyl estradiol 0.02 mg and desogestrel 0.15 mg [21 white tablets]

Day 22-23: 2 inactive light green tablets

Day 24-28: Ethinyl estradiol 0.01 mg [5 light blue tablets] (28s)

Mircette®:

Day 1-21: Ethinyl estradiol 0.02 mg and desogestrel 0.15 mg [21 white tablets]

Day 22-23: 2 inactive green tablets

Day 24-28: Ethinyl estradiol 0.01 mg [5 yellow tablets] (28s)

Tablet, monophasic formulations:

Apri® 28: Ethinyl estradiol 0.03 mg and desogestrel 0.15 mg (28s) [21 rose tablets and 7 white inactive tablets]

Desogen®, Reclipsen®: Ethinyl estradiol 0.03 mg and desogestrel 0.15 mg (28s) [21 white tablets and 7 green inactive tablets]

Ortho-Cept® 28: Ethinyl estradiol 0.03 mg and desogestrel 0.15 mg (28s) [21 light orange tablets and 7 green inactive tablets]

Tablet, triphasic formulations:

Caziant®:

Day 1-7: Ethinyl estradiol 0.025 mg and desogestrel 0.1 mg [7 white tablets]

Day 8-14: Ethinyl estradiol 0.025 mg and desogestrel 0.125 mg [7 light blue tablets]

Day 15-21: Ethinyl estradiol 0.025 mg and desogestrel 0.15 mg [7 blue tablets]

Day 22-28: 7 green inactive tablets (28s)

Cyclessa®:

Day 1-7: Ethinyl estradiol 0.025 mg and desogestrel 0.1 mg [7 light yellow tablets]

Day 8-14: Ethinyl estradiol 0.025 mg and desogestrel 0.125 mg [7 orange tablets]

Day 15-21: Ethinyl estradiol 0.025 mg and desogestrel 0.15 mg [7 red tablets]

Day 22-28: 7 green inactive tablets (28s)

Velivet™:

Day 1-7: Ethinyl estradiol 0.025 mg and desogestrel 0.1 mg [7 beige tablets]

Day 8-14: Ethinyl estradiol 0.025 mg and desogestrel 0.125 mg [7 orange tablets]

Day 15-21: Ethinyl estradiol 0.025 mg and desogestrel 0.15 mg [7 pink tablets]

Day 22-28: 7 white inactive tablets (28s)

Dosing

Adult Females: Contraception: Oral:

Schedule 1 (Sunday starter): Dose begins on first Sunday after onset of menstruation; if the menstrual period starts on Sunday, take first tablet that very same day. **With a Sunday start, an additional method of contraception should be used until after the first 7 days of consecutive administration.**

For 21-tablet package: Dosage is 1 tablet daily for 21 consecutive days, followed by 7 days off of the medication; a new course begins on the 8th day after the last tablet is taken.

For 28-tablet package: Dosage is 1 tablet daily without interruption.

Schedule 2 (Day 1 starter): Dose starts on first day of menstrual cycle taking 1 tablet daily.

For 21-tablet package: Dosage is 1 tablet daily for 21 consecutive days, followed by 7 days off of the medication; a new course begins on the 8th day after the last tablet is taken.

For 28-tablet package: Dosage is 1 tablet daily without interruption.

If all doses have been taken on schedule and one menstrual period is missed, continue dosing cycle. If two consecutive menstrual periods are missed, pregnancy test is required before new dosing cycle is started.

Missed doses **monophasic formulations** (refer to package insert for complete information):

One dose missed: Take as soon as remembered or take 2 tablets next day

Two consecutive doses missed in the first 2 weeks: Take 2 tablets as soon as remembered or 2 tablets next 2 days. **An additional method of contraception should be used for 7 days after missed dose.**

Two consecutive doses missed in week 3 or three consecutive doses missed at any time: Schedule 1 (Sunday starter): Continue to take 1 tablet daily until Sunday, then discard the rest of the pack, and a new pack is started that same day. Schedule 2 (Day 1 starter): Current pack should be discarded, and a new pack started that same day. **An additional method of contraception should be used for 7 days after missed dose.**

Missed doses **biphasic/triphasic formulations** (refer to package insert for complete information):

One dose missed: Take as soon as remembered or take 2 tablets next day.

Two consecutive doses missed in week 1 or week 2 of the pack: Take 2 tablets as soon as remembered and 2 tablets the next day. Resume taking 1 tablet daily until the pack is empty. **An additional method of contraception should be used for 7 days after a missed dose.**

Two consecutive doses missed in week 3 of the pack; **an additional method of contraception must be used for 7 days after a missed dose**:

Schedule 1 (Sunday starter): Take 1 tablet every day until Sunday. Discard the remaining pack and start a new pack of pills on the same day.

Schedule 2 (Day 1 starter): Discard the remaining pack and start a new pack the same day.

Three or more consecutive doses missed; **an additional method of contraception must be used for 7 days after a missed dose**:

Schedule 1 (Sunday starter): Take 1 tablet every day until Sunday; on Sunday, discard the pack and start a new pack.

Schedule 2 (Day 1 starter): Discard the remaining pack and begin new pack of tablets starting on the same day.

Pediatric Females: Contraception: Oral: See adult dosing; not to be used prior to menarche.

Renal Impairment Specific guidelines not available; use with caution and monitor blood pressure closely. Consider other forms of contraception.

Hepatic Impairment Contraindicated in patients with hepatic impairment.

Administration

Oral Administer at the same time each day.

Monitoring and Teaching Issues

Physical Assessment Monitor blood pressure on a regular basis. Teach importance of regular (monthly) blood pressure checks and annual physical assessment, Pap smear, and vision assessment. Teach importance of maintaining prescribed schedule of dosing.

Patient Education Oral contraceptives do not protect against HIV infection or other sexually-transmitted diseases. You are at risk of becoming pregnant if doses are missed. Detailed and complete information on dosing and missed doses can be found in the package insert. Be aware that some medications may reduce the effectiveness of oral contraceptives; an alternate form of contraception may be needed. It is important that you check your blood pressure monthly and that you have an annual physical assessment, Pap smear, and vision exam while taking this medication. Avoid smoking while taking this medication; smoking increases risk of adverse effects, including thromboembolic events and heart attacks. You may experience loss of appetite or constipation. Report immediately pain or muscle soreness; warmth, swelling, pain, or redness in calves; shortness of breath; sudden loss of vision; unresolved leg/foot swelling; change in menstrual pattern (unusual bleeding, amenorrhea, breakthrough spotting); breast tenderness that does not go away; acute abdominal cramping; signs of vaginal infection (drainage, pain, itching); CNS changes (blurred vision, confusion, acute anxiety, or unresolved depression); chest pain; severe headache or vomiting; weakness in arm or leg; severe abdominal pain or tenderness; jaundice; or weight gain. Notify prescriber of changes in contact lens tolerance.

Ethinyl Estradiol and Drospirenone

(ETH in il es tra DYE ole & droh SPYE re none)

U.S. Brand Names Gianvi™; Ocella™; Yasmin®; Yaz®; Zarah®

Index Terms Drospirenone and Ethinyl Estradiol

Generic Availability (U.S.) Yes

Pharmacologic Category Contraceptive; Estrogen and Progestin Combination

Medication Safety Issues

Sound-alike/look-alike issues:

Yasmin® may be confused with Yaz®

Yaz® may be confused with Beyaz™, Yasmin®

Pregnancy Risk Factor X

Lactation Enters breast milk/not recommended

Use Females: Prevention of pregnancy; treatment of premenstrual dysphoric disorder (PMDD); treatment of acne

Unlabeled/Investigational Use Treatment of hypermenorrhea (menorrhagia); pain associated with endometriosis; dysmenorrhea; dysfunctional uterine bleeding

Available Dosage Forms

Tablet:

Gianvi™: Ethinyl estradiol 0.03 mg and drospirenone 3 mg (28s) [24 light pink active tablets and 4 white inactive tablets]

Ocella™, Yasmin®: Ethinyl estradiol 0.03 mg and drospirenone 3 mg (28s) [21 yellow active tablets and 7 white inactive tablets]

Yaz®: Ethinyl estradiol 0.02 mg and drospirenone 3 mg (28s) [24 light pink active tablets and 4 white inactive tablets]

Zarah®: Ethinyl estradiol 0.03 mg and drospirenone 3 mg (28s) [21 blue active tablets and 7 peach inactive tablets]

Dosing

Adult

Acne (Yaz®): Females: Oral: Refer to dosing for contraception.

Contraception (Yasmin®, Yaz®), PMDD (Yaz®): Female: Oral: Dosage is 1 tablet daily for 28 consecutive days. Dosing may be started on the first day of menstrual period (Day 1 starter) or on the first Sunday after the onset of the menstrual period (Sunday starter). **With a Sunday start, an additional method of contraception should be used until after the first 7 days of consecutive administration.**

Day 1 starter: Dose starts on first day of menstrual cycle taking 1 tablet daily.

Sunday starter: Dose begins on first Sunday after onset of menstruation; if the menstrual period starts on Sunday, take first tablet that very same day.

Switching from a different contraceptive:

Oral contraceptive: Start on the same day that a new pack of the previous oral contraceptive would have been taken

Transdermal patch, vaginal ring, injection: Start on the day the next dose would have been due

IUD or implant: Start on the day of removal

Use after childbirth (in women who are not breast-feeding) or after second trimester abortion: Therapy may be started ≥4 weeks postpartum. Pregnancy should be ruled out prior to treatment if menstrual periods have not restarted and an additional method of contraception (nonhormonal) should be used until after the first 7 days of consecutive administration.

Missed doses:

If all doses have been taken on schedule and one menstrual period is missed, continue dosing cycle. If two consecutive menstrual periods are missed, pregnancy test is required before new dosing cycle is started.

If doses have been missed during the first 3 weeks and the menstrual period is missed, pregnancy should be ruled out prior to continuing treatment.

Missed doses (monophasic formulations) (refer to package insert for complete information):

One dose missed: Take as soon as remembered or take 2 tablets next day

Two consecutive doses missed in the first 2 weeks: Take 2 tablets as soon as remembered or 2 tablets next 2 days. **An additional method of contraception should be used for 7 days after missed dose.**

Two consecutive doses missed in week 3 or three consecutive doses missed at any time: **An additional method of contraception must be used for 7 days after a missed dose.**

Day 1 starter: Current pack should be discarded, and a new pack should be started that same day.

Sunday starter: Continue dose of 1 tablet daily until Sunday, then discard the rest of the pack, and a new pack should be started that same day.

Any number of doses missed in week 4: Continue taking one pill each day until pack is empty; no back-up method of contraception is needed

Pediatric Note: Not to be used prior to menarche.

Acne (Yaz®): Females: Children ≥14 years: Oral: Refer to adult dosing.

Contraception (Yasmin®, Yaz®), PMDD (Yaz®): Females: Oral: Refer to adult dosing.

Renal Impairment Contraindicated in patients with renal dysfunction.

Hepatic Impairment Contraindicated in patients with hepatic dysfunction.

Administration

Oral Dose should be taken at the same time each day, either after the evening meal or at bedtime. If severe vomiting or diarrhea occurs, additional contraception (nonhormonal) should be used. If vomiting occurs within 3-4 hours of dosing, consider the dose to be missed.

Monitoring and Teaching Issues

Physical Assessment Monitor blood pressure on a regular (monthly) basis. Teach patient the importance of annual physical examinations (including Pap smear and vision exam) and the importance of maintaining prescribed schedule of dosing.

Patient Education Oral contraceptives do not protect against HIV infection or other sexually-transmitted diseases. You are at risk of becoming pregnant if doses are missed. Detailed and complete information on dosing and missed doses can be found in the package insert. Be aware that some medications may reduce the effectiveness of oral contraceptives; an alternate form of contraception may be needed. It is important that you check your blood pressure monthly and that you have an annual physical assessment, Pap smear, and vision exam while taking this medication. Avoid smoking while taking this medication; smoking increases risk of adverse effects, including thromboembolic events and heart attacks. You may experience loss of appetite or constipation. Report immediately pain or muscle soreness; warmth, swelling, pain, or redness in calves; shortness of breath; sudden loss of vision; unresolved leg/foot swelling; change in menstrual pattern (unusual bleeding, amenorrhea, breakthrough spotting); breast tenderness that does not go away; acute abdominal cramping; signs of vaginal infection (drainage, pain, itching); CNS changes (blurred vision, confusion, acute anxiety, or unresolved depression); chest pain; severe headache or vomiting; weakness in arm or leg; severe abdominal pain or tenderness; jaundice; or weight gain. Notify prescriber of changes in contact lens tolerance.

Ethinyl Estradiol and Ethynodiol Diacetate

(ETH in il es tra DYE ole & e thye noe DYE ole dye AS e tate)

U.S. Brand Names Kelnor™; Zovia®

Index Terms Ethynodiol Diacetate and Ethinyl Estradiol

Generic Availability (U.S.) Yes

Pharmacologic Category Contraceptive; Estrogen and Progestin Combination

Medication Safety Issues

Sound-alike/look-alike issues:

Demulen® may be confused with Dalmane®, Demerol®

Pregnancy Risk Factor X

Lactation Enters breast milk/not recommended

Use Prevention of pregnancy

Unlabeled/Investigational Use Treatment of hypermenorrhea (menorrhagia); pain associated with endometriosis; dysmenorrhea; dysfunctional uterine bleeding

Available Dosage Forms

Tablet, monophasic formulations:

Kelnor™ 1/35: Ethinyl estradiol 0.035 mg and ethynodiol diacetate 1 mg [21 light yellow tablets and 7 white inactive tablets] (28s)

Zovia® 1/35-28: Ethinyl estradiol 0.035 mg and ethynodiol diacetate 1 mg [21 light pink tablets and 7 white inactive tablets] (28s)

Zovia® 1/50-28: Ethinyl estradiol 0.05 mg and ethynodiol diacetate 1 mg [21 pink tablets and 7 white inactive tablets] (28s)

Dosing

Adult

Females: Contraception: Oral:

Schedule 1 (Sunday starter): Dose begins on first Sunday after onset of menstruation; if the menstrual period starts on Sunday, take first tablet that very same day. **With a Sunday start, an additional method of contraception should be used until after the first 7 days of consecutive administration:**

For 21-tablet package: 1 tablet/day for 21 consecutive days, followed by 7 days off of the medication; a new course begins on the 8th day after the last tablet is taken

For 28-tablet package: 1 tablet/day without interruption

Schedule 2 (Day-1 starter): Dose starts on first day of menstrual cycle taking 1 tablet/day:

For 21-tablet package: 1 tablet/day for 21 consecutive days, followed by 7 days off of the medication; a new course begins on the 8th day after the last tablet is taken

For 28-tablet package: 1 tablet/day without interruption

If all doses have been taken on schedule and one menstrual period is missed, continue dosing cycle. If two consecutive menstrual periods are missed, pregnancy test is required before new dosing cycle is started.

Missed doses **monophasic formulations** (refer to package insert for complete information):

One dose missed: Take as soon as remembered or take 2 tablets next day

Two consecutive doses missed in the first 2 weeks: Take 2 tablets as soon as remembered or 2 tablets next 2 days. **An additional method of contraception should be used for 7 days after missed dose.**

Two consecutive doses missed in week 3 or three consecutive doses missed at any time: **An additional method of contraception must be used for 7 days after a missed dose:**

Schedule 1 (Sunday starter): Continue dose of 1 tablet daily until Sunday, then discard the rest of the pack, and a new pack should be started that same day.

Schedule 2 (Day-1 starter): Current pack should be discarded, and a new pack should be started that same day.

Pediatric Females: Contraception: Oral: Refer to adult dosing; not to be used prior to menarche.

Renal Impairment Specific guidelines not available; use with caution and monitor blood pressure closely. Consider other forms of contraception.

Hepatic Impairment Contraindicated in patients with hepatic impairment.

Administration

Oral Administer at the same time each day.

Monitoring and Teaching Issues

Physical Assessment Monitor blood pressure on a regular basis. Teach importance of regular (monthly) blood pressure checks and annual physical assessment, Pap smear, and vision assessment. Teach importance of maintaining prescribed schedule of dosing.

Patient Education Oral contraceptives do not protect against HIV or other sexually-transmitted diseases. You are at risk of becoming pregnant if doses are missed. Be aware that some medications may reduce the effectiveness of oral contraceptives; an alternate form of contraception may be needed. It is important that you check your blood pressure monthly (on same day each month) and that you have an annual physical assessment, Pap smear, and vision assessment while taking this medication. Avoid smoking while taking this medication; smoking increases risk of adverse effects, including thromboembolic events and heart attacks. You may experience loss of appetite or constipation. If you have diabetes, use accurate serum glucose testing to identify any changes in glucose tolerance; notify prescriber of significant changes so antidiabetic medication can be adjusted if necessary. Report immediately pain or muscle soreness; warmth, swelling, pain, or redness in calves; shortness of breath; sudden loss of vision; unresolved leg/foot swelling; change in menstrual pattern (unusual bleeding, amenorrhea, breakthrough spotting); breast tenderness that does not go away; acute abdominal cramping; signs of vaginal infection (drainage, pain, itching); CNS changes (blurred vision, confusion, acute anxiety, or unresolved depression); chest pain; severe headache or vomiting; weakness in arm or leg; severe abdominal pain or tenderness; jaundice; or weight gain. Notify prescriber of changes in contact lens tolerance.

Ethinyl Estradiol and Levonorgestrel

(ETH in il es tra DYE ole & LEE voe nor jes trel)

U.S. Brand Names Aviane™; Enpresse®; Introvale™; Jolessa™; Lessina®; Levora®; LoSeasonique®; Lutera®; Lybrel®; Nordette® 28; Portia®; Quasense®; Seasonale®; Seasonique®; Sronyx®; Trivora®

Index Terms Levonorgestrel and Ethinyl Estradiol

Generic Availability (U.S.) Yes

Pharmacologic Category Contraceptive; Estrogen and Progestin Combination

Medication Safety Issues

Sound-alike/look-alike issues:

Nordette® may be confused with Nicorette®
Seasonale® may be confused with Seasonique®
Seasonique® may be confused with Seasonale®
Tri-Levlen® may be confused with Trilafon®

Pregnancy Risk Factor X

Lactation Enters breast milk/not recommended

Use Prevention of pregnancy; postcoital contraception

Unlabeled/Investigational Use Treatment of hypermenorrhea (menorrhagia); pain associated with endometriosis; dysmenorrhea; dysfunctional uterine bleeding

Available Dosage Forms

Tablet, oral [low-dose formulation]:

Aviane™: Ethinyl estradiol 0.02 mg and levonorgestrel 0.1 mg (28s) [21 orange tablets and 7 light green inactive tablets]

Lutera®, Sronyx®: Ethinyl estradiol 0.02 mg and levonorgestrel 0.1 mg (28s) [21 white tablets and 7 peach inactive tablets]

Tablet, oral [monophasic formulation]:

Levora®: Ethinyl estradiol 0.03 mg and levonorgestrel 0.15 mg (28s) [21 white tablets and 7 peach inactive tablets]

Nordette® 28: Ethinyl estradiol 0.03 mg and levonorgestrel 0.15 mg (28s) [21 light orange tablets and 7 pink inactive tablets]

Portia® 28: Ethinyl estradiol 0.03 mg and levonorgestrel 0.15 mg (28s) [21 pink tablets and 7 white inactive tablets]

Tablet, oral [extended cycle regimen]:

Introvale™: Ethinyl estradiol 0.03 mg and levonorgestrel 0.15 mg (91s) [84 peach tablets and 7 white inactive tablets]

Jolessa™, Seasonale®: Ethinyl estradiol 0.03 mg and levonorgestrel 0.15 mg (91s) [84 pink tablets and 7 white inactive tablets]

LoSeasonique®: Ethinyl estradiol 0.02 mg and levonorgestrel 0.1 mg (91s) [84 orange tablets] and ethinyl estradiol 0.01 mg [7 yellow tablets]

Quasense®: Ethinyl estradiol 0.03 mg and levonorgestrel 0.15 mg] (91s) [84 white tablets and 7 peach inactive tablets]

Seasonique®: Ethinyl estradiol 0.03 mg and levonorgestrel 0.15 mg (91s) [84 light blue-green tablets] and ethinyl estradiol 0.01 mg [7 yellow tablets]

Tablet, oral [noncyclic regimen]:

Lybrel®: Ethinyl estradiol 0.02 mg and levonorgestrel 0.09 mg (28s) [28 yellow tablets]

Tablet, oral [triphasic formulation]:

Enpresse®:

Day 1-6: Ethinyl estradiol 0.03 mg and levonorgestrel 0.05 mg [6 pink tablets]
Day 7-11: Ethinyl estradiol 0.04 mg and levonorgestrel 0.075 mg [5 white tablets]
Day 12-21: Ethinyl estradiol 0.03 mg and levonorgestrel 0.125 mg [10 orange tablets]
Day 22-28: 7 light green inactive tablets (28s)

Trivora®:

Day 1-6: Ethinyl estradiol 0.03 mg and levonorgestrel 0.05 mg [6 blue tablets]

Day 7-11: Ethinyl estradiol 0.04 mg and levonorgestrel 0.075 mg [5 white tablets]

Day 12-21: Ethinyl estradiol 0.03 mg and levonorgestrel 0.125 mg [10 pink tablets]

Day 22-28: 7 peach inactive tablets (28s)

Dosing

Adult Females:

Contraception, 28-day cycle: Oral:

Schedule 1 (Sunday starter): Dose begins on first Sunday after onset of menstruation; if the menstrual period starts on Sunday, take first tablet that very same day. With a Sunday start, an additional method of contraception should be used until after the first 7 days of consecutive administration:

For 21-tablet package: 1 tablet/day for 21 consecutive days, followed by 7 days off of the medication; a new course begins on the 8th day after the last tablet is taken

For 28-tablet package: 1 tablet/day without interruption

Schedule 2 (Day-1 starter): Dose starts on first day of menstrual cycle taking 1 tablet/day:

For 21-tablet package: 1 tablet/day for 21 consecutive days, followed by 7 days off of the medication; a new course begins on the 8th day after the last tablet is taken

For 28-tablet package: 1 tablet/day without interruption

If all doses have been taken on schedule and one menstrual period is missed, continue dosing cycle. If two consecutive menstrual periods are missed, pregnancy test is required before new dosing cycle is started.

Missed doses **monophasic formulations** (refer to package insert for complete information):

One dose missed: Take as soon as remembered or take 2 tablets next day

Two consecutive doses missed in the first 2 weeks: Take 2 tablets as soon as remembered or 2 tablets next 2 days. An additional method of contraception should be used for 7 days after missed dose.

Two consecutive doses missed in week 3 or three consecutive doses missed at any time: An additional method of contraception must be used for 7 days after a missed dose:

Schedule 1 (Sunday starter): Continue dose of 1 tablet daily until Sunday, then discard the rest of the pack, and a new pack should be started that same day.

Schedule 2 (Day-1 starter): Current pack should be discarded, and a new pack should be started that same day.

Missed doses **biphasic/triphasic formulations** (refer to package insert for complete information):

One dose missed: Take as soon as remembered or take 2 tablets next day.

Two consecutive doses missed in week 1 or week 2 of the pack: Take 2 tablets as soon as remembered and 2 tablets the next day. Resume taking 1 tablet daily until the pack is empty. An additional method of contraception should be used for 7 days after a missed dose.

Two consecutive doses missed in week 3 of the pack: An additional method of contraception must be used for 7 days after a missed dose.

Schedule 1 (Sunday starter): Take 1 tablet every day until Sunday. Discard the remaining pack and start a new pack of pills on the same day.

Schedule 2 (Day-1 starter): Discard the remaining pack and start a new pack the same day.

Three or more consecutive doses missed: An additional method of contraception must be used for 7 days after a missed dose.

Schedule 1 (Sunday starter): Take 1 tablet every day until Sunday; on Sunday, discard the pack and start a new pack.

Schedule 2 (Day-1 starter): Discard the remaining pack and begin new pack of tablets starting on the same day.

Contraception, 91-day cycle (extended cycle regimen): Dose begins on first Sunday after onset of menstruation; if the menstrual period starts on Sunday, take first tablet that very same day. An additional method of contraception should be used until after the first 7 days of consecutive administration:

Seasonale®: One active tablet/day for 84 consecutive days, followed by 1 inactive tablet/day for 7 days; if all doses have been taken on schedule and one menstrual period is missed, pregnancy should be ruled out prior to continuing therapy.

Seasonique®, LoSeasonique®: One active tablet/day for 84 consecutive days, followed by 1 low dose estrogen tablet/day for 7 days; if all doses have been taken on schedule and one menstrual period is missed, pregnancy should be ruled out prior to continuing therapy.

Missed doses:

One dose missed: Take as soon as remembered or take 2 tablets the next day

Two consecutive doses missed: Take 2 tablets as soon as remembered or 2 tablets the next 2 days. An additional nonhormonal method of contraception should be used for 7 consecutive days after the missed dose.

Three or more consecutive doses missed: Do not take the missed doses; continue taking 1 tablet/day until pack is complete. Bleeding may occur during the following week. An additional nonhormonal method of contraception should be used for 7 consecutive days after the missed dose.

Any number of pills during week 13: Throw away the missed pills and keep taking scheduled pills until the pack is finished. A back-up method of contraception is not needed

Contraception, continuous use (extended cycle regimen): Oral: Lybrel®: Take one tablet daily, at the same time each day, without a tablet-free interval. Therapy should be initiated as follows:

No previous contraception: Begin on the first day of menstrual cycle. Back-up contraception is not needed.

Previously taking a 21-day or 28-day combination hormonal contraceptive: Begin on day 1 of the withdrawal bleed (at the latest, 7 days after the last active tablet). Back-up contraception is not needed.

Previously using a progestin-only pill: Begin the day after taking a progestin only pill. Back-up contraception is needed for the first 7 days of therapy.

Previously using contraceptive implant: Begin the day of implant removal. Back-up contraception is needed for the first 7 days of therapy.

Previously using contraceptive injection: Begin when the next injection is due. Back-up contraception is needed for the first 7 days of therapy.

Missed doses:

One dose missed: Take as soon as remembered then take the next tablet at the regular time (2 tablets in 1 day). An additional nonhormonal method of contraception should also be used for 7 consecutive days.

Two consecutive doses missed: If remembered the day of the second missed tablet, take 2 tablets as soon as remembered, then 1 tablet the next day. If remembered the day after the second tablet is missed, take 2 tablets the day remembered, then 2 tablets the next day. An additional nonhormonal method of contraception should also be used for 7 consecutive days.

Three or more consecutive doses missed: Take 1 tablet daily and contact healthcare provider; do not take the missed pills. An additional nonhormonal method of contraception should also be used for 7 consecutive days.

Pediatric Females: Contraception or emergency contraception: Oral: Refer to adult dosing; not to be used prior to menarche.

Renal Impairment Specific guidelines not available; use with caution and monitor blood pressure closely. Consider other forms of contraception.

Hepatic Impairment Contraindicated in patients with hepatic impairment.

Administration

Oral Administer at the same time each day.

Monitoring and Teaching Issues

Physical Assessment See individual agents.

Patient Education See individual agents.

Related Information

Levonorgestrel *on page 1097*

◆ **Ethinyl Estradiol and NGM** *see* Ethinyl Estradiol and Norgestimate *on page 704*

Ethinyl Estradiol and Norethindrone (ETH in il es tra DYE ole & nor eth IN drone)

U.S. Brand Names Aranelle®; Balziva™; Brevicon®; Estrostep® Fe; Femcon® Fe; femhrt®; femhrt® Lo; Jinteli™; Junel® 1.5/30; Junel® 1/20; Junel® Fe 1.5/30; Junel® Fe 1/20; Leena®; Lo Loestrin™ Fe; Loestrin® 21 1.5/30; Loestrin® 21 1/20; Loestrin® 24 Fe; Loestrin® Fe 1.5/30; Loestrin® Fe 1/20; Microgestin® 1.5/30; Microgestin® 1/20; Microgestin® Fe 1.5/30; Microgestin® Fe 1/20; Modicon®; Necon® 0.5/35; Necon® 1/35; Necon® 10/11; Necon® 7/7/7; Norinyl® 1+35; Nortrel® 0.5/35; Nortrel® 1/35; Nortrel® 7/7/7; Ortho-Novum® 1/35; Ortho-Novum® 7/7/7; Ovcon® 35; Ovcon® 50; Tilia™ Fe; Tri-Legest™ Fe; Tri-Norinyl®; Zenchent™; Zeosa™

Index Terms Norethindrone Acetate and Ethinyl Estradiol; Ortho Novum

Generic Availability (U.S.) Yes

Pharmacologic Category Contraceptive; Estrogen and Progestin Combination

Medication Safety Issues

Sound-alike/look-alike issues:

femhrt® may be confused with Femara®

Lo Loestrin Fe may be confused with Loestrin® Fe

Modicon® may be confused with Mylicon®

Norinyl® may be confused with Nardil®

Pregnancy Risk Factor X

Lactation Enters breast milk/not recommended

Use Prevention of pregnancy; treatment of acne; moderate-to-severe vasomotor symptoms associated with menopause; prevention of osteoporosis (in women at significant risk only)

Unlabeled/Investigational Use Treatment of hypermenorrhea (menorrhagia); pain associated with endometriosis, dysmenorrhea; dysfunctional uterine bleeding

Available Dosage Forms

Tablet, oral:

femhrt® 1/5: Ethinyl estradiol 0.005 mg and norethindrone acetate 1 mg (28s, 90s) [white tablets]

femhrt® Lo 0.5/2.5: Ethinyl estradiol 0.0025 mg and norethindrone acetate 0.5 mg (28s, 90s) [white tablets]

Jinteli™: Ethinyl estradiol 0.005 mg and norethindrone acetate 1 mg (28s, 90s) [white tablets] ▶

Tablet, oral, monophasic formulations:

Balziva™: Ethinyl estradiol 0.035 mg and norethindrone 0.4 mg (28s) [21 light peach tablets and 7 white inactive tablets]

Brevicon®: Ethinyl estradiol 0.035 mg and norethindrone 0.5 mg (28s) [21 blue tablets and 7 orange inactive tablets]

Junel® 1/20: Ethinyl estradiol 0.02 mg and norethindrone acetate 1 mg (21s) [yellow tablets]

Junel® 1.5/30, Loestrin® 21 1.5/30: Ethinyl estradiol 0.03 mg and norethindrone acetate 1.5 mg (21s) [pink tablets]

Junel® Fe 1/20: Ethinyl estradiol 0.02 mg and norethindrone acetate 1 mg [21 yellow tablets] and ferrous fumarate 75 mg [7 brown tablets] (28s)

Junel® Fe 1.5/30, Loestrin® Fe 21 1.5/30: Ethinyl estradiol 0.03 mg and norethindrone acetate 1.5 mg [21 pink tablets] and ferrous fumarate 75 mg [7 brown tablets] (28s)

Loestrin® 21 1/20: Ethinyl estradiol 0.02 mg and norethindrone acetate 1 mg (21s) [light yellow tablets]

Lo Loestrin Fe: Ethinyl estradiol 0.01 mg and norethindrone acetate 1mg [24 blue tablets] and ethinyl estradiol 0.01 mg [2 white tablets] and ferrous fumarate 75 mg [2 brown tablets] (28s)

Loestrin® 24 Fe: Ethinyl estradiol 0.02 mg and norethindrone acetate 1 mg [24 white tablets] and ferrous fumarate 75 mg [4 brown tablets] (28s)

Loestrin® Fe 1/20: Ethinyl estradiol 0.02 mg and norethindrone acetate 1 mg [21 light yellow tablets] and ferrous fumarate 75 mg [7 brown tablets] (28s)

Loestrin® Fe 1.5/30: Ethinyl estradiol 0.03 mg and norethindrone acetate 1.5 mg [21 pink tablets] and ferrous fumarate 75 mg [7 brown tablets] (28s)

Microgestin® 1/20: Ethinyl estradiol 0.02 mg and norethindrone acetate 1 mg (21s) [white tablets]

Microgestin® 1.5/30: Ethinyl estradiol 0.03 mg and norethindrone acetate 1.5 mg (21s) [green tablets]

Microgestin® Fe 1/20: Ethinyl estradiol 0.02 mg and norethindrone acetate 1 mg [21 white tablets] and ferrous fumarate 75 mg [7 brown tablets] (28s)

Microgestin® Fe 1.5/30: Ethinyl estradiol 0.03 mg and norethindrone acetate 1.5 mg [21 green tablets] and ferrous fumarate 75 mg [7 brown tablets] (28s)

Modicon®: Ethinyl estradiol 0.035 mg and norethindrone 0.5 mg (28s) [21 white tablets and 7 green inactive tablets]

Necon® 0.5/35, Nortrel® 0.5/35: Ethinyl estradiol 0.035 mg and norethindrone 0.5 mg (28s) [21 light yellow tablets and 7 white inactive tablets]

Necon® 1/35: Ethinyl estradiol 0.035 mg and norethindrone 1 mg (28s) [21 dark yellow tablets and 7 white inactive tablets]

Norinyl® 1+35: Ethinyl estradiol 0.035 mg and norethindrone 1 mg (28s) [21 yellow-green tablets and 7 orange inactive tablets]

Nortrel® 1/35:

Ethinyl estradiol 0.035 mg and norethindrone 1 mg (21s) [yellow tablets]

Ethinyl estradiol 0.035 mg and norethindrone 1 mg (28s) [21 yellow tablets and 7 white inactive tablets]

Ortho-Novum® 1/35: Ethinyl estradiol 0.035 mg and norethindrone 1 mg (28s) [21 peach tablets and 7 green inactive tablets]

Ovcon® 35: Ethinyl estradiol 0.035 mg and norethindrone 0.4 mg (28s) [21 light peach tablets and 7 green inactive tablets]

Ovcon® 50: Ethinyl estradiol 0.05 mg and norethindrone 1 mg (28s) [21 yellow tablets and 7 green inactive tablets]

Zenchent™: Ethinyl estradiol 0.035 mg and norethindrone 0.4 mg (28s) [21 orange tablets and 7 white inactive tablets]

Tablet, chewable, oral, monophasic formulations:

Femcon® Fe: Ethinyl estradiol 0.035 mg and norethindrone 0.4 mg [21 white tablets] and ferrous fumarate 75 mg [7 brown tablets] (28s)

Zeosa™: Ethinyl estradiol 0.035 mg and norethindrone 0.4 mg [21 light yellow tablets] and ferrous fumarate 75 mg [7 brown tablets] (28s)

Tablet, oral, biphasic formulations:

Necon® 10/11:

Day 1-10: Ethinyl estradiol 0.035 mg and norethindrone 0.5 mg [10 light yellow tablets]

Day 11-21: Ethinyl estradiol 0.035 mg and norethindrone 1 mg [11 dark yellow tablets]

Day 22-28: 7 white inactive tablets (28s)

Tablet, oral, triphasic formulations:

Aranelle®:

Day 1-7: Ethinyl estradiol 0.035 mg and norethindrone 0.5 mg [7 light yellow tablets]

Day 8-16: Ethinyl estradiol 0.035 mg and norethindrone 1 mg [9 white tablets]

Day 17-21: Ethinyl estradiol 0.035 mg and norethindrone 0.5 mg [5 light yellow tablets]

Day 22-28: 7 peach inactive tablets (28s)

Estrostep® Fe, Tilia™ Fe::

Day 1-5: Ethinyl estradiol 0.02 mg and norethindrone acetate 1 mg [5 white triangular tablets]

Day 6-12: Ethinyl estradiol 0.03 mg and norethindrone acetate 1 mg [7 white square tablets]

Day 13-21: Ethinyl estradiol 0.035 mg and norethindrone acetate 1 mg [9 white round tablets]

Day 22-28: Ferrous fumarate 75 mg [7 brown tablets] (28s)

Leena®:

Day 1-7: Ethinyl estradiol 0.035 mg and norethindrone 0.5 mg [7 light blue tablets]

Day 8-16: Ethinyl estradiol 0.035 mg and norethindrone 1 mg [9 light yellow-green tablets]

Day 17-21: Ethinyl estradiol 0.035 mg and norethindrone 0.5 mg [5 light blue tablets]

Day 22-28: 7 orange inactive tablets (28s)

Necon® 7/7/7, Ortho-Novum® 7/7/7:
Day 1-7: Ethinyl estradiol 0.035 mg and norethindrone 0.5 mg [7 white tablets]
Day 8-14: Ethinyl estradiol 0.035 mg and norethindrone 0.75 mg [7 light peach tablets]
Day 15-21: Ethinyl estradiol 0.035 mg and norethindrone 1 mg [7 peach tablets]
Day 22-28: 7 green inactive tablets (28s)
Nortrel® 7/7/7:
Day 1-7: Ethinyl estradiol 0.035 mg and norethindrone 0.5 mg [7 light yellow tablets]
Day 8-14: Ethinyl estradiol 0.035 mg and norethindrone 0.75 mg [7 blue tablets]
Day 15-21: Ethinyl estradiol 0.035 mg and norethindrone 1 mg [7 peach tablets]
Day 22-28: 7 white inactive tablets (28s)
Tri-Legest™ Fe:
Day 1-5: Ethinyl estradiol 0.02 mg and norethindrone acetate 1 mg [5 light pink tablets]
Day 6-12: Ethinyl estradiol 0.03 mg and norethindrone acetate 1 mg [7 light yellow tablets]
Day 13-21: Ethinyl estradiol 0.035 mg and norethindrone acetate 1 mg [9 light blue tablets]
Day 22-28: Ferrous fumarate 75 mg [7 brown tablets] (28s)
Tri-Norinyl®:
Day 1-7: Ethinyl estradiol 0.035 mg and norethindrone 0.5 mg [7 blue tablets]
Day 8-16: Ethinyl estradiol 0.035 mg and norethindrone 1 mg [9 yellow-green tablets]
Day 17-21: Ethinyl estradiol 0.035 mg and norethindrone 0.5 mg [5 blue tablets]
Day 22-28: 7 orange inactive tablets (28s)

Dosing

Adult & Geriatric

Adolescents ≥15 years and Adults: Females: Acne: Estrostep® Fe: Oral: Refer to dosing for contraception

Moderate-to-severe vasomotor symptoms associated with menopause: Initial: femhrt® 0.5/2.5: Oral: 1 tablet daily; patient should be re-evaluated at 3- to 6-month intervals to determine if treatment is still necessary; patient should be maintained on lowest effective dose

Prevention of osteoporosis: Initial: femhrt® 0.5/2.5: Oral: 1 tablet daily; patient should be maintained on lowest effective dose

Contraception: Oral:

Schedule 1 (Sunday starter): Dose begins on first Sunday after onset of menstruation; if the menstrual period starts on Sunday, take first tablet that very same day. This schedule is not preferred for Lo Loestrin Fe. With a Sunday start, an additional method of contraception should be used until after the first 7 days of consecutive administration (all products).

For 21-tablet package: Dosage is 1 tablet daily for 21 consecutive days, followed by 7 days off of the medication; a new course begins on the 8th day after the last tablet is taken.

For 28-tablet package: Dosage is 1 tablet daily without interruption.

Schedule 2 (Day 1 starter): Dose starts on first day of menstrual cycle taking 1 tablet daily.

For 21-tablet package: Dosage is 1 tablet daily for 21 consecutive days, followed by 7 days off of the medication; a new course begins on the 8th day after the last tablet is taken.

For 28-tablet package: Dosage is 1 tablet daily without interruption.

If all doses have been taken on schedule and one menstrual period is missed, continue dosing cycle. If two consecutive menstrual periods are missed, pregnancy test is required before new dosing cycle is started.

Missed doses **monophasic formulations** (refer to package insert for complete information):

One dose missed: Take as soon as remembered. Take the next tablet at your regular time. You may take 2 tablets in 1 day.

Two consecutive doses missed in the first 2 weeks: Take 2 tablets as soon as remembered and 2 tablets the next day. An additional method of contraception should be used for 7 days after missed dose.

Two consecutive doses missed in week 3 (all products) or in week 4 (Lo Loestrin Fe), or three consecutive doses missed at any time (all products): An additional method of contraception must be used for 7 days after a missed dose.

Schedule 1 (Sunday starter): Continue dose of 1 tablet daily until Sunday, then discard the rest of the pack, and a new pack should be started that same day.

Schedule 2 (Day 1 starter): Current pack should be discarded, and a new pack should be started that same day.

Missed doses **biphasic/triphasic formulations** (refer to package insert for complete information):

One dose missed: Take as soon as remembered. Take the next tablet at your regular time. You may take 2 tablets in 1 day.

Two consecutive doses missed in week 1 or week 2 of the pack: Take 2 tablets as soon as remembered and 2 tablets the next day. Resume taking 1 tablet daily until the pack is empty. An additional method of contraception should be used for 7 days after a missed dose.

Two consecutive doses missed in week 3 of the pack: An additional method of contraception must be used for 7 days after a missed dose.

Schedule 1 (Sunday Starter): Take 1 tablet every day until Sunday. Discard the remaining pack and start a new pack of pills on the same day.

Schedule 2 (Day 1 starter): Discard the remaining pack and start a new pack the same day.

Three or more consecutive doses missed: An additional method of contraception must be used for 7 days after a missed dose.

Schedule 1 (Sunday Starter): Take 1 tablet every day until Sunday; on Sunday, discard the pack and start a new pack.

Schedule 2 (Day 1 Starter): Discard the remaining pack and begin new pack of tablets starting on the same day.

Switching from a different contraceptive:

Oral contraceptive: Start on the same day that a new pack of the previous oral contraceptive would have been taken.

Transdermal patch, vaginal ring, injection: Start on the day the next dose would have been due.

IUD or implant: Start on the day of removal. A backup method of contraception may be required following IUD removal.

Use after childbirth (in women who are not breast-feeding) or after second trimester abortion: Therapy may be started ≥4 weeks postpartum. Pregnancy should be ruled out prior to treatment if menstrual periods have not restarted and an additional method of contraception (nonhormonal) should be used until after the first 7 days of consecutive administration.

Pediatric Females:

Acne: Oral (Estrostep® Fe): For use in females ≥15 years; refer to adult dosing for contraception

Contraception: Oral: Refer to adult dosing; not to be used prior to menarche.

Renal Impairment Specific guidelines not available; use with caution and monitor blood pressure closely. Consider other forms of contraception.

Hepatic Impairment Contraindicated in patients with hepatic impairment.

Administration

Oral Administer at the same time each day; without regard to meals.

Lo Loestrin Fe: If vomiting or diarrhea occurs within 3-4 hours of a dose, consider the dose to be missed.

Monitoring and Teaching Issues

Physical Assessment See individual agents.

Patient Education See individual agents.

Related Information

Norethindrone *on page* 1334

Ethinyl Estradiol and Norgestimate (ETH in il es tra DYE ole & nor JES ti mate)

U.S. Brand Names MonoNessa®; Ortho Tri-Cyclen®; Ortho Tri-Cyclen® Lo; Ortho-Cyclen®; Sprintec®; Tri-Sprintec®; TriNessa®

Index Terms Ethinyl Estradiol and NGM; Norgestimate and Ethinyl Estradiol; Ortho Cyclen; Ortho Tri Cyclen

Generic Availability (U.S.) Yes

Pharmacologic Category Contraceptive; Estrogen and Progestin Combination

Medication Safety Issues

Sound-alike/look-alike issues:

Ortho-Cyclen® may be confused with Ortho-Cept®

Ortho Tri-Cyclen® may be confused with Ortho Tri-Cyclen® Lo

Ortho Tri-Cyclen® Lo may be confused with Ortho Tri-Cyclen®

International issues:

Vivelle: Brand name for ethinyl estradiol/norgestimate [Austria], but also a brand name for estradiol [U.S. (discontinued), Belgium]

Pregnancy Risk Factor X

Lactation Enters breast milk/not recommended

Use Prevention of pregnancy; treatment of acne

Unlabeled/Investigational Use Treatment of hypermenorrhea (menorrhagia); pain associated with endometriosis; dysmenorrhea; dysfunctional uterine bleeding

Available Dosage Forms

Tablet, monophasic formulations:

MonoNessa®, Ortho-Cyclen®: Ethinyl estradiol 0.035 mg and norgestimate 0.25 mg (28s) [21 blue tablets and 7 green inactive tablets]

Sprintec®: Ethinyl estradiol 0.035 mg and norgestimate 0.25 mg (28s) [21 blue tablets and 7 white inactive tablets]

Tablet, triphasic formulations:

Ortho Tri-Cyclen®, TriNessa®:

Day 1-7: Ethinyl estradiol 0.035 mg and norgestimate 0.18 mg [7 white tablets]

Day 8-14: Ethinyl estradiol 0.035 mg and norgestimate 0.215 mg [7 light blue tablets]

Day 15-21: Ethinyl estradiol 0.035 mg and norgestimate 0.25 mg [7 blue tablets]

Day 22-28: 7 green inactive tablets (28s)

Tri-Sprintec®:

Day 1-7: Ethinyl estradiol 0.035 mg and norgestimate 0.18 mg [7 gray tablets]

Day 8-14: Ethinyl estradiol 0.035 mg and norgestimate 0.215 mg [7 light blue tablets]

Day 15-21: Ethinyl estradiol 0.035 mg and norgestimate 0.25 mg [7 blue tablets]

Day 22-28: 7 white inactive tablets (28s)

Ortho Tri-Cyclen® Lo:

Day 1-7: Ethinyl estradiol 0.025 mg and norgestimate 0.18 mg [7 white tablets]

Day 8-14: Ethinyl estradiol 0.025 mg and norgestimate 0.215 mg [7 light blue tablets]

Day 15-21: Ethinyl estradiol 0.025 mg and norgestimate 0.25 mg [7 dark blue tablets]

Day 22-28: 7 green inactive tablets (28s)

Dosing

Adult Females:

Acne (Ortho Tri-Cyclen®): Oral: Refer to dosing for contraception

Contraception: Oral:

Schedule 1 (Sunday starter): Dose begins on first Sunday after onset of menstruation; if the menstrual period starts on Sunday, take first tablet that very same day. **With a Sunday start, an additional method of contraception should be used until after the first 7 days of consecutive administration.**

For 21-tablet package: Dosage is 1 tablet daily for 21 consecutive days, followed by 7 days off of the medication; a new course begins on the 8th day after the last tablet is taken.

For 28-tablet package: Dosage is 1 tablet daily without interruption.

Schedule 2 (Day 1 starter): Dose starts on first day of menstrual cycle taking 1 tablet daily.

For 21-tablet package: Dosage is 1 tablet daily for 21 consecutive days, followed by 7 days off of the medication; a new course begins on the 8th day after the last tablet is taken.

For 28-tablet package: Dosage is 1 tablet daily without interruption.

If all doses have been taken on schedule and one menstrual period is missed, continue dosing cycle. If two consecutive menstrual periods are missed, pregnancy test is required before new dosing cycle is started.

Missed doses **monophasic formulations** (refer to package insert for complete information):

One dose missed: Take as soon as remembered or take 2 tablets next day

Two consecutive doses missed in the first 2 weeks: Take 2 tablets as soon as remembered or 2 tablets next 2 days. **An additional method of contraception should be used for 7 days after missed dose.**

Two consecutive doses missed in week 3 or three consecutive doses missed at any time: **An additional method of contraception must be used for 7 days after a missed dose:**

Schedule 1 (Sunday starter): Continue dose of 1 tablet daily until Sunday, then discard the rest of the pack, and a new pack should be started that same day.

Schedule 2 (Day 1 starter): Current pack should be discarded, and a new pack should be started that same day.

Missed doses **biphasic/triphasic formulations** (refer to package insert for complete information):

One dose missed: Take as soon as remembered or take 2 tablets next day.

Two consecutive doses missed in week 1 or week 2 of the pack: Take 2 tablets as soon as remembered and 2 tablets the next day. Resume taking 1 tablet daily until the pack is empty. **An additional method of contraception must be used for 7 days after a missed dose.**

Two consecutive doses missed in week 3 of the pack. **An additional method of contraception must be used for 7 days after a missed dose.**

Schedule 1 (Sunday starter): Take 1 tablet every day until Sunday. Discard the remaining pack and start a new pack of pills on the same day.

Schedule 2 (Day 1 starter): Discard the remaining pack and start a new pack the same day.

Three or more consecutive doses missed. **An additional method of contraception must be used for 7 days after a missed dose.**

Schedule 1 (Sunday starter): Take 1 tablet every day until Sunday; on Sunday, discard the pack and start a new pack.

Schedule 2 (Day 1 starter): Discard the remaining pack and begin new pack of tablets starting on the same day.

Pediatric Females:

Acne: Oral: Children ≥15 years; refer to adult dosing for contraception

Contraception: Oral: Refer to adult dosing; not to be used prior to menarche.

Renal Impairment Specific guidelines not available; use with caution and monitor blood pressure closely. Consider other forms of contraception.

Hepatic Impairment Contraindicated in patients with hepatic impairment.

Administration

Oral Administer at the same time each day.

Monitoring and Teaching Issues

Physical Assessment Emphasize importance of regular (monthly) blood pressure checks and annual physical assessment, Pap smear, and vision assessment. Teach importance of maintaining prescribed schedule of dosing.

Patient Education Oral contraceptives do not protect against HIV or other sexually-transmitted diseases. You are at risk of becoming pregnant if doses are missed. Be aware that some medications may reduce the effectiveness of oral contraceptives; an alternate form of contraception may be needed. It is important that you check your blood pressure monthly and that you have an annual physical assessment, Pap smear, and vision assessment while taking this medication. Avoid smoking while taking this medication; smoking increases risk of adverse effects, including thromboembolic events and heart attacks. You may experience loss of appetite or constipation. Report immediately pain or muscle soreness; warmth, swelling, pain, or redness in calves; shortness of breath; sudden loss of vision; unresolved leg/foot swelling; change in menstrual pattern (unusual bleeding, amenorrhea, breakthrough spotting); breast tenderness that does not go away; acute abdominal cramping; signs of vaginal infection (drainage, pain, itching); CNS changes (blurred vision, confusion, acute anxiety, or unresolved depression); chest pain; severe headache or vomiting; weakness in arm or leg; severe abdominal pain or tenderness; jaundice; or weight gain. Notify prescriber of changes in contact lens tolerance.

Ethinyl Estradiol, Drospirenone, and Levomefolate

(ETH in il es tra DYE ole, droh SPYE re none, & lee voe me FOE late)

U.S. Brand Names Beyaz™; Safyral™

Index Terms Drospirenone, Ethinyl Estradiol, and Levomefolate Calcium; Ethinyl Estradiol, Drospirenone, and Levomefolate Calcium; Levomefolate Calcium, Drospirenone, and Ethinyl Estradiol; Levomefolate, Drospirenone, and Ethinyl Estradiol

Pharmacologic Category Contraceptive; Estrogen and Progestin Combination

Medication Safety Issues

Sound-alike/look-alike issues:

Beyaz™ may be confused with Yaz®

Lactation Enters breast milk/not recommended

Use Females: Prevention of pregnancy; treatment of premenstrual dysphoric disorder (PMDD); treatment of acne; folate supplementation

Unlabeled/Investigational Use Treatment of hypermenorrhea (menorrhagia); pain associated with endometriosis; dysmenorrhea; dysfunctional uterine bleeding

Available Dosage Forms

Tablet, oral:

Beyaz™: Ethinyl estradiol 0.02 mg, drospirenone 3 mg, and levomefolate calcium 0.451 mg [24 pink tablets] and levomefolate calcium 0.451 mg [4 light orange tablets] (28s)

Safyral™: Ethinyl estradiol 0.03 mg, drospirenone 3 mg, and levomefolate calcium 0.451 mg [21 orange tablets] and levomefolate calcium 0.451 mg [7 light orange tablets] (28s)

Dosing

Adult

Acne, PMDD: Oral: Females: (Beyaz™): Refer to dosing for contraception

Contraception: Oral: Females: (Beyaz™, Safyral™): Dosage is 1 tablet daily

Beyaz™: One pink tablet daily for 24 consecutive days, then one light orange tablet daily on days 25-28

Safyral™: One orange tablet daily for 21 consecutive days, then one light orange tablet daily on days 22-28

Dose should be taken at the same time each day, either after the evening meal or at bedtime. Dosing may be started on the first day of menstrual period (Day 1 starter) or on the first Sunday after the onset of the menstrual period (Sunday starter).

Day 1 starter: Dose starts on first day of menstrual cycle taking 1 tablet daily. If first dose is taken later than the first day of the menstrual cycle, **an additional method of contraception should be used until after the first 7 days of consecutive administration.**

Sunday starter: Dose begins on first Sunday after onset of menstruation; if the menstrual period starts on Sunday, take first tablet that very same day. **With a Sunday start, an additional method of contraception should be used until after the first 7 days of consecutive administration.**

Switching from a different contraceptive:

Oral contraceptive: Start on the same day that a new pack of the previous oral contraceptive would have been taken

Transdermal patch, vaginal ring, injection: Start on the day the next dose would have been due

IUD or implant: Start on the day of removal

Use after childbirth (in women who are not breast-feeding) or after second trimester abortion: Therapy may be started ≥4 weeks postpartum. Pregnancy should be ruled out prior to treatment if menstrual periods have not restarted and an additional method of contraception (nonhormonal) should be used until after the first 7 days of consecutive administration.

Missed doses:

If all doses have been taken on schedule and one menstrual period is missed, continue dosing cycle. If two consecutive menstrual periods are missed, rule out pregnancy and discontinue if pregnancy is confirmed.

If doses have been missed during the first 3 weeks or if active tablets (pink tablets) were started later than as directed and the menstrual period is missed, pregnancy should be ruled out prior to continuing treatment.

Missed doses (monophasic formulations) (refer to package insert for complete information):

One dose missed: Take as soon as remembered or take 2 tablets next day

Two consecutive doses missed in the first 2 weeks: Take 2 tablets as soon as remembered or 2 tablets next 2 days. **An additional method of contraception should be used for 7 days after missed dose.**

Two consecutive doses missed in week 3 or three consecutive doses missed at any time: **An additional method of contraception must be used for 7 days after a missed dose.**

Day 1 starter: Current pack should be discarded, and a new pack should be started that same day.

Sunday starter: Continue dose of 1 tablet daily until Sunday, then discard the rest of the pack, and a new pack should be started that same day.

Any number of doses missed in week 4: Throw away the pills that were missed. Continue taking one pill each day until pack is empty; no back-up method of contraception is needed

Pediatric

Acne: Females: Children ≥14 years: Oral: Refer to adult dosing.

Contraception, PMDD: Females: Oral: Refer to adult dosing; not to be used prior to menarche.

Renal Impairment Contraindicated in patients with renal dysfunction.

Hepatic Impairment Contraindicated in patients with hepatic disease. Exposure to drospirenone is ~3 times higher with moderate liver impairment; information not available for severe impairment.

Administration

Oral May be administered with or without food, but must be taken at the same time each day, preferably after the evening meal or at bedtime. If severe vomiting or diarrhea occurs, additional contraception (nonhormonal) should be used. If vomiting occurs within 3-4 hours of dosing, consider the dose to be missed.

Monitoring and Teaching Issues

Laboratory Monitoring Monitor glycemic control in patients with diabetes; lipid profiles in patients being treated for hyperlipidemias; serum potassium in high-risk patients and those on medications with potassium-retaining properties

◆ **Ethinyl Estradiol, Drospirenone, and Levomefolate Calcium** *see* Ethinyl Estradiol, Drospirenone, and Levomefolate *on page 706*

◆ **Ethoxynaphthamido Penicillin Sodium** *see* Nafcillin *on page 1282*

◆ **Ethyl Esters of Omega-3 Fatty Acids** *see* Omega-3-Acid Ethyl Esters *on page 1355*

◆ **Ethynodiol Diacetate and Ethinyl Estradiol** *see* Ethinyl Estradiol and Ethynodiol Diacetate *on page 698*

Etodolac (ee toe DOE lak)

Index Terms Etodolic Acid; Lodine

Generic Availability (U.S.) Yes

Pharmacologic Category Nonsteroidal Anti-inflammatory Drug (NSAID), Oral

Medication Safety Issues

Sound-alike/look-alike issues:

Lodine® may be confused with codeine, iodine, Iopidine®, Lopid®

Medication Guide Available Yes

Pregnancy Risk Factor C

Lactation Excretion in breast milk unknown/not recommended

Use Acute and long-term use in the management of signs and symptoms of osteoarthritis; rheumatoid arthritis and juvenile idiopathic arthritis (JIA); management of acute pain

Mechanism of Action/Effect Reversibly inhibits cyclooxygenase-1 and 2 (COX-1 and 2) enzymes, which results in decreased formation of prostaglandin precursors; has antipyretic, analgesic, and anti-inflammatory properties

Contraindications Hypersensitivity to etodolac, aspirin, other NSAIDs, or any component of the formulation; perioperative pain in the setting of coronary artery bypass graft (CABG) surgery

Warnings/Precautions [U.S. Boxed Warning]: NSAIDs are associated with an increased risk of adverse cardiovascular thrombotic events, including MI and stroke. Risk may be increased with duration of use or pre-existing cardiovascular risk factors or disease. Carefully evaluate individual cardiovascular risk profiles prior to prescribing. May cause new-onset hypertension or worsening of existing hypertension. Use caution with fluid retention. Avoid use in heart failure. Concurrent administration of ibuprofen, and potentially other nonselective NSAIDs, may interfere with aspirin's cardioprotective effect. **[U.S. Boxed Warning]: Use is contraindicated for treatment of perioperative pain in the setting of coronary artery bypass graft (CABG) surgery.** Risk of MI and stroke may be increased with use following CABG surgery.

[U.S. Boxed Warning]: NSAIDs may increase risk of gastrointestinal irritation, inflammation, ulceration, bleeding, and perforation. These events may occur at any time during therapy and without warning. Use caution with a history of GI disease (bleeding or ulcers), concurrent therapy with aspirin, anticoagulants and/or corticosteroids, smoking, use of alcohol, the elderly or debilitated patients. When used concomitantly with ≤325 mg of aspirin, a substantial increase in the risk of gastrointestinal complications (eg, ulcer) occurs; concomitant gastroprotective therapy (eg, proton pump inhibitors) is recommended (Bhatt, 2008).

Platelet adhesion and aggregation may be decreased; may prolong bleeding time; patients with coagulation disorders or who are receiving anticoagulants should be monitored closely. Anemia may occur; patients on long-term NSAID therapy should be monitored for anemia. Rarely, NSAID use may cause severe blood dyscrasias (eg, agranulocytosis, aplastic anemia, thrombocytopenia).

NSAID use may compromise existing renal function; dose-dependent decreases in prostaglandin synthesis may result from NSAID use, reducing renal blood flow which may cause renal decompensation. NSAID use may increase the risk for hyperkalemia. Patients with impaired renal function, dehydration, heart failure, liver dysfunction, those taking diuretics and ACE inhibitors, and the elderly are at greater risk for renal toxicity and hyperkalemia. Rehydrate patient before starting therapy; monitor renal function closely. Not recommended for use in patients with advanced renal disease. Long-term NSAID use may result in renal papillary necrosis.

Use the lowest effective dose for the shortest duration of time, consistent with individual patient goals, to reduce risk of cardiovascular or GI adverse events. Alternate therapies should be considered for patients at high risk.

NSAIDs may cause serious skin adverse events including exfoliative dermatitis, Stevens-Johnson syndrome (SJS), and toxic epidermal necrolysis (TEN); discontinue use at first sign of skin rash or hypersensitivity. Anaphylactoid reactions may occur, even without prior exposure; patients with "aspirin triad" (bronchial asthma, aspirin intolerance, rhinitis) may be at increased risk. Do not use in patients who experience bronchospasm, asthma, rhinitis, or urticaria with NSAID or aspirin therapy. Use caution in other forms of asthma.

Use with caution in patients with decreased hepatic function. Closely monitor patients with any abnormal LFT. Severe hepatic reactions (eg, fulminant hepatitis, liver failure) have occurred with NSAID use, rarely; discontinue if signs or symptoms of liver disease develop, or if systemic manifestations occur.

NSAIDS may cause drowsiness, dizziness, blurred vision and other neurologic effects which may impair physical or mental abilities; patients must be cautioned about performing tasks which require mental alertness (eg, operating machinery or driving). Discontinue use with blurred or diminished vision and perform ophthalmologic exam. Monitor vision with long-term therapy. The elderly are at increased risk for adverse effects (especially peptic ulceration, CNS effects, renal toxicity) from NSAIDs even at low doses.

Withhold for at least 4-6 half-lives prior to surgical or dental procedures.

Use of extended release product consisting of a nondeformable matrix should be avoided in patients with stricture/narrowing of the GI tract; symptoms of obstruction have been associated with nondeformable products.

Drug Interactions

Avoid Concomitant Use

Avoid concomitant use of Etodolac with any of the following: Ketorolac; Ketorolac (Systemic)

Decreased Effect

Etodolac may decrease the levels/effects of: ACE Inhibitors; Angiotensin II Receptor Blockers; Antiplatelet Agents; Beta-Blockers; Eplerenone; HydrALAZINE; Loop Diuretics; Potassium-Sparing Diuretics; Salicylates; Thiazide Diuretics

The levels/effects of Etodolac may be decreased by: Bile Acid Sequestrants; Nonsteroidal Anti-Inflammatory Agents; Salicylates

Increased Effect/Toxicity

Etodolac may increase the levels/effects of: Aminoglycosides; Anticoagulants; Antiplatelet Agents; Bisphosphonate Derivatives; Collagenase (Systemic); CycloSPORINE; CycloSPORINE (Systemic); Desmopressin; Digoxin; Drotrecogin Alfa; Eplerenone; Haloperidol; Ibritumomab; Lithium; Methotrexate; Nonsteroidal Anti-Inflammatory Agents; PEMEtrexed; Potassium-Sparing Diuretics; PRALAtrexate; Quinolone Antibiotics; Salicylates; Thrombolytic Agents; Tositumomab and Iodine I 131 Tositumomab; Vancomycin; Vitamin K Antagonists

The levels/effects of Etodolac may be increased by: Antidepressants (Tricyclic, Tertiary Amine); Corticosteroids (Systemic); Dasatinib; Glucosamine; Herbs (Anticoagulant/Antiplatelet Properties); Ketorolac; Ketorolac (Systemic); Nonsteroidal Anti-Inflammatory Agents; Omega-3-Acid Ethyl Esters; Pentosan Polysulfate Sodium; Pentoxifylline; Probenecid; Prostacyclin Analogues; Selective Serotonin Reuptake Inhibitors; Serotonin/Norepinephrine Reuptake Inhibitors; Treprostinil

Nutritional/Ethanol Interactions

Ethanol: Avoid ethanol (may enhance gastric mucosal irritation).

Food: Etodolac peak serum levels may be decreased if taken with food.

Herb/Nutraceutical: Avoid alfalfa, anise, bilberry, bladderwrack, bromelain, cat's claw, celery, chamomile, coleus, cordyceps, dong quai, evening primrose, fenugreek, feverfew, garlic, ginger, ginkgo biloba, ginseng (American, Panax, Siberian), grapeseed, green tea, guggul, horse chestnut seed, horseradish, licorice, prickly ash, red clover, reishi, SAMe (S-adenosylmethionine), sweet clover, turmeric, white willow (all have additional antiplatelet activity).

Lab Interactions False-positive for urinary bilirubin and ketone

Adverse Reactions 1% to 10%:

Central nervous system: Dizziness (3% to 9%), chills/fever (1% to 3%), depression (1% to 3%), nervousness (1% to 3%)

Dermatologic: Rash (1% to 3%), pruritus (1% to 3%)

Gastrointestinal: Dyspepsia (10%), abdominal cramps (3% to 9%), diarrhea (3% to 9%), flatulence (3% to 9%), nausea (3% to 9%), vomiting (1% to 3%), constipation (1% to 3%), melena (1% to 3%), gastritis (1% to 3%)

Genitourinary: Dysuria (1% to 3%)

Neuromuscular & skeletal: Weakness (3% to 9%)

Ocular: Blurred vision (1% to 3%)

Otic: Tinnitus (1% to 3%)

Renal: Polyuria (1% to 3%)

Pharmacodynamics/Kinetics

Onset of Action Analgesic: 2-4 hours; Maximum anti-inflammatory effect: A few days

Absorption ≥80%

Bioavailability 100%

Time to Peak Immediate release: Adults: 1-2 hours; Extended release: 5-7 hours, increased 1.4-3.8 hours with food

Protein Binding ≥99%, primarily albumin

Half-Life Elimination Terminal: Adults: 5-8 hours; Extended release: Children (6-16 years): 12 hours

Metabolism Hepatic

Excretion Urine 73% (1% unchanged); feces 16%

Available Dosage Forms

Capsule, oral: 200 mg, 300 mg

Tablet, oral: 400 mg, 500 mg

Tablet, extended release, oral: 400 mg, 500 mg, 600 mg

Dosing

Adult & Geriatric Note: For chronic conditions, response is usually observed within 2 weeks.

Acute pain: Oral: Immediate release formulation: 200-400 mg every 6-8 hours, as needed, not to exceed total daily doses of 1000 mg

Rheumatoid arthritis, osteoarthritis: Oral:

Immediate release formulation: 400 mg 2 times/day **or** 300 mg 2-3 times/day **or** 500 mg 2 times/day (doses >1000 mg/day have not been evaluated)

Extended release formulation: 400-1000 mg once daily

Pediatric Note: For chronic conditions, response is usually observed within 2 weeks.

Juvenile idiopathic arthritis (JIA): Oral: Extended release formulation: Children 6-16 years:

20-30 kg: 400 mg once daily

31-45 kg: 600 mg once daily

46-60 kg: 800 mg once daily

Children >60 kg: 1000 mg once daily

Renal Impairment

Mild-to-moderate: No adjustment required

Severe: Use not recommended; use with caution

Hemodialysis: Not removed

Hepatic Impairment No adjustment required.

Administration

Oral May be administered with food to decrease GI upset.

Stability

Storage Store at 20°C to 25°C (68°F to 77°F). Protect from moisture.

Monitoring and Teaching Issues

Laboratory Monitoring CBC, liver enzymes; in patients receiving diuretics, monitor BUN/serum creatinine.

Physical Assessment Evaluate cardiac risk and potential for GI bleeding prior to prescribing this medication. Monitor blood pressure at the beginning of therapy and periodically during use.

Patient Education Do not crush tablets or break capsules. Take with food or milk to reduce GI distress. Do not use alcohol. You may experience anorexia, nausea, vomiting, heartburn, drowsiness, dizziness, nervousness, headache, or fluid retention; GI bleeding, ulceration, or perforation can occur with or without pain; discontinue medication and contact prescriber if persistent abdominal pain or cramping or blood in stool occurs. Report respiratory difficulty or unusual cough; chest pain, rapid heartbeat, or palpitations; bruising/bleeding; blood in urine, stool, mouth, or vomitus; swollen extremities; skin rash; fever; jaundice; abdominal tenderness; flu-like symptoms; or ringing in ears.

Dietary Considerations May be taken with food to decrease GI upset.

Geriatric Considerations The elderly are a high-risk population for adverse effects from nonsteroidal anti-inflammatory agents. As much as 60% of older adults who experience GI side effects can develop peptic ulceration and/or hemorrhage asymptomatically. The concomitant use of H_2 blockers and sucralfate is not effective as prophylaxis with the exception of NSAID-induced duodenal ulcers which may be prevented by the use of ranitidine. Misoprostol and proton pump inhibitors are the only agents proven to help prevent the development of NSAID-induced ulcers. Also, concomitant disease and drug use contribute to the risk for GI adverse effects. Use lowest effective dose for shortest period possible. Consider renal function decline with age. Use of NSAIDs can compromise existing renal function especially when Cl_{cr} is ≤30 mL/minute.

Tinnitus may be a difficult and unreliable indication of toxicity due to age-related hearing loss or eighth cranial nerve damage. CNS adverse effects such as confusion, agitation, and hallucination are generally seen in overdose or high dose situations, but older adults may demonstrate these adverse effects at lower doses than younger adults. In patients ≥65 years, no substantial differences in the pharmacokinetics or side-effects profile were seen compared with the general population. Studies with etodolac in elderly demonstrated no difference in safety or efficacy compared to younger adults. No dosing adjustment necessary in elderly.

Breast-Feeding Considerations It is not known if etodolac is excreted into breast milk. Use of etodolac while breast-feeding is not recommended by the manufacturer.

Pregnancy Considerations Adverse events were not observed in the initial animal reproduction studies; therefore, the manufacturer classifies etodolac as pregnancy category C. NSAID exposure during the first trimester is not strongly associated with congenital malformations; however, cardiovascular anomalies and cleft palate have been observed following NSAID exposure in some studies. The use of an NSAID close to conception may be associated with an increased risk of miscarriage. Nonteratogenic effects have been observed following NSAID administration during the third trimester including: Myocardial degenerative changes, prenatal constriction of the ductus arteriosus, fetal tricuspid regurgitation, failure of the ductus arteriosus to close postnatally; renal dysfunction or failure, oligohydramnios; gastrointestinal bleeding or perforation, increased risk of necrotizing enterocolitis; intracranial bleeding (including intraventricular hemorrhage), platelet dysfunction with resultant bleeding; pulmonary hypertension. Because they may cause premature closure of the ductus arteriosus, use of NSAIDs late in pregnancy should be avoided (use after 31 or 32 weeks gestation is not recommended by some clinicians). The chronic use of NSAIDs in women of reproductive age may be associated with infertility that is reversible upon discontinuation of the medication.

Related Information

Nonsalicylate / Nonsteroidal Anti-Inflammatory Agents *on page 2002*

◆ **Etodolic Acid** *see* Etodolac *on page 707*

Etonogestrel (e toe noe JES trel)

U.S. Brand Names Implanon™

Index Terms 3-Keto-desogestrel; ENG

Generic Availability (U.S.) No

Pharmacologic Category Contraceptive; Progestin

Prescribing and Access Restrictions Only healthcare providers who have undergone training in the insertion and removal procedures will be able to order Implanon™. Materials related to the insertion and removal of Implanon™ are available from the manufacturer (877-467-5266).

Lactation Enters breast milk/use caution

Use Prevention of pregnancy; for use in women who request long-acting (up to 3 years) contraception

Mechanism of Action/Effect Etonogestrel is the active metabolite of desogestrel. It prevents pregnancy by suppressing ovulation, increasing the viscosity of cervical mucous, and inhibiting endometrial proliferation.

Contraindications Hypersensitivity to etonogestrel or any component of the formulation; undiagnosed abnormal uterine bleeding; active hepatic disease or tumors; active thrombophlebitis or thromboembolic disorders (current or history of); known/suspected or history of carcinoma of the breast; pregnancy

Warnings/Precautions Use does not protect against HIV infection or other sexually-transmitted diseases. Insert intradermally; should be palpable after implanted. Improper insertion may lead to unintended pregnancy or may cause difficult or impossible removal. Failure to properly remove may lead to infertility, ectopic pregnancy, or continued adverse reactions. Menstrual bleeding patterns are likely to be altered; patients should be counseled prior to implant insertion. Abnormal bleeding should be evaluated as required to exclude pathologic conditions or pregnancy. Ectopic pregnancy (rare) may occur more commonly than in women using no contraception. Etonogestrel serum levels and contraceptive efficacy may be significantly decreased by potent hepatic enzyme inducers. The manufacturer does not recommend use in women chronically taking hepatic enzyme inducers. Use caution in overweight women; women >130% of ideal body weight were not included in clinical studies. Use caution with renal disease. Women with renal disease should be encouraged to use a nonhormonal form of contraception. Use in contraindicated with hepatic disease; remove implant if jaundice develops. May increase the risk of thromboembolism. Consider removal during periods of prolonged immobilization

Additional warnings based on combination hormonal (estrogen and progestin) contraceptives: The risk of cardiovascular side effects increases in women who smoke cigarettes, especially those who are >35 years of age; women who use combination hormonal contraceptives should be strongly advised not to smoke. Combination hormonal contraceptives may lead to increased risk of myocardial infarction; use with caution in patients with risk factors for coronary artery disease. Whenever possible, combination hormonal contraceptives should be discontinued at least 4 weeks prior to and for 2 weeks following elective surgery associated with an increased risk of thromboembolism or during periods of prolonged immobilization. Combination hormonal contraceptives may have a dose-related risk of vascular disease, hypertension, and gallbladder disease. Women with hypertension should be encouraged to use another form of contraception. The use of combination hormonal contraceptives has been associated with a slight increase in frequency of breast cancer; however, studies are not consistent. Combination hormonal contraceptives may cause carbohydrate intolerance or effect serum triglyceride and lipoprotein levels. Retinal thrombosis has been reported (rarely). Use caution with conditions that may be aggravated by fluid retention, depression, or history of migraine. Extremely rare adenomas and focal nodular hyperplasia resulting in fatal intra-abdominal hemorrhage have been reported in association with long-term oral contraceptive use. Presentation of an abdominal mass, acute abdominal pain, or intra-abdominal bleeding warrants further evaluation to rule out source. Not for use prior to menarche.

Drug Interactions

Metabolism/Transport Effects Substrate of CYP3A4 (minor)

Avoid Concomitant Use

Avoid concomitant use of Etonogestrel with any of the following: Griseofulvin

Decreased Effect

Etonogestrel may decrease the levels/effects of: Vitamin K Antagonists

The levels/effects of Etonogestrel may be decreased by: Acitretin; Aminoglutethimide; Aprepitant; Artemether; Barbiturates; Bile Acid Sequestrants; Bosentan; CarBAMazepine; Efavirenz; Felbamate; Fosaprepitant; Griseofulvin; LamoTRIgine; Mycophenolate; OXcarbazepine; Phenytoin; Retinoic Acid Derivatives; Rifamycin Derivatives; St Johns Wort; Topiramate

Increased Effect/Toxicity

Etonogestrel may increase the levels/effects of: Benzodiazepines (metabolized by oxidation); Selegiline; Tranexamic Acid; Voriconazole

The levels/effects of Etonogestrel may be increased by: Conivaptan; Herbs (Progestogenic Properties); Voriconazole

Nutritional/Ethanol Interactions

Herb/Nutraceutical: St John's wort (an enzyme inducer) may decrease serum levels of etonogestrel. Concomitant use is not recommended. Bloodroot, chasteberry, damiana, oregano, and yucca may enhance the adverse/toxic effect of progestins.

Adverse Reactions

>10%:

Central nervous system: Headache (25%)

Dermatologic: Acne (14%)

Endocrine & metabolic: Infrequent menstrual bleeding (<3 episodes/90 days: 34%), amenorrhea (no bleeding in 90 days: 22%), prolonged menstrual bleeding (lasting >14 days: 18%), breast pain (13%), menstrual bleeding irregularities requiring discontinuation (11%)

Gastrointestinal: Weight gain (14%), abdominal pain (11%)

Genitourinary: Vaginitis (15%)

Respiratory: Upper respiratory tract infection (13%), pharyngitis (11%)

5% to 10%:

Central nervous system: Dizziness (7%), emotional lability (7%), depression (6%), nervousness (6%), pain (6%)

Endocrine & metabolic: Dysmenorrhea (7%), frequent menstrual bleeding (>5 episodes/90 days: 7%)

Gastrointestinal: Nausea (6%)

Genitourinary: Leukorrhea (10%)

Local: Insertion site pain (5%)

Neuromuscular & skeletal: Back pain (7%)

Respiratory: Sinusitis (6%)

Miscellaneous: Flu-like syndrome (8%)

Pharmacodynamics/Kinetics

Onset of Action Serum levels sufficient to inhibit ovulation: ≤8 hours of implant

Duration of Action Implant: Each rod maintains etonogestrel levels sufficient to inhibit ovulation for 3 years

Bioavailability Implant: 100%

Protein Binding Albumin (66%) and sex hormone binding globulin (32%)

Half-Life Elimination ~25 hours

Metabolism Hepatic via CYP3A4; forms metabolites (activity not known)

Excretion Urine (primarily); feces

Available Dosage Forms

Rod, subdermal:

Implanon™: 68 mg

Dosing

Adult Contraception: Subdermal: Implant 1 rod in the inner side of the upper, nondominant arm. Remove no later than 3 years after the date of insertion. After ruling out pregnancy, timing of insertion is based on the patient's contraceptive history:

No hormonal contraceptives within the past month: Insert between days 1 through 5 of menstruation, even if woman is still bleeding

Switching from combination hormonal contraceptive:

Oral tablet: Insert anytime within 7 days after the last active tablet

Vaginal ring: Insert anytime during the 7-day ring-free period

Transdermal system: Insert anytime during the 7-day patch-free period

Switching from a progestin-only contraceptive:

Oral pill: Any day during the month; do not skip days between the last pill and implant insertion

Implant: Insert on same day as removal of implant

IUD: Insert on same day as removal of IUD

Injection: Insert on day next injection is due

First trimester abortion or miscarriage: Insert immediately. If not inserted within first 5 days follow directions for "no hormonal contraception within the past month"

Following delivery or second trimester abortion: May insert between 21 and 28 days (if not exclusively breast-feeding) or after 4 weeks (if exclusively breast-feeding). Patients should use a second form of contraception for the first 7 days if insertion occurs at >4 weeks.

Note: If following above insertion schedule, no back-up contraception needed. If deviating, use back-up method for 7 days postinsertion.

Geriatric Not for use after menopause

Pediatric Not for use prior to menarche

Renal Impairment Use with caution; formal studies have not been conducted.

Hepatic Impairment Use is contraindicated.

Administration

Other Subdermal: For insertion under local anesthesia by healthcare providers trained in the insertion and removal procedure. Rod must be palpable after insertion. Deep insertion may require surgery to remove. If rod is impalpable, ultrasound should be used to locate the rod; MRI may also be useful if ultrasound is not successful. A pressure bandage should be applied and left in place for 24 hours after insertion to decrease bruising; a small bandage placed over the insertion site should remain in place for 3-5 days.

Stability

Storage Store at controlled room temperature of 25°C (77°F); excursions permitted to 15°C to 30°C (59°F to 86°F). Protect from light.

Monitoring and Teaching Issues

Laboratory Monitoring Before starting therapy, a Papanicolaou smear; pregnancy should be ruled out prior to use; monitor glycemic control in patients with diabetes; lipid profiles in patients being treated for hyperlipidemias

Physical Assessment Assess insertion site.

Patient Education Does not protect against HIV or other sexually transmitted diseases. Regular gynecological and self-breast exams are important. Changes in menstrual periods may occur (change in frequency, length, or spotting between periods). Use of a backup method of birth control is recommended for 7 days after insertion. Periodically check for the presence of the device. If the device cannot be felt, use an alternative form of birth control until your prescriber confirms its presence. You will be given a user card to document the insertion of the device. Keep track of the removal date. You may experience acne, breast pain, weight gain, vaginal discharge, back pain, dizziness, or nausea. Report excessive vaginal bleeding, depression or severe mood swings, persistent or severe headaches, chest pain, coughing up blood, shortness of breath, pain in legs, or abdominal pain.

Breast-Feeding Considerations Etonogestrel was not found to affect the quality or quantity of breast milk. Do not insert <21 days postpartum. Levels of etonogestrel are highest during the first month following insertion (~2.2% of the weight-adjusted maternal daily dose).

Pregnancy Considerations Teratogenic effects were not observed in animal studies. Not for use during pregnancy; rule out pregnancy prior to insertion. Remove implant if pregnancy is detected during use. Ovulation may return within 1 week of implant removal; alternate forms of contraception may be required. In a multicenter clinical trial, 11 out of 46 women no longer using contraception became pregnant between 1 and 18 weeks following removal of the implant. Do not insert <21 days postpartum. Women weighing >130% of their ideal body weight were not included in clinical studies. With oral combination hormonal contraceptives, an increase in contraceptive failure was noted in women with a BMI >27.3. Similar findings were noted in patients weighing ≥90 kg (198 lb) using the contraceptive patch.

Additional Information For subdermal insertion by healthcare providers trained on the insertion and removal procedure. For use in women who request long-acting (up to 3 years) contraception. A User Card (to give to the patient), consent form (to keep on file), and a medication guide (for the patient) are provided with the device. Materials related to the insertion and removal of Implanon™ are available from the manufacturer (877-467-5266).

The rod releases etonogestrel at a rate of 60-70 mcg/day, decreasing to 35-45 mcg/day after the first year, 30-40 mcg/day after the second year, and 25-30 mcg/day at the end of the third year. Following removal of rod, levels decrease rapidly and are less than the level of detection within 1 week.

◆ **ETOP** *see* Etoposide Phosphate *on page 715*

◆ **Etopophos®** *see* Etoposide Phosphate *on page 715*

Etoposide (e toe POE side)

U.S. Brand Names Toposar®

Index Terms EPEG; Epipodophyllotoxin; VePesid; VP-16; VP-16-213

Generic Availability (U.S.) Yes

Pharmacologic Category Antineoplastic Agent, Podophyllotoxin Derivative; Antineoplastic Agent, Topoisomerase II Inhibitor

Medication Safety Issues

Sound-alike/look-alike issues:

- Etoposide may be confused with teniposide
- Etoposide may be confused with etoposide phosphate (a prodrug of etoposide which is rapidly converted in the plasma to etoposide)
- VePesid® may be confused with Versed

High alert medication: This medication is in a class the Institute for Safe Medication Practices (ISMP) includes among its list of drug classes which have a heightened risk of causing significant patient harm when used in error.

Pregnancy Risk Factor D

Lactation Excretion in breast milk unknown/not recommended

Use Treatment of refractory testicular tumors (injectable formulation); treatment of small cell lung cancer

Unlabeled/Investigational Use Treatment of acute lymphocytic leukemia (ALL), refractory acute myeloid leukemia (AML), recurrent or metastatic breast cancer, central nervous system tumors, Ewing's sarcoma, gestational trophoblastic disease, Hodgkin's lymphoma, merkel cell cancer, refractory multiple myeloma, neuroblastoma, neuroendocrine tumors (adrenal gland and carcinoid tumors), non-Hodgkin's lymphomas, nonsmall-cell lung cancer (NSCLC), osteosarcoma, ovarian cancer, prostate cancer, retinoblastoma, metastatic soft tissue sarcoma, thymic malignancies, unknown-primary adenocarcinoma, Wilms' tumor; conditioning regimen for hematopoietic cell transplantation

Mechanism of Action/Effect Inhibits DNA synthesis leading to cell death.

Contraindications Hypersensitivity to etoposide or any component of the formulation

Warnings/Precautions Hazardous agent - use appropriate precautions for handling and disposal. **[U.S. Boxed Warning]: Severe dose-limiting and dose-related myelosuppression with resulting infection or bleeding may occur.** Treatment should be withheld for platelets <50,000/mm^3 or absolute neutrophil count (ANC) <500/mm^3. May cause anaphylactic-like reactions manifested by chills, fever, tachycardia, bronchospasm, dyspnea, and hypotension. In addition, facial/tongue swelling, coughing, chest tightness, cyanosis, laryngospasm, diaphoresis, hypertension, and flushing have also been reported less commonly. Incidence is primarily associated with intravenous administration (up to 2%) compared to oral administration (<1%). Infusion should be interrupted and medications for the treatment of anaphylaxis should be available for immediate use. High drug concentration and rate of infusion, as well as presence of polysorbate 80 and benzyl alcohol in the etoposide intravenous formulation have been suggested as contributing factors to the development of hypersensitivity reactions. Etoposide intravenous formulations may contain polysorbate 80 and/or benzyl alcohol, while etoposide phosphate (the water soluble prodrug of etoposide) intravenous formulation does not contain either vehicle. Case reports have suggested that etoposide phosphate has been used successfully in patients with previous hypersensitivity reactions to etoposide (Collier, 2008; Siderov, 2002). The use of concentrations higher than recommended were associated with higher rates of anaphylactic-like reactions in children.

Secondary acute leukemias have been reported with etoposide, either as monotherapy or in combination with other chemotherapy agents. Must be diluted; do not give I.V. push, infuse over at least 30-60 minutes; hypotension is associated with rapid infusion. If hypotension occurs, interrupt infusion and administer I.V. hydration and supportive care; decrease infusion upon reinitiation. Dosage should be adjusted in patients with hepatic or renal impairment. Use with caution in patients with low serum albumin; may increase risk for toxicities. Use with caution in elderly patients; may be more likely to develop severe myelosuppression and/or GI effects (eg, nausea/vomiting). **[U.S. Boxed Warning]: Should be administered under the supervision of an experienced cancer chemotherapy physician.** Injectable formulation contains polysorbate 80; do not use in premature infants. May contain benzyl alcohol; do not use in newborn infants.

Drug Interactions

Metabolism/Transport Effects **Substrate** of CYP1A2 (minor), CYP2E1 (minor), CYP3A4 (major), P-glycoprotein; **Inhibits** CYP2C9 (weak), 3A4 (weak)

Avoid Concomitant Use

Avoid concomitant use of Etoposide with any of the following: BCG; Natalizumab; Pimecrolimus; Roflumilast; Tacrolimus (Topical); Vaccines (Live)

Decreased Effect

Etoposide may decrease the levels/effects of: BCG; Sipuleucel-T; Vaccines (Inactivated); Vaccines (Live); Vitamin K Antagonists

The levels/effects of Etoposide may be decreased by: Barbiturates; CYP3A4 Inducers (Strong); Deferasirox; Echinacea; Herbs (CYP3A4 Inducers); P-Glycoprotein Inducers; Phenytoin

Increased Effect/Toxicity

Etoposide may increase the levels/effects of: Leflunomide; Natalizumab; Vaccines (Live); Vitamin K Antagonists

The levels/effects of Etoposide may be increased by: Atovaquone; Conivaptan; CycloSPORINE; CycloSPORINE (Systemic); CYP3A4 Inhibitors (Moderate); CYP3A4 Inhibitors (Strong); Dasatinib; Denosumab; P-Glycoprotein Inhibitors; Pimecrolimus; Roflumilast; Tacrolimus (Topical); Trastuzumab

Nutritional/Ethanol Interactions

Ethanol: Avoid ethanol (may increase GI irritation).

Herb/Nutraceutical: Avoid concurrent St John's wort; may decrease etoposide levels.

Adverse Reactions Note: The following may occur with higher doses used in stem cell transplantation: Alopecia, ethanol intoxication, hepatitis, hypotension (infusion-related), metabolic acidosis, mucositis, nausea and vomiting (severe), secondary malignancy, skin lesions (resembling Stevens-Johnson syndrome).

>10%:

- Dermatologic: Alopecia (8% to 66%)
- Gastrointestinal: Nausea/vomiting (31% to 43%), anorexia (10% to 13%), diarrhea (1% to 13%)
- Hematologic: Leukopenia (60% to 91%; grade 4: 3% to 17%; nadir: 7-14 days; recovery: by day 20), thrombocytopenia (22% to 41%; grades 3/4: 1% to 20%; nadir 9-16 days; recovery: by day 20), anemia (≤33%)

1% to 10%:

- Cardiovascular: Hypotension (1% to 2%; due to rapid infusion)
- Gastrointestinal: Stomatitis (1% to 6%), abdominal pain (up to 2%)
- Hepatic: Hepatic toxicity (up to 3%)
- Neuromuscular & skeletal: Peripheral neuropathy (1% to 2%)
- Miscellaneous: Anaphylactic-like reaction (I.V. infusion 1% to 2%; oral capsules <1%; including chills, fever, tachycardia, bronchospasm, dyspnea)

Pharmacodynamics/Kinetics

Absorption Oral: Significant inter- and intrapatient variation

Bioavailability Oral: ~50% (range: 25% to 75%)

Protein Binding 94% to 98%

Half-Life Elimination Terminal: I.V.: 4-11 hours; Children: Normal renal/hepatic function: 6-8 hours

Metabolism Hepatic, via CYP3A4 and 3A5, to various metabolites; in addition, conversion of etoposide to the O-demethylated metabolites (catechol and quinine) via prostaglandin synthases or myeloperoxidase occurs, as well as glutathione and glucuronide conjugation via GSTT1/GSTP1 and UGT1A1 (Yang, 2009)

Excretion

Children: I.V.: Urine (~55% as unchanged drug) in 24 hours

Adults: I.V.: Urine (56%; 45% as unchanged drug) within 120 hours; feces (44%) within 120 hours

Available Dosage Forms

Capsule, softgel, oral: 50 mg

Injection, solution: 20 mg/mL (5 mL, 25 mL, 50 mL, 100 mL)

Toposar®: 20 mg/mL (5 mL, 25 mL, 50 mL)

Dosing

Adult & Geriatric Details concerning dosing in combination regimens should also be consulted:

Small cell lung cancer (in combination with other chemotherapy agents):

I.V.: 35 mg/m²/day for 4 days, up to 50 mg/m²/day for 5 days every 3-4 weeks

Oral: Due to poor bioavailability, oral doses should be twice the I.V. dose (and rounded to the nearest 50 mg)

Small cell lung cancer, limited stage (unlabeled combination chemotherapy dosing): I.V.: 120 mg/m²/day on days 1, 2, and 3 every 3 weeks for 4 courses (Turrisi, 1999) **or** 100 mg/m²/day on days 1, 2, and 3 for induction therapy, followed by consolidation chemotherapy (Saito, 2006) **or** 100 mg/m²/day on days 1, 2, and 3 every 3 weeks up to a maximum of 6 cycles (Skarlos, 2001) **or** 100 mg/m²/day I.V. on day 1, followed by 200 mg/m²/day **orally** on days 2 through 4 every 3 weeks for a maximum of 5 courses (Sundstrom, 2002)

Small cell lung cancer, extensive stage (unlabeled combination chemotherapy dosing): 100 mg/m²/day I.V. on day 1, followed by 200 mg/m²/day **orally** on days 2 through 4 every 3 weeks for a maximum of 5 courses (Sundstrom, 2002) **or** I.V.: 80 mg/m²/day on days 1, 2, and 3 every 3 weeks up to 8 cycles (Ihede, 1994)

Testicular cancer (in combination with other chemotherapy agents): I.V.: 50-100 mg/m²/day for 1-5 days **or** 100 mg/m²/day on days 1, 3, and 5 repeated every 3-4 weeks

Testicular cancer (unlabeled combination chemotherapy dosing):

Nonseminoma: I.V.: 100 mg/m²/day on days 1 through 5 every 21 days for 3-4 courses (Saxman, 1998)

Nonseminoma, metastatic (high-dose regimens): I.V.: 750 mg/m²/day administered 5, 4, and 3 days before peripheral blood stem cell infusion, repeat for a second cycle after recovery of granulocyte and platelet counts (Einhorn, 2007) **or** 400 mg/m²/day (beginning on cycle 3) on days 1, 2, and 3, with peripheral blood stem cell support, administered at 14- to 21-day intervals for 3 cycles (Kondagunta, 2007)

Lymphoid malignancies, conditioning regimen for hematopoietic cell transplantation (unlabeled use): I.V.: 60 mg/kg over 4 hours as a single dose 3 or 4 days prior to transplantation (Horning, 1994; Snyder, 1993; Weaver, 2004)

Pediatric Details concerning dosing in combination regimens should also be consulted:

AML induction (unlabeled use) (Woods, 1996): I.V.:

<3 years: 3.3 mg/kg/day continuous infusion for 4 days

≥3 years: 100 mg/m²/day continuous infusion for 4 days

Brain tumor (unlabeled use): I.V.:

<3 years: 6.5 mg/kg/dose days 3 and 4 of each 28-day "B" treatment cycle (Duffner, 1993)

≥3 years: 100 mg/m²/day on days 1, 2, and 3 of a 3-week treatment cycle (Taylor, 2003)

≥6 years: 150 mg/m²/day on days 3 and 4 of a 3-week treatment course (Kovnar, 1990)

Conditioning regimen for hematopoietic stem cell transplantation: I.V.: 60 mg/kg/dose over 4 hours as a single dose 3 or 4 days prior to transplantation (Horning, 1994; Snyder, 1993)

Hodgkin's lymphoma (unlabeled use): I.V.: 200 mg/m²/day on days 1, 2, and 3 every 3 weeks (Kelly, 2002)

Neuroblastoma (unlabeled use): I.V.:

Induction: 100 mg/m²/day on days 1-5 of each cycle (Kaneko, 2002)

Preconditioning regimen (prior to transplantation): 200 mg/m²/day for 4 days beginning 8 or 9 days prior to transplantation (Kaneko, 2002)

Sarcoma, refractory (unlabeled use): I.V.: 100 mg/m²/day on days 1-5 of cycle; repeat cycle every 21 days (Van Winkle, 2005)

Renal Impairment

The FDA-approved labeling recommends the following adjustments:

Cl_{cr} >50 mL/minute: No adjustment required.

Cl_{cr} 15-50 mL/minute: Administer 75% of dose

Cl_{cr} <15 mL minute: Data not available; consider further dose reductions

The following guidelines have been used by some clinicians:

Aronoff, 2007:

Cl_{cr} 10-50 mL/minute: Children and Adults: Administer 75% of dose

Cl_{cr} <10 mL minute: Children and Adults: Administer 50% of dose

Hemodialysis:

Children: Administer 50% of dose

Adults: Supplemental dose is not necessary

Peritoneal dialysis:

Children: Administer 50% of dose

Adults: Supplemental dose is not necessary

Continuous renal replacement therapy (CRRT):

Children: Administer 75% of dose and reduce for hyperbilirubinemia

Adults: Administer 75% of dose

Kintzel, 1995:

Cl_{cr} 46-60 mL/minute: Administer 85% of dose

Cl_{cr} 31-45 mL/minute: Administer 80% of dose

Cl_{cr} ≤30 mL/minute: Administer 75% of dose

Hepatic Impairment The FDA-approved labeling does not contain dosing adjustment guidelines. The following adjustments have been used by some clinicians:

Donelli, 1998: Liver dysfunction may reduce the metabolism and increase the toxicity of etoposide. Normal doses of I.V. etoposide should be given to patients with liver dysfunction (dose reductions may result in subtherapeutic concentrations); however, use caution with concomitant liver dysfunction (severe) and renal dysfunction as the decreased metabolic clearance cannot be compensated by increased renal clearance.

Floyd, 2006: Bilirubin 1.5-3 mg/dL or AST >3 times ULN: Administer 50% of dose

King, 2001; Koren, 1992: Bilirubin 1.5-3 mg/dL or AST >180 units/L: Administer 50% of dose

Administration

Oral Doses ≤400 mg/day as a single once daily dose; doses >400 mg should be given in 2-4 divided doses. If necessary, the injection may be used for oral administration.

I.M. Do not administer I.M. or SubQ (severe tissue necrosis).

I.V. Irritant.

Administer standard doses over at least 30-60 minutes to minimize the risk of hypotension. Higher (unlabeled) doses used in transplantation may be infused over longer time periods depending on the protocol. Etoposide injection contains polysorbate 80 which may cause leaching of diethylhexyl phthalate (DEHP), a plasticizer contained in polyvinyl chloride (PVC) tubing. Administration through non-PVC (low sorbing) tubing will minimize patient exposure to DEHP.

Concentrations >0.4 mg/mL are very unstable and may precipitate within a few minutes. For large doses, where dilution to ≤0.4 mg/mL is not feasible, consideration should be given to slow infusion of the undiluted drug through a running normal saline, dextrose or saline/dextrose infusion; or use of etoposide phosphate. Etoposide solutions of 0.1-0.4 mg/mL may be filtered through a 0.22 micron filter without damage to the filter; etoposide solutions of 0.2 mg/mL may be filtered through a 0.22 micron filter without significant loss of drug.

Stability

Reconstitution Etoposide should be diluted to a concentration of 0.2-0.4 mg/mL in D_5W or NS for administration. Diluted solutions have concentration-dependent stability: More concentrated solutions have shorter stability times. Precipitation may occur with concentrations >0.4 mg/mL. Use appropriate precautions for handling and disposal.

Storage

Capsules: Store oral capsules under refrigeration at 2°C to 8°C (36°F to 46°F); do not freeze.

Injection: Store intact vials of injection at room temperature of 25°C (77°F); do not freeze. Protect from light. Diluted solutions for infusion, at room temperature, in D_5W or NS in polyvinyl chloride, are stable as follows, depending on the concentration:

0.2 mg/mL: 96 hours

0.4 mg/mL: 24 hours

Etoposide injection contains polysorbate 80 which may cause leaching of diethylhexyl phthalate (DEHP), a plasticizer contained in polyvinyl chloride (PVC) bags and tubing. Higher concentrations and longer storage time after preparation in PVC bags may increase DEHP leaching. Preparation in glass or polyolefin containers will minimize patient exposure to DEHP. When undiluted etoposide injection is stored in acrylic or ABS (acrylonitrile, butadiene and styrene) plastic containers, may crack and leak.

Monitoring and Teaching Issues

Laboratory Monitoring CBC with differential, platelet count, hemoglobin; liver function (bilirubin, ALT, AST), albumin, renal function tests

Physical Assessment Patient should be monitored closely for anaphylactic reaction (chills, fever, tachycardia, bronchospasm, dyspnea, hypotension). Emergency equipment should be available. Assess renal function prior to each treatment and on a regular basis.

Patient Education This medication may be administered by infusion. Report immediately any swelling, pain, burning, or redness at infusion site; swelling of extremities; palpitations, rapid heartbeat, sudden difficulty breathing or swallowing; chest pain; or chills. It is important to maintain adequate nutrition and hydration, unless instructed to restrict fluid intake. You will be more susceptible to infection. May cause nausea, vomiting, diarrhea, loss of hair (reversible), or mouth sores. Report extreme fatigue, pain or numbness in extremities, severe GI upset or diarrhea, bleeding or bruising, fever, sore throat, vaginal discharge, yellowing of eyes or skin, or any changes in color of urine or stool.

Pregnancy Considerations Animal studies have demonstrated teratogenicity and fetal loss. There are no adequate and well-controlled studies in pregnant women. Women of childbearing potential should be advised to avoid pregnancy.

Etoposide Phosphate (e toe POE side FOS fate)

U.S. Brand Names Etopophos®

Index Terms Epipodophyllotoxin; ETOP

Generic Availability (U.S.) No

Pharmacologic Category Antineoplastic Agent, Podophyllotoxin Derivative; Antineoplastic Agent, Topoisomerase II Inhibitor

Medication Safety Issues

Sound-alike/look-alike issues:

Etoposide may be confused with teniposide

Etoposide phosphate is a prodrug of etoposide and is rapidly converted in the plasma to etoposide. To avoid confusion or dosing errors, **dosage should be expressed as the desired etoposide dose,** not as the etoposide phosphate dose (eg, etoposide phosphate equivalent to ____ mg etoposide).

High alert medication: This medication is in a class the Institute for Safe Medication Practices (ISMP) includes among its list of drug classes which have a heightened risk of causing significant patient harm when used in error.

Pregnancy Risk Factor D

Lactation Excretion in breast milk unknown/not recommended

Use Treatment of refractory testicular tumors; treatment of small cell lung cancer

Mechanism of Action/Effect Etoposide phosphate is converted *in vivo* to the active moiety, etoposide, by dephosphorylation. Etoposide inhibits mitotic activity; inhibits cells from entering prophase; inhibits DNA synthesis. Initially thought to be mitotic inhibitors similar to podophyllotoxin, but actually have no effect on microtubule assembly. However, later shown to induce DNA strand breakage and inhibition of topoisomerase II (an enzyme which breaks and repairs DNA); etoposide acts in late S or early G2 phases.

Contraindications Hypersensitivity to etoposide, etoposide phosphate, or any component of the formulation

Warnings/Precautions Hazardous agent - use appropriate precautions for handling and disposal. **[U.S. Boxed Warning]: Severe dose-limiting and dose-related myelosuppression with resulting infection or bleeding may occur.** Treatment should be withheld for platelets <50,000/mm^3 or absolute neutrophil count (ANC) <500/mm^3. May cause anaphylactic-like reactions manifested by chills, fever, tachycardia, bronchospasm, dyspnea, and hypotension. In addition, facial/tongue swelling, coughing, chest tightness, cyanosis, laryngospasm, diaphoresis, hypertension, and flushing have also been reported less commonly. Infusion should be interrupted and medications for the treatment of anaphylaxis should be available for immediate use. Underlying mechanisms behind the development of hypersensitivity reactions is unknown, but have been attributed to high drug concentration and rate of infusion. Another possible mechanism may be due to the differences between available etoposide intravenous formulations. Etoposide intravenous formulation contains polysorbate 80 and benzyl alcohol, while etoposide phosphate (the water soluble prodrug of etoposide) intravenous formulation does not contain either vehicle. Case reports have suggested that etoposide phosphate has been used successfully in patients with previous hypersensitivity reactions to etoposide (Collier, 2008; Siderov, 2002).

Secondary acute leukemias have been reported with etoposide, either as monotherapy or in combination with other chemotherapy agents. Dosage should be adjusted in patients with hepatic or renal impairment. Use with caution in patients with low serum albumin; may increase risk for toxicities. Doses of etoposide phosphate >175 mg/m^2 have not been evaluated. Use caution in elderly patients (may be more likely to develop severe myelosuppression and/or GI effects. Administer by slow I.V. infusion; hypotension has been reported with etoposide phosphate administration, generally associated with rapid I.V. infusion. Injection site reactions may occur; monitor infusion site closely. **[U.S. Boxed Warning]: Should be administered under the supervision of an experienced cancer chemotherapy physician.**

Drug Interactions

Metabolism/Transport Effects Substrate of CYP1A2 (minor), CYP2E1 (minor), CYP3A4 (major), P-glycoprotein; **Inhibits** CYP2C9 (weak), 3A4 (weak)

Avoid Concomitant Use

Avoid concomitant use of Etoposide Phosphate with any of the following: BCG; Natalizumab; Pimecrolimus; Roflumilast; Tacrolimus (Topical); Vaccines (Live)

Decreased Effect

Etoposide Phosphate may decrease the levels/effects of: BCG; Sipuleucel-T; Vaccines (Inactivated); Vaccines (Live)

The levels/effects of Etoposide Phosphate may be decreased by: Barbiturates; CYP3A4 Inducers (Strong); Deferasirox; Echinacea; Herbs (CYP3A4 Inducers); P-Glycoprotein Inducers; Phenytoin

Increased Effect/Toxicity

Etoposide Phosphate may increase the levels/effects of: Leflunomide; Natalizumab; Vaccines (Live)

The levels/effects of Etoposide Phosphate may be increased by: Conivaptan; CycloSPORINE; CycloSPORINE (Systemic); CYP3A4 Inhibitors (Moderate); CYP3A4 Inhibitors (Strong); Dasatinib; Denosumab; P-Glycoprotein Inhibitors; Pimecrolimus; Roflumilast; Tacrolimus (Topical); Trastuzumab

Nutritional/Ethanol Interactions

Ethanol: Avoid ethanol (may increase GI irritation).

Herb/Nutraceutical: Avoid St John's wort (may decrease etoposide levels).

Adverse Reactions Note: Also see adverse reactions for **etoposide;** etoposide phosphate is converted to etoposide, adverse reactions experienced with etoposide would also be expected with etoposide phosphate.

>10%:

Central nervous system: Chills/fever (24%)

Dermatologic: Alopecia (33% to 44%)

Gastrointestinal: Nausea/vomiting (37%), anorexia (16%), mucositis (11%)

Hematologic: Leukopenia (91%; grade 4: 17%; nadir: day 15-22; recovery: usually by day 21), neutropenia (88%; grade 4: 37%; nadir: day 12-19; recovery: usually by day 21), anemia (72%; grades 3/4: 19%), thrombocytopenia (23%; grade 4: 9%; nadir: day 10-15; recovery: usually by day 21)

Neuromuscular & skeletal: Weakness/malaise (39%)

1% to 10%:

Cardiovascular: Hypotension (1% to 5%), hypertension (3%), facial flushing (2%)

Central nervous system: Dizziness (5%)

Dermatologic: Skin rash (3%)

Gastrointestinal: Constipation (8%), abdominal pain (7%), diarrhea (6%), taste perversion (6%)

Local: Extravasation/phlebitis (5%; including swelling, pain, cellulitis, necrosis, and/or skin necrosis at site of infiltration)

Miscellaneous: Anaphylactic-type reactions (3%; including chills, diaphoresis, fever, rigor, tachycardia, bronchospasm, dyspnea, pruritus)

Pharmacodynamics/Kinetics

Protein Binding 94% to 98%

Half-Life Elimination Terminal: 4-11 hours; Children: Normal renal/hepatic function: 6-8 hours

Metabolism

Etoposide phosphate: Rapidly and completely converted to etoposide in plasma

Etoposide: Hepatic, via CYP3A4 and 3A5 to various metabolites; in addition, conversion of etoposide to the O-demethylated metabolites (catechol and quinine) via prostaglandin synthases or myeloperoxidase occurs, as well as glutathione and glucuronide conjugation via GSTT1/GSTP1 and UGT1A1 (Yang, 2009)

Excretion Urine (56%; 45% as etoposide) within 120 hours; feces (44%) within 120 hours

Children: Urine (~55% as etoposide) in 24 hours

Available Dosage Forms

Injection, powder for reconstitution:

Etopophos®: 100 mg

Dosing

Adult & Geriatric Refer to individual protocols. **Note:** Etoposide phosphate is a prodrug of etoposide, doses should be expressed as the desired **ETOPOSIDE** dose; **not** as the etoposide phosphate dose. (eg, etoposide phosphate equivalent to ____ mg etoposide). Etoposide phosphate 113.5 mg is equivalent to etoposide 100 mg.

Small cell lung cancer: I.V. (in combination with other approved chemotherapeutic drugs): Etoposide 35 mg/m^2/day for 4 days up to 50 mg/m^2/day for 5 days. Courses are repeated at 3- to 4-week intervals after adequate recovery from toxicity.

Testicular cancer: I.V. (in combination with other approved chemotherapeutic agents): Etoposide 50-100 mg/m^2/day on days 1-5 to 100 mg/m^2/day on days 1, 3, and 5. Courses are repeated at 3- to 4-week intervals after adequate recovery from toxicity.

Indication-specific unlabeled dosing: Refer to Etoposide monograph.

Renal Impairment Manufacturer recommended guidelines:

Cl_{cr} 15-50 mL/minute: Administer 75% of dose.

Cl_{cr} <15 mL minute: Data are not available; consider further dose reductions.

Etoposide phosphate is rapidly and completely converted to etoposide in plasma, please refer to Etoposide monograph for additional renal dosing adjustments (for etoposide).

Hepatic Impairment The FDA-approved labeling does not contain dosing adjustment guidelines. Etoposide phosphate is rapidly and completely converted to etoposide in plasma; please refer to Etoposide monograph for etoposide hepatic dosing adjustments.

Administration

I.V. Infuse by slow I.V. infusion over 5-210 minutes; risk of hypotension may increase with rate of infusion.

Stability

Reconstitution Reconstitute vials with 5 mL or 10 mL SWFI, D_5W, NS, bacteriostatic SWFI, or bacteriostatic NS to a concentration of 20 mg/mL or 10 mg/mL etoposide equivalent. These solutions may be administered without further dilution or may be diluted in 50-500 mL of D_5W or NS to a concentration as low as 0.1 mg/mL. Use appropriate precautions for handling and disposal.

Storage Store intact vials under refrigeration at 2°C to 8°C (36°F to 46°F). Protect from light. Reconstituted solution is stable refrigerated at 2°C to 8°C (36°F to 46°F) for 7 days. At room temperature of 20°C to 25°C (68°F to 77°F), reconstituted solutions are stable for 24 hours when reconstituted with SWFI, D_5W, or NS, or for 48 hours when reconstituted with bacteriostatic SWFI or bacteriostatic NS. Further diluted solutions for infusion are stable at room temperature 20°C to 25°C (68°F to 77°F) or under refrigeration 2°C to 8°C (36°F to 46°F) for up to 24 hours.

Monitoring and Teaching Issues

Laboratory Monitoring CBC with differential, platelet count, and hemoglobin, bilirubin, AST/ALT, renal function

Physical Assessment Use caution in presence of hepatic or renal impairment. Assess renal function prior to each treatment and on a regular basis.

Patient Education This medication is administered by infusion. Report immediately any swelling, pain, burning, or redness at infusion site. Avoid alcohol. It is important to maintain adequate nutrition and hydration, unless instructed to restrict fluid intake. You will be more susceptible to infection. May cause nausea, vomiting, diarrhea, loss of hair (reversible), or mouth sores. Report immediately chest pain, swelling of extremities, respiratory difficulty, palpitations, or rapid heartbeat. Report extreme fatigue, pain or numbness in extremities, severe GI upset or diarrhea, bleeding or bruising, fever, chills, sore throat, vaginal discharge, respiratory difficulty, yellowing of eyes or skin, or changes in color of urine or stool.

Geriatric Considerations Elderly patients may be more susceptible to severe myelosuppression. Other adverse effects including GI toxicity, infectious complications, weakness, and alopecia may occur more frequently in elderly.

Pregnancy Considerations Animal studies have demonstrated teratogenicity and fetal loss. There are no adequate and well-controlled studies in pregnant women. Women of child-bearing potential should be advised to avoid pregnancy.

Additional Information Etoposide phosphate 113.5 mg is equivalent to etoposide 100 mg. Dosages should always be expressed, and calculated, as the desired **etoposide** dose.

Etravirine (et ra VIR een)

U.S. Brand Names Intelence®

Index Terms TMC125

Generic Availability (U.S.) No

Pharmacologic Category Antiretroviral Agent, Reverse Transcriptase Inhibitor (Non-nucleoside)

Pregnancy Risk Factor B

Lactation Excretion in breast milk unknown/contraindicated

Use Treatment of HIV-1 infection in combination with at least two additional antiretroviral agents in treatment-experienced patients exhibiting viral replication with documented non-nucleoside reverse transcriptase inhibitor (NNRTI) resistance

Mechanism of Action/Effect As a non-nucleoside reverse transcriptase inhibitor, etravirine has activity against HIV-1 by binding to reverse transcriptase. It consequently blocks the RNA-dependent and DNA-dependent DNA polymerase activities, including HIV-1 replication. It does not require intracellular phosphorylation for antiviral activity.

Contraindications There are no contraindications listed in the manufacturer's labeling.

Warnings/Precautions Severe and possibly life-threatening skin reactions (including Stevens-Johnson syndrome, toxic epidermal necrolysis, erythema multiforme, and hypersensitivity reactions [ranging from rash and/or constitutional symptoms to occasional organ dysfunction, including hepatic failure]) have been reported; discontinue immediately with signs or symptoms of severe skin reaction or hypersensitivity. Self-limiting (with continued therapy) mild-to-moderate rashes (higher incidence in women) were also observed in clinical trials, usually during second week of therapy initiation. Not for use in treatment-naive patients, or experienced patients without evidence of viral mutations conferring resistance to NNRTIs and PIs. May cause redistribution of fat (eg, buffalo hump, peripheral wasting with increased abdominal girth, cushingoid appearance). Patients may develop immune reconstitution syndrome resulting in the occurrence of an inflammatory response to an indolent or residual opportunistic infection; further evaluation and treatment may be required.

Use with caution in patients taking major CYP3A4, 2C9 or 2C19 substrates (see Drug Interactions); consider alternative agents that avoid or lessen the potential for CYP-mediated interactions. Not recommended for use with other NNRTIs, unboosted protease inhibitors, high-dose ritonavir, tipranavir/ritonavir, fosamprenavir/ritonavir, atazanavir/ritonavir, enzyme-inducing anticonvulsants, macrolides (except azithromycin), St John's wort, rifampin, or rifapentine.

Drug Interactions

Metabolism/Transport Effects Substrate (major) of CYP3A4, 2C9, 2C19; **Inhibits** CYP2C9 (moderate), 2C19 (moderate); **Induces** CYP3A4 (major)

Avoid Concomitant Use

Avoid concomitant use of Etravirine with any of the following: Atazanavir; CarBAMazepine; Clopidogrel; Dienogest; Dronedarone; Everolimus; Fosamprenavir; Lurasidone; Nilotinib; Nisoldipine; Pazopanib; PHENobarbital; Phenytoin; Praziquantel; Ranolazine; Reverse Transcriptase Inhibitors (Non-Nucleoside); Rifamycin Derivatives; Ritonavir; Roflumilast; RomiDEPsin; St Johns Wort; Tipranavir; Tolvaptan; Vandetanib

Decreased Effect

Etravirine may decrease the levels/effects of: Amiodarone; Antifungal Agents (Azole Derivatives, Systemic); Atazanavir; Bepridil [Off Market]; Clopidogrel; CYP3A4 Substrates; Dienogest; Disopyramide; Dronedarone; Everolimus; Exemestane; Flecainide; Gefitinib; GuanFACINE; HMG-CoA Reductase Inhibitors; Imatinib; Ixabepilone; Lidocaine; Lidocaine (Systemic); Lurasidone; Macrolide Antibiotics; Maraviroc; Methadone; Mexiletine; NIFEdipine; Nilotinib; Nisoldipine; Pazopanib; Phosphodiesterase 5 Inhibitors; Praziquantel; Propafenone; QuiNIDine; Ranolazine; Roflumilast; RomiDEPsin; Saxagliptin; SORAfenib; Tolvaptan; Ulipristal; Vandetanib

The levels/effects of Etravirine may be decreased by: CarBAMazepine; CYP2C19 Inducers (Strong); CYP2C9 Inducers (Highly Effective); CYP3A4 Inducers (Strong); Deferasirox; Peginterferon Alfa-2b; PHENobarbital; Phenytoin; Protease Inhibitors; Reverse Transcriptase Inhibitors (Non-Nucleoside); Rifabutin; Rifamycin Derivatives; Ritonavir; St Johns Wort; Tipranavir

Increased Effect/Toxicity

Etravirine may increase the levels/effects of: Antifungal Agents (Azole Derivatives, Systemic); Carvedilol; CYP2C19 Substrates; CYP2C9 Substrates (High risk); Digoxin; Fosamprenavir; PACLitaxel; Protease Inhibitors

The levels/effects of Etravirine may be increased by: Antifungal Agents (Azole Derivatives, Systemic); Atazanavir; Conivaptan; Reverse Transcriptase Inhibitors (Non-Nucleoside)

Nutritional/Ethanol Interactions

Food: Increases absorption of etravirine by ~50%.

Herb/Nutraceutical: St John's wort (*Hypericum perforatum*) may decrease the levels/effects of etravirine; do not coadminister.

Adverse Reactions

>10%:

Dermatologic: Rash (≥ grade 2: 10%)

Endocrine & metabolic: Cholesterol (total) increased (≤300 mg/dL: 20%; >300 mg/dL: 8%), hyperglycemia (≤250 mg/dL: 15%; 251-500 mg/dL: 4%), LDL increased (≤190 mg/dL: 13%)

Gastrointestinal: Nausea

2% to 10%:

Endocrine & metabolic: Triglycerides increased (≤750 mg/dL: 9%; >750 mg/dL: 4% to 6%)

Hepatic: ALT increased (≤5 x ULN: 6%; >5 x ULN: 3%), AST increased (≤5 x ULN: 6%; >5 x ULN: 3%)

Neuromuscular & skeletal: Peripheral neuropathy (≥ grade 2: 4%)

Renal: Creatinine increased (≤1.8 x ULN: 6%; >1.8 x ULN: 2%)

Pharmacodynamics/Kinetics

Absorption Increased 50% with food

Time to Peak 2.5-4 hours

Protein Binding 99.9%

Half-Life Elimination 41 hours (± 20 hours)

Metabolism Hepatic, primarily by CYP3A4, 2C9, and 2C19; major metabolites exhibit ~10% of parent drug activity against HIV

Excretion Feces (94%, up to 86% as unchanged drug); urine (1%)

Available Dosage Forms

Tablet, oral:

Intelence®: 100 mg, 200 mg

Dosing

Adult Treatment of HIV-1 infection: Oral: 200 mg twice daily after meals

Renal Impairment No dosage adjustment necessary.

Due to extensive protein binding, significant removal by hemodialysis or peritoneal dialysis is unlikely.

Hepatic Impairment No adjustment required for mild-to-moderate (Child-Pugh class A/B) impairment; no data in severe impairment.

Administration

Oral Administer after meals. Dose is given as two 100 mg or one 200 mg tablet. If unable to swallow tablets, may disperse tablets in glass of water; stir well prior to drinking (swallow completely) and rinse glass several times to ensure administration of complete dose.

Stability

Storage Store at USP controlled room temperature of 25°C (77°F); excursions permitted to 15°C to 30°C (59°F to 86°F). Protect from moisture.

Monitoring and Teaching Issues

Laboratory Monitoring Cholesterol, triglycerides, serum glucose, hepatic transaminases (if signs or symptoms of hypersensitivity develop)

Physical Assessment Assess decrease in infections and progression of disease, viral load, and CD4 count. Monitor for skin rash (may be severe and require discontinuing drug) and gastrointestinal upset. Teach patient proper timing of multiple medications.

Patient Education This drug will not cure HIV, nor has it been found to reduce transmission of HIV; use appropriate precautions to prevent spread to other persons. This drug is prescribed as one part of a multi-drug combination; take exactly as directed for full course of therapy. Take after meals. Maintain adequate hydration, unless instructed to restrict fluid intake. Frequent blood tests may be required. You may experience nausea, vomiting, or changes in body fat (increased in upper back and neck and around trunk; decreased from extremities and face). Report immediately any sign of skin rash.

Dietary Considerations Take after meals. May disperse tablets in glass of water; stir well prior to drinking and rinse glass several times to ensure administration of complete dose.

Breast-Feeding Considerations In infants born to mothers who are HIV positive, HAART while breast-feeding may decrease postnatal infection. However, maternal or infant antiretroviral therapy does not completely eliminate the risk of postnatal HIV transmission. In addition, multiclass-resistant virus has been detected in breast-feeding infants despite maternal therapy.

In the United States where formula is accessible, affordable, safe, and sustainable, complete avoidance of breast-feeding by HIV-infected women is recommended to decrease potential transmission of HIV.

Pregnancy Considerations No evidence of fetal toxicity has been noted in animal reproduction studies. However, there are no adequate and well-controlled studies in pregnant women, and use during pregnancy is not recommended unless other alternatives are not available. Healthcare providers are encouraged to enroll pregnant women exposed to antiretroviral medications in the Antiretroviral Pregnancy Registry (1-800-258-4263 or www.-APRegistry.com). Healthcare providers caring for HIV-infected women and their infants may contact the National Perinatal HIV Hotline (888-448-8765) for clinical consultation.

◆ **Eulexin** *see* Flutamide *on page 797*

◆ **Evamist™** *see* Estradiol (Systemic) *on page 670*

Everolimus (e ver OH li mus)

U.S. Brand Names Afinitor®; Zortress®

Index Terms RAD001

Generic Availability (U.S.) No

Pharmacologic Category Antineoplastic Agent, mTOR Kinase Inhibitor; Immunosuppressant Agent; mTOR Kinase Inhibitor

Medication Safety Issues

Sound-alike/look-alike issues:

Everolimus may be confused with sirolimus, tacrolimus, temsirolimus

High alert medication: This medication is in a class the Institute for Safe Medication Practices (ISMP) includes among its list of drug classes which have a heightened risk of causing significant patient harm when used in error.

Medication Guide Available Yes

Pregnancy Risk Factor D (Afinitor®) / C (Zortress®)

Lactation Excretion in breast milk unknown/not recommended

Use Treatment of advanced renal cell cancer (RCC), after sunitinib or sorafenib failure (Afinitor®); treatment of subependymal giant cell astrocytoma (SEGA) associated with tuberous sclerosis, in patients who are not candidates for curative surgical resection (Afinitor®); prophylaxis of organ rejection in patients at low-moderate immunologic risk receiving renal transplants (Zortress®)

Unlabeled/Investigational Use Prophylaxis of organ rejection in heart transplant recipients; treatment of advanced pancreatic neuroendocrine tumors; treatment of relapsed or refractory Waldenström's macroglobulinemia (WM)

Mechanism of Action/Effect Everolimus is a macrolide immunosuppressant and an m-TOR inhibitor which has antiproliferative and antiangiogenic properties; reduces protein synthesis and cell proliferation by binding to the intracellular protein, FK binding protein-12 (FKBP-12) to form a complex that inhibits activation of mTOR (mammalian target of rapamycin) protein kinase activity. Also reduces angiogenesis by inhibiting vascular endothelial growth factor (VEGF) and hypoxia-inducible factor (HIF-1) expression.

Contraindications Hypersensitivity to everolimus, sirolimus, other rapamycin derivatives, or any component of the formulation.

Warnings/Precautions Hazardous agent - use appropriate precautions for handling and disposal. Noninfectious pneumonitis (sometimes fatal) has been observed with mTOR inhibitors including everolimus; symptoms include dyspnea, cough, hypoxia and/or pleural effusion; promptly evaluate worsening respiratory symptoms; may require dosage modification or corticosteroid therapy; severe symptoms may require discontinuation. **[U.S. Boxed Warning]: Everolimus has immunosuppressant properties which may result in infection;** the risk of developing bacterial, viral, fungal and protozoal infections and for local, opportunistic (including polyomavirus infection), systemic infections, and/or sepsis is increased. BK virus-associated nephropathy, which may result in serious cases of deteriorating renal function and renal graft loss, has been observed with use. Reactivation of hepatitis B has been observed in patients with RCC. Resolve pre-existing invasive fungal infections prior to treatment initiation. Monitor for signs and symptoms of infection during treatment. Discontinue if invasive systemic fungal infection is diagnosed (and manage with appropriate antifungal therapy).

[U.S. Boxed Warning]: Immunosuppressant use may result in the development of malignancy, including lymphoma and skin cancer. The risk is associated with treatment intensity and the duration of therapy. To minimize the risk for skin cancer, limit exposure to sunlight and ultraviolet light; wear protective clothing and use effective sunscreen.

[U.S. Boxed Warning]: Due to the increased risk for nephrotoxicity in renal transplantation, avoid standard doses of cyclosporine in combination with everolimus; reduced cyclosporine doses are recommended when everolimus is used in combination with cyclosporine. Therapeutic monitoring of cyclosporine and everolimus concentrations is recommended. Monitor for proteinuria; the risk of proteinuria is increased when everolimus is used in combination with cyclosporine, and with higher serum everolimus concentrations. Everolimus and cyclosporine combination therapy may increase the risk for thrombotic microangiopathy/thrombotic thrombocytopenic purpura/hemolytic uremic syndrome (TMA/TTP/HUS); monitor blood counts. Elevations in serum creatinine (generally mild) have been also observed with everolimus use for renal cell cancer; monitor renal function. Avoid concomitant use with strong CYP3A4 inducers (eg, dexamethasone, phenytoin, carbamazepine, rifampin, rifabutin, rifapentine, phenobarbital) and strong CYP3A4 inhibitors (eg, ketoconazole, itraconazole, voriconazole, clarithromycin, telithromycin, atazanavir, saquinavir, ritonavir, indinavir, delavirdine, fosamprenavir, nelfinavir, nefazodone, grapefruit juice). Dosage modification may be needed if concomitant use with strong CYP3A4 inducers cannot be avoided. Use with caution with concomitant moderate CYP3A4 inhibitors and/or P-gp inhibitors; decreased everolimus doses are recommended. Use is associated with mouth ulcers, mucositis and stomatitis; avoid the use of alcohol or peroxide based mouthwashes (due to the high potential for drug interactions, avoid the use of systemic antifungals unless fungal infection has been diagnosed). In renal transplantation, avoid the use of HMG-CoA reductase inhibitors; may increase the risk for rhabdomyolysis due to the potential interaction with cyclosporine (which is given in combination with everolimus for renal transplantation). **[U.S. Boxed Warning]: An increased risk of renal arterial and venous thrombosis has been reported with use in renal transplantation, generally within the first 30 days after transplant; may result in graft loss.**

Everolimus is associated with the development of angioedema; concomitant use with other agents known to cause angioedema (eg, ACE inhibitors) may increase the risk. Everolimus use may delay wound healing and increase the occurrence of wound-related complications (eg, wound dehiscence, infection, incisional hernia, lymphocele, seroma); may require surgical intervention. Generalized edema, including peripheral edema and lymphedema, and local fluid accumulation (eg, pericardial effusion, pleural effusion, ascites) may also occur.

Everolimus exposure is increased in patients with moderate hepatic impairment; dosage reductions are recommended. Use is not recommended in patients with severe impairment (has not been studied). Use with caution in patients with hyperlipidemia; may increase serum lipids (cholesterol and triglycerides); higher serum concentrations are associated with an increased risk for hyperlipidemia; use has not been studied in patients with baseline cholesterol >350 mg/dL. Decreases in hemoglobin, neutrophils, platelets, and lymphocytes have been reported with use. Increases in serum glucose are common; may alter insulin and/or oral hypoglycemic therapy requirements in patients with diabetes; the risk for new onset diabetes is increased with everolimus use after transplantation. Patients should not be immunized with live viral vaccines during or shortly after treatment and should avoid close contact with recently vaccinated (live vaccine) individuals; consider the timing of routine immunizations prior to the start of therapy in pediatric patients treated for SEGA. Continue treatment with everolimus for renal cell cancer as long as clinical benefit is demonstrated or until occurrence of unacceptable toxicity.

Azoospermia and oligospermia have been observed in males. Avoid use in patients with hereditary galactose intolerance, Lapp lactase deficiency, or glucose-galactose malabsorption; may result in diarrhea and malabsorption. The safety and efficacy of everolimus in patients with high-immunologic risk in renal transplantation or in solid organ transplant other than renal have not been established. **[U.S. Boxed Warning]: In renal transplantation, everolimus should only be used by physicians experienced in immunosuppressive therapy and management of transplant patients. Adequate laboratory and supportive medical resources must be readily available.**

Drug Interactions

Metabolism/Transport Effects Substrate of CYP2C8, 3A4, P-glycoprotein

Avoid Concomitant Use

Avoid concomitant use of Everolimus with any of the following: BCG; CYP3A4 Inducers (Strong); CYP3A4 Inhibitors (Strong); Grapefruit Juice; Natalizumab; Pimecrolimus; Roflumilast; St Johns Wort; Tacrolimus (Topical); Vaccines (Live)

Decreased Effect

Everolimus may decrease the levels/effects of: BCG; Sipuleucel-T; Vaccines (Inactivated); Vaccines (Live)

The levels/effects of Everolimus may be decreased by: CYP3A4 Inducers (Strong); Deferasirox; Echinacea; Efavirenz; P-Glycoprotein Inducers; St Johns Wort

Increased Effect/Toxicity

Everolimus may increase the levels/effects of: ACE Inhibitors; Leflunomide; Natalizumab; Vaccines (Live)

The levels/effects of Everolimus may be increased by: CycloSPORINE; CycloSPORINE (Systemic); CYP3A4 Inhibitors (Moderate); CYP3A4 Inhibitors (Strong); Dasatinib; Denosumab; Grapefruit Juice; P-Glycoprotein Inhibitors; Pimecrolimus; Roflumilast; Tacrolimus (Topical); Trastuzumab

Nutritional/Ethanol Interactions

Food: Avoid grapefruit juice (may increase levels of everolimus).

Herb/Nutraceutical: Avoid St John's wort.

Adverse Reactions

>10%:

Cardiovascular: Peripheral edema (RCC: 25%; renal transplantation: 45%; SEGA: 4%), hypertension (RCC, SEGA: 4%; renal transplant: 30%)

Central nervous system: Fever (19% to 32%), fatigue (RCC: 31%; renal transplant: 9%; SEGA: 7%), seizure (SEGA: 29%), headache (18% to 19%), personality change (SEGA: 18%), insomnia (9% to 17%), dizziness (7% to 14%)

Dermatologic: Rash (18% to 29%), acneiform dermatitis (SEGA: 25%; RCC: 3%), cellulitis (SEGA: 21%), dry skin (13% to 18%), contact dermatitis (14%), excoriation (14%), pruritus (14%), acne (11%)

Endocrine & metabolic: Hypercholesterolemia (RCC: 77%; grade 3: 4%; SEGA: 68%; renal transplant: 17%), hypertriglyceridemia (RCC: 73%; grade 3: <1%; SEGA: 11% to 43%; renal transplant: <10%), hyperglycemia (RCC: 57%; grade 3: 15%; grade 4: <1%; SEGA: 25%; renal transplant: 12%), hypoglycemia (SEGA: 32%), hypophosphatemia (RCC: 37%; grade 3: 6%; renal transplant: 13%), hyperlipidemia (renal transplant: 21%), hyperkalemia (renal transplant: 18%), hypocalcemia (17%), dyslipidemia (renal transplant: 15%), hypomagnesemia (renal transplant: 14%), hypokalemia (renal transplant: 12%)

Gastrointestinal: Stomatitis (SEGA: 86%; grade 3: 4%; RCC: 44%; grade 3: 4%; grade 4: <1%; renal transplant: 8%), constipation (renal transplant: 38%; SEGA: 11%), diarrhea (RCC: 30%; grade 3: 1%; SEGA: 25%; renal transplantation: 19%), nausea (26% to 29%: grade 3: 1%), anorexia (25%), vomiting (15% to 21%; grade 3: 2%), mucosal inflammation (19%; grade 3: 1%), gastroenteritis (SEGA: 18%), abdominal pain (3% to 13%)

Genitourinary: Urinary tract infection (renal transplant: 22%; RCC: 5%), dysuria (renal transplant: 11%)

Hematologic: Anemia (RCC: 92%; grade 3: 12%; grade 4: 1%; SEGA: 39%; renal transplant: 26%), lymphocytopenia (51%; grade 3: 16%; grade 4: 2%), leukopenia (SEGA: 54%; RCC: 26%; renal transplant: 3%), thrombocytopenia (21% to 23%; grade 3: 1%; renal transplant <10%), neutropenia (14%; grade 4: <4%)

Hepatic: AST increased (25% to 89%; grade 3: <4%; grade 4: <1%), ALT increased (21% to 46%; grade 3: 1%)

Neuromuscular & skeletal: Weakness (33%), limb pain (10% to 12%), back pain (renal transplant: 11%)

Otic: Otitis (SEGA: 14% to 36%)

Renal: Creatinine increased (RCC: 50%; grade 3: 1%; renal transplant: 18%; SEGA: 11%), hematuria (renal transplant: 12%)

Respiratory: Upper respiratory infection (SEGA: 82%; renal transplant: 16%), sinusitis (3% to 39%), cough (RCC: 30%; SEGA: 21%; renal transplant: 7%), dyspnea (24%; grade 3: 6%; grade 4: 1%), epistaxis (≤18%), nasal congestion (14%), pneumonitis (includes alveolitis, interstitial lung disease, lung infiltrate, pulmonary alveolar hemorrhage, pulmonary toxicity; 14%; grade 3: 4%), rhinitis (14%), pharyngitis (SEGA: 4% to 11%)

Miscellaneous: Infection (RCC: All infections: 37%; grade 3: 7%; grade 4: 3%; renal transplant: 62%)

1% to 10%:

Cardiovascular: Chest pain (5%), tachycardia (3%), heart failure (1%), angina, atrial fibrillation, chest discomfort, deep vein thrombosis, edema (generalized), hypotension, palpitation, syncope

Central nervous system: Chills (4%), agitation, anxiety, depression, hallucination, hemiparesis, hypesthesia, malaise, somnolence

Dermatologic: Nail disorder (5%), palmar-plantar erythrodysesthesia syndrome ([hand-foot syndrome] 5%), erythema 4%, onychoclasis (4%), pityriasis rosea (4%), skin lesions (4%), alopecia, hirsutism, incision complications, hyperhydrosis, hypertrichosis

Endocrine & metabolic: Diabetes mellitus (exacerbation: 2%; new-onset: <9%), acidosis, cushingoid syndrome, dehydration, gout, hypercalcemia, hyperparathyroidism, hyperphosphatemia, hyperuricemia, hypoglycemia, hyponatremia, iron deficiency, vitamin B_{12} deficiency

Gastrointestinal: Taste alteration (10%), weight loss (9%), xerostomia (8%), gastritis (7%), hemorrhoids (5%), dyspepsia (4%), dysphagia (4%), abdominal distention, epigastric discomfort, flatulence, gastroesophageal reflux, gingival hypertrophy, hematemesis, ileus, peritonitis

Genitourinary: Bladder spasm, erectile dysfunction, ovarian cysts, pollakiuria, polyuria, pyuria, scrotal edema, urinary retention, urinary urgency

Hematologic: Hemorrhage (3%), leukocytosis, lymphadenopathy, thrombocythemia

Hepatic: Bilirubin increased (3%; grade 3: <1%; grade 4: <1%)

Neuromuscular & skeletal: Tremor (8%), paresthesia (5%), jaw pain (3%), arthralgia, joint swelling, muscle spasm, musculoskeletal pain, myalgia, osteonecrosis, osteopenia, osteoporosis, spondylitis

Ocular: Eyelid edema (4%), ocular hyperemia (4%), conjunctivitis (2%), blurred vision, cataract

Renal: Renal failure (3%), BUN increased, hydronephrosis, interstitial nephritis, proteinuria, renal artery thrombosis, renal impairment

Respiratory: Pleural effusion (7%), nasopharyngitis (6%), pneumonia (6%), bronchitis (4%), pharyngolaryngeal pain (4%), rhinorrhea (3%), atelectasis, nasal congestion, pulmonary edema, sinus congestion, wheezing

Miscellaneous: BK virus infection, candidiasis, night sweats

Pharmacodynamics/Kinetics

Absorption Rapid, but moderate

Bioavailability ~30%; systemic exposure reduced by 22% with a high-fat meal and by 32% with a light-fat meal

Time to Peak 1-2 hours

Protein Binding ~74%

Half-Life Elimination ~30 hours

Metabolism Extensively metabolized via CYP3A4; forms 6 weak metabolites

Excretion Feces (80%, based on solid organ transplant studies); Urine (~5%, based on solid organ transplant studies)

Available Dosage Forms

Tablet, oral:

Afinitor®: 2.5 mg, 5 mg, 10 mg

Zortress®: 0.25 mg, 0.5 mg, 0.75 mg

Dosing

Adult & Geriatric

Renal cell cancer, advanced (RCC): Oral: 10 mg once daily

Renal transplantation, rejection prophylaxis: Oral: Initial: 0.75 mg twice daily; adjust maintenance dose if needed at a 4- to 5-day interval (from prior dose adjustment) based on serum concentrations, tolerability, and response

Note: For use in renal transplantation, administer in combination with basiliximab induction and concurrently with cyclosporine (dose adjustment required) and corticosteroids.

Subependymal giant cell astrocytoma (SEGA): Oral: Body surface area based dosing: Initial dose (adjust maintenance dose if needed at 2-week intervals based on serum trough concentrations, tolerability, response and concomitant medications):

0.5 m^2 to 1.2 m^2: 2.5 mg once daily

1.3 m^2 to 2.1 m^2: 5 mg once daily

≥2.2 m^2: 7.5 mg once daily

Note: Assess trough concentrations 2 weeks after initiation or dosage modification; target trough concentration: 5-10 ng/mL. For trough concentration between 10-15 ng/ml, may continue if tolerated; reduce dose for trough concentration >15 ng/mL. If trough <5 ng/mL, increase dose by 2.5 mg/day every 2 weeks if tolerated. Dose reductions may be made in 2.5 mg/day decrements every 2 weeks.

Heart transplantation, rejection prophylaxis (unlabeled use): Oral: Initial: 0.75-1.5 mg twice daily in combination with cyclosporine and prednisone; adjust everolimus dose based on trough concentrations (Eisen, 2003; Vigano, 2007)

Pancreatic neuroendocrine tumors, advanced (unlabeled use): Oral: 10 mg once daily (Yao, 2011) **or** 10 mg once daily (alone or in combination with octreotide LAR) (Yao, 2010)

Waldenström's macroglobulinemia, relapsed or refractory (unlabeled use): Oral: 10 mg once daily (Ghobrial, 2010)

Dosage adjustment for concomitant CYP3A4 inhibitors/inducers:

RCC:

CYP3A4 inducers: Strong inducers: Avoid concomitant administration with strong CYP3A4 inducers; if concomitant use cannot be avoided, consider adjusting everolimus dose upward in 5 mg increments up to 20 mg daily, with careful monitoring. If the strong CYP3A4 enzyme inducer is discontinued, reduce the everolimus to the dose used prior to initiation of the CYP3A4 inducer.

CYP3A4 or P-gp inhibitors:

Strong inhibitors: Avoid concomitant administration with strong CYP3A4 inhibitors.

Moderate CYP3A4 and/or P-gp inhibitors: Reduce dose to 2.5 mg once daily; may consider increasing from 2.5 mg to 5 mg once daily based on patient tolerance. When the moderate inhibitor is discontinued, allow ~2-3 days to elapse prior to adjusting the everolimus upward to the dose used prior to initiation of the moderate inhibitor.

Renal transplantation: Dosage adjustments may be necessary based on everolimus serum concentrations

SEGA:

CYP3A4 inducers: Strong inducers: Avoid concomitant administration with strong CYP3A4 inducers; if concomitant use cannot be avoided, double the everolimus dose; individualize subsequent doses based on therapeutic drug monitoring. If the strong CYP3A4 enzyme inducer is discontinued, reduce the everolimus to the dose used prior to initiation of the CYP3A4 inducer; reassess trough concentration after 2 weeks.

CYP3A4 or P-gp inhibitors:

Strong inhibitors: Avoid concomitant administration with strong CYP3A4 inhibitors.

Moderate CYP3A4 and/or P-gp inhibitors: Reduce dose by 50% to maintain trough concentrations of 5-10 ng/mL (if dose reduction is required for patients receiving 2.5 mg once daily, consider alternate day dosing); assess trough concentrations after 2 weeks; individualize dosing based on therapeutic drug monitoring. When the moderate inhibitor is discontinued, adjust the everolimus upward to the dose used prior to initiation of the moderate inhibitor; reassess trough concentrations after 2 weeks.

Pediatric Subependymal giant cell astrocytoma (SEGA): Children ≥3 years of age: Refer to adult dosing.

Renal Impairment No adjustment necessary.

Hepatic Impairment

Mild hepatic impairment (Child-Pugh class A): No adjustment required.

Moderate hepatic impairment (Child-Pugh class B):

RCC: Reduce dose to 5 mg once daily.

Renal transplantation: Reduce initial dose by 50%; monitor and adjust as appropriate.

SEGA: Adjustment to initial dose may not be required; individualize subsequent dosing based on therapeutic drug monitoring.

Severe hepatic impairment (Child-Pugh class C): Use is not recommended (not studied in severe hepatic impairment).

Adjustment for Toxicity

RCC:

Severe/intolerable adverse reactions: Temporarily reduce dose to 5 mg once daily and/or temporarily interrupt treatment

Noninfectious pneumonitis:

Mild or asymptomatic (radiological changes suggestive of pneumonitis): Continue treatment

Moderate symptoms: Consider interrupting treatment until symptoms improve (may require corticosteroids); may reinitiate at a reduced dose of 5 mg once daily

Severe symptoms: Discontinue treatment and consider corticosteroids until clinical symptoms improve; if appropriate (depending on individual circumstances) may reinitiate at a reduced dose of 5 mg once daily

SEGA:

Severe/intolerable adverse reactions: Temporarily reduce dose and/or temporarily interrupt treatment; if dose reduction is required for patients receiving 2.5 mg once daily, consider alternate day dosing.

Noninfectious pneumonitis:

Mild or asymptomatic (radiological changes suggestive of pneumonitis): Continue treatment

Moderate symptoms: Consider interrupting treatment until symptoms improve (may require corticosteroids); may reinitiate with a 50% dose reduction

Severe symptoms: Discontinue treatment and consider corticosteroids until clinical symptoms improve; if appropriate (depending on individual circumstances) may reinitiate with a 50% dose reduction

Administration

Oral May be taken with or without food; to reduce variability, take consistently with regard to food. Swallow whole with a glass of water. Do not chew or crush. If unable to swallow tablet whole, immediately prior to administration, disperse completely in 30 mL water with gentle stirring; rinse container with additional 30 mL water and swallow. Avoid contact with or exposure to crushed or broken tablets.

Renal cell cancer, subependymal giant cell astrocytoma: Administer at the same time each day.

Renal transplantation: Administer consistently ~12 hours apart; administer at the same time as cyclosporine.

Stability

Storage Store at room temperature of 25°C (77°F); excursions permitted to 15°C to 30°C (59°F to 86°F). Protect from light; protect from moisture.

Monitoring and Teaching Issues

Laboratory Monitoring CBC with differential (baseline and periodic), liver function, serum creatinine and BUN (baseline and periodic), fasting serum glucose and lipid profile (baseline and periodic)

For renal transplantation, monitor everolimus serum concentrations, especially in patients with hepatic impairment, with concomitant CYP3A4 inhibitors and inducers, and when cyclosporine formulations or doses are changed; monitor cyclosporine concentrations; monitor for proteinuria

For SEGA, monitor everolimus trough concentrations approximately 2 weeks after treatment initiation, 2 weeks after dose modifications and after initiation or dose modification of concomitant CYP3A4 and/or P-gp inducers or inhibitors.

Physical Assessment Monitor for hypercholesterolemia, opportunistic infection, interstitial lung disease, gastrointestinal disturbance, and renal failure throughout therapy. Advise patients with diabetes to monitor glucose levels; may cause hyperglycemia.

Patient Education Do not crush or chew tablets; take whole at same time each day with a full glass of water. Avoid grapefruit and grapefruit juice while taking this medication. Maintain adequate nutrition and hydration, unless instructed to restrict fluid intake. You will be required to have regularly scheduled laboratory tests while on this medication. You will be more susceptible to infection. If you have diabetes, check your glucose levels closely and notify prescriber of significant changes; this medication can affect glucose control and diabetic medications may need to be adjusted. You may experience headache, fatigue, loss of appetite, nausea, vomiting, or mouth sores. Report immediately changes in respiratory status (difficulty breathing, dyspnea, unusual cough, fever); swelling of extremities or unusual weight gain; persistent diarrhea, gastrointestinal upset, abdominal pain, or blood in stool; signs or symptoms of any urinary tract infection (difficulty urinating, burning on urination, perineal itching); unusual infection (fever, chills); or delayed wound healing.

Dietary Considerations Avoid grapefruit juice. May be taken with or without food, although should be administered consistently with regard to food.

Breast-Feeding Considerations Due to the potential for serious adverse reactions in the nursing infant, breast-feeding is not recommended.

Pregnancy Considerations Embryotoxicity, fetotoxicity, malformations, and growth retardation were observed in animal studies with exposures lower than expected with human doses. There are no adequate and well-controlled studies in pregnant women. Based on the mechanism of action, may cause fetal harm if administered during pregnancy. Women of childbearing potential should be advised to avoid pregnancy. Women of childbearing potential should use effective birth control during treatment, and continue for 8 weeks after everolimus discontinuation.

◆ **Evista®** *see* Raloxifene *on page 1547*

◆ **Evoclin®** *see* Clindamycin (Topical) *on page 400*

◆ **Evoxac®** *see* Cevimeline *on page 355*

◆ **Exalgo™** *see* HYDROmorphone *on page 922*

◆ **Excedrin® Tension Headache [OTC]** *see* Acetaminophen *on page 38*

◆ **ExeClear-C** *see* Guaifenesin and Codeine *on page 891*

◆ **Exelon®** *see* Rivastigmine *on page 1601*

Exemestane (ex e MES tane)

U.S. Brand Names Aromasin®

Generic Availability (U.S.) No

Pharmacologic Category Antineoplastic Agent, Aromatase Inactivator

Medication Safety Issues

Sound-alike/look-alike issues:

Aromasin® may be confused with Arimidex®

Exemestane may be confused with estramustine.

Pregnancy Risk Factor D

Lactation Excretion in breast milk unknown/use caution

Use Treatment of advanced breast cancer in postmenopausal women whose disease has progressed following tamoxifen therapy; adjuvant treatment of postmenopausal estrogen receptor-positive early breast cancer following 2-3 years of tamoxifen (for a total of 5 years of adjuvant therapy)

Mechanism of Action/Effect Exemestane prevents conversion of androgens to estrogens (aromatase inhibitor) and lowers circulating estrogen levels in postmenopausal breast cancers.

Contraindications Hypersensitivity to exemestane or any component of the formulation

Warnings/Precautions Hazardous agent - use appropriate precautions for handling and disposal. Not indicated for premenopausal women; not to be given with estrogen-containing agents. Dose adjustment recommended with concomitant CYP3A4 inducers.

Drug Interactions

Metabolism/Transport Effects Substrate of CYP3A4 (major)

Avoid Concomitant Use There are no known interactions where it is recommended to avoid concomitant use.

Decreased Effect

Exemestane may decrease the levels/effects of: Saxagliptin

The levels/effects of Exemestane may be decreased by: CYP3A4 Inducers (Strong); Deferasirox; Herbs (CYP3A4 Inducers); Rifampin

Increased Effect/Toxicity

The levels/effects of Exemestane may be increased by: Conivaptan

Nutritional/Ethanol Interactions

Food: Plasma levels increased by 40% when exemestane was taken with a fatty meal.

Herb/Nutraceutical: St John's wort may decrease exemestane levels. Avoid black cohosh, dong quai in estrogen-dependent tumors.

Adverse Reactions

>10%:

Cardiovascular: Hypertension (5% to 15%)

Central nervous system: Fatigue (8% to 22%), insomnia (11% to 14%), pain (13%), headache (7% to 13%), depression (6% to 13%)

Dermatological: Hyperhidrosis (4% to 18%), alopecia (15%)

Endocrine & metabolic: Hot flashes (13% to 33%)

Gastrointestinal: Nausea (9% to 18%), abdominal pain (6% to 11%)

Hepatic: Alkaline phosphatase increased (14% to 15%)

Neuromuscular & skeletal: Arthralgia (15% to 29%)

1% to 10%:

Cardiovascular: Edema (6% to 7%); cardiac ischemic events (2%: MI, angina, myocardial ischemia); chest pain

Central nervous system: Dizziness (8% to 10%), anxiety (4% to 10%), fever (5%), confusion, hypoesthesia

Dermatologic: Dermatitis (8%), itching, rash

Endocrine & metabolic: Weight gain (8%)

Gastrointestinal: Diarrhea (4% to 10%), vomiting (7%), anorexia (6%), constipation (5%), appetite increased (3%), dyspepsia

Genitourinary: Urinary tract infection (2% to 5%)

Hepatic: Bilirubin increased (5% to 7%)

Neuromuscular & skeletal: Back pain (9%), limb pain (9%), myalgia (6%), osteoarthritis (6%), weakness (6%), osteoporosis (5%), pathological fracture (4%), paresthesia (3%), carpal tunnel syndrome (2%), cramps (2%)

Ocular: Visual disturbances (5%)

Renal: Creatinine increased (6%)

Respiratory: Dyspnea (10%), cough (6%), bronchitis, pharyngitis, rhinitis, sinusitis, upper respiratory infection

Miscellaneous: Flu-like syndrome (6%), lymphedema, infection

A dose-dependent decrease in sex hormone-binding globulin has been observed with daily doses of daily doses ≥2.5 mg. Serum luteinizing hormone and follicle-stimulating hormone levels have increased with this medicine.

Pharmacodynamics/Kinetics

Absorption Rapid and moderate (~42%) following oral administration; absorption increases ~40% following high-fat meal

Time to Peak Women with breast cancer: 1.2 hours

Protein Binding 90%, primarily to albumin and α_1-acid glycoprotein

Half-Life Elimination 24 hours

Metabolism Extensively hepatic; oxidation (CYP3A4) of methylene group, reduction of 17-keto group with formation of many secondary metabolites; metabolites are inactive

Excretion Urine (<1% as unchanged drug, 39% to 45% as metabolites); feces (36% to 48%)

Available Dosage Forms

Tablet, oral:

Aromasin®: 25 mg

Dosing

Adult & Geriatric Females: Postmenopausal:

Breast cancer, advanced: Oral: 25 mg once daily; continue until tumor progression

Breast cancer, early (adjuvant treatment): Oral: 25 mg once daily (following 2-3 years of tamoxifen therapy) for a total duration of 5 years of endocrine therapy (in the absence of recurrence or contralateral breast cancer)

Dosage adjustment with CYP3A4 inducers: 50 mg once daily when used with potent inducers (eg, rifampin, phenytoin)

Renal Impairment Safety of chronic dosing in renal impairment has not been established.

Hepatic Impairment Safety of chronic dosing in hepatic impairment has not been established.

Administration

Oral Administer after a meal.

Stability

Storage Store at 25°C (77°F); excursions permitted to 15°C to 30°C (59°F to 86°F).

Monitoring and Teaching Issues

Patient Education Take after meals at approximately the same time each day; may cause indigestion. You may be more susceptible to infection. May cause headache, dizziness, confusion, fatigue, anxiety, insomnia, nausea, vomiting, loss of appetite, or hot flashes. Report chest pain; palpitations; acute headache, visual disturbances; unresolved GI problems; itching or burning on urination, vaginal discharge; acute joint, back, bone, or muscle pain; respiratory difficulty; unusual cough; or respiratory infection.

Dietary Considerations Take after a meal; patients on aromatase inhibitor therapy should receive vitamin D and calcium supplements.

Geriatric Considerations In pharmacokinetic trials, no significant changes were seen in women <68 years of age.

Pregnancy Considerations Exemestane has been associated with prolonged gestation, abnormal or difficult labor, increased resorption, reduced number of live fetuses, decreased fetal weight, and retarded ossification in rats. It is not indicated for premenopausal women, but if exposure occurred during pregnancy, risk to the fetus and potential risk for loss of the pregnancy should be discussed.

Additional Information Oncology Comment: The American Society of Clinical Oncology (ASCO) guidelines for adjuvant endocrine therapy in postmenopausal women with HR-positive breast cancer (Burstein, 2010) recommend considering aromatase inhibitor (AI) therapy at some point in the treatment course (primary, sequentially, or extended). Optimal duration at this time is not known; however, treatment with an AI should not exceed 5 years in primary and extended therapies, and 2-3 years if followed by tamoxifen in sequential therapy (total of 5 years). If initial therapy with AI has been discontinued before the 5 years, consideration should be taken to receive tamoxifen for a total of 5 years. The optimal time to switch to an AI is also not known, but data supports switching after 2-3 years of tamoxifen (sequential) or after 5 years of tamoxifen (extended). If patient becomes intolerant or has poor adherence, consideration should be made to switch to another AI or initiate tamoxifen.

Exenatide (ex EN a tide)

U.S. Brand Names Byetta®

Index Terms AC 2993; AC002993; Exendin-4; LY2148568

Generic Availability (U.S.) No

Pharmacologic Category Antidiabetic Agent, Glucagon-Like Peptide-1 (GLP-1) Receptor Agonist

Medication Guide Available Yes

Pregnancy Risk Factor C

Lactation Excretion in breast milk unknown/use caution

Use Treatment of type 2 diabetes mellitus (noninsulin dependent, NIDDM) to improve glycemic control

Mechanism of Action/Effect Exenatide is an analog of the hormone incretin (glucagon-like peptide 1 or GLP-1) which increases glucose-dependent insulin secretion, decreases inappropriate glucagon secretion, increases B-cell growth/replication, slows gastric emptying, and decreases food intake. Exenatide administration results in decreases in hemoglobin A_{1c} by approximately 0.5% to 1%.

Contraindications Hypersensitivity to exenatide or any component of the formulation

Warnings/Precautions Mechanism requires the presence of insulin, therefore use in type 1 diabetes (insulin dependent, IDDM) or diabetic ketoacidosis is not recommended; it is not a substitute for insulin in insulin-requiring patients. Concurrent use with insulin therapy has not been evaluated. May increase the risk of hypoglycemia in patients receiving concomitant insulin secretagogues (eg, sulfonylureas, meglitinides); dosage reduction of sulfonylureas may be required. Clinicians should note that the risk of hypoglycemia is not increased when exenatide is added to metformin monotherapy.

Exenatide is frequently associated with gastrointestinal adverse effects and is not recommended for use in patients with gastroparesis or severe gastrointestinal disease. Gastrointestinal effects may be dose-related and may decrease in frequency/severity with gradual titration and continued use. Due to its effects on gastric emptying, exenatide may reduce the rate and extent of absorption of orally-administered drugs; use with caution in patients receiving medications with a narrow therapeutic window or require rapid absorption from the GI tract. Administer medications 1 hour prior to the use of exenatide when optimal drug absorption and peak levels are important to the overall therapeutic effect (eg, antibiotics, oral contraceptives). Cases of acute pancreatitis (including hemorrhagic and necrotizing with some fatalities) have been reported; monitor for unexplained severe abdominal pain and if pancreatitis suspected, discontinue use. Do not resume unless an alternative etiology of pancreatitis is confirmed. Consider alternative antidiabetic therapy in patients with a history of pancreatitis. Use may be associated with the development of anti-exenatide antibodies. Low titers are not associated with a loss of efficacy; however, high titers (observed in 6% of patients in clinical studies) may result in an attenuation of response. May be associated with weight loss (due to reduced intake) independent of the change in hemoglobin A_{1c}. Not recommended in severe renal impairment (Cl_{cr} <30 mL/minute) or end-stage renal disease (ESRD). Patients with ESRD receiving dialysis may be more susceptible to GI effects (eg, nausea, vomiting) which may result in hypovolemia and further reductions in renal function. Use with caution in patients with renal transplantation and when initiating or escalating doses in patients with moderate renal impairment (Cl_{cr} 30-50 mL/minute).

Drug Interactions

Avoid Concomitant Use There are no known interactions where it is recommended to avoid concomitant use.

Decreased Effect

The levels/effects of Exenatide may be decreased by: Corticosteroids (Orally Inhaled); Corticosteroids (Systemic); Luteinizing Hormone-Releasing Hormone Analogs; Somatropin; Thiazide Diuretics

Increased Effect/Toxicity

Exenatide may increase the levels/effects of: Sulfonylureas; Vitamin K Antagonists

The levels/effects of Exenatide may be increased by: Pegvisomant

Nutritional/Ethanol Interactions Ethanol: Caution with ethanol (may cause hypoglycemia)

Adverse Reactions Percentages as reported for combination therapy (sulfonylurea and/or metformin; thiazolidinedione and/or metformin) unless otherwise noted:

>10%:

Endocrine & metabolic: Hypoglycemia (monotherapy 4% to 5%; combination therapy: sulfonylurea - 14% to 36%; metformin - similar to placebo; thiazolidinedione - 11%)

Gastrointestinal: Nausea (monotherapy 8%; combination therapy 40% to 44%; dose-dependent), vomiting (monotherapy 4%; combination therapy 13%), diarrhea (monotherapy <2%; combination therapy 6% to 13%)

Miscellaneous: Anti-exenatide antibodies (low titers 38%, high titers 6%)

1% to 10%:

Central nervous system: Dizziness (monotherapy <2%; combination therapy 9%), headache (9%)

Dermatologic: Hyperhidrosis (3%)

Endocrine & metabolic: Appetite decreased (<2%)

Gastrointestinal: Dyspepsia (monotherapy 3%; combination therapy 6% to 7%), GERD (3%)

Neuromuscular & skeletal: Weakness (4%)

Miscellaneous: Feeling jittery (9%)

Pharmacodynamics/Kinetics

Time to Peak SubQ: 2.1 hours

Half-Life Elimination 2.4 hours

Metabolism Minimal systemic metabolism; proteolytic degradation may occur following glomerular filtration

Excretion Urine (majority of dose)

Available Dosage Forms

Injection, solution:

Byetta®: 250 mcg/mL (1.2 mL, 2.4 mL)

Dosing

Adult & Geriatric Adjunctive therapy of type 2 diabetes: SubQ: Initial: 5 mcg twice daily within 60 minutes prior to a meal; after 1 month, may be increased to 10 mcg twice daily (based on response)

Renal Impairment

Cl_{cr} ≥50 mL/minute: No adjustment necessary.

Cl_{cr} 30-50 mL/minute: Use caution when initiating or escalating doses.

Cl_{cr} <30 mL/minute: Not recommended.

Administration

Other SubQ: Use only if clear, colorless, and free of particulate matter. Administer via injection in the upper arm, thigh, or abdomen. Administer within 60 minutes prior to morning and evening meal (or prior to the 2 main meals of the day, approximately ≥6 hours apart). Set up each new pen before the first use by priming it. See pen user manual for further details. Dial the dose into the dose window before each administration.

Stability

Storage Prior to initial use, store under refrigeration at 2°C to 8°C (36°F to 46°F); after initial use, may be stored at a temperature ≤25°C (≤77°F). Do not freeze (discard if freezing occurs). Protect from light. Pen should be discarded 30 days after initial use.

Monitoring and Teaching Issues

Laboratory Monitoring Serum glucose, hemoglobin A_{1c}, and renal function

Physical Assessment Monitor renal function. Teach appropriate injection technique and disposal of needles.

Patient Education Administer injection within 60 minutes of meals. Do not administer after meal. Consume alcohol with caution; may cause hypoglycemia. It is important to follow dietary and lifestyle recommendations of prescriber. You may experience nausea, decreased appetite, dizziness, or lightheadedness. Maintain adequate hydration, unless instructed to restrict fluid intake. Report changes in urination (color, amount); swelling of extremities; unusual weight gain; fatigue; pain in lower back; or persistent nausea, diarrhea, abdominal pain, or dizziness.

Geriatric Considerations Intensive glucose control (Hb A_{1c} <6.5%) has been linked to increased all cause and cardiovascular mortality, hypoglycemia requiring assistance, and weight gain in adult type 2 diabetes. For elderly patients with diabetes who are relatively healthy, attaining target goals for aspirin use, blood pressure, lipids, smoking cessation, and diet and exercise may be more important than normalized glycemic control.

Breast-Feeding Considerations It is not known if exenatide is present in breast milk. The manufacturer recommends that caution be exercised when administering exenatide to nursing women.

Pregnancy Considerations Due to adverse events observed in some animal studies, exenatide is classified as pregnancy category C. Based on *in vitro* data, exenatide has a low potential to cross the placenta. Maternal hyperglycemia can be associated with adverse effects in the fetus, including macrosomia, neonatal hyperglycemia, and hyperbilirubinemia; the risk of congenital malformations is increased when the Hb A_{1c} is above the normal range. Diabetes can also be associated with adverse effects in the mother. Poorly-treated diabetes may cause end-organ damage that may in turn negatively affect obstetric outcomes. Physiologic glucose levels should be maintained prior to and during pregnancy to decrease the risk of adverse events in the mother and the fetus. Until additional safety and efficacy data are obtained, the use of exenatide is generally not recommended in the routine management of diabetes mellitus during pregnancy. Insulin is the drug of choice for the control of diabetes mellitus during pregnancy. A registry has been established for women exposed to exenatide during pregnancy (1-800-633-9081).

Additional Information A dosing strategy which employs progressive dose escalation of exenatide (initiating at 0.02 mcg/kg 3 times daily and increasing in increments of 0.02 mcg/kg every 3 days) has been described, limiting the frequency and severity of gastrointestinal adverse effects. The complexity of this regimen may limit its clinical application.

In animal models, exenatide has been a useful adjunctive therapy when added to immunotherapy protocols, resulting in recovery of beta cell function and sustained remission.

- **Exendin-4** *see* Exenatide *on page* 726
- **Exforge®** *see* Amlodipine and Valsartan *on page* 108
- **Exforge HCT®** *see* Amlodipine, Valsartan, and Hydrochlorothiazide *on page* 109
- **Extavia®** *see* Interferon Beta-1b *on page* 1005
- **Extina®** *see* Ketoconazole (Topical) *on page* 1039

Ezetimibe (ez ET i mibe)

U.S. Brand Names Zetia®

Generic Availability (U.S.) No

Pharmacologic Category Antilipemic Agent, 2-Azetidinone

Medication Safety Issues

Sound-alike/look-alike issues:

Zetia® may be confused with Zebeta®, Zestril®

Pregnancy Risk Factor C

Lactation Excretion in breast milk unknown/not recommended

Use Use in combination with dietary therapy for the treatment of primary hypercholesterolemia (as monotherapy or in combination with HMG-CoA reductase inhibitors); homozygous sitosterolemia; homozygous familial hypercholesterolemia (in combination with atorvastatin or simvastatin); mixed hyperlipidemia (in combination with fenofibrate)

Mechanism of Action/Effect Inhibits absorption of cholesterol at the brush border of the small intestine, leading to a decreased delivery of cholesterol to the liver, reduction of hepatic cholesterol stores and an increased clearance of cholesterol from the blood; decreases total C, LDL-C, ApoB, and triglycerides while increasing HDL-C

Contraindications Hypersensitivity to ezetimibe or any component of the formulation; concomitant use with an HMG-CoA reductase inhibitor in patients with active hepatic disease, unexplained persistent elevations in serum transaminases; pregnancy; breast-feeding

Warnings/Precautions Secondary causes of hyperlipidemia should be ruled out prior to therapy. Use caution with severe renal (Cl_{cr} <30 mL/minute) or mild hepatic impairment (Child-Pugh class A); not recommended for use with moderate or severe hepatic impairment (Child-Pugh classes B and C). Concurrent use of ezetimibe and fibric acid derivatives may increase the risk of cholelithiasis.

Drug Interactions

Metabolism/Transport Effects Substrate of SLCO1B1

Avoid Concomitant Use There are no known interactions where it is recommended to avoid concomitant use.

Decreased Effect

The levels/effects of Ezetimibe may be decreased by: Bile Acid Sequestrants

Increased Effect/Toxicity

Ezetimibe may increase the levels/effects of: CycloSPORINE; CycloSPORINE (Systemic)

The levels/effects of Ezetimibe may be increased by: CycloSPORINE; CycloSPORINE (Systemic); Eltrombopag; Fibric Acid Derivatives

Nutritional/Ethanol Interactions Food: Ezetimibe did not cause meaningful reductions in fat-soluble vitamin concentrations during a 2-week clinical trial. Effects of long-term therapy have not been evaluated.

Adverse Reactions 1% to 10%:

Central nervous system: Fatigue (2%)
Gastrointestinal: Diarrhea (4%)
Hepatic: Transaminases increased (with HMG-CoA reductase inhibitors) (≥3 x ULN, 1%)
Neuromuscular & skeletal: Arthralgia (3%), pain in extremity (3%)

Respiratory: Upper respiratory tract infection (4%), sinusitis (3%)
Miscellaneous: Influenza (2%)

Pharmacodynamics/Kinetics

Bioavailability Variable

Time to Peak Plasma: 4-12 hours

Protein Binding >90% to plasma proteins

Half-Life Elimination 22 hours (ezetimibe and metabolite)

Metabolism Undergoes glucuronide conjugation in the small intestine and liver; forms metabolite (active); may undergo enterohepatic recycling

Excretion Feces (78%, 69% as ezetimibe); urine (11%, 9% as metabolite)

Available Dosage Forms

Tablet, oral:
Zetia®: 10 mg

Dosing

Adult & Geriatric Hyperlipidemias, sitosterolemia: Oral: 10 mg/day

Pediatric Children ≥10 years: Refer to adult dosing.

Renal Impairment AUC increased with severe impairment (Cl_{cr} <30 mL/minute); no dosing adjustment recommended.

Hepatic Impairment AUC increased with hepatic impairment:
Mild impairment (Child-Pugh class A): No dosing adjustment necessary.
Moderate-to-severe impairment (Child-Pugh classes B and C): Use of ezetimibe not recommended.

Administration

Oral May be administered without regard to meals. May be taken at the same time as HMG-CoA reductase inhibitors. Administer ≥2 hours before or ≥4 hours after bile acid sequestrants.

Stability

Storage Store at controlled room temperature of 25°C (77°F). Protect from moisture.

Monitoring and Teaching Issues

Laboratory Monitoring Total cholesterol profile prior to therapy, and when clinically indicated and/or periodically thereafter. When used in combination with fenofibrate, monitor LFTs and signs and symptoms of cholelithiasis.

Physical Assessment Use caution in presence of renal or hepatic impairment. Assess lipid profile at beginning of and at regular intervals during therapy. Teach patient to report signs of hepatic or muscle reactions.

Patient Education Take at the same time of day, without regard for meals. Take 2 hours before or 4 hours after bile acid binding agents (eg, Questran®). This medication does not replace the need for dietary and exercise recommendations of prescriber. May cause headache, dizziness, fatigue, diarrhea, or abdominal pain. Report yellowing of skin or sclera; dark urine or pale stools; excessive tiredness; chest pain or palpitations; muscle, skeletal, or joint pain; twitching or numbness; increased perspiration; or changes in urinary pattern.

Dietary Considerations May be taken without regard to meals. Before initiation of therapy, patients should be placed on a standard cholesterol-lowering diet for 6 weeks and the diet should be continued during drug therapy.

Pregnancy Considerations Safety and efficacy have not been established; use during pregnancy only if the potential benefit to the mother outweighs the possible risk to the fetus.

Additional Information When studied in combination with fenofibrate for mixed hyperlipidemia, the dose of fenofibrate was 160 mg daily.

Related Information

Hyperlipidemia Management *on page 2046*

Ezetimibe and Simvastatin (ez ET i mibe & SIM va stat in)

U.S. Brand Names Vytorin®

Index Terms Simvastatin and Ezetimibe

Generic Availability (U.S.) No

Pharmacologic Category Antilipemic Agent, 2-Azetidinone; Antilipemic Agent, HMG-CoA Reductase Inhibitor

Medication Safety Issues

Sound-alike/look-alike issues:
Vytorin® may be confused with Vyvanse™

Pregnancy Risk Factor X

Lactation Excretion in breast milk unknown/contraindicated

Use Used in combination with dietary modification for the treatment of primary hypercholesterolemia and homozygous familial hypercholesterolemia

Contraindications Hypersensitivity to ezetimibe, simvastatin, or any component of the formulation; acute liver disease; unexplained persistent elevations of serum transaminases; pregnancy; breast-feeding

Warnings/Precautions See individual agents.

Drug Interactions

Metabolism/Transport Effects

Ezetimibe: **Substrate** of SLCO1B1
Simvastatin: **Substrate** of CYP3A4 (major), SLCO1B1; **Inhibits** CYP2C8 (weak), 2C9 (weak), 2D6 (weak)

Avoid Concomitant Use

Avoid concomitant use of Ezetimibe and Simvastatin with any of the following: Protease Inhibitors; Red Yeast Rice

Decreased Effect

The levels/effects of Ezetimibe and Simvastatin may be decreased by: Antacids; Bile Acid Sequestrants; Bosentan; CYP3A4 Inducers (Strong); Deferasirox; Efavirenz; Etravirine; Phenytoin; Rifamycin Derivatives; St Johns Wort

Increased Effect/Toxicity

Ezetimibe and Simvastatin may increase the levels/effects of: CycloSPORINE; CycloSPORINE (Systemic); DAPTOmycin; Diltiazem; Trabectedin; Vitamin K Antagonists

The levels/effects of Ezetimibe and Simvastatin may be increased by: Amiodarone; Antifungal Agents (Azole Derivatives, Systemic); Colchicine; Conivaptan; CycloSPORINE; CycloSPORINE (Systemic); CYP3A4 Inhibitors (Moderate); CYP3A4 Inhibitors (Strong); Danazol; Dasatinib; Diltiazem; Dronedarone; Eltrombopag; Fenofibrate; Fenofibric Acid; Fibric Acid Derivatives; Fluconazole; Fusidic Acid; Gemfibrozil; Grapefruit Juice; Green Tea; Imatinib; Macrolide Antibiotics; Nefazodone; Niacin; Niacinamide; Protease Inhibitors; QuiNINE; Ranolazine; Red Yeast Rice; Rifamycin Derivatives; Sildenafil; Verapamil

Nutritional/Ethanol Interactions

Ethanol: Avoid excessive ethanol consumption (due to potential hepatic effects).

Food: Simvastatin serum concentration may be increased when taken with grapefruit juice; avoid concurrent intake of large quantities (>1 quart/day). Red yeast rice contains an estimated 2.4 mg lovastatin per 600 mg rice. Ezetimibe did not cause meaningful reductions in fat-soluble vitamin concentrations during a 2-week clinical trial. Effects of long-term therapy have not been evaluated.

Herb/Nutraceutical: St John's wort may decrease simvastatin levels.

Adverse Reactions Percentages refer to combination Vytorin®. Also see individual agents.

1% to 10%:

- Central nervous system: Headache (6%)
- Gastrointestinal: Diarrhea (3%)
- Hepatic: ALT increased (4%)
- Neuromuscular & skeletal: Myalgia (4%), pain in extremity (2%)
- Respiratory: Upper respiratory infection (4%)
- Miscellaneous: Influenza (2%)

Pharmacodynamics/Kinetics

Bioavailability Vytorin® is equivalent to coadministered ezetimibe and simvastatin.

Pharmacokinetic Note See individual agents.

Available Dosage Forms

Tablet:

Vytorin®:

- 10/10: Ezetimibe 10 mg and simvastatin 10 mg
- 10/20: Ezetimibe 10 mg and simvastatin 20 mg
- 10/40: Ezetimibe 10 mg and simvastatin 40 mg
- 10/80: Ezetimibe 10 mg and simvastatin 80 mg

Dosing

Adult & Geriatric

Homozygous familial hypercholesterolemia: Ezetimibe 10 mg and simvastatin 40 mg once daily in the evening or ezetimibe 10 mg and simvastatin 80 mg once daily in the evening. Dosing range: Ezetimibe 10 mg and simvastatin 10-80 mg once daily.

Hyperlipidemias: Oral: Initial: Ezetimibe 10 mg and simvastatin 20 mg once daily in the evening; those patients requiring less aggressive LDL-C reductions can start with ezetimibe 10 mg and simvastatin 10 mg once daily

Patients who require less aggressive reduction in LDL-C: Initial: Ezetimibe 10 mg and simvastatin 10 mg once daily in the evening

Patients who require >55% reduction in LDL-C: Initial: Ezetimibe 10 mg and simvastatin 40 mg once daily in the evening

Dosage adjustment with concomitant medications: Oral:

Cyclosporine or danazol: Patient must first demonstrate tolerance to simvastatin ≥5 mg once daily. Dose should **not** exceed ezetimibe 10 mg and simvastatin 10 mg once daily

Gemfibrozil: Although concurrent use is not recommended by manufacturer, dose should **not** exceed ezetimibe 10 mg and simvastatin 10 mg once daily

Amiodarone or verapamil: Dose should **not** exceed ezetimibe 10 mg and simvastatin 20 mg once daily

Diltiazem: Simvastatin dose should **not** exceed 40 mg/day

Dosage adjustment in Chinese patients on niacin doses ≥1 g/day: Oral: Because of an increased risk of myopathy, do not administer ezetimibe 10 mg and simvastatin 80 mg

Renal Impairment Dosage adjustment unnecessary in mild-to-moderate renal dysfunction. In severe dysfunction, start only if patient tolerates 5 mg daily of simvastatin; monitor closely.

Hepatic Impairment Dosage adjustment unnecessary in mild hepatic dysfunction.

Administration

Oral May be administered without regard to meals. Administer in the evening for maximal efficacy.

Stability

Storage Store at 20°C to 25°C (68°F to 77°F).

Monitoring and Teaching Issues

Physical Assessment See individual agents.

Patient Education See individual agents.

Dietary Considerations May be taken without regard to meals. Red yeast rice contains an estimated 2.4 mg lovastatin per 600 mg of rice.

Geriatric Considerations Clinical studies of Vytorin® included a total of 792 patients >65 years of age with 176 of these patients ≥75 years. The safety in this group was similar to the younger patients. No adjustment of dose is necessary for initiation of treatment in the elderly.

Breast-Feeding Considerations See individual agents.

Pregnancy Considerations See individual agents.

Related Information

Hyperlipidemia Management *on page* 2046

◆ **Factive®** *see* Gemifloxacin *on page* 861

Factor VIIa (Recombinant) (FAK ter SEV en aye ree KOM be nant)

U.S. Brand Names NovoSeven® RT

Index Terms Coagulation Factor VIIa; Eptacog Alfa (Activated); rFVIIa

Generic Availability (U.S.) No

Pharmacologic Category Antihemophilic Agent

Medication Safety Issues

Sound-alike/look-alike issues:

NovoSeven® RT may be confused with Novacet®

Pregnancy Risk Factor C

Lactation Excretion in breast milk unknown/not recommended

Use Treatment of bleeding episodes and prevention of bleeding in surgical interventions in patients with either hemophilia A or B with inhibitors to factor VIII or factor IX, acquired hemophilia, or congenital factor VII deficiency

Unlabeled/Investigational Use Reduction of hematoma growth in patients with acute intracerebral hemorrhage, warfarin-related intracerebral hemorrhage

Available Dosage Forms

Injection, powder for reconstitution [preservative free]:

NovoSeven® RT: 1 mg, 2 mg, 5 mg, 8 mg

Dosing

Adult & Geriatric For I.V. administration only:

Hemophilia A or B with inhibitors:

Bleeding episodes: 90 mcg/kg every 2 hours until hemostasis is achieved or until the treatment is judged ineffective. Doses between 35-120 mcg/kg have been used successfully in clinical trials. The dose, interval, and duration of therapy may be adjusted based upon the severity of bleeding and the degree of hemostasis achieved. For patients experiencing severe bleeds, dosing should be continued at 3- to 6-hour intervals after hemostasis has been achieved and the duration of dosing should be minimized.

Surgical interventions: 90 mcg/kg immediately before surgery; repeat at 2-hour intervals for the duration of surgery. Continue every 2 hours for 48 hours, then every 2-6 hours until healed for minor surgery; continue every 2 hours for 5 days, then every 4 hours until healed for major surgery.

Congenital factor VII deficiency: Bleeding episodes and surgical interventions: 15-30 mcg/kg every 4-6 hours until hemostasis is achieved. Doses as low as 10 mcg/kg have been effective.

Acquired hemophilia: 70-90 mcg/kg every 2-3 hours until hemostasis is achieved.

Intracerebral hemorrhage (warfarin-related) (unlabeled use; Freeman, 2004; Ilyas, 2008): 10-100 mcg/kg (see **"Note"** below) administered concurrently with I.V. vitamin K (to correct the nonfactor VII coagulation factors).

Note: Lower doses (10-20 mcg/kg) are generally preferred given the higher risk of thromboembolic complications with higher doses; response is highly variable; monitor INR frequently after administration since rebound increases in INR occur quickly given the short half-life of rFVIIa; duration of INR correction is dose dependent.

Pediatric Refer to adult dosing.

Administration

I.V. I.V. administration only; bolus over 2-5 minutes. Administer within 3 hours after reconstitution.

Monitoring and Teaching Issues

Laboratory Monitoring Although the prothrombin time/INR, aPTT, and factor VII clotting activity have no correlation with achieving hemostasis, these parameters may be useful as adjunct tests to evaluate efficacy and guide dose or interval adjustments

Physical Assessment Assess prothrombin time and factor VII clotting activity. Patient should be monitored closely during and after therapy (vital signs, cardiac and CNS status, hemolytic status, hypersensitivity).

Patient Education This medication can only be administered by infusion. Report immediately any swelling, pain, burning, or itching at infusion site. Report acute headache, visual changes, pain in joints or muscles, respiratory difficulty, chills, back pain, dizziness, or nausea.

◆ **Factor VIII Concentrate** *see* Antihemophilic Factor/von Willebrand Factor Complex (Human) *on page* 134

◆ **Factor VIII (Human)** *see* Antihemophilic Factor (Human) *on page* 132

◆ **Factor VIII (Human)** *see* Antihemophilic Factor/von Willebrand Factor Complex (Human) *on page* 134

◆ **Factor VIII (Recombinant)** *see* Antihemophilic Factor (Recombinant) *on page* 133

Famciclovir (fam SYE kloe veer)

U.S. Brand Names Famvir®

Generic Availability (U.S.) Yes

Pharmacologic Category Antiviral Agent

Medication Safety Issues

Sound-alike/look-alike issues:

Famvir® may be confused with Femara®

Pregnancy Risk Factor B

Lactation Excretion in breast milk unknown/not recommended

Use Treatment of acute herpes zoster (shingles); treatment and suppression of recurrent episodes of genital herpes in immunocompetent patients; treatment of herpes labialis (cold sores) in immunocompetent patients; treatment of recurrent mucocutaneous/genital herpes simplex in HIV-infected patients

Mechanism of Action/Effect The prodrug famciclovir undergoes rapid biotransformation to the active compound, penciclovir, then intracellular conversion to triphosphate which is active against HSV-1, HSV-2, VZV, and EBV infected cells.

Contraindications Hypersensitivity to famciclovir, penciclovir, or any component of the formulation

Warnings/Precautions Has not been studied in immunocompromised patients or patients with ophthalmic, disseminated zoster, or with initial episode of genital herpes. Dosage adjustment is required in patients with renal insufficiency. Tablets contain lactose; do not use with galactose intolerance, severe lactase deficiency, or glucose-galactose malabsorption syndromes.

Drug Interactions

Avoid Concomitant Use

Avoid concomitant use of Famciclovir with any of the following: Zoster Vaccine

Decreased Effect

Famciclovir may decrease the levels/effects of: Zoster Vaccine

Increased Effect/Toxicity There are no known significant interactions involving an increase in effect.

Nutritional/Ethanol Interactions Food: Rate of absorption and/or conversion to penciclovir and peak concentration are reduced with food, but bioavailability is not affected.

Adverse Reactions Note: Frequencies vary with dose and duration. Single-dose treatment (herpes labialis) was associated only with headache (10%), diarrhea (2%), fatigue (1%), and dysmenorrhea (1%).

>10%:

Central nervous system: Headache (14% to 39%)

Gastrointestinal: Nausea (3% to 13%)

1% to 10%:

Central nervous system: Fatigue (1% to 5%), migraine (1% to 3%)

Dermatologic: Pruritus (≤4%), rash (≤3%)

Endocrine & metabolic: Dysmenorrhea (≤8%)

Gastrointestinal: Diarrhea (5% to 9%), abdominal pain (≤8%), flatulence (1% to 5%), vomiting (1% to 5%)

Hematologic: Neutropenia (3%)

Hepatic: Transaminases increased (2% to 3%), bilirubin increased (2%)

Neuromuscular & skeletal: Paresthesia (≤3%)

Pharmacodynamics/Kinetics

Absorption Food decreases maximum peak penciclovir concentration and delays time to penciclovir peak; AUC remains the same

Bioavailability Penciclovir: 69% to 85%

Time to Peak Penciclovir: 0.9 hours; C_{max} and T_{max} are decreased and prolonged with noncompensated hepatic impairment

Protein Binding Penciclovir: ≤20%

Half-Life Elimination Penciclovir: 2-4 hours; Prolonged in renal impairment: Cl_{cr} 20-39 mL/minute: 5-8 hours, Cl_{cr} <20 mL/minute: 3-24 hours

Metabolism Famciclovir is rapidly deacetylated and oxidized to penciclovir (active prodrug); not via CYP

Excretion Urine (73% primarily as penciclovir); feces (27%)

Available Dosage Forms

Tablet, oral: 125 mg, 250 mg, 500 mg

Famvir®: 125 mg, 250 mg, 500 mg

Dosing

Adult & Geriatric

Acute herpes zoster: Oral: 500 mg every 8 hours for 7 days (**Note:** Initiate therapy within 72 hours of rash onset.)

Genital herpes simplex virus (HSV) infection in immunocompetent patients: Oral:

Initial episode: 250 mg 3 times/day for 7-10 days (CDC, 2010)

Recurrence: 1000 mg twice daily for 1 day (**Note:** Initiate therapy within 6 hours of symptoms/lesions)

Alternatively, the following regimens are also recommended: 125 mg twice daily for 5 days or 500 mg as a single dose, followed by 250 mg twice daily for 2 days (CDC, 2010)

Suppressive therapy: 250 mg twice daily for up to 1 year; **Note:** Duration not established, but efficacy/safety have been demonstrated for 1 year (CDC, 2010)

Recurrent herpes labialis (cold sores): Oral: 1500 mg as a single dose; initiate therapy at first sign or symptom such as tingling, burning, or itching (initiated within 1 hour in clinical studies)

Recurrent mucocutaneous/genital HSV infection in HIV patients: Oral: 500 mg twice daily for 7 days or 5-10 days (CDC, 2010)

Prevention of HSV reactivation in HIV patients: Oral: 500 mg twice daily (CDC, 2010)

Renal Impairment

Herpes zoster:

Cl_{cr} 40-59 mL/minute: Administer 500 mg every 12 hours
Cl_{cr} 20-39 mL/minute: Administer 500 mg every 24 hours
Cl_{cr} <20 mL/minute: Administer 250 mg every 24 hours
Hemodialysis: Administer 250 mg after each dialysis session.

Recurrent genital herpes: Treatment (single day regimen):

Cl_{cr} 40-59 mL/minute: Administer 500 mg every 12 hours for 1 day
Cl_{cr} 20-39 mL/minute: Administer 500 mg as a single dose
Cl_{cr} <20 mL/minute: Administer 250 mg as a single dose
Hemodialysis: Administer 250 mg as a single dose after dialysis session.

Recurrent genital herpes: Suppression:

Cl_{cr} 20-39 mL/minute: Administer 125 mg every 12 hours
Cl_{cr} <20 mL/minute: Administer 125 mg every 24 hours
Hemodialysis: Administer 125 mg after each dialysis session.

Recurrent herpes labialis: Treatment (single dose regimen):

Cl_{cr} 40-59 mL/minute: Administer 750 mg as a single dose
Cl_{cr} 20-39 mL/minute: Administer 500 mg as a single dose
Cl_{cr} <20 mL/minute: Administer 250 mg as a single dose
Hemodialysis: Administer 250 mg as a single dose after dialysis session.

Recurrent orolabial or genital herpes in HIV-infected patients:

Cl_{cr} 20-39 mL/minute: Administer 500 mg every 24 hours
Cl_{cr} <20 mL/minute: Administer 250 mg every 24 hours
Hemodialysis: Administer 250 mg after each dialysis session.

Administration

Oral May be administered without regard to meals.

Stability

Storage Store at 25°C (77°F); excursions permitted to 15°C to 30°C (59°F to 86°F).

Monitoring and Teaching Issues

Laboratory Monitoring Periodic CBC during long-term therapy

Physical Assessment Assess periodic CBC during long-term therapy. Monitor for persistent fatigue and gastrointestinal upset.

Patient Education This is not a cure for genital herpes. May cause mild GI disturbances (eg, nausea, vomiting, constipation, diarrhea), fatigue, headache, or muscle aches and pains. If these are severe, contact prescriber.

Dietary Considerations May be taken without regard to meals.

Geriatric Considerations For herpes zoster (shingles) infections, famciclovir should be started within 72 hours of the appearance of the rash to be effective. Famciclovir has been shown to accelerate healing, reduce the duration of viral shedding, and resolve posthepatic neuralgia faster than placebo. Comparison trials to acyclovir or valacyclovir are not available. Adjust dose for estimated renal function.

Breast-Feeding Considerations There is no specific data describing the excretion of famciclovir in breast milk. Breast-feeding is not recommended by the manufacturer unless the potential benefits outweigh any possible risk. If herpes lesions are on breast, breast-feeding should be avoided in order to avoid transmission to infant.

Pregnancy Considerations Teratogenic effects were not observed in animal studies. There are no adequate and well-controlled studies in pregnant women. Use only if benefit outweighs risk. A registry has been established for women exposed to famciclovir during pregnancy (888-669-6682).

Additional Information Most effective for herpes zoster if therapy is initiated within 48 hours of initial lesion. Resistance may occur by alteration of thymidine kinase, resulting in loss of or reduced penciclovir phosphorylation (cross-resistance occurs between acyclovir and famciclovir). When treatment for herpes labialis is initiated within 1 hour of symptom onset, healing time is reduced by ~2 days.

Famotidine (fa MOE ti deen)

U.S. Brand Names Heartburn Relief Maximum Strength [OTC]; Heartburn Relief [OTC]; Pepcid®; Pepcid® AC Maximum Strength [OTC]; Pepcid® AC [OTC]

Generic Availability (U.S.) Yes: Infusion, Injection, oral suspension, tablet

Pharmacologic Category Histamine H_2 Antagonist

Medication Safety Issues

Sound-alike/look-alike issues:

Famotidine may be confused with FLUoxetine, furosemide

Pregnancy Risk Factor B

Lactation Enters breast milk/not recommended

Use Maintenance therapy and treatment of duodenal ulcer; treatment of gastroesophageal reflux disease (GERD), active benign gastric ulcer; pathological hypersecretory conditions

OTC labeling: Relief of heartburn, acid indigestion, and sour stomach

Unlabeled/Investigational Use Part of a multidrug regimen for *H. pylori* eradication to reduce the risk of duodenal ulcer recurrence; stress ulcer prophylaxis in critically-ill patients; symptomatic relief in gastritis

Mechanism of Action/Effect Competitive inhibition of histamine at H_2 receptors of the gastric parietal cells, which inhibits gastric acid secretion

Contraindications Hypersensitivity to famotidine, other H_2 antagonists, or any component of the formulation

Warnings/Precautions Modify dose in patients with moderate-to-severe renal impairment. Relief of symptoms does not preclude the presence of a gastric malignancy. Reversible confusional states, usually clearing within 3-4 days after discontinuation, have been linked to use. Increased age (>50 years) and renal or hepatic impairment are thought to be associated. Multidose vials for injection contain benzyl alcohol.

OTC labeling: When used for self-medication, patients should be instructed not to use if they have difficulty swallowing, are vomiting blood, or have bloody or black stools. Not for use with other acid reducers.

Drug Interactions

Avoid Concomitant Use

Avoid concomitant use of Famotidine with any of the following: Delavirdine; Erlotinib

Decreased Effect

Famotidine may decrease the levels/effects of: Atazanavir; Cefditoren; Cefpodoxime; Cefuroxime; Dasatinib; Delavirdine; Erlotinib; Fosamprenavir; Gefitinib; Indinavir; Iron Salts; Itraconazole; Ketoconazole; Ketoconazole (Systemic); Mesalamine; Nelfinavir; Posaconazole

Increased Effect/Toxicity

Famotidine may increase the levels/effects of: Dexmethylphenidate; Methylphenidate; Saquinavir

Nutritional/Ethanol Interactions

Ethanol: Avoid ethanol (may cause gastric mucosal irritation).

Food: Famotidine bioavailability may be increased if taken with food.

Adverse Reactions

Note: Agitation and vomiting have been reported in up to 14% of pediatric patients <1 year of age.

1% to 10%:

Central nervous system: Headache (5%), dizziness (1%)

Gastrointestinal: Diarrhea (2%), constipation (1%)

Pharmacodynamics/Kinetics

Onset of Action Antisecretory effect: Oral: Within 1 hour; I.V.: Within 30 minutes

Peak effect: Antisecretory effect: Oral: Within 1-3 hours (dose-dependent)

Duration of Action Antisecretory effect: I.V., Oral: 10-12 hours

Absorption Oral: Incompletely absorbed

Bioavailability Oral: 40% to 45%

Time to Peak Serum: Oral: ~1-3 hours

Protein Binding 15% to 20%

Half-Life Elimination

Infants: 0-3 months: ~8-10.5 hours; >3-12 months: ~4.5 hours

Children: 3.4 hours

Adults: 2.5-3.5 hours; prolonged with renal impairment; Oliguria: >20 hours

Metabolism Minimal first-pass metabolism; forms one metabolite (S-oxide)

Excretion Urine (25% to 30% [oral], 65% to 70% [I.V.] as unchanged drug)

Available Dosage Forms

Infusion, premixed in NS [preservative free]: 20 mg (50 mL)

Injection, solution: 10 mg/mL (4 mL, 20 mL, 50 mL)

Injection, solution [preservative free]: 10 mg/mL (2 mL)

Powder for suspension, oral: 40 mg/5 mL (50 mL)

Pepcid®: 40 mg/5 mL (50 mL)

Tablet, oral: 10 mg, 20 mg, 40 mg

Heartburn Relief [OTC]: 10 mg

Heartburn Relief Maximum Strength [OTC]: 20 mg

Pepcid®: 20 mg, 40 mg

Pepcid® AC [OTC]: 10 mg

Pepcid® AC Maximum Strength [OTC]: 20 mg

Tablet, chewable, oral:

Pepcid® AC Maximum Strength [OTC]: 20 mg

Dosing

Adult & Geriatric

Duodenal ulcer: Oral: Acute therapy: 40 mg/day at bedtime (or 20 mg twice daily) for 4-8 weeks; maintenance therapy: 20 mg/day at bedtime

Gastric ulcer: Oral: Acute therapy: 40 mg/day at bedtime

Hypersecretory conditions: Oral: Initial: 20 mg every 6 hours, may increase in increments up to 160 mg every 6 hours

GERD: Oral: 20 mg twice daily for 6 weeks

Esophagitis and accompanying symptoms due to GERD: Oral: 20 mg or 40 mg twice daily for up to 12 weeks

Peptic ulcer disease: Eradication of *Helicobacter pylori* (unlabeled use): Oral: 40 mg once daily; requires combination therapy with antibiotics

Patients unable to take oral medication: I.V.: 20 mg every 12 hours

Heartburn, indigestion, sour stomach: OTC labeling: Oral: 10-20 mg every 12 hours; dose may be taken 15-60 minutes before eating foods known to cause heartburn

Pediatric Treatment duration and dose should be individualized

Peptic ulcer: 1-16 years:

Oral: 0.5 mg/kg/day at bedtime or divided twice daily (maximum dose: 40 mg/day); doses of up to 1 mg/kg/day have been used in clinical studies

I.V.: 0.25 mg/kg every 12 hours (maximum dose: 40 mg/day); doses of up to 0.5 mg/kg have been used in clinical studies

GERD: Oral:

<3 months: 0.5 mg/kg once daily

3-12 months: 0.5 mg/kg twice daily

1-16 years: 1 mg/kg/day divided twice daily (maximum dose: 40 mg twice daily); doses of up to 2 mg/kg/day have been used in clinical studies

Heartburn, indigestion, sour stomach: OTC labeling: Oral: Children ≥12 years: Refer to adult dosing.

Renal Impairment Cl_{cr} <50 mL/minute: Manufacturer recommendation: Administer 50% of dose **or** increase the dosing interval to every 36-48 hours (to limit potential CNS adverse effects).

Administration

Oral May administer with antacids.

Suspension: Shake vigorously before use. May be taken without regard to meals.

Tablet: May be taken without regard to meals.

I.V.

I.V. push: Inject over at least 2 minutes.

Solution for infusion: Administer over 15-30 minutes.

Stability

Reconstitution Solution for injection:

I.V. push: Dilute famotidine with NS (or another compatible solution) to a total of 5-10 mL (some centers also administer undiluted).

Infusion: Dilute with D_5W 100 mL or another compatible solution.

Storage

Oral:

Powder for oral suspension: Prior to mixing, dry powder should be stored at controlled room temperature of 25°C (77°F). Reconstituted oral suspension is stable for 30 days at room temperature; do not freeze.

Tablet: Store controlled room temperature. Protect from moisture.

I.V.:

Solution for injection: Prior to use, store at 2°C to 8°C (36°F to 46°F). If solution freezes, allow to solubilize at controlled room temperature. May be stored at room temperature for up to 3 months (data on file [Bedford Laboratories, 2011]).

I.V. push: Following preparation, solutions for I.V. push should be used immediately, or may be stored in refrigerator and used within 48 hours.

Infusion: Following preparation, the manufacturer states may be stored for up to 48 hours under refrigeration; however, solutions for infusion have been found to be physically and chemically stable for 7 days at room temperature.

Solution for injection, premixed bags: Store at controlled room temperature of 25°C (77°F); avoid excessive heat.

Monitoring and Teaching Issues

Physical Assessment Teach patient proper timing of administration.

Patient Education OTC: Do not use for more than 14 days unless recommended by prescriber. May cause drowsiness, dizziness, constipation, or diarrhea. Report acute headache, unresolved constipation or diarrhea, palpitations, black tarry stools, abdominal pain, rash, worsening of condition being treated, or recurrence of symptoms after therapy is completed.

Dietary Considerations May be taken without regard to meals.

Geriatric Considerations H_2 blockers are the preferred drugs for treating PUD in the elderly due to cost and ease of administration. They are no less or more effective than any other therapy. Famotidine is one of the preferred agents (due to side effects, drug interaction profile, and pharmacokinetics). Treatment for PUD in the elderly is recommended for 12 weeks since their lesions are typically larger; therefore, take longer to heal. Always adjust dose based upon creatinine clearance, since slight accumulation may result in CNS side effects, mainly confusion.

Breast-Feeding Considerations Famotidine is excreted into breast milk with peak concentrations occurring ~6 hours after the maternal dose. According to the manufacturer, the decision to continue or discontinue breast-feeding during therapy should take into account the risk of exposure to the infant and the benefits of treatment to the mother.

Pregnancy Considerations Adverse events have not been observed in animal reproduction studies; therefore, famotidine is classified as pregnancy category B. Famotidine crosses the placenta. An increased risk of congenital malformations or adverse events in the newborn has generally not been observed following maternal use of famotidine during pregnancy. Histamine H_2 antagonists have been evaluated for the treatment of gastroesophageal reflux disease (GERD), as well as gastric and duodenal ulcers, during pregnancy. Although if needed, famotidine is not the agent of choice. Histamine H_2 antagonists may be used for aspiration prophylaxis prior to cesarean delivery.

◆ **Fampridine-SR** *see* Dalfampridine *on page* 458
◆ **Famvir®** *see* Famciclovir *on page* 732
◆ **Fanapt®** *see* Iloperidone *on page* 949
◆ **2F-ara-AMP** *see* Fludarabine *on page* 776
◆ **Fareston®** *see* Toremifene *on page* 1793
◆ **Faslodex®** *see* Fulvestrant *on page* 838

Fat Emulsion (fat e MUL shun)

U.S. Brand Names Intralipid®; Liposyn® II [DSC]; Liposyn® III

Index Terms Intravenous Fat Emulsion

Generic Availability (U.S.) No

Pharmacologic Category Caloric Agent

Pregnancy Risk Factor C

Lactation Excretion in breast milk unknown/compatible

Use Source of calories and essential fatty acids for patients requiring parenteral nutrition of extended duration; prevention and treatment of essential fatty acid deficiency (EFAD)

Unlabeled/Investigational Use Local anesthetic-induced cardiac arrest unresponsive to conventional resuscitation

Available Dosage Forms

Injection, emulsion:

Intralipid®: 20% (100 mL, 250 mL, 500 mL, 1000 mL); 30% (500 mL)

Liposyn® III: 10% (500 mL); 20% (500 mL); 30% (500 mL)

Dosing

Adult & Geriatric

Caloric source: I.V.: Initial dose: 1 g/kg/day, increase by 0.5-1 g/kg/day to a maximum of 2.5-3 g/kg/day

Prevention of essential fatty acid deficiency (EFAD): I.V.: Administer 8% to 10% of total caloric intake as fat emulsion (may be higher in stressed patients with EFAD); may be given 2-3 times weekly to meet essential fatty acid requirements

Local anesthetic toxicity (unlabeled use): 20%: 1.5 mL/kg of lean body weight administered over 1 minute, followed immediately by an infusion of 0.25 mL/kg/minute. Continue chest compressions (lipid must circulate). Repeat bolus 1-2 times as needed for persistent asystole. Continue infusion until hemodynamic stability is restored. Increase the infusion rate to 0.5 mL/kg/minute if BP declines.

Pediatric

Caloric source: I.V.:

Premature infants: Initial dose: 0.25-0.5 g/kg/day, increase by 0.25-0.5 g/kg/day to a maximum of 3 g/kg/day depending on needs/nutritional goals; limit to 1 g/kg/day if on phototherapy; should be administered over 24 hours (A.S.P.E.N. guidelines)

Infants and Children: Initial dose: 0.5-1 g/kg/day, increase by 0.5 g/kg/day to a maximum of 3 g/kg/day depending on needs/nutritional goals; may administer over 24 hours (A.S.P.E.N. guidelines)

Note: Monitor triglycerides while receiving intralipids. If serum triglyceride levels >200 mg/dL, stop infusion and restart at 0.5-1g/kg/day. Intravenous heparin (1 unit/mL of parenteral nutrition) may enhance the clearance of lipid emulsions.

Administration

I.V. Can be administered in a peripheral line or by central venous infusion. At the onset of therapy, the patient should be observed for any immediate allergic reactions such as dyspnea, cyanosis, and fever.

Children: Infuse for 10-15 minutes at a slower rate. Infuse 10% at ≤0.1 mL/minute; can increase to 1 mL/kg/hour if tolerated. Infuse 20% at ≤0.05 mL/minute; can increase to 0.5 mL/kg/hour if tolerated. **Note:** Premature and/or septic infants may need to reduce infusion rate. Do not exceed 1 g fat/kg in 4 hours in this population.

Adults: Infuse for 15-30 minutes at a slower rate. Infuse 10% at 1 mL/minute. If no untoward effects, can double rate. Infuse 20% at 0.5 mL/minute initially; can double rate if tolerated.

Monitoring and Teaching Issues

Laboratory Monitoring Monitor liver function tests periodically. Monitor triglycerides before initiation of lipid therapy and at least weekly during therapy; monitor especially closely in premature infants, septic infants, and patients with pancreatitis or liver disease.

Neonates: Frequent (some advise daily) platelet counts should be performed in neonatal patients receiving parenteral lipids.

Physical Assessment Assess for allergy to eggs prior to initiating therapy. Monitor closely for allergic reactions or fluid overload.

Patient Education Report pain at infusion site or respiratory difficulty.

◆ **FazaClo®** *see* Clozapine *on page* 417
◆ **5-FC** *see* Flucytosine *on page* 775
◆ **FC1157a** *see* Toremifene *on page* 1793
◆ **FE200486** *see* Degarelix *on page* 480

Febuxostat (feb UX oh stat)

U.S. Brand Names Uloric®
Index Terms TEI-6720; TMX-67
Generic Availability (U.S.) No
Pharmacologic Category Xanthine Oxidase Inhibitor
Pregnancy Risk Factor C
Lactation Excretion in breast milk unknown/use caution
Use Chronic management of hyperuricemia in patients with gout
Mechanism of Action/Effect Selectively inhibits xanthine oxidase, the enzyme responsible for the conversion of hypoxanthine to xanthine to uric acid thereby decreasing uric acid.
Contraindications Concurrent use with azathioprine or mercaptopurine

Canadian labeling: Additional contraindications (not in U.S. labeling): Hypersensitivity to febuxostat or any component of the formulation; concomitant administration with theophylline

Warnings/Precautions Administer concurrently with an NSAID or colchicine (up to 6 months) to prevent gout flare upon initiation of therapy. Do not use to treat asymptomatic or secondary hyperuricemia. Significant hepatic transaminase elevations (>3 x ULN), MI, stroke and cardiovascular deaths have been reported in controlled trials (causal relationship not established). Monitor patients for signs/symptoms of MI and stroke. Liver function tests should be monitored 2 and 4 months after initiation of therapy and then periodically. Use with caution in patients with severe hepatic impairment (Child-Pugh class C); not studied. Use with caution in patients with severe renal impairment (Cl_{cr} <30 mL/minute); insufficient data.

Drug Interactions

Avoid Concomitant Use

Avoid concomitant use of Febuxostat with any of the following: AzaTHIOprine; Didanosine; Mercaptopurine

Decreased Effect There are no known significant interactions involving a decrease in effect.

Increased Effect/Toxicity

Febuxostat may increase the levels/effects of: AzaTHIOprine; Didanosine; Mercaptopurine; Theophylline Derivatives

Adverse Reactions 1% to 10%:
Dermatologic: Rash (1% to 2%)
Hepatic: Liver function abnormalities (5% to 7%)
Neuromuscular & skeletal: Arthralgia (1%)

Pharmacodynamics/Kinetics

Absorption ≥49%

Time to Peak Plasma: 1-1.5 hours

Protein Binding ~99%, primarily to albumin

Half-Life Elimination ~5-8 hours

Metabolism Extensive conjugation via uridine diphosphate glucuronosyltransferases (UGTs) 1A1, 1A3, 1A9, and 2B7 and oxidation via cytochrome P450 (CYP) 1A2, 2C8, and 2C9 as well as non-P450 enzymes. Oxidation leads to formation of active metabolites (67M-1, 67M-2, 67M-4)

Excretion Urine (~49% mostly as metabolites, 3% as unchanged drug); feces (~45% mostly as metabolites, 12% as unchanged drug)

Available Dosage Forms

Tablet, oral:
Uloric®: 40 mg, 80 mg

Dosing

Adult & Geriatric Management of hyperuricemia in patients with gout: Note: It is recommended to take an NSAID or colchicine with initiation of therapy and may continue for up to 6 months to help prevent gout flares. If a gout flare occurs, febuxostat does not need to be discontinued.

Oral:
U.S. labeling: Initial: 40 mg once daily; may increase to 80 mg once daily in patients who do not achieve a serum uric acid level <6 mg/dL after 2 weeks
Canadian labeling: 80 mg once daily

Renal Impairment
Mild-to-moderate impairment (Cl_{cr} 30-89 mL/minute): No adjustment needed
Severe impairment (Cl_{cr} <30 mL/minute): Insufficient data; use caution (use not recommended in the Canadian labeling)
Dialysis: Not studied (use not recommended in the Canadian labeling)

Hepatic Impairment
Mild-to-moderate impairment (Child-Pugh classes A and B): No adjustment needed
Severe impairment (Child-Pugh class C): Not studied; use caution (use not recommended in the Canadian labeling)

Administration

Oral Administer with or without meals or antacids.

Stability

Storage Store at 25°C (77°F); excursions permitted to 15°C to 30°C (59°F to 86°F). Protect from light.

Monitoring and Teaching Issues

Laboratory Monitoring Liver function tests 2 and 4 months after initiation and then periodically, serum uric acid levels (as early as 2 weeks after initiation)

Patient Education Report unusual fatigue, easy bruising or bleeding, jaundice, chest pain, shortness of breath, numbness or loss of function in extremities, or change in neurological status.

Dietary Considerations Take with or without meals or antacids.

Geriatric Considerations In clinical trials, no clinically significant differences in safety or effectiveness were observed in elderly subjects. See Renal Impairment.

Pregnancy Considerations Animal studies have demonstrated increased neonatal mortality and reduction in weight gain, but not teratogenic effects. There are no adequate and well-controlled studies in pregnant women. Use during pregnancy only if potential benefit to the mother outweighs potential risk to the fetus.

- **Feiba NF** *see* Anti-inhibitor Coagulant Complex *on page 136*
- **Feiba VH [DSC]** *see* Anti-inhibitor Coagulant Complex *on page 136*
- **Feldene®** *see* Piroxicam *on page 1465*

Felodipine (fe LOE di peen)

Index Terms Plendil

Generic Availability (U.S.) Yes

Pharmacologic Category Calcium Channel Blocker; Calcium Channel Blocker, Dihydropyridine

Medication Safety Issues

Sound-alike/look-alike issues:

Plendil may be confused with Isordil®, pindolol, Pletal®, PriLOSEC®, Prinivil®

Pregnancy Risk Factor C

Lactation Excretion in breast milk unknown/not recommended

Use Treatment of hypertension

Unlabeled/Investigational Use Pediatric hypertension

Mechanism of Action/Effect Inhibits calcium ions from entering the "slow channels" or select voltage-sensitive areas of vascular smooth muscle and myocardium during depolarization

Contraindications Hypersensitivity to felodipine, any component of the formulation, or other calcium channel blocker

Warnings/Precautions Increased angina and/or MI has occurred with initiation or dosage titration of dihydropyridine calcium channel blockers, reflex tachycardia may occur resulting in angina and/or MI in patients with obstructive coronary disease especially in the absence of concurrent beta-blockade. Use with extreme caution in patients with severe aortic stenosis. Use caution in patients with heart failure and/or hypertrophic cardiomyopathy with outflow tract obstruction. Elderly patients and patients with hepatic impairment should start off with a lower dose. Peripheral edema (dose dependent) is the most common side effect (occurs within 2-3 weeks of starting therapy). Symptomatic hypotension with or without syncope can rarely occur; blood pressure must be lowered at a rate appropriate for the patient's clinical condition. Dosage titration should occur after 14 days on a given dose.

Drug Interactions

Metabolism/Transport Effects **Substrate** of CYP3A4 (major); **Inhibits** CYP2C8 (moderate), 2C9 (weak), 2D6 (weak), 3A4 (weak)

Avoid Concomitant Use There are no known interactions where it is recommended to avoid concomitant use.

Decreased Effect

Felodipine may decrease the levels/effects of: Clopidogrel

The levels/effects of Felodipine may be decreased by: Barbiturates; Calcium Salts; CarBAMazepine; CYP3A4 Inducers (Strong); Deferasirox; Herbs (CYP3A4 Inducers); Herbs (Hypertensive Properties); Methylphenidate; Nafcillin; Rifamycin Derivatives; Yohimbine

Increased Effect/Toxicity

Felodipine may increase the levels/effects of: Amifostine; Antihypertensives; Calcium Channel Blockers (Nondihydropyridine); CYP2C8 Substrates (High risk); Hypotensive Agents; Magnesium Salts; Neuromuscular-Blocking Agents (Nondepolarizing); Nitroprusside; Phenytoin; RiTUXimab; Tacrolimus; Tacrolimus (Systemic)

The levels/effects of Felodipine may be increased by: Alpha1-Blockers; Antifungal Agents (Azole Derivatives, Systemic); Calcium Channel Blockers (Nondihydropyridine); Cimetidine; Conivaptan; CycloSPORINE; CycloSPORINE (Systemic); CYP3A4 Inhibitors (Moderate); CYP3A4 Inhibitors (Strong); Dasatinib; Diazoxide; Fluconazole; Grapefruit Juice; Herbs (Hypotensive Properties); Macrolide Antibiotics; Magnesium Salts; MAO Inhibitors; Pentoxifylline; Phosphodiesterase 5 Inhibitors; Prostacyclin Analogues; Protease Inhibitors

Nutritional/Ethanol Interactions

Ethanol: Increases felodipine's absorption; watch for a greater hypotensive effect.

Food: Increased therapeutic and vasodilator side effects, including severe hypotension and myocardial ischemia, may occur if felodipine is taken with grapefruit juice; avoid concurrent use. High-fat/carbohydrate meals will increase C_{max} by 60%; grapefruit juice will increase C_{max} by twofold.

Herb/Nutraceutical: St John's wort may decrease felodipine levels. Avoid dong quai if using for hypertension (has estrogenic activity). Avoid ephedra, yohimbe, ginseng (may worsen hypertension). Avoid garlic (may have increased antihypertensive effect).

Adverse Reactions
>10%: Central nervous system: Headache (11% to 15%)
2% to 10%: Cardiovascular: Peripheral edema (2% to 17%), tachycardia (0.4% to 2.5%), flushing (4% to 7%)

Pharmacodynamics/Kinetics

Onset of Action Antihypertensive: 2-5 hours

Duration of Action Antihypertensive effect: 24 hours

Absorption 100%; absolute: 20% due to first-pass effect

Protein Binding >99%

Half-Life Elimination Immediate release: 11-16 hours

Metabolism Hepatic; CYP3A4 substrate (major); extensive first-pass effect

Excretion Urine (70% as metabolites); feces 10%

Available Dosage Forms

Tablet, extended release, oral: 2.5 mg, 5 mg, 10 mg

Dosing

Adult Hypertension: Oral: 2.5-10 mg once daily; increase by 5 mg at 2-week intervals, as needed, to a maximum of 20 mg/day; usual dose range (JNC 7): 2.5-20 mg once daily.

Geriatric Oral: Initial 2.5 mg/day

Pediatric Hypertension (unlabeled use): Oral: Initial: 2.5 mg once daily; maximum: 10 mg/day

Hepatic Impairment Initial: 2.5 mg/day; monitor blood pressure

Administration

Oral Do not crush or chew extended release tablets; swallow whole. Administer without food.

Monitoring and Teaching Issues

Physical Assessment Use caution in presence of heart failure. When discontinuing, taper dose gradually.

Patient Education Take without food. Avoid concurrent alcohol (may cause dangerous hypotension). Swallow whole; do not crush or chew. May cause headache, constipation, or swelling of ankles. Report irregular heartbeat, chest pain or palpitations, persistent headache, severe constipation, peripheral swelling, weight gain, dyspnea, or respiratory changes.

Dietary Considerations Should be taken without food.

Geriatric Considerations Elderly may experience a greater hypotensive response. Constipation may be more of a problem in the elderly. Calcium channel blockers are no more effective in the elderly than other therapies; however, they do not cause significant CNS effects which is an advantage over some antihypertensive agents.

Pregnancy Considerations Potentially, calcium channel blockers may prolong labor. There are no adequate or well-controlled studies in pregnant women.

Additional Information Felodipine maintains renal and mesenteric blood flow during hemorrhagic shock in animals.

Related Information

Calcium Channel Blockers *on page* 1993

- **Felodipine and Enalapril** *see* Enalapril and Felodipine *on page* 620
- **Femara®** *see* Letrozole *on page* 1078
- **Femcon® Fe** *see* Ethinyl Estradiol and Norethindrone *on page* 701
- **femhrt®** *see* Ethinyl Estradiol and Norethindrone *on page* 701
- **femhrt® Lo** *see* Ethinyl Estradiol and Norethindrone *on page* 701
- **Femring®** *see* Estradiol (Systemic) *on page* 670
- **Femtrace®** *see* Estradiol (Systemic) *on page* 670
- **Fenesin IR [OTC]** *see* GuaiFENesin *on page* 890

Fenofibrate (fen oh FYE brate)

U.S. Brand Names Antara®; Fenoglide®; Lipofen®; Lofibra®; TriCor®; Triglide®

Index Terms Procetofene; Proctofene

Generic Availability (U.S.) Yes: Micronized capsule and tablet

Pharmacologic Category Antilipemic Agent, Fibric Acid

Medication Safety Issues

Sound-alike/look-alike issues:

TriCor® may be confused with Fibricor®, Tracleer®

Pregnancy Risk Factor C

Lactation Excretion in breast milk unknown/not recommended

Use Adjunct to dietary therapy for the treatment of adults with elevations of serum triglyceride levels (types IV and V hyperlipidemia); adjunct to dietary therapy for the reduction of low density lipoprotein cholesterol (LDL-C), total cholesterol (total-C), triglycerides, and apolipoprotein B (apo B), and to increase high density lipoprotein cholesterol (HDL-C) in adult patients with primary hypercholesterolemia or mixed dyslipidemia (Fredrickson types IIa and IIb)

Mechanism of Action/Effect Fenofibric acid increases VLDL catabolism by enhancing the synthesis of lipoprotein lipase; as a result of a decrease in VLDL levels, total plasma triglycerides are reduced by 30% to 60%. Modest increase in HDL occurs in some hypertriglyceridemic patients.

Contraindications Hypersensitivity to fenofibrate or any component of the formulation; hepatic dysfunction including primary biliary cirrhosis and unexplained persistent liver function abnormalities; severe renal dysfunction; pre-existing gallbladder disease; breast-feeding (only Fenoglide®)

Canadian labeling: Additional contraindications (not in U.S. labeling): Pregnancy; breast-feeding; known photoallergy or phototoxic reaction during treatment with fibrates or ketoprofen; allergy to soya lecithin or peanut or arachis oil

Warnings/Precautions Secondary causes of hyperlipidemia should be ruled out prior to therapy. Hepatic transaminases can become significantly elevated (dose-related); hepatocellular, chronic active, and cholestatic hepatitis have been reported. Regular monitoring of liver function tests is required. Increases in serum creatinine (>2 mg/dL) have been observed with use; monitor renal function in patients with renal impairment and consider monitoring patients with increased risk for developing renal impairment. May cause cholelithiasis. Use with caution in patient taking oral anticoagulants (eg, warfarin); adjustments in anticoagulation therapy may be required. Use caution with HMG-CoA reductase inhibitors (may lead to myopathy, rhabdomyolysis). In combination with HMG-CoA reductase inhibitors, fenofibrate is generally regarded as safer than gemfibrozil due to limited pharmacokinetic interaction with statins. Therapy should be withdrawn if an adequate response is not obtained after 2-3 months of therapy at the maximal daily dose. The occurrence of pancreatitis may represent a failure of efficacy in patients with severely elevated triglycerides. May cause mild-to-moderate decreases in hemoglobin, hematocrit, and WBC upon initiation of therapy which usually stabilizes with long-term therapy. Agranulocytosis and thrombocytopenia have rarely been reported. Periodic monitoring of blood counts is recommended during the first year of therapy.

Rare hypersensitivity reactions may occur. Use has been associated with pulmonary embolism (PE) and deep vein thrombosis (DVT). Use with caution in patients with risk factors for VTE. Dose adjustment is required for renal impairment and may be required for elderly patients.

Drug Interactions

Metabolism/Transport Effects **Substrate** of CYP3A4 (minor); **Inhibits** CYP2A6 (weak), 2C8 (weak), 2C9 (weak), 2C19 (weak)

Avoid Concomitant Use There are no known interactions where it is recommended to avoid concomitant use.

Decreased Effect

Fenofibrate may decrease the levels/effects of: Chenodiol; CycloSPORINE; CycloSPORINE (Systemic); Ursodiol

The levels/effects of Fenofibrate may be decreased by: Bile Acid Sequestrants

Increased Effect/Toxicity

Fenofibrate may increase the levels/effects of: Colchicine; Ezetimibe; HMG-CoA Reductase Inhibitors; Sulfonylureas; Vitamin K Antagonists; Warfarin

The levels/effects of Fenofibrate may be increased by: Conivaptan; CycloSPORINE; CycloSPORINE (Systemic)

Adverse Reactions

>10%: Hepatic: Liver function tests increased (dose related; 3% to 13%)

1% to 10%:

- Central nervous system: Headache (3%)
- Gastrointestinal: Abdominal pain (5%), constipation (2%), nausea (2%)
- Neuromuscular & skeletal: Back pain (3%), CPK increased (3%)
- Respiratory: Respiratory disorder (6%), rhinitis (2%)

Pharmacodynamics/Kinetics

Absorption Increased when taken with meals

Time to Peak 3-8 hours

Protein Binding >99%

Half-Life Elimination Half-life elimination: Fenofibric acid: Mean: 20 hours (range: 10-35 hours)

Metabolism Tissue and plasma via esterases to active form, fenofibric acid; undergoes inactivation by glucuronidation hepatically or renally

Excretion Urine (60% as metabolites); feces (25%); hemodialysis has no effect on removal of fenofibric acid from plasma

Available Dosage Forms

Capsule, oral: 67 mg, 134 mg, 200 mg

- Antara®: 43 mg, 130 mg
- Lipofen®: 50 mg, 150 mg
- Lofibra®: 67 mg, 134 mg, 200 mg

Tablet, oral: 54 mg, 160 mg

- Fenoglide®: 40 mg, 120 mg
- Lofibra®: 54 mg, 160 mg
- TriCor®: 48 mg, 145 mg
- Triglide®: 50 mg, 160 mg

Dosing

Adult

Hypertriglyceridemia: Oral Initial:

- Antara® (micronized): 43-130 mg/day; maximum dose: 130 mg/day
- Fenoglide®: 40-120 mg/day; maximum dose: 120 mg/day
- Lipidil EZ® [CAN; not available in U.S.]: 145 mg/day; maximum dose: 145 mg/day
- Lipidil Micro® [CAN; not available in U.S.]: 200 mg/day; maximum dose: 200 mg/day
- Lipidil Supra® [CAN; not available in U.S.]: 160 mg/day; maximum dose: 200 mg/day

Lipofen®: 50-150 mg/day; maximum dose: 150 mg/day
Lofibra® (micronized): 67-200 mg/day with meals; maximum dose: 200 mg/day
Lofibra® (tablets): 54-160 mg/day; maximum dose: 160 mg/day
TriCor®: 48-145 mg/day; maximum dose: 145 mg/day
Triglide®: 50-160 mg/day; maximum dose: 160 mg/day

Hypercholesterolemia or mixed hyperlipidemia: Oral:
Antara® (micronized): 130 mg/day
Fenoglide®: 120 mg/day
Lipidil EZ® [CAN; not available in U.S.]: 145 mg/day; maximum dose: 145 mg/day
Lipidil Micro® [CAN; not available in U.S.]: 200 mg/day; maximum dose: 200 mg/day
Lipidil Supra® [CAN; not available in U.S.]: 160 mg/day; maximum dose: 200 mg/day
Lipofen®: 150 mg/day
Lofibra® (micronized): 200 mg/day
Lofibra® (tablets): 160 mg/day
TriCor®: 145 mg/day
Triglide®: 160 mg/day

Geriatric Oral: Initial:
Antara® (micronized): 43 mg/day
Fenoglide®: Adjust dosage based on creatinine clearance
Lipidil EZ® [CAN; not available in U.S.]: 48 mg/day
Lipidil Micro® [CAN; not available in U.S.]: Adjust dosage based on creatinine clearance
Lipidil Supra® [CAN; not available in U.S.]: Adjust dosage based on creatinine clearance
Lipofen®: 50 mg/day
Lofibra® (micronized): 67 mg/day
Lofibra® (tablets): 54 mg/day
TriCor®: Adjust dosage based on creatinine clearance
Triglide®: 50 mg/day

Renal Impairment Monitor renal function and lipid panel before adjusting. Decrease dose or increase dosing interval for patients with renal failure: **Note:** Use in severe renal impairment is contraindicated (see specific product labeling):
Antara® (micronized): 43 mg/day
Fenoglide®: Cl_{cr} 31-80 mL/minute: 40 mg/day
Lipidil EZ® [CAN; not available in U.S.]: Cl_{cr} ≥20-50 mL/minute: 48 mg/day
Lipidil Micro® [CAN; not available in U.S.]: Cl_{cr} ≥20-100 mL/minute: 67 mg/day; **Note:** Lipidil Micro® 67 mg capsules are discontinued in Canada. Micronized formulation at this dosage strength is available through other manufacturers in Canada.
Lipidil Supra® [CAN; not available in U.S.]: Cl_{cr} ≥20-100 mL/minute: 100 mg/day
Lipofen®: 50 mg/day
Lofibra® (micronized): 67 mg/day
Lofibra® (tablets): 54 mg/day
TriCor®: Cl_{cr} 31-80 mL/minute: 48 mg/day
Triglide®: 50 mg/day

Administration

Oral 6-8 weeks of therapy is required to determine efficacy.
Fenoglide®, Lofibra® (capsules [micronized] and tablets), Lipofen®: Administer with meals.
Antara®, TriCor®: May be administered with or without food.
Triglide®: Do not consume chipped or broken tablets. May be administered with or without food.
Canadian products [not available in U.S.]:
Lipidil Micro®, Lipidil Supra®: Administer with meals.
Lipidil EZ®: May be administered with or without food.

Stability

Storage Store at 15°C to 30°C (59°F to 86°F). Protect from light and moisture. Store tablets in moisture-protective container.

Monitoring and Teaching Issues

Laboratory Monitoring Periodic blood counts during first year of therapy. Total serum cholesterol and triglyceride concentration and CLDL, LDL, and HDL levels should be measured periodically; if only marginal changes are noted in 6-8 weeks, the drug should be discontinued. Serum transaminases should be measured every 3 months; if ALT values increase >100 units/L, therapy should be discontinued. Monitor LFTs prior to initiation, at 6 and 12 weeks after initiation or first dose, then periodically thereafter.

Physical Assessment Use caution and monitor closely in presence of hepatic or renal dysfunction, gallbladder disease, and advanced age. Evaluate results of LFTs and blood counts on a regular basis throughout therapy. Monitor for myopathy, rhabdomyolysis, arrhythmias, gastrointestinal upset, CNS changes, hypoglycemia, and myalgia.

Patient Education Maintain diet and exercise program as prescribed. If you are a diabetic taking a sulfonylurea, monitor blood sugars closely; this medication may alter the effects of your antidiabetic medication. You may experience mild GI disturbances (eg, abdominal pain, constipation, nausea); inform prescriber if these are severe. Report immediately unusual muscle pain or weakness; skin rash or irritation; insomnia; persistent dizziness; chest pain or palpitations; difficult respirations; or pain, swelling, redness, or heat in extremities.

Dietary Considerations
Fenoglide®, Lofibra® (capsules [micronized] and tablets), Lipofen®: Take with meals.
Antara®, TriCor®, Triglide®: May be taken with or without food.
Canadian products [not available in U.S.]:
Lipidil Micro®, Lipidil Supra®: Take with meals.
Lipidil EZ®: May be taken with or without food.

Geriatric Considerations The definition of and, therefore, when to treat hyperlipidemia in the elderly is a controversial issue. The National Cholesterol Education Program recommends that all adults maintain a plasma cholesterol <160 mg/dL. Older adults with one additional risk factor, goal LDL would be <130 mg/dL. It is the authors' belief that pharmacologic treatment be reserved for those who are unable to obtain a desirable plasma cholesterol concentration by diet alone and for whom the benefits of treatment are believed to outweigh the potential adverse effects, drug interactions, and cost of treatment.

Breast-Feeding Considerations Tumor formation was observed in animal studies; nursing is not recommended if the medication cannot be discontinued.

Pregnancy Considerations Animal studies have shown embryocidal and teratogenic effect. There are no adequate and well-controlled studies in pregnant women. Use should be avoided, if possible, in pregnant women since the neonatal glucuronide conjugation pathways are immature.

Related Information

Hyperlipidemia Management *on page 2046*

Fenofibric Acid (fen oh FYE brik AS id)

U.S. Brand Names Fibricor™; TriLipix®

Index Terms ABT-335; Choline Fenofibrate

Generic Availability (U.S.) Yes

Pharmacologic Category Antilipemic Agent, Fibric Acid

Medication Safety Issues

Sound-alike/look-alike issues:

Fibricor™ may be confused with Tricor®

TriLipix™ may be confused with Trileptal®, TriLyte®

Medication Guide Available Yes

Pregnancy Risk Factor C

Lactation Excretion in breast milk unknown/contraindicated

Use Adjunct to dietary therapy for the treatment of severely elevated serum triglyceride levels; adjunct to dietary therapy for the reduction of low density lipoprotein cholesterol (LDL-C), total cholesterol (total-C), triglycerides, and apolipoprotein B (apo B) and to increase high density lipoprotein cholesterol (HDL-C) in patients with primary hypercholesterolemia or mixed dyslipidemia

TriLipix™ is also indicated as adjunct to dietary therapy concomitantly with a statin to reduce triglyceride levels and increase HDL-C levels in patients with mixed dyslipidemia and coronary heart disease (CHD) or at risk for CHD

Mechanism of Action/Effect Fenofibric acid increases VLDL catabolism by enhancing the synthesis of lipoprotein lipase; as a result of a decrease in VLDL levels, total plasma triglycerides are reduced by 30% to 60%; modest increased in HDL occurs in some hypertriglyceridemia patients.

Contraindications Hypersensitivity to fenofibric acid, choline fenofibrate, fenofibrate, or any component of the formulation; hepatic dysfunction including primary biliary cirrhosis and unexplained persistent liver function abnormalities; severe renal dysfunction (including patients on dialysis); pre-existing gallbladder disease; breast-feeding

Warnings/Precautions Secondary causes of hyperlipidemia should be ruled out prior to therapy. Has been associated with rare myositis or rhabdomyolysis; patients should be monitored closely. Risk increased in the elderly, patients with diabetes mellitus, renal failure, or hypothyroidism. Patients should be instructed to report unexplained muscle pain, tenderness, weakness, or brown urine. Hepatic transaminases can become significantly elevated (dose-related); hepatocellular, chronic active, and cholestatic hepatitis have been reported. Regular monitoring of liver function tests is required. Increases in serum creatinine (>2 mg/dL) have been observed with use; monitor renal function in patients with renal impairment and consider monitoring patients with increased risk for developing renal impairment. May cause cholelithiasis discontinue if gallstones found upon gallbladder studies. Use caution with oral anticoagulants; adjustments in therapy may be required.

Use caution with HMG-CoA reductase inhibitors (may lead to myopathy, rhabdomyolysis). In combination with HMG-CoA reductase inhibitors, fenofibric acid derivatives are generally regarded as safer than gemfibrozil due to limited pharmacokinetic interaction. Therapy should be withdrawn if an adequate response is not obtained after 2-3 months of therapy at the maximal daily dose. The occurrence of pancreatitis may represent a failure of efficacy in patients with severely elevated triglycerides. May cause mild-to-moderate decreases in hemoglobin, hematocrit, and WBC upon initiation of therapy, which usually stabilizes with long-term therapy. Rare hypersensitivity reactions may occur. Use has been associated with pulmonary embolism (PE) and deep vein thrombosis (DVT). Use with caution in patients with risk factors for VTE. Dose adjustment is required for renal impairment and elderly patients.

Drug Interactions

Avoid Concomitant Use There are no known interactions where it is recommended to avoid concomitant use.

Decreased Effect

Fenofibric Acid may decrease the levels/effects of: Chenodiol; CycloSPORINE; CycloSPORINE (Systemic); Ursodiol

The levels/effects of Fenofibric Acid may be decreased by: Bile Acid Sequestrants

Increased Effect/Toxicity

Fenofibric Acid may increase the levels/effects of: Carvedilol; Colchicine; CYP2C9 Substrates (High risk); Ezetimibe; HMG-CoA Reductase Inhibitors; Sulfonylureas; Vitamin K Antagonists; Warfarin

The levels/effects of Fenofibric Acid may be increased by: CycloSPORINE; CycloSPORINE (Systemic)

Adverse Reactions Adverse reactions and frequency reported as observed during monotherapy and concurrent administration with a statin (HMG-CoA reductase inhibitor).

>10%: Central nervous system: Headache (12% to 13%)

1% to 10%:

Central nervous system: Dizziness (3% to 4%), pain (1% to 4%), fatigue (2% to 3%)

Gastrointestinal: Nausea (4% to 6%), dyspepsia (3% to 5%), diarrhea (3% to 4%), constipation (3%)

Hepatic: ALT increased (monotherapy: 1%; coadministered with statin: 3%)

Neuromuscular & skeletal: Back pain (4% to 6%), pain in extremities (3% to 5%), arthralgia (4%), myalgia (3% to 4%), muscle spasm (2% to 3%)

Respiratory: Nasopharyngitis (4% to 5%), upper respiratory infection (4% to 5%), sinusitis (3% to 4%)

Additional adverse reactions when fenofibric acid coadministered with a statin (frequency not defined): AST increased, bronchitis, cough, CPK increased, hepatic enzymes increased, hypertension, influenza, insomnia, musculoskeletal pain, pharyngolaryngeal pain, urinary tract infection

Pharmacodynamics/Kinetics

Absorption Well absorbed

Bioavailability TriLipix™: ~81%

Time to Peak Fibricor™: ~2.5 hours; TriLipix™: 4-5 hours

Protein Binding ~99%

Half-Life Elimination ~20 hours

Metabolism Fenofibric acid (active form) undergoes inactivation by glucuronidation. The choline salt dissociates in the GI tract to form fenofibric acid (free acid)

Excretion Urine (as fenofibric acid and fenofibric acid glucuronide)

Available Dosage Forms

Capsule, delayed release, oral:

TriLipix®: 45 mg, 135 mg

Tablet, oral: 35 mg, 105 mg

Fibricor™: 35 mg, 105 mg

Dosing

Adult

Mixed dyslipidemia (coadministered with a statin): Oral: TriLipix™: 135 mg once daily (maximum: 135 mg/day)

Hypertriglyceridemia: Oral:

Fibricor™: Initial: 35-105 mg once daily; Maintenance: Individualize according to patient response (maximum: 105 mg/day)

TriLipix™: Initial: 45-135 mg once daily; Maintenance: Individualize according to patient response (maximum: 135 mg/day)

Primary hypercholesterolemia or mixed dyslipidemia: Oral:

Fibricor™: 105 mg once daily (maximum: 105 mg/day)

TriLipix™: 135 mg once daily (maximum: 135 mg/day)

Geriatric Oral: Dosage based on renal function

Renal Impairment

Mild-to-moderate impairment (Cl_{cr} 30-80 mL/minute): Initial: Fibricor™: 35 mg once daily or TriLipix™: 45 mg once daily; only increase once effects on lipids and renal function evaluated

Severe impairment (Cl_{cr} <30 mL/minute; with or without dialysis): Contraindicated

Administration

Oral May be administered with or without food.

Stability

Storage Store at 25°C (77°F); excursions permitted to 15°C to 30°C (59°F to 86°F). Protect from light and moisture.

Monitoring and Teaching Issues

Laboratory Monitoring Periodic blood counts during first year of therapy; total cholesterol, LDL-C, triglycerides, and HDL-C should be measured periodically; monitor LFTs (including ALT) regularly and discontinue therapy if levels remain >3 times normal limits; serum creatinine (in patients with or at risk for renal impairment)

Physical Assessment Use with caution and monitor closely in presence of hepatic or renal dysfunction, advanced age, diabetes, or hypothyroidism. Teach patient to report signs of myopathy, rhabdomyolysis, and hepatic dysfunction.

Patient Education May take with or without food. Maintain diet and exercise program as prescribed. If you have diabetes and are taking a sulfonylurea, monitor blood sugars closely; this medication may improve the effects of your antidiabetic medication. You will require scheduled blood tests to determine appropriate dosage and to reduce potential for adverse effects; maintaining laboratory testing schedule is vital. May cause mild GI disturbances (eg, gas, diarrhea, constipation, nausea); inform prescriber if these are severe. Report immediately unusual muscle, back, or joint pain, spasms, or weakness; yellowing of skin or eyes; unusual or increased bruising or bleeding; or persistent fatigue.

Dietary Considerations May be taken with or without food. Patients should follow appropriate lipid-lowering diet.

Geriatric Considerations The definition of and, therefore, when to treat hyperlipidemia in the elderly is a controversial issue. The National Cholesterol Education Program recommends that all adults maintain a plasma cholesterol <160 mg/dL. Older adults with one additional risk factor, goal LDL would be <130 mg/dL. It is the authors' belief that pharmacologic treatment be reserved for those who are unable to obtain a desirable plasma cholesterol concentration by diet alone and for whom the benefits of treatment are believed to outweigh the potential adverse effects, drug interactions, and cost of treatment.

Pregnancy Considerations There are no adequate and well-controlled studies in pregnant women. Use only if benefits outweigh the risks.

◆ **Fenoglide®** *see* Fenofibrate *on page* 739

Fenoprofen (fen oh PROE fen)

U.S. Brand Names Nalfon®

Index Terms Fenoprofen Calcium

Generic Availability (U.S.) Yes: Tablet

Pharmacologic Category Nonsteroidal Anti-inflammatory Drug (NSAID), Oral

Medication Safety Issues

Sound-alike/look-alike issues:

Fenoprofen may be confused with flurbiprofen

Nalfon® may be confused with Naldecon®

Medication Guide Available Yes

Pregnancy Risk Factor C

Lactation Enters breast milk/not recommended

Use Symptomatic treatment of acute and chronic rheumatoid arthritis and osteoarthritis; relief of mild-to-moderate pain

Available Dosage Forms

Capsule, oral:

Nalfon®: 200 mg

Tablet, oral: 600 mg

Dosing

Adult & Geriatric

Rheumatoid arthritis, osteoarthritis: Oral: 300-600 mg 3-4 times/day; maximum dose: 3.2 g/day

Mild-to-moderate pain: Oral: 200 mg every 4-6 hours as needed; maximum dose: 3.2 g/day

Renal Impairment Not recommended in patients with advanced renal disease.

Administration

Oral Do not crush tablets. Swallow whole with a full glass of water. Take with food to minimize stomach upset.

Monitoring and Teaching Issues

Laboratory Monitoring CBC, liver enzymes; urine output and BUN/serum creatinine in patients receiving diuretics

Physical Assessment Evaluate cardiac risk and potential for GI bleeding prior to prescribing this medication. Monitor blood pressure at the beginning of therapy and periodically during use.

Patient Education Do not crush tablets or break capsules. Take with food or milk to reduce GI distress. Do not use alcohol. You may experience drowsiness, dizziness, nervousness, headache, anorexia, nausea, vomiting, heartburn, or fluid retention; GI bleeding, ulceration, or perforation can occur with or without pain; discontinue medication and contact prescriber if persistent abdominal pain or cramping or blood in stool occurs. Report respiratory difficulty or unusual cough; chest pain, rapid heartbeat, or palpitations; bruising/bleeding; blood in urine, stool, mouth, or vomitus; swollen extremities; skin rash; weakness in one side or part of body; slurred speech; persistent nausea; yellowing of skin or eyes; abdominal pain; or ringing in ears.

Related Information

Nonsalicylate / Nonsteroidal Anti-Inflammatory Agents *on page* 2002

◆ **Fenoprofen Calcium** *see* Fenoprofen *on page* 744

FentaNYL (FEN ta nil)

U.S. Brand Names Abstral®; Actiq®; Duragesic®; Fentora®; Onsolis™; Sublimaze® [DSC]

Index Terms Fentanyl Citrate; Fentanyl Hydrochloride; Fentanyl Patch; OTFC (Oral Transmucosal Fentanyl Citrate)

Generic Availability (U.S.) Yes: Excludes buccal film, buccal tablet, sublingual tablet

Pharmacologic Category Analgesic, Opioid; Anilidopiperidine Opioid; General Anesthetic

Medication Safety Issues

Sound-alike/look-alike issues:

FentaNYL may be confused with alfentanil, SUFentanil

Dosing of transdermal fentanyl patches may be confusing. Transdermal fentanyl patches should always be prescribed in mcg/hour, not size. Patch dosage form of Duragesic®-12 actually delivers 12.5 mcg/hour of fentanyl. Use caution, as orders may be written as "Duragesic 12.5" which can be erroneously interpreted as a 125 mcg dose.

Fentora®, Onsolis™, Abstral®, and Actiq® are not interchangeable; do not substitute doses on a mcg-per-mcg basis.

High alert medication: The Institute for Safe Medication Practices (ISMP) includes this medication among its list of drug classes which have a heightened risk of causing significant patient harm when used in error.

Fentanyl transdermal system patches: Leakage of fentanyl gel from the patch has been reported; patch may be less effective; do not use. Thoroughly wash any skin surfaces coming into direct contact with gel with water (do not use soap). May contain conducting metal (eg, aluminum); remove patch prior to MRI.

Medication Guide Available Yes

Prescribing and Access Restrictions As a requirement of the REMS program, access is restricted.

Abstral® (fentanyl sublingual tablet) is only available through the ABSTRAL REMS (Risk Evaluation and Mitigation Strategy) program. For outpatient use, enrollment in the ABSTRAL REMS program is required for prescribers, outpatient pharmacies, and patients. For inpatient use, enrollment in the ABSTRAL REMS program is required for inpatient pharmacies; patient and prescriber enrollment is not required for inpatient use. Distributors must also be enrolled in the program. Further information may be obtained by calling the ABSTRAL REMS program at 1-888-227-8725 or online at www.abstralrems.com

Onsolis™ (fentanyl buccal film) is only available through the restricted distribution program (FOCUS™). Enrollment in the FOCUS™ program is required for prescribers, pharmacies, and patients. Further information may be obtained from the manufacturer, Meda Pharmaceuticals, Inc (1-877-466-7654).

Pregnancy Risk Factor C

Lactation Enters breast milk/not recommended (AAP rates "compatible"; AAP 2001 update pending)

Use

Injection: Relief of pain, preoperative medication, adjunct to general or regional anesthesia

Iontophoretic transdermal system (Ionsys™): Short-term, in-hospital management of acute postoperative pain

Transdermal patch (eg, Duragesic®): Management of persistent moderate-to-severe chronic pain

Transmucosal lozenge (eg, Actiq®), buccal tablet (Fentora®), buccal film (Onsolis™), sublingual tablet (Abstral®): Management of breakthrough cancer pain in opioid-tolerant patients

Mechanism of Action/Effect Binds with stereospecific receptors at many sites within the CNS, increases pain threshold, alters pain reception, inhibits ascending pain pathways

Contraindications Hypersensitivity to fentanyl or any component of the formulation

Transdermal system: Severe respiratory disease or depression including acute asthma (unless patient is mechanically ventilated); paralytic ileus; patients requiring short-term therapy, management of intermittent pain

Transmucosal buccal tablets (Fentora®), buccal films (Onsolis™), lozenges (eg, Actiq®), sublingual tablets (Abstral®), and/or transdermal patches (eg, Duragesic®): Contraindicated in the management of acute or postoperative pain (including headache, migraine, dental pain, or use in emergency room), and in patients who are not opioid tolerant

Warnings/Precautions An opioid-containing analgesic regimen should be tailored to each patient's needs and based upon the type of pain being treated (acute versus chronic), the route of administration, degree of tolerance for opioids (naive versus chronic user), age, weight, and medical condition. The optimal analgesic dose varies widely among patients. Doses should be titrated to pain relief/prevention. May cause CNS depression, which may impair physical or mental abilities; patients must be cautioned about performing tasks which require mental alertness (eg, operating machinery or driving). When using with other CNS depressants, reduce dose of one or both agents. Fentanyl shares the toxic potentials of opiate agonists, and precautions of opiate agonist therapy should be observed; use with caution in patients with bradycardia or bradyarrhythmias; rapid I.V. infusion may result in skeletal muscle and chest wall rigidity leading to respiratory distress and/or apnea, bronchoconstriction, laryngospasm; inject slowly over 3-5 minutes. **[U.S. Boxed Warning]: Healthcare provider should be alert to problems of abuse, misuse, and diversion.** Tolerance or drug dependence may result from extended use. The elderly may be particularly susceptible to the CNS depressant and constipating effects of narcotics. Use extreme caution in patients with COPD or other chronic respiratory conditions. Use caution with head injuries, morbid obesity, renal impairment, or hepatic dysfunction. **[U.S. Boxed Warning]: Use with strong or moderate CYP3A4 inhibitors may result in increased effects and potentially fatal respiratory depression.** Use is not recommended with MAO inhibitors or within 14 days of MAO inhibitor use; severe and unpredictable adverse effects may result. Concurrent use of agonist/antagonist analgesics may precipitate withdrawal symptoms and/or reduced analgesic efficacy in patients following prolonged therapy with mu opioid agonists. Abrupt discontinuation following prolonged use may also lead to withdrawal symptoms. Safety and efficacy have not been established in children <16 years of age for the lozenge and <18 years of age for the buccal tablet.

[U.S. Boxed Warning]: Safety and efficacy of the transdermal patch have been limited to children ≥2 years of age who are opioid-tolerant. [U.S. Boxed Warning]: Buccal film (Onsolis™), sublingual tablet (Abstral®): Not indicated for use in opioid-tolerant cancer patients <18 years of age. [U.S. Boxed Warning]: Buccal film, buccal tablet, sublingual tablet, and lozenge preparations contain an amount of medication that can be fatal to children. Keep all units out of the reach of children and discard any open units properly.

Patients and caregivers should be counseled on the dangers to children including the risk of exposure to partially-consumed units.

[U.S. Boxed Warning] Abstral®, Actiq®, Duragesic®, Fentora®, Onsolis™: May cause potentially life-threatening hypoventilation, respiratory depression, and/or death; Abstral®, Actiq®, Duragesic®, Fentora®, or Onsolis™ should only be prescribed for opioid-tolerant patients. Risk of respiratory depression increased in elderly patients, debilitated patients, and patients with conditions associated with hypoxia or hypercapnia; usually occurs after administration of initial dose in nontolerant patients or when given with other drugs that depress respiratory function.

Transmucosal: Lozenge (eg, Actiq®), buccal tablet (Fentora®), buccal film (Onsolis™), sublingual tablet (Abstral®): **[U.S. Boxed Warning]: Should be used only for the care of opioid-tolerant cancer patients with breakthrough pain and is intended for use by specialists who are knowledgeable in treating cancer pain.** Not approved for use in management of acute or postoperative pain.

Transmucosal: Buccal film (eg, Onsolis™): **[U.S. Boxed Warning]: Available only through the FOCUS Program, a restricted distribution program with prescriber, pharmacy, and patient required enrollment. [U.S. Boxed Warning]: Onsolis™ is contraindicated in the management of acute or postoperative pain, including headache/migraine. [U.S. Boxed Warning]: Due to higher bioavailability of fentanyl in the buccal film formulation, do not substitute Onsolis™ on a mcg-per-mcg basis for any other fentanyl product. Serious adverse events, including death, may occur when used inappropriately (improper dose or patient selection). All patients must begin therapy with a 200 mcg dose and titrate, if needed. During therapy, patients must wait at least 2 hours before taking another dose.**

Transmucosal: Buccal tablet (Fentora®): **[U.S. Boxed Warning]: Due to the higher bioavailability of fentanyl in Fentora®, when converting patients from oral transmucosal fentanyl citrate (OTFC, Actiq®) to Fentora®, do not substitute Fentora®): on a mcg-per-mcg basis for any other fentanyl product. [U.S. Boxed Warning]: Fentora® is contraindicated in the management of acute or postoperative pain, including headache/migraine. Serious adverse events, including death, have been reported when used inappropriately (improper dose or patient selection). [U.S. Boxed Warning]: Patients using Fentora® who experience breakthrough pain may only take one additional dose using the same strength and must wait four hours before taking another dose.**

Transmucosal: Lozenge (Actiq®): **[U.S. Boxed Warning]: The substitution of Actiq® for any other fentanyl product may result in a fatal overdose. Do not convert patients on a mcg-per-mcg basis to Actiq® from other fentanyl products. Do not substitute Actiq® for any other fentanyl product. [U.S. Boxed Warning]: Patients using fentanyl lozenges who experience breakthrough pain may only take 1 additional dose using the same strength and must wait 4 hours before taking another dose.**

Transmucosal: Sublingual tablet (Abstral®): **[U.S. Boxed Warning]: Available only through the ABSTRAL REMS program. Prescribers who prescribe to outpatients, outpatients, pharmacies, and distributors are required to enroll in the program. [U.S. Boxed Warning]: Abstral® is contraindicated in opioid nontolerant patients. [U.S. Boxed Warning]: Due to differing pharmacokinetics of fentanyl in the sublingual tablet formulation, do not substitute Abstral® on a mcg-per-mcg basis for any other fentanyl product. Serious adverse events, including death, may occur when used inappropriately (improper dose or patient selection). All patients must begin therapy with a 100 mcg dose. During therapy, patients must wait at least 2 hours before treating another episode of breakthrough pain.**

Transdermal patches (eg, Duragesic®): **[U.S. Boxed Warning]: Indicated for the management of persistent moderate-to-severe pain when around the clock pain control is needed for an extended time period. Should only be used in patients who are already receiving opioid therapy, are opioid tolerant, and who require a total daily dose equivalent to 25 mcg/hour transdermal patch. Contraindicated in patients who are not opioid tolerant, in the management of short-term analgesia, or in the management of postoperative pain. Should be applied only to intact skin. Use of a patch that has been cut, damaged, or altered in any way may result in overdosage.** Serum fentanyl concentrations may increase approximately one-third for patients with a body temperature of 40°C secondary to a temperature-dependent increase in fentanyl release from the patch and increased skin permeability. **[U.S. Boxed Warning]: Avoid exposure of application site and surrounding area to direct external heat sources.** Patients who experience fever or increase in core temperature should be monitored closely. Patients who experience adverse reactions should be monitored for at least 24 hours after removal of the patch. Transdermal patch may contain conducting metal (eg, aluminum); remove patch prior to MRI.

Drug Interactions

Metabolism/Transport Effects Substrate of CYP3A4 (major); **Inhibits** CYP3A4 (weak)

Avoid Concomitant Use

Avoid concomitant use of FentaNYL with any of the following: MAO Inhibitors

Decreased Effect

FentaNYL may decrease the levels/effects of: Pegvisomant

The levels/effects of FentaNYL may be decreased by: Ammonium Chloride; Mixed Agonist / Antagonist Opioids; Rifamycin Derivatives

Increased Effect/Toxicity

FentaNYL may increase the levels/effects of: Alcohol (Ethyl); Alvimopan; Beta-Blockers; Calcium Channel Blockers (Nondihydropyridine); CNS Depressants; Desmopressin; MAO Inhibitors; Selective Serotonin Reuptake Inhibitors; Thiazide Diuretics

The levels/effects of FentaNYL may be increased by: Amphetamines; Antipsychotic Agents (Phenothiazines); CYP3A4 Inhibitors (Moderate); CYP3A4 Inhibitors (Strong); Dasatinib; Droperidol; MAO Inhibitors; Succinylcholine

Nutritional/Ethanol Interactions

Ethanol: Avoid ethanol (may increase CNS depression).

Food: Fentanyl concentrations may be increased by grapefruit juice; avoid concurrent intake of large quantities (>1 quart/day).

Herb/Nutraceutical: St John's wort may decrease fentanyl levels. Avoid valerian, St John's wort, kava kava, gotu kola (may increase CNS depression).

Adverse Reactions

>10%:

Cardiovascular: Bradycardia, edema

Central nervous system: CNS depression, confusion, dizziness, drowsiness, fatigue, headache, sedation

Endocrine & metabolic: Dehydration

Gastrointestinal: Constipation, nausea, vomiting, xerostomia

Local: Application-site reaction erythema

Neuromuscular & skeletal: Chest wall rigidity (high dose I.V.), muscle rigidity, weakness

Ocular: Miosis

Respiratory: Dyspnea, respiratory depression

Miscellaneous: Diaphoresis

1% to 10%:

Cardiovascular: Cardiac arrhythmia, chest pain, DVT, flushing, hyper-/hypotension, orthostatic hypotension, pallor, palpitation, peripheral edema, syncope, tachycardia, vasodilation

Central nervous system: Abnormal dreams, abnormal thinking, agitation, amnesia, anxiety, attention disturbance, DVT, depression, dysphoria, euphoria, fever, hallucinations, hypoesthesia, insomnia, lethargy, malaise, mental status change, migraine, nervousness, paranoid reaction, somnolence, stupor, vertigo

Dermatologic: Alopecia, bruising, cellulitis, erythema, hyperhidrosis, papules, pruritus, rash

Endocrine & metabolic: Breast pain, hot flashes, hyper-/hypocalcemia, hyper-/hypoglycemia, hypoalbuminemia, hypokalemia, hypomagnesemia

Gastrointestinal: Abdominal pain, abnormal taste, anorexia, appetite decreased, biliary tract spasm, diarrhea, dyspepsia, dysphagia (buccal tablet/film), flatulence, GI hemorrhage, gingival pain (buccal tablet), gingivitis (lozenge), glossitis (lozenge), ileus, intestinal obstruction (buccal film), periodontal abscess (lozenge/buccal tablet), stomatitis (lozenge/buccal tablet/sublingual tablet), tongue disorder (sublingual tablet), ulceration (gingival, lip, mouth; transmucosal use), weight loss

Genitourinary: Dysuria, erectile dysfunction, urinary incontinence, urinary retention, vaginitis, vaginal hemorrhage

Hematologic: Anemia, leukopenia, neutropenia, thrombocytopenia

Hepatic: Ascites, jaundice

Local: Application site pain, application site irritation

Neuromuscular & skeletal: Abnormal coordination, abnormal gait, arthralgia, back pain, myalgia, neuropathy, paresthesia, rigors, tremor

Ocular: Blurred vision, diplopia

Renal: Renal failure

Respiratory: Apnea, asthma, bronchitis, cough, epistaxis, hemoptysis, hypoventilation, hypoxia, nasopharyngitis, pharyngolaryngeal pain, pharyngitis, pneumonia, rhinitis, sinusitis, upper respiratory infection, wheezing

Miscellaneous: Flu-like syndrome, hiccups, hypersensitivity, lymphadenopathy, night sweats, parosmia, speech disorder, withdrawal syndrome

Pharmacodynamics/Kinetics

Onset of Action Analgesic: I.M.: 7-8 minutes; I.V.: Almost immediate; Transdermal (initial placement): 6 hours; Transmucosal: 5-15 minutes

Peak effect: Analgesic: Transdermal (initial placement): 12 hours; Transmucosal: 15-30 minutes

Duration of Action I.M.: 1-2 hours; I.V.: 0.5-1 hour; Transdermal (removal of patch/no replacement): 12 hours; Transmucosal: Related to blood level; respiratory depressant effect may last longer than analgesic effect

Absorption

Transdermal: Initial application: Gradually absorbed for the first 12-24 hours, followed by a constant absorption for the remainder of the dosing interval. Absorption is decreased in cachectic patients (compared to normal size patients).

Transmucosal, buccal tablet and buccal film: Rapid, ~50% from the buccal mucosa; remaining 50% swallowed with saliva and slowly absorbed from GI tract.

Transmucosal, lozenge: Rapid, ~25% from the buccal mucosa; 75% swallowed with saliva and slowly absorbed from GI tract

Bioavailability

Buccal film: 71% (mucositis did not have a clinically significant effect on C_{max} and AUC; however, bioavailability is expected to decrease if film is inappropriately chewed and swallowed)

Buccal tablet: 65% (range: 45% to 85%)

Lozenge: 47% (range: 37% to 57%)

Sublingual tablet: 54%

Time to Peak
Buccal film: 0.75-4 hours (median: 1 hour)
Buccal tablet: 20-240 minutes (median: 47 minutes)
Lozenge: 20-480 minutes (median: 20-40 minutes)
Sublingual tablet: 15-240 minutes (median: 30-60 minutes)
Transdermal patch: 24-72 hours, after several sequential 72-hour applications, steady state serum concentrations are reached

Protein Binding 80% to 85%

Half-Life Elimination
I.V.: 2-4 hours
Transdermal patch: 17 hours (13-22 hours, half-life is influenced by absorption rate)
Transmucosal: Lozenge: 7 hours; Buccal film: ~14 hours; Buccal tablet: 100-200 mcg: 3-4 hours, 400-800 mcg: 11-12 hours; Sublingual tablet: 100-200 mcg: 5-7 hours; 400-800 mcg: 10-14 hours

Metabolism Hepatic, primarily via CYP3A4

Excretion Urine 75% (primarily as metabolites, <7% to 10% as unchanged drug); feces ~9%

Controlled Substance C-II

Available Dosage Forms

Film, for buccal application:
Onsolis™: 200 mcg (30s); 400 mcg (30s); 600 mcg (30s); 800 mcg (30s); 1200 mcg (30s)

Injection, solution [preservative free]: 0.05 mg/mL (2 mL, 5 mL, 10 mL, 20 mL, 30 mL, 50 mL)

Lozenge, oral: 200 mcg (30s); 400 mcg (30s); 600 mcg (30s); 800 mcg (30s); 1200 mcg (30s); 1600 mcg (30s)
Actiq®: 200 mcg (30s); 400 mcg (30s); 600 mcg (30s); 800 mcg (30s); 1200 mcg (30s); 1600 mcg (30s)

Patch, transdermal: 12.5 mcg/hr (5s); 25 mcg/hr (5s); 50 mcg/hr (5s); 75 mcg/hr (5s); 100 mcg/hr (5s)
Duragesic®: 12.5 mcg/hr (5s); 25 mcg/hr (5s); 50 mcg/hr (5s); 75 mcg/hr (5s); 100 mcg/hr (5s)

Powder, for prescription compounding: USP: 100% (1 g)

Tablet, for buccal application:
Fentora®: 100 mcg (28s); 200 mcg (28s); 400 mcg (28s); 600 mcg (28s); 800 mcg (28s)

Tablet, sublingual:
Abstral®: 100 mcg (12s, 32s); 200 mcg (12s, 32s); 300 mcg (12s, 32s); 400 mcg (12s, 32s); 600 mcg (32s); 800 mcg (32s)

Dosing

Adult Note: These are guidelines and do not represent the maximum doses that may be required in all patients. Doses and dosage intervals should be titrated to pain relief/prevention. Monitor vital signs routinely. Single I.M. doses have a duration of 1-2 hours, single I.V. doses last 0.5-1 hour.

Surgery:
Premedication: I.M., slow I.V.: 50-100 mcg/dose 30-60 minutes prior to surgery
Adjunct to regional anesthesia: Slow I.V.: 25-100 mcg/dose over 1-2 minutes. **Note:** An I.V. should be in place with regional anesthesia so the I.M. route is rarely used but still maintained as an option in the package labeling.
Adjunct to general anesthesia: Slow I.V.:
Low dose: 0.5-2 mcg/kg/dose depending on the indication.
Moderate dose: Initial: 2-20 mcg/kg/dose; Maintenance (bolus or infusion): 1-2 mcg/kg/**hour**. Discontinuing fentanyl infusion 30-60 minutes prior to the end of surgery will usually allow adequate ventilation upon emergence from anesthesia. For "fast-tracking" and early extubation following major surgery, total fentanyl doses are limited to 10-15 mcg/kg.
High dose: 20-50 mcg/kg/dose; **Note:** High-dose fentanyl as an adjunct to general anesthesia is rarely used, but is still described in the manufacturer's label.

Pain management: Adults:
I.V. (unlabeled use): Bolus at start of infusion: 1-2 mcg/kg **or** 25-100 mcg/dose; continuous infusion rate: 1-2 mcg/kg/**hour or** 25-200 mcg/hour
Severe (unlabeled use): I.M, I.V.: 50-100 mcg/dose every 1-2 hours as needed; patients with prior opiate exposure may tolerate higher initial doses
Patient-controlled analgesia (PCA) (unlabeled use): I.V.:
Usual concentration: 10 mcg/mL
Demand dose: Usual: 20 mcg; range: 10-50 mcg
Lockout interval: 5-8 minutes
Usual basal rate: ≤50 mcg/hour
Critically-ill patients (unlabeled dose): Slow I.V.: 25-100 mcg (based on ~70 kg patient) **or** 0.35-1.5 mcg/kg every 30-60 minutes as needed. **Note:** More frequent dosing may be needed (eg, mechanically-ventilated patients).
Continuous infusion: 50-700 mcg/hour (based on ~70 kg patient) **or** 0.7-10 mcg/kg/**hour**
Intrathecal (I.T.) (unlabeled use; American Pain Society, 2008): **Must be preservative-free.** Doses must be adjusted for age, injection site, and patient's medical condition and degree of opioid tolerance.
Single dose: 5-25 mcg/dose; may provide adequate relief for up to 6 hours
Continuous infusion: Not recommended in acute pain management due to risk of excessive accumulation. For chronic cancer pain, infusion of very small doses may be practical (American Pain Society, 2008).
Epidural (unlabeled use; American Pain Society, 2008): **Must be preservative-free.** Doses must be adjusted for age, injection site, and patient's medical condition and degree of opioid tolerance
Single dose: 25-100 mcg/dose; may provide adequate relief for up to 8 hours

Continuous infusion: 25-100 mcg/hour

Breakthrough cancer pain: For patients who are tolerant to and currently receiving opioid therapy for persistent cancer pain; dosing should be individually titrated to provide adequate analgesia with minimal side effects. Dose titration should be done if patient requires more than 1 dose/breakthrough pain episode for several consecutive episodes. Patients experiencing >4 breakthrough pain episodes/day should have the dose of their long-term opioid re-evaluated.

Lozenge: Initial dose: 200 mcg; the second dose may be started 15 minutes after completion of the first dose if pain unrelieved. A maximum of 1 additional dose can be given per pain episode; must wait at least 4 hours before treating another episode. Consumption should be limited to ≤4 units/day. Additional requirements suggest need for improved baseline therapy.

Buccal film (Onsolis™): Initial dose: 200 mcg for all patients **Note:** Patients previously using another transmucosal product should be initiated at doses of 200 mcg; do **not** switch patients using any other fentanyl product on a mcg-per-mcg basis.

Dose titration: If titration required, increase dose in 200 mcg increments once per episode using multiples of the 200 mcg film; do not redose within a single episode of breakthrough pain and separate single doses by ≥2 hours. During titration, do not exceed 4 simultaneous applications of the 200 mcg films (800 mcg). If >800 mcg required, treat next episode with one 1200 mcg film (maximum dose: 1200 mcg). Once maintenance dose is determined, all other unused films should be disposed of and that strength (using a single film) should be used. During any pain episode, if adequate relief is not achieved after 30 minutes following buccal film application, a rescue medication (as determined by healthcare provider) may be used.

Maintenance: Determined dose applied as a single film once per episode and separated by ≥2 hours (dose range: 200-1200 mcg); limit to 4 applications/day. Consider increasing the around-the-clock opioid therapy in patients experiencing >4 breakthrough pain episodes/day.

Buccal tablet (Fentora®): Initial dose: 100 mcg; a second 100 mcg dose, if needed, may be started 30 minutes after the start of the first dose. **Note:** For patients previously using the transmucosal lozenge (Actiq®), the initial dose should be selected using the conversions listed below (maximum: 2 doses per breakthrough pain episode every 4 hours).

Dose titration, if required, should be done using multiples of the 100 mcg tablets. Patient can take two 100 mcg tablets (one on each side of mouth). If that dose is not successful, can use four 100 mcg tablets (two on each side of mouth). If titration requires >400 mcg/dose, then use 200 mcg tablets.

Conversion from lozenge to buccal tablet (Fentora®):

Lozenge dose 200-400 mcg, then buccal tablet 100 mcg

Lozenge dose 600-800 mcg, then buccal tablet 200 mcg

Lozenge dose 1200-1600 mcg, then buccal tablet 400 mcg

Note: Four 100 mcg buccal tablets deliver approximately 12% and 13% higher values of C_{max} and AUC, respectively, compared to one 400 mcg buccal tablet. To prevent confusion, patient should only have one strength available at a time. Using more than four buccal tablets at a time has not been studied.

Sublingual tablet (Abstral®): Initial dose: 100 mcg for all patients; if pain is unrelieved, a second dose may be given 30 minutes after administration of the first dose. A maximum of 2 doses can be given per breakthrough pain episode; must wait at least 2 hours before treating another episode. **Note:** Patients previously using another fentanyl product should be initiated at a dose of 100 mcg; do not convert patients from other fentanyl products to Abstral® on a mcg-per-mcg basis.

Dose titration: If titration required, increase in 100 mcg increments (up to 400 mcg) over consecutive breakthrough episodes. If titration requires >400 mcg/dose, increase in increments of 200 mcg, starting with 600 mcg dose. During titration, patients may use multiples of 100 mcg and/or 200 mcg tablets for any single dose; do not exceed 4 tablets at one time; safety and efficacy of doses >800 mcg have not been evaluated.

Maintenance dose: Once maintenance dose for breakthrough pain episode has been determined, use only 1 tablet in the appropriate strength per episode (if pain is unrelieved a second dose may be given after 30 minutes; maximum of 2 doses/episode of breakthrough pain); separate treatment of subsequent episodes by ≥2 hours; limit treatment to ≤4 breakthrough episodes/day. Consider increasing the around-the-clock long-acting opioid therapy in patients experiencing >4 breakthrough pain episodes/day; if long-acting opioid therapy dose altered, re-evaluate and retitrate Abstral® dose as needed.

Chronic pain management: Children ≥2 years and Adults (opioid-tolerant patients): Transdermal patch (Duragesic®):

Initial: To convert patients from oral or parenteral opioids to transdermal patch, a 24-hour analgesic requirement should be calculated (based on prior opiate use). Using the tables, the appropriate initial dose can be determined. The initial fentanyl dosage may be approximated from the 24-hour morphine dosage equivalent and titrated to minimize adverse effects and provide analgesia. With the initial application, the absorption of transdermal fentanyl requires several hours to reach plateau; therefore transdermal fentanyl is inappropriate for management of acute pain. Change patch every 72 hours.

Conversion from continuous infusion of fentanyl: In patients who have adequate pain relief with a fentanyl infusion, fentanyl may be converted to transdermal dosing at a rate equivalent to the intravenous rate. A two-step taper of the infusion to be completed over 12 hours has been recommended (Kornick, 2001) after the patch is applied. The infusion is decreased to 50% of the original rate six hours after the application of the first patch, and subsequently discontinued twelve hours after application.

Titration: Short-acting agents may be required until analgesic efficacy is established and/or as supplements for "breakthrough" pain. The amount of supplemental doses should be closely monitored. Appropriate dosage increases may be based on daily supplemental dosage using the ratio of 45 mg/24 hours of oral morphine to a 12.5 mcg/hour increase in fentanyl dosage.

Frequency of adjustment: The dosage should not be titrated more frequently than every 3 days after the initial dose or every 6 days thereafter. Patients should wear a consistent fentanyl dosage through two applications (6 days) before dosage increase based on supplemental opiate dosages can be estimated. **Note:** Upon discontinuation, ~17 hours are required for a 50% decrease in fentanyl levels.

Frequency of application: The majority of patients may be controlled on every 72-hour administration; however, a small number of patients require every 48-hour administration.

Dose conversion guidelines for transdermal fentanyl (see tables).
Note: U.S. and Canadian dose conversion guidelines differ. Consult appropriate table.

U.S. Labeling: Dose Conversion Guidelines: Recommended Initial Duragesic® Dose Based Upon Daily Oral Morphine Dose[1,2]

Oral 24-Hour Morphine (mg/day)	Duragesic® Dose[3] (mcg/h)
60-134	25
135-224	50
225-314	75
315-404	100
405-494	125
495-584	150
585-674	175
675-764	200
765-854	225
855-944	250
945-1034	275
1035-1124	300

[1]The table should NOT be used to convert from transdermal fentanyl (Duragesic®) to other opioid analgesics. Rather, following removal of the patch, titrate the dose of the new opioid until adequate analgesia is achieved.

[2]Recommendations are based on U.S. product labeling for Duragesic®.

[3]Pediatric patients initiating therapy on a 25 mcg/hour Duragesic® system should be opioid-tolerant and receiving at least 60 mg oral morphine equivalents per day.

U.S. Labeling: Dose Conversion Guidelines[1,2]

Current Analgesic	Daily Dosage (mg/day)			
Morphine (I.M./I.V.)	10-22	23-37	38-52	53-67
Oxycodone (oral)	30-67	67.5-112	112.5-157	157.5-202
Oxycodone (I.M./I.V.)	15-33	33.1-56	56.1-78	78.1-101
Codeine (oral)	150-447	448-747	748-1047	1048-1347
Hydromorphone (oral)	8-17	17.1-28	28.1-39	39.1-51
Hydromorphone (I.V.)	1.5-3.4	3.5-5.6	5.7-7.9	8-10
Meperidine (I.M.)	75-165	166-278	279-390	391-503
Methadone (oral)	20-44	45-74	75-104	105-134
Methadone (I.M.)	10-22	23-37	38-52	53-67
Fentanyl transdermal recommended dose (mcg/h)	**25 mcg/h**	**50 mcg/h**	**75 mcg/h**	**100 mcg/h**

[1]The table should NOT be used to convert from transdermal fentanyl (Duragesic®) to other opioid analgesics. Rather, following removal of the patch, titrate the dose of the new opioid until adequate analgesia is achieved.

[2]Recommendations are based on U.S. product labeling for Duragesic®.

Transdermal patch (Duragesic® MAT [Canada; not available in U.S.]): Adults:

Canadian Labeling: Dose Conversion Guidelines (Adults): Recommended Initial Duragesic® MAT Dose Based Upon Daily Oral Morphine Dose[1,2]

Oral 24-Hour Morphine (Current Dose in mg/day)	Duragesic® MAT Dose (Initial Dose in mcg/h)
45-59	12
60-134	25
135-179	37
180-224	50
225-269	62
270-314	75
315-359	87
360-404	100
405-494	125
495-584	150
585-674	175
675-764	200
765-854	225
855-944	250
945-1034	275
1035-1124	300

[1]The table should NOT be used to convert from transdermal fentanyl (Duragesic® MAT) to other opioid analgesics. Rather, following removal of the patch, titrate the dose of the new opioid until adequate analgesia is achieved.

[2]Recommendations are based on Canadian product labeling for Duragesic® MAT.

Note: The 12 mcg/hour dose included in this table is to be used for incremental dose adjustment and is generally not recommended for initial dosing, except for patients in whom lower starting doses are deemed clinically appropriate.

Canadian Labeling: Dosing Conversion Guidelines (Adults)[1,2]

Current Analgesic	Daily Dosage (mg/day)						
Morphine[3] (I.M./I.V.)	20-44	45-60	61-75	76-90	n/a[4]	n/a[4]	n/a[4]
Oxycodone (oral)	30-66	67-90	91-112	113-134	135-157	158-179	180-202
Codeine (oral)	150-447	448-597	598-747	748-897	898-1047	1048-1197	1198-1347
Hydromorphone (oral)	8-16	17-22	23-28	29-33	34-39	40-45	46-51
Hydromorphone (I.V.)	4-8.4	8.5-11.4	11.5-14.4	14.5-16.5	16.6-19.5	19.6-22.5	22.6-25.5
Fentanyl transdermal recommended dose (mcg/h)	**25 mcg/h**	**37 mcg/h**	**50 mcg/h**	**62 mcg/h**	**75 mcg/h**	**87 mcg/h**	**100 mcg/h**

[1]The table should NOT be used to convert from transdermal fentanyl (Duragesic® MAT) to other opioid analgesics. Rather, following removal of the patch, titrate the dose of the new opioid until adequate analgesia is achieved.

[2]Recommendations are based on Canadian product labeling for Duragesic® MAT.

[3]Morphine dose conversion based upon I.M to oral dose ratio of 1:3.

[4]Insufficient data available to provide specific dosing recommendations. Use caution; adjust dose conservatively.

Geriatric Elderly have been found to be twice as sensitive as younger patients to the effects of fentanyl. A wide range of doses may be used. When choosing a dose, take into consideration the following patient factors: age, weight, physical status, underlying disease states, other drugs used, type of anesthesia used, and the surgical procedure to be performed.

Transmucosal lozenge (eg, Actiq®): In clinical trials, patients who were >65 years of age were titrated to a mean dose that was 200 mcg less than that of younger patients.

Pediatric Note: These are guidelines and do not represent the maximum doses that may be required in all patients. Doses and dosage intervals should be titrated to pain relief/prevention. Monitor vital signs routinely. Single I.M. doses have a duration of 1-2 hours, single I.V. doses last 0.5-1 hour.

Adjunct to anesthesia (induction and maintenance): Children ≥2 years: I.V.: 2-3 mcg/kg/dose every 1-2 hours as needed

Pain management (unlabeled use): I.V.: 0.5-2 mcg/kg/dose given every 1-2 hours as needed; continuous infusion: 0.5-2 mcg/kg/**hour**; titrate to desired effects

Patient-controlled analgesia (PCA) (unlabeled use; American Pain Society, 2008): Children <50 kg: **Note:** Opiate-naive: Consider lower end of dosing range:

Usual concentration: 10 mcg/mL

Demand dose: 0.5-1 mcg/kg/dose

Lockout interval: 6-8 minutes

Usual basal rate: 0-0.5 mcg/kg/**hour**

Chronic pain management: Children ≥2 years (opioid-tolerant patients): Transdermal patch (Duragesic®): Refer to adult dosing.

Minor procedures/analgesia (unlabeled use): I.V.:

Children 1-12 years: 0.5-2 mcg/kg/dose given 3 minutes prior to procedure; may repeat every 1-2 hours

Children >12 years: 0.5-2 mcg/kg/dose (maximum: 50 mcg/dose) given 3 minutes prior to procedure; may repeat in 5 minutes if necessary; if more than 2 doses are needed, repeat with a maximum of 25 mcg/dose up to 5 times

Continuous sedation/analgesia: 0.5-2 mcg/kg/**hour**; titrate to desired effect

Breakthrough cancer pain: Children ≥16 years: Transmucosal lozenge: Refer to adult dosing.

Hepatic Impairment Fentanyl kinetics may be altered in hepatic disease.

Administration

Oral

Lozenge: Foil overwrap should be removed just prior to administration. Place the unit in mouth between the cheek and gum and allow it to dissolve. Do not chew. Lozenge may be moved from one side of the mouth to the other. The unit should be consumed over a period of 15 minutes. Handle should be removed after the lozenge is consumed; early removal should be considered if the patient has achieved an adequate response and/or shows signs of respiratory depression.

Buccal film: Foil overwrap should be removed just prior to administration. Prior to placing film, wet inside of cheek using tongue or by rinsing with water. Place film inside mouth with the pink side of the unit against the inside of the moistened cheek. With finger, press the film against cheek and hold for 5 seconds. The film should stick to the inside of cheek after 5 seconds. The film should be left in place until it dissolves (usually within 15-30 minutes after application). Liquids may be consumed after 5 minutes of application. Food can be eaten after film dissolves. If using more than 1 film simultaneously (during titration period), apply films on either side of mouth (do not apply on top of each other). Do not chew or swallow film. Do not cut or tear the film. All patients must initiate therapy using the 200 mcg film.

Buccal tablet: Patient should not open blister until ready to administer. The blister backing should be peeled back to expose the tablet; tablet should not be pushed out through the blister. Immediately use tablet once removed from blister. Place entire tablet in the buccal cavity (above a rear molar, between the upper cheek and gum). Tablet should not be broken, sucked, chewed, or swallowed. Should dissolve in about 14-25 minutes when left between the cheek and the gum. If remnants remain they may be swallowed with water.

Sublingual tablet: Remove from the blister unit immediately prior to administration. Place tablet directly under the tongue on the floor of the mouth and allow to completely dissolve; do not chew, suck, or swallow. Do not eat or drink anything until tablet is completely dissolved. In patients with a dry mouth, water may be used to moisten the buccal mucosa just before administration. All patients must initiate therapy using the 100 mcg tablet.

I.V. Administer as slow I.V. infusion over 1-2 minutes. May also be administered as continuous infusion or PCA (unlabeled use) routes. Muscular rigidity may occur with rapid I.V. administration.

Topical Transdermal patch (eg, Duragesic®): Apply to nonirritated and nonirradiated skin, such as chest, back, flank, or upper arm. Do not shave skin; hair at application site should be clipped. Prior to application, clean site with clear water and allow to dry completely. Do not use damaged, cut or leaking patches; patch may be less effective. Skin exposure from fentanyl gel leaking from patch may lead to serious adverse effects; thoroughly wash affected skin surfaces with water (do not use soap). Firmly press in place and hold for 30 seconds. Change patch every 72 hours. Do **not** use soap, alcohol, or other solvents to remove transdermal gel if it accidentally touches skin; use copious amounts of water. Avoid exposing application site to external heat sources (eg, heating pad, electric blanket, heat lamp, hot tub). If there is difficulty with patch adhesion, the edges of the system may be taped in place with first-aid tape. If there is continued difficulty with adhesion, an adhesive film dressing (eg, Bioclusive®, Tegaderm®) may be applied over the system.

Stability

Storage

Injection formulation: Store at controlled room temperature of 20°C to 25°C (68°F to 77°F). Protect from light.

Transdermal patch: Do not store above 25°C (77°F).

Transmucosal (buccal film, buccal tablet, lozenge, sublingual tablet): Store at controlled room temperature of 20°C to 25°C (68°F to 77°F). Protect from freezing and moisture. Keep out of the reach of children.

Monitoring and Teaching Issues

Physical Assessment Monitor effectiveness of pain relief. Monitor blood pressure, CNS and respiratory status, and degree of sedation prior to treatment and periodically throughout. Monitor closely for signs of withdrawal for 24 hours after transdermal product is removed. Order safety precautions for inpatient use to prevent falls. Assess patient's physical and/or psychological dependence. Discontinue slowly after prolonged use.

Patient Education Do not use alcohol, sedatives, tranquilizers, antihistamines, or pain medications without consulting prescriber. Avoid drinking large quantities of grapefruit juice (eg, >1 quart/day). Keep out of the reach of children. If using oral transmucosal lozenge, you may be at risk for dental carries due to the sugar content. Maintain good oral hygiene. If using patch, avoid exposing application site to external heat sources (eg, heating pad, electric blanket, hot tub, heat lamp). Maintain adequate hydration, unless instructed to restrict fluid intake. May cause hypotension, dizziness, drowsiness, impaired coordination, or blurred vision; nausea or vomiting; or constipation (if unresolved, consult prescriber about use of stool softeners). Report dizziness, chest pain, slow or rapid heartbeat, or headache; confusion or changes in mentation; changes in voiding frequency or amount; swelling of extremities or unusual weight gain; temperature >102°F; shortness of breath or respiratory difficulty; or vision changes.

Transdermal patch: Apply to clean, dry skin immediately after removing from package. Firmly press in place and hold for 30 seconds. Do not use damaged, cut, or leaking patches. If fentanyl gel should leak, wash affected skin surfaces with water; do not use soap. Remove patch while having MRI scan; can cause burns.

Transmucosal lozenge (eg, Actiq®): Contains an amount of medication that can be fatal to children. Keep all units, both used and unused, out of the reach of children and discard any open units properly. Actiq® Child Safety Kits are available which contain educational materials, safe storage, and disposal instructions.

Dietary Considerations Transmucosal lozenge contains 2 g sugar per unit.

Geriatric Considerations The elderly may be particularly susceptible to the CNS depressant and constipating effects of narcotics; therefore, use with caution. The effect of age on the pharmacokinetics of Fentora® (oral transmucosal buccal tablets) has not been studied.

Breast-Feeding Considerations Fentanyl is excreted in low concentrations into breast milk. Breast-feeding is considered acceptable following single doses to the mother; however, limited information is available when used long-term. **Note:** Transdermal patch, transmucosal lozenge, sublingual tablet, buccal tablet (Fentora®), and buccal film (Onsolis™) are not recommended in nursing women due to potential for sedation and/or respiratory depression. Symptoms of opioid withdrawal may occur in infants following the cessation of breast-feeding.

Pregnancy Considerations Teratogenic effects were not observed; however, embryo and fetotoxicity were noted in animal studies. Fentanyl crosses the placenta and the injectable formulation has been used safely during labor. Chronic use during pregnancy has shown detectable serum concentrations in the newborn with transient respiratory depression, behavioral changes, or seizures in the newborn infant characteristic of neonatal abstinence syndrome; transient neonatal muscular rigidity has also been observed. Transdermal patch, transmucosal lozenge, sublingual tablet, buccal tablet (Fentora®), and buccal film (Onsolis™) are not recommended for analgesia during labor and delivery.

Additional Information Fentanyl is 50-100 times as potent as morphine; morphine 10 mg I.M. is equivalent to fentanyl 0.1-0.2 mg I.M.; fentanyl has less hypotensive effects than morphine due to lack of histamine release. However, fentanyl may cause rigidity with high doses. If the patient has required high-dose analgesia or has used for a prolonged period (~7 days), taper dose to prevent withdrawal; monitor for signs and symptoms of withdrawal.

Transmucosal (oral lozenge, Actiq®): Disposal of lozenge units: After consumption of a complete unit, the handle may be disposed of in a trash container that is out of the reach of children. For a partially-consumed unit, or a unit that still has any drug matrix remaining on the handle, the handle should be placed under hot running tap water until the drug matrix has dissolved. Special child-resistant containers are available to temporarily store partially consumed units that cannot be disposed of immediately.

Transmucosal (buccal film, Onsolis™): Disposal of film: Remove foil overwrap from any unused, unneeded films and dispose by flushing in the toilet.

Transmucosal (sublingual tablet, Abstral®): Disposal of tablets: Remove any unused tablets from the blister cards and dispose by flushing in the toilet.

Transdermal patch (Duragesic®): Upon removal of the patch, ~17 hours are required before serum concentrations fall to 50% of their original values. Opioid withdrawal symptoms are possible. Gradual downward titration (potentially by the sequential use of lower-dose patches) is recommended. Keep transdermal patch (both used and unused) out of the reach of children. Do **not** use soap, alcohol, or other solvents to remove transdermal gel if it accidentally touches skin as they may increase transdermal absorption, use copious amounts of water. Avoid exposure of direct external heat sources (eg, heating pads, electric blankets, heat lamps, saunas, hot tubs, heated water beds) to application site.

Related Information

Compatibility of Drugs *on page 1994*
Opioid Analgesics *on page 2003*

◆ **Fentanyl Citrate** *see* FentaNYL *on page 744*
◆ **Fentanyl Hydrochloride** *see* FentaNYL *on page 744*
◆ **Fentanyl Patch** *see* FentaNYL *on page 744*

- ◆ **Fentora®** *see* FentaNYL *on page 744*
- ◆ **Feosol® [OTC]** *see* Ferrous Sulfate *on page 754*
- ◆ **Feraheme®** *see* Ferumoxytol *on page 755*
- ◆ **Ferate [OTC]** *see* Ferrous Gluconate *on page 754*
- ◆ **Fergon® [OTC]** *see* Ferrous Gluconate *on page 754*
- ◆ **Fer-In-Sol® [OTC]** *see* Ferrous Sulfate *on page 754*
- ◆ **Fer-iron [OTC]** *see* Ferrous Sulfate *on page 754*

Ferrous Gluconate (FER us GLOO koe nate)

U.S. Brand Names Ferate [OTC]; Fergon® [OTC]

Index Terms Iron Gluconate

Generic Availability (U.S.) Yes

Pharmacologic Category Iron Salt

Lactation Enters breast milk

Use Prevention and treatment of iron-deficiency anemias

Available Dosage Forms For available OTC formulations, consult specific product labeling.

Dosing

Adult

Dietary Reference Intake: Dose is RDA presented as elemental iron unless otherwise noted:

19-50 years: Male: 8 mg/day; Female: 18 mg/day; Pregnant female: 27 mg/day; Lactating female: 9 mg/day

≥50 years: 8 mg/day

Dose expressed in terms of elemental iron:

Treatment of iron deficiency anemia: Oral: 60 mg twice daily up to 60 mg 4 times/day

Prophylaxis of iron deficiency: Oral: 60 mg/day

Geriatric Lower doses (15-50 mg elemental iron/day) may have similar efficacy and less GI adverse events (eg, nausea, constipation) as compared to higher doses (eg, 150 mg elemental iron/day) (Rimon, 2005).

Pediatric

Dietary Reference Intake: Dose is RDA presented as elemental iron unless otherwise noted:

0-6 months: 0.27 mg/day (adequate intake)

7-12 months: 11 mg/day

1-3 years: 7 mg/day

4-8 years: 10 mg/day

9-13 years: 8 mg/day

14-18 years: Male: 11 mg/day; Female: 15 mg/day; Pregnant female: 27 mg/day; Lactating female: 10 mg/day

Dose expressed in terms of elemental iron:

Treatment of severe iron-deficiency anemia: Oral: 4-6 mg Fe/kg/day in 3 divided doses

Treatment of mild-to-moderate iron-deficiency anemia: Oral: 3 mg Fe/kg/day in 1-2 divided doses

Prophylaxis: Oral: 1-2 mg Fe/kg/day

Administration

Oral Administer 2 hours before or 4 hours after antacids. Administration of iron preparations to premature infants with vitamin E deficiency may cause increased red cell hemolysis and hemolytic anemia, therefore, vitamin E deficiency should be corrected if possible.

Monitoring and Teaching Issues

Laboratory Monitoring Serum iron, total iron binding capacity, reticulocyte count, hemoglobin

Patient Education May color stool black. Take between meals for maximum absorption; take with food if GI upset occurs. Do not take with milk or antacids.

Ferrous Sulfate (FER us SUL fate)

U.S. Brand Names Feosol® [OTC]; Fer-In-Sol® [OTC]; Fer-iron [OTC]; MyKidz Iron 10™ [OTC]; Slow FE® [OTC]

Index Terms $FeSO_4$; Iron Sulfate

Generic Availability (U.S.) Yes

Pharmacologic Category Iron Salt

Medication Safety Issues

Sound-alike/look-alike issues:

Feosol® may be confused with Fer-In-Sol®

Fer-In-Sol® may be confused with Feosol®

Slow FE® may be confused with Slow-K®

Potential for medication errors: Fer-In-Sol® (manufactured by Mead Johnson) and a limited number of generic products are available at a concentration of 15 mg/mL. However, many other generics and brand name products of ferrous sulfate oral liquid drops are available at a concentration of 15 mg/0.6 mL. Check concentration closely prior to dispensing. Prescriptions written in milliliters (mL) should be clarified.

Beers Criteria medication: This drug may be inappropriate for use in geriatric patients (dosage dependent, low severity risk).

Lactation Enters breast milk

Use Prevention and treatment of iron-deficiency anemias

Available Dosage Forms For available OTC formulations, consult specific product labeling.

Dosing

Adult Note: Multiple concentrations of ferrous sulfate oral liquid exist; close attention must be paid to the concentration when ordering and administering ferrous sulfate; incorrect selection or substitution of one ferrous sulfate liquid for another without proper dosage volume adjustment may result in serious over- or underdosing.

Dietary Reference Intake: Dose is RDA presented as elemental iron unless otherwise noted:

19-50 years: Male: 8 mg/day; Female: 18 mg/day; Pregnant female: 27 mg/day; Lactating female: 9 mg/day

≥50 years: 8 mg/day

Dose expressed in terms of ferrous sulfate:

Treatment of iron deficiency anemia: Oral: 300 mg twice daily up to 300 mg 4 times/day or 250 mg (extended release) 1-2 times/day

Prophylaxis of iron deficiency: Oral: 300 mg/day

Geriatric Lower doses (15-50 mg elemental iron/day) may have similar efficacy and less GI adverse events (eg, nausea,constipation) as compared to higher doses (eg, 150 mg elemental iron/day) (Rimon, 2005).

Pediatric Note: Multiple concentrations of ferrous sulfate oral liquid exist; close attention must be paid to the concentration when ordering and administering ferrous sulfate; incorrect selection or substitution of one ferrous sulfate liquid for another without proper dosage volume adjustment may result in serious over- or underdosing.

Dietary Reference Intake: Dose is RDA presented as elemental iron unless otherwise noted:

0-6 months: 0.27 mg/day (adequate intake)

7-12 months: 11 mg/day

1-3 years: 7 mg/day

4-8 years: 10 mg/day

9-13 years: 8 mg/day

14-18 years: Male: 11 mg/day; Female: 15 mg/day; Pregnant female: 27 mg/day; Lactating female: 10 mg/day

Dosage expressed in terms of elemental iron:

Treatment of severe iron-deficiency anemia: Oral: 4-6 mg Fe/kg/day in 3 divided doses

Treatment of mild-to-moderate iron-deficiency anemia: Oral: 3 mg Fe/kg/day in 1-2 divided doses

Prophylaxis: Oral: 1-2 mg Fe/kg/day up to a maximum of 15 mg/day

Administration

Oral Should be taken with water or juice on an empty stomach; administer ferrous sulfate 2 hours prior to, or 4 hours after antacids

Monitoring and Teaching Issues

Laboratory Monitoring Serum iron, total iron binding capacity, reticulocyte count, hemoglobin

Physical Assessment May cause GI irritation. Monitor GI function (observe for epigastric pain, nausea, dark stools, vomiting, stomach cramping, constipation).

Patient Education May color stool black. Take between meals for maximum absorption; take with food if GI upset occurs. Do not take with milk or antacids. You may experience constipation, nausea, vomiting, abdominal pain, and other GI complaints.

Ferumoxytol (fer ue MOX i tol)

U.S. Brand Names Feraheme®

Generic Availability (U.S.) No

Pharmacologic Category Iron Salt

Medication Safety Issues

Sound-alike/look-alike issues:

Ferumoxytol may be confused with ferric gluconate, iron dextran complex, iron sucrose

Pregnancy Risk Factor C

Lactation Excretion in breast milk unknown/not recommended

Use Treatment of iron-deficiency anemia in chronic kidney disease

Mechanism of Action/Effect Iron-carbohydrate complex which releases iron after uptake by the reticuloendothelial system macrophages of the liver, spleen, and bone marrow. The released iron is either transported into storage pools or is transported via plasma transferrin for incorporation into hemoglobin.

Contraindications Hypersensitivity to ferumoxytol or any component of the formulation; evidence of iron overload; anemia not caused by iron deficiency

Warnings/Precautions Hypersensitivity reactions, including rare anaphylactic and anaphylactoid reactions, may occur, presenting with cardiac/cardiorespiratory arrest, clinically significant hypotension, syncope, or unresponsiveness; equipment for resuscitation and trained personnel experienced in handling emergencies should be immediately available during use. Monitor patients for signs/symptoms of hypersensitivity reactions for ≥60 minutes after administration.

Use is contraindicated in the presence of tissue iron overload; periodic monitoring of hemoglobin, serum ferritin, serum iron, and transferrin saturation is recommended. Serum iron and transferrin-bound iron may be overestimated in laboratory assays if level is drawn during the first 24 hours following administration. Administration may alter magnetic resonance (MR) imaging; conduct anticipated MRI studies prior to use. MR imaging alterations may persist for ≤3 months following use, with peak alterations anticipated in the first 2 days following administration. If MR imaging is required within 3 months after administration, use T1- or proton density-weighted MR pulse sequences to decrease effect on imagining. Do not use T2-weighted sequence MR imaging prior to 4 weeks following ferumoxytol administration. Ferumoxytol does not interfere with X-ray, computed tomography (CT), positron emission tomography (PET), single photon emission computed tomography (SPECT), ultrasound or nuclear medicine imaging.

Drug Interactions

Avoid Concomitant Use

Avoid concomitant use of Ferumoxytol with any of the following: Dimercaprol

Decreased Effect There are no known significant interactions involving a decrease in effect.

Increased Effect/Toxicity

The levels/effects of Ferumoxytol may be increased by: Dimercaprol

Lab Interactions May interfere with MR imaging; alterations may persist for ≤3 months following use, with peak alterations anticipated in the first 2 days following administration. If MR imaging is required within 3 months after administration, use T1- or proton density-weighted MR pulse sequences to decrease effect on imaging. Do not use T2-weighted sequence MR imaging prior to 4 weeks following administration.

Serum iron and transferrin-bound iron may be overestimated in laboratory assays if level is drawn during the first 24 hours following administration (due to contribution of iron in ferumoxytol).

Adverse Reactions 1% to 10%:

Cardiovascular: Hypotension (≤3%), edema (2%), peripheral edema (2%), chest pain (1%), hypertension (1%)

Central nervous system: Dizziness (3%), headache (2%), fever (1%)

Dermatologic: Pruritus (1%), rash (1%)

Gastrointestinal: Diarrhea (4%), nausea (3%), constipation (2%), vomiting (2%), abdominal pain (1%)

Neuromuscular & skeletal: Back pain (1%), muscle spasms (1%)

Respiratory: Cough (1%), dyspnea (1%)

Miscellaneous: Hypersensitivity reactions (≤4%; serious reactions: <1%)

Pharmacodynamics/Kinetics

Half-Life Elimination ~15 hours; ferumoxytol is not removed by hemodialysis

Metabolism Iron released from iron-carbohydrate complex after uptake in the reticuloendothelial system macrophages of the liver, spleen, and bone marrow

Available Dosage Forms

Injection, solution:

Feraheme®: Elemental iron 30 mg/mL (17 mL)

Dosing

Adult & Geriatric Doses expressed in mg of **elemental** iron. **Note:** Test dose: Product labeling does not indicate need for a test dose.

Iron-deficiency anemia in chronic kidney disease: I.V.: 510 mg (17 mL) as a single dose, followed by a second 510 mg dose 3-8 days after initial dose. Recommended dose may be readministered in patients with persistent or recurrent iron deficiency anemia.

Renal Impairment Hemodialysis patients should receive injection after at least 1 hour of hemodialysis has been completed and once blood pressure has stabilized.

Administration

I.V. Administer intravenously as an undiluted injection at a rate ≤1 mL/second (30 mg of elemental iron/second). Do not administer if solution has particulate matter or is discolored (solution is black to reddish-brown).

Hemodialysis patients should receive injection after at least 1 hour of hemodialysis has been completed and once blood pressure has stabilized.

Stability

Storage Store vials at controlled room temperature of 20°C to 25°C (68°F to 77°F); excursions permitted to 15°C to 30°C (59°F to 86°F). Do not freeze.

Monitoring and Teaching Issues

Laboratory Monitoring Hemoglobin, serum ferritin, serum iron, transferrin saturation (for at least 1 month following second injection and periodically)

Physical Assessment Monitor closely during administration and for at least 60 minutes following for hypersensitive reactions. Resuscitation equipment should be available. Monitor blood pressure closely; can cause hypotension. May interfere with MR imaging and may persist up to 3 months following administration.

Patient Education You may experience dizziness or lightheadedness. Hypersensitivity reactions can occur. Healthcare personnel will need to monitor you for 60 minutes following the administration of this drug. Report itching, rash, wheezing, or respiratory difficulty immediately.

Geriatric Considerations The manufacturer states that in clinical trials, ferumoxytol was reportedly as safe and effective in patients 65 years and older as younger patients. Anemia in the elderly is most often caused by "anemia of chronic disease", a result of aging effect in bone marrow, or associated with inflammation rather than blood loss. Iron stores are usually normal or increased, with a serum ferritin >50 ng/mL and a decreased total iron binding capacity. Hence, the anemia is not secondary to iron deficiency but the inability of the reticuloendothelial system to use available iron stores. I.V. administration of iron is often preferred over I.M. in the elderly secondary to a decreased muscle mass and the need for daily injections.

Breast-Feeding Considerations Iron is normally found in breast milk. Breast milk or iron-fortified formulas generally provide enough iron to meet the recommended dietary requirements of infants. The amount of iron in breast milk is generally not influenced by maternal iron status.

Pregnancy Considerations Fetal malformations and decreased fetal weights were observed in animal studies at maternally toxic doses. There are no adequate and well-controlled studies in pregnant women. Use in pregnancy only if potential benefit justifies potential risk to fetus. It is recommended that pregnant women meet the dietary requirements of iron with diet and/or supplements in order to prevent adverse events associated with iron-deficiency anemia in pregnancy. Treatment of iron-deficiency anemia in pregnant women is the same as in nonpregnant women and in most cases, oral iron preparations may be used. Except in severe cases of maternal anemia, the fetus achieves normal iron stores regardless of maternal concentrations.

◆ **FESO** *see* Fesoterodine *on page 757*

◆ **$FeSO_4$** *see* Ferrous Sulfate *on page 754*

Fesoterodine (fes oh TER oh deen)

U.S. Brand Names Toviaz™

Index Terms FESO; Fesoterodine Fumarate

Generic Availability (U.S.) No

Pharmacologic Category Anticholinergic Agent

Medication Safety Issues

Sound-alike/look-alike issues:

Fesoterodine may be confused with fexofenadine, tolterodine

Pregnancy Risk Factor C

Lactation Excretion in breast milk unknown/not recommended

Use Treatment of patients with an overactive bladder with symptoms of urinary frequency, urgency, or urge incontinence.

Available Dosage Forms

Tablet, extended release, oral:

Toviaz™: 4 mg, 8 mg

Dosing

Adult & Geriatric Overactive bladder: Oral: 4 mg once daily; dose may be increased to 8 mg once daily based on individual response and tolerability

Dosing adjustment for concomitant CYP3A4 inhibitors: Maximum dose: 4 mg/day when administered concomitantly with potent CYP3A4 inhibitors including (but not limited to) ketoconazole, itraconazole, and clarithromycin. Concurrent therapy of weak or moderate CYP3A4 inhibitors and fesoterodine should be limited to 4 mg/day and increased to 8 mg/day after assessing tolerability.

Renal Impairment

Mild-to-moderate renal impairment (Cl_{cr} 30-80 mL/minute): No dose adjustment is recommended.

Severe renal impairment (Cl_{cr} <30 mL/minute): Maximum dose: 4 mg.

Hepatic Impairment

Moderate hepatic impairment (Child-Pugh class B): No dose adjustment is recommended.

Severe hepatic impairment (Child-Pugh class C): Use is not recommended; not studied in severe impairment.

Administration

Oral May be administered with or without food. Swallow whole; do not chew, crush, or divide.

Monitoring and Teaching Issues

Patient Education You may experience drowsiness. Avoid alcohol; may increase drowsiness. May cause dry mouth or constipation. Report to prescriber problems urinating.

Related Information

Pharmacotherapy of Urinary Incontinence *on page 2071*

◆ **Fesoterodine Fumarate** *see* Fesoterodine *on page 757*

◆ **Feverall® [OTC]** *see* Acetaminophen *on page 38*

◆ **Fexmid®** *see* Cyclobenzaprine *on page 432*

Fexofenadine (feks oh FEN a deen)

U.S. Brand Names Allegra®; Allegra® Allergy 12 Hour [OTC]; Allegra® Allergy 24 Hour [OTC]; Allegra® Children's Allergy ODT [OTC]; Allegra® Children's Allergy [OTC]; Allegra® ODT [DSC]

Index Terms Fexofenadine Hydrochloride

Generic Availability (U.S.) Yes: Excludes orally disintegrating tablet and suspension

Pharmacologic Category Histamine H_1 Antagonist; Histamine H_1 Antagonist, Second Generation; Piperidine Derivative

Medication Safety Issues

Sound-alike/look-alike issues:

Fexofenadine may be confused with fesoterodine

Allegra® may be confused with Viagra®

International issues:

Allegra [U.S, Canada, and multiple international markets] may be confused with Allegro brand name for fluticasone [Israel] and frovatriptan [Germany]

Pregnancy Risk Factor C

Lactation Excretion in breast milk unknown/use caution (AAP rates "compatible"; AAP 2001 update pending)

Use Relief of symptoms associated with seasonal allergic rhinitis; treatment of chronic idiopathic urticaria

OTC labeling: Relief of symptoms associated with allergic rhinitis

Mechanism of Action/Effect Fexofenadine is an active metabolite of terfenadine and like terfenadine it competes with histamine for H_1-receptor sites on effector cells in the GI tract, blood vessels, and respiratory tract; binds to lung receptors significantly greater than it binds to cerebellar receptors, resulting in a greatly reduced sedative potential

Contraindications Hypersensitivity to fexofenadine or any component of the formulation

Warnings/Precautions Use with caution in patients with renal impairment; dosage adjustment recommended. Safety and efficacy in children <6 months of age have not been established; orally disintegrating tablet not recommended for use in children <6 years of age. Orally disintegrating tablet contains phenylalanine.

Drug Interactions

Metabolism/Transport Effects Substrate of CYP3A4 (minor), P-glycoprotein, SLCO1B1; **Inhibits** CYP2D6 (weak)

Avoid Concomitant Use There are no known interactions where it is recommended to avoid concomitant use.

Decreased Effect

Fexofenadine may decrease the levels/effects of: Acetylcholinesterase Inhibitors (Central); Benzylpenicilloyl Polylysine; Betahistine

The levels/effects of Fexofenadine may be decreased by: Acetylcholinesterase Inhibitors (Central); Amphetamines; Antacids; Grapefruit Juice; P-Glycoprotein Inducers; Rifampin

Increased Effect/Toxicity

Fexofenadine may increase the levels/effects of: Alcohol (Ethyl); Anticholinergics; CNS Depressants

The levels/effects of Fexofenadine may be increased by: Conivaptan; Droperidol; Eltrombopag; Erythromycin; Erythromycin (Systemic); Itraconazole; Ketoconazole; Ketoconazole (Systemic); P-Glycoprotein Inhibitors; Pramlintide; Verapamil

Nutritional/Ethanol Interactions

Ethanol: Avoid ethanol (although limited with fexofenadine, may increase risk of sedation).

Food: Fruit juice (apple, grapefruit, orange) may decrease bioavailability of fexofenadine by ~36%.

Herb/Nutraceutical: St John's wort may decrease fexofenadine levels.

Adverse Reactions

>10%:

Central nervous system: Headache (5% to 11%)

Gastrointestinal: Vomiting (children 6 months to 5 years: 4% to 12%)

1% to 10%:

Central nervous system: Fatigue (1% to 3%), somnolence (1% to 3%), dizziness (2%), fever (2%), pain (2%), drowsiness (1%)

Endocrine & metabolic: Dysmenorrhea (2%)

Gastrointestinal: Diarrhea (3% to 4%), nausea (2%), dyspepsia (1% to 2%)

Neuromuscular & skeletal: Myalgia (3%), back pain (2% to 3%), pain in extremities (2%)

Otic: Otitis media (2% to 4%)

Respiratory: Upper respiratory tract infection (3% to 4%), cough (2% to 4%), rhinorrhea (1% to 2%)

Miscellaneous: Viral infection (3%)

Pharmacodynamics/Kinetics

Onset of Action 60 minutes

Duration of Action Antihistaminic effect: ≥12 hours

Time to Peak Serum: ODT: 2 hours (4 hours with high-fat meal); Tablet: ~2.6 hours; Suspension: ~1 hour

Protein Binding 60% to 70%, primarily albumin and alpha$_1$-acid glycoprotein

Half-Life Elimination 14.4 hours (31% to 72% longer in renal impairment)

Metabolism Minimal (~5%)

Excretion Feces (~80%) and urine (~11%) as unchanged drug

Available Dosage Forms

Suspension, oral:

Allegra®: 6 mg/mL (300 mL)

Allegra® Children's Allergy [OTC]: 6 mg/mL (120 mL)

Tablet, oral: 30 mg, 60 mg, 180 mg

Allegra® Allergy 12 Hour [OTC]: 60 mg

Allegra® Allergy 24 Hour [OTC]: 180 mg

Allegra® Children's Allergy [OTC]: 30 mg

Tablet, orally disintegrating, oral:
Allegra® Children's Allergy ODT [OTC]: 30 mg

Dosing

Adult Seasonal allergic rhinitis, idiopathic urticaria, allergic rhinitis (OTC labeling): Oral: 60 mg twice daily **or** 180 mg once daily

Geriatric Chronic idiopathic urticaria, seasonal allergic rhinitis: Oral: Use caution; adjust dose for renal impairment.

Pediatric

Chronic idiopathic urticaria: Oral: Children 6 months to <2 years: 15 mg twice daily

Chronic idiopathic urticaria, seasonal allergic rhinitis: Oral:
Children 2-11 years: 30 mg twice daily
Children ≥12 years: Refer to adult dosing.

Allergic rhinitis (OTC labeling): Oral:
Children 2-11 years: Oral: 30 mg twice daily
Children ≥12 years: Refer to adult dosing.

Renal Impairment

Cl_{cr} <80 mL/minute:
Children 6 months to <2 years: Initial: 15 mg once daily
Children 2-11 years: Initial: 30 mg once daily
Children ≥12 years and Adults: Initial: 60 mg once daily
Hemodialysis: Not effectively removed by hemodialysis.

Administration

Oral

Suspension, tablet: Administer with water only; do not administer with fruit juices. Shake suspension well before use.

Orally disintegrating tablet: Take on an empty stomach. Do not remove from blister pack until administered. Using dry hands, place immediately on tongue. Tablet will dissolve within seconds, and may be swallowed with or without liquid (do not administer with fruit juices). Do not split or chew.

Stability

Storage Store at controlled room temperature of 20°C to 25°C (68°F to 77°F). Protect from excessive moisture.

Monitoring and Teaching Issues

Patient Education Avoid use of alcohol. You may experience mild drowsiness, dizziness, or nausea. Report persistent sedation or drowsiness, lack of improvement, or worsening of condition.

Dietary Considerations Some products may contain phenylalanine and/or sodium. Take suspension and tablets with water only; do not administer with fruit juices.

Geriatric Considerations Plasma levels in the elderly are generally higher than those observed in other age groups. Once daily dosing is recommended when starting therapy in elderly patients or patients with decreased renal function.

Pregnancy Considerations Decreased fetal weight gain and survival were observed in animal studies; teratogenic effects were not observed.

Fexofenadine and Pseudoephedrine (feks oh FEN a deen & soo doe e FED rin)

U.S. Brand Names Allegra-D® 12 Hour; Allegra-D® 24 Hour

Index Terms Pseudoephedrine and Fexofenadine

Generic Availability (U.S.) Yes

Pharmacologic Category Alpha/Beta Agonist; Decongestant; Histamine H_1 Antagonist; Histamine H_1 Antagonist, Second Generation; Piperidine Derivative

Medication Safety Issues

Sound-alike/look-alike issues:
Allegra-D® may be confused with Viagra®

International issues:
Allegra-D [U.S, Canada, and multiple international markets] may be confused with Allegro brand name for fluticasone [Israel] and frovatriptan [Germany]

Pregnancy Risk Factor C

Lactation Enters breast milk/use caution (AAP rates "compatible"; AAP 2001 update pending)

Use Relief of symptoms associated with seasonal allergic rhinitis in adults and children ≥12 years of age

Available Dosage Forms

Tablet, extended release: Fexofenadine 60 mg [immediate release] and pseudoephedrine 120 mg [extended release]
Allegra-D® 12 Hour: Fexofenadine 60 mg [immediate release] and pseudoephedrine 120 mg [extended release]
Allegra-D® 24 Hour: Fexofenadine 180 mg [immediate release] and pseudoephedrine 240 mg [extended release]

Dosing

Adult & Geriatric Allergic symptoms and nasal congestion: Oral:
Allegra-D® 12 Hour: One tablet twice daily
Allegra-D® 24 Hour: One tablet once daily

Pediatric Children ≥12 years: Refer to adult dosing.

Renal Impairment

Allegra-D® 12 Hour: Cl_{cr} <80 mL/minute (based on fexofenadine component): One tablet once daily.

Allegra-D® 24 Hour: Avoid use.

Administration

Oral Tablets should be swallowed whole; do not crush or chew. Administer on an empty stomach with water; avoid administration with food. The inactive ingredients may be eliminated in the feces in a form resembling the original tablet.

Monitoring and Teaching Issues

Physical Assessment See individual agents.

Patient Education See individual agents.

Related Information

Fexofenadine *on page* 757

Pseudoephedrine *on page* 1529

◆ **Fexofenadine Hydrochloride** *see* Fexofenadine *on page* 757

◆ **Fibricor™** *see* Fenofibric Acid *on page* 742

Filgrastim (fil GRA stim)

U.S. Brand Names Neupogen®

Index Terms G-CSF; Granulocyte Colony Stimulating Factor

Generic Availability (U.S.) No

Pharmacologic Category Colony Stimulating Factor

Medication Safety Issues

Sound-alike/look-alike issues:

Neupogen® may be confused with Epogen®, Neulasta®, Neumega®, Neupro®, Nutramigen®

Pregnancy Risk Factor C

Lactation Excretion in breast milk unknown/use caution

Use

Cancer patients (nonmyeloid malignancies) receiving myelosuppressive chemotherapy to decrease the incidence of infection (febrile neutropenia) in regimens associated with a high incidence of neutropenia with fever

Acute myelogenous leukemia (AML) following induction or consolidation chemotherapy to shorten time to neutrophil recovery and reduce the duration of fever

Cancer patients (nonmyeloid malignancies) receiving bone marrow transplant to shorten the duration of neutropenia and neutropenia-related events (eg, neutropenic fever)

Peripheral stem cell transplantation to mobilize hematopoietic progenitor cells for leukapheresis collection

Severe chronic neutropenia (SCN; chronic administration) to reduce the incidence and duration of neutropenic complications (fever, infections, oropharyngeal ulcers) in symptomatic patients with congenital, cyclic, or idiopathic neutropenia

Unlabeled/Investigational Use Treatment of anemia in myelodysplastic syndrome; mobilization of hematopoietic stem cells (HSC) for collection and subsequent autologous transplantation (in combination with plerixafor) in patients with non-Hodgkin's lymphoma (NHL) and multiple myeloma (MM); treatment of neutropenia in HIV-infected patients receiving zidovudine; hepatitis C treatment-associated neutropenia

Mechanism of Action/Effect Stimulates the production, maturation, and activation of neutrophils, filgrastim activates neutrophils to increase both their migration and cytotoxicity. Natural proteins which stimulate hematopoietic stem cells to proliferate, prolong cell survival, stimulate cell differentiation, and stimulate functional activity of mature cells. CSFs are produced by a wide variety of cell types. Specific mechanisms of action are not yet fully understood, but possibly work by a second-messenger pathway with resultant protein production.

Contraindications Hypersensitivity to filgrastim, *E. coli*-derived proteins, or any component of the formulation

Warnings/Precautions Do not use filgrastim in the period 24 hours before to 24 hours after administration of cytotoxic chemotherapy because of the potential sensitivity of rapidly dividing myeloid cells to cytotoxic chemotherapy. May potentially act as a growth factor for any tumor type, particularly myeloid malignancies; caution should be exercised in the usage of filgrastim in any malignancy with myeloid characteristics. Increases circulating leukocytes when used in conjunction with plerixafor for stem cell mobilization; monitor WBC; use with caution in patients with neutrophil count >50,000/mm^3; tumor cells released from marrow could be collected in leukapheresis product; potential effect of tumor cell reinfusion is unknown. Reports of alveolar hemorrhage, manifested as pulmonary infiltrates and hemoptysis, have occurred in healthy donors undergoing PBPC collection (not FDA approved for use in healthy donors); hemoptysis resolved upon discontinuation. Safety and efficacy have not been established with patients receiving radiation therapy (avoid concurrent radiation therapy with filgrastim), or chemotherapy associated with delayed myelosuppression (eg, nitrosoureas, mitomycin C).

Allergic-type reactions (rash, urticaria, facial edema, wheezing, dyspnea, tachycardia, and/or hypotension) have occurred with first or subsequent doses. Reactions tended to involve ≥2 body systems and occur more frequently with intravenous administration and generally within 30 minutes of administration; may recur with rechallenge. Rare cases of acute respiratory distress syndrome (ARDS) have been reported (possibly due to influx of neutrophils to sites of lung inflammation); withhold or discontinue filgrastim if ARDS occurs; patients must be instructed to report respiratory distress; monitor for fever, infiltrates, or respiratory distress.

Rare cases of splenic rupture have been reported (may be fatal); patients must be instructed to report left upper quadrant pain or shoulder tip pain. Cutaneous vasculitis has been reported, generally occurring in severe chronic neutropenia (SCN) patients on long-term therapy; symptoms generally developed with increasing absolute neutrophil count (ANC) and subsided when the ANC decreased; dose reductions may improve symptoms to allow for continued therapy. Use caution in patients with sickle cell disorders; severe sickle cell crises (sometimes resulting in fatalities) have been reported following filgrastim therapy. Filgrastim use prior to appropriate diagnosis of SCN may impair proper evaluation and treatment for neutropenia not due to SCN. Cytogenetic abnormalities, transformation to myelodysplastic syndrome (MDS) and acute myeloid leukemia (AML) have been observed in patients treated with filgrastim for congenital neutropenia; a longer duration of treatment and poorer ANC response appear to increase the risk. Carefully consider the risk of continuing filgrastim in patients who develop abnormal cytogenetics or MDS. The packaging of some forms may contain latex.

Drug Interactions

Avoid Concomitant Use There are no known interactions where it is recommended to avoid concomitant use.

Decreased Effect There are no known significant interactions involving a decrease in effect.

Increased Effect/Toxicity

Filgrastim may increase the levels/effects of: Bleomycin; Topotecan

Lab Interactions May interfere with bone imaging studies; increased hematopoietic activity of the bone marrow may appear as transient positive bone imaging changes

Adverse Reactions

>10%:

Central nervous system: Fever (12%)
Dermatologic: Petechiae (≤17%), rash (≤12%)
Endocrine & metabolic: LDH increased, uric acid increased
Gastrointestinal: Splenomegaly (severe chronic neutropenia: 30%; rare in other patients)
Hepatic: Alkaline phosphatase increased (21%)
Neuromuscular & skeletal: Bone/skeletal pain (22% to 33%; dose related), commonly in the lower back, posterior iliac crest, and sternum
Respiratory: Epistaxis (9% to 15%)

1% to 10%:

Cardiovascular: Hyper-/hypotension (4%), myocardial infarction/arrhythmias (3%)
Central nervous system: Headache (7%)
Gastrointestinal: Nausea (10%), vomiting (7%), peritonitis (≤2%)
Hematologic: Leukocytosis (2%)
Miscellaneous: Transfusion reaction (≤10%)

Pharmacodynamics/Kinetics

Onset of Action ~24 hours; plateaus in 3-5 days

Duration of Action Neutrophil counts generally return to baseline within 4 days

Absorption SubQ: 100%

Time to Peak Serum: SubQ: 2-8 hours

Half-Life Elimination 1.8-3.5 hours

Metabolism Systemically degraded

Available Dosage Forms

Injection, solution [preservative free]:

Neupogen®: 300 mcg/mL (1 mL, 1.6 mL); 600 mcg/mL (0.5 mL, 0.8 mL)

Dosing

Adult & Geriatric Details concerning dosing in combination regimens and institution protocols should also be consulted. Rounding doses to the nearest vial size may enhance patient convenience and reduce costs without compromising clinical response.

Chemotherapy-induced neutropenia SubQ, I.V.: 5 mcg/kg/day; doses may be increased by 5 mcg/kg (for each chemotherapy cycle) according to the duration and severity of the neutropenia; continue for up to 14 days or until the ANC reaches 10,000/mm^3

Bone marrow transplantation (in patients with cancer; to shorten the duration of neutropenia and neutropenia-related events): SubQ, I.V.: 10 mcg/kg/day (administer ≥24 hours after chemotherapy and ≥24 hours after bone marrow infusion); adjust the dose according to the duration and severity of neutropenia; recommended steps based on neutrophil response:

When ANC >1000/mm^3 for 3 consecutive days: Reduce filgrastim dose to 5 mcg/kg/day
If ANC remains >1000/mm^3 for 3 more consecutive days: Discontinue filgrastim
If ANC decreases to <1000/mm^3: Resume at 5 mcg/kg/day.
If ANC decreases to <1000/mm^3 during the 5 mcg/kg/day dose: Increase filgrastim to 10 mcg/kg/day and follow the above steps.

Peripheral blood progenitor cell (PBPC) collection: SubQ: 10 mcg/kg daily, usually for 6-7 days. Begin at least 4 days before the first leukapheresis and continue until the last leukapheresis; consider dose adjustment for WBC >100,000/mm^3

Severe chronic neutropenia: SubQ:

Congenital: Initial: 6 mcg/kg twice daily; adjust the dose based on ANC and clinical response
Idiopathic/cyclic: Initial: 5 mcg/kg/day; adjust the dose based on ANC and clinical response

Anemia in myelodysplastic syndrome (unlabeled use; in combination with epoetin): SubQ: 30 mcg, 75 mcg, or 150 mcg once daily (Hellstrom-Lindberg, 1998) **or** 1 mcg/kg once daily (Greenberg, 2009) **or** 75 mcg, 150 mcg or 300 mcg/dose 3 times/week (Hellstrom-Lindberg, 2003) **or** 1-2 mcg/kg/dose 1-3 times/week (NCCN MDS guidelines v.2.2011)

Hematopoietic stem cell mobilization in autologous transplantation in patients with non-Hodgkin's lymphoma or multiple myeloma (in combination with plerixafor; unlabeled use): SubQ: 10 mcg/kg once daily; begin 4 days before initiation of plerixafor; continue G-CSF on each day prior to apheresis for up to 8 days (DiPersio, *JCO* 2009; DiPersio, *Blood* 2009)

Hepatitis C treatment-associated neutropenia (unlabeled use): SubQ: 150 mcg once weekly to 300 mcg 3 times/week; titrate to maintain ANC between 750-10,000/mm^3 (Younossi, 2008)

Pediatric Details concerning dosing in combination regimens and institution protocols should also be consulted.

Chemotherapy induced neutropenia, bone marrow transplantation, peripheral blood progenitor cell collection, severe chronic neutropenia: Refer to adult dosing.

Neutropenia (ANC <500/mm^3) due to zidovudine treatment for HIV-infection (unlabeled use): SubQ, I.V.: 5-10 mcg/kg once daily (AIDS*info* guidelines, 2010)

Administration

I.V. May be administered by I.V. bolus, or a short infusion over 15-30 minutes in D_5W, or by continuous I.V. infusion. Do not administer earlier than 24 hours after or in the 24 hours prior to cytotoxic chemotherapy.

Other May be administered as a SubQ injection or continuous SubQ infusion.

Stability

Reconstitution Do not dilute with saline at any time; product may precipitate. Filgrastim may be diluted with D_5W to a concentration of 5-15 mcg/mL for I.V. infusion administration (minimum concentration: 5 mcg/mL). Concentrations 5-15 mcg/mL require addition of albumin (final albumin concentration of 2 mg/mL) to prevent adsorption to plastics. Dilution to <5 mcg/mL is not recommended. Do not shake.

Storage Intact vials and prefilled syringes should be stored under refrigeration at 2°C to 8°C (36°F to 46°F) and protected from direct sunlight. Filgrastim should be protected from freezing and temperatures >30°C to avoid aggregation.

Filgrastim vials and prefilled syringes are stable for 24 hours at 9°C to 30°C (47°F to 86°F).

Undiluted filgrastim is stable for 24 hours at 15°C to 30°C (59°F to 86°F) and for up to 14 days at 2°C to 8°C (36°F to 46°F) (data on file, Amgen Medical Information) in BD tuberculin syringes; however, sterility has only been assessed and maintained for up to 7 days when prepared under strict aseptic conditions (Jacobson, 1996; Singh, 1994). The manufacturer recommends using syringes within 24 hours due to the potential for bacterial contamination.

Filgrastim diluted with D_5W for I.V. infusion (5-15 mcg/mL) is stable for 7 days at 2°C to 8°C (36°F to 46°F), however, should be used within 24 hours due to the possibility for bacterial contamination.

Monitoring and Teaching Issues

Laboratory Monitoring CBC with differential and platelets prior to treatment and twice weekly during filgrastim treatment for chemotherapy-induced neutropenia (3 times/week following marrow transplantation). For severe chronic neutropenia, monitor CBC with differential and platelets twice weekly during the first month of therapy and for 2 weeks following dose adjustments; once clinically stable, monthly for 1 year and quarterly thereafter; for congenital neutropenia also monitor bone marrow and karyotype prior to treatment; and monitor marrow and cytogenetics annually throughout treatment.

Physical Assessment Assess for hypersensitivity to *E. coli* products prior to beginning therapy. Allergic-type reactions have occurred in patients receiving G-CSF with first or later doses. If self-administered, teach patient proper storage, administration, and syringe/needle disposal. Instruct patient to report upper quadrant pain, shoulder tip pain, or respiratory distress.

Patient Education If self-administered, follow directions for proper storage and administration of SubQ medication. Never reuse syringes or needles. May cause bone pain, nausea, vomiting, hair loss (reversible), or sore mouth. Report immediately any respiratory difficulty or pain in left shoulder, chest, or back. Report unusual fever or chills; unhealed sores; severe bone pain; pain, redness, or swelling at injection site; unusual swelling of extremities; or chest pain and palpitations.

Dietary Considerations Some products may contain sodium.

Geriatric Considerations No specific data available for the elderly.

Pregnancy Considerations Animal studies have demonstrated adverse effects and fetal loss. Filgrastim has been shown to cross the placenta in humans. There are no adequate and well-controlled studies in pregnant women. Use only if potential benefit to mother justifies risk to the fetus. Women who become pregnant during filgrastim treatment are encouraged to enroll in Amgen's Pregnancy Surveillance Program (1-800-772-6436).

Finasteride (fi NAS teer ide)

U.S. Brand Names Propecia®; Proscar®

Generic Availability (U.S.) Yes

Pharmacologic Category 5 Alpha-Reductase Inhibitor

Medication Safety Issues

Sound-alike/look-alike issues:

Finasteride may be confused with furosemide

Proscar® may be confused with ProSom®, Provera®, PROzac®, Psorcon®

Pregnancy Risk Factor X

Lactation Excretion in breast milk unknown/contraindicated in women of childbearing potential

Use

Propecia®: Treatment of male pattern hair loss in **men only**. Safety and efficacy were demonstrated in men between 18-41 years of age.

Proscar®: Treatment of symptomatic benign prostatic hyperplasia (BPH); can be used in combination with an alpha-blocker, doxazosin

Unlabeled/Investigational Use Prostate cancer prevention (to reduce the incidence); treatment of female hirsutism

Mechanism of Action/Effect Finasteride inhibits conversion of testosterone to dihydrotestosterone and markedly suppresses serum dihydrotestosterone levels

Contraindications Hypersensitivity to finasteride or any component of the formulation; pregnancy; not for use in children

Warnings/Precautions Hazardous agent - use appropriate precautions for handling and disposal. Other urological diseases (including prostate cancer) should be ruled out before initiating. For BPH, a minimum of 6 months of treatment may be necessary to determine whether an individual will respond to finasteride; for male pattern hair loss, daily use for 3 months or longer may be required before benefit is observed. Reduces prostate specific antigen (PSA) by 50%; in patients treated for ≥6 months the PSA should be doubled when comparing to normal ranges in untreated patients. Failure to demonstrate a meaningful PSA response (<50% decrease) or a PSA increase is associated with an increased risk for prostate cancer (NCCN prostate ancer early detection guidelines, v.2.2010). Patients with any increase in PSA levels should be evaluated; may indicate presence of prostate cancer. Use with caution in patients with hepatic dysfunction; finasteride is extensively metabolized in the liver. When compared to placebo, 5-alpha-reductase inhibitors have been shown to reduce the incidence of prostate cancer, although an increase in the incidence of high-grade prostate cancers has been observed (Kramer, 2009; Thompson, 2003). Carefully monitor patients with a large residual urinary volume or severely diminished urinary flow for obstructive uropathy; these patients may not be candidates for finasteride therapy. Patients should promptly report any breast changes, including lumps, pain, or nipple discharge. Active ingredient can be absorbed through the skin; women should always use caution whenever handling. Pregnant women or women trying to conceive should not handle the product; finasteride may negatively impact fetal development.

Drug Interactions

Metabolism/Transport Effects Substrate of CYP3A4 (minor)

Avoid Concomitant Use There are no known interactions where it is recommended to avoid concomitant use.

Decreased Effect There are no known significant interactions involving a decrease in effect.

Increased Effect/Toxicity

The levels/effects of Finasteride may be increased by: Conivaptan

Nutritional/Ethanol Interactions Herb/Nutraceutical: St John's wort may decrease finasteride levels. Avoid saw palmetto (concurrent use has not been adequately studied).

Adverse Reactions Note: "Combination therapy" refers to finasteride and doxazosin.

>10%:

Endocrine & metabolic: Impotence (19%; combination therapy 23%), libido decreased (10%; combination therapy 12%)

Neuromuscular & skeletal: Weakness (5%; combination therapy 17%)

1% to 10%:

Cardiovascular: Postural hypotension (9%; combination therapy 18%), edema (1%, combination therapy 3%)

Central nervous system: Dizziness (7%; combination therapy 23%), somnolence (2%; combination therapy 3%)

Genitourinary: Ejaculation disturbances (7%; combination therapy 14%), decreased volume of ejaculate

Endocrine & metabolic: Gynecomastia (2%)

Respiratory: Dyspnea (1%; combination therapy 2%), rhinitis (1%; combination therapy 2%)

Pharmacodynamics/Kinetics

Onset of Action BPH: 6 months; Male pattern hair loss: ≥3 months of daily use.

Duration of Action

After a single oral dose as small as 0.5 mg: 65% depression of plasma dihydrotestosterone levels persists 5-7 days

After 6 months of treatment with 5 mg/day: Circulating dihydrotestosterone levels are reduced to castrate levels without significant effects on circulating testosterone; levels return to normal within 14 days of discontinuation of treatment

Bioavailability Mean: 63%

Time to Peak Serum: 2-6 hours

Protein Binding ~90%

Half-Life Elimination 6 hours (range: 3-16 hours); Elderly: 8 hours (range: 6-15 hours)

Metabolism Hepatic via CYP3A4; two active metabolites (<20% activity of finasteride)

Excretion Feces (57%) and urine (39%) as metabolites

Available Dosage Forms

Tablet, oral: 5 mg

Propecia®: 1 mg

Proscar®: 5 mg

Dosing

Adult & Geriatric

Benign prostatic hyperplasia (Proscar®): Oral: 5 mg once daily as a single dose; clinical responses occur within 12 weeks to 6 months of initiation of therapy; long-term administration is recommended for maximal response

Male pattern baldness (Propecia®): Oral: 1 mg daily

Prostate cancer prevention (unlabeled use): 5 mg once daily; planned duration of treatment was 7 years (Kramer, 2009; Thompson, 2003)

Female hirsutism (unlabeled use): Oral: 5 mg/day (Moghetti, 2000)

Renal Impairment No adjustment is necessary.

Hepatic Impairment Use with caution in patients with liver function abnormalities because finasteride is metabolized extensively in the liver

Administration

Oral May be administered without regard to meals. Women of childbearing age should not touch or handle broken tablets.

Stability

Storage

Propecia®: Store at 15°C to 30°C (59°F to 86°F). Protect from moisture.

Proscar®: Store below 30°C (86°F). Protect from light.

Monitoring and Teaching Issues

Laboratory Monitoring Finasteride does not interfere with free PSA levels.

Physical Assessment Assess urinary pattern prior to therapy and periodically during therapy. A minimum of 6 months of treatment may be necessary to evaluate response.

Patient Education Take with or without meals. May cause decreased libido or impotence during therapy. Report any changes in urinary pattern (significant increase or decrease in volume or voiding patterns). Report changes in breast condition (pain, lumps, or nipple discharge) in male and female patients.

Dietary Considerations May be taken without regard to meals.

Geriatric Considerations Clearance of finasteride is decreased in the elderly, but no dosage reductions are necessary.

Breast-Feeding Considerations Not indicated for use in women.

Pregnancy Considerations Abnormalities of external male genitalia were reported in animal studies. Pregnant women are advised to avoid contact with crushed or broken tablets.

Fingolimod (fin GOL i mod)

U.S. Brand Names Gilenya™

Index Terms FTY720

Pharmacologic Category Sphingosine 1-Phosphate (S1P) Receptor Modulator

Medication Guide Available Yes

Pregnancy Risk Factor C

Lactation Excretion in breast milk unknown/not recommended

Use Treatment of relapsing forms of multiple sclerosis (MS) to reduce the frequency of clinical exacerbations and delay disability progression

Mechanism of Action/Effect Fingolimod-phosphate, active metabolite of fingolimod, binds to sphingosine 1-phosphate receptors 1, 3, 4, and 5. The amount of lymphocytes available to the central nervous system are decreased which reduces central inflammation.

Contraindications There are no contraindications listed in the manufacturers labeling.

Canadian labeling: Hypersensitivity to fingolimod or any component of the formulation; patients at increased risk for opportunistic infections (eg, immunosuppressed patients); severe active infections, active chronic bacterial, fungal or viral infections; known active malignancy (excluding basal cell carcinoma); severe hepatic impairment (Child-Pugh class C)

Warnings/Precautions Increased blood pressure may occur ~2 months after initiation of therapy; monitor blood pressure throughout treatment. Therapy may result in transient AV conduction delays; recurrence may be observed following discontinuation (>2 weeks) and subsequent resumption of therapy. Decreased heart rate may occur with initiation of therapy. Following the first dose, heart rate may decrease as soon as 1 hour postdose with the maximal decrease occurring ~6 hours postdose. Heart rate typically returns to baseline after 1 month of therapy. All patients should be monitored for 6 hours after the first dose (or in patients where therapy has been interrupted for >2 weeks) for signs and symptoms of bradycardia; in patients who develop bradycardia, initiate appropriate treatment and continue to monitor until symptoms have resolved. Due to the risk of bradycardia and AV conduction delays, ECG is recommended prior to initiation of therapy.

May increase risk of infection due to dose-dependent reduction of lymphocytes; lymphocyte counts may be decreased for up to 2 months following discontinuation of therapy. Do not initiate treatment in patients with acute or chronic infections until the infection has resolved. Use with caution in patients receiving concomitant immunosuppressant, immune modulating, or antineoplastic medications.

Use with caution and closely monitor patients with severe hepatic impairment (contraindicated in the Canadian labeling). Macular edema may occur; use with caution in patients with a history of diabetes mellitus or uveitis. Ophthalmologic exams should be performed prior to therapy and 3-4 months after treatment initiation; more frequent examination is warranted in patients with diabetes or a history of uveitis. Reductions of FEV_1 and diffusion lung capacity for carbon monoxide (DLCO) are dose-dependent and may occur within the first month of therapy. FEV_1 changes may be reversible with drug discontinuation.

Consider varicella zoster virus (VZV) vaccination prior to initiation of treatment in VZV antibody negative patients; postpone fingolimod treatment for 1 month after varicella zoster vaccination.

Drug Interactions

Metabolism/Transport Effects

Substrate of CYP2D6 (minor), 2E1 (minor), 3A4 (minor), 4F2 (major), 4F12 (minor)

Avoid Concomitant Use

Avoid concomitant use of Fingolimod with any of the following: BCG; Natalizumab; Pimecrolimus; Roflumilast; Tacrolimus (Topical); Vaccines (Live)

Decreased Effect

Fingolimod may decrease the levels/effects of: BCG; Sipuleucel-T; Vaccines (Inactivated); Vaccines (Live)

The levels/effects of Fingolimod may be decreased by: Echinacea; Peginterferon Alfa-2b

Increased Effect/Toxicity

Fingolimod may increase the levels/effects of: Antiarrhythmic Agents (Class Ia); Antiarrhythmic Agents (Class III); Leflunomide; Natalizumab; Vaccines (Live)

The levels/effects of Fingolimod may be increased by: Beta-Blockers; Conivaptan; Denosumab; Diltiazem; Ketoconazole; Pimecrolimus; Roflumilast; Tacrolimus (Topical); Trastuzumab; Verapamil

Adverse Reactions

>10%:
- Central nervous system: Headache (25%)
- Gastrointestinal: Diarrhea (12%)
- Hepatic: ALT increased (14%), AST increased (14%)
- Neuromuscular & skeletal: Back pain (12%)
- Miscellaneous: Flu-like syndrome (13%)

1% to 10%:
- Cardiovascular: Hypertension (6%), bradycardia (4%)
- Central nervous system: Depression (8%), dizziness (7%), migraine (5%)
- Dermatologic: Alopecia (4%), eczema (3%), pruritus (3%)
- Endocrine & metabolic: Triglycerides increased (3%)
- Gastrointestinal: Gastroenteritis (5%), weight loss (5%)
- Hematologic: Lymphopenia (4%), leukopenia (3%)
- Hepatic: GGT increased (5%)
- Neuromuscular & skeletal: Paresthesia (5%), weakness (3%)
- Ocular: Blurred vision (4%), eye pain (3%)
- Respiratory: Cough (10%), bronchitis (8%), dyspnea (8%), sinusitis (7%)
- Miscellaneous: Herpes infection (9%), tinea infection (4%)

Pharmacodynamics/Kinetics

Bioavailability 93%

Time to Peak Plasma: 12-16 hours

Protein Binding >99.7% (fingolimod and fingolimod-phosphate)

Half-Life Elimination 6-9 days

Metabolism Hepatic via CYP4F2 to fingolimod-phosphate (active) and other metabolites (inactive); CYP2D6, 2E1, 3A4, and 4F12 also contribute to metabolism

Excretion Urine (~81% as inactive metabolites); feces (fingolimod and fingolimod phosphate: <2.5% of dose)

Available Dosage Forms

Capsule, oral:

Gilenya™: 0.5 mg

Dosing

Adult Multiple sclerosis: Oral: 0.5 mg once daily; doses >0.5 mg/day associated with increased adverse events and no additional benefit

Geriatric Refer to adult dosing.

Hepatic Impairment

Mild-to-moderate hepatic impairment: No dosage adjustment required.

Severe hepatic impairment: Use with caution and closely monitor; exposure is doubled in severe hepatic impairment. Specific dosing recommendations are not provided within the U.S. manufacturer labeling. Use is contraindicated in the Canadian labeling.

Administration

Oral May be administered with or without food.

Stability

Storage Store at 25°C (77°F); excursions permitted to 15°C to 30°C (59°F to 86°F).

Monitoring and Teaching Issues

Laboratory Monitoring CBC (baseline and periodically thereafter); liver enzymes and bilirubin at least 6 months prior to treatment; VZV antibodies (patients with no history of chicken pox or previous VZV vaccination)

Dietary Considerations May be taken with or without food.

Breast-Feeding Considerations Due to the potential for serious adverse reactions in the nursing infant, breast-feeding is not recommended.

Pregnancy Considerations Teratogenic and adverse effects have been observed in animal reproduction studies. Elimination of fingolimod takes approximately 2 months; to avoid potential fetal harm, women of childbearing potential should avoid pregnancy during and for 2 months after discontinuing treatment. Healthcare providers are encouraged to enroll pregnant women, or pregnant women may enroll themselves, in the Gileny™ Pregnancy Registry (1-877-598-7237).

◆ **Fioricet®** *see* Butalbital, Acetaminophen, and Caffeine *on page 260*

- **Fioricet® with Codeine** *see* Butalbital, Acetaminophen, Caffeine, and Codeine *on page 261*
- **Fiorinal®** *see* Butalbital, Aspirin, and Caffeine *on page 262*
- **Fiorinal® with Codeine** *see* Butalbital, Aspirin, Caffeine, and Codeine *on page 262*
- **Firmagon®** *see* Degarelix *on page 480*
- **First™-Progesterone VGS 25** *see* Progesterone *on page 1514*
- **First™-Progesterone VGS 50** *see* Progesterone *on page 1514*
- **First™-Progesterone VGS 100** *see* Progesterone *on page 1514*
- **First™-Progesterone VGS 200** *see* Progesterone *on page 1514*
- **First™-Progesterone VGS 400** *see* Progesterone *on page 1514*
- **First®-Testosterone** *see* Testosterone *on page 1739*
- **First®-Testosterone MC** *see* Testosterone *on page 1739*
- **Fisalamine** *see* Mesalamine *on page 1177*
- **Fish Oil** *see* Omega-3-Acid Ethyl Esters *on page 1355*
- **FK506** *see* Tacrolimus (Systemic) *on page 1695*
- **Flagyl®** *see* MetroNIDAZOLE (Systemic) *on page 1220*
- **Flagyl® 375** *see* MetroNIDAZOLE (Systemic) *on page 1220*
- **Flagyl® ER** *see* MetroNIDAZOLE (Systemic) *on page 1220*
- **Flarex®** *see* Fluorometholone *on page 786*
- **Flebogamma® [DSC]** *see* Immune Globulin *on page 961*
- **Flebogamma® DIF** *see* Immune Globulin *on page 961*

Flecainide (fle KAY nide)

U.S. Brand Names Tambocor™

Index Terms Flecainide Acetate

Generic Availability (U.S.) Yes

Pharmacologic Category Antiarrhythmic Agent, Class Ic

Medication Safety Issues

Sound-alike/look-alike issues:

Flecainide may be confused with fluconazole

Tambocor™ may be confused with Pamelor®, Temodar®, tamoxifen, Tamiflu®

Pregnancy Risk Factor C

Lactation Enters breast milk/compatible

Use Prevention and suppression of documented life-threatening ventricular arrhythmias (eg, sustained ventricular tachycardia); controlling symptomatic, disabling supraventricular tachycardias in patients without structural heart disease in whom other agents fail

Mechanism of Action/Effect Class Ic antiarrhythmic; slows conduction in cardiac tissue by altering transport of ions across cell membranes; causes slight prolongation of refractory periods; decreases the rate of rise of the action potential without affecting its duration; increases electrical stimulation threshold of ventricle, His-Purkinje system; possesses local anesthetic and moderate negative inotropic effects

Contraindications Hypersensitivity to flecainide or any component of the formulation; pre-existing second- or third-degree AV block or with right bundle branch block when associated with a left hemiblock (bifascicular block) (except in patients with a functioning artificial pacemaker); cardiogenic shock; coronary artery disease (based on CAST study results); concurrent use of ritonavir or amprenavir

Warnings/Precautions [U.S. Boxed Warning]: In the Cardiac Arrhythmia Suppression Trial (CAST), recent (>6 days but <2 years ago) myocardial infarction patients with asymptomatic, non-life-threatening ventricular arrhythmias did not benefit and may have been harmed by attempts to suppress the arrhythmia with flecainide or encainide. An increased mortality or nonfatal cardiac arrest rate (7.7%) was seen in the active treatment group compared with patients in the placebo group (3%). The applicability of the CAST results to other populations is unknown. The risks of class 1C agents and the lack of improved survival make use in patients without life-threatening arrhythmias generally unacceptable. **[U.S. Boxed Warning]: Watch for proarrhythmic effects;** monitor and adjust dose to prevent QT_c prolongation. Not recommended for patients with chronic atrial fibrillation. **[U.S. Boxed Warning]: When treating atrial flutter, 1:1 atrioventricular conduction may occur; pre-emptive negative chronotropic therapy (eg, digoxin, beta-blockers) may lower the risk.** Pre-existing hypokalemia or hyperkalemia should be corrected before initiation (can alter drug's effect). A worsening or new arrhythmia may occur (proarrhythmic effect). Use caution in heart failure (may precipitate or exacerbate HF). Dose-related increases in PR, QRS, and QT intervals occur. Use with caution in sick sinus syndrome or with permanent pacemakers or temporary pacing wires (can increase endocardial pacing thresholds). Cautious use in significant hepatic impairment.

Drug Interactions

Metabolism/Transport Effects Substrate of CYP1A2 (minor), 2D6 (major); **Inhibits** CYP2D6 (weak)

Avoid Concomitant Use

Avoid concomitant use of Flecainide with any of the following: Artemether; Dronedarone; Lumefantrine; Nilotinib; Pimozide; QuiNINE; Ritonavir; Saquinavir; Tetrabenazine; Thioridazine; Tipranavir; Toremifene; Vandetanib; Ziprasidone

Decreased Effect

The levels/effects of Flecainide may be decreased by: Etravirine; Peginterferon Alfa-2b; Sodium Bicarbonate

Increased Effect/Toxicity

Flecainide may increase the levels/effects of: Dronedarone; Pimozide; QTc-Prolonging Agents; QuiNINE; Tetrabenazine; Thioridazine; Toremifene; Vandetanib; Ziprasidone

The levels/effects of Flecainide may be increased by: Alfuzosin; Amiodarone; Artemether; Carbonic Anhydrase Inhibitors; Chloroquine; Ciprofloxacin; Ciprofloxacin (Systemic); CYP2D6 Inhibitors (Moderate); CYP2D6 Inhibitors (Strong); Darunavir; Gadobutrol; Lumefantrine; Nilotinib; QuiNINE; Ritonavir; Saquinavir; Sodium Bicarbonate; Sodium Lactate; Tipranavir; Tromethamine; Verapamil

Nutritional/Ethanol Interactions Food: Clearance may be decreased in patients following strict vegetarian diets due to urinary pH ≥8. Dairy products (milk, infant formula, yogurt) may interfere with the absorption of flecainide in infants; there is one case report of a neonate (GA 34 weeks PNA >6 days) who required extremely large doses of oral flecainide when administered every 8 hours with feedings ("milk feeds"); changing the feedings from "milk feeds" to 5% glucose feeds alone resulted in a doubling of the flecainide serum concentration and toxicity.

Adverse Reactions

>10%:

Central nervous system: Dizziness (19% to 30%)
Ocular: Visual disturbances (16%)
Respiratory: Dyspnea (~10%)

1% to 10%:

Cardiovascular: Palpitation (6%), chest pain (5%), edema (3.5%), tachycardia (1% to 3%), proarrhythmic (4% to 12%), sinus node dysfunction (1.2%)
Central nervous system: Headache (4% to 10%), fatigue (8%), nervousness (5%) additional symptoms occurring at a frequency between 1% and 3%: fever, malaise, hypoesthesia, paresis, ataxia, vertigo, syncope, somnolence, tinnitus, anxiety, insomnia, depression
Dermatologic: Rash (1% to 3%)
Gastrointestinal: Nausea (9%), constipation (1%), abdominal pain (3%), anorexia (1% to 3%), diarrhea (0.7% to 3%)
Neuromuscular & skeletal: Tremor (5%), weakness (5%), paresthesia (1%)
Ocular: Diplopia (1% to 3%), blurred vision

Pharmacodynamics/Kinetics

Absorption Oral: Rapid

Bioavailability 85% to 90%

Time to Peak Serum: ~1.5-3 hours

Protein Binding $Alpha_1$ acid glycoprotein: 40% to 50%

Half-Life Elimination Infants: 11-12 hours; Children: 8 hours; Adults: 7-22 hours, increased with congestive heart failure or renal dysfunction; End-stage renal disease: 19-26 hours

Metabolism Hepatic

Excretion Urine (80% to 90%, 10% to 50% as unchanged drug and metabolites)

Available Dosage Forms

Tablet, oral: 50 mg, 100 mg, 150 mg
Tambocor™: 50 mg, 100 mg, 150 mg

Dosing

Adult & Geriatric

Life-threatening ventricular arrhythmias: Oral:

Initial: 100 mg every 12 hours; increase by 50-100 mg/day (given in 2 doses/day) every 4 days; maximum: 400 mg/day

For patients receiving 400 mg/day who are not controlled and have trough concentrations <0.6 mcg/mL, dosage may be increased to 600 mg/day.

Prevention of paroxysmal supraventricular arrhythmias: Oral: (**Note:** In patients with disabling symptoms but no structural heart disease): Initial: 50 mg every 12 hours; increase by 50 mg twice daily at 4-day intervals; maximum: 300 mg/day

Paroxysmal atrial fibrillation: Outpatient: "Pill-in-the-pocket" dose (unlabeled dose): Oral: 200 mg (weight <70 kg), 300 mg (weight ≥70 kg). May not repeat in ≤24 hours. **Note:** An initial inpatient conversion trial should have been successful before sending patient home on this approach. Patient must be taking an AV nodal-blocking agent (eg, beta-blocker, nondihydropyridine calcium channel blocker) prior to initiation of antiarrhythmic.

Pediatric

Life-threatening ventricular arrhythmias: Oral: Children:

Initial: 3 mg/kg/day or 50-100 mg/m²/day in 3 divided doses

Usual maintenance: 3-6 mg/kg/day or 100-150 mg/m²/day in 3 divided doses; up to 11 mg/kg/day or 200 mg/m²/day for uncontrolled patients with subtherapeutic levels

Renal Impairment GFR ≤50 mL/minute: Decrease dose by 50%; dose increases should be made cautiously at intervals >4 days and serum levels monitored frequently.

Hemodialysis: No supplemental dose recommended.

Peritoneal dialysis: No supplemental dose recommended.

Hepatic Impairment Monitoring of plasma levels is recommended because half-life is significantly increased. When transferring from another antiarrhythmic agent, allow for 2-4 half-lives of the agent to pass before initiating flecainide therapy.

Administration

Oral Administer around-the-clock to promote less variation in peak and trough serum levels.

Monitoring and Teaching Issues

Laboratory Monitoring Periodic serum concentrations, especially in patients with renal or hepatic impairment

Physical Assessment Monitor cardiac status. Flecainide has a low toxic:therapeutic ratio and overdose may easily produce severe and life-threatening reactions.

Patient Education Take around-the-clock. You will require frequent monitoring while taking this medication. You may experience dizziness, visual disturbances, or nausea. Report palpitations, chest pain, or excessively slow or rapid heartbeat; acute nervousness, headache, or fatigue; unusual weight gain; unusual cough; respiratory difficulty; swelling of hands or ankles; or muscle tremor, numbness, or weakness.

Geriatric Considerations Decreased clearance and, therefore, prolonged half-life is possible; however, studies have shown no difference in response to usual doses in the elderly despite slight decrease in clearance; calculate or measure GFR since elderly patients may have GFR ≤50 mL/minute.

Related Information

Antiarrhythmic Drugs *on page 1978*

- ◆ **Flecainide Acetate** *see* Flecainide *on page 766*
- ◆ **Flector®** *see* Diclofenac (Topical) *on page 522*
- ◆ **Flexbumin 25%** *see* Albumin *on page 57*
- ◆ **Flexeril®** *see* Cyclobenzaprine *on page 432*
- ◆ **Floctafenina** *see* Floctafenine *on page 768*

Floctafenine (flok ta FEN een)

Index Terms Floctafenina; Floctafeninum

Generic Availability (U.S.) Yes

Pharmacologic Category Nonsteroidal Anti-inflammatory Drug (NSAID), Oral

Lactation Enters breast milk/not recommended

Use Short-term management of acute, mild-to-moderate pain

Mechanism of Action/Effect Reversibly inhibits cyclooxygenase-1 and 2 (COX-1 and 2) enzymes, which results in decreased formation of prostaglandin precursors; has antipyretic, analgesic, and anti-inflammatory properties

Contraindications Hypersensitivity to floctafenine, aspirin, other NSAIDS, or any component of the formulation; active peptic ulcer or a history of ulcerative disease; inflammatory gastrointestinal disease; severe cardiac insufficiency or ischemic cardiomyopathy; significant hepatic impairment or active liver disease; severely impaired (Cl_{cr} <30 mL/minute) or deteriorating renal function; concurrent use with other NSAIDS; severe heart failure, coronary heart disease; concurrent use with beta-blockers; nasal polyp syndrome (complete or partial); patients who experience "aspirin triad" (bronchial asthma, rhinitis complicated by polyps, aspirin intolerance) with aspirin or NSAID therapy

Warnings/Precautions NSAIDs are associated with an increased risk of adverse cardiovascular events, including MI, stroke, and new onset or worsening of pre-existing hypertension. Risk may be increased with duration of use or pre-existing cardiovascular risk factors or disease. Carefully evaluate individual cardiovascular risk profiles prior to prescribing. Use caution with fluid retention. Avoid use in heart failure. Use is contraindicated with severe cardiac insufficiency. Use of NSAIDs is not recommended for treatment of perioperative pain in the setting of coronary artery bypass graft (CABG) surgery. Risk of MI and stroke may be increased with use following CABG surgery.

NSAIDS may increase risk of gastrointestinal irritation, inflammation, ulceration, perforation, and bleeding. These events can sometimes be severe and occasionally fatal, and can occur at any time during therapy and without warning. If ulceration is suspected or confirmed, or if bleeding occurs, discontinue use. Elderly and debilitated patients are more susceptible to adverse GI effects of NSAIDS. Lower dosing and close monitoring of these patients may be required. Use caution with excessive alcohol intake, smoking, concurrent therapy with aspirin, anticoagulants, and/or corticosteroids. Use is contraindicated in patients with active peptic ulcer, history of ulcer disease, or inflammatory GI disease. When used concomitantly with ≤325 mg of aspirin, a substantial increase in the risk of gastrointestinal complications (eg, ulcer) occurs; concomitant gastroprotective therapy (eg, proton pump inhibitors) is recommended (Bhatt, 2008).

Use of lowest effective dose and for shortest duration of time, consistent with individual patient goals, to reduce risk of cardiovascular or GI adverse events. Alternate therapies should be considered for patients at high risk.

Platelet adhesion and aggregation may be decreased; may prolong bleeding time; patients with coagulation disorders or who are receiving anticoagulants should be monitored closely. Anemia may occur; patients on long-term NSAID therapy should be monitored for anemia. Rarely, NSAID use may cause severe blood dyscrasias (eg, agranulocytosis, aplastic anemia, thrombocytopenia).

NSAID use may compromise existing renal function; dose-dependent decreases in prostaglandin synthesis may result from NSAID use, reducing renal blood flow which may cause renal decompensation. NSAID use may increase the risk for hyperkalemia. Patients with impaired renal function, dehydration, heart failure, liver dysfunction, those taking diuretics, and ACE inhibitors, and the elderly are at greater risk of renal toxicity and hyperkalemia. Rehydrate patient before starting therapy; monitor renal function closely. Contraindicated in patients with deteriorating function or severe impairment (Cl_{cr} <30 mL/minute). Long-term NSAID use may result in renal papillary necrosis.

Use caution in hepatic disease; contraindicated in patients with severe or active impairment. Although rare, severe reactions including jaundice and reports of fatal hepatitis have been associated with NSAID use. Closely monitor patients with any abnormal LFT. Discontinue use if signs or symptoms of liver disease develop, or if systemic manifestations occur.

NSAIDS may cause drowsiness, dizziness, blurred vision and other neurologic effects which may impair physical or mental abilities; patients must be cautioned about performing tasks which require mental alertness (eg, operating machinery or driving). Discontinue use with blurred or diminished vision and perform ophthalmologic exam. Monitor vision with long-term therapy.

Symptoms of aseptic meningitis have been observed with NSAID therapy. Patients with autoimmune disorders may be more predisposed. NSAIDS may cause serious skin adverse events including exfoliative dermatitis, Stevens-Johnson syndrome (SJS), and toxic epidermal necrolysis (TEN); discontinue use at first sign of skin rash or hypersensitivity. Anaphylactoid reactions may occur even without prior exposure; patients with "aspirin triad" (bronchial asthma, aspirin intolerance, rhinitis) may be at increased risk. Do not use in patients who experience bronchospasm, asthma, rhinitis, or urticaria with NSAID or aspirin therapy. Use caution in other forms of asthma.

Safety and efficacy in children have not been established.

Withhold for at least 4-6 half-lives prior to surgical or dental procedures.

Drug Interactions

Decreased Effect NSAIDs may decrease the antihypertensive effect of ACE inhibitors, angiotensin II receptor blockers, beta-blockers, hydralazine, loop diuretics and thiazide diuretics. Bile acid sequestrants may decrease the absorption of NSAIDs. NSAIDs may diminish the cardioprotective effect of salicylates. Salicylates may decrease the serum concentration of NSAIDs.

Increased Effect/Toxicity NSAIDs may increase the levels/effects aminoglycosides, cyclosporine, lithium, methotrexate, pemetrexed, and vancomycin. NSAIDs may increase the antiplatelet effect of salicylates. NSAIDs may increase the risk of bleeding with anticoagulants, antiplatelet drugs, treprostinil and warfarin. NSAIDs may enhance the adverse/toxic effects of bisphosphonates (gastrointestinal effects), systemic corticosteroids (gastrointestinal effects), cyclosporine (nephrotoxic effects), and quinolone antibiotics (CNS/seizure effects). Probenecid may increase the levels/effects of NSAIDs. Selective serotonin reuptake inhibitors and tricyclic antidepressants may enhance the antiplatelet effects NSAIDs.

Nutritional/Ethanol Interactions

Ethanol: Avoid ethanol (may enhance gastric mucosal irritation).

Herb/Nutraceutical: Avoid alfalfa, anise, bilberry, bladderwrack, bromelain, cat's claw, celery, chamomile, coleus, cordyceps, dong quai, evening primrose, fenugreek, feverfew, garlic, ginger, ginkgo biloba, ginseng (American, Panax, Siberian), grapeseed, green tea, guggul, horse chestnut seed, horseradish, licorice, prickly ash, red clover, reishi, SAMe (S-adenosylmethionine), sweet clover, turmeric, white willow (all have additional antiplatelet activity).

Adverse Reactions Frequency not defined.

Cardiovascular: Edema, flushing, tachycardia

Central nervous system: Depression, dizziness, drowsiness, fatigue, headache, insomnia, irritability, malaise, nervousness, vertigo

Dermatologic: Angioedema, pruritus, rash, urticaria

Endocrine & metabolic: Fluid retention, hyperkalemia

Gastrointestinal: Abdominal pain, bitter taste, constipation, diarrhea, dyspepsia, flatulence, gastrointestinal bleeding, gastrointestinal ulcer, gross bleeding with perforation, heartburn, nausea, vomiting, xerostomia

Hematologic: Agranulocytosis, aplastic anemia, bleeding, leukopenia, neutropenia, thrombocytopenia

Hepatic: Hepatotoxicity, liver enzymes increased

Ocular: Blurred and/or diminished vision

Otic: Tinnitus

Renal: Burning micturition, cystitis, dysuria, hematuria, interstitial nephritis, polyuria, reversible acute renal insufficiency with or without oliguria/anuria, strong smelling urine, urethritis

Respiratory: Asthmatic-type dyspnea

Miscellaneous: Anaphylaxis, diaphoresis, thirst

Pharmacodynamics/Kinetics

Duration of Action 6-8 hours

Absorption Rapid, well absorbed

Time to Peak 1-2 hours

Half-Life Elimination Initial phase (distribution): 1 hour; second phase (elimination): 8 hours

Metabolism Hepatic

Excretion Feces and bile (60%); urine (40%)

Product Availability Not available in U.S.

Dosing

Adult Pain management: Oral: 200-400 mg every 6-8 hours as needed, up to a maximum of 1200 mg/day

Geriatric Elderly/debilitated: Initiate therapy with lower than usual adult starting dose; adjust dose when necessary under close observation

Pediatric Dosage not established; use not recommended

Renal Impairment Although no specific recommendations are given, initial doses should be lower than usual adult starting doses; individual adjustments to dose should be made when necessary and under close supervision.

Hepatic Impairment Use with caution and under close supervision.

Administration

Oral Administer after food or meal with glass of water.

Stability

Storage Store at 15°C to 30°C (59°F to 86°F). Protect from light.

Monitoring and Teaching Issues

Laboratory Monitoring CBC, liver function tests, renal function (bun and creatinine)

Physical Assessment Assess for allergic reactions to salicylates or other NSAIDs. Monitor blood pressure at the beginning of therapy and periodically throughout. With long-term therapy, periodic ophthalmic exams are recommended.

Patient Education Take with food or milk to avoid GI irritation. Maintain adequate hydration, unless instructed to restrict fluid intake. Do not use alcohol. You may experience drowsiness, dizziness, nausea, vomiting, or gastric discomfort; GI bleeding, ulceration, and perforation can occur with or without pain. Stop taking medication and report occurrence immediately. Report ringing in ears, changes in hearing or vision, unresolved nausea or vomiting, difficulty breathing or shortness of breath, cramping or stomach pain, unusual bruising or bleeding (blood in urine, stool, mouth, or vomitus), unusual swelling of extremities or weight gain, chest pain, rapid heartbeat, or skin rash.

Dietary Considerations Should be taken with food with a glass of water.

Pregnancy Considerations Floctafenic acid (active metabolite) crosses the placenta; therefore, the benefits of use must be weighed against risk to mother and fetus. In late pregnancy, NSAIDs may cause premature closure of the ductus arteriosus.

Additional Information No interactions have been noted with concomitant administration of antacids.

- **Floctafeninum** *see* Floctafenine *on page* *768*
- **Flolan®** *see* Epoprostenol *on page* *643*
- **Flomax®** *see* Tamsulosin *on page* *1706*
- **Flonase®** *see* Fluticasone (Nasal) *on page* *802*
- **Florinef** *see* Fludrocortisone *on page* *780*
- **Flovent** *see* Fluticasone (Oral Inhalation) *on page* *798*
- **Flovent® Diskus®** *see* Fluticasone (Oral Inhalation) *on page* *798*
- **Flovent® HFA** *see* Fluticasone (Oral Inhalation) *on page* *798*
- **Floxin Otic Singles** *see* Ofloxacin (Otic) *on page* *1343*

Floxuridine (floks YOOR i deen)

Index Terms Fluorodeoxyuridine; FUDR

Generic Availability (U.S.) Yes

Pharmacologic Category Antineoplastic Agent, Antimetabolite (Pyrimidine Analog)

Medication Safety Issues

Sound-alike/look-alike issues:

Floxuridine may be confused with Fludara®, fludarabine

FUDR® may be confused with Fludara®

High alert medication: The Institute for Safe Medication Practices (ISMP) includes this medication among its list of drugs which have a heightened risk of causing significant patient harm when used in error.

Pregnancy Risk Factor D

Lactation Excretion in breast milk unknown/contraindicated

Use Management of hepatic metastases of colorectal and gastric cancers

Mechanism of Action/Effect Mechanism of action and pharmacokinetics are very similar to fluorouracil; floxuridine is the deoxyribonucleotide of fluorouracil. Floxuridine is a fluorinated pyrimidine antagonist which inhibits DNA and RNA synthesis and methylation of deoxyuridylic acid to thymidylic acid.

Contraindications Hypersensitivity to floxuridine, fluorouracil, or any component of the formulation; pregnancy

Warnings/Precautions Hazardous agent - use appropriate precautions for handling and disposal. Use caution with impaired kidney or liver function. Discontinue if intractable vomiting, diarrhea, precipitous fall in leukocyte or platelet counts, myocardial ischemia, hemorrhage, gastrointestinal ulcer, or stomatitis occur. Use with caution in patients with poor nutritional status; depressed (leukocyte count $<5000/mm^3$ or platelet count $<100,000/mm^3$) bone marrow function; potentially serious infections. Use with caution in patients who have had high-dose pelvic radiation or previous use of alkylating agents. **[U.S. Boxed Warnings]: Should be administered under the supervision of an experienced cancer chemotherapy physician. Patients should be hospitalized for initiation of the first course of therapy due to the risk for severe toxic reactions.**

Drug Interactions

Avoid Concomitant Use

Avoid concomitant use of Floxuridine with any of the following: BCG; Natalizumab; Pimecrolimus; Roflumilast; Tacrolimus (Topical); Vaccines (Live)

Decreased Effect

Floxuridine may decrease the levels/effects of: BCG; Cardiac Glycosides; Sipuleucel-T; Vaccines (Inactivated); Vaccines (Live); Vitamin K Antagonists

The levels/effects of Floxuridine may be decreased by: Echinacea

Increased Effect/Toxicity

Floxuridine may increase the levels/effects of: Carvedilol; CYP2C9 Substrates (High risk); Leflunomide; Natalizumab; Phenytoin; Vaccines (Live); Vitamin K Antagonists

The levels/effects of Floxuridine may be increased by: Denosumab; Pimecrolimus; Roflumilast; Tacrolimus (Topical); Trastuzumab

Nutritional/Ethanol Interactions Ethanol: Avoid ethanol (due to GI irritation).

Lab Interactions Increased potassium (S)

Adverse Reactions

>10%:

Gastrointestinal: Stomatitis, diarrhea; may be dose limiting

Hematologic: Myelosuppression, may be dose limiting; leukopenia, thrombocytopenia, anemia

Onset: 4-7 days

Nadir: 5-9 days

Recovery: 21 days

1% to 10%:

Dermatologic: Alopecia, photosensitivity, hyperpigmentation of the skin, localized erythema, dermatitis

Gastrointestinal: Anorexia

Hepatic: Biliary sclerosis, cholecystitis, jaundice

Pharmacodynamics/Kinetics

Metabolism Hepatic; Active metabolites: Floxuridine monophosphate (FUDR-MP) and fluorouracil; Inactive metabolites: Urea, CO_2, α-fluoro-β-alanine, α-fluoro-β-guanidopropionic acid, α-fluoro-β-ureidopropionic acid, and dihydrofluorouracil

Excretion Urine: Fluorouracil, urea, α-fluoro-β-alanine, α-fluoro-β-guanidopropionic acid, α-fluoro-β-ureidopropionic acid, and dihydrofluorouracil; exhaled gases (CO_2)

Available Dosage Forms

Injection, powder for reconstitution: 500 mg

Dosing

Adult Refer to individual protocols.

Colorectal or gastric metastases:

Intra-arterial: Primarily by an implantable pump: 0.1-0.6 mg/kg/day continuous intra-arterial administration for 14 days then heparinized saline is given for 14 days; toxicity requires dose reduction.

I.V. (unlabeled use): Many regimens in use, examples:

0.15 mg/kg/day for 7-14 days

0.5-1 mg/kg/day for 6-15 days

30 mg/kg/day for 5 days, then 15 mg/kg/day every other day, up to 11 days

Geriatric Adjust dose since elderly patients are prone to toxicity.

Renal Impairment The FDA-approved labeling does not contain dosing adjustment guidelines; use with extreme caution.

Hepatic Impairment The FDA-approved labeling does not contain dosing adjustment guidelines; use with extreme caution. The following guidelines have been used by some clinicians (Floyd, 2006):

Serum bilirubin 1.2 times ULN or alkaline phosphatase 1.2 times ULN: Administer 80% of dose

Serum bilirubin 1.5 times ULN; transaminases 3 times baseline or alkaline phosphatase 1.5 times ULN: Administer 50% of dose

Serum bilirubin 2 times ULN; transaminases >3 times baseline or alkaline phosphatase 2 times ULN: No recommendation is available

Administration

I.V. Continuous intra-arterial or I.V. infusion (unlabeled use)

Stability

Reconstitution Reconstitute with 5 mL SWFI for a final concentration of 100 mg/mL. Further dilute in 500-1000 mL D_5W or NS for I.V. infusion.

Storage Store intact vials at room temperature of 15°C to 30°C (59°F to 86°F). Reconstituted vials are stable for up to 2 weeks under refrigeration at 2°C to 8°C (36°F to 46°F). Further dilution in 500-1000 mL D_5W or NS is stable for 2 weeks at room temperature. Solutions in 0.9% sodium chloride are stable in some ambulatory infusion pumps for up to 21 days.

Monitoring and Teaching Issues

Laboratory Monitoring CBC, platelet count, liver function

Physical Assessment Use caution with impaired liver or kidney function. Monitor for CNS changes and acute gastrointestinal reactions (intractable vomiting or diarrhea may be dose limiting) on a regular basis. Teach patient or caregiver use and care of implantable pump.

Patient Education This drug can only be administered by infusion. Follow instructions of prescriber for care of implantable pump. Avoid alcohol. It is important to maintain adequate nutrition and hydration, unless instructed to restrict fluid intake. You will be more susceptible to infection. May cause nausea or vomiting, loss of hair (reversible), diarrhea, mouth sores, or sterility. Increased emotional or physical stress will adversely affect the response to this medication. Notify prescriber if you are experiencing unusual or elevated levels of stress. Report extreme fatigue; pain or numbness in extremities; severe GI upset or diarrhea;

bleeding or bruising; fever, chills, or sore throat; vaginal discharge; or signs of fluid retention (eg, swelling of extremities, respiratory difficulty, unusual weight gain).

◆ **Fluarix®** *see* Influenza Virus Vaccine (Inactivated) *on page 978*

◆ **Flubenisolone** *see* Betamethasone *on page 205*

Fluconazole (floo KOE na zole)

U.S. Brand Names Diflucan®

Generic Availability (U.S.) Yes

Pharmacologic Category Antifungal Agent, Oral; Antifungal Agent, Parenteral

Medication Safety Issues

Sound-alike/look-alike issues:

Fluconazole may be confused with flecainide, FLUoxetine, furosemide, itraconazole

Diflucan® may be confused with diclofenac, Diprivan®, disulfiram

International issues:

Canesten [Great Britain] may be confused with Canesten brand name for clotrimazole [multiple international markets]; Cenestin brand name estrogens (conjugated A/synthetic) [U.S., Canada]

Pregnancy Risk Factor C

Lactation Enters breast milk/not recommended (AAP rates "compatible"; AAP 2001 update pending)

Use Treatment of candidiasis (vaginal, oropharyngeal, esophageal, urinary tract infections, peritonitis, pneumonia, and systemic infections); cryptococcal meningitis; antifungal prophylaxis in allogeneic bone marrow transplant recipients

Unlabeled/Investigational Use Cryptococcal pneumonia; candidal intertrigo

Mechanism of Action/Effect Interferes with cytochrome P450 activity, decreasing ergosterol synthesis (principal sterol in fungal cell membrane) and inhibiting cell membrane formation

Contraindications Hypersensitivity to fluconazole or any component of the formulation (cross-reaction with other azole antifungal agents may occur, but has not been established; use caution); concomitant administration with cisapride or terfenadine

Warnings/Precautions Should be used with caution in patients with renal and hepatic dysfunction or previous hepatotoxicity from other azole derivatives. Patients who develop abnormal liver function tests during fluconazole therapy should be monitored closely and discontinued if symptoms consistent with liver disease develop. Rare exfoliative skin disorders have been observed; monitor closely if rash develops and discontinue if lesions progress. The manufacturer reports rare cases of QT_c prolongation and torsade de pointes associated with fluconazole use and advises caution in patients with concomitant medications or conditions which are arrhythmogenic. However, given the limited number of cases and the presence of multiple confounding variables, the likelihood that fluconazole causes conduction abnormalities appears remote.

Drug Interactions

Metabolism/Transport Effects Inhibits CYP1A2 (weak), 2C9 (strong), 2C19 (strong), 3A4 (moderate)

Avoid Concomitant Use

Avoid concomitant use of Fluconazole with any of the following: Artemether; Cisapride; Clopidogrel; Conivaptan; Dofetilide; Dronedarone; Lumefantrine; Nilotinib; Pimozide; QuiNIDine; QuiNINE; Ranolazine; Tetrabenazine; Thioridazine; Tolvaptan; Toremifene; Vandetanib; Ziprasidone

Decreased Effect

Fluconazole may decrease the levels/effects of: Amphotericin B; Clopidogrel; Saccharomyces boulardii

The levels/effects of Fluconazole may be decreased by: Didanosine; Etravirine; Phenytoin; Rifamycin Derivatives; Sucralfate

Increased Effect/Toxicity

Fluconazole may increase the levels/effects of: Alfentanil; Aprepitant; Benzodiazepines (metabolized by oxidation); Bosentan; BusPIRone; Busulfan; Calcium Channel Blockers; CarBAMazepine; Carvedilol; Cilostazol; Cinacalcet; Cisapride; Citalopram; Colchicine; Conivaptan; Corticosteroids (Systemic); CycloSPORINE; CycloSPORINE (Systemic); CYP2C19 Substrates; CYP2C9 Substrates (High risk); CYP3A4 Substrates; DOCEtaxel; Dofetilide; Dronedarone; Eletriptan; Eplerenone; Erlotinib; Eszopiclone; Etravirine; Everolimus; FentaNYL; Fosaprepitant; Gefitinib; HMG-CoA Reductase Inhibitors; Imatinib; Irbesartan; Irinotecan; Losartan; Lurasidone; Macrolide Antibiotics; Methadone; Phenytoin; Phosphodiesterase 5 Inhibitors; Pimecrolimus; Pimozide; Protease Inhibitors; Proton Pump Inhibitors; QTc-Prolonging Agents; QuiNIDine; QuiNINE; Ramelteon; Ranolazine; Repaglinide; Rifamycin Derivatives; Salmeterol; Saxagliptin; Sirolimus; Solifenacin; Sulfonylureas; SUNItinib; Tacrolimus; Tacrolimus (Systemic); Tacrolimus (Topical); Temsirolimus; Tetrabenazine; Thioridazine; Tolterodine; Tolvaptan; Toremifene; Vandetanib; Vilazodone; Vitamin K Antagonists; Zidovudine; Ziprasidone; Zolpidem

The levels/effects of Fluconazole may be increased by: Alfuzosin; Artemether; Chloroquine; Ciprofloxacin; Ciprofloxacin (Systemic); Etravirine; Gadobutrol; Grapefruit Juice; Lumefantrine; Macrolide Antibiotics; Nilotinib; Protease Inhibitors; QuiNINE

Adverse Reactions Frequency not always defined.

Cardiovascular: Angioedema, pallor, QT prolongation (rare, case reports), torsade de pointes (rare, case reports)

Central nervous system: Headache (2% to 13%), dizziness (1%), seizure

Dermatologic: Rash (2%), alopecia, toxic epidermal necrolysis, Stevens-Johnson syndrome

Endocrine & metabolic: Hypercholesterolemia, hypertriglyceridemia, hypokalemia

Gastrointestinal: Nausea (2% to 7%), abdominal pain (2% to 6%), vomiting (2% to 5%), diarrhea (2% to 3%), dyspepsia (1%), taste perversion (1%)

Hematologic: Agranulocytosis, leukopenia, neutropenia, thrombocytopenia

Hepatic: Alkaline phosphatase increased, ALT increased, AST increased, cholestasis, hepatic failure (rare), hepatitis, jaundice

Respiratory: Dyspnea

Miscellaneous: Anaphylactic reactions (rare)

Pharmacodynamics/Kinetics

Bioavailability Oral: >90%

Time to Peak Oral: 1-2 hours

Protein Binding Plasma: 11% to 12%

Half-Life Elimination Normal renal function: ~30 hours

Excretion Urine (80% as unchanged drug)

Available Dosage Forms

Infusion, premixed iso-osmotic dextrose solution: 200 mg (100 mL); 400 mg (200 mL)
Diflucan®: 400 mg (200 mL)

Infusion, premixed iso-osmotic sodium chloride solution: 100 mg (50 mL); 200 mg (100 mL); 400 mg (200 mL)
Diflucan®: 200 mg (100 mL); 400 mg (200 mL)

Infusion, premixed iso-osmotic sodium chloride solution [preservative free]: 200 mg (100 mL); 400 mg (200 mL)

Powder for suspension, oral: 10 mg/mL (35 mL); 40 mg/mL (35 mL)
Diflucan®: 10 mg/mL (35 mL); 40 mg/mL (35 mL)

Tablet, oral: 50 mg, 100 mg, 150 mg, 200 mg
Diflucan®: 50 mg, 100 mg, 150 mg, 200 mg

Dosing

Adult & Geriatric The daily dose of fluconazole is the same for both oral and I.V. administration

Usual dosage range: 150 mg once **or** 200-800 mg/day; duration and dosage depends on severity of infection

Indication-specific dosing:

Candidiasis (Pappas, 2009):

Candidemia (neutropenic and non-neutropenic): Loading dose: 800 mg on first day, then 400 mg/day for 14 days after first negative blood culture and resolution of signs/ symptoms; **Note:** Not recommended for neutropenic patients with recent azole exposure and critical illness

Chronic, disseminated: 400 mg/day until calcification or lesion resolution

CNS candidemia: 400-800 mg/day until CSF/radiological abnormalities resolved

Oropharyngeal: 100-200 mg/day for 7-14 days for uncomplicated, moderate-to-severe disease; chronic therapy of 100 mg 3 times weekly is recommended in immunocompromised patients with history of oropharyngeal candidiasis (OPC)

Osteoarticular: 400 mg/day for 6-12 months (osteomyelitis) or 6 weeks (septic arthritis)

Esophageal: 200-400 mg/day for 14-21 days

Prophylaxis:

Solid organ: 200-400 mg/day for 7-14 days

Neutropenic patients: 400 mg/day for duration of neutropenia

Urinary tract:

Fungus balls: 200-400 mg/day

Pyelonephritis: 200-400 mg/day for 2 weeks

Symptomatic cystitis: 200 mg/day for 2 weeks

Vaginal:

Uncomplicated: 150 mg as a single dose

Complicated: 150 mg every 72 hours for 3 doses

Recurrent: 150 mg daily for 10-14 days, followed by 150 mg once weekly for 6 months

Candidal intertrigo (unlabeled use; Coldiron, 1991; Nozickova, 1998; Stengel, 1994): 50 mg/day **or** 150 mg once weekly

Coccidiomycosis (unlabeled use; Galgiani, 2005): 400-800 mg/day; doses of 800-1000 mg/day have been used for meningeal disease; usual duration of therapy ranges from 3-6 months for primary uncomplicated infections and up to 1 year for pulmonary (chronic and diffuse) infection

Endocarditis, prosthetic valve, early (unlabeled use; Pappas, 2009): 400-800 mg/day for 6 weeks after valve replacement (as step-down in stable, culture-negative patients); long-term suppression in absence of valve replacement: 400-800 mg/day

Endophthalmitis (Pappas, 2009): 400-800 mg/day for 4-6 weeks until examination indicates resolution

Meningitis, cryptococcal (Perfect, 2010):

Induction therapy: Typically consists of an amphotericin product and flucytosine for 2-6 weeks

Consolidation therapy: Fluconazole 400-800 mg/day for 8 weeks

Maintenance therapy: 200 mg/day for 6-12 months (post-transplant patients; non-HIV infected patients) **or** ≥1 year (HIV-infected patients may require lifelong therapy; CDC, 2009)

Pericarditis or myocarditis (Pappas, 2009): 400-800 mg/day

Pneumonia, cryptococcal (mild-to-moderate) (unlabeled use; Perfect, 2010): 400 mg/day for 6-12 months (HIV-infected patients may require lifelong therapy; CDC, 2009)

Pediatric The daily dose of fluconazole is the same for oral and I.V. administration

Usual dosage ranges:

Neonates: First 2 weeks of life, especially premature neonates: Same dose as older children every 72 hours

Children: Loading dose: 6-12 mg/kg; maintenance: 3-12 mg/kg/day; duration and dosage depends on severity of infection

Indication-specific dosing:

Candidiasis:

Oropharyngeal:

Manufacturer's recommendation: Loading dose: 6 mg/kg; maintenance: 3 mg/kg/day once daily for 2 weeks

HIV-exposed/-positive: 3-6 mg/kg/day once daily (maximum: 400 mg/day) (CDC, 2009)

Esophageal:

Manufacturer's recommendation: Loading dose: 6 mg/kg; maintenance: 3-12 mg/kg/day once daily for 21 days and at least 2 weeks following resolution of symptoms

HIV-exposed/-positive: Loading dose: 6 mg/kg once on day 1; maintenance: 3-6 mg/kg/day once daily (maximum: 400 mg/day) (CDC, 2009)

Relapse suppression (HIV-exposed/-positive): 3-6 mg/kg/day once daily (maximum: 200 mg/day) (CDC, 2009)

Invasive disease (independent of HIV status): 5-6 mg/kg every 12 hours for 28 days (maximum: 600 mg/day) (CDC, 2009)

Coccidioidomycosis (CDC, 2009):

Meningeal and disseminated disease (HIV-exposed/-positive): 5-6 mg/kg/dose every 12 hours (maximum: 800 mg/day)

Relapse suppression (HIV-exposed/-positive): 6 mg/kg/day once daily (maximum: 400 mg/day)

Histoplasmosis, relapse suppression (HIV-exposed/-positive): 3-6 mg/kg/day once daily (maximum: 200 mg/day) (CDC, 2009)

Cryptococcal disease (CDC, 2009):

Meningitis (consolidation): Loading dose: 12 mg/kg once on day 1; maintenance: 6-12 mg/kg/day once daily for a minimum of 8 weeks (maximum: 800 mg/day)

Disseminated (non-CNS) or severe pulmonary disease: Loading dose: 12 mg/kg once on day 1; maintenance: 6-12 mg/kg/day once daily (maximum: 600 mg/day)

Relapse suppression (HIV-exposed/-positive): 6 mg/kg/day once daily (maximum: 200 mg/day)

Renal Impairment

No adjustment for vaginal candidiasis single-dose therapy

For multiple dosing, administer usual load then adjust daily doses as follows:

Cl_{cr} ≤50 mL/minute (no dialysis): Administer 50% of recommended dose or administer every 48 hours.

Hemodialysis: 50% is removed by hemodialysis; administer 100% of daily dose (according to indication) after each dialysis treatment.

Continuous renal replacement therapy (CRRT): Drug clearance is highly dependent on the method of renal replacement, filter type, and flow rate. Appropriate dosing requires close monitoring of pharmacologic response, signs of adverse reactions due to drug accumulation, as well as drug levels in relation to target trough (if appropriate). The following are general recommendations only (based on dialysate flow/ultrafiltration rates of 1 L/hour) and should not supersede clinical judgment:

CVVH: 200-400 mg every 24 hours

CVVHD/CVVHDF: 400-800 mg every 24 hours

Note: Higher daily doses of 400 mg (CVVH) and 800 mg (CVVHD/CVVHDF) should be considered when treating resistant organisms and/or when employing combined ultrafiltration and dialysis flow rates of ≥2 L/hour for CVVHD/CVVHDF (Trotman, 2005).

Administration

Oral May be administered without regard to meals.

I.V. Do not use if cloudy or precipitated. Infuse over approximately 1-2 hours; do not exceed 200 mg/hour.

Stability

Storage

Tablet: Store at <30°C (86°F).

Powder for oral suspension: Store dry powder at <30°C (86°F). Following reconstitution, store at 5°C to 30°C (41°F to 86°F). Discard unused portion after 2 weeks. Do not freeze.

Injection: Store injection in glass at 5°C to 30°C (41°F to 86°F). Store injection in Viaflex® at 5°C to 25°C (41°F to 77°F). Do not freeze. Do not unwrap unit until ready for use.

Monitoring and Teaching Issues

Laboratory Monitoring Culture prior to beginning therapy, periodic liver function (AST, ALT, alkaline phosphatase) and renal function, potassium

Physical Assessment Assess results of cultures/sensitivity and patient's allergy history prior to beginning therapy. Assess renal and hepatic function. Monitor for hepatotoxicity (jaundice), skin disorders, and abdominal pain on a regular basis.

Patient Education Frequent blood tests may be required. Maintain adequate hydration, unless instructed to restrict fluid intake. May cause headache, dizziness, drowsiness, nausea, vomiting, or diarrhea. Report skin rash, persistent GI upset, urinary pattern changes, excessively dry eyes or mouth, or changes in color of stool or urine.

Dietary Considerations Take without regard to meals.

Geriatric Considerations Has not been specifically studied in the elderly.

Breast-Feeding Considerations Fluconazole is found in breast milk at concentration similar to plasma.

Pregnancy Considerations When used in high doses, fluconazole is teratogenic in animal studies. Following exposure during the first trimester, case reports have noted similar malformations in humans when used in higher doses (400 mg/day) over extended periods of time. Use of lower doses (150 mg as a single dose or 200 mg/day) may have less risk; however, additional data is needed. Use during pregnancy only if the potential benefit to the mother outweighs any potential risk to the fetus.

Related Information

Compatibility of Drugs *on page 1994*

I.V. to Oral Conversion *on page 1956*

Flucytosine (floo SYE toe seen)

U.S. Brand Names Ancobon®

Index Terms 5-FC; 5-Fluorocytosine; 5-Flurocytosine

Generic Availability (U.S.) No

Pharmacologic Category Antifungal Agent, Oral

Medication Safety Issues

Sound-alike/look-alike issues:

Flucytosine may be confused with fluorouracil

Ancobon® may be confused with Oncovin®

High alert medication: The Institute for Safe Medication Practices (ISMP) includes this medication among its list of drugs which have a heightened risk of causing significant patient harm when used in error.

Pregnancy Risk Factor C

Lactation Excretion in breast milk unknown/not recommended

Use Adjunctive treatment of systemic fungal infections (eg, septicemia, endocarditis, UTI, meningitis, or pulmonary) caused by susceptible strains of *Candida* or *Cryptococcus*

Mechanism of Action/Effect Penetrates fungal cells and interferes with fungal RNA and protein synthesis

Contraindications Hypersensitivity to flucytosine or any component of the formulation

Warnings/Precautions [U.S. Boxed Warning]: Use with extreme caution in patients with renal dysfunction; dosage adjustment required. Avoid use as monotherapy; resistance rapidly develops. Use with caution in patients with bone marrow depression; patients with hematologic disease or who have been treated with radiation or drugs that suppress the bone marrow may be at greatest risk. Bone marrow toxicity can be irreversible. **[U.S. Boxed Warning]: Closely monitor hematologic, renal, and hepatic status.** Hepatotoxicity and bone marrow toxicity appear to be dose related; monitor levels closely and adjust dose accordingly.

Drug Interactions

Avoid Concomitant Use There are no known interactions where it is recommended to avoid concomitant use.

Decreased Effect

Flucytosine may decrease the levels/effects of: Saccharomyces boulardii

The levels/effects of Flucytosine may be decreased by: Cytarabine

Increased Effect/Toxicity

The levels/effects of Flucytosine may be increased by: Amphotericin B

Nutritional/Ethanol Interactions Food: Food decreases the rate, but not the extent of absorption.

Lab Interactions Flucytosine causes markedly false elevations in serum creatinine values when the Ektachem® analyzer is used. The Jaffé reaction is recommended for determining serum creatinine.

Adverse Reactions Frequency not defined.

Cardiovascular: Cardiac arrest, myocardial toxicity, ventricular dysfunction, chest pain

Central nervous system: Ataxia, confusion, dizziness, drowsiness, fatigue, hallucinations, headache, parkinsonism, psychosis, pyrexia, sedation, seizure, vertigo

Dermatologic: Rash, photosensitivity, pruritus, toxic epidermal necrolysis, urticaria

Endocrine & metabolic: Hypoglycemia, hypokalemia

Gastrointestinal: Abdominal pain, diarrhea, dry mouth, duodenal ulcer, hemorrhage, loss of appetite, nausea, ulcerative colitis, vomiting

Hematologic: Agranulocytosis, anemia, aplastic anemia, eosinophilia, leukopenia, pancytopenia, thrombocytopenia

Hepatic: Acute hepatic injury, bilirubin increased, hepatic dysfunction, jaundice, liver enzymes increased

Neuromuscular & skeletal: Paresthesia, peripheral neuropathy, weakness

Otic: Hearing loss

Renal: Azotemia, BUN increased, crystalluria, renal failure, serum creatinine increased

Respiratory: Dyspnea, respiratory arrest

Miscellaneous: Allergic reaction

Pharmacodynamics/Kinetics

Absorption 76% to 89%

Time to Peak Serum: ~1-2 hours

Protein Binding 3% to 4%

Half-Life Elimination Normal renal function: 2-5 hours; Anuria: 85 hours (range: 30-250); End stage renal disease: 75-200 hours

Metabolism Minimally hepatic; deaminated, possibly via gut bacteria, to 5-fluorouracil

Excretion Urine (>90% as unchanged drug)

Available Dosage Forms

Capsule, oral:

Ancobon®: 250 mg, 500 mg

Dosing

Adult & Geriatric

Endocarditis: Oral: 25-37.5 mg/kg every 6 hours (with amphotericin B) for at least 6 weeks after valve replacement

Meningoencephalitis, cryptococcal: Induction: Oral: 25 mg/kg/dose (with amphotericin B) every 6 hours for 2 weeks; if clinical improvement, may discontinue both amphotericin and flucytosine and follow with an extended course of fluconazole (400 mg/day); alternatively, may continue flucytosine for 6-10 weeks (with amphotericin B) without conversion to fluconazole treatment

Pediatric Unlabeled use. Refer to adult dosing.

Renal Impairment Use lower initial dose:

Cl_{cr} 20-40 mL/minute: Administer 37.5 mg/kg every 12 hours

Cl_{cr} 10-20 mL/minute: Administer 37.5 mg/kg every 24 hours

Cl_{cr} <10 mL/minute: Administer 37.5 mg/kg every 24-48 hours, but monitor drug concentrations frequently

Hemodialysis: Dialyzable (50% to 100%); administer dose posthemodialysis

Peritoneal dialysis: Adults: Administer 0.5-1 g every 24 hours

Continuous arteriovenous or venovenous hemodiafiltration effects: Change dosing frequency to every 12-24 hours (monitor serum concentrations and adjust)

Administration

Oral Administer around-the-clock to promote less variation in peak and trough serum levels. To avoid nausea and vomiting, administer a few capsules at a time over 15 minutes until full dose is taken.

Stability

Storage Store at room temperature of 15°C to 30°C (59°F to 86°F). Protect from light.

Monitoring and Teaching Issues

Laboratory Monitoring

Pretreatment: Electrolytes (especially potassium), CBC with differential, BUN, renal function, blood culture

During treatment: CBC with differential, and LFTs (eg, alkaline phosphatase, AST/ALT) frequently, serum flucytosine concentration, renal function

Physical Assessment Hematologic, renal, and hepatic status must be closely monitored; dose adjustments may be necessary. Monitor for cardiac toxicity, CNS changes, bone marrow suppression, jaundice, skin reactions, and hearing loss on a regular basis.

Patient Education Take capsules one at a time over a few minutes with food to reduce GI upset. Frequent blood tests may be required. May cause nausea and vomiting. Report rash; respiratory difficulty; CNS changes (eg, confusion, hallucinations, ataxia, acute headache); yellowing of skin or eyes; changes in frequency of stool or urine; unresolved diarrhea or anorexia; or unusual bleeding, fatigue, or weakness.

Geriatric Considerations Adjust for renal function.

Pregnancy Considerations Teratogenic in some animal studies, however, there are no adequate and well-controlled studies in pregnant women.

◆ **Fludara®** *see* Fludarabine *on page 776*

Fludarabine (floo DARE a been)

U.S. Brand Names Fludara®; Oforta™

Index Terms 2F-ara-AMP; Fludarabine Phosphate

Generic Availability (U.S.) Yes

Pharmacologic Category Antineoplastic Agent, Antimetabolite (Purine Analog)

Medication Safety Issues

Sound-alike/look-alike issues:

Fludarabine may be confused with cladribine, floxuridine, Flumadine®

Fludara® may be confused with FUDR®

High alert medication: This medication is in a class the Institute for Safe Medication Practices (ISMP) includes among its list of drug classes which have a heightened risk of causing significant patient harm when used in error.

Pregnancy Risk Factor D

Lactation Excretion in breast milk unknown/not recommended

Use Treatment of progressive or refractory B-cell chronic lymphocytic leukemia (CLL)

Canadian labeling: Second-line treatment of chronic lymphocytic leukemia (CLL); second-line treatment of low-grade, refractory non-Hodgkin's lymphoma (NHL)

Unlabeled/Investigational Use Treatment of non-Hodgkin's lymphomas (NHL); acute myeloid leukemia (AML), either refractory or in poor risk patients; relapsed acute lymphocytic leukemia (ALL) or AML in pediatric patients; Waldenström's macroglobulinemia (WM); reduced-intensity conditioning regimens prior to allogeneic hematopoietic stem cell transplantation (generally administered in combination with busulfan or cyclophosphamide and antithymocyte globulin or lymphocyte immune globulin, or in combination with melphalan and alemtuzumab)

Mechanism of Action/Effect Inhibits DNA synthesis by inhibition of DNA polymerase and ribonucleotide reductase; also inhibits DNA primase and DNA ligase I

Contraindications Hypersensitivity of fludarabine or any component of the formulation

Canadian labeling: Additional contraindications (not in U.S. labeling): Severe renal impairment (Cl_{cr} <30 mL/minute); decompensated hemolytic anemia; concurrent use with pentostatin

Warnings/Precautions Hazardous agent - use appropriate precautions for handling and disposal. Use with caution in patients with renal insufficiency (clearance of the primary metabolite 2-fluoro-ara-A is reduced); dosage reductions are recommended (monitor closely for excessive toxicity); use of the I.V. formulation is not recommended if Cl_{cr} <30 mL/minute. Use with caution in patients with pre-existing hematological disorders (particularly granulocytopenia) or pre-existing central nervous system disorder (epilepsy), spasticity, or peripheral neuropathy. **[U.S. Boxed Warning]: Higher than recommended doses are associated with severe neurologic toxicity (delayed blindness, coma, death); similar neurotoxicity (agitation, coma, confusion and seizure) has been reported with standard CLL doses.** Neurotoxicity symptoms due to high doses appear from 21-60 days following the last fludarabine dose, although neurotoxicity has been reported as early as 7 days and up to 225 days. Possible neurotoxic effects of chronic administration are unknown. Caution patients about performing tasks which require mental alertness (eg, operating machinery or driving.

[U.S. Boxed Warning]: Life-threatening (and sometimes fatal) autoimmune effects, including hemolytic anemia, autoimmune thrombocytopenia/thrombocytopenic purpura (ITP), Evans syndrome, and acquired hemophilia have occurred; monitor closely for hemolysis; discontinue fludarabine if hemolysis occurs; the hemolytic effects usually recur with fludarabine rechallenge. **[U.S. Boxed Warning]: Severe bone marrow suppression (anemia, thrombocytopenia, and neutropenia) may occur;** may be cumulative. Severe myelosuppression (trilineage bone marrow hypoplasia/aplasia) has been reported (rare) with a duration of significant cytopenias ranging from 2 months to 1 year. First-line combination therapy is associated with prolonged cytopenias, with anemia lasting up to 7 months, neutropenia up to 9 months, and thrombocytopenia up to 10 months; increased age is predictive for prolonged cytopenias (Gill, 2010).

Use with caution in patients with documented infection, fever, immunodeficiency, or with a history of opportunistic infection; prophylactic anti-infectives should be considered for patients with an increased risk for developing opportunistic infections. Progressive multifocal leukoencephalopathy (PML) due to JC virus (usually fatal) has been reported with use; usually in patients who had received prior and/or other concurrent chemotherapy; onset ranges from a few weeks to 1 year; evaluate any neurological change promptly. Avoid vaccination with live vaccines during and after fludarabine treatment. May cause tumor lysis syndrome; risk is increased in patients with large tumor burden prior to treatment. Patients receiving blood products should only receive irradiated blood products due to the potential for transfusion related GVHD. **[U.S. Boxed Warnings]: Do not use in combination with pentostatin; may lead to severe, even fatal pulmonary toxicity. Should be administered under the supervision of an experienced cancer chemotherapy physician.**

Drug Interactions

Avoid Concomitant Use

Avoid concomitant use of Fludarabine with any of the following: BCG; Natalizumab; Pentostatin; Pimecrolimus; Roflumilast; Tacrolimus (Topical); Vaccines (Live)

Decreased Effect

Fludarabine may decrease the levels/effects of: BCG; Sipuleucel-T; Vaccines (Inactivated); Vaccines (Live)

The levels/effects of Fludarabine may be decreased by: Echinacea; Imatinib

Increased Effect/Toxicity

Fludarabine may increase the levels/effects of: Leflunomide; Natalizumab; Pentostatin; Vaccines (Live)

The levels/effects of Fludarabine may be increased by: Denosumab; Pentostatin; Pimecrolimus; Roflumilast; Tacrolimus (Topical); Trastuzumab

Nutritional/Ethanol Interactions Ethanol: Avoid ethanol (due to GI irritation).

Adverse Reactions

>10%:

Cardiovascular: Edema (8% to 19%)

Central nervous system: Fever (11% to 69%), fatigue (10% to 38%), pain (5% to 22%), chills (11% to 19%)

Dermatologic: Rash (4% to 15%)

Gastrointestinal: Nausea/vomiting (1% to 36%), anorexia (≤34%), diarrhea (5% to 15%), gastrointestinal bleeding (3% to 13%)

Genitourinary: Urinary tract infection (2% to 15%)

Hematologic: Myelosuppression (nadir: 10-14 days; recovery: 5-7 weeks; dose-limiting toxicity), anemia (14% to 60%), neutropenia (grade 4: 37% to 59%; nadir: ~13 days), thrombocytopenia (17% to 55%; nadir: ~16 days)
Neuromuscular & skeletal: Weakness (9% to 65%), myalgia (4% to 16%), paresthesia (4% to 12%)
Ocular: Visual disturbance (3% to 15%)
Respiratory: Cough (≤44%), pneumonia (3% to 22%), dyspnea (1% to 22%), upper respiratory infection (2% to 16%), rhinitis (≤11%)
Miscellaneous: Infection (12% to 44%), diaphoresis (≤14%)

1% to 10%:

Cardiovascular: Peripheral edema (≤7%), angina (≤6%), chest pain (≤5%), CHF (≤3%), arrhythmia (≤3%), cerebrovascular accident (≤3%), MI (≤3%), supraventricular tachycardia (≤3%), deep vein thrombosis (1% to 3%), phlebitis (1% to 3%), aneurysm (≤1%), transient ischemic attack (≤1%)
Central nervous system: Headache (≤9%), malaise (6% to 8%), sleep disorder (1% to 3%), cerebellar syndrome (≤1%), depression (≤1%), mentation impaired (≤1%)
Dermatologic: Alopecia (≤3%), pruritus (1% to 3%), seborrhea (≤1%)
Endocrine & metabolic: Hyperglycemia (1% to 6%), LDH increased (≤6%), dehydration (≤1%)
Gastrointestinal: Abdominal pain (≤10%), stomatitis (≤9%), weight loss (≤6%), esophagitis (≤3%), constipation (1% to 3%), mucositis (≤2%), dysphagia (≤1%)
Genitourinary: Dysuria (3% to 4%), hesitancy (≤3%)
Hematologic: Hemorrhage (≤1%), myelodysplastic syndrome/acute myeloid leukemia (usually associated with prior or concurrent treatment with other anticancer agents)
Hepatic: Cholelithiasis (≤3%), liver function tests abnormal (1% to 3%), liver failure (≤1%)
Neuromuscular & skeletal: Back pain (≤9%), osteoporosis (≤2%), arthralgia (≤1%)
Otic: Hearing loss (2% to 6%)
Renal: Hematuria (2% to 3%), renal failure (≤1%), renal function test abnormal (≤1%), proteinuria (≤1%)
Respiratory: Bronchitis (≤9%), pharyngitis (≤9%), allergic pneumonitis (≤6%), hemoptysis (1% to 6%), sinusitis (≤5%), epistaxis (≤1%), hypoxia (≤1%)
Miscellaneous: Flu-like syndrome (5% to 8%), herpes simplex infection (≤8%), anaphylaxis (≤1%), tumor lysis syndrome (1%)

Pharmacodynamics/Kinetics

Bioavailability Oral: 2-fluoro-ara-A: 50% to 65%

Time to Peak Oral: 1-2 hours

Protein Binding 2-fluoro-ara-A: ~19% to 29%

Half-Life Elimination 2-fluoro-ara-A: ~20 hours

Metabolism I.V.: Fludarabine phosphate is rapidly dephosphorylated in the plasma to 2-fluoro-ara-A (active metabolite), which subsequently enters tumor cells and is phosphorylated by deoxycytidine kinase to the active triphosphate derivative (2-fluoro-ara-ATP)

Excretion Urine (60%, 23% as 2-fluoro-ara-A) within 24 hours

Available Dosage Forms

Injection, powder for reconstitution: 50 mg
Fludara®: 50 mg

Injection, solution [preservative free]: 25 mg/mL (2 mL)

Tablet, oral:
Oforta™: 10 mg

Dosing

Adult & Geriatric Details concerning dosing in combination regimens should also be consulted.

Chronic lymphocytic leukemia (CLL):
Oral: 40 mg/m^2 once daily for 5 days every 28 days
I.V.: 25 mg/m^2/day for 5 days every 28 days

CLL combination regimens (unlabeled dosing): I.V.:
CFAR: 20 mg/m^2/day for 3 days every 28 days for 6 cycles (in combination with cyclophosphamide, rituximab and alemtuzumab) (Wierda, 2008)
FC: 30 mg/m^2/day for 3 days every 28 days for 6 cycles (in combination with cyclophosphamide) (Eichhorst, 2006) **or** 20 mg/m^2/day for 5 days every 28 days for 6 cycles (in combination with cyclophosphamide) (Flinn, 2007)
FCR: 25 mg/m^2/day for 3 days every 28 days for 6 cycles (in combination with cyclophosphamide and rituximab) (Keating, 2005; Robak, 2010; Wierda, 2005)
FluCam: 30 mg/m^2/day for 3 days every 28 days for 4-6 cycles (in combination with alemtuzumab) (Elter, 2005)
FR: 25 mg/m^2/day for 5 days every 28 days for 6 cycles (in combination with rituximab) (Byrd, 2003)
OFAR: 30 mg/m^2/day for 2 days every 28 days for 6 cycles (in combination with oxaliplatin, cytarabine, and rituximab) (Tsimberidou, 2008)

AML, high-risk patients (unlabeled use): I.V.: 30 mg/m^2/day for 5 days induction therapy, followed by post remission therapy of 30 mg/m^2/day for 4 days every other cycle (in combination with cytarabine with or without filgrastim) (Borthakur, 2008)

AML, refractory (unlabeled use): I.V.: 30 mg/m^2/day for 5 days (in combination with cytarabine and filgrastim), may repeat once for partial remission (Montillo, 1998) **or** 30 mg/m^2/day for 5 days for 1 or 2 cycles (in combination with cytarabine, idarubicin, and filgrastim) (Virchis, 2004)

Non-hodgkin's lymphomas (unlabeled uses): I.V.:

Follicular lymphoma:

FCR: 25 mg/m^2/day for 3 days every 21 days for 4 cycles (in combination with cyclophosphamide and rituximab) (Sacchi, 2007)

FCMR: 25 mg/m^2/day for 3 days every 28 days for 4 cycles (in combination with cyclophosphamide, mitoxantrone, and rituximab) (Forstpointner, 2004; Forstpointner, 2006)

FND: 25 mg/m^2/day for 3 days every 28 days for up to 8 cycles (in combination with mitoxantrone and dexamethasone) (McLaughlin, 1996; Tsimberidou, 2002)

FNDR: 25 mg/m^2/day for 3 days every 28 days for up to 8 cycles (in combination with mitoxantrone, dexamethasone, and rituximab) (McLaughlin, 2000)

FR: 25 mg/m^2/day for 5 days every 28 days for 6 cycles (in combination with rituximab) (Czuczman, 2005)

Mantle cell lymphoma:

FC: 20 mg/m^2/day for 4-5 days or 25 mg/m^2/day for 3-5 days (in combination with cyclophosphamide) (Cohen, 2001)

FCMR: 25 mg/m^2/day for 3 days every 28 days for 4 cycles (in combination with cyclophosphamide, mitoxantrone, and rituximab) (Forstpointner, 2004; Forstpointner, 2006)

Waldenstron's macroglobulinemia (unlabeled use): I.V.:25 mg/m^2/day for 5 days every 28 days (Foran, 1999) **or** 25 mg/m^2/day for 5 days every 28 days for 6 cycles (in combination with rituximab) (Treon, 2009)

Stem cell transplant (allogeneic) conditioning regimen, reduced-intensity, (unlabeled use): I.V.: 30 mg/m^2/dose for 6 doses beginning 10 days prior to transplant **or** 30 mg/m^2/dose for 5 days beginning 6 days prior to transplant (in combination with busulfan with or without antithymocyte globulin) (Schetelig, 2003)

Stem cell transplant (allogeneic) nonmyeloablative conditioning regimen (unlabeled use): I.V.: 30 mg/m^2/dose for 3 doses beginning 5 days prior to transplant (in combination with cyclophosphamide and rituximab) (Khouri, 2008) **or** 30 mg/m^2/dose for 3 doses beginning 4 days prior to transplant (in combination with total body irradiation) (Rezvani, 2008)

Pediatric

AML (unlabeled use): I.V.: 10.5 mg/m^2 bolus over 15 minutes followed by a continuous infusion of 30.5 mg/m^2/day for 48 hours (Lange, 2008)

ALL or AML, relapsed (unlabeled use): I.V.: 10.5 mg/m^2 bolus over 15 minutes followed by a continuous infusion of 30.5 mg/m^2/day for 48 hours (Avramis, 1998)

Stem cell transplant (allogeneic) conditioning regimen, reduced-intensity (unlabeled use): I.V.: 30 mg/m^2/dose for 6 doses beginning 7-10 days prior to transplant (in combination with busulfan and antithymocyte globulin) (Pulsipher, 2009)

Renal Impairment

FDA-approved labeling contains the following adjustment recommendations: Adults: CLL:

I.V.:

Cl_{cr} 50-79 mL/minute: Decrease dose to 20 mg/m^2.

Cl_{cr} 30-49 mL/minute: Decrease dose to 15 mg/m^2.

Cl_{cr} <30 mL/minute: Avoid use.

Oral:

Cl_{cr} 30-70 mL/minute: Administer 80% of dose.

Cl_{cr} <30 mL/minute: Administer 50% of dose.

Canadian labeling contains the following adjustment recommendations: CLL, NHL:

Cl_{cr} 30-70 mL/minute: Reduce dose by up to 50%.

Cl_{cr} <30 mL/minute: Use is contraindicated.

The following guidelines have been used by some clinicians: Aronoff, 2007: I.V.:

Children:

Cl_{cr} 30-50 mL/minute: Administer 80% of dose.

Cl_{cr} <30 mL/minute: Not recommended.

Hemodialysis: Administer 25% of dose

Continuous ambulatory peritoneal dialysis (CAPD): Not recommended.

Continuous renal replacement therapy (CRRT): Administer 80% of dose.

Adults:

Cl_{cr} 10-50 mL/minute: Administer 75% of dose.

Cl_{cr} <10 mL/minute: Administer 50% of dose.

Hemodialysis: Administer after dialysis

Continuous ambulatory peritoneal dialysis (CAPD): Administer 50% of dose.

Continuous renal replacement therapy (CRRT): Administer 75% of dose.

Adjustment for Toxicity

Hematologic or nonhematologic toxicity (other than neurotoxicity): Consider treatment delay or dosage reduction.

Hemolysis: Discontinue treatment.

Neurotoxicity: Consider treatment delay or discontinuation.

Administration

Oral Tablet may be administered with or without food; should be swallowed whole with water; do not chew, break, or crush.

I.V. Administer I.V. over 30 minutes; continuous infusions (unlabeled administration rate) are occasionally used

Stability

Reconstitution Use appropriate precautions for handling and disposal. Reconstitute vials with SWI, NS, or D_5W to a concentration of 10-25 mg/mL. Standard I.V. dilution: 100-125 mL D_5W or NS.

Storage

I.V.: Store intact vials under refrigeration at 2°C to 8°C (36°F to 46°F). Reconstituted vials are stable for 16 days at room temperature of 15°C to 30°C (59°F to 86°F) or refrigerated, although the manufacturer recommends use within 8 hours. Solutions diluted in saline or dextrose are stable for 48 hours at room temperature or under refrigeration.

Tablet: Store at 25°C (77°F); excursions permitted to 15°C to 30°C (59°F to 86°F); should be kept within packaging until use.

Monitoring and Teaching Issues

Laboratory Monitoring CBC with differential, platelet count, AST, ALT, serum creatinine, serum albumin, uric acid

Physical Assessment Use caution in the presence of infection, fever, or history of opportunistic infection; renal insufficiency; hematological disorders; central nervous system disorders; or peripheral neuropathy.

Patient Education If this drug is administered by infusion, report any burning, pain, redness, or swelling at infusion site. It is important to maintain adequate nutrition and hydration, unless instructed to restrict fluid intake. You will be more susceptible to infection. May cause fatigue, weakness, visual disturbances, nausea, vomiting, loss of hair (reversible), or mouth sores. Report severe or persistent GI upset or diarrhea; extreme fatigue or weakness; pain or numbness in muscles; any unusual bleeding or bruising; fever, chills, or sore throat; vaginal discharge; difficulty or pain on urination; unusual cough or respiratory difficulty; or changes in vision.

Dietary Considerations Tablet may be taken with or without food.

Breast-Feeding Considerations Due to the potential for serious adverse reactions in the nursing infant, breast-feeding is not recommended.

Pregnancy Considerations Teratogenic effects were observed in animal studies. Based on the mechanism of action, fludarabine has the potential to cause fetal harm if administered during pregnancy. There are no adequate and well-controlled studies in pregnant women. Effective contraception is recommended during and for 6 months after treatment for women and men with female partners of reproductive potential.

◆ **Fludarabine Phosphate** *see* Fludarabine *on page 776*

Fludrocortisone (floo droe KOR ti sone)

Index Terms 9α-Fluorohydrocortisone Acetate; Florinef; Fludrocortisone Acetate; Fluohydrisone Acetate; Fluohydrocortisone Acetate

Generic Availability (U.S.) Yes

Pharmacologic Category Corticosteroid, Systemic

Medication Safety Issues

Sound-alike/look-alike issues:

Florinef® may be confused with Fioricet®, Fiorinal®

Pregnancy Risk Factor C

Lactation Excretion in breast milk unknown/use caution

Use Partial replacement therapy for primary and secondary adrenocortical insufficiency in Addison's disease; treatment of salt-losing adrenogenital syndrome

Mechanism of Action/Effect Promotes increased reabsorption of sodium and loss of potassium from renal distal tubules

Contraindications Hypersensitivity to fludrocortisone or any component of the formulation; systemic fungal infections

Warnings/Precautions May cause hypercorticism or suppression of hypothalamic-pituitary-adrenal (HPA) axis, particularly in younger children or in patients receiving high doses for prolonged periods. HPA axis suppression may lead to adrenal crisis. Withdrawal and discontinuation of a corticosteroid should be done slowly and carefully. Fludrocortisone is primarily a mineralocorticoid agonist, but may also inhibit the HPA axis. May increase risk of infection and/or limit response to vaccinations; close observation is required in patients with latent tuberculosis and/or TB reactivity. Restrict use in active TB (only in conjunction with antituberculosis treatment). Use with caution in patients with sodium retention and potassium loss, hepatic impairment, myocardial infarction, osteoporosis, and/or renal impairment. Use with caution in the elderly. Withdraw therapy with gradual tapering of dose.

Drug Interactions

Avoid Concomitant Use

Avoid concomitant use of Fludrocortisone with any of the following: Aldesleukin; BCG; Natalizumab; Pimecrolimus; Roflumilast; Tacrolimus (Topical)

Decreased Effect

Fludrocortisone may decrease the levels/effects of: Aldesleukin; Antidiabetic Agents; BCG; Calcitriol; Corticorelin; Isoniazid; Salicylates; Sipuleucel-T; Vaccines (Inactivated)

The levels/effects of Fludrocortisone may be decreased by: Aminoglutethimide; Antacids; Barbiturates; Bile Acid Sequestrants; Echinacea; Mitotane; Primidone; Rifamycin Derivatives

Increased Effect/Toxicity

Fludrocortisone may increase the levels/effects of: Acetylcholinesterase Inhibitors; Amphotericin B; Leflunomide; Loop Diuretics; Natalizumab; NSAID (COX-2 Inhibitor); NSAID (Nonselective); Thiazide Diuretics; Vaccines (Live); Warfarin

The levels/effects of Fludrocortisone may be increased by: Antifungal Agents (Azole Derivatives, Systemic); Aprepitant; Calcium Channel Blockers (Nondihydropyridine); Denosumab; Estrogen Derivatives; Fluconazole; Fosaprepitant; Macrolide Antibiotics; Neuromuscular-Blocking Agents (Nondepolarizing); Pimecrolimus; Quinolone Antibiotics; Roflumilast; Salicylates; Tacrolimus (Topical); Trastuzumab

Adverse Reactions Frequency not defined.

Cardiovascular: CHF, edema, hypertension
Central nervous system: Dizziness, headache, seizures
Dermatologic: Acne, bruising, rash
Endocrine & metabolic: HPA suppression, hyperglycemia, hypokalemic alkalosis, suppression of growth
Gastrointestinal: Peptic ulcer
Neuromuscular & skeletal: Muscle weakness
Ocular: Cataracts
Miscellaneous: Anaphylaxis (generalized), diaphoresis

Pharmacodynamics/Kinetics

Absorption Rapid and complete

Time to Peak Serum: ~1.7 hours

Protein Binding 42%

Half-Life Elimination Plasma: 30-35 minutes; Biological: 18-36 hours

Metabolism Hepatic

Available Dosage Forms

Tablet, oral: 0.1 mg

Dosing

Adult & Geriatric Mineralocorticoid deficiency: Oral: 0.05-0.2 mg/day with ranges of 0.1 mg 3 times/week to 0.2 mg/day

Pediatric Mineralocorticoid deficiency: Oral: Infants and Children: 0.05-0.1 mg/day

Administration

Oral Administration in conjunction with a glucocorticoid is preferable.

Monitoring and Teaching Issues

Laboratory Monitoring Serum electrolytes, serum renin activity

Physical Assessment Teach patients to report opportunistic infection and adrenal suppression. Instruct patients with diabetes to monitor serum glucose levels closely; corticosteroids can alter glycemic response. Dose may need to be increased if patient is experiencing higher than normal levels of stress. When discontinuing, taper dose and frequency slowly.

Patient Education Take with or after meals. Take once-a-day dose with food in the morning. Limit intake of caffeine or stimulants. Maintain adequate nutrition; consult prescriber for possibility of special dietary recommendations. If you have diabetes, monitor serum glucose closely and notify prescriber of changes; this medication can alter glycemic response. Notify prescriber if you are experiencing higher than normal levels of stress; medication may need adjustment. Periodic ophthalmic examinations will be necessary. You will be susceptible to infection. You may experience insomnia or nervousness. Report weakness, change in menstrual pattern, vision changes, signs of hyperglycemia, signs of infection (eg, fever, chills, mouth sores, perianal itching, vaginal discharge), or worsening of condition.

Dietary Considerations Systemic use of mineralocorticoids/corticosteroids may require a diet with increased potassium, vitamins A, B_6, C, D, folate, calcium, zinc, and phosphorus, and decreased sodium. With fludrocortisone, a decrease in dietary sodium is often not required as the increased retention of sodium is usually the desired therapeutic effect.

Geriatric Considerations The most common use of fludrocortisone in the elderly is orthostatic hypotension that is unresponsive to more conservative measures. Attempt nonpharmacologic measures (hydration, support stockings etc) before starting drug therapy.

Breast-Feeding Considerations Corticosteroids are excreted in human milk; information specific to fludrocortisone has not been located.

Pregnancy Considerations Animal reproduction studies have not been conducted with fludrocortisone; adverse events have been observed with corticosteroids in animal reproduction studies. Some studies have shown an association between first trimester systemic corticosteroid use and oral clefts; adverse events in the fetus/neonate have been noted in case reports following large doses of systemic corticosteroids during pregnancy.

Additional Information In patients with salt-losing forms of congenital adrenogenital syndrome, use along with cortisone or hydrocortisone. Fludrocortisone 0.1 mg has sodium retention activity equal to DOCA® 1 mg.

Related Information

Corticosteroids *on page 1996*

◆ **Fludrocortisone Acetate** *see* Fludrocortisone *on page 780*
◆ **FluLaval®** *see* Influenza Virus Vaccine (Inactivated) *on page 978*
◆ **Flumadine®** *see* Rimantadine *on page 1583*

Flumazenil (FLOO may ze nil)

U.S. Brand Names Romazicon®

Generic Availability (U.S.) Yes

Pharmacologic Category Antidote

Medication Safety Issues

Sound-alike/look-alike issues:

Flumazenil may be confused with influenza virus vaccine

Pregnancy Risk Factor C

Lactation Excretion in breast milk unknown/use caution

Use Benzodiazepine antagonist; reverses sedative effects of benzodiazepines used in conscious sedation and general anesthesia; treatment of benzodiazepine overdose

Mechanism of Action/Effect Competitively inhibits the activity at the benzodiazepine receptor site on the GABA/benzodiazepine receptor complex. Flumazenil does not antagonize the CNS effect of drugs affecting GABA-ergic neurons by means other than the benzodiazepine receptor (ethanol, barbiturates, general anesthetics) and does not reverse the effects of opioids.

Contraindications Hypersensitivity to flumazenil, benzodiazepines, or any component of the formulation; patients given benzodiazepines for control of potentially life-threatening conditions (eg, control of intracranial pressure or status epilepticus); patients who are showing signs of serious cyclic-antidepressant overdosage

Warnings/Precautions **[U.S. Boxed Warning]: Benzodiazepine reversal may result in seizures in some patients.** Patients who may develop seizures include patients on benzodiazepines for long-term sedation, tricyclic antidepressant overdose patients, concurrent major sedative-hypnotic drug withdrawal, recent therapy with repeated doses of parenteral benzodiazepines, myoclonic jerking or seizure activity prior to flumazenil administration. Flumazenil may not reliably reverse respiratory depression/hypoventilation. Flumazenil is not a substitute for evaluation of oxygenation; establishing an airway and assisting ventilation, as necessary, is always the initial step in overdose management. Resedation occurs more frequently in patients where a large single dose or cumulative dose of a benzodiazepine is administered along with a neuromuscular-blocking agent and multiple anesthetic agents. Flumazenil should be used with caution in the intensive care unit because of increased risk of unrecognized benzodiazepine dependence in such settings. Should not be used to diagnose benzodiazepine-induced sedation. Reverse neuromuscular blockade before considering use. Flumazenil does not antagonize the CNS effects of other GABA agonists (such as ethanol, barbiturates, or general anesthetics); nor does it reverse narcotics. Flumazenil does not consistently reverse amnesia; patient may not recall verbal instructions after procedure.

Use with caution in patients with a history of panic disorder; may provoke panic attacks. Use caution in drug and ethanol-dependent patients; these patients may also be dependent on benzodiazepines. Not recommended for treatment of benzodiazepine dependence. Use with caution in head injury patients. Use caution in patients with mixed drug overdoses; toxic effects of other drugs taken may emerge once benzodiazepine effects are reversed. Use caution in hepatic dysfunction and in patients relying on a benzodiazepine for seizure control. Safety and efficacy have not been established in children <1 year of age.

Drug Interactions

Avoid Concomitant Use There are no known interactions where it is recommended to avoid concomitant use.

Decreased Effect

Flumazenil may decrease the levels/effects of: Hypnotics (Nonbenzodiazepine)

Increased Effect/Toxicity There are no known significant interactions involving an increase in effect.

Adverse Reactions

>10%: Gastrointestinal: Vomiting, nausea

1% to 10%:

Cardiovascular: Vasodilation (1% to 3%), palpitation

Central nervous system: Dizziness (10%), agitation (3% to 9%), emotional lability (1% to 3%), fatigue (1% to 3%), headache (1% to 3%)

Gastrointestinal: Xerostomia

Local: Pain at injection site (3% to 9%)

Neuromuscular & skeletal: Tremor, weakness, paresthesia (1% to 3%)

Ocular: Abnormal vision, blurred vision (3% to 9%)

Respiratory: Dyspnea, hyperventilation (3% to 9%)

Miscellaneous: Diaphoresis

Pharmacodynamics/Kinetics

Onset of Action 1-3 minutes; 80% response within 3 minutes; Peak effect: 6-10 minutes

Duration of Action Resedation: ~1 hour; duration related to dose given and benzodiazepine plasma concentrations; reversal effects of flumazenil may wear off before effects of benzodiazepine

Protein Binding 40% to 50%

Half-Life Elimination Adults: Alpha: 7-15 minutes; Terminal: 41-79 minutes; Moderate hepatic dysfunction: 1.3 hours; Severe hepatic impairment: 2.4 hours

Metabolism Hepatic; dependent upon hepatic blood flow

Excretion Feces; urine (0.2% as unchanged drug)

Available Dosage Forms

Injection, solution: 0.1 mg/mL (5 mL, 10 mL)

Romazicon®: 0.1 mg/mL (5 mL, 10 mL)

Dosing

Adult See table.

Flumazenil

Adult dosage for **reversal of conscious sedation and general anesthesia:**	
Initial dose	0.2 mg intravenously over 15 seconds
Repeat doses (maximum: 4 doses)	If desired level of consciousness is not obtained, 0.2 mg may be repeated at 1-minute intervals.
Maximum total cumulative dose	1 mg (usual dose: 0.6-1 mg) **In the event of resedation:** Repeat doses may be given at 20-minute intervals with maximum of 1 mg/dose and 3 mg/hour.
Adult dosage for **suspected benzodiazepine overdose:**	
Initial dose	0.2 mg intravenously over 30 seconds; if the desired level of consciousness is not obtained, 0.3 mg can be given over 30 seconds
Repeat doses	0.5 mg over 30 seconds repeated at 1-minute intervals
Maximum total cumulative dose	3 mg (usual dose: 1-3 mg) Patients with a partial response at 3 mg may require additional titration up to a total dose of 5 mg. If a patient has not responded 5 minutes after cumulative dose of 5 mg, the major cause of sedation is not likely due to benzodiazepines. **In the event of resedation:** May repeat doses at 20-minute intervals with maximum of 1 mg/dose and 3 mg/hour.

Resedation: Repeated doses may be given at 20-minute intervals as needed; repeat treatment doses of 1 mg (at a rate of 0.5 mg/minute) should be given at any time and no more than 3 mg should be given in any hour. After intoxication with high doses of benzodiazepines, the duration of a single dose of flumazenil is not expected to exceed 1 hour; if desired, the period of wakefulness may be prolonged with repeated low intravenous doses of flumazenil, or by an infusion of 0.1-0.4 mg/hour. Most patients with benzodiazepine overdose will respond to a cumulative dose of 1-3 mg and doses >3 mg do not reliably produce additional effects. Rarely, patients with a partial response at 3 mg may require additional titration up to a total dose of 5 mg. **If a patient has not responded 5 minutes after receiving a cumulative dose of 5 mg, the major cause of sedation is not likely to be due to benzodiazepines.**

Geriatric Refer to adult dosing. No differences in safety or efficacy have been reported; however, increased sensitivity may occur in some elderly patients.

Pediatric

Reversal of benzodiazepine when used in conscious sedation or general anesthesia: I.V.: Initial dose: 0.01 mg/kg (maximum dose: 0.2 mg) given over 15 seconds; may repeat 0.01 mg/kg (maximum dose: 0.2 mg) after 45 seconds, and then every minute (maximum: 4 doses) to a maximum of total cumulative dose of 0.05 mg/kg or 1 mg, whichever is lower; usual total dose: 0.08-1 mg (mean: 0.65 mg).

Renal Impairment Not significantly affected by renal failure (Cl_{cr} <10 mL/minute) or hemodialysis beginning 1 hour after drug administration.

Hepatic Impairment Use caution with initial and/or repeat doses in patients with liver disease.

Administration

I.V. Administer in freely-running I.V. into large vein. Inject over 15 seconds for conscious sedation and general anesthesia and over 30 seconds for overdose.

Stability

Reconstitution For I.V. use only. Once drawn up in the syringe or mixed with solution use within 24 hours. Discard any unused solution after 24 hours.

Storage Store at 15°C to 30°C (59°F to 86°F).

Monitoring and Teaching Issues

Physical Assessment Assess level of consciousness frequently. Monitor vital signs and airway closely. Observe continually for resedation, respiratory depression, seizure activity, or other residual benzodiazepine effects.

Patient Education Flumazenil does not consistently reverse amnesia. Do not engage in activities requiring alertness for 18-24 hours after discharge. Avoid alcohol. Resedation may occur in patients on long-acting benzodiazepines.

Pregnancy Considerations Teratogenic effects were not seen in animal studies. Embryocidal effects were seen at large doses. There are no adequate or well-controlled studies in pregnant women. Use only if clearly needed.

◆ **FluMist®** *see* Influenza Virus Vaccine (Live/Attenuated) *on page 980*

Flunisolide (Oral Inhalation) (floo NISS oh lide)

U.S. Brand Names AeroBid® [DSC]; AeroBid®-M [DSC]

Generic Availability (U.S.) No

Pharmacologic Category Corticosteroid, Inhalant (Oral)

Medication Safety Issues

Sound-alike/look-alike issues:

Flunisolide may be confused with Flumadine®, fluocinonide

Pregnancy Risk Factor C

Lactation Excretion in breast milk unknown/use caution

Use Steroid-dependent asthma

Available Dosage Forms

Aerosol, for oral inhalation:

AeroBid®: 250 mcg/actuation (7 g)

AeroBid®-M: 250 mcg/actuation (7 g)

Dosing

Adult & Geriatric Asthma: Oral Inhalation (AeroBid®, AeroBid®-M): 2 inhalations twice daily (morning and evening); up to 8 inhalations/day maximum

NIH Asthma Guidelines (NIH, 2007) (administer in divided doses twice daily):

"Low" dose: 500-1000 mcg/day

"Medium" dose: >1000-2000 mcg/day

"High" dose: >2000 mcg/day

Pediatric Asthma: Oral Inhalation (AeroBid®, AeroBid®-M):

Children 6-15 years: 2 inhalations twice daily (morning and evening); up to 4 inhalations/day

Children ≥16 years and Adults: 2 inhalations twice daily (morning and evening); up to 8 inhalations/day maximum

NIH Asthma Guidelines (NIH, 2007) (administer in divided doses twice daily):

Children 5-11 years:

"Low" dose: 500-750 mcg/day

"Medium" dose: 1000-1250 mcg/day

"High" dose: >1250 mcg/day

Children ≥12 years: Refer to adult dosing.

Administration

Inhalation Aerosol inhalation: Shake well before using. Rinse mouth following use of oral inhalers. Prime inhaler before first use.

Monitoring and Teaching Issues

Physical Assessment Not to be used to treat status asthmaticus. When changing from systemic steroids to inhalational steroid, taper reduction of systemic medication slowly.

Patient Education This medication is not intended to treat an acute asthma attack. Full benefit of regular use may not be seen for 2-4 weeks. Review use of inhaler with prescriber. Keep oral inhaler clean. Always rinse mouth after use of inhaler to prevent infection. If you are also using an inhaled bronchodilator, wait 10 minutes before using this steroid aerosol. You may be susceptible to infections. Avoid measles and chickenpox. You may experience dizziness, anxiety, blurred vision, taste disturbance, or aftertaste. Report palpitations or chest pain; nervousness or inability to sleep; respiratory difficulty, sore throat, hoarseness, or bronchitis; vision changes; loss of taste or smell perception; or worsening of condition or lack of improvement.

Inhaler: Sit when using. Take deep breaths for 3-5 minutes and clear nasal passages before administration (use decongestant as needed). Hold breath for 5-10 seconds after use and wait 1-3 minutes between inhalations. If also using inhaled bronchodilator, use before flunisolide. Rinse mouth and throat after use to reduce aftertaste and prevent candidiasis.

Related Information

Asthma *on page 2015*

Flunisolide (Nasal) (floo NISS oh lide)

Generic Availability (U.S.) Yes

Pharmacologic Category Corticosteroid, Nasal

Medication Safety Issues

Sound-alike/look-alike issues:

Flunisolide may be confused with Flumadine®, fluocinonide

Nasarel may be confused with Nizoral®

Pregnancy Risk Factor C

Lactation Excretion in breast milk unknown/use caution

Use Seasonal or perennial rhinitis

Available Dosage Forms

Solution, intranasal: 25 mcg/actuation (25 mL); 29 mcg/actuation (25 mL)

Dosing

Adult & Geriatric Seasonal allergic rhinitis: Intranasal: 2 sprays each nostril twice daily (morning and evening); may increase to 2 sprays 3 times daily; maximum dose: 8 sprays/day in each nostril (400 mcg/day)

Pediatric Seasonal allergic rhinitis: Intranasal:

Children 6-14 years: 1 spray each nostril 3 times daily **or** 2 sprays in each nostril twice daily; not to exceed 4 sprays/day in each nostril

Children ≥15 years: Refer to adult dosing.

Administration

Inhalation Before first use, prime by pressing pump 5-6 times or until a fine spray appears. Repeat priming if ≥5 days between use, or if dissembled for cleaning. Administer at regular intervals. Blow nose to clear nostrils. Insert applicator into nostril, keeping bottle upright, and close off the other nostril. Breathe in through nose. While inhaling, press pump to release spray.

Monitoring and Teaching Issues

Patient Education Full benefit of regular use may not be seen for 2-4 weeks. Review use of spray with prescriber.

Fluocinolone (Otic) (floo oh SIN oh lone)

U.S. Brand Names DermOtic®

Index Terms Fluocinolone Acetonide

Generic Availability (U.S.) No

Pharmacologic Category Corticosteroid, Otic

Medication Safety Issues

Sound-alike/look-alike issues:

Fluocinolone may be confused with fluocinonide

Pregnancy Risk Factor C

Lactation Excretion in breast milk unknown/use caution

Use Relief of chronic eczematous external otitis

Available Dosage Forms

Oil, otic:

DermOtic®: 0.01% (20 mL)

Dosing

Adult & Geriatric Chronic eczematous external otitis: Otic: 5 drops into the affected ear twice daily for 1-2 weeks

Pediatric Chronic eczematous external otitis: Otic: Children ≥2 years: Refer to adult dosing.

Related Information

Corticosteroids *on page 1996*

Fluocinolone (Topical) (floo oh SIN oh lone)

U.S. Brand Names Capex®; Derma-Smoothe/FS®

Index Terms Fluocinolone Acetonide

Generic Availability (U.S.) Yes: Excludes oil, shampoo

Pharmacologic Category Corticosteroid, Topical

Medication Safety Issues

Sound-alike/look-alike issues:

Fluocinolone may be confused with fluocinonide

Pregnancy Risk Factor C

Lactation Excretion in breast milk unknown/use caution

Use Relief of susceptible inflammatory dermatosis [low, medium corticosteroid]; dermatitis or psoriasis of the scalp; atopic dermatitis in adults and children ≥3 months of age

Available Dosage Forms

Cream, topical: 0.01% (15 g, 60 g); 0.025% (15 g, 60 g)

Oil, topical:

Derma-Smoothe/FS®: 0.01% (120 mL)

Ointment, topical: 0.025% (15 g, 60 g)

Shampoo, topical:

Capex®: 0.01% (120 mL)

Solution, topical: 0.01% (60 mL)

Dosing

Adult & Geriatric

Atopic dermatitis (Derma-Smoothe/FS® body oil): Apply thin film to affected area 3 times/day

Corticosteroid-responsive dermatoses: Topical: Cream, ointment, solution: Apply a thin layer to affected area 2-4 times/day; may use occlusive dressings to manage psoriasis or recalcitrant conditions

Inflammatory and pruritic manifestations (dental use): Topical: Apply to oral lesion 4 times/day, after meals and at bedtime

Scalp psoriasis (Derma-Smoothe/FS® scalp oil): Topical: Massage thoroughly into wet or dampened hair/scalp; cover with shower cap. Leave on overnight (or for at least 4 hours). Remove by washing hair with shampoo and rinsing thoroughly.

Seborrheic dermatitis of the scalp (Capex®): Topical: Apply no more than 1 ounce to scalp once daily; work into lather and allow to remain on scalp for ~5 minutes. Remove from hair and scalp by rinsing thoroughly with water.

Pediatric

Atopic dermatitis: Topical: Children ≥3 months (Derma-Smoothe/FS® body oil): Moisten skin; apply a thin filn to affected area twice daily; do not use for longer than 4 weeks

Corticosteroid-responsive dermatoses: Topical: Refer to adult dosing.

Administration

Topical Apply thin film to affected area; avoid eyes.

Monitoring and Teaching Issues

Patient Education For external use only. Inform prescriber if you are allergic to peanuts. Do not use for eyes, mucous membranes, or open wounds. Before using, wash and dry area gently. Apply in a thin layer (may rub in lightly). Apply light dressing (if necessary) to area being treated. Do not use occlusive dressing unless so advised by prescriber. Avoid prolonged or excessive use around sensitive tissues or genital or rectal areas. Avoid exposing treated area to direct sunlight. Inform prescriber if condition worsens (redness, swelling, irritation, signs of infection, or open sores) or fails to improve after 2 weeks.

Related Information

Corticosteroids *on page* *1996*

◆ **Fluocinolone Acetonide** *see* Fluocinolone (Otic) *on page* *785*

◆ **Fluocinolone Acetonide** *see* Fluocinolone (Topical) *on page* *785*

Fluocinonide (floo oh SIN oh nide)

U.S. Brand Names Vanos™

Index Terms Lidex

Generic Availability (U.S.) Yes

Pharmacologic Category Corticosteroid, Topical

Medication Safety Issues

Sound-alike/look-alike issues:

Fluocinonide may be confused with flunisolide, fluocinolone

Lidex® may be confused with Lasix®, Videx®, Wydase®

Pregnancy Risk Factor C

Use Anti-inflammatory, antipruritic; treatment of plaque-type psoriasis (up to 10% of body surface area) [high-potency topical corticosteroid]

Available Dosage Forms

Cream, topical:

Vanos™: 0.1% (30 g, 60 g)

Cream, anhydrous, emollient, topical: 0.05% (15 g, 30 g, 60 g, 120 g)

Cream, aqueous, emollient, topical: 0.05% (15 g, 30 g, 60 g)

Gel, topical: 0.05% (15 g, 30 g, 60 g)

Ointment, topical: 0.05% (15 g, 30 g, 60 g)

Solution, topical: 0.05% (20 mL, 60 mL)

Dosing

Adult & Geriatric

Pruritus and inflammation: Topical (0.05% cream): Apply thin layer to affected area 2-4 times/day depending on the severity of the condition. Therapy should be discontinued when control is achieved; if no improvement is seen, reassessment of diagnosis may be necessary.

Plaque-type psoriasis (Vanos™): Topical (0.1% cream): Apply a thin layer once or twice daily to affected areas (limited to <10% of body surface area). **Note:** Not recommended for use >2 consecutive weeks or >60 g/week total exposure. Discontinue when control is achieved.

Pediatric

Pruritus and inflammation: Refer to adult dosing.

Plaque-type psoriasis: Children ≥12 years: Refer to adult dosing.

Monitoring and Teaching Issues

Patient Education For external use only. Do not use for eyes, mucous membranes, or open wounds. Before using, wash and dry area gently. Apply in a thin layer (may rub in lightly). Apply light dressing (if necessary) to area being treated. Do not use occlusive dressing unless so advised by prescriber. Avoid prolonged or excessive use around sensitive tissues or genital or rectal areas. Avoid exposing treated area to direct sunlight. Inform prescriber if condition worsens (redness, swelling, irritation, signs of infection, or open sores) or fails to improve.

Related Information

Corticosteroids *on page* *1996*

◆ **Fluohydrisone Acetate** *see* Fludrocortisone *on page* *780*

◆ **Fluohydrocortisone Acetate** *see* Fludrocortisone *on page* *780*

◆ **5-Fluorocytosine** *see* Flucytosine *on page* *775*

◆ **Fluorodeoxyuridine** *see* Floxuridine *on page* *770*

◆ **9α-Fluorohydrocortisone Acetate** *see* Fludrocortisone *on page* *780*

Fluorometholone (flure oh METH oh lone)

U.S. Brand Names Flarex®; FML Forte®; FML®

Generic Availability (U.S.) Yes: Suspension (as base)

Pharmacologic Category Corticosteroid, Ophthalmic

Medication Safety Issues

International issues:

Flarex [U.S., Canada, and multiple international markets] may be confused with Fluarix brand name for influenza virus vaccine (inactivated) [U.S. and multiple international markets] and Fluorex brand name for fluoride [France]

Pregnancy Risk Factor C

Lactation Excretion in breast milk unknown/use caution

Use Treatment of steroid-responsive inflammatory conditions of the eye

Available Dosage Forms

Ointment, ophthalmic:

FML®: 0.1% (3.5 g)

Suspension, ophthalmic: 0.1% (5 mL, 10 mL, 15 mL)

Flarex®: 0.1% (5 mL)

FML Forte®: 0.25% (5 mL, 10 mL)

FML®: 0.1% (5 mL, 10 mL, 15 mL)

Dosing

Adult & Geriatric Ocular inflammation: Ophthalmic:

Ointment (FML®): Apply small amount (~1/2 inch ribbon) to conjunctival sac 1-3 times/day; may increase application to every 4 hours during the initial 24-48 hours

Suspension:

FML®: Instill 1 drop into conjunctival sac 2-4 times/day; may instill 1 drop every 4 hours during initial 24-48 hours

FML® Forte: Instill 1 drop into conjunctival sac 2-4 times/day

Flarex®: Instill 1-2 drops into conjunctival sac 4 times/day; may increase application to 2 drops every 2 hours during initial 24-48 hours. Consult prescriber if no improvement after 14 days.

Note: Re-evaluate therapy if improvement is not seen within 2 days; use care not to discontinue prematurely; in chronic conditions, gradually decrease dosing frequency prior to discontinuing treatment.

Pediatric Children >2 years: Refer to adult dosing.

Administration

Other Contact lenses should be removed before instillation. Shake suspension well before use.

Monitoring and Teaching Issues

Physical Assessment Monitor intraocular pressure in patients with glaucoma or when used for ≥10 days; monitor for presence of secondary infections (including the development of fungal infections and exacerbation of viral infections).

Patient Education For ophthalmic use only. Wash hands before using. Wipe away excess from skin around eye. Do not use any other eye preparation for at least 10 minutes. Do not touch tip of applicator to eye or any other surface. May cause sensitivity to bright light; temporary stinging or blurred vision may occur. Do not wear contacts during administration and for 15 minutes after. Inform prescriber if you experience eye pain, redness, burning, watering, dryness, double vision, puffiness around eye, vision changes, worsening of condition, or lack of improvement.

Ointment: Gently squeeze the tube to apply to inside of lower lid. Close eye for 1-2 minutes and roll eyeball in all directions.

Suspension: Shake well before using. Tilt head back and look upward. Gently pull down lower lid and put drop(s) in inner corner of eye. Close eye and roll eyeball in all directions. Do not blink for 30 seconds. Apply gentle pressure to inner corner of eye for 30 seconds.

◆ **5-Fluorouracil** *see* Fluorouracil (Systemic) *on page* *787*

Fluorouracil (Systemic) (flure oh YOOR a sil)

U.S. Brand Names Adrucil®

Index Terms 5-Fluorouracil; 5-FU; FU

Generic Availability (U.S.) Yes

Pharmacologic Category Antineoplastic Agent, Antimetabolite (Pyrimidine Analog)

Medication Safety Issues

Sound-alike/look-alike issues:

Fluorouracil may be confused with flucytosine

High alert medication: This medication is in a class the Institute for Safe Medication Practices (ISMP) includes among its list of drugs which have a heightened risk of causing significant patient harm when used in error.

Pregnancy Risk Factor D

Lactation Excretion in breast milk unknown/not recommended

Use Treatment of carcinomas of the breast, colon, rectum, pancreas, or stomach

Unlabeled/Investigational Use Treatment of head and neck cancer, esophageal cancer, anal cancer, cervical cancer, bladder cancer, renal cell cancer, and unknown primary cancer

Mechanism of Action/Effect Interferes with DNA synthesis by blocking the methylation of deoxyuricytic acid.

Contraindications Hypersensitivity to fluorouracil or any component of the formulation; poor nutritional states; depressed bone marrow function; potentially serious infections

Warnings/Precautions Hazardous agent - use appropriate precautions for handling and disposal. Use with caution in patients with impaired kidney or liver function. The drug should be discontinued if intractable vomiting or diarrhea, precipitous falls in leukocyte or platelet counts, gastrointestinal ulcer or bleeding, stomatitis, or esophagopharyngitis, hemorrhage, or myocardial ischemia occurs. Use with caution in patients who have had high-dose pelvic radiation or previous use of alkylating agents. Palmar-plantar erythrodysesthesia (hand-foot) syndrome has been associated with use.

Administration to patients with a genetic deficiency of dihydropyrimidine dehydrogenase (DPD) has been associated with prolonged clearance and increased toxicity following administration (diarrhea, neutropenia, and neurotoxicity); rechallenge has resulted in recurrent toxicity (despite dose reduction). **[U.S. Boxed Warning]: Should be administered under the supervision of an experienced cancer chemotherapy physician.**

Drug Interactions

Metabolism/Transport Effects Inhibits CYP2C9 (strong)

Avoid Concomitant Use

Avoid concomitant use of Fluorouracil (Systemic) with any of the following: BCG; Natalizumab; Pimecrolimus; Roflumilast; Tacrolimus (Topical); Vaccines (Live)

Decreased Effect

Fluorouracil (Systemic) may decrease the levels/effects of: BCG; Sipuleucel-T; Vaccines (Inactivated); Vaccines (Live); Vitamin K Antagonists

The levels/effects of Fluorouracil (Systemic) may be decreased by: Echinacea; SORAfenib

Increased Effect/Toxicity

Fluorouracil (Systemic) may increase the levels/effects of: Carvedilol; CYP2C9 Substrates (High risk); Leflunomide; Natalizumab; Phenytoin; Vaccines (Live); Vitamin K Antagonists

The levels/effects of Fluorouracil (Systemic) may be increased by: Denosumab; Gemcitabine; Leucovorin Calcium-Levoleucovorin; Pimecrolimus; Roflumilast; SORAfenib; Tacrolimus (Topical); Trastuzumab

Nutritional/Ethanol Interactions

Ethanol: Avoid ethanol (due to GI irritation).

Herb/Nutraceutical: Avoid black cohosh, dong quai in estrogen-dependent tumors.

Adverse Reactions Toxicity depends on duration of treatment

Cardiovascular: Angina, myocardial ischemia, nail changes

Central nervous system: Acute cerebellar syndrome, confusion, disorientation, euphoria, headache, nystagmus

Dermatologic: Alopecia, dermatitis, dry skin, fissuring, palmar-plantar erythrodysesthesia syndrome, pruritic maculopapular rash, photosensitivity, vein pigmentations

Gastrointestinal: Anorexia, bleeding, diarrhea, esophagopharyngitis, nausea, sloughing, stomatitis, ulceration, vomiting

Hematologic: Myelosuppression (nadir: 9-14 days; recovery by day 30), agranulocytosis, anemia, leukopenia, pancytopenia, thrombocytopenia

Local: Thrombophlebitis

Ocular: Lacrimation, lacrimal duct stenosis, photophobia, visual changes

Respiratory: Epistaxis

Miscellaneous: Anaphylaxis, generalized allergic reactions, nail loss

Pharmacodynamics/Kinetics

Duration of Action ~3 weeks

Half-Life Elimination Biphasic: Initial: 6-20 minutes; two metabolites, FdUMP and FUTP, have prolonged half-lives depending on the type of tissue

Metabolism Hepatic (90%) via dehydrogenase enzyme; FU must be metabolized to be active

Excretion Lung (large amounts as CO_2); urine (5% as unchanged drug) in 6 hours

Available Dosage Forms

Injection, solution: 50 mg/mL (10 mL, 20 mL, 50 mL, 100 mL)

Adrucil®: 50 mg/mL (10 mL, 50 mL, 100 mL)

Dosing

Adult & Geriatric Details concerning dosing in combination regimens should be consulted.

I.V. bolus:

500 mg/m^2 once weekly **or**
500-600 mg/m^2 every 3 weeks **or**
500-600 mg/m^2/dose days 1 and 8 every 4 weeks **or**
500 mg/m^2/dose days 1 and 8 every 3 weeks **or**
500 mg/m^2/dose days 1 and 4 every 3 weeks **or**
500 mg/m^2/dose days 1, 8, 15, 22, 29, and 36 of an 8-week treatment cycle **or**
425 mg/m^2 on days 1-5 every 4 weeks

Continuous I.V. infusion:

500-750 mg/m^2/day for 5 days every 3 weeks **or**
1000 mg/m^2/day for 4-5 days every 3-4 weeks **or**
2600 mg/m^2 on day 1 every week **or**
1600 mg/m^2/day for 2 days every 2 weeks **or**
400 mg/m^2 bolus followed by 1200 mg/m^2/day for 2 days every 2 weeks **or**
200 mg/m^2/day for 21 days; can repeat 21-day cycle up to 8 cycles

Renal Impairment The FDA-approved labeling does not contain specific dosing adjustment guidelines; however, it is stated that extreme caution should be used in patients with renal impairment.

Hemodialysis: Administer dose following hemodialysis.

Aronoff, 2007: Recommends that dosage adjustment is not needed in adult patients with Cl_{cr} <50 mL/minute and patients receiving hemodialysis should be administered 50% of dose.

Hepatic Impairment The FDA-approved labeling does not contain specific dosing adjustment guidelines; however, it is stated that extreme caution should be used in patients with hepatic impairment. The following guidelines have been used by some clinicians:

Floyd, 2006: Bilirubin >5 mg/dL: Avoid use.

Koren, 1992: Hepatic impairment (degree not specified): Administer <50% of dose, then increase if toxicity does not occur.

Administration

I.V. Irritant. Direct I.V. push injection (50 mg/mL solution needs no further dilution) or by I.V. infusion. Doses >1000 mg/m^2 are usually administered as a 24-hour infusion, although some protocols may be continuous infusion with lower doses. Toxicity may be reduced by giving the drug as a constant infusion. Bolus doses may be administered by slow IVP or IVPB.

Stability

Reconstitution Dilute in 50-1000 mL NS, D_5W, or bacteriostatic NS for infusion.

Storage Store intact vials at room temperature. Protect from light. Slight discoloration does not usually denote decomposition. If exposed to cold, a precipitate may form; **gentle** heating to 60°C will dissolve the precipitate without impairing the potency. Solutions in 50-1000 mL NS or D_5W, or undiluted solutions in syringes are stable for 72 hours at room temperature.

Monitoring and Teaching Issues

Laboratory Monitoring CBC with differential, platelet count, renal and liver function

Physical Assessment Assess cardiovascular, respiratory, and renal function prior to each infusion and on a regular basis. Inform prescriber if intractable vomiting or diarrhea, precipitous fall in leukocyte or platelet counts, or myocardial ischemia occurs (drug may be discontinued). Teach patient proper use of oral solution (rinse mouth thoroughly) and importance of adequate hydration.

Patient Education Avoid excessive alcohol (may increase gastrointestinal irritation). Maintain adequate nutrition and hydration, unless instructed to restrict fluid intake. May cause sensitivity to sunlight, susceptibility to infection, nausea, vomiting, diarrhea, loss of appetite, weakness, lethargy, dizziness, decreased vision, or headache. Report signs and symptoms of infection (eg, fever, chills, sore throat, burning urination, vaginal itching or discharge, fatigue, mouth sores); bleeding (eg, black or tarry stools, easy bruising, unusual bleeding); vision changes; unremitting nausea, vomiting, or abdominal pain; CNS changes; respiratory difficulty; or chest pain or palpitations.

Oral solution: May be mixed in water, grape juice, or carbonated beverage. It is generally best to drink undiluted solution, then rinse mouth thoroughly. CocaCola® has been recommended as the best rinse following oral fluorouracil.

Dietary Considerations Increase dietary intake of thiamine.

Pregnancy Considerations Teratogenic effects have been observed with parenteral administration in animal studies; fetal defects and miscarriages have been reported following use of intravenous products in humans.

Additional Information Oncology Comment: An investigational uridine prodrug, uridine triacetate (formerly called vistonuridine), has been studied in a limited number of cases of fluorouracil overdose. Of 17 patients receiving uridine triacetate beginning within 8-96 hours after fluorouracil overdose, all patients fully recovered (von Borstel, 2009). Updated data has described a total of 28 patients treated with uridine triacetate for fluorouracil overdose (including overdoses related to continuous infusions delivering fluorouracil at rates faster than prescribed), all of whom recovered fully (Bamat, 2010).

FLUoxetine (floo OKS e teen)

U.S. Brand Names PROzac®; PROzac® Weekly™; Sarafem®; Selfemra® [DSC]

Index Terms Fluoxetine Hydrochloride

Generic Availability (U.S.) Yes

Pharmacologic Category Antidepressant, Selective Serotonin Reuptake Inhibitor

Medication Safety Issues

Sound-alike/look-alike issues:

FLUoxetine may be confused with DULoxetine, famotidine, Feldene®, fluconazole, fluvastatin, fluvoxaMINE, fosinopril, furosemide, PARoxetine, thiothixene

PROzac® may be confused with Paxil®, Prelone®, PriLOSEC®, Prograf®, Proscar®, ProSom®, ProStep®, Provera®

Sarafem® may be confused with Serophene®

Beers Criteria medication: This drug may be inappropriate for use in geriatric patients (high severity risk).

International issues:

Reneuron [Spain] may be confused with Remeron brand name for mirtazapine [U.S., Canada, and multiple international markets]

Medication Guide Available Yes

Pregnancy Risk Factor C

Lactation Enters breast milk/not recommended (AAP rates "of concern"; AAP 2001 update pending)

Use Treatment of major depressive disorder (MDD); treatment of binge-eating and vomiting in patients with moderate-to-severe bulimia nervosa; obsessive-compulsive disorder (OCD); premenstrual dysphoric disorder (PMDD); panic disorder with or without agoraphobia; in combination with olanzapine for treatment-resistant or bipolar I depression

Unlabeled/Investigational Use Selective mutism; treatment of mild dementia-associated agitation in nonpsychotic patients; post-traumatic stress disorder (PTSD); social anxiety disorder; chronic neuropathic pain, fibromyalgia; Raynaud's phenomenon

Mechanism of Action/Effect Inhibits CNS neuron serotonin reuptake; minimal or no effect on reuptake of norepinephrine or dopamine; does not significantly bind to alpha-adrenergic, histamine or cholinergic receptors

Contraindications Hypersensitivity to fluoxetine or any component of the formulation; patients currently receiving MAO inhibitors, pimozide, or thioridazine

Note: MAO inhibitor therapy must be stopped for 14 days before fluoxetine is initiated. Treatment with MAO inhibitors or thioridazine should not be initiated until 5 weeks after the discontinuation of fluoxetine.

Warnings/Precautions [U.S. Boxed Warning]: Antidepressants increase the risk of suicidal thinking and behavior in children, adolescents, and young adults (18-24 years of age) with major depressive disorder (MDD) and other psychiatric disorders; consider risk prior to prescribing. Short-term studies did not show an increased risk in patients >24 years of age and showed a decreased risk in patients ≥65 years. Closely monitor patients for clinical worsening, suicidality, or unusual changes in behavior, particularly during the initial 1-2 months of therapy or during periods of dosage adjustments (increases or decreases); the patient's family or caregiver should be instructed to closely observe the patient and communicate condition with healthcare provider. A medication guide concerning the use of antidepressants should be dispensed with each prescription. **Fluoxetine is FDA approved for the treatment of OCD in children ≥7 years of age and MDD in children ≥8 years of age.**

The possibility of a suicide attempt is inherent in major depression and may persist until remission occurs. Use caution in high-risk patients. Worsening depression and severe abrupt suicidality that are not part of the presenting symptoms may require discontinuation or modification of drug therapy. The patient's family or caregiver should be alerted to monitor patients for the emergence of suicidality and associated behaviors (such as agitation, irritability, hostility, impulsivity, and hypomania) and call healthcare provider.

May worsen psychosis in some patients or precipitate a shift to mania or hypomania in patients with bipolar disorder. Patients presenting with depressive symptoms should be screened for bipolar disorder. Monotherapy in patients with bipolar disorder should be avoided. **Fluoxetine monotherapy is not FDA approved for the treatment of bipolar depression.** May cause insomnia, anxiety, nervousness, or anorexia. Use with caution in patients where weight loss is undesirable. May impair cognitive or motor performance; caution operating hazardous machinery or driving.

Serotonin syndrome and neuroleptic malignant syndrome (NMS)-like reactions have occurred with serotonin/norepinephrine reuptake inhibitors (SNRIs) and selective serotonin reuptake inhibitors (SSRIs) when used alone, and particularly when used in combination with serotonergic agents (eg, triptans) or antidopaminergic agents (eg, antipsychotics). Concurrent use with MAO inhibitors is contraindicated. Fluoxetine may elevate plasma levels of thioridazine or pimozide and increase the risk of QT_c interval prolongation. This may lead to serious ventricular arrhythmias, such as torsade de pointes-type arrhythmias, and sudden death. Fluoxetine use has been associated with occurrences of significant rash and allergic events, including vasculitis, lupus-like syndrome, laryngospasm, anaphylactoid reactions, and pulmonary inflammatory disease. Discontinue if underlying cause of rash cannot be identified.

Use caution in patients with a previous seizure disorder or condition predisposing to seizures such as brain damage, alcoholism, or concurrent therapy with other drugs which lower the seizure threshold. Use with caution in patients with hepatic or severe renal dysfunction and in elderly patients. Fluoxetine (daily) may be inappropriate for use in the elderly due to risk of agitation, sleep disturbances, and excessive CNS stimulation, attributed to this drug's long half-life (Beers Criteria). May cause hyponatremia/SIADH (elderly at increased risk); volume depletion (diuretics may increase risk). May increase the risks associated with electroconvulsive treatment. Use caution with concomitant use of NSAIDs, ASA, or other drugs that affect coagulation; the risk of bleeding may be potentiated. Use caution with history of MI or unstable heart disease; use in these patients is limited. May alter glycemic control in patients with diabetes. Due to the long half-life of fluoxetine and its metabolites, the effects and interactions noted may persist for prolonged periods following discontinuation. May cause or exacerbate sexual dysfunction. Discontinuation symptoms (eg, dysphoric mood, irritability, agitation, confusion, anxiety, insomnia, hypomania) may occur upon abrupt discontinuation. Taper dose when discontinuing therapy.

Drug Interactions

Metabolism/Transport Effects Substrate of CYP1A2 (minor), 2B6 (minor), 2C9 (major), 2C19 (minor), 2D6 (major), 2E1 (minor), 3A4 (minor); **Inhibits** CYP1A2 (moderate), 2B6 (weak), 2C9 (weak), 2C19 (moderate), 2D6 (strong), 3A4 (weak)

Avoid Concomitant Use

Avoid concomitant use of FLUoxetine with any of the following: Artemether; Clopidogrel; Dronedarone; Iobenguane I 123; Lumefantrine; MAO Inhibitors; Methylene Blue; Nilotinib; Pimozide; QuiNINE; Sibutramine; Tamoxifen; Tetrabenazine; Thioridazine; Toremifene; Tryptophan; Vandetanib; Ziprasidone

Decreased Effect

FLUoxetine may decrease the levels/effects of: Clopidogrel; Iobenguane I 123

The levels/effects of FLUoxetine may be decreased by: CarBAMazepine; CYP2C9 Inducers (Highly Effective); Cyproheptadine; Peginterferon Alfa-2b

Increased Effect/Toxicity

FLUoxetine may increase the levels/effects of: Alcohol (Ethyl); Alpha-/Beta-Blockers; Anticoagulants; Antidepressants (Serotonin Reuptake Inhibitor/Antagonist); Antiplatelet Agents; Aspirin; Atomoxetine; Benzodiazepines (metabolized by oxidation); Beta-Blockers; BusPIRone; CarBAMazepine; CloZAPine; CNS Depressants; Collagenase (Systemic); CYP1A2 Substrates; CYP2C19 Substrates; CYP2D6 Substrates; Desmopressin; Dextromethorphan; Dronedarone; Drotrecogin Alfa; Fesoterodine; Galantamine; Haloperidol; Ibritumomab; Lithium; Methadone; Methylene Blue; Mexiletine; NSAID (COX-2 Inhibitor); NSAID (Nonselective); Phenytoin; Pimozide; Propafenone; QTc-Prolonging Agents; QuiNIDine; QuiNINE; RisperiDONE; Salicylates; Serotonin Modulators; Tamoxifen; Tetrabenazine; Thioridazine; Thrombolytic Agents; Toremifene; Tositumomab and Iodine I 131 Tositumomab; TraMADol; Tricyclic Antidepressants; Vandetanib; Vitamin K Antagonists; Ziprasidone

The levels/effects of FLUoxetine may be increased by: Alfuzosin; Analgesics (Opioid); Artemether; BusPIRone; Chloroquine; Cimetidine; Ciprofloxacin; Ciprofloxacin (Systemic); Conivaptan; CYP2C9 Inhibitors (Moderate); CYP2C9 Inhibitors (Strong); CYP2D6 Inhibitors (Moderate); CYP2D6 Inhibitors (Strong); Darunavir; Gadobutrol; Glucosamine; Herbs (Anticoagulant/Antiplatelet Properties); Lumefantrine; Macrolide Antibiotics; MAO Inhibitors; Metoclopramide; Nilotinib; Omega-3-Acid Ethyl Esters; Pentosan Polysulfate Sodium; Pentoxifylline; Prostacyclin Analogues; QuiNINE; Sibutramine; TraMADol; Tryptophan

Nutritional/Ethanol Interactions

Ethanol: Avoid ethanol (may increase CNS depression). Depressed patients should avoid/limit intake.

Herb/Nutraceutical: Avoid valerian, St John's wort, kava kava, gotu kola (may increase CNS depression).

Lab Interactions Increased albumin in urine

Adverse Reactions Percentages listed for adverse effects as reported in placebo-controlled trials and were generally similar in adults and children; actual frequency may be dependent upon diagnosis and in some cases the range presented may be lower than or equal to placebo for a particular disorder.

>10%:

- Central nervous system: Insomnia (10% to 33%), headache (21%), somnolence (5% to 17%), anxiety (6% to 15%), nervousness (8% to 14%)
- Endocrine & metabolic: Libido decreased (1% to 11%)
- Gastrointestinal: Nausea (12% to 29%), diarrhea (8% to 18%), anorexia (4% to 17%), xerostomia (4% to 12%)
- Neuromuscular & skeletal: Weakness (7% to 21%), tremor (3% to 13%)
- Respiratory: Pharyngitis (3% to 11%), yawn (≤11%)

1% to 10%:

- Cardiovascular: Vasodilation (1% to 5%), chest pain, hemorrhage, hypertension, palpitation
- Central nervous system: Dizziness (9%), abnormal dreams (1% to 5%), abnormal thinking (2%), agitation, amnesia, chills, confusion, emotional lability, sleep disorder
- Dermatologic: Rash (2% to 6%), pruritus (4%)
- Endocrine & metabolic: Ejaculation abnormal (≤7%), impotence (≤7%), menorrhagia (≥2%)
- Gastrointestinal: Dyspepsia (6% to 10%), constipation (5%), flatulence (3%), vomiting (3%), thirst (≥2%), weight loss (2%), appetite increased, taste perversion, weight gain
- Genitourinary: Urinary frequency
- Neuromuscular & skeletal: Hyperkinesia (≥2%)
- Ocular: Vision abnormal (2%)
- Otic: Ear pain, tinnitus
- Respiratory: Sinusitis (1% to 6%)
- Miscellaneous: Flu-like syndrome (3% to 10%), diaphoresis (2% to 8%), epistaxis (≥2%)

Pharmacodynamics/Kinetics

Onset of Action Depression: The onset of action is within a week; however, individual response varies greatly and full response may not be seen until 8-12 weeks after initiation of treatment.

Absorption Well absorbed; delayed 1-2 hours with weekly formulation

Time to Peak Serum: 6-8 hours

Protein Binding 95% to albumin and alpha$_1$ glycoprotein

Half-Life Elimination Adults: Parent drug: 1-3 days (acute), 4-6 days (chronic), 7.6 days (cirrhosis); Metabolite (norfluoxetine): 9.3 days (range: 4-16 days), 12 days (cirrhosis)

Metabolism Hepatic, via CYP2C19 and 2D6, to norfluoxetine (activity equal to fluoxetine)

Excretion Urine (10% as norfluoxetine, 2.5% to 5% as fluoxetine)

Pharmacokinetic Note The once-weekly formulation results in greater fluctuations between peak and trough concentrations of fluoxetine and norfluoxetine compared to once-daily dosing (24% daily/164% weekly; 17% daily/43% weekly, respectively). Trough concentrations are 76% lower for fluoxetine and 47% lower for norfluoxetine than the concentrations maintained by 20 mg once-daily dosing. Steady-state fluoxetine concentrations are ~50% lower following the once-weekly regimen compared to 20 mg once daily. Average steady-state concentrations of once-daily dosing were highest in children ages 6 to <13 (fluoxetine 171 ng/mL; norfluoxetine 195 ng/mL), followed by adolescents ages 13 to <18 (fluoxetine 86 ng/mL; norfluoxetine 113 ng/mL); concentrations were considered to be within the ranges reported in adults (fluoxetine 91-302 ng/mL; norfluoxetine 72-258 ng/mL).

Available Dosage Forms

Capsule, oral: 10 mg, 20 mg, 40 mg
PROzac®: 10 mg, 20 mg, 40 mg

Capsule, delayed release, enteric coated pellets, oral: 90 mg
PROzac® Weekly™: 90 mg

Solution, oral: 20 mg/5 mL (5 mL, 120 mL)

Tablet, oral: 10 mg, 20 mg
Sarafem®: 10 mg, 15 mg, 20 mg

Dosing

Adult

Depression, obsessive-compulsive disorder, premenstrual dysphoric disorder, bulimia: Oral: 20 mg/day in the morning; may increase after several weeks by 20 mg/day increments; maximum: 80 mg/day; doses >20 mg may be given once daily or divided twice daily. **Note:** Lower doses of 5-10 mg/day have been used for initial treatment.

Usual dosage range:

Bulimia nervosa: Oral:60 mg/day

Depression: Oral: Initial: 20 mg/day; may increase after several weeks if inadequate response (maximum: 80 mg/day). Patients maintained on Prozac® 20 mg/day may be changed to Prozac® Weekly™ 90 mg/week, starting dose 7 days after the last 20 mg/day dose

Depression associated with bipolar disorder (in combination with olanzapine): Oral: Initial: 20 mg in the evening; adjust as tolerated to usual range of 20-50 mg/day. See **"Note"** below.

Fibromyalgia (unlabeled use): Oral: Range: 20-80 mg/day (Arnold, 2002)

Obsessive-compulsive disorder: Oral: Initial: 20 mg/day; may increase after several weeks if inadequate response; recommended range: 20-60 mg/day (maximum: 80 mg/day)

Panic disorder: Oral: Initial: 10 mg/day; after 1 week, increase to 20 mg/day; may increase after several weeks; doses >60 mg/day have not been evaluated

Post-traumatic stress disorder (PTSD) (unlabeled use): Oral: 20-40 mg/day

Premenstrual dysphoric disorder (Sarafem®): Oral: 20 mg/day continuously, **or** 20 mg/day starting 14 days prior to menstruation and through first full day of menses (repeat with each cycle)

Raynaud's phenomena (unlabeled use): Oral: 20 mg/day (Coleiro, 2001)

Social anxiety disorder (unlabeled use): Oral: Target dose: 40 mg/day; range 30-60 mg/day (Davidson, 2004)

Treatment-resistant depression (in combination with olanzapine): Oral: Initial: 20 mg in the evening; adjust as tolerated to usual range of 20-50 mg/day. See **"Note."**

Note: When using individual components of fluoxetine with olanzapine rather than fixed dose combination product (Symbyax®), approximate dosage correspondence is as follows:
Olanzapine 2.5 mg + fluoxetine 20 mg = Symbyax® 3/25
Olanzapine 5 mg + fluoxetine 20 mg = Symbyax® 6/25
Olanzapine 12.5 mg + fluoxetine 20 mg = Symbyax® 12/25
Olanzapine 5 mg + fluoxetine 50 mg = Symbyax® 6/50
Olanzapine 12.5 mg + fluoxetine 50 mg = Symbyax® 12/50

Note: Upon discontinuation of fluoxetine therapy, gradually taper dose. If intolerable symptoms occur following a dose reduction, consider resuming the previously prescribed dose and/or decrease dose at a more gradual rate.

Geriatric Oral: Some patients may require an initial dose of 10 mg/day with dosage increases of 10 mg and 20 mg every several weeks as tolerated; should not be taken at night unless patient experiences sedation.

Pediatric

Depression: Oral: 8-18 years: 10-20 mg/day; lower-weight children can be started at 10 mg/day, may increase to 20 mg/day after 1 week if needed

Obsessive-compulsive disorder: Oral: 7-17 years: Initial: 10 mg/day; may increase after 2 weeks if inadequate clinical response to 20 mg/day; further increases may be considered after several weeks to recommended range of 20-30 mg/day (lower weight children) or 20-60 mg/day (adolescents and higher weight children)

Selective mutism (unlabeled use): Oral: 5-18 years: Initial: 5-10 mg/day; titrate upwards as needed (usual maximum dose: 60 mg/day)

Note: Upon discontinuation of fluoxetine therapy, gradually taper dose. If intolerable symptoms occur following a dose reduction, consider resuming the previously prescribed dose and/or decrease dose at a more gradual rate.

Renal Impairment

Single dose studies: Pharmacokinetics of fluoxetine and norfluoxetine were similar among subjects with all levels of impaired renal function, including anephric patients on chronic hemodialysis.

Chronic administration: Additional accumulation of fluoxetine or norfluoxetine may occur in patients with severely impaired renal function.

Not removed by hemodialysis; use of lower dose or less frequent dosing is not usually necessary.

Hepatic Impairment Elimination half-life of fluoxetine is prolonged in patients with hepatic impairment. A lower dose or less frequent dosing of fluoxetine should be used in these patients.

Cirrhosis patient: Administer a lower dose or less frequent dosing interval.

Compensated cirrhosis without ascites: Administer 50% of normal dose.

Administration

Oral Administer without regard to meals.

Bipolar I disorder and treatment-resistant depression: Take once daily in the evening.

Major depressive disorder and obsessive compulsive disorder: Once daily doses should be taken in the morning, or twice daily (morning and noon).

Bulimia: Take once daily in the morning.

Stability

Storage All dosage forms should be stored at controlled room temperature of 15°C to 30°C (50°F to 86°F). Oral liquid should be dispensed in a light-resistant container.

Monitoring and Teaching Issues

Laboratory Monitoring Blood glucose (for diabetic patients), baseline liver function before beginning drug therapy

Physical Assessment Taper dosage slowly when discontinuing. Assess mental status for depression, signs of clinical worsening, suicide ideation, anxiety, social functioning, mania, or panic attack.

Patient Education It may take 2-3 weeks to achieve desired results. Take once-a-day dose in the morning to reduce incidence of insomnia. Avoid alcohol. Maintain adequate hydration, unless instructed to restrict fluid intake. You may experience drowsiness, lightheadedness, weakness, impaired coordination, dizziness, blurred vision, constipation, anorexia, or postural hypotension. Report persistent CNS effects (nervousness, restlessness, insomnia, anxiety, excitation, headache, sedation); suicide ideation; rash or skin irritation; muscle cramping, tremors, or change in gait; respiratory depression or respiratory difficulty; or worsening of condition.

Dietary Considerations May be taken without regard to meals.

Geriatric Considerations Fluoxetine's favorable side effect profile makes it a useful alternative to the traditional tricyclic antidepressants. Its potential stimulating and anorexic effects may be bothersome to some patients and has not been shown to be superior in efficacy to the traditional tricyclic antidepressants or other SSRIs. The long half-life in the elderly makes it less attractive compared to other SSRIs. Data from a clinical trial comparing fluoxetine to tricyclics suggest that fluoxetine is significantly less effective than nortriptyline in hospitalized elderly patients with unipolar major affective disorder, especially those with melancholia and concurrent cardiovascular diseases. The elderly are more prone to SSRI/SNRI-induced hyponatremia.

Daily fluoxetine is considered to be potentially inappropriate in this patient population (Beers Criteria severity: High).

Breast-Feeding Considerations Fluoxetine and its metabolite are excreted into breast milk and can be detected in the serum of breast-feeding infants. Concentrations in breast milk are variable. Colic, irritability, slow weight gain, and feeding and sleep disorders have been reported in nursing infants. Breast-feeding is not recommended by the manufacturer.

Because the long-term effects on development and behavior have not been studied and adverse effects have been noted in some infants exposed, one should prescribe fluoxetine to a mother who is breast-feeding only when the benefits outweigh the potential risks.

Pregnancy Considerations Due to adverse effects observed in animal studies, fluoxetine is classified as pregnancy category C. Fluoxetine and its metabolite cross the human placenta. Nonteratogenic effects in the newborn following SSRIs exposure late in the third trimester include respiratory distress, cyanosis, apnea, seizures, temperature instability, feeding difficulty, vomiting, hypoglycemia, hypo- or hypertonia, hyper-reflexia, jitteriness, irritability, constant crying, and tremor. An increased risk of low birth weight, lower APGAR scores, and blunted behavioral response to pain for a prolonged period after delivery have also been reported. Exposure to SSRIs after the twentieth week of gestation has been associated with persistent pulmonary hypertension of the newborn (PPHN). Adverse effects may be due to toxic effects of the SSRI or drug withdrawal without a taper. The long term effects of *in utero* SSRI exposure on infant development and behavior are not known.

Due to pregnancy-induced physiologic changes, women who are pregnant may require increased doses of fluoxetine to achieve euthymia. Women treated for major depression and who are euthymic prior to pregnancy are more likely to experience a relapse when medication is discontinued as compared to pregnant women who continue taking antidepressant medications. The ACOG recommends that therapy with SSRIs or SNRIs during pregnancy be individualized; treatment of depression during pregnancy should incorporate the clinical expertise of the mental health clinician, obstetrician, primary healthcare provider, and pediatrician. If treatment during pregnancy is required, consider tapering therapy during the third trimester in order to prevent withdrawal symptoms in the infant. If this is done and the woman is considered to be at risk of relapse from her major depressive disorder, the medication can be restarted following delivery, although the dose should be readjusted to that required before pregnancy. Treatment algorithms have been developed by the ACOG and the APA for the management of depression in women prior to conception and during pregnancy (Yonkers, 2009).

Additional Information ECG may reveal S-T segment depression. Not shown to be teratogenic in rodents; 15-60 mg/day, buspirone and cyproheptadine, may be useful in treatment of sexual dysfunction during treatment with a selective serotonin reuptake inhibitor.

Weekly capsules are a delayed release formulation containing enteric-coated pellets of fluoxetine hydrochloride, equivalent to 90 mg fluoxetine. Therapeutic equivalence of weekly formulation with daily formulation for delaying time to relapse has not been established.

Related Information

Antidepressant Agents *on page 1982*

◆ **Fluoxetine and Olanzapine** *see* Olanzapine and Fluoxetine *on page 1348*

◆ **Fluoxetine Hydrochloride** *see* FLUoxetine *on page 789*

Fluphenazine (floo FEN a zeen)

Index Terms Fluphenazine Decanoate; Fluphenazine Hydrochloride

Generic Availability (U.S.) Yes

Pharmacologic Category Antipsychotic Agent, Typical, Phenothiazine

Medication Safety Issues

Sound-alike/look-alike issues:

FluPHENAZine may be confused with fluvoxaMINE

International issues:

Prolixin [Turkey] may be confused with Prolixan brand name for azapropazone [Greece]

Use Management of manifestations of psychotic disorders and schizophrenia; depot formulation may offer improved outcome in individuals with psychosis who are nonadherent with oral antipsychotics

Unlabeled/Investigational Use Psychosis/agitation related to Alzheimer's dementia

Mechanism of Action/Effect Fluphenazine is a piperazine phenothiazine antipsychotic which blocks postsynaptic mesolimbic dopaminergic D_1 and D_2 receptors in the brain; depresses the release of hypothalamic and hypophyseal hormones; believed to depress the reticular activating system, thus affecting basal metabolism, body temperature, wakefulness, vasomotor tone, and emesis

Contraindications Hypersensitivity to fluphenazine or any component of the formulation (cross-reactivity between phenothiazines may occur); severe CNS depression; coma; subcortical brain damage; in patients receiving large doses of hypnotics; blood dyscrasias; hepatic disease

Warnings/Precautions [U.S. Boxed Warning]: Elderly patients with dementia-related psychosis treated with antipsychotics are at an increased risk of death compared to placebo. Most deaths appeared to be either cardiovascular (eg, heart failure, sudden death) or infectious (eg, pneumonia) in nature. Fluphenazine is not approved for the treatment of dementia-related psychosis. May be sedating; use with caution in disorders where CNS depression is a feature. Use with caution in Parkinson's disease. Caution in patients with hemodynamic instability; predisposition to seizures; or severe cardiac disease. Use caution in renal impairment; discontinue therapy if BUN abnormal. Use caution in hepatic impairment; use contraindicated in patients with liver damage. Esophageal dysmotility and aspiration have been associated with antipsychotic use; use with caution in patients at risk of pneumonia (ie, Alzheimer's disease). May alter temperature regulation or mask toxicity of other drugs due to antiemetic effects. May alter cardiac conduction; life-threatening arrhythmias have occurred with therapeutic doses of phenothiazines. Hypotension may occur, particularly with I.M. administration. May cause orthostatic hypotension; use with caution in patients at risk of this effect or those who would not tolerate transient hypotensive episodes (cerebrovascular disease, cardiovascular disease, or other medications which may predispose). Adverse effects of depot injections may be prolonged. Use associated with increased prolactin levels; clinical significance of hyperprolactinemia in patients with breast cancer or other prolactin-dependent tumors is unknown. May cause pigmentary retinopathy, and lenticular and corneal deposits, particularly with prolonged therapy.

Leukopenia, neutropenia, and agranulocytosis (sometimes fatal) have been reported in clinical trials and postmarketing reports with antipsychotic use; presence of risk factors (eg, pre-existing low WBC or history of drug-induced leuko-/neutropenia) should prompt periodic blood count assessment. Discontinue therapy at first signs of blood dyscrasias or if absolute neutrophil count $<1000/mm^3$.

Due to anticholinergic effects, use caution in patients with decreased gastrointestinal motility, urinary retention, BPH, xerostomia, visual problems, narrow-angle glaucoma, and myasthenia gravis. Relative to other antipsychotics, fluphenazine has a low potency of cholinergic blockade.

May cause extrapyramidal symptoms, including pseudoparkinsonism, acute dystonic reactions, akathisia, and tardive dyskinesia (risk of these reactions is high relative to other antipsychotics). Risk of dystonia (and possibly other EPS) may be greater with increased doses, use of conventional antipsychotics, males, and younger patients. May also be associated with neuroleptic malignant syndrome (NMS). Use caution in the elderly.

Drug Interactions

Metabolism/Transport Effects Substrate of CYP2D6 (major); **Inhibits** CYP1A2 (weak), 2C9 (weak), 2D6 (weak), 2E1 (weak)

Avoid Concomitant Use

Avoid concomitant use of FluPHENAZine with any of the following: Metoclopramide

Decreased Effect

FluPHENAZine may decrease the levels/effects of: Amphetamines; Quinagolide

The levels/effects of FluPHENAZine may be decreased by: Antacids; Anti-Parkinson's Agents (Dopamine Agonist); Lithium formulations; Peginterferon Alfa-2b

Increased Effect/Toxicity

FluPHENAZine may increase the levels/effects of: Alcohol (Ethyl); Analgesics (Opioid); Anticholinergics; Anti-Parkinson's Agents (Dopamine Agonist); Beta-Blockers; CNS Depressants; Methotrimeprazine; Methylphenidate

The levels/effects of FluPHENAZine may be increased by: Acetylcholinesterase Inhibitors (Central); Antimalarial Agents; Beta-Blockers; CYP2D6 Inhibitors (Moderate); CYP2D6 Inhibitors (Strong); Darunavir; Droperidol; Lithium formulations; Methotrimeprazine; Methylphenidate; Metoclopramide; Pramlintide; Tetrabenazine

Nutritional/Ethanol Interactions

Ethanol: Avoid ethanol (may increase CNS depression).

Herb/Nutraceutical: Avoid dong quai, St John's wort (may also cause photosensitization). Avoid kava kava, gotu kola, valerian, St John's wort (may increase CNS depression).

Lab Interactions Increased cholesterol (S), glucose; decreased uric acid (S)

Adverse Reactions Frequency not defined.

Cardiovascular: Hyper-/hypotension, tachycardia, fluctuations in blood pressure, arrhythmia, edema

Central nervous system: Parkinsonian symptoms, akathisia, dystonias, tardive dyskinesia, dizziness, hyper-reflexia, headache, cerebral edema, drowsiness, lethargy, restlessness, excitement, bizarre dreams, EEG changes, depression, seizure, NMS, altered central temperature regulation

Dermatologic: Dermatitis, eczema, erythema, itching, photosensitivity, rash, seborrhea, skin pigmentation, urticaria

Endocrine & metabolic: Menstrual cycle changes, breast pain, amenorrhea, galactorrhea, gynecomastia, libido changes, prolactin increased, SIADH

Gastrointestinal: Weight gain, appetite loss, salivation, xerostomia, constipation, paralytic ileus, laryngeal edema

Genitourinary: Ejaculatory disturbances, impotence, polyuria, bladder paralysis, enuresis

Hematologic: Agranulocytosis, leukopenia, thrombocytopenia, nonthrombocytopenic purpura, eosinophilia, pancytopenia

Hepatic: Cholestatic jaundice, hepatotoxicity

Neuromuscular & skeletal: Trembling of fingers, SLE, facial hemispasm

Ocular: Pigmentary retinopathy, cornea and lens changes, blurred vision, glaucoma

Respiratory: Nasal congestion, asthma

Pharmacodynamics/Kinetics

Onset of Action Decanoate: 24-72 hours; Peak effect: Neuroleptic: Decanoate: 48-96 hours

Duration of Action Hydrochloride salt: 6-8 hours; Decanoate: ~4 weeks

Absorption Oral: Erratic and variable

Time to Peak Serum: Hydrochloride: Oral: 2 hours; Decanoate: 8-10 hours

Half-Life Elimination Derivative dependent: Hydrochloride: ~14-16.4 hours; Decanoate: ~14 days

Available Dosage Forms

Elixir, oral: 2.5 mg/5 mL (60 mL, 473 mL)

Injection, oil: 25 mg/mL (5 mL)

Injection, solution: 2.5 mg/mL (10 mL)

Solution, oral: 5 mg/mL (118 mL)

Tablet, oral: 1 mg, 2.5 mg, 5 mg, 10 mg

Dosing

Adult

Psychosis:

Oral: Initial: 2.5-10 mg/day in divided doses at 6- to 8-hour intervals; Maintenance: 1-5 mg/day; **Note:** Some patients may require up to 40 mg/day for symptom control (long-term safety of higher doses not established)

PORT guidelines: Acute therapy: 6-20 mg/day for up to 6 weeks; Maintenance: 6-12 mg/day (Buchanan, 2009)

I.M. (hydrochloride): Initial: 1.25 mg as a single dose; depending on severity and duration, may need 2.5-10 mg/day in divided doses at 6- to 8-hour intervals (4 mg I.M. fluphenazine HCl is approximately equivalent to 10 mg oral fluphenazine HCl); use caution with doses >10 mg/day; once symptoms stabilized, transition to oral maintenance therapy

Long-acting maintenance injections (decanoate):

I.M., SubQ (decanoate): Initial: 12.5-25 mg every 2-4 weeks; response may last up to 6 weeks in some patients; titrate dose cautiously, if doses >50 mg are needed, increase in 12.5 mg increments (maximum dose: 100 mg)

Conversion from hydrochloride dosage forms to decanoate I.M.: 12.5 mg of decanoate every 2-4 weeks is approximately equivalent to 10 mg of oral hydrochloride/day; **Note:** Clinically, an every-2-week interval is frequently utilized

PORT guidelines: 6.25-25 mg every 2 weeks (Buchanan, 2009)

Geriatric Oral: Initial: 1-2.5 mg daily; titrated gradually based on patient response.

Renal Impairment Use with caution; not dialyzable (0% to 5%).

Hepatic Impairment Use with caution.

Administration

Oral Avoid contact of oral solution or injection with skin (contact dermatitis). Oral liquid should be diluted into at least 60 mL (2 fl oz) of the following **only**: Water, saline, homogenized milk, carbonated orange beverages, pineapple, apricot, prune, orange, tomato, and grapefruit juices. Do **not** dilute in beverages containing caffeine, tannics (eg, tea), or pectinate (eg, apple juice).

I.M. The hydrochloride or decanoate formulation may be administered intramuscularly. Watch for hypotension when administering I.M. Use a dry syringe and needle of ≥21 gauge to administer the fluphenazine decanoate; a wet needle/syringe may cause the solution to become cloudy.

Other SubQ: Only the decanoate formulation may be administered subcutaneously. Use a dry syringe and needle of ≥21 gauge to administer the fluphenazine decanoate; a wet needle/syringe may cause the solution to become cloudy.

Stability

Storage Store at room temperature; avoid freezing and excessive heat. Protect all dosage forms from light. Clear or slightly yellow solutions may be used. Should be dispensed in amber or opaque vials/bottles. Solutions may be diluted or mixed with fruit juices or other liquids, but must be administered immediately after mixing. Do not prepare bulk dilutions or store bulk dilutions.

Monitoring and Teaching Issues

Laboratory Monitoring CBC prior to and regularly during therapy, lipid profile, liver and kidney function, fasting blood glucose/Hgb A_{1c}; BMI

Physical Assessment Review ophthalmic screening at beginning of therapy and periodically throughout. With I.M. or SubQ use, monitor closely for hypotension. Initiate at lower doses and taper dosage slowly when discontinuing.

Patient Education Dilute with water, milk, orange juice, or grapefruit juice; do not dilute with beverages containing caffeine, tannin, or pectinate (eg, coffee, colas, tea, or apple juice). Avoid alcohol. Avoid skin contact with liquid medication; may cause contact dermatitis (wash immediately with warm, soapy water). Maintain adequate hydration, unless instructed to restrict fluid intake. You may experience excess drowsiness, lightheadedness, dizziness, blurred vision, dry mouth, upset stomach, nausea, vomiting, constipation, urinary retention, ejaculatory dysfunction (reversible), decreased perspiration, or photosensitivity. Report persistent CNS effects (eg, trembling fingers, altered gait or balance, excessive sedation, seizures, unusual movements, anxiety, confusion); chest pain or palpitations; severe dizziness; unresolved urinary retention; altered menstrual pattern; change in libido; swelling or pain in breasts (male or female); vision changes; skin rash or yellowing of skin; or worsening of condition.

Geriatric Considerations Any changes in disease status in any organ system can result in behavior changes.

Many elderly patients receive antipsychotic medications for inappropriate nonpsychotic behavior. Before initiating antipsychotic medication, the clinician should investigate any possible reversible cause; any stress or stress from any disease can cause acute "confusion" or worsening of baseline nonpsychotic behavior. Most commonly, acute changes in behavior are due to increases in drug dose or addition of a new drug to regimen, fluid electrolyte loss, infections, and changes in environment.

In the treatment of agitated, demented, and elderly patients, authors of meta-analysis of controlled trials of the response to the traditional antipsychotics (phenothiazines, butyrophenones) in controlling agitation have concluded that the use of neuroleptics results in a response rate of 18%. Clearly, neuroleptic therapy for behavior control should be limited with frequent attempts to withdraw the agent given for behavior control.

Breast-Feeding Considerations Other phenothiazines are excreted in human milk; excretion of fluphenazine is not known.

Pregnancy Considerations Jaundice or hyper-/hyporeflexia have been reported in newborn infants following maternal use of phenothiazines. Antipsychotic use during the third trimester of pregnancy has a risk for abnormal muscle movements (extrapyramidal symptoms [EPS]) and withdrawal symptoms in newborns following delivery. Symptoms in the newborn may include agitation, feeding disorder, hypertonia, hypotonia, respiratory distress, somnolence, and tremor; these effects may be self-limiting or require hospitalization.

Additional Information Less sedative and hypotensive effects than chlorpromazine.

Related Information

Antipsychotic Agents *on page* 1986

◆ **Fluphenazine Decanoate** *see* Fluphenazine *on page* 794

◆ **Fluphenazine Hydrochloride** *see* Fluphenazine *on page* 794

Flurazepam (flure AZ e pam)

Index Terms Flurazepam Hydrochloride

Generic Availability (U.S.) Yes

Pharmacologic Category Hypnotic, Benzodiazepine

Medication Safety Issues

Sound-alike/look-alike issues:

Flurazepam may be confused with temazepam

Dalmane® may be confused with Demulen®, Dialume®

Beers Criteria medication: This drug may be inappropriate for use in geriatric patients (high severity risk).

Medication Guide Available Yes

Lactation Excretion in breast milk unknown

Use Short-term treatment of insomnia

Controlled Substance C-IV

Available Dosage Forms

Capsule, oral: 15 mg, 30 mg

Dosing

Adult Insomnia (short-term treatment): Oral: 15-30 mg at bedtime

Geriatric Oral: 15 mg at bedtime. Avoid use if possible.

Pediatric Hypnotic: Oral:

<15 years: Dose not established

≥15 years: 15 mg at bedtime

Monitoring and Teaching Issues

Physical Assessment Assess for history of addiction; long-term use can result in dependence, abuse, or tolerance. Evaluate periodically need for continued use. Monitor for CNS changes. For inpatient use, institute safety measures to prevent falls.

Patient Education Drug may cause physical and/or psychological dependence. While using this medication, do not use alcohol. You may experience drowsiness, dizziness, lightheadedness, blurred vision, dry mouth, nausea, vomiting, difficulty urinating, or altered libido (resolves when medication is discontinued). Report CNS changes (confusion, depression, increased sedation, excitation, headache, abnormal thinking, insomnia, or nightmares, memory impairment, impaired coordination); muscle pain or weakness; respiratory difficulty; persistent dizziness, chest pain, or palpitations; unusual swelling, especially on face or neck; alterations in normal gait; vision changes; ringing in ears; or ineffectiveness of medication.

Related Information

Benzodiazepines *on page* 1988

◆ **Flurazepam Hydrochloride** *see* Flurazepam *on page* 796

◆ **5-Flurocytosine** *see* Flucytosine *on page* 775

Flutamide (FLOO ta mide)

Index Terms 4'-Nitro-3'-Trifluoromethylisobutyrantide; Eulexin; Niftolid; NSC-147834; SCH 13521

Generic Availability (U.S.) Yes

Pharmacologic Category Antineoplastic Agent, Antiandrogen

Medication Safety Issues

Sound-alike/look-alike issues:

Flutamide may be confused with Flumadine®, thalidomide

Eulexin may be confused with Edecrin®, Eurax®

Pregnancy Risk Factor D

Lactation Excretion in breast milk unknown/not recommended

Use Treatment of metastatic prostatic carcinoma in combination therapy with LHRH agonist analogues

Unlabeled/Investigational Use Female hirsutism

Mechanism of Action/Effect Nonsteroidal antiandrogen that inhibits androgen uptake or inhibits binding of androgen in target tissues

Contraindications Hypersensitivity to flutamide or any component of the formulation; severe hepatic impairment; pregnancy

Warnings/Precautions Hazardous agent - use appropriate precautions for handling and disposal. **[U.S. Boxed Warning]: Hospitalization and, rarely, death due to liver failure have been reported in patients taking flutamide.** Elevated serum transaminase levels, jaundice, hepatic encephalopathy, and acute hepatic failure have been reported. Androgen-deprivation therapy may increase the risk for cardiovascular disease (Levine, 2010). Product labeling states flutamide is not for use in women, particularly for non-life-threatening conditions. In some patients, the toxicity reverses after discontinuation of therapy. About 50% of the cases occur within the first 3 months of treatment. Serum transaminase levels should be measured prior to starting treatment, monthly for 4 months, and periodically thereafter. Liver function tests should be obtained at the first suggestion of liver dysfunction (nausea, vomiting, abdominal pain, fatigue, anorexia, "flu-like" symptoms, hyperbilirubinuria, jaundice, or right upper quadrant tenderness). Flutamide should be immediately discontinued any time a patient has jaundice, and/or an ALT level greater than twice the upper limit of normal. Flutamide should not be used in patients whose ALT values are greater than twice the upper limit of normal.

Patients with glucose-6 phosphate dehydrogenase deficiency or hemoglobin M disease or smokers are at risk of toxicities associated with aniline exposure, including methemoglobinemia, hemolytic anemia, and cholestatic jaundice. Monitor methemoglobin levels.

Drug Interactions

Metabolism/Transport Effects Substrate (major) of CYP1A2, 3A4; **Inhibits** CYP1A2 (weak)

Avoid Concomitant Use There are no known interactions where it is recommended to avoid concomitant use.

Decreased Effect

The levels/effects of Flutamide may be decreased by: CYP1A2 Inducers (Strong); CYP3A4 Inducers (Strong); Deferasirox; Herbs (CYP3A4 Inducers)

Increased Effect/Toxicity

The levels/effects of Flutamide may be increased by: Conivaptan; CYP1A2 Inhibitors (Moderate); CYP1A2 Inhibitors (Strong); CYP3A4 Inhibitors (Moderate); CYP3A4 Inhibitors (Strong); Dasatinib

Nutritional/Ethanol Interactions

Food: No effect on bioavailability of flutamide.

Herb/Nutraceutical: St John's wort may decrease flutamide levels.

Adverse Reactions

>10%:

Endocrine & metabolic: Gynecomastia, hot flashes, breast tenderness, galactorrhea (9% to 42%), impotence, libido decreased, tumor flare

Gastrointestinal: Nausea, vomiting (11% to 12%)

Hepatic: AST increased (transient; mild), LDH increased (transient; mild)

1% to 10%:

Cardiovascular: Hypertension (1%), edema

Central nervous system: Drowsiness, confusion, depression, anxiety, nervousness, headache, dizziness, insomnia

Dermatologic: Ecchymosis, photosensitivity, pruritus

Gastrointestinal: Anorexia, appetite increased, constipation, indigestion, upset stomach (4% to 6%); diarrhea

Hematologic: Anemia (6%), leukopenia (3%), thrombocytopenia (1%)

Neuromuscular & skeletal: Weakness (1%)

Miscellaneous: Herpes zoster

Pharmacodynamics/Kinetics

Absorption Oral: Rapid and complete

Protein Binding Parent drug: 94% to 96%; 2-hydroxyflutamide: 92% to 94%

Half-Life Elimination 5-6 hours (2-hydroxyflutamide)

Metabolism Extensively hepatic to more than 10 metabolites, primarily 2-hydroxyflutamide (active)

Excretion Primarily urine (as metabolites)

Available Dosage Forms

Capsule, oral: 125 mg

Dosing

Adult & Geriatric Refer to individual protocols.

Prostate carcinoma: Oral: 250 mg 3 times/day; alternatively, once-daily doses of 0.5-1.5 g have been used (unlabeled dosing)

Female hirsutism (unlabeled use): Oral: 250 mg daily

Administration

Oral Usually administered orally in 3 divided doses. Contents of capsule may be opened and mixed with applesauce, pudding, or other soft foods. Mixing with a beverage is not recommended.

Stability

Storage Store at room temperature.

Monitoring and Teaching Issues

Laboratory Monitoring Serum transaminase levels should be obtained at baseline and repeated monthly for the first 4 months of therapy, and periodically thereafter. LFTs should be checked at the first sign or symptom of liver dysfunction. Other parameters include tumor reduction, testosterone/estrogen, prostate specific antigen, and phosphatase serum levels.

Physical Assessment Assess serum transaminase levels prior to and periodically during therapy. Monitor for galactorrhea, CNS changes, ataxia, anorexia, vomiting, lacrimation, and anemia on a regular basis. Monitor liver function. Teach patient to report chest pain, respiratory difficulty, abdominal pain, and signs of liver dysfunction.

Patient Education This medication will be prescribed in conjunction with another medication; take both exactly as directed; do not discontinue without consulting prescriber. May cause decreased libido, impotence, swelling of breasts, hot flashes, decreased appetite, or diarrhea. Report chest pain or palpitation; acute abdominal pain; pain, tingling, or numbness of extremities; swelling of extremities or unusual weight gain; respiratory difficulty; yellowing of skin or sclera; dark urine; pale stool; or unusual fatigue.

Geriatric Considerations A study has shown that the addition of flutamide to leuprolide therapy in patients with advanced prostatic cancer increased median actuarial survival time to 34.9 months versus 27.9 months with leuprolide alone. No specific dose alterations are necessary in the elderly.

Fluticasone (Oral Inhalation) (floo TIK a sone)

U.S. Brand Names Flovent® Diskus®; Flovent® HFA

Index Terms Flovent; Fluticasone Propionate

Generic Availability (U.S.) No

Pharmacologic Category Corticosteroid, Inhalant (Oral)

Medication Safety Issues

Sound-alike/look-alike issues:

Flovent® may be confused with Flonase®

International issues:

Allegro: Brand name for fluticasone [Israel], but also the brand name for frovatriptan [Germany]

Allegro [Israel] may be confused with Allegra and Allegra-D brand names for fexofenadine and fexofenadine/pseudoephedrine, respectively, [U.S., Canada, and multiple international markets]

Flovent® [U.S., Canada] may be confused with Flogen brand name for naproxen [Mexico]

Pregnancy Risk Factor C

Lactation Excretion in breast milk unknown/use caution

Use Maintenance treatment of asthma as prophylactic therapy; also indicated for patients requiring oral corticosteroid therapy for asthma to assist in total discontinuation or reduction of total oral dose

Mechanism of Action/Effect Fluticasone belongs to a group of corticosteroids which utilizes a fluorocarbothioate ester linkage at the 17 carbon position; extremely potent vasoconstrictive and anti-inflammatory activity. The effectiveness of inhaled fluticasone is due to its direct local effect.

Contraindications Hypersensitivity to fluticasone or any component of the formulation; primary treatment of status asthmaticus or acute bronchospasm

Warnings/Precautions May cause hypercorticism or suppression of hypothalamic-pituitary-adrenal (HPA) axis, particularly in younger children or in patients receiving high doses for prolonged periods. HPA axis suppression may lead to adrenal crisis. Withdrawal and discontinuation of a corticosteroid should be done slowly and carefully. Particular care is required when patients are transferred from systemic corticosteroids to inhaled products due to possible adrenal insufficiency or withdrawal from steroids, including an increase in allergic symptoms. Patients receiving ≥20 mg per day of prednisone (or equivalent) may be most susceptible. Concurrent use of ritonavir (and potentially other strong inhibitors of CYP3A4) may increase fluticasone levels and effects on HPA suppression. Fatalities have occurred due to adrenal insufficiency in asthmatic patients during and after transfer from systemic corticosteroids to aerosol steroids; aerosol steroids do **not** provide the systemic steroid needed to treat patients having trauma, surgery, or infections.

Bronchospasm may occur with wheezing after inhalation; if this occurs, stop steroid and treat with a fast-acting bronchodilator. Supplemental steroids (oral or parenteral) may be needed during stress or severe asthma attacks. Corticosteroid use may cause psychiatric disturbances, including depression, euphoria, insomnia, mood swings, and personality changes. Pre-existing psychiatric conditions may be exacerbated by corticosteroid use. Prolonged use of corticosteroids may also increase the incidence of secondary infection, mask acute infection (including fungal infections), prolong or exacerbate viral infections, or limit response to vaccines. Exposure to chickenpox should be avoided; corticosteroids should not be used to treat ocular herpes simplex. Corticosteroids should not be used for cerebral malaria. Close observation is required in patients with latent tuberculosis and/or TB reactivity; restrict use in active TB (only in conjunction with antituberculosis treatment). Rare cases of vasculitis (Churg-Strauss syndrome) or other eosinophilic conditions can occur. Prolonged treatment with corticosteroids has been associated with the development of Kaposi's sarcoma (case reports); if noted, discontinuation of therapy should be considered.

Use with caution in patients with thyroid disease, hepatic impairment, renal impairment, cardiovascular disease, diabetes, glaucoma, cataracts, myasthenia gravis, patients at risk for osteoporosis, patients at risk for seizures, or GI diseases (diverticulitis, peptic ulcer, ulcerative colitis) due to perforation risk. Use caution following acute MI (corticosteroids have been associated with myocardial rupture). Because of the risk of adverse effects, systemic corticosteroids should be used cautiously in the elderly in the smallest possible effective dose for the shortest duration.

Orally-inhaled corticosteroids may cause a reduction in growth velocity in pediatric patients (~1 centimeter per year [range: 0.3-1.8 cm per year] and related to dose and duration of exposure). To minimize the systemic effects of orally-inhaled corticosteroids, each patient should be titrated to the lowest effective dose. Growth should be routinely monitored in pediatric patients.

Not to be used in status asthmaticus or for the relief of acute bronchospasm. Flovent® Diskus® contains lactose; very rare anaphylactic reactions have been reported in patients with severe milk protein allergy. There have been reports of systemic corticosteroid withdrawal symptoms (eg, joint/muscle pain, lassitude, depression) when withdrawing oral inhalation therapy. Local yeast infections (eg, oral pharyngeal candidiasis) may occur. Lower respiratory tract infections, including pneumonia, have been reported in patients with COPD with an even higher incidence in the elderly.

Drug Interactions

Metabolism/Transport Effects Substrate of CYP3A4 (major)

Avoid Concomitant Use

Avoid concomitant use of Fluticasone (Oral Inhalation) with any of the following: Aldesleukin; BCG; Natalizumab; Pimecrolimus; Roflumilast; Tacrolimus (Topical)

Decreased Effect

Fluticasone (Oral Inhalation) may decrease the levels/effects of: Aldesleukin; Antidiabetic Agents; BCG; Corticorelin; Sipuleucel-T; Vaccines (Inactivated)

The levels/effects of Fluticasone (Oral Inhalation) may be decreased by: Echinacea

Increased Effect/Toxicity

Fluticasone (Oral Inhalation) may increase the levels/effects of: Amphotericin B; Leflunomide; Loop Diuretics; Natalizumab; Thiazide Diuretics

The levels/effects of Fluticasone (Oral Inhalation) may be increased by: CYP3A4 Inhibitors (Moderate); CYP3A4 Inhibitors (Strong); Dasatinib; Denosumab; Pimecrolimus; Roflumilast; Tacrolimus (Topical); Trastuzumab

Nutritional/Ethanol Interactions Herb/Nutraceutical: In theory, St John's wort may decrease serum levels of fluticasone by inducing CYP3A4 isoenzymes.

Adverse Reactions

>10%:

Central nervous system: Headache (2% to 14%)

Respiratory: Upper respiratory tract infection (14% to 21%), throat irritation (3% to 22%)

3% to 10%:

Central nervous system: Fever (1% to 7%)

Gastrointestinal: Oral candidiasis (≤9%), nausea/vomiting (1% to 8%), gastrointestinal infection (including viral; 1% to 5%), gastrointestinal discomfort/pain (1% to 4%)

Neuromuscular & skeletal: Musculoskeletal pain (2% to 5%), muscle injury (1% to 5%)

Respiratory: Sinusitis/sinus infection (4% to 10%), lower respiratory tract infections/pneumonia (1% to 7%; COPD diagnosis and age >65 years increase risk), cough (1% to 6%), bronchitis (≤8%), hoarseness/dysphonia (2% to 6%), upper respiratory tract inflammation (≤5%), viral respiratory infection (1% to 5%), rhinitis (1% to 4%)

Miscellaneous: Viral infection (≤5%)

1% to 3%:

Cardiovascular: Chest symptoms, edema, palpitation

Central nervous system: Cranial nerve paralysis, dizziness, fatigue, malaise, migraine, mood disorders, pain, sleep disorder

Dermatologic: Acne, dermatitis/dermatosis, eczema, folliculitis, photodermatitis, infection (fungal, viral), pruritus, rash, urticaria

Endocrine & metabolic: Fluid disturbance, goiter, uric acid metabolism disturbance

Gastrointestinal: Abdominal discomfort/pain, appetite changes, dental discomfort/pain, diarrhea, dyspepsia, gastroenteritis, hyposalivation, oral discomfort/pain, oral erythema/rash, oral ulcerations, oropharyngeal plaques, tooth decay, weight gain

Genitourinary: Reproductive organ infections (bacterial), urinary tract infection

Hematologic: Hematoma

Hepatic: Cholecystitis

Neuromuscular & skeletal: Arthralgia, articular rheumatism, muscle cramps/spasms, muscle pain, muscle stiffness/tightness/rigidity, musculoskeletal inflammation

Ocular: Blepharoconjunctivitis, conjunctivitis, keratitis

Otic: Otitis

Respiratory: Epistaxis, hoarseness/dysphonia, laryngitis, nasal sinus disorder, pharyngitis/throat infection, rhinorrhea/postnasal drip, throat constriction

Miscellaneous: Infection (bacterial, fungal); injuries (including muscle, soft tissue); polyps (ear, nose, throat); tonsillitis

Pharmacodynamics/Kinetics

Onset of Action Maximal benefit may take 1-2 weeks or longer

Absorption Absorbed systemically (Flovent® Diskus®: ~18%) primarily via lungs, minimal GI absorption (<1%) due to presystemic metabolism

Bioavailability ~18% to 21%

Protein Binding 91% to >99%

Metabolism Hepatic via CYP3A4 to 17β-carboxylic acid (negligible activity)

Excretion Feces (as parent drug and metabolites); urine (<5% as metabolites)

Available Dosage Forms

Aerosol, for oral inhalation:

Flovent® HFA: 44 mcg/inhalation (10.6 g); 110 mcg/inhalation (12 g); 220 mcg/inhalation (12 g)

Powder, for oral inhalation:

Flovent® Diskus®: 50 mcg (60s); 100 mcg (60s); 250 mcg (60s)

Dosing

Adult & Geriatric Asthma: Inhalation, oral: **Note:** Titrate to the lowest effective dose once asthma stability is achieved

Flovent® HFA: Manufacturers labeling: Dosing based on previous therapy

Bronchodilator alone: Recommended starting dose: 88 mcg twice daily; highest recommended dose: 440 mcg twice daily

Inhaled corticosteroids: Recommended starting dose: 88-220 mcg twice daily; highest recommended dose: 440 mcg twice daily; a higher starting dose may be considered in patients previously requiring higher doses of inhaled corticosteroids

Oral corticosteroids:

Recommended starting dose: 440 mcg twice daily

Highest recommended dose: 880 mcg twice daily; starting dose is patient dependent. In patients on chronic oral corticosteroids therapy, reduce prednisone dose no faster than 2.5-5 mg/day on a weekly basis; begin taper after 1 week of fluticasone therapy.

NIH Asthma Guidelines (NIH, 2007) (administer in divided doses twice daily):

"Low" dose: 88-264 mcg/day

"Medium" dose: 264-440 mcg/day

"High" dose: >440 mcg/day

Flovent® Diskus® *(U.S. labeling)*: **Note:** May increase dose after 2 weeks of therapy in patients not adequately controlled. Higher starting doses may be considered in patients with poorer asthma control or those requiring high ranges of inhaled corticosteroids. Titrate to the lowest effective dose once asthma stability is achieved.

Bronchodilator alone: Recommended starting dose: 100 mcg twice daily; maximum recommended dose: 500 mcg twice daily

Inhaled corticosteroids: Recommended starting dose: 100-250 mcg twice daily; maximum recommended dose: 500 mcg twice daily

Oral corticosteroids: Recommended starting dose: 500-1000 mcg twice daily; maximum recommended dose: 1000 mcg twice daily. Starting dose is patient dependent. In patients on chronic oral corticosteroids therapy, reduce prednisone dose no faster than 2.5 mg/day on a weekly basis; begin taper after 1 week of fluticasone therapy.

Flovent® Diskus® *(Canadian labeling)*:

Mild asthma: 100-250 mcg twice daily

Moderate asthma: 250-500 mcg twice daily

Severe asthma: 500 mcg twice daily; may increase to 1000 mcg twice daily in very severe patients requiring high doses of corticosteroids

Pediatric Asthma: Inhalation, oral:

Flovent® HFA:

Children 4-11 years: 88 mcg twice daily

Children ≥12 years: Refer to adult dosing.

NIH Asthma Guidelines (NIH, 2007) (administer in divided doses twice daily):

"Low" dose:

0-4 years: 176 mcg/day

5-11 years: 88-176 mcg/day

≥12 years: 88-264 mcg/day

"Medium" dose:

0-4 years: >176-352 mcg/day

5-11 years: >176-352 mcg/day

≥12 years: >264-440 mcg/day

"High" dose:

0-4 years: >352 mcg/day

5-11 years: >352 mcg/day

≥12 years: >440 mcg/day

Flovent® Diskus® *(U.S. labeling)*:

Children 4-11 years: Usual starting dose: 50 mcg twice daily; may increase to 100 mcg twice daily in patients not adequately controlled after 2 weeks of therapy. Higher starting doses may be considered in patients with poorer asthma control or those requiring high ranges of inhaled corticosteroids. Titrate to the lowest effective dose once asthma stability is achieved (maximum dose: 100 mcg twice daily)

Children >11 years: Refer to adult dosing.

Flovent® Diskus® *(Canadian labeling)*:

Children 4-16 years: Usual starting dose: 50-100 mcg twice daily; may increase to 200 mcg twice daily in patients not adequately controlled; titrate to the lowest effective dose once asthma stability is achieved

Children ≥16 years: Refer to adult dosing.

Hepatic Impairment Fluticasone is primarily cleared in the liver. Fluticasone plasma levels may be increased in patients with hepatic impairment, use with caution; monitor.

Administration

Inhalation

Aerosol inhalation: Flovent® HFA: Shake container thoroughly before using. Take 3-5 deep breaths. Use inhaler on inspiration. Allow 1 full minute between inhalations. Rinse mouth with water after use to reduce aftertaste and incidence of candidiasis; do not swallow. Flovent® HFA inhaler must be primed before first use, when not used for 7 days, or if dropped. To prime the first time, release 4 sprays into air; shake well before each spray and spray away from face. If dropped or not used for 7 days, prime by releasing a single test spray. Patient should contact pharmacy for refill when the dose counter reads "020". Discard device when the dose counter reads "000". Do not use "float" test to determine contents.

Powder for oral inhalation: Flovent® Diskus®: Do not use with a spacer device. Do not exhale into Diskus®. Do not wash or take apart. Use in horizontal position. Mouth should be rinsed with water after use (do not swallow). Discard after 6 weeks once removed from protective pouch or when the dose counter reads "0", whichever comes first (device is not reusable).

Stability

Storage

Flovent® HFA: Store at 15°C to 30°C (59°F to 86°F). Discard device when the dose counter reads "000". Store with mouthpiece down.

Flovent® Diskus®: Store at 20°C to 25°C (68°F to 77°F) in a dry place away from direct heat or sunlight. Discard after 6 weeks from removal from protective foil pouch or when the dose counter reads "0" (whichever comes first); device is not reusable.

Monitoring and Teaching Issues

Physical Assessment May take as long as 2 weeks before full benefit of medication is known. Encourage regular eye exams with long-term use. Monitor for possible eosinophilic conditions (including Churg-Strauss syndrome) and signs/symptoms of HPA axis suppression/adrenal insufficiency. Assess growth in adolescents and children.

Patient Education Although you may see improvement within a few hours of use, the full benefit of the medication may not be achieved for several days. Avoid exposure to chickenpox or measles. If exposed, inform your prescriber as soon as possible. May cause headache. Report signs of infection or change in vision to prescriber.

Metered-dose inhalation: Sit when using. Take deep breaths for 3-5 minutes and clear nasal passages before administration (use decongestant as needed). Hold breath for 5-10 seconds after use and wait 1-3 minutes between inhalations. If also using inhaled bronchodilator, use before fluticasone. Rinse mouth and throat after use to reduce aftertaste and prevent candidiasis.

Powder for oral inhalation: Flovent® Diskus®: Do not attempt to take device apart. Do not use with a spacer device. Do not exhale into the Diskus®; use in a level horizontal position. Do not wash the mouthpiece.

Dietary Considerations Flovent® Diskus® contains lactose; very rare anaphylactic reactions have been reported in patients with severe milk protein allergy.

Geriatric Considerations No specific geriatric information is available. No differences in safety have been observed in the elderly when compared to younger patients. Based on current data, no dosage adjustment is needed based on age.

Breast-Feeding Considerations Systemic corticosteroids are excreted in human milk. It is not known if sufficient quantities of fluticasone are absorbed following inhalation to produce detectable amounts in breast milk. The use of inhaled corticosteroids is not considered a contraindication to breast feeding.

Pregnancy Considerations Adverse events have been observed with systemic corticosteroids in animal reproduction studies. A decrease in fetal growth has not been observed with inhaled corticosteroid use during pregnancy. Inhaled corticosteroids are recommended for the treatment of asthma (most information available using budesonide) during pregnancy.

Additional Information Effects of inhaled steroids on growth have been observed in the absence of laboratory evidence of HPA axis suppression, suggesting that growth velocity is a more sensitive indicator of systemic corticosteroid exposure in pediatric patients than some commonly used tests of HPA axis function. The long-term effects of this reduction in growth velocity associated with orally-inhaled corticosteroids, including the impact on final adult height, are unknown. The potential for "catch up" growth following discontinuation of treatment with inhaled corticosteroids has not been adequately studied.

In the United States, dosage for the metered dose inhaler (Flovent® HFA) is expressed as the amount of drug which leaves the actuater and is delivered to the patient. This differs from other countries, which express the dosage as the amount of drug which leaves the valve.

Related Information

Asthma *on page 2015*
Corticosteroids *on page 1996*

Fluticasone (Nasal) (floo TIK a sone)

U.S. Brand Names Flonase®; Veramyst®

Index Terms Fluticasone Furoate; Fluticasone Propionate

Generic Availability (U.S.) Yes: Propionate spray

Pharmacologic Category Corticosteroid, Nasal

Medication Safety Issues

Sound-alike/look-alike issues:

Flonase® may be confused with Flovent®

International issues:

Allegro: Brand name for fluticasone [Israel], but also the brand name for frovatriptan [Germany]

Allegro [Israel] may be confused with Allegra and Allegra-D brand names for fexofenadine and fexofenadine/pseudoephedrine, respectively, [U.S., Canada, and multiple international markets]

Pregnancy Risk Factor C

Lactation Excretion in breast milk unknown/use caution

Use

Flonase®: Management of seasonal and perennial allergic rhinitis and nonallergic rhinitis
Veramyst®, Avamys® [CAN]: Management of seasonal and perennial allergic rhinitis

Available Dosage Forms

Suspension, intranasal: 50 mcg/inhalation (16 g)
Flonase®: 50 mcg/inhalation (16 g)
Veramyst®: 27.5 mcg/inhalation (10 g)

Dosing

Adult & Geriatric Rhinitis: Intranasal:

Flonase® (fluticasone propionate): Initial: 2 sprays (50 mcg/spray) per nostril once daily; may also be divided into 100 mcg twice a day. After the first few days, dosage may be reduced to 1 spray per nostril once daily for maintenance therapy.

Veramyst® (fluticasone furoate): Initial: 2 sprays (27.5 mcg/spray) per nostril once daily (110 mcg/day). Once symptoms are controlled, may reduce dosage to 1 spray per nostril once daily (55 mcg/day) for maintenance therapy.

Avamys® [CAN] (fluticasone furoate): 2 sprays (27.5 mcg/spray) in each nostril once daily (110 mcg/day). Total daily dosage should not exceed 2 sprays in each nostril (110 mcg)/day.

Pediatric Rhinitis: Intranasal:

Flonase® (fluticasone propionate): Children ≥4 years and Adolescents: Initial: 1 spray (50 mcg/spray) per nostril once daily; patients not adequately responding or patients with more severe symptoms may use 2 sprays (100 mcg) per nostril. Depending on response, dosage may be reduced to 100 mcg daily. Total daily dosage should not exceed 2 sprays in each nostril (200 mcg)/day. Dosing should be at regular intervals.

Veramyst® (fluticasone furoate):

Children 2-11 years: Initial: 1 spray (27.5 mcg/spray) per nostril once daily (55 mcg/day); patients not adequately responding may use 2 sprays per nostril once daily (110 mcg/day). Once symptoms are controlled, dosage may be reduced to 55 mcg once daily. Total daily dosage should not exceed 2 sprays in each nostril (110 mcg)/day.

Children ≥12 years and Adolescents: Initial: 2 sprays (27.5 mcg/spray) per nostril once daily (110 mcg/day). Once symptoms are controlled, dosage may be reduced to 1 spray per nostril once daily (55 mcg/day). Total daily dosage should not exceed 2 sprays in each nostril (110 mcg)/day.

Avamys® [CAN] (fluticasone furoate):

Children 2-11 years: Initial: 1 spray (27.5 mcg/spray) per nostril once daily (55 mcg/day); patients not adequately responding may use 2 sprays per nostril once daily (110 mcg/day). Once symptoms are controlled, dosage may be reduced to 55 mcg once daily. Total daily dosage should not exceed 2 sprays in each nostril (110 mcg)/day.

Children ≥12 years and Adolescents: Initial: 2 sprays (27.5 mcg/spray) per nostril once daily (110 mcg/day). Total daily dosage should not exceed 2 sprays in each nostril (110 mcg)/day.

Administration

Inhalation Nasal spray: Administer at regular intervals. Shake bottle gently before using. Blow nose to clear nostrils. Insert applicator into nostril, keeping bottle upright, and close off the other nostril. Breathe in through nose. While inhaling, press pump to release spray. Discard after labeled number of doses has been used, even if bottle is not completely empty.

Flonase®: Prime pump (press 6 times until fine spray appears) prior to first use or if spray unused for ≥7 days. Once weekly, nasal applicator may be removed and rinsed with warm water to clean.

Veramyst®, Avamys® [CAN]: Prime pump (press 6 times until fine spray appears) prior to first use, if spray unused for ≥30 days, or if cap left off bottle for ≥5 days. After each use, nozzle should be wiped with a clean, dry tissue. Once weekly, inside of cap should be cleaned with a clean, dry tissue.

Monitoring and Teaching Issues

Physical Assessment May take as long as 2 weeks before full benefit of medication is known. Encourage regular eye exams with long-term use. Monitor growth in adolescents and children. Assess for signs/symptoms of HPA axis suppression/adrenal insufficiency.

Patient Education Shake gently before use. Report unusual cough; persistent nasal bleeding, burning, or irritation; or worsening of condition.

Fluticasone (Topical) (floo TIK a sone)

U.S. Brand Names Cutivate®

Index Terms Fluticasone Propionate

Generic Availability (U.S.) Yes: Cream, ointment

Pharmacologic Category Corticosteroid, Topical

Medication Safety Issues

Sound-alike/look-alike issues:

Cutivate® may be confused with Ultravate®

International issues:

Allegro: Brand name for fluticasone [Israel], but also the brand name for frovatriptan [Germany]

Allegro [Israel] may be confused with Allegra and Allegra-D brand names for fexofenadine and fexofenadine/pseudoephedrine, respectively, [U.S., Canada, and multiple international markets]

Pregnancy Risk Factor C

Lactation Excretion in breast milk unknown/use caution

Use Relief of inflammation and pruritus associated with corticosteroid-responsive dermatoses; atopic dermatitis

Available Dosage Forms

Cream, topical: 0.05% (15 g, 30 g, 60 g)

Cutivate®: 0.05% (30 g, 60 g)

Lotion, topical:

Cutivate®: 0.05% (120 mL)

Ointment, topical: 0.005% (15 g, 30 g, 60 g)

Cutivate®: 0.005% (30 g, 60 g)

Dosing

Adult & Geriatric

Corticosteroid-responsive dermatoses: Topical: Cream, lotion, ointment: Apply sparingly to affected area twice daily. If no improvement is seen within 2 weeks, reassessment of diagnosis may be necessary.

Atopic dermatitis: Topical: Cream, lotion: Apply sparingly to affected area once or twice daily. If no improvement is seen within 2 weeks, reassessment of diagnosis may be necessary.

Pediatric

Corticosteroid-responsive dermatoses: Topical: Children ≥3 months: Cream: Apply sparingly to affected area twice daily. If no improvement is seen within 2 weeks, reassessment of diagnosis may be necessary.

Atopic dermatitis: Topical:

Children ≥3 months: Cream: Apply sparingly to affected area 1-2 times/day. If no improvement is seen within 2 weeks, reassessment of diagnosis may be necessary.

Children ≥1 year: Lotion: Apply sparingly to affected area once daily.

Administration

Topical Apply sparingly in a thin film. Rub in lightly. Unless otherwise directed by healthcare professional, do not use with occlusive dressing; do not use on children's skin covered by diapers or plastic pants.

Monitoring and Teaching Issues

Physical Assessment May take as long as 2 weeks before full benefit of medication is known. Monitor for possible eosinophilic conditions (including Churg-Strauss syndrome) and signs/symptoms of HPA axis suppression/adrenal insufficiency. Assess growth in adolescents and children.

Patient Education For external use only. Apply thin film to affected area only; rub in lightly. Do not apply occlusive covering unless advised by prescriber. Wash hand thoroughly after use; avoid contact with eyes. Notify prescriber if skin condition persists or worsens. Do not use for treatment of diaper dermatitis or under diapers or plastic pants.

Related Information

Corticosteroids *on page 1996*

Fluticasone and Salmeterol (floo TIK a sone & sal ME te role)

U.S. Brand Names Advair Diskus®; Advair® HFA

Index Terms Fluticasone Propionate and Salmeterol Xinafoate; Salmeterol and Fluticasone

Generic Availability (U.S.) No

Pharmacologic Category Beta$_2$-Adrenergic Agonist; Beta$_2$-Adrenergic Agonist, Long-Acting; Corticosteroid, Inhalant (Oral)

Medication Safety Issues

Sound-alike/look-alike issues:

Advair® may be confused with Adcirca®, Advicor®

Medication Guide Available Yes

Pregnancy Risk Factor C

Lactation

Fluticasone: Excretion in breast milk unknown/use caution

Salmeterol: Enters breast milk/use caution

Use Maintenance treatment of asthma; maintenance treatment of COPD

Contraindications Hypersensitivity to fluticasone, salmeterol, or any component of the formulation; status asthmaticus; acute episodes of asthma or COPD; severe hypersensitivity to milk proteins (Advair Diskus®)

Warnings/Precautions See individual agents.

Drug Interactions

Metabolism/Transport Effects Fluticasone: **Substrate** of CYP3A4 (major); Salmeterol: **Substrate** of CYP3A4 (major)

Avoid Concomitant Use

Avoid concomitant use of Fluticasone and Salmeterol with any of the following: Aldesleukin; BCG; CYP3A4 Inhibitors (Strong); Iobenguane I 123; Natalizumab; Pimecrolimus; Roflumilast; Tacrolimus (Topical)

Decreased Effect

Fluticasone and Salmeterol may decrease the levels/effects of: Aldesleukin; Antidiabetic Agents; BCG; Corticorelin; Iobenguane I 123; Sipuleucel-T; Vaccines (Inactivated)

The levels/effects of Fluticasone and Salmeterol may be decreased by: Alpha-/Beta-Blockers; Beta-Blockers (Beta1 Selective); Beta-Blockers (Nonselective); Betahistine; Echinacea

Increased Effect/Toxicity

Fluticasone and Salmeterol may increase the levels/effects of: Amphotericin B; Leflunomide; Loop Diuretics; Natalizumab; Sympathomimetics; Thiazide Diuretics

The levels/effects of Fluticasone and Salmeterol may be increased by: Atomoxetine; Cannabinoids; CYP3A4 Inhibitors (Moderate); CYP3A4 Inhibitors (Strong); Dasatinib; Denosumab; MAO Inhibitors; Pimecrolimus; Roflumilast; Tacrolimus (Topical); Trastuzumab; Tricyclic Antidepressants

Adverse Reactions Percentages reported in patients with asthma; also see individual agents:

>10%:

Central nervous system: Headache (12% to 21%)

Respiratory: Upper respiratory tract infection (16% to 27%), pharyngitis (9% to 13%)

>3% to 10%:

Central nervous system: Dizziness (1% to 4%)

Endocrine & metabolic: Menstruation symptoms (3% to 5%)

Gastrointestinal: Nausea/vomiting (3% to 6%), diarrhea (2% to 4%), pain/discomfort (1% to 4%), oral candidiasis (1% to 4%), gastrointestinal infections (including viral, ≤4%)

Neuromuscular & skeletal: Musculoskeletal pain (2% to 7%), muscle pain (≤4%)

Respiratory: Throat irritation (7% to 9%), bronchitis (2% to 8%), upper respiratory tract inflammation (4% to 7%), lower respiratory tract infections/pneumonia (1% to 7%; COPD diagnosis and age >65 years increase risk), cough (3% to 6%), sinusitis (4% to 5%), hoarseness/dysphonia (1% to 5%), viral respiratory tract infection (3% to 5%)

1% to 3%:

Cardiovascular: Arrhythmia, chest symptoms, fluid retention, MI, palpitation, syncope, tachycardia

Central nervous system: Compressed nerve syndromes, hypnagogic effects, migraine, pain, sleep disorders, tremor

Dermatologic: Dermatitis, dermatosis, eczema, hives, skin flakiness, urticaria, viral skin infection

Endocrine & metabolic: Hypothyroidism

Gastrointestinal: Constipation, dental discomfort/pain, gastrointestinal infection, hemorrhoids, oral discomfort/pain, oral erythema/rash, oral ulcerations, unusual taste, weight gain

Genitourinary: Urinary tract infection
Hematologic: Contusions/hematomas
Hepatic: Abnormal liver function tests
Neuromuscular & skeletal: Arthralgia, articular rheumatism, bone/cartilage disorders, bone pain, cramps, fractures, muscle injuries (≤3%), muscle spasm, muscle stiffness, tightness/rigidity
Ocular: Conjunctivitis, edema, eye redness, keratitis, xerophthalmia
Respiratory: Blood in nasal mucosa, congestion, ear/nose/throat infection, epistaxis, laryngitis, lower respiratory hemorrhage, nasal irritation, rhinitis, rhinorrhea/postnasal drip, sneezing
Miscellaneous: Allergies/allergic reactions, bacterial infection, burns, candidiasis (≤3%), diaphoresis, sweat/sebum disorders, viral infection, wounds and lacerations

Pharmacodynamics/Kinetics

Pharmacokinetic Note See individual agents.

Available Dosage Forms

Aerosol, for oral inhalation:

Advair® HFA:

45/21: Fluticasone propionate 45 mcg and salmeterol 21 mcg (8 g, 12 g) [chlorofluorocarbon free]

115/21: Fluticasone propionate 115 mcg and salmeterol 21 mcg (8 g, 12 g) [chlorofluorocarbon free]

230/21: Fluticasone propionate 230 mcg and salmeterol 21 mcg (8 g, 12 g) [chlorofluorocarbon free]

Powder, for oral inhalation:

Advair Diskus®:

100/50: Fluticasone propionate 100 mcg and salmeterol 50 mcg (14s, 60s)
250/50: Fluticasone propionate 250 mcg and salmeterol 50 mcg (60s)
500/50: Fluticasone propionate 500 mcg and salmeterol 50 mcg (60s)

Dosing

Adult & Geriatric Do not use to transfer patients from systemic corticosteroid therapy.

COPD: Oral Inhalation:

Advair Diskus®: Fluticasone 250 mcg/salmeterol 50 mcg twice daily, 12 hours apart. **Note:** This is the maximum dose.

Advair Diskus® [Canadian labeling; not in approved U.S. labeling]: Fluticasone 250 mcg/salmeterol 50 mcg **or** fluticasone 500 mcg/salmeterol 50 mcg twice daily, 12 hours apart. Maximum dose: Fluticasone 500 mcg/salmeterol 50 mcg per inhalation (2 inhalations/day)

Asthma (maintenance): Oral inhalation:

Advair Diskus®: One inhalation twice daily, morning and evening, 12 hours apart
Maximum dose: Fluticasone 500 mcg/salmeterol 50 mcg per inhalation (2 inhalations/day)

Advair® HFA: Two inhalations twice daily, morning and evening, 12 hours apart
Maximum dose: Fluticasone 230 mcg/salmeterol 21 mcg per inhalation (4 inhalations/day)

Advair® 125 or Advair® 250 [Canadian labeling; not in approved U.S. labeling]: Two inhalations twice daily, morning and evening, 12 hours apart
Maximum dose: Fluticasone 250 mcg/salmeterol 25 mcg per inhalation (4 inhalations/day)

Note: Initial dose prescribed should be based upon previous dose of inhaled-steroid asthma therapy. Dose should be increased after 2 weeks if adequate response is not achieved. Patients should be titrated to lowest effective dose once stable. Each suggestion below specifies the product strength to use; remember to **use 1 inhalation for Diskus® and 2 inhalations for HFA.**

Patients not currently on inhaled corticosteroids:

Advair Diskus®: Fluticasone 100 mcg/salmeterol 50 mcg **or** fluticasone 250 mcg/salmeterol 50 mcg

Advair® HFA: Fluticasone 45 mcg/salmeterol 21 mcg **or** fluticasone 115 mcg/salmeterol 21 mcg

Patients currently using inhaled beclomethasone dipropionate:

≤160 mcg/day: Fluticasone 100 mcg/salmeterol 50 mcg **or** Advair® HFA: Fluticasone 45 mcg/salmeterol 21 mcg

320 mcg/day: Fluticasone 250 mcg/salmeterol 50 mcg **or** Advair® HFA: Fluticasone 115 mcg/salmeterol 21 mcg

640 mcg/day: Fluticasone 500 mcg/salmeterol 50 mcg **or** Advair® HFA: Fluticasone 230 mcg/salmeterol 21 mcg

Patients currently using inhaled budesonide:

≤400 mcg/day: Fluticasone 100 mcg/salmeterol 50 mcg **or** Advair® HFA: Fluticasone 45 mcg/salmeterol 21 mcg

800-1200 mcg/day: Fluticasone 250 mcg/salmeterol 50 mcg **or** Advair® HFA: Fluticasone 115 mcg/salmeterol 21mcg

1600 mcg/day: Fluticasone 500 mcg/salmeterol 50 mcg **or** Advair® HFA: Fluticasone 230 mcg/salmeterol 21 mcg

Patients currently using inhaled flunisolide CFC aerosol:

≤1000 mcg/day: Fluticasone 100 mcg/salmeterol 50 mcg **or** Advair® HFA: Fluticasone 45 mcg/salmeterol 21 mcg

1250-2000 mcg/day: Fluticasone 250 mcg/salmeterol 50 mcg **or** Advair® HFA: Fluticasone 115 mcg/salmeterol 21 mcg

Patients currently using inhaled flunisolide HFA inhalation aerosol:

≤320 mcg/day: Fluticasone 100 mcg/salmeterol 50 mcg **or** Advair® HFA: Fluticasone 45 mcg/salmeterol 21 mcg

640 mcg/day: Fluticasone 250 mcg/salmeterol 50 mcg **or** Advair® HFA: Fluticasone 115 mcg/salmeterol 21 mcg

Patients currently using inhaled fluticasone HFA aerosol:

≤176 mcg/day: Fluticasone 100 mcg/salmeterol 50 mcg **or** Advair® HFA: Fluticasone 45 mcg/salmeterol 21 mcg

440 mcg/day: Fluticasone 250 mcg/salmeterol 50 mcg **or** Advair® HFA: Fluticasone 115 mcg/salmeterol 21 mcg

660-880 mcg/day: Fluticasone 500 mcg/salmeterol 50 mcg **or** Advair® HFA: Fluticasone 230 mcg/salmeterol 21 mcg

Patients currently using inhaled fluticasone propionate powder:

≤200 mcg/day: Fluticasone 100 mcg/salmeterol 50 mcg **or** Advair® HFA: Fluticasone 45 mcg/salmeterol 21 mcg

500 mcg/day: Fluticasone 250 mcg/salmeterol 50 mcg **or** Advair® HFA: Fluticasone 115 mcg/salmeterol 21 mcg

1000 mcg/day: Fluticasone 500 mcg/salmeterol 50 mcg **or** Advair® HFA: Fluticasone 230 mcg/salmeterol 21 mcg

Patients currently using inhaled mometasone furoate powder:

220 mcg/day: Fluticasone 100 mcg/salmeterol 50 mcg **or** Advair® HFA: Fluticasone 45 mcg/salmeterol 21 mcg

440 mcg/day: Fluticasone 250 mcg/salmeterol 50 mcg **or** Advair® HFA: Fluticasone 115 mcg/salmeterol 21 mcg

880 mcg/day: Fluticasone 500 mcg/salmeterol 50 mcg **or** Advair® HFA: Fluticasone 230 mcg/salmeterol 21 mcg

Patients currently using inhaled triamcinolone acetonide:

≤1000 mcg/day: Fluticasone 100 mcg/salmeterol 50 mcg **or** Advair® HFA: Fluticasone 45 mcg/salmeterol 21 mcg

1100-1600 mcg/day: Fluticasone 250 mcg/salmeterol 50 mcg **or** Advair® HFA: Fluticasone 115 mcg/salmeterol 21 mcg

Pediatric Asthma: Oral inhalation:

Children 4-11 years: Advair Diskus®: Fluticasone 100 mcg/salmeterol 50 mcg twice daily, 12 hours apart. **Note:** This is the maximum dose.

Children ≥12 years: Refer to adult dosing.

Hepatic Impairment No dosage adjustment required; manufacturer suggests close monitoring of patients with hepatic impairment.

Administration

Inhalation

Advair Diskus®: After removing from box and foil pouch, write the "Pouch opened" and "Use by" dates on the label on top of the Diskus®. The "Use by" date is 1 month from date of opening the pouch. Every time the lever is pushed back, a dose is ready to be inhaled. Do not close or tilt the Diskus® after the lever is pushed back. Do not play with the lever or move the lever more than once. The dose indicator tells you how many doses are left. When the numbers 5 to 0 appear in red, only a few doses remain. Discard device 1 month after you remove it from the foil pouch or when the dose counter reads "0" (whichever comes first). Rinse mouth with water after use and spit to reduce risk of oral candidiasis.

Advair® HFA: Shake well for 5 seconds before each spray. Prime with 4 test sprays (into air and away from face) before using for the first time. If canister is dropped or not used for >4 weeks, prime with 2 sprays. Patient should contact pharmacy for refill when the dose counter reads "020". Discard device when the dose counter reads "000". Do not spray in eyes. Rinse mouth with water after use and spit to reduce risk of oral candidiasis.

Stability

Storage

Advair Diskus®: Store at controlled room temperature of 20°C to 25°C (68°F to 77°F). Store in a dry place out of direct heat or sunlight. Diskus® device should be discarded 1 month after removal from foil pouch, or when dosing indicator reads "0" (whichever comes first); device is not reusable.

Advair® HFA: Store at controlled room temperature of 25°C (77°F). Store with mouthpiece down. Discard after 120 inhalations. Discard device when the dose counter reads "000". Device is not reusable.

Monitoring and Teaching Issues

Laboratory Monitoring FEV_1, peak flow, and/or other pulmonary function tests

Physical Assessment See individual agents.

Patient Education See individual agents.

Dietary Considerations Advair Diskus® powder for oral inhalation contains lactose; very rare anaphylactic reactions have been reported in patients with severe milk protein allergy.

Geriatric Considerations No differences in safety or effectiveness have been seen in studies of patients ≥65 years of age. However, increased sensitivity may be seen in the elderly. Use with caution in patients with concomitant cardiovascular disease.

Pregnancy Considerations See individual agents.

Additional Information Effects of inhaled/intranasal steroids on growth have been observed in the absence of laboratory evidence of HPA axis suppression, suggesting that growth velocity is a more sensitive indicator of systemic corticosteroid exposure in pediatric patients than some commonly used tests of HPA axis function. The long-term effects of this reduction in growth velocity associated with orally-inhaled and intranasal corticosteroids, including the impact on final adult height, are unknown. The potential for "catch up" growth following discontinuation of treatment with inhaled corticosteroids has not been adequately studied.

Advair® HFA: Salmeterol (base) 21 mcg is equivalent to 30.45 mcg of salmeterol xinafoate.

Related Information

Fluticasone (Oral Inhalation) *on page 798*

Salmeterol *on page 1618*

◆ **Fluticasone Furoate** *see* Fluticasone (Nasal) *on page 802*

◆ **Fluticasone Propionate** *see* Fluticasone (Nasal) *on page 802*

◆ **Fluticasone Propionate** *see* Fluticasone (Oral Inhalation) *on page 798*

◆ **Fluticasone Propionate** *see* Fluticasone (Topical) *on page 803*

◆ **Fluticasone Propionate and Salmeterol Xinafoate** *see* Fluticasone and Salmeterol *on page 804*

Fluvastatin (FLOO va sta tin)

U.S. Brand Names Lescol®; Lescol® XL

Generic Availability (U.S.) No

Pharmacologic Category Antilipemic Agent, HMG-CoA Reductase Inhibitor

Medication Safety Issues

Sound-alike/look-alike issues:

Fluvastatin may be confused with fluoxetine, nystatin, pitavastatin

Pregnancy Risk Factor X

Lactation Enters breast milk/contraindicated

Use To be used as a component of multiple risk factor intervention in patients at risk for atherosclerosis vascular disease due to hypercholesterolemia

Adjunct to dietary therapy to reduce elevated total cholesterol (total-C), LDL-C, triglyceride, and apolipoprotein B (apo-B) levels and to increase HDL-C in primary hypercholesterolemia and mixed dyslipidemia (Fredrickson types IIa and IIb); to slow the progression of coronary atherosclerosis in patients with coronary heart disease; reduce risk of coronary revascularization procedures in patients with coronary heart disease

Mechanism of Action/Effect Acts by competitively inhibiting 3-hydroxyl-3-methylglutaryl-coenzyme A (HMG-CoA) reductase, the enzyme that catalyzes the reduction of HMG-CoA to mevalonate; this is an early rate-limiting step in cholesterol biosynthesis. HDL is increased while total, LDL, and VLDL cholesterols; apolipoprotein B; and plasma triglycerides are decreased.

Contraindications Hypersensitivity to fluvastatin or any component of the formulation; active liver disease; unexplained persistent elevations of serum transaminases; pregnancy; breast-feeding

Warnings/Precautions Secondary causes of hyperlipidemia should be ruled out prior to therapy. Liver function must be monitored by periodic laboratory assessment. Rhabdomyolysis with acute renal failure has occurred with fluvastatin and other HMG-CoA reductase inhibitors. Risk may be increased with concurrent use of other drugs which may cause rhabdomyolysis (including colchicine, gemfibrozil, fibric acid derivatives, or niacin at doses ≥1 g/day). Temporarily discontinue in any patient experiencing markedly elevated CPK levels, myopathy, or an acute/serious condition predisposing to renal failure secondary to rhabdomyolysis. Based upon current evidence, HMG-CoA reductase inhibitor therapy should be continued in the perioperative period unless risk outweighs cardioprotective benefit. Use with caution in patients with advanced age; these patients are predisposed to myopathy. Use caution in patients with previous liver disease or heavy ethanol use. Use caution in patients with concurrent medications or conditions which reduce steroidogenesis.

Drug Interactions

Metabolism/Transport Effects Substrate of CYP2C9 (major), CYP2C8 (minor), CYP2D6 (minor), CYP3A4 (minor), SLCO1B1; **Inhibits** CYP1A2 (weak), 2C8 (weak), 2C9 (moderate), 2D6 (weak), 3A4 (weak)

Avoid Concomitant Use

Avoid concomitant use of Fluvastatin with any of the following: Red Yeast Rice

Decreased Effect

The levels/effects of Fluvastatin may be decreased by: Antacids; Cholestyramine Resin; Etravirine; Peginterferon Alfa-2b; Phenytoin; Rifamycin Derivatives

Increased Effect/Toxicity

Fluvastatin may increase the levels/effects of: Carvedilol; CYP2C9 Substrates (High risk); DAPTOmycin; Trabectedin; Vitamin K Antagonists

The levels/effects of Fluvastatin may be increased by: Amiodarone; Colchicine; Conivaptan; Eltrombopag; Fenofibrate; Fenofibric Acid; Fluconazole; Gemfibrozil; Niacin; Niacinamide; Red Yeast Rice; Rifamycin Derivatives

Nutritional/Ethanol Interactions

Ethanol: Avoid excessive ethanol consumption (due to potential hepatic effects).

Food: Reduces rate but not the extent of absorption. Red yeast rice contains an estimated 2.4 mg lovastatin per 600 mg rice.

Lab Interactions Increased serum transaminases, CPK, alkaline phosphatase, and bilirubin and thyroid function tests

Adverse Reactions As reported with fluvastatin capsules; in general, adverse reactions reported with fluvastatin extended release tablet were similar, but the incidence was less.

1% to 10%:

Central nervous system: Headache (9%), fatigue (3%), insomnia (3%)

Gastrointestinal: Dyspepsia (8%), diarrhea (5%), abdominal pain (5%), nausea (3%)

Genitourinary: Urinary tract infection (2%)
Neuromuscular & skeletal: Myalgia (5%)
Respiratory: Sinusitis (3%), bronchitis (2%)

Pharmacodynamics/Kinetics

Onset of Action Peak effect: Maximal LDL-C reductions achieved within 4 weeks

Bioavailability Absolute: Capsule: 24%; Extended release tablet: 29%

Time to Peak Capsule: 1 hour; Extended release tablet: 3 hours

Protein Binding >98%

Half-Life Elimination Capsule: <3 hours; Extended release tablet: 9 hours

Metabolism To inactive and active metabolites (oxidative metabolism via CYP2C9 [75%], 2C8 [~5%], and 3A4 [~20%] isoenzymes); active forms do not circulate systemically; extensive (saturable) first-pass hepatic extraction

Excretion Feces (90%): urine (5%)

Available Dosage Forms

Capsule, oral:
Lescol®: 20 mg, 40 mg

Tablet, extended release, oral:
Lescol® XL: 80 mg

Dosing

Adult & Geriatric

Dyslipidemia (also delay in progression of CAD): Oral:

Patients requiring ≥25% decrease in LDL-C: 40 mg capsule once daily in the evening, 80 mg extended release tablet once daily (anytime), or 40 mg capsule twice daily

Patients requiring <25% decrease in LDL-C: Initial: 20 mg capsule once daily in the evening; may increase based on tolerability and response to a maximum recommended dose of 80 mg/day, given in 2 divided doses (immediate release capsule) or as a single daily dose (extended release tablet)

Pediatric

Heterozygous familial hypercholesterolemia: Adolescents 10-16 years: Oral: Initial: 20 mg once daily; may increase every 6 weeks based on tolerability and response to a maximum recommended dose of 80 mg/day, given in 2 divided doses (immediate release capsule) or as a single daily dose (extended release tablet)

Note: Indicated only for adjunctive therapy when diet alone cannot reduce LDL-C below 190 mg/dL, or 160 mg/dL (with cardiovascular risk factors). Female patients must be 1 year postmenarche.

Renal Impairment Less than 6% is excreted renally. No dosage adjustment needed with mild-to-moderate renal impairment; use with caution in severe impairment.

Hepatic Impairment Levels may accumulate in patients with liver disease (increased AUC and C_{max}). Use caution with severe hepatic impairment or heavy ethanol ingestion. Contraindicated in active liver disease or unexplained transaminase elevations. Decrease dose and monitor effects carefully in patients with hepatic insufficiency.

Administration

Oral Patient should be placed on a standard cholesterol-lowering diet before and during treatment. Fluvastatin may be taken without regard to meals. Adjust dosage as needed in response to periodic lipid determinations during the first 4 weeks after a dosage change; lipid-lowering effects are additive when fluvastatin is combined with a bile-acid binding resin or niacin, however, it must be administered at least 2 hours following these drugs. Do not break, chew, or crush extended release tablets; do not open capsules.

Stability

Storage Store at 15°C to 30°C (59°F to 86°F). Protect from light.

Monitoring and Teaching Issues

Laboratory Monitoring Obtain baseline LFTs and total cholesterol profile. Repeat tests at 12 weeks after initiation of therapy or elevation in dose, and periodically thereafter; baseline CPK (recheck CPK in any patient with symptoms suggestive of myopathy). Monitor LDL-C at intervals no less than 4 weeks.

Physical Assessment Rule out secondary causes of hyperlipidemia prior to initiation. Assess risk potential for interactions with other prescriptions or herbal products patient may be taking that may increase risk of rhabdomyolysis. Assess LFTs and cholesterol profile prior to treatment and at regular intervals.

Patient Education Take as directed, with or without food. If taking other chloesterol-lowering medication, check with prescriber for appropriate timing. Do not chew, crush, or dissolve extended release tablets; swallow whole. Follow prescribed diet and exercise regimen. You will need periodic laboratory tests to evaluate response. Avoid excessive alcohol. Report unusual muscle cramping or weakness, yellowing of skin or eyes, easy bruising or bleeding, or unusual fatigue.

Dietary Considerations Generally, patients should be placed on a standard cholesterol-lowering diet and other lifestyle modifications for 3-6 months prior to the initiation of drug therapy. The diet should be continued during drug therapy. However, for patients with advanced risk factors (eg, known coronary heart disease), drug therapy may be initiated concurrently with diet modification. May be taken without regard to meals. Red yeast rice contains an estimated 2.4 mg lovastatin per 600 mg rice.

Geriatric Considerations The definition of and, therefore, when to treat hyperlipidemia in the elderly is a controversial issue. The National Cholesterol Education Program recommends that all adults maintain a plasma cholesterol <160 mg/dL. In elderly patients with one additional risk factor, goal LDL would decrease to <130 mg/dL. Pharmacologic treatment should be reserved for those who are unable to obtain a desirable plasma cholesterol concentration by diet alone and for whom the benefits of treatment are believed to outweigh the potential adverse effects, drug interactions, and cost of treatment.

Breast-Feeding Considerations Fluvastatin is excreted in human breast milk (milk plasma ratio 2:1); do not use in breast-feeding women.

Pregnancy Considerations Cholesterol biosynthesis may be important in fetal development. Contraindicated in pregnancy. Administer to women of childbearing potential only when conception is highly unlikely and patients have been informed of potential hazards.

Related Information

Hyperlipidemia Management *on page 2046*

◆ **Fluvirin®** *see* Influenza Virus Vaccine (Inactivated) *on page 978*

Fluvoxamine (floo VOKS a meen)

U.S. Brand Names Luvox® CR

Index Terms Luvox

Generic Availability (U.S.) Yes: Excludes extended release capsule

Pharmacologic Category Antidepressant, Selective Serotonin Reuptake Inhibitor

Medication Safety Issues

Sound-alike/look-alike issues:

FluvoxaMINE may be confused with flavoxATE, FLUoxetine, fluPHENAZine

Luvox may be confused with Lasix®, Levoxyl®, Lovenox®

Medication Guide Available Yes

Pregnancy Risk Factor C

Lactation Enters breast milk/consider risk:benefit (AAP rates "of concern"; AAP 2001 update pending)

Use Treatment of obsessive-compulsive disorder (OCD); treatment of social anxiety disorder

Unlabeled/Investigational Use Treatment of major depression; panic disorder; anxiety disorders in children; treatment of mild dementia-associated agitation in nonpsychotic patients; post-traumatic stress disorder (PTSD)

Mechanism of Action/Effect Inhibits CNS neuron serotonin uptake; minimal or no effect on reuptake of norepinephrine or dopamine; does not significantly bind to alpha-adrenergic, histamine or cholinergic receptors

Contraindications Hypersensitivity to fluvoxamine or any component of the formulation; concurrent use with alosetron, pimozide, thioridazine, or tizanidine; use with or within 14 days of MAO inhibitors

Warnings/Precautions [U.S. Boxed Warning]: Antidepressants increase the risk of suicidal thinking and behavior in children, adolescents, and young adults (18-24 years of age) with major depressive disorder (MDD) and other psychiatric disorders; consider risk prior to prescribing. Short-term studies did not show an increased risk in patients >24 years of age and showed a decreased risk in patients ≥65 years. Closely monitor patients for clinical worsening, suicidality, or unusual changes in behavior, particularly during the initial 1-2 months of therapy or during periods of dosage adjustments (increases or decreases); the patient's family or caregiver should be instructed to closely observe the patient and communicate condition with healthcare provider. A medication guide concerning the use of antidepressants should be dispensed with each prescription. **Fluvoxamine is FDA approved for the treatment of OCD in children ≥8 years of age; extended release capsules are not FDA approved for use in children.**

The possibility of a suicide attempt is inherent in major depression and may persist until remission occurs. Use caution in high-risk patients. Worsening depression and severe abrupt suicidality that are not part of the presenting symptoms may require discontinuation or modification of drug therapy. The patient's family or caregiver should be alerted to monitor patients for the emergence of suicidality and associated behaviors (such as agitation, irritability, hostility, impulsivity, and hypomania) and call healthcare provider.

May worsen psychosis in some patients or precipitate a shift to mania or hypomania in patients with bipolar disorder. Patients presenting with depressive symptoms should be screened for bipolar disorder. Monotherapy in patients with bipolar disorder should be avoided. **Fluvoxamine is not FDA approved for the treatment of bipolar depression.**

Serotonin syndrome and neuroleptic malignant syndrome (NMS)-like reactions have occurred with serotonin/norepinephrine reuptake inhibitors (SNRIs) and selective serotonin reuptake inhibitors (SSRIs) when used alone, and particularly when used in combination with serotonergic agents (eg, triptans) or antidopaminergic agents (eg, antipsychotics). Concurrent use with MAO inhibitors is contraindicated. Fluvoxamine has a low potential to impair cognitive or motor performance; caution operating hazardous machinery or driving. Use caution in patients with a previous seizure disorder or condition predisposing to seizures such as brain damage, alcoholism, or concurrent therapy with other drugs which lower the seizure threshold. Fluvoxamine may significantly increase alosetron concentrations; concurrent use **contraindicated.** Potential for QT_c prolongation and arrhythmia with thioridazine and pimozide; concurrent use of fluvoxamine with either of these agents is **contraindicated.** Concomitant use with tizanidine may cause a significant decrease in blood pressure and increase in drowsiness; concurrent use is **contraindicated.** Fluvoxamine levels may be lower in patients who smoke.

May increase the risks associated with electroconvulsive therapy. Use with caution in patients with hepatic dysfunction and in elderly patients. May cause hyponatremia/SIADH (elderly at increased risk); volume depletion (diuretics may increase risk). Use with caution in patients at risk of bleeding or receiving concurrent anticoagulant therapy, although not consistently noted, fluvoxamine may cause impairment in platelet function. May cause or exacerbate sexual dysfunction.

Drug Interactions

Metabolism/Transport Effects Substrate (major) of CYP1A2, 2D6; **Inhibits** CYP1A2 (strong), 2B6 (weak), 2C9 (weak), 2C19 (strong), 2D6 (weak), 3A4 (weak)

Avoid Concomitant Use

Avoid concomitant use of FluvoxaMINE with any of the following: Alosetron; Clopidogrel; Iobenguane I 123; MAO Inhibitors; Methylene Blue; Pimozide; Ramelteon; Sibutramine; Thioridazine; TiZANidine; Tryptophan

Decreased Effect

FluvoxaMINE may decrease the levels/effects of: Clopidogrel; Iobenguane I 123

The levels/effects of FluvoxaMINE may be decreased by: CarBAMazepine; CYP1A2 Inducers (Strong); Cyproheptadine; Peginterferon Alfa-2b

Increased Effect/Toxicity

FluvoxaMINE may increase the levels/effects of: Alcohol (Ethyl); Alosetron; Anticoagulants; Antidepressants (Serotonin Reuptake Inhibitor/Antagonist); Antiplatelet Agents; Asenapine; Aspirin; Bendamustine; Benzodiazepines (metabolized by oxidation); Bromazepam; BusPIRone; CarBAMazepine; CloZAPine; CNS Depressants; Collagenase (Systemic); CYP1A2 Substrates; CYP2C19 Substrates; Desmopressin; Drotrecogin Alfa; DULoxetine; Erlotinib; Haloperidol; Ibritumomab; Lithium; Methadone; Methotrimeprazine; Methylene Blue; Mexiletine; NSAID (COX-2 Inhibitor); NSAID (Nonselective); OLANZapine; Phenytoin; Pimozide; Propafenone; Propranolol; QuiNIDine; Ramelteon; Roflumilast; Ropivacaine; Salicylates; Serotonin Modulators; Theophylline Derivatives; Thioridazine; Thrombolytic Agents; TiZANidine; Tositumomab and Iodine I 131 Tositumomab; TraMADol; Tricyclic Antidepressants; Vitamin K Antagonists

The levels/effects of FluvoxaMINE may be increased by: Analgesics (Opioid); BusPIRone; Cimetidine; CYP1A2 Inhibitors (Moderate); CYP1A2 Inhibitors (Strong); CYP2D6 Inhibitors (Moderate); CYP2D6 Inhibitors (Strong); Darunavir; Dasatinib; Droperidol; Glucosamine; Herbs (Anticoagulant/Antiplatelet Properties); MAO Inhibitors; Methotrimeprazine; Metoclopramide; Omega-3-Acid Ethyl Esters; Pentosan Polysulfate Sodium; Pentoxifylline; Prostacyclin Analogues; Sibutramine; TraMADol; Tryptophan

Nutritional/Ethanol Interactions

Ethanol: Avoid ethanol. Patients with depression should avoid/limit intake.

Food: The bioavailability of melatonin has been reported to be increased by fluvoxamine.

Herb/Nutraceutical: Avoid valerian, St John's wort, SAMe, kava kava (may increase risk of serotonin syndrome and/or excessive sedation). Avoid alfalfa, anise, bilberry, bladderwrack, bromelain, cat's claw, celery, chamomile, coleus, cordyceps, dong quai, evening primrose, fenugreek, feverfew, garlic, ginger, ginkgo biloba, ginseng (American), ginseng (Panax), ginseng (Siberian), grape seed, green tea, guggul, horse chestnuts, horseradish, licorice, prickly ash, red clover, reishi, SAMe (S-adenosylmethionine), sweet clover, turmeric, white willow (all have additional antiplatelet activity).

Adverse Reactions Frequency varies by dosage form and indication. Adverse reactions reported as a composite of all indications.

>10%:

Central nervous system: Headache (22% to 35%), insomnia (21% to 35%), somnolence (22% to 27%), dizziness (11% to 15%), nervousness (10% to 12%)

Gastrointestinal: Nausea (34% to 40%), diarrhea (11% to 18%), xerostomia (10% to 14%), anorexia (6% to 14%)

Genitourinary: Ejaculation abnormal (8% to 11%)

Neuromuscular & skeletal: Weakness (14% to 26%)

1% to 10%:

Cardiovascular: Chest pain (3%), palpitation (3%), vasodilation (2% to 3%), hypertension (1% to 2%), edema (≤1%), hypotension (≤1%), syncope (≤1%), tachycardia (≤1%)

Central nervous system: Pain (10%), anxiety (5% to 8%), abnormal dreams (3%), abnormal thinking (3%), agitation (2% to 3%), apathy (≥1% to 3%), chills (2%), CNS stimulation (2%), depression (2%), neurosis (2%), amnesia, malaise, manic reaction, psychotic reaction

Dermatologic: Bruising (4%), acne (2%)

Endocrine & metabolic: Libido decreased (2% to 10%; incidence higher in males), anorgasmia (2% to 5%), sexual function abnormal (2% to 4%), menorrhagia (3%)

Gastrointestinal: Dyspepsia (8% to 10%), constipation (4% to 10%), vomiting (4% to 6%), abdominal pain (5%), flatulence (4%), taste perversion (2% to 3%), tooth disorder (2% to 3%), dysphagia (2%), gingivitis (2%), weight loss (≤1% to 2%), weight gain

Genitourinary: Polyuria (2% to 3%), impotence (2%), urinary tract infection (2%), urinary retention (1%)

Hepatic: Liver function tests abnormal (≥1% to 2%)

Neuromuscular & skeletal: Tremor (5% to 8%), myalgia (5%), paresthesia (3%), hypertonia (2%), twitching (2%), hyper-/hypokinesia, myoclonus

Ocular: Amblyopia (2% to 3%)

Respiratory: Upper respiratory infection (9%), pharyngitis (6%), yawn (2% to 5%), laryngitis (3%), bronchitis (2%), dyspnea (2%), epistaxis (2%), cough increased, sinusitis

Miscellaneous: Diaphoresis (6% to 7%), flu-like syndrome (3%), viral infection (2%)

Pharmacodynamics/Kinetics

Onset of Action Depression: The onset of action is within a week; however, individual response varies greatly and full response may not be seen until 8-12 weeks after initiation of treatment.

Absorption Steady-state plasma concentrations have been noted to be 2-3 times higher in children than those in adolescents; female children demonstrated a significantly higher AUC than males

Bioavailability Immediate release: 53%; not significantly affected by food

Time to Peak Plasma: 3-8 hours

Protein Binding ~80%, primarily to albumin

Half-Life Elimination 15-16 hours; 17-26 hours in the elderly

Metabolism Extensively hepatic via oxidative demethylation and deamination

Excretion Urine (~85% as metabolites; ~2% as unchanged drug)

Available Dosage Forms

Capsule, extended release, oral:

Luvox® CR: 100 mg, 150 mg

Tablet, oral: 25 mg, 50 mg, 100 mg

Dosing

Adult

Obsessive-compulsive disorder: Oral:

Immediate release: Initial: 50 mg once daily at bedtime; may be increased in 50 mg increments at 4- to 7-day intervals, as tolerated; usual dose range: 100-300 mg/day; maximum dose: 300 mg/day. **Note:** When total daily dose exceeds 100 mg, the dose should be given in 2 divided doses with larger portion administered at bedtime.

Extended release: Initial: 100 mg once daily at bedtime; may be increased in 50 mg increments at intervals of at least 1 week; usual dosage range: 100-300 mg/day; maximum dose: 300 mg/day

Social anxiety disorder: Extended release: Oral: Initial: 100 mg once daily at bedtime; may be increased in 50 mg increments at intervals of at least 1 week; usual dosage range: 100-300 mg/day; maximum dose: 300 mg/day

Post-traumatic stress disorder (PTSD) (unlabeled use): Immediate release: Oral: 75 mg twice daily

Geriatric Reduce dose; titrate slowly.

Pediatric Obsessive-compulsive disorder: Oral:

Children 8-17 years: Immediate release: Initial: 25 mg once daily at bedtime; may be increased in 25 mg increments at 4- to 7-day intervals, as tolerated, to maximum therapeutic benefit; usual dose range: 50-200 mg/day. **Note:** When total daily dose of immediate release exceeds 50 mg, the dose should be given in 2 divided doses with larger portion administered at bedtime.

Maximum dose: Children: 8-11 years: 200 mg/day; Adolescents: 300 mg/day; lower doses may be effective in female versus male patients

Hepatic Impairment Reduce dose; titrate slowly.

Administration

Oral May be administered with or without food. Do not crush, open, or chew extended release capsules.

Stability

Storage Protect from high humidity and store at controlled room temperature 25°C (77°F).

Monitoring and Teaching Issues

Laboratory Monitoring Liver function assessment prior to beginning drug therapy

Physical Assessment Taper dosage slowly when discontinuing. Assess mental status for depression, signs of clinical worsening, suicide ideation, anxiety, social functioning, mania, or panic attack.

Patient Education It may take 2-3 weeks to achieve desired results. Avoid alcohol. Maintain adequate hydration, unless instructed to restrict fluid intake. You may experience drowsiness, lightheadedness, impaired coordination, dizziness, weakness, blurred vision, nausea, vomiting, dry mouth, anorexia, diarrhea, postural hypotension, or decreased sexual function or libido (reversible). Report persistent CNS effects (insomnia, anxiety, suicide ideation, sedation, seizures, mania, abnormal thinking); rash; tremors; chest pain or palpitations; or worsening of condition.

Dietary Considerations May be taken with or without food.

Geriatric Considerations Given fluvoxamine's approved indication (OCD), the number of drug interactions, and the limited information available on its use in the elderly, it may be best to select a different agent when treating depression. The elderly are more prone to SSRI/SNRI-induced hyponatremia.

Breast-Feeding Considerations Fluvoxamine is excreted in breast milk. Based on case reports, the dose the infant receives is relatively small and adverse events have not been observed. According to the manufacturer, the decision to continue or discontinue breast-feeding during therapy should take into account the risk of exposure to the infant and the benefits of treatment to the mother.

The long-term effects on development and behavior have not been studied; therefore, fluvoxamine should be prescribed to a mother who is breast-feeding only when the benefits outweigh the potential risks.

Pregnancy Considerations Due to adverse effects observed in animal studies, fluvoxamine is classified as pregnancy category C. Fluvoxamine crosses the human placenta. Non-teratogenic effects in the newborn following SSRI exposure late in the third trimester include respiratory distress, cyanosis, apnea, seizures, temperature instability, feeding difficulty, vomiting, hypoglycemia, hypo- or hypertonia, hyper-reflexia, jitteriness, irritability, constant crying, and tremor. An increased risk of low birth weight and low Apgar scores has also been reported. Exposure to SSRIs after the twentieth week of gestation has been associated with persistent pulmonary hypertension of the newborn (PPHN). Adverse effects may be due to toxic effects of the SSRI or drug withdrawal due to discontinuation. The long-term effects of *in utero* SSRI exposure on infant development and behavior are not known.

Women treated for major depression and who are euthymic prior to pregnancy are more likely to experience a relapse when medication is discontinued as compared to pregnant women who continue taking antidepressant medications. The ACOG recommends that therapy with SSRIs or SNRIs during pregnancy be individualized; treatment of depression during pregnancy should incorporate the clinical expertise of the mental health clinician, obstetrician, primary healthcare provider, and pediatrician. If treatment during pregnancy is required, consider tapering therapy during the third trimester in order to prevent withdrawal symptoms in the infant. If this is done and the woman is considered to be at risk of relapse from her major depressive disorder, the medication can be restarted following delivery, although the dose should be readjusted to that required before pregnancy. Treatment algorithms have been developed by the ACOG and the APA for the management of depression in women prior to conception and during pregnancy (Yonkers, 2009).

Related Information

Antidepressant Agents *on page* *1982*

- **Fluzone®** *see* Influenza Virus Vaccine (Inactivated) *on page* *978*
- **Fluzone® High-Dose** *see* Influenza Virus Vaccine (Inactivated) *on page* *978*
- **FML®** *see* Fluorometholone *on page* *786*
- **FML Forte®** *see* Fluorometholone *on page* *786*
- **Focalin®** *see* Dexmethylphenidate *on page* *506*
- **Focalin® XR** *see* Dexmethylphenidate *on page* *506*
- **Folacin** *see* Folic Acid *on page* *812*
- **Folacin-800 [OTC]** *see* Folic Acid *on page* *812*
- **Folate** *see* Folic Acid *on page* *812*

Folic Acid (FOE lik AS id)

U.S. Brand Names Folacin-800 [OTC]

Index Terms Folacin; Folate; Pteroylglutamic Acid

Generic Availability (U.S.) Yes

Pharmacologic Category Vitamin, Water Soluble

Medication Safety Issues

Sound-alike/look-alike issues:

Folic acid may be confused with folinic acid

Pregnancy Risk Factor A

Lactation Enters breast milk/compatible

Use Treatment of megaloblastic and macrocytic anemias due to folate deficiency; dietary supplement to prevent neural tube defects

Unlabeled/Investigational Use Adjunctive cofactor therapy in methanol toxicity (alternative to leucovorin calcium)

Available Dosage Forms

Injection, solution: 5 mg/mL (10 mL)

Tablet, oral: 0.4 mg, 0.8 mg, 1 mg

Folacin-800 [OTC]: 0.8 mg

Dosing

Adult

Anemia: Oral, I.M., I.V., SubQ: 0.4 mg/day

Pregnant and lactating women: 0.8 mg/day

RDA: Expressed as dietary folate equivalents: 400 mcg/day

Prevention of neural tube defects: Oral:

Females of childbearing potential: 400-800 mcg/day (USPSTF)

Females at high risk or with family history of neural tube defects: 4 mg/day

Geriatric Refer to adult dosing. Vitamin B_{12} deficiency must be ruled out before initiating folate therapy due to frequency of combined nutritional deficiencies: RDA requirements (1999): 400 mcg/day (0.4 mg) minimum.

Pediatric

Anemia: Oral, I.M., I.V., SubQ:

Infants: 0.1 mg/day

Children <4 years: Up to 0.3 mg/day

Children >4 years and Adults: Refer to adult dosing.

RDA: Expressed as dietary folate equivalents: Oral: Children:

1-3 years: 150 mcg/day

4-8 years: 200 mcg/day

9-13 years: 300 mcg/day

≥14 years: Refer to adult dosing.

Administration

I.M. May also be administered by deep I.M. injection.

Monitoring and Teaching Issues

Patient Education Increased intake of foods high in folic acid may be recommended by prescriber. Excessive use of alcohol increases requirement for folic acid. Report skin rash.

- **Folinic Acid (error prone synonym)** *see* Leucovorin Calcium *on page* *1080*

- ◆ **Follicle Stimulating Hormone, Recombinant** *see* Follitropin Alfa *on page* 813
- ◆ **Follicle Stimulating Hormone, Recombinant** *see* Follitropin Beta *on page* 815
- ◆ **Follistim® AQ** *see* Follitropin Beta *on page* 815
- ◆ **Follistim® AQ Cartridge** *see* Follitropin Beta *on page* 815

Follitropin Alfa (foe li TRO pin AL fa)

U.S. Brand Names Gonal-f®; Gonal-f® RFF; Gonal-f® RFF Pen

Index Terms Follicle Stimulating Hormone, Recombinant; FSH; rFSH-alpha; rhFSH-alpha

Generic Availability (U.S.) No

Pharmacologic Category Gonadotropin; Ovulation Stimulator

Pregnancy Risk Factor X

Lactation Excretion in breast milk unknown/not recommended

Use

Gonal-f®: Ovulation induction in patients in whom the cause of infertility is functional and not caused by primary ovarian failure; development of multiple follicles with Assisted Reproductive Technology (ART); spermatogenesis induction

Gonal-f® RFF: Ovulation induction in patients in whom the cause of infertility is functional and not caused by primary ovarian failure; development of multiple follicles with ART

Mechanism of Action/Effect Follitropin alfa is a human FSH preparation of recombinant DNA origin. Follitropins stimulate ovarian follicular growth in women who do not have primary ovarian failure, and stimulate spermatogenesis in men with hypogonadotrophic hypogonadism. FSH is required for normal follicular growth, maturation, gonadal steroid production, and spermatogenesis.

Contraindications Hypersensitivity to follitropins or any component of the formulation; high levels of FSH indicating primary gonadal failure (ovarian or testicular); uncontrolled thyroid or adrenal dysfunction; tumor of the ovary, breast, uterus, hypothalamus, testis, or pituitary gland; abnormal vaginal bleeding of undetermined origin; ovarian cysts or enlargement not due to polycystic ovary syndrome; pregnancy

Warnings/Precautions These medications should only be used by physicians who are thoroughly familiar with infertility problems and their management. To minimize risks, use only at the lowest effective dose. Monitor ovarian response with serum estradiol and vaginal ultrasound on a regular basis.

Ovarian enlargement, which may be accompanied by abdominal distention or abdominal pain, occurs in ~20% of those treated with urofollitropin and hCG, and generally regresses without treatment within 2-3 weeks. If ovaries are abnormally enlarged on the last day of treatment, withhold hCG to reduce the risk of ovarian hyperstimulation syndrome (OHSS). OHSS is reported in about 7% of patients; it is characterized by severe ovarian enlargement, abdominal pain/distention, nausea, vomiting, diarrhea, dyspnea, and oliguria, and may be accompanied by ascites, pleural effusion, hypovolemia, electrolyte imbalance, hemoperitoneum, and thromboembolic events. If hyperstimulation occurs, stop treatment and hospitalize patient. This syndrome develops rapidly within 24 hours to several days and generally occurs during the 7-10 days immediately following treatment. Hemoconcentration associated with fluid loss into the abdominal cavity has occurred and should be assessed by fluid intake and output, weight, hematocrit, serum and urinary electrolytes, urine specific gravity, BUN and creatinine, and abdominal girth. Determinations should be performed daily or more often if the need arises. Treatment is primarily symptomatic and consists of bedrest, fluid and electrolyte replacement, and analgesics. The ascitic, pleural, and pericardial fluids should not be removed unless needed to relieve symptoms of cardiopulmonary distress.

Serious pulmonary conditions (atelectasis, acute respiratory distress syndrome, and exacerbation of asthma) have been reported. Thromboembolic events, both in association with and separate from ovarian hyperstimulation syndrome, have been reported.

Multiple births may result from the use of these medications; advise patient of the potential risk of multiple births before starting the treatment. Safety and efficacy have not been established in children.

Drug Interactions

Avoid Concomitant Use There are no known interactions where it is recommended to avoid concomitant use.

Decreased Effect There are no known significant interactions involving a decrease in effect.

Increased Effect/Toxicity There are no known significant interactions involving an increase in effect.

Adverse Reactions Percentage may vary by indication, product formulation

>10%:

Central nervous system: Headache
Endocrine & metabolic: Ovarian cyst
Gastrointestinal: Abdomen enlarged, abdominal pain, nausea
Miscellaneous: Upper respiratory infection

1% to 10%:

Central nervous system: Dizziness, emotional lability, fever, malaise, migraine, pain
Dermatologic: Acne

Endocrine & metabolic: Breast pain, cervix lesion, hot flashes, intermenstrual bleeding, menstrual disorder, ovarian disorder, ovarian hyperstimulation

Gastrointestinal: Constipation, diarrhea, dyspepsia, flatulence, pelvic pain, stomatitis (ulcerative), toothache, vomiting, weight gain

Genitourinary: Cystitis, leukorrhea, micturition frequency, urinary tract infection, uterine hemorrhage, vaginal hemorrhage

Local: Injection site bruising, edema, inflammation, pain, reaction

Neuromuscular & skeletal: Back pain

Respiratory: Cough, flu-like symptoms, pharyngitis, rhinitis, sinusitis

Miscellaneous: Infection, moniliasis

Pharmacodynamics/Kinetics

Onset of Action Peak effect:

Spermatogenesis, median: 6.8-12.4 months (range: 2.7-15.7 months)

Follicle development: Within cycle

Absorption I.M., SubQ: Absorption rate is slower than the elimination rate

Bioavailability ~66% to 76% in healthy female volunteers

Time to Peak In healthy volunteers:

Females: SubQ: 8-16 hours; I.M.: 25 hours

Males: SubQ: 11-20 hours

Half-Life Elimination

I.M.: 50 hours in healthy female volunteers

SubQ: 24 hours in healthy female volunteers; 32 hours with *in vitro* fertilization/embryo transfer patients; 32-41 hours in healthy male volunteers

Excretion Clearance: I.V.: 0.6 L/hour in healthy female volunteers

Available Dosage Forms

Injection, powder for reconstitution:

Gonal-f®: 450 int. units, 1050 int. units

Gonal-f® RFF: 75 int. units

Injection, solution:

Gonal-f® RFF Pen: 300 int. units/0.5 mL (0.5 mL); 450 int. units/0.75 mL (0.75 mL); 900 int. units/1.5 mL (1.5 mL)

Dosing

Adult Note: Dose should be individualized. Use the lowest dose consistent with the expectation of good results. Over the course of treatment, doses may vary depending on individual patient response.

Ovulation induction: *Gonal-f®, Gonal-f® RFF:* Females: SubQ: Initial: 75 int. units/day; incremental dose adjustments of up to 37.5 int. units may be considered after 14 days; further dose increases of the same magnitude can be made, if necessary, every 7 days (maximum dose: 300 int. units/day). If response to follitropin is appropriate, hCG is given 1 day following the last dose. Withhold hCG if serum estradiol is >2000 pg/mL, if the ovaries are abnormally enlarged, or if abdominal pain occurs. In general, therapy should not exceed 35 days.

ART: *Gonal-f®, Gonal-f® RFF:* Females: SubQ: Initiate therapy with follitropin alfa in the early follicular phase (cycle day 2 or day 3) at a dose of 150 int. units/day, until sufficient follicular development is attained. In most cases, therapy should not exceed 10 days. In patients ≥35 years whose endogenous gonadotropin levels are suppressed, initiate follitropin alfa at a dose of 225 int. units/day. Continue treatment until adequate follicular development is indicated as determined by ultrasound in combination with measurement of serum estradiol levels. Consider adjustments to dose after 5 days based on the patient's response; adjust subsequent dosage every 3-5 days by ≤75-150 int. units additionally at each adjustment. Doses >450 int. units/day are not recommended. Once adequate follicular development is evident, administer hCG to induce final follicular maturation in preparation for oocyte. Withhold hCG if the ovaries are abnormally enlarged.

Spermatogenesis induction: *Gonal-f®:* Males: SubQ: Therapy should begin with hCG pretreatment until serum testosterone is in normal range, then 150 int. units 3 times/week with hCG 3 times/week; continue with lowest dose needed to induce spermatogenesis (maximum dose: 300 int. units 3 times/week); may be given for up to 18 months

Geriatric Refer to adult dosing. Clinical studies did not include patients >65 years.

Administration

Other Gonal-f®, Gonal-f® RFF: Administer SubQ. Contents of multidose vials should be administered using the calibrated syringes provided by the manufacturer. Do not shake solution; allow any bubbles to settle prior to administration.

Stability

Reconstitution

Gonal-f®: Dissolve the contents of vial by slowly injecting provided diluent; do not shake. If bubbles appear, allow to settle prior to use. Final concentration: 600 int. units/mL.

Gonal-f® RFF: Powder: Dissolve contents of one or more vials using diluent provided in prefilled syringe. (Total concentration should not exceed 450 int. units/mL.) Slowly inject diluent into vial, and gently rotate vial until powder is dissolved; do not shake vial. If bubbles appear, allow to settle prior to use. Use immediately after reconstitution.

Storage

Gonal-f®: Store powder refrigerated or at room temperature of 2°C to 25°C (36°F to 77°F). Protect from light. Following reconstitution, multidose vials may be stored under refrigeration or at room temperature for up to 28 days. Protect from light.

Gonal-f® RFF:

Powder: Store at room temperature or under refrigeration of 2°C to 25°C (36°F to 77°F). Protect from light.

Solution: Prior to dispensing, store under refrigeration at 2°C to 8°C (36°F to 46°F). Upon dispensing, patient may store under refrigeration until product expiration date or at room temperature of 20°C to 25°C (68°F to 77°F) for up to 3 months. Do not freeze. Protect from light. After first use, discard unused portion after 28 days.

Monitoring and Teaching Issues

Laboratory Monitoring Monitor sufficient follicular maturation. This may be directly estimated by sonographic visualization of the ovaries and endometrial lining or measuring serum estradiol levels. The combination of both ultrasonography and measurement of estradiol levels is useful for monitoring for the growth and development of follicles and timing hCG administration.

Spermatogenesis: Monitor serum testosterone levels, sperm count.

Physical Assessment Teach patient appropriate injection technique and syringe disposal.

Patient Education This medication can only be administered by injection. If you are using this medication at home, follow exact instructions for administering injections and disposal of syringes. Frequent laboratory tests will be required while you are on this therapy; do not miss appointments for laboratory tests or ultrasound. You may experience headache, dizziness, fever, nausea, or vomiting. Report immediately abdominal pain/distension or bloating; persistent nausea, vomiting, or diarrhea; dyspnea; respiratory difficulty or exacerbation of asthma; swelling, pain, or redness of extremities; itching or burning on urination; menstrual irregularity, acute backache; or rash, pain, or inflammation at injection site.

Pregnancy Considerations Ectopic pregnancy, congenital abnormalities, spontaneous abortion, and multiple births have been reported. The incidence of congenital abnormality may be slightly higher after ART than with spontaneous conception; higher incidence may be related to parenteral characteristics (maternal age, sperm characteristics).

Additional Information The currently available recombinant follitropin products are structurally identical to native follicle-stimulating hormone. The "alpha" and "beta" nomenclature refers to their differences in purification and order of marketing. Follitropin alpha was marketed first, followed by follitropin beta. RFF for the Gonal-f® product signifies "revised formula female."

Follitropin Beta (foe li TRO pin BAY ta)

U.S. Brand Names Follistim® AQ; Follistim® AQ Cartridge

Index Terms Follicle Stimulating Hormone, Recombinant; FSH; rFSH-beta; rhFSH-beta

Generic Availability (U.S.) No

Pharmacologic Category Gonadotropin; Ovulation Stimulator

Pregnancy Risk Factor X

Lactation Excretion in breast milk unknown/not recommended

Use Ovulation induction in patients in whom the cause of infertility is functional and not caused by primary ovarian failure; development of multiple follicles with Assisted Reproductive Technology (ART)

Mechanism of Action/Effect Follitropin beta is a human FSH preparation of recombinant DNA origin. Follitropins stimulate ovarian follicular growth in women who do not have primary ovarian failure. FSH is required for normal follicular growth, maturation, gonadal steroid production, and spermatogenesis.

Contraindications Hypersensitivity to follitropins or any component of the formulation; high levels of FSH indicating primary ovarian failure; uncontrolled thyroid or adrenal dysfunction; tumor of the ovary, breast, uterus, hypothalamus, or pituitary gland; abnormal vaginal bleeding of undetermined origin; ovarian cysts or enlargement not due to polycystic ovary syndrome; pregnancy

Warnings/Precautions These medications should only be used by physicians who are thoroughly familiar with infertility problems and their management. To minimize risks, use only at the lowest effective dose. Monitor ovarian response with serum estradiol and vaginal ultrasound on a regular basis.

Ovarian enlargement, which may be accompanied by abdominal distention or abdominal pain, occurs in ~20% of those treated with urofollitropin and hCG, and generally regresses without treatment within 2-3 weeks. If ovaries are abnormally enlarged on the last day of treatment, withhold hCG to reduce the risk of ovarian hyperstimulation syndrome (OHSS). OHSS is characterized by severe ovarian enlargement, abdominal pain/distention, nausea, vomiting, diarrhea, dyspnea, and oliguria, and may be accompanied by ascites, pleural effusion, hypovolemia, electrolyte imbalance, hemoperitoneum, and thromboembolic events. If hyperstimulation occurs, stop treatment and hospitalize patient. This syndrome develops rapidly within 24 hours to several days and generally occurs during the 7-10 days immediately following treatment. Hemoconcentration associated with fluid loss into the abdominal cavity has occurred and should be assessed by fluid intake and output, weight, hematocrit, serum and urinary electrolytes, urine specific gravity, BUN and creatinine, and abdominal girth. Determinations should be performed daily or more often if the need arises. Treatment is primarily symptomatic and consists of bedrest, fluid and electrolyte replacement, and analgesics. The ascitic, pleural, and pericardial fluids should not be removed unless needed to relieve symptoms of cardiopulmonary distress.

Serious pulmonary conditions (atelectasis, acute respiratory distress syndrome, and exacerbation of asthma) have been reported. Thromboembolic events, both in association with and separate from ovarian hyperstimulation syndrome, have been reported.

Multiple births may result from the use of these medications; advise patient of the potential risk of multiple births before starting the treatment. May contain trace amounts of neomycin or streptomycin. Safety and efficacy have not been established in children and the elderly.

Drug Interactions

Avoid Concomitant Use There are no known interactions where it is recommended to avoid concomitant use.

Decreased Effect There are no known significant interactions involving a decrease in effect.

Increased Effect/Toxicity There are no known significant interactions involving an increase in effect.

Adverse Reactions Percentage may vary by indication, product formulation

>10%:

Endocrine & metabolic: Breast pain
Gastrointestinal: Abdominal pain, flatulence, nausea
Miscellaneous: Miscarriage

1% to 10%:

Central nervous system: Headache
Endocrine & metabolic: Ovarian hyperstimulation syndrome, ovarian pain
Gastrointestinal: Abdomen enlarged, constipation
Local: Injection site reaction
Neuromuscular & skeletal: Back pain
Respiratory: Sinusitis, upper respiratory tract infection

Pharmacodynamics/Kinetics

Onset of Action Peak effect: Follicle development: Within cycle

Absorption I.M.: 76%; SubQ: 78%

Time to Peak SubQ: 13 hours

Half-Life Elimination I.M.: 44 hours (single dose), 27-30 hours (multiple doses); SubQ: 33 hours (single dose)

Available Dosage Forms

Injection, solution:

Follistim® AQ: 75 int. units/0.5 mL (0.5 mL); 150 int. units/0.5 mL (0.5 mL)
Follistim® AQ Cartridge: 350 int. units/0.42 mL (0.42 mL); 650 int. units/0.78 mL (0.78 mL); 975 int. units/1.17 mL (1.17 mL)

Dosing

Adult Note: Dose should be individualized. Use the lowest dose consistent with the expectation of good results. Over the course of treatment, doses may vary depending on individual patient response.

Ovulation induction: Females:

Follistim® AQ: I.M., SubQ: Stepwise approach: Initiate therapy with 75 int. units/day for up to 14 days. Increase by 37.5 int. units at weekly intervals until follicular growth or serum estradiol levels indicate an adequate response. The maximum (individualized) daily dose that has been safely used for ovulation induction in patients during clinical trials is 300 int. units. If response to follitropin is appropriate, hCG is given 1 day following the last dose. Withhold hCG if the ovaries are abnormally enlarged, or if abdominal pain occurs.

Follistim® AQ Cartridge: SubQ: Stepwise approach: Initiate therapy with 75 int. units/day for up to 7 days. Increase by 25 or 50 int. units at weekly intervals until follicular growth or serum estradiol levels indicate an adequate response. The maximum (individualized) daily dose that has been safely used for ovulation induction in patients during clinical trials is 175 int. units. If response to follitropin is appropriate, hCG is given 1 day following the last dose. Withhold hCG if the ovaries are abnormally enlarged, or if abdominal pain occurs. See **"Note"** for dosage adjustment for this product.

ART: Females:

Follistim® AQ: I.M., SubQ: A starting dose of 150-225 int. units is recommended for at least the first 4 days of treatment. The dose may be adjusted for the individual patient based upon their ovarian response. The usual maintenance dose was 75-300 int. units for 6-12 days; 375-600 int. units in patients who were poor responders. The maximum daily dose used in clinical studies is 600 int. units. When a sufficient number of follicles of adequate size are present, the final maturation of the follicles is induced by administering hCG. Oocyte retrieval is performed 34-36 hours later. Withhold hCG in cases where the ovaries are abnormally enlarged on the last day of follitropin beta therapy.

Follistim® AQ Cartridge: SubQ: A starting dose of 150-225 int. units is recommended for at least the first 5 days of treatment. The dose may be adjusted for the individual patient based upon their ovarian response. The maximum daily dose used in clinical studies is 450 int. units. When a sufficient number of follicles of adequate size are present, the final maturation of the follicles is induced by administering hCG. Oocyte retrieval is performed 34-36 hours later. Withhold hCG in cases where the ovaries are abnormally enlarged on the last day of follitropin beta therapy. See **"Note"** for dosage adjustment for this product.

Note: Dose adjustment for Follistim® AQ Cartridge: When administered using the Follistim Pen®, the Follistim® AQ Cartridge delivers 18% more follitropin beta when compared to dissolved lyophilized follitropin beta administered by a conventional syringe. If the above starting doses were previously used when administering a recombinant lyophilized gonadotropin product via a conventional syringe, lower starting and maintenance doses should be considered when switching to Follistim® AQ Cartridge. The following dose conversion may be used:

Follistim® AQ Dosing Conversion

Dose Administered Using Powder for Solution/Conventional Syringe	Follistim® AQ Dose Administered Using Follistim Pen®
75 int. units	50 int. units
150 int. units	125 int. units
225 int. units	175 int. units
300 int. units	250 int. units
375 int. units	300 int. units
450 int. units	375 int. units

Administration

I.M. Follistim® AQ may be administered by I.M. or SubQ injection.

Other Follistim® AQ may be administered by I.M. or SubQ injection. Follistim® AQ cartridge may be administered only by SubQ injection using the Follistim Pen® which can be set to deliver the appropriate dose.

Stability

Storage Prior to dispensing, store refrigerated at 2°C to 8°C (36°F to 46°F). After dispensed, may be stored under refrigeration or ≤25°C (77°F) for up to 3 months. Once cartridge is pierced, must be stored in refrigerator and used within 28 days. Do not freeze. Protect from light.

Monitoring and Teaching Issues

Laboratory Monitoring Monitor sufficient follicular maturation. This may be directly estimated by sonographic visualization of the ovaries and endometrial lining or measuring serum estradiol levels. The combination of both ultrasonography and measurement of estradiol levels is useful for monitoring for the growth and development of follicles and timing hCG administration.

Physical Assessment Teach patient appropriate injection technique and syringe disposal.

Patient Education This medication can only be administered by injection. If you are using this medication at home, follow exact instruction for administering injections and disposal of syringes. Frequent laboratory tests will be required while you are on this therapy; do not miss appointments for laboratory tests or ultrasound. You may experience headache, dizziness, fever, nausea, or vomiting. Report immediately abdominal pain/distension or bloating; persistent nausea, vomiting, or diarrhea; dyspnea; respiratory difficulty; swelling, pain, or redness of extremities; acute backache; or rash, pain, or inflammation at injection site.

Pregnancy Considerations Ectopic pregnancy, congenital abnormalities, and multiple births have been reported. The incidence of congenital abnormality may be slightly higher after ART than with spontaneous conception; higher incidence may be related to parenteral characteristics (maternal age, sperm characteristics).

Additional Information The currently available recombinant follitropin products are structurally identical to native follicle-stimulating hormone. The "alpha" and "beta" nomenclature refers to their differences in purification and order of marketing. Follitropin alpha was marketed first, followed by follitropin beta.

◆ **Folotyn®** *see* Pralatrexate *on page 1487*

Fondaparinux (fon da PARE i nuks)

U.S. Brand Names Arixtra®

Index Terms Fondaparinux Sodium

Generic Availability (U.S.) No

Pharmacologic Category Factor Xa Inhibitor

Medication Safety Issues

High alert medication: The Institute for Safe Medication Practices (ISMP) includes this medication among its list of drugs which have a heightened risk of causing significant patient harm when used in error.

Pregnancy Risk Factor B

Lactation Excretion in breast milk unknown/use caution

Use Prophylaxis of deep vein thrombosis (DVT) in patients undergoing surgery for hip replacement, knee replacement, hip fracture (including extended prophylaxis following hip fracture surgery), or abdominal surgery (in patients at risk for thromboembolic complications); treatment of acute pulmonary embolism (PE); treatment of acute DVT without PE

Canadian labeling: Additional uses (not approved in U.S.): Unstable angina or non-ST segment elevation myocardial infarction (UA/NSTEMI) for the prevention of death and subsequent MI; ST segment elevation MI (STEMI) for the prevention of death and myocardial reinfarction

Unlabeled/Investigational Use Prophylaxis of DVT in patients with a history of heparin-induced thrombocytopenia (HIT)

Mechanism of Action/Effect Fondaparinux prevents factor Xa from binding with antithrombin III and inhibits thrombin formation and thrombus development.

Contraindications Hypersensitivity to fondaparinux or any component of the formulation; severe renal impairment (Cl_{cr} <30 mL/minute); body weight <50 kg (prophylaxis); active major bleeding; bacterial endocarditis; thrombocytopenia associated with a positive *in vitro* test for antiplatelet antibody in the presence of fondaparinux

Warnings/Precautions **[U.S. Boxed Warning]: Spinal or epidural hematomas, including subsequent paralysis, may occur with recent or anticipated neuraxial anesthesia (epidural or spinal anesthesia) or spinal puncture in patients anticoagulated with LMWH, heparinoids, or fondaparinux.** Consider risk versus benefit prior to spinal procedures; risk is increased by the use of concomitant agents which may alter hemostasis, the use of indwelling epidural catheters for analgesia, a history of spinal deformity or spinal surgery, as well as a history of traumatic or repeated epidural or spinal punctures. Patient should be observed closely for bleeding and signs and symptoms of neurological impairment if therapy is administered during or immediately following diagnostic lumbar puncture, epidural anesthesia, or spinal anesthesia.

Not to be used interchangeably (unit-for-unit) with heparin, low molecular weight heparins (LMWHs), or heparinoids. Use caution in patients with moderate renal dysfunction (Cl_{cr} 30-50 mL/minute); contraindicated in patients with Cl_{cr} <30 mL/minute. Discontinue if severe dysfunction or labile function develops.

Use caution in congenital or acquired bleeding disorders; bacterial endocarditis; renal impairment; hepatic impairment; active ulcerative or angiodysplastic gastrointestinal disease; hemorrhagic stroke; shortly after brain, spinal, or ophthalmologic surgery; or in patients taking platelet inhibitors. Risk of major bleeding may be increased if initial dose is administered earlier than recommended (initiation recommended at 6-8 hours following surgery). Discontinue agents that may enhance the risk of hemorrhage if possible. Although considered an insensitive measure of fondaparinux activity, there have been postmarketing reports of bleeding associated with elevated aPTT. Thrombocytopenia has occurred with administration, including reports of thrombocytopenia with thrombosis similar to heparin-induced thrombocytopenia. Monitor patients closely and discontinue therapy if platelets fall to <100,000/mm^3.

For subcutaneous administration; not for I.M. administration. Do not use interchangeably (unit for unit) with low molecular weight heparins, heparin, or heparinoids. Use caution in patients <50 kg who are being treated for DVT/PE; dosage reduction recommended. Contraindicated in patients <50 kg when used for prophylactic therapy. Use with caution in the elderly. The needle guard contains natural latex rubber.

The administration of fondaparinux is **not recommended** prior to and during primary PCI in patients with STEMI, due to an increased risk for guiding-catheter thrombosis. Patients with UA/NSTEMI or STEMI undergoing any PCI should not receive fondaparinux as the sole anticoagulant. Use of an anticoagulant with antithrombin activity (eg, unfractionated heparin) is recommended as adjunctive therapy to PCI even if prior treatment with fondaparinux (must take into account whether GP IIb/IIIa antagonists have been administered) (King, 2008). Do not administer with other agents that increase the risk of hemorrhage unless they are essential for the management of the underlying condition (eg, warfarin for treatment of VTE).

Additional Canadian labeling warnings: Following sheath removal, fondaparinux therapy should not resume for at least 2 hours in patients with UA/NSTEMI and 3 hours in patients with STEMI. Avoid administration 24 hours before and 48 hours after coronary artery bypass graft (CABG) surgery.

Drug Interactions

Avoid Concomitant Use There are no known interactions where it is recommended to avoid concomitant use.

Decreased Effect There are no known significant interactions involving a decrease in effect.

Increased Effect/Toxicity

Fondaparinux may increase the levels/effects of: Anticoagulants; Collagenase (Systemic); Ibritumomab; Tositumomab and Iodine I 131 Tositumomab

The levels/effects of Fondaparinux may be increased by: Antiplatelet Agents; Dasatinib; Drotrecogin Alfa; Herbs (Anticoagulant/Antiplatelet Properties); Nonsteroidal Anti-Inflammatory Agents; Pentosan Polysulfate Sodium; Prostacyclin Analogues; Salicylates; Thrombolytic Agents

Nutritional/Ethanol Interactions Herb/Nutraceutical: Avoid alfalfa, anise, bilberry, bladderwrack, bromelain, cat's claw, celery, coleus, cordyceps, dong quai, evening primrose oil, fenugreek, feverfew, garlic, ginger, ginkgo biloba, ginseng (American/Panax/Siberian), grapeseed, green tea, guggul, horse chestnut seed, horseradish, licorice, prickly ash, red clover, reishi, sweet clover, turmeric, white willow (all possess anticoagulant or antiplatelet activity and as such, may enhance the anticoagulant effects of fondaparinux).

Lab Interactions International standards of heparin or LMWH are not the appropriate calibrators for antifactor Xa activity of fondaparinux.

Adverse Reactions As with all anticoagulants, bleeding is the major adverse effect. Hemorrhage may occur at any site. Risk appears increased by a number of factors including renal dysfunction, age (>75 years), and weight (<50 kg).

>10%:

Central nervous system: Fever (4% to 14%)
Gastrointestinal: Nausea (11%)
Hematologic: Anemia (20%)

1% to 10%:

Cardiovascular: Edema (9%), hypotension (4%), thrombosis PCI catheter (without heparin 1%)

Central nervous system: Insomnia (5%), dizziness (4%), headache (2% to 5%), confusion (3%), pain (2%)

Dermatologic: Rash (8%), purpura (4%), bullous eruption (3%)

Endocrine & metabolic: Hypokalemia (1% to 4%)

Gastrointestinal: Constipation (5% to 9%), nausea (3%), vomiting (6%), diarrhea (3%), dyspepsia (2%)

Genitourinary: Urinary tract infection (4%), urinary retention (3%)

Hematologic: Moderate thrombocytopenia (50,000-100,000/mm^3: 3%), major bleeding (1% to 3%), minor bleeding (2% to 4%), hematoma (3%); risk of major bleeding increased as high as 5% in patients receiving initial dose <6 hours following surgery

Hepatic: ALT increased (≤3%), AST increased (≤2%)

Local: Injection site reaction (bleeding, rash, pruritus)

Miscellaneous: Wound drainage increased (5%)

Pharmacodynamics/Kinetics

Absorption SubQ: Rapid and complete

Bioavailability SubQ: 100%

Time to Peak SubQ: 2-3 hours

Protein Binding ≥94% to antithrombin III

Half-Life Elimination 17-21 hours; prolonged with renal impairment

Excretion Urine (~77%, unchanged drug)

Available Dosage Forms

Injection, solution [preservative free]:

Arixtra®: 2.5 mg/0.5 mL (0.5 mL); 5 mg/0.4 mL (0.4 mL); 7.5 mg/0.6 mL (0.6 mL); 10 mg/0.8 mL (0.8 mL)

Dosing

Adult & Geriatric

DVT prophylaxis: SubQ: Adults ≥50 kg: 2.5 mg once daily.

DVT prophylaxis with history of HIT (unlabeled use): 2.5 mg once daily.

Note: Initiate dose after hemostasis has been established, 6-8 hours postoperatively.

Usual duration: 5-9 days (up to 10 days following abdominal surgery or up to 11 days following hip replacement or knee replacement).

Extended prophylaxis is recommended following hip fracture surgery (has been tolerated for up to 32 days total).

Acute DVT/PE treatment: SubQ: **Note:** Start warfarin on the first treatment day and continue fondaparinux until INR is between 2 and 3 (usually 5-7 days) (Hirsh, 2008):

<50 kg: 5 mg once daily

50-100 kg: 7.5 mg once daily

>100 kg: 10 mg once daily

Usual duration: 5-9 days (has been administered up to 26 days)

Canadian labeling only: Adults:

UA/NSTEMI: SubQ: 2.5 mg once daily; initiate as soon as possible after diagnosis; treat for up to 8 days or until hospital discharge.

STEMI: I.V.: 2.5 mg once; subsequent doses: SubQ: 2.5 mg once daily; treat for up to 8 days or until hospital discharge

Renal Impairment

Cl_{cr} 30-50 mL/minute: Use caution

Cl_{cr} <30 mL/minute: Contraindicated

Hepatic Impairment

Mild-to-moderate impairment: Dosage adjustment not required; monitor for signs of bleeding.

Severe impairment: No data.

Administration

I.M. Do **not** administer I.M.

I.V. Canadian labeling only: STEMI patients: I.V. push or mixed in 25-50 mL of NS and infused over 2 minutes. Flush tubing with NS after infusion to ensure complete administration of fondaparinux. Infusion bag should not be mixed with other agents.

Other For SubQ administration only. Do not mix with other injections or infusions. Do not expel air bubble from syringe before injection. Administer according to recommended regimen; early initiation (before 6 hours after surgery) has been associated with increased bleeding.

To convert from I.V. unfractionated heparin (UFH) infusion to SubQ fondaparinux (Nutescu, 2007): Calculate specific dose for fondaparinux based on indication, discontinue UFH, and begin fondaparinux within 1 hour

To convert from SubQ fondaparinux to I.V. UFH infusion (Nutescu, 2007): Discontinue fondaparinux; calculate specific dose for I.V. UFH infusion based on indication; omit heparin bolus/loading dose

For subQ fondaparinux dosed every 24 hours: Start I.V. UFH infusion 22-23 hours after last dose of fondaparinux

Stability

Reconstitution Canadian labeling: For I.V. administration: May mix with 25 mL or 50 mL NS

Storage Store at 25°C (77°F); excursions permitted to 15°C to 30°C (59°F to 86°F).

Canadian labeling: For I.V. administration: Manufacturer recommends immediate use once diluted in NS, but is stable for up to 24 hours at 15°C to 30°C (59°F to 86°F).

Monitoring and Teaching Issues

Laboratory Monitoring CBC, platelet count, serum creatinine; stool occult blood tests

Physical Assessment Assess closely for bleeding; bleeding precautions should be observed. Teach appropriate injection technique, syringe/needle disposal, and bleeding precautions.

Patient Education This drug can only be administered by injection. Report pain, burning, redness, or swelling at injection site. You may have a tendency to bleed easily while taking this drug. May cause bleeding problems, anemia, nausea, and fever. Report unusual bleeding or bruising (bleeding gums, nosebleed, blood in urine, dark stool), pain in joints or back, CNS changes (severe headache, confusion), any falls or accidents, or rash.

Geriatric Considerations Patients studied for DVT prophylaxis following elective knee or hip fracture surgery averaged 67.5 and 77 years of age, respectively. Use with caution in patients with estimated or actual creatinine clearance between 30-50 mL/minute. Contraindicated in patients with Cl_{cr} <30 mL/minute.

Pregnancy Considerations Reproductive animal studies have not shown fetal harm. Based on case reports, small amounts of fondaparinux have been detected in the umbilical cord following multiple doses during pregnancy. There are no adequate and well-controlled studies in pregnant women; use only if clearly needed.

◆ **Fondaparinux Sodium** *see* Fondaparinux *on page* *817*

◆ **Foradil® Aerolizer®** *see* Formoterol *on page* *820*

Formoterol (for MOH te rol)

U.S. Brand Names Foradil® Aerolizer®; Perforomist™

Index Terms Formoterol Fumarate; Formoterol Fumarate Dihydrate

Generic Availability (U.S.) No

Pharmacologic Category $Beta_2$-Adrenergic Agonist; $Beta_2$-Adrenergic Agonist, Long-Acting

Medication Safety Issues

Sound-alike/look-alike issues:

Foradil® may be confused with Toradol®

Foradil® capsules for inhalation are for administration via Aerolizer™ inhaler and are **not** for oral use.

International issues:

Foradil [U.S., Canada, and multiple international markets] may be confused with Theradol brand name for tramadol [Netherlands]

Medication Guide Available Yes

Pregnancy Risk Factor C

Lactation Excretion in breast milk unknown/use caution

Use Maintenance treatment of asthma and prevention of bronchospasm (as concomitant therapy) in patients ≥5 years of age with reversible obstructive airway disease, including patients with symptoms of nocturnal asthma; maintenance treatment of bronchoconstriction in patients with COPD; prevention of exercise-induced bronchospasm in patients ≥5 years of age (monotherapy may be indicated in patients without persistent asthma)

Canadian labeling: Oxeze®: Also approved for acute relief of symptoms ("on demand" treatment) in patients ≥6 years of age

Mechanism of Action/Effect Relaxes bronchial smooth muscle

Contraindications Hypersensitivity to formoterol or any component of the formulation (Foradil® only); monotherapy in the treatment of asthma (ie, use without a concomitant long-term asthma control medication, such as an inhaled corticosteroid)

Canadian labeling: Oxeze®: Hypersensitivity to formoterol, inhaled lactose, or any component of the formulation; presence of tachyarrhythmias

Warnings/Precautions [U.S. Boxed Warning]: Long-acting $beta_2$-agonists (LABAs) increase the risk of asthma-related deaths. Formoterol should only be used in asthma patients as adjuvant therapy in patients who are currently receiving but are not adequately controlled on a long-term asthma control medication (ie, an inhaled corticosteroid). Monotherapy with an LABA is contraindicated in the treatment of asthma. In a large, randomized, placebo-controlled U.S. clinical trial (SMART, 2006), salmeterol was associated with an increase in asthma-related deaths (when added to usual asthma therapy); risk is considered a class effect among all LABAs. Data are not available to determine if the addition of an inhaled corticosteroid lessens this increased risk of death associated with LABA use. Assess patients at regular intervals once asthma control is maintained on combination therapy to determine if step-down therapy is appropriate and the LABA can be discontinued (without loss of asthma control), and the patient can be maintained on an inhaled corticosteroid. LABAs are not appropriate in patients whose asthma is adequately controlled on low- or medium-dose inhaled corticosteroids. Do **not** use for acute bronchospasm. Short-acting $beta_2$-agonist (eg, albuterol) should be used for acute symptoms and symptoms occurring between treatments. Do **not** initiate in patients with significantly worsening or acutely deteriorating asthma; reports of severe (sometimes fatal) respiratory events have been reported when formoterol has been initiated in this situation. Corticosteroids should not be stopped or reduced when formoterol is initiated. Formoterol is not a substitute for inhaled or systemic corticosteroids and should not be used as monotherapy. During initiation, watch for signs of worsening asthma. **[U.S. Boxed Warning]: LABAs may increase the risk of asthma-related hospitalization in pediatric and**

adolescent patients. In general, a combination product containing a LABA and an inhaled corticosteroid is preferred in patients <18 years of age to ensure compliance.

Because LABAs may disguise poorly controlled persistent asthma, frequent or chronic use of LABAs for exercise-induced bronchospasm is discouraged by the NIH Asthma Guidelines (NIH, 2007). The safety and efficacy of Perforomist™ in the treatment of asthma have not been established. Oxeze® is a formulation of formoterol (available outside the U.S. [eg, Canada]) approved for acute treatment of asthmatic symptoms. The labelings for U.S. approved formulations (Foradil®, Perforomist™) state that formoterol is not meant to relieve acute asthmatic symptoms.

Do **not** use for acute episodes of COPD. Do **not** initiate in patients with significantly worsening or acutely deteriorating COPD. Data are not available to determine if LABA use increases the risk of death in patients with COPD. Increased use and/or ineffectiveness of short-acting $beta_2$-agonists may indicate rapidly deteriorating disease and should prompt re-evaluation of the patient's condition.

Immediate hypersensitivity reactions (urticaria, angioedema, rash, bronchospasm) have been reported. Do not exceed recommended dose or frequency; serious adverse events (including serious asthma exacerbations and fatalities) have been associated with excessive use of inhaled sympathomimetics. $Beta_2$-agonists may increase risk of arrhythmias, decrease serum potassium, prolong QT_c interval, or increase serum glucose. These effects may be exacerbated in hypoxemia. Use caution in patients with cardiovascular disease (arrhythmia, coronary insufficiency, hypertension, or HF), seizures, diabetes, hyperthyroidism, or hypokalemia. Beta-agonists may cause elevation in blood pressure and heart rate, and result in CNS stimulation/excitation. Tolerance to the bronchodilator effect, measured by FEV_1, has been observed in studies.

Powder for oral inhalation contains lactose; very rare anaphylactic reactions have been reported in patients with severe milk protein allergy. The contents of the Foradil® capsules are for inhalation via the Aerolizer™ device. There have been reports of incorrect administration (swallowing of the capsules).

Drug Interactions

Metabolism/Transport Effects Substrate (minor) of CYP2A6, 2C9, 2C19, 2D6

Avoid Concomitant Use

Avoid concomitant use of Formoterol with any of the following: Iobenguane I 123

Decreased Effect

Formoterol may decrease the levels/effects of: Iobenguane I 123

The levels/effects of Formoterol may be decreased by: Alpha-/Beta-Blockers; Beta-Blockers (Beta1 Selective); Beta-Blockers (Nonselective); Betahistine

Increased Effect/Toxicity

Formoterol may increase the levels/effects of: Loop Diuretics; Sympathomimetics

The levels/effects of Formoterol may be increased by: Atomoxetine; Caffeine; Cannabinoids; MAO Inhibitors; Theophylline Derivatives; Tricyclic Antidepressants

Adverse Reactions

1% to 10%:

Cardiovascular: Chest pain (2% to 3%), palpitation

Central nervous system: Anxiety (2%), dizziness (2%), fever (2%), insomnia (2%), dysphonia (1%), headache

Dermatologic: Pruritus (2%), rash (1%)

Gastrointestinal: Diarrhea (5%), nausea (5%), xerostomia (1% to 3%), vomiting (2%), abdominal pain, dyspepsia, gastroenteritis

Neuromuscular & skeletal: Muscle cramps (2%), tremor

Respiratory: Infection (3% to 7%), asthma exacerbation (age 5-12 years: 5% to 6%; age >12 years: <4%), bronchitis (5%), pharyngitis (3% to 4%), sinusitis (3%), dyspnea (2%), tonsillitis (1%)

Pharmacodynamics/Kinetics

Onset of Action Powder for inhalation: Within 3 minutes

Peak effect: Powder for inhalation: 80% of peak effect within 15 minutes; Solution for nebulization: 2 hours

Duration of Action Improvement in FEV_1 observed for 12 hours in most patients

Absorption Rapidly into plasma

Time to Peak Maximum improvement in FEV_1 in 1-3 hours

Protein Binding 61% to 64% *in vitro* at higher concentrations than achieved with usual dosing

Half-Life Elimination Powder: ~10-14 hours; Nebulized solution: ~7 hours

Metabolism Hepatic via direct glucuronidation and O-demethylation; CYP2D6, CYP2C19, CYP2C8/9, CYP2A6 involved in O-demethylation

Excretion

Children 5-12 years: Urine (6% as unchanged drug, 7% to 9% as direct glucuronide metabolites)

Adults: Urine (15% to 18% as direct glucuronide metabolites, 2% to 10% as unchanged drug)

Available Dosage Forms

Powder, for oral inhalation:

Foradil® Aerolizer®: 12 mcg/capsule (12s, 60s)

Solution, for nebulization:

Perforomist™: 20 mcg/2 mL (60s)

Dosing

Adult & Geriatric

Asthma, maintenance: Inhalation: **Note:** For asthma control, long-acting beta$_2$-agonists (LABAs) should be used in combination with inhaled corticosteroids and **not** as monotherapy

Foradil®: 12 mcg capsule inhaled every 12 hours via Aerolizer™ device (maximum: 24 mcg/day)

Oxeze® (CAN): **Note:** Not labeled for use in the U.S.: Inhalation: 6 mcg or 12 mcg every 12 hours (maximum dose: Children: 24 mcg/day; Adults: 48 mcg/day)

Exercise-induced bronchospasm: Inhalation:

Foradil®: 12 mcg capsule inhaled via Aerolizer™ device at least 15 minutes before exercise on an "as needed" basis; additional doses should not be used for another 12 hours. **Note:** If already using for asthma maintenance then should not use additional doses for exercise-induced bronchospasm. Because LABAs may disguise poorly controlled persistent asthma, frequent or chronic use of LABAs for exercise-induced bronchospasm is discouraged by the NIH Asthma Guidelines (NIH, 2007).

Oxeze® (CAN): **Note:** Not labeled for use in the U.S.: Children ≥6 years and Adults: Inhalation: 6 mcg or 12 mcg at least 15 minutes before exercise.

COPD (maintenance): Inhalation:

Foradil®: 12 mcg capsule inhaled every 12 hours via Aerolizer™ device (maximum: 24 mcg/day)

Perforomist™: 20 mcg twice daily (maximum dose: 40 mcg/day)

Acute ("on demand") relief of bronchoconstriction: *Indication for Oxeze® approved in Canada:* 6 mcg or 12 mcg as a single dose (maximum dose: Children: 48 mcg/24-hour period; Adults: 72 mcg/24-hour period). The prolonged use of high dosages (48 mcg/day for ≥3 consecutive days) may be a sign of suboptimal control, and should prompt the re-evaluation of therapy.

Pediatric

Asthma maintenance (Foradil®): Inhalation: Children ≥5 years: Refer to adult dosing.

Exercise-induced bronchospasm: Inhalation:

Foradil®: Children ≥5 years: Refer to adult dosing.

Oxeze® [CAN]: Children ≥6 years: Refer to adult dosing.

Acute "on demand" treatment of bronchospasm (Oxeze® [CAN]): Inhalation: Refer to adult dosing.

Renal Impairment Not studied

Administration

Inhalation

Foradil®: Remove capsule from foil blister **immediately** before use. Place capsule in the capsule-chamber in the base of the Aerolizer™ Inhaler. Must only use the Aerolizer™ Inhaler. Press both buttons **once only** and then release. Keep inhaler in a level, horizontal position. Exhale fully. Do not exhale into inhaler. Tilt head slightly back and inhale (rapidly, steadily, and deeply). Hold breath as long as possible. If any powder remains in capsule, exhale and inhale again. Repeat until capsule is empty. Throw away empty capsule; do not leave in inhaler. Do not use a spacer with the Aerolizer™ Inhaler. Always keep capsules and inhaler dry.

Perforomist™: Remove unit-dose vial from foil pouch **immediately** before use. Solution does not require dilution prior to administration; do not mix other medications with formoterol solution. Place contents of unit-dose vial into the reservoir of a standard jet nebulizer connected to an air compressor; assemble nebulizer based on the manufacturer's instructions and turn nebulizer on; breathe deeply and evenly until all of the medication has been inhaled. Discard any unused medication immediately; do not ingest contents of vial. Clean nebulizer after use.

Oxeze® Turbuhaler® [CAN; not available in U.S.]: Hold inhaler upright. Turn colored grip as far as it will go in one direction and then turn back to original position; a clicking sound should be heard which means the inhaler is ready for use. Exhale fully. Do not exhale into mouthpiece of inhaler. Place mouthpiece to lips and inhale forcefully and deeply. Do not chew or bite on mouthpiece. Clean outside of mouthpiece once weekly with a dry tissue. Avoid getting inhaler wet.

Stability

Storage

Foradil®: Prior to dispensing, store in refrigerator at 2°C to 8°C (36°F to 46°F). After dispensing, store at room temperature at 20°C to 25°C (68°F to 77°F). Protect from heat and moisture. Capsules should always be stored in the blister and only removed immediately before use. Always check expiration date. Use within 4 months of purchase date or product expiration date, whichever comes first.

Perforomist™: Prior to dispensing, store in refrigerator at 2°C to 8°C (36°F to 46°F). After dispensing, store at 2°C to 25°C (36°F to 77°F) for up to 3 months. Protect from heat. Unit-dose vials should always be stored in the foil pouch and only removed immediately before use.

Monitoring and Teaching Issues

Laboratory Monitoring FEV$_1$, peak flow, and/or other pulmonary function tests; serum potassium, serum glucose (in selected patients)

Patient Education Do not swallow capsules; this medication can only be used in the Aerolizer™ Inhaler. It is recommended that you wear identification (Med-Alert bracelet) if you have asthma. You may experience nervousness, dizziness, insomnia, dry mouth, nausea, or GI discomfort. Report any unresolved GI upset, nervousness or dizziness, muscle cramping, chest pain or palpitations, skin rash, or worsening of condition.

Administration: Wash hands prior to treatment and sit in comfortable position for treatment. Place capsule in the capsule-chamber in the base of the Aerolizer™ Inhaler. Press both buttons once only and then release. Hold inhaler in a level, horizontal position, exhale fully. Tilt head slightly back and inhale from inhaler rapidly, steadily, and deeply. Hold breath as long as possible. If any powder remains in capsule, exhale and inhale again. Repeat until capsule is empty. Throw away empty capsule. Do not use a spacer with Aerolizer™. Do not wash inhaler; store in dry place.

Geriatric Considerations Elderly patients should be specifically counseled about the proper use of this inhaler/spacing of doses and/or the proper use of a nebulizer system. No significant difference in both safety and effectiveness was seen between elderly and younger patients.

Pregnancy Considerations When given orally to rats throughout organogenesis, formoterol caused delayed ossification and decreased fetal weight, but no malformations. There were no adverse events when given to pregnant rats in late pregnancy. Doses used were ≥70 times the recommended daily inhalation dose in humans. There are no adequate and well-controlled studies in pregnant women. Use only if benefit outweighs risk to the fetus. Beta-agonists interfere with uterine contractility so use during labor only if benefit outweighs risk to the fetus.

- ◆ **Formoterol and Budesonide** *see* Budesonide and Formoterol *on page 239*
- ◆ **Formoterol Fumarate** *see* Formoterol *on page 820*
- ◆ **Formoterol Fumarate Dihydrate** *see* Formoterol *on page 820*
- ◆ **Formoterol Fumarate Dihydrate and Budesonide** *see* Budesonide and Formoterol *on page 239*
- ◆ **5-Formyl Tetrahydrofolate** *see* Leucovorin Calcium *on page 1080*
- ◆ **Fortamet®** *see* MetFORMIN *on page 1182*
- ◆ **Fortaz®** *see* Ceftazidime *on page 332*
- ◆ **Forteo®** *see* Teriparatide *on page 1736*
- ◆ **Fortesta™** *see* Testosterone *on page 1739*
- ◆ **Fortical®** *see* Calcitonin *on page 269*
- ◆ **Fosamax®** *see* Alendronate *on page 67*

Fosamprenavir (FOS am pren a veer)

U.S. Brand Names Lexiva®

Index Terms Fosamprenavir Calcium; GW433908G

Generic Availability (U.S.) No

Pharmacologic Category Antiretroviral Agent, Protease Inhibitor

Medication Safety Issues

Sound-alike/look-alike issues:

Lexiva® may be confused with Levitra®

Pregnancy Risk Factor C

Lactation Excretion in breast milk unknown/contraindicated

Use Treatment of HIV infections in combination with at least two other antiretroviral agents

Mechanism of Action/Effect Fosamprenavir is rapidly and almost completely converted to amprenavir *in vivo*. Amprenavir blocks the site of HIV-1 protease activity, resulting in the formation of immature, noninfectious viral particles.

Contraindications Clinically-significant hypersensitivity (eg, Stevens-Johnson syndrome) to fosamprenavir, amprenavir, or any component of the formulation; concurrent therapy with CYP3A4 substrates with a narrow therapeutic window; concomitant use with alfuzosin, cisapride, delavirdine, ergot derivatives, lovastatin, midazolam, pimozide, rifampin, simvastatin, St John's wort, and triazolam; use of flecainide and propafenone with concomitant ritonavir therapy; sildenafil (when used for pulmonary artery hypertension [eg, Revatio®])

Warnings/Precautions Use with caution in patients taking strong CYP3A4 inhibitors, moderate or strong CYP3A4 inducers, and major CYP3A4 substrates (see Drug Interactions); consider alternative agents that avoid or lessen the potential for CYP-mediated interactions. Do not use with hormonal contraceptives. Do not coadminister colchicine in patient with renal or hepatic impairment; avoid concurrent use with salmeterol.

Use with caution in patients with diabetes mellitus or sulfonamide allergy. Use caution with hepatic impairment (dosage adjustment required) or underlying hepatitis B or C. Redistribution of fat may occur (eg, buffalo hump, peripheral wasting, cushingoid appearance). Dosage adjustment is required for combination therapies (ritonavir and/or efavirenz); in addition, the risk of hyperlipidemia may be increased during concurrent therapy. Protease inhibitors have been associated with a variety of hypersensitivity events (some severe), including rash, anaphylaxis (rare), angioedema, bronchospasm, erythema multiforme, and/or Stevens-Johnson syndrome (rare). It is generally recommended to discontinue treatment if severe rash or moderate symptoms accompanied by other systemic symptoms occur. Acute hemolytic anemia has been reported in association with amprenavir use. Cases of nephrolithiasis have been reported in postmarketing surveillance; temporary or permanent discontinuation of therapy should be considered if symptoms develop. Spontaneous bleeding has been reported in patients with hemophilia A or B following treatment with protease inhibitors; use caution. Immune reconstitution syndrome may develop resulting in the occurrence of an inflammatory response to an indolent or residual opportunistic infection; further evaluation and treatment may be necessary. Safety and efficacy have not been established in children <2 years of age.

Drug Interactions

Metabolism/Transport Effects As amprenavir: **Substrate** of CYP2C9 (minor), 3A4 (major), P-glycoprotein; **Inhibits** CYP2C19 (weak), 3A4 (strong)

Avoid Concomitant Use

Avoid concomitant use of Fosamprenavir with any of the following: Alfuzosin; Amiodarone; Cisapride; Conivaptan; Delavirdine; Dronedarone; Eplerenone; Ergot Derivatives; Etravirine; Everolimus; Halofantrine; Lovastatin; Lurasidone; Midazolam; Nilotinib; Nisoldipine; Pimozide; QuiNIDine; Ranolazine; Rifampin; Rivaroxaban; RomiDEPsin; Salmeterol; Silodosin; Simvastatin; St Johns Wort; Tamsulosin; Tolvaptan; Toremifene; Triazolam

Decreased Effect

Fosamprenavir may decrease the levels/effects of: Abacavir; Clarithromycin; Contraceptives (Estrogens); Delavirdine; Divalproex; Lopinavir; Meperidine; Methadone; PARoxetine; Phenytoin; Posaconazole; Prasugrel; Valproic Acid; Zidovudine

The levels/effects of Fosamprenavir may be decreased by: Antacids; CarBAMazepine; Contraceptives (Estrogens); CYP3A4 Inducers (Strong); Deferasirox; Efavirenz; Garlic; H2-Antagonists; Nevirapine; Peginterferon Alfa-2b; P-Glycoprotein Inducers; Rifampin; St Johns Wort; Tenofovir

Increased Effect/Toxicity

Fosamprenavir may increase the levels/effects of: Alfuzosin; Almotriptan; Alosetron; ALPRAZolam; Amiodarone; Antifungal Agents (Azole Derivatives, Systemic); Bortezomib; Brinzolamide; Calcium Channel Blockers (Dihydropyridine); Calcium Channel Blockers (Nondihydropyridine); CarBAMazepine; Ciclesonide; Cisapride; Clarithromycin; Clorazepate; Colchicine; Conivaptan; Corticosteroids (Orally Inhaled); CycloSPORINE; CycloSPORINE (Systemic); CYP3A4 Substrates; Diazepam; Dienogest; Digoxin; Dronedarone; Dutasteride; Enfuvirtide; Eplerenone; Ergot Derivatives; Everolimus; FentaNYL; Fesoterodine; Flurazepam; Fusidic Acid; GuanFACINE; Halofantrine; HMG-CoA Reductase Inhibitors; Ixabepilone; Lovastatin; Lumefantrine; Lurasidone; Maraviroc; Meperidine; MethylPREDNISolone; Midazolam; Nefazodone; Nilotinib; Nisoldipine; Paricalcitol; Pazopanib; Pimecrolimus; Pimozide; Protease Inhibitors; QuiNIDine; Ranolazine; Rifabutin; Rivaroxaban; RomiDEPsin; Salmeterol; Saxagliptin; Sildenafil; Silodosin; Simvastatin; Sirolimus; SORAfenib; Tacrolimus; Tacrolimus (Systemic); Tacrolimus (Topical); Tadalafil; Tamsulosin; Temsirolimus; Tenofovir; Tolvaptan; Toremifene; TraZODone; Triazolam; Tricyclic Antidepressants; Vardenafil; Vilazodone; Warfarin

The levels/effects of Fosamprenavir may be increased by: Antifungal Agents (Azole Derivatives, Systemic); Clarithromycin; CycloSPORINE; CycloSPORINE (Systemic); Delavirdine; Efavirenz; Enfuvirtide; Etravirine; Fusidic Acid; P-Glycoprotein Inhibitors; Phenytoin; Posaconazole; Rifabutin

Nutritional/Ethanol Interactions Herb/Nutraceutical: Amprenavir serum concentration may be decreased by St John's wort; concurrent use contraindicated.

Adverse Reactions Frequency not defined: Diabetes mellitus, fat redistribution, and immune reconstitution syndrome have been associated with protease inhibitor therapy. Spontaneous bleeding has been reported in patients with hemophilia A or B following treatment with protease inhibitors. Acute hemolytic anemia has been reported in association with amprenavir use.

>10%:

- Dermatologic: Rash (≤19%; onset: ~11 days; duration: ~13 days)
- Endocrine & metabolic: Hypertriglyceridemia (>750 mg/dL: ≤11%)
- Gastrointestinal: Diarrhea (moderate-to-severe; 5% to 13%)

1% to 10%:

- Central nervous system: Headache (moderate-to-severe; 2% to 4%), fatigue (moderate-to-severe; 2% to 4%)
- Dermatologic: Pruritus (7% to 8%)
- Endocrine & metabolic: Hyperglycemia (>251 mg/dL: ≤2%)
- Gastrointestinal: Serum lipase increased (>2 times ULN: 5% to 8%), nausea (moderate-to-severe; 3% to 7%), vomiting (moderate-to-severe; 2% to 6%), abdominal pain (moderate-to-severe; ≤2%)
- Hematologic: Neutropenia (<750 cells/mm^3: 3%)
- Hepatic: Transaminases increased (>5 times ULN: 4% to 8%)

Pharmacodynamics/Kinetics

Absorption 63%

Bioavailability Not established; food does not have a significant effect on absorption of tablets. Administration of oral suspension with food reduced C_{max} by 46% and AUC by 28%.

Time to Peak 1.5-4 hours (median: 2.5 hours)

Protein Binding ~90% (to alpha$_1$-acid glycoprotein); decreased in hepatic impairment

Half-Life Elimination ~7.7 hours (amprenavir)

Metabolism Fosamprenavir is rapidly and almost completely converted to amprenavir by cellular phosphatases in gut epithelium; amprenavir is hepatically metabolized via CYP isoenzymes (primarily CYP3A4)

Excretion Feces (75% as metabolites, <1% as unchanged drug); urine (14% as metabolites, ~1% as unchanged drug)

Available Dosage Forms

Suspension, oral:

Lexiva®: 50 mg/mL (225 mL)

Tablet, oral:

Lexiva®: 700 mg

Dosing

Adult & Geriatric

HIV infection: Oral:

Antiretroviral therapy-naive patients: Oral: **Note:** Caution when using without ritonavir; may promote viral strains cross-resistant to darunavir:

Unboosted regimen: 1400 mg twice daily (without ritonavir)

Ritonavir-boosted regimens:

Once-daily regimen: Fosamprenavir 1400 mg plus ritonavir 100-200 mg once daily

Twice-daily regimen: Fosamprenavir 700 mg plus ritonavir 100 mg twice daily

Protease inhibitor (PI)-experienced patients: Fosamprenavir 700 mg plus ritonavir 100 mg twice daily. **Note:** Once-daily administration is not recommended in protease inhibitor-experienced patients.

Dosage adjustments for concomitant therapy: Oral:

Coadministration with bosentan:

Coadministration of bosentan in patients currently receiving fosamprenavir: For patients receiving fosamprenavir for at least 10 days, begin with bosentan 62.5 mg once daily or every other day based on tolerability

Coadministration of fosamprenavir in patients currently receiving bosentan: Discontinue bosentan 36 hours prior to the initiation of fosamprenavir. After at least 10 days of fosamprenavir, resume bosentan 62.5 mg once daily or every other day based on tolerability.

Coadministration with colchicine:

Familial Mediterranean fever (FMF):

Fosamprenavir: Maximum colchicine dose: 1.2 mg/day (0.6 mg twice daily)

Fosamprenavir with ritonavir: Maximum colchicine dose: 0.6 mg/day (0.3 mg twice daily)

Gout prophylaxis:

Fosamprenavir:

If original colchicine dose is 0.6 mg twice daily, adjust dose to 0.3 mg twice daily or 0.6 mg once daily

If original colchicine dose is 0.6 mg once daily, adjust dose to 0.3 mg once daily

Fosamprenavir with ritonavir:

If original colchicine dose is 0.6 mg twice daily, adjust dose to 0.3 mg once daily

If original colchicine dose is 0.6 mg once daily, adjust dose to 0.3 mg every other day

Gout flare treatment:

Fosamprenavir: Initial: Colchicine 1.2 mg; do not repeat for at least 3 days

Fosamprenavir with ritonavir: Initial: Colchicine 0.6 mg, followed in 1 hour by a single dose of 0.3 mg; do not repeat for at least 3 days

Combination therapy with efavirenz (ritonavir-boosted regimen):

Once-daily regimen (PI-naive patients only): Fosamprenavir 1400 mg plus ritonavir 300 mg plus efavirenz 600 mg once daily

Twice-daily regimen: Fosamprenavir 700 mg plus ritonavir 100 mg twice daily plus efavirenz 600 mg once daily

Combination therapy with maraviroc: Fosamprenavir 700 mg plus ritonavir 100 mg plus maraviroc 150 mg twice daily

Coadministration with phosphodiesterase-5 enzyme (PDE-5) inhibitor:

Pulmonary arterial hypertension: Fosamprenavir coadministered with tadalafil:

Patient receiving fosamprenavir for at least 1 week: Initiate tadalafil at 20 mg once daily; increase to 40 mg once daily based on individual tolerability

Patient receiving tadalafil when initiating fosamprenavir: Stop tadalafil at least 24 hours prior to starting fosamprenavir. After at least 1 week following the initiation of fosamprenavir, resume tadalafil at 20 mg once daily; increase to 40 mg once daily based on individual tolerability.

Erectile dysfunction:

Fosamprenavir coadministered with or without ritonavir:

Sildenafil (Viagra®): Maximum sildenafil dose: 25 mg in a 48-hour period

Tadalafil (Cialis®): Maximum tadalafil dose: 10 mg in a 72-hour period

Vardenafil:

Fosamprenavir: Maximum vardenafil dose: 2.5 mg in a 24-hour period

Fosamprenavir coadministered with ritonavir and vardenafil: Maximum vardenafil dose: 2.5 mg in a 72-hour period

Pediatric

HIV infection: Oral:

Antiretroviral therapy-naive patients:

Children 2-5 years of age: Fosamprenavir 30 mg/kg/dose twice daily (not to exceed adult dosage of 1400 mg twice daily without ritonavir)

Children ≥6 years of age:

Unboosted regimen: Fosamprenavir 30 mg/kg/dose twice daily (not to exceed adult dosage of 1400 mg twice daily without ritonavir)

Ritonavir-boosted regimen: Fosamprenavir 18 mg/kg/dose twice daily plus ritonavir 3 mg/kg/dose twice daily (not to exceed the adult dose of fosamprenavir 700 mg plus ritonavir 100 mg twice daily)

Protease inhibitor (PI)-experienced patients: Children ≥6 years: Fosamprenavir 18 mg/kg/dose plus ritonavir 3 mg/kg/dose twice daily (not to exceed the adult dose of fosamprenavir 700 mg plus ritonavir 100 mg twice daily)

Notes: The adult unboosted regimen of 1400 mg twice daily may be used for pediatric patients who weigh ≥47 kg. When combined with ritonavir, the adult regimen of fosamprenavir 700 mg plus ritonavir 100 mg twice daily can be used in children who weigh ≥39 kg while ritonavir capsules may be used for pediatric patients who weigh ≥33 kg.

Renal Impairment No dosage adjustment required.

Hepatic Impairment

Mild impairment (Child-Pugh score 5-6): Reduce dosage of fosamprenavir to 700 mg twice daily without concurrent ritonavir (therapy naive) **or** fosamprenavir 700 mg twice daily plus ritonavir 100 mg once daily (therapy naive or PI experienced).

Moderate impairment (Child-Pugh score 7-9): Reduce dosage of fosamprenavir to 700 mg twice daily without concurrent ritonavir (therapy naive) **or** fosamprenavir 450 mg twice daily plus ritonavir 100 mg once daily (therapy naive or PI experienced).

Severe impairment (Child-Pugh score 10-15): Reduce dosage of fosamprenavir to 350 mg twice daily without concurrent ritonavir (therapy naive) **or** fosamprenavir 300 mg twice daily plus ritonavir 100 mg once daily (therapy naïve or PI experienced).

Administration

Oral

Oral suspension: Administer **without** food to adults; administer **with** food to pediatric patients. Readminister dose of suspension if emesis occurs within 30 minutes after dosing. Shake suspension vigorously prior to use.

Tablet: Administer with food if taken with ritonavir. May be administered without regard to food if not taken with ritonavir.

Stability

Storage

Lexiva®: Store tablets at 25°C (77°F); excursions permitted to 15°C to 30°C (59°F to 86°F). Store oral suspension at 5°C to 30°C (41°F to 86°F). Do not freeze.

Telzir®: Store tablets 2°C to 30°C; do not freeze and discard 25 days after opening.

Monitoring and Teaching Issues

Laboratory Monitoring Monitor viral load, CD4 count, glucose; triglycerides and cholesterol (prior to initiation and periodically during therapy)

Physical Assessment Assess CD4 count and hepatic function at regular intervals during therapy. Monitor for hypersensitivity, gastrointestinal disturbance, and hyperglycemia. Monitor cardiac status. Caution patients to monitor glucose levels closely; protease inhibitors may cause hyperglycemia or new-onset diabetes. Teach patient proper timing of multiple medications. Instruct patient on glucose testing (protease inhibitors may cause hyperglycemia), exacerbation or new-onset diabetes.

Patient Education This is not a cure for HIV, nor has it been found to reduce transmission of HIV; use appropriate precautions to prevent spread to other persons. Maintain adequate hydration, unless instructed to restrict fluid intake. This medication will be prescribed with a combination of other medications; time these medications as directed by prescriber. You may be advised to check your glucose levels; this class of drugs can cause hyperglycemia. Frequent blood tests may be required. May cause body changes due to redistribution of body fat (buffalo hump, peripheral wasting, cushingoid appearance may occur), dizziness or fatigue, nausea or vomiting, diarrhea, back pain, or arthralgia. Inform prescriber if you experience muscle numbness or tingling; unresolved persistent vomiting, diarrhea, or abdominal pain; respiratory difficulty or chest pain; unusual skin rash; or change in color of stool or urine.

Dietary Considerations Tablets may be taken with or without food. Adults should take oral suspension **without** food; however, children should take oral suspension **with** food.

Breast-Feeding Considerations In infants born to mothers who are HIV positive, HAART while breast-feeding may decrease postnatal infection. However, maternal or infant antiretroviral therapy does not completely eliminate the risk of postnatal HIV transmission. In addition, multiclass-resistant virus has been detected in breast-feeding infants despite maternal therapy.

In the United States where formula is accessible, affordable, safe, and sustainable, complete avoidance of breast-feeding by HIV-infected women is recommended to decrease potential transmission of HIV.

Pregnancy Considerations Animal data showed some abortifacient and minor skeletal abnormalities with amprenavir. It is not known if amprenavir crosses the human placenta. There are no adequate and well-controlled studies in pregnant women. Pregnancy and protease inhibitors are both associated with an increased risk of hyperglycemia. Glucose levels should be closely monitored. The Perinatal HIV Guidelines Working Group notes there is insufficient data to recommend use during pregnancy; however, if used, they recommend that fosamprenavir be given with low-dose ritonavir boosting. Healthcare providers are encouraged to enroll pregnant women exposed to antiretroviral medications in the Antiretroviral Pregnancy Registry (1-800-258-4263 or www.APRegistry.com). Healthcare providers caring for HIV-infected women and their infants may contact the National Perinatal HIV Hotline (888-448-8765) for clinical consultation.

◆ **Fosamprenavir Calcium** *see* Fosamprenavir *on page* 823

Fosaprepitant (fos a PRE pi tant)

U.S. Brand Names Emend® for Injection

Index Terms Aprepitant Injection; Fosaprepitant Dimeglumine; L-758,298; MK 0517

Generic Availability (U.S.) No

Pharmacologic Category Antiemetic; Substance P/Neurokinin 1 Receptor Antagonist

Medication Safety Issues

Sound-alike/look-alike issues:

Fosaprepitant may be confused with aprepitant, fosamprenavir, fospropofol

Emend® for Injection (fosaprepitant) may be confused with Emend® (aprepitant) which is an oral capsule formulation.

Pregnancy Risk Factor B

Lactation Excretion in breast milk unknown/not recommended

Use Prevention of acute and delayed nausea and vomiting associated with moderately- and highly-emetogenic chemotherapy (in combination with other antiemetics)

Mechanism of Action/Effect Fosaprepitant is a prodrug of aprepitant, a substance P/neurokinin 1 (NK1) receptor antagonist. It is rapidly converted to aprepitant which prevents acute and delayed vomiting by inhibiting the substance P/neurokinin 1 (NK1) receptor; augments the antiemetic activity of the 5-HT_3 receptor antagonist and corticosteroid activity and inhibits chemotherapy-induced emesis.

Contraindications Hypersensitivity to fosaprepitant, aprepitant, polysorbate 80, or any component of the formulation; concurrent use with pimozide or cisapride

Warnings/Precautions Fosaprepitant is rapidly converted to aprepitant, which has a high potential for drug interactions. Use caution with agents primarily metabolized via CYP3A4; aprepitant is a 3A4 inhibitor. Effect on orally administered 3A4 substrates is greater than those administered intravenously. Immediate hypersensitivity has been reported (rarely) with fosaprepitant; stop infusion with hypersensitivity symptoms (dyspnea, erythema, flushing, or anaphylaxis); do not reinitiate. Use caution with hepatic impairment; has not been studied in patients with severe hepatic impairment (Child-Pugh class C). Not studied for treatment of existing nausea and vomiting. Chronic continuous administration of fosaprepitant is not recommended.

Drug Interactions

Metabolism/Transport Effects Substrate of CYP1A2 (minor), 2C19 (minor), 3A4 (major); **Inhibits** CYP2C9 (weak), 2C19 (weak), 3A4 (moderate); **Induces** CYP2C9 (weak), 3A4 (weak)

Avoid Concomitant Use

Avoid concomitant use of Fosaprepitant with any of the following: Cisapride; Pimozide; Tolvaptan

Decreased Effect

Fosaprepitant may decrease the levels/effects of: Contraceptives (Estrogens); Contraceptives (Progestins); PARoxetine; Saxagliptin; TOLBUTamide; Warfarin

The levels/effects of Fosaprepitant may be decreased by: CYP3A4 Inducers (Strong); Deferasirox; Herbs (CYP3A4 Inducers); PARoxetine; Rifampin

Increased Effect/Toxicity

Fosaprepitant may increase the levels/effects of: Benzodiazepines (metabolized by oxidation); Cisapride; Colchicine; Corticosteroids (Systemic); CYP3A4 Substrates; Diltiazem; Eplerenone; Everolimus; FentaNYL; Halofantrine; Lurasidone; Pimecrolimus; Pimozide; Ranolazine; Salmeterol; Saxagliptin; Tolvaptan; Vilazodone

The levels/effects of Fosaprepitant may be increased by: Antifungal Agents (Azole Derivatives, Systemic); Conivaptan; CYP3A4 Inhibitors (Moderate); CYP3A4 Inhibitors (Strong); Dasatinib; Diltiazem

Nutritional/Ethanol Interactions

Food: Aprepitant serum concentration may be increased when taken with grapefruit juice; avoid concurrent use.

Herb/Nutraceutical: Avoid St John's wort (may decrease aprepitant levels).

Adverse Reactions Adverse reactions reported with aprepitant and fosaprepitant (as part of a combination chemotherapy regimen) occurring at a higher frequency than standard antiemetic therapy:

1% to 10%:

Central nervous system: Fatigue (1% to 3%), headache (2%)

Gastrointestinal: Anorexia (2%), constipation 2%), dyspepsia (2%), diarrhea (1%), eructation (1%)

Hepatic: ALT increased (1% to 3%), AST increased (1%)

Local: Injection site reactions (3%; includes erythema, induration, pain, pruritus, or thrombophlebitis)

Neuromuscular & skeletal: Weakness (3%)

Miscellaneous: Hiccups (5%)

Pharmacodynamics/Kinetics

Time to Peak Fosaprepitant is converted to aprepitant within 30 minutes after the end of infusion

Protein Binding Aprepitant: >95%

Half-Life Elimination

Half-life elimination: Fosaprepitant: ~2 minutes; Aprepitant: ~9-13 hours

Metabolism

Fosaprepitant: Hepatic and extrahepatic; rapidly (within 30 minutes after the end of infusion) converted to aprepitant (nearly complete conversion)

Aprepitant: Hepatic via CYP3A4 (major); CYP1A2 and CYP2C19 (minor); forms 7 weakly-active metabolites

Excretion Urine (57%); feces (45%)

Available Dosage Forms

Injection, powder for reconstitution:

Emend® for Injection: 150 mg

Dosing

Adult & Geriatric Prevention of chemotherapy-induced nausea/vomiting: I.V.:

Single-dose regimen (for highly-emetogenic chemotherapy): 150 mg over 20-30 minutes ~30 minutes prior to chemotherapy on day 1 only (in combination with a 5-HT_3 antagonist on day 1 and dexamethasone on days 1 to 4)

3-day regimen (for highly-emetogenic chemotherapy): 115 mg over 15 minutes 30 minutes prior to chemotherapy on day 1, followed by aprepitant 80 mg orally on days 2 and 3 (in combination with a 5-HT_3 antagonist on day 1 and dexamethasone on days 1 to 4)

3-day regimen (for moderately-emetogenic chemotherapy): 115 mg over 15 minutes 30 minutes prior to chemotherapy on day 1, followed by aprepitant 80 mg orally on days 2 and 3 (in combination with a 5-HT_3 antagonist and dexamethasone on day 1)

Renal Impairment

Mild, moderate, or severe impairment: No adjustment required.

Dialysis-dependent end-stage renal disease (ESRD): No adjustment required.

Hepatic Impairment

Child-Pugh class A and B: No adjustment required.

Child-Pugh class C: Has not been evaluated; use with caution.

Administration

I.V.

115 mg: Infuse over 15 minutes 30 minutes prior to chemotherapy

150 mg: Infuse over 20-30 minutes ~30 minutes prior to chemotherapy

Stability

Reconstitution Reconstitute either vial size with 5 mL of sodium chloride 0.9%, directing diluent down side of vial to avoid foaming; swirl gently. Add reconstituted contents of the 150 mg vial to 145 mL sodium chloride 0.9% (add 115 mg vial to 110 mL), resulting in a final concentration of 1 mg/mL; gently invert bag to mix.

Storage Store intact vials at 2°C to 8°C (36°F to 46°F). Solutions diluted for infusion are stable for 24 hours at room temperature of ≤25°C (≤77°F).

Monitoring and Teaching Issues

Physical Assessment Use with caution in presence of severe hepatic impairment. Patient must be monitored for immediate hypersensitivity reaction (dyspnea, erythema, and/or flushing); if reaction occurs, infusion should be stopped and not restarted.

Patient Education This medication is intended to prevent or treat nausea/vomiting. Report immediately any pain or burning at infusion site, swelling of mouth, difficulty swallowing, difficulty breathing, or flushing.

Geriatric Considerations Prior studies with aprepitant by the manufacturer were demonstrated in a total of 544 patients, 31% were >65 years of age, while 5% were >75 years. No differences in safety and efficacy were noted between elderly subjects and younger adults. No dosing adjustment is necessary.

Pregnancy Considerations Teratogenic effects were not observed in animal studies. There are no adequate and well-controlled studies in pregnant women; use only if clearly needed. Efficacy of hormonal contraceptive may be reduced; alternative or additional methods of contraception should be used both during treatment with fosaprepitant or aprepitant and for at least 1 month following the last fosaprepitant/aprepitant dose.

Additional Information Oncology Comment: Fosaprepitant is recommended in the National Comprehensive Cancer Network® (NCCN) Clinical Practice Guidelines in Oncology for Antiemesis (version 1.2011) for use on day 1 in combination with a serotonin receptor antagonist and dexamethasone for chemotherapy with high emetic risk and for select moderately emetogenic regimens (carboplatin, cisplatin, doxorubicin, epirubicin, ifosfamide, irinotecan, or methotrexate). Either fosaprepitant 115 mg or aprepitant (125 mg orally) are administered on day 1; for day 2 and 3, patients should receive aprepitant 80 mg orally. The 1-day regimen (fosaprepitant 150 mg on day 1 only) is listed in the guidelines for highly emetogenic treatments.

◆ **Fosaprepitant Dimeglumine** *see* Fosaprepitant *on page 826*

Foscarnet (fos KAR net)

Index Terms PFA; Phosphonoformate; Phosphonoformic Acid

Generic Availability (U.S.) Yes

Pharmacologic Category Antiviral Agent

Pregnancy Risk Factor C

Lactation Excretion in breast milk unknown/contraindicated

Use Treatment of acyclovir-resistant mucocutaneous herpes simplex virus (HSV) infections in immunocompromised persons (eg, with advanced AIDS); treatment of CMV retinitis in persons with HIV

Unlabeled/Investigational Use Other CMV infections (eg, colitis, esophagitis, neurological disease); CMV prophylaxis for cancer patients receiving alemtuzumab therapy or allogeneic stem cell transplant

Mechanism of Action/Effect Pyrophosphate analogue which acts as a noncompetitive inhibitor of many viral RNA and DNA polymerases as well as HIV reverse transcriptase. Inhibitory effects occur at concentrations which do not affect host cellular DNA polymerases; however, some human cell growth suppression has been observed with high *in vitro* concentrations. Similar to ganciclovir, foscarnet is a virostatic agent. Foscarnet does not require activation by thymidine kinase.

Contraindications Hypersensitivity to foscarnet or any component of the formulation

Warnings/Precautions [U.S. Boxed Warning]: Indicated only for immunocompromised patients with CMV retinitis and mucocutaneous acyclovir-resistant HSV infection. [U.S. Boxed Warning]: Renal impairment occurs to some degree in the majority of patients treated with foscarnet; renal impairment may occur at any time and is usually reversible within 1 week following dose adjustment or discontinuation of therapy, however, several patients have died with renal failure within 4 weeks of stopping foscarnet; therefore, renal function should be closely monitored. To reduce the risk of nephrotoxicity and the potential to administer a relative overdose, always calculate the creatine clearance even if serum creatinine is within the normal range. Adequate hydration may reduce the risk of nephrotoxicity; the manufacturer makes specific recommendations regarding this (see Administration).

Imbalance of serum electrolytes or minerals occurs in at least 15% of patients (hypocalcemia, low ionized calcium, hyper/hypophosphatemia, hypomagnesemia, or hypokalemia). Correct electrolytes before initiating therapy. Use caution when administering other medications that cause electrolyte imbalances. Patients who experience signs or symptoms of an electrolyte imbalance should be assessed immediately. **[U.S. Boxed Warning]: Seizures related to plasma electrolyte/mineral imbalance may occur;** incidence has been reported in up to 10% of HIV patients. Risk factors for seizures include impaired baseline renal function, low total serum calcium, and underlying CNS conditions. May cause anemia and granulocytopenia. May cause genital/vascular tissue irritation/ulceration; adequately hydrate and administer only into vein with adequate blood flow to minimize risk. Foscarnet is deposited in teeth and bone of young, growing animals; it has adversely affected tooth enamel development in rats.

Drug Interactions

Avoid Concomitant Use

Avoid concomitant use of Foscarnet with any of the following: Artemether; Dronedarone; Lumefantrine; Nilotinib; Pimozide; QuiNINE; Tetrabenazine; Thioridazine; Toremifene; Vandetanib; Ziprasidone

Decreased Effect There are no known significant interactions involving a decrease in effect.

Increased Effect/Toxicity

Foscarnet may increase the levels/effects of: Dronedarone; Pimozide; QTc-Prolonging Agents; QuiNINE; Tetrabenazine; Thioridazine; Toremifene; Vandetanib; Ziprasidone

The levels/effects of Foscarnet may be increased by: Alfuzosin; Artemether; Chloroquine; Ciprofloxacin; Ciprofloxacin (Systemic); Gadobutrol; Lumefantrine; Nilotinib; QuiNINE

Adverse Reactions

>10%:

Central nervous system: Fever (65%), headache (26%)

Endocrine & metabolic: Hypokalemia (16% to 48%), hypocalcemia (15% to 30%), hypomagnesemia (15% to 30%), hypophosphatemia (8% to 26%)

Gastrointestinal: Nausea (47%), diarrhea (30%), vomiting (26%)

Hematologic: Anemia (33%), granulocytopenia (17%)

Renal: Abnormal renal function/decreased creatinine clearance (12%; without adequate hydration: 33%)

1% to 10%:

Cardiovascular: Chest pain (1% to 5%), edema (1% to 5%), facial edema (1% to 5%), flushing (1% to 5%), hyper-/hypotension (1% to 5%), palpitation (1% to 5%), ECG changes (1% to 5%)

Central nervous system: Seizure (includes grand mal; 8%), anxiety (≥5%), confusion (≥5%), depression (≥5%), dizziness (≥5%), fatigue (≥5%), hypoesthesia (≥5%), malaise (≥5%), pain (≥5%), aggressiveness (1% to 5%), agitation (1% to 5%), amnesia (1% to 5%), aphasia (1% to 5%), ataxia (1% to 5%), coordination abnormal (1% to 5%), dementia (1% to 5%), EEG abnormal (1% to 5%), hallucination (1% to 5%), insomnia (1% to 5%), meningitis (1% to 5%), nervousness (1% to 5%), somnolence (1% to 5%), stupor (1% to 5%)

Dermatologic: Rash (≥5%), erythematous rash (1% to 5%), maculopapular rash (1% to 5%), pruritus (1% to 5%), seborrhea (1% to 5%), skin discoloration (1% to 5%), skin ulceration (1% to 5%)

Endocrine & metabolic: Hyperphosphatemia (6%), acidosis (1% to 5%), hyponatremia (1% to 5%)

Gastrointestinal: Abdominal pain (≥5%), anorexia (≥5%), constipation (1% to 5%), dyspepsia (1% to 5%), dysphasia (1% to 5%), flatulence (1% to 5%), melena (1% to 5%), pancreatitis (1% to 5%), rectal hemorrhage (1% to 5%), taste perversion (1% to 5%), ulcerative stomatitis (1% to 5%), weight loss (1% to 5%), xerostomia (1% to 5%)

Genitourinary: Dysuria (1% to 5%), nocturia (1% to 5%), urinary retention (1% to 5%)

Hematologic: Leukopenia (≥5%), lymphadenopathy (1% to 5%), thrombocytopenia (1% to 5%), thrombosis (1% to 5%)

Hepatic: Alkaline phosphatase increased (1% to 5%), ALT increased (1% to 5%), AST increased (1% to 5%), hepatic function abnormal (1% to 5%), LDH increased (1% to 5%)

Local: Injection site pain/inflammation (1% to 5%)

Neuromuscular & skeletal: Paresthesia (≥5%), involuntary muscle contractions (≥5%), rigors (≥5%), neuropathy (peripheral; ≥5%), weakness (≥5%), arthralgia (1% to 5%), back pain (1% to 5%), leg cramps (1% to 5%), myalgia (1% to 5%), tremor (1% to 5%)

Ocular: Vision abnormalities (≥5%), conjunctivitis (1% to 5%), eye pain (1% to 5%)

Renal: Acute renal failure (1% to 5%), albuminuria (1% to 5%), BUN increased (1% to 5%), polyuria (1% to 5%), urinary tract infection (1% to 5%)

Respiratory: Cough (≥5%), dyspnea (≥5%), bronchospasm (1% to 5%), hemoptysis (1% to 5%), pharyngitis (1% to 5%), pneumonia (1% to 5%), pneumothorax (1% to 5%), rhinitis (1% to 5%), sinusitis (1% to 5%), stridor (1% to 5%)

Miscellaneous: Diaphoresis (≥5%), sepsis (≥5%), infection (includes bacterial and fungal; ≥5%), flu-like syndrome (1% to 5%), malignancies (lymphoma/sarcoma 1% to 5%), thirst (1% to 5%)

Pharmacodynamics/Kinetics

Protein Binding 14% to 17%

Half-Life Elimination Elimination: ~3-4 hours; terminal: ~88 hours (due to bone deposition)

Metabolism Biotransformation does not occur

Excretion Urine (≤28% as unchanged drug)

Available Dosage Forms

Injection, solution [preservative free]: 24 mg/mL (250 mL, 500 mL)

Dosing

Adult & Geriatric

CMV retinitis: I.V.:

Induction treatment: 60 mg/kg/dose every 8 hours for 14-21 days **or** 90 mg/kg every 12 hours for 14-21 days

Maintenance therapy: 90-120 mg/kg/day as a single daily infusion

Acyclovir-resistant HSV induction treatment: I.V.: 40 mg/kg/dose every 8-12 hours for 14-21 days

Therapy of CMV infection in cancer patients (unlabeled use): I.V.:

Prophylaxis: 60 mg/kg every 8-12 hours for 7 days, followed by 90-120 mg/kg daily until day 100 after HSCT

Pre-emptive treatment: 60 mg/kg every 12 hours for 14 days; if CMV still detectable, continue with 90 mg/kg daily for 5 days/week for 2 additional weeks

Treatment: 90 mg/kg every 12 hours for 2 weeks, followed by 120 mg/kg daily for ≥2 weeks

Pediatric Adolescents: Refer to adult dosing.

Renal Impairment See tables.

Induction Dosing of Foscarnet in Patients With Abnormal Renal Function

Cl_{cr} (mL/min/kg)	HSV	HSV	CMV	CMV
	Equivalent to 40 mg/kg q12h	**Equivalent to 40 mg/kg q8h**	**Equivalent to 60 mg/kg q8h**	**Equivalent to 90 mg/kg q12h**
<0.4	Not recommended	Not recommended	Not recommended	Not recommended
≥0.4-0.5	20 mg/kg every 24 hours	35 mg/kg every 24 hours	50 mg/kg every 24 hours	50 mg/kg every 24 hours
>0.5-0.6	25 mg/kg every 24 hours	40 mg/kg every 24 hours	60 mg/kg every 24 hours	60 mg/kg every 24 hours
>0.6-0.8	35 mg/kg every 24 hours	25 mg/kg every 12 hours	40 mg/kg every 12 hours	80 mg/kg every 24 hours
>0.8-1.0	20 mg/kg every 12 hours	35 mg/kg every 12 hours	50 mg/kg every 12 hours	50 mg/kg every 12 hours
>1.0-1.4	30 mg/kg every 12 hours	30 mg/kg every 8 hours	45 mg/kg every 8 hours	70 mg/kg every 12 hours
>1.4	40 mg/kg every 12 hours	40 mg/kg every 8 hours	60 mg/kg every 8 hours	90 mg/kg every 12 hours

Maintenance Dosing of Foscarnet in Patients With Abnormal Renal Function

Cl_{cr} (mL/min/kg)	CMV	CMV
	Equivalent to 90 mg/kg q24h	**Equivalent to 120 mg/kg q24h**
<0.4	Not recommended	Not recommended
≥0.4-0.5	50 mg/kg every 48 hours	65 mg/kg every 48 hours
>0.5-0.6	60 mg/kg every 48 hours	80 mg/kg every 48 hours
>0.6-0.8	80 mg/kg every 48 hours	105 mg/kg every 48 hours
>0.8-1.0	50 mg/kg every 24 hours	65 mg/kg every 24 hours
>1.0-1.4	70 mg/kg every 24 hours	90 mg/kg every 24 hours
>1.4	90 mg/kg every 24 hours	120 mg/kg every 24 hours

Hemodialysis:

Foscarnet is highly removed by hemodialysis (up to ~38% in 2.5 hours HD with high-flux membrane)

Doses of 50 mg/kg/dose posthemodialysis have been found to produce similar serum concentrations as doses of 90 mg/kg twice daily in patients with normal renal function

Doses of 60-90 mg/kg/dose loading dose (posthemodialysis) followed by 45-60 mg/kg/dose posthemodialysis (3 times/week) with the monitoring of weekly plasma concentrations to maintain peak plasma concentrations in the range of 400-800 µMolar have been recommended by some clinicians

Continuous arteriovenous or venovenous hemodiafiltration effects: Dose as for Cl_{cr} 10-50 mL/minute

Administration

I.V. Use an infusion pump, at a rate not exceeding 1 mg/kg/minute. Adult induction doses of 60 mg/kg are administered over 1 hour. Adult maintenance doses of 90-120 mg/kg are infused over 2 hours. The manufacturer recommends 750-1000 mL of NS or D_5W be administered prior to first infusion to establish diuresis. With subsequent infusions of 90-120 mg/kg, this volume would be repeated. If the dose were 40-60 mg/kg, then the volume could be reduced to 500 mL. After the first dose, the hydration fluid should be administered concurrently with foscarnet.

Stability

Reconstitution Foscarnet should be diluted in D_5W or NS. For peripheral line administration, foscarnet **must** be diluted to ≤12 mg/mL with D_5W or NS. For central line administration, foscarnet may be administered undiluted.

Storage Foscarnet injection is a clear, colorless solution. Store intact bottles at room temperature of 15°C to 30°C (59°F to 86°F) and protect from temperatures >40°C and from freezing. Diluted solution is stable for 24 hours at room temperature or under refrigeration.

Monitoring and Teaching Issues

Laboratory Monitoring Renal function, CBC, electrolytes, calcium, magnesium

Physical Assessment Evaluate electrolytes, renal status, and dental status prior to beginning therapy. Monitor for nephrotoxicity, electrolyte imbalance, and seizures. Teach patient need for regular dental evaluations.

Patient Education While on therapy, it is important to maintain adequate nutrition and hydration, unless instructed to restrict fluid intake. Regular dental check-ups are recommended. May cause dizziness, confusion, nausea, vomiting, or diarrhea. Report any change in sensorium or seizures; unresolved diarrhea or vomiting; unusual fever, chills, or sore throat; unhealed sores; swollen lymph glands; or malaise.

Geriatric Considerations Information on the use of foscarnet is lacking in the elderly. Dose adjustments and proper monitoring must be performed because of the decreased renal function common in older patients.

Breast-Feeding Considerations The CDC recommends **not** to breast-feed if diagnosed with HIV to avoid postnatal transmission of the virus.

Pregnancy Considerations Associated with an increase in skeletal anomalies in animal studies at approximately the equivalent of 13% to 33% of the maximal daily human dose. There are no adequate and well controlled studies in pregnant women. A single case report of use during the third trimester with normal infant outcome was observed. Monitoring of amniotic fluid volumes by ultrasound is recommended weekly after 20 weeks of gestation to detect oligohydramnios.

Additional Information CMV retinitis maintenance treatment may be discontinued if immune reconstitution occurs as a result of ART.

Fosinopril (foe SIN oh pril)

Index Terms Fosinopril Sodium; Monopril

Generic Availability (U.S.) Yes

Pharmacologic Category Angiotensin-Converting Enzyme (ACE) Inhibitor

Medication Safety Issues

Sound-alike/look-alike issues:

Fosinopril may be confused with FLUoxetine, Fosamax®, furosemide, lisinopril

Monopril may be confused with Accupril®, minoxidil, moexipril, Monoket®, Monurol®, ramipril

Pregnancy Risk Factor C (1st trimester); D (2nd and 3rd trimesters)

Lactation Enters breast milk/not recommended

Use Treatment of hypertension, either alone or in combination with other antihypertensive agents; treatment of heart failure (HF)

Mechanism of Action/Effect Competitive inhibitor of angiotensin-converting enzyme (ACE); prevents conversion of angiotensin I to angiotensin II, a potent vasoconstrictor; results in lower levels of angiotensin II which causes an increase in plasma renin activity and a reduction in aldosterone secretion; a CNS mechanism may also be involved in hypotensive effect as angiotensin II increases adrenergic outflow from CNS; vasoactive kallikreins may be decreased in conversion to active hormones by ACE inhibitors, thus reducing blood pressure

Contraindications Hypersensitivity to fosinopril, any other ACE inhibitor, or any component of the formulation; angioedema related to previous treatment with an ACE inhibitor

Warnings/Precautions Anaphylactic reactions may occur rarely with ACE inhibitors. At any time during treatment (especially following first dose), angioedema may occur rarely with ACE inhibitors; it may involve the head and neck (potentially compromising airway) or the intestine (presenting with abdominal pain). African-Americans may be at an increased risk and patients with idiopathic or hereditary angioedema may be at an increased risk. Prolonged frequent monitoring may be required especially if tongue, glottis, or larynx are involved as they are associated with airway obstruction. Patients with a history of airway surgery may have a higher risk of airway obstruction. Aggressive early and appropriate management is critical. Use in patients with previous angioedema associated with ACE inhibitor therapy is contraindicated. Severe anaphylactoid reactions may be seen during hemodialysis (eg, CVVHD) with high-flux dialysis membranes (eg, AN69), and rarely, during low density lipoprotein apheresis with dextran sulfate cellulose. Rare cases of anaphylactoid reactions have been reported in patients undergoing sensitization treatment with hymenoptera (bee, wasp) venom while receiving ACE inhibitors.

Symptomatic hypotension with or without syncope can occur with ACE inhibitors (usually with the first several doses); effects are most often observed in volume-depleted patients; correct volume depletion prior to initiation; close monitoring of patient is required especially with initial dosing and dosing increases; blood pressure must be lowered at a rate appropriate for the patient's clinical condition. Initiation of therapy in patients with ischemic heart disease or cerebrovascular disease warrants close observation due to the potential consequences posed by falling blood pressure (eg, MI, stroke). Use with caution in hypertrophic cardiomyopathy with outflow tract obstruction, severe aortic stenosis, or before, during, or immediately after major surgery. **[U.S. Boxed Warning]: Based on human data, ACEIs can cause injury and death to the developing fetus when used in the second and third trimesters. ACEIs should be discontinued as soon as possible once pregnancy is detected.**

Hyperkalemia may occur with ACE inhibitors; risk factors include renal dysfunction, diabetes mellitus, concomitant use of potassium-sparing diuretics, potassium supplements, and/or potassium-containing salts. Use cautiously, if at all, with these agents and monitor potassium closely. Cough may occur with ACE inhibitors. Other causes of cough should be considered (eg, pulmonary congestion in patients with heart failure) and excluded prior to discontinuation.

May be associated with deterioration of renal function and/or increases in serum creatinine, particularly in patients with low renal blood flow (eg, renal artery stenosis, heart failure) whose glomerular filtration rate (GFR) is dependent on efferent arteriolar vasoconstriction by angiotensin II; deterioration may result in oliguria, acute renal failure, and progressive azotemia. Small increases in serum creatinine may occur following initiation; consider discontinuation only in patients with progressive and/or significant deterioration in renal function. Use with caution in patients with unstented unilateral/bilateral renal artery stenosis. When unstented bilateral renal artery stenosis is present, use is generally avoided due to the elevated risk of deterioration in renal function unless possible benefits outweigh risks. Concurrent use of angiotensin receptor blockers may increase the risk of clinically-significant adverse events (eg, renal dysfunction, hyperkalemia).

Rare toxicities associated with ACE inhibitors include cholestatic jaundice (which may progress to fulminant hepatic necrosis), agranulocytosis, neutropenia or leukopenia with myeloid hypoplasia. Patients with collagen vascular diseases (especially with concomitant renal impairment) or renal impairment alone may be at increased risk for hematologic toxicity; periodically monitor CBC with differential in these patients.

Drug Interactions

Avoid Concomitant Use There are no known interactions where it is recommended to avoid concomitant use.

Decreased Effect

The levels/effects of Fosinopril may be decreased by: Antacids; Aprotinin; Herbs (Hypertensive Properties); Methylphenidate; Nonsteroidal Anti-Inflammatory Agents; Salicylates; Yohimbine

Increased Effect/Toxicity

Fosinopril may increase the levels/effects of: Allopurinol; Amifostine; Antihypertensives; AzaTHIOprine; CycloSPORINE; CycloSPORINE (Systemic); Ferric Gluconate; Gold Sodium Thiomalate; Hypotensive Agents; Iron Dextran Complex; Lithium; RiTUXimab

The levels/effects of Fosinopril may be increased by: Angiotensin II Receptor Blockers; Diazoxide; DPP-IV Inhibitors; Eplerenone; Everolimus; Herbs (Hypotensive Properties); Loop Diuretics; MAO Inhibitors; Pentoxifylline; Phosphodiesterase 5 Inhibitors; Potassium Salts; Potassium-Sparing Diuretics; Prostacyclin Analogues; Sirolimus; Temsirolimus; Thiazide Diuretics; TiZANidine; Tolvaptan; Trimethoprim

Nutritional/Ethanol Interactions Herb/Nutraceutical: Avoid bayberry, blue cohosh, cayenne, ephedra, ginger, ginseng (American), kola, licorice (may worsen hypertension). Avoid black cohosh, california poppy, coleus, golden seal, hawthorn, mistletoe, periwinkle, quinine, shepherd's purse (may have increased antihypertensive effect).

Lab Interactions Positive Coombs' (direct); may cause false-positive results in urine acetone determinations using sodium nitroprusside reagent; may cause false low serum digoxin levels with the Digi-Tab RIA kit for digoxin.

Adverse Reactions Note: Frequency ranges include data from hypertension and heart failure trials. Higher rates of adverse reactions have generally been noted in patients with CHF. However, the frequency of adverse effects associated with placebo is also increased in this population.

>10%: Central nervous system: Dizziness (2% to 12%)

1% to 10%:

- Cardiovascular: Orthostatic hypotension (1% to 2%), palpitation (1%)
- Central nervous system: Dizziness (1% to 2%; up to 12% in CHF patients), headache (3%), fatigue (1% to 2%)
- Endocrine & metabolic: Hyperkalemia (2.6%)
- Gastrointestinal: Diarrhea (2%), nausea/vomiting (1.2% to 2.2%)
- Hepatic: Transaminases increased
- Neuromuscular & skeletal: Musculoskeletal pain (<1% to 3%), noncardiac chest pain (<1% to 2%), weakness (1%)
- Renal: Serum creatinine increased, renal function worsening (in patients with bilateral renal artery stenosis or hypovolemia)
- Respiratory: Cough (2% to 10%)
- Miscellaneous: Upper respiratory infection (2%)

>1% but ≤ frequency in patients receiving placebo: Sexual dysfunction, fever, flu-like syndrome, dyspnea, rash, headache, insomnia

Other events reported with ACE inhibitors: Neutropenia, agranulocytosis, eosinophilic pneumonitis, cardiac arrest, pancytopenia, hemolytic anemia, anemia, aplastic anemia, thrombocytopenia, acute renal failure, hepatic failure, jaundice, symptomatic hyponatremia, bullous pemphigus, exfoliative dermatitis, Stevens-Johnson syndrome. In addition, a syndrome which may include fever, myalgia, arthralgia, interstitial nephritis, vasculitis, rash, eosinophilia and positive ANA, and elevated ESR has been reported for other ACE inhibitors.

Pharmacodynamics/Kinetics

Onset of Action 1 hour

Duration of Action 24 hours

Absorption 36%

Bioavailability 36%

Time to Peak Serum: ~3 hours

Protein Binding 95%

Half-Life Elimination Serum (fosinoprilat): 12 hours

Metabolism Prodrug, hydrolyzed to its active metabolite fosinoprilat by intestinal wall and hepatic esterases

Excretion Urine and feces (as fosinoprilat and other metabolites in roughly equal proportions, 45% to 50%)

Available Dosage Forms

Tablet, oral: 10 mg, 20 mg, 40 mg

Dosing

Adult & Geriatric

Heart failure: Oral: Initial: 10 mg/day (5 mg if renal dysfunction present) and increase, as needed, to a maximum of 40 mg once daily over several weeks. Usual dose: 20-40 mg/day. If hypotension, orthostasis, or azotemia occurs during titration, consider decreasing concomitant diuretic dose, if any.

Hypertension: Oral: Initial: 10 mg/day; increase to a maximum dose of 80 mg/day. Most patients are maintained on 20-40 mg/day. May need to divide the dose into two if trough effect is inadequate. Discontinue the diuretic, if possible 2-3 days before initiation of therapy. Resume diuretic therapy carefully, if needed.

Pediatric Hypertension: Children ≥6 years and >50 kg: Oral: Initial: 5-10 mg once daily (maximum: 40 mg/day)

Renal Impairment None needed since hepatobiliary elimination compensates adequately diminished renal elimination.

Hemodialysis: Moderately dialyzable (20% to 50%)

Hepatic Impairment Decrease dose and monitor effects

Stability

Storage Store at 25°C (77°F); excursions permitted to 15°C to 30°C (59°F to 86°F). Protect from moisture by keeping bottle tightly closed.

Monitoring and Teaching Issues

Laboratory Monitoring Serum creatinine and potassium; if patient has collagen vascular disease and/or renal impairment, periodically monitor CBC with differential

Physical Assessment Use with caution in presence of renal impairment, hypovolemia, aortic stenosis, and before, during, and after major surgery. Assess potential for interactions with other pharmacological agents or herbal products that may impact fluid balance or cardiac status. Monitor for anaphylactic reactions, hypovolemia, angioedema, and postural hypotension.

Patient Education Do not use potassium supplement or salt substitutes without consulting prescriber. This drug does not eliminate need for diet or exercise regimen as recommended by prescriber. May cause dizziness, fainting, lightheadedness, postural hypotension, nausea, vomiting, abdominal pain, dry mouth, or loss of appetite - report if these persist. Report chest pain or palpitations; mouth sores; fever or chills; swelling of extremities, face, mouth, or tongue; skin rash; numbness, tingling, or pain in muscles; respiratory difficulty; or unusual cough.

Dietary Considerations Should not take a potassium salt supplement without the advice of healthcare provider.

Geriatric Considerations Due to frequent decreases in glomerular filtration (also creatinine clearance) with aging, elderly patients may have exaggerated responses to ACE inhibitors. Differences in clinical response due to hepatic changes are not observed. ACE inhibitors may be preferred agents in elderly patients with congestive heart failure and diabetes mellitus. Diabetic proteinuria is reduced and insulin sensitivity is enhanced. In general, the side effect profile is favorable in the elderly and causes little or no CNS confusion; use lowest dose recommendations initially. Many elderly may be volume depleted due to diuretic use and/or blunted thirst reflex resulting in inadequate fluid intake.

Breast-Feeding Considerations Fosinoprilat is excreted in breast milk. Breast-feeding is not recommended by the manufacturer.

Pregnancy Considerations Due to adverse events observed in some animal studies, fosinopril is considered pregnancy category C during the first trimester. Based on human data, fosinopril is considered pregnancy category D if used during the second and third trimesters (per the manufacturer; however, one study suggests that fetal injury may occur at anytime during pregnancy). First trimester exposure to ACE inhibitors may cause major congenital malformations. An increased risk of cardiovascular and/or central nervous system malformations was observed in one study; however, an increased risk of teratogenic events was not observed in other studies. Second and third trimester use of an ACE inhibitor is associated with oligohydramnios. Oligohydramnios due to decreased fetal renal function may lead to fetal limb contractures, craniofacial deformation, and hypoplastic lung development.

The use of ACE inhibitors during the second and third trimesters is also associated with anuria, hypotension, renal failure (reversible or irreversible), skull hypoplasia, and death in the fetus/neonate. Chronic maternal hypertension itself is also associated with adverse events in the fetus/infant. ACE inhibitors are not recommended during pregnancy to treat maternal hypertension or heart failure. Those who are planning a pregnancy should be considered for other medication options if an ACE inhibitor is currently prescribed or the ACE inhibitor should be discontinued as soon as possible once pregnancy is detected. The exposed fetus should be monitored for fetal growth, amniotic fluid volume, and organ formation. Infants exposed to an ACE inhibitor *in utero*, especially during the second and third trimester, should be monitored for hyperkalemia, hypotension, and oliguria.

[U.S. Boxed Warning]: Based on human data, ACE inhibitors can cause injury and death to the developing fetus when used in the second and third trimesters. ACE inhibitors should be discontinued as soon as possible once pregnancy is detected.

Related Information

Angiotensin Agents *on page 1974*
Heart Failure (Systolic) *on page 2040*

◆ **Fosinopril Sodium** *see* Fosinopril *on page 831*

Fosphenytoin (FOS fen i toyn)

U.S. Brand Names Cerebyx®

Index Terms Fosphenytoin Sodium

Generic Availability (U.S.) Yes

Pharmacologic Category Anticonvulsant, Hydantoin

Medication Safety Issues

Sound-alike/look-alike issues:

Cerebyx® may be confused with Celebrex®, Celexa™, Cerezyme®, Cervarix®
Fosphenytoin may be confused with fospropofol

Overdoses have occurred due to confusion between the **mg per mL concentration** of fosphenytoin (50 mg PE/mL) and **total drug content per vial** (either 100 mg PE/2 mL vial or 500 mg PE/10 mL vial). ISMP recommends that the total drug content per container is identified instead of the concentration in mg per mL to avoid confusion and potential overdosages. Additionally, since most errors have occurred with overdoses in children, they recommend that pediatric hospitals should consider stocking only the 2 mL vial.

Pregnancy Risk Factor D

Lactation Excretion in breast milk unknown/not recommended

Use Used for the control of generalized convulsive status epilepticus and prevention and treatment of seizures occurring during neurosurgery; indicated for short-term parenteral administration when other means of phenytoin administration are unavailable, inappropriate, or deemed less advantageous (the safety and effectiveness of fosphenytoin use for more than 5 days has not been systematically evaluated)

Mechanism of Action/Effect Diphosphate ester salt of phenytoin which acts as a water soluble prodrug of phenytoin; after administration, plasma esterases convert fosphenytoin to phosphate, formaldehyde, and phenytoin as the active moiety; phenytoin works by stabilizing neuronal membranes and decreasing seizure activity by increasing efflux or decreasing influx of sodium ions across cell membranes in the motor cortex during generation of nerve impulses

Contraindications Hypersensitivity to phenytoin, other hydantoins, or any component of the formulation; patients with sinus bradycardia, sinoatrial block, second- and third-degree AV block, or Adams-Stokes syndrome; occurrence of rash during treatment (should not be resumed if rash is exfoliative, purpuric, or bullous); treatment of absence seizures

Warnings/Precautions Doses of fosphenytoin are expressed as their phenytoin sodium equivalent (PE). Antiepileptic drugs should not be abruptly discontinued. Hypotension may occur, especially after I.V. administration at high doses and high rates of administration. Administration of phenytoin has been associated with atrial and ventricular conduction depression and ventricular fibrillation. Careful cardiac monitoring is needed when administering I.V. loading doses of fosphenytoin. Acute hepatotoxicity associated with a hypersensitivity syndrome characterized by fever, skin eruptions, and lymphadenopathy has been reported to occur within the first 2 months of treatment. Discontinue if skin rash or lymphadenopathy occurs. A spectrum of hematologic effects have been reported with use (eg, neutropenia, leukopenia, thrombocytopenia, pancytopenia, and anemias). Use with caution in patients with hypotension, severe myocardial insufficiency, diabetes mellitus, porphyria, hypoalbuminemia, hypothyroidism, fever, or hepatic or renal dysfunction. Effects with other sedative drugs or ethanol may be potentiated. Severe reactions, including toxic epidermal necrolysis and Stevens-Johnson syndromes, although rarely reported, have resulted in fatalities; drug should be discontinued if there are any signs of rash. Patients of Asian descent with the variant *HLA-B*1502* may be at an increased risk of developing Stevens-Johnson syndrome and/or toxic epidermal necrolysis.

Drug Interactions

Metabolism/Transport Effects As phenytoin: **Substrate** of CYP2C9 (major), 2C19 (major), 3A4 (minor); **Induces** CYP2B6 (strong), 2C8 (strong), 2C9 (strong), 2C19 (strong), 3A4 (strong)

Avoid Concomitant Use

Avoid concomitant use of Fosphenytoin with any of the following: Dienogest; Dronedarone; Everolimus; Lurasidone; Nilotinib; Nisoldipine; Pazopanib; Praziquantel; Ranolazine; Roflumilast; RomiDEPsin; Tolvaptan; Vandetanib

Decreased Effect

Fosphenytoin may decrease the levels/effects of: Acetaminophen; Chloramphenicol; CYP2B6 Substrates; CYP2C19 Substrates; CYP2C8 Substrates (High risk); CYP2C9 Substrates (High risk); CYP3A4 Substrates; Dienogest; Dronedarone; Everolimus; Exemestane; Gefitinib; GuanFACINE; Imatinib; Ixabepilone; Lurasidone; Maraviroc; NIFEdipine; Nilotinib; Nisoldipine; Pazopanib; Praziquantel; Ranolazine; Roflumilast; RomiDEPsin; Saxagliptin; SORAfenib; Tadalafil; Tolvaptan; Treprostinil; Ulipristal; Vandetanib

The levels/effects of Fosphenytoin may be decreased by: Antacids; CYP2C19 Inducers (Strong); CYP2C9 Inducers (Highly Effective); Ketorolac; Ketorolac (Systemic); Mefloquine; Peginterferon Alfa-2b

Increased Effect/Toxicity

Fosphenytoin may increase the levels/effects of: Alcohol (Ethyl); CNS Depressants; Methotrimeprazine

The levels/effects of Fosphenytoin may be increased by: Allopurinol; Carbonic Anhydrase Inhibitors; Chloramphenicol; Cimetidine; Conivaptan; CYP2C19 Inhibitors (Moderate); CYP2C19 Inhibitors (Strong); CYP2C9 Inhibitors (Moderate); CYP2C9 Inhibitors (Strong); Droperidol; Methotrimeprazine

Nutritional/Ethanol Interactions Ethanol:

Acute use: Avoid or limit ethanol (inhibits metabolism of phenytoin); watch for sedation.
Chronic use: Avoid or limit ethanol (stimulates metabolism of phenytoin).

Lab Interactions May decrease serum concentrations of thyroxine; may produce artifactually low results in dexamethasone or metyrapone tests; may cause increase serum concentrations of glucose, alkaline phosphatase, and gamma glutamyl transpeptidase (GGT)

Adverse Reactions The more important adverse clinical events caused by the I.V. use of fosphenytoin or phenytoin are cardiovascular collapse and/or central nervous system depression. Hypotension can occur when either drug is administered rapidly by the I.V. route. Do not exceed a rate of 150 mg phenytoin equivalent/minute when administering fosphenytoin.

The adverse clinical events most commonly observed with the use of fosphenytoin in clinical trials were nystagmus, dizziness, pruritus, paresthesia, headache, somnolence, and ataxia. Paresthesia and pruritus were seen more often following fosphenytoin (versus phenytoin) administration and occurred more often with I.V. fosphenytoin than with I.M. administration. These events were dose and rate related (doses ≥15 mg/kg at a rate of 150 mg/minute). These sensations, generally described as itching, burning, or tingling are usually not at the infusion site. The location of the discomfort varied with the groin mentioned most frequently. The paresthesia and pruritus were transient events that occurred within several minutes of the start of infusion and generally resolved within 10 minutes after completion of infusion.

Transient pruritus, tinnitus, nystagmus, somnolence, and ataxia occurred 2-3 times more often at doses ≥15 mg/kg and rates ≥150 mg/minute.

I.V. administration (maximum dose/rate):

>10%:

- Central nervous system: Nystagmus, dizziness, somnolence, ataxia
- Dermatologic: Pruritus

1% to 10%:

- Cardiovascular: Hypotension, vasodilation, tachycardia
- Central nervous system: Stupor, incoordination, paresthesia, extrapyramidal syndrome, tremor, agitation, hypoesthesia, dysarthria, vertigo, brain edema, headache
- Gastrointestinal: Nausea, tongue disorder, dry mouth, vomiting
- Neuromuscular & skeletal: Pelvic pain, muscle weakness, back pain
- Ocular: Diplopia, amblyopia
- Otic: Tinnitus, deafness
- Miscellaneous: Taste perversion

I.M. administration (substitute for oral phenytoin):

1% to 10%:

- Central nervous system: Nystagmus, tremor, ataxia, headache, incoordination, somnolence, dizziness, paresthesia, reflexes decreased
- Dermatologic: Pruritus
- Gastrointestinal: Nausea, vomiting
- Hematologic/lymphatic: Ecchymosis
- Neuromuscular & skeletal: Muscle weakness

Pharmacodynamics/Kinetics

Bioavailability I.M.: Fosphenytoin: 100%

Time to Peak Conversion to phenytoin: Following I.V. administration (maximum rate of administration): 15 minutes; following I.M. administration, peak phenytoin levels are reached in 3 hours

Protein Binding Fosphenytoin: 95% to 99% to albumin; can displace phenytoin and increase free fraction (up to 30% unbound) during the period required for conversion of fosphenytoin to phenytoin

Half-Life Elimination Fosphenytoin: 15 minutes; Phenytoin: Variable (mean: 12-29 hours); kinetics of phenytoin are saturable

Metabolism Fosphenytoin is rapidly converted via hydrolysis to phenytoin; phenytoin is metabolized in the liver and forms metabolites

Excretion Phenytoin: Urine (as inactive metabolites)

Pharmacokinetic Note Refer to Phenytoin monograph for additional information.

Available Dosage Forms

Injection, solution: 75 mg/mL (2 mL, 10 mL)
Cerebyx®: 75 mg/mL (2 mL)
Injection, solution [preservative free]: 75 mg/mL (2 mL)

Dosing

Adult

The dose, concentration in solutions, and infusion rates for fosphenytoin are expressed as phenytoin sodium equivalents (PE); fosphenytoin should always be prescribed and dispensed in phenytoin sodium equivalents (PE)

Status epilepticus: I.V.: Loading dose: 15-20 mg PE/kg I.V. administered at 100-150 mg PE/minute

Nonemergent loading and maintenance dosing: I.V. or I.M.:
Loading dose: 10-20 mg PE/kg I.V. or I.M. (maximum I.V. rate: 150 mg PE/minute)
Initial daily maintenance dose: 4-6 mg PE/kg/day I.V. or I.M.

Substitution for oral phenytoin therapy: I.M. or I.V.: May be substituted for oral phenytoin sodium at the same total daily dose; however, Dilantin® capsules are ~90% bioavailable by the oral route; phenytoin, supplied as fosphenytoin, is 100% bioavailable by both the I.M. and I.V. routes; for this reason, plasma phenytoin concentrations may increase when I.M. or I.V. fosphenytoin is substituted for oral phenytoin sodium therapy; in clinical trials, I.M. fosphenytoin was administered as a single daily dose utilizing either 1 or 2 injection sites; some patients may require more frequent dosing

Geriatric Phenytoin clearance is decreased in geriatric patients; lower doses may be required. In addition, older adults may have lower serum albumin which may increase the free fraction and, therefore, pharmacologic response. Refer to adult dosing.

Pediatric

Note: The dose, concentration in solutions, and infusion rates for fosphenytoin are expressed as phenytoin sodium equivalents (PE); fosphenytoin should always be prescribed and dispensed in phenytoin sodium equivalents (PE).

Infants and Children (unlabeled use): I.V.:
Loading dose: 15-20 mg PE/kg for the treatment of generalized convulsive status epilepticus.
Maintenance dosing: Phenytoin dosing guidelines in pediatric patients are used when dosing fosphenytoin using doses in PE equal to the phenytoin doses (ie, phenytoin 1 mg = fosphenytoin 1 PE); maintenance doses may be started 8-12 hours after a loading dose

Renal Impairment Free phenytoin levels should be monitored closely in patients with renal disease or in those with hypoalbuminemia; furthermore, fosphenytoin clearance to phenytoin may be increased without a similar increase in phenytoin clearance in these patients leading to increase frequency and severity of adverse events.

Hepatic Impairment Phenytoin clearance may be substantially reduced in cirrhosis and plasma level monitoring with dose adjustment advisable. Free phenytoin levels should be monitored closely in patients with hepatic disease or in those with hypoalbuminemia; furthermore, fosphenytoin clearance to phenytoin may be increased without a similar increase in phenytoin clearance in these patients leading to increased frequency and severity of adverse events.

Administration

I.M. I.M. may be administered as a single daily dose using either 1 or 2 injection sites.

I.V. Rates of infusion:
Children: 1-3 mg PE/kg/minute
Adults: Should not exceed 150 mg PE/minute

Stability

Reconstitution Must be diluted to concentrations of 1.5-25 mg PE/mL, in normal saline or D_5W, for I.V. infusion.

Storage Refrigerate at 2°C to 8°C (36°F to 46°F). Do not store at room temperature for more than 48 hours. Do not use vials that develop particulate matter.

Monitoring and Teaching Issues

Laboratory Monitoring Serum phenytoin, renal function, albumin

Physical Assessment Continuous monitoring is essential during infusion and for 30 minutes following infusion. Monitor closely for adverse reactions during and following infusion.

Patient Education Patients may not be in a position to evaluate their response. If conscious or alert, advise patient to report signs or symptoms of palpitations, slow heartbeat, respiratory difficulty, faintness, CNS disturbances (eg, somnolence, ataxia), and visual disturbances.

Dietary Considerations Provides phosphate 0.0037 mmol/mg PE fosphenytoin

Geriatric Considerations No significant changes in fosphenytoin pharmacokinetics with age have been noted. Phenytoin clearance is decreased in the elderly and lower doses may be needed. Elderly may have reduced hepatic clearance due to age decline in Phase I metabolism. Elderly may have low albumin which will increase free fraction and, therefore, pharmacologic response. Monitor closely in those who are hypoalbuminemic. Free fraction measurements advised, also elderly may display a higher incidence of adverse effects (cardiovascular) when using the I.V. loading regimen; therefore, it is recommended to decrease loading I.V. dose to 25 mg/minute.

Breast-Feeding Considerations Fosphenytoin is the prodrug of phenytoin. It is not known if fosphenytoin is excreted in breast milk prior to conversion to phenytoin. Refer to Phenytoin monograph for additional information.

Pregnancy Considerations Fosphenytoin is the prodrug of phenytoin. Refer to Phenytoin on page 1453 for additional information.

Additional Information 1.5 mg fosphenytoin is approximately equivalent to 1 mg phenytoin. Equimolar fosphenytoin dose is 375 mg (75 mg/mL solution) to phenytoin 250 mg (50 mg/mL).

◆ **Fosphenytoin Sodium** *see* Fosphenytoin *on page 834*

◆ **Fragmin®** *see* Dalteparin *on page 459*

◆ **Frova®** *see* Frovatriptan *on page 837*

Frovatriptan (froe va TRIP tan)

U.S. Brand Names Frova®

Index Terms Frovatriptan Succinate

Generic Availability (U.S.) No

Pharmacologic Category Antimigraine Agent; Serotonin 5-$HT_{1B,\ 1D}$ Receptor Agonist

Medication Safety Issues

International issues:

Allegro: Brand name for frovatriptan [Germany], but also the brand name for fluticasone [Israel]

Allegro [Germany] may be confused with Allegra and Allegra-D brand names for fexofenadine and fexofenadine/pseudoehedrine, respectively, in the [U.S., Canada, and multiple international markets]

Pregnancy Risk Factor C

Lactation Excretion in breast milk unknown/use caution

Use Acute treatment of migraine with or without aura

Mechanism of Action/Effect Selective agonist for serotonin receptor in cranial arteries; causes vasoconstriction and relief of migraine

Contraindications Hypersensitivity to frovatriptan or any component of the formulation; patients with ischemic heart disease or signs or symptoms of ischemic heart disease (including Prinzmetal's angina, angina pectoris, myocardial infarction, silent myocardial ischemia); cerebrovascular syndromes (including strokes, transient ischemic attacks); peripheral vascular syndromes (including ischemic bowel disease); uncontrolled hypertension; use within 24 hours of ergotamine derivatives; use within 24 hours of another 5-HT_1 agonist; management of hemiplegic or basilar migraine

Canadian labeling: Additional contraindications (not in U.S. labeling): Cardiac arrhythmias, valvular heart disease, congenital heart disease, atherosclerotic disease; management of ophthalmoplegic migraine; severe hepatic impairment

Warnings/Precautions Not intended for migraine prophylaxis, or treatment of cluster headaches, hemiplegic or basilar migraines. Rule out underlying neurologic disease in patients with atypical headache, migraine (with no prior history of migraine) or inadequate clinical response to initial dosing. Cardiac events (coronary artery vasospasm, transient ischemia, MI, ventricular tachycardia/fibrillation, cardiac arrest, and death), cerebral/subarachnoid hemorrhage, stroke, peripheral vascular ischemia, and colonic ischemia have been reported with 5-HT_1 agonist administration. May cause vasospastic reactions resulting in colonic, peripheral, or coronary ischemia. Do not give to patients with risk factors for CAD until a cardiovascular evaluation has been performed; if evaluation is satisfactory, the healthcare provider should administer the first dose and cardiovascular status should be periodically evaluated. Significant elevation in blood pressure, including hypertensive crisis, has also been reported on rare occasions in patients using other 5-HT_{1D} agonists with and without a history of hypertension. May lower seizure threshold, use caution in epilepsy or structural brain lesions. Symptoms of agitation, confusion, hallucinations, hyper-reflexia, myoclonus, shivering, and tachycardia (serotonin syndrome) may occur with concomitant proserotonergic drugs (ie, SSRIs/SNRIs or triptans) or agents which reduce frovatriptan's metabolism. Safety and efficacy in pediatric patients have not been established.

Drug Interactions

Metabolism/Transport Effects Substrate of CYP1A2 (minor)

Avoid Concomitant Use

Avoid concomitant use of Frovatriptan with any of the following: Ergot Derivatives; Sibutramine

Decreased Effect There are no known significant interactions involving a decrease in effect.

Increased Effect/Toxicity

Frovatriptan may increase the levels/effects of: Ergot Derivatives; Serotonin Modulators

The levels/effects of Frovatriptan may be increased by: Ergot Derivatives; Sibutramine

Nutritional/Ethanol Interactions Food: Food does not affect frovatriptan bioavailability.

Adverse Reactions 1% to 10%:

Cardiovascular: Flushing (4%), chest pain (2%), palpitation (1%)

Central nervous system: Dizziness (8%), fatigue (5%), headache (4%), hot or cold sensation (3%), somnolence (≥2%), anxiety (1%), dysesthesia (1%), hypoesthesia (1%), insomnia (1%), pain (1%)

Gastrointestinal: Xerostomia (3%), nausea (≥2%), dyspepsia (2%), abdominal pain (1%), diarrhea (1%), vomiting (1%)

Neuromuscular & skeletal: Paresthesia (4%), skeletal pain (3%)

Ocular: Vision abnormal (1%)

Otic: Tinnitus (1%)

Respiratory: Rhinitis (1%), sinusitis (1%)

Miscellaneous: Diaphoresis (1%)

Pharmacodynamics/Kinetics

Bioavailability Male: ~20%; Female: ~30%

Time to Peak 2-4 hours

Protein Binding ~15%

Half-Life Elimination ~26 hours

Metabolism Primarily hepatic via CYP1A2

Excretion Feces (62%); urine (32%; <10% as unchanged drug)

Available Dosage Forms

Tablet, oral:

Frova®: 2.5 mg

Dosing

Adult & Geriatric Migraine: Oral:

U.S. labeling: 2.5 mg; if headache recurs, a second dose may be given if first dose provided relief and at least 2 hours have elapsed since the first dose (maximum daily dose: 7.5 mg)

Canadian labeling: 2.5 mg; if headache recurs, a second dose may be given if first dose provided relief and at least 4 hours have elapsed since the first dose (maximum daily dose: 5 mg)

Note: The safety of treating more than 4 migraines/month has not been established.

Renal Impairment No adjustment necessary.

Hepatic Impairment No adjustment necessary in mild-to-moderate hepatic impairment; use with caution in severe impairment (has not been studied in severe impairment).

Canadian labeling (not in U.S. labeling): Use is contraindicated in severe hepatic impairment.

Administration

Oral Administer with fluids.

Stability

Storage Store at controlled room temperature of 25°C (77°F); excursions permitted to 15°C to 30°C (59°F to 86°F). Protect from moisture.

Monitoring and Teaching Issues

Physical Assessment Cardiovascular status should be evaluated prior to initiating medication and periodically thereafter.

Patient Education This drug is to be used to reduce your migraine, not to prevent or reduce the number of attacks. If first dose brings relief, a second dose may be taken anytime after 2 hours if migraine returns. May cause dizziness, fatigue, insomnia, drowsiness, dry mouth, skin flushing or hot flashes, mild abdominal discomfort, or vomiting. Report immediately any chest pain, palpitations, or irregular heartbeat; severe dizziness; acute headache; stiff or painful neck; facial swelling; muscle weakness or pain; feeling of tingling in extremities; changes in mental acuity; blurred vision, eye pain, or ringing in ears; changes in urinary pattern; or respiratory difficulty.

Geriatric Considerations Migraine headaches occur infrequently in elderly; however, since elderly often have cardiovascular disease, careful evaluation of the use of 5-HT agonists is needed to avoid complications with the use of these agents. The pharmacokinetic disposition of these agents is similar to that seen in younger adults.

Pregnancy Considerations There are no adequate and well-controlled studies using frovatriptan in pregnant women. Use only if potential benefit to the mother outweighs the potential risk to the fetus.

Related Information

Antimigraine Drugs: 5-HT_1 Receptor Agonists *on page* 1985

- **Frovatriptan Succinate** *see* Frovatriptan *on page* 837
- **Frusemide** *see* Furosemide *on page* 840
- **FSH** *see* Follitropin Alfa *on page* 813
- **FSH** *see* Follitropin Beta *on page* 815
- **FTC** *see* Emtricitabine *on page* 613
- **FTC, TDF, and EFV** *see* Efavirenz, Emtricitabine, and Tenofovir *on page* 606
- **FTY720** *see* Fingolimod *on page* 764
- **FU** *see* Fluorouracil (Systemic) *on page* 787
- **5-FU** *see* Fluorouracil (Systemic) *on page* 787
- **FUDR** *see* Floxuridine *on page* 770

Fulvestrant (fool VES trant)

U.S. Brand Names Faslodex®

Index Terms ICI-182,780; ZD9238

Generic Availability (U.S.) No

Pharmacologic Category Antineoplastic Agent, Estrogen Receptor Antagonist

Pregnancy Risk Factor D

Lactation Excretion in breast milk unknown/not recommended

Use Treatment of hormone receptor positive metastatic breast cancer in postmenopausal women with disease progression following antiestrogen therapy

Mechanism of Action/Effect Estrogen receptor antagonist; competitively binds to estrogen receptors on tumors and other tissue targets, producing a nuclear complex that causes a dose-related down-regulation of estrogen receptors and inhibits tumor growth.

Contraindications Hypersensitivity to fulvestrant or any component of the formulation

Warnings/Precautions Hazardous agent - use appropriate precautions for handling and disposal. Use caution in hepatic impairment; dosage adjustment is recommended in patients with moderate hepatic impairment. Safety and efficacy have not been established in severe hepatic impairment. Use with caution in patients with a history of bleeding disorders (including thrombocytopenia) and/or patients on anticoagulant therapy; bleeding/hematoma may occur from I.M. administration.

Drug Interactions

Metabolism/Transport Effects **Substrate** of CYP3A4 (minor)

Avoid Concomitant Use There are no known interactions where it is recommended to avoid concomitant use.

Decreased Effect There are no known significant interactions involving a decrease in effect.

Increased Effect/Toxicity

The levels/effects of Fulvestrant may be increased by: Conivaptan

Adverse Reactions Adverse reactions reported with 500 mg dose.

>10%:

Endocrine & metabolic: Hot flushes (7% to 13%)

Hepatic: Alkaline phosphatase increased (>15%; grades 3/4: 1 to 2%), transaminases increased (>15%; grades 3/4: 1 to 2%)

Local: Injection site pain (12% to 14%)

Neuromuscular & skeletal: Joint disorders (14% to 19%)

1% to 10%:

Cardiovascular: Ischemic disorder (1%)

Central nervous system: Fatigue (8%), headache (8%)

Gastrointestinal: Nausea (10%), anorexia (6%), vomiting (6%), constipation (5%), weight gain (≤1%)

Genitourinary: Urinary tract infection (2% to 4%)

Neuromuscular & skeletal: Bone pain (9%), arthralgia (8%), back pain (8%), extremity pain (7%), musculoskeletal pain (6%), weakness (6%)

Respiratory: Cough (5%), dyspnea (4%)

<1%, postmarketing, and/or case reports (reported with 250 mg or 500 mg dose): Angioedema, hypersensitivity reactions, leukopenia, myalgia, osteoporosis, thrombosis, urticaria, vaginal bleeding, vertigo

Pharmacodynamics/Kinetics

Duration of Action I.M.: Steady state concentrations reached within first month, when administered with additional dose given 2 weeks following the initial dose; plasma levels maintained for at least 1 month

Protein Binding 99%; to plasma proteins (VLDL, LDL and HDL lipoprotein fractions)

Half-Life Elimination 250 mg: ~40 days

Metabolism Hepatic via multiple biotransformation pathways (CYP3A4 substrate involved in oxidation pathway, although relative contribution to metabolism unknown); metabolites formed are either less active or have similar activity to parent compound

Excretion Feces (~90%); urine (<1%)

Available Dosage Forms

Injection, solution:

Faslodex®: 50 mg/mL (5 mL)

Dosing

Adult & Geriatric **Breast cancer, metastatic (postmenopausal women):** I.M.: Initial: 500 mg on days 1, 15, and 29; Maintenance: 500 mg once monthly

Hepatic Impairment

Moderate impairment (Child-Pugh class B): Decrease initial and maintenance dose to 250 mg

Severe impairment (Child-Pugh class C): Use has not been evaluated.

Administration

I.M. **For I.M. administration only; do not administer I.V., SubQ, or intra-arterially.** Administer 500 mg dose as two 5 mL injections (one in each buttocks) slowly over 1-2 minutes per injection.

Stability

Storage Store in original carton under refrigeration at 2°C to 8°C (36°F to 46°F). Protect from light.

Monitoring and Teaching Issues

Physical Assessment Use caution in presence of hepatic impairment; dosage adjustment may be necessary. Monitor for thromboembolism, vasodilation, edema, gastrointestinal disturbances, dyspnea, and pain on a regular basis throughout.

Patient Education This medication is administered by injection; report immediately any redness, swelling, burning, or pain at injection site. You may experience bone or muscle pain, back pain, or headache; nausea, vomiting, or loss of appetite; dizziness; or hot flashes. Report any chest pain or palpitations, swelling of extremities or weight gain, cough, or respiratory difficulty.

Breast-Feeding Considerations Approved for use only in postmenopausal women.

Pregnancy Considerations Fetal loss and abnormalities were observed in animal studies. Approved for use only in postmenopausal women. If used prior to confirmed menopause, women of reproductive potential should be advised not to become pregnant.

◆ **Fungoid® [OTC]** *see* Miconazole (Topical) *on page* 1224

◆ **Furadantin®** *see* Nitrofurantoin *on page* 1325

Furosemide (fyoor OH se mide)

U.S. Brand Names Lasix®

Index Terms Frusemide

Generic Availability (U.S.) Yes

Pharmacologic Category Diuretic, Loop

Medication Safety Issues

Sound-alike/look-alike issues:

Furosemide may be confused with famotidine, finasteride, fluconazole, FLUoxetine, fosinopril, loperamide, torsemide

Lasix® may be confused with Esidrix®, Lanoxin®, Lidex®, Lomotil®, Lovenox®, Luvox®, Luxiq®

International issues:

Diuril: Brand name for furosemide [Philippines], but also the brand name for chlorothiazide [U.S., Canada]

Urex: Brand name for furosemide [Australia], but is also brand name for methenamine [multiple international markets]

Urex [Australia] may be confused with Eurax brand name for crotamiton [U.S., Canada, and multiple international markets]

Pregnancy Risk Factor C

Lactation Enters breast milk/use caution

Use Management of edema associated with heart failure and hepatic or renal disease; acute pulmonary edema; treatment of hypertension (alone or in combination with other antihypertensives)

Mechanism of Action/Effect Inhibits reabsorption of sodium and chloride in the ascending loop of Henle and distal renal tubule, interfering with the chloride-binding cotransport system, thus causing increased excretion of water, sodium, chloride, magnesium, and calcium

Contraindications Hypersensitivity to furosemide or any component of the formulation; anuria

Warnings/Precautions [U.S. Boxed Warning]: If given in excessive amounts, furosemide, similar to other loop diuretics, can lead to profound diuresis, resulting in fluid and electrolyte depletion; close medical supervision and dose evaluation are required. Watch for and correct electrolyte disturbances; adjust dose to avoid dehydration. When electrolyte depletion is present, therapy should not be initiated unless serum electrolytes, especially potassium, are normalized. In cirrhosis, avoid electrolyte and acid/base imbalances that might lead to hepatic encephalopathy; correct electrolyte and acid/base imbalances prior to initiation when hepatic coma is present. Coadministration of antihypertensives may increase the risk of hypotension.

Monitor fluid status and renal function in an attempt to prevent oliguria, azotemia, and reversible increases in BUN and creatinine; close medical supervision of aggressive diuresis is required. May increase risk of contrast-induced nephropathy. Rapid I.V. administration, renal impairment, excessive doses, hypoproteinemia, and concurrent use of other ototoxins is associated with ototoxicity. Asymptomatic hyperuricemia has been reported with use; rarely, gout may precipitate. Photosensitization may occur.

Use with caution in patients with prediabetes or diabetes mellitus; may see a change in glucose control. Use with caution in patients with systemic lupus erythematosus (SLE); may cause SLE exacerbation or activation. Use with caution in patients with prostatic hyperplasia/urinary stricture; may cause urinary retention. May lead to nephrocalcinosis or nephrolithiasis in premature infants or in children <4 years of age with chronic use. May prevent closure of patent ductus arteriosus in premature infants. Chemical similarities are present among sulfonamides, sulfonylureas, carbonic anhydrase inhibitors, thiazides, and loop diuretics (except ethacrynic acid). A risk of cross-reaction exists in patients with allergy to any of these compounds; avoid use when previous reaction has been severe. Discontinue if signs of hypersensitivity are noted.

Drug Interactions

Avoid Concomitant Use

Avoid concomitant use of Furosemide with any of the following: Ethacrynic Acid

Decreased Effect

Furosemide may decrease the levels/effects of: Lithium; Neuromuscular-Blocking Agents

The levels/effects of Furosemide may be decreased by: Aliskiren; Bile Acid Sequestrants; Herbs (Hypertensive Properties); Methylphenidate; Nonsteroidal Anti-Inflammatory Agents; Phenytoin; Probenecid; Salicylates; Yohimbine

Increased Effect/Toxicity

Furosemide may increase the levels/effects of: ACE Inhibitors; Allopurinol; Amifostine; Aminoglycosides; Antihypertensives; CISplatin; Dofetilide; Ethacrynic Acid; Hypotensive Agents; Lithium; Neuromuscular-Blocking Agents; RiTUXimab; Salicylates

The levels/effects of Furosemide may be increased by: Beta2-Agonists; Corticosteroids (Orally Inhaled); Corticosteroids (Systemic); Diazoxide; Herbs (Hypotensive Properties); Licorice; MAO Inhibitors; Pentoxifylline; Phosphodiesterase 5 Inhibitors; Probenecid; Prostacyclin Analogues

Nutritional/Ethanol Interactions

Food: Furosemide serum levels may be decreased if taken with food.

Herb/Nutraceutical: Avoid bayberry, blue cohosh, cayenne, ephedra, ginger, ginseng (American), kola, licorice (may worsen hypertension). Avoid black cohosh, California poppy, coleus, golden seal, hawthorn, mistletoe, periwinkle, quinine, shepherd's purse (may increase antihypertensive effect). Licorice may also cause or worsen hypokalemia.

Adverse Reactions Frequency not defined.

Cardiovascular: Acute hypotension, chronic aortitis, necrotizing angiitis, orthostatic hypotension, vasculitis

Central nervous system: Dizziness, fever, headache, hepatic encephalopathy, lightheadedness, restlessness, vertigo

Dermatologic: Bullous pemphigoid, cutaneous vasculitis, erythema multiforme, exfoliative dermatitis, photosensitivity, pruritus, purpura, rash, Stevens-Johnson syndrome, toxic epidermal necrolysis, urticaria

Endocrine & metabolic: Cholesterol and triglycerides increased, glucose tolerance test altered, gout, hyperglycemia, hyperuricemia, hypocalcemia, hypochloremia, hypokalemia, hypomagnesemia, hyponatremia, metabolic alkalosis

Gastrointestinal: Anorexia, constipation, cramping, diarrhea, nausea, oral and gastric irritation, pancreatitis, vomiting

Genitourinary: Urinary bladder spasm, urinary frequency

Hematological: Agranulocytosis (rare), anemia, aplastic anemia (rare), eosinophilia, hemolytic anemia, leukopenia, thrombocytopenia

Hepatic: Intrahepatic cholestatic jaundice, ischemic hepatitis, liver enzymes increased

Local: Injection site pain (following I.M. injection), thrombophlebitis

Neuromuscular & skeletal: Muscle spasm, paresthesia, weakness

Ocular: Blurred vision, xanthopsia

Otic: Hearing impairment (reversible or permanent with rapid I.V. or I.M. administration), tinnitus

Renal: Allergic interstitial nephritis, fall in glomerular filtration rate and renal blood flow (due to overdiuresis), glycosuria, transient rise in BUN

Miscellaneous: Anaphylaxis (rare), exacerbate or activate systemic lupus erythematosus

Pharmacodynamics/Kinetics

Onset of Action Diuresis: Oral, S.L.: 30-60 minutes; I.M.: 30 minutes; I.V.: ~5 minutes

Symptomatic improvement with acute pulmonary edema: Within 15-20 minutes; occurs prior to diuretic effect

Peak effect: Oral: 1-2 hours

Duration of Action Oral, S.L.: 6-8 hours; I.V.: 2 hours

Bioavailability Oral tablet: 47-64%; Oral solution: 60%; S.L. administration of tablet: ~60%; results of a small comparative study (n=11) showed bioavailability of SL administration of tablet was ~12% higher than oral administration of tablet (Haegeli, 2007).

Protein Binding 91% to 99%; primarily to albumin

Half-Life Elimination Normal renal function: 0.5-2 hours; End-stage renal disease: 9 hours

Metabolism Minimally hepatic

Excretion Urine (Oral: 50%, I.V.: 80%) within 24 hours; feces (as unchanged drug); nonrenal clearance prolonged with renal impairment

Available Dosage Forms

Injection, solution [preservative free]: 10 mg/mL (2 mL, 4 mL, 10 mL)

Solution, oral: 40 mg/5 mL (5 mL, 500 mL); 10 mg/mL (4 mL, 60 mL, 120 mL)

Tablet, oral: 20 mg, 40 mg, 80 mg

Lasix®: 20 mg, 40 mg, 80 mg

Dosing

Adult

Edema, heart failure:

Oral: Initial: 20-80 mg/dose; if response not adequate, may repeat the same dose or increase dose in increments of 20-40 mg/dose at intervals of 6-8 hours; usual maintenance dose interval is once or twice daily; may be titrated up to 600 mg/day with severe edematous states. **Note:** May also be given on 2-4 consecutive days every week.

I.M., I.V.: Initial: 20-40 mg/dose; if response not adequate, may repeat the same dose or increase dose in increments of 20 mg/dose and administer 1-2 hours after previous dose (maximum dose: 200 mg/dose). Individually determined dose should then be given once or twice daily although some patients may initially require dosing as frequent as every 6 hours. **Note:** ACC/AHA 2009 guidelines for heart failure recommend a maximum single dose of 160-200 mg.

Continuous I.V. infusion (Howard, 2001; Hunt, 2009): Initial: I.V. bolus dose 20-40 mg over 1-2 minutes, followed by continuous I.V. infusion doses of 10-40 mg/hour. If urine output is <1 mL/kg/hour, double as necessary to a maximum of 80-160 mg/hour. The risk associated with higher infusion rates (80-160 mg/hour) must be weighed against alternative strategies. **Note:** ACC/AHA 2009 guidelines for heart failure recommend 40 mg I.V. load, then 10-40 mg/hour infusion.

Acute pulmonary edema: *I.V.:* 40 mg over 1-2 minutes. If response not adequate within 1 hour, may increase dose to 80 mg. **Note:** ACC/AHA 2009 guidelines for heart failure recommend a maximum single dose of 160-200 mg.

Hypertension, resistant (Chobanian, 2003; JNC 7): *Oral:* 20-80 mg/day in 2 divided doses

Refractory heart failure: *Oral, I.V.:* Doses up to 8 g/day have been used.

Geriatric Oral, I.M., I.V.: Initial: 20 mg/day; increase slowly to desired response.

Pediatric

Edema, heart failure: Infants and Children:

Oral: Initial: 2 mg/kg/dose increased in increments of 1-2 mg/kg/dose with each succeeding dose at intervals of 6-8 hours until a satisfactory response is achieved; maximum dose: 6 mg/kg/dose

I.M., I.V.: Initial: 1 mg/kg/dose; if response not adequate, may increase dose in increments of 1 mg/kg/dose and administer not sooner than 2 hours after previous dose, until a satisfactory response is achieved; may administer maintenance dose at intervals of every 6-12 hours; maximum dose: 6 mg/kg/dose

Hypertension, resistant (unlabeled; AAP, 2004): Children 1-17 years: *Oral:* Initial: 0.5-2 mg/kg/dose once or twice daily; maximum dose: 6 mg/kg/dose

Renal Impairment

Acute renal failure: Doses up to 1-3 g/day may be necessary to initiate desired response; avoid use in oliguric states.

Not removed by hemo- or peritoneal dialysis; supplemental dose is not necessary.

Hepatic Impairment Diminished natriuretic effect with increased sensitivity to hypokalemia and volume depletion in cirrhosis. Monitor effects, particularly with high doses.

Administration

Oral Administer on an empty stomach (Bard, 2004). May be administered with food or milk if GI distress occurs; however, this may reduce diuretic efficacy.

I.V. I.V. injections should be given slowly. In adults, undiluted direct I.V. injections may be administered at a rate of 20-40 mg per minute; maximum rate of administration for short-term intermittent infusion is 4 mg/minute; exceeding this rate increases the risk of ototoxicity. In children, a maximum rate of 0.5 mg/kg/minute has been recommended.

Other When I.V. or oral administration is not possible, the sublingual route may be used. Place 1 tablet under tongue for at least 5 minutes to allow for maximal absorption. Patients should be advised not to swallow during disintegration time (Haegeli, 2007).

Stability

Reconstitution I.V. infusion solution mixed in NS or D_5W solution is stable for 24 hours at room temperature. May also be diluted for infusion to 1-2 mg/mL (maximum: 10 mg/mL).

Storage

Injection: Store at room temperature of 15°C to 30°C (59°F to 86°F). Protect from light. Exposure to light may cause discoloration; do not use furosemide solutions if they have a yellow color. Furosemide solutions are unstable in acidic media, but very stable in basic media. Refrigeration may result in precipitation or crystallization; however, resolubilization at room temperature or warming may be performed without affecting the drug's stability.

Tablet: Store at 25°C (77°F); excursions permitted to 15°C to 30°C (59°F to 89°F). Protect from light.

Monitoring and Teaching Issues

Laboratory Monitoring Serum electrolytes, renal function

Physical Assessment Assess for allergy to sulfonylurea before beginning therapy. For intravenous use. Monitor for dehydration, electrolyte imbalance, and postural hypotension on a regular basis during therapy.

Patient Education For daily administration, may be taken with food or milk early in the day to reduce GI distress; if taken twice daily, take last dose in early afternoon in order to avoid sleep disturbance and to achieve maximum therapeutic effect. Follow dietary advice of prescriber; include potassium-rich foods in daily diet. Do not take potassium supplements without advice of prescriber. Weigh yourself each day at the same time when beginning therapy and weekly for long-term therapy. Report unusual or unanticipated weight gain or loss. May cause dizziness, blurred vision, drowsiness, or sensitivity to sunlight. Report signs of edema (eg, weight gain; swollen ankles, feet, or hands), trembling, numbness or fatigue, cramping or muscle weakness, chest pain or palpitations, unresolved nausea or vomiting, or any change in hearing.

Dietary Considerations May cause potassium loss; potassium supplement or dietary changes may be required.

Geriatric Considerations Loop diuretics are potent diuretics; excess amounts can lead to profound diuresis with fluid and electrolyte loss; close medical supervision and dose evaluation is required, particularly in the elderly. Severe loss of sodium and/or increase in BUN can cause confusion. For any change in mental status in patients on furosemide, monitor electrolytes and renal function.

Breast-Feeding Considerations Crosses into breast milk; may suppress lactation

Pregnancy Considerations Animal studies have demonstrated maternal death, fetal toxicity, and fetal loss. There are no adequate and well-controlled studies in pregnant women. Crosses the placenta. Increased fetal urine production, electrolyte disturbances reported. Generally, use of diuretics during pregnancy is avoided due to risk of decreased placental perfusion. Monitor fetal growth if used during pregnancy; may increase birth weight.

Related Information

Compatibility of Drugs *on page* 1994

Heart Failure (Systolic) *on page* 2040

◆ **Fusilev™** *see* LEVOleucovorin *on page* 1096

◆ **Fuzeon®** *see* Enfuvirtide *on page* 621

◆ **FVIII/vWF** *see* Antihemophilic Factor/von Willebrand Factor Complex (Human) *on page* 134

Gabapentin (GA ba pen tin)

U.S. Brand Names Neurontin®

Generic Availability (U.S.) Yes

Pharmacologic Category Anticonvulsant, Miscellaneous

Medication Safety Issues

Sound-alike/look-alike issues:

Neurontin® may be confused with Motrin®, Neoral®, nitrofurantoin, Noroxin®, Zarontin®

Medication Guide Available Yes

Pregnancy Risk Factor C

Lactation Enters breast milk/use caution

Use Adjunct for treatment of partial seizures with and without secondary generalized seizures in patients >12 years of age with epilepsy; adjunct for treatment of partial seizures in pediatric patients 3-12 years of age; management of postherpetic neuralgia (PHN) in adults

Unlabeled/Investigational Use Neuropathic pain, diabetic peripheral neuropathy, fibromyalgia, postoperative pain, bipolar disorder, restlesslegs syndrome (RLS), social phobia, vasomotor symptoms

Mechanism of Action/Effect Although structurally related to GABA, it does not interact with GABA receptors. Interacts with calcium channels to inhibit neurotransmission related to seizure activity and pain perception.

Contraindications Hypersensitivity to gabapentin or any component of the formulation

Warnings/Precautions Antiepileptics are associated with an increased risk of suicidal behavior/thoughts with use (regardless of indication); patients should be monitored for signs/symptoms of depression, suicidal tendencies, and other unusual behavior changes during therapy and instructed to inform their healthcare provider immediately if symptoms occur. Avoid abrupt withdrawal, may precipitate seizures; use cautiously in patients with severe renal dysfunction; male rat studies demonstrated an association with pancreatic adenocarcinoma (clinical implication unknown). May cause CNS depression, which may impair physical or mental abilities. Patients must be cautioned about performing tasks which require mental alertness (eg, operating machinery or driving). Effects with other sedative drugs or ethanol may be potentiated. Pediatric patients (3-12 years of age) have shown increased incidence of CNS-related adverse effects, including emotional lability, hostility, thought disorder, and hyperkinesia.

Drug Interactions

Avoid Concomitant Use There are no known interactions where it is recommended to avoid concomitant use.

Decreased Effect

The levels/effects of Gabapentin may be decreased by: Ketorolac; Ketorolac (Systemic); Mefloquine

Increased Effect/Toxicity

Gabapentin may increase the levels/effects of: Alcohol (Ethyl); CNS Depressants; Methotrimeprazine

The levels/effects of Gabapentin may be increased by: Droperidol; Methotrimeprazine

Nutritional/Ethanol Interactions

Ethanol: Avoid ethanol (may increase CNS depression).

Food: Does not change rate or extent of absorption.

Herb/Nutraceutical: Avoid evening primrose (seizure threshold decreased). Avoid valerian, St John's wort, kava kava, gotu kola (may increase CNS depression).

Lab Interactions False positives have been reported with the Ames N-Multistix SG® dipstick test for urine protein

Adverse Reactions As reported in patients >12 years of age, unless otherwise noted in children (3-12 years)

>10%:

Central nervous system: Somnolence (20%; children 8%), dizziness (17% to 28%; children 3%), ataxia (13%), fatigue (11%)

Miscellaneous: Viral infection (children 11%)

1% to 10%:

Cardiovascular: Peripheral edema (2% to 8%), vasodilatation (1%)

Central nervous system: Fever (children 10%), hostility (children 8%), emotional lability (children 4%), fatigue (children 3%), headache (3%), ataxia (3%), abnormal thinking (2% to 3%; children 2%), amnesia (2%), depression (2%), dysarthria (2%), nervousness (2%), abnormal coordination (1% to 2%), twitching (1%), hyperesthesia (1%)

Dermatologic: Pruritus (1%), rash (1%)

Endocrine & metabolic: Hyperglycemia (1%)

Gastrointestinal: Diarrhea (6%), nausea/vomiting (3% to 4%; children 8%), abdominal pain (3%), xerostomia (2% to 5%), constipation (2% to 4%), weight gain (adults and children 2% to 3%), dyspepsia (2%), flatulence (2%), dry throat (2%), dental abnormalities (2%), appetite stimulation (1%)

Genitourinary: Impotence (2%)

Hematologic: Leukopenia (1%), decreased WBC (1%)

Neuromuscular & skeletal: Tremor (7%), weakness (6%), hyperkinesia (children 3%), abnormal gait (2%), back pain (2%), myalgia (2%), fracture (1%)

Ocular: Nystagmus (8%), diplopia (1% to 6%), blurred vision (3% to 4%), conjunctivitis (1%)

Otic: Otitis media (1%)

Respiratory: Rhinitis (4%), bronchitis (children 3%), respiratory infection (children 3%), pharyngitis (1% to 3%), cough (2%)
Miscellaneous: Infection (5%)

Pharmacodynamics/Kinetics

Absorption 50% to 60% from proximal small bowel by L-amino transport system

Bioavailability Inversely proportional to dose due to saturable absorption:
900 mg/day: 60%
1200 mg/day: 47%
2400 mg/day: 34%
3600 mg/day: 33%
4800 mg/day: 27%

Protein Binding 0%

Half-Life Elimination 5-7 hours; anuria 132 hours; during dialysis 3.8 hours

Excretion Proportional to renal function; urine (as unchanged drug)

Product Availability

Gralise™: FDA approved January 2011; availability expected in late 2011
Gralise™ is a once-daily formulation of gabapentin approved for the treatment of postherpetic neuralgia.

Available Dosage Forms

Capsule, oral: 100 mg, 300 mg, 400 mg
Neurontin®: 100 mg, 300 mg, 400 mg
Solution, oral: 250 mg/5 mL (470 mL)
Neurontin®: 250 mg/5 mL (470 mL)
Tablet, oral: 600 mg, 800 mg
Neurontin®: 600 mg, 800 mg

Dosing

Adult

Anticonvulsant: Oral:
Initial: 300 mg 3 times/day, if necessary the dose may be increased up to 1800 mg/day
Maintenance: 900-1800 mg/day administered in 3 divided doses; doses of up to 2400 mg/day have been tolerated in long-term clinical studies; up to 3600 mg/day has been tolerated in short-term studies
Note: If gabapentin is discontinued or if another anticonvulsant is added to therapy, it should be done slowly over a minimum of 1 week.

Chronic pain (unlabeled use): Oral: 300-1800 mg/day given in 3 divided doses has been the most common dosage range

Postoperative pain (unlabeled use): 300-1200 mg 1-2 hours before surgery

Postherpetic neuralgia: Day 1: 300 mg, Day 2: 300 mg twice daily, Day 3: 300 mg 3 times/day; dose may be titrated as needed for pain relief (range: 1800-3600 mg/day, daily doses >1800 mg do not generally show greater benefit)

Restless legs syndrome (RLS) (unlabeled use): Oral: Initial: 300 mg once daily 2 hours before bedtime. Doses ≥600 mg/day have been given in 2 divided doses (late afternoon and 2 hours before bedtime). Dose may be titrated every 2 weeks until symptom relief achieved (range: 300-1800 mg/day). Suggested maintenance dosing schedule: One-third of total daily dose given at 12 pm, remaining two-thirds total daily dose given at 8 pm. (Garcia-Borreguero, 2002; Happe, 2003; Saletu, 2010; Vignatelli, 2006)

Vasomotor symptoms associated with menopause (unlabeled use; Butt, 2008): 300 mg 3 times/day

Geriatric Studies in elderly patients have shown a decrease in clearance as age increases. This is most likely due to age-related decreases in renal function; dose reductions may be needed.

Pediatric

Anticonvulsant: Oral
Children 3-12 years: Initial: 10-15 mg/kg/day in 3 divided doses; titrate to effective dose over ~3 days; dosages of up to 50 mg/kg/day have been tolerated in clinical studies
Children 3-4 years: Effective dose: 40 mg/kg/day in 3 divided doses
Children 5-12 years: Effective dose: 25-35 mg/kg/day in 3 divided doses
Children >12 years: Refer to adult dosing.
Note: If gabapentin is discontinued or if another anticonvulsant is added to therapy, it should be done slowly over a minimum of 1 week

Renal Impairment Children ≥12 years and Adults: See table.
Hemodialysis: Dialyzable

Gabapentin Dosing Adjustments in Renal Impairment

Creatinine Clearance (mL/min)	Daily Dose Range
≥60	300-1200 mg tid
>30-59	200-700 mg bid
>15-29	200-700 mg daily
15[1]	100-300 mg daily
Hemodialysis[2]	125-350 mg

[1]Cl_{cr}<15 mL/minute: Reduce daily dose in proportion to creatinine clearance.
[2]Single supplemental dose administered after each 4 hours of hemodialysis

Administration

Oral Administer first dose on first day at bedtime to avoid somnolence and dizziness. Dosage must be adjusted for renal function; when given 3 times daily, the maximum time between doses should not exceed 12 hours.

Stability

Storage Store at 25°C (77°F); excursions permitted to 15°C to 30°C (59°F to 86°F).

Monitoring and Teaching Issues

Laboratory Monitoring Monitor serum levels of concomitant anticonvulsant therapy. Routine monitoring of gabapentin levels is not mandatory.

Physical Assessment Assess for CNS depression. Taper dosage slowly when discontinuing. Teach patient safety and seizure precautions.

Patient Education It may take 2-3 weeks to achieve desired results. If prescribed once-a-day, take dose at bedtime. Do not stop medication abruptly, may lead to increased seizure activity. Avoid alcohol. Maintain adequate hydration, unless instructed to restrict fluid intake. You may experience drowsiness, lightheadedness, impaired coordination, dizziness, blurred vision, nausea, vomiting, anorexia, constipation, diarrhea, postural hypotension, or decreased sexual function or libido (reversible). Report persistent CNS effects (nervousness, restlessness, insomnia, anxiety, excitation, headache, sedation, seizures, mania, abnormal thinking); suicide ideation or depression; rash or skin irritation; muscle cramping, tremors, or change in gait; chest pain or palpitations; change in urinary pattern; or worsening of condition.

Dietary Considerations May be taken without regard to meals.

Geriatric Considerations Studies in the elderly have shown a decrease in clearance as age increases. This is most likely due to age-related decreases in renal function; calculations of Cl_{cr} recommended since dose reductions may be needed.

Breast-Feeding Considerations Gabapentin is excreted in human breast milk. A nursed infant could be exposed to ~1 mg/kg/day of gabapentin; the effect on the child is not known. Use in breast-feeding women only if the benefits to the mother outweigh the potential risk to the infant.

Pregnancy Considerations Animal studies have documented teratogenic effects. There are no adequate and well-controlled studies in pregnant women. Use during pregnancy only if the potential benefit to the mother outweighs the potential risk to the fetus.

Patients exposed to gabapentin during pregnancy are encouraged to enroll themselves into the AED Pregnancy Registry by calling 1-888-233-2334. Additional information is available at www.aedpregnancyregistry.org.

Related Information

Anticonvulsant Drugs of Choice *on page 1981*

◆ **Gabitril®** *see* TiaGABine *on page 1758*

◆ **Gablofen®** *see* Baclofen *on page 187*

Gadofosveset (gad oh FOS ve set)

U.S. Brand Names Ablavar™

Index Terms Gadofosveset Trisodium

Generic Availability (U.S.) No

Pharmacologic Category Gadolinium-Containing Contrast Agent; Radiological/Contrast Media, Nonionic (Low Osmolality); Radiological/Contrast Media, Paramagnetic Agent

Medication Safety Issues

Sound-alike/look-alike issues:

Vasovist® may be confused with Magnevist®, Gadovist®

High alert medication: The Institute for Safe Medication Practices (ISMP) includes this medication among its list of drug classes which have a heightened risk of causing significant patient harm when used in error.

Pregnancy Risk Factor C

Lactation Excretion in breast milk unknown/use caution

Use Contrast medium used in magnetic resonance angiography (MRA) to evaluate or better define aortoiliac occlusive disease

Mechanism of Action/Effect Gadofosveset is a contrasting agent used as a diagnostic aid in MRA.

Contraindications Hypersensitivity to gadofosveset, gadolinium, or any component of the formulation

Warnings/Precautions [U.S. Boxed Warning]: Gadolinium-based contrast agent (GBCA) exposure may increase the risk for NSF development in patients with acute or chronic severe renal insufficiency (GFR <30 mL/minute/1.73 m^2) or acute renal insufficiency, of any severity, due to hepatorenal syndrome or in patients during the perioperative liver transplantation period. Avoid use in those high risk patients unless use of GBCA enhanced imaging is essential for diagnostic purposes. NSF, a potentially fatal disease, affects the skin, muscle, and internal organs and can occur days to months after exposure. The potential risk of NSF development, if any, in patients with mild-to-moderate renal insufficiency or normal function is unknown; all patients should be screened for renal dysfunction prior to administration; consider follow-up monitoring in patients with renal dysfunction. Additional risk factors may include repeated exposure and exceeding dosage recommendations. Allow adequate time for drug elimination prior to readministration.

Use caution in renal impairment. Acute renal failure (ARF) also has been reported with the use of similar agents in renally impaired patients. Dose reductions may be necessary. Rare cases of QT_c prolongation have been observed. Data from pooled safety studies have demonstrated minimal changes to the QT_c interval as compared to placebo (means of 2.8 msec and 3.2 msec respectively). Consider baseline and follow up ECG in patients at increased risk of arrhythmias due to QT_c prolongation (eg, underlying cardiac disease, concurrent medications). Patients should be monitored for at least one hour after the administration of gadofosveset.

Use caution with history of allergy, drug reactions, hypersensitivity disorders, and asthma. Elimination of gadofosveset may be quicker in patients with decreased levels of serum albumin. Use with caution in patients who have received iodine-containing contrast agents within 72 hours prior to administration of gadofosveset or other gadolinium based-agents within 24 hours prior to administration of gadofosveset. Safety and efficacy have not been established in patients <18 years of age.

Drug Interactions

Avoid Concomitant Use

Avoid concomitant use of Gadofosveset with any of the following: Artemether; Dronedarone; Lumefantrine; Nilotinib; Pimozide; QuiNINE; Tetrabenazine; Thioridazine; Toremifene; Vandetanib; Ziprasidone

Decreased Effect There are no known significant interactions involving a decrease in effect.

Increased Effect/Toxicity

Gadofosveset may increase the levels/effects of: Dronedarone; Pimozide; QTc-Prolonging Agents; QuiNINE; Tetrabenazine; Thioridazine; Toremifene; Vandetanib; Ziprasidone

The levels/effects of Gadofosveset may be increased by: Alfuzosin; Artemether; Chloroquine; Ciprofloxacin; Ciprofloxacin (Systemic); Gadobutrol; Lumefantrine; Nilotinib; QuiNINE

Adverse Reactions 1% to 10% (observed with 0.03 mmol/kg dose):

Cardiovascular: Vasodilatation (3%), hypertension (1%)
Central nervous system: Headache (4%), dizziness (1%)
Dermatologic: Pruritus (5%)
Gastrointestinal: Nausea (4%), taste disturbance (2%)
Local: Injection site: Bruising (2%)
Neuromuscular & skeletal: Paresthesia (3%)
Miscellaneous: Burning sensation (2%), cold feeling (1%)

Pharmacodynamics/Kinetics

Onset of Action ~15 minutes

Duration of Action ~1 hour

Protein Binding 80% to 87% (predominantly to albumin)

Half-Life Elimination ~16 hours; increases with moderate-to-severe renal impairment (Cl_{cr} <50 mL/minute)

Metabolism Negligible

Excretion Urine (84% as unchanged drug); feces (~5%)

Available Dosage Forms

Injection, solution [preservative free]:
Ablavar™: 0.25 mmol/mL (10 mL, 15 mL)

Dosing

Adult & Geriatric

MRA: I.V.: 0.03 mmol/kg (0.12 mL/kg)

Renal Impairment Use with caution in renal impairment; specific dosing recommendations are not provided in the approved labeling.

Hepatic Impairment No dosage adjustment necessary for Child-Pugh class A and B. Use caution for Child-Pugh class C; specific dosing recommendations are not provided in the approved labeling

Administration

I.V. Administer as an intravenous bolus injection over a period up to 30 seconds or at a rate not exceeding 1.5 mL/sec through a dedicated I.V. line separate from other medications. Flush line with 25-30 mL NS after administration to ensure complete injection of medium. Imaging should be completed within 1 hour of injection.

Stability

Storage Store at 15°C to 30°C (59°F to 86°F); do not freeze. Protect from light.

Monitoring and Teaching Issues

Laboratory Monitoring Baseline electrolytes (including potassium, calcium and magnesium), baseline renal function and follow-up evaluation in patients with renal dysfunction

Physical Assessment Use caution in the presence of severe renal impairment (dose reduction may be necessary), history of QT prolongation, allergies, or asthma. Monitor closely for anaphylactic reaction; equipment and trained personnel for resuscitation should be immediately available during infusion.

Patient Education This medication can only be administered by infusion; you will be closely monitored during treatment. Report immediately headache, itching, or shortness of breath.

Breast-Feeding Considerations Low amounts of gadolinium (0.01% to 0.04%) are excreted into breast milk. The manufacturer does not recommend use in breast-feeding women unless diagnostic imaging is essential and cannot be obtained by noncontrast MRA.

Pregnancy Considerations Animal studies suggest increased fetal loss but no teratogenic effects were observed. There are no adequate and well-controlled studies in pregnant women. Use during pregnancy only if clearly needed.

◆ **Gadofosveset Trisodium** *see* Gadofosveset *on page 845*

Galantamine (ga LAN ta meen)

U.S. Brand Names Razadyne®; Razadyne® ER

Index Terms Galantamine Hydrobromide

Generic Availability (U.S.) Yes

Pharmacologic Category Acetylcholinesterase Inhibitor (Central)

Medication Safety Issues

Sound-alike/look-alike issues:

Razadyne® may be confused with Rozerem™

Reminyl® may be confused with Amaryl®, Robinul®

Due to patient safety concerns regarding prescribing and dispensing errors between Reminyl® and Amaryl®, Reminyl® (galantamine) is being renamed to Razadyne® (immediate-release) and Razadyne® ER (extended-release). The brand name Reminyl® was discontinued with the July, 2005 distribution of Razadyne®.

International issues:

Reminyl [multiple international markets] may be confused with Amarel [France] and Amaryl [U.S., Canada, and multiple international markets], brand names for glimepiride

Pregnancy Risk Factor B

Lactation Excretion in breast milk unknown/not recommended

Use Treatment of mild-to-moderate dementia of Alzheimer's disease

Unlabeled/Investigational Use Severe dementia associated with Alzheimer's disease; mild-to-moderate dementia associated with Parkinson's disease; Lewy body dementia

Mechanism of Action/Effect Increases the concentration of acetylcholine in the brain by slowing its metabolism.

Contraindications Hypersensitivity to galantamine or any component of the formulation; severe liver dysfunction (Child-Pugh score 10-15); severe renal dysfunction (Cl_{cr} <9 mL/minute)

Warnings/Precautions Use caution in patients with supraventricular conduction delays (without a functional pacemaker in place); Alzheimer's treatment guidelines consider bradycardia to be a relative contraindication for use of centrally-active cholinesterase inhibitors. Use caution in patients taking medicines that slow conduction through SA or AV node. Use caution in peptic ulcer disease (or in patients at risk); seizure disorder; asthma; COPD; mild-to-moderate liver dysfunction; moderate renal dysfunction. May cause bladder outflow obstruction. May exaggerate neuromuscular blockade effects of succinylcholine and like agents. May cause nausea, vomiting, diarrhea, weight loss, and anorexia.

Drug Interactions

Metabolism/Transport Effects Substrate (minor) of CYP2D6, 3A4

Avoid Concomitant Use There are no known interactions where it is recommended to avoid concomitant use.

Decreased Effect

Galantamine may decrease the levels/effects of: Anticholinergics; Neuromuscular-Blocking Agents (Nondepolarizing)

The levels/effects of Galantamine may be decreased by: Anticholinergics; Peginterferon Alfa-2b

Increased Effect/Toxicity

Galantamine may increase the levels/effects of: Antipsychotics; Beta-Blockers; Cholinergic Agonists; Succinylcholine

The levels/effects of Galantamine may be increased by: Conivaptan; Corticosteroids (Systemic); Selective Serotonin Reuptake Inhibitors

Nutritional/Ethanol Interactions

Ethanol: Avoid ethanol (may increase CNS adverse events).

Herb/Nutraceutical: St John's wort may decrease galantamine serum levels; avoid concurrent use.

Adverse Reactions

>10%: Gastrointestinal: Nausea (6% to 24%), vomiting (4% to 13%), diarrhea (6% to 12%)

1% to 10%:

Cardiovascular: Bradycardia (2% to 3%), syncope (0.4% to 2.2%: dose related), chest pain (≥1%)

Central nervous system: Dizziness (9%), headache (8%), depression (7%), fatigue (5%), insomnia (5%), somnolence (4%)

Gastrointestinal: Anorexia (7% to 9%), weight loss (5% to 7%), abdominal pain (5%), dyspepsia (5%), flatulence (≥1%)

Genitourinary: Urinary tract infection (8%), hematuria (<1% to 3%), incontinence (≥1%)

Hematologic: Anemia (3%)

Neuromuscular & skeletal: Tremor (3%)

Respiratory: Rhinitis (4%)

Pharmacodynamics/Kinetics

Duration of Action 3 hours; maximum inhibition of erythrocyte acetylcholinesterase ~40% at 1 hour post 8 mg oral dose; levels return to baseline at 30 hours

Absorption Rapid and complete

Bioavailability ~90%

Time to Peak Immediate release: 1 hour (2.5 hours with food); extended release: 4.5-5 hours

Protein Binding 18%

Half-Life Elimination 7 hours

Metabolism Hepatic; linear, CYP2D6 and 3A4; metabolized to epigalanthaminone and galanthaminone both of which have acetylcholinesterase inhibitory activity 130 times less than galantamine

Excretion Urine (25%)

Available Dosage Forms

Capsule, extended release, oral: 8 mg, 16 mg, 24 mg
Razadyne® ER: 8 mg, 16 mg, 24 mg

Solution, oral: 4 mg/mL (100 mL)
Razadyne®: 4 mg/mL (100 mL)

Tablet, oral: 4 mg, 8 mg, 12 mg
Razadyne®: 4 mg, 8 mg, 12 mg

Dosing

Adult & Geriatric

Alzheimer's dementia (mild-to-moderate): Oral:

Immediate release tablet or solution: Mild-to-moderate dementia of Alzheimer's: Initial: 4 mg twice a day for 4 weeks; if tolerated, increase to 8 mg twice daily for ≥4 weeks; if tolerated, increase to 12 mg twice daily
Range: 16-24 mg/day in 2 divided doses

Extended-release capsule: Initial: 8 mg once daily for 4 weeks; if tolerated, increase to 16 mg once daily for ≥4 weeks; if tolerated, increase to 24 mg once daily
Range: 16-24 mg once daily

Note: Oral solution and tablet should be taken with breakfast and dinner; capsule should be taken with breakfast. If therapy is interrupted for ≥3 days, restart at the lowest dose and increase to current dose.

Conversion to galantamine from other cholinesterase inhibitors: Patients experiencing poor tolerability with donepezil or rivastigmine should wait until side effects subside or allow a 7-day washout period prior to beginning galantamine. Patients not experiencing side effects with donepezil or rivastigmine may begin galantamine therapy the day immediately following discontinuation of previous therapy (Morris, 2001).

Renal Impairment
Moderate renal impairment: Maximum dose: 16 mg/day.
Severe renal dysfunction (Cl_{cr} <9 mL/minute): Use is not recommended

Hepatic Impairment
Moderate liver dysfunction (Child-Pugh score 7-9): Maximum dose: 16 mg/day
Severe liver dysfunction (Child-Pugh score 10-15): Use is not recommended

Administration

Oral Administer oral solution or tablet with breakfast and dinner; administer extended release capsule with breakfast. If therapy is interrupted for ≥3 days, restart at the lowest dose and increase to current dose. If using oral solution, mix dose with 3-4 ounces of any nonalcoholic beverage; mix well and drink immediately.

Stability

Storage Store at 15°C to 30°C (59°F to 86°F). Do not freeze oral solution; protect from light.

Monitoring and Teaching Issues

Physical Assessment Assess bladder and sphincter adequacy prior to treatment. Assess other medications patient may be taking that are dependent on CYP450 metabolism. Monitor for cholinergic crisis.

Patient Education This medication will not cure Alzheimer's disease, but may help reduce symptoms. May cause dizziness, sedation, hypotension, or tremor; diarrhea; or nausea or vomiting. Report persistent GI disturbances; significantly increased salivation, sweating, or tearing; excessive fatigue, insomnia, dizziness, or depression; increased muscle, joint, or body pain or spasms; vision changes; respiratory changes, wheezing, or signs of dyspnea; chest pain or palpitations; or other adverse reactions.

Dietary Considerations Administration with food is preferred, but not required; should be taken with breakfast and dinner (tablet or solution) or with breakfast (capsule).

Geriatric Considerations No dosage adjustment needed.

Pregnancy Considerations In animal studies, there was a slight increased in the incident of skeletal variations when given during organogenesis. Adequate, well-controlled studies in pregnant women do not exist. Should be used in pregnancy only if benefit outweighs potential risk to the fetus.

◆ **Galantamine Hydrobromide** *see* Galantamine *on page* 847

Gallium Nitrate (GAL ee um NYE trate)

U.S. Brand Names Ganite™

Index Terms NSC-15200

Generic Availability (U.S.) No

Pharmacologic Category Calcium-Lowering Agent

Pregnancy Risk Factor C

Lactation Excretion in breast milk unknown/not recommended

Use Treatment of symptomatic cancer-related hypercalcemia

Available Dosage Forms

Injection, solution [preservative free]:
Ganite™: 25 mg/mL (20 mL)

Dosing

Adult & Geriatric Note: Initiate I.V. hydration prior to treatment; maintain throughout treatment.

Hypercalcemia: I.V.: 200 mg/m^2/day for 5 days; duration may be shortened during a course if normocalcemia is achieved. If hypercalcemia is mild and with very few symptoms, 100 mg/m^2/day may be used.

Renal Impairment

Serum creatinine >2.5 mg/dL: Contraindicated

Serum creatinine 2 to ≤2.5 mg/dL: No guidelines exist; frequent monitoring is recommended.

Administration

I.V. The manufacturer recommends continuous I.V. infusion over 24 hours.

Monitoring and Teaching Issues

Laboratory Monitoring Renal function (BUN, serum creatinine); serum calcium (baseline, then daily); serum phosphorus (baseline, then twice weekly)

Physical Assessment Use with caution in presence of renal impairment. Assess renal function and calcium levels. Monitor for hypotension, tachycardia, gastrointestinal upset, central nervous system changes, hypocalcemia, and renal impairment on a regular basis throughout therapy.

Patient Education This medication is given only by intravenous infusion: Report immediately any redness, swelling, or pain at infusion site. Inform prescriber if you experience persistent nausea or vomiting, rash, or are unable to pass urine.

- **GamaSTAN™ S/D** *see* Immune Globulin *on page 961*
- **Gamma Benzene Hexachloride** *see* Lindane *on page 1110*
- **Gammagard® Liquid** *see* Immune Globulin *on page 961*
- **Gammagard S/D®** *see* Immune Globulin *on page 961*
- **Gamma Globulin** *see* Immune Globulin *on page 961*
- **Gammaplex®** *see* Immune Globulin *on page 961*
- **Gamunex®** *see* Immune Globulin *on page 961*
- **Gamunex®-C** *see* Immune Globulin *on page 961*

Ganciclovir (Systemic) (gan SYE kloe veer)

U.S. Brand Names Cytovene®-IV

Index Terms DHPG Sodium; GCV Sodium; Nordeoxyguanosine

Generic Availability (U.S.) Yes

Pharmacologic Category Antiviral Agent

Medication Safety Issues

Sound-alike/look-alike issues:

Cytovene® may be confused with Cytosar®, Cytosar-U®

Ganciclovir may be confused with acyclovir

Pregnancy Risk Factor C

Lactation Excretion in breast milk unknown/not recommended

Use Treatment of CMV retinitis in immunocompromised individuals, including patients with acquired immunodeficiency syndrome; prophylaxis of CMV infection in transplant patients

Unlabeled/Investigational Use CMV retinitis: May be given in combination with foscarnet in patients who relapse after monotherapy with either drug

Mechanism of Action/Effect Ganciclovir is phosphorylated to a substrate which competitively inhibits the binding of deoxyguanosine triphosphate to DNA polymerase resulting in inhibition of viral DNA synthesis.

Contraindications Hypersensitivity to ganciclovir, acyclovir, or any component of the formulation

Warnings/Precautions Hazardous agent - use appropriate precautions for handling and disposal. **[U.S. Boxed Warning]: Granulocytopenia (neutropenia), anemia, and thrombocytopenia may occur.** Dosage adjustment or interruption of ganciclovir therapy may be necessary in patients with neutropenia and/or thrombocytopenia and patients with impaired renal function. **[U.S. Boxed Warning]: Animal studies have demonstrated carcinogenic and teratogenic effects, and inhibition of spermatogenesis;** contraceptive precautions for female and male patients need to be followed during and for at least 90 days after therapy with the drug; take care to administer only into veins with good blood flow. **[U.S. Boxed Warning]: Indicated only for treatment of CMV retinitis in the immunocompromised patient and CMV prevention in transplant patients at risk.**

Drug Interactions

Avoid Concomitant Use

Avoid concomitant use of Ganciclovir (Systemic) with any of the following: Imipenem

Decreased Effect There are no known significant interactions involving a decrease in effect.

Increased Effect/Toxicity

Ganciclovir (Systemic) may increase the levels/effects of: Imipenem; Mycophenolate; Reverse Transcriptase Inhibitors (Nucleoside); Tenofovir

The levels/effects of Ganciclovir (Systemic) may be increased by: Mycophenolate; Probenecid; Tenofovir

Adverse Reactions

>10%:

Central nervous system: Fever (48%)
Gastrointestinal: Diarrhea (44%), anorexia (14%), vomiting (13%)
Hematologic: Thrombocytopenia (57%), leukopenia (41%), anemia (16% to 26%), neutropenia with ANC <500/mm^3 (12% to 14%)
Ocular: Retinal detachment (11%; relationship to ganciclovir not established)
Renal: Serum creatinine increased (2% to 14%)
Miscellaneous: Sepsis (15%), diaphoresis (12%)

1% to 10%:

Central nervous system: Chills (10%), neuropathy (9%)
Dermatologic: Pruritus (5%)

<1%, postmarketing, and/or case reports (limited to important or life-threatening): Allergic reaction (including anaphylaxis), alopecia, arrhythmia, bronchospasm, cardiac arrest, cataracts, cholestasis, coma, dyspnea, edema, encephalopathy, exfoliative dermatitis, extrapyramidal symptoms, hepatitis, hepatic failure, pancreatitis, pancytopenia, pulmonary fibrosis, psychosis, rhabdomyolysis, seizure, alopecia, urticaria, eosinophilia, hemorrhage, Stevens-Johnson syndrome, torsade de pointes, renal failure, SIADH, visual loss

Pharmacodynamics/Kinetics

Protein Binding 1% to 2%

Half-Life Elimination 1.7-5.8 hours; prolonged with renal impairment; End-stage renal disease: 5-28 hours

Excretion Urine (80% to 99% as unchanged drug)

Available Dosage Forms

Injection, powder for reconstitution: 500 mg
Cytovene®-IV: 500 mg

Dosing

Adult

CMV retinitis: *I.V. (slow infusion):*

Induction therapy: 5 mg/kg/dose every 12 hours for 14-21 days followed by maintenance therapy

Maintenance therapy: 5 mg/kg/day as a single daily dose for 7 days/week or 6 mg/kg/day for 5 days/week

Prevention of CMV disease in transplant patients: *I.V. (slow infusion):* Same initial and maintenance dose as CMV retinitis except duration of initial course is 7-14 days, duration of maintenance therapy is dependent on clinical condition and degree of immunosuppression

Geriatric Refer to adult dosing. In general, dose selection should be cautious, reflecting greater frequency of organ impairment.

Pediatric

CMV CNS infection in HIV-exposed/-infected patients (unlabeled use; CDC, 2009): I.V.: Infants and Children: 5 mg/kg/dose every 12 hours plus foscarnet until symptoms improve followed by chronic suppression

CMV retinitis: *I.V. (slow infusion):* Refer to adult dosing.

Prevention of CMV disease in HIV-exposed/-infected patients (unlabeled use; CDC, 2009): I.V.: Infants and Children: 5 mg/kg/dose daily

Prevention of CMV disease in transplant patients: *I.V. (slow infusion):* Refer to adult dosing.

Varicella zoster: Progressive outer retinal necrosis in HIV-exposed/-infected patients (unlabeled use; CDC, 2009): Infants and Children: I.V.: 5 mg/kg/dose every 12 hours plus systemic foscarnet and intravitreal ganciclovir or intravitreal foscarnet

Renal Impairment

I.V. (Induction):

Cl_{cr} 50-69 mL/minute: Administer 2.5 mg/kg/dose every 12 hours.
Cl_{cr} 25-49 mL/minute: Administer 2.5 mg/kg/dose every 24 hours.
Cl_{cr} 10-24 mL/minute: Administer 1.25 mg/kg/dose every 24 hours.
Cl_{cr} <10 mL/minute: Administer 1.25 mg/kg/dose 3 times/week following hemodialysis.

I.V. (Maintenance):

Cl_{cr} 50-69 mL/minute: Administer 2.5 mg/kg/dose every 24 hours.
Cl_{cr} 25-49 mL/minute: Administer 1.25 mg/kg/dose every 24 hours.
Cl_{cr} 10-24 mL/minute: Administer 0.625 mg/kg/dose every 24 hours
Cl_{cr} <10 mL/minute: Administer 0.625 mg/kg/dose 3 times/week following hemodialysis.

Hemodialysis effects: Dialyzable (50%) following hemodialysis; administer dose postdialysis. During peritoneal dialysis, dose as for Cl_{cr} <10 mL/minute. During continuous arteriovenous or venovenous hemofiltration, administer 2.5 mg/kg/dose every 24 hours.

Administration

I.V. Should not be administered by I.M., SubQ, or rapid IVP. Administer by slow I.V. infusion over at least 1 hour. Too rapid infusion can cause increased toxicity and excessive plasma levels.

Stability

Reconstitution Reconstitute powder with unpreserved sterile water not bacteriostatic water because parabens may cause precipitation. Dilute in 250-1000 mL D_5W or NS to a concentration ≤10 mg/mL for infusion.

Storage Intact vials should be stored at room temperature and protected from temperatures >40°C. Reconstituted solution is stable for 12 hours at room temperature, however, conflicting data indicates that reconstituted solution is stable for 60 days under refrigeration (4°C). Stability of parenteral admixture at room temperature (25°C) and at refrigeration temperature (4°C) is 5 days.

Monitoring and Teaching Issues

Laboratory Monitoring CBC with differential and platelet count, serum creatinine

Physical Assessment I.V.: Monitor for paresthesia, neutropenia, anemia, and nephrotoxicity throughout therapy. Teach patient importance of contraceptive precautions during and for 90 days following therapy.

Patient Education Ganciclovir is not a cure for CMV retinitis. You will need frequent blood tests and regular ophthalmic exams while taking this drug. You may experience increased susceptibility to infection. You may experience confusion, headache, nausea, vomiting, anorexia, diarrhea, or photosensitivity. Report rash, infection (fever, chills, unusual bleeding or bruising, or unhealed sores or white plaques in mouth); abdominal pain; tingling, weakness, or pain in extremities; or pain, redness, or swelling at injection site.

Dietary Considerations Some products may contain sodium.

Geriatric Considerations Adjust dose based upon renal function.

Breast-Feeding Considerations Due to the carcinogenic and teratogenic effects observed in animal studies, the possibility of adverse events in a nursing infant is considered likely. Therefore, nursing should be discontinued during therapy. In addition, the CDC recommends **not** to breast-feed if diagnosed with HIV to avoid postnatal transmission of the virus.

Pregnancy Considerations [U.S. Boxed Warning]: Animal studies have demonstrated carcinogenic and teratogenic effects, and inhibition of spermatogenesis. Female patients should use effective contraception during therapy; male patients should use a barrier contraceptive during and for at least 90 days after therapy.

◆ **Ganidin® NR [OTC] [DSC]** *see* GuaiFENesin *on page 890*

Ganirelix (ga ni REL ix)

Index Terms Antagon; Ganirelix Acetate

Generic Availability (U.S.) No

Pharmacologic Category Gonadotropin Releasing Hormone Antagonist

Medication Safety Issues

International issues:

Antagon® (former U.S. brand name for ganirelix): Brand name for astemizole in Mexico; brand name for ranitidine in Brazil

Pregnancy Risk Factor X

Lactation Excretion in breast milk unknown/not recommended

Use Inhibits premature luteinizing hormone (LH) surges in women undergoing controlled ovarian hyperstimulation

Mechanism of Action/Effect Suppresses gonadotropin secretion and luteinizing hormone secretion to prevent ovulation until the follicles are of adequate size.

Contraindications Hypersensitivity to ganirelix or any component of the formulation; hypersensitivity to gonadotropin-releasing hormone (GnRH) or any other GnRH analog; known or suspected pregnancy

Warnings/Precautions Should only be prescribed by fertility specialists. Hypersensitivity reactions, including anaphylactoid reactions, have been reported; may occur with the first dose. The packaging contains natural rubber latex (may cause allergic reactions). Pregnancy must be excluded before starting medication.

Drug Interactions

Avoid Concomitant Use There are no known interactions where it is recommended to avoid concomitant use.

Decreased Effect There are no known significant interactions involving a decrease in effect.

Increased Effect/Toxicity There are no known significant interactions involving an increase in effect.

Adverse Reactions 1% to 10%:

Central nervous system: Headache (3%)

Endocrine & metabolic: Ovarian hyperstimulation syndrome (2%)

Gastrointestinal: Abdominal pain (1%), nausea (1%)

Genitourinary: Pelvic pain (5%), vaginal bleeding (2%)

Local: Injection site reaction (1%)

Pharmacodynamics/Kinetics

Duration of Action <48 hours

Absorption SubQ: Rapid

Bioavailability SubQ: 91.1%

Time to Peak 1.1 hours

Protein Binding 81.9%

Half-Life Elimination Single dose: 12.8 hours; Multiple dosing: 16.2 hours

Metabolism Hepatic to two primary metabolites (1-4 and 1-6 peptide)

Excretion Feces (75%) within 288 hours; urine (22%) within 24 hours

Available Dosage Forms

Injection, solution: 250 mcg/0.5 mL (0.5 mL)

Dosing

Adult & Geriatric Adjunct to controlled ovarian hyperstimulation: SubQ: 250 mcg/day during the mid-to-late phase after initiating follicle-stimulating hormone on day 2 or 3 of cycle. Treatment should be continued daily until the day of chorionic gonadotropin administration.

Administration

Other Administer SubQ in abdomen (around upper navel) or upper thigh; rotate injection site.

Stability

Storage Store at controlled room temperature of 25°C (77°F); excursions permitted to 15°C to 30°C (59°F to 86°F). Protect from light.

Monitoring and Teaching Issues

Laboratory Monitoring Ultrasound to assess follicle size

Physical Assessment Teach patient proper injection procedures and syringe disposal.

Patient Education This drug can only be given by injection. You must keep all scheduled ultrasound appointments. You may experience headache or nausea. Report immediately any sudden or acute abdominal pain; vaginal bleeding; or pain, itching, or signs of infection at injection site.

Pregnancy Considerations Fetal resorption occurred in pregnant rats and rabbits. These effects are results of hormonal alterations and could result in fetal loss in humans. The drug should not be used in pregnant women.

- **Ganirelix Acetate** *see* Ganirelix *on page* 851
- **Ganite™** *see* Gallium Nitrate *on page* 848
- **Gani-Tuss® NR** *see* Guaifenesin and Codeine *on page* 891
- **GAR-936** *see* Tigecycline *on page* 1761
- **Garamycin™** *see* Gentamicin (Ophthalmic) *on page* 868
- **Gardasil®** *see* Papillomavirus (Types 6, 11, 16, 18) Vaccine (Human, Recombinant) *on page* 1408
- **Gastrocrom®** *see* Cromolyn (Systemic, Oral Inhalation) *on page* 429

Gatifloxacin (gat i FLOKS a sin)

U.S. Brand Names Zymar® [DSC]; Zymaxid™

Generic Availability (U.S.) No

Pharmacologic Category Antibiotic, Ophthalmic; Antibiotic, Quinolone

Pregnancy Risk Factor C

Lactation Excretion in breast milk unknown/use caution

Use Treatment of bacterial conjunctivitis

Mechanism of Action/Effect Inhibits bacterial DNA

Contraindications

Zymar®: Hypersensitivity to gatifloxacin, other quinolone antibiotics, or any component of the formulation

Zymaxid™: There are no contraindications listed in the manufacturer's labeling.

Warnings/Precautions Severe hypersensitivity reactions, including anaphylaxis, have occurred with systemic quinolone therapy. Reactions may present as typical allergic symptoms after a single dose, or may manifest as severe idiosyncratic dermatologic, vascular, pulmonary, renal, hepatic, and/or hematologic events, usually after multiple doses. Prompt discontinuation of drug should occur if skin rash or other symptoms arise. Prolonged use may result in fungal or bacterial superinfection. For topical ophthalmic use only. Do not inject ophthalmic solution subconjunctivally or introduce directly into the anterior chamber of the eye. Contact lenses should not be worn during treatment of ophthalmic infections.

Drug Interactions

Avoid Concomitant Use There are no known interactions where it is recommended to avoid concomitant use.

Decreased Effect There are no known significant interactions involving a decrease in effect.

Increased Effect/Toxicity There are no known significant interactions involving an increase in effect.

Lab Interactions Some quinolones may produce a false-positive urine screening result for opiates using commercially-available immunoassay kits. This has been demonstrated most consistently for levofloxacin and ofloxacin, but other quinolones have shown cross-reactivity in certain assay kits. Confirmation of positive opiate screens by more specific methods should be considered.

Adverse Reactions 1% to 10%:

Central nervous system: Headache

Gastrointestinal: Taste disturbance

Ocular: Chemosis, conjunctival hemorrhage, conjunctival irritation, discharge, dry eye, edema, irritation, keratitis, lacrimation increased, pain, papillary conjunctivitis, visual acuity decreased

Available Dosage Forms

Solution, ophthalmic:

Zymaxid™: 0.5% (2.5 mL)

Dosing

Adult & Geriatric Bacterial conjunctivitis: Ophthalmic:

Zymar®:

Days 1 and 2: Instill 1 drop into affected eye(s) every 2 hours while awake (maximum: 8 times/day)

Days 3-7: Instill 1 drop into affected eye(s) up to 4 times/day while awake

Zymaxid™:

Day 1: Instill 1 drop into affected eye(s) every 2 hours while awake (maximum: 8 times/day)

Days 2-7: Instill 1 drop into affected eye(s) 2-4 times/day while awake

Pediatric Bacterial conjunctivitis: Children ≥1 year: Ophthalmic: Refer to adult dosing.

Administration

Other For topical ophthalmic use only; avoid touching tip of applicator to eye, fingers, or other surfaces.

Stability

Storage Store between 15°C to 25°C (59°F to 77°F); do not freeze.

Monitoring and Teaching Issues

Patient Education Tilt head back and instill prescribed number of drops in affected eye as often as directed for length of time prescribed. Do not allow dropper to touch any surface, including the eyes or hands. Apply light pressure to the inside corner of the eye (near the nose) after each drop. Avoid wearing contact lenses during treatment. May cause headache or dizziness. May cause temporary eye discomfort (stinging, burning, itching, pain, tearing) or a bad taste in mouth after instillation. Report persistent adverse reactions, visual disturbances, or if condition worsens. If you experience signs of allergic reaction (eg, itching, rash, respiratory difficulty, facial edema, difficulty swallowing), discontinue use immediately and report to prescriber.

Geriatric Considerations Evaluate the patient's ability to self-administer the ophthalmic product.

Breast-Feeding Considerations Other quinolones are known to be excreted in breast milk. The manufacturer recommends using caution if gatifloxacin is administered while nursing.

Pregnancy Considerations Gatifloxacin has been show to be fetotoxic in animal studies. Quinolone exposure during human pregnancy has been reported with other agents (refer to Ciprofloxacin (Systemic) monograph). Following ophthalmic administration, serum concentrations of gatifloxacin are below the limits of quantification (<5 ng/mL). Systemic absorption would be required in order for gatifloxacin to cross the placenta.

Related Information

Antimicrobial Drugs of Choice *on page 2008*

Community-Acquired Pneumonia in Adults *on page 2021*

I.V. to Oral Conversion *on page 1956*

◆ **GaviLyte™-C** *see* Polyethylene Glycol-Electrolyte Solution *on page 1474*

◆ **GaviLyte™-G** *see* Polyethylene Glycol-Electrolyte Solution *on page 1474*

◆ **GaviLyte™-N** *see* Polyethylene Glycol-Electrolyte Solution *on page 1474*

◆ **G-CSF** *see* Filgrastim *on page 760*

◆ **GCV Sodium** *see* Ganciclovir (Systemic) *on page 849*

Gefitinib (ge FI tye nib)

U.S. Brand Names Iressa®

Index Terms ZD1839

Generic Availability (U.S.) No

Pharmacologic Category Antineoplastic Agent, Tyrosine Kinase Inhibitor

Medication Safety Issues

Sound-alike/look-alike issues:

Gefitinib may be confused with erlotinib, imatinib, SORAfenib, SUNItinib, vandetanib

High alert medication: This medication is in a class the Institute for Safe Medication Practices (ISMP) includes among its list of drug classes which have a heightened risk of causing significant patient harm when used in error.

Prescribing and Access Restrictions As of September 15, 2005, distribution of gefitinib (IRESSA®) is limited to patients enrolled in the IRESSA® Access Program. Under this program, access to gefitinib will be limited to the following groups:

Patients who are currently receiving and benefiting from gefitinib

Patients who have previously received and benefited from gefitinib

Previously-enrolled patients or new patients in non-Investigational New Drug (IND) clinical trials involving gefitinib if these protocols were approved by an IRB prior to June 17, 2005

New patients may also receive gefitinib if the manufacturer (AstraZeneca) decides to make it available under IND, and the patients meet the criteria for enrollment under the IND

Additional information on the IRESSA® Access Program, including enrollment forms, may be obtained by calling AstraZeneca at 1-800-601-8933 or via the web at www.Iressa-access.com

Pregnancy Risk Factor D

Lactation Excretion in breast milk unknown/not recommended

Use Treatment of locally advanced or metastatic nonsmall cell lung cancer (NSCLC) after failure of platinum-based and docetaxel therapies. Treatment is limited to patients who are benefiting or have benefited from treatment with gefitinib.

Note: Due to the lack of improved survival data from clinical trials of gefitinib, and in response to positive survival data with another EGFR inhibitor, according to the U.S. labeling, physicians are advised to use treatment options other than gefitinib in patients with advanced nonsmall cell lung cancer following one or two prior chemotherapy regimens when they are refractory/intolerant to their most recent regimen.

Canada labeling: First-line treatment of locally advanced or metastatic NSCLC with activating mutations of EGFR-TK

Unlabeled/Investigational Use First-line treatment of NSCLC with known EGFR mutation

Mechanism of Action/Effect Gefitinib inhibits tyrosine kinase activity, particularly in the epidermal growth factor receptor (EGFR), resulting in inhibition of cell growth and reproduction.

Contraindications Hypersensitivity to gefitinib or any component of the formulation

Warnings/Precautions Hazardous agent - use appropriate precautions for handling and disposal. Rare, sometimes fatal, pulmonary toxicity, including interstitial lung disease (ILD) (eg, alveolitis, interstitial pneumonia, pneumonitis) has occurred. ILD has occurred in patients with prior radiation therapy, prior chemotherapy, and less commonly in treatment naïve patients. Therapy should be interrupted in patients with acute onset or worsening pulmonary symptoms (dyspnea, cough, fever); discontinue if interstitial pneumonitis is confirmed. An increase in mortality was observed in patients with concurrent idiopathic pulmonary fibrosis. Asymptomatic increases in transaminases have been reported; monitor liver function periodically and discontinue if elevations/changes are severe. Gefitinib exposure may be increased in patients with hepatic impairment. Interruption of therapy may be required in patients with poorly tolerated diarrhea or adverse skin reactions. Eye irritation should be promptly evaluated and therapy may be interrupted based on appropriate medical evaluation; may be reinitiated following resolution of symptoms or eye changes.

EGFR mutations, specifically exon 19 deletions and exon 21 mutation (L858R), are associated with better response to gefitinib in patients with NSCLC (Riely, 2006). There is a high potential for CYP3A4 mediated interactions with gefitinib. Concurrent use with CYP3A4 inducers may decrease gefitinib levels; consider increased gefitinib doses (to 500 mg) with close monitoring if concurrent use with inducers cannot be avoided. CYP3A4 inhibitors may increase gefitinib levels, use caution with concurrent administration.

Drug Interactions

Metabolism/Transport Effects Substrate of CYP3A4 (major); **Inhibits** CYP2C19 (weak), CYP2D6 (weak), ABCG2

Avoid Concomitant Use

Avoid concomitant use of Gefitinib with any of the following: BCG; Natalizumab; Pimecrolimus; Roflumilast; Tacrolimus (Topical); Vaccines (Live)

Decreased Effect

Gefitinib may decrease the levels/effects of: BCG; Cardiac Glycosides; Sipuleucel-T; Vaccines (Inactivated); Vaccines (Live); Vitamin K Antagonists

The levels/effects of Gefitinib may be decreased by: CYP3A4 Inducers (Strong); Deferasirox; Echinacea; H2-Antagonists; Herbs (CYP3A4 Inducers); Peginterferon Alfa-2b; Proton Pump Inhibitors; Rifamycin Derivatives

Increased Effect/Toxicity

Gefitinib may increase the levels/effects of: Leflunomide; Natalizumab; Topotecan; Vaccines (Live); Vinorelbine; Vitamin K Antagonists

The levels/effects of Gefitinib may be increased by: Antifungal Agents (Azole Derivatives, Systemic); Conivaptan; CYP2D6 Inhibitors (Moderate); CYP2D6 Inhibitors (Strong); CYP3A4 Inhibitors (Moderate); CYP3A4 Inhibitors (Strong); Darunavir; Dasatinib; Denosumab; Pimecrolimus; Roflumilast; Tacrolimus (Topical); Trastuzumab

Nutritional/Ethanol Interactions

Food: Grapefruit juice may increase serum gefitinib concentrations.

Herb/Nutraceutical: St John's wort may decrease serum gefitinib concentrations.

Adverse Reactions

>10%:

Dermatologic: Rash (43% to 54%), acne (25% to 33%), dry skin (13% to 26%), paronychia (14%)

Gastrointestinal: Diarrhea (48% to 67%; grade 3: 1%), nausea (13% to 18%), vomiting (9% to 12%)

1% to 10%:

Cardiovascular: Peripheral edema (2%)

Dermatologic: Pruritus (8% to 9%)

Gastrointestinal: Anorexia (7% to 10%), weight loss (3% to 5%), mouth ulceration (1%)

Neuromuscular & skeletal: Weakness (4% to 6%)

Ocular: Amblyopia (2%), conjunctivitis (1%)

Respiratory: Dyspnea (2%), interstitial lung disease (1% to 2%; includes alveolitis, interstitial pneumonia, pneumonitis)

Pharmacodynamics/Kinetics

Absorption Oral: Slow

Bioavailability 60%

Time to Peak Plasma: Oral: 3-7 hours

Protein Binding 90%, albumin and alpha$_1$-acid glycoprotein

Half-Life Elimination Oral: 41 hours

Metabolism Hepatic, primarily via CYP3A4; forms metabolites

Excretion Feces (86%); urine (<4%)

Available Dosage Forms

Tablet, oral:

Iressa®: 250 mg

Dosing

Adult

Nonsmall cell lung cancer (NSCLC): Oral: 250 mg once daily

NSCLC, first-line therapy in patients with EGFR mutations (unlabeled use): Oral: 250 mg once daily (Maemondo, 2010; Mok, 2009; Sequist, 2008)

Dosage adjustment for concomitant CYP3A4 inducers (eg, phenytoin, rifampin): Consider increasing gefitinib dose to 500 mg once daily with close monitoring

Geriatric No adjustment necessary. Refer to adult dosing.

Renal Impairment No adjustment necessary.

Hepatic Impairment

Moderate-to-severe impairment due to metastases: No adjustment necessary.

Hepatotoxicity during treatment (elevations in transaminases): Discontinue if severe.

Adjustment for Toxicity

Worsening pulmonary symptoms (cough dyspnea, fever): Interrupt treatment and evaluate promptly; discontinue if interstitial lung disease is confirmed.

Diarrhea (poorly tolerated or associated with dehydration) or skin toxicity: Interrupt treatment for up to 14 days; may reinitiate at 250 mg once daily.

Ocular symptoms (eye pain): Evaluate and interrupt treatment based on symptoms; once symptoms or eye changes have resolved, may consider reinitiating at 250 mg once daily.

Administration

Oral May administer with or without food.

For patients unable to swallow tablets or for administration via NG tube: Tablets may be dispersed in noncarbonated drinking water. Drop whole tablet (do not crush) into 1/2 glass of water; stir until tablet is dispersed (~10 minutes). Drink immediately. Rinse glass with 1/2 glass of water and drink.

Stability

Storage Store tablets at controlled room temperature of 20°C to 25°C (68°F to 77°F). Protect from light and moisture.

Monitoring and Teaching Issues

Laboratory Monitoring Periodic liver function tests (ALT, AST, bilirubin and alkaline phosphatase), INR or prothrombin time (with concurrently warfarin treatment)

Physical Assessment Assess results of liver function tests on a regular basis.

Patient Education Take with or without food. Do not take with grapefruit juice. You will need periodic laboratory tests while taking this medication. Maintain adequate hydration, unless instructed to restrict fluid intake. You may experience loss of appetite, nausea, vomiting, or diarrhea. Report immediately persistent diarrhea; skin rash; unusual or persistent respiratory difficulty or wheezing; chest pain or cough; any change in vision, eye pain, or signs of eye infection; unusual weakness; or joint pain.

Dietary Considerations Food does not affect gefitinib absorption.

Breast-Feeding Considerations Due to the potential for serious adverse reactions in the nursing infant, breast-feeding is not recommended.

Pregnancy Considerations Animal studies have demonstrated fetal harm; there are no well-controlled studies in pregnant women. The risk of fetal harm should be carefully weighed. Women of childbearing potential should be advised to avoid pregnancy.

Additional Information Oncology Comment: Recent studies have demonstrated a subset of patients who are more likely to respond to treatment with gefitinib. This subset includes: patients of Asian origin, never-smokers, women, patients with bronchoalveolar adenocarcinoma, and patients with EGFR-mutated tumors. Deletion in exon 19 and mutation in exon 21 are the two most commonly found EGFR mutations; both mutations correlate with clinical response, resulting in increased response rates in patients with the mutation (Riely, 2006). Studies have compared gefitinib in treatment naïve patients to combination chemotherapy in the subsets of patients described above, resulting in a longer progression free survival in the gefitinib arm (Mok, 2009). Based on these data, the 2009 ASCO guidelines recommend the first-line use of gefitinib in stage IV with the known EGFR mutation (Azzoli, 2009). The NCCN guidelines recommend erlotinib as first-line therapy for EGFR mutation positive patients with stage IV NSCLC, and also states that gefitinib could be used in place of erlotinib in areas of the world where available. In patients with a kras mutation, however, EGFR-TKI therapy is not recommended.

◆ **Gelnique™** *see* Oxybutynin *on page 1378*

Gemcitabine (jem SITE a been)

U.S. Brand Names Gemzar®

Index Terms dFdC; dFdCyd; Difluorodeoxycytidine Hydrochlorothiazide; Gemcitabine Hydrochloride; LY-188011

Generic Availability (U.S.) Yes

Pharmacologic Category Antineoplastic Agent, Antimetabolite (Pyrimidine Analog)

Medication Safety Issues

Sound-alike/look-alike issues:

Gemcitabine may be confused with gemtuzumab

Gemzar® may be confused with Zinecard®

High alert medication: This medication is in a class the Institute for Safe Medication Practices (ISMP) includes among its list of drug classes which have a heightened risk of causing significant patient harm when used in error.

Pregnancy Risk Factor D

Lactation Excretion in breast milk unknown/not recommended

Use Treatment of metastatic breast cancer; inoperable locally-advanced or metastatic nonsmall cell lung cancer (NSCLC); locally advanced or metastatic pancreatic cancer; advanced, relapsed ovarian cancer

Unlabeled/Investigational Use Treatment of biliary tract cancers (advanced), bladder cancer, cervical cancer (recurrent or persistent), Ewing's sarcoma (refractory), head and neck cancer (nasopharyngeal), Hodgkin's lymphoma (relapsed), non-Hodgkin's lymphomas (refractory), malignant pleural mesothelioma, osteosarcoma (refractory), renal cell cancer (metastatic), small cell lung cancer (refractory or relapsed), soft tissue sarcoma (advanced), testicular cancer (refractory germ cell tumors), thymic malignancies, uterine sarcoma, and unknown-primary adenocarcinoma

Mechanism of Action/Effect A pyrimidine antimetabolite that inhibits DNA synthesis by inhibition of DNA polymerase and ribonucleotide reductase, specific for the S-phase of the cycle.

Contraindications Hypersensitivity to gemcitabine or any component of the formulation

Warnings/Precautions Hazardous agent - use appropriate precautions for handling and disposal. Prolongation of the infusion time >60 minutes and more frequent than weekly dosing have been shown to increase toxicity. Gemcitabine can suppress bone marrow function (leukopenia, thrombocytopenia, and anemia); myelosuppression is usually the dose-limiting toxicity. Gemcitabine may cause fever in the absence of clinical infection. Pulmonary toxicity has occurred; discontinue if severe and institute supportive measures.

Hemolytic uremic syndrome has been reported; monitor for evidence of microangiopathic hemolysis (elevation of bilirubin or LDH, reticulocytosis, severe thrombocytopenia, and/or renal failure); use with caution in patients with pre-existing renal impairment. Serious hepatotoxicity (including liver failure and death) has been reported when used in combination with other chemotherapy. Use with caution in patients with hepatic impairment (history of cirrhosis, hepatitis, or alcoholism) or in patients with hepatic metastases; may lead to exacerbation of hepatic impairment; dose adjustments may be recommended with elevated bilirubin. Use caution with concurrent radiation therapy; radiation toxicity has been reported with concurrent and nonconcurrent administration; may have radiosensitizing activity when gemcitabine and radiation therapy are given ≤7 days apart; optimum regimen for combination therapy has not been determined for all tumor types. Use caution in the elderly; clearance is affected by age.

Drug Interactions

Avoid Concomitant Use

Avoid concomitant use of Gemcitabine with any of the following: BCG; Natalizumab; Pimecrolimus; Roflumilast; Tacrolimus (Topical); Vaccines (Live)

Decreased Effect

Gemcitabine may decrease the levels/effects of: BCG; Sipuleucel-T; Vaccines (Inactivated); Vaccines (Live); Vitamin K Antagonists

The levels/effects of Gemcitabine may be decreased by: Echinacea

Increased Effect/Toxicity

Gemcitabine may increase the levels/effects of: Bleomycin; Fluorouracil; Fluorouracil (Systemic); Fluorouracil (Topical); Leflunomide; Natalizumab; Vaccines (Live); Vitamin K Antagonists

The levels/effects of Gemcitabine may be increased by: Denosumab; Pimecrolimus; Roflumilast; Tacrolimus (Topical); Trastuzumab

Nutritional/Ethanol Interactions Ethanol: Avoid ethanol (due to GI irritation).

Adverse Reactions Frequency of adverse reactions reported for single-agent use of gemcitabine only.

>10%:

Cardiovascular: Peripheral edema (20%), edema (13%)

Central nervous system: Fever (38% to 41%), somnolence (11%)

Dermatologic: Rash (28% to 30%), alopecia (15% to 16%), pruritus (13%)

Gastrointestinal: Nausea/vomiting (69% to 71%; grade 3: 10% to 13%; grade 4: 1% to 2%), diarrhea (19% to 30%), stomatitis (10% to 11%)

Hematologic: Anemia (68% to 73%; grade 4: 1% to 2%), leukopenia (62% to 64%; grade 4: ≤1%), neutropenia (61% to 63%; grade 4: 6% to 7%), thrombocytopenia (24% to 36%; grade 4: ≤1%), hemorrhage (4% to 17%; grades 3: ≤2%; grade 4: <1%); myelosuppression is the dose-limiting toxicity

Hepatic: AST increased (67% to 78%; grade 3: 6% to 12%; grade 4: 2% to 5%), alkaline phosphatase increased (55% to 77%; grade 3: 7% to 16%; grade 4: 2% to 4%), ALT increased (68% to 72%; grade 3: 8% to 10%; grade 4: 1% to 2%), bilirubin increased (13% to 26%; grade 3: 2% to 6%; grade 4: ≤2%)

Renal: (32% to 45%; grades 3/4: <1%), hematuria (23% to 35%; grades 3/4: <1%), BUN increased (15% to 16%)

Respiratory: Dyspnea (10% to 23%)

Miscellaneous: Flu-like syndrome (19%), infection (10% to 16%; grade 3: 1% to 2%; grade 4: <1%)

1% to 10%:

Local: Injection site reactions (4%)

Neuromuscular & skeletal: Paresthesia (10%)

Renal: Creatinine increased (6% to 8%)

Respiratory: Bronchospasm (<2%)

Pharmacodynamics/Kinetics

Time to Peak 30 minutes after completion of infusion

Protein Binding Low

Half-Life Elimination

Gemcitabine: Infusion time ≤70 minutes: 42-94 minutes; infusion time 3-4 hours: 4-10.5 hours

Metabolite (gemcitabine triphosphate), terminal phase: 1.7-19.4 hours

Metabolism Metabolized intracellularly by nucleoside kinases to the active diphosphate (dFdCDP) and triphosphate (dFdCTP) nucleoside metabolites

Excretion Urine (92% to 98%; primarily as inactive uracil metabolite); feces (<1%)

Available Dosage Forms

Injection, powder for reconstitution: 200 mg, 1 g, 2 g

Gemzar®: 200 mg, 1 g

Dosing

Adult & Geriatric Details concerning dosing in combination regimens should also be consulted. **Note**: Prolongation of the infusion time >60 minutes and administration more frequently than once weekly have been shown to increase toxicity.

Pancreatic cancer, locally advanced or metastatic: I.V.: Initial: 1000 mg/m^2 weekly for up to 7 weeks followed by 1 week rest; then weekly for 3 weeks out of every 4 weeks

Dose adjustment: Patients who complete an entire cycle of therapy may have the dose in subsequent cycles increased by 25% as long as the absolute granulocyte count (AGC) nadir is >1500 x 10^6/L, platelet nadir is >100,000 x 10^6/L, and nonhematologic toxicity is less than WHO Grade 1. If the increased dose is tolerated (with the same parameters) the dose in subsequent cycles may again be increased by 20%.

Pancreatic cancer, advanced (unlabeled dosing/combinations): I.V.: 1000 mg/m^2 weekly for up to 7 weeks followed by 1 week rest; then weekly for 3 weeks out of every 4 weeks (in combination with erlotinib) (Moore, 2007) **or** 1000 mg/m^2 days 1, 8, and 15 every 4 weeks (in combination with capecitabine) (Cunningham, 2009) **or** 1000 mg/m^2 days 1 and 15 every 4 weeks (in combination with cisplatin) (Heinemann, 2006) **or** 1000 mg/m^2 every 2 weeks (in combination with oxaliplatin) (Louvet, 2005)

Nonsmall cell lung cancer (in combination with cisplatin): I.V.: 1000 mg/m^2 days 1, 8, and 15; repeat cycle every 28 days **or** 1250 mg/m^2 days 1 and 8; repeat cycle every 21 days

Breast cancer, metastatic: I.V.: 1250 mg/m^2 days 1 and 8; repeat cycle every 21 days in combination with paclitaxel **or** (unlabeled dosing) as a single agent: 800 mg/m^2 days 1, 8, and 15 of a 28-day treatment cycle (Carmichael, 1995)

Ovarian cancer, advanced: I.V.: 1000 mg/m^2 days 1 and 8; repeat cycle every 21 days (in combination with carboplatin)

Biliary tract cancer, advanced (unlabeled use): I.V.: 1000 mg/m^2 days 1 and 8; repeat cycle every 21 days (in combination with cisplatin) (Valle, 2010) **or** 1000 mg/m^2 days 1 and 8; repeat cycle every 21 days (in combination with capecitabine) (Knox, 2005) **or** 1000 mg/m^2 over 100 minutes every 2 weeks (in combination with oxaliplatin) (Andre, 2004)

Bladder cancer (unlabeled use):

I.V.: 1000 mg/m^2 once weekly for 3 weeks; repeat cycle every 4 weeks (in combination with cisplatin) (von der Maase, 2000)

Intravesicular instillation: 2000 mg (in 100 mL NS; retain for 1 hour) twice weekly for 3 weeks; repeat cycle every 4 weeks for at least 2 cycles (Dalbagni, 2006)

Cervical cancer, recurrent or persistent (unlabeled use): I.V.: 1000 mg/m^2 days 1 and 8; repeat cycle every 21 days (in combination with cisplatin) (Monk, 2009) **or** 1250 mg/m^2 days 1 and 8; repeat cycle every 21 days (in combination with cisplatin) (Burnett, 2000) **or** 800 mg/m^2 days 1, 8, and 15; repeat cycle every 28 days (as a single-agent) (Schilder, 2005)

Head and neck cancer, nasopharyngeal (unlabeled use): I.V.: 1000 mg/m^2 days 1, 8, and 15 every 4 weeks (Zhang, 2008)

Hodgkin's lymphoma, relapsed (unlabeled use): I.V.: 1000 mg/m^2 (800 mg/m^2 for post-transplant patients) days 1 and 8; repeat cycle every 21 days (in combination with vinorelbine and doxorubicin liposomal) (Bartlett, 2007) **or** 800 mg/m^2 days 1 and 4; repeat cycle every 21 days (in combination with ifosfamide, mesna, vinorelbine, and prednisolone) (Santoro, 2007)

Malignant pleural mesothelioma (unlabeled use; in combination with cisplatin): I.V.: 1000 mg/m^2/dose days 1, 8 and 15 every 4 weeks (Nowak, 2002) **or** 1250 mg/m^2/dose days 1 and 8 every 3 weeks (van Haarst, 2002)

Non-Hodgkin's lymphoma, refractory (unlabeled use): I.V.: 1000 mg/m^2 days 1 and 8; repeat cycle every 21 days (in combination with cisplatin and dexamethasone) (Crump, 2004) **or** 1000 mg/m^2 every 15-21days (in combination with oxaliplatin and rituximab) (Lopez, 2008)

Sarcoma (unlabeled uses): I.V.:

Ewing's sarcoma, refractory: 675 mg/m^2 days 1 and 8; repeat cycle every 21 days (in combination with docetaxel) (Navid, 2008)

Osteosarcoma, refractory: 675 mg/m^2 days 1 and 8; repeat cycle every 21 days (in combination with docetaxel) (Navid, 2008) **or** 1000 mg/m^2 weekly for 7 weeks followed by 1 week rest; then weekly for 3 weeks out of every 4 weeks (Merimsky, 2000)

Soft tissue sarcoma, advanced: I.V.: 800 mg/m^2 days 1 and 8; repeat cycle every 21 days (in combination with vinorelbine) (Dileo, 2007) **or** 675 mg/m^2 days 1 and 8; repeat cycle every 21 days (in combination with docetaxel) (Leu, 2004) **or** 900 mg/m^2 days 1 and 8; repeat cycle every 21 days (fixed dose rate infusion; in combination with docetaxel) (Maki, 2007)

Small cell lung cancer, refractory or relapsed (unlabeled use): I.V.: 1000-1250 mg/m^2 days 1, 8, and 15 every 4 weeks (as a single agent) (Masters, 2003)

Testicular cancer, refractory germ cell (unlabeled use): I.V.: 1000 mg/m^2 days 1 and 8 every 3 weeks (in combination with oxaliplatin) (Kohllmannsberger, 2004; Pectasides, 2004) **or** 1250 mg/m^2 days 1 and 8 every 3 weeks (in combination with oxaliplatin) (De Giorgi, 2006) **or** 1000 mg/m^2/dose days 1, 8 and 15 every 4 weeks (in combination with paclitaxel) (Hinton, 2002)

Unknown-primary, adenocarcinoma (unlabeled use): I.V.: 1250 mg/m^2 days 1 and 8 every 3 weeks (in combination with cisplatin) (Culine, 2003) **or** 1000 mg/m^2 days 1 and 8 every 3 weeks (in combination with docetaxel) (Pouessel, 2004)

Uterine cancer (unlabeled use): I.V.: 900 mg/m^2 days 1 and 8 every 3 weeks (in combination with docetaxel) (Hensley, 2008) **or** 1000 mg/m^2 days 1, 8, and 15 every 4 weeks (Look, 2004)

Pediatric Details concerning dosing in combination regimens should also be consulted. **Note**: Prolongation of the infusion time >60 minutes and administration more frequently than once weekly have been shown to increase toxicity. Refer to specific references for ages of populations studied):

Germ cell tumor, refractory (unlabeled use): I.V.: 1000 mg/m^2/dose days 1, 8, and 15 every 4 weeks (in combination with paclitaxel) (Hinton, 2002)

Hodgkin's lymphoma, relapsed (unlabeled use): I.V.: 1000 mg/m^2 days 1 and 8; repeat cycle every 21 days (in combination with vinorelbine) (Cole; 2009) **or** 800 mg/m^2 days 1 and 4; repeat cycle every 21 days (in combination with ifosfamide, mesna, vinorelbine, and prednisolone) (Santoro, 2007)

Sarcomas (unlabeled use): I.V.:

Ewing's sarcoma, refractory: 675 mg/m^2 days 1 and 8; repeat cycle every 21 days (in combination with docetaxel) (Navid, 2008)

Osteosarcoma, refractory: 675 mg/m^2 days 1 and 8; repeat cycle every 21 days (in combination with docetaxel) (Navid, 2008) **or** 1000 mg/m^2 weekly for 7 weeks followed by 1 week rest; then weekly for 3 weeks out of every 4 weeks (Merimsky, 2000)

Renal Impairment The FDA-approved labeling does not contain dosing adjustment guidelines; use with caution in patients with pre-existing renal dysfunction. Discontinue if severe renal toxicity or hemolytic uremic syndrome (HUS) occur during gemcitabine treatment.

Mild-to-severe renal impairment: No adjustment required (Janus, 2010; Li, 2007).

ESRD (on hemodialysis): Hemodialysis should begin 6-12 hours after gemcitabine infusion (Janus 2010; Li, 2007).

Hepatic Impairment The FDA-approved labeling does not contain dosing adjustment guidelines; use with caution. Discontinue if severe hepatotoxicity occurs during treatment with gemcitabine. The following guidelines have been used by some clinicians:

Transaminases elevated (with normal bilirubin): No adjustment required (Venook, 2000).

Serum bilirubin >1.6 mg/dL: Use initial dose of 800 mg/m^2; may escalate if tolerated (Ecklund, 2005; Floyd, 2006; Venook, 2000).

Adjustment for Toxicity

Pancreatic cancer: Hematologic toxicity:

AGC ≥1000 x 10^6/L and platelet count ≥100,000 x 10^6/L: Administer 100% of full dose

AGC 500-999 x 10^6/L or platelet count 50,000-90,000 x 10^6/L: Administer 75% of full dose

AGC <500 x 10^6/L or platelet count <50,000 x 10^6/L: Hold dose

Nonsmall cell lung cancer:

Hematologic toxicity: Refer to guidelines for pancreatic cancer. Cisplatin dosage may also need adjusted.

Severe (grades 3 or 4) nonhematologic toxicity (except alopecia, nausea, and vomiting): Hold or decrease dose by 50%.

Breast cancer:

Hematologic toxicity: Adjustments based on granulocyte and platelet counts on day 8:

AGC ≥1200 x 10^6/L and platelet count >75,000 x 10^6/L: Administer 100% of full dose

AGC 1000-1199 x 10^6/L or platelet count 50,000-75,000 x 10^6/L: Administer 75% of full dose

AGC 700-999 x 10^6/L and platelet count ≥50,000 x 10^6/L: Administer 50% of full dose

AGC <700 x 10^6/L or platelet count <50,000 x 10^6/L: Hold dose

Severe (grades 3 or 4) nonhematologic toxicity (except alopecia, nausea, and vomiting): Hold or decrease dose by 50%. Paclitaxel dose may also need adjusted.

Ovarian cancer:

Hematologic toxicity: Adjustments based on granulocyte and platelet counts on day 8:

AGC ≥1500 x 10^6/L and platelet count ≥100,000 x 10^6/L: Administer 100% of full dose

AGC 1000-1499 x 10^6/L and/or platelet count 75,000-99,999 x 10^6/L: Administer 50% of full dose

AGC <1000 x 10^6/L and/or platelet count <75,000 x 10^6/L: Hold dose

Severe (grades 3 or 4) nonhematologic toxicity (except nausea and vomiting): Hold or decrease dose by 50%. Carboplatin dose may also need adjusted.

Dose adjustment for subsequent cycles:

AGC < 500 x 10^6/L for >5 days, AGC <100 x 10^6/L for >3 days, febrile neutropenia, platelet count <25,000 x 10^6/L, cycle delay >1 week due to toxicity: Reduce gemcitabine to 800 mg/m^2 on days 1 and 8.

For recurrence of any of the above toxicities after initial dose reduction: Administer gemcitabine 800 mg/m^2 on day 1 only for the subsequent cycle

Administration

I.V. Infuse over 30 minutes. **Note**: Prolongation of the infusion time >60 minutes has been shown to increase toxicity (some unlabeled protocols may include infusion times >30 minutes). Gemcitabine is being investigated in clinical trials for fixed dose rate (FDR) infusion administration at doses from 1000-2200 mg/m^2 at a rate of 10 mg/m^2/minute. Prolonged infusion times increase the accumulation of the active metabolite, gemcitabine triphosphate. Patients who receive gemcitabine FDR experience more grade 3/4 hematologic toxicity.

Other For intravesicular (bladder) instillation, gemcitabine was diluted in 50-100 mL normal saline; patients were instructed to retain in the bladder for 1 hour (Addeo, 2010; Dalbaghi, 2006)

Stability

Reconstitution Use appropriate precautions for handling and disposal. Reconstitute with preservative free 0.9% NaCl; add 5 mL to the 200 mg vial, add 25 mL to the 1000 mg vial, or add 50 mL to the 2000 mg vial, resulting in a reconstituted concentration of 38 mg/mL (solutions must be reconstituted to ≤40 mg/mL to completely dissolve). Further dilute (for infusion) in 50-500 mL 0.9% sodium chloride injection; to concentrations as low as 0.1 mg/mL.

Storage Store intact vials at room temperature of 20°C to 25°C (68°F to 77°F); excursions permitted to 15°C to 30°C (59°F to 86°F). Reconstituted vials are stable for up to 35 days and infusion solutions diluted in 0.9% sodium chloride are stable up to 7 days at 23°C when protected from light; however, the manufacturers recommend use within 24 hours for both reconstituted vials and infusion solutions. Do not refrigerate.

Monitoring and Teaching Issues

Laboratory Monitoring CBC with differential and platelet count (prior to each dose); hepatic and renal function (prior to initiation of therapy and periodically, thereafter); monitor electrolytes, including potassium, magnesium, and calcium (when in combination therapy with cisplatin)

Physical Assessment Use caution in presence of renal or hepatic impairment. Assess CBC with differential and platelet count prior to each dose. Monitor hepatic and renal function. Monitor for fever, CNS changes, rash, gastrointestinal upset, myelosuppression, anemia, dyspnea, and infection prior to each treatment and on a regular basis.

Patient Education You will be monitored during infusion. Report immediately any pain, burning, or swelling at infusion site; sudden chest pain or palpitations; difficulty breathing or swallowing; or chills. Between infusions, maintain adequate nutrition and hydration, unless instructed to restrict fluid intake. You may be more susceptible to infection. You may experience new fatigue, lethargy, somnolence, nausea, vomiting, loss of hair (reversible), or mouth sores. Report extreme fatigue; severe GI upset, constipation, or diarrhea; unusual bleeding or bruising; fever, chills, or sore throat; vaginal discharge; signs of fluid retention (swelling of extremities, respiratory difficulty, unusual weight gain); yellowing of skin or eyes; change in color of urine or stool; or muscle or skeletal pain or weakness.

Geriatric Considerations Clearance is affected by age. There is no evidence; however, that unusual dose adjustment is necessary in patients older than 65 years of age. In general, adverse reaction rates were similar to patients older and younger than 65 years. Grade 3/4 thrombocytopenia was more common in the elderly. Older women were more likely to experience grade 3/4 neutropenia and thrombocytopenia.

Breast-Feeding Considerations Due to the potential for serious adverse reactions in nursing the infant, breast-feeding is not recommended.

Pregnancy Considerations Embryotoxicity and fetal malformations (cleft palate, incomplete ossification, fused pulmonary artery, absence of gallbladder) have been reported in animal studies. There are no adequate and well-controlled studies in pregnant women. If patient becomes pregnant, she should be informed of risks.

◆ **Gemcitabine Hydrochloride** *see* Gemcitabine *on page* 855

Gemfibrozil (jem FI broe zil)

U.S. Brand Names Lopid®

Index Terms CI-719

Generic Availability (U.S.) Yes

Pharmacologic Category Antilipemic Agent, Fibric Acid

Medication Safety Issues

Sound-alike/look-alike issues:

Lopid® may be confused with Levbid®, Lipitor®, Lodine®, Lorabid®, Slo-bid™

Pregnancy Risk Factor C

Lactation Excretion in breast milk unknown/not recommended

Use Treatment of hypertriglyceridemia in Fredrickson types IV and V hyperlipidemia for patients who are at greater risk for pancreatitis and who have not responded to dietary intervention; to reduce the risk of CHD development in Fredrickson type IIb patients without a history or symptoms of existing CHD who have not responded to dietary and other interventions (including pharmacologic treatment) and who have decreased HDL, increased LDL, and increased triglycerides

Mechanism of Action/Effect Inhibits lipolysis and decreases subsequent hepatic fatty acid uptake and hepatic secretion of VLDL; decreases serum levels of VLDL and increases HDL levels

Contraindications Hypersensitivity to gemfibrozil or any component of the formulation; hepatic or severe renal dysfunction; primary biliary cirrhosis; pre-existing gallbladder disease; concurrent use with repaglinide

Warnings/Precautions Secondary causes of hyperlipidemia should be ruled out prior to therapy. Possible increased risk of malignancy and cholelithiasis. Anemia, leukopenia, thrombocytopenia, and bone marrow hypoplasia have rarely been reported. Periodic monitoring recommended during the first year of therapy. Elevations in serum transaminases can be seen. Discontinue if lipid response not seen. Be careful in patient selection; this is not a first- or second-line choice. Other agents may be more suitable. Adjustments in warfarin therapy may be required with concurrent use. Has been associated with rare myositis or rhabdomyolysis; patients should be monitored closely. Patients should be instructed to report unexplained muscle pain, tenderness, weakness, or brown urine. Use caution when combining gemfibrozil with HMG-CoA reductase inhibitors (may lead to myopathy, rhabdomyolysis). Use with caution in patients with mild-to-moderate renal impairment; contraindicated in patients with severe ▶

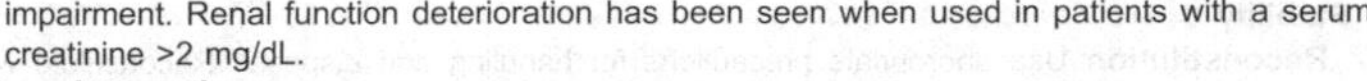

impairment. Renal function deterioration has been seen when used in patients with a serum creatinine >2 mg/dL.

Drug Interactions

Metabolism/Transport Effects Substrate of CYP3A4 (minor); **Inhibits** CYP1A2 (moderate), 2C8 (strong), 2C9 (strong), 2C19 (strong)

Avoid Concomitant Use

Avoid concomitant use of Gemfibrozil with any of the following: Clopidogrel; Repaglinide

Decreased Effect

Gemfibrozil may decrease the levels/effects of: Chenodiol; Clopidogrel; CycloSPORINE; CycloSPORINE (Systemic); Ursodiol

The levels/effects of Gemfibrozil may be decreased by: Bile Acid Sequestrants

Increased Effect/Toxicity

Gemfibrozil may increase the levels/effects of: Antidiabetic Agents (Thiazolidinedione); Atorvastatin; Carvedilol; Colchicine; CYP1A2 Substrates; CYP2C19 Substrates; CYP2C8 Substrates (High risk); CYP2C9 Substrates (High risk); Ezetimibe; Fluvastatin; Lovastatin; Pitavastatin; Pravastatin; Repaglinide; Rosuvastatin; Simvastatin; Sulfonylureas; Treprostinil; Vitamin K Antagonists

The levels/effects of Gemfibrozil may be increased by: Conivaptan; CycloSPORINE; CycloSPORINE (Systemic)

Nutritional/Ethanol Interactions

Ethanol: Avoid ethanol to decrease triglycerides.

Food: When given after meals, the AUC of gemfibrozil is decreased.

Adverse Reactions

>10%: Gastrointestinal: Dyspepsia (20%)

1% to 10%:

Cardiovascular: Atrial fibrillation (1%)

Central nervous system: Fatigue (4%), vertigo (2%)

Dermatologic: Eczema (2%), rash (2%)

Gastrointestinal: Abdominal pain (10%), nausea/vomiting (3%)

Reports where causal relationship has not been established: Alopecia, anaphylaxis, cataracts, colitis, confusion, decreased fertility (male), drug-induced lupus-like syndrome, extrasystoles, hepatoma, intracranial hemorrhage, pancreatitis, peripheral vascular disease, photosensitivity, positive ANA, renal dysfunction, retinal edema, seizure, syncope, thrombocytopenia, vasculitis, weight loss

Pharmacodynamics/Kinetics

Onset of Action May require several days

Absorption Well absorbed

Time to Peak Serum: 1-2 hours

Protein Binding 99%

Half-Life Elimination 1.5 hours

Metabolism Hepatic via oxidation to two inactive metabolites; undergoes enterohepatic recycling

Excretion Urine (~70% primarily as conjugated drug); feces (6%)

Available Dosage Forms

Tablet, oral: 600 mg

Lopid®: 600 mg

Dosing

Adult & Geriatric Hyperlipidemia/hypertriglyceridemia: Oral: 600 mg twice daily; administer 30 minutes before breakfast and dinner

Renal Impairment

Mild-to-moderate impairment: Use caution; deterioration of renal function has been reported in patients with baseline serum creatinine >2 mg/dL

Severe impairment: Use is contraindicated

Hemodialysis: Not removed by hemodialysis; supplemental dose is not necessary

Hepatic Impairment Use is contraindicated.

Administration

Oral Administer 30 minutes prior to breakfast and dinner.

Stability

Storage Store at controlled room temperature of 20°C to 25°C (68°F to 77°F). Protect from light and moisture.

Monitoring and Teaching Issues

Laboratory Monitoring Serum cholesterol, LFTs periodically, CBC periodically (first year)

Physical Assessment Assess serum cholesterol and LFTs. Monitor for gastrointestinal disturbances periodically during therapy.

Patient Education Should be taken 30 minutes before meals. Take with milk or meals if GI upset occurs. Avoid alcohol. Follow dietary recommendations of prescriber. You will need check-ups and blood work to assess effectiveness of therapy. You may experience loss of appetite, flatulence, or diarrhea. Report severe stomach pain, nausea, and vomiting.

Dietary Considerations Before initiation of therapy, patients should be placed on a standard cholesterol-lowering diet for 3-6 months and the diet should be continued during drug therapy. Should be taken 30 minutes prior to breakfast and dinner

Geriatric Considerations Gemfibrozil is the drug of choice for the treatment of hypertriglyceridemia and hypoalphaproteinemia in the elderly; it is usually well tolerated; myositis may be more common in patients with poor renal function. The definition of and, therefore, when to treat hyperlipidemia in the elderly is a controversial issue. The National Cholesterol Education Program recommends that all adults maintain a plasma cholesterol <160 mg/dL. Older adults with one additional risk factor, goal LDL would be <130 mg/dL. It is the authors' belief that pharmacologic treatment be reserved for those who are unable to obtain a desirable plasma cholesterol concentration by diet alone and for whom the benefits of treatment are believed to outweigh the potential adverse effects, drug interactions, and cost of treatment.

Pregnancy Considerations Adverse events were observed in animal reproduction studies. There are no adequate and well-controlled studies in pregnant women. Use only if benefits outweigh the risks.

Related Information

Hyperlipidemia Management *on page 2046*

Gemifloxacin (je mi FLOKS a sin)

U.S. Brand Names Factive®

Index Terms DW286; Gemifloxacin Mesylate; LA 20304a; SB-265805

Generic Availability (U.S.) No

Pharmacologic Category Antibiotic, Quinolone; Respiratory Fluoroquinolone

Medication Guide Available Yes

Pregnancy Risk Factor C

Lactation Excretion in breast milk unknown/not recommended

Use Treatment of acute exacerbation of chronic bronchitis; treatment of community-acquired pneumonia (CAP), including pneumonia caused by multidrug-resistant strains of *S. pneumoniae* (MDRSP)

Unlabeled/Investigational Use Acute sinusitis

Mechanism of Action/Effect Gemifloxacin is a DNA gyrase inhibitor and also inhibits topoisomerase IV. These enzymes are required for DNA replication and transcription, DNA repair, recombination, and transposition; quinolones are bactericidal

Contraindications Hypersensitivity to gemifloxacin, other fluoroquinolones, or any component of the formulation

Warnings/Precautions **[U.S. Boxed Warning]: There have been reports of tendon inflammation and/or rupture with quinolone antibiotics; risk may be increased with concurrent corticosteroids, organ transplant recipients, and in patients >60 years of age.** Rupture of the Achilles tendon sometimes requiring surgical repair has been reported most frequently; but other tendon sites (eg, rotator cuff, biceps) have also been reported. Strenuous physical activity, rheumatoid arthritis, and renal impairment may be an independent risk factor for tendonitis. Discontinue at first sign of tendon inflammation or pain. May occur even after discontinuation of therapy. Use with caution in patients with rheumatoid arthritis; may increase risk of tendon rupture. Fluoroquinolones may prolong QT_c interval; avoid use of gemifloxacin in patients with a history of QT_c prolongation, uncorrected hypokalemia, hypomagnesemia, or concurrent administration of other medications known to prolong the QT interval (including Class Ia and Class III antiarrhythmics, cisapride, erythromycin, antipsychotics, and tricyclic antidepressants). Use with caution in patients with significant bradycardia or acute myocardial ischemia. Use with caution in individuals at risk of seizures (CNS disorders or concurrent therapy with medications which may lower seizure threshold). Potential for seizures, although very rare, may be increased with concomitant NSAID therapy. Discontinue in patients who experience significant CNS adverse effects (dizziness, hallucinations, suicidal ideation or actions). Use caution in renal dysfunction; dosage adjustment required for Cl_{cr} ≤40 mL/minute.

Fluoroquinolones have been associated with the development of serious, and sometimes fatal, hypoglycemia, most often in elderly diabetics, but also in patients without diabetes. This occurred most frequently with gatifloxacin (no longer available systemically) but may occur at a lower frequency with other quinolones.

Severe hypersensitivity reactions, including anaphylaxis, have occurred with quinolone therapy. Reactions may present as typical allergic symptoms after a single dose, or may manifest as severe idiosyncratic dermatologic, vascular, pulmonary, renal, hepatic, and/or hematologic events, usually after multiple doses. May cause maculopapular rash, usually 8-10 days after treatment initiation; risk factors may include age <40 years, female gender (including postmenopausal women on HRT), and treatment duration >7 days. Prompt discontinuation of drug should occur if skin rash or other symptoms arise. **[U.S. Boxed Warning]: Quinolones may exacerbate myasthenia gravis; avoid use (rare, potentially life-threatening weakness of respiratory muscles may occur).** Avoid excessive sunlight and take precautions to limit exposure (eg, loose fitting clothing, sunscreen); may cause moderate-to-severe phototoxicity reactions. Discontinue use if photosensitivity occurs. Prolonged use may result in fungal or bacterial superinfection, including *C. difficile*-associated diarrhea (CDAD) and pseudomembranous colitis; CDAD has been observed >2 months postantibiotic treatment. Peripheral neuropathy has been linked to the use of quinolones; these cases were rare. Hemolytic reactions may (rarely) occur with quinolone use in patients with latent or actual G6PD deficiency.

Drug Interactions

Avoid Concomitant Use

Avoid concomitant use of Gemifloxacin with any of the following: BCG

Decreased Effect

Gemifloxacin may decrease the levels/effects of: BCG; Mycophenolate; Sulfonylureas; Typhoid Vaccine

The levels/effects of Gemifloxacin may be decreased by: Antacids; Calcium Salts; Didanosine; Iron Salts; Magnesium Salts; Quinapril; Sevelamer; Sucralfate; Zinc Salts

Increased Effect/Toxicity

Gemifloxacin may increase the levels/effects of: Corticosteroids (Systemic); Sulfonylureas; Vitamin K Antagonists

The levels/effects of Gemifloxacin may be increased by: Insulin; Nonsteroidal Anti-Inflammatory Agents; Probenecid

Nutritional/Ethanol Interactions Herb/Nutraceutical: Avoid dong quai, St John's wort (may also cause photosensitization).

Adverse Reactions 1% to 10%:

Central nervous system: Headache (4%), dizziness (2%)
Dermatologic: Rash (4%)
Gastrointestinal: Diarrhea (5%), nausea (4%), abdominal pain (2%), vomiting (2%)
Hepatic: Transaminases increased (1% to 4%)

Important adverse effects reported with other agents in this drug class include (not reported for gemifloxacin): Allergic reactions, CNS stimulation, hepatitis, jaundice, peripheral neuropathy, pneumonitis (eosinophilic), seizure; sensorimotor-axonal neuropathy (paresthesia, hypoesthesias, dysesthesias, weakness); severe dermatologic reactions (toxic epidermal necrolysis, Stevens-Johnson syndrome); torsade de pointes, vasculitis

Pharmacodynamics/Kinetics

Absorption Well absorbed from the GI tract

Bioavailability ~71%

Time to Peak Plasma: 0.5-2 hours

Protein Binding ~60% to 70%

Half-Life Elimination 7 hours (range 4-12 hours)

Metabolism Hepatic (minor); forms metabolites (CYP isoenzymes are not involved)

Excretion Feces (61%); urine (36%)

Available Dosage Forms

Tablet, oral:

Factive®: 320 mg

Dosing

Adult & Geriatric

Susceptible infections: Oral: 320 mg once daily

Acute exacerbations of chronic bronchitis: Oral: 320 mg once daily for 5 days

Community-acquired pneumonia (mild-to-moderate): Oral: 320 mg once daily for 5 or 7 days (decision to use 5- or 7-day regimen should be guided by initial sputum culture; 7 days are recommended for MDRSP, *Klebsiella*, or *M. catarrhalis* infection)

Sinusitis (unlabeled use): Oral: 320 mg once daily for 10 days

Renal Impairment

Cl_{cr} >40 mL/minute: No adjustment required.

Cl_{cr} ≤40 mL/minute (or patients on hemodialysis/CAPD): 160 mg once daily (administer dose following hemodialysis).

Hepatic Impairment No adjustment required.

Administration

Oral May be administered with or without food, milk, or calcium supplements. Gemifloxacin should be taken 3 hours before or 2 hours after supplements (including multivitamins) containing iron, zinc, or magnesium.

Stability

Storage Store at 25°C (77°F). Protect from light.

Monitoring and Teaching Issues

Laboratory Monitoring WBC, renal function

Physical Assessment Assess allergy history before initiating therapy. Use caution in presence of bradycardia, CNS disorders, renal dysfunction, or colitis. Teach patient proper use (timing of meals, supplements, or other medications). Monitor for allergic reaction, tendon pain, and opportunistic infection.

Patient Education Should be taken at least 3 hours before or 2 hours after antacids or other products containing aluminum, iron, magnesium, or zinc (including multivitamins). Maintain adequate hydration, unless instructed to restrict fluid intake. May cause headache, dizziness, nausea, vomiting, abdominal discomfort, or diarrhea. Discontinue use immediately and report to prescriber if signs of tendon inflammation or pain occur or if you experience signs of allergic reaction (eg, itching, rash, respiratory difficulty, facial edema, difficulty swallowing). Report CNS changes (eg, hallucinations, suicide ideation, seizures) or signs of opportunistic infection (unusual fever or chills, vaginal itching or foul-smelling vaginal discharge, easy bruising or bleeding).

Dietary Considerations May take tablets with or without food, milk, or calcium supplements. Gemifloxacin should be taken 3 hours before or 2 hours after supplements (including multivitamins) containing iron, zinc, or magnesium.

Geriatric Considerations The risk of torsade de pointes and tendon inflammation and/or rupture associated with the concomitant use of corticosteroids and quinolones is increased in the elderly population. See Warnings/Precautions regarding tendon rupture in patients >60 years of age.

Breast-Feeding Considerations It is not known if gemifloxacin is excreted in breast milk. Breast-feeding is not recommended by the manufacturer. Nondose-related effects could include modification of bowel flora.

Pregnancy Considerations Adverse events have been observed in some animal studies; therefore, the manufacturer classifies gemifloxacin as pregnancy category C. Quinolone exposure during human pregnancy has been reported with other agents (see Ciprofloxacin (Systemic) monograph). To date, no specific teratogenic effect or increased pregnancy risk has been identified; however, because of concerns of cartilage damage in immature animals exposed to quinolones and the limited gemifloxacin specific data, gemifloxacin should only be used during pregnancy if a safer option is not available.

◆ **Gemifloxacin Mesylate** *see* Gemifloxacin *on page 861*

Gemtuzumab Ozogamicin (gem TOO zoo mab oh zog a MY sin)

U.S. Brand Names Mylotarg® [DSC]

Index Terms CMA-676

Generic Availability (U.S.) No

Pharmacologic Category Antineoplastic Agent, Monoclonal Antibody

Medication Safety Issues

Sound-alike/look-alike issues:

Gemtuzumab may be confused with gemcitabine

High alert medication: This medication is in a class the Institute for Safe Medication Practices (ISMP) includes among its list of drug classes which have a heightened risk of causing significant patient harm when used in error.

Prescribing and Access Restrictions As of June 2010, gemtuzumab has been withdrawn from the U.S. market and is no longer commercially available to new patients; thereafter, gemtuzumab will only be available in the U.S. under an Investigational New Drug (IND) protocol.

Pregnancy Risk Factor D

Lactation Excretion in breast milk unknown/not recommended

Use Treatment of relapsed CD33 positive acute myeloid leukemia (AML) in patients ≥60 years of age who are not candidates for cytotoxic chemotherapy

Note: Due to safety concerns as well as lack of clinical benefit demonstrated in a post-approval clinical trial, gemtuzumab was withdrawn from the U.S. commercial market.

Unlabeled/Investigational Use Salvage therapy for acute promyelocytic leukemia (APL), relapsed/ refractory CD33 positive acute myeloid leukemia in children and adults <60 years

Mechanism of Action/Effect Antibody to CD33 antigen, which is expressed on leukemic blasts in 80% of AML patients. Binds to the CD33 antigen, resulting in internalization of the antibody-antigen complex. Following internalization, the calicheamicin derivative is released inside the myeloid cell. The calicheamicin derivative binds to DNA resulting in double strand breaks and cell death. Pluripotent stem cells and nonhematopoietic cells are not affected.

Contraindications Hypersensitivity to gemtuzumab ozogamicin, calicheamicin derivatives, or any component of the formulation; patients with anti-CD33 antibody

Warnings/Precautions Hazardous agent - use appropriate precautions for handling and disposal.

[U.S. Boxed Warning]: Gemtuzumab has been associated with hepatotoxicity, including severe hepatic veno-occlusive disease (VOD). Symptoms of VOD include right upper quadrant pain, rapid weight gain, ascites, hepatomegaly, and bilirubin/transaminase elevations. Risk may be increased by combination chemotherapy, underlying hepatic disease, or hematopoietic stem cell transplant. Use with caution in patients with hepatic impairment; has not been studied in patients with serum bilirubin >2 mg/dL.

[U.S. Boxed Warning]: Severe hypersensitivity reactions (including anaphylaxis) and other infusion-related reactions may occur. Infusion-related events are common, generally reported to occur with the first dose after the end of the 2-hour intravenous infusion. These symptoms usually resolved after 2-4 hours with a supportive therapy of acetaminophen, diphenhydramine, and intravenous fluids. Other severe and potentially fatal infusion related pulmonary events (including dyspnea and hypoxia) have been reported infrequently. Symptomatic intrinsic lung disease or high peripheral blast counts may increase the risk of severe reactions. Fewer infusion-related events were observed after the second dose. Postinfusion reactions (may include fever, chills, hypotension, or dyspnea) may occur during the first 24 hours after administration. Consider discontinuation in patients who develop severe infusion-related reactions. In addition to infusion-related pulmonary events, gemtuzumab therapy is also associated with acute respiratory distress syndrome, pulmonary infiltrates, pleural effusion, noncardiogenic pulmonary edema, and pulmonary insufficiency.

[U.S. Boxed Warning]: Severe myelosuppression occurs in all patients at recommended dosages. Use caution in patients with renal impairment. Tumor lysis syndrome may occur as a consequence of leukemia treatment, adequate hydration and prophylactic allopurinol must be instituted prior to use. Other methods to lower WBC <30,000 cells/mm^3 may be considered (hydroxyurea or leukapheresis) to minimize the risk of tumor lysis syndrome, and/or severe infusion reactions. **[U.S. Boxed Warning]: Should be administered under the supervision of an experienced cancer chemotherapy physician. Should only be administered in facilities equipped to monitor and treat patients with leukemia. [U.S. Boxed Warning]: Safety and efficacy have not been established in combination with other chemotherapy**

agents, in pediatric patients, or in patients with poor performance status. Gemtuzumab is not FDA-approved for use in children.

Drug Interactions

Avoid Concomitant Use

Avoid concomitant use of Gemtuzumab Ozogamicin with any of the following: BCG; Belimumab; Natalizumab; Pimecrolimus; Roflumilast; Tacrolimus (Topical); Vaccines (Live)

Decreased Effect

Gemtuzumab Ozogamicin may decrease the levels/effects of: BCG; Sipuleucel-T; Vaccines (Inactivated); Vaccines (Live)

The levels/effects of Gemtuzumab Ozogamicin may be decreased by: Echinacea

Increased Effect/Toxicity

Gemtuzumab Ozogamicin may increase the levels/effects of: Belimumab; Leflunomide; Natalizumab; Vaccines (Live)

The levels/effects of Gemtuzumab Ozogamicin may be increased by: Abciximab; Denosumab; Pimecrolimus; Roflumilast; Tacrolimus (Topical); Trastuzumab

Nutritional/Ethanol Interactions Ethanol: Avoid ethanol (due to GI irritation).

Lab Interactions None known

Adverse Reactions Adverse reactions reported for adults of all ages. **Note:** A postinfusion symptom complex (fever, chills, less commonly hypertension, and/or dyspnea) may occur within 24 hours of administration; the incidence of infusion-related events decreases with repeat administration.

>10%:

- Cardiovascular: Hypotension (20%), hypertension (16%), peripheral edema (14%)
- Central nervous system: Fever (82%), chills (66%), headache (37%), pain (18%), dizziness (12%), insomnia (12%)
- Dermatologic: Petechiae (19%), rash (18%)
- Endocrine & metabolic: Hypokalemia (26%)
- Gastrointestinal: Nausea (68%), vomiting (58%), abdominal pain (32%), diarrhea (32%), anorexia (25%), mucositis/stomatitis (25%), constipation (23%)
- Hematologic: Thrombocytopenia (grades 3/4: 49% to 99%; median recovery 36-51 days), neutropenia (grades 3/4: 98%; median recovery 40-51 days), leukopenia (grades 3/4: 46% to 96%), lymphopenia (grades 3/4: 94%), anemia/hemoglobin decreased (grades 3/4: 14% to 52%), neutropenic fever (17%), hemorrhage (11% to 13%)
- Hepatic: Hyperbilirubinemia (grades 3/4: 29%), veno-occlusive disease (1% to 20%; higher frequency in patients with prior history of or subsequent hematopoietic stem cell transplant), AST increased (grades 3/4: 18%), LDH increased (16%)
- Local: Local reaction (22%)
- Neuromuscular & skeletal: Weakness (36%), back pain (14%)
- Respiratory: Epistaxis (28%; grade 3/4: 3%), dyspnea (26%), cough (17%), pneumonia (13%; grades 3/4: 8%), pharyngitis (12%)
- Miscellaneous: Infection (grades 3/4: 30%), sepsis (26%; grades 3/4: 17%), cutaneous herpes simplex (21%)

1% to 10%:

- Cardiovascular: Tachycardia (10%), cerebral hemorrhage (2%)
- Central nervous system: Depression (9%), anxiety (8%), intracranial hemorrhage (1%)
- Dermatologic: Bruising (10%), pruritus (6%)
- Endocrine & metabolic: Hyperglycemia (10%), hypocalcemia (10%), hypophosphatemia (8%) hypomagnesemia (6%)
- Gastrointestinal: Dyspepsia (10%), gingival hemorrhage (9%), melena (1%)
- Genitourinary: Vaginal hemorrhage (4%), vaginal bleeding (3%), hematuria (grade 3/4: 1%)
- Hematologic: Disseminated intravascular coagulation (DIC) (1%)
- Hepatic: ALT increased (grades 3/4: 9%), prothrombin time increased (grades 3/4: 9%), alkaline phosphatase increased (8%; grades 3/4: 4%), ascites (3%), PTT increased (grades 3/4: 2%)
- Neuromuscular & skeletal: Arthralgia (10%), myalgia (6%)
- Renal: Creatinine increased (2%)
- Respiratory: Rhinitis (8%), hypoxia (5%)

Pharmacodynamics/Kinetics

Time to Peak Immediate; higher concentrations observed after repeat dose

Half-Life Elimination Total calicheamicin: Initial: 41-45 hours, Repeat dose: 60-64 hours; Unconjugated: 100-143 hours (no change noted in repeat dosing)

Product Availability As of June 2010, no longer commercially available in the U.S. market for new patients.

Available Dosage Forms

Injection, powder for reconstitution [preservative free]:

Mylotarg®: 5 mg

Dosing

Adult & Geriatric Refer to individual protocols. **Note:** Patients should receive diphenhydramine 50 mg orally and acetaminophen 650-1000 mg orally 1 hour prior to administration of each dose. Acetaminophen dosage should be repeated as needed every 4 hours for 2 additional doses. Pretreatment with methylprednisolone may ameliorate infusion-related symptoms.

AML: I.V.:

≥60 years: 9 mg/m^2 infused over 2 hours. A full treatment course is a total of 2 doses administered with 14 days between doses. Full hematologic recovery is not necessary for administration of the second dose. There has been only limited experience with repeat courses of gemtuzumab ozogamicin.

<60 years (unlabeled use): 9 mg/m^2 infused over 2 hours. A full treatment course is a total of 2 doses administered with 14 days between doses.

APL (unlabeled use): I.V.: 6 mg/m^2 infused over 2 hours. A full treatment course is a total of 2 doses administered with 15 days between doses.

Pediatric Note: Patients should receive diphenhydramine (1 mg/kg) 1 hour prior to infusion and acetaminophen 15 mg/kg 1 hour prior to infusion and every 4 hours for 2 additional doses.

AML (unlabeled use): I.V.: 4-9 mg/m^2 infused over 2 hours every 2 weeks for a total of 1-3 doses per treatment course. Patients received the second and third doses and/or dose escalation if no dose-limiting toxicities were observed. (**Note:** Higher incidences of liver toxicities were observed in children at the 9 mg/m^2 dose level.)

or

Children <3 years: 0.2 mg/kg infused over 2 hours every 2 weeks for a total of 2 doses

Children ≥3 years: 6 mg/m^2 infused over 2 hours every 2 weeks for a total of 2 doses

Renal Impairment No recommendation (not studied).

Hepatic Impairment Use extra caution; has not been studied in patients with bilirubin >2 mg/dL.

Adjustment for Toxicity

Dyspnea or significant hypotension: Interrupt infusion; monitor

Anaphylaxis, pulmonary edema, acute respiratory distress syndrome: Strongly consider discontinuing treatment

Administration

I.V. Do not administer as I.V. push or bolus. Administer via I.V. infusion, over at least 2 hours through a low protein-binding (0.2-1.2 micron) in-line filter. Protect from light during infusion. Premedicate with acetaminophen and diphenhydramine prior to each infusion.

Stability

Reconstitution Protect from light during preparation (and administration). Prepare in biologic safety hood with shielded fluorescent light; (some institutions prepare in a darkened room with the lights in the biologic safety cabinet turned off). Allow to warm to room temperature prior to reconstitution. Reconstitute vial with sterile water for injection to a concentration of 1 mg/mL. Dilute in 100 mL of 0.9% sodium chloride injection. Hazardous agent - use appropriate precautions for handling and disposal.

Storage Light sensitive; protect from light (including direct and indirect sunlight, and unshielded fluorescent light). The infusion container should be placed in a UV protectant bag immediately after preparation. Store intact vials under refrigeration at 2°C to 8°C (36°F to 46°F). Reconstituted solutions may be stored for up to 2 hours at room temperature or under refrigeration. Following dilution for infusion, solutions are stable for up to 16 hours at room temperature. Administration requires 2 hours; therefore, the maximum elapsed time from initial reconstitution to completion of infusion should be 20 hours.

Monitoring and Teaching Issues

Laboratory Monitoring Monitor electrolytes, liver function, CBC with differential, and platelet counts frequently.

Physical Assessment Infusion reactions can be severe; premedicate with acetaminophen and diphenhydramine prior to each infusion and acetaminophen as needed following each infusion. Patient must be monitored closely during and for 4 hours following treatment for infusion-related reactions (eg, anaphylaxis, pulmonary edema, or ARDS). Monitor for post-infusion symptom complex for immediate 24 hours following infusion. Monitor for tachycardia, hyper- or hypotension, CNS changes, gastrointestinal disturbance, and hepatic reaction regularly between infusions.

Patient Education This medication can only be administered intravenously. During and immediately following infusion, you will be closely monitored; report immediately any burning, pain, or swelling at infusion site; difficulty breathing or swallowing; chest pain; chills; or sudden headache. You will need frequent laboratory tests during course of therapy. Do not use alcohol or aspirin-containing medications between treatments without consulting your prescriber. It is important to maintain adequate nutrition and hydration, unless instructed to restrict fluid intake. You will be susceptible to infection. You may experience nausea, vomiting, or mouth sores. Report immediately any difficulty breathing, unusual cough, nosebleed, fever, chills, unusual bleeding or bruising, signs of infection (eg, sore throat, cough, white plaques in mouth or perianal area, burning on urination), chest pain or palpitations, yellowing of the eyes or skin, swelling of extremities, rapid weight gain, right upper quadrant pain, or rash.

Breast-Feeding Considerations Due to the potential for serious adverse reactions in the nursing infant, breast-feeding is not recommended.

Pregnancy Considerations Animal studies have demonstrated teratogenic effects, fetal loss, and maternal toxicity. There are no adequate and well-controlled studies in pregnant women. May cause fetal harm when administered to a pregnant woman. Women of child-bearing potential should avoid becoming pregnant while receiving treatment.

- **Gemzar®** *see* Gemcitabine *on page 855*
- **Genahist™ [OTC] [DSC]** *see* DiphenhydrAMINE (Systemic) *on page 543*
- **Genaphed™ [OTC]** *see* Pseudoephedrine *on page 1529*
- **Genebs Extra Strength [OTC] [DSC]** *see* Acetaminophen *on page 38*
- **Generlac** *see* Lactulose *on page 1053*

- **Gengraf®** *see* CycloSPORINE (Systemic) *on page* 437
- **Genotropin®** *see* Somatropin *on page* 1664
- **Genotropin Miniquick®** *see* Somatropin *on page* 1664
- **Gentak®** *see* Gentamicin (Ophthalmic) *on page* 868

Gentamicin (Systemic) (jen ta MYE sin)

Index Terms Gentamicin Sulfate

Generic Availability (U.S.) Yes

Pharmacologic Category Antibiotic, Aminoglycoside

Medication Safety Issues

Sound-alike/look-alike issues:

Gentamicin may be confused with gentian violet, kanamycin, vancomycin

High alert medication: The Institute for Safe Medication Practices (ISMP) includes this medication (intrathecal administration) among its list of drug classes which have a heightened risk of causing significant patient harm when used in error.

Pregnancy Risk Factor D

Lactation Enters breast milk/use caution (AAP rates "compatible"; AAP 2001 update pending)

Use Treatment of susceptible bacterial infections, normally gram-negative organisms, including *Pseudomonas*, *Proteus*, *Serratia*, and gram-positive *Staphylococcus*; treatment of bone infections, respiratory tract infections, skin and soft tissue infections, as well as abdominal and urinary tract infections, and septicemia; treatment of infective endocarditis

Mechanism of Action/Effect Bactericidal; interferes with bacterial protein synthesis resulting in cell death

Contraindications Hypersensitivity to gentamicin or other aminoglycosides

Warnings/Precautions [U.S. Boxed Warning]: Aminoglycosides may cause neurotoxicity and/or nephrotoxicity; usual risk factors include pre-existing renal impairment, concomitant neuro-/nephrotoxic medications, advanced age and dehydration. Ototoxicity may be directly proportional to the amount of drug given and the duration of treatment; tinnitus or vertigo are indications of vestibular injury and impending hearing loss; renal damage is usually reversible. May cause neuromuscular blockade and respiratory paralysis; especially when given soon after anesthesia or muscle relaxants.

Not intended for long-term therapy due to toxic hazards associated with extended administration; use caution in pre-existing renal insufficiency, vestibular or cochlear impairment, myasthenia gravis, hypocalcemia, conditions which depress neuromuscular transmission. Dosage modification required in patients with impaired renal function. Prolonged use may result in fungal or bacterial superinfection, including *C. difficile*-associated diarrhea (CDAD) and pseudomembranous colitis; CDAD has been observed >2 months postantibiotic treatment.

Drug Interactions

Avoid Concomitant Use

Avoid concomitant use of Gentamicin (Systemic) with any of the following: Agalsidase Beta; BCG; Gallium Nitrate

Decreased Effect

Gentamicin (Systemic) may decrease the levels/effects of: Agalsidase Beta; BCG; Typhoid Vaccine

The levels/effects of Gentamicin (Systemic) may be decreased by: Penicillins

Increased Effect/Toxicity

Gentamicin (Systemic) may increase the levels/effects of: AbobotulinumtoxinA; Bisphosphonate Derivatives; CARBOplatin; Colistimethate; CycloSPORINE; CycloSPORINE (Systemic); Gallium Nitrate; Neuromuscular-Blocking Agents; OnabotulinumtoxinA; RimabotulinumtoxinB

The levels/effects of Gentamicin (Systemic) may be increased by: Amphotericin B; Capreomycin; CISplatin; Loop Diuretics; Nonsteroidal Anti-Inflammatory Agents; Vancomycin

Lab Interactions Some penicillin derivatives may accelerate the degradation of aminoglycosides *in vitro*, leading to a potential underestimation of aminoglycoside serum concentration.

Adverse Reactions

>10%:

Central nervous system: Neurotoxicity (vertigo, ataxia)

Neuromuscular & skeletal: Gait instability

Otic: Ototoxicity (auditory), ototoxicity (vestibular)

Renal: Nephrotoxicity, decreased creatinine clearance

1% to 10%: Cardiovascular: Edema

Pharmacodynamics/Kinetics

Absorption

Intramuscular: Rapid and complete

Oral: None

Time to Peak Serum: I.M.: 30-90 minutes; I.V.: 30 minutes after 30-minute infusion

Protein Binding <30%

Half-Life Elimination

Infants: <1 week: 3-11.5 hours; 1 week to 6 months: 3-3.5 hours

Adults: 1.5-3 hours; End-stage renal disease: 36-70 hours

Excretion Urine (as unchanged drug)

Clearance: Directly related to renal function

Available Dosage Forms

Infusion, premixed in NS: 60 mg (50 mL, 100 mL); 80 mg (50 mL, 100 mL); 100 mg (50 mL, 100 mL); 120 mg (50 mL, 100 mL)

Injection, solution: 10 mg/mL (2 mL, 6 mL, 8 mL, 10 mL); 40 mg/mL (2 mL, 20 mL, 50 mL)

Injection, solution [preservative free]: 10 mg/mL (2 mL)

Dosing

Adult & Geriatric Individualization is **critical** because of the low therapeutic index.

Use of ideal body weight (IBW) for determining the mg/kg/dose appears to be more accurate than dosing on the basis of total body weight (TBW). In morbid obesity, dosage requirement may best be estimated using a dosing weight of IBW + 0.4 (TBW - IBW).

Initial and periodic plasma drug levels (eg, peak and trough with conventional dosing) should be determined, particularly in critically-ill patients with serious infections or in disease states known to significantly alter aminoglycoside pharmacokinetics (eg, cystic fibrosis, burns, or major surgery).

Usual dosage ranges:

I.M., I.V.:

Conventional: 1-2.5 mg/kg/dose every 8-12 hours; to ensure adequate peak concentrations early in therapy, higher initial dosage may be considered in selected patients when extracellular water is increased (edema, septic shock, postsurgical, or trauma)

Once daily: 4-7 mg/kg/dose once daily; some clinicians recommend this approach for all patients with normal renal function; this dose is at least as efficacious with similar, if not less, toxicity than conventional dosing

Intrathecal: 4-8 mg/day

Indication-specific dosing: I.M., I.V.:

Brucellosis: 240 mg (I.M.) daily or 5 mg/kg (I.V.) daily for 7 days; either regimen recommended in combination with doxycycline

Cholangitis: 4-6 mg/kg once daily with ampicillin

Diverticulitis (complicated): 1.5-2 mg/kg every 8 hours (with ampicillin and metronidazole)

Endocarditis: Treatment: 3 mg/kg/day in 1-3 divided doses

Meningitis *Enterococcus* sp or *Pseudomonas aeruginosa*: I.V.: Loading dose 2 mg/kg, then 1.7 mg/kg/dose every 8 hours (administered with another bacteriocidal drug)

Pelvic inflammatory disease: Loading dose: 2 mg/kg, then 1.5 mg/kg every 8 hours

Alternate therapy: 4.5 mg/kg once daily

Plague (*Yersinia pestis*): Treatment: 5 mg/kg/day, followed by postexposure prophylaxis with doxycycline

Pneumonia, hospital- or ventilator-associated: 7 mg/kg/day (with antipseudomonal beta-lactam or carbapenem)

Synergy (for gram-positive infections): 3 mg/kg/day in 1-3 divided doses (with ampicillin)

Tularemia: 5 mg/kg/day divided every 8 hours for 1-2 weeks

Urinary tract infection: 1.5 mg/kg/dose every 8 hours

Pediatric Individualization is **critical** because of the low therapeutic index.

Use of ideal body weight (IBW) for determining the mg/kg/dose appears to be more accurate than dosing on the basis of total body weight (TBW). In morbid obesity, dosage requirement may best be estimated using a dosing weight of IBW + 0.4 (TBW - IBW).

Initial and periodic plasma drug levels (eg, peak and trough with conventional dosing) should be determined, particularly in critically-ill patients with serious infections or in disease states known to significantly alter aminoglycoside pharmacokinetics (eg, cystic fibrosis, burns, or major surgery).

Usual dosage ranges: I.M., I.V.:

Infants and Children <5 years: 2.5 mg/kg/dose every 8 hours*

Children ≥5 years: 2-2.5 mg/kg/dose every 8 hours*

***Note:** Higher individual doses and/or more frequent intervals (eg, every 6 hours) may be required in selected clinical situations (cystic fibrosis) or serum levels document the need.

Indication-specific dosing:

Meningitis: Neonates: I.V.:

0-7 days of age: <2000 g: 2.5 mg/kg every 18-24 hours; >2000 g: 2.5 mg/kg every 12 hours

8-28 days of age: <2000 g: 2.5 mg/kg every 8-12 hours; >2000 g: 2.5 mg/kg every 8 hours

Renal Impairment

Conventional dosing:

Cl_{cr} ≥60 mL/minute: Administer every 8 hours

Cl_{cr} 40-60 mL/minute: Administer every 12 hours

Cl_{cr} 20-40 mL/minute: Administer every 24 hours

Cl_{cr} <20 mL/minute: Loading dose, then monitor levels

High-dose therapy: Interval may be extended (eg, every 48 hours) in patients with moderate renal impairment (Cl_{cr} 30-59 mL/minute) and/or adjusted based on serum level determinations.

Hemodialysis: Dialyzable; removal by hemodialysis: 30% removal of aminoglycosides occurs during 4 hours of HD; administer dose after dialysis and follow levels

Removal by continuous ambulatory peritoneal dialysis (CAPD):

Administration via CAPD fluid:

Gram-negative infection: 4-8 mg/L (4-8 mcg/mL) of CAPD fluid

Gram-positive infection (eg, synergy): 3-4 mg/L (3-4 mcg/mL) of CAPD fluid

Administration via I.V., I.M. route during CAPD: Dose as for Cl_{cr} <10 mL/minute and follow levels

Removal via continuous arteriovenous or venovenous hemofiltration: Dose as for Cl_{cr} 10-40 mL/minute and follow levels

Hepatic Impairment Monitor plasma concentrations.

Administration

I.M. Administer by deep I.M. route if possible. Slower absorption and lower peak concentrations, probably due to poor circulation in the atrophic muscle, may occur following I.M. injection; in paralyzed patients, suggest I.V. route.

I.V. Some penicillins (eg, carbenicillin, ticarcillin, and piperacillin) have been shown to inactivate aminoglycosides *in vitro*. This has been observed to a greater extent with tobramycin and gentamicin, while amikacin has shown greater stability against inactivation. Concurrent use of these agents may pose a risk of reduced antibacterial efficacy *in vivo*, particularly in the setting of profound renal impairment. However, definitive clinical evidence is lacking. If combination penicillin/aminoglycoside therapy is desired in a patient with renal dysfunction, separation of doses (if feasible), and routine monitoring of aminoglycoside levels, CBC, and clinical response should be considered.

Stability

Storage Gentamicin is a colorless to slightly yellow solution which should be stored between 2°C to 30°C, but refrigeration is not recommended. I.V. infusion solutions mixed in NS or D_5W solution are stable for 24 hours at room temperature and refrigeration. Premixed bag: Manufacturer expiration date; remove from overwrap stability: 30 days.

Monitoring and Teaching Issues

Laboratory Monitoring Urinalysis, BUN, serum creatinine, plasma gentamicin levels (as appropriate to dosing method). Peak levels are drawn 30 minutes after the end of a 30-minute infusion or 1 hour after initiation of infusion or I.M. injection. The trough is drawn just before the next dose. Levels are typically obtained after the third dose in conventional dosing. Perform culture and sensitivity studies prior to initiating therapy to determine the causative organism and its susceptibility to gentamicin. Some penicillin derivatives may accelerate the degradation of aminoglycosides.

Physical Assessment Assess kidney function and hearing before, during, and following therapy. Monitor for decreased renal function, ototoxicity, and neurotoxicity. Perform hearing tests prior to initiating treatment and periodically during therapy (>2 weeks) if at high risk.

Patient Education Drink adequate amounts of water unless instructed to restrict fluid intake. You may experience ringing in ears, dizziness, blurred vision, GI upset, loss of appetite, or photosensitivity. Report severe headache, changes in hearing acuity, ringing in ears, change in balance, changes in urine pattern, persistent diarrhea, respiratory difficulty, rash, fever, unhealed sores, sores in mouth, vaginal drainage, muscle or bone pain, change in gait, or worsening of condition.

Dietary Considerations Calcium, magnesium, potassium: Renal wasting may cause hypocalcemia, hypomagnesemia, and/or hypokalemia.

Geriatric Considerations The aminoglycosides are important therapeutic interventions for infections due to susceptible organisms and as empiric therapy in seriously ill patients. Their use is not without risk of toxicity, however, these risks can be minimized if initial dosing is adjusted for estimated renal function and appropriate monitoring performed. High dose, once daily aminoglycosides have been advocated as an alternative to traditional dosing regimens. Once daily or extended interval dosing is as effective and may be safer than traditional dosing. The interval must be adjusted for renal function.

Breast-Feeding Considerations Gentamicin is excreted into breast milk; however, it is not well absorbed when taken orally. This limited oral absorption may minimize exposure to the nursing infant. Nondose-related effects could include modification of bowel flora.

Pregnancy Considerations Gentamicin crosses the placenta and produces detectable serum levels in the fetus. Renal toxicity has been described in two case reports following first trimester exposure. There are several reports of total irreversible bilateral congenital deafness in children whose mothers received streptomycin during pregnancy; therefore, the manufacturer classifies gentamicin as pregnancy category D. Although ototoxicity has not been reported following maternal use of gentamicin, a potential for harm exists. **[U.S. Boxed Warning]: Aminoglycosides may cause fetal harm if administered to a pregnant woman.**

Due to pregnancy induced physiologic changes, some pharmacokinetic parameters of gentamicin may be altered. Pregnant women have an average-to-larger volume of distribution which may result in lower serum peak levels than for the same dose in nonpregnant women. Serum half-life is also shorter.

Related Information

Antimicrobial Drugs of Choice *on page* 2008

Peak and Trough Guidelines *on page* 1958

Gentamicin (Ophthalmic) (jen ta MYE sin)

U.S. Brand Names Garamycin™; Gentak®

Index Terms Gentamicin Sulfate

Generic Availability (U.S.) Yes

Pharmacologic Category Antibiotic, Aminoglycoside; Antibiotic, Ophthalmic

Medication Safety Issues

Sound-alike/look-alike issues:

Gentamicin may be confused with gentian violet, kanamycin, vancomycin

Pregnancy Risk Factor C

Use Treatment of ophthalmic infections caused by susceptible bacteria

Available Dosage Forms

Ointment, ophthalmic:
Gentak®: 0.3% (3.5 g)

Ointment, ophthalmic [preservative free]:
Garamycin™: 0.3% (3.5 g)

Solution, ophthalmic: 0.3% (5 mL, 15 mL)
Gentak®: 0.3% (5 mL)

Dosing

Adult & Geriatric Ophthalmic infections: Ophthalmic:
Ointment: Instill 1/2" (1.25 cm) 2-3 times/day to every 3-4 hours
Solution: Instill 1-2 drops every 2-4 hours, up to 2 drops every hour for severe infections

Pediatric Ophthalmic infections: Children: Refer to adult dosing.

Administration

Other Administer any other ophthalmics 10 minutes before or after gentamicin preparations.

Monitoring and Teaching Issues

Patient Education Wash hands before instilling. Sit or lie down to instill. Open eye, look at ceiling, and instill prescribed amount of solution; for ointment, pull lower lid down gently, instill thin ribbon of ointment inside lid. Close eye, roll eye in all directions, and apply gentle pressure to inner corner of eye. Do not let tip of applicator touch eye; do not contaminate tip of applicator (may cause eye infection, eye damage, or vision loss). Temporary stinging or blurred vision may occur. Report persistent pain, burning, vision changes, swelling, itching, or worsening of condition.

- ◆ **Gentamicin Sulfate** *see* Gentamicin (Ophthalmic) *on page 868*
- ◆ **Gentamicin Sulfate** *see* Gentamicin (Systemic) *on page 866*
- ◆ **Geodon®** *see* Ziprasidone *on page 1896*
- ◆ **GF196960** *see* Tadalafil *on page 1700*
- ◆ **GG** *see* GuaiFENesin *on page 890*
- ◆ **Gianvi™** *see* Ethinyl Estradiol and Drospirenone *on page 696*
- ◆ **Gilenya™** *see* Fingolimod *on page 764*
- ◆ **Glargine Insulin** *see* Insulin Glargine *on page 986*

Glatiramer Acetate (gla TIR a mer AS e tate)

U.S. Brand Names Copaxone®

Index Terms Copolymer-1

Generic Availability (U.S.) No

Pharmacologic Category Biological, Miscellaneous

Medication Safety Issues
Sound-alike/look-alike issues:
Copaxone® may be confused with Compazine®

Pregnancy Risk Factor B

Lactation Excretion in breast milk unknown/use caution

Use Management of relapsing-remitting type multiple sclerosis, including patients with a first clinical episode with MRI features consistent with multiple sclerosis

Mechanism of Action/Effect Glatiramer is a mixture of random polymers of four amino acids; L-alanine, L-glutamic acid, L-lysine, and L-tyrosine, the resulting mixture is antigenically similar to myelin basic protein, which is an important component of the myelin sheath of nerves; glatiramer is thought to induce and activate T-lymphocyte suppressor cells specific for a myelin antigen, it is also proposed that glatiramer interferes with the antigen-presenting function of certain immune cells opposing pathogenic T-cell function

Contraindications Hypersensitivity to glatiramer acetate, mannitol, or any component of the formulation

Warnings/Precautions For SubQ use only, **not for I.V. administration**. Glatiramer acetate is antigenic, and may interfere with recognition of foreign antigens affecting tumor surveillance and infection defense systems. Immediate postinjection systemic reactions occur in a substantial percentage of patients (~16% in studies); symptoms may begin within minutes of injection and are usually self-limiting. Most patients only have one reaction despite repeated administration. Chest pain (transient pain resolving in minutes) may occur as part of the postinjection systemic reaction, but can also occur alone. Lipoatrophy may occur at injection site; proper injection site rotation may prevent. Safety and efficacy has not been established in patients with renal impairment, in the elderly, or in patients <18 years of age.

Drug Interactions

Avoid Concomitant Use

Avoid concomitant use of Glatiramer Acetate with any of the following: BCG; Natalizumab; Pimecrolimus; Roflumilast; Tacrolimus (Topical); Vaccines (Live)

Decreased Effect

Glatiramer Acetate may decrease the levels/effects of: BCG; Sipuleucel-T; Vaccines (Inactivated); Vaccines (Live)

The levels/effects of Glatiramer Acetate may be decreased by: Echinacea

Increased Effect/Toxicity

Glatiramer Acetate may increase the levels/effects of: Leflunomide; Natalizumab; Vaccines (Live)

The levels/effects of Glatiramer Acetate may be increased by: Denosumab; Pimecrolimus; Roflumilast; Tacrolimus (Topical); Trastuzumab

Adverse Reactions

>10%:

Cardiovascular: Vasodilation (20%), chest pain (13%)
Central nervous system: Pain (20%), anxiety (13%)
Dermatologic: Rash (19%)
Gastrointestinal: Nausea (15%)
Local: Injection site reactions: Inflammation (49%), erythema (43%), pain (40%), pruritus (27%), mass (27%)
Neuromuscular & skeletal: Weakness (22%), back pain (12%)
Respiratory: Dyspnea (14%)
Miscellaneous: Infection (30%), flu-like syndrome (14%), diaphoresis (15%)

1% to 10%:

Cardiovascular: Edema (8%; includes peripheral and facial), palpitation (7%), tachycardia (5%), syncope (3%), hypertension (1%)
Central nervous system: Fever (6%), migraine (4%), chills (3%), nervousness (2%), speech disorder (2%), abnormal dreams (1%), emotional lability (1%), stupor (1%)
Dermatologic: Bruising (8%), pruritus (5%), erythema (4%), urticaria (3%), skin nodule (2%), eczema (1%), pustular rash (1%)
Endocrine & metabolic: Amenorrhea (1%), impotence (1%), menorrhagia (1%)
Gastrointestinal: Vomiting (7%), gastroenteritis (6%), weight gain (3%), dysphagia (2%), dental caries (1%)
Genitourinary: Urinary urgency (5%), vaginal moniliasis (4%)
Local: Injection site reactions: Hemorrhage (5%), hypersensitivity (4%), fibrosis (2%), lipoatrophy (2%), abscess (1%), edema (1%)
Neuromuscular & skeletal: Neck pain (8%), tremor (4%)
Ocular: Diplopia (3%), visual field defect (1%)
Respiratory: Rhinitis (7%), bronchitis (6%), cough (6%), laryngismus (5%), hyperventilation (1%)
Miscellaneous: Lymphadenopathy (7%), hypersensitivity (3%)

Pharmacodynamics/Kinetics

Metabolism SubQ: Large percentage hydrolyzed locally

Available Dosage Forms

Injection, solution [preservative free]:
Copaxone®: 20 mg/mL (1 mL)

Dosing

Adult & Geriatric Multiple sclerosis (relapsing-remitting): SubQ: 20 mg daily

Administration

Other For SubQ administration in the arms, abdomen, hips, or thighs; rotate injection sites to prevent lipoatrophy. Bring to room temperature prior to use. Visually inspect the solution; discard if solution is cloudy or contains any particulate matter.

Stability

Storage Store in refrigerator at 2°C to 8°C (36°F to 46°F); excursions to room temperature for up to 1 month do not have a negative impact on potency. Avoid heat; protect from intense light.

Monitoring and Teaching Issues

Physical Assessment Monitor for postinjection reactions (eg, self-resolving flushing, chest tightness, dyspnea, and palpitations). Teach patient proper use (reconstitution, injection technique, and syringe/needle disposal).

Patient Education This drug will not cure MS, but may help relieve the severity and frequency of attacks. This drug can only be given by subcutaneous injection. Your prescriber will instruct you in proper injection technique and syringe/needle disposal. May cause a transient reaction after injection, including flushing, chest tightness, dyspnea, or palpitations. May cause weakness, dizziness, confusion, nervousness, anxiety, nausea, or vomiting. Report chest pain or pounding heartbeat; persistent diarrhea or GI upset; infection (vaginal itching or drainage, sores in mouth, unusual fever or chills) or flu-like symptoms (swollen glands, chills, excessive sweating); bruising, rash, or skin irritation; joint pain or neck pain; swelling of puffiness of face; vision changes or ear pain; unusual cough or respiratory difficulty; alterations in menstrual pattern; or redness, pain, or swelling at injection site.

Pregnancy Considerations Adverse events were not observed in animal studies. There are no adequate and well-controlled studies in pregnant women. Use in pregnancy only if clearly necessary.

◆ **Gleevec®** *see* Imatinib *on page* 951
◆ **Gliadel®** *see* Carmustine *on page* 302
◆ **Glibenclamide** *see* GlyBURIDE *on page* 877

Glimepiride (GLYE me pye ride)

U.S. Brand Names Amaryl®
Generic Availability (U.S.) Yes
Pharmacologic Category Antidiabetic Agent, Sulfonylurea

Medication Safety Issues

Sound-alike/look-alike issues:

Glimepiride may be confused with glipiZIDE

Amaryl® may be confused with Altace®, Amerge®, Reminyl®

International issues:

Amarel [France], Amaryl [U.S., Canada, and multiple international markets] may be confused with Reminyl brand name for galantamine [multiple international markets]

Amaryl [U.S., Canada, and multiple international markets] may be confused with Almarl brand name for arotinolol [Japan]

High alert medication: The Institute for Safe Medication Practices (ISMP) includes this medication among its list of drugs which have a heightened risk of causing significant patient harm when used in error.

Pregnancy Risk Factor C

Lactation Excretion in breast milk unknown/not recommended

Use Management of type 2 diabetes mellitus (noninsulin dependent, NIDDM) as an adjunct to diet and exercise to lower blood glucose; may be used in combination with metformin or insulin in patients whose hyperglycemia cannot be controlled by diet and exercise in conjunction with a single oral hypoglycemic agent

Mechanism of Action/Effect Stimulates insulin release from the pancreatic beta cells; reduces glucose output from the liver; insulin sensitivity is increased at peripheral target sites

Contraindications Hypersensitivity to glimepiride, any component of the formulation, or sulfonamides; diabetic ketoacidosis (with or without coma)

Warnings/Precautions All sulfonylurea drugs are capable of producing severe hypoglycemia. Hypoglycemia is more likely to occur when caloric intake is deficient, after severe or prolonged exercise, when ethanol is ingested, or when more than one glucose-lowering drug is used. It is also more likely in elderly patients, malnourished patients and in patients with impaired renal or hepatic function; use with caution. Autonomic neuropathy, advanced age, and concomitant use of beta-blockers or other sympatholytic agents may impair the patient's ability to recognize the signs and symptoms of hypoglycemia; use with caution.

Chemical similarities are present among sulfonamides, sulfonylureas, carbonic anhydrase inhibitors, thiazides, and loop diuretics (except ethacrynic acid). Use in patients with sulfonamide allergy is not specifically contraindicated in product labeling, however, a risk of cross-reaction exists in patients with allergy to any of these compounds; avoid use when previous reaction has been severe.

Product labeling states oral hypoglycemic drugs may be associated with an increased cardiovascular mortality as compared to treatment with diet alone or diet plus insulin. Data to support this association are limited, and several studies, including a large prospective trial (UKPDS) have not supported an association.

It may be necessary to discontinue therapy and administer insulin if the patient is exposed to stress (fever, trauma, infection, surgery).

Drug Interactions

Metabolism/Transport Effects Substrate of CYP2C9 (major)

Avoid Concomitant Use There are no known interactions where it is recommended to avoid concomitant use.

Decreased Effect

The levels/effects of Glimepiride may be decreased by: Corticosteroids (Orally Inhaled); Corticosteroids (Systemic); CYP2C9 Inducers (Highly Effective); Luteinizing Hormone-Releasing Hormone Analogs; Peginterferon Alfa-2b; Quinolone Antibiotics; Rifampin; Somatropin; Thiazide Diuretics

Increased Effect/Toxicity

Glimepiride may increase the levels/effects of: Alcohol (Ethyl); Hypoglycemic Agents

The levels/effects of Glimepiride may be increased by: Beta-Blockers; Chloramphenicol; Cimetidine; Cyclic Antidepressants; CYP2C9 Inhibitors (Moderate); CYP2C9 Inhibitors (Strong); Fibric Acid Derivatives; Fluconazole; GLP-1 Agonists; Herbs (Hypoglycemic Properties); Pegvisomant; Quinolone Antibiotics; Ranitidine; Salicylates; Sulfonamide Derivatives; Voriconazole

Nutritional/Ethanol Interactions

Ethanol: Caution with ethanol (may cause hypoglycemia).

Herb/Nutraceutical: Caution with chromium, garlic, gymnema (may cause hypoglycemia).

Adverse Reactions 1% to 10%:

Central nervous system: Dizziness (2%), headache (2%)

Endocrine & metabolic: Hypoglycemia (1% to 2%)

Gastrointestinal: Nausea (1%)

Neuromuscular & skeletal: Weakness (2%)

Pharmacodynamics/Kinetics

Onset of Action Peak effect: Blood glucose reductions: 2-3 hours

Duration of Action 24 hours

Absorption 100%; delayed when given with food

Time to Peak 2-3 hours

Protein Binding >99.5%

Half-Life Elimination 5-9 hours

Metabolism Hepatic oxidation via CYP2C9 to M1 metabolite (~33% activity of parent compound); further oxidative metabolism to inactive M2 metabolite

Excretion Urine (60%, 80% to 90% as M1 and M2); feces (40%, 70% as M1 and M2)

Available Dosage Forms

Tablet, oral: 1 mg, 2 mg, 4 mg

Amaryl®: 1 mg, 2 mg, 4 mg

Dosing

Adult

Type 2 diabetes: Oral:

Initial: 1-2 mg once daily, administered with breakfast or the first main meal

Adjustment: Allow several days between dose titrations: usual maintenance dose: 1-4 mg once daily; after a dose of 2 mg once daily, increase in increments of 2 mg at 1- to 2-week intervals based upon the patient's blood glucose response to a maximum of 8 mg once daily. If inadequate response to maximal dose, combination therapy with metformin may be considered.

Combination with insulin therapy:

Note: Fasting glucose level for instituting combination therapy is in the range of >150 mg/dL in plasma or serum depending on the patient)

Initial: 8 mg once daily with the first main meal

Adjustment: After starting with low-dose insulin, upward adjustments of insulin can be done approximately weekly as guided by frequent measurements of fasting blood glucose. Once stable, combination-therapy patients should monitor their capillary blood glucose on an ongoing basis, preferably daily.

Conversion from therapy with long half-life agents: Observe patient carefully for 1-2 weeks when converting from a longer half-life agent (eg, chlorpropamide) to glimepiride due to overlapping hypoglycemic effects.

Geriatric Initial: 1 mg/day; dose titration and maintenance dosing should be conservative to avoid hypoglycemia

Pediatric Type 2 diabetes: Oral: Children 10-18 years (unlabeled use): Initial: 1 mg once daily; maintenance: 1-4 mg once daily

Renal Impairment Cl_{cr} <22 mL/minute: Initial starting dose should be 1 mg and dosage increments should be based on fasting blood glucose levels.

Administration

Oral Administer once daily with breakfast or first main meal of the day. Patients that are NPO or require decreased caloric intake may need doses held to avoid hypoglycemia.

Monitoring and Teaching Issues

Laboratory Monitoring Fasting blood glucose, hemoglobin A_{1c}

Physical Assessment Assess any allergies prior to beginning therapy.

Patient Education This medication is used to control diabetes; it is not a cure. Monitor glucose as recommended by prescriber. Other important components of treatment plan may include prescribed diet and exercise regimen (consult prescriber or diabetic educator). Always carry quick source of sugar with you. Take with breakfast or the first main meal of the day. Avoid alcohol while taking this medication; could cause severe reaction. If you experience hypoglycemic reaction, contact prescriber immediately. You may experience side effects during first weeks of therapy (eg, headache, nausea); consult prescriber if these persist. Report severe or persistent side effects (eg, hypoglycemia: palpitations, sweaty palms, lightheadedness; extended vomiting or flu-like symptoms; skin rash; easy bruising or bleeding; or change in color of urine or stool).

Dietary Considerations Administer with breakfast or the first main meal of the day. Individualized medical nutrition therapy (MNT) based on ADA recommendations is an integral part of therapy.

Geriatric Considerations Rapid and prolonged hypoglycemia (>12 hours) despite hypertonic glucose injections have been reported with glimepiride. Age, hepatic impairment, and renal impairment are independent risk factors for hypoglycemia; dosage titration should be made at weekly intervals. How "tightly" a geriatric patient's blood glucose should be controlled is controversial; however, a fasting blood sugar of <150 mg/dL is now an acceptable endpoint. Such a decision should be based on the patient's functional and cognitive status, how well they recognize hypoglycemic or hyperglycemic symptoms, and how to respond to them and their other disease states. Intensive glucose control (Hb A_{1c} <6.5%) has been linked to increased all cause and cardiovascular mortality, hypoglycemia requiring assistance, and weight gain in adult type 2 diabetes. For elderly patients with diabetes who are relatively healthy, attaining target goals for aspirin use, blood pressure, lipids, smoking cessation, and diet and exercise may be more important than normalized glycemic control.

Breast-Feeding Considerations It is not known if glimepiride is excreted in breast milk. Breast-feeding is not recommended by the manufacturer. Potentially, hypoglycemia may occur in a nursing infant exposed to a sulfonylurea via breast milk.

Pregnancy Considerations Adverse events have been observed in animal studies; therefore, glimepiride is classified as pregnancy category C. Severe hypoglycemia lasting 4-10 days has been noted in infants born to mothers taking a sulfonylurea at the time of delivery. The manufacturer recommends that patients be switched to insulin during pregnancy. Maternal hyperglycemia can be associated with adverse effects in the fetus, including macrosomia, neonatal hyperglycemia, and hyperbilirubinemia; the risk of congenital malformations is increased when the Hb A_{1c} is above the normal range. Diabetes can also be associated with adverse effects in the mother. Poorly-treated diabetes may cause end-organ damage that may in turn negatively affect obstetric outcomes. Physiologic glucose levels should be maintained prior to and during pregnancy to decrease the risk of adverse events in the mother and the fetus. Until additional safety and efficacy data are obtained, the use of oral agents is generally not recommended as routine management of GDM or type 2 diabetes mellitus during pregnancy. Insulin is the drug of choice for the control of diabetes mellitus during pregnancy.

Related Information

Diabetes Mellitus Management, Adults *on page 2026*

◆ **Glimepiride and Pioglitazone** *see* Pioglitazone and Glimepiride *on page 1462*

◆ **Glimepiride and Pioglitazone Hydrochloride** *see* Pioglitazone and Glimepiride *on page 1462*

◆ **Glimepiride and Rosiglitazone Maleate** *see* Rosiglitazone and Glimepiride *on page 1611*

GlipiZIDE (GLIP i zide)

U.S. Brand Names Glucotrol XL®; Glucotrol®

Index Terms Glydiazinamide

Generic Availability (U.S.) Yes

Pharmacologic Category Antidiabetic Agent, Sulfonylurea

Medication Safety Issues

Sound-alike/look-alike issues:

GlipiZIDE may be confused with glimepiride, glyBURIDE
Glucotrol® may be confused with Glucophage®, Glucotrol® XL, glyBURIDE
Glucotrol XL® may be confused with Glucotrol®

High alert medication: The Institute for Safe Medication Practices (ISMP) includes this medication among its list of drugs which have a heightened risk of causing significant patient harm when used in error.

Pregnancy Risk Factor C

Lactation Excretion in breast milk unknown/not recommended

Use Management of type 2 diabetes mellitus (noninsulin dependent, NIDDM)

Mechanism of Action/Effect Stimulates insulin release from the pancreatic beta cells; reduces glucose output from the liver; insulin sensitivity is increased at peripheral target sites

Contraindications Hypersensitivity to glipizide or any component of the formulation, other sulfonamides; type 1 diabetes mellitus (insulin dependent, IDDM); diabetic ketoacidosis

Warnings/Precautions All sulfonylurea drugs are capable of producing severe hypoglycemia. Hypoglycemia is more likely to occur when caloric intake is deficient, after severe or prolonged exercise, when ethanol is ingested, or when more than one glucose-lowering drug is used. It is also more likely in elderly patients, malnourished patients and in patients with impaired renal or hepatic function; use with caution.

Chemical similarities are present among sulfonamides, sulfonylureas, carbonic anhydrase inhibitors, thiazides, and loop diuretics (except ethacrynic acid). Use in patients with sulfonamide allergy is specifically contraindicated in product labeling, however, a risk of cross-reaction exists in patients with allergy to any of these compounds; avoid use when previous reaction has been severe.

Product labeling states oral hypoglycemic drugs may be associated with an increased cardiovascular mortality as compared to treatment with diet alone or diet plus insulin. Data to support this association are limited, and several studies, including a large prospective trial (UKPDS) have not supported an association.

Use with caution in patients with severe hepatic disease. It may be necessary to discontinue therapy and administer insulin if the patient is exposed to stress (fever, trauma, infection, surgery).

Avoid use of extended release tablets (Glucotrol XL®) in patients with known stricture/ narrowing of the GI tract.

Drug Interactions

Metabolism/Transport Effects Substrate of 2C9 (major)

Avoid Concomitant Use There are no known interactions where it is recommended to avoid concomitant use.

Decreased Effect

The levels/effects of GlipiZIDE may be decreased by: Corticosteroids (Orally Inhaled); Corticosteroids (Systemic); CYP2C9 Inducers (Highly Effective); Luteinizing Hormone-Releasing Hormone Analogs; Peginterferon Alfa-2b; Quinolone Antibiotics; Rifampin; Somatropin; Thiazide Diuretics

Increased Effect/Toxicity

GlipiZIDE may increase the levels/effects of: Alcohol (Ethyl); Hypoglycemic Agents

The levels/effects of GlipiZIDE may be increased by: Beta-Blockers; Chloramphenicol; Cimetidine; Clarithromycin; Cyclic Antidepressants; CYP2C9 Inhibitors (Moderate); CYP2C9 Inhibitors (Strong); Fibric Acid Derivatives; Fluconazole; GLP-1 Agonists; Herbs (Hypoglycemic Properties); Pegvisomant; Posaconazole; Quinolone Antibiotics; Ranitidine; Salicylates; Sulfonamide Derivatives; Voriconazole

Nutritional/Ethanol Interactions

Ethanol: Caution with ethanol (may cause hypoglycemia or rare disulfiram reaction).

Food: A delayed release of insulin may occur if glipizide is taken with food. Immediate release tablets should be administered 30 minutes before meals to avoid erratic absorption.

Herb/Nutraceutical: Herbs with hypoglycemic properties may enhance the hypoglycemic effect of glipizide. This includes alfalfa, aloe, bilberry, bitter melon, burdock, celery, damiana, fenugreek, garcinia, garlic, ginger, ginseng (American), gymnema, marshmallow, stinging nettle

Adverse Reactions Frequency not defined.

Cardiovascular: Edema, syncope

Central nervous system: Anxiety, depression, dizziness, drowsiness, headache, hypoesthesia, insomnia, nervousness, pain

Dermatologic: Eczema, erythema, maculopapular eruptions, morbilliform eruptions, photosensitivity, pruritus, rash, urticaria

Endocrine & metabolic: Disulfiram-like reaction, hypoglycemia, hyponatremia, SIADH (rare)

Gastrointestinal: Anorexia, constipation, diarrhea, epigastric fullness, flatulence, gastralgia, heartburn, nausea, vomiting

Hematologic: Agranulocytopenia, aplastic anemia, blood dyscrasias, hemolytic anemia, leukopenia, pancytopenia, porphyria cutanea tarda, thrombocytopenia

Hepatic: Hepatic porphyria

Neuromuscular & skeletal: Arthralgia, leg cramps, myalgia, paresthesia, tremor

Ocular: Blurred vision

Renal: Diuretic effect (minor)

Respiratory: Rhinitis

Miscellaneous: Diaphoresis

Pharmacodynamics/Kinetics

Duration of Action 12-24 hours

Absorption Rapid and complete; delayed with food

Bioavailability 90% to 100%

Time to Peak 1-3 hours; extended release tablets: 6-12 hours

Protein Binding 98% to 99%; primarily to albumin

Half-Life Elimination 2-5 hours

Metabolism Hepatic via CYP2C9; forms metabolites (inactive)

Excretion Urine (60% to 80%, 91% to 97% as metabolites); feces (11%)

Available Dosage Forms

Tablet, oral: 5 mg, 10 mg

Glucotrol®: 5 mg, 10 mg

Tablet, extended release, oral: 2.5 mg, 5 mg, 10 mg

Glucotrol XL®: 2.5 mg, 5 mg, 10 mg

Dosing

Adult

Type 2 diabetes: Oral (allow several days between dose titrations): Initial: 5 mg/day; adjust dosage at 2.5-5 mg daily increments as determined by blood glucose response at intervals of several days.

Immediate release tablet: Maximum recommended once-daily dose: 15 mg; maximum recommended total daily dose: 40 mg. Doses >15 mg/day should be administered in divided doses.

Extended release tablet (Glucotrol XL®): Maximum recommended dose: 20 mg

When transferring from insulin to glipizide:

Current insulin requirement ≤20 units: Discontinue insulin and initiate glipizide at usual dose

Current insulin requirement >20 units: Decrease insulin by 50% and initiate glipizide at usual dose; gradually decrease insulin dose based on patient response. Several days should elapse between dosage changes.

Geriatric Initial: 2.5 mg/day; increase by 2.5-5 mg/day at 1- to 2-week intervals.

Renal Impairment Cl_{cr} <10 mL/minute: Some investigators recommend not using.

Hepatic Impairment Initial dosage should be 2.5 mg/day.

Administration

Oral Administer immediate release tablets 30 minutes before a meal to achieve greatest reduction in postprandial hyperglycemia. Extended release tablets should be given with breakfast. Patients that are NPO or require decreased caloric intake may need doses held to avoid hypoglycemia.

Monitoring and Teaching Issues

Laboratory Monitoring Blood glucose, hemoglobin A_{1c}

Physical Assessment Monitor for hypoglycemia during therapy.

Patient Education This medication is used to control diabetes; it is not a cure. Monitor glucose as recommended by prescriber. Other important components of treatment plan may include prescribed diet and exercise regimen (consult prescriber or diabetic educator). Always carry quick source of sugar with you. Immediate release tablets should be taken 30 minutes before meals, at the same time each day. Extended release tablets should be taken with breakfast. Do not chew or crush extended release tablets. Avoid alcohol while taking this medication; could cause severe reaction. If you experience hypoglycemic reaction, contact prescriber immediately. You may experience more sensitivity to sunlight, headache, or nausea. Report severe or persistent side effects (eg, hypoglycemia: palpitations, sweaty palms, lightheadedness; extended vomiting; diarrhea or constipation; flu-like symptoms; skin rash; easy bruising or bleeding; or change in color of urine or stool).

Dietary Considerations Take immediate release tablets 30 minutes before meals; extended release tablets should be taken with breakfast. Individualized medical nutrition therapy (MNT) based on ADA recommendations is an integral part of therapy.

Geriatric Considerations Glipizide is a useful agent since there are few drug-to-drug interactions and elimination of the active drug is not dependent upon renal function. How "tightly" a geriatric patient's blood glucose should be controlled is controversial; however, a fasting blood sugar <150 mg/dL is now an acceptable endpoint. Such a decision should be based on the patient's functional and cognitive status, how well they recognize hypoglycemic or hyperglycemic symptoms, and how to respond to them and their other disease states. Intensive glucose control (Hb A_{1c} <6.5%) has been linked to increased all cause and cardiovascular mortality, hypoglycemia requiring assistance, and weight gain in adult type 2 diabetes. For elderly patients with diabetes who are relatively healthy, attaining target goals for aspirin use, blood pressure, lipids, smoking cessation, and diet and exercise may be more important than normalized glycemic control.

Breast-Feeding Considerations Data from initial studies note that glipizide was not detected in breast milk. Breast-feeding is not recommended by the manufacturer. Potentially, hypoglycemia may occur in a nursing infant exposed to a sulfonylurea via breast milk.

Pregnancy Considerations Adverse events have been observed in animal studies; therefore, glipizide is classified as pregnancy category C. Glipizide crosses the placenta. Severe hypoglycemia lasting 4-10 days has been noted in infants born to mothers taking a sulfonylurea at the time of delivery. Maternal hyperglycemia can be associated with adverse effects in the fetus, including macrosomia, neonatal hyperglycemia, and hyperbilirubinemia; the risk of congenital malformations is increased when the Hb A_{1c} is above the normal range. Diabetes can also be associated with adverse effects in the mother. Poorly-treated diabetes may cause end-organ damage that may in turn negatively affect obstetric outcomes. Physiologic glucose levels should be maintained prior to and during pregnancy to decrease the risk of adverse events in the mother and the fetus. Until additional safety and efficacy data are obtained, the use of oral agents is generally not recommended as routine management of GDM or type 2 diabetes mellitus during pregnancy. The manufacturer recommends if glipizide is used during pregnancy it should be discontinued at least 1 month before the expected delivery date. Insulin is the drug of choice for the control of diabetes mellitus during pregnancy.

Related Information

Diabetes Mellitus Management, Adults *on page 2026*

Glipizide and Metformin (GLIP i zide & met FOR min)

U.S. Brand Names Metaglip™

Index Terms Glipizide and Metformin Hydrochloride; Metformin and Glipizide

Generic Availability (U.S.) Yes

Pharmacologic Category Antidiabetic Agent, Biguanide; Antidiabetic Agent, Sulfonylurea

Medication Safety Issues

High alert medication: The Institute for Safe Medication Practices (ISMP) includes this medication among its list of drugs which have a heightened risk of causing significant patient harm when used in error.

Pregnancy Risk Factor C

Lactation

Glipizide: Excretion in breast milk unknown/not recommended

Metformin: Enters breast milk/not recommended

Use Indicated as an adjunct to diet and exercise to improve glycemic control in adults with type 2 diabetes mellitus (noninsulin dependent, NIDDM)

Available Dosage Forms

Tablet, oral: 2.5/250: Glipizide 2.5 mg and metformin 250 mg; 2.5/500: Glipizide 2.5 mg and metformin 500 mg; 5/500: Glipizide 5 mg and metformin 500 mg

Metaglip™: 2.5/500: Glipizide 2.5 mg and metformin 500 mg; 5/500: Glipizide 5 mg and metformin 500 mg

Dosing

Adult Type 2 diabetes:

Patients inadequately controlled on diet and exercise alone: Initial dose: Glipizide 2.5 mg/metformin 250 mg once daily with a meal. In patients with fasting plasma glucose (FPG) 280-320 mg/dL, initiate therapy with glipizide 2.5 mg/metformin 500 mg twice daily.

Note: Increase dose by 1 tablet/day every 2 weeks (maximum daily dose: Glipizide 10 mg/metformin 2000 mg in divided doses)

Patients inadequately controlled on a sulfonylurea and/or metformin: Initial dose: Glipizide 2.5 mg/metformin 500 mg or glipizide 5 mg/metformin 500 mg twice daily with morning and evening meals; starting dose should not exceed current daily dose of glipizide (or sulfonylurea equivalent) and/or metformin.

Note: Increase dose in increments of no more than glipizide 5 mg/metformin 500 mg (maximum daily dose: Glipizide 20 mg/metformin 2000 mg)

Geriatric Conservative doses are recommended in the elderly due to potentially decreased renal function; **do not titrate to maximum dose**; should not be used in patients ≥80 years unless renal function is verified as normal

Renal Impairment Contraindicated in the presence of renal disease or renal dysfunction (serum creatinine ≥1.5 mg/dL [males], ≥1.4 mg/dL [females], or abnormal creatinine clearance).

Hepatic Impairment Avoid use in patients with impaired liver function.

Administration

Oral All doses should be administered with a meal. Twice-daily dosing should be administered with the morning and evening meals. Patients that are NPO or require decreased caloric intake may need doses held to avoid hypoglycemia.

Monitoring and Teaching Issues

Laboratory Monitoring See individual agents.

Physical Assessment See individual agents.

Patient Education See individual agents.

Related Information

GlipiZIDE *on page 873*

MetFORMIN *on page 1182*

◆ **Glipizide and Metformin Hydrochloride** *see* Glipizide and Metformin *on page 875*

◆ **Glivec** *see* Imatinib *on page 951*

◆ **GlucaGen®** *see* Glucagon *on page 876*

◆ **GlucaGen® Diagnostic Kit** *see* Glucagon *on page 876*

◆ **GlucaGen® HypoKit®** *see* Glucagon *on page 876*

Glucagon (GLOO ka gon)

U.S. Brand Names GlucaGen®; GlucaGen® Diagnostic Kit; GlucaGen® HypoKit®; Glucagon Emergency Kit

Index Terms Glucagon Hydrochloride

Generic Availability (U.S.) No

Pharmacologic Category Antidote; Diagnostic Agent

Medication Safety Issues

Sound-alike/look-alike issues:

Glucagon may be confused with Glaucon®

Pregnancy Risk Factor B

Lactation Excretion in breast milk unknown/compatible

Use Management of hypoglycemia; diagnostic aid in radiologic examinations to temporarily inhibit GI tract movement

Unlabeled/Investigational Use Beta-blocker- or calcium channel blocker-induced myocardial depression (with or without hypotension) unresponsive to standard measures; suspected or documented hypoglycemia secondary to insulin or sulfonylurea overdose (as adjunct to dextrose)

Mechanism of Action/Effect Stimulates adenylate cyclase to produce increased cyclic AMP, which promotes hepatic glycogenolysis and gluconeogenesis, causing a raise in blood glucose levels

Contraindications Hypersensitivity to glucagon or any component of the formulation; insulinoma; pheochromocytoma

Warnings/Precautions Use of glucagon is contraindicated in insulinoma; exogenous glucagon may cause an initial rise in blood glucose followed by rebound hypoglycemia. Use of glucagon is contraindicated in pheochromocytoma; exogenous glucagon may cause the release of catecholamines, resulting in an increase in blood pressure. Use caution with prolonged fasting, starvation, adrenal insufficiency or chronic hypoglycemia; levels of glucose stores in liver may be decreased. Supplemental carbohydrates should be given to patients who respond to glucagon for severe hypoglycemia to prevent secondary hypoglycemia. Monitor blood glucose levels closely.

In patients with hypoglycemia secondary to insulin or sulfonylurea overdose, dextrose should be immediately administered; if I.V. access cannot be established or if dextrose is not available, glucagon may be considered as alternative acute treatment until dextrose can be administered.

May contain lactose; avoid administration in hereditary galactose intolerance, Lapp lactase deficiency, or glucose-galactose malabsorption.

Drug Interactions

Avoid Concomitant Use There are no known interactions where it is recommended to avoid concomitant use.

Decreased Effect There are no known significant interactions involving a decrease in effect.

Increased Effect/Toxicity

Glucagon may increase the levels/effects of: Vitamin K Antagonists

Nutritional/Ethanol Interactions Glucagon depletes glycogen stores.

Adverse Reactions Frequency not defined.

Cardiovascular: Hypotension (up to 2 hours after GI procedures), hypertension, tachycardia

Gastrointestinal: Nausea, vomiting (high incidence with rapid administration of high doses)

Miscellaneous: Hypersensitivity reactions, anaphylaxis

Pharmacodynamics/Kinetics

Onset of Action Peak effect: Blood glucose levels: Parenteral: I.V.: 5-20 minutes; I.M.: 30 minutes; SubQ: 30-45 minutes

Duration of Action Glucose elevation: SubQ: 60-90 minutes; I.V.: 30 minutes

Half-Life Elimination Plasma: 8-18 minutes

Metabolism Primarily hepatic; some inactivation occurring renally and in plasma

Available Dosage Forms

Injection, powder for reconstitution:

GlucaGen®: 1 mg

GlucaGen® Diagnostic Kit: 1 mg

GlucaGen® HypoKit®: 1 mg

Glucagon Emergency Kit: 1 mg

Dosing

Adult & Geriatric

Hypoglycemia: I.M., I.V., SubQ: 1 mg; may repeat in 20 minutes as needed

Note: I.V. dextrose should be administered as soon as it is available; if patient fails to respond to glucagon, I.V. dextrose must be given.

Beta-blocker- or calcium channel blocker-induced myocardial depression (with or without hypotension) unresponsive to standard measures (unlabeled use): I.V.: 3-10 mg (or 0.05-0.15 mg/kg) bolus followed by an infusion of 3-5 mg/hour (or 0.05-0.1 mg/kg/hour); titrate infusion rate to achieve adequate hemodynamic response (ACLS, 2010)

Diagnostic aid:

I.M.: 1-2 mg 10 minutes prior to procedure

I.V.: 0.25-2 mg 10 minutes prior to procedure

Pediatric

Hypoglycemia: I.M., I.V., SubQ:

Children <20 kg: 0.5 mg or 20-30 mcg/kg/dose; repeated in 20 minutes as needed

Children ≥20 kg: Refer to adult dosing.

Note: I.V. dextrose should be administered as soon as it is available; if patient fails to respond to glucagon, I.V. dextrose must be given.

Beta-blocker- or calcium channel blocker-induced myocardial depression (with or without hypotension) unresponsive to standard measures (unlabeled use): I.V.:

Children: Initial bolus of 30-150 mcg/kg followed by an infusion of 70 mcg/kg/hour (maximum: 5 mg/hour) (Hegenbarth, 2008)

Adolescents: Initial: 5-10 mg over several minutes followed by infusion of 1-5 mg/hour (Hegenbarth, 2008)

Administration

I.V. Bolus may be associated with nausea and vomiting.

Beta-blocker/calcium channel blocker toxicity: Administer bolus over 3-5 minutes; continuous infusions may be used. Ensure adequate supply available to continue therapy.

Stability

Reconstitution Reconstitute powder for injection by adding 1 mL of sterile diluent to a vial containing 1 unit of the drug, to provide solutions containing 1 mg of glucagon/mL. Gently roll vial to dissolve.

Storage Prior to reconstitution, store at controlled room temperature of 20°C to 25° (69°F to 77°F); do not freeze. Use reconstituted solution immediately. May be kept at 5°C for up to 48 hours if necessary.

Monitoring and Teaching Issues

Laboratory Monitoring Blood glucose

Physical Assessment Arouse patient from hypoglycemic or insulin shock as soon as possible and administer carbohydrates. Instruct patient (or significant other) in appropriate administration procedures for emergency use of glucagon.

Patient Education Identify appropriate support person to administer glucagon if necessary.

Dietary Considerations Administer carbohydrates to patient as soon as possible after response to treatment.

Geriatric Considerations No specific recommendations needed.

Additional Information 1 unit = 1 mg

- ◆ **Glucagon Emergency Kit** *see* Glucagon *on page 876*
- ◆ **Glucagon Hydrochloride** *see* Glucagon *on page 876*
- ◆ **Glucophage®** *see* MetFORMIN *on page 1182*
- ◆ **Glucophage® XR** *see* MetFORMIN *on page 1182*
- ◆ **Glucotrol®** *see* GlipiZIDE *on page 873*
- ◆ **Glucotrol XL®** *see* GlipiZIDE *on page 873*
- ◆ **Glucovance®** *see* Glyburide and Metformin *on page 880*
- ◆ **Glulisine Insulin** *see* Insulin Glulisine *on page 988*
- ◆ **Glumetza®** *see* MetFORMIN *on page 1182*
- ◆ **Glybenclamide** *see* GlyBURIDE *on page 877*
- ◆ **Glybenzcyclamide** *see* GlyBURIDE *on page 877*

GlyBURIDE (GLYE byoor ide)

U.S. Brand Names DiaBeta®; Glynase® PresTab®

Index Terms Diabeta; Glibenclamide; Glybenclamide; Glybenzcyclamide; Micronase

Generic Availability (U.S.) Yes

Pharmacologic Category Antidiabetic Agent, Sulfonylurea

Medication Safety Issues

Sound-alike/look-alike issues:

GlyBURIDE may be confused with glipiZIDE, Glucotrol®

Diaβeta® may be confused with Diabinese®, Zebeta®

Micronase may be confused with microK®, miconazole, Micronor®, Microzide™

High alert medication: The Institute for Safe Medication Practices (ISMP) includes this medication among its list of drugs which have a heightened risk of causing significant patient harm when used in error.

Pregnancy Risk Factor B/C (manufacturer dependent)

Lactation Does not enter breast milk/use caution

Use Adjunct to diet and exercise for the management of type 2 diabetes mellitus (noninsulin dependent, NIDDM)

Unlabeled/Investigational Use Alternative to insulin in women for the treatment of gestational diabetes mellitus (GDM) (11-33 weeks gestation)

Mechanism of Action/Effect Stimulates insulin release from the pancreatic beta cells; reduces glucose output from the liver; insulin sensitivity is increased at peripheral target sites

Contraindications Hypersensitivity to glyburide or any component of the formulation; type 1 diabetes mellitus (insulin dependent, IDDM), diabetic ketoacidosis; concomitant use with bosentan

Warnings/Precautions All sulfonylurea drugs are capable of producing severe hypoglycemia. Hypoglycemia is more likely to occur when caloric intake is deficient, after severe or prolonged exercise, when ethanol is ingested, or when more than one glucose-lowering drug is used. It is also more likely in elderly patients, malnourished patients and in patients with impaired renal or hepatic function; use with caution.

Elderly: Rapid and prolonged hypoglycemia (>12 hours) despite hypertonic glucose injections have been reported; age and hepatic and renal impairment are independent risk factors for hypoglycemia; dosage titration should be made at weekly intervals.

Chemical similarities are present among sulfonamides, sulfonylureas, carbonic anhydrase inhibitors, thiazides, and loop diuretics (except ethacrynic acid). Use in patients with sulfonamide allergy is not specifically contraindicated in product labeling, however, a risk of cross-reaction exists in patients with allergy to any of these compounds; avoid use when previous reaction has been severe.

Product labeling states oral hypoglycemic drugs may be associated with an increased cardiovascular mortality as compared to treatment with diet alone or diet plus insulin. Data to support this association are limited, and several studies, including a large prospective trial (UKPDS) have not supported an association.

Patients with G6PD deficiency may be at an increased risk of sulfonylurea-induced hemolytic anemia; however, cases have also been described in patients without G6PD deficiency during postmarketing surveillance. Use with caution and consider a nonsulfonylurea alternative in patients with G6PD deficiency.

Micronized glyburide tablets are **not** bioequivalent to *conventional* glyburide tablets; retitration should occur if patients are being transferred to a different glyburide formulation (eg, micronized-to-conventional or vice versa) or from other hypoglycemic agents.

It may be necessary to discontinue therapy and administer insulin if the patient is exposed to stress (fever, trauma, infection, surgery).

Drug Interactions

Metabolism/Transport Effects **Substrate** of CYP2C9 (major), 3A4 (minor); **Inhibits** CYP2C8 (weak), 3A4 (weak)

Avoid Concomitant Use

Avoid concomitant use of GlyBURIDE with any of the following: Bosentan

Decreased Effect

GlyBURIDE may decrease the levels/effects of: Bosentan

The levels/effects of GlyBURIDE may be decreased by: Bosentan; Colesevelam; Corticosteroids (Orally Inhaled); Corticosteroids (Systemic); CycloSPORINE; CycloSPORINE (Systemic); CYP2C9 Inducers (Highly Effective); Luteinizing Hormone-Releasing Hormone Analogs; Peginterferon Alfa-2b; Quinolone Antibiotics; Rifampin; Somatropin; Thiazide Diuretics

Increased Effect/Toxicity

GlyBURIDE may increase the levels/effects of: Alcohol (Ethyl); Bosentan; CycloSPORINE; CycloSPORINE (Systemic); Hypoglycemic Agents

The levels/effects of GlyBURIDE may be increased by: Beta-Blockers; Chloramphenicol; Cimetidine; Clarithromycin; Cyclic Antidepressants; CYP2C9 Inhibitors (Moderate); CYP2C9 Inhibitors (Strong); Fibric Acid Derivatives; Fluconazole; GLP-1 Agonists; Herbs (Hypoglycemic Properties); Pegvisomant; Quinolone Antibiotics; Ranitidine; Salicylates; Sulfonamide Derivatives; Voriconazole

Nutritional/Ethanol Interactions

Ethanol: Caution with ethanol (may cause hypoglycemia).

Herb/Nutraceutical: Herbs with hypoglycemic properties may enhance the hypoglycemic effect of glyburide. This includes alfalfa, aloe, bilberry, bitter melon, burdock, celery, damiana, fenugreek, garcinia, garlic, ginger, ginseng (American), gymnema, marshmallow, stinging nettle

Adverse Reactions Frequency not defined.

Cardiovascular: Vasculitis

Central nervous system: Dizziness, headache

Dermatologic: Angioedema, erythema, maculopapular eruptions, morbilliform eruptions, photosensitivity reaction, pruritus, purpura, rash, urticaria

Endocrine & metabolic: Disulfiram-like reaction, hypoglycemia, hyponatremia (SIADH reported with other sulfonylureas)

Gastrointestinal: Anorexia, constipation, diarrhea, epigastric fullness, heartburn, nausea

Genitourinary: Nocturia

Hematologic: Agranulocytosis, aplastic anemia, hemolytic anemia, leukopenia, pancytopenia, porphyria cutanea tarda, thrombocytopenia
Hepatic: Cholestatic jaundice, hepatitis, liver failure, transaminase increased
Neuromuscular & skeletal: Arthralgia, myalgia, paresthesia
Ocular: Blurred vision
Renal: Diuretic effect (minor)
Miscellaneous: Allergic reaction

Pharmacodynamics/Kinetics

Onset of Action Serum insulin levels begin to increase 15-60 minutes after a single dose

Duration of Action ≤24 hours

Absorption Significant within 1 hour

Bioavailability Variable among oral dosage forms

Time to Peak Serum: Adults: 2-4 hours

Protein Binding Plasma: >99% primarily to albumin

Half-Life Elimination Diabeta®: 10 hours; Glynase® PresTab®: ~4 hours; may be prolonged with renal or hepatic impairment

Metabolism Hepatic; forms metabolites (weakly active)

Excretion Feces (50%) and urine (50%) as metabolites

Available Dosage Forms

Tablet, oral: 1.25 mg, 1.5 mg, 2.5 mg, 3 mg, 5 mg, 6 mg
DiaBeta®: 1.25 mg, 2.5 mg, 5 mg
Glynase® PresTab®: 1.5 mg, 3 mg, 6 mg

Dosing

Adult Micronized glyburide tablets are **not** bioequivalent to conventional glyburide tablets; retitration should occur if patients are being transferred to a different glyburide formulation (eg, micronized-to-conventional or vice versa) or from other hypoglycemic agents.

Type 2 diabetes: Oral:

Note: Regular tablets cannot be used interchangeably with micronized tablet formulations

Regular tablets (Diaβeta®):

Initial: 2.5-5 mg/day, administered with breakfast or the first main meal of the day. In patients who are more sensitive to hypoglycemic drugs, start at 1.25 mg/day.

Adjustment: Increase in increments of no more than 2.5 mg/day at weekly intervals based on the patient's blood glucose response

Maintenance: 1.25-20 mg/day given as single or divided doses. Some patients (especially those receiving >10 mg/day) may have a more satisfactory response with twice-daily dosing. Maximum: 20 mg/day

Micronized tablets (Glynase® PresTab®):

Initial: 1.5-3 mg/day, administered with breakfast or the first main meal of the day in patients who are more sensitive to hypoglycemic drugs, start at 0.75 mg/day. Increase in increments of no more than 1.5 mg/day in weekly intervals based on the patient's blood glucose response.

Maintenance: 0.75-12 mg/day given as a single dose or in divided doses. Some patients (especially those receiving >6 mg/day) may have a more satisfactory response with twice-daily dosing. Maximum: 12 mg/day

Management of noninsulin-dependent diabetes mellitus in patients previously maintained on insulin: Oral: Initial dosage dependent upon previous insulin dosage, see table.

Dose Conversion: Insulin to Glyburide

Previous Daily Insulin Dosage (units/day)	Initial Glyburide Dosage *Conventional Formulation* (mg/day)	Initial Glyburide Dosage *Micronized Formulation* (mg/day)	Insulin Dosage Change (after glyburide started)
<20	2.5-5	1.5-3	Discontinue
20-40	5	3	Discontinue
>40	5 (increase in increments of 1.25-2.5 mg every 2-10 days)	3 (increase in increments of 0.75-1.5 mg every 2-10 days)	Reduce insulin dosage by 50% (gradually taper off insulin as glyburide dosage increased)

Geriatric Regular tablets (Diaβeta®): Oral: Initial: 1.25-2.5 mg/day, increase by 1.25-2.5 mg/day every 1-3 weeks. Refer to adult dosing.

Renal Impairment Cl_{cr} <50 mL/minute: Not recommended

Hepatic Impairment Use conservative initial and maintenance doses and avoid use in severe disease.

Administration

Oral Administer with meals at the same time each day (twice-daily dosing may be beneficial if conventional glyburide doses are >10 mg or micronized glyburide doses are >6 mg). Patients that are NPO or require decreased caloric intake may need doses held to avoid hypoglycemia.

Monitoring and Teaching Issues

Laboratory Monitoring Fasting blood glucose, hemoglobin A_{1c}

Physical Assessment Assess allergy history prior to beginning treatment. Monitor for hypoglycemia during therapy.

Patient Education This medication is used to control diabetes; it is not a cure. Monitor glucose as recommended by prescriber. Other important components of treatment plan may include prescribed diet and exercise regimen (consult prescriber or diabetic educator). If you experience hypoglycemic reaction, contact prescriber immediately. Always carry quick source of sugar with you. Take 30 minutes before meals at the same time each day. Avoid alcohol while taking this medication; could cause severe reaction. You may experience more sensitivity to sunlight, headache, or nausea. Report hypoglycemia (palpitations, sweaty palms, lightheadedness); extended vomiting, diarrhea, or constipation; flu-like symptoms; skin rash; easy bruising or bleeding; or change in color of urine or stool.

Dietary Considerations Should be taken with meals at the same time each day (twice-daily dosing may be beneficial if conventional glyburide doses are >10 mg or micronized glyburide doses are >6 mg). Individualized medical nutrition therapy (MNT) based on ADA recommendations is an integral part of therapy.

Geriatric Considerations Rapid and prolonged hypoglycemia (>12 hours) despite hypertonic glucose injections has been reported; age, hepatic, and renal impairment are independent risk factors for hypoglycemia; dosage titration should be made at weekly intervals. How "tightly" a geriatric patient's blood glucose should be controlled is controversial; however, a fasting blood sugar <150 mg/dL is now an acceptable endpoint. Such a decision should be based on the patient's functional and cognitive status, how well they recognize hypoglycemic or hyperglycemic symptoms, and how to respond to them and their other disease states. Use with caution in the elderly with renal insufficiency.

Breast-Feeding Considerations Data from initial studies note that glyburide was not detected in breast milk. Breast-feeding is not recommended by the manufacturer. Potentially, hypoglycemia may occur in a nursing infant exposed to a sulfonylurea via breast milk.

Pregnancy Considerations Reproduction studies differ by manufacturer labeling. Because adverse events were not observed in animal reproduction studies, one manufacturer classifies glyburide as pregnancy category B. Because adverse events were noted in animal studies during the period of lactation, another manufacturer classifies glyburide as pregnancy category C.

Glyburide was not found to significantly cross the placenta *in vitro* and was not found in the cord serum infants of mothers taking glyburide for gestational diabetes mellitus (GDM). Nonteratogenic effects such as hypoglycemia in the neonate have been associated with maternal glyburide use. Maternal hyperglycemia can be associated with adverse effects in the fetus, including macrosomia, neonatal hyperglycemia, and hyperbilirubinemia; the risk of congenital malformations is increased when the Hb A_{1c} is above the normal range. Diabetes can also be associated with adverse effects in the mother. Poorly-treated diabetes may cause end-organ damage that may in turn negatively affect obstetric outcomes. Physiologic glucose levels should be maintained prior to and during pregnancy to decrease the risk of adverse events in the mother and the fetus. The manufacturer recommends that if glyburide is used during pregnancy, it should be discontinued at least 2 weeks before the expected delivery date. Although studies have shown positive outcomes using glyburide for the treatment of GDM, use may not be appropriate for all women. Until additional safety and efficacy data are obtained, the use of oral agents is generally not recommended as routine management of type 2 diabetes mellitus during pregnancy. Insulin is considered the drug of choice for the control of diabetes mellitus during pregnancy.

Related Information

Diabetes Mellitus Management, Adults *on page 2026*

Glyburide and Metformin (GLYE byoor ide & met FOR min)

U.S. Brand Names Glucovance®

Index Terms Glyburide and Metformin Hydrochloride; Metformin and Glyburide

Generic Availability (U.S.) Yes

Pharmacologic Category Antidiabetic Agent, Biguanide; Antidiabetic Agent, Sulfonylurea

Medication Safety Issues

Sound-alike/look-alike issues:

Glucovance® may be confused with Vyvanse™

High alert medication: The Institute for Safe Medication Practices (ISMP) includes this medication among its list of drugs which have a heightened risk of causing significant patient harm when used in error.

Pregnancy Risk Factor B

Lactation Excretion in breast milk unknown/not recommended

Use Adjunct to diet and exercise for the management of type 2 diabetes mellitus (noninsulin dependent, NIDDM)

Available Dosage Forms

Tablet: Glyburide 1.25 mg and metformin 250 mg; glyburide 2.5 mg and metformin 500 mg; glyburide 5 mg and metformin 500 mg

Glucovance®: 2.5 mg/500 mg: Glyburide 2.5 mg and metformin 500 mg; 5 mg/500 mg: Glyburide 5 mg and metformin 500 mg

Dosing

Adult Note: Dose must be individualized. All doses should be taken with a meal. Twice daily dosage should be taken with the morning and evening meals. Dosages expressed as glyburide/metformin components.

Type 2 diabetes: Oral:

No prior treatment with sulfonylurea or metformin: Initial: 1.25 mg/250 mg once daily with a meal; patients with Hb A_{1c} >9% or fasting plasma glucose (FPG) >200 mg/dL may start with 1.25 mg/250 mg twice daily with meals. Adjustment: Dosage may be increased in increments of 1.25 mg/250 mg, at intervals of not less than 2 weeks; maximum daily dose: 10 mg/2000 mg (limited experience with higher doses); **Note:** Doses of 5 mg/500 mg should not be used as initial therapy, due to risk of hypoglycemia.

Previously treated with a sulfonylurea or metformin alone: Initial: 2.5 mg/500 mg or 5 mg/500 mg twice daily with meals; increase in increments no greater than 5 mg/500 mg; maximum daily dose: 20 mg/2000 mg

Note: When switching patients previously on a sulfonylurea and metformin together, do not exceed the daily dose of glyburide (or glyburide equivalent) or metformin. When adding thiazolidinedione, continue glyburide and metformin at current dose and initiate thiazolidinedione at recommended starting dose.

Combination with thiazolidinedione: May be combined with a thiazolidinedione in patients with an inadequate response to glyburide/metformin therapy, however the risk of hypoglycemia may be increased.

Geriatric Refer to adult dosing. Adjust carefully to renal function. Should not be used in patients ≥80 years of age unless renal function is verified as normal. Do not titrate to maximum dose.

Administration

Oral All doses should be administered with a meal. Twice-daily dosing should be administered with the morning and evening meals. Patients that are NPO or require decreased caloric intake may need doses held to avoid hypoglycemia.

Monitoring and Teaching Issues

Physical Assessment See individual agents.

Patient Education See individual agents.

Related Information

GlyBURIDE *on page 877*

MetFORMIN *on page 1182*

◆ **Glyburide and Metformin Hydrochloride** *see* Glyburide and Metformin *on page 880*

◆ **Glycerol Guaiacolate** *see* GuaiFENesin *on page 890*

◆ **Glyceryl Trinitrate** *see* Nitroglycerin *on page 1327*

Glycopyrrolate (glye koe PYE roe late)

U.S. Brand Names Cuvposa™; Robinul®; Robinul® Forte

Index Terms Glycopyrronium Bromide

Generic Availability (U.S.) Yes: Excludes oral solution

Pharmacologic Category Anticholinergic Agent

Medication Safety Issues

Sound-alike/look-alike issues:

Robinul® may be confused with Reminyl®

Pregnancy Risk Factor B (injection) / C (oral solution)

Lactation Excretion in breast milk unknown/use caution

Use Inhibit salivation and excessive secretions of the respiratory tract preoperatively; control of upper airway secretions; intraoperatively to counteract drug-induced or vagal mediated bradyarrhythmias; adjunct in treatment of peptic ulcer (indication listed in product labeling but currently has no place in management of peptic ulcer disease)

Cuvposa™: Reduce chronic, severe drooling in those with neurologic conditions (eg, cerebral palsy) associated with drooling

Unlabeled/Investigational Use Adjunct with acetylcholinesterase inhibitors (eg, neostigmine, edrophonium, pyridostigmine) to antagonize cholinergic effects

Mechanism of Action/Effect Blocks the action of acetylcholine at parasympathetic sites in smooth muscle, secretory glands, and the CNS; reduces saliva and thus drooling

Contraindications Hypersensitivity to glycopyrrolate or any component of the formulation; medical conditions that preclude use of anticholinergic medication; severe ulcerative colitis, toxic megacolon complicating ulcerative colitis, paralytic ileus, obstructive disease of GI tract (eg, pyloric stenosis), intestinal atony in the elderly or debilitated patient; unstable cardiovascular status in acute hemorrhage; narrow-angle glaucoma; acute hemorrhage; tachycardia; obstructive uropathy; myasthenia gravis

Oral solution: Additional contraindication: Concomitant use of potassium chloride in a solid oral dosage form

Warnings/Precautions Diarrhea may be a sign of incomplete intestinal obstruction, treatment should be discontinued if this occurs. Use caution in elderly and in patients with autonomic neuropathy, renal disease, or ulcerative colitis; may precipitate/aggravate ileus or toxic megacolon, hyperthyroidism, CAD, CHF, arrhythmias, tachycardia, BPH, or hiatal hernia with reflux. Use of anticholinergics in gastric ulcer treatment may cause a delay in gastric emptying. Caution should be used in individuals demonstrating decreased pigmentation (skin and iris coloration, dark versus light) since there has been some evidence that these individuals have an enhanced sensitivity to the anticholinergic response. May cause drowsiness, eye sensitivity to light, or blurred vision; caution should be used when performing tasks which require mental alertness, such as driving. The risk of heat stroke with this medication may be increased during ▶

exercise or hot weather. Injection contains benzyl alcohol (associated with gasping syndrome in neonates).

Drug Interactions

Avoid Concomitant Use

Avoid concomitant use of Glycopyrrolate with any of the following: Potassium Chloride

Decreased Effect

Glycopyrrolate may decrease the levels/effects of: Acetylcholinesterase Inhibitors (Central); Haloperidol; Levodopa; Secretin

The levels/effects of Glycopyrrolate may be decreased by: Acetylcholinesterase Inhibitors (Central)

Increased Effect/Toxicity

Glycopyrrolate may increase the levels/effects of: AbobotulinumtoxinA; Anticholinergics; Atenolol; Cannabinoids; Digoxin; MetFORMIN; OnabotulinumtoxinA; Potassium Chloride; RimabotulinumtoxinB

The levels/effects of Glycopyrrolate may be increased by: Amantadine; MAO Inhibitors; Pramlintide

Nutritional/Ethanol Interactions Food: Administration with a high-fat meal significantly reduced absorption; administer on an empty stomach.

Adverse Reactions

>10% (as reported with Cuvposa™):

Cardiovascular: Flushing (30%)

Central nervous system: Headache (15%)

Gastrointestinal: Vomiting (40%), xerostomia (40%), constipation (35%)

Genitourinary: Urinary retention (15%)

Respiratory: Nasal congestion (30%), sinusitis (15%), upper respiratory tract infection (15%)

<10% (frequency not always defined):

Cardiovascular: Pallor (≤2%), arrhythmias, cardiac arrest, heart block, hyper-/hypotension, malignant hyperthermia, palpitation, QT_c-interval prolongation, tachycardia

Central nervous system: Aggressiveness (≤2%), agitation (≤2%), crying (abnormal; ≤2%), irritability (≤2%), mood changes (≤2%), pain (≤2%), restlessness (≤2%), confusion, dizziness, drowsiness, excitement, insomnia, nervousness, seizure

Dermatologic: Dry skin (≤2%), pruritus (≤2%), rash (≤2%), urticaria

Endocrine & metabolic: Dehydration (≤2%), lactation suppression

Gastrointestinal: Abdominal distention (≤2%), abdominal pain (≤2%), flatulence (≤2%), retching (≤2%), bloated feeling, intestinal obstruction, loss of taste, nausea, pseudo-obstruction

Genitourinary: Urinary tract infection (≤2%), impotence, urinary hesitancy

Local: Injection site reactions (edema, erythema, pain)

Neuromuscular & skeletal: Weakness

Ocular: Nystagmus (≤2%), blurred vision, cycloplegia, mydriasis, ocular tension increased, photophobia, sensitivity to light increased

Respiratory: Bronchial secretion (thickening; ≤2%), nasal dryness (≤2%), pneumonia (≤2%), respiratory depression

Miscellaneous: Anaphylactoid reactions, diaphoresis decreased, hypersensitivity reactions

Pharmacodynamics/Kinetics

Onset of Action Oral: 50 minutes; I.M.: 15-30 minutes; I.V.: ~1 minute

Peak effect: Oral: ~1 hour; I.M.: 30-45 minutes

Duration of Action Vagal effect: 2-3 hours; Inhibition of salivation: Up to 7 hours; Anticholinergic: Oral: 8-12 hours

Absorption Oral tablet: Poor and erratic; Oral solution: 23% lower compared to tablet

Bioavailability Tablet: ~1% to 13%

Half-Life Elimination Infants: 22-130 minutes; Children 19-99 minutes; Adults: ~60-75 minutes; Oral solution: Adults: 3 hours

Metabolism Hepatic (minimal)

Excretion Urine (as unchanged drug, I.M.: 80%, I.V.: 85%); bile (as unchanged drug)

Available Dosage Forms

Injection, solution: 0.2 mg/mL (1 mL, 2 mL, 5 mL, 20 mL)

Robinul®: 0.2 mg/mL (1 mL, 2 mL, 5 mL, 20 mL)

Solution, oral:

Cuvposa™: 1 mg/5 mL (473 mL)

Tablet, oral: 1 mg, 2 mg

Robinul®: 1 mg

Robinul® Forte: 2 mg

Dosing

Adult & Geriatric

Reduction of secretions:

Preoperative: I.M.: 4 mcg/kg 30-60 minutes before procedure

Intraoperative: I.V.: 0.1 mg repeated as needed at 2- to 3-minute intervals

Reversal of neuromuscular blockade: I.V.: 0.2 mg for each 1 mg of neostigmine or 5 mg of pyridostigmine administered or 5-15 mcg/kg glycopyrrolate with 25-70 mcg/kg of neostigmine or 0.1-0.3 mg/kg of pyridostigmine (agents usually administered simultaneously, but glycopyrrolate may be administered first if bradycardia is present)

Pediatric

Reduction of secretions:

Preoperative: I.M.:

<2 years: 4-9 mcg/kg 30-60 minutes before procedure

>2 years: 4 mcg/kg 30-60 minutes before procedure

Intraoperative: I.V.: 4 mcg/kg not to exceed 0.1 mg; repeat at 2- to 3-minute intervals as needed.

Chronic (unlabeled):

Oral: 40-100 mcg/kg/dose 3-4 times/day

I.M., I.V.: 4-10 mcg/kg/dose every 3-4 hours; maximum: 0.2 mg/dose or 0.8 mg/24 hours

Drooling, chronic: Children 3-16 years: Oral solution (Cuvposa™): 0.02 mg/kg 3 times/day; titrate in increments of 0.02 mg/kg every 5-7 days as tolerated, up to a maximum dose of 0.1 mg/kg 3 times/day, not to exceed 1.5-3 mg/dose

Reversal of neuromuscular blockade: Refer to adult dosing.

Administration

Oral Administer oral solution on an empty stomach, 1 hour before or 2 hours after meals

I.V. Administer at a rate of 0.2 mg over 1-2 minutes.

Stability

Storage Store at 20°C to 25°C (68°F to 77°F).

Monitoring and Teaching Issues

Physical Assessment Assess potential for interactions with any drugs that may add to anticholinergic effects. Monitor for excessive dryness of eyes, nose, mouth, and throat.

Patient Education Take before meals. Void before taking medication. You may experience dizziness, blurred vision, dry mouth, photosensitivity, decreased ability to sweat, or impotence (temporary). Report excessive and persistent anticholinergic effects (blurred vision, headache, flushing, tachycardia, nervousness, constipation, dizziness, insomnia, mental confusion or excitement, dry mouth, altered taste perception, dysphagia, palpitations, bradycardia, urinary hesitancy or retention, impotence, decreased sweating).

Geriatric Considerations Anticholinergic agents are generally not well tolerated in the elderly and their use should be avoided when possible.

Breast-Feeding Considerations May suppress lactation

Pregnancy Considerations Teratogenic effects were not observed in animal studies. Small amounts of glycopyrrolate cross the human placenta.

◆ **Glycopyrronium Bromide** *see* Glycopyrrolate *on page* 881

◆ **Glydiazinamide** *see* GlipiZIDE *on page* 873

◆ **Glynase® PresTab®** *see* GlyBURIDE *on page* 877

◆ **Glyset®** *see* Miglitol *on page* 1231

◆ **GM-CSF** *see* Sargramostim *on page* 1624

Golimumab (goe LIM ue mab)

U.S. Brand Names Simponi™

Index Terms CNTO-148

Generic Availability (U.S.) No

Pharmacologic Category Antipsoriatic Agent; Antirheumatic, Disease Modifying; Monoclonal Antibody; Tumor Necrosis Factor (TNF) Blocking Agent

Medication Guide Available Yes

Pregnancy Risk Factor B

Lactation Excretion in breast milk unknown/not recommended

Use Treatment of active rheumatoid arthritis (moderate-to-severe), active psoriatic arthritis, and active ankylosing spondylitis

Mechanism of Action/Effect Monoclonal antibody that binds to human tumor necrosis factor alpha (TNFα), thereby decreasing inflammatory and other responses

Contraindications There are no contraindications listed in the FDA-approved manufacturer's labeling.

Canadian labeling: Hypersensitivity to golimumab, latex, or any other component of formulation or packaging; patients with severe infections (eg, sepsis, tuberculosis, opportunistic infections)

Warnings/Precautions [U.S. Boxed Warning]: Patients receiving golimumab are at increased risk for serious infections which may result in hospitalization and/or fatality; infections usually developed in patients receiving concomitant immunosuppressive agents (eg, methotrexate or corticosteroids); infection may be disseminated, rather than localized, upon presentation. Active tuberculosis (or reactivation of latent tuberculosis), invasive fungal (including aspergillosis, candidiasis, coccidioidomycosis, histoplasmosis, and pneumocystosis), bacterial, viral, and other opportunistic infections have been reported in patients receiving TNF-blocking agents, including golimumab. Monitor closely for signs/symptoms of infection. Discontinue for serious infection, opportunistic infection, or sepsis. Consider risks versus benefits prior to use in patients with a history of chronic or recurrent infection. Caution should be exercised when considering the use in patients with concomitant immunosuppressive therapy or predisposition to infection (eg, diabetes or residence/travel from areas of endemic mycoses). Do not administer to patients with an active chronic or localized infection. Patients who develop a new infection while undergoing treatment should be monitored closely. If a patient develops a serious infection, therapy should be discontinued.

[U.S. Boxed Warning]: Tuberculosis (disseminated or extrapulmonary) has been reported in patients receiving golimumab; both reactivation of latent infection and new infections have been reported. Patients should be evaluated for tuberculosis risk factors and latent tuberculosis infection (with a tuberculin skin test) prior to therapy. Treatment of latent tuberculosis should be initiated before use. Patients with initial negative tuberculin skin tests should receive continued monitoring for tuberculosis throughout treatment; active tuberculosis has developed in this population during treatment with TNF-blocking agents. Use with caution in patients who have resided in regions where tuberculosis is endemic. Consider antituberculosis therapy if an adequate course of treatment cannot be confirmed in patients with a history of latent or active tuberculosis or for patients with risk factors despite negative skin test.

Rare reactivation of HBV has occurred in chronic carriers of the virus usually in patients receiving concomitant immunosuppressants; evaluate prior to initiation and during treatment in patients at risk for HBV infection. If resumption of therapy is deemed necessary, exercise caution and monitor closely. Patients should be brought up to date with all immunizations before initiating therapy. Live vaccines should not be given concurrently. In clinical trials, humoral response to pneumococcal vaccine was not suppressed in psoriatic arthritis patients.

[U.S. Boxed Warning]: Lymphoma and other malignancies have been reported in children and adolescent patients receiving TNF-blocking agents. Half of the malignancies reported in children were lymphomas (Hodgkin's and non-Hodgkin's) while other cases varied and included malignancies not typically observed in this population. The impact of golimumab on the development and course of malignancy is not fully defined. Compared to the general population, an increased risk of lymphoma has been noted in clinical trials; however, rheumatoid arthritis alone has been previously associated with an increased rate of lymphoma. Lymphomas and other malignancies were also observed (at rates higher than expected for the general population) in adult patients receiving TNF-blocking agents. Treatment may result in the formation of autoimmune antibodies; cases of autoimmune disease have not been described. Neutralizing antibodies to golimumab may also be formed. Rarely, a reversible lupus-like syndrome has occurred with use of TNF blockers.

Use with caution in patients with pre-existing or recent onset CNS demyelinating disorders; rare cases of new onset or exacerbation of CNS demyelinating disorders have occurred; may present with mental status changes and some may be associated with permanent disability. Optic neuritis, transverse myelitis, multiple sclerosis, and new onset or exacerbation of seizures has been reported. Use with caution in patients with heart failure or decreased left ventricular function and discontinue use with new onset or worsening of symptoms. Use caution in patients with a history of significant hematologic abnormalities (cytopenias).

Avoid concomitant use with abatacept (increased incidence of serious infections) or anakinra (increased incidence of neutropenia and serious infection). Use with caution in the elderly (general incidence of infection is higher). Packaging (prefilled syringe and needle cover) contains dry natural rubber (latex). Some dosage forms may contain dry natural rubber (latex) and/or polysorbate 80.

Drug Interactions

Avoid Concomitant Use

Avoid concomitant use of Golimumab with any of the following: Abatacept; Anakinra; BCG; Belimumab; Canakinumab; Certolizumab Pegol; Natalizumab; Pimecrolimus; Rilonacept; Roflumilast; Tacrolimus (Topical); Vaccines (Live)

Decreased Effect

Golimumab may decrease the levels/effects of: BCG; Sipuleucel-T; Vaccines (Inactivated); Vaccines (Live)

The levels/effects of Golimumab may be decreased by: Echinacea

Increased Effect/Toxicity

Golimumab may increase the levels/effects of: Abatacept; Anakinra; Belimumab; Canakinumab; Certolizumab Pegol; Leflunomide; Natalizumab; Rilonacept; Vaccines (Live)

The levels/effects of Golimumab may be increased by: Abciximab; Denosumab; Pimecrolimus; Roflumilast; Tacrolimus (Topical); Trastuzumab

Adverse Reactions

>10%: Miscellaneous: Infection (28%)

1% to 10%:

- Cardiovascular: Hypertension (3%)
- Central nervous system: Dizziness (2%), fever (1%)
- Hepatic: ALT increased (4%), AST increased (3%)
- Local: Injection site reactions (6%), erythema (3%)
- Neuromuscular & skeletal: Paresthesia (1%)
- Respiratory: Upper respiratory tract infection (7%), nasopharyngitis (6%), bronchitis (2%), sinusitis (2%), rhinitis (1%)
- Miscellaneous: Antibody formation (4%), influenza (2%), oral herpes (1%)

Pharmacodynamics/Kinetics

Bioavailability SubQ: ~53%

Time to Peak SubQ: 2-6 days

Half-Life Elimination ~2 weeks

Available Dosage Forms

Injection, solution [preservative free]:

Simponi™: 50 mg/0.5 mL (0.5 mL)

Dosing

Adult & Geriatric Note: Should be administered in conjunction with methotrexate in rheumatoid arthritis; may administer with or without methotrexate or other nonbiologic disease-modifying antirheumatic drugs (DMARDs) in psoriatic arthritis or ankylosing spondylitis.

Rheumatoid arthritis, psoriatic arthritis, ankylosing spondylitis: SubQ: 50 mg once per month

Administration

Other Subcutaneous injection: Prior to administration, allow syringe to sit at room temperature for 30 minutes. Solution should be clear to slightly opalescent and colorless to light yellow. Discard if solution is cloudy, discolored, or has foreign particles. Hold autoinjector firmly against skin and inject subcutaneously into thigh, lower abdomen (below navel), or upper arm. A loud click is heard when injection has begun. Continue to hold autoinjector against skin until second click is heard (may take 3-15 seconds). Following second click, lift autoinjector from injection site. Discard any unused portion. Rotate injection sites and avoid injecting into tender, red, hard, or bruised skin.

Stability

Storage Store under refrigeration at 2°C to 8°C (36°F to 46°F); do not freeze. Do not shake. Protect from light.

Monitoring and Teaching Issues

Laboratory Monitoring CBC with differential

Physical Assessment Perform tuberculin skin test prior to initiating therapy. Monitor for signs of tuberculosis throughout therapy. Do not initiate therapy if active infection is present. Monitor closely for signs and symptoms of infection. Identify history of latex allergy; some dosage containers may contain latex. Assess for liver dysfunction. Assess results of laboratory tests (PDD) at regular intervals during treatment. If self-injected, teach patient appropriate injection technique and syringe/needle disposal.

Patient Education Inform prescriber of any allergies, history of tuberculosis, or any kind of infection you have. If self-administered, follow directions for injection and needle/syringe disposal exactly. You may be more susceptible to infection. May cause dizziness. Report persistent fever; increased bruising or bleeding; respiratory tract infection; unhealed or infected wounds; urinary tract infection; flu-like symptoms; unexplained weight loss; persistent cough; respiratory difficulty; unusual bump or sore that does not heal; weight gain; swelling of extremities; or redness, swelling, or pain at injection site.

Geriatric Considerations Phase three trials did not demonstrate any significant differences in adverse drug reactions, infections, or in the side effects profile in elderly compared to younger adults. However, since elderly experience a higher incidence of inffections, use with caution and close monitoring in the elderly patient.

Breast-Feeding Considerations It is not known whether golimumab is secreted in human milk. Because many immunoglobulins are secreted in milk and the potential for serious adverse reactions exists, a decision should be made whether to discontinue nursing or discontinue the drug, taking into account the importance of the drug to the mother.

Pregnancy Considerations In animal studies, no evidence of fetal harm has been demonstrated. There are no adequate and well-controlled studies in pregnant women. Use during pregnancy only if clearly needed.

◆ **GoLYTELY®** *see* Polyethylene Glycol-Electrolyte Solution *on page* 1474

◆ **Gonal-f®** *see* Follitropin Alfa *on page* 813

◆ **Gonal-f® RFF** *see* Follitropin Alfa *on page* 813

◆ **Gonal-f® RFF Pen** *see* Follitropin Alfa *on page* 813

Goserelin (GOE se rel in)

U.S. Brand Names Zoladex®

Index Terms Goserelin Acetate; ICI-118630; ZDX

Generic Availability (U.S.) No

Pharmacologic Category Antineoplastic Agent, Gonadotropin-Releasing Hormone Agonist; Gonadotropin Releasing Hormone Agonist

Pregnancy Risk Factor X (endometriosis, endometrial thinning); D (advanced breast cancer)

Lactation Excretion in breast milk unknown/not recommended

Use Treatment of locally confined prostate cancer; palliative treatment of advanced prostate cancer; palliative treatment of advanced breast cancer in pre- and perimenopausal women; treatment of endometriosis, including pain relief and reduction of endometriotic lesions; endometrial thinning agent as part of treatment for dysfunctional uterine bleeding

Mechanism of Action/Effect LHRH synthetic analog of luteinizing hormone-releasing hormone also known as gonadotropin-releasing hormone (GnRH)

Contraindications Hypersensitivity to goserelin, GnRH, GnRH agonist analogues, or any component of the formulation; pregnancy (except if using for palliative treatment of advanced breast cancer)

Warnings/Precautions Hazardous agent - use appropriate precautions for handling and disposal. Allergic hypersensitivity reactions (including anaphylaxis) and antibody formation may occur; monitor. Androgen-deprivation therapy may increase the risk for cardiovascular disease (Levine, 2010). Transient increases in serum testosterone (in men with prostate cancer) and estrogen (in women with breast cancer) may result in a worsening of disease signs and symptoms (tumor flare) during the first few weeks of treatment. Urinary tract obstruction or spinal cord compression have been reported when used for prostate cancer; ▶

closely observe patients for weakness, paresthesias, and urinary tract obstruction in first few weeks of therapy. Decreased bone density has been reported in women and may be irreversible; use caution if other risk factors are present; evaluate and institute preventative treatment if necessary.

Women of childbearing potential should not receive therapy until pregnancy has been excluded. Nonhormonal contraception is recommended for premenopausal women during therapy and for 12 weeks after therapy is discontinued. Cervical resistance may be increased; use caution when dilating the cervix. The 3-month implant currently has no approved indications for use in women. Rare cases of pituitary apoplexy (frequently secondary to pituitary adenoma) have been observed with GnRH administration (onset from 1 hour to usually <2 weeks); may present as sudden headache, vomiting, visual or mental status changes, and infrequently cardiovascular collapse; immediate medical attention required. Hyperglycemia has been reported in males and may manifest as diabetes or worsening of pre-existing diabetes. Decreased AUC may be observed when using the 3-month implant in obese patients. Monitor testosterone levels if desired clinical response is not observed. Safety and efficacy have not been established in pediatric patients.

Drug Interactions

Avoid Concomitant Use There are no known interactions where it is recommended to avoid concomitant use.

Decreased Effect

Goserelin may decrease the levels/effects of: Antidiabetic Agents

Increased Effect/Toxicity There are no known significant interactions involving an increase in effect.

Lab Interactions Interferes with pituitary gonadotropic and gonadal function tests during and for up to 12 weeks after discontinued

Adverse Reactions Percentages reported with the 1-month implant:

>10%:

Cardiovascular: Peripheral edema (female 21%)

Central nervous system: Headache (female 32% to 75%; male 1% to 5%), emotional lability (female 60%), depression (female 54%; male 1% to 5%), pain (female 17%; male 8%), insomnia (female 11%; male 5%)

Dermatologic: Acne (female 42%), seborrhea (female 26%)

Endocrine & metabolic: Hot flashes (female 57% to 96%; male 62%), libido decreased (female 48% to 61%), sexual dysfunction (male 21%), breast atrophy (female 33%), breast enlargement (female 18%), erections decreased (18%), libido increased (female 12%)

Gastrointestinal: Nausea (female 8% to 11%; male 5%), abdominal pain (female 7% to 11%)

Genitourinary: Vaginitis (75%), pelvic symptoms (female 9% to 18%), dyspareunia (female 14%), lower urinary symptoms (male 13%)

Neuromuscular & skeletal: Bone mineral density decreased (female 23%; ~4% decrease from baseline in 6 months; postmarketing reports in males), weakness (female 11%)

Miscellaneous: Diaphoresis (female 16% to 45%; male 6%), tumor flare (female: 23%), infection (female 13%)

1% to 10%:

Cardiovascular: Arrhythmia, cerebrovascular accident, chest pain, edema, heart failure, hypertension, MI, palpitation, peripheral vascular disorder, tachycardia

Central nervous system: Abnormal thinking, anxiety, chills, dizziness, fever, lethargy, malaise, migraine, nervousness, somnolence

Dermatologic: Alopecia, bruising, dry skin, hair disorder, hirsutism, pruritus, rash, skin discoloration

Endocrine & metabolic: Breast pain, breast swelling/tenderness, dysmenorrhea, gout, hyperglycemia

Gastrointestinal: Anorexia, appetite increased, constipation, diarrhea, dyspepsia, flatulence, ulcer, vomiting, weight gain/loss, xerostomia

Genitourinary: Urinary frequency, urinary obstruction, urinary tract infection, vaginal hemorrhage, vulvovaginitis

Hematologic: Anemia, hemorrhage

Local: Application site reaction

Neuromuscular & skeletal: Arthralgia, back pain, hypertonia, joint disorder, leg cramps, myalgia, paresthesia

Ocular: Amblyopia, dry eyes

Renal: Renal insufficiency

Respiratory: Bronchitis, COPD, cough, epistaxis, pharyngitis, rhinitis, sinusitis, upper respiratory tract infection

Miscellaneous: Allergic reaction, flu-like syndrome, voice alteration

Pharmacodynamics/Kinetics

Onset of Action

Females: Estradiol suppression reaches postmenopausal levels within 3 weeks and FSH and LH are suppressed to follicular phase levels within 4 weeks of initiation.

Males: Testosterone suppression reaches castrate levels within 2-4 weeks after initiation.

Duration of Action

Females: Estradiol, LH and FSH generally return to baseline levels within 12 weeks following the last monthly implant.

Males: Testosterone levels maintained at castrate levels throughout the duration of therapy.

Absorption SubQ: Rapid and can be detected in serum in 30-60 minutes; 3.6 mg: released slowly in first 8 days, then rapid and continuous release for 28 days

Time to Peak SubQ: Male: 12-15 days, Female: 8-22 days

Protein Binding 27%

Half-Life Elimination SubQ: Male: ~4 hours, Female: ~2 hours; Renal impairment: Male: 12 hours

Excretion Urine (>90%; 20% as unchanged drug)

Available Dosage Forms

Implant, subcutaneous:

Zoladex®: 3.6 mg (1s); 10.8 mg (1s)

Dosing

Adult & Geriatric

Prostate cancer, advanced: SubQ:

28-day implant: 3.6 mg every 28 days

12-week implant: 10.8 mg every 12 weeks

Prostate cancer, locally confined (in combination with an antiandrogen and radiotherapy; begin 8 weeks prior to radiotherapy): SubQ:

Combination 28-day/12-week implant: 3.6 mg implant, followed in 28 days by 10.8 mg implant

28-day implant (alternate dosing): 3.6 mg; repeated every 28 days for a total of 4 doses

Breast cancer, advanced: SubQ: 3.6 mg every 28 days

Endometriosis: SubQ: 3.6 mg every 28 days for 6 months

Endometrial thinning: SubQ: 3.6 mg every 28 days for 1 or 2 doses

Renal Impairment No adjustment is necessary.

Hepatic Impairment No adjustment is necessary.

Administration

Other SubQ: Administer implant by inserting needle at a 30-45 degree angle into the anterior abdominal wall below the navel line. Goserelin is an implant; therefore, do not attempt to eliminate air bubbles prior to injection (may displace implant). Do not attempt to aspirate prior to injection; if a large vessel is penetrated, blood will be visualized in the syringe chamber (if vessel is penetrated, withdraw needle and inject elsewhere with a new syringe). Do not penetrate into muscle or peritoneum. Implant may be detected by ultrasound if removal is required.

Stability

Storage Zoladex® should be stored at room temperature not to exceed 25°C (77°F). Protect from light.

Monitoring and Teaching Issues

Laboratory Monitoring Serum calcium, cholesterol/lipids

Prostate cancer: Screen for diabetes

Physical Assessment Monitor patients for development of diabetes; manage cardiovascular risk factors.

Patient Education This drug must be implanted under the skin of your abdomen every 28 days or every 3 months; it is important to maintain appointment schedule. If you have diabetes, monitor blood sugar frequently; can cause loss of glycemic control/hyperglycemia. Males or females, you may experience systemic hot flashes; headache; depression; mood swings; insomnia; acne; increased sweating, especially in women; constipation; sexual dysfunction (decreased libido, decreased erection for males, vaginal dryness for females); or bone pain. Symptoms may worsen temporarily during first weeks of therapy. Report chest pain, palpitations, or respiratory difficulty; swelling of extremities; unusual persistent nausea, vomiting, or constipation; infections; unresolved dizziness; skin rash; or paresthesias or muscle weakness.

Geriatric Considerations No dosage adjustments are needed in the elderly. Monitoring for bone density changes, serum lipid, hemoglobin A_{1c}, blood pressure, and serum calcium changes is recommended.

Breast-Feeding Considerations Goserelin is inactivated when used orally. Breast-feeding is not recommended by the manufacturer.

Pregnancy Considerations Goserelin has been found to be teratogenic and increases pregnancy loss in animal studies. Goserelin induces hormonal changes which increase the risk for fetal loss and use is contraindicated in pregnancy unless being used for palliative treatment of advanced breast cancer.

Breast cancer: If used for the palliative treatment of breast cancer during pregnancy, the potential for increased fetal loss should be discussed with the patient.

Endometriosis, endometrial thinning: Women of childbearing potential should not receive therapy until pregnancy has been excluded. Nonhormonal contraception is recommended for premenopausal women during therapy and for 12 weeks after therapy is discontinued. Although ovulation is usually inhibited and menstruation may stop, pregnancy prevention is not ensured during goserelin therapy. Changes in reproductive function may occur following chronic administration.

Additional Information If removal is necessary, implant may be located by ultrasound.

◆ **Goserelin Acetate** *see* Goserelin *on page* *885*

◆ **GP 47680** *see* OXcarbazepine *on page* *1375*

◆ **GR38032R** *see* Ondansetron *on page* *1360*

Granisetron (gra NI se tron)

U.S. Brand Names Granisol™; Kytril®; Sancuso®

Index Terms BRL 43694

Generic Availability (U.S.) Yes: Injection, tablet

Pharmacologic Category Antiemetic; Selective 5-HT_3 Receptor Antagonist

Medication Safety Issues

Sound-alike/look-alike issues:

Granisetron may be confused with dolasetron, ondansetron, palonosetron

Pregnancy Risk Factor B

Lactation Excretion in breast milk unknown/use caution

Use Prophylaxis of nausea and vomiting associated with emetogenic chemotherapy and radiation therapy; prophylaxis and treatment of postoperative nausea and vomiting (PONV)

Unlabeled/Investigational Use Breakthrough treatment of nausea and vomiting associated with chemotherapy

Mechanism of Action/Effect Selective 5-HT_3 receptor antagonist, blocking serotonin, both peripherally on vagal nerve terminals and centrally in the chemoreceptor trigger zone.

Contraindications Hypersensitivity to granisetron or any component of the formulation

Warnings/Precautions Use with caution in patients with congenital long QT syndrome or other risk factors for QT prolongation (eg, medications known to prolong QT interval, electrolyte abnormalities, and cumulative high-dose anthracycline therapy). 5-HT_3 antagonists have been associated with a number of dose-dependent increases in ECG intervals (eg, PR, QRS duration, QT/QT_c, JT), usually occurring 1-2 hours after I.V. administration. In general, these changes are not clinically relevant, however, when used in conjunction with other agents that prolong these intervals, arrhythmia may occur. When used with agents that prolong the QT interval (eg, Class I and III antiarrhythmics), clinically relevant QT interval prolongation may occur resulting in torsade de pointes. I.V. formulations of 5-HT_3 antagonists have more association with ECG interval changes, compared to oral formulations.

For chemotherapy-related emesis, **granisetron should be used on a scheduled basis, not on an "as needed" (PRN) basis**, since data support the use of this drug in the prevention of nausea and vomiting and not in the rescue of nausea and vomiting. Granisetron should be used only in the first 24-48 hours of receiving chemotherapy or radiation. Data do not support any increased efficacy of granisetron in delayed nausea and vomiting.

Use with caution in patients allergic to other 5-HT_3 receptor antagonists; cross-reactivity has been reported. Routine prophylaxis for PONV is not recommended in patients where there is little expectation of nausea and vomiting postoperatively. In patients where nausea and vomiting must be avoided postoperatively, administer to all patients even when expected incidence of nausea and vomiting is low. Use caution following abdominal surgery or in chemotherapy-induced nausea and vomiting; may mask progressive ileus or gastric distention. Application site reactions, generally mild, have occurred with transdermal patch use; if skin reaction is severe or generalized, remove patch. Cover patch application site with clothing to protect from natural or artificial sunlight exposure while patch is applied and for 10 days following removal; granisetron may potentially be affected by natural or artificial sunlight. Do not apply patch to red, irritated, or damaged skin. Injection contains benzyl alcohol (1 mg/mL) and should not be used in neonates.

Drug Interactions

Metabolism/Transport Effects Substrate of CYP3A4 (minor)

Avoid Concomitant Use

Avoid concomitant use of Granisetron with any of the following: Apomorphine

Decreased Effect There are no known significant interactions involving a decrease in effect.

Increased Effect/Toxicity

Granisetron may increase the levels/effects of: Apomorphine

The levels/effects of Granisetron may be increased by: Conivaptan

Adverse Reactions

>10%:

Central nervous system: Headache (3% to 21%; transdermal patch: 1%)
Gastrointestinal: Constipation (3% to 18%)
Neuromuscular & skeletal: Weakness (5% to 18%)

1% to 10%:

Cardiovascular: QT_c prolongation (1% to 3%), hypertension (1% to 2%)
Central nervous system: Pain (10%), fever (3% to 9%), dizziness (4% to 5%), insomnia (<2% to 5%), somnolence (1% to 4%), anxiety (2%), agitation (<2%), CNS stimulation (<2%)
Dermatologic: Rash (1%)
Gastrointestinal: Diarrhea (3% to 9%), abdominal pain (4% to 6%), dyspepsia (3% to 6%), taste perversion (2%)
Hepatic: Liver enzymes increased (5% to 6%)
Renal: Oliguria (2%)
Respiratory: Cough (2%)
Miscellaneous: Infection (3%)

Pharmacodynamics/Kinetics

Duration of Action Oral, I.V.: Generally up to 24 hours

Absorption Oral: Tablets and oral solution are bioequivalent; Transdermal patch: ~66% over 7 days

Time to Peak Transdermal patch: Maximum systemic concentrations: ~48 hours after application (range: 24-168 hours)

Protein Binding 65%

Half-Life Elimination Oral: 6 hours; I.V.: 9 hours

Metabolism Hepatic via N-demethylation, oxidation, and conjugation; some metabolites may have 5-HT_3 antagonist activity

Excretion Urine (12% as unchanged drug, 48% to 49% as metabolites); feces (34% to 38% as metabolites)

Available Dosage Forms

Injection, solution: 1 mg/mL (1 mL, 4 mL)

Injection, solution [preservative free]: 0.1 mg/mL (1 mL); 1 mg/mL (1 mL)

Patch, transdermal:

Sancuso®: 3.1 mg/24 hours (1s)

Solution, oral:

Granisol™: 2 mg/10 mL (30 mL)

Tablet, oral: 1 mg

Kytril®: 1 mg

Dosing

Adult & Geriatric

Prophylaxis of chemotherapy-related emesis:

Oral: 2 mg once daily up to 1 hour before chemotherapy or 1 mg twice daily; the first 1 mg dose should be given up to 1 hour before chemotherapy.

I.V.:

Within U.S.: 10 mcg/kg/dose (maximum: 1 mg/dose) given 30 minutes prior to chemotherapy; for some drugs (eg, carboplatin, cyclophosphamide) with a later onset of emetic action, 10 mcg/kg every 12 hours may be necessary.

Outside U.S.: 40 mcg/kg/dose (or 3 mg/dose); maximum: 9 mg/24 hours

Breakthrough: Granisetron has not been shown to be effective in terminating nausea or vomiting once it occurs and should not be used for this purpose.

Transdermal patch: Prophylaxis of chemotherapy-related emesis: Apply 1 patch at least 24 hours prior to chemotherapy; do not apply ≥48 hours before chemotherapy. Remove patch a minimum of 24 hours after chemotherapy completion. Maximum duration: Patch may be worn up to 7 days, depending on chemotherapy regimen duration.

Prophylaxis of radiation therapy-associated emesis: Oral: 2 mg once daily given 1 hour before radiation therapy.

Postoperative nausea and vomiting (PONV): I.V.:

Prevention: 1 mg given undiluted over 30 seconds; the manufacturer recommends administration before induction of anesthesia or immediately before reversal of anesthesia. **Note:** The Society for Ambulatory Anesthesia (SAMBA) Guidelines recommend a dosage range of 0.35-1.5 mg administered at the end of surgery (Gan, 2007). However, doses ≤1 mg are generally used since doses >1 mg are not more effective. Of note, 5 mcg/kg (~0.35 mg in a 70 kg adult) has been shown to be effective; doses >5 mcg/kg were not more effective (Mikawa, 1997).

Treatment: 1 mg given undiluted over 30 seconds

Pediatric Prophylaxis associated with cancer chemotherapy: Children >2 years: Refer to adult dosing.

Renal Impairment No dosage adjustment required.

Hepatic Impairment Kinetic studies in patients with hepatic impairment showed that total clearance was approximately halved; however, standard doses were very well tolerated, and dose adjustments are not necessary.

Administration

Oral Doses should be given up to 1 hour prior to initiation of chemotherapy/radiation

I.V. Administer I.V. push over 30 seconds or as a 5- to 10-minute infusion

Prevention of PONV: Administer before induction of anesthesia or immediately before reversal of anesthesia.

Treatment of PONV: Administer undiluted over 30 seconds.

Topical Transdermal (Sancuso®): Apply patch to clean, dry, intact skin on upper outer arm. Do not use on red, irritated or damaged skin. Remove patch from pouch immediately before application. Do not cut patch.

Stability

Storage

I.V.: Store at 15°C to 30°C (59°F to 86°F). Protect from light. Do not freeze vials. Stable when mixed in NS or D_5W for 7 days under refrigeration and for 3 days at room temperature.

Oral: Store tablet or oral solution at 15°C to 30°C (59°F to 86°F). Protect from light.

Transdermal patch: Store at 20°C to 25°C (68°F to 77°F). Keep patch in original packaging until immediately prior to use.

Monitoring and Teaching Issues

Physical Assessment Assess allergy history (selective 5-HT_3 receptor antagonists) prior to administering. Use with caution in presence of, or potential for, cardiac conduction abnormalities (eg, QT prolongation, medication known to prolong QT interval, electrolyte abnormalities). Oral, I.V., and transdermal formulations have different doses and schedules and should not be administered on a PRN basis.

Patient Education This drug is given to prevent nausea and vomiting. If this medication is given by intravenous infusion you will be monitored during infusion. Report immediately any chest pain, respiratory difficulty, or pain or itching at infusion site. Remove patch from packaging pouch immediately before application; do not cut patch. Apply to clean, dry, intact skin on upper outer arm. You may experience headache, drowsiness, or dizziness. Report chest pain or palpitations, persistent headache, excessive drowsiness, fever, or changes in elimination patterns (constipation or diarrhea).

Geriatric Considerations Clinical trials with patients older than 65 years of age are limited; however, the data indicates that safety and efficacy are similar to that observed in younger adults. No adjustment in dose necessary for elderly.

Pregnancy Considerations There are no adequate or well-controlled studies in pregnant women. Teratogenic effects were not observed in animal studies. Injection (1 mg/mL strength) contains benzyl alcohol which may cross the placenta. Use only if benefit exceeds the risk.

◆ **Granisol™** *see* Granisetron *on page 887*

◆ **Granulocyte Colony Stimulating Factor** *see* Filgrastim *on page 760*

◆ **Granulocyte-Macrophage Colony Stimulating Factor** *see* Sargramostim *on page 1624*

◆ **Green Tea Extract** *see* Sinecatechins *on page 1647*

◆ **Grifulvin V®** *see* Griseofulvin *on page 890*

Griseofulvin (gri see oh FUL vin)

U.S. Brand Names Grifulvin V®; Gris-PEG®

Index Terms Griseofulvin Microsize; Griseofulvin Ultramicrosize

Generic Availability (U.S.) Yes: Suspension, ultramicrosized product

Pharmacologic Category Antifungal Agent, Oral

Medication Safety Issues

Sound-alike/look-alike issues:

International issues: Fulvicin® (brand name used in international markets) may be confused with Furacin®

Pregnancy Risk Factor C

Lactation Excretion in breast milk unknown/use caution

Use Treatment of susceptible tinea infections of the skin, hair, and nails

Available Dosage Forms

Suspension, oral: 125 mg/5 mL (120 mL)

Tablet, oral:

Grifulvin V®: 500 mg

Gris-PEG®: 125 mg, 250 mg

Dosing

Adult & Geriatric

Tinea infections: Oral:

Microsize: 500-1000 mg/day in single or divided doses

Ultramicrosize: 375 mg/day in single or divided doses; doses up to 750 mg/day have been used for infections more difficult to eradicate such as tinea unguium and tinea pedis.

Note: Duration of therapy depends on the site of infection:

Tinea corporis: 2-4 weeks

Tinea capitis: 4-6 weeks or longer (up to 8-12 weeks)

Tinea pedis: 4-8 weeks

Tinea unguium: 4-6 months

Pediatric

Tinea infections: Oral: Children >2 years:

Microsize: 10-20 mg/kg/day in single or divided doses. In the treatment of tinea capitis, higher dosages (20-25 mg/kg/day for 8-12 weeks) have been recommended by some authors (unlabeled).

Ultramicrosize: Usual: 7.3 mg/kg/day in single dose or 2 divided doses; range: 5-15 mg/kg/day in single dose or 2 divided doses (maximum: 750 mg/day)

Administration

Oral Administer with a fatty meal (peanuts or ice cream) to increase absorption, or with food or milk to avoid GI upset

Gris-PEG® tablets: May be swallowed whole or crushed and sprinkled onto 1 tablespoonful of applesauce and swallowed immediately without chewing.

Monitoring and Teaching Issues

Laboratory Monitoring Periodic renal, hepatic, and hematopoietic function especially with long-term use

Physical Assessment Assess renal and hepatic function with long-term use. Monitor for CNS changes, gastrointestinal upset, rash, and opportunistic infection periodically during therapy.

Patient Education Avoid alcohol while taking this drug (disulfiram reactions). You may experience confusion, dizziness, drowsiness, nausea, vomiting, diarrhea, or increased sensitivity to sun. Report skin rash, respiratory difficulty, CNS changes (confusion, dizziness, acute headache), changes in color of stool or urine, or worsening of condition.

◆ **Griseofulvin Microsize** *see* Griseofulvin *on page 890*

◆ **Griseofulvin Ultramicrosize** *see* Griseofulvin *on page 890*

◆ **Gris-PEG®** *see* Griseofulvin *on page 890*

◆ **Growth Hormone, Human** *see* Somatropin *on page 1664*

◆ **GSK-580299** *see* Papillomavirus (Types 16, 18) Vaccine (Human, Recombinant) *on page 1409*

GuaiFENesin (gwye FEN e sin)

U.S. Brand Names Allfen [OTC]; Bidex®-400 [OTC]; Diabetic Siltussin DAS-Na [OTC]; Diabetic Tussin® EX [OTC]; Fenesin IR [OTC]; Ganidin® NR [OTC] [DSC]; Humibid® Maximum Strength [OTC]; Mucinex® Kid's Mini-Melts™ [OTC]; Mucinex® Kid's [OTC]; Mucinex® Maximum Strength [OTC]; Mucinex® [OTC]; Mucus Relief [OTC]; Organidin® NR [OTC] [DSC]; Phanasin® Diabetic Choice® [OTC] [DSC]; Phanasin® [OTC] [DSC]; Refenesen™ 400 [OTC]; Refenesen™ [OTC]; Robafen [OTC]; Robitussin® Chest Congestion [OTC] [DSC]; Scot-Tussin® Expectorant [OTC]; Siltussin DAS [OTC] [DSC]; Siltussin SA [OTC]; Vicks® Casero™ Chest Congestion Relief [OTC]; Vicks® DayQuil® Mucus Control [OTC]; Xpect™ [OTC]

Index Terms Cheratussin; GG; Glycerol Guaiacolate
Generic Availability (U.S.) Yes: Excludes extended release and granules
Pharmacologic Category Expectorant
Medication Safety Issues
Sound-alike/look-alike issues:
GuaiFENesin may be confused with guanFACINE
Mucinex® may be confused with Mucomyst®
Naldecon® may be confused with Nalfon®

International issues:
Mucolex® [Hong Kong] may be confused with Mycelex® which is a brand name for clotrimazole in the U.S.

Pregnancy Risk Factor C
Lactation Excretion in breast milk unknown/use caution
Use Help loosen phlegm and thin bronchial secretions to make coughs more productive
Available Dosage Forms
Caplet, oral:
Fenesin IR [OTC]: 400 mg
Refenesen™ 400 [OTC]: 400 mg
Granules, oral:
Mucinex® Kid's Mini-Melts™ [OTC]: 50 mg/packet (12s); 100 mg/packet (12s)
Liquid, oral:
Diabetic Tussin® EX [OTC]: 100 mg/5 mL (118 mL)
Mucinex® Kid's [OTC]: 100 mg/5 mL (118 mL)
Scot-Tussin® Expectorant [OTC]: 100 mg/5 mL (120 mL)
Vicks® Casero™ Chest Congestion Relief [OTC]: 100 mg/6.25 mL (120 mL, 240 mL)
Vicks® DayQuil® Mucus Control [OTC]: 200 mg/15 mL (295 mL)
Syrup, oral: 100 mg/5 mL (5 mL, 10 mL, 15 mL, 118 mL, 120 mL, 240 mL, 473 mL, 480 mL)
Diabetic Siltussin DAS-Na [OTC]: 100 mg/5 mL (118 mL)
Robafen [OTC]: 100 mg/5 mL (120 mL, 240 mL, 480 mL)
Siltussin SA [OTC]: 100 mg/5 mL (120 mL, 240 mL, 480 mL)
Tablet, oral: 400 mg
Allfen [OTC]: 400 mg
Bidex®-400 [OTC]: 400 mg
Mucus Relief [OTC]: 400 mg
Refenesen™ [OTC]: 200 mg
Xpect™ [OTC]: 400 mg
Tablet, extended release, oral:
Humibid® Maximum Strength [OTC]: 1200 mg
Mucinex® [OTC]: 600 mg
Mucinex® Maximum Strength [OTC]: 1200 mg

Dosing
Adult & Geriatric
Cough (expectorant): Oral: 200-400 mg every 4 hours to a maximum of 2.4 g/day
Extended release tablet: 600-1200 mg every 12 hours, not to exceed 2.4 g/day
Pediatric
Cough (expectorant): Oral: Children:
6 months to 2 years: 25-50 mg every 4 hours, not to exceed 300 mg/day
2-5 years: 50-100 mg every 4 hours, not to exceed 600 mg/day
6-11 years: 100-200 mg every 4 hours, not to exceed 1.2 g/day
>12 years: Refer to adult dosing.

Administration
Oral Do not crush, chew, or break extended release tablets. Administer with a full glass of water.

Monitoring and Teaching Issues
Patient Education Do not chew or crush extended release tablet; take with a full glass of water. Maintain adequate hydration, unless instructed to restrict fluid intake. Report excessive drowsiness, respiratory difficulty, lack of improvement, or worsening of condition.

Guaifenesin and Codeine (gwye FEN e sin & KOE deen)

U.S. Brand Names Allfen CD; Allfen CDX; Dex-Tuss; ExeClear-C; Gani-Tuss® NR; Mar-Cof® CG; Robafen AC; Tusso-C™
Index Terms Codeine and Guaifenesin; Robitussin AC
Generic Availability (U.S.) Yes: Oral solution, syrup
Pharmacologic Category Antitussive; Cough Preparation; Expectorant
Pregnancy Risk Factor C
Lactation Excretion in breast milk unknown/use caution
Use Temporary control of cough due to minor throat and bronchial irritation
Controlled Substance C-V
Available Dosage Forms
Liquid, oral:
Dex-Tuss: Guaifenesin 300 mg and codeine 10 mg per 5 mL
Gani-Tuss® NR: Guaifenesin 100 mg and codeine 10 mg per 5 mL

Solution, oral: Guaifenesin 100 mg and codeine 10 mg per 5 mL
Mar-Cof® CG: Guaifenesin 225 mg and codeine 7.5 mg per 5 mL
Syrup, oral: Guaifenesin 100 mg and codeine 10 mg per 5 mL (473 mL)
ExeClear-C, Tusso-C™: Guaifenesin 200 mg and codeine 10 mg per 5 mL
Robafen AC: Guaifenesin 100 mg and codeine 10 mg per 5 mL
Tablet, oral:
Allfen CD: Guaifenesin 400 mg and codeine 10 mg
Allfen CDX: Guaifenesin 400 mg and codeine 20 mg

Dosing

Adult & Geriatric Cough (antitussive/expectorant): Oral:
ExeClear-C: 10 mL every 4-6 hours; maximum: 60 mL/24 hours
Dex-Tuss, Gani-Tuss® NR: 5 mL every 4-6 hours; maximum 40 mL/24 hours
Note: Also refer to specific product labeling.

Pediatric Cough (antitussive/expectorant): Oral:
Children 6-11 years:
ExeClear-C: 5 mL every 4-6 hours; maximum: 30 mL/24 hours
Dex-Tuss, Gani-Tuss® NR: 2.5 mL every 4-6 hours; maximum: 20 mL/24 hours
Children ≥12 years: Refer to adult dosing.
Note: Also refer to specific product labeling.

Monitoring and Teaching Issues

Physical Assessment See individual agents.

Patient Education See individual agents.

Related Information

Codeine *on page* 421
GuaiFENesin *on page* 890

◆ **GW433908G** *see* Fosamprenavir *on page* 823

◆ **GW572016** *see* Lapatinib *on page* 1064

◆ **GW786034** *see* Pazopanib *on page* 1418

◆ **H1N1 Influenza Vaccine** *see* Influenza Virus Vaccine (Inactivated) *on page* 978

◆ **H1N1 Influenza Vaccine** *see* Influenza Virus Vaccine (Live/Attenuated) *on page* 980

◆ **H5N1 Influenza Vaccine** *see* Influenza Virus Vaccine (H5N1) *on page* 977

◆ **Habitrol** *see* Nicotine *on page* 1312

Haemophilus b Conjugate and Hepatitis B Vaccine

(he MOF i lus bee KON joo gate & hep a TYE tis bee vak SEEN)

U.S. Brand Names Comvax®

Index Terms *Haemophilus* b (meningococcal protein conjugate) Conjugate Vaccine; Hepatitis B Vaccine (Recombinant); Hib Conjugate Vaccine; Hib-HepB

Generic Availability (U.S.) No

Pharmacologic Category Vaccine, Inactivated (Bacterial); Vaccine, Inactivated (Viral)

Medication Safety Issues

Sound-alike/look-alike issues:
Comvax® may be confused with Recombivax [Recombivax HB®]

Pregnancy Risk Factor C

Use

Immunization against invasive disease caused by *H. influenzae* type b and against infection caused by all known subtypes of hepatitis B virus in infants 6 weeks to 15 months of age born of hepatitis B surface antigen (HB_sAg)-negative mothers

Infants born of HB_sAg-positive mothers or mothers of unknown HB_sAg status should receive hepatitis B vaccine (recombinant) at birth and should complete the hepatitis B vaccination series given according to a particular schedule (refer to current ACIP recommendations).

Available Dosage Forms

Injection, suspension [preservative free]:
Comvax®: *Haemophilus* b capsular polysaccharide 7.5 mcg and hepatitis B surface antigen 5 mcg per 0.5 mL (0.5 mL)

Dosing

Pediatric

Immunization: Infants: I.M.: 0.5 mL/dose; one dose at 2, 4, and 12-15 months of age (total of 3 doses). **Note:** If the recommended schedule cannot be followed, the interval between the first two doses should be at least 6 weeks and the interval between the second and third dose should be as close as possible to 8-11 months. Minimum age for first dose is 6 weeks.

Modified Schedule: Children who receive one dose of hepatitis B vaccine at or shortly after birth may receive Comvax® on a schedule of 2, 4, and 12-15 months of age

Administration

I.M. Shake well prior to use. Administer 0.5 mL I.M. into anterolateral thigh [data suggests that injections given in the buttocks frequently are given into fatty tissue instead of into muscle and result in lower seroconversion rates]; **do not administer intravenously, intradermally, or subcutaneously.**

For patients at risk of hemorrhage following intramuscular injection, the ACIP recommends "it should be administered intramuscularly if, in the opinion of the physician familiar with the patients bleeding risk, the vaccine can be administered with by this route with reasonable safety. If the patient receives antihemophilia or other similar therapy, intramuscular vaccination can be scheduled shortly after such therapy is administered. A fine needle (23 gauge or smaller) can be used for the vaccination and firm pressure applied to the site (without rubbing) for at least 2 minutes. The patient should be instructed concerning the risk of hematoma from the injection." Patients on anticoagulant therapy should be considered to have the same bleeding risks and treated as those with clotting factor disorders (CDC, 2011).

Simultaneous administration of vaccines helps ensure the patients will be fully vaccinated by the appropriate age. Simultaneous administration of vaccines is defined as administering >1 vaccine on the same day at different anatomic sites. The use of licensed combination vaccines is generally preferred over separate injections of the equivalent components. Separate vaccines should not be combined in the same syringe unless indicated by product specific labeling. Separate needles and syringes should be used for each injection. The ACIP prefers each dose of a specific vaccine in a series come from the same manufacturer when possible. Adolescents and adults should be vaccinated while seated or lying down. In general, preterm infants should be vaccinated at the same chronological age as full-term infants (CDC, 2011).

Antipyretics have not been shown to prevent febrile seizures. Antipyretics may be used to treat fever or discomfort following vaccination (CDC, 2011). One study reported that routine prophylactic administration of acetaminophen to prevent fever prior to vaccination decreased the immune response of some vaccines; the clinical significance of this reduction in immune response has not been established (Prymula, 2009).

Monitoring and Teaching Issues

Physical Assessment Federal law requires entry into the patient's medical record.

Related Information

Immunization Recommendations *on page 1941*

◆ ***Haemophilus* B Conjugate (Hib)** *see* Diphtheria and Tetanus Toxoids, Acellular Pertussis, Poliovirus and *Haemophilus* b Conjugate Vaccine *on page 550*

Haemophilus b Conjugate Vaccine (he MOF fi lus bee KON joo gate vak SEEN)

U.S. Brand Names ActHIB®; Hiberix®; PedvaxHIB®

Index Terms *Haemophilus* b Oligosaccharide Conjugate Vaccine; *Haemophilus* b Polysaccharide Vaccine; Diphtheria Toxoid Conjugate; HbCV; Hib; Hib Conjugate Vaccine; Hib Polysaccharide Conjugate; PRP-OMP; PRP-T

Generic Availability (U.S.) No

Pharmacologic Category Vaccine, Inactivated (Bacterial)

Medication Safety Issues

Sound-alike/look-alike issues:

International issues:

Hiberix is also a brand name for influenza virus vaccine in multiple international markets

Pregnancy Risk Factor C

Use Routine immunization of children against invasive disease caused by *H. influenzae* type b

The Advisory Committee on Immunization Practices (ACIP) recommends routine vaccination of all children through age 59 months. Efficacy data are not available for use in older children and adults with chronic conditions associated with an increased risk of Hib disease. However, a single dose may also be considered for older children, adolescents, and adults who did not receive the childhood series and who have had splenectomies or who have sickle cell disease, leukemia, or HIV infection.

Available Dosage Forms

Injection, powder for reconstitution [preservative free]:

ActHIB® *Haemophilus* b capsular polysaccharide 10 mcg per 0.5 mL

Hiberix®: *Haemophilus* b capsular polysaccharide 10 mcg per 0.5 mL

Injection, suspension:

PedvaxHIB®: *Haemophilus* b capsular polysaccharide 7.5 mcg

Dosing

Pediatric Immunization: I.M.: 0.5 mL as a single dose should be administered to previously unvaccinated children according to one of the following "brand-specific" schedules; number of doses in series is dependent upon age at first dose. ActHIB® and PedvaxHIB® are approved for a complete vaccine series; Hiberix® is approved only as a booster (final) dose in children who have received primary immunization.

ActHIB®: *Age at first dose:*

2 months of age: Immunization consists of 3 doses (0.5 mL/dose) administered at 2-, 4-, and 6 months of age (may reconstitute with provided diluent or DTP vaccine). A booster dose is given at 15-18 months of age (may reconstitute with provided diluent or Tripedia® vaccine).

7-11 months of age: Two doses (0.5 mL/dose) administered 8 weeks apart, with a booster dose at 15-18 months of age

12-14 months of age: One dose (0.5 mL) followed by a booster dose 2 months later

PedvaxHIB®: *Age at first dose:*

2-10 months of age: Two doses (0.5 mL/dose) administered 2 months apart; booster dose at 12-15 months of age

11-14 months of age: Two doses (0.5 mL/dose) administered 2 months apart

15-71 months of age: One 0.5 mL dose

Hiberix®: 15-59 months: One 0.5 mL booster dose (per manufacturer). The ACIP recommends booster dose administration at 12-15 months

Administration

I.M. For I.M. administration; do not inject I.V.

Hiberix®: Shake well prior to use. Administer into the anterolateral thigh or deltoid. If Hiberix® is inadvertently administered during the primary vaccination series, the dose can be counted as a valid PRP-T dose that does not need to be repeated if administered according to schedule. In this case, a total of 3 doses completes the primary series.

ActHIB®, PedvaxHIB®: Shake well prior to use. Administer into the anterolateral thigh or deltoid. Do not administer into buttocks due to potential risk of injury to sciatic nerve.

For patients at risk of hemorrhage following intramuscular injection, the ACIP recommends "it should be administered intramuscularly if, in the opinion of the physician familiar with the patients bleeding risk, the vaccine can be administered by this route with reasonable safety. If the patient receives antihemophilia or other similar therapy, intramuscular vaccination can be scheduled shortly after such therapy is administered. A fine needle (23 gauge or smaller) can be used for the vaccination and firm pressure applied to the site (without rubbing) for at least 2 minutes. The patient should be instructed concerning the risk of hematoma from the injection." Patients on anticoagulant therapy should be considered to have the same bleeding risks and treated as those with clotting factor disorders (CDC, 2011).

Simultaneous administration of vaccines helps ensure the patients will be fully vaccinated by the appropriate age. Simultaneous administration of vaccines is defined as administering >1 vaccine on the same day at different anatomic sites. The use of licensed combination vaccines is generally preferred over separate injections of the equivalent components. Separate vaccines should not be combined in the same syringe unless indicated by product specific labeling. Separate needles and syringes should be used for each injection. The ACIP prefers each dose of a specific vaccine in a series come from the same manufacturer when possible. Adolescents and adults should be vaccinated while seated or lying down. In general, preterm infants should be vaccinated at the same chronological age as full-term infants (CDC, 2011).

Antipyretics have not been shown to prevent febrile seizures. Antipyretics may be used to treat fever or discomfort following vaccination (CDC, 2011). One study reported that routine prophylactic administration of acetaminophen to prevent fever prior to vaccination decreased the immune response of some vaccines; the clinical significance of this reduction in immune response has not been established (Prymula, 2009).

Monitoring and Teaching Issues

Physical Assessment Federal law requires entry into the patient's medical record.

Related Information

Immunization Recommendations *on page 1941*

- ***Haemophilus* b (meningococcal protein conjugate) Conjugate Vaccine** *see Haemophilus* b Conjugate and Hepatitis B Vaccine *on page 892*
- ***Haemophilus* b Oligosaccharide Conjugate Vaccine** *see Haemophilus* b Conjugate Vaccine *on page 893*
- ***Haemophilus* B Polysaccharide** *see* Diphtheria and Tetanus Toxoids, Acellular Pertussis, Poliovirus and *Haemophilus* b Conjugate Vaccine *on page 550*
- ***Haemophilus* b Polysaccharide Vaccine** *see Haemophilus* b Conjugate Vaccine *on page 893*
- ***Haemophilus influenzae* b Conjugate Vaccine and Diphtheria, Tetanus Toxoids, and Acellular Pertussis Vaccine** *see* Diphtheria and Tetanus Toxoids, Acellular Pertussis and *Haemophilus influenzae* b Conjugate Vaccine *on page 548*
- **Halaven™** *see* Eribulin *on page 652*

Halcinonide (hal SIN oh nide)

U.S. Brand Names Halog®

Generic Availability (U.S.) No

Pharmacologic Category Corticosteroid, Topical

Medication Safety Issues

Sound-alike/look-alike issues:

Halcinonide may be confused with Halcion®

Halog® may be confused with Haldol®, Mycolog®

Pregnancy Risk Factor C

Use Inflammation of corticosteroid-responsive dermatoses [high potency topical corticosteroid]

Available Dosage Forms

Cream, topical:

Halog®: 0.1% (30 g, 60 g)

Ointment, topical:

Halog®: 0.1% (30 g, 60 g)

Dosing

Adult & Geriatric Steroid-responsive dermatoses: Topical: Apply sparingly 1-3 times/day, occlusive dressing may be used for severe or resistant dermatoses; a thin film is effective; do not overuse. Therapy should be discontinued when control is achieved; if no improvement is seen, reassessment of diagnosis may be necessary.

Pediatric Refer to adult dosing.

Monitoring and Teaching Issues

Patient Education For external use only. Do not use for eyes, mucous membranes, or open wounds. Before using, wash and dry area gently. Apply in a thin layer (may rub in lightly). Apply light dressing (if necessary) to area being treated. Do not use occlusive dressing unless so advised by prescriber. Avoid prolonged or excessive use around sensitive tissues or genital or rectal areas. Avoid exposing treated area to direct sunlight. Inform prescriber if condition worsens (redness, swelling, irritation, signs of infection, or open sores) or fails to improve.

Related Information

Corticosteroids *on page 1996*

- **Halcion®** *see* Triazolam *on page 1817*
- **Haldol®** *see* Haloperidol *on page 895*
- **Haldol® Decanoate** *see* Haloperidol *on page 895*
- **HalfLytely® and Bisacodyl** *see* Polyethylene Glycol-Electrolyte Solution and Bisacodyl *on page 1475*
- **Halfprin® [OTC]** *see* Aspirin *on page 155*
- **Halichondrin B Analog** *see* Eribulin *on page 652*
- **Halog®** *see* Halcinonide *on page 894*

Haloperidol (ha loe PER i dole)

U.S. Brand Names Haldol®; Haldol® Decanoate

Index Terms Haloperidol Decanoate; Haloperidol Lactate

Generic Availability (U.S.) Yes

Pharmacologic Category Antipsychotic Agent, Typical

Medication Safety Issues

Sound-alike/look-alike issues:

Haloperidol may be confused Halotestin®

Haldol® may be confused with Halcion®, Halenol®, Halog®, Halotestin®, Stadol®

Pregnancy Risk Factor C

Lactation Enters breast milk/not recommended (AAP rates "of concern"; AAP 2001 update pending)

Use Management of schizophrenia; control of tics and vocal utterances of Tourette's disorder in children and adults; severe behavioral problems in children

Unlabeled/Investigational Use Treatment of non-schizophrenia psychosis; may be used for the emergency sedation of severely-agitated or delirious patients; adjunctive treatment of ethanol dependence; postoperative nausea and vomiting (alternative therapy); psychosis/agitation related to Alzheimer's dementia

Mechanism of Action/Effect Haloperidol is a butyrophenone antipsychotic which blocks postsynaptic mesolimbic dopaminergic D_1 and D_2 receptors in the brain; depresses the release of hypothalamic and hypophyseal hormones; believed to depress the reticular activating system thus affecting basal metabolism, body temperature, wakefulness, vasomotor tone, and emesis

Contraindications Hypersensitivity to haloperidol or any component of the formulation; Parkinson's disease; severe CNS depression; coma

Warnings/Precautions [U.S. Boxed Warning]: Elderly patients with dementia-related psychosis treated with antipsychotics are at an increased risk of death compared to placebo. Most deaths appeared to be either cardiovascular (eg, heart failure, sudden death) or infectious (eg, pneumonia) in nature. Haloperidol is not approved for the treatment of dementia-related psychosis. Hypotension may occur, particularly with parenteral administration. Although the short-acting form (lactate) is used clinically, the I.V. use of the injection is not an FDA-approved route of administration; the decanoate form should never be administered intravenously.

May alter cardiac conduction and prolong QT interval; life-threatening arrhythmias have occurred with therapeutic doses of antipsychotics but risk may be increased with doses exceeding recommendations and/or intravenous administration (unlabeled route). Use caution or avoid use in patients with electrolyte abnormalities (eg, hypokalemia, hypomagnesemia), hypothyroidism, familial long QT syndrome, concomitant medications which may augment QT prolongation, or any underlying cardiac abnormality which may also potentiate risk. Monitor ECG closely for dose-related QT effects. Adverse effects of decanoate may be prolonged. Avoid in thyrotoxicosis.

Leukopenia, neutropenia, and agranulocytosis (sometimes fatal) have been reported in clinical trials and postmarketing reports with antipsychotic use; presence of risk factors (eg, pre-existing low WBC or history of drug-induced leuko-/neutropenia) should prompt periodic blood count assessment. Discontinue therapy at first signs of blood dyscrasias or if absolute neutrophil count $<1000/mm^3$.

May be sedating, use with caution in disorders where CNS depression is a feature. Effects may be potentiated when used with other sedative drugs or ethanol. Caution in patients with severe cardiovascular disease, predisposition to seizures, subcortical brain damage, or renal disease. Esophageal dysmotility and aspiration have been associated with antipsychotic use - use with caution in patients at risk of pneumonia (eg, Alzheimer's disease). Use associated with increased prolactin levels; clinical significance of hyperprolactinemia in patients with breast cancer or other prolactin-dependent tumors is unknown. May alter temperature regulation or mask toxicity of other drugs due to antiemetic effects. May cause orthostatic hypotension; use with caution in patients at risk of this effect or those who would tolerate transient hypotensive episodes (cerebrovascular disease, cardiovascular disease, or other medications which may predispose). Some tablets contain tartrazine. Antipsychotics have been associated with pigmentary retinopathy.

May cause anticholinergic effects (confusion, agitation, constipation, xerostomia, blurred vision, urinary retention). Therefore, they should be used with caution in patients with decreased gastrointestinal motility, urinary retention, BPH, xerostomia, or visual problems. Conditions which also may be exacerbated by cholinergic blockade include narrow-angle glaucoma and worsening of myasthenia gravis. Relative to other neuroleptics, haloperidol has a low potency of cholinergic blockade.

May cause extrapyramidal symptoms (EPS), including pseudoparkinsonism, acute dystonic reactions, akathisia, and tardive dyskinesia. Risk of dystonia (and possibly other EPS) may be greater with increased doses, use of conventional antipsychotics, males, and younger patients. May be associated with neuroleptic malignant syndrome (NMS). Use with caution in the elderly.

Drug Interactions

Metabolism/Transport Effects Substrate of CYP1A2 (minor), 2D6 (major), 3A4 (major); **Inhibits** CYP2D6 (moderate), 3A4 (moderate)

Avoid Concomitant Use

Avoid concomitant use of Haloperidol with any of the following: Artemether; Dronedarone; Lumefantrine; Metoclopramide; Nilotinib; Pimozide; QuiNINE; Tetrabenazine; Thioridazine; Tolvaptan; Toremifene; Vandetanib; Ziprasidone

Decreased Effect

Haloperidol may decrease the levels/effects of: Amphetamines; Codeine; Quinagolide; TraMADol

The levels/effects of Haloperidol may be decreased by: Anti-Parkinson's Agents (Dopamine Agonist); CarBAMazepine; CYP3A4 Inducers (Strong); Deferasirox; Glycopyrrolate; Herbs (CYP3A4 Inducers); Lithium formulations; Peginterferon Alfa-2b

Increased Effect/Toxicity

Haloperidol may increase the levels/effects of: Alcohol (Ethyl); Anticholinergics; Anti-Parkinson's Agents (Dopamine Agonist); ChlorproMAZINE; CNS Depressants; Colchicine; CYP2D6 Substrates; CYP3A4 Substrates; Dronedarone; Eplerenone; Everolimus; FentaNYL; Fesoterodine; Lurasidone; Methylphenidate; Nebivolol; Pimecrolimus; Pimozide; QTc-Prolonging Agents; QuiNIDine; QuiNINE; Salmeterol; Saxagliptin; Tamoxifen; Tetrabenazine; Thioridazine; Tolvaptan; Toremifene; Vandetanib; Ziprasidone

The levels/effects of Haloperidol may be increased by: Acetylcholinesterase Inhibitors (Central); Alfuzosin; Artemether; Chloroquine; ChlorproMAZINE; Ciprofloxacin; Ciprofloxacin (Systemic); Conivaptan; CYP2D6 Inhibitors (Moderate); CYP2D6 Inhibitors (Strong); CYP3A4 Inhibitors (Moderate); CYP3A4 Inhibitors (Strong); Darunavir; Gadobutrol; Lithium formulations; Lumefantrine; Methylphenidate; Metoclopramide; Nilotinib; Nonsteroidal Anti-Inflammatory Agents; Pramlintide; QuiNIDine; QuiNINE; Selective Serotonin Reuptake Inhibitors; Tetrabenazine

Nutritional/Ethanol Interactions

Ethanol: Avoid ethanol (may increase CNS depression).

Herb/Nutraceutical: Avoid valerian, St John's wort, kava kava, gotu kola (may increase CNS depression).

Lab Interactions decreased cholesterol (S)

Adverse Reactions Frequency not defined.

Cardiovascular: Abnormal T waves with prolonged ventricular repolarization, arrhythmia, hyper-/hypotension, QT prolongation, sudden death, tachycardia, torsade de pointes

Central nervous system: Agitation, akathisia, altered central temperature regulation, anxiety, confusion, depression, drowsiness, dystonic reactions, euphoria, extrapyramidal reactions, headache, insomnia, lethargy, neuroleptic malignant syndrome (NMS), pseudoparkinsonian signs and symptoms, restlessness, seizure, tardive dyskinesia, tardive dystonia, vertigo

Dermatologic: Alopecia, contact dermatitis, hyperpigmentation, photosensitivity (rare), pruritus, rash

Endocrine & metabolic: Amenorrhea, breast engorgement, galactorrhea, gynecomastia, hyper-/hypoglycemia, hyponatremia, lactation, mastalgia, menstrual irregularities, sexual dysfunction

Gastrointestinal: Anorexia, constipation, diarrhea, dyspepsia, hypersalivation, nausea, vomiting, xerostomia

Genitourinary: Priapism, urinary retention

Hematologic: Cholestatic jaundice, obstructive jaundice

Ocular: Blurred vision

Respiratory: Bronchospasm, laryngospasm

Miscellaneous: Diaphoresis, heat stroke

Pharmacodynamics/Kinetics

Onset of Action Sedation: I.M., I.V.: 30-60 minutes

Duration of Action Decanoate: ~3 weeks

Bioavailability Oral: 60% to 70%

Time to Peak Oral: 2-6 hours; I.M.: 20 minutes; decanoate: 7 days

Protein Binding 90%

Half-Life Elimination 18 hours; Decanoate: 21 days

Metabolism Hepatic: 50% to 60% glucuronidation (inactive); 23% CYP3A4-mediated reduction to inactive metabolites (some back-oxidation to haloperidol); and 20% to 30% CYP3A4-mediated N-dealkylation, including minor oxidation pathway to toxic pyridinium derivative (Kudo, 1999)

Excretion Urine (30%, 1% as unchanged drug); feces (15%)

Available Dosage Forms

Injection, oil: 50 mg/mL (1 mL, 5 mL); 100 mg/mL (1 mL, 5 mL)
Haldol® Decanoate: 50 mg/mL (1 mL); 100 mg/mL (1 mL)

Injection, solution: 5 mg/mL (1 mL, 10 mL)
Haldol®: 5 mg/mL (1 mL)

Solution, oral: 2 mg/mL (5 mL, 15 mL, 120 mL)

Tablet, oral: 0.5 mg, 1 mg, 2 mg, 5 mg, 10 mg, 20 mg

Dosing

Adult

Psychosis:

Oral: 0.5-5 mg 2-3 times/day; usual maximum: 30 mg/day

I.M. (as lactate): 2-5 mg every 4-8 hours as needed

I.M. (as decanoate): Initial: 10-20 times the daily oral dose administered at 4-week intervals. Maintenance dose: 10-15 times initial oral dose; used to stabilize psychiatric symptoms

Delirium in the intensive care unit (unlabeled use, unlabeled route; Jacobi, 2002):

I.V.: Initial: 2-10 mg depending on degree of agitation; if inadequate response, may repeat bolus dose (with sequential doubling of initial bolus dose) every 15-30 minutes until calm achieved, then administer 25% of the last bolus dose every 6 hours; monitor ECG and QT_c interval. After the patient is controlled, haloperidol therapy should be tapered over several days. **Note:** QT_c prolongation may occur with cumulative doses ≥35 mg and torsade de pointes has been reported with single doses of ≥20 mg. The optimal dose and regimen of haloperidol for the treatment of severe agitation and/or delirium has not been established.

Continuous I.V. infusion (100 mg/100 mL D_5W): Rates of 3-25 mg/hour have been used

Rapid tranquilization of severely-agitated patient (unlabeled use; administer every 30-60 minutes):

Oral: 5-10 mg

I.M. (as lactate): 5 mg

Average total dose (oral or I.M.) for tranquilization: 10-20 mg

Postoperative nausea and vomiting (PONV) (unlabeled use): I.M., I.V.: 0.5-2 mg (Gan, 2007)

Geriatric Nonpsychotic patient, dementia behavior (unlabeled use): Initial: Oral: 0.25-0.5 mg 1-2 times/day; increase dose at 4- to 7-day intervals by 0.25-0.5 mg/day. Increase dosing intervals (twice daily, 3 times/day, etc) as necessary to control response or side effects.

Pediatric

Sedation/psychotic disorders: Oral:

Children 3-12 years (15-40 kg): Initial: 0.05 mg/kg/day or 0.25-0.5 mg/day given in 2-3 divided doses; increase by 0.25-0.5 mg every 5-7 days; maximum: 0.15 mg/kg/day

Usual maintenance:

Agitation or hyperkinesia: 0.01-0.03 mg/kg/day once daily

Nonpsychotic disorders: 0.05-0.075 mg/kg/day in 2-3 divided doses

Psychotic disorders: 0.05-0.15 mg/kg/day in 2-3 divided doses

Children 6-12 years: Sedation/psychotic disorders: I.M. (as lactate): 1-3 mg/dose every 4-8 hours to a maximum of 0.15 mg/kg/day; change over to oral therapy as soon as able.

Renal Impairment Hemodialysis/peritoneal dialysis: Supplemental dose is not necessary.

Administration

Oral Dilute the oral concentrate with water or juice before administration. **Note:** Avoid skin contact with oral medication; may cause contact dermatitis.

I.M. The decanoate injectable formulation should be administered I.M. only; **do not give decanoate I.V.**

I.V.

Decanoate: Do **not** administer I.V.

Lactate: Although not an FDA-approved route of administration, Haldol® has been administered by this route in many acute care settings.

Stability

Reconstitution Haloperidol lactate may be administered IVPB or I.V. infusion in D_5W solutions. NS solutions should not be used due to reports of decreased stability and incompatibility.

Standardized dose: 0.5-100 mg/50-100 mL D_5W.

Storage Protect oral dosage forms from light. Haloperidol lactate injection should be stored at controlled room temperature; do not freeze or expose to temperatures >40°C. Protect from light; exposure to light may cause discoloration and the development of a grayish-red precipitate over several weeks. Stability of standardized solutions is 38 days at room temperature (24°C).

Monitoring and Teaching Issues

Laboratory Monitoring Lipid profile, fasting blood glucose/Hgb A_{1c}; BMI

Physical Assessment With I.M. or I.V. use, monitor for hypotension and cardiac irregularities. Initiate at lower doses and taper dosage slowly when discontinuing.

Patient Education It may take 2-3 weeks to achieve desired results. Dilute oral concentration with water or juice. Avoid alcohol. Maintain adequate hydration, unless instructed to restrict fluid intake. Avoid skin contact with medication; may cause contact dermatitis (wash immediately with warm, soapy water). You may experience excess drowsiness, restlessness, dizziness, blurred vision, nausea, vomiting, constipation, postural hypotension, urinary retention, or decreased perspiration. Report persistent CNS effects (eg, trembling fingers, altered gait or balance, excessive sedation, seizures, unusual movements, anxiety, abnormal thoughts, confusion, personality changes), chest pain, palpitations, rapid heartbeat, severe dizziness, unresolved urinary retention or changes in urinary pattern, vision changes, skin rash or yellowing of skin, respiratory difficulty, or worsening of condition.

Geriatric Considerations Many elderly patients receive antipsychotic medications for inappropriate nonpsychotic behavior. Before initiating antipsychotic medication, the clinician should investigate any possible reversible cause; any stress or stress from any disease can cause acute "confusion" or worsening of baseline nonpsychotic behavior. Most commonly acute changes in behavior are due to increases in drug dose or addition of new drug to regimen; fluid electrolyte loss; infections; and changes in environment.

Any changes in disease status in any organ system can result in behavior changes.

In the treatment of agitated, demented, elderly patients, authors of meta-analysis of controlled trials of the response to the traditional antipsychotics (phenothiazines, butyrophenones) in controlling agitation have concluded that the use of neuroleptics results in a response rate of 18%. Clearly neuroleptic therapy for behavior control should be limited with frequent attempts to withdraw the agent given for behavior control.

Clinical studies of haloperidol did not include sufficient numbers of subjects ≥65 years of age to determine whether they respond differently from younger subjects. Other reported clinical experience has not consistently identified differences between the elderly and younger patients. However, the prevalence of tardive dyskinesia appears to be highest among the elderly, especially elderly women. Also, the pharmacokinetics of haloperidol in geriatric patients generally warrants the use of lower doses.

Breast-Feeding Considerations Haloperidol is found in breast milk and has been detected in the plasma and urine of nursing infants. Developmental decline was observed in 3 nursing infants following maternal use of haloperidol in combination with chlorpromazine. Breast engorgement, gynecomastia, and lactation are known side effects with the use of haloperidol.

Pregnancy Considerations Adverse events were observed in animal studies. Haloperidol crosses the placenta. There are case reports of limb malformations following first trimester exposure in humans. Antipsychotic use during the third trimester of pregnancy has a risk for abnormal muscle movements (extrapyramidal symptoms [EPS]) and withdrawal symptoms in newborns following delivery. Symptoms in the newborn may include agitation, feeding disorder, hypertonia, hypotonia, respiratory distress, somnolence, and tremor; these effects may be self-limiting or require hospitalization.

Related Information

Antipsychotic Agents *on page* 1986

◆ **Haloperidol Decanoate** *see* Haloperidol *on page* 895
◆ **Haloperidol Lactate** *see* Haloperidol *on page* 895
◆ **Harkoseride** *see* Lacosamide *on page* 1051
◆ **Havrix®** *see* Hepatitis A Vaccine *on page* 904
◆ **Havrix® and Engerix-B®** *see* Hepatitis A and Hepatitis B Recombinant Vaccine *on page* 903
◆ **HbCV** *see* *Haemophilus* b Conjugate Vaccine *on page* 893
◆ **hBNP** *see* Nesiritide *on page* 1299
◆ **hCG** *see* Chorionic Gonadotropin (Human) *on page* 364
◆ **HCTZ (error-prone abbreviation)** *see* Hydrochlorothiazide *on page* 912
◆ **HDCV** *see* Rabies Vaccine *on page* 1546
◆ **Heartburn Relief [OTC]** *see* Famotidine *on page* 733
◆ **Heartburn Relief Maximum Strength [OTC]** *see* Famotidine *on page* 733
◆ **Heather** *see* Norethindrone *on page* 1334
◆ **Hectorol®** *see* Doxercalciferol *on page* 579
◆ **Helixate® FS** *see* Antihemophilic Factor (Recombinant) *on page* 133
◆ **Hemabate®** *see* Carboprost Tromethamine *on page* 299
◆ **Hemofil M** *see* Antihemophilic Factor (Human) *on page* 132
◆ **Hemorrhoidal HC** *see* Hydrocortisone (Topical) *on page* 920
◆ **Hemorrhoidal HC [DSC]** *see* Hydrocortisone (Topical) *on page* 920
◆ **Hemril® -30** *see* Hydrocortisone (Topical) *on page* 920
◆ **HepA** *see* Hepatitis A Vaccine *on page* 904
◆ **HepA-HepB** *see* Hepatitis A and Hepatitis B Recombinant Vaccine *on page* 903

Heparin (HEP a rin)

U.S. Brand Names Hep-Lock; Hep-Lock U/P; HepFlush®-10

Index Terms Heparin Calcium; Heparin Lock Flush; Heparin Sodium

Generic Availability (U.S.) Yes

Pharmacologic Category Anticoagulant

Medication Safety Issues

Sound-alike/look-alike issues:

Heparin may be confused with Hespan®

High alert medication: The Institute for Safe Medication Practices (ISMP) includes this medication among its list of drugs which have a heightened risk of causing significant patient harm when used in error.

Heparin sodium injection 10,000 units/mL and Hep-Lock U/P 10 units/mL have been confused with each other. Fatal medication errors have occurred between the two whose labels are both blue. **Never rely on color as a sole indicator to differentiate product identity.**

Heparin lock flush solution is intended only to maintain patency of I.V. devices and is **not** to be used for anticoagulant therapy.

Note: The 100 unit/mL concentration should not be used to flush heparin locks, I.V. lines, or intra-arterial lines in neonates or infants <10 kg (systemic anticoagulation may occur). The 10 unit/mL flush concentration may inadvertently cause systemic anticoagulation in infants <1 kg who receive frequent flushes.

2009 National Patient Safety Goals: The Joint Commission (TJC) requires healthcare organizations that provide anticoagulant therapy to have a process in place to reduce the risk of anticoagulant-associated patient harm. Patients receiving anticoagulants should receive individualized care through a defined process that includes standardized ordering, dispensing, administration, monitoring and education. This does not apply to routine short-term use of anticoagulants for prevention of venous thromboembolism when the expectation is that the patient's laboratory values will remain within or close to normal values (NPSG.03.05.01).

Pregnancy Risk Factor C

Lactation Does not enter breast milk

Use Prophylaxis and treatment of thromboembolic disorders; as an anticoagulant for extracorporeal and dialysis procedures

Note: Heparin lock flush solution is intended only to maintain patency of I.V. devices and is **not** to be used for systemic anticoagulant therapy.

Unlabeled/Investigational Use ST-elevation myocardial infarction (STEMI) as an adjunct to thrombolysis; unstable angina/non-STEMI (UA/NSTEMI); anticoagulant used during percutaneous coronary intervention (PCI)

Mechanism of Action/Effect Potentiates the action of antithrombin III and thereby inactivates thrombin (as well as activated coagulation factors IX, X, XI, XII, and plasmin) and prevents the conversion of fibrinogen to fibrin; heparin also stimulates release of lipoprotein lipase (lipoprotein lipase hydrolyzes triglycerides to glycerol and free fatty acids)

Contraindications Hypersensitivity to heparin or any component of the formulation (unless a life-threatening situation necessitates use and use of an alternative anticoagulant is not possible); severe thrombocytopenia; uncontrolled active bleeding except when due to disseminated intravascular coagulation (DIC); not for use when appropriate blood coagulation tests cannot be obtained at appropriate intervals (applies to full-dose heparin only)

Note: Some products contain benzyl alcohol as a preservative; their use in neonates, infants, or pregnant or nursing mothers is contraindicated by some manufacturers.

Warnings/Precautions Hypersensitivity reactions can occur. Only in life-threatening situations when use of an alternative anticoagulant is not possible should heparin be cautiously used in patients with a documented hypersensitivity reaction. Hemorrhage is the most common complication. Monitor for signs and symptoms of bleeding. Certain patients are at increased risk of bleeding. Risk factors for bleeding include bacterial endocarditis; congenital or acquired bleeding disorders; active ulcerative or angiodysplastic GI diseases; continuous GI tube drainage; severe uncontrolled hypertension; history of hemorrhagic stroke; or use shortly after brain, spinal, or ophthalmology surgery; patient treated concomitantly with platelet inhibitors; conditions associated with increased bleeding tendencies (hemophilia, vascular purpura); recent GI bleeding; thrombocytopenia or platelet defects; severe liver disease; hypertensive or diabetic retinopathy; renal failure; or in patients undergoing invasive procedures including spinal tap or spinal anesthesia. Many concentrations of heparin are available ranging from 1 unit/mL to 20,000 units/mL. Clinicians **must** carefully examine each prefilled syringe or vial prior to use ensuring that the correct concentration is chosen; fatal hemorrhages have occurred related to heparin overdose especially in pediatric patients. A higher incidence of bleeding has been reported in patients >60 years of age, particularly women. They are also more sensitive to the dose. Discontinue heparin if hemorrhage occurs; severe hemorrhage or overdosage may require protamine.

May cause thrombocytopenia; monitor platelet count closely. Patients who develop HIT may be at risk of developing a new thrombus (heparin-induced thrombocytopenia and thrombosis [HITT]). Discontinue therapy and consider alternatives if platelets are <100,000/mm^3 and/or thrombosis develops. HIT or HITT may be delayed and can occur up to several weeks after discontinuation of heparin. Osteoporosis may occur with prolonged use (>6 months) due to a reduction in bone mineral density. Monitor for hyperkalemia; can cause hyperkalemia by suppressing aldosterone production. Patients >60 years of age may require lower doses of heparin.

[U.S. Boxed Warning]: Some products contain benzyl alcohol as a preservative; use of these products is contraindicated in neonates. In neonates, large amounts of benzyl alcohol (>100 mg/kg/day) have been associated with fatal toxicity (gasping syndrome). Use in neonates, infants, or pregnant or nursing mothers is contraindicated by some manufacturers; the use of preservative-free heparin is, therefore, recommended in these populations. Some preparations contain sulfite which may cause allergic reactions.

Heparin resistance may occur in patients with antithrombin deficiency, increased heparin clearance, elevations in heparin-binding proteins, elevations in factor VIII and/or fibrinogen; frequently encountered in patients with fever, thrombosis, thrombophlebitis, infections with thrombosing tendencies, MI, cancer, and in postsurgical patients; measurement of anticoagulant effects using antifactor Xa levels may be of benefit.

Drug Interactions

Avoid Concomitant Use

Avoid concomitant use of Heparin with any of the following: Corticorelin

Decreased Effect

The levels/effects of Heparin may be decreased by: Nitroglycerin

Increased Effect/Toxicity

Heparin may increase the levels/effects of: Anticoagulants; Collagenase (Systemic); Corticorelin; Drotrecogin Alfa; Ibritumomab; Tositumomab and Iodine I 131 Tositumomab

The levels/effects of Heparin may be increased by: 5-ASA Derivatives; Antiplatelet Agents; Aspirin; Dasatinib; Herbs (Anticoagulant/Antiplatelet Properties); Nonsteroidal Anti-Inflammatory Agents; Pentosan Polysulfate Sodium; Pentoxifylline; Prostacyclin Analogues; Salicylates; Thrombolytic Agents

Nutritional/Ethanol Interactions Herb/Nutraceutical: Avoid cat's claw, dong quai, evening primrose, feverfew, red clover, horse chestnut, garlic, green tea, ginseng, ginkgo (all have additional antiplatelet activity).

Lab Interactions Increased thyroxine (competitive protein binding methods); increased PT

Aprotinin significantly increases aPTT and celite Activated Clotting Time (ACT) which may not reflect the actual degree of anticoagulation by heparin. Kaolin-based ACTs are not affected by aprotinin to the same degree as celite ACTs. While institutional protocols may vary, a minimal celite ACT of 750 seconds or kaolin-ACT of 480 seconds is recommended in the presence of aprotinin. Consult the manufacturer's information on specific ACT test interpretation in the presence of aprotinin.

Adverse Reactions Frequency not defined.

Cardiovascular: Allergic vasospastic reaction (possibly related to thrombosis), chest pain, hemorrhagic shock, shock, thrombosis

Central nervous system: Chills, fever, headache

Dermatologic: Alopecia (delayed, transient), bruising (unexplained), cutaneous necrosis, dysesthesia pedis, erythematous plaques (case reports), eczema, urticaria, purpura

Endocrine & metabolic: Adrenal hemorrhage, hyperkalemia (suppression of aldosterone synthesis), ovarian hemorrhage, rebound hyperlipidemia on discontinuation

Gastrointestinal: Constipation, hematemesis, nausea, tarry stools, vomiting

Genitourinary: Frequent or persistent erection

Hematologic: Bleeding from gums, epistaxis, hemorrhage, ovarian hemorrhage, retroperitoneal hemorrhage, thrombocytopenia (see note)

Hepatic: Liver enzymes increased

Local: Irritation, erythema, pain, hematoma, and ulceration have been rarely reported with deep SubQ injections; I.M. injection (not recommended) is associated with a high incidence of these effects

Neuromuscular & skeletal: Peripheral neuropathy, osteoporosis (chronic therapy effect)

Ocular: Conjunctivitis (allergic reaction), lacrimation

Renal: Hematuria

Respiratory: Asthma, bronchospasm (case reports), hemoptysis, pulmonary hemorrhage, rhinitis

Miscellaneous: Allergic reactions, anaphylactoid reactions, heparin resistance, hypersensitivity (including chills, fever, and urticaria)

Note: Thrombocytopenia has been reported to occur at an incidence between 0% and 30%. It is often of no clinical significance. However, immunologically mediated heparin-induced thrombocytopenia (HIT) has been estimated to occur in 1% to 2% of patients, and is marked by a progressive fall in platelet counts and, in some cases, thromboembolic complications (skin necrosis, pulmonary embolism, gangrene of the extremities, stroke, or MI). For recommendations regarding platelet monitoring during heparin therapy, see Laboratory Monitoring.

Pharmacodynamics/Kinetics

Onset of Action Anticoagulation: I.V.: Immediate; SubQ: ~20-30 minutes

Absorption Oral, rectal: Erratic at best from these routes of administration; SubQ absorption is also erratic, but considered acceptable for prophylactic use

Half-Life Elimination

Dose-dependent: I.V. bolus: 25 units/kg: 30 minutes; 100 units/kg: 60 minutes; 400 units/kg: 150 minutes (Hirsh, 2008)

Mean: 1.5 hours; Range: 1-2 hours; affected by obesity, renal function, malignancy, presence of pulmonary embolism, and infections

Note: At therapeutic doses, elimination occurs rapidly via nonrenal mechanisms. With very high doses, renal elimination may play more of a role; however, dosage adjustment remains unnecessary for patients with renal impairment (Hirsh, 2008).

Metabolism Hepatic; may be partially metabolized in the reticuloendothelial system

Excretion Urine (small amounts as unchanged drug)

Available Dosage Forms

Infusion, premixed in 1/2 NS: 25,000 units (250 mL, 500 mL)

Infusion, premixed in D_5W: 10,000 units (100 mL, 250 mL); 12,500 units (250 mL); 20,000 units (500 mL); 25,000 units (250 mL, 500 mL)

Infusion, premixed in NS: 1000 units (500 mL); 2000 units (1000 mL)

Infusion, premixed in NS [preservative free]: 1000 units (500 mL); 2000 units (1000 mL)

Injection, solution: 10 units/mL (1 mL, 2 mL, 3 mL, 5 mL, 10 mL, 30 mL); 100 units/mL (1 mL, 2 mL, 3 mL, 5 mL, 10 mL, 30 mL); 1000 units/mL (1 mL, 10 mL, 30 mL); 5000 units/mL (1 mL, 10 mL); 10,000 units/mL (1 mL, 4 mL, 5 mL); 20,000 units/mL (1 mL)

Hep-Lock: 10 units/mL (1 mL, 2 mL, 10 mL, 30 mL); 100 units/mL (1 mL, 2 mL, 10 mL, 30 mL)

Injection, solution [preservative free]: 1 units/mL (2 mL, 3 mL, 5 mL); 2 units/mL (3 mL); 10 units/mL (1 mL, 2 mL, 2.5 mL, 3 mL, 5 mL, 6 mL, 10 mL); 100 units/mL (1 mL, 2 mL, 2.5 mL, 3 mL, 5 mL, 10 mL); 1000 units/mL (2 mL); 10,000 units/mL (0.5 mL)

Hep-Lock U/P: 10 units/mL (1 mL); 100 units/mL (1 mL)

HepFlush®-10: 10 units/mL (10 mL)

Dosing

Adult Note: Many concentrations of heparin are available ranging from 1 unit/mL to 20,000 units/mL. Carefully examine each prefilled syringe or vial prior to use ensuring that the correct concentration is chosen. Heparin lock flush solution is intended only to maintain patency of I.V. devices and is not to be used for anticoagulant therapy.

DVT Prophylaxis (low-dose heparin): SubQ: 5000 units every 8-12 hours

Systemic anticoagulation: I.V. infusion (weight-based dosing per institutional nomogram recommended):

Acute coronary syndromes: I.V. infusion:

Percutaneous coronary intervention:

If no concurrent GPIIb/IIIa inhibitor: Initial bolus of 70-100 units/kg (target ACT 250-300 seconds for HemoTec®, 300-350 seconds for Hemochron®) (Kushner, 2009)

or

If receiving GPIIb/IIIa inhibitor: Initial bolus of 50-70 units/kg (target ACT 200-250 seconds)

STEMI: Fibrinolytic therapy:

Full-dose alteplase, reteplase, or tenecteplase with dosing as follows: Concurrent bolus of 60 units/kg (maximum: 4000 units), then 12 units/kg/hour (maximum: 1000 units/hour) as continuous infusion. Check aPTT every 4-6 hours; adjust to target of 1.5-2 times the upper limit of control (50-70 seconds in clinical trials); usual range: 10-30 units/kg/hour. Duration of heparin therapy depends on concurrent therapy and the specific patient risks for systemic or venous thromboembolism.

Combination regimen (unlabeled): Half-dose tenecteplase (15-25 mg based on weight) and abciximab 0.25 mg/kg bolus then 0.125 mcg/kg/minute (maximum: 10 mcg/minute) for 12 hours with heparin dosing as follows: Concurrent bolus of 40 units/kg (maximum: 3000 units), then 7 units/kg/hour (maximum: 800 units/hour) as continuous infusion. Adjust to a aPTT target of 50-70 seconds.

Unstable angina/Non-ST-elevation myocardial infarction (NSTEMI): Initial bolus of 60 units/kg (maximum: 4000 units), followed by an initial infusion of 12 units/kg/hour (maximum: 1000 units/hour). The American College of Chest Physicians consensus conference has recommended dosage adjustments to correspond to a therapeutic range equivalent to heparin levels of 0.3-0.7 units/mL by antifactor Xa determinations.

Treatment of venous thromboembolism:

DVT/PE: I.V.: 80 units/kg (or alternatively 5000 units) I.V. push followed by continuous infusion of 18 units/kg/hour (or alternatively 1300 units/hour). The American College of Chest Physicians consensus conference has recommended dosage adjustments to correspond to a therapeutic range equivalent to heparin levels of 0.3-0.7 units/mL by antifactor Xa determinations.

DVT/PE: SubQ:

Monitored dosing regimen: Initial: 17,500 units or 250 units/kg then 250 units/kg every 12 hours. The American College of Chest Physicians consensus conference has recommended dosage adjustments to correspond to a therapeutic range equivalent to heparin levels of 0.3-0.7 units/mL by antifactor Xa determinations.

Unmonitored dosing regimen: Initial: 333 units/kg then 250 units/kg every 12 hours

Intermittent I.V. Anticoagulation: Intermittent I.V.: Initial: 10,000 units, then 50-70 units/kg (5000-10,000 units) every 4-6 hours

Maintenance of line patency (line flushing): When using daily flushes of heparin to maintain patency of single and double lumen central catheters, 10 units/mL is commonly used for younger infants (eg, <10 kg) while 100 units/mL is used for older infants, children, and adults. Capped PVC catheters and peripheral heparin locks require flushing more frequently (eg, every 6-8 hours). Volume of heparin flush is usually similar to volume of catheter (or slightly greater). Additional flushes should be given when stagnant blood is observed in catheter, after catheter is used for drug or blood administration, and after blood withdrawal from catheter.

Parenteral nutrition: Addition of heparin (0.5-3 unit/mL) to peripheral and central parenteral nutrition has not been shown to decrease catheter-related thrombosis. The final concentration of heparin used for TPN solutions may need to be decreased to 0.5 units/mL in small infants receiving larger amounts of volume in order to avoid approaching therapeutic amounts. Arterial lines are heparinized with a final concentration of 1 unit/mL.

Geriatric Patients >60 years of age may have higher serum levels and clinical response (longer aPTTs) as compared to younger patients receiving similar dosages. Lower dosages may be required.

Pediatric Note: Many concentrations of heparin are available ranging from 1 unit/mL to 20,000 units/mL. Carefully examine each prefilled syringe or vial prior to use ensuring that the correct concentration is chosen. Heparin lock flush solution is intended only to maintain patency of I.V. devices and is not to be used for anticoagulant therapy.

Prophylaxis for cardiac catheterization (arterial approach): I.V.: Bolus: 100-150 units/kg (Monagle, 2008)

Systemic heparinization:

Intermittent I.V.: Initial: 50-100 units/kg, then 50-100 units/kg every 4 hours (**Note:** Continuous I.V. infusion is preferred)

I.V. infusion: Initial loading dose: 75 units/kg given over 10 minutes, then initial maintenance dose: 20 units/kg/hour; adjust dose to maintain aPTT of 60-85 seconds (assuming this reflects an antifactor Xa level of 0.35-0.7 units/mL); see table on next page.

Pediatric Protocol For Systemic Heparin Adjustment

To be used after initial loading dose and maintenance I.V. infusion dose (see usual dosage listed above) to maintain aPTT of 60-85 seconds (assuming this reflects antifactor Xa level of 0.35-0.7 units/mL).

Obtain blood for aPTT 4 hours after heparin loading dose and 4 hours after every infusion rate change.

Obtain daily CBC and aPTT after aPTT is therapeutic.

aPTT (seconds)	Dosage Adjustment	Time to Repeat aPTT
<50	Give 50 units/kg bolus and increase infusion rate by 10%	4 h after rate change
50-59	Increase infusion rate by 10%	4 h after rate change
60-85	Keep rate the same	Next day
86-95	Decrease infusion rate by 10%	4 h after rate change
96-120	Hold infusion for 30 minutes and decrease infusion rate by 10%	4 h after rate change
>120	Hold infusion for 60 minutes and decrease infusion rate by 15%	4 h after rate change

Modified from Monagle P, Chalmers E, Chan A, et al, "Antithrombotic Therapy in Neonates and Children," *Chest*, 2008, 133(6 Suppl):887-968.

Note: Refer to adult dosing for notes on line flushing and TPN.

Renal Impairment No dosage adjustment required; adjust therapeutic heparin according to aPTT or anti-Xa activity.

Hepatic Impairment No dosage adjustment required; adjust therapeutic heparin according to aPTT or anti-Xa activity.

Administration

I.M. Do not administer I.M. due to pain, irritation, and hematoma formation.

I.V.

Continuous infusion: Infuse via infusion pump.

Heparin lock: Inject via injection cap using positive pressure flushing technique. Heparin lock flush solution is intended only to maintain patency of I.V. devices and is **not** to be used for anticoagulant therapy.

Other SubQ: Inject in subcutaneous tissue only (not muscle tissue). Injection sites should be rotated (usually left and right portions of the abdomen, above iliac crest).

Stability

Reconstitution

Standard concentration/diluent: 25,000 units/500 mL D_5W (premixed). If preparing solution, mix thoroughly prior to administration.

Minimum volume: 250 mL D_5W.

Storage Heparin solutions are colorless to slightly yellow. Minor color variations do not affect therapeutic efficacy. Heparin should be stored at controlled room temperature. Protect from freezing and temperatures >40°C.

Stability at room temperature and refrigeration:

Prepared bag: 24-72 hours (specific to solution, concentration, and/or study conditions)

Premixed bag: After seal is broken. 4 days.

Out of overwrap stability: 30 days.

Monitoring and Teaching Issues

Laboratory Monitoring Hemoglobin, hematocrit; fecal occult blood test; aPTT (or antifactor Xa activity levels) or ACT depending upon indication

Platelet counts should be routinely monitored when the risk of HIT is >0.1% (eg, receiving therapeutic dose heparin, postoperative antithrombotic prophylaxis), if the patient has received heparin or low molecular weight heparin (eg, enoxaparin) within the past 100 days, if pre-exposure history is uncertain, or if anaphylactoid reaction to heparin occurs. When the risk of HIT is <0.1% (eg, medical/obstetrical patients receiving heparin flushes), routine platelet count monitoring is not recommended (Hirsh, 2008).

For intermittent I.V. injections, aPTT is measured 3.5-4 hours after I.V. injection.

For SubQ injections, when used for treatment (eg, monitored dosing regimen), aPTT is measured 6 hours after injection.

Heparin infusion dose adjustment: A number of dose-adjustment nomograms have been developed which target an aPTT range of 1.5-2.5 times control (Cruickshank, 1991; Flaker, 1994; Hull, 1992; Raschke, 1993). However, institution-specific and indication-specific nomograms should be consulted for dose adjustment. **Note:** aPTT values vary throughout the day with maximum values occurring during the night (Decousus, 1985).

Physical Assessment Assess for risk factors for increased bleeding prior to starting therapy. Note specific infusion directions in Administration. Bleeding precautions should be observed at all times during heparin therapy. Monitor for hypersensitivity reaction, bleeding, chest pain, hyperkalemia, and peripheral neuropathy. For I.V. bolus administration, emergency treatment for hypersensitivity reactions should be immediately available. Teach patient bleeding precautions.

Patient Education This drug can only be administered by infusion or injection. You may have a tendency to bleed easily while taking this drug (brush teeth with soft brush, floss with waxed floss, use electric razor, avoid scissors or sharp knives and potentially harmful activities). Report immediately any chest pain; difficulty breathing or unusual cough; bleeding or bruising (bleeding gums, nosebleed, blood in urine, dark stool); pain in joints or back; CNS changes (fever, confusion); unusual fever; persistent nausea or GI upset; change in vision, or swelling, pain, or redness at injection site.

Geriatric Considerations In the clinical setting, age has not been shown to be a reliable predictor of a patient's anticoagulant response to heparin. However, it is common for the elderly to have a "standard" response for the first 24-48 hours after a loading dose (5000 units) and a maintenance infusion of 800-1000 units/hour. After this period, they then have an exaggerated response (ie, elevated aPTT), requiring a lower infusion rate. Hence, monitor closely during this period of therapy. Elderly women are more likely to have bleeding complications and osteoporosis may be a problem when used >3 months or total daily dose exceeds 30,000 units.

Breast-Feeding Considerations Some products contain benzyl alcohol as a preservative; their use in breast-feeding women is contraindicated by some manufacturers due to the association of gasping syndrome in premature infants.

Pregnancy Considerations Animal reproduction studies have not been conducted. Heparin does not cross the placenta. Some products contain benzyl alcohol as a preservative; their use in pregnant women is contraindicated by some manufacturers.

Related Information

Compatibility of Drugs *on page 1994*

◆ **Heparin Calcium** *see* Heparin *on page 898*

◆ **Heparin Lock Flush** *see* Heparin *on page 898*

◆ **Heparin Sodium** *see* Heparin *on page 898*

Hepatitis A and Hepatitis B Recombinant Vaccine

(hep a TYE tis aye & hep a TYE tis bee ree KOM be nant vak SEEN)

U.S. Brand Names Twinrix®

Index Terms Engerix-B® and Havrix®; Havrix® and Engerix-B®; HepA-HepB; Hepatitis B and Hepatitis A Vaccine

Generic Availability (U.S.) No

Pharmacologic Category Vaccine, Inactivated (Viral)

Pregnancy Risk Factor C

Lactation Excretion in breast milk unknown/use caution

Use Active immunization against disease caused by hepatitis A virus and hepatitis B virus (all known subtypes) in populations desiring protection against or at high risk of exposure to these viruses.

Populations include travelers or people living in or relocating to areas of intermediate/high endemicity for **both** HAV and HBV and are at increased risk of HBV infection due to behavioral or occupational factors; patients with chronic liver disease; laboratory workers who handle live HAV and HBV; healthcare workers, police, and other personnel who render first-aid or medical assistance; workers who come in contact with sewage; employees of day care centers and correctional facilities; patients/staff of hemodialysis units; men who have sex with men; patients frequently receiving blood products; military personnel; users of injectable illicit drugs; close household contacts of patients with hepatitis A and hepatitis B infection; residents of drug and alcohol treatment centers

Available Dosage Forms

Injection, suspension [preservative free]:

Twinrix®: Hepatitis A virus antigen 720 ELISA units and hepatitis B surface antigen 20 mcg per mL (1 mL)

Dosing

Adult & Geriatric Primary immunization: I.M.: Three doses (1 mL each) given on a 0-, 1-, and 6-month schedule

Alternative regimen: Accelerated regimen: Four doses (1 mL each) on day 0, 7, and 21-30, followed by a booster at 12 months

Pediatric *Canadian labeling (not in U.S. labeling):*

Primary immunization: I.M.: Children 1-18 years: Twinrix® Junior [(CAN); not available in U.S.]: Three doses (0.5 mL each) given on a 0-, 1-, and 6-month schedule

Alternative regimen: Children 1-15 years: Twinrix®: One dose (1 mL) given on elected date followed by second dose (1 mL) 6-12 months later

Administration

I.M. Shake well prior to use. Do not dilute prior to administration. Discard if the suspension is discolored or does not appear homogenous after shaking or if there are cracks in the vial or syringe. Administer in the deltoid region; do not administer in the gluteal region (may give suboptimal response). Administer in the anterolateral thigh in infants (Canadian labeling). Do not administer at the same site, or using the same syringe, as additional vaccines or immunoglobulins.

For patients at risk of hemorrhage following intramuscular injection, the ACIP recommends "it should be administered intramuscularly if, in the opinion of the physician familiar with the patients bleeding risk, the vaccine can be administered by this route with reasonable safety. If the patient receives antihemophilia or other similar therapy, intramuscular vaccination can be ▶

scheduled shortly after such therapy is administered. A fine needle (23 gauge or smaller) can be used for the vaccination and firm pressure applied to the site (without rubbing) for at least 2 minutes. The patient should be instructed concerning the risk of hematoma from the injection." Patients on anticoagulant therapy should be considered to have the same bleeding risks and treated as those with clotting factor disorders (CDC, 2011).

Simultaneous administration of vaccines helps ensure the patients will be fully vaccinated by the appropriate age. Simultaneous administration of vaccines is defined as administering >1 vaccine on the same day at different anatomic sites. The use of licensed combination vaccines is generally preferred over separate injections of the equivalent components. Separate vaccines should not be combined in the same syringe unless indicated by product specific labeling. Separate needles and syringes should be used for each injection. The ACIP prefers each dose of a specific vaccine in a series come from the same manufacturer when possible. Adolescents and adults should be vaccinated while seated or lying down. In general, preterm infants should be vaccinated at the same chronological age as full-term infants (CDC, 2011).

Antipyretics have not been shown to prevent febrile seizures. Antipyretics may be used to treat fever or discomfort following vaccination (CDC, 2011). One study reported that routine prophylactic administration of acetaminophen to prevent fever prior to vaccination decreased the immune response of some vaccines; the clinical significance of this reduction in immune response has not been established (Prymula, 2009).

Monitoring and Teaching Issues

Physical Assessment Have emergency treatment for anaphylactoid or hypersensitivity reaction available. Observe patient for 15 minutes following administration. All serious adverse reactions must be reported to the U.S. DHHS. Federal law also requires entry into the patient's medical record.

Patient Education You may experience fever, fatigue, nausea, vomiting, diarrhea, and redness and tenderness at injection site. Notify prescriber if symptoms persist.

Related Information

Immunization Recommendations *on page 1941*

Hepatitis A Vaccine (hep a TYE tis aye vak SEEN)

U.S. Brand Names Havrix®; VAQTA®

Index Terms HepA

Generic Availability (U.S.) No

Pharmacologic Category Vaccine, Inactivated (Viral)

Medication Safety Issues

International issues:

Avaxim [Canada and multiple international markets] may be confused with Avastin brand name for bevacizumab [U.S., Canada, and multiple international markets]

Pregnancy Risk Factor C

Lactation Excretion in breast milk unknown/use caution

Use

Active immunization against disease caused by hepatitis A virus (HAV)

The Advisory Committee on Immunization Practices (ACIP) recommends routine vaccination for:

- All children ≥12 months of age
- All unvaccinated adults requesting protection from HAV infection
- All unvaccinated adults at risk for HAV infection, such as:
  - Behavioral risks: Men who have sex with men; injection drug users
  - Occupational risks: Persons who work with HAV-infected primates or with HAV in a research laboratory setting
  - Medical risks: Persons with chronic liver disease; patients who receive clotting-factor concentrates
- Other risks: International travelers to regions with high or intermediate levels of endemic HAV infection (a list of countries is available at http://wwwn.cdc.gov/travel/contentdiseases.aspx)
- Unvaccinated persons who anticipate close personal contact with international adoptee from a country of intermediate to high endemicity of HAV, during their first 60 days of arrival into the United States (eg, household contacts, babysitters)

Available Dosage Forms

Injection, suspension [preservative free]:

Havrix®: Hepatitis A virus antigen 720 ELISA units/0.5 mL (0.5 mL); Hepatitis A virus antigen 1440 ELISA units/mL (1 mL)

VAQTA®: Hepatitis A virus antigen 25 units/0.5 mL (0.5 mL); Hepatitis A virus antigen 50 units/mL (1 mL)

Dosing

Adult & Geriatric Immunization: I.M.: **Note:** When used for primary immunization, the vaccine should be given at least 2 weeks prior to expected HAV exposure. When used prior to an international adoption, the vaccination series should begin when adoption is being planned, but ideally ≥2 weeks prior to expected arrival of adoptee. When used for postexposure prophylaxis, the vaccine should be given as soon as possible.

HAVRIX®: 1440 ELISA units (1 mL) with a booster dose of 1440 ELISA units to be given 6-12 months following primary immunization

VAQTA®: 50 units (1 mL) with a booster dose of 50 units (1 mL) to be given 6-18 months after primary immunization (6-12 months if initial dose was with HAVRIX®)

Pediatric Immunization: I.M.: **Note:** When used for primary immunization, the vaccine should be given at least 2 weeks prior to expected HAV exposure. When used prior to an international adoption, the vaccination series should begin when adoption is being planned, but ideally ≥2 weeks prior to expected arrival of adoptee. When used for postexposure prophylaxis, the vaccine should be given as soon as possible.

HAVRIX®: Children 12 months to 18 years: 720 ELISA units (0.5 mL) with a booster dose of 720 ELISA units to be given 6-12 months following primary immunization

VAQTA®: Children 12 months to 18 years: 25 units (0.5 mL) with a booster dose of 25 units (0.5 mL) to be given 6-18 months after primary immunization (6-12 months if initial dose was with HAVRIX®)

Administration

I.M. The deltoid muscle is the preferred site for injection for older children and adults; administer to the anterolateral aspect of the thigh in infants and young children. Do not administer to the gluteal region; may decrease efficacy. Do not administer intravenously, intradermally, or subcutaneously. Shake well prior to use; discard if the suspension is discolored or does not appear homogenous after shaking, or if there are cracks in the vial or syringe. When used for primary immunization, the vaccine should be given at least 2 weeks prior to expected HAV exposure. When used for postexposure prophylaxis, the vaccine should be given as soon as possible. For patients at risk of hemorrhage following intramuscular injection, the ACIP recommends "it should be administered intramuscularly if, in the opinion of the physician familiar with the patients bleeding risk, the vaccine can be administered by this route with reasonable safety. If the patient receives antihemophilia or other similar therapy, intramuscular vaccination can be scheduled shortly after such therapy is administered. A fine needle (23 gauge or smaller) can be used for the vaccination and firm pressure applied to the site (without rubbing) for at least 2 minutes. The patient should be instructed concerning the risk of hematoma from the injection." Patients on anticoagulant therapy should be considered to have the same bleeding risks and treated as those with clotting factor disorders (CDC, 2011).

Simultaneous administration of vaccines helps ensure the patients will be fully vaccinated by the appropriate age. Simultaneous administration of vaccines is defined as administering >1 vaccine on the same day at different anatomic sites. The use of licensed combination vaccines is generally preferred over separate injections of the equivalent components. Separate vaccines should not be combined in the same syringe unless indicated by product specific labeling. Separate needles and syringes should be used for each injection. The ACIP prefers each dose of a specific vaccine in a series come from the same manufacturer when possible. Adolescents and adults should be vaccinated while seated or lying down. In general, preterm infants should be vaccinated at the same chronological age as full-term infants (CDC 2011).

Antipyretics have not been shown to prevent febrile seizures. Antipyretics may be used to treat fever or discomfort following vaccination (CDC, 2011). One study reported that routine prophylactic administration of acetaminophen to prevent fever prior to vaccination decreased the immune response of some vaccines; the clinical significance of this reduction in immune response has not been established (Prymula, 2009).

Monitoring and Teaching Issues

Physical Assessment All serious adverse reactions must be reported to the U.S. DHHS. Federal law also requires entry into the patient's medical record.

Patient Education Inform healthcare provider if you have a high fever, change in behavior, or a rash.

Related Information

Immunization Recommendations *on page 1941*

Prophylaxis for Patients Exposed to Common Communicable Diseases *on page 2073*

◆ **Hepatitis B and Hepatitis A Vaccine** *see* Hepatitis A and Hepatitis B Recombinant Vaccine *on page 903*

◆ **Hepatitis B Inactivated Virus Vaccine (recombinant DNA)** *see* Hepatitis B Vaccine (Recombinant) *on page 905*

Hepatitis B Vaccine (Recombinant)

(hep a TYE tis bee vak SEEN ree KOM be nant)

U.S. Brand Names Engerix-B®; Recombivax HB®

Index Terms Hepatitis B Inactivated Virus Vaccine (recombinant DNA); HepB

Generic Availability (U.S.) No

Pharmacologic Category Vaccine, Inactivated (Viral)

Medication Safety Issues

Sound-alike/look-alike issues:

Engerix-B® adult may be confused with Engerix-B® pediatric/adolescent

Recombivax HB® may be confused with Comvax®

Pregnancy Risk Factor C

Lactation Excretion in breast milk unknown/use caution

Use Immunization against infection caused by all known subtypes of hepatitis B virus (HBV)

The Advisory Committee on Immunization Practices (ACIP) recommends routine vaccination for the following (CDC 2006; CDC 2005):

- All infants at birth
- All infants and children (post-birth dose; refer to recommended vaccination schedule)
- All unvaccinated adults requesting protection from HBV infection

- All unvaccinated adults at risk for HBV infection such as those with:
  Behavioral risks: Sexually-active persons with >1 partner in a 6-month period; persons seeking evaluation or treatment for a sexually-transmitted disease; men who have sex with men; injection drug users
  Occupational risks: Healthcare and public safety workers with reasonably anticipated risk for exposure to blood or blood contaminated body fluids
  Medical risks: Persons with end-stage renal disease (including predialysis, hemodialysis, peritoneal dialysis, and home dialysis); persons with HIV infection; persons with chronic liver disease
  Other risks: Household contacts and sex partners of persons with chronic HBV infection; residents and staff of facilities for developmentally disabled persons; international travelers to regions with high or intermediate levels of endemic HBV infection

In addition, the ACIP recommends vaccination for any persons who are wounded in bombings or similar mass casualty events who have penetrating injuries or nonintact skin exposure, or who have contact with mucous membranes (exception - superficial contact with intact skin), and who cannot confirm receipt of a hepatitis B vaccination (CDC, 2008).

Available Dosage Forms

Injection, suspension [preservative free]:

Engerix-B®: Hepatitis B surface antigen 10 mcg/0.5 mL (0.5 mL); Hepatitis B surface antigen 20 mcg/mL (1 mL)

Recombivax HB®: Hepatitis B surface antigen 5 mcg/0.5 mL (0.5 mL); Hepatitis B surface antigen 10 mcg/mL (1 mL); Hepatitis B surface antigen 40 mcg/mL (1 mL)

Dosing

Adult & Geriatric

Primary immunization: I.M.: 1 mL/dose (adult formulation) for 3 total doses administered at 0, 1, and 6 months

Note: Adult formulations of hepatitis B vaccine products differ by concentration (mcg/mL) but when dosed in terms of volume (mL), the dose of Engerix-B® and Recombivax HB® are the same (both 1 mL).

Alternate dosing schedules (selection of schedule should optimize compliance with vaccination): All regimens use the adult formulation administered as one dose at the following intervals (three schedules presented):

0, 1, and 4 months (CDC, 2005)
0, 2, and 4 months (CDC, 2005)
0, 12, and 24 months (CDC, 2005)

Bombings or similar mass casualty events: I.M.: In persons without a reliable history of vaccination against HepB and who have no known contraindications to the vaccine, vaccination should begin within 24 hours (but no later than 7 days) following the event (CDC, 2008).

Pediatric

Primary immunization: I.M.:

Infants: 0.5 mL/dose (pediatric/adolescent formulation) for 3 total doses administered at 0, 1 and 6 months. Alternate dosing regimens are also available for children who begin vaccination ≥1 year of age.

Note: Doses are presented using the pediatric/adolescent formulations. Pediatric/adolescent formulations of hepatitis B vaccine products differ by concentration (mcg/mL). However, when dosed in terms of volume (mL), the dose of Engerix-B® and Recombivax HB® are the same (both 0.5 mL).

Note: Combination vaccines (eg, vaccines containing HepB with DTaP, HIB) should not be used for the "birth" dose but may be used to complete the course beginning after the infant is ≥6 weeks of age (CDC, 2005). Please see combination vaccine monographs for dose and schedule details.

Infants (HB_sAg-**negative** mothers):

First dose: 0.5 mL at birth or before discharge (may be delayed in certain cases)
Second dose: 0.5 mL at 1-2 months of age
Third dose: 0.5 mL at 6-18 months of age, but no sooner than 24 weeks of age

Note: Premature neonates <2 kg may have the initial dose deferred up to 30 days of chronological age or at hospital discharge (CDC, 2005).

Infants (HB_sAg-**positive** mothers):

First dose: 0.5 mL within first 12 hours of life, even if premature and regardless of birth weight (hepatitis immune globulin should also be administered at the same time at a different site)
Second dose: 0.5 mL at 1-2 months of age
Third dose: 0.5 mL at 6 months of age but no sooner than 24 weeks of age

Note: Anti-HB_s and HB_sAg levels should be checked at 9-18 months of age (ie, next well-child visit after series completion). If HB_sAg negative and anti-HB_s levels <10 mIU/mL, reimmunize with 3 doses and reassess 1-2 months after the third dose.

Note: In premature neonates <2 kg, the birth dose should not be counted as part of the 3-dose vaccine series (CDC, 2005).

Infants (mother's HB_sAg status **unknown**):

First dose: 0.5 mL within 12 hours of birth even if premature and regardless of birth weight
Second dose: 0.5 mL at 1-2 months of age
Third dose: 0.5 mL at 6 months of age but no sooner than 24 weeks of age

Note: If mother is later determined to be HB_sAg-positive, the infant should receive hepatitis immune globulin as soon as possible (no later than age 1 week).

Note: In premature neonates <2 kg, the birth dose should not be counted as part of the 3-dose vaccine series (CDC, 2005).

Children: 0.5 mL/dose (pediatric/adolescent formulation) administered at 0, 1, and 6 months (for 3 total doses). Alternate dosing regimens are also available for children who begin vaccination ≥1 year of age.

Alternate dosing schedules (selection of schedule should optimize compliance with vaccination):

Children 1-10 years: 0.5 mL (pediatric/adolescent formulation) at the following intervals (two schedules presented):

0, 2, and 4 months (CDC, 2005)

0, 1, 2, and 12 months (Engerix-B®)

Children 5-10 years: 0.5 mL (pediatric/adolescent formulation) at 0, 12, and 24 months (Engerix-B®)

Children 11-15 years: 1 mL (adult formulation) at 0 and 4-6 months (Recombivax HB®)

Children 11-16 years: 0.5 mL (pediatric/adolescent formulation) at 0, 12, and 24 months (Engerix-B®)

Children 11-18 years: 0.5 mL (pediatric/adolescent formulation) at the following intervals (three schedules presented):

0, 1, and 4 months (CDC, 2005)

0, 2, and 4 months (CDC, 2005)

0, 12, and 24 months (CDC, 2005)

Children 11-18 years: 1 mL (adult formulation) at 0, 1, 2, and 12 months (Engerix-B®)

Bombings or similar mass casualty events: Refer to adult dosing.

Renal Impairment Adults on dialysis:

Engerix-B® 20 mcg/mL: Administer 2 mL per dose at 0, 1, 2, and 6 months

Recombivax HB® 40 mcg/mL: Administer 1 mL per dose at 0, 1, and 6 months

Note: Serologic testing is recommended 1-2 months after the final dose of the primary vaccine series and annually to determine the need for booster doses. Persons with anti-HB_s concentrations of <10 mIU/mL should be revaccinated with 3 doses of the vaccine (CDC, 2006).

Administration

I.M. Pediatric/adolescent formulations of hepatitis B vaccine products differ by concentration (mcg/mL). However, when dosed in terms of volume (mL), the dose of Engerix-B® and Recombivax HB® are the same (both 0.5 mL). Adult formulations of hepatitis B vaccine products also differ by concentration (mcg/mL), but when dosed in terms of volume (mL), the dose of Engerix-B® and Recombivax HB® are the same (both 1 mL). It is possible to interchange the vaccines for completion of a series or for booster doses; the antibody produced in response to each type of vaccine is comparable, however, the quantity of the vaccine will vary

I.M. injection only; in adults, the deltoid muscle is the preferred site; the anterolateral thigh is the recommended site in infants and young children. Not for gluteal administration. Shake well prior to withdrawal and use.

For patients at risk of hemorrhage following intramuscular injection, hepatitis B vaccine may be administered subcutaneously although lower titers and/or increased incidence of local reactions may result. The ACIP recommends "it should be administered intramuscularly if, in the opinion of the physician familiar with the patients bleeding risk, the vaccine can be administered by this route with reasonable safety. If the patient receives antihemophilia or other similar therapy, intramuscular vaccination can be scheduled shortly after such therapy is administered. A fine needle (23 gauge or smaller) can be used for the vaccination and firm pressure applied to the site (without rubbing) for at least 2 minutes. The patient should be instructed concerning the risk of hematoma from the injection." Patients on anticoagulant therapy should be considered to have the same bleeding risks and treated as those with clotting factor disorders (CDC, 2011).

Simultaneous administration of vaccines helps ensure the patients will be fully vaccinated by the appropriate age. Simultaneous administration of vaccines is defined as administering >1 vaccine on the same day at different anatomic sites. The use of licensed combination vaccines is generally preferred over separate injections of the equivalent components. Separate vaccines should not be combined in the same syringe unless indicated by product specific labeling. Separate needles and syringes should be used for each injection. The ACIP prefers each dose of a specific vaccine in a series come from the same manufacturer when possible. Adolescents and adults should be vaccinated while seated or lying down. In general, preterm infants should be vaccinated at the same chronological age as full-term infants (CDC, 2011).

Antipyretics have not been shown to prevent febrile seizures. Antipyretics may be used to treat fever or discomfort following vaccination (CDC, 2011). One study reported that routine prophylactic administration of acetaminophen to prevent fever prior to vaccination decreased the immune response of some vaccines; the clinical significance of this reduction in immune response has not been established (Prymula, 2009).

Vaccination at the time of HB_sAg testing: For persons in whom vaccination is recommended, the first dose of hepatitis B vaccine can be given after blood is drawn to test for HB_sAg.

Monitoring and Teaching Issues

Physical Assessment All serious adverse reactions must be reported to the U.S. DHHS. Federal law also requires entry into the patient's medical record.

Patient Education All serious adverse reactions must be reported to the U.S. DHHS. Federal law also requires entry into the patient's medical record.

Related Information

Immunization Recommendations *on page* 1941

Prophylaxis for Patients Exposed to Common Communicable Diseases *on page* 2073

◆ **Hepatitis B Vaccine (Recombinant)** *see Haemophilus* b Conjugate and Hepatitis B Vaccine *on page* 892

◆ **HepB** *see* Hepatitis B Vaccine (Recombinant) *on page* 905

◆ **HepFlush®-10** *see* Heparin *on page* 898

◆ **Hep-Lock** *see* Heparin *on page* 898

◆ **Hep-Lock U/P** *see* Heparin *on page* 898

◆ **Hepsera®** *see* Adefovir *on page* 52

◆ **Herceptin®** *see* Trastuzumab *on page* 1804

◆ **HES** *see* Hetastarch *on page* 908

◆ **Hespan®** *see* Hetastarch *on page* 908

Hetastarch (HET a starch)

U.S. Brand Names Hespan®; Hextend®

Index Terms HES; Hydroxyethyl Starch

Generic Availability (U.S.) Yes: Sodium chloride infusion

Pharmacologic Category Plasma Volume Expander, Colloid

Medication Safety Issues

Sound-alike/look-alike issues:

Hespan® may be confused with heparin

Pregnancy Risk Factor C

Lactation Excretion in breast milk unknown/use caution

Use Blood volume expander used in treatment of hypovolemia; adjunct in leukapheresis to improve harvesting and increase the yield of granulocytes by centrifugation (Hespan®)

Unlabeled/Investigational Use Priming fluid in pump oxygenators during cardiopulmonary bypass; plasma volume expansion during cardiopulmonary bypass

Available Dosage Forms

Infusion:

Hextend®: 6% (500 mL)

Infusion, premixed in NS: 6% (500 mL)

Hespan®: 6% (500 mL)

Dosing

Adult & Geriatric

Volume expansion: I.V. infusion: 500-1000 mL (up to 1500 mL/day) or 20 mL/kg/day (up to 1500 mL/day); larger volumes (15,000 mL/24 hours) have been used safely in small numbers of patients

Leukapheresis (Hespan®): I.V. infusion: 250-700 mL; **Note:** Citrate anticoagulant is added before use.

Renal Impairment Cl_{cr} <10 mL/minute: Initial dose is the same but subsequent doses should be reduced by 20% to 50% of normal.

Administration

I.V. Administer I.V. only; infusion pump is required. May administer up to 1.2 g/kg/hour (20 mL/kg/hour). Change I.V. tubing or flush copiously with normal saline before administering blood through the same line. Change I.V. tubing at least every 24 hours. Do not administer Hextend® with blood through the same administration set. Anaphylactoid reactions can occur, have epinephrine and resuscitative equipment available.

Other Leukapheresis: Mix Hespan® and citrate well. Administer to the input line of the centrifuge apparatus at a ration of 1:8 to 1:13 to venous whole blood.

Monitoring and Teaching Issues

Laboratory Monitoring

Volume expansion: Hemoglobin, hematocrit, serum electrolytes, renal function, acid-base balance, coagulation parameters

Leukapheresis: CBC, total leukocyte and platelet counts, leukocyte differential count, hemoglobin, hematocrit, PT, PTT

Physical Assessment Assess patient's allergy history prior to therapy (patients allergic to corn may have a cross allergy to hetastarch). Assess contraindications: Coagulation or bleeding disorder, intracranial bleeding, dialysis, renal failure, severe hepatic disease, fluid overload condition. Patient must be monitored closely for hypersensitivity reaction and circulatory overload. Vital signs, CVP, and urine output should be monitored frequently (every 5-15 minutes) during first hour and at regular intervals thereafter.

Patient Education Report immediately any chest pain or palpitations, respiratory difficulty, acute headache, chills, or itching.

◆ **Hexachlorocyclohexane** *see* Lindane *on page* 1110

◆ **Hexalen®** *see* Altretamine *on page* 89

◆ **Hexamethylmelamine** *see* Altretamine *on page* 89

◆ **HEXM** *see* Altretamine *on page* 89

◆ **Hextend®** *see* Hetastarch *on page* 908

◆ **hGH** *see* Somatropin *on page* 1664

- **Hib** *see Haemophilus* b Conjugate Vaccine *on page 893*
- **Hib Conjugate Vaccine** *see Haemophilus* b Conjugate and Hepatitis B Vaccine *on page 892*
- **Hib Conjugate Vaccine** *see Haemophilus* b Conjugate Vaccine *on page 893*
- **Hiberix®** *see Haemophilus* b Conjugate Vaccine *on page 893*
- **Hib-HepB** *see Haemophilus* b Conjugate and Hepatitis B Vaccine *on page 892*
- **Hib Polysaccharide Conjugate** *see Haemophilus* b Conjugate Vaccine *on page 893*
- **High-Molecular-Weight Iron Dextran (DexFerrum®)** *see* Iron Dextran Complex *on page 1021*
- **Histaprin [OTC]** *see* DiphenhydrAMINE (Systemic) *on page 543*
- **Hizentra®** *see* Immune Globulin *on page 961*
- **hMG** *see* Menotropins *on page 1170*
- **HMM** *see* Altretamine *on page 89*
- **HMR 3647** *see* Telithromycin *on page 1715*
- **Horse Antihuman Thymocyte Gamma Globulin** *see* Antithymocyte Globulin (Equine) *on page 136*
- **HPV2** *see* Papillomavirus (Types 16, 18) Vaccine (Human, Recombinant) *on page 1409*
- **HPV4** *see* Papillomavirus (Types 6, 11, 16, 18) Vaccine (Human, Recombinant) *on page 1408*
- **HPV 16/18 L1 VLP/AS04 VAC** *see* Papillomavirus (Types 16, 18) Vaccine (Human, Recombinant) *on page 1409*
- **HPV Vaccine** *see* Papillomavirus (Types 6, 11, 16, 18) Vaccine (Human, Recombinant) *on page 1408*
- **HPV Vaccine** *see* Papillomavirus (Types 16, 18) Vaccine (Human, Recombinant) *on page 1409*
- **HTF919** *see* Tegaserod *on page 1712*
- **HumaLOG®** *see* Insulin Lispro *on page 989*
- **HumaLOG® KwikPen™** *see* Insulin Lispro *on page 989*
- **HumaLOG® Mix 50/50™** *see* Insulin Lispro Protamine and Insulin Lispro *on page 991*
- **HumaLOG® Mix 50/50™ KwikPen™** *see* Insulin Lispro Protamine and Insulin Lispro *on page 991*
- **HumaLOG® Mix 75/25™** *see* Insulin Lispro Protamine and Insulin Lispro *on page 991*
- **HumaLOG® Mix 75/25™ KwikPen™** *see* Insulin Lispro Protamine and Insulin Lispro *on page 991*
- **Human Albumin Grifols® 25%** *see* Albumin *on page 57*
- **Human Antitumor Necrosis Factor Alpha** *see* Adalimumab *on page 48*
- **Human Diploid Cell Cultures Rabies Vaccine** *see* Rabies Vaccine *on page 1546*
- **Human Growth Hormone** *see* Somatropin *on page 1664*
- **Human LFA-3/IgG(1) Fusion Protein** *see* Alefacept *on page 65*
- **Human Menopausal Gonadotropin** *see* Menotropins *on page 1170*
- **Human Papillomavirus Vaccine** *see* Papillomavirus (Types 6, 11, 16, 18) Vaccine (Human, Recombinant) *on page 1408*
- **Human Papillomavirus Vaccine** *see* Papillomavirus (Types 16, 18) Vaccine (Human, Recombinant) *on page 1409*
- **Human Rotavirus Vaccine, Attenuated (HRV)** *see* Rotavirus Vaccine *on page 1616*
- **Humate-P®** *see* Antihemophilic Factor/von Willebrand Factor Complex (Human) *on page 134*
- **Humatrope®** *see* Somatropin *on page 1664*
- **HuMax-CD20** *see* Ofatumumab *on page 1342*
- **Humibid® Maximum Strength [OTC]** *see* GuaiFENesin *on page 890*
- **Humira®** *see* Adalimumab *on page 48*
- **Humira® Pen** *see* Adalimumab *on page 48*
- **HumuLIN® 70/30** *see* Insulin NPH and Insulin Regular *on page 993*
- **HumuLIN® N** *see* Insulin NPH *on page 992*
- **HumuLIN® R** *see* Insulin Regular *on page 994*
- **HumuLIN® R U-500** *see* Insulin Regular *on page 994*
- **HXM** *see* Altretamine *on page 89*
- **Hycamptamine** *see* Topotecan *on page 1790*
- **Hycamtin®** *see* Topotecan *on page 1790*
- **hycet®** *see* Hydrocodone and Acetaminophen *on page 915*

HydrALAZINE (hye DRAL a zeen)

Index Terms Apresoline [DSC]; Hydralazine Hydrochloride
Generic Availability (U.S.) Yes
Pharmacologic Category Vasodilator

Medication Safety Issues

Sound-alike/look-alike issues:

HydrALAZINE may be confused with hydrOXYzine

Pregnancy Risk Factor C

Lactation Enters breast milk/use caution (AAP rates "compatible"; AAP 2001 update pending)

Use Management of moderate-to-severe hypertension

Unlabeled/Investigational Use Heart failure; hypertension secondary to pre-eclampsia/ eclampsia

Mechanism of Action/Effect Direct vasodilation of arterioles (with little effect on veins) with decreased systemic resistance

Contraindications Hypersensitivity to hydralazine or any component of the formulation; mitral valve rheumatic heart disease

Warnings/Precautions May cause peripheral neuritis or a drug-induced lupus-like syndrome (more likely on larger doses, longer duration). Discontinue hydralazine in patients who develop SLE-like syndrome or positive ANA. Use with caution in patients with severe renal disease or cerebral vascular accidents or with known or suspected coronary artery disease; monitor blood pressure closely with I.V. use. Slow acetylators, patients with decreased renal function, and patients receiving >200 mg/day (chronically) are at higher risk for SLE. Titrate dosage cautiously to patient's response. Hypotensive effect after I.V. administration may be delayed and unpredictable in some patients. Usually administered with diuretic and a beta-blocker to counteract side effects of sodium and water retention and reflex tachycardia.

Adjust dose in severe renal dysfunction. Use with caution in CAD (increase in tachycardia may increase myocardial oxygen demand). Use with caution in pulmonary hypertension (may cause hypotension). Patients may be poorly compliant because of frequent dosing. Hydralazine-induced fluid and sodium retention may require addition or increased dosage of a diuretic.

Drug Interactions

Metabolism/Transport Effects Inhibits CYP3A4 (weak)

Avoid Concomitant Use There are no known interactions where it is recommended to avoid concomitant use.

Decreased Effect

The levels/effects of HydrALAZINE may be decreased by: Herbs (Hypertensive Properties); Methylphenidate; Nonsteroidal Anti-Inflammatory Agents; Yohimbine

Increased Effect/Toxicity

HydrALAZINE may increase the levels/effects of: Amifostine; Antihypertensives; Hypotensive Agents; RiTUXimab

The levels/effects of HydrALAZINE may be increased by: Diazoxide; Herbs (Hypotensive Properties); MAO Inhibitors; Pentoxifylline; Phosphodiesterase 5 Inhibitors; Prostacyclin Analogues

Nutritional/Ethanol Interactions

Ethanol: Avoid ethanol (may increase CNS depression).

Food: Food enhances bioavailability of hydralazine.

Herb/Nutraceutical: Avoid dong quai if using for hypertension (has estrogenic activity). Avoid ephedra, yohimbe, ginseng (may worsen hypertension). Avoid garlic (may have increased antihypertensive effect).

Adverse Reactions Frequency not defined.

Cardiovascular: Angina pectoris, flushing, orthostatic hypotension, palpitations, paradoxical hypertension, peripheral edema, tachycardia, vascular collapse

Central nervous system: Anxiety, chills, depression, disorientation, dizziness, fever, headache, increased intracranial pressure (I.V.; in patient with pre-existing increased intracranial pressure), psychotic reaction

Dermatologic: Pruritus, rash, urticaria

Gastrointestinal: Anorexia, constipation, diarrhea, nausea, paralytic ileus, vomiting

Genitourinary: Dysuria, impotence

Hematologic: Agranulocytosis, eosinophilia, erythrocyte count reduced, hemoglobin decreased, hemolytic anemia, leukopenia, thrombocytopenia (rare)

Neuromuscular & skeletal: Muscle cramps, peripheral neuritis, rheumatoid arthritis, tremor, weakness

Ocular: Conjunctivitis, lacrimation

Respiratory: Dyspnea, nasal congestion

Miscellaneous: Diaphoresis, drug-induced lupus-like syndrome (dose related; fever, arthralgia, splenomegaly, lymphadenopathy, asthenia, myalgia, malaise, pleuritic chest pain, edema, positive ANA, positive LE cells, maculopapular facial rash, positive direct Coombs' test, pericarditis, pericardial tamponade)

Pharmacodynamics/Kinetics

Onset of Action Oral: 20-30 minutes; I.V.: 5-20 minutes

Duration of Action Oral: Up to 8 hours; I.V.: 1-4 hours; **Note:** May vary depending on acetylator status of patient

Bioavailability 30% to 50%; increased with food

Protein Binding 85% to 90%

Half-Life Elimination Normal renal function: 2-8 hours; End-stage renal disease: 7-16 hours

Metabolism Hepatically acetylated; extensive first-pass effect (oral)

Excretion Urine (14% as unchanged drug)

Available Dosage Forms

Injection, solution: 20 mg/mL (1 mL)

Tablet, oral: 10 mg, 25 mg, 50 mg, 100 mg

Dosing

Adult

Hypertension: Oral: Initial: 10 mg 4 times/day; increase by 10-25 mg/dose every 2-5 days (maximum: 300 mg/day); usual dose range (JNC 7): 25-100 mg/day in 2 divided doses

Acute hypertension: I.M., I.V.: Initial: 10-20 mg/dose every 4-6 hours as needed, may increase to 40 mg/dose; change to oral therapy as soon as possible.

Pre-eclampsia/eclampsia: I.M., I.V.: 5 mg/dose then 5-10 mg every 20-30 minutes as needed

Congestive heart failure: Oral:

Initial dose: 10-25 mg 3-4 times/day

Adjustment: Dosage must be adjusted based on individual response

Target dose: 225-300 mg/day in divided doses; use in combination with isosorbide dinitrate

Geriatric Oral: Initial: 10 mg 2-3 times/day; increase by 10-25 mg/day every 2-5 days.

Pediatric

Hypertension: Oral: Initial: 0.75-1 mg/kg/day in 2-4 divided doses; increase over 3-4 weeks to maximum of 7.5 mg/kg/day in 2-4 divided doses; maximum daily dose: 200 mg/day

Acute hypertension: I.M., I.V.: 0.1-0.2 mg/kg/dose (not to exceed 20 mg) every 4-6 hours as needed, up to 1.7-3.5 mg/kg/day in 4-6 divided doses

Renal Impairment

Cl_{cr} 10-50 mL/minute: Administer every 8 hours.

Cl_{cr} <10 mL/minute: Administer every 8-16 hours in fast acetylators and every 12-24 hours in slow acetylators.

Hemodialysis effects: Supplemental dose is not necessary.

Peritoneal dialysis effects: Supplemental dose is not necessary.

Administration

I.V. Solution for injection: Administer as a slow I.V. push; maximum rate: 5 mg/minute

Stability

Reconstitution Hydralazine should be diluted in NS for IVPB administration due to decreased stability in D_5W. Stability of IVPB solution in NS is 4 days at room temperature.

Storage Intact ampuls/vials of hydralazine should not be stored under refrigeration because of possible precipitation or crystallization.

Monitoring and Teaching Issues

Laboratory Monitoring ANA titer

Physical Assessment Orthostatic precautions should be observed and patient monitored closely during and following infusion. Monitor for hypotension and fluid retention periodically during therapy.

Patient Education Take with meals. Avoid alcohol. This medication does not replace other antihypertensive interventions; follow prescriber's instructions for diet and lifestyle changes. Weigh daily for the first 2 weeks and weekly thereafter. Report weight gain or swelling of feet or ankles. May cause dizziness, weakness, nausea, vomiting, or headache. Report skin rash, severe dizziness or loss of consciousness, significant weight gain, joint pain or swelling, or persistent GI problems.

Dietary Considerations Administer tablet with meals.

Breast-Feeding Considerations In a case report, following a maternal dose of hydralazine 50 mg three times daily, exposure to the infant was calculated to be 0.013 mg per 75mL breast milk.

Pregnancy Considerations Teratogenic effects were observed in animal studies at 20-30 times the maximun daily human dose. Hydralazine crosses the placenta. Hydralazine is recommended for use in the management of hypertension associated with pre-eclampsia.

Related Information

Heart Failure (Systolic) *on page 2040*

Hyperlipidemia Management *on page 2046*

Hydralazine and Hydrochlorothiazide

(hye DRAL a zeen & hye droe klor oh THYE a zide)

Index Terms Apresazide [DSC]; Hydrochlorothiazide and Hydralazine

Generic Availability (U.S.) Yes

Pharmacologic Category Diuretic, Thiazide; Vasodilator, Direct-Acting

Pregnancy Risk Factor C

Lactation Enters breast milk/compatible

Use Management of moderate-to-severe hypertension and treatment of congestive heart failure

Dosing

Adult Hypertension: Oral: Hydralazine 25-100 mg/day and hydrochlorothiazide 25-50 mg/day in 2 divided doses (maximum: Hydrochlorothiazide: 50 mg/day)

Geriatric Refer to dosing in individual monographs.

Monitoring and Teaching Issues

Physical Assessment See individual agents.

Patient Education See individual agents.

Related Information

HydrALAZINE *on page 909*

Hydrochlorothiazide *on page 912*

◆ **Hydralazine Hydrochloride** *see* HydrALAZINE *on page 909*

◆ **Hydrated Chloral** *see* Chloral Hydrate *on page 356*

◆ **Hydrea®** *see* Hydroxyurea *on page 931*

Hydrochlorothiazide (hye droe klor oh THYE a zide)

U.S. Brand Names Microzide®

Index Terms HCTZ (error-prone abbreviation); Hydrodiuril

Generic Availability (U.S.) Yes

Pharmacologic Category Diuretic, Thiazide

Medication Safety Issues

Sound-alike/look-alike issues:

Esidrix may be confused with Lasix®

HCTZ is an error-prone abbreviation (mistaken as hydrocortisone)

Hydrochlorothiazide may be confused with hydrocortisone, hydroflumethiazide, Viskazide®

Microzide™ may be confused with Maxzide®, Micronase®

Pregnancy Risk Factor B

Lactation Enters breast milk/not recommended (AAP rates "compatible"; AAP 2001 update pending)

Use Management of mild-to-moderate hypertension; treatment of edema in heart failure and nephrotic syndrome

Unlabeled/Investigational Use Treatment of lithium-induced diabetes insipidus

Mechanism of Action/Effect Inhibits sodium reabsorption in the distal tubules causing increased excretion of sodium and water as well as potassium and hydrogen ions

Contraindications Hypersensitivity to hydrochlorothiazide or any component of the formulation, thiazides, or sulfonamide-derived drugs; anuria; renal decompensation; pregnancy

Warnings/Precautions Avoid in severe renal disease (ineffective as a diuretic). Electrolyte disturbances (hypokalemia, hypochloremic alkalosis, hyponatremia) can occur. Use with caution in severe hepatic dysfunction; hepatic encephalopathy can be caused by electrolyte disturbances. Gout may be precipitated in certain patients with a history of gout, a familial predisposition to gout, or chronic renal failure. Thiazide diuretics reduce calcium excretion; pathologic changes in the parathyroid glands with hypercalcemia and hypophosphatemia have been observed with prolonged use. Use with caution in patients with prediabetes and diabetes; may alter glucose control. May cause SLE exacerbation or activation. Use with caution in patients with moderate or high cholesterol concentrations. Photosensitization may occur. Correct hypokalemia before initiating therapy. Thiazide diuretics may decrease renal calcium excretion; consider avoiding use in patients with hypercalcemia.

Chemical similarities are present among sulfonamides, sulfonylureas, carbonic anhydrase inhibitors, thiazides, and loop diuretics (except ethacrynic acid). Use in patients with sulfonamide allergy is specifically contraindicated in product labeling, however, a risk of cross-reaction exists in patients with allergy to any of these compounds; avoid use when previous reaction has been severe. Discontinue if signs of hypersensitivity are noted.

Drug Interactions

Avoid Concomitant Use

Avoid concomitant use of Hydrochlorothiazide with any of the following: Dofetilide

Decreased Effect

Hydrochlorothiazide may decrease the levels/effects of: Antidiabetic Agents

The levels/effects of Hydrochlorothiazide may be decreased by: Bile Acid Sequestrants; Herbs (Hypertensive Properties); Methylphenidate; Nonsteroidal Anti-Inflammatory Agents; Yohimbine

Increased Effect/Toxicity

Hydrochlorothiazide may increase the levels/effects of: ACE Inhibitors; Allopurinol; Amifostine; Antihypertensives; Calcium Salts; CarBAMazepine; Dofetilide; Hypotensive Agents; Lithium; OXcarbazepine; RiTUXimab; Topiramate; Toremifene; Vitamin D Analogs

The levels/effects of Hydrochlorothiazide may be increased by: Alcohol (Ethyl); Analgesics (Opioid); Barbiturates; Corticosteroids (Orally Inhaled); Corticosteroids (Systemic); Herbs (Hypotensive Properties); Licorice; MAO Inhibitors; Pentoxifylline; Phosphodiesterase 5 Inhibitors; Prostacyclin Analogues

Nutritional/Ethanol Interactions

Food: Hydrochlorothiazide peak serum levels may be decreased if taken with food. This product may deplete potassium, sodium, and magnesium.

Herb/Nutraceutical: Avoid herbs with *hypertensive* properties (bayberry, blue cohosh, cayenne, ephedra, ginger, ginseng [American], kola, licorice); may diminish the antihypertensive effect of hydrochlorothiazide. Avoid herbs with *hypotensive* properties (black cohosh, California poppy, coleus, golden seal, hawthorn, mistletoe, periwinkle, quinine, shepherd's purse); may enhance the hypotensive effect of hydrochlorothiazide.

Lab Interactions May interfere with parathyroid function tests. Tyramine and phentolamine tests, histamine tests for pheochromocytoma

Adverse Reactions 1% to 10%:

Cardiovascular: Orthostatic hypotension, hypotension

Dermatologic: Photosensitivity

Endocrine & metabolic: Hypokalemia

Gastrointestinal: Anorexia, epigastric distress

Pharmacodynamics/Kinetics

Onset of Action Diuresis: ~2 hours; Peak effect: 4-6 hours

Duration of Action 6-12 hours
Absorption ~50% to 80%
Bioavailability 50% to 80%
Time to Peak 1-2.5 hours
Protein Binding 68%
Half-Life Elimination 5.6-14.8 hours
Metabolism Not metabolized
Excretion Urine (as unchanged drug)

Available Dosage Forms

Capsule, oral: 12.5 mg
Microzide®: 12.5 mg
Tablet, oral: 12.5 mg, 25 mg, 50 mg

Dosing

Adult

Edema (diuresis): Oral: 25-100 mg/day in 1-2 doses; maximum: 200 mg/day
Hypertension: Oral: 12.5-50 mg/day; minimal increase in response and more electrolyte disturbances are seen with doses >50 mg/day

Geriatric Oral: 12.5-25 mg once daily; minimal increase in response and more electrolyte disturbances are seen with doses >50 mg/day.

Pediatric

Hypertension, edema (diuretic): Oral (effect of drug may be decreased when used every day):
<6 months: 1-3 mg/kg/day in 2 divided doses
>6 months to 2 years: 1-3 mg/kg/day in 2 divided doses; maximum: 37.5 mg/day
>2-17 years: Initial: 1 mg/kg/day; maximum: 3 mg/kg/day (50 mg/day)

Note: In pediatric patients, chlorothiazide may be preferred over hydrochlorothiazide as there are more dosage formulations (eg, suspension) available.

Renal Impairment Cl_{cr} <10 mL/minute: Avoid use. Usually ineffective with GFR <30 mL/minute. Effective at lower GFR in combination with a loop diuretic.

Note: ACC/AHA 2009 Heart Failure guidelines suggest that thiazides lose their efficacy when Cl_{cr} <40 mL/minute.

Administration

Oral May be administered with food or milk. Take early in day to avoid nocturia. Take the last dose of multiple doses no later than 6 PM unless instructed otherwise.

Monitoring and Teaching Issues

Laboratory Monitoring Serum electrolytes, BUN, creatinine

Physical Assessment Assess allergy history prior to beginning therapy (sulfonamides). Assess electrolytes, BUN, and creatinine regularly during therapy. Monitor for hypotension, hypokalemia, and confusion regularly. Caution patients with diabetes to monitor glucose levels closely; may alter glucose control.

Patient Education Follow prescriber's instructions for diet and lifestyle changes. Take with meals early in the day to avoid nocturia. Your physician may prescribe a potassium supplement or recommend that you eat foods high in potassium. Do not change your diet on your own while taking this medication, especially if you are taking potassium supplements or medications to reduce potassium loss. May cause dizziness, postural hypotension, or photosensitivity. Report palpitations, muscle cramping, or skin rash.

Dietary Considerations May be taken with food or milk.

Geriatric Considerations Hydrochlorothiazide is not effective in patients with a Cl_{cr} <30 mL/minute, therefore, it may not be a useful agent in many elderly patients.

Breast-Feeding Considerations Thiazide diuretics are found in breast milk. Following a single oral maternal dose of hydrochlorothiazide 50 mg, the mean breast milk concentration was 80 ng/mL (samples collected over 24 hours) and hydrochlorothiazide was not detected in the blood of the breast feeding infant (limit of detection 20 ng/mL). Peak plasma concentrations reported in adults following hydrochlorothiazide 12.5-100 mg are 70-490 ng/mL.

Pregnancy Considerations Adverse events were not observed in animal reproduction studies. Thiazide diuretics cross the placenta and are found in cord blood. Maternal use may cause may cause fetal or neonatal jaundice, thrombocytopenia, or other adverse events observed in adults. Use of thiazide diuretics during normal pregnancies is not appropriate; use may be considered when edema is due to pathologic causes (as in the nonpregnant patient); monitor.

Additional Information If given the morning of surgery, hydrochlorothiazide may render the patient volume depleted and blood pressure may be labile during general anesthesia. Effect of drug may be decreased when used every day.

Related Information

Heart Failure (Systolic) *on page 2040*

◆ **Hydrochlorothiazide, Aliskiren, and Amlodipine** *see* Aliskiren, Amlodipine, and Hydrochlorothiazide *on page 73*

◆ **Hydrochlorothiazide, Amlodipine, and Aliskiren** *see* Aliskiren, Amlodipine, and Hydrochlorothiazide *on page 73*

◆ **Hydrochlorothiazide, Amlodipine, and Valsartan** *see* Amlodipine, Valsartan, and Hydrochlorothiazide *on page 109*

◆ **Hydrochlorothiazide and Aliskiren** *see* Aliskiren and Hydrochlorothiazide *on page 74*

◆ **Hydrochlorothiazide and Amiloride** *see* Amiloride and Hydrochlorothiazide *on page 98*

◆ **Hydrochlorothiazide and Benazepril** *see* Benazepril and Hydrochlorothiazide *on page 198*

◆ **Hydrochlorothiazide and Bisoprolol** *see* Bisoprolol and Hydrochlorothiazide *on page 223*

◆ **Hydrochlorothiazide and Captopril** *see* Captopril and Hydrochlorothiazide *on page 287*

◆ **Hydrochlorothiazide and Enalapril** *see* Enalapril and Hydrochlorothiazide *on page 620*

◆ **Hydrochlorothiazide and Eprosartan** *see* Eprosartan and Hydrochlorothiazide *on page 648*

◆ **Hydrochlorothiazide and Hydralazine** *see* Hydralazine and Hydrochlorothiazide *on page 911*

◆ **Hydrochlorothiazide and Irbesartan** *see* Irbesartan and Hydrochlorothiazide *on page 1014*

◆ **Hydrochlorothiazide and Lisinopril** *see* Lisinopril and Hydrochlorothiazide *on page 1122*

◆ **Hydrochlorothiazide and Losartan** *see* Losartan and Hydrochlorothiazide *on page 1135*

◆ **Hydrochlorothiazide and Moexipril** *see* Moexipril and Hydrochlorothiazide *on page 1252*

◆ **Hydrochlorothiazide and Olmesartan Medoxomil** *see* Olmesartan and Hydrochlorothiazide *on page 1351*

◆ **Hydrochlorothiazide and Propranolol** *see* Propranolol and Hydrochlorothiazide *on page 1526*

◆ **Hydrochlorothiazide and Quinapril** *see* Quinapril and Hydrochlorothiazide *on page 1540*

Hydrochlorothiazide and Spironolactone

(hye droe klor oh THYE a zide & speer on oh LAK tone)

U.S. Brand Names Aldactazide®

Index Terms Spironolactone and Hydrochlorothiazide

Generic Availability (U.S.) Yes

Pharmacologic Category Diuretic, Thiazide; Selective Aldosterone Blocker

Medication Safety Issues

Sound-alike/look-alike issues:

Aldactazide® may be confused with Aldactone®

Pregnancy Risk Factor C

Lactation Enters breast milk/use caution

Use Management of mild-to-moderate hypertension; treatment of edema in congestive heart failure and nephrotic syndrome, and cirrhosis of the liver accompanied by edema and/or ascites

Available Dosage Forms

Tablet: Hydrochlorothiazide 25 mg and spironolactone 25 mg

Aldactazide®: 25/25: Hydrochlorothiazide 25 mg and spironolactone 25 mg; 50/50: Hydrochlorothiazide 50 mg and spironolactone 50 mg

Dosing

Adult Hypertension, edema: Oral: Hydrochlorothiazide 12.5-50 mg/day and spironolactone 12.5-50 mg/day; manufacturer labeling states hydrochlorothiazide maximum 200 mg/day, however, usual dose in JNC-7 is 12.5-50 mg/day

Geriatric Oral: Initial: 1 tablet/day; increase as necessary.

Pediatric Edema: Oral: 1.5-3 mg/kg/day in 2-4 divided doses (maximum: 200 mg/day)

Renal Impairment Efficacy of hydrochlorothiazide is limited in patients with Cl_{cr} <30 mL/minute.

Monitoring and Teaching Issues

Physical Assessment See individual agents.

Patient Education See individual agents.

Related Information

Hydrochlorothiazide *on page 912*

Spironolactone *on page 1678*

◆ **Hydrochlorothiazide and Telmisartan** *see* Telmisartan and Hydrochlorothiazide *on page 1719*

Hydrochlorothiazide and Triamterene

(hye droe klor oh THYE a zide & trye AM ter een)

U.S. Brand Names Dyazide®; Maxzide®; Maxzide®-25

Index Terms Triamterene and Hydrochlorothiazide

Generic Availability (U.S.) Yes

Pharmacologic Category Diuretic, Potassium-Sparing; Diuretic, Thiazide

Medication Safety Issues

Sound-alike/look-alike issues:

Dyazide® may be confused with diazoxide, Dynacin®

Maxzide® may be confused with Maxidex®, Microzide®

Pregnancy Risk Factor C

Lactation Enters breast milk/not recommended

Use Treatment of hypertension or edema (not recommended for initial treatment) when hypokalemia has developed on hydrochlorothiazide alone or when the development of hypokalemia must be avoided

Available Dosage Forms

Capsule: Hydrochlorothiazide 25 mg and triamterene 37.5 mg; hydrochlorothiazide 25 mg and triamterene 50 mg

Dyazide®: Hydrochlorothiazide 25 mg and triamterene 37.5 mg

Tablet: Hydrochlorothiazide 25 mg and triamterene 37.5 mg; hydrochlorothiazide 50 mg and triamterene 75 mg

Maxzide®: Hydrochlorothiazide 50 mg and triamterene 75 mg [scored]

Maxzide®-25: Hydrochlorothiazide 25 mg and triamterene 37.5 mg [scored]

Dosing

Adult & Geriatric Hypertension, edema: Oral:

Hydrochlorothiazide 25 mg and triamterene 37.5 mg: 1-2 tablets/capsules once daily

Hydrochlorothiazide 50 mg and triamterene 75 mg: 1/2-1 tablet daily

Monitoring and Teaching Issues

Laboratory Monitoring Serum electrolytes, BUN, creatinine, liver function tests

Physical Assessment See individual agents.

Patient Education See individual agents.

Related Information

Hydrochlorothiazide *on page 912*

◆ **Hydrochlorothiazide and Valsartan** *see* Valsartan and Hydrochlorothiazide *on page 1840*

Hydrocodone and Acetaminophen (hye droe KOE done & a seet a MIN oh fen)

U.S. Brand Names hycet®; Lorcet® 10/650; Lorcet® Plus; Lortab®; Margesic® H; Maxidone®; Norco®; Stagesic™; Vicodin®; Vicodin® ES; Vicodin® HP; Xodol® 10/300; Xodol® 5/300; Xodol® 7.5/300; Zamicet™; Zolvit™; Zydone®

Index Terms Acetaminophen and Hydrocodone

Generic Availability (U.S.) Yes: Oral solution, tablet

Pharmacologic Category Analgesic Combination (Opioid)

Medication Safety Issues

Sound-alike/look-alike issues:

Lorcet® may be confused with Fioricet®

Lortab® may be confused with Cortef®, Lorabid®

Vicodin® may be confused with Hycodan®, Hycomine®, Indocin®, Uridon®

Zydone® may be confused with Vytone®

High alert medication: The Institute for Safe Medication Practices (ISMP) includes this medication among its list of drug classes which have a heightened risk of causing significant patient harm when used in error.

Duplicate therapy issues: This product contains acetaminophen, which may be a component of other combination products. Do not exceed the maximum recommended daily dose of acetaminophen.

Pregnancy Risk Factor C

Lactation Enters breast milk/not recommended

Use Relief of moderate-to-severe pain

Controlled Substance C-III

Available Dosage Forms

Capsule, oral: Hydrocodone 5 mg and acetaminophen 500 mg

Margesic® H, Stagesic™: Hydrocodone 5 mg and acetaminophen 500 mg

Elixir, oral:

Lortab®: Hydrocodone 7.5 mg and acetaminophen 500 mg per 15 mL

Solution, oral: Hydrocodone 7.5 mg and acetaminophen 500 mg per 15 mL; hydrocodone 10 mg and acetaminophen 325 mg per 15 mL

hycet®: Hydrocodone 7.5 mg and acetaminophen 325 mg per 15 mL

Zamicet™: Hydrocodone 10 mg and acetaminophen 325 mg per 15 mL

Zolvit™: Hydrocodone 10 mg and acetaminophen 300 mg per 15 mL (480 mL)

Tablet, oral:

Generics:

Hydrocodone 2.5 mg and acetaminophen 500 mg
Hydrocodone 5 mg and acetaminophen 300 mg
Hydrocodone 5 mg and acetaminophen 325 mg
Hydrocodone 5 mg and acetaminophen 500 mg
Hydrocodone 7.5 mg and acetaminophen 300 mg
Hydrocodone 7.5 mg and acetaminophen 325 mg
Hydrocodone 7.5 mg and acetaminophen 500 mg
Hydrocodone 7.5 mg and acetaminophen 650 mg
Hydrocodone 7.5 mg and acetaminophen 750 mg
Hydrocodone 10 mg and acetaminophen 300 mg
Hydrocodone 10 mg and acetaminophen 325 mg
Hydrocodone 10 mg and acetaminophen 500 mg
Hydrocodone 10 mg and acetaminophen 650 mg
Hydrocodone 10 mg and acetaminophen 660 mg
Hydrocodone 10 mg and acetaminophen 750 mg

Brands:

Lorcet® 10/650: Hydrocodone 10 mg and acetaminophen 650 mg

Lorcet® Plus: Hydrocodone 7.5 mg and acetaminophen 650 mg

Lortab®: 5/500: Hydrocodone 5 mg and acetaminophen 500 mg; 7.5/500: Hydrocodone 7.5 mg and acetaminophen 500 mg; 10/500: Hydrocodone 10 mg and acetaminophen 500 mg

Maxidone®: Hydrocodone 10 mg and acetaminophen 750 mg

Norco®: Hydrocodone 5 mg and acetaminophen 325 mg; hydrocodone 7.5 mg and acetaminophen 325 mg; hydrocodone 10 mg and acetaminophen 325 mg

Vicodin®: Hydrocodone 5 mg and acetaminophen 500 mg

Vicodin® ES: Hydrocodone 7.5 mg and acetaminophen 750 mg

Vicodin® HP: Hydrocodone 10 mg and acetaminophen 660 mg

Xodol®: 5/300: Hydrocodone 5 mg and acetaminophen 300 mg; 7.5/300: Hydrocodone 7.5 mg and acetaminophen 300 mg; 10/300: Hydrocodone 10 mg and acetaminophen 300 mg

Zydone®: Hydrocodone 5 mg and acetaminophen 400 mg; hydrocodone 7.5 mg and acetaminophen 400 mg; hydrocodone 10 mg and acetaminophen 400 mg

Dosing

Adult Pain management (analgesic): Oral (doses should be titrated to appropriate analgesic effect): Average starting dose in opioid naive patients: Hydrocodone 5-10 mg 4 times/day; the dosage of acetaminophen should be limited to ≤4 g/day (and possibly less in patients with hepatic impairment or ethanol use).

Dosage ranges (based on specific product labeling): Hydrocodone 2.5-10 mg every 4-6 hours (maximum dose of hydrocodone may be limited by the acetaminophen content of specific product)

Geriatric Doses should be titrated to appropriate analgesic effect; 2.5-5 mg of the hydrocodone component every 4-6 hours. Do not exceed 4 g/day of acetaminophen.

Pediatric Pain management (analgesic): Oral (doses should be titrated to appropriate analgesic effect):

Children 2-13 years or <50 kg: Hydrocodone 0.1-0.2 mg/kg/dose every 4-6 hours; do not exceed 6 doses/day or the maximum recommended dose of acetaminophen

Children ≥50 kg: Refer to adult dosing.

Hepatic Impairment Use with caution. Limited, low-dose therapy usually well tolerated in hepatic disease/cirrhosis; however, cases of hepatotoxicity at daily acetaminophen dosages <4 g/day have been reported. Avoid chronic use in hepatic impairment.

Monitoring and Teaching Issues

Physical Assessment See individual agents.

Patient Education See individual agents.

Related Information

Acetaminophen *on page* 38

Hydrocodone and Ibuprofen (hye droe KOE done & eye byoo PROE fen)

U.S. Brand Names Ibudone™; Reprexain™; Vicoprofen®

Index Terms Hydrocodone Bitartrate and Ibuprofen; Ibuprofen and Hydrocodone

Generic Availability (U.S.) Yes

Pharmacologic Category Analgesic, Opioid; Nonsteroidal Anti-inflammatory Drug (NSAID), Oral

Medication Safety Issues

Sound-alike/look-alike issues:

Reprexain™ may be confused with ZyPREXA®

High alert medication: The Institute for Safe Medication Practices (ISMP) includes this medication among its list of drug classes which have a heightened risk of causing significant patient harm when used in error.

Medication Guide Available Yes

Pregnancy Risk Factor C/D (3rd trimester)

Lactation Enters breast milk/not recommended

Use Short-term (generally <10 days) management of moderate-to-severe acute pain; is not indicated for treatment of such conditions as osteoarthritis or rheumatoid arthritis

Controlled Substance C-III

Available Dosage Forms

Tablet: Hydrocodone 5 mg and ibuprofen 200 mg; hydrocodone 7.5 mg and ibuprofen 200 mg

Ibudone™: 5/200: Hydrocodone 5 mg and ibuprofen 200 mg; 10/200: Hydrocodone 10 mg and ibuprofen 200 mg

Reprexain™: 2.5/200: Hydrocodone 2.5 mg and ibuprofen 200 mg; 5/200: Hydrocodone 5 mg and ibuprofen 200 mg; 10/200: Hydrocodone 10 mg and ibuprofen 200 mg

Vicoprofen®: 7.5/200: Hydrocodone 7.5 mg and ibuprofen 200 mg

Dosing

Adult Analgesic: Oral: 1 tablet every 4-6 hours as needed for pain; maximum: 5 tablets/day. **Note:** Short-term use is recommended (<10 days).

Geriatric Use with caution; consider reduced doses. Refer to dosing in individual monographs.

Monitoring and Teaching Issues

Laboratory Monitoring Periodic CBC and chemistry profile with long-term use

Physical Assessment See individual agents.

Patient Education See individual agents.

Related Information

Ibuprofen *on page 938*

◆ **Hydrocodone Bitartrate and Ibuprofen** *see* Hydrocodone and Ibuprofen *on page 916*

Hydrocortisone (Systemic) (hye droe KOR ti sone)

U.S. Brand Names A-Hydrocort®; Cortef®; Solu-CORTEF®

Index Terms A-hydroCort; Compound F; Cortisol; Hydrocortisone Sodium Succinate

Generic Availability (U.S.) Yes: Tablet

Pharmacologic Category Corticosteroid, Systemic

Medication Safety Issues

Sound-alike/look-alike issues:

Hydrocortisone may be confused with hydrocodone, hydroxychloroquine, hydrochlorothiazide

Cortef® may be confused with Coreg®, Lortab®

HCT (occasional abbreviation for hydrocortisone) is an error-prone abbreviation (mistaken as hydrochlorothiazide)

Solu-CORTEF® may be confused with Solu-MEDROL®

Pregnancy Risk Factor C

Lactation Enters breast milk/use caution

Use Management of adrenocortical insufficiency

Unlabeled/Investigational Use Management of septic shock when blood pressure is poorly responsive to fluid resuscitation and vasopressor therapy

Mechanism of Action/Effect Decreases inflammation by suppression of migration of polymorphonuclear leukocytes and reversal of increased capillary permeability

Contraindications Hypersensitivity to hydrocortisone or any component of the formulation; serious infections, except septic shock or tuberculous meningitis; viral, fungal, or tubercular skin lesions; I.M. administration contraindicated in idiopathic thrombocytopenia purpura; intrathecal administration of injection

Warnings/Precautions Use with caution in patients with thyroid disease, hepatic impairment, renal impairment, heart failure, hypertension, diabetes, glaucoma, cataracts, myasthenia gravis, patients at risk for osteoporosis, patients at risk for seizures, or GI diseases (diverticulitis, peptic ulcer, ulcerative colitis) due to perforation risk. Use caution following acute MI (corticosteroids have been associated with myocardial rupture). Because of the risk of adverse effects, systemic corticosteroids should be used cautiously in the elderly in the smallest possible effective dose for the shortest duration. May affect growth velocity; growth should be routinely monitored in pediatric patients. Withdraw therapy with gradual tapering of dose.

May cause hypercorticism or suppression of hypothalamic-pituitary-adrenal (HPA) axis, particularly in younger children or in patients receiving high doses for prolonged periods. HPA axis suppression may lead to adrenal crisis. Withdrawal and discontinuation of a corticosteroid should be done slowly and carefully. Particular care is required when patients are transferred from systemic corticosteroids to inhaled products due to possible adrenal insufficiency or withdrawal from steroids, including an increase in allergic symptoms. Patients receiving >20 mg per day of prednisone (or equivalent) may be most susceptible. Fatalities have occurred due to adrenal insufficiency in asthmatic patients during and after transfer from systemic corticosteroids to aerosol steroids; aerosol steroids do not provide the systemic steroid needed to treat patients having trauma, surgery, or infections.

Acute myopathy has been reported with high dose corticosteroids, usually in patients with neuromuscular transmission disorders; may involve ocular and/or respiratory muscles; monitor creatine kinase; recovery may be delayed. Corticosteroid use may cause psychiatric disturbances, including depression, euphoria, insomnia, mood swings, and personality changes. Pre-existing psychiatric conditions may be exacerbated by corticosteroid use. Prolonged use of corticosteroids may also increase the incidence of secondary infection, mask acute infection (including fungal infections), prolong or exacerbate viral infections, or limit response to vaccines. Exposure to chickenpox should be avoided; corticosteroids should not be used to treat ocular herpes simplex. Corticosteroids should not be used for cerebral malaria or viral hepatitis. Oral steroid treatment is not recommended for the treatment of acute optic neuritis. Close observation is required in patients with latent tuberculosis and/or TB reactivity; restrict use in active TB (only in conjunction with antituberculosis treatment). Prolonged treatment with corticosteroids has been associated with the development of Kaposi's sarcoma (case reports); if noted, discontinuation of therapy should be considered. High-dose corticosteroids should not be used to manage acute head injury.

Drug Interactions

Metabolism/Transport Effects **Substrate** of CYP3A4 (minor), P-glycoprotein; **Induces** CYP3A4 (weak)

Avoid Concomitant Use

Avoid concomitant use of Hydrocortisone (Systemic) with any of the following: Aldesleukin; BCG; Natalizumab; Pimecrolimus; Roflumilast; Tacrolimus (Topical)

Decreased Effect

Hydrocortisone (Systemic) may decrease the levels/effects of: Aldesleukin; Antidiabetic Agents; BCG; Calcitriol; Corticorelin; Isoniazid; Salicylates; Sipuleucel-T; Vaccines (Inactivated)

The levels/effects of Hydrocortisone (Systemic) may be decreased by: Aminoglutethimide; Antacids; Barbiturates; Bile Acid Sequestrants; Echinacea; Mitotane; P-Glycoprotein Inducers; Primidone; Rifamycin Derivatives

Increased Effect/Toxicity

Hydrocortisone (Systemic) may increase the levels/effects of: Acetylcholinesterase Inhibitors; Amphotericin B; Leflunomide; Loop Diuretics; Natalizumab; NSAID (COX-2 Inhibitor); NSAID (Nonselective); Thiazide Diuretics; Vaccines (Live); Warfarin

The levels/effects of Hydrocortisone (Systemic) may be increased by: Antifungal Agents (Azole Derivatives, Systemic); Aprepitant; Calcium Channel Blockers (Nondihydropyridine); Conivaptan; Denosumab; Estrogen Derivatives; Fluconazole; Fosaprepitant; Macrolide Antibiotics; Neuromuscular-Blocking Agents (Nondepolarizing); P-Glycoprotein Inhibitors; Pimecrolimus; Quinolone Antibiotics; Roflumilast; Salicylates; Tacrolimus (Topical); Trastuzumab

Nutritional/Ethanol Interactions

Ethanol: Avoid ethanol (may enhance gastric mucosal irritation).

Food: Hydrocortisone interferes with calcium absorption.

Herb/Nutraceutical: St John's wort may decrease hydrocortisone levels. Avoid cat's claw, echinacea (have immunostimulant properties).

Lab Interactions Interferes with skin tests

Adverse Reactions Frequency not defined.

Cardiovascular: Arrhythmias, bradycardia, cardiac arrest, cardiomegaly, circulatory collapse, congestive heart failure, edema, fat embolism, hypertension, hypertrophic cardiomyopathy (premature infants), myocardial rupture (post MI), syncope, tachycardia, thromboembolism, vasculitis

Central nervous system: Delirium, depression, emotional instability, euphoria, hallucinations, headache, insomnia, intracranial pressure increased, malaise, mood swings, nervousness, neuritis, neuropathy, personality changes, pseudotumor cerebri, psychic disorders, psychoses, seizure, vertigo

Dermatologic: Acne, allergic dermatitis, alopecia, bruising, burning/tingling, dry scaly skin, edema, erythema, hirsutism, hyper-/hypopigmentation, impaired wound healing, petechiae, rash, skin atrophy, skin test reaction impaired, sterile abscess, striae, urticaria

Endocrine & metabolic: Adrenal suppression, alkalosis, amenorrhea, carbohydrate intolerance increased, Cushing's syndrome, diabetes mellitus, glucose intolerance, growth suppression, hyperglycemia, hyperlipidemia, hypokalemia, hypokalemic alkalosis, menstrual irregularities, negative nitrogen balance, pituitary-adrenal axis suppression, potassium loss, protein catabolism, sodium and water retention, sperm motility increased/decreased, spermatogenesis increased/decreased

Gastrointestinal: Abdominal distention, appetite increased, bowel dysfunction (intrathecal administration), indigestion, nausea, pancreatitis, peptic ulcer, gastrointestinal perforation, ulcerative esophagitis, vomiting, weight gain

Genitourinary: Bladder dysfunction (intrathecal administration)

Hematologic: Leukocytosis (transient)

Hepatic: Hepatomegaly, transaminases increased

Local: Atrophy (at injection site), postinjection flare (intra-articular use), thrombophlebitis

Neuromuscular & skeletal: Arthralgia, necrosis (femoral and humoral heads), Charcot-like arthropathy, fractures, muscle mass loss, muscle weakness, myopathy, osteoporosis, tendon rupture, vertebral compression fractures

Ocular: Cataracts, exophthalmoses, glaucoma, intraocular pressure increased

Miscellaneous: Abnormal fat deposits, anaphylaxis, avascular necrosis, diaphoresis, hiccups, hypersensitivity reactions, infection, secondary malignancy

Pharmacodynamics/Kinetics

Onset of Action Hydrocortisone sodium succinate (water soluble): Rapid

Absorption Rapid

Half-Life Elimination Biologic: 8-12 hours

Metabolism Hepatic

Excretion Urine (primarily as 17-hydroxysteroids and 17-ketosteroids)

Available Dosage Forms

Injection, powder for reconstitution:

A-Hydrocort®: 100 mg

Solu-CORTEF®: 100 mg, 250 mg, 500 mg, 1000 mg

Tablet, oral: 5 mg, 10 mg, 20 mg

Cortef®: 5 mg, 10 mg, 20 mg

Dosing

Adult & Geriatric Dose should be based on severity of disease and patient response.

Adrenal hyperplasia (congenital): Oral: Initial: 10-20 mg/m^2/day in 3 divided doses; a variety of dosing schedules have been used. **Note:** Inconsistencies have occurred with liquid formulations; tablets may provide more reliable levels. Doses must be individualized by monitoring growth, bone age, and hormonal levels. Mineralocorticoid and sodium supplementation may be required based upon electrolyte regulation and plasma renin activity.

Adrenal insufficiency (acute): I.M., I.V.: Succinate: 100 mg I.V. bolus, then 300 mg/day in divided doses every 8 hours or as a continuous infusion for 48 hours. Once patient is stable change to oral, 50 mg every 8 hours for 6 doses, then taper to 30-50 mg/day in divided doses.

Adrenal insufficiency (chronic)/physiologic replacement: Oral: 20-30 mg/day

Anti-inflammatory or immunosuppressive: Oral, I.M., I.V.: Succinate: 15-240 mg every 12 hours

Septic shock (unlabeled use): I.V.: Succinate: 50 mg every 6 hours (Annane, 2002; Marik, 2008); not to exceed 300 mg/day (Dellinger, 2008). Practice guidelines also recommend alternative dosing of 100 mg bolus, followed by continuous infusion of 10 mg/hour (240 mg/day). Taper slowly (for total of 11 days) and do not stop abruptly. **Note:** Fludrocortisone is optional with use of hydrocortisone.

Status asthmaticus: I.V.: Succinate: 1-2 mg/kg/dose every 6 hours for 24 hours, then maintenance of 0.5-1 mg/kg every 6 hours

Stress dosing (surgery) in patients known to be adrenally-suppressed or on chronic systemic steroids: I.V.:

Minor stress (ie, inguinal herniorrhaphy): 25 mg/day for 1 day

Moderate stress (ie, joint replacement, cholecystectomy): 50-75 mg/day (25 mg every 8-12 hours) for 1-2 days

Major stress (pancreatoduodenectomy, esophagogastrectomy, cardiac surgery): 100-150 mg/day (50 mg every 8-12 hours) for 2-3 days

Pediatric Dose should be based on severity of disease and patient response.

Adrenal hyperplasia (congenital): Oral: Initial: 10-20 mg/m²/day in 3 divided doses; a variety of dosing schedules have been used. **Note:** Inconsistencies have occurred with liquid formulations; tablets may provide more reliable levels. Doses must be individualized by monitoring growth, bone age, and hormonal levels. Mineralocorticoid and sodium supplementation may be required based upon electrolyte regulation and plasma renin activity

Adrenal insufficiency (acute): I.M., I.V.:

Infants and young Children: Succinate: 1-2 mg/kg/dose bolus, then 25-150 mg/day in divided doses every 6-8 hours

Older Children: Succinate: 1-2 mg/kg bolus then 150-250 mg/day in divided doses every 6-8 hours

Anti-inflammatory or immunosuppressive:

Infants and Children:

Oral: 2.5-10 mg/kg/day **or** 75-300 mg/m²/day every 6-8 hours

I.M., I.V.: Succinate: 1-5 mg/kg/day **or** 30-150 mg/m²/day divided every 12-24 hours

Adolescents: Oral, I.M., I.V.: Succinate: 15-240 mg every 12 hours

Physiologic replacement: Children:

Oral: 0.5-0.75 mg/kg/day **or** 20-25 mg/m²/day every 8 hours

I.M.: Succinate: 0.25-0.35 mg/kg/day **or** 12-15 mg/m²/day once daily

Septic shock (unlabeled use): Children: I.V.: Succinate: Initial: 1-2 mg/kg/day (intermittent or as continuous infusion); may titrate up to 50 mg/kg/day for shock reversal (Brierley, 2009); alternative dosing suggests 50 mg/m²/day (Dellinger, 2008). **Note:** Use recommended only in catecholamine-resistant shock and suspected or proven adrenal insufficiency.

Status asthmaticus: Children: I.V.: Succinate: 1-2 mg/kg/dose every 6 hours for 24 hours, then maintenance of 0.5-1 mg/kg every 6 hours.

Administration

Oral Administer with food or milk to decrease GI upset.

I.V.

Parenteral: Hydrocortisone sodium succinate may be administered by I.M. or I.V. routes. Dermal and/or subdermal skin depression may occur at the site of injection. Avoid injection into deltoid muscle (high incidence of subcutaneous atrophy).

I.V. bolus: Dilute to 50 mg/mL and administer over 30 seconds or over 10 minutes for doses ≥500 mg

I.V. intermittent infusion: Dilute to 1 mg/mL and give over 20-30 minutes.

Note: Should be administered in a 0.1-1 mg/mL concentration due to stability problems.

Stability

Reconstitution

Sodium succinate: Reconstitute 100 mg vials with bacteriostatic water (not >2 mL). Act-O-Vial (self-contained powder for injection plus diluent) may be reconstituted by pressing the activator to force diluent into the powder compartment. Following gentle agitation, solution may be withdrawn via syringe through a needle inserted into the center of the stopper. May be administered (I.V. or I.M.) without further dilution.

Solutions for I.V. infusion: Reconstituted solutions may be added to an appropriate volume of compatible solution for infusion. Concentration should generally not exceed 1 mg/mL. However, in cases where administration of a small volume of fluid is desirable, 100-3000 mg may be added to 50 mL of D_5W or NS (stability limited to 4 hours).

Storage Store at controlled room temperature 20°C to 25°C (68°F to 77°F). Protect from light. Hydrocortisone sodium phosphate and hydrocortisone sodium succinate are clear, light yellow solutions which are heat labile.

Sodium succinate: After initial reconstitution, hydrocortisone sodium succinate solutions are stable for 3 days at room temperature or under refrigeration when protected from light. Stability of parenteral admixture (Solu-Cortef®) at room temperature (25°C) and at refrigeration temperature (4°C) is concentration-dependent:

Stability of concentration 1 mg/mL: 24 hours.

Stability of concentration 2 mg/mL to 60 mg/mL: At least 4 hours.

Monitoring and Teaching Issues

Laboratory Monitoring Serum glucose, electrolytes

Physical Assessment Teach patients to report opportunistic infection and adrenal suppression. Instruct patients with diabetes to monitor serum glucose levels closely; corticosteroids can alter glycemic response. Dose may need to be increased if patient is experiencing higher than normal levels of stress. When discontinuing, taper dose and frequency slowly.

Patient Education Dosage is usually tapered off gradually. Take oral dose with food to reduce GI upset. Avoid alcohol. Hydrocortisone may cause immunosuppression and mask symptoms of infection; avoid exposure to contagion and notify prescriber of any signs of infection (eg, fever, chills, sore throat, injury) and notify dentist or surgeon (if necessary) that you are taking this medication. You may experience increased appetite, indigestion, or increased nervousness. Report weight gain, swelling of extremities or respiratory difficulty, abdominal pain, severe vomiting, black or tarry stools, fatigue, anorexia, weakness, or unusual mood swings.

Dietary Considerations Systemic use of corticosteroids may require a diet with increased potassium, vitamins A, B_6, C, D, folate, calcium, zinc, phosphorus, and decreased sodium. Some products may contain sodium.

Geriatric Considerations Because of the risk of adverse effects, systemic corticosteroids should be used cautiously in the elderly, in the smallest possible dose, and for the shortest possible time.

Breast-Feeding Considerations Corticosteroids are excreted in breast milk and endogenous hydrocortisone is also found in human milk; the effect of maternal hydrocortisone intake is not known.

Pregnancy Considerations Adverse events have been observed with corticosteroids in animal reproduction studies. Hydrocortisone crosses the placenta. Some studies have shown an association between first trimester systemic corticosteroid use and oral clefts; adverse events in the fetus/neonate have been noted in case reports following large doses of systemic corticosteroids during pregnancy.

Related Information

Corticosteroids *on page* 1996

Hydrocortisone (Topical) (hye droe KOR ti sone)

U.S. Brand Names Ala-Cort; Ala-Scalp; Anu-med HC; Anucort-HC™; Anusol-HC®; Aquanil HC® [OTC]; Beta-HC® [OTC]; Caldecort® [OTC]; Colocort®; Cortaid® Advanced [OTC]; Cortaid® Intensive Therapy [OTC]; Cortaid® Maximum Strength [OTC]; Cortenema®; Corti-Cool® [OTC]; Cortifoam®; Cortizone-10® Hydratensive Healing [OTC]; Cortizone-10® Hydratensive Soothing [OTC]; Cortizone-10® Intensive Healing Eczema [OTC]; Cortizone-10® Maximum Strength Cooling Relief [OTC]; Cortizone-10® Maximum Strength Easy Relief [OTC]; Cortizone-10® Maximum Strength Intensive Healing Formula [OTC]; Cortizone-10® Maximum Strength [OTC]; Cortizone-10® Plus Maximum Strength [OTC]; Dermarest® Eczema Medicated [OTC]; Hemorrhoidal HC [DSC]; Hemril® -30; HYDRO-Rx [DSC]; Hydrocortisone Plus [OTC]; Hydroskin® [OTC]; HydroZone Plus [OTC] [DSC]; Ivy Soothe® [OTC] [DSC]; Locoid Lipocream®; Locoid®; Pandel®; Preparation H® Hydrocortisone [OTC]; Procto-Kit™ [DSC]; Procto-Pak™; Proctocort®; ProctoCream®-HC; Proctosol-HC®; Proctozone-HC 2.5%™; Recort [OTC]; Scalpana [OTC]; Texacort®; Tucks® Anti-Itch [OTC] [DSC]; U-Cort™; Westcort®

Index Terms A-hydroCort; Compound F; Cortisol; Hemorrhoidal HC; Hydrocortisone Acetate; Hydrocortisone Butyrate; Hydrocortisone Probutate; Hydrocortisone Valerate

Generic Availability (U.S.) Yes: Excludes aerosol (acetate), cream (probutate), gel (base), liquid (base), lotion (base), solution (base)

Pharmacologic Category Corticosteroid, Rectal; Corticosteroid, Topical

Medication Safety Issues

Sound-alike/look-alike issues:

- Hydrocortisone may be confused with hydrocodone, hydroxychloroquine, hydrochlorothiazide
- Anusol® may be confused with Anusol-HC®, Aplisol®, Aquasol®
- Anusol-HC® may be confused with Anusol®
- Cortizone® may be confused with cortisone
- HCT (occasional abbreviation for hydrocortisone) is an error-prone abbreviation (mistaken as hydrochlorothiazide)
- Hytone® may be confused with Vytone®
- Proctocort® may be confused with ProctoCream®
- ProctoCream® may be confused with Proctocort®

International issues:

- Nutracort [U.S. and multiple international markets] may be confused with Nitrocor brand name of nitroglycerin [Italy, Russia, and Venezuela]

Pregnancy Risk Factor C

Lactation Enters breast milk/use caution

Use Relief of inflammation of corticosteroid-responsive dermatoses (low and medium potency topical corticosteroid); adjunctive treatment of ulcerative colitis

Available Dosage Forms

Aerosol, rectal:
Cortifoam®: 10% (15 g)

Cream, topical: 0.1% (15 g, 45 g); 0.2% (15 g, 45 g, 60 g); 0.5% (0.9 g, 15 g, 30 g, 60 g); 1% (0.9 g, 1 g, 1.5 g, 15 g, 20 g, 28.35 g, 28.4 g, 30 g, 114 g, 120 g, 454 g); 2% (43 g); 2.5% (20 g, 28 g, 28.35 g, 30 g, 454 g)
Ala-Cort: 1% (28.4 g, 85.2 g)
Anusol-HC®: 2.5% (30 g)
Caldecort® [OTC]: 1% (28.4 g)
Cortaid® Advanced [OTC]: 1% (42 g)
Cortaid® Intensive Therapy [OTC]: 1% (37 g, 56 g)
Cortaid® Maximum Strength [OTC]: 1% (14 g, 28 g, 37 g, 56 g)
Cortizone-10® Maximum Strength [OTC]: 1% (15 g, 28 g, 56 g)
Cortizone-10® Maximum Strength Intensive Healing Formula [OTC]: 1% (28 g, 56 g)
Cortizone-10® Plus Maximum Strength [OTC]: 1% (28 g, 56 g)
Hydrocortisone Plus [OTC]: 1% (28.4 g)
Hydroskin® [OTC]: 1% (28 g)
Locoid Lipocream®: 0.1% (15 g, 45 g, 60 g)
Locoid®: 0.1% (15 g, 45 g)
Pandel®: 0.1% (15 g, 45 g, 80 g)
Preparation H® Hydrocortisone [OTC]: 1% (26 g)
Procto-Pak™: 1% (28.4 g)
Proctocort®: 1% (28.35 g)
ProctoCream®-HC: 2.5% (30 g)
Proctosol-HC®: 2.5% (28.35 g)
Proctozone-HC 2.5%™: 2.5% (30 g)
Recort [OTC]: 1% (30 g)
U-Cort™: 1% (28 g)

Gel, topical:
CortiCool® [OTC]: 1% (0.9 g, 42.5 g)
Cortizone-10® Maximum Strength Cooling Relief [OTC]: 1% (28 g)

Liquid, topical:
Cortizone-10® Maximum Strength Easy Relief [OTC]: 1% (36 mL)
Scalpana [OTC]: 1% (85.5 mL)

Lotion, topical: 1% (114 g, 118 mL, 120 mL); 2.5% (59 mL, 60 mL, 118 mL)
Ala-Scalp: 2% (29.6 mL)
Aquanil HC® [OTC]: 1% (120 mL)
Beta-HC® [OTC]: 1% (60 mL)
Cortaid® Intensive Therapy [OTC]: 1% (98 g)
Cortizone-10® Hydratensive Healing [OTC]: 1% (113 g)
Cortizone-10® Hydratensive Soothing [OTC]: 1% (113 g)
Cortizone-10® Intensive Healing Eczema [OTC]: 1% (99 g)
Dermarest® Eczema Medicated [OTC]: 1% (118 mL)
Hydroskin® [OTC]: 1% (118 mL)
Locoid®: 0.1% (60 mL)

Ointment, topical: 0.1% (15 g, 45 g); 0.2% (15 g, 45 g, 60 g); 0.5% (30 g); 1% (25 g, 28.4 g, 30 g, 110 g, 430 g, 454 g); 2.5% (20 g, 28.35 g, 30 g, 454 g)
Cortaid® Maximum Strength [OTC]: 1% (28 g, 37 g)
Cortizone-10® Maximum Strength [OTC]: 1% (28 g, 56 g)
Locoid®: 0.1% (15 g, 45 g)
Westcort®: 0.2% (15 g, 45 g, 60 g)

Powder, for prescription compounding: USP: 100% (10 g, 25 g, 50 g, 100 g, 1000 g)

Solution, topical: 0.1% (20 mL, 60 mL)
Cortaid® Intensive Therapy [OTC]: 1% (59 mL)
Locoid®: 0.1% (20 mL, 60 mL)
Texacort®: 2.5% (30 mL)

Suppository, rectal: 25 mg (12s, 24s, 1000s); 30 mg (12s)
Anu-med HC: 25 mg (12s)
Anucort-HC™: 25 mg (12s, 24s, 100s)
Anusol-HC®: 25 mg (12s, 24s)
Hemril® -30: 30 mg (12s, 24s)
Proctocort®: 30 mg (12s, 24s)

Suspension, rectal: 100 mg/60 mL (60 mL)
Colocort®: 100 mg/60 mL (60 mL)
Cortenema®: 100 mg/60 mL (60 mL)

Dosing

Adult & Geriatric

Dermatosis: Topical: Apply to affected area 2-4 times/day.

Ulcerative colitis: Rectal: 10-100 mg 1-2 times/day for 2-3 weeks

Pediatric Dermatosis: Topical: Children >2 years: Apply to affected area 2-4 times/day

Administration

Topical

Topical cream, lotion, ointment: Apply a thin film to clean, dry skin and rub in gently.

Rectal suppository: Remove foil from rectal suppository and insert pointed end first. Avoid handling unwrapped suppository for too long.

Rectal suspension: Shake bottle well. Remove protective sheath from applicator tip. Lie on left side with left leg extended and right leg flexed forward. Gently insert lubricated applicator tip into rectum, pointed slightly toward navel. Grasp bottle firmly and squeeze slowly to instill the medication. After administering, withdraw and discard the used unit. Remain in position for at least 30 minutes. Retain the enema all night if possible.

Monitoring and Teaching Issues

Physical Assessment Topical absorption may be minimal.

Patient Education

Topical: Before applying, wash area gently and thoroughly. Apply a thin film to cleansed area and rub in gently until medication vanishes. Avoid use of occlusive dressings over topical application unless directed by a prescriber. Avoid use on weeping or exudative lesions. Avoid exposing affected area to sunlight; you will be more sensitive and severe sunburn may occur.

Rectal: Gently insert suppository as high as possible with gloved finger while lying down. Remain in resting position for 10 minutes after insertion.

Enema: When patient is in the proper position, insert applicator tip rectally. Slowly squeeze to instill medication. Maintain patient in position for at least 30 minutes.

- ◆ **Hydrocortisone Acetate** *see* Hydrocortisone (Topical) *on page 920*
- ◆ **Hydrocortisone, Acetic Acid, and Propylene Glycol Diacetate** *see* Acetic Acid, Propylene Glycol Diacetate, and Hydrocortisone *on page 43*
- ◆ **Hydrocortisone and Acyclovir** *see* Acyclovir and Hydrocortisone *on page 48*
- ◆ **Hydrocortisone and Ciprofloxacin** *see* Ciprofloxacin and Hydrocortisone *on page 381*
- ◆ **Hydrocortisone Butyrate** *see* Hydrocortisone (Topical) *on page 920*
- ◆ **Hydrocortisone Plus [OTC]** *see* Hydrocortisone (Topical) *on page 920*
- ◆ **Hydrocortisone Probutate** *see* Hydrocortisone (Topical) *on page 920*
- ◆ **Hydrocortisone Sodium Succinate** *see* Hydrocortisone (Systemic) *on page 917*
- ◆ **Hydrocortisone Valerate** *see* Hydrocortisone (Topical) *on page 920*
- ◆ **Hydrodiuril** *see* Hydrochlorothiazide *on page 912*

HYDROmorphone (hye droe MOR fone)

U.S. Brand Names Dilaudid-HP®; Dilaudid®; Exalgo™

Index Terms Dihydromorphinone; Hydromorphone Hydrochloride

Generic Availability (U.S.) Yes: Excludes extended release tablet, liquid, powder for injection

Pharmacologic Category Analgesic, Opioid

Medication Safety Issues

Sound-alike/look-alike issues:

Dilaudid® may be confused with Demerol®, Dilantin®

HYDROmorphone may be confused with morphine; significant overdoses have occurred when hydromorphone products have been inadvertently administered instead of morphine sulfate. Commercially available prefilled syringes of both products looks similar and are often stored in close proximity to each other. **Note:** Hydromorphone 1 mg oral is approximately equal to morphine 4 mg oral; hydromorphone 1 mg I.V. is approximately equal to morphine 5 mg I.V.

High alert medication: The Institute for Safe Medication Practices (ISMP) includes this medication among its list of drug classes which have a heightened risk of causing significant patient harm when used in error.

Dilaudid®, Dilaudid-HP®: Extreme caution should be taken to avoid confusing the highly-concentrated (Dilaudid-HP®) injection with the less-concentrated (Dilaudid®) injectable product.

Exalgo™: Extreme caution should be taken to avoid confusing the extended release Exalgo™ 8 mg tablets with immediate release hydromorphone 8 mg tablets

Significant differences exist between oral and I.V. dosing. Use caution when converting from one route of administration to another.

Medication Guide Available Yes

Prescribing and Access Restrictions Exalgo™: As a requirement of the REMS program, healthcare providers who prescribe Exalgo™ need to receive training on the proper use and potential risks of Exalgo™. For training, please refer to http://www.exalgorems.com. Prescribers will need retraining every 2 years or following any significant changes to the Exalgo™ REMS program.

Pregnancy Risk Factor C

Lactation Enters breast milk/not recommended

Use Management of moderate-to-severe pain

Exalgo™: Management of moderate-to-severe pain in opioid-tolerant patients (requiring around-the-clock analgesia for an extended period of time)

Mechanism of Action/Effect Binds to opiate receptors in the CNS, causing inhibition of ascending pain pathways, altering the perception of and response to pain; causes cough supression by direct central action in the medulla; produces generalized CNS depression

Contraindications Hypersensitivity to hydromorphone, any component of the formulation; acute or severe asthma, severe respiratory depression (in absence of resuscitative equipment or ventilatory support); severe CNS depression

Additional product-specific contraindications:

Dilaudid®, Dilaudid-HP®: Obstetrical analgesia

Exalgo™: Opioid nontolerant patients, paralytic ileus, preexisting GI surgery or diseases resulting in narrowing of GI tract, loops in the GI tract or GI obstruction

Warnings/Precautions Use with caution in patients with hypersensitivity reactions to other phenanthrene derivative opioid agonists (codeine, hydrocodone, levorphanol, oxycodone, oxymorphone). Hydromorphone shares toxic potential of opiate agonists, including CNS depression and respiratory depression. Precautions associated with opiate agonist therapy should be observed. May cause CNS depression, which may impair physical or mental abilities; patients must be cautioned about performing tasks which require mental alertness (eg, operating machinery or driving). Myoclonus and seizures have been reported with high doses. Critical respiratory depression may occur, even at therapeutic dosages, particularly in elderly or debilitated patients or in patients with pre-existing respiratory compromise (hypoxia and/or hypercapnia). Use caution in COPD or other obstructive pulmonary disease. Use with caution in patients with hypersensitivity to other phenanthrene opiates, kyphoscoliosis, cardiovascular disease, morbid obesity, adrenocortical insufficiency, hypothyroidism, acute alcoholism, delirium tremens, toxic psychoses, prostatic hyperplasia and/or urinary stricture, or severe liver or renal failure. Use with caution in patients with biliary tract dysfunction. Hydromorphone may increase biliary tract pressure following spasm in sphincter of Oddi. Use caution in patients with inflammatory or obstructive bowel disorder, acute pancreatitis secondary to biliary tract disease, and patients undergoing biliary surgery. Use extreme caution in patients with head injury, intracranial lesions, or elevated intracranial pressure; exaggerated elevation of ICP may occur (in addition, hydromorphone may complicate neurologic evaluation due to pupillary dilation and CNS depressant effects). Use with caution in patients with depleted blood volume or drugs which may exaggerate hypotensive effects (including phenothiazines or general anesthetics). May obscure diagnosis or clinical course of patients with acute abdominal conditions.

[U.S. Boxed Warning]: Hydromorphone has a high potential for abuse. Those at risk for opioid abuse include patients with a history of substance abuse or mental illness. Tolerance or drug dependence may result from extended use; however, concerns for abuse should not prevent effective management of pain. In general, abrupt discontinuation of therapy in dependent patients should be avoided.

An opioid-containing analgesic regimen should be tailored to each patient's needs and based upon the type of pain being treated (acute versus chronic), the route of administration, degree of tolerance for opioids (naive versus chronic user), age, weight, and medical condition. The optimal analgesic dose varies widely among patients. Doses should be titrated to pain relief/ prevention. I.M. use may result in variable absorption and a lag time to peak effect.

Dosage form specific warnings:

[U.S. Boxed Warning]: Dilaudid-HP®: Extreme caution should be taken to avoid confusing the highly-concentrated (Dilaudid-HP®) injection with the less-concentrated (Dilaudid®) injectable product. Dilaudid-HP® should only be used in patients who are opioid-tolerant.

Controlled release: Capsules should only be used when continuous analgesia is required over an extended period of time. Controlled release products are not to be used on an "as needed" (PRN) basis.

Extended release tablets (Exalgo™): **[U.S. Boxed Warning]: For use in opioid tolerant patients only; fatal respiratory depression may occur in patient who are not opioid tolerant. Indicated for the management of moderate-to-severe pain when around the clock pain control is needed for an extended time period. Not for use as an as-needed analgesic or for the management of acute or postoperative pain. Tablets should be swallowed whole; do not crush, break, chew, dissolve or inject; doing so may lead to rapid release and absorption of a potentially fatal dose of hydromorphone. Accidental consumption may lead to fatal overdose, especially in children.** Exalgo™ tablets are nondeformable; do not administer to patients with preexisting severe gastrointestinal narrowing (eg, esophageal motility, small bowel inflammatory disease, short gut syndrome, history of peritonitis, cystic fibrosis, chronic intestinal pseudo-obstruction, Meckel's diverticulum); obstruction may occur. Exalgo™ is not recommended for use within 14 days of MAO inhibitors; severe and unpredictable potentiation by MAO inhibitors has been reported with opioid analgesics

Some dosage forms contain trace amounts of sodium metabisulfite which may cause allergic reactions in susceptible individuals.

Drug Interactions

Avoid Concomitant Use

Avoid concomitant use of HYDROmorphone with any of the following: MAO Inhibitors

Decreased Effect

HYDROmorphone may decrease the levels/effects of: Pegvisomant

The levels/effects of HYDROmorphone may be decreased by: Ammonium Chloride; Mixed Agonist / Antagonist Opioids

Increased Effect/Toxicity

HYDROmorphone may increase the levels/effects of: Alcohol (Ethyl); Alvimopan; CNS Depressants; Desmopressin; Selective Serotonin Reuptake Inhibitors; Thiazide Diuretics

The levels/effects of HYDROmorphone may be increased by: Amphetamines; Antipsychotic Agents (Phenothiazines); Droperidol; MAO Inhibitors; Succinylcholine

Nutritional/Ethanol Interactions

Ethanol: Avoid ethanol (may increase CNS depression).

Herb/Nutraceutical: Avoid valerian, St John's wort, kava kava, gotu kola (may increase CNS depression).

Lab Interactions Some quinolones may produce a false-positive urine screening result for opiates using commercially-available immunoassay kits. This has been demonstrated most consistently for levofloxacin and ofloxacin, but other quinolones have shown cross-reactivity in certain assay kits. Confirmation of positive opiate screens by more specific methods should be considered.

Adverse Reactions Frequency not defined.

Cardiovascular: Bradycardia, extrasystoles, flushing of face, hyper-/hypotension, palpitation, peripheral edema, peripheral vasodilation, syncope, tachycardia

Central nervous system: Abnormal dreams, abnormal feelings, agitation, aggression, apprehension, attention disturbances, chills, coordination impaired, CNS depression, confusion, cognitive disorder, crying, dizziness, drowsiness, dysphoria, encephalopathy, euphoria, fatigue, hallucinations, headache, hyper-reflexia, hypo/hyperesthesia, hypothermia, increased intracranial pressure, insomnia, lightheadedness, listlessness, malaise, memory impairment, mental depression, mood alterations, nervousness, panic attacks, paranoia, psychomotor hyperactivity, restlessness, sedation, seizure, somnolence, suicide ideation, vertigo

Dermatologic: Hyperhidrosis, pruritus, rash, urticaria

Endocrine & metabolic: Amylase decreased, dehydration, erectile dysfunction, fluid retention, hyperuricemia, hypogonadism, hypokalemia, libido decreased, sexual dysfunction, testosterone decreased

Gastrointestinal: Abdominal distention, anal fissure, anorexia, appetite increased, bezoar (Exalgo™), biliary tract spasm, constipation, diarrhea, diverticulum, diverticulitis, duodenitis, dysgeusia, dysphagia, eructation, flatulence, gastric emptying impaired, gastrointestinal motility disorder (Exalgo™), gastroenteritis, hematochezia, ileus, intestinal obstruction (Exalgo™), large intestine perforation (Exalgo™), nausea, painful defecation, paralytic ileus, stomach cramps, taste perversion, vomiting, weight loss, xerostomia

Genitourinary: Dysuria, micturition disorder, ureteral spasm, urinary frequency, urinary hesitation, urinary retention, urinary tract spasm, urination decreased

Hepatic: LFTs increased

Local: Pain at injection site (I.M.), wheal/flare over vein (I.V.)

Neuromuscular & skeletal: Arthralgia, dysarthria, dyskinesia, muscle rigidity, muscle spasms, myalgia, myoclonus, paresthesia, trembling, tremor, uncoordinated muscle movements, weakness

Ocular: Blurred vision, diplopia, dry eyes, miosis, nystagmus

Otic: Tinnitus

Respiratory: Apnea, bronchospasm, dyspnea, hyperventilation, hypoxia, laryngospasm, oxygen saturation decreased, respiratory depression/distress, rhinorrhea

Miscellaneous: Antidiuretic effects, balance disorder, diaphoresis, difficulty walking, histamine release, physical and psychological dependence

Pharmacodynamics/Kinetics

Onset of Action Analgesic: Immediate release formulations:

Oral: 15-30 minutes; Peak effect: 30-60 minutes

I.V.: 5 minutes; Peak effect: 10-20 minutes

Duration of Action Immediate release formulations: Oral, I.V.: 4-5 hours

Absorption I.M.: Variable and delayed

Bioavailability 62%

Protein Binding ~8% to 19%

Half-Life Elimination

Immediate release formulations: 2-3 hours

Extended release tablets (Exalgo™): ~11 hours

Metabolism Hepatic via glucuronidation; to inactive metabolites

Excretion Urine (primarily as glucuronide conjugates)

Controlled Substance C-II

Available Dosage Forms

Injection, powder for reconstitution:

Dilaudid-HP®: 250 mg

Injection, solution: 1 mg/mL (1 mL); 2 mg/mL (1 mL, 20 mL); 4 mg/mL (1 mL)

Dilaudid-HP®: 10 mg/mL (1 mL, 5 mL, 50 mL)

Dilaudid®: 1 mg/mL (1 mL); 2 mg/mL (1 mL); 4 mg/mL (1 mL)

Injection, solution [preservative free]: 10 mg/mL (1 mL, 5 mL, 50 mL)

Liquid, oral:

Dilaudid®: 1 mg/mL (473 mL)

Powder, for prescription compounding: USP: 100% (972 mg)

Suppository, rectal: 3 mg (6s)

Tablet, oral: 2 mg, 4 mg, 8 mg

Dilaudid®: 2 mg, 4 mg, 8 mg

Tablet, extended release, oral:

Exalgo™: 8 mg, 12 mg, 16 mg

Dosing

Adult

Acute pain (moderate-to-severe): Note: These are guidelines and do not represent the maximum doses that may be required in all patients. Doses should be titrated to provide adequate pain relief. When changing routes of administration, oral doses and parenteral doses are **NOT** equivalent; parenteral doses are up to 5 times more potent. Therefore, when administered parenterally, one-fifth of the oral dose will provide similar analgesia.

Oral:

Initial: Opiate-naive: 2-4 mg every 4-6 hours as needed; elderly/debilitated patients may require lower doses; patients with prior opiate exposure may require higher initial doses

Usual dosage range: 2-8 mg every 3-4 hours as needed

Note: The American Pain Society recommends an initial dose of 4-8 mg for severe pain in adults.

I.V.: Initial: Opiate-naive: 0.2-0.6 mg every 2-3 hours as needed; patients with prior opiate exposure may tolerate higher initial doses.

Critically-ill patients (unlabeled dose): 0.7-2 mg (based on 70 kg patient) every 1-2 hours as needed. **Note:** More frequent dosing may be needed (eg, mechanically-ventilated patients).

Continuous infusion: Usual dosage range: 0.5-1 mg/hour (based on 70 kg patient) or 7-15 mcg/kg/**hour**

Patient-controlled analgesia (PCA): **Note:** Opiate-naive: Consider lower end of dosing range:

Usual concentration: 0.2 mg/mL

Demand dose: Usual: 0.1-0.2 mg; range: 0.05-0.4 mg

Lockout interval: 5-10 minutes

Epidural:

Bolus dose: 1-1.5 mg

Infusion concentration: 0.05-0.075 mg/mL

Infusion rate: 0.04-0.4 mg/hour

Demand dose: 0.15 mg

Lockout interval: 30 minutes

I.M., SubQ: **Note:** I.M. use may result in variable absorption and a lag time to peak effect.

Initial: Opiate-naive: 0.8-1 mg every 4-6 hours as needed; patients with prior opiate exposure may require higher initial doses

Usual dosage range: 1-2 mg every 4-6 hours as needed

Rectal: 3 mg every 4-8 hours as needed

Chronic pain: Note: Patients taking opioids chronically may become tolerant and require doses higher than the usual dosage range to maintain the desired effect. Tolerance can be managed by appropriate dose titration. There is no optimal or maximal dose for hydromorphone in chronic pain. The appropriate dose is one that relieves pain throughout its dosing interval without causing unmanageable side effects.

Controlled release formulation (Hydromorph Contin®, not available in U.S.): Oral: 3-30 mg every 12 hours. **Note:** A patient's hydromorphone requirement should be established using prompt release formulations; conversion to long acting products may be considered when chronic, continuous treatment is required. Higher dosages should be reserved for use only in opioid-tolerant patients.

Extended release formulation (Exalgo™): Dosing range: 8-64 mg every 24 hours. For use in opioid tolerant patients only; discontinue all other extended release opioids when starting therapy. Suggested recommendations for converting to Exalgo™ from other analgesics are presented, but when selecting the initial dose, other characteristics (eg, patient status, degree of opioid tolerance, concurrent medications, type of pain, risk factors for addiction or diversion, etc) should also be considered.

Individualization of dose: Pain relief and adverse events should be assessed frequently. Dose increases may occur not more often than every 3-4 days; consider titrating with increases of 25% to 50% of the current daily dose. If more than 2 doses of rescue medications are needed within 24 hours for 2 consecutive days, consider increasing the dose of Exalgo™. Do not administer more frequently than every 24 hours.

Discontinuing Exalgo™: Taper by gradually decreasing the dose by 25% to 50% every 2-3 days to a dose of 8 mg every 24 hours before discontinuing therapy.

Conversion from other oral hydromorphone formulations to Exalgo™: Start with the equivalent total daily dose of hydromorphone administered once daily. May titrate every 3-4 days until adequate pain relief with tolerable side effects have been achieved.

Conversion from other opioids to Exalgo™: Refer to published potency data to determine approximate conversion ratio. In general, start Exalgo™ at 50% of the calculated total daily dose every 24 hours. Titrate until adequate pain relief with tolerable side effects has been achieved. The following conversion ratios may be used to convert from **oral** opioid therapy to Exalgo™. Close observation and titration is required.

Conversion ratios to Exalgo™ (see table): Select the opioid, sum the total daily dose, then multiply by the conversion ratio to calculate the *approximate* oral hydromorphone equivalent; start Exalgo™ at 50% of the calculated total daily dose every 24 hours. (**Note:** The conversion ratios and approximate equivalent doses in this conversion table are only to be used for the conversion from current opioid therapy to Exalgo™).

Conversion Ratios to Exalgo™[1]

Previous Opioid	Approximate Equivalent Oral Dose	Oral Conversion Ratio[2]
Hydromorphone	12 mg	1
Codeine	200 mg	0.06
Hydrocodone	30 mg	0.4
Methadone[3]	20 mg	0.6
Morphine	60 mg	0.2
Oxycodone	30 mg	0.4
Oxymorphone	20 mg	0.6

[1] *Approximate* equivalent doses for conversion from current opioid therapy to Exalgo™.

[2]Ratio for converting oral opioid dose to approximate hydromorphone equivalent dose.

[3]Monitor closely; ratio between methadone and other opioid agonists may vary widely as a function of previous drug exposure. Methadone has a long half-life and may accumulate in the plasma.

Conversion from transdermal fentanyl to Exalgo™: Treatment with Exalgo™ can be started 18 hours after the removal of the transdermal fentanyl patch. For every fentanyl 25 mcg/hour transdermal dose, the equianalgesic dose of Exalgo™ is 12 mg every 24 hours. An appropriate starting dose is 50% of the calculated total daily dose given every 24 hours.

Geriatric Doses should be titrated to appropriate analgesic effects. When changing routes of administration, oral doses and parenteral doses are **NOT** equivalent; parenteral doses are up to 5 times more potent. Therefore, when administered parenterally, one-fifth of the oral dose will provide similar analgesia.

Pain: Oral: 1-2 mg every 4-6 hours

Pediatric Acute pain (moderate-to-severe): Note: These are guidelines and do not represent the maximum doses that may be required in all patients. Doses should be titrated to pain relief/prevention.

Children ≥6 months and <50 kg:

Oral: 0.03-0.08 mg/kg/dose every 3-4 hours as needed. **Note:** The American Pain Society recommends an initial dose of 0.06 mg/kg for severe pain in children.

I.V.: 0.015 mg/kg/dose every 3-6 hours as needed

Patient-controlled analgesia (PCA) (American Pain Society, 2008): **Note:** Opiate-naive: Consider lower end of dosing range:

Usual concentration: 0.2 mg/mL

Demand dose: Usual: 0.003-0.004 mg/kg/dose; range: 0.003-0.005 mg/kg/dose

Lockout interval: 6-10 minutes

Usual basal rate: 0-0.004 mg/kg/hour

Children >50 kg: Refer to adult dosing.

Renal Impairment Exalgo™:

Moderate impairment: Start with a reduced dose and monitor closely.

Severe impairment: Consider use of an alternate analgesic with better dosing flexibility.

Hepatic Impairment Dose adjustment should be considered.

Exalgo™: In patients with moderate and severe hepatic impairment, start with a reduced dose and monitor closely. Consider use of an alternate analgesic with better dosing flexibility.

Administration

Oral Hydromorphone is available in an 8 mg immediate release tablet and an 8 mg extended release tablet. Extreme caution should be taken to avoid confusing dosage forms.

Exalgo™: Tablets should be swallowed whole; do not crush, break, chew, dissolve or inject. May be taken with or without food.

Hydromorph Contin®: Capsule should be swallowed whole; do not crush or chew; contents may be sprinkled on soft food and swallowed

I.M. May be given SubQ or I.M.; vial stopper contains latex

I.V. For IVP, must be given slowly over 2-3 minutes (rapid IVP has been associated with an increase in side effects, especially respiratory depression and hypotension)

Other May be given SubQ or I.M.

Stability

Storage Store injection and oral dosage forms at 15°C to 30°C (59°F to 86°F). Protect tablets from light. A slightly yellowish discoloration has not been associated with a loss of potency.

Monitoring and Teaching Issues

Physical Assessment Monitor for effectiveness of pain relief. Assess patient's physical and/or psychological dependence. Monitor blood pressure, CNS and respiratory status, and degree of sedation prior to treatment and periodically throughout. For inpatients, implement safety measures to prevent falls. Discontinue slowly after prolonged use.

Patient Education Exalgo™ tablets should be swallowed whole; do not crush, break, chew, dissolve, or inject. May cause physical and/or psychological dependence. Do not use alcohol, sedatives, tranquilizers, antihistamines, or pain medications without consulting prescriber. Maintain adequate hydration, unless instructed to restrict fluid intake. May cause dizziness, drowsiness, impaired coordination, or blurred vision; loss of appetite, nausea, or vomiting; or constipation (if unresolved, consult prescriber about use of stool softeners). Report chest pain, slow or rapid heartbeat, dizziness, or persistent headache; confusion or respiratory difficulties; or severe constipation.

Geriatric Considerations Elderly may be particularly susceptible to the CNS depressant and constipating effects of narcotics.

Breast-Feeding Considerations Low concentrations of hydromorphone can be found in breast milk. Withdrawal symptoms may be observed in breast-feeding infants when opioid analgesics are discontinued. Breast-feeding is not recommended.

Pregnancy Considerations Hydromorphone was teratogenic in some, but not all, animal studies; however, maternal toxicity was also reported. Hydromorphone crosses the placenta. Chronic opioid use during pregnancy may lead to a withdrawal syndrome in the neonate. Symptoms include irritability, hyperactivity, loss of sleep pattern, abnormal crying, tremor, vomiting, diarrhea, weight loss, or failure to gain weight.

Additional Information Equianalgesic doses: Morphine 10 mg I.M. = hydromorphone 1.5 mg I.M.

Exalgo™ is indicated for the management of moderate-to-severe pain in opioid-tolerant patients (requiring around-the-clock analgesia for an extended period of time). Patients are considered to be opioid tolerant if they have been taking oral morphine ≥60 mg/day, fentanyl transdermal ≥25 mcg/hour, oral oxycodone ≥30 mg/day, oral hydromorphone ≥8 mg/day, oral oxymorphone ≥25 mg/day, or an equianalgesic dose of another opioid for ≥1 week.

Related Information

Opioid Analgesics *on page 2003*

◆ **Hydromorphone Hydrochloride** *see* HYDROmorphone *on page 922*

◆ **Hydroquinol** *see* Hydroquinone *on page 927*

Hydroquinone (HYE droe kwin one)

U.S. Brand Names Aclaro PD®; Aclaro®; Alphaquin HP®; Eldopaque Forte®; Eldopaque® [OTC]; Eldoquin Forte®; Eldoquin® [OTC]; EpiQuin® Micro; Esoterica® Daytime [OTC]; Esoterica® Nighttime [OTC]; Lustra-AF®; Lustra-Ultra™; Lustra®; Melanex® [DSC]; Melpaque HP®; Melquin HP®; Melquin-3®; NeoStrata® HQ Skin Lightening [OTC]; Nuquin HP®; Palmer's® Skin Success® Eventone® Fade Cream [OTC]; Palmer's® Skin Success® Eventone® Fade Milk [OTC]; Palmer's® Skin Success® Eventone® Ultra Fade Serum [OTC]

Index Terms Hydroquinol; Quinol

Generic Availability (U.S.) Yes

Pharmacologic Category Depigmenting Agent

Medication Safety Issues

Sound-alike/look-alike issues:

- Eldopaque® may be confused with Eldoquin®
- Eldoquin® may be confused with Eldopaque®
- Eldopaque Forte® may be confused with Eldoquin Forte®
- Eldoquin Forte® may be confused with Eldopaque Forte®

Pregnancy Risk Factor C

Lactation Excretion in breast milk unknown

Use Gradual bleaching of hyperpigmented skin conditions

Available Dosage Forms

Cream, topical: 4% (28.35 g, 28.4 g, 30 g)

- Alphaquin HP®: 4% (28.4 g, 56.7 g)
- Eldopaque Forte®: 4% (28.35 g)
- Eldopaque® [OTC]: 2% (28.35 g)
- Eldoquin Forte®: 4% (28.4 g)
- Eldoquin® [OTC]: 2% (28.35 g)
- EpiQuin® Micro: 4% (40 g)
- Esoterica® Daytime [OTC]: 2% (70 g, 85 g)
- Esoterica® Nighttime [OTC]: 2% (85 g)
- Lustra-AF®: 4% (56.8 g)
- Lustra-Ultra™: 4% (56.8 g)
- Lustra®: 4% (56.8 g)
- Melpaque HP®: 4% (14.2 g, 28.4 g)
- Melquin HP®: 4% (14.2 g, 28.4 g)
- Nuquin HP®: 4% (14.2 g, 28.4 g, 56.7 g)
- Palmer's® Skin Success® Eventone® Fade Cream [OTC]: 2% (75 g, 125 g)

Emulsion, topical:

- Aclaro PD®: 4% (42.5 g)
- Aclaro®: 4% (48.2 g)

Gel, topical: 4% (28.35 g, 30 g)

- NeoStrata® HQ Skin Lightening [OTC]: 2% (30 g)
- Nuquin HP®: 4% (14.2 g, 28.4 g)

Lotion, topical:

- Palmer's® Skin Success® Eventone® Fade Milk [OTC]: 2% (250 mL)

Solution, topical:
Melquin-3®: 3% (29.57 mL)
Palmer's® Skin Success® Eventone® Ultra Fade Serum [OTC]: 2% (30 mL)

Dosing

Adult & Geriatric Bleaching: Topical: Apply a thin layer and rub in twice daily.

Pediatric Refer to adult dosing.

Administration

Topical For external use only; avoid contact with eyes

Monitoring and Teaching Issues

Physical Assessment When applied to large areas or for extensive periods of time, monitor for skin irritation.

Patient Education Therapeutic effect may take several weeks. Test response by applying to small area of unbroken skin and check in 24 hours; if irritation or blistering occurs do not use. Avoid contact with eyes. Do not apply to open wounds or weeping areas. Before using, wash and dry area gently. Apply a thin film to affected area and rub in gently. Avoid direct sunlight or use sunblock or protective clothing to prevent repigmentation. Report rash, itching, or worsening of condition.

◆ **HYDRO-Rx [DSC]** *see* Hydrocortisone (Topical) *on page* 920

◆ **Hydroskin® [OTC]** *see* Hydrocortisone (Topical) *on page* 920

Hydroxocobalamin (hye droks oh koe BAL a min)

U.S. Brand Names Cyanokit®

Index Terms Vitamin B_{12a}

Generic Availability (U.S.) Yes: Excludes powder for injection

Pharmacologic Category Antidote; Vitamin, Water Soluble

Pregnancy Risk Factor C

Lactation Excretion in breast milk unknown/use caution

Use Treatment of pernicious anemia, vitamin B_{12} deficiency due to dietary deficiencies or malabsorption diseases, inadequate secretion of intrinsic factor, and inadequate utilization of B_{12} (eg, during neoplastic treatment); diagnostic agent for Schilling test

Cyanokit®: Treatment of cyanide poisoning (known or suspected)

Unlabeled/Investigational Use Neuropathies

Mechanism of Action/Effect Hydroxocobalamin (vitamin B_{12a}) is a precursor to cyanocobalamin (vitamin B_{12}). Cyanocobalamin acts as a coenzyme for various metabolic functions, including fat and carbohydrate metabolism and protein synthesis, used in cell replication and hematopoiesis. In the presence of cyanide, each hydroxocobalamin molecule can bind one cyanide ion by displacing it for the hydroxo ligand linked to the trivalent cobalt ion, forming cyanocobalamin.

Contraindications Hypersensitivity to hydroxocobalamin, cyanocobalamin, cobalt, or any component of the formulation

Warnings/Precautions

Solution for I.M. injection: Treatment of severe vitamin B_{12} megaloblastic anemia may result in thrombocytosis and severe hypokalemia, sometimes fatal, due to intracellular potassium shift upon anemia resolution. Use caution in folic acid deficient megaloblastic anemia; administration of vitamin B_{12} alone is not a substitute for folic acid and might mask true diagnosis. Vitamin B_{12} deficiency masks signs of polycythemia vera; vitamin B_{12} administration may unmask this condition. Neurologic manifestations of vitamin B_{12} deficiency will not be prevented with folic acid unless vitamin B_{12} is also given; spinal cord degeneration might also occur when folic acid is used as a substitute for vitamin B_{12} in anemia prevention. Blunted therapeutic response to vitamin B_{12} may occur in certain conditions (eg, infection, uremia, concurrent iron or folic acid deficiency) or in patients on medications with bone marrow suppressant properties (eg, chloramphenicol). Approved for use as I.M. injection only.

Cyanokit®: Use caution or consider alternatives in patients with known allergic reactions, including anaphylaxis, to hydroxocobalamin or cyanocobalamin. Increased blood pressure (≥180 mm Hg systolic or ≥110 mm Hg diastolic) is associated with infusion; elevations usually noted at beginning of infusion, peak toward the end of infusion and return to baseline within 4 hours of infusion. Collection of pretreatment blood cyanide concentrations does not preclude administration and should not delay administration in the emergency management of highly suspected or confirmed cyanide toxicity. Pretreatment levels may be useful as post infusion levels may be inaccurate. Treatment of cyanide poisoning should include decontamination and supportive therapy. Use caution with concurrent use of other cyanide antidotes; safety has not been established. Photosensitivity is a potential concern; avoid direct sunlight while skin remains discolored.

Drug Interactions

Avoid Concomitant Use There are no known interactions where it is recommended to avoid concomitant use.

Decreased Effect There are no known significant interactions involving a decrease in effect.

Increased Effect/Toxicity There are no known significant interactions involving an increase in effect.

Lab Interactions The following values may be affected, *in vitro*, following hydroxocobalamin 5 g dose. Interference following hydroxocobalamin 10 g dose can be expected to last up to an additional 24 hours. **Note:** Extent and duration of interference dependant on analyzer used and patient variability.

Falsely elevated:

Basophils, hemoglobin, MCH, and MCHC [duration: 12-16 hours]

Albumin, alkaline phosphatase, cholesterol, creatinine, glucose, total protein, and triglycerides [duration: 24 hours]

Bilirubin [duration: up to 4 days]

Urinalysis: Glucose, protein, erythrocytes, leukocytes, ketones, bilirubin, urobilinogen, nitrite [duration: 2-8 days]

Falsely decreased: ALT and amylase [duration: 24 hours]

Unpredictable:

AST, CK, CKMB, LDH, phosphate, and uric acid [duration: 24 hours]

PT (quick or INR) and aPTT [duration: 24-48 hours]

Urine pH [duration: 2-8 days]

May also interfere with colorimetric tests and cause hemodialysis machines to shut down due to false detection of a blood leak from the blood-like appearance of the solution.

Adverse Reactions

I.M. injection: Frequency not defined:

Dermatologic: Exanthema (transient), itching

Gastrointestinal: Diarrhea (mild, transient)

Local: Injection site pain

Miscellaneous: Anaphylaxis

I.V. infusion (Cyanokit®):

>10%:

Cardiovascular: Blood pressure increased (18% to 28%; systolic ≥180 mm Hg or diastolic ≥110 mm Hg)

Central nervous system: Headache (6% to 33%)

Dermatologic: Erythema (94% to 100%; may last up to 2 weeks), rash (predominantly acneiform; 20% to 44%; can appear 7-28 days after administration and usually resolves within a few weeks)

Gastrointestinal: Nausea (6% to 11%)

Genitourinary: Chromaturia (100%; may last up to 5 weeks after administration)

Hematologic: Lymphocytes decreased (8% to 17%)

Local: Infusion site reaction (6% to 39%)

Frequency not defined:

Cardiovascular: Chest discomfort, hot flashes, peripheral edema

Central nervous system: Dizziness, memory impairment, restlessness

Dermatologic: Pruritus, urticaria

Gastrointestinal: Abdominal discomfort, diarrhea, dyspepsia, dysphagia, hematochezia, vomiting

Ocular: Irritation, redness, swelling

Respiratory: Dry throat, dyspnea, throat tightness

Miscellaneous: Allergic reaction (including anaphylaxis)

Pharmacodynamics/Kinetics

Protein Binding Significant; forms various cobalamin-(III) complexes

Half-Life Elimination 26-31 hours

Excretion Urine (50% to 60% within initial 72 hours)

Available Dosage Forms

Injection, powder for reconstitution:

Cyanokit®: 2.5 g

Injection, solution: 1000 mcg/mL (30 mL)

Dosing

Adult & Geriatric

Vitamin B_{12} deficiency: I.M.: 30 mcg/day for 5-10 days, followed by 100-200 mcg/month

Note: Larger doses may be required in critically-ill patients or if patient has neurologic disease, an infectious disease, or hyperthyroidism.

Schilling test: I.M.: 1000 mcg

Cyanide toxicity (Cyanokit®): I.V.: Initial: 5 g as single infusion; may repeat a second 5 g dose depending on severity of poisoning and clinical response. Maximum cumulative dose: 10 g. **Note:** If suspected, antidotal therapy must be given immediately.

Pediatric Vitamin B_{12} deficiency: I.M.: 100 mcg once daily for 2 or more weeks (total dose: 1-5 mg); maintenance: 30-50 mcg/month

Administration

I.M. Solution for I.M. injection: Administer 1000 mcg/mL solution I.M. only

I.V. Cyanokit®: Administer by I.V. infusion over 15 minutes; if repeat dose needed, administer second dose over 15 minutes to 2 hours

Stability

Reconstitution I.V. infusion (Cyanokit®): Reconstitute each 2.5 g vial with 100 mL of NS using provided sterile transfer spike. If NS unavailable, may use LR or D_5W. Invert or rock each vial for at least 30 seconds prior to infusion; do not shake. Do not use if solution is **not** dark red.

Storage

Solution for I.M. injection: Store at 20°C to 25°C (68°F to 77°F). Protect from light.

I.V. infusion (Cyanokit®): Prior to reconstitution, store at 25°C (77°F): excursions permitted to 15°C to 30°C (59°F to 86°F).

Temperature variation exposure allowed for transport of lyophilized form:

Usual transport: ≤15 days at 5°C to 40°C (41°F to 104°F)

Desert transport: ≤4 days at 5°C to 60°C (41°F to 140°F)

Freezing/defrosting cycles: ≤15 days at -20°C to 40°C (-4°F to 104°F)

Following reconstitution, store up to 6 hours at ≤40°C (104°F); do not freeze. Discard any remaining solution after 6 hours.

Monitoring and Teaching Issues

Laboratory Monitoring Vitamin B_{12}, hematocrit, hemoglobin, reticulocyte count, red blood cell counts, folate and iron levels should be obtained prior to treatment and periodically during treatment.

Cyanide toxicity: Blood pressure and heart rate during and after infusion, serum lactate levels, venous-arterial PO_2 gradient. Pretreatment levels may be useful as post infusion levels may be inaccurate.

Megaloblastic anemia: In addition to normal hematological parameters, serum potassium and platelet counts should be monitored during therapy, particularly in the first 48 hours of treatment.

Physical Assessment Teach patient appropriate injection technique and needle disposal and appropriate nutrition. Cyanide toxicity: Monitor blood pressure and heart rate during infusion.

Patient Education Pernicious anemia may require monthly injections for life. Report skin rash; swelling, pain, or redness in extremities; or acute persistent diarrhea. Cyanokit®: May cause headache, redness of skin (can last up to 2 weeks; avoid exposure to sun while skin is red), skin lesions (can appear 7-28 days after infusion), and red urine (can last for 5 weeks).

Geriatric Considerations Evidence exists that people, particularly elderly, whose serum cobalamin concentrations are <500 pg/mL, should receive replacement parenteral therapy. This recommendation is based upon neuropsychiatric disorders and cardiovascular disorders associated with lower sodium cobalamin concentrations.

Pregnancy Considerations Animal studies are insufficient to determine the effect, if any, on pregnancy or fetal development. There are no adequate and well-controlled studies in pregnant women. Data on the use of hydroxocobalamin in pregnancy for the treatment of cyanide poisoning and cobalamin defects are limited.

Additional Information Expert advice from a regional poison control center for appropriate use may be obtained (1-800-222-1222). Cyanide is a clear colorless gas or liquid with a faint bitter almond odor. Cyanide reacts with trivalent ions in cytochrome oxidase in the mitochondria leading to histotoxic hypoxia and lactic acidosis. Signs and symptoms of cyanide toxicity include headache, altered mental status, dyspnea, mydriasis, chest tightness, nausea, vomiting, tachycardia/hypertension (initially), bradycardia/hypotension (later), seizures, cardiovascular collapse, or coma.

◆ **Hydroxycarbamide** *see* Hydroxyurea *on page 931*

Hydroxychloroquine (hye droks ee KLOR oh kwin)

U.S. Brand Names Plaquenil®

Index Terms Hydroxychloroquine Sulfate

Generic Availability (U.S.) Yes

Pharmacologic Category Aminoquinoline (Antimalarial)

Medication Safety Issues

Sound-alike/look-alike issues:

Hydroxychloroquine may be confused with hydrocortisone

Plaquenil® may be confused with Platinol®

Lactation Enters breast milk (AAP considers "compatible"; AAP 2001 update pending)

Use Suppression and treatment of acute attacks of malaria; treatment of systemic lupus erythematosus (SLE) and rheumatoid arthritis

Unlabeled/Investigational Use Porphyria cutanea tarda, polymorphous light eruptions

Available Dosage Forms

Tablet, oral: 200 mg

Plaquenil®: 200 mg

Dosing

Adult & Geriatric Note: Hydroxychloroquine sulfate 200 mg is equivalent to 155 mg hydroxychloroquine base and 250 mg chloroquine phosphate. All doses below expressed as hydroxychloroquine sulfate. Second-line alternative treatment for malaria (chloroquine is preferred).

Malaria, chemoprophylaxis: Oral: 400 mg weekly on same day each week; begin 2 weeks before exposure; continue for 4 weeks (per CDC guidelines) after leaving endemic area; if suppressive therapy is not begun prior to the exposure, double the initial dose and give in 2 doses, 6 hours apart and continue treatment for 8 weeks

Malaria, acute attack: Oral: 800 mg initially, followed by 400 mg at 6, 24, and 48 hours

Rheumatoid arthritis: Oral: Initial: 400-600 mg/day taken with food or milk; increase dose gradually until optimum response level is reached; usually after 4-12 weeks dose should be reduced by ½ to a maintenance dose of 200-400 mg/day

Lupus erythematosus: Oral: 400 mg every day or twice daily for several weeks-months depending on response; 200-400 mg/day for prolonged maintenance therapy

Pediatric Note: Hydroxychloroquine sulfate 200 mg is equivalent to 155 mg hydroxychloroquine base and 250 mg chloroquine phosphate. All doses below expressed as hydroxychloroquine sulfate. Second-line alternative treatment for malaria (chloroquine is preferred).

Malaria, chemoprophylaxis: Oral: 6.5 mg/kg once weekly (not to exceed 400 mg/dose); begin 2 weeks before exposure; continue for 4 weeks (per CDC guidelines) after leaving endemic area; if suppressive therapy is not begun prior to the exposure, double the initial dose and give in 2 doses, 6 hours apart and continue treatment for 8 weeks

Malaria, acute attack: Oral: 13 mg/kg initially (not to exceed 800 mg/dose), followed by 6.5 mg/kg (not to exceed 400 mg/dose) at 6, 24, and 48 hours

Renal Impairment Use with caution; dosage adjustment may be necessary in severe dysfunction (Bernstein, 1992); specific guidelines not available.

Hepatic Impairment Use with caution; dosage adjustment may be necessary.

Administration

Oral Administer with food or milk.

Monitoring and Teaching Issues

Laboratory Monitoring CBC, liver function

Physical Assessment Evaluate results of CBC, liver function tests, and ophthalmic exam prior to treatment and periodically throughout. Monitor for dermatologic, neuromuscular, or ocular changes.

Patient Education It is important to complete full course of therapy. May be taken with meals to decrease GI upset and bitter aftertaste. Avoid excessive alcohol. You should have regular ophthalmic exams (every 3 months) if using this medication over extended periods. You may experience skin discoloration (blue/black), hair bleaching, or skin rash. If you have psoriasis, you may experience exacerbation. You may experience dizziness, headache, nervousness, abnormal color vision, lightheadedness, nausea, vomiting, loss of appetite, or increased sensitivity to sunlight. Report any changes in hearing acuity or ringing in ears, any changes in vision (visual disturbances, blurred vision), weakness, numbness, tingling, tremors in muscles, skin rash or itching, persistent GI disturbances, chest pain or palpitation, CNS changes, unusual fatigue, or easy bruising or bleeding.

◆ **Hydroxychloroquine Sulfate** *see* Hydroxychloroquine *on page* 930

◆ **Hydroxydaunomycin Hydrochloride** *see* DOXOrubicin *on page* 579

◆ **Hydroxyethyl Starch** *see* Hetastarch *on page* 908

◆ **Hydroxyldaunorubicin Hydrochloride** *see* DOXOrubicin *on page* 579

◆ **9-hydroxy-risperidone** *see* Paliperidone *on page* 1391

Hydroxyurea (hye droks ee yoor EE a)

U.S. Brand Names Droxia®; Hydrea®

Index Terms Hydroxycarbamide; Hydurea

Generic Availability (U.S.) Yes

Pharmacologic Category Antineoplastic Agent, Antimetabolite

Medication Safety Issues

Sound-alike/look-alike issues:

Hydroxyurea may be confused with hydrOXYzine

High alert medication: This medication is in a class the Institute for Safe Medication Practices (ISMP) includes among its list of drugs which have a heightened risk of causing significant patient harm when used in error.

International issues:

Hydrea [U.S., Canada, and multiple international markets] may be confused with Hydra brand name for isoniazid [Japan]

Pregnancy Risk Factor D

Lactation Enters breast milk/not recommended

Use Treatment of melanoma, refractory chronic myelocytic leukemia (CML); recurrent, metastatic, or inoperable ovarian cancer; radiosensitizing agent in the treatment of squamous cell head and neck cancer (excluding lip cancer); adjunct in the management of sickle cell patients who have had at least three painful crises in the previous 12 months (to reduce frequency of these crises and the need for blood transfusions)

Unlabeled/Investigational Use Treatment of essential thrombocythemia, polycythemia vera, hypereosinophilic syndrome; management of hyperleukocytosis due to acute myeloid leukemia; treatment of cervical cancer, treatment of meningiomas

Mechanism of Action/Effect Antimetabolite which selectively inhibits ribonucleoside diphosphate reductase, preventing the conversion of ribonucleotides to deoxyribonucleotides, halting the cell cycle at the G1/S phase and therefore has radiation sensitizing activity by maintaining cells in the G_1 phase and interfering with DNA repair. In sickle cell anemia, hydroxyurea increases red blood cell (RBC) hemoglobin F levels, RBC water content, deformability of sickled cells, and alters adhesion of RBCs to endothelium.

Contraindications Hypersensitivity to hydroxyurea or any component of the formulation; severe bone marrow suppression (WBC <2500/mm^3 or platelet count <100,000/mm^3) or severe anemia (in patients with sickle cell anemia; use is not recommended if neutrophils <2000/mm^3, platelets <80,000/mm^3, hemoglobin <4.5 g/dL, or reticulocytes <80,000/mm^3 when hemoglobin <9 g/dL)

Warnings/Precautions Hazardous agent - use appropriate precautions for handling and disposal; to decrease risk of exposure, wear gloves when handling and wash hands before and after contact. Leukopenia may commonly occur (thrombocytopenia and anemia are less common; reversible with treatment interruption. Use with caution in patients with a history of prior chemotherapy or radiation therapy; myelosuppression is more common. Correct severe anemia prior to initiating treatment. Patients with a history of radiation therapy are also at risk for exacerbation of post irradiation erythema. Self-limiting megaloblastic erythropoiesis may be seen early in treatment (may resemble pernicious anemia, but is unrelated to vitamin B_{12} or folic acid deficiency). Plasma iron clearance may be delayed and iron utilization rate (by erythrocytes) may be reduced. When treated concurrently with hydroxyurea and antiretroviral agents (including didanosine), HIV-infected patients are at higher risk for potentially fatal pancreatitis, hepatotoxicity, hepatic failure, and severe peripheral neuropathy. Hyperuricemia may occur with treatment; adequate hydration and initiation or dosage adjustment of uricosuric agents (eg, allopurinol) may be necessary.

In patients with sickle cell anemia, use is not recommended if neutrophils <2000/mm^3, platelets <80,000/mm^3, hemoglobin <4.5 g/dL, or reticulocytes <80,000/mm^3 when hemoglobin <9 g/dL. May cause macrocytosis, which can mask folic acid deficiency; prophylactic fold acid supplementation is recommended. **[U.S. Boxed Warning]: Hydroxyurea is mutagenic and clastogenic. Treatment of myeloproliferative disorders (eg, polycythemia vera, thrombocythemia) with long-term hydroxyurea is associated with secondary leukemia;** it is unknown if this is drug-related or disease-related. Cutaneous vasculitic toxicities (vasculitic ulceration and gangrene) have been reported with hydroxyurea treatment, most often in patients with a history of or receiving concurrent interferon therapy; discontinue hydroxyurea and consider alternate cytoreductive therapy if cutaneous vasculitic toxicity develops. Use caution with renal dysfunction; may require dose reductions. Elderly patients may be more sensitive to the effects of hydroxyurea; may require lower doses. **[U.S. Boxed Warning]: Should be administered under the supervision of a physician experienced in the treatment of sickle cell anemia** or in cancer chemotherapy.

Drug Interactions

Avoid Concomitant Use

Avoid concomitant use of Hydroxyurea with any of the following: BCG; Didanosine; Natalizumab; Pimecrolimus; Roflumilast; Stavudine; Tacrolimus (Topical); Vaccines (Live)

Decreased Effect

Hydroxyurea may decrease the levels/effects of: BCG; Sipuleucel-T; Vaccines (Inactivated); Vaccines (Live)

The levels/effects of Hydroxyurea may be decreased by: Echinacea

Increased Effect/Toxicity

Hydroxyurea may increase the levels/effects of: Didanosine; Leflunomide; Natalizumab; Stavudine; Vaccines (Live)

The levels/effects of Hydroxyurea may be increased by: Denosumab; Didanosine; Pimecrolimus; Roflumilast; Stavudine; Tacrolimus (Topical); Trastuzumab

Adverse Reactions Frequency not defined.

Cardiovascular: Edema

Central nervous system: Chills, disorientation, dizziness, drowsiness (dose-related), fever, hallucinations, headache, malaise, seizure

Dermatologic: Alopecia, cutaneous vasculitic toxicities, dermatomyositis-like skin changes, facial erythema, gangrene, hyperpigmentation, maculopapular rash, nail atrophy, nail discoloration, peripheral erythema, scaling, skin atrophy, skin cancer, skin ulcer, vasculitis ulcerations, violet papules

Endocrine & metabolic: Hyperuricemia

Gastrointestinal: Anorexia, constipation, diarrhea, gastrointestinal irritation and mucositis, (potentiated with radiation therapy), nausea, pancreatitis, stomatitis, vomiting

Genitourinary: Dysuria

Hematologic: Myelosuppression (anemia, leukopenia [common; reversal of WBC count occurs rapidly], thrombocytopenia); macrocytosis, megaloblastic erythropoiesis, secondary leukemias (long-term use)

Hepatic: Hepatic enzymes increased, hepatotoxicity

Neuromuscular & skeletal: Peripheral neuropathy, weakness

Renal: BUN increased, creatinine increased

Respiratory: Acute diffuse pulmonary infiltrates (rare), dyspnea, pulmonary fibrosis (rare)

Pharmacodynamics/Kinetics

Onset of Action Sickle cell anemia: Fetal hemoglobin increase: 4-12 weeks

Absorption Readily (≥80%)

Time to Peak 1-4 hours

Half-Life Elimination 3-4 hours

Metabolism 60% via hepatic and GI tract

Excretion Urine (sickle cell anemia: 40% of administered dose)

Available Dosage Forms

Capsule, oral: 500 mg

Droxia®: 200 mg, 300 mg, 400 mg

Hydrea®: 500 mg

Dosing

Adult & Geriatric

Antineoplastic uses: Titrate dose to patient response; if WBC count falls to <2500/mm^3, or the platelet count to <100,000/mm^3, therapy should be stopped for at least 3 days and resumed when values rise toward normal

Chronic myeloid leukemia (resistant): Oral: Continuous therapy: 20-30 mg/kg once daily

Solid tumors: Oral:

Intermittent therapy: 80 mg/kg as a single dose every third day

Continuous therapy: 20-30 mg/kg once daily

Concomitant therapy with irradiation (head and neck cancer): 80 mg/kg as a single dose every third day starting at least 7 days before initiation of irradiation

Sickle cell anemia: Oral: Initial: 15 mg/kg/day; if blood counts are in an acceptable range, may increase by 5 mg/kg every 12 weeks until the maximum tolerated dose of 35 mg/kg/day is achieved or the dose that does not produce toxic effects (do not increase dose if blood counts are between acceptable and toxic ranges). Monitor for toxicity every 2 weeks; if toxicity occurs, withhold treatment until the bone marrow recovers, then restart with a dose reduction of 2.5 mg/kg/day; if no toxicity occurs over the next 12 weeks, then the subsequent dose may be increased by 2.5 mg/kg/day every 12 weeks to a maximum tolerated dose (dose which does not produce hematologic toxicity for 24 consecutive weeks). If hematologic toxicity recurs a second time at a specific dose, do not retry that dose.

Acceptable hematologic ranges: Neutrophils ≥2500/mm^3; platelets ≥95,000/mm^3; hemoglobin >5.3 g/dL, and reticulocytes ≥95,000/mm^3 if the hemoglobin concentration is <9 g/dL

Toxic hematologic ranges: Neutrophils <2000/mm^3; platelets <80,000/mm^3; hemoglobin <4.5 g/dL; and reticulocytes <80,000/mm^3 if the hemoglobin concentration is <9 g/dL

Cervical cancer (unlabeled use; with concurrent radiation therapy, cisplatin and fluorouracil): Oral: 2000 mg/m^2 (2 hours prior to radiation treatment) twice a week for 6 weeks (Rose, 2007)

Essential thrombocythemia, high-risk (unlabeled use): Oral: 500-1000 mg daily; adjust dose to maintain platelets <400,000/mm^3 (Harrison, 2005)

Head and neck cancer (unlabeled dosing; with concurrent radiation therapy and fluorouracil): Oral: 1000 mg every 12 hours for 11 doses (Garden, 2004)

Hypereosinophilic syndrome (unlabeled use): Oral: 1000-3000 mg/day (Klion, 2006)

Meningioma (unlabeled use): Oral: 20 mg/kg once daily (Newton, 2000; Rosenthal, 2002)

Polycythemia vera, high-risk (unlabeled use): Oral: 15-20 mg/kg/day (Finazzi, 2007)

Pediatric Note: Doses should be based on ideal or actual body weight, whichever is less.

Sickle cell anemia (unlabeled use): Oral: 20 mg/kg once daily; increase by 5 mg/kg/day every 2-6 months to a maximum dose of 30 mg/kg/day (Ferster, 2001; Hankins, 2005; Thornburg, 2009; Wang, 2001; Zimmerman, 2004)

Renal Impairment

The FDA-approved labeling recommends the following adjustment:

Sickle cell anemia:

Cl_{cr} ≥60 mL/minute: No adjustment (of initial dose) required.

Cl_{cr} <60 mL/minute: Reduce initial dose to 7.5 mg/kg/day; titrate to response/avoidance of toxicity (refer to usual dosing).

ESRD: Reduce initial dose to 7.5 mg/kg/dose (administer after dialysis on dialysis days); titrate to response/avoidance of toxicity.

Other approved indications: It is recommended to reduce the initial dose; however, no specific guidelines are available.

The following guidelines have been used by some clinicians:

Aronoff, 2007: Adults:

Cl_{cr} 10-50 mL/minute: Administer 50% of dose.

Cl_{cr} <10 mL/minute: Administer 20% of dose.

Hemodialysis: Administer dose after dialysis on dialysis days; supplemental dose is not necessary. Hydroxyurea is a low molecular weight compound with high aqueous solubility that may be freely dialyzable, however, clinical studies confirming this hypothesis have not been performed.

Continuous renal replacement therapy (CRRT): Administer 50% of dose.

Kintzel, 1995:

Cl_{cr} 46-60 mL/minute: Administer 85% of dose.

Cl_{cr} 31-45 mL/minute: Administer 80% of dose.

Cl_{cr} <30 mL/minute: Administer 75% of dose.

Hepatic Impairment Specific guidelines are not available for dosage adjustment in hepatic impairment. The FDA-approved labeling recommends closely monitoring for bone marrow toxicity in patients with hepatic impairment.

Administration

Oral The manufacturer does not recommend opening the capsules; observe proper handling procedures (eg, wear gloves)

Stability

Storage Store at room temperature of 25°C (77°F); excursions permitted between 15°C and 30°C (59°F and 86°F).

Monitoring and Teaching Issues

Laboratory Monitoring CBC with differential and platelets, renal function and liver function tests, serum uric acid

Sickle cell disease: Monitor for toxicity every 2 weeks. If toxicity occurs, stop treatment until the bone marrow recovers; restart at 2.5 mg/kg/day less than the dose at which toxicity occurs. If no toxicity occurs over the next 12 weeks, then the subsequent dose should be ▶

increased by 2.5 mg/kg/day. Reduced dosage of hydroxyurea alternating with erythropoietin may decrease myelotoxicity and increase levels of fetal hemoglobin in patients who have not been helped by hydroxyurea alone.

Acceptable range: Neutrophils ≥2500 cells/mm^3, platelets ≥95,000/mm^3, hemoglobin >5.3 g/dL, and reticulocytes ≥95,000/mm^3 if the hemoglobin concentration is <9 g/dL

Toxic range: Neutrophils <2000 cells/mm^3, platelets <80,000/mm^3, hemoglobin <4.5 g/dL, and reticulocytes <80,000/mm^3 if the hemoglobin concentration is <9 g/dL

Physical Assessment Assess results of CBC, renal function, and LFTs. Monitor for CNS changes, gastrointestinal upset. hepatotoxicity, and peripheral neuropathy. Teach proper use and need for frequent monitoring.

Patient Education Take capsules exactly as directed by prescriber (dosage and timing will be specific to purpose of therapy). Contents of capsule may be emptied into a glass of water and taken immediately. You will require frequent monitoring and blood tests while taking this medication to assess effectiveness and monitor adverse reactions. You will be susceptible to infection. May cause nausea, vomiting, loss of appetite, constipation, diarrhea, or mouth sores. Report persistent vomiting, diarrhea, constipation, stomach pain, or mouth sores; skin rash, redness, irritation, or sores; painful or difficult urination; anemia (unusual fatigue, lethargy), CNS changes (increased confusion, depression, hallucinations, or seizures); opportunistic infection (persistent fever or chills, white plaques in mouth, vaginal discharge, or unhealed sores); unusual lassitude, muscle tremors or weakness; easy bruising/bleeding; or blood in vomitus, stool, or urine. People not taking hydroxyurea should not be exposed to it. If powder from capsule is spilled, wipe up with damp, disposable towel immediately, and discard the towel in a closed container, such as a plastic bag. Wash hands thoroughly.

Dietary Considerations In sickle cell patients, supplemental administration of folic acid is recommended; hydroxyurea may mask development of folic acid deficiency.

Geriatric Considerations Elderly may be more sensitive to the effects of this drug and may require a lower dosage regimen; advance dose slowly and adjust dose for renal function with careful monitoring.

Breast-Feeding Considerations Due to the potential for serious adverse reactions in the nursing infant, breast-feeding is not recommended.

Pregnancy Considerations Animal studies have demonstrated teratogenicity and embryotoxicity at doses lower than the usual human dose. Women of childbearing potential should be advised to avoid becoming pregnant during treatment.

HydrOXYzine (hye DROKS i zeen)

U.S. Brand Names Vistaril®

Index Terms Hydroxyzine Hydrochloride; Hydroxyzine Pamoate

Generic Availability (U.S.) Yes

Pharmacologic Category Antiemetic; Histamine H_1 Antagonist; Histamine H_1 Antagonist, First Generation; Piperazine Derivative

Medication Safety Issues

Sound-alike/look-alike issues:

HydrOXYzine may be confused with hydrALAZINE, hydroxyurea

Atarax® may be confused with Ativan®

Vistaril® may be confused with Restoril™, Versed, Zestril®

Beers Criteria medication: This drug may be inappropriate for use in geriatric patients (high severity risk).

International issues:

Vistaril [U.S. and Turkey] may be confused with Vastarel brand name for trimetazidine [multiple international markets]

Pregnancy Risk Factor C

Lactation Excretion in breast milk unknown/not recommended

Use Treatment of anxiety; preoperative sedative; antipruritic

Unlabeled/Investigational Use Antiemetic; ethanol withdrawal symptoms

Mechanism of Action/Effect Competes with histamine for H_1-receptor sites on effector cells in the gastrointestinal tract, blood vessels, and respiratory tract. Possesses skeletal muscle relaxing, bronchodilator, antihistamine, antiemetic, and analgesic properties.

Contraindications Hypersensitivity to hydroxyzine or any component of the formulation; early pregnancy; SubQ, intra-arterial, or I.V. administration of injection

Warnings/Precautions Causes sedation, caution must be used in performing tasks which require alertness (eg, operating machinery or driving). Sedative effects of CNS depressants or ethanol are potentiated. SubQ, I.V., and intra-arterial administration are contraindicated since tissue damage, intravascular hemolysis, thrombosis, and digital gangrene can occur. Use with caution with narrow-angle glaucoma, prostatic hyperplasia, bladder neck obstruction, asthma, or COPD. May be inappropriate for use in the elderly due to potent anticholinergic effects; nonanticholinergic antihistamines preferred for treating allergic reactions (Beers Criteria).

Drug Interactions

Metabolism/Transport Effects Inhibits CYP2D6 (weak)

Avoid Concomitant Use There are no known interactions where it is recommended to avoid concomitant use.

Decreased Effect
HydrOXYzine may decrease the levels/effects of: Acetylcholinesterase Inhibitors (Central); Benzylpenicilloyl Polylysine; Betahistine

The levels/effects of HydrOXYzine may be decreased by: Acetylcholinesterase Inhibitors (Central); Amphetamines

Increased Effect/Toxicity
HydrOXYzine may increase the levels/effects of: Alcohol (Ethyl); Anticholinergics; CNS Depressants

The levels/effects of HydrOXYzine may be increased by: Droperidol; Pramlintide

Nutritional/Ethanol Interactions
Ethanol: Avoid ethanol (may increase CNS depression).
Herb/Nutraceutical: Avoid valerian, St John's wort, kava kava, gotu kola (may increase CNS depression).

Lab Interactions May cause false-positive serum TCA screen.

Adverse Reactions Frequency not defined.
Central nervous system: Dizziness, drowsiness, fatigue, hallucination, headache, nervousness, seizure
Dermatologic: Pruritus, rash, urticaria
Gastrointestinal: Xerostomia
Neuromuscular & skeletal: Involuntary movements, paresthesia, tremor
Ocular: Blurred vision
Respiratory: Thickening of bronchial secretions
Miscellaneous: Allergic reaction

Pharmacodynamics/Kinetics
Onset of Action Oral: 15-30 minutes
Duration of Action 4-6 hours
Absorption Oral: Rapid
Time to Peak ~2 hours
Half-Life Elimination 3-7 hours
Metabolism Forms metabolites
Excretion Urine

Available Dosage Forms
Capsule, oral: 25 mg, 50 mg, 100 mg
Vistaril®: 25 mg, 50 mg
Injection, solution: 25 mg/mL (1 mL); 50 mg/mL (1 mL, 2 mL, 10 mL)
Solution, oral: 10 mg/5 mL (473 mL)
Syrup, oral: 10 mg/5 mL (118 mL, 473 mL, 480 mL)
Tablet, oral: 10 mg, 25 mg, 50 mg

Dosing
Adult
Antiemetic (unlabeled use): I.M.: 25-100 mg/dose every 4-6 hours as needed
Anxiety: Oral, I.M.: 50-100 mg 4 times/day
Preoperative sedation:
Oral: 50-100 mg
I.M.: 25-100 mg
Pruritus: Oral, I.M.: 25 mg 3-4 times/day

Geriatric Management of pruritus: 10 mg 3-4 times/day; increase to 25 mg 3-4 times/day if necessary.

Pediatric
Preoperative sedation:
Oral: 0.6 mg/kg/dose
I.M.: 0.5-1 mg/kg/dose
Pruritus, anxiety: Oral:
<6 years: 50 mg daily in divided doses
≥6 years: 50-100 mg daily in divided doses

Hepatic Impairment Change dosing interval to every 24 hours in patients with primary biliary cirrhosis.

Administration
I.M. Do not administer SubQ or intra-arterially. Administer I.M. deep in large muscle.
I.V. Extravasation can result in sterile abscess and marked tissue induration.

Stability
Storage Injection: Store at 15°C to 30°C. Protect from light.

Monitoring and Teaching Issues
Physical Assessment Institute precautions to prevent falls.
Patient Education Will cause drowsiness. Do not use alcohol. Report hallucinations, seizure activity, tremors or involuntary movements, or loss of sensation.
Geriatric Considerations Anticholinergic effects are not well tolerated in the elderly and frequently result in bowel, bladder, and mental status changes (ie, constipation, confusion, and urinary retention). Hydroxyzine may be useful as a short-term antipruritic, but it is not recommended for use as a sedative or anxiolytic in the elderly.

This medication is considered to be potentially inappropriate in this patient population (Beers Criteria severity: High).

Pregnancy Considerations Hydroxyzine-induced fetal abnormalities at high dosages in animal studies. Neonatal withdrawal symptoms have been reported following long-term maternal use or the use of large doses near term. Use in early pregnancy is contraindicated by the manufacturer.

- **Hydroxyzine Hydrochloride** *see* HydrOXYzine *on page 934*
- **Hydroxyzine Pamoate** *see* HydrOXYzine *on page 934*
- **HydroZone Plus [OTC] [DSC]** *see* Hydrocortisone (Topical) *on page 920*
- **Hydurea** *see* Hydroxyurea *on page 931*
- **Hygroton** *see* Chlorthalidone *on page 361*
- **Hyoscine Butylbromide** *see* Scopolamine (Systemic) *on page 1627*
- **HyperRHO™ S/D Full Dose** *see* Rh_o(D) Immune Globulin *on page 1569*
- **HyperRHO™ S/D Mini-Dose** *see* Rh_o(D) Immune Globulin *on page 1569*
- **Hytrin** *see* Terazosin *on page 1731*
- **Hyzaar®** *see* Losartan and Hydrochlorothiazide *on page 1135*

Ibandronate (eye BAN droh nate)

U.S. Brand Names Boniva®

Index Terms Ibandronate Sodium; Ibandronic Acid

Generic Availability (U.S.) No

Pharmacologic Category Bisphosphonate Derivative

Medication Guide Available Yes

Pregnancy Risk Factor C

Lactation Excretion in breast milk unknown/use caution

Use Treatment and prevention of osteoporosis in postmenopausal females

Unlabeled/Investigational Use Hypercalcemia of malignancy; corticosteroid-induced osteoporosis; Paget's disease; reduce bone pain and skeletal complications from metastatic bone disease

Mechanism of Action/Effect A bisphosphonate which inhibits bone resorption via actions on osteoclasts or on osteoclast precursors; decreases the rate of bone resorption, leading to an indirect increase in bone mineral density.

Contraindications Hypersensitivity to ibandronate or any component of the formulation; hypocalcemia; oral tablets are also contraindicated in patients unable to stand or sit upright for at least 60 minutes and in patients with abnormalities of the esophagus which delay esophageal emptying, such as stricture or achalasia

Warnings/Precautions Hypocalcemia must be corrected before therapy initiation. Ensure adequate calcium and vitamin D intake. Osteonecrosis of the jaw (ONJ) has been reported in patients receiving bisphosphonates. Risk factors include invasive dental procedures (eg, tooth extraction, dental implants, boney surgery); a diagnosis of cancer, with concomitant chemotherapy or corticosteroids; poor oral hygiene, ill-fitting dentures; and comorbid disorders (anemia, coagulopathy, infection, pre-existing dental disease). Most reported cases occurred after I.V. bisphosphonate therapy; however, cases have been reported following oral therapy. A dental exam and preventative dentistry should be performed prior to placing patients with risk factors on chronic bisphosphonate therapy. The manufacturer's labeling states that discontinuing bisphosphonates in patients requiring invasive dental procedures may reduce the risk of ONJ. However, other experts suggest that there is no evidence that discontinuing therapy reduces the risk of developing ONJ (Assael, 2009). The benefit/risk must be assessed by the treating physician and/or dentist/surgeon prior to any invasive dental procedure. Patients developing ONJ while on bisphosphonates should receive care by an oral surgeon.

Atypical femur fractures have been reported in patients receiving bisphosphonates for treatment/prevention of osteoporosis. The fractures include subtrochanteric femur (bone just below the hip joint) and diaphyseal femur (long segment of the thigh bone). Some patients experience prodromal pain weeks or months before the fracture occurs. It is unclear if bisphosphonate therapy is the cause for these fractures, although the majority have been reported in patients taking bisphosphonates. Patients receiving long-term (>3-5 years) therapy may be at an increased risk. Discontinue bisphosphonate therapy in patients who develop a femoral shaft fracture.

Infrequently, severe (and occasionally debilitating) bone, joint, and/or muscle pain have been reported during bisphosphonate treatment. The onset of pain ranged from a single day to several months. Consider discontinuing therapy in patients who experience severe symptoms; symptoms usually resolve upon discontinuation. Some patients experienced recurrence when rechallenged with same drug or another bisphosphonate; avoid use in patients with a history of these symptoms in association with bisphosphonate therapy.

Oral bisphosphonates may cause dysphagia, esophagitis, esophageal or gastric ulcer; risk may increase in patients unable to comply with dosing instructions; discontinue use if new or worsening symptoms develop. Intravenous bisphosphonates may cause transient decreases in serum calcium and have also been associated with renal toxicity.

Use not recommended with severe renal impairment (Cl_{cr} <30 mL/minute).

Drug Interactions

Avoid Concomitant Use There are no known interactions where it is recommended to avoid concomitant use.

Decreased Effect

The levels/effects of Ibandronate may be decreased by: Antacids; Calcium Salts; Iron Salts; Magnesium Salts; Proton Pump Inhibitors

Increased Effect/Toxicity

Ibandronate may increase the levels/effects of: Phosphate Supplements

The levels/effects of Ibandronate may be increased by: Aminoglycosides; Nonsteroidal Anti-Inflammatory Agents

Nutritional/Ethanol Interactions

Ethanol: Avoid ethanol (may increase risk of osteoporosis).

Food: May reduce absorption; mean oral bioavailability is decreased up to 90% when given with food.

Lab Interactions Bisphosphonates may interfere with diagnostic imaging agents such as technetium-99m-diphosphonate in bone scans.

Adverse Reactions Percentages vary based on frequency of administration (daily vs monthly). Unless specified, percentages are reported with oral use.

>10%:

Gastrointestinal: Dyspepsia (6% to 12%)

Neuromuscular & skeletal: Back pain (4% to 14%)

1% to 10%:

Cardiovascular: Hypertension (6% to 7%)

Central nervous system: Headache (3% to 7%), dizziness (1% to 4%), insomnia (1% to 2%)

Dermatologic: Rash (1% to 2%)

Endocrine & metabolic: Hypercholesterolemia (5%)

Gastrointestinal: Abdominal pain (5% to 8%), diarrhea (4% to 7%), nausea (5%), tooth disorder (4%), constipation (3% to 4%), vomiting (3%)

Genitourinary: Urinary tract infection (2% to 6%)

Hepatic: Alkaline phosphatase decreased (frequency not defined)

Local: Injection site reaction (<2%)

Neuromuscular & skeletal: Pain in extremity (1% to 8%), arthralgia (4% to 6%), myalgia (1% to 6%), joint disorder (4%), weakness (4%), osteoarthritis (localized; 1% to 3%), muscle cramp (2%)

Respiratory: Bronchitis (3% to 10%), pneumonia (6%), pharyngitis/nasopharyngitis (3% to 4%), upper respiratory infection (2%)

Miscellaneous: Acute phase reaction (I.V. 10%; oral 3% to 9%), infection (4%), flu-like syndrome (1% to 4%), allergic reaction (3%)

Pharmacodynamics/Kinetics

Bioavailability Oral: 2.5 mg tablet: 0.6%; Reduced by 90% following standard breakfast

Time to Peak Oral: 0.5-2 hours

Protein Binding 85.7% to 99.5%

Half-Life Elimination

Oral: 150 mg dose: Terminal: 37-157 hours

I.V.: Terminal: ~5-25 hours

Metabolism Not metabolized

Excretion Urine (50% to 60% of absorbed dose, excreted as unchanged drug); feces (unabsorbed drug)

Available Dosage Forms

Injection, solution:

Boniva®: 1 mg/mL (3 mL)

Tablet, oral:

Boniva®: 150 mg

Dosing

Adult & Geriatric

Treatment of postmenopausal osteoporosis: Patients should receive supplemental calcium and vitamin D if dietary intake is inadequate

Oral: 2.5 mg once daily **or** 150 mg once a month

I.V.: 3 mg every 3 months

Prevention of postmenopausal osteoporosis: Patients should receive supplemental calcium and vitamin D if dietary intake is inadequate: Oral: 2.5 mg once daily **or** 150 mg once a month

Hypercalcemia of malignancy (unlabeled use): I.V.: 2-4 mg over 2 hours

Metastatic bone disease (unlabeled use):

Oral: 50 mg once daily

I.V.: 6 mg over 1 hour every 3-4 weeks

Renal Impairment

Mild or moderate impairment: Dosing adjustment not needed.

Severe impairment (Cl_{cr} <30 mL/minute): Use not recommended.

Dosage adjustment in renal impairment for oncologic uses (unlabeled): Severe impairment (Cl_{cr} <30 mL/minute):

Oral: 50 mg once weekly

I.V.: 2 mg over 1 hour every 3-4 weeks

Hepatic Impairment Dosing adjustment not needed.

Administration

Oral Should be administered 60 minutes before the first food or drink of the day (other than water) and prior to taking any oral medications or supplements (eg, calcium, antacids, vitamins). Ibandronate should be taken in an upright position with a full glass (6-8 oz) of plain water and the patient should avoid lying down for 60 minutes to minimize the possibility of GI side effects. Mineral water with a high calcium content should be avoided. The tablet should be swallowed whole; do not chew or suck. Do not eat or drink anything (except water) for 60 minutes following administration of ibandronate.

Once-monthly dosing: The 150 mg tablet should be taken on the same date each month. In case of a missed dose, do not take two 150 mg tablets within the same week. If the next scheduled dose is 1-7 days away, wait until the next scheduled dose to take the tablet. If the next scheduled dose is >7 days away, take the dose the morning it is remembered, and then resume taking the once-monthly dose on the originally scheduled day.

I.V. Administer as a 15-30 second bolus. Do not mix with calcium-containing solutions or other drugs. For osteoporosis, do not administer more frequently than every 3 months. Infuse over 1 hour for metastatic bone disease and over 2 hours for hypercalcemia of malignancy.

Stability

Storage Store at controlled room temperature of 25°C (77°F); excursions permitted to 15°C to 30°C (59°F to 86°F).

Monitoring and Teaching Issues

Laboratory Monitoring

Osteoporosis: Bone mineral density as measured by central dual-energy x-ray absorptiometry (DXA) of the hip or spine (prior to initiation of therapy and at least every 2 years); biochemical markers of bone turnover (optional); serum calcium and 25(OH)D

Serum creatinine prior to each I.V. dose

Physical Assessment Assess history for any previous adverse response to bisphosphonates and ability to comply with administration instructions. Use caution with renal impairment. Correct any hypocalcemia prior to beginning treatment. Patients at risk for osteonecrosis of the jaw (eg, chemotherapy, corticosteroids, poor oral hygiene) should have dental exams; necessary preventive dentistry should be done before beginning bisphosphonate therapy. Monitor for immediate or long-term musculoskeletal pain. Teach patient specific administration directions. Instruct patient in lifestyle and dietary changes.

Patient Education Oral: Take with a full glass of water first thing in the morning and at least 60 minutes before the first food or beverage of the day. Wait at least 60 minutes after taking Ibandronate before taking anything else. Stay in sitting or standing position for 60 minutes following administration and until after the first food of the day to reduce potential for esophageal irritation. Consult prescriber to determine necessity of lifestyle changes (eg, decreased smoking, decreased alcohol intake). Certain dental procedures should be avoided if possible while you are taking this medication. You may experience temporary flatulence, bloating, nausea, acid regurgitation, or temporary bone pain. Report persistent muscle or bone pain, leg cramps, acute headache, persistent gastric pain or unresolved GI upset, unusual fever, chills, rash, or pain in mouth.

Dietary Considerations Ensure adequate calcium and vitamin D intake; women and men >50 years of age should consume 1200-1500 mg/day of elemental calcium and 800-1000 int. units/day of vitamin D. Ibandronate tablet should be taken with a full glass (6-8 oz) of plain water, at least 60 minutes prior to any food, beverages, or medications. Mineral water with a high calcium content should be avoided.

Geriatric Considerations Studies with elderly found no difference between younger adults and the elderly. No special dosage changes are necessary.

Pregnancy Considerations Adverse effects were demonstrated in animal studies. There are no adequate and well-controlled studies in pregnant women. Bisphosphonates are incorporated into the bone matrix and are gradually released over time. Theoretically, there may be a risk of fetal harm when pregnancy follows the completion of therapy. Based on limited case reports with pamidronate, serum calcium levels in the newborn may be altered if administered during pregnancy.

◆ **Ibandronate Sodium** *see* Ibandronate *on page 936*

◆ **Ibandronic Acid** *see* Ibandronate *on page 936*

◆ **Ibidomide Hydrochloride** *see* Labetalol *on page 1048*

◆ **Ibu®** *see* Ibuprofen *on page 938*

◆ **Ibu-200 [OTC]** *see* Ibuprofen *on page 938*

◆ **Ibudone™** *see* Hydrocodone and Ibuprofen *on page 916*

Ibuprofen (eye byoo PROE fen)

U.S. Brand Names Addaprin [OTC]; Advil® Children's [OTC]; Advil® Infants' [OTC]; Advil® Migraine [OTC]; Advil® [OTC]; Caldolor™; I-Prin [OTC]; Ibu-200 [OTC]; Ibu®; Midol® Cramps & Body Aches [OTC]; Motrin® Children's [OTC]; Motrin® IB [OTC]; Motrin® Infants' [OTC]; Motrin® Junior [OTC]; NeoProfen®; Proprinal® [OTC]; TopCare® Junior Strength [OTC]; Ultraprin [OTC]

Index Terms *p*-Isobutylhydratropic Acid; Ibuprofen Lysine

Generic Availability (U.S.) Yes: Caplet, softgel capsule, suspension, tablet

Pharmacologic Category Nonsteroidal Anti-inflammatory Drug (NSAID), Oral; Nonsteroidal Anti-inflammatory Drug (NSAID), Parenteral

Medication Safety Issues

Sound-alike/look-alike issues:

Haltran® may be confused with Halfprin®

Motrin® may be confused with Neurontin®

Injectable formulations: Both ibuprofen and ibuprofen lysine are available for parenteral use. Ibuprofen lysine is **only** indicated for closure of a clinically-significant patent ductus arteriosus.

Medication Guide Available Yes

Pregnancy Risk Factor C/D ≥30 weeks gestation

Lactation Enters breast milk/not recommended (AAP rates "compatible"; AAP 2001 update pending)

Use

Oral: Inflammatory diseases and rheumatoid disorders including juvenile idiopathic arthritis (JIA), mild-to-moderate pain, fever, dysmenorrhea, osteoarthritis

Ibuprofen injection (Caldolor™): Management of mild-to-moderate pain; management moderate-to-severe pain when used concurrently with an opioid analgesic; reduction of fever

Ibuprofen lysine injection (NeoProfen®): To induce closure of a clinically-significant patent ductus arteriosus (PDA) in premature infants weighing between 500-1500 g and who are ≤32 weeks gestational age (GA) when usual treatments are ineffective

Unlabeled/Investigational Use Cystic fibrosis, gout, ankylosing spondylitis, acute migraine headache

Mechanism of Action/Effect Reversibly inhibits cyclooxygenase-1 and 2 (COX-1 and 2) enzymes, which results in decreased formation of prostaglandin precursors; has antipyretic, analgesic, and anti-inflammatory properties

Contraindications Hypersensitivity to ibuprofen; history of asthma, urticaria, or allergic-type reaction to aspirin or other NSAIDs; aspirin triad (eg, bronchial asthma, aspirin intolerance, rhinitis); perioperative pain in the setting of coronary artery bypass graft (CABG) surgery

Ibuprofen lysine (NeoProfen®): Preterm infants with untreated proven or suspected infection; congenital heart disease where patency of the PDA is necessary for pulmonary or systemic blood flow; bleeding (especially with active intracranial hemorrhage or GI bleed); thrombocytopenia; coagulation defects; proven or suspected necrotizing enterocolitis (NEC); significant renal dysfunction

Warnings/Precautions [U.S. Boxed Warning]: NSAIDs are associated with an increased risk of adverse cardiovascular thrombotic events, including fatal MI and stroke. Risk may be increased with duration of use or pre-existing cardiovascular risk factors or disease. Carefully evaluate individual cardiovascular risk profiles prior to prescribing. May cause new-onset hypertension or worsening of existing hypertension. Response to ACE inhibitors, thiazides, or loop diuretics may be impaired with concurrent use of NSAIDs. Use caution with fluid retention. Avoid use in heart failure. Concurrent administration of ibuprofen, and potentially other nonselective NSAIDs, may interfere with aspirin's cardioprotective effect. **[U.S. Boxed Warning]: Use is contraindicated for treatment of perioperative pain in the setting of coronary artery bypass graft (CABG) surgery.** Risk of MI and stroke may be increased with use following CABG surgery.

May increase the risk of aseptic meningitis, especially in patients with systemic lupus erythematosus (SLE) and mixed connective tissue disorders. Platelet adhesion and aggregation may be decreased; may prolong bleeding time; patients with coagulation disorders or who are receiving anticoagulants should be monitored closely. Anemia may occur; patients on long-term NSAID therapy should be monitored for anemia. Rarely, NSAID use may cause severe blood dyscrasias (eg, agranulocytosis, aplastic anemia, thrombocytopenia).

NSAID use may compromise existing renal function; dose-dependent decreases in prostaglandin synthesis may result from NSAID use, reducing renal blood flow which may cause renal decompensation. NSAID use may increase the risk for hyperkalemia. Patients with impaired renal function, dehydration, heart failure, liver dysfunction, those taking diuretics, and ACE inhibitors, and the elderly are at greater risk of renal toxicity and hyperkalemia. Rehydrate patient before starting therapy; monitor renal function closely. Not recommended for use in patients with advanced renal disease. Long-term NSAID use may result in renal papillary necrosis.

NSAIDs may increase risk of gastrointestinal irritation, inflammation, ulceration, bleeding, and perforation. These events can be fatal and may occur at any time during therapy and without warning. Use caution with a history of GI disease (bleeding or ulcers), concurrent therapy with aspirin, anticoagulants and/or corticosteroids, smoking, use of ethanol, the elderly or debilitated patients. When used concomitantly with ≤325 mg of aspirin, a substantial increase in the risk of gastrointestinal complications (eg, ulcer) occurs; concomitant gastroprotective therapy (eg, proton pump inhibitors) is recommended (Bhatt, 2008).

Use the lowest effective dose for the shortest duration of time, consistent with individual patient goals, to reduce risk of cardiovascular or GI adverse events. Alternate therapies should be considered for patients at high risk.

NSAIDs may cause serious skin adverse events including exfoliative dermatitis, Stevens-Johnson Syndrome (SJS) and toxic epidermal necrolysis (TEN); discontinue use at first sign of skin rash or hypersensitivity. Anaphylactoid reactions may occur, even without prior exposure; patients with "aspirin triad" (bronchial asthma, aspirin intolerance, rhinitis) may be at increased risk. Do not use in patients who experience bronchospasm, asthma, rhinitis, or urticaria with NSAID or aspirin therapy. Use caution in other forms of asthma.

NSAIDS may cause drowsiness, dizziness, blurred vision and other neurologic effects which may impair physical or mental abilities; patients must be cautioned about performing tasks which require mental alertness (eg, operating machinery or driving). Monitor vision with long-term therapy. Blurred/diminished vision, scotomata, and changes in color vision have been reported. Discontinue use with altered vision and perform ophthalmologic exam.

Use with caution in patients with decreased hepatic function. Closely monitor patients with any abnormal LFT. Severe hepatic reactions (eg, fulminant hepatitis, liver failure) have occurred with NSAID use, rarely; discontinue if signs or symptoms of liver disease develop, or if systemic manifestations occur.

The elderly are at increased risk for adverse effects (especially serious gastrointestinal events, CNS effects, renal toxicity) from NSAIDs even at low doses.

Withhold for at least 4-6 half-lives prior to surgical or dental procedures. Some products may contain phenylalanine. Ibuprofen injection (Caldolor™) must be diluted prior to administration; hemolysis can occur if not diluted.

Ibuprofen lysine injection (NeoProfen®): Hold second or third doses if urinary output is <0.6 mL/kg/hour. May alter signs of infection. May inhibit platelet aggregation; monitor for signs of bleeding. May displace bilirubin; use caution when total bilirubin is elevated. Long-term evaluations of neurodevelopment, growth, or diseases associated with prematurity following treatment have not been conducted. A second course of treatment, alternative pharmacologic therapy or surgery may be needed if the ductus arteriosus fails to close or reopens following the initial course of therapy.

Self medication (OTC use): Prior to self-medication, patients should contact healthcare provider if they have had recurring stomach pain or upset, ulcers, bleeding problems, high blood pressure, heart or kidney disease, other serious medical problems, are currently taking a diuretic, aspirin, anticoagulant, or are ≥60 years of age. If patients are using for migraines, they should also contact healthcare provider if they have not had a migraine diagnosis by healthcare provider, a headache that is different from usual migraine, worst headache of life, fever and neck stiffness, headache from head injury or coughing, first headache at ≥50 years of age, daily headache, or migraine requiring bed rest. Recommended dosages should not be exceeded, due to an increased risk of GI bleeding. Stop use and consult a healthcare provider if symptoms get worse, newly appear, fever lasts for >3 days or pain lasts >3 days (children) and >10 days (adults). Do not give for >10 days unless instructed by healthcare provider. Consuming ≥3 alcoholic beverages/day or taking longer than recommended may increase the risk of GI bleeding.

Drug Interactions

Metabolism/Transport Effects **Substrate** (minor) of CYP2C9, 2C19; **Inhibits** CYP2C9 (strong)

Avoid Concomitant Use

Avoid concomitant use of Ibuprofen with any of the following: Ketorolac; Ketorolac (Systemic)

Decreased Effect

Ibuprofen may decrease the levels/effects of: ACE Inhibitors; Angiotensin II Receptor Blockers; Antiplatelet Agents; Beta-Blockers; Eplerenone; HydrALAZINE; Loop Diuretics; Potassium-Sparing Diuretics; Salicylates; Thiazide Diuretics

The levels/effects of Ibuprofen may be decreased by: Bile Acid Sequestrants; Nonsteroidal Anti-Inflammatory Agents; Salicylates

Increased Effect/Toxicity

Ibuprofen may increase the levels/effects of: Aminoglycosides; Anticoagulants; Antiplatelet Agents; Bisphosphonate Derivatives; Collagenase (Systemic); CycloSPORINE; CycloSPORINE (Systemic); Desmopressin; Digoxin; Drotrecogin Alfa; Eplerenone; Haloperidol; Ibritumomab; Lithium; Methotrexate; Nonsteroidal Anti-Inflammatory Agents; PEMEtrexed; Potassium-Sparing Diuretics; PRALAtrexate; Quinolone Antibiotics; Salicylates; Thrombolytic Agents; Tositumomab and Iodine I 131 Tositumomab; Vancomycin; Vitamin K Antagonists

The levels/effects of Ibuprofen may be increased by: Antidepressants (Tricyclic, Tertiary Amine); Corticosteroids (Systemic); Dasatinib; Glucosamine; Herbs (Anticoagulant/Antiplatelet Properties); Ketorolac; Ketorolac (Systemic); Nonsteroidal Anti-Inflammatory Agents; Omega-3-Acid Ethyl Esters; Pentosan Polysulfate Sodium; Pentoxifylline; Probenecid; Prostacyclin Analogues; Selective Serotonin Reuptake Inhibitors; Serotonin/Norepinephrine Reuptake Inhibitors; Treprostinil; Voriconazole

Nutritional/Ethanol Interactions

Ethanol: Avoid ethanol (may enhance gastric mucosal irritation).

Food: Ibuprofen peak serum levels may be decreased if taken with food.

Herb/Nutraceutical: Avoid alfalfa, anise, bilberry, bladderwrack, bromelain, cat's claw, celery, chamomile, coleus, cordyceps, dong quai, evening primrose, fenugreek, feverfew, garlic, ginger, ginkgo biloba, ginseng (American, Panax, Siberian), grapeseed, green tea, guggul, horse chestnut seed, horseradish, licorice, prickly ash, red clover, reishi, SAMe (S-adenosylmethionine), sweet clover, turmeric, white willow (all have additional antiplatelet activity).

Lab Interactions Increased serum chloride, serum sodium, bleeding time; may interfere with urine detection of PCP, cannabinoids, and barbiturates (false-positives)

Adverse Reactions

Oral:

1% to 10%:

Cardiovascular: Edema (1% to 3%)

Central nervous system: Dizziness (3% to 9%), headache (1% to 3%), nervousness (1% to 3%)

Dermatologic: Rash (3% to 9%), itching (1% to 3%)
Endocrine & metabolic: Fluid retention (1% to 3%)
Gastrointestinal: Epigastric pain (3% to 9%), heartburn (3% to 9%), nausea (3% to 9%), abdominal pain/cramps/distress (1% to 3%), appetite decreased (1% to 3%), constipation (1% to 3%), diarrhea (1% to 3%), dyspepsia (1% to 3%), flatulence (1% to 3%), vomiting (1% to 3%)
Otic: Tinnitus (3% to 9%)

Injection: Ibuprofen (Caldolor™): Abdominal pain, anemia, BUN increased, cough, dizziness, dyspepsia, edema, flatulence, headache, hemorrhage, hypokalemia, hypernatremia, hypertension, nausea, neutropenia, pruritus, urinary retention, vomiting

Injection: Ibuprofen lysine (NeoProfen®):
>10%:
Cardiovascular: Intraventricular hemorrhage (29%; grade 3/4: 15%)
Dermatologic: Skin irritation (16%)
Endocrine & metabolic: Hypocalcemia (12%), hypoglycemia (12%)
Gastrointestinal: GI disorders, non NEC (22%)
Hematologic: Anemia (32%)
Respiratory: Apnea (28%), respiratory infection (19%)
Miscellaneous: Sepsis (43%)
1% to 10%:
Cardiovascular: Edema (4%)
Endocrine & metabolic: Adrenal insufficiency (7%), hypernatremia (7%)
Genitourinary: Urinary tract infection (9%)
Renal: Urea increased (7%), renal impairment (6%), creatinine increased (3%), urine output decreased (3%; small decrease reported on days 2-6 with compensatory increase in output on day 9), renal failure (1%)
Respiratory: Respiratory failure (10%), atelectasis (4%)
Frequency not defined: Abdominal distension, cholestasis, feeding problems, gastritis, GI reflux, heart failure, hyperglycemia, hypotension, ileus, infection, inguinal hernia, injection site reaction, jaundice, neutropenia, seizure, tachycardia, thrombocytopenia

Pharmacodynamics/Kinetics

Onset of Action Oral: Analgesic: 30-60 minutes; Anti-inflammatory: ≤7 days
Duration of Action Oral: 4-6 hours
Absorption Oral: Rapid (85%)
Time to Peak Oral: ~1-2 hours
Protein Binding 90% to 99%
Half-Life Elimination
Premature infants (highly variable between studies):
Day 3: 35-51 hours
Day 5: 20-33 hours
Children 3 months to 10 years: 1.6 ± 0.7 hours
Adults: 2-4 hours; End-stage renal disease: Unchanged
Metabolism Hepatic via oxidation
Excretion Urine (primarily as metabolites; 1% as unchanged drug); some feces

Available Dosage Forms

Caplet, oral: 200 mg
Advil® [OTC]: 200 mg
Motrin® IB [OTC]: 200 mg
Motrin® Junior [OTC]: 100 mg
Capsule, liquid filled, oral:
Advil® [OTC]: 200 mg
Advil® Migraine [OTC]: 200 mg
Capsule, softgel, oral: 200 mg
Gelcap, oral:
Advil® [OTC]: 200 mg
Injection, solution:
Caldolor™: 100 mg/mL (4 mL, 8 mL)
Injection, solution [preservative free]:
NeoProfen®: 17.1 mg/mL (2 mL)
Suspension, oral: 100 mg/5 mL (5 mL, 10 mL, 120 mL, 240 mL, 480 mL); 40 mg/mL (15 mL)
Advil® Children's [OTC]: 100 mg/5 mL (120 mL)
Advil® Infants' [OTC]: 40 mg/mL (15 mL)
Motrin® Children's [OTC]: 100 mg/5 mL (60 mL, 120 mL)
Motrin® Infants' [OTC]: 40 mg/mL (15 mL)
Tablet, oral: 200 mg, 400 mg, 600 mg, 800 mg
Addaprin [OTC]: 200 mg
Advil® [OTC]: 200 mg
I-Prin [OTC]: 200 mg
Ibu-200 [OTC]: 200 mg
Ibu®: 400 mg, 600 mg, 800 mg
Midol® Cramps & Body Aches [OTC]: 200 mg
Motrin® IB [OTC]: 200 mg
Proprinal® [OTC]: 200 mg
Ultraprin [OTC]: 200 mg
Tablet, chewable, oral:
Motrin® Junior [OTC]: 100 mg
TopCare® Junior Strength [OTC]: 100 mg

Dosing

Adult & Geriatric

Inflammatory disease: Oral: 400-800 mg/dose 3-4 times/day (maximum: 3.2 g/day)

Analgesia/pain/fever/dysmenorrhea: Oral: 200-400 mg/dose every 4-6 hours (maximum daily dose: 1.2 g, unless directed by physician; under physician supervision daily doses ≤2.4 g may be used)

Analgesic: I.V. (Caldolor™): 400-800 mg every 6 hours as needed (maximum: 3.2 g/day). **Note**: Patients should be well hydrated prior to administration.

Antipyretic: I.V. (Caldolor™): Initial: 400 mg, then every 4-6 hours or 100-200 mg every 4 hours as needed (maximum: 3.2 g/day). **Note**: Patients should be well hydrated prior to administration.

OTC labeling (analgesic, antipyretic): Oral: 200 mg every 4-6 hours as needed (maximum: 1200 mg/24 hours); treatment for >10 days is not recommended unless directed by healthcare provider.

Migraine: 2 capsules at onset of symptoms (maximum: 400 mg/24 hours unless directed by healthcare provider)

Pediatric

Antipyretic: Oral: 6 months to 12 years: Temperature <102.5°F (39°C): 5 mg/kg/dose; temperature >102.5°F: 10 mg/kg/dose given every 6-8 hours; maximum daily dose: 40 mg/kg/day

Juvenile idiopathic arthritis (JIA): Oral: 30-50 mg/kg/24 hours divided every 8 hours; start at lower end of dosing range and titrate upward (maximum: 2.4 g/day)

Analgesic: Oral: 4-10 mg/kg/dose every 6-8 hours

Cystic fibrosis (unlabeled use): Oral: Chronic (>4 years) twice daily dosing adjusted to maintain serum concentration of 50-100 mcg/mL has been associated with slowing of disease progression in younger patients with mild lung disease

Patent ductus arteriosus: I.V. (ibuprofen lysine [NeoProfen®]): Infants between 500-1500 g and ≤32 weeks GA: Initial dose: Ibuprofen 10 mg/kg, followed by two doses of 5 mg/kg at 24 and 48 hours. Dose should be based on birth weight.

OTC labeling (analgesic, antipyretic): Oral: **Note:** Treatment for >10 days is not recommended unless directed by healthcare provider.

Children 6 months to 11 years: See table; use of weight to select dose is preferred; doses may be repeated every 6-8 hours (maximum: 4 doses/day)

Children ≥12 years: Refer to adult dosing.

Ibuprofen Dosing

Weight (lb)	Age	Dosage (mg)
12-17	6-11 mo	50
18-23	12-23 mo	75
24-35	2-3 y	100
36-47	4-5 y	150
48-59	6-8 y	200
60-71	9-10 y	250
72-95	11 y	300

Renal Impairment If anuria or oliguria evident, hold dose until renal function returns to normal.

Hepatic Impairment Avoid use in severe hepatic impairment.

Administration

Oral Administer with food.

I.V.

Caldolor™: For I.V. administration only; must be diluted to a final concentration of ≤4 mg/mL prior to administration; infuse over at least 30 minutes

NeoProfen® (ibuprofen lysine): For I.V. administration only; administration via umbilical arterial line has not been evaluated. Infuse over 15 minutes through port closest to insertion site. Avoid extravasation. Do not administer simultaneously via same line with TPN. If needed, interrupt TPN for 15 minutes prior to and after ibuprofen administration, keeping line open with dextrose or saline.

Stability

Reconstitution

Ibuprofen injection (Caldolor™): Must be diluted prior to use. Dilute with D_5W, NS or LR to a final concentration ≤4 mg/mL.

Ibuprofen lysine injection (NeoProfen®): Dilute with dextrose or saline to an appropriate volume.

Storage

Ibuprofen injection (Caldolor™): Store intact vials at room temperature of 20°C to 25°C (68°F to 77°F). Must be diluted prior to use. Diluted solutions stable for 24 hours at room temperature.

Ibuprofen lysine injection (NeoProfen®): Store at room temperature of 20°C to 25°C (68°F to 77°F). Protect from light. Following dilution, administer within 30 minutes of preparation.

Monitoring and Teaching Issues

Laboratory Monitoring CBC, chemistry profile, periodic liver function, renal function (serum BUN and creatinine)

Physical Assessment Evaluate cardiac risk and potential for GI bleeding prior to prescribing this medication. Assess patient for allergic reaction to salicylates or other NSAIDs. Monitor blood pressure prior to treatment and periodically throughout. Periodic ophthalmic exams are recommended.

Patient Education Consult your prescriber before use if you have hypertension or heart failure. Do not take longer than 3 days for fever or 10 days for pain without consulting prescriber. Take with food or milk. Do not use alcohol. Maintain adequate hydration, unless instructed to restrict fluid intake. You may experience nausea, vomiting, or gastric discomfort. GI bleeding, ulceration, or perforation can occur with or without pain. Stop taking medication and report ringing in ears, persistent cramping or stomach pain, unresolved nausea or vomiting, respiratory difficulty or shortness of breath, unusual bruising or bleeding (mouth, urine, stool), skin rash, unusual swelling of extremities, chest pain, or palpitations.

Dietary Considerations Should be taken with food. Some products may contain phenylalanine and/or potassium.

Geriatric Considerations Elderly are a high-risk population for adverse effects from NSAIDs. As much as 60% of elderly can develop peptic ulceration and/or hemorrhage asymptomatically. The concomitant use of H_2 blockers and sucralfate is not effective as prophylaxis with the exception of NSAID-induced duodenal ulcers which may be prevented by the use of ranitidine. Misoprostol and proton pump inhibitors are the only agents proven to help prevent the development of NSAID-induced ulcers. Also, concomitant disease and drug use contribute to the risk for GI adverse effects. Use lowest effective dose for shortest period possible. Consider renal function decline with age. Use of NSAIDs can compromise existing renal function especially when Cl_{cr} is ≤30 mL/minute. Tinnitus may be a difficult and unreliable indication of toxicity due to age-related hearing loss or eighth cranial nerve damage. CNS adverse effects such as confusion, agitation, and hallucination are generally seen in overdose or high dose situations, but the elderly may demonstrate these adverse effects at lower doses than younger adults.

Breast-Feeding Considerations Based on limited data, only very small amounts of ibuprofen are excreted into breast milk. Adverse events have not been reported in nursing infants. Because there is a potential for adverse events to occur in nursing infants, the manufacturer does not recommend the use of ibuprofen while breast-feeding. Use with caution in nursing women with hypertensive disorders of pregnancy or pre-existing renal disease.

Pregnancy Considerations

Adverse events were not observed in the initial animal reproduction studies; therefore, the manufacturer classifies ibuprofen as pregnancy category C (category D: ≥30 weeks gestation). NSAID exposure during the first trimester is not strongly associated with congenital malformations; however, cardiovascular anomalies and cleft palate have been observed following NSAID exposure in some studies. The use of a NSAID close to conception may be associated with an increased risk of miscarriage. Nonteratogenic effects have been observed following NSAID administration during the third trimester including: Myocardial degenerative changes, prenatal constriction of the ductus arteriosus, fetal tricuspid regurgitation, failure of the ductus arteriosus to close postnatally; renal dysfunction or failure, oligohydramnios; gastrointestinal bleeding or perforation, increased risk of necrotizing enterocolitis; intracranial bleeding (including intraventricular hemorrhage), platelet dysfunction with resultant bleeding; pulmonary hypertension. Because they may cause premature closure of the ductus arteriosus, use of NSAIDs late in pregnancy should be avoided (use after 31 or 32 weeks gestation is not recommended by some clinicians). Product labeling for Caldolor™ specifically notes that use at ≥30 weeks gestation should be avoided and therefore classifies ibuprofen as pregnancy category D at this time. The chronic use of NSAIDs in women of reproductive age may be associated with infertility that is reversible upon discontinuation of the medication. A registry is available for pregnant women exposed to autoimmune medications including ibuprofen. For additional information contact the Organization of Teratology Information Specialists, OTIS Autoimmune Diseases Study, at 877-311-8972.

Related Information

Nonsalicylate / Nonsteroidal Anti-Inflammatory Agents *on page 2002*

◆ **Ibuprofen and Hydrocodone** *see* Hydrocodone and Ibuprofen *on page 916*

◆ **Ibuprofen and Oxycodone** *see* Oxycodone and Ibuprofen *on page 1384*

◆ **Ibuprofen Lysine** *see* Ibuprofen *on page 938*

Ibutilide (i BYOO ti lide)

U.S. Brand Names Corvert®

Index Terms Ibutilide Fumarate

Generic Availability (U.S.) Yes

Pharmacologic Category Antiarrhythmic Agent, Class III

Medication Safety Issues

High alert medication: The Institute for Safe Medication Practices (ISMP) includes this medication among its list of drugs which have a heightened risk of causing significant patient harm when used in error.

Pregnancy Risk Factor C

Lactation Enters breast milk/contraindicated

Use Acute termination of atrial fibrillation or flutter of recent onset; the effectiveness of ibutilide has not been determined in patients with arrhythmias >90 days in duration

Mechanism of Action/Effect Exact mechanism of action is unknown; prolongs the action potential in cardiac tissue

Contraindications Hypersensitivity to ibutilide or any component of the formulation; QT_c >440 msec

Warnings/Precautions [U.S. Boxed Warning]: Potentially fatal arrhythmias (eg, polymorphic ventricular tachycardia) can occur with ibutilide, usually in association with torsade de pointes (QT prolongation). Studies indicate a 1.7% incidence of arrhythmias in treated patients. The drug should be given in a setting of continuous ECG monitoring and by personnel trained in treating arrhythmias particularly polymorphic ventricular tachycardia. **[U.S. Boxed Warning]: Patients with chronic atrial fibrillation may not be the best candidates for ibutilide since they often revert after conversion and the risks of treatment may not be justified when compared to alternative management.** Dosing adjustments are not required in patients with renal or hepatic dysfunction. Safety and efficacy in children have not been established. Use caution in elderly patients. Avoid concurrent use of any drug that can prolong QT interval. Correct hyperkalemia and hypomagnesemia before using. Monitor for heart block.

Drug Interactions

Avoid Concomitant Use

Avoid concomitant use of Ibutilide with any of the following: Artemether; Dronedarone; Lumefantrine; Nilotinib; Pimozide; QuiNINE; Tetrabenazine; Thioridazine; Toremifene; Vandetanib; Ziprasidone

Decreased Effect There are no known significant interactions involving a decrease in effect.

Increased Effect/Toxicity

Ibutilide may increase the levels/effects of: Dronedarone; Pimozide; QTc-Prolonging Agents; QuiNINE; Tetrabenazine; Thioridazine; Toremifene; Vandetanib; Ziprasidone

The levels/effects of Ibutilide may be increased by: Alfuzosin; Artemether; Chloroquine; Ciprofloxacin; Ciprofloxacin (Systemic); Eribulin; Fingolimod; Gadobutrol; Lumefantrine; Nilotinib; QuiNINE

Adverse Reactions 1% to 10%:

Cardiovascular: Ventricular extrasystoles (5.1%), nonsustained monomorphic ventricular tachycardia (4.9%), nonsustained polymorphic ventricular tachycardia (2.7%), tachycardia/supraventricular tachycardia (2.7%), hypotension (2%), bundle branch block (1.9%), sustained polymorphic ventricular tachycardia (eg, torsade de pointes) (1.7%, often requiring cardioversion), AV block (1.5%), bradycardia (1.2%), QT segment prolongation, hypertension (1.2%), palpitation (1%)

Central nervous system: Headache (3.6%)

Gastrointestinal: Nausea (>1%)

Pharmacodynamics/Kinetics

Onset of Action ~90 minutes after start of infusion (1/2 of conversions to sinus rhythm occur during infusion)

Protein Binding 40%

Half-Life Elimination 2-12 hours (average: 6 hours)

Metabolism Extensively hepatic; oxidation

Excretion Urine (82%; 7% as unchanged drug and metabolites); feces (19%)

Available Dosage Forms

Injection, solution: 0.1 mg/mL (10 mL)

Corvert®: 0.1 mg/mL (10 mL)

Dosing

Adult

Atrial fibrillation/flutter: I.V.:

<60 kg: 0.01 mg/kg over 10 minutes

≥60 kg: 1 mg over 10 minutes

If the arrhythmia does not terminate within 10 minutes after the end of the initial infusion, a second infusion of equal strength may be infused over a 10-minute period.

Geriatric Refer to adult dosing. Dose selection should be cautious, usually starting at the lower end of the dosing range.

Administration

I.V. May be administered undiluted or diluted in 50 mL diluent (0.9% NS or D_5W). Infuse over 10 minutes.

Stability

Reconstitution May be administered undiluted or diluted in 50 mL diluent (0.9% NS or D_5W).

Storage Admixtures are chemically and physically stable for 24 hours at room temperature and for 48 hours at refrigerated temperatures.

Monitoring and Teaching Issues

Laboratory Monitoring Electrolytes

Physical Assessment Requires infusion pump and continuous cardiac and hemodynamic monitoring during and for 4 hours following infusion.

Patient Education This drug is only given I.V. and you will be on continuous cardiac monitoring during and for several hours following administration. You may experience headache or irregular heartbeat during infusion. Report chest pain or respiratory difficulty immediately.

Pregnancy Considerations Teratogenic and embryocidal in rats; avoid use in pregnancy

Related Information

Antiarrhythmic Drugs *on page 1978*

◆ **Ibutilide Fumarate** *see* Ibutilide *on page 943*

- ◆ **ICI-182,780** *see* Fulvestrant *on page 838*
- ◆ **ICI-204,219** *see* Zafirlukast *on page 1882*
- ◆ **ICI-46474** *see* Tamoxifen *on page 1703*
- ◆ **ICI-118630** *see* Goserelin *on page 885*
- ◆ **ICI-176334** *see* Bicalutamide *on page 217*
- ◆ **ICI-D1033** *see* Anastrozole *on page 128*
- ◆ **ICRF-187** *see* Dexrazoxane *on page 508*
- ◆ **Idamycin PFS®** *see* IDArubicin *on page 945*

IDArubicin (eye da ROO bi sin)

U.S. Brand Names Idamycin PFS®

Index Terms 4-Demethoxydaunorubicin; 4-DMDR; Idarubicin Hydrochloride; IDR; IMI 30; SC 33428

Generic Availability (U.S.) Yes

Pharmacologic Category Antineoplastic Agent, Anthracycline; Antineoplastic Agent, Antibiotic

Medication Safety Issues

Sound-alike/look-alike issues:

IDArubicin may be confused with DOXOrubicin, DAUNOrubicin, epirubicin
Idamycin PFS® may be confused with Adriamycin

High alert medication: The Institute for Safe Medication Practices (ISMP) includes this medication among its list of drugs which have a heightened risk of causing significant patient harm when used in error.

Pregnancy Risk Factor D

Lactation Excretion in breast milk unknown

Use Treatment of acute myeloid leukemia (AML)

Unlabeled/Investigational Use Acute lymphocytic leukemia (ALL)

Mechanism of Action/Effect Similar to daunorubicin, idarubicin exhibits inhibitory effects on DNA and RNA polymerase.

Contraindications Hypersensitivity to idarubicin, other anthracyclines, or any component of the formulation; bilirubin >5 mg/dL; pregnancy

Warnings/Precautions Hazardous agent - use appropriate precautions for handling and disposal. **[U.S. Boxed Warning]: May cause myocardial toxicity (HF, arrhythmias or cardiomyopathies) and is more common in patients who have previously received anthracyclines or have pre-existing cardiac disease.** The risk of myocardial toxicity is also increased in patients with concomitant or prior mediastinal/pericardial irradiation, patients with anemia, bone marrow depression, infections, leukemic pericarditis or myocarditis. Monitor cardiac function during treatment.

[U.S. Boxed Warnings]: May cause severe myelosuppression; use caution in patients with pre-existing myelosuppression from prior treatment or radiation. Use caution with renal or hepatic impairment; may required dosage reductions. For I.V. administration only; may cause severe local tissue damage and necrosis if extravasation occurs. Rapid lysis of leukemic cells may lead to hyperuricemia. Systemic infections should be managed prior to initiation of treatment. **[U.S. Boxed Warning]: Should be administered under the supervision of an experienced cancer chemotherapy physician. Safety and efficacy in children have not been established.**

Drug Interactions

Metabolism/Transport Effects Substrate of P-glycoprotein

Avoid Concomitant Use

Avoid concomitant use of IDArubicin with any of the following: BCG; Natalizumab; Pimecrolimus; Roflumilast; Tacrolimus (Topical); Vaccines (Live)

Decreased Effect

IDArubicin may decrease the levels/effects of: BCG; Cardiac Glycosides; Sipuleucel-T; Vaccines (Inactivated); Vaccines (Live)

The levels/effects of IDArubicin may be decreased by: Cardiac Glycosides; Echinacea; P-Glycoprotein Inducers

Increased Effect/Toxicity

IDArubicin may increase the levels/effects of: Leflunomide; Natalizumab; Vaccines (Live)

The levels/effects of IDArubicin may be increased by: Bevacizumab; Denosumab; P-Glycoprotein Inhibitors; Pimecrolimus; Roflumilast; Tacrolimus (Topical); Taxane Derivatives; Trastuzumab

Adverse Reactions

>10%:

Cardiovascular: Transient ECG abnormalities (supraventricular tachycardia, S-T wave changes, atrial or ventricular extrasystoles); generally asymptomatic and self-limiting. CHF, dose related. The relative cardiotoxicity of idarubicin compared to doxorubicin is unclear. Some investigators report no increase in cardiac toxicity at cumulative oral idarubicin doses up to 540 mg/m^2; other reports suggest a maximum cumulative intravenous dose of 150 mg/m^2.

Central nervous system: Headache

Dermatologic: Alopecia (25% to 30%), radiation recall, skin rash (11%), urticaria
Gastrointestinal: Nausea, vomiting (30% to 60%); diarrhea (9% to 22%); stomatitis (11%); GI hemorrhage (30%)
Genitourinary: Discoloration of urine (darker yellow)
Hematologic: Myelosuppression, primarily leukopenia; thrombocytopenia and anemia. Effects are generally less severe with oral dosing.
Nadir: 10-15 days
Recovery: 21-28 days
Hepatic: Bilirubin and transaminases increased (44%)

1% to 10%:
Central nervous system: Seizure
Neuromuscular & skeletal: Peripheral neuropathy

Pharmacodynamics/Kinetics

Absorption Oral: Variable (4% to 77%; mean: ~30%)

Time to Peak Serum: 1-5 hours

Protein Binding 94% to 97%

Half-Life Elimination Oral: 14-35 hours; I.V.: 12-27 hours

Metabolism Hepatic to idarubicinol (pharmacologically active)

Excretion
Oral: Urine (~5% of dose; 0.5% to 0.7% as unchanged drug, 4% as idarubicinol); hepatic (8%)
I.V.: Urine (13% as idarubicinol, 3% as unchanged drug); hepatic (17%)

Available Dosage Forms

Injection, solution [preservative free]: 1 mg/mL (5 mL, 10 mL, 20 mL)
Idamycin PFS®: 1 mg/mL (5 mL, 10 mL, 20 mL)

Dosing

Adult & Geriatric Refer to individual protocols.

AML: I.V.:
Induction: 12 mg/m^2/day for 3 days
Consolidation: 10-12 mg/m^2/day for 2 days

Pediatric AML (unlabeled use): I.V.: 10-12 mg/m^2 once daily for 3 days every 3 weeks.

Renal Impairment The FDA-approved labeling does not contain specific dosing adjustment guidelines; however, it does reccomend that dosage reductions be made. Patients with S_{cr}: ≥2 mg/dL did not receive treatment in many clinical trials. The following guidelines have been used by some clinicians (Aronoff, 2007):

Children:
Cl_{cr} <50 mL/minute: Administer 75% of dose.
Hemodialysis: Administer 75% of dose.
Continuous ambulatory peritoneal dialysis (CAPD): Administer 75% of dose.
Continuous renal replacement therapy (CRRT): Administer 75% of dose.

Adults:
Cl_{cr} 10-50 mL/minute: Administer 75% of dose.
Cl_{cr} <10 mL/minute: Administer 50% of dose.
Hemodialysis: Supplemental dose not needed.
Continuous ambulatory peritoneal dialysis (CAPD): Supplemental dose not needed.

Hepatic Impairment
Bilirubin 2.6-5 mg/dL: Administer 50% of dose
Bilirubin >5 mg/dL: Avoid use

Administration

I.V. Do not administer I.M. or SubQ; administer as slow push over 3-5 minutes, preferably into the side of a freely-running saline or dextrose infusion **or** as intermittent infusion over 10-15 minutes into a free-flowing I.V. solution of NS or D_5W; also occasionally administered as a bladder lavage.

Stability

Storage Store intact vials of solution under refrigeration at 2°C to 8°C (36°F to 46°F). Protect from light. Solutions diluted in D_5W or NS for infusion are stable for 4 weeks at room temperature, protected from light. Syringe and IVPB solutions are stable for 72 hours at room temperature and 7 days under refrigeration.

Monitoring and Teaching Issues

Laboratory Monitoring CBC with differential, platelet count, cardiac function, serum electrolytes, creatinine, uric acid, ALT, AST, bilirubin

Physical Assessment Infusion site must be closely monitored; extravasation can cause severe cellulitis or tissue necrosis (eg, do not apply heat). Monitor for cardiac toxicity, myelosuppression, and peripheral neuropathy frequently during therapy.

Patient Education This medication is only administered by intravenous infusion; report immediately any swelling, pain, burning, or redness at infusion site or sudden onset of chest pain, breathing or swallowing difficulty, or chills. It is important to maintain adequate nutrition and hydration, unless instructed to restrict fluid intake. You will be more susceptible to infection. You may experience nausea or vomiting, diarrhea, or loss of hair (reversible). Urine may turn darker color (normal). Report immediately chest pain, swelling of extremities, respiratory difficulty, palpitations, or rapid heartbeat. Report unresolved nausea, vomiting, or diarrhea; alterations in urinary pattern (increased or decreased); opportunistic infection (eg, fever, chills, unusual bruising or bleeding, signs of infection fatigue, purulent vaginal discharge, unhealed mouth sores); abdominal pain or blood in stools; excessive fatigue; yellowing of eyes or skin; swelling of extremities; respiratory difficulty; or unresolved diarrhea.

Geriatric Considerations During induction therapy, patients >60 years of age experience CHF, arrhythmias, MI, and decline in LVEF more frequently than younger populations.

◆ **Idarubicin Hydrochloride** *see* IDArubicin *on page 945*
◆ **IDEC-C2B8** *see* RITUXimab *on page 1596*
◆ **IDR** *see* IDArubicin *on page 945*
◆ **Ifex** *see* Ifosfamide *on page 947*

Ifosfamide (eye FOSS fa mide)

U.S. Brand Names Ifex

Index Terms Isophosphamide; Z4942

Generic Availability (U.S.) Yes

Pharmacologic Category Antineoplastic Agent, Alkylating Agent; Antineoplastic Agent, Alkylating Agent (Nitrogen Mustard)

Medication Safety Issues

Sound-alike/look-alike issues:

Ifosfamide may be confused with cyclophosphamide

High alert medication: The Institute for Safe Medication Practices (ISMP) includes this medication among its list of drugs which have a heightened risk of causing significant patient harm when used in error.

Pregnancy Risk Factor D

Lactation Enters breast milk/not recommended

Use Treatment of testicular cancer

Unlabeled/Investigational Use Treatment of bladder cancer, cervical cancer, ovarian cancer, nonsmall cell lung cancer, small cell lung cancer, Hodgkin's and non-Hodgkin's lymphoma; acute lymphocytic leukemia; Ewing's sarcoma, osteosarcoma, and soft tissue sarcomas

Mechanism of Action/Effect Inhibits protein synthesis and DNA synthesis

Contraindications Hypersensitivity to ifosfamide or any component of the formulation; patients with severely depressed bone marrow function

Warnings/Precautions Hazardous agent - use appropriate precautions for handling and disposal. **[U.S. Boxed Warning]: Urotoxic side effects, primarily hemorrhagic cystitis, may occur (dose-limiting toxicity).** Hydration (at least 2 L/day) and/or mesna administration will protect against hemorrhagic cystitis. **[U.S. Boxed Warning]: Severe bone marrow suppression may occur (dose-limiting toxicity);** use is contraindicated in patients with severely depressed bone marrow function. **[U.S. Boxed Warning]: May cause CNS toxicity, including confusion and coma;** usually reversible upon discontinuation of treatment. Encephalopathy, ranging from mild somnolence to hallucinations and/or coma may occur; risk factors may include hypoalbuminemia, renal dysfunction and prior history of ifosfamide-induced encephalopathy. Use with caution in patients with impaired renal function or those with compromised bone marrow reserve. May interfere with wound healing. **[U.S. Boxed Warning]: Should be administered under the supervision of an experienced cancer chemotherapy physician.** Safety and efficacy in children have not been established.

Drug Interactions

Metabolism/Transport Effects Substrate of CYP2A6 (major), 2B6 (minor), 2C8 (minor), 2C9 (minor), 2C19 (major), 3A4 (major); **Inhibits** CYP3A4 (weak); **Induces** CYP2C8 (weak), 2C9 (weak)

Avoid Concomitant Use

Avoid concomitant use of Ifosfamide with any of the following: BCG; Natalizumab; Pimecrolimus; Roflumilast; Tacrolimus (Topical); Vaccines (Live)

Decreased Effect

Ifosfamide may decrease the levels/effects of: BCG; Sipuleucel-T; Vaccines (Inactivated); Vaccines (Live); Vitamin K Antagonists

The levels/effects of Ifosfamide may be decreased by: CYP2A6 Inducers (Strong); CYP2C19 Inducers (Strong); CYP3A4 Inducers (Strong); Deferasirox; Echinacea; Herbs (CYP3A4 Inducers)

Increased Effect/Toxicity

Ifosfamide may increase the levels/effects of: Leflunomide; Natalizumab; Vaccines (Live); Vitamin K Antagonists

The levels/effects of Ifosfamide may be increased by: Conivaptan; CYP2A6 Inhibitors (Moderate); CYP2A6 Inhibitors (Strong); CYP2C19 Inhibitors (Moderate); CYP2C19 Inhibitors (Strong); CYP3A4 Inhibitors (Moderate); CYP3A4 Inhibitors (Strong); Dasatinib; Denosumab; Pimecrolimus; Roflumilast; Tacrolimus (Topical); Trastuzumab

Nutritional/Ethanol Interactions Herb/Nutraceutical: St John's wort may decrease ifosfamide levels.

Adverse Reactions

>10%:

Central nervous system: CNS toxicity or encephalopathy (10% to 30%; includes somnolence, agitation, confusion, delirium, hallucinations, depressive psychosis, incontinence, palsy, diplopia, aphasia, or coma)

Dermatologic: Alopecia (83%)

Endocrine & metabolic: Metabolic acidosis (31%)

Gastrointestinal: Nausea/vomiting (58%), may be more common with higher doses or bolus infusion

Hematologic: Myelosuppression (onset: 7-14 days; nadir: 21-28 days; recovery: 21-28 days), leukopenia (50% to ≤100%; grade 4: ≤50%), thrombocytopenia (20%; grades 3/4: 8%)

Renal: Hematuria (6% to 92%; grade 2 [gross hematuria]: 8% to 12%)

1% to 10%:

Central nervous system: Fever

Hepatic: Bilirubin increased (3%), liver dysfunction (3%), transaminases increased (3%)

Local: Phlebitis (2%)

Renal: Renal impairment (6%)

Miscellaneous: Infection (8%)

Pharmacodynamics/Kinetics

Protein Binding Negligible

Half-Life Elimination

High dose (3800-5000 mg/m^2): ~15 hours

Lower dose (1600-2400 mg/m^2): ~7 hours

Metabolism Hepatic to active metabolites isofosforamide mustard, 4-hydroxy-ifosfamide, acrolein, and inactive dichloroethylated and carboxy metabolites; acrolein is the agent implicated in development of hemorrhagic cystitis

Excretion

High dose (5000 mg/m^2): Urine (70% to 86%; 61% as unchanged drug)

Lower dose (1600-2400 mg/m^2): Urine (12% to 18% as unchanged drug)

Pharmacokinetic Note Pharmacokinetics are dose dependent.

Available Dosage Forms

Injection, powder for reconstitution: 1 g, 3 g

Ifex: 1 g, 3 g

Injection, solution: 50 mg/mL (20 mL, 60 mL)

Dosing

Adult & Geriatric Refer to individual protocols.

Antineoplastic: I.V.:

Testicular cancer: 1200 mg/m^2/day for 5 days every 3 weeks

Dose ranges used in other cancers (unlabeled uses):

4000-5000 mg/m^2/day for 1 day every 14-28 days **or**

1000-3000 mg/m^2/day for 2-5 days every 21-28 days

Note: To prevent bladder toxicity, ifosfamide should be given with extensive hydration consisting of at least 2 L of oral or I.V. fluid per day. The dose-limiting toxicity is hemorrhagic cystitis and, therefore, ifosfamide should be used in conjunction with a uroprotective agent, such as mesna.

Pediatric Refer to individual protocols.

Antineoplastic (unlabeled use): I.V.:

1200-1800 mg/m^2/day for 3-5 days every 21-28 days **or**

5 g/m^2 once every 21-28 days **or**

3 g/m^2/day for 2 days every 21-28 days

See "Note" in adult dosing.

Renal Impairment The FDA-approved labeling does not contain dosage adjustment guidelines (has not been studied). The following guidelines have been used by some clinicians:

Aronoff, 2007:

Cl_{cr} <10 mL/minute: Children and Adults: Administer 75% of dose

Hemodialysis:

Children: 1 g/m^2 followed by hemodialysis 6-8 hours later

Adults: No supplemental dose needed

Kintzel, 1995:

Cl_{cr} 46-60 mL/minute: Administer 80% of dose

Cl_{cr} 31-45 mL/minute: Administer 75% of dose

Cl_{cr} <30 mL/minute: Administer 70% of dose

Hepatic Impairment The FDA-approved labeling does not contain dosage adjustment guidelines (has not been studied). The following guidelines have been used by some clinicians (Floyd, 2006): Bilirubin >3 mg/dL: Administer 25% of dose

Administration

I.V. Administer I.V. over 30 minutes to several hours or continuous intravenous infusion over 5 days.

Stability

Reconstitution Dilute powder with SWFI or bacteriostatic SWFI to a concentration of 50 mg/mL. Further dilution in 50-1000 mL D_5W or NS (to a final concentration of 0.6-20 mg/mL) is recommended for I.V. infusion.

Storage Store intact vials of powder for injection at room temperature of 20°C to 25°C (68°F to 77°F). Store intact vials of solution under refrigeration at 2°C to 8°C (36°F to 46°F). Reconstituted solutions may be stored under refrigeration for up to 21 days. Solutions diluted for administration are stable for 7 days at room temperature and for 6 weeks under refrigeration.

Monitoring and Teaching Issues

Laboratory Monitoring CBC with differential, platelet count, urinalysis (prior to each dose), liver and renal function

Physical Assessment Use caution in presence of impaired renal function or compromised bone marrow reserve. To prevent bladder toxicity, maintain adequate hydration for 72 hours prior to infusion to minimize risk of hemorrhagic cystitis. Premedication with antiemetic may be advisable prior to each infusion. Assess vital signs prior to each infusion and regularly during therapy. Monitor for CNS depression or psychoses, hematuria (hemorrhagic cystitis), and myelosuppression (anemia) throughout therapy. Teach patient importance of adequate hydration.

Patient Education This drug can only be administered by infusion. Report immediately any swelling, redness, or pain at infusion site. Maintain adequate hydration, unless instructed to restrict fluid intake, for at least 3 days prior to infusion and each day of therapy. You will be more susceptible to infection. May cause loss of hair (reversible, although regrowth hair may be different color or texture), fertility or amenorrhea, nausea or vomiting, headache, or mouth sores. Report any difficulty or pain with urination, chest pain, rapid heartbeat, palpitations, CNS changes (eg, hallucinations, confusion, somnolence), unusual rash, persistent nausea or vomiting, swelling of extremities, respiratory difficulty, unusual fatigue, or opportunistic infection (eg, fever, chills, easy bruising, or unusual bleeding).

Pregnancy Considerations Increased resorptions and embryotoxic effects have been observed in animal studies.

- ◆ **IG** *see* Immune Globulin *on page 961*
- ◆ **IgG4-Kappa Monoclonal Antibody** *see* Natalizumab *on page 1292*
- ◆ **IGIM** *see* Immune Globulin *on page 961*
- ◆ **IGIV** *see* Immune Globulin *on page 961*
- ◆ **IL-2** *see* Aldesleukin *on page 62*

Iloperidone (eye loe PER i done)

U.S. Brand Names Fanapt®

Generic Availability (U.S.) No

Pharmacologic Category Antipsychotic Agent, Atypical

Medication Safety Issues

Sound-alike/look-alike issues:

Fanapt® may be confused with Xanax®

Iloperidone may be confused with domperidone

Pregnancy Risk Factor C

Lactation Excretion in breast milk unknown/not recommended

Use Acute treatment of schizophrenia

Mechanism of Action/Effect Iloperidone is an atypical antipsychotic which blocks serotonin and dopamine receptors. Results in improvement of psychoses with lower incidence of extrapyramidal side effects.

Contraindications Hypersensitivity to iloperidone or any component of the formulation

Warnings/Precautions [U.S. Boxed Warning]: Elderly patients with dementia-related psychosis treated with antipsychotics are at an increased risk of death compared to placebo. Most deaths appeared to be either cardiovascular (eg, heart failure, sudden death) or infectious (eg, pneumonia) in nature. In addition, an increased incidence of cerebrovascular effects (eg, transient ischemic attack, cerebrovascular accidents) has been reported in studies of placebo-controlled trials of antipsychotics in elderly patients with dementia-related psychosis. Iloperidone is not approved for the treatment of dementia-related psychosis.

May be sedating; use with caution in disorders where CNS depression is a feature. Caution in patients with predisposition to seizures. Use is not recommended in patients with hepatic impairment. Esophageal dysmotility and aspiration have been associated with antipsychotic use; use with caution in patients at risk of aspiration pneumonia (ie, Alzheimer's disease). Use is associated with increased prolactin levels; clinical significance of hyperprolactinemia in patients with breast cancer or other prolactin-dependent tumors is unknown. May alter temperature regulation. Leukopenia, neutropenia, and agranulocytosis (sometimes fatal) have been reported in clinical trials and postmarketing reports; presence of risk factors (eg, pre-existing low WBC or history of drug-induced leuko-/neutropenia) should prompt periodic blood count assessment and discontinuation at first signs of blood dyscrasias.

May alter cardiac conduction and prolong the QT_c interval; life-threatening arrhythmias have occurred with therapeutic doses of antipsychotics. Risks may be increased by conditions or concomitant medications which cause bradycardia, hypokalemia, and/or hypomagnesemia. Avoid use in combination with QT_c-prolonging drugs and in patients with congenital long QT syndrome, history of cardiac arrhythmia, recent MI, or uncompensated heart failure. Discontinue treatment in patients found to have persistent QT_c intervals >500 msec. Further cardiac evaluation is warranted in patients with symptoms of dizziness, palpitations, or syncope. May cause orthostatic hypotension; use with caution in patients at risk of this effect (eg, concurrent medication use which may predispose to hypotension/bradycardia or presence of hypovolemia) or in those who would not tolerate transient hypotensive episodes. Use with caution in patients with cardiovascular diseases (eg, heart failure, history of myocardial infarction or ischemia, cerebrovascular disease, conduction abnormalities).

May cause anticholinergic effects (confusion, agitation, constipation, xerostomia, blurred vision, urinary retention); therefore, use with caution in patients with decreased gastrointestinal motility, urinary retention, BPH, xerostomia, or visual problems (including narrow-angle glaucoma). May cause extrapyramidal symptoms (EPS), including pseudoparkinsonism, acute dystonic reactions, akathisia, and tardive dyskinesia. Risk of dystonia (and probably other EPS) may be greater with increased doses, use of conventional antipsychotics, males, and younger patients. Risk of neuroleptic malignant syndrome (NMS) may be increased in patients with Parkinson's disease or Lewy body dementia. May cause hyperglycemia; in some cases may be extreme and associated with ketoacidosis, hyperosmolar coma, or death. Use with caution in patients with diabetes or other disorders of glucose regulation; monitor for worsening of glucose control. Significant weight gain has been observed with antipsychotic therapy; incidence varies with product. Monitor waist circumference and BMI. Rare cases of priapism have been reported. ▶

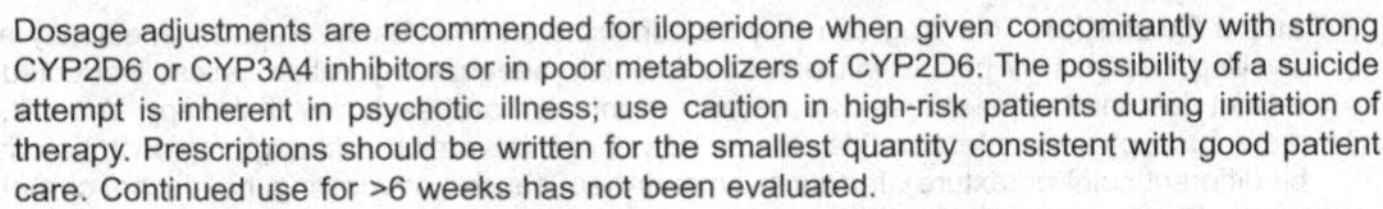

Dosage adjustments are recommended for iloperidone when given concomitantly with strong CYP2D6 or CYP3A4 inhibitors or in poor metabolizers of CYP2D6. The possibility of a suicide attempt is inherent in psychotic illness; use caution in high-risk patients during initiation of therapy. Prescriptions should be written for the smallest quantity consistent with good patient care. Continued use for >6 weeks has not been evaluated.

Drug Interactions

Metabolism/Transport Effects Substrate of CYP2D6 (major)

Avoid Concomitant Use

Avoid concomitant use of Iloperidone with any of the following: Artemether; Dronedarone; Lumefantrine; Metoclopramide; Nilotinib; Pimozide; QuiNINE; Tetrabenazine; Thioridazine; Toremifene; Vandetanib; Ziprasidone

Decreased Effect

Iloperidone may decrease the levels/effects of: Amphetamines; Anti-Parkinson's Agents (Dopamine Agonist); Quinagolide

The levels/effects of Iloperidone may be decreased by: Lithium formulations; Peginterferon Alfa-2b

Increased Effect/Toxicity

Iloperidone may increase the levels/effects of: Alcohol (Ethyl); CNS Depressants; Dronedarone; Methylphenidate; Pimozide; QTc-Prolonging Agents; QuiNINE; Tetrabenazine; Thioridazine; Toremifene; Vandetanib; Ziprasidone

The levels/effects of Iloperidone may be increased by: Acetylcholinesterase Inhibitors (Central); Alfuzosin; Artemether; Chloroquine; Ciprofloxacin; Ciprofloxacin (Systemic); Conivaptan; CYP2D6 Inhibitors (Moderate); CYP2D6 Inhibitors (Strong); Darunavir; Gadobutrol; Lithium formulations; Lumefantrine; MAO Inhibitors; Methylphenidate; Metoclopramide; Nilotinib; QuiNINE; Tetrabenazine

Nutritional/Ethanol Interactions

Ethanol: Avoid ethanol (may increase CNS depression).

Herb/Nutraceutical: Avoid St John's wort (may decrease serum levels of iloperidone). Avoid kava kava, gotu kola, valerian, St John's wort (may increase CNS depression).

Adverse Reactions

>10%:

Cardiovascular: Tachycardia (3% to 12%; dose related)

Central nervous system: Dizziness (10% to 20%; dose related), somnolence (9% to 15%)

1% to 10%:

Cardiovascular: Orthostatic hypotension (3% to 5%), hypotension (1% to 3%; dose related), palpitations (≥1%)

Central nervous system: Fatigue (4% to 6%), extrapyramidal symptoms (≤5%), tremor (3%), lethargy (≤3%), akathisia (2%), aggression (≥1%), delusion (≥1%), restlessness (≥1%)

Dermatologic: Rash (≤3%)

Gastrointestinal: Nausea (≤10%), xerostomia (8% to 10%), weight gain (1% to 9%; dose related), diarrhea (5% to 7%), abdominal discomfort (1% to 3%; dose related), weight loss (≥1%)

Genitourinary: Ejaculation failure (2%), urinary incontinence (≥1%), erectile dysfunction (≥1%)

Neuromuscular & skeletal: Arthralgia (3%), stiffness (1% to 3%; dose related), dyskinesia (<2%), muscle spasm (≥1%), myalgia (≥1%)

Ocular: Blurred vision (≤3%), conjunctivitis (≥1%)

Respiratory: Nasal congestion (5% to 8%), nasopharyngitis (≤4%), upper respiratory tract infection (2% to 3%), dyspnea (2%)

Pharmacodynamics/Kinetics

Absorption Well absorbed

Bioavailability Oral: Tablet (relative to solution): 96%

Time to Peak Plasma: 2-4 hours

Protein Binding ~95% (iloperidone and active metabolites)

Half-Life Elimination

Extensive metabolizers: Iloperidone: 18 hours; P88: 26 hours; P95: 23 hours

Poor metabolizers: Iloperidone: 33 hours; P88: 37 hours; P95: 31 hours

Metabolism Hepatic via carbonyl reduction, hydroxylation (CYP2D6) and O-demethylation (CYP3A4); forms active metabolites (P88 and P95)

Excretion Urine (58% extensive metabolizers, 45% poor metabolizers); feces (20% extensive metabolizers, 22% poor metabolizers)

Available Dosage Forms

Tablet, oral:

Fanapt®: 1 mg, 2 mg, 4 mg, 6 mg, 8 mg, 10 mg, 12 mg, 1 mg (2s), 2 mg (2s), 4 mg (2s), and 6 mg (2s)

Dosing

Adult & Geriatric Schizophrenia: Oral: Initial: 1 mg twice daily; recommended dosage range: 6-12 mg twice daily (maximum: 24 mg/day)

Recommended titration schedule: Increase in 2 mg increments every 24 hours on days 2-7 (eg, Day 2: 2 mg twice daily; Day 3: 4 mg twice daily; Day 4: 6 mg twice daily; Day 5: 8 mg twice daily; Day 6: 10 mg twice daily; Day 7: 12 mg twice daily)

Note: Titrate dose to effect (to avoid orthostatic hypotensive effects); treatment >6 weeks has not been evaluated; when reinitiating treatment after discontinuation (>3 days), the initial titration schedule should be followed.

Dosage adjustment in patients receiving strong CYP2D6 inhibitors (eg, paroxetine, fluoxetine, quinidine): Decrease iloperidone dose by 50%; when the CYP2D6 inhibitor is discontinued, return to previous dose.

Dosage adjustment in patients receiving strong CYP3A4 inhibitors (eg, ketoconazole, clarithromycin): Decrease iloperidone dose by 50%; when the CYP3A4 inhibitor is discontinued, return to previous dose.

Dosage adjustment in poor metabolizers of CYP2D6: Decrease iloperidone dose by 50%.

Hepatic Impairment Not recommended in patients with hepatic impairment due to lack of data.

Administration

Oral May be administered with or without food.

Stability

Storage Store at 25°C (77°F); excursions permitted to 15°C to 30°C (59°F to 86°F). Protect from light and moisture.

Monitoring and Teaching Issues

Laboratory Monitoring Fasting blood glucose/Hgb A_{1c} (prior to treatment and periodically during treatment); CBC (frequently during first few months of therapy); serum potassium and magnesium levels (prior to treatment and periodically during treatment)

Physical Assessment Monitor weight prior to initiating therapy and at least monthly; can cause weight gain. Be alert to the potential for suicide ideation and orthostatic hypotension, especially during the titration phase. Initiate at lower doses and titrate to target dose. Taper dosage slowly when discontinuing.

Patient Education It may take several weeks to achieve desired results. Avoid alcohol. Maintain adequate hydration. Avoid overheating. If you have diabetes, you may experience increased blood sugars; monitor blood sugars closely. You may experience excess sedation, drowsiness, restlessness, dizziness, or blurred vision; dry mouth, nausea, or GI upset; postural hypotension; or urinary retention. Report persistent CNS effects (eg, trembling fingers, altered gait or balance, excessive sedation, seizures, unusual muscle or skeletal movements, anxiety, abnormal thoughts [especially suicide ideation], confusion, personality changes); chest pain, palpitations, irregular or rapid heartbeat, feeling faint, or severe dizziness; signs of infection or fever; vision changes; respiratory difficulty; or worsening of condition.

Dietary Considerations May be given with or without food.

Geriatric Considerations Any change in disease status in any organ system may result in behavior changes. EPS appears significantly less than with the other agents in this class. Many elderly patients receive antipsychotic medications for inappropriate nonpsychotic behavior. Before initiating antipsychotic medication, the clinician should investigate any reversible cause; any stress or stress from any disease can cause acute "confusion" or worsening of baseline nonpsychotic behavior. Most commonly, acute changes in behavior are due to increases in drug dose or addition of a new medication to the regimen, fluid and electrolyte loss, infection, or changes in their environment.

Studies of elderly patients with psychosis associated with Alzheimer's disease, treated with antipsychotics, have demonstrated an increased risk of mortality and cardiovascular events as compared to younger patient populations.

Pregnancy Considerations Animal studies have shown an increased risk of developmental toxicity and fetal mortality. Antipsychotic use during the third trimester of pregnancy has a risk for abnormal muscle movements (extrapyramidal symptoms [EPS]) and withdrawal symptoms in newborns following delivery. Symptoms in the newborn may include agitation, feeding disorder, hypertonia, hypotonia, respiratory distress, somnolence, and tremor; these effects may be self-limiting or require hospitalization.

Related Information

Antipsychotic Agents *on page 1986*

Imatinib (eye MAT eh nib)

U.S. Brand Names Gleevec®

Index Terms CGP-57148B; Glivec; Imatinib Mesylate; STI-571

Generic Availability (U.S.) No

Pharmacologic Category Antineoplastic Agent, Tyrosine Kinase Inhibitor

Medication Safety Issues

Sound-alike/look-alike issues:

Imatinib may be confused with dasatinib, erlotinib, gefitinib, nilotinib, SORAfenib, SUNItinib, vandetanib

High alert medication: The Institute for Safe Medication Practices (ISMP) includes this medication among its list of drug classes which have a heightened risk of causing significant patient harm when used in error.

Pregnancy Risk Factor D

Lactation Enters breast milk/not recommended

Use Treatment of:

Gastrointestinal stromal tumors (GIST) kit-positive (CD117), including unresectable and/or metastatic malignant and adjuvant treatment following complete resection

Philadelphia chromosome-positive (Ph+) chronic myeloid leukemia (CML) in chronic phase (newly-diagnosed)

Ph+ CML in chronic phase in pediatric patients recurring following stem cell transplant or who are resistant to interferon-alpha therapy (**not** an approved use in Canada)
Ph+ CML in blast crisis, accelerated phase, or chronic phase after failure of interferon therapy
Ph+ acute lymphoblastic leukemia (ALL) (relapsed or refractory)
Aggressive systemic mastocytosis (ASM) without D816V c-Kit mutation (or c-Kit mutation status unknown)
Dermatofibrosarcoma protuberans (DFSP) (unresectable, recurrent and/or metastatic)
Hypereosinophilic syndrome (HES) and/or chronic eosinophilic leukemia (CEL)
Myelodysplastic/myeloproliferative disease (MDS/MPD) associated with platelet-derived growth factor receptor (PDGFR) gene rearrangements

Canada labeling (not an approved indication in the U.S.): Ph+ ALL induction therapy (newly diagnosed)

Unlabeled/Investigational Use Treatment of desmoid tumors (soft tissue sarcoma); post-stem cell transplant (allogeneic) follow-up treatment in CML

Mechanism of Action/Effect Inhibits a specific enzyme (Bcr-Abl tyrosine kinase) produced by the Philadelphia chromosome found in many patients with chronic myeloid leukemia (CML). Inhibition of this enzyme blocks proliferation and induces cell death in leukemic cells. Also inhibits tyrosine kinase for platelet-derived growth factor (SCF), c-Kit, and cellular events mediated by PDGF and SCF.

Contraindications There are no contraindications listed within the FDA-approved manufacturer's labeling.

Canadian labeling: Hypersensitivity to imatinib or any component of the formulation

Warnings/Precautions Hazardous agent - use appropriate precautions for handling and disposal. Often associated with fluid retention, weight gain, and edema (probability increases with higher doses and age >65 years); occasionally leading to significant complications, including pleural effusion, pericardial effusion, pulmonary edema, and ascites. Use with caution in patients where fluid accumulation may be poorly tolerated, such as in cardiovascular disease (heart failure [HF] or hypertension) and pulmonary disease. Severe HF and left ventricular dysfunction (LVD) have been reported rarely, usually in patients with comorbidities and/or risk factors; carefully monitor patients with pre-existing cardiac disease or risk factors for HF. With initiation of imatinib treatment, cardiogenic shock and/or LVD have been reported in patients with hypereosinophilic syndrome and cardiac involvement (reversible with systemic steroids, circulatory support and temporary cessation of imatinib). Patients with high eosinophil levels and an abnormal echocardiogram or abnormal serum troponin level may benefit from prophylactic systemic steroids with the initiation of imatinib.

Severe bullous dermatologic reactions (including erythema multiforme and Stevens-Johnson syndrome) have been reported; reintroduction has been attempted following resolution. Successful resumption at a lower dose (with corticosteroids and/or antihistamine) has been described; however, some patients may experience recurrent reactions.

Hepatotoxicity may occur (may be severe); monitor; therapy interruption or dose reduction may be necessary. Transaminase and bilirubin elevations, and acute liver failure have been observed with imatinib in combination with chemotherapy. Use with caution in patients with pre-existing hepatic impairment; may require dosage adjustment. Use with caution in renal impairment; may require dosage adjustment.

May cause GI irritation, severe hemorrhage (grades 3 and 4; including gastrointestinal hemorrhage and/or tumor hemorrhage; hemorrhage incidence is higher in patients with GIST), or hematologic toxicity (anemia, neutropenia, and thrombocytopenia); median duration of neutropenia is 2-3 weeks; median duration of thrombocytopenia is 3-4 weeks. Hypothyroidism has been reported in thyroidectomy patients (receiving thyroid hormone replacement therapy) during imatinib therapy; monitor. Has been associated with development of opportunistic infections. Use with caution in patients receiving concurrent therapy with drugs which alter cytochrome P450 activity or require metabolism by these isoenzymes; avoid concomitant use of strong CYP3A4 inducers. Safety and efficacy in patients <2 years of age have not been established.

Drug Interactions

Metabolism/Transport Effects Substrate of CYP1A2 (minor), CYP2D6 (minor), CYP2C9 (minor), CYP2C19 (minor), CYP3A4 (major), P-glycoprotein; **Inhibits** CYP2C9 (weak), CYP2D6 (moderate), CYP3A4 (strong), ABCG2

Avoid Concomitant Use

Avoid concomitant use of Imatinib with any of the following: Alfuzosin; BCG; Conivaptan; Dronedarone; Eplerenone; Everolimus; Halofantrine; Lurasidone; Natalizumab; Nilotinib; Nisoldipine; Pimecrolimus; Ranolazine; Rivaroxaban; Roflumilast; RomiDEPsin; Salmeterol; Silodosin; Tacrolimus (Topical); Tamsulosin; Thioridazine; Tolvaptan; Toremifene; Vaccines (Live)

Decreased Effect

Imatinib may decrease the levels/effects of: BCG; Cardiac Glycosides; Codeine; Fludarabine; Prasugrel; Sipuleucel-T; TraMADol; Vaccines (Inactivated); Vaccines (Live); Vitamin K Antagonists

The levels/effects of Imatinib may be decreased by: CYP3A4 Inducers (Strong); Deferasirox; Echinacea; Peginterferon Alfa-2b; P-Glycoprotein Inducers; Rifamycin Derivatives; St Johns Wort

Increased Effect/Toxicity

Imatinib may increase the levels/effects of: Acetaminophen; Alfuzosin; Almotriptan; Alosetron; Bortezomib; Brinzolamide; Ciclesonide; Colchicine; Conivaptan; Corticosteroids (Orally Inhaled); CycloSPORINE; CycloSPORINE (Systemic); CYP2D6 Substrates; CYP3A4 Substrates; Dienogest; Dronedarone; Dutasteride; Eplerenone; Everolimus; FentaNYL; Fesoterodine; GuanFACINE; Halofantrine; Ixabepilone; Leflunomide; Lumefantrine; Lurasidone; Maraviroc; MethylPREDNISolone; Natalizumab; Nebivolol; Nilotinib; Nisoldipine; Paricalcitol; Pazopanib; Pimecrolimus; Ranolazine; Rivaroxaban; RomiDEPsin; Salmeterol; Saxagliptin; Silodosin; Simvastatin; SORAfenib; Tadalafil; Tamoxifen; Tamsulosin; Thioridazine; Tolvaptan; Topotecan; Toremifene; Vaccines (Live); Vilazodone; Vitamin K Antagonists; Warfarin

The levels/effects of Imatinib may be increased by: Acetaminophen; Antifungal Agents (Azole Derivatives, Systemic); CYP3A4 Inhibitors (Moderate); CYP3A4 Inhibitors (Strong); Dasatinib; Denosumab; Lansoprazole; P-Glycoprotein Inhibitors; Pimecrolimus; Roflumilast; Tacrolimus (Topical); Trastuzumab

Nutritional/Ethanol Interactions

Ethanol: Avoid ethanol.

Food: Food may reduce gastrointestinal irritation. Avoid grapefruit juice (may increase imatinib plasma concentration).

Herb/Nutraceutical: Avoid St John's wort (may increase metabolism and decrease imatinib plasma concentration).

Adverse Reactions Note: Adverse reactions listed as a composite of data across many trials, except where noted for a specific cancer type.

>10%:

Cardiovascular: Edema/fluid retention (33% to 86%; grades 3/4: 3% to 13%; includes aggravated edema, anasarca, ascites, pericardial effusion, peripheral edema, pleural effusion, pulmonary edema and superficial edema); facial edema (DFSP 17%), chest pain (GIST ≤7%, CML 7% to 11%)

Central nervous system: Fatigue (29% to 75%), fever (13% to 41%), headache (19% to 37%), dizziness (10% to 19%), insomnia (10% to 19%), depression (≤15%), anxiety (7% to 12%), chills (≤11%)

Dermatologic: Rash (9% to 50%; grades 3/4: 1% to 9%), pruritus (8% to 19%), alopecia (GIST 10% to 15%)

Endocrine & metabolic: Hypokalemia (6% to 13%)

Gastrointestinal: Nausea (42% to 73%), diarrhea (25% to 59%), vomiting (23% to 58%), abdominal pain (6% to 57%), anorexia (≤36%), weight gain (5% to 32%), dyspepsia (11% to 27%), constipation (9% to 16%)

Hematologic: Hemorrhage (12% to 53%; grades 3/4: 2% to 19%), neutropenia (grade 3: 7% to 27%; grade 4: 3% to 48%), thrombocytopenia (grade 3: 1% to 31%; grade 4: <1% to 33%), anemia (grade 3: 1% to 42%; grade 4: 1% to 11%), leukopenia (GIST 5% to 20%)

Hepatic: ALT increased (≤17%; grade 3: 2% to 7%; grade 4: <3%), hepatotoxicity (6% to 12%; grades 3/4: 3% to 8%)

Neuromuscular & skeletal: Muscle cramps (16% to 62%), arthralgia (≤40%), joint pain (11% to 31%), myalgia (9% to 32%), weakness (≤21%), musculoskeletal pain (children 21%; adults 12% to 49%), rigors (10% to 12%), bone pain (≤11%)

Ocular: Periorbital edema (DFSP 33%; MPD 29%; GIST ≤47%), lacrimation increased (DFSP 25%; GIST ≤10%)

Renal: Serum creatinine increased (≤12%; grade 3: ≤3%; DFSP: grade 4: 8%)

Respiratory: Nasopharyngitis (10% to 31%), cough (11% to 27%), dyspnea (≤21%), upper respiratory tract infection (3% to 21%), pharyngolaryngeal pain (7% to 18%), rhinitis (DFSP 17%), pharyngitis (CML 10% to 15%), pneumonia (CML 4% to 13%), sinusitis (4% to 11%)

Miscellaneous: Night sweats (CML 13% to 17%), infection without neutropenia (GIST ≤17%), influenza (1% to 14%), diaphoresis (GIST ≤13%)

1% to 10%:

Cardiovascular: Flushing

Central nervous system: CNS/cerebral hemorrhage (≤9%), hypoesthesia

Dermatologic: Dry skin, erythema, photosensitivity reaction

Endocrine & metabolic: Hyperglycemia (≤10%), hypocalcemia (GIST ≤6%), albumin decreased (grade 3: ≤4%)

Gastrointestinal: Flatulence (≤10%), stomatitis/mucositis (≤10%), weight loss (≤10%), gastrointestinal hemorrhage (2% to 8%), abdominal distension, gastritis, gastroesophageal reflux, mouth ulceration, taste disturbance, xerostomia

Hematologic: Lymphopenia (GIST ≤10%), neutropenic fever, pancytopenia

Hepatic: Alkaline phosphatase increased (grade 3: ≤6%; grade 4: <1%), AST increased (grade 3: 2% to 4%; grade 4: ≤3%), bilirubin increased (grade 3: 1% to 4%; grade 4: ≤3%)

Neuromuscular & skeletal: Back pain (GIST ≤7%), limb pain (GIST ≤7%), peripheral neuropathy, joint swelling, paresthesia

Ocular: Blurred vision, conjunctival hemorrhage, conjunctivitis, dry eyes, eyelid edema

Respiratory: Epistaxis

Pharmacodynamics/Kinetics

Absorption Rapid

Bioavailability 98%

Time to Peak 2-4 hours

Protein Binding Parent drug and metabolite: ~95% to albumin and alpha$_1$-acid glycoprotein

Half-Life Elimination Adults: Parent drug: ~18 hours; N-desmethyl metabolite: ~40 hours; Children: Parent drug: ~15 hours

Metabolism Hepatic via CYP3A4 (minor metabolism via CYP1A2, CYP2D6, CYP2C9, CYP2C19); primary metabolite (active): N-demethylated piperazine derivative (CGP74588); severe hepatic impairment (bilirubin >3-10 times ULN) increases AUC by 45% to 55% for imatinib and its active metabolite, respectively

Excretion Feces (68% primarily as metabolites, 20% as unchanged drug); urine (13% primarily as metabolites, 5% as unchanged drug)

Available Dosage Forms

Tablet, oral:

Gleevec®: 100 mg, 400 mg

Dosing

Adult & Geriatric Note: For concurrent use with a strong CYP3A4 enzyme-inducing agent (eg, rifampin, phenytoin), imatinib dosage should be increased by at least 50%. Doses ≤600 mg should be administered once daily, 800 mg doses should be administered as 400 mg twice a day. The optimal duration of therapy for CML is not yet determined, discontinuing treatment is not recommended after achieving remission due to the potential for relapse (NCCN CML guidelines v.2.2010).

Ph+ CML: Oral:

Chronic phase: 400 mg once daily; may be increased to 600 mg/day, if tolerated, for disease progression, lack of hematologic response after 3 months, lack of cytogenetic response after 6-12 months, or loss of previous hematologic or cytogenetic response

Canadian labeling and NCCN CML guidelines (v.2.2010): Includes range up to 800 mg/day (400 mg twice daily)

Accelerated phase or blast crisis: 600 mg once daily; may be increased to 800 mg/day (400 mg twice daily), if tolerated, for disease progression, lack of hematologic response after 3 months, lack of cytogenetic response after 6-12 months, or loss of previous hematologic or cytogenetic response

Ph+ ALL (relapsed or refractory): Oral: 600 mg once daily

GIST (adjuvant treatment following complete resection): 400 mg once daily

GIST (unresectable and/or metastatic malignant): 400 mg once daily; may be increased up to 800 mg/day (400 mg twice daily), if tolerated, for disease progression. **Note:** Significant improvement (progression-free survival, objective response rate) was demonstrated in patients with KIT exon 9 mutation with 800 mg (versus 400 mg), although overall survival (OS) was not impacted. The higher dose did not demonstrate a difference in time to progression or OS patients with Kit exon 11 mutation or wild-type status (Debiec-Rychter, 2006; Heinrich, 2009).

ASM with eosinophilia: Oral: Initiate at 100 mg once daily; titrate up to a maximum of 400 mg once daily (if tolerated) for insufficient response to lower dose

ASM without D816V c-Kit mutation or c-Kit mutation status unknown: Oral: 400 mg once daily

DFSP: Oral: 400 mg twice daily

HES/CEL: Oral: 400 mg once daily

HES/CEL with FIP1L1-PDGFRα fusion kinase: Oral: Initiate at 100 mg once daily; titrate up to a maximum of 400 mg once daily (if tolerated) if insufficient response to lower dose

MDS/MPD: Oral: 400 mg once daily

Ph+ ALL (induction, newly diagnosed): *Canadian labeling (not an approved use in the U.S.):* Oral: 600 mg once daily

Dosage adjustment with concomitant strong CYP3A4 inducers: Avoid concomitant use of strong CYP3A4 inducers (eg, dexamethasone, carbamazepine, phenobarbital, phenytoin, rifampin); if concomitant use can not be avoided, increase imatinib dose by at least 50% with careful monitoring.

Pediatric Notes: May be administered once daily or in 2 divided doses. Dosage should be increased by at least 50% when used concurrently with a potent CYP3A4 enzyme-inducing agent (ie, rifampin, phenytoin). The optimal duration of therapy for CML is not yet determined, discontinuing treatment is not recommended after achieving remission due to the potential for relapse (NCCN CML guidelines v.2.2010).

Ph+ CML: Children ≥2 years: Oral:

Chronic phase, recurrent or resistant: 260 mg/m^2/day

Chronic phase, newly diagnosed: 340 mg/m^2/day; maximum: 600 mg /day

Dosage adjustment for hepatotoxicity or other nonhematologic adverse reactions: Refer to Dosing: Hepatic Impairment.

Dosage adjustment for hematologic adverse reactions: Refer to Dosing: Adjustment for Toxicity.

Renal Impairment

Recommendation in the FDA-approved labeling:

Mild impairment (Cl_{cr} 40-59 mL/minute): Maximum recommended dose: 600 mg

Moderate impairment (Cl_{cr} 20-39 mL/minute): Decrease recommended starting dose by 50%; dose may be increased as tolerated; maximum recommended dose: 400 mg

Severe impairment (Cl_{cr} <20 mL/minute): Use caution; a dose of 100 mg/day has been tolerated in severe impairment (Gibbons, 2008)

Canadian labeling recommendation:

Mild impairment (Cl_{cr} 40-59 mL/minute): Use caution; usual minimum recommended effective dose: 400 mg once daily; titrate to efficacy and tolerability

Moderate impairment (Cl_{cr} 20-39 mL/minute): Use caution; usual minimum recommended effective dose: 400 mg once daily; titrate to efficacy and tolerability; the use of 800 mg dose is not recommended

Severe impairment (Cl_{cr} <20 mL/minute): Use is not recommended

Hepatic Impairment

Mild-to-moderate impairment: No adjustment necessary

Canadian labeling: GIST: Minimum effective dose: 400 mg once daily

Severe impairment:

Manufacturer's FDA-approved labeling: Reduce dose by 25%

Canadian labeling: GIST: 200 mg dose once daily with titration to 300 mg once daily in the absence of severe toxicity

NCCN soft tissue sarcoma guidelines (v.2.2009): GIST: Reduce dose by 25% to 50%

Hepatotoxicity (during therapy) or other nonhematologic adverse reactions: Withhold treatment until toxicity resolves; may resume if appropriate (depending on initial severity of adverse event)

NCCN soft tissue sarcoma guidelines (v.2.2009): GIST: Superficial edema: Manage with supportive care, diuretics, or dosage reduction

If elevations of bilirubin >3 times upper limit of normal (ULN) or transaminases >5 times ULN occur, withhold treatment until bilirubin <1.5 times ULN and transaminases <2.5 times ULN. Resume treatment at a reduced dose as follows:

Children ≥2 years:

If current dose 260 mg/m²/day, reduce dose to 200 mg/m²/day

If current dose 340 mg/m²/day, reduce dose to 260 mg/m²/day

Adults:

If current dose 400 mg, reduce dose to 300 mg

If current dose 600 mg, reduce dose to 400 mg

If current dose 800 mg, reduce dose to 600 mg

Adjustment for Toxicity Dosage adjustment for hematologic adverse reactions:

Chronic phase CML (initial dose 400 mg/day in adults or 260-340 mg/m²/day in children), ASM, MDS/MPD, and HES/CEL (initial dose 400 mg/day), or GIST (initial dose 400 mg): If ANC <1 x 10^9/L and/or platelets <50 x 10^9/L: Withhold until ANC ≥1.5 x 10^9/L and platelets ≥75 x 10^9/L; resume treatment at original starting dose. For recurrent neutropenia or thrombocytopenia, withhold until recovery, and reinstitute treatment at a reduced dose as follows:

Children ≥2 years:

If initial dose 260 mg/m²/day, reduce dose to 200 mg/m²/day

If initial dose 340 mg/m²/day, reduce dose to 260 mg/m²/day

Adults: If initial dose 400 mg, reduce dose to 300 mg

CML (accelerated phase or blast crisis) and PH+ ALL: Adults (initial dose 600 mg): If ANC <0.5 x 10^9/L and/or platelets <10 x 10^9/L, establish whether cytopenia is related to leukemia (bone marrow aspirate or biopsy). If unrelated to leukemia, reduce dose to 400 mg. If cytopenia persists for an additional 2 weeks, further reduce dose to 300 mg. If cytopenia persists for 4 weeks and is still unrelated to leukemia, withhold treatment until ANC ≥1 x 10^9/L and platelets ≥20 x 10^9/L, then resume treatment at 300 mg.

ASM associated with eosinophilia and HES/CEL with FIP1L1-PDGFRα fusion kinase (starting dose 100 mg/day): If ANC <1 x 10^9/L and/or platelets <50 x 10^9/L: Withhold until ANC ≥1.5 x 10^9/L and platelets ≥75 x 10^9/L; resume treatment at previous dose.

DFSP (initial dose 800 mg/day): If ANC <1 x 10^9/L and/or platelets <50 x 10^9/L, withhold until ANC ≥1.5 x 10^9/L and platelets ≥75 x 10^9/L; resume treatment at reduced dose of 600 mg/day. If depression in neutrophils or platelets recurs, withhold until recovery, and reinstitute treatment with a further dose reduction to 400 mg/day.

Administration

Oral Should be administered with a meal and a large glass of water. Tablets may be dispersed in water or apple juice (using ~50 mL for 100 mg tablet, ~200 mL for 400 mg tablet); stir until dissolved and use immediately. For daily dosing ≥800 mg, the 400 mg tablets should be used in order to reduce iron exposure.

Stability

Storage Store at 25°C (77°F); excursions permitted between 15°C to 30°C (59°F to 86°F). Protect from moisture.

Monitoring and Teaching Issues

Laboratory Monitoring CBC (weekly for first month, biweekly for second month, then periodically thereafter), liver function tests (at baseline and monthly or as clinically indicated; more frequently [at least weekly] in patients with moderate-to-severe hepatic impairment [Ramanathan, 2008]), renal function, serum electrolytes (including calcium, phosphorus, potassium and sodium levels); thyroid function tests (in thyroidectomy patients); consider echocardiogram and serum troponin levels in patients with HES/CEL, and in patients with MDS/MPD or ASM with high eosinophil levels; in pediatric patients, also monitor serum glucose and albumin

In Canada, a baseline evaluation of left ventricular ejection fraction is recommended prior to initiation of imatinib therapy in all patients with known underlying heart disease or in elderly patients.

Physical Assessment Use caution when fluid accumulation may be poorly tolerated (CHF, hypertension) or with renal or hepatic impairment. Evaluate CBC, serum electrolytes, LFTs, and renal and thyroid function tests on a regular basis. Monitor weight and fluid status. Monitor for hemorrhage, paresthesia, and respiratory or CNS changes.

Patient Education Avoid chronic use of acetaminophen or aspirin unless approved by prescriber. Take with food or a large glass of water. If you have difficulty swallowing tablets, tablet may be dispersed in water or apple juice (using ~50 mL for 100 mg tablet or ~200 mL for 400 mg tablet); stir until dissolved and use immediately. Maintain adequate hydration, unless instructed to restrict fluid intake. You will be required to have regularly scheduled laboratory tests while on this medication. You will be more susceptible to infection. You may experience headache, dizziness, fatigue, loss of appetite, nausea, vomiting, mouth sores, or constipation. Report chest pain, palpitations, or swelling of extremities; cough, difficulty breathing, or wheezing; weight gain; skin rash; muscle or bone pain, tremors, or cramping; persistent fatigue or weakness; easy bruising or unusual bleeding (eg, tarry stools, blood in vomitus, stool, urine, or mouth); or persistent GI problems or pain.

Dietary Considerations Should be taken with food and a large glass of water to decrease gastrointestinal irritation. Avoid grapefruit juice.

Geriatric Considerations Incidence of edema and edema-related adverse effects is increased in elderly patients.

Breast-Feeding Considerations Imatinib and its active metabolite are found in human breast milk; the milk/plasma ratio is 0.5 for imatinib and 0.9 for the active metabolite. Based on body weight, up to 10% of a therapeutic maternal dose could potentially be received by a breastfed infant. Due to the potential for serious adverse reactions in the nursing infant, breast-feeding is not recommended.

Pregnancy Considerations There are no adequate and well-controlled studies in pregnant women. Animal studies have demonstrated teratogenic effects and fetal loss. Women of childbearing potential are advised not to become pregnant (female patients and female partners of male patients). Adequate contraception is recommended. Case reports of pregnancies while on therapy (both males and females) include reports of spontaneous abortion, minor abnormalities (hypospadias, pyloric stenosis, and small intestine rotation) at or shortly after birth, and other congenital abnormalities including skeletal malformations, hypoplastic lungs, exomphalos, kidney abnormalities, hydrocephalus, cerebellar hypoplasia, and cardiac defects.

Retrospective case reports of women with CML in complete hematologic response (CHR) with cytogenic response (partial or complete) who interrupted imatinib therapy due to pregnancy, demonstrated a loss of response in some patients while off treatment. At 18 months after treatment reinitiation following delivery, CHR was again achieved in all patients and cytogenic response was achieved in some patients. Cytogenetic response rates may not be at as high as compared to patients with 18 months of uninterrupted therapy (Ault, 2006; Pye, 2008).

Additional Information Patients with HES/CEL, MDS/MPD or ASM with an abnormal echocardiogram or abnormal serum troponin level may benefit from prophylactic systemic steroids (1-2 mg/kg for 1-2 weeks) with the initiation of imatinib.

◆ **Imatinib Mesylate** *see* Imatinib *on page 951*

◆ **IMC-C225** *see* Cetuximab *on page 352*

◆ **Imdur®** *see* Isosorbide Mononitrate *on page 1029*

◆ **Imferon** *see* Iron Dextran Complex *on page 1021*

◆ **IMI 30** *see* IDArubicin *on page 945*

◆ **IMid-1** *see* Lenalidomide *on page 1071*

◆ **Imidazole Carboxamide** *see* Dacarbazine *on page 452*

◆ **Imidazole Carboxamide Dimethyltriazene** *see* Dacarbazine *on page 452*

◆ **Imipemide** *see* Imipenem and Cilastatin *on page 956*

Imipenem and Cilastatin (i mi PEN em & sye la STAT in)

U.S. Brand Names Primaxin® I.M. [DSC]; Primaxin® I.V.

Index Terms Imipemide

Generic Availability (U.S.) No

Pharmacologic Category Antibiotic, Carbapenem

Medication Safety Issues

Sound-alike/look-alike issues:

Imipenem may be confused with ertapenem, meropenem

Primaxin® may be confused with Premarin®, Primacor®

Pregnancy Risk Factor C

Lactation Enters breast milk/use caution

Use Treatment of lower respiratory tract, urinary tract, intra-abdominal, gynecologic, bone and joint, skin and skin structure, and polymicrobic infections as well as bacterial septicemia and endocarditis. Antibacterial activity includes resistant gram-negative bacilli (*Pseudomonas aeruginosa* and *Enterobacter* sp), gram-positive bacteria (methicillin-sensitive *Staphylococcus aureus* and *Streptococcus* sp) and anaerobes.

Unlabeled/Investigational Use Hepatic abscess; neutropenic fever; melioidosis

Available Dosage Forms

Injection, powder for reconstitution:

Primaxin® I.V.: Imipenem 250 mg and cilastatin 250 mg; imipenem 500 mg and cilastatin 500 mg

Dosing

Adult & Geriatric Doses based on **imipenem** content. **Note:** I.M. administration is not intended for severe or life-threatening infections (eg, septicemia, endocarditis, shock), UTI, bone/joint or polymicrobic infections. For adults weighing <70 kg, refer to Dosing: Renal Impairment

***Burkholderia mallei* (melioidosis) (unlabeled use):** 25 mg/kg (up to 1 g) every 6 hours for at least 10 days (Currie, 2003)

Intra-abdominal infections:

I.V.:

Mild infection: 250-500 mg every 6 hours

Severe infection: 500 mg every 6 hours **or** 1 g every 8 hours for 4-7 days (provided source controlled). **Note:** Not recommended for mild-to-moderate, community-acquired intra-abdominal infections due to risk of toxicity and the development of resistant organisms (Solomkin, 2010)

I.M.: Mild-to-moderate infection: 750 mg every 12 hours

Liver abscess (unlabeled use): I.V.: 500 mg every 6 hours for 4-6 weeks (Ulug, 2010)

Lower respiratory tract, skin/skin structure, gynecologic infections: I.M.: Mild/moderate: 500-750 mg every 12 hours

Moderate infections:

I.M.: 750 mg every 12 hours

I.V.:

Fully-susceptible organisms: 500 mg every 6-8 hours

Moderately-susceptible organisms: 500 mg every 6 hours or 1 g every 8 hours

Neutropenic fever (unlabeled use): I.V.: 500 mg every 6 hours (Paul, 2006)

***Pseudomonas* infections:** I.V.: 500 mg every 6 hours; **Note:** Higher doses may be required based on organism sensitivity.

Severe infections: I.V.: **Note:** I.M. administration is not intended for severe or life-threatening infections (eg, septicemia, endocarditis, shock):

Fully-susceptible organisms: 500 mg every 6 hours

Moderately-susceptible organisms: 1 g every 6-8 hours

Maximum daily dose should not exceed 50 mg/kg or 4 g/day, whichever is lower

Urinary tract infection, uncomplicated: I.V.: 250 mg every 6 hours

Urinary tract infection, complicated: I.V.: 500 mg every 6 hours

Mild infections: Note: Rarely a suitable option in mild infections; normally reserved for moderate-severe cases:

I.M.: 500 mg every 12 hours

I.V.:

Fully-susceptible organisms: 250 mg every 6 hours

Moderately-susceptible organisms: 500 mg every 6 hours

Pediatric Dosage based on **imipenem** content:

Non-CNS infections: I.V.:

Neonates ≤3 months and weight ≥1500 g:

<1 week: 25 mg/kg every 12 hours

1-4 weeks: 25 mg/kg every 8 hours

4 weeks to 3 months: 25 mg/kg every 6 hours

Children: >3 months: 15-25 mg/kg every 6 hours

Maximum dosage: Susceptible infections: 2 g/day; moderately-susceptible organisms: 4 g/day

Burkholderia mallei (melioidosis) (unlabeled use): 20 mg/kg every 8 hours for 10 days

Cystic fibrosis: Doses up to 90 mg/kg/day have been used

Renal Impairment I.V.: **Note:** Adjustments have not been established for I.M. dosing:

Patients with a Cl_{cr} ≤5 mL/minute/1.73 m^2 should not receive imipenem/cilastatin unless hemodialysis is instituted within 48 hours.

Patients weighing <30 kg with impaired renal function should not receive imipenem/cilastatin.

Hemodialysis: Use the dosing recommendation for patients with a Cl_{cr} 6-20 mL/minute; administer dose after dialysis session and every 12 hours thereafter

Peritoneal dialysis: Dose as for Cl_{cr} 6-20 mL/minute.

Continuous renal replacement therapy (CRRT): Drug clearance is highly dependent on the method of renal replacement, filter type, and flow rate. Appropriate dosing requires close monitoring of pharmacologic response, signs of adverse reactions due to drug accumulation, as well as drug levels in relation to target trough (if appropriate). The following are general recommendations only (based on dialysate flow/ultrafiltration rates of 1 L/hour) and should not supersede clinical judgment:

CVVH: 250 mg every 6 hours or 500 mg every 8 hours

CVVHD/CVVHDF: 250 mg every 6 hours or 500 mg every 6-8 hours

Note: Data suggest that 500 mg every 12 hours may provide sufficient T>MIC to cover organisms with MIC values ≤2 mg/L; however, a higher dose of 500 mg every 6 hours is recommended for resistant organisms (particularly *Pseudomonas*) with MIC ≥4 mg/L (Fish, 2005).

See table.

Imipenem and Cilastatin Dosage in Renal Impairment

Reduced I.V. Dosage Regimen Based on Creatinine Clearance (mL/minute/1.73 m²) and/or Body Weight <70 kg					
	Body Weight (kg)				
	≥70	60	50	40	30
Total daily dose for normal renal function: 1 g/day					
Cl_{cr} ≥71	250 mg q6h	250 mg q8h	125 mg q6h	125 mg q6h	125 mg q8h
Cl_{cr} 41-70	250 mg q8h	125 mg q6h	125 mg q6h	125 mg q8h	125 mg q8h
Cl_{cr} 21-40	250 mg q12h	250 mg q12h	125 mg q8h	125 mg q12h	125 mg q12h
Cl_{cr} 6-20	250 mg q12h	125 mg q12h	125 mg q12h	125 mg q12h	125 mg q12h
Total daily dose for normal renal function: 1.5 g/day					
Cl_{cr} ≥71	500 mg q8h	250 mg q6h	250 mg q6h	250 mg q8h	125 mg q6h
Cl_{cr} 41-70	250 mg q6h	250 mg q8h	250 mg q8h	125 mg q6h	125 mg q8h
Cl_{cr} 21-40	250 mg q8h	250 mg q8h	250 mg q12h	125 mg q8h	125 mg q8h
Cl_{cr} 6-20	250 mg q12h	250 mg q12h	250 mg q12h	125 mg q12h	125 mg q12h
Total daily dose for normal renal function: 2 g/day					
Cl_{cr} ≥71	500 mg q6h	500 mg q8h	250 mg q6h	250 mg q6h	250 mg q8h
Cl_{cr} 41-70	500 mg q8h	250 mg q6h	250 mg q6h	250 mg q8h	125 mg q6h
Cl_{cr} 21-40	250 mg q6h	250 mg q8h	250 mg q8h	250 mg q12h	125 mg q8h
Cl_{cr} 6-20	250 mg q12h	250 mg q12h	250 mg q12h	250 mg q12h	125 mg q12h
Total daily dose for normal renal function: 3 g/day					
Cl_{cr} ≥71	1000 mg q8h	750 mg q8h	500 mg q6h	500 mg q8h	250 mg q6h
Cl_{cr} 41-70	500 mg q6h	500 mg q8h	500 mg q8h	250 mg q6h	250 mg q8h
Cl_{cr} 21-40	500 mg q8h	500 mg q8h	250 mg q6h	250 mg q8h	250 mg q8h
Cl_{cr} 6-20	500 mg q12h	500 mg q12h	250 mg q12h	250 mg q12h	250 mg q12h
Total daily dose for normal renal function: 4 g/day					
Cl_{cr} ≥71	1000 mg q6h	1000 mg q8h	750 mg q8h	500 mg q6h	500 mg q8h
Cl_{cr} 41-70	750 mg q8h	750 mg q8h	500 mg q6h	500 mg q8h	250 mg q6h
Cl_{cr} 21-40	500 mg q6h	500 mg q8h	500 mg q8h	250 mg q6h	250 mg q8h
Cl_{cr} 6-20	500 mg q12h	500 mg q12h	500 mg q12h	250 mg q12h	250 mg q12h

Hepatic Impairment Hepatic dysfunction may further impair cilastatin clearance in patients receiving chronic renal replacement therapy; consider decreasing the dosing frequency.

Administration

I.M. Note: I.M. administration is not intended for severe or life-threatening infections (eg, septicemia, endocarditis, shock). Administer by deep injection into a large muscle (gluteal or lateral thigh). **Only the I.M. formulation can be used for I.M. administration.**

I.V. I.V.: Do not administer I.V. push. Infuse doses ≤500 mg over 20-30 minutes; infuse doses ≥750 mg over 40-60 minutes. **Only the I.V. formulation can be used for I.V. administration.**

Monitoring and Teaching Issues

Laboratory Monitoring Perform culture and sensitivity studies prior to initiating therapy. Periodically monitor renal, hepatic, and hematologic function.

Physical Assessment Assess results of culture and sensitivity tests and patient's allergy history prior to beginning therapy. Note Administration for I.M. and I.V. specifics. Advise patients with diabetes about use of Clinitest®.

Patient Education This medication can only be administered by injection or infusion. Report immediately any warmth, swelling, pain, or redness at infusion or injection site. Maintain adequate hydration, unless instructed to restrict fluid intake, and nutrition. May cause false test results with Clinitest®; use of another type of glucose testing is preferable. Report immediately any CNS changes (dizziness, hallucinations, anxiety, visual disturbances); swelling of throat, tongue, lips, or face; chills or fever; persistent diarrhea; or unusual discharge or foul-smelling urine.

Related Information

Antimicrobial Drugs of Choice *on page 2008*
Community-Acquired Pneumonia in Adults *on page 2021*

Imipramine (im IP ra meen)

U.S. Brand Names Tofranil-PM®; Tofranil®
Index Terms Imipramine Hydrochloride; Imipramine Pamoate
Generic Availability (U.S.) Yes

Pharmacologic Category Antidepressant, Tricyclic (Tertiary Amine)

Medication Safety Issues

Sound-alike/look-alike issues:

Imipramine may be confused with amitriptyline, desipramine, Norpramin®

Medication Guide Available Yes

Lactation Enters breast milk/not recommended (AAP rates "of concern"; AAP 2001 update pending)

Use Treatment of depression; treatment of nocturnal enuresis in children

Unlabeled/Investigational Use Analgesic for certain chronic and neuropathic pain; panic disorder; attention-deficit/hyperactivity disorder (ADHD); post-traumatic stress disorder (PTSD)

Available Dosage Forms

Capsule, oral: 75 mg, 100 mg, 125 mg, 150 mg

Tofranil-PM®: 75 mg, 100 mg, 125 mg, 150 mg

Tablet, oral: 10 mg, 25 mg, 50 mg

Tofranil®: 10 mg, 25 mg, 50 mg

Dosing

Adult

Depression:

Outpatients: Initial: 75 mg/day; may increase gradually to 150 mg/day. May be given in divided doses or as a single bedtime dose; maximum: 200 mg/day

Inpatients: Initial: 100-150 mg/day; may increase gradually to 200 mg/day; if no response after 2 weeks, may further increase to 250-300 mg/day. May be given in divided doses or as a single bedtime dose; maximum: 300 mg/day.

Note: Maximum antidepressant effect may not be seen for 2 or more weeks after initiation of therapy.

Post-traumatic stress disorder (PTSD) (unlabeled use): Oral: 75-200 mg/day

Geriatric

Depression: Initial: 25-50 mg at bedtime; may increase every 3 days for inpatients and weekly for outpatients if tolerated to a recommended maximum of 100 mg/day.

Pediatric

Depression: Oral:

Children (unlabeled use): 1.5 mg/kg/day with dosage increments of 1 mg/kg every 3-4 days to a maximum dose of 5 mg/kg/day in 1-4 divided doses; monitor carefully especially with doses ≥3.5 mg/kg/day.

Adolescents: Initial: 30-40 mg/day; increase gradually; maximum: 100 mg/day in single or divided doses.

Enuresis: Oral: Children ≥6 years: Initial: 25 mg at bedtime, if inadequate response still seen after 1 week of therapy, increase by 25 mg/day; dose should not exceed 2.5 mg/kg/day or 50 mg at bedtime if 6-12 years of age or 75 mg at bedtime if ≥12 years of age.

Adjunct in the treatment of cancer pain (unlabeled use): Oral: Children: Initial: 0.2-0.4 mg/kg at bedtime; dose may be increased by 50% every 2-3 days up to 1-3 mg/kg/dose at bedtime.

Monitoring and Teaching Issues

Laboratory Monitoring ECG, CBC

Physical Assessment Perform careful cardiovascular assessment prior to initiating therapy. Assess CNS status and clinical worsening and be alert for suicide ideation. Taper dosage slowly when discontinuing.

Patient Education It may take 2-3 weeks to achieve desired results. Take in the evening. Avoid alcohol. Maintain adequate hydration, unless instructed to restrict fluid intake. You may experience drowsiness, lightheadedness, impaired coordination, dizziness, blurred vision, nausea, vomiting, altered taste, dry mouth, constipation, diarrhea, postural hypotension, or urinary retention. Report persistent insomnia; muscle cramping or tremors; chest pain, palpitations, rapid heartbeat, swelling of extremities, or severe dizziness; unresolved urinary retention; rash or skin irritation; yellowing of eyes or skin; pale stools/dark urine; worsening of condition; and suicide ideation.

Related Information

Antidepressant Agents *on page 1982*

Peak and Trough Guidelines *on page 1958*

Pharmacotherapy of Urinary Incontinence *on page 2071*

◆ **Imipramine Hydrochloride** *see* Imipramine *on page 958*

◆ **Imipramine Pamoate** *see* Imipramine *on page 958*

Imiquimod (i mi KWI mod)

U.S. Brand Names Aldara®; Zyclara™

Generic Availability (U.S.) Yes

Pharmacologic Category Skin and Mucous Membrane Agent; Topical Skin Product

Medication Safety Issues

Sound-alike/look-alike issues:

Aldara® may be confused with Alora®, Lialda™

Pregnancy Risk Factor C

Lactation Excretion in breast milk unknown/use caution

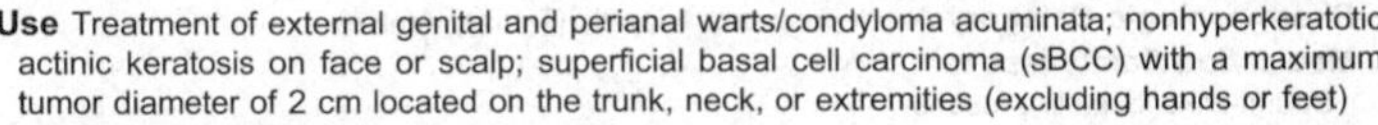

Use Treatment of external genital and perianal warts/condyloma acuminata; nonhyperkeratotic actinic keratosis on face or scalp; superficial basal cell carcinoma (sBCC) with a maximum tumor diameter of 2 cm located on the trunk, neck, or extremities (excluding hands or feet)

Unlabeled/Investigational Use Treatment of common warts

Available Dosage Forms

Cream, topical: 5% (24s)

Aldara®: 5% (24s)

Zyclara™: 3.75% (28s)

Dosing

Adult & Geriatric Note: A rest period of several days may be taken if required by the patient's discomfort or severity of the local skin reaction. Treatment may resume once the reaction subsides. Imiquimod treatment should not be prolonged beyond recommended period due to missed doses or rest periods.

Perianal warts/condyloma acuminata: Topical (Aldara®): Apply a thin layer 3 times/week on alternative days prior to bedtime and leave on skin for 6-10 hours. Remove by washing with mild soap and water. Continue imiquimod treatment until there is total clearance of the genital/perianal warts (maximum duration of therapy: 16 weeks)

Actinic keratosis: Topical:

Aldara®: Apply twice weekly for 16 weeks to a treatment area on face or scalp (but not both concurrently); no more than 1 packet should be applied at each application and no more than 36 packets applied per 16 weeks; apply prior to bedtime and leave on skin for 8 hours. Remove with mild soap and water.

Zyclara™: Treatment consists of 2 cycles (14 days each) separated by 1 rest period (14 days) with no treatment. Apply up to 2 packets once daily at bedtime to affected area on either face or balding scalp (but not both concurrently); apply no more than 2 packets at each application and no more than 56 packets per 2 cycles of treatment. Leave on skin for 8 hours. Remove with mild soap and water. **Note:** Canadian labeling recommends avoiding application to areas larger than the face or balding scalp (~200 cm^2).

Common warts (unlabeled use): Topical (Aldara®): Apply once daily prior to bedtime for 5 days/week for up to 16 weeks (Hengge, 2000) or apply twice daily for up to 24 weeks (Grussendorf-Conen, 2002)

Superficial basal cell carcinoma: Topical (Aldara®): Apply once daily prior to bedtime, 5 days/week for 6 weeks. No more than 36 packets should be used during the 6-week treatment period. Treatment area should include a 1 cm margin of skin around the tumor. Leave on skin for 8 hours. Remove with mild soap and water.

Pediatric Perianal warts/condyloma acuminata: Topical (Aldara®): Children ≥12 years: Refer to adult dosing.

Note: A rest period of several days may be taken if required by the patient's discomfort or severity of the local skin reaction. Treatment may resume once the reaction subsides. Imiquimod treatment should not be prolonged beyond recommended period due to missed doses or rest periods.

Administration

Topical Topical: Wash hands prior to and following application. Do not occlude the application site. Partially used packets should be discarded and not reused.

Actinic keratosis: Apply Aldara® over a single contiguous area (approximately 25 cm^2) on the face or scalp or Zyclara™ over an area <200 cm^2 on the face or scalp; the treatment area should be washed and thoroughly dried prior to application. Both areas should not be treated concurrently. Apply a thin layer to the affected area and rub in until the cream is no longer visible. Avoid contact with the eyes, lips, and nostrils.

External genital warts: Aldara®: Instruct patients to apply to external or perianal warts; not for vaginal use. Apply a thin layer to the wart area and rub in until the cream is no longer visible. Single-use packets contain sufficient cream to cover a wart area of up to 20 cm^2; avoid use of excessive amounts of cream. Nonocclusive dressings (such as cotton gauze or cotton underwear) may be used in the management of skin reactions.

Superficial basal cell carcinoma: Aldara®: Treatment area should have a maximum diameter no more than 2 cm on the trunk, neck, or extremities (excluding the hands, feet, and anogenital skin). Treatment area should include a 1 cm margin around the tumor. Wash and thoroughly dry treatment area prior to application; apply a thin layer to the affected area (and margin) and rub in until the cream is no longer visible. Avoid contact with the eyes, lips, and nostrils.

Monitoring and Teaching Issues

Patient Education This medication will not eliminate nor prevent the transmission of the virus. For external use only; avoid contact with eyes, mouth, nostrils, or vagina. Exposure to sun should be avoided or minimized. Use sunscreen or wear protective clothing if sun exposure is unavoidable. Sexual contact (vaginal, anal, or oral) should be avoided while cream is on skin. May cause pain, itching, redness, burning, flaking, swelling, or scabbing in treated area. If these effects persist or become severe or open sores develop, stop treatment and notify prescriber. Report fever, malaise, myalgia, or flu-like symptoms. Prescriber may recommend a rest period of several days before resuming treatment. Apply treatment just prior to sleeping and leave on 6-10 hours. Wash hands thoroughly before and after application. Wash and dry area to be treated before applying cream. After treatment period, remove cream with mild soap and water. Apply a thin layer to external warts and rub in until cream is no longer visible. Avoid use of excessive cream. May cover area with light gauze dressing or cotton underwear; do not apply occlusive dressing.

◆ **Imitrex®** *see* SUMAtriptan *on page* 1691

Immune Globulin (i MYUN GLOB yoo lin)

U.S. Brand Names Carimune® NF; Flebogamma® DIF; Flebogamma® [DSC]; GamaSTAN™ S/D; Gammagard S/D®; Gammagard® Liquid; Gammaplex®; Gamunex®; Gamunex®-C; Hizentra®; Octagam®; Privigen®; Vivaglobin® [DSC]

Index Terms Gamma Globulin; IG; IGIM; IGIV; Immune Globulin Subcutaneous (Human); Immune Serum Globulin; ISG; IV Immune Globulin; IVIG; Panglobulin; SCIG

Generic Availability (U.S.) No

Pharmacologic Category Blood Product Derivative; Immune Globulin

Medication Safety Issues

Sound-alike/look-alike issues:

Gamimune® N may be confused with CytoGam®

Immune globulin (intravenous) may be confused with hepatitis B immune globulin

Pregnancy Risk Factor C

Lactation Excretion in breast milk unknown/use caution

Use

Treatment of primary humoral immunodeficiency syndromes (congenital agammaglobulinemia, severe combined immunodeficiency syndromes [SCIDS], common variable immunodeficiency, X-linked immunodeficiency, Wiskott-Aldrich syndrome) (Carimune® NF, Flebogamma® DIF, Gammagard® Liquid, Gammagard S/D®, Gammaplex®, Gamunex®, Gamunex®-C, Hizentra®, Octagam®, Privigen®, Vivaglobin®)

Treatment of acute and chronic immune (idiopathic) thrombocytopenic purpura (ITP) (Carimune® NF, Gammagard S/D®, Gamunex®, Gamunex®-C, Privigen® [chronic only])

Treatment of chronic inflammatory demyelinating polyneuropathy (CIDP) (Gamunex®, Gamunex®-C)

Prevention of coronary artery aneurysms associated with Kawasaki syndrome (in combination with aspirin) (Gammagard S/D®)

Prevention of bacterial infection in patients with hypogammaglobulinemia and/or recurrent bacterial infections with B-cell chronic lymphocytic leukemia (CLL) (Gammagard S/D®)

Prevention of serious infection in immunoglobulin deficiency (select agammaglobulinemias) (GamaSTAN™ S/D)

Provision of passive immunity in the following susceptible individuals (GamaSTAN™ S/D):

Hepatitis A: Pre-exposure prophylaxis; postexposure: within 14 days and/or prior to manifestation of disease

Measles: For use within 6 days of exposure in an unvaccinated person, who has not previously had measles

Rubella: Postexposure prophylaxis (within 72 hours) to reduce the risk of infection and fetal damage in exposed pregnant women who will not consider therapeutic abortion

Varicella: For immunosuppressed patients when varicella zoster immune globulin is not available

Unlabeled/Investigational Use Acquired hypogammaglobulinemia secondary to malignancy; Guillain-Barré syndrome; hematopoietic stem cell transplantation (HSCT), to prevent bacterial infections among allogeneic recipients with severe hypogammaglobulinemia (IgG <400 mg/dL) at <100 days post transplant (CDC guidelines); HIV-associated thrombocytopenia; multiple sclerosis (relapsing, remitting when other therapies cannot be used); myasthenia gravis; refractory dermatomyositis/polymyositis

Mechanism of Action/Effect Replacement therapy for primary and secondary immunodeficiencies, and IgG antibodies against bacteria, viral, parasitic and mycoplasma antigens; interference with F_c receptors on the cells of the reticuloendothelial system for autoimmune cytopenias and ITP; provides passive immunity by increasing the antibody titer and antigen-antibody reaction potential

Contraindications Hypersensitivity to immune globulin or any component of the formulation; selective IgA deficiency; hyperprolinemia (Hizentra®, Privigen®); severe thrombocytopenia or coagulation disorders; severe thrombocytopenia or coagulation disorders where IM injections are contraindicated

Warnings/Precautions **[U.S. Boxed Warning]: I.V. formulation only: Acute renal dysfunction (increased serum creatinine, oliguria, acute renal failure, osmotic nephrosis) can rarely occur; usually within 7 days of use (more likely with products stabilized with sucrose). Use with caution in the elderly, patients with renal disease, diabetes mellitus, volume depletion, sepsis, paraproteinemia, and nephrotoxic medications due to risk of renal dysfunction.** In patients at risk of renal dysfunction, the rate of infusion and concentration of solution should be minimized. Discontinue if renal function deteriorates. High-dose regimens (1 g/kg for 1-2 days) are not recommended for individuals with fluid overload or where fluid volume may be of concern. Hypersensitivity and anaphylactic reactions can occur; a severe fall in blood pressure may rarely occur with anaphylactic reaction; immediate treatment (including epinephrine 1:1000) should be available. Product of human plasma; may potentially contain infectious agents which could transmit disease. Screening of donors, as well as testing and/or inactivation or removal of certain viruses, reduces the risk. Infections thought to be transmitted by this product should be reported to the manufacturer. Aseptic meningitis may occur with high doses (≥1-2 g/kg [product-dependent]) and/or rapid infusion; syndrome usually appears within several hours to 2 days following treatment; usually resolves within several days after IVIG is discontinued; patients with a migraine history may be at higher risk for AMS. Increased risk of hypersensitivity, especially in patients with anti-IgA antibodies. Increased risk of hematoma formation when administered subcutaneously for the treatment of ITP.

Intravenous immune globulin has been associated with antiglobulin hemolysis; monitor for signs of hemolytic anemia. Patients should be adequately hydrated prior to initiation of therapy.

Hyperproteinemia, increased serum viscosity and hyponatremia may occur; distinguish hyponatremia from pseudohyponatremia to prevent volume depletion, a further increase in serum viscosity, and a higher risk of thrombotic events. Use caution in patients with a history of thrombotic events or a history of atherosclerosis or cardiovascular disease or patients with known/suspected hyperviscosity; there is clinical evidence of a possible association between thrombotic events and administration of intravenous immune globulin and subcutaneous immune globulin. Consider a baseline assessment of blood viscosity in patients at risk for hyperviscosity. Patients should be monitored for adverse events during and after the infusion. Stop administration with signs of infusion reaction (fever, chills, nausea, vomiting, and rarely shock). Risk may be increased with initial treatment, when switching brands of immune globulin, and with treatment interruptions of >8 weeks. Monitor for transfusion-related acute lung injury (TRALI); noncardiogenic pulmonary edema has been reported with intravenous immune globulin use. TRALI is characterized by severe respiratory distress, pulmonary edema, hypoxemia, and fever (in the presence of normal left ventricular function) and usually occurs within 1-6 hours after infusion. Response to live vaccinations may be impaired. Some clinicians may administer intravenous immune globulin products as a subcutaneous infusion based on patient tolerability and clinical judgement. SubQ infusion should begin 1 week after the last I.V. dose; dose should be individualized based on clinical response and serum IgG trough concentrations; consider premedicating with acetaminophen and diphenhydramine.

Some products may contain maltose, which may result in falsely-elevated blood glucose readings; maltose-containing products are contraindicated in patients with an allergy to corn. Some products may contain polysorbate 80, sodium, and/or sucrose. Some products may contain sorbitol; do not use in patients with fructose intolerance. Hizentra® and Privigen® contain the stabilizer L-proline and are contraindicated in patients with hyperprolinemia. Packaging of some products may contain natural latex/natural rubber; skin testing should not be performed with GamaSTAN™ S/D as local irritation can occur and be misinterpreted as a positive reaction.

Drug Interactions

Avoid Concomitant Use There are no known interactions where it is recommended to avoid concomitant use.

Decreased Effect

Immune Globulin may decrease the levels/effects of: Vaccines (Live)

Increased Effect/Toxicity There are no known significant interactions involving an increase in effect.

Lab Interactions Octagam® contains maltose. Falsely-elevated blood glucose levels may occur when glucose monitoring devices and test strips utilizing the glucose dehydrogenase pyrroloquinolinequinone (GDH-PQQ) based methods are used. Glucose monitoring devices and test strips which utilize the glucose-specific method are recommended. Passively-transferred antibodies may yield false-positive serologic testing results; may yield false-positive direct and indirect Coombs' test. Skin testing should not be performed with GamaSTAN™ S/D as local irritation can occur and be misinterpreted as a positive reaction.

Adverse Reactions Frequency not defined.

Cardiovascular: Angioedema, chest tightness, edema, flushing of the face, hyper-/hypotension, palpitation, tachycardia

Central nervous system: Anxiety, aseptic meningitis syndrome, chills, dizziness, drowsiness, fatigue, fever, headache, irritability, lethargy, lightheadedness, malaise, migraine, pain

Dermatologic: Bruising, contact dermatitis, eczema, erythema, hyperhidrosis, petechiae, pruritus, purpura, rash, urticaria

Gastrointestinal: Abdominal cramps, abdominal pain, diarrhea, discomfort, dyspepsia, gastroenteritis, nausea, sore throat, toothache, vomiting

Hematologic: Anemia, autoimmune hemolytic anemia, hematocrit decreased, hemolysis (mild), hemorrhage, thrombocytopenia

Hepatic: Bilirubin increased, LDH increased, liver function test increased

Local: Muscle stiffness at I.M. site, pain or irritation at the infusion site

Neuromuscular & skeletal: Arthralgia, back or hip pain, leg cramps, muscle cramps, myalgia, neck pain, rigors, weakness

Ocular: Conjunctivitis

Otic: Ear pain

Renal: Acute renal failure, acute tubular necrosis, anuria, BUN increased, creatinine increased, oliguria, proximal tubular nephropathy, osmotic nephrosis

Respiratory: Asthma aggravated, bronchitis, cough, dyspnea, epistaxis, nasal congestion, pharyngeal pain, pharyngitis, rhinitis, rhinorrhea, sinus headache, sinusitis, upper respiratory infection, wheezing

Miscellaneous: Anaphylaxis, diaphoresis, flu-like syndrome, hypersensitivity reactions, infusion reaction, thermal burn

Pharmacodynamics/Kinetics

Onset of Action I.V.: Provides immediate antibody levels

Duration of Action I.M., I.V.: Immune effects: 3-4 weeks (variable)

Bioavailability SubQ: Vivaglobin®: 73%

Time to Peak

Plasma: SubQ: Hizentra®: 2.9 days; Vivaglobin®: 2.5 days

Serum: I.M.: ~48 hours

Half-Life Elimination I.M.: ~23 days; I.V.: IgG (variable among patients): Healthy subjects: 14-24 days; Patients with congenital humoral immunodeficiencies: 26-40 days; hypermetabolism associated with fever and infection have coincided with a shortened half-life

Available Dosage Forms

Injection, powder for reconstitution [preservative free]:

Carimune® NF: 3 g, 6 g, 12 g

Gammagard S/D®: 2.5 g, 5 g, 10 g

Injection, solution [preservative free]:

Flebogamma® DIF: 5% [50 mg/mL] (10 mL, 50 mL, 100 mL, 200 mL, 400 mL); 10% [100 mg/mL] (100 mL, 200 mL)

GamaSTAN™ S/D: 15% to 18% (2 mL, 10 mL)

Gammagard® Liquid: 10% [100 mg/mL] (10 mL, 25 mL, 50 mL, 100 mL, 200 mL)

Gammaplex®: 5% [50 mg/mL] (50 mL, 100 mL, 200 mL)

Gamunex®: 10% [100 mg/mL] (10 mL, 25 mL, 50 mL, 100 mL, 200 mL)

Gamunex®-C: 10% [100 mg/mL] (10 mL, 25 mL, 50 mL, 100 mL, 200 mL)

Hizentra®: 200 mg/mL (5 mL, 10 mL, 20 mL)

Octagam®: 5% [50 mg/mL] (20 mL, 50 mL, 100 mL, 200 mL)

Privigen®: 10% [100 mg/mL] (50 mL, 100 mL, 200 mL)

Dosing

Adult & Geriatric According to manufacturer product labeling, intravenous formulations are for intravenous administration only. However, some clinicians may administer intravenous formulations as a subcutaneous infusion based on clinical judgment and patient tolerability. Some clinicians dose IVIG on ideal body weight or an adjusted ideal body weight in morbidly-obese patients (Siegel, 2010).

B-cell chronic lymphocytic leukemia (CLL) (Gammagard S/D®): I.V.: 400 mg/kg every 3-4 weeks

Chronic inflammatory demyelinating polyneuropathy (CIDP) (Gamunex®, Gamunex-C®): I.V.: Loading dose: 2000 mg/kg (given in divided doses over 2-4 consecutive days); Maintenance: 1000 mg/kg every 3 weeks. Alternatively, administer 500 mg/kg/day for 2 consecutive days every 3 weeks.

Hepatitis A (GamaSTAN™ S/D): I.M.:

Pre-exposure prophylaxis upon travel into endemic areas (hepatitis A vaccine preferred):

0.02 mL/kg for anticipated risk of exposure <3 months

0.06 mL/kg for anticipated risk of exposure ≥3 months; repeat every 4-6 months.

Postexposure prophylaxis: 0.02 mL/kg given within 14 days of exposure and/or prior to manifestation of disease; not needed if at least 1 dose of hepatitis A vaccine was given at ≥1 month before exposure

Immunoglobulin deficiency (GamaSTAN™ S/D): I.M.: 0.66 mL/kg (minimum dose should be 100 mg/kg) every 3-4 weeks. Administer a double dose at onset of therapy; some patients may require more frequent injections.

Immune (idiopathic) thrombocytopenic purpura (ITP):

Carimune® NF: I.V.: Initial: 400 mg/kg/day for 2-5 days; Maintenance: 400 mg/kg as needed to maintain platelet count ≥30,000/mm^3 and/or to control significant bleeding; may increase dose if needed (range: 800-1000 mg/kg)

Gammagard S/D®: I.V.: 1000 mg/kg; up to 3 additional doses may be given based on patient response and/or platelet count. **Note:** Additional doses should be given on alternate days.

Gamunex®, Gamunex-C®: I.V.: 1000 mg/kg/day for 2 consecutive days (second dose may be withheld if adequate platelet response in 24 hours) **or** 400 mg/kg once daily for 5 consecutive days

Privigen®: I.V.: 1000 mg/kg/day for 2 consecutive days

Kawasaki syndrome (Gammagard S/D®): I.V.:

Gammagard S/D®: 1000 mg/kg as a single dose **or** 400 mg/kg/day for 4 consecutive days. Begin within 7 days of onset of fever.

AHA guidelines (2004): 2000 mg/kg as a single dose within 10 days of disease onset

Note: Must be used in combination with aspirin: 80-100 mg/kg/day orally, divided every 6 hours for up to 14 days (until fever resolves for at least 48 hours); then decrease dose to 3-5 mg/kg/day once daily. In patients without coronary artery abnormalities, give lower dose for 6-8 weeks. In patients with coronary artery abnormalities, low-dose aspirin should be continued indefinitely.

Measles:

GamaSTAN™ S/D: I.M.:

Immunocompetent: 0.25 mL/kg given within 6 days of exposure followed by live attenuated measles vaccine in 5-6 months when indicated (Watson, 1998)

Immunocompromised children: 0.5 mL/kg (maximum dose: 15 mL) immediately following exposure

Gamunex-C®, Octagam®: I.V.:

Prophylaxis in patients with primary humoral immunodeficiency (**ONLY** if routine dose is <400 mg/kg): ≥400 mg/kg immediately before expected exposure

Treatment in patients with primary immunodeficiency: 400 mg/kg administered as soon as possible after exposure

Hizentra®: SubQ infusion: Measles exposure in patients with primary humoral immunodeficiency: Weekly dose: ≥200 mg/kg for 2 consecutive weeks for patients at risk of measles exposure (eg, during an outbreak; travel to endemic area). In patients who have been exposed to measles, administer the minimum dose as soon as possible following exposure.

Primary humoral immunodeficiency disorders:

Carimune® NF: I.V.: 400-800 mg/kg every 3-4 weeks

Flebogamma® DIF, Gammagard® Liquid, Gammagard S/D®, Gamunex®, Gamunex-C®, Octagam®: I.V.: 300-600 mg/kg every 3-4 weeks; adjusted based on dosage and interval in conjunction with monitored serum IgG concentrations and clinical response

Gammaplex®: I.V.: 300-800 mg/kg every 3-4 weeks

Gamunex-C®: SubQ infusion: Begin 1 week after last I.V. dose. Use the following equation to calculate initial dose:

Initial weekly dose (grams) = [1.37 x IGIV dose (grams)] divided by [I.V. dose interval (weeks)]

Note: For subsequent dose adjustments, refer to product labeling.

Hizentra®: SubQ infusion: Begin 1 week after last I.V. dose. Use the following equation to calculate initial dose:

Initial weekly dose (grams) = [1.53 x IGIV dose (grams)] divided by [I.V. dose interval (weeks)]

Note: For subsequent dose adjustments, refer to product labeling.

Privigen®: I.V.: 200-800 mg/kg every 3-4 weeks; adjusted based on dosage and interval in conjunction with monitored serum IgG concentrations and clinical response

Vivaglobin®: SubQ infusion: Begin 1 week after last I.V. dose; **Note:** Patient should have received an I.V. immune globulin routinely for at least 3 months before switching to SubQ. Use the following equation to calculate initial dose:

Initial weekly dose (grams) = [1.37 x IGIV dose (grams)] divided by [I.V. dose interval (weeks)]

Note: For subsequent dose adjustments, refer to product labeling.

Rubella (GamaSTAN™ S/D): I.M.: Prophylaxis during pregnancy: 0.55 mL/kg within 72 hours of exposure (Watson, 1998)

Varicella (GamaSTAN™ S/D): I.M.: Prophylaxis: 0.6-1.2 mL/kg (varicella zoster immune globulin preferred) within 72 hours of exposure

Unlabeled uses: I.V.:

Acquired hypogammaglobulinemia secondary to malignancy (unlabeled use): Adults: 400 mg/kg/dose every 3 weeks; reevaluate every 4-6 months (Anderson, 2007)

Guillain-Barré syndrome (unlabeled use): Children and Adults: Various regimens have been used, including:

400 mg/kg/day for 5 days (Hughes, 2003)

or

2000 mg/kg in divided doses administered over 2-5 days (Feasby, 2007)

Hematopoietic stem cell transplantation with hypogammaglobulinemia (CDC guidelines, 2000; unlabeled use):

Children: 400 mg/kg per month; increase dose or frequency to maintain IgG levels >400 mg/dL

Adolescents and Adults: 500 mg/kg/week

HIV-associated thrombocytopenia (unlabeled use): Adults: 1000 mg/kg/day for 2 days (Anderson, 2007)

Multiple sclerosis (relapsing-remitting, when other therapies cannot be used) (unlabeled use): Children and Adults: 1000 mg/kg per month, with or without an induction of 400 mg/kg/day for 5 days (Feasby, 2007)

Myasthenia gravis (severe exacerbation) (unlabeled use): Children and Adults: Total dose of 2000 mg/kg over 2-5 days (Feasby, 2007)

Refractory dermatomyositis/polymyositis (unlabeled uses): Children and Adults: 2000 mg/kg per treatment course administered over 2-5 days (Feasby, 2007)

Dosing adjustment/comments in renal impairment: Cl_{cr} <10 mL/minute: Avoid use; in patients at risk of renal dysfunction, consider infusion at a rate less than maximum.

Pediatric Refer to adult dosing.

Renal Impairment I.V.: Cl_{cr} <10 mL/minute: Avoid use; in patients at risk of renal dysfunction, consider infusion at a rate less than maximum.

Administration

I.M. Administer I.M. in the anterolateral aspects of the upper thigh or deltoid muscle of the upper arm. Avoid gluteal region due to risk of injury to sciatic nerve. Divide doses >10 mL and inject in multiple sites.

GamaSTAN™ S/D is for I.M. administration only.

I.V. Infuse over 2-24 hours; administer in separate infusion line from other medications; if using primary line, flush with saline prior to administration. Decrease dose, rate and/or concentration of infusion in patients who may be at risk of renal failure. Decreasing the rate or stopping the infusion may help relieve some adverse effects (flushing, changes in pulse rate, changes in blood pressure). Epinephrine should be available during administration.

For initial treatment or in the elderly, a lower concentration and/or a slower rate of infusion should be used. Initial rate of administration and titration is specific to each IVIG product. Consult specific product prescribing information for detailed recommendations. Refrigerated product should be warmed to room temperature prior to infusion. Some products require filtration; refer to individual product labeling. Antecubital veins should be used, especially with concentrations ≥10% to prevent injection site discomfort.

Other SubQ infusion: Initial dose should be administered in a healthcare setting capable of providing monitoring and treatment in the event of hypersensitivity. Using aseptic technique, follow the infusion device manufacturer's instructions for filling the reservoir and preparing the pump. Remove air from administration set and needle by priming. Appropriate injection sites include the abdomen, thigh, upper arm, and/or lateral hip; dose may be infused into multiple sites (spaced ≥2 inches apart) simultaneously. After the sites are clean and dry, insert subcutaneous needle and prime administration set. Attach sterile needle to administration set, gently pull back on the syringe to assure a blood vessel has not been inadvertently accessed (do not use needle and tubing if blood present). Repeat for each injection site; deliver the dose following instructions for the infusion device. Rotate the site(s) weekly. Treatment may be transitioned to the home/home care setting in the absence of adverse reactions.

Gamunex-C®:
Injection sites: ≤8 simultaneous injection sites
Recommended infusion rate: 20 mL/hour per injection site
Hizentra®:
Injection sites: ≤4 simultaneous injection sites
Maximum infusion rate: First infusion: 15 mL/hour per injection site; subsequent infusions: 25 mL/hour per injection site (maximum: 50 mL/hour for all simultaneous sites combined)
Maximum infusion volume: First 4 infusions: 15 mL per injection site; subsequent infusions: 20 mL per injection site (maximum: 25 mL per site as tolerated)
Vivaglobin®:
Injection sites: Children <45 kg: ≤3 simultaneous injection sites; Adults ≤65 years: ≤6 simultaneous injection sites; Adults >65 years: ≤4 simultaneous injection sites
Maximum infusion rate: 20 mL/hour per injection site (maximum: 3 mg/kg/minute [1.13 mL/kg/hour] for all simultaneous sites combined)
Maximum infusion volume: 15 mL per injection site

Stability

Reconstitution Dilution is dependent upon the manufacturer and brand. Gently swirl; do not shake; avoid foaming. Do not mix products from different manufacturers together. Discard unused portion of vials.

Carimune® NF: In a sterile laminar air flow environment, reconstitute with NS, D_5W, or SWFI. Complete dissolution may take up to 20 minutes. Begin infusion within 24 hours.
Flebogamma® DIF: Dilution is not recommended.
Gammagard® Liquid: May dilute in D_5W only.
Gammagard S/D®: Reconstitute with SWFI.
Gamunex®, Gamunex®-C: May dilute in D_5W only.
Privigen®: If necessary to further dilute, D_5W may be used.

Storage Stability is dependent upon the manufacturer and brand. Do not freeze.

Carimune® NF: Prior to reconstitution, store at or below 30°C (86°F). Reconstitute with NS, D_5W, or SWFI. Following reconstitution in a sterile laminar air flow environment, store under refrigeration. Begin infusion within 24 hours.
Flebogamma® DIF: Store at 2°C to 25°C (36°F to 77°F)); do not freeze.
GamaSTAN™ S/D: Store under refrigeration at 2°C to 8°C (36°F to 46°F). The following stability information has also been reported for GamaSTAN™ S/D: May be exposed to room temperature for a cumulative 7 days (Cohen, 2007).
Gammagard® Liquid: Prior to use, store at 2°C to 8°C (36°F to 46°F); do not freeze. May store at room temperature of 25°C (77°F) within the first 24 months of manufacturing. Storage time at room temperature varies with length of time previously refrigerated; refer to product labeling for details.
Gammagard S/D®: Store at ≤25°C (≤77°F). May store diluted solution under refrigeration at 2°C to 8°C (36°F to 46°F) for up to 24 hours if originally prepared in a sterile laminar air flow environment.
Gammaplex®: Store at 2°C to 25°C (36°F to 77°F); do not freeze. Protect from light.
Gamunex®, Gamunex®-C: Store at 2°C to 8°C (36°F to 46°F); may be stored at ≤25°C (≤77°F) for up to 6 months.
Hizentra®: Store at ≤25°C (≤77°F); do not freeze or use product if previously frozen. Do not shake.
Octagam®: Store at 2°C to 25°C (36°F to 77°F).
Privigen®: Store at ≤25°C (≤77°F); do not freeze (do not use if previously frozen). Protect from light.
Vivaglobin®: Store at 2°C to 8°C (36°F to 46°F); do not freeze or use product if previously frozen. Do not shake.

Monitoring and Teaching Issues

Laboratory Monitoring Renal function, IgG concentrations, hemoglobin and hematocrit, platelets (in patients with ITP); presence of antineutrophil antibodies (if TRALI is suspected)

SubQ infusion: Monitor IgG trough levels every 2-3 months before/after conversion from I.V.; subcutaneous infusions provide more constant IgG levels than usual I.V. immune globulin treatments.

Physical Assessment Assess for history of previous allergic reactions. Patient should be monitored during infusion or injection for vital sign changes and adverse or allergic reactions. Hypersensitivity and anaphylaxis can occur. Medications for the treatment of hypersensitivity reactions should be available for immediate use. Teach patient adverse symptoms to report.

Patient Education This medication can be administered I.M., I.V. or SubQ. You will be monitored closely during the I.V. or SubQ infusion. If you experience nausea ask for assistance, do not get up alone. Immediately report chills; chest pain, tightness, or rapid heartbeat; acute back pain; or respiratory difficulty during infusion. Also report decrease in urine output, swelling of extremities, or weight gain; fever and other signs of infection; trouble breathing; increased heart rate, yellowing of skin or eyes, dark urine; stiff neck, severe headache, unexplained drowsiness, or sensitivity to light.

Dietary Considerations Some products may contain sodium.

Pregnancy Considerations Reproduction studies have not been conducted. Immune globulins cross the placenta in increased amounts after 30 weeks gestation. Intravenous immune globulin has been recommended for use in fetal-neonatal alloimmune thrombocytopenia and pregnancy-associated ITP.

Additional Information I.M.: When administering immune globulin for hepatitis A prophylaxis, use should be considered for the following close contacts of persons with confirmed hepatitis A: unvaccinated household and sexual contacts, persons who have shared illicit drugs, regular babysitters, staff and attendees of child care centers, food handlers within the same establishment (*MMWR*, 2006).

All household contacts of measles patients should be evaluated to receive immune globulin unless the measles vaccine has been given on or after the first birthday, unless immunocompromised (*MMWR*, 1998).

For travelers, immune globulin is not an alternative to careful selection of foods and water; immune globulin can interfere with the antibody response to parenterally administered live virus vaccines. Frequent travelers should be tested for hepatitis A antibody, immune hemolytic anemia, and neutropenia (with ITP, I.V. route is usually used).

IgA content:
Carimune® NF: 720 mcg/mL
Flebogamma® 5% DIF: 2.9 ± 0.1 mcg/mL
Flebogamma® 10% DIF: <100 mcg/mL
Gammagard® Liquid: 37 mcg/mL
Gammagard S/D® 5% solution: <1 mcg/mL or <2.2 mcg/mL(product dependent)
Gammaplex®: <10 mcg/mL
Gamunex-C®: 46 mcg/mL
Hizentra®: ≤50 mcg/mL
Octagam®: ≤200 mcg/mL
Privigen®: ≤25 mcg/mL
Vivaglobin®: ≤1700 mcg/mL

Related Information
Immunization Recommendations *on page* 1941
Intravenous Immune Globulin *on page* 1999

◆ **Immune Globulin Subcutaneous (Human)** *see* Immune Globulin *on page* 961
◆ **Immune Serum Globulin** *see* Immune Globulin *on page* 961
◆ **Imodium® A-D [OTC]** *see* Loperamide *on page* 1126
◆ **Imodium® A-D for children [OTC]** *see* Loperamide *on page* 1126
◆ **Imovax® Rabies** *see* Rabies Vaccine *on page* 1546
◆ **Implanon™** *see* Etonogestrel *on page* 710
◆ **Imuran®** *see* AzaTHIOprine *on page* 178

Indapamide (in DAP a mide)

Generic Availability (U.S.) Yes
Pharmacologic Category Diuretic, Thiazide-Related
Medication Safety Issues
Sound-alike/look-alike issues:
Indapamide may be confused with Iopidine®
International issues:
Pretanix [Hungary] may be confused with Protonix brand name for pantoprazole [U.S., Canada]
Pregnancy Risk Factor B (manufacturer); D (expert analysis)
Lactation Excretion in breast milk unknown
Use Management of mild-to-moderate hypertension; treatment of edema in heart failure and nephrotic syndrome
Available Dosage Forms
Tablet, oral: 1.25 mg, 2.5 mg
Dosing
Adult & Geriatric
Edema: Oral: 2.5-5 mg/day. **Note:** There is little therapeutic benefit to increasing the dose >5 mg/day; there is, however, an increased risk of electrolyte disturbances.
Hypertension: Oral: 1.25 mg in the morning, may increase to 5 mg/day by increments of 1.25-2.5 mg; consider adding another antihypertensive and decreasing the dose if response is not adequate.
Administration
Oral May be taken with food or milk. Take early in day to avoid nocturia. Take the last dose of multiple doses no later than 6 PM unless instructed otherwise.
Monitoring and Teaching Issues
Laboratory Monitoring Serum electrolytes, renal function
Physical Assessment Assess allergy history prior to beginning therapy (sulfonamides, thiazides). Monitor for hypotension, hypokalemia, and photosensitivity at regular intervals during therapy.
Patient Education Take early in the day. Follow prescriber's instructions for diet and lifestyle changes. Monitor weight on a regular basis. Report weight gain, swelling of ankles or hands, or respiratory difficulty. You may experience dizziness, weakness, sensitivity to sunlight, or dry mouth.

◆ **Inderal® LA** *see* Propranolol *on page* 1522

◆ **Inderide** *see* Propranolol and Hydrochlorothiazide *on page* 1526

Indinavir (in DIN a veer)

U.S. Brand Names Crixivan®

Index Terms Indinavir Sulfate

Generic Availability (U.S.) No

Pharmacologic Category Antiretroviral Agent, Protease Inhibitor

Medication Safety Issues

Sound-alike/look-alike issues:

Indinavir may be confused with Denavir™

Pregnancy Risk Factor C

Lactation Excretion in breast milk unknown/contraindicated

Use Treatment of HIV infection; should always be used as part of a multidrug regimen (at least three antiretroviral agents)

Mechanism of Action/Effect Blocks the site of HIV-1 protease activity, resulting in the formation of immature, noninfectious viral particles.

Contraindications Hypersensitivity to indinavir or any component of the formulation; concurrent use of alfuzosin, alprazolam, amiodarone, cisapride, triazolam, midazolam (oral), pimozide, or ergot alkaloids; sildenafil (when used for pulmonary artery hypertension [eg, Revatio®]), simvastatin, St John's wort, or triazolam

Warnings/Precautions Because indinavir may cause nephrolithiasis/urolithiasis the drug should be discontinued if signs and symptoms occur. Adequate hydration is recommended. May cause tubulointerstitial nephritis (rare); severe asymptomatic leukocyturia may warrant evaluation. Use with caution in patients taking strong CYP3A4 inhibitors, moderate or strong CYP3A4 inducers and major CYP3A4 substrates (see Drug Interactions); consider alternative agents that avoid or lessen the potential for CYP-mediated interactions. Do not coadminister colchicine in patient with renal or hepatic impairment; avoid concurrent use with salmeterol.

Patients with hepatic insufficiency due to cirrhosis should have dose reduction. Warn patients about fat redistribution that can occur. Indinavir has been associated with hemolytic anemia (discontinue if diagnosed), hepatitis, hyperbilirubinemia, and hyperglycemia (exacerbation or new-onset diabetes). Treatment may result in immune reconstitution syndrome (acute inflammatory response to indolent or residual opportunistic infections). Use caution in patients with hemophilia; spontaneous bleeding has been reported.

Drug Interactions

Metabolism/Transport Effects Substrate of CYP2D6 (minor), CYP3A4 (major), P-glycoprotein; **Inhibits** CYP2C9 (weak), 2C19 (weak), 2D6 (weak), 3A4 (strong)

Avoid Concomitant Use

Avoid concomitant use of Indinavir with any of the following: Alfuzosin; ALPRAZolam; Amiodarone; Atazanavir; Cisapride; Conivaptan; Dronedarone; Eplerenone; Ergot Derivatives; Everolimus; Halofantrine; Lovastatin; Lurasidone; Midazolam; Nilotinib; Nisoldipine; Pimozide; QuiNIDine; Ranolazine; Rifampin; Rivaroxaban; RomiDEPsin; Salmeterol; Silodosin; Simvastatin; St Johns Wort; Tamsulosin; Tolvaptan; Toremifene; Triazolam

Decreased Effect

Indinavir may decrease the levels/effects of: Abacavir; Clarithromycin; Contraceptives (Estrogens); Delavirdine; Divalproex; Etravirine; Meperidine; Prasugrel; Theophylline Derivatives; Valproic Acid; Zidovudine

The levels/effects of Indinavir may be decreased by: Antacids; Atovaquone; Bosentan; CarBAMazepine; Contraceptives (Estrogens); CYP3A4 Inducers (Strong); Deferasirox; Didanosine; Efavirenz; Garlic; H2-Antagonists; Nevirapine; Peginterferon Alfa-2b; P-Glycoprotein Inducers; Proton Pump Inhibitors; Rifabutin; Rifampin; St Johns Wort; Tenofovir; Venlafaxine

Increased Effect/Toxicity

Indinavir may increase the levels/effects of: Alfuzosin; Almotriptan; Alosetron; ALPRAZolam; Amiodarone; Antifungal Agents (Azole Derivatives, Systemic); Atazanavir; Bortezomib; Bosentan; Brinzolamide; Calcium Channel Blockers (Dihydropyridine); Calcium Channel Blockers (Nondihydropyridine); CarBAMazepine; Ciclesonide; Cisapride; Clarithromycin; Colchicine; Conivaptan; Corticosteroids (Orally Inhaled); CycloSPORINE; CycloSPORINE (Systemic); CYP3A4 Substrates; Dienogest; Digoxin; Dronedarone; Dutasteride; Enfuvirtide; Eplerenone; Ergot Derivatives; Everolimus; FentaNYL; Fesoterodine; Fusidic Acid; GuanFACINE; Halofantrine; HMG-CoA Reductase Inhibitors; Ixabepilone; Lovastatin; Lumefantrine; Lurasidone; Maraviroc; Meperidine; MethylPREDNISolone; Midazolam; Nefazodone; Nilotinib; Nisoldipine; Paricalcitol; Pazopanib; Pimecrolimus; Pimozide; Protease Inhibitors; QuiNIDine; Ranolazine; Rifabutin; Rivaroxaban; RomiDEPsin; Salmeterol; Saxagliptin; Sildenafil; Silodosin; Simvastatin; Sirolimus; SORAfenib; Tacrolimus; Tacrolimus (Systemic); Tacrolimus (Topical); Tadalafil; Tamsulosin; Temsirolimus; Tenofovir; Tolvaptan; Toremifene; TraZODone; Triazolam; Tricyclic Antidepressants; Vardenafil; Vilazodone

The levels/effects of Indinavir may be increased by: Antifungal Agents (Azole Derivatives, Systemic); Atazanavir; Clarithromycin; CycloSPORINE; CycloSPORINE (Systemic); Delavirdine; Efavirenz; Enfuvirtide; Etravirine; Fusidic Acid; P-Glycoprotein Inhibitors

Nutritional/Ethanol Interactions

Food: Indinavir bioavailability may be decreased if taken with food. Meals high in calories, fat, and protein result in a significant decrease in drug levels. Indinavir serum concentrations may be decreased by grapefruit juice.

Herb/Nutraceutical: Garlic may decrease the levels/effects of protease inhibitors. St John's wort *(Hypericum)* appears to induce CYP3A enzymes and has lead to 57% reductions in indinavir AUCs and 81% reductions in trough serum concentrations, which may lead to treatment failures; should not be used concurrently with indinavir.

Adverse Reactions

>10%:

Gastrointestinal: Abdominal pain (17%), nausea (12%)

Hepatic: Hyperbilirubinemia (14%; dose dependent)

Renal: Nephrolithiasis/urolithiasis, including flank pain with/without hematuria (29%, pediatric patients; 12% adult patients; dose dependent)

1% to 10%:

Central nervous system: Headache (5%), dizziness (3%), somnolence (2%), fever (2%), malaise (2%), fatigue (2%)

Dermatologic: Pruritus (4%), rash (1%)

Endocrine & metabolic: Hyperglycemia (1%)

Gastrointestinal: Vomiting (8%), diarrhea (3%), taste perversion (3%), acid reflux (3%), anorexia (3%), appetite increased (2%), dyspepsia (2%), serum amylase increased (2%)

Hematologic: Neutropenia (2%), anemia (1%), thrombocytopenia (1%)

Hepatic: Transaminases increased (4% to 5%), jaundice (2%)

Neuromuscular & skeletal: Back pain (8%), weakness (2%)

Renal: Dysuria (2%)

Respiratory: Cough (2%)

Pharmacodynamics/Kinetics

Absorption Administration with a high fat, high calorie diet resulted in a reduction in AUC and in maximum serum concentration (77% and 84% respectively); lighter meal resulted in little or no change in these parameters.

Bioavailability Good

Time to Peak 0.8 ± 0.3 hour

Protein Binding Plasma: 60%

Half-Life Elimination 1.8 ± 0.4 hour; hepatic insufficiency: 2.8 ± 0.5 hour

Metabolism Hepatic via CYP3A4 enzymes; seven metabolites of indinavir identified

Excretion Feces (83%; 19% as unchanged drug); urine (19%; 9% as unchanged drug)

Available Dosage Forms

Capsule, oral:

Crixivan®: 100 mg, 200 mg, 400 mg

Dosing

Adult & Geriatric HIV infection: Oral:

Unboosted regimen: 800 mg every 8 hours

Ritonavir-boosted regimen: Ritonavir 100-200 mg twice daily plus indinavir 800 mg twice daily

Dosage adjustments for indinavir when administered in combination therapy:

Delavirdine, itraconazole, or ketoconazole: Reduce indinavir dose to 600 mg every 8 hours

Efavirenz: Increase indinavir dose to 1000 mg every 8 hours

Lopinavir and ritonavir (Kaletra™): Indinavir 600 mg twice daily

Nelfinavir: Increase indinavir dose to 1200 mg twice daily

Nevirapine: Increase indinavir dose to 1000 mg every 8 hours

Rifabutin: Reduce rifabutin to 1/2 the standard dose plus increase indinavir to 1000 mg every 8 hours

Dosage adjustments for concomitant therapy: Oral:

Coadministration with bosentan:

Coadministration of bosentan in patients currently receiving indinavir: Begin with bosentan 62.5 mg once daily or every other day based on tolerability

Coadministration of indinavir in patients currently receiving bosentan: Adjust bosentan to 62.5 mg once daily or every other day based on tolerability

Coadministration with colchicine:

Familial Mediterranean fever (FMF): Maximum colchicine dose: 0.6 mg/day (0.3 mg twice daily)

Gout prophylaxis:

If original colchicine dose is 0.6 mg twice daily, adjust dose to 0.3 mg once daily

If original colchicine dose is 0.6 mg once daily, adjust dose to 0.3 mg every other day

Gout flare treatment: Initial: Colchicine 0.6 mg, followed in 1 hour by a single dose of 0.3 mg; do not repeat for at least 3 days

Coadministration with phosphodiesterase-5 enzyme (PDE-5) inhibitor:

Pulmonary arterial hypertension: Indinavir coadministered with tadalafil:

Patient receiving indinavir when initiating tadalafil: Initiate tadalafil at 20 mg once daily; increase to 40 mg once daily based on individual tolerability

Patient receiving tadalafil when initiating indinavir: Adjust tadalafil to 20 mg once daily; increase to 40 mg once daily based on individual tolerability.

Erectile dysfunction: Indinavir coadministered with:

Sildenafil (Viagra®): Maximum sildenafil dose: 25 mg in a 48-hour period

Tadalafil (Cialis®): Maximum tadalafil dose: 10 mg in a 72-hour period

Vardenafil: Maximum vardenafil dose: 2.5 mg in a 24-hour period

Pediatric HIV: Children 4-15 years (investigational): 500 mg/m^2 every 8 hours

Hepatic Impairment 600 mg every 8 hours with mild/medium impairment due to cirrhosis

Administration

Oral Drink at least 48 oz of water daily. Administer with water, 1 hour before or 2 hours after a meal. May also be administered with other liquids (eg, skim milk, juice, coffee, tea) or a light meal (eg, toast, corn flakes). Administer around-the-clock to avoid significant fluctuation in serum levels. May be taken with food when administered in combination with ritonavir.

Stability

Storage Medication should be stored at 15°C to 30°C (59°F to 86°F), and used in the original container and the desiccant should remain in the bottle. Capsules are sensitive to moisture.

Monitoring and Teaching Issues

Laboratory Monitoring Monitor viral load, CD4 count, triglycerides, cholesterol, glucose, liver function tests, CBC, urinalysis (severe leukocyturia should be monitored frequently).

Physical Assessment Assess CD4 count and hepatic function. Monitor for gastrointestinal disturbance (nausea, vomiting, diarrhea) that can lead to dehydration and weight loss, hyperlipidemia and redistribution of body fat, rash, CNS effects (malaise, insomnia, abnormal thinking), and electrolyte imbalance at regular intervals during therapy. Caution patients to monitor glucose levels closely; protease inhibitors may cause hyperglycemia or new-onset diabetes. Teach patient proper timing of multiple medications. Instruct patient on glucose testing.

Patient Education This is not a cure for HIV, nor has it been found to reduce transmission of HIV; use appropriate precautions to prevent spread to other persons. Take with meals. Maintain adequate hydration, unless instructed to restrict fluid intake. This medication will be prescribed with a combination of other medications; time these medications as directed by prescriber. You may be advised to check your glucose levels; this class of drug can cause hyperglycemia. Frequent blood tests may be required. May cause body changes due to redistribution of body fat, facial atrophy, or breast enlargement (normal effects of drug); headache, dizziness, or fatigue; nausea or vomiting; diarrhea; back pain, or arthralgia. Inform prescriber if you experience muscle numbness or tingling; unresolved persistent vomiting, diarrhea, or abdominal pain; respiratory difficulty or chest pain; unusual skin rash; or change in color of stool or urine.

Dietary Considerations Should be taken without food but with water 1 hour before or 2 hours after a meal. Administration with lighter meals (eg, dry toast, skim milk, corn flakes) resulted in little/no change in indinavir concentration. If taking with ritonavir, may take with food. Patient should drink at least 48 oz of water daily.

Breast-Feeding Considerations In infants born to mothers who are HIV positive, HAART while breast-feeding may decrease postnatal infection. However, maternal or infant antiretroviral therapy does not completely eliminate the risk of postnatal HIV transmission. In addition, multiclass-resistant virus has been detected in breast-feeding infants despite maternal therapy.

In the United States where formula is accessible, affordable, safe, and sustainable, complete avoidance of breast-feeding by HIV-infected women is recommended to decrease potential transmission of HIV.

Pregnancy Considerations Adverse events were observed in some animal reproduction studies. No increased risk of overall birth defects has been observed according to data collected by the antiretroviral pregnancy registry. Plasma levels of indinavir were 74% lower at weeks 30-32 of gestation when compared to the same women at 14-28 weeks of gestation. Plasma levels were not measurable in some patients 8 hours post dose. It is not known if indinavir will exacerbate hyperbilirubinemia in neonates. Pregnancy and protease inhibitors are both associated with an increased risk of hyperglycemia. Glucose levels should be closely monitored. Until optimal dosing during pregnancy has been established, the manufacturer does not recommend indinavir use in pregnant patients. The AIDS*info* guidelines consider indinavir an alternative agent if lopinavir/ritonavir cannot be used, however, indinavir should be used in combination with low-dose ritonavir during pregnancy (with ritonavir boosting, 82% of pregnant women reached target trough concentrations). Healthcare providers are encouraged to enroll pregnant women exposed to antiretroviral medications in the Antiretroviral Pregnancy Registry (1-800-258-4263 or www.APRegistry.com). Healthcare providers caring for HIV-infected women and their infants may contact the National Perinatal HIV Hotline (888-448-8765) for clinical consultation.

◆ **Indinavir Sulfate** *see* Indinavir *on page 967*

◆ **Indocin®** *see* Indomethacin *on page 969*

◆ **Indocin® I.V.** *see* Indomethacin *on page 969*

◆ **Indometacin** *see* Indomethacin *on page 969*

Indomethacin (in doe METH a sin)

U.S. Brand Names Indocin®; Indocin® I.V.

Index Terms Indometacin; Indomethacin Sodium Trihydrate

Generic Availability (U.S.) Yes: Excludes oral suspension

Pharmacologic Category Nonsteroidal Anti-inflammatory Drug (NSAID), Oral; Nonsteroidal Anti-inflammatory Drug (NSAID), Parenteral

Medication Safety Issues

Sound-alike/look-alike issues:

Indocin® may be confused with Imodium®, Lincocin®, Minocin®, Vicodin®

Beers Criteria medication: This drug may be inappropriate for use in geriatric patients (high severity risk).

International issues:

Flexin® [Great Britain] may be confused with Floxin® which is a brand name for ofloxacin in the U.S.

Flexin® [Great Britain]: Brand name for orphenadrine in Israel

Medication Guide Available Yes

Pregnancy Risk Factor C

Lactation Enters breast milk/not recommended (AAP rates "compatible"; AAP 2001 update pending)

Use Acute gouty arthritis, acute bursitis/tendonitis, moderate-to-severe osteoarthritis, rheumatoid arthritis, ankylosing spondylitis; I.V. form used as alternative to surgery for closure of patent ductus arteriosus in neonates

Unlabeled/Investigational Use Management of preterm labor

Mechanism of Action/Effect Reversibly inhibits cyclooxygenase-1 and 2 (COX-1 and 2) enzymes, which results in decreased formation of prostaglandin precursors; has antipyretic, analgesic, and anti-inflammatory properties

Contraindications Hypersensitivity to indomethacin, aspirin, other NSAIDs, or any component of the formulation; perioperative pain in the setting of coronary artery bypass graft (CABG) surgery; patients with a history of proctitis or recent rectal bleeding (suppositories)

Neonates: Necrotizing enterocolitis; impaired renal function; active bleeding (including intracranial hemorrhage and gastrointestinal bleeding), thrombocytopenia, coagulation defects; untreated infection; congenital heart disease where patent ductus arteriosus is necessary

Warnings/Precautions [U.S. Boxed Warning]: NSAIDs are associated with an increased risk of adverse cardiovascular thrombotic events, including MI and stroke. Risk may be increased with duration of use or pre-existing cardiovascular risk factors or disease. May cause new-onset hypertension or worsening of existing hypertension. Use caution with fluid retention. Avoid use in heart failure. Concurrent administration of ibuprofen, and potentially other nonselective NSAIDs, may interfere with aspirin's cardioprotective effect. **[U.S. Boxed Warning]: Use is contraindicated for treatment of perioperative pain in the setting of coronary artery bypass graft (CABG) surgery.** Risk of MI and stroke may be increased with use following CABG surgery.

Platelet adhesion and aggregation may be decreased; may prolong bleeding time; patients with coagulation disorders or who are receiving anticoagulants should be monitored closely. Anemia may occur; patients on long-term NSAID therapy should be monitored for anemia. Rarely, NSAID use may cause severe blood dyscrasias (eg, agranulocytosis, aplastic anemia, thrombocytopenia).

NSAID use may compromise existing renal function; dose-dependent decreases in prostaglandin synthesis may result from NSAID use, reducing renal blood flow which may cause renal decompensation. NSAID use may increase the risk for hyperkalemia. Patients with impaired renal function, dehydration, heart failure, liver dysfunction, those taking diuretics, and ACE inhibitors are at greater risk of renal toxicity and hyperkalemia. Rehydrate patient before starting therapy; monitor renal function closely. Not recommended for use in patients with advanced renal disease. Long-term NSAID use may result in renal papillary necrosis.

The elderly are at increased risk for adverse effects (especially peptic ulceration, CNS effects, renal toxicity) from NSAIDs even at low doses. Risk of CNS adverse events may be higher with indomethacin compared to other NSAIDs; avoid use in this age group (Beers Criteria).

[U.S. Boxed Warning]: NSAIDs may increase risk of gastrointestinal irritation, inflammation, ulceration, bleeding, and perforation. Use caution with a history of GI disease (bleeding or ulcers), concurrent therapy with aspirin, anticoagulants and/or corticosteroids, smoking, use of alcohol, the elderly or debilitated patients. When used concomitantly with ≤325 mg of aspirin, a substantial increase in the risk of gastrointestinal complications (eg, ulcer) occurs; concomitant gastroprotective therapy (eg, proton pump inhibitors) is recommended (Bhatt, 2008).

Use the lowest effective dose for the shortest duration of time, consistent with individual patient goals, to reduce risk of cardiovascular or GI adverse events. Alternate therapies should be considered for patients at high risk.

NSAIDS may cause drowsiness, dizziness, blurred vision and other neurologic effects which may impair physical or mental abilities; patients must be cautioned about performing tasks which require mental alertness (eg, operating machinery or driving). Discontinue use with blurred or diminished vision and perform ophthalmologic exam. Monitor vision with long-term therapy.

NSAIDs may cause serious skin adverse events including exfoliative dermatitis, Stevens-Johnson syndrome (SJS) and toxic epidermal necrolysis (TEN); discontinue use at first sign of skin rash or hypersensitivity. Anaphylactoid reactions may occur, even without prior exposure; patients with "aspirin triad" (bronchial asthma, aspirin intolerance, rhinitis) may be at increased risk. Do not use in patients who experience bronchospasm, asthma, rhinitis, or urticaria with NSAID or aspirin therapy. Use caution in other forms of asthma.

Use with caution in patients with decreased hepatic function. Closely monitor patients with any abnormal LFT. Severe hepatic reactions (eg, fulminant hepatitis, liver failure) have occurred with NSAID use, rarely; discontinue if signs or symptoms of liver disease develop, or if systemic manifestations occur. The elderly are at increased risk for adverse effects (especially peptic ulceration, CNS effects, renal toxicity) from NSAIDs even at low doses. Prolonged use may cause corneal deposits and retinal disturbances; discontinue if visual changes are observed. Use caution with depression, epilepsy, or Parkinson's disease.

Withhold for at least 4-6 half-lives prior to surgical or dental procedures.

Oral: Safety and efficacy have not been established in children <14 years of age. Hepatotoxicity has been reported in younger children treated for juvenile idiopathic arthritis (JIA). Closely monitor if use is needed in children ≥2 years of age.

Drug Interactions

Metabolism/Transport Effects Substrate (minor) of CYP2C9, 2C19; **Inhibits** CYP2C9 (strong), 2C19 (weak)

Avoid Concomitant Use

Avoid concomitant use of Indomethacin with any of the following: Ketorolac; Ketorolac (Systemic)

Decreased Effect

Indomethacin may decrease the levels/effects of: ACE Inhibitors; Angiotensin II Receptor Blockers; Antiplatelet Agents; Beta-Blockers; Eplerenone; HydrALAZINE; Loop Diuretics; Potassium-Sparing Diuretics; Salicylates; Thiazide Diuretics

The levels/effects of Indomethacin may be decreased by: Bile Acid Sequestrants; Nonsteroidal Anti-Inflammatory Agents; Salicylates

Increased Effect/Toxicity

Indomethacin may increase the levels/effects of: Aminoglycosides; Anticoagulants; Antiplatelet Agents; Bisphosphonate Derivatives; Collagenase (Systemic); CycloSPORINE; CycloSPORINE (Systemic); Desmopressin; Digoxin; Drotrecogin Alfa; Eplerenone; Haloperidol; Ibritumomab; Lithium; Methotrexate; Nonsteroidal Anti-Inflammatory Agents; PEMEtrexed; Potassium-Sparing Diuretics; PRALAtrexate; Quinolone Antibiotics; Salicylates; Thrombolytic Agents; Tiludronate; Tositumomab and Iodine I 131 Tositumomab; Triamterene; Vancomycin; Vitamin K Antagonists

The levels/effects of Indomethacin may be increased by: Antidepressants (Tricyclic, Tertiary Amine); Corticosteroids (Systemic); Dasatinib; Glucosamine; Herbs (Anticoagulant/Antiplatelet Properties); Ketorolac; Ketorolac (Systemic); Nonsteroidal Anti-Inflammatory Agents; Omega-3-Acid Ethyl Esters; Pentosan Polysulfate Sodium; Pentoxifylline; Probenecid; Prostacyclin Analogues; Selective Serotonin Reuptake Inhibitors; Serotonin/Norepinephrine Reuptake Inhibitors; Treprostinil

Nutritional/Ethanol Interactions

Ethanol: Avoid ethanol (may enhance gastric mucosal irritation).

Food: Food may decrease the rate but not the extent of absorption. Indomethacin peak serum levels may be delayed if taken with food.

Herb/Nutraceutical: Avoid alfalfa, anise, bilberry, bladderwrack, bromelain, cat's claw, celery, chamomile, coleus, cordyceps, dong quai, evening primrose, fenugreek, feverfew, garlic, ginger, ginkgo biloba, ginseng (American, Panax, Siberian), grapeseed, green tea, guggul, horse chestnut seed, horseradish, licorice, prickly ash, red clover, reishi, SAMe (S-adenosylmethionine), sweet clover, turmeric, white willow (all have additional antiplatelet activity).

Lab Interactions False-negative dexamethasone suppression test

Adverse Reactions

>10%: Central nervous system: Headache (12%)

1% to 10%:

Central nervous system: Dizziness (3% to 9%), depression (<3%), fatigue (<3%), malaise (<3%), somnolence (<3%), vertigo (<3%)

Gastrointestinal: Dyspepsia (3% to 9%), epigastric pain (3% to 9%), heartburn (3% to 9%), indigestion (3% to 9%), nausea (3% to 9%), abdominal pain/cramps/distress (<3%), constipation (<3%), diarrhea (<3%), rectal irritation (suppository), tenesmus (suppository), vomiting

Otic: Tinnitus (<3%)

Pharmacodynamics/Kinetics

Onset of Action ~30 minutes

Duration of Action 4-6 hours

Absorption Oral: Immediate release: Prompt and extensive; Extended release: 90% over 12 hours

Bioavailability 100%

Time to Peak Oral: Immediate release: 2 hours

Protein Binding 99%

Half-Life Elimination 4.5 hours; prolonged with neonates

Metabolism Hepatic; significant enterohepatic recirculation

Excretion Urine (60%, primarily as glucuronide conjugates); feces (33%, primarily as metabolites)

Available Dosage Forms

Capsule, oral: 25 mg, 50 mg

Capsule, extended release, oral: 75 mg

Injection, powder for reconstitution: 1 mg

Indocin® I.V.: 1 mg

Suppository, rectal: 50 mg (30s)

Suspension, oral:

Indocin®: 25 mg/5 mL (237 mL)

Dosing

Adult

Inflammatory/rheumatoid disorders (use lowest effective dose): Oral: 25-50 mg/dose 2-3 times/day; maximum dose: 200 mg/day; extended release capsule should be given on a 1-2 times/day schedule (maximum dose for extended release: 150 mg/day). In patients with arthritis and persistent night pain and/or morning stiffness, may give the larger portion (up to 100 mg) of the total daily dose at bedtime.

Bursitis/tendonitis: Oral: Initial dose: 75-150 mg/day in 3-4 divided doses **or** 1-2 divided doses for extended release; usual treatment is 7-14 days

Acute gouty arthritis: Oral: 50 mg 3 times daily until pain is tolerable then reduce dose; usual treatment <3-5 days

Geriatric Refer to adult dosing. Use lowest recommended dose and frequency in elderly to initiate therapy for indications listed in adult dosing.

Pediatric

Patent ductus arteriosus:

Neonates: I.V.: Initial: 0.2 mg/kg, followed by 2 doses depending on postnatal age (PNA):

PNA at time of FIRST dose <48 hours: 0.1 mg/kg at 12- to 24-hour intervals

PNA at time of FIRST dose 2-7 days: 0.2 mg/kg at 12- to 24-hour intervals

PNA at time of FIRST dose >7 days: 0.25 mg/kg at 12- to 24-hour intervals

Note: In general, may use 12-hour dosing interval if urine output >1 mL/kg/hour after prior dose; use 24-hour dosing interval if urine output is <1 mL/kg/hour but >0.6 mL/kg/hour; doses should be withheld if patient has oliguria (urine output <0.6 mL/kg/hour) or anuria

Inflammatory/rheumatoid disorders: Children ≥2 years: Oral: 1-2 mg/kg/day in 2-4 divided doses; maximum dose: 4 mg/kg/day; not to exceed 150-200 mg/day

Renal Impairment Not recommended with advanced renal disease.

Administration

Oral Administer with food, milk, or antacids to decrease GI adverse effects. Extended release capsules must be swallowed whole; do not crush.

I.V. Administer over 20-30 minutes. Reconstitute I.V. formulation just prior to administration; discard any unused portion; avoid I.V. bolus administration or infusion via an umbilical catheter into vessels near the superior mesenteric artery as these may cause vasoconstriction and can compromise blood flow to the intestines. Do not administer intra-arterially.

Stability

Reconstitution Reconstitute with 1-2 mL preservative free NS or SWFI just prior to administration. Discard any unused portion. Do not use preservative-containing diluents for reconstitution.

Storage I.V.: Store below 30°C (86°F). Protect from light.

Monitoring and Teaching Issues

Laboratory Monitoring Renal function (serum creatinine and BUN), CBC, liver function (particularly with pediatric use)

Physical Assessment Evaluate cardiac risk and potential for GI bleeding prior to prescribing this medication. Monitor blood pressure prior to treatment and periodically throughout. Regular ophthalmic evaluations are recommended.

Patient Education Do not crush, break, or chew extended-release capsules. Take with food or milk to reduce GI distress. Maintain adequate hydration, unless instructed to restrict fluid intake. May cause drowsiness, dizziness, nervousness, headache, anorexia, nausea, vomiting, heartburn, or fluid retention (weigh yourself weekly and report unusual weight gain). GI bleeding, ulceration, or perforation can occur with or without pain; discontinue medication and contact prescriber if persistent abdominal pain or cramping or blood in stool occurs. Report difficult breathing or unusual cough; chest pain, rapid heartbeat, or palpitations; unusual bruising or bleeding; blood in urine, gums, or vomitus; swollen extremities; skin rash, irritation, or itching; acute persistent fatigue; vision changes; or ringing in ears.

Dietary Considerations May cause GI upset; take with food or milk to minimize

Geriatric Considerations Elderly are a high-risk population for adverse effects from NSAIDs. As much as 60% of elderly can develop peptic ulceration and/or hemorrhage asymptomatically. The concomitant use of H_2 blockers and sucralfate is not effective as prophylaxis with the exception of NSAID-induced duodenal ulcers which may be prevented by the use of ranitidine. Misoprostol and proton pump inhibitors are the only agents proven to help prevent the development of NSAID-induced ulcers. Also, concomitant disease and drug use contribute to the risk for GI adverse effects. Use lowest effective dose for shortest period possible. Consider renal function decline with age. Use of NSAIDs may compromise existing renal function especially when Cl_{cr} is ≤30 mL/minute. Tinnitus may be a difficult and unreliable indication of toxicity due to age-related hearing loss or eighth cranial nerve damage. CNS adverse effects such as confusion, agitation, and hallucination are generally seen in overdose or high-dose situations, but the elderly may demonstrate these adverse effects at lower doses than younger adults. Indomethacin frequently causes confusion at recommended doses in the elderly.

This medication is considered to be potentially inappropriate in this patient population (Beers Criteria severity: High).

Breast-Feeding Considerations Indomethacin is excreted into breast milk and low amounts have been measured in the plasma of nursing infants. Seizures in a nursing infant were observed in one case report, although adverse events have not been noted in other cases. Breast-feeding is not recommended by the manufacturer. (The therapeutic use of indomethacin is contraindicated in neonates with significant renal failure.) Hypertensive crisis and psychiatric side effects have been noted in case reports following use of indomethacin for analgesia in postpartum women. Use with caution in nursing women with hypertensive disorders of pregnancy or pre-existing renal disease.

Pregnancy Considerations Adverse events have been observed in animal reproduction studies; therefore, the manufacturer classifies indomethacin as pregnancy category C. Indomethacin crosses the placenta and can be detected in fetal plasma and amniotic fluid. Indomethacin exposure during the first trimester is not strongly associated with congenital malformations; however, cardiovascular anomalies and cleft palate have been observed following NSAID exposure in some studies. The use of an NSAID close to conception may be associated with an increased risk of miscarriage. Nonteratogenic effects have been observed following NSAID administration during the third trimester, including myocardial degenerative changes, prenatal constriction of the ductus arteriosus, failure of the ductus arteriosus to close postnatally, and fetal tricuspid regurgitation; renal dysfunction or failure, oligohydramnios; gastrointestinal bleeding or perforation, increased risk of necrotizing enterocolitis; intracranial bleeding (including intraventricular hemorrhage), platelet dysfunction with resultant bleeding; and pulmonary hypertension. The risk of fetal ductal constriction following maternal use of indomethacin is increased with gestational age and duration of therapy. Because they may cause premature closure of the ductus arteriosus, use of NSAIDs late in pregnancy should be avoided (use after 31 or 32 weeks gestation is not recommended by some clinicians). Indomethacin has been used in the management of preterm labor. Indomethacin should be used with caution in pregnant women with hypertension. The chronic use of NSAIDs in women of reproductive age may be associated with infertility that is reversible upon discontinuation of the medication.

Related Information

Nonsalicylate / Nonsteroidal Anti-Inflammatory Agents *on page 2002*

- **Indomethacin Sodium Trihydrate** *see* Indomethacin *on page 969*
- **INF-alpha 2** *see* Interferon Alfa-2b *on page 1000*
- **Infanrix®** *see* Diphtheria and Tetanus Toxoids, and Acellular Pertussis Vaccine *on page 552*
- **Infantaire [OTC]** *see* Acetaminophen *on page 38*
- **INFeD®** *see* Iron Dextran Complex *on page 1021*
- **Infergen®** *see* Interferon Alfacon-1 *on page 1002*

InFLIXimab (in FLIKS e mab)

U.S. Brand Names Remicade®

Index Terms Avakine; Infliximab, Recombinant

Generic Availability (U.S.) No

Pharmacologic Category Antirheumatic, Disease Modifying; Gastrointestinal Agent, Miscellaneous; Immunosuppressant Agent; Monoclonal Antibody; Tumor Necrosis Factor (TNF) Blocking Agent

Medication Safety Issues

Sound-alike/look-alike issues:

InFLIXimab may be confused with riTUXimab

Remicade® may be confused with Renacidin®, Rituxan®

Medication Guide Available Yes

Pregnancy Risk Factor B

Lactation Excretion in breast milk unknown/not recommended

Use

Treatment of moderately- to severely-active rheumatoid arthritis (with methotrexate)

Treatment of moderately- to severely-active Crohn's disease with inadequate response to conventional therapy (to reduce signs/symptoms and induce and maintain clinical remission) or to reduce the number of draining enterocutaneous and rectovaginal fistulas and maintain fistula closure

Treatment of psoriatic arthritis (to reduce signs/symptoms of active arthritis and inhibit progression of structural damage and improve physical function)

Treatment of chronic severe plaque psoriasis

Treatment of active ankylosing spondylitis (reduce signs/symptoms)

Treatment of moderately- to severely-active ulcerative colitis with inadequate response to conventional therapy (reduce signs/symptoms and induce and maintain clinical remission, mucosal healing and eliminate corticosteroid use)

Mechanism of Action/Effect Infliximab is a monoclonal antibody that binds to human tumor necrosis factor alpha (TNFα), thereby decreasing inflammatory and other responses.

Contraindications Hypersensitivity to infliximab, murine proteins or any component of the formulation; doses >5 mg/kg in patients with moderate or severe heart failure (NYHA Class III/IV)

Canadian labeling: Additional contraindications (not in U.S. labeling): Severe infections (eg, sepsis, abscesses, tuberculosis, and opportunistic infections)

Warnings/Precautions [U.S. Boxed Warning]: Patients receiving infliximab are at increased risk for serious infections which may result in hospitalization and/or fatality; infections usually developed in patients receiving concomitant immunosuppressive agents (eg, methotrexate or corticosteroids) and may present as disseminated (rather than local) disease. Active tuberculosis (or reactivation of latent tuberculosis), invasive fungal (including aspergillosis, blastomycosis, candidiasis, coccidioidomycosis, histoplasmosis, and pneumocystosis) and bacterial, viral or other opportunistic infections have been reported in patients receiving TNF-blocking agents, including infliximab. Monitor closely for signs/symptoms of infection. Discontinue for serious infection or sepsis. Consider risks versus benefits prior to use in patients with a history of chronic or

recurrent infection. Consider empiric antifungal therapy in patients who are at risk for invasive fungal infection and develop severe systemic illness. Other opportunistic infections (eg, invasive fungal infections, listeriosis, *Pneumocystis*) have occurred during therapy. Caution should be exercised when considering the use in patients with conditions that predispose them to infections (eg, diabetes) or residence/travel from areas of endemic mycoses (blastomycosis, coccidioidomycosis, histoplasmosis), or with latent or localized infections. Do not give with clinically important active infection. Patients who develop a new infection while undergoing treatment should be monitored closely. Serious infections have been reported when anakinra or abatacept have been used concurrently with other TNF-blocking agents; concurrent use of infliximab with anakinra or abatacept is not recommended. Use caution when switching from one biologic disease-modifying antirheumatic drug (DMARD) to another; overlapping biological activities may further increase the risk of infection.

[U.S. Boxed Warning]: Infliximab treatment has been associated with active tuberculosis (may be disseminated or extrapulmonary) or reactivation of latent infections; evaluate patients for tuberculosis risk factors and latent tuberculosis infection (with a tuberculin skin test) prior to and during therapy; treatment of latent tuberculosis should be initiated before use. Patients with initial negative tuberculin skin tests should receive continued monitoring for tuberculosis throughout treatment. Most cases of reactivation have been reported within the first 3-6 months of treatment. Caution should be exercised when considering the use of infliximab in patients who have been exposed to tuberculosis.

Patients should be brought up to date with all immunizations before initiating therapy. Live vaccines should not be given concurrently; there is no data available concerning secondary transmission of live vaccines in patients receiving therapy. Rare reactivation of hepatitis B virus (HBV) has occurred in chronic virus carriers; use with caution; evaluate prior to initiation and during treatment.

[U.S. Boxed Warning]: Lymphoma and other malignancies have been reported in children and adolescent patients receiving TNF-blocking agents including infliximab. Half the cases are lymphomas (Hodgkin's and non-Hodgkin's). **[U.S. Boxed Warning]: Hepatosplenic T-cell lymphoma has been reported in patients with Crohn's disease or ulcerative colitis treated with infliximab and concurrent or prior azathioprine or mercaptopurine use, usually reported in adolescent and young adult males.** The impact of infliximab on the development and course of malignancies is not fully defined, but may be dose dependent. As compared to the general population, an increased risk of lymphoma has been noted in clinical trials; however, rheumatoid arthritis alone has been previously associated with an increased rate of lymphoma. Use caution in patients with a history of COPD, higher rates of malignancy were reported in COPD patients treated with infliximab. Psoriasis patients with a history of phototherapy had a higher incidence of nonmelanoma skin cancers.

Severe hepatic reactions (including hepatitis, jaundice, acute hepatic failure, and cholestasis) have been reported during treatment; discontinue with jaundice or marked increase in liver enzymes (≥5 times ULN). Use caution with heart failure; if a decision is made to use with heart failure, monitor closely and discontinue if exacerbated or new symptoms occur. Doses >5 mg/kg should not be administered in patients with moderate-to-severe heart failure (NYHA Class III/IV). Use caution with history of hematologic abnormalities; hematologic toxicities (eg, leukopenia, neutropenia, thrombocytopenia, pancytopenia) have been reported; discontinue if significant abnormalities occur. Autoimmune antibodies and a lupus-like syndrome have been reported. If antibodies to double-stranded DNA are confirmed in a patient with lupus-like symptoms, infliximab should be discontinued. Rare cases of optic neuritis and demyelinating disease (including multiple sclerosis, systemic vasculitis, and Guillain-Barré syndrome) have been reported; use with caution in patients with pre-existing or recent onset CNS demyelinating disorders, or seizures; discontinue if significant CNS adverse reactions develop.

Acute infusion reactions may occur. Hypersensitivity reaction may occur within 2 hours of infusion. Medication and equipment for management of hypersensitivity reaction should be available for immediate use. Interruptions and/or reinstitution at a slower rate may be required (consult protocols). Pretreatment may be considered, and may be warranted in all patients with prior infusion reactions. Serum sickness-like reactions have occurred; may be associated with a decreased response to treatment. The development of antibodies to infliximab may increase the risk of hypersensitivity and/or infusion reactions; concomitant use of immunosuppressants may lessen the development of anti-infliximab antibodies. The risk of infusion reactions may be increased with retreatment after an interruption or discontinuation of prior maintenance therapy. Retreatment in psoriasis patients should be resumed as a scheduled maintenance regimen without any induction doses; use of an induction regimen should be used cautiously for retreatment of all other patients.

Efficacy was not established in a study to evaluate infliximab use in juvenile idiopathic arthritis (JIA). Safety and efficacy for use in pediatric plaque psoriasis or pediatric ulcerative colitis have not been established. **Note:** For use in Crohn's disease: Safety and efficacy have not been established in children <6 years of age (U.S. labeling) and in children <9 years of age (Canadian labeling).

Drug Interactions

Avoid Concomitant Use

Avoid concomitant use of InFLIXimab with any of the following: Abatacept; Anakinra; BCG; Belimumab; Canakinumab; Certolizumab Pegol; Natalizumab; Pimecrolimus; Rilonacept; Roflumilast; Tacrolimus (Topical); Vaccines (Live)

Decreased Effect

InFLIXimab may decrease the levels/effects of: BCG; Sipuleucel-T; Vaccines (Inactivated); Vaccines (Live)

The levels/effects of InFLIXimab may be decreased by: Echinacea

Increased Effect/Toxicity

InFLIXimab may increase the levels/effects of: Abatacept; Anakinra; Belimumab; Canakinumab; Certolizumab Pegol; Leflunomide; Natalizumab; Rilonacept; Vaccines (Live)

The levels/effects of InFLIXimab may be increased by: Abciximab; Denosumab; Pimecrolimus; Roflumilast; Tacrolimus (Topical); Trastuzumab

Nutritional/Ethanol Interactions Herb/Nutraceutical: Avoid echinacea (may diminish the therapeutic effect of infliximab).

Adverse Reactions Although profile is similar, frequency of adverse effects may vary with disease state. Except where noted, percentages reported in adults with rheumatoid arthritis:

>10%:

Central nervous system: Headache (18%)

Gastrointestinal: Nausea (21%), diarrhea (12%), abdominal pain (12%, Crohn's 26%)

Hepatic: ALT increased (risk increased with concomitant methotrexate)

Respiratory: Upper respiratory tract infection (32%), sinusitis (14%), cough (12%), pharyngitis (12%)

Miscellaneous: Development of antinuclear antibodies (~50%), infection (36%), infusion reactions (20%; severe <1%), development of antibodies to double-stranded DNA (20%), development of new abscess (Crohn's patients with fistulizing disease: 15%), anti-infliximab antibodies (variable; ~10% to 15% [range: 6% to 61%]; Mayer, 2006)

5% to 10%:

Cardiovascular: Hypertension (7%)

Central nervous system: Fatigue (9%), pain (8%), fever (7%)

Dermatologic: Rash (1% to 10%), pruritus (7%)

Gastrointestinal: Dyspepsia (10%)

Genitourinary: Urinary tract infection (8%)

Neuromuscular & skeletal: Arthralgia (1% to 8%), back pain (8%)

Respiratory: Bronchitis (10%), rhinitis (8%), dyspnea (6%)

Miscellaneous: Moniliasis (5%)

The following adverse events were reported in children with Crohn's disease and were found more frequently in children than adults:

>10%:

Hepatic: Liver enzymes increased (18%; ≥5 times ULN: 1%)

Hematologic: Anemia (11%)

Miscellaneous: Infections (56%; more common with every 8-week versus every 12-week infusions)

1% to 10%:

Central nervous system: Flushing (9%)

Gastrointestinal: Blood in stool (10%)

Hematologic: Leukopenia (9%), neutropenia (7%)

Neuromuscular & skeletal: Bone fracture (7%)

Respiratory: Respiratory tract allergic reaction (6%)

Miscellaneous: Viral infection (8%), bacterial infection (6%), antibodies to infliximab (3%)

Pharmacodynamics/Kinetics

Onset of Action Crohn's disease: ~2 weeks

Half-Life Elimination 7-12 days

Available Dosage Forms

Injection, powder for reconstitution:

Remicade®: 100 mg

Dosing

Adult & Geriatric Note: Premedication with antihistamines (H_1-antagonist +/- H_2-antagonist), acetaminophen, and/or corticosteroids may be considered to prevent and/or manage infusion-related reactions.

Crohn's disease: I.V.: 5 mg/kg at 0, 2, and 6 weeks, followed by 5 mg/kg every 8 weeks thereafter; dose may be increased to 10 mg/kg in patients who respond but then lose their response. If no response by week 14, consider discontinuing therapy.

Psoriatic arthritis (with or without methotrexate): I.V.: 5 mg/kg at 0,2, and 6 weeks, followed by 5 mg/kg every 8 weeks thereafter

Rheumatoid arthritis (in combination with methotrexate therapy): I.V. 3 mg/kg at 0, 2, and 6 weeks, followed by 3 mg/kg every 8 weeks thereafter; doses have ranged from 3-10 mg/kg repeated at 4- to 8-week intervals

Ankylosing spondylitis: I.V.: 5 mg/kg at 0, 2, and 6 weeks, followed by 5 mg/kg every 6 weeks thereafter (Canadian labeling recommends every 6-8 weeks thereafter)

Plaque psoriasis: I.V.: 5 mg/kg at 0, 2, and 6 weeks, followed by 5 mg/kg every 8 weeks thereafter

Ulcerative colitis: I.V.: 5 mg/kg at 0, 2, and 6 weeks, followed by 5 mg/kg every 8 weeks thereafter

Dosage adjustment with heart failure (HF): Weigh risk versus benefits for individual patient: *Moderate-to-severe (NYHA Class III or IV):* ≤5 mg/kg

Pediatric Note: Premedication with antihistamines (H_1-antagonist +/- H_2-antagonist), acetaminophen, and/or corticosteroids may be considered to prevent and/or manage infusion-related reactions:

Crohn's disease: I.V.: Children: U.S. labeling ≥6 years, Canadian labeling ≥9 years: 5 mg/kg at 0, 2, and 6 weeks, followed by 5 mg/kg every 8 weeks thereafter; if no response by week 14, consider discontinuing therapy

Renal Impairment No adjustment is recommended.

Hepatic Impairment No adjustment necessary.

Administration

I.V. Infuse over at least 2 hours; do not infuse with other agents; use in-line low protein binding filter (≤1.2 micron). Temporarily discontinue or decrease infusion rate with infusion-related reactions. Antihistamines (H_1-antagonist +/- H_2-antagonist), acetaminophen and/or corticosteroids may be used to manage reactions. Infusion may be reinitiated at a lower rate upon resolution of mild-to-moderate symptoms.

Canadian labeling (not approved in U.S. labeling): Infusion of doses ≤6 mg/kg over not less than 1 hour may be considered in patients treated for rheumatoid arthritis who have initially tolerated 3 infusions each over 2 hours. Safety of shortened infusion has not been studied with doses >6 mg/kg.

Guidelines for the treatment and prophylaxis of infusion reactions: (**Note:** Limited to adult patients and dosages used in Crohn's; prospective data for other populations [pediatrics, other indications/dosing] are not available).

A protocol for the treatment of infusion reactions, as well as prophylactic therapy for repeat infusions, has been published (Mayer, 2006).

Treatment of infusion reactions: Medications for the treatment of hypersensitivity reactions should be available for immediate use. For mild reactions, the rate of infusion should be decreased to 10 mL/hour. Initiate a normal saline infusion (500-1000 mL/hour) and appropriate symptomatic treatment (eg, acetaminophen and diphenhydramine); monitor vital signs every 10 minutes until normal. After 20 minutes, the infusion may be increased at 15-minute intervals, as tolerated, to completion (initial increase to 20 mL/hour, then 40 mL/hour, then 80 mL/hour, etc [maximum of 125 mL/hour]). For moderate reactions, the infusion should be stopped or slowed. Initiate a normal saline infusion (500-1000 mL/hour) and appropriate symptomatic treatment. Monitor vital signs every 5 minutes until normal. After 20 minutes, the infusion may be reinstituted at 10 mL/hour; then increased at 15-minute intervals, as tolerated, to completion (initial increase 20 mL/hour, then 40 mL/hour, then 80 mL/hour, etc [maximum of 125 mL/hour]). For severe reactions, the infusion should be stopped with administration of appropriate symptomatic treatment (eg, hydrocortisone/methylprednisolone, diphenhydramine and epinephrine) and frequent monitoring of vitals (consult institutional policies, if available). Retreatment after a severe reaction should only be done if the benefits outweigh the risks and with appropriate prophylaxis. Delayed infusion reactions typically occur 1-7 days after an infusion. Treatment should consist of appropriate symptomatic treatment (eg. acetaminophen, antihistamine, methylprednisolone).

Prophylaxis of infusion reactions: Premedication with acetaminophen and diphenhydramine 90 minutes prior to infusion may be considered in all patients with prior infusion reactions, and in patients with severe reactions corticosteroid administration is recommended. Steroid dosing may be oral (prednisone 50 mg orally every 12 hours for 3 doses prior to infusion) or intravenous (a single dose of hydrocortisone 100 mg or methylprednisolone 20-40 mg administered 20 minutes prior to the infusion). On initiation of the infusion, begin with a test dose at 10 mL/hour for 15 minutes. Thereafter, the infusion may be increased at 15-minute intervals, as tolerated, to completion (initial increase 20 mL/hour, then 40 mL/hour, then 80 mL/hour, etc). A maximum rate of 125 mL/hour is recommended in patients who experienced prior mild-moderate reactions and 100 mL/hour is recommended in patients who experienced prior severe reactions. In patients with cutaneous flushing, aspirin may be considered (Becker, 2004). For delayed infusion reactions, premedicate with acetaminophen and diphenhydramine 90 minutes prior to infusion. On initiation of the infusion, begin with a test dose at 10 mL/hour for 15 minutes. Thereafter, the infusion may be increased to infuse over 3 hours. Postinfusion therapy with acetaminophen for 3 days and an antihistamine for 7 days is recommended.

Stability

Reconstitution Reconstitute vials with 10 mL sterile water for injection. Swirl vial gently to dissolve powder; do not shake. Allow solution to stand for 5 minutes. Total dose of reconstituted product should be further diluted to 250 mL of 0.9% sodium chloride injection to a final concentration of 0.4-4 mg/mL. Infusion of dose should begin within 3 hours of preparation.

Storage Store vials at 2°C to 8°C (36°F to 46°F).

Monitoring and Teaching Issues

Physical Assessment Infusion reactions may occur. Premedication may be helpful. Treatment for hypersensitivity reactions should be available. Place and read PPD before initiation of therapy. Treatment of latent TB infection should be initiated prior to treatment with infliximab. Monitor for signs or symptoms of infection. Assess for signs of liver dysfunction (eg, unusual fatigue, easy bruising or bleeding, jaundice).

Patient Education This drug can only be administered by infusion. You will be more prone to infection. Report headache or unusual fatigue; increased nausea or abdominal pain; bruising or bleeding easily; cough, runny nose, respiratory difficulty; chest pain or persistent dizziness; fatigue, muscle pain or weakness, back pain; fever or chills; mouth sores; vaginal itching or discharge; sore throat; unhealed sores; or frequent infections.

Breast-Feeding Considerations It is not known whether infliximab is secreted in human milk. Because many immunoglobulins are secreted in milk and the potential for serious adverse reactions exists, a decision should be made whether to discontinue nursing or discontinue the drug, taking into account the importance of the drug to the mother.

Pregnancy Considerations Reproduction studies have not been conducted. Use during pregnancy only if clearly needed. A Rheumatoid Arthritis and Pregnancy Registry has been established for women exposed to infliximab during pregnancy (Organization of Teratology Information Services, 877-311-8972).

◆ **Infliximab, Recombinant** *see* InFLIXimab *on page 973*

◆ **Influenza Vaccine** *see* Influenza Virus Vaccine (Inactivated) *on page 978*

◆ **Influenza Vaccine** *see* Influenza Virus Vaccine (Live/Attenuated) *on page 980*

Influenza Virus Vaccine (H5N1) (in floo EN za VYE rus vak SEEN H5N1)

Index Terms Avian Influenza Virus Vaccine; Bird Flu Vaccine; H5N1 Influenza Vaccine; Influenza Virus Vaccine (Monovalent)

Generic Availability (U.S.) No

Pharmacologic Category Vaccine, Inactivated (Viral)

Medication Safety Issues

Sound-alike/look-alike issues:

Influenza virus vaccine (H5N1) may be confused with the nonavian strain of influenza virus vaccine

Prescribing and Access Restrictions Commercial distribution is not planned. The vaccine will be included as part of the U.S. Strategic National Stockpile. It will be distributed by public health officials if needed.

Pregnancy Risk Factor C

Lactation Excretion in breast milk unknown/use caution

Use Active immunization of adults at increased risk of exposure to the H5N1 viral subtype of influenza

Available Dosage Forms

Injection, suspension: Hemagglutinin (H5N1strain) 90 mcg/mL (5 mL)

Dosing

Adult Immunization: Adults 18-64 years: I.M.: 1 mL, followed by second 1 mL dose given 28 days later (acceptable range: 21-35 days)

Administration

I.M. For I.M. administration only. Inspect for particulate matter and discoloration prior to administration. Vaccinate in the deltoid muscle using a ≥1 inch needle length. Suspension should be shaken well prior to use. **Note:** For patients at risk of hemorrhage following intramuscular injection, the ACIP recommends "it should be administered intramuscularly if, in the opinion of the physician familiar with the patients bleeding risk, the vaccine can be administered by this route with reasonable safety. If the patient receives antihemophilia or other similar therapy, intramuscular vaccination can be scheduled shortly after such therapy is administered. A fine needle (23 gauge or smaller) can be used for the vaccination and firm pressure applied to the site (without rubbing) for at least 2 minutes. The patient should be instructed concerning the risk of hematoma from the injection." Patients on anticoagulant therapy should be considered to have the same bleeding risks and treated as those with clotting factor disorders (CDC, 2011).

Simultaneous administration of vaccines helps ensure the patients will be fully vaccinated by the appropriate age. Simultaneous administration of vaccines is defined as administering >1 vaccine on the same day at different anatomic sites. Separate vaccines should not be combined in the same syringe unless indicated by product specific labeling. Separate needles and syringes should be used for each injection. The ACIP prefers each dose of a specific vaccine in a series come from the same manufacturer when possible. Adolescents and adults should be vaccinated while seated or lying down. In general, preterm infants should be vaccinated at the same chronological age as full-term infants (CDC, 2011).

Antipyretics have not been shown to prevent febrile seizures. Antipyretics may be used to treat fever or discomfort following vaccination (CDC, 2011). One study reported that routine prophylactic administration of acetaminophen to prevent fever prior to vaccination decreased the immune response of some vaccines; the clinical significance of this reduction in immune response has not been established (Prymula, 2009).

Monitoring and Teaching Issues

Physical Assessment Carefully evaluate patient for contraindications and prior immunization history for possible adverse events. Treatment for anaphylactic/anaphylactoid reaction should be immediately available during vaccine use. All serious adverse reactions must be reported to the U.S. DHHS. Federal law also requires entry into the patient's medical record.

Patient Education Notify prescriber immediately of any acute reaction to vaccination (eg, difficulty breathing, chest pain, acute headache, rash, difficulty swallowing). May cause mild headache, fever, muscle pain, or some redness, pain, or swelling at injection site; consult prescriber if excessive or persisting. All serious adverse reactions must be reported to the U.S. DHHS. Federal law also requires entry into the patient's medical record.

Related Information

Immunization Recommendations *on page 1941*

Influenza Virus Vaccine (Inactivated)

(in floo EN za VYE rus vak SEEN, in ak ti VAY ted)

U.S. Brand Names Afluria®; Agriflu®; Fluarix®; FluLaval®; Fluvirin®; Fluzone®; Fluzone® High-Dose

Index Terms H1N1 Influenza Vaccine; Influenza Vaccine; Influenza Virus Vaccine (Purified Surface Antigen); Influenza Virus Vaccine (Split-Virus); Trivalent Inactivated Influenza Vaccine (TIV)

Generic Availability (U.S.) No

Pharmacologic Category Vaccine, Inactivated (Viral)

Medication Safety Issues

Sound-alike/look-alike issues:

Fluarix® may be confused with Flarex®

Influenza virus vaccine may be confused with flumazenil

Influenza virus vaccine may be confused with tetanus toxoid and tuberculin products. Medication errors have occurred when tuberculin skin tests (PPD) have been inadvertently administered instead of tetanus toxoid products and influenza virus vaccine. These products are refrigerated and often stored in close proximity to each other.

International issues:

Fluarix [U.S., Canada, and multiple international markets] may be confused with Flarex brand name for fluorometholone [U.S. and multiple international markets] and Fluorex brand name for fluoride [France]

Pregnancy Risk Factor B/C (manufacturer specific)

Lactation Excretion in breast milk unknown/use caution

Use Provide active immunity to influenza virus strains contained in the vaccine

The Advisory Committee on Immunization Practices (ACIP) recommends annual vaccination with the seasonal trivalent inactivated influenza vaccine (TIV) (injection) for all persons ≥6 months of age.

When vaccine supply is limited, target groups for vaccination (those at higher risk of complications from influenza infection and their close contacts) include the following:

- Persons ≥50 years of age
- Residents of nursing homes and other chronic-care facilities that house persons of any age with chronic medical conditions
- Adults and children with chronic disorders of the pulmonary or cardiovascular systems (except hypertension), including asthma
- Adults and children who have chronic metabolic diseases (including diabetes mellitus), hepatic disease, renal dysfunction, hematologic disorders, or immunosuppression (including immunosuppression caused by medications or HIV)
- Adults and children with cognitive or neurologic/neuromuscular conditions (including conditions such as spinal cord injuries or seizure disorders) which may compromise respiratory function, the handling of respiratory secretions, or that can increase the risk of aspiration
- Children and adolescents (6 months to 18 years of age) who are receiving long-term aspirin therapy, and therefore, may be at risk for developing Reye's syndrome after influenza
- Women who are or will be pregnant during the influenza season
- Children 6-59 months of age
- Healthcare personnel
- Household contacts and caregivers of children <5 years (particularly children <6 months) and adults ≥50 years
- Household contacts and caregivers of persons with medical conditions which put them at high risk of complications from influenza infection
- American Indians/Alaska Natives
- Morbidly obese (BMI ≥40)

The Advisory Committee on Immunization Practices (ACIP) states that healthy, nonpregnant persons aged 2-49 years may receive vaccination with either the seasonal live, attenuated influenza vaccine (LAIV) (nasal spray) or the seasonal trivalent inactivated influenza vaccine (TIV) (injection).

Available Dosage Forms

Injection, suspension:

Afluria®: Hemagglutinin 45 mcg/0.5 mL (5 mL)
FluLaval®: Hemagglutinin 45 mcg/0.5 mL (5 mL)
Fluvirin®: Hemagglutinin 45 mcg/0.5 mL (5 mL)
Fluzone®: Hemagglutinin 45 mcg/0.5 mL (5 mL)

Injection, suspension [preservative free]:

Afluria®: Hemagglutinin 45 mcg/0.5 mL (0.5 mL)
Agriflu®: Hemagglutinin 45 mcg/0.5 mL (0.5 mL)
Fluarix®: Hemagglutinin 45 mcg/0.5 mL (0.5 mL)
Fluvirin®: Hemagglutinin 45 mcg/0.5 mL (0.5 mL)

Fluzone®: Hemagglutinin 22.5 mcg/0.25 mL (0.25 mL); Hemagglutinin 45 mcg/0.5 mL (0.5 mL)
Fluzone® High-Dose: Hemagglutinin 180 mcg/0.5 mL (0.5 mL)

Dosing

Adult It is important to note that influenza seasons vary in their timing and duration from year to year. In general, vaccination should begin soon after the vaccine becomes available and if possible, prior to October. However, vaccination should continue throughout the influenza season as long as vaccine is available.

Immunization: I.M.: *Afluria®, Agriflu®, Fluarix®, FluLaval®, Fluvirin®, Fluzone®:* 0.5 mL/dose (1 dose per season)

Geriatric It is important to note that influenza seasons vary in their timing and duration from year to year. In general, vaccination should begin soon after the vaccine becomes available and if possible, prior to October. However, vaccination should continue throughout the influenza season as long as vaccine is available.

Immunization: I.M.: Adults ≥ 65 years: *Afluria®, Agriflu®, Fluarix®, FluLaval®, Fluvirin®, Fluzone®, Fluzone® High-Dose:* 0.5 mL/dose (1 dose per season) The ACIP considers Fluzone® High-Dose an alternative vaccine for this age group

Pediatric It is important to note that influenza seasons vary in their timing and duration from year to year. In general, vaccination should begin soon after the vaccine becomes available and if possible, prior to October. However, vaccination should continue throughout the influenza season as long as vaccine is available.

Immunization: I.M.:

Afluria®: The ACIP does not recommend use of Afluria® in children 6 months to 8 years of age during the 2010-11 influenza season in the United States. If other age-appropriate vaccines are not available, children 5-8 years of age who are also considered at risk for influenza complications may be given Afluria®. The benefits and risks of this vaccine should be discussed with parents or caregivers prior to administration.
Children 6-35 months: 0.25 mL/dose (1 or 2 doses per season; see **Note**)
Children 3-8 years: 0.5 mL/dose (1 or 2 doses per season; see **Note**)
Children ≥9 years: Refer to adult dosing.

Fluarix®:
Children 3-8 years: 0.5 mL/dose (1 or 2 doses per season; see **Note**)
Children ≥9 years: Refer to adult dosing.

Fluzone®:
Children 6-35 months: 0.25 mL/dose (1 or 2 doses per season; see **Note**)
Children 3-8 years: 0.5 mL/dose (1 or 2 doses per season; see **Note**)
Children ≥9 years: Refer to adult dosing.

Fluvirin®:
Children 4-8 years: 0.5 mL/dose (1 or 2 doses per season; see **Note**)
Children ≥9 years: Refer to adult dosing.

Note: Children <9 years who are not previously vaccinated or who received only 1 dose of vaccine during the previous season (if it was their first year of vaccination) should receive 2 doses separated by ≥4 weeks, in order to achieve satisfactory antibody response per ACIP recommendations. In addition, for the 2010-11 influenza season, children who did not receive at least 1 dose of the influenza A (H1N1) 2009 monovalent vaccine during the 2009-10 season should receive 2 doses of the 2010-11 seasonal influenza vaccine, regardless of previous influenza vaccination history. If vaccine history for either the influenza A (H1N1) 2009 monovalent vaccine or the 2009-10 seasonal influenza vaccine cannot be determined, the child should receive 2 doses of the 2010-11 seasonal influenza vaccine.

Administration

I.M. For I.M. administration only. Inspect for particulate matter and discoloration prior to administration. Adults and older children should be vaccinated in the deltoid muscle using a ≥1 inch needle length. Infants and young children <12 months of age should be vaccinated in the anterolateral aspect of the thigh using a 7/8 inch to 1 inch needle length. Young children with adequate deltoid muscle mass should be vaccinated using a 7/8 inch to 1.25 inch needle. Do not inject into the gluteal region or areas where there may be a major nerve trunk. Suspensions should be shaken well prior to use.

If a pediatric vaccine (0.25 mL) is inadvertently administered to an adult, an additional 0.25 mL should be administered to provide the full adult dose (0.5 mL). If the error is discovered after the patient has left, an adult dose should be given as soon as the patient can return. If an adult vaccine (0.5 mL) is inadvertently given to a child, no action needs to be taken.

Note: For patients at risk of hemorrhage following intramuscular injection, the ACIP recommends "it should be administered intramuscularly if, in the opinion of the physician familiar with the patients bleeding risk, the vaccine can be administered by this route with reasonable safety. If the patient receives antihemophilia or other similar therapy, intramuscular vaccination can be scheduled shortly after such therapy is administered. A fine needle (23 gauge or smaller) can be used for the vaccination and firm pressure applied to the site (without rubbing) for at least 2 minutes. The patient should be instructed concerning the risk of hematoma from the injection." Patients on anticoagulant therapy should be considered to have the same bleeding risks and treated as those with clotting factor disorders (CDC, 2011).

Simultaneous administration of vaccines helps ensure the patients will be fully vaccinated by the appropriate age. Simultaneous administration of vaccines is defined as administering >1 vaccine on the same day at different anatomic sites. Separate vaccines should not be combined in the same syringe unless indicated by product specific labeling. Separate needles and syringes should be used for each injection. However, in general, vaccination should not be deferred if the brand name or route of the previous dose is not available or not known (CDC, 2011). Adolescents and adults should be vaccinated while seated or lying down. In general, preterm infants should be vaccinated at the same chronological age as full-term infants (CDC, 2011).

Antipyretics have not been shown to prevent febrile seizures. Antipyretics may be used to treat fever or discomfort following vaccination (CDC, 2011). One study reported that routine prophylactic administration of acetaminophen to prevent fever prior to vaccination decreased the immune response of some vaccines; the clinical significance of this reduction in immune response has not been established (Prymula, 2009).

Monitoring and Teaching Issues

Physical Assessment Have emergency treatment for anaphylactoid or hypersensitivity reaction available. Evaluate for allergies (some products are manufactured with chicken egg protein, gentamicin, neomycin, polymyxin, and/or thimerosal), previous adverse reactions (especially Guillain-Barré syndrome), bleeding disorders, presence of acute illness, and immunosuppressed status. All serious adverse reactions must be reported to the U.S. DHHS. Federal law also requires entry into the patient's medical record.

Patient Education The vaccination is not effective immediately. The full effect of the vaccine is generally reached approximately 3 weeks after vaccination. You may experience nausea, vomiting, diarrhea, flu-like symptoms (eg, cough, rhinitis, fever, muscle or joint pain, fatigue, headache), and redness and tenderness at injection site. Notify prescriber if symptoms persist.

Related Information

Immunization Recommendations *on page 1941*

Influenza Virus Vaccine (Live/Attenuated) (in floo EN za VYE rus vak SEEN)

U.S. Brand Names FluMist®

Index Terms H1N1 Influenza Vaccine; Influenza Vaccine; Influenza Virus Vaccine (Trivalent, Live); Live Attenuated Influenza Vaccine (LAIV)

Generic Availability (U.S.) No

Pharmacologic Category Vaccine, Live (Viral)

Medication Safety Issues

Sound-alike/look-alike issues:

Influenza virus vaccine may be confused with flumazenil

Pregnancy Risk Factor C

Lactation Excretion in breast milk unknown/use caution

Use Provide active immunity to influenza virus strains contained in the vaccine

The Advisory Committee on Immunization Practices (ACIP) states that healthy, nonpregnant persons aged 2-49 years may receive vaccination with either the seasonal live, attenuated influenza vaccine (LAIV) (nasal spray) or the seasonal trivalent inactivated influenza vaccine (TIV) (injection).

Available Dosage Forms

Solution, intranasal [preservative free]:

FluMist®: (0.2 mL)

Dosing

Adult It is important to note that influenza seasons vary in their timing and duration from year to year. In general, vaccination should begin soon after the vaccine becomes available and if possible, prior to October. However, vaccination should continue throughout the influenza season as long as vaccine is available.

Immunization: Intranasal (FluMist®):

U.S. labeling: Adults ≤49 years: 0.2 mL/dose (1 dose per season)

Canadian labeling: Adults ≤59 years: 0.2 mL/dose (1 dose per season)

Geriatric Not indicated for use in patients ≥50 years (U.S. labeling) or ≥60 years (Canadian labeling).

Pediatric It is important to note that influenza seasons vary in their timing and duration from year to year. In general, vaccination should begin soon after the vaccine becomes available and if possible, prior to October. However, vaccination should continue throughout the influenza season as long as vaccine is available.

Immunization: Intranasal: *FluMist®*:

Children 2-8 years, previously **not vaccinated** with influenza vaccine: Two doses (0.2 mL/dose) separated by at least 4 weeks (see **"Note"**)

Children 2-8 years, previously **vaccinated** with influenza vaccine: 0.2 mL/dose (1 dose per season; see **"Note"**)

Children ≥9 years: Refer to adult dosing.

Note: Children <9 years who are not previously vaccinated or who received only 1 dose of vaccine during the previous season (if it was their first year of vaccination) should receive 2 doses separated by ≥4 weeks, in order to achieve satisfactory antibody response per ACIP recommendations. In addition, for the 2010-11 influenza season, children who did not receive at least 1 dose of the influenza A (H1N1) 2009 monovalent vaccine during the 2009-10 season should receive 2 doses of the 2010-11 seasonal influenza vaccine, regardless of previous influenza vaccination history. If vaccine history for either the influenza A (H1N1) 2009 monovalent vaccine or the 2009-10 seasonal influenza vaccine cannot be determined, the child should receive 2 doses of the 2010-11 seasonal influenza vaccine.

Administration

Other LAIV: Intranasal: Half the dose (0.1 mL) is administered to each nostril; patient should be in upright position. A dose divider clip is provided. Severely-immunocompromised persons should not administer the live vaccine. If recipient sneezes following administration, the dose should not be repeated.

Simultaneous administration of vaccines helps ensure the patients will be fully vaccinated by the appropriate age. Simultaneous administration of vaccines is defined as administering >1 vaccine on the same day at different anatomic sites. The ACIP prefers each dose of a specific vaccine in a series come from the same manufacturer when possible. However, in general, vaccination should not be deferred if the brand name or route of the previous dose is not available or not known (CDC, 2011).

Antipyretics have not been shown to prevent febrile seizures. Antipyretics may be used to treat fever or discomfort following vaccination (CDC, 2011). One study reported that routine prophylactic administration of acetaminophen to prevent fever prior to vaccination decreased the immune response of some vaccines; the clinical significance of this reduction in immune response has not been established (Prymula, 2009).

Vaccine administration with oral influenza antiviral medications: Live influenza virus vaccine (LAIV) should not be given until 48 hours after the completion of influenza antiviral therapy (influenza A and B). Influenza antiviral therapy (influenza A and B) should not be administered for 2 weeks after receiving LAIV.

Monitoring and Teaching Issues

Physical Assessment Federal law requires entry into the patient's medical record.

Related Information

Immunization Recommendations *on page 1941*

- ◆ **Influenza Virus Vaccine (Monovalent)** *see* Influenza Virus Vaccine (H5N1) *on page 977*
- ◆ **Influenza Virus Vaccine (Purified Surface Antigen)** *see* Influenza Virus Vaccine (Inactivated) *on page 978*
- ◆ **Influenza Virus Vaccine (Split-Virus)** *see* Influenza Virus Vaccine (Inactivated) *on page 978*
- ◆ **Influenza Virus Vaccine (Trivalent, Live)** *see* Influenza Virus Vaccine (Live/Attenuated) *on page 980*
- ◆ **Infumorph 200** *see* Morphine (Systemic) *on page 1258*
- ◆ **Infumorph 500** *see* Morphine (Systemic) *on page 1258*
- ◆ **INH** *see* Isoniazid *on page 1024*
- ◆ **Innohep®** *see* Tinzaparin *on page 1766*
- ◆ **InnoPran XL®** *see* Propranolol *on page 1522*
- ◆ **Inspra™** *see* Eplerenone *on page 636*

Insulin Aspart (IN soo lin AS part)

U.S. Brand Names NovoLOG®; NovoLOG® FlexPen®; NovoLOG® Penfill®

Index Terms Aspart Insulin

Generic Availability (U.S.) No

Pharmacologic Category Antidiabetic Agent, Insulin

Medication Safety Issues

Sound-alike/look-alike issues:

NovoLOG® may be confused with HumaLOG®, HumuLIN® R, NovoLIN® N, NovoLIN® R, NovoLOG® Mix 70/30

High alert medication: The Institute for Safe Medication Practices (ISMP) includes this medication among its list of drugs which have a heightened risk of causing significant patient harm when used in error. ***Due to the number of insulin preparations, it is essential to identify/clarify the type of insulin to be used.***

Cross-contamination may occur if insulin pens are shared among multiple patients. Steps should be taken to prohibit sharing of insulin pens.

Pregnancy Risk Factor B

Lactation Excretion in breast milk unknown/compatible

Use Treatment of type 1 diabetes mellitus (insulin dependent, IDDM) and type 2 diabetes mellitus (noninsulin dependent, NIDDM) to improve glycemic control

Unlabeled/Investigational Use Gestational diabetes mellitus (GDM); mild-to-moderate diabetic ketoacidosis (DKA); mild-to-moderate hyperosmolar hyperglycemic state (HHS)

Mechanism of Action/Effect Insulin aspart is a rapid-acting insulin analog.

Refer to Insulin Regular on page 994.

Contraindications Hypersensitivity to insulin aspart or any component of the formulation; during episodes of hypoglycemia

Warnings/Precautions Refer to Insulin Regular on page 994.

Due to short duration of action, a longer acting insulin is needed to maintain adequate glucose control. Administration should be immediately followed by a meal. Insulin aspart may be administered I.V. in selected clinical situations to control hyperglycemia.

Drug Interactions

Metabolism/Transport Effects Induces CYP1A2 (weak)

Avoid Concomitant Use There are no known interactions where it is recommended to avoid concomitant use.

Decreased Effect

The levels/effects of Insulin Aspart may be decreased by: Corticosteroids (Orally Inhaled); Corticosteroids (Systemic); Luteinizing Hormone-Releasing Hormone Analogs; Somatropin; Thiazide Diuretics

Increased Effect/Toxicity Refer to Insulin Regular on page 994.

Nutritional/Ethanol Interactions Refer to Insulin Regular on page 994.

Pharmacodynamics/Kinetics

Onset of Action 0.2-0.3 hours; Peak effect: 1-3 hours

Duration of Action 3-5 hours

Time to Peak Plasma: 40-50 minutes

Protein Binding <10%

Half-Life Elimination SubQ: 81 minutes

Excretion Urine

Pharmacokinetic Note Rate of absorption, onset, and duration of activity may be affected by site of injection, exercise, presence of lipodystrophy, local blood supply, and/or temperature.

Available Dosage Forms

Injection, solution:

NovoLOG®: 100 units/mL (10 mL)

NovoLOG® FlexPen®: 100 units/mL (3 mL)

NovoLOG® Penfill®: 100 units/mL (3 mL)

Dosing

Adult & Geriatric Refer to Insulin Regular on page 994. Insulin aspart is a rapid-acting insulin analog which is normally administered as a premeal component of the insulin regimen. It is normally used along with a long-acting (basal) form of insulin.

SubQ: When used in a meal-related treatment regimen, 50% to 70% of total daily insulin requirement may be provided by insulin aspart and the remainder provided by an intermediate or long-acting insulin. Due to rapid onset and short duration, some patients may require more basal insulin to prevent premeal hypoglycemia when using insulin aspart as opposed to regular insulin.

SubQ infusion pump: ~50% of total dose given as meal related bolus and ~50% of total dose given as basal infusion; adjust dose as necessary

Pediatric Refer to Insulin Regular on page 994.

Renal Impairment Refer to Insulin Regular on page 994.

Hepatic Impairment Refer to Insulin Regular on page 994.

Administration

I.V. Do not use if solution is viscous or cloudy; use only if clear and colorless. May be administered I.V. with close monitoring of blood glucose and serum potassium; appropriate medical supervision is required. **Do not administer insulin mixtures intravenously.**

Other

SubQ administration: Do not use if solution is viscous or cloudy; use only if clear and colorless. Insulin aspart should be administered immediately (within 5-10 minutes) before a meal. Cold injections should be avoided. SubQ administration is usually made into the thighs, arms, buttocks, or abdomen; rotate injection sites. When mixing insulin aspart with other preparations of insulin (eg, insulin NPH), insulin aspart should be drawn into syringe first. Do not dilute or mix other insulin formulations with insulin aspart contained in a cartridge or prefilled pen.

CSII administration: Do not use if solution is viscous or cloudy; use only if clear and colorless. Patients should be trained in the proper use of their external insulin pump and in intensive insulin therapy. Infusion sets and infusion set insertion sites should be changed at least every 3 days; rotate infusion sites. Do not dilute or mix other insulin formulations with insulin aspart that is to be used in an external insulin pump.

Stability

Reconstitution

For SubQ administration: *NovoLog® vials:* May be diluted with Insulin Diluting Medium for NovoLog® to a concentration of 10 units/mL (U-10) or 50 units/mL (U-50). Do not dilute insulin contained in a cartridge, prefilled pen, or external insulin pump.

For I.V. infusion: May be diluted in NS, D_5W, or $D_{10}W$ to concentrations of 0.05-1 unit/mL.

Storage Unopened vials, cartridges, and prefilled pens may be stored under refrigeration between 2°C and 8°C (36°F to 46°F) until the expiration date or at room temperature <30°C (<86°F) for 28 days; do not freeze; keep away from heat and sunlight. Once punctured (in use), vials may be stored under refrigeration or at room temperature <30°C (<86°F); use within 28 days. Cartridges and prefilled pens that have been punctured (in use) should be stored at temperatures <30°C (<86°F) and used within 28 days; do not freeze or refrigerate. When used for CSII, insulin aspart contained within an external insulin pump reservoir should be replaced at least every 6 days; discard if exposed to temperatures >37°C (>98.6°F).

For SubQ administration: *NovoLog® vials:* According to the manufacturer, diluted insulin should be stored at temperatures <30°C (<86°F) and used within 28 days.

For I.V. infusion: Stable for 24 hours at room temperature.

Monitoring and Teaching Issues

Laboratory Monitoring

Diabetes mellitus: Plasma glucose, electrolytes, Hb A_{1c}

I.V. administration: Close monitoring of blood glucose and serum potassium

Physical Assessment Monitor for hypoglycemia at regular intervals during therapy. Teach patient proper use, including appropriate injection technique and syringe/needle disposal, and monitoring requirements.

Patient Education Do not share pens, cartridges, or needles with others. This medication is used to control diabetes; it is not a cure. It is imperative to follow other components of prescribed treatment (eg, diet and exercise regimen). With insulin aspart (NovoLog®), you must start eating within 5-10 minutes after injection. If you experience hypoglycemic reaction, contact prescriber immediately. Always carry quick source of sugar with you. Monitor glucose levels as directed by prescriber. Report adverse side effects, including chest pain or palpitations; persistent fatigue, confusion, headache; skin rash or redness; numbness of mouth, lips, or tongue; muscle weakness or tremors; vision changes; respiratory difficulty; or nausea, vomiting, or flu-like symptoms.

Dietary Considerations Individualized medical nutrition therapy (MNT) based on ADA recommendations is an integral part of therapy.

Geriatric Considerations How "tightly" a geriatric patient's blood glucose should be controlled is controversial; however, a fasting blood sugar <150 mg/dL is now an acceptable endpoint. Such a decision should be based on the patient's functional and cognitive status, how well he/she recognizes hypoglycemic or hyperglycemic symptoms, and how to respond to them and any other disease states. Patients who are unable to accurately draw up their dose will need assistance such as prefilled syringes. Initial doses may require considerations for renal function in the elderly with dosing adjusted subsequently based on blood glucose monitoring. Intensive glucose control (Hb A_{1c} <6.5%) has been linked to increased all cause and cardiovascular mortality, hypoglycemia requiring assistance, and weight gain in adult type 2 diabetes. For elderly patients with diabetes who are relatively healthy, attaining target goals for aspirin use, blood pressure, lipids, smoking cessation, and diet and exercise may be more important than normalized glycemic control.

Breast-Feeding Considerations It is not known if insulin aspart is found in breast milk. Endogenous insulin can be found in breast milk. Plasma glucose concentrations in the mother affect glucose concentrations in breast milk. The gastrointestinal tract destroys insulin when administered orally; therefore, insulin is not expected to be absorbed intact by the breast-feeding infant. All types of insulin are safe for use while breast-feeding. Due to increased calorie expenditure, women with diabetes may require less insulin while nursing.

Pregnancy Considerations Adverse events have generally not been observed in animal reproduction studies; therefore, the manufacturer classifies insulin aspart as pregnancy category B. When compared to regular insulin, the use of insulin aspart during pregnancy has not been found to increase the risk of adverse events to the fetus. Maternal hyperglycemia can be associated with adverse effects in the fetus, including macrosomia, neonatal hyperglycemia, and hyperbilirubinemia; the risk of congenital malformations is increased when the Hb A_{1c} is above the normal range.

Insulin requirements tend to fall during the first trimester of pregnancy and increase in the later trimesters, peaking at 28-32 weeks of gestation. Following delivery, insulin requirements decrease rapidly. Diabetes can be associated with adverse effects in the mother. Poorly-treated diabetes may cause end-organ damage that may in turn negatively affect obstetric outcomes. Physiologic glucose levels should be maintained prior to and during pregnancy to decrease the risk of adverse events in the fetus and the mother. Insulin is the drug of choice for the control of diabetes mellitus during pregnancy. Insulin aspart has been demonstrated to be as safe and effective as regular human insulin when used during pregnancy and may have advantages over regular insulin during pregnancy.

Additional Information Refer to Insulin Regular on page 994.

Related Information

Diabetes Mellitus and Pregnancy *on page* 2035

Diabetes Mellitus Management, Adults *on page* 2026

Insulin Regular *on page* 994

◆ **Insulin Aspart and Insulin Aspart Protamine** *see* Insulin Aspart Protamine and Insulin Aspart *on page* 983

Insulin Aspart Protamine and Insulin Aspart

(IN soo lin AS part PROE ta meen & IN soo lin AS part)

U.S. Brand Names NovoLOG® Mix 70/30; NovoLOG® Mix 70/30 FlexPen®

Index Terms Insulin Aspart and Insulin Aspart Protamine; NovoLog 70/30

Generic Availability (U.S.) No

Pharmacologic Category Antidiabetic Agent, Insulin

Medication Safety Issues

Sound-alike/look-alike issues:

NovoLOG® Mix 70/30 may be confused with HumaLOG® Mix 75/25™, HumuLIN® 70/30, NovoLIN® 70/30, NovoLOG®

High alert medication: The Institute for Safe Medication Practices (ISMP) includes this medication among its list of drugs which have a heightened risk of causing significant patient harm when used in error. ***Due to the number of insulin preparations, it is essential to identify/clarify the type of insulin to be used.***

Cross-contamination may occur if insulin pens are shared among multiple patients. Steps should be taken to prohibit sharing of insulin pens.

Pregnancy Risk Factor B

Lactation Refer to Insulin Aspart on page 981.

Use Treatment of type 1 diabetes mellitus (insulin dependent, IDDM) and type 2 diabetes mellitus (noninsulin dependent, NIDDM) to improve glycemic control

Available Dosage Forms

Injection, suspension:

NovoLOG® Mix 70/30: Insulin aspart protamine suspension 70% [intermediate acting] and insulin aspart solution 30% [rapid acting]: 100 units/mL (10 mL)

NovoLOG® Mix 70/30 FlexPen®: Insulin aspart protamine suspension 70% [intermediate acting] and insulin aspart solution 30% [rapid acting]: 100 units/mL (3 mL)

Dosing

Adult & Geriatric Refer to Insulin Regular on page 994. Fixed ratio insulins (such as insulin aspart protamine and insulin aspart combination) are normally administered in 2 daily doses.

Renal Impairment Refer to Insulin Regular on page 994.

Hepatic Impairment Refer to Insulin Regular on page 994.

Administration

Other SubQ administration: In order to properly resuspend the insulin, vials and prefilled pens should be gently rolled between the palms ten times; in addition, prefilled pens should be inverted 180° ten times. Properly resuspended insulin should look uniformly cloudy or milky; do not use if any white insulin substance remains at the bottom of the container, if any clumps are present, if the insulin remains clear after adequate mixing, or if white particles are stuck to the bottom or wall of the container. Cold injections should be avoided. Insulin aspart protamine and insulin aspart combination products should be administered within 15 minutes before a meal (type 1 diabetes) or 15 minutes before or after a meal (type 2 diabetes); typically given twice daily. SubQ administration is usually made into the thighs, arms, buttocks, or abdomen; rotate injection sites. Do not dilute or mix with any other insulin formulation or solution; not recommended for use in external SubQ insulin infusion pump.

Monitoring and Teaching Issues

Laboratory Monitoring Diabetes mellitus: Plasma glucose, electrolytes, Hb A_{1c}

Physical Assessment See individual agents.

Patient Education See individual agents.

Related Information

Diabetes Mellitus and Pregnancy *on page* 2035

Diabetes Mellitus Management, Adults *on page* 2026

Insulin Regular *on page* 994

Insulin Detemir (IN soo lin DE te mir)

U.S. Brand Names Levemir®; Levemir® FlexPen®

Index Terms Detemir Insulin

Generic Availability (U.S.) No

Pharmacologic Category Antidiabetic Agent, Insulin

Medication Safety Issues

High alert medication: The Institute for Safe Medication Practices (ISMP) includes this medication among its list of drugs which have a heightened risk of causing significant patient harm when used in error. ***Due to the number of insulin preparations, it is essential to identify/clarify the type of insulin to be used.***

Note: Insulin detemir is a clear solution, but it is NOT intended for I.V. or I.M. administration.

Cross-contamination may occur if insulin pens are shared among multiple patients. Steps should be taken to prohibit sharing of insulin pens.

Pregnancy Risk Factor C

Lactation Excretion in breast milk unknown/compatible

Use Treatment of type 1 diabetes mellitus (insulin dependent, IDDM) and type 2 diabetes mellitus (noninsulin dependent, NIDDM) to improve glycemic control

Mechanism of Action/Effect Insulin detemir is an intermediate- to long-acting insulin analog. Refer to Insulin Regular on page 994.

Contraindications Hypersensitivity to insulin detemir or any component of the formulation

Warnings/Precautions Refer to Insulin Regular on page 994. Safety and efficacy not established in children <6 years of age.

Careful adjustment of dosage and timing is required to achieve glycemic targets. Adjustment of other antidiabetic therapy (short-acting or oral antidiabetic agents) may be required. The duration of of action of insulin detemir is dose-dependent and this factor must be considered during dosage adjustment and titration. Insulin detemir is a clear solution, but it is not for intravenous administration.

Drug Interactions

Metabolism/Transport Effects Refer to Insulin Regular on page 994.

Avoid Concomitant Use There are no known interactions where it is recommended to avoid concomitant use.

Decreased Effect

The levels/effects of Insulin Detemir may be decreased by: Corticosteroids (Orally Inhaled); Corticosteroids (Systemic); Luteinizing Hormone-Releasing Hormone Analogs; Somatropin; Thiazide Diuretics

Increased Effect/Toxicity Refer to Insulin Regular on page 994.

Nutritional/Ethanol Interactions Refer to Insulin Regular on page 994.

Adverse Reactions Refer to Insulin Regular on page 994.

Pharmacodynamics/Kinetics

Onset of Action 3-4 hours; Peak effect: 3-9 hours (Plank, 2005)

Duration of Action Dose dependent: 6-23 hours; **Note:** Duration is dose-dependent. At lower dosages (0.1-0.2 units/kg), mean duration is variable (5.7-12.1 hours). At 0.4 units/kg, the mean duration was 19.9 hours. At high dosages (≥0.8 units/kg) the duration is longer and less variable (mean of 22-23 hours) (Plank, 2005).

Bioavailability 60%

Time to Peak Plasma: 6-8 hours

Protein Binding 98% (albumin)

Half-Life Elimination 5-7 hours (dose-dependent)

Excretion Urine

Pharmacokinetic Note Rate of absorption, onset, and duration of activity may be affected by site of injection, exercise, presence of lipodystrophy, local blood supply, and/or temperature.

Available Dosage Forms

Injection, solution:

Levemir®: 100 units/mL (10 mL)

Levemir® FlexPen®: 100 units/mL (3 mL)

Dosing

Adult & Geriatric Also refer to Insulin Regular on page 994.

Note: Duration is dose-dependent. Dosage must be carefully titrated (adjustment of dose and timing. Adjustment of concomitant antidiabetic treatment (short-acting insulins or oral antidiabetic agents) may be required.

Type 1 or type 2 diabetes:

Basal insulin or basal-bolus: May be substituted on a unit-per-unit basis. Adjust dose to achieve glycemic targets.

Insulin-naive patients (type 2 diabetes only): 0.1-0.2 units/kg once daily in the evening or 10 units once or twice daily. Adjust dose to achieve glycemic targets. Note: Canadian labeling recommends 10 units once daily (twice daily dosing is not included).

Pediatric Note: When compared to insulin NPH, insulin detemir has a slower, more prolonged absorption; duration is dose-dependent. Insulin detemir may be given once or twice daily when used as the basal insulin component of therapy.

Diabetes mellitus:

Type 1: SubQ: Children ≥6 years: Refer to Insulin Regular on page 994

Renal Impairment Refer to Insulin Regular on page 994.

Hepatic Impairment Refer to Insulin Regular on page 994.

Administration

Other SubQ administration: Do not use if solution is viscous or cloudy; use only if clear and colorless with no visible particles. Insulin detemir should be administered once or twice daily. When given once daily, administer with the evening meal or at bedtime. When given twice daily, administer the evening dose with the evening meal, at bedtime, or 12 hours following the morning dose. Cold injections should be avoided. SubQ administration is usually made into the thighs, arms, buttocks, or abdomen; rotate injection sites. Do not dilute or mix insulin detemir with any other insulin formulation or solution; **not** recommended for use in external SubQ insulin infusion pump.

Stability

Storage Unopened vials, cartridges, and prefilled pens may be stored under refrigeration between 2°C and 8°C (36°F to 46°F) until the expiration date or at room temperature <30°C (<86°F) for 42 days; do not freeze; keep away from heat and sunlight. Once punctured (in use), vials may be stored under refrigeration or at room temperature <30°C (<86°F); use within 42 days. Cartridges and prefilled pens that have been punctured (in use) should be stored at temperatures <30°C (<86°F) and used within 42 days; do not freeze or refrigerate.

Monitoring and Teaching Issues

Laboratory Monitoring Diabetes mellitus: Plasma glucose, electrolytes, Hb A_{1c}, lipid profile

Physical Assessment Monitor for hypoglycemia at regular intervals during therapy. Teach patient proper use, including appropriate injection technique and syringe/needle disposal, and monitoring requirements.

Patient Education Do not share pens, cartridges, or needles with others. This medication is used to control diabetes; it is not a cure. It is imperative to follow other components of prescribed treatment (eg, diet and exercise regimen). If you experience hypoglycemic reaction, contact prescriber immediately. Always carry quick source of sugar with you. Monitor glucose levels as directed by prescriber. Report adverse side effects, including chest pain or palpitations; persistent fatigue, confusion, headache; skin rash or redness; numbness of mouth, lips, or tongue; muscle weakness or tremors; vision changes; respiratory difficulty; or nausea, vomiting, or flu-like symptoms.

Dietary Considerations Individualized medical nutrition therapy (MNT) based on ADA recommendations is an integral part of therapy.

Geriatric Considerations How "tightly" a geriatric patient's blood glucose should be controlled is controversial; however, a fasting blood sugar <150 mg/dL is now an acceptable endpoint. Such a decision should be based on the patient's functional and cognitive status, how well he/she recognizes hypoglycemic or hyperglycemic symptoms, and how to respond to them and any other disease states. Patients who are unable to accurately draw up their dose will need assistance such as prefilled syringes. Initial doses may require considerations for renal function in the elderly with dosing adjusted subsequently based on blood glucose monitoring. Intensive glucose control (Hb A_{1c} <6.5%) has been linked to increased all cause and cardiovascular mortality, hypoglycemia requiring assistance, and weight gain in adult type 2 diabetes. For elderly patients with diabetes who are relatively healthy, attaining target goals for aspirin use, blood pressure, lipids, smoking cessation, and diet and exercise may be more important than normalized glycemic control.

Breast-Feeding Considerations It is not known if insulin detemir is found in breast milk. Endogenous insulin can be found in breast milk. Plasma glucose concentrations in the mother affect glucose concentrations in breast milk. The gastrointestinal tract destroys insulin when administered orally; therefore, insulin is not expected to be absorbed intact by the breast-feeding infant. All types of insulin are safe for use while breast-feeding. Due to increased calorie expenditure, women with diabetes may require less insulin while nursing.

Pregnancy Considerations Adverse events were observed in animal reproduction studies; therefore, the manufacturer classifies insulin detemir as pregnancy category C. Maternal hyperglycemia can be associated with adverse effects in the fetus, including macrosomia, neonatal hyperglycemia, and hyperbilirubinemia; the risk of congenital malformations is increased when the Hb A_{1c} is above the normal range. Insulin requirements tend to fall during the first trimester of pregnancy and increase in the later trimesters, peaking at 28-32 weeks of gestation. Following delivery, insulin requirements decrease rapidly. Diabetes can be associated with adverse effects in the mother. Poorly-treated diabetes may cause end-organ damage that may in turn negatively affect obstetric outcomes. Physiologic glucose levels should be maintained prior to and during pregnancy to decrease the risk of adverse events in the fetus and the mother. Insulin is the drug of choice for the control of diabetes mellitus during pregnancy. Pregnant women using insulin detemir should be switched to NPH insulin pending additional safety information with this agent.

Additional Information Insulin detemir differs from human insulin by a single amino acid omission (threonine at B30) and the addition of a 14-carbon fatty acid chain attached at the B29 position. On injection, the fatty acid chain facilitates self-association between the molecules as well as binding to albumin. The delayed release of insulin from the injection site and albumin binding sites result in more prolonged action and limits variability in the amount of free insulin at steady-state. Insulin detemir has a duration of action which is dose-dependent. The FDA-approved product labeling identifies this product as a long-acting insulin analog; however, at lower dosages (<0.4 units/kg) published data regarding its duration of action is consistent with an intermediate insulin form (12-20 hours) (Plank, 2005). In clinical trials it has been compared primarily with NPH insulin and dosed in a similar manner. In some patients, or at higher dosages, it may have a duration of action up to 24 hours, which is consistent with a long-acting insulin (Le Floch, 2009; Plank, 2005; Porcellati, 2007).

Refer to Insulin Regular on page 994

Related Information

Diabetes Mellitus and Pregnancy *on page 2035*

Diabetes Mellitus Management, Adults *on page 2026*

Insulin Regular *on page 994*

Insulin Glargine (IN soo lin GLAR jeen)

U.S. Brand Names Lantus®; Lantus® Solostar®

Index Terms Glargine Insulin

Generic Availability (U.S.) No

Pharmacologic Category Antidiabetic Agent, Insulin

Medication Safety Issues

Sound-alike/look-alike issues:

Insulin glargine may be confused with insulin glulisine

Lantus® may be confused with latanoprost, Xalatan®

International issues:

Lantus [U.S., Canada, and multiple international markets] may be confused with Lanvis brand name for thioguanine [Canada and multiple international markets]

High alert medication: The Institute for Safe Medication Practices (ISMP) includes this medication among its list of drugs which have a heightened risk of causing significant patient harm when used in error. ***Due to the number of insulin preparations, it is essential to identify/clarify the type of insulin to be used.***

Note: Insulin glargine is a clear solution, but it is NOT intended for I.V. or I.M. administration.

Cross-contamination may occur if insulin pens are shared among multiple patients. Steps should be taken to prohibit sharing of insulin pens.

Pregnancy Risk Factor C

Lactation Excretion in breast milk unknown/compatible

Use Treatment of type 1 diabetes mellitus (insulin dependent, IDDM) and type 2 diabetes mellitus (noninsulin dependent, NIDDM) to improve glycemic control

Mechanism of Action/Effect Insulin glargine is a long-acting insulin analog.

Refer to Insulin Regular on page 994.

Contraindications Hypersensitivity to insulin glargine or any component of the formulation

Warnings/Precautions Refer to Insulin Regular on page 994. Safety and efficacy not established in children <6 years of age.

In type 1 diabetes mellitus (insulin dependent, IDDM), insulin lispro (Humalog®) and insulin glulisine (Apidra™) should be used in combination with a long-acting insulin. However, in type 2 diabetes mellitus (noninsulin dependent, NIDDM), insulin lispro (Humalog®) may be used without a long-acting insulin when used in combination with a sulfonylurea.

Drug Interactions

Metabolism/Transport Effects Refer to Insulin Regular on page 994.

Avoid Concomitant Use There are no known interactions where it is recommended to avoid concomitant use.

Decreased Effect

The levels/effects of Insulin Glargine may be decreased by: Corticosteroids (Orally Inhaled); Corticosteroids (Systemic); Luteinizing Hormone-Releasing Hormone Analogs; Somatropin; Thiazide Diuretics

Increased Effect/Toxicity Refer to Insulin Regular on page 994.

Nutritional/Ethanol Interactions Refer to Insulin Regular on page 994.

Adverse Reactions Refer to Insulin Regular on page 994.

Pharmacodynamics/Kinetics

Onset of Action 3-4 hours; Peak effect: No pronounced peak

Duration of Action Generally 24 hours or longer; reported range: 10.8 to >24 hours (up to 32 hours documented in some studies)

Absorption Slow; upon injection into the subcutaneous tissue, microprecipitates form which allow small amounts of insulin glargine to release over time

Time to Peak Plasma: No pronounced peak

Metabolism Partially metabolized in the skin to form two active metabolites

Excretion Urine

Pharmacokinetic Note Rate of absorption, onset, and duration of activity may be affected by site of injection, exercise, presence of lipodystrophy, local blood supply, and/or temperature.

Available Dosage Forms

Injection, solution:

Lantus®: 100 units/mL (3 mL, 10 mL)

Lantus® Solostar®: 100 units/mL (3 mL)

Dosing

Adult & Geriatric SubQ:

Type 1 diabetes: Refer to Insulin Regular on page 994.

Type 2 diabetes:

Patient not already on insulin: 10 units once daily, adjusted according to patient response (range in clinical study: 2-100 units/day)

Patient already receiving insulin: In clinical studies, when changing to insulin glargine from once-daily NPH or Ultralente® insulin, the initial dose was not changed; when changing from twice-daily NPH to once-daily insulin glargine, the total daily dose was reduced by 20% and adjusted according to patient response

Pediatric Note: Insulin glargine is approximately equipotent to human insulin, but has a slower onset, no pronounced peak, and a longer duration of activity. Changing the basal insulin component from another insulin to insulin glargine can be done on a unit-to-unit basis.

Diabetes mellitus:

Type 1: SubQ:

Children <6 years (unlabeled use): Refer to Insulin Regular on page 994.

Children ≥6 years: Refer to Insulin Regular on page 994.

Type 2: SubQ: Children (unlabeled use): Refer to Insulin Regular on page 994.

Renal Impairment Refer to Insulin Regular on page 994.

Hepatic Impairment Refer to Insulin Regular on page 994.

Administration

Other SubQ administration: Do not use if solution is viscous or cloudy; use only if clear and colorless with no visible particles. Insulin glargine should be administered once daily, at any time of day; however, administer at the same time each day. Cold injections should be avoided. SubQ administration is usually made into the thighs, arms, buttocks, or abdomen; rotate injection sites. Do not dilute or mix insulin glargine with any other insulin formulation or solution.

Stability

Storage Unopened vials, cartridges, and prefilled pens may be stored under refrigeration between 2°C and 8°C (36°F to 46°F) until the expiration date or at room temperature <30°C (<86°F) for 28 days; do not freeze; keep away from heat and sunlight. Once punctured (in use), vials may be stored under refrigeration or at room temperature <30°C (<86°F); use within 28 days. Cartridges within the OptiClik® system and prefilled pens (SoloStar®) that have been punctured (in use) should be stored at temperatures <30°C (<86°F) and used within 28 days; do not freeze or refrigerate.

Monitoring and Teaching Issues

Laboratory Monitoring Diabetes mellitus: Plasma glucose, electrolytes, Hb A_{1c}

Physical Assessment Monitor for hypoglycemia at regular intervals during therapy. Teach patient proper use, including appropriate injection technique and syringe/needle disposal, and monitoring requirements.

Patient Education Do not share pens, cartridges, or needles with others. This medication is used to control diabetes; it is not a cure. It is imperative to follow other components of prescribed treatment (eg, diet and exercise regimen). If you experience hypoglycemic reaction, contact prescriber immediately. Always carry quick source of sugar with you. Monitor glucose levels as directed by prescriber. Report adverse side effects, including chest pain or palpitations; persistent fatigue, confusion, headache; skin rash or redness; numbness of mouth, lips, or tongue; muscle weakness or tremors; vision changes; respiratory difficulty; or nausea, vomiting, or flu-like symptoms.

Dietary Considerations Individualized medical nutrition therapy (MNT) based on ADA recommendations is an integral part of therapy.

Geriatric Considerations Intensive glucose control (Hb A_{1c} <6.5%) has been linked to increased all cause and cardiovascular mortality, hypoglycemia requiring assistance, and weight gain in adult type 2 diabetes. For elderly patients with diabetes who are relatively healthy, attaining target goals for aspirin use, blood pressure, lipids, smoking cessation, and diet and exercise may be more important than normalized glycemic control.

Breast-Feeding Considerations It is not known if significant amounts of insulin glargine are found in breast milk. Endogenous insulin can be found in breast milk. Plasma glucose concentrations in the mother affect glucose concentrations in breast milk. The gastrointestinal tract destroys insulin when administered orally; therefore, insulin is not expected to be absorbed intact by the breast-feeding infant. All types of insulin are safe for use while breast-feeding. Due to increased calorie expenditure, women with diabetes may require less insulin while nursing.

Pregnancy Considerations Adverse events have been shown in some animal studies; therefore, the manufacturer classifies insulin glargine as pregnancy category C. Maternal hyperglycemia can be associated with adverse effects in the fetus, including macrosomia, neonatal hyperglycemia, and hyperbilirubinemia; the risk of congenital malformations is increased when Hb A_{1c} is above the normal range.

Insulin requirements tend to fall during the first trimester of pregnancy and increase in the later trimesters, peaking at 28-32 weeks of gestation. Following delivery, insulin requirements decrease rapidly. Diabetes can be associated with adverse effects in the mother. Poorly-treated diabetes may cause end-organ damage that may in turn negatively affect obstetric outcomes. Physiologic glucose levels should be maintained prior to and during pregnancy to decrease the risk of adverse events in the fetus and the mother. Insulin is the drug of choice for the control of diabetes mellitus during pregnancy. Pregnancy outcome information following the use of insulin glargine is available from case reports and small studies. Current reports indicate that insulin glargine is effective when used during pregnancy and may be an option for pregnant women with significantly uncontrolled diabetes; however, pregnant women using insulin glargine should be switched to NPH insulin pending additional safety information with this agent.

Additional Information The duration of action of insulin glargine is generally 24 hours or longer with a relatively flat action profile throughout this interval. Many pharmacokinetic and pharmacodynamic studies were terminated at 24 hours despite the fact that insulin glargine continued to exhibit hypoglycemic activity beyond 24 hours; therefore, it is difficult to determine the absolute duration of action.

Clinicians should be aware that, in rare cases, patients may exhibit hypoglycemic activity beyond 24 hours and that accumulation of insulin glargine is possible. Adequate monitoring and subsequent dosage adjustments should be made in patients who are requiring less insulin to maintain euglycemia after several days of therapy.

On the other hand, insulin glargine has a reported duration of action that ranges from 10.8 to >24 hours. On rare occasions, patients may require twice-daily injections of insulin glargine to deliver adequate basal insulin coverage over 24 hours. Some clinicians may also switch to twice-daily dosing in patients who require >100 units of insulin glargine per day to allow for complete absorption. Dosing insulin glargine 3 times daily is not recommended.

Also, refer to Insulin Regular on page 994.

Related Information

Diabetes Mellitus and Pregnancy *on page 2035*
Diabetes Mellitus Management, Adults *on page 2026*
Insulin Regular *on page 994*

Insulin Glulisine (IN soo lin gloo LIS een)

U.S. Brand Names Apidra®; Apidra® SoloStar®

Index Terms Glulisine Insulin

Generic Availability (U.S.) No

Pharmacologic Category Antidiabetic Agent, Insulin

Medication Safety Issues

Sound-alike/look-alike issues:

Insulin glulisine may be confused with insulin glargine

High alert medication: The Institute for Safe Medication Practices (ISMP) includes this medication among its list of drugs which have a heightened risk of causing significant patient harm when used in error. ***Due to the number of insulin preparations, it is essential to identify/clarify the type of insulin to be used.***

Cross-contamination may occur if insulin pens are shared among multiple patients. Steps should be taken to prohibit sharing of insulin pens.

Pregnancy Risk Factor C

Lactation Excretion in breast milk unknown/compatible

Use Treatment of type 1 diabetes mellitus (insulin dependent, IDDM) and type 2 diabetes mellitus (noninsulin dependent, NIDDM) to improve glycemic control

Available Dosage Forms

Injection, solution:

Apidra®: 100 units/mL (3 mL, 10 mL)

Apidra® SoloStar®: 100 units/mL (3 mL)

Dosing

Adult & Geriatric Refer to Insulin Regular on page 994.

Pediatric Refer to Insulin Regular on page 994.

Renal Impairment Refer to Insulin Regular on page 994.

Hepatic Impairment Refer to Insulin Regular on page 994.

Administration

I.V. Do not use if solution is viscous or cloudy; use only if clear and colorless. May be administered I.V. with close monitoring of blood glucose and serum potassium; appropriate medical supervision is required. **Do not administer insulin mixtures intravenously.**

Other

SubQ administration: Do not use if solution is viscous or cloudy; use only if clear and colorless. Insulin glulisine should be administered within 15 minutes before or within 20 minutes after starting a meal. Cold injections should be avoided. SubQ administration is usually made into the thighs, arms, buttocks, or abdomen; rotate injection sites. When mixing insulin glulisine with other preparations of insulin (eg, insulin NPH), insulin glulisine should be drawn into syringe first. Do not mix other insulin formulations with insulin glulisine contained in a cartridge or prefilled pen.

CSII administration: Do not use if solution is viscous or cloudy; use only if clear and colorless. Patients should be trained in the proper use of their external insulin pump and in intensive insulin therapy. Infusion sets, reservoirs, and infusion set insertion sites should be changed every 48 hours; rotate infusion sites. Do not dilute or mix other insulin formulations with insulin glulisine that is to be used in an external insulin pump.

Monitoring and Teaching Issues

Laboratory Monitoring

Diabetes mellitus: Plasma glucose, electrolytes, Hb A_{1c}

I.V. administration: Close monitoring of blood glucose and serum potassium

Physical Assessment Monitor for hypoglycemia at regular intervals during therapy. Teach patient proper use, including appropriate injection technique and syringe/needle disposal, and monitoring requirements.

Patient Education Do not share pens, cartridges, or needles with others. This medication is used to control diabetes; it is not a cure. It is imperative to follow other components of prescribed treatment (eg, diet and exercise regimen). Insulin glulisine (Apidra®) should be administered within 15 minutes before or within 20 minutes after start of a meal. If you experience hypoglycemic reaction, contact prescriber immediately. Always carry quick source of sugar with you. Monitor glucose levels as directed by prescriber. Report adverse side effects, including chest pain or palpitations; persistent fatigue, confusion, headache; skin rash or redness; numbness of mouth, lips, or tongue; muscle weakness or tremors; vision changes; respiratory difficulty; or nausea, vomiting, or flu-like symptoms.

Related Information

Diabetes Mellitus and Pregnancy *on page 2035*

Diabetes Mellitus Management, Adults *on page 2026*

Insulin Regular *on page 994*

Insulin Lispro (IN soo lin LYE sproe)

U.S. Brand Names HumaLOG®; HumaLOG® KwikPen™

Index Terms Lispro Insulin

Generic Availability (U.S.) No

Pharmacologic Category Antidiabetic Agent, Insulin

Medication Safety Issues

Sound-alike/look-alike issues:

HumaLOG® may be confused with HumaLOG® Mix 50/50, Humira®, HumuLIN® N, HumuLIN® R, NovoLOG®

High alert medication: The Institute for Safe Medication Practices (ISMP) includes this medication among its list of drugs which have a heightened risk of causing significant patient harm when used in error. ***Due to the number of insulin preparations, it is essential to identify/clarify the type of insulin to be used.***

Cross-contamination may occur if insulin pens are shared among multiple patients. Steps should be taken to prohibit sharing of insulin pens.

Pregnancy Risk Factor B

Lactation Excretion in breast milk unknown/compatible

Use Treatment of type 1 diabetes mellitus (insulin dependent, IDDM) and type 2 diabetes mellitus (noninsulin dependent, NIDDM) to improve glycemic control

Unlabeled/Investigational Use Gestational diabetes mellitus (GDM); mild-to-moderate diabetic ketoacidosis (DKA); mild-to-moderate hyperosmolar hyperglycemic state (HHS)

Mechanism of Action/Effect Refer to Insulin Regular on page 994. Insulin lispro is a rapid-acting form of insulin.

Contraindications Hypersensitivity to insulin lispro or any component of the formulation; during episodes of hypoglycemia

Warnings/Precautions Refer to Insulin Regular on page 994.

In type 1 diabetes mellitus (insulin dependent, IDDM), insulin lispro (Humalog®) and insulin glulisine (Apidra™) should be used in combination with a long-acting insulin. However, in type 2 diabetes mellitus (noninsulin dependent, NIDDM), insulin lispro (Humalog®) may be used without a long-acting insulin when used in combination with a sulfonylurea.

Drug Interactions

Metabolism/Transport Effects Refer to Insulin Regular on page 994.

Avoid Concomitant Use There are no known interactions where it is recommended to avoid concomitant use.

Decreased Effect

The levels/effects of Insulin Lispro may be decreased by: Corticosteroids (Orally Inhaled); Corticosteroids (Systemic); Luteinizing Hormone-Releasing Hormone Analogs; Somatropin; Thiazide Diuretics

Increased Effect/Toxicity Refer to Insulin Regular on page 994.

Nutritional/Ethanol Interactions Refer to Insulin Regular on page 994.

Adverse Reactions Refer to Insulin Regular on page 994.

Pharmacodynamics/Kinetics

Onset of Action 0.25-0.5 hours; Peak effect: 0.5-2.5 hours

Duration of Action ≤5 hours

Bioavailability 55% to 77%

Time to Peak Plasma: 0.5-1.5 hours

Half-Life Elimination

I.V.: ~0.5-1 hour (dose-dependent)

SubQ: 1 hour

Excretion Urine

Pharmacokinetic Note Rate of absorption, onset, and duration of activity may be affected by site of injection, exercise, presence of lipodystrophy, local blood supply, and/or temperature.

Available Dosage Forms

Injection, solution:

HumaLOG®: 100 units/mL (3 mL, 10 mL)

HumaLOG® KwikPen™: 100 units/mL (3 mL)

Dosing

Adult & Geriatric Refer to Insulin Regular on page 994. Insulin lispro is equipotent to insulin regular, but has a more rapid onset.

Pediatric Refer to Insulin Regular on page 994. Insulin lispro is equipotent to insulin regular, but has a more rapid onset.

Renal Impairment Refer to Insulin Regular on page 994.

Hepatic Impairment Refer to Insulin Regular on page 994.

Administration

I.V. I.V. administration (unlabeled use): Do not use if solution is viscous or cloudy; use only if clear and colorless. May be administered I.V. with close monitoring of blood glucose and serum potassium; appropriate medical supervision is required. Do not administer insulin mixtures intravenously.

Other

SubQ administration: Do not use if solution is viscous or cloudy; use only if clear and colorless. Insulin lispro should be administered within 15 minutes before or immediately after a meal. Cold injections should be avoided. SubQ administration is usually made into the thighs, arms, buttocks, or abdomen; rotate injection sites. When mixing insulin lispro with other preparations of insulin (eg, insulin NPH), insulin lispro should be drawn into syringe first. Do not dilute or mix other insulin formulations with insulin lispro contained in a cartridge or prefilled pen.

CSII administration: Do not use if solution is viscous or cloudy; use only if clear and colorless. Patients should be trained in the proper use of their external insulin pump and in intensive insulin therapy. Infusion sets, reservoirs, and infusion set insertion sites should be changed every 48 hours; rotate infusion sites. Do not dilute or mix other insulin formulations with insulin lispro contained in an external insulin pump.

Stability

Reconstitution

For SubQ administration: *Humalog® vials:* May be diluted with the universal diluent, Sterile Diluent for Humalog®, Humulin® N, Humulin® R, Humulin® 70/30, and Humulin® R U-500, to a concentration of 10 units/mL (U-10) or 50 units/mL (U-50). Do not dilute insulin contained in a cartridge, prefilled pen, or external insulin pump.

For I.V. infusion (unlabeled use): May be diluted in NS or D_5W to concentrations of 0.025-2 units/mL.

Storage Unopened vials, cartridges, and prefilled pens may be stored under refrigeration between 2°C and 8°C (36°F to 46°F) until the expiration date or at room temperature <30°C (<86°F) for 28 days; do not freeze; keep away from heat and sunlight. Once punctured (in use), vials may be stored under refrigeration or at room temperature <30°C (<86°F); use within 28 days. Cartridges and prefilled pens that have been punctured (in use) should be stored at temperatures <30°C (<86°F) and used within 28 days; do not freeze or refrigerate. When used for CSII, insulin lispro contained within an external insulin pump reservoir should be replaced every 48 hours and insulin lispro contained within a 3 mL cartridge should be discarded after 7 days; discard if exposed to temperatures >37°C (>98.6°F).

For SubQ administration: *Humalog® vials:* According to the manufacturer, diluted insulin should be stored at 30°C (86°F) and used within 14 days or 5°C (41°F) and used within 28 days.

For I.V. infusion (unlabeled use): Stable for 48 hours at room temperature.

Monitoring and Teaching Issues

Laboratory Monitoring

Diabetes mellitus: Plasma glucose, electrolytes, Hb A_{1c}

I.V. administration (unlabeled use): Close monitoring of blood glucose and serum potassium

Physical Assessment Monitor for hypoglycemia at regular intervals during therapy. Teach patient proper use, including appropriate injection technique and syringe/needle disposal, and monitoring requirements.

Patient Education Do not share pens, cartridges, or needles with others. This medication is used to control diabetes; it is not a cure. It is imperative to follow other components of prescribed treatment (eg, diet and exercise regimen). If you experience hypoglycemic reaction, contact prescriber immediately. Always carry quick source of sugar with you. Monitor glucose levels as directed by prescriber. Report adverse side effects, including chest pain or palpitations; persistent fatigue, confusion, headache; skin rash or redness; numbness of mouth, lips, or tongue; muscle weakness or tremors; vision changes; respiratory difficulty; or nausea, vomiting, or flu-like symptoms.

Dietary Considerations Individualized medical nutrition therapy (MNT) based on ADA recommendations is an integral part of therapy.

Geriatric Considerations How "tightly" a geriatric patient's blood glucose should be controlled is controversial; however, a fasting blood sugar <150 mg/dL is now an acceptable endpoint. Such a decision should be based on the patient's functional and cognitive status, how well he/she recognizes hypoglycemic or hyperglycemic symptoms, and how to respond to them and any other disease states. Patients who are unable to accurately draw up their dose will need assistance such as prefilled syringes. Initial doses may require considerations for renal function in the elderly with dosing adjusted subsequently based on blood glucose monitoring. Intensive glucose control (Hb A_{1c} <6.5%) has been linked to increased all cause and cardiovascular mortality, hypoglycemia requiring assistance, and weight gain in adult type 2 diabetes. For elderly patients with diabetes who are relatively healthy, attaining target goals for aspirin use, blood pressure, lipids, smoking cessation, and diet and exercise may be more important than normalized glycemic control.

Breast-Feeding Considerations It is not known if significant amounts of insulin lispro are found in breast milk. Endogenous insulin can be found in breast milk. Plasma glucose concentrations in the mother affect glucose concentrations in breast milk. The gastrointestinal tract destroys insulin when administered orally; therefore, insulin is not expected to be absorbed intact by the breast-feeding infant. All types of insulin are safe for use while breast-feeding. Due to increased calorie expenditure, women with diabetes may require less insulin while nursing.

Pregnancy Considerations Adverse events have not been observed in animal reproduction studies; therefore, the manufacturer classifies insulin lispro as pregnancy category B. Insulin lispro has not been shown to cross the placenta at standard clinical doses. Although congenital anomalies have been noted in case reports, when compared to regular insulin, insulin lispro has not been found to increase the risk of adverse events to the fetus in larger studies. Maternal hyperglycemia can be associated with adverse effects in the fetus, including macrosomia, neonatal hyperglycemia, and hyperbilirubinemia; the risk of congenital malformations is increased when Hb A_{1c} is above the normal range.

Insulin requirements tend to fall during the first trimester of pregnancy and increase in the later trimesters, peaking at 28-32 weeks of gestation. Following delivery, insulin requirements decrease rapidly. Diabetes can be associated with adverse effects in the mother. Poorly-treated diabetes may cause end-organ damage that may in turn negatively affect obstetric outcomes. Physiologic glucose levels should be maintained prior to and during pregnancy to decrease the risk of adverse events in the fetus and mother. Insulin is the drug of choice for the control of diabetes mellitus during pregnancy. The use of insulin lispro has been shown to be as effective as regular insulin to treat diabetes in pregnancy and may have advantages over regular insulin during pregnancy.

Additional Information Refer to Insulin Regular on page 994.

Related Information

Diabetes Mellitus and Pregnancy *on page 2035*

Diabetes Mellitus Management, Adults *on page 2026*

Insulin Regular *on page 994*

◆ **Insulin Lispro and Insulin Lispro Protamine** *see* Insulin Lispro Protamine and Insulin Lispro *on page 991*

Insulin Lispro Protamine and Insulin Lispro

(IN soo lin LYE sproe PROE ta meen & IN soo lin LYE sproe)

U.S. Brand Names HumaLOG® Mix 50/50™; HumaLOG® Mix 50/50™ KwikPen™; HumaLOG® Mix 75/25™; HumaLOG® Mix 75/25™ KwikPen™

Index Terms Insulin Lispro and Insulin Lispro Protamine

Generic Availability (U.S.) No

Pharmacologic Category Antidiabetic Agent, Insulin

Medication Safety Issues

Sound-alike/look-alike issues:

HumaLOG® Mix 50/50™ may be confused with HumaLOG®

HumaLOG® Mix 75/25™ may be confused with HumuLIN® 70/30, NovoLIN® 70/30, and NovoLOG® Mix 70/30

High alert medication: The Institute for Safe Medication Practices (ISMP) includes this medication among its list of drugs which have a heightened risk of causing significant patient harm when used in error. ***Due to the number of insulin preparations, it is essential to identify/clarify the type of insulin to be used.***

Cross-contamination may occur if insulin pens are shared among multiple patients. Steps should be taken to prohibit sharing of insulin pens.

Pregnancy Risk Factor B

Lactation Refer to Insulin Lispro on page 989.

Use Treatment of type 1 diabetes mellitus (insulin dependent, IDDM) and type 2 diabetes mellitus (noninsulin dependent, NIDDM) to improve glycemic control

Available Dosage Forms

Injection, suspension:

HumaLOG® Mix 50/50™: Insulin lispro protamine suspension 50% [intermediate acting] and insulin lispro solution 50% [rapid acting]: 100 units/mL (10 mL)

HumaLOG® Mix 50/50™ KwikPen™: Insulin lispro protamine suspension 50% [intermediate acting] and insulin lispro solution 50% [rapid acting]: 100 units/mL (3 mL)

HumaLOG® Mix 75/25™: Insulin lispro protamine suspension 75% [intermediate acting] and insulin lispro solution 25% [rapid acting]: 100 units/mL (10 mL)

HumaLOG® Mix 75/25™ KwikPen™: Insulin lispro protamine suspension 75% [intermediate acting] and insulin lispro solution 25% [rapid acting]: 100 units/mL (3 mL)

Dosing

Adult & Geriatric Refer to Insulin Regular on page 994. Fixed ratio insulins (such as insulin lispro protamine and insulin lispro) are normally administered in 2 daily doses.

Renal Impairment Refer to Insulin Regular on page 994.

Hepatic Impairment Refer to Insulin Regular on page 994.

Administration

Other SubQ administration: In order to properly resuspend the insulin, vials should be carefully shaken or rolled several times and prefilled pens should be rolled between the palms ten times and inverted 180° ten times. Properly resuspended insulin should look uniformly cloudy or milky; do not use if any white insulin substance remains at the bottom of the container, if any clumps are present, if the insulin remains clear after adequate mixing, or if white particles are stuck to the bottom or wall of the container. Cold injections should be avoided. Insulin lispro protamine and insulin lispro combination products should be administered within 15 minutes before a meal; typically given once- or twice daily. SubQ administration is usually made into the thighs, arms, buttocks, or abdomen; rotate injection sites. Do not dilute or mix with any other insulin formulation or solution; **not** recommended for use in external SubQ insulin infusion pump.

Monitoring and Teaching Issues

Laboratory Monitoring Diabetes mellitus: Plasma glucose, electrolytes, Hb A_{1c}

Physical Assessment See individual agents.

Patient Education See individual agents.

Related Information

Diabetes Mellitus and Pregnancy *on page 2035*

Diabetes Mellitus Management, Adults *on page 2026*

Insulin Regular *on page 994*

Insulin NPH (IN soo lin N P H)

U.S. Brand Names HumuLIN® N; NovoLIN® N

Index Terms Isophane Insulin; NPH Insulin

Generic Availability (U.S.) No

Pharmacologic Category Antidiabetic Agent, Insulin

Medication Safety Issues

Sound-alike/look-alike issues:

HumuLIN® N may be confused with HumuLIN® R, HumaLOG®, Humira®

NovoLIN® N may be confused with NovoLIN® R, NovoLOG®

High alert medication: The Institute for Safe Medication Practices (ISMP) includes this medication among its list of drugs which have a heightened risk of causing significant patient harm when used in error. ***Due to the number of insulin preparations, it is essential to identify/clarify the type of insulin to be used.***

Cross-contamination may occur if insulin pens are shared among multiple patients. Steps should be taken to prohibit sharing of insulin pens.

Lactation Excretion in breast milk unknown/compatible

Use Treatment of type 1 diabetes mellitus (insulin dependent, IDDM) and type 2 diabetes mellitus (noninsulin dependent, NIDDM) to improve glycemic control

Unlabeled/Investigational Use Gestational diabetes mellitus (GDM)

Available Dosage Forms

Injection, suspension:

HumuLIN® N: 100 units/mL (3 mL, 10 mL)

NovoLIN® N: 100 units/mL (10 mL)

Dosing

Adult & Geriatric Refer to Insulin Regular on page 994. Insulin NPH is usually administered 1-2 times daily.

Pediatric Refer to Insulin Regular on page 994. Insulin NPH is usually administered 1-2 times daily.

Renal Impairment Refer to Insulin Regular on page 994.

Hepatic Impairment Refer to Insulin Regular on page 994.

Administration

Other SubQ administration: In order to properly resuspend the insulin, vials should be carefully shaken or rolled several times, prefilled pens should be rolled between the palms ten times and inverted 180° ten times, and cartridges should be inverted 180° at least ten times. Properly resuspended insulin NPH should look uniformly cloudy or milky; do not use if any white insulin substance remains at the bottom of the container, if any clumps are present, or if white particles are stuck to the bottom or wall of the container. Cold injections should be avoided. SubQ administration is usually made into the thighs, arms, buttocks, or abdomen; rotate injection sites. When mixing insulin NPH with other preparations of insulin (eg, insulin aspart, insulin glulisine, insulin lispro, insulin regular), insulin NPH should be drawn into the syringe **after** the other insulin preparations. Do not dilute or mix other insulin formulations with insulin NPH contained in a cartridge or prefilled pen. Insulin NPH is **not** recommended for use in external SubQ insulin infusion pump.

Monitoring and Teaching Issues

Laboratory Monitoring Diabetes mellitus: Plasma glucose, electrolytes, Hb A_{1c}

Physical Assessment Monitor for hypoglycemia at regular intervals during therapy. Teach patient proper use, including appropriate injection technique and syringe/needle disposal, and monitoring requirements.

Patient Education Do not share pens, cartridges, or needles with others. This medication is used to control diabetes; it is not a cure. It is imperative to follow other components of prescribed treatment (eg, diet and exercise regimen). If you experience hypoglycemic reaction, contact prescriber immediately. Always carry quick source of sugar with you. Monitor glucose levels as directed by prescriber. Report adverse side effects, including chest pain or palpitations; persistent fatigue, confusion, headache; skin rash or redness; numbness of mouth, lips, or tongue; muscle weakness or tremors; vision changes; respiratory difficulty; or nausea, vomiting, or flu-like symptoms.

Related Information

Diabetes Mellitus and Pregnancy *on page 2035*

Diabetes Mellitus Management, Adults *on page 2026*

Insulin Regular *on page 994*

Insulin NPH and Insulin Regular (IN soo lin N P H & IN soo lin REG yoo ler)

U.S. Brand Names HumuLIN® 70/30; NovoLIN® 70/30

Index Terms Insulin Regular and Insulin NPH; Isophane Insulin and Regular Insulin; NPH Insulin and Regular Insulin

Generic Availability (U.S.) No

Pharmacologic Category Antidiabetic Agent, Insulin

Medication Safety Issues

Sound-alike/look-alike issues:

HumuLIN® 70/30 may be confused with HumaLOG® Mix 75/25, HumuLIN® R, NovoLIN® 70/30, NovoLOG® Mix 70/30

NovoLIN® 70/30 may be confused with HumaLOG® Mix 75/25, HumuLIN® 70/30, HumuLIN® R, NovoLIN® R, and NovoLOG® Mix 70/30

High alert medication: The Institute for Safe Medication Practices (ISMP) includes this medication among its list of drugs which have a heightened risk of causing significant patient harm when used in error. ***Due to the number of insulin preparations, it is essential to identify/clarify the type of insulin to be used.***

Cross-contamination may occur if insulin pens are shared among multiple patients. Steps should be taken to prohibit sharing of insulin pens.

Use Treatment of type 1 diabetes mellitus (insulin dependent, IDDM) and type 2 diabetes mellitus (noninsulin dependent, NIDDM) to improve glycemic control

Unlabeled/Investigational Use Gestational diabetes mellitus (GDM)

Available Dosage Forms

Injection, suspension:

HumuLIN® 70/30: Insulin NPH suspension 70% [intermediate acting] and insulin regular solution 30% [short acting]: 100 units/mL (3 mL, 10 mL)

NovoLIN® 70/30: Insulin NPH suspension 70% [intermediate acting] and insulin regular solution 30% [short acting]: 100 units/mL (10 mL)

Dosing

Adult & Geriatric Refer to Insulin Regular on page 994. Fixed ratio insulins are normally administered in 1-2 daily doses.

Pediatric Refer to Insulin Regular on page 994. Fixed ratio insulins are normally administered in 1-2 daily doses.

Renal Impairment Refer to Insulin Regular on page 994.

Hepatic Impairment Refer to Insulin Regular on page 994.

Administration

Other SubQ administration: In order to properly resuspend the insulin, vials should be carefully shaken or rolled several times, prefilled pens should be rolled between the palms ten times and inverted 180° ten times, and cartridges should be inverted 180° at least ten times.

Properly resuspended insulin should look uniformly cloudy or milky; do not use if any white insulin substance remains at the bottom of the container, if any clumps are present, if the insulin remains clear after adequate mixing, or if white particles are stuck to the bottom or wall of the container. Cold injections should be avoided. Insulin NPH and insulin regular combination products should be administered within 30 minutes before a meal; typically given once- or twice daily. SubQ administration is usually made into the thighs, arms, buttocks, or abdomen; rotate injection sites. Do not mix with any other insulin formulation. Do not dilute combination product (insulin NPH and insulin regular) contained in a cartridge or prefilled pen. Combination insulin products are not recommended for use in an external SubQ insulin infusion pump.

Monitoring and Teaching Issues

Laboratory Monitoring Diabetes mellitus: Plasma glucose, electrolytes, Hb A_{1c}

Physical Assessment See individual agents.

Patient Education See individual agents.

Related Information

Diabetes Mellitus and Pregnancy *on page 2035*

Diabetes Mellitus Management, Adults *on page 2026*

Insulin Regular *on page 994*

Insulin Regular (IN soo lin REG yoo ler)

U.S. Brand Names HumuLIN® R; HumuLIN® R U-500; NovoLIN® R

Index Terms Regular Insulin

Generic Availability (U.S.) No

Pharmacologic Category Antidiabetic Agent, Insulin

Medication Safety Issues

Sound-alike/look-alike issues:

HumuLIN® R may be confused with HumaLOG®, Humira®, HumuLIN® 70/30, HumuLIN® N, NovoLIN® 70/30, NovoLIN® R, NovoLOG®

NovoLIN® R may be confused with HumuLIN® R, NovoLIN® 70/30, NovoLIN® N, NovoLOG®

High alert medication: The Institute for Safe Medication Practices (ISMP) includes this medication among its list of drugs which have a heightened risk of causing significant patient harm when used in error. ***Due to the number of insulin preparations, it is essential to identify/clarify the type of insulin to be used.***

Concentrated solutions (eg, U-500) should not be available in patient care areas. U-500 regular insulin should be stored, dispensed, and administered separately from U-100 regular insulin. For patients who receive U-500 insulin in the hospital setting, highlighting the strength prominently on the patient's medical chart and medication record may help to reduce dispensing errors.

Cross-contamination may occur if insulin pens are shared among multiple patients. Steps should be taken to prohibit sharing of insulin pens.

Lactation Excretion in breast milk unknown/compatible

Use Treatment of type 1 diabetes mellitus (insulin dependent, IDDM) and type 2 diabetes mellitus (noninsulin dependent, NIDDM) to improve glycemic control

Unlabeled/Investigational Use Hyperkalemia; gestational diabetes mellitus (GDM), diabetic ketoacidosis (DKA); hyperosmolar hyperglycemic state (HHS); adjunct of parenteral nutrition

Mechanism of Action/Effect Insulin acts via specific membrane-bound receptors on target tissues to regulate metabolism of carbohydrate, protein, and fats. Target organs for insulin include the liver, skeletal muscle, and adipose tissue.

Within the liver, insulin stimulates hepatic glycogen synthesis. Insulin promotes hepatic synthesis of fatty acids, which are released into the circulation as lipoproteins. Skeletal muscle effects of insulin include increased protein synthesis and increased glycogen synthesis. Within adipose tissue, insulin stimulates the processing of circulating lipoproteins to provide free fatty acids, facilitating triglyceride synthesis and storage by adipocytes; also directly inhibits the hydrolysis of triglycerides. In addition, insulin stimulates the cellular uptake of amino acids and increases cellular permeability to several ions, including potassium, magnesium, and phosphate. By activating sodium-potassium ATPases, insulin promotes the intracellular movement of potassium.

Insulins are categorized based on the onset, peak, and duration of effect (eg, rapid-, short-, intermediate-, and long-acting insulin).

Contraindications Hypersensitivity to regular insulin or any component of the formulation; during episodes of hypoglycemia

Warnings/Precautions Hypoglycemia is the most common adverse effect of insulin. The timing of hypoglycemia differs among various insulin formulations. Hypoglycemia may result from increased work or exercise without eating; use of long-acting insulin preparations (eg, insulin detemir, insulin glargine) may delay recovery from hypoglycemia. Profound and prolonged episodes of hypoglycemia may result in convulsions, unconsciousness, temporary or permanent brain damage or even death. Insulin requirements may be altered during illness, emotional disturbances or other stressors. Insulin may produce hypokalemia which, if left untreated, may result in respiratory paralysis, ventricular arrhythmia and even death. Use with caution in patients at risk for hypokalemia (eg, I.V. insulin use). Use with caution in renal or hepatic impairment.

Human insulin differs from animal-source insulin. Any change of insulin should be made cautiously; changing manufacturers, type, and/or method of manufacture may result in the need for a change of dosage. U-500 regular insulin is a concentrated insulin formulation which contains 500 units of insulin per mL; for SubQ administration only using a U-100 insulin syringe or tuberculin syringe; **not for I.V. administration**. To avoid dosing errors when using a U-100 insulin syringe, the prescribed dose should be written in actual insulin units and as unit markings on the U-100 insulin syringe (eg, 50 units [10 units on a U-100 insulin syringe]). To avoid dosing errors when using a tuberculin syringe, the prescribed dose should be written in actual insulin units and as a volume (eg, 50 units [0.1 mL]). Mixing U-500 regular insulin with other insulin formulations is not recommended.

Regular insulin may be administered I.V. or I.M. in selected clinical situations; close monitoring of blood glucose and serum potassium, as well as medical supervision, is required.

The general objective of exogenous insulin therapy is to approximate the physiologic pattern of insulin secretion which is characterized by two distinct phases. Phase 1 insulin secretion suppresses hepatic glucose production and phase 2 insulin secretion occurs in response to carbohydrate ingestion; therefore, exogenous insulin therapy may consist of basal insulin (eg, intermediate- or long-acting insulin or via continuous subcutaneous insulin infusion [CSII]) and/or preprandial insulin (eg, short- or rapid-acting insulin). Patients with type 1 diabetes do not produce endogenous insulin; therefore, these patients require both basal and preprandial insulin administration. Patients with type 2 diabetes retain some beta-cell function in the early stages of their disease; however, as the disease progresses, phase 1 insulin secretion may become completely impaired and phase 2 insulin secretion becomes delayed and/or inadequate in response to meals. Therefore, patients with type 2 diabetes may be treated with oral antidiabetic agents, basal insulin, and/or preprandial insulin depending on the stage of disease and current glycemic control. Since treatment regimens often consist of multiple agents, dosage adjustments must address the specific phase of insulin release that is primarily contributing to the patient's impaired glycemic control. Diabetes self-management education (DSME) is essential to maximize the effectiveness of therapy. Treatment and monitoring regimens must be individualized.

Drug Interactions

Metabolism/Transport Effects Induces CYP1A2 (weak)

Avoid Concomitant Use There are no known interactions where it is recommended to avoid concomitant use.

Decreased Effect

The levels/effects of Insulin Regular may be decreased by: Corticosteroids (Orally Inhaled); Corticosteroids (Systemic); Luteinizing Hormone-Releasing Hormone Analogs; Somatropin; Thiazide Diuretics

Increased Effect/Toxicity

Insulin Regular may increase the levels/effects of: Antidiabetic Agents (Thiazolidinedione); Hypoglycemic Agents; Quinolone Antibiotics

The levels/effects of Insulin Regular may be increased by: Beta-Blockers; Edetate CALCIUM Disodium; Edetate Disodium; Herbs (Hypoglycemic Properties); Pegvisomant

Nutritional/Ethanol Interactions

Ethanol: Use caution with ethanol; may increase risk of hypoglycemia.

Herb/Nutraceutical: Use caution with alfalfa, aloe, bilberry, bitter melon, burdock, celery, damiana, fenugreek, garcinia, garlic, ginger, ginseng (American), gymnema, marshmallow, stinging nettle; may increase risk of hypoglycemia.

Adverse Reactions Frequency not defined.

Cardiovascular: Palpitation, pallor, peripheral edema, tachycardia

Central nervous system: Fatigue, headache, hypothermia, loss of consciousness, mental confusion

Dermatologic: Pruritus, rash, redness, urticaria

Endocrine & metabolic: Hypoglycemia, hypokalemia

Gastrointestinal: Hunger, nausea, numbness of mouth, weight gain

Local: Injection site reaction (including edema, itching, pain or warmth, stinging), lipoatrophy, lipodystrophy

Neuromuscular & skeletal: Muscle weakness, paresthesia, tremor

Ocular: Transient presbyopia or blurred vision

Miscellaneous: Anaphylaxis, antibodies to insulin (no change in efficacy), diaphoresis, local allergy, systemic allergic symptoms

Pharmacodynamics/Kinetics

Onset of Action SubQ: 0.5 hours; Peak effect: SubQ: 2.5-5 hours

Duration of Action SubQ:

U-100: 4-12 hours (may increase with dose)

U-500: Up to 24 hours

Bioavailability SubQ: 55% to 77%

Time to Peak Plasma: SubQ: 0.8-2 hours

Half-Life Elimination I.V.: ~0.5-1 hour (dose-dependent); SubQ: 1 hour

Excretion Urine

Pharmacokinetic Note Rate of absorption, onset, and duration of activity may be affected by site of injection, exercise, presence of lipodystrophy, local blood supply, and/or temperature.

Available Dosage Forms

Injection, solution:

HumuLIN® R: 100 units/mL (3 mL, 10 mL)

HumuLIN® R U-500: 500 units/mL (20 mL)

NovoLIN® R: 100 units/mL (10 mL)

Dosing

Adult & Geriatric

Diabetes mellitus: SubQ: **Note:** Insulin requirements vary dramatically between patients and therapy requires dosage adjustments with careful medical supervision. Specific formulations may require distinct administration procedures; please see individual agents.

Type 1: **Note:** Multiple daily injections (MDI) guided by blood glucose monitoring or the use of continuous subcutaneous insulin infusions (CSII) is the standard of care for patients with type 1 diabetes. Combinations of insulin formulations are commonly used.

Initial dose: 0.5-1.0 units/kg/day in divided doses. Conservative initial doses of 0.2-0.4 units/kg/day may be recommended to avoid the potential for hypoglycemia.

Division of daily insulin requirement: Generally, 50% to 75% of the total daily dose (TDD) is given as an intermediate- or long-acting form of insulin (in 1-2 daily injections). The remaining portion of the TDD is then divided and administered before or at mealtimes (depending on the formulation) as a rapid-acting or short-acting form of insulin. Premixed combinations are available that deliver the rapid- or short-acting component at the same time as the intermediate- or long-acting component. Some patients may benefit from the use of CSII which delivers rapid-acting insulin as a continuous infusion throughout the day and as boluses at mealtimes via an external pump device.

Adjustment of dose: Dosage must be titrated to achieve glucose control and avoid hypoglycemia. Adjust dose to maintain preprandial plasma glucose between 70-130 mg/dL for most patients. Since treatment regimens often consist of multiple formulations, dosage adjustments must address the specific phase of insulin release that is primarily contributing to the patient's impaired glycemic control. Treatment and monitoring regimens must be individualized. Also see Additional Information.

Usual maintenance range: 0.5-1.2 units/kg/day in divided doses. Insulin requirements are patient-specific and may vary based on age, body weight, and/or activity factors:

Adolescents: May require as much as 1.5 units/kg/day during puberty (Silverstein, 2005)

Prepuberty: 0.7-1 unit/kg/day

Type 2: The goal of therapy is to achieve an Hb A_{1c} <7% as quickly as possible using the safe titration of medications. According to a consensus statement by the ADA and European Association for the Study of Diabetes (EASD), basal insulin therapy (eg, intermediate- or long-acting insulin) should be considered in patients with type 2 diabetes who fail to achieve glycemic goals with lifestyle interventions and metformin ± a sulfonylurea. Pioglitazone or a GLP-1 agonist may also be considered prior to initiation of basal insulin therapy. In patients who continue to fail to achieve glycemic goals despite the addition of basal insulin, intensification of insulin therapy should be considered; this generally consists of multiple daily injections with a combination of insulin formulations (Nathan, 2009).

Initial basal insulin dose: 0.2 units/kg or 10 units/day (Nathan, 2009). **Note:** Current guidelines recommend that insulin therapy begin with intermediate- or long-acting insulin given at bedtime or long-acting insulin given in the morning (Nathan, 2009).

Adjustment of basal insulin dose: Increase dose by 2 units/day every 3 days until fasting glucose levels are consistently within target range (70-130 mg/dL); may increase dose in larger increments (eg, 4 units/day) if fasting glucose levels are >180 mg/dL (Nathan, 2009)

Note: If the patient experiences hypoglycemia following adjustment, reduce dose by 4 units/day or 10% of total daily dose, whichever is greater (Nathan, 2009). Additional algorithms, such as the "1-1-100", "2-4-6-8", "3-0-3", and "3-2-1" algorithms, exist to aid in the titration of basal insulin (Davies, 2005; Gerstein, 2006; Meneghini, 2007; Riddle, 2003); therapy should be individualized and based on patient-specific details.

Intensification of therapy: Add a second injection of a short-, rapid-, or intermediate-acting insulin as needed based on blood glucose monitoring; the timing of administration and type of insulin added for intensification of therapy depends on the blood glucose level that is consistently out of the target range (eg, preprandial glucose levels before lunch or dinner, postprandial glucose levels, and/or bedtime glucose levels). Additional injections and subsequent dosage adjustments must address the specific phase of insulin release that is primarily contributing to the patient's impaired glycemic control. Intensification of therapy can usually begin with a second injection of ~4 units/day followed by adjustments of ~2 units/day every 3 days until the targeted blood glucose is within range (Nathan, 2009).

In the setting of glucose toxicity (loss of beta-cell sensitivity to glucose concentrations), insulin therapy may be used for short-term management to restore sensitivity of beta-cells; in these cases, the dose may need to be rapidly reduced/withdrawn when sensitivity is re-established.

Diabetic ketoacidosis (DKA) (unlabeled use): Only I.V. regular insulin should be used for severe DKA; use of SubQ rapid-acting insulin analogs (eg, aspart, lispro) may be appropriate for mild-moderate DKA (Kitabchi, 2009). Treatment should continue until reversal of acid-base derangement/ketonemia. Serum glucose is not a direct indicator of these abnormalities, and may decrease more rapidly than correction of the metabolic abnormalities. Also, refer to institution-specific protocols where appropriate.

Adults <20 years (Kitabchi, 2004):

I.V. infusion: 0.1 units/kg/hour

Adjustment: If serum glucose does not fall by 50 mg/dL in the first hour, check hydration status; if acceptable, double insulin dose hourly until glucose levels fall at rate of 50-75 mg/dL per hour. Once serum glucose reaches 250 mg/dL, decrease dose to 0.05-0.1 units/kg/hour; dextrose-containing I.V. fluids should be administered to maintain serum glucose between 150-250 mg/dL until the acidosis clears. After resolution of DKA, supplement I.V. insulin with SubQ insulin as needed until the patient is able to eat and transition fully to a SubQ insulin regimen. An overlap of ~1-2 hours between discontinuation of I.V. insulin and administration of SubQ insulin is recommended to ensure adequate plasma insulin levels.

SubQ, I.M. (**Note:** Only use the SubQ and I.M route if I.V. infusion access is unavailable): 0.1-0.3 units/kg SubQ bolus, followed by 0.1 units/kg given every hour SubQ or I.M. or 0.15-0.2 units/kg every 2 hours SubQ; continue until acidosis clears, then decrease to 0.05 units/kg given every hour until SubQ replacement dosing can be initiated (Kitabchi, 2004; Wolfsdorf, 2007)

Adults ≥20 years (Kitabchi, 2009):

I.V.:

Bolus: 0.1 units/kg (optional)

Infusion: 0.1-0.14 units/kg/hour. **Note:** If no I.V. bolus was administered, patients should receive a continuous infusion of 0.14 units/kg/hour; lower doses may not achieve adequate insulin concentrations to suppress hepatic ketone body production.

Adjustment: If serum glucose does not fall by at least 10% in the first hour, give an I.V. bolus of 0.14 units/kg and continue previous regimen. In addition, if serum glucose does not fall by 50-70 mg/dL in the first hour, the insulin infusion dose should be increased hourly until a steady glucose decline is achieved Once serum glucose reaches 200 mg/dL, decrease infusion dose to 0.02-0.05 units/kg/hour or switch to SubQ rapid-acting insulin (eg, aspart, lispro) at 0.1 units/kg every 2 hours; dextrose-containing I.V. fluids should be administered to maintain serum glucose between 150-250 mg/dL until the acidosis clears. After resolution of DKA, supplement I.V. insulin with SubQ insulin as needed until the patient is able to eat and transition fully to a SubQ insulin regimen. An overlap of ~1-2 hours between discontinuation of I.V. insulin and administration of SubQ insulin is recommended to ensure adequate plasma insulin levels.

SubQ, I.M.: According to the 2009 ADA consensus statement on hyperglycemic crises, a rapid-acting insulin analog (eg, aspart, lispro) given every 1-2 hours via the SubQ route may be appropriate for mild-moderate DKA; however, specific dosing recommendations are not provided (Kitabchi, 2009). If using the I.V. route for severe DKA, consider switching to SubQ rapid-acting insulin once serum glucose reaches 200 mg/dL (Kitabchi, 2009). The following dosing regimen from the 2004 ADA position statement recommends regular insulin (Kitabchi, 2004):

Bolus: 0.4 units/kg; **Note:** Give half of the dose (0.2 units/kg) as an I.V. bolus and half of the dose (0.2 units/kg) as SubQ or I.M.

Intermittent: 0.1 units/kg given every hour SubQ or I.M.

Adjustment: If serum glucose does not fall by 50-70 mg/dL in the first hour, administer 10 units hourly by I.V. bolus until glucose levels fall at a rate of 50-70 mg/dL per hour. Once serum glucose reaches 250 mg/dL, decrease dose to 5-10 units SubQ every 2 hours; dextrose-containing I.V. fluids should be administered to maintain serum glucose between 150-250 mg/dL until the acidosis clears.

Gestational diabetes mellitus (unlabeled use): Insulin therapy should be considered when medical nutrition therapy has not achieved GDM glycemic goals (fasting plasma glucose: <95 mg/dL; 1-hour postprandial levels: <130-140 mg/dL; 2-hour postprandial levels: <120 mg/dL); dose and timing of administration should be based on frequent monitoring of plasma glucose levels (ACOG, 2001; ADA, 2004). Human insulin may be preferred (ADA, 2004); however, rapid-acting insulin analogues may also be considered (ACOG, 2001).

Hyperkalemia, moderate-to-severe (unlabeled use): I.V.: 10 units regular insulin mixed with 25 g dextrose (50 mL $D_{50}W$) given over 15-30 minutes (ACLS, 2010); alternatively, 50 mL $D_{50}W$ over 5 minutes followed by 10 units regular insulin I.V. push over seconds may be administered in the setting of imminent cardiac arrest. In patients with ongoing cardiac arrest (eg, PEA with presumed hyperkalemia), administration of $D_{50}W$ over <5 minutes is routine. Effects on potassium are temporary. As appropriate, consider methods of enhancing potassium removal/excretion.

Hyperosmolar hyperglycemic state (HHS) (unlabeled use): Only regular insulin should be used. Infusion should continue until reversal of mental status changes and hyperosmolality. Serum glucose is not a direct indicator of these abnormalities, and may decrease more rapidly than correction of the metabolic abnormalities. Also, refer to institution-specific protocols where appropriate.

Adults <20 years (Kitabchi, 2004):

I.V.:

Infusion: 0.1 units/kg/hour

Adjustment: If serum glucose does not fall by 50 mg/dL in the first hour, check hydration status; if acceptable, double insulin dose hourly until glucose levels fall at rate of 50-75 mg/dL per hour. Once serum glucose reaches 300 mg/dL, decrease dose to 0.05-0.1 units/kg/hour; dextrose-containing I.V. fluids should be administered to maintain serum glucose between 250-300 mg/dL until hyperosmolality clears and mental status returns to normal. After resolution of HHS, supplement I.V. insulin with SubQ insulin as needed until the patient is able to eat and transition fully to a SubQ insulin regimen. An overlap of ~1-2 hours between discontinuation of I.V. insulin and administration of SubQ insulin is recommended to ensure adequate plasma insulin levels.

SubQ, I.M. (**Note:** Only use the SubQ and I.M route if I.V. infusion access is unavailable): 0.1-0.3 units/kg SubQ bolus, followed by 0.1 units/kg given every hour SubQ or I.M. or 0.15-0.2 units/kg every 2 hours SubQ; continue until resolution of hyperosmolality, then decrease to 0.05 units/kg given every hour until SubQ replacement dosing can be initiated (Kitabchi, 2004; Wolfsdorf, 2007)

Adults ≥20 years (Kitabchi, 2009):

I.V.:

Bolus: 0.1 units/kg bolus (optional)

Infusion: 0.1-0.14 units/kg/hour. **Note:** If no I.V. bolus was administered, patients should receive a continuous infusion of 0.14 units/kg/hour.

Adjustment: If serum glucose does not fall by at least 10% in the first hour, give an I.V. bolus of 0.14 units/kg and continue previous regimen. In addition, if serum glucose does not fall by 50-70 mg/dL in the first hour, the insulin infusion dose should be increased hourly until a steady glucose decline is achieved. Once serum glucose reaches 300 mg/dL, decrease dose to 0.02-0.05 units/kg/hour; dextrose-containing I.V. fluids should be administered to maintain serum glucose between 200-300 mg/dL until the patient is mentally alert. After resolution of HHS, supplement I.V. insulin with SubQ insulin as needed until the patient is able to eat and transition fully to a SubQ insulin regimen. An overlap of ~1-2 hours between discontinuation of I.V. insulin and administration of SubQ insulin is recommended to ensure adequate plasma insulin levels.

Pediatric Diabetes mellitus: Refer to adult dosing.

Diabetic ketoacidosis (DKA) (unlabeled use): Only I.V. regular insulin should be used for severe DKA; use of SubQ rapid-acting insulin analogs (eg, aspart, lispro) may be appropriate for mild-moderate DKA (Kitabchi, 2009). Treatment should continue until reversal of acid-base derangement/ketonemia. Serum glucose is not a direct indicator of these abnormalities, and may decrease more rapidly than correction of the metabolic abnormalities. Also, refer to institution-specific protocols where appropriate.

I.V.: (Kitabchi, 2004):

Infusion: 0.1 units/kg/hour

Adjustment: If serum glucose does not fall by 50 mg/dL in the first hour, check hydration status; if acceptable, double insulin dose hourly until glucose levels fall at rate of 50-75 mg/dL per hour. Once serum glucose reaches 250 mg/dL, decrease dose to 0.05-0.1 units/kg/hour; dextrose-containing I.V. fluids should be administered to maintain serum glucose between 150-250 mg/dL until the acidosis clears. After resolution of DKA, supplement I.V. insulin with SubQ insulin as needed until the patient is able to eat and transition fully to a SubQ insulin regimen. An overlap of ~1-2 hours between discontinuation of I.V. insulin and administration of SubQ insulin is recommended to ensure adequate plasma insulin levels.

SubQ, I.M. (**Note:** Only use the SubQ and I.M route if I.V. infusion access is unavailable): 0.1-0.3 units/kg SubQ bolus, followed by 0.1 units/kg given every hour SubQ or I.M. or 0.15-0.2 units/kg every 2 hours SubQ; continue until acidosis clears, then decrease to 0.05 units/kg given every hour until SubQ replacement dosing can be initiated (Kitabchi, 2004; Wolfsdorf, 2007)

Hyperkalemia, moderate-to-severe (unlabeled use): I.V.: 0.1 units/kg regular insulin with dextrose 400 mg/kg infused over 15-30 minutes; ratio of ~1 unit of insulin to every 4 g of dextrose (Hegenbarth, 2008). **Note:** Dextrose monotherapy may be sufficient to correct hyperkalemia.

Hyperosmolar hyperglycemic state (HHS) (unlabeled use): Only regular insulin should be used. Infusion should continue until reversal of mental status changes and hyperosmolality. Serum glucose is not a direct indicator of these abnormalities, and may decrease more rapidly than correction of the metabolic abnormalities. Also, refer to institution-specific protocols where appropriate.

I.V. (Kitabchi, 2004):

Infusion: 0.1 units/kg/hour

Adjustment: If serum glucose does not fall by 50 mg/dL in the first hour, check hydration status; if acceptable, double insulin dose hourly until glucose levels fall at rate of 50-75 mg/dL per hour. Once serum glucose reaches 300 mg/dL, decrease dose to 0.05-0.1 units/kg/hour; dextrose-containing I.V. fluids should be administered to maintain serum glucose between 250-300 mg/dL until hyperosmolality clears and mental status returns to normal. After resolution of HHS, supplement I.V. insulin with SubQ insulin as needed until the patient is able to eat and transition fully to a SubQ insulin regimen. An overlap of ~1-2 hours between discontinuation of I.V. insulin and administration of SubQ insulin is recommended to ensure adequate plasma insulin levels.

SubQ, I.M. (**Note:** Only use the SubQ and I.M route if I.V. infusion access is unavailable): 0.1-0.3 units/kg SubQ bolus, followed by 0.1 units/kg given every hour SubQ or I.M. or 0.15-0.2 units/kg every 2 hours SubQ; continue until resolution of hyperosmolality, then decrease to 0.05 units/kg given every hour until SubQ replacement dosing can be initiated (Kitabchi, 2004; Wolfsdorf, 2007)

Renal Impairment Insulin requirements are reduced due to changes in insulin clearance or metabolism. Close monitoring of blood glucose and adjustment of therapy is required in renal impairment.

Cl_{cr} 10-50 mL/minute: Administer at 75% of normal dose and monitor glucose closely

Cl_{cr} <10 mL/minute: Administer at 25% to 50% of normal dose and monitor glucose closely

Hemodialysis: Because of a large molecular weight (6000 daltons), insulin is not significantly removed by hemodialysis; supplemental dose is not necessary.

Peritoneal dialysis: Because of a large molecular weight (6000 daltons), insulin is not significantly removed by peritoneal dialysis; supplemental dose is not necessary.

Continuous renal replacement therapy: Administer 75% of normal dose and monitor glucose closely; supplemental dose is not necessary.

Hepatic Impairment Insulin requirements may be reduced. Close monitoring of blood glucose and adjustment of therapy is required in hepatic impairment.

Administration

I.M. Do not use if solution is viscous or cloudy; use only if clear and colorless. May be administered I.M. in selected clinical situations; close monitoring of blood glucose and serum potassium as well as medical supervision is required.

I.V. Do not use if solution is viscous or cloudy; use only if clear and colorless. May be administered I.V. with close monitoring of blood glucose and serum potassium; appropriate medical supervision is required. If possible, avoid I.V. bolus administration in pediatric patients with DKA; may increase risk of cerebral edema. **Do not administer mixtures of insulin formulations intravenously.** I.V. administration of U-500 regular insulin is not recommended.

Other SubQ administration: Do not use if solution is viscous or cloudy; use only if clear and colorless. Regular insulin should be administered within 30-60 minutes before a meal. Cold injections should be avoided. SubQ administration is usually made into the thighs, arms, buttocks, or abdomen; rotate injection sites. When mixing regular insulin with other preparations of insulin, regular insulin should be drawn into syringe first. Regular insulin is not recommended for use in external SubQ insulin infusion pump.

Stability

Reconstitution

For SubQ administration:

Humulin® R: May be diluted with the universal diluent, Sterile Diluent for Humalog®, Humulin® N, Humulin® R, Humulin® 70/30, and Humulin® R U-500, to a concentration of 10 units/mL (U-10) or 50 units/mL (U-50).

Novolin® R: Insulin Diluting Medium for NovoLog® is **not** intended for use with Novolin® R or any insulin product other than insulin aspart.

For I.V. infusion:

Humulin® R: May be diluted in NS or D_5W to concentrations of 0.1-1 unit/mL.

Novolin® R: May be diluted in NS, D_5W, or $D_{10}W$ with 40 mEq/L potassium chloride at concentrations of 0.05-1 unit/mL.

Storage Store unopened vials in refrigerator between 2°C and 8°C (36°F to 46°F); do not freeze; keep away from heat and sunlight. Once punctured (in use), vials may be stored under refrigeration or at room temperature. If refrigeration is not possible, unopened Novolin® R vials may be kept at room temperature ≤25°C (≤77°F) for up to 42 days. Punctured (in use) Novolin® R vials may be stored at room temperature <25°C (<77°F); use within 42 days.

For SubQ administration:

Humulin® R: According to the manufacturer, diluted insulin should be stored at 30°C (86°F) and used within 14 days **or** at 5°C (41°F) and used within 28 days.

For I.V. infusion:

Humulin® R: Stable for 48 hours at room temperature, 96 hours under refrigeration, or for 48 hours under refrigeration followed by 48 hours at room temperature.

Novolin® R: Stable for 24 hours at room temperature

Monitoring and Teaching Issues

Laboratory Monitoring

Diabetes mellitus: Plasma glucose, electrolytes, Hb A_{1c}

DKA/HHS: Serum electrolytes, glucose, BUN, creatinine, osmolality, venous pH (repeat arterial blood gases are generally unnecessary), anion gap; urine output, urinalysis

Hyperkalemia: Serum potassium and glucose must be closely monitored to avoid hypokalemia, rebound hyperkalemia, and hypoglycemia.

Physical Assessment Monitor for hypoglycemia at regular intervals during therapy. Teach patient proper use, including appropriate injection technique and syringe/needle disposal, and monitoring requirements.

Patient Education Do not share pens, cartridges, or needles with others. This medication is used to control diabetes; it is not a cure. It is imperative to follow other components of prescribed treatment (eg, diet and exercise regimen). If you experience hypoglycemic reaction, contact prescriber immediately. Always carry quick source of sugar with you. Monitor glucose levels as directed by prescriber. Report adverse side effects, including chest pain or palpitations; persistent fatigue, confusion, headache; skin rash or redness; numbness of mouth, lips, or tongue; muscle weakness or tremors; vision changes; respiratory difficulty; or nausea, vomiting, or flu-like symptoms.

Dietary Considerations Individualized medical nutrition therapy (MNT) based on ADA recommendations is an integral part of therapy.

Geriatric Considerations How "tightly" a geriatric patient's blood glucose should be controlled is controversial; however, a fasting blood sugar <150 mg/dL is now an acceptable endpoint. Such a decision should be based on the patient's functional and cognitive status, how well he/she recognizes hypoglycemic or hyperglycemic symptoms, and how to respond to them and any other disease states. Patients who are unable to accurately draw up their dose will need assistance such as prefilled syringes. Initial doses may require considerations for renal function in the elderly with dosing adjusted subsequently based on blood glucose monitoring. Intensive glucose control (Hb A_{1c} <6.5%) has been linked to increased all cause and cardiovascular mortality, hypoglycemia requiring assistance, and weight gain in adult type 2 diabetes. For elderly patients with diabetes who are relatively healthy, attaining target goals for aspirin use, blood pressure, lipids, smoking cessation, and diet and exercise may be more important than normalized glycemic control.

Breast-Feeding Considerations Endogenous insulin can be found in breast milk. Plasma glucose concentrations in the mother affect glucose concentrations in breast milk. The gastrointestinal tract destroys insulin when administered orally; therefore, insulin is not expected to be absorbed intact by the breast-feeding infant. All types of insulin are safe for use while breast-feeding. Due to increased calorie expenditure, women with diabetes may require less insulin while nursing.

Pregnancy Considerations Insulin has not been found to cross the placenta, but insulin bound to anti-insulin antibodies has been detected in cord blood. Maternal hyperglycemia can be associated with adverse effects in the fetus, including macrosomia, neonatal hyperglycemia, and hyperbilirubinemia; the risk of congenital malformations is increased when the Hb A_{1c} is above the normal range. Insulin requirements tend to fall during the first trimester of pregnancy and increase in the later trimesters, peaking at 28-32 weeks of gestation. Following delivery, insulin requirements decrease rapidly. Diabetes can be associated with adverse effects in the mother. Poorly-treated diabetes may cause end-organ damage that may in turn negatively affect obstetric outcomes. Physiologic glucose levels should be maintained prior to and during pregnancy to decrease the risk of adverse events in the fetus and the mother. Insulin is the drug of choice for the control of diabetes mellitus during pregnancy.

Additional Information

Split-mixed or basal-bolus regimens: Combination regimens which optimize differences in the onset and duration of different insulin products are commonly used to approximate physiologic secretion. In split-mixed regimens, an intermediate-acting insulin (eg, NPH insulin) is administered once or twice daily and supplemented by short-acting (regular) or rapid-acting (lispro, aspart, or glulisine) insulin. Blood glucose measurements are completed several times daily. Dosages are adjusted emphasizing the individual component of the regimen which most directly influences the blood sugar in question (either the intermediate-acting component or the shorter-acting component). Fixed-ratio formulations (eg, 70/30 mix) may be used as twice daily injections in this scenario; however, the ability to titrate the dosage of an individual component is limited. A example of a "split-mixed" regimen would be 21 units of NPH plus 9 units of regular insulin in the morning and an evening meal dose consisting of 14 units of NPH plus 6 units of regular insulin.

Basal-bolus regimens are designed to more closely mimic physiologic secretion. These regimens employ a long-acting insulin (eg, glargine) to simulate basal insulin secretion. The basal component is frequently administered at bedtime or in the early morning. This is supplemented by multiple daily injections of rapid-acting products (lispro, aspart, or glulisine) immediately prior to a meal, which provides insulin at the time when nutrients are absorbed. An example of a basal-bolus regimen would be 30 units of glargine at bedtime and 12 units of lispro insulin prior to each meal.

Estimation of the effect per unit: A "Rule of 1500" has been frequently used as a means to estimate the change in blood sugar relative to each unit of insulin administered. In fact, the recommended values used in these calculations may vary from 1500-2200 (a value of 1500 is generally recommended for regular insulin while 1800 is recommended for "rapid-acting insulins"). The higher values lead to more conservative estimates of the effect per unit of insulin, and therefore lead to more cautious adjustments. The effect per unit of insulin is approximated by dividing the selected numerical value (eg, 1500-2200) by the number of units/day received by the patient. This may be used as a crude approximation of the patient's insulin sensitivity as adjustments to individual components of the regimen are made. Each additional unit of insulin added to the corresponding insulin dose may be expected to lower the blood glucose by this amount.

To illustrate, in the "basal-bolus" regimen example presented above, the rule of 1800 would indicate an expected change of 27 mg/dL per unit of lispro insulin (the total daily insulin dose is 66 units; using the formula: 1800/66 = 27). A patient may be instructed to add additional insulin if the preprandial glucose is >125 mg/dL. For a prelunch glucose of 195 mg/dL, this would mean the patient would administer the scheduled 12 units of lispro along with an additional "correctional" 3 units for a total of 15 units prior to the meal. If correctional doses are required on a consistent basis, an adjustment of the patients diet and/or scheduled insulin dose may be necessary.

Related Information

Diabetes Mellitus and Pregnancy *on page* 2035
Diabetes Mellitus Management, Adults *on page* 2026
Insulin Aspart *on page* 981
Insulin Aspart Protamine and Insulin Aspart *on page* 983
Insulin Detemir *on page* 984
Insulin Glargine *on page* 986
Insulin Glulisine *on page* 988
Insulin Lispro *on page* 989
Insulin Lispro Protamine and Insulin Lispro *on page* 991
Insulin NPH *on page* 992
Insulin NPH and Insulin Regular *on page* 993

◆ **Insulin Regular and Insulin NPH** *see* Insulin NPH and Insulin Regular *on page* 993
◆ **Integrilin®** *see* Eptifibatide *on page* 648
◆ **Intelence®** *see* Etravirine *on page* 718
◆ **α-2-interferon** *see* Interferon Alfa-2b *on page* 1000
◆ **Interferon Alfa-2a (PEG Conjugate)** *see* Peginterferon Alfa-2a *on page* 1423

Interferon Alfa-2b (in ter FEER on AL fa too bee)

U.S. Brand Names Intron® A
Index Terms INF-alpha 2; Interferon Alpha-2b; rLFN-α2; α-2-interferon
Generic Availability (U.S.) No
Pharmacologic Category Interferon

Medication Safety Issues

Sound-alike/look-alike issues:

Interferon alfa-2b may be confused with interferon alfa-2a, interferon alfa-n3, pegylated interferon alfa-2b

Intron® A may be confused with PEG-Intron®

International issues:

Interferon alfa-2b may be confused with interferon alpha multi-subtype which is available in international markets

Medication Guide Available Yes

Pregnancy Risk Factor C / X in combination with ribavirin

Lactation Enters breast milk/not recommended (AAP rates "compatible"; AAP 2001 update pending)

Use

Patients ≥1 year of age: Chronic hepatitis B

Patients ≥3 years of age: Chronic hepatitis C (in combination with ribavirin)

Patients ≥18 years of age: Condyloma acuminata, chronic hepatitis B, chronic hepatitis C, hairy cell leukemia, malignant melanoma, AIDS-related Kaposi's sarcoma, follicular non-Hodgkin's lymphoma

Unlabeled/Investigational Use AIDS-related thrombocytopenia, cutaneous ulcerations of Behçet's disease, neuroendocrine tumors (including carcinoid syndrome and islet cell tumor), cutaneous T-cell lymphoma, desmoid tumor, lymphomatoid granulomatosis, hepatitis D, chronic myelogenous leukemia (CML), non-Hodgkin's lymphomas (other than follicular lymphoma, see approved use), multiple myeloma, renal cell carcinoma, West Nile virus

Available Dosage Forms

Injection, powder for reconstitution [preservative free]:

Intron® A: 10 million int. units, 18 million int. units, 50 million int. units

Injection, solution:

Intron® A: 6 million int. units/mL (3 mL); 10 million int. units/mL (2.5 mL); 3 million int. units/0.2 mL (1.2 mL); 5 million int. units/0.2 mL (1.2 mL); 10 million int. units/0.2 mL (1.2 mL)

Dosing

Adult & Geriatric Details concerning dosing in combination regimens should also be consulted. **Note:** Withhold treatment for ANC <500/mm^3 or platelets <25,000/mm^3. Consider premedication with acetaminophen prior to administration to reduce the incidence of some adverse reactions. Not all dosage forms and strengths are appropriate for all indications; refer to product labeling for details.

Hairy cell leukemia: I.M., SubQ: 2 million units/m^2 3 times/week for up to 6 months (may continue treatment with continued treatment response)

Lymphoma (follicular): SubQ: 5 million units 3 times/week for up to 18 months

Malignant melanoma: Induction: 20 million units/m^2 I.V. for 5 consecutive days per week for 4 weeks, followed by maintenance dosing of 10 million units/m^2 SubQ 3 times/week for 48 weeks

AIDS-related Kaposi's sarcoma: I.M., SubQ: 30 million units/m^2 3 times/week

Chronic hepatitis B: I.M., SubQ: 5 million units/day or 10 million units 3 times/week for 16 weeks

Chronic hepatitis C: I.M., SubQ: 3 million units 3 times/week. In patients with normalization of ALT at 16 weeks, continue treatment (if tolerated) for 18-24 months; consider discontinuation if normalization does not occur at 16 weeks. **Note:** May be used in combination therapy with ribavirin in previously untreated patients or in patients who relapse following alpha interferon therapy.

Condyloma acuminata: Intralesionally: 1 million units/lesion (maximum: 5 lesions/treatment) 3 times/week (on alternate days) for 3 weeks. May administer a second course at 12-16 weeks.

Pediatric Details concerning dosing in combination regimens should also be consulted.

Note: The following dosing may also be used in **infants** in the setting of HIV-exposure/-infection (CDC, 2009).

Chronic hepatitis B (including HIV coinfection): SubQ: Children 1-17 years: 3 million units/m^2 3 times/week for 1 week, followed by 6 million units/m^2 3 times/week (maximum: 10 million units/dose) total duration of therapy 16-24 weeks (treat for 24 weeks in HIV-exposure/-infection)

Chronic hepatitis C with HIV coinfection: I.M., SubQ: Children 1-17 years: 3-5 million units/m^2 3 times/week (maximum: 3 million units/dose) with ribavirin for 48 weeks, regardless of HCV genotype (CDC, 2009)

Renal Impairment Combination therapy with ribavirin (hepatitis C) should not be used in patients with reduced renal function (Cl_{cr} <50 mL/minute).

Adjustment for Toxicity

Hypersensitivity reaction (acute, serious), ophthalmic disorders (new or worsening), thyroid abnormality development (which cannot be normalized with medication), signs or symptoms of liver failure: Discontinue treatment

Liver function abnormality, pulmonary infiltrate development, evidence of pulmonary function impairment, or autoimmune disorder development: Monitor closely and discontinue if appropriate

Neuropsychiatric disorders (during treatment):
Clinical depression or other psychiatric problem: Monitor closely during and for 6 months after treatment
Severe depression or other psychiatric disorder: Discontinue treatment
Persistent or worsening psychiatric symptoms, suicidal ideation, aggression towards others: Discontinue treatment and follow with appropriate psychiatric intervention

Manufacturer-recommended adjustments, listed according to indication:
Lymphoma (follicular):
Neutrophils >1000/mm^3 to <1500/mm^3: Reduce dose by 50%; may re-escalate to starting dose when neutrophils return to >1500/mm^3
Severe toxicity (neutrophils <1000/mm^3 or platelets <50,000/mm^3): Temporarily withhold
AST >5 times ULN or serum creatinine >2 mg/dL: Permanently discontinue
Hairy cell leukemia: Severe toxicity: Reduce dose by 50% or temporarily withhold and resume with 50% dose reduction; permanently discontinue if persistent or recurrent severe toxicity is noted
Chronic hepatitis B:
WBC <1500/mm^3, granulocytes <750/mm^3, or platelet count <50,000/mm^3, or other laboratory abnormality or severe adverse reaction: Reduce dose by 50%; may re-escalate to starting dose upon resolution of hematologic toxicity. Discontinue for persistent intolerance.
WBC <1000/mm^3, granulocytes <500/mm^3, or platelet count <25,000/mm^3: Permanently discontinue
Chronic hepatitis C: Severe toxicity: Reduce dose by 50% or temporarily withhold until subsides; permanently discontinue for persistent toxicities after dosage reduction
AIDS-related Kaposi sarcoma: Severe toxicity: Reduce dose by 50% or temporarily withhold; may resume at reduced dose with toxicity resolution; permanently discontinue for persistent/recurrent toxicities
Malignant melanoma:
Severe toxicity (neutrophils >250/mm^3 to <500/mm^3 or ALT/AST >5-10 times ULN): Temporarily withhold; resume with a 50% dose reduction when adverse reaction abates
Neutrophils <250/mm^3, ALT/AST >10 times ULN, or severe/persistent adverse reactions: Permanently discontinue

Administration

I.M. Administer in evening (if possible)

I.V. Infuse over ~20 minutes

Other

SubQ: SubQ administration is suggested for those who are at risk for bleeding or are thrombocytopenic. Rotate SubQ injection site. Administer in evening (if possible). Patient should be well hydrated. Reconstitute with recommended amount of SWFI and agitate gently; do not shake. **Note:** Different vial strengths require different amounts of diluent. Not every dosage form is appropriate for every indication; refer to manufacturer's labeling.
Intralesional: Inject at an angle nearly parallel to the plane of the skin, directing the needle to center of the base of the wart to infiltrate the lesion core and cause a small wheal. Only infiltrate the keratinized layer; avoid administration which is too deep or shallow.

Monitoring and Teaching Issues

Laboratory Monitoring CBC with differential and platelets (baseline and routinely during treatment), liver function tests, serum creatinine, electrolytes, triglycerides, thyroid function tests (baseline and periodically during treatment)

Physical Assessment Patients with pre-existing cardiac abnormalities or in advanced stages of cancer should have ECGs taken before and during treatment. Monitor for neuropsychiatric changes, especially depression, suicidal or homicidal ideation, psychosis, or mania; decreased pulmonary function; or ophthalmic changes. Evaluate immediately any reported changes in vision. Teach appropriate reconstitution, injection, and needle disposal.

Patient Education Maintain adequate hydration, unless instructed to restrict fluid intake. You may experience flu-like syndrome, nausea, vomiting, dizziness, or abnormal thinking. Inform prescriber immediately if you feel depressed or have any thoughts of suicide or homicide. Report unusual bruising or bleeding; persistent abdominal disturbances; unusual fatigue; muscle pain or tremors; fever; chest pain or palpitation; swelling of extremities or unusual weight gain; respiratory difficulty; pain, swelling, or redness at injection site; or sudden change in vision.

Interferon Alfacon-1 (in ter FEER on AL fa con one)

U.S. Brand Names Infergen®

Generic Availability (U.S.) No

Pharmacologic Category Interferon

Medication Safety Issues

Sound-alike/look-alike issues:
Interferon alfacon-1 may be confused with interferon alfa-2a, interferon alfa-2b, interferon alfa-n3, peginterferon alfa-2b
International issues:
Interferon alfacon-1 may be confused with interferon alpha multi-subtype which is available in international markets

Medication Guide Available Yes

Pregnancy Risk Factor C

Lactation Excretion in breast milk unknown/use caution (AAP rates "compatible"; AAP 2001 update pending)

Use Treatment of chronic hepatitis C virus (HCV) infection in patients ≥18 years of age with compensated liver disease and anti-HCV serum antibodies or HCV RNA; concurrent use with ribavirin in HCV-infected patients who have failed treatment with pegylated interferon/ribavirin (Bacon, 2009)

Available Dosage Forms

Injection, solution [preservative free]:
Infergen®: 30 mcg/mL (0.3 mL, 0.5 mL)

Dosing

Adult & Geriatric Chronic HCV infection: SubQ: 9 mcg 3 times/week for 24 weeks; allow 48 hours between doses.

Combination therapy with ribavirin: SubQ: 15 mcg/day with ribavirin for up to 48 weeks

Patients who have previously tolerated interferon therapy but did not respond or relapsed: 15 mcg 3 times/week week for up to 48 weeks

Pediatric Not indicated for patients <18 years of age.

Renal Impairment Cl_{cr} <50 mL/minute: Hepatitis C: Avoid combination therapy with ribavirin.

Hepatic Impairment Use in decompensated hepatic disease (Child-Pugh class B and C) is contraindicated.

Adjustment for Toxicity Dose should be held in patients who experience a severe adverse reaction, and treatment should be stopped or decreased if the reaction does not become tolerable.

Doses were reduced from 9 mcg to 7.5 mcg in the pivotal study.

For patients receiving 15 mcg/dose, doses were reduced in 3 mcg decrements. Efficacy is decreased with doses <7.5 mcg.

Administration

Other Interferon alfacon-1 is given by SubQ injection, 3 times/week, with at least 48 hours between doses. Allow to reach room temperature just prior to administration.

Monitoring and Teaching Issues

Laboratory Monitoring Hemoglobin and hematocrit, white blood cell count, platelets, triglycerides, and thyroid function. Laboratory tests should be taken prior to therapy, 2 weeks after therapy has begun, and periodically during treatment. HCV RNA, and ALT to determine success/response to therapy.

The following guidelines were used during the clinical studies as acceptable baseline values:

Platelet count ≥75 x 10^9/L
Hemoglobin ≥100 g/L
ANC ≥1500 x 10^6/L
S_{cr} <180 μmol/L (<2 mg/dL) or Cl_{cr} >0.83 mL/second (>50 mL/minute)
Serum albumin ≥25 g/L
Bilirubin ≤1.4 mg/dL (except for patients with Gilbert's syndrome)
TSH and T_4 WNL

Physical Assessment Monitor for signs of depression and suicide ideation. Patient with pre-existing diabetes mellitus or hypertension should have an ophthalmic exam prior to beginning treatment. If self-administered, instruct patient in appropriate storage, injection technique, and syringe disposal.

Patient Education If self-administered, follow exact instructions for injection and syringe disposal. You will need frequent laboratory tests during course of therapy. If you have diabetes or hypertension, you should have ophthalmic exam prior to beginning therapy. You may experience dizziness; nausea, vomiting, or diarrhea; flu-like symptoms, such as headache, fatigue, or muscle or joint pain; or hair loss. Promptly report any persistent GI upset, depression or suicide ideation, chest pain or palpitations, respiratory difficulties, unusual bruising or bleeding, yellowing of skin, or vision changes.

◆ **Interferon Alpha-2b** *see* Interferon Alfa-2b *on page* 1000

Interferon Beta-1a (in ter FEER on BAY ta won aye)

U.S. Brand Names Avonex®; Rebif®

Index Terms rIFN beta-1a

Generic Availability (U.S.) No

Pharmacologic Category Interferon

Medication Safety Issues

Sound-alike/look-alike issues:
Avonex® may be confused with Avelox®

Medication Guide Available Yes

Pregnancy Risk Factor C

Lactation Excretion in breast milk unknown/not recommended

Use Treatment of relapsing forms of multiple sclerosis (MS)

Mechanism of Action/Effect Mechanism in the treatment of MS is unknown; slows the accumulation of physical disability and decreases frequency of clinical MS exacerbations

Contraindications Hypersensitivity to natural or recombinant interferons, human albumin, or any other component of the formulation

Warnings/Precautions Interferons have been associated with severe psychiatric adverse events (psychosis, mania, depression, suicidal behavior/ideation) in patients with and without previous psychiatric symptoms, avoid use in severe psychiatric disorders and use caution in patients with a history of depression; patients exhibiting depressive symptoms should be closely monitored and discontinuation of therapy should be considered.

Autoimmune disorders including idiopathic thrombocytopenia, hyper- and hypothyroidism and rarely autoimmune hepatitis have been reported. Allergic reactions, including anaphylaxis, have been reported. Caution should be used in patients with hepatic impairment or in those who abuse alcohol. Rare cases of severe hepatic injury, including hepatic failure, have been reported in patients receiving interferon beta-1a; risk may be increased by ethanol use or concurrent therapy with hepatotoxic drugs. Treatment should be suspended if jaundice or symptoms of hepatic dysfunction occur. Transaminase elevations may be asymptomatic, so monitoring is important. Dose adjustment may be necessary with hepatic impairment. Hematologic effects, including pancytopenia (rare) and thrombocytopenia, have been reported. Associated with a high incidence of flu-like adverse effects; use of analgesics and/or antipyretics on treatment days may be helpful. Use caution in patients with pre-existing cardiovascular disease, including angina, HF, and/or arrythmia. Rare cases of new-onset cardiomyopathy and/or HF have been reported. Use caution in patients with seizure disorders, or myelosuppression. Safety and efficacy in patients with chronic progressive MS or in patients <18 years of age have not been established. Albumin is a component of some formulations (contraindicated in albumin-sensitive patients); rare risk of CJD or viral transmission.

Drug Interactions

Avoid Concomitant Use There are no known interactions where it is recommended to avoid concomitant use.

Decreased Effect There are no known significant interactions involving a decrease in effect.

Increased Effect/Toxicity

Interferon Beta-1a may increase the levels/effects of: Theophylline Derivatives; Zidovudine

Adverse Reactions Note: Adverse reactions reported as a composite of both commercially-available products. Spectrum and incidence of reactions is generally similar between products, but consult individual product labels for specific incidence.

>10%:

- Central nervous system: Headache (58% to 70%), fatigue (33% to 41%), fever (20% to 28%), pain (23%), chills (19%), depression (18% to 25%), dizziness (14%)
- Gastrointestinal: Nausea (23%), abdominal pain (8% to 22%)
- Genitourinary: Urinary tract infection (17%)
- Hematologic: Leukopenia (28% to 36%)
- Hepatic: ALT increased (20% to 27%), AST increased (10% to 17%)
- Local: Injection site reaction (3% to 92%)
- Neuromuscular & skeletal: Myalgia (25% to 29%), back pain (23% to 25%), weakness (24%), skeletal pain (10% to 15%), rigors (6% to 13%)
- Ocular: Vision abnormal (7% to 13%)
- Respiratory: Sinusitis (14%), upper respiratory tract infection (14%)
- Miscellaneous: Flu-like syndrome (49% to 59%), neutralizing antibodies (significance not known; Avonex® 5%; Rebif® 24%), lymphadenopathy (11% to 12%)

1% to 10%:

- Cardiovascular: Chest pain (5% to 6%), vasodilation (2%)
- Central nervous system: Migraine (5%), somnolence (4% to 5%), malaise (4% to 5%), seizure (1% to 5%)
- Dermatologic: Erythematous rash (5% to 7%), maculopapular rash (4% to 5%), alopecia (4%), urticaria
- Endocrine & metabolic: Thyroid disorder (4% to 6%)
- Gastrointestinal: Xerostomia (1% to 5%), toothache (3%)
- Genitourinary: Micturition frequency (2% to 7%), urinary incontinence (2% to 4%)
- Hematologic: Thrombocytopenia (2% to 8%), anemia (3% to 5%)
- Hepatic: Bilirubinemia (2% to 3%)
- Local: Injection site pain (8%), injection site bruising (6%), injection site necrosis (1% to 3%), injection site inflammation
- Neuromuscular & skeletal: Arthralgia (9%), hypertonia (6% to 7%), coordination abnormal (4% to 5%)
- Ocular: Eye disorder (4%), xerophthalmia (1% to 3%)
- Respiratory: Bronchitis (8%)
- Miscellaneous: Infection (7%)

Pharmacodynamics/Kinetics

Onset of Action Avonex®: 12 hours (based on biological response markers)

Duration of Action Avonex®: 4 days (based on biological response markers)

Time to Peak Serum: Avonex® (I.M.): 3-15 hours; Rebif® (SubQ): 16 hours

Half-Life Elimination Avonex®: 10 hours; Rebif®: 69 hours

Pharmacokinetic Note Limited data due to small doses used.

Available Dosage Forms

Injection, powder for reconstitution [preservative free]:

Avonex®: 33 mcg [contains albumin (human); 6.6 million units; provides 30 mcg/mL following reconstitution; supplied with diluent]

Injection, solution:

Avonex®: 30 mcg/0.5 mL (0.5 mL)

Injection, solution [preservative free]:

Rebif®: 22 mcg/0.5 mL (0.5 mL), 44 mcg/0.5 mL (0.5 mL)

Injection, solution [preservative free, combination package]:

Rebif®: Titration Pack: 22 mcg/0.5 mL (6s) and 8.8 mcg/0.2 mL (6s)

Dosing

Adult & Geriatric Multiple sclerosis: **Note:** Analgesics and/or antipyretics may help decrease flu-like symptoms on treatment days:

I.M. (Avonex®): 30 mcg once weekly

SubQ (Rebif®): Doses should be separated by at least 48 hours:

Target dose 44 mcg 3 times/week:

Initial: 8.8 mcg (20 % of final dose) 3 times/week for 2 weeks

Titration: 22 mcg (50% of final dose) 3 times/week for 2 weeks

Final dose: 44 mcg 3 times/week

Target dose 22 mcg 3 times/week:

Initial: 4.4 mcg (20 % of final dose) 3 times/week for 2 weeks

Titration: 11 mcg (50% of final dose) 3 times/week for 2 weeks

Final dose: 22 mcg 3 times/week

Hepatic Impairment Rebif®: If liver function tests increase or in case of leukopenia: Decrease dose 20% to 50% until toxicity resolves

Administration

I.M. Avonex®: Must be given by I.M. injection.

Other Rebif®: Administer SubQ at the same time of day on the same 3 days each week (ie, late afternoon/evening Mon, Wed, Fri). Rotate injection sites.

Stability

Reconstitution Avonex®: Reconstitute with 1.1 mL of diluent and swirl gently to dissolve. Do not shake. The reconstituted product contains no preservative and is for single-use only; discard unused portion.

Storage

Avonex®:

Prefilled syringe: Store at 2°C to 8°C (36°F to 46°F); do not freeze. Protect from light. Allow to warm to room temperature prior to use (do not use external heat source). If refrigeration is not available, product may be stored at ≤25°C (77°F) for up to 7 days.

Vial: Store unreconstituted vial at 2°C to 8°C (36°F to 46°F). If refrigeration is not available, may be stored at 25°C (77°F) for up to 30 days; do not freeze. Protect from light. Following reconstitution, use immediately, but may be stored up to 6 hours at 2°C to 8°C (36°F to 46°F); do not freeze.

Rebif®: Store at 2°C to 8°C (36°F to 46°F); do not freeze. Protect from light. May also be stored ≤25°C (77°F) for up to 30 days if protected from heat and light.

Monitoring and Teaching Issues

Laboratory Monitoring Thyroid function, transaminase levels, blood chemistries, CBC and differential, BUN, creatinine

Avonex®: Frequency of monitoring has not been specifically defined; in clinical trials, monitoring was at 6-month intervals.

Rebif®: CBC and liver function testing at 1-, 3-, and 6 months, then periodically thereafter; thyroid function every 6 months (in patients with pre-existing abnormalities and/or clinical indications)

Physical Assessment Monitor for signs of depression and suicide ideation. Instruct patient/caregiver on appropriate reconstitution, injection, and needle disposal.

Patient Education This is not a cure for MS; you will continue to receive regular treatment and follow-up for MS. Maintain adequate hydration, unless instructed to restrict fluid intake. You may experience flu-like syndrome, nausea, vomiting, dizziness, or abnormal thinking. Inform prescriber immediately if you feel depressed or have suicide ideation. Report unusual bruising or bleeding; persistent abdominal disturbances; chest pain or palpitations; shortness of breath; swelling of extremities; visual disturbances; or pain, swelling, or redness at injection site.

Breast-Feeding Considerations Potential for serious adverse reactions. Because its use has not been evaluated during lactation, a decision should be made to either discontinue breast-feeding or discontinue the drug.

Pregnancy Considerations There are no adequate and well-controlled studies in pregnant women. Consideration should be given to discontinue treatment if a woman becomes pregnant, or plans to become pregnant during therapy. A dose-related abortifacient activity was reported in Rhesus monkeys.

Healthcare providers are encouraged to register pregnant women receiving Rebif® during pregnancy online at www.rebifpregnancyregistry.com or by telephone at MS LifeLines 1-877-44-REBIF. A registry has been established for women who become pregnant while receiving Avonex®. Women may be enrolled in the registry by calling 1-800-456-2255.

Interferon Beta-1b (in ter FEER on BAY ta won bee)

U.S. Brand Names Betaseron®; Extavia®

Index Terms rIFN beta-1b

Generic Availability (U.S.) No

Pharmacologic Category Interferon

Medication Guide Available Yes

Pregnancy Risk Factor C

Lactation Excretion in breast milk unknown/not recommended

Use Treatment of relapsing forms of multiple sclerosis (MS); treatment of first clinical episode with MRI features consistent with MS

Canadian labeling: Additional use (not in U.S. labeling): Treatment of secondary-progressive MS

Mechanism of Action/Effect Alters the expression and response to cell surface antigens and can enhance immune cell activities; mechanism in MS in unknown

Contraindications Hypersensitivity to *E. coli*-derived products, natural or recombinant interferon beta, albumin human or any other component of the formulation

Canadian labeling: Additional contraindication (not in U.S. labeling): Pregnancy

Warnings/Precautions Anaphylaxis has been reported rarely with use. Associated with a high incidence of flu-like adverse effects; improvement in symptoms occurs over time. Hepatotoxicity has been reported with beta interferons, including rare reports of hepatitis (autoimmune) and hepatic failure requiring transplant. Interferons have been associated with severe psychiatric adverse events (psychosis, mania, depression, suicidal behavior/ideation) in patients with and without previous psychiatric symptoms, avoid use in severe psychiatric disorders and use caution in patients with a history of depression; patients exhibiting symptoms of depression should be closely monitored and discontinuation of therapy should be considered. Use caution in patients with pre-existing cardiovascular disease, pulmonary disease, seizure disorders, renal impairment or hepatic impairment. Use caution in myelosuppression; routine monitoring for leukopenia is recommended; dose reduction may be required. Thyroid dysfunction has rarely been reported with use. Severe injection site reactions (necrosis) may occur, which may or may not heal with continued therapy; patient and/or caregiver competency in injection technique should be confirmed and periodically re-evaluated. Contains albumin, which may carry a remote risk of transmitting viral diseases.

Drug Interactions

Avoid Concomitant Use There are no known interactions where it is recommended to avoid concomitant use.

Decreased Effect There are no known significant interactions involving a decrease in effect.

Increased Effect/Toxicity

Interferon Beta-1b may increase the levels/effects of: Theophylline Derivatives; Zidovudine

Adverse Reactions Note: Flu-like syndrome (including at least two of the following - headache, fever, chills, malaise, diaphoresis, and myalgia) are reported in the majority of patients (60%) and decrease over time (average duration ~1 week).

>10%:

- Cardiovascular: Peripheral edema (15%), chest pain (11%)
- Central nervous system: Headache (57%), fever (36%), pain (51%), chills (25%), dizziness (24%), insomnia (24%)
- Dermatologic: Rash (24%), skin disorder (12%)
- Endocrine & metabolic: Metrorrhagia (11%)
- Gastrointestinal: Nausea (27%), diarrhea (19%), abdominal pain (19%), constipation (20%), dyspepsia (14%)
- Genitourinary: Urinary urgency (13%)
- Hematologic: Lymphopenia (88%), neutropenia (14%), leukopenia (14%)
- Local: Injection site reaction (85%), inflammation (53%), pain (18%)
- Neuromuscular & skeletal: Weakness (61%), myalgia (27%), hypertonia (50%), myasthenia (46%), arthralgia (31%), incoordination (21%)
- Miscellaneous: Flu-like syndrome (decreases over treatment course; 60%), neutralizing antibodies (≤45%; significance not known)

1% to 10%:

- Cardiovascular: Palpitation (4%), vasodilation (8%), hypertension (7%), tachycardia (4%), peripheral vascular disorder (6%)
- Central nervous system: Anxiety (10%), malaise (8%), nervousness (7%)
- Dermatologic: Alopecia (4%)
- Endocrine & metabolic: Menorrhagia (8%), dysmenorrhea (7%)
- Gastrointestinal: Weight gain (7%)
- Genitourinary: Impotence (9%), pelvic pain (6%), cystitis (8%), urinary frequency (7%), prostatic disorder (3%)
- Hematologic: Lymphadenopathy (8%)
- Hepatic: ALT increased >5x baseline (10%), AST increased >5x baseline (3%)
- Local: Injection site necrosis (4% to 5%), edema (3%), mass (2%)
- Neuromuscular & skeletal: Leg cramps (4%)
- Respiratory: Dyspnea (7%)
- Miscellaneous: Diaphoresis (8%), hypersensitivity (3%)

Pharmacodynamics/Kinetics

Time to Peak 1-8 hours

Half-Life Elimination 8 minutes to 4.3 hours

Pharmacokinetic Note Limited data due to small doses used.

Available Dosage Forms

Injection, powder for reconstitution:

Betaseron®: 0.3 mg [~9.6 million int. units]

Injection, powder for reconstitution [preservative free]:

Extavia®: 0.3 mg [~9.6 million int. units]

Dosing

Adult & Geriatric Note: Gradual dose-titration, analgesics, and/or antipyretics may help decrease flu-like symptoms on treatment days.

Multiple sclerosis (relapsing): Initial: 0.0625 mg (2 million units [0.25 mL]) every other day; gradually increase dose by 0.0625 every 2 weeks

Target dose: 0.25 mg (8 million units [1 mL]) every other day

Multiple sclerosis (secondary-progressive) [Canadian labeling; not in U.S. labeling]: Initial: 0.125 mg (4 million units [0.5 mL]) every other day for 2 weeks

Target dose: 0.25 mg (8 million units [1 mL]) every other day

Pediatric Not recommended in children <18 years of age

Administration

Other SubQ: Withdraw 1 mL of reconstituted solution from the vial into a sterile syringe fitted with a 27-gauge needle and inject the solution subcutaneously. Sites for self-injection include outer surface of the arms, abdomen, hips, and thighs. Rotate SubQ injection site. Patient should be well hydrated.

Stability

Reconstitution To reconstitute solution, inject 1.2 mL of diluent (provided); gently swirl to dissolve, do not shake. Reconstituted solution provides 0.25 mg/mL (8 million units). Use product within 3 hours of reconstitution. Discard unused portion of vial.

Storage Store at room temperature of 25°C (77°F); excursions permitted to 15°C to 30°C (59°F to 86°F). If not used immediately following reconstitution, refrigerate solution at 2°C to 8°C (36°F to 46°F) and use within 3 hours; do not freeze or shake solution. Discard unused portion of vial.

Monitoring and Teaching Issues

Laboratory Monitoring Hemoglobin, liver function, blood chemistries, thyroid function tests in those with history of thyroid dysfunction

Canadian labeling: Additional monitoring recommendations (not in U.S. labeling): Baseline pregnancy test

Physical Assessment Assess for psychiatric or suicide histories. Monitor injection sites for signs of necrosis. Teach proper administration for SubQ injections and disposal of needles if appropriate. Emphasize the need for adequate hydration. Monitor for opportunistic infection.

Patient Education This is not a cure for MS; you will continue to receive regular treatment and follow-up for MS. Rotate injection site with each injection. Maintain adequate hydration, unless instructed to restrict fluid intake. You may experience flu-like syndrome, nausea, vomiting, diarrhea, dizziness, or abnormal thinking. Inform prescriber immediately if you feel depressed or have suicide ideation. Report unusual bruising or bleeding; persistent abdominal disturbances; chest pain or palpitations; swelling of extremities; visual disturbances; or pain, swelling, or redness at injection site.

Geriatric Considerations No specific recommendations necessary for use in the elderly. Monitor for CNS adverse effects which may be significant in the elderly.

Breast-Feeding Considerations Because its use has not been evaluated during lactation, breast-feeding is not recommended.

Pregnancy Considerations A dose-related abortifacient activity was reported in Rhesus monkeys. There are no adequate and well-controlled studies in pregnant women. Treatment should be discontinued if a woman becomes pregnant, or plans to become pregnant during therapy.

Additional Information American Academy of Neurology and MS Council guidelines suggest that, based upon published data, 6 million units of Avonex® (interferon beta-1a) (30 mcg) is equivalent to approximately 7-9 million units of Betaseron® (220-280 mcg).

Interferon Gamma-1b (in ter FEER on GAM ah won bee)

U.S. Brand Names Actimmune®

Generic Availability (U.S.) No

Pharmacologic Category Interferon

Pregnancy Risk Factor C

Lactation Excretion in breast milk unknown/not recommended

Use Reduce frequency and severity of serious infections associated with chronic granulomatous disease; delay time to disease progression in patients with severe, malignant osteopetrosis

Mechanism of Action/Effect Interferon gamma participates in immunoregulation. The exact mechanism of action for the treatment of chronic granulomatous disease or osteopetrosis has not been defined.

Contraindications Hypersensitivity to interferon gamma, *E. coli* derived proteins, or any component of the formulation

Warnings/Precautions Hypersensitivity reactions have been reported (rarely). Transient cutaneous rashes may occur. Dose-related bone marrow toxicity has been reported; use caution in patients with myelosuppression. May cause hepatotoxicity and the incidence may be increased in children <1 year of age. Doses >10 times the weekly recommended dose (used in studies for unlabeled indications) have been associated with a different pattern/frequency of adverse effects. Flu-like symptoms which may exacerbate pre-existing cardiovascular disorders (including ischemia, HF, or arrhythmias) and the development of neurologic disorders have been noted at the higher doses. Caution should also be used in patients with seizure disorders or compromised CNS function.

Drug Interactions

Metabolism/Transport Effects Inhibits CYP1A2 (weak), 2E1 (weak)

Avoid Concomitant Use There are no known interactions where it is recommended to avoid concomitant use.

Decreased Effect There are no known significant interactions involving a decrease in effect.

Increased Effect/Toxicity

Interferon Gamma-1b may increase the levels/effects of: Theophylline Derivatives; Zidovudine

Adverse Reactions Based on 50 mcg/m^2 dose administered 3 times weekly for chronic granulomatous disease

>10%:

Central nervous system: Fever (52%), headache (33%), chills (14%), fatigue (14%)
Dermatologic: Rash (17%)
Gastrointestinal: Diarrhea (14%), vomiting (13%)
Local: Injection site erythema or tenderness (14%)

1% to 10%:

Central nervous system: Depression (3%)
Gastrointestinal: Nausea (10%), abdominal pain (8%)
Neuromuscular & skeletal: Myalgia (6%), arthralgia (2%), back pain (2%)

Additional adverse reactions noted at doses >100 mcg/m^2 administered 3 times weekly: ALT increased, AST increased, autoantibodies increased, bronchospasm, chest discomfort, confusion, dermatomyositis exacerbation, disorientation, DVT, gait disturbance, GI bleeding, hallucinations, heart block, heart failure, hepatic insufficiency, hyperglycemia, hypertriglyceridemia, hyponatremia, hypotension, interstitial pneumonitis, lupus-like syndrome, MI, neutropenia, pancreatitis (may be fatal), Parkinsonian symptoms, PE, proteinuria, renal insufficiency (reversible), seizure, syncope, tachyarrhythmia, tachypnea, thrombocytopenia, TIA

Pharmacodynamics/Kinetics

Absorption I.M., SubQ: >89%

Time to Peak Plasma: I.M.: 4 hours (1.5 ng/mL); SubQ: 7 hours (0.6 ng/mL)

Half-Life Elimination I.V.: 38 minutes; I.M.: ~3 hours, SubQ: ~6 hours

Available Dosage Forms

Injection, solution [preservative free]:
Actimmune®: 100 mcg (0.5 mL)

Dosing

Adult & Geriatric If severe reactions occur, modify dose (50% reduction) or therapy should be discontinued until adverse reactions abate.

Chronic granulomatous disease: SubQ:
BSA ≤0.5 m^2: 1.5 mcg/kg/dose 3 times/week
BSA >0.5 m^2: 50 mcg/m^2 (1 million int. units/m^2) 3 times/week

Note: Previously expressed as 1.5 million units/m^2; 50 mcg is equivalent to 1 million int. units/m^2.

Pediatric

Chronic granulomatous disease: Refer to adult dosing.
Severe, malignant osteopetrosis: SubQ:
BSA ≤0.5 m^2: 1.5 mcg/kg/dose 3 times/week
BSA >0.5 m^2: 50 mcg/m^2 (1 million int. units/m^2) 3 times/week

Adjustment for Toxicity If severe reactions occur, reduce dose by 50% or therapy should be interrupted until adverse reaction abates.

Administration

Other Administer by SubQ injection into the right and left deltoid or anterior thigh.

Stability

Storage Store in refrigerator at 2°C to 8°C (36°F to 46°F); do not freeze. Do not shake. Discard if left unrefrigerated for >12 hours.

Monitoring and Teaching Issues

Laboratory Monitoring CBC with differential, platelets, LFTs (monthly in children <1 year), electrolytes, BUN, creatinine, and urinalysis prior to therapy and at 3-month intervals

Physical Assessment Teach patient/caregiver appropriate reconstitution, injection, and needle disposal.

Patient Education Maintain adequate hydration, unless instructed to restrict fluid intake. You may experience flu-like syndrome, nausea, vomiting, or abnormal thinking. Report unusual bruising or bleeding; persistent abdominal disturbances; unusual fatigue; muscle pain or tremors; chest pain or palpitations; swelling of extremities; visual disturbances; or pain, swelling, or redness at injection site.

Breast-Feeding Considerations Potential for serious adverse reactions. Because its use has not been evaluated during lactation, breast-feeding is not recommended

Pregnancy Considerations Teratogenic effects were not observed in animal studies. A dose-related abortifacient activity was reported in Rhesus monkeys. Safety and efficacy in pregnant women has not been established.

◆ **Interleukin 2** *see* Aldesleukin *on page* 62

◆ **Intralipid®** *see* Fat Emulsion *on page* 736

◆ **Intravenous Fat Emulsion** *see* Fat Emulsion *on page* 736

◆ **Intrifiban** *see* Eptifibatide *on page* 648

◆ **Intron® A** *see* Interferon Alfa-2b *on page* 1000

- **Intropin** *see* DOPamine *on page* 571
- **Introvale™** *see* Ethinyl Estradiol and Levonorgestrel *on page* 699
- **INVanz®** *see* Ertapenem *on page* 656
- **Invega®** *see* Paliperidone *on page* 1391
- **Invega® Sustenna®** *see* Paliperidone *on page* 1391
- **Invirase®** *see* Saquinavir *on page* 1621
- **Iodine and Potassium Iodide** *see* Potassium Iodide and Iodine *on page* 1484
- **Iopidine®** *see* Apraclonidine *on page* 139
- **iOSAT™ [OTC]** *see* Potassium Iodide *on page* 1483
- **IPOL®** *see* Poliovirus Vaccine (Inactivated) *on page* 1473

Ipratropium (Oral Inhalation) (i pra TROE pee um)

U.S. Brand Names Atrovent® HFA

Index Terms Ipratropium Bromide

Generic Availability (U.S.) Yes: Solution for nebulization

Pharmacologic Category Anticholinergic Agent

Medication Safety Issues

Sound-alike/look-alike issues:

Atrovent® may be confused with Alupent®, Serevent®

Ipratropium may be confused with tiotropium

Pregnancy Risk Factor B

Lactation Excretion in breast milk unknown/use caution

Use Anticholinergic bronchodilator used in bronchospasm associated with COPD, bronchitis, and emphysema

Mechanism of Action/Effect Blocks the action of acetylcholine at parasympathetic sites in bronchial smooth muscle causing bronchodilation; local application to nasal mucosa inhibits serous and seromucous gland secretions.

Contraindications Hypersensitivity to ipratropium, atropine (and its derivatives), or any component of the formulation

Warnings/Precautions Immediate hypersensitivity reactions (urticaria, angioedema, rash, bronchospasm) have been reported. Rarely, paradoxical bronchospasm may occur with use of inhaled bronchodilating agents; this should be distinguished from inadequate response. Not indicated for the initial treatment of acute episodes of bronchospasm where rescue therapy is required for rapid response. Should only be used in acute exacerbations of asthma in conjunction with short-acting beta-adrenergic agonists for acute episodes. Use with caution in patients with myasthenia gravis, narrow-angle glaucoma, benign prostatic hyperplasia (BPH), or bladder neck obstruction

Drug Interactions

Avoid Concomitant Use There are no known interactions where it is recommended to avoid concomitant use.

Decreased Effect

Ipratropium (Oral Inhalation) may decrease the levels/effects of: Acetylcholinesterase Inhibitors (Central); Secretin

The levels/effects of Ipratropium (Oral Inhalation) may be decreased by: Acetylcholinesterase Inhibitors (Central)

Increased Effect/Toxicity

Ipratropium (Oral Inhalation) may increase the levels/effects of: AbobotulinumtoxinA; Anticholinergics; Cannabinoids; OnabotulinumtoxinA; Potassium Chloride; RimabotulinumtoxinB

The levels/effects of Ipratropium (Oral Inhalation) may be increased by: Pramlintide

Adverse Reactions

>10%: Respiratory: Upper respiratory tract infection (9% to 34%), bronchitis (10% to 23%), sinusitis (1% to 11%)

1% to 10%:

Cardiovascular: Chest pain (3%), palpitation

Central nervous system: Headache (6% to 7%), dizziness (2% to 3%)

Gastrointestinal: Dyspepsia (1% to 5%), nausea (4%), xerostomia (2% to 4%)

Genitourinary: Urinary tract infection (2% to 10%)

Neuromuscular & skeletal: Back pain (2% to 7%)

Respiratory: Dyspnea (7% to 10%), rhinitis (2% to 6%), cough (3% to 5%), pharyngitis (4%), bronchospasm (2%), sputum increased (1%)

Miscellaneous: Flu-like syndrome (4% to 8%)

Pharmacodynamics/Kinetics

Onset of Action Bronchodilation: Within 15 minutes; Peak effect: 1-2 hours

Duration of Action 2-5 hours

Absorption Negligible

Protein Binding ≤9%

Half-Life Elimination 2 hours

Excretion Urine

Available Dosage Forms

Aerosol, for oral inhalation:

Atrovent® HFA: 17 mcg/actuation (12.9 g)

Solution, for nebulization: 0.02% [500 mcg/2.5 mL] (2 mL, 2.5 mL, 25s, 30s, 60s)

Solution, for nebulization [preservative free]: 0.02% [500 mcg/2.5 mL] (25s, 30s, 60s)

Dosing

Adult & Geriatric

Asthma exacerbation, acute (*NIH Asthma Guidelines, 2007*):

Nebulization: 500 mcg every 20 minutes for 3 doses, then as needed. **Note:** Should be given in combination with a short-acting beta-adrenergic agonist.

Metered-dose inhaler: 8 inhalations every 20 minutes as needed for up to 3 hours. **Note:** Should be given in combination with a short-acting beta-adrenergic agonist.

Bronchospasm associated with COPD:

Nebulization: 500 mcg (one unit-dose vial) 3-4 times/day with doses 6-8 hours apart

Metered-dose inhaler: 2 inhalations 4 times/day, up to 12 inhalations/24 hours

Pediatric Asthma exacerbation, acute (*NIH Asthma Guidelines, 2007*):

Nebulization:

Children ≤12 years: 250-500 mcg every 20 minutes for 3 doses, then as needed. **Note:** Should be given in combination with a short-acting beta-adrenergic agonist.

Children >12 years: Refer to adult dosing.

Metered-dose inhaler:

Children ≤12 years: 4-8 inhalations every 20 minutes as needed for up to 3 hours. **Note:** Should be given in combination with a short-acting beta-adrenergic agonist.

Children >12 years: Refer to adult dosing.

Administration

Inhalation Atrovent® HFA: Prior to initial use, prime inhaler by releasing 2 test sprays into the air. If the inhaler has not been used for >3 days, reprime.

Stability

Storage

Aerosol: Store at controlled room temperature of 25°C (77°F). Do not store near heat or open flame.

Solution: Store at 15°C to 30°C (59°F to 86°F). Protect from light.

Monitoring and Teaching Issues

Physical Assessment Teach patient importance of proper administration.

Patient Education Use care to avoid direct contact with eyes. Do not use more often than recommended. Maintain adequate hydration, unless instructed to restrict fluid intake. May cause sensitivity to heat, nervousness, dizziness, fatigue, dry mouth, unpleasant taste, stomach upset, or difficulty urinating (always void before treatment). Report unresolved GI upset, dizziness or fatigue, vision changes, palpitations, persistent inability to void, nervousness, or insomnia.

Inhaler: Close eyes when administering ipratropium; blurred vision may result if sprayed into eyes. Effects are enhanced by holding breath 10 seconds after inhalation; wait at least 1 full minute between inhalations.

Nebulizer: Wash hands before and after treatment. Wash and dry nebulizer after each treatment. Twist open the top of one unit dose vial and squeeze the contents into the nebulizer reservoir. Connect the nebulizer reservoir to the mouthpiece or face mask. Connect nebulizer to compressor. Sit in a comfortable, upright position. Place mouthpiece in your mouth or put on the face mask and turn on the compressor. If a face mask is used, avoid leakage around the mask (temporary blurring of vision, worsening of narrow-angle glaucoma, or eye pain may occur if mist gets into eyes). Breathe calmly and deeply until no more mist is formed in the nebulizer (about 5 minutes). At this point, treatment is finished.

Geriatric Considerations The elderly may find it difficult to use the metered dose inhaler. A spacer device may be useful. Ipratropium has not been specifically studied in the elderly, but it is poorly absorbed from the airways and appears to be safe in this population.

Pregnancy Considerations Teratogenic effects were not observed in animal studies. Inhaled ipratropium is recommended for use as additional therapy for pregnant women with severe asthma exacerbations.

Ipratropium (Nasal) (i pra TROE pee um)

U.S. Brand Names Atrovent®

Index Terms Ipratropium Bromide

Generic Availability (U.S.) Yes

Pharmacologic Category Anticholinergic Agent

Medication Safety Issues

Sound-alike/look-alike issues:

Ipratropium may be confused with tiotropium

Atrovent® may be confused with Alupent®, Serevent®

Pregnancy Risk Factor B

Lactation Excretion in breast milk unknown/use caution

Use Symptomatic relief of rhinorrhea associated with the common cold and allergic and nonallergic rhinitis

Available Dosage Forms

Solution, intranasal: 0.03% (30 mL); 0.06% (15 mL)

Atrovent®: 0.03% (30 mL); 0.06% (15 mL)

Dosing

Adult & Geriatric

Colds (symptomatic relief of rhinorrhea): Safety and efficacy of use beyond 4 days not established: *Intranasal:* Nasal spray (0.06%): 2 sprays in each nostril 3-4 times/day

Allergic/nonallergic rhinitis: *Intranasal:* Nasal spray (0.03%): 2 sprays in each nostril 2-3 times/day

Seasonal allergic rhinitis (safety and efficacy of use beyond 3 weeks in patients with seasonal allergic rhinitis has not been established): *Intranasal:* Nasal spray (0.06%): 2 sprays in each nostril 4 times/day

Pediatric

Colds (symptomatic relief of rhinorrhea): Intranasal: Safety and efficacy of use beyond 4 days in patients with the common cold have not been established:

Children 5-11 years: 0.06%: 2 sprays in each nostril 3 times/day

Children ≥12 years and Adults: 0.06%: 2 sprays in each nostril 3-4 times/day

Allergic/nonallergic rhinitis: Intranasal: Children ≥6 years: Refer to adult dosing.

Seasonal allergic rhinitis: Intranasal: Children ≥5 years: Refer to adult dosing.

Administration

Inhalation Prior to initial use, prime inhaler by releasing 7 test sprays into the air. If the inhaler has not been used for >24 hours, reprime by releasing 2 test sprays into the air.

Monitoring and Teaching Issues

Physical Assessment Teach patient importance of proper administration.

Patient Education Use care to avoid direct contact with eyes. Do not use more often than recommended. Store solution away from light. May cause dry mouth, unpleasant taste, or stomach upset. Report unresolved GI upset or persistent inability to void.

Ipratropium and Albuterol (i pra TROE pee um & al BYOO ter ole)

U.S. Brand Names Combivent®; DuoNeb®

Index Terms Albuterol and Ipratropium; Salbutamol and Ipratropium

Generic Availability (U.S.) Yes: Solution for nebulization

Pharmacologic Category Anticholinergic Agent; Beta$_2$-Adrenergic Agonist

Medication Safety Issues

Sound-alike/look-alike issues:

Combivent® may be confused with Combivir®, Serevent®

International issues:

DuoNeb® may be confused with DuoTrav™ which is a brand name for travoprost/timolol combination product in Canada or may be confused with Duovent® UDV which is a brand name for ipratropium/fenoterol combination product in Canada

Pregnancy Risk Factor C

Use Treatment of COPD in those patients who are currently on a regular bronchodilator who continue to have bronchospasms and require a second bronchodilator

Contraindications Hypersensitivity to ipratropium, albuterol, atropine (and its derivatives) or any component of the formulation

Warnings/Precautions See individual agents. The aerosol dosage form of this combination contains soya lecithin; may cause allergic reactions in patients with allergy to soya lecithin or related food products (eg, soybean and peanut)

Drug Interactions

Avoid Concomitant Use

Avoid concomitant use of Ipratropium and Albuterol with any of the following: Iobenguane I 123

Decreased Effect

Ipratropium and Albuterol may decrease the levels/effects of: Acetylcholinesterase Inhibitors (Central); Iobenguane I 123; Secretin

The levels/effects of Ipratropium and Albuterol may be decreased by: Acetylcholinesterase Inhibitors (Central); Alpha-/Beta-Blockers; Beta-Blockers (Beta1 Selective); Beta-Blockers (Nonselective); Betahistine

Increased Effect/Toxicity

Ipratropium and Albuterol may increase the levels/effects of: AbobotulinumtoxinA; Anticholinergics; Cannabinoids; Loop Diuretics; OnabotulinumtoxinA; Potassium Chloride; RimabotulinumtoxinB; Sympathomimetics

The levels/effects of Ipratropium and Albuterol may be increased by: Atomoxetine; MAO Inhibitors; Pramlintide; Tricyclic Antidepressants

Adverse Reactions

Percentages reported with either combination product (not versus placebo). Also see individual agents.

>10%: Respiratory: Bronchitis (2% to 12%), upper respiratory tract infection (11%)

1% to 10%:

Cardiovascular: Chest pain (≤3%), angina (<2%), arrhythmia (<2%), edema (<2%), hypertension (<2%), palpitation (<2%), tachycardia (<2%)

Central nervous system: Headache (6%), pain (1% to 3%), dizziness (<2%), fatigue (<2%), insomnia (<2%), nervousness (<2%), tremor (<2%)

Gastrointestinal: Diarrhea (≤2%), dyspepsia (≤2%), nausea (1% to 2%), sputum increased (<2%), taste perversion (<2%), vomiting (<2%), xerostomia (<2%)

Genitourinary: Urinary tract infection (≤2%)

Neuromuscular & skeletal: Arthralgia (<2%), paresthesia (<2%), leg cramps (1%)

Respiratory: Lung disease (6%), dyspnea (5%), cough (4%), pharyngitis (2% to 4%), respiratory disorder (3%), sinusitis (2%), pneumonia (1%), rhinitis (1%)

Miscellaneous: Dysphonia (<2%), flu-like syndrome (1%)

Pharmacodynamics/Kinetics

Pharmacokinetic Note See individual agents.

Available Dosage Forms

Aerosol for oral inhalation:

Combivent®: Ipratropium bromide 18 mcg and albuterol (base) 90 mcg per inhalation (14.7 g) [200 metered actuations]

Solution for nebulization: Ipratropium 0.5 mg and albuterol (base) 2.5 mg per 3 mL (30s, 60s)

DuoNeb®: Ipratropium 0.5 mg and albuterol (base) 2.5 mg per 3 mL (30s, 60s)

Dosing

Adult & Geriatric

COPD:

Aerosol for inhalation: 2 metered-dose inhalations 4 times/day; may receive additional doses as necessary, but total number of doses in 24 hours should not exceed 12 inhalations.

Solution for nebulization: Initial: 3 mL every 6 hours (maximum: 3 mL every 4 hours)

Administration

Inhalation Nebulization: Administer via jet nebulizer to an air compressor with an adequate air flow, equipped with a mouthpiece or face mask. MDI: Shake canister vigorously for ≥10 seconds. Prior to first use (or if not used for >24 hours) a test spray of 3 sprays is recommended. Avoid spraying into eyes.

Stability

Storage

DuoNeb®: Store at 2°C to 30°C (36°F to 86°F). Protect from light.

Combivent®: Store at 15°C to 30°C (59°F to 86°F). Avoid excessive humidity. Do not store near heat or open flame.

Monitoring and Teaching Issues

Physical Assessment See individual agents.

Patient Education See individual agents.

Dietary Considerations The aerosol dosage form contains soya lecithin. Do not use in patients allergic to soya lecithin or related food products such as soybean and peanut.

Breast-Feeding Considerations See individual agents.

Pregnancy Considerations Reproduction studies have not been conducted with this combination. See individual agents.

Related Information

Albuterol *on page 58*

Ipratropium (Oral Inhalation) *on page 1009*

◆ **Ipratropium Bromide** *see* Ipratropium (Nasal) *on page 1010*

◆ **Ipratropium Bromide** *see* Ipratropium (Oral Inhalation) *on page 1009*

◆ **I-Prin [OTC]** *see* Ibuprofen *on page 938*

◆ **Iprivask®** *see* Desirudin *on page 490*

◆ **Iproveratril Hydrochloride** *see* Verapamil *on page 1858*

◆ **IPV** *see* Poliovirus Vaccine (Inactivated) *on page 1473*

Irbesartan (ir be SAR tan)

U.S. Brand Names Avapro®

Generic Availability (U.S.) No

Pharmacologic Category Angiotensin II Receptor Blocker

Medication Safety Issues

Sound-alike/look-alike issues:

Avapro® may be confused with Anaprox®

Pregnancy Risk Factor C (1st trimester); D (2nd and 3rd trimesters)

Lactation Excretion in breast milk unknown/contraindicated

Use Treatment of hypertension alone or in combination with other antihypertensives; treatment of diabetic nephropathy in patients with type 2 diabetes mellitus (noninsulin dependent, NIDDM) and hypertension

Unlabeled/Investigational Use To slow the rate of progression of aortic-root dilation in pediatric patients with Marfan's syndrome

Mechanism of Action/Effect Irbesartan is an angiotensin receptor antagonist. Angiotensin II acts as a vasoconstrictor and stimulates the release of aldosterone, which results in reabsorption of sodium and water. These effects result in an elevation in blood pressure. Irbesartan blocks the AT1 angiotensin II receptor, thereby blocking the vasoconstriction and the aldosterone secreting effects of angiotensin II.

Contraindications Hypersensitivity to irbesartan or any component of the formulation

Warnings/Precautions [U.S. Boxed Warning]: Based on human data, drugs that act on the angiotensin system can cause injury and death to the developing fetus when used in the second and third trimesters. Angiotensin receptor blockers should be discontinued as soon as possible once pregnancy is detected. May cause hyperkalemia; avoid potassium supplementation unless specifically required by healthcare provider. May be associated with deterioration of renal function and/or increases in serum creatinine, particularly in patients with low renal blood flow (eg, renal artery stenosis, heart failure) whose glomerular filtration rate (GFR) is dependent on efferent arteriolar vasoconstriction by angiotensin II. Avoid use or use a much smaller dose in patients who are intravascularly volume-depleted; use caution in patients with unstented unilateral or bilateral renal artery stenosis. When unstented bilateral renal artery stenosis is present, use is generally avoided due to the elevated risk of deterioration in renal function unless possible benefits outweigh risks. AUCs of irbesartan (not the active metabolite) are about 50% greater in patients with Cl_{cr} <30 mL/minute and are doubled in hemodialysis patients. Concurrent use of ACE inhibitors may increase the risk of clinically-significant adverse events (eg, renal dysfunction, hyperkalemia).

Drug Interactions

Metabolism/Transport Effects Substrate of CYP2C9 (minor); **Inhibits** CYP2C8 (moderate), 2C9 (moderate), 2D6 (weak), 3A4 (weak)

Avoid Concomitant Use There are no known interactions where it is recommended to avoid concomitant use.

Decreased Effect

The levels/effects of Irbesartan may be decreased by: Herbs (Hypertensive Properties); Methylphenidate; Nonsteroidal Anti-Inflammatory Agents; Rifamycin Derivatives; Yohimbine

Increased Effect/Toxicity

Irbesartan may increase the levels/effects of: ACE Inhibitors; Amifostine; Antihypertensives; Carvedilol; CYP2C8 Substrates (High risk); CYP2C9 Substrates (High risk); Hypotensive Agents; Lithium; Potassium-Sparing Diuretics; RiTUXimab

The levels/effects of Irbesartan may be increased by: Diazoxide; Eplerenone; Fluconazole; Herbs (Hypotensive Properties); MAO Inhibitors; Pentoxifylline; Phosphodiesterase 5 Inhibitors; Potassium Salts; Prostacyclin Analogues; Tolvaptan; Trimethoprim

Nutritional/Ethanol Interactions Herb/Nutraceutical: Avoid dong quai if using for hypertension (has estrogenic activity). Avoid ephedra, yohimbe, ginseng (may worsen hypertension). Avoid garlic (may have increased antihypertensive effect).

Adverse Reactions Unless otherwise indicated, percentage of incidence is reported for patients with hypertension.

>10%: Endocrine & metabolic: Hyperkalemia (19%, diabetic nephropathy; rarely seen in HTN)

1% to 10%:

- Cardiovascular: Orthostatic hypotension (5%, diabetic nephropathy)
- Central nervous system: Fatigue (4%), dizziness (10%, diabetic nephropathy)
- Gastrointestinal: Diarrhea (3%), dyspepsia (2%)
- Respiratory: Upper respiratory infection (9%), cough (2.8% versus 2.7% in placebo)

>1% but frequency ≤ placebo: Abdominal pain, anxiety, chest pain, edema, headache, influenza, musculoskeletal pain, nausea, nervousness, pharyngitis, rash, rhinitis, sinus abnormality, syncope, tachycardia, urinary tract infection, vertigo, vomiting

Pharmacodynamics/Kinetics

Onset of Action Peak levels in 1-2 hours

Duration of Action >24 hours

Bioavailability 60% to 80%

Time to Peak Serum: 1.5-2 hours

Protein Binding Plasma: 90%

Half-Life Elimination Terminal: 11-15 hours

Metabolism Hepatic, primarily CYP2C9

Excretion Feces (80%); urine (20%)

Available Dosage Forms

Tablet, oral:

Avapro®: 75 mg, 150 mg, 300 mg

Dosing

Adult & Geriatric

Hypertension: Oral: 150 mg once daily; patients may be titrated to 300 mg once daily. **Note:** Starting dose in volume-depleted patients should be 75 mg.

Nephropathy in patients with type 2 diabetes and hypertension: Oral: Target dose: 300 mg once daily

Pediatric

Hypertension: Oral:

<6 years: Safety and efficacy have not been established.

≥6-12 years: Initial: 75 mg once daily; may be titrated to a maximum of 150 mg once daily

13-16 years: Refer to adult dosing.

Aortic-root dilation with Marfan's syndrome (unlabeled use): Children 14 months to 16 years: Initial: 1.4 mg/kg/day; can be increased to a maximum of 2 mg/kg/day (not to exceed adult maximum of 300 mg/day)

Renal Impairment No dosage adjustment necessary with mild to severe impairment unless the patient is also volume depleted.

Stability

Storage Store at room temperature of 15°C to 30°C (59°F to 86°F).

Monitoring and Teaching Issues

Laboratory Monitoring Electrolytes, serum creatinine, BUN, urinalysis

Physical Assessment Use caution in presence of renal insufficiency or aortic/mitral stenosis. Assess potential for interactions with other pharmacological agents or herbal products (risk of hyperkalemia or toxicity). Monitor for hypotension at regular intervals during therapy.

Patient Education May be taken with or without food. Take first dose at bedtime. This medication does not replace other antihypertensive interventions; follow prescriber's instructions for diet and lifestyle changes. May cause dizziness, fainting, lightheadedness, nausea, vomiting, abdominal pain, or diarrhea. Report chest pain or palpitations, skin rash, fluid retention (swelling of extremities), or respiratory difficulty or unusual cough.

Dietary Considerations May be taken with or without food.

Geriatric Considerations No dosage adjustment is necessary when initiating angiotensin II receptor antagonists in the elderly. In clinical studies, no differences between younger adults and the elderly were demonstrated. Many elderly may be volume depleted due to diuretic use and/or blunted thirst reflex resulting in inadequate fluid intake.

Pregnancy Considerations Medications which act on the renin-angiotensin system are reported to have the following fetal/neonatal effects: Hypotension, neonatal skull hypoplasia, anuria, renal failure, and death; oligohydramnios is also reported. These effects are reported to occur with exposure during the second and third trimesters. There are no adequate and well-controlled studies in pregnant women. **[U.S. Boxed Warning]: Based on human data, drugs that act on the angiotensin system can cause injury and death to the developing fetus when used in the second and third trimesters. Angiotensin receptor blockers should be discontinued as soon as possible once pregnancy is detected.**

Related Information

Angiotensin Agents *on page 1974*

Irbesartan and Hydrochlorothiazide

(ir be SAR tan & hye droe klor oh THYE a zide)

U.S. Brand Names Avalide®

Index Terms Avapro® HCT; Hydrochlorothiazide and Irbesartan

Generic Availability (U.S.) No

Pharmacologic Category Angiotensin II Receptor Blocker; Diuretic, Thiazide

Medication Safety Issues

Sound-alike/look-alike issues:

Avalide® may be confused with Avandia®

Pregnancy Risk Factor D

Lactation Enters breast milk/not recommended

Use Combination therapy for the management of hypertension; may be used as initial therapy in patients likely to need multiple drugs to achieve blood pressure goals

Contraindications Hypersensitivity to irbesartan, hydrochlorothiazide, or any component of the formulation; sulfonamide-derived drugs; anuria

Warnings/Precautions See individual agents.

Drug Interactions

Metabolism/Transport Effects Irbesartan: **Substrate** of CYP2C9 (minor); **Inhibits** CYP2C8 (moderate), 2C9 (moderate), 2D6 (weak), 3A4 (weak)

Avoid Concomitant Use

Avoid concomitant use of Irbesartan and Hydrochlorothiazide with any of the following: Dofetilide

Decreased Effect

Irbesartan and Hydrochlorothiazide may decrease the levels/effects of: Antidiabetic Agents

The levels/effects of Irbesartan and Hydrochlorothiazide may be decreased by: Bile Acid Sequestrants; Herbs (Hypertensive Properties); Methylphenidate; Nonsteroidal Anti-Inflammatory Agents; Rifamycin Derivatives; Yohimbine

Increased Effect/Toxicity

Irbesartan and Hydrochlorothiazide may increase the levels/effects of: ACE Inhibitors; Allopurinol; Amifostine; Antihypertensives; Calcium Salts; CarBAMazepine; Carvedilol; CYP2C8 Substrates (High risk); CYP2C9 Substrates (High risk); Dofetilide; Hypotensive Agents; Lithium; OXcarbazepine; Potassium-Sparing Diuretics; RiTUXimab; Topiramate; Toremifene; Vitamin D Analogs

The levels/effects of Irbesartan and Hydrochlorothiazide may be increased by: Alcohol (Ethyl); Analgesics (Opioid); Barbiturates; Corticosteroids (Orally Inhaled); Corticosteroids (Systemic); Eplerenone; Fluconazole; Herbs (Hypotensive Properties); Licorice; MAO Inhibitors; Pentoxifylline; Phosphodiesterase 5 Inhibitors; Potassium Salts; Prostacyclin Analogues; Tolvaptan; Trimethoprim

Adverse Reactions Reactions/percentages reported with combination product; also refer to individual agents.

1% to 10%:

Cardiovascular: Edema (3%), chest pain (2%), tachycardia (1%)

Central nervous system: Dizziness (8%; orthostatic: 1%), fatigue (6%)

Gastrointestinal: Nausea/vomiting (3%), abdominal pain (2%), dyspepsia (2%)

Genitourinary: Urination abnormal (2%)

Neuromuscular & skeletal: Musculoskeletal pain (6%)

Renal: BUN increased (2%), creatinine increased (1%)

Miscellaneous: Flu-like syndrome (3%)

Pharmacodynamics/Kinetics

Pharmacokinetic Note See individual agents.

Available Dosage Forms

Tablet:

Avalide®: Irbesartan 150 mg and hydrochlorothiazide 12.5 mg; irbesartan 300 mg and hydrochlorothiazide 12.5 mg; irbesartan 300 mg and hydrochlorothiazide 25 mg

Dosing

Adult & Geriatric Dose must be individualized.

Hypertension: Oral: **Note:** Maximum antihypertensive effects are attained within 2-4 weeks after initiation or a change in dose; however, if necessary, may carefully titrate dose as soon as after 1 week of treatment.

Add-on therapy: A patient who is not controlled with either agent alone may be switched to the combination product. The lowest dosage available is irbesartan 150 mg/hydrochlorothiazide 12.5 mg.

Initial therapy: Irbesartan 150 mg/hydrochlorothiazide 12.5 mg once daily. If initial response is inadequate, may titrate dose after 1-2 weeks, to a maximum dose of irbesartan 300 mg/hydrochlorothiazide 25 mg once daily.

Renal Impairment Not recommended in patients with Cl_{cr} ≤30 mL/minute.

Hepatic Impairment Use with caution.

Stability

Storage Store at 25°C (77°F); excursions permitted to 15°C to 30°C (59°F to 86°F).

Monitoring and Teaching Issues

Laboratory Monitoring Serum electrolytes, BUN, creatinine

Physical Assessment See individual agents.

Patient Education See individual agents.

Dietary Considerations May be taken without regard to meals.

Pregnancy Considerations [U.S. Boxed Warning]: Based on human data, drugs that act on the angiotensin system can cause injury and death to the developing fetus when used in the second and third trimesters. Angiotensin receptor blockers should be discontinued as soon as possible once pregnancy is detected. Also see individual agents.

Related Information

Hydrochlorothiazide *on page 912*

Irbesartan *on page 1012*

◆ **Iressa®** *see* Gefitinib *on page 853*

Irinotecan (eye rye no TEE kan)

U.S. Brand Names Camptosar®

Index Terms Camptothecin-11; CPT-11; Irinotecan HCl; Irinotecan Hydrochloride

Generic Availability (U.S.) Yes

Pharmacologic Category Antineoplastic Agent, Camptothecin; Antineoplastic Agent, Natural Source (Plant) Derivative; Antineoplastic Agent, Topoisomerase I Inhibitor

Medication Safety Issues

High alert medication: This medication is in a class the Institute for Safe Medication Practices (ISMP) includes among its list of drug classes which have a heightened risk of causing significant patient harm when used in error.

Pregnancy Risk Factor D

Lactation Excretion in breast milk unknown/not recommended

Use Treatment of metastatic carcinoma of the colon or rectum

Unlabeled/Investigational Use Treatment of cervical cancer (recurrent or metastatic), central nervous system tumors (recurrent glioblastoma), esophageal cancer, Ewing's sarcoma (recurrent or progressive), gastric cancer (metastatic or locally advanced), nonsmall cell lung cancer (advanced), ovarian cancer (recurrent), pancreatic cancer (advanced), small cell lung cancer (extensive stage)

Mechanism of Action/Effect Irinotecan and its active metabolite (SN-38) bind reversibly to topoisomerase I-DNA complex preventing religation of the cleaved DNA strand. This results in the accumulation of cleavable complexes and double-strand DNA breaks. As mammalian cells cannot efficiently repair these breaks, cell death consistent with S-phase cell cycle specificity occurs, leading to termination of cellular replication.

Contraindications Hypersensitivity to irinotecan or any component of the formulation

Warnings/Precautions Hazardous agent - use appropriate precautions for handling and disposal. Severe hypersensitivity reactions (including anaphylaxis) have occurred. For I.V. use only; monitor infusion site; may cause local tissue necrosis or thrombophlebitis if extravasation occurs.

[U.S. Boxed Warning]: Severe diarrhea may be dose-limiting and potentially fatal; early-onset and late-onset diarrhea may occur. Early diarrhea occurs during or within 24 hours of receiving irinotecan and is characterized by cholinergic symptoms (eg, increased salivation, diaphoresis, flushing, abdominal cramping, lacrimation); may be prevented or treated with atropine. Late diarrhea occurs more than 24 hours after treatment which may lead to dehydration, electrolyte imbalance, or sepsis; may be life-threatening and should be promptly treated with loperamide; dose reductions may be recommended for future doses within the current cycle. Antibiotics may be necessary if patient develops ileus, fever, or severe neutropenia. Patients with diarrhea should be carefully monitored and treated promptly; may require fluid and electrolyte therapy. Colitis, complicated by ulceration, bleeding, ileus, and infection has been reported; initiate antibiotics promptly in patients with ileus.

[U.S. Boxed Warning]: May cause severe myelosuppression. Deaths due to sepsis following severe neutropenia have been reported. Complications due to neutropenia should be promptly managed with antibiotics. Therapy should be temporarily discontinued if neutropenic fever occurs or if the absolute neutrophil count is <1000/mm^3. The dose of irinotecan should be reduced if there is a clinically significant decrease in the total WBC (<200/mm^3), neutrophil count (<1500/mm^3), hemoglobin (<8 g/dL), or platelet count (<100,000/mm^3). Routine administration of a colony-stimulating factor is generally not necessary, but may be considered for patients experiencing significant neutropenia. Fatal cases of Interstitial Pulmonary Disease (IPD)-like events have been reported with single-agent and combination therapy. Promptly evaluate changes in baseline pulmonary symptoms or any new-onset pulmonary symptoms. Discontinue therapy if IPD is diagnosed.

Patients with even modest elevations in total serum bilirubin levels (1-2 mg/dL) have a significantly greater likelihood of experiencing first-course grade 3 or 4 neutropenia than those with bilirubin levels that were <1 mg/dL. Patients with abnormal glucuronidation of bilirubin, such as those with Gilbert's syndrome, may also be at greater risk of myelosuppression when receiving therapy with irinotecan. Use caution when treating patients with known hepatic dysfunction or hyperbilirubinemia exposure to the active metabolite (SN-38) is increased; toxicities may be increased. Dosage adjustments should be considered.

Patients homozygous for the UGT1A1*28 allele are at increased risk of neutropenia; initial one-level dose reduction should be considered for both single-agent and combination regimens. Heterozygous carriers of the UGT1A1*28 allele may also be at increased risk; however, most patients have tolerated normal starting doses. Avoid vaccination with live vaccines during treatment (risk of infection may be increased due to immunosuppression). Although the response to vaccines may be diminished, inactivated vaccines may be administered during treatment.

Renal impairment and acute renal failure have been reported, possibly due to dehydration secondary to diarrhea. Use with caution in patients with renal impairment; not recommended in patients on dialysis. Patients with bowel obstruction should not be treated with irinotecan until resolution of obstruction. Use caution in patients who previously received pelvic/abdominal radiation, elderly patients with comorbid conditions, or baseline performance status of 2; close monitoring and dosage adjustments are recommended. Contains sorbitol; do not use in patients with hereditary fructose intolerance. **[U.S. Boxed Warning]: Should be administered under the supervision of an experienced cancer chemotherapy physician.** Except as part of a clinical trial, use in combination with fluorouracil and leucovorin "Mayo Clinic" regimen is not recommended. Increased toxicity has also been noted in patients with a baseline performance status of 2 in other combination regimens containing irinotecan, leucovorin, and fluorouracil. High potential for CYP-mediated drug interactions; enzyme inducers may decrease exposure to irinotecan and SN-38 (active metabolite); enzyme inhibitors may increase exposure; for use in patients with CNS tumors (unlabeled use), selection of antiseizure medications which are not enzyme inducers is preferred.

Drug Interactions

Metabolism/Transport Effects Substrate (major) of CYP2B6, CYP3A4, P-glycoprotein, SLCO1B1, UGT1A1

Avoid Concomitant Use

Avoid concomitant use of Irinotecan with any of the following: Atazanavir; BCG; Natalizumab; Pimecrolimus; Roflumilast; St Johns Wort; Tacrolimus (Topical); Vaccines (Live)

Decreased Effect

Irinotecan may decrease the levels/effects of: BCG; Sipuleucel-T; Vaccines (Inactivated); Vaccines (Live)

The levels/effects of Irinotecan may be decreased by: CarBAMazepine; CYP2B6 Inducers (Strong); CYP3A4 Inducers (Strong); Deferasirox; Echinacea; P-Glycoprotein Inducers; PHENobarbital; Phenytoin; St Johns Wort

Increased Effect/Toxicity

Irinotecan may increase the levels/effects of: Leflunomide; Natalizumab; Vaccines (Live)

The levels/effects of Irinotecan may be increased by: Antifungal Agents (Azole Derivatives, Systemic); Atazanavir; Bevacizumab; Conivaptan; CYP2B6 Inhibitors (Moderate); CYP2B6 Inhibitors (Strong); CYP3A4 Inhibitors (Moderate); CYP3A4 Inhibitors (Strong); Dasatinib; Denosumab; Eltrombopag; P-Glycoprotein Inhibitors; Pimecrolimus; Quazepam; Roflumilast; SORAfenib; Tacrolimus (Topical); Trastuzumab

Nutritional/Ethanol Interactions Herb/Nutraceutical: Avoid St John's wort (decreases the efficacy of irinotecan).

Adverse Reactions Frequency of adverse reactions reported for single-agent use of irinotecan only.

>10%:

Cardiovascular: Vasodilation (9% to 11%)

Central nervous system: Cholinergic toxicity (47% - includes rhinitis, increased salivation, miosis, lacrimation, diaphoresis, flushing and intestinal hyperperistalsis); fever (44% to 45%), pain (23% to 24%), dizziness (15% to 21%), insomnia (19%), headache (17%), chills (14%)

Dermatologic: Alopecia (46% to 72%), rash (13% to 14%)

Endocrine & metabolic: Dehydration (15%)

Gastrointestinal: Diarrhea, late (83% to 88%; grade 3/4: 14% to 31%), diarrhea, early (43% to 51%; grade 3/4: 7% to 22%), nausea (70% to 86%), abdominal pain (57% to 68%), vomiting (62% to 67%), cramps (57%), anorexia (44% to 55%), constipation (30% to 32%), mucositis (30%), weight loss (30%), flatulence (12%), stomatitis (12%)

Hematologic: Anemia (60% to 97%; grades 3/4: 5% to 7%), leukopenia (63% to 96%, grades 3/4: 14% to 28%), thrombocytopenia (96%, grades 3/4: 1% to 4%), neutropenia (30% to 96%; grades 3/4: 14% to 31%)

Hepatic: Bilirubin increased (84%), alkaline phosphatase increased (13%)

Neuromuscular & skeletal: Weakness (69% to 76%), back pain (14%)

Respiratory: Dyspnea (22%), cough (17% to 20%), rhinitis (16%)

Miscellaneous: Diaphoresis (16%), infection (14%)

1% to 10%:

Cardiovascular: Edema (10%), hypotension (6%), thromboembolic events (5%)

Central nervous system: Somnolence (9%), confusion (3%)

Gastrointestinal: Abdominal fullness (10%), dyspepsia (10%)

Hematologic: Neutropenic fever (grades 3/4: 2% to 6%), hemorrhage (grades 3/4: 1% to 5%), neutropenic infection (grades 3/4: 1% to 2%)

Hepatic: AST increased (10%), ascites and/or jaundice (grades 3/4: 9%)

Respiratory: Pneumonia (4%)

Note: In limited pediatric experience, dehydration (often associated with severe hypokalemia and hyponatremia) was among the most significant grade 3/4 adverse events, with a frequency up to 29%. In addition, grade 3/4 infection was reported in 24%.

Pharmacodynamics/Kinetics

Time to Peak SN-38: Following 90-minute infusion: ~1 hour

Protein Binding Plasma: Predominantly albumin; Irinotecan: 30% to 68%, SN-38 (active metabolite): ~95%

Half-Life Elimination Irinotecan: 6-12 hours; SN-38: ~10-20 hours

Metabolism Primarily hepatic to SN-38 (active metabolite) by carboxylesterase enzymes; SN-38 undergoes conjugation by UDP- glucuronosyl transferase 1A1 (UGT1A1) to form a glucuronide metabolite. Conversion of irinotecan to SN-38 is decreased and glucuronidation of SN-38 is increased patients who smoke cigarettes, resulting in lower levels of the metabolite and overall decreased systemic exposure. SN-38 is increased by UGT1A1*28 polymorphism (10% of North Americans are homozygous for UGT1A1*28 allele). The lactones of both irinotecan and SN-38 undergo hydrolysis to inactive hydroxy acid forms.

Excretion Urine: Irinotecan (11% to 20%), metabolites (SN-38 <1%, SN-38 glucuronide, 3%)

Available Dosage Forms

Injection, solution: 20 mg/mL (2 mL, 5 mL, 25 mL)

Camptosar®: 20 mg/mL (2 mL, 5 mL, 15 mL)

Dosing

Adult Note: A reduction in the starting dose by one dose level should be considered for prior pelvic/abdominal radiotherapy, performance status of 2, or known homozygosity for UGT1A1*28 allele. Consider premedication of atropine 0.25-1 mg I.V. or SubQ in patients with cholinergic symptoms (eg, increased salivation, diaphoresis, abdominal cramping) or diarrhea. Details concerning dosage in combination regimens should also be consulted.

Colorectal cancer, metastatic (single-agent therapy): I.V.:

Weekly regimen: 125 mg/m^2 over 90 minutes on days 1, 8, 15, and 22 of a 6-week treatment cycle (may adjust upward to 150 mg/m^2 if tolerated)

Adjusted dose level -1: 100 mg/m^2

Adjusted dose level -2: 75 mg/m^2

Further adjust to 50 mg/m^2 (in decrements of 25-50 mg/m^2) if needed

Once-every-3-week regimen: 350 mg/m^2 over 90 minutes, once every 3 weeks

Adjusted dose level -1: 300 mg/m^2

Adjusted dose level -2: 250 mg/m^2

Further adjust to 200 mg/m^2 (in decrements of 25-50 mg/m^2) if needed

Colorectal cancer, metastatic (in combination with fluorouracil and leucovorin): I.V.: Six-week (42-day) cycle:

Regimen 1: 125 mg/m^2 over 90 minutes on days 1, 8, 15, and 22; to be given in combination with bolus leucovorin and fluorouracil (leucovorin administered immediately following irinotecan; fluorouracil immediately following leucovorin)

Adjusted dose level -1: 100 mg/m^2

Adjusted dose level -2: 75 mg/m^2

Further adjust if needed in decrements of ~20%

Regimen 2: 180 mg/m^2 over 90 minutes on days 1, 15, and 29; to be given in combination with infusional leucovorin and bolus/infusion fluorouracil (leucovorin administered immediately following irinotecan; fluorouracil immediately following leucovorin)

Adjusted dose level -1: 150 mg/m^2

Adjusted dose level -2: 120 mg/m^2

Further adjust if needed in decrements of ~20%

Colorectal cancer, metastatic (unlabeled dosing): I.V.: FOLFOXIRI regimen: 165 mg/m^2 over 1 hour once every 2 weeks (Falcone, 2007)

Cervical cancer, recurrent or metastatic (unlabeled use): I.V.: 125 mg/m^2 over 90 minutes once weekly for 4 consecutive weeks followed by a 2-week rest during each 6 week treatment cycle (Verschraegen, 1997)

CNS tumor, recurrent glioblastoma (unlabeled use): I.V.: 125 mg/m^2 over 90 minutes once every 2 weeks (in combination with bevacizumab). **NOTE:** in patients taking concurrent antiepileptic enzyme-inducing medications irinotecan dose was increased to 340 mg/m^2 (Friedman, 2009; Vredenburgh, 2007).

Esophageal cancer, metastatic or locally advanced (unlabeled use): I.V.: 65 mg/m^2/dose over 90 minutes days 1, 8, 15, and 22 of a 6-week treatment cycle (in combination with cisplatin) (Ajani, 2002; Ilson, 1999) **or** 80 mg/m^2/dose weekly for 6 weeks of a 7-week treatment cycle (in combination with leucovorin and fluorouracil) (Dank, 2008) **or** 250 mg/m^2/dose every 3 weeks (in combination with capecitabine) (Leary, 2009; Moehler, 2010)

Ewing's sarcoma, recurrent or progressive (unlabeled use): I.V.: 20 mg/m^2/dose days 1-5 and days 8-12 every 3 weeks (in combination with temozolomide) (Casey, 2009)

Gastric cancer, metastatic or locally advanced (unlabeled use): 65 mg/m^2/dose over 90 minutes days 1, 8, 15, and 22 of a 6-week treatment cycle (in combination with cisplatin) (Ajani, 2002) **or** 180 mg/m^2/dose over 90 minutes every 2 weeks (in combination with leucovorin and fluorouracil) (Bouche, 2004) **or** 80 mg/m^2/dose weekly for 6 weeks of a 7-week treatment cycle (in combination with leucovorin and fluorouracil) (Dank, 2008) **or** 250 mg/m^2/dose every 3 weeks (in combination with capecitabine) (Moehler, 2010)

Nonsmall cell lung cancer, advanced (unlabeled use): I.V.: 60 mg/m^2 days 1, 8, and 15 every 4 weeks (in combination with cisplatin) (Ohe, 2007)

Pancreatic cancer, advanced (unlabeled use): I.V.: FOLFIRINOX regimen: 180 mg/m^2/dose over 90 minutes every 2 weeks (Conroy, 2005; Conroy, 2010)

Small cell lung cancer, extensive stage (unlabeled use): I.V.: 60 mg/m^2 days 1, 8, and 15 every 4 weeks (in combination with cisplatin) (Noda, 2002) **or** 65 mg/m^2 days 1 and 8 every 3 weeks (in combination with cisplatin) (Hanna, 2006) **or** 175 mg/m^2 day 1 every 3 weeks (in combination with carboplatin) (Hermes, 2008) **or** 50 mg/m^2 days 1, 8 and 15 every 4 weeks (in combination with carboplatin) (Schmittel, 2006)

Geriatric

Weekly dosing schedule: No dosing adjustment is recommended

Every 3-week dosing colorectal cancer schedule: Recommended initial dose is 300 mg/m^2/dose for patients ≥70 years

Pediatric Ewing's sarcoma, recurrent or progressive (unlabeled use): I.V.: Refer to adult dosing.

Renal Impairment Effects have not been evaluated; use caution; not recommended for use in patients on dialysis.

Hepatic Impairment

Liver metastases with normal hepatic function: No adjustment required.

Bilirubin >ULN to ≤2 mg/dL: Consider reducing initial dose by one dose level.

Bilirubin >2 mg/dL: Use is not recommended.

The following guidelines have been used by some clinicians: Bilirubin 1.5-3 mg/dL: Administer 75% of dose (Floyd, 2006).

Adjustment for Toxicity It is recommended that new courses begin only after the granulocyte count recovers to ≥1500/mm^3, the platelet counts recover to ≥100,000/mm^3, and treatment-related diarrhea has fully resolved. Depending on the patient's ability to tolerate therapy, doses should be adjusted in increments of 25-50 mg/m^2. Treatment should be delayed 1-2 weeks to allow for recovery from treatment-related toxicities. If the patient has not recovered after a 2-week delay, consider discontinuing irinotecan. See tables.

Colorectal Cancer: Single-Agent Schedule: Recommended Dosage Modifications[1]

Toxicity NCI Grade[2] (Value)	During a Cycle of Therapy	At Start of Subsequent Cycles of Therapy (After Adequate Recovery), Compared to Starting Dose in Previous Cycle[1]	
	Weekly	Weekly	Once Every 3 Weeks
No toxicity	Maintain dose level	↑ 25 mg/m^2 up to a maximum dose of 150 mg/m^2	Maintain dose level
Neutropenia			
1 (1500-1999/mm^3)	Maintain dose level	Maintain dose level	Maintain dose level
2 (1000-1499/mm^3)	↓ 25 mg/m^2	Maintain dose level	Maintain dose level
3 (500-999/mm^3)	Omit dose until resolved to ≤ grade 2, then ↓ 25 mg/m^2	↓ 25 mg/m^2	↓ 50 mg/m^2
4 (<500/mm^3)	Omit dose until resolved to ≤ grade 2, then ↓ 50 mg/m^2	↓ 50 mg/m^2	↓ 50 mg/m^2
Neutropenic Fever (grade 4 neutropenia and ≥ grade 2 fever)	Omit dose until resolved, then ↓ 50 mg/m^2	↓ 50 mg/m^2	↓ 50 mg/m^2
Other Hematologic Toxicities	Dose modifications for leukopenia, thrombocytopenia, and anemia during a course of therapy and at the start of subsequent courses of therapy are also based on NCI toxicity criteria and are the same as recommended for neutropenia above.		
Diarrhea			
1 (2-3 stools/day > pretreatment)	Maintain dose level	Maintain dose level	Maintain dose level
2 (4-6 stools/day > pretreatment)	↓ 25 mg/m^2	Maintain dose level	Maintain dose level
3 (7-9 stools/day > pretreatment)	Omit dose until resolved to ≤ grade 2, then ↓ 25 mg/m^2	↓ 25 mg/m^2	↓ 50 mg/m^2
4 (≥10 stools/day > pretreatment)	Omit dose until resolved to ≤ grade 2, then ↓ 50 mg/m^2	↓ 50 mg/m^2	↓ 50 mg/m^2
Other Nonhematologic Toxicities[3]			
1	Maintain dose level	Maintain dose level	Maintain dose level
2	↓ 25 mg/m^2	↓ 25 mg/m^2	↓ 50 mg/m^2
3	Omit dose until resolved to ≤ grade 2, then ↓ 25 mg/m^2	↓ 25 mg/m^2	↓ 50 mg/m^2
4	Omit dose until resolved to ≤ grade 2, then ↓ 50 mg/m^2	↓ 50 mg/m^2	↓ 50 mg/m^2

[1]All dose modifications should be based on the worst preceding toxicity.

[2]National Cancer Institute Common Toxicity Criteria (version 1.0).

[3]Excludes alopecia, anorexia, asthenia.

Colorectal Cancer: Combination Schedules: Recommended Dosage Modifications[1]

Toxicity NCI[2] Grade (Value)	During a Cycle of Therapy	At the Start of Subsequent Cycles of Therapy (After Adequate Recovery), Compared to the Starting Dose in the Previous Cycle[1]
No toxicity	Maintain dose level	Maintain dose level
Neutropenia		
1 (1500-1999/mm³)	Maintain dose level	Maintain dose level
2 (1000-1499/mm³)	↓ 1 dose level	Maintain dose level
3 (500-999/mm³)	Omit dose until resolved to ≤ grade 2, then ↓ 1 dose level	↓ 1 dose level
4 (<500/mm³)	Omit dose until resolved to ≤ grade 2, then ↓ 2 dose levels	↓ 2 dose levels
Neutropenic Fever (grade 4 neutropenia and ≥ grade 2 fever)	Omit dose until resolved, then ↓ 2 dose levels	
Other Hematologic Toxicities	Dose modifications for leukopenia or thrombocytopenia during a course of therapy and at the start of subsequent courses of therapy are also based on NCI toxicity criteria and are the same as recommended for neutropenia above.	
Diarrhea		
1 (2-3 stools/day > pretreatment)	Delay dose until resolved to baseline, then give same dose	Maintain dose level
2 (4-6 stools/day > pretreatment)	Omit dose until resolved to baseline, then ↓ 1 dose level	Maintain dose level
3 (7-9 stools/day > pretreatment)	Omit dose until resolved to baseline, then ↓ by 1 dose level	↓ 1 dose level
4 (≥10 stools/day > pretreatment)	Omit dose until resolved to baseline, then ↓ 2 dose levels	↓ 2 dose levels
Other Nonhematologic Toxicities[3]		
1	Maintain dose level	Maintain dose level
2	Omit dose until resolved to ≤ grade 1, then ↓ 1 dose level	Maintain dose level
3	Omit dose until resolved to ≤ grade 2, then ↓ 1 dose level	↓ 1 dose level
4	Omit dose until resolved to ≤ grade 2, then ↓ 2 dose levels	↓ 2 dose levels
Mucositis and/or stomatitis	Decrease only 5-FU, not irinotecan	Decrease only 5-FU, not irinotecan

[1]All dose modifications should be based on the worst preceding toxicity.

[2]National Cancer Institute Common Toxicity Criteria (version 1.0).

[3]Excludes alopecia, anorexia, asthenia.

Administration

I.V. Administer by I.V. infusion, usually over 90 minutes. Premedication with dexamethasone and a 5-HT_3 blocker is recommended 30 minutes prior to administration; prochlorperazine may be considered for subsequent use. Consider premedication of atropine 0.25-1 mg I.V. or SubQ in patients with cholinergic symptoms (eg, increased salivation, diaphoresis, abdominal cramping) or diarrhea.

The recommended regimen to manage late diarrhea is loperamide 4 mg orally at onset of late diarrhea, followed by 2 mg every 2 hours (or 4 mg every 4 hours at night) until 12 hours have passed without a bowel movement. If diarrhea recurs, then repeat administration. Loperamide should not be used for more than 48 consecutive hours.

Stability

Reconstitution Use appropriate precautions for handling and disposal. Dilute in 250-500 mL D_5W or NS to a final concentration of 0.12-2.8 mg/mL. Due to the relatively acidic pH, irinotecan appears to be more stable in D_5W than NS.

Storage Store intact vials of injection at room temperature. Protect from light. Solutions diluted in NS may precipitate if refrigerated. Solutions diluted in D_5W are stable for 24 hours at room temperature or 48 hours under refrigeration at 2°C to 8°C, although the manufacturer recommends use within 6 hours at room temperature and 24 hours if refrigerated. Do not freeze.

Monitoring and Teaching Issues

Laboratory Monitoring CBC with differential and platelet count, bilirubin, electrolytes (with severe diarrhea)

A test is available for genotyping of UGT1A1; however, guidelines for use are not established and not recommended in patients who have experienced toxicity as a dose reduction is already recommended (NCCN Colon Cancer Guidelines v.1.2011)

Physical Assessment Use caution and closely monitor use for patients with increased risk of neutropenia, previous pelvic or abdominal radiation, and elderly patients with comorbid conditions. Premedicate with antiemetic (emetic potential moderate). Infusion site must be monitored to prevent extravasation. Assess CBC with differential and platelet count. Monitor for neutropenia, immediate or delayed diarrhea (can be fatal), sepsis, mucositis, and/or stomatitis.

Patient Education This drug can only be administered by infusion. Report immediately any burning, pain, redness, or swelling at infusion site. Maintain adequate hydration, unless instructed to restrict fluid intake. May cause severe diarrhea; follow instructions for taking antidiarrheal medication (do not use antidiarrheal medication for longer than 48 consecutive hours). Report immediately if diarrhea persists or you experience signs of dehydration (eg, fainting, dizziness, lightheadedness). You may be more susceptible to infection. You may experience nausea, vomiting, or hair loss (will regrow after treatment is completed). Report immediately persistent diarrhea, unresolved nausea or vomiting, alterations in urinary pattern (increased or decreased), opportunistic infection (fever, chills, unusual bruising or bleeding, fatigue, purulent vaginal discharge, unhealed mouth sores), chest pain, or respiratory difficulty.

Dietary Considerations Contains sorbitol; do not use in patients with hereditary fructose intolerance.

Breast-Feeding Considerations Due to the potential for serious adverse reactions in the nursing infant, breast-feeding is not recommended.

Pregnancy Considerations Teratogenic effects were noted in animal studies. There are no adequate and well-controlled studies in pregnant women. Women of childbearing potential should avoid becoming pregnant while receiving treatment.

Additional Information Patients who are homozygous for the UGT1A1*28 allele are at increased risk for neutropenia; a decreased dose is recommended. Clinical research of patients who are heterozygous for UGT1A1*28 have been variable for increased neutropenic risk and such patients have tolerated normal starting doses. An FDA-approved test (Invader® Molecular Assay) is available for clinical determination of UGT phenotype.

◆ **Irinotecan HCl** *see* Irinotecan *on page* 1015

◆ **Irinotecan Hydrochloride** *see* Irinotecan *on page* 1015

◆ **Iron Dextran** *see* Iron Dextran Complex *on page* 1021

Iron Dextran Complex (EYE ern DEKS tran KOM pleks)

U.S. Brand Names Dexferrum®; INFeD®

Index Terms High-Molecular-Weight Iron Dextran (DexFerrum®); Imferon; Iron Dextran; Low-Molecular-Weight Iron Dextran (INFeD®)

Generic Availability (U.S.) No

Pharmacologic Category Iron Salt

Medication Safety Issues

Sound-alike/look-alike issues:

Dexferrum® may be confused with Desferal®

Iron dextran complex may be confused with ferumoxytol

Pregnancy Risk Factor C

Lactation Enters breast milk/use caution

Use Treatment of iron deficiency in patients in whom oral administration is infeasible or ineffective

Unlabeled/Investigational Use Cancer-/chemotherapy-associated anemia

Available Dosage Forms

Injection, solution:

Dexferrum®: Elemental iron 50 mg/mL (1 mL, 2 mL)

INFeD®: Elemental iron 50 mg/mL (2 mL)

Dosing

Adult & Geriatric

Note: A 0.5 mL test dose should be given prior to starting iron dextran therapy.

Iron-deficiency anemia: I.M. (INFeD®), I.V. (Dexferrum®, INFeD®):

Dose (mL) = 0.0442 (desired Hgb - observed Hgb) x LBW + (0.26 x LBW)

Desired hemoglobin: Usually 14.8 g/dL

LBW = Lean body weight in kg

Iron replacement therapy for blood loss: (INFeD®), I.V. (Dexferrum®, INFeD®): Replacement iron (mg) = blood loss (mL) x Hct

Maximum daily dosage: Manufacturer's labeling: **Note:** Replacement of larger estimated iron deficits may be achieved by serial administration of smaller incremental dosages. Daily dosages should be limited to 100 mg iron (2 mL)

Total dose infusion (unlabeled): The entire dose (estimated iron deficit) may be diluted and administered as a one-time I.V. infusion.

Cancer-/chemotherapy-associated anemia (NCCN guidelines v.2.2010) (unlabeled use): I.V.: Test dose: 25 mg slow I.V. slow push, followed 1 hour later by 100 mg over 5 minutes; larger doses (unlabeled), up to total dose infusion (over several hours) may be administered. Low-molecular-weight iron dextran preferred.

Pediatric Note: A 0.5 mL test dose (0.25 mL in infants) should be given prior to starting iron dextran therapy.

Iron-deficiency anemia: I.M. (INFeD®), I.V. (Dexferrum®, INFeD®):

Children 5-15 kg: Should not normally be given in the first 4 months of life:

Dose (mL) = 0.0442 (desired Hgb - observed Hgb) x W + (0.26 x W)

Desired hemoglobin: Usually 12 g/dL

W = Total body weight in kg

Children >15 kg: Refer to adult dosing.

Iron replacement therapy for blood loss: Refer to adult dosing.

Maximum daily dose:

Children <5 kg: 25 mg iron (0.5 mL)

Children 5-10 kg: 50 mg iron (1 mL)

Children ≥10 kg: Refer to adult dosing.

Administration

I.M. Note: Test dose: A test dose should be given on the first day of therapy; patient should be observed for 1 hour for hypersensitivity reaction, then the remaining dose (dose minus test dose) should be given. Resuscitation equipment and trained personnel should be available. An uneventful test dose does not ensure an anaphylactic-type reaction will not occur during administration of the therapeutic dose.

I.M. (INFeD®): Use Z-track technique (displacement of the skin laterally prior to injection); injection should be deep into the upper outer quadrant of buttock; alternate buttocks with subsequent injections. Administer test dose at same recommended site using the same technique.

I.V. Test dose should be given gradually over at least 30 seconds (INFeD®) or 5 minutes (Dexferrum®). Subsequent dose(s) may be administered by I.V. bolus undiluted at a rate not to exceed 50 mg/minute or diluted in 250-1000 mL NS and infused over 1-6 hours (initial 25 mL should be given slowly and patient should be observed for allergic reactions); avoid dilutions with dextrose (increased incidence of local pain and phlebitis). Resuscitation equipment and trained personnel should be available. An uneventful test dose does not ensure an anaphylactic-type reaction will not occur during administration of the therapeutic dose.

Monitoring and Teaching Issues

Laboratory Monitoring Hemoglobin, hematocrit, reticulocyte count, serum ferritin

Physical Assessment Be alert to the potential for anaphylaxis. Resuscitation equipment should be available. Note that adverse response may occur some time (1-4 days) after administration. Assess patients with rheumatoid arthritis for exacerbated swelling and joint pain; adjust medications as needed.

Patient Education You will need frequent blood tests while on this therapy. If you have rheumatoid arthritis, you may experience increased swelling or joint pain; consult prescriber for medication adjustment. You may experience dizziness, severe headache, nausea, metallic taste, or increased sweating. Large doses can sometimes be associated with a delayed reaction (muscle pain, backache, headache, chills, fever, nausea, or vomiting) occurring 24-48 hours after administration and usually lasting 3-4 days. Report acute GI problems, fever, respiratory difficulty, rapid heartbeat, yellowing of skin or eyes, or swelling of hands and feet.

◆ **Iron Gluconate** *see* Ferrous Gluconate *on page* 754

Iron Sucrose (EYE ern SOO krose)

U.S. Brand Names Venofer®

Generic Availability (U.S.) No

Pharmacologic Category Iron Salt

Medication Safety Issues

Sound-alike/look-alike issues:

Iron sucrose may be confused with ferumoxytol

Pregnancy Risk Factor B

Lactation Excretion in breast milk unknown/use caution

Use Treatment of iron-deficiency anemia in chronic renal failure, including nondialysis-dependent patients (with or without erythropoietin therapy) and dialysis-dependent patients receiving erythropoietin therapy

Unlabeled/Investigational Use Cancer-/chemotherapy-associated anemia

Mechanism of Action/Effect Iron sucrose is dissociated by the reticuloendothelial system into iron and sucrose. The released iron increases serum iron concentrations and is incorporated into hemoglobin.

Contraindications Hypersensitivity to iron sucrose or any component of the formulation; evidence of iron overload; anemia not caused by iron deficiency

Warnings/Precautions Hypersensitivity reactions, including rare postmarketing anaphylactic and anaphylactoid reactions, have been reported. Hypotension has been reported frequently in hemodialysis-dependent patients. Hypotension has also been reported in peritoneal dialysis and nondialysis patients. Hypotension may be related to total dose or rate of administration (avoid rapid I.V. injection), follow recommended guidelines. Withhold iron in the presence of tissue iron overload; periodic monitoring of hemoglobin, hematocrit, serum ferritin, and transferrin saturation is recommended.

Drug Interactions

Avoid Concomitant Use

Avoid concomitant use of Iron Sucrose with any of the following: Dimercaprol

Decreased Effect There are no known significant interactions involving a decrease in effect.

Increased Effect/Toxicity

The levels/effects of Iron Sucrose may be increased by: Dimercaprol

Adverse Reactions

>10%:

Cardiovascular: Hypotension (1% to 7%; 39% in hemodialysis patients; may be related to total dose or rate of administration), peripheral edema (2% to 17%)

Central nervous system: Headache (3% to 13%)

Gastrointestinal: Diarrhea (1% to 17%), nausea (1% to 15%), vomiting (3% to 12%)

Neuromuscular & skeletal: Muscle cramps (1% to 3%; 29% in hemodialysis patients)

1% to 10%:

Cardiovascular: Hypertension (6% to 8%), edema (1% to 7%), chest pain (1% to 6%), murmur (<1% to 3%), heart failure (2%), myocardial infarction (1%)

Central nervous system: Dizziness (1% to 10%), fatigue (2% to 5%), fever (1% to 3%), stroke (1%)
Dermatologic: Pruritus (1% to 7%), rash (≤1%)
Endocrine & metabolic: Gout (2% to 7%), hypoglycemia (<1% to 4%), hyperglycemia (3% to 4%), fluid overload (1% to 3%)
Gastrointestinal: Taste perversion (1% to 9%), peritoneal infection (≤8%), constipation (1% to 7%), abdominal pain (1% to 4%), positive fecal occult blood (1% to 3%)
Genitourinary: Urinary tract infection (≤1%)
Local: Injection site reaction (2% to 6%), catheter site infection (≤4%)
Neuromuscular & skeletal: Arthralgia (1% to 8%), back pain (1% to 8%), muscle pain (1% to 7%), extremity pain (3% to 6%), weakness (1% to 3%)
Ocular: Conjunctivitis (<1% to 3%)
Otic: Ear pain (1% to 7%)
Respiratory: Dyspnea (1% to 10%), pharyngitis (<1% to 7%), cough (1% to 7%), sinusitis (1% to 4%), nasopharyngitis (≤3%), upper respiratory infection (1% to 3%), nasal congestion (1%), pneumonia (1%), pulmonary edema (1%), rhinitis (≤1%)
Miscellaneous: Graft complication (1% to 10%), sepsis (2%)

Pharmacodynamics/Kinetics

Half-Life Elimination Healthy adults: 6 hours

Metabolism Dissociated into iron and sucrose by the reticuloendothelial system

Excretion Healthy adults: Urine (5%) within 24 hours

Available Dosage Forms

Injection, solution [preservative free]:
Venofer®: Elemental iron 20 mg/mL (5 mL, 10 mL)

Dosing

Adult Doses expressed in mg of **elemental** iron. **Note:** Test dose: Product labeling does not indicate need for a test dose in product-naive patients.

Iron-deficiency anemia in chronic renal disease: I.V.:

Hemodialysis-dependent patient: 100 mg over 2-5 minutes administered 1-3 times/week during dialysis; administer no more than 3 times/week to a cumulative total dose of 1000 mg (10 doses); may continue to administer at lowest dose necessary to maintain target hemoglobin, hematocrit, and iron storage parameters

Peritoneal dialysis-dependent patient: Two infusions of 300 mg each over 1.5 hours 14 days apart, followed by a single 400 mg infusion over 2.5 hours 14 days later (total cumulative dose of 1000 mg in 3 divided doses)

Nondialysis-dependent patient: 200 mg slow injection (over 2-5 minutes) on 5 different occasions within a 14-day period. Total cumulative dose: 1000 mg in 14-day period. **Note:** Dosage has also been administered as two infusions of 500 mg in a maximum of 250 mL normal saline infused over 3.5-4 hours on day 1 and day 14 (limited experience)

Cancer-/chemotherapy-associated anemia (unlabeled use): I.V. infusion: 200 mg over 1 hour; maximum 300-400 mg/infusion. Repeat dose every 2-3 weeks. Test doses (25 mg slow I.V. push) are recommended in patients with iron dextran hypersensitivity or those with other drug allergies (NCCN guidelines, v.2.2010)

Geriatric Insufficient data to identify differences between elderly and other adults; use caution.

Pediatric Doses expressed in mg of **elemental** iron. **Note:** Test dose: Product labeling does not indicate need for a test dose in product-naive patients.

Iron-deficiency anemia in chronic renal disease (hemodialysis-dependent patients): Children ≥2 years (unlabeled use): I.V.:

Correction: 1 mg/kg/dose per dialysis session (maximum: 100 mg)

Maintenance therapy: 0.3 mg/kg/dose per dialysis session (maximum: 100 mg). **Note:** Dosing based on limited data from a study (Leijn, 2004); study used only 14 patients (2-14 years of age) with ESRD on hemodialysis. Study initially used an iron repletion dose of 3 mg/kg/dose per dialysis session which resulted in possible iron overload (ferritin >400 mcg/L); protocol dose subsequently lowered to 1 mg/kg/dose per dialysis session which resulted in a gradual increase in ferritin levels >100 mcg/L; maintenance therapy resulted in median ferritin levels between 193-250 mcg/L.

Administration

I.V. Not for rapid I.V. injection; inject slowly over 2-5 minutes. Can be administered through dialysis line. Do not mix with other medications or parenteral nutrient solutions.

Slow I.V. injection: May administer undiluted by slow I.V. injection (100 mg over 2-5 minutes in hemodialysis-dependent patients **or** 200 mg over 2-5 minutes in nondialysis-dependent patients)

Infusion: Dilute 100 mg in maximum of 100 mL normal saline; infuse over at least 15 minutes; 300 mg/250 mL should be infused over at least 1.5 hours; 400 mg/250 mL should be infused over at least 2.5 hours; 500 mg/250 mL should be infused over at least 3.5 hours

Stability

Reconstitution May be administered via the dialysis line as an undiluted solution or by diluting 100 mg (5 mL) in a maximum of 100 mL normal saline. Doses ≥200 mg should be diluted in a maximum of 250 mL normal saline.

Storage Store vials at controlled room temperature of 25°C (77°F); do not freeze. Iron sucrose is stable for 7 days at room temperature or under refrigeration when undiluted in a plastic syringe or following dilution in normal saline in a plastic syringe (2-10 mg/mL) or I.V. bag (1-2 mg/mL) (data on file [American Regent, Inc, 2010]).

Monitoring and Teaching Issues

Laboratory Monitoring Hematocrit, hemoglobin, serum ferritin, transferrin, percent transferrin saturation, TIBC; takes about 4 weeks of treatment to see increased serum iron and ferritin, and decreased TIBC. Serum iron concentrations should be drawn 48 hours after last dose.

Physical Assessment Facilities for cardiopulmonary resuscitation must be available during administration. Monitor blood pressure closely during infusion. Teach patient dangers of iron overdosing.

Patient Education You will be watched closely during infusion. You will need frequent blood tests while on this therapy. You may experience hypotension, black stools, nausea, vomiting, or constipation. Report immediately severe unresolved nausea, headache, dizziness, leg cramps, chest pain or palpations, or swelling of extremities.

Geriatric Considerations Anemia in the elderly is most often caused by "anemia of chronic disease," a result of aging effect in bone marrow, or associated with inflammation rather than blood loss. Iron stores are usually normal or increased, with a serum ferritin >50 ng/mL and a decreased total iron binding capacity. Hence, the anemia is not secondary to iron deficiency but the inability of the reticuloendothelial system to use available iron stores. I.V. administration of iron is often preferred over I.M. in the elderly secondary to a decreased muscle mass and the need for daily injections.

Breast-Feeding Considerations Iron is normally found in breast milk. Breast milk or iron fortified formulas generally provide enough iron to meet the recommended dietary requirements of infants. The amount of iron in breast milk is generally not influenced by maternal iron status.

Pregnancy Considerations Teratogenic effects were not observed in animal studies. There are no adequate and well-controlled studies in pregnant women. Based on limited data, iron sucrose may be effective for the treatment of iron-deficiency anemia in pregnancy. It is recommended that pregnant women meet the dietary requirements of iron with diet and/or supplements in order to prevent adverse events associated with iron deficiency anemia in pregnancy. Treatment of iron deficiency anemia in pregnant women is the same as in nonpregnant women and in most cases, oral iron preparations may be used. Except in severe cases of maternal anemia, the fetus achieves normal iron stores regardless of maternal concentrations.

◆ **Iron Sulfate** *see* Ferrous Sulfate *on page* 754
◆ **ISD** *see* Isosorbide Dinitrate *on page* 1028
◆ **ISDN** *see* Isosorbide Dinitrate *on page* 1028
◆ **Isentress®** *see* Raltegravir *on page* 1549
◆ **ISG** *see* Immune Globulin *on page* 961
◆ **ISMN** *see* Isosorbide Mononitrate *on page* 1029
◆ **Ismo®** *see* Isosorbide Mononitrate *on page* 1029
◆ **Isobamate** *see* Carisoprodol *on page* 300
◆ **IsonaRif™** *see* Rifampin and Isoniazid *on page* 1580

Isoniazid (eye soe NYE a zid)

Index Terms INH; Isonicotinic Acid Hydrazide

Generic Availability (U.S.) Yes

Pharmacologic Category Antitubercular Agent

Medication Safety Issues

International issues:

Hydra [Japan] may be confused with Hydrea brand name for hydroxyurea [U.S., Canada, and multiple international markets]

Pregnancy Risk Factor C

Lactation Enters breast milk/compatible

Use Treatment of susceptible tuberculosis infections; treatment of latent tuberculosis infection (LTBI)

Mechanism of Action/Effect Unknown, but may include the inhibition of mycolic acid synthesis resulting in disruption of the bacterial cell wall

Contraindications Hypersensitivity to isoniazid or any component of the formulation; acute liver disease; previous history of hepatic damage during isoniazid therapy; previous severe adverse reaction (drug fever, chills, arthritis) to isoniazid

Warnings/Precautions Use with caution in patients with severe renal impairment and liver disease. **[U.S. Boxed Warning]: Severe and sometimes fatal hepatitis may occur; usually occurs within the first 3 months of treatment, although may develop even after many months of treatment.** The risk of developing hepatitis is age-related, although isoniazid-induced hepatotoxicity has been reported in children; daily ethanol consumption may also increase the risk. Patients must report any prodromal symptoms of hepatitis, such as fatigue, weakness, malaise, anorexia, nausea, abdominal pain, jaundice, or vomiting. Patients should be instructed to immediately discontinue therapy if any of these symptoms occur, even if a clinical evaluation has yet to be conducted. Treatment with isoniazid for latent tuberculosis infection should be deferred in patients with acute hepatic diseases. Periodic ophthalmic examinations are recommended even when usual symptoms do not occur. Pyridoxine (10-50 mg/day) is recommended in individuals at risk for development of peripheral neuropathies (eg, HIV infection, nutritional deficiency, diabetes, pregnancy). Children with low milk and low meat intake should receive concomitant pyridoxine therapy. Multidrug regimens should be utilized for the treatment of active tuberculosis to prevent the emergence of drug resistance.

Drug Interactions

Metabolism/Transport Effects Substrate of CYP2E1 (major); **Inhibits** CYP1A2 (weak), 2A6 (moderate), 2C9 (weak), 2C19 (strong), 2D6 (moderate), 2E1 (moderate), 3A4 (strong); **Induces** CYP2E1 (after discontinuation) (weak)

Avoid Concomitant Use

Avoid concomitant use of Isoniazid with any of the following: Alfuzosin; Clopidogrel; Conivaptan; Dronedarone; Eplerenone; Everolimus; Halofantrine; Lurasidone; Nilotinib; Nisoldipine; Ranolazine; Rivaroxaban; RomiDEPsin; Salmeterol; Silodosin; Tamsulosin; Thioridazine; Tolvaptan; Toremifene

Decreased Effect

Isoniazid may decrease the levels/effects of: Clopidogrel; Codeine; Prasugrel; TraMADol

The levels/effects of Isoniazid may be decreased by: Antacids; Corticosteroids (Systemic)

Increased Effect/Toxicity

Isoniazid may increase the levels/effects of: Acetaminophen; Alfuzosin; Almotriptan; Alosetron; Benzodiazepines (metabolized by oxidation); Bortezomib; Brinzolamide; CarBAMazepine; Chlorzoxazone; Ciclesonide; Colchicine; Conivaptan; Corticosteroids (Orally Inhaled); CycloSERINE; CYP2A6 Substrates; CYP2C19 Substrates; CYP2D6 Substrates; CYP2E1 Substrates; CYP3A4 Substrates; Dienogest; Dronedarone; Dutasteride; Eplerenone; Everolimus; FentaNYL; Fesoterodine; GuanFACINE; Halofantrine; Ixabepilone; Lumefantrine; Lurasidone; Maraviroc; MethylPREDNISolone; Nebivolol; Nilotinib; Nisoldipine; Paricalcitol; Pazopanib; Phenytoin; Pimecrolimus; Ranolazine; Rivaroxaban; RomiDEPsin; Salmeterol; Saxagliptin; Silodosin; SORAfenib; Tadalafil; Tamoxifen; Tamsulosin; Theophylline Derivatives; Thioridazine; Tolvaptan; Toremifene; Vilazodone

The levels/effects of Isoniazid may be increased by: Rifamycin Derivatives

Nutritional/Ethanol Interactions

Ethanol: Avoid ethanol (increases the risk of hepatitis).

Food: Isoniazid should not be taken with food; serum levels may be decreased if taken with food. Has some ability to inhibit tyramine metabolism; several case reports of mild reactions (flushing, palpitations) after ingestion of cheese (with or without wine). Reactions resembling allergic symptoms following ingestion of fish high in histamine content have been reported. Isoniazid decreases folic acid absorption. Isoniazid alters pyridoxine metabolism.

Lab Interactions False-positive urinary glucose with Clinitest®

Adverse Reactions Frequency not defined.

Cardiovascular: Hypertension, palpitation, tachycardia, vasculitis

Central nervous system: Depression, dizziness, encephalopathy, fever, lethargy, memory impairment, psychosis, seizure, slurred speech, toxic encephalopathy

Dermatologic: Flushing, rash (morbilliform, maculopapular, pruritic, or exfoliative)

Endocrine & metabolic: Gynecomastia, hyperglycemia, metabolic acidosis, pellagra, pyridoxine deficiency

Gastrointestinal: Anorexia, epigastric distress, nausea, stomach pain, vomiting

Hematologic: Agranulocytosis, anemia (sideroblastic, hemolytic, or aplastic), eosinophilia, thrombocytopenia

Hepatic: LFTs mildly increased (10% to 20%), hyperbilirubinemia, bilirubinuria, jaundice, hepatic dysfunction, hepatitis (may involve progressive liver damage; risk increases with age; 2.3% in patients >50 years)

Neuromuscular & skeletal: Arthralgia, hyper-reflexia, paresthesia, peripheral neuropathy (dose-related incidence, 10% to 20% incidence with 10 mg/kg/day), weakness

Ocular: Blurred vision, loss of vision, optic neuritis and atrophy

Miscellaneous: Lupus-like syndrome, lymphadenopathy, rheumatic syndrome

Pharmacodynamics/Kinetics

Absorption Rapid and complete; rate can be slowed with food

Time to Peak Serum: 1-2 hours

Protein Binding 10% to 15%

Half-Life Elimination Fast acetylators: 30-100 minutes; Slow acetylators: 2-5 hours; may be prolonged with hepatic or severe renal impairment

Metabolism Hepatic with decay rate determined genetically by acetylation phenotype

Excretion Urine (75% to 95%); feces; saliva

Available Dosage Forms

Injection, solution: 100 mg/mL (10 mL)

Solution, oral: 50 mg/5 mL (473 mL)

Tablet, oral: 100 mg, 300 mg

Dosing

Adult & Geriatric Recommendations often change due to resistant strains and newly-developed information; consult *MMWR* for current CDC recommendations. Intramuscular injection is available for patients who are unable to either take or absorb oral therapy.

Nontuberculous mycobacterium *(M. kansasii)* (unlabeled use): Oral, I.M.: 5 mg/kg/day (maximum: 300 mg/day) for duration to include 12 months of culture-negative sputum; typically used in combination with ethambutol and rifampin

Treatment of latent tuberculosis infection (LTBI): Oral, I.M.: CDC recommendations: 5 mg/kg (maximum: 300 mg/dose) once daily or 15 mg/kg (maximum: 900 mg/dose) twice weekly by directly observed therapy (DOT) for 6-9 months in patients who do not have HIV infection (9 months is optimal, 6 months may be considered to reduce costs of therapy) and 9 months in patients who have HIV infection. Extend to 12 months of therapy if interruptions in treatment occur. (*MMWR*, 2000)

Treatment of active TB infection (drug susceptible): Oral, I.M.:

Daily therapy: CDC recommendations: 5 mg/kg/day once daily (usual dose: 300 mg/day) (*MMWR*, 2003)

Directly observed therapy (DOT): CDC recommendations: 15 mg/kg (maximum: 900 mg/dose) twice weekly or 3 times/week; **Note:** CDC guidelines state that once-weekly therapy (15 mg/kg/dose) may be considered, but only after the first 2 months of initial therapy in HIV-negative patients, and only in combination with rifapentine. (*MMWR*, 2003)

Note: Treatment may be defined by the number of doses administered (eg, "six-month" therapy involves 182 doses of INH and rifampin, and 56 doses of pyrazinamide). Six months is the shortest interval of time over which these doses may be administered, assuming no interruption of therapy.

Note: Concomitant administration of 10-50 mg/day pyridoxine is recommended in malnourished patients or those prone to neuropathy (eg, alcoholics, patients with diabetes)

Pediatric Recommendations often change due to resistant strains and newly-developed information; consult *MMWR* for current CDC recommendations. Intramuscular injection is available for patients who are unable to either take or absorb oral therapy.

Treatment of latent TB infection (LTBI): Infants and Children: Oral, I.M.:

Daily therapy: CDC recommendations: 10-20 mg/kg/day once daily (maximum: 300 mg/dose) (*MMWR*, 2000); Manufacturer's labeling: 10 mg/kg/day once daily (maximum: 300 mg/dose)

Directly observed therapy (DOT): CDC recommendations: 20-40 mg/kg (maximum: 900 mg/dose) twice weekly for 9 months (*MMWR*, 2000); Manufacturer's labeling: 20-30 mg/kg twice weekly (maximum: 900 mg/dose)

Treatment of active TB infection: Infants and Children: Oral, I.M.:

Daily therapy: CDC recommendations: 10-15 mg/kg/day once daily (maximum: 300 mg/day) (*MMWR*, 2003)

Directly observed therapy (DOT): CDC recommendations: 20-30 mg/kg (maximum: 900 mg/dose) twice weekly (*MMWR*, 2003); Manufacturer's labeling: 20-40 mg/kg (maximum: 900 mg/dose) twice weekly or 3 times/week

Renal Impairment No adjustment necessary

Hemodialysis: Dialyzable (50% to 100%); administer dose postdialysis

Hepatic Impairment No adjustment required, however, use with caution, may accumulate and additional liver damage may occur in patients with pre-existing liver disease. For ALT or AST >3 times the ULN: discontinue or temporarily withhold treatment. Treatment with isoniazid for latent tuberculosis infection should be deferred in patients with acute hepatic diseases.

Administration

Oral Should be administered 1 hour before or 2 hours after meals on an empty stomach.

Stability

Storage

Tablet: Store at 20°C to 25°C (68°F to 77°F). Protect from light.

Oral solution: Store at 15°C to 30°C (59°F to 86°F). Protect from light.

Monitoring and Teaching Issues

Laboratory Monitoring Baseline and periodic (more frequently in patients with higher risk for hepatitis) liver function tests (ALT and AST); sputum cultures monthly (until 2 consecutive negative cultures reported)

LTBI therapy: American Thoracic Society/Centers for Disease Control (ATS/CDC) recommendations: Baseline serum AST or ALT and bilirubin should be considered for patients at higher risk for adverse events (eg, history of liver disease, chronic ethanol use, HIV-infected patients, women who are pregnant or postpartum ≤3 months, older adults with concomitant medications or diseases).

Physical Assessment Use caution with pre-existing renal impairment or hepatic disease. Monitor for liver damage, nausea, vomiting, peripheral neuropathy, and CNS changes at regular intervals during therapy. Teach patient importance of proper diet and ophthalmic examinations.

Patient Education Best if taken on an empty stomach, 1 hour before or 2 hours after meals. Avoid excessive alcohol and tyramine-containing foods. Increase dietary intake of folate, niacin, and magnesium. You will need to have frequent ophthalmic exams and periodic medical check-ups to evaluate drug effects. If you experience nausea, vomiting, loss of appetite, weakness, fatigue, abdominal pain, dark-colored urine or change in color of stool, or yellowing of eyes/skin, discontinue and contact prescriber as soon as possible. Report chest pain, rapid heart beat, or palpitations; tingling, numbness, or loss of sensation in hands or feet; CNS changes (depression, dizziness, memory impairment, slurred speech, seizure); unusual weakness or fatigue; persistent gastrointestinal upset; change in vision; or skin rash.

Dietary Considerations Should be taken 1 hour before or 2 hours after meals on an empty stomach; increase dietary intake of folate, niacin, magnesium. Avoid tyramine-containing foods; some examples include aged or matured cheese, air-dried or cured meats (including sausages and salamis), fava or broad bean pods, tap/draft beers, Marmite concentrate, sauerkraut, soy sauce and other soybean condiments. Avoid histamine-containing foods.

Geriatric Considerations Age has not been shown to affect the pharmacokinetics of INH since acetylation phenotype determines clearance and half-life, acetylation rate does not change significantly with age. Most strains of *M. tuberculosis* found the elderly should be susceptible to INH since most acquired their initial infection prior to INH's introduction.

Breast-Feeding Considerations Small amounts of isoniazid are excreted in breast milk. However, women with tuberculosis should not be discouraged from breast-feeding. Pyridoxine supplementation is recommended for the mother and infant.

Pregnancy Considerations Isoniazid was found to be embryocidal in animal studies; teratogenic effects were not noted. Isoniazid crosses the human placenta. Due to the risk of tuberculosis to the fetus, treatment is recommended when the probability of maternal disease is moderate to high. The CDC recommends isoniazid as part of the initial treatment regimen (CDC, 2003). Pyridoxine supplementation is recommended (25 mg/day).

Additional Information The AAP recommends that pyridoxine supplementation (1-2 mg/kg/day) should be administered to malnourished patients, children or adolescents on meat or milk-deficient diets, breast-feeding infants, and those predisposed to neuritis to prevent peripheral neuropathy; administration of isoniazid syrup has been associated with diarrhea

◆ **Isoniazid and Rifampin** *see* Rifampin and Isoniazid *on page 1580*

◆ **Isonicotinic Acid Hydrazide** *see* Isoniazid *on page 1024*

◆ **Isonipecaine Hydrochloride** *see* Meperidine *on page 1172*

◆ **Isophane Insulin** *see* Insulin NPH *on page 992*

◆ **Isophane Insulin and Regular Insulin** *see* Insulin NPH and Insulin Regular *on page 993*

◆ **Isophosphamide** *see* Ifosfamide *on page 947*

Isoproterenol (eye soe proe TER e nole)

U.S. Brand Names Isuprel®

Index Terms Isoproterenol Hydrochloride

Generic Availability (U.S.) No

Pharmacologic Category $Beta_1$- & $Beta_2$-Adrenergic Agonist Agent

Medication Safety Issues

Sound-alike/look-alike issues:

Isuprel® may be confused with Disophrol®, Ismelin®, Isordil®

Pregnancy Risk Factor C

Lactation Excretion in breast milk unknown

Use Manufacturer's labeled indications (see **"Note"**): Mild or transient episodes of heart block that do not require electric shock or pacemaker therapy; serious episodes of heart block and Adams-Stokes attacks (except when caused by ventricular tachycardia or fibrillation); cardiac arrest until electric shock or pacemaker therapy is available; bronchospasm during anesthesia; adjunct to fluid and electrolyte replacement therapy and other drugs and procedures in the treatment of hypovolemic or septic shock and low cardiac output states (eg, decompensated heart failure, cardiogenic shock)

Note: The use of isoproterenol in advanced cardiac life support (ACLS) has largely been supplanted by the use of other adrenergic agents (eg, epinephrine and dopamine). The use of isoproterenol for bronchospasm during anesthesia and cardiogenic, hypovolemic, or septic shock is no longer recommended. See *Unlabeled/Investigational Use* for more appropriate, yet unlabeled, uses.

Unlabeled/Investigational Use Pharmacologic overdrive pacing for refractory torsade de pointes; pharmacologic provocation during tilt table testing for syncope; temporary control of bradycardia in denervated heart transplant patients unresponsive to atropine; ventricular arrhythmias due to AV nodal block; beta-blocker overdose

Available Dosage Forms

Injection, solution:

Isuprel®: 0.2 mg/mL (1 mL, 5 mL)

Dosing

Adult & Geriatric

Bradyarrhythmias, AV nodal block, or refractory torsade de pointes: Continuous I.V. infusion: 2-10 mcg/minute; titrate to patient response

Tilt table testing for syncope (Benditt, 1996; Brignole, 2004): Continuous I.V infusion: Initial: 1 mcg/minute; increase as necessary based on response to a maximum dose of 5 mcg/minute. **Note:** Timing of initiation and dose adjustment during test may be institution specific.

Pediatric Bradyarrhythmias, AV nodal block, or refractory torsade de pointes: Continuous I.V. infusion: 0.05-2 mcg/kg/minute; titrate to patient response

Administration

I.V. I.V. infusion administration requires the use of an infusion pump.

Monitoring and Teaching Issues

Laboratory Monitoring Arterial blood gas, serum magnesium, serum potassium, serum glucose (in selected patients)

Physical Assessment Assess cardiac, respiratory, and hemodynamic status when used in acute or emergency situations.

Patient Education You may experience nervousness, dizziness, fatigue, dry mouth, nausea, or vomiting. Report chest pain, rapid heartbeat or palpitations, unresolved/persistent GI upset, dizziness, fatigue, trembling, increased anxiety, sleeplessness, or respiratory difficulty.

◆ **Isoproterenol Hydrochloride** *see* Isoproterenol *on page 1027*

◆ **Isoptin® SR** *see* Verapamil *on page 1858*

◆ **Isopto® Atropine** *see* Atropine *on page 172*

◆ **Isordil® Titradose™** *see* Isosorbide Dinitrate *on page 1028*

Isosorbide Dinitrate (eye soe SOR bide dye NYE trate)

U.S. Brand Names Dilatrate®-SR; Isordil® Titradose™

Index Terms ISD; ISDN

Generic Availability (U.S.) Yes: Excludes capsule

Pharmacologic Category Vasodilator

Medication Safety Issues

Sound-alike/look-alike issues:

Isordil® may be confused with Inderal®, Isuprel®, Plendil®

Pregnancy Risk Factor C

Lactation Excretion in breast milk unknown

Use Prevention and treatment of angina pectoris

Note: Due to slower onset of action, not the drug of choice to abort an acute anginal episode.

Unlabeled/Investigational Use Patients with heart failure (HF) who do not tolerate an ACE inhibitor or an angiotensin receptor blocker (ARB); African-American (self-identified) patients with HF remaining symptomatic despite optimal standard therapy; esophageal spastic disorders

Mechanism of Action/Effect Relaxes vascular smooth muscles, decreases arterial resistance and venous return which reduces cardiac oxygen demand. Additionally, coronary artery dilation improves collateral flow to ischemic regions.

Contraindications Hypersensitivity to isosorbide dinitrate or any component of the formulation; hypersensitivity to organic nitrates; concurrent use with phosphodiesterase-5 (PDE-5) inhibitors (sildenafil, tadalafil, or vardenafil)

Warnings/Precautions Severe hypotension can occur; paradoxical bradycardia and increased angina pectoris can accompany hypotension. Postural hypotension can also occur; ethanol may potentiate this effect. Use with caution in volume depletion and moderate hypotension, and use with extreme caution with inferior wall MI and suspected right ventricular infarctions. Nitrates may reduce preload, exacerbating obstruction and cause hypotension or syncope and/or worsening of heart failure (Gibbons, 2003). Avoid use in patients with hypertrophic cardiomyopathy (HCM).

Use of isosorbide dinitrate sublingual tablets to treat acute angina attacks is recommended only in patients unresponsive to sublingual nitroglycerin; however, current clinical practice guidelines do not recommend use during an acute anginal episode. Avoid use of extended release formulations in acute MI or acute HF; cannot easily reverse effects if adverse events develop. Nitrates may precipitate or aggravate increased intracranial pressure and subsequently may worsen clinical outcomes in patients with neurologic injury (eg, intracranial hemorrhage, traumatic brain injury). Appropriate dosing intervals are needed to minimize tolerance development. Tolerance can only be overcome by short periods of nitrate absence from the body. Dose escalation does not overcome this effect. When used for HF in combination with hydralazine, tolerance is less of a concern (Gogia, 1995).

Avoid concurrent use with PDE-5 inhibitors (eg, sildenafil, tadalafil, vardenafil). When nitrate administration becomes medically necessary, may administer nitrates only if 24 hours have elapsed after use of sildenafil or vardenafil (48 hours after tadalafil use) (Trujillo, 2007).

Drug Interactions

Metabolism/Transport Effects Substrate of CYP3A4 (major)

Avoid Concomitant Use

Avoid concomitant use of Isosorbide Dinitrate with any of the following: Phosphodiesterase 5 Inhibitors

Decreased Effect

The levels/effects of Isosorbide Dinitrate may be decreased by: CYP3A4 Inducers (Strong); Deferasirox; Herbs (CYP3A4 Inducers)

Increased Effect/Toxicity

Isosorbide Dinitrate may increase the levels/effects of: Hypotensive Agents; Rosiglitazone

The levels/effects of Isosorbide Dinitrate may be increased by: Conivaptan; CYP3A4 Inhibitors (Moderate); CYP3A4 Inhibitors (Strong); Dasatinib; Phosphodiesterase 5 Inhibitors

Nutritional/Ethanol Interactions

Ethanol: Caution with ethanol (may increase risk of hypotension).

Herb/Nutraceutical: Avoid black cohosh, California poppy, coleus, golden seal, hawthorn, mistletoe, periwinkle, quinine, shepherd's purse (may cause hypotension).

Adverse Reactions Frequency not defined.

Cardiovascular: Crescendo angina (uncommon), hypotension, postural hypotension, rebound hypertension (uncommon), syncope (uncommon)

Central nervous system: Headache (most common), lightheadedness (related to blood pressure changes)

Hematologic: Methemoglobinemia (rare, overdose)

Pharmacodynamics/Kinetics

Onset of Action Sublingual tablet: ~3 minutes; Oral tablet and capsule (includes extended-release formulations): ~1 hour

Duration of Action Sublingual tablet: 1-2 hours; Oral tablet and capsule (includes extended-release formulations): Up to 8 hours

Bioavailability Sublingual tablet: 40% to 50%; Oral immediate release formulations: Highly variable (10% to 90%); increases with chronic therapy

Half-Life Elimination Parent drug: ~1 hour; Metabolites (5-mononitrate: 5 hours; 2-mononitrate: 2 hours)

Metabolism Extensively hepatic to conjugated metabolites, including isosorbide 5-mononitrate (active) and 2-mononitrate (active)

Excretion Urine and feces

Available Dosage Forms

Capsule, sustained release, oral:
Dilatrate®-SR: 40 mg

Tablet, oral: 5 mg, 10 mg, 20 mg, 30 mg
Isordil® Titradose™: 5 mg, 40 mg

Tablet, sublingual: 2.5 mg, 5 mg

Tablet, extended release, oral: 40 mg

Dosing

Adult

Angina:

Oral:

Immediate release: Initial: 5-20 mg 2-3 times/day; Maintenance: 10-40 mg 2-3 times/day **or** 5-80 mg 2-3 times/day (Anderson, 2007; Gibbons, 2002)

Sustained release: 40-160 mg/day has been used in clinical trials (a nitrate free interval of at least 18 hours is recommended; however, a clinically efficacious dosage interval has not been clearly established) **or** 40 mg 1-2 times/day (Anderson, 2007; Gibbons, 2002)

Sublingual:

Prophylactic use: 2.5-5 mg administered 15 minutes prior to activities which may provoke an anginal episode

Treatment of acute anginal episode (use only if patient has failed sublingual nitroglycerin): 2.5-5 mg every 5-10 minutes for maximum of 3 doses in 15-30 minutes

Heart failure (unlabeled use; Cohn, 1991; HFSA, 2010; Hunt, 2009): *Oral:*

Immediate release (**Note:** Use in combination with hydralazine):

Initial dose: 20 mg 3-4 times per day

Target dose: 160 mg/day in 4 divided doses

Esophageal spastic disorders (unlabeled use; Goyal, 1998): *Oral, sublingual:* Immediate release: 10-30 mg before meals

Geriatric Elderly patients should be given lowest recommended adult daily doses initially and titrate upward.

Renal Impairment

Hemodialysis: Supplemental dose is not necessary

Peritoneal dialysis: Supplemental dose is not necessary

Administration

Oral May consider administration of first dose in physician office; observe for maximal cardiovascular dynamic effects and adverse effects (orthostatic hypotension, headache). Do not administer around the clock; allow nitrate-free interval ≥14 hours (immediate release products) and >18 hours (sustained release products). Do not crush sublingual tablets or extended release formulations.

Immediate release products: When prescribed twice daily, consider administering at 8 AM and 1 PM). For 3 times/day dosing, consider 8 AM, 1 PM, and 6 PM)

Sustained release products: Consider once daily in morning or twice-daily dosing at 8 AM and between 1-2 PM.

Monitoring and Teaching Issues

Physical Assessment Assess patient closely for volume depletion, hypotension, and right ventricular infarction. Tolerance to nitrates develops and appropriate dosing intervals are needed to minimize tolerance. Teach patient importance of maintaining dosing schedule.

Patient Education Take at the same time each day, with last dose in early evening. Do not chew or swallow sublingual tablets; allow them to dissolve under your tongue. Do not crush or chew sustained release or extended release products; swallow whole with water. Avoid excessive alcohol; combination may cause severe hypotension. May cause headache, dizziness, and flushed feeling. If chest pain occurs, seek emergency medical help at once. Report severe headache, dizziness, loss of consciousness, or any rash.

Geriatric Considerations The first dose of nitrates (sublingual, chewable, oral) should be taken in a physician's office to observe for maximal cardiovascular dynamic effects and adverse effects (eg, orthostatic blood pressure drop, headache). The use of nitrates for angina may occasionally promote reflux esophagitis. This may require dose adjustments or changing therapeutic agents to correct this adverse effect.

Pregnancy Considerations

Increased fetal mortality has been observed in animal studies using isosorbide dinitrate at doses much higher than those used in humans. There are no adequate and well-controlled studies in pregnant women.

Related Information

Heart Failure (Systolic) *on page 2040*

Isosorbide Mononitrate (eye soe SOR bide mon oh NYE trate)

U.S. Brand Names Imdur®; Ismo®; Monoket®

Index Terms ISMN

Generic Availability (U.S.) Yes

Pharmacologic Category Vasodilator

Medication Safety Issues

Sound-alike/look-alike issues:

Imdur® may be confused with Imuran®, Inderal LA®, K-Dur®

Monoket® may be confused with Monopril®

Pregnancy Risk Factor B/C (manufacturer dependent)

Lactation Excretion in breast milk unknown/use caution

Use Prevention of angina pectoris

Available Dosage Forms

Tablet, oral: 10 mg, 20 mg

Ismo®: 20 mg

Monoket®: 10 mg, 20 mg

Tablet, extended release, oral: 30 mg, 60 mg, 120 mg

Imdur®: 30 mg, 60 mg, 120 mg

Dosing

Adult

Angina: Oral:

Regular release tablet: Initial: 5-20 mg twice daily with the 2 doses given 7 hours apart (eg, 8 AM and 3 PM) to decrease tolerance development; patients initiating therapy with 5 mg twice daily (eg, small stature) should be titrated up to 10 mg twice daily in first 2-3 days.

Extended release tablet: Initial: 30-60 mg given once daily in the morning; titrate upward as needed, giving at least 3 days between increases; maximum daily single dose: 240 mg

Note: Tolerance to nitrate effects develops with chronic exposure. Dose escalation does not overcome this effect. Tolerance can only be overcome by short periods of nitrate absence from the body. Short periods of nitrate withdrawal may help minimize tolerance. Recommended twice daily dosage regimens incorporate this interval. Administer sustained release tablet once daily in the morning.

Geriatric Start with lowest recommended adult dose.

Renal Impairment Dose adjustment not necessary.

Hemodialysis: Dose supplementation is not necessary.

Peritoneal dialysis: Dose supplementation is not necessary.

Hepatic Impairment Dose adjustment not necessary.

Administration

Oral Do not administer around-the-clock. Immediate release tablet should be scheduled twice daily with doses 7 hours apart (8 AM and 3 PM); extended release tablet may be administered once daily in the morning upon rising with a half-glassful of fluid and should not be chewed or crushed.

Monitoring and Teaching Issues

Physical Assessment Assess patient closely for previous hypersensitivity. Use caution in presence of volume depletion, hypotension, right ventricular infarction, and hypertrophic cardiomyopathy. Tolerance to nitrates will develop and proper timing of doses is needed to minimize tolerance. Monitor for hypotension and GI disturbance when beginning therapy, adjusting dosage, and at regular intervals during therapy. Teach patient importance of maintaining dosing schedule.

Patient Education Take at same time(s) each day. Do not crush or chew extended release tablets; swallow whole with water. Avoid excess alcohol intake; combination may cause severe hypotension. May cause dizziness, headache, and flushed feeling. Report severe headache, persistent dizziness, loss of consciousness, or any rash. If chest pain occurs, seek emergency medical help at once.

Isotretinoin (eye soe TRET i noyn)

U.S. Brand Names Amnesteem®; Claravis™; Sotret®

Index Terms 13-*cis*-Retinoic Acid

Generic Availability (U.S.) No

Pharmacologic Category Acne Products; Retinoic Acid Derivative

Medication Safety Issues

Sound-alike/look-alike issues:

Accutane® may be confused with Accolate®, Accupril®

Claravis™ may be confused with Cleviprex™

ISOtretinoin may be confused with tretinoin

Medication Guide Available Yes

Prescribing and Access Restrictions As a requirement of the REMS program, access to this medication is restricted. All patients (male and female), prescribers, wholesalers, and dispensing pharmacists must register and be active in the iPLEDGE™ risk management program, designed to eliminate fetal exposures to isotretinoin. This program covers all isotretinoin products (brand and generic). The iPLEDGE™ program requires that all patients meet qualification criteria and monthly program requirements (eg, pregnancy testing). Healthcare providers can only prescribe a maximum 30-day supply at each monthly visit and must counsel patients on the iPLEDGE™ program requirements and confirm counseling via the iPLEDGE™ automated system. Registration, activation, and additional information are provided at www.-ipledgeprogram.com or by calling 866-495-0654.

Pregnancy Risk Factor X

Lactation Excretion in breast milk unknown/contraindicated

Use Treatment of severe recalcitrant nodular acne unresponsive to conventional therapy

Unlabeled/Investigational Use Investigational: Treatment of children with metastatic neuroblastoma or leukemia that does not respond to conventional therapy

Mechanism of Action/Effect Reduces sebaceous gland size and reduces sebum production; regulates cell proliferation and differentiation

Contraindications Hypersensitivity to isotretinoin or any component of the formulation; sensitivity to parabens, vitamin A, or other retinoids; pregnancy

Warnings/Precautions This medication should only be prescribed by prescribers competent in treating severe recalcitrant nodular acne and experienced with the use of systemic retinoids. **[U.S. Boxed Warning]: Because of the high likelihood of teratogenic effects, all patients (male and female), prescribers, wholesalers, and dispensing pharmacists must register and be active in the iPLEDGE™ risk management program; do not prescribe isotretinoin for women who are or who are likely to become pregnant while using the drug (see Additional Information for details).** Women of childbearing potential must be capable of complying with effective contraceptive measures. Patients must select and commit to two forms of contraception. Therapy is begun after two negative pregnancy tests; effective contraception must be used for at least 1 month before beginning therapy, during therapy, and for 1 month after discontinuation of therapy. Prescriptions should be written for no more than a 30-day supply, and pregnancy testing and counseling should be repeated monthly.

May cause depression, psychosis, aggressive or violent behavior, and changes in mood; use with extreme caution in patients with psychiatric disorders. Rarely, suicidal thoughts and actions have been reported during isotretinoin usage. All patients should be observed closely for symptoms of depression or suicidal thoughts. Discontinuation of treatment alone may not be sufficient, further evaluation may be necessary. Cases of pseudotumor cerebri (benign intracranial hypertension) have been reported, some with concomitant use of tetracycline (avoid using together). Patients with papilledema, headache, nausea, vomiting, and visual disturbances should be referred to a neurologist and treatment with isotretinoin discontinued. Hearing impairment, which can continue after therapy is discontinued, may occur. Clinical hepatitis, elevated liver enzymes, inflammatory bowel disease, skeletal hyperostosis, premature epiphyseal closure, vision impairment, corneal opacities, and decreased night vision have also been reported with the use of isotretinoin. Rare postmarketing cases of severe skin reactions (eg, Stevens-Johnson syndrome, erythema multiforme) have been reported with use.

Use with caution in patients with diabetes mellitus; impaired glucose control has been reported. Use caution in patients with hypertriglyceridemia; acute pancreatitis and fatal hemorrhagic pancreatitis (rare) have been reported. Bone mineral density may decrease; use caution in patients with a genetic predisposition to bone disorders (ie osteoporosis, osteomalacia) and with disease states or concomitant medications that can induce bone disorders. Patients may be at risk when participating in activities with repetitive impact (such as sports). Patients should be instructed not to donate blood during therapy and for 1 month following discontinuation of therapy due to risk of donated blood being given to a pregnant female. Safety of long-term use is not established and is not recommended. Safety and efficacy have not been established in children <12 years of age.

Drug Interactions

Avoid Concomitant Use

Avoid concomitant use of ISOtretinoin with any of the following: Tetracycline Derivatives; Vitamin A

Decreased Effect

ISOtretinoin may decrease the levels/effects of: Contraceptives (Estrogens); Contraceptives (Progestins)

Increased Effect/Toxicity

ISOtretinoin may increase the levels/effects of: Vitamin A

The levels/effects of ISOtretinoin may be increased by: Alcohol (Ethyl); Tetracycline Derivatives

Nutritional/Ethanol Interactions

Ethanol: Avoid or limit ethanol (may increase triglyceride levels if taken in excess).

Food: Isotretinoin bioavailability increased if taken with food or milk.

Herb/Nutraceutical: Avoid dong quai, St John's wort (may also cause photosensitization and may decrease the effectiveness of oral contraceptives). Additional vitamin A supplements may lead to vitamin A toxicity (dry skin, irritation, arthralgias, myalgias, abdominal pain, hepatic changes); avoid use.

Adverse Reactions Frequency not always defined.

Cardiovascular: Chest pain, edema, flushing, palpitation, stroke, syncope, tachycardia, vascular thrombotic disease

Central nervous system: Aggressive behavior, depression, dizziness, drowsiness, emotional instability, fatigue, headache, insomnia, lethargy, malaise, nervousness, paresthesia, pseudotumor cerebri, psychosis, seizure, stroke, suicidal ideation, suicide attempts, suicide, violent behavior

Dermatologic: Abnormal wound healing acne fulminans, alopecia, bruising, cheilitis, cutaneous allergic reactions, dry nose, dry skin, eczema, eruptive xanthomas, facial erythema, fragility of skin, hair abnormalities, hirsutism, hyperpigmentation, hypopigmentation, increased sunburn susceptibility, nail dystrophy, paronychia, peeling of palms, peeling of soles, photoallergic reactions, photosensitizing reactions, pruritus, purpura, rash

Endocrine & metabolic: Triglycerides increased (25%), abnormal menses, blood glucose increased, cholesterol increased, HDL decreased, hyperuricemia

Gastrointestinal: Bleeding and inflammation of the gums, colitis, esophagitis, esophageal ulceration, inflammatory bowel disease, nausea, nonspecific gastrointestinal symptoms, pancreatitis, weight loss, xerostomia

Genitourinary: Nonspecific urogenital findings

Hematologic: Agranulocytosis (rare), anemia, neutropenia, pyogenic granuloma, thrombocytopenia

Hepatic: Alkaline phosphatase increased, ALT increased, AST increased, GGTP increased, hepatitis, LDH increased

Neuromuscular & skeletal: Back pain (29% in pediatric patients), arthralgia, arthritis, bone abnormalities, bone mineral density decreased, calcification of tendons and ligaments, CPK increased, myalgia, premature epiphyseal closure, skeletal hyperostosis, tendonitis, weakness

Ocular: Cataracts, color vision disorder, conjunctivitis, corneal opacities, dry eyes, eyelid inflammation, keratitis, night vision decreased, optic neuritis, photophobia, visual disturbances

Otic: Hearing impairment, tinnitus

Renal: Glomerulonephritis, hematuria, proteinuria, pyuria, vasculitis

Respiratory: Bronchospasms, epistaxis, respiratory infection, voice alteration, Wegener's granulomatosis

Miscellaneous: Allergic reactions, anaphylactic reactions, disseminated herpes simplex, diaphoresis, infection, lymphadenopathy

Pharmacodynamics/Kinetics

Time to Peak Serum: 3-5 hours

Protein Binding 99% to 100%; primarily albumin

Half-Life Elimination Terminal: Parent drug: 21 hours; Metabolite: 21-24 hours

Metabolism Hepatic via CYP2B6, 2C8, 2C9, 2D6, 3A4; forms metabolites; major metabolite: 4-oxo-isotretinoin (active)

Excretion Urine and feces (equal amounts)

Available Dosage Forms

Capsule, oral:

Claravis™: 10 mg, 20 mg, 30 mg, 40 mg

Capsule, softgel, oral:

Amnesteem®: 10 mg, 20 mg, 40 mg

Sotret®: 10 mg, 20 mg, 30 mg, 40 mg

Dosing

Adult & Geriatric Severe recalcitrant nodular acne: Oral: 0.5-1 mg/kg/day in 2 divided doses (dosages as low as 0.05 mg/kg/day have been reported to be beneficial) for 15-20 weeks or until the total cyst count decreases by 70%, whichever is sooner. Adults with very severe disease/scarring or primarily involves the trunk may require dosage adjustment up to 2 mg/kg/day. A second course of therapy may be initiated after a period of ≥2 months off therapy.

Pediatric

Neuroblastoma (investigational): Oral: Children: Maintenance therapy for neuroblastoma: 100-250 mg/m^2/day in 2 divided doses

Acne (severe recalcitrant nodular): Oral: Children 12-17 years: 0.5-1 mg/kg/day in 2 divided doses (dosages as low as 0.05 mg/kg/day have been reported to be beneficial) for 15-20 weeks or until the total cyst count decreases by 70%, whichever is sooner. A second course of therapy may be initiated after a period of ≥2 months off therapy.

Hepatic Impairment Empiric dose reductions are recommended in patient with hepatitis.

Administration

Oral Administer with food. Capsules should be swallowed whole with a full glass of water. For patients unable to swallow, the Accutane® capsule may be pierced with a large-gauge needle and the contents placed in food (cottage cheese, ice cream, pudding, or oatmeal with butter) for immediate consumption (Accutane® data on file, Roche Pharmaceuticals). Use appropriate precautions for handling teratogenic capsule contents.

Stability

Storage Store at room temperature of 59°F to 86°F (15°C to 30°C). Protect from light.

Monitoring and Teaching Issues

Laboratory Monitoring CBC with differential and platelet count, baseline sedimentation rate, serum triglycerides, liver enzymes

Must have two negative pregnancy tests prior to beginning therapy (for all female patients of childbearing potential): Two negative tests with a sensitivity of at least 25 mIU/mL prior to beginning therapy (the second performed at least 19 days after the first test and performed during the first 5 days of the menstrual period immediately preceding the start of therapy); monthly tests to rule out pregnancy prior to refilling prescription.

Physical Assessment Monitor patients with diabetes closely; monitor skin for unusual reactions. Observe for depression or suicide ideation.

Patient Education A patient information/consent form must be signed before this medication is prescribed. Do not sign (and do not take this medication) if you do not understand all of the information on the form. Prescriptions will be written for a 1-month supply and must be filled within 7 days; they will not be honored if filled after that time or if they do not have the appropriate yellow qualification sticker attached. Capsule can be chewed and swallowed, swallowed, or opened with a large needle and contents sprinkled on applesauce or ice cream. Whole capsules should be swallowed with a full glass of liquid. Do not take any other vitamin A products, limit vitamin A intake, and increase exercise during therapy. Limit or avoid alcohol intake. Exacerbations of acne may occur during first weeks of therapy. You may experience headache; loss of night vision; muscle aches; lethargy; visual disturbances; photosensitivity; dry mouth; nausea; dryness, redness, or itching of skin; eye irritation; or increased sensitivity to contact lenses. Report depression, suicide ideation, or severe skin reactions. Discontinue therapy and report acute vision changes, ringing in the ears or changes in hearing, rectal bleeding, abdominal cramping, or unresolved diarrhea.

Dietary Considerations Should be taken with food. Limit intake of vitamin A; avoid use of other vitamin A products. Some formulations may contain soybean oil.

Pregnancy Considerations Major fetal abnormalities (both internal and external), spontaneous abortion, premature births and low IQ scores in surviving infants have been reported. **[U.S. Boxed Warning]: Because of the high likelihood of teratogenic effects, all patients (male and female), prescribers, wholesalers, and dispensing pharmacists must register and be active in the iPLEDGE™ risk management program; do not prescribe isotretinoin for women who are or who are likely to become pregnant while using the drug.** This medication is contraindicated in females of childbearing potential unless they are able to comply with the guidelines of the iPLEDGE™ pregnancy prevention program. Females of childbearing potential should not become pregnant during therapy or for 1 month following discontinuation of isotretinoin. Upon discontinuation of treatment, females of childbearing potential should have a pregnancy test after their last dose and again one month after their last dose. Two forms of contraception should be continued during this time. Any pregnancies should be reported to the iPLEDGE™ program (www.ipledgeprogram.com or 866-495-0654).

Additional Information All patients (male and female), must be registered in the iPLEDGE™ risk management program. Females of childbearing potential must receive oral and written information reviewing the hazards of therapy and the effects that isotretinoin can have on a fetus. Therapy should not begin without two negative pregnancy tests at least 19 days apart. Two forms of contraception (a primary and secondary form as described in the iPLEDGE™ program materials) must be used simultaneously beginning 1 month prior to treatment, during treatment, and for 1 month after therapy is discontinued; limitations to their use must be explained. Prescriptions should be written for no more than a 30-day supply, and pregnancy testing and counseling should be repeated monthly. During therapy, pregnancy tests must be conducted by a CLIA-certified laboratory. Prescriptions must be filled and picked up from the pharmacy within 7 days of specimen collection for pregnancy test for women of childbearing potential. Prescriptions for males and females of non-childbearing potential must be filled and picked up within 30 days of prescribing.

Any cases of accidental pregnancy should be reported to the iPLEDGE™ program or FDA MedWatch. All patients (male and female) must read and sign the informed consent material provided in the pregnancy prevention program.

Isradipine (iz RA di peen)

U.S. Brand Names DynaCirc CR®

Generic Availability (U.S.) Yes: Capsule

Pharmacologic Category Calcium Channel Blocker; Calcium Channel Blocker, Dihydropyridine

Medication Safety Issues

Sound-alike/look-alike issues:

DynaCirc® may be confused with Dynabac®, Dynacin®

Pregnancy Risk Factor C

Lactation Excretion in breast milk unknown/not recommended

Use Treatment of hypertension

Unlabeled/Investigational Use Pediatric hypertension

Available Dosage Forms

Capsule, oral: 2.5 mg, 5 mg

Tablet, controlled release, oral:

DynaCirc CR®: 5 mg, 10 mg

Dosing

Adult Hypertension: Oral:

Capsule: 2.5 mg twice daily; antihypertensive response occurs in 2-3 hours; maximal response in 2-4 weeks; increase dose at 2- to 4-week intervals at 2.5-5 mg increments; usual dose range (JNC 7): 2.5-10 mg/day in 2 divided doses. **Note:** Most patients show no improvement with doses >10 mg/day except adverse reaction rate increases; therefore, maximal dose in older adults should be 10 mg/day.

Controlled release tablet: 5 mg once daily; antihypertensive response occurs in 2 hours. Adjust dose in increments of 5 mg at 2-4 week intervals. Maximum dose: 20 mg/day; adverse events are increased at doses >10 mg/day.

Geriatric

Capsule: Refer to adult dosing.

Controlled release tablet: Initial dose: 5 mg once daily

Pediatric Hypertension (unlabeled use): Capsule: Oral: Initial: 0.15-0.2 mg/kg/day in 2-3 divided doses; maximum 0.8 mg/kg/day, up to 20 mg/day. **Note:** Controlled release formulation is administered once daily or in 2 divided doses.

Renal Impairment

Cl_{cr} 30-80 mL/minute: Bioavailability increased by 45%

Cl_{cr} <10 mL/minute on hemodialysis: Bioavailability decreased by 20% to 50%

Capsule: Refer to adult dosing.

Controlled release tablet: Initial dose: 5 mg once daily

Hepatic Impairment

Peak serum concentrations are increased by 32% and bioavailability is increased by 52%.

Capsule: Refer to adult dosing.

Controlled release tablet: Initial dose: 5 mg once daily

Administration

Oral May be administered without regard to meals. Controlled release tablets should be swallowed whole; do not divide or chew

Monitoring and Teaching Issues

Physical Assessment Monitor for tachycardia, hypotension, edema, and dyspnea at regular intervals during therapy. When discontinuing, taper dose slowly.

Patient Education Take with or without food. Do not crush extended release tablets. Follow prescriber's instructions for diet and lifestyle changes. You may experience headache, constipation, dizziness, or ankle swelling. Report unrelieved headache, severe constipation, chest pain, palpitations, swelling of feet or weight gain, or chest pain or pressure.

Related Information

Calcium Channel Blockers *on page 1993*

◆ **Istalol®** *see* Timolol (Ophthalmic) *on page 1763*

◆ **Isuprel®** *see* Isoproterenol *on page 1027*

Itraconazole (i tra KOE na zole)

U.S. Brand Names Sporanox®

Generic Availability (U.S.) Yes: Capsule

Pharmacologic Category Antifungal Agent, Oral

Medication Safety Issues

Sound-alike/look-alike issues:

Itraconazole may be confused with fluconazole

Sporanox® may be confused with Suprax®, Topamax®

Pregnancy Risk Factor C

Lactation Enters breast milk/not recommended

Use

Oral capsules: Treatment of susceptible fungal infections in immunocompromised and immunocompetent patients including blastomycosis and histoplasmosis; indicated for aspergillosis (in patients intolerant/refractory to amphotericin B), and onychomycosis of the toenail and fingernail (in nonimmunocompromised patients)

Oral solution: Treatment of oral and esophageal candidiasis

Mechanism of Action/Effect Interferes with cytochrome P450 activity, decreasing ergosterol synthesis (principal sterol in fungal cell membrane) and inhibiting cell membrane formation

Contraindications Hypersensitivity to itraconazole (use caution in patients with a history of hypersensitivity to other azoles), any component of the formulation; concurrent administration with cisapride, dofetilide, ergot derivatives, levomethadyl, lovastatin, midazolam (oral), nisoldipine, pimozide, quinidine, simvastatin, or triazolam; treatment of onychomycosis (or other non-life-threatening indications) in patients with evidence of ventricular dysfunction, heart failure (HF) or a history of HF; treatment of onychomycosis in patients who are pregnant or intend on becoming pregnant

Warnings/Precautions [U.S. Boxed Warning]: Negative inotropic effects have been observed following intravenous administration. Discontinue or reassess use if signs or symptoms of HF (heart failure) occur during treatment. [U.S. Boxed Warning]: Not recommended for treatment of onychomycosis in patients with ventricular dysfunction or a history of HF. HF has been reported, particularly in patients receiving a total daily oral dose of 400 mg. Use with caution in patients with risk factors for HF (COPD, renal failure, edematous disorders, ischemic or valvular disease). Discontinue if signs or symptoms of HF or neuropathy occur during treatment. **[U.S. Boxed Warning]: Serious cardiovascular adverse events including, QT prolongation, ventricular tachycardia, torsade de pointes, cardiac arrest and/or sudden death have been observed due to increased cisapride, pimozide, quinidine or levomethadyl concentrations induced by itraconazole; concurrent use contraindicated.** Additionally, the following drugs metabolized by the CYP 3A4 isoenzyme system are also contraindicated: Ergot derivatives, lovastatin, midazolam (oral), simvastatin, and triazolam.

Calcium channel blockers (CCBs) may cause additive negative inotropic effects when used concurrently with itraconazole. Itraconazole may also inhibit the metabolism of CCBs. Use caution with concurrent use of itraconazole and CCBs due to an increased risk of HF. Concurrent use of itraconazole and nisoldipine is contraindicated.

Use with caution in patients with renal impairment. Rare cases of serious hepatotoxicity (including liver failure and death) have been reported (including some cases occurring within the first week of therapy); hepatotoxicity was reported in some patients without pre-existing liver disease or risk factors. Use with caution in patients with pre-existing hepatic impairment; monitor liver function closely and dosage adjustment may be warranted. Not recommended for use in patients with active liver disease, elevated liver enzymes, or prior hepatotoxic reactions to other drugs unless the expected benefit exceeds the risk of hepatotoxicity. Transient or permanent hearing loss has been reported. Quinidine (a contraindicated drug) was used concurrently in several of these cases. Hearing loss usually resolves after discontinuation, but may persist in some patients.

Large differences in itraconazole pharmacokinetic parameters have been observed in cystic fibrosis patients receiving the solution; if a patient with cystic fibrosis does not respond to therapy, alternate therapies should be considered. Due to differences in bioavailability, oral capsules and oral solution cannot be used interchangeably. Only the oral solution has proven efficacy for oral and esophageal candidiasis. Initiation of treatment with oral solution is not recommended in patients at immediate risk for systemic candidiasis (eg, patients with severe neutropenia).

Drug Interactions

Metabolism/Transport Effects **Substrate** of CYP3A4 (major); **Inhibits** CYP3A4 (strong), P-glycoprotein

Avoid Concomitant Use

Avoid concomitant use of Itraconazole with any of the following: Alfuzosin; Cisapride; Conivaptan; Dofetilide; Dronedarone; Eplerenone; Ergot Derivatives; Everolimus; Halofantrine; Lurasidone; Nilotinib; Nisoldipine; Pimozide; QuiNIDine; Ranolazine; Rivaroxaban; RomiDEPsin; Salmeterol; Silodosin; Tamsulosin; Tolvaptan; Topotecan; Toremifene

Decreased Effect

Itraconazole may decrease the levels/effects of: Amphotericin B; Prasugrel; Saccharomyces boulardii

The levels/effects of Itraconazole may be decreased by: Antacids; CYP3A4 Inducers (Strong); Deferasirox; Didanosine; Efavirenz; Etravirine; H2-Antagonists; Herbs (CYP3A4 Inducers); Phenytoin; Proton Pump Inhibitors; Rifamycin Derivatives; Sucralfate

Increased Effect/Toxicity

Itraconazole may increase the levels/effects of: Alfentanil; Alfuzosin; Aliskiren; Almotriptan; Alosetron; Aprepitant; Benzodiazepines (metabolized by oxidation); Bortezomib; Bosentan; Brinzolamide; BusPIRone; Busulfan; Calcium Channel Blockers; CarBAMazepine; Cardiac Glycosides; Ciclesonide; Cilostazol; Cisapride; Colchicine; Conivaptan; Corticosteroids (Orally Inhaled); Corticosteroids (Systemic); CycloSPORINE; CycloSPORINE (Systemic); CYP3A4 Substrates; Dabigatran Etexilate; Dienogest; DOCEtaxel; Dofetilide; Dronedarone; Dutasteride; Eletriptan; Eplerenone; Ergot Derivatives; Erlotinib; Eszopiclone; Etravirine; Everolimus; FentaNYL; Fesoterodine; Fexofenadine; Fosaprepitant; Gefitinib; GuanFACINE; Halofantrine; HMG-CoA Reductase Inhibitors; Imatinib; Irinotecan; Ixabepilone; Losartan; Lumefantrine; Lurasidone; Macrolide Antibiotics; Maraviroc; Methadone; MethylPREDNISolone; Nilotinib; Nisoldipine; Paliperidone; Paricalcitol; Pazopanib; P-Glycoprotein Substrates; Phenytoin; Phosphodiesterase 5 Inhibitors; Pimecrolimus; Pimozide; Protease Inhibitors; QuiNIDine; Ramelteon; Ranolazine; Repaglinide; Rifamycin Derivatives; Rivaroxaban; RomiDEPsin; Salmeterol; Saxagliptin; Silodosin; Sirolimus; Solifenacin; SORAfenib; SUNItinib; Tacrolimus; Tacrolimus (Systemic); Tacrolimus (Topical); Tadalafil; Tamsulosin; Temsirolimus; Tolterodine; Tolvaptan; Topotecan; Toremifene; Vilazodone; VinBLAStine; VinCRIStine; Vinorelbine; Vitamin K Antagonists; Ziprasidone; Zolpidem

The levels/effects of Itraconazole may be increased by: Etravirine; Grapefruit Juice; Macrolide Antibiotics; Protease Inhibitors

Nutritional/Ethanol Interactions

Food:

Capsules: Absorption enhanced by food and possibly by gastric acidity. Cola drinks have been shown to increase the absorption of the capsules in patients with achlorhydria or those taking H_2-receptor antagonists or other gastric acid suppressors. Avoid grapefruit juice.

Solution: Food decreases the bioavailability and increases the time to peak concentration.

Herb/Nutraceutical: St John's wort may decrease itraconazole levels.

Adverse Reactions

>10%: Gastrointestinal: Nausea (11%), diarrhea (3% to 11%)

1% to 10%:

Cardiovascular: Edema (4%), hypertension (3%), chest pain (3%)

Central nervous system: Fever (3% to 7%), headache (4%), fatigue (2% to 3%), dizziness (2%), depression (2%)

Dermatologic: Rash (4% to 9%), pruritus (3%)

Endocrine & metabolic: Hypokalemia (2%)

Gastrointestinal: Vomiting (5% to 7%), abdominal pain (2% to 6%), constipation (2%)

Hepatic: LFTs abnormal (3%)

Respiratory: Rhinitis (5% to 9%), cough (4%), dyspnea (2%), pneumonia (2%), sinusitis (2%), sputum increased (2%)

Miscellaneous: Diaphoresis increased (3%)

Pharmacodynamics/Kinetics

Absorption Requires gastric acidity; capsule better absorbed with food, solution better absorbed on empty stomach

Bioavailability Variable, ~55% (oral solution) in 1 small study; **Note:** Oral solution has a higher degree of bioavailability (149% ± 68%) relative to oral capsules; should not be interchanged

Time to Peak Plasma: Capsules: 3-5 hours; Oral solution: 2-3 hours

Protein Binding Plasma: 99.8%; metabolite hydroxy-itraconazole: 99.5%

Half-Life Elimination Oral: Single dose: ~21 hours, steady state: 64 hours; Cirrhosis (single dose): 37 hours (range 20-54 hours)

Metabolism Extensively hepatic via CYP3A4 into >30 metabolites including hydroxy-itraconazole (major metabolite); appears to have *in vitro* antifungal activity. Main metabolic pathway is oxidation; may undergo saturation metabolism with multiple dosing.

Excretion Urine (<0.03% active drug, 40% as inactive metabolites); feces (~3% to 18%)

Available Dosage Forms

Capsule, oral: 100 mg

Sporanox®: 100 mg

Solution, oral:

Sporanox®: 10 mg/mL (150 mL)

Dosing

Adult & Geriatric

Aspergillosis, invasive (salvage therapy): Duration of therapy should be a minimum of 6-12 weeks or throughout period of immunosuppression: Oral: 200-400 mg/day; **Note:** 2008 IDSA guidelines recommend 600 mg/day for 3 days, followed by 400 mg/day.

Appropriate use: Itraconazole should **NOT** be used for voriconazole-refractory aspergillosis since the same antifungal and/or resistance mechanism(s) may be shared by both agents. Itraconazole oral solution and capsule formulations are not bioequivalent or interchangeable. Due to variable bioavailability of oral preparations, therapeutic drug monitoring advisable.

Aspergillosis, allergic (ABPA, sinusitis): Oral: 200 mg/day; may be used in conjunction with corticosteroids

Blastomycosis: Oral: 200 mg 3 times/day for 3 days, then 200 mg twice daily for 6-12 months; in moderately-severe to severe infection, therapy should be initiated with ~2 weeks of amphotericin B (Chapman, 2008)

Brain abscess: Cerebral phaeohyphomycosis (dematiaceous): Oral: 200 mg twice daily for at least 6 months with amphotericin

Candidiasis: Oral:

Oropharyngeal: Oral solution: 200 mg once daily for 1-2 weeks; in patients unresponsive or refractory to fluconazole: 100 mg twice daily (clinical response expected in 1-2 weeks)

Esophageal: Oral solution: 100-200 mg once daily for a minimum of 3 weeks; continue dosing for 2 weeks after resolution of symptoms

Coccidioidomycosis: Oral: 200 mg twice daily

Histoplasmosis: Oral: 200 mg 3 times/day for 3 days, then 200 mg twice daily (or once daily in mild-moderate disease) for 6-12 weeks in mild-moderate disease or ≥12 months in progressive disseminated or chronic cavitary pulmonary histoplasmosis; in moderately-severe to severe infection, therapy should be initiated with ~2 weeks of a lipid formation of amphotericin B (Wheat, 2007)

Long-term suppression therapy: 200 mg/day (AIDS*info* guidelines, 2008)

Meningitis: Oral:

Coccidioides: 400-800 mg/day

Coccidioides, HIV-positive (unlabeled use): 200 mg 3 times/day for 3 days, then 200 mg twice daily; maintenance: 200 mg twice daily life-long (AIDS*info* guidelines, 2008)

Appropriate use: Fluconazole is preferred for meningeal infections.

Onychomycosis: Oral: 200 mg once daily for 12 consecutive weeks; alternative "pulse-dosing" may be considering for fingernail involvement only: 200 mg twice daily for 1 week; repeat 1-week course after 3-week off-time

Penicilliosis, HIV-positive (unlabeled use): Oral: 200 mg twice daily for 8-10 weeks (in severely-ill patients, initiate therapy with 2 weeks of amphotericin B); maintenance: 200 mg/day (AIDS*info* guidelines, 2008)

Pneumonia: Oral:

Coccidioides: Mild-to-moderate: 200 mg twice daily

Coccidioides, HIV-positive (focal pneumonia): 200 mg 3 times/day for 3 days, then 200 mg twice daily (AIDS*info* guidelines, 2008)

Protothecal infection: Oral: 200 mg once daily for 2 months

Sporotrichosis: Oral:

Lymphocutaneous: 100-200 mg/day for 3-6 months

Osteoarticular and pulmonary: 200 mg twice daily for 1-2 years (may use amphotericin B initially for stabilization)

Pediatric

Infants and Children (HIV-exposed/-positive; unlabeled use; CDC, 2009):

Candidiasis:

Oropharyngeal: Oral solution: 2.5 mg/kg/dose twice daily (maximum: 200 mg/day [400 mg/day if fluconazole-refractory]) for 7-14 days

Esophageal: Oral solution: 5 mg/kg/day once daily or divided twice daily for 4-21 days

Coccidioidomycosis:

Treatment: Oral: 5-10 mg/kg/dose twice daily for 3 days, followed by 2-5 mg/kg/dose orally twice daily (maximum: 400 mg/day)

Relapse prevention: Oral: 2-5 mg/kg/dose twice daily (maximum: 400 mg/day)

Cryptococcus: *Relapse prevention:* Oral solution: 5 mg/kg/dose once daily (maximum: 200 mg/day)

Histoplasmosis:

Treatment of mild disseminated disease: Oral solution: 2-5 mg/kg/dose 3 times daily for 3 days (9 doses), followed by twice daily for 12 months (maximum: 200 mg/dose)

Consolidation treatment for moderate-severe to severe disseminated disease, including CNS infection (following appropriate induction therapy): 2-5 mg/kg/dose 3 times daily for 3 days, followed by 2-5 mg/kg/dose (maximum: 200 mg/dose) twice daily for 12 months for non-CNS-disseminated disease or for ≥12 months for CNS infection

Relapse prevention: Oral solution: 5 mg/kg/dose twice daily (maximum: 400 mg/day)

Renal Impairment The FDA-approved labeling states to use with caution in patients with renal impairment. The following guidelines have been used by some clinicians:

Aronoff, 2007:

Cl_{cr} >10 mL/minute: No adjustment recommended.

Cl_{cr} <10 mL/minute: Administer 50% of normal dose.

Continuous renal replacement therapy (CRRT)/hemodialysis: 200 mg every 12 hours for 4 doses, then 200 mg every 24 hours (Heintz, 2009).

Hemodialysis: Not dialyzable.

Hepatic Impairment Use caution in patients with hepatic impairment.

Administration

Oral Doses >200 mg/day are given in 2 divided doses; do not administer with antacids. Capsule and oral solution formulations are not bioequivalent and thus are not interchangeable. Capsule absorption is best if taken with food, therefore, it is best to administer itraconazole after meals; solution should be taken on an empty stomach. When treating oropharyngeal and esophageal candidiasis, solution should be swished vigorously in mouth, then swallowed.

Stability

Storage

Capsule: Store at room temperature, 15°C to 25°C (59°F to 77°F). Protect from light and moisture.

Oral solution: Store at ≤25°C (77°F); do not freeze.

Monitoring and Teaching Issues

Laboratory Monitoring Liver function in patients with pre-existing hepatic dysfunction, and in all patients being treated for longer than 1 month; serum concentrations particularly for oral therapy (due to erratic bioavailability with capsule formulation); renal function

Physical Assessment Evaluate hepatic status and hypersensitivity history prior to treatment. Assess results of LFTs.

Patient Education Treatment for some fungal infections may take several weeks or months. Take capsule immediately after meals; take solution on empty stomach (1 hour before or 2 hours after meals). Frequent blood tests may be required with prolonged therapy. May cause dizziness, drowsiness, nausea, vomiting, or anorexia. Report any rash, any change in hearing acuity, difficulty breathing, or chest pain. Report any signs and symptoms of liver dysfunction (eg, unusual fatigue, anorexia, nausea and/or vomiting, jaundice [yellowing of skin or sclera], dark urine, pale stool) so that the appropriate laboratory testing can be done.

Dietary Considerations

Capsule: Take with food.

Solution: Take without food, if possible.

Geriatric Considerations No specific data for the elderly. Transient or permanent hearing loss reported in the elderly; several reports include concurrent administration of quinidine.

Pregnancy Considerations Should not be used to treat onychomycosis during pregnancy. Effective contraception should be used during treatment and for 2 months following treatment. Congenital abnormalities have been reported during postmarketing surveillance, but a causal relationship has not been established.

Additional Information Due to potential toxicity, the manufacturer recommends confirmation of diagnosis testing of nail specimens prior to treatment of onychomycosis.

- **IVIG** *see* Immune Globulin *on page 961*
- **IV Immune Globulin** *see* Immune Globulin *on page 961*
- **Ivy Soothe® [OTC] [DSC]** *see* Hydrocortisone (Topical) *on page 920*
- **Jalyn™** *see* Dutasteride and Tamsulosin *on page 600*
- **Jantoven®** *see* Warfarin *on page 1877*
- **Janumet®** *see* Sitagliptin and Metformin *on page 1654*
- **Januvia®** *see* SitaGLIPtin *on page 1652*
- **Jevtana®** *see* Cabazitaxel *on page 264*
- **Jinteli™** *see* Ethinyl Estradiol and Norethindrone *on page 701*
- **Jolessa™** *see* Ethinyl Estradiol and Levonorgestrel *on page 699*
- **Jolivette®** *see* Norethindrone *on page 1334*
- **Junel® 1.5/30** *see* Ethinyl Estradiol and Norethindrone *on page 701*
- **Junel® 1/20** *see* Ethinyl Estradiol and Norethindrone *on page 701*
- **Junel® Fe 1.5/30** *see* Ethinyl Estradiol and Norethindrone *on page 701*
- **Junel® Fe 1/20** *see* Ethinyl Estradiol and Norethindrone *on page 701*
- **Kadian®** *see* Morphine (Systemic) *on page 1258*
- **Kaletra®** *see* Lopinavir and Ritonavir *on page 1127*
- **Kalexate** *see* Sodium Polystyrene Sulfonate *on page 1660*
- **Kaon-CL® 10** *see* Potassium Chloride *on page 1480*
- **Kao Paverin® [OTC] [DSC]** *see* Loperamide *on page 1126*
- **Kaopectate® [OTC]** *see* Bismuth *on page 221*
- **Kaopectate® Extra Strength [OTC]** *see* Bismuth *on page 221*
- **Kao-Tin [OTC]** *see* Bismuth *on page 221*
- **Kapidex** *see* Dexlansoprazole *on page 504*
- **Kapidex™ [DSC]** *see* Dexlansoprazole *on page 504*
- **Kapvay™** *see* CloNIDine *on page 408*
- **Kariva®** *see* Ethinyl Estradiol and Desogestrel *on page 695*
- **Kayexalate®** *see* Sodium Polystyrene Sulfonate *on page 1660*
- **KCl** *see* Potassium Chloride *on page 1480*
- **Kdur** *see* Potassium Chloride *on page 1480*
- **Keflex®** *see* Cephalexin *on page 346*
- **Kelnor™** *see* Ethinyl Estradiol and Ethynodiol Diacetate *on page 698*

- ◆ **Kenalog®** *see* Triamcinolone (Topical) *on page* *1816*
- ◆ **Kenalog®-10** *see* Triamcinolone (Systemic) *on page* *1812*
- ◆ **Kenalog®-40** *see* Triamcinolone (Systemic) *on page* *1812*
- ◆ **Keoxifene Hydrochloride** *see* Raloxifene *on page* *1547*
- ◆ **Keppra®** *see* Levetiracetam *on page* *1087*
- ◆ **Keppra XR™** *see* Levetiracetam *on page* *1087*
- ◆ **Kerlone®** *see* Betaxolol (Systemic) *on page* *208*
- ◆ **Ketek®** *see* Telithromycin *on page* *1715*

Ketoconazole (Systemic) (kee toe KOE na zole)

Generic Availability (U.S.) Yes

Pharmacologic Category Antifungal Agent, Oral

Medication Safety Issues

Sound-alike/look-alike issues:

Nizoral® may be confused with Nasarel, Neoral®, Nitrol®

Pregnancy Risk Factor C

Lactation Enters breast milk/not recommended

Use Treatment of susceptible fungal infections, including candidiasis, oral thrush, blastomycosis, histoplasmosis, paracoccidioidomycosis, coccidioidomycosis, chromomycosis, candiduria, chronic mucocutaneous candidiasis, as well as certain recalcitrant cutaneous dermatophytoses

Unlabeled/Investigational Use Treatment of prostate cancer (androgen synthesis inhibitor)

Mechanism of Action/Effect Inhibits several fungal enzymes that results in a build-up of toxic concentrations of hydrogen peroxide resulting in cell death; inhibits androgen synthesis

Contraindications Hypersensitivity to ketoconazole or any component of the formulation; CNS fungal infections (due to poor CNS penetration); coadministration with ergot derivatives, cisapride, or triazolam is contraindicated due to risk of potentially fatal cardiac arrhythmias

Warnings/Precautions [U.S. Boxed Warning]: Ketoconazole has been associated with hepatotoxicity, including some fatalities; use with caution in patients with impaired hepatic function and perform periodic liver function tests. **[U.S. Boxed Warning]: Concomitant use with cisapride is contraindicated due to the occurrence of ventricular arrhythmias.** High doses of ketoconazole may depress adrenocortical function.

Drug Interactions

Metabolism/Transport Effects Substrate of CYP3A4 (major); **Inhibits** CYP1A2 (strong), CYP2A6 (moderate), CYP2B6 (weak), CYP2C8 (weak), CYP2C9 (strong), CYP2C19 (moderate), CYP2D6 (moderate), CYP3A4 (strong), P-glycoprotein

Avoid Concomitant Use

Avoid concomitant use of Ketoconazole (Systemic) with any of the following: Alfuzosin; Cisapride; Clopidogrel; Conivaptan; Dofetilide; Dronedarone; Eplerenone; Everolimus; Halofantrine; Lurasidone; Nilotinib; Nisoldipine; Pimozide; QuiNIDine; Ranolazine; Rivaroxaban; RomiDEPsin; Salmeterol; Silodosin; Tamsulosin; Thioridazine; Tolvaptan; Topotecan; Toremifene

Decreased Effect

Ketoconazole (Systemic) may decrease the levels/effects of: Amphotericin B; Clopidogrel; Codeine; Prasugrel; Saccharomyces boulardii; TraMADol

The levels/effects of Ketoconazole (Systemic) may be decreased by: Antacids; CYP3A4 Inducers (Strong); Deferasirox; Didanosine; Etravirine; H2-Antagonists; Herbs (CYP3A4 Inducers); Phenytoin; Proton Pump Inhibitors; Rifamycin Derivatives; Sucralfate

Increased Effect/Toxicity

Ketoconazole (Systemic) may increase the levels/effects of: Alfentanil; Alfuzosin; Aliskiren; Almotriptan; Alosetron; Aprepitant; Bendamustine; Benzodiazepines (metabolized by oxidation); Bortezomib; Bosentan; Brinzolamide; BusPIRone; Busulfan; Calcium Channel Blockers; CarBAMazepine; Carvedilol; Ciclesonide; Cilostazol; Cinacalcet; Cisapride; Colchicine; Conivaptan; Corticosteroids (Orally Inhaled); Corticosteroids (Systemic); CycloSPORINE; CycloSPORINE (Systemic); CYP1A2 Substrates; CYP2A6 Substrates; CYP2C19 Substrates; CYP2C9 Substrates (High risk); CYP2D6 Substrates; CYP3A4 Substrates; Dabigatran Etexilate; Dienogest; DOCEtaxel; Dofetilide; Dronedarone; Dutasteride; Eletriptan; Eplerenone; Erlotinib; Eszopiclone; Etravirine; Everolimus; FentaNYL; Fesoterodine; Fexofenadine; Fosaprepitant; Gefitinib; GuanFACINE; Halofantrine; HMG-CoA Reductase Inhibitors; Imatinib; Irinotecan; Ixabepilone; Losartan; Lumefantrine; Lurasidone; Macrolide Antibiotics; Maraviroc; Methadone; MethylPREDNISolone; Nebivolol; Nilotinib; Nisoldipine; Paricalcitol; Pazopanib; P-Glycoprotein Substrates; Phenytoin; Phosphodiesterase 5 Inhibitors; Pimecrolimus; Pimozide; Praziquantel; Protease Inhibitors; Proton Pump Inhibitors; QuiNIDine; Ramelteon; Ranolazine; Repaglinide; Rifamycin Derivatives; Rivaroxaban; RomiDEPsin; Salmeterol; Saxagliptin; Silodosin; Sirolimus; Solifenacin; SORAfenib; SUNItinib; Tacrolimus; Tacrolimus (Systemic); Tacrolimus (Topical); Tadalafil; Tamoxifen; Tamsulosin; Temsirolimus; Thioridazine; Tolterodine; Tolvaptan; Topotecan; Toremifene; Vilazodone; Vitamin K Antagonists; Ziprasidone; Zolpidem

The levels/effects of Ketoconazole (Systemic) may be increased by: Etravirine; Grapefruit Juice; Macrolide Antibiotics; Protease Inhibitors

Nutritional/Ethanol Interactions

Food: Ketoconazole peak serum levels may be prolonged if taken with food.

Herb/Nutraceutical: St John's wort may decrease ketoconazole levels.

Adverse Reactions 1% to 10%:

Dermatologic: Pruritus (2%)

Gastrointestinal: Nausea/vomiting (3% to 10%), abdominal pain (1%)

Pharmacodynamics/Kinetics

Absorption Rapid (~75%)

Bioavailability Decreases as gastric pH increases

Time to Peak Serum: 1-2 hours

Protein Binding 93% to 96%

Half-Life Elimination Biphasic: Initial: 2 hours; Terminal: 8 hours

Metabolism Partially hepatic via CYP3A4 to inactive compounds

Excretion Feces (57%); urine (13%)

Available Dosage Forms

Tablet, oral: 200 mg

Dosing

Adult & Geriatric

Fungal infections: Oral: 200-400 mg/day as a single daily dose

Prostate cancer (unlabeled use): Oral: 400 mg 3 times/day

Pediatric Fungal infections: Oral: Children ≥2 years: 3.3-6.6 mg/kg/day as a single dose for 1-2 weeks for candidiasis, for at least 4 weeks in recalcitrant dermatophyte infections, and for up to 6 months for other systemic mycoses

Renal Impairment Hemodialysis: Not dialyzable (0% to 5%)

Hepatic Impairment Dose reductions should be considered in patients with severe liver disease.

Administration

Oral Administer oral tablets 2 hours prior to antacids to prevent decreased absorption due to the high pH of gastric contents.

Stability

Storage Store at 15°C to 25°C (59°F to 77°F).

Monitoring and Teaching Issues

Laboratory Monitoring Liver function

Physical Assessment Evaluate hepatic function prior to beginning therapy. Assess liver function on a regular basis. Teach patient necessity of completing full therapy and importance of adequate hydration.

Patient Education Maintain adequate hydration unless instructed to restrict fluid intake. Cream, foam, gel, and shampoo are for external use only. Use full course of medication; some infections may require long periods of therapy. May cause nausea and vomiting. Report unresolved headache, rash or itching, yellowing of eyes or skin, changes in color of urine or stool, chest pain or palpitations, sense of fullness or ringing in ears, or if condition worsens.

Dietary Considerations May be taken with food or milk to decrease GI adverse effects.

Geriatric Considerations No specific recommendations.

Breast-Feeding Considerations In a case report, ketoconazole in concentrations of ≤0.22 mcg/mL were detected in the breast milk of a woman 1 month post-partum. She had been taking oral ketoconazole 200 mg/day for 5 days at the time of sampling. The maximum milk concentration occurred 3.25 hours after the dose and concentrations were undetectable 24 hours after the dose. Based on the highest milk concentration, the estimated dose to the nursing infant was 1.4% of the maternal dose. Breast-feeding is not recommended by the manufacturer.

Pregnancy Considerations Adverse effects were noted in animal reproduction studies.

Ketoconazole (Topical) (kee toe KOE na zole)

U.S. Brand Names Extina®; Nizoral®; Nizoral® A-D [OTC]; Xolegel®

Generic Availability (U.S.) Yes: Cream, shampoo

Pharmacologic Category Antifungal Agent, Topical

Medication Safety Issues

Sound-alike/look-alike issues:

Nizoral® may be confused with Nasarel, Neoral®, Nitrol®

Pregnancy Risk Factor C

Lactation Excretion in breast milk unknown/use caution

Use

Cream: Treatment of tinea corporis, tinea cruris, tinea versicolor, cutaneous candidiasis, seborrheic dermatitis

Foam, gel: Treatment of seborrheic dermatitis

Shampoo: Treatment of dandruff, seborrheic dermatitis, tinea versicolor

Available Dosage Forms

Aerosol, topical:

Extina®: 2% (50 g, 100 g)

Cream, topical: 2% (15 g, 30 g, 60 g)

Gel, topical:

Xolegel®: 2% (45 g)

Shampoo, topical: 2% (120 mL)

Nizoral®: 2% (120 mL)

Nizoral® A-D [OTC]: 1% (120 mL, 210 mL)

Dosing

Adult & Geriatric

Fungal infections: *Topical:*

Cream: Tinea infections: Rub gently into the affected area once daily. Duration of treatment: Tinea corporis, cruris: 2 weeks; tinea pedis: 6 weeks

Shampoo (ketoconazole 2%): Tinea versicolor: Apply to damp skin, lather, leave on 5 minutes, and rinse (one application should be sufficient)

Seborrheic dermatitis: *Topical:*

Cream: Rub gently into the affected area twice daily for 4 weeks or until clinical response is noted.

Foam: Apply to affected area twice daily for 4 weeks

Gel: Rub gently into the affected area once daily for 2 weeks.

Shampoo (ketoconazole 1%): Apply twice weekly for up to 8 weeks with at least 3 days between each shampoo

Pediatric Seborrheic dermatitis: *Topical (cream/foam/gel, shampoo):* Children ≥12 years: Refer to adult dosing.

Administration

Topical Cream, foam, gel, and shampoo are for external use only. Avoid exposure to flame or smoking immediately following application of gel or foam; do not apply directly to hands.

Monitoring and Teaching Issues

Physical Assessment Teach patient proper administration or application and necessity of completing full therapy.

Patient Education Cream, foam, gel, and shampoo are for external use only.

Cream, foam, and gel: Wash hands thoroughly before and after applying; keep away from eyes or mouth. Keep Extina foam can away from open fire, flame, or direct heat (Extina foam is flammable). You may experience some burning, dryness, irritation, or rash at site of application. Report severe or persistent adverse effects or if condition worsens.

Shampoo: May cause some temporary hair loss, scalp irritation, itching, or change in hair texture. Report severe or persistent adverse effects or if condition worsens.

◆ **3-Keto-desogestrel** *see* Etonogestrel *on page* 710

Ketoprofen (kee toe PROE fen)

Generic Availability (U.S.) Yes

Pharmacologic Category Nonsteroidal Anti-inflammatory Drug (NSAID), Oral

Medication Safety Issues

Sound-alike/look-alike issues:

Ketoprofen may be confused with ketotifen

Medication Guide Available Yes

Pregnancy Risk Factor C

Lactation Enters breast milk

Use Acute and long-term treatment of rheumatoid arthritis and osteoarthritis; primary dysmenorrhea; mild-to-moderate pain

Mechanism of Action/Effect Reversibly inhibits cyclooxygenase-1 and 2 (COX-1 and 2) enzymes, which results in decreased formation of prostaglandin precursors; has antipyretic, analgesic, and anti-inflammatory properties

Contraindications Hypersensitivity to ketoprofen, aspirin, other NSAIDs, or any component of the formulation; perioperative pain in the setting of coronary artery bypass graft (CABG) surgery

Warnings/Precautions [U.S. Boxed Warning]: NSAIDs are associated with an increased risk of adverse cardiovascular thrombotic events, including MI and stroke Risk may be increased with duration of use or pre-existing cardiovascular risk factors or disease. Carefully evaluate individual cardiovascular risk profiles prior to prescribing. May cause new-onset hypertension or worsening of existing hypertension. Use caution with fluid retention. Avoid use in heart failure. Concurrent administration of ibuprofen, and potentially other nonselective NSAIDs, may interfere with aspirin's cardioprotective effect. **[U.S. Boxed Warning]: Use is contraindicated for treatment of perioperative pain in the setting of coronary artery bypass graft (CABG) surgery.** Risk of MI and stroke may be increased with use following CABG surgery.

NSAID use may compromise existing renal function; dose-dependent decreases in prostaglandin synthesis may result from NSAID use, reducing renal blood flow which may cause renal decompensation. NSAID use may increase the risk for hyperkalemia. Patients with impaired renal function, dehydration, heart failure, liver dysfunction, those taking diuretics, and ACE inhibitors, and the elderly are at greater risk of renal toxicity and hyperkalemia. Rehydrate patient before starting therapy; monitor renal function closely. Not recommended for use in patients with advanced renal disease. Long-term NSAID use may result in renal papillary necrosis.

[U.S. Boxed Warning]: NSAIDs may increase risk of gastrointestinal irritation, inflammation, ulceration, bleeding, and perforation. These events may occur at any time during therapy and without warning. Use caution with a history of GI disease (bleeding or ulcers), concurrent therapy with aspirin, anticoagulants and/or corticosteroids, smoking, use of alcohol, the elderly or debilitated patients. When used concomitantly with ≤325 mg of aspirin, a substantial increase in the risk of gastrointestinal complications (eg, ulcer) occurs; concomitant gastroprotective therapy (eg, proton pump inhibitors) is recommended (Bhatt, 2008). Platelet adhesion and aggregation may be decreased; may prolong bleeding time; patients with coagulation disorders or who are receiving anticoagulants should be monitored closely. Anemia may occur; patients on long-term NSAID therapy should be monitored for anemia. Rarely, NSAID use may cause severe blood dyscrasias (eg, agranulocytosis, aplastic anemia, thrombocytopenia).

Use the lowest effective dose for the shortest duration of time, consistent with individual patient goals, to reduce risk of cardiovascular or GI adverse events. Alternate therapies should be considered for patients at high risk.

NSAIDS may cause drowsiness, dizziness, blurred vision and other neurologic effects which may impair physical or mental abilities; patients must be cautioned about performing tasks which require mental alertness (eg, operating machinery or driving). Discontinue use with blurred or diminished vision and perform ophthalmologic exam. Monitor vision with long-term therapy.

NSAIDs may cause serious skin adverse events including exfoliative dermatitis, Stevens-Johnson syndrome (SJS), and toxic epidermal necrolysis (TEN); discontinue use at first sign of skin rash or hypersensitivity. Anaphylactoid reactions may occur, even without prior exposure; patients with "aspirin triad" (bronchial asthma, aspirin intolerance, rhinitis) may be at increased risk. Do not use in patients who experience bronchospasm, asthma, rhinitis, or urticaria with NSAID or aspirin therapy. Use caution in other forms of asthma.

Use with caution in patients with decreased hepatic function. Closely monitor patients with any abnormal LFT. Severe hepatic reactions (eg, fulminant hepatitis, liver failure) have occurred with NSAID use, rarely; discontinue if signs or symptoms of liver disease develop, or if systemic manifestations occur. The elderly are at increased risk for adverse effects (especially peptic ulceration, CNS effects, renal toxicity) from NSAIDs, even at low doses.

Withhold for at least 4-6 half-lives prior to surgical or dental procedures. Safety and efficacy have not been established in pediatric patients.

Drug Interactions

Metabolism/Transport Effects Inhibits CYP2C9 (weak)

Avoid Concomitant Use

Avoid concomitant use of Ketoprofen with any of the following: Ketorolac; Ketorolac (Systemic)

Decreased Effect

Ketoprofen may decrease the levels/effects of: ACE Inhibitors; Angiotensin II Receptor Blockers; Antiplatelet Agents; Beta-Blockers; Eplerenone; HydrALAZINE; Loop Diuretics; Potassium-Sparing Diuretics; Salicylates; Thiazide Diuretics

The levels/effects of Ketoprofen may be decreased by: Bile Acid Sequestrants; Nonsteroidal Anti-Inflammatory Agents; Salicylates

Increased Effect/Toxicity

Ketoprofen may increase the levels/effects of: Aminoglycosides; Anticoagulants; Antiplatelet Agents; Bisphosphonate Derivatives; Collagenase (Systemic); CycloSPORINE; CycloSPORINE (Systemic); Desmopressin; Digoxin; Drotrecogin Alfa; Eplerenone; Haloperidol; Ibritumomab; Lithium; Methotrexate; Nonsteroidal Anti-Inflammatory Agents; PEMEtrexed; Potassium-Sparing Diuretics; PRALAtrexate; Quinolone Antibiotics; Salicylates; Thrombolytic Agents; Tositumomab and Iodine I 131 Tositumomab; Vancomycin; Vitamin K Antagonists

The levels/effects of Ketoprofen may be increased by: Antidepressants (Tricyclic, Tertiary Amine); Corticosteroids (Systemic); Dasatinib; Glucosamine; Herbs (Anticoagulant/Antiplatelet Properties); Ketorolac; Ketorolac (Systemic); Nonsteroidal Anti-Inflammatory Agents; Omega-3-Acid Ethyl Esters; Pentosan Polysulfate Sodium; Pentoxifylline; Probenecid; Prostacyclin Analogues; Selective Serotonin Reuptake Inhibitors; Serotonin/Norepinephrine Reuptake Inhibitors; Treprostinil

Nutritional/Ethanol Interactions

Ethanol: Avoid ethanol (due to GI irritation).

Food: Food slows rate of absorption resulting in delayed and reduced peak serum concentrations; total bioavailability is not affected by food.

Herb/Nutraceutical: Avoid alfalfa, anise, bilberry, bladderwrack, bromelain, cat's claw, celery, chamomile, coleus, cordyceps, dong quai, evening primrose, fenugreek, feverfew, garlic, ginger, ginkgo biloba, ginseng (American, Panax, Siberian), grapeseed, green tea, guggul, horse chestnut seed, horseradish, licorice, prickly ash, red clover, reishi, SAMe (S-adenosylmethionine), sweet clover, turmeric, and white willow (all have additional antiplatelet activity).

Adverse Reactions

>10%:

Gastrointestinal: Dyspepsia (11%)

Hepatic: Liver function test abnormal (≤15%)

1% to 10%:

Cardiovascular: Peripheral edema (2%)

Central nervous system: Headache (3% to 9%), depression, dizziness (>1%), dreams, insomnia, malaise, nervousness, somnolence

Dermatologic: Rash (>1%)

Gastrointestinal: Abdominal pain (3% to 9%), constipation (3% to 9%), diarrhea (3% to 9%), flatulence (3% to 9%), nausea (3% to 9%), gastrointestinal bleeding (>2%), peptic ulcer (>2%), anorexia (>1%), stomatitis (>1%), vomiting (>1%)

Genitourinary: Urinary tract irritation (>1%)

Ocular: Visual disturbances (>1%)
Otic: Tinnitus (>1%)
Renal: Renal dysfunction (3% to 9%)

Pharmacodynamics/Kinetics

Onset of Action Regular release: <30 minutes

Duration of Action Regular release: Up to 6 hours

Absorption Almost complete

Bioavailability ~90%

Time to Peak Regular release: 0.5-2 hours; Extended release: 6-7 hours

Protein Binding >99%, primarily to albumin; Hepatic impairment: Unbound fraction is approximately doubled

Half-Life Elimination

Regular release: 2-4 hours; Renal impairment: Mild: 3 hours; moderate-to-severe: 5-9 hours
Extended release: ~3-7.5 hours

Metabolism Hepatic via glucuronidation; metabolite (inactive) can be converted back to parent compound; may have enterohepatic recirculation

Excretion Urine (~80%, primarily as glucuronide conjugates)

Available Dosage Forms

Capsule, oral: 50 mg, 75 mg
Capsule, extended release, oral: 200 mg

Dosing

Adult Note: The extended release formulation is not recommended for the treatment of acute pain.

Rheumatoid arthritis or osteoarthritis: Oral:
Regular release: 50 mg 4 times/day **or** 75 mg 3 times/day; up to a maximum of 300 mg/day
Extended release: 200 mg once daily
Note: Lower doses may be used in small patients or in the elderly, or debilitated.

Dysmenorrhea, mild-to-moderate pain: Oral: Regular release: 25-50 mg every 6-8 hours up to a maximum of 300 mg/day

Geriatric Initial: 25-50 mg 3-4 times/day; increase up to 150-300 mg/day (maximum daily dose: 300 mg)

Renal Impairment In general, NSAIDs are not recommended for use in patients with advanced renal disease, but the manufacturer of ketoprofen does provide some guidelines for adjustment in renal dysfunction:
Mild impairment: Maximum dose: 150 mg/day
Severe impairment: Cl_{cr} <25 mL/minute: Maximum dose: 100 mg/day

Hepatic Impairment Hepatic impairment and serum albumin <3.5 g/dL: Maximum dose: 100 mg/day

Administration

Oral May take with food to reduce GI upset. Do not crush or break extended release capsules.

Stability

Storage Store at room temperature of 25°C (77°F). Protect from light; avoid excessive heat and humidity.

Monitoring and Teaching Issues

Laboratory Monitoring CBC, chemistry profile, occult blood loss, periodic liver function; renal function (urine output, serum BUN, creatinine)

Physical Assessment Evaluate cardiac risk and potential for GI bleeding prior to prescribing this medication. Monitor blood pressure at the beginning of therapy and periodically during use. Schedule ophthalmic evaluations for patients who develop eye complaints during long-term NSAID therapy.

Patient Education Do not break capsules. Take with food or milk to reduce GI distress. Do not use alcohol. You may experience drowsiness, dizziness, nervousness, headache, anorexia, nausea, vomiting, heartburn, or fluid retention; GI bleeding, ulceration, or perforation can occur with or without pain; discontinue medication and contact prescriber if persistent abdominal pain or cramping or blood in stool occurs. Report respiratory difficulty or unusual cough; chest pain or rapid heartbeat; bruising/bleeding; blood in urine, stool, mouth, or vomitus; swollen extremities; skin rash or itching; hearing changes (ringing in ears); jaundice; right upper quadrant tenderness; or flu-like symptoms.

Dietary Considerations In order to minimize gastrointestinal effects, ketoprofen can be prescribed to be taken with food or milk.

Geriatric Considerations Elderly are a high-risk population for adverse effects from NSAIDs. As much as 60% of the elderly can develop peptic ulceration and/or hemorrhage asymptomatically. The concomitant use of H_2 blockers and sucralfate is not effective as prophylaxis with the exception of NSAID-induced duodenal ulcers which may be prevented by the use of ranitidine. Misoprostol and proton pump inhibitors are the only agents proven to help prevent the development of NSAID-induced ulcers. Also, concomitant disease and drug use contribute to the risk for GI adverse effects. Use lowest effective dose for shortest period possible. Consider renal function decline with age. Use of NSAIDs can compromise existing renal function especially when Cl_{cr} is ≤30 mL/minute. Tinnitus may be a difficult and unreliable indication of toxicity due to age-related hearing loss or eighth cranial nerve damage. CNS adverse effects such as confusion, agitation, and hallucination are generally seen in overdose or high dose situations, but elderly may demonstrate these adverse effects at lower doses than younger adults.

Breast-Feeding Considerations Small amounts of ketoprofen are found in breast milk. Breast-feeding is not recommended by the manufacturer.

Pregnancy Considerations Adverse events were not observed in the initial animal reproduction studies; therefore, the manufacturer classifies ketoprofen as pregnancy category C. Ketoprofen crosses the placenta. NSAID exposure during the first trimester is not strongly associated with congenital malformations; however, cardiovascular anomalies and cleft palate have been observed following NSAID exposure in some studies. The use of an NSAID close to conception may be associated with an increased risk of miscarriage. Nonteratogenic effects have been observed following NSAID administration during the third trimester including myocardial degenerative changes, prenatal constriction of the ductus arteriosus, fetal tricuspid regurgitation, failure of the ductus arteriosus to close postnatally; renal dysfunction or failure, oligohydramnios; gastrointestinal bleeding or perforation, increased risk of necrotizing enterocolitis; intracranial bleeding (including intraventricular hemorrhage), platelet dysfunction with resultant bleeding; pulmonary hypertension. Because they may cause premature closure of the ductus arteriosus, use of NSAIDs late in pregnancy should be avoided (use after 31or 32 weeks gestation is not recommended by some clinicians). The chronic use of NSAIDs in women of reproductive age may be associated with infertility that is reversible upon discontinuation of the medication.

Related Information

Nonsalicylate / Nonsteroidal Anti-Inflammatory Agents *on page* 2002

Ketorolac (Systemic) (KEE toe role ak)

Index Terms Ketorolac Tromethamine; Toradol

Generic Availability (U.S.) Yes

Pharmacologic Category Nonsteroidal Anti-inflammatory Drug (NSAID), Oral; Nonsteroidal Anti-inflammatory Drug (NSAID), Parenteral

Medication Safety Issues

Sound-alike/look-alike issues:

Ketorolac may be confused with Ketalar®

Toradol® may be confused with Foradil®, Inderal®, TEGretol®, Torecan®, traMADol, tromethamine

Beers Criteria medication: This drug may be inappropriate for use in geriatric patients (high severity risk).

International issues:

Toradol [Canada and multiple international markets] may be confused with Theradol brand name for tramadol [Netherlands]

Medication Guide Available Yes

Pregnancy Risk Factor C

Lactation Enters breast milk/contraindicated (per manufacturer)

Use Short-term (≤5 days) management of moderate-to-severe acute pain requiring analgesia at the opioid level

Mechanism of Action/Effect Reversibly inhibits cyclooxygenase-1 and 2 (COX-1 and 2) enzymes, which results in decreased formation of prostaglandin precursors; has antipyretic, analgesic, and anti-inflammatory properties

Contraindications Hypersensitivity to ketorolac, aspirin, other NSAIDs, or any component of the formulation; active or history of peptic ulcer disease; recent or history of GI bleeding or perforation; patients with advanced renal disease or risk of renal failure (due to volume depletion); prophylaxis before major surgery; suspected or confirmed cerebrovascular bleeding; hemorrhagic diathesis, incomplete hemostasis, or high risk of bleeding; concurrent ASA or other NSAIDs; concomitant probenecid or pentoxifylline; epidural or intrathecal administration; perioperative pain in the setting of coronary artery bypass graft (CABG) surgery; labor and delivery; breast-feeding

Warnings/Precautions [U.S. Boxed Warning]: May inhibit platelet function; contraindicated in patients with cerebrovascular bleeding (suspected or confirmed), hemorrhagic diathesis, incomplete hemostasis and patients at high risk for bleeding. Effects on platelet adhesion and aggregation may prolong bleeding time. Anemia may occur; patients on long-term NSAID therapy should be monitored for anemia. Rarely, NSAID use has been associated with potentially severe blood dyscrasias (eg, agranulocytosis, thrombocytopenia, aplastic anemia).

[U.S. Boxed Warning]: NSAIDs are associated with an increased risk of adverse cardiovascular thrombotic events, including MI and stroke. Risk may be increased with duration of use or pre-existing cardiovascular risk factors or disease. Carefully evaluate individual cardiovascular risk profiles prior to prescribing. May cause new-onset hypertension or worsening of existing hypertension. Use caution with fluid retention. Avoid use in heart failure. Concurrent administration of ibuprofen, and potentially other nonselective NSAIDs, may interfere with aspirin's cardioprotective effect. **[U.S. Boxed Warning]: Use is contraindicated as prophylactic analgesic before any major surgery and is contraindicated for treatment of perioperative pain in the setting of coronary artery bypass graft (CABG) surgery.** Risk of MI and stroke may be increased with use following CABG surgery. Wound bleeding and postoperative hematomas have been associated with ketorolac use in the perioperative setting. Withhold for at least 4-6 half-lives prior to surgical or dental procedures.

[U.S. Boxed Warning]: Ketorolac is contraindicated in patients with advanced renal impairment and in patients at risk for renal failure due to volume depletion. NSAID use may compromise existing renal function; dose-dependent decreases in prostaglandin synthesis may result from NSAID use, reducing renal blood flow which may cause renal decompensation. NSAID use may increase the risk for hyperkalemia. Patients with impaired renal function, dehydration, heart failure, liver dysfunction, those taking diuretics and ACE inhibitors, and the elderly are at greater risk of renal toxicity. Use with caution in patients with impaired renal function or history of kidney disease; dosage adjustment is required in patients with moderate elevation in serum creatinine. Monitor renal function closely. Acute renal failure, interstitial nephritis, and nephrotic syndrome have been reported with ketorolac use; papillary necrosis and renal injury have been reported with the use of NSAIDs. Use of NSAIDs can compromise existing renal function. Rehydrate patient before starting therapy.

[U.S. Boxed Warning]: NSAIDs may increase risk of gastrointestinal irritation, inflammation, ulceration, bleeding, and perforation. These events may occur at any time during therapy and without warning. Use caution with a history of GI disease (bleeding, ulcers, inflammatory bowel disease), concurrent therapy with aspirin, anticoagulants and/or corticosteroids, smoking, use of alcohol, the elderly, or debilitated patients. When used concomitantly with ≤325 mg of aspirin, a substantial increase in the risk of gastrointestinal complications (eg, ulcer) occurs; concomitant gastroprotective therapy (eg, proton pump inhibitors) is recommended (Bhatt, 2008).

NSAIDs may cause serious skin adverse events including exfoliative dermatitis, Stevens-Johnson syndrome (SJS), and toxic epidermal necrolysis (TEN); discontinue use at first sign of skin rash or hypersensitivity. Hypersensitivity or anaphylactoid reactions may occur, even without prior exposure; patients with "aspirin triad" (bronchial asthma, aspirin intolerance, rhinitis) may be at increased risk. Do not use in patients who experience bronchospasm, asthma, rhinitis, or urticaria with NSAID or aspirin therapy. **[U.S. Boxed Warning]: Ketorolac injection is contraindicated in patients with prior hypersensitivity reaction to aspirin or NSAIDs**. Use caution in other forms of asthma.

Use with caution in patients with hepatic impairment or a history of liver disease. Closely monitor patients with any abnormal LFT. Rarely, severe hepatic reactions (eg, fulminant hepatitis, hepatic necrosis, liver failure) have occurred with NSAID use; discontinue if signs or symptoms of liver disease develop, or if systemic manifestations occur.

[U.S. Boxed Warning]: Dosage adjustment is required for patients ≥65 years of age. The elderly are at increased risk for adverse effects (especially peptic ulceration, CNS effects, renal toxicity) from NSAIDs, even at low doses. Avoid immediate and long-term use (Beers Criteria). **[U.S. Boxed Warning]: Dosage adjustment is required for patients weighing <50 kg (<110 pounds). [U.S. Boxed Warning]: May inhibit uterine contractions and affect fetal circulation; inhibits prostaglandin synthesis in neonates; use is contraindicated in labor and delivery and breast-feeding women.** Avoid use in late pregnancy. **[U.S. Boxed Warning]: Concurrent use of ketorolac with aspirin or other NSAIDs is contraindicated due to the increased risk of adverse reactions.**

[U.S. Boxed Warning]: Contraindicated for epidural or intrathecal administration. [U.S. Boxed Warning]: Systemic ketorolac is indicated for short term (≤5 days) use in adults for treatment of moderately severe acute pain requiring opioid-level analgesia. Low doses of narcotics may be needed for breakthrough pain. **[U.S. Boxed Warning]: Oral therapy is only indicated for use as continuation treatment, following parenteral ketorolac and is not indicated for minor or chronic painful conditions. The maximum daily oral dose is 40 mg (adults); doses above 40 mg/day do not improve efficacy but may increase the risk of serious adverse effects.** The combined therapy duration (oral and parenteral) should not exceed 5 days. Use the lowest effective dose for the shortest duration of time, consistent with individual patient goals, to reduce risk of cardiovascular or GI adverse events. Alternate therapies should be considered for patients at high risk. **[U.S. Boxed Warning]: Oral ketorolac is not indicated for use in children.**

NSAIDS may cause drowsiness, dizziness, blurred vision and other neurologic effects which may impair physical or mental abilities; patients must be cautioned about performing tasks which require mental alertness (eg, operating machinery or driving). Discontinue use with blurred or diminished vision and perform ophthalmologic exam. Monitor vision with long-term therapy.

Drug Interactions

Avoid Concomitant Use

Avoid concomitant use of Ketorolac (Systemic) with any of the following: Aspirin; Ketorolac; Nonsteroidal Anti-Inflammatory Agents; Pentoxifylline; Probenecid

Decreased Effect

Ketorolac (Systemic) may decrease the levels/effects of: ACE Inhibitors; Angiotensin II Receptor Blockers; Anticonvulsants; Antiplatelet Agents; Beta-Blockers; Eplerenone; HydrALAZINE; Loop Diuretics; Potassium-Sparing Diuretics; Salicylates; Thiazide Diuretics

The levels/effects of Ketorolac (Systemic) may be decreased by: Bile Acid Sequestrants; Salicylates

Increased Effect/Toxicity

Ketorolac (Systemic) may increase the levels/effects of: Aminoglycosides; Anticoagulants; Antiplatelet Agents; Aspirin; Bisphosphonate Derivatives; Collagenase (Systemic); CycloSPORINE; CycloSPORINE (Systemic); Desmopressin; Digoxin; Drotrecogin Alfa; Eplerenone; Haloperidol; Ibritumomab; Lithium; Methotrexate; Neuromuscular-Blocking Agents (Nondepolarizing); Nonsteroidal Anti-Inflammatory Agents; PEMEtrexed; Pentoxifylline;

Potassium-Sparing Diuretics; PRALAtrexate; Quinolone Antibiotics; Salicylates; Thrombolytic Agents; Tositumomab and Iodine I 131 Tositumomab; Vancomycin; Vitamin K Antagonists

The levels/effects of Ketorolac (Systemic) may be increased by: Antidepressants (Tricyclic, Tertiary Amine); Corticosteroids (Systemic); Dasatinib; Glucosamine; Herbs (Anticoagulant/Antiplatelet Properties); Ketorolac; Omega-3-Acid Ethyl Esters; Pentosan Polysulfate Sodium; Probenecid; Prostacyclin Analogues; Selective Serotonin Reuptake Inhibitors; Serotonin/Norepinephrine Reuptake Inhibitors; Treprostinil

Nutritional/Ethanol Interactions

Ethanol: Avoid ethanol (may enhance gastric mucosal irritation).

Food: Oral: High-fat meals may delay time to peak (by ~1 hour) and decrease peak concentrations.

Herb/Nutraceutical: Avoid alfalfa, anise, bilberry, bladderwrack, bromelain, cat's claw, celery, chamomile, coleus, cordyceps, dong quai, evening primrose, fenugreek, feverfew, garlic, ginger, ginkgo biloba, ginseng (American, Panax, Siberian), grapeseed, green tea, guggul, horse chestnut seed, horseradish, licorice, prickly ash, red clover, reishi, SAMe (S-adenosylmethionine), sweet clover, turmeric, and white willow (all have additional antiplatelet activity).

Adverse Reactions

Frequencies noted for parenteral administration:

>10%:

Central nervous system: Headache (17%)

Gastrointestinal: Gastrointestinal pain (13%), dyspepsia (12%), nausea (12%)

>1% to 10%:

Cardiovascular: Edema (4%), hypertension

Central nervous system: Dizziness (7%), drowsiness (6%)

Dermatologic: Pruritus, purpura, rash

Gastrointestinal: Diarrhea (7%), constipation, flatulence, GI bleeding, GI fullness, GI perforation, GI ulcer, heartburn, stomatitis, vomiting

Hematologic: Anemia, bleeding time increased

Hepatic: Liver enzymes increased

Local: Injection site pain (2%)

Otic: Tinnitus

Renal: Renal function abnormal

Miscellaneous: Diaphoresis

Pharmacodynamics/Kinetics

Onset of Action Analgesic: I.M.: ~10 minutes; Peak effect: Analgesic: 2-3 hours

Duration of Action Analgesic: 6-8 hours

Absorption Oral: Well absorbed (100%)

Time to Peak Serum: I.M.: 30-60 minutes

Protein Binding 99%

Half-Life Elimination 2-6 hours; increased 30% to 50% in elderly; up to 19 hours in renal impairment

Metabolism Hepatic

Excretion Urine (92%, ~60% as unchanged drug); feces ~6%

Available Dosage Forms

Injection, solution: 15 mg/mL (1 mL, 2 mL); 30 mg/mL (1 mL, 2 mL, 10 mL)

Tablet, oral: 10 mg

Dosing

Adult Pain management (acute; moderately-severe): Note: The maximum combined duration of treatment (for parenteral and oral) is 5 days; do not increase dose or frequency; supplement with low dose opioids if needed for breakthrough pain. For patients <50 kg and/or ≥65 years of age, see Geriatric dosing.

I.M.: 60 mg as a single dose or 30 mg every 6 hours (maximum daily dose: 120 mg)

I.V.: 30 mg as a single dose or 30 mg every 6 hours (maximum daily dose: 120 mg)

Oral: 20 mg, followed by 10 mg every 4-6 hours; do not exceed 40 mg/day; oral dosing is intended to be a continuation of I.M. or I.V. therapy only

Geriatric Dosage adjustments in elderly (≥65 years), renal insufficiency, or low body weight (<50 kg): **Note:** These groups have an increased incidence of GI bleeding, ulceration, and perforation. The maximum combined duration of treatment (for parenteral and oral) is 5 days.

I.M.: 30 mg as a single dose or 15 mg every 6 hours (maximum daily dose: 60 mg)

I.V.: 15 mg as a single dose or 15 mg every 6 hours (maximum daily dose: 60 mg)

Oral: 10 mg, followed by 10 mg every 4-6 hours; do not exceed 40 mg/day; oral dosing is intended to be a continuation of I.M. or I.V. therapy only

Pediatric Pain management (acute; moderately-severe):

Children ≥16 years and <50 kg: *I.V.:* Refer to Dosing: Geriatric.

Children ≥16 years and ≥50 kg: *I.V.:* Refer to adult dosing.

Children ≥17 years and <50 kg: *Oral:* Refer to Dosing: Geriatric.

Children ≥17 years and ≥50 kg: *Oral:* Refer to adult dosing.

Renal Impairment Contraindicated in patients with advanced renal impairment. Patients with moderately-elevated serum creatinine should use half the recommended dose, not to exceed 60 mg/day I.M./I.V.

Hepatic Impairment Use with caution, may cause elevation of liver enzymes; discontinue if clinical signs and symptoms of liver disease develop.

Administration

Oral May take with food to reduce GI upset.

I.M. Administer slowly and deeply into the muscle. Analgesia begins in 30 minutes and maximum effect within 2 hours.

I.V. Administer I.V. bolus over a minimum of 15 seconds; onset within 30 minutes; peak analgesia within 2 hours.

Stability

Storage

Injection: Store at room temperature of 15°C to 30°C (59°F to 86°F). Protect from light. Injection is clear and has a slight yellow color. Precipitation may occur at relatively low pH values.

Tablet: Store at room temperature of 15°C to 30°C (59°F to 86°F).

Monitoring and Teaching Issues

Laboratory Monitoring CBC and platelets, liver function, platelets; renal function (serum creatinine, BUN, urine output)

Physical Assessment Evaluate cardiac risk and potential for GI bleeding prior to prescribing this medication. Assess allergy history prior to treatment. I.V./I.M.: Vital signs should be monitored on a regular basis during infusion or following injection. Oral: Monitor blood pressure prior to treatment and periodically throughout.

Patient Education Do not take aspirin-containing products or any other NSAIDs during therapy unless approved by prescriber. Oral doses may be taken with food or milk. Avoid alcohol. Maintain adequate hydration unless instructed to restrict fluid intake. May cause nausea or vomiting. Report blood in vomitus or stool or other signs of unusual bleeding, abdominal pain, weakness, slurring of speech, ringing in ears, unresolved nausea or vomiting, respiratory difficulty or shortness of breath, skin rash, unusual swelling of extremities, unexplained weight gain, chest pain, or palpitations.

Dietary Considerations Administer tablet with food or milk to decrease gastrointestinal distress.

Geriatric Considerations Ketorolac is cleared more slowly in the elderly. It is recommended to use lower doses in the elderly. Elderly are a high-risk population for adverse effects from NSAIDs. As much as 60% of elderly can develop peptic ulceration and/or hemorrhage asymptomatically. The concomitant use of H_2 blockers and sucralfate is not effective as prophylaxis with the exception of NSAID-induced duodenal ulcers which may be prevented by the use of ranitidine. Misoprostol and proton pump inhibitors are the only agents proven to help prevent the development of NSAID-induced ulcers. Also, concomitant disease and drug use contribute to the risk for GI adverse effects. Use lowest effective dose for shortest period possible. Consider renal function decline with age. Use of NSAIDs can compromise existing renal function especially when Cl_{cr} is ≤30 mL/minute or weight <50 kg. Tinnitus may be a difficult and unreliable indication of toxicity due to age-related hearing loss or eighth cranial nerve damage. CNS adverse effects such as confusion, agitation, and hallucination are generally seen in overdose or high dose situations, but elderly may demonstrate these adverse effects at lower doses than younger adults.

This medication is considered to be potentially inappropriate in this patient population (Beers Criteria severity: High).

Breast-Feeding Considerations Low concentrations of ketorolac are found in breast milk. **[U.S. Boxed Warning]: Inhibition of prostaglandin synthesis may adversely affect neonates; use of systemic ketorolac is contraindicated in breast-feeding women.** The manufacturer of the ophthalmic product recommends that caution be used if administered to a breast-feeding woman. The maternal pharmacokinetics of ketorolac were not found to change immediately postpartum.

Pregnancy Considerations Adverse events were not observed in the initial animal reproduction studies; therefore, the manufacturer classifies ketorolac as pregnancy category C. Ketorolac crosses the placenta. NSAID exposure during the first trimester is not strongly associated with congenital malformations; however, cardiovascular anomalies and cleft palate have been observed following NSAID exposure in some studies. The use of an NSAID close to conception may be associated with an increased risk of miscarriage. Nonteratogenic effects have been observed following NSAID administration during the third trimester including myocardial degenerative changes, prenatal constriction of the ductus arteriosus, fetal tricuspid regurgitation, failure of the ductus arteriosus to close postnatally; renal dysfunction or failure, oligohydramnios; gastrointestinal bleeding or perforation, increased risk of necrotizing enterocolitis; intracranial bleeding (including intraventricular hemorrhage), platelet dysfunction with resultant bleeding; pulmonary hypertension. Because they may cause premature closure of the ductus arteriosus, use of NSAIDs late in pregnancy should be avoided (use after 31 or 32 weeks gestation is not recommended by some clinicians). **[U.S. Boxed Warning]: Ketorolac is contraindicated during labor and delivery (may inhibit uterine contractions and adversely affect fetal circulation).** The chronic use of NSAIDs in women of reproductive age may be associated with infertility that is reversible upon discontinuation of the medication.

Additional Information First parenteral NSAID for analgesia; 30 mg provides the analgesia comparable to 12 mg of morphine or 100 mg of meperidine.

Related Information

Nonsalicylate / Nonsteroidal Anti-Inflammatory Agents *on page* 2002

Ketorolac (Ophthalmic) (KEE toe role ak)

U.S. Brand Names Acular LS®; Acular®; Acuvail®

Index Terms Ketorolac Tromethamine

Generic Availability (U.S.) Yes

Pharmacologic Category Nonsteroidal Anti-inflammatory Drug (NSAID), Ophthalmic

Medication Safety Issues

Sound-alike/look-alike issues:

Acular® may be confused with Acthar®, Ocular®

Ketorolac may be confused with Ketalar®

Pregnancy Risk Factor C

Lactation Use caution

Use Temporary relief of ocular itching due to seasonal allergic conjunctivitis; postoperative inflammation following cataract extraction; reduction of ocular pain and photophobia following incisional refractive surgery; reduction of ocular pain, burning, and stinging following corneal refractive surgery

Available Dosage Forms

Solution, ophthalmic: 0.4% (5 mL); 0.5% (3 mL, 5 mL, 10 mL)

Acular LS®: 0.4% (5 mL)

Acular®: 0.5% (5 mL)

Solution, ophthalmic [preservative free]:

Acuvail®: 0.45% (0.4 mL)

Dosing

Adult

Seasonal allergic conjunctivitis (relief of ocular itching) (Acular®): *Ophthalmic:* Instill 1 drop (0.25 mg) 4 times/day

Inflammation following cataract extraction (Acular®): *Ophthalmic:* Instill 1 drop (0.25 mg) to affected eye(s) 4 times/day beginning 24 hours after surgery; continue for 2 weeks

Pain following corneal refractive surgery (Acular LS®): *Ophthalmic:* Instill 1 drop 4 times/day as needed to affected eye for up to 4 days

Pediatric Ophthalmic uses: Children ≥3 years: Refer to adult dosing.

Administration

Other Contact lenses should be removed before instillation. Acular® and Acular LS® have been safely administered with other ophthalmic medications including antibiotics, beta-blockers, carbonic anhydrase inhibitors, cycloplegics, and mydriatics.

Monitoring and Teaching Issues

Patient Education Wash hands before instilling. Sit or lie down to instill. Open eye, look at ceiling, and instill prescribed amount of solution. Close eye and roll eye in all directions. Apply gentle pressure to inner corner of eye for 1-2 minutes after instillation. Do not let tip of applicator touch eye; do not contaminate tip of applicator (may cause eye infection, eye damage, or vision loss). Temporary stinging or blurred vision may occur. Do not wear soft contact lenses. Report persistent pain, burning, double vision, swelling, itching, or worsening of condition.

Related Information

Nonsalicylate / Nonsteroidal Anti-Inflammatory Agents *on page 2002*

- ◆ **Ketorolac Tromethamine** *see* Ketorolac (Ophthalmic) *on page 1046*
- ◆ **Ketorolac Tromethamine** *see* Ketorolac (Systemic) *on page 1043*
- ◆ **Khloditan** *see* Mitotane *on page 1242*
- ◆ **KI** *see* Potassium Iodide *on page 1483*
- ◆ **Kinrix®** *see* Diphtheria and Tetanus Toxoids, Acellular Pertussis, and Poliovirus Vaccine *on page 548*
- ◆ **Kionex®** *see* Sodium Polystyrene Sulfonate *on page 1660*
- ◆ **KlonoPIN®** *see* ClonazePAM *on page 406*
- ◆ **Klor-Con®** *see* Potassium Chloride *on page 1480*
- ◆ **Klor-Con® 8** *see* Potassium Chloride *on page 1480*
- ◆ **Klor-Con® 10** *see* Potassium Chloride *on page 1480*
- ◆ **Klor-Con®/25** *see* Potassium Chloride *on page 1480*
- ◆ **Klor-Con®/EF** *see* Potassium Bicarbonate and Potassium Citrate *on page 1479*
- ◆ **Klor-Con® M10** *see* Potassium Chloride *on page 1480*
- ◆ **Klor-Con® M15** *see* Potassium Chloride *on page 1480*
- ◆ **Klor-Con® M20** *see* Potassium Chloride *on page 1480*
- ◆ **K-Lyte/Cl** *see* Potassium Bicarbonate and Potassium Chloride *on page 1479*
- ◆ **KMD 3213** *see* Silodosin *on page 1643*
- ◆ **Kogenate® FS** *see* Antihemophilic Factor (Recombinant) *on page 133*
- ◆ **Kombiglyze™ XR** *see* Saxagliptin and Metformin *on page 1626*
- ◆ **Koāte®-DVI** *see* Antihemophilic Factor (Human) *on page 132*
- ◆ **K-Phos® MF** *see* Potassium Phosphate and Sodium Phosphate *on page 1486*
- ◆ **K-Phos® Neutral** *see* Potassium Phosphate and Sodium Phosphate *on page 1486*
- ◆ **K-Phos® No. 2** *see* Potassium Phosphate and Sodium Phosphate *on page 1486*
- ◆ **Kristalose®** *see* Lactulose *on page 1053*
- ◆ **Krystexxa™** *see* Pegloticase *on page 1427*
- ◆ **K-Tab®** *see* Potassium Chloride *on page 1480*

- ◆ **Kunecatechins** *see* Sinecatechins *on page 1647*
- ◆ **Kytril®** *see* Granisetron *on page 887*
- ◆ **L-749,345** *see* Ertapenem *on page 656*
- ◆ **L-758,298** *see* Fosaprepitant *on page 826*
- ◆ **L-M-X® 4 [OTC]** *see* Lidocaine (Topical) *on page 1107*
- ◆ **L-M-X® 5 [OTC]** *see* Lidocaine (Topical) *on page 1107*
- ◆ **L 754030** *see* Aprepitant *on page 139*
- ◆ **LA 20304a** *see* Gemifloxacin *on page 861*

Labetalol (la BET a lole)

U.S. Brand Names Trandate®

Index Terms Ibidomide Hydrochloride; Labetalol Hydrochloride

Generic Availability (U.S.) Yes

Pharmacologic Category Beta Blocker With Alpha-Blocking Activity

Medication Safety Issues

Sound-alike/look-alike issues:

Labetalol may be confused with betaxolol, Hexadrol®, lamoTRIgine, Lipitor®

Normodyne® may be confused with Norpramin®

Trandate® may be confused with traMADol, Trendar®, Trental®, Tridrate®

High alert medication: The Institute for Safe Medication Practices (ISMP) includes this medication among its list of drugs which have a heightened risk of causing significant patient harm when used in error.

Significant differences exist between oral and I.V. dosing. Use caution when converting from one route of administration to another.

Pregnancy Risk Factor C

Lactation Enters breast milk/use caution (AAP rates "compatible"; AAP 2001 update pending)

Use Treatment of mild-to-severe hypertension; I.V. for severe hypertension (eg, hypertensive emergencies)

Unlabeled/Investigational Use Pediatric hypertension; management of pre-eclampsia; severe hypertension in pregnancy; hypertension during acute ischemic stroke

Mechanism of Action/Effect Blocks alpha-, $beta_1$-, and $beta_2$-adrenergic receptor sites; elevated renins are reduced. The ratios of alpha- to beta-blockade differ depending on the route of administration: 1:3 (oral) and 1:7 (I.V.).

Contraindications Hypersensitivity to labetalol or any component of the formulation; severe bradycardia; heart block greater than first degree (except in patients with a functioning artificial pacemaker); cardiogenic shock; bronchial asthma; uncompensated cardiac failure; conditions associated with severe and prolonged hypotension

Warnings/Precautions Consider pre-existing conditions such as sick sinus syndrome before initiating. Symptomatic hypotension with or without syncope may occur with labetalol; close monitoring of patient is required especially with initial dosing and dosing increases; blood pressure must be lowered at a rate appropriate for the patient's clinical condition. Initiation with a low dose and gradual up-titration may help to decrease the occurrence of hypotension or syncope. Patients should be advised to avoid driving or other hazardous tasks during initiation of therapy due to the risk of syncope. Orthostatic hypotension may occur with I.V. administration; patient should remain supine during and for up to 3 hours after I.V. administration. Use with caution in impaired hepatic function; bioavailability is increased due to decreased first-pass metabolism. Severe hepatic injury including some fatalities have also been rarely reported with use: periodically monitor LFTs with prolonged use. Use with caution in patients with diabetes mellitus; may potentiate hypoglycemia and/or mask signs and symptoms. May also reduce release of insulin in response to hyperglycemia; dosage of antidiabetic agents may need to be adjusted. Elimination of labetalol is reduced in elderly patients; lower maintenance doses may be required.

Use only with extreme caution in compensated heart failure and monitor for a worsening of the condition. Beta-blocker therapy should not be withdrawn abruptly (particularly in patients with CAD), but gradually tapered to avoid acute tachycardia, hypertension, and/or ischemia. Use caution with concurrent use of beta-blockers and either verapamil or diltiazem; bradycardia or heart block can occur. Patients with bronchospastic disease should not receive beta-blockers; if used at all, should be used cautiously with close monitoring. Use with caution in patients with myasthenia gravis, psychiatric disease (may cause or exacerbate CNS depression), or peripheral vascular disease. If possible, obtain diagnostic tests for pheochromocytoma prior to use. May induce or exacerbate psoriasis. Labetalol has been shown to be effective in lowering blood pressure and relieving symptoms in patients with pheochromocytoma. However, some patients have experienced paradoxical hypertensive responses; use with caution in patients with pheochromocytoma. Additional alpha-blockade may be required during use of labetalol. Use caution with history of severe anaphylaxis to allergens; patients taking beta-blockers may become more sensitive to repeated challenges. Treatment of anaphylaxis (eg, epinephrine) in patients taking beta-blockers may be ineffective or promote undesirable effects. Use with caution in patients receiving anesthetic agents which decrease myocardial function.

Drug Interactions

Avoid Concomitant Use

Avoid concomitant use of Labetalol with any of the following: Methacholine

Decreased Effect

Labetalol may decrease the levels/effects of: Beta2-Agonists; Theophylline Derivatives

The levels/effects of Labetalol may be decreased by: Barbiturates; Herbs (Hypertensive Properties); Methylphenidate; Nonsteroidal Anti-Inflammatory Agents; Rifamycin Derivatives; Yohimbine

Increased Effect/Toxicity

Labetalol may increase the levels/effects of: Alpha-/Beta-Agonists (Direct-Acting); Alpha1-Blockers; Alpha2-Agonists; Amifostine; Antihypertensives; Antipsychotic Agents (Phenothiazines); Bupivacaine; Cardiac Glycosides; Fingolimod; Hypotensive Agents; Insulin; Lidocaine; Lidocaine (Systemic); Lidocaine (Topical); Mepivacaine; Methacholine; Midodrine; RiTUXimab; Sulfonylureas

The levels/effects of Labetalol may be increased by: Acetylcholinesterase Inhibitors; Aminoquinolines (Antimalarial); Amiodarone; Anilidopiperidine Opioids; Antipsychotic Agents (Phenothiazines); Calcium Channel Blockers (Nondihydropyridine); Diazoxide; Dipyridamole; Disopyramide; Dronedarone; Herbs (Hypotensive Properties); MAO Inhibitors; Pentoxifylline; Phosphodiesterase 5 Inhibitors; Propafenone; Propoxyphene; Prostacyclin Analogues; QuiNIDine; Reserpine; Selective Serotonin Reuptake Inhibitors

Nutritional/Ethanol Interactions

Food: Labetalol serum concentrations may be increased if taken with food.

Herb/Nutraceutical: Avoid dong quai if using for hypertension (has estrogenic activity). Avoid ephedra, yohimbe, ginseng (may worsen hypertension). Avoid natural licorice (causes sodium and water retention and increases potassium loss). Avoid garlic (may have increased antihypertensive effect).

Lab Interactions False-positive urine catecholamines, vanillylmandelic acid (VMA) if measured by fluorometric or photometric methods; use HPLC or specific catecholamine radioenzymatic technique; false-positive amphetamine if measured by thin-layer chromatography or radioenzymatic assay (gas chromatographic-mass spectrometer technique should be used)

Adverse Reactions

>10%:

Cardiovascular: Postural hypotension (I.V. use; ≤58%)

Central nervous system: Dizziness (1% to 20%), fatigue (1% to 11%)

Gastrointestinal: Nausea (≤19%)

1% to 10%:

Cardiovascular: Hypotension (1% to 5%), edema (≤2%), flushing (1%), ventricular arrhythmia (I.V. use; 1%)

Central nervous system: Somnolence (3%), headache (2%), vertigo (1% to 2%)

Dermatologic: Scalp tingling (≤7%), pruritus (1%), rash (1%)

Gastrointestinal: Dyspepsia (≤4%), vomiting (≤3%), taste disturbance (1%)

Genitourinary: Ejaculatory failure (≤5%), impotence (1% to 4%)

Hepatic: Transaminases increased (4%)

Neuromuscular & skeletal: Paresthesia (≤5%), weakness (1%)

Ocular: Vision abnormal (1%)

Renal: BUN increased (≤8%)

Respiratory: Nasal congestion (1% to 6%), dyspnea (2%)

Miscellaneous: Diaphoresis (≤4%)

Other adverse reactions noted with beta-adrenergic blocking agents include mental depression, catatonia, disorientation, short-term memory loss, emotional lability, clouded sensorium, intensification of pre-existing AV block, laryngospasm, respiratory distress, agranulocytosis, thrombocytopenic purpura, nonthrombocytopenic purpura, mesenteric artery thrombosis, and ischemic colitis.

Pharmacodynamics/Kinetics

Onset of Action Oral: 20 minutes to 2 hours; I.V.: 2-5 minutes; Peak effect: Oral: 1-4 hours; I.V.: 5-15 minutes

Duration of Action Blood pressure response:

Oral: 8-12 hours (dose dependent)

I.V.: 2-18 hours (dose dependent; based on single and multiple sequential doses of 0.25-0.5 mg/kg with cumulative dosing up to 3.25 mg/kg)

Absorption Complete

Bioavailability Oral: 25%; increased with liver disease, elderly, and concurrent cimetidine

Time to Peak Plasma: Oral: 1-2 hours

Protein Binding 50%

Half-Life Elimination Oral: 6-8 hours; I.V.: ~5.5 hours

Metabolism Hepatic, primarily via glucuronide conjugation; extensive first-pass effect

Excretion Urine (55% to 60% as glucuronide conjugates, <5% as unchanged drug)

Clearance: Possibly decreased in neonates/infants

Available Dosage Forms

Injection, solution: 5 mg/mL (4 mL, 8 mL, 20 mL, 40 mL)

Trandate®: 5 mg/mL (20 mL, 40 mL)

Tablet, oral: 100 mg, 200 mg, 300 mg

Trandate®: 100 mg, 200 mg, 300 mg

Dosing

Adult

Hypertension: Oral: Initial: 100 mg twice daily, may increase as needed every 2-3 days by 100 mg twice daily (titration increments not to exceed 200 mg twice daily) until desired response is obtained; usual dose: 200-400 mg twice daily; may require up to 2.4 g/day.

Usual dose range (JNC 7): 200-800 mg/day in 2 divided doses

Acute hypertension (hypertensive emergency/urgency):

I.V. bolus: Per the manufacturer: Initial: 20 mg I.V. push over 2 minutes; may administer 40-80 mg at 10-minute intervals, up to 300 mg total cumulative dose; as appropriate, follow with oral antihypertensive regimen

I.V. infusion (acute loading): Per the manufacturer: Initial: 2 mg/minute; titrate to response up to 300 mg total cumulative dose (eg, discontinue after 2.5 hours of 2 mg/minute); as appropriate, follow with oral antihypertensive regimen

Note: Although loading infusions are well described in the product labeling, the labeling is silent in specific clinical situations, such as in the patient who has an initial response to labetalol infusions but cannot be converted to an oral route for subsequent dosing. There is limited documentation of prolonged continuous infusions (ie, >300 mg/day). In rare clinical situations, higher continuous infusion doses up to 6 mg/minute have been used in the critical care setting (eg, aortic dissection) and up to 8 mg/minute (eg, hypertension with ongoing acute ischemic stroke). At these doses, it may be best to consider an alternative agent if the labetalol infusion is not meeting the goals of therapy. At the other extreme, continuous infusions at relatively low doses (0.03-0.1 mg/minute) have been used in some settings (following loading infusion in patients who are unable to be converted to oral regimens or in some cases as a continuation of outpatient oral regimens). These prolonged infusions should not be confused with loading infusions. Because of wide variation in the use of infusions, an awareness of institutional policies and practices is extremely important. Careful clarification of orders and specific infusion rates/units is required to avoid confusion. Due to the prolonged duration of action, careful monitoring should be extended for the duration of the infusion and for several hours after the infusion. Excessive administration may result in prolonged hypotension and/or bradycardia.

Arterial hypertension in acute ischemic stroke (unlabeled use [Adams, 2007; Jauch, 2010]): I.V.:

Patient otherwise eligible for reperfusion treatment (eg, alteplase): Blood pressure (BP): Systolic >185 mm Hg or diastolic >110 mm Hg: 10-20 mg over 1-2 minutes; may repeat once. If BP does not decline and remains >185/110 mm Hg, alteplase should not be administered.

Management of BP during and after reperfusion treatment (eg, alteplase): BP: Systolic ≥180 mm Hg or diastolic ≥105 mm Hg: 10 mg over 1-2 minutes; may repeat every 10-20 minutes (maximum dose: 300 mg) **or** 10 mg followed by an infusion of 2-8 mg/minute. If hypertension is refractory, consider other I.V. antihypertensives (eg, nitroprusside)

Geriatric Oral: Initial dose: Refer to adult dosing. Usual maintenance: 100-200 mg twice daily

Pediatric Note: Due to limited documentation of its use, labetalol should be initiated cautiously in pediatric patients with careful dosage adjustment and blood pressure monitoring.

Hypertension:

Oral: Hypertension (unlabeled use): Initial: 1-3 mg/kg/day, in 2 divided doses; maximum: 10-12 mg/kg/day, up to 1200 mg/day

I.V.: Intermittent bolus doses of 0.3-1 mg/kg/dose have been reported.

Pediatric hypertensive emergencies: Initial continuous infusions of 0.4-1 mg/kg/hour with a maximum of 3 mg/kg/hour have been used; administration requires the use of an infusion pump.

Renal Impairment Not removed by hemo- or peritoneal dialysis; supplemental dose is not necessary.

Hepatic Impairment Dosage reduction may be necessary.

Administration

I.V. Bolus dose may be administered I.V. push at a rate of 10 mg/minute; may follow with continuous I.V. infusion

Stability

Reconstitution

Standard concentration: 500 mg/250 mL D_5W.

Minimum volume: 250 mL D_5W.

Storage

Tablets: Store tablets at 2°C to 30°C (36°F to 86°F). Protect from light and excessive moisture.

Vials: Store unopened injectable vials at 20°C to 25°C (68°F to 77°F); do not freeze. Protect from light. The solution is clear to slightly yellow.

Parenteral admixture: Stability of parenteral admixture at room temperature (25°C) and refrigeration temperature (4°C): 3 days.

Monitoring and Teaching Issues

Physical Assessment Blood pressure and heart rate should be assessed prior to and following first dose and any change in dosage. Caution patients with diabetes to monitor glucose levels closely; beta-blockers may alter glucose tolerance. Monitor for CHF.

Patient Education Take with meals. This medication does not replace other antihypertensive interventions; follow prescriber's instructions for diet and lifestyle changes. If you have diabetes, monitor serum glucose closely and notify prescriber of changes (this medication can alter glycemic response). You may experience drowsiness, dizziness, postural hypotension, or dry mouth. Report altered CNS status (eg, fatigue, depression, numbness or tingling of fingers, toes, or skin), palpitations or slowed heartbeat, respiratory difficulty, edema, or cold extremities.

Geriatric Considerations Due to alterations in the beta-adrenergic autonomic nervous system, beta-adrenergic blockade may result in less hemodynamic response than seen in younger adults. Studies indicate that despite decreased sensitivity to the chronotropic effects of beta-blockade with age, there appears to be an increased myocardial sensitivity to the negative inotropic effect during stress (ie, exercise). Controlled trials have shown the overall response rate for propranolol to be only 20% to 50% in elderly populations. Therefore, all beta-adrenergic blocking drugs may result in a decreased response as compared to younger adults.

Breast-Feeding Considerations Low amounts of labetalol are found in breast milk and can be detected in the serum of nursing infants. The manufacturer recommends that caution be exercised when administering labetalol to nursing women.

Pregnancy Considerations Because adverse events were observed in some animal reproduction studies, labetalol is classified as pregnancy category C. Labetalol crosses the placenta and can be detected in cord blood and infant serum after delivery. It has been shown to decrease maternal blood pressure without significantly effecting placental blood flow. In a cohort study, an increased risk of cardiovascular defects was observed following maternal use of beta-blockers during pregnancy. Intrauterine growth restriction (IUGR), small placentas, as well as fetal/neonatal bradycardia, hypoglycemia, and/or respiratory depression have been observed following *in utero* exposure to beta-blockers as a class. Adequate facilities for monitoring infants at birth should be available. Untreated chronic maternal hypertension and pre-eclampsia are also associated with adverse events in the fetus, infant, and mother. The pharmacokinetics of labetalol are not significantly changed during the third trimester of pregnancy. Labetalol is considered an appropriate agent for the treatment of hypertension in pregnancy; intravenous labetalol is also used for the management of pre-eclampsia.

Related Information

Beta-Blockers *on page 1990*

Hyperlipidemia Management *on page 2046*

◆ **Labetalol Hydrochloride** *see* Labetalol *on page 1048*

Lacosamide (la KOE sa mide)

U.S. Brand Names Vimpat®

Index Terms ADD 234037; Harkoseride; LCM; SPM 927

Generic Availability (U.S.) No

Pharmacologic Category Anticonvulsant, Miscellaneous

Medication Safety Issues

Sound-alike/look-alike issues:

Lacosamide may be confused with zonisamide

Vimpat® may be confused with Vimovo™

Medication Guide Available Yes

Pregnancy Risk Factor C

Lactation Excretion in breast milk unknown/not recommended

Use Adjunctive therapy in the treatment of partial-onset seizures

Mechanism of Action/Effect Lacosamide stabilizes hyperexcitable neuronal membranes and inhibits repetitive neuronal firing to decrease epileptiform activity.

Contraindications There are no contraindications listed in manufacturer's labeling.

Warnings/Precautions Antiepileptics are associated with an increased risk of suicidal behavior/thoughts with use (regardless of indication); patients should be monitored for signs/symptoms of depression, suicidal tendencies, and other unusual behavior changes during therapy and instructed to inform their healthcare provider immediately if symptoms occur. CNS effects may occur; patients should be cautioned about performing tasks which require alertness (eg, operating machinery or driving). Lacosamide may prolong PR interval; use caution in patients with conduction problems (eg, first/second degree atrioventricular block and sick sinus syndrome without pacemaker), myocardial ischemia, heart failure, or if concurrent use with other drugs that prolong the PR interval; ECG is recommended prior to initiating therapy and when at steady state. During investigational trials, atrial fibrillation/flutter, or syncope occurred slightly more often in patients with diabetic neuropathy and/or cardiovascular disease. Use caution with renal or hepatic impairment; dosage adjustment may be necessary. Multiorgan hypersensitivity reactions can occur (rare); monitor patient and discontinue therapy if necessary. Withdraw therapy gradually (≥1 week) to minimize the potential of increased seizure frequency. Effects with ethanol may be potentiated. Some products may contain phenylalanine.

Drug Interactions

Avoid Concomitant Use There are no known interactions where it is recommended to avoid concomitant use.

Decreased Effect

The levels/effects of Lacosamide may be decreased by: CarBAMazepine; PHENobarbital; Phenytoin

Increased Effect/Toxicity There are no known significant interactions involving an increase in effect.

Nutritional/Ethanol Interactions Ethanol: Avoid ethanol (may increase CNS depression).

Adverse Reactions

>10%:

Central nervous system: Dizziness (31%), headache (13%)

Gastrointestinal: Nausea (11%)

Ocular: Diplopia (11%)

1% to 10%:

Cardiovascular: Syncope (1%; dose-related: >400 mg/day)

Central nervous system: Fatigue (9%), ataxia (8%), somnolence (7%), coordination impaired (4%), vertigo (4%), depression (2%), memory impairment (2%)

Dermatologic: Pruritus (2%)

Gastrointestinal: Vomiting (9%), diarrhea (4%)

Hepatic: ALT increased (1%)

Local: Contusion (3%), skin laceration (3%), injection site pain/discomfort (2.5%), irritation (1%)

Neuromuscular & skeletal: Tremor (7%), gait instability (2%), weakness (2%)

Ocular: Blurred vision (8%), nystagmus (5%)

Pharmacodynamics/Kinetics

Absorption Oral: Completely

Bioavailability ~100%

Time to Peak Oral: 1-4 hours postdose

Protein Binding <15%

Half-Life Elimination ~13 hours

Metabolism Hepatic; forms metabolite, O-desmethyl-lacosamide (inactive)

Excretion Urine (95%; 40% as unchanged drug, 30% as inactive metabolite, 20% as uncharacterized metabolite); feces (<0.5%)

Controlled Substance C-V

Available Dosage Forms

Injection, solution:

Vimpat®: 10 mg/mL (20 mL)

Solution, oral:

Vimpat®: 10 mg/mL (20 mL)

Tablet, oral:

Vimpat®: 50 mg, 100 mg, 150 mg, 200 mg

Dosing

Adult & Geriatric Partial onset seizure: Oral, I.V.:

Initial: 50 mg twice daily; may be increased at weekly intervals by 100 mg/day

Maintenance dose: 200-400 mg/day

Note: When switching from oral to I.V. formulations, the total daily dose and frequency should be the same; I.V. therapy should only be used temporarily.

Pediatric Adolescents ≥17 years: Refer to adult dosing.

Renal Impairment Use caution when titrating dose.

Mild-to-moderate renal impairment: No dose adjustment necessary.

Severe renal impairment (Cl_{cr} ≤30 mL/minute): Maximum dose: 300 mg/day.

Hemodialysis: Removed by hemodialysis; after 4-hour HD treatment, a supplemental dose of up to 50% should be considered.

Hepatic Impairment Use caution when titrating dose.

Mild-to-moderate hepatic impairment: Maximum dose: 300 mg/day.

Severe hepatic impairment: Use is not recommended.

Administration

Oral Oral solution, tablets: May be administered with or without food. Oral solution should be administered with a calibrated measuring device (not a household teaspoon or tablespoon).

I.V. Administer over 30-60 minutes. Twice daily I.V. infusions have been used for up to 5 days.

Stability

Reconstitution Injection solution: Can be administered without further dilution or may be mixed with compatible diluents (NS, LR, D_5W).

Storage

Injection: Store at 20°C to 25°C (68°F to 77°F); excursions permitted between 15°C to 30°C (59°F to 86°F). Do not freeze. Stable when mixed with compatible diluents for ≤24 hours in glass or PVC at room temperature of 15°C to 30°C (59°F to 86°F). Any unused portion should be discarded.

Oral solution, tablets: Store at 20°C to 25°C (68°F to 77°F); excursions permitted between 15°C to 30°C (59°F to 86°F). Do not freeze oral solution. Discard any unused portion of oral solution after 7 weeks.

Monitoring and Teaching Issues

Laboratory Monitoring ECG

Physical Assessment Taper dosage slowly when discontinuing. Do not discontinue abruptly. Monitor for depression. Be alert to suicide ideation. Teach patient safety and seizure precautions.

Patient Education Avoid alcohol. You may experience dizziness, lightheadedness, excessive drowsiness, headaches, nausea, vomiting, tremors, or change in vision. Contact prescriber if symptoms persist. Report signs of suicide ideation or depression.

Dietary Considerations Oral solution and tablets may be taken with or without food. Some products may contain phenylalanine.

Geriatric Considerations Elderly often have compromised renal function with creatinine clearance <30 mL/minute. Evaluate (calculate) creatinine clearance in elderly before initiating lacosamide therapy. Monitor closely those elderly with cardiac disease and/or conduction disease. No specific data in studies related to elderly to date.

Breast-Feeding Considerations It is unknown if lacosamide is excreted in human milk. Use during lactation only if the potential benefits to the mother outweigh the potential risks to the infant.

Pregnancy Considerations Developmental toxicities were observed in animal studies. There are no adequate and well-controlled studies in pregnant women; only use during pregnancy if potential benefit justifies the potential risk to the fetus. Two registries are available for women exposed to lacosamide during pregnancy:

Antiepileptic Drug Pregnancy Registry (888-233-2334 or http://www.aedpregnancyregistry.org)

UCB AED Pregnancy Registry (888-537-7734)

Related Information

Anticonvulsant Drugs of Choice *on page 1981*

Lactulose (LAK tyoo lose)

U.S. Brand Names Constulose; Enulose; Generlac; Kristalose®

Generic Availability (U.S.) Yes: Excludes crystals for solution

Pharmacologic Category Ammonium Detoxicant; Laxative, Osmotic

Medication Safety Issues

Sound-alike/look-alike issues:

Lactulose may be confused with lactose

Pregnancy Risk Factor B

Lactation Excretion in breast milk unknown/use caution

Use Prevention and treatment of portal-systemic encephalopathy (including hepatic precoma and coma); treatment of constipation

Available Dosage Forms

Crystals for solution, oral:

Kristalose®: 10 g/packet (30s); 20 g/packet (30s)

Solution, oral: 10 g/15 mL (15 mL, 30 mL, 237 mL, 473 mL, 500 mL, 946 mL,1892 mL)

Constulose: 10 g/15 mL (237 mL, 946 mL)

Enulose: 10 g/15 mL (473 mL)

Solution, oral/rectal: 10 g/15 mL (237 mL, 473 mL, 946 mL)

Generlac: 10 g/15 mL (473 mL, 1892 mL)

Dosing

Adult & Geriatric

Constipation: Oral: 10-20 g (15-30 mL) daily; may increase to 40 g (60 mL) daily if necessary

Prevention of portal systemic encephalopathy (PSE): Oral: 20-30 g (30-45 mL) 3-4 times/day; adjust dose every 1-2 days to produce 2-3 soft stools/day

Treatment of acute PSE:

Oral: 20-30 g (30-45 mL) every 1 hour to induce rapid laxation; reduce to 20-30 g (30-45 mL) 3-4 times/day after laxation is achieved titrate to produce 2-3 soft stools/day

Rectal administration (retention enema): 200 g (300 mL) diluted with 700 mL of water or NS via rectal balloon catheter; retain for 30-60 minutes; may repeat every 4-6 hours; transition to oral treatment prior to discontinuing rectal administration

Pediatric

Prevention of portal systemic encephalopathy (PSE): Oral:

Infants: 1.7-6.7 g/day (2.5-10 mL/day) in divided doses; adjust dosage to produce 2-3 stools/day

Children: 26.7-60 g/day (40-90 mL/day) in divided doses; adjust dosage to produce 2-3 stools/day

Constipation (unlabeled use): Oral: 0.7-2 g/kg/day (1-3 mL/kg/day) in divided doses, maximum 40 g/day (60 mL/day) (NASPGHAN, 2006)

Administration

Oral

Oral solution: May mix with fruit juice, water, or milk.

Crystals for oral solution: Dissolve contents of packet in 120 mL water.

Other Rectal: Mix with water or normal saline; administer as retention enema using a rectal balloon catheter; retain for 30-60 minutes. Transition to oral lactulose when appropriate (able to take oral medication and no longer a risk for aspiration) prior to discontinuing rectal administration.

Monitoring and Teaching Issues

Laboratory Monitoring Serum electrolytes, serum ammonia

Physical Assessment Assess therapeutic effectiveness (soft formed stools or resolution of CNS status). Monitor frequency/consistency of stools. May need to adjust dose for severe diarrhea.

Patient Education Not for long-term use. Take alone or diluted with water, juice or milk, or take with food. Laxative results may not occur for 24-48 hours; do not take more often than recommended or for a longer time than recommended. Do not use any other laxatives while taking lactulose. Do not use if experiencing abdominal pain, nausea, or vomiting. Diarrhea may indicate need to decrease dose. May cause flatulence, belching, or abdominal cramping. Report persistent or severe diarrhea or abdominal cramping.

◆ **Ladakamycin** *see* AzaCITIDine *on page 175*

◆ **L-AmB** *see* Amphotericin B (Liposomal) *on page 121*

◆ **LaMICtal®** *see* LamoTRIgine *on page 1057*

◆ **LaMICtal® ODT™** *see* LamoTRIgine *on page* 1057

◆ **LaMICtal® XR™** *see* LamoTRIgine *on page* 1057

◆ **LamISIL®** *see* Terbinafine (Systemic) *on page* 1733

LamiVUDine (la MI vyoo deen)

U.S. Brand Names Epivir-HBV®; Epivir®

Index Terms 3TC

Generic Availability (U.S.) No

Pharmacologic Category Antiretroviral Agent, Reverse Transcriptase Inhibitor (Nucleoside)

Medication Safety Issues

Sound-alike/look-alike issues:

LamiVUDine may be confused with lamoTRIgine

Epivir® may be confused with Combivir®

Pregnancy Risk Factor C

Lactation Enters breast milk/contraindicated

Use

Epivir®: Treatment of HIV infection when antiretroviral therapy is warranted; should always be used as part of a multidrug regimen (at least three antiretroviral agents)

Epivir-HBV®: Treatment of chronic hepatitis B associated with evidence of hepatitis B viral replication and active liver inflammation

Unlabeled/Investigational Use Postexposure prophylaxis for HIV exposure as part of a multidrug regimen

Mechanism of Action/Effect Lamivudine is a cytosine analog. *In vitro*, lamivudine is phosphorylated to its active 5′-triphosphate metabolite (L-TP), which inhibits HIV reverse transcription via viral DNA chain termination; L-TP also inhibits the RNA- and DNA-dependent DNA polymerase activities of reverse transcriptase. The monophosphate form is incorporated into viral DNA by hepatitis B polymerase, resulting in DNA chain termination.

Contraindications Hypersensitivity to lamivudine or any component of the formulation

Warnings/Precautions Use caution with renal impairment; dosage reduction recommended. Use with extreme caution in children with history of pancreatitis or risk factors for development of pancreatitis. Pancreatitis has been reported, particularly in HIV-infected children with a history of nucleoside use. Do not use as monotherapy in treatment of HIV. Treatment of HBV in patients with unrecognized/untreated HIV may lead to rapid HIV resistance. In addition, treatment of HIV in patients with unrecognized/untreated HBV may lead to rapid HBV resistance. Use with caution in combination with interferon alfa with or without ribavirin in HIV/HBV coinfected patients; monitor closely for hepatic decompensation, anemia, or neutropenia; dose reduction or discontinuation of interferon and/or ribavirin may be required if toxicity evident. **[U.S. Boxed Warning]: Do not use Epivir-HBV® tablets or Epivir-HBV® oral solution for the treatment of HIV.**

[U.S. Boxed Warning]: Lactic acidosis and severe hepatomegaly with steatosis have been reported, including fatal cases. Use caution in hepatic impairment. Pregnancy, obesity, and/or prolonged therapy may increase the risk of lactic acidosis and liver damage.

Immune reconstitution syndrome may develop resulting in the occurrence of an inflammatory response to an indolent or residual opportunistic infection. May be associated with fat redistribution.

[U.S. Boxed Warning]: Monitor patients closely for several months following discontinuation of therapy for chronic hepatitis B; clinical exacerbations may occur.

Not recommended as first line therapy of chronic HBV due to high rate of resistance. May be appropriate for short-term treatment of acute HBV (Lok, 2009). Potential compliance problems, frequency of administration, and adverse effects should be discussed with patients before initiating therapy to help prevent the emergence of resistance.

Drug Interactions

Avoid Concomitant Use

Avoid concomitant use of LamiVUDine with any of the following: Emtricitabine

Decreased Effect There are no known significant interactions involving a decrease in effect.

Increased Effect/Toxicity

LamiVUDine may increase the levels/effects of: Emtricitabine

The levels/effects of LamiVUDine may be increased by: Ganciclovir-Valganciclovir; Ribavirin; Trimethoprim

Nutritional/Ethanol Interactions Food: Food decreases the rate of absorption and C_{max}; however, there is no change in the systemic AUC. Therefore, may be taken with or without food.

Adverse Reactions Reported for treatment of HIV or HBV in adults. Incidence data includes patients on combination therapy with other antiretroviral agents.

>10%:

Central nervous system: Headache (21% to 35%), fatigue (24% to 27%), insomnia (11%)

Gastrointestinal: Nausea (15% to 33%), diarrhea (14% to 18%), pancreatitis (range: 0.3% to 18%; higher percentage in pediatric patients), abdominal pain (9% to 16%), vomiting (13% to 15%)

Hematologic: Neutropenia (7% to 15%)

Hepatic: Transaminases increased (2% to 11%)

Neuromuscular & skeletal: Myalgia (8% to 14%), neuropathy (12%), musculoskeletal pain (12%)
Respiratory: Nasal signs and symptoms (20%), cough (18%), sore throat (13%)
Miscellaneous: Infections (25%; includes ear, nose, and throat)

1% to 10%:

Central nervous system: Dizziness (10%), depression (9%), fever (7% to 10%), chills (7% to 10%)
Dermatologic: Rash (5% to 9%)
Gastrointestinal: Anorexia (10%), lipase increased (10%), abdominal cramps (6%), dyspepsia (5%), amylase increased (<1% to 4%), heartburn
Hematologic: Thrombocytopenia (1% to 4%), hemoglobinemia (2% to 3%)
Neuromuscular & skeletal: Creatine phosphokinase increased (9%), arthralgia (5% to 7%)

Pharmacodynamics/Kinetics

Absorption Rapid

Bioavailability Absolute: Cp_{max} decreased with food although AUC not significantly affected
Children: 66%
Adults: 86% to 87%

Time to Peak Fed: 3.2 hours; Fasted: 0.9 hours

Protein Binding Plasma: <36%

Half-Life Elimination Children: 2 hours; Adults: 5-7 hours

Metabolism 4.2% to trans-sulfoxide metabolite

Excretion Primarily urine (as unchanged drug)

Available Dosage Forms

Solution, oral:
Epivir-HBV®: 5 mg/mL
Epivir®: 10 mg/mL

Tablet, oral:
Epivir-HBV®: 100 mg
Epivir®: 150 mg, 300 mg

Dosing

Adult & Geriatric Note: The formulation and dosage of Epivir-HBV® are not appropriate for patients infected with both HBV and HIV.

HIV: Oral (use with at least two other antiretroviral agents): 150 mg twice daily **or** 300 mg once daily
<50 kg: 4 mg/kg twice daily (maximum: 150 mg twice daily)

Postexposure prophylaxis for HIV exposure: Oral: 150 mg twice daily (with zidovudine with or without a protease inhibitor, depending on risk)

Prevention of maternal-fetal HIV transmission (AIDS*info* guidelines): Note: Lamivudine may be used in combination with zidovudine and nevirapine in select situations (eg, infants born to mothers with suboptimal viral suppression at delivery, infants born to mothers with only intrapartum therapy or no therapy, or infants born to mothers with known antiretroviral drug-resistant virus). Lamivudine is used in this situation to reduce the development of nevirapine resistant virus:
Mother: 150 mg twice daily starting at onset of labor and continuing through 1 week postpartum

Treatment of hepatitis B (Epivir-HBV®): Oral: 100 mg/day
Treatment duration (AASLD practice guidelines):
Hepatitis Be antigen (HBeAg) positive chronic hepatitis: Treat ≥1 year until HBeAg seroconversion and undetectable serum HBV DNA; continue therapy for ≥6 months after HBeAg seroconversion
HBeAg negative chronic hepatitis: Treat >1 year until hepatitis B surface antigen (HBsAg) clearance
Note: Patients achieving <2 log decrease in serum HBV DNA after at least 6 months of therapy should either receive additional treatment or be switched to an alternative therapy (Lok, 2009).

Pediatric Note: The formulation and dosage of Epivir-HBV® are not appropriate for patients infected with both HBV and HIV.

HIV: Oral (use with at least two other antiretroviral agents)
Neonates <30 days (AIDS*info* guidelines): 2 mg/kg/dose twice daily
Infants 1-3 months (AIDS*info* guidelines): 4 mg/kg/dose twice daily
Infants and Children 3 months to 16 years: 4 mg/kg/dose twice daily (maximum: 150 mg/dose twice daily)
Alternate weight-based dosing using scored 150 mg tablets (AIDSinfo guidelines):
14-21 kg: 75 mg/dose twice daily (150 mg/day)
22-29 kg: 75 mg in the morning, 150 mg in the evening (225 mg/day)
≥30 kg: 150 mg/dose twice daily (300 mg/day)
Children >16 years: Refer to adult dosing.

Treatment of hepatitis B/HIV coinfection (in patients with both infections requiring treatment): Oral: Infants and Children: 4 mg/kg/dose (maximum: 150 mg/dose) twice daily, in combination with other antiretrovirals in a HAART regimen (CDC, 2009)

Prevention of maternal-fetal HIV transmission (AIDS*info* guidelines): Note: Lamivudine may be used in combination with zidovudine and nevirapine in select situations (eg, infants born to mothers with suboptimal viral suppression at delivery, infants born to mothers with only intrapartum therapy or no therapy, or infants born to mothers with known antiretroviral drug-resistant virus). Lamivudine is used in this situation to reduce the development of nevirapine resistant virus:
Neonate: 2 mg/kg/dose twice daily given at birth through 1 week of age

Treatment of hepatitis B: Oral: Children 2-17 years: 3 mg/kg/dose once daily (maximum: 100 mg/day).

Treatment duration (AASLD practice guidelines):

Hepatitis Be antigen (HBeAg) positive chronic hepatitis: Treat ≥1 year until HBeAg seroconversion and undetectable serum HBV DNA; continue therapy for ≥6 months after HBeAg seroconversion

HBeAg negative chronic hepatitis: Treat >1 year until hepatitis B surface antigen (HBsAg) clearance

Note: Patients achieving <2 log decrease in serum HBV DNA after at least 6 months of therapy should either receive additional treatment or be switched to an alternative therapy (Lok, 2009).

Renal Impairment

HIV:

Patients ≤16 years: Insufficient data; however, dose reduction should be considered.

Patients >16 years:

Cl_{cr} 30-49 mL/minute: Administer 150 mg once daily

Cl_{cr} 15-29 mL/minute: Administer 150 mg first dose, then 100 mg once daily

Cl_{cr} 5-14 mL/minute: Administer 150 mg first dose, then 50 mg once daily

Cl_{cr} <5 mL/minute: Administer 50 mg first dose, then 25 mg once daily

Treatment of hepatitis B patients: Adults:

Cl_{cr} 30-49 mL/minute: Administer 100 mg first dose, then 50 mg once daily.

Cl_{cr} 15-29 mL/minute: Administer 100 mg first dose, then 25 mg once daily.

Cl_{cr} 5-14 mL/minute: Administer 35 mg first dose, then 15 mg once daily.

Cl_{cr} <5 mL/minute: Administer 35 mg first dose, then 10 mg once daily.

Dialysis: Negligible amounts are removed by 4-hour hemodialysis or peritoneal dialysis. Supplemental dosing is not required.

Administration

Oral May be administered without regard to meals. Adjust dosage in renal failure.

Stability

Storage

Oral solution:

Epivir®: Store at 25°C (77°F) tightly closed.

Epivir-HBV®: Store at 20°C to 25°C (68°F to 77°F) tightly closed.

Tablet: Store at 25°C (77°F); excursions permitted to 15°C to 30°C (59°F to 86°F).

Monitoring and Teaching Issues

Laboratory Monitoring Amylase, bilirubin, liver enzymes (every 3 months during therapy), hematologic parameters, HIV viral load, and CD4 count; HBV DNA (every 3-6 months during therapy); HBeAg and anti-HBe (after 1 year of therapy and every 3-6 months thereafter)

Physical Assessment Use caution in presence of impaired renal function. Monitor for headache, fatigue, and insomnia on a regular basis throughout therapy. Monitor patients closely for several months following discontinuation of therapy for chronic hepatitis B. Teach patient proper timing of multiple medications.

Patient Education Maintain adequate hydration unless instructed to restrict fluid intake. This medication may be prescribed with a combination of other medications; time these medications as directed by prescriber. Take with or without food. Frequent blood tests may be required. May cause nausea, vomiting, abdominal pain, diarrhea, dizziness, insomnia, headache, fever, or muscle pain. Report persistent lethargy or unusual fatigue, yellowing of eyes, pale stool and dark urine, acute headache, severe nausea or vomiting, respiratory difficulty, loss of sensation, or rash.

Dietary Considerations May be taken without regard to meals. Some products may contain sucrose.

Breast-Feeding Considerations In infants born to mothers who are HIV positive, HAART while breast-feeding may decrease postnatal infection. However, maternal or infant antiretroviral therapy does not completely eliminate the risk of postnatal HIV transmission. In addition, multiclass-resistant virus has been detected in breast-feeding infants despite maternal therapy.

In the United States where formula is accessible, affordable, safe, and sustainable, complete avoidance of breast-feeding by HIV-infected women is recommended to decrease potential transmission of HIV.

Pregnancy Considerations Adverse events were observed in some animal reproduction studies. Lamivudine crosses the human placenta. No increased risk of overall birth defects has been observed following first trimester exposure according to data collected by the antiretroviral pregnancy registry. The pharmacokinetics of lamivudine during pregnancy are not significantly altered and dosage adjustment is not required. The Perinatal HIV Guidelines Working Group recommends lamivudine for use during pregnancy; the combination of lamivudine with zidovudine is the recommended dual combination NRTI in pregnancy. It may also be used in combination with zidovudine in HIV-infected women who are in labor, but have had no prior antiretroviral therapy, in order to reduce the maternal-fetal transmission of HIV. Cases of lactic acidosis/hepatic steatosis syndrome related to mitochondrial toxicity have been reported in pregnant women receiving nucleoside analogues. It is not known if pregnancy itself potentiates this known side effect; however, women may be at increased risk of lactic acidosis and liver damage. In addition, these adverse events are similar to other rare but life-threatening syndromes which occur during pregnancy (eg, HELLP syndrome). Hepatic enzymes and electrolytes should be monitored frequently during the third trimester of pregnancy in women receiving nucleoside analogues and clinicians should watch for early signs of the syndrome. Use caution with hepatitis B coinfection; hepatitis B flare may occur if lamivudine is discontinued postpartum. Healthcare providers are encouraged to enroll pregnant women exposed to antiretroviral medications in the Antiretroviral Pregnancy Registry (1-800-258-4263 or www.APRegistry.com). Healthcare providers caring for HIV-infected women and their infants may contact the National Perinatal HIV Hotline (888-448-8765) for clinical consultation.

- **Lamivudine, Abacavir, and Zidovudine** *see* Abacavir, Lamivudine, and Zidovudine *on page 32*
- **Lamivudine and Abacavir** *see* Abacavir and Lamivudine *on page 32*
- **Lamivudine and Zidovudine** *see* Zidovudine and Lamivudine *on page 1894*

LamoTRIgine (la MOE tri jeen)

U.S. Brand Names LaMICtal®; LaMICtal® ODT™; LaMICtal® XR™

Index Terms BW-430C; LTG

Generic Availability (U.S.) Yes; excludes extended release tablet, orally disintegrating tablet

Pharmacologic Category Anticonvulsant, Miscellaneous

Medication Safety Issues

Sound-alike/look-alike issues:

LamoTRIgine may be confused with labetalol, Lamisil®, lamiVUDine, levothyroxine, Lomotil®, ludiomil

LaMICtal® may be confused with LamISIL®, Lomotil®, ludiomil

Potential exists for medication errors to occur among different formulations of Lamictal® (tablets, extended release tablets, orally disintegrating tablets, and chewable/dispersible tablets). Patients should be instructed to visually inspect tablets dispensed to verify receiving the correct medication and formulation. The medication guide includes illustrations to aid in tablet verification.

Medication Guide Available Yes

Pregnancy Risk Factor C

Lactation Enters breast milk/not recommended (AAP rates "of concern"; AAP 2001 update pending)

Use Adjunctive therapy in the treatment of generalized seizures of Lennox-Gastaut syndrome, primary generalized tonic-clonic seizures, and partial seizures in adults and children ≥2 years of age; conversion to monotherapy in adults (≥16 years of age) with partial seizures who are receiving treatment with valproic acid or a single enzyme-inducing antiepileptic drug (specifically carbamazepine, phenytoin, phenobarbital or primidone); maintenance treatment of bipolar I disorder in adults

Mechanism of Action/Effect A triazine derivative which inhibits release of glutamate (an excitatory amino acid) and inhibits voltage-sensitive sodium channels, which stabilizes neuronal membranes. Lamotrigine has weak inhibitory effect on the $5HT_3$ receptor; *in vitro* inhibits dihydrofolate reductase.

Contraindications Hypersensitivity to lamotrigine or any component of the formulation

Warnings/Precautions [U.S. Boxed Warning]: Severe and potentially life-threatening skin rashes requiring hospitalization have been reported; risk may be increased by coadministration with valproic acid, higher than recommended starting doses, and rapid dose titration. The majority of cases occur in the first 8 weeks; however, isolated cases may occur after prolonged treatment or in patients without these risk factors. Discontinue at first sign of rash unless rash is clearly not drug related. Rare cases of Stevens-Johnson syndrome, toxic epidermal necrolysis, and angioedema have been reported.

Antiepileptics are associated with an increased risk of suicidal behavior/thoughts with use (regardless of indication); patients should be monitored for signs/symptoms of depression, suicidal tendencies, and other unusual behavior changes during therapy and instructed to inform their healthcare provider immediately if symptoms occur.

Acute multiorgan failure has also been reported. A spectrum of hematologic effects have been reported with use (eg, neutropenia, leukopenia, thrombocytopenia, pancytopenia, anemias, and rarely, aplastic anemia and pure red cell aplasia); patients with a previous history of adverse hematologic reaction to any drug may be at increased risk. Early detection of hematologic change is important; advise patients of early signs and symptoms including fever, sore throat, mouth ulcers, infections, easy bruising, petechial or purpuric hemorrhage. May be associated with hypersensitivity syndrome. Use caution in patients with impaired renal, hepatic, or cardiac function. Avoid abrupt cessation, taper over at least 2 weeks if possible. May cause CNS depression, which may impair physical or mental abilities. Patients must be cautioned about performing tasks which require mental alertness (eg, operating machinery or driving). Effects with other sedative drugs or ethanol may be potentiated. Binds to melanin and may accumulate in the eye and other melanin-rich tissues; the clinical significance of this is not known. Safety and efficacy have not been established for use as initial monotherapy, conversion to monotherapy from antiepileptic drugs (AED) other than carbamazepine, phenytoin, phenobarbital, primidone or valproic acid or conversion to monotherapy from two or more AEDs. Patients treated for bipolar disorder should be monitored closely for clinical worsening or suicidality; prescriptions should be written for the smallest quantity consistent with good patient care. Hormonal contraceptives may cause a decrease in lamotrigine levels; dose adjustment of the lamotrigine maintenance dose may be required when initiating or discontinuing estrogen-containing oral contraceptives. Valproic acid may cause an increase in lamotrigine levels requiring dose adjustment. There is a potential for medication errors with similar-sounding medications and among different lamotrigine formulations; medication errors have occurred.

Drug Interactions

Avoid Concomitant Use There are no known interactions where it is recommended to avoid concomitant use.

Decreased Effect

LamoTRIgine may decrease the levels/effects of: Contraceptives (Progestins)

The levels/effects of LamoTRIgine may be decreased by: Barbiturates; CarBAMazepine; Contraceptives (Estrogens); Ketorolac; Ketorolac (Systemic); Mefloquine; Phenytoin; Primidone; Rifampin; Ritonavir

Increased Effect/Toxicity

LamoTRIgine may increase the levels/effects of: Alcohol (Ethyl); CarBAMazepine; CNS Depressants; Desmopressin; Methotrimeprazine; OLANZapine

The levels/effects of LamoTRIgine may be increased by: Divalproex; Droperidol; Methotrimeprazine; Valproic Acid

Nutritional/Ethanol Interactions

Ethanol: Avoid ethanol (may increase CNS depression).
Food: Has no effect on absorption.
Herb/Nutraceutical: Avoid evening primrose (seizure threshold decreased).

Adverse Reactions Percentages reported in adults on monotherapy for epilepsy or bipolar disorder.

>10%: Gastrointestinal: Nausea (7% to 14%)

1% to 10%:

Cardiovascular: Chest pain (5%), peripheral edema (2% to 5%), edema (1% to 5%)

Central nervous system: Insomnia (5% to 10%), somnolence (9%), fatigue (8%), coordination impaired (7%), dizziness (7%), anxiety (5%), pain (5%), ataxia (2% to 5%), irritability (2% to 5%), suicidal ideation (2% to 5%), agitation (1% to 5%), amnesia (1% to 5%), depression (1% to 5%), dream abnormality (1% to 5%), emotional lability (1% to 5%), fever (1% to 5%), hypoesthesia (1% to 5%), migraine (1% to 5%), thought abnormality (1% to 5%), confusion (1%)

Dermatologic: Rash (nonserious: 7%), dermatitis (2% to 5%), dry skin (2% to 5%)

Endocrine & metabolic: Dysmenorrhea (5%), libido increased (2% to 5%)

Gastrointestinal: Vomiting (5% to 9%), dyspepsia (7%), abdominal pain (6%), xerostomia (2% to 6%), constipation (5%), weight loss (5%), anorexia (2% to 5%), peptic ulcer (2% to 5%), rectal hemorrhage (2% to 5%), flatulence (1% to 5%), weight gain (1% to 5%)

Genitourinary: Urinary frequency (1% to 5%)

Neuromuscular & skeletal: Back pain (8%), weakness (2% to 5%), arthralgia (1% to 5%), myalgia (1% to 5%), neck pain (1% to 5%), paresthesia (1%)

Ocular: Nystagmus (2% to 5%), vision abnormal (2% to 5%), amblyopia (1%)

Respiratory: Rhinitis (7%), cough (5%), pharyngitis (5%), bronchitis (2% to 5%), dyspnea (2% to 5%), epistaxis (2% to 5%), sinusitis (1% to 5%)

Miscellaneous: Infection (5%), diaphoresis (2% to 5%), reflexes increased/decreased (2% to 5%), dyspraxia (1% to 5%)

Pharmacodynamics/Kinetics

Absorption Immediate release: Rapid and complete

Bioavailability Immediate release: 98%; Extended release: ~77%

Time to Peak Plasma: Immediate release: 1-1.5 hours; Extended release: 4-11 hours (dependent on adjunct therapy)

Protein Binding ~55%

Half-Life Elimination Immediate release: Adults: 25-33 hours, Elderly: 25-43 hours;

Extended release: Similar to immediate release
Concomitant valproic acid therapy: 48-70 hours
Concomitant phenytoin, phenobarbital, primidone, or carbamazepine therapy: 13-14 hours
Chronic renal failure: 43 hours
Hemodialysis: 13 hours during dialysis; 57 hours between dialysis (~20% of a dose is eliminated in a 4-hour dialysis session)
Hepatic impairment:
Mild: 26-66 hours
Moderate: 28-116 hours
Severe without ascites: 56-78 hours
Severe with ascites: 52-148 hours

Metabolism Hepatic and renal; metabolized primarily by glucuronic acid conjugation to inactive metabolites

Excretion Urine (94%, ~90% as glucuronide conjugates and ~10% unchanged); feces (2%)

Available Dosage Forms

Tablet, oral: 25 mg, 100 mg, 150 mg, 200 mg

LaMICtal®: 25 mg, 100 mg, 150 mg, 200 mg, 25 mg (42s) [white tablets] and 100 mg (7s) [peach tablets], 25 mg (84s) [white tablets] and 100 mg (14s) [peach tablets]

Tablet, chewable/dispersible, oral: 5 mg, 25 mg

LaMICtal®: 2 mg, 5 mg, 25 mg

Tablet, extended release, oral:

LaMICtal® XR™: 25 mg, 50 mg, 100 mg, 200 mg, 25 mg (21s) [yellow/white tablets] and 50 mg (7s) [green/white tablets], 50 mg (14s) [green/white tablets], 100 mg (14s) [orange/white tablets], and 200 mg (7s) [blue/white tablets], 25 mg (14s) [yellow/white tablets], 50 mg (14s) [green/white tablets], and 100 mg (7s) [orange/white tablets]

Tablet, orally disintegrating, oral:

LaMICtal® ODT™: 25 mg, 50 mg, 100 mg, 200 mg, 25 mg (21s) and 50 mg (7s), 50 mg (42s) and 100 mg (14s), 25 mg (14s), 50 mg (14s), and 100 mg (7s)

Dosing

Adult & Geriatric Note: Only whole tablets should be used for dosing, round calculated dose down to the nearest whole tablet. Enzyme-inducing regimens specifically refer to those containing carbamazepine, phenytoin, phenobarbital, or primidone. Oral:

Lennox-Gastaut (adjunctive), primary generalized tonic-clonic seizures (adjunctive) or partial seizures (adjunctive): Immediate release formulations: Initial: 25 mg/day for weeks 1 and 2, then increase to 50 mg/day for weeks 3 and 4; maintenance: titrate dose to effect; after week 4 increase daily dose every 1-2 weeks by 50 mg/day; usual maintenance: 225-375 mg/day in 2 divided doses.

Adjustment for AED regimens **containing** valproic acid (see "**Note**" below): Initial: 25 mg every other day for weeks 1 and 2, then increase to 25 mg every day for weeks 3 and 4. Maintenance: Titrate dose to effect; after week 4 increase daily dose every 1-2 weeks by 25-50 mg/day; usual maintenance: 100-400 mg/day in 1 or 2 divided doses.

Note: For patients taking lamotrigine with valproic acid alone, the usual maintenance dose is 100-200 mg/day.

Adjustment for **enzyme-inducing** AED regimens **without** valproic acid: Initial: 50 mg/day for weeks 1 and 2, then increase to 100 mg/day in 2 divided doses for weeks 3 and 4. Maintenance: Titrate dose to effects; after week 4 increase daily dose every 1-2 weeks by 100 mg/day; usual maintenance: 300-500 mg/day in 2 divided doses. Doses as high as 700 mg/day have been used, though additional benefit has not been established.

Conversion to monotherapy with lamotrigine:

Conversion from adjunctive therapy with valproic acid: Initiate and titrate as per recommendations to a lamotrigine dose of 200 mg/day. Then taper valproic acid dose in decrements of not >500 mg/day at intervals of 1 week (or longer) to a valproic acid dosage of 500 mg/day; this dosage should be maintained for 1 week. The lamotrigine dosage should then be increased to 300 mg/day while valproic acid is decreased to 250 mg/day; this dosage should be maintained for 1 week. Valproic acid may then be discontinued, while the lamotrigine dose is increased by 100 mg/day at weekly intervals to achieve a lamotrigine maintenance dose of 500 mg/day.

Conversion from adjunctive therapy with carbamazepine, phenytoin, phenobarbital, or primidone: Initiate and titrate as per recommendations to a lamotrigine dose of 500 mg/day. Concomitant enzyme-inducing AED should then be withdrawn by 20% decrements each week over a 4-week period. Patients should be monitored for rash.

Conversion from adjunctive therapy with AED other than carbamazepine, phenytoin, phenobarbital, primidone or valproic acid: No specific guidelines available.

Partial seizures (adjunctive) and primary generalized tonic-clonic seizures (adjunctive): Extended release formulation: **Note:** Dose increases after week 8 should not exceed 100 mg/day at weekly intervals

Regimens **containing** valproic acid: Initial: Week 1 and 2: 25 mg every other day; Week 3 and 4: 25 mg once daily; Week 5: 50 mg once daily; Week 6: 100 mg once daily; Week 7: 150 mg once daily; Maintenance: 200-250 mg once daily

Regimens **containing** carbamazepine, phenytoin, phenobarbital, or primidone and **without** valproic acid: Initial: Week 1 and 2: 50 mg once daily; Week 3 and 4: 100 mg once daily; Week 5: 200 mg once daily; Week 6: 300 mg once daily; Week 7: 400 mg once daily; Maintenance: 400-600 mg once daily

Regimens **not containing** carbamazepine, phenytoin, phenobarbital, primidone, or valproic acid: Initial: Week 1 and 2: 25 mg once daily; Week 3 and 4: 50 mg once daily; Week 5: 100 mg once daily; Week 6: 150 mg once daily; Week 7: 200 mg once daily; Maintenance: 300-400 mg once daily

Bipolar disorder: Initial: 25 mg/day for weeks 1 and 2, then increase to 50 mg/day for weeks 3 and 4, then increase to 100 mg/day for week 5; Maintenance: Increase dose to 200 mg/day beginning week 6.

Adjustment for regimens **containing** valproic acid: Initial: 25 mg every other day for weeks 1 and 2, then increase to 25 mg every day for weeks 3 and 4, then increase to 50 mg/day for week 5. Maintenance: 100 mg/day beginning week 6.

Adjustment for **enzyme-inducing** regimens **without** valproic acid: Initial: 50 mg/day for weeks 1 and 2, then increase to 100 mg/day in divided doses for weeks 3 and 4, then increase to 200 mg/day in divided doses for week 5, then increase to 300 mg/day in divided dose for week 6. Maintenance: 400 mg/day in divided doses beginning week 7.

Adjustment following discontinuation of psychotropic medication:

Discontinuing valproic acid with current dose of lamotrigine 100 mg/day: 150 mg/day for week 1, then increase to 200 mg/day beginning week 2.

Discontinuing carbamazepine, phenytoin, phenobarbital, primidone, or rifampin with current dose of lamotrigine 400 mg/day: 400 mg/day for week 1, then decrease to 300 mg/day for week 2, then decrease to 200 mg/day beginning week 3.

Conversion from immediate release to extended release (Lamictal® XR™): Initial dose of the extended release tablet should match the total daily dose of the immediate-release formulation; monitor for seizure control, especially in patients on AED agents. Adjust dose as needed within the recommended dosing guidelines.

Discontinuing therapy: Decrease dose by ~50% per week, over at least 2 weeks unless safety concerns require a more rapid withdrawal. Discontinuing carbamazepine, phenytoin, phenobarbital, primidone, or rifampin should prolong the half-life of lamotrigine; discontinuing valproic acid should shorten the half-life of lamotrigine

Restarting therapy after discontinuation: If lamotrigine has been withheld for >5 half-lives, consider restarting according to initial dosing recommendations.

Dosage adjustment with estrogen-containing hormonal contraceptives: Follow initial lamotrigine dosing guidelines, maintenance dose should be adjusted as follows:

Patients taking concomitant carbamazepine, phenytoin, phenobarbital, primidone or rifampin: No dosing adjustment required

Patients **not** taking concomitant carbamazepine, phenytoin, phenobarbital, primidone or rifampin: Lamotrigine maintenance dose may need increased by twofold over target dose. If already taking a stable dose of lamotrigine and starting contraceptive, maintenance dose may need increased by twofold. Dose increases should start when contraceptive is started and titrated to clinical response increasing no more rapidly than 50-100 mg/day every week. Gradual increases of lamotrigine plasma levels may occur during the inactive "pill-free" week and will be greater when dose increases are made the week before. If increased adverse events consistently occur during "pill-free" week, overall maintenance dose adjustments may be required. When discontinuing estrogen-containing hormonal contraceptive, dose of lamotrigine may need decreased by as much as 50%; do not decrease by more than 25% of total daily dose over a 2-week period unless clinical response or plasma levels indicate otherwise. Dose adjustments during "pill-free" week are not recommended.

Pediatric Note: Only whole tablets should be used for dosing, round calculated dose down to the nearest whole tablet. Extended release tablets not approved for use in children ≤12 years of age. Enzyme-inducing regimens specifically refer to those containing carbamazepine, phenytoin, phenobarbital, or primidone.

Lennox-Gastaut (adjunctive), primary generalized tonic-clonic seizures (adjunctive), or partial seizures (adjunctive): Oral: **Note:** Children <30 kg will likely require maintenance doses to be increased as much as 50% based on clinical response regardless of regimen below:

Children 2-12 years: Immediate release formulations: Initial: 0.3 mg/kg/day in 1-2 divided doses for weeks 1 and 2, then increase to 0.6 mg/kg/day in 2 divided doses for weeks 3 and 4; maintenance: titrate dose to effect; after week 4, increase daily dose every 1-2 weeks by 0.6 mg/kg/day; usual maintenance: 4.5-7.5 mg/kg/day in 2 divided doses; maximum: 300 mg/day in 2 divided doses.

Adjustment for AED regimens **containing** valproic acid (see **"Note"** below): Initial: 0.15 mg/kg/day in 1-2 divided doses for weeks 1 and 2, then increase to 0.3 mg/kg/day in 1-2 divided doses for weeks 3 and 4; maintenance: titrate dose to effect; after week 4, increase daily dose every 1-2 weeks by 0.3 mg/kg/day; usual maintenance: 1-5 mg/kg/day in 2 divided doses; maximum: 200 mg/day in 1-2 divided doses

Note: For patients >6.7 kg and <14 kg, initial dosing should be 2 mg every other day for first 2 weeks, then increased to 2 mg daily for weeks 3-4. For patients taking lamotrigine with valproic acid alone, the usual maintenance dose is 1-3 mg/kg/day in 2 divided doses

Adjustment for **enzyme-inducing** AED regimens **without** valproic acid: Initial: 0.6 mg/kg/day in 2 divided doses for weeks 1 and 2, then increase to 1.2 mg/kg/day in 2 divided doses for weeks 3 and 4; maintenance: titrate dose to effect; after week 4, increase daily dose every 1-2 weeks by 1.2 mg/kg/day; usual maintenance: 5-15 mg/kg/day in 2 divided doses; maximum: 400 mg/day in 2 divided doses

Children >12 years: Refer to adult dosing.

Conversion from single enzyme-inducing AED regimen to monotherapy: Children ≥16 years: Refer to adult dosing.

Discontinuing therapy: Refer to adult dosing.

Restarting therapy after discontinuation: Refer to adult dosing.

Dosage adjustment with estrogen-containing hormonal contraceptives: Refer to adult dosing.

Renal Impairment Decreased maintenance dosage may be effective in patients with significant renal impairment; has not been adequately studied; use with caution.

Hepatic Impairment

Mild impairment: No adjustment required.

Moderate-to-severe impairment without ascites: Decrease initial, escalation, and maintenance doses by ~25%; adjust as clinically indicated.

Moderate-to-severe impairment with ascites: Decrease initial, escalation, and maintenance doses by ~50%; adjust according to clinical response.

Administration

Oral Doses should be rounded down to the nearest whole tablet.

Lamictal® chewable/dispersible tablets: May be chewed, dispersed in water or diluted fruit juice, or swallowed whole. To disperse tablets, add to a small amount of liquid (just enough to cover tablet); let sit ~1 minute until dispersed; swirl solution and consume immediately. Do not administer partial amounts of liquid. If tablets are chewed, a small amount of water or diluted fruit juice should be used to aid in swallowing.

Lamictal® ODT™: Place tablets on tongue and move around in the mouth. Tablets will dissolve rapidly and can be swallowed with or without food or water.

Lamictal® XR™: Administer without regard to meals. Swallow whole; do not chew, crush, or cut.

Stability

Storage Store at 25°C (77°F); excursions permitted to 15°C to 30°C (59°F to 86°F). Protect from light.

Monitoring and Teaching Issues

Laboratory Monitoring Serum levels of concurrent anticonvulsants, LFTs, renal function

Physical Assessment Monitor for skin rash. Discontinue at the first sign of rash, unless clearly not drug-related. Monitor for suicide ideation, depression, or unusual behavior changes. Taper dosage slowly when discontinuing. Observe and teach seizure/safety precautions.

Patient Education Only whole tablets should be used for dosing, rounded down to the nearest whole tablet. While using this medication, do not use alcohol. Maintain adequate hydration unless instructed to restrict fluid intake. You may experience drowsiness, dizziness, blurred vision, nausea, vomiting, loss of appetite, heartburn, or dry mouth. Wear identification of epileptic status and medications. Report CNS changes, mentation changes, suicide ideation, depression, or changes in cognition; persistent GI symptoms (cramping, constipation, vomiting, anorexia); swelling of face, lips, or tongue; easy bruising or bleeding (mouth, urine, stool); vision changes; worsening of seizure activity, or loss of seizure control. A skin rash may indicate a serious medical problem; contact prescriber immediately if rash noted.

Geriatric Considerations No pharmacokinetic differences noted between young adults and the elderly. Use with caution in the elderly with significant renal decline.

Breast-Feeding Considerations Lamotrigine is found in breast milk. In one study, the relative dose to the infant was 9% (range: 2% to 20%) of the weight-adjusted maternal dose. Lamotrigine was measurable in the plasma of nursing infants; adverse events were not observed.

Pregnancy Considerations Lamotrigine has been found to decrease folate concentrations in animal studies. Teratogenic effects in animals were not observed. Lamotrigine crosses the human placenta and can be measured in the plasma of exposed newborns. Preliminary data from the North American Antiepileptic Drug Pregnancy Registry (NAAED) suggest an increased incidence of cleft lip and/or cleft palate following first trimester exposure. Healthcare providers may enroll patients in the Lamotrigine Pregnancy Registry by calling (800) 336-2176. Patients may enroll themselves in the NAAED registry by calling (888) 233-2334. Additional information is available at www.aedpregnancyregistry.org. Dose of lamotrigine may need adjustment during pregnancy to maintain clinical response; lamotrigine serum levels may decrease during pregnancy and return to prepartum levels following delivery. Monitor frequently during pregnancy, following delivery, and when adding or discontinuing combination hormonal contraceptives.

Related Information

Anticonvulsant Drugs of Choice *on page 1981*

◆ **Lanoxin®** *see* Digoxin *on page 529*

Lansoprazole (lan SOE pra zole)

U.S. Brand Names Prevacid®; Prevacid® 24 HR [OTC]; Prevacid® SoluTab™

Generic Availability (U.S.) Yes

Pharmacologic Category Proton Pump Inhibitor; Substituted Benzimidazole

Medication Safety Issues

Sound-alike/look-alike issues:

Lansoprazole may be confused with aripiprazole, dexlansoprazole

Prevacid® may be confused with Pravachol®, Prevpac®, PriLOSEC®, Prinivil®

Pregnancy Risk Factor B

Lactation Excretion in breast milk unknown/not recommended

Use Short-term treatment of active duodenal ulcers; maintenance treatment of healed duodenal ulcers; as part of a multidrug regimen for *H. pylori* eradication to reduce the risk of duodenal ulcer recurrence; short-term treatment of active benign gastric ulcer; treatment of NSAID-associated gastric ulcer; to reduce the risk of NSAID-associated gastric ulcer in patients with a history of gastric ulcer who require an NSAID; short-term treatment of symptomatic GERD; short-term treatment for all grades of erosive esophagitis; to maintain healing of erosive esophagitis; long-term treatment of pathological hypersecretory conditions, including Zollinger-Ellison syndrome

OTC labeling: Relief of frequent heartburn (≥2 days/week)

Mechanism of Action/Effect A proton pump inhibitor which decreases acid secretion in gastric parietal cells

Contraindications Hypersensitivity to lansoprazole or any component of the formulation

Warnings/Precautions Use of proton pump inhibitors may increase the risk of gastrointestinal infections (eg, *Salmonella, Campylobacter*). Relief of symptoms does not preclude the presence of a gastric malignancy. Atrophic gastritis (by biopsy) has been noted with long-term omeprazole therapy; this may also occur with lansoprazole. No reports of enterochromaffin-like (ECL) cell carcinoids, dysplasia, or neoplasia have occurred. Severe liver dysfunction may require dosage reductions. Decreased *H. pylori* eradication rates have been observed with short-term (≤7 days) combination therapy. The American College of Gastroenterology recommends 10-14 days of therapy (triple or quadruple) for eradication of *H. pylori* (Chey, 2007). Proton pump inhibitors may diminish the therapeutic effect of clopidogrel thought to be due to reduced formation of the active metabolite of clopidogrel; an increase in the risk of cardiovascular events may occur. The manufacturer of clopidogrel recommends avoidance of concomitant administration of another PPI (ie, omeprazole); given the potency of lansoprazole's CYP2C19 inhibitory activity, similar recommendations would appear prudent. Lansoprazole has been shown to be ineffective for the treatment of symptomatic GERD in children 1 month to <1 year.

Increased incidence of osteoporosis-related bone fractures of the hip, spine, or wrist may occur with proton pump inhibitor therapy. Patients on high-dose or long-term therapy should be monitored. Use the lowest effective dose for the shortest duration of time, use vitamin D and calcium supplementation, and follow appropriate guidelines to reduce risk of fractures in patients at risk.

When used for self-medication, patients should be instructed not to use if they have difficulty swallowing, are vomiting blood, or have bloody or black stools. Prior to use, patients should contact healthcare provider if they have liver disease, heartburn for >3 months, heartburn with dizziness, lightheadedness, or sweating, MI symptoms, frequent chest pain, frequent wheezing (especially with heartburn), unexplained weight loss, nausea/vomiting, stomach pain, or are taking antifungals, atazanavir, digoxin, tacrolimus, theophylline, or warfarin. Patients should stop use and consult a healthcare provider if heartburn continues or worsens, or if they need to take for >14 days or more often than every 4 months. Patients should be informed that it may take 1-4 days for full effect to be seen; should not be used for immediate relief.

Drug Interactions

Metabolism/Transport Effects Substrate of CYP2C9 (minor), 2C19 (major), 3A4 (major); **Inhibits** CYP2C9 (weak), 2C19 (moderate), 2D6 (weak), 3A4 (weak); **Induces** CYP1A2 (weak)

Avoid Concomitant Use

Avoid concomitant use of Lansoprazole with any of the following: Delavirdine; Erlotinib; Nelfinavir; Posaconazole

Decreased Effect

Lansoprazole may decrease the levels/effects of: Atazanavir; Bisphosphonate Derivatives; Cefditoren; Clopidogrel; Dabigatran Etexilate; Dasatinib; Delavirdine; Erlotinib; Gefitinib; Indinavir; Iron Salts; Itraconazole; Ketoconazole; Ketoconazole (Systemic); Mesalamine; Mycophenolate; Nelfinavir; Posaconazole

The levels/effects of Lansoprazole may be decreased by: CYP2C19 Inducers (Strong); CYP3A4 Inducers (Strong); Deferasirox; Herbs (CYP3A4 Inducers); Tipranavir

Increased Effect/Toxicity

Lansoprazole may increase the levels/effects of: Amphetamines; CYP2C19 Substrates; Dexmethylphenidate; Imatinib; Methotrexate; Methylphenidate; Raltegravir; Saquinavir; Tacrolimus; Tacrolimus (Systemic); Vitamin K Antagonists; Voriconazole

The levels/effects of Lansoprazole may be increased by: Conivaptan; Fluconazole; Ketoconazole; Ketoconazole (Systemic)

Nutritional/Ethanol Interactions

Ethanol: Avoid ethanol (may cause gastric mucosal irritation).

Food: Lansoprazole serum concentrations may be decreased if taken with food.

Herb/Nutraceutical: Avoid St John's wort (may decrease the levels/effect of lansoprazole).

Adverse Reactions 1% to 10%:

Central nervous system: Headache (children 1-11 years 3%, 12-17 years 7%), dizziness (children 12-17 years 3%; adults <1%)

Gastrointestinal: Diarrhea (1% to 5%; 60 mg/day: 7%), abdominal pain (children 12-17 years 5%; adults 2%), constipation (children 1-11 years 5%; adults 1%), nausea (children 12-17 years 3%; adults 1%)

Pharmacodynamics/Kinetics

Onset of Action Gastric acid suppression: Oral: 1-3 hours

Duration of Action Gastric acid suppression: Oral: >1 day

Absorption Rapid

Bioavailability ≥80%; decreased 50% to 70% if given 30 minutes after food

Time to Peak Plasma: 1.7 hours

Protein Binding 97%

Half-Life Elimination 1.5 ± 1 hours; Elderly: 2-3 hours; Hepatic impairment: 3-7 hours

Metabolism Hepatic via CYP2C19 and 3A4, and in parietal cells to two active metabolites that are not present in systemic circulation

Excretion Feces (67%); urine (33%)

Available Dosage Forms

Capsule, delayed release, oral: 15 mg, 30 mg

Prevacid®: 15 mg, 30 mg

Prevacid® 24 HR [OTC]: 15 mg

Tablet, delayed release, orally disintegrating, oral: 15 mg, 30 mg

Prevacid® SoluTab™: 15 mg, 30 mg

Dosing

Adult & Geriatric

Symptomatic GERD: Oral: Short-term treatment: 15 mg once daily for up to 8 weeks

Erosive esophagitis: Oral: Short-term treatment: 30 mg once daily for up to 8 weeks; continued treatment for an additional 8 weeks may be considered for recurrence or for patients who do not heal after the first 8 weeks of therapy; maintenance therapy: 15 mg once daily

Hypersecretory conditions: Oral: Initial: 60 mg once daily; adjust dose based upon patient response and to reduce acid secretion to <10 mEq/hour (5 mEq/hour in patients with prior gastric surgery); doses of 90 mg twice daily have been used; administer doses >120 mg/day in divided doses

Duodenal ulcer: Oral: Short-term treatment: 15 mg once daily for 4 weeks; maintenance therapy: 15 mg once daily

***Helicobacter pylori* eradication:**

Manufacturer labeling: 30 mg 3 times/day administered with amoxicillin 1000 mg 3 times/day for 14 days **or** 30 mg twice daily administered with amoxicillin 1000 mg *and* clarithromycin 500 mg twice daily for 10-14 days

American College of Gastroenterology guidelines (Chey, 2007):

Nonpenicillin allergy: 30 mg twice daily administered with amoxicillin 1000 mg *and* clarithromycin 500 mg twice daily for 10-14 days

Penicillin allergy: 30 mg twice daily administered with clarithromycin 500 mg *and* metronidazole 500 mg twice daily for 10-14 days **or** 30 mg once or twice daily administered with bismuth subsalicylate 525 mg *and* metronidazole 250 mg *plus* tetracycline 500 mg 4 times/day for 10-14 days

Gastric ulcer: Oral: Short-term treatment: 30 mg once daily for up to 8 weeks

NSAID-associated gastric ulcer (healing): Oral: 30 mg once daily for 8 weeks; controlled studies did not extend past 8 weeks

NSAID-associated gastric ulcer (to reduce risk): Oral: 15 mg once daily for up to 12 weeks; controlled studies did not extend past 12 weeks

Heartburn (OTC labeling): Oral: 15 mg once daily for 14 days; may repeat 14 days of therapy every 4 months. Do not take for >14 days or more often than every 4 months, unless instructed by healthcare provider.

Pediatric

GERD, erosive esophagitis: Oral: Children 1-11 years:

≤30 kg: 15 mg once daily for up to 12 weeks

>30 kg: 30 mg once daily for up to 12 weeks

Note: Doses were increased in some pediatric patients if still symptomatic after 2 or more weeks of treatment (maximum dose: 30 mg twice daily)

Erosive esophagitis: Children 12-17 years: Oral: 30 mg once daily for up to 8 weeks

Nonerosive GERD: Children 12-17 years: Oral: 15 mg once daily for up to 8 weeks

Renal Impairment No adjustment is necessary.

Hepatic Impairment Severe hepatic impairment: Consider a dose reduction.

Administration

Oral

Administer before food; best if taken before breakfast. The intact granules should not be chewed or crushed; however, several options are available for those patients unable to swallow capsules:

Capsules may be opened and the intact granules sprinkled on 1 tablespoon of applesauce, Ensure® pudding, cottage cheese, yogurt, or strained pears. The granules should then be swallowed immediately.

Capsules may be opened and emptied into ~60 mL orange juice, apple juice, or tomato juice; mix and swallow immediately. Rinse the glass with additional juice and swallow to assure complete delivery of the dose.

Orally-disintegrating tablets: Should not be swallowed whole, broken, cut, or chewed. Place tablet on tongue; allow to dissolve (with or without water) until particles can be swallowed. Orally-disintegrating tablets may also be administered via an oral syringe: Place the 15 mg tablet in an oral syringe and draw up ~4 mL water, or place the 30 mg tablet in an oral syringe and draw up ~10 mL water. After tablet has dispersed, administer within 15 minutes. Refill the syringe with water (2 mL for the 15 mg tablet; 5 mL for the 30 mg tablet), shake gently, then administer any remaining contents.

Other Nasogastric tube administration:

Capsule: Capsule can be opened, the granules mixed (not crushed) with 40 mL of apple juice and then injected through the NG tube into the stomach, then flush tube with additional apple juice. Do not mix with other liquids.

Orally-disintegrating tablet: Nasogastric tube ≥8 French: Place a 15 mg tablet in a syringe and draw up ~4 mL water, or place the 30 mg tablet in a syringe and draw up ~10 mL water. After tablet has dispersed, administer within 15 minutes. Refill the syringe with ~5 mL water, shake gently, and then flush the nasogastric tube.

Stability

Storage Store at 25°C (77°F); excursions permitted to 15°C to 30°C (59°F to 86°F).

Monitoring and Teaching Issues

Laboratory Monitoring CBC, liver function, renal function, and serum gastrin levels. Patients with Zollinger-Ellison syndrome should be monitored for gastric acid output, which should be maintained at ≤10 mEq/hour during the last hour before the next lansoprazole dose.

Physical Assessment Assess periodic laboratory results and effectiveness of medications that require an acid medium for absorption (eg, ketoconazole, itraconazole). Monitor effectiveness of ulcer symptom relief.

Patient Education Take before eating. Do not crush or chew granules. Patients who may have difficulty swallowing capsules may open the delayed-release capsules and sprinkle the contents on applesauce, pudding, cottage cheese, or yogurt. Avoid alcohol. Report unresolved diarrhea, persistent heartburn, or abdominal pain.

Dietary Considerations Should be taken before eating; best if taken before breakfast. Some products may contain phenylalanine.

Geriatric Considerations The clearance of lansoprazole is decreased in the elderly; however, the half-life is only increased by 50% to 100%, resulting in a continued short half-life with no accumulation in the elderly. No dosage adjustment is required with normal hepatic function. The rate of healing and side effects are similar to younger adults.

An increased risk of fractures of the hip, spine, or wrist has been observed in epidemiologic studies with proton pump inhibitor (PPI) use, primarily in older adults ≥50 years of age. The greatest risk was seen in patients receiving high doses or on long-term therapy (≥1 year). Calcium and vitamin D supplementation and close monitoring are recommended to reduce the risk of fracture in high-risk patients.

Pregnancy Considerations Animal studies have not shown teratogenic effects to the fetus. However, there are no adequate and well-controlled studies in pregnant women; use during pregnancy only if clearly needed.

Related Information

Compatibility of Drugs *on page* 1994
Helicobacter pylori Treatment *on page* 2045

Lansoprazole, Amoxicillin, and Clarithromycin

(lan SOE pra zole, a moks i SIL in, & kla RITH roe mye sin)

U.S. Brand Names Prevpac®

Index Terms Amoxicillin, Clarithromycin, and Lansoprazole; Clarithromycin, Lansoprazole, and Amoxicillin; Lansoprazole, Amoxicillin, and Clarithromycin

Generic Availability (U.S.) No

Pharmacologic Category Antibiotic, Macrolide Combination; Antibiotic, Penicillin; Gastrointestinal Agent, Miscellaneous; Proton Pump Inhibitor; Substituted Benzimidazole

Medication Safety Issues

Sound-alike/look-alike issues:

Prevpac® may be confused with Prevacid®

Pregnancy Risk Factor C (clarithromycin)

Lactation Excretion in breast milk unknown/not recommended

Use Eradication of *H. pylori* to reduce the risk of recurrent duodenal ulcer

Available Dosage Forms

Combination package [each administration card contains]:

Prevpac®:

Capsule: Amoxicillin 500 mg (4 capsules/day)

Capsule, delayed release (Prevacid®): Lansoprazole 30 mg (2 capsules/day)

Tablet (Biaxin®): Clarithromycin 500 mg (2 tablets/day)

Dosing

Adult & Geriatric *H. pylori* eradication: Oral: Lansoprazole 30 mg, amoxicillin 1 g, and clarithromycin 500 mg taken together twice daily for 10 or 14 days

Renal Impairment

Cl_{cr} <30 mL/minute: Use is not recommended.

Monitoring and Teaching Issues

Laboratory Monitoring CBC with differential, BUN, creatinine, liver function test periodically with prolonged use

Physical Assessment See individual agents.

Patient Education See individual agents.

Related Information

Amoxicillin *on page* 110
Clarithromycin *on page* 391
Lansoprazole *on page* 1061

◆ **Lansoprazole, Amoxicillin, and Clarithromycin** *see* Lansoprazole, Amoxicillin, and Clarithromycin *on page* 1064

◆ **Lantus®** *see* Insulin Glargine *on page* 986

◆ **Lantus® Solostar®** *see* Insulin Glargine *on page* 986

Lapatinib (la PA ti nib)

U.S. Brand Names Tykerb®

Index Terms GW572016; Lapatinib Ditosylate

Generic Availability (U.S.) No

Pharmacologic Category Antineoplastic Agent, Tyrosine Kinase Inhibitor; Epidermal Growth Factor Receptor (EGFR) Inhibitor

Medication Safety Issues

Sound-alike/look-alike issues:

Lapatinib may be confused with dasatinib, erlotinib, imatinib, SUNItinib, vandetanib

High alert medication: This medication is in a class of medications the Institute for Safe Medication Practices (ISMP) includes among its list of drug classes which have a heightened risk of causing significant patient harm when used in error.

Prescribing and Access Restrictions Lapatinib is available **only** at specialty pharmacies through a restricted-access program, Tykerb® CARES. Information is available at www.tykerbcares.com or 1-866-489-5372.

Pregnancy Risk Factor D

Lactation Excretion in breast milk unknown/not recommended

Use Treatment of HER2 overexpressing advanced or metastatic breast cancer (in combination with capecitabine) in patients who have received prior therapy (with an anthracycline, a taxane, and trastuzumab) and HER2 overexpressing hormone receptor positive metastatic breast cancer in postmenopausal women (in combination with letrozole)

Unlabeled/Investigational Use Treatment (in combination with trastuzumab) of HER2 overexpressing metastatic breast cancer which had progressed on prior trastuzumab containing therapy

Mechanism of Action/Effect Tyrosine kinase (dual kinase) inhibitor that blocks HER2 and EGFR pathways.

Contraindications Hypersensitivity to lapatinib or any component of the formulation

Warnings/Precautions Decreases in left ventricular ejection fraction (LVEF) have been reported (usually within the first 3 months of treatment); baseline and periodic LVEF evaluations are recommended; interrupt therapy or decrease dose with decreased LVEF ≥ grade 2 or LVEF < LLN. QT_c prolongation has been observed; use caution in patients with a history of QT_c prolongation or with medications known to prolong the QT interval; a baseline and periodic 12-lead ECG should be considered; correct electrolyte (potassium, calcium and magnesium) abnormalities prior to and during treatment. Use with caution in conditions which may impair left ventricular function and in patients with a history of or predisposed (prior treatment with anthracyclines, chest wall irradiation) to left ventricular dysfunction. Interstitial lung disease (ILD) and pneumonitis have been reported (with lapatinib monotherapy and with combination chemotherapy); monitor for pulmonary symptoms which may indicate ILD or pneumonitis; discontinue therapy for grade 3 (or higher) pulmonary symptoms indicative of ILD or pneumonitis (eg, dyspnea, dry cough).

[U.S. Boxed Warning]: Hepatotoxicity (ALT or AST >3 times ULN and total bilirubin >2 times ULN) has been reported with lapatinib; may be severe and/or fatal. Onset of hepatotoxicity may occur within days to several months after treatment initiation; monitor (at baseline and during treatment); discontinue with severe changes in liver function; do not retreat. Use caution in patients with hepatic dysfunction; Dose reductions should be considered in patients with severe (Child-Pugh class C) preexisting hepatic impairment. Avoid concurrent use with strong CYP3A4 inhibitors or inducers; if concomitant therapy cannot be avoided, lapatinib dosage adjustments should be considered. May cause diarrhea (may be severe); manage with antidiarrheal agents; severe diarrhea may require hydration, electrolytes, and or interruption of therapy.

Drug Interactions

Metabolism/Transport Effects Substrate of CYP2C8 (minor), 3A4 (major), P-glycoprotein (P-gp, ABCB1); **Inhibits** CYP2C8 (moderate), CYP3A4 (moderate), ABCG2, P-glycoprotein

Avoid Concomitant Use

Avoid concomitant use of Lapatinib with any of the following: Artemether; BCG; Dronedarone; Lumefantrine; Natalizumab; Nilotinib; Pimecrolimus; Pimozide; QuiNINE; Roflumilast; Silodosin; Tacrolimus (Topical); Tetrabenazine; Thioridazine; Tolvaptan; Toremifene; Vaccines (Live); Vandetanib; Ziprasidone

Decreased Effect

Lapatinib may decrease the levels/effects of: BCG; Cardiac Glycosides; Sipuleucel-T; Vaccines (Inactivated); Vaccines (Live); Vitamin K Antagonists

The levels/effects of Lapatinib may be decreased by: CYP3A4 Inducers (Strong); Deferasirox; Echinacea; Herbs (CYP3A4 Inducers); P-Glycoprotein Inducers

Increased Effect/Toxicity

Lapatinib may increase the levels/effects of: Colchicine; CYP2C8 Substrates (High risk); CYP3A4 Substrates; Dabigatran Etexilate; Dronedarone; Eplerenone; Everolimus; FentaNYL; Leflunomide; Lurasidone; Natalizumab; Pazopanib; P-Glycoprotein Substrates; Pimozide; QTc-Prolonging Agents; QuiNINE; Rivaroxaban; Salmeterol; Saxagliptin; Silodosin; Tetrabenazine; Thioridazine; Tolvaptan; Topotecan; Toremifene; Vaccines (Live); Vandetanib; Vilazodone; Vitamin K Antagonists; Ziprasidone

The levels/effects of Lapatinib may be increased by: Alfuzosin; Artemether; Chloroquine; Ciprofloxacin; Ciprofloxacin (Systemic); Conivaptan; CYP3A4 Inhibitors (Moderate); CYP3A4 Inhibitors (Strong); Denosumab; Gadobutrol; Lumefantrine; Nilotinib; P-Glycoprotein Inhibitors; Pimecrolimus; QuiNINE; Roflumilast; Tacrolimus (Topical); Trastuzumab

Nutritional/Ethanol Interactions

Food: Systemic exposure of lapatinib is increased when administered with food (AUC three- to fourfold higher). Avoid grapefruit juice (may increase the levels/effects of lapatinib).

Herb/Nutraceutical: Avoid St John's wort (may increase metabolism and decrease lapatinib concentrations).

Adverse Reactions Percentages reported for combination therapy.

>10%:

Central nervous system: Fatigue (10% to 20%), headache (≤14%)

Dermatologic: Palmar-plantar erythrodysesthesia (hand-and-foot syndrome) (with capecitabine: 53%; grade 3: 12%), rash (28% to 44%), dry skin (10% to 13%), alopecia (≤13%), pruritus (≤12%), nail disorder (≤11%)

Gastrointestinal: Diarrhea (64% to 65%; grade 3: 9% to 13%; grade 4: ≤1%), nausea (31% to 44%), vomiting (17% to 26%), abdominal pain (≤15%), mucosal inflammation (≤15%), stomatitis (≤14%), anorexia (≤11%), dyspepsia (≤11%)

Hematologic: Anemia (with capecitabine: 56%; grade 3: <1%), neutropenia (with capecitabine: 22%; grade 3: 3%; grade 4: <1%), thrombocytopenia (with capecitabine: 18%; grade 3: <1%)

Hepatic: AST increased (49% to 53%; grade 3: 2% to 6%; grade 4: <1%), ALT increased (37% to 46%; grade 3: 2% to 5%; grade 4<1%) total bilirubin increased (22% to 45%; grade 3: ≤4%; grade 4: <1%)

Neuromuscular & skeletal: Limb pain (≤12%), weakness (≤12%), back pain (≤11%)

Respiratory:Dyspnea (≤12%), epistaxis (≤11%)

1% to 10%:

Cardiovascular: LVEF decreased (grades 1/2: 2% to 4%; grades 3/4: <1%)

Central nervous system: Insomnia (≤10%)

Pharmacodynamics/Kinetics

Absorption Incomplete and variable

Time to Peak 3-6 hours

Protein Binding >99% to albumin and alpha$_1$-acid glycoprotein

Half-Life Elimination ~24 hours

Metabolism Hepatic; extensive via CYP3A4 and 3A5, and to a lesser extent via CYP2C19 and 2C8 to oxidized metabolites

Excretion Feces (27% as unchanged drug; range 3% to 67%); urine (<2%)

Available Dosage Forms

Tablet, oral:

Tykerb®: 250 mg

Dosing

Adult & Geriatric Details concerning dosing in combination regimens should also be consulted. **Note:** Dose reductions are likely to be needed when lapatinib is administered concomitantly with a strong CYP3A4 inhibitor (an alternate medication for CYP3A4 enzyme inhibitors should be investigated first).

Breast cancer: oral:

In combination with capecitabine: 1250 mg once daily

In combination with letrozole: 1500 mg once daily

In combination with trastuzumab (unlabeled use): 1000 mg once daily (O'Shaughnessy, 2008)

Dosage adjustment for concomitant CYP3A4 inhibitors/inducers:

CYP3A4 inhibitors: Dose reductions are likely to be needed when lapatinib is administered concomitantly with a strong CYP3A4 inhibitor (an alternate medication for CYP3A4 enzyme inhibitors should be investigated first); in the event that lapatinib must be administered concomitantly with a potent enzyme inhibitor, consider reducing lapatinib to 500 mg once daily with careful monitoring. When a strong CYP3A4 inhibitor is discontinued, allow ~1 week to elapse prior to adjusting the lapatinib dose upward.

CYP3A4 inducers: Concomitant administration with CYP3A4 inducers may require increased lapatinib doses (alternatives to the enzyme-inducing agent should be utilized first); consider titrating gradually from 1250 mg/day up to 4500 mg/day (in combination with capecitabine) **or** from 1500 mg/day up to 5500 mg/day (in combination with letrozole), with careful monitoring. (If the strong CYP3A4 enzyme inducer is discontinued, reduce the lapatinib dose to the indicated dose.)

Renal Impairment Not studied in renal dysfunction, however, due to the minimal renal elimination (<2%), dosage adjustments for renal dysfunction may not be necessary.

Hepatic Impairment

Severe preexisting hepatic impairment (Child-Pugh class C):

In combination with capecitabine: Reduce dose from 1250 mg once daily to 750 mg once daily.

In combination with letrozole: Reduce dose from 1500 mg once daily to 1000 mg once daily.

Severe hepatotoxicity during treatment: Discontinue treatment; do not retreat.

Adjustment for Toxicity

Cardiac toxicity: Discontinue treatment for decreased LVEF ≥ grade 2 or LVEF < LLN; may be restarted after at least 2 weeks at 1000 mg once daily (in combination with capecitabine) **or** 1250 mg once daily (in combination with letrozole) if LVEF recovers to normal and patient is asymptomatic.

Pulmonary toxicity: Discontinue treatment with pulmonary symptoms indicative of interstitial lung disease or pneumonitis which are ≥ grade 3

Other toxicities: Withhold for any toxicity (other than cardiac) ≥ grade 2 until toxicity resolves to ≤ grade 1 and re-initiate at 1250 mg once daily; for persistent toxicity, reduce dosage to 1000 mg once daily (in combination with capecitabine) **or** 1250 mg once daily (in combination with letrozole)

Administration

Oral Administer once daily, on an empty stomach, 1 hour before or 1 hour after a meal. Take at the same time each day; dividing doses is not recommended.

Stability

Storage Store at room temperature of 25°C (77°F); excursions permitted between 15°C and 30°C (59°F and 86°F).

Monitoring and Teaching Issues

Laboratory Monitoring CBC with differential, liver function tests, including transaminases, bilirubin, and alkaline phosphatase (baseline and every 4-6 weeks during treatment); electrolytes including calcium, potassium, magnesium

Physical Assessment Use caution in presence of hepatic or left ventricular dysfunction. Evaluate CBC, LFTs, electrolytes, and left ventricular ejection fraction at baseline and on a regular basis. Monitor for cardiac changes, gastrointestinal disturbance (diarrhea may become severe), interstitial lung disease, and pneumonitis.

Patient Education Take on an empty stomach 1 hour before or 1 hour after a meal. Avoid grapefruit or grapefruit juice while taking this medication. Maintain adequate hydration unless instructed to restrict fluid intake. You may be required to have regularly scheduled laboratory tests while on this medication. You will be more susceptible to infection. You may experience diarrhea (contact prescriber if persistent or severe); insomnia or fatigue; nausea, vomiting, stomach pain, or dyspepsia; red, painful hands, feet, or limbs; or back pain. Report chest pain or palpitations, any unusual cough, respiratory difficulty or wheezing, easy bruising, or unusual bleeding.

Dietary Considerations Take on an empty stomach, 1 hour before or 1 hour after a meal. (**Note:** For combination with capecitabine treatment, capecitabine should be taken with food, or within 30 minutes after a meal.) Avoid grapefruit juice.

Geriatric Considerations No differences in safety or effectiveness were observed between elderly and younger patients.

Breast-Feeding Considerations Due to the potential for serious adverse reactions in the nursing infant, breast-feeding is not recommended.

Pregnancy Considerations Increased pup deaths were demonstrated in animal studies. There are no adequate and well-controlled studies in pregnant women. Lapatinib may cause fetal harm if administered during pregnancy. Women of childbearing potential should be advised to avoid pregnancy during treatment.

Additional Information Oncology Comment: The National Comprehensive Cancer Network (NCCN) breast cancer guidelines list lapatinib (in combination with capecitabine) as an option for the treatment of HER2-positive breast cancer in patients who are refractory to anthracycline, taxane, and trastuzumab treatment. In a randomized phase III study (Geyer, 2006) of lapatinib plus capecitabine versus capecitabine alone in HER2-positive advanced breast cancer, the addition of lapatinib was associated with a 51% reduction in the risk of disease progression in heavily pretreated patients. Lapatinib shows activity in HER2-positive metastatic breast cancer that has progressed after trastuzumab treatment. The NCCN breast cancer guidelines also list lapatinib in combination with trastuzumab in metastatic HER2+ breast cancer which has progressed on trastuzumab therapy; the combination of lapatinib and trastuzumab should not be given with concurrent chemotherapy.

◆ **Lapatinib Ditosylate** *see* Lapatinib *on page 1064*
◆ **Lasix®** *see* Furosemide *on page 840*
◆ **L-asparaginase** *see* Asparaginase *on page 152*
◆ **L-asparaginase with Polyethylene Glycol** *see* Pegaspargase *on page 1421*
◆ **Lastacaft™** *see* Alcaftadine *on page 62*

Latanoprost (la TA noe prost)

U.S. Brand Names Xalatan®

Generic Availability (U.S.) No

Pharmacologic Category Ophthalmic Agent, Antiglaucoma; Prostaglandin, Ophthalmic

Medication Safety Issues

Sound-alike/look-alike issues:

Latanoprost may be confused with Lantus®

Xalatan® may be confused with Lantus®, Travatan®, Xalacom™, Zarontin®

Pregnancy Risk Factor C

Use Reduction of elevated intraocular pressure in patients with open-angle glaucoma or ocular hypertension

Contraindications Hypersensitivity to latanoprost or any component of the formulation

Warnings/Precautions May permanently change/increase brown pigmentation of the iris, the eyelid skin, and eyelashes. In addition, may increase the length and/or number of eyelashes (may vary between eyes); changes occur slowly and may not be noticeable for months or years. Long-term consequences and potential injury to eye are not known. Use with caution in patients with intraocular inflammation, aphakic patients, pseudophakic patients with a torn posterior lens capsule, or patients with risk factors for macular edema. Safety and efficacy have not been determined for use in patients with angle-closure-, inflammatory-, or neovascular glaucoma.

There have been reports of bacterial keratitis associated with the use of multiple-dose containers of topical ophthalmic products. Contains benzalkonium chloride which may be adsorbed by contact lenses; remove contacts prior to administration and wait 15 minutes before reinserting.

Drug Interactions

Avoid Concomitant Use There are no known interactions where it is recommended to avoid concomitant use.

Decreased Effect

The levels/effects of Latanoprost may be decreased by: NSAID (Ophthalmic)

Increased Effect/Toxicity

Latanoprost may increase the levels/effects of: Bimatoprost

Adverse Reactions

>10%: Ocular: Blurred vision, burning and stinging, conjunctival hyperemia, foreign body sensation, itching, increased pigmentation of the iris, and punctate epithelial keratopathy

1% to 10%:

Cardiovascular: Chest pain, angina pectoris

Dermatologic: Rash, allergic skin reaction

Neuromuscular & skeletal: Myalgia, arthralgia, back pain

Ocular: Dry eye, excessive tearing, eye pain, lid crusting, lid edema, lid erythema, lid discomfort/pain, photophobia

Respiratory: Upper respiratory tract infection, cold, flu

Pharmacodynamics/Kinetics

Onset of Action 3-4 hours; Peak effect: Maximum: 8-12 hours

Absorption Through the cornea where the isopropyl ester prodrug is hydrolyzed by esterases to the biologically active acid. Peak concentration is reached in 2 hours after topical administration in the aqueous humor.

Half-Life Elimination 17 minutes

Metabolism Primarily hepatic via fatty acid beta-oxidation

Excretion Urine (as metabolites)

Available Dosage Forms

Solution, ophthalmic:

Xalatan®: 0.005% (2.5 mL)

Dosing

Adult & Geriatric Glaucoma: Ophthalmic: 1 drop (1.5 mcg) in the affected eye(s) once daily in the evening; do not exceed the once daily dosage because it has been shown that more frequent administration may decrease the IOP lowering effect

Note: A medication delivery device (Xal-Ease™) is available for use with Xalatan®.

Administration

Other If more than one topical ophthalmic drug is being used, administer the drugs at least 5 minutes apart. A delivery aid, Xal-Ease™, is available for administering Xalatan®.

Stability

Storage Store intact bottles under refrigeration (2°C to 8°C/36°F to 46°F). Protect from light. Once opened, the container may be stored at room temperature up to 25°C (77°F) for 6 weeks.

Monitoring and Teaching Issues

Physical Assessment Monitor for blurred vision, burning and stinging, conjunctival hyperemia, foreign body sensation, itching, increased pigmentation of the iris, and punctate epithelial keratopathy.

Patient Education For use in eyes only. Iris color may change because of an increase of the brown pigment. Iris pigmentation changes may be more noticeable in patients with green-brown, blue/gray-brown, or yellow-brown irides. If any ocular reaction develops, particularly conjunctivitis and lid reactions, immediately notify prescriber. If more than one topical ophthalmic drug is being used, administer the drugs at least 5 minutes apart. Latanoprost contains benzalkonium chloride, which may be absorbed by contact lenses. Remove contact lenses prior to administration; lenses may be reinserted after 15 minutes. Do not let tip of applicator touch eye; do not contaminate tip of applicator (may cause eye infection, eye damage, or vision loss).

Geriatric Considerations Evaluate patient's ability to self-administer eye drops

- ◆ **Latisse®** *see* Bimatoprost *on page* 219
- ◆ **Latuda®** *see* Lurasidone *on page* 1140
- ◆ **LCM** *see* Lacosamide *on page* 1051
- ◆ **L-Deoxythymidine** *see* Telbivudine *on page* 1714
- ◆ **L-Deprenyl** *see* Selegiline *on page* 1630
- ◆ **LDP-341** *see* Bortezomib *on page* 226
- ◆ **LdT** *see* Telbivudine *on page* 1714
- ◆ **Leena®** *see* Ethinyl Estradiol and Norethindrone *on page* 701

Leflunomide (le FLOO noh mide)

U.S. Brand Names Arava®

Generic Availability (U.S.) Yes

Pharmacologic Category Antirheumatic, Disease Modifying

Pregnancy Risk Factor X

Lactation Excretion in breast milk unknown/not recommended

Use Treatment of active rheumatoid arthritis; indicated to reduce signs and symptoms, and to inhibit structural damage and improve physical function

Unlabeled/Investigational Use Treatment of cytomegalovirus (CMV) disease in transplant recipients resistant to standard antivirals; prevention of acute and chronic rejection in recipients of solid organ transplants

Mechanism of Action/Effect Leflunomide is an immunodulatory agent that inhibits pyrimidine synthesis, resulting in antiproliferative and anti-inflammatory effects. Leflunomide is a prodrug; the active metabolite is responsible for activity. For CMV, may interfere with virion assembly.

Contraindications Hypersensitivity to leflunomide or any component of the formulation; pregnancy

Warnings/Precautions Hazardous agent - use appropriate precautions for handling and disposal. **[U.S. Boxed Warning]: Use has been associated with rare reports of hepatotoxicity, hepatic failure, and death. Treatment should not be initiated in patients with pre-existing acute or chronic liver disease or ALT >2 x ULN. Use caution in patients with concurrent exposure to potentially hepatotoxic drugs. Monitor ALT levels during therapy; discontinue if ALT >3 x ULN occurs and, if hepatotoxicity is likely leflunomide-induced, start drug elimination procedures** (eg, cholestyramine, charcoal).

Use has been associated (rarely) with interstitial lung disease; discontinue in patients who develop new onset or worsening of pulmonary symptoms. Drug elimination procedures should be considered if interstitial lung disease occurs; fatal outcomes have been reported. May increase susceptibility to infection, including opportunistic pathogens. Severe infections, sepsis, and fatalities have been reported. Not recommended in patients with severe immunodeficiency, bone marrow dysplasia, or severe, uncontrolled infections. Caution should be exercised when considering the use in patients with a history of new/recurrent infections, with conditions that predispose them to infections, or with chronic, latent, or localized infections. Patients who develop a new infection while undergoing treatment should be monitored closely; consider discontinuation of therapy and drug elimination procedures if infection is serious.

Use may affect defenses against malignancies; impact on the development and course of malignancies is not fully defined. As compared to the general population, an increased risk of lymphoma has been noted in clinical trials; however, rheumatoid arthritis has been previously associated with an increased rate of lymphoma. Use with caution in patients with a prior history of significant hematologic abnormalities; avoid use with bone marrow dysplasia. Use has been associated with rare pancytopenia, agranulocytosis, and thrombocytopenia, generally when given concurrently or recently with methotrexate or other immunosuppressive agents. Monitoring of hematologic function is required; discontinue if evidence of bone marrow suppression and begin drug elimination procedures (eg, cholestyramine or activated charcoal). Rare cases of dermatologic reactions (including Stevens-Johnson syndrome and toxic epidermal necrolysis) have been reported; discontinue if evidence of severe dermatologic reaction occurs, and begin drug elimination procedures (eg, cholestyramine or activated charcoal).

Safety has not been established in patients with latent tuberculosis infection. Patients should be screened for tuberculosis and if necessary, treated prior to initiating therapy. Use with caution in patients with renal impairment. **[U.S. Boxed Warning]: Women of childbearing potential should not receive therapy until pregnancy has been excluded,** they have been counseled concerning fetal risk and reliable contraceptive measures have been confirmed. Women of childbearing potential should also undergo drug elimination procedures (eg, cholestyramine, charcoal) following discontinuation of therapy. Patients should be brought up to date with all immunizations before initiating therapy. Live vaccines should not be given concurrently; there is no data available concerning secondary transmission of live vaccines in patients receiving therapy. Due to variations in clearance, it may take up to 2 years to reach low levels of leflunomide metabolite serum concentrations. A drug elimination procedure using cholestyramine or activated charcoal is recommended when a more rapid elimination is needed.

Drug Interactions

Metabolism/Transport Effects Inhibits CYP2C9 (weak)

Avoid Concomitant Use

Avoid concomitant use of Leflunomide with any of the following: BCG; Natalizumab; Pimecrolimus; Roflumilast; Tacrolimus (Topical)

Decreased Effect

Leflunomide may decrease the levels/effects of: BCG; Sipuleucel-T; Vaccines (Inactivated)

The levels/effects of Leflunomide may be decreased by: Bile Acid Sequestrants; Charcoal, Activated; Echinacea

Increased Effect/Toxicity

Leflunomide may increase the levels/effects of: Carvedilol; CYP2C9 Substrates (High risk); Natalizumab; TOLBUTamide; Vaccines (Live); Vitamin K Antagonists

The levels/effects of Leflunomide may be increased by: Denosumab; Immunosuppressants; Methotrexate; Pimecrolimus; Rifampin; Roflumilast; Tacrolimus (Topical); TOLBUTamide; Trastuzumab

Nutritional/Ethanol Interactions

Food: No interactions with food have been noted.

Herb/Nutraceutical: Echinacea may diminish the therapeutic effect of leflunomide.

Adverse Reactions

>10%:

Gastrointestinal: Diarrhea (17%)

Respiratory: Respiratory tract infection (4% to 15%)

1% to 10%:

Cardiovascular: Hypertension (10%), chest pain (2%), edema (peripheral), palpitation, tachycardia, vasodilation, varicose vein, vasculitis

Central nervous system: Headache (7%), dizziness (4%), pain (2%), anxiety, depression, fever, insomnia, malaise, migraine, sleep disorder, vertigo

Dermatologic: Alopecia (10%), rash (10%), pruritus (4%), dry skin (2%), eczema (2%), acne, bruising, dermatitis, hair discoloration, hematoma, nail disorder, skin disorder/discoloration, skin ulcer, subcutaneous nodule

Endocrine & metabolic: Hypokalemia (1%), diabetes mellitus, hyperglycemia, hyperlipidemia, hyperthyroidism, menstrual disorder

Gastrointestinal: Nausea (9%), abdominal pain (5% to 6%), dyspepsia (5%), weight loss (4%), anorexia (3%), gastroenteritis (3%), mouth ulceration (3%), vomiting (3%), candidiasis (oral), colitis, constipation, esophagitis, flatulence, gastritis, gingivitis, melena, salivary gland enlarged, stomatitis, taste disturbance, tooth disorder, xerostomia

Genitourinary: Urinary tract infection (5%), albuminuria, cystitis, dysuria, prostate disorder, urinary frequency, vaginal candidiasis

Hematologic: Anemia

Hepatic: Abnormal LFTs (5%), cholelithiasis

Local: Abscess

Neuromuscular & skeletal: Back pain (5%), joint disorder (4%), weakness (3%), tenosynovitis (3%), synovitis (2%), paresthesia (2%), arthralgia (1%), leg cramps (1%), arthrosis, bone necrosis, bone pain, bursitis, CPK increased, myalgia, neck pain, neuralgia, neuritis, pelvic pain, tendon rupture

Ocular: Blurred vision, cataract, conjunctivitis, eye disorder

Renal: Hematuria

Respiratory: Bronchitis (7%), cough (3%), pharyngitis (3%), pneumonia (2%), rhinitis (2%), sinusitis (2%), asthma, dyspnea, epistaxis

Miscellaneous: Accidental injury (5%), allergic reactions (2%), flu-like syndrome (2%), cyst, diaphoresis, hernia, herpes infection

Pharmacodynamics/Kinetics

Bioavailability 80% (relative to oral solution)

Time to Peak M1: 6-12 hours

Protein Binding M1: >99% to albumin

Half-Life Elimination M1: Mean: 14-15 days; enterohepatic recycling appears to contribute to the long half-life of this agent, since activated charcoal and cholestyramine substantially reduce plasma half-life

Metabolism Hepatic to an active metabolite M1 (also known as A77 1726 or teriflunomide), which accounts for nearly all pharmacologic activity; further metabolism to multiple inactive metabolites; undergoes enterohepatic recirculation

Excretion Feces (48%); urine (43%)

Available Dosage Forms

Tablet, oral: 10 mg, 20 mg

Arava®: 10 mg, 20 mg

Dosing

Adult & Geriatric

Rheumatoid arthritis: Oral: Loading dose: 100 mg/day for 3 days, followed by 20 mg/day; **Note:** The loading dose may be omitted in patients at increased risk of hepatic or hematologic toxicity (eg, recent concomitant methotrexate). Dosage may be decreased to 10 mg/day in patients who have difficulty tolerating the 20 mg dose. Due to the long half-life of the active metabolite, serum concentrations may require a prolonged period to decline after dosage reduction.

CMV disease, resistant to standard antivirals (unlabeled use): Oral: Some authors recommend 100-200 mg/day for 5-7 days, followed by 40-60 mg/day (Avery, 2004; Avery, 2010). Others have utilized the standard rheumatoid arthritis dosing (John, 2004). Adjust dose based on serum concentrations of metabolite and adverse events (Avery, 2008; Avery, 2010; Williams, 2002).

Renal Impairment No specific dosage adjustment is recommended. There is no clinical experience in the use of leflunomide in patients with renal impairment. The free fraction of M1 is doubled in dialysis patients. Patients should be monitored closely for adverse effects requiring dosage adjustment.

Hepatic Impairment Not recommended for use in patients with pre-existing liver disease or in patients with significant hepatic impairment (ALT >2 times ULN). Patients should have LFTs monitored closely. Discontinue leflunomide if ALT >3 times ULN.

Adjustment for Toxicity

ALT elevations >3 times ULN: Discontinue leflunomide and initiate cholestyramine to enhance elimination.

Drug elimination procedure: To achieve nondetectable serum concentrations (<0.02 mg/L) of the active metabolite (M1) of leflunomide administer the following:

Cholestyramine: 8 g administered 3 times/day for 11 days. The 11 days do not need to be consecutive unless plasma concentrations need to be lowered rapidly. Verify serum concentrations by 2 separate tests ≥14 days apart. If plasma concentrations are still high, additional cholestyramine treatment may be considered. In healthy volunteers, cholestyramine 8 g administered 3 times/day for 24 hours decreased M1 concentrations by 40% in 24 hours and 49% to 65% in 48 hours.

Activated charcoal: 50 g every 6 hours for 24 hours was shown to decrease plasma concentrations of M1 by 37% in 24 hours and 48% in 48 hours.

Administration

Oral Administer without regard to meals.

Stability

Storage Store at 25°C (77°F); excursions permitted to 15°C to 30°C (59°F to 86°F). Protect from light.

Monitoring and Teaching Issues

Laboratory Monitoring A complete blood count (WBC, platelet count, hemoglobin or hematocrit), serum phosphate, as well as serum transaminase determinations, should be monitored at baseline and monthly during the initial 6 months of treatment; if stable, monitoring frequency may be decreased to every 6-8 weeks thereafter (continue monthly when used in combination with other immunosuppressive agents). ALT should be monitored at least monthly for the first 6 months of treatment, then every 6-8 weeks thereafter (discontinue if ALT >3 x ULN, treat with cholestyramine, and monitor liver function at least weekly until normal). If coadministered with methotrexate, monthly transaminases (ALT, AST) and serum albumin levels are recommended. Screen for tuberculosis and pregnancy prior to therapy. When used for CMV disease, monitor serum trough concentrations of active metabolite.

Physical Assessment Place and read PPD prior to initiating. Monitor for signs and symptoms of severe infection, hypertension, or hepatic dysfunction. Monitor for new onset or worsening of pulmonary symptoms.

Patient Education Maintain adequate hydration unless instructed to restrict fluid intake. You will be more prone to infections. You may experience diarrhea, nausea, vomiting, loss of appetite, flatulence, or dizziness. If you have diabetes, monitor blood sugars closely; this medication may alter glucose levels. If you experience symptoms such as nausea, vomiting, stomach pain or swelling, jaundice, dark urine, or unusual tiredness, report these to your prescriber immediately. Report chest pain, palpitations, rapid heartbeat, or swelling of extremities; persistent GI problems; skin rash; mucous membrane lesions; frequent, painful, or difficult urination; genital itching; depression; acute headache; muscle tremors, cramping, or weakness; back pain; altered gait; cough, cold symptoms, wheezing, or respiratory difficulty; easy bruising/bleeding; or blood in vomitus, stool, or urine.

Dietary Considerations May be taken without regard to meals.

Geriatric Considerations In Phase III studies, no difference in safety and effectiveness were seen between older and younger adults. No dosage reduction necessary based on age alone; monitor in renal and hepatic impairment.

Breast-Feeding Considerations It is not known whether leflunomide is secreted in human milk. Because the potential for serious adverse reactions exists in the nursing infant, a decision should be made whether to discontinue nursing or discontinue the drug, taking into account the importance of the drug to the mother.

Pregnancy Considerations Has been associated with teratogenic and embryolethal effects in animal models at low doses. Leflunomide is contraindicated in pregnant women or women of childbearing potential who are not using reliable contraception. Pregnancy must be excluded prior to initiating treatment. **[U.S. Boxed Warning]: Women of childbearing potential should not receive therapy until pregnancy has been excluded,** they have been counseled concerning fetal risk, and reliable contraceptive measures have been confirmed. Following treatment, pregnancy should be avoided until undetectable serum concentrations (<0.02 mg/L) are verified. This may be accomplished by the use of an enhanced drug elimination procedure using cholestyramine. Serum concentrations <0.02 mg/L should be verified by two separate tests performed at least 14 days apart. If serum concentrations are >0.02 mg/L, additional cholestyramine treatment should be considered. Pregnant women exposed to leflunomide should be registered with the pregnancy registry (877-311-8972). It is not known if males taking leflunomide may contribute to fetal toxicity. Males taking leflunomide who wish to father a child should consider discontinuing therapy and using the cholestyramine procedure to eliminate the medication.

Lenalidomide (le na LID oh mide)

U.S. Brand Names Revlimid®

Index Terms CC-5013; IMid-1

Generic Availability (U.S.) No

Pharmacologic Category Angiogenesis Inhibitor; Antineoplastic Agent; Immunomodulator, Systemic

Medication Safety Issues

Sound-alike/look-alike issues:

Lenalidomide may be confused with thalidomide

High alert medication: This medication is in a class the Institute for Safe Medication Practices (ISMP) includes among its list of drug classes which have a heightened risk of causing significant patient harm when used in error.

Medication Guide Available Yes

Prescribing and Access Restrictions As a requirement of the REMS program, access to this medication is restricted. Lenalidomide is approved for marketing in the U.S. only under a Food and Drug Administration (FDA) approved, restricted distribution program called RevAssist® (www.REVLIMID.com or 1-888-423-5436). In Canada, distribution is restricted through RevAid® (www.RevAid.ca or 1-888-738-2431). Physicians, pharmacies, and patients must be registered; a maximum 28-day supply may be dispensed; a new prescription is required each time it is filled; pregnancy testing is required for females of childbearing potential.

Pregnancy Risk Factor X

Lactation Excretion in breast milk unknown/not recommended

Use Treatment of low- or intermediate-risk myelodysplastic syndrome (MDS) in patients with deletion 5q (del 5q) cytogenetic abnormality with transfusion-dependent anemia (with or without other cytogenetic abnormalities); treatment of multiple myeloma (in combination with dexamethasone) in patients who have received at least one prior therapy

Unlabeled/Investigational Use Treatment of non-Hodgkin's lymphomas; systemic amyloidosis (light chain); lower-risk myelodysplastic syndrome (MDS) in transfusion-dependent patients without deletion 5q (del 5q); maintenance treatment for multiple myeloma (following autologous stem cell transplant)

Mechanism of Action/Effect Immune system modulator with antiangiogenic and antineoplastic properties

Contraindications Hypersensitivity to lenalidomide or any component of the formulation; pregnancy or women capable of becoming pregnant

Canadian labeling: Additional contraindications (not in U.S. labeling): Platelet count <50,000/mm^3; hypersensitivity to thalidomide; breast-feeding women

Warnings/Precautions Hazardous agent - use appropriate precautions for handling and disposal. **[U.S. Boxed Warning]: Hematologic toxicity (neutropenia and thrombocytopenia) occurs in a majority of patients (grade 3/4: 80% in patients with del 5q myelodysplastic syndrome) and may require dose reductions and/or delays; the use of blood**

product support and/or growth factors may be needed. CBC should be monitored weekly for the first 8 weeks and at least monthly thereafter in patients being treated for del 5q myelodysplastic syndromes. In patients being treated for multiple myeloma, monitor CBC every 2 weeks for 12 weeks and monthly thereafter. **[U.S. Boxed Warning]: Lenalidomide has been associated with a significant increase in risk for thrombosis and embolism in multiple myeloma patients treated with combination therapy. Deep vein thrombosis (DVT) and pulmonary embolism (PE) have occurred; monitor for signs and symptoms of thromboembolism (shortness of breath, chest pain, or arm or leg swelling) and seek prompt medical attention with development of these symptoms.** Use caution in renal impairment; may experience an increased rate of toxicities. The NCCN multiple myeloma guidelines (v1.2011) recommend anticoagulant prophylaxis when used in combination with dexamethasone. Anticoagulant prophylaxis should be individualized and selected based on the venous thromboembolism risk of the combination treatment regimen, using the safest and easiest to administer (Palumbo, 2008).

Angioedema, Stevens-Johnson syndrome (SJS), and toxic epidermal necrolysis (TEN) have been reported; may be fatal. Consider interrupting or discontinuing treatment with grade 2 or 3 skin rash; discontinue and do not reinitiate treatment with grade 4 rash, exfoliative or bullous rash, or for suspected SJS or TEN. Patients with a history of grade 4 rash with thalidomide should not receive lenalidomide. Discontinue treatment with angioedema. Use caution in renal impairment; may experience an increased rate of toxicities (due to reduced clearance and increased half-life); initial dosage adjustments are recommended for moderate-to-severe and dialysis-dependent renal impairment. Patients with a high tumor burden may be at risk for tumor lysis syndrome.

[U.S. Boxed Warning]: Lenalidomide is an analogue of thalidomide (a human teratogen) and could potentially cause birth defects in humans; avoid pregnancy while taking lenalidomide. Distribution is restricted; physicians, pharmacists, and patients must be registered with the RevAssist® program. Patients should be advised not to donate blood during therapy and for 4 weeks following completion of therapy. May cause dizziness or fatigue; caution patients about performing tasks which require mental alertness (eg, operating machinery or driving). Formulation contains lactose; avoid use in patients with Lapp lactase deficiency, glucose-galactose malabsorption, or glucose intolerance. Lenalidomide should only be prescribed to patients (male and female) who can understand and comply with the conditions of the RevAssist® program. If used in patients between 12-18 years of age, the parent or legal guardian must agree to ensure compliance with the RevAssist® program.

Drug Interactions

Avoid Concomitant Use

Avoid concomitant use of Lenalidomide with any of the following: Abatacept; Anakinra; BCG; Canakinumab; Certolizumab Pegol; Natalizumab; Pimecrolimus; Rilonacept; Roflumilast; Tacrolimus (Topical); Vaccines (Live)

Decreased Effect

Lenalidomide may decrease the levels/effects of: BCG; Sipuleucel-T; Vaccines (Inactivated); Vaccines (Live)

The levels/effects of Lenalidomide may be decreased by: Echinacea

Increased Effect/Toxicity

Lenalidomide may increase the levels/effects of: Abatacept; Anakinra; Canakinumab; Certolizumab Pegol; Leflunomide; Natalizumab; Rilonacept; Vaccines (Live)

The levels/effects of Lenalidomide may be increased by: Denosumab; Dexamethasone; Dexamethasone (Systemic); Pimecrolimus; Roflumilast; Tacrolimus (Topical); Trastuzumab

Nutritional/Ethanol Interactions Herb/Nutraceutical: Avoid echinacea (has immunostimulant properties; consider therapy modifications).

Adverse Reactions

>10%:

Cardiovascular: Peripheral edema (8% to 21%)

Central nervous system: Fatigue (31% to 38%), insomnia (10% to 32%), fever (21% to 23%), dizziness (20% to 21%), headache (20% to 21%)

Dermatologic: Pruritus (42%), rash (16% to 36%; grades 3/4: 7%), dry skin (14%)

Endocrine & metabolic: Hyperglycemia (15%), hypokalemia (11%)

Gastrointestinal: Diarrhea (29% to 49%), constipation (24% to 39%), nausea (22% to 24%), weight loss (18%), dyspepsia (14%), anorexia (10% to 14%), taste perversion (6% to 13%), abdominal pain (8% to 12%)

Genitourinary: Urinary tract infection (11%)

Hematologic: Thrombocytopenia (17% to 62%; grades 3/4: 10% to 50%; onset [MDS]: 28 days [range 8-290 days]; recovery [MDS]: 22 days [range: 5-224 days]), neutropenia (28% to 59%; grades 3/4: 21% to 53%; onset [MDS]: 42 days [range 14-411 days]; recovery [MDS]: 17 days [range: 2-170 days]), anemia (12% to 24%; grades 3/4: 6% to 8%); myelosuppression is dose-dependent and reversible with treatment interruption and/or dose reduction

Neuromuscular & skeletal: Muscle cramp (18% to 30%), weakness (15% to 23%), arthralgia (10% to 22%), back pain (15% to 21%), tremor (20%), paresthesia (12%), limb pain (11%)

Ocular: Blurred vision (15%)

Respiratory: Nasopharyngitis (23%), cough (15% to 20%), dyspnea (7% to 20%), pharyngitis (16%), epistaxis (15%), upper respiratory infection (14% to 15%), pneumonia (11% to 12%)

1% to 10%:

Cardiovascular: Edema (10%), deep vein thrombosis (≤8%; grades 3/4: ≤7%), hypertension (6%), chest pain (5%), palpitation (5%), atrial fibrillation (grades 3/4: ≤3%), syncope (grade 3: 1% to 2%)

Central nervous system: Hypoesthesia (7%), pain (7%), depression (5%)

Dermatologic: Bruising (5% to 8%), cellulitis (5%), erythema (5%)

Endocrine & metabolic: Hypothyroidism (7%), hypomagnesemia (6%), hypocalcemia (grades 3/4: 4%)

Gastrointestinal: Vomiting (10%), xerostomia (7%), loose stools (6%)

Genitourinary: Dysuria (7%)

Hematologic: Leukopenia (8%; grade 3/4: ≤5%), febrile neutropenia (5%; grades 3/4: 4%), granulocytopenia (grades 3/4: 2%), lymphopenia (grade 3: 2%), pancytopenia (grades 3/4: 2%)

Hepatic: ALT increased (8%)

Neuromuscular & skeletal: Myalgia (9%), rigors (6%), peripheral neuropathy (5%)

Respiratory: Sinusitis (8%), rhinitis (7%), bronchitis (6%), pulmonary embolism (≤3%; grades 3/4: 1% to 3%), respiratory distress (grades 3/4: 2%), hypoxia (grades 3/4: 1%), pleural effusion (grades 3/4: 1%), pneumonitis (grades 3/4: 1%), pulmonary hypertension (grades 3/4: 1%)

Miscellaneous: Night sweats (8%), diaphoresis (7%), sepsis (grades 3/4: 3%)

Pharmacodynamics/Kinetics

Absorption Rapid

Time to Peak Healthy volunteers: ~0.6-1.5 hours; Myeloma patients: 0.5-4 hours

Protein Binding ~30%

Half-Life Elimination ~3 hours; moderate-to-severe renal impairment: ~9 hours; hemodialysis patients: ~13.5 hours

Excretion Urine (~67% as unchanged drug); Hemodialysis effect: ~40% of a dose is removed in a single dialysis session

Available Dosage Forms

Capsule, oral:

Revlimid®: 5 mg, 10 mg, 15 mg, 25 mg

Dosing

Adult

Multiple myeloma: Oral: 25 mg once daily for 21 days of a 28-day treatment cycle (in combination with dexamethasone)

Myelodysplastic syndrome (MDS) with deletion 5q: Oral: 10 mg once daily

Diffuse large B-cell lymphoma (unlabeled use): Oral: 25 mg once daily for 21 days of a 28-day treatment cycle for up to 1 year (Wiernik, 2008)

Mantle cell lymphoma, relapsed or refractory (unlabeled use): Oral: 25 mg once daily for 21 days of a 28-day treatment cycle for up to 1 year (Habermann, 2009)

Multiple myeloma, maintenance (following autologous stem cell transplant; unlabeled use): Oral: 10-15 mg once daily until relapse (Attal, 2009; McCarthy, 2009) **or** 10 mg once daily for 21 days of a 28-day treatment cycle until relapse (Palumbo, 2010)

Myelodysplastic syndrome (MDS), lower risk, without deletion 5q (unlabeled use): Oral: 10 mg once daily (Raza, 2008)

Geriatric Refer to adult dosing. Due to the potential for decreased renal function in the elderly, select dose carefully and closely monitor renal function.

Renal Impairment

Recommended initial dose adjustment in the FDA-approved labeling:

MDS:

- Cl_{cr} ≥60 mL/minute: No adjustment required.
- Cl_{cr} 30-59 mL/minute: 5 mg once daily.
- Cl_{cr} <30 mL/minute (nondialysis dependent): 5 mg every 48 hours.
- Cl_{cr} <30 mL/minute (dialysis dependent): 5 mg 3 times/week (administer following each dialysis).

Multiple myeloma:

- Cl_{cr} ≥60 mL/minute: No adjustment required.
- Cl_{cr} 30-59 mL/minute: 10 mg once daily.
- Cl_{cr} <30 mL/minute (nondialysis dependent): 15 mg every 48 hours.
- Cl_{cr} <30 mL/minute (dialysis dependent): 5 mg once daily (administer after dialysis on dialysis days).

Recommended adjustment in Canadian labeling:

MDS:

- Cl_{cr} ≥50 mL/minute: No adjustment required.
- Cl_{cr} 30-49 mL/minute: 5 mg once daily.
- Cl_{cr} <30 mL/minute (nondialysis dependent): 5 mg every 48 hours.
- Cl_{cr} <30 mL/minute (dialysis dependent): 5 mg 3 times/week (administer following each dialysis).

Multiple myeloma:

- Cl_{cr} ≥50 mL/minute: No adjustment required.
- Cl_{cr} 30-49 mL/minute: 10 mg once daily; (may increase to 15 mg once daily after 2 cycles if nonresponsive but tolerating treatment; Chen, 2007)
- Cl_{cr} <30 mL/minute (nondialysis dependent): 15 mg every 48 hours.
- Cl_{cr} <30 mL/minute (dialysis dependent): 15 mg 3 times/week (administer following each dialysis).

Adjustment for Toxicity

NONHEMATOLOGIC toxicities:

Dermatologic toxicities:

Skin rash, grade 2 or 3: Consider interrupting or discontinuing treatment

Angioedema, grade 4 rash, exfoliative or bullous rash, or suspected Stevens-Johnson syndrome or toxic epidermal necrolysis: Discontinue treatment

Other toxicities: For additional treatment-related grade 3/4 toxicities, hold treatment and restart at next lower dose level when toxicity has resolved to ≤ grade 2.

HEMATOLOGIC toxicities:

Adjustment for thrombocytopenia in MDS:

Thrombocytopenia developing within 4 weeks of beginning treatment at 10 mg/day:

Baseline platelets ≥100,000/mm^3:

If platelets <50,000/mm^3: Hold treatment

When platelets return to ≥50,000/mm^3: Resume treatment at 5 mg/day

Baseline platelets <100,000/mm^3:

If platelets fall to 50% of baseline: Hold treatment

If baseline ≥60,000/mm^3 and platelet level returns to ≥50,000/mm^3: Resume at 5 mg/day

If baseline <60,000/mm^3 and platelet level returns to ≥30,000/mm^3: Resume at 5 mg/day

Thrombocytopenia developing after 4 weeks of beginning treatment at 10 mg/day:

Platelets <30,000/mm^3 **or** <50,000/mm^3 with platelet transfusions: Hold treatment

Platelets ≥30,000/mm^3 (without hemostatic failure): Resume at 5 mg/day

Thrombocytopenia developing with treatment at 5 mg/day:

Platelets <30,000/mm^3 **or** <50,000/mm^3 with platelet transfusions: Hold treatment

Platelets ≥30,000/mm^3 (without hemostatic failure): Resume at 5 mg every other day

Adjustment for neutropenia in MDS:

Neutropenia developing within 4 weeks of beginning treatment at 10 mg/day:

For baseline absolute neutrophil count (ANC) ≥1000/mm^3:

ANC <750/mm^3: Hold treatment

When ANC returns to ≥1000/mm^3: Resume at 5 mg/day

For baseline absolute neutrophil count (ANC) <1000/mm^3:

ANC <500/mm^3: Hold treatment

When ANC returns to ≥500/mm^3: Resume at 5 mg/day

Neutropenia developing after 4 weeks of beginning treatment at 10 mg/day:

ANC <500/mm^3 for ≥7 days or associated with fever: Hold treatment

When ≥500/mm^3: Resume at 5 mg/day

Neutropenia developing with treatment at 5 mg/day:

ANC <500/mm^3 for ≥7 days or associated with fever: Hold treatment

When ≥500/mm^3: Resume at 5 mg every other day

Adjustment for thrombocytopenia in multiple myeloma:

Platelets <30,000/mm^3: Hold treatment, check CBC weekly

When platelets ≥30,000/mm^3: Resume at 15 mg daily

Additional occurrence of platelets <30,000/mm^3: Hold treatment

When platelets ≥30,000/mm^3: Resume treatment at 5 mg below previous dose; do not dose below 5 mg daily

Adjustment for neutropenia in multiple myeloma:

ANC <1000/mm^3: Hold treatment, add G-CSF, check CBC weekly

When ≥1000/mm^3 (with neutropenia as only toxicity): Resume at 25 mg/day

When ≥1000/mm^3 (with additional toxicities): Resume at 15 mg/day

Additional occurrence of ANC <1000/mm^3: Hold treatment

When ≥1000/mm^3: Resume treatment at 5 mg below previous dose; do not dose below 5 mg daily.

Administration

Oral Administer with water. Swallow capsule whole; do not break, open, or chew.

Stability

Storage Store at 25°C (77°F); excursions permitted to 15°C and 30°C (59°F and 86°F).

Monitoring and Teaching Issues

Laboratory Monitoring CBC with differential (MDS: weekly for first 8 weeks; multiple myeloma: every 2 weeks for the first 3 months), then monthly thereafter; serum creatinine, liver function tests, thyroid function tests. Women of childbearing potential: Pregnancy test 10-14 days **and** 24 hours prior to initiating therapy, weekly during the first 4 weeks of treatment, then every 2-4 weeks through 4 weeks after therapy discontinued

Physical Assessment Verify that patient is not pregnant prior to initiating therapy. Instruct patient on the need to use two reliable forms of contraception beginning 4 weeks prior to, during, and for 4 weeks after therapy and during therapy interruptions. Monitor for signs of thromboembolism (shortness of breath, chest pain, or arm or leg swelling), deep vein thrombosis (swelling and tenderness of extremities), rash, angioedema, infection, or bleeding.

Patient Education You will need frequent blood tests while taking this medication. Maintain adequate hydration unless instructed to restrict intake by prescriber. If you have diabetes, monitor blood glucose closely. Can cause hyperglycemia. You may be susceptible to infections. Avoid vaccinations unless approved by prescriber. Do not donate blood during treatment or for 4 weeks following completion of therapy. You may experience headache, fever, insomnia, fatigue, dizziness, swelling of extremities, rash, itching, nausea, diarrhea, constipation, abdominal pain, loss of appetite, change in taste, upper respiratory infections, urinary tract infection, or sore throat. Report rash, shortness of breath, chest pain, arm or leg swelling and tenderness, weight gain, extreme weakness or fatigue, muscle cramping, unusual bleeding or bruising, or nosebleeds.

Geriatric Considerations The manufacturer reports that the frequency of serious adverse effects was higher in patients >65 years of age compared to younger patients (54% vs 33%). More older patients withdrew from the clinical studies because of side effects. There was no significant difference in efficacy in older versus younger patients.

Breast-Feeding Considerations Due to the potential for adverse reactions in nursing infants, breast-feeding is not recommended.

Pregnancy Considerations [U.S. Boxed Warning]: Lenalidomide is an analogue of thalidomide (a human teratogen) and could potentially cause birth defects in humans; avoid pregnancy while taking lenalidomide. Distribution is restricted; physicians, pharmacists, and patients must be registered with the RevAssist® program. Animal studies with lenalidomide in nonhuman primates have demonstrated malformations similar to those observed with thalidomide; there are no adequate and well-controlled studies in pregnant women. Women of childbearing potential should be treated only if they are able to comply with the conditions of the RevAssist® program. Female patients must commit either to abstain continuously or two forms of effective contraception are required beginning 4 weeks prior to, during, and for 4 weeks after therapy and during therapy interruptions. Pregnancy tests (sensitivity of at least 50 mIU/mL) should be performed 10-14 days and 24 hours prior to beginning therapy; weekly for the first 4 weeks and every 4 weeks (every 2 weeks if menstrual cycle irregular) thereafter and during therapy interruptions. Lenalidomide must be immediately discontinued and the patient referred to a reproductive toxicity specialist if pregnancy occurs during treatment. Males (even those vasectomized) should use a latex condom during any sexual contact with women of childbearing age. Risk to the fetus from semen of male patients is unknown. The parent or legal guardian for patients between 12 and 18 years of age must agree to ensure compliance with the required guidelines. Any suspected fetal exposure should be reported to the FDA via the MedWatch program (1-800-FDA-1088) and to Celgene Corporation (1-888-423-5436)

Additional Information Pregnancy tests are required prior to beginning therapy, throughout treatment and during therapy interruptions for all women of childbearing age. The pregnancy test must be verified by the prescriber and the pharmacist prior to dispensing. Effective contraception with at least two reliable forms of contraception (IUD, hormonal contraception, tubal ligation or partner's vasectomy plus latex condom, diaphragm, or cervical cap) should be used for 4 weeks prior to beginning therapy, during therapy, and for 4 weeks following discontinuance of therapy. Women who have undergone a hysterectomy or have been postmenopausal for at least 24 consecutive months are the only exception. Do not prescribe, administer, or dispense to women of childbearing age or males who may have intercourse with women of childbearing age unless both female and male are capable of complying with contraceptive measures. Even males who have undergone vasectomy must acknowledge these risks in writing, and must use a latex condom during any sexual contact with women of childbearing age. Oral and written warnings concerning contraception and the hazards of thalidomide must be conveyed to females and males and they must acknowledge their understanding in writing. Parents or guardians must consent and sign acknowledgment for patients 12-18 years of age following therapy. A maximum 28-day supply should be dispensed.

Lepirudin (leh puh ROO din)

U.S. Brand Names Refludan®

Index Terms Lepirudin (rDNA); Recombinant Hirudin

Generic Availability (U.S.) No

Pharmacologic Category Anticoagulant, Thrombin Inhibitor

Medication Safety Issues

High alert medication: The Institute for Safe Medication Practices (ISMP) includes this medication among its list of drugs which have a heightened risk of causing significant patient harm when used in error.

Pregnancy Risk Factor B

Lactation Enters breast milk/consult prescriber

Use Indicated for anticoagulation in patients with heparin-induced thrombocytopenia (HIT) and associated thromboembolic disease in order to prevent further thromboembolic complications

Unlabeled/Investigational Use Investigational: Prevention or reduction of ischemic complications associated with unstable angina

Mechanism of Action/Effect Lepirudin is a highly specific direct thrombin inhibitor. Each molecule is capable of binding one molecule of thrombin and inhibiting its thrombogenic activity.

Contraindications Hypersensitivity to hirudins or any component of the formulation

Warnings/Precautions Hemorrhagic events: Intracranial bleeding following concomitant thrombolytic therapy with rt-PA or streptokinase may be life threatening. For patients with an increased risk of bleeding, a careful assessment weighing the risk of lepirudin administration versus its anticipated benefit has to be made by the treating physician. In particular, this includes the following conditions: Recent puncture of large vessels or organ biopsy; anomaly of vessels or organs; recent cerebrovascular accident, stroke, intracerebral surgery, or other neuroaxial procedures; severe uncontrolled hypertension; bacterial endocarditis; advanced renal impairment; hemorrhagic diathesis; recent major surgery; and recent major bleeding (eg, intracranial, gastrointestinal, intraocular, or pulmonary bleeding). With renal impairment, relative overdose might occur even with standard dosage regimen. The bolus dose and rate of infusion must be reduced in patients with known or suspected renal insufficiency.

Formation of antihirudin antibodies may increase the anticoagulant effect of lepirudin possibly due to delayed renal elimination of active lepirudin-antihirudin complexes. Therefore, strict monitoring of aPTT is necessary also during prolonged therapy. No evidence of neutralization of lepirudin or of allergic reactions associated with positive antibody test results was found. Allergic and hypersensitivity reactions, including anaphylaxis have been reported and may occur frequently in patients treated concomitantly with streptokinase; caution is warranted during re-exposure (anaphylaxis has been reported).

Serious liver injury (eg, liver cirrhosis) may enhance the anticoagulant effect of lepirudin due to coagulation defects secondary to reduced generation of vitamin K-dependent clotting factors.

Clinical trials have provided limited information to support any recommendations for re-exposure to lepirudin (anaphylaxis has been reported). Safety and efficacy have not been established in children.

Drug Interactions

Avoid Concomitant Use There are no known interactions where it is recommended to avoid concomitant use.

Decreased Effect There are no known significant interactions involving a decrease in effect.

Increased Effect/Toxicity

Lepirudin may increase the levels/effects of: Anticoagulants; Collagenase (Systemic); Ibritumomab; Tositumomab and Iodine I 131 Tositumomab

The levels/effects of Lepirudin may be increased by: Antiplatelet Agents; Dasatinib; Herbs (Anticoagulant/Antiplatelet Properties); Nonsteroidal Anti-Inflammatory Agents; Pentosan Polysulfate Sodium; Prostacyclin Analogues; Salicylates; Thrombolytic Agents

Nutritional/Ethanol Interactions Herb/Nutraceutical: Avoid cat's claw, dong quai, evening primrose, feverfew, garlic, ginger, ginkgo, red clover, horse chestnut, green tea, ginseng (all have additional antiplatelet activity)

Lab Interactions PT/INR levels may become elevated in the absence of warfarin. If warfarin is initiated, initial PT/INR goals while on lepirudin may require modification.

Adverse Reactions As with all anticoagulants, bleeding is the most common adverse event associated with lepirudin. Hemorrhage may occur at virtually any site. Risk is dependent on multiple variables.

HIT patients:

>10%: Hematologic: Anemia (12%), bleeding from puncture sites (11%), hematoma (11%)

1% to 10%:

- Cardiovascular: Heart failure (3%), pericardial effusion (1%), ventricular fibrillation (1%)
- Central nervous system: Fever (7%)
- Dermatologic: Maculopapular rash (4%), eczema (3%)
- Gastrointestinal: GI bleeding/rectal bleeding (5%)
- Genitourinary: Vaginal bleeding (2%)
- Hepatic: Transaminases increased (6%)
- Renal: Hematuria (4%)
- Respiratory: Epistaxis (4%)

Non-HIT populations (including those receiving thrombolytics and/or contrast media):

1% to 10%: Respiratory: Bronchospasm/stridor/dyspnea/cough

Pharmacodynamics/Kinetics

Half-Life Elimination Initial: ~10 minutes: Terminal: Healthy volunteers: 1.3 hours; Significant renal impairment (Cl_{cr} <15 mL/minute and on hemodialysis): ≤2 days

Metabolism Via release of amino acids via catabolic hydrolysis of parent drug

Excretion Urine (~48%, 35% as unchanged drug and unchanged drug fragments of parent drug); systemic clearance is proportional to glomerular filtration rate or creatinine clearance

Available Dosage Forms

Injection, powder for reconstitution:

Refludan®: 50 mg

Dosing

Adult & Geriatric Note: Maximum infusion dose: Do not exceed 0.21 mg/kg/hour unless an evaluation of coagulation abnormalities limiting response has been completed.

Heparin-induced thrombocytopenia: Bolus dose: 0.4 mg/kg IVP (over 15-20 seconds), followed by continuous infusion at 0.15 mg/kg/hour (maximum initial bolus dose: 44 mg; maximum initial infusion dose: 16.5 mg/hour); bolus and infusion must be reduced in renal insufficiency

or

Alternate dosing regimen (unlabeled dose; Selleng, 2007; Warkentin, 2008): Bolus dose: 0.2 mg/kg (use only if life- or limb-threatening thrombosis present) followed by continuous infusion of 0.05-0.1 mg/kg/hour. Further dosage reduction may be required in patients with renal dysfunction. This alternate dosing regimen has been recommended due to higher rates of bleeding associated with the FDA-approved dosing regimen.

Concomitant use with thrombolytic therapy: I.V.: Bolus dose: 0.2 mg/kg IVP (over 15-20 seconds), followed by continuous infusion at 0.1 mg/kg/hour

Dosing adjustments during infusions: Monitor first aPTT 4 hours after the start of the infusion. Subsequent determinations of aPTT should be obtained at least once daily during treatment. More frequent monitoring is recommended in renally- or hepatically-impaired patients. Any aPTT ratio measurement out of range (1.5-2.5) should be confirmed prior to adjusting dose, unless a clinical need for immediate reaction exists. If the aPTT is below target range, increase infusion by 20%. If the aPTT is in excess of the target range, stop infusion for 2 hours and when restarted the infusion rate should be decreased by 50%. A repeat aPTT should be obtained 4 hours after any dosing change.

Transition to oral anticoagulants: Once platelets normalize, reduce lepirudin dose gradually to reach aPTT ratio just above 1.5 before starting warfarin therapy. Monitor PT/INR closely until results stabilize in therapeutic range. When lepirudin is discontinued, there may be a small reduction in INR.

Renal Impairment All patients with a creatinine clearance of <60 mL/minute or a serum creatinine of >1.5 mg/dL require dosage reduction; there is only limited information on the therapeutic use of lepirudin in patients with HIT and significant renal impairment; the following dosage recommendations are mainly based on single-dose studies in a small number of patients with renal impairment. An alternate dosing regimen has also been recommended for patients with serum creatinine >1 mg/dL (Warkentin, 2008).

Initial: Bolus dose: 0.2 mg/kg IVP (over 15-20 seconds), followed by adjusted infusion based on renal function; refer to the following infusion rate adjustments based on creatinine clearance (mL/minute) and serum creatinine (mg/dL):

Note: Acute renal failure or hemodialysis: Infusion is to be avoided or stopped. Following the bolus dose, additional bolus doses of 0.1 mg/kg may be administered every other day only if aPTT falls below lower therapeutic limit (1.5-times patient baseline [or mean laboratory] aPTT).

Lepirudin infusion rates in patients with renal impairment: See tables.

Lepirudin Infusion Rates in Patients With Renal Impairment

Creatinine Clearance (mL/min)	Serum Creatinine (mg/dL)	Adjusted Infusion Rate	
		% of Standard Initial Infusion Rate	mg/kg/h
45-60	1.6-2.0	50%	0.075
30-44	2.1-3.0	30%	0.045
15-29	3.1-6.0	15%	0.0225
<15	>6.0	***Avoid or STOP infusion***	

Alternate Dosing Regimen for Renal Impairment (based on *Chest* 2008 guidelines[1])

Serum Creatinine (mg/dL)	Adjusted Infusion Rate	
	% of Standard Initial Infusion Rate[2]	mg/kg/h
1.0-1.6	50%	0.05
1.7-4.5	10%	0.01
>4.5-6.0	5%	0.005
>6.0	***Avoid or STOP infusion[3]***	

[1]Recommendation based on low or very low-quality evidence.

[2]Recommended standard initial infusion rate: 0.1 mg/kg/hour

[3]Recommendation based on manufacturer's labeling.

Note: The initial bolus should either be omitted, or in the case of perceived life- or limb-threatening thrombosis, be given at a reduced dose of 0.2 mg/kg.

Administration

Oral Administer **only** intravenously

I.V. I.V. bolus: Inject slowly for continuous infusion; solutions with 0.2 or 0.4 mg/mL may be used.

Stability

Reconstitution

Intravenous bolus: Use a solution with a concentration of 5 mg/mL: Reconstitute one vial (50 mg) of lepirudin with 1 mL of sterile water for injection or 0.9% sodium chloride injection. The final concentration of 5 mg/mL is obtained by transferring the contents of the vial into a sterile, single-use syringe (of at least 10 mL capacity) and diluting the solution to a total volume of 10 mL using sterile water for injection, 0.9% sodium chloride, or 5% dextrose in water.

Intravenous infusion: For continuous intravenous infusion, solutions with concentrations of 0.2 or 0.4 mg/mL may be used. Reconstitute 2 vials (50 mg each) of lepirudin with 1 mL each using either sterile water for injection or 0.9% sodium chloride injection. The final concentration of 0.2 mg/mL or 0.4 mg/mL is obtained by transferring the contents of both vials into an infusion bag containing 500 mL or 250 mL of 0.9% sodium chloride injection or 5% dextrose injection.

Storage

Intact vials should be stored at 2°C to 25°C (36°F to 77°F). Manufacturer recommends using reconstituted solution immediately after preparation. Reconstituted solutions of lepirudin are stable for 24 hours at room temperature.

Monitoring and Teaching Issues

Laboratory Monitoring Monitor aPTT levels; obtain baseline aPTT, then monitor first aPTT 4 hours after the start of the infusion and every 4 hours until steady state is reached (2 consecutive aPTTs in the same range) (Warkentin, 2008). Subsequent determinations of aPTT should be obtained at least once daily during treatment. More frequent monitoring is recommended in renally- or hepatically-impaired patients. Any aPTT ratio measurement out of range (1.5-2.5) should be confirmed prior to adjusting dose, unless a clinical need for immediate reaction exists

Physical Assessment Note Administration for infusion specifics. Bleeding precautions should be observed. Monitor for hypersensitivity reaction, bleeding, chest pain, and rash. Teach patient bleeding precautions.

Patient Education This drug can only be administered by infusion. Report immediately any pain, swelling, burning, or bleeding at infusion site. You may have a tendency to bleed easily while taking this drug (brush teeth with soft brush, floss with waxed floss, use electric razor, avoid scissors or sharp knives, and avoid potentially harmful activities). Report unusual bleeding or bruising (bleeding gums, nosebleed, blood in urine, dark stool), pain in joints or back, CNS changes (fever, confusion), unusual fever, persistent nausea or GI upset, or swelling or pain at injection site.

Pregnancy Considerations Lepirudin crosses the placenta in pregnant rats; however, it is not known if lepirudin crosses the placenta in humans.

- **Lepirudin (rDNA)** *see* Lepirudin *on page* 1075
- **Lescol®** *see* Fluvastatin *on page* 807
- **Lescol® XL** *see* Fluvastatin *on page* 807
- **Lessina®** *see* Ethinyl Estradiol and Levonorgestrel *on page* 699
- **Letairis®** *see* Ambrisentan *on page* 93

Letrozole (LET roe zole)

U.S. Brand Names Femara®

Index Terms CGS-20267

Generic Availability (U.S.) No

Pharmacologic Category Antineoplastic Agent, Aromatase Inhibitor

Medication Safety Issues

Sound-alike/look-alike issues:

Femara® may be confused with Famvir®, femhrt®, Provera®

Letrozole may be confused with anastrozole

Pregnancy Risk Factor X

Lactation Excretion in breast milk unknown/not recommended

Use For use in postmenopausal women in the adjuvant treatment of hormone receptor positive early breast cancer, extended adjuvant treatment of early breast cancer after 5 years of tamoxifen, advanced breast cancer with disease progression following antiestrogen therapy, hormone receptor positive or hormone receptor unknown, locally-advanced, or first-line (or second-line) treatment of advanced or metastatic breast cancer

Unlabeled/Investigational Use Treatment of ovarian (epithelial) cancer, endometrial cancer

Mechanism of Action/Effect Nonsteroidal competitive inhibitor of the aromatase enzyme system, which catalyzes conversion of androgens to estrogens. Inhibition leads to a significant reduction in plasma estrogen levels. Does not affect synthesis of adrenal or thyroid hormones, aldosterone, or androgens.

Contraindications Use in women who are or may become pregnant

Warnings/Precautions Hazardous agent - use appropriate precautions for handling and disposal. Use caution with hepatic impairment; dose adjustment recommended in patients with cirrhosis or severe hepatic dysfunction. May cause dizziness, fatigue, and somnolence; patients should be cautioned before performing tasks which require mental alertness (eg, operating machinery or driving). May increase total serum cholesterol; in patients treated with adjuvant therapy and cholesterol levels within normal limits, an increase of >1.5 x ULN in total cholesterol has been demonstrated in 8.2% of letrozole-treated patients (25% requiring lipid-lowering medications) vs 3.2% of tamoxifen-treated patients (16% requiring medications); monitor cholesterol panel; may require antihyperlipidemics. May cause decreases in bone mineral density (BMD); a decrease in hip BMD by 3.8% from baseline in letrozole-treated patients vs 2% in placebo at 2 years has been demonstrated; however, there was no statistical difference in changes to the lumbar spine BMD scores; monitor BMD.

Drug Interactions

Metabolism/Transport Effects Substrate (minor) of CYP2A6, 3A4; **Inhibits** CYP2A6 (strong), 2C19 (weak)

Avoid Concomitant Use There are no known interactions where it is recommended to avoid concomitant use.

Decreased Effect

The levels/effects of Letrozole may be decreased by: Tamoxifen

Increased Effect/Toxicity

Letrozole may increase the levels/effects of: CYP2A6 Substrates

The levels/effects of Letrozole may be increased by: Conivaptan

Adverse Reactions

>10%:

Cardiovascular: Edema (7% to 18%)

Central nervous system: Headache (4% to 20%), dizziness (3% to 14%), fatigue (8% to 13%)

Endocrine & metabolic: Hypercholesterolemia (3% to 52%), hot flashes (6% to 50%)

Gastrointestinal: Nausea (9% to 17%), weight gain (2% to 13%), constipation (2% to 11%)

Neuromuscular & skeletal: Weakness (4% to 34%), arthralgia (8% to 25%), arthritis (7% to 25%), bone pain (5% to 22%), back pain (5% to 18%), bone mineral density decreased/ osteoporosis (5% to 15%), bone fracture (10% to 14%)
Respiratory: Dyspnea (6% to 18%), cough (6% to 13%)
Miscellaneous: Diaphoresis (≤24%), night sweats (15%)

1% to 10%:

Cardiovascular: Chest pain (6% to 8%), hypertension (5% to 8%), chest wall pain (6%), peripheral edema (5%), cerebrovascular accident (2% to 3%), thromboembolic event (2% to 3%), MI (1% to 2%), angina (1%)
Central nervous system: Insomnia (6% to 7%), pain (5%), anxiety (<5%), depression (<5%), vertigo (<5%),somnolence (3%)
Dermatologic: Rash (5%), alopecia (3% to 5%), pruritus (1%)
Endocrine & metabolic: Breast pain (2% to 7%), hypercalcemia (<5%)
Gastrointestinal: Diarrhea (5% to 8%), vomiting (3% to 7%), weight loss (6% to 7%), abdominal pain (6%), anorexia (1% to 5%), dyspepsia (3%)
Genitourinary: Urinary tract infection (6%), vaginal bleeding (5%), vaginal dryness (5%), vaginal hemorrhage (5%), vaginal irritation (5%)
Neuromuscular & skeletal: Limb pain (4% to 10%), myalgia (7% to 9%)
Ocular: Cataract (2%)
Renal: Renal disorder (5%)
Respiratory: Pleural effusion (<5%)
Miscellaneous: Infection (7%), influenza (6%), viral infection (6%), secondary malignancy (2% to 4%)

Pharmacodynamics/Kinetics

Absorption Rapid and well absorbed; not affected by food

Time to Peak Steady state, plasma: 2-6 weeks

Protein Binding Plasma: Weak

Half-Life Elimination Terminal: ~2 days

Metabolism Hepatic via CYP3A4 and 2A6 to an inactive carbinol metabolite

Excretion Urine (90%; 6% as unchanged drug, 75% as glucuronide carbinol metabolite, 9% as unidentified metabolites)

Available Dosage Forms

Tablet, oral:
Femara®: 2.5 mg

Dosing

Adult & Geriatric Females: Postmenopausal:

Breast cancer, advanced (first- or second-line treatment): Oral: 2.5 mg once daily; continue until tumor progression

Breast cancer, early (adjuvant treatment): Oral: 2.5 mg once daily; optimal duration unknown, duration in clinical trial is 5 years; discontinue at relapse

Breast cancer, early (extended adjuvant treatment): Oral: 2.5 mg once daily; optimal duration unknown, duration in clinical trials is 5 years (after 5 years of tamoxifen); discontinue at relapse

Ovarian (epithelial) cancer (unlabeled use): Oral: 2.5 mg once daily; continue until disease progression (Ramirez, 2008)

Renal Impairment No dosage adjustment is required in patients with renal impairment if Cl_{cr} is ≥10 mL/minute.

Hepatic Impairment

Mild-to-moderate impairment (Child-Pugh class A and B): No adjustment recommended.
Severe impairment (Child-Pugh class C) and cirrhosis: 2.5 mg every other day.

Administration

Oral Administer with or without food.

Stability

Storage Store at room temperature of 25°C (77°F); excursions permitted to 15°C to 30°C (59°F to 86°F).

Monitoring and Teaching Issues

Laboratory Monitoring CBC, cholesterol, thyroid function tests, serum electrolytes, serum transaminases, serum creatinine

Physical Assessment For use in postmenopausal women only. Monitor for hypertension, pain, gastrointestinal upset, and hot flashes on a regular basis.

Patient Education You may experience nausea, vomiting, hot flashes, loss of appetite, musculoskeletal pain, headache, sleepiness, fatigue, dizziness, constipation, diarrhea, or loss of hair (will grow back). Report chest pain, pressure, palpitations, or swollen extremities; weakness, severe headache, numbness, or loss of strength in any part of the body; difficulty speaking; vaginal bleeding; unusual signs of bleeding or bruising; respiratory difficulty; severe nausea; muscle pain; or skin rash.

Dietary Considerations May be taken without regard to meals. Calcium and vitamin D supplementation are recommended.

Geriatric Considerations No dosage adjustment recommended.

Pregnancy Considerations Letrozole may cause fetal harm when administered to pregnant women. Animal studies have demonstrated embryotoxicity and fetotoxicity. There are no adequate and well-controlled studies in pregnant women. If used in pregnancy, or if patient becomes pregnant during treatment, the patient should be apprised of potential hazard to the fetus. Letrozole is FDA indicated for postmenopausal women only (no clinical benefit for breast cancer has been demonstrated in premenopausal women). Women who are peri-menopausal or recently postmenopausal should use adequate contraception until post-menopausal status is fully established.

Additional Information Oncology Comment: The American Society of Clinical Oncology (ASCO) guidelines for adjuvant endocrine therapy in postmenopausal women with HR-positive breast cancer (Burstein, 2010) recommend considering aromatase inhibitor (AI) therapy at some point in the treatment course (primary, sequentially, or extended). Optimal duration at this time is not known; however, treatment with an AI should not exceed 5 years in primary and extended therapies, and 2-3 years if followed by tamoxifen in sequential therapy (total of 5 years). If initial therapy with AI has been discontinued before the 5 years, consideration should be taken to receive tamoxifen for a total of 5 years. The optimal time to switch to an AI is also not known, but data supports switching after 2-3 years of tamoxifen (sequential) or after 5 years of tamoxifen (extended). If patient becomes intolerant or has poor adherence, consideration should be made to switch to another AI or initiate tamoxifen.

◆ **Leucovorin** *see* Leucovorin Calcium *on page 1080*

Leucovorin Calcium (loo koe VOR in)

Index Terms 5-Formyl Tetrahydrofolate; Calcium Leucovorin; Citrovorum Factor; Folinic Acid (error prone synonym); Leucovorin

Generic Availability (U.S.) Yes

Pharmacologic Category Antidote; Chemotherapy Modulating Agent; Rescue Agent (Chemotherapy); Vitamin, Water Soluble

Medication Safety Issues

Sound-alike/look-alike issues:

Leucovorin may be confused with Leukeran®, Leukine®, LEVOleucovorin
Folinic acid may be confused with folic acid
Folinic acid is an error prone synonym and should not be used

Pregnancy Risk Factor C

Lactation Excretion in breast milk unknown/use caution

Use Antidote for folic acid antagonists (methotrexate, trimethoprim, pyrimethamine) and rescue therapy following high-dose methotrexate; in combination with fluorouracil in the treatment of colon cancer; treatment of megaloblastic anemias when folate is deficient as in infancy, sprue, pregnancy, and nutritional deficiency when oral folate therapy is not possible

Unlabeled/Investigational Use Adjunctive cofactor therapy in methanol toxicity

Mechanism of Action/Effect A reduced form of folic acid, leucovorin supplies the necessary cofactor blocked by methotrexate. Leucovorin actively competes with methotrexate for transport sites, displaces methotrexate from intracellular binding sites, and restores active folate stores required for DNA/RNA synthesis. Stabilizes the binding of 5-dUMP and thymidylate synthetase, enhancing the activity of fluorouracil.

Methanol toxicity treatment: Formic acid (methanol's toxic metabolite) is normally metabolized to carbon dioxide and water by 10-formyltetrahydrofolate dehydrogenase after being bound to tetrahydrofolate. Administering a source of tetrahydrofolate may aid the body in eliminating formic acid.

Contraindications Pernicious anemia or vitamin B_{12}-deficient megaloblastic anemias

Warnings/Precautions When used for the treatment of accidental weak folic acid antagonist overdose, administer as soon as possible. When used for the treatment of a methotrexate overdose, administer as soon as possible. Do not wait for the results of a methotrexate level before initiating therapy. It is important to adjust the leucovorin dose once a methotrexate level is known. When used for methotrexate rescue therapy, methotrexate serum concentrations should be monitored to determine dose and duration of leucovorin therapy. The dose may need to be increased or administration prolonged in situations where methotrexate excretion may be delayed (eg, ascites, pleural effusion, renal insufficiency, inadequate hydration); **never administer leucovorin intrathecally.** Combination of leucovorin and sulfamethoxazole-trimethoprim for the acute treatment of PCP in patients with HIV infection has been reported to cause increased rates of treatment failure. Leucovorin may increase the toxicity of 5-fluorouracil; dose of 5-fluorouracil may need decreased.

Powder for injection: When doses >10 mg/m^2 are required, reconstitute using sterile water for injection, not a solution containing benzyl alcohol.

Injection: Due to calcium content, do not administer I.V. solutions at a rate >160 mg/minute. Not intended for intrathecal use.

Drug Interactions

Avoid Concomitant Use

Avoid concomitant use of Leucovorin Calcium with any of the following: Raltitrexed

Decreased Effect

Leucovorin Calcium may decrease the levels/effects of: PHENobarbital; Phenytoin; Primidone; Raltitrexed; Trimethoprim

Increased Effect/Toxicity

Leucovorin Calcium may increase the levels/effects of: Capecitabine; Fluorouracil; Fluorouracil (Systemic); Fluorouracil (Topical)

Adverse Reactions Frequency not defined. Toxicities (especially gastrointestinal toxicity) of fluorouracil is higher when used in combination with leucovorin.

Dermatologic: Rash, pruritus, erythema, urticaria
Hematologic: Thrombocytosis
Respiratory: Wheezing
Miscellaneous: Allergic reactions, anaphylactoid reactions

Pharmacodynamics/Kinetics

Absorption Oral, I.M.: Well absorbed

Bioavailability Saturable at oral doses >25 mg; 25 mg (97%), 50 mg (75%), 100 mg (37%)

Time to Peak Oral: ~2 hours; I.V.: Total folates: 10 minutes; 5MTHF: ~1 hour

Half-Life Elimination ~4-8 hours

Metabolism Intestinal mucosa and hepatically to 5-methyl-tetrahydrofolate (5MTHF; active)

Excretion Urine (primarily); feces

Available Dosage Forms

Injection, powder for reconstitution: 50 mg, 100 mg, 200 mg, 350 mg

Injection, solution [preservative free]: 10 mg/mL (50 mL)

Tablet, oral: 5 mg, 10 mg, 15 mg, 25 mg

Dosing

Adult & Geriatric

Treatment of weak folic acid antagonist overdosage (eg, trimethoprim, pyrimethamine): Oral: 5-15 mg/day

Folate-deficient megaloblastic anemia: I.M.: ≤1 mg/day

High-dose methotrexate-rescue dose: Initial: Oral, I.M., I.V.: 15 mg (~10 mg/m^2); start 24 hours after beginning methotrexate infusion; continue every 6 hours for 10 doses, until methotrexate level is <0.05 micromole/L. Adjust dose as follows:

Normal methotrexate elimination: Oral, I.M., I.V.: 15 mg every 6 hours

Delayed early methotrexate elimination: I.V.: 150 mg every 3 hours until methotrexate level is <1 micromole/L, then 15 mg every 3 hours until methotrexate level is <0.05 micromole/L

Colorectal cancer :

I.V.: 200 mg/m^2 over at least 3 minutes (used in combination with fluorouracil 370 mg/m^2)

or

I.V.: 20 mg/m^2 (used in combination with fluorouracil 425 mg/m^2)

Methotrexate overdose: Note: The amount of leucovorin administered should equal the amount of methotrexate inadvertently administered.

I.V.: 1 mg per mg of methotrexate inadvertently administered; 100-1000 mg/m^2 every 3-6 hours has been used; administer until methotrexate levels decrease to goal level or longer if methotrexate levels are unavailable or if patient has renal dysfunction or third-space storage (ascites, pleural effusion)

A nomogram for leucovorin rescue in cancer patients receiving high-dose methotrexate based upon a 48-hour methotrexate level may be helpful (Widemann, 2006). Methotrexate level:

≥80 micromole/L: 1000 mg/m^2 every 6 hours

≥8 to <80 micromole/L: 100 mg/m^2 every 3 hours

≥2 to <8 micromole/L: 10 mg/m^2 every 3 hours

≥0.1 to <2 micromole/L: 10 mg/m^2 every 6 hours

Use of I.T. leucovorin is not advised (Jardine, 1996; Smith, 2008).

Pemetrexed toxicity (unlabeled dose): I.V.: 100 mg/m^2 once, followed by 50 mg/m^2 every 6 hours for 8 days was used in clinical trial for CTC grade 4 leukopenia ≥3 days; CTC grade 4 neutropenia ≥3 days; immediately for CTC grade 4 thrombocytopenia, bleeding associated with grade 3 thrombocytopenia, or grade 3 or 4 mucositis

Cofactor therapy in methanol toxicity (unlabeled use): I.V.: 1 mg/kg (maximum dose: 50 mg) over 30-60 minutes every 4-6 hours. Therapy should continue until methanol and formic acid have been completely eliminated (Barceloux, 2002)

Pediatric

Treatment of weak folic acid antagonist overdosage (eg, trimethoprim, pyrimethamine): Refer to adult dosing.

Folate-deficient megaloblastic anemia: Refer to adult dosing.

High-dose methotrexate-rescue dose: Refer to adult dosing.

Cofactor therapy in methanol toxicity (unlabeled use): Refer to adult dosing.

Administration

Oral Do not administer orally in the presence of nausea or vomiting. Doses >25 mg should be administered parenterally.

I.V. Due to calcium content, do not administer I.V. solutions at a rate >160 mg/minute; not intended for intrathecal use.

Refer to individual protocols. Should be administered I.M., I.V. push, or I.V. infusion (15 minutes to 2 hours). Leucovorin should not be administered concurrently with methotrexate. It is commonly initiated 24 hours after the start of methotrexate. Toxicity to normal tissues may be irreversible if leucovorin is not initiated by ~40 hours after the start of methotrexate.

As a rescue after folate antagonists: Administer by I.V. bolus, I.M., or orally.

In combination with fluorouracil: Fluorouracil activity, the fluorouracil is usually given after, or at the midpoint, of the leucovorin infusion. Leucovorin is usually administered by I.V. bolus injection or short (10-120 minutes) I.V. infusion. Other administration schedules have been used; refer to individual protocols.

Stability

Reconstitution Powder for injection: Reconstitute with SWFI or BWFI; dilute in 100-1000 mL NS, D_5W for infusion. When doses >10 mg/m^2 are required, reconstitute using sterile water for injection, not a solution containing benzyl alcohol.

Storage

Powder for injection: Store at room temperature of 25°C (77°F). Protect from light. Solutions reconstituted with bacteriostatic water for injection U.S.P., must be used within 7 days. Solutions reconstituted with SWFI must be used immediately. Parenteral admixture is stable for 24 hours stored at room temperature (25°C) and for 4 days when stored under refrigeration (4°C).

Solution for injection: Prior to dilution, store vials under refrigeration at 2°C to 8°C (36°F to 46°F). Protect from light.

Tablet: Store at room temperature of 15°C to 30°C (59°F to 86°F).

Monitoring and Teaching Issues

Laboratory Monitoring

High-dose methotrexate therapy: Plasma methotrexate concentration; leucovorin is continued until the plasma methotrexate level <0.05 micromole/L. With 4- to 6-hour high-dose methotrexate infusions, plasma drug values in excess of 50 and 1 micromole/L at 24 and 48 hours after starting the infusion, respectively, are often predictive of delayed methotrexate clearance.

Fluorouracil therapy: CBC with differential and platelets, liver function tests, electrolytes

Patient Education Maintain hydration. Report respiratory difficulty, lethargy, rash, or itching.

Dietary Considerations Solutions for injection contain calcium 0.004 mEq per leucovorin 1 mg

Breast-Feeding Considerations Leucovorin is a biologically active form of folic acid. Adequate amounts of folic acid are recommended in breast-feeding women. Refer to Folic Acid monograph.

Pregnancy Considerations Animal reproduction studies have not been conducted. Leucovorin is a biologically active form of folic acid. Adequate amounts of folic acid are recommended during pregnancy. Refer to Folic Acid monograph.

◆ **Leukeran®** *see* Chlorambucil *on page* 357

◆ **Leukine®** *see* Sargramostim *on page* 1624

Leuprolide (loo PROE lide)

U.S. Brand Names Eligard®; Lupron Depot-Ped®; Lupron Depot®; Lupron Depot®-3 Month; Lupron Depot®-4 Month; Lupron®

Index Terms Abbott-43818; Leuprolide Acetate; Leuprorelin Acetate; TAP-144

Generic Availability (U.S.) Yes: Injection (solution)

Pharmacologic Category Antineoplastic Agent, Gonadotropin-Releasing Hormone Agonist; Gonadotropin Releasing Hormone Agonist

Medication Safety Issues

Sound-alike/look-alike issues:

Lupron® may be confused with Nuprin®

Lupron Depot®-3 Month may be confused with Lupron Depot-Ped®

Pregnancy Risk Factor X

Lactation Excretion in breast milk unknown/contraindicated

Use Palliative treatment of advanced prostate cancer; management of endometriosis; treatment of anemia caused by uterine leiomyomata (fibroids); central precocious puberty

Unlabeled/Investigational Use Treatment of breast cancer; infertility; prostatic hyperplasia

Mechanism of Action/Effect Leuprolide, is an agonist of luteinizing hormone-releasing hormone (LHRH). Acting as a potent inhibitor of gonadotropin secretion; continuous administration results in suppression of ovarian and testicular steroidogenesis due to decreased levels of LH and FSH with subsequent decrease in testosterone (male) and estrogen (female) levels. In males, testosterone levels are reduced to below castrate levels. Leuprolide may also have a direct inhibitory effect on the testes, and act by a different mechanism not directly related to reduction in serum testosterone.

Contraindications Hypersensitivity to leuprolide, GnRH, GnRH-agonist analogs, or any component of the formulation; undiagnosed abnormal vaginal bleeding; pregnancy; breast-feeding

Lupron Depot®-4 month (30 mg) is not indicated for use in women

Eligard® is contraindicated in women and children

Warnings/Precautions Hazardous agent - use appropriate precautions for handling and disposal. Transient increases in testosterone serum levels occur at the start of treatment. Androgen-deprivation therapy may increase the risk for cardiovascular disease (Levine, 2010). Tumor flare, bone pain, neuropathy, urinary tract obstruction, and spinal cord compression have been reported when used for prostate cancer; closely observe patients for weakness, paresthesias, hematuria, and urinary tract obstruction in first few weeks of therapy. Observe patients with metastatic vertebral lesions or urinary obstruction closely. Exacerbation of endometriosis or uterine leiomyomata may occur initially. Decreased bone density has been reported when used for ≥6 months; use caution in patients with additional risk factors for bone loss (eg, chronic alcohol use, corticosteroid therapy). In patients with prostate cancer, androgen deprivation therapy may increase the risk for cardiovascular disease, diabetes, insulin resistance, obesity, alterations in lipids, and fractures. Use caution in patients with a history of psychiatric illness; alteration in mood, memory impairment, and depression have been associated with use. Rare cases of pituitary apoplexy (frequently secondary to pituitary adenoma) have been observed with leuprolide administration (onset from 1 hour to usually <2 weeks); may present as sudden headache, vomiting, visual or mental status changes, and infrequently cardiovascular collapse; immediate medical attention required. Females treated for precocious puberty may experience menses or spotting during the first 2 months of treatment; notify healthcare provider if bleeding continues after the second month.

Some dosage forms may contain benzyl alcohol which has been associated with "gasping syndrome" in neonates; patients with benzyl alcohol allergy may demonstrate a hypersensitivity reaction (usually local) in the form of erythema and induration at the injection site. Vehicle used in injectable (polylactide-co-glycolide microspheres) has rarely been associated with retinal artery occlusion in patients with abnormal arteriovenous anastomosis.

Drug Interactions

Avoid Concomitant Use There are no known interactions where it is recommended to avoid concomitant use.

Decreased Effect

Leuprolide may decrease the levels/effects of: Antidiabetic Agents

Increased Effect/Toxicity There are no known significant interactions involving an increase in effect.

Lab Interactions Interferes with pituitary gonadotropic and gonadal function tests during and up to 3 months after monthly administration of leuprolide therapy.

Adverse Reactions

Children: 2% to 10%:

Central nervous system: Pain (2%)
Dermatologic: Acne (2%), rash (2% including erythema multiforme), seborrhea (2%)
Genitourinary: Vaginitis (2%), vaginal bleeding (2%), vaginal discharge (2%)
Local: Injection site reaction (5%)

Adults: Note: For prostate cancer treatment, an initial rise in serum testosterone concentrations may cause "tumor flare" or worsening of symptoms, including bone pain, neuropathy, hematuria, or ureteral or bladder outlet obstruction during the first 2 weeks. Similarly, an initial increase in estradiol levels, with a temporary worsening of symptoms, may occur in women treated with leuprolide.

Delayed release formulations:

10%:

Cardiovascular: Edema (≤14%)
Central nervous system: Headache (≤65%), pain (<2% to 33%), depression (≤31%), insomnia (≤31%), fatigue (≤17%), dizziness/vertigo (≤16%)
Dermatologic: Skin reaction (≤12%)
Endocrine & metabolic: Hot flashes (25% to 98%), testicular atrophy (≤20%), hyperlipidemia (≤12%), libido decreased (≤11%)
Gastrointestinal: Nausea/vomiting (≤25%), bowel function altered (≤14%), weight gain/loss (≤13%)
Genitourinary: Vaginitis (11% to 28%), urinary disorder (13% to 15%)
Local: Injection site burning/stinging (transient: ≤35%)
Neuromuscular & skeletal: Weakness (≤18%), joint disorder (≤12%)
Miscellaneous: Flu-like syndrome (≤12%)

1% to 10% (limited to important or life-threatening):

Cardiovascular: Angina (<5%), arrhythmia (<5%), atrial fibrillation (<5%), bradycardia (<5%), CHF (<5%), deep thrombophlebitis (<5%), hyper-/hypotension (<5%), palpitation (<5%), syncope (<5%), tachycardia (<5%)
Central nervous system: Nervousness (≤8%), anxiety (≤6%), confusion (<5%), delusions (<5%), dementia (<5%), fever (<5%), seizure (<5%)
Dermatologic: Acne (≤10%), alopecia (≤5%), bruising (≤5%), cellulitis (<5%), pruritus (≤3%), hirsutism (<2%), rash (<2%)
Endocrine & metabolic: Dehydration (≤8%), gynecomastia (≤7%), breast tenderness/pain (≤6%), bicarbonate decreased (≥5%), hyper-/hypocholesterolemia (≥5%), hyperglycemia (≥5%), hyperphosphatemia (≥5%), hyperuricemia (≥5%), hypoalbuminemia (≥5%), hypoproteinemia (≥5%), lactation (<5%), testicular pain (≤4%), menstrual disorder (≤2%)
Gastrointestinal: Dysphagia (<5%), gastrointestinal hemorrhage (<5%), intestinal obstruction (<5%), ulcer (<5%), gastroenteritis/colitis (≤3%), diarrhea (≤2%), constipation (≤2%)
Genitourinary: Prostatic acid phosphatase increased/decreased (≥5%), urine specific gravity increased/decreased (≥5%), impotence (≤5%), balanitis (<5%), incontinence (<5%), penile/testis disorder (<5%), urinary tract infection (<5%), nocturia (≤4%), polyuria (2% to 4%), bladder spasm (<2%), dysuria (<2%), erectile dysfunction (<2%), hematuria (<2%), urinary retention (<2%), urinary urgency (<2%)
Hematologic: Eosinophilia (≥5%), leukopenia (≥5%), platelets increased (≥5%), anemia
Hepatic: Liver function tests abnormal (≥5%), partial thromboplastin time increased (≥5%), prothrombin time increased (≥5%), hepatomegaly (<5%)
Local: Injection site pain (2% to 5%), injection site erythema (1% to 3%)
Neuromuscular & skeletal: Myalgia (≤8%), paresthesia (≤8%), neuropathy (<5%), paralysis (<5%), pathologic fracture (<5%), bone pain (<2%)
Renal: BUN increased (≥5%), creatinine increased (≥5%)
Respiratory: Emphysema (<5%), epistaxis (<5%), hemoptysis (<5%), pleural effusion (<5%), pulmonary edema (<5%), dyspnea (≤2%)
Miscellaneous: Diaphoresis (≤5%), allergic reaction (<5%), infection (5%), lymphadenopathy (<5%)

Immediate release formulation:

>10%:

Cardiovascular: ECG changes/ischemia (19%), peripheral edema (12%)
Central nervous system: Pain (13%)
Endocrine & metabolic: Hot flashes (55%)

1% to 10% (limited to important or life-threatening):

Cardiovascular: Hypertension (8%), murmur (3%), thrombosis/phlebitis (2%), CHF (1%), angina, arrhythmia, MI, syncope
Central nervous system: Headache (7%), insomnia (7%), dizziness/lightheadedness (5%), anxiety, depression, fatigue, fever, nervousness
Dermatologic: Dermatitis (5%), alopecia, bruising, itching, lesions, pigmentation

Endocrine & metabolic: Gynecomastia/breast tenderness/pain (7%), testicular size decreased (7%), diabetes, hypercalcemia, hypoglycemia, libido decreased, thyroid enlarged
Gastrointestinal: Constipation (7%), anorexia (6%), nausea/vomiting (5%), diarrhea, dysphagia, gastrointestinal bleeding, peptic ulcer, rectal polyps
Genitourinary: Urinary frequency/urgency (6%), impotence (4%), urinary tract infection (3%), bladder spasm, dysuria, incontinence, testicular pain, urinary obstruction
Hematologic: Anemia (5%)
Local: Injection site reaction
Neuromuscular & skeletal: Weakness (10%), bone pain (5%), peripheral neuropathy
Ocular: Blurred vision
Renal: Hematuria (6%), BUN increased, creatinine increased
Respiratory: Dyspnea (2%), cough, pneumonia, pulmonary embolus, pulmonary fibrosis
Miscellaneous: Infection, inflammation

Pharmacodynamics/Kinetics

Onset of Action Following transient increase, testosterone suppression occurs in ~2-4 weeks of continued therapy

Bioavailability Oral: None; SubQ: 94%

Protein Binding 43% to 49%

Metabolism Major metabolite, pentapeptide (M-1)

Excretion Urine (<5% as parent and major metabolite)

Available Dosage Forms

Injection, powder for reconstitution:
Eligard®: 7.5 mg, 22.5 mg, 30 mg, 45 mg
Lupron Depot-Ped®: 7.5 mg, 11.25 mg, 15 mg
Lupron Depot®: 3.75 mg, 7.5 mg
Lupron Depot®-3 Month: 11.25 mg, 22.5 mg
Lupron Depot®-4 Month: 30 mg

Injection, solution: 5 mg/mL (2.8 mL)
Lupron®: 5 mg/mL (2.8 mL)

Dosing

Adult & Geriatric

Advanced prostate cancer:
SubQ:
Eligard®: 7.5 mg monthly **or** 22.5 mg every 3 months **or** 30 mg every 4 months **or** 45 mg every 6 months
Lupron®: 1 mg/day
I.M.:
Lupron Depot®: 7.5 mg/dose given monthly (every 28-33 days) **or**
Lupron Depot®-3: 22.5 mg every 3 months **or**
Lupron Depot®-4: 30 mg every 4 months

Breast cancer, premenopausal ovarian ablation (unlabeled use; Boccardo, 1999): I.M.:
Lupron Depot®: 3.75 mg every 28 days **or**
Lupron Depot®-3: 11.25 mg every 3 months

Endometriosis: I.M.: Initial therapy may be with leuprolide alone or in combination with norethindrone; if retreatment for an additional 6 months is necessary, norethindrone should be used. Retreatment is not recommended for longer than one additional 6-month course.
Lupron Depot®: 3.75 mg/month for up to 6 months **or**
Lupron Depot®-3: 11.25 mg every 3 months for up to 2 doses (6 months total duration of treatment)

Uterine leiomyomata (fibroids): I.M. (in combination with iron):
Lupron Depot®: 3.75 mg/month for up to 3 months **or**
Lupron Depot®-3: 11.25 mg as a single injection

Pediatric

Precocious puberty (consider discontinuing by age 11 for females and by age 12 for males):
SubQ (Lupron®): Initial: 50 mcg/kg/day (per manufacturer, doses of 20-45 mcg/kg/day have also been reported); titrate dose upward by 10 mcg/kg/day if down-regulation is not achieved. **Note:** Higher mg/kg doses may be required in younger children.
I.M. (Lupron Depot-Ped®): 0.3 mg/kg/dose given every 28 days (minimum dose: 7.5 mg)
≤25 kg: 7.5 mg
>25-37.5 kg: 11.25 mg
>37.5 kg: 15 mg
Titrate dose upward in increments of 3.75 mg every 4 weeks if down-regulation is not achieved.

Administration

I.M. Lupron Depot®: Vary injection site periodically

Other SubQ:
Eligard®: Vary injection site; choose site with adequate subcutaneous tissue (eg, abdomen, upper buttocks)
Lupron®: Vary injection site; if an alternate syringe from the syringe provided is required, insulin syringes should be used

Stability

Reconstitution
Eligard®: Packaged in two syringes; one contains the Atrigel® polymer system and the second contains leuprolide acetate powder; follow package instructions for mixing
Lupron Depot®: Reconstitute only with diluent provided

Storage

Lupron®: Lupron®: Store below 25°C (77°F). Protect from light and store vial in carton until use. Do not freeze.

Eligard®: Store at 2°C to 8°C (36°F to 46°C). Allow to reach room temperature prior to using; once mixed, must be administered within 30 minutes.

Lupron Depot® may be stored at room temperature of 15°C to 30°C (59°F to 86°F). Upon reconstitution, the suspension does not contain a preservative and should be used immediately.

Monitoring and Teaching Issues

Laboratory Monitoring Precocious puberty: GnRH testing (blood LH and FSH levels), testosterone in males and estradiol in females

Physical Assessment Assess carefully for use-related cautions prior to therapy. If self-administered, teach patient or caregiver proper storage, injection technique, and syringe/needle disposal. Monitor patients for development of diabetes; manage cardiovascular risk factors.

Patient Education This medication may be administered on a regular schedule; keep all appointments. If you have diabetes, monitor blood sugar frequently; can cause alteration in glycemic control. You may experience disease flare (increased bone pain) and urinary retention during early treatment (usually resolves); dizziness, headache, lethargy, or faintness; nausea or vomiting; constipation; hot flashes or flushing; breast swelling or tenderness; or decreased libido or impotence. Report chest pain; palpitations; irregular heart beat; swelling of extremities; weight gain; shortness of breath; difficulty urinating; weakness or numbness in hands, feet, or legs; CNS changes (depression, mood swings, insomnia); continuation of menstruation; pain, swelling, or redness at injection site; or paresthesias or muscle weakness.

Geriatric Considerations No dosage adjustments are needed in the elderly. Monitoring for bone density changes, serum lipid, hemoglobin A_{1c}, blood pressure, and serum calcium changes is recommended.

Pregnancy Considerations Pregnancy must be excluded prior to the start of treatment. Although leuprolide usually inhibits ovulation and stops menstruation, contraception is not ensured and a nonhormonal contraceptive should be used. Fetal abnormalities and increased fetal mortality have been noted in animal studies.

Additional Information

Eligard® Atrigel®: A nongelatin-based, biodegradable, polymer matrix

Oncology Comment: Guidelines from the American Society of Clinical Oncology (ASCO) for hormonal management of advanced prostate cancer which is androgen-sensitive (Loblaw, 2007) recommend either orchiectomy or luteinizing hormone-releasing hormone (LHRH) agonists as initial treatment for androgen deprivation.

◆ **Leuprolide Acetate** *see* Leuprolide *on page* 1082

◆ **Leuprorelin Acetate** *see* Leuprolide *on page* 1082

◆ **Leurocristine Sulfate** *see* VinCRIStine *on page* 1865

◆ **Leustatin®** *see* Cladribine *on page* 389

Levalbuterol (leve al BYOO ter ole)

U.S. Brand Names Xopenex HFA™; Xopenex®

Index Terms Levalbuterol Hydrochloride; Levalbuterol Tartrate; R-albuterol

Generic Availability (U.S.) Yes: Excludes aerosol

Pharmacologic Category $Beta_2$-Adrenergic Agonist

Medication Safety Issues

Sound-alike/look-alike issues:

Xopenex® may be confused with Xanax®

Pregnancy Risk Factor C

Lactation Excretion in breast milk unknown/use caution

Use Treatment or prevention of bronchospasm in children and adults with reversible obstructive airway disease

Mechanism of Action/Effect Relaxes bronchial smooth muscle by action on $beta_2$-receptors with little effect on heart rate

Contraindications Hypersensitivity to levalbuterol, albuterol, or any component of the formulation

Warnings/Precautions Optimize anti-inflammatory treatment before initiating maintenance treatment with levalbuterol. Do not use as a component of chronic therapy without an anti-inflammatory agent. Only the mildest form of asthma (Step 1 and/or exercise-induced) would not require concurrent use based upon asthma guidelines. Patient must be instructed to seek medical attention in cases where acute symptoms are not relieved or a previous level of response is diminished. The need to increase frequency of use may indicate deterioration of asthma, and treatment must not be delayed. A spacer device or valved holding chamber is recommended when using a metered-dose inhaler.

Use caution in patients with cardiovascular disease (arrhythmia or hypertension or HF), convulsive disorders, diabetes, glaucoma, hyperthyroidism, or hypokalemia. Beta-agonists may cause elevation in blood pressure, heart rate, and result in CNS stimulation/excitation. $Beta_2$-agonists may increase risk of arrhythmia, increase serum glucose, or decrease serum potassium.

Immediate hypersensitivity reactions (urticaria, angioedema, rash, bronchospasm) have been reported. Do not exceed recommended dose; serious adverse events including fatalities, have been associated with excessive use of inhaled sympathomimetics. Rarely, paradoxical bronchospasm may occur with use of inhaled bronchodilating agents; this should be distinguished from inadequate response. Use with caution during labor and delivery. Safety and efficacy have not been established in patients <4 years of age.

Drug Interactions

Avoid Concomitant Use

Avoid concomitant use of Levalbuterol with any of the following: Iobenguane I 123

Decreased Effect

Levalbuterol may decrease the levels/effects of: Iobenguane I 123

The levels/effects of Levalbuterol may be decreased by: Alpha-/Beta-Blockers; Beta-Blockers (Beta1 Selective); Beta-Blockers (Nonselective); Betahistine

Increased Effect/Toxicity

Levalbuterol may increase the levels/effects of: Loop Diuretics; Sympathomimetics

The levels/effects of Levalbuterol may be increased by: Atomoxetine; Cannabinoids; MAO Inhibitors; Tricyclic Antidepressants

Adverse Reactions

>10%:

Endocrine & metabolic: Serum glucose increased, serum potassium decreased
Neuromuscular & skeletal: Tremor (≤7%)
Respiratory: Rhinitis (3% to 11%)
Miscellaneous: Viral infection (7% to 12%)

>2% to 10%:

Central nervous system: Headache (8% to 12%), nervousness (3% to 10%), dizziness (1% to 3%), anxiety (≤3%), migraine (≤3%), weakness (3%)
Cardiovascular: Tachycardia (~3%)
Dermatologic: Rash (≤8%)
Gastrointestinal: Diarrhea (2% to 6%), dyspepsia (1% to 3%)
Neuromuscular & skeletal: Leg cramps (≤3%)
Respiratory: Asthma (9%), pharyngitis (3% to 10%), cough (1% to 4%), sinusitis (1% to 4%), nasal edema (1% to 3%)
Miscellaneous: Flu-like syndrome (1% to 4%), accidental injury (≤3%)

Note: Immediate hypersensitivity reactions have occurred (including angioedema, oropharyngeal edema, urticaria, and anaphylaxis).

Pharmacodynamics/Kinetics

Onset of Action Measured as a 15% increase in FEV_1:
Aerosol: 5.5-10.2 minutes; Peak effect: ~77 minutes
Nebulization: 10-17 minutes; Peak effect: 1.5 hours

Duration of Action Measured as a 15% increase in FEV_1:
Aerosol: 3-4 hours (up to 6 hours in some patients)
Nebulization: 5-6 hours (up to 8 hours in some patients)

Absorption A portion of inhaled dose is absorbed to systemic circulation

Time to Peak
Aerosol: Children: 0.8 hours, Adults: 0.5 hours
Nebulization: Children: 0.3-0.6 hours, Adults: 0.2 hours

Half-Life Elimination 3.3-4 hours

Available Dosage Forms

Aerosol, for oral inhalation:
Xopenex HFA™: 45 mcg/actuation (15 g)

Solution, for nebulization [preservative free]: 1.25 mg/0.5 mL (30s)
Xopenex®: 0.31 mg/3 mL (24s); 0.63 mg/3 mL (24s); 1.25 mg/3 mL (24s)

Dosing

Adult

Bronchospasm:

Metered-dose inhaler: 2 puffs every 4-6 hours
Solution for nebulization: 0.63 mg 3 times/day at intervals of 6-8 hours; dosage may be increased to 1.25 mg 3 times/day with close monitoring for adverse effects

Exacerbation of asthma (acute, severe) *(NIH Guidelines, 2007):*

Metered-dose inhaler: 4-8 puffs every 20 minutes for up to 4 hours, then every 1-4 hours as needed
Solution for nebulization: 1.25-2.5 mg every 20 minutes for 3 doses, then 1.25-5 mg every 1-4 hours as needed

Geriatric Only a small number of patients have been studied. Although greater sensitivity of some elderly patients cannot be ruled out, no overall differences in safety or effectiveness were observed. An initial dose of 0.63 mg should be used in all patients >65 years of age.

Pediatric

Bronchospasm:

Metered-dose inhaler: Children ≥4 years: 2 puffs every 4-6 hours as needed
Solution for nebulization:
Children ≤4 years (NIH Guidelines, 2007): 0.31-1.25 mg every 4-6 hours as needed
Children 5-11 years (NIH Guidelines, 2007): 0.31-0.63 mg 3 times/day as needed
Children ≥12 years: 0.63-1.25 mg every 8 hours as needed

Exacerbation of asthma (acute, severe) ***(NIH Guidelines, 2007):***
Metered-dose inhaler: Children ≥4 years: 4-8 puffs every 20 minutes for 3 doses, then every 1-4 hours as needed
Solution for nebulization:
Children <12 years: 0.075 mg/kg (minimum: 1.25 mg) every 20 minutes for 3 doses, then 0.075-0.15 mg/kg (maximum: 5 mg) every 1-4 hours as needed
Children ≥12 years: 1.25-2.5 mg every 20 minutes for 3 doses, then 1.25-5 mg every 1-4 hours as needed

Administration

Inhalation

Metered-dose inhaler: Shake well before use; prime with 4 test sprays prior to first use or if inhaler has not been use of more than 3 days. Clean actuator (mouthpiece) weekly. A spacer device or valved holding chamber is recommended when using a metered-dose inhaler.

Solution for nebulization: Safety and efficacy were established when administered with the following nebulizers: PARI LC Jet™, PARI LC Plus™, as well as the following compressors: PARI Master®, Dura-Neb® 2000, and Dura-Neb® 3000. Concentrated solution should be diluted prior to use. Blow-by administration is not recommended, use a mask device if patient unable to hold mouthpiece in mouth for administration.

Stability

Reconstitution Concentrated solution should be diluted with 2.5 mL NS prior to use.

Storage

Aerosol: Store at room temperature of 20°C to 25°C (68°F to 77°F); protect from freezing and direct sunlight. Store with mouthpiece down. Discard after 200 actuations.

Solution for nebulization: Store in protective foil pouch at room temperature of 20°C to 25°C (68°F to 77°F). Protect from light and excessive heat. Vials should be used within 2 weeks after opening protective pouch. Use within 1 week and protect from light if removed from pouch. Vials of concentrated solution should be used immediately after removing from protective pouch.

Monitoring and Teaching Issues

Laboratory Monitoring FEV_1 and/or peak expiratory flow rate, arterial blood gases (if condition warrants); serum potassium, serum glucose (in selected patients)

Physical Assessment Teach patient safe use of nebulizer.

Patient Education Stress or excessive exercising may exacerbate wheezing or bronchospasm. You may experience tremor, anxiety, dizziness, headache, upset stomach, nausea, or vomiting. Paradoxical bronchospasm can occur. Notify prescriber if any of the following occur: Chest pain, tightness, palpitations, severe headache, increased nervousness, restlessness, trembling, or muscle cramps. Report unusual signs of flu or infection, leg or muscle cramps, unusual cough, persistent GI problems, or vision changes.

Geriatric Considerations For aerosol formulation, start with low end of dosage range. Refer to dosing information for nebulization dosing specifics.

Breast-Feeding Considerations It is not known whether levalbuterol is excreted in human milk. Plasma levels following oral inhalation are low. Racemic albuterol was shown to be tumorigenic in animal studies.

Pregnancy Considerations Teratogenic effects were not observed in animal studies; however, racemic albuterol was teratogenic in some species. There are no adequate and well-controlled studies in pregnant women. This drug should be used during pregnancy only if benefit exceeds risk. Use caution if needed for bronchospasm during labor and delivery; has potential to interfere with uterine contractions.

- ◆ **Levalbuterol Hydrochloride** *see* Levalbuterol *on page 1085*
- ◆ **Levalbuterol Tartrate** *see* Levalbuterol *on page 1085*
- ◆ **Levaquin®** *see* Levofloxacin (Systemic) *on page 1092*
- ◆ **Levarterenol Bitartrate** *see* Norepinephrine *on page 1333*
- ◆ **Levemir®** *see* Insulin Detemir *on page 984*
- ◆ **Levemir® FlexPen®** *see* Insulin Detemir *on page 984*

Levetiracetam (lee va tye RA se tam)

U.S. Brand Names Keppra XR™; Keppra®

Generic Availability (U.S.) Yes: Excludes extended release tablet

Pharmacologic Category Anticonvulsant, Miscellaneous

Medication Safety Issues

Sound-alike/look-alike issues:
Keppra® may be confused with Keflex®, Keppra XR™
LevETIRAcetam may be confused with levOCARNitine, levofloxacin
Potential for dispensing errors between Keppra® and Kaletra® (lopinavir/ritonavir)

Medication Guide Available Yes

Pregnancy Risk Factor C

Lactation Enters breast milk/not recommended

Use Adjunctive therapy in the treatment of partial onset, myoclonic, and/or primary generalized tonic-clonic seizures

Unlabeled/Investigational Use Bipolar disorder

Mechanism of Action/Effect The precise mechanism by which levetiracetam exerts its antiepileptic effect is unknown. However, several studies have suggested the mechanism may involve one or more central pharmacologic effects.

Contraindications Hypersensitivity to levetiracetam or any component of the formulation

Warnings/Precautions Antiepileptics are associated with an increased risk of suicidal behavior/thoughts with use (regardless of indication); patients should be monitored for signs/symptoms of depression, suicidal tendencies, and other unusual behavior changes during therapy and instructed to inform their healthcare provider immediately if symptoms occur.

Psychotic symptoms (psychosis, hallucinations) and behavioral symptoms (including aggression, anger, anxiety, depersonalization, depression, personality disorder) may occur; incidence may be increased in children. Dose reduction may be required. Levetiracetam should be withdrawn gradually to minimize the potential of increased seizure frequency. Use caution with renal impairment; dosage adjustment may be necessary. Weakness, dizziness, and somnolence occur mostly during the first month of therapy. Although rare, decreases in red blood cell counts, hemoglobin, hematocrit, white blood cell counts and neutrophils have been observed. Safety and efficacy in children <4 years of age (oral formulation) or <16 years (I.V. formulation and extended release tablets) have not been established.

Drug Interactions

Avoid Concomitant Use There are no known interactions where it is recommended to avoid concomitant use.

Decreased Effect

The levels/effects of LevETIRAcetam may be decreased by: Ketorolac; Ketorolac (Systemic); Mefloquine

Increased Effect/Toxicity

LevETIRAcetam may increase the levels/effects of: Alcohol (Ethyl); CNS Depressants; Methotrimeprazine

The levels/effects of LevETIRAcetam may be increased by: Droperidol; Methotrimeprazine

Nutritional/Ethanol Interactions

Ethanol: Avoid ethanol (may increase CNS depression).

Food: Food may delay, but does not affect the extent of absorption.

Adverse Reactions

>10%:

Central nervous system: Behavioral symptoms (agitation, aggression, anger, anxiety, apathy, depersonalization, depression, emotional lability, hostility, hyperkinesias, irritability, nervousness, neurosis and personality disorder: adults 5% to 13%; children 5% to 38%), somnolence (8% to 23%), headache (14%), hostility (2% to 12%)

Gastrointestinal: Vomiting (15%), anorexia (3% to 13%)

Neuromuscular & skeletal: Weakness (9% to 15%)

Respiratory: Pharyngitis (6% to 14%), rhinitis (4% to 13%), cough (2% to 11%)

Miscellaneous: Accidental injury (17%), infection (2% to 13%)

1% to 10%:

Cardiovascular: Facial edema (2%)

Central nervous system: Fatigue (10%), nervousness (4% to 10%), dizziness (5% to 9%), personality disorder (8%), pain (6% to 7%), agitation (6%), irritability (6% to 7%), emotional lability (2% to 6%), mood swings (5%), depression (3% to 5%), vertigo (3% to 5%), ataxia (3%), amnesia (2%), anxiety (2%), confusion (2%)

Dermatologic: Bruising (4%), pruritus (2%), rash (2%), skin discoloration (2%)

Endocrine & metabolic: Dehydration (2%)

Gastrointestinal: Diarrhea (8%), nausea (5%), gastroenteritis (4%), constipation (3%)

Genitourinary: Urine abnormality (2%)

Hematologic: Leukocytes decreased (2% to 3%)

Neuromuscular & skeletal: Neck pain (2% to 8%), paresthesia (2%), reflexes increased (2%)

Ocular: Conjunctivitis (3%), diplopia (2%), amblyopia (2%)

Otic: Ear pain (2%)

Renal: Albuminuria (4%)

Respiratory: Influenza (5%), asthma (2%), sinusitis (2%)

Miscellaneous: Flu-like syndrome (3% to 8%), viral infection (2%)

Pharmacodynamics/Kinetics

Onset of Action Peak effect: Oral: 1 hour

Absorption Oral: Rapid and almost complete

Bioavailability 100%

Time to Peak Oral: Immediate release: ~1 hour; Extended release: ~4 hours

Protein Binding <10%

Half-Life Elimination ~6-8 hours; extended release tablet: ~7 hours; half-life increased in renal dysfunction

Metabolism Not extensive; primarily by enzymatic hydrolysis; forms metabolites (inactive)

Excretion Urine (66% as unchanged drug)

Available Dosage Forms

Injection, solution: 100 mg/mL (5 mL)

Keppra®: 100 mg/mL (5 mL)

Solution, oral: 100 mg/mL (5 mL, 472 mL, 473 mL, 480 mL, 500 mL)

Keppra®: 100 mg/mL (480 mL)

Tablet, oral: 250 mg, 500 mg, 750 mg, 1000 mg

Keppra®: 250 mg, 500 mg, 750 mg

Tablet, extended release, oral:

Keppra XR™: 500 mg, 750 mg

Dosing

Adult & Geriatric

Myoclonic seizures: Oral: Immediate release: Initial: 500 mg twice daily; may increase every 2 weeks by 500 mg/dose to the recommended dose of 1500 mg twice daily. Efficacy of doses >3000 mg/day has not been established.

Partial onset seizures:

Oral:

Immediate release: Initial: 500 mg twice daily; may increase every 2 weeks by 500 mg/dose to a maximum of 1500 mg twice daily. Doses >3000 mg/day have been used in trials; however, there is no evidence of increased benefit.

Extended release: Initial: 1000 mg once daily; may increase every 2 weeks by 1000 mg/day to a maximum of 3000 mg once daily.

I.V.: Initial: 500 mg twice daily; may increase every 2 weeks by 500 mg/dose to a maximum of 1500 mg twice daily. Doses >3000 mg/day have been used in trials; however, there is no evidence of increased benefit.

Note: When switching from oral to I.V. formulations, the total daily dose should be the same.

Tonic-clonic seizures: Oral: Immediate release: Initial: 500 mg twice daily; may increase every 2 weeks by 500 mg/dose to the recommended dose of 1500 mg twice daily. Efficacy of doses >3000 mg/day has not been established.

Bipolar disorder (unlabeled use): Oral: Immediate release: Initial: 500 mg twice daily; if tolerated, increase by 500 mg twice daily; dose may be increased every 3 days until target dose of 3000 mg/day is reached; maximum: 4000 mg/day

Loading dose (unlabeled): Immediate release: Initial doses of 1500-2000 mg have been well-tolerated (Betts, 2000; Koubeissi, 2008), although the necessity of a loading dose has not been established

Pediatric

Myoclonic seizures: Oral: Children ≥12 years: Immediate release: Initial: 500 mg twice daily; may increase every 2 weeks by 500 mg/dose to the recommended dose of 1500 mg twice daily. Efficacy of doses >3000 mg/day has not been established.

Partial onset seizures: Oral:

Children 4-15 years: Partial onset seizures: Immediate release: 10 mg/kg/dose given twice daily; may increase every 2 weeks by 10 mg/kg/dose to a maximum of 30 mg/kg/dose twice daily

Children ≥16 years: Refer to adult dosing.

Tonic-clonic seizures: Oral:

Children 6-15 years: Immediate release: Initial: 10 mg/kg dose given twice daily; may increase every 2 weeks by 10 mg/kg/dose to the recommended dose of 30 mg/kg twice daily. Efficacy of doses >60 mg/kg/day has not been established.

Children ≥16 years: Refer to adult dosing.

Bipolar disorder (unlabeled use): Oral: Children ≥16 years: Refer to adult dosing.

Renal Impairment Adults:

Immediate release and I.V. formulations:

Cl_{cr} >80 mL/minute: 500-1500 mg every 12 hours

Cl_{cr} 50-80 mL/minute: 500-1000 mg every 12 hours

Cl_{cr} 30-50 mL/minute: 250-750 mg every 12 hours

Cl_{cr} <30 mL/minute: 250-500 mg every 12 hours

End-stage renal disease patients using dialysis: 500-1000 mg every 24 hours; a supplemental dose of 250-500 mg following dialysis is recommended

Extended release tablets:

Cl_{cr} >80 mL/minute: 1000-3000 mg every 24 hours

Cl_{cr} 50-80 mL/minute: 1000-2000 mg every 24 hours

Cl_{cr} 30-50 mL/minute: 500-1500 mg every 24 hours

Cl_{cr} <30 mL/minute: 500-1000 mg every 24 hours

Hepatic Impairment No adjustment required

Administration

Oral

May be administered without regard to meals.

Oral solution: Should be administered with a calibrated measuring device (not a household teaspoon or tablespoon)

Tablet (immediate release and extended release): Only administer as whole tablet; do not crush, break or chew.

I.V. Infuse over 15 minutes

Stability

Reconstitution Injection solution: Must dilute dose in 100 mL of NS, LR, or D_5W.

Storage

Oral solution, tablets: Store at 25°C (77°F); excursions permitted to 15°C to 30°C (59°F to 86°F).

Injection solution: Store at 25°C (77°F); excursions permitted to 15°C to 30°C (59°F to 86°F). Admixed solution is stable for 24 hours in PVC bags kept at room temperature.

Monitoring and Teaching Issues

Physical Assessment Monitor for CNS depression (somnolence and fatigue), behavioral abnormalities (psychosis, hallucinations, psychotic depression), and other behavioral symptoms (agitation, anger, aggression, irritability, hostility, anxiety, apathy, emotional lability, depersonalization, and depression). Taper dosage slowly when discontinuing. Observe and teach seizure/safety precautions.

Patient Education While using this medication, do not use alcohol. Maintain adequate hydration unless instructed to restrict fluid intake. You may experience drowsiness, dizziness, blurred vision, nausea, vomiting, loss of appetite, or dry mouth. Wear identification of epileptic status and medications. Report CNS changes, mentation changes, suicide ideation, depression, or changes in cognition; muscle cramping, weakness, tremors, changes in gait; persistent GI symptoms (cramping, constipation, vomiting, anorexia); rash or skin irritations; unusual bruising or bleeding (mouth, urine, stool); or worsening of seizure activity or loss of seizure control.

Dietary Considerations May be taken without regard to meals.

Geriatric Considerations In a study of 16 older adults (61-88 years of age) receiving levetiracetam daily and with creatinine clearances ranging from 30-74 mL/minute, a decrease in creatinine clearance (38%) and a 2.5 hour longer half-life were recorded in the elderly compared to younger adults. The authors concluded that the difference was due to renal function. Other studies show no overall difference in safety and efficacy, although larger numbers in studies are needed to verify efficacy. Levetiracetam has demonstrated a low incidence of cognitive effects. When using the drug in elderly, it is essential to base the dose on estimated creatinine clearance and adjust appropriately.

Pregnancy Considerations Developmental toxicities were observed in animal studies. There are no adequate and well-controlled studies in pregnant women. Two registries are available for women exposed to levetiracetam during pregnancy:

Antiepileptic Drug Pregnancy Registry (888-233-2334 or http://www.mgh.harvard.edu/aed/)
UCB AED Pregnancy Registry (888-537-7734)

Related Information

Anticonvulsant Drugs of Choice *on page 1981*

◆ **Levitra®** *see* Vardenafil *on page 1846*

◆ **Levocabastine Hydrochloride** *see* Levocabastine (Nasal) *on page 1090*

◆ **Levocabastine Hydrochloride** *see* Levocabastine (Ophthalmic) *on page 1090*

Levocabastine (Nasal) (LEE voe kab as teen)

Index Terms Levocabastine Hydrochloride

Generic Availability (U.S.) No

Pharmacologic Category Histamine H_1 Antagonist; Histamine H_1 Antagonist, Second Generation; Piperidine Derivative

Medication Safety Issues

Sound-alike/look-alike issues:

Levocabastine may be confused with levobunolol, levOCARNitine
Livostin® may be confused with lovastatin

Use Symptomatic treatment of allergic rhinitis

Product Availability Not available in U.S.

Dosing

Adult Allergic rhinitis: Intranasal: Adults ≤65 years: Two sprays in each nostril twice daily; if necessary, may increase dose to 2 sprays 3-4 times daily; consider therapy discontinuation if no response within 3 days. Continuous treatment >10 weeks has not been evaluated.

Pediatric Allergic rhinitis: Intranasal: Children ≥12 years: Refer to adult dosing.

Renal Impairment Use caution; manufacturer labeling provides no specific dosing recommendations.

Administration

Other Intranasal: Shake bottle well before each use. Prior to initial use, bottle should be primed until a fine spray is delivered. Instruct patients to blow nose and clear nasal passages before administering spray and to inhale nasally while spraying.

Levocabastine (Ophthalmic) (LEE voe kab as teen)

Index Terms Levocabastine Hydrochloride

Generic Availability (U.S.) No

Pharmacologic Category Histamine H_1 Antagonist; Histamine H_1 Antagonist, Second Generation; Piperidine Derivative

Medication Safety Issues

Sound-alike/look-alike issues:

Levocabastine may be confused with levobunolol, levOCARNitine
Livostin® may be confused with lovastatin

International issues:

Livostin [Canada and multiple international markets] may be confused with Limoxin brand name for ambroxol [Indonesia] and amoxicillin [Mexico]; Lovastin brand name for lovastatin [Malaysia, Poland, Singapore]

Use Treatment of seasonal allergic conjunctivitis

Product Availability Not available in U.S.

Dosing

Adult Allergic conjunctivitis: Adults ≤65 years: Ophthalmic: Usual dose: Instill 1 drop in affected eye(s) 2 times/day; may increase to 1 drop 3-4 times/day. If no improvement within 3 days, consider discontinuation of therapy. Continuous therapy >16 weeks has not been studied.

Pediatric Allergic conjunctivitis: Ophthalmic: Children ≥12 years: Refer to adult dosing.

Administration

Other For topical ophthalmic use only. Shake bottle well. Wash hands prior to use. Avoid touching the dropper tip to surfaces to avoid contamination.

Monitoring and Teaching Issues

Patient Education For use in eyes only. Shake well before using. Do not let tip of applicator touch eye; do not contaminate tip of applicator (may cause eye infection, eye damage, or vision loss). Do not wear contact lenses during treatment. This medication may cause drowsiness in some patients.

Levocetirizine (LEE vo se TI ra zeen)

U.S. Brand Names Xyzal®

Index Terms Levocetirizine Dihydrochloride

Generic Availability (U.S.) Yes: Tablet

Pharmacologic Category Histamine H_1 Antagonist; Histamine H_1 Antagonist, Second Generation; Piperazine Derivative

Medication Safety Issues

Sound-alike/look-alike issues:

Levocetirizine may be confused with cetirizine

Pregnancy Risk Factor B

Lactation Excretion in breast milk unknown/not recommended

Use Relief of symptoms of perennial and seasonal allergic rhinitis; treatment of skin manifestations (uncomplicated) of chronic idiopathic urticaria

Available Dosage Forms

Solution, oral:

Xyzal®: 0.5 mg/mL (150 mL)

Tablet, oral: 5 mg

Xyzal®: 5 mg

Dosing

Adult Allergic rhinitis, chronic urticaria: Oral: 5 mg once daily (in the evening); some patients may experience relief of symptoms with 2.5 mg once daily

Geriatric Refer to adult dosing; dosing should begin at the lower end of the dosing range.

Pediatric

Perennial allergic rhinitis, chronic urticaria: Oral:

Children 6 months to 5 years: 1.25 mg once daily (in the evening); maximum: 1.25 mg

Children 6-11 years: 2.5 mg once daily (in the evening); maximum: 2.5 mg/day

Children ≥12 years: Refer to adult dosing.

Seasonal allergic rhinitis: Oral:

Children 2-5 years: 1.25 mg once daily (in the evening); maximum: 1.25 mg

Children 6-11 years: 2.5 mg once daily (in the evening); maximum: 2.5 mg/day

Children ≥12 years: Refer to adult dosing.

Renal Impairment

Children 6 months to 11 years with renal impairment: Contraindicated

Children ≥12 and Adults:

Cl_{cr} 50-80 mL/minute: 2.5 mg once daily

Cl_{cr} 30-50 mL/minute: 2.5 mg once every other day

Cl_{cr} 10-30 mL/minute: 2.5 mg twice weekly (every 3 or 4 days)

Cl_{cr} <10 mL/minute, hemodialysis patients: Contraindicated

Hepatic Impairment No adjustment required.

Administration

Oral Administer in the evening. May be administered without regard to meals.

Monitoring and Teaching Issues

Laboratory Monitoring Creatinine clearance (prior to treatment for dosing adjustment)

Patient Education You may experience drowsiness. Avoid alcohol; may increase drowsiness. Children may experience diarrhea or constipation. Report excessive sedation.

◆ **Levocetirizine Dihydrochloride** *see* Levocetirizine *on page 1091*

◆ **Levodopa and Carbidopa** *see* Carbidopa and Levodopa *on page 291*

Levodopa, Carbidopa, and Entacapone

(lee voe DOE pa, kar bi DOE pa, & en TA ka pone)

U.S. Brand Names Stalevo®

Index Terms Carbidopa, Entacapone, and Levodopa; Carbidopa, Levodopa, and Entacapone; Entacapone, Carbidopa, and Levodopa

Generic Availability (U.S.) No

Pharmacologic Category Anti-Parkinson's Agent, COMT Inhibitor; Anti-Parkinson's Agent, Decarboxylase Inhibitor; Anti-Parkinson's Agent, Dopamine Precursor

Pregnancy Risk Factor C

Lactation Excretion in breast milk unknown/use caution

Use Treatment of idiopathic Parkinson's disease

Available Dosage Forms

Tablet:

Stalevo®: 50: Levodopa 50 mg, carbidopa 12.5 mg, and entacapone 200 mg; 75: Levodopa 75 mg, carbidopa 18.75 mg, and entacapone 200 mg; 100: Levodopa 100 mg, carbidopa 25 mg, and entacapone 200 mg; 125: Levodopa 125 mg, carbidopa 31.25 mg, and entacapone 200 mg; 150: Levodopa 150 mg, carbidopa 37.5 mg, and entacapone 200 mg; 200: Levodopa 200 mg, carbidopa 50 mg, and entacapone 200 mg

Dosing

Adult & Geriatric

Note: All strengths of Stalevo® contain a carbidopa/levodopa ratio of 1:4 plus entacapone 200 mg.

Parkinson's disease: Oral: Dose should be individualized based on therapeutic response; doses may be adjusted by changing strength or adjusting interval. Fractionated doses are not recommended and only 1 tablet should be given at each dosing interval; maximum daily dose: 8 tablets of Stalevo® 50, 75, 100, 125, or 150, **or** 6 tablets of Stalevo® 200.

Patients previously treated with carbidopa/levodopa immediate release tablets (ratio of 1:4):

With current entacapone therapy: May switch directly to corresponding strength of combination tablet. No data available on transferring patients from controlled release preparations or products with a 1:10 ratio of carbidopa/levodopa.

Without entacapone therapy:

If current levodopa dose is >600 mg/day: Levodopa dose reduction may be required when adding entacapone to therapy; therefore, titrate dose using individual products first (carbidopa/levodopa immediate release with a ratio of 1:4 plus entacapone 200 mg); then transfer to combination product once stabilized.

If current levodopa dose is <600 mg without dyskinesias: May transfer to corresponding dose of combination product; monitor, dose reduction of levodopa may be required.

Patients previously treated with benserazide/levodopa immediate release tablets (Canadian labeling, not in U.S. labeling): *With current entacapone therapy:* Prior to switching to combination product (carbidopa/levodopa/entacapone), withhold treatment for 1 night, then initiate (carbidopa/levodopa/entacapone) therapy the following morning at a dose that provides either an equivalent amount or ~5% to 10% more levodopa.

Renal Impairment Use caution with severe renal impairment; specific dosing recommendations not available.

Hepatic Impairment Use with caution; specific dosing recommendations not available.

Administration

Oral Swallow tablet whole; do not crush, break, or chew. Only 1 tablet should be administered at each dosing interval. May be administered without regard to meals.

Monitoring and Teaching Issues

Laboratory Monitoring CBC, liver function tests, renal function tests, serum iron (if signs of anemia)

Physical Assessment See individual agents.

Patient Education See individual agents.

Related Information

Entacapone *on page 627*

◆ **Levo-Dromoran** *see* Levorphanol *on page 1100*

Levofloxacin (Systemic) (lee voe FLOKS a sin)

U.S. Brand Names Levaquin®

Generic Availability (U.S.) No

Pharmacologic Category Antibiotic, Quinolone; Respiratory Fluoroquinolone

Medication Safety Issues

Sound-alike/look-alike issues:

Levaquin® may be confused with Levoxyl®, Levsin/SL®, Lovenox®

Levofloxacin may be confused with levETIRAcetam, levodopa, Levophed®, levothyroxine

Medication Guide Available Yes

Pregnancy Risk Factor C

Lactation Enters breast milk/not recommended

Use Treatment of community-acquired pneumonia, including multidrug resistant strains of *S. pneumoniae* (MDRSP); nosocomial pneumonia; chronic bronchitis (acute bacterial exacerbation); acute bacterial sinusitis; prostatitis, urinary tract infection (uncomplicated or complicated); acute pyelonephritis; skin or skin structure infections (uncomplicated or complicated); reduce incidence or disease progression of inhalational anthrax (postexposure)

Unlabeled/Investigational Use Diverticulitis, enterocolitis (*Shigella* spp), epididymitis (nongonococcal), gonococcal infections, complicated intra-abdominal infections (in combination with metronidazole), Legionnaires' disease, peritonitis, PID

Note: As of April 2007, the CDC no longer recommends the use of fluoroquinolones for the treatment of gonococcal disease.

Mechanism of Action/Effect Levofloxacin, a fluorinated quinolone, exerts a broad spectrum bactericidal effect. It inhibits DNA gyrase which is required for DNA replication and transcription, DNA repair, recombination, and transposition within the bacteria.

Contraindications Hypersensitivity to levofloxacin, any component of the formulation, or other quinolones

Warnings/Precautions

[U.S. Boxed Warning]: There have been reports of tendon inflammation and/or rupture with quinolone antibiotics; risk may be increased with concurrent corticosteroids, organ transplant recipients, and in patients >60 years of age. Rupture of the Achilles tendon sometimes requiring surgical repair has been reported most frequently; but other tendon sites (eg, rotator cuff, biceps) have also been reported. Strenuous physical activity, rheumatoid arthritis, and renal impairment may be an independent risk factor for tendonitis. Discontinue at first sign of tendon inflammation or pain. May occur even after discontinuation of therapy. Use with caution in patients with rheumatoid arthritis; may increase risk of tendon rupture. Systemic use is only recommended in children <18 years of age for the prevention of inhalational anthrax (postexposure); increased incidence of musculoskeletal disorders (eg, arthralgia, tendon rupture) has been observed in children; CNS stimulation may occur (tremor, restlessness, confusion, and very rarely hallucinations or seizures). Potential for seizures, although very rare, may be increased with concomitant NSAID therapy. Use with caution in individuals at risk of seizures, with known or suspected CNS disorders or renal dysfunction. Avoid excessive sunlight and take precautions to limit exposure (eg, loose fitting clothing, sunscreen); may cause moderate-to-severe phototoxicity reactions. Discontinue use if photosensitivity occurs.

Rare cases of torsade de pointes have been reported in patients receiving levofloxacin. Use caution in patients with known prolongation of QT interval, bradycardia, hypokalemia, hypomagnesemia, or in those receiving concurrent therapy with Class Ia or Class III antiarrhythmics.

Severe hypersensitivity reactions, including anaphylaxis, have occurred with quinolone therapy. Reactions may present as typical allergic symptoms after a single dose, or may manifest as severe idiosyncratic dermatologic, vascular, pulmonary, renal, hepatic, and/or hematologic events, usually after multiple doses. Prompt discontinuation of drug should occur if skin rash or other symptoms arise. Prolonged use may result in fungal or bacterial superinfection, including *C. difficile*-associated diarrhea (CDAD) and pseudomembranous colitis; CDAD has been observed >2 months postantibiotic treatment. Peripheral neuropathies have been linked to levofloxacin use; discontinue if numbness, tingling, or weakness develops. **[U.S. Boxed Warning]: Quinolones may exacerbate myasthenia gravis; avoid use (rare, potentially life-threatening weakness of respiratory muscles may occur).** Unrelated to hypersensitivity, severe hepatotoxicity (including acute hepatitis and fatalities) has been reported. Elderly patients may be at greater risk. Discontinue therapy immediately if signs and symptoms of hepatitis occur. Hemolytic reactions may (rarely) occur with quinolone use in patients with latent or actual G6PD deficiency.

Fluoroquinolones have been associated with the development of serious, and sometimes fatal, hypoglycemia, most often in elderly diabetics, but also in patients without diabetes. This occurred most frequently with gatifloxacin (no longer available systemically) but may occur at a lower frequency with other quinolones.

Drug Interactions

Avoid Concomitant Use

Avoid concomitant use of Levofloxacin (Systemic) with any of the following: Artemether; BCG; Dronedarone; Lumefantrine; Nilotinib; Pimozide; QuiNINE; Tetrabenazine; Thioridazine; Toremifene; Vandetanib; Ziprasidone

Decreased Effect

Levofloxacin (Systemic) may decrease the levels/effects of: BCG; Mycophenolate; Sulfonylureas; Typhoid Vaccine

The levels/effects of Levofloxacin (Systemic) may be decreased by: Antacids; Calcium Salts; Didanosine; Iron Salts; Magnesium Salts; Quinapril; Sevelamer; Sucralfate; Zinc Salts

Increased Effect/Toxicity

Levofloxacin (Systemic) may increase the levels/effects of: Corticosteroids (Systemic); Dronedarone; Pimozide; QTc-Prolonging Agents; QuiNINE; Sulfonylureas; Tetrabenazine; Thioridazine; Toremifene; Vandetanib; Vitamin K Antagonists; Ziprasidone

The levels/effects of Levofloxacin (Systemic) may be increased by: Alfuzosin; Artemether; Chloroquine; Ciprofloxacin; Ciprofloxacin (Systemic); Gadobutrol; Insulin; Lumefantrine; Nilotinib; Nonsteroidal Anti-Inflammatory Agents; Probenecid; QuiNINE

Lab Interactions Some quinolones may produce a false-positive urine screening result for opiates using commercially-available immunoassay kits. This has been demonstrated most consistently for levofloxacin and ofloxacin, but other quinolones have shown cross-reactivity in certain assay kits. Confirmation of positive opiate screens by more specific methods should be considered.

Adverse Reactions 1% to 10%:

Cardiovascular: Chest pain (1%), edema (1%)

Central nervous system: Headache (6%), insomnia (4%), dizziness (3%), fatigue (1%), pain (1%)

Dermatologic: Rash (2%), pruritus (1%)

Gastrointestinal: Nausea (7%), diarrhea (5%), constipation (3%), abdominal pain (2%), dyspepsia (2%), vomiting (2%)

Genitourinary: Vaginitis (1%)

Local: Injection site reaction (1%)

Respiratory: Pharyngitis (4%), dyspnea (1%)

Miscellaneous: Moniliasis (1%)

Pharmacodynamics/Kinetics

Absorption Rapid and complete

Bioavailability ~99%

Time to Peak 1-2 hours

Protein Binding ~24% to 38%; primarily to albumin

Half-Life Elimination ~6-8 hours

Metabolism Minimally hepatic

Excretion Urine (~87% as unchanged drug, <5% as metabolites); feces (<4%)

Available Dosage Forms

Infusion, premixed in D_5W [preservative free]:
Levaquin®: 250 mg (50 mL); 500 mg (100 mL); 750 mg (150 mL)

Injection, solution [preservative free]:
Levaquin®: 25 mg/mL (20 mL, 30 mL)

Solution, oral:
Levaquin®: 25 mg/mL (480 mL)

Tablet, oral:
Levaquin®: 250 mg, 500 mg, 750 mg

Dosing

Adult & Geriatric Note: Sequential therapy (intravenous to oral) may be instituted based on prescriber's discretion.

Anthrax (inhalational): 500 mg every 24 hours for 60 days, beginning as soon as possible after exposure

Chronic bronchitis (acute bacterial exacerbation): Oral, I.V.: 500 mg every 24 hours for at least 7 days

Diverticulitis, peritonitis (unlabeled use): Oral, I.V.: 750 mg every 24 hours for 7-10 days; use adjunctive metronidazole therapy

Dysenteric enterocolitis, *Shigella spp.* (unlabeled use): Oral, I.V.: 500 mg every 24 hours for 3-5 days

Epididymitis, nongonococcal (unlabeled use): 500 mg once daily for 10 days

Gonococcal infection (unlabeled use): Oral, I.V.:

Cervicitis, urethritis: 250 mg for one dose with azithromycin or doxycycline; **Note:** As of April 2007, the CDC no longer recommends the use of fluoroquinolones for the treatment of uncomplicated gonococcal disease.

Disseminated infection: 250 mg I.V. once daily; 24 hours after symptoms improve may change to 500 mg orally every 24 hours to complete total therapy of 7 days; **Note:** As of April 2007, the CDC no longer recommends the use of fluoroquinolones for the treatment of more serious gonococcal disease, unless no other options exist and susceptibility can be confirmed via culture.

Intra-abdominal infection, complicated, community-acquired (in combination with metronidazole) (unlabeled use): I.V.: 750 mg once daily for 4-7 days (provided source controlled). **Note:** Avoid using in settings where *E. coli* susceptibility to fluoroquinolones is <90%.

Pelvic inflammatory disease (unlabeled use): 500 mg once daily for 14 days with or without adjunctive metronidazole; **Note:** The CDC recommends use only if standard cephalosporin therapy is not feasible and community prevalence of quinolone-resistant gonococcal organisms is low. Culture sensitivity must be confirmed.

Pneumonia: Oral, I.V.:

Community-acquired: 500 mg every 24 hours for 7-14 days or 750 mg every 24 hours for 5 days (efficacy of 5-day regimen for MDRSP not established)

Nosocomial: 750 mg every 24 hours for 7-14 days

Prostatitis (chronic bacterial): Oral, I.V.: 500 mg every 24 hours for 28 days

Sinusitis (acute bacterial): Oral, I.V.: 500 mg every 24 hours for 10-14 days or 750 mg every 24 hours for 5 days

Skin and skin structure infections: Oral, I.V.:

Uncomplicated: 500 mg every 24 hours for 7-10 days

Complicated: 750 mg every 24 hours for 7-14 days

Traveler's diarrhea (unlabeled use): Oral, I.V.: 500 mg for one dose

Urinary tract infections: Oral, I.V.:

Uncomplicated: 250 mg once daily for 3 days

Complicated, including acute pyelonephritis: 250 mg once daily for 10 days **or** 750 mg once daily for 5 days

Pediatric Anthrax (inhalational, postexposure): Oral, I.V.:

Children ≥6 months and ≤50 kg: 8 mg/kg every 12 hours for 60 days (do not exceed 250 mg/dose), beginning as soon as possible after exposure

Children >50 kg: 500 mg every 24 hours for 60 days, beginning as soon as possible after exposure

Renal Impairment

Normal renal function dosing of 750 mg/day:

Cl_{cr} 20-49 mL/minute: Administer 750 mg every 48 hours

Cl_{cr} 10-19 mL/minute: Administer 750 mg initial dose, followed by 500 mg every 48 hours

Hemodialysis/CAPD: Administer 750 mg initial dose, followed by 500 mg every 48 hours

Normal renal function dosing of 500 mg/day:

Cl_{cr} 20-49 mL/minute: Administer 500 mg initial dose, followed by 250 mg every 24 hours

Cl_{cr} 10-19 mL/minute: Administer 500 mg initial dose, followed by 250 mg every 48 hours

Hemodialysis/CAPD: Administer 500 mg initial dose, followed by 250 mg every 48 hours

Normal renal function dosing of 250 mg/day:

Cl_{cr} 20-49 mL/minute: No dosage adjustment required

Cl_{cr} 10-19 mL/minute: Administer 250 mg every 48 hours (except in uncomplicated UTI, where no dosage adjustment is required)

Hemodialysis/CAPD: No information available

CRRT: **Note:** Clearance dependent on filter type, flow rates, and other variables.

CVVH/CVVHD/CVVHDF: Alternative recommendations exist:

500 mg every 48 hours **or**

250 mg every 24 hours (**Note:** This regimen has been shown to be equivalent to 500 mg/day in normal renal function. Appropriateness of this regimen for target dosing equal to 750 mg/day is not known.)

Administration

Oral Tablets may be administered without regard to meals. Oral solution should be administered 1 hour before or 2 hours after meals. Maintain adequate hydration of patient to prevent crystalluria.

I.V. Infuse 250-500 mg I.V. solution over 60 minutes; infuse 750 mg I.V. solution over 90 minutes. Too rapid of infusion can lead to hypotension. Avoid administration through an intravenous line with a solution containing multivalent cations (eg, magnesium, calcium). Maintain adequate hydration of patient to prevent crystalluria.

Stability

Reconstitution Solution for injection: Single-use vials must be further diluted in compatible solution to a final concentration of 5 mg/mL prior to infusion.

Storage

Solution for injection:

Vial: Store at room temperature. Protect from light. Diluted solution is stable for 72 hours when stored at room temperature; stable for 14 days when stored under refrigeration. When frozen, stable for 6 months; do not refreeze. Do not thaw in microwave or by bath immersion.

Premixed: Store at ≤25°C (77°F); do not freeze. Brief exposure to 40°C (104°F) does not affect product. Protect from light.

Tablet, oral solution: Store at 25°C (77°F); excursions permitted to 15°C to 30°C (59°F to 86°F).

Monitoring and Teaching Issues

Laboratory Monitoring Perform culture and sensitivity studies prior to initiating drug therapy. Monitor CBC periodically during therapy. Monitor renal or hepatic function if therapy is prolonged.

Physical Assessment Assess results of culture and sensitivity tests prior to beginning therapy. Use caution in patients with known or suspected CNS disorder, current or potential for QT prolongation, renal or hepatic impairment, or diabetes. Patient should be monitored closely; if an allergic reaction occurs (itching, urticaria, dyspnea or facial edema, loss of consciousness, tingling, cardiovascular collapse), drug should be discontinued immediately and prescriber notified. Monitor for hypersensitivity reactions (severe reactions, including anaphylaxis, have occurred with quinolone therapy), opportunistic infection, tendon rupture, or persistent diarrhea (*C. difficile*-associated colitis can occur post-treatment).

Patient Education If administered by infusion, report immediately any chest or back pain; tightness in chest; difficulty swallowing; swelling of face or mouth; or redness, swelling, or pain at infusion site.

Oral: Take exactly as directed (timing with meals, dairy products, antacids, or products containing calcium, iron, or zinc differs with each formulation). If you have diabetes, monitor glucose levels closely; may cause hypoglycemia. May cause dizziness, lightheadedness, confusion, nausea, vomiting, or photosensitivity. Report chest pain or palpitations; persistent diarrhea, abdominal pain, or constipation; signs of infection (unusual fever or chills, vaginal itching, or foul-smelling vaginal discharge); or unusual bruising or bleeding. If tendon inflammation or pain occurs or you experience signs of an allergic reaction (eg, itching, skin rash, respiratory difficulty, facial edema, difficulty swallowing, chest pain, palpitations), discontinue use and contact prescriber immediately.

Dietary Considerations Tablets may be taken without regard to meals. Oral solution should be administered on an empty stomach (1 hour before or 2 hours after a meal). Take 2 hours before or 2 hours after multiple vitamins, antacids, or other products containing magnesium, aluminum, iron, or zinc.

Geriatric Considerations The risk of torsade de pointes and tendon inflammation and/or rupture associated with the concomitant use of corticosteroids and quinolones is increased in the elderly population. See Warnings/Precautions regarding tendon rupture in patients >60 years of age. Adjust dose for renal function.

Breast-Feeding Considerations Based on data from a case report, small amounts of levofloxacin are excreted in breast milk. Breast-feeding is not recommended by the manufacturer. Levofloxacin is the L-isomer of ofloxacin. Ofloxacin has also been shown to have minimal concentrations in human milk. Nondose-related effects could include modification of bowel flora.

Pregnancy Considerations Adverse events have been observed in some animal studies; therefore, the manufacturer classifies levofloxacin as pregnancy category C. Levofloxacin crosses the placenta. Quinolone exposure during human pregnancy has been reported with other agents (see Ciprofloxacin (Systemic) monograph). To date, no specific teratogenic effect or increased pregnancy risk has been identified; however, because of concerns of cartilage damage in immature animals exposed to quinolones and the limited levofloxacin specific data, levofloxacin should only be used during pregnancy if a safer option is not available.

Related Information

Antimicrobial Drugs of Choice *on page 2008*

Community-Acquired Pneumonia in Adults *on page 2021*

Compatibility of Drugs *on page 1994*

I.V. to Oral Conversion *on page 1956*

◆ **Levo-folinic Acid** *see* LEVOleucovorin *on page 1096*

LEVOleucovorin (lee voe loo koe VOR in)

U.S. Brand Names Fusilev™

Index Terms 6S-leucovorin; Calcium Levoleucovorin; L-leucovorin; Levo-folinic Acid; Levo-leucovorin; Levoleucovorin Calcium Pentahydrate; S-leucovorin

Generic Availability (U.S.) No

Pharmacologic Category Antidote; Rescue Agent (Chemotherapy)

Medication Safety Issues

Sound-alike/look-alike issues:

LEVOleucovorin may be confused with leucovorin calcium, Leukeran®, Leukine®

Pregnancy Risk Factor C

Lactation Excretion in breast milk unknown/use caution

Use Rescue agent after high-dose methotrexate therapy in osteosarcoma; antidote for impaired methotrexate elimination and for inadvertent overdosage of folic acid antagonists

Unlabeled/Investigational Use Treatment of colorectal cancer (in combination with fluorouracil)

Available Dosage Forms

Injection, powder for reconstitution:

Fusilev™: 50 mg

Dosing

Adult & Geriatric Note: Levoleucovorin is dosed at **one-half** the usual dose of the racemic form (leucovorin calcium):

High-dose methotrexate rescue: I.V.: Usual dose: 7.5 mg (~5 mg/m^2) every 6 hours for 10 doses, beginning 24 hours after the start of the methotrexate infusion (based on a methotrexate dose of 12 g/m^2 I.V. over 4 hours). Levoleucovorin (and hydration and urinary alkalinization) should be continued and/or adjusted until the methotrexate level is <0.05 micromolar (5 x 10^{-8} M) as follows:

Normal methotrexate elimination (serum methotrexate levels ~10 micromolar at 24 hours post administration, 1 micromolar at 48 hours and <0.2 micromolar at 72 hours post infusion): 7.5 mg I.V. every 6 hours for 10 doses

Delayed late methotrexate elimination (serum methotrexate levels >0.2 micromolar at 72 hours and >0.05 micromolar at 96 hours post methotrexate infusion): Continue 7.5 mg I.V. every 6 hours until methotrexate level is <0.05 micromolar

Delayed early methotrexate elimination and/or evidence of acute renal injury (serum methotrexate level ≥50 micromolar at 24 hours, ≥5 micromolar at 48 hours or a doubling or more of the serum creatinine level at 24 hours post methotrexate infusion): 75 mg I.V. every 3 hours until methotrexate level is <1 micromolar, followed by 7.5 mg I.V. every 3 hours until methotrexate level is <0.05 micromolar

Significant clinical toxicity in the presence of less severe abnormalities in methotrexate elimination or renal function (as described above): Extend levoleucovorin treatment for an additional 24 hours (total of 14 doses) in subsequent treatment cycles.

Delayed methotrexate elimination due to third space fluid accumulation, renal insufficiency, or inadequate hydration: May require higher levoleucovorin doses or prolonged administration.

Methotrexate overdose (inadvertent): I.V.: 7.5 mg (~5 mg/m^2) every 6 hours; continue until the methotrexate level is <0.01 micromolar (10^{-8} M). Initiate treatment as soon as possible after methotrexate overdose. Increase the levoleucovorin dose to 50 mg/m^2 I.V. every 3 hours if the 24-hour serum creatinine has increased 50% over baseline, or if the 24 hour methotrexate level is >5 micromolar (5 x 10^{-6} M), or if the 48-hour methotrexate level is >0.9 micromolar (9 x 10^{-7} M); continue levoleucovorin until the methotrexate level is <0.01 micromolar (10^{-8} M). Hydration (aggressive) and urinary alkalinization (with sodium bicarbonate) should also be maintained.

Treatment of colorectal cancer (in combination with fluorouracil; unlabeled use): I.V.: Levoleucovorin is dosed at **one-half** the usual dose of the racemic form (leucovorin calcium)

Pediatric Note: Levoleucovorin is dosed at **one-half** the usual dose of the racemic form (leucovorin calcium):

High-dose methotrexate rescue: Refer to adult dosing.

Methotrexate overdose (inadvertent): Refer to adult dosing.

Administration

I.V. For I.V. administration only; do not administer intrathecally. Due to calcium content, do not administer I.V. solutions at a rate >160 mg/minute.

For colorectal cancer (unlabeled use): Levoleucovorin has been administered as I.V. push and as I.V. infusion over 2 hours in clinical trials.

Other Do not administer intrathecally.

Monitoring and Teaching Issues

Laboratory Monitoring High-dose methotrexate therapy: Serum methotrexate and creatinine levels at least once daily. Monitor fluid and electrolyte status in patients with delayed methotrexate elimination (likely to experience renal toxicity).

Patient Education You may experience nausea, vomiting, diarrhea, heartburn, change in taste, or sores in mouth or on skin. Report respiratory difficulty, confusion, decreased urine output, swelling of extremities and unusual weight gain, or lethargy.

◆ **Levo-leucovorin** *see* LEVOleucovorin *on page* 1096

◆ **Levoleucovorin Calcium Pentahydrate** *see* LEVOleucovorin *on page* 1096

◆ **Levomefolate Calcium, Drospirenone, and Ethinyl Estradiol** *see* Ethinyl Estradiol, Drospirenone, and Levomefolate *on page* 706

◆ **Levomefolate, Drospirenone, and Ethinyl Estradiol** *see* Ethinyl Estradiol, Drospirenone, and Levomefolate *on page 706*

Levonorgestrel (LEE voe nor jes trel)

U.S. Brand Names Mirena®; Next Choice™; Plan B® One Step

Index Terms LNg 20; Plan B

Generic Availability (U.S.) Yes: Tablet

Pharmacologic Category Contraceptive; Progestin

Prescribing and Access Restrictions Plan B® One-Step will be limited to pharmacies or healthcare clinics with a valid license to distribute prescription products. Because there will be one package for both OTC and prescription use, pharmacies are required to keep the product behind the counter.

Lactation Enters breast milk/use caution

Use

Intrauterine device (IUD): Prevention of pregnancy; treatment of heavy menstrual bleeding in women who also choose to use an IUD for contraception

Oral: Emergency contraception following unprotected intercourse or possible contraceptive failure

Plan B® One-Step is approved for OTC use by women ≥17 years of age and available by prescription only for women <17 years of age. Next Choice™ (generic of the original Plan-B® 2-dose regimen) is also approved for OTC use by women ≥17 years of age and by prescription only for women <17 years of age.

Mechanism of Action/Effect Levonorgestrel prevents pregnancy by thickening the cervical mucus (which inhibits sperm passage and survival) and inhibiting implantation.

Contraindications Hypersensitivity to levonorgestrel or any component of the formulation; pregnancy

Additional product-specific contraindications:

Intrauterine device: Congenital or acquired uterine anomaly, acute pelvic inflammatory disease, history of pelvic inflammatory disease (unless there has been a subsequent intrauterine pregnancy), postpartum endometritis or infected abortion within past 3 months, known or suspected uterine or cervical neoplasia, unresolved/abnormal Pap smear, untreated acute cervicitis or vaginitis, conditions which increase susceptibility to pelvic infections, unremoved IUD, undiagnosed abnormal uterine bleeding, active hepatic disease or hepatic tumors, current or history of known or suspected carcinoma of the breast

Oral: It is not known if the same contraindications associated with long term progestin only contraceptives apply to the use of levonorgestrel and the emergency 2-dose regimen. A history of ectopic pregnancy is not a contraindication to use in emergency contraception.

Warnings/Precautions These products do not protect against HIV infection or other sexually-transmitted diseases. Menstrual bleeding patterns may be altered with use of the intrauterine device; the possibility of pregnancy should be considered if menstruation does not occur within 6 weeks of the previous menstrual period. If bleeding irregularities continue with prolonged use, appropriate diagnostic measures should be taken to rule out endometrial pathology. An increase in menstrual bleeding may indicate a partial or complete expulsion of the IUD. If expulsion occurs, device may be replaced within 7 days once pregnancy is ruled out. When using the oral tablet, spotting may occur following use; the possibility of pregnancy should be considered if menstruation is delayed for >7 days of the expected menstrual period.

Patients taking progestin-only contraceptives and presenting with lower abdominal pain should be evaluated for follicular atresia and ectopic pregnancy. Use caution in patients with previous ectopic pregnancy. Women with history of ectopic pregnancy were excluded from clinical trials; women with previous ectopic pregnancy, tubal surgery, or pelvic infection may be at increased risk ectopic pregnancy. The possibility of ectopic pregnancy should be considered in patients with abdominal pain or vaginal bleeding in women with prior amenorrhea. Patients receiving hepatic enzyme-inducing medications should be evaluated for an alternative method of contraception. May have adverse effects on glucose tolerance; use caution in women with diabetes. Safety and efficacy for use in renal impairment has not been established. Not indicated for use in postmenopausal women.

The use of combination hormonal contraceptives has been associated with a slight increase in the frequency of breast cancer, however, studies are not consistent. Data is insufficient to determine if progestin only contraceptives also increase this risk. Use of the intrauterine device is contraindicated in patients who have or who have had breast cancer. The risk of cardiovascular side effects increases in women using estrogen containing combined hormonal contraceptives and who smoke cigarettes, especially those who are >35 years of age. This risk relative to progestin-only contraceptives has not been established. Women who take contraceptives should be advised not to smoke

Additional formulation-specific warnings:

Intrauterine device: Insertion should be done by a trained healthcare provider. Increased incidence of group A streptococcal sepsis and pelvic inflammatory disease (may be asymptomatic). The highest risk of pelvic inflammatory disease is within 20 days of insertion; risk is increased with multiple sexual partners. May perforate uterus or cervix; risk of perforation is increased in lactating women. Pregnancy may result if perforation occurs; delayed detection of perforation may result in migration of IUD outside of uterine cavity. Partial penetration or embedment in the myometrium may decrease effectiveness and lead to difficult removal. Use caution in patients with coagulopathy or receiving anticoagulants. Use caution in patients with congenital heart disease or other heart conditions which may increase the risk of infective ▶

endocarditis during insertion of the device (prophylactic antibiotics may be required at time of insertion). Bradycardia or syncope may occur during insertion or removal of the intrauterine device. The device should be removed for the following reasons: Bleeding which causes anemia; if the patient or her partner become HIV positive or acquire a sexually-transmitted disease; pelvic infection, endometritis, symptomatic genital actinomycosis; intractable pelvic pain, pain during intercourse; endometrial or cervical cancer; uterine or cervical perforation; pregnancy. Embedded devices should also be removed. Use caution with or consider removal of the intrauterine device if any of the following conditions occur for the first time during therapy: Migraine, severe headache, jaundice, marked increase in blood pressure, severe arterial disease (eg, stroke, MI). Use is contraindicated in patients with vaginitis or cervicitis. Postpone insertion until after treatment for infection is complete and cause of the cervicitis is proven not to be due to gonorrhea or chlamydia. Not effective for emergency contraception.

Oral tablet: Not intended to be used for routine contraception and will not terminate an existing pregnancy

Drug Interactions

Metabolism/Transport Effects Substrate of CYP3A4 (major)

Avoid Concomitant Use

Avoid concomitant use of Levonorgestrel with any of the following: Griseofulvin

Decreased Effect

Levonorgestrel may decrease the levels/effects of: Vitamin K Antagonists

The levels/effects of Levonorgestrel may be decreased by: Acitretin; Aminoglutethimide; Aprepitant; Artemether; Barbiturates; Bile Acid Sequestrants; Bosentan; CarBAMazepine; CYP3A4 Inducers (Strong); Deferasirox; Felbamate; Fosaprepitant; Griseofulvin; LamoTRIgine; Mycophenolate; OXcarbazepine; Phenytoin; Retinoic Acid Derivatives; Rifamycin Derivatives; St Johns Wort; Topiramate

Increased Effect/Toxicity

Levonorgestrel may increase the levels/effects of: Benzodiazepines (metabolized by oxidation); Selegiline; Tranexamic Acid; Voriconazole

The levels/effects of Levonorgestrel may be increased by: Conivaptan; Herbs (Progestogenic Properties); Voriconazole

Nutritional/Ethanol Interactions Herb/Nutraceutical: St John's wort (an enzyme inducer) may decrease serum levels of levonorgestrel.

Lab Interactions Increased triiodothyronine uptake; decreased concentrations of sex hormone-binding globulin, thyroxine concentrations (slight)

Adverse Reactions

Intrauterine device:

>5%:

Central nervous system: Headache/migraine (8%), depression (6%)

Dermatologic: Acne (7%)

Endocrine & metabolic: Amenorrhea (24%; 20% at 1 year), enlarged follicles (12%), menorrhagia (6%), breast pain/tenderness (5%), ovarian cysts

Gastrointestinal: Abdominal pain (12%)

Genitourinary: Uterine/vaginal bleeding alterations (52%), intermenstrual bleeding/spotting (23%), pelvic pain (13%), leukorrhea (5%)

Miscellaneous: Ectopic pregnancy (≤50%), IUD expulsion (5%)

Oral tablets:

>10%:

Central nervous system: Fatigue (13% to 17%), headache (10% to 17%), dizziness (10% to 11%)

Endocrine & metabolic: Heavier menstrual bleeding (14% to 31%), lighter menstrual bleeding (12%), breast tenderness (8% to 11%)

Gastrointestinal: Nausea (14% to 23%), abdominal pain (13% to 18%)

1% to 10%:

Endocrine & metabolic: Menses delayed (5%)

Gastrointestinal: Vomiting (6%), diarrhea (5%)

Pharmacodynamics/Kinetics

Duration of Action Intrauterine device: Up to 5 years

Absorption Oral: Rapid and complete

Time to Peak Oral: ~2 hours

Protein Binding Highly bound to albumin (~50%) and sex hormone-binding globulin (~47%)

Half-Life Elimination Oral: ~24 hours

Metabolism To inactive metabolites

Excretion Urine (45%); feces (32%)

Available Dosage Forms

Intrauterine device, intrauterine:

Mirena®: 52 mg/device

Tablet, oral:

Next Choice™: 0.75 mg

Plan B® One Step: 1.5 mg

Dosing

Adult Females:

Long-term prevention of pregnancy, treatment of heavy menstrual bleeding: Intrauterine device (Mirena®): To be inserted into uterine cavity; should be inserted within 7 days of onset of menstruation or immediately after 1st trimester abortion. Releases 20 mcg levonorgestrel/day over 5 years. May be removed and replaced with a new unit at anytime during menstrual cycle. Do not leave any one system in place for >5 years.

Emergency contraception: Oral: May be used at any time during menstrual cycle:

Next Choice™: One 0.75 mg tablet as soon as possible within 72 hours of unprotected sexual intercourse; a second 0.75 mg tablet should be taken 12 hours after the first dose

Plan B® One-Step: One 1.5 mg tablet as soon as possible within 72 hours of unprotected sexual intercourse

Geriatric Not indicated for use in postmenopausal women.

Renal Impairment Safety and efficacy have not been established.

Hepatic Impairment Safety and efficacy have not been established; use of the intrauterine device is contraindicated with active hepatic disease or hepatic tumor.

Administration

Oral Oral (Plan B® One Step): Consider repeating the dose if vomiting occurs within 2 hours. If severe vomiting occurs, may consider administering the oral tablets vaginally (ACOG, 2010).

Other

Intrauterine device: Inserted in the uterine cavity, to a depth of 6-10 cm, with the provided insertion device; should not be forced into the uterus

Oral tablets: If severe vomiting occurs, may consider administering the oral tablets vaginally (ACOG, 2010).

Stability

Storage Store at room temperature of 20°C to 25°C (68°F to 77°F).

Monitoring and Teaching Issues

Laboratory Monitoring IUD: Monitor serum glucose in patients with diabetes, LDL levels in patients with hyperlipidemias

Physical Assessment Pregnancy should be ruled out prior to insertion of IUD. Monitor for prolonged menstrual bleeding, amenorrhea, and irregularity of menses. Caution patient about need for annual medical exams.

Patient Education This drug does not protect against HIV infection or other sexually-transmitted diseases. Cigarette smoking is not recommended. You may experience cramping, headache, abdominal discomfort, hair loss, weight changes, or unusual menses (break-through bleeding, irregularity, excessive bleeding). Report sudden acute headache or visual disturbance, unusual nausea or vomiting, any loss of feeling in arms or legs, or lower abdominal pain.

Intrauterine device: This method provides up to 5 years of birth control. It will be inserted and removed by your prescriber. Notify your prescriber if the system comes out by itself or if you have heavy bleeding, unusual vaginal discharge, low abdominal pain, painful sexual inter-course, chills, or fever. There is an increased risk of ectopic pregnancy with this product. Thread placement should be checked following each menstrual cycle; do not pull thread.

Tablet: This method provides emergency contraception. It is used after your normal form of birth control has failed or following unprotected sexual intercourse. It should be used within 72 hours. Contact prescriber if you vomit within 2 hours of taking either dose.

Breast-Feeding Considerations Levonorgestrel is found in breast milk. Following long-term use of oral levonorgestrel, infant serum levels range from 1% to 6% of the maternal level; detectable levels may be found in nursing infants. Isolated cases of decreased milk production have been reported. Risk of perforation with IUD is increased in lactating women. Following pregnancy, insertion of the device should not take place until 6 weeks postpartum or until involution of the uterus is complete. Consider waiting until 12 weeks postpartum if involution is substantially delayed. Women who are breast-feeding may use levonorgestrel for emergency contraception.

Pregnancy Considerations Epidemiologic studies have not shown an increased risk of birth defects when used prior to pregnancy or inadvertently during early pregnancy, although rare reports of congenital anomalies have been reported. In doses larger than those used for oral contraception, progestins have been reported to increase the risk of masculinization of female genitalia.

Intrauterine device: Pregnancy should be ruled out prior to insertion. Women who become pregnant with an IUD in place risk septic abortion (septic shock and death may occur). Removal of the device is recommended, however, removal or manipulation of IUD may result in pregnancy loss. In addition, miscarriage, premature labor, and premature delivery may occur if pregnancy is continued with IUD in place. Following pregnancy, insertion of the device should not take place until 6 weeks postpartum or until involution of the uterus is complete. Consider waiting until 12 weeks postpartum if involution is substantially delayed. The device may be inserted immediately following a first trimester abortion. Following removal of the device, ~80% of women who wished to conceive became pregnant within 12 months.

Oral tablet: A rapid return of fertility is expected following use for emergency contraception; routine contraceptive measures should be initiated or continued following use to ensure ongoing prevention of pregnancy. Barrier contraception is recommended immediately follow-ing emergency contraception. Short-term contraception (eg, oral hormonal contraceptive pills, patches, rings) may be started with barrier contraception or after the next menstrual period. Long term contraception (eg, IUD, depot medroxyprogesterone, progestin implant) should be started after the next menstrual period.

Additional Information

Intrauterine device: The cumulative 5-year pregnancy rate is ~0.7 pregnancies/100 users. Over 70% of women in the trials had previously used IUDs. The reported pregnancy rate after 12 months was ≤0.2 pregnancies/100 users. Approximately 80% of women who wish to conceive have become pregnant within 12 months of device removal. The recommended patient profile for this product: A woman who has at least one child, is in a stable and mutually-monogamous relationship, no history of pelvic inflammatory disease, and no history of ectopic pregnancy or predisposition to ectopic pregnancy. Keep a copy of the consent form and record lot number of device.

Oral tablet: Treatment for emergency contraception should begin as soon as possible; however, treatment is still moderately effective if used within 5 days and should be made available to women up to 5 days after unprotected or inadequately protected intercourse. May be used in women with contraindications to conventional oral contraceptive agents (eg, cardiovascular disease, migraines, liver disease). When used as directed for emergency contraception, the expected pregnancy rate is decreased from 8% to 1%. Approximately 87% of women have their next menstrual period at approximately the expected time. A rapid return to fertility following use is expected. When using the two-dose emergency contraceptive regimen, the second dose is equally effective if taken 12-24 hours after the first.

◆ **Levonorgestrel and Ethinyl Estradiol** *see* Ethinyl Estradiol and Levonorgestrel *on page* 699

◆ **Levophed®** *see* Norepinephrine *on page* 1333

◆ **Levora®** *see* Ethinyl Estradiol and Levonorgestrel *on page* 699

Levorphanol (lee VOR fa nole)

Index Terms Levo-Dromoran; Levorphan Tartrate; Levorphanol Tartrate

Generic Availability (U.S.) Yes: Tablet

Pharmacologic Category Analgesic, Opioid

Medication Safety Issues

High alert medication: The Institute for Safe Medication Practices (ISMP) includes this medication among its list of drug classes which have a heightened risk of causing significant patient harm when used in error.

Pregnancy Risk Factor B/D (prolonged use or high doses at term)

Lactation Excretion in breast milk unknown/not recommended

Use Relief of moderate-to-severe pain; preoperative sedation/analgesia; management of chronic pain (eg, cancer) requiring opioid therapy

Controlled Substance C-II

Available Dosage Forms

Tablet, oral: 2 mg

Dosing

Adult & Geriatric Note: These are guidelines and do not represent the maximum doses that may be required in all patients. Doses should be titrated to pain relief/prevention.

Acute pain (moderate-to-severe): *Oral:* Initial: Opiate-naive: 2 mg every 6-8 hours as needed; patients with prior opiate exposure may require higher initial doses; usual dosage range: 2-4 mg every 6-8 hours as needed

Note: The American Pain Society recommends an initial dose of 4 mg for severe pain in adults (APS, 6th ed)

Chronic pain: Patients taking opioids chronically may become tolerant and require doses higher than the usual dosage range to maintain the desired effect. Tolerance can be managed by appropriate dose titration. **There is no optimal or maximal dose for levorphanol in chronic pain. The appropriate dose is one that relieves pain throughout its dosing interval without causing unmanageable side effects.**

Renal Impairment Use with caution; initial dose should be reduced in severe renal impairment.

Hepatic Impairment Use with caution; initial dose should be reduced in severe hepatic impairment.

Monitoring and Teaching Issues

Physical Assessment Assess patient's physical and/or psychological dependence. Safety measures required for inpatients to prevent falls. Discontinue slowly after prolonged use.

Patient Education Drug may cause physical and/or psychological dependence. While using this medication, do not use alcohol and other prescription or OTC medications (especially sedatives, tranquilizers, antihistamines, or pain medications) without consulting prescriber. Maintain adequate hydration, unless instructed to restrict fluid intake. May cause hypotension, dizziness, drowsiness, impaired coordination, or blurred vision; loss of appetite, nausea, or vomiting; or constipation. Report chest pain, slow or rapid heartbeat, dizziness, or persistent headache; confusion or respiratory difficulties; or severe constipation.

Related Information

Opioid Analgesics *on page* 2003

◆ **Levorphanol Tartrate** *see* Levorphanol *on page* 1100

◆ **Levorphan Tartrate** *see* Levorphanol *on page* 1100

◆ **Levothroid®** *see* Levothyroxine *on page* 1101

Levothyroxine (lee voe thye ROKS een)

U.S. Brand Names Levothroid®; Levoxyl®; Synthroid®; Tirosint®; Unithroid®

Index Terms *L*-Thyroxine Sodium; Levothyroxine Sodium; T_4

Generic Availability (U.S.) Yes

Pharmacologic Category Thyroid Product

Medication Safety Issues

Sound-alike/look-alike issues:

Levothyroxine may be confused with lamoTRIgine, Lanoxin®, levofloxacin, liothyronine

Levoxyl® may be confused with Lanoxin®, Levaquin®, Luvox®

Synthroid® may be confused with Symmetrel

To avoid errors due to misinterpretation of a decimal point, always express dosage in mcg (**not** mg).

Significant differences exist between oral and I.V. dosing. Use caution when converting from one route of administration to another.

Pregnancy Risk Factor A

Lactation Enters breast milk/compatible

Use Replacement or supplemental therapy in hypothyroidism; pituitary TSH suppression

Unlabeled/Investigational Use Management of hemodynamically unstable potential organ donors increasing the quantity of organs available for transplantation

Mechanism of Action/Effect It is believed the thyroid hormone exerts its many metabolic effects through control of DNA transcription and protein synthesis

Contraindications Hypersensitivity to levothyroxine sodium or any component of the formulation; acute MI; thyrotoxicosis of any etiology; uncorrected adrenal insufficiency

Capsule: Additional contraindication: Inability to swallow capsules

Warnings/Precautions [U.S. Boxed Warning]: Thyroid supplements are ineffective and potentially toxic when used for the treatment of obesity or for weight reduction, especially in euthyroid patients. High doses may produce serious or even life-threatening toxic effects particularly when used with some anorectic drugs (eg, sympathomimetic amines). Routine use of T_4 for TSH suppression is not recommended in patients with benign thyroid nodules. In patients deemed appropriate candidates, treatment should never be fully suppressive (TSH <0.1 mIU/L). Use with caution and reduce dosage in patients with angina pectoris or other cardiovascular disease; decrease initial dose. Use cautiously in the elderly since they may be more likely to have compromised cardiovascular functions. Patients with adrenal insufficiency, myxedema, diabetes mellitus and insipidus may have symptoms exaggerated or aggravated. Chronic hypothyroidism predisposes patients to coronary artery disease. Long-term therapy can decrease bone mineral density. Levoxyl® may rapidly swell and disintegrate causing choking or gagging (should be administered with a full glass of water); use caution in patients with dysphagia or other swallowing disorders.

Drug Interactions

Avoid Concomitant Use

Avoid concomitant use of Levothyroxine with any of the following: Sodium Iodide I131

Decreased Effect

Levothyroxine may decrease the levels/effects of: Sodium Iodide I131; Theophylline Derivatives

The levels/effects of Levothyroxine may be decreased by: Aluminum Hydroxide; Bile Acid Sequestrants; Calcium Polystyrene Sulfonate; Calcium Salts; CarBAMazepine; Estrogen Derivatives; Iron Salts; Orlistat; Phenytoin; Raloxifene; Rifampin; Sevelamer; Sodium Polystyrene Sulfonate; Sucralfate

Increased Effect/Toxicity

Levothyroxine may increase the levels/effects of: Vitamin K Antagonists

Nutritional/Ethanol Interactions Food: Taking levothyroxine with enteral nutrition may cause reduced bioavailability and may lower serum thyroxine levels leading to signs or symptoms of hypothyroidism. Soybean flour (infant formula), cottonseed meal, walnuts, and dietary fiber may decrease absorption of levothyroxine from the GI tract.

Lab Interactions Many drugs may have effects on thyroid function tests (see Additional Information). Pregnancy, infectious hepatitis, and acute intermittent porphyria may increase TBG concentrations; nephrosis, severe hypoproteinemia, severe liver disease, and acromegaly may decrease TBG concentrations.

Adverse Reactions Frequency not defined.

Cardiovascular: Angina, arrhythmia, cardiac arrest, flushing, heart failure, hypertension, MI, palpitation, pulse increased, tachycardia

Central nervous system: Anxiety, emotional lability, fatigue, fever, headache, hyperactivity, insomnia, irritability, nervousness, pseudotumor cerebri (children), seizure (rare)

Dermatologic: Alopecia

Endocrine & metabolic: Fertility impaired, menstrual irregularities

Gastrointestinal: Abdominal cramps, appetite increased, diarrhea, vomiting, weight loss

Hepatic: Liver function tests increased

Neuromuscular & skeletal: Bone mineral density decreased, muscle weakness, tremor, slipped capital femoral epiphysis (children)

Respiratory: Dyspnea

Miscellaneous: Diaphoresis, heat intolerance, hypersensitivity (to inactive ingredients, symptoms include urticaria, pruritus, rash, flushing, angioedema, GI symptoms, fever, arthralgia, serum sickness, wheezing)

Levoxyl®: Choking, dysphagia, gagging

Pharmacodynamics/Kinetics

Onset of Action Therapeutic: Oral: 3-5 days; I.V. 6-8 hours; Peak effect: I.V.: 24 hours

Absorption Oral: Erratic (40% to 80%); may be decreased by age and specific foods and drugs

Time to Peak Serum: 2-4 hours

Protein Binding >99% bound to plasma proteins including thyroxine-binding globulin, thyroxine-binding prealbumin, and albumin

Half-Life Elimination Euthyroid: 6-7 days; Hypothyroid: 9-10 days; Hyperthyroid: 3-4 days

Metabolism Hepatic to triiodothyronine (active); T_4 deiodination in kidney and periphery; glucuronidation/conjugation also occurs; undergoes enterohepatic recirculation

Excretion Urine (major route of elimination; decreases with age); feces (~20%)

Available Dosage Forms

Capsule, soft gelatin, oral:

Tirosint®: 13 mcg, 25 mcg, 50 mcg, 75 mcg, 88 mcg, 100 mcg, 112 mcg, 125 mcg, 137 mcg, 150 mcg

Injection, powder for reconstitution: 200 mcg, 500 mcg

Tablet, oral: 25 mcg, 50 mcg, 75 mcg, 88 mcg, 100 mcg, 112 mcg, 125 mcg, 137 mcg, 150 mcg, 175 mcg, 200 mcg, 300 mcg

Levothroid®: 25 mcg, 50 mcg, 75 mcg, 88 mcg, 100 mcg, 112 mcg, 125 mcg, 137 mcg, 150 mcg, 175 mcg, 200 mcg, 300 mcg

Levoxyl®: 25 mcg, 50 mcg, 75 mcg, 88 mcg, 100 mcg, 112 mcg, 125 mcg, 137 mcg, 150 mcg, 175 mcg, 200 mcg

Synthroid®: 25 mcg, 50 mcg, 75 mcg, 88 mcg, 100 mcg, 112 mcg, 125 mcg, 137 mcg, 150 mcg, 175 mcg, 200 mcg, 300 mcg

Unithroid®: 25 mcg, 50 mcg, 75 mcg, 88 mcg, 100 mcg, 112 mcg, 125 mcg, 150 mcg, 175 mcg, 200 mcg, 300 mcg

Dosing

Adult Doses should be adjusted based on clinical response and laboratory parameters.

Hypothyroidism: Adults, healthy adults <50 years of age, children in whom growth and puberty are complete, and older adults who have been recently treated for hyperthyroidism or who have been hypothyroid for only a few months):

Oral: ~1.7 mcg/kg/day; usual doses are ≤200 mcg/day (range: 100-125 mcg/day for a 70 kg adult); doses ≥300 mcg/day are rare (consider poor compliance, malabsorption, and/or drug interactions). Titrate dose every 6 weeks.

Patients >50 years or patients with cardiac disease: Refer to elderly dosing.

I.M., I.V.: 50% of the oral dose

Severe hypothyroidism: Oral: Initial: 12.5-25 mcg/day; adjust dose by 25 mcg/day every 2-4 weeks as appropriate

Subclinical hypothyroidism (if treated): Oral: 1 mcg/kg/day

TSH suppression: Oral:

Well-differentiated thyroid cancer: Highly individualized; Doses >2 mcg/kg/day may be needed to suppress TSH to <0.1 mIU/L in intermediate- to high-risk tumors. Low-risk tumors may be maintained at or slightly below the lower limit of normal (0.1-0.5 mIU/L) (Cooper, 2009).

Benign nodules and nontoxic multinodular goiter: Routine use of T_4 for TSH suppression is not recommended in patients with benign thyroid nodules. In patients deemed appropriate candidates, treatment should never be fully suppressive (TSH <0.1 mIU/L) (Cooper, 2009; Gharib, 2010). Avoid use if TSH is already suppressed.

Myxedema coma or stupor: I.V.: 200-500 mcg, then 100-300 mcg the next day if necessary; smaller doses should be considered in patients with cardiovascular disease

Geriatric Doses should be adjusted based on clinical response and laboratory parameters.

Hypothyroidism: Elderly patients may require <1 mcg/kg/day:

Oral:

>50 years without cardiac disease **or** <50 years with cardiac disease: Initial: 25-50 mcg/day; adjust dose at 6- to 8-week intervals as needed

>50 years with cardiac disease: Initial: 12.5-25 mcg/day; adjust dose by 12.5-25 mcg increments at 4- to 6-week intervals (many clinicians prefer to adjust at 6- to 8-week intervals).

Note: Patients with combined hypothyroidism and cardiac disease should be monitored carefully for changes in stability.

I.M., I.V.: 50% of the oral dose

Myxedema coma: *I.V.*: Refer to adult dosing; lower doses may be needed.

Pediatric Hypothyroidism: Neonates, Infants, and Children: Doses should be adjusted based on clinical response and laboratory parameters.

Oral: Daily dosage based on body weight and age as listed below:

0-3 months: 10-15 mcg/kg/day; if the infant is at risk for development of cardiac failure, use a lower starting dose of 25 mcg/day; if the initial serum T_4 is very low (<5 mcg/dL) begin treatment at a higher dosage of 50 mcg/day

3-6 months: 8-10 mcg/kg/day **or** 25-50 mcg/day

6-12 months: 6-8 mcg/kg/day **or** 50-75 mcg/day

1-5 years: 5-6 mcg/kg/day **or** 75-100 mcg/day

6-12 years: 4-5 mcg/kg/day **or** 100-125 mcg/day

>12 years: 2-3 mcg/kg/day **or** ≥150 mcg/day

Growth and puberty complete: 1.7 mcg/kg/day; refer to adult dosing.

Note: Hyperactivity in older children may be minimized by starting at 1/4 of the recommended dose and increasing each week by that amount until the full dose is achieved (4 weeks). Children with severe or chronic hypothyroidism should be started at 25 mcg/day; adjust dose by 25 mcg every 2-4 weeks.

I.M., I.V.: 50% of the oral dose

Administration

Oral Administer in the morning on an empty stomach, at least 30 minutes before food.

Capsule: Must be swallowed whole; do not cut, crush, or attempt to dissolve capsules in water to prepare a suspension

Tablet: May be crushed and suspended in 1-2 teaspoonfuls of water; suspension should be used immediately. Levoxyl® should be administered with a full glass of water to prevent gagging (due to tablet swelling).

I.V. Dilute vial with 5 mL normal saline; use immediately after reconstitution; do not mix with other I.V. fluids

Other Nasogastric tube: Bioavailability of levothyroxine is reduced if administered with enteral tube feeds. Since holding feedings for at least 1 hour before and after levothyroxine administration may not completely resolve the interaction, an increase in dose (eg, additional 25 mcg) may be necessary (Dickerson, 2010).

Stability

Reconstitution Dilute vial for injection with 5 mL normal saline. Reconstituted concentrations for the 200 mcg and 500 mcg vials are 40 mcg/mL and 100 mcg/mL, respectively. Shake well and use immediately after reconstitution (manufacturer recommendation); discard any unused portions.

Storage Store capsules, tablets, and injection at room temperature; excursions permitted to 15°C to 30°C (59°F to 86°F). Protect from light and moisture.

Additional stability data:

Stability in polypropylene syringes (100 mcg/mL in NS) at 5°C ± 1°C is 7 days (Gupta, 2000).

Stability in latex-free, PVC minibags protected from light and stored at 15°C to 30°C (59°F to 86°F) was 12 hours for a 2 mcg/mL concentration or 18 hours for a 0.4 mcg/mL concentration in NS. May be exposed to light; however, stability time is significantly reduced, especially for the 2 mcg/mL concentration (Strong, 2010).

Monitoring and Teaching Issues

Laboratory Monitoring Thyroid function (serum thyroxine, thyrotropin concentrations), resin triiodothyronine uptake (rT_3U), free thyroxine index (FTI), T_4, TSH, TSH may be elevated during the first few months of thyroid replacement despite patients being clinically euthyroid. In cases where T_4 remains low and TSH is within normal limits, an evaluation of "free" (unbound) T_4 is needed to evaluate further increase in dosage.

Physical Assessment Use with caution in presence of cardiovascular disease, adrenal insufficiency, and diabetes mellitus. Monitor for hyper-/hypothyroidism on a regular basis during therapy.

Patient Education Thyroid replacement therapy is generally for life. Take in the morning, 30 minutes before breakfast. Do not take antacids or iron preparations within 4 hours of thyroid medication. Report chest pain, rapid heart rate, palpitations, heat intolerance, excessive sweating, increased nervousness, agitation, or lethargy.

Dietary Considerations Should be taken on an empty stomach, at least 30 minutes before food.

Geriatric Considerations Elderly do not have a change in serum thyroxine associated with aging; however, plasma T_3 concentrations are decreased 25% to 40% in the elderly. There is not a compensatory rise in thyrotropin suggesting that lower T_3 is not reacted upon as a deficiency by the pituitary. This indicates a slightly lower than normal dosage of thyroid hormone replacement is usually sufficient in elderly patients than in younger adult patients. TSH must be monitored since insufficient thyroid replacement (elevated TSH) is a risk for coronary artery disease and excessive replacement (low TSH) may cause signs of hyperthyroidism and excessive bone loss. Some clinicians suggest levothyroxine is the drug of choice for replacement therapy.

Breast-Feeding Considerations Minimally excreted in human milk; adequate levels are needed to maintain normal lactation

Pregnancy Considerations Untreated maternal hypothyroidism may have adverse effects on fetal growth and development and is associated with higher rate of complications (spontaneous abortion, pre-eclampsia, stillbirth, premature delivery). Treatment should not be discontinued during pregnancy. TSH levels should be monitored during each trimester and 6-8 weeks postpartum. Increased doses may be needed during pregnancy.

Additional Information Equivalent doses: The following statement on relative potency of thyroid products is included in a joint statement by American Thyroid Association (ATA), American Association of Clinical Endocrinologists (AACE) and The Endocrine Society (TES): For purposes of conversion, levothyroxine sodium (T_4) 100 mcg is usually considered equivalent to desiccated thyroid 60 mg, thyroglobulin 60 mg, or liothyronine sodium (T_3) 25 mcg. However, these are rough guidelines only and do not obviate the careful re-evaluation of a patient when switching thyroid hormone preparations, including a change from one brand of levothyroxine to another. Joint position statement is available at http://www.thyroid.org/professionals/advocacy/04_12_08_thyroxine.html.

Note: Several medications have effects on thyroid production or conversion. The impact in thyroid replacement has not been specifically evaluated, but patient response should be monitored:

Methimazole: Decreases thyroid hormone secretion, while propylthiouracil decrease thyroid hormone secretion and decreases conversion of T_4 to T_3.

Beta-adrenergic antagonists: Decrease conversion of T_4 to T_3 (dose related, propranolol ≥160 mg/day); patients may be clinically euthyroid.

Iodide, iodine-containing radiographic contrast agents may decrease thyroid hormone secretion; may also increase thyroid hormone secretion, especially in patients with Graves' disease.

Other agents reported to impact on thyroid production/conversion include aminoglutethimide, amiodarone, chloral hydrate, diazepam, ethionamide, interferon-alpha, interleukin-2, lithium, lovastatin (case report), glucocorticoids (dose-related), mercaptopurine, sulfonamides, thiazide diuretics, and tolbutamide.

In addition, a number of medications have been noted to cause transient depression in TSH secretion, which may complicate interpretation of monitoring tests for levothyroxine, including corticosteroids, octreotide, and dopamine. Metoclopramide may increase TSH secretion

◆ **Levothyroxine Sodium** *see* Levothyroxine *on page 1101*
◆ **Levoxyl®** *see* Levothyroxine *on page 1101*
◆ **Lexapro®** *see* Escitalopram *on page 662*
◆ **Lexiva®** *see* Fosamprenavir *on page 823*
◆ **Lexxel® [DSC]** *see* Enalapril and Felodipine *on page 620*
◆ **LFA-3/IgG(1) Fusion Protein, Human** *see* Alefacept *on page 65*
◆ **Lialda®** *see* Mesalamine *on page 1177*
◆ **Librax® *[original formulation]*** *see* Clidinium and Chlordiazepoxide *on page 396*
◆ **Librium** *see* ChlordiazePOXIDE *on page 358*
◆ **Licide® [OTC]** *see* Pyrethrins and Piperonyl Butoxide *on page 1530*
◆ **LidaMantle®** *see* Lidocaine (Topical) *on page 1107*
◆ **Lidex** *see* Fluocinonide *on page 786*

Lidocaine (Systemic) (LYE doe kane)

U.S. Brand Names Xylocaine®; Xylocaine® Dental; Xylocaine® MPF

Index Terms Lidocaine Hydrochloride; Lignocaine Hydrochloride

Generic Availability (U.S.) Yes

Pharmacologic Category Antiarrhythmic Agent, Class Ib; Local Anesthetic

Medication Safety Issues

High alert medication: The Institute for Safe Medication Practices (ISMP) includes this medication (epidural administration; I.V. formulation) among its list of drugs which have a heightened risk of causing significant patient harm when used in error.

International issues:

Lidosen [Italy] may be confused with Lincocin brand name for lincomycin [U.S., Canada, and multiple international markets]; Linoten brand name for pamidronate [Spain]; Lodosyn brand name for carbidopa [U.S.]

Pregnancy Risk Factor B

Lactation Enters breast milk/use caution (AAP rates "compatible"; AAP 2001 update pending)

Use Local and regional anesthesia by infiltration, nerve block, epidural, or spinal techniques; acute treatment of ventricular arrhythmias from myocardial infarction or cardiac manipulation

Unlabeled/Investigational Use

ACLS guidelines: Hemodynamically stable monomorphic ventricular tachycardia (VT) (preserved ventricular function); polymorphic VT (preserved ventricular function); drug-induced monomorphic VT; when amiodarone is not available, pulseless VT or ventricular fibrillation (VF) (unresponsive to defibrillation, CPR, and vasopressor administration)

PALS guidelines: When amiodarone is not available, pulseless VT or VF (unresponsive to defibrillation, CPR, and epinephrine administration); consider in patients with cocaine overdose to prevent arrhythmias secondary to MI

I.V. infusion for chronic pain syndrome

Mechanism of Action/Effect Class Ib antiarrhythmic; suppresses automaticity of conduction tissue by increasing electrical stimulation threshold of ventricles, His-Purkinje system, and spontaneous depolarization of ventricles during diastole by direct action on tissues; blocks both initiation and conduction of nerve impulses by decreasing the neuronal membrane's permeability to sodium ions, which results in inhibition of depolarization with resultant blockade of conduction

Contraindications Hypersensitivity to lidocaine or any component of the formulation; hypersensitivity to another local anesthetic of the amide type; Adam-Stokes syndrome; severe degrees of SA, AV, or intraventricular heart block (except in patients with a functioning artificial pacemaker); premixed injection may contain corn-derived dextrose and its use is contraindicated in patients with allergy to corn-related products

Warnings/Precautions Use caution in patients with severe hepatic dysfunction or pseudocholinesterase deficiency; may have increased risk of lidocaine toxicity.

Intravenous: Constant ECG monitoring is necessary during I.V. administration. Use cautiously in hepatic impairment, any degree of heart block, Wolff-Parkinson-White syndrome, HF, marked hypoxia, severe respiratory depression, hypovolemia, history of malignant hyperthermia, or shock. Increased ventricular rate may be seen when administered to a patient with atrial fibrillation. Correct electrolyte disturbances, especially hypokalemia or hypomagnesemia, prior to use and throughout therapy. Correct any underlying causes of ventricular arrhythmias.

Monitor closely for signs and symptoms of CNS toxicity. The elderly may be prone to increased CNS and cardiovascular side effects. Reduce dose in hepatic dysfunction and CHF.

Injectable anesthetic: Follow appropriate administration techniques so as not to administer any intravascularly. Continuous intra-articular infusion of local anesthetics after arthroscopic or other surgical procedures is **not** an approved use; chondrolysis (primarily in the shoulder joint) has occurred following infusion, with some cases requiring arthroplasty or shoulder replacement. Solutions containing antimicrobial preservatives should not be used for epidural or spinal anesthesia. Some solutions contain a bisulfite; avoid in patients who are allergic to bisulfite. Resuscitative equipment, medicine and oxygen should be available in case of emergency. Use products containing epinephrine cautiously in patients with significant vascular disease, compromised blood flow, or during or following general anesthesia (increased risk of arrhythmias). Adjust the dose for the elderly, pediatric, acutely ill, and debilitated patients.

Drug Interactions

Metabolism/Transport Effects **Substrate** of CYP1A2 (minor), CYP2A6 (minor), CYP2B6 (minor), CYP2C9 (minor), CYP2D6 (major), CYP3A4 (major), P-glycoprotein; **Inhibits** CYP1A2 (strong), 2D6 (moderate), 3A4 (moderate)

Avoid Concomitant Use

Avoid concomitant use of Lidocaine (Systemic) with any of the following: Saquinavir; Thioridazine; Tolvaptan

Decreased Effect

The levels/effects of Lidocaine (Systemic) may be decreased by: CYP3A4 Inducers (Strong); Deferasirox; Etravirine; Herbs (CYP3A4 Inducers); Peginterferon Alfa-2b; P-Glycoprotein Inducers

Increased Effect/Toxicity

Lidocaine (Systemic) may increase the levels/effects of: Bendamustine; Colchicine; CYP1A2 Substrates; CYP2D6 Substrates; CYP3A4 Substrates; Eplerenone; Everolimus; Fesoterodine; Halofantrine; Lurasidone; Pimecrolimus; Ranolazine; Salmeterol; Saxagliptin; Tamoxifen; Thioridazine; Tolvaptan; Vilazodone

The levels/effects of Lidocaine (Systemic) may be increased by: Amiodarone; Beta-Blockers; Conivaptan; CYP2D6 Inhibitors (Moderate); CYP2D6 Inhibitors (Strong); CYP3A4 Inhibitors (Moderate); CYP3A4 Inhibitors (Strong); Darunavir; Dasatinib; Disopyramide; P-Glycoprotein Inhibitors; Saquinavir

Nutritional/Ethanol Interactions Herb/Nutraceutical: St John's wort may decrease lidocaine levels; avoid concurrent use.

Adverse Reactions Effects vary with route of administration. Many effects are dose related.

Frequency not defined.

Cardiovascular: Arrhythmia, bradycardia, arterial spasms, cardiovascular collapse, defibrillator threshold increased, edema, flushing, heart block, hypotension, sinus node supression, vascular insufficiency (periarticular injections)

Central nervous system: Agitation, anxiety, apprehension, coma, confusion, disorientation, dizziness, drowsiness, euphoria, hallucinations, headache, hyperesthesia, hypoesthesia, lethargy, lightheadedness, nervousness, psychosis, seizure, slurred speech, somnolence, unconsciousness

Gastrointestinal: Metallic taste, nausea, vomiting

Local: Thrombophlebitis

Neuromuscular & skeletal: Paresthesia, transient radicular pain (subarachnoid administration; up to 1.9%), tremor, twitching, weakness

Otic: Tinnitus

Respiratory: Bronchospasm, dyspnea, respiratory depression or arrest

Miscellaneous: Allergic reactions, anaphylactoid reaction, sensitivity to temperature extremes

Following spinal anesthesia: Positional headache (3%), shivering (2%) nausea, peripheral nerve symptoms, respiratory inadequacy and double vision (<1%), hypotension, cauda equina syndrome

Pharmacodynamics/Kinetics

Onset of Action Single bolus dose: 45-90 seconds

Duration of Action 10-20 minutes

Protein Binding 60% to 80% to alpha$_1$ acid glycoprotein

Half-Life Elimination Biphasic: Prolonged with congestive heart failure, liver disease, shock, severe renal disease; Initial: 7-30 minutes; Terminal: Infants, premature: 3.2 hours, Adults: 1.5-2 hours

Metabolism 90% hepatic; active metabolites monoethylglycinexylidide (MEGX) and glycinexylidide (GX) can accumulate and may cause CNS toxicity

Excretion Urine (<10% as unchanged drug, ~90% as metabolites)

Available Dosage Forms

Infusion, premixed in D_5W: 0.4% [4 mg/mL] (250 mL, 500 mL); 0.8% [8 mg/mL] (250 mL, 500 mL)

Injection, solution: 0.5% [5 mg/mL] (50 mL); 1% [10 mg/mL] (2 mL, 10 mL, 20 mL, 30 mL, 50 mL); 2% [20 mg/mL] (2 mL, 5 mL, 20 mL, 50 mL)

Xylocaine®: 0.5% [5 mg/mL] (50 mL); 1% [10 mg/mL] (10 mL, 20 mL, 50 mL); 2% [20 mg/mL] (10 mL, 20 mL, 50 mL)

Xylocaine® Dental: 2% [20 mg/mL] (1.8 mL)

Injection, solution [preservative free]: 0.5% [5 mg/mL] (50 mL); 1% [10 mg/mL] (2 mL, 5 mL, 30 mL); 1.5% [15 mg/mL] (20 mL); 2% [20 mg/mL] (2 mL, 5 mL, 10 mL); 4% [40 mg/mL] (5 mL)

Xylocaine®: 2% [20 mg/mL] (5 mL)

Xylocaine® MPF: 0.5% [5 mg/mL] (50 mL); 1% [10 mg/mL] (2 mL, 5 mL, 10 mL, 30 mL); 1.5% [15 mg/mL] (10 mL, 20 mL); 2% [20 mg/mL] (2 mL, 5 mL, 10 mL); 4% [40 mg/mL] (5 mL)

Dosing

Adult & Geriatric

Antiarrhythmic (ACLS, 2010):

VF or pulseless VT (after defibrillation attempts, CPR, and vasopressor administration) if amiodarone is not available: I.V., intraosseous (I.O.): Initial: 1-1.5 mg/kg. If refractory VF or pulseless VT, repeat 0.5-0.75 mg/kg bolus every 5-10 minutes (maximum cumulative dose: 3 mg/kg). Follow with continuous infusion (1-4 mg/minute) after return of perfusion. Reappearance of arrhythmia during constant infusion: 0.5 mg/kg bolus and reassessment of infusion (Zipes, 2000)

Intratracheal (loading dose only): 2-3.75 mg/kg (2-2.5 times the recommended I.V. dose); dilute in 5-10 mL NS or sterile water. **Note:** Absorption is greater with sterile water and results in less impairment of PaO_2.

Hemodynamically stable monomorphic VT: I.V.: 1-1.5 mg/kg; repeat with 0.5-0.75 mg/kg every 5-10 minutes as necessary (maximum cumulative dose: 3 mg/kg). Follow with continuous infusion of 1-4 mg/minute or 30-50 mcg/kg/minute

Note: Dose reduction (eg, of maintenance infusion) necessary in patients with CHF, shock, or hepatic disease.

Anesthesia, local injectable: Varies with procedure, degree of anesthesia needed, vascularity of tissue, duration of anesthesia required, and physical condition of patient; maximum: 4.5 mg/kg/dose not to exceed 300 mg; do not repeat within 2 hours.

Pediatric

Antiarrhythmic (PALS, 2010):

I.V., intraosseous (I.O.): **Note:** For use in VF or pulseless VT if amiodarone is not available; give after defibrillation attempts, CPR, and epinephrine:

Loading dose: 1 mg/kg; follow with continuous infusion; may administer second bolus of 0.5-1 mg/kg if delay between bolus and start of infusion is >15 minutes (PALS, 2000)

Continuous infusion: 20-50 mcg/kg/minute. Per the manufacturer, use a maximum of 20 mcg/kg/minute in patients with shock, hepatic disease, cardiac arrest, or CHF

Intratracheal: 2-3 mg/kg; flush with 5 mL of NS and follow with 5 assisted manual ventilations

Anesthesia, local injectable: Refer to adult dosing.

Renal Impairment Not dialyzable (0% to 5%) by hemo- or peritoneal dialysis; supplemental dose is not necessary.

Hepatic Impairment Dose reduction (eg, of maintenance infusion) necessary in patients with hepatic impairment; monitor lidocaine concentrations closely.

Administration

I.V. Continuous I.V. infusion rates: 2 g/250 mL D_5W:

1 mg/minute: 7.5 mL/hour
2 mg/minute: 15 mL/hour
3 mg/minute: 22.5 mL/hour
4 mg/minute: 30 mL/hour

Other

Intraosseous (I.O.; unlabeled administration route): Intraosseous administration is a safe and effective alternative to venous access in children with cardiac arrest; the onset for most medications is similar to that of I.V. administration (PALS, 2010). In adults, I.O. administration is a reasonable alternative when quick I.V. access is not feasible (ACLS, 2010).

Intratracheal (unlabeled administration route): Dilute in NS or sterile water. Absorption is greater with sterile water and results in less impairment of PaO_2 (Hahnel, 1990). Pass catheter beyond tip of tracheal tube, stop compressions, spray drug quickly down tube. Flush with 5 mL of NS and follow immediately with several quick insufflations and continue chest compressions.

Local infiltration: Buffered lidocaine for injectable local anesthetic may be prepared: Add 2 mL of sodium bicarbonate 8.4% to 18 mL of lidocaine 1% (Christoph, 1988)

Stability

Reconstitution Standard diluent: 2 g/250 mL D_5W.

Storage Injection: Stable at room temperature. Stability of parenteral admixture at room temperature (25°C) is the expiration date on premixed bag; out of overwrap stability is 30 days.

Monitoring and Teaching Issues

Laboratory Monitoring I.V.: Serum lidocaine levels. Therapeutic levels range from 1.5-5 mcg/mL; >6 mcg/mL is associated with toxicity.

Physical Assessment Dental/local anesthetic: Use caution to prevent gagging or choking. Avoid food or drink for 1 hour. **Antiarrhythmic: I.V.:** ECG and vital signs must be closely and continually monitored. Keep patient supine to reduce hypotensive effects. Assess frequently for adverse reactions or signs of CNS toxicity.

Patient Education I.V.: You will be monitored during infusion. Do not get up without assistance. Report dizziness, numbness, double vision, nausea, pain or burning at infusion site, nightmares, hearing strange noises, seeing unusual visions, or respiratory difficulty.

Dietary Considerations Premixed injection may contain corn-derived dextrose and its use is contraindicated in patients with allergy to corn-related products.

Geriatric Considerations Due to decreases in Phase I metabolism and possibly decrease in splanchnic perfusion with age, there may be a decreased clearance or increased half-life in the elderly and increased risk for CNS side effects and cardiac effects.

Breast-Feeding Considerations Small amounts of lidocaine and the MEGX metabolite are found in breast milk. The actual amount may depend on route and duration of administration. When administered topically at recommended doses, the amount of lidocaine available to the nursing infant would not be expected to cause adverse events. Cumulative exposure from all routes of administration should be considered.

Pregnancy Considerations Animal studies with lidocaine have not shown teratogenic effects. Lidocaine and the MEGX metabolite cross the placenta. Use is not contraindicated during labor and delivery. Topical lidocaine is used locally to provide analgesia prior to episiotomy and during repair of obstetric lacerations. Administration by the perineal route may result in greater absorption than administration by the epidural route. Adverse events have been reported in the infant following maternal administration, however, when used in appropriate doses, the risk to the fetus is low. Cumulative exposure from all routes of administration should be considered.

Related Information

Antiarrhythmic Drugs *on page 1978*

Lidocaine (Topical) (LYE doe kane)

U.S. Brand Names AneCream™ [OTC]; Anestafoam™ [OTC]; Band-Aid® Hurt Free™ Antiseptic Wash [OTC]; Burn Jel Plus [OTC]; Burn Jel® [OTC]; L-M-X® 4 [OTC]; L-M-X® 5 [OTC]; LidaMantle®; Lidoderm®; LTA® 360; Premjact®; Regenecare®; Regenecare® HA [OTC]; Solarcaine® cool aloe Burn Relief [OTC]; Topicaine® [OTC]; Unburn® [OTC]; Xylocaine®

Index Terms Lidocaine Hydrochloride; Lidocaine Patch; Lignocaine Hydrochloride; Viscous Lidocaine; Xylocaine Viscous

Generic Availability (U.S.) Yes: Hydrochloride cream, jelly, ointment, solution

Pharmacologic Category Analgesic, Topical; Local Anesthetic

Pregnancy Risk Factor B

Lactation Enters breast milk/use caution (AAP rates "compatible"; AAP 2001 update pending)

Use

Rectal: Temporary relief of pain and itching due to anorectal disorders

Topical: Local anesthetic for oral mucous membrane; use in laser/cosmetic surgeries; minor burns, cuts, and abrasions of the skin

Oral solution (viscous): Topical anesthesia of irritated oral mucous membranes and pharyngeal tissue

Patch (Lidoderm®): Relief of allodynia (painful hypersensitivity) and chronic pain in postherpetic neuralgia

Mechanism of Action/Effect Local anesthetics block both initiation and conduction of nerve impulses by decreasing the neuronal membrane's permeability to sodium ions, which results in inhibition of depolarization with resultant blockade of conduction

Contraindications Hypersensitivity to lidocaine or any component of the formulation; hypersensitivity to another local anesthetic of the amide type

Warnings/Precautions Potentially life-threatening side effects (eg, irregular heart beat, seizures, coma, respiratory depression, death) have occurred when used prior to cosmetic procedures. Excessive dosing (application to large areas, application to denuded skin, or wearing of device for longer than recommended) may lead to increased absorption and systemic toxicity. Application to broken or inflamed skin may lead to increased systemic absorption; use caution. Use caution in patients with severe hepatic disease due to diminished ability to metabolize systemically-absorbed lidocaine.

When topical anesthetics are used prior to cosmetic or medical procedures, the lowest amount of anesthetic necessary for pain relief should be applied. High systemic levels and toxic effects (eg, methemoglobinemia, irregular heart beats, respiratory depression, seizures, death) have been reported in patients who (without supervision of a trained professional) have applied topical anesthetics in large amounts (or to large areas of the skin), left these products on for prolonged periods of time, or have used wraps/dressings to cover the skin following application.

Topical cream, liquid, gel, and ointment: Do not leave on large body areas for >2 hours. Not for ophthalmic use. Some products are not recommended for use on mucous membranes; consult specific product labeling.

Topical patch: To avoid accidental ingestion by children, store and dispose of products out of the reach of children.

Drug Interactions

Metabolism/Transport Effects Substrate of CYP1A2 (minor), CYP2A6 (minor), CYP2B6 (minor), CYP2C9 (minor), CYP2D6 (major), CYP3A4 (major), P-glycoprotein; **Inhibits** CYP1A2 (strong), 2D6 (moderate), 3A4 (moderate)

Avoid Concomitant Use

Avoid concomitant use of Lidocaine (Topical) with any of the following: Thioridazine; Tolvaptan

Decreased Effect

The levels/effects of Lidocaine (Topical) may be decreased by: CYP3A4 Inducers (Strong); Deferasirox; Herbs (CYP3A4 Inducers); Peginterferon Alfa-2b; P-Glycoprotein Inducers

Increased Effect/Toxicity

Lidocaine (Topical) may increase the levels/effects of: Bendamustine; Colchicine; CYP1A2 Substrates; CYP2D6 Substrates; CYP3A4 Substrates; Eplerenone; Everolimus; Fesoterodine; Halofantrine; Lurasidone; Pimecrolimus; Ranolazine; Salmeterol; Saxagliptin; Tamoxifen; Thioridazine; Tolvaptan; Vilazodone

The levels/effects of Lidocaine (Topical) may be increased by: Amiodarone; Beta-Blockers; Conivaptan; CYP2D6 Inhibitors (Moderate); CYP2D6 Inhibitors (Strong); CYP3A4 Inhibitors (Moderate); CYP3A4 Inhibitors (Strong); Darunavir; Dasatinib; P-Glycoprotein Inhibitors

Adverse Reactions Frequency not defined.

Cardiovascular: Cyanosis, tachycardia
Central nervous system: Anxiety, confusion, dizziness, lethargy, lightheadedness, somnolence
Dermatologic: Angioedema, bruising (topical patch), contact dermatitis, depigmentation (topical patch), edema of the skin, itching, petechia (topical patch), pruritus, rash, urticaria
Hematologic: Methemoglobinemia
Local: Irritation (topical patch)
Neuromuscular & skeletal: Pain exacerbation (topical patch), paresthesia, weakness
Respiratory: Hypoxia

Available Dosage Forms

Aerosol, topical:
Anestafoam™ [OTC]: 4% (30 g)
Solarcaine® cool aloe Burn Relief [OTC]: 0.5% (127 g)
Cream, rectal:
L-M-X® 5 [OTC]: 5% (15 g, 30 g)
Cream, topical: 0.5% (0.9 g)
AneCream™ [OTC]: 4% (5 g, 15 g, 30 g)
L-M-X® 4 [OTC]: 4% (5 g, 15 g, 30 g)
LidaMantle®: 3% (85 g)
Gel, topical:
Burn Jel Plus [OTC]: 2.5% (118 mL)
Burn Jel® [OTC]: 2% (59 mL, 118 mL); 2% (3.5 g)
Regenecare®: 2% (14 g, 85 g)
Regenecare® HA [OTC]: 2% (85 g)
Solarcaine® cool aloe Burn Relief [OTC]: 0.5% (113 g, 226 g)
Topicaine® [OTC]: 4% (10 g, 30 g, 113 g); 5% (10 g, 30 g, 113 g)
Unburn® [OTC]: 2.5% (59 mL)
Jelly, topical: 2% (5 mL, 30 mL)
Xylocaine®: 2% (5 mL, 30 mL)
Jelly, topical [preservative free]: 2% (5 mL, 10 mL, 20 mL)
Lotion, topical:
LidaMantle®: 3% (177 mL)
Ointment, topical: 5% (30 g, 35.4 g, 50 g)
Patch, topical:
Lidoderm®: 5% (30s)
Solution, topical: 4% [40 mg/mL] (50 mL)
Band-Aid® Hurt Free™ Antiseptic Wash [OTC]: 2% [20 mg/mL] (177 mL)
LTA® 360: 4% [40 mg/mL] (4 mL)
Premjact®: 9.6% (13 mL)
Xylocaine®: 4% [40 mg/mL] (50 mL)
Solution, topical [preservative free]: 4% [40 mg/mL] (4 mL)
Solution, viscous, oral: 2% [20 mg/mL] (20 mL, 100 mL, 500 mL)

Dosing

Adult & Geriatric Anesthesia, topical:

Cream:
LidaMantle®: Skin irritation: Apply a thin film to affected area 2-3 times/day as needed
L-M-X® 4: Skin irritation: Apply up to 3-4 times daily to intact skin
L-M-X® 5: Relief of anorectal pain and itching: Apply to affected area up to 6 times/day

Gel, ointment: Apply to affected area ≤4 times/day as needed (maximum dose: 4.5 mg/kg, not to exceed 300 mg)

Topical solution: Apply 1-5 mL (40-200 mg) to affected area

Jelly: Maximum dose: 30 mL (600 mg) in any 12-hour period:
Anesthesia of male urethra: 5-30 mL (100-600 mg)
Anesthesia of female urethra: 3-5 mL (60-100 mg)
Lubrication of endotracheal tube: Apply a moderate amount to external surface only

Oral solution (viscous):
Anesthesia of the mouth: 15 mL swished in the mouth and spit out no more frequently than every 3 hours (maximum: 8 doses per 24-hour period)
Anesthesia of the pharynx: 15 mL gargled no more frequently than every 3 hours (maximum: 8 doses per 24-hour period); may be swallowed

Patch: Postherpetic neuralgia: Apply patch to most painful area. Up to 3 patches may be applied in a single application. Patch(es) may remain in place for up to 12 hours in any 24-hour period.

Pediatric Anesthesia, topical:

Cream:
LidaMantle®: Skin irritation: Refer to adult dosing.
L-M-X® 4: Skin irritation: Children ≥2 years: Refer to adult dosing.
L-M-X® 5: Relief of anorectal pain and itching: Children ≥12 years: Refer to adult dosing.

Jelly: Children: Dose varies with age and weight (maximum dose: 4.5 mg/kg)

Oral solution (viscous):

Infants and Children <3 years: 1.25 mL applied to area with a cotton-tipped applicator no more frequently than every 3 hours (maximum: 4 doses per 12-hour period)

Children ≥3 years: Should not exceed 4.5 mg/kg/dose (or 300 mg/dose); swished in the mouth and spit out no more frequently than every 3 hours (maximum: 4 doses per 12-hour period)

Administration

Topical

Gel (Topicaine®): Apply a moderately thick layer to affected area (~1/8 inch thick). Allow time for numbness to develop (~20-60 minutes after application). When used prior to laser surgery, avoid mucous membranes and remove prior to laser treatment.

Oral solution (viscous): Have patient swish medication around mouth and then spit it out; for pharyngeal anesthesia, patient should gargle and may swallow medication.

Patch: Apply to most painful area of skin immediately after removal from protective envelope. May be cut (with scissors, prior to removal of release liner) to appropriate size. Clothing may be worn over application area. After removal from skin, fold used patches so the adhesive side sticks to itself. Remove immediately if burning sensation occurs. Wash hands after application. Avoid exposing application site to external heat sources (eg, heating pad, electric blanket, heat lamp, hot tub).

Stability

Storage All formulations: Store at controlled room temperature; see product-specific labeling for any additional storage requirements.

Monitoring and Teaching Issues

Patient Education

Dermatologic: You will experience decreased sensation to pain, heat, or cold in the area and/or decreased muscle strength (depending on area of application) until effects wear off; use necessary caution to reduce incidence of possible injury until full sensation returns. Report irritation, pain, persistent numbness, tingling, swelling, restlessness, dizziness, acute weakness, blurred vision, ringing in ears, or respiratory difficulty.

Topical patch: Patch may be cut to appropriate size. Apply patch to most painful area. Up to 3 patches may be applied in a single application. Patch may remain in place for up to 12 hours in any 24-hour period. Remove immediately if burning sensation occurs. Wash hands after application. Remove patch while having MRI scan; can cause burns.

Oral (solution): Instruct patient to swish medication around mouth and then spit it out; if unable to spit, can apply with cotton tip to painful area.

Breast-Feeding Considerations When administered topically at recommended doses, the amount of lidocaine available to the nursing infant would not be expected to cause adverse events. Cumulative exposure from all routes of administration should be considered.

Pregnancy Considerations Animal studies with systemic lidocaine have not shown teratogenic effects. Lidocaine and the MEGX metabolite cross the placenta. Topical lidocaine is used locally to provide analgesia prior to episiotomy and during repair of obstetric lacerations. Cumulative exposure from all routes of administration should be considered.

Lidocaine and Epinephrine (LYE doe kane & ep i NEF rin)

U.S. Brand Names Lignospan® Forte; Lignospan® Standard; Xylocaine® MPF With Epinephrine; Xylocaine® With Epinephrine

Index Terms Epinephrine and Lidocaine

Generic Availability (U.S.) Yes

Pharmacologic Category Local Anesthetic

Pregnancy Risk Factor B

Lactation Lidocaine enters breast milk/use caution

Use Local infiltration anesthesia; AVS for nerve block

Available Dosage Forms

Injection, solution:

Generics:

0.5% / 1:200,000: Lidocaine hydrochloride 0.5% and epinephrine 1:200,000 (50 mL)

1% / 1:100,000: Lidocaine hydrochloride 1% and epinephrine 1:100,000 (20 mL, 30 mL, 50 mL)

2% / 1:100,000: Lidocaine hydrochloride 2% and epinephrine 1:100,000 (30 mL, 50 mL)

Brands:

Xylocaine® with Epinephrine:

0.5% / 1:200,000: Lidocaine hydrochloride 0.5% and epinephrine 1:200,000 (50 mL)

1% / 1:100,000: Lidocaine hydrochloride 1% and epinephrine 1:100,000 (10 mL, 20 mL, 50 mL)

2% / 1:100,000: Lidocaine hydrochloride 2% and epinephrine 1:100,000 (10 mL, 20 mL, 50 mL)

Injection, solution [preservative free]:

Generics:

1% / 1:200,000: Lidocaine hydrochloride 1% and epinephrine 1:200,000 (30 mL)

1.5% / 1:200,000: Lidocaine hydrochloride 1.5% and epinephrine 1:200,000 (5 mL, 30 mL)

2% / 1:200,000: Lidocaine hydrochloride 2% and epinephrine 1:200,000 (20 mL)

Brands:

Xylocaine®-MPF with Epinephrine:

1% / 1:200,000: Lidocaine hydrochloride 1% and epinephrine 1:200,000 (5 mL, 10 mL, 30 mL)

1.5% / 1:200,000: Lidocaine hydrochloride 1.5% and epinephrine 1:200,000 (5 mL, 10 mL, 30 mL)

2% / 1:200,000: Lidocaine hydrochloride 2% and epinephrine 1:200,000 (5 mL, 10 mL, 20 mL)

Injection, solution [for dental use]:

Generics:

2% / 1:50,000: Lidocaine hydrochloride 2% and epinephrine 1:50,000 (1.7 mL, 1.8 mL)

2% / 1:100,000: Lidocaine hydrochloride 2% and epinephrine 1:100,000 (1.7 mL, 1.8 mL)

Brands:

Lignospan® Forte: 2% / 1:50,000: Lidocaine hydrochloride 2% and epinephrine 1:50,000 (1.7 mL)

Lignospan® Standard: 2% / 1:100,000: Lidocaine hydrochloride 2% and epinephrine 1:100,000 (1.7 mL)

Dosing

Adult & Geriatric Dosage varies with the anesthetic procedure, degree of anesthesia needed, vascularity of tissue, duration of anesthesia required, and physical condition of patient.

Dental anesthesia, infiltration, or conduction block:

Children <12 years: 20-30 mg (1-1.5 mL) of lidocaine hydrochloride as a 2% solution with epinephrine 1:100,000; maximum: 4.5 mg of lidocaine hydrochloride/kg of body weight or 100-150 mg as a single dose

Children ≥12 years and Adults: Do not exceed 7 mg/kg body weight up to a maximum range of 300 mg (usual dental practice) to 500 mg (approved product labeling) of lidocaine hydrochloride and 3 mcg (0.003 mg) of epinephrine/kg of body weight or 0.2 mg epinephrine per dental appointment. The effective anesthetic dose varies with procedure, intensity of anesthesia needed, duration of anesthesia required, and physical condition of the patient. Always use the lowest effective dose along with careful aspiration.

Note: For most routine dental procedures, lidocaine hydrochloride 2% with epinephrine 1:100,000 is preferred. When a more pronounced hemostasis is required, a 1:50,000 epinephrine concentration should be used.

Pediatric Dosage varies with the anesthetic procedure, degree of anesthesia needed, vascularity of tissue, duration of anesthesia required, and physical condition of patient.

Dental anesthesia, infiltration, or conduction block:

Children <12 years: 20-30 mg (1-1.5 mL) of lidocaine hydrochloride as a 2% solution with epinephrine 1:100,000; maximum: 4.5 mg of lidocaine hydrochloride/kg of body weight or 100-150 mg as a single dose

Children ≥12 years: Refer to adult dosing.

Note: For most routine dental procedures, lidocaine hydrochloride 2% with epinephrine 1:100,000 is preferred. When a more pronounced hemostasis is required, a 1:50,000 epinephrine concentration should be used.

Administration

Other Injection solution for infiltration: Before injecting, withdraw syringe plunger to ensure injection is not into vein or artery. Aspirate the syringe after tissue penetration and before injection to minimize chance of direct vascular injection.

Monitoring and Teaching Issues

Physical Assessment See individual agents.

Patient Education See individual agents.

Related Information

EPINEPHrine (Systemic, Oral Inhalation) *on page 629*

Lidocaine (Systemic) *on page 1104*

◆ **Lidocaine Hydrochloride** *see* Lidocaine (Systemic) *on page 1104*

◆ **Lidocaine Hydrochloride** *see* Lidocaine (Topical) *on page 1107*

◆ **Lidocaine Patch** *see* Lidocaine (Topical) *on page 1107*

◆ **Lidoderm®** *see* Lidocaine (Topical) *on page 1107*

◆ **Lignocaine Hydrochloride** *see* Lidocaine (Systemic) *on page 1104*

◆ **Lignocaine Hydrochloride** *see* Lidocaine (Topical) *on page 1107*

◆ **Lignospan® Forte** *see* Lidocaine and Epinephrine *on page 1109*

◆ **Lignospan® Standard** *see* Lidocaine and Epinephrine *on page 1109*

Lindane (LIN dane)

Index Terms Benzene Hexachloride; Gamma Benzene Hexachloride; Hexachlorocyclohexane

Generic Availability (U.S.) Yes

Pharmacologic Category Antiparasitic Agent, Topical; Pediculocide; Scabicidal Agent

Medication Guide Available Yes

Pregnancy Risk Factor C

Lactation Enters breast milk/contraindicated

Use Treatment of *Sarcoptes scabiei* (scabies), *Pediculus capitis* (head lice), and *Phthirus pubis* (crab lice); FDA recommends reserving lindane as a second-line agent or with inadequate response to other therapies

Mechanism of Action/Effect Directly absorbed by parasites and ova through the exoskeleton; stimulates the nervous system resulting in seizures and death of parasitic arthropods

Contraindications Hypersensitivity to lindane or any component of the formulation; uncontrolled seizure disorders; crusted (Norwegian) scabies, acutely-inflamed skin or raw, weeping surfaces or other skin conditions which may increase systemic absorption

Warnings/Precautions Hazardous agent - use appropriate precautions for handling and disposal. **[U.S. Boxed Warning]: Not considered a drug of first choice; use only in patients who have failed first-line treatments, or in patients who cannot tolerate these agents.** Because of the potential for systemic absorption and CNS side effects, lindane should be used with caution; consider permethrin or crotamiton agent first. Oil-based hair dressing may increase toxic potential.

[U.S. Boxed Warning]: May be associated with severe neurologic toxicities (contraindicated in premature infants and uncontrolled seizure disorders). Seizures and death have been reported with use; use with caution in infants, small children, patients <50 kg, or patients with a history of seizures; use caution with conditions which may increase risk of seizures or medications which decrease seizure threshold; use caution with hepatic impairment; avoid contact with face, eyes, mucous membranes, and urethral meatus.

[U.S. Boxed Warning]: A lindane medication use guide must be given to all patients along with instructions for proper use. Patients should be informed that itching may occur following successful killing of lice and re-treatment may not be indicated. Should be used as a part of an overall lice management program.

Drug Interactions

Avoid Concomitant Use There are no known interactions where it is recommended to avoid concomitant use.

Decreased Effect There are no known significant interactions involving a decrease in effect.

Increased Effect/Toxicity There are no known significant interactions involving an increase in effect.

Adverse Reactions Frequency not defined (includes postmarketing and/or case reports).

Cardiovascular: Cardiac arrhythmia

Central nervous system: Ataxia, dizziness, headache, restlessness, seizure, pain

Dermatologic: Alopecia, contact dermatitis, skin and adipose tissue may act as repositories, eczematous eruptions, pruritus, urticaria

Gastrointestinal: Nausea, vomiting

Hematologic: Aplastic anemia

Hepatic: Hepatitis

Local: Burning and stinging

Neuromuscular & skeletal: Paresthesia

Renal: Hematuria

Respiratory: Pulmonary edema

Pharmacodynamics/Kinetics

Absorption ≤13% systemically

Time to Peak Serum: Children: 6 hours

Half-Life Elimination Children: 17-22 hours

Metabolism Hepatic

Excretion Urine and feces

Available Dosage Forms

Lotion, topical: 1% (60 mL, 480 mL)

Shampoo, topical: 1% (60 mL, 480 mL)

Dosing

Adult & Geriatric

Scabies: Topical: Apply a thin layer of lotion and massage it on skin from the neck to the toes; after 8-12 hours, bathe and remove the drug

Head lice, crab lice: Topical: Apply shampoo to dry hair and massage into hair for 4 minutes; add small quantities of water to hair until lather forms, then rinse hair thoroughly and comb with a fine tooth comb to remove nits. Amount of shampoo needed is based on length and density of hair; most patients will require 30 mL (maximum: 60 mL).

Pediatric Refer to adult dosing.

Administration

Oral Never administer orally.

Topical For topical use only. Caregivers should apply with gloves (avoid natural latex, may be permeable to lindane). Rinse off with warm (not hot) water.

Lotion: Apply to dry, cool skin; do not apply to face or eyes. Wait at least 1 hour after bathing or showering (wet or warm skin increases absorption). Skin should be clean and free of any other lotions, creams, or oil prior to lindane application.

Shampoo: Apply to clean, dry hair. Wait at least 1 hour after washing hair before applying lindane shampoo. Hair should be washed with a shampoo not containing a conditioner; hair and skin of head and neck should be free of any lotions, oils, or creams prior to lindane application.

Monitoring and Teaching Issues

Physical Assessment Assess head, hair, and skin surfaces for presence of lice and nits. Teach patient appropriate application.

Patient Education For external use only. Caregivers should apply with gloves on. Do not apply to face and avoid getting in eyes. Do not apply immediately after hot, soapy bath. For scabies, apply from neck to toes. For head lice or crab lice, massage into dry hair for 4 minutes; add water to hair to form lather, then rinse thoroughly. Clothing and bedding must be washed in hot water or dry cleaned to kill nits. Wash combs and brushes with lindane shampoo and thoroughly rinse. May need to treat all members of household and all sexual contacts concurrently. Report if condition persists or infection occurs.

Geriatric Considerations Because of the potential for systemic absorption and CNS side effects, lindane should be used with caution. Not considered a drug of first choice; consider permethrin or crotamiton agent first.

Breast-Feeding Considerations Nursing mothers should interrupt breast-feeding, express and discard milk for at least 24 hours following use.

Pregnancy Considerations There are no well-controlled studies in pregnant women.

Linezolid (li NE zoh lid)

U.S. Brand Names Zyvox®

Generic Availability (U.S.) No

Pharmacologic Category Antibiotic, Oxazolidinone

Medication Safety Issues

Sound-alike/look-alike issues:

Zyvox® may be confused with Ziox™, Zosyn®, Zovirax®

Pregnancy Risk Factor C

Lactation Excretion in breast milk unknown/use caution

Use Treatment of vancomycin-resistant *Enterococcus faecium* (VRE) infections, nosocomial pneumonia caused by *Staphylococcus aureus* (including MRSA) or *Streptococcus pneumoniae* (including multidrug-resistant strains [MDRSP]), complicated and uncomplicated skin and skin structure infections (including diabetic foot infections without concomitant osteomyelitis), and community-acquired pneumonia caused by susceptible gram-positive organisms

Mechanism of Action/Effect Inhibits bacterial protein synthesis by binding to bacterial 23S ribosomal RNA of the 50S subunit. This prevents the formation of a functional 70S initiation complex that is essential for the bacterial translation process. Linezolid is bacteriostatic against enterococci and staphylococci and bactericidal against most strains of streptococci.

Contraindications Hypersensitivity to linezolid or any other component of the formulation; concurrent use or within 2 weeks of MAO inhibitors; patients with uncontrolled hypertension, pheochromocytoma, thyrotoxicosis, and/or taking sympathomimetics (eg, pseudoephedrine), vasopressive agents (eg, epinephrine, norepinephrine), or dopaminergic agents (eg, dopamine, dobutamine) unless closely monitored for increased blood pressure; patients with carcinoid syndrome and/or taking SSRIs, tricyclic antidepressants, serotonin 5-$HT_{1B,1D}$ receptor agonists, meperidine, or buspirone unless closely monitored for sign/symptoms of serotonin syndrome

Warnings/Precautions Myelosuppression has been reported and may be dependent on duration of therapy (generally >2 weeks of treatment); use with caution in patients with pre-existing myelosuppression, in patients receiving other drugs which may cause bone marrow suppression, or in chronic infection (previous or concurrent antibiotic therapy). Weekly CBC monitoring is recommended. Consider discontinuation in patients developing myelosuppression (or in whom myelosuppression worsens during treatment).

Lactic acidosis has been reported with use. Linezolid exhibits mild MAO inhibitor properties and has the potential to have the same interactions as other MAO inhibitors; use with caution and monitor closely in patients with uncontrolled hypertension, pheochromocytoma, carcinoid syndrome, or untreated hyperthyroidism; use is contraindicated in the absence of close monitoring. Symptoms of agitation, confusion, hallucinations, hyper-reflexia, myoclonus, shivering, and tachycardia may occur with concomitant proserotonergic drugs (eg, SSRIs/SNRIs or triptans) or agents which reduce linezolid's metabolism; concurrent use with these medications is contraindicated unless patient is closely monitored for signs/symptoms of serotonin syndrome. Unnecessary use may lead to the development of resistance to linezolid; consider alternatives before initiating outpatient treatment.

Peripheral and optic neuropathy (with vision loss) has been reported and may occur primarily with extended courses of therapy >28 days; any symptoms of visual change or impairment warrant immediate ophthalmic evaluation and possible discontinuation of therapy. Seizures have been reported; use with caution in patients with a history of seizures. Prolonged use may result in fungal or bacterial superinfection, including *C. difficile*-associated diarrhea (CDAD) and pseudomembranous colitis; CDAD has been observed >2 months postantibiotic treatment.

Due to inconsistent concentrations in the CSF, empiric use in pediatric patients with CNS infections is not recommended by the manufacturer; however, there are multiple case reports describing successful treatment of documented VRE and *Staphylococcus aureus* CNS and shunt infections in the literature. Linezolid should not be used in the empiric treatment of catheter-related bloodstream infection (CRBSI), but may be appropriate for targeted therapy (Mermel, 2009). Oral suspension contains phenylalanine.

Drug Interactions

Avoid Concomitant Use

Avoid concomitant use of Linezolid with any of the following: Alpha-/Beta-Agonists (Indirect-Acting); Alpha1-Agonists; Alpha2-Agonists (Ophthalmic); Amphetamines; Anilidopiperidine Opioids; Atomoxetine; Bezafibrate; Buprenorphine; BuPROPion; BusPIRone; CarBAMazepine; Cyclobenzaprine; Dexmethylphenidate; Dextromethorphan; Diethylpropion;

HYDROmorphone; MAO Inhibitors; Maprotiline; Meperidine; Methyldopa; Methylphenidate; Mirtazapine; Propoxyphene; Selective Serotonin Reuptake Inhibitors; Serotonin 5-HT1D Receptor Agonists; Serotonin/Norepinephrine Reuptake Inhibitors; Sibutramine; Tapentadol; Tetrabenazine; Tetrahydrozoline; Tetrahydrozoline (Nasal); Tricyclic Antidepressants; Tryptophan

Decreased Effect There are no known significant interactions involving a decrease in effect.

Increased Effect/Toxicity

Linezolid may increase the levels/effects of: Alpha-/Beta-Agonists (Direct-Acting); Alpha-/Beta-Agonists (Indirect-Acting); Alpha1-Agonists; Alpha2-Agonists (Ophthalmic); Amphetamines; Antihypertensives; Atomoxetine; Beta2-Agonists; Bezafibrate; BuPROPion; Dexmethylphenidate; Dextromethorphan; Diethylpropion; Doxapram; HYDROmorphone; Lithium; Meperidine; Methadone; Methyldopa; Methylphenidate; Mirtazapine; Orthostatic Hypotension Producing Agents; Reserpine; Selective Serotonin Reuptake Inhibitors; Serotonin 5-HT1D Receptor Agonists; Serotonin Modulators; Serotonin/Norepinephrine Reuptake Inhibitors; Tetrahydrozoline; Tetrahydrozoline (Nasal); Tricyclic Antidepressants

The levels/effects of Linezolid may be increased by: Altretamine; Anilidopiperidine Opioids; Buprenorphine; BusPIRone; CarBAMazepine; COMT Inhibitors; Cyclobenzaprine; Levodopa; MAO Inhibitors; Maprotiline; Propoxyphene; Sibutramine; Tapentadol; Tetrabenazine; TraMADol; Tryptophan

Nutritional/Ethanol Interactions

Ethanol: Avoid ethanol (based on CNS depressant effects and potential tyramine content)

Food: Concurrent ingestion of foods rich in tyramine may cause sudden and severe high blood pressure (hypertensive crisis). Avoid tyramine-containing foods with MAOIs. Food's freshness is also an important concern; improperly stored or spoiled food can create an environment where tyramine concentrations may increase.

Herb/Nutraceutical: Avoid supplements containing caffeine, tyrosine, tryptophan or phenylalanine. Ingestion of large quantities may increase the risk of severe side effects (eg, hypertensive reactions, serotonin syndrome).

Adverse Reactions Percentages as reported in adults; frequency similar in pediatric patients

>10%:

- Central nervous system: Headache (<1% to 11%)
- Gastrointestinal: Diarrhea (3% to 11%)

1% to 10%:

- Central nervous system: Insomnia (3%), dizziness (≤2%), fever (2%)
- Dermatologic: Rash (2%)
- Gastrointestinal: Nausea (3% to 10%), lipase increased (3% to 4%), vomiting (1% to 4%), constipation (2%), taste alteration (1% to 2%), amylase increased (<1% to 2%), tongue discoloration (≤1%), oral moniliasis (≤1%), pancreatitis
- Genitourinary: Vaginal moniliasis (1% to 2%)
- Hematologic: Thrombocytopenia (<1% to 10%), hemoglobin decreased (1% to 7%), leukopenia (<1% to 2%), neutropenia (≤1%)
- Hepatic: ALT increased (2% to 10%), AST increased (2% to 5%), alkaline phosphatase increased (<1% to 4%), bilirubin increased (≤1%)
- Renal: BUN increased (≤2%)
- Miscellaneous: Fungal infection (≤1% to 2%), lactate dehydrogenase increased (<1% to 2%)

Pharmacodynamics/Kinetics

Absorption Rapid and extensive

Bioavailability Oral: ~100%

Time to Peak Adults: Oral: 1-2 hours

Protein Binding Adults: 31%

Half-Life Elimination Children ≥1 week (full-term) to 11 years: 1.5-3 hours; Adults: 4-5 hours

Metabolism Hepatic via oxidation of the morpholine ring, resulting in two inactive metabolites (aminoethoxyacetic acid, hydroxyethyl glycine); minimally metabolized, may be mediated by cytochrome P450

Excretion Urine (~30% of total dose as parent drug, ~50% of total dose as metabolites); feces (~9% of total dose as metabolites)

Nonrenal clearance: Adults: ~65%

Available Dosage Forms

Infusion, premixed:

Zyvox®: 200 mg (100 mL); 600 mg (300 mL)

Powder for suspension, oral:

Zyvox®: 100 mg/5 mL (150 mL)

Tablet, oral:

Zyvox®: 600 mg

Dosing

Adult & Geriatric

Usual dosage: Oral, I.V.: 600 mg every 12 hours

Indication-specific dosing:

VRE infections including concurrent bacteremia: Oral, I.V.: 600 mg every 12 hours for 14-28 days

MRSA infections:

Brain abscess, subdural empyema, spinal epidural abscess (unlabeled use; Liu, 2011): Oral, I.V.: 600 mg every 12 hours for 4-6 weeks

Meningitis (unlabeled use; Liu, 2011): Oral, I.V.: 600 mg every 12 hours for 2 weeks

Osteomyelitis (unlabeled use; Liu, 2011): Oral, I.V.: 600 mg every 12 hours for a minimum of 8 weeks (some experts combine with rifampin)

Pneumonia (healthcare associated or community acquired) (Liu, 2011): Oral, I.V.: 600 mg every 12 hours for 7-21 days
Septic arthritis (unlabeled use; Liu, 2011): Oral, I.V.: 600 mg every 12 hours for 3-4 weeks
Septic thrombosis of cavernous or dural venous sinus (unlabeled use; Liu, 2011): Oral, I.V.: 600 mg every 12 hours for 4-6 weeks

Nosocomial pneumonia, complicated skin and skin structure infections, community-acquired pneumonia including concurrent bacteremia: Oral, I.V.: 600 mg every 12 hours for 10-14 days. **Note:** May consider 7-day treatment course (versus manufacturer recommended 10-14 days) in patients with healthcare-, hospital-, and ventilator- associated pneumonia who have demonstrated good clinical response (ATS/IDSA, 2005).

Uncomplicated skin and skin structure infections: Oral: 400 mg every 12 hours for 10-14 days. **Note:** 400 mg dose is recommended in the product labeling; however, 600 mg dose is commonly employed clinically (Stevens, 2005)

Pediatric

Usual dosage: Oral, I.V.:
Preterm neonates (<34 weeks gestational age): 10 mg/kg every 12 hours; neonates with a suboptimal clinical response can be advanced to 10 mg/kg every 8 hours. By day 7 of life, all neonates should receive 10 mg/kg every 8 hours.
Children ≤11 years: 10 mg/kg (maximum: 600 mg/dose) every 8 hours
Children ≥12 years: Refer to adult dosing.

Indication-specific dosing:

Nosocomial pneumonia, complicated skin and skin structure infections, community acquired pneumonia including concurrent bacteremia: Oral, I.V.:
Preterm neonates (<34 weeks gestational age): 10 mg/kg every 12 hours; neonates with a suboptimal clinical response can be advanced to 10 mg/kg every 8 hours. By day 7 of life, all neonates should receive 10 mg/kg every 8 hours.
Infants (excluding preterm neonates <1 week) and Children ≤11 years: 10 mg/kg every 8 hours for 10-14 days

VRE infections including concurrent bacteremia: Oral, I.V.:
Preterm neonates (<34 weeks gestational age): 10 mg/kg every 12 hours; neonates with a suboptimal clinical response can be advanced to 10 mg/kg every 8 hours. By day 7 of life, all neonates should receive 10 mg/kg every 8 hours.
Infants (excluding preterm neonates <1 week) and Children ≤11 years: 10 mg/kg every 8 hours for 14-28 days
Children ≥12 years: Refer to adult dosing.

MRSA infections:

Brain abscess, subdural empyema, spinal epidural abscess (unlabeled use; Liu, 2011): Oral, I.V.:
Neonates: 10 mg/kg every 12 hours; neonates with a suboptimal clinical response can advance to 10 mg/kg every 8 hours. By day 7 of life, all neonates should receive 10 mg/kg every 8 hours. Total duration of therapy: 6 weeks
Children ≤ 11 years: 10 mg/kg every 8 hours for 4-6 weeks (maximum: 600 mg/dose)
Children ≥12 years: Refer to adult dosing.

Meningitis (unlabeled use; Liu, 2011): Oral, I.V.: Children ≥12 years: Refer to adult dosing.

Osteomyelitis (unlabeled use; Liu, 2011): Oral, I.V.:
Infants (excluding preterm neonates <1 week) and Children ≤11 years: 10 mg/kg every 8 hours for a minimum of 4-6 weeks (maximum: 600 mg/dose)
Children ≥12 years: Refer to adult dosing.

Pneumonia (healthcare associated or community acquired) (Liu, 2011): Oral, I.V.:
Children ≤11 years: 10 mg/kg every 8 hours for 7-21 days (maximum: 600 mg/dose)
Children ≥12 years: Refer to adult dosing.

Septic arthritis (unlabeled use; Liu, 2011): Oral, I.V.:
Infants (excluding preterm neonates <1 week) and Children ≤11 years: 10 mg/kg every 8 hours for 3-4 weeks (maximum: 600 mg/dose
Children ≥12 years: Refer to adult dosing.

Septic thrombosis of cavernous or dural venous sinus (unlabeled use; Liu, 2011): Oral, I.V.:
Children ≤11 years: 10 mg/kg every 8 hours for 4-6 weeks (maximum: 600 mg/dose)
Children ≥12 years and Adults: 600 mg every 12 hours for 4-6 weeks

Children ≥12 years: Refer to adult dosing.

Uncomplicated skin and skin structure infections: Oral:
Preterm neonates (<34 weeks gestational age): 10 mg/kg every 12 hours; neonates with a suboptimal clinical response can be advanced to 10 mg/kg every 8 hours. By day 7 of life, all neonates should receive 10 mg/kg every 8 hours.
Infants (excluding preterm neonates <1 week) and Children <5 years: 10 mg/kg every 8 hours for 10-14 days
Children 5-11 years: 10 mg/kg every 12 hours for 10-14 days
Children ≥12-18 years: 600 mg every 12 hours for 10-14 days

Renal Impairment No adjustment is recommended. The two primary metabolites may accumulate in patients with renal impairment but the clinical significance is unknown. Weigh the risk of accumulation of metabolites versus the benefit of therapy. Monitor for hematopoietic (eg, anemia, leukopenia, thrombocytopenia) and neuropathic (eg, peripheral neuropathy) adverse events when administering for extended periods.

Intermittent hemodialysis: Both linezolid and the two metabolites are eliminated by dialysis. Linezolid should be given after hemodialysis.
Continuous renal replacement therapy (CRRT): No adjustment needed.

Hepatic Impairment

Mild-to-moderate hepatic impairment (Child-Pugh class A or B): No dosage adjustment required.

Severe hepatic impairment (Child-Pugh class C): Use has not been adequately evaluated.

Administration

Oral Oral suspension: Invert gently to mix prior to administration, do not shake. Administer without regard to meals.

I.V. Administer intravenous infusion over 30-120 minutes. Do not mix or infuse with other medications. When the same intravenous line is used for sequential infusion of other medications, flush line with D_5W, NS, or LR before and after infusing linezolid. The yellow color of the injection may intensify over time without affecting potency.

Stability

Reconstitution Oral suspension: Reconstitute with 123 mL of distilled water (in 2 portions); shake vigorously. Concentration is 100 mg/5 mL. Prior to administration mix gently by inverting bottle; do not shake.

Storage

Infusion: Store at 25°C (77°F); excursions permitted to 15°C to 30°C (59°F to 86°F). Protect from light. Keep infusion bags in overwrap until ready for use. Protect infusion bags from freezing.

Oral suspension: Following reconstitution, store at 25°C (77°F); excursions permitted to 15°C to 30°C (59°F to 86°F). Use reconstituted suspension within 21 days. Protect from light.

Tablet: Store at 25°C (77°F); excursions permitted to 15°C to 30°C (59°F to 86°F). Protect from light; protect from moisture.

Monitoring and Teaching Issues

Laboratory Monitoring Weekly CBC, particularly in patients at increased risk of bleeding, with pre-existing myelosuppression, on concomitant medications that cause bone marrow suppression, in those who require >2 weeks of therapy, or in those with chronic infection who have received previous or concomitant antibiotic therapy.

Physical Assessment Assess for previous drug allergies before administering first dose. Assess other pharmacological agents patient may be taking for effectiveness and interactions (eg, serotonergic agents may increase resistance to linezolid and increase risk of serotonin syndrome, increased risk of hypertension with adrenergic agents). Assess results of laboratory tests, therapeutic effectiveness (resolution of infection), and adverse reactions (eg, myelosuppression, anemia, leukopenia, pancytopenia, and thrombocytopenia; may be more common in patients receiving linezolid for >2 weeks; lactic acidosis) on a regular basis during therapy. Teach patient proper use (oral), possible side effects/appropriate interventions (eg, tyramine-free diet), and adverse reactions to report.

Patient Education

Oral suspension: Store at room temperature and use within 21 days. Maintain adequate hydration unless instructed to restrict fluid intake. Avoid alcohol. Avoid tyramine-containing foods (eg, pickles, aged cheese, wine).

Oral/I.V.: You may experience mild headache, GI discomfort, nausea, vomiting, taste alteration, or constipation. Report immediately unresolved, white plaques in mouth; skin rash or irritation; acute headache, dizziness, blurred vision, or changes in visual acuity; tingling or numbness in extremities; or persistent diarrhea.

Dietary Considerations Take without regard to meals. Some products may contain sodium and/or phenylalanine. Avoid consuming large amounts of tyramine-containing foods/beverages. Some examples include aged or matured cheese, air-dried or cured meats (including sausages and salamis), fava or broad bean pods, tap/draft beers, Marmite concentrate, sauerkraut, soy sauce, and other soybean condiments.

Geriatric Considerations According to the manufacturer the pharmacokinetics of linezolid are not significantly altered in patients ≥65 years of age.

Breast-Feeding Considerations It is not known if linezolid is excreted in human milk. Linezolid has low protein binding and is 100% bioavailable orally which may increase the exposure to a nursing infant. The manufacturer advises caution if administering linezolid to a breast-feeding woman. Linezolid is used therapeutically in infants. Nondose-related effects could include modification of bowel flora.

Pregnancy Considerations Because adverse effects were observed in some animal studies, linezolid is classified pregnancy category C. There are no adequate and well-controlled studies in pregnant women.

Related Information

Antimicrobial Drugs of Choice *on page 2008*

Community-Acquired Pneumonia in Adults *on page 2021*

◆ **Lioresal®** *see* Baclofen *on page 187*

◆ **Lipancreatin** *see* Pancrelipase *on page 1400*

◆ **Lipase, Protease, and Amylase** *see* Pancrelipase *on page 1400*

◆ **Lipitor®** *see* Atorvastatin *on page 166*

◆ **Lipofen®** *see* Fenofibrate *on page 739*

◆ **Liposomal DAUNOrubicin** *see* DAUNOrubicin Citrate (Liposomal) *on page 472*

◆ **Liposomal DOXOrubicin** *see* DOXOrubicin (Liposomal) *on page 582*

◆ **Liposyn® II [DSC]** *see* Fat Emulsion *on page 736*

◆ **Liposyn® III** *see* Fat Emulsion *on page 736*

Liraglutide (lir a GLOO tide)

U.S. Brand Names Victoza®

Index Terms NN2211

Generic Availability (U.S.) No

Pharmacologic Category Antidiabetic Agent, Glucagon-Like Peptide-1 (GLP-1) Receptor Agonist

Medication Safety Issues Cross-contamination may occur if pens are shared among multiple patients. Steps should be taken to prohibit sharing of pens.

Medication Guide Available Yes

Pregnancy Risk Factor C

Lactation Excretion in breast milk unknown/not recommended

Use Treatment of type 2 diabetes mellitus (noninsulin dependent, NIDDM) to improve glycemic control

Mechanism of Action/Effect Liraglutide is a long acting analog of human glucagon-like peptide-1 (GLP-1) (an incretin hormone) which increases glucose-dependent insulin secretion, decreases inappropriate glucagon secretion, increases B-cell growth/replication, slows gastric emptying, and decreases food intake. Liraglutide administration results in decreases in hemoglobin A_{1c} by approximately 1%.

Contraindications History of or family history of medullary thyroid carcinoma (MTC); patients with multiple endocrine neoplasia syndrome type 2 (MEN2)

Warnings/Precautions [U.S. Boxed Warning] Dose and duration dependent thyroid C-cell tumors have developed in animal studies with liraglutide therapy; relevance in humans unknown. During clinical studies a few cases of thyroid C-cell hyperplasia were reported. Due to the finding in animal studies, patients were monitored with serum calcitonin or thyroid ultrasound during clinical trials; however it us unknown if this is beneficial in decreasing the risk of thyroid tumors. Consultation with an endocrinologist is recommended in patients who develop elevated calcitonin concentrations. Patients should be counseled on the risk and symptoms of thyroid tumors. Use is contraindicated in patients with or a family history of medullary thyroid cancer and in patients with multiple endocrine neoplasia syndrome type 2 (MEN2). Cases of acute and chronic pancreatitis (including one case of fatal necrotizing pancreatitis) have been reported although conclusive evidence to liraglutide therapy has not been established; monitor for unexplained severe abdominal pain, and if pancreatitis is suspected, discontinue use. Do not resume unless an alternative etiology of pancreatitis is confirmed. Use with caution in patients with a history of pancreatitis, cholelithiasis, and/or alcohol abuse. Most common reactions are gastrointestinal related; these symptoms may be dose-related and may decrease in frequency/severity with gradual titration and continued use. Use may be associated with weight loss (likely due to reduced intake) independent of the change in hemoglobin A_{1c}. Use with caution in patients with hepatic or renal impairment.

Concurrent use with insulin therapy has not been evaluated. Concomitant use of an insulin secretagogue (eg, sulfonylurea, meglitinide) may increase the risk of hypoglycemia; dosage reduction of secretagogues may be required during initiation of liraglutide. Due to its effects on gastric emptying, liraglutide may reduce the rate and extent of absorption of orally-administered drugs; use with caution in patients receiving medications with a narrow therapeutic window or require rapid absorption from the GI tract. Not recommended for first-line therapy; use as adjunct to diet and exercise. Do not use in patients with type 1 diabetes mellitus or for the treatment of diabetic ketoacidosis; not a substitute for insulin. Diabetes self-management education (DSME) is essential to maximize the effectiveness of therapy.

Drug Interactions

Avoid Concomitant Use There are no known interactions where it is recommended to avoid concomitant use.

Decreased Effect

The levels/effects of Liraglutide may be decreased by: Corticosteroids (Orally Inhaled); Corticosteroids (Systemic); Luteinizing Hormone-Releasing Hormone Analogs; Somatropin; Thiazide Diuretics

Increased Effect/Toxicity

Liraglutide may increase the levels/effects of: Sulfonylureas

The levels/effects of Liraglutide may be increased by: Pegvisomant

Nutritional/Ethanol Interactions Ethanol: Caution with ethanol (may cause hypoglycemia).

Adverse Reactions Percentages are as reported for monotherapy.

>10%: Gastrointestinal: Nausea (28%), diarrhea (17%), vomiting (11%)

1% to 10%:

Cardiovascular: Hypertension (3%)
Central nervous system: Headache (9%), dizziness (6%)
Gastrointestinal: Constipation (10%)
Genitourinary: Urinary tract infection (6%)
Hepatic: Hyperbilirubinemia (4%)
Local: Injection site reactions (2%; includes rash, erythema)
Neuromuscular & skeletal: Back pain (5%)
Respiratory: Upper respiratory infection (10%), sinusitis (6%), nasopharyngitis (5%)
Miscellaneous: Anti-liraglutide antibodies (low titers 9%, cross-reacting 7%), influenza (7%)

Pharmacodynamics/Kinetics

Bioavailability SubQ: ~55%

Time to Peak Plasma: 8-12 hours

Protein Binding >98%

Half-Life Elimination ~13 hours

Metabolism Endogenously metabolized by dipeptidyl peptidase IV (DPP-IV) and endogenous endopeptidases (Croom, 2009); metabolism occurs slower than that seen with native GLP-1

Excretion Urine (6%, as metabolites); feces (5%, as metabolites)

Available Dosage Forms

Injection, solution:

Victoza®: 6 mg/mL (3 mL)

Dosing

Adult & Geriatric Note: Initial dose is intended to reduce GI symptoms; does not provide effective glycemic control.

Treatment of type 2 diabetes: SubQ: Initial: 0.6 mg once daily for 1 week; then increase to 1.2 mg once daily; may increase further to 1.8 mg once daily if optimal glycemic response not achieved with 1.2 mg/day

Renal Impairment No dosage adjustment recommended; use caution, limited experience.

Hepatic Impairment No dosage adjustment recommended; use caution, limited experience.

Administration

Other SubQ: Use only if clear, colorless, and free of particulate matter. Administer via injection in the upper arm, thigh, or abdomen. Administer without regard to meals or time of day. Change needle with each administration. Do not share pens between patients even if needle is changed.

Stability

Storage Prior to initial use, store under refrigeration at 2°C to 8°C (36°F to 46°F); after initial use, may be stored in refrigerator or at room temperature of 15°C to 30°C (59°F to 86°F). Do not freeze (discard if freezing occurs). Protect from heat and light. Pen should be discarded 30 days after initial use.

Monitoring and Teaching Issues

Laboratory Monitoring Plasma glucose, Hb A_{1c}

Physical Assessment Assess for use-related cautions (eg, renal or hepatic impairment, history of patient or familial medullary thyroid cancer, multiple endocrine neoplasia syndrome type 2 [MEN 2]). Teach patient diabetes self-management and proper injection techniques and syringe/needle disposal.

Patient Education This medication is used to help control diabetes; it is not a cure. It is imperative that you follow other components of prescribed treatment regimen (eg, diet, regular exercise, glucose monitoring, laboratory testing). Follow directions for disposal of needles. May cause dizziness, headache, constipation, nausea, vomiting, or loss of appetite. Report persistent vomiting or diarrhea, severe or persistent abdominal pain, unusual lump or swelling of neck, difficulty swallowing, or unusual hoarseness.

Dietary Considerations Individualized medical nutrition therapy (MNT) based on ADA recommendations is an integral part of therapy.

Geriatric Considerations In clinical trials liraglutide's pharmacokinetics did not differ between younger and older participants. The manufacturer reports that the safety and efficacy of liraglutide did not differ in older diabetics. How "tightly" a geriatric patient's blood glucose should be controlled is controversial; however, a fasting blood sugar of <150 mg/dL is now an acceptable endpoint. Such a decision should be based on the patient's functional and cognitive status, how well they recognize hypoglycemic or hyperglycemic symptoms, and how to respond to them and their other disease states.

Intensive glucose control (Hb A_{1c} <6.5%) has been linked to increased all cause and cardiovascular mortality, hypoglycemia requiring assistance, and weight gain in adult type 2 diabetes. For elderly patients with diabetes who are relatively healthy, attaining target goals for aspirin use, blood pressure, lipids, smoking cessation, and diet and exercise may be more important than normalized glycemic control.

Pregnancy Considerations Teratogenic in animal studies. There are no adequate or well-controlled studies in pregnant women; use only if potential benefit outweighs possible risk to the fetus.

Lisdexamfetamine (lis dex am FET a meen)

U.S. Brand Names Vyvanse®

Index Terms Lisdexamfetamine Dimesylate; Lisdexamphetamine; NRP104

Generic Availability (U.S.) No

Pharmacologic Category Stimulant

Medication Safety Issues

Sound-alike/look-alike issues:

Vyvanse™ may be confused with Vytorin®, Glucovance®, Vivactil®

Beers Criteria medication: This drug may be inappropriate for use in geriatric patients (high severity risk).

Medication Guide Available Yes

Pregnancy Risk Factor C

Lactation Enters breast milk/not recommended

Use Treatment of attention-deficit/hyperactivity disorder (ADHD)

Mechanism of Action/Effect Lisdexamfetamine dimesylate is a prodrug that is converted to the active component dextroamphetamine. Amphetamines release catecholamines from storage sites in the nerve terminals.

Contraindications Known hypersensitivity or idiosyncratic reaction sympathomimetic amines; advanced arteriosclerosis, symptomatic cardiovascular disease, moderate-to-severe hypertension; hyperthyroidism; glaucoma; agitated states; history of drug abuse; concurrent use or within 2 weeks of use of MAO inhibitors

Warnings/Precautions [U.S. Boxed Warning]: Use has been associated with serious cardiovascular events including sudden death in patients with pre-existing structural cardiac abnormalities or other serious heart problems (sudden death in children and adolescents; sudden death, stroke and MI in adults. Use of this product should be avoided in the patients with known serious structural cardiac abnormalities, cardiomyopathy, serious heart rhythm abnormalities, coronary artery disease (adults), or other serious cardiac problems that could increase the risk of sudden death that these conditions alone carry. Patients should be carefully evaluated for these cardiac disorders prior to initiation of therapy.

Use with caution in patients with psychiatric or seizure disorders. May exacerbate symptoms of behavior and thought disorder in psychotic patients. Stimulants may unmask tics in individuals with coexisting Tourette's syndrome. **[U.S. Boxed Warning]: Potential for drug dependency exists; prolonged use may lead to drug dependency.** Use is contraindicated is patients with history of ethanol or drug abuse. Prescriptions should be written for the smallest quantity consistent with good patient care to minimize the possibility of overdose. Abrupt discontinuation following high doses or for prolonged periods may result in symptoms for withdrawal. Recommended to be used as part of a comprehensive treatment program for attention deficit disorders.

May be inappropriate for use in the elderly due to CNS stimulant adverse effects (Beers Criteria). Safety and efficacy of long-term use have not yet been established. Safety and efficacy in children <6 years of age have not been established. Appetite suppression may occur; monitor weight during therapy, particularly in children. Use of stimulants has been associated with slowing of growth rate; monitor growth rate during treatment. Treatment interruption may be necessary in patients who are not growing or gaining weight as expected.

Drug Interactions

Avoid Concomitant Use

Avoid concomitant use of Lisdexamfetamine with any of the following: Iobenguane I 123; MAO Inhibitors

Decreased Effect

Lisdexamfetamine may decrease the levels/effects of: Antihistamines; Ethosuximide; Iobenguane I 123; PHENobarbital; Phenytoin

The levels/effects of Lisdexamfetamine may be decreased by: Ammonium Chloride; Antipsychotics; Gastrointestinal Acidifying Agents; Lithium; Methenamine

Increased Effect/Toxicity

Lisdexamfetamine may increase the levels/effects of: Analgesics (Opioid); Sympathomimetics

The levels/effects of Lisdexamfetamine may be increased by: Alkalinizing Agents; Antacids; Atomoxetine; Cannabinoids; Carbonic Anhydrase Inhibitors; MAO Inhibitors; Proton Pump Inhibitors; Tricyclic Antidepressants

Nutritional/Ethanol Interactions

Ethanol: Avoid ethanol (may increase CNS depression).
Food: High-fat meal prolongs T_{max} by ~1 hour.

Lab Interactions Amphetamines may elevate plasma corticosteroid levels; may interfere with urinary steroid determinations.

Adverse Reactions

>10%:

Central nervous system: Headache (children 12%), insomnia (19% to 27%; 4% [initially])
Gastrointestinal: Appetite decreased (27% to 39%), xerostomia (children 5%; adults 26%), abdominal pain (children 12%)

1% to 10%:

Cardiovascular: Blood pressure increased (adults 3%), heart rate increased (adults 2%)
Central nervous system: Irritability (children 10%), anxiety (adults 6%), dizziness (children 5%), jitteriness (adults 4%), affect lability (children 3%), agitation (adults 3%), restlessness (adults 3%), fever (children 2%), somnolence (children 2%), tic (children 2%)
Dermatologic: Hyperhidrosis (adults 3%), rash (children 3%)
Gastrointestinal: Vomiting (children 9%), weight loss (children 9%), diarrhea (adults 7%), nausea (6% to 7%), anorexia (adult: 5%)
Genitourinary: Erectile dysfunction (adults <2%), libido decreased (adults <2%)
Neuromuscular & skeletal: Tremor (adults 2%)
Respiratory: Dyspnea (adults 2%)

Additional adverse reaction associated with amphetamines; frequency not defined.

Cardiovascular: Cardiomyopathy, hypertension, MI, sudden death, tachycardia
Central nervous system: Exacerbation of motor and phonic tics, overstimulation, stroke, Tourette's syndrome
Dermatologic: Stevens-Johnson syndrome, toxic epidermal necrolysis
Gastrointestinal: Abnormal taste, constipation

Pharmacodynamics/Kinetics

Absorption Rapid

Time to Peak T_{max}: Lisdexamfetamine: ~1 hour; dextroamphetamine: ~3.5 hours

Half-Life Elimination Lisdexamfetamine: <1 hour; Dextroamphetamine: 10-13 hours

Metabolism Non-CYP-mediated hepatic or intestinal metabolism to dextroamphetamine and l-lysine

Excretion Urine (96%, 42% as amphetamine-related compounds, 2% as lisdexamfetamine, 25% hippuric acid); feces (minimal)

Controlled Substance C-II

Available Dosage Forms

Capsule, oral:

Vyvanse®: 20 mg, 30 mg, 40 mg, 50 mg, 60 mg, 70 mg

Dosing

Adult ADHD: Oral: Initial: 30 mg once daily in the morning; may increase in increments of 10 mg or 20 mg/day at weekly intervals until optimal response is obtained; maximum: 70 mg/day

Note: Individualize dosage based on patient need and response to therapy. Administer at the lowest effective dose.

Pediatric ADHD: Oral: Children ≥6 years: Refer to adult dosing.

Administration

Oral Administer in the morning without regard to meals; swallow capsule whole, do not chew; capsule may be opened and the contents dissolved in glass of water; consume the resulting solution immediately; do not store solution.

Stability

Storage Store at controlled room temperature of 25°C (77°F) excursions permitted to 15°C to 30°C (59°F to 86°F). Protect from light.

Monitoring and Teaching Issues

Physical Assessment Perform careful cardiovascular assessment prior to initiating therapy. Monitor weight, blood pressure, and vital signs at beginning of therapy and periodically throughout. Taper dose when discontinuing.

Patient Education Avoid alcohol and caffeine use. May cause problems with sleeping, headache, irritability, dizziness, nausea, vomiting, abdominal pain, and decreased appetite. Report chest pain, difficulty breathing, fainting, abnormal thinking or behavior, increased aggression, hallucinations, or weight loss.

Dietary Considerations May be taken without regard to meals.

Geriatric Considerations This medication is considered to be potentially inappropriate in this patient population (Beers Criteria severity: High).

Breast-Feeding Considerations Manufacturer advises nursing mothers taking amphetamines to refrain from breast-feeding.

Pregnancy Considerations Animal studies have shown that amphetamines may cause embryotoxic and teratogenic effects and that pre- or early postnatal exposure to amphetamines may lead to lasting changes in behavior, including impaired learning, memory, and motor skills, as well as changes to libido. There are no adequate and well-controlled studies in pregnant women. No reproductive studies have been performed with lisdexamfetamine. Infants born to mothers dependent on amphetamines are more likely to arrive prematurely with low birth weight and may experience withdrawal symptoms including irritation, restlessness, anxiousness, weakness, listlessness, or lethargy.

◆ **Lisdexamfetamine Dimesylate** *see* Lisdexamfetamine *on page 1117*

◆ **Lisdexamphetamine** *see* Lisdexamfetamine *on page 1117*

Lisinopril (lyse IN oh pril)

U.S. Brand Names Prinivil®; Zestril®

Generic Availability (U.S.) Yes

Pharmacologic Category Angiotensin-Converting Enzyme (ACE) Inhibitor

Medication Safety Issues

Sound-alike/look-alike issues:

Lisinopril may be confused with fosinopril, Lioresal®, Lipitor®, RisperDAL®

Prinivil® may be confused with Plendil®, Pravachol®, Prevacid®, PriLOSEC®, Proventil®

Zestril® may be confused with Desyrel, Restoril™, Vistaril®, Zegerid®, Zerit®, Zetia®, Zostrix®, ZyPREXA®

International issues:

Acepril [Malaysia] may be confused with Accupril which is a brand name for quinapril [U.S.]

Acepril: Brand name for lisinopril [Malaysia], but also the brand name for captopril [Great Britain]; enalapril [Hungary, Switzerland]

Carace [Ireland] may be confused with Carac which is a brand name for fluorouracil [U.S.]

Pregnancy Risk Factor C (1st trimester); D (2nd and 3rd trimesters)

Lactation Excretion in breast milk unknown/not recommended

Use Treatment of hypertension, either alone or in combination with other antihypertensive agents; adjunctive therapy in treatment of heart failure (afterload reduction); treatment of acute myocardial infarction within 24 hours in hemodynamically-stable patients to improve survival; treatment of left ventricular dysfunction after myocardial infarction

Mechanism of Action/Effect Competitive inhibitor of angiotensin-converting enzyme (ACE); prevents conversion of angiotensin I to angiotensin II, a potent vasoconstrictor; results in lower levels of angiotensin II which causes an increase in plasma renin activity and a reduction in aldosterone secretion

Contraindications Hypersensitivity to lisinopril or any component of the formulation; angioedema related to previous treatment with an ACE inhibitor; patients with idiopathic or hereditary angioedema

Warnings/Precautions Anaphylactic reactions may occur rarely with ACE inhibitors. At any time during treatment (especially following first dose), angioedema may occur rarely with ACE inhibitors; it may involve the head and neck (potentially compromising airway) or the intestine (presenting with abdominal pain). African-Americans may be at an increased risk. Prolonged frequent monitoring may be required especially if tongue, glottis, or larynx are involved as they are associated with airway obstruction. Patients with a history of airway surgery may have a higher risk of airway obstruction. Aggressive early and appropriate management is critical. Use in patients with idiopathic or hereditary angioedema or previous angioedema associated with ACE inhibitor therapy is contraindicated. Severe anaphylactoid reactions may be seen during hemodialysis (eg, CVVHD) with high-flux dialysis membranes (eg, AN69), and rarely, during low density lipoprotein apheresis with dextran sulfate cellulose. Rare cases of anaphylactoid reactions have been reported in patients undergoing sensitization treatment with hymenoptera (bee, wasp) venom while receiving ACE inhibitors.

Symptomatic hypotension with or without syncope can occur with ACE inhibitors (usually with the first several doses); effects are most often observed in volume depleted patients; correct volume depletion prior to initiation; close monitoring of patient is required especially with initial dosing and dosing increases; blood pressure must be lowered at a rate appropriate for the patient's clinical condition. Initiation of therapy in patients with ischemic heart disease or cerebrovascular disease warrants close observation due to the potential consequences posed by falling blood pressure (eg, MI, stroke). Use with caution in hypertrophic cardiomyopathy with outflow tract obstruction, severe aortic stenosis, or before, during, or immediately after major surgery. **[U.S. Boxed Warning]: Based on human data, ACEIs can cause injury and death to the developing fetus when used in the second and third trimesters. ACEIs should be discontinued as soon as possible once pregnancy is detected.**

Hyperkalemia may occur with ACE inhibitors; risk factors include renal dysfunction, diabetes mellitus, concomitant use of potassium-sparing diuretics, potassium supplements, and/or potassium-containing salts. Use cautiously, if at all, with these agents and monitor potassium closely. Cough may occur with ACE inhibitors. Other causes of cough should be considered (eg, pulmonary congestion in patients with heart failure) and excluded prior to discontinuation.

May be associated with deterioration of renal function and/or increases in serum creatinine, particularly in patients with low renal blood flow (eg, renal artery stenosis, heart failure) whose glomerular filtration rate (GFR) is dependent on efferent arteriolar vasoconstriction by angiotensin II; deterioration may result in oliguria, acute renal failure, and progressive azotemia. Small increases in serum creatinine may occur following initiation; consider discontinuation only in patients with progressive and/or significant deterioration in renal function. Use with caution in patients with unstented unilateral/bilateral renal artery stenosis. When unstented bilateral renal artery stenosis is present, use is generally avoided due to the elevated risk of deterioration in renal function unless possible benefits outweigh risks. Concurrent use of angiotensin receptor blockers may increase the risk of clinically-significant adverse events (eg, renal dysfunction, hyperkalemia).

Rare toxicities associated with ACE inhibitors include cholestatic jaundice (which may progress to fulminant hepatic necrosis), agranulocytosis, neutropenia, or leukopenia with myeloid hypoplasia. Patients with collagen vascular diseases (especially with concomitant renal impairment) or renal impairment alone may be at increased risk for hematologic toxicity; periodically monitor CBC with differential in these patients. Safety and efficacy have not been established in children <6 years of age or children with a Cl_{cr} ≤30 mL/minute.

Drug Interactions

Avoid Concomitant Use There are no known interactions where it is recommended to avoid concomitant use.

Decreased Effect

The levels/effects of Lisinopril may be decreased by: Antacids; Aprotinin; Herbs (Hypertensive Properties); Methylphenidate; Nonsteroidal Anti-Inflammatory Agents; Salicylates; Yohimbine

Increased Effect/Toxicity

Lisinopril may increase the levels/effects of: Allopurinol; Amifostine; Antihypertensives; AzaTHIOprine; CycloSPORINE; CycloSPORINE (Systemic); Ferric Gluconate; Gold Sodium Thiomalate; Hypotensive Agents; Iron Dextran Complex; Lithium; RiTUXimab

The levels/effects of Lisinopril may be increased by: Angiotensin II Receptor Blockers; Diazoxide; DPP-IV Inhibitors; Eplerenone; Everolimus; Herbs (Hypotensive Properties); Loop Diuretics; MAO Inhibitors; Pentoxifylline; Phosphodiesterase 5 Inhibitors; Potassium Salts; Potassium-Sparing Diuretics; Prostacyclin Analogues; Sirolimus; Temsirolimus; Thiazide Diuretics; TiZANidine; Tolvaptan; Trimethoprim

Nutritional/Ethanol Interactions

Food: Potassium-containing salt substitutes may increase risk of hyperkalemia.

Herb/Nutraceutical: Avoid bayberry, blue cohosh, cayenne, ephedra, ginger, ginseng (American), kola, licorice (may worsen hypertension). Avoid black cohosh, California poppy, coleus, golden seal, hawthorn, mistletoe, periwinkle, quinine, shepherd's purse (may have increased antihypertensive effect).

Lab Interactions May cause false-positive results in urine acetone determinations using sodium nitroprusside reagent

Adverse Reactions Note: Frequency ranges include data from hypertension and heart failure trials. Higher rates of adverse reactions have generally been noted in patients with CHF. However, the frequency of adverse effects associated with placebo is also increased in this population.

1% to 10%:

Cardiovascular: Orthostatic effects (1%), hypotension (1% to 4%)

Central nervous system: Headache (4% to 6%), dizziness (5% to 12%), fatigue (3%)
Dermatologic: Rash (1% to 2%)
Endocrine & metabolic: Hyperkalemia (2% to 5%)
Gastrointestinal: Diarrhea (3% to 4%), nausea (2%), vomiting (1%), abdominal pain (2%)
Genitourinary: Impotence (1%)
Hematologic: Decreased hemoglobin (small)
Neuromuscular & skeletal: Chest pain (3%), weakness (1%)
Renal: BUN increased (2%); deterioration in renal function (in patients with bilateral renal artery stenosis or hypovolemia); serum creatinine increased (often transient)
Respiratory: Cough (4% to 9%), upper respiratory infection (1% to 2%)

Pharmacodynamics/Kinetics

Onset of Action 1 hour; Peak effect: Hypotensive: Oral: ~6 hours

Duration of Action 24 hours

Absorption Well absorbed; unaffected by food

Bioavailability Decreased with NYHA Class II-IV heart failure

Time to Peak ~7 hours

Protein Binding 25%

Half-Life Elimination 11-12 hours

Metabolism Not metabolized

Excretion Primarily urine (as unchanged drug)

Available Dosage Forms

Tablet, oral: 2.5 mg, 5 mg, 10 mg, 20 mg, 30 mg, 40 mg
Prinivil®: 5 mg, 10 mg, 20 mg
Zestril®: 2.5 mg, 5 mg, 10 mg, 20 mg, 30 mg, 40 mg

Dosing

Adult

Heart failure: Oral: Initial: 2.5-5 mg once daily; then increase by no more than 10 mg increments at intervals no less than 2 weeks to a maximum daily dose of 40 mg. Usual maintenance: 5-40 mg/day as a single dose. Target dose: 20-40 mg once daily (ACC/AHA 2009 Heart Failure Guidelines)

Note: If patient has hyponatremia (serum sodium <130 mEq/L) or renal impairment (Cl_{cr} <30 mL/minute or creatinine >3 mg/dL), then initial dose should be 2.5 mg/day

Hypertension: Oral: Usual dosage range (JNC 7): 10-40 mg/day
Not maintained on diuretic: Initial: 10 mg/day
Maintained on diuretic: Initial: 5 mg/day

Note: Antihypertensive effect may diminish toward the end of the dosing interval especially with doses of 10 mg/day. An increased dose may aid in extending the duration of antihypertensive effect. Doses up to 80 mg/day have been used, but do not appear to give greater effect.

Patients taking diuretics should have them discontinued 2-3 days prior to initiating lisinopril if possible. Restart diuretic after blood pressure is stable if needed. If diuretic cannot be discontinued prior to therapy, begin with 5 mg with close supervision until stable blood pressure. In patients with hyponatremia (<130 mEq/L), start dose at 2.5 mg/day.

Acute myocardial infarction (within 24 hours in hemodynamically stable patients): Oral: 5 mg immediately, then 5 mg at 24 hours, 10 mg at 48 hours, and 10 mg every day thereafter for 6 weeks. Patients should continue to receive standard treatments such as thrombolytics, aspirin, and beta-blockers.

Geriatric Oral: Initial: 2.5-5 mg/day; increase doses 2.5-5 mg/day at 1- to 2-week intervals; maximum daily dose: 40 mg

Patients taking diuretics should have them discontinued 2-3 days prior to initiating lisinopril if possible. Restart diuretic after blood pressure is stable if needed. In patients with hyponatremia (<130 mEq/L), start dose at 2.5 mg/day (see Renal Impairment).

Pediatric

Hypertension: Children ≥6 years: Oral: Initial: 0.07 mg/kg once daily (up to 5 mg); increase dose at 1- to 2-week intervals; doses >0.61 mg/kg or >40 mg have not been evaluated.

Renal Impairment

Heart failure: Adults: Cl_{cr} <30 mL/minute or creatinine >3 mg/dL: Initial: 2.5 mg/day
Hypertension:
Adults: Initial doses should be modified and upward titration should be cautious, based on response (maximum: 40 mg/day)
Cl_{cr} >30 mL/minute: Initial: 10 mg/day
Cl_{cr} 10-30 mL/minute: Initial: 5 mg/day
Hemodialysis: Initial: 2.5 mg/day; dialyzable (50%)
Children: Use in not recommended in pediatric patients with GFR <30 mL/minute/1.73 m^2

Administration

Oral Watch for hypotensive effects within 1-3 hours of first dose or new higher dose.

Monitoring and Teaching Issues

Laboratory Monitoring BUN, serum creatinine, renal function, WBC, and potassium; if patient has collagen vascular disease and/or renal impairment, periodically monitor CBC with differential

Physical Assessment Assess patient carefully for use cautions prior to beginning therapy. Assess potential for interactions with other pharmacological agents or herbal products that may impact fluid balance or cardiac status. Patient should be monitored for angioedema that may potentially affect airway or intestine, hypovolemia, postural hypotension, and anaphylactic reaction following first dose, any increase in dose, and regularly during therapy.

Patient Education Take first dose at bedtime. Do not use potassium supplement or salt substitutes without consulting prescriber. This drug does not eliminate need for diet or exercise regimen as recommended by prescriber. May cause dizziness, fainting, lightheadedness, postural hypotension, nausea, vomiting, abdominal pain, dry mouth, or transient loss of appetite; report if these persist. Report chest pain or palpitations; mouth sores; fever or chills; swelling of extremities, face, mouth, or tongue; skin rash; numbness, tingling, or pain in muscles; or respiratory difficulty or unusual cough.

Dietary Considerations Use potassium-containing salt substitutes cautiously in patients with diabetes, patients with renal dysfunction, or those maintained on potassium supplements or potassium-sparing diuretics.

Geriatric Considerations Due to frequent decreases in glomerular filtration (also creatinine clearance) with aging, elderly patients may have exaggerated responses to ACE inhibitors. Differences in clinical response due to hepatic changes are not observed. ACE inhibitors may be preferred agents in elderly patients with congestive heart failure and diabetes mellitus. Diabetic proteinuria is reduced and insulin sensitivity is enhanced. In general, the side effect profile is favorable in the elderly and causes little or no CNS confusion. Use lowest dose recommendations initially. Many elderly may be volume depleted due to diuretic use and/or blunted thirst reflex resulting in inadequate fluid intake.

Breast-Feeding Considerations It is not known if lisinopril is excreted in breast milk. Breast-feeding is not recommended by the manufacturer.

Pregnancy Considerations Due to adverse events observed in some animal studies, lisinopril is considered pregnancy category C during the first trimester. Based on human data, lisinopril is considered pregnancy category D if used during the second and third trimesters (per the manufacturer; however, one study suggests that fetal injury may occur at anytime during pregnancy). Lisinopril crosses the placenta. First trimester exposure to ACE inhibitors may cause major congenital malformations. An increased risk of cardiovascular and/or central nervous system malformations was observed in one study; however, an increased risk of teratogenic events was not observed in other studies. Second and third trimester use of an ACE inhibitor is associated with oligohydramnios. Oligohydramnios due to decreased fetal renal function may lead to fetal limb contractures, craniofacial deformation, and hypoplastic lung development. The use of ACE inhibitors during the second and third trimesters is also associated with anuria, hypotension, renal failure (reversible or irreversible), skull hypoplasia, and death in the fetus/neonate. Chronic maternal hypertension itself is also associated with adverse events in the fetus/infant. ACE inhibitors are not recommended during pregnancy to treat maternal hypertension or heart failure. Those who are planning a pregnancy should be considered for other medication options if an ACE inhibitor is currently prescribed or the ACE inhibitor should be discontinued as soon as possible once pregnancy is detected. The exposed fetus should be monitored for fetal growth, amniotic fluid volume, and organ formation. Infants exposed to an ACE inhibitor *in utero*, especially during the second and third trimester, should be monitored for hyperkalemia, hypotension, and oliguria.

[U.S. Boxed Warning]: Based on human data, ACE inhibitors can cause injury and death to the developing fetus when used in the second and third trimesters. ACE inhibitors should be discontinued as soon as possible once pregnancy is detected.

Related Information

Angiotensin Agents *on page 1974*
Heart Failure (Systolic) *on page 2040*

Lisinopril and Hydrochlorothiazide (lyse IN oh pril & hye droe klor oh THYE a zide)

U.S. Brand Names Prinzide®; Zestoretic®

Index Terms Hydrochlorothiazide and Lisinopril

Generic Availability (U.S.) Yes

Pharmacologic Category Angiotensin-Converting Enzyme (ACE) Inhibitor; Diuretic, Thiazide

Pregnancy Risk Factor C/D (2nd and 3rd trimesters)

Lactation Enters breast milk/not recommended

Use Treatment of hypertension

Available Dosage Forms

Tablet, oral: 10/12.5: Lisinopril 10 mg and hydrochlorothiazide 12.5 mg; 20/12.5: Lisinopril 20 mg and hydrochlorothiazide 12.5 mg; 20/25: Lisinopril 20 mg and hydrochlorothiazide 25 mg

Prinzide®:
- 10/12.5: Lisinopril 10 mg and hydrochlorothiazide 12.5 mg
- 20/12.5: Lisinopril 20 mg and hydrochlorothiazide 12.5 mg

Zestoretic®:
- 10/12.5: Lisinopril 10 mg and hydrochlorothiazide 12.5 mg
- 20/12.5: Lisinopril 20 mg and hydrochlorothiazide 12.5 mg
- 20/25: Lisinopril 20 mg and hydrochlorothiazide 25 mg

Dosing

Adult & Geriatric Hypertension: Oral: Initial: Lisinopril 10 mg/hydrochlorothiazide 12.5 mg or lisinopril 20 mg/hydrochlorothiazide 12.5 mg with further increases of either or both components could depend on clinical response. Doses >80 mg/day lisinopril or >50 mg/day hydrochlorothiazide are not recommended.

Renal Impairment Dosage adjustments should be made with caution. Usual regimens of therapy need not be adjusted as long as patient's Cl_{cr} >30 mL/minute. In patients with more severe renal impairment, loop diuretics are preferred.

Monitoring and Teaching Issues

Laboratory Monitoring BUN, serum creatinine, and electrolytes; if patient has collagen vascular disease and/or renal impairment, periodically monitor CBC with differential

Physical Assessment See individual agents.

Patient Education See individual agents.

Related Information

Hydrochlorothiazide *on page 912*
Lisinopril *on page 1119*

◆ **Lispro Insulin** *see* Insulin Lispro *on page 989*

Lithium (LITH ee um)

U.S. Brand Names Lithobid®

Index Terms Eskalith; Lithium Carbonate; Lithium Citrate

Generic Availability (U.S.) Yes

Pharmacologic Category Antimanic Agent

Medication Safety Issues

Sound-alike/look-alike issues:

Eskalith® may be confused with Estratest®
Lithium may be confused with lanthanum
Lithobid® may be confused with Levbid®, Lithostat®

Do not confuse **mEq** (milliequivalent) with **mg** (milligram). **Note:** 300 mg lithium carbonate or citrate contain 8 mEq lithium. Dosage should be written in **mg** (milligrams) to avoid confusion. Check prescriptions for unusually high volumes of the syrup for dosing errors.

Pregnancy Risk Factor D

Lactation Enters breast milk/contraindicated

Use Management of bipolar disorders; treatment of mania in individuals with bipolar disorder (maintenance treatment prevents or diminishes intensity of subsequent episodes)

Unlabeled/Investigational Use Potential augmenting agent for antidepressants; aggression, post-traumatic stress disorder, conduct disorder in children

Mechanism of Action/Effect Stabilizes mood by actions on nerve cells of the central nervous system; involves serotonin, phosphatidylinositol cycle, and dopamine receptor sensitivity

Contraindications Hypersensitivity to lithium or any component of the formulation; avoid use in patients with severe cardiovascular or renal disease, or with severe debilitation, dehydration, or sodium depletion; pregnancy

Warnings/Precautions [U.S. Boxed Warning]: Lithium toxicity is closely related to serum levels and can occur at therapeutic doses; serum lithium determinations are required to monitor therapy. Use with caution in patients with thyroid disease, mild-moderate renal impairment, or mild-moderate cardiovascular disease. Use caution in patients receiving medications which alter sodium excretion (eg, diuretics, ACE inhibitors, NSAIDs), or in patients with significant fluid loss (protracted sweating, diarrhea, or prolonged fever); temporary reduction or cessation of therapy may be warranted. Some elderly patients may be extremely sensitive to the effects of lithium, see Dosing. Chronic therapy results in diminished renal concentrating ability (nephrogenic DI); this is usually reversible when lithium is discontinued. Changes in renal function should be monitored, and re-evaluation of treatment may be necessary. Use caution in patients at risk of suicide (suicidal thoughts or behavior).

Use with caution in patients receiving neuroleptic medications - a syndrome resembling NMS has been associated with concurrent therapy. Lithium may impair the patient's alertness, affecting the ability to operate machinery or driving a vehicle. Neuromuscular-blocking agents should be administered with caution; the response may be prolonged.

Higher serum concentrations may be required and tolerated during an acute manic phase; however, the tolerance decreases when symptoms subside. Normal fluid and salt intake must be maintained during therapy.

Drug Interactions

Avoid Concomitant Use

Avoid concomitant use of Lithium with any of the following: Sibutramine

Decreased Effect

Lithium may decrease the levels/effects of: Amphetamines; Antipsychotics; Desmopressin

The levels/effects of Lithium may be decreased by: Calcitonin; Calcium Polystyrene Sulfonate; Carbonic Anhydrase Inhibitors; Loop Diuretics; Sodium Bicarbonate; Sodium Chloride; Sodium Polystyrene Sulfonate; Theophylline Derivatives

Increased Effect/Toxicity

Lithium may increase the levels/effects of: Antipsychotics; Neuromuscular-Blocking Agents; Serotonin Modulators; Tricyclic Antidepressants

The levels/effects of Lithium may be increased by: ACE Inhibitors; Angiotensin II Receptor Blockers; Calcium Channel Blockers (Nondihydropyridine); CarBAMazepine; Desmopressin; Loop Diuretics; MAO Inhibitors; Methyldopa; Nonsteroidal Anti-Inflammatory Agents; Phenytoin; Potassium Iodide; Selective Serotonin Reuptake Inhibitors; Sibutramine; Thiazide Diuretics; Topiramate

Nutritional/Ethanol Interactions Food: Limit caffeine.

Lab Interactions Increased calcium (S), glucose, magnesium, potassium (S); decreased thyroxine (S)

Adverse Reactions Frequency not defined.

Cardiovascular: Cardiac arrhythmia, hypotension, sinus node dysfunction, flattened or inverted T waves (reversible), edema, bradycardia, syncope

Central nervous system: Blackout spells, coma, confusion, dizziness, dystonia, fatigue, headache, lethargy, pseudotumor cerebri, psychomotor retardation, restlessness, sedation, seizure, slowed intellectual functioning, slurred speech, stupor, tics, vertigo

Dermatologic: Dry or thinning of hair, folliculitis, alopecia, exacerbation of psoriasis, rash

Endocrine & metabolic: Euthyroid goiter and/or hypothyroidism, hyperthyroidism, hyperglycemia, diabetes insipidus

Gastrointestinal: Polydipsia, anorexia, nausea, vomiting, diarrhea, xerostomia, metallic taste, weight gain, salivary gland swelling, excessive salivation

Genitourinary: Incontinence, polyuria, glycosuria, oliguria, albuminuria

Hematologic: Leukocytosis

Neuromuscular & skeletal: Tremor, muscle hyperirritability, ataxia, choreoathetoid movements, hyperactive deep tendon reflexes, myasthenia gravis (rare)

Ocular: Nystagmus, blurred vision, transient scotoma

Miscellaneous: Coldness and painful discoloration of fingers and toes

Postmarketing and/or case reports: Drug-induced Brugada syndrome

Pharmacodynamics/Kinetics

Absorption Rapid and complete

Bioavailability Not affected by food; Capsule, immediate release tablet: 95% to 100%; Extended release tablet: 60% to 90%; Syrup: 100%

Time to Peak Serum: Nonsustained release: ~0.5-2 hours; extended release: 4-12 hours; syrup: 15-60 minutes

Protein Binding Not protein bound

Half-Life Elimination 18-24 hours; can increase to more than 36 hours in elderly or with renal impairment

Metabolism Not metabolized

Excretion Urine (90% to 98% as unchanged drug); sweat (4% to 5%); feces (1%)

Clearance: 80% of filtered lithium is reabsorbed in the proximal convoluted tubules; therefore, clearance approximates 20% of GFR or 20-40 mL/minute

Available Dosage Forms

Capsule, oral: 150 mg, 300 mg, 600 mg

Solution, oral: 300 mg/5 mL (5 mL, 473 mL, 500 mL)

Tablet, oral: 300 mg, 600 mg

Tablet, extended release, oral: 300 mg, 450 mg

Lithobid®: 300 mg

Dosing

Adult

Bipolar disorders: Oral: 900-2400 mg/day in 3-4 divided doses or 900-1800 mg/day in two divided doses of extended release

Note: Monitor serum concentrations and clinical response (efficacy and toxicity) to determine proper dose

Geriatric Bipolar disorders: Oral: Initial: 300 mg twice daily; increase weekly in increments of 300 mg/day, monitoring levels; rarely need >900-1200 mg/day.

Pediatric

Bipolar disorders (unlabeled use): Oral: Children 6-12 years: 15-60 mg/kg/day in 3-4 divided doses; dose not to exceed usual adult dosage. **Note:** Monitor serum concentrations and clinical response (efficacy and toxicity) to determine proper dose.

Conduct disorder (unlabeled use): Oral: Children 6-12 years: 15-30 mg/kg/day in 3-4 divided doses; dose not to exceed usual adult dosage

Renal Impairment

Cl_{cr} 10-50 mL/minute: Administer 50% to 75% of normal dose.

Cl_{cr} <10 mL/minute: Administer 25% to 50% of normal dose.

Dialyzable (50% to 100%); 4-7 times more efficient than peritoneal dialysis

Administration

Oral Administer with meals to decrease GI upset. Extended release tablets must be swallowed whole; do not crush or chew.

Monitoring and Teaching Issues

Laboratory Monitoring Serum lithium every 4-5 days during initial therapy. Monitor renal and thyroid; serum electrolytes; CBC with differential, urinalysis.

Levels should be obtained twice weekly until both patient's clinical status and levels are stable then levels may be obtained every 1-3 months.

Timing of serum samples: Draw trough just before next dose (8-12 hours after previous dose).

Therapeutic levels:

Acute mania: 0.6-1.2 mEq/L (SI: 0.6-1.2 mmol/L)

Protection against future episodes in most patients with bipolar disorder: 0.8-1 mEq/L (SI: 0.8-1.0 mmol/L); a higher rate of relapse is described in subjects who are maintained at <0.4 mEq/L (SI: 0.4 mmol/L).

Elderly patients can usually be maintained at lower end of therapeutic range (0.6-0.8 mEq/L).

Toxic concentration: >1.5 mEq/L (SI: >2 mmol/L)

Adverse effect levels:
GI complaints/tremor: 1.5-2 mEq/L
Confusion/somnolence: 2-2.5 mEq/L
Seizures/death: >2.5 mEq/L

Physical Assessment Monitor cardiovascular status; assess for fluid retention. Educate patient about risks of toxicity and how to minimize.

Patient Education Do not crush or chew extended release tablets or capsules. Maintain adequate hydration unless instructed to restrict fluid intake. Avoid changes in sodium content (eg, low sodium diets); reduction of sodium can increase lithium toxicity. Frequent blood tests and monitoring will be necessary. You may experience decreased appetite, altered taste sensation, drowsiness, or dizziness, especially during early therapy. Immediately report unresolved diarrhea, abrupt changes in weight, muscular tremors or lack of coordination, fever, or changes in urinary volume.

Dietary Considerations May be taken with meals to avoid GI upset; maintain adequate fluid intake.

Geriatric Considerations Some elderly patients may be extremely sensitive to the effects of lithium. Initial doses need to be adjusted for renal function in the elderly; thereafter, adjust doses based upon serum concentrations and response.

Pregnancy Considerations Cardiac malformations in the infant, including Ebstein's anomaly, are associated with use of lithium during the first trimester of pregnancy. Nontoxic effects to the newborn include shallow respiration, hypotonia, lethargy, cyanosis, diabetes insipidus, thyroid depression, and nontoxic goiter when lithium is used near term. Efforts should be made to avoid lithium use during the first trimester; if an alternative therapy is not appropriate, the lowest possible dose of lithium should be used throughout the pregnancy. Fetal echocardiography and ultrasound to screen for anomalies should be conducted between 16-20 weeks of gestation. Lithium levels should be monitored in the mother and may need to be adjusted following delivery.

Related Information

Peak and Trough Guidelines *on page 1958*

- **Lithium Carbonate** *see* Lithium *on page 1123*
- **Lithium Citrate** *see* Lithium *on page 1123*
- **Lithobid®** *see* Lithium *on page 1123*
- **Little Fevers™ [OTC]** *see* Acetaminophen *on page 38*
- **Little Noses® Decongestant [OTC]** *see* Phenylephrine (Nasal) *on page 1451*
- **Livalo®** *see* Pitavastatin *on page 1466*
- **Live Attenuated Influenza Vaccine (LAIV)** *see* Influenza Virus Vaccine (Live/Attenuated) *on page 980*
- **L-leucovorin** *see* LEVOleucovorin *on page 1096*
- **LM3100** *see* Plerixafor *on page 1468*
- **LNg 20** *see* Levonorgestrel *on page 1097*
- **Locoid®** *see* Hydrocortisone (Topical) *on page 920*
- **Locoid Lipocream®** *see* Hydrocortisone (Topical) *on page 920*
- **Lodine** *see* Etodolac *on page 707*

Lodoxamide (loe DOKS a mide)

U.S. Brand Names Alomide®

Index Terms Lodoxamide Tromethamine

Generic Availability (U.S.) No

Pharmacologic Category Mast Cell Stabilizer

Medication Safety Issues

International issues:
Thilomide [Greece, Turkey] may be confused with Thalomid brand name for thalidomide [U.S., Canada]

Pregnancy Risk Factor B

Use Treatment of vernal keratoconjunctivitis, vernal conjunctivitis, and vernal keratitis

Available Dosage Forms

Solution, ophthalmic:
Alomide®: 0.1% (10 mL)

Dosing

Adult & Geriatric Vernal conjunctivitis, keratitis: Ophthalmic: Children ≥2 years and Adults: Instill 1-2 drops in eye(s) 4 times/day for up to 3 months

Pediatric Children ≥2 years: Refer to adult dosing.

Monitoring and Teaching Issues

Patient Education For use in eyes only. Avoid wearing soft contact lenses while using this medication. Wash hands before using. Lie down or tilt your head back and look upward. Hold dropper tip as near as possible to your eyelid without touching it. Pull the lower lid of eye down to form a pocket. Drop the prescribed number of drops into the pocket made by the lower lid and the eye (placing drops on the surface of the eyeball can cause stinging). Do not blink or rub eye. Close your eye and press lightly against the inside corner of your eye for about 1 minute. Repeat in other eye if directed by prescriber. You may experience temporary stinging or burning in the eyes, headache, increased eye tearing or dry eye, sneezing, or blurred vision. Inform prescriber if you experience eye pain, disturbance of vision, skin rash, swelling in or around the eyes, or if condition worsens or fails to improve. Do not use if solution has changed color, is cloudy, or contains particles.

- **Lodoxamide Tromethamine** *see* Lodoxamide *on page 1125*
- **Lodrane® 24 [DSC]** *see* Brompheniramine *on page 234*
- **Loestrin® 21 1.5/30** *see* Ethinyl Estradiol and Norethindrone *on page 701*
- **Loestrin® 21 1/20** *see* Ethinyl Estradiol and Norethindrone *on page 701*
- **Loestrin® 24 Fe** *see* Ethinyl Estradiol and Norethindrone *on page 701*
- **Loestrin® Fe 1.5/30** *see* Ethinyl Estradiol and Norethindrone *on page 701*
- **Loestrin® Fe 1/20** *see* Ethinyl Estradiol and Norethindrone *on page 701*
- **Lofibra®** *see* Fenofibrate *on page 739*
- **LoHist-12** *see* Brompheniramine *on page 234*
- **L-OHP** *see* Oxaliplatin *on page 1370*
- **Lo Loestrin™ Fe** *see* Ethinyl Estradiol and Norethindrone *on page 701*
- **Lomotil®** *see* Diphenoxylate and Atropine *on page 547*
- **Longastatin** *see* Octreotide *on page 1339*

Loperamide (loe PER a mide)

U.S. Brand Names Anti-Diarrheal [OTC]; Diamode [OTC]; Imodium® A-D for children [OTC]; Imodium® A-D [OTC]; Kao Paverin® [OTC] [DSC]

Index Terms Loperamide Hydrochloride

Generic Availability (U.S.) Yes

Pharmacologic Category Antidiarrheal

Medication Safety Issues

Sound-alike/look-alike issues:

Imodium® A-D may be confused with Indocin®
Loperamide may be confused with furosemide

International issues:

Indiaral [France] may be confused with Inderal and Inderal LA brand names for propranolol [U.S., Canada, and multiple international markets]

Pregnancy Risk Factor C

Lactation Enters breast milk/not recommended.

Use Treatment of chronic diarrhea associated with inflammatory bowel disease; acute nonspecific diarrhea; increased volume of ileostomy discharge

OTC labeling: Control of symptoms of diarrhea, including Traveler's diarrhea

Unlabeled/Investigational Use Cancer treatment-induced diarrhea (eg, irinotecan induced); chronic diarrhea caused by bowel resection

Available Dosage Forms For available OTC formulations, consult specific product labeling.

Dosing

Adult & Geriatric

Acute diarrhea: Oral: Initial: 4 mg, followed by 2 mg after each loose stool, up to 16 mg/day

Chronic diarrhea: Oral: Initial: Follow acute diarrhea; maintenance dose should be slowly titrated downward to minimum required to control symptoms (typically, 4-8 mg/day in divided doses)

Traveler's diarrhea: Oral: Initial: 4 mg after first loose stool, followed by 2 mg after each subsequent stool (maximum dose: 8 mg/day)

Irinotecan-induced diarrhea (unlabeled use): Oral: 4 mg after first loose or frequent bowel movement, then 2 mg every 2 hours until 12 hours have passed without a bowel movement. If diarrhea recurs, then repeat administration

Pediatric

Acute diarrhea: Initial doses (in first 24 hours):

2-5 years (13-20 kg): 1 mg 3 times/day
6-8 years (20-30 kg): 2 mg twice daily
8-12 years (>30 kg): 2 mg 3 times/day
Maintenance: After initial dosing, 0.1 mg/kg doses after each loose stool, but not exceeding initial dosage

Traveler's diarrhea:

6-8 years: 2 mg after first loose stool, followed by 1 mg after each subsequent stool (maximum dose: 4 mg/day)
9-11 years: 2 mg after first loose stool, followed by 1 mg after each subsequent stool (maximum dose: 6 mg/day)
≥12 years: Refer to adult dosing.

Hepatic Impairment No specific guidelines available.

Monitoring and Teaching Issues

Physical Assessment Assess for cause of diarrhea before administering first dose.

Patient Education May cause drowsiness. If acute diarrhea lasts longer than 48 hours, consult prescriber. Do not take if diarrhea is bloody.

- **Loperamide Hydrochloride** *see* Loperamide *on page 1126*
- **Lopid®** *see* Gemfibrozil *on page 859*

Lopinavir and Ritonavir (loe PIN a veer & rit ON uh veer)

U.S. Brand Names Kaletra®
Index Terms Ritonavir and Lopinavir
Generic Availability (U.S.) No
Pharmacologic Category Antiretroviral Agent, Protease Inhibitor
Medication Safety Issues
Sound-alike/look-alike issues:
Potential for dispensing errors between Kaletra® and Keppra® (levETIRAcetam)

Administration issues:
Children's doses are based on weight and calculated by milligrams of lopinavir. Care should be taken to accurately calculate the dose. The oral solution contains lopinavir 80 mg and ritonavir 20 mg per one mL. Children <12 years of age (and ≤40 kg) who are not taking certain concomitant antiretroviral medications will receive <5 mL of solution per dose.
Medication Guide Available Yes
Pregnancy Risk Factor C
Lactation Excretion in breast milk unknown/contraindicated
Use Treatment of HIV infection in combination with other antiretroviral agents
Available Dosage Forms
Solution, oral:
Kaletra®: Lopinavir 80 mg and ritonavir 20 mg per mL
Tablet:
Kaletra®:
Lopinavir 100 mg and ritonavir 25 mg
Lopinavir 200 mg and ritonavir 50 mg
Dosing
Adult
HIV infection (as a component of combination therapy): Oral:
Twice-daily dosing:
Therapy-naive or therapy-experienced: Lopinavir 400 mg/ritonavir 100 mg twice daily. **Note:** This regimen is preferred (with zidovudine and lamivudine or zidovudine and emtricitabine) in pregnant therapy-naive patients (DHHS, 2011)
Therapy-naive or therapy-experienced patients receiving efavirenz, fosamprenavir, nelfinavir, nevirapine: Lopinavir 500 mg/ritonavir 125 mg twice daily **or** lopinavir 533 mg/ritonavir 133 mg solution twice daily
Once-daily dosing: Therapy-naive or experienced patients with <3 lopinavir resistance-associated substitutions: Lopinavir 800 mg/ritonavir 200 mg once daily

Dosage adjustment for combination therapy with efavirenz, fosamprenavir, nelfinavir, or nevirapine: Oral:
Twice-daily dosing: Therapy-naive and therapy-experienced patients:
Solution: Lopinavir 533 mg/ritonavir 133 mg (6.5 mL) twice daily
Tablet: Lopinavir 500 mg/ritonavir 125 mg twice daily
Once-daily dosing: Not recommended in those receiving efavirenz, fosamprenavir, nevirapine, nelfinavir, carbamazepine, phenobarbital, phenytoin.

Dosage adjustments for concomitant therapy: Adults:
Combination therapy with bosentan:
Coadministration of bosentan in patients currently receiving lopinavir/ritonavir: For patients receiving lopinavir/ritonavir for at least 10 days, begin with bosentan 62.5 mg once daily or every other day based on tolerability
Coadministration of lopinavir/ritonavir in patients currently receiving bosentan: Discontinue bosentan 36 hours prior to the initiation of lopinavir/ritonavir. After at least 10 days of lopinavir/ritonavir, resume bosentan 62.5 mg once daily or every other day based on tolerability
Combination therapy with colchicine:
Familial Mediterranean fever (FMF): Maximum colchicine dose: 0.6 mg/day (0.3 mg twice daily)
Gout prophylaxis:
If original colchicine dose is 0.6 mg twice daily, adjust dose to 0.3 mg once daily
If original colchicine dose is 0.6 mg once daily, adjust dose to 0.3 mg every other day
Gout flare treatment: Initial: Colchicine 0.6 mg, followed in 1 hour by a single dose of 0.3 mg; do not repeat for at least 3 days
Coadministration with phosphodiesterase-5 enzyme (PDE-5) inhibitor:
Pulmonary arterial hypertension: Lopinavir/ritonavir coadministered with tadalafil:
Patient receiving lopinavir/ritonavir for at least 1 week: Initiate tadalafil at 20 mg once daily; increase to 40 mg once daily based on individual tolerability
Patient receiving tadalafil when initiating lopinavir/ritonavir: Stop tadalafil at least 24 hours prior to starting lopinavir/ritonavir. After at least 1 week following the initiation of lopinavir/ritonavir, resume tadalafil at 20 mg once daily; increase to 40 mg once daily based on individual tolerability.
Erectile dysfunction: Lopinavir/ritonavir coadministered with:
Sildenafil (Viagra®): Maximum sildenafil dose: 25 mg in a 48-hour period
Tadalafil (Cialis®): Maximum tadalafil dose: 10 mg in a 72-hour period
Vardenafil: Maximum vardenafil dose: 2.5 mg in a 72-hour period
Geriatric Initial studies did not include enough elderly patients to determine effects based on age. Use with caution due to possible decreased hepatic, renal, and cardiac function.

Pediatric

HIV infection (component of combination therapy): Oral: Dosage based on weight or body surface area (BSA), **presented based on lopinavir component** (maximum dose: Lopinavir 400 mg/ritonavir 100 mg).

14 days to 6 months: 16 mg/kg or 300 mg/m^2 twice daily; **Note:** Should not be administered to neonates age <14 days (defined as postmenstrual age of 42 weeks [first day of mother's last menstrual period to birth plus postnatal age]) and a postnatal age of at least 14 days

6 months to 18 years: **Note:** FDA-approved dose is approximately equivalent to lopinavir 230 mg/m^2 per dose.

<15 kg: 12 mg/kg twice daily

15-40 kg: 10 mg/kg twice daily

>40 kg: Lopinavir 400 mg/ritonavir 100 mg twice daily

Dosage adjustment for combination therapy with efavirenz, fosamprenavir, nelfinavir, or nevirapine: Oral:

Twice-daily dosing:

Children 14 days to 6 months: Combination therapy with these agents is not recommended due to lack of data.

Children 6 months to 18 years: Solution or tablet (**based on mg of lopinavir component**): FDA-approved dose is approximately equivalent to lopinavir 300 mg/m^2 per dose:

<15 kg: 13 mg/kg twice daily (**Note:** Tablets are not recommended)

15-45 kg: 11 mg/kg twice daily

>45 kg: Refer to adult dosing.

Once-daily dosing: Not recommended in children.

Renal Impairment Has not been studied in patients with renal impairment; however, a decrease in clearance is not expected.

Hemodialysis: Do not use once-daily dosing in hemodialysis patients (DHHS, 2011)

Hepatic Impairment Use caution in hepatic impairment (metabolized primarily by the liver).

Mild-to-moderate impairment: Lopinavir AUC may be increased ~30%

Severe impairment: No data available

Administration

Oral

Solution: Administer with food; if using didanosine, take didanosine 1 hour before or 2 hours after lopinavir/ritonavir. Administer using calibrated dosing syringe.

Tablet: May be taken with or without food. Swallow whole, do not break, crush, or chew. May be taken with didanosine when taken without food. Tablets are not recommended in patients <15 kg.

Monitoring and Teaching Issues

Physical Assessment See individual agents.

Patient Education See individual agents.

Related Information

Ritonavir *on page* 1593

◆ **Lopressor®** *see* Metoprolol *on page* 1217

◆ **Loradamed [OTC]** *see* Loratadine *on page* 1128

Loratadine (lor AT a deen)

U.S. Brand Names Alavert® Allergy 24 Hour [OTC]; Alavert® Children's Allergy [OTC]; Claritin® 24 Hour Allergy [OTC]; Claritin® Children's Allergy [OTC]; Claritin® Liqui-Gels® 24 Hour Allergy [OTC]; Claritin® RediTabs® 24 Hour Allergy [OTC]; Loradamed [OTC]; Tavist® ND Allergy [OTC]

Generic Availability (U.S.) Yes

Pharmacologic Category Histamine H_1 Antagonist; Histamine H_1 Antagonist, Second Generation; Piperidine Derivative

Medication Safety Issues

Sound-alike/look-alike issues:

Claritin® may be confused with clarithromycin

Claritin® (loratadine) may be confused with Claritin™ Eye (ketotifen)

Use Relief of nasal and non-nasal symptoms of seasonal allergic rhinitis; treatment of chronic idiopathic urticaria

Mechanism of Action/Effect Long-acting tricyclic antihistamine with selective peripheral histamine H_1 receptor antagonistic properties; management of idiopathic chronic urticaria

Contraindications Hypersensitivity to loratadine or any component of the formulation

Warnings/Precautions Use with caution in patients with liver or renal impairment; dosage adjustment recommended. Some products may contain phenylalanine.

Drug Interactions

Metabolism/Transport Effects Substrate of CYP2D6 (minor), CYP3A4 (minor), P-glycoprotein; **Inhibits** CYP2C8 (weak), 2C19 (moderate), 2D6 (weak)

Avoid Concomitant Use There are no known interactions where it is recommended to avoid concomitant use.

Decreased Effect

Loratadine may decrease the levels/effects of: Acetylcholinesterase Inhibitors (Central); Benzylpenicilloyl Polylysine; Betahistine

The levels/effects of Loratadine may be decreased by: Acetylcholinesterase Inhibitors (Central); Amphetamines; Peginterferon Alfa-2b; P-Glycoprotein Inducers

Increased Effect/Toxicity

Loratadine may increase the levels/effects of: Alcohol (Ethyl); Anticholinergics; CNS Depressants

The levels/effects of Loratadine may be increased by: Amiodarone; Conivaptan; Droperidol; P-Glycoprotein Inhibitors; Pramlintide

Nutritional/Ethanol Interactions

Ethanol: Avoid ethanol (although sedation is limited with loratadine, may increase risk of CNS depression).

Food: Increases bioavailability and delays peak.

Herb/Nutraceutical: St John's wort may decrease loratadine levels.

Adverse Reactions

Adults:

Central nervous system: Headache (12%), somnolence (8%), fatigue (4%)

Gastrointestinal: Xerostomia (3%)

Children:

Central nervous system: Nervousness (4% ages 6-12 years), fatigue (3% ages 6-12 years, 2% to 3% ages 2-5 years), malaise (2% ages 6-12 years)

Dermatologic: Rash (2% to 3% ages 2-5 years)

Gastrointestinal: Abdominal pain (2% ages 6-12 years), stomatitis (2% to 3% ages 2-5 years)

Neuromuscular & skeletal: Hyperkinesia (3% ages 6-12 years)

Ocular: Conjunctivitis (2% ages 6-12 years)

Respiratory: Wheezing (4% ages 6-12 years), dysphonia (2% ages 6-12 years), upper respiratory infection (2% ages 6-12 years), epistaxis (2% to 3% ages 2-5 years), pharyngitis (2% to 3% ages 2-5 years)

Miscellaneous: Flu-like syndrome (2% to 3% ages 2-5 years), viral infection (2% to 3% ages 2-5 years)

Pharmacodynamics/Kinetics

Onset of Action 1-3 hours; Peak effect: 8-12 hours

Duration of Action >24 hours

Absorption Rapid

Half-Life Elimination 12-15 hours

Metabolism Extensively hepatic via CYP2D6 and 3A4 to active metabolite

Excretion Urine (40%) and feces (40%) as metabolites

Available Dosage Forms For available OTC formulations, consult specific product labeling.

Dosing

Adult & Geriatric Seasonal allergic rhinitis, chronic idiopathic urticaria: Oral: 10 mg/day

Pediatric

Children 2-5 years: Seasonal allergic rhinitis, chronic idiopathic urticaria: Oral: 5 mg once daily

Children ≥6 years: Refer to adult dosing.

Renal Impairment Cl_{cr} ≤30 mL/minute:

Children 2-5 years: 5 mg every other day.

Children ≥6 years and Adults: 10 mg every other day.

Hepatic Impairment Elimination half-life increases with severity of disease.

Children 2-5 years: 5 mg every other day.

Children ≥6 years and Adults: 10 mg every other day.

Administration

Oral Administer on an empty stomach.

Stability

Storage Store at 2°C to 25°C (36°F to 77°F).

Rapidly-disintegrating tablets: Use within 6 months of opening foil pouch, and immediately after opening individual tablet blister. Store in a dry place.

Monitoring and Teaching Issues

Patient Education Avoid use of alcohol. You may experience drowsiness, dizziness, dry mouth, or nausea. Report persistent dizziness or sedation; swelling of face, mouth, lips, or tongue; respiratory difficulty; lack of improvement; or worsening of condition.

Rapidly-disintegrating tablets: Place tablet on tongue; it dissolves rapidly. May be used with or without water. Use within 6 months of opening foil pouch and immediately after opening individual tablet blister.

Dietary Considerations Take on an empty stomach. Some products may contain phenylalanine and/or sodium.

Geriatric Considerations Loratadine is a nonsedating antihistamines; because of its low incidence of side effects, it seems to be a good choice in the elderly. However, there is a wide variation in loratadine half-life reported in the elderly and this should be kept in mind when initiating dosing. Because of its new OTC status, patients should be advised of appropriate use.

Loratadine and Pseudoephedrine (lor AT a deen & soo doe e FED rin)

U.S. Brand Names Alavert™ Allergy and Sinus [OTC]; Claritin-D® 12 Hour Allergy & Congestion [OTC]; Claritin-D® 24 Hour Allergy & Congestion [OTC]

Index Terms Pseudoephedrine and Loratadine

Generic Availability (U.S.) Yes

Pharmacologic Category Alpha/Beta Agonist; Decongestant; Histamine H_1 Antagonist; Histamine H_1 Antagonist, Second Generation; Piperidine Derivative

Medication Safety Issues

Sound-alike/look-alike issues:

Claritin-D® may be confused with Claritin-D® 24

Claritin-D® 24 may be confused with Claritin-D®

Use Temporary relief of symptoms of seasonal allergic rhinitis, other upper respiratory allergies, or the common cold

Available Dosage Forms For available OTC formulations, consult specific product labeling.

Dosing

Adult & Geriatric Seasonal allergic rhinitis/nasal congestion:

Oral: 1 tablet every 12 hours

Extended release: 1 tablet daily

Pediatric Seasonal allergic rhinitis/nasal congestion: Children ≥12 years: Refer to adult dosing.

Renal Impairment Cl_{cr} <30 mL/minute:

Claritin-D® 12-Hour: 1 tablet daily

Claritin-D® 24-Hour: 1 tablet every other day

Hepatic Impairment Should be avoided.

Monitoring and Teaching Issues

Physical Assessment See individual agents.

Patient Education See individual agents.

Related Information

Loratadine *on page 1128*

Pseudoephedrine *on page 1529*

LORazepam (lor A ze pam)

U.S. Brand Names Ativan®; Lorazepam Intensol™

Generic Availability (U.S.) Yes

Pharmacologic Category Benzodiazepine

Medication Safety Issues

Sound-alike/look-alike issues:

LORazepam may be confused with ALPRAZolam, clonazePAM, diazepam, KlonoPIN®, Lovaza®, temazepam, zolpidem

Ativan® may be confused with Ambien®, Atarax®, Atgam®, Avitene®

Injection dosage form contains propylene glycol. Monitor for toxicity when administering continuous lorazepam infusions.

Beers Criteria medication: This drug may be inappropriate for use in geriatric patients (high severity risk).

Pregnancy Risk Factor D

Lactation Enters breast milk/not recommended (AAP rates "of concern"; AAP 2001 update pending)

Use

Oral: Management of anxiety disorders or short-term (≤4 months) relief of the symptoms of anxiety or anxiety associated with depressive symptoms

I.V.: Status epilepticus, amnesia, sedation

Unlabeled/Investigational Use Ethanol detoxification; insomnia; psychogenic catatonia; partial complex seizures; agitation (I.V.); antiemetic adjunct

Mechanism of Action/Effect Binds to stereospecific benzodiazepine receptors on the postsynaptic GABA neuron at several sites within the central nervous system, including the limbic system, reticular formation. Enhancement of the inhibitory effect of GABA on neuronal excitability results by increased neuronal membrane permeability to chloride ions. This shift in chloride ions results in hyperpolarization (a less excitable state) and stabilization.

Contraindications Hypersensitivity to lorazepam or any component of the formulation (cross-sensitivity with other benzodiazepines may exist); acute narrow-angle glaucoma; sleep apnea (parenteral); intra-arterial injection of parenteral formulation; severe respiratory insufficiency (except during mechanical ventilation)

Warnings/Precautions Use with caution in elderly or debilitated patients, patients with hepatic disease (including alcoholics) or renal impairment. Due to increased sensitivity in the elderly, smaller doses of benzodiazepines may be safer and as effective; in this age group, avoid using doses >3 mg daily of lorazepam (Beers Criteria). Use with caution in patients with respiratory disease (COPD or sleep apnea) or limited pulmonary reserve, or impaired gag reflex. Initial doses in elderly or debilitated patients should be at the lower end of the dosing range. May worsen hepatic encephalopathy.

Causes CNS depression (dose-related) resulting in sedation, dizziness, confusion, or ataxia which may impair physical and mental capabilities. Patients must be cautioned about performing tasks which require mental alertness (eg, operating machinery or driving). Use with caution in patients receiving other CNS depressants or psychoactive agents. Effects with other sedative drugs or ethanol may be potentiated. Benzodiazepines have been associated with falls and traumatic injury and should be used with extreme caution in patients who are at risk of these events (especially the elderly).

Lorazepam may cause anterograde amnesia. Paradoxical reactions, including hyperactive or aggressive behavior have been reported with benzodiazepines, particularly in adolescent/pediatric or psychiatric patients. Does not have analgesic, antidepressant, or antipsychotic properties.

Use caution in patients with depression, particularly if suicidal risk may be present. Pre-existing depression may worsen or emerge during therapy. Not recommended for use in primary depressive or psychotic disorders. Use with caution in patients with a history of drug dependence, alcoholism, or significant personality disorders. Benzodiazepines have been associated with dependence and acute withdrawal symptoms on discontinuation or reduction in dose. Acute withdrawal, including seizures, may be precipitated after administration of flumazenil to patients receiving long-term benzodiazepine therapy.

As a hypnotic agent, should be used only after evaluation of potential causes of sleep disturbance. Failure of sleep disturbance to resolve after 7-10 days may indicate psychiatric or medical illness. A worsening of insomnia or the emergence of new abnormalities of thought or behavior may represent unrecognized psychiatric or medical illness and requires immediate and careful evaluation.

Parenteral formulation of lorazepam contains polyethylene glycol which has resulted in toxicity during high-dose and/or longer-term infusions. Parenteral formulation also contains propylene glycol (PG); may be associated with dose-related toxicity and can occur ≥48 hours after initiation of lorazepam. Limited data suggest increased risk of PG accumulation at doses of ≥6 mg/hour for 48 hours or more (Nelson, 2008). Consider monitoring for signs of toxicity which may include acute renal failure, lactic acidosis, and/or osmol gap. In high-risk patients requiring higher doses/extended treatment durations, use of enteral delivery of lorazepam tablets may be beneficial (Jacobi, 2002). Also contains benzyl alcohol; avoid in neonates.

Drug Interactions

Avoid Concomitant Use

Avoid concomitant use of LORazepam with any of the following: OLANZapine

Decreased Effect

The levels/effects of LORazepam may be decreased by: Theophylline Derivatives; Yohimbine

Increased Effect/Toxicity

LORazepam may increase the levels/effects of: Alcohol (Ethyl); CloZAPine; CNS Depressants; Methotrimeprazine; Phenytoin

The levels/effects of LORazepam may be increased by: Divalproex; Droperidol; Loxapine; Methotrimeprazine; OLANZapine; Probenecid; Valproic Acid

Nutritional/Ethanol Interactions

Ethanol: Avoid or limit ethanol (may increase CNS depression).

Herb/Nutraceutical: Avoid valerian, St John's wort, kava kava, gotu kola (may increase CNS depression).

Lab Interactions May result in elevated liver function tests

Adverse Reactions

>10%:

Central nervous system: Sedation

Respiratory: Respiratory depression

1% to 10%:

Cardiovascular: Hypotension

Central nervous system: Akathisia, amnesia, ataxia, confusion, depression, disorientation, dizziness, headache

Dermatologic: Dermatitis, rash

Gastrointestinal: Changes in appetite, nausea, weight gain/loss

Neuromuscular & skeletal: Weakness

Ocular: Visual disturbances

Respiratory: Apnea, hyperventilation, nasal congestion

Pharmacodynamics/Kinetics

Onset of Action Hypnosis: I.M.: 20-30 minutes; Sedation: I.V.: 5-20 minutes; Anticonvulsant: I.V.: 5 minutes, oral: 30-60 minutes

Duration of Action 6-8 hours

Absorption Oral, I.M.: Prompt

Bioavailability Oral: 90%

Time to Peak Oral: 2 hours

Protein Binding 85%; free fraction may be significantly higher in elderly

Half-Life Elimination Neonates: 40.2 hours; Older children: 10.5 hours; Adults: 12.9 hours; Elderly: 15.9 hours; End-stage renal disease: 32-70 hours

Metabolism Hepatic to inactive compounds

Excretion Urine; feces (minimal)

Controlled Substance C-IV

Available Dosage Forms

Injection, solution: 2 mg/mL (1 mL, 10 mL); 4 mg/mL (1 mL, 10 mL)

Ativan®: 2 mg/mL (1 mL, 10 mL); 4 mg/mL (1 mL, 10 mL)

Injection, solution [preservative free]: 2 mg/mL (1 mL); 4 mg/mL (1 mL)

Solution, oral: 2 mg/mL (30 mL)

Lorazepam Intensol™: 2 mg/mL (30 mL)

Tablet, oral: 0.5 mg, 1 mg, 2 mg

Ativan®: 0.5 mg, 1 mg, 2 mg

Dosing

Adult

Antiemetic: Oral, I.V. (**Note:** May be administered sublingually; not a labeled route): 0.5-2 mg every 4-6 hours as needed

Anxiety and sedation: Oral: 1-10 mg/day in 2-3 divided doses; usual dose: 2-6 mg/day in divided doses; initial dose should not exceed 2 mg in debilitated patients

Insomnia: Oral: 2-4 mg at bedtime

Preoperative:

I.M.: 0.05 mg/kg administered 2 hours before surgery; maximum: 4 mg/dose

I.V.: 0.044 mg/kg 15-20 minutes before surgery; usual maximum: 2 mg/dose

Operative amnesia: I.V.: Up to 0.05 mg/kg; maximum: 4 mg/dose

Status epilepticus: I.V.: 4 mg/dose slow I.V. (maximum rate: 2 mg/minute); may repeat in 10-15 minutes; usual maximum dose: 8 mg

Rapid tranquilization of agitated patient (administer every 30-60 minutes):

Oral: 1-2 mg

I.M.: 0.5-1 mg

Average total dose for tranquilization: 4-8 mg

Agitation in the ICU patient (unlabeled):

I.V.: 0.02-0.06 mg/kg every 2-6 hours

I.V. infusion: 0.01-0.1 mg/kg/hour

Concurrent use of probenecid or valproic acid: Reduce lorazepam dose by 50%

Geriatric Anxiety and sedation: Oral, I.V.: 0.5-4 mg/day; refer to adult dosing for other indications. Dose selection should generally be on the low end of the dosage range (ie, initial dose not to exceed 2 mg)

Beers Criteria: Avoid doses >3 mg/day

Pediatric

Antiemetic: Children 2-15 years (unlabeled): I.V.: 0.05 mg/kg (up to 2 mg/dose) prior to chemotherapy

Anxiety and sedation: Infants and Children (unlabeled except for oral use in children >12 years): Oral, I.V.: Usual: 0.05 mg/kg/dose (range: 0.02-0.09 mg/kg) every 4-8 hours

Sedation (preprocedure): Infants and Children (unlabeled):

Oral, I.M., I.V.: Usual: 0.05 mg/kg; range: 0.02-0.09 mg/kg

I.V.: May use smaller doses (eg, 0.01-0.03 mg/kg) and repeat every 20 minutes, as needed to titrate to effect

Status epilepticus: I.V.:

Infants and Children (unlabeled): 0.05-0.1 mg/kg (maximum: 4 mg/dose) slow I.V. (maximum rate: 2 mg/minute); may repeat every 10-15 minutes as needed (Hegenbarth, 2008; Sabo-Graham, 1998)

Adolescents: Refer to adult dosing.

Renal Impairment I.V.: Risk of propylene glycol toxicity. Monitor closely if using for prolonged periods or at high doses.

Hepatic Impairment Use cautiously.

Administration

I.M. Should be administered deep into the muscle mass.

I.V. Continuous infusion solutions should have an in-line filter and the solution should be checked frequently for possible precipitation. Avoid intra-arterial administration. Monitor I.V. site for extravasation.

Stability

Reconstitution

Injection: Dilute with equal volume of compatible diluent (D_5W, NS, SWFI).

Infusion: Use 2 mg/mL injectable vial to prepare; there may be decreased stability when using 4 mg/mL vial. Dilute ≤1 mg/mL and mix in glass bottle. Precipitation may develop. Can also be administered undiluted via infusion.

Storage

I.V.: Intact vials should be refrigerated. Protect from light. Do not use discolored or precipitate-containing solutions. May be stored at room temperature for up to 3 months [data on file (Hospira Inc, 2010)]. Parenteral admixture is stable at room temperature (25°C) for 24 hours.

Tablet: Store at room temperature.

Monitoring and Teaching Issues

Physical Assessment Oral: Assess for history of addiction; long-term use can result in dependence, abuse, or tolerance; periodically evaluate need for continued use. For inpatient use, institute safety measures to prevent falls. Taper dosage slowly when discontinuing. **I.V./I.M.:** Monitor vital signs, CNS status, and ability to void.

Patient Education Oral: Drug may cause physical and/or psychological dependence. Do not use alcohol. You may experience drowsiness, lightheadedness, impaired coordination, dizziness, blurred vision, nausea, vomiting, dry mouth, constipation, altered sexual drive or ability (reversible), or photosensitivity. Report persistent CNS effects (eg, confusion, depression, increased sedation, excitation, headache, agitation, insomnia or nightmares, dizziness, fatigue, impaired coordination, changes in personality, or changes in cognition); changes in urinary pattern; chest pain, palpitations, or rapid heartbeat; muscle cramping, weakness, tremors, or rigidity; ringing in ears or visual disturbances; excessive perspiration; excessive GI symptoms (cramping, constipation, vomiting, anorexia); or worsening of condition.

Geriatric Considerations Because lorazepam is relatively short-acting with an inactive metabolite, it is a preferred agent to use in elderly patients when a benzodiazepine is indicated.

This medication is considered to be potentially inappropriate in this patient population (Beers Criteria severity: High).

Breast-Feeding Considerations Drowsiness, lethargy, or weight loss in nursing infants have been observed in case reports following maternal use of some benzodiazepines.

Pregnancy Considerations Teratogenic effects have been observed in some animal studies. Lorazepam and its metabolite cross the human placenta. Teratogenic effects in humans have been observed with some benzodiazepines (including lorazepam); however, additional studies are needed. The incidence of premature birth and low birth weights may be increased following maternal use of benzodiazepines; hypoglycemia and respiratory problems in the neonate may occur following exposure late in pregnancy. Neonatal withdrawal symptoms may occur within days to weeks after birth and "floppy infant syndrome" (which also includes withdrawal symptoms) have been reported with some benzodiazepines (including lorazepam). Elimination of lorazepam in the newborn infant is slow; following *in utero* exposure, term infants may excrete lorazepam for up to 8 days.

Other Issues Taper dosage gradually after long-term therapy, especially in epileptic patients. Abrupt withdrawal may cause tremors, nausea, vomiting, abdominal and/or muscle cramps.

Additional Information Oral doses >0.09 mg/kg produced increased ataxia without increased sedative benefit vs lower doses; preferred anxiolytic when I.M. route needed. Abrupt discontinuation after sustained use (generally >10 days) may cause withdrawal symptoms.

Related Information

Benzodiazepines *on page 1988*

Compatibility of Drugs *on page 1994*

◆ **Lorazepam Intensol™** *see* LORazepam *on page 1130*

◆ **Lorcet® 10/650** *see* Hydrocodone and Acetaminophen *on page 915*

◆ **Lorcet® Plus** *see* Hydrocodone and Acetaminophen *on page 915*

◆ **Lortab®** *see* Hydrocodone and Acetaminophen *on page 915*

Losartan (loe SAR tan)

U.S. Brand Names Cozaar®

Index Terms DuP 753; Losartan Potassium; MK594

Generic Availability (U.S.) Yes

Pharmacologic Category Angiotensin II Receptor Blocker

Medication Safety Issues

Sound-alike/look-alike issues:

Cozaar® may be confused with Colace®, Coreg®, Hyzaar®, Zocor®

Losartan may be confused with valsartan

Pregnancy Risk Factor C (1st trimester); D (2nd and 3rd trimesters)

Lactation Excretion in breast milk unknown/not recommended

Use Treatment of hypertension (HTN); treatment of diabetic nephropathy in patients with type 2 diabetes mellitus (noninsulin dependent, NIDDM) and a history of hypertension; stroke risk reduction in patients with HTN and left ventricular hypertrophy (LVH)

Unlabeled/Investigational Use To slow the rate of progression of aortic-root dilation in pediatric patients with Marfan's syndrome

Mechanism of Action/Effect As a selective and competitive, nonpeptide angiotensin II receptor antagonist, losartan blocks the vasoconstrictor and aldosterone-secreting effects of angiotensin II. Losartan increases urinary flow rate and in addition to being natriuretic and kaliuretic, increases excretion of chloride, magnesium, uric acid, calcium, and phosphate.

Contraindications Hypersensitivity to losartan or any component of the formulation

Warnings/Precautions [U.S. Boxed Warning]: Based on human data, drugs that act on the angiotensin system can cause injury and death to the developing fetus when used in the second and third trimesters. Angiotensin receptor blockers should be discontinued as soon as possible once pregnancy is detected. Avoid use or use a much smaller dose in patients who are volume-depleted; correct depletion first. Use with caution in patients with significant aortic/mitral stenosis. May cause hyperkalemia; avoid potassium supplementation unless specifically required by healthcare provider. May be associated with deterioration of renal function and/or increases in serum creatinine, particularly in patients with low renal blood flow (eg, renal artery stenosis, heart failure) whose glomerular filtration rate (GFR) is dependent on efferent arteriolar vasoconstriction by angiotensin II. Use caution in patients with unstented unilateral/bilateral renal artery stenosis. When unstented bilateral renal artery stenosis is present, use is generally avoided due to the elevated risk of deterioration in renal function unless possible benefits outweigh risks. Use with caution with pre-existing renal insufficiency. AUCs of losartan (not the active metabolite) are about 50% greater in patients with Cl_{cr} <30 mL/minute and are doubled in hemodialysis patients. Concurrent use of ACE inhibitors may increase the risk of clinically-significant adverse events (eg, renal dysfunction, hyperkalemia).

At any time during treatment (especially following first dose), angioedema may occur rarely; may involve the head and neck (potentially compromising airway) or the intestine (presenting with abdominal pain). Patients with idiopathic or hereditary angioedema or previous angioedema associated with ACE-inhibitor therapy may be at an increased risk. Prolonged frequent monitoring may be required, especially if tongue, glottis, or larynx are involved, as they are associated with airway obstruction. Patients with a history of airway surgery may have a higher risk of airway obstruction. Aggressive early management is critical; intramuscular (I.M.) administration of epinephrine may be necessary.

When used to reduce the risk of stroke in patients with HTN and LVH, may not be effective in African-American population. Use caution with hepatic dysfunction, dose adjustment may be needed.

Drug Interactions

Metabolism/Transport Effects Substrate (major) of CYP2C9, 3A4; **Inhibits** CYP1A2 (weak), 2C8 (moderate), 2C9 (moderate), 2C19 (weak), 3A4 (weak)

Avoid Concomitant Use There are no known interactions where it is recommended to avoid concomitant use.

Decreased Effect

The levels/effects of Losartan may be decreased by: CYP2C9 Inducers (Highly Effective); CYP3A4 Inducers (Strong); Deferasirox; Herbs (CYP3A4 Inducers); Herbs (Hypertensive Properties); Methylphenidate; Nonsteroidal Anti-Inflammatory Agents; Peginterferon Alfa-2b; Rifamycin Derivatives; Yohimbine

Increased Effect/Toxicity

Losartan may increase the levels/effects of: ACE Inhibitors; Amifostine; Antihypertensives; Carvedilol; CYP2C8 Substrates (High risk); CYP2C9 Substrates (High risk); Hypoglycemic Agents; Hypotensive Agents; Lithium; Potassium-Sparing Diuretics; RiTUXimab

The levels/effects of Losartan may be increased by: Antifungal Agents (Azole Derivatives, Systemic); Conivaptan; CYP2C9 Inhibitors (Moderate); CYP2C9 Inhibitors (Strong); Diazoxide; Eplerenone; Fluconazole; Herbs (Hypoglycemic Properties); Herbs (Hypotensive Properties); MAO Inhibitors; Milk Thistle; Pentoxifylline; Phosphodiesterase 5 Inhibitors; Potassium Salts; Prostacyclin Analogues; Tolvaptan; Trimethoprim

Nutritional/Ethanol Interactions Herb/Nutraceutical: St John's wort may decrease levels of losartan. Avoid bayberry, blue cohosh, ginseng (American), kola, licorice (may worsen hypertension). Avoid black cohosh; california poppy; coleus; golden seal; hawthorn; mistletoe; periwinkle; quinine; shepherd's purse (may increase risk for hypotension). Hypoglycemic effects of losartan may be enhanced by alfalfa; aloe; bilberry; bitter melon; burdock; celery; damiana; fenugreek; garcinia; garlic; ginger; ginseng (American); gymnema; marshmallow; stinging nettle.

Adverse Reactions Note: The incidence of some adverse reactions varied based on the underlying disease state. Notations are made, where applicable, for data derived from trials conducted in diabetic nephropathy and hypertensive patients, respectively.

>10%:

- Cardiovascular: Chest pain (12% diabetic nephropathy)
- Central nervous system: Fatigue (14% diabetic nephropathy)
- Endocrine: Hypoglycemia (14% diabetic nephropathy)
- Gastrointestinal: Diarrhea (2% hypertension to 15% diabetic nephropathy)
- Genitourinary: Urinary tract infection (13% diabetic nephropathy)
- Hematologic: Anemia (14% diabetic nephropathy)
- Neuromuscular & skeletal: Weakness (14% diabetic nephropathy), back pain (2% hypertension to 12% diabetic nephropathy)
- Respiratory: Cough (≤3% to 11%; similar to placebo; incidence higher in patients with previous cough related to ACE inhibitor therapy)

1% to 10%:

- Cardiovascular: Hypotension (7% diabetic nephropathy), orthostatic hypotension (4% hypertension to 4% diabetic nephropathy), first-dose hypotension (dose related: <1% with 50 mg, 2% with 100 mg)
- Central nervous system: Dizziness (4%), hypoesthesia (5% diabetic nephropathy), fever (4% diabetic nephropathy), insomnia (1%)
- Dermatology: Cellulitis (7% diabetic nephropathy)
- Endocrine: Hyperkalemia (<1% hypertension to 7% diabetic nephropathy)
- Gastrointestinal: Gastritis (5% diabetic nephropathy), weight gain (4% diabetic nephropathy), dyspepsia (1% to 4%), abdominal pain (2%), nausea (2%)
- Neuromuscular & skeletal: Muscular weakness (7% diabetic nephropathy), knee pain (5% diabetic nephropathy), leg pain (1% to 5%), muscle cramps (1%), myalgia (1%)
- Respiratory: Bronchitis (10% diabetic nephropathy), upper respiratory infection (8%), nasal congestion (2%), sinusitis (1% hypertension to 6% diabetic nephropathy)
- Miscellaneous: Infection (5% diabetic nephropathy), flu-like syndrome (10% diabetic nephropathy)

Pharmacodynamics/Kinetics

Onset of Action 6 hours

Bioavailability 25% to 33%; AUC of E-3174 is four times greater than that of losartan

Time to Peak Serum: Losartan: 1 hour; E-3174: 3-4 hours

Protein Binding Plasma: High

Half-Life Elimination Losartan: 1.5-2 hours; E-3174: 6-9 hours

Metabolism Hepatic (14%) via CYP2C9 and 3A4 to an active metabolite E-3174 (40 times more potent than losartan); extensive first-pass effect

Excretion Excretion: Urine (4% as unchanged drug, 6% as active metabolite)

Clearance: Plasma: Losartan: 600 mL/minute; Active metabolite: 50 mL/minute

Available Dosage Forms

Tablet, oral: 25 mg, 50 mg, 100 mg

Cozaar®: 25 mg, 50 mg, 100 mg

Dosing

Adult & Geriatric

Hypertension: Oral: Usual starting dose: 50 mg once daily; can be administered once or twice daily with total daily doses ranging from 25-100 mg

Usual initial doses in patients receiving diuretics or those with intravascular volume depletion: 25 mg once daily

Nephropathy in patients with type 2 diabetes and hypertension: Oral: Initial: 50 mg once daily; can be increased to 100 mg once daily based on blood pressure response

Stroke reduction (HTN with LVH): Oral: 50 mg once daily (maximum daily dose: 100 mg); may be used in combination with a thiazide diuretic

Pediatric Hypertension: Oral: Children 6-16 years:

U.S. labeling: 0.7 mg/kg once daily (maximum: 50 mg/day); doses >1.4 mg/kg (maximum: 100 mg) have not been studied

Canadian labeling:

≥20 kg to <50 kg: 25 mg once daily (maximum: 50 mg once daily)

≥50 kg: 50 mg once daily (maximum: 100 mg once daily)

Aortic-root dilation with Marfan's syndrome (unlabeled use): Children 14 months to 16 years: Initial: 0.6 mg/kg/day; can be increased to a maximum of 1.4 mg/kg/day (not to exceed adult maximum of 100 mg/day)

Renal Impairment

Children: Use is not recommended if GFR <30 mL/minute/1.73 m^2

Adults: No adjustment necessary.

Hepatic Impairment

Children 6-16 years:

U.S. labeling: No specific dosing recommendations are provided in the approved labeling, however it may be advisable to initiate therapy at a reduced dosage.

Canadian labeling: Use is not recommended.

Adults: Reduce the initial dose to 25 mg/day

Administration

Oral May be administered without regard to meals.

Stability

Storage Store at 15°C to 30°C (59°F to 86°F). Protect from light.

Monitoring and Teaching Issues

Laboratory Monitoring Electrolytes, serum creatinine, BUN, urinalysis, CBC

Physical Assessment Use caution in presence of impaired renal function, significant aortic/mitral stenosis, or history of angioedema and airway surgery. Monitor for hypotension on a regular basis during therapy. Caution patients with diabetes to monitor glucose levels closely; may alter glucose control.

Patient Education Preferable to take at same time each day without regard to meals. This drug does not eliminate need for diet or exercise regimen as recommended by prescriber. Do not use potassium supplement or salt substitutes without consulting prescriber. If you have diabetes, you may be cautioned to monitor glucose levels closely; may alter glucose control. May cause dizziness, fainting, lightheadedness, postural hypotension, or diarrhea. Report immediately swelling of face, lips, or mouth; difficulty swallowing; chest pain or palpitations; unrelenting headache; or CNS changes (delusions or depression).

Dietary Considerations May be taken without regard to meals. Some products may contain potassium.

Geriatric Considerations Serum concentrations of losartan and its metabolites are not significantly different and no initial dose adjustment is necessary even in low creatinine clearance states (<30 mL/minute). Many elderly may be volume depleted due to diuretic use and/or blunted thirst reflex resulting in inadequate fluid intake.

Breast-Feeding Considerations It is not known if losartan is found in breast milk; the manufacturer recommends discontinuing the drug or discontinuing nursing based on the importance of the drug to the mother.

Pregnancy Considerations Medications which act on the renin-angiotensin system are reported to have the following fetal/neonatal effects: Hypotension, neonatal skull hypoplasia, anuria, renal failure, and death; oligohydramnios is also reported. These effects are reported to occur with exposure during the second and third trimesters. There are no adequate and well-controlled studies in pregnant women. **[U.S. Boxed Warning]: Based on human data, drugs that act on the angiotensin system can cause injury and death to the developing fetus when used in the second and third trimesters. Angiotensin receptor blockers should be discontinued as soon as possible once pregnancy is detected.**

Related Information

Angiotensin Agents *on page 1974*

Heart Failure (Systolic) *on page 2040*

Losartan and Hydrochlorothiazide (loe SAR tan & hye droe klor oh THYE a zide)

U.S. Brand Names Hyzaar®

Index Terms Hydrochlorothiazide and Losartan

Generic Availability (U.S.) Yes

Pharmacologic Category Angiotensin II Receptor Blocker; Diuretic, Thiazide

Medication Safety Issues

Sound-alike/look-alike issues:

Hyzaar® may be confused with Cozaar®

Pregnancy Risk Factor C/D (2nd and 3rd trimesters)

Lactation Enters breast milk/contraindicated

Use Treatment of hypertension; stroke risk reduction in patients with HTN and left ventricular hypertrophy (LVH)

Contraindications Hypersensitivity to losartan, hydrochlorothiazide, or any component of the formulation; sulfonamide-derived drugs; anuria

Warnings/Precautions See individual agents.

Drug Interactions

Metabolism/Transport Effects Losartan: **Substrate** (major) of CYP2C9, 3A4; **Inhibits** CYP1A2 (weak), 2C8 (moderate), 2C9 (moderate), 2C19 (weak), 3A4 (weak)

Avoid Concomitant Use

Avoid concomitant use of Losartan and Hydrochlorothiazide with any of the following: Dofetilide

Decreased Effect

Losartan and Hydrochlorothiazide may decrease the levels/effects of: Antidiabetic Agents

The levels/effects of Losartan and Hydrochlorothiazide may be decreased by: Bile Acid Sequestrants; CYP2C9 Inducers (Highly Effective); CYP3A4 Inducers (Strong); Deferasirox; Herbs (CYP3A4 Inducers); Herbs (Hypertensive Properties); Methylphenidate; Nonsteroidal Anti-Inflammatory Agents; Peginterferon Alfa-2b; Rifamycin Derivatives; Yohimbine

Increased Effect/Toxicity

Losartan and Hydrochlorothiazide may increase the levels/effects of: ACE Inhibitors; Allopurinol; Amifostine; Antihypertensives; Calcium Salts; CarBAMazepine; Carvedilol; CYP2C8 Substrates (High risk); CYP2C9 Substrates (High risk); Dofetilide; Hypoglycemic Agents; Hypotensive Agents; Lithium; OXcarbazepine; Potassium-Sparing Diuretics; RiTUXimab; Topiramate; Toremifene; Vitamin D Analogs

The levels/effects of Losartan and Hydrochlorothiazide may be increased by: Alcohol (Ethyl); Analgesics (Opioid); Antifungal Agents (Azole Derivatives, Systemic); Barbiturates; Conivaptan; Corticosteroids (Orally Inhaled); Corticosteroids (Systemic); CYP2C9 Inhibitors (Moderate); CYP2C9 Inhibitors (Strong); Eplerenone; Fluconazole; Herbs (Hypoglycemic Properties); Herbs (Hypotensive Properties); Licorice; MAO Inhibitors; Milk Thistle; Pentoxifylline; Phosphodiesterase 5 Inhibitors; Potassium Salts; Prostacyclin Analogues; Tolvaptan; Trimethoprim

Adverse Reactions Based on clinical trials of the combination product in patients with essential hypertension. Also see individual agents.

1% to 10%:

Cardiovascular: Edema (1%), palpitation (1%)
Central nervous system: Dizziness (6%)
Dermatologic: Skin rash (1%)
Gastrointestinal: Abdominal pain (1%)
Neuromuscular & skeletal: Back pain (2%)
Respiratory: Upper respiratory infection (6%), cough (3%), sinusitis (1%)

Pharmacodynamics/Kinetics

Pharmacokinetic Note See individual agents.

Available Dosage Forms

Tablet: 50/12.5: Losartan 50 mg and hydrochlorothiazide 12.5 mg; 100/12.5: Losartan 100 mg and hydrochlorothiazide 12.5 mg; 100/25: Losartan 100 mg and hydrochlorothiazide 25 mg

Hyzaar®: 50/12.5: Losartan 50 mg and hydrochlorothiazide 12.5 mg; 100/12.5: Losartan 100 mg and hydrochlorothiazide 12.5 mg; 100/25: Losartan 100 mg and hydrochlorothiazide 25 mg

Dosing

Adult Note: Dose is individualized (combination substituted for individual components); dose may be titrated after 2-4 weeks of therapy

Hypertension/stroke reduction in hypertension (with LVH): Usual recommended starting dose of losartan: 50 mg once daily when used as monotherapy in patients who are not volume depleted

Geriatric Refer to dosing in individual monographs.

Renal Impairment Cl_{cr} ≤30 mL/minute: Use of combination formulation is not recommended.

Hepatic Impairment Use is not recommended.

Monitoring and Teaching Issues

Physical Assessment See individual agents.

Patient Education See individual agents.

Dietary Considerations Some products may contain potassium.

Pregnancy Considerations See individual agents.

Related Information

Hydrochlorothiazide *on page 912*
Losartan *on page 1133*

◆ **Losartan Potassium** *see* Losartan *on page 1133*
◆ **LoSeasonique®** *see* Ethinyl Estradiol and Levonorgestrel *on page 699*
◆ **Lotemax®** *see* Loteprednol *on page 1136*
◆ **Lotensin®** *see* Benazepril *on page 195*
◆ **Lotensin HCT®** *see* Benazepril and Hydrochlorothiazide *on page 198*

Loteprednol (loe te PRED nol)

U.S. Brand Names Alrex®; Lotemax®

Index Terms Loteprednol Etabonate

Generic Availability (U.S.) No

Pharmacologic Category Corticosteroid, Ophthalmic

Pregnancy Risk Factor C

Lactation Excretion in breast milk unknown/use caution

Use

Suspension, 0.2% (Alrex®): Temporary relief of signs and symptoms of seasonal allergic conjunctivitis

Suspension, 0.5% (Lotemax®): Inflammatory conditions (treatment of steroid-responsive inflammatory conditions of the palpebral and bulbar conjunctiva, cornea, and anterior segment of the globe such as allergic conjunctivitis, acne rosacea, superficial punctate keratitis, herpes zoster keratitis, iritis, cyclitis, selected infective conjunctivitis, when the inherent hazard of steroid use is accepted to obtain an advisable diminution in edema and inflammation) and treatment of postoperative inflammation following ocular surgery

Product Availability

Lotemax® 0.5% ointment: FDA approved April 2011; expected availability undetermined

Lotemax® 0.5% ointment is a topical corticosteroid approved for the treatment of postoperative inflammation and pain following ocular surgery.

Available Dosage Forms

Suspension, ophthalmic:

Alrex®: 0.2% (5 mL, 10 mL)

Lotemax®: 0.5% (2.5 mL, 5 mL, 10 mL, 15 mL)

Dosing

Adult & Geriatric

Seasonal allergic conjunctivitis: Ophthalmic: 0.2% suspension (Alrex®): Instill 1 drop into affected eye(s) 4 times/day.

Inflammatory conditions: Ophthalmic: 0.5% suspension (Lotemax®): Apply 1-2 drops into the conjunctival sac of the affected eye(s) 4 times/day. During the initial treatment within the first week, the dosing may be increased up to 1 drop every hour. Advise patients not to discontinue therapy prematurely. If signs and symptoms fail to improve after 2 days, re-evaluate the patient.

Postoperative inflammation: Ophthalmic: 0.5% suspension (Lotemax®): Apply 1-2 drops into the conjunctival sac of the operated eye(s) 4 times/day beginning 24 hours after surgery and continuing throughout the first 2 weeks of the postoperative period.

Administration

Other Shake well before using.

Monitoring and Teaching Issues

Patient Education For use in eyes only. Shake well before using. Do not let tip of applicator touch eye; do not contaminate tip of applicator (may cause eye infection, eye damage, or vision loss). Tilt head back, place medication in conjunctival sac, and close eyes. Apply finger pressure at corner of eye for 1 minute following application. May cause temporary sensitivity to bright light, blurring or stinging, changes in visual acuity, headache, runny nose, or sore throat. If improvement is not noted within 2 days, notify prescriber. Report persistent vision changes, signs of infection, swollen eyelids, or inflammation.

Loteprednol and Tobramycin (loe te PRED nol & toe bra MYE sin)

U.S. Brand Names Zylet®

Index Terms Loteprednol Etabonate and Tobramycin; Tobramycin and Loteprednol Etabonate

Generic Availability (U.S.) No

Pharmacologic Category Antibiotic/Corticosteroid, Ophthalmic

Pregnancy Risk Factor C

Lactation Excretion in breast milk unknown/use caution

Use Treatment of steroid-responsive ocular inflammatory conditions where either a superficial bacterial ocular infection or the risk of a superficial bacterial ocular infection exists

Available Dosage Forms

Suspension, ophthalmic [drops]:

Zylet®: Loteprednol 0.5% and tobramycin 0.3% (2.5 mL, 5 mL, 10 mL)

Dosing

Adult & Geriatric Ophthalmic: Instill 1-2 drops into the affected eye(s) every 4-6 hours; may increase frequency during the first 24-48 hours to every 1-2 hours. Interval should increase as signs and symptoms improve. Further evaluation should occur for use of greater than 20 mL.

Pediatric Refer to adult dosing.

Administration

Other Contact lenses should not be worn during therapy. Shake well before using; Tilt head back, instill suspension in conjunctival sac and close eye(s). Do not touch dropper to eye. Apply light finger pressure on lacrimal sac for 1 minute following instillation.

Monitoring and Teaching Issues

Physical Assessment See individual agents.

Patient Education See individual agents.

- ◆ **Loteprednol Etabonate** *see* Loteprednol *on page 1136*
- ◆ **Loteprednol Etabonate and Tobramycin** *see* Loteprednol and Tobramycin *on page 1137*
- ◆ **Lotrel®** *see* Amlodipine and Benazepril *on page 107*
- ◆ **Lotrimin AF® [OTC]** *see* Miconazole (Topical) *on page 1224*
- ◆ **Lotrisone®** *see* Betamethasone and Clotrimazole *on page 208*

Lovastatin (LOE va sta tin)

U.S. Brand Names Altoprev®; Mevacor®

Index Terms Mevinolin; Monacolin K

Generic Availability (U.S.) Yes: Exludes extended release tablet

Pharmacologic Category Antilipemic Agent, HMG-CoA Reductase Inhibitor

Medication Safety Issues

Sound-alike/look-alike issues:

Lovastatin may be confused with atorvastatin, Leustatin®, Livostin®, Lotensin®, nystatin, pitavastatin

Mevacor® may be confused with Benicar®, Lipitor®, Mivacron®

International issues:

Lovacol [Chile and Finland] may be confused with Levatol brand name for penbutolol [U.S.]

Lovastin [Malaysia, Poland, and Singapore] may be confused with Livostin brand name for levocabastine [multiple international markets]

Pregnancy Risk Factor X

Lactation Excretion in breast milk unknown/contraindicated

Use

Adjunct to dietary therapy to decrease elevated serum total and LDL-cholesterol concentrations in primary hypercholesterolemia

Primary prevention of coronary artery disease (patients without symptomatic disease with average to moderately elevated total and LDL-cholesterol and below average HDL-cholesterol); slow progression of coronary atherosclerosis in patients with coronary heart disease

Adjunct to dietary therapy in adolescent patients (10-17 years of age, females >1 year postmenarche) with heterozygous familial hypercholesterolemia having LDL >189 mg/dL, **or** LDL >160 mg/dL with positive family history of premature cardiovascular disease (CVD), **or** LDL >160 mg/dL with the presence of at least two other CVD risk factors

Available Dosage Forms

Tablet, oral: 10 mg, 20 mg, 40 mg

Mevacor®: 20 mg, 40 mg

Tablet, extended release, oral:

Altoprev®: 20 mg, 40 mg, 60 mg

Dosing

Adult & Geriatric

Dyslipidemia and primary prevention of CAD: Oral: Initial: 20 mg with evening meal, then adjust at 4-week intervals; maximum: 80 mg/day immediate release tablet **or** 60 mg/day extended release tablet.

Note: Doses should be individualized according to the baseline LDL-cholesterol levels, the recommended goal of therapy, and patient response.

Dosage modification/limits based on concurrent therapy:

Cyclosporine or danazol: Initial dose: 10 mg/day with a maximum recommended dose of 20 mg/day

Concurrent therapy with fibrates and/or lipid-lowering doses of niacin (≥1 g/day): Maximum recommended dose: 20 mg/day. Concurrent use with fibrates should be avoided unless risk to benefit favors use.

Concurrent therapy with amiodarone or verapamil: Maximum recommended dose: 40 mg/day of immediate release or 20 mg/day with extended release.

Dosage adjustment in renal impairment: Cl_{cr} <30 mL/minute: Use doses >20 mg/day with caution.

Pediatric

Heterozygous familial hypercholesterolemia: Oral (immediate release tablet): Adolescents 10-17 years:

LDL reduction <20%: Initial: 10 mg/day with evening meal

LDL reduction ≥20%: Initial: 20 mg/day with evening meal

Usual range: 10-40 mg with evening meal, then adjust dose at 4-week intervals; maximum dose per manufacturer: 40 mg/day

Renal Impairment Cl_{cr} <30 mL/minute: Use with caution and carefully consider doses >20 mg/day.

Administration

Oral Administer immediate release tablet with the evening meal. Administer extended release tablet at bedtime; do not crush or chew.

Monitoring and Teaching Issues

Laboratory Monitoring Obtain baseline LFTs and total cholesterol profile. LFTs should be performed before initiation of therapy, at 6 and 12 weeks after initiation or first dose, and periodically thereafter; baseline CPK (recheck CPK in any patient with symptoms suggestive of myopathy). Monitor LDL-C at intervals no less than 4 weeks.

Physical Assessment Use caution with history of hepatic disease. Assess risk potential for interactions with other prescriptions or herbal products patient may be taking that may increase risk of myopathy or rhabdomyolysis. Evaluate LFTs and lipid profile prior to treatment and at regular intervals. Teach proper diet and exercise program.

Patient Education Take with food at evening meal. Follow prescribed diet and exercise regimen. You will have periodic blood tests to assess effectiveness. Avoid excessive alcohol. Report unusual muscle cramping or weakness, yellowing of skin or eyes, easy bruising or bleeding, or unusual fatigue.

Related Information

Hyperlipidemia Management *on page 2046*

◆ **Lovaza®** *see* Omega-3-Acid Ethyl Esters *on page 1355*

◆ **Lovenox®** *see* Enoxaparin *on page 622*

◆ **Low-Molecular-Weight Iron Dextran (INFeD®)** *see* Iron Dextran Complex *on page 1021*

◆ **L-PAM** *see* Melphalan *on page 1162*

◆ **L-Phenylalanine Mustard** *see* Melphalan *on page 1162*

◆ **L-Sarcolysin** *see* Melphalan *on page 1162*

◆ **LTA® 360** *see* Lidocaine (Topical) *on page 1107*

◆ **LTG** *see* LamoTRIgine *on page 1057*

◆ ***L*-Thyroxine Sodium** *see* Levothyroxine *on page 1101*

◆ **Lu-26-054** *see* Escitalopram *on page 662*

Lubiprostone (loo bi PROS tone)

U.S. Brand Names Amitiza®

Index Terms RU 0211; SPI 0211

Generic Availability (U.S.) No

Pharmacologic Category Chloride Channel Activator; Gastrointestinal Agent, Miscellaneous

Pregnancy Risk Factor C

Lactation Excretion in breast milk unknown/not recommended

Use Treatment of chronic idiopathic constipation; treatment of irritable bowel syndrome with constipation in adult women

Mechanism of Action/Effect Increases intestinal fluid and intestinal motility

Contraindications Known or suspected mechanical bowel obstruction

Warnings/Precautions Symptoms of mechanical gastrointestinal obstruction should be evaluated before prescribing this medicine; use is contraindicated in patients with bowel obstruction. Avoid use in patients with severe diarrhea. Nausea may occur; administer with food to reduce symptoms. In long-term clinical studies for chronic idiopathic constipation, patients were allowed to reduce the dose to 24 mcg once daily if nausea was severe. Dyspnea, often described as chest tightness, has been observed with use, including postmarketing reports; generally occurs following the first dose with an acute onset (within 30-60 minutes) and resolves within a few hours; however, has been frequently reported with subsequent dosing. Use caution in renal or hepatic dysfunction; has not been studied in renal or hepatic impairment. Not approved for use in males with irritable bowel syndrome with constipation.

Drug Interactions

Avoid Concomitant Use There are no known interactions where it is recommended to avoid concomitant use.

Decreased Effect There are no known significant interactions involving a decrease in effect.

Increased Effect/Toxicity There are no known significant interactions involving an increase in effect.

Adverse Reactions

>10%:

Central nervous system: Headache (11%)

Gastrointestinal: Nausea (8% to 29%; severe: 4%; dose related), diarrhea (7% to 12%; severe 2%)

1% to 10%:

Cardiovascular: Edema (3%), chest discomfort/pain (2%), hypertension (1%)

Central nervous system: Dizziness (3%), fatigue (2%), fever (1%), insomnia (1%)

Gastrointestinal: Abdominal pain (5% to 8%), abdominal distention (3% to 6%), flatulence (6%), vomiting (3%), loose stools (3%), dyspepsia (2%), stomach/abdominal discomfort (1% to 2%), xerostomia (1%), weight gain (1%)

Neuromuscular & skeletal: Arthralgia (3%), back pain (2%)

Renal: Urinary tract infection (4%)

Respiratory: Sinusitis (5%), upper respiratory tract infection (4%), nasopharyngitis (3%), bronchitis (2%), dyspnea (2%)

Pharmacodynamics/Kinetics

Absorption Systemic: Parent drug: Poor (below levels of detection); Active metabolite (M3): Low

Bioavailability Minimal

Half-Life Elimination M3: 0.9-1.4 hours

Metabolism Rapid and extensive within stomach and jejunum by carbonyl reductase to M3 (active metabolite) and others

Excretion Parent drug and M3: Feces (trace amounts)

Available Dosage Forms

Capsule, softgel, oral:

Amitiza®: 8 mcg, 24 mcg

Dosing

Adult & Geriatric

Chronic idiopathic constipation: Adults: 24 mcg twice daily

Irritable bowel syndrome with constipation: Females ≥18 years: 8 mcg twice daily

Renal Impairment Has not been studied.

Hepatic Impairment Has not been studied.

Adjustment for Toxicity

Chronic idiopathic constipation: May decrease dose to 24 mcg once daily in case of severe nausea

Administration

Oral Administer with food and water. Swallow whole; do not break or chew.

Stability

Storage Store at controlled room temperature of 25°C (77°F).

Monitoring and Teaching Issues

Dietary Considerations May take with food to decrease nausea.

Geriatric Considerations No studies have been done in elderly populations to date. Data in subpopulation analysis demonstrate lubiprostone is safe and well tolerated in all sexes, races, and age groups.

Pregnancy Considerations Animal studies suggest that lubiprostone may cause fetal loss, teratogenic effects were not observed. There are no adequate and well-controlled studies in pregnant women. Women of childbearing potential should have a negative pregnancy test prior to starting therapy and should be capable of complying with effective contraception.

- ◆ **Lugol's Solution** *see* Potassium Iodide and Iodine *on page* 1484
- ◆ **Lumigan®** *see* Bimatoprost *on page* 219
- ◆ **Luminal® Sodium [DSC]** *see* PHENobarbital *on page* 1447
- ◆ **Lunesta®** *see* Eszopiclone *on page* 688
- ◆ **Lupron®** *see* Leuprolide *on page* 1082
- ◆ **Lupron Depot®** *see* Leuprolide *on page* 1082
- ◆ **Lupron Depot®-3 Month** *see* Leuprolide *on page* 1082
- ◆ **Lupron Depot®-4 Month** *see* Leuprolide *on page* 1082
- ◆ **Lupron Depot-Ped®** *see* Leuprolide *on page* 1082

Lurasidone (loo RAS i done)

U.S. Brand Names Latuda®

Index Terms Lurasidone Hydrochloride; SM-13496

Generic Availability (U.S.) No

Pharmacologic Category Antipsychotic Agent, Atypical

Pregnancy Risk Factor B

Lactation Excretion in breast milk unknown/not recommended

Use Treatment of schizophrenia

Mechanism of Action/Effect Atypical antipsychotic with high affinity for serotonin, dopamine, and moderate affinity for alpha$_2$-adrenergic receptors; no significant affinity for muscarinic or histamine receptors. Results in improvement of psychotic symptoms and reduction of extrapyramidal and antimuscarinic side effects as compared to typical antipsychotics.

Contraindications Hypersensitivity to lurasidone or any component of the formulation; concomitant use with potent CYP3A4 inhibitors (eg, ketoconazole) and inducers (eg, rifampin)

Warnings/Precautions **[U.S. Boxed Warning]: Elderly patients with dementia-related psychosis treated with antipsychotics are at an increased risk of death compared to placebo.** Most deaths appeared to be either cardiovascular (eg, heart failure, sudden death) or infectious (eg, pneumonia) in nature. Lurasidone is not approved for the treatment of dementia-related psychosis. An increased incidence of cerebrovascular effects (eg, transient ischemic attack, stroke), including fatalities, has been reported in placebo-controlled trials of antipsychotics for the unapproved use in elderly patients with dementia-related psychosis.

Leukopenia, neutropenia, and agranulocytosis (sometimes fatal) have been reported in clinical trials and postmarketing reports with antipsychotic use; presence of risk factors (eg, pre-existing low WBC or history of drug-induced leuko-/neutropenia) should prompt periodic blood count assessment. Discontinue therapy at first signs of blood dyscrasias or if absolute neutrophil count <1000/mm^3.

Low to moderately sedating, use with caution in disorders where CNS depression is a feature. Use with caution in Parkinson's disease. Caution in patients with predisposition to seizures. Use with caution in renal or hepatic dysfunction; dose reduction recommended in moderate-to-severe impairment. Esophageal dysmotility and aspiration have been associated with antipsychotic use; use with caution in patients at risk of aspiration pneumonia (ie, Alzheimer's disease). Use is associated with increased prolactin levels; clinical significance of hyperprolactinemia in patients with breast cancer or other prolactin-dependent tumors is unknown. May alter temperature regulation.

Use with caution in patients with severe cardiac disease, hemodynamic instability, prior myocardial infarction or ischemic heart disease. May cause orthostatic hypotension; use with caution in patients at risk of this effect (eg, concurrent medication use which may predispose to hypotension/bradycardia or presence of hypovolemia) or in those who would not tolerate transient hypotensive episodes. Antipsychotics may alter cardiac conduction; life-threatening arrhythmias have occurred with therapeutic doses of antipsychotics. Relative to other antipsychotics, lurasidone has minimal effects on the QT$_c$ interval and therefore, risk for arrhythmias is low. Increases in total cholesterol and triglyceride concentrations have been observed with atypical antipsychotic use; during clinical trials of lurasidone, there were no significant changes in total cholesterol or triglycerides observed. Concurrent use with strong inhibitors/inducers of CYP3A4 is contraindicated; dosage adjustment is recommended with concurrent use of moderate CYP3A4 inhibitors (eg, diltiazem).

May cause extrapyramidal symptoms (EPS), including pseudoparkinsonism, acute dystonic reactions, akathisia, and tardive dyskinesia (potentially irreversible). Risk of tardive dyskinesia may be increased in elderly patients, particularly elderly women. Risk of dystonia (and probably other EPS) may be greater with increased doses, use of conventional antipsychotics, males, and younger patients. Use may be associated with neuroleptic malignant syndrome (NMS); monitor for mental status changes, fever, muscle rigidity and/or autonomic instability (risk may be increased in patients with Parkinson's disease or Lewy body dementia). May cause hyperglycemia; in some cases may be extreme and associated with ketoacidosis, hyperosmolar coma, or death. Use with caution in patients with diabetes or other disorders of glucose regulation; monitor for worsening of glucose control. Significant weight gain has been observed with antipsychotic therapy; incidence varies with product. Monitor waist circumference and BMI.

The possibility of a suicide attempt is inherent in psychotic illness or bipolar disorder; use caution in high-risk patients during initiation of therapy. Prescriptions should be written for the smallest quantity consistent with good patient care.

Drug Interactions

Metabolism/Transport Effects

Substrate of CYP3A4 (major); **Inhibits** CYP3A4 (weak)

Avoid Concomitant Use

Avoid concomitant use of Lurasidone with any of the following: CYP3A4 Inducers (Strong); CYP3A4 Inhibitors (Strong); DOPamine; EPINEPHrine; EPINEPHrine (Systemic, Oral Inhalation); Metoclopramide

Decreased Effect

Lurasidone may decrease the levels/effects of: Amphetamines; Anti-Parkinson's Agents (Dopamine Agonist); Quinagolide

The levels/effects of Lurasidone may be decreased by: CYP3A4 Inducers (Strong); Deferasirox; Herbs (CYP3A4 Inducers); Lithium formulations

Increased Effect/Toxicity

Lurasidone may increase the levels/effects of: Alcohol (Ethyl); CNS Depressants; Disopyramide; Methotrimeprazine; Methylphenidate; Procainamide; QuiNIDine

The levels/effects of Lurasidone may be increased by: Acetylcholinesterase Inhibitors (Central); CYP3A4 Inhibitors (Moderate); CYP3A4 Inhibitors (Strong); Dasatinib; DOPamine; Droperidol; EPINEPHrine; EPINEPHrine (Systemic, Oral Inhalation); Lithium formulations; MAO Inhibitors; Methotrimeprazine; Methylphenidate; Metoclopramide; Tetrabenazine

Nutritional/Ethanol Interactions

Ethanol: Avoid ethanol (may increase CNS depression).

Food: Administration with food (≥350 calories) increased C_{max} and AUC of lurasidone ~3 times and 2 times, respectively, compared to administration under fasting conditions. Lurasidone exposure was not affected by the fat content of the meal.

Adverse Reactions

10%:

- Central nervous system: Somnolence (dose-related: 19% to 23%), akathisia (dose-related: 11% to 15%)
- Endocrine & metabolic: Fasting glucose increased (10% to 14%)
- Gastrointestinal: Nausea (12%)
- Neuromuscular & skeletal: Extrapyramidal symptoms (24% to 26%), parkinsonism (11%)

1% to 10%:

- Cardiovascular: Tachycardia
- Central nervous system: Insomnia (8%), agitation (6%), anxiety (6%), dizziness (5%), dystonia (5%), fatigue (4%), restlessness (3%)
- Dermatologic: Pruritus, rash
- Endocrine & metabolic: Prolactin increased (≥5 x ULN: females: 8%; males: 2%)
- Gastrointestinal: Dyspepsia (8%), vomiting (8%), weight gain (≥7% increase in baseline body weight: 6%), salivary hypersecretion (2%), abdominal pain, appetite decreased, diarrhea
- Neuromuscular & skeletal: Back pain (4%), CPK increased
- Ocular: Blurred vision
- Renal: Creatinine increased (3%)

Pharmacodynamics/Kinetics

Bioavailability 9% to 19%

Time to Peak 1-3 hours; steady state concentrations achieved within 7 days

Protein Binding ~99%

Half-Life Elimination 18 hours; Main active metabolite, ID-14283 (exo-hydroxy metabolite), exhibits a half-life of 7.5-10 hours

Metabolism Primarily via CYP3A4; two active metabolites (ID-14283 and ID-14326) and two major nonactive metabolites (ID-20219 and ID-20220) produced

Excretion Urine (~9%); feces (~80%)

Available Dosage Forms

Tablet, oral:

Latuda®: 40 mg, 80 mg

Dosing

Adult & Geriatric Schizophrenia: Oral: Initial: 40 mg once daily; titration is not required; maximum recommended dose: 80 mg/day

Concomitant CYP3A4 inhibitors/inducers:

CYP3A4 inhibitors: If concomitant administration with a moderate CYP3A4 inhibitor (eg, diltiazem) is necessary, do not exceed 40 mg/day of lurasidone. Concomitant administration with a strong CYP3A4 inhibitor (eg, ketoconazole) is contraindicated.

CYP3A4 inducers: Concomitant administration with a strong CYP3A4 inducer (eg, rifampin) is contraindicated.

Renal Impairment Exposure is increased in renal impairment; use caution.

Cl_{cr} ≥50 mL/minute: No dosage adjustment required.

Cl_{cr} 10-49 mL/minute: Do not exceed 40 mg/day.

Hepatic Impairment Exposure is increased in hepatic impairment; use caution.

Mild hepatic impairment (Child-Pugh class A): No dosage adjustment required.

Moderate-to-severe hepatic impairment (Child-Pugh class B or C): Do not exceed 40 mg/day.

Administration

Oral Administer with food (≥350 calories).

Stability

Storage Store at controlled room temperature of 25°C (77°F).

Monitoring and Teaching Issues

Laboratory Monitoring Fasting lipid profile and fasting blood glucose/Hgb A_{1c} (baseline and periodically); CBC frequently during first few months of therapy in patients with pre-existing low WBC or a history of drug-induced leukopenia/neutropenia

Physical Assessment Monitor weight prior to treatment and periodically throughout. Be alert to the potential for orthostatic hypotension, especially during the titration phase. Initiate at lower doses and titrate to target dose. Taper dosage slowly when discontinuing.

Patient Education It may take several weeks to achieve desired results. Avoid alcohol. Maintain adequate hydration. If you have diabetes, you may experience increased blood sugars; monitor closely. You may experience excess sedation, drowsiness, problems sleeping, restlessness, dizziness, or blurred vision; dry mouth, nausea, or GI upset; postural hypotension; or urinary retention. Report persistent CNS effects; diaphoresis, chest pain, palpitations, rapid heartbeat, or severe dizziness; or worsening of condition.

Dietary Considerations Should be taken with food (≥350 calories).

Geriatric Considerations Clinical studies of schizophrenic patients did not include sufficient numbers of elderly to determine a difference in response compared to younger adults. Elderly with psychosis had similar serum concentrations to younger adults; therefore, no dosage adjustments are recommended for elderly patients with psychosis. This drug is not recommended/indicated for use in elderly patients with dementia-related psychosis. Such patients are at an increased risk of death compared to placebo. Most deaths were cardiovascular (eg, heart failure, sudden death) or infectious (eg, pneumonia) in nature.

Pregnancy Considerations No teratogenic or adverse developmental effects were observed in animal studies. Antipsychotic use during the third trimester of pregnancy has a risk for abnormal muscle movements (extrapyramidal symptoms [EPS]) and withdrawal symptoms in newborns following delivery. Symptoms in the newborn may include agitation, feeding disorder, hypertonia, hypotonia, respiratory distress, somnolence, and tremor; these effects may be self-limiting or require hospitalization. There are no adequate and well-controlled studies in pregnant women. Use in pregnancy only when potential benefit to mother outweighs possible risk to the fetus.

- **Lurasidone Hydrochloride** *see* Lurasidone *on page* 1140
- **LuSonal™ [DSC]** *see* Phenylephrine (Systemic) *on page* 1449
- **Lustra®** *see* Hydroquinone *on page* 927
- **Lustra-AF®** *see* Hydroquinone *on page* 927
- **Lustra-Ultra™** *see* Hydroquinone *on page* 927
- **Lutera®** *see* Ethinyl Estradiol and Levonorgestrel *on page* 699

Lutropin Alfa (LOO troe pin AL fa)

U.S. Brand Names Luveris®

Index Terms r-hLH; Recombinant Human Luteinizing Hormone

Generic Availability (U.S.) No

Pharmacologic Category Gonadotropin; Ovulation Stimulator

Pregnancy Risk Factor X

Lactation Excretion in breast milk unknown/use caution

Use Stimulation of follicular development in infertile hypogonadotropic hypogonadal (HH) women with profound luteinizing hormone (LH) deficiency; to be used in combination with follitropin alfa

Available Dosage Forms

Injection, powder for reconstitution:

Luveris®: 75 int. units

Dosing

Adult Infertility: Females: SubQ: 75 int. units daily until adequate follicular development is noted; maximum duration of treatment: 14 days; to be used concomitantly with follitropin alfa

Administration

Other SubQ: Administer on the stomach, a few inches above or below the navel.

Monitoring and Teaching Issues

Physical Assessment For subcutaneous use only. Administer around navel area. Instruct patient in appropriate administration technique and disposal of used needles and syringes.

Patient Education For subcutaneous injection only. Follow administration schedule as directed by prescriber. You may experience headache, nausea, fatigue, constipation, or diarrhea. Report immediately abdominal pain/distension or persistent nausea.

- ◆ **Luveris®** *see* Lutropin Alfa *on page* 1142
- ◆ **Luvox** *see* Fluvoxamine *on page* 809
- ◆ **Luvox® CR** *see* Fluvoxamine *on page* 809
- ◆ **Luxiq®** *see* Betamethasone *on page* 205
- ◆ **LY139603** *see* Atomoxetine *on page* 164
- ◆ **LY170053** *see* OLANZapine *on page* 1344
- ◆ **LY-188011** *see* Gemcitabine *on page* 855
- ◆ **LY231514** *see* Pemetrexed *on page* 1429
- ◆ **LY246736** *see* Alvimopan *on page* 90
- ◆ **LY248686** *see* DULoxetine *on page* 596
- ◆ **LY303366** *see* Anidulafungin *on page* 130
- ◆ **LY-640315** *see* Prasugrel *on page* 1493
- ◆ **LY2148568** *see* Exenatide *on page* 726
- ◆ **Lybrel®** *see* Ethinyl Estradiol and Levonorgestrel *on page* 699
- ◆ **Lymphocyte Immune Globulin** *see* Antithymocyte Globulin (Equine) *on page* 136
- ◆ **Lymphocyte Mitogenic Factor** *see* Aldesleukin *on page* 62
- ◆ **Lyrica®** *see* Pregabalin *on page* 1504
- ◆ **Lysodren®** *see* Mitotane *on page* 1242
- ◆ **Maalox® Total Relief® [OTC] [DSC]** *see* Bismuth *on page* 221
- ◆ **Macrobid®** *see* Nitrofurantoin *on page* 1325
- ◆ **Macrodantin®** *see* Nitrofurantoin *on page* 1325
- ◆ **Mag 64™ [OTC]** *see* Magnesium Chloride *on page* 1143
- ◆ **Mag Delay [OTC]** *see* Magnesium Chloride *on page* 1143
- ◆ **Mag®-G [OTC]** *see* Magnesium Gluconate *on page* 1144

Magnesium Chloride (mag NEE zhum KLOR ide)

U.S. Brand Names Chloromag®; Mag 64™ [OTC]; Mag Delay [OTC]; Mag-SR with Calcium [OTC] [DSC]; Slow-Mag® [OTC]

Generic Availability (U.S.) Yes

Pharmacologic Category Electrolyte Supplement, Oral; Electrolyte Supplement, Parenteral; Magnesium Salt

Pregnancy Risk Factor C

Lactation Enters breast milk/compatible

Use Correction or prevention of hypomagnesemia; dietary supplement

Available Dosage Forms

Injection, solution: 200 mg/mL (50 mL)
Chloromag®: 200 mg/mL (50 mL)

Tablet, delayed release, enteric coated, oral:
Mag 64™ [OTC]: Elemental magnesium 64 mg
Mag Delay [OTC]: Elemental magnesium 64 mg

Tablet, enteric coated, oral:
Slow-Mag® [OTC]: Elemental magnesium 64 mg

Dosing

Adult & Geriatric Note: Serum magnesium is poor reflection of repletional status as the majority of magnesium is intracellular; serum levels may be transiently normal for a few hours after a dose is given; therefore, aim for consistently high normal serum levels in patients with normal renal function for most efficient repletion.

Dietary supplement: Oral (Mag 64™, Mag Delay®, Slow-Mag®): 2 tablets once daily

Parenteral nutrition supplementation: I.V. (elemental magnesium): 8-24 mEq/day

RDA (elemental magnesium):

19-30 years:
Female: 310 mg/day
Pregnant female: 350 mg/day
Male: 400 mg/day

≥31 years:
Female: 320 mg/day
Pregnant female: 360 mg/day
Male: 420 mg/day

Pediatric Note: Serum magnesium is poor reflection of repletional status as the majority of magnesium is intracellular; serum levels may be transiently normal for a few hours after a dose is given; therefore, aim for consistently high normal serum levels in patients with normal renal function for most efficient repletion.

Parenteral nutrition supplementation: I.V. (elemental magnesium):
- <50 kg: 0.3-0.5 mEq/kg/day
- >50 kg: 10-30 mEq/day

RDA (elemental magnesium):
- 1-3 years: 80 mg/day
- 4-8 years: 130 mg/day
- 9-13 years: 240 mg/day
- 14-18 years:
  - Female: 360 mg/day
  - Pregnant female: 400 mg/day
  - Male: 410 mg/day

Renal Impairment Cl_{cr} <30 mL/minute: Use with caution; monitor for hypermagnesemia

Monitoring and Teaching Issues

Laboratory Monitoring Magnesium, calcium, potassium, and renal function

Magnesium Gluconate (mag NEE zhum GLOO koe nate)

U.S. Brand Names Magonate® [OTC]; Magtrate® [OTC]; Mag®-G [OTC]

Generic Availability (U.S.) Yes: Tablet

Pharmacologic Category Electrolyte Supplement, Oral; Magnesium Salt

Lactation Enters breast milk/compatible

Use Dietary supplement

Available Dosage Forms For available OTC formulations, consult specific product labeling.

Dosing

Adult & Geriatric RDA (elemental magnesium): Oral:
- 19-30 years:
  - Female: 310 mg/day
  - Pregnant female: 350 mg/day
  - Male: 400 mg/day
- ≥31 years:
  - Female: 320 mg/day
  - Pregnant female: 360 mg/day
  - Male: 420 mg/day

Pediatric RDA (elemental magnesium): Oral:
- 1-3 years: 80 mg/day
- 4-8 years: 130 mg/day
- 9-13 years: 240 mg/day
- 14-18 years:
  - Female: 360 mg/day
  - Pregnant female: 400 mg/day
  - Male: 410 mg/day

Renal Impairment Cl_{cr} <30 mL/minute: Use with caution; monitor for hypermagnesemia

Administration

Oral Administer on an empty stomach

Magnesium Sulfate (mag NEE zhum SUL fate)

Index Terms Epsom Salts; $MgSO_4$ (error-prone abbreviation)

Generic Availability (U.S.) Yes

Pharmacologic Category Anticonvulsant, Miscellaneous; Electrolyte Supplement, Parenteral; Magnesium Salt

Medication Safety Issues

Sound-alike/look-alike issues:

Magnesium sulfate may be confused with manganese sulfate, morphine sulfate

$MgSO_4$ is an error-prone abbreviation (mistaken as morphine sulfate)

High alert medication: The Institute for Safe Medication Practices (ISMP) includes this medication (I.V. formulation) among its list of drugs which have a heightened risk of causing significant patient harm when used in error.

Pregnancy Risk Factor A/C (manufacturer dependent)

Lactation Enters breast milk/compatible

Use Treatment and prevention of hypomagnesemia; prevention and treatment of seizures in severe pre-eclampsia or eclampsia, pediatric acute nephritis; torsade de pointes; treatment of cardiac arrhythmias (VT/VF) caused by hypomagnesemia; soaking aid

Unlabeled/Investigational Use Asthma exacerbation (life-threatening)

Available Dosage Forms

Infusion, premixed in D_5W: 10 mg/mL (100 mL); 20 mg/mL (500 mL)

Infusion, premixed in water for injection: 40 mg/mL (50 mL, 100 mL, 500 mL, 1000 mL); 80 mg/mL (50 mL)

Injection, solution: 500 mg/mL (5 mL, 10 mL, 20 mL, 25 mL, 50 mL)

Injection, solution [preservative free]: 500 mg/mL (2 mL, 5 mL, 10 mL, 20 mL, 50 mL)

Powder, oral/topical: USP: 100% (227 g, 454 g, 1810 g, 2720 g)

Dosing

Adult & Geriatric Dose represented as magnesium sulfate unless stated otherwise. **Note:** Serum magnesium is poor reflection of repletional status as the majority of magnesium is intracellular; serum concentrations may be transiently normal for a few hours after a dose is given, therefore, aim for consistently high normal serum concentrations in patients with normal renal function for most efficient repletion.

Note: 1 g of magnesium sulfate = 98.6 mg elemental magnesium = 8.12 mEq elemental magnesium

Hypomagnesemia: Note: Treatment depends on severity and clinical status:

Mild deficiency: I.M.: 1 g every 6 hours for 4 doses, or as indicated by serum magnesium concentrations

Severe deficiency:

I.M.: Up to 250 mg/kg within a 4-hour period

I.V.: Severe, non-life-threatening: 1-2 g/hour for 3-6 hours then 0.5-1 g/hour as needed to correct deficiency

Symptomatic deficiency: I.V.: 1-2 g over 5-60 minutes; maintenance infusion may be required to correct deficiency (0.5-1 g/hour).

With polymorphic VT (including torsade de pointes): I.V. push: 1-2 g (ACLS, 2010)

With seizures: I.V.: 2 g over 10 minutes; calcium administration may also be appropriate as many patients are also hypocalcemic

Asthma (life-threatening or severe exacerbation after 1 hour of intensive conventional therapy; unlabeled use): I.V.: 2 g

Eclampsia:

I.V.: 4-5 g infusion; followed by a 1-2 g/hour continuous infusion; or may follow with I.M. doses of 4-5 g in each buttock every 4 hours. **Note:** Initial infusion may be given over 3-4 minutes if eclampsia is severe; maximum: 40 g/24 hours

ACOG Practice Bulletin 2002: 4-6 g over 15-20 minutes followed by 2 g/hour continuous infusion

Pre-eclampsia (severe): I.V. 4-5 g infusion; followed by a 1-2 g/hour continuous infusion; or may follow with I.M. doses of 4-5 g in each buttock every 4 hours; maximum: 40 g/24 hour

Torsade de pointes or VF/pulseless VT associated with torsade de pointes: I.V., I.O.: 1-2 g over 15 minutes or faster with cardiac arrest (ACLS, 2010)

Parenteral nutrition supplementation: I.V.: 8-24 mEq elemental magnesium/day

Soaking aid: Topical: Dissolve 2 cupfuls of powder per gallon of warm water

RDA:

19-30 years:

Female: 310 mg elemental magnesium/day

Pregnant female: 350 mg elemental magnesium/day

Male: 400 mg elemental magnesium/day

≥31 years:

Female: 320 mg elemental magnesium/day

Pregnant female: 360 mg elemental magnesium/day

Male: 420 mg elemental magnesium/day

Pediatric Dose represented as magnesium sulfate unless stated otherwise. **Note:** Serum magnesium is poor reflection of repletional status as the majority of magnesium is intracellular; serum concentrations may be transiently normal for a few hours after a dose is given, therefore, aim for consistently high normal serum concentrations in patients with normal renal function for most efficient repletion.

Note: 1 g of magnesium sulfate = 98.6 mg elemental magnesium = 8.12 mEq elemental magnesium

Hypomagnesemia: Note: Treatment depends on severity and clinical status: I.V., I.O.: 25-50 mg/kg/dose over 10-20 minutes (over several minutes for torsade de pointes); maximum single dose: 2000 mg (PALS, 2010)

Asthma (life-threatening or severe exacerbation after 1 hour of intensive conventional therapy; unlabeled use): I.V.: 25-75 mg/kg (maximum: 2 g)

Parenteral nutrition supplementation: I.V.:

<50 kg: 0.3-0.5 mEq elemental magnesium/kg/day

>50 kg: 10-30 mEq elemental magnesium/day

RDA: Children:

1-3 years: 80 mg elemental magnesium/day

4-8 years: 130 mg elemental magnesium/day

9-13 years: 240 mg elemental magnesium/day

14-18 years:
Female: 360 mg elemental magnesium/day
Pregnant female: 400 mg elemental magnesium/day
Male: 410 mg elemental magnesium/day

Renal Impairment Cl_{cr} <30 mL/minute: Use with caution; monitor for hypermagnesemia; do not exceed 20 g/48 hours as per manufacturer. Close monitoring is required.

Administration

I.M. A 25% or 50% concentration may be used for adults and dilution to a ≤20% solution is recommended for children

I.V. Magnesium should be diluted to a ≤20% solution for I.V. infusion and may be administered I.V. push, IVPB, or continuous I.V. infusion. When giving I.V. push, must dilute first and should not be given any faster than 150 mg/minute; may administer over 1-2 minutes in patients with persistent pulseless VT or VF with known hypomagnesemia (Dager, 2006). ACLS guidelines recommend administration over 15 minutes in patients with torsade de pointes (ACLS, 2010). In patients not in cardiac arrest, hypotension and asystole may occur with rapid administration.

Maximal rate of infusion: 2 g/hour to avoid hypotension; doses of 4 g/hour have been given in emergencies (eclampsia, seizures); optimally, should add magnesium to I.V. fluids, but bolus doses are also effective

Topical Dissolve 2 cups of powder per gallon of warm water to use as a soaking aid. To make a compress, dissolve 2 cups of powder per 2 cups of hot water and use a towel to apply as a wet dressing.

Monitoring and Teaching Issues

Laboratory Monitoring I.V.: Rapid administration: ECG monitoring, vital signs, deep tendon reflexes; magnesium concentrations if frequent or prolonged dosing required particularly in patients with renal dysfunction, calcium, and potassium concentrations

Physical Assessment When administered parenterally, monitor serum magnesium concentration, respiratory rate, deep tendon reflex, and renal function.

Patient Education Take in divided doses. Report diarrhea (>5 stools/day) or changes in mental function to prescriber.

Related Information

Compatibility of Drugs *on page* 1994

◆ **Magonate® [OTC]** *see* Magnesium Gluconate *on page* 1144

◆ **Mag-SR with Calcium [OTC] [DSC]** *see* Magnesium Chloride *on page* 1143

◆ **Magtrate® [OTC]** *see* Magnesium Gluconate *on page* 1144

Mannitol (MAN i tole)

U.S. Brand Names Aridol™; Osmitrol

Index Terms *D*-Mannitol

Generic Availability (U.S.) Yes: Excludes powder for inhalation

Pharmacologic Category Diagnostic Agent; Diuretic, Osmotic; Genitourinary Irrigant

Medication Safety Issues

Sound-alike/look-alike issues:
Osmitrol® may be confused with esmolol

Pregnancy Risk Factor C

Lactation Excretion in breast milk unknown/use caution

Use

Injection: Reduction of increased intracranial pressure associated with cerebral edema; reduction of increased intraocular pressure; promoting urinary excretion of toxic substances; genitourinary irrigant in transurethral prostatic resection or other transurethral surgical procedures

Note: Although FDA-labeled indications, the use of mannitol for the prevention of acute renal failure and/or promotion of diuresis is not routinely recommended (Kellum, 2008).

Genitourinary irrigation solution: Irrigation in transurethral prostatic resection or other transurethral surgical procedures

Powder for inhalation: Assessment of bronchial hyper-responsiveness

Available Dosage Forms

Injection, solution: 20% [200 mg/mL] (250 mL, 500 mL); 25% [250 mg/mL] (50 mL)
Osmitrol: 5% [50 mg/mL] (1000 mL); 10% [100 mg/mL] (500 mL); 15% [150 mg/mL] (500 mL); 20% [200 mg/mL] (250 mL, 500 mL)

Injection, solution [preservative free]: 25% [250 mg/mL] (50 mL)

Powder, for oral inhalation:
Aridol™: 0 mg (1s) [empty], 5 mg (1s), 10 mg (1s), 20 mg (1s), 40 mg (15s) (19s)

Solution, genitourinary irrigation: 5% [50 mg/mL] (2000 mL)

Dosing

Adult

Assessment of bronchial hyper-responsiveness: Inhalation: Administer in a stepwise fashion (measuring FEV_1 in duplicate after each administration) until the patient has a positive response or 635 mg of mannitol has been administered (whichever comes first).

Positive test: 15% reduction in FEV_1 from baseline or 10% incremental reduction in FEV_1 between consecutive doses

Negative test: Administration of full dose (635 mg) without reduction in FEV_1 sufficient to meet criteria for a positive test

Administration should be as follows:

Stepwise Administration Schedule

Dose #	Dose (mg)	Cumulative Dose (mg)	Capsules/Dose
1	0	0	1
2	5	5	1
3	10	15	1
4	20	35	1
5	40	75	1
6	80	155	2 x 40 mg caps
7	160	315	4 x 40 mg caps
8	160	475	4 x 40 mg caps
9	160	635	4 x 40 mg caps

Increased intracranial pressure: I.V.: 0.25 g/kg/dose; may repeat every 6-8 hours as needed. Reported dosing range: 0.25-1 g/kg/dose (Adelson, 2003); maintain serum osmolality <300-320 mOsm/kg (Adelson, 2003; Broderick, 2007)

Reduction of intraocular pressure: I.V.: 1.5-2 g/kg administered over 30 minutes

Severe traumatic brain injury (unlabeled use): I.V.: ~1.4 g/kg as initial management prior to neurosurgery with concurrent fluid replacement (Cruz, 2001; Cruz, 2002; Cruz, 2004)

Transurethral: Irrigation: Use urogenital solution as required for irrigation.

Geriatric Refer to adult dosing. Consider initiation at lower end of dosing range.

Pediatric

Assessment of bronchial hyper-responsiveness: Inhalation: Children ≥6 years: Refer to adult dosing.

Increased intracranial pressure (unlabeled use): I.V.: 0.25-1 g/kg/dose; repeat as needed to maintain serum osmolality <300-320 mOsm/kg (Adelson, 2003; Broderick, 2007; Hegenbarth, 2008)

Additional indications: I.V.: Children ≥12 years: Refer to adult dosing.

Renal Impairment Contraindicated in severe renal impairment. Use caution in patients with underlying renal disease.

Hepatic Impairment No adjustment required.

Administration

I.V. Vesicant; avoid extravasation. Do not administer with blood. Crenation and agglutination of red blood cells may occur if administered with whole blood. Inspect for crystals prior to administration. If crystals present redissolve by warming solution. Use filter-type administration set for infusion solutions containing mannitol ≥20%. For cerebral edema or elevated ICP, administer over 20-30 minutes.

Other

Inhalation (Aridol™): Administer using supplied single patient use inhaler; do not puncture capsule more than once; do not swallow capsules. A nose clip may be used if preferred. The patient should exhale completely, followed by a controlled rapid deep inspiration from the device; hold breath for 5 seconds and exhale through the mouth. Measure FEV_1 in duplicate 60 seconds after inhalation; repeat process until positive response or full dose (635 mg) has been administered.

Irrigation: Administer using only the appropriate transurethral urologic instrumentation.

Monitoring and Teaching Issues

Laboratory Monitoring Renal function, serum electrolytes, serum and urine osmolality. For treatment of elevated intracranial pressure, maintain serum osmolality <300-320 mOsm/kg.

Physical Assessment Assess for adequate renal function and urine flow prior to administration. Infusion site must be closely monitored for extravasation; this is a vesicant. Renal and cardiovascular status should be monitored during infusion. Monitor for circulatory overload, CHF, rash, and water intoxication.

Patient Education Report immediately any nausea, dizziness, respiratory difficulty, chest pain, or pain at infusion site.

◆ **Mapap® [OTC]** *see* Acetaminophen *on page* 38

◆ **Mapap® Arthritis Pain [OTC]** *see* Acetaminophen *on page* 38

◆ **Mapap® Children's [OTC]** *see* Acetaminophen *on page* 38

◆ **Mapap® Extra Strength [OTC]** *see* Acetaminophen *on page* 38

◆ **Mapap® Infant's [OTC]** *see* Acetaminophen *on page* 38

◆ **Mapap® Junior Rapid Tabs [OTC]** *see* Acetaminophen *on page* 38

Maraviroc (mah RAV er rock)

U.S. Brand Names Selzentry™

Index Terms UK-427,857

Generic Availability (U.S.) No

Pharmacologic Category Antiretroviral Agent, CCR5 Antagonist

Medication Guide Available Yes

Pregnancy Risk Factor B

Lactation Excretion in breast milk unknown/contraindicated

Use Treatment of CCR5-tropic HIV-1 infection, in combination with other antiretroviral agents

Mechanism of Action/Effect Inhibits CCR5-tropic HIV-1 virus from entering into CD4 cells

Contraindications Patients with severe renal impairment (Cl_{cr} <30 mL/minute) or end-stage renal disease (ESRD) who are taking potent CYP3A4 inhibitors or inducers

Warnings/Precautions [U.S. Boxed Warning] Possible drug-induced hepatotoxicity with allergic type features has been reported; hepatotoxicity may be preceded by allergic type reactions (eg, pruritic rash, eosinophilia, or increased IgE) and/or hepatic adverse events (transaminase increases or signs/symptoms of hepatitis); immediately evaluate patients with signs and symptoms of allergic reaction or hepatitis. Consider discontinuation in any patient with possible hepatitis or with elevated transaminases combined with systemic allergic events. Patients may develop immune reconstitution syndrome resulting in the occurrence of an inflammatory response to an indolent or residual opportunistic infection; further evaluation and treatment may be required. Monitor closely for signs/symptoms of developing infections; use associated with a small increase of certain upper respiratory tract infections and herpes virus infections during clinical trials. Use with caution in patients with cardiovascular disease or cardiac risk factors. During trials, a small increase in cardiovascular events (myocardial ischemia and/or infarction) occurred in treated patients compared to placebo, although a contributory relationship relative to therapy is unknown. Symptomatic postural hypotension has occurred; use caution in patients at risk for postural hypotension due to concomitant medication or history of condition. Adjust dose in patients with severe renal dysfunction if postural hypotension experienced.

Use caution in patients with mild-to-moderate hepatic impairment; maraviroc concentrations are increased; no dosage adjustment recommended. Maraviroc concentrations are further increased in patients with moderate hepatic impairment receiving concomitant strong CYP3A inhibitors; monitor closely for adverse events. Renal impairment may increase maraviroc concentrations. Use with caution in patients with mild-to-moderate renal impairment. Use with caution in patients taking strong CYP3A4/P-glycoprotein inhibitors and moderate or strong CYP3A4/P-glycoprotein inducers; may require dosage adjustments; avoid concurrent use in severe renal dysfunction (Cl_{cr} <30 mL/minute). Prior to therapy, tropism testing should be performed for presence of CCR5-tropic only virus HIV-1 infection. Therapy not recommended for use in patients with CXCR4- or dual/mixed tropic HIV-1 infection; efficacy not demonstrated in this population. In studies with treatment-naive patients, virologic failure and emergent lamivudine resistance was more common in maraviroc-treated patients compared to patients receiving efavirenz.

Drug Interactions

Metabolism/Transport Effects Substrate of CYP3A4 (major), P-glycoprotein

Avoid Concomitant Use

Avoid concomitant use of Maraviroc with any of the following: St Johns Wort

Decreased Effect

The levels/effects of Maraviroc may be decreased by: CYP3A4 Inducers (Strong); Deferasirox; St Johns Wort

Increased Effect/Toxicity

The levels/effects of Maraviroc may be increased by: CYP3A4 Inhibitors (Moderate); CYP3A4 Inhibitors (Strong); Dasatinib

Nutritional/Ethanol Interactions Herb/Nutraceutical: St. John's wort may decrease maraviroc concentrations leading to loss of therapeutic efficacy and potentially increased risk of resistance; concomitant use not recommended.

Adverse Reactions

>10%:

- Central nervous system: Fever (13%)
- Dermatologic: Rash (11%)
- Respiratory: Upper respiratory tract infection (23%), cough (14%)

2% to 10%:

- Cardiovascular: Vascular hypertensive disorder (3%)
- Central nervous system: Dizziness (9%; including postural dizziness), insomnia (8%), anxiety (4%), consciousness disturbances (4%), depression (4%), pain (4%)
- Dermatologic: Folliculitis (4%), pruritus (4%), skin neoplasms (benign; 3%), erythema (2%)
- Endocrine & metabolic: Lipodystrophy (3%)
- Gastrointestinal: Appetite disorders (8%), constipation (6%)
- Genitourinary: Urinary tract/bladder symptoms (3% to 5%), genital warts (2%)
- Hematologic: Neutropenia (grades 3/4: 4%)
- Hepatic: Transaminases increased (grades 3/4: 3% to 5%), bilirubin increased (grades 3/4: 6%)
- Neuromuscular & skeletal: Joint disorders (7%), paresthesia (5%), peripheral neuropathy (4%), sensory abnormality (4%), muscle pain (3%)
- Ocular: Conjunctivitis (2%), infection/inflammation (2%)
- Otic: Otitis media (2%)
- Respiratory: Bronchitis (7%), sinusitis (7%), respiratory tract/sinus disorder (3% to 6%), breathing abnormality (4%)
- Miscellaneous: Herpes infection (8%), sweat gland disturbances (5%), influenza (2%)

Pharmacodynamics/Kinetics

Bioavailability 23% to 33%

Time to Peak Plasma: 0.5-4 hours

Protein Binding ~76%

Half-Life Elimination 14-18 hours

Metabolism Hepatic, via CYP3A to inactive metabolites

Excretion Urine (~20%, 8% as unchanged drug); feces (76%, 25% as unchanged drug)

Available Dosage Forms

Tablet, oral:

Selzentry™: 150 mg, 300 mg

Dosing

Adult HIV treatment: Oral: 300 mg twice daily

Dosage adjustment for concomitant CYP3A4 inhibitors/inducers:

CYP3A inhibitors (with or without a CYP3A4 inducer): 150 mg twice daily; dose recommended when maraviroc administered concomitantly with strong CYP3A inhibitors including (but not limited to) protease inhibitors (excluding tipranavir/ritonavir), delavirdine, ketoconazole, itraconazole, clarithromycin, nefazodone, and telithromycin.

CYP3A inducers (without a strong CYP3A4 inhibitor): 600 mg twice daily; dose recommended when maraviroc administered concomitantly with CYP3A inducers including (but not limited to) efavirenz, etravirine, rifampin, carbamazepine, phenobarbital, and phenytoin

Pediatric HIV treatment: Oral: Adolescents ≥16 years: Refer to adult dosing.

Renal Impairment

Cl_{cr} ≥30 mL/minute:

Cl_{cr} ≥30 mL/minute and concomitant potent CYP3A4 inhibitors (with or without a CYP3A4 inducer): 150 mg twice daily.

Cl_{cr} ≥30 mL/minute and concomitant potent CYP3A4 inducer (without a CYP3A4 inhibitor): 600 mg twice daily.

Cl_{cr} ≥30 mL/minute and concomitant medications (eg, tipranavir/ritonavir, nevirapine, raltegravir, all NRTIs, and enfuvirtide): 300 mg twice daily.

Cl_{cr} <30 mL/minute:

Cl_{cr} <30 mL/minute or ESRD and concomitant potent CYP3A4 inhibitors (with or without a CYP3A4 inducer) or concomitant potent CYP3A inducer (without a CYP3A4 inhibitor): Not recommended.

Cl_{cr} <30 mL/minute or ESRD and concomitant medications (eg, tipranavir/ritonavir, nevirapine, raltegravir, all NRTIs, and enfuvirtide): 300 mg twice daily. If postural hypotension occurs, reduce dose to 150 mg twice daily.

Cl_{cr} <30 mL/minute and experiencing postural hypotension: Reduce dose to 150 mg twice daily.

Hemodialysis has minimal effect on clearance.

Hepatic Impairment

Mild-to-moderate impairment: Use caution; maraviroc concentrations are increased although dosage adjustment is not recommended.

Moderate impairment (with concomitant strong CYP3A4 inhibitor): Use caution; monitor closely for adverse events.

Severe impairment: Patient population has not been studied.

Administration

Oral Administer without regards to meals.

Stability

Storage Store at 25°C (77°F); excursions permitted to 15°C to 30°C (59°F to 86°F).

Monitoring and Teaching Issues

Laboratory Monitoring Viral load, CD4 count, transaminases; tropism testing (prior to initiation)

Physical Assessment Evaluate renal or hepatic impairment, cardiovascular disease, and cardiac risk factors prior to prescribing. Evaluate viral load, CD4 count, and transaminase levels. Monitor for cardiotoxicity, hepatotoxicity, hypotension, dizziness, insomnia, and rash periodically during therapy. Teach patient proper timing of multiple medications.

Patient Education You will be provided with a medication guide with each prescription. This drug will not cure HIV, nor has it been found to reduce transmission of HIV; use appropriate precautions to prevent spread to other persons. This drug is prescribed as one part of a multidrug combination; take exactly as directed for full course of therapy. May be taken with or without food. Maintain adequate hydration unless advised by prescriber to restrict fluids. May cause dizziness, insomnia, constipation, or muscle or joint pain. Report skin rash, persistent muscle pain, unusual cough, fever, cold symptoms, abdominal pain, yellow eyes or skin, or fatigue.

Dietary Considerations May be taken without regards to meals.

Breast-Feeding Considerations In infants born to mothers who are HIV positive, HAART while breast-feeding may decrease postnatal infection. However, maternal or infant antiretroviral therapy does not completely eliminate the risk of postnatal HIV transmission. In addition, multiclass-resistant virus has been detected in breast-feeding infants despite maternal therapy.

In the United States where formula is accessible, affordable, safe, and sustainable, complete avoidance of breast-feeding by HIV-infected women is recommended to decrease potential transmission of HIV.

Pregnancy Considerations Adverse fetal effects were not observed in animal studies. There are no adequate and well-controlled studies in pregnant women and available data is insufficient to recommend use in pregnancy. An antiretroviral registry has been established to monitor maternal and fetal outcomes in women receiving antiretroviral drugs. Healthcare providers are encouraged to enroll pregnant women exposed to antiretroviral medications in the Antiretroviral Pregnancy Registry (1-800-258-4263 or www.APRegistry.com). Healthcare providers caring for HIV-infected women and their infants may contact the National Perinatal HIV Hotline (888-448-8765) for clinical consultation.

Additional Information Maraviroc should only be used in patients with documented CCR5-tropic only virus; if it is used in mixed tropism patients, eg, with CCR5-tropic and CXCR4-tropic, the CCR5-tropic virus will be suppressed and the CXCR4-tropic virus will continue to proliferate. If a patient is receiving a stable antiretroviral regimen and their viral loads are undetectable, no routine, validated test currently exists to evaluate viral status and potential success of maraviroc therapy (DHHS, 2011).

- ◆ **Marcaine®** *see* Bupivacaine *on page 244*
- ◆ **Marcaine® Spinal** *see* Bupivacaine *on page 244*
- ◆ **Mar-Cof® CG** *see* Guaifenesin and Codeine *on page 891*
- ◆ **Margesic** *see* Butalbital, Acetaminophen, and Caffeine *on page 260*
- ◆ **Margesic® H** *see* Hydrocodone and Acetaminophen *on page 915*
- ◆ **Marinol®** *see* Dronabinol *on page 590*
- ◆ **Matulane®** *see* Procarbazine *on page 1510*
- ◆ **Matzim™ LA** *see* Diltiazem *on page 536*
- ◆ **Mavik®** *see* Trandolapril *on page 1800*
- ◆ **Maxalt®** *see* Rizatriptan *on page 1603*
- ◆ **Maxalt-MLT®** *see* Rizatriptan *on page 1603*
- ◆ **Maxidex®** *see* Dexamethasone (Ophthalmic) *on page 503*
- ◆ **Maxidone®** *see* Hydrocodone and Acetaminophen *on page 915*
- ◆ **Maxipime®** *see* Cefepime *on page 318*
- ◆ **Maxzide®** *see* Hydrochlorothiazide and Triamterene *on page 914*
- ◆ **Maxzide®-25** *see* Hydrochlorothiazide and Triamterene *on page 914*
- ◆ **3M™ Cavilon™ Antifungal [OTC]** *see* Miconazole (Topical) *on page 1224*
- ◆ **MCV** *see* Meningococcal (Groups A / C / Y and W-135) Diphtheria Conjugate Vaccine *on page 1168*
- ◆ **MCV4** *see* Meningococcal (Groups A / C / Y and W-135) Diphtheria Conjugate Vaccine *on page 1168*
- ◆ **MDL 73,147EF** *see* Dolasetron *on page 567*
- ◆ **ME-609** *see* Acyclovir and Hydrocortisone *on page 48*

Measles, Mumps, and Rubella Virus Vaccine

(MEE zels, mumpz & roo BEL a VYE rus vak SEEN)

U.S. Brand Names M-M-R® II

Index Terms MMR; Mumps, Measles and Rubella Vaccines; Rubella, Measles and Mumps Vaccines

Generic Availability (U.S.) No

Pharmacologic Category Vaccine, Live (Viral)

Medication Safety Issues

Sound-alike/look-alike issues:

MMR (measles, mumps and rubella virus vaccine) may be confused with MMRV (measles, mumps, rubella, and varicella) vaccine

Pregnancy Risk Factor C

Lactation

Measles/mumps: Excretion in breast milk unknown/use caution

Rubella: Enters breast milk/use caution

Use Measles, mumps, and rubella prophylaxis

The Advisory Committee on Immunization Practices (ACIP) recommends routine vaccination for the following:

- All children (first dose given at 12-15 months of age)
- Adults born 1957 or later (without evidence of immunity or documentation of vaccination).
- Adults at higher risk for exposure to and transmission of measles mumps and rubella should receive special consideration for vaccination, unless an acceptable evidence of immunity exists. This includes international travelers, persons attending colleges and other post-high school education, persons working in healthcare facilities.

Available Dosage Forms

Injection, powder for reconstitution [preservative free]:

M-M-R® II: Measles virus ≥1000 $TCID_{50}$, mumps virus ≥20,000 $TCID_{50}$, and rubella virus ≥1000 $TCID_{50}$

Dosing

Adult

Immunization: SubQ: 0.5 mL

Birth year in or after 1957 without evidence of immunity: 1 or 2 doses (0.5 mL/dose); minimum interval between doses is 28 days

Adults born in or after 1957 without documentation of live vaccine on or after first birthday, or without physician-diagnosed measles or mumps, or without laboratory evidence of immunity, should be vaccinated with at least one dose; a second dose, separated by no less than 1 month, is indicated for those previously vaccinated with one dose of measles vaccine, students entering institutions of higher learning, recently exposed in an outbreak setting, healthcare workers at time of employment, and for travelers to endemic areas (CDC, 1998).

Persons vaccinated between 1963 and 1967 with a killed measles vaccine, followed by live vaccine within 3 months, or with a vaccine of unknown type should be revaccinated with live measles virus vaccine (CDC, 1998).

Women of childbearing potential, without documentation of rubella immunity, regardless of birth year, should also receive one dose of vaccine. Do not administer rubella to women who are or who may become pregnant within 1 month of receiving vaccine; administer following completion or termination of pregnancy (CDC, 1998).

Healthcare personnel (unvaccinated) born prior to 1957 and who are without laboratory evidence of measles, mumps and/or rubella immunity or laboratory confirmation of disease: Consider 2 doses of MMR vaccine at the appropriate interval. Two doses of the MMR vaccine are needed for measles and mumps, one dose is needed for rubella (CDC, 2006).

Pediatric

Immunization: SubQ: *Children ≥12 months:* 0.5 mL

Primary immunization is recommended at 12-15 months of age and repeated at 4-6 years of age; the second dose is recommended prior to elementary school. If the second dose was not received, the schedule should be completed by the 11- to 12-year old visit. (The second dose may be administered at any time provided at least 4 weeks have elapsed since the first dose.) For older children not previously vaccinated, at least 28 days should elapse between doses (CDC, 1998).

Measles outbreak: SubQ:

Infants 6-11 months: If there is risk of exposure to measles, single-antigen measles vaccine should be administered. If single-antigen vaccine is not readily available, MMR is an acceptable alternative. Children should be revaccinated at ≥12 months with standard 2-dose series (CDC, 1998).

Children ≥12 months: Revaccination with MMR is recommended for attendees and siblings of daycare facilities or schools if they cannot provide adequate documentation of 2 previous doses of a measles-containing vaccine after their first birthday or evidence of measles immunity (CDC, 1998).

Mumps outbreak: SubQ: *Children ≥12 months:* During a mumps outbreak, children ages 1-4 years should consider a second dose of a live mumps virus vaccine; minimum interval between doses is 28 days (CDC, 2006).

Administration

I.V. Not for I.V. administration.

Other Administer SubQ in outer aspect of the upper arm in patients ≥12 months

Simultaneous administration of vaccines helps ensure the patients will be fully vaccinated by the appropriate age. Simultaneous administration of vaccines is defined as administering >1 vaccine on the same day at different anatomic sites. The use of licensed combination vaccines is generally preferred over separate injections of the equivalent components. Separate vaccines should not be combined in the same syringe unless indicated by product specific labeling. Separate needles and syringes should be used for each injection. The ACIP prefers each dose of a specific vaccine in a series come from the same manufacturer when possible. Adolescents and adults should be vaccinated while seated or lying down. In general, preterm infants should be vaccinated at the same chronological age as full-term infants (CDC, 2011).

Antipyretics have not been shown to prevent febrile seizures. Antipyretics may be used to treat fever or discomfort following vaccination (CDC, 2011). One study reported that routine prophylactic administration of acetaminophen to prevent fever prior to vaccination decreased the immune response of some vaccines; the clinical significance of this reduction in immune response has not been established (Prymula, 2009).

Monitoring and Teaching Issues

Physical Assessment Federal law requires entry into the patient's medical record.

Related Information

Immunization Recommendations *on page 1941*

Measles, Mumps, Rubella, and Varicella Virus Vaccine

(MEE zels, mumpz, roo BEL a, & var i SEL a VYE rus vak SEEN)

U.S. Brand Names ProQuad®

Index Terms MMR-V; MMRV; Mumps, Rubella, Varicella, and Measles Vaccine; Rubella, Varicella, Measles, and Mumps Vaccine; Varicella, Measles, Mumps, and Rubella Vaccine

Generic Availability (U.S.) No

Pharmacologic Category Vaccine, Live (Viral)

Pregnancy Risk Factor C

Lactation

Measles, mumps, varicella: Excretion in breast milk unknown/use caution

Rubella: Enters breast milk/use caution

Use To provide simultaneous active immunization against measles, mumps, rubella, and varicella

The Advisory Committee on Immunization Practices (ACIP) recommends routine vaccination against measles, mumps, rubella, and varicella in healthy children 12 months to 12 years of age. For children receiving their first dose at 12-47 months of age, either the MMRV combination vaccine or separate MMR and varicella vaccines can be used. (The ACIP prefers administration of separate MMR and varicella vaccines as the first dose in this age group unless the parent or caregiver expresses preference for the MMRV combination.) For children receiving the first dose at ≥48 months or their second dose at any age, use of MMRV is preferred.

Canadian labeling (not in U.S. labeling): MMRV combination vaccine is approved for use in healthy children 9 months to 6 years; may consider use in healthy children ≤12 years of age based upon prior experience with the separate component (live-attenuated MMR or live-attenuated varicella [OKA-strain]) vaccines.

Available Dosage Forms

Injection, powder for reconstitution [preservative free]:

ProQuad®: Measles virus ≥3.00 $\log_{10}$ $TCID_{50}$, mumps virus ≥4.30 $\log_{10}$ $TCID_{50}$, rubella virus ≥3.00 $\log_{10}$ $TCID_{50}$, and varicella virus ≥3.99 $\log_{10}$ PFU

Dosing

Pediatric Immunization:

U.S. labeling: Children 12 months to 12 years: SubQ: One dose (0.5 mL). The first dose is usually administered at 12-15 months of age. If a second dose of measles, mumps, rubella, and varicella vaccine is needed, ProQuad® can be used with the second dose usually administered at 4-6 years of age. (The second dose may be administered before age 4 if needed, as long as ≥3 months have elapsed since the first dose.)

Administer on or after the first birthday, as soon as child becomes eligible for vaccination. It may be used whenever all components of the vaccine are needed in children within this age group. (Refer to current CDC Recommended Immunization Schedule)

ACIP recommendations: For children receiving their first dose at 12-47 months of age, either the MMRV combination vaccine or separate MMR and varicella vaccines can be used. (The ACIP prefers administration of separate MMR and varicella vaccines as the first dose in this age group unless the parent or caregiver expresses preference for the MMRV combination.) For children receiving the first dose at ≥48 months or their second dose at any age, use of MMRV is preferred. The ACIP recommends that children with a personal or family history of seizures be vaccinated with separate MMR and varicella vaccines, as opposed to the MMRV combination vaccine (CDC, 2010).

Canadian labeling: I.M., SubQ: Children 9 months to 6 years: Two doses (0.5 mL each dose) administered at least 4-6 weeks apart (minimum interval between doses: 4 weeks)

Administration

Other Disinfectants (eg, alcohol) may inactivate the attenuated viruses in the vaccine. Allow disinfectant adequate time to evaporate from skin prior to administration.

U.S labeling: For SubQ injection only; inject in the outer aspect of the deltoid region of the upper arm or in the higher anterolateral area of the thigh. Administer immediately following reconstitution.

Canadian labeling: For SubQ or I.M. injection only; inject in the deltoid region of upper arm. Do not administer by I.M. injection in patients with bleeding disorders.

Note: The Canadian labeling states that Priorix-Tetra™ (MMRV) may be given simultaneously (at different injection sites) with the combination vaccine Infanrix-hexa™ (contains diphtheria-tetanus-acellular pertussis-hepatitis B-inactivated polio virus-*Haemophilus* influenzae type B [DTaP-HBV-IPV/Hib]) and with monovalent vaccines DTaP, Hib, IPV, HBV.

Simultaneous administration of vaccines helps ensure the patients will be fully vaccinated by the appropriate age. Simultaneous administration of vaccines is defined as administering >1 vaccine on the same day at different anatomic sites. The use of licensed combination vaccines is generally preferred over separate injections of the equivalent components. Separate vaccines should not be combined in the same syringe unless indicated by product specific labeling. Separate needles and syringes should be used for each injection. The ACIP prefers each dose of a specific vaccine in a series come from the same manufacturer when possible. Adolescents and adults should be vaccinated while seated or lying down. In general, preterm infants should be vaccinated at the same chronological age as full-term infants (CDC, 2011).

Antipyretics have not been shown to prevent febrile seizures. Antipyretics may be used to treat fever or discomfort following vaccination (CDC, 2011). One study reported that routine prophylactic administration of acetaminophen to prevent fever prior to vaccination decreased the immune response of some vaccines; the clinical significance of this reduction in immune response has not been established (Prymula, 2009).

Monitoring and Teaching Issues

Physical Assessment Assess hypersensitivity history and health status prior to administration. Treatment must be immediately available in event of anaphylactic or serious allergic reactions. Federal law requires entry into the patient's medical record.

Patient Education Children who are moderately-to-severely ill should not get this vaccination until they have recovered. You may experience fever; mild pain, redness, or swelling at injection site; headache; mild gastrointestinal upset; irritability; mild rash; or upper respiratory tract infection. Report immediately any severe reaction at injection site, any chills or fever, persistent diarrhea, or severe rash.

Related Information

Immunization Recommendations *on page 1941*

Mebendazole (me BEN da zole)

Index Terms Vermox

Generic Availability (U.S.) Yes

Pharmacologic Category Anthelmintic

Medication Safety Issues

Sound-alike/look-alike issues:

Mebendazole may be confused with metroNIDAZOLE

Pregnancy Risk Factor C

Lactation Excretion in breast milk unknown/use caution

Use Treatment of *Enterobius vermicularis* (pinworms), *Trichuris trichiura* (whipworms), *Ascaris lumbricoides* (roundworms), and *Ancylostoma duodenale* or *Necator amiericanus* (hookworms)

Unlabeled/Investigational Use Treatment of *Ancylostoma caninum* (eosinophilic enterocolitis), *Capillaria philippinensis* (capillariasis), *Giardia duodenalis* (giardiasis), *Mansonella perstans* (filariasis), visceral larva migrans (toxocariasis)

Available Dosage Forms

Tablet, chewable, oral: 100 mg

Dosing

Adult & Geriatric

***Ancylostoma duodenale* (hookworm), *Necator americanus* (hookworm):** 100 mg twice daily for 3 days **or** (unlabeled dosing) 500 mg as a single dose

***Ascaris lumbricoides* (roundworm):** 100 mg twice daily for 3 days **or** (unlabeled dosing) 500 mg as a single dose

***Enterobius vermicularis* (pinworm):** 100 mg as a single dose; may repeat in 2-3 weeks; treatment should include family members in close contact with patient

***Trichuris trichiura* (whipworm):** 100 mg twice daily for 3 days **or** (unlabeled dosing) 500 mg as a single dose

***Ancylostoma caninum* (unlabeled use):** 100 mg twice daily for 3 days

***Capillaria philippinensis* (capillariasis) (unlabeled use):** 200 mg twice daily for 20 days

***Giardia duodenalis* (giardiasis) (unlabeled use):** 200 mg three times a day for 5 days (Canete, 2006; Chandy, 2009)

***Mansonella perstans* (filariasis) (unlabeled use):** 100 mg twice daily for 30 days

Visceral larva migrans (toxocariasis) (unlabeled use): 100-200 mg twice daily for 5 days

Pediatric Children ≥2 years: Refer to adult dosing.

Administration

Oral Tablets may be chewed, swallowed whole, or crushed and mixed with food.

Monitoring and Teaching Issues

Laboratory Monitoring Check for helminth ova in feces within 3-4 weeks following the initial therapy. Periodically assess hematologic and hepatic function.

Physical Assessment Since worm infestations are easily transmitted, all persons sharing same household should be treated. Teach transmission prevention.

Patient Education Tablets may be chewed, swallowed whole, or crushed and mixed with food. Increase dietary intake of fruit juices. All family members and close friends should also be treated. To reduce possibility of reinfection, wash hands and scrub nails carefully with soap and hot water before handling food, before eating, and before and after toileting. Keep hands out of mouth. Disinfect toilet daily and launder bed linens, undergarments, and nightclothes daily with hot water and soap. Do not go barefoot and do not sit directly on grass or ground. May cause abdominal pain, nausea, vomiting, or hair loss (reversible). Report skin rash or itching, unusual fatigue or sore throat, unresolved diarrhea or vomiting, or CNS changes.

Meclizine (MEK li zeen)

U.S. Brand Names Antivert®; Bonine® [OTC]; Dramamine® Less Drowsy Formula [OTC]; Medi-Meclizine [OTC]; Trav-L-Tabs® [OTC]

Index Terms Meclizine Hydrochloride; Meclozine Hydrochloride

Generic Availability (U.S.) Yes

Pharmacologic Category Antiemetic; Histamine H_1 Antagonist; Histamine H_1 Antagonist, First Generation; Piperazine Derivative

Medication Safety Issues

Sound-alike/look-alike issues:

Antivert® may be confused with Anzemet®, Axert®

Pregnancy Risk Factor B

Lactation Excretion in breast milk unknown/not recommended

Use Prevention and treatment of symptoms of motion sickness; management of vertigo with diseases affecting the vestibular system

Mechanism of Action/Effect Has central anticholinergic action by blocking chemoreceptor trigger zone; decreases excitability of the middle ear labyrinth and blocks conduction in the middle ear vestibular-cerebellar pathways

Contraindications Hypersensitivity to meclizine or any component of the formulation

Warnings/Precautions Use with caution in patients with asthma, angle-closure glaucoma, prostatic hyperplasia, pyloric or duodenal obstruction, or bladder neck obstruction. Elderly may be at risk for anticholinergic side effects such as glaucoma, prostatic hyperplasia, constipation, GI obstructive disease. If vertigo does not respond in 1-2 weeks, it is advised to discontinue use. May be sedating, use with caution in disorders where CNS depression is a feature; patients must be cautioned about performing tasks which require mental alertness (eg, operating machinery or driving). Effects may be potentiated when used with other sedative drugs or ethanol.

Drug Interactions

Avoid Concomitant Use There are no known interactions where it is recommended to avoid concomitant use.

Decreased Effect

Meclizine may decrease the levels/effects of: Acetylcholinesterase Inhibitors (Central); Benzylpenicilloyl Polylysine; Betahistine

The levels/effects of Meclizine may be decreased by: Acetylcholinesterase Inhibitors (Central); Amphetamines

Increased Effect/Toxicity

Meclizine may increase the levels/effects of: Alcohol (Ethyl); Anticholinergics; CNS Depressants

The levels/effects of Meclizine may be increased by: Droperidol; Pramlintide

Nutritional/Ethanol Interactions Ethanol: Avoid ethanol (may increase CNS depression).

Adverse Reactions

>10%:

Central nervous system: Slight to moderate drowsiness
Respiratory: Thickening of bronchial secretions

1% to 10%:

Central nervous system: Headache, fatigue, nervousness, dizziness
Gastrointestinal: Appetite increase, weight gain, nausea, diarrhea, abdominal pain, xerostomia
Respiratory: Pharyngitis

Pharmacodynamics/Kinetics

Onset of Action ~1 hour

Duration of Action 8-24 hours

Half-Life Elimination 6 hours

Metabolism Hepatic

Excretion Urine (as metabolites); feces (as unchanged drug)

Available Dosage Forms

Caplet, oral: 12.5 mg

Tablet, oral: 12.5 mg, 25 mg
Antivert®: 12.5 mg, 25 mg, 50 mg
Dramamine® Less Drowsy Formula [OTC]: 25 mg
Medi-Meclizine [OTC]: 25 mg
Trav-L-Tabs® [OTC]: 25 mg

Tablet, chewable, oral: 25 mg
Bonine® [OTC]: 25 mg

Dosing

Adult & Geriatric

Motion sickness: Oral: 12.5-25 mg 1 hour before travel, repeat dose every 12-24 hours if needed; doses up to 50 mg may be needed

Vertigo: Oral: 25-100 mg/day in divided doses

Pediatric Children >12 years: Refer to adult dosing.

Monitoring and Teaching Issues

Patient Education Avoid alcohol. You may experience dizziness, drowsiness, blurred vision, dry mouth, constipation, or heat intolerance. Report CNS change (hallucination, confusion, nervousness), sudden or unusual weight gain, unresolved nausea or diarrhea, chest pain or palpitations, muscle pain, or changes in urinary pattern.

Geriatric Considerations Due to anticholinergic action, use lowest dose in divided doses to avoid side effects and their inconvenience. Limit use if possible. May cause confusion or aggravate symptoms of confusion in those with dementia. If vertigo does not respond in 1-2 weeks, discontinue use.

Pregnancy Considerations No data available on crossing the placenta. Probably no effect on the fetus (insufficient data). Available evidence suggests safe use during pregnancy.

◆ **Meclizine Hydrochloride** *see* Meclizine *on page* 1153

◆ **Meclozine Hydrochloride** *see* Meclizine *on page* 1153

◆ **Medi-First® Sinus Decongestant [OTC]** *see* Phenylephrine (Systemic) *on page* 1449

◆ **Medi-Meclizine [OTC]** *see* Meclizine *on page* 1153

◆ **Medi-Phenyl [OTC]** *see* Phenylephrine (Systemic) *on page* 1449

◆ **Mediproxen [OTC]** *see* Naproxen *on page* 1289

◆ **Medrol®** *see* MethylPREDNISolone *on page* 1208

◆ **Medrol Dose Pack** *see* MethylPREDNISolone *on page* 1208

◆ **Medrol® Dosepak™** *see* MethylPREDNISolone *on page* 1208

MedroxyPROGESTERone (me DROKS ee proe JES te rone)

U.S. Brand Names Depo-Provera®; Depo-Provera® Contraceptive; depo-subQ provera 104®; Provera®

Index Terms Acetoxymethylprogesterone; Medroxyprogesterone Acetate; Methylacetoxyprogesterone; MPA

Generic Availability (U.S.) Yes

Pharmacologic Category Contraceptive; Progestin

Medication Safety Issues

Sound-alike/look-alike issues:

Depo-Provera® may be confused with depo-subQ provera 104™

depo-subQ provera 104™ may be confused with Depo-Provera®

MedroxyPROGESTERone may be confused with hydroxyprogesterone caproate, methylPREDNISolone, methylTESTOSTERone

Provera® may be confused with Covera®, Femara®, Parlodel®, Premarin®, Proscar®, PROzac®

The injection dosage form is available in different formulations. Carefully review prescriptions to assure the correct formulation and route of administration.

Pregnancy Risk Factor X

Lactation Enters breast milk

Use Secondary amenorrhea or abnormal uterine bleeding due to hormonal imbalance; reduction of endometrial hyperplasia in nonhysterectomized postmenopausal women receiving conjugated estrogens; prevention of pregnancy; management of endometriosis-associated pain; adjunctive therapy and palliative treatment of recurrent and metastatic endometrial carcinoma

Unlabeled/Investigational Use Treatment of low-grade endometrial stromal sarcoma

Mechanism of Action/Effect Inhibits secretion of pituitary gonadotropins, which prevents follicular maturation and ovulation; causes endometrial thinning

Contraindications Hypersensitivity to medroxyprogesterone or any component of the formulation; history of or current thrombophlebitis or venous thromboembolic disorders (including DVT, PE); cerebral vascular disease; severe hepatic dysfunction or disease; carcinoma of the breast or other estrogen- or progesterone-dependent neoplasia; undiagnosed vaginal bleeding; missed abortion, diagnostic test for pregnancy, pregnancy

Warnings/Precautions **[U.S. Boxed Warning]: Prolonged use of medroxyprogesterone contraceptive injection may result in a loss of bone mineral density (BMD). It is not known if use during adolescence or early adulthood will decrease peak bone mass accretion or increase the risk for osteoporotic fractures later in life. Loss is related to the duration of use, may not be completely reversible on discontinuation of the drug,** and incidence is not significantly different between the SubQ and I.M. dosage forms. The impact on peak bone mass in adolescents should be weighed against the potential for unintended pregnancies in treatment decision. Consider alternative contraceptive methods in patients at risk for osteoporosis (eg, metabolic bone disease, family history of osteoporosis, chronic use of medications associated with osteoporosis such as corticosteroids). **[U.S. Boxed Warning]: Long-term use (ie, >2 years) should be limited to situations where other birth control methods are inadequate.** Consider other methods of birth control in women with (or at risk for) osteoporosis. **[U.S. Boxed Warning]: Inform patients that injectable contraceptives do not protect against HIV infection or other sexually-transmitted diseases.** When used for contraception, the possibility of ectopic pregnancy should be considered in patients with abdominal pain. Anaphylaxis or anaphylactoid reactions have been reported with use of the injection; medication for the treatment of hypersensitivity reactions should be available for immediate use.

[U.S. Boxed Warning]: Estrogens with or without progestin should not be used to prevent coronary heart disease. Use caution with cardiovascular disease or dysfunction. MPA used in combination with estrogen may increase the risks of hypertension, myocardial infarction (MI), stroke, pulmonary emboli (PE), and deep vein thrombosis; incidence of these effects was shown to be significantly increased in postmenopausal women using conjugated equine estrogens (CEE) in combination with MPA.

[U.S. Boxed Warning]: The risk of dementia may be increased in postmenopausal women; increased incidence was observed in women ≥65 years of age taking MPA in combination with CEE. An increased risk of invasive breast cancer was observed in postmenopausal women using MPA in combination with CEE. An increase in abnormal mammograms has also been reported with estrogen and progestin therapy. Use is contraindicated in patients with known or suspected breast cancer, Whenever possible, progestins in combination with estrogens should be discontinued at least 4-6 weeks prior to surgeries associated with an increased risk of thromboembolism or during periods of prolonged immobilization. If thrombosis develops with contraceptive treatment, discontinue treatment (unless no other acceptable contraceptive alternative). Progestins used in combination with estrogen should be used for shortest duration possible consistent with treatment goals. Conduct periodic risk:benefit assessments.

Discontinue pending examination in cases of sudden partial or complete vision loss, sudden onset of proptosis, diplopia, or migraine; discontinue permanently if papilledema or retinal vascular lesions are observed on examination. Use with caution in patients with diseases that may be exacerbated by fluid retention (including asthma, epilepsy, migraine, cardiac, or renal dysfunction). Contraceptive therapy with medroxyprogesterone commonly results in an average weight gain of ~2.5 kg after 1 year and ~3.7 kg after 2 years of treatment. Use caution with history of depression.

May have adverse effects on glucose tolerance; use caution in women with diabetes. MPA is extensively metabolized in the liver. Discontinue if jaundice develops or if acute or chronic hepatic disturbances occur. Use is contraindicated with severe hepatic disease. Unscheduled bleeding/spotting may occur. Presentation of irregular, unresolving vaginal bleeding following previously regular cycles warrants further evaluation including endometrial sampling, if indicated, to rule out malignancy. Not for use prior to menarche.

Drug Interactions

Metabolism/Transport Effects Substrate of CYP3A4 (major); **Induces** CYP3A4 (weak)

Avoid Concomitant Use

Avoid concomitant use of MedroxyPROGESTERone with any of the following: Griseofulvin

Decreased Effect

MedroxyPROGESTERone may decrease the levels/effects of: Saxagliptin; Vitamin K Antagonists

The levels/effects of MedroxyPROGESTERone may be decreased by: Acitretin; Aminoglutethimide; Aprepitant; Artemether; Barbiturates; Bile Acid Sequestrants; Bosentan; CarBAMazepine; CYP3A4 Inducers (Strong); Deferasirox; Felbamate; Fosaprepitant; Griseofulvin; LamoTRIgine; Mycophenolate; OXcarbazepine; Phenytoin; Retinoic Acid Derivatives; Rifamycin Derivatives; St Johns Wort; Topiramate

Increased Effect/Toxicity

MedroxyPROGESTERone may increase the levels/effects of: Benzodiazepines (metabolized by oxidation); Selegiline; Tranexamic Acid; Voriconazole

The levels/effects of MedroxyPROGESTERone may be increased by: Conivaptan; Herbs (Progestogenic Properties); Voriconazole

Nutritional/Ethanol Interactions

Ethanol: Avoid ethanol (may increase risk of osteoporosis).

Food: Bioavailability of the oral tablet is increased when taken with food; half-life is unchanged.

Herb/Nutraceutical: St John's wort may diminish the therapeutic effect of progestin contraceptives (contraceptive failure is possible).

Lab Interactions

The following tests may be decreased: Steroid levels (plasma and urinary), gonadotropin levels, SHBG concentration, T_3 uptake

The following tests may be increased: Protein-bound iodine, butanol extractable protein-bound iodine, Factors II, VII, VIII, IX, X

Pathologist should be advised of estrogen/progesterone therapy when specimens are submitted.

Adverse Reactions Adverse effects as reported with any dosage form; percent ranges presented are noted with the MPA I.M. contraceptive injection:

>5%:

Central nervous system: Dizziness, headache, nervousness

Endocrine & metabolic: Libido decreased, menstrual irregularities (includes bleeding, amenorrhea, or both)

Gastrointestinal: Abdominal pain/discomfort, weight gain (>10 lbs at 24 months: 38%)

1% to 5%:

Cardiovascular: Edema

Central nervous system: Depression, fatigue, insomnia

Dermatologic: Acne, alopecia, rash

Endocrine & metabolic: Breast pain, hot flashes

Gastrointestinal: Bloating, nausea

Genitourinary: Dysmenorrhea, leukorrhea, vaginitis

Local: Injection site reaction (SubQ administration): Atrophy, induration, pain

Neuromuscular & skeletal: Arthralgia, backache, leg cramp, weakness

<1%, postmarketing, and/or case reports: Allergic reaction, anaphylaxis, anaphylactoid reactions, anemia, angioedema, anxiety, appetite changes, asthma, axillary swelling, blood dyscrasia, body odor, BMD loss, breast cancer, breast changes, cervical cancer, chest pain, chills, chloasma, cholestatic jaundice, deep vein thrombosis, diaphoresis, diarrhea, drowsiness, dry skin, dyspareunia, dyspnea, facial palsy, fainting, fever, galactorrhea, genitourinary infections, glucose tolerance decreased, hirsutism, hoarseness, jaundice, lack of return to fertility, lactation decreased, libido increased, melasma, nipple bleeding, oligomenorrhea, optic neuritis, osteoporosis, osteoporotic fractures, paralysis, paresthesia, pruritus, pulmonary embolus, rectal bleeding, retinal thrombosis, scleroderma, seizure, somnolence, syncope, tachycardia, thirst, thrombophlebitis, urticaria, uterine hyperplasia, vaginal cysts, varicose veins

In addition: Depo-Provera® aqueous suspension: Residual lump, sterile abscess, or skin discoloration at the injection

Pharmacodynamics/Kinetics

Absorption Oral: Well absorbed; I.M.: Slow

Time to Peak Oral: 2-4 hours; I.M. (Depo-Provera® Contraceptive): ~3 weeks; SubQ: ~1 week

Protein Binding 86% to 90% primarily to albumin; does not bind to sex hormone-binding globulin

Half-Life Elimination Oral: 12-17 hours; I.M. (Depo-Provera® Contraceptive): ~50 days; SubQ: ~40 days

Metabolism Extensively hepatic via hydroxylation and conjugation; forms metabolites

Excretion Urine

Available Dosage Forms

Injection, suspension: 150 mg/mL (1 mL)

Depo-Provera®: 400 mg/mL (2.5 mL)

Depo-Provera® Contraceptive: 150 mg/mL (1 mL)

depo-subQ provera 104®: 104 mg/0.65 mL (0.65 mL)

Tablet, oral: 2.5 mg, 5 mg, 10 mg

Provera®: 2.5 mg, 5 mg, 10 mg

Dosing

Adult & Geriatric

Amenorrhea: Oral: 5-10 mg/day for 5-10 days

Abnormal uterine bleeding: Oral: 5-10 mg for 5-10 days starting on day 16 or 21 of cycle

Contraception:

Depo-Provera® Contraceptive: I.M.: 150 mg every 3 months

depo-subQ provera 104™: SubQ: 104 mg every 3 months (every 12-14 weeks)

Endometriosis (depo-subQ provera 104™): SubQ: 104 mg every 3 months (every 12-14 weeks)

Endometrial carcinoma, recurrent or metastatic (adjunctive/palliative treatment) (Depo-Provera®): I.M.: 400-1000 mg/week

Accompanying cyclic estrogen therapy, postmenopausal: Oral: 5-10 mg for 12-14 consecutive days each month, starting on day 1 or day 16 of the cycle; lower doses may be used if given with estrogen continuously throughout the cycle

Pediatric Adolescents:

Amenorrhea: Refer to adult dosing.

Abnormal uterine bleeding: Refer to adult dosing.

Contraception: Refer to adult dosing.

Endometriosis: Refer to adult dosing.

Hepatic Impairment Use is contraindicated with severe impairment. Discontinue with jaundice or if liver function disturbances occur. Consider lower dose or less frequent administration with mild-to-moderate impairment. Use of the contraceptive injection has not been studied in patients with hepatic impairment; consideration should be given to not readminister if jaundice develops

Administration

I.M. Depo-Provera® Contraceptive: Administer first dose during the first 5 days of menstrual period, or within the first 5 days postpartum if not breast-feeding, or at the sixth week postpartum if breast-feeding exclusively. Shake vigorously prior to administration. Administer by deep I.M. injection in the gluteal or deltoid muscle. When switching from combined hormonal contraceptives (estrogen plus progestin), the first injection should be on the day after the last active tablet or (at the latest) the day after the final inactive tablet. When switching from other contraceptive methods, ensure continuous contraceptive coverage.

Other SubQ: depo-subQ provera 104™: Administer first dose during the first 5 days of menstrual period, or at the sixth week postpartum if breast-feeding. Shake vigorously prior to administration. Administer by SubQ injection in the anterior thigh or abdomen; avoid boney areas and the umbilicus. Administer over 5-7 seconds. Do not rub the injection area. When switching from combined hormonal contraceptives (estrogen plus progestin), the first injection should be within 7 days after the last active pill, or removal of patch or ring. If switching from the I.M. to SubQ formulation, the next dose should be given within the prescribed dosing period for the I.M. injection to assure continuous coverage.

Stability

Storage Store at controlled room temperature.

Monitoring and Teaching Issues

Laboratory Monitoring Must have pregnancy test prior to beginning therapy.

Physical Assessment Instruct patient on appropriate dose scheduling.

Patient Education You may experience sensitivity to sunlight, dizziness, anxiety, depression, changes in appetite, hot flashes, or decreased libido or increased body hair (reversible when drug is discontinued). Maintain adequate hydration, unless instructed to restrict fluid intake. Report swelling of face, lips, or mouth; absent or altered menses; abdominal pain; vaginal itching, irritation, or discharge; heat, warmth, redness, or swelling of extremities; or sudden onset change in vision.

Dietary Considerations Ensure adequate calcium and vitamin D intake

Breast-Feeding Considerations Composition, quality, and quantity of breast milk are not affected; adverse developmental and behavioral effects have not been noted following exposure of infant to MPA while breast-feeding. The manufacturer does not recommend the use of MPA tablets in breastfeeding mothers.

Pregnancy Considerations In general, there is not an increased risk of birth defects following inadvertent use of the injectable medroxyprogesterone contraceptives early in pregnancy. There is an increased risk of minor birth defects in children whose mothers take progesterones during the first 4 months of pregnancy. Hypospadias has been reported in male babies and mild masculinization of the external genitalia has been reported in female babies exposed during the first trimester. High doses are used to impair fertility. Ectopic pregnancies have been reported with use of the MPA contraceptive injection. Median time to conception/return to ovulation following discontinuation of MPA contraceptive injection is 10 months following the last injection.

◆ **Medroxyprogesterone Acetate** *see* MedroxyPROGESTERone *on page* 1154

◆ **Medroxyprogesterone and Estrogens (Conjugated)** *see* Estrogens (Conjugated/Equine) and Medroxyprogesterone *on page* 686

Mefloquine (ME floe kwin)

Index Terms Mefloquine Hydrochloride

Generic Availability (U.S.) Yes

Pharmacologic Category Antimalarial Agent

Medication Guide Available Yes

Pregnancy Risk Factor C

Lactation Enters breast milk/not recommended

Use Treatment of mild-to-moderate acute malarial infections (including treatment of chloroquine-resistant malaria) and prevention of malaria caused by *Plasmodium falciparum* or *P. vivax*

Available Dosage Forms

Tablet, oral: 250 mg

Dosing

Adult & Geriatric Dose expressed as mg of mefloquine hydrochloride:

Malaria treatment (mild-to-moderate infection): Oral: 5 tablets (1250 mg) as a single dose. If clinical improvement is not seen within 48-72 hours, an alternative therapy should be used for retreatment.

Malaria prophylaxis: Oral: 1 tablet (250 mg) weekly starting 1 week before arrival in endemic area, continuing weekly during travel and for 4 weeks after leaving endemic area. **Note:** Prophylaxis may begin 2-3 weeks prior to travel to ensure tolerance.

Pediatric Dose expressed as mg of mefloquine hydrochloride: Children ≥6 months:

Malaria treatment (mild-to-moderate infection): Note: If clinical improvement is not seen within 48-72 hours, an alternative therapy should be used for retreatment.

Manufacturer's labeling: 20-25 mg/kg/day in 2 divided doses, taken 6-8 hours apart (maximum: 1250 mg)

Unlabeled dosing (CDC): 15 mg/kg followed 12 hours later by 10 mg/kg/dose

Malaria prophylaxis: 5 mg/kg/dose once weekly (maximum dose: 250 mg) starting 1-2 weeks before arrival in endemic area, continuing weekly during travel and for 4 weeks after leaving endemic area. **Note:** Prophylaxis may begin 2-3 weeks prior to travel to ensure tolerance.

Manufacturer's labeling:

20-30 kg: 1/2 of 250 mg tablet (125 mg) once weekly
30-45 kg: 3/4 of 250 mg tablet (187.5 mg) once weekly
>45 kg: 1 tablet (250 mg) once weekly

Unlabeled dosing (CDC):

≤9 kg: 5 mg/kg/dose once weekly
10-19 kg: 1/4 of 250 mg tablet (62.5 mg) once weekly
20-30 kg: 1/2 of 250 mg tablet (125 mg) once weekly
31-45 kg: 3/4 of 250 mg tablet (187.5 mg) once weekly
≥46 kg: 1 tablet (250 mg) once weekly

Renal Impairment No dosage adjustment needed in patients with renal impairment or on dialysis.

Hepatic Impairment Half-life may be prolonged and plasma levels may be higher. Specific dosing adjustments are not available.

Administration

Oral Administer with food and with at least 8 oz of water. When used for malaria prophylaxis, dose should be taken once weekly on the same day each week. If vomiting occurs within 30 minutes after the dose, an additional full dose should be given; if it occurs within 30-60 minutes after dose, an additional half-dose should be given. Tablets may be crushed and suspended in a small amount of water, milk, or another beverage for persons unable to swallow tablets.

Monitoring and Teaching Issues

Laboratory Monitoring When use is prolonged, periodically monitor liver function tests.

Physical Assessment Monitor for hypertension, cardiomyopathy, hyperglycemia, and hepatotoxicity on a regular basis throughout therapy. Monitor patient closely for any development of psychiatric symptoms (anxiety, paranoia, depression, hallucinations, and psychosis); may persist long after mefloquine has been discontinued. Advise patient about the importance of carrying medication guide and wallet provided when mefloquine is dispensed for malaria. Teach patient importance of adequate hydration.

Patient Education Take with food and at least 8 oz of water. Maintain adequate nutrition and hydration unless instructed to restrict fluid intake. Carry drug information card in wallet for as long as you are taking this drug. May cause dizziness, anxiety, loss of balance, nausea, vomiting, or decreased appetite. Report immediately any anxiety, confusion, agitation, restlessness, paranoia, depression, hallucinations, or suicide ideation.

- ◆ **Mefloquine Hydrochloride** *see* Mefloquine *on page* 1157
- ◆ **Mefoxin®** *see* Cefoxitin *on page* 326
- ◆ **Megace®** *see* Megestrol *on page* 1158
- ◆ **Megace® ES** *see* Megestrol *on page* 1158

Megestrol (me JES trole)

U.S. Brand Names Megace®; Megace® ES

Index Terms 5071-1DL(6); Megestrol Acetate; NSC-71423

Generic Availability (U.S.) Yes: Excludes Megace® ES

Pharmacologic Category Antineoplastic Agent, Hormone; Appetite Stimulant; Progestin

Medication Safety Issues

Sound-alike/look-alike issues:

Megace® may be confused with Reglan®
Megestrol may be confused with mesalamine

Pregnancy Risk Factor D (tablet) / X (suspension)

Lactation Enters breast milk/not recommended

Use Palliative treatment of breast and endometrial carcinoma; treatment of anorexia, cachexia, or unexplained significant weight loss in patients with AIDS

Available Dosage Forms

Suspension, oral: 40 mg/mL (10 mL, 20 mL, 237 mL, 240 mL, 473 mL, 480 mL)
Megace®: 40 mg/mL (240 mL)
Megace® ES: 125 mg/mL (150 mL)

Tablet, oral: 20 mg, 40 mg

Dosing

Adult & Geriatric Note: Megace® ES suspension is not equivalent to other formulations on a mg-per-mg basis.

Breast carcinoma (females): Refer to individual protocols: Oral: Tablet: 40 mg 4 times/day

Endometrial carcinoma: Refer to individual protocols: Oral: Tablet: 40-320 mg/day in divided doses; use for 2 months to determine efficacy; maximum doses used have been up to 800 mg/day.

HIV-related cachexia (males/females): Oral: Suspension:
Megace®: Initial dose: 800 mg/day; daily doses of 400 and 800 mg/day were found to be clinically effective
Megace® ES: 625 mg/day

Renal Impairment No data available; however, the urinary excretion of megestrol acetate administered in doses of 4-90 mg ranged from 57% to 78% within 10 days.

Administration

Oral Megestrol acetate (Megace®) oral suspension is compatible with water, orange juice, apple juice, or Sustacal H.C. for immediate consumption. Shake suspension well before use.

Monitoring and Teaching Issues

Laboratory Monitoring Serum glucose

Physical Assessment Monitor for hypertension, CNS changes (confusion, insomnia), rash, changes in menses, gastrointestinal upset, jaundice, and thrombophlebitis regularly during therapy. Teach patient importance of adequate hydration and importance of avoiding pregnancy.

Patient Education May cause sensitivity to sunlight, dizziness, anxiety, depression, change in appetite, decreased libido or increased body hair (reversible when drug is discontinued), or hot flashes. Report swelling of face, lips, or mouth; absent or altered menses; abdominal pain; vaginal itching, irritation, or discharge; heat, warmth, redness, or swelling of extremities; or sudden onset change in vision.

◆ **Megestrol Acetate** *see* Megestrol *on page* 1158

◆ **Melanex® [DSC]** *see* Hydroquinone *on page* 927

Meloxicam (mel OKS i kam)

U.S. Brand Names Mobic®

Generic Availability (U.S.) Yes:

Pharmacologic Category Nonsteroidal Anti-inflammatory Drug (NSAID), Oral

Medication Guide Available Yes

Pregnancy Risk Factor C / D ≥30 weeks gestation

Lactation Excretion in breast milk unknown/not recommended

Use Relief of signs and symptoms of osteoarthritis, rheumatoid arthritis, and juvenile idiopathic arthritis (JIA)

Mechanism of Action/Effect Reversibly inhibits cyclooxygenase-1 and 2 (COX-1 and 2) enzymes, which results in decreased formation of prostaglandin precursors; has antipyretic, analgesic, and anti-inflammatory properties

Contraindications Hypersensitivity (eg, asthma, urticaria, allergic-type reactions) to meloxicam, aspirin, other NSAIDs, or any component of the formulation; perioperative pain in the setting of coronary artery bypass graft (CABG) surgery

Warnings/Precautions [U.S. Boxed Warning]: NSAIDs are associated with an increased risk of adverse cardiovascular thrombotic events, including MI and stroke. Risk may be increased with duration of use or pre-existing cardiovascular risk factors or disease. Carefully evaluate individual cardiovascular risk profiles prior to prescribing. May cause new-onset hypertension or worsening of existing hypertension. Use caution with fluid retention. Avoid use in heart failure. Concurrent administration of ibuprofen, and potentially other nonselective NSAIDs, may interfere with aspirin's cardioprotective effect. **[U.S. Boxed Warning]: Use is contraindicated for treatment of perioperative pain in the setting of coronary artery bypass graft (CABG) surgery.** Risk of MI and stroke may be increased with use within the first 10-14 days following CABG surgery.

Platelet adhesion and aggregation may be decreased; may prolong bleeding time; patients with coagulation disorders or who are receiving anticoagulants should be monitored closely. Anemia may occur; patients on long-term NSAID therapy should be monitored for anemia. Rarely, NSAID use may cause severe blood dyscrasias (eg, agranulocytosis, aplastic anemia, thrombocytopenia).

NSAID use may compromise existing renal function; dose-dependent decreases in prostaglandin synthesis may result from NSAID use, reducing renal blood flow which may cause renal decompensation. NSAID use may increase the risk for hyperkalemia. Patients with impaired renal function, dehydration, heart failure, liver dysfunction, those taking diuretics, and ACE inhibitors, and the elderly are at greater risk of renal toxicity and hyperkalemia. Rehydrate patient before starting therapy; monitor renal function closely. Not recommended for use in patients with advanced renal disease. Long-term NSAID use may result in renal papillary necrosis.

[U.S. Boxed Warning]: NSAIDs may increase risk of gastrointestinal irritation, inflammation, ulceration, bleeding, and perforation. These events may occur at any time during therapy and without warning. Use caution with a history of GI disease (bleeding or ulcers), concurrent therapy with aspirin, anticoagulants and/or corticosteroids, smoking, use of alcohol, the elderly or debilitated patients. When used concomitantly with ≤325 mg of aspirin, a substantial increase in the risk of gastrointestinal complications (eg, ulcer) occurs; concomitant gastroprotective therapy (eg, proton pump inhibitors) is recommended (Bhatt, 2008).

Use the lowest effective dose for the shortest duration of time, consistent with individual patient goals, to reduce risk of cardiovascular or GI adverse events. Alternate therapies should be considered for patients at high risk.

NSAIDs may cause serious skin adverse events including exfoliative dermatitis, Stevens-Johnson syndrome (SJS) and toxic epidermal necrolysis (TEN); discontinue use at first sign of skin rash or hypersensitivity. Anaphylactoid reactions may occur, even without prior exposure; patients with "aspirin triad" (bronchial asthma, aspirin intolerance, rhinitis) may be at increased risk. Do not use in patients who experience bronchospasm, asthma, rhinitis, or urticaria with NSAID or aspirin therapy. Use caution in other forms of asthma.

Use with caution in patients with decreased hepatic function. Closely monitor patients with any abnormal LFT. Severe hepatic reactions (eg, fulminant hepatitis, liver failure) have occurred with NSAID use, rarely; discontinue if signs or symptoms of liver disease develop, or if systemic manifestations occur.

NSAIDS may cause drowsiness, dizziness, blurred vision and other neurologic effects which may impair physical or mental abilities; patients must be cautioned about performing tasks which require mental alertness (eg, operating machinery or driving). Discontinue use with blurred or diminished vision and perform ophthalmologic exam. Monitor vision with long-term therapy.

The elderly are at increased risk for adverse effects (especially peptic ulceration, CNS effects, renal toxicity) from NSAIDs even at low doses.

Withhold for at least 4-6 half-lives prior to surgical or dental procedures.

Drug Interactions

Metabolism/Transport Effects Substrate (minor) of CYP2C9, 3A4; **Inhibits** CYP2C9 (weak)

Avoid Concomitant Use

Avoid concomitant use of Meloxicam with any of the following: Ketorolac; Ketorolac (Systemic)

Decreased Effect

Meloxicam may decrease the levels/effects of: ACE Inhibitors; Angiotensin II Receptor Blockers; Antiplatelet Agents; Beta-Blockers; Eplerenone; HydrALAZINE; Loop Diuretics; Potassium-Sparing Diuretics; Salicylates; Thiazide Diuretics

The levels/effects of Meloxicam may be decreased by: Bile Acid Sequestrants; Nonsteroidal Anti-Inflammatory Agents; Salicylates

Increased Effect/Toxicity

Meloxicam may increase the levels/effects of: Aminoglycosides; Anticoagulants; Antiplatelet Agents; Bisphosphonate Derivatives; Collagenase (Systemic); CycloSPORINE; CycloSPORINE (Systemic); Desmopressin; Digoxin; Drotrecogin Alfa; Eplerenone; Haloperidol; Ibritumomab; Lithium; Methotrexate; Nonsteroidal Anti-Inflammatory Agents; PEMEtrexed; Potassium-Sparing Diuretics; PRALAtrexate; Quinolone Antibiotics; Salicylates; Thrombolytic Agents; Tositumomab and Iodine I 131 Tositumomab; Vancomycin; Vitamin K Antagonists

The levels/effects of Meloxicam may be increased by: Antidepressants (Tricyclic, Tertiary Amine); Conivaptan; Corticosteroids (Systemic); Dasatinib; Glucosamine; Herbs (Anticoagulant/Antiplatelet Properties); Ketorolac; Ketorolac (Systemic); Nonsteroidal Anti-Inflammatory Agents; Omega-3-Acid Ethyl Esters; Pentosan Polysulfate Sodium; Pentoxifylline; Probenecid; Prostacyclin Analogues; Selective Serotonin Reuptake Inhibitors; Serotonin/Norepinephrine Reuptake Inhibitors; Treprostinil; Voriconazole

Nutritional/Ethanol Interactions

Ethanol: Avoid ethanol (may enhance gastric mucosal irritation).

Herb/Nutraceutical: Avoid alfalfa, anise, bilberry, bladderwrack, bromelain, cat's claw, celery, chamomile, coleus, cordyceps, dong quai, evening primrose, fenugreek, feverfew, garlic, ginger, ginkgo biloba, ginseng (American, Panax, Siberian), grapeseed, green tea, guggul, horse chestnut seed, horseradish, licorice, prickly ash, red clover, reishi, SAMe (S-adenosylmethionine), sweet clover, turmeric, white willow (all have additional antiplatelet activity).

Adverse Reactions Percentages reported in adult patients; abdominal pain, diarrhea, fever, headache, pyrexia, and vomiting were reported more commonly in pediatric patients

2% to 10%:

Cardiovascular: Edema (≤5%)

Central nervous system: Headache (2% to 8%), pain (1% to 5%), dizziness (≤4%), insomnia (≤4%)

Dermatologic: Pruritus (≤2%), rash (≤3%)

Gastrointestinal: Dyspepsia (4% to 10%), diarrhea (2% to 8%), nausea (2% to 7%), abdominal pain (2% to 5%), constipation (≤3%), flatulence (≤3%), vomiting (≤3%)

Genitourinary: Urinary tract infection (≤7%), micturition (≤2%)

Hematologic: Anemia (≤4%)
Neuromuscular & skeletal: Arthralgia (≤5%), back pain (≤3%)
Respiratory: Upper respiratory infection (≤8%), cough (≤2%), pharyngitis (≤3%)
Miscellaneous: Flu-like syndrome (2% to 6%), falls (≤3%)

Pharmacodynamics/Kinetics

Bioavailability 89%

Time to Peak Initial: 4-5 hours; Secondary: 12-14 hours

Protein Binding ~99%, primarily to albumin

Half-Life Elimination Adults: 15-20 hours

Metabolism Hepatic via CYP2C9 and CYP3A4 (minor); forms 4 metabolites (inactive)

Excretion Urine and feces (as inactive metabolites)

Available Dosage Forms

Suspension, oral: 7.5 mg/5 mL (100 mL)
Mobic®: 7.5 mg/5 mL (100 mL)

Tablet, oral: 7.5 mg, 15 mg
Mobic®: 7.5 mg, 15 mg

Dosing

Adult & Geriatric Osteoarthritis, rheumatoid arthritis: Oral: Initial: 7.5 mg once daily; some patients may receive additional benefit from increasing dose to 15 mg once daily; maximum dose: 15 mg/day.

Pediatric Juvenile idiopathic arthritis (JIA): Oral: Children ≥2 years: 0.125 mg/kg/day; maximum dose: 7.5 mg/day

Renal Impairment

Mild-to-moderate impairment: No specific dosage recommendations

Significant impairment (Cl_{cr} ≤20 mL/minute): Patients with severe renal impairment have not been adequately studied; use not recommended.

Hemodialysis: Maximum dose: 7.5 mg/day

Hepatic Impairment

Mild (Child-Pugh class A) to moderate (Child-Pugh class B) hepatic dysfunction: No dosage adjustment is necessary

Severe hepatic impairment: Patients with severe hepatic impairment have not been adequately studied

Administration

Oral May be administered with or without meals; take with food or milk to minimize gastrointestinal irritation. Oral suspension: Shake gently prior to use.

Stability

Storage Store at 25°C (77°F). Protect tablets from moisture.

Monitoring and Teaching Issues

Laboratory Monitoring Periodic CBC, serum chemistries, liver function, renal function (serum BUN and creatinine) with long-term use

Physical Assessment Evaluate cardiac risk and potential for GI bleeding prior to prescribing this medication. Monitor blood pressure at the beginning of therapy and periodically during use.

Patient Education Take with food or milk to reduce GI distress. Avoid alcohol. You may experience anorexia, nausea, vomiting, heartburn, drowsiness, dizziness, nervousness, headache, or fluid retention; GI bleeding, ulceration, or perforation can occur with or without pain; discontinue medication and contact prescriber if persistent abdominal pain or cramping or blood in stool occurs. Report breathlessness, respiratory difficulty, or unusual cough; chest pain, rapid heartbeat, or palpitations; slurring of speech; unusual bruising/bleeding; blood in urine, stool, mouth, or vomitus; swollen extremities; skin blisters, rash, or itching; acute fatigue; jaundice; flu-like symptoms; or hearing changes (ringing in ears).

Dietary Considerations Should be taken with food or milk to minimize gastrointestinal irritation.

Geriatric Considerations Men ≥65 years of age exhibited steady-state plasma concentrations and pharmacokinetics similar to younger men. Elderly women (≥65 years of age) had nearly a 50% greater AUC and 32% higher C_{max} compared to younger women.

Breast-Feeding Considerations It is not known whether meloxicam is excreted in human milk. Breast-feeding is not recommended by the manufacturer.

Pregnancy Considerations Adverse events were not observed in the initial animal reproduction studies; therefore, the manufacturer classifies meloxicam as pregnancy category C (category D: ≥30 weeks gestation). Meloxicam crosses the placenta. NSAID exposure during the first trimester is not strongly associated with congenital malformations; however, cardiovascular anomalies and cleft palate have been observed following NSAID exposure in some studies. The use of an NSAID close to conception may be associated with an increased risk of miscarriage. Nonteratogenic effects have been observed following NSAID administration during the third trimester including myocardial degenerative changes, prenatal constriction of the ductus arteriosus, fetal tricuspid regurgitation, failure of the ductus arteriosus to close postnatally; renal dysfunction or failure, oligohydramnios; gastrointestinal bleeding or perforation, increased risk of necrotizing enterocolitis; intracranial bleeding (including intraventricular hemorrhage), platelet dysfunction with resultant bleeding; pulmonary hypertension. Because they may cause premature closure of the ductus arteriosus, use of NSAIDs late in pregnancy should be avoided (use after 31 or 32 weeks gestation is not recommended by some clinicians). Product labeling for Mobic® specifically notes that use at ≥30 weeks gestation should be avoided and therefore classifies meloxicam as pregnancy category D at this time. The chronic use of NSAIDs in women of reproductive age may be associated with infertility that is reversible upon discontinuation of the medication.

Related Information

Nonsalicylate / Nonsteroidal Anti-Inflammatory Agents *on page* 2002

◆ **Melpaque HP®** *see* Hydroquinone *on page* 927

Melphalan (MEL fa lan)

U.S. Brand Names Alkeran®

Index Terms L-PAM; L-Phenylalanine Mustard; L-Sarcolysin; Phenylalanine Mustard

Generic Availability (U.S.) Yes: Excludes tablet

Pharmacologic Category Antineoplastic Agent, Alkylating Agent

Medication Safety Issues

Sound-alike/look-alike issues:

Melphalan may be confused with Mephyton®, Myleran®

Alkeran® may be confused with Alferon®, Leukeran®, Myleran®

High alert medication: This medication is in a class of medications the Institute for Safe Medication Practices (ISMP) includes among its list of drug classes which have a heightened risk of causing significant patient harm when used in error.

Pregnancy Risk Factor D

Lactation Excretion in breast milk unknown/not recommended

Use Palliative treatment of multiple myeloma and nonresectable epithelial ovarian carcinoma

Unlabeled/Investigational Use Treatment of Hodgkin's disease, amyloidosis; conditioning regimen for autologous hematopoietic stem cell transplantation in adults with hematologic disorders (eg, multiple myeloma) and autologous marrow or stem cell transplantation in pediatric neuroblastoma and Ewing's sarcoma

Mechanism of Action/Effect Alkylating agent which is a derivative of mechlorethamine that inhibits DNA and RNA synthesis via formation of carbonium ions; cross-links strands of DNA; acts on both resting and rapidly dividing tumor cells.

Contraindications Hypersensitivity to melphalan or any component of the formulation; patients whose disease was resistant to prior melphalan therapy

Warnings/Precautions [U.S. Boxed Warning]: Bone marrow suppression is common; may be severe and result in infection or bleeding; myelosuppression is dose-related. Monitor blood counts; may require treatment delay or dose modification for thrombocytopenia or neutropenia. Use with caution in patients with prior bone marrow suppression, impaired renal function (consider dose reduction), or who have received prior (or concurrent) chemotherapy or irradiation. Myelotoxicity is generally reversible, although irreversible bone marrow failure has been reported. In patients who are candidates for autologous transplantation, avoid melphalan-containing regimens prior to transplant (due to the effects on stem cell reserve). Myelosuppression has been demonstrated more with the I.V. formulation (compared to oral); may be dose-related. Signs of infection, such as fever and WBC rise, may not occur; lethargy and confusion may be more prominent signs of infection.

[U.S. Boxed Warning]: Hypersensitivity reactions have occurred in ~2% of patients receiving I.V. melphalan, usually after multiple treatment cycles. Discontinue infusion and treat symptomatically. Hypersensitivity may also occur (rarely) with oral melphalan. Do not readminister (oral or I.V.) in patients who experience hypersensitivity to melphalan.

Gastrointestinal toxicities, including nausea, vomiting, diarrhea and mucositis, are common. When administering high-dose melphalan in autologous transplantation, cryotherapy is recommended to prevent mucositis (Keefe, 2007). Abnormal liver function tests may occur; hepatitis and jaundice have also been reported; hepatic veno-occlusive disease (VOD) has been reported with I.V. melphalan. Pulmonary fibrosis (some fatal) and interstitial pneumonitis have been observed with treatment. Dosage reduction is recommended with I.V. melphalan in patients with renal impairment; reduced initial doses may also be recommended with oral melphalan. Closely monitor patients with azotemia.

[U.S. Boxed Warning]: Produces chromosomal changes and is potentially mutagenic and leukemogenic; secondary malignancies (including acute myeloid leukemia, myeloproliferative disease, and carcinoma) have been reported reported (some patients were receiving combination chemotherapy or radiation therapy); the risk is increased with increased treatment duration and cumulative doses. Suppresses ovarian function and produces amenorrhea; may also cause testicular suppression.

Extravasation may cause local tissue damage; administration by slow injection into a fast running I.V. solution into an injection port or via a central line is recommended; do not administer directly into a peripheral vein. **[U.S. Boxed Warning]: Should be administered under the supervision of an experienced cancer chemotherapy physician.** Avoid vaccination with live vaccines during treatment if immunocompromised. Toxicity may be increased in elderly; start with lowest recommended adult doses.

Drug Interactions

Avoid Concomitant Use

Avoid concomitant use of Melphalan with any of the following: BCG; Nalidixic Acid; Natalizumab; Pimecrolimus; Roflumilast; Tacrolimus (Topical); Vaccines (Live)

Decreased Effect

Melphalan may decrease the levels/effects of: BCG; Cardiac Glycosides; Sipuleucel-T; Vaccines (Inactivated); Vaccines (Live); Vitamin K Antagonists

The levels/effects of Melphalan may be decreased by: Echinacea

Increased Effect/Toxicity

Melphalan may increase the levels/effects of: Carmustine; CycloSPORINE; CycloSPORINE (Systemic); Leflunomide; Natalizumab; Vaccines (Live); Vitamin K Antagonists

The levels/effects of Melphalan may be increased by: Denosumab; Nalidixic Acid; Pimecrolimus; Roflumilast; Tacrolimus (Topical); Trastuzumab

Nutritional/Ethanol Interactions

Ethanol: Avoid ethanol (due to GI irritation).

Food: Food interferes with oral absorption.

Lab Interactions False-positive Coombs' test [direct]

Adverse Reactions

>10%:

Gastrointestinal: Nausea/vomiting (oral low-dose: <10%; I.V.: 30% to 90%), oral ulceration

Hematologic: Myelosuppression, leukopenia (nadir: 14-21 days; recovery: 28-35 days), thrombocytopenia (nadir: 14-21 days; recovery: 28-35 days), anemia

Miscellaneous: Secondary malignancy (<2% to 20%; cumulative dose and duration dependent, includes acute myeloid leukemia, myeloproliferative syndrome, carcinoma)

1% to 10%: Miscellaneous: Hypersensitivity (I.V.: 2%; includes bronchospasm, dyspnea, edema, hypotension, pruritus, rash, tachycardia, urticaria)

Pharmacodynamics/Kinetics

Absorption Oral: Variable and incomplete

Bioavailability Unpredictable; 61% ± 26%, decreasing with repeated doses

Time to Peak Serum: ~1-2 hours

Protein Binding 60% to 90%; primarily to albumin, 20% to α_1-acid glycoprotein

Half-Life Elimination Terminal: I.V.: 75 minutes; Oral: 1-2 hours

Metabolism Hepatic; chemical hydrolysis to monohydroxymelphalan and dihydroxymelphalan

Excretion Oral: Feces (20% to 50%); urine (~10% as unchanged drug)

Pharmacokinetic Note Pharmacokinetics listed are for FDA-approved doses.

Available Dosage Forms

Injection, powder for reconstitution: 50 mg

Alkeran®: 50 mg

Tablet, oral:

Alkeran®: 2 mg

Dosing

Adult

Details regarding dosing in combination regimens should also be consulted. Adjust dose based on patient response and weekly blood counts.

Multiple myeloma (palliative treatment): Note: Response is gradual; may require repeated courses to realize benefit:

I.V.: 16 mg/m^2 administered at 2-week intervals for 4 doses, then administer at 4-week intervals after adequate hematologic recovery.

Oral: Usual dose (as described in the manufacturer's labeling):

6 mg once daily for 2-3 weeks initially, followed by up to 4 weeks rest, then a maintenance dose of 2 mg daily as hematologic recovery begins **or**

10 mg daily for 7-10 days; institute 2 mg daily maintenance dose after WBC >4000 cells/mm^3 and platelets >100,000 cells/mm^3 (~4-8 weeks); titrate maintenance dose to hematologic response **or**

0.15 mg/kg/day for 7 days, with a 2-6 week rest, followed by a maintenance dose of ≤0.05 mg/kg/day as hematologic recovery begins **or**

0.25 mg/kg/day for 4 days (or 0.2 mg/kg/day for 5 days); repeat at 4- to 6-week intervals as ANC and platelet counts return to normal

Other dosing regimens in combination therapy (unlabeled doses):

4 mg/m^2/day for 7 days every 4 weeks (Palumbo, 2006; Palumbo, 2008) **or**

6 mg/m^2/day for 7 days every 4 weeks (Palumbo, 2004) **or**

0.25 mg/kg/day for 4 days every 6 weeks (Facon, 2006; Facon, 2007) **or**

9 mg/m^2/day for 4 days every 6 weeks (Dimopoulos, 2009; San Miguel, 2008)

Ovarian carcinoma: Oral: 0.2 mg/kg/day for 5 days, repeat every 4-5 weeks **or**

Unlabeled dosing: 7 mg/m^2/day in 2 divided doses for 5 days, repeat every 28 days (Wadler, 1996)

Amyloidosis (unlabeled use): Oral: 0.22 mg/kg/day for 4 days every 28 days in combination with oral dexamethasone (Palladini, 2004)

Hodgkin's disease (unlabeled use): I.V.: 30 mg/m^2 on day 6 of combination chemotherapy (mini-BEAM) regimen (Colwill, 1995; Martin, 2001)

Conditioning regimen for autologous hematopoietic stem cell transplantation (unlabeled use): I.V.:

200 mg/m^2 alone 2 days prior to transplantation (Fermand, 2005; Moreau, 2002) **or**

140 mg/m^2 2 days prior to transplantation (combined with busulfan) (Fermand, 2005) **or**

140 mg/m^2 2 days prior to transplantation (combined with total body irradiation [TBI]) (Moreau, 2002) **or**

140 mg/m^2 5 days prior to transplantation (combined with TBI) (Barlogie, 2006)

Geriatric Refer to adult dosing. Use caution and begin at the lower end of dosing range.

Pediatric Details regarding dosing in combination regimens should also be consulted.

Conditioning regimen for autologous hematopoietic stem cell transplantation (unlabeled use):

140 mg/m^2 2 days prior to transplantation (combined with busulfan) (Canete, 2009; Oberlin, 2006) **or**

180 mg/m^2 (with pre- and posthydration) 12-30 hours prior to transplantation (Pritchard, 2005) **or**

45 mg/m^2/day for 4 days starting 8 days prior to transplantation (combined with busulfan or etoposide and carboplatin) (Berthold, 2005)

Renal Impairment

The FDA-approved labeling contains the following adjustment recommendations (for approved dosing levels) based on route of administration:

Oral: Moderate-to-severe renal impairment: Consider a reduced dose initially.

I.V.: BUN ≥30 mg/dL: Reduce dose by up to 50%.

The following guidelines have been used by some clinicians:

Aronoff, 2007 (route of administration not specified): Adults (based on a 6 mg once-daily dose):

Cl_{cr} 10-50 mL/minute: Administer 75% of dose.

Cl_{cr} <10 mL/minute: Administer 50% of dose.

Hemodialysis: Administer dose after hemodialysis.

Continuous ambulatory peritoneal dialysis (CAPD): Administer 50% of dose.

Continuous renal replacement therapy (CRRT): Administer 75% of dose.

Badros, 2001: I.V.: Autologous stem cell transplant: Serum creatinine >2 mg/dL: Reduce dose from 200 mg/m^2 to 140 mg/m^2

Carlson, 2005: Oral (for melphalan-prednisone combination therapy; based on a study evaluating toxicity with melphalan dosed at 0.25 mg/kg/day for 4 days/cycle):

Cl_{cr} >10 to <30 mL/minute: Administer 75% of dose

Cl_{cr} ≤10 mL/minute: Data is insufficient for a recommendation

Kintzel, 1995:

Oral: Adjust dose in the presence of hematologic toxicity

I.V.:

Cl_{cr} 46-60 mL/minute: Administer 85% of normal dose.

Cl_{cr} 31-45 mL/minute: Administer 75% of normal dose.

Cl_{cr} <30 mL/minute: Administer 70% of normal dose.

Hepatic Impairment Melphalan is hepatically metabolized; however, dosage adjustment does not appear to be necessary (King, 2001).

Adjustment for Toxicity Oral:

WBC <3000/mm^3: Withhold treatment until recovery

Platelets <100,000/mm^3: Withhold treatment until recovery

Administration

Oral Administer on an empty stomach.

I.V. Due to limited stability, complete administration of I.V. dose should occur within 60 minutes of reconstitution. Infuse over 15-30 minutes. Extravasation may cause local tissue damage; administration by slow injection into a fast running I.V. solution into an injection port or via a central line is recommended; do not administer by direct injection into a peripheral vein.

BMT only: Saline-based hydration preceding (2-4 hours), during, and following (6-12 hours) administration reduces risk of drug precipitation in renal tubules. Hydrolysis causes loss of 1% melphalan injection per 10 minutes.

Stability

Reconstitution Injection: Use appropriate precautions for handling and disposal. Stability is limited; must be prepared fresh. **The time between reconstitution/dilution and administration of parenteral melphalan must be kept to a minimum (manufacturer recommends <60 minutes) because reconstituted and diluted solutions are unstable.** Dissolve powder initially with 10 mL of supplied diluent to a concentration of 5 mg/mL; shake immediately and vigorously to dissolve. **Immediately** dilute dose in NS to a concentration of ≤0.45 mg/mL (manufacturer recommended concentration). Do not refrigerate solution; precipitation occurs. The manufacturer recommends administration within 60 minutes of reconstitution.

Storage

Tablet: Store in refrigerator at 2°C to 8°C (36°F to 46°F). Protect from light.

Injection: Store at room temperature of 15°C to 30°C (59°F to 86°F). Protect from light. Stability is limited; must be prepared fresh. A 5 mg/mL concentration is chemically and physically stable for ≤90 minutes when stored at room temperature, although the manufacturer recommends administration be completed within 60 minutes of reconstitution; **immediately** dilute dose in NS. Do not refrigerate solution; precipitation occurs.

Monitoring and Teaching Issues

Laboratory Monitoring CBC with differential, platelet count, serum electrolytes, serum uric acid

Physical Assessment Evaluate patient for use-related cautions prior to beginning treatment. Assess hematologic parameters at baseline and at regular intervals. I.V.: Follow administration specifics and monitor infusion site carefully to prevent extravasation. Monitor for pulmonary toxicity, gastrointestinal upset, myelosuppression (leukopenia), diarrhea, and hypersensitivity reaction on a regular basis.

Patient Education I.V.: Report immediately any burning, swelling, pain, or redness at infusion or injection site. Oral: Preferable to take oral doses on an empty stomach, 1 hour before or 2 hours after meals. Avoid excessive alcohol (may increase gastric irritation). Maintain adequate nutrition and adequate hydration, unless instructed to restrict fluid intake. You may be more susceptible to infection. May cause nausea, vomiting, hair loss (reversible), or easy bleeding or bruising. Report unusual lethargy, confusion, or fever; persistent or severe nausea or vomiting; diarrhea or abdominal pain; chest pain or palpitations; difficulty or pain on urination; unusual bruising/bleeding; or respiratory difficulty.

Dietary Considerations Should be taken on an empty stomach (1 hour prior to or 2 hours after meals).

Geriatric Considerations Toxicity to immunosuppressives is increased in the elderly. Start with lowest recommended adult doses. Signs of infection, such as fever and WBC rise, may not occur. Lethargy and confusion may be more prominent signs of infection.

Pregnancy Considerations Animal studies have demonstrated embryotoxicity and teratogenicity. Therapy may suppress ovarian function leading to amenorrhea. There are no adequate and well-controlled studies in pregnant women. Women of childbearing potential should be advised to avoid pregnancy while on melphalan therapy.

◆ **Melquin-3®** *see* Hydroquinone *on page 927*

◆ **Melquin HP®** *see* Hydroquinone *on page 927*

Memantine (me MAN teen)

U.S. Brand Names Namenda®

Index Terms Memantine Hydrochloride; Namenda XR

Generic Availability (U.S.) No

Pharmacologic Category N-Methyl-D-Aspartate Receptor Antagonist

Medication Safety Issues

Sound-alike/look-alike issues:

Memantine may be confused with mesalamine

Pregnancy Risk Factor B

Lactation Excretion in breast milk unknown/use caution

Use Treatment of moderate-to-severe dementia of the Alzheimer's type

Unlabeled/Investigational Use Treatment of mild-to-moderate vascular dementia

Mechanism of Action/Effect Memantine reduces the decline in function in Alzheimer's disease; it has not been shown to prevent or slow neurodegeneration associated with this disease.

Contraindications Hypersensitivity to memantine or any component of the formulation

Warnings/Precautions Use with caution in patients with cardiovascular disease; an increased incidence of cardiac failure, angina, bradycardia, and hypertension (compared with placebo) was observed in clinical trials. Use caution with seizure disorders or severe hepatic impairment. Use with caution in moderate-to-severe renal impairment; dose adjustments may be required. Worsening of corneal condition has been observed in a clinical trial; periodic ophthalmic exams during use have been recommended (Canadian labeling). Clearance is significantly reduced by alkaline urine; use caution with medications, dietary changes, or patient conditions which may alter urine pH.

Drug Interactions

Avoid Concomitant Use There are no known interactions where it is recommended to avoid concomitant use.

Decreased Effect There are no known significant interactions involving a decrease in effect.

Increased Effect/Toxicity

Memantine may increase the levels/effects of: Trimethoprim

The levels/effects of Memantine may be increased by: Carbonic Anhydrase Inhibitors; Sodium Bicarbonate; Trimethoprim

Adverse Reactions 1% to 10%:

Cardiovascular: Hypertension (4%), hypotension (2%), cardiac failure, cerebrovascular accident, syncope, transient ischemic attack

Central nervous system: Dizziness (5% to 7%), confusion (6%), headache (6%), anxiety (4%), depression (3%), hallucinations (3%), pain (3%), somnolence (3%), fatigue (2%), aggressive reaction (1% to 2%), ataxia, vertigo

Dermatologic: Rash

Gastrointestinal: Constipation (3% to 5%), diarrhea (5%), weight gain (3%), vomiting (2% to 3%), abdominal pain (2%), weight loss

Genitourinary: Urinary incontinence (2%), micturition

Hematologic: Anemia

Hepatic: Alkaline phosphatase increased

Neuromuscular & skeletal: Back pain (3%), hypokinesia

Ocular: Cataract, conjunctivitis

Respiratory: Cough (4%), dyspnea (2%), pneumonia

Miscellaneous: Influenza (4%)

Pharmacodynamics/Kinetics

Time to Peak Serum: Immediate release: 3-7 hours; Extended release: 9-12 hours

Protein Binding 45%

Half-Life Elimination Terminal: ~60-80 hours; severe renal impairment (Cl_{cr} 5-29 mL/minute): 117-156 hours

Metabolism Partially hepatic, primarily independent of the CYP enzyme system; forms 3 metabolites (minimal activity)

Excretion Urine (74%; ~48% of the total dose as unchanged drug; undergoes active tubular secretion moderated by pH-dependent tubular reabsorption; excretion reduced by alkaline urine pH)

Product Availability

Namenda XR™: FDA approved in June 2010; anticipated availability is currently undetermined

Namenda XR™ is an extended release capsule (once-daily administration) approved for the treatment of moderate-to-severe dementia associated with Alzheimer's disease

Available Dosage Forms

Combination package, oral:

Namenda®: Tablet: 5 mg (28s) and Tablet: 10 mg (21s)

Solution, oral:

Namenda®: 2 mg/mL (360 mL)

Tablet, oral:

Namenda®: 5 mg, 10 mg

Dosing

Adult & Geriatric

Alzheimer's disease: Oral:

Immediate release: Initial: 5 mg/day; increase dose by 5 mg/day to a target dose of 20 mg/day; wait ≥1 week between dosage changes. Doses >5 mg/day should be given in 2 divided doses.

Suggested titration: 5 mg/day for ≥1 week; 5 mg twice daily for ≥1 week; 15 mg/day given in 5 mg and 10 mg separated doses for ≥1 week; then 10 mg twice daily

Extended release: Initial: 7 mg once daily, increase dose by 7 mg/day to a target maximum dose of 28 mg/day; wait ≥1 week between dosage changes

Note: When switching from the immediate release product to the extended release product, begin the extended release product the day after the last dose of the immediate release product. Patients on immediate release 10 mg twice daily should be switched to extended release 28 mg once daily.

Mild-to-moderate vascular dementia (unlabeled use): Oral: Immediate release: Initial: 5 mg/day, titrated by 5 mg/day weekly to a target dose of 10 mg twice daily (Orgogozo, 2002)

Renal Impairment

Mild impairment: No adjustment required.

Moderate impairment:

U.S. labeling: No adjustment required.

Canadian labeling: (Cl_{cr} 30-49 mL/minute): Initial: 5 mg once daily; after at least 1 week of therapy and if tolerated, may titrate up to 5 mg twice daily; may further titrate dosage upward in weekly increments to 20 mg/day according to suggested titration schedule.

Severe impairment:

U.S. labeling: Cl_{cr} 5-29 mL/minute: Immediate release: Initial: 5 mg once daily; after at least 1 week of therapy and if tolerated, may titrate up to 5 mg twice daily; Extended release: Target dose of 14 mg/day

Note: When switching from the immediate release product to the extended release product, begin the extended release product the day after the last dose of the immediate release product. Patients on immediate release 5 mg twice daily should be switched to extended release 14 mg once daily.

Canadian labeling: Cl_{cr} 15-29 mL/minute: Initial: 5 mg once daily; after at least 1 week of therapy and if tolerated, may titrate up to 5 mg twice daily.

Hepatic Impairment

Mild-to-moderate impairment: No adjustment required.

Severe impairment: Use caution.

U.S. labeling: No specific dosing recommendations.

Canadian labeling: Avoid use.

Administration

Oral Administer without regard to meals. Extended release capsules may be swallowed whole or entire contents of capsule may be sprinkled on applesauce and swallowed immediately. Do not chew, crush, or divide.

Stability

Storage Store at 25°C (77°C); excursions permitted to 15°C to 30°C (59°F to 86°F).

Monitoring and Teaching Issues

Physical Assessment Monitor for hypertension, CNS changes, rash, and constipation on a regular basis throughout therapy.

Patient Education Take with or without food. May cause hypertension or headache. Report increase or changes in CNS symptoms (confusion, hallucinations, fatigue, aggressive reaction), chest pain or palpitations, dizziness or fainting, difficulty breathing or tightness in chest, or rash.

Dietary Considerations May be taken without regard to meals.

Geriatric Considerations In clinical trials, patients on memantine had less of a decline in cognitive function and activities of daily living (ADL) as compared to placebo. This was true for monotherapy with memantine, as well as combination therapy with donepezil, an acetylcholinesterase inhibitor.

Pregnancy Considerations Teratogenic effects were not observed in animal studies. There are no studies in pregnant women.

◆ **Memantine Hydrochloride** *see* Memantine *on page 1165*

◆ **Menactra®** *see* Meningococcal (Groups A / C / Y and W-135) Diphtheria Conjugate Vaccine *on page 1168*

◆ **MenACWY-D (Menactra®)** *see* Meningococcal (Groups A / C / Y and W-135) Diphtheria Conjugate Vaccine *on page 1168*

◆ **MenACWY-CRM (Menveo®)** *see* Meningococcal (Groups A / C / Y and W-135) Diphtheria Conjugate Vaccine *on page 1168*

◆ **MenCC** *see* Meningococcal Group C-CRM197 Conjugate Vaccine *on page 1167*

◆ **MenC-CRM197** *see* Meningococcal Group C-CRM197 Conjugate Vaccine *on page 1167*

◆ **Menest®** *see* Estrogens (Esterified) *on page 687*

◆ **Meningococcal Conjugate Vaccine** *see* Meningococcal (Groups A / C / Y and W-135) Diphtheria Conjugate Vaccine *on page 1168*

Meningococcal Group C-CRM197 Conjugate Vaccine

(me NIN joe kok al groop see see ahr em wuhn nahyn tee sev uhn KON joo gate vak SEEN)

Index Terms MenC-CRM197; MenCC

Generic Availability (U.S.) No

Pharmacologic Category Vaccine

Lactation Excretion in breast milk unknown/use caution

Use To provide active immunization against invasive meningococcal disease caused by *N. meningitidis* serogroup C, in children ≥2 months and adults

The National Advisory Committee on Immunization (NACI) recommendations for persons considered at an increased risk for meningococcal disease:

Chemoprophylaxis and immunoprophylaxis: Selection of meningococcal vaccination to be based upon serogroup(s):

Individuals living in the same household or with close contact (eg, kissing, shared cigarettes, shared eating or drinking utensils) of infected patient

Employees and children of nursery schools or day care

Immunoprophylaxis: Selection of meningococcal vaccination to be based upon serogroup(s):

Adolescents and young adults

Laboratory workers routinely exposed to isolates of *N. meningitidis*

Military recruits

Persons traveling to or who reside in countries where *N. meningitidis* is hyperendemic or epidemic, particularly if contact with local population will be prolonged

Persons with terminal complement component deficiencies

Persons with anatomic or functional asplenia

Note: Use is also recommended during meningococcal outbreaks caused by serogroup C.

Chemoprophylaxis:

Healthcare workers with intensive unprotected contact with infected patients

Airline passengers sitting directly next to an infected patient for duration of at least 8 hours

See NACI guidelines for specific drug treatment at http://www.phac-aspc.gc.ca/naci-ccni

Product Availability Not available in U.S.

Dosing

Adult & Geriatric Immunization: I.M.: 0.5 mL as a single dose

Pediatric Immunization: I.M.:

Infants:

≥2-12 months: 0.5 mL as a single dose for a total of 3 doses administered at least 4 weeks apart

≥4-11 months without prior vaccination: 0.5 mL as a single dose for a total of 2 doses administered at least 4 weeks apart

Note: The NACI recommends at least 1 of the 3 sequential doses for infants ≥2-12 months be administered beyond 5 months of age.

Children ≥1 year: Refer to adult dosing.

Administration

I.M. Administer by deep intramuscular injection only into the anterolateral thigh in infants and the deltoid area in older children, adolescents, and adults. Use separate injection sites if administering multiple vaccinations on the same day.

Acetaminophen may be used when needed to provide comfort; however, routine prophylactic administration of acetaminophen to prevent fever due to vaccine use is not recommended. There is evidence of a decreased immune response to some vaccines associated with acetaminophen administration; the clinical significance of this reduction in immune response has not been established.

I.V. Do not administer via I.V., SubQ, or I.D. routes.

Monitoring and Teaching Issues

Physical Assessment Use caution in immunocompromised patients, patients with bleeding disorders, or those taking anticoagulants. Anaphylactoid and/or hypersensitivity reactions may occur; treatment should be available for immediate use. All serious adverse reactions must be reported to the U.S. DHHS. Federal law also requires entry into the patient's medical record.

Patient Education You may experience mild headache, fever or chills, nausea or vomiting, or unusual sleepiness. Report persistent pain, redness, or swelling at injection site.

Meningococcal (Groups A / C / Y and W-135) Diphtheria Conjugate Vaccine

(me NIN joe kok al groops aye, see, why & dubl yoo won thur tee fyve dif THEER ee a KON joo gate vak SEEN)

U.S. Brand Names Menactra®; Menveo®

Index Terms MCV; MCV4; MenACWY-CRM (Menveo®); MenACWY-D (Menactra®); Meningococcal Conjugate Vaccine

Generic Availability (U.S.) No

Pharmacologic Category Vaccine, Inactivated (Bacterial)

Medication Safety Issues

Administration issue:

Menactra® (MCV4) should be administered by intramuscular (I.M.) injection only. Inadvertent subcutaneous (SubQ) administration has been reported; possibly due to confusion of this product with Menomume® (MPSV4), also a meningococcal polysaccharide vaccine, which is administered by the SubQ route.

Pregnancy Risk Factor B/C (manufacturer dependent)

Lactation Excretion in breast milk unknown/use caution

Use Provide active immunization of children and adults against invasive meningococcal disease caused by *N. meningitidis* serogroups A, C, Y, and W-135.

The Advisory Committee on Immunization Practices (ACIP) recommends routine vaccination of all persons at age 11 or 12 years of age, followed by a booster at age 16 years of age (CDC, 60[3], 2011).

The ACIP also recommends vaccination for persons 2 through 55 years of age at increased risk for meningococcal disease (CDC, 60[3], 2011). Meningococcal conjugate vaccine (MCV4) is preferred for persons aged 2-55 years; meningococcal polysaccharide vaccine (MPSV4) is preferred in adults ≥56 years of age (CDC, 2005).

Persons at increased risk include:

- Previously unvaccinated college freshmen living in dormitories
- Microbiologists routinely exposed to isolates of *N. meningitidis*
- Military recruits
- Persons traveling to or who reside in countries where *N. meningitidis* is hyperendemic or epidemic, particularly if contact with local population will be prolonged
- Persons with persistent complement component deficiencies (eg, C5-C9, properidin, factor H, or factor D)
- Persons with anatomic or functional asplenia
- Persons with HIV infection

Use is also recommended during meningococcal outbreaks caused by vaccine preventable serogroups.

Available Dosage Forms

Injection, solution [preservative free]:

Menactra®: 4 mcg each of polysaccharide antigen groups A, C, Y, and W-135 [bound to diphtheria toxoid 48 mcg] per 0.5 mL

Menveo®: MenA oligosaccharide 10 mcg, MenC oligosaccharide 5 mcg, MenY oligosaccharide 5 mcg, and MenW-135 oligosaccharide 5 mcg [bound to CRM_{197} protein 32.7-64.1 mcg] per 0.5 mL

Dosing

Adult Immunization: I.M.:

Menactra®, Menveo®: Adults ≤55 years: 0.5 mL/dose

ACIP recommendations (CDC, 60[3], 2011):

Adults ≤55 years with persistent complement component deficiency, or functional or anatomic asplenia: Two doses, 2 months apart. A booster dose should be given every 5 years.

Adults ≤55 years with HIV infection and another indication for vaccination: Two doses, 2 months apart. A booster dose should be given every 5 years if still at risk for meningococcal disease.

Adults ≤55 years with prolonged increased risk of exposure: One dose. If still at risk for meningococcal disease, a booster dose should be given based on the age at first dose.

College students: Persons ≤21 years of age should have documentation of vaccination ≤5 years prior to enrollment. If the primary dose was given at <16 years of age, a booster dose should be given anytime after the 16th birthday and prior to college enrollment. The minimum interval between doses is 8 weeks.

Geriatric Safety and efficacy not established in patients >55 years.

Pediatric Immunization: I.M.:

Menactra®, Menveo®: Children ≥2 years: 0.5 mL/dose

ACIP recommendations (CDC, 60[3], 2011):

Children 11-18 years of age: Routine vaccination: One dose at 11 or 12 years of age with a booster dose at age 16. If primary dose was given at age 13-15 years, 1 booster dose should be given at 16-18 years of age. If primary dose was given ≥16 years of age, no booster dose is needed.

Children ≥2 years with persistent complement component deficiency, or functional or anatomic asplenia: Two doses, 2 months apart. A booster dose should be given every 5 years.

Children ≥2 years with HIV infection and another indication for vaccination: Two doses, 2 months apart. A booster dose should be given every 5 years if still at risk for meningococcal disease.

Children ≥2 years with prolonged increased risk of exposure: One dose. If still at risk for meningococcal disease, a booster dose should be given based on the age at first dose:

If first dose received at 2-6 years of age: Repeat dose 3 years after primary vaccination, and every 5 years thereafter if the person remains at increased risk.

If first dose received at ≥7 years of age: Repeat dose 5 years after primary vaccination, and every 5 years thereafter if the person remains at increased risk.

College students: Refer to adult dosing.

Administration

I.M. Administer by I.M. route, preferably into the upper deltoid region. Do not administer via I.V., SubQ or I.D. route. For patients at risk of hemorrhage, the ACIP recommends "it should be administered intramuscularly if, in the opinion of a physician familiar with the patient's bleeding risk, the vaccine can be administered by this route with reasonable safety. If the patient receives antihemophilia or other similar therapy, intramuscular vaccination can be scheduled shortly after such therapy is administered. A fine needle (23 gauge or smaller) can be used for the vaccination and firm pressure applied to the site (without rubbing) for at least 2 minutes. The patient or family should be instructed concerning the risk of hematoma from the injection." Patients on anticoagulant therapy should be considered to have the same bleeding risks and treated as those with clotting factor disorders (CDC, 60[2], 2011).

For I.M. administration only. Based on limited data, inadvertent SubQ administration provides a lower serologic response, however, the response is still considered to be protective. If inadvertently administered by the SubQ route, revaccination is not necessary.

Simultaneous administration of vaccines helps ensure the patients will be fully vaccinated by the appropriate age. Simultaneous administration of vaccines is defined as administering >1 vaccine on the same day at different anatomic sites. Separate vaccines should not be combined in the same syringe unless indicated by product specific labeling. Separate needles and syringes should be used for each injection. The ACIP prefers each dose of a specific vaccine in a series come from the same manufacturer when possible. Adolescents and adults should be vaccinated while seated or lying down. In general, preterm infants should be vaccinated at the same chronological age as full-term infants (CDC, 60[2], 2011).

Antipyretics have not been shown to prevent febrile seizures. Antipyretics may be used to treat fever or discomfort following vaccination (CDC, 2011). One study reported that routine prophylactic administration of acetaminophen to prevent fever prior to vaccination decreased the immune response of some vaccines; the clinical significance of this reduction in immune response has not been established (Prymula, 2009).

I.V. Do not administer via I.V., SubQ or I.D. route.

Other For I.M. administration only. Based on limited data, inadvertent SubQ administration provides a lower serologic response, however the response is still considered to be protective. If inadvertently administered by the SubQ route, revaccination is not necessary.

Monitoring and Teaching Issues

Physical Assessment Federal law requires entry into the patient's medical record.

◆ **Meningococcal Polysaccharide Vaccine** *see* Meningococcal Polysaccharide Vaccine (Groups A / C / Y and W-135) *on page 1169*

Meningococcal Polysaccharide Vaccine (Groups A / C / Y and W-135)

(me NIN joe kok al pol i SAK a ride vak SEEN groops aye, see, why & dubl yoo won thur tee fyve)

U.S. Brand Names Menomune®-A/C/Y/W-135

Index Terms Meningococcal Polysaccharide Vaccine; MPSV; MPSV4

Generic Availability (U.S.) No

Pharmacologic Category Vaccine, Inactivated (Bacterial)

Medication Safety Issues

Administration issue:

Menomume® (MPSV4) should be administered by subcutaneous (SubQ) injection. Menactra® (MCV4), also a meningococcal polysaccharide vaccine, is to be administered by intramuscular (I.M.) injection only.

Pregnancy Risk Factor C

Lactation Excretion in breast milk unknown/use caution

Use Provide active immunity to meningococcal serogroups contained in the vaccine

The Advisory Committee on Immunization Practices (ACIP) recommends routine vaccination for persons at increased risk for meningococcal disease. Meningococcal conjugate vaccine (MCV4) is preferred for persons aged 2-55 years; meningococcal polysaccharide vaccine (MPSV4) is preferred in adults ≥56 years of age (CDC, 2005).

Persons at increased risk include:

- Previously unvaccinated college freshmen living in dormitories
- Microbiologists routinely exposed to isolates of *N. meningitidis*
- Military recruits
- Persons traveling to or who reside in countries where *N. meningitidis* is hyperendemic or epidemic, particularly if contact with local population will be prolonged
- Persons with persistent complement component deficiencies (eg, C5-C9, properidin, factor H, or factor D)
- Persons with anatomic or functional asplenia
- Persons with HIV infection

Use is also recommended during meningococcal outbreaks caused by vaccine preventable serogroups.

Available Dosage Forms

Injection, powder for reconstitution [MPSV4]:

Menomune®-A/C/Y/W-135: 50 mcg each of polysaccharide antigen groups A, C, Y, and W-135 per 0.5 mL dose

Dosing

Adult & Geriatric Immunization: SubQ: 0.5 mL/dose

ACIP recommendations:

Adults ≤55 years: 0.5 mL/dose; however, use is not generally recommended; meningococcal conjugate vaccine (MCV4) is preferred (CDC, 2011); If MCV4 is unavailable, meningococcal polysaccharide vaccine (MPSV4) is an acceptable alternative (CDC, 2005). Persons at prolonged increased risk for meningococcal disease should be revaccinated with MCV4 (CDC, 2009).

Adults >55 years: 0.5 mL/dose (MPSV4 preferred in this population) (CDC, 2005)

Pediatric Immunization: SubQ: *ACIP recommendations:*

Children <2 years: Not usually recommended. Two doses (0.5 mL/dose), 3 months apart, may be considered in children 3-18 months to elicit short-term protection against serogroup A disease. A single dose may be considered in children 19-23 months (CDC, 2005).

Children ≥2 years: 0.5 mL/dose; however, use is not generally recommended; meningococcal conjugate vaccine (MCV4) is preferred (CDC, 2011); If MCV4 is unavailable, meningococcal polysaccharide vaccine (MPSV4) is an acceptable alternative (CDC, 2005) Persons at prolonged increased risk for meningococcal disease should be revaccinated with MCV4 (CDC, 2009).

Administration

Other Administer by SubQ injection to the deltoid region; do not administer intradermally, I.M., or I.V.

Simultaneous administration of vaccines helps ensure the patients will be fully vaccinated by the appropriate age. Simultaneous administration of vaccines is defined as administering ≥1 vaccine on the same day at different anatomic sites. Separate vaccines should not be combined in the same syringe unless indicated by product specific labeling. Separate needles and syringes should be used for each injection. The ACIP prefers each dose of a specific vaccine in a series come from the same manufacturer when possible. Adolescents and adults should be vaccinated while seated or lying down. In general, preterm infants should be vaccinated at the same chronological age as full-term infants (CDC, 2011).

Antipyretics have not been shown to prevent febrile seizures. Antipyretics may be used to treat fever or discomfort following vaccination (CDC, 2011). One study reported that routine prophylactic administration of acetaminophen to prevent fever prior to vaccination decreased the immune response of some vaccines; the clinical significance of this reduction in immune response has not been established (Prymula, 2009).

Monitoring and Teaching Issues

Physical Assessment Federal law requires entry into the patient's medical record.

Related Information

Immunization Recommendations *on page 1941*

- **Menomune®-A/C/Y/W-135** *see* Meningococcal Polysaccharide Vaccine (Groups A / C / Y and W-135) *on page 1169*
- **Menopur®** *see* Menotropins *on page 1170*
- **Menostar®** *see* Estradiol (Systemic) *on page 670*

Menotropins (men oh TROE pins)

U.S. Brand Names Menopur®; Repronex®

Index Terms hMG; Human Menopausal Gonadotropin

Generic Availability (U.S.) No

Pharmacologic Category Gonadotropin; Ovulation Stimulator

Medication Safety Issues

Sound-alike/look-alike issues:

Repronex® may be confused with Regranex®

Pregnancy Risk Factor X

Lactation Excretion in breast milk unknown/use caution

Use Female:

In conjunction with hCG to induce ovulation and pregnancy in infertile females experiencing oligoanovulation or anovulation when the cause of anovulation is functional and not caused by primary ovarian failure (Repronex®)

Stimulation of multiple follicle development in ovulatory patients as part of an assisted reproductive technology (ART) (Menopur®, Repronex®)

Unlabeled/Investigational Use Male: Stimulation of spermatogenesis in primary or secondary hypogonadotropic hypogonadism

Mechanism of Action/Effect Actions occur as a result of both follicle stimulating hormone (FSH) effects and luteinizing hormone (LH) effects; menotropins stimulate the development and maturation of the ovarian follicle (FSH), cause ovulation (LH), and stimulate the development of the corpus luteum (LH); in males it stimulates spermatogenesis (LH)

Contraindications Hypersensitivity to menotropins or any component of the formulation; primary ovarian failure as indicated by a high follicle-stimulating hormone (FSH) level; uncontrolled thyroid and adrenal dysfunction; abnormal bleeding of undetermined origin; intracranial lesion (ie, pituitary tumor); ovarian cyst or enlargement not due to polycystic ovary syndrome; infertility due to any cause other than anovulation (except candidates for *in vitro* fertilization); sex hormone-dependent tumors of the reproductive tract and accessory organs; pregnancy

Warnings/Precautions These medications should only be used by physicians who are thoroughly familiar with infertility problems and their management. Advise patient of frequency and potential hazards of multiple pregnancy. May cause ovarian hyperstimulation syndrome (OHSS); if severe, treatment should be discontinued and patient should be hospitalized (may become more severe if pregnancy occurs). Monitor for ovarian enlargement; to minimize the hazard of abnormal ovarian enlargement, use the lowest possible dose. Serious pulmonary conditions (atelectasis, acute respiratory distress syndrome) and arterial thromboembolism have been reported. Safety and efficacy have not been established in renal or hepatic impairment, or in pediatric and geriatric patients. Use may lead to multiple births. Products may contain lactose.

Drug Interactions

Avoid Concomitant Use There are no known interactions where it is recommended to avoid concomitant use.

Decreased Effect There are no known significant interactions involving a decrease in effect.

Increased Effect/Toxicity There are no known significant interactions involving an increase in effect.

Adverse Reactions Adverse effects may vary according to specific product, route, and/or dosage.

>10%:

Central nervous system: Headache (up to 34%)
Gastrointestinal: Abdominal pain (up to 18%), nausea (up to 12%)
Genitourinary: OHSS (up to 13%, dose related)
Local: Injection site reaction (4% to 12%)

1% to 10%:

Cardiovascular: Flushing
Central nervous system: Dizziness, malaise, migraine
Endocrine & metabolic: Breast tenderness, hot flashes, menstrual irregularities
Gastrointestinal: Abdominal cramping, abdominal fullness, constipation, diarrhea, enlarged abdomen, vomiting
Genitourinary: Ectopic pregnancy, ovarian disease, vaginal hemorrhage
Local: Injection site edema/pain
Neuromuscular & skeletal: Back pain
Respiratory: Cough increased, respiratory disorder
Miscellaneous: Infection, flu-like syndrome

Frequency not defined:

Cardiovascular: Stroke, tachycardia, thrombosis (venous or arterial)
Dermatologic: Angioedema, rash, urticaria
Genitourinary: Adnexal torsion, hemoperitoneum, ovarian enlargement
Neuromuscular & skeletal: Limb necrosis
Respiratory: Acute respiratory distress syndrome, atelectasis, dyspnea, embolism, laryngeal edema, pulmonary infarction, tachypnea
Miscellaneous: Allergic reaction, anaphylaxis

Pharmacodynamics/Kinetics

Excretion Urine (~10% as unchanged drug)

Available Dosage Forms

Injection, powder for reconstitution:

Menopur®, Repronex®: Follicle stimulating hormone activity 75 int. units and luteinizing hormone activity 75 int. units

Dosing

Adult

Repronex®: I.M., SubQ:

Induction of ovulation in patients with oligoanovulation (Female): Initial: 150 int. units daily for the first 5 days of treatment. Adjustments should not be made more frequently than once every 2 days and should not exceed 75-150 int. units per adjustment. Maximum daily dose should not exceed 450 int. units and dosing beyond 12 days is not recommended. If patient's response is appropriate, hCG 5000-10,000 units should be given one day following the last dose of Repronex®. Hold dose if serum estradiol is >2000 pg/mL, if the ovaries are abnormally enlarged, or if abdominal pain occurs; the patient should also be advised to refrain from intercourse. May repeat process if follicular development is inadequate or if pregnancy does not occur.

Assisted reproductive technologies (Female): Initial (in patients who have received GnRH agonist or antagonist pituitary suppression): 225 int. units; adjustments in dose should not be made more frequently than once every 2 days and should not exceed more than 75-150 int. units per adjustment. The maximum daily doses of Repronex® given should not exceed 450 int. units and dosing beyond 12 days is not recommended. Once adequate follicular development is evident, hCG (5000-10,000 units) should be administered to induce final follicular maturation in preparation for oocyte retrieval. Withhold treatment when ovaries are abnormally enlarged on last day of therapy (to reduce chance of developing OHSS).

Menopur®: SubQ: *Assisted reproductive technologies (ART):* Initial (in patients who have received GnRH agonist for pituitary suppression): 225 int. units; adjustments in dose should not be made more frequently than once every 2 days and should not exceed more than 150 int. units per adjustment. The maximum daily dose given should not exceed 450 int. units and dosing beyond 20 days is not recommended. Once adequate follicular development is evident, hCG should be administered to induce final follicular maturation in preparation for oocyte retrieval. Withhold treatment when ovaries are abnormally enlarged on last day of therapy (to reduce chance of developing OHSS).

Spermatogenesis (Male) (unlabeled use): I.M.: Following pretreatment with hCG: 75 int. units 3 times/week and hCG 2000 units twice weekly until sperm is detected in the ejaculate (4-6 months); may then be increased to menotropins 150 int. units 3 times/week

Administration

I.M. Repronex®: Administer deep in a large muscle.

Other SubQ:

Menopur®: Administer to alternating sites of the abdomen. When administration to the lower abdomen is not possible, the injection may be given into the thigh.

Repronex®: Administer to alternating sites of the lower abdomen.

Stability

Reconstitution After reconstitution inject immediately; discard any unused portion.

Storage Lyophilized powder may be refrigerated or stored at room temperature. Protect from light.

Monitoring and Teaching Issues

Physical Assessment Teach appropriate method for measuring basal body temperature to indicate ovulation. Stress importance of following prescriber's instructions for timing intercourse. If self-administered, teach appropriate injection technique and needle disposal.

Patient Education Self injection: Follow prescriber's recommended schedule for injections. You may experience headache, nausea, abdominal pain, flushing, dizziness, or menstrual irregularities. Report pain at injection site; enlarged breasts (male); respiratory difficulty; nosebleeds; acute abdominal discomfort; abdominal distention; fever; or warmth, swelling, weight gain, pain, or redness in calves.

Pregnancy Considerations Ectopic pregnancy and congenital abnormalities have been reported. The incidence of congenital abnormality is similar during natural conception.

◆ **Menveo®** *see* Meningococcal (Groups A / C / Y and W-135) Diphtheria Conjugate Vaccine *on page 1168*

Meperidine (me PER i deen)

U.S. Brand Names Demerol®

Index Terms Isonipecaine Hydrochloride; Meperidine Hydrochloride; Pethidine Hydrochloride

Generic Availability (U.S.) Yes

Pharmacologic Category Analgesic, Opioid

Medication Safety Issues

Avoid the use of meperidine for pain control, especially in elderly and renally-compromised patients because of the risk of neurotoxicity (American Pain Society, 2008; Institute for Safe Medication Practices [ISMP], 2007)

Sound-alike/look-alike issues:

Meperidine may be confused with meprobamate

Demerol® may be confused with Demulen®, Desyrel, dicumarol, Dilaudid®, Dymelor®, Pamelor®

High alert medication: The Institute for Safe Medication Practices (ISMP) includes this medication among its list of drug classes which have a heightened risk of causing significant patient harm when used in error.

Beers Criteria medication: This drug may be inappropriate for use in geriatric patients (high severity risk).

Pregnancy Risk Factor C

Lactation Enters breast milk/not recommended (AAP rates "compatible"; AAP 2001 update pending)

Use Management of moderate-to-severe pain; adjunct to anesthesia and preoperative sedation

Unlabeled/Investigational Use Reduce postoperative shivering; reduce rigors from amphotericin B (conventional)

Controlled Substance C-II

Available Dosage Forms

Injection, solution: 10 mg/mL (30 mL, 50 mL, 60 mL); 25 mg/mL (1 mL); 50 mg/mL (1 mL); 100 mg/mL (1 mL)

Demerol®: 25 mg/mL (1 mL); 25 mg/0.5 mL (0.5 mL); 50 mg/mL (1 mL, 1.5 mL, 2 mL, 30 mL); 75 mg/mL (1 mL); 100 mg/mL (1 mL, 20 mL)

Solution, oral: 50 mg/5 mL (500 mL)

Tablet, oral: 50 mg, 100 mg

Demerol®: 50 mg, 100 mg

Dosing

Adult Note: The American Pain Society (2008) and ISMP (2007) do not recommend meperidine's use as an analgesic. If use in acute pain (in patients without renal or CNS disease) cannot be avoided, treatment should be limited to ≤48 hours and doses should not exceed 600 mg/24 hours.

Pain (analgesic):

Oral: Initial: Opiate-naive: 50 mg every 3-4 hours as needed; usual dosage range: 50-150 mg every 2-4 hours as needed (manufacturers recommendation; oral route is not recommended for acute pain)

I.M., SubQ: Initial: Opiate-naive: 50-75 mg every 3-4 hours as needed; patients with prior opiate exposure may require higher initial doses.

Preoperatively: 50-100 mg given 30-90 minutes before the beginning of anesthesia

Slow I.V.: Initial: 5-10 mg every 5 minutes as needed

Postoperative shivering (unlabeled use): *I.V.:* 25-50 mg once (Crowley, 2008; Kranke, 2002; Mercandante, 1994; Wang, 1999)

Geriatric Note: The American Pain Society (2008) and ISMP (2007) do not recommend meperidine's use as an analgesic.

Oral: 50 mg every 4 hours
I.M.: 25 mg every 4 hours

Pediatric Note: The American Pain Society (2008) and ISMP (2007) do not recommend meperidine's use as an analgesic.

Pain (analgesic): Oral, I.M., I.V., SubQ: Children: 1-1.5 mg/kg/dose every 3-4 hours as needed; 1-2 mg/kg as a single dose preoperative medication may be used; maximum 100 mg/dose. (Oral route is not recommended for acute pain.)

Renal Impairment Avoid use in renal impairment.

Hepatic Impairment Increased narcotic effect in cirrhosis; reduction in dose is more important for oral than I.V. route.

Administration

Oral Oral solution: Administer solution in 1/2 glass of water; undiluted solution may exert topical anesthetic effect on mucous membranes

I.V. Meperidine may be administered I.M., SubQ, or I.V. IVP should be given slowly, use of a 10 mg/mL concentration has been recommended. For continuous I.V. infusions, a more dilute solution (eg, 1 mg/mL) should be used.

Monitoring and Teaching Issues

Physical Assessment Monitor frequently for need; assess patient's physical and/or psychological dependence. For inpatients, implement safety measures to prevent falls. Discontinue slowly after prolonged use.

Patient Education Drug may cause physical and/or psychological dependence. While using this medication, do not use alcohol and other prescription or OTC medications (especially sedatives, tranquilizers, antihistamines, or pain medications) without consulting prescriber. Maintain adequate hydration, unless instructed to restrict fluid intake. May cause hypotension, dizziness, drowsiness, impaired coordination, or blurred vision; loss of appetite, nausea, or vomiting; or constipation. Report chest pain, slow or rapid heartbeat, dizziness, or persistent headache; changes in mental status; seizures; changes in renal function; skin rash; or shortness of breath.

Related Information

Opioid Analgesics *on page 2003*

◆ **Meperidine Hydrochloride** *see* Meperidine *on page 1172*

◆ **Mephyton®** *see* Phytonadione *on page 1457*

◆ **Mepron®** *see* Atovaquone *on page 169*

◆ **Mercaptoethane Sulfonate** *see* Mesna *on page 1180*

Mercaptopurine (mer kap toe PYOOR een)

U.S. Brand Names Purinethol®

Index Terms 6-Mercaptopurine (error-prone abbreviation); 6-MP (error-prone abbreviation); NSC-755

Generic Availability (U.S.) Yes

Pharmacologic Category Antineoplastic Agent, Antimetabolite; Antineoplastic Agent, Antimetabolite (Purine Analog); Immunosuppressant Agent

Medication Safety Issues

Sound-alike/look-alike issues:

Mercaptopurine may be confused with methotrexate
Purinethol® may be confused with propylthiouracil

High alert medication: The Institute for Safe Medication Practices (ISMP) includes this medication among its list of drugs which have a heightened risk of causing significant patient harm when used in error.

To avoid potentially serious dosage errors, the terms "6-mercaptopurine" or "6-MP" should be avoided; use of these terms has been associated with sixfold overdosages.

Azathioprine is metabolized to mercaptopurine; concurrent use of these commercially-available products has resulted in profound myelosuppression.

Pregnancy Risk Factor D

Lactation Enters breast milk/contraindicated

Use Treatment (maintenance and induction) of acute lymphoblastic leukemia (ALL)

Unlabeled/Investigational Use Steroid-sparing agent for corticosteroid-dependent Crohn's disease (CD) and ulcerative colitis (UC); maintenance of remission in CD; fistulizing Crohn's disease

Mechanism of Action/Effect Purine antagonist which inhibits DNA and RNA synthesis

Contraindications Hypersensitivity to mercaptopurine or any component of the formulation; patients whose disease showed prior resistance to mercaptopurine or thioguanine; severe liver disease, severe bone marrow suppression; pregnancy

Warnings/Precautions Hazardous agent - use appropriate precautions for handling and disposal. Consider adjusting dosage in patients with renal impairment or hepatic failure; use with caution in patients with prior bone marrow suppression. Toxicity to immunosuppressives is increased in elderly. Start with lowest recommended adult doses. Signs of infection, such as fever and WBC rise, may not occur. Lethargy and confusion may be more prominent signs of infection. Use caution with other hepatotoxic drugs or in dosages >2.5 mg/kg/day; hepatotoxicity may occur. Patients with genetic deficiency of thiopurine methyltransferase (TPMT) or concurrent therapy with drugs which may inhibit TPMT (eg, olsalazine) or xanthine oxidase (eg, allopurinol) may be sensitive to myelosuppressive effects. Azathioprine is metabolized to mercaptopurine; concomitant use may result in profound myelosuppression and should be avoided. Immune response to vaccines may be diminished.

To avoid potentially serious dosage errors, the terms "6-mercaptopurine" or "6-MP" should be avoided; use of these terms has been associated with sixfold overdosages.

Drug Interactions

Avoid Concomitant Use

Avoid concomitant use of Mercaptopurine with any of the following: BCG; Febuxostat; Natalizumab; Pimecrolimus; Roflumilast; Tacrolimus (Topical)

Decreased Effect

Mercaptopurine may decrease the levels/effects of: BCG; Sipuleucel-T; Vaccines (Inactivated); Vitamin K Antagonists

The levels/effects of Mercaptopurine may be decreased by: Echinacea

Increased Effect/Toxicity

Mercaptopurine may increase the levels/effects of: Leflunomide; Natalizumab; Vaccines (Live); Vitamin K Antagonists

The levels/effects of Mercaptopurine may be increased by: 5-ASA Derivatives; Allopurinol; AzaTHIOprine; Denosumab; Febuxostat; Pimecrolimus; Roflumilast; Tacrolimus (Topical); Trastuzumab

Adverse Reactions

>10%:

Hematologic: Myelosuppression; leukopenia, thrombocytopenia, anemia
- Onset: 7-10 days
- Nadir: 14-16 days
- Recovery: 21-28 days

Hepatic: Intrahepatic cholestasis and focal centralobular necrosis (40%), characterized by hyperbilirubinemia, increased alkaline phosphatase and AST, jaundice, ascites, encephalopathy; more common at doses >2.5 mg/kg/day. Usually occurs within 2 months of therapy but may occur within 1 week, or be delayed up to 8 years.

1% to 10%:

Central nervous system: Drug fever
Dermatologic: Hyperpigmentation, rash
Endocrine & metabolic: Hyperuricemia
Gastrointestinal: Anorexia, diarrhea, mucositis, nausea, pancreatitis, stomach pain, stomatitis, vomiting
Renal: Renal toxicity

Pharmacodynamics/Kinetics

Absorption Variable and incomplete (16% to 50%)

Time to Peak Serum: ~2 hours

Protein Binding 19%

Half-Life Elimination Age dependent: Children: 21 minutes; Adults: 47 minutes

Metabolism Hepatic and via GI mucosa; hepatically via xanthine oxidase and methylation via TPMT to sulfate conjugates, 6-thiouric acid, and other inactive compounds; first-pass effect

Excretion Urine (46% as mercaptopurine and metabolites)

Available Dosage Forms

Tablet, oral: 50 mg
Purinethol®: 50 mg

Dosing

Adult Refer to individual protocols.

ALL:

Induction: Oral: 2.5-5 mg/kg/day (100-200 mg)
Maintenance: Oral: 1.5-2.5 mg/kg/day **or** 80-100 mg/m²/day given once daily

Note: In ALL, administration in the evening (vs morning administration) may lower the risk of relapse.

Reduction of steroid use in CD or UC, maintenance of remission in CD or fistulizing disease (unlabeled uses): Oral: Initial: 50 mg daily; may increase by 25 mg/day every 1-2 weeks as tolerated to target dose of 1-1.5 mg/kg/day

Dosage adjustment with concurrent allopurinol: Reduce mercaptopurine dosage to 1/4 to 1/3 the usual dose.

Dosage adjustment in TPMT-deficiency: Not established; substantial reductions are generally required only in homozygous deficiency.

Geriatric Due to renal decline with age, start with lower recommended doses for adults.

Pediatric ALL: Refer to individual protocols: Oral:

Induction: 2.5-5 mg/kg/day **or** 70-100 mg/m^2/day given once daily

Maintenance: 1.5-2.5 mg/kg/day **or** 50-75 mg/m^2/day given once daily

Note: In ALL, administration in the evening (vs morning administration) may lower the risk of relapse.

Renal Impairment The FDA-approved labeling recommends starting with reduced doses in patients with renal impairment to avoid accumulation; however, specific guidelines are not available. The following guidelines have been used by some clinicians (Aronoff, 2007): Children:

Cl_{cr} <50 mL/minute: Administer every 48 hours

Hemodialysis: Administer every 48 hours

Continuous ambulatory peritoneal dialysis (CAPD): Administer every 48 hours

Continuous renal replacement therapy (CRRT): Administer every 48 hours

Hepatic Impairment The FDA-approved labeling recommends considering a reduced dose in patients with hepatic impairment; however, specific guidelines are not available.

Administration

Oral Preferably on an empty stomach (1 hour before or 2 hours after meals)

Stability

Storage Store at room temperature of 15°C to 25°C (59°F to 77°F). Protect from moisture.

Monitoring and Teaching Issues

Laboratory Monitoring CBC with differential, platelet count, liver function, uric acid, renal function

For use as immunomodulatory therapy in CD or UC, monitor CBC with differential weekly for 1 month, then biweekly for 1 month, followed by monitoring every 1-2 months throughout the course of therapy. LFTs should be assessed every 3 months.

Physical Assessment Do not use the terms "6-mercaptopurine" or "6-MP" when writing prescriptions; use of these terms has been associated with sixfold overdosage. Assess hepatic function; jaundice, ascites, and encephalopathy can occur some time following therapy. Monitor nutritional status and renal status. Monitor for dehydration, myelosuppression, anemia, and leukopenia on a regular basis. Teach patient importance of adequate hydration.

Patient Education Take daily dose at the same time each day. Preferable to take an on empty stomach, 1 hour before or 2 hours after meals. Maintain adequate hydration unless instructed to restrict fluid intake. You may be more susceptible to infection. May cause nausea, vomiting, diarrhea, loss of appetite, weakness or lethargy, mouth sores, or headache. Report signs of persistent fever, opportunistic infection (eg, fever, chills, sore throat, burning urination, fatigue), bleeding (eg, tarry stools, easy bruising), unresolved mouth sores, nausea or vomiting, swelling of extremities, respiratory difficulty, unusual weight gain, or changes in urinary pattern.

Dietary Considerations Should not be administered with meals.

Geriatric Considerations Toxicity to immunosuppressives is increased in the elderly. Start with lowest recommended adult doses. Signs of infection, such as fever and WBC rise, may not occur. Lethargy and confusion may be more prominent signs of infection.

◆ **6-Mercaptopurine (error-prone abbreviation)** *see* Mercaptopurine *on page 1173*

◆ **Meridia® [DSC]** *see* Sibutramine *on page 1638*

Meropenem (mer oh PEN em)

U.S. Brand Names Merrem® I.V.

Generic Availability (U.S.) Yes

Pharmacologic Category Antibiotic, Carbapenem

Medication Safety Issues

Sound-alike/look-alike issues:

Meropenem may be confused with ertapenem, imipenem, metronidazole.

Pregnancy Risk Factor B

Lactation Excretion in breast milk unknown/use caution

Use Treatment of intra-abdominal infections (complicated appendicitis and peritonitis); treatment of bacterial meningitis in pediatric patients ≥3 months of age caused by *S. pneumoniae*, *H. influenzae*, and *N. meningitidis*; treatment of complicated skin and skin structure infections caused by susceptible organisms

Unlabeled/Investigational Use *Burkholderia pseudomallei* (melioidosis), febrile neutropenia, liver abscess, meningitis (adults), otitis externa, pneumonia, urinary tract infections

Mechanism of Action/Effect Inhibits cell wall synthesis in susceptible bacteria

Contraindications Hypersensitivity to meropenem, any component of the formulation, or other carbapenems (eg, imipenem); patients who have experienced anaphylactic reactions to other beta-lactams

Warnings/Precautions Serious hypersensitivity reactions, including anaphylaxis, have been reported (some without a history of previous allergic reactions to beta-lactams). Has been associated with CNS adverse effects, including confusional states and seizures; use caution with CNS disorders (eg, brain lesions, history of seizures, or renal impairment). Prolonged use may result in fungal or bacterial superinfection, including *C. difficile*-associated diarrhea (CDAD) and pseudomembranous colitis; CDAD has been observed >2 months postantibiotic treatment. Use with caution in patients with renal impairment; dosage adjustment required in patients with moderate-to-severe renal dysfunction. Thrombocytopenia has been reported in patients with renal dysfunction. Lower doses (based upon renal function) are often required in the elderly. May decrease divalproex sodium/valproic acid concentrations leading to breakthrough seizures; concomitant use not recommended. Alternative antimicrobial agents should be considered; if concurrent meropenem is necessary, consider additional antiseizure medication.

Drug Interactions

Avoid Concomitant Use

Avoid concomitant use of Meropenem with any of the following: BCG; Probenecid

Decreased Effect

Meropenem may decrease the levels/effects of: BCG; Divalproex; Typhoid Vaccine; Valproic Acid

Increased Effect/Toxicity

The levels/effects of Meropenem may be increased by: Probenecid

Lab Interactions Increased AST/ALT, alkaline phosphatase, LDH, bilirubin, platelets, eosinophils, BUN, creatinine; decreased platelets, hemoglobin/hematocrit, WBC; prolonged or shortened PT; prolonged PTT; positive direct or indirect Coombs' test; presence of urine red blood cells

Adverse Reactions 1% to 10%:

Central nervous system: Headache (2% to 8%), pain (≤5%)
Dermatologic: Rash (2% to 3%, includes diaper-area moniliasis in pediatrics), pruritus (1%)
Endocrine & metabolic: Hypoglycemia
Gastrointestinal: Diarrhea (4% to 7%), nausea/vomiting (1% to 8%), constipation (1% to 7%), oral moniliasis (up to 2% in pediatric patients), glossitis (1%)
Hematologic: Anemia (≤6%)
Local: Inflammation at the injection site (2%), phlebitis/thrombophlebitis (1%), injection site reaction (1%)
Respiratory: Apnea (1%), pharyngitis, pneumonia
Miscellaneous: Sepsis (2%), shock (1%)

Pharmacodynamics/Kinetics

Time to Peak Tissue: 1 hour following infusion

Protein Binding ~2%

Half-Life Elimination

Normal renal function: 1-1.5 hours
Cl_{cr} 30-80 mL/minute: 1.9-3.3 hours
Cl_{cr} 2-30 mL/minute: 3.82-5.7 hours

Metabolism Hepatic; metabolized to open beta-lactam form (inactive)

Excretion Urine (~70% as unchanged drug)

Available Dosage Forms

Injection, powder for reconstitution: 500 mg, 1 g
Merrem® I.V.: 500 mg, 1 g

Dosing

Adult & Geriatric

Burkholderia pseudomallei* (melioidosis) (unlabeled use), *Pseudomonas: I.V.: 1 g every 8 hours

Cholangitis, intra-abdominal infections, severe: I.V.: 1 g every 8 hours. **Note:** 2010 IDSA guidelines recommend a treatment duration of 4-7 days (provided source controlled). Not recommended for mild-to-moderate, community-acquired intra-abdominal infections due to risk of toxicity and the development of resistant organisms (Solomkin, 2010).

Febrile neutropenia, otitis externa, pneumonia (unlabeled uses): I.V.: 1 g every 8 hours

Liver abscess (unlabeled use): I.V.: 1 g every 8 hours for 2-3 weeks, then oral therapy for duration of 4-6 weeks

Meningitis (unlabeled use): I.V.: 2 g every 8 hours

Mild-to-moderate infection, other severe infections (unlabeled use): I.V.: 1.5-3 g/day divided every 8 hours

Skin and skin structure infections (complicated): I.V.: 500 mg every 8 hours; diabetic foot: 1 g every 8 hours

Urinary tract infections, complicated (unlabeled use): I.V.: 500 mg to 1 g every 8 hours

Pediatric

Febrile neutropenia (unlabeled use): I.V.:
Children ≥3 months (<50 kg): 20 mg/kg every 8 hours (maximum dose: 1 g every 8 hours)
Children >50 kg: Refer to adult dosing.

Intra-abdominal infections: I.V.:
Children ≥3 months (<50 kg): 20 mg/kg every 8 hours (maximum dose: 1 g every 8 hours)
Children >50 kg: 1 g every 8 hours

Meningitis: I.V.: Children ≥3 months (<50 kg): 40 mg/kg every 8 hours (maximum dose: 2 g every 8 hours)

Skin and skin structure infections (complicated): I.V.:
Children ≥3 months (<50 kg): 10 mg/kg every 8 hours (maximum dose: 500 mg every 8 hours)
Children >50 kg: Refer to adult dosing.

Renal Impairment

Cl_{cr} 26-50 mL/minute: Administer recommended dose based on indication every 12 hours

Cl_{cr} 10-25 mL/minute: Administer one-half recommended dose based on indication every 12 hours

Cl_{cr} <10 mL/minute: Administer one-half recommended dose based on indication every 24 hours

Intermittent hemodialysis: Meropenem and its metabolite are readily dialyzable; administer dose after dialysis session

Continuous renal replacement therapy (CRRT): Drug clearance is highly dependent on the method of renal replacement, filter type, and flow rate. Appropriate dosing requires close monitoring of pharmacologic response, signs of adverse reactions due to drug accumulation, as well as drug levels in relation to target trough (if appropriate). The following are general recommendations only (based on dialysate flow/ultrafiltration rates of 1 L/hour) and should not supersede clinical judgment:

CVVH or CVVHD/CVVHDF: 1 g every 12 hours achieves target trough of ~4 mg/L; 500 mg every 12 hours may be considered for highly sensitive organisms. **Note:** Substantial variability exists in various published recommendations, ranging from 1-3 g/day given in 2-3 divided doses.

Administration

I.V. Administer I.V. infusion over 15-30 minutes; I.V. bolus injection over 3-5 minutes.

Stability

Reconstitution Meropenem infusion vials may be reconstituted with SWFI or a compatible diluent (eg, NS). The 500 mg vials should be reconstituted with 10 mL, and 1 g vials with 20 mL. May be further diluted with compatible solutions for infusion. Consult detailed reference/product labeling for compatibility.

Storage Dry powder should be stored at controlled room temperature 20°C to 25°C (68°F to 77°F).

Injection reconstitution: Stability in vial when constituted (up to 50 mg/mL) with:

SWFI: Stable for up to 2 hours at controlled room temperature of 15°C to 25°C (59°F to 77°F) or for up to 12 hours under refrigeration.

Sodium chloride: Stable for up to 2 hours at controlled room temperature of 15°C to 25°C (59°F to 77°F) or for up to 18 hours under refrigeration.

Dextrose 5% injection: Stable for 1 hour at controlled room temperature of 15°C to 25°C (59°F to 77°F) or for 8 hours under refrigeration.

Infusion admixture (1-20 mg/mL): Solution stability when diluted in NS is 4 hours at controlled room temperature of 15°C to 25°C (59°F to 77°F) or 24 hours under refrigeration. Stability in D_5W is 1 hour at controlled room temperature of 15°C to 25°C (59°F to 77°F) or for 4 hours under refrigeration. For other diluents, see prescribing information.

Monitoring and Teaching Issues

Laboratory Monitoring Perform culture and sensitivity testing prior to initiating therapy. During prolonged therapy, monitor renal function, liver function, CBC.

Physical Assessment Assess results of culture and sensitivity tests and patient's allergy history prior to beginning treatment. Use caution in presence of renal impairment or neurologic disorder. Infusion site should be monitored closely for phlebitis/thrombophlebitis. Assess renal and hepatic function and CBC. Teach patient importance of adequate hydration.

Patient Education This medication can only be given by infusion. Report immediately any burning, pain, swelling, or redness at infusion site. Maintain adequate hydration unless instructed to restrict fluid intake. May cause nausea, vomiting, diarrhea, or headache. Report persistent GI distress, persistent diarrhea, mouth sores, respiratory difficulty, headache, or CNS changes (agitation, delirium).

Dietary Considerations Some products may contain sodium.

Geriatric Considerations Adjust dose based on renal function.

Breast-Feeding Considerations It is not known if meropenem is excreted in breast milk. The manufacturer recommends that caution be exercised when administering meropenem to breast-feeding women. Most penicillins and carbapenems are safe for use in breast-feeding. Nondose-related effects could include modification of bowel flora.

Pregnancy Considerations Meropenem is classified as pregnancy category B because no evidence of impaired fertility or fetal harm has been found in animals. Adequate and well-controlled studies have not been conducted in pregnant women and it is not known whether meropenem can cause fetal harm.

Related Information

Antimicrobial Drugs of Choice *on page 2008*

Community-Acquired Pneumonia in Adults *on page 2021*

◆ **Merrem® I.V.** *see* Meropenem *on page 1175*

Mesalamine (me SAL a meen)

U.S. Brand Names Apriso™; Asacol®; Asacol® HD; Canasa®; Lialda®; Pentasa®; Rowasa®; sfRowasa™

Index Terms 5-Aminosalicylic Acid; 5-ASA; Fisalamine; Mesalazine

Generic Availability (U.S.) Yes: Rectal suspension

Pharmacologic Category 5-Aminosalicylic Acid Derivative

Medication Safety Issues

Sound-alike/look-alike issues:

Mesalamine may be confused with mecamylamine, megestrol, memantine, metaxalone, methenamine

Apriso™ may be confused with Apri®

Asacol® may be confused with Ansaid®, Os-Cal®, Visicol®

Lialda™ may be confused with Aldara®

Pentasa® may be confused with Pancrease®, Pangestyme™

Pregnancy Risk Factor B/C (product specific)

Lactation Enters breast milk/use caution

Use

Oral:

Asacol®, Pentasa®: Treatment and maintenance of remission of mildly- to moderately-active ulcerative colitis

Apriso™: Maintenance of remission of ulcerative colitis

Asacol® HD: Treatment of moderately-active ulcerative colitis

Lialda™: Treatment of mildly- to moderately-active ulcerative colitis

Rectal: Treatment of active mild-to-moderate distal ulcerative colitis, proctosigmoiditis, or proctitis

Mechanism of Action/Effect Mesalamine (5-aminosalicylic acid) is the active component of sulfasalazine; the specific mechanism of action of mesalamine is unknown; however, it is thought that it modulates local chemical mediators of the inflammatory response, especially leukotrienes, and is also postulated to be a free radical scavenger or an inhibitor of tumor necrosis factor (TNF); action appears topical rather than systemic

Contraindications Hypersensitivity to mesalamine, aminosalicylates, salicylates, or any component of the formulation

Warnings/Precautions May cause an acute intolerance syndrome (cramping, acute abdominal pain, bloody diarrhea; sometimes fever, headache, rash); discontinue if this occurs. Use caution in patients with active peptic ulcers. Patients with pyloric stenosis may have prolonged gastric retention of tablets, delaying the release of mesalamine in the colon. Pericarditis or myocarditis should be considered in patients with chest pain; use with caution in patients predisposed to these conditions. Pancreatitis should be considered in patients with new abdominal discomfort. Symptomatic worsening of colitis/IBD may occur following initiation of therapy. Oligospermia (rare, reversible) has been reported in males. Use caution in patients with sulfasalazine hypersensitivity. Use caution in patients with impaired hepatic function; hepatic failure has been reported. Renal impairment (including minimal change nephropathy and acute/chronic interstitial nephritis) and rarely failure have been reported; use caution in patients with renal impairment. Use caution with other medications converted to mesalamine. Postmarketing reports suggest an increased incidence of blood dyscrasias in patients >65 years of age. In addition, elderly may have difficulty administering and retaining rectal suppositories or may have decreased renal function; use with caution and monitor.

Apriso™ contains phenylalanine. The Asacol® HD 800 mg tablet has not been shown to be bioequivalent to 2 Asacol® 400 mg tablets. Canasa® suppositories contain saturated vegetable fatty acid esters (contraindicated in patients with allergy to these components). Rowasa® enema contains potassium metabisulfite; may cause severe hypersensitivity reactions (ie, anaphylaxis) in patients with sulfite allergies.

Drug Interactions

Avoid Concomitant Use There are no known interactions where it is recommended to avoid concomitant use.

Decreased Effect

Mesalamine may decrease the levels/effects of: Cardiac Glycosides

The levels/effects of Mesalamine may be decreased by: Antacids; H2-Antagonists; Proton Pump Inhibitors

Increased Effect/Toxicity

Mesalamine may increase the levels/effects of: Heparin; Heparin (Low Molecular Weight); Thiopurine Analogs; Varicella Virus-Containing Vaccines

Adverse Reactions Adverse effects vary depending upon dosage form. Incidence usually on lower end with enema and suppository dosage forms.

>10%:

Central nervous system: Headache (2% to 35%), pain (≤14%)

Gastrointestinal: Abdominal pain (1% to 18%), eructation (16%), nausea (3% to 13%)

Respiratory: Pharyngitis (11%)

1% to 10%:

Cardiovascular: Chest pain (3%), peripheral edema (3%), vasodilation (≥2%)

Central nervous system: Dizziness (2% to 8%), fever (1% to 6%), chills (3%), malaise (2% to 3%), fatigue (<3%), vertigo (<3%), anxiety (≥2%), migraine (≥2%), nervousness (≥2%), insomnia (2%),

Dermatologic: Rash (1% to 6%), pruritus (1% to 3%), alopecia (<3%), acne (1% to 2%)

Endocrine & metabolic: Triglyceride increased (<3%)

Gastrointestinal: Diarrhea (2% to 8%), dyspepsia (1% to 6%), flatulence (1% to 6%), constipation (5%), vomiting (1% to 5%), colitis exacerbation (1% to 3%), rectal bleeding (<3%), abdominal distention (≥2%), gastroenteritis (≥2%), gastrointestinal bleeding (≥2%), stool abnormalities (≥2%), tenesmus (≥2%), rectal pain (1% to 2%), hemorrhoids (1%)

Genitourinary: Polyuria (≥2%)

Hematologic: Hematocrit/hemoglobin decreased (<3%)

Hepatic: Cholestatic hepatitis (<3%), transaminases increased (<3%), ALT increased (1%)

Local: Pain on insertion of enema tip (1%)

Neuromuscular & skeletal: Back pain (1% to 7%), arthralgia (≤5%), hypertonia (5%), myalgia (3%), paresthesia (≥2%), weakness (≥2%), arthritis (2%), leg/joint pain (2%)

Ocular: Vision abnormalities (≥2%), conjunctivitis (2%)

Otic: Tinnitus (<3%), ear pain (≥2%)

Renal: Creatinine clearance decreased (<3%), hematuria (<3%)

Respiratory: Nasopharyngitis (1% to 4%), dyspnea (<3%), bronchitis (≥2%), sinusitis (≥2%), cough (≤2%)

Miscellaneous: Flu-like syndrome (1% to 5%), infection (≥2%), diaphoresis (3%), intolerance syndrome (3%)

Pharmacodynamics/Kinetics

Absorption Rectal: Variable and dependent upon retention time, underlying GI disease, and colonic pH; Oral: Tablet: ~20% to 28%, Capsule: ~20% to 40%

Time to Peak

Capsule: Apriso™: ~4 hours; Pentasa®: 3 hours

Rectal: 4-7 hours

Tablet: Asacol®: 4-12 hours; Asacol® HD: 10-16 hours; Lialda™: 9-12 hours; Mezavant®: 8 hours

Protein Binding Mesalamine (5-ASA): ~43%; N-acetyl-5-ASA: ~78%

Half-Life Elimination 5-ASA: 0.5-10 hours; N-acetyl-5-ASA: 2-15 hours

Metabolism Hepatic and via GI tract to N-acetyl-5-aminosalicylic acid

Excretion Urine (primarily as metabolites, <8% as unchanged drug); feces (<2%)

Available Dosage Forms

Capsule, controlled release, oral:

Pentasa®: 250 mg, 500 mg

Capsule, delayed and extended release, oral:

Apriso™: 0.375 g

Suppository, rectal:

Canasa®: 1000 mg (30s, 42s)

Suspension, rectal: 4 g/60 mL (7s, 28s)

Rowasa®: 4 g/60 mL (7s, 28s)

sfRowasa™: 4 g/60 mL (7s, 28s)

Tablet, delayed release, enteric coated, oral:

Asacol®: 400 mg

Asacol® HD: 800 mg

Lialda®: 1.2 g

Dosing

Adult & Geriatric

Treatment of ulcerative colitis: Oral: Usual course of therapy is 3-8 weeks:

Capsule (Pentasa®): 1 g 4 times/day; **Note:** Apriso™ capsules are approved for maintenance of remission only.

Tablet: Initial:

Asacol®: 800 mg 3 times/day for 6 weeks

Asacol® HD: 1.6 g 3 times/day for 6 weeks

Lialda™, Mezavant®: 2.4-4.8 g once daily for up to 8 weeks

Maintenance of remission of ulcerative colitis: Oral:

Capsule:

Apriso™: 1.5 g once daily in the morning

Pentasa®: 1 g 4 times/day

Tablet (Asacol®): 1.6 g/day in divided doses; **Note:** Asacol® HD, Lialda™ and Mezavant® tablets are approved for treatment only.

Active mild-to-moderate distal ulcerative colitis, proctosigmoiditis, or proctitis: Retention enema: 60 mL (4 g) at bedtime, retained overnight, approximately 8 hours

Active ulcerative proctitis: Rectal suppository (Canasa®): Insert one 1000 mg suppository in rectum daily at bedtime; retained for at least 1-3 hours to achieve maximum benefit

Note: Duration of rectal therapy is 3-6 weeks; some patients may require rectal and oral therapy concurrently.

Administration

Oral Swallow capsules or tablets whole, do not break, chew, or crush.

Apriso™: Administer with or without food; do not administer with antacids

Asacol®: Do not break outer coating.

Asacol® HD: Do not break outer coating; administer with or without food.

Lialda™: Do not break outer coating; should be administered once daily with a meal

Mezavant®: Do not break outer coating; should be administered once daily with a meal

Other

Rectal enema: Shake bottle well. Retain enemas for 8 hours or as long as practical.

Suppository: Remove foil wrapper; avoid excessive handling. Should be retained for at least 1-3 hours to achieve maximum benefit.

Stability

Storage

Capsule:

Apriso™: Store at controlled room temperature of 20°C to 25°C (68°F to 77°F)

Pentasa®: Store at controlled room temperature of 15°C to 30°C (59°F to 86°F). Protect from light.

Enema: Store at controlled room temperature. Use promptly once foil wrap is removed. Contents may darken with time (do not use if dark brown).

Suppository: Store below 25°C (below 77°F). May store under refrigeration; do not freeze. Protect from direct heat, light, and humidity.

Tablet: Store at controlled room temperature:

Asacol®, Asacol® HD: 20°C to 25°C (68°F to 77°F)

Lialda™: 15°C to 30°C (59°F to 86°F)

Mezavant®: 15°C to 25°C (59°F to 77°F)

Monitoring and Teaching Issues

Laboratory Monitoring Renal function (prior to and periodically during therapy); CBC (particularly in elderly patients)

Physical Assessment Assess history of hypersensitivity to salicylates prior to beginning treatment. Use caution in presence of impaired hepatic or renal function, predisposition to pericarditis or myocarditis, or active peptic ulcers. Assess potential for interactions or toxicity with other pharmacological agents or herbal products the patient may be taking (eg, other medications converted to mesalamine). Assess results of laboratory tests (CBC and renal function), therapeutic effectiveness, and adverse reactions on a regular basis throughout therapy (acute intolerance syndrome may necessitate discontinuing). Teach patient proper use (according to formulation), possible side effects/appropriate interventions (eg, importance of adequate hydration), and adverse symptoms to report.

Patient Education Do not take any new prescriptions, OTC medications, or herbal products during therapy unless approved by prescriber. Take exactly as directed. Symptomatic exacerbation of colitis/IBD may occur when beginning treatment; this should resolve in a short time. May cause fatigue, dizziness, or insomnia (avoid driving or engaging in tasks requiring alertness until response to drug is known); mild gastrointestinal disturbance (eg, gas, constipation, nausea); back, joint, or muscle pain; or flu-like syndrome or cough (consult prescriber if persistent). Report immediately severe new abdominal pain or diarrhea; chest pain or rapid heartbeat; unusual pain (back, joint, muscle, or chest) or swelling of extremities; rash; ringing in ears or change in hearing; or other persistent adverse effects or lack of improvement.

Oral: Swallow tablets or capsules whole; do not break, crush, or chew. Notify prescriber if whole or partial tablets are repeatedly found in stool; should be taken with a meal.

Enema: Follow package insert direction for administering enema. Shake well before using; retain for 8 hours or as long as possible. May cause staining of clothing and undergarments. Do not use if solution is dark brown.

Suppository: Do not refrigerate; store at room temperature. After removing foil wrapper, insert high in rectum without excessive handling (warmth will melt suppository). Lubricating gel may be used if needed to assist insertion. Retain suppositories for at least 1-3 hours to achieve maximum benefit. May cause staining of clothing and undergarments.

Dietary Considerations Some products may contain phenylalanine.

Apriso™: Take with or without food; do not administer with antacids.

Asacol® HD: Take with or without food.

Canasa® rectal suppository contains saturated vegetable fatty acid esters.

Geriatric Considerations Use with caution. Elderly may have difficulty administering and retaining rectal suppositories. Given renal function decline with aging, monitor serum creatinine often during therapy.

Breast-Feeding Considerations Adverse effects (diarrhea) in a nursing infant have been reported while the mother received rectal administration of mesalamine within 12 hours after the first dose. Low concentrations of the parent drug and higher concentrations of the N-acetyl metabolite of the parent drug have been detected in human breast milk.

Pregnancy Considerations Animal reproduction studies with mesalamine have not demonstrated teratogenicity or fertility impairment. Dibutyl phthalate (DBP) is an inactive ingredient in the enteric coating of Asacol® and Asacol® HD; adverse effects in male rats were noted at doses greater than the recommended human dose. Mesalamine is known to cross the placenta. An increased rate of congenital malformations has not been observed in human studies. Preterm birth, still birth and decreased birth weight have been observed; however, these events may also be due to maternal disease.

◆ **Mesalazine** *see* Mesalamine *on page* 1177

Mesna (MES na)

U.S. Brand Names Mesnex®

Index Terms Mercaptoethane Sulfonate; Sodium 2-Mercaptoethane Sulfonate

Generic Availability (U.S.) Yes: Solution for injection

Pharmacologic Category Antidote; Uroprotectant

Pregnancy Risk Factor B

Lactation Excretion in breast milk unknown/not recommended

Use Preventative agent to reduce the incidence of ifosfamide-induced hemorrhagic cystitis

Unlabeled/Investigational Use Preventative agent to reduce the incidence of cyclophosphamide-induced hemorrhagic cystitis with high-dose cyclophosphamide

Available Dosage Forms

Injection, solution: 100 mg/mL (10 mL)

Mesnex®: 100 mg/mL (10 mL)

Tablet, oral:

Mesnex®: 400 mg

Dosing

Adult & Geriatric Note: Details concerning dosing in combination regimens should also be consulted. Mesna dosing schedule should be repeated each day ifosfamide is received. If ifosfamide dose is adjusted, the mesna dose should also be modified to maintain the mesna-to-ifosfamide ratio.

Prevention of ifosfamide-induced hemorrhagic cystitis:

I.V.:

Short infusion standard-dose ifosfamide (<2.5 g/m^2/day): Mesna dose is equal to 60% of the ifosfamide dose given in 3 divided doses (0, 4, and 8 hours after the start of ifosfamide)

Continuous infusion standard-dose ifosfamide (<2.5 g/m^2/day): ASCO guidelines: Mesna dose (as an I.V. bolus) is equal to 20% of the ifosfamide dose, followed by a continuous infusion of mesna at 40% of the ifosfamide dose, continue mesna infusion for 12-24 hours after completion of ifosfamide infusion (Hensley, 2008)

High-dose ifosfamide (>2.5 g/m^2/day): ASCO guidelines: Evidence for use is inadequate; more frequent and prolonged mesna administration regimens may be required.

I.V. followed by oral (for ifosfamide doses ≤2 g/m^2/day): Mesna dose is equal to 100% of the ifosfamide dose, given as 20% of the ifosfamide dose I.V. at hour 0, followed by 40% of the ifosfamide dose given orally 2- and 6 hours after start of ifosfamide

Pediatric Refer to adult dosing.

Administration

Oral Administer orally in tablet formulation or parenteral solution diluted in water, milk, juice, or carbonated beverages; patients who vomit within 2 hours after taking oral mesna should repeat the dose or receive I.V. mesna

I.V. Administer by short (15-30 minutes) infusion or continuous infusion (maintain continuous infusion for 12-24 after completion of ifosfamide infusion) (Hensley, 2008)

Monitoring and Teaching Issues

Laboratory Monitoring Urinalysis

Physical Assessment Assess frequently for hematuria/bladder hemorrhage. Hypersensitive reactions have been reported, ranging from mild hypersensitivity to systemic anaphylactic reactions. Monitor closely.

Patient Education This drug is given to help prevent side effects of other chemotherapeutic agents you are taking. Drink at least a quart of liquid each day. Report urine turning pink or red. You may experience a bad taste in your mouth, nausea, and/or vomiting with oral administration.

- ◆ **Mesnex®** *see* Mesna *on page* *1180*
- ◆ **Mestinon®** *see* Pyridostigmine *on page* *1531*
- ◆ **Mestinon® Timespan®** *see* Pyridostigmine *on page* *1531*
- ◆ **Mestranol and Norethindrone** *see* Norethindrone and Mestranol *on page* *1335*
- ◆ **Metadate CD®** *see* Methylphenidate *on page* *1204*
- ◆ **Metadate® ER** *see* Methylphenidate *on page* *1204*
- ◆ **Metaglip™** *see* Glipizide and Metformin *on page* *875*

Metaxalone (me TAKS a lone)

U.S. Brand Names Skelaxin®

Generic Availability (U.S.) Yes

Pharmacologic Category Skeletal Muscle Relaxant

Medication Safety Issues

Sound-alike/look-alike issues:

Metaxalone may be confused with mesalamine, metolazone

Skelaxin® may be confused with Robaxin®

Beers Criteria medication: This drug may be inappropriate for use in geriatric patients (high severity risk).

Lactation Excretion in breast milk unknown/not recommended

Use Relief of discomfort associated with acute, painful musculoskeletal conditions

Mechanism of Action/Effect Precise mechanism has not been established; however, efficacy appears to result from disruption of the spasm-pain-spasm cycle, probably by a general CNS depressant effect. Does not have a direct effect on skeletal muscle.

Contraindications Hypersensitivity to metaxalone or any component of the formulation; significantly impaired hepatic or renal function, history of drug-induced hemolytic anemias or other anemias

Warnings/Precautions May cause CNS depression. CNS depressant effects may be augmented when used in conjunction with other depressants (eg, barbiturates, ethanol), when taken with food, or in the elderly. May impair mental and/or physical ability to perform hazardous tasks such as operating machinery or driving a motor vehicle. Use with caution in patients with impaired renal or hepatic function (contraindicated if significant impairment); routine monitoring of transaminases is recommended. An increase in bioavailability and half-life have been observed in female patients. This class of medication is poorly tolerated by the elderly due to anticholinergic effects, sedation, and weakness. Efficacy is questionable at dosages tolerated by elderly patients (Beers Criteria). Safety and efficacy have not been established in children ≤12 years of age.

Drug Interactions

Metabolism/Transport Effects

Substrate of CYP1A2, 2C8, 2C9, 2C19, 2D6, 2E1, 3A4

Avoid Concomitant Use There are no known interactions where it is recommended to avoid concomitant use.

Decreased Effect

The levels/effects of Metaxalone may be decreased by: Peginterferon Alfa-2b

Increased Effect/Toxicity

Metaxalone may increase the levels/effects of: Alcohol (Ethyl); CNS Depressants; Methotrimeprazine

The levels/effects of Metaxalone may be increased by: Conivaptan; Droperidol; Methotrimeprazine

Nutritional/Ethanol Interactions

Ethanol: Avoid ethanol (may increase CNS depression).
Food: Bioavailability may be increased (may increase CNS depression).
Herb/Nutraceutical: Avoid valerian, St John's wort, kava kava, gotu kola (may increase CNS depression).

Lab Interactions False-positive Benedict's test

Adverse Reactions Frequency not defined.

Central nervous system: Dizziness, drowsiness, headache, irritability, nervousness
Dermatologic: Rash (with or without pruritus)
Gastrointestinal: Gastrointestinal upset, nausea, vomiting
Hematologic: Hemolytic anemia, leukopenia
Hepatic: Jaundice
Miscellaneous: Hypersensitivity (including rare anaphylactoid reactions)

Pharmacodynamics/Kinetics

Onset of Action ~1 hour

Duration of Action ~4-6 hours

Bioavailability Not established; food may increase

Time to Peak T_{max}: ~3 hours

Half-Life Elimination 4-14 hours

Metabolism Hepatic via CYP1A2, CYP2D6, CYP2E1, CYP3A4 and to lesser extent CYP2C8, CPY2C9, and CYP2C19

Excretion Urine (as metabolites)

Available Dosage Forms

Tablet, oral: 800 mg
Skelaxin®: 800 mg

Dosing

Adult & Geriatric Muscle discomfort: Oral: 800 mg 3-4 times/day

Pediatric Children >12 years: Refer to adult dosing.

Renal Impairment Use caution in patients with mild-to-moderate renal impairment; contraindicated with significant impairment. No specific recommendation are provided in approved labeling.

Hepatic Impairment Use caution in patients with mild-to-moderate hepatic impairment; contraindicated with significant impairment. No specific recommendation are provided in approved labeling.

Administration

Oral May be administered with or without food. However, serum concentrations may be increased when administered with food; clinical significance has not been established. Patients should be monitored.

Stability

Storage Store at controlled room temperature of 15°C to 30°C (59°F to 86°F).

Monitoring and Teaching Issues

Dietary Considerations Administration with food may increase serum concentrations.

Geriatric Considerations This medication is considered to be potentially inappropriate in this patient population (Beers Criteria severity: High).

Pregnancy Considerations Teratogenic effects were not observed in animal studies. There are no adequate and well-controlled studies in pregnant women. Use during pregnancy (especially first trimester) only if benefits outweigh risks.

MetFORMIN (met FOR min)

U.S. Brand Names Fortamet®; Glucophage®; Glucophage® XR; Glumetza®; Riomet®

Index Terms Metformin Hydrochloride

Generic Availability (U.S.) Yes: Excludes solution

Pharmacologic Category Antidiabetic Agent, Biguanide

Medication Safety Issues

Sound-alike/look-alike issues:
MetFORMIN may be confused with metroNIDAZOLE
Glucophage® may be confused with Glucotrol®, Glutofac®

International issues:
Dianben [Spain] may be confused with Diovan brand name for valsartan [U.S., Canada, and multiple international markets]

Pregnancy Risk Factor B

Lactation Enters breast milk/not recommended

Use Management of type 2 diabetes mellitus (noninsulin dependent, NIDDM) when hyperglycemia cannot be managed with diet and exercise alone.

Unlabeled/Investigational Use Gestational diabetes mellitus (GDM); polycystic ovary syndrome (PCOS); prevention of type 2 diabetes mellitus

Mechanism of Action/Effect Decreases hepatic glucose production, decreasing intestinal absorption of glucose and improves insulin sensitivity (increases peripheral glucose uptake and utilization)

Contraindications Hypersensitivity to metformin or any component of the formulation; renal disease or renal dysfunction (serum creatinine ≥1.5 mg/dL in males or ≥1.4 mg/dL in females) or abnormal creatinine clearance from any cause, including shock, acute myocardial infarction, or septicemia; acute or chronic metabolic acidosis with or without coma (including diabetic ketoacidosis)

Note: Temporarily discontinue in patients undergoing radiologic studies in which intravascular iodinated contrast media are utilized.

Warnings/Precautions [U.S. Boxed Warning]: Lactic acidosis is a rare, but potentially severe consequence of therapy with metformin. Lactic acidosis should be suspected in any patient with diabetes receiving metformin with evidence of acidosis but without evidence of ketoacidosis. Discontinue metformin in clinical situations predisposing to hypoxemia, including conditions such as cardiovascular collapse, respiratory failure, acute myocardial infarction, acute congestive heart failure, and septicemia. Use caution in patients with congestive heart failure requiring pharmacologic management, particularly in patients with unstable or acute CHF; risk of lactic acidosis may be increased secondary to hypoperfusion.

Metformin is substantially excreted by the kidney. The risk of accumulation and lactic acidosis increases with the degree of impairment of renal function. Patients with renal function below the limit of normal for their age should not receive metformin. In elderly patients, renal function should be monitored regularly; should not be initiated in patients ≥80 years of age unless normal renal function is confirmed. Use of concomitant medications that may affect renal function (ie, affect tubular secretion) may also affect metformin disposition. Metformin should be withheld in patients with dehydration and/or prerenal azotemia. Therapy should be suspended for any surgical procedures (resume only after normal oral intake resumed and normal renal function is verified). Therapy should be temporarily discontinued prior to or at the time of intravascular administration of iodinated contrast media (potential for acute alteration in renal function). Metformin should be withheld for 48 hours after the radiologic study and restarted only after renal function has been confirmed as normal. It may be necessary to discontinue metformin and administer insulin if the patient is exposed to stress (fever, trauma, infection, surgery).

Avoid use in patients with impaired liver function. Patient must be instructed to avoid excessive acute or chronic ethanol use; ethanol may potentiate metformin's effect on lactate metabolism. Administration of oral antidiabetic drugs has been reported to be associated with increased cardiovascular mortality; metformin does not appear to share this risk. Insoluble tablet shell of Glumetza® 1000 mg extended release tablet may remain intact and be visible in the stool. Other extended released tablets (Fortamet®, Glucophage® XR, Glumetza® 500 mg) may appear in the stool as a soft mass resembling the tablet.

Drug Interactions

Avoid Concomitant Use There are no known interactions where it is recommended to avoid concomitant use.

Decreased Effect

The levels/effects of MetFORMIN may be decreased by: Corticosteroids (Orally Inhaled); Corticosteroids (Systemic); Luteinizing Hormone-Releasing Hormone Analogs; Somatropin; Thiazide Diuretics

Increased Effect/Toxicity

The levels/effects of MetFORMIN may be increased by: Cephalexin; Cimetidine; Glycopyrrolate; Iodinated Contrast Agents; Pegvisomant

Nutritional/Ethanol Interactions

Ethanol: Avoid or limit ethanol (incidence of lactic acidosis may be increased; may cause hypoglycemia).

Food: Food decreases the extent and slightly delays the absorption. May decrease absorption of vitamin B_{12} and/or folic acid.

Herb/Nutraceutical: Caution with chromium, garlic, gymnema (may cause hypoglycemia).

Adverse Reactions

>10%:

- Gastrointestinal: Diarrhea (10% to 53%), nausea/vomiting (7% to 26%), flatulence (12%)
- Neuromuscular & skeletal: Weakness (9%)

1% to 10%:

- Cardiovascular: Chest discomfort, flushing, palpitation
- Central nervous system: Headache (6%), chills, dizziness, lightheadedness
- Dermatologic: Rash
- Endocrine & metabolic: Hypoglycemia
- Gastrointestinal: Indigestion (7%), abdominal discomfort (6%), abdominal distention, abnormal stools, constipation, dyspepsia/ heartburn, taste disorder
- Neuromuscular & skeletal: Myalgia
- Respiratory: Dyspnea, upper respiratory tract infection
- Miscellaneous: Decreased vitamin B_{12} levels (7%), increased diaphoresis, flu-like syndrome, nail disorder

Pharmacodynamics/Kinetics

Onset of Action Within days; maximum effects up to 2 weeks

Bioavailability Absolute: Fasting: 50% to 60%

Time to Peak Immediate release: 2-3 hours; Extended release: 7 hours (range: 4-8 hours)

Protein Binding Negligible

Half-Life Elimination Plasma: 4-9 hours

Metabolism Not metabolized by the liver

Excretion Urine (90% as unchanged drug; active secretion)

Available Dosage Forms

Solution, oral:
Riomet®: 100 mg/mL (118 mL, 473 mL)

Tablet, oral: 500 mg, 850 mg, 1000 mg
Glucophage®: 500 mg, 850 mg, 1000 mg

Tablet, extended release, oral: 500 mg, 750 mg
Fortamet®: 500 mg, 1000 mg
Glucophage® XR: 500 mg, 750 mg
Glumetza®: 500 mg, 1000 mg

Dosing

Adult

Management of type 2 diabetes mellitus: Oral: **Note:** Allow 1-2 weeks between dose titrations: Generally, clinically significant responses are not seen at doses <1500 mg daily; however, a lower recommended starting dose and gradual increased dosage is recommended to minimize gastrointestinal symptoms.

Immediate release tablet or solution: Adults ≥17 years: Initial: 500 mg twice daily **or** 850 mg once daily; titrate in increments of 500 mg weekly or 850 mg every other week; may also titrate from 500 mg twice a day to 850 mg twice a day after 2 weeks

Doses of up to 2000 mg/day may be given twice daily. If a dose >2000 mg/day is required, it may be better tolerated in three divided doses. Maximum recommended dose 2550 mg/day.

Extended release tablet: **Note:** If glycemic control is not achieved at maximum dose, may divide dose and administer twice daily.

Fortamet®: Initial: 500-1000 mg once daily;dosage may be increased by 500 mg weekly; maximum dose: 2500 mg once daily

Glucophage® XR: Initial: 500 mg once daily; dosage may be increased by 500 mg weekly; maximum dose: 2000 mg once daily

Glumetza®: Initial: 1000 mg once daily; dosage may be increased by 500 mg weekly; maximum dose: 2000 mg once daily

Transfer from other antidiabetic agents: No transition period is generally necessary except when transferring from chlorpropamide. When transferring from chlorpropamide, care should be exercised during the first 2 weeks because of the prolonged retention of chlorpropamide in the body, leading to overlapping drug effects and possible hypoglycemia.

Concomitant metformin and oral sulfonylurea therapy: If patients have not responded to 4 weeks of the maximum dose of metformin monotherapy, consider a gradual addition of an oral sulfonylurea, even if prior primary or secondary failure to a sulfonylurea has occurred. Continue metformin at the maximum dose. If adequate response has not occurred following 3 months of metformin and sulfonylurea combination therapy, consider switching to insulin with or without metformin.

Failed sulfonylurea therapy: Patients with prior failure on glyburide may be treated by gradual addition of metformin. Initiate with glyburide 20 mg and metformin 500 mg daily. Metformin dosage may be increased by 500 mg/day at weekly intervals, up to a maximum metformin dose (dosage of glyburide maintained at 20 mg/day).

Concomitant metformin and insulin therapy: Initial: 500 mg metformin once daily, continue current insulin dose; increase by 500 mg metformin weekly until adequate glycemic control is achieved

Maximum daily dose: Immediate release and solution: 2550 mg metformin; Extended release: 2000-2500 mg (varies by product)

Decrease insulin dose 10% to 25% when FPG <120 mg/dL; monitor and make further adjustments as needed

Type 2 diabetes prevention (unlabeled use): *Immediate release tablet or solution:* Oral: Initial: 850 mg once daily; Target: 850 mg twice daily (Knowler, 2002)

Geriatric The initial and maintenance dosing should be conservative, due to the potential for decreased renal function. Generally, elderly patients should **not** be titrated to the maximum dose of metformin. Do not use in patients ≥80 years of age unless normal renal function has been established.

Pediatric Management of type 2 diabetes mellitus: Oral: **Note:** Allow 1-2 weeks between dose titrations: Generally, clinically significant responses are not seen at doses <1500 mg daily; however, a lower recommended starting dose and gradual increased dosage is recommended to minimize gastrointestinal symptoms.

Immediate release tablet or solution:

Children 10-16 years: Initial: 500 mg twice daily; increases in daily dosage should be made in increments of 500 mg at weekly intervals, given in divided doses, up to a maximum of 2000 mg/day

Children ≥17 years: Refer to adult dosing.

Extended release tablet: Children ≥17 years: **Note:** If glycemic control is not achieved at maximum dose, may divide dose and administer twice daily.

Fortamet®: Initial: 500-1000 mg once daily; dosage may be increased by 500 mg weekly; maximum dose: 2500 mg once daily

Glucophage® XR: Initial: 500 mg once daily; dosage may be increased by 500 mg weekly; maximum dose: 2000 mg once daily

Renal Impairment The plasma and blood half-life of metformin is prolonged and the renal clearance is decreased in proportion to the decrease in creatinine clearance. Per the manufacturer, metformin is contraindicated in the presence of renal dysfunction defined as a serum creatinine ≥1.5 mg/dL in males, or ≥1.4 mg/dL in females and in patients with abnormal clearance. The Canadian labeling recommends that metformin be avoided in patients with Cl_{cr} <60 mL/minute.

Hepatic Impairment Avoid metformin; liver disease is a risk factor for the development of lactic acidosis during metformin therapy.

Administration

Oral Administer with a meal (to decrease GI upset).

Extended release: Swallow whole; do not crush, break, or chew. Administer once daily doses with the evening meal. Fortamet® should also be administered with a full glass of water.

Stability

Storage

Oral solution: Store at 15°C to 30°C (59°F to 86°F).

Tablets: Store at 20°C to 25°C (68°F to 77°F); excursion permitted to 15°C to 30°C (59°F to 86°F). Protect from light and moisture.

Monitoring and Teaching Issues

Laboratory Monitoring Urine for glucose and ketones, fasting blood glucose, hemoglobin A_{1c}, and fructosamine. Initial and periodic monitoring of hematologic parameters (eg, hemoglobin/hematocrit and red blood cell indices) and renal function should be performed, at least annually. While megaloblastic anemia has been rarely seen with metformin, if suspected, vitamin B_{12} deficiency should be excluded.

Physical Assessment Assess for signs and symptoms of vitamin B_{12} and/or folic acid deficiency during therapy; supplementation may be required. Refer patient to diabetes educator for instruction if needed.

Patient Education Take with food to decrease GI upset. Do not chew or crush extended release tablets. Parts of extended-release tablets may be excreted in the stool (normal). Avoid alcohol; could cause severe reaction. Follow prescribed diet and lifestyle recommendations. You will be instructed in signs of hyper-/hypoglycemia by prescriber or diabetes educator. May cause weakness, nausea, vomiting, flatulence, or diarrhea. Report unusual weakness or fatigue, unusual muscle pain, persistent GI discomfort, dizziness or lightheadedness, unusual somnolence, poor glucose control, or chest discomfort.

Dietary Considerations Drug may cause GI upset; take with food (to decrease GI upset). Take at the same time(s) each day. Dietary modification based on ADA recommendations is a part of therapy. Monitor for signs and symptoms of vitamin B_{12} and/or folic acid deficiency; supplementation may be required.

Geriatric Considerations Limited data suggest that metformin's total body clearance may be decreased and AUC and half-life increased in elderly patients; presumably due to decreased renal clearance. Metformin has been well tolerated by the elderly but lower doses and frequent monitoring are recommended. In one study of elderly subjects, its effects could not be distinguished from tolbutamide, except for weight loss. The initial and maintenance dosing should be conservative, due to the potential for decreased renal function. Generally, elderly patients should not be titrated to the maximum dose of metformin. Do not use in patients ≥80 years of age unless normal renal function has been established. Intensive glucose control (Hb A_{1c} <6.5%) has been linked to increased all cause and cardiovascular mortality, hypoglycemia requiring assistance, and weight gain in adult type 2 diabetes. For elderly patients with diabetes who are relatively healthy, attaining target goals for aspirin use, blood pressure, lipids, smoking cessation, and diet and exercise may be more important than normalized glycemic control.

Breast-Feeding Considerations Low amounts of metformin (generally ≤1% of the weight-adjusted maternal dose) are excreted into breast milk. Breast-feeding is not recommended by the manufacturer. Because breast milk concentrations of metformin stay relatively constant, avoiding nursing around peak plasma concentrations in the mother would not be helpful in reducing metformin exposure to the infant. Growth and development were not affected in infants born to mothers with PCOS and who took metformin while breast-feeding.

Pregnancy Considerations Adverse events have not been observed in animal studies; therefore, metformin is classified as pregnancy category B. Metformin has been found to cross the placenta in concentrations which may be comparable to those found in the maternal plasma. Pharmacokinetic studies suggest that clearance of metformin may be increased during pregnancy and dosing may need adjusted in some women when used during the third trimester.

Fetal, neonatal, and maternal outcomes have been evaluated following maternal use of metformin for the treatment of GDM and type 2 diabetes. Available information suggests that metformin use during pregnancy may be safe as long as good glycemic control is maintained; however, many studies used metformin during the second or third trimester only. Maternal hyperglycemia can be associated with adverse effects in the fetus, including macrosomia, neonatal hyperglycemia, and hyperbilirubinemia; the risk of congenital malformations is increased when the Hb A_{1c} is above the normal range. Diabetes can also be associated with adverse effects in the mother. Poorly-treated diabetes may cause end-organ damage that may negatively affect obstetric outcomes. Physiologic glucose levels should be maintained prior to and during pregnancy to decrease the risk of adverse events in the mother and the fetus. Until additional safety and efficacy data are obtained, the use of oral agents is generally not recommended as routine management of GDM or type 2 diabetes mellitus during pregnancy. Insulin is the drug of choice for the control of diabetes mellitus during pregnancy.

Metformin has also been evaluated for the treatment of PCOS, a syndrome which may exhibit oligomenorrhea and, in some women, hyperinsulinemia. It is not recommended as first-line therapy; when used to treat infertility related to PCOS, current guidelines restrict the use of metformin to women with glucose intolerance. Because ovulation rates will likely improve in women with PCOS who are taking metformin, appropriate contraceptive measures should be discussed in women who are not attempting to conceive.

Related Information

Diabetes Mellitus Management, Adults *on page 2026*

- **Metformin and Glipizide** *see* Glipizide and Metformin *on page 875*
- **Metformin and Glyburide** *see* Glyburide and Metformin *on page 880*
- **Metformin and Repaglinide** *see* Repaglinide and Metformin *on page 1566*
- **Metformin and Rosiglitazone** *see* Rosiglitazone and Metformin *on page 1612*
- **Metformin and Saxagliptin** *see* Saxagliptin and Metformin *on page 1626*
- **Metformin and Sitagliptin** *see* Sitagliptin and Metformin *on page 1654*
- **Metformin Hydrochloride** *see* MetFORMIN *on page 1182*
- **Metformin Hydrochloride and Pioglitazone Hydrochloride** *see* Pioglitazone and Metformin *on page 1463*
- **Metformin Hydrochloride and Rosiglitazone Maleate** *see* Rosiglitazone and Metformin *on page 1612*
- **Metformin Hydrochloride and Saxagliptin** *see* Saxagliptin and Metformin *on page 1626*

Methadone (METH a done)

U.S. Brand Names Dolophine®; Methadone Diskets®; Methadone Intensol™; Methadose®

Index Terms Methadone Hydrochloride

Generic Availability (U.S.) Yes

Pharmacologic Category Analgesic, Opioid

Medication Safety Issues

Sound-alike/look-alike issues:

Methadone may be confused with dexmethylphenidate, Mephyton®, methylphenidate, Metadate® CD, Metadate® ER, morphine

High alert medication: The Institute for Safe Medication Practices (ISMP) includes this medication among its list of drug classes which have a heightened risk of causing significant patient harm when used in error.

Prescribing and Access Restrictions When used for treatment of opioid addiction: May only be dispensed in accordance to guidelines established by the Substance Abuse and Mental Health Services Administration's (SAMHSA) Center for Substance Abuse Treatment (CSAT). Regulations regarding methadone use may vary by state and/or country. Obtain advice from appropriate regulatory agencies and/or consult with pain management/palliative care specialists.

Note: Regulatory Exceptions to the General Requirement to Provide Opioid Agonist Treatment (per manufacturer's labeling):

1. During inpatient care, when the patient was admitted for any condition other than concurrent opioid addiction, to facilitate the treatment of the primary admitting diagnosis.
2. During an emergency period of no longer than 3 days while definitive care for the addiction is being sought in an appropriately licensed facility.

Pregnancy Risk Factor C

Lactation Enters breast milk/not recommended (AAP rates "compatible"; AAP 2001 update pending)

Use Management of moderate-to-severe pain; detoxification and maintenance treatment of opioid addiction as part of an FDA-approved program

Mechanism of Action/Effect Binds to opiate receptors in the CNS, causing inhibition of ascending pain pathways, altering the perception of and response to pain; produces generalized CNS depression

Contraindications Hypersensitivity to methadone or any component of the formulation; respiratory depression (in the absence of resuscitative equipment or in an unmonitored setting); acute bronchial asthma or hypercarbia; paralytic ileus; concurrent use of selegiline

Warnings/Precautions An opioid-containing analgesic regimen should be tailored to each patient's needs and based upon the type of pain being treated (acute versus chronic), the route of administration, degree of tolerance for opioids (naive versus chronic user), age, weight, and medical condition. The optimal analgesic dose varies widely among patients. Doses should be titrated to pain relief/prevention. Patients maintained on stable doses of methadone may need higher and/or more frequent doses in case of acute pain (eg, postoperative pain, physical trauma). Methadone is ineffective for the relief of anxiety.

[U.S. Boxed Warning]: May prolong the QT_c interval and increase risk for torsade de pointes. Patients should be informed of the potential arrhythmia risk, evaluated for any history of structural heart disease, arrhythmia, syncope, and for existence of potential drug interactions including drugs that possess QT_c interval-prolonging properties, promote hypokalemia, hypomagnesemia, or hypocalcemia, or reduce elimination of methadone (eg, CYP3A4 inhibitors). Obtain baseline ECG for all patients and risk stratify according to QT_c interval (see Laboratory Monitoring). Use with caution in patients at risk for QT_c prolongation, with medications known to prolong the QT_c interval, promote electrolyte depletion, or inhibit CYP3A4, or history of conduction abnormalities. QT_c interval prolongation and torsade de pointes may be associated with doses >100 mg/day, but have also been observed with lower doses. May cause severe hypotension; use caution with severe volume depletion or other conditions which may compromise maintenance of normal blood pressure. Use caution with cardiovascular disease or patients predisposed to dysrhythmias.

[U.S. Boxed Warning]: May cause respiratory depression. Use caution in patients with respiratory disease or pre-existing respiratory conditions (eg, severe obesity, asthma, COPD, sleep apnea, CNS depression). Because the respiratory effects last longer than the analgesic effects, slow titration is required. Use extreme caution during treatment initiation, dose titration and conversion from other opioid agonists. Incomplete cross tolerance may occur; patients tolerant to other mu opioid agonists may not be tolerant to methadone. Abrupt cessation may precipitate withdrawal symptoms.

May cause CNS depression, which may impair physical or mental abilities. Patients must be cautioned about performing tasks which require mental alertness (eg, operating machinery or driving). Effects with other sedative drugs or ethanol may be potentiated. Use with caution in patients with depression or suicidal tendencies, or in patients with a history of drug abuse. Tolerance or psychological and physical dependence may occur with prolonged use.

Use with caution in patients with head injury or increased intracranial pressure. May obscure diagnosis or clinical course of patients with acute abdominal conditions. Elderly may be more susceptible to adverse effects (eg, CNS, respiratory, gastrointestinal). Decrease initial dose and use caution in the elderly or debilitated; with hyper/hypothyroidism, morbid obesity, adrenal insufficiency, prostatic hyperplasia, or urethral stricture; or with severe renal or hepatic failure. Use with caution in patients with biliary tract dysfunction; acute pancreatitis may cause constriction of sphincter of Oddi. Safety and efficacy have not been established in children. **[U.S. Boxed Warning]: For oral administration only;** excipients to deter use by injection are contained in tablets.

[U.S. Boxed Warning]: When used for treatment of narcotic addiction: May only be dispensed by opioid treatment programs certified by the Substance Abuse and Mental Health Services Administration (SAMHSA) and certified by the designated state authority. Exceptions include inpatient treatment of other conditions and emergency period (not >3 days) while definitive substance abuse treatment is being sought.

Drug Interactions

Metabolism/Transport Effects Substrate of CYP2B6 (major), 2C9 (minor), 2C19 (minor), 2D6 (minor), 3A4 (major); **Inhibits** CYP2D6 (moderate), 3A4 (weak)

Avoid Concomitant Use

Avoid concomitant use of Methadone with any of the following: Artemether; Dronedarone; Lumefantrine; Nilotinib; Pimozide; QuiNINE; Tetrabenazine; Thioridazine; Toremifene; Vandetanib; Ziprasidone

Decreased Effect

Methadone may decrease the levels/effects of: Codeine; Didanosine; Pegvisomant; TraMADol

The levels/effects of Methadone may be decreased by: Ammonium Chloride; Barbiturates; CarBAMazepine; CYP2B6 Inducers (Strong); CYP3A4 Inducers (Strong); Deferasirox; Etravirine; Herbs (CYP3A4 Inducers); Mixed Agonist / Antagonist Opioids; Phenytoin; Protease Inhibitors; Reverse Transcriptase Inhibitors (Non-Nucleoside); Rifamycin Derivatives

Increased Effect/Toxicity

Methadone may increase the levels/effects of: Alcohol (Ethyl); Alvimopan; CNS Depressants; CYP2D6 Substrates; Desmopressin; Dronedarone; Fesoterodine; Nebivolol; Pimozide; QTc-Prolonging Agents; QuiNINE; Selective Serotonin Reuptake Inhibitors; Tamoxifen; Tetrabenazine; Thiazide Diuretics; Thioridazine; Toremifene; Vandetanib; Zidovudine; Ziprasidone

The levels/effects of Methadone may be increased by: Alfuzosin; Amphetamines; Antifungal Agents (Azole Derivatives, Systemic); Antipsychotic Agents (Phenothiazines); Artemether; Chloroquine; Ciprofloxacin; Ciprofloxacin (Systemic); Conivaptan; CYP2B6 Inhibitors (Moderate); CYP2B6 Inhibitors (Strong); CYP3A4 Inhibitors (Moderate); CYP3A4 Inhibitors (Strong); Gadobutrol; Interferons (Alfa); Lumefantrine; MAO Inhibitors; Nilotinib; Quazepam; QuiNINE; Selective Serotonin Reuptake Inhibitors; Succinylcholine

Nutritional/Ethanol Interactions

Ethanol: Avoid ethanol (may increase CNS effects). Watch for sedation.

Herb/Nutraceutical: Avoid St John's wort (may decrease methadone levels; may increase CNS depression). Avoid valerian, kava kava, gotu kola (may increase CNS depression). Methadone is metabolized by CYP3A4 in the intestines; avoid concurrent use of grapefruit juice.

Lab Interactions Some quinolones may produce a false-positive urine screening result for opiates using commercially-available immunoassay kits. This has been demonstrated most consistently for levofloxacin and ofloxacin, but other quinolones have shown cross-reactivity in certain assay kits. Confirmation of positive opiate screens by more specific methods should be considered.

Adverse Reactions Frequency not defined. During prolonged administration, adverse effects may decrease over several weeks; however, constipation and sweating may persist.

Cardiovascular: Arrhythmia, bigeminal rhythms, bradycardia, cardiac arrest, cardiomyopathy, ECG changes, edema, extrasystoles, faintness, flushing, heart failure, hypotension, palpitation,peripheral vasodilation, phlebitis, orthostatic hypotension, QT interval prolonged, shock, syncope, tachycardia, torsade de pointes, T-wave inversion, ventricular fibrillation, ventricular tachycardia,

Central nervous system: Agitation, confusion, disorientation, dizziness, drowsiness, dysphoria, euphoria, hallucination, headache, insomnia, lightheadedness, sedation, seizure

Dermatologic: Hemorrhagic urticaria, pruritus, rash, urticaria

Endocrine & metabolic: Antidiuretic effect, amenorrhea, hypokalemia, hypomagnesemia, libido decreased

Gastrointestinal: Abdominal pain, anorexia, biliary tract spasm, constipation, glossitis, nausea, stomach cramps, vomiting, weight gain, xerostomia

Genitourinary: Impotence, urinary retention or hesitancy

Hematologic: Thrombocytopenia (reversible, reported in patients with chronic hepatitis)

Neuromuscular & skeletal: Weakness

Local: I.M./SubQ injection: Erythema, pain, swelling; I.V. injection: Hemorrhagic urticaria (rare), pruritus, urticaria, rash

Ocular: Miosis, visual disturbances

Respiratory: Pulmonary edema, respiratory depression, respiratory arrest

Miscellaneous: Death, diaphoresis, physical and psychological dependence

Pharmacodynamics/Kinetics

Onset of Action Oral: Analgesic: 0.5-1 hour; Parenteral: 10-20 minutes; Peak effect: Parenteral: 1-2 hours; Oral: Continuous dosing: 3-5 days

Duration of Action Analgesia: Oral: 4-8 hours, increases to 22-48 hours with repeated doses

Bioavailability Oral: 36% to 100%

Time to Peak 1-7.5 hours

Protein Binding 85% to 90%

Half-Life Elimination 8-59 hours; may be prolonged with alkaline pH, decreased during pregnancy

Metabolism Hepatic; N-demethylation primarily via CYP3A4, CYP2B6, and CYP2C19 to inactive metabolites

Excretion Urine (<10% as unchanged drug); increased with urine pH <6

Controlled Substance C-II

Available Dosage Forms

Injection, solution: 10 mg/mL (20 mL)

Solution, oral: 5 mg/5 mL (500 mL); 10 mg/5 mL (500 mL); 10 mg/mL (946 mL, 960 mL, 1000 mL, 1000s)

Methadone Intensol™: 10 mg/mL (30 mL)

Methadose®: 10 mg/mL (1000 mL)

Tablet, oral: 5 mg, 10 mg

Dolophine®: 5 mg, 10 mg

Tablet, dispersible, oral: 40 mg

Methadone Diskets®: 40 mg

Methadose®: 40 mg

Dosing

Adult Regulations regarding methadone use may vary by state and/or country. Obtain advice from appropriate regulatory agencies and/or consult with pain management/palliative care specialists. **Note:** These are guidelines and do not represent the maximum doses that may be required in all patients. Methadone accumulates with repeated doses and dosage may need reduction after 3-5 days to prevent CNS depressant effects. Some patients may benefit from every 8-12 hour dosing interval for chronic pain management. Doses should be titrated to appropriate effects.

Acute pain (moderate-to-severe):

Opioid-naive: *Oral:* Initial: 2.5-10 mg every 8-12 hours; more frequent administration may be required during initiation to maintain adequate analgesia. Dosage interval may range from 4-12 hours, since duration of analgesia is relatively short during the first days of therapy, but increases substantially with continued administration.

Chronic pain (opioid-tolerant): Conversion from oral morphine to oral methadone:

Daily oral morphine dose <100 mg: Estimated daily oral methadone dose: 20% to 30% of total daily morphine dose

Daily oral morphine dose 100-300 mg: Estimated daily oral methadone dose: 10% to 20% of total daily morphine dose

Daily oral morphine dose 300-600 mg: Estimated daily oral methadone dose: 8% to 12% of total daily morphine dose

Daily oral morphine dose 600-1000 mg: Estimated daily oral methadone dose: 5% to 10% of total daily morphine dose.

Daily oral morphine dose >1000 mg: Estimated daily oral methadone dose: <5% of total daily morphine dose.

Note: The total daily methadone dose should then be divided to reflect the intended dosing schedule.

Or, per American Pain Society:

Daily oral morphine or equivalent dose per day <90 mg: Estimated daily oral methadone dose: 25% of total daily morphine dose

Daily oral morphine or equivalent dose per day 90-300 mg: Estimated daily oral methadone dose: 12% of total daily morphine dose

Daily oral morphine or equivalent dose per day >300 mg: Estimated daily oral methadone dose: 8% of total daily morphine dose

Note: The estimated total daily methadone dose should then be divided by 3 and administered every 8 hours.

I.V.: Manufacturers labeling: Initial: 2.5-10 mg every 8-12 hours in opioid-naive patients; titrate slowly to effect; may also be administered by SubQ or I.M. injection

Conversion from oral to parenteral dose: Initial dose: Parenteral: Oral ratio: 1:2 (eg, 5 mg parenteral methadone equals 10 mg oral methadone)

Detoxification: *Oral:*

Initial: A single dose of 20-30 mg is usually sufficient to suppress symptoms. Should not exceed 30 mg; lower doses should be considered in patients with low tolerance at initiation (eg, absence of opioids ≥5 days); an additional 5-10 mg of methadone may be provided if withdrawal symptoms have not been suppressed or if symptoms reappear after 2-4 hours; total daily dose on the first day should not exceed 40 mg, unless the program physician documents in the patient's record that 40 mg did not control opiate abstinence symptoms.

Maintenance: Titrate to a dosage which prevents craving, attenuates euphoric effect of self-administered opiates, and tolerance to sedative effects of methadone. Usual range: 80-120 mg/day (titration should occur cautiously)

Withdrawal: Dose reductions should be <10% of the maintenance dose, every 10-14 days

Detoxification (short-term): *Oral:*

Initial: Titrate to ~40 mg/day in divided doses to achieve stabilization. May continue 40 mg dose for 2-3 days

Maintenance: Titrate to a dosage which prevents/attenuates euphoric effects of self-administered opioids, reduces drug craving, and withdrawal symptoms are prevented for 24 hours.

Withdrawal: Requires individualization. Decrease daily or every other day, keeping withdrawal symptoms tolerable; hospitalized patients may tolerate a 20% reduction/day; ambulatory patients may require a slower reduction

Dosage adjustment during pregnancy: Methadone dose may need to be increased, or the dosing interval decreased; see Pregnancy Considerations - use should be reserved for cases where the benefits clearly outweigh the risks

Geriatric Oral, I.M.: 2.5 mg every 8-12 hours; refer to adult dosing.

Pediatric Regulations regarding methadone use may vary by state and/or country. Obtain advice from appropriate regulatory agencies and/or consult with pain management/palliative care specialists. **Note:** These are guidelines and do not represent the maximum doses that may be required in all patients. Methadone accumulates with repeated doses and dosage may need reduction after 3-5 days to prevent CNS depressant effects. Some patients may benefit from every 8-12 hour dosing interval for chronic pain management. Doses should be titrated to appropriate effects.

Pain (analgesia) (unlabeled use):

Oral: Initial: 0.1-0.2 mg/kg 4-8 hours initially for 2-3 doses, then every 6-12 hours as needed. Dosing interval may range from 4-12 hours during initial therapy; decrease in dose or frequency may be required (~days 2-5) due to accumulation with repeated doses (maximum dose: 5-10 mg)

I.V. (unlabeled use): 0.1 mg/kg every 4-8 hours initially for 2-3 doses, then every 6-12 hours as needed. Dosing interval may range from 4-12 hours during initial therapy; decrease in dose or frequency may be required (~days 2-5) due to accumulation with repeated doses (maximum dose: 5-8 mg)

Iatrogenic narcotic dependency (unlabeled use): Oral: General guidelines: Initial: 0.05-0.1 mg/kg/dose every 6 hours; increase by 0.05 mg/kg/dose until withdrawal symptoms are controlled; after 24-48 hours, the dosing interval can be lengthened to every 12-24 hours; to taper dose, wean by 0.05 mg/kg/day; if withdrawal symptoms recur, taper at a slower rate

Renal Impairment Cl_{cr} <10 mL/minute: Administer 50% to 75% of normal dose.

Hepatic Impairment Avoid in severe liver disease.

Adjustment for Toxicity

QT_c >450-499 msecs: Monitor QT_c more frequently

QT_c ≥500 msecs: Consider discontinuation or reducing methadone dose **or** eliminate factors promoting QT_c prolongation (eg, potassium-wasting drugs) **or** use alternative therapy (eg, buprenorphine)

Administration

Oral Oral dose for detoxification and maintenance may be administered in fruit juice or water. Dispersible tablet should not be chewed or swallowed; add to liquid and allow to dissolve before administering. May rinse if residual remains.

Stability

Storage

Injection: Store at controlled room temperature of 15°C to 30°C (59°F to 86°F). Protect from light.

Oral concentrate, oral solution, tablet: Store at controlled room temperature of 15°C to 30°C (59°F to 86°F).

Monitoring and Teaching Issues

Laboratory Monitoring Obtain baseline ECG (evaluate QT_c interval) within 30 days of initiation

Physical Assessment Assess patient's physical and/or psychological dependence. Monitor QT_c, blood pressure, CNS and respiratory status, and degree of sedation. For inpatients, implement safety measures to prevent falls. Discontinue slowly after prolonged use.

Patient Education May cause physical and/or psychological dependence. While using this medication, do not use alcohol and other prescription or OTC medications (especially sedatives, tranquilizers, antihistamines, or pain medications) without consulting prescriber. Maintain adequate hydration, unless instructed to restrict fluid intake. May cause hypotension, dizziness, drowsiness, impaired coordination, or blurred vision; loss of appetite, nausea, or vomiting; or constipation. Report chest pain, slow or rapid heartbeat, dizziness, or persistent headache; confusion or respiratory difficulties; or severe constipation.

Geriatric Considerations Because of it's long half-life and risk of accumulation, methadone is difficult to titrate and is not considered a drug of first choice. It should be prescribed only by physicians who are experienced in using it. Elderly may be particularly susceptible to the CNS depressant and constipating effects of narcotics.

Breast-Feeding Considerations Peak methadone levels appear in breast milk 4-5 hours after an oral dose. Methadone has been detected in the plasma of some breast-fed infants whose mothers are taking methadone. Use during breast-feeding is not recommended, and the manufacturer recommends that women on high dose methadone maintenance who already are breast-feeding be instructed to wean breast-feeding gradually to avoid neonatal abstinence syndrome. Sedation and respiratory depression have been reported in nursing infants.

Pregnancy Considerations Teratogenic effects have been observed in some, but not all, animal studies. Data collected by the Teratogen Information System are complicated by maternal use of illicit drugs, nutrition, infection, and psychosocial circumstances. However, pregnant women in methadone treatment programs are reported to have improved fetal outcomes compared to pregnant women using illicit drugs. Methadone can be detected in the amniotic fluid, cord plasma, and newborn urine. Fetal growth, birth weight, length, and/or head circumference may be decreased in infants born to narcotic-addicted mothers treated with methadone during pregnancy. Growth deficits do not appear to persist; however, decreased performance on psychometric and behavioral tests has been found to continue into childhood. Abnormal fetal nonstress tests have also been reported. Withdrawal symptoms in the neonate may be observed up to 2-4 weeks after delivery. The manufacturer states that methadone should be used during pregnancy only if clearly needed. Because methadone clearance in pregnant women is increased and half-life is decreased during the 2nd and 3rd trimesters of pregnancy, withdrawal symptoms may be observed in the mother; dosage of methadone may need increased or dosing interval decreased during pregnancy.

Related Information

Opioid Analgesics *on page 2003*

- ◆ **Methadone Diskets®** *see* Methadone *on page 1186*
- ◆ **Methadone Hydrochloride** *see* Methadone *on page 1186*
- ◆ **Methadone Intensol™** *see* Methadone *on page 1186*
- ◆ **Methadose®** *see* Methadone *on page 1186*
- ◆ **Methaminodiazepoxide Hydrochloride** *see* ChlordiazePOXIDE *on page 358*

Methamphetamine (meth am FET a meen)

U.S. Brand Names Desoxyn®

Index Terms Desoxyephedrine Hydrochloride; Methamphetamine Hydrochloride

Generic Availability (U.S.) Yes

Pharmacologic Category Anorexiant; Stimulant; Sympathomimetic

Medication Safety Issues

Sound-alike/look-alike issues:

Desoxyn® may be confused with digoxin

Beers Criteria medication: This drug may be inappropriate for use in geriatric patients (high severity risk).

Medication Guide Available Yes

Pregnancy Risk Factor C

Lactation Enters breast milk/contraindicated

Use Treatment of attention-deficit/hyperactivity disorder (ADHD); exogenous obesity (short-term adjunct)

Pharmacotherapy for weight loss is recommended only for obese patients with a body mass index ≥30 kg/m^2, or ≥27 kg/m^2 in the presence of other risk factors such as hypertension, diabetes, and/or dyslipidemia or a high waist circumference; therapy should be used in conjunction with a comprehensive weight management program.

Unlabeled/Investigational Use Narcolepsy

Mechanism of Action/Effect A sympathomimetic amine related to ephedrine and amphetamine with CNS stimulant activity; causes release of catecholamines (primarily dopamine and other catecholamines) from storage sites in the nerve terminals.

Contraindications Hypersensitivity to methamphetamine, any component of the formulation, or idiosyncrasy to amphetamines or other sympathomimetic amines; patients with advanced arteriosclerosis, symptomatic cardiovascular disease, moderate-to-severe hypertension, hyperthyroidism, glaucoma, agitated states; patients with a history of drug abuse; use during or within 14 days following MAO inhibitor therapy; stimulant medications are contraindicated for use in children with attention-deficit/hyperactivity disorders and concomitant Tourette's syndrome or tics

Warnings/Precautions Use has been associated with serious cardiovascular events including sudden death in patients with pre-existing structural cardiac abnormalities or other serious heart problems (sudden death in children and adolescents; sudden death, stroke and MI in adults). These products should be avoided in the patients with known serious structural cardiac abnormalities, cardiomyopathy, serious heart rhythm abnormalities, or other serious cardiac problems that could increase the risk of sudden death that these conditions alone carry. Patients should be carefully evaluated for cardiac disease prior to initiation of therapy. Use with caution in patients with hypertension and other cardiovascular conditions that might be exacerbated by increases in blood pressure or heart rate. Use is contraindicated in patients with moderate-to-severe hypertension. Amphetamines may impair the ability to engage in potentially hazardous activities. Difficulty in accommodation and blurred vision has been reported with the use of stimulants.

Use with caution in patients with psychiatric disorders, diabetes, or seizure disorders,. May exacerbate symptoms of behavior and thought disorder in psychotic patients. Stimulants may unmask tics in individuals with coexisting Tourette's syndrome **[U.S. Boxed Warning]: Potential for drug dependency exists; prolonged use may lead to drug dependency.** Use is contraindicated in patients with history of ethanol or drug abuse. Prescriptions should be written for the smallest quantity consistent with good patient care to minimize possibility of overdose. **[U.S. Boxed Warning]: Use in weight reduction programs only when alternative therapy has been ineffective.** Abrupt discontinuation following high doses or for prolonged periods may result in symptoms for withdrawal. Discontinue if satisfactory weight loss has not occurred within the first 4 weeks of treatment, or if tolerance develops.

May be inappropriate for use in the elderly due to the risk for causing dependence, hypertension, angina, and myocardial infarction (Beers Criteria). Safety and efficacy have not been established in children <12 years of age for obesity. Use of stimulants has been associated with suppression of growth; monitor growth rate during treatment.

Drug Interactions

Metabolism/Transport Effects Substrate of CYP2D6 (major)

Avoid Concomitant Use

Avoid concomitant use of Methamphetamine with any of the following: Iobenguane I 123; MAO Inhibitors

Decreased Effect

Methamphetamine may decrease the levels/effects of: Antihistamines; Ethosuximide; Iobenguane I 123; PHENobarbital; Phenytoin

The levels/effects of Methamphetamine may be decreased by: Ammonium Chloride; Antipsychotics; Gastrointestinal Acidifying Agents; Lithium; Methenamine; Peginterferon Alfa-2b

Increased Effect/Toxicity

Methamphetamine may increase the levels/effects of: Analgesics (Opioid); Sympathomimetics

The levels/effects of Methamphetamine may be increased by: Alkalinizing Agents; Antacids; Atomoxetine; Cannabinoids; Carbonic Anhydrase Inhibitors; CYP2D6 Inhibitors (Moderate); CYP2D6 Inhibitors (Strong); Darunavir; MAO Inhibitors; Proton Pump Inhibitors; Tricyclic Antidepressants

Nutritional/Ethanol Interactions

Ethanol: Avoid ethanol (may cause CNS depression).

Food: Amphetamine serum levels may be altered if taken with acidic food, juices, or vitamin C. Avoid caffeine.

Herb/Nutraceutical: Avoid ephedra (may cause hypertension or arrhythmias).

Adverse Reactions Frequency not defined.

Cardiovascular: Hypertension, tachycardia, palpitation

Central nervous system: Restlessness, headache, exacerbation of motor and phonic tics and Tourette's syndrome, dizziness, psychosis, dysphoria, overstimulation, euphoria, insomnia

Dermatologic: Rash, urticaria

Endocrine & metabolic: Change in libido

Gastrointestinal: Diarrhea, nausea, vomiting, stomach cramps, constipation, anorexia, weight loss, xerostomia, unpleasant taste

Genitourinary: Impotence

Neuromuscular & skeletal: Tremor

Miscellaneous: Suppression of growth in children, tolerance and withdrawal with prolonged use

Pharmacodynamics/Kinetics

Absorption Rapid from GI tract

Half-Life Elimination 4-5 hours

Metabolism Hepatic; forms metabolite

Excretion Urine primarily (dependent on urine pH)

Controlled Substance C-II

Available Dosage Forms

Tablet, oral: 5 mg

Desoxyn®: 5 mg

Dosing

Adult & Geriatric

ADHD: Oral: 5 mg 1-2 times/day, may increase by 5 mg increments weekly until optimum response is achieved, usually 20-25 mg/day

Exogenous obesity: Oral: 5 mg, 30 minutes before each meal; treatment duration should not exceed a few weeks

Pediatric

ADHD: Oral: Children ≥6 years: Refer to adult dosing.

Exogenous obesity: Oral: Children ≥12 years: Refer to adult dosing.

Stability

Storage Store below 30°C (86°F). Protect from light.

Monitoring and Teaching Issues

Physical Assessment Monitor vital signs at beginning of therapy and periodically during therapy.

Patient Education Report chest pain, difficulty breathing, fainting, and visual disturbances.

Dietary Considerations Most effective when combined with a low calorie diet and behavior modification counseling.

Geriatric Considerations This medication is considered to be potentially inappropriate in this patient population (Beers Criteria severity: High).

Pregnancy Considerations Teratogenic and embryocidal effects have been observed in animal studies. Infants may deliver prematurely and suffer withdrawal symptoms. There are no adequate and well-controlled studies in pregnant women.

Additional Information Illicit methamphetamine may contain lead; alkalinizing urine can result in longer methamphetamine half-life and elevated blood level; ephedrine is a precursor in the illicit manufacture of methamphetamine; ephedrine is extracted by dissolving ephedrine tablets in water or alcohol (50,000 tablets can result in 1 kg of ephedrine); conversion to methamphetamine occurs at a rate of 50% to 70% of the weight of ephedrine. 3,4-methylene dioxymethamphetamine (slang: XTC, Ecstasy, Adam) affects the serotonergic, dopaminergic, and noradrenergic pathways. As such, it can cause the serotonin syndrome associated with malignant hyperthermia and rhabdomyolysis.

Related Information

Obesity Treatment Guidelines *on page 2064*

◆ **Methamphetamine Hydrochloride** *see* Methamphetamine *on page 1190*

◆ **Methergine®** *see* Methylergonovine *on page 1201*

Methimazole (meth IM a zole)

U.S. Brand Names Tapazole®

Index Terms Thiamazole

Generic Availability (U.S.) Yes

Pharmacologic Category Antithyroid Agent; Thioamide

Medication Safety Issues

Sound-alike/look-alike issues:

Methimazole may be confused with metolazone

Pregnancy Risk Factor D

Lactation Enters breast milk/contraindicated (per manufacturer) (AAP rates "compatible"; AAP 2001 update pending)

Use Treatment of hyperthyroidism; improve hyperthyroidism prior to thyroidectomy or radioactive iodine therapy

Available Dosage Forms

Tablet, oral: 5 mg, 10 mg

Tapazole®: 5 mg, 10 mg

Dosing

Adult & Geriatric

Hyperthyroidism: Oral: Initial: 15 mg/day in 3 divided doses (approximately every 8 hours) for mild hyperthyroidism; 30-40 mg/day in moderately severe hyperthyroidism; 60 mg/day in severe hyperthyroidism; maintenance: 5-15 mg/day (may be given as a single daily dose in many cases)

Adjust dosage as required to achieve and maintain serum T_3, T_4, and TSH levels in the normal range. An elevated T_3 may be the sole indicator of inadequate treatment. An elevated TSH indicates excessive antithyroid treatment.

Thyrotoxic crisis (unlabeled use): Note: Recommendations vary; use in combination with other specific agents. Dosages of 20-25 mg every 6 hours have been used; once stable, dosing frequency may be reduced to once or twice daily (Nayak, 2006). Rectal administration has been described (Nabil, 1982).

Pediatric Note: Administer in 3 equally divided doses at approximately 8-hour intervals.

Hyperthyroidism: Oral: Initial: 0.4 mg/kg/day in 3 divided doses; maintenance: 0.2 mg/kg/day in 3 divided doses

Administration

Other Administer consistently in relation to meals every day. In thyrotoxic crisis, rectal administration has been described (Nabil, 1982).

Monitoring and Teaching Issues

Laboratory Monitoring T_4, T_3, CBC with differential, liver function (baseline and as needed), serum thyroxine, free thyroxine index; prothrombin time

Patient Education Take at the same time each day, around-the-clock (eg, every 8 hours). This drug will need to be taken for an extended period of time to achieve appropriate results. May cause nausea, vomiting, abdominal pain, abnormal taste, dizziness, drowsiness, or unusual CNS stimulation. Report rash, fever, unusual bleeding or bruising, unresolved headache, yellowing of eyes or skin, changes in color of urine or feces, or unresolved malaise.

◆ **Methitest™** *see* MethylTESTOSTERone *on page 1212*

Methocarbamol (meth oh KAR ba mole)

U.S. Brand Names Robaxin®; Robaxin®-750

Generic Availability (U.S.) Yes: Tablet

Pharmacologic Category Skeletal Muscle Relaxant

Medication Safety Issues

Sound-alike/look-alike issues:

Methocarbamol may be confused with mephobarbital

Robaxin® may be confused with ribavirin, Rubex®, Skelaxin®

Beers Criteria medication: This drug may be inappropriate for use in geriatric patients (high severity risk).

Pregnancy Risk Factor C

Lactation Excretion in breast milk unknown/use caution

Use Adjunctive treatment of muscle spasm associated with acute painful musculoskeletal conditions (eg, tetanus)

Available Dosage Forms

Injection, solution:

Robaxin®: 100 mg/mL (10 mL)

Tablet, oral: 500 mg, 750 mg

Robaxin®: 500 mg

Robaxin®-750: 750 mg

Dosing

Adult

Muscle spasm:

Oral: 1.5 g 4 times/day for 2-3 days (up to 8 g/day may be given in severe conditions), then decrease to 4-4.5 g/day in 3-6 divided doses

I.M., I.V.: Initial: 1 g; may repeat every 8 hours if oral administration not possible; maximum dose: 3 g/day for no more than 3 consecutive days. If condition persists, may repeat course of therapy after a drug-free interval of 48 hours.

Tetanus: I.V.: Initial dose: 1-2 g by direct I.V. injection, which may be followed by an additional 1-2 g by infusion (maximum initial dose: 3 g total); may repeat initial dose every 6 hours until NG tube or oral therapy possible; total oral daily dose of up to 24 g may be needed; injection should not be used for more than 3 consecutive days

Pediatric

Tetanus (recommended **only** for use in tetanus): I.V.: 15 mg/kg/dose or 500 mg/m^2/dose, may repeat every 6 hours if needed; maximum dose: 1.8 g/m^2/day for 3 days only

Muscle spasm: Oral: Children ≥16 years: Refer to adult dosing.

Renal Impairment Administration of the parenteral formulation is contraindicated in patients with renal dysfunction due to the presence of polyethylene glycol.

Hepatic Impairment Specific dosing guidelines are not available.

Administration

Oral Tablets may be crushed and mixed with food or liquid if needed.

I.M. A maximum of 5 mL can be administered into each gluteal region.

I.V. Maximum rate: 3 mL/minute; may be administered undiluted or mixed with 5% dextrose or 0.9% saline (1 vial/≤250 mL diluent)

Monitoring and Teaching Issues

Physical Assessment Monitor I.V. site closely to prevent extravasation.

Patient Education Do not use alcohol. You may experience drowsiness, dizziness, or lightheadedness. Report excessive drowsiness.

Methotrexate (meth oh TREKS ate)

U.S. Brand Names Rheumatrex®; Trexall™

Index Terms Amethopterin; Methotrexate Sodium; Methotrexatum; MTX (error-prone abbreviation)

Generic Availability (U.S.) Yes

Pharmacologic Category Antineoplastic Agent, Antimetabolite (Antifolate); Antirheumatic, Disease Modifying; Immunosuppressant Agent

Medication Safety Issues

Sound-alike/look-alike issues:

Methotrexate may be confused with mercaptopurine, methylPREDNISolone sodium succinate, metolazone, metroNIDAZOLE, mitoXANtrone, PRALAtrexate

MTX is an error-prone abbreviation (mistaken as mitoxantrone)

High alert medication: The Institute for Safe Medication Practices (ISMP) includes this medication among its list of drugs which have a heightened risk of causing significant patient harm when used in error.

Intrathecal medication safety: The American Society of Clinical Oncology (ASCO)/Oncology Nursing Society (ONS) chemotherapy administration safety standards (Jacobson, 2009) encourage the following safety measures for intrathecal chemotherapy:

- Intrathecal medication should not be prepared during the preparation of any other agents
- After preparation, store in an isolated location or container clearly marked with a label identifying as "intrathecal" use only

- Delivery to the patient should only be with other medications intended for administration into the central nervous system

Errors have occurred (resulting in death) when methotrexate was administered as "daily" dose instead of the recommended "weekly" dose.

International issues:

Trexall [U.S.] may be confused with Trexol brand name for tamadol [Mexico]; Truxal brand name for chlorprothixene [multiple international markets]

Pregnancy Risk Factor X (psoriasis, rheumatoid arthritis)

Lactation Enters breast milk/contraindicated

Use

Oncology-related uses: Treatment of trophoblastic neoplasms (gestational choriocarcinoma, chorioadenoma destruens and hydatidiform mole), acute lymphocytic leukemia (ALL), meningeal leukemia, breast cancer, head and neck cancer (epidermoid), cutaneous T-Cell lymphoma (advanced mycosis fungoides), lung cancer (squamous cell and small cell), advanced non-Hodgkin's lymphomas (NHL), osteosarcoma

Nononcology uses: Treatment of psoriasis (severe, recalcitrant, disabling) and severe rheumatoid arthritis (RA), including polyarticular-course juvenile idiopathic arthritis (JIA)

Unlabeled/Investigational Use Treatment and maintenance of remission in Crohn's disease; ectopic pregnancy; dermatomyositis/polymyositis; bladder cancer, central nervous system tumors (including nonleukemic meningeal cancers), acute promyelocytic leukemia (maintenance treatment), soft tissue sarcoma (desmoid tumors); acute graft-versus-host disease (GVHD) prophylaxis; medical management of abortion; systemic lupus erythematosus; Takayasu arteritis

Mechanism of Action/Effect Methotrexate is a folate antimetabolite that inhibits DNA synthesis. Methotrexate irreversibly binds to dihydrofolate reductase, inhibiting the formation of reduced folates, and thymidylate synthetase, resulting in inhibition of purine and thymidylic acid synthesis. Methotrexate is cell cycle specific for the S phase of the cycle.

The MOA in the treatment of rheumatoid arthritis is unknown, but may affect immune function. In psoriasis, methotrexate is thought to target rapidly proliferating epithelial cells in the skin.

In Crohn's disease, it may have immune modulator and anti-inflammatory activity

Contraindications Hypersensitivity to methotrexate or any component of the formulation; breast-feeding

Additional contraindications for patients with psoriasis or rheumatoid arthritis: Pregnancy, alcoholism, alcoholic liver disease or other chronic liver disease, immunodeficiency syndrome (overt or laboratory evidence); pre-existing blood dyscrasias (eg, bone marrow hypoplasia, leukopenia, thrombocytopenia, significant anemia)

Warnings/Precautions Hazardous agent - use appropriate precautions for handling and disposal.

[U.S. Boxed Warning]: Methotrexate has been associated with acute (elevated transaminases) and potentially fatal chronic (fibrosis, cirrhosis) hepatotoxicity. Risk is related to cumulative dose and prolonged exposure. Monitor closely (with liver function tests, including serum albumin) for liver toxicities. Liver enzyme elevations may be noted, but may not be predictive of hepatic disease in long term treatment for psoriasis (but generally is predictive in rheumatoid arthritis [RA] treatment). With long-term use, liver biopsy may show histologic changes, fibrosis, or cirrhosis; periodic liver biopsy is recommended with long-term use for psoriasis patients with risk factors for hepatotoxicity and for persistent abnormal liver function tests in psoriasis patients without risk factors for hepatotoxicity and in RA patients; discontinue methotrexate with moderate-to-severe change in liver biopsy. Risk factors for hepatotoxicity include history of above moderate ethanol consumption, persistent abnormal liver chemistries, history of chronic liver disease (including hepatitis B or C), family history of inheritable liver disease, diabetes, obesity, hyperlipidemia, lack of folate supplementation during methotrexate therapy, and history of significant exposure to hepatotoxic drugs. Use caution with preexisting liver impairment; may require dosage reduction. Use caution when used with other hepatotoxic agents (azathioprine, retinoids, sulfasalazine). **[U.S. Boxed Warning]: Methotrexate elimination is reduced in patients with ascites;** may require dose reduction or discontinuation. Monitor closely for toxicity.

[U.S. Boxed Warning]: May cause renal damage leading to acute renal failure, especially with high-dose methotrexate; monitor renal function and methotrexate levels closely, maintain adequate hydration and urinary alkalinization. Use caution in osteosarcoma patients treated with high-dose methotrexate in combination with nephrotoxic chemotherapy (eg, cisplatin). **[U.S. Boxed Warning]: Methotrexate elimination is reduced in patients with renal impairment;** may require dose reduction or discontinuation; monitor closely for toxicity. **[U.S. Boxed Warning]: Tumor lysis syndrome may occur in patients with high tumor burden;** use appropriate prevention and treatment.

[U.S. Boxed Warning]: May cause potentially life-threatening pneumonitis (may occur at any time during therapy and at any dosage); monitor closely for pulmonary symptoms, particularly dry, nonproductive cough. Other potential symptoms include fever, dyspnea, hypoxemia, or pulmonary infiltrate. **[U.S. Boxed Warning]: Methotrexate elimination is reduced in patients with pleural effusions;** may require dose reduction or discontinuation. Monitor closely for toxicity.

[U.S. Boxed Warning]: Bone marrow suppression may occur, resulting in anemia, aplastic anemia, pancytopenia, leukopenia, neutropenia, and/or thrombocytopenia. Use caution in patients with pre-existing bone marrow suppression. Discontinue therapy in RA or psoriasis if a significant decrease in hematologic components is noted. **[U.S. Boxed Warning]: Use of low dose methotrexate has been associated with the development of malignant lymphomas;** may regress upon discontinuation of therapy; treat lymphoma appropriately if regression is not induced by cessation of methotrexate.

[U.S. Boxed Warning]: Diarrhea and ulcerative stomatitis may require interruption of therapy; death from hemorrhagic enteritis or intestinal perforation has been reported. Use with caution in patients with peptic ulcer disease, ulcerative colitis.

May cause neurotoxicity including seizures (usually in pediatric ALL patients), leukoencephalopathy (usually with concurrent cranial irradiation) and stroke-like encephalopathy (usually with high-dose regimens). Chemical arachnoiditis (headache, back pain, nuchal rigidity, fever), myelopathy and chronic leukoencephalopathy may result from intrathecal administration.

[U.S. Boxed Warning]: Any dose level or route of administration may cause severe and potentially fatal dermatologic reactions, including toxic epidermal necrolysis, Stevens-Johnson syndrome, exfoliative dermatitis, skin necrosis, and erythema multiforme. Radiation dermatitis and sunburn may be precipitated by methotrexate administration. Psoriatic lesions may be worsened by concomitant exposure to ultraviolet radiation.

[U.S. Boxed Warning]: Concomitant administration with NSAIDs may cause severe bone marrow suppression, aplastic anemia, and GI toxicity. Do not administer NSAIDs prior to or during high dose methotrexate therapy; may increase and prolong serum methotrexate levels. Doses used for psoriasis may still lead to unexpected toxicities; use caution when administering NSAIDs or salicylates with lower doses of methotrexate for RA. Methotrexate may increase the levels and effects of mercaptopurine; may require dosage adjustments. Vitamins containing folate may decrease response to systemic methotrexate; folate deficiency may increase methotrexate toxicity. **[U.S. Boxed Warning]: Concomitant methotrexate administration with radiotherapy may increase the risk of soft tissue necrosis and osteonecrosis.**

[U.S. Boxed Warnings]: Should be administered under the supervision of a physician experienced in the use of antimetabolite therapy; serious and fatal toxicities have occurred at all dose levels. Immune suppression may lead to potentially fatal opportunistic infections. For rheumatoid arthritis and psoriasis, immunosuppressive therapy should only be used when disease is active and less toxic, traditional therapy is ineffective. Methotrexate formulations and/or diluents containing preservatives should not be used for intrathecal or high-dose therapy. May cause fetal death or congenital abnormalities; do not use for psoriasis or RA treatment in pregnant women. May cause impairment of fertility, oligospermia, and menstrual dysfunction. Toxicity from methotrexate or any immunosuppressive is increased in the elderly. Methotrexate injection may contain benzyl alcohol and should not be used in neonates.

When used for intrathecal administration, should not be prepared during the preparation of any other agents; after preparation, store intrathecal medications in an isolated location or container clearly marked with a label identifying as "intrathecal" use only; delivery of intrathecal medications to the patient should only be with other medications intended for administration into the central nervous system (Jacobson, 2009).

Drug Interactions

Metabolism/Transport Effects Substrate of P-glycoprotein, SLCO1B1

Avoid Concomitant Use

Avoid concomitant use of Methotrexate with any of the following: Acitretin; BCG; Natalizumab; Pimecrolimus; Roflumilast; Tacrolimus (Topical)

Decreased Effect

Methotrexate may decrease the levels/effects of: BCG; Cardiac Glycosides; Sapropterin; Sipuleucel-T; Vaccines (Inactivated); Vitamin K Antagonists

The levels/effects of Methotrexate may be decreased by: Bile Acid Sequestrants; Echinacea; P-Glycoprotein Inducers

Increased Effect/Toxicity

Methotrexate may increase the levels/effects of: CycloSPORINE; CycloSPORINE (Systemic); Leflunomide; Natalizumab; Theophylline Derivatives; Vaccines (Live); Vitamin K Antagonists

The levels/effects of Methotrexate may be increased by: Acitretin; Ciprofloxacin; Ciprofloxacin (Systemic); CycloSPORINE; CycloSPORINE (Systemic); Denosumab; Eltrombopag; Non-steroidal Anti-Inflammatory Agents; Penicillins; P-Glycoprotein Inhibitors; Pimecrolimus; Probenecid; Proton Pump Inhibitors; Roflumilast; Salicylates; Sulfonamide Derivatives; Tacrolimus (Topical); Trastuzumab; Trimethoprim

Nutritional/Ethanol Interactions

Ethanol: Avoid ethanol (may be associated with increased liver injury).

Food: Methotrexate peak serum levels may be decreased if taken with food. Milk-rich foods may decrease methotrexate absorption. Folate may decrease drug response.

Herb/Nutraceutical: Avoid echinacea (has immunostimulant properties).

Adverse Reactions Note: Adverse reactions vary by route and dosage. Hematologic and/or gastrointestinal toxicities may be common at dosages used in chemotherapy; these reactions are much less frequent when used at typical dosages for rheumatic diseases.

>10%:

Central nervous system (with I.T. administration or very high-dose therapy):

Arachnoiditis: Acute reaction manifested as severe headache, nuchal rigidity, vomiting, and fever; may be alleviated by reducing the dose

Subacute toxicity: 10% of patients treated with 12-15 mg/m^2 of I.T. methotrexate may develop this in the second or third week of therapy; consists of motor paralysis of extremities, cranial nerve palsy, seizure, or coma. This has also been seen in pediatric cases receiving very high-dose I.V. methotrexate.

Demyelinating encephalopathy: Seen months or years after receiving methotrexate; usually in association with cranial irradiation or other systemic chemotherapy

Dermatologic: Reddening of skin

Endocrine & metabolic: Hyperuricemia, defective oogenesis or spermatogenesis

Gastrointestinal: Ulcerative stomatitis, glossitis, gingivitis, nausea, vomiting, diarrhea, anorexia, intestinal perforation, mucositis (dose dependent; appears in 3-7 days after therapy, resolving within 2 weeks)

Hematologic: Leukopenia, myelosuppression (nadir: 7-10 days), thrombocytopenia

Renal: Renal failure, azotemia, nephropathy

Respiratory: Pharyngitis

1% to 10%:

Cardiovascular: Vasculitis

Central nervous system: Dizziness, malaise, encephalopathy, seizure, fever, chills

Dermatologic: Alopecia, rash, photosensitivity, depigmentation or hyperpigmentation of skin

Endocrine & metabolic: Diabetes

Genitourinary: Cystitis

Hematologic: Hemorrhage

Hepatic: Cirrhosis and portal fibrosis have been associated with chronic methotrexate therapy; acute elevation of liver enzymes are common after high-dose methotrexate, and usually resolve within 10 days.

Neuromuscular & skeletal: Arthralgia

Ocular: Blurred vision

Renal: Renal dysfunction: Manifested by an abrupt rise in serum creatinine and BUN and a fall in urine output; more common with high-dose methotrexate, and may be due to precipitation of the drug.

Respiratory: Pneumonitis: Associated with fever, cough, and interstitial pulmonary infiltrates; treatment is to withhold methotrexate during the acute reaction; interstitial pneumonitis has been reported to occur with an incidence of 1% in patients with RA (dose 7.5-15 mg/week)

Pharmacodynamics/Kinetics

Onset of Action Antirheumatic: 3-6 weeks; additional improvement may continue longer than 12 weeks

Absorption Oral: Dose dependant; well absorbed at low doses (<30 mg/m^2), incomplete after higher doses; I.M. injection: Complete

Bioavailability Dose dependent; ~60% at low doses

Time to Peak Serum: Oral: 1-2 hours; I.M.: 30-60 minutes

Protein Binding ~50%

Half-Life Elimination Low dose: 3-10 hours; High dose: 8-15 hours

Metabolism <10%; degraded by intestinal flora to DAMPA by carboxypeptidase; hepatic aldehyde oxidase converts methotrexate to 7-OH methotrexate; polyglutamates are produced intracellularly and are just as potent as methotrexate; their production is dose- and duration-dependent and they are slowly eliminated by the cell once formed. Polyglutamated forms can be converted back to methotrexate.

Excretion Urine (44% to 100%); feces (small amounts)

Available Dosage Forms

Injection, powder for reconstitution: 1 g

Injection, solution: 25 mg/mL (2 mL, 10 mL)

Injection, solution [preservative free]: 25 mg/mL (2 mL, 4 mL, 8 mL, 10 mL, 20 mL, 40 mL, 100 mL)

Tablet, oral: 2.5 mg

Rheumatrex®: 2.5 mg

Trexall™: 5 mg, 7.5 mg, 10 mg, 15 mg

Dosing

Adult Details concerning dosing in combination regimens should also be consulted.

Note: Doses between 100-500 mg/m^2 **may require** leucovorin calcium rescue. Doses >500 mg/m^2 **require** leucovorin calcium rescue: I.V., I.M., Oral: Leucovorin calcium 10-15 mg/m^2 every 6 hours for 8 or 10 doses, starting 24 hours after the start of methotrexate infusion. Continue until the methotrexate level is ≤0.1 micromolar (10^{-7} M). Some clinicians continue leucovorin calcium until the methotrexate level is <0.05 micromolar (5×10^{-8} M) or 0.01 micromolar (10^{-8} M).

If the 48-hour methotrexate level is >1 micromolar (10^{-6} M) or the 72-hour methotrexate level is >0.2 micromolar (2×10^{-7} M): I.V., I.M, Oral: Leucovorin calcium 100 mg/m^2 every 6 hours until the methotrexate level is ≤0.1 micromolar (10^{-7} M). Some clinicians continue leucovorin calcium until the methotrexate level is <0.05 micromolar (5×10^{-8} M) or 0.01 micromolar (10^{-8} M).

Antineoplastic dosage range: I.V.: Range is wide from 30-40 mg/m^2/week to 100-12,000 mg/m^2 with leucovorin calcium rescue

Breast cancer: I.V.: 30-60 mg/m^2 Day 1 and 8 every 3-4 weeks

Head and neck cancer: Oral, I.M., I.V.: 25-50 mg/m^2 once weekly

Lymphoma, non-Hodgkin's: I.V.:
30 mg/m^2 days 3 and 10 every 3 weeks **or**
120 mg/m^2 day 8 and 15 every 3-4 weeks **or**
200 mg/m^2 day 8 and 15 every 3 weeks **or**
400 mg/m^2 every 4 weeks for 3 cycles **or**
1 g/m^2 every 3 weeks **or**
1.5 g/m^2 every 4 weeks

Meningeal leukemia: I.T.: Usual dose: 12 mg/dose. **Note:** Optimal intrathecal chemotherapy dosing should be based on age rather than on body surface area (BSA); CSF volume correlates with age and not to BSA (Bleyer, 1983; Kerr, 2001).

Mycosis fungoides (cutaneous T-cell lymphoma): Oral, I.M.: Initial (early stages):
5-50 mg once weekly **or**
15-37.5 mg twice weekly

Osteosarcoma: I.V.: 8-12 g/m^2 weekly for 2-4 weeks

Psoriasis: Some experts recommend concomitant folic acid 1-5 mg/day (except the day of methotrexate) to reduce hematologic, gastrointestinal, and hepatic adverse events related to methotrexate.
Oral: 2.5-5 mg/dose every 12 hours for 3 doses given weekly **or**
Oral, I.M., SubQ: 10-25 mg/dose given once weekly; titrate to lowest effective dose
Note: An initial test dose of 2.5-5 mg is recommended in patients with risk factors for hematologic toxicity or renal impairment. (Kalb, 2009).

Rheumatoid arthritis: Some experts recommend concomitant folic acid at a dose of least 5 mg/week (except the day of methotrexate) to reduce hematologic, gastrointestinal, and hepatic adverse events related to methotrexate.
Oral (manufacturer labeling): 7.5 mg once weekly or 2.5 mg every 12 hours for 3 doses/week (dosage exceeding 20 mg/week may cause a higher incidence and severity of adverse events); *alternatively,* 10-15 mg once weekly, increased by 5 mg every 2-4 weeks to a maximum of 20-30 mg once weekly has been recommended by some experts (Visser, 2009)
I.M., SubQ (unlabeled route): 15 mg once weekly (dosage varies, similar to oral) (Braun, 2008)

Trophoblastic neoplasms:
Oral, I.M.: 15-30 mg/day for 5 days; repeat in 7 days for 3-5 courses
I.V.: 11 mg/m^2 days 1 through 5 every 3 weeks

Unlabeled uses:

Active Crohn's disease (unlabeled use): Induction of remission: I.M., SubQ: 15-25 mg once weekly; remission maintenance: 15 mg once weekly
Note: Oral dosing has been reported as effective but oral absorption is highly variable. If patient relapses after a switch to oral, may consider returning to injectable.

Bladder cancer (unlabeled use): I.V.:
30 mg/m^2 day 1 and 8 every 3 weeks **or**
30 mg/m^2 day 1, 15, and 22 every 4 weeks

Dermatomyositis/polymyositis (unlabeled uses):
Oral: Initial: 7.5-15 mg/week, often adjunctively with high-dose corticosteroid therapy; may increase in weekly 2.5 mg increments to target dose of 10-25 mg/week (**Note:** Administration of folate 5-7 mg/week has been used to reduce side effects). (Briemberg, 2003; Newman, 1995; Wiendl, 2008)
I.V., I.M.: Doses of 20-60 mg/week have been employed if failure with oral therapy (doses >50 mg/week may require leucovorin calcium rescue) (Briemberg, 2003)

Ectopic pregnancy (unlabeled use): I.M.:
Single-dose regimen: Methotrexate 50 mg/m^2 on day 1; Measure serum hCG levels on days 4 and 7; if needed, repeat dose on day 7 (Barnhart, 2009)
Two-dose regimen: Methotrexate 50 mg/m^2 on day 1; Measure serum hCG levels on day 4 and administer a second dose of methotrexate 50 mg/m^2; Measure serum hCG levels on day 7 and if needed, administer a third dose of 50 mg/m^2 (Barnhart, 2009)
Multidose regimen: Methotrexate 1 mg/kg on day 1; leucovorin calcium 0.1 mg/kg I.M. on day 2; measure serum hCG on day 2; methotrexate 1 mg/kg on day 3; leucovorin calcium 0.1 mg/kg on day 4; measure serum hCG on day 4; continue up to a total of 4 courses based on hCG concentrations (Barnhart, 2009)

GVHD (acute) prophylaxis: I.V.: 15 mg/m^2/dose on day 1 and 10 mg/m^2/dose on days 3 and 6 after allogeneic transplant (in combination with cyclosporine and prednisone) (Chao, 1993; Chao, 2000; Ross, 1999) **or** 15 mg/m^2/dose on day 1 and 10 mg/m^2/dose on days 3, 6, and 11 after allogeneic transplant (in combination with cyclosporine) (Chao, 2000)

Nonleukemic meningeal cancer (unlabeled uses): I.T.: 10-12 mg/dose twice weekly for 4 weeks, then weekly for 4 weeks, then monthly (NCCN CNS cancer guidelines v.2.2009) **or** 12 mg/dose twice weekly for 4 weeks, then weekly for 4 doses, then monthly for 4 doses (Glantz, 1998) **or** 10 mg twice weekly for 4 weeks, then weekly for 1 month, then every 2 weeks for 2 months (Glantz, 1999)

Takayasu arteritis, refractory or relapsing disease (unlabeled use): Oral: Initial dose: 0.3 mg/kg/week (maximum: 15 mg/week), titrated by 2.5 mg increments every 1-2 weeks until reaching a maximum tolerated weekly dose of 25 mg (use in combination with a corticosteroid; Hoffman, 1994)

Geriatric Refer to individual protocols; adjust for renal impairment.

Meningeal leukemia: I.T.: Consider a dose reduction (CSF volume and turnover may decrease with age)

Rheumatoid arthritis/psoriasis: Oral: Initial: 5-7.5 mg/week, not to exceed 20 mg/week

Pediatric Details concerning dosing in combination regimens should also be consulted.

Note: Doses between 100-500 mg/m^2 **may require** leucovorin calcium rescue. Doses >500 mg/m^2 **require** leucovorin calcium rescue: I.V., I.M., Oral: Leucovorin calcium 10-15 mg/m^2 every 6 hours for 8 or 10 doses, starting 24 hours after the start of methotrexate infusion. Continue until the methotrexate level is ≤0.1 micromolar (10^{-7} M). Some clinicians continue leucovorin calcium until the methotrexate level is <0.05 micromolar (5 x 10^{-8} M) or 0.01 micromolar (10^{-8} M).

If the 48-hour methotrexate level is >1 micromolar (10^{-6} M) or the 72-hour methotrexate level is >0.2 micromolar (2 x 10^{-7} M): I.V., I.M, Oral: Leucovorin calcium 100 mg/m^2 every 6 hours until the methotrexate level is ≤0.1 micromolar (10^{-7} M). Some clinicians continue leucovorin calcium until the methotrexate level is <0.05 micromolar (5 x 10^{-8} M) or 0.01 micromolar (10^{-8} M).

Dermatomyositis (unlabeled use): Oral: 15-20 mg/m^2/week as a single dose once weekly **or** 0.3-1 mg/kg/dose once weekly

GVHD (acute) prophylaxis (unlabeled use): I.V.: Refer to adult dosing.

Juvenile idiopathic arthritis (JIA): Oral, I.M.:10 mg/m^2 once weekly, then 5-15 mg/m^2/week as a single dose **or** as 3 divided doses given 12 hours apart

Antineoplastic dosage range:

Oral, I.M.: 7.5-30 mg/m^2/week **or** every 2 weeks

I.V.: 10-18,000 mg/m^2 bolus dosing **or** continuous infusion over 6-42 hours

Pediatric solid tumors (high-dose): I.V.:

<12 years: 12-25 g/m^2

≥12 years: 8 g/m^2

Acute lymphocytic leukemia (intermediate-dose): I.V.: Loading: 100 mg/m^2 bolus dose, followed by 900 mg/m^2/day infusion over 23-41 hours.

Meningeal leukemia: I.T.: 6-12 mg/dose based on age. **Note**: Optimal intrathecal chemotherapy dosing should be based on age rather than on body surface area (BSA); CSF volume correlates with age and not to BSA (Bleyer, 1983; Kerr, 2001):

<1 year: 6 mg/dose

1 year: 8 mg/dose

2 years: 10 mg/dose

≥3 years: 12 mg/dose

Renal Impairment The FDA-approved labeling does not contain dosage adjustment guidelines.

The following guidelines have been used by some clinicians:

Cl_{cr} 61-80 mL/minute: Administer 75% of dose

Cl_{cr} 51-60 mL/minute: Administer 70% of dose

Cl_{cr} 10-50 mL/minute: Administer 30% to 50% of dose

Cl_{cr} <10 mL/minute: Avoid use

Hemodialysis: Not dialyzable (0% to 5%); supplemental dose is not necessary

Peritoneal dialysis effects: Supplemental dose is not necessary

CAVH effects: Unknown

Aronoff, 2007:

Children:

Cl_{cr} 10-50 mL/minute: Administer 50% of dose

Cl_{cr} <10 mL/minute: Administer 30% of dose

Hemodialysis: Administer 30% of dose

Continuous ambulatory peritoneal dialysis (CAPD): Administer 30% of dose

Continuous renal replacement therapy (CRRT): Administer 50% of dose

Adults:

Cl_{cr} 10-50 mL/minute: Administer 50% of dose

Cl_{cr} <10 mL/minute: Avoid use

Hemodialysis: Administer 50% of dose

Continuous renal replacement therapy (CRRT): Administer 50% of dose

Kintzel, 1995:

Cl_{cr} 46-60 mL/minute: Administer 65% of normal dose

Cl_{cr} 31-45 mL/minute: Administer 50% of normal dose

Cl_{cr} <30 mL/minute: Avoid use

Hepatic Impairment The FDA-approved labeling does not contain dosage adjustment guidelines. The following guidelines have been used by some clinicians (Floyd, 2006):

Bilirubin 3.1-5 mg/dL **or** transaminases >3 times ULN: Administer 75% of dose

Bilirubin >5 mg/dL: Avoid use

Administration

I.M. May be administered I.M.

I.V. May be administered I.V.; I.V. administration may be as slow push, short bolus infusion, or 24- to 42-hour continuous infusion

Specific dosing schemes vary, but high dose should be followed by leucovorin calcium to prevent toxicity; refer to Leucovorin Calcium monograph on page 1080

Other May be administered I.T or SubQ.

Stability

Reconstitution Use appropriate precautions for handling and disposal. **Use preservative-free preparations for intrathecal or high-dose methotrexate administration.**

I.M., I.V., SubQ: Dilute powder with D_5W or NS to a concentration of ≤25 mg/mL (20 mg and 50 mg vials) and 50 mg/mL (1 g vial). May further dilute in D_5W or NS.

Intrathecal: Prepare intrathecal solutions with preservative-free NS, lactated Ringer's, or Elliot's B solution to a final volume of up to 12 mL (volume generally based on institution or practitioner preference). Intrathecal methotrexate concentrations may be institution specific or based on practitioner preference, generally ranging from a final concentration of 1 mg/mL (per prescribing information; Grossman, 1993; Lin, 2008) up to ~2-4 mg/mL (de Lemos, 2009; Glantz, 1999). For triple intrathecal therapy (methotrexate 12 mg/hydrocortisone 24 mg/cytarabine 36 mg), preparation to final volume of 12 mL is reported (Lin, 2008). Intrathecal medications should **NOT** be prepared during the preparation of any other agents.

Storage Store tablets and intact vials at room temperature (15°C to 25°C). Protect from light.

I.M., I.V., SubQ: Solution diluted in D_5W or NS is stable for 24 hours at room temperature (21°C to 25°C). Reconstituted solutions with a preservative may be stored under refrigeration for up to 3 months, and up to 4 weeks at room temperature.

Intrathecal: Intrathecal dilutions are preservative free and should be used as soon as possible after preparation. After preparation, store intrathecal medications (until use) in an isolated location or container clearly marked with a label identifying as "intrathecal" use only.

Monitoring and Teaching Issues

Laboratory Monitoring

Laboratory tests should be performed on day 5 or day 6 of the weekly methotrexate cycle (eg, psoriasis, RA) to detect the leukopenia nadir and to avoid elevated LFTs 1-2 days after taking dose.

Patients with psoriasis: CBC with differential and platelets (baseline, 7-14 days after initiating therapy or dosage increase, every 2-4 weeks for first few months, then every 1-3 months); BUN and serum creatinine (baseline and every 2-3 months); consider PPD for latent TB screening (baseline); LFTs (baseline, monthly for first 6 months, then every 1-2 months)

Patients with RA: CBC with differential and platelets, serum creatinine and LFTs (baseline then every 2-4 weeks for initial 3 months of therapy, then every 8-12 weeks for 3-6 months of therapy and then every 12 weeks after 6 months of therapy); chest x-ray (baseline); pulmonary function test (if methotrexate-induced lung disease suspected); hepatitis B or C testing (baseline)

Patients with cancer: Baseline and frequently during treatment: CBC with differential and platelets, serum creatinine, LFTs; methotrexate levels and urine pH (with high-dose therapy)

Ectopic pregnancy (unlabeled use): Prior to therapy, measure serum hCG, CBC with differential, liver function tests, serum creatinine. Serum hCG concentrations should decrease between treatment days 4 and 7. If hCG decreases by >15%, additional courses are not needed however, continue to measure hCG weekly until no longer detectable. If <15% decrease is observed, repeat dose per regimen (Barnhart 2009).

Physical Assessment Monitor closely if used in presence of preexisting conditions that increase potential for toxicity (eg, renal impairment, peptic ulcer disease, ulcerative colitis, hepatic impairment, bone marrow suppression). Evaluate for additional contraindications with psoriasis or rheumatoid arthritis. Patient should be monitored closely for hyper-/hypothyroidism, pneumonitis (dry, nonproductive cough), gastrointestinal disturbance (ulcerative stomatitis, pain, intestinal perforation), dermatological reactions, and renal failure (decreased urine output).

Patient Education You will be more susceptible to infection. May cause sensitivity to sunlight, nausea, vomiting, drowsiness, dizziness, numbness, blurred vision, loss of hair (may be reversible), color change of skin, permanent sterility, or mouth sores. Report immediately any new skin rash, eruptions, redness, or peeling; respiratory difficulty, fever, or cough; rapid heartbeat or palpitations; black or tarry stools; fever; chills; unusual bleeding or bruising; persistent GI disturbances (abdominal pain, diarrhea, constipation); or pain on urination or change in urinary patterns. Oral: It is very important to maintain adequate nutrition and hydration. Avoid alcohol. Infusion/injection: Report immediately any redness, swelling, pain, or burning at infusion/injection site.

Dietary Considerations Some products may contain sodium.

Geriatric Considerations Toxicity to methotrexate or any immunosuppressive is increased in the elderly. Must monitor carefully. For rheumatoid arthritis and psoriasis, immunosuppressive therapy should only be used when disease is active and less toxic, traditional therapy is ineffective. Recommended doses should be reduced when initiating therapy in the elderly due to possible decreased metabolism, reduced renal function, and presence of interacting diseases and drugs. Adjust dose as needed for renal function (Cl_{cr}).

Breast-Feeding Considerations Low amounts of methotrexate are excreted into breast milk. Due to the potential for serious adverse reactions in a breast-feeding infant, use is contraindicated in nursing mothers.

Pregnancy Considerations [U.S. Boxed Warning]: Methotrexate may cause fetal death and/or congenital abnormalities. Studies in animals and pregnant women have shown evidence of fetal abnormalities; therefore, the manufacturer classifies methotrexate as pregnancy category X (for psoriasis or RA). A pattern of congenital malformations associated with maternal methotrexate use is referred to as the aminopterin/methotrexate syndrome. Features of the syndrome include CNS, skeletal, and cardiac abnormalities. Low birth weight and developmental delay have also been reported. The use of methotrexate may impair fertility and cause menstrual irregularities or oligospermia during treatment and following therapy. Methotrexate is approved for the treatment of trophoblastic neoplasms (gestational choriocarcinoma, chorioadenoma destruens, and hydatidiform mole) and has been used for the medical management of ectopic pregnancy and the medical management of abortion. **[U.S. Boxed Warning]: Use is contraindicated for the treatment of psoriasis or RA in pregnant women.** Pregnancy should be excluded prior to therapy in women of childbearing potential. Use for the treatment of neoplastic diseases only when the potential benefit to the mother outweighs the possible risk to the fetus. Pregnancy should be avoided for ≥3 months following treatment in male patients and ≥1 ovulatory cycle in female patients. A registry is available for pregnant women exposed to autoimmune medications including methotrexate. For additional information contact the Organization of Teratology Information Specialists, OTIS Autoimmune Diseases Study, at 877-311-8972.

Additional Information Oncology Comment: Methotrexate overexposure: The investigational rescue agent, glucarpidase, is an enzyme which rapidly hydrolyzes extracellular methotrexate into inactive metabolites, resulting in a rapid reduction of methotrexate concentrations. Glucarpidase is available for intrathecal (IT) use through an Emergency Use IND and for I.V. use under an Open-Label Treatment protocol.

◆ **Methotrexate Sodium** *see* Methotrexate *on page* 1193

◆ **Methotrexatum** *see* Methotrexate *on page* 1193

Methoxsalen (Topical) (meth OKS a len)

U.S. Brand Names Oxsoralen®

Index Terms Methoxypsoralen

Generic Availability (U.S.) No

Pharmacologic Category Psoralen

Pregnancy Risk Factor C

Lactation Excretion in breast milk unknown/not recommended

Use Repigmentation of idiopathic vitiligo

Available Dosage Forms

Lotion, topical:

Oxsoralen®: 1% (29.57 mL)

Dosing

Adult & Geriatric Note: Refer to treatment protocols for UVA exposure guidelines.

Vitiligo: Topical: Lotion is applied by healthcare provider prior to UVA light exposure, usually no more than once weekly; frequency is determined by erythema response

Pediatric Vitiligo: Topical: Children ≥12 years: Refer to adult dosing.

Administration

Topical Hands and fingers of person applying the lotion should be protected to prevent possible photosensitization and/or burns.

Monitoring and Teaching Issues

Physical Assessment This drug is administered in conjunction with ultraviolet light or ultraviolet radiation therapy. Teach patient sunlight precautions.

Patient Education This medication is used in conjunction with specific ultraviolet treatment. Control exposure to direct sunlight as per prescriber's instructions. Consult prescriber immediately if burning, blistering, or skin irritation occur.

◆ **Methoxypsoralen** *see* Methoxsalen (Topical) *on page* 1200

◆ **Methylacetoxyprogesterone** *see* MedroxyPROGESTERone *on page* 1154

Methyldopa (meth il DOE pa)

Index Terms Aldomet; Methyldopate Hydrochloride

Generic Availability (U.S.) Yes

Pharmacologic Category Alpha-Adrenergic Inhibitor; Alpha$_2$-Adrenergic Agonist

Medication Safety Issues

Sound-alike/look-alike issues:

Methyldopa may be confused with L-dopa, levodopa

Beers Criteria medication: This drug may be inappropriate for use in geriatric patients (high severity risk).

Pregnancy Risk Factor B

Lactation Enters breast milk/use caution (AAP rates "compatible"; AAP 2001 update pending)

Use Management of moderate-to-severe hypertension

Available Dosage Forms

Injection, solution: 50 mg/mL (5 mL)

Tablet, oral: 250 mg, 500 mg

Dosing

Adult Hypertension:

Oral: Initial: 250 mg 2-3 times/day; increase every 2 days as needed (maximum dose: 3 g/day); usual dose range (JNC 7): 250-1000 mg/day in 2 divided doses

I.V.: 250-1000 mg every 6-8 hours; maximum: 1 g every 6 hours

Geriatric Oral: Initial: 125 mg 1-2 times/day; increase by 125 mg every 2-3 days as needed. Adjust for renal impairment.

Pediatric Hypertension:

Oral: Initial: 10 mg/kg/day in 2-4 divided doses; increase every 2 days as needed to maximum dose of 65 mg/kg/day. Do not exceed 3 g/day.

I.V.: 5-10 mg/kg/dose every 6-8 hours up to a total dose of 65 mg/kg/24 hours or 3 g/24 hours

Renal Impairment

Cl_{cr} >50 mL/minute: Administer every 8 hours.

Cl_{cr} 10-50 mL/minute: Administer every 8-12 hours.

Cl_{cr} <10 mL/minute: Administer every 12-24 hours.

Slightly dialyzable (5% to 20%)

Administration

I.V. Infuse over 30 minutes.

Monitoring and Teaching Issues

Laboratory Monitoring CBC, liver enzymes, Coombs' test (direct)

Physical Assessment Evaluate hepatic and renal status prior to treatment. Monitor for hypotension, bradycardia, or CNS changes on a regular basis.

Patient Education Oral: Follow recommended diet and exercise program. Periodic laboratory tests may be required. This medication may cause altered color of urine (normal), drowsiness, dizziness, impaired judgment, postural hypotension, dry mouth, or nausea. Report altered CNS status (eg, nightmares, depression, anxiety, increased nervousness); sudden weight gain; unusual or persistent swelling of ankles, feet, or extremities; palpitations or rapid heartbeat; persistent weakness or fatigue; or unusual bleeding.

◆ **Methyldopate Hydrochloride** *see* Methyldopa *on page* 1200

◆ **Methylergometrine Maleate** *see* Methylergonovine *on page* 1201

Methylergonovine (meth il er goe NOE veen)

U.S. Brand Names Methergine®

Index Terms Methylergometrine Maleate; Methylergonovine Maleate

Generic Availability (U.S.) Yes: Injection

Pharmacologic Category Ergot Derivative

Medication Safety Issues

Sound-alike/look-alike issues:

Methergine® may be confused with Brethine

Methylergonovine and terbutaline parenteral dosage forms look similar. Due to their contrasting indications, use care when administering these agents.

Pregnancy Risk Factor C

Lactation Enters breast milk/use caution

Use Prevention and treatment of postpartum and postabortion hemorrhage caused by uterine atony or subinvolution

Mechanism of Action/Effect Similar smooth muscle actions as seen with ergotamine; however, it affects primarily uterine smooth muscles producing sustained contractions and thereby shortens the third stage of labor and reduces blood loss.

Contraindications Hypersensitivity to methylergonovine or any component of the formulation; ergot alkaloids are contraindicated with potent inhibitors of CYP3A4 (includes protease inhibitors, azole antifungals, and some macrolide antibiotics); hypertension; toxemia; pregnancy

Warnings/Precautions Use caution in patients with sepsis, obliterative vascular disease, cardiovascular disease, hepatic or renal involvement, or second stage of labor; administer with extreme caution if using intravenously. Pleural and peritoneal fibrosis have been reported with prolonged daily use of other ergot alkaloids. Cardiac valvular fibrosis has also been associated with ergot alkaloids. Ergot alkaloid use may result in ergotism (intense vasoconstriction) resulting in peripheral vascular ischemia and possible gangrene. Concomitant use with potent inhibitors of CYP3A4 (includes protease inhibitors, azole antifungals, and some macrolide antibiotics) and ergot alkaloids has been associated with acute ergot toxicity (ergotism); concurrent use of certain ergot alkaloids (eg, ergotamine and dihydroergotamine) are not recommended by the manufacturer. Use with caution in the elderly. Safety and efficacy have not been established in children.

Drug Interactions

Metabolism/Transport Effects Substrate of CYP3A4 (major)

Avoid Concomitant Use

Avoid concomitant use of Methylergonovine with any of the following: Efavirenz; Itraconazole; Nitroglycerin; Posaconazole; Protease Inhibitors; Serotonin 5-HT1D Receptor Agonists; Sibutramine; Voriconazole

Decreased Effect

Methylergonovine may decrease the levels/effects of: Nitroglycerin

Increased Effect/Toxicity

Methylergonovine may increase the levels/effects of: Serotonin 5-HT1D Receptor Agonists; Serotonin Modulators

The levels/effects of Methylergonovine may be increased by: Conivaptan; CYP3A4 Inhibitors (Moderate); CYP3A4 Inhibitors (Strong); Dasatinib; Efavirenz; Itraconazole; Macrolide Antibiotics; Nitroglycerin; Posaconazole; Protease Inhibitors; Serotonin 5-HT1D Receptor Agonists; Sibutramine; Voriconazole

Adverse Reactions Frequency not defined.

Cardiovascular: Acute MI, arterial spasm, bradycardia, hyper-/hypotension, palpitation, tachycardia, temporary chest pain

Central nervous system: Dizziness, hallucinations, headache, seizure

Dermatologic: Rash

Endocrine & metabolic: Water intoxication

Gastrointestinal: Diarrhea, foul taste, nausea, vomiting
Local: Thrombophlebitis
Neuromuscular & skeletal: Leg cramps
Otic: Tinnitus
Renal: Hematuria
Respiratory: Dyspnea, nasal congestion
Miscellaneous: Anaphylaxis, diaphoresis

Pharmacodynamics/Kinetics

Onset of Action Oxytocic: Oral: 5-10 minutes; I.M.: 2-5 minutes; I.V.: Immediately

Duration of Action Oral: ~3 hours; I.M.: ~3 hours; I.V.: 45 minutes

Absorption Rapid

Bioavailability Oral: 60%; I.M.: 78%

Time to Peak Serum: Oral: 0.3-2 hours; I.M.: 0.2-0.6 hours

Half-Life Elimination Biphasic: Initial: 1-5 minutes; Terminal: 0.5-2 hours

Metabolism Hepatic

Excretion Urine and feces

Available Dosage Forms

Injection, solution: 0.2 mg/mL (1 mL)
Methergine®: 0.2 mg/mL (1 mL)

Tablet, oral:
Methergine®: 0.2 mg

Dosing

Adult & Geriatric Prevention of hemorrhage:
Oral: 0.2 mg 3-4 times/day in the puerperium for 2-7 days
I.M., I.V.: 0.2 mg after delivery of anterior shoulder, after delivery of placenta, or during puerperium; may be repeated as required at intervals of 2-4 hours

Administration

I.V. Administer over ≥60 seconds. Should not be routinely administered I.V. because of possibility of inducing sudden hypertension and cerebrovascular accident.

Stability

Storage
Injection: Store under refrigeration at 2°C to 8°C (36°F to 46°F). Protect from light. The following stability information has also been reported: May be stored at room temperature for up to 14 days (Cohen, 2007).
Tablet: Store below 25°C (77°F).

Monitoring and Teaching Issues

Physical Assessment Blood pressure, CNS status, and vaginal bleeding should be monitored on a regular basis.

Patient Education May cause nausea, vomiting, dizziness, or headache. Report immediately any chest pain or tightness; jaw, shoulder, or midback pain; difficulty breathing; headache; cold extremities; or severe abdominal cramping.

Breast-Feeding Considerations At normal doses used to control postpartum uterine bleeding, small amounts are excreted in breast milk.

Pregnancy Considerations Prolonged constriction of the uterine vessels and/or increased myometrial tone may lead to reduced placental blood flow. This has contributed to fetal growth retardation in animals. Methylergonovine is intended for use after delivery of the infant.

◆ **Methylergonovine Maleate** *see* Methylergonovine *on page* 1201
◆ **Methylin®** *see* Methylphenidate *on page* 1204
◆ **Methylin® ER** *see* Methylphenidate *on page* 1204
◆ **Methylmorphine** *see* Codeine *on page* 421

Methylnaltrexone (meth il nal TREKS one)

U.S. Brand Names Relistor®

Index Terms Methylnaltrexone Bromide; N-methylnaltrexone Bromide

Generic Availability (U.S.) No

Pharmacologic Category Gastrointestinal Agent, Miscellaneous; Opioid Antagonist, Peripherally-Acting

Medication Safety Issues
Sound-alike/look-alike issues:
Methylnaltrexone may be confused with naltrexone

Pregnancy Risk Factor B

Lactation Excretion in breast milk unknown/use caution

Use Treatment of opioid-induced constipation in patients with advanced illness receiving palliative care with inadequate response to conventional laxative regimens

Mechanism of Action/Effect Peripherally-acting mu-opioid receptor antagonist which decreases opioid-induced constipation without affecting opioid analgesic effects or inducing opioid withdrawal symptom

Contraindications Known or suspected mechanical bowel obstruction

Canadian labeling: Additional contraindications (not in U.S. labeling): Hypersensitivity to methylnaltrexone or any component of the formulation

Warnings/Precautions Discontinue treatment for severe or persistent diarrhea. Gastrointestinal perforation of the colon, duodenum, and stomach has been reported (rarely) in patients with advanced illnesses associated with impaired structural integrity of the GI wall (eg, cancer, Ogilvie's syndrome, peptic ulcer). Use caution in patients with known or history of GI tract lesions; discontinue therapy if persistent, severe, or worsening abdominal symptoms occur. Use with caution in patients with renal impairment; dosage adjustment recommended for severe renal impairment (Cl_{cr} <30 mL/minute). Has not been studied in patients with end-stage renal impairment requiring dialysis. Discontinue methylnaltrexone if opioids are discontinued. Use has not been studied in patients with peritoneal catheters. Use beyond 4 months has not been studied.

Drug Interactions

Metabolism/Transport Effects Inhibits CYP2D6 (weak)

Avoid Concomitant Use There are no known interactions where it is recommended to avoid concomitant use.

Decreased Effect

The levels/effects of Methylnaltrexone may be decreased by: Peginterferon Alfa-2b

Increased Effect/Toxicity There are no known significant interactions involving an increase in effect.

Adverse Reactions

>10%: Gastrointestinal: Abdominal pain (29%), flatulence (13%), nausea (12%)

1% to 10%:

Central nervous system: Dizziness (7%)

Dermatologic: Hyperhidrosis (7%)

Gastrointestinal: Diarrhea (6%)

Pharmacodynamics/Kinetics

Onset of Action Usually within 30-60 minutes (in responding patients)

Absorption SubQ: Rapid

Time to Peak SubQ: 30 minutes

Protein Binding 11% to 15%

Half-Life Elimination Terminal: ~8 hours

Metabolism Metabolized to methyl-6-naltrexol isomers, methylnaltrexone sulfate, and other minor metabolites

Excretion Urine (~50%, primarily as unchanged drug); feces (<50%, primarily as unchanged drug)

Available Dosage Forms

Injection, solution:

Relistor®: 12 mg/0.6 mL (0.6 mL)

Dosing

Adult & Geriatric Opioid-induced constipation: SubQ: Dosing is according to body weight: Administer 1 dose every other day as needed; maximum: 1 dose/24 hours

<38 kg: 0.15 mg/kg (round dose up to nearest 0.1 mL of volume)

38 to <62 kg: 8 mg

62-114 kg: 12 mg

>114 kg: 0.15 mg/kg (round dose up to nearest 0.1 mL of volume)

Renal Impairment

Mild-to-moderate renal impairment: No adjustment required.

Severe renal impairment (Cl_{cr} <30 mL/minute): Administer 50% of normal dose.

End-stage renal impairment (dialysis-dependent): Has not been studied.

Hepatic Impairment

Mild-to-moderate hepatic impairment (Child-Pugh class A and B): No adjustment required.

Severe hepatic impairment: Has not been studied.

Administration

Other SubQ: Administer subcutaneously into upper arm, abdomen, or thigh. Rotate injection site. Do not use tender, bruised, red, or hard areas.

Stability

Storage Store intact vials at room temperature of 20°C to 25°C (68°F to 77°F); excursions permitted to 15°C to 30°C (59°F to 86°F); do not freeze. Protect from light. Solution for injection is stable in a syringe for 24 hours at room temperature (protection from light during this 24 hours is not necessary).

Monitoring and Teaching Issues

Physical Assessment Use caution in presence of renal impairment; dosage adjustment may be necessary. Discontinue if severe or persistent diarrhea occurs. Must be discontinued if opioids are discontinued. Teach patient appropriate injection technique and syringe/needle disposal.

Patient Education This medication can only be administered via injection. If self-administered, follow instructions for injection and syringe/needle disposal. May cause dizziness. Report immediately any severe or persistent diarrhea or gastrointestinal upset (pain, nausea, vomiting).

Geriatric Considerations In small studies (Phase 2 and 3), no differences in safety and efficacy were noted between elderly and young adults. No dose adjustment is required in elderly.

Pregnancy Considerations Adverse effects were not observed in animal studies. There are no adequate and well-controlled studies in pregnant women.

Additional Information In some clinical trials, patients who received methylnaltrexone were on a palliative opioid therapy equivalent to a mean daily oral morphine dose of 172 mg, at a stable dose for ≥3 days. Constipation was defined as <3 bowel movements/week or no bowel movement for >2 days. Patients maintained their regular laxative regimen for at least 3 days prior to treatment and throughout the study.

◆ **Methylnaltrexone Bromide** *see* Methylnaltrexone *on page 1202*

Methylphenidate (meth il FEN i date)

U.S. Brand Names Concerta®; Daytrana™; Metadate CD®; Metadate® ER; Methylin®; Methylin® ER; Ritalin LA®; Ritalin-SR®; Ritalin®

Index Terms Methylphenidate Hydrochloride

Generic Availability (U.S.) Yes: Immediate release tablet, oral solution, sustained release tablet

Pharmacologic Category Central Nervous System Stimulant

Medication Safety Issues

Sound-alike/look-alike issues:

Metadate CD® may be confused with Metadate® ER
Metadate® ER may be confused with Metadate CD®, methadone
Methylphenidate may be confused with methadone
Ritalin® may be confused with Ismelin®, Rifadin®, ritodrine
Ritalin LA® may be confused with Ritalin-SR®
Ritalin-SR® may be confused with Ritalin LA®

Medication Guide Available Yes

Pregnancy Risk Factor C

Lactation Enters breast milk/use caution

Use Treatment of attention-deficit/hyperactivity disorder (ADHD); symptomatic management of narcolepsy

Unlabeled/Investigational Use Depression (especially elderly or medically ill)

Mechanism of Action/Effect Mild CNS stimulant; blocks the reuptake of norepinephrine and dopamine into presynaptic neurons; appears to stimulate the cerebral cortex and subcortical structures similar to amphetamines

Contraindications Hypersensitivity to methylphenidate, any component of the formulation, or idiosyncratic reactions to sympathomimetic amines; marked anxiety, tension, and agitation; glaucoma; use during or within 14 days following MAO inhibitor therapy; family history or diagnosis of Tourette's syndrome or tics

Metadate CD® and Metadate® ER: Additional contraindications: Severe hypertension, heart failure, arrhythmia, hyperthyroidism, recent MI or angina; concomitant use of halogenated anesthetics

Warnings/Precautions CNS stimulant use has been associated with serious cardiovascular events (eg, sudden death in children and adolescents; sudden death, stroke, and MI in adults) in patients with pre-existing structural cardiac abnormalities or other serious heart problems. These products should be avoided in patients with known serious structural cardiac abnormalities, cardiomyopathy, serious heart rhythm abnormalities, or other serious cardiac problems that could further increase their risk of sudden death. Patients should be carefully evaluated for cardiac disease prior to initiation of therapy. Use of stimulants can cause an increase in blood pressure (average 2-4 mm Hg) and increases in heart rate (average 3-6 bpm), although some patients may have larger than average increases. Use caution with hypertension, hyperthyroidism, or other cardiovascular conditions that might be exacerbated by increases in blood pressure or heart rate. Some products are contraindicated in patients with heart failure, arrhythmias, severe hypertension, hyperthyroidism, angina, or recent MI.

Has demonstrated value as part of a comprehensive treatment program for ADHD. Use with caution in patients with bipolar disorder (may induce mixed/manic episode). May exacerbate symptoms of behavior and thought disorder in psychotic patients; new-onset psychosis or mania may occur with stimulant use; observe for symptoms of aggression and/or hostility. Use caution with seizure disorders (may reduce seizure threshold). Use caution in patients with history of ethanol or drug abuse. May exacerbate symptoms of behavior and thought disorder in psychotic patients. **[U.S. Boxed Warning]: Potential for drug dependency exists - avoid abrupt discontinuation in patients who have received for prolonged periods.** Visual disturbances have been reported (rare). Not labeled for use in children <6 years of age. Use of stimulants has been associated with suppression of growth in children; monitor growth rate during treatment.

Concerta® should not be used in patients with esophageal motility disorders or pre-existing severe gastrointestinal narrowing (small bowel disease, short gut syndrome, history of peritonitis, cystic fibrosis, chronic intestinal pseudo-obstruction, Meckel's diverticulum). Metadate CD® and Metadate® ER contain sucrose and lactose, respectively; avoid administration in hereditary galactose intolerance, Lapp lactase deficiency, or glucose-galactose malabsorption. Concomitant use with halogenated anesthetics is contraindicated; may cause sudden elevations in blood pressure; if surgery is planned, do not administer Metadate CD® or Metadate® ER on the day of surgery. Transdermal system may cause allergic contact sensitization, characterized by intense local reactions (edema, papules) that may spread beyond the patch site; sensitization may subsequently manifest systemically with other routes of methylphenidate administration; monitor closely. Avoid exposure of application site to any direct external heat sources (eg, hair dryers, heating pads, electric blankets); may increase the rate and extent of absorption and risk of overdose. Efficacy of transdermal methylphenidate therapy for >7 weeks has not been established.

Drug Interactions

Metabolism/Transport Effects Inhibits CYP2D6 (weak)

Avoid Concomitant Use

Avoid concomitant use of Methylphenidate with any of the following: Inhalational Anesthetics; Iobenguane I 123; MAO Inhibitors

Decreased Effect

Methylphenidate may decrease the levels/effects of: Antihypertensives; Iobenguane I 123

Increased Effect/Toxicity

Methylphenidate may increase the levels/effects of: Anti-Parkinson's Agents (Dopamine Agonist); Antipsychotics; CloNIDine; Inhalational Anesthetics; PHENobarbital; Phenytoin; Primidone; Sympathomimetics; Tricyclic Antidepressants; Vitamin K Antagonists

The levels/effects of Methylphenidate may be increased by: Antacids; Antipsychotics; Atomoxetine; Cannabinoids; H2-Antagonists; MAO Inhibitors; Proton Pump Inhibitors

Nutritional/Ethanol Interactions

Ethanol: Avoid ethanol (may cause CNS depression).

Food: Food may increase oral absorption; Concerta® formulation is not affected. Food delays early peak and high-fat meals increase C_{max} and AUC of Metadate CD® formulation.

Herb/Nutraceutical: Avoid ephedra (may cause hypertension or arrhythmias) and yohimbe (also has CNS stimulatory activity).

Lab Interactions May interfere with urine detection of amphetamines/methamphetamines (false-positive).

Adverse Reactions

Transdermal system: Frequency of adverse events as reported in trials of 7-week duration. Incidence of some events higher with extended use.

>10%:

Central nervous system: Headache (≤15%; long-term use in children: 28%), insomnia (6% to 13%; long-term use in children: 30%), irritability (7% to 11%)

Gastrointestinal: Appetite decreased (26%), nausea (10% to 12%)

Miscellaneous: Viral infection (long-term use in children: 28%)

1% to 10%:

Cardiovascular: Tachycardia (≤1%)

Central nervous system: Tic (7%), dizziness (adolescents 6%), emotional instability (6%)

Gastrointestinal: Vomiting (3% to 10%), weight loss (6% to 9%), abdominal pain (5% to 7%), anorexia (5%; long-term use in children: 46%)

Local: Application site reaction

Respiratory: Nasal congestion (6%) nasopharyngitis (5%)

Postmarketing and/or case reports (limited to important or life-threatening): Allergic contact dermatitis/sensitization, anaphylaxis, angioedema, hallucinations, seizures

All dosage forms: Frequency not defined:

Cardiovascular: Angina, cardiac arrhythmia, cerebral arteritis, cerebral hemorrhage, cerebral occlusion, cerebrovascular accidents, vasculitis, hyper-/hypotension, MI, murmur, palpitation, pulse increased/decreased, Raynaud's phenomenon, tachycardia

Central nervous system: Aggression, agitation, anger, anxiety, confusional state, depression, dizziness, drowsiness, fatigue, fever, headache, hypervigilance, insomnia, irritability, lethargy, mood alterations, nervousness, neuroleptic malignant syndrome (NMS) (rare), restlessness, stroke, tension, Tourette's syndrome (rare), toxic psychosis, tremor, vertigo

Dermatologic: Alopecia, erythema multiforme, exfoliative dermatitis, hyperhidrosis, rash, urticaria

Endocrine & metabolic: Dysmenorrhea, growth retardation, libido decreased

Gastrointestinal: Abdominal pain, anorexia, appetite decreased, bruxism, constipation, diarrhea, dyspepsia, nausea, vomiting, weight loss, xerostomia

Genitourinary: Erectile dysfunction

Hematologic: Anemia, leukopenia, pancytopenia, thrombocytopenic purpura, thrombocytopenia

Hepatic: Bilirubin increased, liver function tests abnormal, hepatic coma, transaminases increased

Neuromuscular & skeletal: Arthralgia, dyskinesia, muscle tightness, paresthesia

Ocular: Blurred vision, dry eyes, mydriasis, visual accommodation disturbance

Renal: Necrotizing vasculitis

Respiratory: Cough increased, dyspnea, pharyngitis, pharyngolaryngeal pain, rhinitis, sinusitis, upper respiratory tract infection

Miscellaneous: Accidental injury, hypersensitivity reactions

Pharmacodynamics/Kinetics

Onset of Action Peak effect:

Immediate release tablet: Cerebral stimulation: ~2 hours

Extended release capsule (Metadate CD®, Ritalin LA®): Biphasic; initial peak similar to immediate release product, followed by second rising portion (corresponding to extended release portion)

Sustained release tablet: 4-7 hours

Osmotic release tablet (Concerta®): Initial: 1-2 hours

Transdermal: ~2 hours; may be expedited by the application of external heat

Duration of Action Immediate release tablet: 3-6 hours; Sustained release tablet: 8 hours; Extended release tablet: Methylin® ER, Metadate® ER: 8 hours; Concerta®: 12 hours

Absorption
Oral: Readily absorbed
Transdermal: Absorption increased when applied to inflamed skin or exposed to heat. Absorption is continuous for 9 hours after application.

Time to Peak Concerta®: C_{max}: 6-8 hours; Daytrana™: 7.5-10.5 hours

Protein Binding 10% to 33%

Half-Life Elimination *d*-methylphenidate: 3-4 hours; *l*-methylphenidate: 1-3 hours

Metabolism Hepatic via carboxylesterase CES1A1 to minimally active metabolite

Excretion Urine (90%; 80% as metabolite)

Controlled Substance C-II

Available Dosage Forms

Capsule, extended release, oral:
Metadate CD®: 10 mg, 20 mg, 30 mg, 40 mg, 50 mg, 60 mg
Ritalin LA®: 10 mg, 20 mg, 30 mg, 40 mg

Patch, transdermal:
Daytrana™: 10 mg/9 hours (30s); 15 mg/9 hours (30s); 20 mg/9 hours (30s); 30 mg/9 hours (30s)

Solution, oral:
Methylin®: 5 mg/5 mL (500 mL); 10 mg/5 mL (500 mL)

Tablet, oral: 5 mg, 10 mg, 20 mg
Methylin®: 5 mg, 10 mg, 20 mg
Ritalin®: 5 mg, 10 mg, 20 mg

Tablet, chewable, oral:
Methylin®: 2.5 mg, 5 mg, 10 mg

Tablet, extended release, oral:
Concerta®: 18 mg, 27 mg, 36 mg, 54 mg
Metadate® ER: 20 mg
Methylin® ER: 10 mg, 20 mg

Tablet, sustained release, oral: 20 mg
Ritalin-SR®: 20 mg

Dosing

Adult & Geriatric

ADHD: Oral:

Concerta®:

Patients not currently taking methylphenidate: Initial dose: 18-36 mg once daily in the morning

Patients currently taking methylphenidate: **Note:** Initial dose: Dosing based on current regimen and clinical judgment; suggested dosing listed below:
- Patients taking methylphenidate 5 mg 2-3 times/day: 18 mg once every morning
- Patients taking methylphenidate 10 mg 2-3 times/day: 36 mg once every morning
- Patients taking methylphenidate 15 mg 2-3 times/day: 54 mg once every morning
- Patients taking methylphenidate 20 mg 2-3 times/day: 72 mg once every morning

Metadate® ER, Methylin® ER, Ritalin® SR: May be given in place of immediate release products, once the daily dose is titrated and the titrated 8-hour dosage corresponds to sustained or extended release tablet size; maximum: 60 mg/day

Metadate CD®, Ritalin LA®: Initial: 20 mg once daily; may be adjusted in 10-20 mg increments at weekly intervals; maximum: 60 mg/day

Narcolepsy: Oral: 10 mg 2-3 times/day, up to 60 mg/day

Depression (unlabeled use): Oral: Initial: 2.5 mg every morning before 9 AM; dosage may be increased by 2.5-5 mg every 2-3 days as tolerated to a maximum of 20 mg/day; may be divided (ie, 7 AM and 12 noon), but should not be given after noon; do not use sustained release product

Note: Discontinue periodically to re-evaluate or if no improvement occurs within 1 month.

Pediatric ADHD:

Immediate release products Oral: Children ≥6 years: Initial: 5 mg/dose (~0.3 mg/kg/dose) given twice daily before breakfast and lunch; increase by 5-10 mg/day (0.2 mg/kg/day) at weekly intervals; maximum dose: 60 mg/day (2 mg/kg/day). **Note:** Discontinue periodically to re-evaluate or if no improvement occurs within 1 month.

Extended release products: Oral:

Children ≥6 years:

Metadate® ER, Methylin® ER, Ritalin® SR: May be given in place of immediate release products, once the daily dose is titrated and the titrated 8-hour dosage corresponds to sustained or extended release tablet size; maximum: 60 mg/day

Metadate CD®, Ritalin LA®: Initial: 20 mg once daily; may be adjusted in 10-20 mg increments at weekly intervals; maximum: 60 mg/day

Children 6-12 years and Adolescents 13-17 years: *Concerta®:*

Patients not currently taking methylphenidate: Initial dose: 18 mg once daily in the morning

Patients currently taking methylphenidate: **Note:** Initial dose: Dosing based on current regimen and clinical judgment; suggested dosing listed below:
- Patients taking methylphenidate 5 mg 2-3 times/day **or** 20 mg/day sustained release formulation: 18 mg once every morning
- Patients taking methylphenidate 10 mg 2-3 times/day **or** 40 mg/day sustained release formulation: 36 mg once every morning
- Patients taking methylphenidate 15 mg 2-3 times/day **or** 60 mg/day sustained release formulation: 54 mg once every morning

Dose adjustment: May increase dose in increments of 18 mg; dose may be adjusted at weekly intervals. A dosage strength of 27 mg is available for situations in which a dosage between 18-36 mg is desired. Maximum dose should not exceed 2 mg/kg/day **or** 54 mg/day in children 6-12 years or 72 mg/day in children 13-17 years.

Transdermal (Daytrana™): Children 6-17 years: Initial: 10 mg patch once daily; remove up to 9 hours after application. Titrate based on response and tolerability; may increase to next transdermal dose no more frequently than every week. **Note:** Application should occur 2 hours prior to desired effect. Drug absorption may continue for a period of time after patch removal; patients converting from another formulation of methylphenidate should be initiated at 10 mg regardless of their previous dose and titrated as needed due to the differences in bioavailability of the transdermal formulation.

Administration

Oral Do not crush or allow patient to chew sustained or extended release dosage form. To effectively avoid insomnia, dosing should be completed by noon.

Concerta®: Administer dose once daily in the morning. May be taken with or without food, but must be taken with water, milk, or juice.

Metadate CD®, Ritalin LA®: Capsules may be opened and the contents sprinkled onto a small amount (equal to 1 tablespoon) of cold applesauce. Swallow applesauce without chewing. Do not crush or chew capsule contents.

Methylin® chewable tablet: Administer with at least 8 ounces of water or other fluid.

Topical Transdermal (Daytrana™): Apply to clean, dry, non-oily, intact skin to the hip area, avoiding the waistline; do not premedicate the patch site with hydrocortisone or other solutions, creams, ointments, or emollients. Apply at the same time each day to alternating hips. Press firmly for 30 seconds to ensure proper adherence. Avoid exposure of application site to external heat source, which may increase the amount of drug absorbed. If difficulty is experienced when separating the patch from the liner or if any medication (sticky substance) remains on the liner after separation; discard that patch and apply a new patch. Do not use a patch that has been damaged or torn; do not cut patch. If patch should dislodge, may replace with new patch (to different site) but total wear time should not exceed 9 hours; do not reapply with dressings, tape, or common adhesives. Patch may be removed early if a shorter duration of effect is desired or if late day side effects occur. Wash hands with soap and water after handling. Avoid touching the sticky side of the patch. If patch removal is difficult, an oil-based product (eg, petroleum jelly, olive oil) may be applied to the patch edges to aid removal; never apply acetone-based products (eg, nail polish remover) to patch. Dispose of used patch by folding adhesive side onto itself, and discard in toilet or appropriate lidded container.

Stability

Storage

Capsule: *Extended release:* Store at 25°C (77°F); excursions permitted to 15°C to 30°C (59°F to 86°F). Protect from light.

Solution: Store at controlled room temperature of 20°C to 25°C (68°F to 77°F).

Tablet:

Chewable: Store at controlled room temperature of 20°C to 25°C (68°F to 77°F). Protect from light and moisture.

Extended and sustained release: Store at controlled room temperature of 20°C to 25°C (68°F to 77°F). Protect from light and moisture.

Immediate release: Store at controlled room temperature of 20°C to 25°C (68°F to 77°F). Protect from light and moisture.

Osmotic controlled release (Concerta®): Store at controlled room temperature of 25°C; excursions permitted to 15°C to 30°C (59°F to 86°F). Protect from humidity.

Transdermal system: Store at 25°C (77°F); excursions permitted to 15°C to 30°C (59°F to 86°F). Keep patches stored in protective pouch. Once tray is opened, use patches within 2 months; once an individual patch has been removed from the pouch and the protective liner removed, use immediately. Do not refrigerate or freeze.

Monitoring and Teaching Issues

Laboratory Monitoring Periodic CBC, differential, and platelet counts with prolonged use; liver function tests

Physical Assessment Assess for history of addiction; long-term use can result in dependence, abuse, or tolerance. Evaluate periodically for need for continued use. After long-term use, taper dosage slowly when discontinuing. In children, monitor growth pattern. If growth/weight gain is not as expected, may need to discontinue medication. Perform careful cardiovascular assessment prior to initiating therapy. Assess vital signs at beginning of therapy and periodically throughout.

Patient Education Response may take some time. Do not crush or chew long-acting forms. Tablets and sustained release tablets should be taken 30-45 minutes before meals. Concerta® may be taken with or without food, but must be taken with water, milk, or juice. Metadate CD® and Ritalin LA® capsules may be opened and the contents sprinkled onto a small amount (equal to 1 tablespoon) of applesauce; swallow applesauce without chewing. Transdermal: Apply to clean, dry skin, immediately after removing from package. Firmly press in place and hold for 30 seconds. Avoid exposing application site to external heat sources. Total wear time should not exceed 9 hours. Avoid alcohol and caffeine. You may experience decreased appetite or weight loss, restlessness, impaired judgment, or dizziness, especially during early therapy. Report unresolved rapid heartbeat, chest pain, difficulty breathing, and fainting; excessive agitation or nervousness; insomnia, tremors, or dizziness; or skin rash.

Dietary Considerations Should be taken 30-45 minutes before meals. Concerta® is not affected by food. Some products may contain phenylalanine.

Geriatric Considerations Methylphenidate is often useful in treating elderly patients who are discouraged, withdrawn, apathetic, or disinterested in their activities. In particular, it is useful in patients who are starting a rehabilitation program but have resigned themselves to fail; these patients may not have a major depressive disorder; will not improve memory or cognitive function; use with caution in patients with dementia who may have increased agitation and confusion.

Breast-Feeding Considerations Methylphenidate excretion into breast milk has been noted in case reports. In both cases, the authors calculated the relative infant dose to be ≤0.2% of the weight adjusted maternal dose. Adverse events were not noted in either infant, however, both were older (6 months of age and 11 months of age) and exposure was limited.

Pregnancy Considerations Animal studies have shown teratogenic effects to the fetus. There are no adequate and well-controlled studies in pregnant women. Do not use in women of childbearing age unless the potential benefit outweighs the possible risk.

Additional Information Treatment with methylphenidate may include "drug holidays" or periodic discontinuation in order to assess the patient's requirements and to decrease tolerance and limit suppression of linear growth and weight. Specific patients may require 3 doses/day for treatment of ADHD (ie, additional dose at 4 PM).

Concerta® is an osmotic controlled release formulation (OROS®) of methylphenidate. The tablet has an immediate-release overcoat that provides an initial dose of methylphenidate within 1 hour. The overcoat covers a trilayer core. The trilayer core is composed of two layers containing the drug and excipients, and one layer of osmotic components. As water from the gastrointestinal tract enters the core, the osmotic components expand and methylphenidate is released.

Metadate CD® capsules contain a mixture of immediate release and extended release beads, designed to release 30% of the dose immediately and 70% over an extended period.

Ritalin LA® uses a combination of immediate release and enteric coated, delayed release beads.

◆ **Methylphenidate Hydrochloride** *see* Methylphenidate *on page* 1204

◆ **Methylphenoxy-Benzene Propanamine** *see* Atomoxetine *on page* 164

◆ **Methylphytyl Napthoquinone** *see* Phytonadione *on page* 1457

MethylPREDNISolone (meth il pred NIS oh lone)

U.S. Brand Names A-Methapred®; Depo-Medrol®; Medrol®; Medrol® Dosepak™; Solu-MEDROL®

Index Terms 6-α-Methylprednisolone; A-Methapred; Medrol Dose Pack; Methylprednisolone Acetate; Methylprednisolone Sodium Succinate; Solumedrol

Generic Availability (U.S.) Yes: Excludes preservative free injection, suspension

Pharmacologic Category Corticosteroid, Systemic

Medication Safety Issues

Sound-alike/look-alike issues:

MethylPREDNISolone may be confused with medroxyPROGESTERone, methotrexate, methylTESTOSTERone, predniSONE
Depo-Medrol® may be confused with Solu-Medrol®
Medrol® may be confused with Mebaral®
Solu-MEDROL® may be confused with Depo-Medrol®, salmeterol, Solu-CORTEF®

International issues:

Medrol [U.S., Canada, and multiple international markets] may be confused with Medral brand name for omeprazole [Mexico]

Lactation Enters breast milk/use caution

Use Primarily as an anti-inflammatory or immunosuppressant agent in the treatment of a variety of diseases including those of hematologic, allergic, inflammatory, neoplastic, and autoimmune origin. Prevention and treatment of graft-versus-host disease following allogeneic bone marrow transplantation.

Unlabeled/Investigational Use Acute spinal cord injury

Mechanism of Action/Effect In a tissue-specific manner, corticosteroids regulate gene expression subsequent to binding specific intracellular receptors and translocation into the nucleus. Corticosteroids exert a wide array of physiologic effects, including modulation of carbohydrate, protein, and lipid metabolism, and maintenance of fluid and electrolyte homeostasis. Moreover, cardiovascular, immunologic, musculoskeletal, endocrine, and neurologic physiology are influenced by corticosteroids.

Contraindications Hypersensitivity to methylprednisolone or any component of the formulation; systemic fungal infection (except intra-articular injection in localized joint conditions); administration of live virus vaccines. methylprednisolone formulations containing benzyl alcohol preservative are contraindicated in premature infants; I.M. administration in idiopathic thrombocytopenia purpura; intrathecal administration

Warnings/Precautions Use with caution in patients with thyroid disease, hepatic impairment, renal impairment, cardiovascular disease, diabetes, glaucoma, cataracts, myasthenia gravis, patients at risk for osteoporosis, patients at risk for seizures, or GI diseases (diverticulitis, peptic ulcer, ulcerative colitis) due to perforation risk. Not recommended for the treatment of optic neuritis; may increase frequency of new episodes. Use caution following acute MI (corticosteroids have been associated with myocardial rupture). Cardiomegaly and congestive heart failure have been reported following concurrent use of amphotericin B and hydrocortisone for the management of fungal infections.

Because of the risk of adverse effects, systemic corticosteroids should be used cautiously in the elderly in the smallest possible effective dose for the shortest duration. May affect growth velocity; growth should be routinely monitored in pediatric patients. Withdraw therapy with gradual tapering of dose.

May cause hypercorticism or suppression of hypothalamic-pituitary-adrenal (HPA) axis, particularly in younger children or in patients receiving high doses for prolonged periods. HPA axis suppression may lead to adrenal crisis. Withdrawal and discontinuation of a corticosteroid should be done slowly and carefully. Particular care is required when patients are transferred from systemic corticosteroids to inhaled products due to possible adrenal insufficiency or withdrawal from steroids, including an increase in allergic symptoms. Patients receiving >20 mg per day of prednisone (or equivalent) may be most susceptible. Fatalities have occurred due to adrenal insufficiency in asthmatic patients during and after transfer from systemic corticosteroids to aerosol steroids; aerosol steroids do not provide the systemic steroid needed to treat patients having trauma, surgery, or infections.

Acute myopathy has been reported with high dose corticosteroids, usually in patients with neuromuscular transmission disorders; may involve ocular and/or respiratory muscles; monitor creatine kinase; recovery may be delayed. Corticosteroid use may cause psychiatric disturbances, including depression, euphoria, insomnia, mood swings, and personality changes. Pre-existing psychiatric conditions may be exacerbated by corticosteroid use. Prolonged use of corticosteroids may also increase the incidence of secondary infection, cause activation of latent infections, mask acute infection (including fungal infections), prolong or exacerbate viral or parasitic infections, or limit response to vaccines. Exposure to chickenpox or measles should be avoided; corticosteroids should not be used to treat ocular herpes simplex. Corticosteroids should not be used for cerebral malaria or viral hepatitis. Close observation is required in patients with latent tuberculosis and/or TB reactivity; restrict use in active TB (only in conjunction with antituberculosis treatment). Amebiasis should be ruled out in any patient with recent travel to tropic climates or unexplained diarrhea prior to initiation of corticosteroids. Prolonged treatment with corticosteroids has been associated with the development of Kaposi's sarcoma (case reports); discontinuation may result in clinical improvement.

High-dose corticosteroids should not be used to manage acute head injury. Rare cases of anaphylactoid reactions have been observed in patients receiving corticosteroids. Avoid injection or leakage into the dermis; dermal and/or subdermal skin depression may occur at the site of injection. Avoid deltoid muscle injection; subcutaneous atrophy may occur. Some dosage forms contain benzyl alcohol which has been associated with "gasping syndrome" in neonates.

Drug Interactions

Metabolism/Transport Effects Substrate of CYP3A4 (major); **Inhibits** CYP2C8 (weak), 3A4 (weak)

Avoid Concomitant Use

Avoid concomitant use of MethylPREDNISolone with any of the following: Aldesleukin; BCG; Natalizumab; Pimecrolimus; Roflumilast; Tacrolimus (Topical)

Decreased Effect

MethylPREDNISolone may decrease the levels/effects of: Aldesleukin; Antidiabetic Agents; BCG; Calcitriol; Corticorelin; CycloSPORINE; CycloSPORINE (Systemic); Isoniazid; Salicylates; Sipuleucel-T; Vaccines (Inactivated)

The levels/effects of MethylPREDNISolone may be decreased by: Aminoglutethimide; Antacids; Barbiturates; Bile Acid Sequestrants; Echinacea; Mitotane; Primidone; Rifamycin Derivatives

Increased Effect/Toxicity

MethylPREDNISolone may increase the levels/effects of: Acetylcholinesterase Inhibitors; Amphotericin B; CycloSPORINE; CycloSPORINE (Systemic); Leflunomide; Loop Diuretics; Natalizumab; NSAID (COX-2 Inhibitor); NSAID (Nonselective); Thiazide Diuretics; Vaccines (Live); Warfarin

The levels/effects of MethylPREDNISolone may be increased by: Antifungal Agents (Azole Derivatives, Systemic); Aprepitant; Calcium Channel Blockers (Nondihydropyridine); CycloSPORINE; CycloSPORINE (Systemic); CYP3A4 Inhibitors (Strong); Denosumab; Estrogen Derivatives; Fluconazole; Fosaprepitant; Macrolide Antibiotics; Neuromuscular-Blocking Agents (Nondepolarizing); Pimecrolimus; Quinolone Antibiotics; Roflumilast; Salicylates; Tacrolimus (Topical); Trastuzumab

Nutritional/Ethanol Interactions

Ethanol: Avoid ethanol (may increase gastric mucosal irritation).

Food: Methylprednisolone interferes with calcium absorption. Limit caffeine.

Herb/Nutraceutical: St John's wort may decrease methylprednisolone levels. Avoid cat's claw, echinacea (have immunostimulant properties).

Lab Interactions Interferes with skin tests

Adverse Reactions Frequency not defined.

Cardiovascular: Arrhythmias, bradycardia, cardiac arrest, cardiomegaly, circulatory collapse, congestive heart failure, edema, fat embolism, hypertension, hypertrophic cardiomyopathy in premature infants, myocardial rupture (post MI), syncope, tachycardia, thromboembolism, vasculitis

Central nervous system: Delirium, depression, emotional instability, euphoria, hallucinations, headache, intracranial pressure increased, insomnia, malaise, mood swings, nervousness, neuritis, personality changes, psychic disorders, pseudotumor cerebri (usually following discontinuation), seizure, vertigo

Dermatologic: Acne, allergic dermatitis, alopecia, dry scaly skin, ecchymoses, edema, erythema, hirsutism, hyper-/hypopigmentation, hypertrichosis, impaired wound healing, petechiae, rash, skin atrophy, sterile abscess, skin test reaction impaired, striae, urticaria

Endocrine & metabolic: Adrenal suppression, amenorrhea, carbohydrate intolerance increased, Cushing's syndrome, diabetes mellitus, fluid retention, glucose intolerance, growth suppression (children), hyperglycemia, hyperlipidemia, hypokalemia, hypokalemic alkalosis, menstrual irregularities, negative nitrogen balance, pituitary-adrenal axis suppression, protein catabolism, sodium and water retention

Gastrointestinal: Abdominal distention, appetite increased, bowel/bladder dysfunction (after intrathecal administration), gastrointestinal hemorrhage, gastrointestinal perforation, nausea, pancreatitis, peptic ulcer, perforation of the small and large intestine, ulcerative esophagitis, vomiting, weight gain

Hematologic: Leukocytosis (transient)

Hepatic: Hepatomegaly, transaminases increased

Local: Postinjection flare (intra-articular use), thrombophlebitis

Neuromuscular & skeletal: Arthralgia, arthropathy, aseptic necrosis (femoral and humoral heads), fractures, muscle mass loss, muscle weakness, myopathy (particularly in conjunction with neuromuscular disease or neuromuscular-blocking agents), neuropathy, osteoporosis, parasthesia, tendon rupture, vertebral compression fractures, weakness

Ocular: Cataracts, exophthalmoses, glaucoma, intraocular pressure increased

Renal: Glycosuria

Respiratory: Pulmonary edema

Miscellaneous: Abnormal fat disposition, anaphylactoid reaction, anaphylaxis, angioedema, avascular necrosis, diaphoresis, hiccups, hypersensitivity reactions, infections, secondary malignancy

Pharmacodynamics/Kinetics

Onset of Action Peak effect (route dependent): Oral: 1-2 hours; I.M.: 4-8 days; Intra-articular: 1 week; methylprednisolone sodium succinate is highly soluble and has a rapid effect by I.M. and I.V. routes

Duration of Action Route dependent: Oral: 30-36 hours; I.M.: 1-4 weeks; Intra-articular: 1-5 weeks; methylprednisolone acetate has a low solubility and has a sustained I.M. effect

Half-Life Elimination 3-3.5 hours; reduced in obese

Excretion Clearance: Reduced in obese

Available Dosage Forms

Injection, powder for reconstitution: 40 mg, 125 mg, 500 mg, 1 g
A-Methapred®: 40 mg
Solu-MEDROL®: 500 mg, 1 g, 2 g

Injection, powder for reconstitution [preservative free]:
Solu-MEDROL®: 40 mg, 125 mg, 500 mg, 1 g

Injection, suspension: 40 mg/mL (1 mL, 5 mL, 10 mL); 80 mg/mL (1 mL, 5 mL)
Depo-Medrol®: 20 mg/mL (5 mL); 40 mg/mL (5 mL, 10 mL); 80 mg/mL (5 mL)

Injection, suspension [preservative free]:
Depo-Medrol®: 40 mg/mL (1 mL); 80 mg/mL (1 mL)

Tablet, oral: 4 mg, 8 mg, 16 mg, 32 mg
Medrol®: 2 mg, 4 mg, 8 mg, 16 mg, 32 mg
Medrol® Dosepak™: 4 mg

Dosing

Adult & Geriatric Only sodium succinate may be given I.V.; methylprednisolone sodium succinate is highly soluble and has a rapid effect by I.M. and I.V. routes. Methylprednisolone acetate has a low solubility and has a sustained I.M. effect.

Acute spinal cord injury (unlabeled use): I.V. (sodium succinate): 30 mg/kg over 15 minutes, followed in 45 minutes by a continuous infusion of 5.4 mg/kg/hour for 23 hours. **Note:** Due to insufficient evidence of clinical efficacy (ie, preserving or improving spinal cord function), the routine use of methylprednisolone in the treatment of acute spinal cord injury is no longer recommended. If used in this setting, methylprednisolone should not be initiated >8 hours after the injury; not effective in penetrating trauma (eg, gunshot) (Consortium for Spinal Cord Medicine, 2008).

Allergic conditions: Oral: Tapered-dosage schedule:

Day 1: 24 mg on day 1 administered as 8 mg before breakfast, 4 mg after lunch, 4 mg after supper, and 8 mg at bedtime **OR** 24 mg as a single dose or divided into 2 or 3 doses upon initiation (regardless of time of day)

Day 2: 20 mg on day 2 administered as 4 mg before breakfast, 4 mg after lunch, 4 mg after supper, and 8 mg at bedtime

Day 3: 16 mg on day 3 administered as 4 mg before breakfast, 4 mg after lunch, 4 mg after supper, and 4 mg at bedtime

Day 4: 12 mg on day 4 administered as 4 mg before breakfast, 4 mg after lunch, and 4 mg at bedtime

Day 5: 8 mg on day 5 administered as 4 mg before breakfast and 4 mg at bedtime

Day 6: 4 mg on day 6 administered as 4 mg before breakfast

Anti-inflammatory or immunosuppressive:

Oral: 2-60 mg/day in 1-4 divided doses to start, followed by gradual reduction in dosage to the lowest possible level consistent with maintaining an adequate clinical response.

I.M. (sodium succinate): 10-80 mg/day once daily

I.M. (acetate): 10-80 mg every 1-2 weeks

I.V. (sodium succinate): 10-40 mg over a period of several minutes and repeated I.V. or I.M. at intervals depending on clinical response; when high dosages are needed, give 30 mg/kg over a period ≥30 minutes and may be repeated every 4-6 hours for 48 hours.

Arthritis: Intra-articular (acetate): Administer every 1-5 weeks.

Large joints (eg, knee, ankle): 20-80 mg

Medium joints (eg, elbow, wrist): 10-40 mg

Small joints: 4-10 mg

Asthma exacerbations, including status asthmaticus (emergency medical care or hospital doses): Oral, I.V.: 40-80 mg/day in 1- 2 divided doses until peak expiratory flow is 70% of predicted or personal best (NIH Asthma Guidelines, NAEPP, 2007)

Asthma, severe persistent, long-term control: Oral: 7.5-60 mg/day (or on alternate days) (NIH Asthma Guidelines, NAEPP, 2007)

Dermatitis, acute severe: I.M. (acetate): 80-120 mg as a single dose

Dermatitis, chronic: I.M. (acetate): 40-120 mg every 5-10 days

Dermatologic conditions (eg, keloids, lichen planus): Intralesional (acetate): 20-60 mg

Dermatomyositis/polymyositis: I.V. (sodium succinate): 1 g/day for 3-5 days for severe muscle weakness, followed by conversion to oral prednisone (Drake, 1996)

Lupus nephritis: High-dose "pulse" therapy: I.V. (sodium succinate): 0.5-1 g/day for 3 days (Ponticelli, 2010)

***Pneumocystis* pneumonia in AIDS patients:** I.V.: 30 mg twice daily for 5 days, then 30 mg once daily for 5 days, then 15 mg once daily for 11 days

Pediatric Dosing should be based on the lesser of ideal body weight or actual body weight. **Only sodium succinate may be given I.V.;** methylprednisolone sodium succinate is highly soluble and has a rapid effect by I.M. and I.V. routes. Methylprednisolone acetate has a low solubility and has a sustained I.M. effect.

Acute spinal cord injury (unlabeled use): I.V. (sodium succinate): 30 mg/kg over 15 minutes, followed in 45 minutes by a continuous infusion of 5.4 mg/kg/hour for 23 hours. **Note:** Due to insufficient evidence of clinical efficacy (ie, preserving or improving spinal cord function), the routine use of methylprednisolone in the treatment of acute spinal cord injury is no longer recommended. If used in this setting, methylprednisolone should not be initiated >8 hours after the injury; not effective in penetrating trauma (eg, gunshot) (Consortium for Spinal Cord Medicine, 2008).

Anti-inflammatory or immunosuppressive: Oral, I.M., I.V. (sodium succinate): 0.5-1.7 mg/kg/day **or** 5-25 mg/m^2/day in divided doses every 6-12 hours; "Pulse" therapy: 15-30 mg/kg/dose over ≥30 minutes given once daily for 3 days

Asthma exacerbations, including status asthmaticus (emergency medical care or hospital doses) (NIH Asthma Guidelines, NAEPP, 2007): Children <12 years: Oral, I.V.: 1-2 mg/kg/day in 2 divided doses (maximum: 60 mg/day) until peak expiratory flow is 70% of predicted or personal best

Lupus nephritis: I.V. (sodium succinate): 30 mg/kg over ≥30 minutes every other day for 6 doses

Renal Impairment

Hemodialysis effects: Slightly dialyzable (5% to 20%)

Administer dose posthemodialysis.

Administration

Oral Administer with meals to decrease GI upset. Give daily dose in the morning to mimic normal peak blood levels.

I.V. Only sodium succinate formulation may be given I.V. Acetate salt should not be given I.V.

Parenteral: Methylprednisolone sodium succinate may be administered I.M. or I.V.; I.V. administration may be IVP over one to several minutes or IVPB or continuous I.V. infusion. Avoid injection or leakage into the dermis; dermal and/or subdermal skin depression may occur at the site of injection.

I.V.: Succinate:

Low dose: ≤1.8 mg/kg or ≤125 mg/dose: I.V. push over 3-15 minutes

Moderate dose: ≥2 mg/kg or 250 mg/dose: I.V. over 15-30 minutes

High dose: 15 mg/kg or ≥500 mg/dose: I.V. over ≥30 minutes

Doses >15 mg/kg or ≥1 g: Administer over 1 hour

Do **not** administer high-dose I.V. push; hypotension, cardiac arrhythmia, and sudden death have been reported in patients given high-dose methylprednisolone I.V. push (>0.5 g over <10 minutes). Intermittent infusion over 15-60 minutes; maximum concentration: I.V. push 125 mg/mL.

I.M.: Avoid injection into the deltoid muscle due to a high incidence of subcutaneous atrophy. Avoid injection or leakage into the dermis; dermal and/or subdermal skin depression may occur at the site of injection. Do not inject into areas that have evidence of acute local infection.

Topical For external use only. Apply sparingly.

Stability

Reconstitution

Standard diluent (Solu-Medrol®): 40 mg/50 mL D_5W; 125 mg/50 mL D_5W.

Minimum volume (Solu-Medrol®): 50 mL D_5W.

Storage Intact vials of methylprednisolone sodium succinate should be stored at controlled room temperature of 20°C to 25°C (68°F to 77°F). Protect from light. Reconstituted solutions of methylprednisolone sodium succinate should be stored at room temperature of 20°C to 25°C (68°F to 77°F) and used within 48 hours. Stability of parenteral admixture at room temperature (25°C) and at refrigeration temperature (4°C) is 48 hours.

Monitoring and Teaching Issues

Laboratory Monitoring Blood glucose, electrolytes

Physical Assessment Teach patients to report opportunistic infection and adrenal suppression. Instruct patients with diabetes to monitor serum glucose levels closely; corticosteroids can alter glycemic response. Dose may need to be increased if patient is experiencing higher than normal levels of stress. When discontinuing, taper dose and frequency slowly.

Patient Education Maintain adequate nutritional intake; consult prescriber for possibility of special dietary instructions. If you have diabetes, monitor serum glucose closely and notify prescriber of any changes; this medication can alter glycemic response. Avoid alcohol. Inform prescriber if you are experiencing unusual stress; dosage may need to be adjusted. You will be susceptible to infection. You may experience insomnia or nervousness. Report increased pain, swelling, or redness in area being treated; excessive or sudden weight gain; swelling of extremities; muscle pain or weakness; change in menstrual pattern; vision changes; signs of hyperglycemia; signs of infection (eg, fever, chills, mouth sores, perianal itching, vaginal discharge); blackened stool; or worsening of condition.

Oral: Take with food or milk.

Intra-articular: Refrain from excessive use of joint following therapy, even if pain is gone.

Dietary Considerations Take with meals to decrease GI upset.; need diet rich in pyridoxine, vitamin C, vitamin D, folate, calcium, phosphorus, and protein.

Geriatric Considerations Because of the risk of adverse effects, systemic corticosteroids should be used cautiously in the elderly, in the smallest possible dose, and for the shortest possible time.

Breast-Feeding Considerations Low levels of methylprednisolone are excreted in breast milk

Pregnancy Considerations Adverse events have been observed with corticosteroids in animal reproduction studies. Methylprednisolone crosses the placenta. Some studies have shown an association between first trimester systemic corticosteroid use and oral clefts; adverse events in the fetus/neonate have been noted in case reports following large doses of systemic corticosteroids during pregnancy. Pregnant women exposed to methylprednisolone for antirejection therapy following a transplant may contact the National Transplantation Pregnancy Registry (NTPR) at 215-955-4820. Women exposed to methylprednisolone during pregnancy for the treatment of an autoimmune disease may contact the OTIS Autoimmune Diseases Study at 877-311-8972.

Additional Information Sodium content of 1 g sodium succinate injection: 2.01 mEq; 53 mg of sodium succinate salt is equivalent to 40 mg of methylprednisolone base

Methylprednisolone acetate: Depo-Medrol®

Methylprednisolone sodium succinate: Solu-Medrol®

Related Information

Compatibility of Drugs *on page 1994*

Corticosteroids *on page 1996*

◆ **6-α-Methylprednisolone** *see* MethylPREDNISolone *on page 1208*

◆ **Methylprednisolone Acetate** *see* MethylPREDNISolone *on page 1208*

◆ **Methylprednisolone Sodium Succinate** *see* MethylPREDNISolone *on page 1208*

MethylTESTOSTERone (meth il tes TOS te rone)

U.S. Brand Names Android®; Methitest™; Testred®

Generic Availability (U.S.) No

Pharmacologic Category Androgen

Medication Safety Issues

Sound-alike/look-alike issues:

MethylTESTOSTERone may be confused with medroxyPROGESTERone, methylPREDNISolone

Virilon® may be confused with Verelan®

Beers Criteria medication: This drug may be inappropriate for use in geriatric patients (high severity risk).

Pregnancy Risk Factor X

Lactation Excretion in breast milk unknown/contraindicated

Use

Male: Hypogonadism; delayed puberty; impotence and climacteric symptoms

Female: Palliative treatment of metastatic breast cancer

Unlabeled/Investigational Use Hypogonadism (male); delayed puberty (male)

Controlled Substance C-III

Available Dosage Forms

Capsule, oral:

Android®: 10 mg

Testred®: 10 mg

Tablet, oral:

Methitest™: 10 mg

Dosing

Adult & Geriatric

Hypogonadism (male), delayed puberty (male): Oral: Individualize dose based on response and tolerability.

Androgen deficiency (Male): Oral: 10-50 mg/day

Breast cancer (Female): Oral: 50-200 mg/day

Monitoring and Teaching Issues

Physical Assessment Use extreme caution in presence of hepatic, renal, or cardiovascular disease. Monitor for virilism (male and female), edema, CNS changes (anxiety, depression), acne, baldness, GI irritation, leukopenia, and hepatic dysfunction frequently during therapy. Caution patients with diabetes; effects of hypoglycemic agents may be increased.

Patient Education If you have diabetes, monitor serum glucose closely and notify prescriber of changes; this medication can alter hypoglycemic requirements. May cause acne, growth of body hair, loss of libido, impotence, menstrual irregularity (usually reversible), nausea, or vomiting. Report changes in menstrual pattern, deepening of voice or unusual growth of body hair, gynecomastia or breast soreness, priapism, fluid retention (swelling of ankles, feet, or hands, respiratory difficulty, or sudden weight gain), change in color of urine or stool, yellowing of eyes or skin, unusual bruising or bleeding, or unusual fatigue or weakness.

Metoclopramide (met oh KLOE pra mide)

U.S. Brand Names Metozolv™ ODT; Reglan®

Generic Availability (U.S.) Yes: Excludes oral-disintegrating tablet

Pharmacologic Category Antiemetic; Gastrointestinal Agent, Prokinetic

Medication Safety Issues

Sound-alike/look-alike issues:

Metoclopramide may be confused with metolazone, metoprolol, metroNIDAZOLE

Reglan® may be confused with Megace®, Regonol®, Renagel®

Medication Guide Available Yes

Pregnancy Risk Factor B

Lactation Enters breast milk/use caution

Use

Oral: Symptomatic treatment of diabetic gastroparesis; gastroesophageal reflux

I.V., I.M.: Symptomatic treatment of diabetic gastroparesis; postpyloric placement of enteral feeding tubes; prevention and/or treatment of nausea and vomiting associated with chemotherapy, or postsurgery; to stimulate gastric emptying and intestinal transit of barium during radiological examination of the stomach/small intestine

Mechanism of Action/Effect Blocks dopamine receptors and (when given in higher doses) also blocks serotonin receptors in chemoreceptor trigger zone of the CNS; enhances the response to acetylcholine of tissue in upper GI tract causing enhanced motility and accelerated gastric emptying without stimulating gastric, biliary, or pancreatic secretions; increases lower esophageal sphincter tone

Contraindications Hypersensitivity to metoclopramide or any component of the formulation; GI obstruction, perforation or hemorrhage; pheochromocytoma; history of seizures or concomitant use of other agents likely to increase extrapyramidal reactions

Warnings/Precautions [U.S. Boxed Warning]: May cause tardive dyskinesia, which is often irreversible; duration of treatment and total cumulative dose are associated with an increased risk. Therapy durations >12 weeks should be avoided (except in rare cases following risk:benefit assessment). Risk appears to be increased in the elderly, women, and diabetics; however, it is not possible to predict which patients will develop tardive dyskinesia. Therapy should be discontinued in any patient if signs/symptoms of tardive dyskinesia appear.

May cause extrapyramidal symptoms, generally manifested as acute dystonic reactions within the initial 24-48 hours of use. Risk of these reactions is increased at higher doses, and in pediatric patients, and adults <30 years of age. Pseudoparkinsonism (eg, bradykinesia, tremor, rigidity) may also occur (usually within first 6 months of therapy) and is generally reversible following discontinuation. Use with caution or avoid in patients with Parkinson's disease. Use caution in the elderly; may have increased risk of tardive dyskinesia, particularly older women. Neuroleptic malignant syndrome (NMS) has been reported (rarely) with metoclopramide.

May cause transient increase in serum aldosterone; use caution in patients who are at risk of fluid overload (HF, cirrhosis). Use caution in patients with hypertension or following surgical anastomosis/closure. Use caution with a history of mental illness; has been associated with depression. Abrupt discontinuation may (rarely) result in withdrawal symptoms (dizziness, headache, nervousness). Use caution and adjust dose in renal impairment. Patients with NADH-cytochrome b5 reductase deficiency are at increased risk of methemoglobinemia and/or sulfhemoglobinemia. Neonates may have an increased risk of methemoglobinemia due to decreased levels of NADH-cytochrome b5 reductase deficiency and prolonged clearance of metoclopramide.

Drug Interactions

Metabolism/Transport Effects Substrate (minor) of CYP1A2, 2D6; **Inhibits** CYP2D6 (weak)

Avoid Concomitant Use

Avoid concomitant use of Metoclopramide with any of the following: Antipsychotics; Droperidol; Promethazine; Tetrabenazine

Decreased Effect

Metoclopramide may decrease the levels/effects of: Anti-Parkinson's Agents (Dopamine Agonist); Posaconazole; Quinagolide

The levels/effects of Metoclopramide may be decreased by: Peginterferon Alfa-2b

Increased Effect/Toxicity

Metoclopramide may increase the levels/effects of: Antipsychotics; CycloSPORINE; CycloSPORINE (Systemic); Promethazine; Selective Serotonin Reuptake Inhibitors; Tetrabenazine; Tricyclic Antidepressants; Venlafaxine

The levels/effects of Metoclopramide may be increased by: Droperidol

Nutritional/Ethanol Interactions Ethanol: Avoid ethanol (may increase CNS depression).

Lab Interactions Increased aminotransferase [ALT/AST] (S), amylase (S)

Adverse Reactions Frequency not always defined.

Cardiovascular: AV block, bradycardia, HF, fluid retention, flushing (following high I.V. doses), hyper-/hypotension, supraventricular tachycardia

Central nervous system: Drowsiness (~10% to 70%; dose related), acute dystonic reactions (<1% to 25%; dose and age related), fatigue (2% to 10%), lassitude (~10%), restlessness (~10%), headache (4% to 5%), dizziness (1% to 4%), somnolence (2% to 3%), akathisia, confusion, depression, hallucinations (rare), insomnia, neuroleptic malignant syndrome (rare), Parkinsonian-like symptoms, suicidal ideation, seizure, tardive dyskinesia

Dermatologic: Angioneurotic edema (rare), rash, urticaria

Endocrine & metabolic: Amenorrhea, galactorrhea, gynecomastia, hyperprolactinemia, impotence

Gastrointestinal: Nausea (4% to 6%), vomiting (1% to 2%), diarrhea

Hematologic: Agranulocytosis, leukopenia, neutropenia, porphyria

Hepatic: Hepatotoxicity (rare)

Ocular: Visual disturbance

Respiratory: Bronchospasm, laryngeal edema (rare), laryngospasm (rare)

Miscellaneous: Allergic reactions, methemoglobinemia, sulfhemoglobinemia

Pharmacodynamics/Kinetics

Onset of Action Oral: 30-60 minutes; I.V.: 1-3 minutes; I.M.: 10-15 minutes

Duration of Action Therapeutic: 1-2 hours, regardless of route

Absorption Oral: Rapid

Bioavailability Oral: Range: 65% to 95%

Time to Peak Serum: Oral: 1-2 hours

Protein Binding ~30%

Half-Life Elimination Normal renal function: Children: ~4 hours; Adults: 5-6 hours (may be dose dependent)

Excretion Urine (~85%)

Available Dosage Forms

Injection, solution [preservative free]: 5 mg/mL (2 mL)

Reglan®: 5 mg/mL (2 mL, 10 mL, 30 mL)

Solution, oral: 5 mg/5 mL (10 mL, 473 mL)

Tablet, oral: 5 mg, 10 mg

Reglan®: 5 mg, 10 mg

Tablet, orally disintegrating, oral:

Metozolv™ ODT: 5 mg, 10 mg

Dosing

Adult

Gastroesophageal reflux: Oral: 10-15 mg/dose up to 4 times/day 30 minutes before meals or food and at bedtime; single doses of 20 mg are occasionally needed prior to provoking situations. Treatment >12 weeks is not recommended.

Diabetic gastroparesis:

Oral: 10 mg/dose up to 4 times/day 30 minutes before meals or food and at bedtime for 2-8 weeks

I.M., I.V. (for severe symptoms): 10 mg over 1-2 minutes; 10 days of I.V. therapy may be necessary before symptoms are controlled to allow transition to oral administration

Chemotherapy-induced emesis prophylaxis: I.V.: 1-2 mg/kg 30 minutes before chemotherapy and repeated every 2 hours for 2 doses, then every 3 hours for 3 doses (manufacturer labeling); pretreatment with diphenhydramine will decrease risk of extrapyramidal reactions

Alternate dosing: **Note:** Metoclopramide is considered an antiemetic with a low therapeutic index; use is generally reserved for agents with low emetogenic potential or in patients intolerant/refractory to first line antiemetics.

Low-risk chemotherapy (unlabeled): I.V., Oral: 10-40 mg prior to dose, then every 4-6 hours as needed (NCCN Antiemesis guidelines, v.4.2009)

Breakthrough treatment (unlabeled): I.V., Oral: 10-40 mg every 4-6 hours (NCCN Antiemesis guidelines, v.4.2009)

Delayed-emesis prophylaxis (unlabeled): Oral: 20-40 mg/dose (or 0.5 mg/kg/dose) 2-4 times/day for 3-4 days (in combination with dexamethasone [ASCO guidelines, 2006])

Refractory or intolerant to antiemetics with a higher therapeutic index (unlabeled; Hesketh, 2008):

I.V.: 1-2 mg/kg/dose before chemotherapy and repeat 2 hours after chemotherapy

Oral: 0.5 mg/kg every 6 hours on days 2-4

Postoperative nausea and vomiting prophylaxis: I.M., I.V. (unlabeled route): 10-20 mg near end of surgery. **Note:** Guidelines discourage use of 10 mg metoclopramide as being ineffective (Gan, 2007); comparative study indicates higher dose (20 mg) may be efficacious (Quaynor, 2002).

Postpyloric feeding tube placement, radiological exam: I.V.: 10 mg as a single dose

Geriatric Initial: Dose at the lower end of the recommended range. Refer to adult dosing.

Pediatric

Gastroesophageal reflux (unlabeled use): Oral: 0.1-0.2 mg/kg/dose 4 times/day (maximum: 5 doses/day); pretreatment with diphenhydramine will decrease risk of extrapyramidal reactions to this dosage

Chemotherapy-induced emesis (unlabeled use): I.V.: 1-2 mg/kg 30 minutes before chemotherapy and every 2-4 hours

Postpyloric feeding tube placement: I.V.:

<6 years: 0.1 mg/kg as a single dose

6-14 years: 2.5-5 mg as a single dose

>14 years: Refer to adult dosing.

Renal Impairment

Cl_{cr} <40 mL/minute: Administer 50% of normal dose.

Not dialyzable (0% to 5%); supplemental dose is not necessary.

Administration

Oral Orally-disintegrating tablets: Administer on an empty stomach at least 30 minutes prior to food. Do not remove from packaging until time of administration. If tablet breaks or crumbles while handling, discard and remove new tablet. Using dry hands, place tablet on tongue and allow to dissolve. Swallow with saliva.

I.M. May be administered I.M.

I.V. Injection solution may be given I.M., direct I.V. push, short infusion (15-30 minutes), or continuous infusion; lower doses (≤10 mg) of metoclopramide can be given I.V. push undiluted over 1-2 minutes; higher doses (>10 mg) to be diluted in 50 mL of compatible solution (preferably NS) and given IVPB over at least 15 minutes; continuous SubQ infusion and rectal administration have been reported. **Note:** Rapid I.V. administration may be associated with a transient (but intense) feeling of anxiety and restlessness, followed by drowsiness.

Other Continuous SubQ infusion and rectal administration have been reported

Stability

Storage

Injection: Store intact vial at controlled room temperature; injection is photosensitive and should be protected from light during storage; parenteral admixtures in D_5W or NS are stable for at least 24 hours and do not require light protection if used within 24 hours.

Tablet: Store at controlled room temperature of 20°C to 25°C (68°F to 77°F).

Monitoring and Teaching Issues

Laboratory Monitoring Periodic renal function

Physical Assessment Vital signs should be monitored during intravenous administration. Inpatients should use safety measures to prevent falls (eg, side rails up, call light within reach) and caution patient to call for assistance with ambulation. Monitor for CNS changes (sedation, extrapyramidal effects, Parkinsonian-like reactions).

Patient Education Oral: Take 30 minutes prior to eating. Avoid alcohol; may increase adverse effects. May cause dizziness, drowsiness, insomnia, or blurred vision. Report persistent CNS changes (restlessness, anxiety, depression), spasticity or involuntary movements, unresolved diarrhea, or visual disturbances.

Geriatric Considerations Elderly are more likely to develop tardive dyskinesia syndrome (especially elderly females) reactions than younger adults. Use lowest recommended doses initially. Must consider renal function (estimate creatinine clearance). It is recommended to do involuntary movement assessments on elderly using this medication at high doses and for long-term therapy.

Breast-Feeding Considerations Enters breast milk; may increase milk production

Pregnancy Considerations Teratogenic effects were not observed in animal studies; however, there are no adequate and well-controlled studies in pregnant women. Crosses the placenta; available evidence suggests safe use during pregnancy.

Metolazone (me TOLE a zone)

U.S. Brand Names Zaroxolyn®

Generic Availability (U.S.) Yes

Pharmacologic Category Diuretic, Thiazide-Related

Medication Safety Issues

Sound-alike/look-alike issues:

Metolazone may be confused with metaxalone, methazolamide, methimazole, methotrexate, metoclopramide, metoprolol, minoxidil

Zaroxolyn® may be confused with Zarontin®

Pregnancy Risk Factor B

Lactation Enters breast milk/not recommended

Use Management of mild-to-moderate hypertension; treatment of edema in heart failure and nephrotic syndrome, impaired renal function

Mechanism of Action/Effect Inhibits sodium reabsorption in the distal tubules causing increased excretion of sodium and water, as well as, potassium and hydrogen ions

Contraindications Hypersensitivity to metolazone, any component of the formulation, other thiazides, and sulfonamide derivatives; anuria; hepatic coma; pregnancy (expert analysis)

Warnings/Precautions Electrolyte disturbances (hypokalemia, hypochloremic alkalosis, hyponatremia) can occur. Large or prolonged fluid and electrolyte losses may occur with concomitant furosemide administration. Use with caution in severe hepatic dysfunction; hepatic encephalopathy can be caused by electrolyte disturbances. Gout can be precipitate in certain patients with a history of gout, a familial predisposition to gout, or chronic renal failure. Cautious use in patients with prediabetes or diabetes; may see a change in glucose control. Can cause SLE exacerbation or activation. Use caution in severe renal impairment. Use with caution in patients with moderate or high cholesterol concentrations. Photosensitization may occur.

Chemical similarities are present among sulfonamides, sulfonylureas, carbonic anhydrase inhibitors, thiazides, and loop diuretics (except ethacrynic acid). Use in patients with thiazide or sulfonamide allergy is specifically contraindicated in product labeling, however, a risk of cross-reaction exists in patients with allergy to any of these compounds; avoid use when previous reaction has been severe. Discontinue if signs of hypersensitivity are noted.

Drug Interactions

Avoid Concomitant Use

Avoid concomitant use of Metolazone with any of the following: Dofetilide

Decreased Effect

Metolazone may decrease the levels/effects of: Antidiabetic Agents

The levels/effects of Metolazone may be decreased by: Bile Acid Sequestrants; Herbs (Hypertensive Properties); Methylphenidate; Nonsteroidal Anti-Inflammatory Agents; Yohimbine

Increased Effect/Toxicity

Metolazone may increase the levels/effects of: ACE Inhibitors; Allopurinol; Amifostine; Antihypertensives; Calcium Salts; CarBAMazepine; Dofetilide; Hypotensive Agents; Lithium; OXcarbazepine; RiTUXimab; Topiramate; Toremifene; Vitamin D Analogs

The levels/effects of Metolazone may be increased by: Alcohol (Ethyl); Analgesics (Opioid); Barbiturates; Corticosteroids (Orally Inhaled); Corticosteroids (Systemic); Herbs (Hypotensive Properties); Licorice; MAO Inhibitors; Pentoxifylline; Phosphodiesterase 5 Inhibitors; Prostacyclin Analogues

Nutritional/Ethanol Interactions

Ethanol: May potentiate hypotensive effect of metazolone.

Herb/Nutraceutical: Avoid herbs with *hypertensive* properties (bayberry, blue cohosh, cayenne, ephedra, ginger, ginseng [American], kola, licorice); may diminish the antihypertensive effect of metolazone. Avoid herbs with *hypotensive* properties (black cohosh, California poppy, coleus, golden seal, hawthorn, mistletoe, periwinkle, quinine, shepherd's purse); may enhance the hypotensive effect of metolazone.

Adverse Reactions

Frequency not defined.

Cardiovascular: Chest pain/discomfort, necrotizing angiitis, orthostatic hypotension, palpitation, syncope, venous thrombosis, vertigo, volume depletion

Central nervous system: Chills, depression, dizziness, drowsiness, fatigue, headache, lightheadedness, restlessness

Dermatologic: Petechiae, photosensitivity, pruritus, purpura, rash, skin necrosis, Stevens-Johnson syndrome, toxic epidermal necrolysis, urticaria

Endocrine & metabolic: Gout attacks, hypercalcemia, hyperglycemia, hyperuricemia, hypochloremia, hypochloremic alkalosis, hypokalemia, hypomagnesemia, hyponatremia, hypophosphatemia

Gastrointestinal: Abdominal bloating, abdominal pain, anorexia, constipation, diarrhea, epigastric distress, nausea, pancreatitis, vomiting, xerostomia

Genitourinary: Impotence

Hematologic: Agranulocytosis, aplastic/hypoplastic anemia, hemoconcentration, leukopenia, thrombocytopenia

Hepatic: Cholestatic jaundice, hepatitis

Neuromuscular & skeletal: Joint pain, muscle cramps/spasm, neuropathy, paresthesia, weakness

Ocular: Blurred vision (transient)

Renal: BUN increased, glucosuria

Pharmacodynamics/Kinetics

Onset of Action Diuresis: ~60 minutes

Duration of Action ≥24 hours

Absorption Incomplete

Protein Binding 95%

Half-Life Elimination 20 hours

Excretion Urine (80%); bile (10%)

Available Dosage Forms

Tablet, oral: 2.5 mg, 5 mg, 10 mg

Zaroxolyn®: 2.5 mg, 5 mg

Dosing

Adult

Edema: Oral: Initial: 2.5-10 mg once daily; may increase as necessary to 20 mg once daily (ACC/AHA 2009 Heart Failure Guidelines)

Hypertension: Oral: 2.5-5 mg/dose every 24 hours

Geriatric Oral: Initial: 2.5 mg/day or every other day

Renal Impairment Not dialyzable (0% to 5%) via hemo- or peritoneal dialysis; supplemental dose is not necessary

Administration

Oral May be taken with food or milk. Take early in day to avoid nocturia. Take the last dose of multiple doses no later than 6 PM unless instructed otherwise.

Monitoring and Teaching Issues

Laboratory Monitoring Serum electrolytes (potassium, sodium, chloride, bicarbonate), renal function

Physical Assessment Evaluate patient's renal status and allergy history (thiazides and sulfonamide derivatives) prior to beginning therapy. Assess electrolytes and renal function. Monitor for hypersensitivity reactions, electrolyte imbalance, and hypotension on a regular basis during therapy. Patients with diabetes may see a change in glucose control.

Patient Education Take after breakfast. Include bananas or orange juice in daily diet, but do not take potassium supplements without advice of prescriber. Follow prescriber's instructions for diet and lifestyle changes. Weigh yourself weekly and report weight gain. May cause dizziness, weakness, nausea, or photosensitivity. Report chest pain or palpitations, dizziness, headache, pain, weakness, skin rash, excessive fatigue, or swelling of extremities.

Dietary Considerations Should be taken after breakfast; may require potassium supplementation

Geriatric Considerations When metolazone is used in combination with other diuretics, there is an increased risk of azotemia and electrolyte depletion, particularly in the elderly, monitor closely. May be effective in patients with glomerular filtration rate <20 mL/minute. Metolazone is often used in combination with a loop diuretic in patients who are unresponsive to the loop diuretic alone.

Pregnancy Considerations Teratogenic effects were not observed in animal studies. Metolazone crosses the placenta and appears in cord blood. Hypoglycemia, hypokalemia, hyponatremia, jaundice, and thrombocytopenia are reported as complications to the fetus or newborn following maternal use of thiazide diuretics.

Additional Information Metolazone 5 mg is approximately equivalent to hydrochlorothiazide 50 mg.

Related Information

Heart Failure (Systolic) *on page 2040*

Metoprolol (me toe PROE lole)

U.S. Brand Names Lopressor®; Toprol-XL®

Index Terms Metoprolol Succinate; Metoprolol Tartrate

Generic Availability (U.S.) Yes

Pharmacologic Category Beta Blocker, Beta-1 Selective

Medication Safety Issues

Sound-alike/look-alike issues:

Lopressor® may be confused with Lyrica®
Metoprolol may be confused with metaproterenol, metoclopramide, metolazone, misoprostol
Metoprolol succinate may be confused with metoprolol tartrate
Toprol-XL® may be confused with TEGretol®, TEGretol®-XR, Topamax®

High alert medication: The Institute for Safe Medication Practices (ISMP) includes this medication among its list of drugs which have a heightened risk of causing significant patient harm when used in error.

Significant differences exist between oral and I.V. dosing. Use caution when converting from one route of administration to another.

Pregnancy Risk Factor C

Lactation Enters breast milk/use caution (AAP rates "compatible"; AAP 2001 update pending)

Use Treatment of angina pectoris, hypertension, or hemodynamically-stable acute myocardial infarction

Extended release: Treatment of angina pectoris or hypertension; to reduce mortality/hospitalization in patients with heart failure (stable NYHA Class II or III) already receiving ACE inhibitors, diuretics, and/or digoxin

Unlabeled/Investigational Use Treatment of ventricular arrhythmias, atrial ectopy; migraine prophylaxis, essential tremor, aggressive behavior (not recommended for dementia-associated aggression); prevention of reinfarction and sudden death after myocardial infarction; prevention and treatment of atrial fibrillation and atrial flutter; multifocal atrial tachycardia; symptomatic treatment of hypertrophic obstructive cardiomyopathy

Mechanism of Action/Effect Due to inhibition of $beta_1$-receptors, metoprolol reduces myocardial contractility, heart rate, and blood pressure.

Contraindications

Hypersensitivity to metoprolol, any component of the formulation, or other beta-blockers

Note: Additional contraindications are formulation and/or indication specific.

Immediate release tablets/injectable formulation:

Hypertension and angina: Sinus bradycardia; second- and third-degree heart block; cardiogenic shock; overt heart failure; sick sinus syndrome (except in patients with a functioning artificial pacemaker); severe peripheral arterial disease; pheochromocytoma (without alpha blockade)

Myocardial infarction: Severe sinus bradycardia (heart rate <45 beats/minute); significant first-degree heart block (P-R interval ≥0.24 seconds); second- and third-degree heart block; systolic blood pressure <100 mm Hg; moderate-to-severe cardiac failure

Extended release tablet: Severe bradycardia, second- and third degree heart block; cardiogenic shock; decompensated heart failure; sick sinus syndrome (except in patients with a functioning artificial pacemaker)

Warnings/Precautions [U.S. Boxed Warning]: Beta-blocker therapy should not be withdrawn abruptly (particularly in patients with CAD), but gradually tapered over 1-2 weeks to avoid acute tachycardia, hypertension, and/or ischemia. Consider pre-existing conditions such as sick sinus syndrome before initiating. Metoprolol commonly produces mild first-degree heart block (P-R interval >0.2-0.24 sec). May also produce severe first- (P-R interval ≥0.26 sec), second-, or third-degree heart block. Patients with acute MI (especially right ventricular MI) have a high risk of developing heart block of varying degrees. If severe heart block occurs, metoprolol should be discontinued and measures to increase heart rate should be employed. Symptomatic hypotension may occur with use. Use caution in patients with PVD (can aggravate arterial insufficiency). Use caution with concurrent use of beta-blockers and either verapamil or diltiazem; bradycardia or heart block can occur; avoid concurrent I.V. use of both agents. Use with caution in patients receiving CYP2D6 inhibitors (eg, bupropion, chlorpromazine, cimetidine, diphenhydramine, hydroxychloroquine, fluoxetine, paroxetine, propafenone, propoxyphene, quinidine, ritonavir, terbinafine, thioridazine); concurrent use may increase metoprolol plasma concentrations.

In general, beta-blockers should be avoided in patients with bronchospastic disease. Metoprolol, with B_1 selectivity, should be used cautiously in bronchospastic disease with close monitoring. Use cautiously in patients with diabetes because it can mask prominent hypoglycemic symptoms. Use caution in hyperthyroidism since beta-blockade may mask signs of thyrotoxicosis. Use caution with hepatic dysfunction. Use with caution in patients with myasthenia gravis or psychiatric disease (may cause CNS depression). Use caution with inhalation anesthetic agents which may decrease myocardial function. Although perioperative beta-blocker therapy is recommended prior to elective surgery in selected patients, use of high-dose extended release metoprolol in patients naïve to beta-blocker therapy undergoing noncardiac surgery has been associated with bradycardia, hypotension, stroke, and death. Chronic beta-blocker therapy should not be routinely withdrawn prior to major surgery. Use of beta-blockers may unmask cardiac failure in patients without a history of dysfunction. Adequate alpha-blockade is required prior to use of any beta-blocker for patients with untreated pheochromocytoma. May induce or exacerbate psoriasis. Use caution with history of severe anaphylaxis to allergens; patients taking beta-blockers may become more sensitive to repeated allergen challenges. Treatment of anaphylaxis (eg, epinephrine) in patients taking beta-blockers may be ineffective or promote undesirable effects.

Extended release: Use with caution in patients with compensated heart failure; monitor for a worsening of heart failure.

Drug Interactions

Metabolism/Transport Effects Substrate of CYP2C19 (minor), 2D6 (major); **Inhibits** CYP2D6 (weak)

Avoid Concomitant Use

Avoid concomitant use of Metoprolol with any of the following: Methacholine

Decreased Effect

Metoprolol may decrease the levels/effects of: Beta2-Agonists; Theophylline Derivatives

The levels/effects of Metoprolol may be decreased by: Barbiturates; Herbs (Hypertensive Properties); Methylphenidate; Nonsteroidal Anti-Inflammatory Agents; Peginterferon Alfa-2b; Rifamycin Derivatives; Yohimbine

Increased Effect/Toxicity

Metoprolol may increase the levels/effects of: Alpha-/Beta-Agonists (Direct-Acting); Alpha1-Blockers; Alpha2-Agonists; Amifostine; Antihypertensives; Antipsychotic Agents (Phenothiazines); Bupivacaine; Cardiac Glycosides; Fingolimod; Hypotensive Agents; Insulin; Lidocaine; Lidocaine (Systemic); Lidocaine (Topical); Mepivacaine; Methacholine; Midodrine; RiTUXimab; Sulfonylureas

The levels/effects of Metoprolol may be increased by: Acetylcholinesterase Inhibitors; Aminoquinolines (Antimalarial); Amiodarone; Anilidopiperidine Opioids; Antipsychotic Agents (Phenothiazines); Calcium Channel Blockers (Nondihydropyridine); CYP2D6 Inhibitors (Moderate); CYP2D6 Inhibitors (Strong); Darunavir; Diazoxide; Dipyridamole; Disopyramide; Dronedarone; Herbs (Hypotensive Properties); MAO Inhibitors; Pentoxifylline; Phosphodiesterase 5 Inhibitors; Propafenone; Propoxyphene; Prostacyclin Analogues; QuiNIDine; Reserpine; Selective Serotonin Reuptake Inhibitors

Nutritional/Ethanol Interactions

Food: Food increases absorption. Metoprolol serum levels may be increased if taken with food.

Herb/Nutraceutical: Avoid bayberry, blue cohosh, cayenne, ephedra, ginger, ginseng (American), gotu kola, licorice, (may worsen hypertension). Avoid black cohosh, California poppy, coleus, golden seal, hawthorn, mistletoe, periwinkle, quinine, shepherd's purse (may have increased antihypertensive effect).

Adverse Reactions Frequency may not be defined.

Cardiovascular: Hypotension (1% to 27%), bradycardia (2% to 16%), first-degree heart block (P-R interval ≥0.26 sec; 5%), arterial insufficiency (usually Raynaud type; 1%), chest pain (1%), CHF (1%), edema (peripheral; 1%), palpitation (1%), syncope (1%)

Central nervous system: Dizziness (2% to 10%), fatigue (1% to 10%), depression (5%), confusion, hallucinations, headache, insomnia, memory loss (short-term), nightmares, sleep disturbances, somnolence, vertigo

Dermatology: Pruritus (5%), rash (5%), photosensitivity, psoriasis exacerbated

Endocrine & metabolic: Libido decreased, Peyronie's disease (<1%), diabetes exacerbated

Gastrointestinal: Diarrhea (5%), constipation (1%), flatulence (1%), gastrointestinal pain (1%), heartburn (1%), nausea (1%), xerostomia (1%), vomiting

Hematologic: Claudication

Neuromuscular & skeletal: Musculoskeletal pain

Ocular: Blurred vision, visual disturbances

Otic: Tinnitus

Respiratory: Dyspnea (1% to 3%), bronchospasm (1%), wheezing (1%), rhinitis, shortness of breath

Miscellaneous: Cold extremities (1%)

Other events reported with beta-blockers: Catatonia, emotional lability, fever, hypersensitivity reactions, laryngospasm, nonthrombocytopenic purpura, respiratory distress, thrombocytopenic purpura

Pharmacodynamics/Kinetics

Onset of Action Peak effect: Oral: 1.5-4 hours; I.V.: 20 minutes (when infused over 10 minutes)

Duration of Action Oral: Immediate release: 10-20 hours, Extended release: ~24 hours; I.V.: 5-8 hours

Absorption 95%, rapid and complete

Bioavailability Oral: ~50%

Protein Binding 12% to albumin

Half-Life Elimination 3-8 hours (dependent on rate of CYP2D6 metabolism)

Metabolism Extensively hepatic via CYP2D6; significant first-pass effect (~50%)

Excretion Urine (<5% to 10% as unchanged drug)

Available Dosage Forms

Injection, solution: 1 mg/mL (5 mL)

Lopressor®: 1 mg/mL (5 mL)

Injection, solution [preservative free]: 1 mg/mL (5 mL)

Tablet, oral: 25 mg, 50 mg, 100 mg

Lopressor®: 50 mg, 100 mg

Tablet, extended release, oral: 25 mg, 50 mg, 100 mg, 200 mg

Toprol-XL®: 25 mg, 50 mg, 100 mg, 200 mg

Dosing

Adult

Angina: Oral:

Immediate release: Initial: 50 mg twice daily; usual dosage range: 50-200 mg twice daily; maximum: 400 mg/day; increase dose at weekly intervals to desired effect

Extended release: Initial: 100 mg/day (maximum: 400 mg/day)

Atrial fibrillation/flutter (ventricular rate control), supraventricular tachycardia (SVT) (acute treatment; unlabeled use; Antman, 2004; Fuster, 2006; Neumar, 2010): I.V.: 2.5-5 mg every 2-5 minutes (maximum total dose: 15 mg over a 10-15 minute period). **Note:** Initiate cautiously in patients with concomitant heart failure; avoid in patients with decompensated heart failure.

Maintenance: Oral (immediate release): 25-100 mg twice daily

Heart failure: Oral: *Extended release:* Initial: 25 mg once daily (reduce to 12.5 mg once daily in NYHA class higher than class II); may double dosage every 2 weeks as tolerated (maximum: 200 mg/day)

Hypertension: Oral:

Immediate release: Initial: 50 mg twice daily; effective dosage range: 100-450 mg/day in 2-3 divided doses; increase dose at weekly intervals to desired effect; maximum: 450 mg/day; usual dosage range (JNC 7): 50-100 mg/day

Extended release: Initial: 25-100 mg once daily; increase doses at weekly (or longer) intervals to desired effect; maximum: 400 mg/day; usual dosage range (JNC 7): 50-100 mg/day

Hypertension/ventricular rate control: I.V. (in patients having nonfunctioning GI tract): Initial: 1.25-5 mg every 6-12 hours; titrate initial dose to response. Initially, low doses may be appropriate to establish response; however, although not routine, up to 15 mg administered as frequently as every 3 hours has been employed in patients with refractory tachycardia.

Myocardial infarction:

Acute: I.V.: 5 mg every 2 minutes for 3 doses in early treatment of myocardial infarction; thereafter, give 50 mg orally every 6 hours beginning 15 minutes after last I.V. dose and continue for 48 hours; then administer a maintenance dose of 100 mg twice daily. **Note:** If initial I.V. dosing is not tolerated, may give 25-50 mg orally (depending on degree of intolerance) every 6 hours beginning 15 minutes after the last I.V. dose or as soon as clinical condition permits.

Secondary prevention (unlabeled use; Olsson, 1992): Oral: Immediate release: 25-100 mg twice daily; optimize dose based on heart rate and blood pressure; continue indefinitely.

Note: Switching dosage forms:

When switching from immediate release metoprolol to extended release, the same total daily dose of metoprolol should be used.

When switching between oral and intravenous dosage forms, equivalent beta-blocking effect is achieved when doses in a 2.5:1 (Oral:I.V.) ratio is used. For example, if the patient is receiving an oral dose of 25 mg twice daily (50 mg/day), this would translate to 5 mg I.V. every 6 hours; consider reducing initial I.V. dose to evaluate patient response.

Geriatric Refer to adult dosing. Select dose cautiously, starting at the lower end of the dosing range.

Pediatric

Hypertension: Oral:

Immediate release tablet: Children: 1-17 years (National High Blood Pressure Education Program Working Group on High Blood Pressure in Children and Adolescents, 2004): Initial: 1-2 mg/kg/day; maximum 6 mg/kg/day (≤200 mg/day); administer in 2 divided doses

Extended release tablet: Children ≥6 years: Initial: 1 mg/kg once daily (maximum initial dose: 50 mg/day). Adjust dose based on patient response (maximum: 2 mg/kg/day or 200 mg/day)

Renal Impairment No adjustment required.

Hepatic Impairment Reduced dose may be necessary.

Administration

Oral Extended release tablets may be divided in half; do not crush or chew.

I.V. I.V. dose is much smaller than oral dose. When administered acutely for cardiac treatment, monitor ECG and blood pressure; may administer by rapid infusion (I.V. push) over 1 minute. May also be administered by slow infusion (ie, 5-10 mg of metoprolol in 50 mL of fluid) over ~30-60 minutes during less urgent situations (eg, substitution for oral metoprolol).

Stability

Storage

Injection: Store at 25°C (77°F); excursions permitted to 15°C to 30°C (59°F to 86°F). Protect from light.

Tablet: Store at 25°C (77°F); excursions permitted to 15°C to 30°C (59°F to 86°F). Protect from moisture.

Monitoring and Teaching Issues

Physical Assessment Monitor blood pressure and cardiac status. Assess for fluid balance, heart failure symptoms, and postural hypotension. Taper dosage slowly when discontinuing. Advise patients with diabetes to monitor glucose levels closely; beta-blockers may alter glucose tolerance.

Patient Education

I.V. use in emergency situations: Patient information is appropriate to patient condition.

Oral: Take pulse daily prior to medication and follow prescriber's instruction about holding medication. If you have diabetes, monitor serum sugar closely; drug may alter glucose tolerance or mask signs of hypoglycemia. May cause fatigue, dizziness, postural hypotension, or alteration in sexual performance (reversible). Report unresolved swelling of extremities, respiratory difficulty or new cough, unresolved fatigue, unusual weight gain, unresolved constipation, or unusual muscle weakness.

Dietary Considerations Regular tablets should be taken with food. Extended release tablets may be taken without regard to meals.

Geriatric Considerations Due to alterations in the beta-adrenergic autonomic nervous system, beta-adrenergic blockade may result in less hemodynamic response than seen in younger adults. Studies indicate that despite decreased sensitivity to the chronotropic effects of beta-blockade with age, there appears to be an increased myocardial sensitivity to the negative inotropic effect during stress (ie, exercise). Controlled trials have shown the overall response rate for propranolol to be only 20% to 50% in the elderly populations. Therefore, all beta-adrenergic blocking drugs may result in a decreased response as compared to younger adults.

Breast-Feeding Considerations Small amounts of metoprolol can be detected in breast milk. The manufacturer recommends that caution be exercised when administering metoprolol to nursing women.

Pregnancy Considerations Adverse events were observed in animal studies; therefore, the manufacturer classifies metoprolol as pregnancy category C. Metoprolol crosses the placenta and can be detected in cord blood, amniotic fluid, and the serum of newborn infants. In a cohort study, an increased risk of cardiovascular defects was observed following maternal use of beta-blockers during pregnancy. Intrauterine growth restriction (IUGR), small placentas, as well as fetal/neonatal bradycardia, hypoglycemia, and/or respiratory depression have been observed following *in utero* exposure to beta-blockers as a class. Adequate facilities for monitoring infants at birth should be available. Untreated chronic maternal hypertension and pre-eclampsia are also associated with adverse events in the fetus, infant, and mother. The clearance of metoprolol is increased and serum concentrations and AUC of metoprolol are decreased during pregnancy. Metoprolol has been evaluated for the treatment of hypertension in pregnancy, but other agents may be more appropriate for use.

Related Information

Beta-Blockers *on page 1990*

Heart Failure (Systolic) *on page 2040*

◆ **Metoprolol Succinate** *see* Metoprolol *on page 1217*

◆ **Metoprolol Tartrate** *see* Metoprolol *on page 1217*

◆ **Metozolv™ ODT** *see* Metoclopramide *on page 1213*

MetroNIDAZOLE (Systemic) (met roe NYE da zole)

U.S. Brand Names Flagyl®; Flagyl® 375; Flagyl® ER

Index Terms Metronidazole Hydrochloride

Generic Availability (U.S.) Yes: Excludes extended release tablet

Pharmacologic Category Amebicide; Antibiotic, Miscellaneous; Antiprotozoal, Nitroimidazole

Medication Safety Issues

Sound-alike/look-alike issues:

MetroNIDAZOLE may be confused with mebendazole, meropenem, metFORMIN, methotrexate, metoclopramide, miconazole

Pregnancy Risk Factor B

Lactation Enters breast milk/not recommended (AAP rates "of concern"; AAP 2001 update pending)

Use Treatment of susceptible anaerobic bacterial and protozoal infections in the following conditions: Amebiasis, symptomatic and asymptomatic trichomoniasis; skin and skin structure infections, bone and joint infections, CNS infections, endocarditis, gynecologic infections, intra-abdominal infections (as part of combination regimen), respiratory tract infections (lower), systemic anaerobic infections; treatment of antibiotic-associated pseudomembranous colitis (AAPC); as part of a multidrug regimen for *H. pylori* eradication to reduce the risk of duodenal ulcer recurrence; surgical prophylaxis (colorectal)

Unlabeled/Investigational Use Crohn's disease

Mechanism of Action/Effect Inhibits DNA synthesis in susceptible organisms

Contraindications Hypersensitivity to metronidazole, nitroimidazole derivatives, or any component of the formulation; pregnancy (first trimester)

Warnings/Precautions Use with caution in patients with severe liver impairment due to potential accumulation, blood dyscrasias; history of seizures, CHF or other sodium-retaining states; reduce dosage in patients with severe liver impairment, CNS disease, and consider dosage reduction in longer-term therapy with severe renal failure (Cl_{cr} <10 mL/minute); if *H. pylori* is not eradicated in patients being treated with metronidazole in a regimen, it should be assumed that metronidazole-resistance has occurred and it should not again be used; aseptic meningitis, encephalopathy, seizures, and neuropathies have been reported especially with increased doses and chronic treatment; monitor and consider discontinuation of therapy if symptoms occur. **[U.S. Boxed Warning]: Possibly carcinogenic based on animal data.** Prolonged use may result in fungal or bacterial superinfection, including *C. difficile*-associated diarrhea (CDAD) and pseudomembranous colitis; CDAD has been observed >2 months postantibiotic treatment. The Infectious Disease Society of America (IDSA) recommends the use of oral metronidazole for initial treatment of mild-to-moderate *C. difficile* infection and the use of oral vancomycin for initial treatment of severe *C. difficile* infection with or without I.V. metronidazole depending on the presence of complications. May treat recurrent mild-to-moderate infection once with oral metronidazole; avoid use beyond first reoccurrence due to potential cumulative neurotoxicity (Cohen, 2010). Candidiasis infection (known or unknown) maybe more prominent during metronidazole treatment, antifungal treatment required. Disulfiram-like reactions to ethanol have been reported with oral metronidazole; avoid alcoholic beverages during therapy

Drug Interactions

Metabolism/Transport Effects Inhibits CYP2C9 (weak), 3A4 (moderate)

Avoid Concomitant Use

Avoid concomitant use of MetroNIDAZOLE (Systemic) with any of the following: BCG; Tolvaptan

Decreased Effect

MetroNIDAZOLE (Systemic) may decrease the levels/effects of: BCG; Mycophenolate; Typhoid Vaccine

The levels/effects of MetroNIDAZOLE (Systemic) may be decreased by: PHENobarbital; Phenytoin

Increased Effect/Toxicity

MetroNIDAZOLE (Systemic) may increase the levels/effects of: Alcohol (Ethyl); Busulfan; Calcineurin Inhibitors; Colchicine; CYP3A4 Substrates; Eplerenone; Everolimus; FentaNYL; Halofantrine; Lurasidone; Phenytoin; Pimecrolimus; Ranolazine; Salmeterol; Saxagliptin; Tipranavir; Tolvaptan; Vilazodone; Vitamin K Antagonists

The levels/effects of MetroNIDAZOLE (Systemic) may be increased by: Disulfiram; Mebendazole

Nutritional/Ethanol Interactions

Ethanol: The manufacturer recommends to avoid all ethanol or any ethanol-containing drugs (may cause disulfiram-like reaction characterized by flushing, headache, nausea, vomiting, sweating, or tachycardia).

Food: Peak antibiotic serum concentration lowered and delayed, but total drug absorbed not affected.

Lab Interactions May cause falsely decreased AST and ALT levels.

Adverse Reactions Frequency not always defined.

Cardiovascular: Flattening of the T-wave, flushing, syncope

Central nervous system: Aseptic meningitis, ataxia, confusion, coordination impaired, depression, dizziness, encephalopathy, fever, headache, insomnia, irritability, seizure, vertigo

Dermatologic: Erythematous rash, pruritus, Stevens-Johnson syndrome, toxic epidermal necrolysis, urticaria

Endocrine & metabolic: Disulfiram-like reaction, dysmenorrhea

Gastrointestinal: Nausea (~12%), anorexia, abdominal cramping, constipation, diarrhea, epigastric distress, furry tongue, glossitis, pancreatitis (rare), proctitis, stomatitis, unusual/metallic taste, vomiting, xerostomia

Genitourinary: Cystitis, darkened urine (rare), dyspareunia, dysuria, incontinence, libido decreased, pelvic pressure, polyuria, vaginal dryness, vaginitis

Hematologic: Neutropenia (reversible), thrombocytopenia (reversible, rare)
Local: Thrombophlebitis
Neuromuscular & skeletal: Dysarthria, peripheral neuropathy, weakness
Ocular: Optic neuropathy
Respiratory: Nasal congestion, pharyngitis, rhinitis, sinusitis, pharyngitis
Miscellaneous: Flu-like syndrome, joint pains resembling serum sickness, moniliasis

Pharmacodynamics/Kinetics

Absorption Oral: Well absorbed

Time to Peak Serum: Oral: Immediate release: 1-2 hours

Protein Binding <20%

Half-Life Elimination Neonates: 25-75 hours; Others: 6-8 hours, prolonged with hepatic impairment; End-stage renal disease: 21 hours

Metabolism Hepatic (30% to 60%)

Excretion Urine (60% to 80% as unchanged drug); feces (6% to 15%)

Available Dosage Forms

Capsule, oral: 375 mg
Flagyl® 375: 375 mg

Infusion, premixed iso-osmotic sodium chloride solution: 500 mg (100 mL)

Tablet, oral: 250 mg, 500 mg
Flagyl®: 250 mg, 500 mg

Tablet, extended release, oral:
Flagyl® ER: 750 mg

Dosing

Adult

Anaerobic infections (diverticulitis, intra-abdominal, peritonitis, cholangitis, or abscess): Oral, I.V.: 500 mg every 6-8 hours, not to exceed 4 g/day; **Note:** Initial: 1 g I.V. loading dose may be administered

Amebiasis: Oral: 500-750 mg every 8 hours for 5-10 days

Antibiotic-associated pseudomembranous colitis: IDSA Guidelines (Cohen, 2010):
Mild-to-moderate infection: Oral: 500 mg 3 times/day for 10-14 days
Severe complicated infection: I.V.: 500 mg 3 times/day with oral vancomycin (recommended agent) for 10-14 days
Note: Due to the emergence of a new strain of *C. difficile*, some clinicians recommend converting to oral vancomycin therapy if the patient does not show a clear clinical response after 2 days of metronidazole therapy.

Giardiasis: 500 mg twice daily for 5-7 days

Intra-abdominal infection, complicated, community-acquired, mild-to-moderate (in combination with cephalosporin or fluoroquinolone): I.V.: 500 mg every 8-12 hours **or** 1.5 g every 24 hours for for 4-7 days (provided source controlled)

Peptic ulcer disease: *Helicobacter pylori* eradication: Oral: 250-500 mg with meals and at bedtime for 14 days; requires combination therapy with at least one other antibiotic and an acid-suppressing agent (proton pump inhibitor or H_2 blocker)

Bacterial vaginosis or vaginitis due to *Gardnerella*, *Mobiluncus*: Oral: 500 mg twice daily (regular release) or 750 mg once daily (extended release tablet) for 7 days

Pelvic inflammatory disease (unlabeled use): Oral: 500 mg twice daily for 14 days (in combination with a cephalosporin and doxycycline) (CDC, 2010)

Trichomoniasis: Oral: 250 mg every 8 hours for 7 days **or** 375 mg twice daily for 7 days **or** 2 g as a single dose **or** 1 g twice daily for 2 doses (on same day)

Urethritis (unlabeled use): Oral: 2 g as a single dose with azithromycin (CDC, 2010)

Surgical prophylaxis (colorectal): I.V. 15 mg/kg 1 hour prior to surgery; followed by 7.5 mg/kg 6 and 12 hours after initial dose

Geriatric Refer to adult dosing. Use the lower end of the dosing recommendations for adults; do not administer as single dose as efficacy has not been established.

Pediatric Infants and Children:

Anaerobic infections:
Oral: 15-35 mg/kg/day in divided doses every 8 hours
I.V.: 30 mg/kg/day in divided doses every 6 hours

Colitis due to *Clostridium difficile*: Oral: 20 mg/kg/day divided every 6 hours. Maximum dose: 2 g/day

Amebiasis: Oral: 35-50 mg/kg/day in divided doses every 8 hours for 10 days

Trichomoniasis: Oral: 15-30 mg/kg/day in divided doses every 8 hours for 7 days

Renal Impairment

Cl_{cr} <10 mL/minute, but not on dialysis: Recommendations vary: To reduce possible accumulation in patients receiving multiple doses, consider reduction to 50% of dose or every 12 hours; **Note:** Dosage reduction is unnecessary in short courses of therapy. Clinical recommendations and practice vary. Some references do not recommend reduction at any level of renal impairment (Lamp, 1999).

Hemodialysis effects: Extensively removed by hemodialysis and peritoneal dialysis (50% to 100%); dosage reduction not recommended; administer full dose posthemodialysis. During peritoneal dialysis, dose as for Cl_{cr} <10 mL/minute.

Continuous arteriovenous or venovenous hemofiltration: Dose as for normal renal function

Hepatic Impairment Unchanged in mild liver disease; reduce dosage in severe liver disease.

Administration

Oral May be taken with food to minimize stomach upset. Extended release tablets should be taken on an empty stomach (1 hour before or 2 hours after meals).

I.V. Infuse intravenously over 30-60 minutes. Avoid contact of drug solution with equipment containing aluminum.

Stability

Reconstitution Standard diluent: 500 mg/100 mL NS.

Storage

Injection: Store at controlled room temperature of 15°C to 30°C (59°F to 8F°C). Protect from light. Keep in overwrap until ready to use. Product may be refrigerated but crystals may form. Crystals redissolve on warming to room temperature. Prolonged exposure to light will cause a darkening of the product. However, short-term exposure to normal room light does not adversely affect metronidazole stability. Direct sunlight should be avoided. Stability of parenteral admixture at room temperature (25°C); Out of overwrap stability: 30 days.

Tablets: Store at room temperature. Protect from light and moisture.

Monitoring and Teaching Issues

Patient Education May take with or without food. Take with food if medication causes upset stomach. Extended release tablets should be taken on an empty stomach. Avoid alcohol during therapy. With alcohol you may experience severe flushing, headache, nausea, vomiting, or chest and abdominal pain. May discolor urine (brown/black/dark). You may experience "metallic" taste disturbance, nausea, or vomiting. Report unresolved or severe fatigue; weakness; fever or chills; mouth or vaginal sores; numbness, tingling, or swelling of extremities; respiratory difficulty; or lack of improvement or worsening of condition.

Dietary Considerations Take on an empty stomach. Drug may cause GI upset; if GI upset occurs, take with food. Extended release tablets should be taken on an empty stomach (1 hour before or 2 hours after meals). Some products may contain sodium. The manufacturer recommends that ethanol be avoided during treatment and for 3 days after therapy is complete.

Geriatric Considerations Adjust dose based on renal function.

Breast-Feeding Considerations Metronidazole and its active metabolite are measurable in the breast milk and infant plasma. Milk concentrations are similar to those in the maternal plasma and are highly variable. Peak concentrations of metronidazole in breast milk occur ~2-4 hours after the oral dose. In studies, the calculated relative infant doses have ranged from 0.13% to 36% of the weight-adjusted maternal dose. Use of metronidazole in a lactating patient is not recommended by the manufacturer. If metronidazole is given, breast-feeding should be withheld for 12-24 hours after the dose.

Pregnancy Considerations Teratogenic effects have not been observed in animal reproduction studies; therefore, the manufacturer classifies metronidazole as pregnancy category B. Metronidazole crosses the placenta and rapidly distributes into the fetal circulation. Although there have been a few reports of facial anomalies after *in utero* exposure, most studies have not found an increased risk of congenital abnormalities following maternal use of metronidazole during the first trimester of pregnancy. In studies that included women taking metronidazole during all trimesters of pregnancy, an increased risk of adverse fetal and neonatal outcomes has not been observed. Because metronidazole has been carcinogenic in some animal species, concern has been raised whether metronidazole should be used during pregnancy; however, a strong carcinogenic potential in humans has not been observed, including one study of prenatal exposure.

Metronidazole pharmacokinetics are similar between pregnant and nonpregnant patients. Bacterial vaginosis has been associated with adverse pregnancy outcomes (including preterm labor); metronidazole is recommended for the treatment of symptomatic bacterial vaginosis in pregnant patients. Vaginal trichomoniasis has been also associated with adverse pregnancy outcomes (including preterm labor). Treatment may relieve symptoms and prevent further sexual transmission; however, metronidazole has not resulted in reduced perinatal morbidity and should not be used solely to prevent preterm delivery. Some clinicians consider deferring therapy in asymptomatic women until >37 weeks gestation. Use of oral metronidazole is contraindicated during the first trimester (per the FDA approved labeling). Consult current CDC guidelines for appropriate use in pregnant women.

Related Information

Antimicrobial Drugs of Choice *on page 2008*

Compatibility of Drugs *on page 1994*

Helicobacter pylori Treatment *on page 2045*

I.V. to Oral Conversion *on page 1956*

◆ **Metronidazole Hydrochloride** *see* MetroNIDAZOLE (Systemic) *on page 1220*

◆ **Mevacor®** *see* Lovastatin *on page 1138*

◆ **Mevinolin** *see* Lovastatin *on page 1138*

◆ **$MgSO_4$ (error-prone abbreviation)** *see* Magnesium Sulfate *on page 1144*

◆ **Miacalcin®** *see* Calcitonin *on page 269*

◆ **Micaderm® [OTC]** *see* Miconazole (Topical) *on page 1224*

◆ **Micardis®** *see* Telmisartan *on page 1717*

◆ **Micardis® HCT** *see* Telmisartan and Hydrochlorothiazide *on page 1719*

◆ **Micatin® [OTC]** *see* Miconazole (Topical) *on page 1224*

Miconazole (Topical) (mi KON a zole)

U.S. Brand Names 3M™ Cavilon™ Antifungal [OTC]; Aloe Vesta® Antifungal [OTC]; Baza® Antifungal [OTC]; Carrington® Antifungal [OTC]; Critic-Aid® Clear AF [OTC]; DermaFungal [OTC]; Dermagran® AF [OTC]; DiabetAid® Antifungal Foot Bath [OTC]; Fungoid® [OTC]; Lotrimin AF® [OTC]; Micaderm® [OTC]; Micatin® [OTC]; Micro-Guard® [OTC]; Miranel AF™ [OTC]; Mitrazol® [OTC]; Monistat® 1 Day or Night [OTC]; Monistat® 1 [OTC]; Monistat® 3 [OTC]; Monistat® 7 [OTC]; Neosporin® AF [OTC]; Podactin Cream [OTC]; Secura® Antifungal Extra Thick [OTC]; Secura® Antifungal Greaseless [OTC]; Ting® Spray Powder [OTC]; Zeasorb®-AF [OTC]

Index Terms Miconazole Nitrate

Generic Availability (U.S.) Yes: Combination package (topical/vaginal), cream (topical and vaginal), vaginal suppository

Pharmacologic Category Antifungal Agent, Topical; Antifungal Agent, Vaginal

Medication Safety Issues

Sound-alike/look-alike issues:

Miconazole may be confused with metroNIDAZOLE, Micronase®, Micronor®

Lotrimin® may be confused with Lotrisone®, Otrivin®

Micatin® may be confused with Miacalcin®

Pregnancy Risk Factor C

Lactation Excretion in breast milk unknown/use caution

Use Treatment of vulvovaginal candidiasis and a variety of skin and mucous membrane fungal infections

Available Dosage Forms For available OTC formulations, consult specific product labeling.

Dosing

Adult & Geriatric

Tinea corporis: Topical: Apply twice daily for 4 weeks

Tinea pedis: Topical: Apply twice daily for 4 weeks

Effervescent tablet: Dissolve 1 tablet in ~1 gallon of water; soak feet for 15-30 minutes; pat dry

Tinea cruris: Topical: Apply twice daily for 2 weeks

Vulvovaginal candidiasis: Vaginal:

Cream, 2%: Insert 1 applicatorful at bedtime for 7 days

Cream, 4%: Insert 1 applicatorful at bedtime for 3 days

Suppository, 100 mg: Insert 1 suppository at bedtime for 7 days

Suppository, 200 mg: Insert 1 suppository at bedtime for 3 days

Suppository, 1200 mg: Insert 1 suppository (a one-time dose); may be used at bedtime or during the day

Note: Many products are available as a combination pack, with a suppository for vaginal instillation and cream to relieve external symptoms. External cream may be used twice daily, as needed, for up to 7 days.

Pediatric

Tinea corporis, tinea pedis, tinea cruris: Topical: **Note:** Not for OTC use in children <2 years: Refer to adult dosing.

Vulvovaginal candidiasis: Vaginal: Children ≥12 years: Refer to adult dosing.

Monitoring and Teaching Issues

Physical Assessment Caution patients with diabetes to test serum glucose regularly; may inhibit the metabolism of oral sulfonylureas. Teach patient bleeding precautions.

Patient Education Some infections may require long periods of therapy. Report persistent burning, itching, or irritation to healthcare provider.

Topical: Wash and dry area before applying medication; apply thinly. Do not get in or near eyes.

Vaginal: Consult with healthcare provider if using for a vaginal yeast infection for the first time. Insert high in vagina. Refrain from intercourse during treatment. Condoms and diaphragms may not be effective during therapy. Do not use tampons, douches, spermicides, or other vaginal products during treatment. Deodorant-free pads or panty shields may be used to protect clothing during use.

- ◆ **Miconazole Nitrate** *see* Miconazole (Topical) *on page 1224*
- ◆ **MICRhoGAM® UF Plus** *see* Rh_o(D) Immune Globulin *on page 1569*
- ◆ **Microgestin® 1.5/30** *see* Ethinyl Estradiol and Norethindrone *on page 701*
- ◆ **Microgestin® 1/20** *see* Ethinyl Estradiol and Norethindrone *on page 701*
- ◆ **Microgestin® Fe 1.5/30** *see* Ethinyl Estradiol and Norethindrone *on page 701*
- ◆ **Microgestin® Fe 1/20** *see* Ethinyl Estradiol and Norethindrone *on page 701*
- ◆ **Micro-Guard® [OTC]** *see* Miconazole (Topical) *on page 1224*
- ◆ **microK®** *see* Potassium Chloride *on page 1480*
- ◆ **microK® 10** *see* Potassium Chloride *on page 1480*
- ◆ **Micronase** *see* GlyBURIDE *on page 877*
- ◆ **Microzide®** *see* Hydrochlorothiazide *on page 912*

Midazolam (MID aye zoe lam)

Index Terms Midazolam Hydrochloride; Versed
Generic Availability (U.S.) Yes
Pharmacologic Category Benzodiazepine
Medication Safety Issues
Sound-alike/look-alike issues:
Versed may be confused with VePesid®, Vistaril®

High alert medication: The Institute for Safe Medication Practices (ISMP) includes this medication among its list of drugs which have a heightened risk of causing significant patient harm when used in error.

Pregnancy Risk Factor D

Lactation Enters breast milk/use caution (AAP rates "of concern"; AAP 2001 update pending)

Use Preoperative sedation; moderate sedation prior to diagnostic or radiographic procedures; ICU sedation (continuous infusion); induction and maintenance of general anesthesia

Unlabeled/Investigational Use Anxiety, status epilepticus

Mechanism of Action/Effect Binds to stereospecific benzodiazepine receptors on the postsynaptic GABA neuron at several sites within the central nervous system, including the limbic system, reticular formation. Enhancement of the inhibitory effect of GABA on neuronal excitability results by increased neuronal membrane permeability to chloride ions. This shift in chloride ions results in hyperpolarization (a less excitable state) and stabilization.

Contraindications Hypersensitivity to midazolam or any component of the formulation, including benzyl alcohol (cross-sensitivity with other benzodiazepines may exist); parenteral form is not for intrathecal or epidural injection; narrow-angle glaucoma; concurrent use of potent inhibitors of CYP3A4 (amprenavir, atazanavir, or ritonavir); pregnancy

Warnings/Precautions [U.S. Boxed Warning]: May cause severe respiratory depression, respiratory arrest, or apnea. Use with extreme caution, particularly in noncritical care settings. Appropriate resuscitative equipment and qualified personnel must be available for administration and monitoring. Initial dosing must be cautiously titrated and individualized, particularly in elderly or debilitated patients, patients with hepatic impairment (including alcoholics), or in renal impairment, particularly if other CNS depressants (including opiates) are used concurrently. **[U.S. Boxed Warning]: Initial doses in elderly or debilitated patients should be conservative; as little as 1 mg, but not to exceed 2.5 mg.** Use with caution in patients with respiratory disease or impaired gag reflex. Use during upper airway procedures may increase risk of hypoventilation. Prolonged responses have been noted following extended administration by continuous infusion (possibly due to metabolite accumulation) or in the presence of drugs which inhibit midazolam metabolism.

Causes CNS depression (dose-related) resulting in sedation, dizziness, confusion, or ataxia which may impair physical and mental capabilities. Patients must be cautioned about performing tasks which require mental alertness (eg, operating machinery or driving). A minimum of 1 day should elapse after midazolam administration before attempting these tasks. Use with caution in patients receiving other CNS depressants or psychoactive agents. Effects with other sedative drugs or ethanol may be potentiated. Benzodiazepines have been associated with falls and traumatic injury and should be used with extreme caution in patients who are at risk of these events (especially the elderly).

May cause hypotension - hemodynamic events are more common in pediatric patients or patients with hemodynamic instability. Hypotension and/or respiratory depression may occur more frequently in patients who have received opioid analgesics. Use with caution in obese patients, chronic renal failure, and HF. Does not protect against increases in heart rate or blood pressure during intubation. Should not be used in shock, coma, or acute alcohol intoxication. **[U.S. Boxed Warning]: Parenteral form contains benzyl alcohol; avoid rapid injection in neonates or prolonged infusions.** Avoid intra-arterial administration or extravasation of parenteral formulation.

Midazolam causes anterograde amnesia. Paradoxical reactions, including hyperactive or aggressive behavior have been reported with benzodiazepines, particularly in adolescent/pediatric or psychiatric patients. Does not have analgesic, antidepressant, or antipsychotic properties.

Benzodiazepines have been associated with dependence and acute withdrawal symptoms on discontinuation or reduction in dose. Acute withdrawal, including seizures, may be precipitated after administration of flumazenil to patients receiving long-term benzodiazepine therapy.

Drug Interactions

Metabolism/Transport Effects Substrate of CYP2B6 (minor), 3A4 (major); **Inhibits** CYP2C8 (weak), 2C9 (weak), 3A4 (weak)

Avoid Concomitant Use

Avoid concomitant use of Midazolam with any of the following: Efavirenz; OLANZapine; Protease Inhibitors

Decreased Effect

The levels/effects of Midazolam may be decreased by: CarBAMazepine; CYP3A4 Inducers (Strong); Deferasirox; Ginkgo Biloba; Rifamycin Derivatives; St Johns Wort; Theophylline Derivatives; Yohimbine

Increased Effect/Toxicity

Midazolam may increase the levels/effects of: Alcohol (Ethyl); CloZAPine; CNS Depressants; Methotrimeprazine; Phenytoin; Propofol

The levels/effects of Midazolam may be increased by: Antifungal Agents (Azole Derivatives, Systemic); Aprepitant; Atorvastatin; Calcium Channel Blockers (Nondihydropyridine); Cimetidine; Conivaptan; Contraceptives (Estrogens); Contraceptives (Progestins); CYP3A4 Inhibitors (Moderate); CYP3A4 Inhibitors (Strong); Dasatinib; Droperidol; Efavirenz; Fluconazole; Fosaprepitant; Grapefruit Juice; Isoniazid; Macrolide Antibiotics; Methotrimeprazine; Nefazodone; OLANZapine; Propofol; Protease Inhibitors; Proton Pump Inhibitors; Selective Serotonin Reuptake Inhibitors

Nutritional/Ethanol Interactions

Ethanol: Avoid ethanol (may increase CNS depression).

Food: Grapefruit juice may increase serum concentrations of midazolam; avoid concurrent use with oral form.

Herb/Nutraceutical: Avoid concurrent use with St John's wort (may decrease midazolam levels, may increase CNS depression). Avoid concurrent use with valerian, kava kava, gotu kola (may increase CNS depression).

Adverse Reactions As reported in adults unless otherwise noted:

>10%: Respiratory: Decreased tidal volume and/or respiratory rate decrease, apnea (3% children)

1% to 10%:

- Cardiovascular: Hypotension (3% children)
- Central nervous system: Drowsiness (1%), oversedation, headache (1%), seizure-like activity (1% children)
- Gastrointestinal: Nausea (3%), vomiting (3%)
- Local: Pain and local reactions at injection site (4% I.M., 5% I.V.; severity less than diazepam)
- Ocular: Nystagmus (1% children)
- Respiratory: Cough (1%)
- Miscellaneous: Physical and psychological dependence with prolonged use, hiccups (4%, 1% children), paradoxical reaction (2% children)

Pharmacodynamics/Kinetics

Onset of Action I.M.: Sedation: ~15 minutes; I.V.: 1-5 minutes; Peak effect: I.M.: 0.5-1 hour

Duration of Action I.M.: Up to 6 hours; Mean: 2 hours

Absorption Oral: Rapid

Bioavailability Mean: 45%

Protein Binding 95%

Half-Life Elimination 1-4 hours; prolonged with cirrhosis, congestive heart failure, obesity, elderly

Metabolism Extensively hepatic via CYP3A4

Excretion Urine (as glucuronide conjugated metabolites); feces (~2% to 10%)

Controlled Substance C-IV

Available Dosage Forms

Injection, solution: 1 mg/mL (2 mL, 5 mL, 10 mL); 5 mg/mL (1 mL, 2 mL, 5 mL, 10 mL)

Injection, solution [preservative free]: 1 mg/mL (2 mL, 5 mL); 5 mg/mL (1 mL, 2 mL)

Syrup, oral: 2 mg/mL (118 mL)

Dosing

Adult

Note: The dose of midazolam needs to be individualized based on the patient's age, underlying diseases, and concurrent medications. Decrease dose (by ~30%) if narcotics or other CNS depressants are administered concomitantly. **Personnel and equipment needed for standard respiratory resuscitation should be immediately available during midazolam administration.**

Preoperative sedation:

I.M.: 0.07-0.08 mg/kg 30-60 minutes prior to surgery/procedure; usual dose: 5 mg; **Note:** Reduce dose in patients with COPD, high-risk patients, patients ≥60 years of age, and patients receiving other narcotics or CNS depressants

I.V.: 0.02-0.04 mg/kg; repeat every 5 minutes as needed to desired effect or up to 0.1-0.2 mg/kg

Intranasal (not an approved route): 0.2 mg/kg (up to 0.4 mg/kg in some studies); administer 30-45 minutes prior to surgery/procedure

Conscious sedation: I.V.: Initial: 0.5-2 mg slow I.V. over at least 2 minutes; slowly titrate to effect by repeating doses every 2-3 minutes if needed; usual total dose: 2.5-5 mg; use decreased doses in elderly.

Healthy Adults <60 years:

Initial: Some patients respond to doses as low as 1 mg; no more than 2.5 mg should be administered over a period of 2 minutes. Additional doses of midazolam may be administered after a 2-minute waiting period and evaluation of sedation after each dose increment. A total dose >5 mg is generally not needed. If narcotics or other CNS depressants are administered concomitantly, the midazolam dose should be reduced by 30%. *Refer to Dosing: Geriatric for patients ≥60 years, debilitated, or chronically ill.*

Maintenance: 25% of dose used to reach sedative effect

Anesthesia: I.V.:

Induction:

Unpremedicated patients: 0.3-0.35 mg/kg (up to 0.6 mg/kg in resistant cases)

Premedicated patients: 0.15-0.35 mg/kg

Maintenance: 0.05-0.3 mg/kg as needed, or continuous infusion 0.25-1.5 mcg/kg/minute

Sedation in mechanically-ventilated patients: I.V. continuous infusion: 100 mg in 250 mL D_5W or NS (if patient is fluid-restricted, may concentrate up to a maximum of 0.5 mg/mL); initial dose: 0.02-0.08 mg/kg (~1-5 mg in 70 kg adult) initially and repeated at 5- to 15-minute intervals until adequate sedation is achieved; may use continuous infusion to maintain sedation; usual dosage range for continuous infusion: 0.04-0.2 mg/kg/hour (Jacobi, 2002). Titrate to reach desired level of sedation.

Refractory status epilepticus (unlabeled use): I.V.: 0.15-0.3 mg/kg (usual dose: 5-15 mg); may repeat every 10-15 minutes as needed **or** continuous infusion of 0.05-0.6 mg/kg/hour

Geriatric The dose of midazolam needs to be individualized based on the patient's age, underlying diseases, and concurrent medications. Decrease dose (by ~30%) if narcotics or other CNS depressants are administered concomitantly. **Personnel and equipment needed for standard respiratory resuscitation should be immediately available during midazolam administration.**

I.V.: Conscious sedation: Initial: 0.5 mg slow I.V.; give no more than 1.5 mg in a 2-minute period. If additional titration is needed, give no more than 1 mg over 2 minutes, waiting another 2 or more minutes to evaluate sedative effect. A total dose >3.5 mg is rarely necessary.

Pediatric

Notes: The dose of midazolam needs to be individualized based on the patient's age, underlying diseases, and concurrent medications. Decrease dose (by ~30%) if narcotics or other CNS depressants are administered concomitantly. **Personnel and equipment needed for standard respiratory resuscitation should be immediately available during midazolam administration.** Children <6 years may require higher doses and closer monitoring than older children; calculate dose on ideal body weight

Conscious sedation for procedures or preoperative sedation:

Oral: 0.25-0.5 mg/kg as a single dose preprocedure, up to a maximum of 20 mg; administer 30-40 minutes prior to procedure. Children <6 years, or less cooperative patients may require as much as 1 mg/kg as a single dose; 0.25 mg/kg may suffice for children 6-16 years of age.

Intranasal (not an approved route): 0.2 mg/kg (up to 0.4 mg/kg in some studies), administered 30-45 minutes prior to procedure

I.M.: 0.1-0.15 mg/kg 30-60 minutes before surgery or procedure; range: 0.05-0.15 mg/kg; doses up to 0.5 mg/kg have been used in more anxious patients; maximum total dose: 10 mg

I.V.:

Infants <6 months: Limited information is available in nonintubated infants; dosing recommendations not clear; infants <6 months are at higher risk for airway obstruction and hypoventilation; titrate dose in small increments to desired effect; monitor carefully

Infants 6 months to Children 5 years: Initial: 0.05-0.1 mg/kg; titrate dose carefully; total dose of 0.6 mg/kg may be required; usual maximum total dose: 6 mg

Children 6-12 years: Initial: 0.025-0.05 mg/kg; titrate dose carefully; total doses of 0.4 mg/kg may be required; usual maximum total dose: 10 mg

Children 12-16 years: Dose as adults; usual maximum total dose: 10 mg

Conscious sedation during mechanical ventilation: I.V.: Children: Loading dose: 0.05-0.2 mg/kg, followed by initial continuous infusion: 1-2 mcg/kg/minute; titrate to the desired effect; usual range: 0.4-6 mcg/kg/minute

Status epilepticus refractory to standard therapy (unlabeled use): I.V.: Infants >2 months and Children: Loading dose: 0.15 mg/kg followed by a continuous infusion of 0.06 mg/kg/hour (1 mcg/kg/minute); titrate dose upward every 5 minutes until clinical seizure activity is controlled; mean infusion rate required in 24 children was 0.14 mg/kg/hour (2.3 mcg/kg/minute) with a range of 0.06-1.1 mg/kg/hour (Rivera, 1993)

Renal Impairment

Hemodialysis: Supplemental dose is not necessary.

Peritoneal dialysis: Significant drug removal is unlikely based on physiochemical characteristics.

Administration

Oral Do not mix with any liquid (such as grapefruit juice) prior to administration.

I.M. Give deep I.M. into large muscle.

I.V. Administer by slow I.V. injection over at least 2-5 minutes at a concentration of 1-5 mg/mL or by I.V. infusion. Continuous infusions should be administered via an infusion pump.

Other Intranasal: Administer using a 1 mL needleless syringe into the nares over 15 seconds; use the 5 mg/mL injection; 1/2 of the dose may be administered to each nare

Stability

Storage The manufacturer states that midazolam, at a final concentration of 0.5 mg/mL, is stable for up to 24 hours when diluted with D_5W or NS. A final concentration of 1 mg/mL in NS has been documented to be stable for up to 10 days (McMullen, 1995). Admixtures do not require protection from light for short-term storage.

Monitoring and Teaching Issues

Physical Assessment For inpatient use, institute safety measures. I.V.: Monitor cardiac and respiratory status continuously. Monitor I.V. infusion site carefully for extravasation. I.V./I.M.: Monitor closely following administration. Bedrest and assistance with ambulation necessary for several hours.

Patient Education Avoid use of alcohol.

Dietary Considerations Avoid grapefruit juice with oral syrup.

Geriatric Considerations In the elderly if concomitant CNS depressant medications are used, the midazolam dose will be at least 50% less than doses used in healthy, young, unpremedicated patients.

Breast-Feeding Considerations Midazolam and hydroxymidazolam can be detected in breast milk. Based on information from two women, 2-3 months postpartum, the half-life of midazolam in breast milk is ~1 hour. Milk concentrations were below the limit of detection (<5 nmol/L) 4 hours after a single maternal dose of midazolam 15 mg. Drowsiness, lethargy, or weight loss in nursing infants have been observed in case reports following maternal use of some benzodiazepines.

Pregnancy Considerations Adverse events were not observed in animal teratology studies. Midazolam has been found to cross the human placenta and can be detected in the serum of the umbilical vein and artery, as well as the amniotic fluid. Teratogenic effects have been observed with some benzodiazepines; however, additional studies are needed. The incidence of premature birth and low birth weights may be increased following maternal use of benzodiazepines; hypoglycemia and respiratory problems in the neonate may occur following exposure late in pregnancy. Neonatal withdrawal symptoms may occur within days to weeks after birth and "floppy infant syndrome" (which also includes withdrawal symptoms) have been reported with some benzodiazepines.

Additional Information Abrupt discontinuation after sustained use (generally >10 days) may cause withdrawal symptoms. For neonates, since both concentrations of the injection contain 1% benzyl alcohol, use the 5 mg/mL injection and dilute to 0.5 mg/mL with SWI without preservatives to decrease the amount of benzyl alcohol delivered to the neonate; with continuous infusion, midazolam may accumulate in peripheral tissues; use lowest effective infusion rate to reduce accumulation effects; midazolam is 3-4 times as potent as diazepam; paradoxical reactions associated with midazolam use in children (eg, agitation, restlessness, combativeness) have been successfully treated with flumazenil (Massanari, 1997).

Related Information

Benzodiazepines *on page 1988*

Compatibility of Drugs *on page 1994*

◆ **Midazolam Hydrochloride** *see* Midazolam *on page 1225*

Midodrine (MI doe dreen)

U.S. Brand Names ProAmatine® [DSC]

Index Terms Midodrine Hydrochloride

Generic Availability (U.S.) Yes

Pharmacologic Category Alpha$_1$ Agonist

Medication Safety Issues

Sound-alike/look-alike issues:

Midodrine may be confused with Midrin®, minoxidil

ProAmatine® may be confused with protamine

Pregnancy Risk Factor C

Lactation Excretion in breast milk is unknown/use caution

Use Orphan drug: Treatment of symptomatic orthostatic hypotension

Unlabeled/Investigational Use Management of urinary incontinence; vasovagal syncope; prevention of dialysis-induced hypotension

Available Dosage Forms

Tablet, oral: 2.5 mg, 5 mg, 10 mg

Dosing

Adult & Geriatric

Orthostatic hypotension: Oral: 10 mg 3 times/day during daytime hours (every 3-4 hours) when patient is upright (maximum: 40 mg/day)

Prevention of hemodialysis-induced hypotension (unlabeled use): Oral: 2.5-10 mg given 15-30 minutes prior to dialysis session (Cruz, 1998; KDOQI, 2005; Prakash, 2004)

Vasovagal syncope (unlabeled use): Oral: Initial: 5 mg 3 times/day during daytime hours (every 6 hours) increased up to 15 mg/dose if necessary (Perez-Lugones, 2001; Ward, 1998)

Renal Impairment Orthostatic hypotension: 2.5 mg 3 times/day; gradually increase as tolerated.

Hemodialysis: Dialyzable; dose after hemodialysis unless used for prevention of hemodialysis-induced hypotension.

Administration

Oral Doses may be given in approximately 3- to 4-hour intervals (eg, shortly before or upon rising in the morning, at midday, in the late afternoon not later than 6 PM). Avoid dosing after the evening meal or within 4 hours of bedtime. Continue therapy only in patients who appear to attain symptomatic improvement during initial treatment. Standing systolic blood pressure may be elevated 15-30 mm Hg at 1 hour after a 10 mg dose. Some effect may persist for 2-3 hours.

Monitoring and Teaching Issues

Laboratory Monitoring Kidney and liver function tests

Physical Assessment Assess for reduction of hypotension and adverse reactions (eg, supine hypertension, urinary urgency/retention, rash) prior to treatment and periodically thereafter. Standing blood pressure may be elevated 1 hour after administration and remain slightly elevated 3-4 hours.

Patient Education Take when sitting upright. Do not take within 4 hours of bedtime or when lying down for any length of time. Follow instructions for checking blood pressure and pulse routinely (same time of day; for 1 week at least). May cause urinary urgency or retention, dizziness, drowsiness, or headache. Report skin rash, severe gastric upset or pain, or muscle weakness or pain.

◆ **Midodrine Hydrochloride** *see* Midodrine *on page 1228*

◆ **Midol® Cramps & Body Aches [OTC]** *see* Ibuprofen *on page 938*

◆ **Midol® Extended Relief [OTC]** *see* Naproxen *on page 1289*

◆ **Mifeprex®** *see* Mifepristone *on page 1229*

Mifepristone (mi FE pris tone)

U.S. Brand Names Mifeprex®

Index Terms RU-38486; RU-486

Generic Availability (U.S.) No

Pharmacologic Category Abortifacient; Antineoplastic Agent, Hormone Antagonist; Antiprogestin

Medication Safety Issues

Sound-alike/look-alike issues:

Mifeprex® may be confused with Mirapex®

Mifepristone may be confused with misoprostol

High alert medication: The Institute for Safe Medication Practices (ISMP) includes this medication among its list of drug classes which have a heightened risk of causing significant patient harm when used in error.

Medication Guide Available Yes

Prescribing and Access Restrictions Mifepristone is deemed to have an approved REMS program. As a requirement of the REMS program, a medication guide must be given to the patient prior to receiving the medication. In addition, the manufacturer recommends distributing a patient agreement form which must be signed by the patient and prescriber confirming the patient's agreement to terminate her pregnancy. A signed copy of the patient agreement should be kept in the patient's medical record.

Mifeprex® is only available direct from Danco Laboratories' distributor. To obtain the product, please refer to, http://www.earlyoptionpill.com, or call 1-877-432-7596.

Investigators wishing to obtain the agent for use in oncology patients must apply for a patient-specific IND from the FDA.

Pregnancy Risk Factor X

Lactation Excretion in breast milk unknown/contraindicated

Use Medical termination of intrauterine pregnancy, through day 49 of pregnancy. Patients may need treatment with misoprostol and possibly surgery to complete therapy

Unlabeled/Investigational Use Treatment of unresectable meningioma; has been studied in the treatment of breast cancer, ovarian cancer, and adrenal cortical carcinoma

Mechanism of Action/Effect Mifepristone, a synthetic steroid, competitively binds to the intracellular progesterone receptor, blocking the effects of progesterone. When used for the termination of pregnancy, this leads to contraction-inducing activity in the myometrium. In the absence of progesterone, mifepristone acts as a partial progesterone agonist. Mifepristone also has weak antiglucocorticoid and antiandrogenic properties; it blocks the feedback effect of cortisol on corticotropin secretion.

Contraindications Hypersensitivity to mifepristone, misoprostol, other prostaglandins, or any component of the formulation; chronic adrenal failure; porphyrias; hemorrhagic disorder or concurrent anticoagulant therapy; pregnancy termination >49 days; intrauterine device (IUD) in place; ectopic pregnancy or undiagnosed adnexal mass; concurrent long-term corticosteroid therapy; inadequate or lack of access to emergency medical services; inability to understand effects and/or comply with treatment

Warnings/Precautions [U.S. Boxed Warning]: Patient must be instructed of the treatment procedure and expected effects. A signed agreement form must be kept in the patient's file. Physicians may obtain patient agreement forms, physician enrollment forms, and medical consultation directly from Danco Laboratories at 1-877-432-7596. Adverse effects (including blood transfusions, hospitalization, ongoing pregnancy, and other major complications) must be reported in writing to the medication distributor. To be administered only by physicians who can date pregnancy, diagnose ectopic pregnancies, provide access to surgical abortion (if needed), and can provide access to emergency care. Medication will be distributed directly to these physicians following signed agreement with the distributor. Must be administered under supervision by the qualified physician. Pregnancy is dated from day 1 of last menstrual period (presuming a 28-day cycle, ovulation occurring midcycle). Pregnancy duration can be determined using menstrual history and clinical examination. Ultrasound should be used if an ectopic pregnancy is suspected or if duration of pregnancy is uncertain. Ultrasonography may not identify all ectopic pregnancies, and healthcare providers should be alert for signs and symptoms which may be related to undiagnosed ectopic pregnancy in any patient who receives mifepristone

[U.S. Boxed Warning]: Patients should be counseled to seek medical attention in cases of excessive bleeding. Bleeding occurs and should be expected (average 9-16 days, may be ≥30 days). In some cases, bleeding may be prolonged and heavy, potentially leading to hypovolemic shock; the manufacturer cites soaking through two thick sanitary pads per hour for two consecutive hours as an example of excessive bleeding. Bleeding may require blood transfusion (rare), curettage, saline infusions, and/or vasoconstrictors. Use caution in patients with severe anemia. Confirmation of pregnancy termination by clinical exam or ultrasound must be made 14 days following treatment. Manufacturer recommends surgical termination of pregnancy when medical termination fails or is not complete. Prescriber should determine in advance whether they will provide such care themselves or through other providers. Preventative measures to prevent rhesus immunization must be taken prior to surgical abortion. Prescriber should also give the patient clear instructions on whom to call and what to do in the event of an emergency following administration of mifepristone.

[U.S. Boxed Warning]: Bacterial infections have been reported following use of this product. In rare cases, these infections may be serious and/or fatal, with septic shock as a potential complication. A causal relationship has not been established. Sustained fever, abdominal pain, or pelvic tenderness should prompt evaluation; however, healthcare professionals are warned that atypical presentations of serious infection without these symptoms have also been noted. Patients presenting with nausea, vomiting, diarrhea, or weakness, with or without abdominal pain or fever, should be evaluated for serious bacterial infection when symptoms occur >24 hours after taking misoprostol. Treatment with antibiotics, including coverage for anaerobic bacteria (eg, *Clostridium sordellii*) should be initiated. **[U.S. Boxed Warning]: Patients undergoing treatment with mifepristone should be instructed to bring their Medication Guide with them when an obtaining treatment from an emergency room or healthcare provider that did not prescribe the medication initially in order to identify that they are undergoing a medical abortion.**

Safety and efficacy have not been established for use in women with chronic cardiovascular, hypertensive, hepatic, respiratory, or renal disease, insulin-dependent diabetes mellitus, severe anemia, or heavy smokers. Women >35 years of age and smokers (>10 cigarettes/day) were excluded from clinical trials. Safety and efficacy in pediatric patients have not been established.

Drug Interactions

Metabolism/Transport Effects Substrate of CYP3A4 (minor); **Inhibits** CYP2D6 (weak), 3A4 (weak)

Avoid Concomitant Use There are no known interactions where it is recommended to avoid concomitant use.

Decreased Effect There are no known significant interactions involving a decrease in effect.

Increased Effect/Toxicity

The levels/effects of Mifepristone may be increased by: Conivaptan

Nutritional/Ethanol Interactions

Food: Do not take with grapefruit juice; grapefruit juice may inhibit mifepristone metabolism leading to increased levels.

Herb/Nutraceutical: Avoid St John's wort (may induce mifepristone metabolism, leading to decreased levels).

Lab Interactions hCG levels will not be useful to confirm pregnancy termination until at least 10 days following mifepristone treatment.

Adverse Reactions Vaginal bleeding and uterine cramping are expected to occur when this medication is used to terminate a pregnancy; 90% of women using this medication for this purpose also report adverse reactions. Bleeding or spotting occurs in most women for a period of 9-16 days. Up to 8% of women will experience some degree of bleeding or spotting for 30 days or more. In some cases, bleeding may be prolonged and heavy, potentially leading to hypovolemic shock.

>10%:

Central nervous system: Headache (2% to 31%), dizziness (1% to 12%)

Gastrointestinal: Abdominal pain (cramping) (96%), nausea (43% to 61%), vomiting (18% to 26%), diarrhea (12% to 20%)

Genitourinary: Uterine cramping (83%)

1% to 10%:

Cardiovascular: Syncope (1%)

Central nervous system: Fatigue (10%), fever (4%), insomnia (3%), anxiety (2%), fainting (2%)

Gastrointestinal: Dyspepsia (3%)

Genitourinary: Uterine hemorrhage (5%), vaginitis (3%), pelvic pain (2%), endometriosis/salpingitis/pelvic inflammatory disease (1%)

Hematologic: Decreased hemoglobin >2 g/dL (6%), anemia (2%), leukorrhea (2%)

Neuromuscular & skeletal: Back pain (9%), rigors (3%), leg pain (2%), weakness (2%)

Respiratory: Sinusitis (2%)

Miscellaneous: Viral infection (4%)

Pharmacodynamics/Kinetics

Absorption Oral: Rapid

Bioavailability Oral: 69%

Time to Peak Oral: 90 minutes

Protein Binding 98% to albumin and α_1-acid glycoprotein

Half-Life Elimination Terminal: 18 hours following a slower phase where 50% eliminated between 12-72 hours

Metabolism Hepatic via CYP3A4 to three metabolites (may possess some antiprogestin and antiglucocorticoid activity)

Excretion Feces (83%); urine (9%)

Available Dosage Forms

Tablet, oral:

Mifeprex®: 200 mg

Dosing

Adult

Termination of pregnancy: Oral: Treatment consists of three office visits by the patient; the patient must read medication guide and sign patient agreement prior to treatment:

Day 1: 600 mg (three 200 mg tablets) taken as a single dose under physician supervision

Day 3: Patient must return to the healthcare provider 2 days following administration of mifepristone; unless abortion has occurred (confirmed using ultrasound or clinical examination): 400 mcg (two 200 mcg tablets) of misoprostol; patient may need treatment for cramps or gastrointestinal symptoms at this time

Day 14: Patient must return to the healthcare provider ~14 days after administration of mifepristone; confirm complete termination of pregnancy by ultrasound or clinical exam. Surgical termination is recommended to manage treatment failures.

Dosing for unlabeled uses: Refer to individual protocols. The dose used in meningioma is usually 200 mg/day, continued based on toxicity and response.

Geriatric Safety and efficacy have not been established.

Renal Impairment Safety and efficacy have not been established.

Hepatic Impairment Safety and efficacy have not been established; use with caution due to CYP3A4 metabolism.

Stability

Storage Store at room temperature of 25°C (77°F).

Monitoring and Teaching Issues

Laboratory Monitoring Consider CBC in any patient who reports nausea, vomiting, diarrhea, or weakness with or without abdominal pain, but without fever or other signs of infection, more than 24 hours after administration of misoprostol.

Physical Assessment May only be administered under supervision of a qualified physician. Patient must be instructed in procedure and sign patient consent forms. Monitor for excessive bleeding. Monitor vital signs.

Patient Education This medication is used to terminate pregnancy under 7 weeks. It must be administered under direction of a qualified physician. You will need follow-up visits as directed by your prescriber (approximately 3 days and 14 days after treatment). Surgical termination of pregnancy may be required if medication fails; there is a risk of fetal malformation if treatment fails. You may experience vaginal bleeding and cramping that is heavier than a normal menstrual period; report immediately if severe or persistent. You may experience nausea, vomiting, and diarrhea. It is possible to get pregnant before your next period. Once the pregnancy has proved to be ended, contraception should be started before having sexual intercourse.

Breast-Feeding Considerations Breast milk should be discarded for a few days following use of this medication.

Pregnancy Considerations This medication is used to terminate pregnancy; there are no approved treatment indications for its use during pregnancy. Prostaglandins (including mifepristone and misoprostol) may have teratogenic effects when used during pregnancy. If treatment fails, there is a risk of fetal malformation. In sexually active women, pregnancy can occur prior to the first menstrual period following treatment. Appropriate contraception can be started as soon as termination of pregnancy is confirmed or before sexual intercourse is resumed.

Additional Information Medication will be distributed directly to qualified physicians following signed agreement with the distributor, Danco Laboratories. It will not be available through pharmacies. Major adverse reactions (hospitalization, blood transfusion, ongoing pregnancy, etc) should be reported to Danco Laboratories.

Miglitol (MIG li tol)

U.S. Brand Names Glyset®

Generic Availability (U.S.) No

Pharmacologic Category Antidiabetic Agent, Alpha-Glucosidase Inhibitor

Medication Safety Issues

Sound-alike/look-alike issues:

Glyset® may be confused with Cycloset®

Pregnancy Risk Factor B

Lactation Enters breast milk (small amounts)/not recommended

Use Type 2 diabetes mellitus (noninsulin-dependent, NIDDM):

Monotherapy as an adjunct to diet to improve glycemic control in patients with type 2 diabetes mellitus (noninsulin-dependent, NIDDM) whose hyperglycemia cannot be managed with diet alone

Combination therapy with a sulfonylurea when diet plus either miglitol or a sulfonylurea alone do not result in adequate glycemic control. The effect of miglitol to enhance glycemic control is additive to that of sulfonylureas when used in combination.

Mechanism of Action/Effect In contrast to sulfonylureas, miglitol does not enhance insulin secretion. The antihyperglycemic action of miglitol results from a reversible inhibition of membrane-bound intestinal alpha-glucosidases which hydrolyze oligosaccharides and disaccharides to glucose and other monosaccharides in the brush border of the small intestine. In patients with diabetes, this enzyme inhibition results in delayed glucose absorption and lowering of postprandial hyperglycemia.

Contraindications Hypersensitivity to miglitol or any of component of the formulation; diabetic ketoacidosis; inflammatory bowel disease; colonic ulceration; partial intestinal obstruction or predisposition to intestinal obstruction; chronic intestinal diseases associated with marked disorders of digestion or absorption or with conditions that may deteriorate as a result of increased gas formation in the intestine

Warnings/Precautions GI symptoms are the most common reactions. The incidence of abdominal pain and diarrhea tend to diminish considerably with continued treatment. Use with caution in patients with mild-to-moderate renal impairment; not recommended in severe impairment (serum creatinine >2 mg/dL); studies have not been conducted. In combination with a sulfonylurea will cause a further lowering of blood glucose and may increase the hypoglycemic potential of the sulfonylurea. It may be necessary to discontinue miglitol and administer insulin if the patient is exposed to stress (ie, fever, trauma, infection, surgery).

Drug Interactions

Avoid Concomitant Use There are no known interactions where it is recommended to avoid concomitant use.

Decreased Effect

The levels/effects of Miglitol may be decreased by: Corticosteroids (Orally Inhaled); Corticosteroids (Systemic); Luteinizing Hormone-Releasing Hormone Analogs; Somatropin; Thiazide Diuretics

Increased Effect/Toxicity

Miglitol may increase the levels/effects of: Hypoglycemic Agents

The levels/effects of Miglitol may be increased by: Herbs (Hypoglycemic Properties); Pegvisomant

Adverse Reactions

>10%: Gastrointestinal: Flatulence (42%), diarrhea (29%), abdominal pain (12%)

1% to 10%: Dermatologic: Rash (4%)

Pharmacodynamics/Kinetics

Absorption Saturable at high doses: 25 mg dose: Completely absorbed; 100 mg dose: 50% to 70% absorbed

Time to Peak 2-3 hours

Protein Binding <4%

Half-Life Elimination ~2 hours

Metabolism None

Excretion Urine (as unchanged drug)

Available Dosage Forms

Tablet, oral:

Glyset®: 25 mg, 50 mg, 100 mg

Dosing

Adult & Geriatric Type 2 diabetes (noninsulin dependent, NIDDM): Oral: Initial: 25 mg 3 times/day with the first bite of food at each meal; the dose may be increased to 50 mg 3 times/day after 4-8 weeks; maximum recommended dose: 100 mg 3 times/day

Renal Impairment Miglitol is primarily excreted by the kidneys; no dosage adjustment recommended in mild-moderate impairment. Not recommended in patients with a S_{cr} >2 mg/dL; studies have not been conducted.

Hepatic Impairment No adjustment necessary.

Administration

Oral Should be taken orally at the start (with the first bite) of each main meal.

Stability

Storage Store at 25°C (77°F); excursions permitted to 15°C to 30°C (59°F to 86°F).

Monitoring and Teaching Issues

Laboratory Monitoring Blood glucose tests; measurement of glycosylated hemoglobin is recommended for the monitoring of long-term glycemic control.

Physical Assessment Teach patient importance of adequate diabetic control.

Patient Education Take with the first bite of each main meal. Avoid alcohol. It is important to follow dietary and lifestyle recommendations of prescriber. You will be instructed in signs of hyper-/hypoglycemia. If combining this medication with other diabetic medication (eg, sulfonylureas, insulin), keep source of glucose in the form of dextrose (NOT table sugar, candy, or cookies) on hand in case hypoglycemia occurs. May cause mild side effects during first weeks of therapy (eg, bloating, flatulence, diarrhea, abdominal discomfort); these should diminish over time. Report severe or persistent side effects, fever, extended vomiting or flu, or change in color of urine or stool.

Geriatric Considerations In a double-blind randomized, placebo-controlled trial, glyburide caused significantly greater reductions in hemoglobin A_{1c} compared to miglitol 25 mg or 50 mg three times per day, but was associated with more weight gain. Diarrhea, soft stools, and flatulence were more common with miglitol. Intensive glucose control (Hb A_{1c} <6.5%) has been linked to increased all cause and cardiovascular mortality, hypoglycemia requiring assistance, and weight gain in adult type 2 diabetes. For elderly patients with diabetes who are relatively healthy, attaining target goals for aspirin use, blood pressure, lipids, smoking cessation, and diet and exercise may be more important than normalized glycemic control.

Breast-Feeding Considerations Miglitol is found in breast milk. The exposure to a nursing infant is ~0.4% of a 100 mg maternal dose. Breast-feeding is not recommended by the manufacturer.

Pregnancy Considerations Adverse events have not been reported in animal reproduction studies; therefore, miglitol is classified as pregnancy category B. Information specific to the use of miglitol during pregnancy has not been located. Maternal hyperglycemia can be associated with adverse effects in the fetus, including macrosomia, neonatal hyperglycemia, and hyperbilirubinemia; the risk of congenital malformations is increased when the Hb A_{1c} is above the normal range. Diabetes can also be associated with adverse effects in the mother. Poorly-treated diabetes may cause end-organ damage that may in turn negatively affect obstetric outcomes. Physiologic glucose levels should be maintained prior to and during pregnancy to decrease the risk of adverse events in the mother and the fetus. Until additional safety and efficacy data are obtained, the use of oral agents is generally not recommended as routine management of GDM or type 2 diabetes mellitus during pregnancy. Insulin is the drug of choice for the control of diabetes mellitus during pregnancy.

Related Information

Diabetes Mellitus Management, Adults *on page 2026*

◆ **Migranal®** *see* Dihydroergotamine *on page 535*

◆ **Millipred™** *see* PrednisoLONE (Systemic) *on page 1497*

Milnacipran (mil NAY ci pran)

U.S. Brand Names Savella®

Generic Availability (U.S.) No

Pharmacologic Category Antidepressant, Serotonin/Norepinephrine Reuptake Inhibitor

Medication Safety Issues

Sound-alike/look-alike issues:

Savella® may be confused with cevimeline, sevelamer

Medication Guide Available Yes

Pregnancy Risk Factor C

Lactation Excretion in breast milk unknown/not recommended

Use Management of fibromyalgia

Mechanism of Action/Effect Inhibits norepinephrine and serotonin reuptake; improves symptoms associated with fibromyalgia

Contraindications Concomitant use or within 2 weeks of MAO inhibitors; uncontrolled narrow-angle glaucoma

Warnings/Precautions [U.S. Boxed Warning]: Milnacipran is a serotonin/norepinephrine reuptake inhibitor (SNRI) similar to SNRIs used to treat depression and other psychiatric disorders. **Antidepressants increase the risk of suicidal thinking and behavior in children, adolescents, and young adults (18-24 years of age) with major depressive disorder (MDD) and other psychiatric disorders**; consider risk prior to prescribing. Short-term studies did not show an increased risk in patients >24 years of age and showed a decreased risk in patients ≥65 years. Closely monitor for clinical worsening, suicidality, or unusual changes in behavior; the patient's family or caregiver should be instructed to closely observe the patient and communicate condition with healthcare provider. A medication guide should be dispensed with each prescription. **Milnacipran is not FDA approved for the treatment of major depressive disorder or for use in children.**

Suicide risks should be monitored in patients treated with SNRIs regardless of the indication. The possibility of a suicide attempt is inherent in major depression and may persist until remission occurs. Monitor for worsening of depression or suicidality, especially during initiation of therapy (generally first 1-2 months) or with dose increases or decreases. Use caution in high-risk patients. Worsening depression and severe abrupt suicidality that are not part of the presenting symptoms may require discontinuation or modification of drug therapy. The patient's family or caregiver should be alerted to monitor patients for the emergence of suicidality and associated behaviors (such as agitation, irritability, hostility, impulsivity, and hypomania) and call healthcare provider.

Patients with major depressive disorder were excluded from clinical trials evaluating milnacipran for fibromyalgia; however, mania has been reported in patients with mood disorders taking similar medications. May worsen psychosis in some patients or precipitate a shift to mania or hypomania in patients with bipolar disorder. Patients presenting with depressive symptoms should be screened for bipolar disorder. Monotherapy in patients with bipolar disorder should be avoided. **Milnacipran is not FDA approved for the treatment of bipolar depression.**

Serotonin syndrome and neuroleptic malignant syndrome (NMS)-like reactions have occurred with serotonin/norepinephrine reuptake inhibitors (SNRIs) and selective serotonin reuptake inhibitors (SSRIs) when used alone, and particularly when used in combination with serotonergic agents (eg, triptans) or antidopaminergic agents (eg, antipsychotics). Concurrent use with MAO inhibitors is contraindicated. May cause sustained increase in blood pressure or heart rate. Control pre-existing hypertension and cardiovascular disease prior to initiation of milnacipran. Use caution in patients with renal impairment; dose reduction required in severe renal impairment. Use caution in patients with hepatic impairment. Avoid ethanol use. May cause hyponatremia/SIADH (elderly at increased risk); volume depletion (diuretics may increase risk). Use cautiously in patients with a history of seizures. May impair platelet aggregation, resulting in bleeding. May cause increased urinary resistance. Use caution in patients with controlled narrow-angle glaucoma; use is contraindicated with uncontrolled narrow-angle glaucoma.

Abrupt discontinuation or dosage reduction after extended therapy may lead to agitation, dysphoria, anxiety, and other symptoms. When discontinuing therapy, dosage should be tapered gradually. If intolerable symptoms occur following a decrease in dosage or upon discontinuation of therapy, then resuming the previous dose with a more gradual taper should be considered.

Drug Interactions

Avoid Concomitant Use

Avoid concomitant use of Milnacipran with any of the following: Iobenguane I 123; MAO Inhibitors; Methylene Blue; Sibutramine

Decreased Effect

Milnacipran may decrease the levels/effects of: Alpha2-Agonists; Iobenguane I 123

Increased Effect/Toxicity

Milnacipran may increase the levels/effects of: Alcohol (Ethyl); Alpha-/Beta-Agonists; Aspirin; CNS Depressants; Digoxin; Methotrimeprazine; Methylene Blue; NSAID (Nonselective); Serotonin Modulators; Vitamin K Antagonists

The levels/effects of Milnacipran may be increased by: ClomiPRAMINE; Droperidol; MAO Inhibitors; Methotrimeprazine; Sibutramine

Nutritional/Ethanol Interactions

Ethanol: Avoid ethanol use.

Herb/Nutraceutical: Avoid valerian, St John's wort, SAMe, kava kava, tryptophan (may increase risk of serotonin syndrome and/or excessive sedation).

Adverse Reactions

>10%:

- Central nervous system: Headache (18%), insomnia (12%)
- Endocrine & metabolic: Hot flashes (12%)
- Gastrointestinal: Nausea (37%), constipation (16%)

1% to 10%:

- Cardiovascular: Palpitation (7%), heart rate increased (6%), hypertension (5%), flushing (3%), blood pressure increased (3%), tachycardia (2%), peripheral edema (≥1%)
- Central nervous system: Dizziness (10%), migraine (5%), chills (2%), tremor (2%), depression (≥1%), fatigue (≥1%), fever (≥1%), irritability (≥1%), somnolence (≥1%)
- Dermatologic: Hyperhidrosis (9%), rash (3%)
- Endocrine & metabolic: Hypercholesterolemia (≥1%)
- Gastrointestinal: Vomiting (7%), xerostomia (5%), abdominal pain (3%), appetite decreased (2%), abdominal distension (≥1%), abnormal taste (≥1%), diarrhea (≥1%), dyspepsia (≥1%), flatulence (≥1%), gastroesophageal reflux disease (≥1%), weight changes (≥1%)
- Genitourinary: Dysuria (≥2%), ejaculation disorder/failure (≥2%), erectile dysfunction (≥2%), libido decreased (≥2%), prostatitis (≥2%), scrotal pain (≥2%), testicular pain (≥2%), testicular swelling (≥2%), urethral pain (≥2%), urinary hesitation (≥2%), urinary retention (≥2%), urine flow decreased (≥2%), cystitis (≥1%), urinary tract infection (≥1%)
- Neuromuscular & skeletal: Falling (≥1%)
- Ocular: Blurred vision (2%)
- Respiratory: Dyspnea (2%)
- Miscellaneous: Night sweats (≥1%)

Pharmacodynamics/Kinetics

Absorption Well absorbed

Bioavailability 85% to 90%

Time to Peak Plasma: Oral: 2-4 hours

Protein Binding 13%

Half-Life Elimination 6-8 hours

Metabolism Hepatic to inactive metabolites

Excretion Urine (55% as unchanged drug)

Available Dosage Forms

Combination package, oral:

Savella®: Tablet: 12.5 mg (5s), Tablet: 25 mg (8s), and Tablet: 50 mg (42s)

Tablet, oral:

Savella®: 12.5 mg, 25 mg, 50 mg, 100 mg

Dosing

Adult & Geriatric Fibromyalgia: Oral: 50 mg twice daily (maximum dose: 200 mg/day).

Titration schedule: 12.5 mg once on day 1, then 12.5 mg twice daily on days 2-3, 25 mg twice daily on days 4-7, then 50 mg twice daily thereafter. Dose may be increased to 100 mg twice daily, based on individual response. Doses >200 mg/day have not been studied.

Discontinuation of therapy: Gradually taper dose. If intolerable symptoms occur following a dose reduction, consider resuming the previously prescribed dose and/or decrease dose at a more gradual rate.

Renal Impairment

Mild renal impairment: No dose adjustment is recommended.

Moderate renal impairment: Use with caution.

Severe renal impairment (Cl_{cr} ≤29 mL/minute): Reduce maintenance dose to 25 mg twice daily; dose may be increased to 50 mg twice daily, based on individual tolerance.

End-stage renal disease (ESRD): Use not recommended.

Hepatic Impairment

Mild-to-moderate hepatic impairment: No dose adjustment is recommended.

Severe hepatic impairment: Use with caution.

Administration

Oral May be administered with or without food; food may improve tolerability.

Stability

Storage Store at 25°C (77°F); excursions permitted between 15°C to 30°C (59°F to 86°F).

Monitoring and Teaching Issues

Laboratory Monitoring Renal function should be monitored for dosing purposes

Physical Assessment Monitor blood pressure and heart rate prior to initiating therapy and periodically throughout. Monitor for signs and symptoms of suicide ideation (eg, anxiety, depression, clinical worsening, behavior changes). Taper dosage when discontinuing.

Patient Education Avoid use of alcohol. You may experience headaches, trouble sleeping, hot flashes, nausea, constipation, dizziness, increased perspiration, and dry mouth. Report unusual bleeding or bruising; blood in stool, vomitus, or urine; nosebleeds; bleeding gums; pain in joints or back; new or worsening depression; changes in mood; aggressive or violent behavior; panic attacks; or suicide ideation.

Dietary Considerations May be taken with or without food; food may improve tolerability.

Geriatric Considerations According to the manufacturer of milnacipran, 402 participants in the clinical trials were age 60 years and older; no difference in efficacy or safety were reported compared to younger participants. Milnacipran should be used cautiously in patients with moderate renal impairment and its dose reduced in patients with Cl_{cr} 5-29 mL/minute. Like SSRIs and SNRIs, the risk of hyponatremia may be greater in the elderly.

Breast-Feeding Considerations It is unknown if milnacipran is excreted in human milk; there are no adequate and well-controlled studies in nursing mothers.

Pregnancy Considerations Milnacipran was fetotoxic in some animal reproduction studies; teratogenic effects or embryotoxicity were not observed in other species.

Nonteratogenic effects in the newborn following SSRI/SNRI exposure late in the third trimester include respiratory distress, cyanosis, apnea, seizures, temperature instability, feeding difficulty, vomiting, hypoglycemia, hyper- or hypotonia, hyper-reflexia, jitteriness, irritability, constant crying, and tremor. The long-term effects on neurobehavior have not been studied.

Women inadvertently exposed to milnacipran during pregnancy may be enrolled in the Savella Pregnancy Registry (877-643-3010 or http://www.savellapregnancyregistry.com).

Related Information

Antidepressant Agents *on page 1982*

Milrinone (MIL ri none)

Index Terms Milrinone Lactate

Generic Availability (U.S.) Yes

Pharmacologic Category Phosphodiesterase Enzyme Inhibitor

Medication Safety Issues

Sound-alike/look-alike issues:

Primacor® may be confused with Primaxin®

High alert medication: The Institute for Safe Medication Practices (ISMP) includes this medication among its list of drugs which have a heightened risk of causing significant patient harm when used in error.

Pregnancy Risk Factor C

Lactation Excretion in breast milk unknown/use caution

Use Short-term I.V. therapy of acutely-decompensated heart failure

Unlabeled/Investigational Use Inotropic therapy for patients unresponsive to other acute heart failure therapies (eg, dobutamine); outpatient inotropic therapy for heart transplant candidates; palliation of symptoms in end-stage heart failure patients who cannot otherwise be discharged from the hospital and are not transplant candidates

Mechanism of Action/Effect Phosphodiesterase inhibitor resulting in vasodilation

Contraindications Hypersensitivity to milrinone, inamrinone, or any component of the formulation; concurrent use of inamrinone

Warnings/Precautions Monitor closely for hypotension. Avoid in severe obstructive aortic or pulmonic valvular disease. Milrinone may aggravate outflow tract obstruction in hypertrophic subaortic stenosis. Supraventricular and ventricular arrhythmias have developed in high-risk patients. Ensure that ventricular rate controlled in atrial fibrillation/flutter prior to initiating milrinone. Not recommended for use in acute MI patients. Monitor and correct fluid and electrolyte problems. Adjust dose in renal dysfunction. Discontinue therapy if dose-related elevations in LFTs and clinical symptoms of hepatotoxicity occur.

Drug Interactions

Avoid Concomitant Use There are no known interactions where it is recommended to avoid concomitant use.

Decreased Effect There are no known significant interactions involving a decrease in effect.

Increased Effect/Toxicity There are no known significant interactions involving an increase in effect.

Adverse Reactions

>10%: Cardiovascular: Ventricular arrhythmia (ectopy 9%, NSVT 3%, sustained ventricular tachycardia 1%, ventricular fibrillation <1%)

1% to 10%:

Cardiovascular: Supraventricular arrhythmia (4%), hypotension (3%), angina/chest pain (1%)

Central nervous system: Headache (3%)

Pharmacodynamics/Kinetics

Onset of Action I.V.: 5-15 minutes

Protein Binding Plasma: ~70%

Half-Life Elimination Normal renal function: ~2.5 hours; CVVH: 20.1 hours (Taniguchi, 2000)

Metabolism Hepatic (12%)

Excretion Urine (85% as unchanged drug) within 24 hours; active tubular secretion is a major elimination pathway for milrinone

Available Dosage Forms

Infusion, premixed in D_5W: 200 mcg/mL (100 mL, 200 mL)

Injection, solution: 1 mg/mL (10 mL, 20 mL, 50 mL)

Injection, solution [preservative free]: 1 mg/mL (10 mL, 20 mL)

Dosing

Adult & Geriatric CHF/Hemodynamic support: I.V.: Loading dose (optional): 50 mcg/kg administered over 10 minutes followed by a maintenance dose titrated according to the hemodynamic and clinical response; Maintenance dose: I.V. infusion: 0.375-0.75 mcg/kg/minute.

Renal Impairment

Cl_{cr} 50 mL/minute: Administer 0.43 mcg/kg/minute.
Cl_{cr} 40 mL/minute: Administer 0.38 mcg/kg/minute.
Cl_{cr} 30 mL/minute: Administer 0.33 mcg/kg/minute.
Cl_{cr} 20 mL/minute: Administer 0.28 mcg/kg/minute.
Cl_{cr} 10 mL/minute: Administer 0.23 mcg/kg/minute.
Cl_{cr} 5 mL/minute: Administer 0.2 mcg/kg/minute.

Administration

I.V. Infuse via infusion pump.

Stability

Reconstitution Standard dilution: For a final concentration of 0.2 mg/mL: Dilute Primacor® 1 mg/mL (20 mL) with 80 mL diluent (final volume: 100 mL) of 1/2 NS, NS or D_5W. May also dilute 1 mg/mL (10 mL) with 40 mL diluent (final volume: 50 mL).

Storage Store at 15°C to 30°C (59°F to 86°F); avoid freezing. Stable at 0.2 mg/mL in 1/2NS, NS, or D_5W for 72 hours at room temperature in normal light.

Monitoring and Teaching Issues

Laboratory Monitoring Platelet count, CBC, electrolytes (especially potassium and magnesium), liver function and renal function tests

Physical Assessment Monitor cardiac/hemodynamic status continuously during therapy and serum potassium at regular intervals. Monitor for fluid retention.

Patient Education This drug can only be given intravenously. Weigh daily and report weight gain. Report pain at infusion site; numbness, tingling, or swelling of extremities; or respiratory difficulty.

- **Milrinone Lactate** *see* Milrinone *on page 1235*
- **Mimvey™** *see* Estradiol and Norethindrone *on page 674*
- **Minitran™** *see* Nitroglycerin *on page 1327*
- **Minocin®** *see* Minocycline *on page 1236*
- **Minocin® PAC** *see* Minocycline *on page 1236*

Minocycline (mi noe SYE kleen)

U.S. Brand Names Dynacin®; Minocin®; Minocin® PAC; Solodyn®

Index Terms Minocycline Hydrochloride

Generic Availability (U.S.) Yes: Excludes extended release tablet, injection, pellet-filled capsule

Pharmacologic Category Antibiotic, Tetracycline Derivative

Medication Safety Issues

Sound-alike/look-alike issues:

Dynacin® may be confused with Dyazide®, Dynabac®, DynaCirc®, Dynapen®
Minocin® may be confused with Indocin®, Lincocin®, Minizide®, Mithracin®, niacin

Pregnancy Risk Factor D

Lactation Enters breast milk/not recommended

Use Treatment of susceptible bacterial infections of both gram-negative and gram-positive organisms; treatment of anthrax (inhalational, cutaneous, and gastrointestinal); moderate-to-severe acne; meningococcal (asymptomatic) carrier state; Rickettsial diseases (including Rocky Mountain spotted fever, Q fever); nongonococcal urethritis, gonorrhea; acute intestinal amebiasis; respiratory tract infection; skin/soft tissue infections; chlamydial infections

Extended release (Solodyn®): Only indicated for treatment of inflammatory lesions of non-nodular moderate-to-severe acne

Unlabeled/Investigational Use Rheumatoid arthritis (patients with low disease activity of short duration); nocardiosis; alternative treatment for community-acquired MRSA infection

Mechanism of Action/Effect Inhibits bacterial protein synthesis by binding with the 30S and possibly the 50S ribosomal subunit(s) of susceptible bacteria; cell wall synthesis is not affected

Rheumatoid arthritis: The mechanism of action of minocycline in rheumatoid arthritis is not completely understood. It is thought to have antimicrobial, anti-inflammatory, immunomodulatory, and chondroprotective effects. More specifically, it is thought to be a potent inhibitor of metalloproteinases, which are active in rheumatoid arthritis joint destruction.

Contraindications Hypersensitivity to minocycline, other tetracyclines, or any component of the formulation

Warnings/Precautions May be associated with increases in BUN secondary to antianabolic effects; use caution in patients with renal impairment (Cl_{cr} <80 mL/minute). Hepatotoxicity has been reported; use caution in patients with hepatic insufficiency. Autoimmune syndromes (eg, lupus-like, hepatitis, and vasculitis) have been reported; discontinue if symptoms occur. CNS effects (lightheadedness, vertigo) may occur; patients must be cautioned about performing tasks which require mental alertness (eg, operating machinery or driving). Pseudotumor cerebri has been (rarely) reported with tetracycline use; usually resolves with discontinuation. May cause photosensitivity; discontinue if skin erythema occurs. Prolonged use may result in fungal or bacterial superinfection, including *C. difficile*-associated diarrhea (CDAD) and pseudomembranous colitis; CDAD has been observed >2 months postantibiotic treatment. May cause tissue hyperpigmentation, enamel hypoplasia, or permanent tooth discoloration; use of tetracyclines should be avoided during tooth development (children ≤8 years of age) unless other drugs are not likely to be effective or are contraindicated. However, use is recommended in treatment of anthrax exposure. Do not use during pregnancy. In addition to affecting tooth development, tetracycline use has been associated with retardation of skeletal development and reduced bone growth. Rash, along with eosinophilia, fever, and organ failure (Drug Rash with Eosinophilia and Systemic Symptoms [DRESS] syndrome) has been reported; discontinue treatment immediately if DRESS syndrome is suspected.

Drug Interactions

Avoid Concomitant Use

Avoid concomitant use of Minocycline with any of the following: BCG; Retinoic Acid Derivatives

Decreased Effect

Minocycline may decrease the levels/effects of: Atazanavir; BCG; Penicillins; Typhoid Vaccine

The levels/effects of Minocycline may be decreased by: Antacids; Bile Acid Sequestrants; Bismuth; Bismuth Subsalicylate; Iron Salts; Magnesium Salts; Quinapril; Sucralfate; Zinc Salts

Increased Effect/Toxicity

Minocycline may increase the levels/effects of: Neuromuscular-Blocking Agents; Retinoic Acid Derivatives; Vitamin K Antagonists

Nutritional/Ethanol Interactions

Food: Minocycline serum concentrations are not significantly altered if taken with food or dairy products.

Herb/Nutraceutical: Avoid dong quai, St John's wort (may also cause photosensitization).

Lab Interactions May cause interference with fluorescence test for urinary catecholamines (false elevations)

Adverse Reactions Frequency not defined.

Cardiovascular: Myocarditis, pericarditis, vasculitis

Central nervous system: Bulging fontanels, dizziness, fatigue, fever, headache, hypoesthesia, malaise, mood changes, paresthesia, pseudotumor cerebri, sedation, seizure, somnolence, vertigo

Dermatologic: Alopecia, angioedema, DRESS (Drug Rash with Eosinophilia and Systemic Symptoms) syndrome, erythema multiforme, erythema nodosum, erythematous rash, exfoliative dermatitis, hyperpigmentation of nails, maculopapular rash, photosensitivity, pigmentation of the skin and mucous membranes, pruritus, Stevens-Johnson syndrome, toxic epidermal necrolysis, urticaria

Endocrine & metabolic: Thyroid cancer, thyroid discoloration, thyroid dysfunction

Gastrointestinal: Anorexia, diarrhea, dyspepsia, dysphagia, enamel hypoplasia, enterocolitis, esophageal ulcerations, esophagitis, glossitis, inflammatory lesions (oral/anogenital), moniliasis, nausea, oral cavity discoloration, pancreatitis, pseudomembranous colitis, stomatitis, tooth discoloration, vomiting, xerostomia

Genitourinary: Balanitis, vulvovaginitis

Hematologic: Agranulocytosis, eosinophilia, hemolytic anemia, leukopenia, neutropenia, pancytopenia, thrombocytopenia

Hepatic: Autoimmune hepatitis, hepatic cholestasis, hepatic failure, hepatitis, hyperbilirubinemia, jaundice, liver enzyme increases

Local: Injection site reaction (I.V. administration)

Neuromuscular & skeletal: Arthralgia, arthritis, bone discoloration, joint stiffness, joint swelling, myalgia

Otic: Hearing loss, tinnitus

Renal: Acute renal failure, BUN increased, interstitial nephritis

Respiratory: Asthma, bronchospasm, cough, dyspnea, pneumonitis, pulmonary infiltrate (with eosinophilia)

Miscellaneous: Anaphylaxis, hypersensitivity, lupus erythematosus, lupus-like syndrome, serum sickness

Pharmacodynamics/Kinetics

Absorption Oral: Well absorbed

Time to Peak Capsule, pellet filled: 1-4 hours; Extended release tablet: 3.5-4 hours

Protein Binding 70% to 75%

Half-Life Elimination I.V.: 15-23 hours; Oral: 16 hours (range: 11-22 hours)

Metabolism Hepatic to inactive metabolites

Excretion Urine, feces

Available Dosage Forms

Capsule, oral: 50 mg, 75 mg, 100 mg

Capsule, pellet filled, oral:

Minocin®: 50 mg, 100 mg

Minocin® PAC: 50 mg, 100 mg

Injection, powder for reconstitution:
Minocin®: 100 mg
Tablet, oral: 50 mg, 75 mg, 100 mg
Dynacin®: 50 mg, 75 mg, 100 mg
Tablet, extended release, oral:
Solodyn®: 45 mg, 65 mg, 90 mg, 115 mg, 135 mg

Dosing

Adult & Geriatric

Usual dosage range:
I.V.: Initial: 200 mg, followed by 100 mg every 12 hours (maximum: 400 mg/day)
Oral: Initial: 200 mg, followed by 100 mg every 12 hours; more frequent dosing intervals may be used (100-200 mg initially, followed by 50 mg 4 times daily)

Acne: Oral: Capsule or immediate-release tablet: 50-100 mg twice daily
Inflammatory, non-nodular, moderate-to-severe acne (Solodyn®):
45-54 kg: 45 mg once daily
55-77 kg: 65 mg once daily
78-102 kg: 90 mg once daily
103-125 kg: 115 mg once daily
126-136 kg: 135 mg once daily
Note: Therapy should be continued for 12 weeks. Higher doses do not confer greater efficacy and may be associated with more acute vestibular side effects. Safety of use beyond 12 weeks has not been established.

Cellulitis (purulent) due to community-acquired MRSA (unlabeled use): Oral: Initial: 200 mg; Maintenance: 100 mg twice daily for 5-10 days (Liu, 2011)

Chlamydial or *Ureaplasma urealyticum* infection, uncomplicated: Oral, I.V.: Urethral, endocervical, or rectal: Oral: 100 mg every 12 hours for at least 7 days

Gonococcal infection, uncomplicated (males): Oral, I.V.:
Without urethritis or anorectal infection: Initial: 200 mg, followed by 100 mg every 12 hours for at least 4 days (cultures 2-3 days post-therapy)
Urethritis: 100 mg every 12 hours for 5 days

Meningococcal carrier state (manufacturer's labeling): Oral: 100 mg every 12 hours for 5 days. **Note:** CDC recommendations do not mention use of minocycline for eradicating nasopharyngeal carriage of meningococcal

Mycobacterium marinum: Oral: 100 mg every 12 hours for 6-8 weeks

Nocardiosis, cutaneous (non-CNS) (unlabeled use): Oral: 100-200 mg every 12 hours

Rheumatoid arthritis (unlabeled use): Oral: 100 mg twice daily (O'Dell, 2001)

Syphilis: Oral, I.V.: Initial: 200 mg, followed by 100 mg every 12 hours for 10-15 days

Pediatric

Usual dosage range: Children >8 years: Oral, I.V.: Initial: 4 mg/kg followed by 2 mg/kg/dose every 12 hours

Inflammatory, non-nodular, moderate-to-severe acne (Solodyn®): Children ≥12 years: Oral: Refer to adult dosing.

Cellulitis (purulent) infection due to community-acquired MRSA (unlabeled use): Oral: Children >8 years: Initial: 4 mg/kg (maximum: 200 mg); Maintenance: 2 mg/kg/dose (maximum: 100 mg) every 12 hours for 5-10 days (Liu, 2011);

Renal Impairment Use with caution; monitor BUN and creatinine clearance. Consider decreasing dose or increasing dosing interval (extended release).
Cl_{cr} <80 mL/minute: Do not exceed 200 mg/day

Administration

Oral May be administered with or without food. Administer with adequate fluid to decrease the risk of esophageal irritation and ulceration. Swallow pellet-filled capsule and extended release tablet whole; do not chew, crush, or split.

I.V. I.V.: Infuse slowly; avoid rapid administration. The manufacturer's labeling does not provide a recommended administration rate. The injectable route should be used only if the oral route is not feasible or adequate. Prolonged intravenous therapy may be associated with thrombophlebitis.

Stability

Reconstitution Injection: Reconstitute with 5 mL of sterile water for injection, and further dilute in 500-1000 mL of NS, D_5W, D_5NS, Ringer's injection, or LR.

Storage
Capsule (including pellet-filled), tablet: Store at 20°C to 25°C (68°F to 77°F); protect from heat. Protect from light and moisture.
Extended release tablet: Store at 15°C to 30°C (59°F to 86°F); protect from heat. Protect from light and moisture.
Injection: Store vials at 20°C to 25°C (68°F to 77°F) prior to reconstitution. Reconstituted solution is stable at room temperature for 24 hours. Final dilutions should be administered immediately.

Monitoring and Teaching Issues

Laboratory Monitoring LFTs, BUN, renal function with long-term treatment; if symptomatic for autoimmune disorder, include ANA, CBC monitoring.

Physical Assessment Assess results of culture and sensitivity tests and allergy history before beginning therapy. Teach patient importance of adequate hydration.

Patient Education May cause photosensitivity reaction, nausea, fatigue, headache, dizziness, sedation, or diarrhea. Report rash or itching, unresolved nausea or diarrhea, change in urinary output (excess), and opportunistic infection (eg, fever, chills, sore throat, burning urination, fatigue).

I.V.: Report immediately any pain, burning, or swelling at infusion site or any signs of allergic reaction (eg, respiratory difficulty or swallowing, back pain, chest tightness, rash, hives, swelling of lips or mouth).

Oral: May be taken with or without food.

Dietary Considerations May be taken with or without food.

Geriatric Considerations Minocycline has not been studied in the elderly but its CNS effects may limit its use. Dose reduction for renal function not necessary.

Breast-Feeding Considerations Small amounts of minocycline are excreted in breast milk and therefore, breast-feeding is not recommended by the manufacturer. Minocycline absorption is not affected by dairy products. This may lead to increased absorption from maternal milk when compared to other tetracyclines which are bound by the calcium in the maternal milk. Nondose-related effects could include modification of bowel flora. There have been case reports of black discoloration of breast milk in women taking minocycline.

Pregnancy Considerations Tetracyclines, including minocycline, cross the placenta, enter fetal circulation, and may cause permanent discoloration of teeth if used during the second or third trimester. Congenital anomalies after minocycline use have been reported postmarketing. Because use during pregnancy may cause fetal harm, minocycline is classified as pregnancy category D.

Related Information

Antimicrobial Drugs of Choice *on page 2008*

◆ **Minocycline Hydrochloride** *see* Minocycline *on page 1236*
◆ **Miranel AF™ [OTC]** *see* Miconazole (Topical) *on page 1224*
◆ **Mirapex®** *see* Pramipexole *on page 1489*
◆ **Mirapex® ER™** *see* Pramipexole *on page 1489*
◆ **Mircette®** *see* Ethinyl Estradiol and Desogestrel *on page 695*
◆ **Mirena®** *see* Levonorgestrel *on page 1097*

Mirtazapine (mir TAZ a peen)

U.S. Brand Names Remeron SolTab®; Remeron®

Generic Availability (U.S.) Yes

Pharmacologic Category Antidepressant, Alpha-2 Antagonist

Medication Safety Issues

Sound-alike/look-alike issues:

Remeron® may be confused with Premarin®, ramelteon, Rozerem®, Zemuron®

International issues:

Avanza [Australia] may be confused with Albenza brand name for albendazole [U.S.]; Avandia brand name for rosiglitazone [U.S., Canada, and multiple international markets]

Remeron [U.S., Canada, and multiple international markets] may be confused with Reneuron which is a brand name for fluoxetine [Spain]

Medication Guide Available Yes

Pregnancy Risk Factor C

Lactation Excreted in breast milk/use caution

Use Treatment of depression

Unlabeled/Investigational Use Post-traumatic stress disorder (PTSD)

Mechanism of Action/Effect Mirtazapine is a tetracyclic antidepressant that works by its central presynaptic alpha$_2$-adrenergic antagonist effects, which results in increased release of norepinephrine and serotonin. It is also a potent antagonist of 5-HT$_2$ and 5-HT$_3$ serotonin receptors and H1 histamine receptors and a moderate peripheral alpha$_1$-adrenergic and muscarinic antagonist; it does not inhibit the reuptake of norepinephrine or serotonin.

Contraindications Hypersensitivity to mirtazapine or any component of the formulation; use of MAO inhibitors within 14 days

Warnings/Precautions [U.S. Boxed Warning]: Antidepressants increase the risk of suicidal thinking and behavior in children, adolescents, and young adults (18-24 years of age) with major depressive disorder (MDD) and other psychiatric disorders; consider risk prior to prescribing. Short-term studies did not show an increased risk in patients >24 years of age and showed a decreased risk in patients ≥65 years. Closely monitor for clinical worsening, suicidality, or unusual changes in behavior; the patient's family or caregiver should be instructed to closely observe the patient and communicate condition with healthcare provider. A medication guide should be dispensed with each prescription. **Mirtazapine is not FDA approved for use in children.**

The possibility of a suicide attempt is inherent in major depression and may persist until remission occurs. Monitor for worsening of depression or suicidality, especially during initiation of therapy (generally first 1-2 months) or with dose increases or decreases. Use caution in high-risk patients. Worsening depression and severe abrupt suicidality that are not part of the presenting symptoms may require discontinuation or modification of drug therapy. The patient's family or caregiver should be alerted to monitor patients for the emergence of suicidality and associated behaviors (such as agitation, irritability, hostility, impulsivity, and hypomania) and call healthcare provider.

May worsen psychosis in some patients or precipitate a shift to mania or hypomania in patients with bipolar disorder. Patients presenting with depressive symptoms should be screened for bipolar disorder. Monotherapy in patients with bipolar disorder should be avoided. **Mirtazapine is not FDA approved for the treatment of bipolar depression.**

Patients should not discontinue treatment abruptly, unless significant life-threatening event, due to risk of withdrawal symptoms. A gradual reduction in the dose over several weeks is recommended.

Discontinue immediately if signs and symptoms of neutropenia/agranulocytosis occur. May cause sedation, resulting in impaired performance of tasks requiring alertness (eg, operating machinery or driving). Sedative effects may be additive with other CNS depressants and/or ethanol. The degree of sedation is moderate-high relative to other antidepressants. Conversely, may increase psychomotor restlessness within first few weeks of therapy. The risks of orthostatic hypotension or anticholinergic effects are low relative to other antidepressants. The incidence of sexual dysfunction with mirtazapine is generally lower than with SSRIs. Potential for severe reaction when used with MAO inhibitors; autonomic instability, coma, death, delirium, diaphoresis, hyperthermia, mental status changes/agitation, muscular rigidity, myoclonus, neuroleptic malignant syndrome features, and seizures may occur.

May increase appetite and stimulate weight gain. Weight gain of >7% of body weight reported in 7.5% of patients treated with mirtazapine compared to 0% for placebo; 8% of patients receiving mirtazapine discontinued treatment due to the weight gain. In an 8-week pediatric clinical trial, 49% of mirtazapine-treated patients had a weight gain of at least 7% (mean increase 4 kg) as compared to 5.7% of placebo-treated patients (mean increase 1 kg). May increase serum cholesterol and triglyceride levels.

Use caution in patients with a previous seizure disorder or condition predisposing to seizures such as brain damage, alcoholism, or concurrent therapy with other drugs which lower the seizure threshold. May cause hyponatremia.Use with caution in patients with hepatic or renal dysfunction and in elderly patients. Clinically significant transaminase elevations have been observed. SolTab® formulation contains phenylalanine.

Drug Interactions

Metabolism/Transport Effects Substrate of CYP1A2 (major), 2C9 (minor), 2D6 (major), 3A4 (major); **Inhibits** CYP1A2 (weak), 3A4 (weak)

Avoid Concomitant Use

Avoid concomitant use of Mirtazapine with any of the following: MAO Inhibitors; Methylene Blue; Sibutramine

Decreased Effect

Mirtazapine may decrease the levels/effects of: Alpha2-Agonists

The levels/effects of Mirtazapine may be decreased by: CYP1A2 Inducers (Strong); CYP3A4 Inducers (Strong); Deferasirox; Peginterferon Alfa-2b

Increased Effect/Toxicity

Mirtazapine may increase the levels/effects of: Alcohol (Ethyl); CNS Depressants; Methotrimeprazine; Methylene Blue; Serotonin Modulators; Warfarin

The levels/effects of Mirtazapine may be increased by: Conivaptan; CYP1A2 Inhibitors (Moderate); CYP1A2 Inhibitors (Strong); CYP2D6 Inhibitors (Moderate); CYP2D6 Inhibitors (Strong); CYP3A4 Inhibitors (Moderate); CYP3A4 Inhibitors (Strong); Darunavir; Dasatinib; Droperidol; MAO Inhibitors; Methotrimeprazine; Sibutramine

Nutritional/Ethanol Interactions

Ethanol: Avoid ethanol (may increase CNS depression).

Herb/Nutraceutical: Avoid St John's wort (may decrease mirtazapine levels). Avoid valerian, St John's wort, SAMe, kava kava (may increase CNS depression).

Adverse Reactions

>10%:

Central nervous system: Somnolence (54%)

Endocrine & metabolic: Increased cholesterol

Gastrointestinal: Constipation (13%), xerostomia (25%), increased appetite (17%), weight gain (12%; weight gain of >7% reported in 8% of adults, ≤49% of pediatric patients)

1% to 10%:

Cardiovascular: Hypertension, vasodilatation, peripheral edema (2%), edema (1%)

Central nervous system: Dizziness (7%), abnormal dreams (4%), abnormal thoughts (3%), confusion (2%), malaise

Endocrine & metabolic: Increased triglycerides

Gastrointestinal: Vomiting, anorexia, abdominal pain

Genitourinary: Urinary frequency (2%)

Hepatic: SGPT increased (≥3 times ULN: 2%)

Neuromuscular & skeletal: Myalgia (2%), back pain (2%), arthralgia, tremor (2%), weakness (8%)

Respiratory: Dyspnea (1%)

Miscellaneous: Flu-like syndrome (5%), thirst

Pharmacodynamics/Kinetics

Absorption Rapid and complete

Bioavailability 50%

Time to Peak Serum: 2 hours

Protein Binding 85%

Half-Life Elimination 20-40 hours; hampered with renal or hepatic impairment

Metabolism Extensively hepatic via CYP1A2, 2C9, 2D6, 3A4 and via demethylation (forms demethylmirtazapine, an active metabolite) and hydroxylation (forms inactive metabolites)

Excretion Urine (75%) and feces (15%) as metabolites

Available Dosage Forms

Tablet, oral: 7.5 mg, 15 mg, 30 mg, 45 mg
Remeron®: 15 mg, 30 mg, 45 mg

Tablet, orally disintegrating, oral: 15 mg, 30 mg, 45 mg
Remeron SolTab®: 15 mg, 30 mg, 45 mg

Dosing

Adult

Depression: Oral: Initial: 15 mg nightly, titrate up to 15-45 mg/day with dose increases made no more frequently than every 1-2 weeks. There is an inverse relationship between dose and sedation.

Post-traumatic stress disorder (PTSD) (unlabeled use): Oral: 30-60 mg/day

Geriatric Initial: 7.5 mg/day as a single bedtime dose; increase by 7.5-15 mg/day every 1-2 weeks; usual dose: 15-30 mg/day; maximum dose: 45 mg/day

Alzheimer's dementia-related depression: Initial: 7.5 mg at bedtime; may increase at 7.5-15 mg increments to 45-60 mg/day

Renal Impairment

Cl_{cr} 11-39 mL/minute: 30% decreased clearance

Cl_{cr} <10 mL/minute: 50% decreased clearance

Hepatic Impairment Clearance is decreased by 30%.

Administration

Oral SolTab®: Open blister pack and place tablet on the tongue. Do not split tablet. Tablet is formulated to dissolve on the tongue without water.

Stability

Storage Store at controlled room temperature of 25°C (77°F); excursions permitted to 15°C to 30°C (59°F to 86°F). Protect from light and moisture.

SolTab®: Protect from light and moisture. Use immediately upon opening tablet blister.

Monitoring and Teaching Issues

Laboratory Monitoring CBC

Physical Assessment Monitor for CNS depression/sedation. Monitor for clinical worsening and suicide ideation. Taper dosage slowly when discontinuing.

Patient Education It may take 2-3 weeks to achieve desired results. Take once-a-day dose at bedtime. Avoid alcohol. Maintain adequate hydration unless instructed to restrict fluid intake. You may experience drowsiness, dizziness, lightheadedness, nausea, vomiting, anorexia, dry mouth, or orthostatic hypotension. Report persistent insomnia, agitation, or confusion; suicide ideation; muscle cramping, tremors, weakness, or change in gait; breathlessness or respiratory difficulty; chest pain, palpitations, or rapid heartbeat; change in urinary pattern; vision changes or eye pain; yellowing of eyes or skin; pale stools/dark urine; or worsening of condition.

SolTab®: Tablet is formulated to dissolve on the tongue without water.

Dietary Considerations Some products may contain phenylalanine.

Geriatric Considerations Limited published data specifically in the elderly or addressing *in vivo* drug interactions.

Breast-Feeding Considerations Mirtazapine and its active metabolite are found in breast milk, with higher levels in the hindmilk than foremilk. Adverse events have not been observed in nursing infants. The manufacturer recommends that caution be used if administered to a breast-feeding woman.

Pregnancy Considerations Adverse events were observed in some animal studies; therefore, the manufacturer classifies mirtazapine as pregnancy category C. A significant increase in major teratogenic effects has not been observed in humans following exposure to mirtazapine during pregnancy; however, some nonteratogenic adverse events (similar to those observed with SSRI agents) have been reported. Mirtazapine was found to cross the placenta following a maternal overdose. Pregnancy itself does not provide "protection" against depression. Women treated for major depression and who are euthymic prior to pregnancy are more likely to experience a relapse when medication is discontinued as compared to pregnant women who continue taking antidepressant medications. The ACOG recommends that therapy with antidepressants during pregnancy be individualized. According to their recommendations, treatment of depression during pregnancy should incorporate the clinical expertise of the mental health clinician, obstetrician, primary care provider, and pediatrician. If treatment during pregnancy is required, consider tapering therapy during the third trimester in order to prevent withdrawal symptoms in the infant. If this is done, and the woman is considered to be at risk of relapse from her major depressive disorder, the medication can be restarted following delivery, although the dose should be readjusted to that required before pregnancy. Treatment algorithms have been developed by the ACOG and the APA for the management of depression in women prior to conception and during pregnancy (Yonkers, 2009).

Additional Information Note: At least 14 days should elapse between discontinuation of an MAO inhibitor and initiation of therapy with mirtazapine; at least 14 days should be allowed after discontinuing mirtazapine before starting an MAO inhibitor.

Related Information

Antidepressant Agents *on page* 1982

Misoprostol (mye soe PROST ole)

U.S. Brand Names Cytotec®

Generic Availability (U.S.) Yes

Pharmacologic Category Prostaglandin

Medication Safety Issues

Sound-alike/look-alike issues:

Cytotec® may be confused with Cytoxan, Sytobex®

Misoprostol may be confused with metoprolol, mifepristone

Pregnancy Risk Factor X

Lactation Enters breast milk/use caution

Use Prevention of NSAID-induced gastric ulcers; medical termination of pregnancy of ≤49 days (in conjunction with mifepristone)

Unlabeled/Investigational Use Cervical ripening and labor induction (except in women with prior cesarean delivery or major uterine surgery); fat malabsorption in cystic fibrosis

Available Dosage Forms

Tablet, oral: 100 mcg, 200 mcg

Cytotec®: 100 mcg, 200 mcg

Dosing

Adult

Prevention of NSAID-induced ulcers: Oral: 200 mcg 4 times/day with food; if not tolerated, may decrease dose to 100 mcg 4 times/day with food. Last dose of the day should be taken at bedtime.

Labor induction or cervical ripening (unlabeled uses): Intravaginal: 25 mcg (1/4 of 100 mcg tablet); may repeat at intervals no more frequent than every 3-6 hours. Do not use in patients with previous cesarean delivery or prior major uterine surgery.

Medical termination of pregnancy: Oral: Refer to Mifepristone monograph.

Geriatric Oral: 100-200 mcg 4 times/day with food; if 200 mcg 4 times/day not tolerated, reduce to 100 mcg 4 times/day. **Note:** To avoid the diarrhea potential, doses can be initiated at 100 mcg/day and increased 100 mcg/day at 3-day intervals until desired dose is achieved; also, recommend administering with food to decrease diarrhea incidence.

Pediatric Fat absorption in cystic fibrosis (unlabeled use): Oral: Children 8-16 years: 100 mcg 4 times/day

Renal Impairment Half-life, maximum plasma concentration, and bioavailability may be increased; however, a correlation has not been observed with degree of dysfunction. Decrease dose if recommended dose is not tolerated. It is not known if misoprostol is removed by dialysis.

Administration

Oral Incidence of diarrhea may be lessened by having patient take dose right after meals and avoiding magnesium-containing antacids. When used for the prevention of NSAID-induced ulcers, therapy is usually begun on the second or third day of the next normal menstrual period in women of childbearing potential.

Monitoring and Teaching Issues

Physical Assessment Teach appropriate diet and lifestyle if being used to prevent ulcers.

Patient Education Take with meals or after meals to prevent nausea, diarrhea, and flatulence. You may experience increased menstrual pain or cramping. Report abnormal menstrual periods, spotting (may occur even in postmenstrual women), or severe menstrual bleeding.

◆ **Misoprostol and Diclofenac** *see* Diclofenac and Misoprostol *on page* 523

Mitotane (MYE toe tane)

U.S. Brand Names Lysodren®

Index Terms Chloditan; Chlodithane; Khloditan; Mytotan; o,p′-DDD; Ortho,para-DDD

Generic Availability (U.S.) No

Pharmacologic Category Antineoplastic Agent, Miscellaneous

Medication Safety Issues

Sound-alike/look-alike issues:

Mitotane may be confused with mitoMYcin, mitoXANtrone

High alert medication: The Institute for Safe Medication Practices (ISMP) includes this medication among its list of drug classes which have a heightened risk of causing significant patient harm when used in error.

Pregnancy Risk Factor C

Lactation Excretion in breast milk unknown/not recommended

Use Treatment of inoperable adrenocortical carcinoma

Unlabeled/Investigational Use Treatment of Cushing's syndrome

Mechanism of Action/Effect Adrenolytic agent which causes adrenal cortical atrophy; affects mitochondria in adrenal cortical cells and decreases production of cortisol; also alters the peripheral metabolism of steroids

Contraindications Hypersensitivity to mitotane or any component of the formulation

Warnings/Precautions Hazardous agent - use appropriate precautions for handling and disposal. Patients treated with mitotane may develop adrenal insufficiency; steroid replacement with glucocorticoid, and sometimes mineralocorticoid, is necessary. It has been recommended that steroid replacement therapy be initiated at the start of therapy, rather than waiting for evidence of adrenal insufficiency. **[U.S. Boxed Warning]: Because the primary action of mitotane is through adrenal suppression, discontinue mitotane temporarily with onset of shock or severe trauma; administer appropriate steroid coverage.** Because mitotane can increase the metabolism of exogenous steroids, higher than usual replacement steroid doses may be required. Surgically remove tumor tissues from metastatic masses prior to initiation of treatment; rapid cytotoxic effect may cause tumor hemorrhage. Observe patients for neurotoxicity with long-term (>2 years) use. Use caution with hepatic impairment; metabolism may be decreased. Other CNS adverse effects, including lethargy, sedation, and vertigo may occur; patients must be cautioned about performing tasks which require mental alertness (eg, operating machinery or driving). The manufacturer recommends initiating treatment within a hospital environment until a stabilized dose is achieved. Continue treatment as long as clinical benefit (maintenance of clinical status or metastatic lesion grown slowing) is observed. Clinical benefit is usually observed within 3 months at maximum tolerated dose, although 10% of patients may require more than 3 months for benefit. Continuous treatment at the maximum tolerated dose is generally the best approach. Some patients have been treated intermittently, restarting when severe symptoms reappear, although often response is no longer observed after 3 or 4 courses of intermittent treatment. **[U.S. Boxed Warnings]: Should be administered under the supervision of an experienced cancer chemotherapy physician.** Safety and efficacy in children have not been established.

Drug Interactions

Avoid Concomitant Use There are no known interactions where it is recommended to avoid concomitant use.

Decreased Effect

Mitotane may decrease the levels/effects of: Corticosteroids (Systemic); Vitamin K Antagonists

The levels/effects of Mitotane may be decreased by: Spironolactone

Increased Effect/Toxicity

Mitotane may increase the levels/effects of: Vitamin K Antagonists

The levels/effects of Mitotane may be increased by: MAO Inhibitors

Nutritional/Ethanol Interactions Ethanol: Avoid ethanol (may increase CNS depression).

Adverse Reactions The majority of adverse events are dose-dependent.

>10%:

Central nervous system: CNS depression (32%), lethargy/somnolence (25%), dizziness/vertigo (15%)

Dermatologic: Skin rash (15%)

Gastrointestinal: Anorexia (24%), nausea (39%), vomiting (37%), diarrhea (13%)

Neuromuscular & skeletal: Weakness (12%)

1% to 10%:

Central nervous system: Headache (5%), confusion (3%)

Neuromuscular & skeletal: Muscle tremor (3%)

Pharmacodynamics/Kinetics

Absorption Oral: ~35% to 40%

Time to Peak Serum: 3-5 hours

Half-Life Elimination 18-159 days

Metabolism Hepatic and other tissues

Excretion Urine (~10%, as metabolites); feces (1% to 17%, as metabolites)

Available Dosage Forms

Tablet, oral:

Lysodren®: 500 mg

Dosing

Adult & Geriatric

Adrenocortical carcinoma: Oral: Start at 2-6 g/day in 3-4 divided doses, then increase incrementally to 9-10 g/day in 3-4 divided doses (maximum tolerated range: 2-16 g/day, usually 9-10 g/day; maximum dose studied: 18-19 g/day)

Cushing's syndrome (unlabeled use): Oral: Initial dose: 500 mg 3 times/day; maximum dose: 3000 mg 3 times/day (Biller, 2008)

Pediatric Adrenocortical carcinoma (unlabeled use): Oral: 1-2 g/day in divided doses, increasing gradually to a maximum of 5-7 g/day

Hepatic Impairment Dose may need to be decreased in patients with liver disease.

Adjustment for Toxicity

Severe side effects: Reduce dose until achieve a maximum tolerated dose.

Significant neuropsychiatric adverse effects: Withhold treatment for at least 1 week and restart at a lower dose (Allolio, 2006).

Administration

Oral Administer in 3-4 divided doses/day. Do not crush tablets; wear gloves when handling; avoid exposure to crushed or broken tablets.

Stability

Storage Store at room temperature of 25°C (77°F); excursions permitted to 15°C to 30°C (59°F to 86°F).

Monitoring and Teaching Issues

Patient Education Do not crush tablets or allow other people to handle crushed or broken tablets. Desired effects of this drug may not be seen for 2-3 months. Maintain adequate nutrition and hydration, unless instructed to restrict fluid intake. Avoid alcohol; may increase CNS depression. May cause dizziness, headache, confusion, nausea, vomiting, or loss of appetite. Report severe or persistent vomiting or diarrhea; CNS changes (depression, lethargy, dizziness); rash; or muscular twitching, tremor, numbness, or weakness.

Breast-Feeding Considerations Due to the potential for serious adverse reactions in the nursing infant, breast-feeding is not recommended.

Pregnancy Considerations Animal studies have not been conducted. There are no adequate and well-controlled studies in pregnant women. Use during pregnancy only if clearly needed.

Mitoxantrone (mye toe ZAN trone)

U.S. Brand Names Novantrone®

Index Terms CL-232315; DHAD; DHAQ; Dihydroxyanthracenedione; Dihydroxyanthracenedione Dihydrochloride; Mitoxantrone Dihydrochloride; Mitoxantrone HCl; Mitoxantrone Hydrochloride; Mitozantrone

Generic Availability (U.S.) Yes

Pharmacologic Category Antineoplastic Agent, Anthracenedione

Medication Safety Issues

Sound-alike/look-alike issues:

MitoXANtrone may be confused with methotrexate, mitoMYcin, mitotane, Mutamycin®

High alert medication: This medication is in a class the Institute for Safe Medication Practices (ISMP) includes among its list of drug classes which have a heightened risk of causing significant patient harm when used in error.

Pregnancy Risk Factor D

Lactation Enters breast milk/not recommended

Use Treatment of acute nonlymphocytic leukemias (ANLL [includes myelogenous, promyelocytic, monocytic and erythroid leukemias]); advanced hormone-refractory prostate cancer; secondary progressive or relapsing-remitting multiple sclerosis (MS)

Unlabeled/Investigational Use Treatment of Hodgkin's lymphoma, non-Hodgkin's lymphomas (NHL), acute lymphocytic leukemia (ALL), myelodysplastic syndrome, breast cancer, pediatric acute myelogenous leukemia (AML), pediatric acute promyelocytic leukemia (APL); part of a conditioning regimen for autologous hematopoietic stem cell transplantation (HSCT)

Mechanism of Action/Effect Related to the anthracyclines, mitoxantrone intercalates into DNA resulting in cross-links and strand breaks; also interferes with RNA and inhibits topoisomerase II; active throughout entire cell cycle (cell-cycle nonspecific)

Contraindications Hypersensitivity to mitoxantrone or any component of the formulation

Warnings/Precautions Hazardous agent - use appropriate precautions for handling and disposal.

[U.S. Boxed Warning]: Usually should not be administered if baseline neutrophil count <1500 cells/mm^3 (except for treatment of ANLL). Monitor blood counts and monitor for infection due to neutropenia. Treatment may lead to severe myelosuppression; unless the expected benefit outweighs the risk, use is generally not recommended in patients with pre-existing myelosuppression from prior chemotherapy.

[U.S. Boxed Warning]: May cause myocardial toxicity and potentially-fatal heart failure (HF); risk increases with cumulative dosing. Effects may occur during therapy or may be delayed (months or years after completion of therapy). Predisposing factors for mitoxantrone-induced cardiotoxicity include prior anthracycline or anthracenedione therapy, prior cardiovascular disease, concomitant use of cardiotoxic drugs, and mediastinal/pericardial irradiation, although may also occur in patients without risk factors. Prior to therapy initiation, evaluate all patients for cardiac-related signs/symptoms, including history, physical exam, and ECG; and evaluate baseline left ventricular ejection fraction (LVEF) with echocardiogram or multigated radionuclide angiography (MUGA) or MRI. Not recommended for use in MS patients when LVEF <50%, or baseline LVEF below the lower limit of normal (LLN). Evaluate for cardiac signs/symptoms (by history, physical exam, and ECG) and evaluate LVEF (using same method as baseline LVEF) in MS patients prior to each dose and if signs/symptoms of HF develop. Use in MS should be limited to a cumulative dose of ≤140 mg/m^2, and discontinued if LVEF falls below LLN or a significant decrease in LVEF is observed; decreases in LVEF and HF have been observed in patients with MS who have received cumulative doses <100 mg/m^2. Patients with MS should undergo annual LVEF evaluation following discontinuation of therapy to monitor for delayed cardiotoxicity.

[U.S. Boxed Warnings]: For I.V. administration only, into a free-flowing I.V.; may cause severe local tissue damage if extravasation occurs; do not administer subcutaneously, intramuscularly, or intra-arterially. Do not administer intrathecally; may cause serious and permanent neurologic damage. Extravasation resulting in burning, erythema, pain, swelling and skin discoloration (blue) has been reported; extravasation may result in tissue necrosis and require debridement for skin graft. May cause urine, saliva, tears, and sweat to turn blue-green for 24 hours postinfusion. Whites of eyes may have blue-green tinge. **[U.S. Boxed Warning]: Treatment with mitoxantrone increases the risk of developing secondary acute myelogenous leukemia (AML) in patients with cancer and in patients with MS;** acute promyelocytic leukemia (APL) has also been observed. Symptoms of acute leukemia include excessive bruising, bleeding and recurrent infections. The risk for secondary leukemia is increased in patients who are heavily pretreated, with higher doses, and with combination chemotherapy.

[U.S. Boxed Warning]: Should be administered under the supervision of a physician experienced in cancer chemotherapy agents. Dosage should be reduced in patients with impaired hepatobiliary function (clearance is reduced); not for treatment of multiple sclerosis in patients with concurrent hepatic impairment. Not for treatment of primary progressive multiple sclerosis. Rapid lysis of tumor cells may lead to hyperuricemia.

Drug Interactions

Metabolism/Transport Effects Inhibits CYP3A4 (weak)

Avoid Concomitant Use

Avoid concomitant use of MitoXANtrone with any of the following: BCG; Natalizumab; Pimecrolimus; Roflumilast; Tacrolimus (Topical); Vaccines (Live)

Decreased Effect

MitoXANtrone may decrease the levels/effects of: BCG; Sipuleucel-T; Vaccines (Inactivated); Vaccines (Live)

The levels/effects of MitoXANtrone may be decreased by: Echinacea

Increased Effect/Toxicity

MitoXANtrone may increase the levels/effects of: Leflunomide; Natalizumab; Vaccines (Live)

The levels/effects of MitoXANtrone may be increased by: Denosumab; Pimecrolimus; Roflumilast; Tacrolimus (Topical); Trastuzumab

Nutritional/Ethanol Interactions Herb/Nutraceutical: Avoid echinacea (may diminish the immunosuppressant effect).

Adverse Reactions Includes events reported with any indication; incidence varies based on treatment, dose, and/or concomitant medications

>10%:

Cardiovascular: Edema (10% to 30%), arrhythmia (3% to 18%), cardiac function changes (≤18%), ECG changes (≤11%)

Central nervous system: Fever (6% to 78%), pain (8% to 41%), fatigue (≤39%), headache (6% to 13%)

Dermatologic: Alopecia (20% to 61%), nail bed changes (≤11%), petechiae/bruising (6% to 11%)

Endocrine & metabolic: Menstrual disorder (26% to 61%), amenorrhea (28% to 53%), hyperglycemia (10% to 31%)

Gastrointestinal: Nausea (26% to 76%), vomiting (6% to 72%), diarrhea (14% to 47%), mucositis (10% to 29%; onset: ≤1 week), stomatitis (8% to 29%; onset: ≤1 week), anorexia (22% to 25%), weight gain/loss (13% to 17%), constipation (10% to 16%), GI bleeding (2% to 16%), abdominal pain (9% to 15%), dyspepsia (5% to 14%)

Genitourinary: Urinary tract infection (7% to 32%), abnormal urine (5% to 11%)

Hematologic: Neutropenia (79% to 100%; onset: ≤3 weeks; grade 4: 23% to 54%), leukopenia (9% to 100%), lymphopenia (72% to 95%), anemia/hemoglobin decreased (5% to 75%) thrombocytopenia (33% to 39%; grades 3/4: 3% to 4%), neutropenic fever (≤11%)

Hepatic: Alkaline phosphatase increased (≤37%), transaminases increased (5% to 20%), GGT increased (3% to 15%)

Neuromuscular & skeletal: Weakness (≤24%)

Renal: BUN increased (≤22%), creatinine increased (≤13%), hematuria (≤11%)

Respiratory: Upper respiratory tract infection (7% to 53%), pharyngitis (≤19%), dyspnea (6% to 18%), cough (5% to 13%)

Miscellaneous: Infection (4% to 60%), sepsis (ANLL 31% to 34%), fungal infection (9% to 15%)

1% to 10%:

Cardiovascular: CHF (≤5%), ischemia (≤5%), LVEF decreased (≤5%), hypertension (≤4%)

Central nervous system: Chills (≤5%), anxiety (5%), depression (5%), seizure (2% to 4%)

Dermatologic: Cutaneous mycosis (≤10%), skin infection (≤5%)

Endocrine & metabolic: Hypocalcemia (10%), hypokalemia (7% to 10%), hyponatremia (9%), menorrhagia (7%)

Gastrointestinal: Aphthosis (≤10%)

Genitourinary: Impotence (≤7%), sterility (≤5%)

Hematologic: Granulocytopenia (6%), hemorrhage (5% to 6%), secondary acute leukemias (≤3%; includes AML, APL)

Hepatic: Jaundice (3% to 7%)

Neuromuscular & skeletal: Back pain (6% to 8%), myalgia (≤5%), arthralgia (≤5%)

Ocular: Conjunctivitis (≤5%), blurred vision (≤3%)

Renal: Renal failure (≤8%), proteinuria (≤6%)

Respiratory: Rhinitis (10%), pneumonia (≤9%), sinusitis (≤6%)

Miscellaneous: Systemic infection (≤10%), diaphoresis (≤9%)

Pharmacodynamics/Kinetics

Absorption Oral: Poor

Protein Binding >95%, 76% to 78% to albumin

Half-Life Elimination Terminal: 23-215 hours (median: ~75 hours); may be prolonged with hepatic impairment

Metabolism Hepatic; pathway not determined

Excretion Feces (25%); urine (6% to 11%; 65% as unchanged drug)

Available Dosage Forms

Injection, solution [preservative free]: 2 mg/mL (10 mL, 12.5 mL, 15 mL, 20 mL)
Novantrone®: 2 mg/mL (10 mL)

Dosing

Adult & Geriatric Details concerning dosing in combination regimens should also be consulted.

Acute nonlymphocytic leukemias: I.V.:
AML induction: 12 mg/m^2 once daily for 3 days (in combination with cytarabine); for incomplete response, may repeat at 12 mg/m^2 once daily for 2 days
AML consolidation: 12 mg/m^2 once daily for 2 days (in combination with cytarabine), repeat in 4 weeks
APL consolidation phase (second course; unlabeled dosing): 10 mg/m^2 once daily for 5 days (Sanz, 2004)

Multiple sclerosis: I.V.: 12 mg/m^2 every 3 months (maximum lifetime cumulative dose: 140 mg/m^2; discontinue use with LVEF <50% or clinically significant reduction in LVEF)

Prostate cancer (advanced, hormone-refractory): I.V.: 12-14 mg/m^2 every 3 weeks (in combination with corticosteroids)

Hodgkin's lymphoma (unlabeled use): I.V.: 10 mg/m^2 every 28 days as part of a combination chemotherapy regimen (Phillips, 1990)

Non-Hodgkin's lymphoma (unlabeled use; as part of combination chemotherapy regimens): I.V.:
CNOP regimen: 10 mg/m^2 every 21 days (Bessell, 2003)
FCMR regimen: 8 mg/m^2 every 28 days (Forstpointner, 2004)
FMR regimen: 10 mg/m^2 every 21 days (Zinzani, 2004)
FND regimen: 10 mg/m^2 every 28 days (Tsimberidou, 2002)
MINE regimen: 8 mg/m^2 every 21 days (Rodriguez, 1995)

Stem cell transplantation, autologous (unlabeled use): I.V.: 60 mg/m^2 administered 4-5 days prior to autografting (in combination with other chemotherapeutic agent[s]) (Oyan, 2006; Tarella, 2001)

Pediatric Details concerning dosing in combination regimens should also be consulted.

Acute nonlymphocytic leukemias: I.V.:
AML consolidation phase (second course; unlabeled use): 10 mg/m^2 once daily for 5 days (Stevens, 1998)
APL consolidation phase (second course; unlabeled use): 10 mg/m^2 once daily for 5 days (Ortega, 2005; Sanz, 2004)

Renal Impairment Safety and efficacy have not been established.
Hemodialysis: Supplemental dose is not necessary
Peritoneal dialysis: Supplemental dose is not necessary
Elderly: Clearance is decreased in elderly patients; use with caution

Hepatic Impairment Official dosage adjustment recommendations have not been established. Clearance is reduced in hepatic dysfunction; patients with severe hepatic dysfunction (bilirubin >3.4 mg/dL) have an AUC of 3 times greater than patients with normal hepatic function. Consider dose adjustments. **Note:** MS patients with hepatic impairment should not receive mitoxantrone.

Adjustment for Toxicity
ANLL patients: Severe or life-threatening nonhematologic toxicity: Withhold treatment until toxicity resolves
MS patients:
Neutrophils <1500/mm^3: Use is not recommended.
Signs/symptoms of HF: Evaluate for cardiac signs/symptoms and LVEF.
LVEF <50% or baseline LVEF below the lower limit of normal (LLN): Use is not recommended.

Administration

I.V. Irritant (is considered a vesicant by some institutions). For I.V. administration only; do not administer intrathecally, subcutaneously, intramuscularly or intra-arterially. Must be diluted prior to use. Avoid extravasation; may cause severe local tissue damage if extravasation occurs. Usually administered as a short I.V. infusion over 5-15 minutes; do not infuse over less then 3 minutes. High doses for bone marrow transplant (unlabeled use) are usually given as 1- to 3-hour infusions.

Stability

Reconstitution Dilute in at least 50 mL of NS or D_5W.

Storage Store intact vials at 15°C to 25°C (59°F to 77°F); do not freeze. Opened vials may be stored at room temperature for 7 days or under refrigeration for up to 14 days. Solutions diluted for administration are stable for 7 days at room temperature or under refrigeration, although the manufacturer recommends immediate use.

Monitoring and Teaching Issues

Laboratory Monitoring CBC with differential, serum uric acid (for leukemia treatment), liver function tests; for the treatment of multiple sclerosis, obtain pregnancy test; monitor injection site for extravasation

Cardiac monitoring: Prior to initiation, evaluate ECG, baseline and periodic left ventricular ejection fraction (LVEF) with echocardiogram or multigated radionuclide angiography (MUGA) or MRI. In patients with MS, evaluate LVEF (using same method as baseline LVEF) prior to each dose and if signs/symptoms of HF develop. Patients with MS should undergo annual LVEF evaluation following discontinuation of therapy to monitor for delayed cardiotoxicity.

Physical Assessment Evaluate patient carefully for use-related cautions and contraindications. Infusion site must be monitored closely to prevent extravasation, which may cause severe local tissue damage. Monitor for cardiotoxicity, hypersensitivity reactions, myelosuppression, gastrointestinal upset, and opportunistic infection with each dose and throughout therapy; dosage adjustment may be necessary. Caution patients with diabetes to monitor glucose levels closely; may cause hyperglycemia.

Patient Education This drug is only administered by infusion; report any redness, swelling, burning, or pain at infusion site. Maintain adequate nutrition and hydration unless instructed to restrict fluid intake. You will be more susceptible to infection. If you have diabetes, check your glucose levels closely; may cause hyperglycemia. May cause urine, saliva, tears, sweat, and whites of eyes to turn blue-green for 24 hours postinfusion (this is normal). May cause nausea, vomiting, GI upset, mouth sores, headache, dizziness, blurred vision, or loss of hair (may be reversible). Report chest pain or palpitations, rapid or erratic heartbeat, difficulty breathing or constant cough, swelling of extremities or sudden weight gain, persistent gastrointestinal response (nausea, vomiting, diarrhea, constipation, abdominal pain), signs of opportunistic infection (eg, fever, chills, sore throat, burning on urination), or changed or decreased urine output.

Breast-Feeding Considerations Mitoxantrone is excreted in human milk and significant concentrations (18 ng/mL) have been reported for 28 days after the last administration. Because of the potential for serious adverse reactions in infants from mitoxantrone, breast-feeding should be discontinued before starting treatment.

Pregnancy Considerations Adverse effects were noted in animal studies. May cause fetal harm if administered to a pregnant woman. There are no adequate and well-controlled studies in pregnant women. Pregnancy should be avoided while on treatment. Women with multiple sclerosis and who are biologically capable of becoming pregnant should have a pregnancy test prior to each dose.

- **Mitoxantrone Dihydrochloride** *see* Mitoxantrone *on page 1244*
- **Mitoxantrone HCl** *see* Mitoxantrone *on page 1244*
- **Mitoxantrone Hydrochloride** *see* Mitoxantrone *on page 1244*
- **Mitozantrone** *see* Mitoxantrone *on page 1244*
- **Mitrazol® [OTC]** *see* Miconazole (Topical) *on page 1224*
- **MK-217** *see* Alendronate *on page 67*
- **MK383** *see* Tirofiban *on page 1774*
- **MK-0431** *see* SitaGLIPtin *on page 1652*
- **MK462** *see* Rizatriptan *on page 1603*
- **MK 0517** *see* Fosaprepitant *on page 826*
- **MK-0518** *see* Raltegravir *on page 1549*
- **MK594** *see* Losartan *on page 1133*
- **MK0826** *see* Ertapenem *on page 656*
- **MK 869** *see* Aprepitant *on page 139*
- **MLN341** *see* Bortezomib *on page 226*
- **MMF** *see* Mycophenolate *on page 1270*
- **MMR** *see* Measles, Mumps, and Rubella Virus Vaccine *on page 1150*
- **M-M-R® II** *see* Measles, Mumps, and Rubella Virus Vaccine *on page 1150*
- **MMR-V** *see* Measles, Mumps, Rubella, and Varicella Virus Vaccine *on page 1151*
- **MMRV** *see* Measles, Mumps, Rubella, and Varicella Virus Vaccine *on page 1151*
- **MOAB ABX-EGF** *see* Panitumumab *on page 1403*
- **MOAB anti-Tac** *see* Daclizumab *on page 453*
- **MOAB C225** *see* Cetuximab *on page 352*
- **MOAB HER2** *see* Trastuzumab *on page 1804*
- **Mobic®** *see* Meloxicam *on page 1159*

Modafinil (moe DAF i nil)

U.S. Brand Names Provigil®

Generic Availability (U.S.) No

Pharmacologic Category Stimulant

Medication Guide Available Yes

Pregnancy Risk Factor C

Lactation Excretion in breast milk unknown/use caution

Use Improve wakefulness in patients with excessive daytime sleepiness associated with narcolepsy and shift work sleep disorder (SWSD); adjunctive therapy for obstructive sleep apnea/hypopnea syndrome (OSAHS)

Unlabeled/Investigational Use Attention-deficit/hyperactivity disorder (ADHD); treatment of fatigue in MS and other disorders

Mechanism of Action/Effect The exact mechanism of action is unclear, it does not appear to alter the release of dopamine or norepinephrine, it may exert its stimulant effects by decreasing GABA-mediated neurotransmission, although this theory has not yet been fully evaluated; several studies also suggest that an intact central alpha-adrenergic system is required for modafinil's activity; the drug increases high-frequency alpha waves while decreasing both delta ▶

and theta wave activity, and these effects are consistent with generalized increases in mental alertness

Contraindications Hypersensitivity to modafinil, armodafinil, or any component of the formulation

Warnings/Precautions For use following complete evaluation of sleepiness and in conjunction with other standard treatments (eg, CPAP). The degree of sleepiness should be reassessed frequently; some patients may not return to a normal level of wakefulness. Use is not recommended with a history of angina, cardiac ischemia, recent history of myocardial infarction, left ventricular hypertrophy, or patients with mitral valve prolapse who have developed mitral valve prolapse syndrome with previous CNS stimulant use.

Serious and life-threatening rashes (including Stevens-Johnson syndrome and toxic epidermal necrolysis) have been reported with modafinil. Most cases have occurred within the first 5 weeks of therapy; however, rare cases have occurred after long-term use. No risk factors have been identified to predict occurrence or severity. Patients should be advised to discontinue at first sign of rash. The serious nature of these dermatologic adverse effects, as well reports of psychiatric events, resulted in the FDA's Pediatric Advisory Committee unanimously recommending that a specific warning against the use of modafinil in children be added to the manufacturer's labeling. Modafinil is not FDA-approved for use in pediatrics for any indication.

In addition, rare cases of multiorgan hypersensitivity reactions in association with modafinil use, and lone cases of angioedema and anaphylactoid reactions with armodafinil, have been reported. Signs and symptoms are diverse, reflecting the involvement of specific organs. Patients typically present with fever and rash associated with organ-system dysfunction. Patients should be advised to report any signs and symptoms related to these effects; discontinuation of therapy is recommended.

Caution should be exercised when modafinil is given to patients with a history of psychosis; may impair the ability to engage in potentially hazardous activities. Stimulants may unmask tics in individuals with coexisting Tourette's syndrome. Use caution with renal or hepatic impairment (dosage adjustment in severe hepatic dysfunction is recommended).

Drug Interactions

Metabolism/Transport Effects Substrate of CYP3A4 (major); **Inhibits** CYP1A2 (weak), 2A6 (weak), 2C9 (weak), 2C19 (strong), 2E1 (weak), 3A4 (weak); **Induces** CYP1A2 (weak), 2B6 (weak), 3A4 (weak)

Avoid Concomitant Use

Avoid concomitant use of Modafinil with any of the following: Clopidogrel; Iobenguane I 123

Decreased Effect

Modafinil may decrease the levels/effects of: Clopidogrel; Contraceptives (Estrogens); CycloSPORINE; CycloSPORINE (Systemic); Iobenguane I 123; Saxagliptin

The levels/effects of Modafinil may be decreased by: CYP3A4 Inducers (Strong); Deferasirox; Herbs (CYP3A4 Inducers)

Increased Effect/Toxicity

Modafinil may increase the levels/effects of: CYP2C19 Substrates; Sympathomimetics

The levels/effects of Modafinil may be increased by: Atomoxetine; Cannabinoids; Conivaptan; CYP3A4 Inhibitors (Moderate); CYP3A4 Inhibitors (Strong); Dasatinib

Nutritional/Ethanol Interactions

Ethanol: Avoid or limit ethanol.

Food: Delays absorption, but does not affect bioavailability.

Adverse Reactions

>10%:

Central nervous system: Headache (34%, dose related)

Gastrointestinal: Nausea (11%)

1% to 10%:

Cardiovascular: Chest pain (3%), hypertension (3%), palpitation (2%), tachycardia (2%), vasodilation (2%), edema (1%)

Central nervous system: Nervousness (7%), dizziness (5%), anxiety (5%; dose related), insomnia (5%), depression (2%), somnolence (2%), chills (1%), agitation (1%), confusion (1%), emotional lability (1%), vertigo (1%)

Dermatologic: Rash (1%; includes some severe cases requiring hospitalization)

Gastrointestinal: Diarrhea (6%), dyspepsia (5%), xerostomia (4%), anorexia (4%), constipation (2%), flatulence (1%), mouth ulceration (1%), taste perversion (1%)

Genitourinary: Abnormal urine (1%), hematuria (1%), pyuria (1%)

Hematologic: Eosinophilia (1%)

Hepatic: LFTs abnormal (2%)

Neuromuscular & skeletal: Back pain (6%), paresthesia (2%), dyskinesia (1%), hyperkinesia (1%), hypertonia (1%), neck rigidity (1%), tremor (1%)

Ocular: Amblyopia (1%), eye pain (1%), vision abnormal (1%)

Respiratory: Rhinitis (7%), pharyngitis (4%), lung disorder (2%), asthma (1%), epistaxis (1%)

Miscellaneous: Flu-like syndrome (4%), thirst (1%), diaphoresis (1%), herpes simplex infection (1%)

Pharmacodynamics/Kinetics

Time to Peak Serum: 2-4 hours

Protein Binding ~60%, primarily to albumin

Half-Life Elimination Effective half-life: 15 hours

Metabolism Hepatic; multiple pathways including CYP3A4

Excretion Urine (as metabolites, <10% as unchanged drug)

Pharmacokinetic Note Modafinil is a racemic compound (10% *d*-isomer and 90% *l*-isomer at steady state), whose enantiomers have different pharmacokinetics.

Controlled Substance C-IV

Available Dosage Forms

Tablet, oral:

Provigil®: 100 mg, 200 mg

Dosing

Adult

ADHD (unlabeled use): Oral: 100-400 mg/day (Taylor, 2000)

Narcolepsy, obstructive sleep apnea/hypopnea syndrome (OSAHS): Oral: Initial: 200 mg as a single daily dose in the morning.

Shift work sleep disorder (SWSD): Oral: Initial: 200 mg as a single dose taken ~1 hour prior to start of work shift.

Note: Doses of 400 mg/day, given as a single dose, have been well tolerated, but there is no consistent evidence that this dose confers additional benefit.

Geriatric Elimination of modafinil and its metabolites may be reduced as a consequence of aging and as a result, consider initiating at lower doses in this patient population.

Renal Impairment Safety and efficacy have not been established in severe renal impairment.

Hepatic Impairment Severe hepatic impairment: Dose should be reduced to one-half of that recommended for patients with normal liver function.

Administration

Oral For the treatment of narcolepsy and obstructive sleep apnea/hypopnea syndrome (OSAHS), administer dose in the morning. For the treatment of shift work sleep disorder (SWSD), administer dose ~1 hour prior to start of work shift.

Stability

Storage Store at 20°C to 25°C (68°F to 77°F).

Monitoring and Teaching Issues

Physical Assessment Perform careful cardiovascular assessment prior to initiating therapy.

Patient Education Avoid alcohol or caffeine. You may experience headache, nervousness, dizziness, diarrhea, dry mouth, or loss of appetite. If you have diabetes, monitor glucose levels closely. Report chest pain or palpitations, respiratory difficulty, insomnia, agitation, depression, rash, or weight loss.

Geriatric Considerations Clearance of modafinil may be reduced in the elderly. Safety and effectiveness in persons >65 years of age have not been established. In the limited number of elderly patients studied, the incidence of adverse events was similar to younger patients.

Pregnancy Considerations Embryotoxic effects have been observed in some, but not all animal studies. There are no adequate and well-controlled studies in pregnant women; use only when the potential risk of drug therapy is outweighed by the drug's benefits.

Healthcare providers are encouraged to register pregnant patients exposed to modafinil by calling 1-866-404-4106.

Efficacy of steroidal contraceptives (including depot and implantable contraceptives) may be decreased; alternate means of contraception should be considered during therapy and for 1 month after modafinil is discontinued.

◆ **Modicon®** *see* Ethinyl Estradiol and Norethindrone *on page 701*

◆ **Modified Shohl's Solution** *see* Sodium Citrate and Citric Acid *on page 1660*

Moexipril (mo EKS i pril)

U.S. Brand Names Univasc®

Index Terms Moexipril Hydrochloride

Generic Availability (U.S.) Yes

Pharmacologic Category Angiotensin-Converting Enzyme (ACE) Inhibitor

Medication Safety Issues

Sound-alike/look-alike issues:

Moexipril may be confused with Monopril®

Pregnancy Risk Factor C (1st trimester); D (2nd and 3rd trimesters)

Lactation Excretion in breast milk unknown/use caution

Use Treatment of hypertension, alone or in combination with thiazide diuretics

Mechanism of Action/Effect Competitive inhibitor of angiotensin-converting enzyme (ACE); prevents conversion of angiotensin I to angiotensin II, a potent vasoconstrictor; results in lower levels of angiotensin II which causes an increase in plasma renin activity and a reduction in aldosterone secretion

Contraindications Hypersensitivity to moexipril or any component of the formulation; angioedema related to previous treatment with an ACE inhibitor

Warnings/Precautions Anaphylactic reactions may occur rarely with ACE inhibitors. At any time during treatment (especially following first dose) angioedema may occur rarely with ACE inhibitors; it may involve the head and neck (potentially compromising airway) or the intestine (presenting with abdominal pain). African-Americans and patients with idiopathic or hereditary angioedema may be at an increased risk. Prolonged frequent monitoring may be required especially if tongue, glottis, or larynx are involved as they are associated with airway obstruction. Patients with a history of airway surgery may have a higher risk of airway obstruction. Aggressive early and appropriate management is critical. Use in patients with previous angioedema associated with ACE inhibitor therapy is contraindicated. Severe anaphylactoid reactions may be seen during hemodialysis (eg, CVVHD) with high-flux dialysis membranes (eg, AN69), and rarely, during low density lipoprotein apheresis with dextran sulfate cellulose. Rare cases of anaphylactoid reactions have been reported in patients undergoing sensitization treatment with hymenoptera (bee, wasp) venom while receiving ACE inhibitors.

Symptomatic hypotension with or without syncope can occur with ACE inhibitors (usually with the first several doses); effects are most often observed in volume depleted patients; correct volume depletion prior to initiation; close monitoring of patient is required especially with initial dosing and dosing increases; blood pressure must be lowered at a rate appropriate for the patient's clinical condition. Initiation of therapy in patients with ischemic heart disease or cerebrovascular disease warrants close observation due to the potential consequences posed by falling blood pressure (eg, MI, stroke). Use with caution in hypertrophic cardiomyopathy with outflow tract obstruction, severe aortic stenosis, or before, during, or immediately after major surgery. **[U.S. Boxed Warning]: Based on human data, ACEIs can cause injury and death to the developing fetus when used in the second and third trimesters. ACEIs should be discontinued as soon as possible once pregnancy is detected.**

Hyperkalemia may occur with ACE inhibitors; risk factors include renal dysfunction, diabetes mellitus, concomitant use of potassium-sparing diuretics, potassium supplements, and/or potassium-containing salts. Use cautiously, if at all, with these agents and monitor potassium closely. Cough may occur with ACE inhibitors. Other causes of cough should be considered (eg, pulmonary congestion in patients with heart failure) and excluded prior to discontinuation.

May be associated with deterioration of renal function and/or increases in serum creatinine, particularly in patients with low renal blood flow (eg, renal artery stenosis, heart failure) whose glomerular filtration rate (GFR) is dependent on efferent arteriolar vasoconstriction by angiotensin II; deterioration may result in oliguria, acute renal failure, and progressive azotemia. Small increases in serum creatinine may occur following initiation; consider discontinuation only in patients with progressive and/or significant deterioration in renal function. Use with caution in patients with unstented unilateral/bilateral renal artery stenosis. When unstented bilateral renal artery stenosis is present, use is generally avoided due to the elevated risk of deterioration in renal function unless possible benefits outweigh risks. Concurrent use of angiotensin receptor blockers may increase the risk of clinically-significant adverse events (eg, renal dysfunction, hyperkalemia).

Rare toxicities associated with ACE inhibitors include cholestatic jaundice (which may progress to fulminant hepatic necrosis), agranulocytosis, neutropenia, or leukopenia with myeloid hypoplasia. Patients with collagen vascular diseases (especially with concomitant renal impairment) or renal impairment alone may be at increased risk for hematologic toxicity; periodically monitor CBC with differential in these patients.

Drug Interactions

Avoid Concomitant Use There are no known interactions where it is recommended to avoid concomitant use.

Decreased Effect

The levels/effects of Moexipril may be decreased by: Antacids; Aprotinin; Herbs (Hypertensive Properties); Methylphenidate; Nonsteroidal Anti-Inflammatory Agents; Salicylates; Yohimbine

Increased Effect/Toxicity

Moexipril may increase the levels/effects of: Allopurinol; Amifostine; Antihypertensives; AzaTHIOprine; CycloSPORINE; CycloSPORINE (Systemic); Ferric Gluconate; Gold Sodium Thiomalate; Hypotensive Agents; Iron Dextran Complex; Lithium; RiTUXimab

The levels/effects of Moexipril may be increased by: Angiotensin II Receptor Blockers; Diazoxide; DPP-IV Inhibitors; Eplerenone; Everolimus; Herbs (Hypotensive Properties); Loop Diuretics; MAO Inhibitors; Pentoxifylline; Phosphodiesterase 5 Inhibitors; Potassium Salts; Potassium-Sparing Diuretics; Prostacyclin Analogues; Sirolimus; Temsirolimus; Thiazide Diuretics; TiZANidine; Tolvaptan; Trimethoprim

Nutritional/Ethanol Interactions

Food: Food may delay and reduce peak serum levels.

Herb/Nutraceutical: Avoid bayberry, blue cohosh, cayenne, ephedra, ginger, ginseng (American), kola, licorice (may worsen hypertension). Avoid black cohosh, California poppy, coleus, golden seal, hawthorn, mistletoe, periwinkle, quinine, shepherd's purse (may have increased antihypertensive effect).

Lab Interactions Increased BUN, creatinine, potassium, positive Coombs' [direct]; decreased cholesterol (S); may cause false-positive results in urine acetone determinations using sodium nitroprusside reagent

Adverse Reactions 1% to 10%:

Cardiovascular: Hypotension, peripheral edema
Central nervous system: Headache, dizziness, fatigue
Dermatologic: Flushing, rash
Endocrine & metabolic: Hyperkalemia, hyponatremia
Gastrointestinal: Diarrhea, nausea, heartburn
Genitourinary: Polyuria
Neuromuscular & skeletal: Myalgia
Renal: Reversible increases in creatinine or BUN
Respiratory: Cough, pharyngitis, upper respiratory infection, sinusitis

Pharmacodynamics/Kinetics

Onset of Action Peak effect: 1-2 hours

Duration of Action >24 hours

Absorption Incomplete

Bioavailability Moexiprilat: 13%; reduced with food (AUC decreased by ~40%)

Time to Peak 1.5 hours

Protein Binding Plasma: Moexipril: 90%; Moexiprilat: 50% to 70%

Half-Life Elimination Moexipril: 1 hour; Moexiprilat: 2-9 hours

Metabolism Parent drug: Hepatic and via GI tract to moexiprilat, 1000 times more potent than parent

Excretion Feces (50%)

Available Dosage Forms

Tablet, oral: 7.5 mg, 15 mg

Univasc®: 7.5 mg, 15 mg

Dosing

Adult Hypertension: Oral: Initial: 7.5 mg once daily (in patients **not** receiving diuretics), 1 hour prior to a meal **or** 3.75 mg once daily (when combined with thiazide diuretics); maintenance dose: 7.5-30 mg/day in 1 or 2 divided doses 1 hour before meals

Geriatric Dose the same as adults; adjust for renal impairment. Tablet may be cut in half (3.75 mg) for starting therapy (see Renal Impairment).

Renal Impairment Cl_{cr} ≤40 mL/minute: Patients may be cautiously placed on 3.75 mg once daily, then upwardly titrated to a maximum of 15 mg/day.

Administration

Oral Administer on an empty stomach.

Monitoring and Teaching Issues

Laboratory Monitoring Serum creatinine and potassium; if patient has collagen vascular disease and/or renal impairment, periodically monitor CBC with differential

Physical Assessment Assess potential for interactions with other pharmacological agents or herbal products that may impact fluid balance or cardiac status. Patient should be monitored closely for anaphylactic reaction or angioedema which can occur at any time during treatment and may involve head and neck. Evaluate blood pressure. Monitor for hypotension, rash, diarrhea, myalgia, and electrolyte imbalance regularly during therapy.

Patient Education Do not use potassium supplements or salt substitutes without consulting prescriber. Take first dose at bedtime. Take all doses on an empty stomach, 1 hour before or 2 hours after meals. This drug does not eliminate need for diet or exercise regimen as recommended by prescriber. May cause dizziness, fainting, lightheadedness, postural hypotension, nausea, vomiting, abdominal pain, dry mouth, or transient loss of appetite. Report immediately unusual swelling of mouth, tongue, face, or throat. Report respiratory difficulty or unusual cough, rash, excessive urination, chest pain or palpitations, mouth sores, fever or chills, numbness, or tingling or pain in muscles.

Dietary Considerations Take on an empty stomach.

Geriatric Considerations Due to frequent decreases in glomerular filtration (also creatinine clearance) with aging, elderly patients may have exaggerated responses to ACE inhibitors; differences in clinical response due to hepatic changes are not observed. ACE inhibitors may be preferred agents in elderly patients with congestive heart failure and diabetes mellitus. Diabetic proteinuria is reduced and insulin sensitivity is enhanced. In general, the side effect profile is favorable in the elderly and causes little or no CNS confusion; use lowest dose recommendations initially; adjust dose for renal function in the elderly. Many elderly may be volume depleted due to diuretic use and/or blunted thirst reflex resulting in inadequate fluid intake.

Breast-Feeding Considerations It is not known if moexipril is excreted into breast milk. The manufacturer recommends that caution be exercised when administering moexipril to nursing women.

Pregnancy Considerations Due to adverse events observed in some animal studies, moexipril is considered pregnancy category C during the first trimester. Based on human data, moexipril is considered pregnancy category D if used during the second and third trimesters (per the manufacturer; however, one study suggests that fetal injury may occur at anytime during pregnancy). First trimester exposure to ACE inhibitors may cause major congenital malformations. An increased risk of cardiovascular and/or central nervous system malformations was observed in one study; however, an increased risk of teratogenic events was not observed in other studies. Second and third trimester use of an ACE inhibitor is associated with oligohydramnios. Oligohydramnios due to decreased fetal renal function may lead to fetal limb contractures, craniofacial deformation, and hypoplastic lung development. The use of ACE inhibitors during the second and third trimesters is also associated with anuria, hypotension, renal failure (reversible or irreversible), skull hypoplasia, and death in the fetus/neonate. Chronic maternal hypertension itself is also associated with adverse events in the fetus/infant. ACE inhibitors are not recommended during pregnancy to treat maternal hypertension or heart failure. Those who are planning a pregnancy should be considered for other medication options if an ACE inhibitor is currently prescribed or the ACE inhibitor should be discontinued as soon as possible once pregnancy is detected. The exposed fetus should be monitored for fetal growth, amniotic fluid volume, and organ formation. Infants exposed to an ACE inhibitor *in utero*, especially during the second and third trimester, should be monitored for hyperkalemia, hypotension, and oliguria

[U.S. Boxed Warning]: Based on human data, ACE inhibitors can cause injury and death to the developing fetus when used in the second and third trimesters. ACE inhibitors should be discontinued as soon as possible once pregnancy is detected.

Related Information

Angiotensin Agents *on page* 1974

Moexipril and Hydrochlorothiazide (mo EKS i pril & hye droe klor oh THYE a zide)

U.S. Brand Names Uniretic®

Index Terms Hydrochlorothiazide and Moexipril

Generic Availability (U.S.) Yes

Pharmacologic Category Angiotensin-Converting Enzyme (ACE) Inhibitor; Diuretic, Thiazide

Pregnancy Risk Factor C/D (2nd and 3rd trimesters)

Lactation Enters breast milk/use caution

Use Treatment of hypertension; not indicated for initial treatment of hypertension

Available Dosage Forms

Tablet, oral: 7.5/12.5: Moexipril 7.5 mg and hydrochlorothiazide 12.5; 15/12.5: Moexipril 15 mg and hydrochlorothiazide 12.5; 15/25: Moexipril 15 mg and hydrochlorothiazide 25

Uniretic®: 7.5/12.5: Moexipril 7.5 mg and hydrochlorothiazide 12.5 mg [scored]; 15/12.5: Moexipril 15 mg and hydrochlorothiazide 12.5 mg [scored]; 15/25: Moexipril 15 mg and hydrochlorothiazide 25 mg [scored]

Dosing

Adult Hypertension: Oral: 7.5-30 mg of moexipril, taken either in a single or divided dose 1 hour before meals; hydrochlorothiazide dose should be ≤50 mg/day

Geriatric Overall safety and efficacy are not different in elderly patients, although a higher moexipril AUC was observed in elderly patients. Greater sensitivity to effects may be observed in some older individuals. Refer to adult dosing.

Monitoring and Teaching Issues

Laboratory Monitoring BUN, serum creatinine, and electrolytes; if patient has collagen vascular disease and/or renal impairment, periodically monitor CBC with differential

Physical Assessment See individual agents.

Patient Education See individual agents.

Related Information

Hydrochlorothiazide *on page* 912

Moexipril *on page* 1249

◆ **Moexipril Hydrochloride** *see* Moexipril *on page* 1249

Mometasone (Oral Inhalation) (moe MET a sone)

U.S. Brand Names Asmanex® Twisthaler®

Index Terms Mometasone Furoate

Generic Availability (U.S.) No

Pharmacologic Category Corticosteroid, Inhalant (Oral)

Pregnancy Risk Factor C

Lactation Excretion in breast milk unknown/use caution

Use Maintenance treatment of asthma as prophylactic therapy

Mechanism of Action/Effect Blocks inflammation; reverses capillary permeability and release of inflammatory mediators (leukotrienes and prostaglandins); suppresses migration of polymorphonuclear leukocytes.

Contraindications Hypersensitivity to mometasone or any component of the formulation; hypersensitivity to milk proteins; primary treatment of status asthmaticus or acute bronchospasm

Warnings/Precautions May cause hypercorticism or suppression of hypothalamic-pituitary-adrenal (HPA) axis, particularly in younger children or in patients receiving high doses for prolonged periods. HPA axis suppression may lead to adrenal crisis. Withdrawal and discontinuation of a corticosteroid should be done slowly and carefully. Particular care is required when patients are transferred from systemic corticosteroids to inhaled products due to possible adrenal insufficiency or withdrawal from steroids, including an increase in allergic symptoms. Patients receiving >20 mg per day of prednisone (or equivalent) may be most susceptible. Fatalities have occurred due to adrenal insufficiency in asthmatic patients during and after transfer from systemic corticosteroids to aerosol steroids; aerosol steroids do not provide the systemic steroid needed to treat patients having trauma, surgery, or infections. When transferring to oral inhaler, previously-suppressed allergic conditions (rhinitis, conjunctivitis, eczema) may be unmasked.

Bronchospasm may occur with wheezing after inhalation; if this occurs, stop steroid and treat with a fast-acting bronchodilator. Supplemental steroids (oral or parenteral) may be needed during stress or severe asthma attacks. Not to be used in status asthmaticus or for the relief of acute bronchospasm. Corticosteroid use may cause psychiatric disturbances, including depression, euphoria, insomnia, mood swings, and personality changes. Pre-existing psychiatric conditions may be exacerbated by corticosteroid use. Prolonged use of corticosteroids may also increase the incidence of secondary infection, mask acute infection (including fungal infections), prolong or exacerbate viral infections, or limit response to vaccines. Exposure to chickenpox should be avoided; corticosteroids should not be used to treat ocular herpes simplex. Corticosteroids should not be used for cerebral malaria or viral hepatitis. Close observation is required in patients with latent tuberculosis and/or TB reactivity; restrict use in active TB (only in conjunction with antituberculosis treatment). Prolonged treatment with corticosteroids has been associated with the development of Kaposi's sarcoma (case reports); if noted, discontinuation of therapy should be considered. Local oropharyngeal *Candida* infections have been reported; if occurs treat appropriately while continuing mometasone therapy. Patients should be instructed to rinse mouth after each use.

Reactions including, anaphylaxis, angioedema, pruritus, and rash have been reported; if these symptoms occur discontinue use. Use with caution in patients with thyroid disease, hepatic impairment, renal impairment, cardiovascular disease, diabetes, glaucoma, cataracts, myasthenia gravis, patients with or who are at risk for osteoporosis, patients at risk for seizures, or GI diseases (diverticulitis, peptic ulcer, ulcerative colitis) due to perforation risk. Use caution following acute MI (corticosteroids have been associated with myocardial rupture). Because of the risk of adverse effects, systemic corticosteroids should be used cautiously in the elderly in the smallest possible effective dose for the shortest duration.

Orally-inhaled corticosteroids may cause a reduction in growth velocity in pediatric patients (~1 centimeter per year [range: 0.3-1.8 cm per year] and related to dose and duration of exposure). To minimize the systemic effects of orally-inhaled corticosteroids, each patient should be titrated to the lowest effective dose. Growth should be routinely monitored in pediatric patients. Prior to use, the dose and duration of treatment should be based on the risk versus benefit for each individual patient. In general, use the smallest effective dose for the shortest duration of time to minimize adverse events. A gradual tapering of dose may be required prior to discontinuing therapy. There have been reports of systemic corticosteroid withdrawal symptoms (eg, joint/ muscle pain, lassitude, depression) when withdrawing inhalation therapy. May contain lactose; very rare anaphylactic reactions have been reported in patients with severe milk protein allergy.

Drug Interactions

Metabolism/Transport Effects Substrate of CYP3A4 (minor)

Avoid Concomitant Use

Avoid concomitant use of Mometasone (Oral Inhalation) with any of the following: Aldesleukin

Decreased Effect

Mometasone (Oral Inhalation) may decrease the levels/effects of: Aldesleukin; Antidiabetic Agents; Corticorelin

Increased Effect/Toxicity

Mometasone (Oral Inhalation) may increase the levels/effects of: Amphotericin B; Loop Diuretics; Thiazide Diuretics

The levels/effects of Mometasone (Oral Inhalation) may be increased by: CYP3A4 Inhibitors (Strong)

Adverse Reactions

>10%:

Central nervous system: Headache (17% to 22%), fatigue (1% to 13%), depression (11%)
Neuromuscular & skeletal: Musculoskeletal pain (4% to 22%), arthralgia (13%)
Respiratory: Sinusitis (5% to 22%), rhinitis (4% to 20%), upper respiratory infection (8% to 15%), pharyngitis (8% to 13%)
Miscellaneous: Oral candidiasis (4% to 22%)

1% to 10%:

Central nervous system: Fever (children 7%), pain (1% to <3%)
Dermatologic: Bruising (children 2%)
Gastrointestinal: Abdominal pain (2% to 6%), dyspepsia (3% to 5%), nausea (1% to 3%), vomiting (1% to ≤3%), anorexia (1% to <3%), dry throat (1% to <3%), gastroenteritis (1% to <3%)
Genitourinary: Dysmenorrhea (4% to 9%), urinary tract infection (children 2%)
Neuromuscular & skeletal: Back pain (3% to 6%), myalgia (2% to 3%)
Ocular: Ocular pressure increased (3%), cataracts (1%)
Otic: Earache (1% to <3%)
Respiratory: Sinus congestion (9%), dysphonia (1% to <3%), epistaxis (1% to <3%), nasal irritation (1% to <3%)
Miscellaneous: Flu-like syndrome (1% to <3%), infection (1% to <3%)

Pharmacodynamics/Kinetics

Absorption <1%

Protein Binding 98% to 99%

Half-Life Elimination 5 hours

Metabolism Hepatic via CYP3A4; forms metabolite

Excretion Feces, bile, urine

Available Dosage Forms

Powder, for oral inhalation:

Asmanex® Twisthaler®: 110 mcg (30 units); 220 mcg (14 units, 30 units, 60 units, 120 units)

Dosing

Adult & Geriatric Asthma: Oral inhalation:

Bronchodilators or inhaled corticosteroids: Initial: 1 inhalation (220 mcg) daily (maximum: 2 inhalations or 440 mcg/day); may be given in the evening or in divided doses twice daily
Oral corticosteroids: Initial: 440 mcg twice daily (maximum: 880 mcg/day); prednisone should be reduced no faster than 2.5 mg/day on a weekly basis, beginning after at least 1 week of mometasone furoate use

NIH Asthma Guidelines (NIH, 2007):
"Low" dose: 220 mcg/day
"Medium" dose: 440 mcg/day
"High" dose: >440 mcg/day

Note: Maximum effects may not be evident for 1-2 weeks or longer; dose should be titrated to effect, using the lowest possible dose

Pediatric Asthma: Oral inhalation:
Children 4-11 years: 110 mcg once daily in the evening (maximum 110 mcg/day)
Children ≥12 years: Refer to adult dosing.

Administration

Inhalation Exhale fully prior to bringing the Twisthaler® up to the mouth. Place between lips and inhale quickly and deeply. Do not breathe out through the inhaler. Remove inhaler and hold breath for 10 seconds if possible. Rinse mouth after use.

Stability

Storage Store at 25°C (77°F); excursions permitted to 15°C to 30°C (59°F to 86°F). Discard when oral dose counter reads "00" (or 45 days after opening the foil pouch).

Monitoring and Teaching Issues

Physical Assessment Long-term use: Assess for glaucoma and cataracts periodically. Monitor growth in pediatric patients.

Patient Education Not a bronchodilator and not indicated for the acute relief of bronchospasm. May take 1-2 weeks before effects of medication are seen. Avoid exposure to chickenpox or measles. Consult prescriber immediately if exposure does occur. Discard inhaler 45 days after opening foil pouch or when dose counter reads "00." Rinse mouth after using. Keep the inhaler clean and dry.

Dietary Considerations Asmanex® Twisthaler® contains lactose.

Breast-Feeding Considerations Systemic corticosteroids are excreted in human milk; however, information for mometasone is not available. The use of inhaled corticosteroids is not considered a contraindication to breast-feeding.

Pregnancy Considerations Adverse events were observed in animal studies following topical and SubQ administration. Hypoadrenalism may occur in infants born to women receiving corticosteroids during pregnancy. Monitor these infants closely after birth. A decrease in fetal growth has not been observed with inhaled corticosteroid use during pregnancy. Inhaled corticosteroids are recommended for the treatment of asthma (most information available using budesonide) during pregnancy.

Related Information

Asthma *on page 2015*
Corticosteroids *on page 1996*

Mometasone (Nasal) (moe MET a sone)

U.S. Brand Names Nasonex®

Index Terms Mometasone Furoate

Generic Availability (U.S.) No

Pharmacologic Category Corticosteroid, Nasal

Pregnancy Risk Factor C

Lactation Excretion in breast milk unknown/use caution

Use Treatment of nasal symptoms of seasonal and perennial allergic rhinitis; prevention of nasal symptoms associated with seasonal allergic rhinitis; treatment of nasal polyps in adults

Mechanism of Action/Effect Reverses capillary permeability and release of inflammatory mediators (leukotrienes and prostaglandins); suppresses migration of polymorphonuclear leukocytes.

Contraindications Hypersensitivity to mometasone or any component of the formulation

Warnings/Precautions Avoid nasal corticosteroid use in patients with recent nasal septal ulcers, nasal surgery or nasal trauma until healing has occurred. Prolonged use of corticosteroids may also increase the incidence of secondary infection, mask acute infection (including fungal infections), prolong or exacerbate viral infections, or limit response to vaccines. Exposure to chickenpox should be avoided.

Prior to use, the dose and duration of treatment should be based on the risk versus benefit for each individual patient. In general, use the smallest effective dose for the shortest duration of time to minimize adverse events. A gradual tapering of dose may be required prior to discontinuing therapy. When recommended doses are exceeded, or in extremely sensitive individuals may cause hypercorticism or suppression of hypothalamic-pituitary-adrenal (HPA) axis. Reports consistent with hypercorticism are rare. HPA axis suppression may lead to adrenal crisis. Withdrawal and discontinuation of a corticosteroid should be done slowly and carefully. Fatalities have occurred due to adrenal insufficiency in asthmatic patients during and after transfer from systemic corticosteroids to aerosol steroids; aerosol steroids do **not** provide the systemic steroid needed to treat patients having trauma, surgery, or infections. Use with caution in patients with cataracts and/or glaucoma; increased intraocular pressure, open-angle glaucoma, and cataracts have occurred with prolonged use. Consider routine eye exams in chronic users.

Orally-inhaled and intranasal corticosteroids may cause a reduction in growth velocity in pediatric patients (~1 centimeter per year [range: 0.3-1.8 cm per year] and related to dose and duration of exposure). To minimize the systemic effects of orally-inhaled and intranasal corticosteroids, each patient should be titrated to the lowest effective dose. Growth should be routinely monitored in pediatric patients.

Drug Interactions

Metabolism/Transport Effects Substrate of CYP3A4 (minor)

Avoid Concomitant Use There are no known interactions where it is recommended to avoid concomitant use.

Decreased Effect

Mometasone (Nasal) may decrease the levels/effects of: Corticorelin

Increased Effect/Toxicity

The levels/effects of Mometasone (Nasal) may be increased by: Conivaptan

Adverse Reactions

>10%:

Central nervous system: Headache (17% to 26%)

Respiratory: Pharyngitis (8% to 13%), cough (nasal inhalation 7% to 13%), epistaxis (1% to 11%)

Miscellaneous: Viral infection (nasal inhalation 8% to 14%)

1% to 10%:

Gastrointestinal: Diarrhea, dyspepsia, vomiting

Genitourinary: Dysmenorrhea

Neuromuscular & skeletal: Musculoskeletal pain, myalgia

Ocular: Conjunctivitis

Otic: Otitis media

Respiratory: Asthma, nasal irritation, rhinitis, sinusitis, upper respiratory infection, wheezing

Miscellaneous: Flu-like syndrome

Available Dosage Forms

Suspension, intranasal:

Nasonex®: 50 mcg/spray (17 g)

Dosing

Adult & Geriatric

Seasonal and perennial allergic rhinitis: Intranasal:

Treatment: 2 sprays (100 mcg) in each nostril daily

Prevention: 2 sprays (100 mcg) in each nostril daily beginning 2-4 weeks prior to pollen season

Treatment of nasal polyps: Intranasal: 2 sprays (100 mcg) in each nostril twice daily; 2 sprays (100 mcg) once daily may be effective in some patients

Pediatric Treatment of seasonal and perennial allergic rhinitis treatment: Intranasal:

Children 2-11 years: 1 spray (50 mcg) in each nostril daily

Children ≥12 years: Refer to adult dosing.

Administration

Inhalation Shake well prior to use. Prior to first use, prime pump by actuating 10 times or until fine spray appears; may store for a maximum of 1 week without repriming. Spray should be administered once or twice daily, at a regular interval.

Stability

Storage Store at room temperature of 15°C to 30°C (59°F to 86°F). Protect from light.

Monitoring and Teaching Issues

Physical Assessment Monitor growth with long-term use in pediatric patients.

Patient Education Gently blow your nose to clear nostrils prior to use. You may experience headache, cough, or nosebleed. Report unusual chest pain, gastrointestinal upset, muscle pain, flu-like symptoms, worsening of condition, or failure to improve.

Breast-Feeding Considerations Systemic corticosteroids are excreted in human milk; however, information for mometasone is not available. The use of inhaled corticosteroids is not considered a contraindication to breast-feeding.

Pregnancy Considerations Adverse events were observed in animal studies following topical and SubQ administration. Hypoadrenalism may occur in infants born to women receiving corticosteroids during pregnancy. Monitor these infants closely after birth. A decrease in fetal growth has not been observed with inhaled corticosteroid use during pregnancy. Inhaled corticosteroids are recommended for the treatment of allergic rhinitis during pregnancy.

Related Information

Corticosteroids *on page 1996*

Mometasone (Topical) (moe MET a sone)

U.S. Brand Names Elocon®

Index Terms Mometasone Furoate

Generic Availability (U.S.) Yes

Pharmacologic Category Corticosteroid, Topical

Medication Safety Issues

Sound-alike/look-alike issues:

Elocon® lotion may be confused with ophthalmic solutions. Manufacturer's labeling emphasizes the product is **NOT** for use in the eyes.

Pregnancy Risk Factor C

Lactation Excretion in breast milk unknown/use caution

Use Relief of the inflammatory and pruritic manifestations of corticosteroid-responsive dermatoses (medium potency topical corticosteroid)

Available Dosage Forms

Cream, topical: 0.1% (15 g, 45 g)
Elocon®: 0.1% (15 g, 45 g)

Lotion, topical: 0.1% (30 mL, 60 mL)
Elocon®: 0.1% (30 mL, 60 mL)

Ointment, topical: 0.1% (15 g, 45 g)
Elocon®: 0.1% (15 g, 45 g)

Dosing

Adult & Geriatric Treatment of corticosteroid-responsive dermatoses: Topical: Apply sparingly, do not use occlusive dressings. Therapy should be discontinued when control is achieved; if no improvement is seen in 2 weeks, reassessment of diagnosis may be necessary.

Cream, ointment: Apply a thin film to affected area once daily

Lotion: Apply a few drops to affected area once daily

Pediatric Treatment of corticosteroid-responsive dermatoses: Topical:

Cream, ointment: Children ≥2 years: Refer to adult dosing. Do not use in pediatric patients for longer than 3 weeks.

Lotion: Children ≥12 years: Refer to adult dosing.

Administration

Topical Apply sparingly; avoid eyes, face, underarms, and groin. Do not wrap or bandage affected area.

Monitoring and Teaching Issues

Patient Education Do not use for eyes, mucous membranes, or open wounds. Before using, wash and dry area gently. Apply in a thin layer (cream, ointment) or a few drops (lotion) and rub in lightly. Apply light dressing (if necessary) to area being treated. Do not use occlusive dressing unless so advised by prescriber. Avoid prolonged or excessive use around sensitive tissues, underarms, genital, or rectal areas. Avoid exposing treated area to direct sunlight (severe sunburn may occur). Inform prescriber if condition worsens (redness, swelling, irritation, signs of infection, or open sores) or fails to improve.

Related Information

Corticosteroids *on page 1996*

- **Mometasone Furoate** *see* Mometasone (Nasal) *on page 1254*
- **Mometasone Furoate** *see* Mometasone (Oral Inhalation) *on page 1252*
- **Mometasone Furoate** *see* Mometasone (Topical) *on page 1255*
- **Monacolin K** *see* Lovastatin *on page 1138*
- **Monarc-M™** *see* Antihemophilic Factor (Human) *on page 132*
- **Monistat® 1 [OTC]** *see* Miconazole (Topical) *on page 1224*
- **Monistat® 1 Day or Night [OTC]** *see* Miconazole (Topical) *on page 1224*
- **Monistat® 3 [OTC]** *see* Miconazole (Topical) *on page 1224*
- **Monistat® 7 [OTC]** *see* Miconazole (Topical) *on page 1224*
- **Monoclate-P®** *see* Antihemophilic Factor (Human) *on page 132*
- **Monoclonal Antibody** *see* Muromonab-CD3 *on page 1268*
- **Monoclonal Antibody ABX-EGF** *see* Panitumumab *on page 1403*
- **Monodox®** *see* Doxycycline *on page 586*
- **Monoket®** *see* Isosorbide Mononitrate *on page 1029*
- **MonoNessa®** *see* Ethinyl Estradiol and Norgestimate *on page 704*
- **Monopril** *see* Fosinopril *on page 831*

Montelukast (mon te LOO kast)

U.S. Brand Names Singulair®

Index Terms Montelukast Sodium

Generic Availability (U.S.) No

Pharmacologic Category Leukotriene-Receptor Antagonist

Medication Safety Issues

Sound-alike/look-alike issues:
Singulair® may be confused with SINEquan®

Pregnancy Risk Factor B

Lactation Excretion in breast milk unknown/use caution

Use Prophylaxis and chronic treatment of asthma; relief of symptoms of seasonal allergic rhinitis and perennial allergic rhinitis; prevention of exercise-induced bronchospasm

Unlabeled/Investigational Use Acute asthma

Mechanism of Action/Effect Montelukast is a selective leukotriene receptor antagonist which inhibits cysteinyl leukotriene. Leukotrienes are responsible for edema and smooth muscle contraction that is felt to be associated with the signs and symptoms of asthma. Cysteinyl leukotrienes are also released following allergen exposure leading to symptoms associated with allergic rhinitis.

Contraindications Hypersensitivity to montelukast or any component of the formulation

Warnings/Precautions Montelukast is not FDA approved for use in the reversal of bronchospasm in acute asthma attacks, including status asthmaticus; some clinicians, however, support its use as adjunctive therapy (Camargo, 2003; Cylly, 2003; Ferreira, 2001; Harmancik 2006). Appropriate rescue medication should be available. Appropriate clinical monitoring and caution are recommended when systemic corticosteroid reduction is considered in patients receiving montelukast. Patients should be instructed to notify prescriber if behavioral changes occur. Inform phenylketonuric patients that the chewable tablet contains phenylalanine.

In rare cases, patients on therapy with montelukast may present with systemic eosinophilia, sometimes presenting with clinical features of vasculitis consistent with Churg-Strauss syndrome, a condition which is often treated with systemic corticosteroid therapy. Healthcare providers should be alert to eosinophilia, vasculitic rash, worsening pulmonary symptoms, cardiac complications, and/or neuropathy presenting in their patients. A causal association between montelukast and these underlying conditions has not been established. Montelukast will not interrupt bronchoconstrictor response to aspirin or other NSAIDs; aspirin sensitive asthmatics should continue to avoid these agents. Postmarketing reports of behavior changes (agitation, aggression, depression, insomnia) have been noted in children and adults.

Drug Interactions

Metabolism/Transport Effects Substrate (major) of CYP2C9, 3A4; **Inhibits** CYP2C8 (weak), 2C9 (weak)

Avoid Concomitant Use There are no known interactions where it is recommended to avoid concomitant use.

Decreased Effect

The levels/effects of Montelukast may be decreased by: CYP2C9 Inducers (Highly Effective); CYP3A4 Inducers (Strong); Deferasirox; Herbs (CYP3A4 Inducers); Peginterferon Alfa-2b

Increased Effect/Toxicity

The levels/effects of Montelukast may be increased by: Conivaptan; CYP2C9 Inhibitors (Moderate); CYP2C9 Inhibitors (Strong)

Nutritional/Ethanol Interactions Herb/Nutraceutical: St John's wort may decrease montelukast levels.

Adverse Reactions Note: Percentages and adverse events as reported in adults: 1% to 10%:

Central nervous system: Dizziness (2%), fatigue (2%), fever (2%), headache (≥1%)
Dermatologic: Rash (2%)
Gastrointestinal: Dyspepsia (2%), dental pain (2%), gastroenteritis (2%)
Hepatic: AST increased (2%), ALT increased (≥1%)
Neuromuscular & skeletal: Weakness (2%)
Respiratory: Cough (≥1%), nasal congestion (2%), epistaxis (≥1%), sinusitis (≥1%), upper respiratory infection (≥1%)

Pharmacodynamics/Kinetics

Duration of Action >24 hours

Absorption Rapid

Bioavailability Tablet: 10 mg: Mean: 64%; 5 mg: 63% to 73%

Time to Peak Serum: Tablet: 10 mg: 3-4 hours; 5 mg: 2-2.5 hours; 4 mg: 2 hours

Protein Binding Plasma: >99%

Half-Life Elimination Plasma: Mean: 2.7-5.5 hours

Metabolism Extensively hepatic via CYP3A4 and 2C9

Excretion Feces (86%); urine (<0.2%)

Available Dosage Forms

Granules, oral:
Singulair®: 4 mg/packet (30s)

Tablet, oral:
Singulair®: 10 mg

Tablet, chewable, oral:
Singulair®: 4 mg, 5 mg

Dosing

Adult & Geriatric

Asthma, allergic seasonal or perennial rhinitis: Oral: 10 mg once daily

Asthma, acute (unlabeled use): 10 mg as a single dose administered with first-line therapy (Camargo, 2003; Cylly, 2003)

Bronchoconstriction, exercise-induced (prevention): 10 mg at least 2 hours prior to exercise; additional doses should not be administered within 24 hours. Daily administration to prevent exercise-induced bronchoconstriction has not been evaluated.

Pediatric

Asthma: Oral: *12-23 months:* 4 mg (oral granules) once daily, taken in the evening

Seasonal or perennial allergic rhinitis: Oral: *6-23 months:* 4 mg (oral granules) once daily

Asthma, seasonal or perennial allergic rhinitis: Oral:
2-5 years: 4 mg (chewable tablet or oral granules) once daily
6-14 years: 5 mg (chewable tablet) once daily
≥15 years: Refer to adult dosing.

Renal Impairment No adjustment is necessary.

Hepatic Impairment No adjustment necessary in mild-to-moderate hepatic disease. Patients with severe hepatic disease were **not** studied.

Administration

Oral When treating asthma, administer dose in the evening. Patients with allergic rhinitis may individualize administration time (morning or evening). Patients with both asthma and allergic rhinitis should take their dose in the evening. Granules may be administered directly in the mouth or mixed with a spoonful of applesauce, carrots, rice, ice cream, baby formula, or breast milk; do not add to any other liquids or foods. Administer within 15 minutes of opening packet. May administer without regard to meals.

Stability

Storage Store at room temperature of 25°C (77°F); excursions permitted to 15°C to 30°C (59°F to 86°F).

Granules: Store in original package; use within 15 minutes of opening packet.

Monitoring and Teaching Issues

Physical Assessment Not for use in acute asthma attacks, including status asthmaticus. Monitor mental and mood status. Be alert to signs of depression, hallucinations, irritability, agitation, and suicide ideation.

Patient Education Do not stop other asthma medication unless advised by prescriber. Chewable tablet contains phenylalanine. Granules may be administered directly in the mouth or mixed with applesauce, carrots, rice, ice cream, baby formula, or breast milk (do not add to any other liquids); administer within 15 minutes of opening packet. You may experience mild headache, fatigue, or dizziness. Report skin rash or itching, abdominal pain or persistent GI upset, unusual cough or congestion, behavior and mood changes including depression and suicide ideation, feeling of numbness in arms or legs, flu-like illness, or worsening of asthmatic condition.

Dietary Considerations Some products may contain phenylalanine.

Geriatric Considerations The pharmacokinetic profile in the elderly is similar to younger adults except the half-life is slightly longer in the elderly. Despite this difference, no adjustment in dose is necessary in the elderly. Elimination is mostly fecal and bile with insignificant amounts from renal elimination, which is an advantage for the elderly.

Pregnancy Considerations Montelukast was not teratogenic in animal studies, however, there are no adequate and well-controlled studies in pregnant women. Based on limited data, structural defects have been reported in neonates exposed to montelukast *in utero*; however, a specific pattern and relationship to montelukast has not been established. Healthcare providers should report any prenatal exposures to the montelukast pregnancy registry at (800) 986-8999.

◆ **Montelukast Sodium** *see* Montelukast *on page* 1256

Morphine (Systemic) (MOR feen)

U.S. Brand Names Astramorph®/PF; AVINza®; Duramorph; Infumorph 200; Infumorph 500; Kadian®; MS Contin®; Oramorph® SR

Index Terms MS (error-prone abbreviation and should not be used); MSO_4 (error-prone abbreviation and should not be used); Roxanol

Generic Availability (U.S.) Yes: Excludes capsule, sustained release tablet

Pharmacologic Category Analgesic, Opioid

Medication Safety Issues

Sound-alike/look-alike issues:

Morphine may be confused with HYDROmorphone, methadone
Morphine sulfate may be confused with magnesium sulfate
Kadian® may be confused with Kapidex™ [DSC]
MS Contin® may be confused with OxyCONTIN®
MSO_4 and MS are error-prone abbreviations (mistaken as magnesium sulfate)
AVINza® may be confused with Evista®, INVanz®
Roxanol may be confused with OxyFast®, Roxicet™, Roxicodone®

High alert medication: The Institute for Safe Medication Practices (ISMP) includes this medication (I.V. formulation) among its list of drug classes which have a heightened risk of causing significant patient harm when used in error.

Use care when prescribing and/or administering morphine solutions. These products are available in different concentrations. Always prescribe dosage in mg; **not** by volume (mL).

Use caution when selecting a morphine formulation for use in neurologic infusion pumps (eg, Medtronic delivery systems). The product should be appropriately labeled as "preservative-free" and suitable for intraspinal use via continuous infusion. In addition, the product should be formulated in a pH range that is compatible with the device operation specifications.

Significant differences exist between oral and I.V. dosing. Use caution when converting from one route of administration to another.

Medication Guide Available Yes

Pregnancy Risk Factor C

Lactation Enters breast milk/use caution (AAP rates "compatible"; AAP 2001 update pending)

Use Relief of moderate-to-severe acute and chronic pain; relief of pain of myocardial infarction; relief of dyspnea of acute left ventricular failure and pulmonary edema; preanesthetic medication

Infumorph®: Used in continuous microinfusion devices for intrathecal or epidural administration in treatment of intractable chronic pain

Controlled, extended, or sustained release products: Only intended/indicated for use when repeated doses for an extended period of time are required. The 100 mg and 200 mg tablets or capsules of Kadian®, MS Contin®, and morphine sulfate controlled-release tablets and the 60 mg, 90 mg, and 120 mg capsules of Avinza® should only be used in opioid-tolerant patients.

Mechanism of Action/Effect Binds to opiate receptors in the CNS, causing inhibition of ascending pain pathways, altering the perception of and response to pain; produces generalized CNS depression

Contraindications Note: Some contraindications are product specific. For details, please see detailed product prescribing information.

Hypersensitivity to morphine sulfate or any component of the formulation; severe respiratory depression (without resuscitative equipment); acute or severe asthma; known or suspected paralytic ileus; sustained release products are not recommended with gastrointestinal obstruction or in acute/postoperative pain. Oral solutions contraindicated in patients with heart failure due to chronic lung disease, cardiac arrhythmias, head injuries, brain tumors, acute alcoholism, deliriums tremens, seizure disorders, Injectable solution contraindicated during labor when a premature birth is anticipated. Some products contraindicated in patients with head injuries or increased intracranial pressure. MS Contin® and Kadian® contraindicated in patients with hypercarbia. Some immediate release formulations (tablets and solution) contraindicated in post biliary tract surgery, suspected surgical abdomen, surgical anastomosis, MAO inhibitor use (concurrent or within 14 days), general CNS depression.

Warnings/Precautions An opioid-containing analgesic regimen should be tailored to each patient's needs and based upon the type of pain being treated (acute versus chronic), the route of administration, degree of tolerance for opioids (naive versus chronic user), age, weight, and medical condition. The optimal analgesic dose varies widely among patients. Doses should be titrated to pain relief/prevention. When used as an epidural injection, monitor for delayed sedation. **[U.S. Boxed Warning]: Healthcare provider should be alert to problems of abuse, misuse, and diversion.**

May cause respiratory depression; use with caution in patients (particularly elderly or debilitated) with impaired respiratory function, morbid obesity, adrenal insufficiency, prostatic hyperplasia, urinary stricture, renal impairment, or severe hepatic dysfunction and in patients with hypersensitivity reactions to other phenanthrene derivative opioid agonists (codeine, hydrocodone, hydromorphone, levorphanol, oxycodone, oxymorphone). Use with caution in patients with biliary tract dysfunction; acute pancreatitis may cause constriction of sphincter of Oddi. Some preparations contain sulfites which may cause allergic reactions; infants <3 months of age are more susceptible to respiratory depression, use with caution and generally in reduced doses in this age group.

May cause CNS depression, which may impair physical or mental abilities; patients must be cautioned about performing tasks which require mental alertness (eg, operating machinery or driving). Effects may be potentiated when used with other sedative drugs or ethanol. May cause hypotension in patients with acute myocardial infarction, volume depletion, or concurrent drug therapy which may exaggerate vasodilation. Use with extreme caution in patients with head injury, intracranial lesions, or elevated intracranial pressure; exaggerated elevation of ICP may occur. May cause seizures if high doses are used; use with caution in patients with seizure disorders. Tolerance or drug dependence may result from extended use. Concurrent use of agonist/antagonist analgesics may precipitate withdrawal symptoms and/or reduced analgesic efficacy in patients following prolonged therapy with mu opioid agonists. Abrupt discontinuation following prolonged use may also lead to withdrawal symptoms. Elderly may be particularly susceptible to adverse effects of narcotics. May obscure diagnosis or clinical course of patients with acute abdominal conditions.

Extended or sustained-release formulations:

[U.S. Boxed Warning]: Extended or sustained release dosage forms should not be crushed or chewed. Controlled-, extended-, or sustained-release products are not intended for "as needed (PRN)" use. **MS Contin® 100 or 200 mg tablets and Kadian® 100 mg or 200 mg capsules are for use only in opioid-tolerant patients.** Avinza®, Kadian®, MS Contin®: **[U.S. Boxed Warning]: Indicated for the management of moderate-to-severe pain when around the clock pain control is needed for an extended time period.**

[U.S. Boxed Warning]: Avinza®: Do not administer with alcoholic beverages or ethanol-containing products, which may disrupt extended-release characteristic of product.

Highly concentrated oral solutions: [U.S. Boxed Warning]: Check doses carefully when using highly concentrated oral solutions.

Injections: Note: Products are designed for administration by specific routes (I.V., intrathecal, epidural). Use caution when prescribing, dispensing, or administering to use formulations only by intended route(s).

[U.S. Boxed Warning]: Duramorph®: Due to the risk of severe and/or sustained cardiopulmonary depressant effects of Duramorph® must be administered in a fully equipped and staffed environment. Naloxone injection should be immediately available. Patient should remain in this environment for at least 24 hours following the initial dose.

[U.S. Boxed Warning]: Intrathecal dosage is usually $^{1}/_{10}$ that of epidural dosage.

Infumorph® solutions are **for use in microinfusion devices only**; not for I.V., I.M., or SubQ administration, or for single-dose administration.

When used as an epidural injection, monitor for delayed sedation.

Drug Interactions

Metabolism/Transport Effects Substrate of CYP2D6 (minor)

Avoid Concomitant Use There are no known interactions where it is recommended to avoid concomitant use.

Decreased Effect

Morphine (Systemic) may decrease the levels/effects of: Pegvisomant

The levels/effects of Morphine (Systemic) may be decreased by: Ammonium Chloride; Mixed Agonist / Antagonist Opioids; Peginterferon Alfa-2b; Rifamycin Derivatives

Increased Effect/Toxicity

Morphine (Systemic) may increase the levels/effects of: Alcohol (Ethyl); Alvimopan; CNS Depressants; Desmopressin; Selective Serotonin Reuptake Inhibitors; Thiazide Diuretics

The levels/effects of Morphine (Systemic) may be increased by: Amphetamines; Antipsychotic Agents (Phenothiazines); Droperidol; Succinylcholine

Nutritional/Ethanol Interactions

Ethanol: Avoid ethanol, including alcoholic beverages or ethanol-containing products (may increase CNS depression).

Avinza®: Alcoholic beverages or ethanol-containing products may disrupt extended-release formulation resulting in rapid release of entire morphine dose.

Food: Administration of oral morphine solution with food may increase bioavailability (ie, a report of 34% increase in morphine AUC when morphine oral solution followed a high-fat meal). The bioavailability of Avinza®, Oramorph SR®, or Kadian® does not appear to be affected by food.

Herb/Nutraceutical: Avoid valerian, St John's wort, kava kava, gotu kola (may increase CNS depression).

Lab Interactions Some quinolones may produce a false-positive urine screening result for opiates using commercially-available immunoassay kits. This has been demonstrated most consistently for levofloxacin and ofloxacin, but other quinolones have shown cross-reactivity in certain assay kits. Confirmation of positive opiate screens by more specific methods should be considered.

Adverse Reactions Note: Individual patient differences are unpredictable, and percentage may differ in acute pain (surgical) treatment. Reactions may be dose, formulation, and/or route dependent.

Frequency not defined:
- Cardiovascular: Circulatory depression, flushing, shock
- Central nervous system: Dysphonia, physical and psychological dependence, sedation
- Endocrine & metabolic: Antidiuretic hormone release

>10%:
- Cardiovascular: Bradycardia, hypotension
- Central nervous system: Drowsiness (9% to 48%; tolerance usually develops to drowsiness with regular dosing for 1-2 weeks), dizziness (6% to 20%), fever (<3% to >10%), confusion, headache (following epidural or intrathecal use)
- Dermatologic: Pruritus (may be dose related)
- Gastrointestinal: Xerostomia (78%), constipation (9% to 40%; tolerance develops very slowly if at all), nausea (7% to 28%; tolerance usually develops to nausea and vomiting with chronic use), vomiting
- Genitourinary: Urinary retention (16%; may be prolonged, up to 20 hours, following epidural or intrathecal use)
- Hematologic: Anemia (following intrathecal use)
- Local: Pain at injection site
- Neuromuscular & skeletal: Weakness
- Respiratory: Oxygen saturation decreased
- Miscellaneous: Histamine release

1% to 10%:
- Cardiovascular: Atrial fibrillation (<3%), chest pain (<3%), edema, hypertension, palpitation, peripheral edema, syncope, tachycardia, vasodilation
- Central nervous system: Amnesia, agitation, anxiety, apathy, apprehension, ataxia, chills, coma, delirium, depression, dream abnormalities, euphoria, false sense of well being, hallucination, hypoesthesia, insomnia, lethargy, malaise, nervousness, restlessness, seizure, slurred speech, somnolence, vertigo
- Dermatologic: Dry skin, rash, urticaria
- Endocrine & metabolic: Gynecomastia (<3%), hypokalemia, hyponatremia, libido decreased
- Gastrointestinal: Abdominal distension, abdominal pain, anorexia, biliary colic, diarrhea, dyspepsia, dysphagia, flatulence, gastroenteritis, GERD, GI irritation, paralytic ileus, rectal disorder, taste perversion, weight loss
- Genitourinary: Bladder spasm, dysuria, ejaculation abnormal, impotence, urination decreased
- Hematologic: Leukopenia (<3%), thrombocytopenia (<3%), hematocrit decreased
- Hepatic: Liver function tests increased
- Neuromuscular & skeletal: Arthralgia, back pain, bone pain, foot drop, gait abnormalities, paresthesia, rigors, skeletal muscle rigidity, tremor
- Ocular: Amblyopia, conjunctivitis, eye pain, vision problems/disturbance
- Renal: Oliguria
- Respiratory: Asthma, atelectasis, dyspnea, hiccups, hypercapnia, hypoxia, pulmonary edema (noncardiogenic), respiratory depression, rhinitis
- Miscellaneous: Diaphoresis, flu-like syndrome, infection, thirst, voice alteration, withdrawal syndrome

Pharmacodynamics/Kinetics

Onset of Action Patient dependent; dosing must be individualized: Oral (immediate release): ~30 minutes; I.V.: 5-10 minutes

Duration of Action Patient dependent; dosing must be individualized: Pain relief:
- Immediate release formulations: 4 hours
- Extended release capsule and tablet: 8-24 hours (formulation dependent)

Absorption Oral: Variable

Bioavailability Oral: 17% to 33% (first-pass effect limits oral bioavailability; oral:parenteral effectiveness reportedly varies from 1:6 in opioid naive patients to 1:3 with chronic use)

Time to Peak Avinza®: 30 minutes (maintained for 24 hours); Kadian®: ~10 hours; Oramorph® SR: ~4 hours

Protein Binding 30% to 35%

Half-Life Elimination Adults: 2-4 hours (immediate release forms)

Metabolism Hepatic via conjugation with glucuronic acid primarily to morphine-6-glucoronide (active analgesic) morphine-3-glucuronide (inactive as analgesic); minor metabolites include morphine-3-6-diglucuronide; other minor metabolites include normorphine (active) and morphine 3-ethereal sulfate

Excretion Urine (primarily as morphine-3-glucuronide, ~2% to 12% excreted unchanged); feces (~7% to 10%). It has been suggested that accumulation of morphine-6-glucuronide might cause toxicity with renal insufficiency. All of the metabolites (ie, morphine-3-glucuronide, morphine-6-glucuronide, and normorphine) have been suggested as possible causes of neurotoxicity (eg, myoclonus).

Controlled Substance C-II

Available Dosage Forms

Capsule, extended release, oral:
AVINza®: 30 mg, 45 mg, 60 mg, 75 mg, 90 mg, 120 mg
Kadian®: 10 mg, 20 mg, 30 mg, 50 mg, 60 mg, 80 mg, 100 mg, 200 mg

Injection, solution: 1 mg/mL (10 mL, 30 mL, 50 mL); 2 mg/mL (1 mL); 4 mg/mL (1 mL); 5 mg/mL (1 mL, 30 mL, 50 mL); 8 mg/mL (1 mL); 10 mg/mL (1 mL, 10 mL); 10 mg/0.7 mL (0.7 mL); 15 mg/mL (1 mL, 20 mL); 25 mg/mL (4 mL, 10 mL, 20 mL); 50 mg/mL (20 mL, 40 mL, 50 mL)

Injection, solution [preservative free]: 0.5 mg/mL (10 mL, 30 mL); 1 mg/mL (10 mL, 30 mL); 5 mg/mL (30 mL); 25 mg/mL (4 mL, 10 mL, 20 mL)
Astramorph®/PF: 0.5 mg/mL (2 mL, 10 mL); 1 mg/mL (2 mL, 10 mL)
Duramorph: 0.5 mg/mL (10 mL); 1 mg/mL (10 mL)
Infumorph 200: 10 mg/mL (20 mL)
Infumorph 500: 25 mg/mL (20 mL)

Solution, oral: 10 mg/5 mL (5 mL, 10 mL, 100 mL, 500 mL); 20 mg/5 mL (100 mL, 500 mL); 100 mg/5 mL (1 mL, 15 mL, 30 mL, 120 mL, 240 mL)

Suppository, rectal: 5 mg (12s); 10 mg (12s); 20 mg (12s); 30 mg (12s)

Tablet, oral: 15 mg, 30 mg

Tablet, controlled release, oral:
MS Contin®: 15 mg, 30 mg, 60 mg, 100 mg, 200 mg

Tablet, extended release, oral: 15 mg, 30 mg, 60 mg, 100 mg, 200 mg

Tablet, sustained release, oral:
Oramorph® SR: 15 mg, 30 mg, 60 mg, 100 mg

Dosing

Adult These are guidelines and do not represent the doses that may be required in all patients. Doses and dosage intervals should be titrated to pain relief/prevention.

Acute pain (moderate-to-severe):

Oral (immediate release formulations: Opiate-naive: Initial: 10 mg every 4 hours as needed; patients with prior opiate exposure may require higher initial doses: usual dosage range: 10-30 mg every 4 hours as needed

I.M., SubQ: **Note:** Repeated SubQ administration causes local tissue irritation, pain, and induration.

Initial: Opiate-naive: 5-10 mg every 4 hours as needed; patients with prior opiate exposure may require higher initial doses; usual dosage range: 5-20 mg every 4 hours as needed

Rectal: 10-20 mg every 3-4 hours

I.V.: Initial: Opiate-naive: 2.5-5 mg every 3-4 hours; patients with prior opiate exposure may require higher initial doses. **Note:** Repeated doses (up to every 5 minutes if needed) in small increments (eg, 1-4 mg) may be preferred to larger and less frequent doses.

Acute myocardial infarction, analgesia (ACC/AHA 2004 Guidelines): Initial management: 2-4 mg, give 2-8 mg every 5-15 minutes as needed

Critically-ill patients (unlabeled dose): 0.7-10 mg (based on 70 kg patient) **or** 0.01-0.15 mg/kg every 1-2 hours as needed. **Note:** More frequent dosing may be needed (eg, mechanically-ventilated patients).

I.V., SubQ continuous infusion: 0.8-10 mg/hour; usual range: Up to 80 mg/hour

Continuous infusion: Usual dosage range: 5-35 mg/hour (based on 70 kg patient) **or** 0.07-0.5 mg/kg/hour

Patient-controlled analgesia (PCA): (Opiate-naive: Consider lower end of dosing range):
Usual concentration: 1 mg/mL
Demand dose: Usual: 1 mg; range: 0.5-2.5 mg
Lockout interval: 5-10 minutes

Intrathecal (I.T.): **Note: Must be preservative-free.** Administer with extreme caution and in reduced dosage to geriatric or debilitated patients. I.T. dose is usually 1/10 that of epidural dosage.

Opioid-naive: 0.2-1 mg/dose (may provide adequate relief for up to 24 hours); repeat doses are **not** recommended. **Note:** The American Pain Society recommends 0.1-0.3 mg/dose; adjust dose for age, injection site, and patient's medical condition and degree of opioid tolerance.

Continuous microinfusion (Infumorph®): Initial: 0.2-1 mg/day

Opioid-tolerant: 1-10 mg/day
Continuous microinfusion (Infumorph®): Initial: 1-10 mg/day, titrate to effect; usual maximum is ~20 mg/day

Epidural: Pain management: **Note: Must be preservative-free.** Administer with extreme caution and in reduced dosage to geriatric or debilitated patients. Vigilant monitoring is particularly important in these patients.

Single-dose (Astromorph/PF™, Duramorph®): Initial: 5 mg, if pain relief not achieved in 1 hour, careful administration of 1-2 mg at intervals sufficient to assess effectiveness may be given; maximum: 10 mg/24 hours (single doses may provide adequate relief for up to 24 hours)

Infusion: Bolus dose: 1-6 mg; infusion rate: 0.1-0.2 mg/hour; maximum dose: 10 mg/24 hours.

Note: The American Pain Society recommends 1-6 mg/dose as a single dose or an infusion of 0.1-1 mg/hour; adjust dose for age, injection site, and patient's medical condition and degree of opioid tolerance.

Continuous microinfusion (Infumorph®):
Opioid-naive: Initial: 0.2-1 mg/day
Opioid-tolerant: Initial: 1-10 mg/day, titrate to effect; usual maximum is ~20 mg/day

Chronic pain: Note: Patients taking opioids chronically may become tolerant and require doses higher than the usual dosage range to maintain the desired effect. Tolerance can be managed by appropriate dose titration. There is no optimal or maximal dose for morphine in chronic pain. The appropriate dose is one that relieves pain throughout its dosing interval without causing unmanageable side effects.

Oral: Controlled-, extended-, or sustained-release formulations: A patient's morphine requirement should be established using prompt-release formulations. Conversion to long-acting products may be considered when chronic, continuous treatment is required. Higher dosages should be reserved for use only in opioid-tolerant patients.

Capsules, extended release (Avinza®): Daily dose administered once daily (for best results, administer at same time each day)

Capsules, sustained release (Kadian®): Daily dose administered once daily or in 2 divided doses daily (every 12 hours)

Tablets, controlled release (MS Contin®), sustained release (Oramorph SR®), or extended release: Daily dose divided and administered every 8 or every 12 hours

Geriatric Refer to adult dosing. Use with caution; may require reduced dosage in the elderly and debilitated patients.

Pediatric These are guidelines and do not represent the doses that may be required in all patients. Doses and dosage intervals should be titrated to pain relief/prevention.

Acute pain (moderate-to-severe): Children >6 months and <50 kg:
Oral (prompt release): 0.15-0.2 mg/kg every 3-4 hours as needed
I.M., I.V.: 0.1-0.2 mg/kg every 3-4 hours as needed
I.V. infusion: Range: 10-60 mcg/kg/**hour**

Renal Impairment

Cl_{cr} 10-50 mL/minute: Children and Adults: Administer at 75% of normal dose
Cl_{cr} <10 mL/minute: Children and Adults: Administer at 50% of normal dose
Intermittent HD:
Children: Administer 50% of normal dose
Adults: No dosage adjustment necessary
Peritoneal dialysis: Children: Administer 50% of normal dose
CRRT: Children and Adults: Administer 75% of normal dose, titrate

Hepatic Impairment Unchanged in mild liver disease; substantial extrahepatic metabolism may occur. Excessive sedation may occur in cirrhosis.

Administration

Oral Do not crush controlled release drug product, swallow whole. Kadian® and Avinza® can be opened and sprinkled on applesauce; do not crush or chew the beads. Contents of Kadian® capsules may be opened and sprinkled over 10 mL water and flushed through prewetted 16F gastrostomy tube; do not administer Kadian® through nasogastric tube.

I.V. When giving morphine I.V. push, it is best to first dilute with sterile water or NS for a final concentration of 1-2 mg/mL and then administer slowly.

Other Use preservative-free solutions for intrathecal or epidural use.

Stability

Reconstitution Injection: Usual concentration for continuous I.V. infusion: 0.1-1 mg/mL in D_5W.

Storage

Capsule, sustained release (Avinza®, Kadian®): Store at 25°C (77°F); excursions permitted to 15°C to 30°C (59°F to 86°F). Protect from light and moisture.

Injection: Store at controlled room temperature of 20°C to 25°C (68°F to 77°F); do not freeze. Protect from light. Degradation depends on pH and presence of oxygen; relatively stable in pH ≤4; darkening of solutions indicate degradation.

Oral solution: Store at controlled room temperature of 25°C (68°F to 77°F); do not freeze.

Suppositories: Store at controlled room temperature 25°C (77°F). Protect from light.

Tablet, extended release: Store at controlled room temperature of 25°C (77°F).

Tablet, immediate release: Store at controlled room temperature of 25°C (77°F). Protect from moisture.

Monitoring and Teaching Issues

Physical Assessment Monitor respiratory and CNS status periodically. Assess patient's physical and/or psychological dependence. For inpatients, implement safety measures to prevent falls. Discontinue slowly after prolonged use.

Patient Education Do not crush or chew controlled release tablet or capsule. May cause physical and/or psychological dependence. While using this medication, do not use alcohol (especially if using Avinza®) and other prescription or OTC medications (especially sedatives, tranquilizers, antihistamines, or pain medications) without consulting prescriber. Maintain adequate hydration, unless instructed to restrict fluid intake. May cause itching, hypotension, dizziness, drowsiness, impaired coordination, or blurred vision; loss of appetite, dry mouth, nausea, or vomiting; or constipation. Report chest pain, slow or rapid heartbeat, dizziness, or persistent headache; confusion or respiratory difficulties; or severe constipation.

Dietary Considerations Morphine may cause GI upset; take with food if GI upset occurs. Be consistent when taking morphine with or without meals.

Geriatric Considerations The elderly may be particularly susceptible to the CNS depressant and constipating effects of narcotics. For chronic administration of narcotic analgesics, morphine is preferable in the elderly due to its pharmacokinetics and side effect profile as compared to meperidine and methadone.

Breast-Feeding Considerations Morphine concentrates in breast milk, with a milk to plasma AUC ratio of 2.5:1. Detectable serum levels of morphine can be found in infants following morphine administration to nursing mothers. Treatment of the mother with single doses of morphine is not expected to cause detrimental effects in nursing infants. Breast-feeding following chronic use or in neonates with hepatic or renal dysfunction may lead to higher levels of morphine in the infant and a risk of adverse effects.

Pregnancy Considerations Teratogenic effects were not observed in animal studies; however reduced growth and behavioral abnormalities in offspring have been observed. Morphine crosses the human placenta. The frequency of congenital malformations has not been reported to be greater than expected in children from mothers treated with morphine during pregnancy. However, following *in utero* exposure, infants may exhibit withdrawal, decreased brain volume (reversible), small size, decreased ventilatory response to CO_2, and increased risk of sudden infant death syndrome. In patients with chronic, noncancer pain, minimal (if any) opioids should be used during pregnancy. Neonates born to mothers receiving chronic opioids during pregnancy should be monitored for neonatal withdrawal syndrome.

Related Information

Compatibility of Drugs *on page 1994*

Opioid Analgesics *on page 2003*

Morphine and Naltrexone (MOR feen & nal TREKS one)

U.S. Brand Names Embeda™

Index Terms Morphine Sulfate and Naltrexone Hydrochloride; MS (error-prone abbreviation and should not be used); MSO_4 (error-prone abbreviation and should not be used); Naltrexone and Morphine

Generic Availability (U.S.) No

Pharmacologic Category Analgesic, Opioid; Opioid Antagonist

Medication Safety Issues

Sound-alike/look-alike issues:

- Morphine may be confused with HYDROmorphone
- Morphine sulfate may be confused with magnesium sulfate
- Naltrexone may be confused with methylnaltrexone, naloxone
- MSO_4 and MS are error-prone abbreviations (mistaken as magnesium sulfate)

Medication Guide Available Yes

Pregnancy Risk Factor C

Lactation Enters breast milk/not recommended

Use Relief of moderate-to-severe pain when continual, around-the-clock therapy is needed for an extended period of time

Controlled Substance C-II

Available Dosage Forms

Capsule, extended release, oral:

- Embeda™ 20/0.8: Morphine 20 mg and naltrexone 0.8 mg
- Embeda™ 30/1.2: Morphine 30 mg and naltrexone 1.2 mg
- Embeda™ 50/2: Morphine 50 mg and naltrexone 2 mg
- Embeda™ 80/3.2: Morphine 80 mg and naltrexone 3.2 mg
- Embeda™ 100/4: Morphine 100 mg and naltrexone 4 mg

Dosing

Adult Note: These are guidelines and do not represent the doses that may be required in all patients. Treatment should be individualized based on patient's prior analgesic treatment experience/tolerance and pain relief. Not intended for use as a PRN medication.

Moderate-to-severe pain: Oral: Opiate-naive: Initial: 20 mg/0.8 mg once or twice daily; 100 mg/4 mg strength for use in opioid-tolerant patients only

Titration: Do not increase dose more frequently than every other day. May supplement dose with a short-acting analgesic (<20% of total daily dose) for breakthrough pain. If once-daily dosing is inadequate may switch to twice daily dosing.

Conversion from other oral morphine products to Embeda™: Administer one-half of the patient's total daily oral morphine dose as Embeda™ every 12 hours or all of the patient's total daily oral morphine dose as Embeda™ once daily.

Conversion from other oral/parenteral opioids or parenteral morphine to Embeda™: Must first convert to oral morphine equivalent.

Conversion from parenteral to oral morphine: It may take 2-6 mg of oral morphine to provide pain relief equivalent to 1 mg of parenteral morphine. An oral dose 3 times the daily parenteral dose may be sufficient in chronic pain settings.

Conversion from other oral/parenteral opioids to oral morphine: Specific recommendations are not available; refer to published relative potency data realizing that such ratios are only approximations. It is generally safest to give half the estimated daily morphine requirement as the initial dose and manage inadequate relief with immediate release morphine.

Note: When converting from other opioid analgesics it is better to underestimate the patient's 24-hour oral requirement and provide breakthrough treatment than to overestimate and manage an adverse event.

Geriatric Refer to adult dosing. Use with caution; may require reduced dosage in the elderly and debilitated patients.

Renal Impairment Use with caution in patients with severe impairment; no specific dosing recommendations are provided by the manufacturer.

Hepatic Impairment Use with caution in patients with severe impairment; no specific dosing recommendations are provided by the manufacturer.

Administration

Oral Capsule should be swallowed whole. Contents of the capsule may be sprinkled on applesauce (do not divide in separate doses) and swallowed immediately. Rinse mouth to ensure all contents have been swallowed. Do not crush, chew, or dissolve pellets in the capsule prior to swallowing. Not for nasogastric/gastric tube administration. First dose may be taken at the same time as the last dose of immediate release opioid medication.

Monitoring and Teaching Issues

Physical Assessment See individual agents.

Patient Education See individual agents.

- ◆ **Morphine Sulfate and Naltrexone Hydrochloride** *see* Morphine and Naltrexone *on page* 1263
- ◆ **Motofen®** *see* Difenoxin and Atropine *on page* 528
- ◆ **Motrin® Children's [OTC]** *see* Ibuprofen *on page* 938
- ◆ **Motrin® IB [OTC]** *see* Ibuprofen *on page* 938
- ◆ **Motrin® Infants' [OTC]** *see* Ibuprofen *on page* 938
- ◆ **Motrin® Junior [OTC]** *see* Ibuprofen *on page* 938
- ◆ **MoviPrep®** *see* Polyethylene Glycol-Electrolyte Solution *on page* 1474
- ◆ **Moxatag™** *see* Amoxicillin *on page* 110
- ◆ **Moxeza™** *see* Moxifloxacin (Ophthalmic) *on page* 1267

Moxifloxacin (Systemic) (moxs i FLOKS a sin)

U.S. Brand Names Avelox®; Avelox® ABC Pack; Avelox® I.V.

Index Terms Moxifloxacin Hydrochloride

Generic Availability (U.S.) No

Pharmacologic Category Antibiotic, Quinolone; Respiratory Fluoroquinolone

Medication Safety Issues

Sound-alike/look-alike issues:

Avelox® may be confused with Avonex®

Medication Guide Available Yes

Pregnancy Risk Factor C

Lactation Excretion in breast milk unknown/not recommended

Use Treatment of mild-to-moderate community-acquired pneumonia, including multidrug-resistant *Streptococcus pneumoniae* (MDRSP); acute bacterial exacerbation of chronic bronchitis; acute bacterial sinusitis; complicated and uncomplicated skin and skin structure infections; complicated intra-abdominal infections

Unlabeled/Investigational Use Treatment of *Legionella* pneumonia

Mechanism of Action/Effect Moxifloxacin is a quinolone antibiotic with bactericidal activity against susceptible gram-negative and gram-positive microorganisms.

Contraindications Hypersensitivity to moxifloxacin, other quinolone antibiotics, or any component of the formulation

Warnings/Precautions [U.S. Boxed Warning]: There have been reports of tendon inflammation and/or rupture with quinolone antibiotics; risk may be increased with concurrent corticosteroids, organ transplant recipients, and in patients >60 years of age. Rupture of the Achilles tendon sometimes requiring surgical repair has been reported most frequently; but other tendon sites (eg, rotator cuff, biceps) have also been reported. Strenuous physical activity, rheumatoid arthritis, and renal impairment may be an independent risk factor for tendonitis. Discontinue at first sign of tendon inflammation or pain. Tendon rupture may occur even after discontinuation of therapy. Use with caution in patients with rheumatoid arthritis or renal impairment; may increase risk of tendon rupture.

Use with caution in patients with significant bradycardia or acute myocardial ischemia. Moxifloxacin causes a concentration-dependent QT prolongation. Do not exceed recommended dose or infusion rate. Avoid use with uncorrected hypokalemia, with other drugs that prolong the QT interval or induce bradycardia, or with class Ia or III antiarrhythmic agents. Use with caution in individuals at risk of seizures (CNS disorders or concurrent therapy with medications which may lower seizure threshold). Potential for seizures, although very rare, may be increased with concomitant NSAID therapy. Discontinue in patients who experience significant CNS adverse effects (dizziness, hallucinations, suicidal ideation or actions). Use with caution in patients with mild, moderate, or severe hepatic impairment or liver cirrhosis; may increase the risk of QT prolongation. Fulminant hepatitis potentially leading to liver failure (including fatalities) has been reported with use. Use with caution in diabetes; glucose regulation may be altered.

Fluoroquinolones have been associated with the development of serious, and sometimes fatal, hypoglycemia, most often in elderly diabetics, but also in patients without diabetes. This occurred most frequently with gatifloxacin (no longer available systemically) but may occur at a lower frequency with other quinolones.

Severe hypersensitivity reactions, including anaphylaxis, have occurred with quinolone therapy. Reactions may present as typical allergic symptoms after a single dose, or may manifest as severe idiosyncratic dermatologic, vascular, pulmonary, renal, hepatic, and/or hematologic events, usually after multiple doses. Prompt discontinuation of drug should occur if skin rash or other symptoms arise. Avoid excessive sunlight and take precautions to limit exposure (eg, loose fitting clothing, sunscreen); may cause moderate-to-severe phototoxicity reactions. Discontinue use if photosensitivity occurs. Prolonged use may result in fungal or bacterial superinfection, including *C. difficile*-associated diarrhea (CDAD) and pseudomembranous colitis; CDAD has been observed >2 months postantibiotic treatment. **[U.S. Boxed Warning]: Quinolones may exacerbate myasthenia gravis; avoid use (rare, potentially life-threatening weakness of respiratory muscles may occur).** Peripheral neuropathy may rarely occur. Hemolytic reactions may (rarely) occur with quinolone use in patients with latent or actual G6PD deficiency. Adverse effects (eg, tendon rupture, QT changes) may be increased in the elderly. Some quinolones may exacerbate myasthenia gravis, use with caution (rare, potentially life-threatening weakness of respiratory muscles may occur). Safety and efficacy of systemically administered moxifloxacin (oral, intravenous) in patients <18 years of age have not been established.

Drug Interactions

Avoid Concomitant Use

Avoid concomitant use of Moxifloxacin (Systemic) with any of the following: Artemether; BCG; Dronedarone; Lumefantrine; Nilotinib; Pimozide; QuiNINE; Tetrabenazine; Thioridazine; Toremifene; Vandetanib; Ziprasidone

Decreased Effect

Moxifloxacin (Systemic) may decrease the levels/effects of: BCG; Mycophenolate; Sulfonylureas; Typhoid Vaccine

The levels/effects of Moxifloxacin (Systemic) may be decreased by: Antacids; Didanosine; Iron Salts; Magnesium Salts; Quinapril; Sevelamer; Sucralfate; Zinc Salts

Increased Effect/Toxicity

Moxifloxacin (Systemic) may increase the levels/effects of: Corticosteroids (Systemic); Dronedarone; Pimozide; QTc-Prolonging Agents; QuiNINE; Sulfonylureas; Tetrabenazine; Thioridazine; Toremifene; Vandetanib; Vitamin K Antagonists; Ziprasidone

The levels/effects of Moxifloxacin (Systemic) may be increased by: Alfuzosin; Artemether; Chloroquine; Ciprofloxacin; Ciprofloxacin (Systemic); Gadobutrol; Insulin; Lumefantrine; Nilotinib; Nonsteroidal Anti-Inflammatory Agents; Probenecid; QuiNINE

Nutritional/Ethanol Interactions Food: Absorption is not affected by administration with a high-fat meal or yogurt.

Lab Interactions Some quinolones may produce a false-positive urine screening result for opiates using commercially-available immunoassay kits. This has been demonstrated most consistently for levofloxacin and ofloxacin, but other quinolones have shown cross-reactivity in certain assay kits. Confirmation of positive opiate screens by more specific methods should be considered.

Adverse Reactions

2% to 10%:

- Central nervous system: Dizziness (2%)
- Endocrine & metabolic: Serum chloride increased (≥2%), serum ionized calcium increased (≥2%), serum glucose decreased (≥2%)
- Gastrointestinal: Nausea (6%), diarrhea (5%), amylase decreased (≥2%)
- Hematologic: Decreased serum levels of the following (≥2%): Basophils, eosinophils, hemoglobin, RBC, neutrophils; increased serum levels of the following (≥2%): MCH, neutrophils, WBC
- Hepatic: Bilirubin decreased/increased (≥2%)
- Renal: Serum albumin increased (≥2%)
- Respiratory: PO_2 decreased (≥2%)

0.1% to <2%:

- Cardiovascular: Cardiac arrhythmias, palpitation, QT_c prolongation, tachycardia, vasodilation
- Central nervous system: Anxiety, headache, insomnia, malaise, nervousness, pain, somnolence, vertigo
- Dermatologic: Pruritus, rash (maculopapular, purpuric, pustular), urticaria
- Gastrointestinal: Abdominal pain, amylase increased, anorexia, constipation, dyspepsia, flatulence, glossitis, lactic dehydrogenase increased, stomatitis, taste perversion, vomiting, xerostomia
- Genitourinary: Vaginal moniliasis, vaginitis
- Hematologic: Eosinophilia, leukopenia, prothrombin time prolonged, increased INR, thrombocythemia
- Hepatic: GGTP increased, liver function test abnormal
- Local: Injection site reaction

Neuromuscular & skeletal: Arthralgia, myalgia, tremor, weakness
Respiratory: Pharyngitis, pneumonia, rhinitis, sinusitis
Miscellaneous: Allergic reaction, infection, diaphoresis, oral moniliasis

Pharmacodynamics/Kinetics

Absorption Well absorbed; not affected by high-fat meal or yogurt

Bioavailability ~90%

Protein Binding ~30% to 50%

Half-Life Elimination Single dose: Oral: 12-16 hours; I.V.: 8-15 hours

Metabolism Hepatic (~52% of dose) via glucuronide (~14%) and sulfate (~38%) conjugation

Excretion Urine (as unchanged drug [20%] and glucuronide conjugates); feces (as unchanged drug [25%] and sulfate conjugates)

Available Dosage Forms

Infusion, premixed in sodium chloride 0.8% [preservative free]:
Avelox® I.V.: 400 mg (250 mL)

Tablet, oral:
Avelox®: 400 mg
Avelox® ABC Pack: 400 mg

Dosing

Adult & Geriatric

Acute bacterial sinusitis: Oral, I.V.: 400 mg every 24 hours for 10 days

Chronic bronchitis, acute bacterial exacerbation: Oral, I.V.: 400 mg every 24 hours for 5 days

Intra-abdominal infections, complicated: 400 mg every 24 hours for 5-14 days (initiate with I.V.); **Note:** 2010 IDSA guidelines recommend a treatment duration of 4-7 days (provided source controlled) for community-acquired, mild-to-moderate IAI

Pneumonia, community-acquired (including MDRSP): Oral, I.V.: 400 mg every 24 hours for 7-14 days

Skin and skin structure infections: Oral, I.V.:
Complicated: 400 mg every 24 hours for 7-21 days
Uncomplicated: 400 mg every 24 hours for 7 days

Renal Impairment No adjustment is necessary, including patients on hemodialysis, CRRT, or CAPD.

Hepatic Impairment No dosage adjustment is required in mild, moderate, or severe hepatic insufficiency (Child-Pugh class A, B, or C); however, use with caution in this patient population secondary to the risk of QT prolongation.

Administration

I.V. Infuse over 60 minutes; do not infuse by rapid or bolus intravenous infusion

Stability

Storage Store at controlled room temperature of 25°C (77°F). Do not refrigerate infusion solution.

Monitoring and Teaching Issues

Laboratory Monitoring WBC

Physical Assessment Assess results of culture and sensitivity tests and patient's allergy history before initiating therapy. Use caution with known or suspected CNS disorders, myasthenia gravis, current or potential for QT prolongation, hepatic impairment, or diabetes. Patient should be monitored closely; if an allergic reaction occurs (itching, urticaria, dyspnea or facial edema, loss of consciousness, tingling, cardiovascular collapse), drug should be discontinued immediately and prescriber notified. Monitor for hypersensitivity reactions (severe reactions, including anaphylaxis, have occurred with quinolone therapy), opportunistic infection, tendon rupture, and persistent diarrhea (*C. difficile*-associated colitis can occur post-treatment).

Patient Education If administered by infusion: Report immediately any redness, swelling, or pain at infusion site; any swelling of mouth, lips, tongue, or throat; chest pain or tightness; respiratory difficulty; back pain; itching; skin rash; tingling; tendon pain; dizziness; abnormal thinking; or anxiety. May cause dizziness, lightheadedness, confusion, nausea, or vomiting (request antiemetic from prescriber). Report any tendon pain, chest pain, or palpitations.

Oral: Do not take antacids 4 hours before or 8 hours after taking this medication. Maintain adequate hydration unless instructed to restrict fluid intake. Consult prescriber before having any vaccinations. May cause nausea, vomiting, taste perversion, headache, dizziness, insomnia, or anxiety. Avoid excessive sunlight and wear sunscreen during therapy. If you develop severe sunburn or sensitivity to sunlight, if tendon inflammation or pain occurs, or if you experience signs of an allergic reaction (eg, itching, urticaria, respiratory difficulty, facial edema or difficulty swallowing, loss of consciousness, tingling, chest pain, palpitations), discontinue use and contact prescriber immediately. Report persistent GI disturbances, CNS changes (eg, excessive sleepiness, agitation, tremors), skin rash, vision changes, respiratory difficulty, signs of opportunistic infection (eg, sore throat, chills, fever, burning, itching on urination, vaginal discharge, white plaques in mouth), persistent diarrhea (especially if it lasts after completing prescription); or worsening of condition.

Dietary Considerations May be taken without regard to meals. Take 4 hours before or 8 hours after multiple vitamins, antacids, or other products containing magnesium, aluminum, iron, or zinc.

Avelox® I.V. infusion (premixed in sodium chloride 0.8%) contains sodium 34.2 mEq (~787 mg)/250 mL.

Geriatric Considerations See Warnings/Precautions regarding tendon rupture in patients >60 years of age. No dosage adjustments are required based on age.

Breast-Feeding Considerations It is not known if moxifloxacin is excreted into breast milk. Breast-feeding is not recommended by the manufacturer. Although there is no information on the use of moxifloxacin during breast-feeding, other quinolones are considered compatible. Nondose-related effects could include modification of bowel flora.

Pregnancy Considerations Adverse events have been observed in some animal studies; therefore, the manufacturer classifies moxifloxacin as pregnancy category C. Quinolone exposure during human pregnancy has been reported with other agents (see Ciprofloxacin (Systemic) monograph). To date, no specific teratogenic effect or increased pregnancy risk has been identified; however, because of concerns of cartilage damage in immature animals exposed to quinolones and the limited moxifloxacin specific data, moxifloxacin should only be used during pregnancy if a safer option is not available.

Related Information

Antimicrobial Drugs of Choice *on page 2008*

Community-Acquired Pneumonia in Adults *on page 2021*

Moxifloxacin (Ophthalmic) (moxs i FLOKS a sin)

U.S. Brand Names Moxeza™; Vigamox®

Index Terms Moxifloxacin Hydrochloride

Generic Availability (U.S.) No

Pharmacologic Category Antibiotic, Ophthalmic; Antibiotic, Quinolone

Medication Safety Issues

International issues:

Vigamox [U.S., Canada, and multiple international markets] may be confused with Fisamox brand name for amoxicillin [Australia]

Pregnancy Risk Factor C

Lactation Use caution

Use Treatment of bacterial conjunctivitis caused by susceptible organisms

Available Dosage Forms

Solution, ophthalmic:

Moxeza™: 0.5% (3 mL)

Vigamox®: 0.5% (3 mL)

Dosing

Adult & Geriatric Bacterial conjunctivitis: Ophthalmic:

Moxeza™: Instill 1 drop into affected eye(s) 2 times/day for 7 days

Vigamox®: Instill 1 drop into affected eye(s) 3 times/day for 7 days

Pediatric Bacterial conjunctivitis: Ophthalmic:

Children ≥4 months (Moxeza™): Refer to adult dosing.

Children ≥1 year (Vigamox®): Refer to adult dosing.

Administration

Other For topical ophthalmic use only; avoid touching tip of applicator to eye or other surfaces.

Monitoring and Teaching Issues

Patient Education Wash hands before instilling solution. Sit or lie down to instill. Open eye, look at ceiling, and instill prescribed amount of solution as directed. Do not touch tip of applicator or let tip of applicator touch eye. Do not wear contact lenses during therapy. Temporary stinging, blurred vision, or dry eyes may occur. Report persistent pain, burning, excessive tearing, decreased visual acuity, swelling, itching, or worsening of condition.

- ◆ **Moxifloxacin Hydrochloride** *see* Moxifloxacin (Ophthalmic) *on page 1267*
- ◆ **Moxifloxacin Hydrochloride** *see* Moxifloxacin (Systemic) *on page 1264*
- ◆ **Mozobil™** *see* Plerixafor *on page 1468*
- ◆ **MPA** *see* MedroxyPROGESTERone *on page 1154*
- ◆ **MPA** *see* Mycophenolate *on page 1270*
- ◆ **MPA and Estrogens (Conjugated)** *see* Estrogens (Conjugated/Equine) and Medroxyprogesterone *on page 686*
- ◆ **6-MP (error-prone abbreviation)** *see* Mercaptopurine *on page 1173*
- ◆ **MPSV** *see* Meningococcal Polysaccharide Vaccine (Groups A / C / Y and W-135) *on page 1169*
- ◆ **MPSV4** *see* Meningococcal Polysaccharide Vaccine (Groups A / C / Y and W-135) *on page 1169*
- ◆ **MS Contin®** *see* Morphine (Systemic) *on page 1258*
- ◆ **MS (error-prone abbreviation and should not be used)** *see* Morphine and Naltrexone *on page 1263*
- ◆ **MS (error-prone abbreviation and should not be used)** *see* Morphine (Systemic) *on page 1258*
- ◆ **MSO_4 (error-prone abbreviation and should not be used)** *see* Morphine and Naltrexone *on page 1263*
- ◆ **MSO_4 (error-prone abbreviation and should not be used)** *see* Morphine (Systemic) *on page 1258*
- ◆ **MTX (error-prone abbreviation)** *see* Methotrexate *on page 1193*
- ◆ **Mucinex® [OTC]** *see* GuaiFENesin *on page 890*
- ◆ **Mucinex® Kid's [OTC]** *see* GuaiFENesin *on page 890*

◆ **Mucinex® Kid's Mini-Melts™ [OTC]** *see* GuaiFENesin *on page 890*

◆ **Mucinex® Maximum Strength [OTC]** *see* GuaiFENesin *on page 890*

◆ **Mucus Relief [OTC]** *see* GuaiFENesin *on page 890*

◆ **Multaq®** *see* Dronedarone *on page 591*

◆ **Mumps, Measles and Rubella Vaccines** *see* Measles, Mumps, and Rubella Virus Vaccine *on page 1150*

◆ **Mumps, Rubella, Varicella, and Measles Vaccine** *see* Measles, Mumps, Rubella, and Varicella Virus Vaccine *on page 1151*

Muromonab-CD3 (myoo roe MOE nab see dee three)

U.S. Brand Names Orthoclone OKT® 3 [DSC]

Index Terms Monoclonal Antibody; OKT3

Generic Availability (U.S.) No

Pharmacologic Category Immunosuppressant Agent; Monoclonal Antibody

Pregnancy Risk Factor C

Lactation Excretion in breast milk unknown/contraindicated

Use Treatment of acute allograft rejection in renal transplant patients; treatment of steroid-resistant acute allograft rejection in cardiac or hepatic transplantation

Unlabeled/Investigational Use Treatment of acute pancreas rejection episodes resistant to conventional treatment

Mechanism of Action/Effect Reverses graft rejection by binding to T cells and interfering with their function

Contraindications Hypersensitivity to OKT3 or any murine product; patients with uncompensated heart failure or uncontrolled hypertension, in fluid overload or those with >3% weight gain within 1 week prior to start of OKT3; mouse antibody titers >1:1000; history of seizures; known or suspected pregnancy; breast-feeding

Warnings/Precautions It is imperative, especially prior to the first few doses, that there be no clinical evidence of volume overload, uncontrolled hypertension, or uncompensated heart failure, including a clear chest x-ray and weight restriction of ≤3% above the patient's minimum weight during the week prior to injection.

Risk of development of lymphoproliferative disorders (particularly of the skin) is increased. May result in an increased susceptibility to infection; dosage of concomitant immunosuppressants should be reduced during OKT3 therapy; cyclosporine should be decreased to 50% usual maintenance dose and maintenance therapy resumed about 4 days before stopping OKT3.

Severe pulmonary edema has occurred in patients with fluid overload. Seizures, encephalopathy, cerebral edema, aseptic meningitis, and headache have been reported following muromonab-CD3. Contraindicated for use in patients with a history of seizures or those who are predisposed to seizures. Arterial, venous, and capillary thrombosis of allografts and other vascular beds have been reported with use; use with caution in patients with history of thrombosis or underlying vascular disease.

[U.S. Boxed Warning]: Anaphylactic and anaphylactoid reactions may occur after administration of any dose of muromonab-CD3; acute hypersensitivity reactions may be characterized by cardiovascular collapse, cardiorespiratory arrest, loss of consciousness, shock, tachycardia, tingling, angioedema, airway obstruction, bronchospasm, dyspnea, urticaria, and pruritus. These reactions may be difficult to differentiate from the cytokine release syndrome associated with use; however, hypersensitivity reactions are more likely to occur within the first 10 minutes after administration. Cytokine release syndrome may occur in a significant proportion of patients following the first couple of doses of muromonab-CD3; symptoms usually begin 30-60 minutes after administration of dose and may persist for several hours; symptoms range from a mild, self-limiting "flu-like reaction" to severe, life-threatening shock-like reaction. Patients at higher risk for serious complications include those with unstable angina, recent MI or ischemic heart disease, heart failure, pulmonary edema, COPD, intravascular volume overload or depletion, cerebrovascular disease, patients with advanced symptomatic vascular disease or neuropathy, history of seizures, and septic shock. Pretreatment with corticosteroids may decrease serum levels of cytokines and manifestations of the syndrome, but it is not known if this decreases organ damage and sequelae associated with it.

Cardiopulmonary resuscitation may be needed. If the patient's temperature is >37.8°C, reduce before administering OKT3. **[U.S. Boxed Warning]: Should be administered under the supervision of a physician experienced in immunosuppressive therapy in a facility appropriate for monitoring and resuscitation.**

Drug Interactions

Avoid Concomitant Use

Avoid concomitant use of Muromonab-CD3 with any of the following: BCG; Natalizumab; Pimecrolimus; Roflumilast; Tacrolimus (Topical); Vaccines (Live)

Decreased Effect

Muromonab-CD3 may decrease the levels/effects of: BCG; Sipuleucel-T; Vaccines (Inactivated); Vaccines (Live)

The levels/effects of Muromonab-CD3 may be decreased by: Echinacea

Increased Effect/Toxicity

Muromonab-CD3 may increase the levels/effects of: Leflunomide; Natalizumab; Vaccines (Live)

The levels/effects of Muromonab-CD3 may be increased by: Denosumab; Pimecrolimus; Roflumilast; Tacrolimus (Topical); Trastuzumab

Adverse Reactions Note: Signs and symptoms of cytokine release syndrome (characterized by pyrexia, chills, dyspnea, nausea, vomiting, chest pain, diarrhea, tremor, wheezing, headache, tachycardia, rigor, hypertension, pulmonary edema and/or other cardiorespiratory manifestations) occurs in a significant proportion of patients following the first couple of doses of muromonab-CD3. See Warnings/Precautions. Additionally, some patients have experienced immediate hypersensitivity reactions to muromonab-CD3 (characterized by cardiovascular collapse, cardiorespiratory arrest, loss of consciousness, hypotension/shock, tachycardia, tingling, angioedema (including laryngeal, pharyngeal, or facial edema), airway obstruction, bronchospasm, dyspnea, urticaria, and/or pruritus) upon initial exposure and re-exposure.

>10%:

Cardiovascular: Tachycardia (26%), hypotension (25%), hypertension (19%), edema (12%)
Central nervous system: Pyrexia (77%), chills (43%), headache (28%)
Dermatologic: Rash (14%; erythematous 2%)
Gastrointestinal: Diarrhea (37%), nausea (32%), vomiting (25%)
Respiratory: Dyspnea (16%)

1% to 10%:

Cardiovascular: Chest pain (9%), vasodilation (7%), arrhythmia (4%), bradycardia (4%), vascular occlusion (2%)
Central nervous system: Fatigue (9%), confusion (6%), dizziness (6%), lethargy (6%), pain trunk (6%), malaise (5%), nervousness (5%), depression (3%), somnolence (2%), meningitis (1%), seizure (1%)
Dermatologic: Pruritus (7%)
Gastrointestinal: Gastrointestinal pain (7%), abdominal pain (6%), anorexia (4%)
Hematologic: Leukopenia (7%), anemia (2%), thrombocytopenia (2%), leukocytosis (1%)
Neuromuscular & skeletal: Weakness (10%), arthralgia (7%), myalgia (1%), tremor (14%)
Ocular: Photophobia (1%)
Otic: Tinnitus (1%)
Renal: Renal dysfunction (3%)
Respiratory: Abnormal chest sound (10%), hyperventilation (7%), wheezing (6%), respiratory congestion (4%), pulmonary edema (2%), hypoxia (1%), pneumonia (1%)
Miscellaneous: Diaphoresis (7%), infections (various)

Pharmacodynamics/Kinetics

Duration of Action 7 days after discontinuation

Time to Peak Steady-state: Trough: 3-14 days

Product Availability Orthoclone OKT® 3: Due to diminishing use, the manufacturer of muromonab is discontinuing production; supplies are expected to be available through the end of 2010.

Dosing

Adult & Geriatric Treatment of acute allograft rejection: I.V. (refer to individual protocols): 5 mg/day once daily for 10-14 days

Note: Suggested prevention/treatment of muromonab-CD3 first-dose effects (grouped by adverse reaction):

Severe pulmonary edema:

- Effective prevention or palliation: Clear chest x-ray within 24 hours preinjection; weight restriction to ≤3% gain over 7days preinjection
- Supportive treatment: Prompt intubation and oxygenation; 24 hours close observation

Fever, chills:

- Effective prevention or palliation: 15 mg/kg methylprednisolone sodium succinate 1 hour preinjection; fever reduction to <37.8°C (100°F) 1 hour preinjection; acetaminophen (1 g orally) and diphenhydramine(50 mg orally) 1 hour preinjection
- Supportive treatment: Cooling blanket; acetaminophen as needed

Respiratory effects:

- Effective prevention or palliation: 100 mg hydrocortisone sodium succinate 30 minutes postinjection
- Supportive treatment: Additional 100 mg hydrocortisone sodium succinate as needed for wheezing; if respiratory distress, give epinephrine 1:1000 (0.3 mL SubQ)

Pediatric Refer to individual protocols.

Treatment of acute allograft rejection: I.V.

Children ≤30 kg: 2.5 mg/day once daily for 10-14 days
Children >30 kg: 5 mg/day once daily for 10-14 days

or

Children <12 years (unlabeled dosing): 0.1 mg/kg/day once daily for 10-14 days
Children ≥12 years: Refer to adult dosing.

Note: Suggested prevention/treatment of muromonab-CD3 first-dose effects (grouped by adverse reaction): Refer to adult dosing.

Renal Impairment Removal by dialysis: Molecular size of OKT3 is 150,000 daltons. Not dialyzed by most standard dialyzers; however, may be dialyzed by high flux dialysis. OKT3 will be removed by plasmapheresis. Administer following dialysis treatments.

Administration

I.V. Not for I.M. administration. Give I.V. push over <1 minute at a final concentration of 1 mg/mL. Methylprednisolone sodium succinate 1 mg/kg I.V. given prior to first muromonab-CD3 administration, and I.V. hydrocortisone sodium succinate 50-100 mg, given 30 minutes after administration are strongly recommended to decrease the incidence of reactions to the first dose.

Stability

Storage Refrigerate; do not freeze. Do not shake. Stable in Becton Dickinson syringe for 16 hours at room temperature or refrigeration.

Monitoring and Teaching Issues

Laboratory Monitoring Chest x-ray, CBC with differential, immunologic monitoring of T cells, serum levels of OKT3

Physical Assessment Monitor closely for pulmonary, cardiac, and anaphylactic-type reactions during and for 24 hours following first infusion. Monitor vital signs on a regular basis. Instruct patient to report infection.

Patient Education There may be a severe reaction to the first infusion of this medication. You may experience high fever, chills, respiratory difficulty, or congestion. Effects are substantially reduced with subsequent infusions. You will be susceptible to infection. You may experience dizziness, nausea, vomiting, sensitivity to direct sunlight, headache, fever, chills, rash, and diarrhea. Report chest pain or tightness, symptoms of infection, respiratory difficulty, vision change, swelling of the extremities, or weight gain.

Dietary Considerations Some products may contain sodium.

◆ **Muse®** *see* Alprostadil *on page 83*

◆ **Myambutol®** *see* Ethambutol *on page 693*

◆ **Mycelex** *see* Clotrimazole (Oral) *on page 416*

◆ **Mycobutin®** *see* Rifabutin *on page 1576*

Mycophenolate (mye koe FEN oh late)

U.S. Brand Names CellCept®; Myfortic®

Index Terms MMF; MPA; Mycophenolate Mofetil; Mycophenolate Sodium; Mycophenolic Acid

Generic Availability (U.S.) Yes: Capsule, tablet

Pharmacologic Category Immunosuppressant Agent

Medication Guide Available Yes

Pregnancy Risk Factor D

Lactation Excretion in breast milk unknown/not recommended

Use Prophylaxis of organ rejection concomitantly with cyclosporine and corticosteroids in patients receiving allogeneic renal (CellCept®, Myfortic®), cardiac (CellCept®), or hepatic (CellCept®) transplants

Unlabeled/Investigational Use Treatment of rejection in liver transplant patients unable to tolerate tacrolimus or cyclosporine due to neurotoxicity; mild rejection in heart transplant patients; treatment of moderate-severe psoriasis; treatment of proliferative lupus nephritis; treatment of myasthenia gravis; prevention and treatment of graft-versus-host disease (GVHD)

Mechanism of Action/Effect Inhibition of purine synthesis of human lymphocytes and proliferation of human lymphocytes

Contraindications Hypersensitivity to mycophenolate mofetil, mycophenolic acid, mycophenolate sodium, or any component of the formulation; intravenous formulation is contraindicated in patients who are allergic to polysorbate 80

Warnings/Precautions Hazardous agent - use appropriate precautions for handling and disposal. **[U.S. Boxed Warning]: Risk for infection and development of lymphoma and skin malignancy is increased.** Opportunistic infections, sepsis, and/or fatal infections may occur with immunosuppressive therapy. Patients should be monitored appropriately. Instruct patients to limit exposure to sunlight/UV light and give supportive treatment should these conditions occur. Pure red cell aplasia (PRCA), progressive multifocal leukoencephalopathy (PML), or BK virus-associated nephropathy (BKVAN) may occur rarely, particularly in immunosuppressed patients or those receiving immunosuppressant therapy; monitor for signs of PRCA (anemia, fatigue, lethargy, pallor, dyspnea), PML (neurologic impairment, apathy, ataxia, cognitive deficiencies, confusion, and hemiparesis), or BKVAN (deterioration of renal function, renal graft loss); may require dosage reduction or discontinuation of therapy. Neutropenia (including severe neutropenia) may occur, requiring dose reduction or interruption of treatment (risk greater from day 31-180 post-transplant). Use caution with active peptic ulcer disease; may be associated with gastric or duodenal ulcers, GI bleeding and/or perforation. Use caution in renal impairment as toxicity may be increased; may require dosage adjustment in severe impairment.

[U.S. Boxed Warning]: Mycophenolate is associated with an increased risk of congenital malformations and spontaneous abortions when used during pregnancy. Females of childbearing potential should have a negative pregnancy test within 1 week prior to beginning therapy. Two reliable forms of contraception should be used beginning 4 weeks prior to, during, and for 6 weeks after therapy. Because mycophenolate mofetil has demonstrated teratogenic effects in rats and rabbits, tablets should not be crushed, and capsules should not be opened or crushed. Avoid inhalation or direct contact with skin or mucous membranes of the powder contained in the capsules and the powder for oral suspension. Caution should be exercised in the handling and preparation of solutions of intravenous mycophenolate. Avoid skin contact with the intravenous solution and reconstituted suspension. If such contact occurs, wash thoroughly with soap and water, rinse eyes with plain water.

Theoretically, use should be avoided in patients with the rare hereditary deficiency of hypoxanthine-guanine phosphoribosyltransferase (such as Lesch-Nyhan or Kelley-Seegmiller syndrome). Intravenous solutions should be given over at least 2 hours; never administer intravenous solution by rapid or bolus injection. **[U.S. Boxed Warning]: Should be administered under the supervision of a physician experienced in immunosuppressive therapy.**

Note: CellCept® and Myfortic® dosage forms should not be used interchangeably due to differences in absorption. Some dosage forms may contain phenylalanine.

Drug Interactions

Avoid Concomitant Use

Avoid concomitant use of Mycophenolate with any of the following: BCG; Cholestyramine Resin; Natalizumab; Pimecrolimus; Rifamycin Derivatives; Roflumilast; Tacrolimus (Topical); Vaccines (Live)

Decreased Effect

Mycophenolate may decrease the levels/effects of: BCG; Contraceptives (Estrogens); Contraceptives (Progestins); Sipuleucel-T; Vaccines (Inactivated); Vaccines (Live)

The levels/effects of Mycophenolate may be decreased by: Antacids; Cholestyramine Resin; CycloSPORINE; CycloSPORINE (Systemic); Echinacea; Magnesium Salts; MetroNIDAZOLE; MetroNIDAZOLE (Systemic); Penicillins; Proton Pump Inhibitors; Quinolone Antibiotics; Rifamycin Derivatives; Sevelamer

Increased Effect/Toxicity

Mycophenolate may increase the levels/effects of: Acyclovir-Valacyclovir; Ganciclovir-Valganciclovir; Leflunomide; Natalizumab; Vaccines (Live)

The levels/effects of Mycophenolate may be increased by: Acyclovir-Valacyclovir; Denosumab; Ganciclovir-Valganciclovir; Pimecrolimus; Probenecid; Roflumilast; Tacrolimus (Topical); Trastuzumab

Nutritional/Ethanol Interactions

Food: Decreases C_{max} of MPA by 40% following CellCept® administration and 33% following Myfortic® use; the extent of absorption is not changed

Herb/Nutraceutical: Avoid cat's claw, echinacea (have immunostimulant properties)

Adverse Reactions Data for incidence >20% as reported in adults following oral dosing of CellCept® alone in renal, cardiac, and hepatic allograft rejection studies. Profile in 3% to <20% range reflects use in combination with cyclosporine and corticosteroids. In general, lower doses used in renal rejection patients had less adverse effects than higher doses. Rates of adverse effects were similar for each indication, except for those unique to the specific organ involved. The type of adverse effects observed in pediatric patients was similar to those seen in adults; abdominal pain, anemia, diarrhea, fever, hypertension, infection, pharyngitis, respiratory tract infection, sepsis, and vomiting were seen in higher proportion; lymphoproliferative disorder was the only type of malignancy observed. Percentages of adverse reactions were similar in studies comparing CellCept® to Myfortic® in patients following renal transplant.

>20%:

- Cardiovascular: Hypertension (28% to 78%), hypotension (33%), peripheral edema (27% to 64%), edema (27% to 28%), chest pain (26%), tachycardia (20% to 22%)
- Central nervous system: Pain (31% to 76%), headache (16% to 54%), insomnia (41% to 52%), fever (21% to 52%), dizziness (29%), anxiety (28%)
- Dermatologic: Rash (22%)
- Endocrine & metabolic: Hyperglycemia (44% to 47%), hypercholesterolemia (41%), hypomagnesemia (39%), hypokalemia (32% to 37%), hypocalcemia (30%), hyperkalemia (22%)
- Gastrointestinal: Abdominal pain (25% to 63%), nausea (20% to 55%), diarrhea (31% to 51%), constipation (19% to 41%), vomiting (33% to 34%), anorexia (25%), dyspepsia (22%)
- Genitourinary: Urinary tract infection (37%)
- Hematologic: Leukopenia (23% to 46%), anemia (26% to 43%; hypochromic 25%), leukocytosis (22% to 41%), thrombocytopenia (24% to 38%)
- Hepatic: Liver function tests abnormal (25%), ascites (24%)
- Neuromuscular & skeletal: Back pain (35% to 47%), weakness (35% to 43%), tremor (24% to 34%), paresthesia (21%)
- Renal: Creatinine increased (39%), BUN increased (35%), kidney function abnormal (22% to 26%)
- Respiratory: Dyspnea (31% to 37%), respiratory tract infection (22% to 37%), pleural effusion (34%), cough (31%), lung disorder (22% to 30%), sinusitis (26%)
- Miscellaneous: Infection (18% to 27%), sepsis (27%), lactate dehydrogenase increased (23%), *Candida* (17% to 22%), herpes simplex (10% to 21%)

3% to <20%:

- Cardiovascular: Angina, arrhythmia, arterial thrombosis, atrial fibrillation, atrial flutter, bradycardia, cardiac arrest, cardiac failure, CHF, extrasystole, facial edema, hyper-/hypovolemia, pallor, palpitation, pericardial effusion, peripheral vascular disorder, postural hypotension, supraventricular extrasystoles, supraventricular tachycardia, syncope, thrombosis, vasodilation, vasospasm, venous pressure increased, ventricular extrasystole, ventricular tachycardia
- Central nervous system: Agitation, chills with fever, confusion, delirium, depression, emotional lability, hallucinations, hypoesthesia, malaise, nervousness, psychosis, seizure, somnolence, thinking abnormal, vertigo
- Dermatologic: Acne, alopecia, bruising, cellulitis, fungal dermatitis, hirsutism, petechia, pruritus, skin carcinoma, skin hypertrophy, skin ulcer, vesiculobullous rash

Endocrine & metabolic: Acidosis, alkalosis, Cushing's syndrome, dehydration, diabetes mellitus, gout, hypercalcemia, hyper-hypophosphatemia, hyperlipemia, hyperuricemia, hypochloremia, hypoglycemia, hyponatremia, hypoproteinemia, hypothyroidism, parathyroid disorder

Gastrointestinal: Abdomen enlarged, dysphagia, esophagitis, flatulence, gastritis, gastroenteritis, gastrointestinal hemorrhage, gastrointestinal moniliasis, gingivitis, gum hyperplasia, ileus, melena, mouth ulceration, oral moniliasis, stomach disorder, stomach ulcer, stomatitis, xerostomia, weight gain/loss

Genitourinary: Impotence, nocturia, pelvic pain, prostatic disorder, scrotal edema, urinary frequency, urinary incontinence, urinary retention, urinary tract disorder

Hematologic: Coagulation disorder, hemorrhage, neutropenia, pancytopenia, polycythemia, prothrombin time increased, thromboplastin time increased

Hepatic: Alkaline phosphatase increased, bilirubinemia, cholangitis, cholestatic jaundice, GGT increased, hepatitis, jaundice, liver damage, transaminases increased

Local: Abscess

Neuromuscular & skeletal: Arthralgia, hypertonia, joint disorder, leg cramps, myalgia, myasthenia, neck pain, neuropathy, osteoporosis

Ocular: Amblyopia, cataract, conjunctivitis, eye hemorrhage, lacrimation disorder, vision abnormal

Otic: Deafness, ear disorder, ear pain, tinnitus

Renal: Albuminuria, creatinine increased, dysuria, hematuria, hydronephrosis, oliguria, pyelonephritis, renal failure, renal tubular necrosis

Respiratory: Apnea, asthma, atelectasis, bronchitis, epistaxis, hemoptysis, hiccup, hyperventilation, hypoxia, respiratory acidosis, pharyngitis, pneumonia, pneumothorax, pulmonary edema, pulmonary hypertension, respiratory moniliasis, rhinitis, sputum increased, voice alteration

Miscellaneous: *Candida* (mucocutaneous 16% to 18%), CMV viremia/syndrome (12% to 14%), CMV tissue invasive disease (6% to 12%), herpes zoster cutaneous disease (4% to 10%), cyst, diaphoresis, flu-like syndrome, healing abnormal, hernia, ileus infection, neoplasm, peritonitis, thirst

Pharmacodynamics/Kinetics

Onset of Action Peak effect: Correlation of toxicity or efficacy is still being developed, however, one study indicated that 12-hour AUCs >40 mcg/mL/hour were correlated with efficacy and decreased episodes of rejection

Absorption AUC values for MPA are lower in the early post-transplant period versus later (>3 months) post-transplant period. The extent of absorption in pediatrics is similar to that seen in adults, although there was wide variability reported.

Oral: Myfortic®: 93%

Bioavailability Oral: CellCept®: 94%; Myfortic®: 72%

Time to Peak Plasma: Oral: MPA:

CellCept®: 1-1.5 hours

Myfortic®: 1.5-2.75 hours

Protein Binding MPA: >97%, MPAG 82%

Half-Life Elimination

CellCept®: MPA: Oral: 18 hours; I.V.: 17 hours

Myfortic®: MPA: Oral: 8-16 hours; MPAG: 13-17 hours

Metabolism Hepatic and via GI tract; CellCept® is completely hydrolyzed in the liver to mycophenolic acid (MPA; active metabolite); enterohepatic recirculation of MPA may occur; MPA is glucuronidated to MPAG (inactive metabolite)

Excretion

CellCept®: MPA: Urine (<1%), feces (6%); MPAG: Urine (87%)

Myfortic®: MPA: Urine (3%), feces; MPAG: Urine (>60%)

Available Dosage Forms

Capsule, oral: 250 mg

CellCept®: 250 mg

Injection, powder for reconstitution:

CellCept®: 500 mg

Powder for suspension, oral:

CellCept®: 200 mg/mL (175 mL)

Tablet, oral: 500 mg

CellCept®: 500 mg

Tablet, delayed release, oral:

Myfortic®: 180 mg, 360 mg

Dosing

Adult Note: May be used I.V. for up to 14 days; transition to oral therapy as soon as tolerated.

Renal transplant:

CellCept®:

Oral: 1 g twice daily. Doses >2 g/day are not recommended.

I.V.: 1 g twice daily

Myfortic®: Oral: 720 mg twice daily (1440 mg/day)

Cardiac transplantation:

Oral (CellCept®): 1.5 g twice daily

I.V. (CellCept®): 1.5 g twice daily

Hepatic transplantation:

Oral (CellCept®): 1.5 g twice daily

I.V. (CellCept®): 1 g twice daily

Lupus nephritis (unlabeled use): Oral: 0.5-3 g/day (Contreras, 2004; Ong, 2005)

Myasthenia gravis (unlabeled use): Oral (CellCept®): 1 g twice daily (range: 1-3 g/day) (Cahoon, 2006; Ciafaloni, 2001; Merriggioli, 2003)

Psoriasis (unlabeled use): Oral: 2-3 g/day (Menter, 2009)

Geriatric Dosage is the same as younger patients, however, dosing should be cautious due to possibility of increased hepatic, renal, or cardiac dysfunction. Elderly patients may be at an increased risk of certain infections, gastrointestinal hemorrhage, and pulmonary edema, as compared to younger patients.

Pediatric

Renal transplant: Oral:

CellCept® suspension: 600 mg/m^2/dose twice daily; maximum dose: 1 g twice daily

Alternatively, may use solid dosage forms according to BSA as follows:

BSA 1.25-1.5 m^2: 750 mg capsule twice daily

BSA >1.5 m^2: 1 g capsule or tablet twice daily

Myfortic®: 400 mg/m^2/dose twice daily; maximum dose: 720 mg twice daily

BSA <1.19 m^2: Use of this formulation is not recommended

BSA 1.19-1.58 m^2: 540 mg twice daily (maximum: 1080 mg/day)

BSA >1.58 m^2: 720 mg twice daily (maximum: 1440 mg/day)

Renal Impairment

Renal transplant: GFR <25 mL/minute/1.73 m^2 in patients outside the immediate post-transplant period:

CellCept®: Doses of >1 g administered twice daily should be avoided; patients should also be carefully observed; no dose adjustments are needed in renal transplant patients experiencing delayed graft function postoperatively

Myfortic®: No dose adjustments are needed in renal transplant patients experiencing delayed graft function postoperatively; however, monitor carefully for potential concentration dependent adverse events

Cardiac or liver transplant: No data available; mycophenolate may be used in cardiac or hepatic transplant patients with severe chronic renal impairment if the potential benefit outweighs the potential risk.

Hemodialysis: Not removed; supplemental dose is not necessary.

Peritoneal dialysis: Supplemental dose is not necessary.

Hepatic Impairment No dosage adjustment is recommended for renal patients with severe hepatic parenchymal disease; however, it is not currently known whether dosage adjustments are necessary for hepatic disease with other etiologies.

Adjustment for Toxicity Neutropenia (ANC <1.3 x 10^3/µL): Dosing should be interrupted or the dose reduced, appropriate diagnostic tests performed and patients managed appropriately

Administration

Oral Oral dosage formulations (tablet, capsule, suspension) should be administered on an empty stomach to avoid variability in MPA absorption. The oral solution may be administered via a nasogastric tube (minimum 8 French, 1.7 mm interior diameter); oral suspension should not be mixed with other medications. Delayed release tablets should not be crushed, cut, or chewed.

I.V. Intravenous solutions should be given over at least 2 hours. Do not administer intravenous solution by rapid or bolus injection.

Stability

Reconstitution

Oral suspension: Should be constituted prior to dispensing to the patient and **not** mixed with any other medication. Add 47 mL of water to the bottle and shake well for ~1 minute. Add another 47 mL of water to the bottle and shake well for an additional minute. Final concentration is 200 mg/mL of mycophenolate mofetil.

I.V.: Reconstitute the contents of each vial with 14 mL of 5% dextrose injection; dilute the contents of a vial with 5% dextrose in water to a final concentration of 6 mg mycophenolate mofetil per mL. **Note:** Vial is vacuum-sealed; if a lack of vacuum is noted during preparation, the vial should not be used.

Storage

Capsules: Store at 25°C (77°F); excursions permitted to 15°C to 30°C (59°F to 86°F).

Tablets: Store at 25°C (77°F); excursions permitted to 15°C to 30°C (59°F to 86°F). Protect from moisture and light.

Oral suspension: Store powder for oral suspension at 25°C (77°F); excursions permitted to 15°C to 30°C (59°F to 86°F). Once reconstituted, the oral solution may be stored at room temperature or under refrigeration. Do not freeze. The mixed suspension is stable for 60 days.

Injection: Store intact vials and diluted solutions at 25°C (77°F); excursions permitted to 15°C to 30°C (59°F to 86°F). Begin infusion within 4 hours of reconstitution.

Monitoring and Teaching Issues

Laboratory Monitoring Complete blood count (weekly for first month, twice monthly during months 2 and 3, then monthly thereafter through the first year); renal and liver function; pregnancy test (prior to initiation in females of childbearing potential)

Physical Assessment Monitor blood pressure periodically while receiving this medication. Assess for peripheral edema and other signs of fluid retention. Patients with diabetes should monitor glucose levels closely (this medication may alter glucose levels). Monitor for signs of opportunistic infection. Patient is at risk for lymphoproliferative disease and certain other malignancies; monitor closely.

Patient Education Take oral formulations as directed, preferably 1 hour before or 2 hours after meals. Do not cut, chew, or crush delayed-release tablets. You will be susceptible to infection. You may be at increased risk for skin cancer. If you have diabetes, monitor glucose levels closely (drug may alter glucose levels). You may experience dizziness or trembling, trouble sleeping, nausea or vomiting, diarrhea, sores or white plaques in mouth, or muscle or back pain. Report chest pain; irregular or rapid heartbeat; acute headache or dizziness; swelling of extremities; unusual weight gain; symptoms of respiratory infection, cough, or respiratory difficulty; abdominal pain or unresolved GI effects; unusual weakness; fatigue, chills, or fever; unhealed sores or white plaques in mouth; irritation in genital area or unusual discharge; change in mental status, memory loss, or loss of coordination or clumsiness; weakness in legs; difficulty speaking or understanding what others say; or unusual bruising or bleeding.

Dietary Considerations Oral dosage formulations should be taken on an empty stomach to avoid variability in MPA absorption. However, in stable renal transplant patients, may be administered with food if necessary. Some products may contain phenylalanine.

Breast-Feeding Considerations It is unknown if mycophenolate is excreted in human milk. Due to potentially serious adverse reactions, the decision to discontinue the drug or discontinue breast-feeding should be considered. Breast-feeding is not recommended during therapy or for 6 weeks after treatment is complete.

Pregnancy Considerations [U.S. Boxed Warning]: Mycophenolate is associated with an increased risk of congenital malformations and spontaneous abortions when used during pregnancy. Adverse events have been reported in animal studies at doses less than the equivalent recommended human dose. Data from the National Transplantation Pregnancy Registry (NTPR) have observed an increase in structural malformations (including ear malformations) in infants born to mothers taking mycophenolate during pregnancy. Spontaneous abortions have also been noted. Females of childbearing potential should have a negative pregnancy test within 1 week prior to beginning therapy. Two reliable forms of contraception should be used beginning 4 weeks prior to, during, and for 6 weeks after therapy. The effectiveness of hormonal contraceptive agents may be affected by mycophenolate.

The National Transplantation Pregnancy Registry (NTPR, Temple University) is a registry for pregnant women taking immunosuppressants following any solid organ transplant. The NTPR encourages reporting of all immunosuppressant exposures during pregnancy in transplant recipients at 877-955-6877.

- **Mycophenolate Mofetil** *see* Mycophenolate *on page* 1270
- **Mycophenolate Sodium** *see* Mycophenolate *on page* 1270
- **Mycophenolic Acid** *see* Mycophenolate *on page* 1270
- **Mydfrin®** *see* Phenylephrine (Ophthalmic) *on page* 1452
- **Myfortic®** *see* Mycophenolate *on page* 1270
- **MyKidz Iron 10™ [OTC]** *see* Ferrous Sulfate *on page* 754
- **Myleran®** *see* Busulfan *on page* 257
- **Mylotarg® [DSC]** *see* Gemtuzumab Ozogamicin *on page* 863
- **Mysoline®** *see* Primidone *on page* 1507
- **Mytelase®** *see* Ambenonium *on page* 92
- **Mytotan** *see* Mitotane *on page* 1242

Nabilone (NA bi lone)

U.S. Brand Names Cesamet®

Generic Availability (U.S.) No

Pharmacologic Category Antiemetic

Pregnancy Risk Factor C

Lactation Excretion in breast milk unknown/not recommended

Use Treatment of refractory nausea and vomiting associated with cancer chemotherapy

Mechanism of Action/Effect Not fully characterized; antiemetic activity may be due to effect on cannabinoid receptors (CB1) within the central nervous system.

Contraindications Hypersensitivity to nabilone, cannabinoids, tetrahydrocannabinol, or any component of the formulation

Warnings/Precautions May affect CNS function; use with caution in the elderly and those with pre-existing CNS depression. May cause additive CNS effects with sedatives, hypnotics, or other psychoactive agents; patients must be cautioned about performing tasks which require mental alertness (eg, operating machinery or driving). Use caution with current or previous history of mental illness; cannabinoid use may reveal symptoms of psychiatric disorders. Psychiatric adverse reactions may persist for up to 3 days after discontinuing treatment. Has potential for abuse and or dependence, use caution in patients with substance abuse history or potential. May cause tachycardia and orthostatic hypotension; use caution with cardiovascular disease. Safety and efficacy in children have not been established.

Drug Interactions

Avoid Concomitant Use There are no known interactions where it is recommended to avoid concomitant use.

Decreased Effect There are no known significant interactions involving a decrease in effect.

Increased Effect/Toxicity

Nabilone may increase the levels/effects of: Alcohol (Ethyl); CNS Depressants; Methotrimeprazine; Sympathomimetics

The levels/effects of Nabilone may be increased by: Anticholinergic Agents; Cocaine; Droperidol; Methotrimeprazine

Nutritional/Ethanol Interactions Ethanol: Avoid ethanol (may increase CNS depression).

Adverse Reactions

>10%:

Central nervous system: Drowsiness (52% to 66%), dizziness (59%), vertigo (52% to 59%), euphoria (11% to 38%), ataxia (13% to 14%), depression (14%), concentration decreased (12%), sleep disturbance (11%)

Gastrointestinal: Xerostomia (22% to 36%)

Ocular: Visual disturbance (13%)

1% to 10%:

Cardiovascular: Hypotension (8%)

Central nervous system: Dysphoria (9%), headache (6% to 7%), sedation (3%), depersonalization (2%), disorientation (2%)

Gastrointestinal: Anorexia (8%), nausea (4%), appetite increased (2%)

Neuromuscular & skeletal: Weakness (8%)

Pharmacodynamics/Kinetics

Absorption Rapid and complete

Time to Peak Serum: Within 2 hours

Half-Life Elimination Parent compound: 2 hours; Metabolites: 35 hours

Metabolism To several active metabolites by oxidation and stereospecific enzyme reduction; CYP450 enzymes may also be involved

Excretion Feces (~60%); renal (~24%)

Controlled Substance C-II

Available Dosage Forms

Capsule, oral:

Cesamet®: 1 mg

Dosing

Adult & Geriatric Refer to individual protocols.

Nausea and vomiting associated with cancer chemotherapy: Oral: 1-2 mg twice daily (maximum: 6 mg divided in 3 doses daily)

Pediatric Refer to individual protocols.

Nausea and vomiting associated with cancer chemotherapy (unlabeled use): Oral: Children >4 years:

<18 kg: 0.5 mg twice daily

18-30 kg: 1 mg twice daily

>30 kg: 1 mg 3 times/day

Renal Impairment No adjustment required.

Administration

Oral Initial dose should be given 1-3 hours before chemotherapy; may be given 2-3 times a day during the entire chemotherapy course and for up to 48 hours after the last dose of chemotherapy; a dose of 1-2 mg the night before chemotherapy may be useful.

Stability

Storage Store at room temperature between 15°C and 30°C (59°F and 86°F).

Monitoring and Teaching Issues

Physical Assessment For use when other antiemetic agents have proved ineffective. Use caution with history of substance abuse or mental illness. Assess effectiveness of therapy and monitor closely for adverse psychotic reactions which may persist for up to 3 days following discontinuation; this drug has the psychoactive properties of marijuana and has the potential for abuse or dependence.

Patient Education Avoid alcohol. May cause psychotic reaction, impaired coordination or judgment, faintness, dizziness, drowsiness, unsteadiness, sleep disturbance or visual disturbances, orthostatic hypotension, dry mouth, or decreased appetite. Report excessive or persistent CNS changes (euphoria, anxiety, depression, memory lapse, bizarre thought patterns, excitability, inability to control thoughts or behavior, fainting), respiratory difficulties, or rapid heartbeat.

Breast-Feeding Considerations Because some cannabinoids are excreted in breast milk, use in breast-feeding is not recommended.

Pregnancy Considerations Animal studies did not demonstrate teratogenic effects; however, dose-related decreased fetal weights and increased fetal resorptions were observed. There are no adequate and well-controlled studies in pregnant women. Use during pregnancy only if clearly needed.

◆ **nab-Paclitaxel** *see* Paclitaxel (Protein Bound) *on page* 1390

Nabumetone (na BYOO me tone)

Index Terms Relafen

Generic Availability (U.S.) Yes

Pharmacologic Category Nonsteroidal Anti-inflammatory Drug (NSAID), Oral

Medication Guide Available Yes

Pregnancy Risk Factor C

Lactation Excretion in breast milk unknown/not recommended

Use Management of osteoarthritis and rheumatoid arthritis

Unlabeled/Investigational Use Moderate pain

Mechanism of Action/Effect Reversibly inhibits cyclooxygenase-1 and 2 (COX-1 and 2) enzymes, which results in decreased formation of prostaglandin precursors; has antipyretic, analgesic, and anti-inflammatory properties

Contraindications Hypersensitivity to nabumetone, aspirin, other NSAIDs, or any component of the formulation; perioperative pain in the setting of coronary artery bypass graft (CABG) surgery

Warnings/Precautions [U.S. Boxed Warning]: NSAIDs are associated with an increased risk of adverse cardiovascular thrombotic events, including MI and stroke. Risk may be increased with duration of use or pre-existing cardiovascular risk factors or disease. Carefully evaluate individual cardiovascular risk profiles prior to prescribing. May cause new-onset hypertension or worsening of existing hypertension. Use caution with fluid retention. Avoid use in heart failure. Concurrent administration of ibuprofen, and potentially other nonselective NSAIDs, may interfere with aspirin's cardioprotective effect. **[U.S. Boxed Warning]: Use is contraindicated for treatment of perioperative pain in the setting of coronary artery bypass graft (CABG) surgery.** Risk of MI and stroke may be increased with use following CABG surgery.

Platelet adhesion and aggregation may be decreased; may prolong bleeding time; patients with coagulation disorders or who are receiving anticoagulants should be monitored closely. Anemia may occur; patients on long-term NSAID therapy should be monitored for anemia. Rarely, NSAID use may cause severe blood dyscrasias (eg, agranulocytosis, aplastic anemia, thrombocytopenia).

NSAID use may compromise existing renal function; dose-dependent decreases in prostaglandin synthesis may result from NSAID use, reducing renal blood flow which may cause renal decompensation. NSAID use may increase the risk for hyperkalemia. Patients with impaired renal function, dehydration, heart failure, liver dysfunction, those taking diuretics, and ACE inhibitors, and the elderly are at greater risk of renal toxicity and hyperkalemia. Rehydrate patient before starting therapy; monitor renal function closely. Not recommended for use in patients with advanced renal disease. Long-term NSAID use may result in renal papillary necrosis.

[U.S. Boxed Warning]: NSAIDs may increase risk of gastrointestinal irritation, inflammation, ulceration, bleeding, and perforation. These events may occur at any time during therapy and without warning. Use caution with a history of GI disease (bleeding or ulcers), concurrent therapy with aspirin, anticoagulants and/or corticosteroids, smoking, use of alcohol, the elderly or debilitated patients. When used concomitantly with ≤325 mg of aspirin, a substantial increase in the risk of gastrointestinal complications (eg, ulcer) occurs; concomitant gastroprotective therapy (eg, proton pump inhibitors) is recommended (Bhatt, 2008).

Use the lowest effective dose for the shortest duration of time, consistent with individual patient goals, to reduce risk of cardiovascular or GI adverse events. Alternate therapies should be considered for patients at high risk.

NSAIDs may cause serious skin adverse events including exfoliative dermatitis, Stevens-Johnson syndrome (SJS) and toxic epidermal necrolysis (TEN); discontinue use at first sign of skin rash or hypersensitivity. Anaphylactoid reactions may occur, even without prior exposure; patients with "aspirin triad" (bronchial asthma, aspirin intolerance, rhinitis) may be at increased risk. Do not use in patients who experience bronchospasm, asthma, rhinitis, or urticaria with NSAID or aspirin therapy. Use caution in other forms of asthma.

Use with caution in patients with decreased hepatic function. Closely monitor patients with any abnormal LFT. Severe hepatic reactions (eg, fulminant hepatitis, liver failure) have occurred with NSAID use, rarely; discontinue if signs or symptoms of liver disease develop, or if systemic manifestations occur.

NSAIDS may cause drowsiness, dizziness, blurred vision and other neurologic effects which may impair physical or mental abilities; patients must be cautioned about performing tasks which require mental alertness (eg, operating machinery or driving). Discontinue use with blurred or diminished vision and perform ophthalmologic exam. Monitor vision with long-term therapy.

The elderly are at increased risk for adverse effects (especially peptic ulceration, CNS effects, renal toxicity) from NSAIDs even at low doses.

Withhold for at least 4-6 half-lives prior to surgical or dental procedures. May cause photosensitivity reactions.

Drug Interactions

Avoid Concomitant Use

Avoid concomitant use of Nabumetone with any of the following: Ketorolac; Ketorolac (Systemic)

Decreased Effect

Nabumetone may decrease the levels/effects of: ACE Inhibitors; Angiotensin II Receptor Blockers; Antiplatelet Agents; Beta-Blockers; Eplerenone; HydrALAZINE; Loop Diuretics; Potassium-Sparing Diuretics; Salicylates; Thiazide Diuretics

The levels/effects of Nabumetone may be decreased by: Bile Acid Sequestrants; Nonsteroidal Anti-Inflammatory Agents; Salicylates

Increased Effect/Toxicity

Nabumetone may increase the levels/effects of: Aminoglycosides; Anticoagulants; Antiplatelet Agents; Bisphosphonate Derivatives; Collagenase (Systemic); CycloSPORINE; CycloSPORINE (Systemic); Desmopressin; Digoxin; Drotrecogin Alfa; Eplerenone; Haloperidol; Ibritumomab; Lithium; Methotrexate; Nonsteroidal Anti-Inflammatory Agents; PEMEtrexed; Potassium-Sparing Diuretics; PRALAtrexate; Quinolone Antibiotics; Salicylates; Thrombolytic Agents; Tositumomab and Iodine I 131 Tositumomab; Vancomycin; Vitamin K Antagonists

The levels/effects of Nabumetone may be increased by: Antidepressants (Tricyclic, Tertiary Amine); Corticosteroids (Systemic); Dasatinib; Glucosamine; Herbs (Anticoagulant/Antiplatelet Properties); Ketorolac; Ketorolac (Systemic); Nonsteroidal Anti-Inflammatory Agents; Omega-3-Acid Ethyl Esters; Pentosan Polysulfate Sodium; Pentoxifylline; Probenecid; Prostacyclin Analogues; Selective Serotonin Reuptake Inhibitors; Serotonin/Norepinephrine Reuptake Inhibitors; Treprostinil

Nutritional/Ethanol Interactions

Ethanol: Avoid ethanol (may enhance gastric mucosal irritation).

Food: Nabumetone peak serum concentrations may be increased if taken with food or dairy products.

Herb/Nutraceutical: Avoid alfalfa, anise, bilberry, bladderwrack, bromelain, cat's claw, celery, chamomile, coleus, cordyceps, dong quai, evening primrose, fenugreek, feverfew, garlic, ginger, ginkgo biloba, ginseng (American, Panax, Siberian), grapeseed, green tea, guggul, horse chestnut seed, horseradish, licorice, prickly ash, red clover, reishi, SAMe (S-adenosylmethionine), sweet clover, turmeric, white willow (all have additional antiplatelet activity).

Adverse Reactions

>10%: Gastrointestinal: Diarrhea (14%), dyspepsia (13%), abdominal pain (12%)

1% to 10%:

Cardiovascular: Edema (3% to 9%)

Central nervous system: Dizziness (3% to 9%), headache (3% to 9%), fatigue (1% to 3%), insomnia (1% to 3%), nervousness (1% to 3%), somnolence (1% to 3%)

Dermatologic: Pruritus (3% to 9%), rash (3% to 9%)

Gastrointestinal: Constipation (3% to 9%), flatulence (3% to 9%), guaiac positive (3% to 9%), nausea (3% to 9%), gastritis (1% to 3%), stomatitis (1% to 3%), vomiting (1% to 3%), xerostomia (1% to 3%)

Otic: Tinnitus

Miscellaneous: Diaphoresis (1% to 3%)

Pharmacodynamics/Kinetics

Onset of Action Several days

Time to Peak Serum: 6MNA: Oral: 2.5-4 hours; Synovial fluid: 4-12 hours

Protein Binding 6MNA: >99%

Half-Life Elimination 6MNA: ~24 hours

Metabolism Prodrug, rapidly metabolized in the liver to an active metabolite [6-methoxy-2-naphthylacetic acid (6MNA)] and inactive metabolites; extensive first-pass effect

Excretion 6MNA: Urine (80%) and feces (9%)

Available Dosage Forms

Tablet, oral: 500 mg, 750 mg

Dosing

Adult Osteoarthritis, rheumatoid arthritis: Oral: 1000 mg/day; an additional 500-1000 mg may be needed in some patients to obtain more symptomatic relief; may be administered once or twice daily; maximum dose: 2000 mg/day

Note: Patients <50 kg are less likely to require doses >1000 mg/day.

Geriatric Refer to adult dosing; do not exceed 2000 mg/day.

Renal Impairment In general, NSAIDs are not recommended for use in patients with advanced renal disease, but the manufacturer of nabumetone does provide some guidelines for adjustment in renal dysfunction:

Moderate impairment (Cl_{cr} 30-49 mL/minute): Initial dose: 750 mg/day; maximum dose: 1500 mg/day

Severe impairment (Cl_{cr} <30 mL/minute): Initial dose: 500 mg/day; maximum dose: 1000 mg/day

Monitoring and Teaching Issues

Laboratory Monitoring Patients with renal insufficiency: Baseline renal function followed by repeat test within weeks (to determine if renal function has deteriorated)

Physical Assessment Evaluate cardiac risk and potential for GI bleeding prior to prescribing this medication. Monitor blood pressure at the beginning of therapy and periodically during use. Monitor for GI effects, hepatotoxicity, and ototoxicity at beginning of therapy and periodically throughout. Schedule ophthalmic evaluations for patients who develop eye complaints during long-term NSAID therapy.

Patient Education Do not crush tablets. Take with food or milk to reduce GI distress. Do not use alcohol. You may experience drowsiness, dizziness, nervousness, headache, anorexia, nausea, vomiting, heartburn, or fluid retention; GI bleeding, ulceration, or perforation can occur with or without pain; discontinue medication and contact prescriber if persistent abdominal pain or cramping or blood in stool occurs. Report respiratory difficulty or unusual cough; chest pain, rapid heartbeat, or palpitations; bruising/bleeding; blood in urine, stool, mouth, or vomitus; swollen extremities; skin rash or itching; or hearing changes (ringing in ears).

Geriatric Considerations In trials with nabumetone, no significant differences were noted between young and the elderly in regards to efficacy and safety. However, the elderly are a high-risk population for adverse effects from NSAIDs. As much as 60% of elderly can develop peptic ulceration and/or hemorrhage asymptomatically. The concomitant use of H_2 blockers and sucralfate is not effective as prophylaxis with the exception of NSAID-induced duodenal ulcers which may be prevented by the use of ranitidine. Misoprostol and proton pump inhibitors are the only agents proven to help prevent the development of NSAID-induced ulcers. Also, concomitant disease and drug use contribute to the risk for GI adverse effects. Use lowest effective dose for shortest period possible. Consider renal function decline with age. Use of NSAIDs can compromise existing renal function especially when Cl_{cr} is ≤30 mL/minute. Tinnitus may be a difficult and unreliable indication of toxicity due to age-related hearing loss or eighth cranial nerve damage. CNS adverse effects such as confusion, agitation, and hallucination are generally seen in overdose or high dose situations, but the elderly may demonstrate these adverse effects at lower doses than younger adults.

Breast-Feeding Considerations It is not known if nabumetone or 6MNA are excreted into breast milk. Breast-feeding is not recommended by the manufacturer.

Pregnancy Considerations Adverse events were not observed in the initial animal reproduction studies; therefore, the manufacturer classifies nabumetone as pregnancy category C. NSAID exposure during the first trimester is not strongly associated with congenital malformations; however, cardiovascular anomalies and cleft palate have been observed following NSAID exposure in some studies. The use of an NSAID close to conception may be associated with an increased risk of miscarriage. Nonteratogenic effects have been observed following NSAID administration during the third trimester including myocardial degenerative changes, prenatal constriction of the ductus arteriosus, fetal tricuspid regurgitation, failure of the ductus arteriosus to close postnatally; renal dysfunction or failure, oligohydramnios; gastrointestinal bleeding or perforation, increased risk of necrotizing enterocolitis; intracranial bleeding (including intraventricular hemorrhage), platelet dysfunction with resultant bleeding; pulmonary hypertension. Because they may cause premature closure of the ductus arteriosus, use of NSAIDs late in pregnancy should be avoided (use after 31 or 32 weeks gestation is not recommended by some clinicians). The chronic use of NSAIDs in women of reproductive age may be associated with infertility that is reversible upon discontinuation of the medication. A registry is available for pregnant women exposed to autoimmune medications including nabumetone. For additional information contact the Organization of Teratology Information Specialists, OTIS Autoimmune Diseases Study, at 877-311-8972.

Related Information

Nonsalicylate / Nonsteroidal Anti-Inflammatory Agents *on page 2002*

◆ **N-Acetyl-P-Aminophenol** *see* Acetaminophen *on page 38*

Nadolol (NAY doe lol)

U.S. Brand Names Corgard®

Generic Availability (U.S.) Yes

Pharmacologic Category Beta-Adrenergic Blocker, Nonselective

Medication Safety Issues

Sound-alike/look-alike issues:

Nadolol may be confused with Mandol®

Corgard® may be confused with Cognex®, Coreg®

Pregnancy Risk Factor C

Lactation Enters breast milk/use caution consider risk:benefit (AAP rates "compatible"; AAP 2001 update pending)

Use Treatment of hypertension and angina pectoris; prophylaxis of migraine headaches

Unlabeled/Investigational Use Primary and secondary prophylaxis of variceal hemorrhage

Mechanism of Action/Effect Competitively blocks response to $beta_1$- and $beta_2$-adrenergic stimulation; does not exhibit any membrane stabilizing or intrinsic sympathomimetic activity; reduces portal pressure

Contraindications Hypersensitivity to nadolol or any component of the formulation; bronchial asthma; sinus bradycardia; sinus node dysfunction; heart block greater than first degree (except in patients with a functioning artificial pacemaker); cardiogenic shock; uncompensated cardiac failure

Warnings/Precautions Consider pre-existing conditions such as sick sinus syndrome before initiating. Administer only with extreme caution in patients with compensated heart failure, monitor for a worsening of the condition. Efficacy in heart failure has not been established for nadolol. **[U.S. Boxed Warning]: Beta-blocker therapy should not be withdrawn abruptly (particularly in patients with CAD), but gradually tapered to avoid acute tachycardia, hypertension, and/or ischemia.** Use caution with concurrent use of beta-blockers and either verapamil or diltiazem; bradycardia or heart block can occur. In general, patients with bronchospastic disease should not receive beta-blockers. Nadolol, if used at all, should be used cautiously in bronchospastic disease with close monitoring. Use cautiously in diabetics because it can mask prominent hypoglycemic symptoms. Use cautiously in the renally impaired (dosage adjustments are required). Use with caution in patients with myasthenia gravis, peripheral vascular disease, or psychiatric disease (may cause CNS depression). Use care with anesthetic agents which decrease myocardial function. Adequate alpha-blockade is required prior to use of any beta-blocker for patients with untreated pheochromocytoma. May induce or exacerbate psoriasis. Use caution with history of severe anaphylaxis to allergens; patients taking beta-blockers may become more sensitive to repeated challenges. Treatment of anaphylaxis (eg, epinephrine) in patients taking beta-blockers may be ineffective or promote undesirable effects.

Drug Interactions

Metabolism/Transport Effects **Substrate** of P-glycoprotein

Avoid Concomitant Use

Avoid concomitant use of Nadolol with any of the following: Methacholine

Decreased Effect

Nadolol may decrease the levels/effects of: Beta2-Agonists; Theophylline Derivatives

The levels/effects of Nadolol may be decreased by: Herbs (Hypertensive Properties); Methylphenidate; Nonsteroidal Anti-Inflammatory Agents; P-Glycoprotein Inducers; Yohimbine

Increased Effect/Toxicity

Nadolol may increase the levels/effects of: Alpha-/Beta-Agonists (Direct-Acting); Alpha1-Blockers; Alpha2-Agonists; Amifostine; Antihypertensives; Bupivacaine; Cardiac Glycosides; Fingolimod; Hypotensive Agents; Insulin; Lidocaine; Lidocaine (Systemic); Lidocaine (Topical); Mepivacaine; Methacholine; Midodrine; RiTUXimab; Sulfonylureas

The levels/effects of Nadolol may be increased by: Acetylcholinesterase Inhibitors; Amiodarone; Anilidopiperidine Opioids; Calcium Channel Blockers (Nondihydropyridine); Diazoxide; Dipyridamole; Disopyramide; Dronedarone; Herbs (Hypotensive Properties); MAO Inhibitors; Pentoxifylline; P-Glycoprotein Inhibitors; Phosphodiesterase 5 Inhibitors; Prostacyclin Analogues; Reserpine

Nutritional/Ethanol Interactions Herb/Nutraceutical: Avoid dong quai if using for hypertension (has estrogenic activity). Avoid ephedra, garlic, yohimbe, ginseng (may worsen hypertension). Avoid natural licorice (causes sodium and water retention and increases potassium loss).

Adverse Reactions

>10%:

Central nervous system: Drowsiness, insomnia

Endocrine & metabolic: Decreased sexual ability

1% to 10%:

Cardiovascular: Bradycardia, palpitation, edema, CHF, reduced peripheral circulation

Central nervous system: Mental depression

Gastrointestinal: Diarrhea or constipation, nausea, vomiting, stomach discomfort

Respiratory: Bronchospasm

Miscellaneous: Cold extremities

Pharmacodynamics/Kinetics

Duration of Action 17-24 hours

Absorption 30% to 40%

Time to Peak Serum: 2-4 hours

Protein Binding 30%

Half-Life Elimination Adults: 10-24 hours, prolonged with renal impairment; End-stage renal disease: 45 hours

Metabolism Not metabolized

Excretion Urine (as unchanged drug)

Available Dosage Forms

Tablet, oral: 20 mg, 40 mg, 80 mg

Corgard®: 20 mg, 40 mg, 80 mg

Dosing

Adult

Hypertension, angina: Oral: Initial: 40-80 mg/day, increase dosage gradually by 40-80 mg increments at 3- to 7-day intervals until optimum clinical response is obtained with profound slowing of heart rate. Doses up to 160-240 mg/day in angina and 240-320 mg/day in hypertension may be necessary. Doses as high as 640 mg/day have been used.

Usual dosage range (JNC 7): 40-120 mg once daily

Variceal hemorrhage prophylaxis (unlabeled use) (Garcia-Tsao, 2007): Oral:

Primary prophylaxis: Initial: 40 mg once daily; adjust to maximal tolerated dose. **Note:** Risk factors for hemorrhage include Child-Pugh class B/C or variceal red wale markings on endoscopy.

Secondary prophylaxis: Initial: 40 mg once daily; adjust to maximal tolerated dose

Geriatric Oral: Initial: 20 mg/day; increase doses by 20 mg increments at 3- to 7-day intervals; usual dosage range: 20-240 mg/day. Adjust for renal impairment.

Renal Impairment

Cl_{cr} 31-40 mL/minute: Administer every 24-36 hours or administer 50% of normal dose.

Cl_{cr} 10-30 mL/minute: Administer every 24-48 hours or administer 50% of normal dose.

Cl_{cr} <10 mL/minute: Administer every 40-60 hours or administer 25% of normal dose.

Hemodialysis effects: Moderately dialyzable (20% to 50%) via hemodialysis. Administer dose postdialysis or administer 40 mg supplemental dose. Supplemental dose is not necessary following peritoneal dialysis.

Hepatic Impairment Reduced dose is probably necessary.

Administration

Oral May be administered without regard to meals.

Monitoring and Teaching Issues

Physical Assessment Assess blood pressure and heart rate prior to and following first dose, any change in dosage, and periodically thereafter. Monitor or advise patient to monitor weight, fluid balance, and signs of CHF. Monitor serum glucose levels of patients with diabetes since beta-blockers may alter glucose tolerance.

Patient Education Check pulse daily prior to taking medication. If pulse is <50, hold medication and consult prescriber. May cause dizziness, fatigue, blurred vision, or constipation. If you have diabetes, monitor serum glucose closely (the drug may mask symptoms of hypoglycemia). Report swelling in feet or legs, respiratory difficulty or persistent cough, unresolved fatigue, or unusual weight gain.

Dietary Considerations May be taken without regard to meals.

Geriatric Considerations Due to alterations in the beta-adrenergic autonomic nervous system, beta-adrenergic blockade may result in less hemodynamic response than seen in younger adults. Studies indicate that despite decreased sensitivity to the chronotropic effects of beta-blockade with age, there appears to be an increased myocardial sensitivity to the negative inotropic effect during stress (ie, exercise). Controlled trials have shown the overall response rate for propranolol to be only 20% to 50% in elderly populations. Therefore, all beta-adrenergic blocking drugs may result in a decreased response as compared to younger adults. Must adjust dose for renal function.

Breast-Feeding Considerations Nadolol is excreted into breast milk in concentrations higher than the maternal serum. According to the manufacturer, the decision to continue or discontinue breast-feeding during therapy should take into account the risk of exposure to the infant and the benefits of treatment to the mother. The time to peak milk concentration is 6 hours after the oral dose, the half-life of nadolol in breast milk is similar to that in the maternal serum, and nadolol can still be detected in breast milk for several days after the last maternal dose.

Pregnancy Considerations Adverse events were observed in some animal reproduction studies; therefore, the manufacturer classifies nadolol as pregnancy category C. Nadolol crosses the placenta and is measurable in infant serum after birth. In a cohort study, an increased risk of cardiovascular defects was observed following maternal use of beta-blockers during pregnancy. Intrauterine growth restriction (IUGR), small placentas, as well as fetal/neonatal bradycardia, hypoglycemia, and/or respiratory depression have been observed following *in utero* exposure to beta-blockers as a class. Adequate facilities for monitoring infants at birth should be available. Untreated chronic maternal hypertension and pre-eclampsia are also associated with adverse events in the fetus, infant, and mother. Nadolol is indicated for the treatment of hypertension, but due to its long half-life and potential effects to the fetus, other agents may be more appropriate for use during pregnancy.

Related Information

Beta-Blockers *on page 1990*

Nafarelin (naf a REL in)

U.S. Brand Names Synarel®

Index Terms Nafarelin Acetate

Generic Availability (U.S.) No

Pharmacologic Category Gonadotropin Releasing Hormone Agonist

Medication Safety Issues

Sound-alike/look-alike issues:

Nafarelin may be confused with Anafranil®, enalapril

Pregnancy Risk Factor X

Lactation Excretion in breast milk unknown/contraindicated

Use Treatment of endometriosis, including pain and reduction of lesions; treatment of central precocious puberty (CPP; gonadotropin-dependent precocious puberty) in children of both sexes

Mechanism of Action/Effect Potent synthetic decapeptide analogue of gonadotropin-releasing hormone (GnRH; LHRH) which is approximately 200 times more potent than GnRH in terms of pituitary release of luteinizing hormone (LH) and follicle-stimulating hormone (FSH)

Contraindications Hypersensitivity to gonadotropin-releasing hormone (GnRH), GnRH-agonist analogs, or any component of the formulation; undiagnosed abnormal vaginal bleeding; pregnancy; breast-feeding

Warnings/Precautions Hazardous agent - use appropriate precautions for handling and disposal. Use with caution in patients with risk factors for decreased bone mineral density, nafarelin therapy may pose an additional risk. Ovarian cysts may occur within the first 2 months of therapy and may occur more commonly in women with polycystic ovarian disease. When used for the treatment of CPP, some signs of puberty (eg vaginal bleeding, breast enlargement) may occur but should resolve within the first 2 months of therapy.

Drug Interactions

Avoid Concomitant Use There are no known interactions where it is recommended to avoid concomitant use.

Decreased Effect

Nafarelin may decrease the levels/effects of: Antidiabetic Agents

Increased Effect/Toxicity There are no known significant interactions involving an increase in effect.

Lab Interactions Diagnostic tests of pituitary gonadotropic and gonadal functions during and up to 4-8 weeks after discontinuing treatment may be misleading.

Adverse Reactions Note: Adverse events may be more frequent in the first 6 weeks of treatment due to stimulation of the pituitary-gonadal axis. Sensitivity reactions included chest pain, pruritus, shortness of breath, rash.

CPP: 1% to 10%:

Central nervous system: Emotional lability (6%)

Dermatologic: Acne (10%), seborrhea (3%)

Endocrine & metabolic: Breast enlargement (8%; transient), vaginal bleeding (8%), hot flashes (3%; transient), vaginal discharge (3%)

Respiratory: Rhinitis (5%)

Miscellaneous: Pubic hair increased (5%; transient), body odor (4%), sensitivity reactions (3%)

Endometriosis:

>10%:

Central nervous system: Headache, emotional lability

Dermatologic: Acne

Endocrine & metabolic: Hot flashes (90%), hyperphosphatemia, hypertriglyceridemia, hypocalcemia, libido decreased

Genitourinary: Vaginal dryness

Hematologic: Leukopenia

1% to 10%:

Cardiovascular: Edema

Central nervous system: Depression, insomnia

Dermatologic: Hirsutism, seborrhea

Endocrine & metabolic: Breast size reduced, cholesterol increased, hyperlipidemia, libido increased

Gastrointestinal: Weight gain/loss

Neuromuscular & skeletal: Bone mineral density decreased, myalgia

Respiratory: Nasal irritation

Pharmacodynamics/Kinetics

Bioavailability ~1% to 6%

Time to Peak Serum: 10-45 minutes

Protein Binding Plasma: 80%

Half-Life Elimination ~3 hours; Metabolites: ~86 hours

Metabolism Degraded by peptidase; forms metabolites

Excretion Urine (44% to 55%, ~3% as unchanged drug); feces (19% to 44%)

Available Dosage Forms

Solution, intranasal:

Synarel®: 2 mg/mL (8 mL)

Dosing

Adult & Geriatric Endometriosis: Intranasal: Female: 1 spray (200 mcg) in 1 nostril each morning and the other nostril each evening starting on days 2-4 of menstrual cycle (total: 2 sprays/day). Dose may be increased to 2 sprays (400 mcg; 1 spray in each nostril) in the morning and evening if amenorrhea is not achieved (total: 4 sprays [800 mcg]/day). Total duration of therapy should not exceed 6 months due to decreases in bone mineral density; retreatment is not recommended by the manufacturer.

Pediatric Central precocious puberty: Intranasal: Male/Female: 2 sprays (400 mcg) into each nostril in the morning and 2 sprays (400 mcg) into each nostril in the evening (total: 8 sprays [1600 mcg]/day). If inadequate suppression, may increase dose to 3 sprays (600 mcg) into alternating nostrils 3 times/day (total: 9 sprays [1800 mcg]/day).

Administration

Inhalation Nasal spray: Do not use topical nasal decongestant for at least 2 hours after nafarelin use. Allow ~30 seconds to elapse between sprays. Sneezing during or immediately after dosing should be avoided (may decrease drug absorption).

Stability

Storage Store at room temperature of 15°C to 30°C (59°F to 86°F). Protect from light.

Monitoring and Teaching Issues

Laboratory Monitoring CPP: GnRH testing (blood LH and FSH levels)

Physical Assessment For treatment of precocious puberty. Teach patient or caregiver correct timing and administration of nasal spray.

Patient Education Endometriosis: You will begin this treatment between days 2-4 of your regular menstrual cycle. Use daily at the same time (arising and bedtime) and rotate nostrils. Maintain regular follow-up schedule. May cause hot flashes, flushing, or redness; decreased or increased libido; emotional lability; weight gain; decreased breast size; or hirsutism. Report any breakthrough bleeding or continuing menstruation or musculoskeletal pain. Do not use a nasal decongestant within 2 hours after nafarelin.

Pregnancy Considerations Major fetal abnormalities have been reported in some animal studies; a dose-related increase in fetal mortality and decrease in fetal weight was also observed. Ovulation is inhibited and menstruation is stopped when used appropriately for the treatment of endometriosis, however contraception is not assured. Nonhormonal contraception is recommended. Pregnancy should be excluded prior to initiating treatment. There is no evidence that pregnancy rates are enhanced or adversely affected by use.

◆ **Nafarelin Acetate** *see* Nafarelin *on page 1280*

Nafcillin (naf SIL in)

Index Terms Ethoxynaphthamido Penicillin Sodium; Nafcillin Sodium; Nallpen; Sodium Nafcillin

Generic Availability (U.S.) Yes

Pharmacologic Category Antibiotic, Penicillin

Pregnancy Risk Factor B

Lactation Enters breast milk/use caution

Use Treatment of infections such as osteomyelitis, septicemia, endocarditis, and CNS infections caused by susceptible strains of staphylococci species

Available Dosage Forms

Infusion, premixed iso-osmotic dextrose solution: 1 g (50 mL); 2 g (100 mL)

Injection, powder for reconstitution: 1 g, 2 g, 10 g

Dosing

Adult & Geriatric

Susceptible infections:

I.M.: 500 mg every 4-6 hours

I.V.: 500-2000 mg every 4-6 hours

Endocarditis: MSSA:

Native valve: I.V.: 12 g/24 hours in 4-6 divided doses for 6 weeks

Prosthetic valve: I.V.: 12 g/24 hours in 6 divided doses for ≥6 weeks (use with rifampin and gentamicin)

Joint:

Bursitis, septic: I.V.: 2 g every 4 hours

Prosthetic: I.V.: 2 g every 4-6 hours with rifampin for 6 weeks

***Staphylococcus aureus*, methicillin-susceptible infections, including brain abscess, empyema, erysipelas, mastitis, myositis, orbital cellulitis, osteomyelitis, pneumonia, splenic abscess, toxic shock, urinary tract (perinephric abscess)**: I.V.: 2 g every 4 hours

Pediatric

Neonates:

Usual dosage range: I.M., I.V.:

1200-2000 g, <7 days: 50 mg/kg/day divided every 12 hours

>2000 g, <7 days: 75 mg/kg/day divided every 8 hours

1200-2000 g, ≥7 days: 75 mg/kg/day divided every 8 hours

>2000 g, ≥7 days: 100-140 mg/kg/day divided every 6 hours

Children:

I.M.: 25 mg/kg twice daily

I.V.:

Mild-to-moderate infections: 50-100 mg/kg/day in divided doses every 6 hours

Severe infections: 100-200 mg/kg/day in divided doses every 4-6 hours (maximum: 12 g/day)

Staphylococcal endocarditis:

Native valve: 200 mg/kg/day in divided doses every 4-6 hours for 6 weeks

Prosthetic valve: 200 mg/kg/day in divided doses every 4-6 hours for ≥6 weeks (use with rifampin and gentamicin)

Renal Impairment Not necessary unless renal impairment is in the setting of concomitant hepatic impairment.

Hemodialysis effects: Not dialyzable (0% to 5%) via hemodialysis. Supplemental dose is not necessary with hemo- or peritoneal dialysis or continuous arteriovenous or venovenous hemofiltration.

Hepatic Impairment In patients with both hepatic and renal impairment, modification of dosage may be necessary; no data available.

Administration

I.M. Rotate injection sites.

I.V. Vesicant. Administer around-the-clock to promote less variation in peak and trough serum levels. Infuse over 30-60 minutes.

Monitoring and Teaching Issues

Laboratory Monitoring Perform culture and sensitivity studies prior to initiating drug therapy. Monitor renal, hepatic, CBC with prolonged therapy.

Physical Assessment Assess results of culture and sensitivity tests and allergy history prior to starting therapy. Infusion/Injection site must be monitored closely to prevent extravasation (use ice packs). Monitor for hypersensitivity and opportunistic infection (eg, fever, chills, unhealed sores, white plaques in mouth or vagina, purulent vaginal discharge).

Patient Education This medication can only be administered by infusion or injection. Report immediately any redness, swelling, burning, or pain at injection/infusion site; respiratory difficulty or swallowing; chest pain; persistent diarrhea; or rash. May cause nausea or opportunistic infection (eg, fever, chills, sore throat, burning urination). Report persistent side effects or if condition does not respond to treatment.

◆ **Nafcillin Sodium** *see* Nafcillin *on page* 1282

◆ **$NaHCO_3$** *see* Sodium Bicarbonate *on page* 1658

Nalbuphine (NAL byoo feen)

Index Terms Nalbuphine Hydrochloride; Nubain

Generic Availability (U.S.) Yes

Pharmacologic Category Analgesic, Opioid; Analgesic, Opioid Partial Agonist

Medication Safety Issues

Sound-alike/look-alike issues:

Nubain may be confused with Navane®, Nebcin®

High alert medication: The Institute for Safe Medication Practices (ISMP) includes this medication among its list of drug classes which have a heightened risk of causing significant patient harm when used in error.

Pregnancy Risk Factor C

Lactation Enters breast milk/use caution

Use Relief of moderate-to-severe pain; preoperative analgesia, postoperative and surgical anesthesia, and obstetrical analgesia during labor and delivery

Unlabeled/Investigational Use Opioid-induced pruritus

Mechanism of Action/Effect Binds to opiate receptors in the CNS, causing inhibition of ascending pain pathways, altering the perception of and response to pain; produces generalized CNS depression

Contraindications Hypersensitivity to nalbuphine or any component of the formulation

Warnings/Precautions Use caution in CNS depression. Sedation and psychomotor impairment are likely, and are additive with other CNS depressants or ethanol. May cause respiratory depression. Ambulatory patients must be cautioned about performing tasks which require mental alertness (eg, operating machinery or driving). Effects may be potentiated when used with other sedative drugs or ethanol. Use with caution in patients with recent myocardial infarction, biliary tract impairment, morbid obesity, thyroid dysfunction, head trauma, or increased intracranial pressure. Use caution in patients with prostatic hyperplasia and/or urinary stricture, adrenal insufficiency, decreased hepatic or renal function. Use with caution in patients with pre-existing respiratory compromise (hypoxia and/or hypercapnia), COPD or other obstructive pulmonary disease; critical respiratory depression may occur, even at therapeutic dosages. May cause hypotension; use with caution in patients with hypovolemia, cardiovascular disease (including acute MI), or drugs which may exaggerate hypotensive effects (including phenothiazines or general anesthetics). May obscure diagnosis or clinical course of patients with acute abdominal conditions. May result in tolerance and/or drug dependence with chronic use; use with caution in patients with a history of drug dependence. Abrupt discontinuation following prolonged use may lead to withdrawal symptoms. May precipitate withdrawal symptoms in patients following prolonged therapy with mu opioid agonists. Use with caution in pregnancy (close neonatal monitoring required when used in labor and delivery). Use with caution in the elderly and debilitated patients; may be more sensitive to adverse effects. Safety and efficacy in children have not been established.

Drug Interactions

Avoid Concomitant Use There are no known interactions where it is recommended to avoid concomitant use.

Decreased Effect

Nalbuphine may decrease the levels/effects of: Analgesics (Opioid); Pegvisomant

The levels/effects of Nalbuphine may be decreased by: Ammonium Chloride; Mixed Agonist / Antagonist Opioids

Increased Effect/Toxicity

Nalbuphine may increase the levels/effects of: Alcohol (Ethyl); Alvimopan; CNS Depressants; Desmopressin; Selective Serotonin Reuptake Inhibitors; Thiazide Diuretics

The levels/effects of Nalbuphine may be increased by: Amphetamines; Antipsychotic Agents (Phenothiazines); Droperidol; Succinylcholine

Nutritional/Ethanol Interactions

Ethanol: Avoid ethanol (may increase CNS depression).

Herb/Nutraceutical: Avoid valerian, St John's wort, kava kava, gotu kola (may increase CNS depression).

Adverse Reactions

>10%: Central nervous system: Sedation (36%)

1% to 10%:

Central nervous system: Dizziness (5%), headache (3%)

Gastrointestinal: Nausea/vomiting (6%), xerostomia (4%)

Miscellaneous: Clamminess (9%)

Pharmacodynamics/Kinetics

Onset of Action Peak effect: SubQ, I.M.: <15 minutes; I.V.: 2-3 minutes

Half-Life Elimination 5 hours

Metabolism Hepatic

Excretion Feces; urine (~7% as metabolites)

Available Dosage Forms

Injection, solution: 10 mg/mL (10 mL); 20 mg/mL (10 mL)

Injection, solution [preservative free]: 10 mg/mL (1 mL); 20 mg/mL (1 mL)

Dosing

Adult

Pain management: I.M., I.V., SubQ: 10 mg/70 kg every 3-6 hours; maximum single dose in nonopioid-tolerant patients: 20 mg; maximum daily dose: 160 mg

Surgical anesthesia supplement: I.V.: Induction: 0.3-3 mg/kg over 10-15 minutes; maintenance doses of 0.25-0.5 mg/kg may be given as required

Opioid-induced pruritus (unlabeled use): I.V. 2.5-5 mg; may repeat dose

Geriatric Refer to adult dosing; use with caution.

Pediatric Pain management (unlabeled use): Children ≥1 year: I.M., I.V., SubQ: 0.1-0.2 mg/kg every 3-4 hours as needed; maximum: 20 mg/dose and/or 160 mg/day

Renal Impairment Use with caution and reduce dose. Monitor.

Hepatic Impairment Use with caution and reduce dose.

Stability

Storage Store at room temperature of 15°C to 30°C (59°F to 86°F). Protect from light.

Monitoring and Teaching Issues

Physical Assessment Monitor for effectiveness of pain relief. Monitor blood pressure, CNS and respiratory status, and degree of sedation at beginning of therapy and periodically thereafter. For inpatients, implement safety measures to prevent falls. Assess patient's physical and/or psychological dependence. Discontinue slowly after prolonged use.

Patient Education May cause physical and/or psychological dependence. While using this medication, do not use alcohol and other prescription or OTC medications (especially sedatives, tranquilizers, antihistamines, or pain medications) without consulting prescriber. Maintain adequate hydration, unless instructed to restrict fluid intake. May cause hypotension, dizziness, drowsiness, impaired coordination, or blurred vision; loss of appetite, nausea, or vomiting; or constipation. Report chest pain, slow or rapid heartbeat, dizziness, or persistent headache; confusion or respiratory difficulties; or severe constipation.

Geriatric Considerations The elderly may be particularly susceptible to CNS effects; monitor closely.

Pregnancy Considerations Severe fetal bradycardia has been reported following use in labor/delivery. Fetal bradycardia may occur when administered earlier in pregnancy (not documented). Use only if clearly needed, with monitoring to detect and manage possible adverse fetal effects. Naloxone has been reported to reverse bradycardia. Newborn should be monitored for respiratory depression or bradycardia following nalbuphine use in labor.

Related Information

Opioid Analgesics *on page* 2003

◆ **Nalbuphine Hydrochloride** *see* Nalbuphine *on page* 1283

◆ **Nalfon®** *see* Fenoprofen *on page* 744

◆ **Nallpen** *see* Nafcillin *on page* 1282

◆ ***N*-allylnoroxymorphine Hydrochloride** *see* Naloxone *on page* 1284

Naloxone (nal OKS one)

Index Terms *N*-allylnoroxymorphine Hydrochloride; Naloxone Hydrochloride; Narcan

Generic Availability (U.S.) Yes

Pharmacologic Category Antidote; Opioid Antagonist

Medication Safety Issues

Sound-alike/look-alike issues:

Naloxone may be confused with Lanoxin®, naltrexone

Narcan® may be confused with Marcaine®, Norcuron®

International issues:

Narcan [multiple international markets] may be confused with Marcen brand name for ketazolam [Spain]

Pregnancy Risk Factor C

Lactation Excretion in breast milk unknown/not recommended

Use Complete or partial reversal of opioid drug effects, including respiratory depression; management of known or suspected opioid overdose; diagnosis of suspected opioid dependence or acute opioid overdose

Unlabeled/Investigational Use Opioid-induced pruritus

Mechanism of Action/Effect Pure opioid antagonist that competes and displaces narcotics at opioid receptor sites

Contraindications Hypersensitivity to naloxone or any component of the formulation

Warnings/Precautions Due to an association between naloxone and acute pulmonary edema, use with caution in patients with cardiovascular disease or in patients receiving medications with potential adverse cardiovascular effects (eg, hypotension, pulmonary edema, or arrhythmias). Administration of naloxone causes the release of catecholamines; may precipitate acute withdrawal or unmask pain in those who regularly take opioids. Excessive dosages should be avoided after use of opiates in surgery. Abrupt postoperative reversal may result in nausea, vomiting, sweating, tachycardia, hypertension, seizures, and other cardiovascular events (including pulmonary edema and arrhythmias). May precipitate withdrawal symptoms in patients addicted to opiates, including pain, hypertension, sweating, agitation, irritability; in neonates: shrill cry, failure to feed; carefully titrate dose to reverse hypoventilation; do not fully awaken patient or reverse analgesic effect (postoperative patient). Use caution in patients with history of seizures; avoid use in treatment of meperidine-induced seizures. Recurrence of respiratory depression is possible if the opioid involved is long-acting; observe patients until there is no reasonable risk of recurrent respiratory depression.

Drug Interactions

Avoid Concomitant Use There are no known interactions where it is recommended to avoid concomitant use.

Decreased Effect There are no known significant interactions involving a decrease in effect.

Increased Effect/Toxicity There are no known significant interactions involving an increase in effect.

Adverse Reactions Adverse reactions are related to reversing dependency and precipitating withdrawal. Withdrawal symptoms are the result of sympathetic excess. Adverse events occur secondarily to reversal (withdrawal) of narcotic analgesia and sedation.

Central nervous system: Narcotic withdrawal

Pharmacodynamics/Kinetics

Onset of Action Endotracheal, I.M., SubQ: 2-5 minutes; Intranasal: ~8-13 minutes (Kelley, 2005; Robertson, 2009); I.V.: ~2 minutes

Duration of Action Depending on route of administration, ~30-120 minutes; I.V. has a shorter duration of action than I.M. administration; since naloxone's action is shorter than that of most opioids, repeated doses are usually needed

Half-Life Elimination Neonates: 3-4 hours; Adults: 0.5-1.5 hours

Metabolism Primarily hepatic via glucuronidation

Excretion Urine (as metabolites)

Available Dosage Forms

Injection, solution: 0.4 mg/mL (1 mL, 10 mL)

Injection, solution [preservative free]: 0.4 mg/mL (1 mL); 1 mg/mL (2 mL)

Dosing

Adult & Geriatric Note: I.M., I.V. (preferred), intranasal (adults only), and SubQ routes may be used. Intratracheal administration is the least desirable and is supported by only anecdotal evidence (case report) (ACLS, 2010):

Opioid intoxication: Respiratory depression:

I.V.: 0.4-2 mg; may need to repeat doses every 2-3 minutes; after reversal, may need to readminister dose(s) at a later interval (ie, 20-60 minutes) depending on type/duration of opioid. If no response is observed after 10 mg, consider other causes of respiratory depression. **Note:** Opioid-dependent patients may require lower doses (0.1 mg) titrated incrementally to avoid precipitating acute withdrawal.

Intranasal administration (unlabeled route): 2 mg (1 mg per nostril); may repeat in 5 minutes if respiratory depression persists. **Note:** Onset of action is slightly delayed compared to I.M. or I.V. routes (ACLS, 2010; Kelly, 2005; Robertson, 2009).

Opioid intoxication: Respiratory depression: Opioid-dependent patient: Initial: 0.04-0.4 mg; may repeat or escalate dose up to 2 mg if initial response inadequate. **Note:** Atypical opioids (eg, propoxyphene) or massive opioid overdoses may require much higher doses (ACLS, 2010).

Continuous infusion (unlabeled dosing): I.V.: Calculate dosage/hour based on effective intermittent dose used and duration of adequate response seen **or** use two-thirds ($^{2}/_{3}$) of the initial effective naloxone bolus on an hourly basis (typically 0.25-6.25 mg/hour); one-half ($^{1}/_{2}$) of the initial bolus dose should be readministered 15 minutes after initiation of the continuous infusion to prevent a drop in naloxone levels; adjust infusion rate as needed to assure adequate ventilation and prevent withdrawal symptoms

Opioid-dependent patients being treated for cancer pain (NCCN guidelines, v.1.2010): I.V.: 0.04-0.08 mg (40-80 mcg) slow I.V. push; administer every 30-60 seconds until improvement in symptoms, if no response is observed after total naloxone dose 1 mg, consider other causes of respiratory depression. **Note:** May dilute 0.4 mg/mL (1 mL) ampule into 9 mL of normal saline for a total volume of 10 mL to achieve a 0.04 mg/mL (40 mcg/mL) concentration.

Postoperative reversal: I.V.: 0.1-0.2 mg every 2-3 minutes until desired response (adequate ventilation and alertness without significant pain). **Note:** Repeat doses may be needed within 1-2 hour intervals depending on type, dose, and timing of the last dose of opioid administered.

Opioid-induced pruritus (unlabeled use): I.V. infusion: 0.25 mcg/kg/**hour**; **Note:** Monitor pain control; verify that the naloxone is not reversing analgesia (Gan, 1997).

Pediatric Note: I.M., I.V. (preferred), and SubQ routes may be used. Intratracheal administration is the least desirable and is supported by only anecdotal evidence (case report) (ACLS, 2010):

Opiate intoxication: Respiratory depression: I.V., intraosseous (I.O), intratracheal:

Birth (including premature infants) to 5 years or ≤20 kg (unlabeled dose): Acute: Initial: 0.1 mg/kg (maximum dose: 2 mg); repeat every 2-3 minutes if needed; consider lower initial doses of 0.01 mg/kg for non-acute situations (eg, respiratory depression during pain management) (*Drugs for Pediatric Emergencies*, 1998)

>5 years or >20 kg: Minimum dose: 2 mg/dose; if no response, repeat every 2-3 minutes (*Drugs for Pediatric Emergencies*, 1998)

Note: I.O. and Intratracheal routes are alternative routes recommended by PALS 2010 guidelines. Consider using lower doses to reverse respiratory depression associated with therapeutic opioid use: 1-5 mcg/kg, titrate to effect (PALS, 2010)

Continuous infusion (unlabeled dosing): I.V.: If continuous infusion is required, calculate dosage/hour based on effective intermittent dose used and duration of adequate response seen **or** use two-thirds ($^{2}/_{3}$) of the initial effective naloxone bolus on an hourly basis; titrate dose (typically 0.04-0.16 mg/kg/hour for 2-5 days in children); one-half ($^{1}/_{2}$) of the initial bolus dose should be readministered 15 minutes after initiation of the continuous infusion to prevent a drop in naloxone levels; increase infusion rate as needed to assure adequate ventilation and prevent withdrawal symptoms

Postoperative reversal: Infants and Children: I.V.: 0.01 mg/kg; may repeat every 2-3 minutes as needed based on response (adequate ventilation without significant pain)

Administration

I.M. May administer I.M. if unable to obtain I.V. access.

I.V.

I.V. push: Administer over 30 seconds as undiluted preparation **or** (unlabeled) administer as diluted preparation slow I.V. push by diluting 0.4 mg (1 mL) ampul with 9 mL of normal saline for a total volume of 10 mL to achieve a concentration of 0.04 mg/mL

I.V. continuous infusion: Dilute to 4 mcg/mL in D_5W or normal saline

Other

Intratracheal (unlabeled route): There is only anecdotal support for this route of administration. May require a slightly higher dose than used in other routes. Dilute to 1-2 mL with normal saline; flush with 5 cc of saline and then administer 5 ventilations

Intranasal (unlabeled route): Administer total dose equally divided into each nostril using a mucosal atomizer device (MAD) (ACLS, 2010; Kelly, 2005; Robertson, 2009)

SubQ: May administer SubQ if unable to obtain I.V. access

Stability

Reconstitution Stable in 0.9% sodium chloride and D_5W at 4 mcg/mL for 24 hours.

Storage Store at 25°C (77°F). Protect from light.

Monitoring and Teaching Issues

Physical Assessment Assess patient for opioid dependency. Monitor vital signs and cardiorespiratory status continuously during infusion; maintain patent airway.

Patient Education Report respiratory difficulty, palpitations, or tremors.

Geriatric Considerations In small trials, naloxone has shown temporary improvement in Alzheimer's disease; however, is not recommended for treatment.

Breast-Feeding Considerations No data reported. Since naloxone is used for opiate reversal the concern should be on opiate drug levels in a breast-feeding mother and transfer to the infant rather than naloxone exposure. The safest approach would be **not** to breast-feed.

Pregnancy Considerations Consider benefit to the mother and the risk to the fetus before administering to a pregnant woman who is known or suspected to be opioid dependent. May precipitate withdrawal in both the mother and fetus.

Additional Information May contain methyl and propylparabens

- ◆ **Naloxone and Buprenorphine** *see* Buprenorphine and Naloxone *on page 249*
- ◆ **Naloxone Hydrochloride** *see* Naloxone *on page 1284*
- ◆ **Naloxone Hydrochloride and Pentazocine** *see* Pentazocine and Naloxone *on page 1439*
- ◆ **Naloxone Hydrochloride Dihydrate and Buprenorphine Hydrochloride** *see* Buprenorphine and Naloxone *on page 249*

Naltrexone (nal TREKS one)

U.S. Brand Names ReVia®; Vivitrol®

Index Terms Naltrexone Hydrochloride

Generic Availability (U.S.) Yes: Tablet

Pharmacologic Category Antidote; Opioid Antagonist

Medication Safety Issues

Sound-alike/look-alike issues:

Naltrexone may be confused with methylnaltrexone, naloxone

ReVia® may be confused with Revatio®, Revex®

Administration issues: Vivitrol®: For intramuscular (I.M.) gluteal injection only

Medication Guide Available Yes

Pregnancy Risk Factor C

Lactation Enters breast milk/not recommended

Use Treatment of ethanol dependence; prevention of relapse in opioid dependent patients, following opioid detoxification

Mechanism of Action/Effect Naltrexone (a pure opioid antagonist) is a cyclopropyl derivative of oxymorphone similar in structure to naloxone and nalorphine (a morphine derivative); it acts as a competitive antagonist at opioid receptor sites, showing the highest affinity for mu receptors.

Contraindications Hypersensitivity to naltrexone or any component of the formulation; narcotic dependence or current use of opioid analgesics; acute opioid withdrawal; failure to pass naloxone challenge or positive urine screen for opioids; acute hepatitis; liver failure

Warnings/Precautions

[U.S. Boxed Warning]: Dose-related hepatocellular injury is possible; the margin of separation between the apparent safe and hepatotoxic doses appears to be ≤ fivefold. Discontinue therapy if signs/symptoms of acute hepatitis develop. Therapy may precipitate withdrawal symptoms in patients addicted to opiates; patients should be opioid-free for a minimum of 7-10 days; use naloxone challenge test to confirm patient is opioid-free prior to therapy if there is any suspicion since urinary opioid screen may not be sufficient proof. Use of naltrexone does not eliminate or diminish withdrawal symptoms. Patients who had been treated with naltrexone may respond to lower opioid doses than previously used. This could result in potentially life-threatening opioid intoxication. Patients should be aware that they may be more sensitive to lower doses of opioids after naltrexone treatment is discontinued, after a missed dose, or near the end of the dosing interval. Warn patients that any attempt to overcome opioid blockade during naltrexone therapy, could potentially lead to fatal opioid overdose; the opioid competitive receptor blockade produced by naltrexone is potentially surmountable in the presence of large amounts of opioids. In naltrexone-treated patients requiring emergency pain management, consider alternatives to opioid therapy (eg, regional analgesia, nonopioid analgesics, general anesthesia). If opioid therapy is required for pain therapy, patients should be under the direct care of a trained anesthesia provider.

Suicidal thoughts and depression have been reported in both alcohol- and opioid-dependent patients; monitor closely. Hypersensitivity, including anaphylaxis, has been reported. Cases of eosinophilic pneumonia have been reported and should be considered in patients presenting with progressive hypoxia and dyspnea. Use with caution in patients with a history of bleeding disorders (including thrombocytopenia) and/or patients on anticoagulant therapy; bleeding/ hematoma may occur from I.M. administration. Serious injection site reactions (eg, cellulitis, induration, hematoma, abscess, necrosis) have been reported with use, including severe cases requiring surgical debridement. Females appear to be at a higher risk. Patients should report any injection site pain, swelling, bruising, pruritus, or redness that does not improve (or worsens). For I.M. use only in the gluteal muscle; do **not** administer I.V., SubQ, or into fatty tissue; incorrect administration may increase the risk of injection site reactions. Use with caution in patients with hepatic or renal impairment; not studied in moderate-to-severe renal impairment or in severe hepatic impairment. Use is contraindicated in patients with acute hepatitis or hepatic failure. Vehicle used in the injectable naltrexone formulation (polylactide-co-glycolide microspheres) has rarely been associated with retinal artery occlusion in patients with abnormal arteriovenous anastomosis following injection of other drug products that also use the polylactide-co-glycolide microspheres vehicle.

Drug Interactions

Avoid Concomitant Use There are no known interactions where it is recommended to avoid concomitant use.

Decreased Effect There are no known significant interactions involving a decrease in effect.

Increased Effect/Toxicity There are no known significant interactions involving an increase in effect.

Lab Interactions May cause cross-reactivity with some opioid immunoassay methods.

Adverse Reactions Combined reporting of adverse events from oral and injectable formulations:

>10%:

Cardiovascular: Syncope (13%)

Central nervous system: Headache (3% to 25%), insomnia (3% to 14%), dizziness (4% to 13%), anxiety (2% to 12%), nervousness (4% to >10%)

Gastrointestinal: Nausea (10% to 33%), vomiting (3% to 14%), appetite decreased (14%), diarrhea (13%), abdominal pain (11%), abdominal cramping

Hepatic: ALT increased (13%)

Local: Injection site reaction (≤69%; includes bruising, induration, nodules, pain, pruritus, swelling, tenderness)

Neuromuscular & skeletal: Arthralgia (12%), CPK increased (11% to 39%)

Respiratory: Pharyngitis (7% to 11%)

1% to 10%:

Cardiovascular: Hypertension (5%)

Central nervous system: Suicidal thoughts (≤10%), depression (8%), somnolence (2% to 4%), fatigue (4%), chills, energy increased, feeling down, irritability

Dermatologic: Rash (6%)

Endocrine & metabolic: Polydipsia

Gastrointestinal: Dry mouth (5%), toothache (4%)

Genitourinary: Delayed ejaculation, impotency

Hepatic: AST increased (2% to 10%), GGT increased (7%)

Neuromuscular & skeletal: Muscle cramps (8%), back pain (6%)

Miscellaneous: Influenza (5%)

Pharmacodynamics/Kinetics

Duration of Action Oral: 50 mg: 24 hours; 100 mg: 48 hours; 150 mg: 72 hours; I.M.: 4 weeks

Absorption Oral: Almost complete

Bioavailability Oral: Variable range (5% to 40%)

Time to Peak Serum: Oral: ~60 minutes; I.M.: Biphasic: ~2 hours (first peak), ~2-3 days (second peak)

Protein Binding 21%

Half-Life Elimination Oral: 4 hours; 6-beta-naltrexol: 13 hours; I.M.: naltrexone and 6-beta-naltrexol: 5-10 days

Metabolism Extensively metabolized via noncytochrome-mediated dehydrogenase conversion to 6-beta-naltrexol (primary metabolite) and related minor metabolites; glucuronide conjugates are also formed from naltrexone and its metabolites

Oral: Extensive first-pass effect

Excretion Primarily urine (as metabolites and small amounts of unchanged drug)

Available Dosage Forms

Injection, microspheres for suspension, extended release:

Vivitrol®: 380 mg

Tablet, oral: 50 mg

ReVia®: 50 mg

Dosing

Adult & Geriatric Alcohol dependence, opioid dependence: Note: Do not initiate therapy until patient is opioid-free for at least 7-10 days as determined by urinalysis; consider naloxone challenge test to confirm patient is opioid-free if there is any suspicion since urinary opioid screen may not be sufficient proof.

Oral: Initial: 25 mg; if no withdrawal signs occur, administer 50 mg on day 2; maintenance regimen: 50 mg/day; alternative maintenance regimens may be used and include: 50 mg on weekdays with a 100 mg dose on Saturday; 100 mg every other day; or 150 mg every 3 days (degree of blockade may be reduced with extended dosing interval regimens and doses >50 mg may increase risk of hepatocellular injury)

I.M.: 380 mg once every 4 weeks

Renal Impairment Use caution. No adjustment needed in mild impairment. Not adequately studied in moderate-to-severe renal impairment.

Hepatic Impairment Use caution. An increase in naltrexone AUC of approximately five- and 10-fold in patients with compensated or decompensated liver cirrhosis respectively, compared with normal liver function has been reported No adjustment required with mild-to-moderate hepatic impairment. Not adequately studied in severe hepatic impairment. Use is contraindicated in patients with acute hepatitis or hepatic failure.

Administration

Oral May be administered with or without food. Administration with food or after meals may minimize adverse gastrointestinal effects. Advise patient not to self-administer opiates while receiving naltrexone therapy.

I.M. Vivitrol®: Administer I.M. into the upper outer quadrant of the gluteal area; must inject dose using one of the provided needles for administration. Use either the 1.5-inch 20-gauge needle or the 2-inch 20-gauge needle (for patients with a larger amount of subcutaneous tissue overlying the gluteal muscle). Avoid inadvertent injection into a blood vessel; do not administer I.V., SubQ, or into fatty tissue (the risk of serious injection site reaction is increased if given incorrectly as a SubQ injection or into fatty tissue instead of the gluteal muscle). Injection should alternate between the 2 buttocks. Do not substitute any components of the dose-pack.

Stability

Reconstitution Injection: Prior to reconstitution, allow drug vial and provided diluent to reach room temperature (~45 minutes). Using the provided 1-inch *preparation* needle, reconstitute with 3.4 mL of the diluent and allow to dissolve by vigorously shaking the vial for ~1 minute. Mixed suspension will be milky white, free of clumps, and will move freely down the walls of the vial. Immediately after suspension, withdraw 4.2 mL of the suspension using the same preparation needle.

Prior to administration, replace the preparation needle with the appropriate size provided *administration* needle (1.5-inch Terumo® needle or 2-inch Needle-Pro® needle). Prior to injection, remove any air bubbles and push on the plunger until 4 mL of the suspension remains in the syringe. Following reconstitution of the suspension, administer immediately.

Storage

Injection: Store unopened kit at 2°C to 8°C (36°F to 46°F). Kit may be kept at room temperature of ≤25°C (77°F) for ≤7 days prior to use; do not freeze. Following reconstitution of the suspension, administer immediately.

Tablet: Store at room temperature. Protect from light.

Monitoring and Teaching Issues

Laboratory Monitoring Periodic LFTs

Physical Assessment Do not use until patient has been opioid-free for 7-10 days. Assess carefully for several days following start of therapy for narcotic withdrawal symptoms or severe adverse reactions. Monitor injection site for reaction. Use non-narcotic analgesics for pain. Monitor for suicide ideation.

Patient Education This medication will help you achieve abstinence from opiates if taken as directed. Do not use opiates. Carry documentation to alert medical personnel you are taking medication in the event of an emergency. You may experience drowsiness, dizziness, or blurred vision; trouble sleeping; decreased appetite; abdominal cramping, nausea or vomiting; low energy; or decreased sexual function (reversible when drug is discontinued). Report yellowing of skin or eyes; change in color of stool or urine; suicide ideation; increased perspiration or chills; acute headache; palpitations; unusual joint pain; signs and symptoms of pneumonia (trouble breathing, coughing, or wheezing); or injection site pain, swelling, or unresolved redness.

Pregnancy Considerations Evidence of early fetal loss has been observed in animal studies with oral naltrexone. Reproduction studies have not been conduced using the sustained release I.M formulation. There are no adequate and well-controlled studies of naltrexone in pregnant women.

- **Naltrexone and Morphine** *see* Morphine and Naltrexone *on page* 1263
- **Naltrexone Hydrochloride** *see* Naltrexone *on page* 1286
- **Namenda®** *see* Memantine *on page* 1165
- **Namenda XR** *see* Memantine *on page* 1165
- **Nanoparticle Albumin-Bound Paclitaxel** *see* Paclitaxel (Protein Bound) *on page* 1390
- **Naprelan®** *see* Naproxen *on page* 1289
- **Naprosyn®** *see* Naproxen *on page* 1289

Naproxen (na PROKS en)

U.S. Brand Names Aleve® [OTC]; Anaprox®; Anaprox® DS; EC-Naprosyn®; Mediproxen [OTC]; Midol® Extended Relief [OTC]; Naprelan®; Naprosyn®; Pamprin® Maximum Strength All Day Relief [OTC]

Index Terms Naproxen Sodium

Generic Availability (U.S.) Yes: Caplet, suspension, tablet

Pharmacologic Category Nonsteroidal Anti-inflammatory Drug (NSAID), Oral

Medication Safety Issues

Sound-alike/look-alike issues:

Naproxen may be confused with Natacyn®, Nebcin®
Anaprox® may be confused with Anaspaz®, Avapro®
Naprelan® may be confused with Naprosyn®
Naprosyn® may be confused with Naprelan®, Natacyn®, Nebcin®

Beers Criteria medication: This drug may be inappropriate for use in geriatric patients (high severity risk).

International issues:

Flogen [Mexico] may be confused with Flovent brand name for fluticasone [U.S., Canada]
Flogen [Mexico] may be confused with Floxin brand name for flunarizine [Thailand], norfloxacin [South Africa], ofloxacin [U.S., Canada], and perfloxacin [Philippines]

Medication Guide Available Yes

Pregnancy Risk Factor C

Lactation Enters breast milk/not recommended (AAP rates "compatible"; AAP 2001 update pending)

Use Management of ankylosing spondylitis, osteoarthritis, and rheumatoid disorders (including juvenile idiopathic arthritis [JIA]); acute gout; mild-to-moderate pain; tendonitis, bursitis; dysmenorrhea; fever

Available Dosage Forms

Caplet, oral: 220 mg
Aleve® [OTC]: 220 mg
Midol® Extended Relief [OTC]: 220 mg
Pamprin® Maximum Strength All Day Relief [OTC]: 220 mg

Capsule, liquid gel, oral:
Aleve® [OTC]: 220 mg

Combination package, oral:
Naprelan®: Day 1-3: Tablet, controlled release: 825 mg [equivalent to naproxen base 750 mg] (6s) [contains sodium 75 mg] and Day 4-10: Tablet, controlled release: 550 mg [equivalent to naproxen base 500 mg] (14s) [contains sodium 50 mg]

Gelcap, oral:
Aleve® [OTC]: 220 mg

Suspension, oral: 125 mg/5 mL (500 mL)
Naprosyn®: 125 mg/5 mL (473 mL)

Tablet, oral: 220 mg, 250 mg, 275 mg, 375 mg, 500 mg, 550 mg
Aleve® [OTC]: 220 mg
Anaprox®: 275 mg
Anaprox® DS: 550 mg
Mediproxen [OTC]: 220 mg
Naprosyn®: 250 mg, 375 mg, 500 mg

Tablet, controlled release, oral:
Naprelan®: 412.5 mg, 550 mg, 825 mg

Tablet, delayed release, enteric coated, oral: 375 mg, 500 mg
EC-Naprosyn®: 375 mg, 500 mg

Dosing

Adult & Geriatric Note: Dosage expressed as naproxen base; 200 mg naproxen base is equivalent to 220 mg naproxen sodium.

Gout, acute: Oral: Initial: 750 mg, followed by 250 mg every 8 hours until attack subsides. **Note:** EC-Naprosyn® is not recommended.

Migraine, acute (unlabeled use): Initial: 500-750 mg; an additional 250-500 mg may be given if needed (maximum: 1250 mg in 24 hours). **Note:** EC-Naprosyn® is not recommended.

Pain (mild-to-moderate), dysmenorrhea, acute tendonitis, bursitis: Oral: Initial: 500 mg, then 250 mg every 6-8 hours; maximum: 1250 mg/day naproxen base

Rheumatoid arthritis, osteoarthritis, and ankylosing spondylitis: 500-1000 mg/day in 2 divided doses; may increase to 1.5 g/day of naproxen base for limited time period

OTC labeling: Pain/fever: 200 mg naproxen base every 8-12 hours; if needed, may take 400 mg naproxen base for the initial dose; maximum: 400 mg naproxen base in any 8- to 12-hour period or 600 mg naproxen base/24 hours

Pediatric Note: Dosage expressed as naproxen base; 200 mg naproxen base is equivalent to 220 mg naproxen sodium.

Juvenile idiopathic arthritis: Oral: Children >2 years: 10 mg/kg/day in 2 divided doses

OTC labeling: Pain/fever: Oral: Children ≥12 years: Refer to adult dosing.

Renal Impairment Cl_{cr} <30 mL/minute: use is not recommended.

Administration

Oral Administer with food, milk, or antacids to decrease GI adverse effects

Suspension: Shake suspension well before administration.

Tablet, extended release: Swallow tablet whole; do not break, crush, or chew.

Monitoring and Teaching Issues

Laboratory Monitoring Periodic liver function, CBC, BUN, serum creatinine

Physical Assessment Evaluate cardiac risk and potential for GI bleeding prior to prescribing this medication. Monitor blood pressure at the beginning of therapy and periodically during use. Monitor for GI effects, hepatotoxicity, and ototoxicity at beginning of therapy and periodically throughout. Schedule ophthalmic evaluations for patients who develop eye complaints during long-term NSAID therapy.

Patient Education Do not crush tablets. Take with food or milk to reduce GI distress. Do not use alcohol. You may experience drowsiness, dizziness, lightheadedness, headache, anorexia, nausea, vomiting, heartburn, or fluid retention; GI bleeding, ulceration, or perforation can occur with or without pain; discontinue medication and contact prescriber if persistent abdominal pain or cramping or blood in stool occurs. Report breathlessness, respiratory difficulty, or unusual cough; chest pain, rapid heartbeat, or palpitations; bruising/bleeding; blood in urine, stool, mouth, or vomitus; swollen extremities; skin rash; changes in eyesight (double vision, color changes, blurred vision) or hearing; or ringing in ears.

Related Information

Nonsalicylate / Nonsteroidal Anti-Inflammatory Agents *on page 2002*

Naproxen and Esomeprazole (na PROKS en & es oh ME pray zol)

U.S. Brand Names Vimovo™

Index Terms Esomeprazole and Naproxen

Generic Availability (U.S.) No

Pharmacologic Category Nonsteroidal Anti-inflammatory Drug (NSAID), Oral; Proton Pump Inhibitor; Substituted Benzimidazole

Medication Safety Issues

Sound-alike/look-alike issues:

Vimovo™ may be confused with Vimpat®

Medication Guide Available Yes

Pregnancy Risk Factor C; Naproxen: D/3rd trimester)

Lactation Enters breast milk/not recommended

Use Reduction of the risk of NSAID-associated gastric ulcers in patients at risk of developing gastric ulcers who require an NSAID for the treatment of rheumatoid arthritis, osteoarthritis, and ankylosing spondylitis

Available Dosage Forms

Tablet, variable release, oral:

Vimovo™: Naproxen [delayed release] 375 mg and esomeprazole [immediate release] 20 mg, Naproxen [delayed release] 500 mg and esomeprazole [immediate release] 20 mg

Dosing

Adult Reduce NSAID-associated gastric ulcers during treatment for arthritis: Oral: One tablet (375 mg naproxen/20 mg esomeprazole or 500 mg naproxen/20 mg esomeprazole) twice daily; maximum daily esomeprazole dose: 40 mg.

Note: If a daily dose of esomeprazole <40 mg/day is necessary, alternate treatment should be considered.

Geriatric Naproxen: Dosing adjustment should be considered; use lowest effective dose. Refer to adult dosing.

Renal Impairment Moderate-to-severe renal impairment (Cl_{cr} <30 mL/minute): Use is not recommended.

Hepatic Impairment Severe liver disease: Use of this combination product not recommended since esomeprazole dose will exceed 20 mg/day.

Administration

Oral Administer dose at least 30 minutes prior to meals. Tablets should be swallowed whole; do not chew, crush, dissolve, or split tablet.

Monitoring and Teaching Issues

Laboratory Monitoring Occult blood loss; periodic liver function test, CBC, BUN, serum creatinine

Physical Assessment See individual agents.

Patient Education See individual agents.

Related Information

Esomeprazole *on page 667*

Naproxen *on page 1289*

◆ **Naproxen and Sumatriptan** *see* Sumatriptan and Naproxen *on page 1694*

◆ **Naproxen Sodium** *see* Naproxen *on page 1289*

◆ **Naproxen Sodium and Sumatriptan** *see* Sumatriptan and Naproxen *on page 1694*

◆ **Naproxen Sodium and Sumatriptan Succinate** *see* Sumatriptan and Naproxen *on page 1694*

Naratriptan (NAR a trip tan)

U.S. Brand Names Amerge®

Index Terms Naratriptan Hydrochloride

Generic Availability (U.S.) Yes

Pharmacologic Category Antimigraine Agent; Serotonin 5-$HT_{1B, 1D}$ Receptor Agonist

Medication Safety Issues

Sound-alike/look-alike issues:

Amerge® may be confused with Altace®, Amaryl®

Pregnancy Risk Factor C

Lactation Excretion in breast milk unknown/use caution

Use Treatment of acute migraine headache with or without aura

Mechanism of Action/Effect Selective agonist for serotonin receptor in cranial arteries; causes vasoconstriction and relief of migraine

Contraindications Hypersensitivity to naratriptan or any component of the formulation; cerebrovascular, peripheral vascular disease (ischemic bowel disease), ischemic heart disease (angina pectoris, history of myocardial infarction, or proven silent ischemia); or in patients with symptoms consistent with ischemic heart disease, coronary artery vasospasm, or Prinzmetal's angina; uncontrolled hypertension or patients who have received within 24 hours another 5-HT agonist (sumatriptan, zolmitriptan) or ergotamine-containing product; patients with known risk factors associated with coronary artery disease; patients with severe hepatic (Child-Pugh grade C) or renal disease (Cl_{cr} <15 mL/minute); do not administer naratriptan to patients with hemiplegic or basilar migraine

Warnings/Precautions Use only if there is a clear diagnosis of migraine. Dosage reduction is required in mild-to-moderate hepatic impairment and moderate renal impairment; use is contraindicated in patients with severe hepatic or renal impairment. Do not give to patients with risk factors for CAD until a cardiovascular evaluation has been performed; if evaluation is satisfactory, the healthcare provider should administer the first dose and cardiovascular status should be periodically re-evaluated. Cardiac events (coronary artery vasospasm, transient ischemia, myocardial infarction, ventricular tachycardia/fibrillation, cardiac arrest, and death), cerebral/subarachnoid hemorrhage, stroke, peripheral vascular ischemia, and colonic ischemia have been reported with 5-HT_1 agonist administration. Significant elevation in blood pressure, including hypertensive crisis, has also been reported on rare occasions in patients with and without a history of hypertension. Only indicated for the acute treatment of migraine; not indicated for migraine prophylaxis, or for the treatment of cluster headache, hemiplegic or basilar migraine. If a patient does not respond to the first dose, the diagnosis of migraine should be reconsidered; rule out underlying neurologic disease in patients with atypical headache and in patients with no prior history of migraine.

Drug Interactions

Avoid Concomitant Use

Avoid concomitant use of Naratriptan with any of the following: Ergot Derivatives; Sibutramine

Decreased Effect There are no known significant interactions involving a decrease in effect.

Increased Effect/Toxicity

Naratriptan may increase the levels/effects of: Ergot Derivatives; Serotonin Modulators

The levels/effects of Naratriptan may be increased by: Ergot Derivatives; Sibutramine

Adverse Reactions 1% to 10%:

Central nervous system: Pain/pressure (2% to 4%), malaise/fatigue (2%), dizziness (1% to 2%), drowsiness (1% to 2%), vertigo (1%)

Gastrointestinal: Nausea (4% to 5%), hyposalivation (1%), vomiting (1%)

Neuromuscular & skeletal: Paresthesia (1% to 2%)

Ocular: Photophobia (1%)

Miscellaneous: Ear/nose/throat infection (1%), pressure/tightness/heaviness sensations (1%), warm/cold temperature sensations (1%)

Pharmacodynamics/Kinetics

Onset of Action ~1-2 hours (Bomhof, 1999; Tfelt-Hansen, 2000)

Absorption Well absorbed

Bioavailability ~70%

Time to Peak 2-3 hours

Protein Binding Plasma: 28% to 31%

Half-Life Elimination 6 hours; increased in renal impairment (moderate impairment; mean: 11 hours; range 7-20 hours); increased in hepatic impairment (moderate impairment: 8-16 hours)

Metabolism Hepatic via CYP

Excretion Urine (50% of total dose as unchanged drug; 30% of total dose as metabolites)

Available Dosage Forms

Tablet, oral: 1 mg, 2.5 mg

Amerge®: 1 mg, 2.5 mg

Dosing

Adult Migraine: Oral: 1 mg to 2.5 mg at the onset of headache. It is recommended to use the lowest possible dose to minimize adverse effects. If headache returns or does not fully resolve, the dose may be repeated after 4 hours. Do not exceed 5 mg in 24 hours.

Geriatric Not recommended for use in the elderly.

Renal Impairment

Mild-to-moderate renal impairment: Initial: 1 mg; do not exceed 2.5 mg in 24 hours.

Severe renal impairment (Cl_{cr} <15 mL/minute): Use is contraindicated.

Hepatic Impairment

Mild-to-moderate hepatic impairment (Child-Pugh grade A or B): Initial: 1 mg; do not exceed 2.5 mg in 24 hours

Severe hepatic impairment (Child-Pugh grade C): Use is contraindicated.

Administration

Oral Do **not** crush or chew tablet; swallow whole with water.

Stability

Storage Store at 20°C to 25°C (68°F to 77°F).

Monitoring and Teaching Issues

Physical Assessment Assess for clear diagnosis of migraine prior to beginning therapy. Cardiovascular status should be evaluated prior to initiating medication and periodically thereafter. Assess potential for interactions with ergot-containing drugs and SSRIs patient may be taking. Monitor closely, especially after the first dose. Monitor for drowsiness, nausea/vomiting, paresthesias, and hypertension. If no response to first dose, diagnosis of migraine should be re-evaluated.

Patient Education Do not crush or chew tablet; swallow whole with water. This drug is to be used to reduce your migraine, not to prevent or reduce the number of attacks. If headache returns or is not fully resolved, the dose may be repeated after 4 hours. If you have no relief with first dose, do not take a second dose without consulting prescriber. **Do not exceed 5 mg in 24 hours. Do not take within 24 hours of any other migraine medication without first consulting prescriber.** May cause dizziness, fatigue, drowsiness, nausea, or vomiting. Report immediately any chest pain, palpitations, or rapid heartbeat; tightness in throat or neck; or rash, itching, or hives.

Geriatric Considerations Naratriptan was not studied in patients >65 years of age. Use in elderly patients is not recommended because of the presence of risk factors associated with adverse effects. These include the presence of coronary artery disease, decreased liver or renal function, and the risk of pronounced blood pressure increases.

Pregnancy Considerations There are no adequate and well-controlled studies using naratriptan in pregnant women. Use only if potential benefit to the mother outweighs the potential risk to the fetus. A pregnancy registry has been established to monitor outcomes of women exposed to naratriptan during pregnancy (800-336-2176). In animal studies, administration was associated with embryolethality, fetal abnormalities, and pup mortality and growth retardation. Tremors were observed in the offspring of female rats when exposed to naratriptan late in gestation.

Related Information

Antimigraine Drugs: 5-HT_1 Receptor Agonists *on page 1985*

- ◆ **Naratriptan Hydrochloride** *see* Naratriptan *on page 1291*
- ◆ **Narcan** *see* Naloxone *on page 1284*
- ◆ **Nardil®** *see* Phenelzine *on page 1446*
- ◆ **Nasacort® AQ** *see* Triamcinolone (Nasal) *on page 1815*
- ◆ **Nascobal®** *see* Cyanocobalamin *on page 431*
- ◆ **Nasonex®** *see* Mometasone (Nasal) *on page 1254*

Natalizumab (na ta LIZ u mab)

U.S. Brand Names Tysabri®

Index Terms AN100226; Anti-4 Alpha Integrin; IgG4-Kappa Monoclonal Antibody

Generic Availability (U.S.) No

Pharmacologic Category Gastrointestinal Agent, Miscellaneous; Monoclonal Antibody, Selective Adhesion-Molecule Inhibitor

Medication Guide Available Yes

Prescribing and Access Restrictions

U.S.: Tysabri® is deemed to have an approved REMS program. As a requirement of the REMS program, access to this medication is restricted. Patients must be enrolled in the Tysabri® Outreach Unified Commitment to Health (TOUCH™) Prescribing Program (800-456-2255) to receive natalizumab (MS-TOUCH™ for multiple sclerosis or CD-TOUCH™ for Crohn's disease). Healthcare providers must also register with the program in order to prescribe, dispense or administer natalizumab. Treatment must be reauthorized every 6 months. Natalizumab is available only through infusion centers registered with the TOUCH™ program; infusion center information is available at 1-800-456-2255.

Canada: Patients receiving natalizumab therapy for multiple sclerosis are to be enrolled in the Tysabri Care Program™ (888-827-2827). This program is associated with the prescribing, administration, and monitoring of Canadian patients receiving natalizumab. Clinicians are educated on the appropriate use of natalizumab and are expected to discuss the benefits/risks of therapy. Clinicians should evaluate patients every 6 months during treatment.

Pregnancy Risk Factor C

Lactation Excretion in breast milk unknown/not recommended

Use Monotherapy for the treatment of relapsing forms of multiple sclerosis; treatment of moderately- to severely-active Crohn's disease

Canada labeling: Treatment of relapsing forms of multiple sclerosis

Available Dosage Forms

Injection, solution [preservative free]:

Tysabri®: 300 mg/15 mL (15 mL)

Dosing

Adult & Geriatric

Multiple sclerosis: I.V.: 300 mg infused over 1 hour every 4 weeks

Crohn's disease: I.V.: 300 mg infused over 1 hour every 4 weeks; discontinue if therapeutic benefit is not observed within initial 12 weeks of therapy

Concomitant use with corticosteroids: For patients who begin treatment while on chronic oral corticosteroids, begin tapering oral steroids when the onset of natalizumab therapeutic benefit is observed; discontinue use if patient cannot be tapered off of oral corticosteroids within 6 months of therapy initiation. If additional concomitant corticosteroids are required and exceed 3 months/year (in addition to initial corticosteroid taper), consider discontinuing therapy.

Renal Impairment Not studied.

Hepatic Impairment Not studied. Discontinue use with jaundice or signs/symptoms of hepatic injury.

Administration

I.V. Solution may be warmed to room temperature prior to administration. Diluted solution should be infused over 1 hour; do not administer by I.V. bolus or push. Patients should be closely monitored for signs and symptoms of hypersensitivity during the infusion and for at least 1 hour after the infusion is complete. The infusion should be discontinued if a reaction occurs, and treatment of the reaction should be instituted. Following infusion, flush line with NS.

Monitoring and Teaching Issues

Laboratory Monitoring Liver enzymes, bilirubin; when indicated, obtain antibody testing, CSF analysis, and MRI scan

Physical Assessment Patient should be monitored closely for infusion-related reactions during and for 1 hour following infusion. If hypersensitivity reaction occurs, infusion should be promptly discontinued; retreatment is not recommended. Monitor for hepatotoxicity, opportunistic infection (including herpes), excessive fatigue, depression or anxiety, and progressive multifocal leukoencephalopathy (hemiparesis, visual field deficits, cognitive impairment, aphasia, ataxia, and/or cranial nerve deficits).

Patient Education This drug can only be administered by intravenous infusion. You will be monitored closely during and following infusion. Report immediately any skin rash; dizziness; nausea; flushing; difficulty breathing; chest pain or tightness; redness, swelling, or pain at infusion site; signs of urinary tract infection (itching, pain, discharge); dark urine or altered frequency of urination; lower respiratory infection (cough, difficulty breathing, chest tightness); unusual sores or unhealed sores; chest discomfort or pain; back pain; unusual depression or anxiety; changes in speech or movement; vision changes; or worsening symptoms. Following infusion, you may experience headache, joint pain, or unusual fatigue.

◆ **Natazia™** *see* Estradiol and Dienogest *on page* 673

Nateglinide (na te GLYE nide)

U.S. Brand Names Starlix®

Generic Availability (U.S.) Yes

Pharmacologic Category Antidiabetic Agent, Meglitinide Derivative

Medication Safety Issues

High alert medication: The Institute for Safe Medication Practices (ISMP) includes this medication among its list of drug classes which have a heightened risk of causing significant patient harm when used in error.

Pregnancy Risk Factor C

Lactation Excretion in breast milk unknown/not recommended

Use Management of type 2 diabetes mellitus (noninsulin dependent, NIDDM) as monotherapy when hyperglycemia cannot be managed by diet and exercise alone; in combination with metformin or a thiazolidinedione to lower blood glucose in patients whose hyperglycemia cannot be controlled by exercise, diet, or a single agent alone

Mechanism of Action/Effect Increases insulin release from pancreatic beta cells; decreases postprandial hyperglycemia; not a sulfonylurea

Contraindications Hypersensitivity to nateglinide or any component of the formulation; diabetic ketoacidosis, with or without coma (treat with insulin); type 1 diabetes mellitus (insulin dependent, IDDM)

Warnings/Precautions Use with caution in patients with moderate-to-severe hepatic impairment. Use caution in severe renal dysfunction, elderly, malnourished, or patients with adrenal/pituitary dysfunction; may be more susceptible to glucose-lowering effects. All oral hypoglycemic agents are capable of producing hypoglycemia. Proper patient selection, dosage, and instructions to the patients are important to avoid hypoglycemic episodes. It may be necessary to discontinue nateglinide and administer insulin if the patient is exposed to stress (ie, fever, trauma, infection, surgery). Indicated for adjunctive therapy with metformin; not to be used as a substitute for metformin monotherapy. Combination treatment with sulfonylureas is not recommended (no additional benefit). Patients not adequately controlled on oral agents which stimulate insulin release (eg, glyburide) should not be switched to nateglinide or have nateglinide added to therapy.

Drug Interactions

Metabolism/Transport Effects Substrate (major) of CYP2C9, CYP3A4, SLCO1B1; **Inhibits** CYP2C9 (weak)

Avoid Concomitant Use There are no known interactions where it is recommended to avoid concomitant use.

Decreased Effect

The levels/effects of Nateglinide may be decreased by: Corticosteroids (Orally Inhaled); Corticosteroids (Systemic); CYP2C9 Inducers (Highly Effective); CYP3A4 Inducers (Strong); Deferasirox; Herbs (CYP3A4 Inducers); Luteinizing Hormone-Releasing Hormone Analogs; Peginterferon Alfa-2b; Somatropin; Thiazide Diuretics

Increased Effect/Toxicity

Nateglinide may increase the levels/effects of: Hypoglycemic Agents

The levels/effects of Nateglinide may be increased by: Conivaptan; CYP2C9 Inhibitors (Moderate); CYP2C9 Inhibitors (Strong); CYP3A4 Inhibitors (Moderate); CYP3A4 Inhibitors (Strong); Dasatinib; Eltrombopag; Herbs (Hypoglycemic Properties); Pegvisomant

Nutritional/Ethanol Interactions

Ethanol: Avoid ethanol (increased risk of hypoglycemia).

Food: Rate of absorption is decreased and time to T_{max} is delayed when taken with food. Food does not affect AUC. Multiple peak plasma concentrations may be observed if fasting. Not affected by composition of meal.

Herb/Nutraceutical: Avoid alfalfa, aloe, bilberry, bitter melon, burdock, celery, damiana, fenugreek, garcinia, garlic, ginger, ginseng (American), gymnema, marshmallow, and stinging nettle (may enhance the hypoglycemic effects of antidiabetic agents). St. John's wort may decrease the levels/effect of nateglinide.

Adverse Reactions As reported with nateglinide monotherapy: 1% to 10%:

Central nervous system: Dizziness (4%)
Endocrine & metabolic: Hypoglycemia (2%), increased uric acid
Gastrointestinal: Weight gain
Neuromuscular & skeletal: Arthropathy (3%)
Respiratory: Upper respiratory infection (10%)
Miscellaneous: Flu-like syndrome (4%)

Pharmacodynamics/Kinetics

Onset of Action Insulin secretion: ~20 minutes; Peak effect: 1 hour

Duration of Action 4 hours

Absorption Rapid

Bioavailability 73%

Time to Peak ≤1 hour

Protein Binding 98%, primarily to albumin

Half-Life Elimination 1.5 hours

Metabolism Hepatic via hydroxylation followed by glucuronide conjugation via CYP2C9 (70%) and CYP3A4 (30%) to metabolites

Excretion Urine (83%, 16% as unchanged drug); feces (10%)

Available Dosage Forms

Tablet, oral: 60 mg, 120 mg
Starlix®: 60 mg, 120 mg

Dosing

Adult & Geriatric Management of type 2 diabetes mellitus: Oral: Initial and maintenance dose: 120 mg 3 times/day, 1-30 minutes before meals; may be given alone or in combination with metformin or a thiazolidinedione; patients close to Hb A_{1c} goal may be started at 60 mg 3 times/day

Renal Impairment No specific dosage adjustment is recommended for patients with mild-to-severe renal disease. Patients on dialysis showed reduced medication exposure and plasma protein binding. Patients with severe renal dysfunction are more susceptible to glucose-lowering effect; use with caution.

Hepatic Impairment Increased serum levels are seen with mild hepatic insufficiency; no dosage adjustment is needed. Has not been studied in patients with moderate-to-severe liver disease; use with caution.

Stability

Storage Store at 25°C (77°F).

Monitoring and Teaching Issues

Laboratory Monitoring Glucose and Hb A_{1c} levels, lipid profile

Physical Assessment Teach patient importance of proper diabetic monitoring.

Patient Education Take 1-30 minutes before a meal. If you skip a meal, skip a dose for that meal. Follow dietary and lifestyle recommendations of provider. You will be instructed in signs of hyper-/hypoglycemia by prescriber or diabetic educator; be alert for adverse hypoglycemia (tachycardia, profuse perspiration, tingling of lips and tongue, seizures, or change in sensorium) and follow prescriber's instructions for intervention. Note that unusual strenuous exercise, excessive alcohol intake, or acute reduction in caloric intake may increase risk of hypoglycemia. Persistent nausea or vomiting, or severely decreased dietary intake may increase risk of hyperglycemia. May cause mild side effects during first weeks of therapy (dizziness, weight gain, mild muscle aches or pain, or flu-like symptoms); if these do not diminish, notify prescriber. Report signs of respiratory infection.

Dietary Considerations Nateglinide should be taken 1-30 minutes prior to meals. Scheduled dose should not be taken if meal is missed. Dietary modification based on ADA recommendations is a part of therapy. Decreases blood glucose concentration. Hypoglycemia may occur. Must be able to recognize symptoms of hypoglycemia (palpitations, sweaty palms, lightheadedness).

Geriatric Considerations No changes in safety and efficacy were seen in patients ≥65 years; however, some older adults may show increased sensitivity to dosing. How "tightly" a geriatric patient's blood glucose should be controlled is controversial; however, a fasting blood sugar of <150 mg/dL is now an acceptable endpoint. Such a decision should be based on the patient's functional and cognitive status, how well they recognize hypoglycemic or hyperglycemic symptoms, and how to respond to them and their other disease states. Intensive glucose control (Hb A_{1c} <6.5%) has been linked to increased all cause and cardiovascular mortality, hypoglycemia requiring assistance, and weight gain in adult type 2 diabetes. For elderly patients with diabetes who are relatively healthy, attaining target goals for aspirin use, blood pressure, lipids, smoking cessation, and diet and exercise may be more important than normalized glycemic control.

Breast-Feeding Considerations It is not known if nateglinide is excreted in breast milk. Breast-feeding is not recommended by the manufacturer.

Pregnancy Considerations Adverse events have been observed in animal reproduction studies; therefore, nateglinide is classified as pregnancy category C. Information describing the effects of nateglinide on pregnancy outcomes is limited. Maternal hyperglycemia can be associated with adverse effects in the fetus, including macrosomia, neonatal hyperglycemia, and hyperbilirubinemia; the risk of congenital malformations is increased when the Hb A_{1c} is above the normal range. Diabetes can also be associated with adverse effects in the mother. Poorly-treated diabetes may cause end-organ damage that may in turn negatively affect obstetric outcomes. Physiologic glucose levels should be maintained prior to and during pregnancy to decrease the risk of adverse events in the mother and the fetus. Until additional safety and efficacy data are obtained, the use of oral agents is generally not recommended as routine management of GDM or type 2 diabetes mellitus during pregnancy. Insulin is the drug of choice for the control of diabetes mellitus during pregnancy.

Additional Information An increase in weight was seen in nateglinide monotherapy, which was not seen when used in combination with metformin.

Related Information

Diabetes Mellitus Management, Adults *on page 2026*

- **Natrecor®** *see* Nesiritide *on page 1299*
- **Natriuretic Peptide** *see* Nesiritide *on page 1299*
- **Nature-Throid™** *see* Thyroid, Desiccated *on page 1757*
- **Navane®** *see* Thiothixene *on page 1756*
- **Navelbine®** *see* Vinorelbine *on page 1868*

Nebivolol (ne BIV oh lole)

U.S. Brand Names Bystolic®

Index Terms Nebivolol Hydrochloride

Generic Availability (U.S.) No

Pharmacologic Category Beta Blocker, Beta-1 Selective

Pregnancy Risk Factor C

Lactation Excretion in breast milk unknown/not recommended

Use Treatment of hypertension, alone or in combination with other agents

Unlabeled/Investigational Use Heart failure

Available Dosage Forms

Tablet, oral:

Bystolic®: 2.5 mg, 5 mg, 10 mg, 20 mg

Dosing

Adult & Geriatric

Hypertension: Oral: Initial: 5 mg once daily; if initial response is inadequate, may be increased at 2-week intervals to a maximum dose of 40 mg once daily

Heart failure (unlabeled use): Adults ≥70 years: Oral: Initial: 1.25 mg once daily; if tolerated, may increase by 2.5 mg at 1- to 2-week intervals to a maximum dose of 10 mg once daily (Flather, 2005). **Note:** Nebivolol has not been shown to reduce morbidity or mortality in the general HF population.

Renal Impairment Severe impairment (Cl_{cr} <30 mL/minute): Initial: 2.5 mg/day; increase cautiously.

Hepatic Impairment Moderate impairment (Child-Pugh class B): Initial: 2.5 mg/day; increase cautiously.

Administration

Oral May be administered with or without food.

Monitoring and Teaching Issues

Laboratory Monitoring Serum glucose (regularly in patients with diabetes)

Physical Assessment Monitor therapeutic response, especially pulse rate and blood pressure, prior to initiation and periodically thereafter. Taper dosage slowly when discontinuing. Advise patients with diabetes to monitor glucose levels closely; beta-blockers may alter glucose tolerance.

Patient Education If you have diabetes, monitor serum sugar closely; drug may alter glucose tolerance or mask signs of hypoglycemia. May cause postural hypotension. Use caution when climbing stairs or changing position. Report signs of fluid retention (unusual weight gain, swelling of the extremities), shortness of breath, or chest pain.

- **Nebivolol Hydrochloride** *see* Nebivolol *on page 1295*

- ◆ **Nebupent®** *see* Pentamidine *on page 1438*
- ◆ **Necon® 0.5/35** *see* Ethinyl Estradiol and Norethindrone *on page 701*
- ◆ **Necon® 1/35** *see* Ethinyl Estradiol and Norethindrone *on page 701*
- ◆ **Necon® 1/50** *see* Norethindrone and Mestranol *on page 1335*
- ◆ **Necon® 7/7/7** *see* Ethinyl Estradiol and Norethindrone *on page 701*
- ◆ **Necon® 10/11** *see* Ethinyl Estradiol and Norethindrone *on page 701*

Nefazodone (nef AY zoe done)

Index Terms Nefazodone Hydrochloride; Serzone

Generic Availability (U.S.) Yes

Pharmacologic Category Antidepressant, Serotonin Reuptake Inhibitor/Antagonist

Medication Safety Issues

Sound-alike/look-alike issues:

Serzone® may be confused with selegiline, Serentil®, SEROquel®, sertraline

Medication Guide Available Yes

Pregnancy Risk Factor C

Lactation Enters breast milk/use caution

Use Treatment of depression

Unlabeled/Investigational Use Post-traumatic stress disorder (PTSD)

Available Dosage Forms

Tablet, oral: 50 mg, 100 mg, 150 mg, 200 mg, 250 mg

Dosing

Adult

Depression: Oral: 200 mg/day, administered in two divided doses initially, with a range of 300-600 mg/day in 2 divided doses thereafter.

Post-traumatic stress disorder (PTSD) (unlabeled use): Oral: Initial: 100 mg twice daily; target dose: 600 mg/day (average daily dose: 463 mg).

Geriatric Oral: Initial: 50 mg twice daily; increase dose to 100 mg twice daily in 2 weeks; usual maintenance dose: 200-400 mg/day

Pediatric Depression (unlabeled use): Oral: Children and Adolescents: Target dose: 300-400 mg/day (mean: 3.4 mg/kg)

Administration

Oral Dosing after meals may decrease lightheadedness and postural hypotension, but may also decrease absorption and therefore effectiveness.

Monitoring and Teaching Issues

Laboratory Monitoring If AST/ALT increase >3 times ULN, the drug should be discontinued and not reintroduced.

Physical Assessment Monitor for clinical worsening and suicide ideation. Taper dosage slowly when discontinuing.

Patient Education It may take 2-3 weeks to achieve desired results. Avoid alcohol. Maintain adequate hydration unless instructed to restrict fluid intake. You may experience drowsiness, dizziness, lightheadedness, nausea, vomiting, or orthostatic hypotension. Report persistent insomnia or excessive daytime sedation; suicide ideation; muscle cramping, tremors, weakness, tiredness, or change in gait; chest pain, palpitations, or rapid heartbeat; vision changes or eye pain; respiratory difficulty or breathlessness; malaise, loss of appetite, GI complaints, abdominal pain, or blood in stool; yellowing of skin or eyes (jaundice); or worsening of condition.

Related Information

Antidepressant Agents *on page 1982*

- ◆ **Nefazodone Hydrochloride** *see* Nefazodone *on page 1296*

Nelfinavir (nel FIN a veer)

U.S. Brand Names Viracept®

Index Terms NFV

Generic Availability (U.S.) No

Pharmacologic Category Antiretroviral Agent, Protease Inhibitor

Medication Safety Issues

Sound-alike/look-alike issues:

Nelfinavir may be confused with nevirapine

Viracept® may be confused with Viramune®, Viramune® XR™

Pregnancy Risk Factor B

Lactation Excretion in breast milk unknown/contraindicated

Use In combination with other antiretroviral therapy in the treatment of HIV infection

Mechanism of Action/Effect Blocks the site of HIV-1 protease activity, resulting in the formation of immature, noninfectious viral particles.

Contraindications Hypersensitivity to nelfinavir or any component of the formulation; concurrent therapy with alfuzosin, amiodarone, ergot derivatives, midazolam, pimozide, quinidine, sildenafil (when used for pulmonary artery hypertension [eg, Revatio®]), triazolam

Warnings/Precautions Use with caution in patients taking strong CYP3A4 inhibitors, moderate or strong CYP3A4 inducers and major CYP3A4 substrates and if coadministered with QT-prolonging drugs that are metabolized by CYP3A (see Drug Interactions); consider alternative agents that avoid or lessen the potential for CYP-mediated interactions. Not recommended for use with rifampin, St John's wort, lovastatin, simvastatin, phosphodiesterase-5 (PDE-5) inhibitors, or proton pump inhibitors (based on omeprazole data). Do not coadminister colchicine in patient with renal or hepatic impairment; avoid concurrent use with salmeterol.

Use caution with hepatic impairment; use not recommended with moderate-to-severe impairment. Warn patients that redistribution of body fat can occur. New-onset diabetes mellitus, exacerbation of diabetes, and hyperglycemia have been reported in HIV-infected patients receiving protease inhibitors. Use with caution in patients with hemophilia A or B; increased bleeding during protease inhibitor therapy has been reported. Immune reconstitution syndrome has been reported; may require additional evaluation and treatment. The oral powder contains phenylalanine. Safety and efficacy have not been established in children <2 years of age.

Drug Interactions

Metabolism/Transport Effects Substrate of CYP2C9 (minor), CYP2C19 (major), CYP2D6 (minor), CYP3A4 (major), P-glycoprotein; **Inhibits** CYP1A2 (weak), CYP2B6 (weak), CYP2C9 (weak), CYP2C19 (weak), CYP2D6 (weak), CYP3A4 (strong), P-glycoprotein

Avoid Concomitant Use

Avoid concomitant use of Nelfinavir with any of the following: Alfuzosin; Amiodarone; Cisapride; Conivaptan; Dronedarone; Eplerenone; Ergot Derivatives; Everolimus; Halofantrine; Lovastatin; Lurasidone; Midazolam; Nilotinib; Nisoldipine; Pimozide; Proton Pump Inhibitors; QuiNIDine; Ranolazine; Rifampin; Rivaroxaban; RomiDEPsin; Salmeterol; Silodosin; Simvastatin; St Johns Wort; Tamsulosin; Tolvaptan; Topotecan; Toremifene; Triazolam

Decreased Effect

Nelfinavir may decrease the levels/effects of: Abacavir; Clarithromycin; Contraceptives (Estrogens); Delavirdine; Divalproex; Etravirine; Lopinavir; Meperidine; Methadone; Prasugrel; Theophylline Derivatives; Valproic Acid; Warfarin; Zidovudine

The levels/effects of Nelfinavir may be decreased by: Antacids; Bosentan; CarBAMazepine; Contraceptives (Estrogens); CYP2C19 Inducers (Strong); CYP3A4 Inducers (Strong); Deferasirox; Efavirenz; Garlic; H2-Antagonists; Nevirapine; Peginterferon Alfa-2b; P-Glycoprotein Inducers; Proton Pump Inhibitors; Rifabutin; Rifampin; St Johns Wort; Tenofovir

Increased Effect/Toxicity

Nelfinavir may increase the levels/effects of: Alfuzosin; Almotriptan; Alosetron; ALPRAZolam; Amiodarone; Antifungal Agents (Azole Derivatives, Systemic); Azithromycin; Azithromycin (Systemic); Bortezomib; Bosentan; Brinzolamide; Calcium Channel Blockers (Dihydropyridine); Calcium Channel Blockers (Nondihydropyridine); CarBAMazepine; Ciclesonide; Cisapride; Clarithromycin; Colchicine; Conivaptan; Corticosteroids (Orally Inhaled); CycloSPORINE; CycloSPORINE (Systemic); CYP3A4 Substrates; Dabigatran Etexilate; Dienogest; Digoxin; Dronedarone; Dutasteride; Enfuvirtide; Eplerenone; Ergot Derivatives; Everolimus; FentaNYL; Fesoterodine; Fusidic Acid; GuanFACINE; Halofantrine; HMG-CoA Reductase Inhibitors; Ixabepilone; Lovastatin; Lumefantrine; Lurasidone; Maraviroc; Meperidine; MethylPREDNISolone; Midazolam; Nefazodone; Nilotinib; Nisoldipine; Paricalcitol; Pazopanib; P-Glycoprotein Substrates; Pimecrolimus; Pimozide; Protease Inhibitors; QuiNIDine; Ranolazine; Rifabutin; Rivaroxaban; RomiDEPsin; Salmeterol; Saxagliptin; Sildenafil; Silodosin; Simvastatin; Sirolimus; SORAfenib; Tacrolimus; Tacrolimus (Systemic); Tacrolimus (Topical); Tadalafil; Tamsulosin; Temsirolimus; Tenofovir; Tolvaptan; Topotecan; Toremifene; TraZODone; Triazolam; Tricyclic Antidepressants; Vardenafil; Vilazodone; Warfarin

The levels/effects of Nelfinavir may be increased by: Antifungal Agents (Azole Derivatives, Systemic); Clarithromycin; CycloSPORINE; CycloSPORINE (Systemic); Delavirdine; Efavirenz; Enfuvirtide; Etravirine; Fusidic Acid; Lopinavir; P-Glycoprotein Inhibitors

Nutritional/Ethanol Interactions

Food: Nelfinavir taken with food increases plasma concentration time curve (AUC) by two- to threefold. Do not administer with acidic food or juice (orange juice, apple juice, or applesauce) since the combination may have a bitter taste.

Herb/Nutraceutical: St John's wort may decrease the levels/effects of protease inhibitors; concurrent use should probably be avoided.

Adverse Reactions Data presented on experience in adults, unless otherwise noted.

>10%: Gastrointestinal: Diarrhea (14% to 20%; children: 39% to 47%)

2% to 10%:

Dermatologic: Rash (1% to 3%)

Gastrointestinal: Nausea (3% to 7%), flatulence (1% to 5%)

Hematologic: Lymphocytes decreased (1% to 6%), neutrophils decreased (1% to 5%)

Pharmacodynamics/Kinetics

Absorption Food increases AUC of nelfinavir by two- to fivefold

Time to Peak Serum: 2-4 hours

Protein Binding >98%

Half-Life Elimination 3.5-5 hours

Metabolism Hepatic via CYP2C19 and 3A4; major metabolite has activity comparable to parent drug

Excretion Feces (98% to 99%, 78% as metabolites, 22% as unchanged drug); urine (1% to 2%)

Available Dosage Forms

Powder, oral:
Viracept®: 50 mg/g (144 g)

Tablet, oral:
Viracept®: 250 mg, 625 mg

Dosing

Adult & Geriatric HIV infection: Oral: 750 mg 3 times/day or 1250 mg twice daily with meals in combination with other antiretroviral therapies

Dosage adjustments for concomitant therapy: Oral:

Coadministration with bosentan:

Coadministration of bosentan in patients currently receiving nelfinavir: Begin with bosentan 62.5 mg once daily or every other day based on tolerability

Coadministration of nelfinavir in patients currently receiving bosentan: Adjust bosentan to 62.5 mg once daily or every other day based on tolerability

Coadministration with colchicine:

Familial Mediterranean fever (FMF): Maximum colchicine dose: 0.6 mg/day (0.3 mg twice daily)

Gout prophylaxis:

If original colchicine dose is 0.6 mg twice daily, adjust dose to 0.3 mg once daily

If original colchicine dose is 0.6 mg once daily, adjust dose to 0.3 mg every other day

Gout flare treatment: Initial: Colchicine 0.6 mg, followed in 1 hour by a single dose of 0.3 mg; do not repeat for at least 3 days

Coadministration with phosphodiesterase-5 enzyme (PDE-5) inhibitor:

Pulmonary arterial hypertension: Nelfinavir coadministered with tadalafil:

Patient receiving nelfinavir: Initiate tadalafil at 20 mg once daily; increase to 40 mg once daily based on individual tolerability

Patient receiving tadalafil when initiating nelfinavir: Adjust tadalafil to 20 mg once daily; increase to 40 mg once daily based on individual tolerability

Erectile dysfunction: Nelfinavir coadministered with:

Sildenafil (Viagra®): Maximum sildenafil dose: 25 mg in a 48-hour period

Tadalafil (Cialis®): Maximum tadalafil dose: 10 mg in a 72-hour period

Vardenafil: Maximum vardenafil dose: 2.5 mg in a 24-hour period

Pediatric HIV infection: Oral: Children 2-13 years: 45-55 mg/kg twice daily **or** 25-35 mg/kg 3 times/day (maximum: 2500 mg/day). If tablets are unable to be taken, use oral powder in small amount of water, milk (cow's or soy), formula, or dietary supplements; do not use acidic food/juice or store for >6 hours.

Renal Impairment No pharmacokinetic data in patients with renal impairment. However, <2% of dose excreted in urine; no dose adjustment is needed.

Hepatic Impairment No dose adjustment necessary in mild impairment (Child-Pugh class A); not recommended in patients with moderate-to-severe impairment (Child-Pugh class B or C)

Administration

Oral

Oral powder: Administer with a meal. Mix powder in a small amount of water, milk, formula, soy milk, soy formula, pudding, ice cream, or dietary supplement. Do not reconstitute the oral powder in its original container. Be sure entire contents is consumed to receive full dose. Do not use acidic food/juice to dilute due to bitter taste. Once mixed, solution should be used immediately, but may be stored for up to 6 hours if refrigerated.

Tablets: Administer with a meal. If unable to swallow tablets, may dissolve tablets in a small amount of water; mix cloudy liquid well and consume immediately. Rinse glass with water to ensure receiving full dose. Tablets may also be crushed and mixed with pudding.

Stability

Storage Store at room temperature of 15°C to 30°C (59°F to 86°F). Oral powder (or dissolved tablets) diluted in nonacidic liquid is stable for 6 hours under refrigeration.

Monitoring and Teaching Issues

Laboratory Monitoring Liver function tests, blood glucose levels, CBC with differential, CD4 cell count, plasma levels of HIV RNA

Physical Assessment Assess CD4 count, hepatic function, CBC, and serum glucose at regular intervals during therapy. Caution patients to monitor glucose levels closely; may cause hyperglycemia or new-onset diabetes. Teach patient proper timing of multiple medications.

Patient Education This is not a cure for HIV, nor has it been found to reduce transmission of HIV; use appropriate precautions to prevent spread to other people. Take with food. Mix powder with water, formula, or dairy products. Maintain adequate hydration unless instructed to restrict fluid intake. This medication will be prescribed with a combination of other medications; time these medications as directed by prescriber. You may be advised to check your glucose levels; this drug can cause hyperglycemia. Frequent blood tests may be required. May cause body changes due to redistribution of body fat, facial atrophy, or breast enlargement (normal effects of drug); diarrhea; or nausea.

Dietary Considerations Should be taken as scheduled with a meal. Some products may contain phenylalanine.

Breast-Feeding Considerations In infants born to mothers who are HIV positive, HAART while breast-feeding may decrease postnatal infection. However, maternal or infant antiretroviral therapy does not completely eliminate the risk of postnatal HIV transmission. In addition, multiclass-resistant virus has been detected in breast-feeding infants despite maternal therapy.

In the United States where formula is accessible, affordable, safe, and sustainable, complete avoidance of breast-feeding by HIV-infected women is recommended to decrease potential transmission of HIV.

Pregnancy Considerations Adverse events were not observed in animal studies and no increased risk of overall birth defects has been observed following 1st trimester exposure in humans according to data collected by the antiretroviral pregnancy registry. Nelfinavir crosses the placenta. The Perinatal HIV Guidelines Working Group recommends nelfinavir as an alternative PI in combination regimens during pregnancy with HAART for perinatal prophylaxis. A dose of 1250 mg twice daily has been shown to provide adequate plasma concentrations although lower and variable levels may occur late in pregnancy. Pregnancy and protease inhibitors are both associated with an increased risk of hyperglycemia. Glucose levels should be closely monitored. Healthcare providers are encouraged to enroll pregnant women exposed to antiretroviral medications in the Antiretroviral Pregnancy Registry (1-800-258-4263 or www.APRegistry.com). Healthcare providers caring for HIV-infected women and their infants may contact the National Perinatal HIV Hotline (888-448-8765) for clinical consultation.

Additional Information Nelfinavir (alone or in combination) is not recommended as initial therapy in the treatment of HIV infection due to inferior virologic efficacy and a high incidence of diarrhea (DHHS, 2011).

- **Neofrin** *see* Phenylephrine (Ophthalmic) *on page 1452*
- **NeoProfen®** *see* Ibuprofen *on page 938*
- **Neoral®** *see* CycloSPORINE (Systemic) *on page 437*
- **Neosar** *see* Cyclophosphamide *on page 434*
- **Neosporin® AF [OTC]** *see* Miconazole (Topical) *on page 1224*
- **NeoStrata® HQ Skin Lightening [OTC]** *see* Hydroquinone *on page 927*
- **Neo-Synephrine® Extra Strength [OTC]** *see* Phenylephrine (Nasal) *on page 1451*
- **Neo-Synephrine® Mild Formula [OTC]** *see* Phenylephrine (Nasal) *on page 1451*
- **Neo-Synephrine® Regular Strength [OTC]** *see* Phenylephrine (Nasal) *on page 1451*

Nepafenac (ne pa FEN ak)

U.S. Brand Names Nevanac™

Generic Availability (U.S.) No

Pharmacologic Category Nonsteroidal Anti-inflammatory Drug (NSAID), Ophthalmic

Pregnancy Risk Factor C/D (3rd trimester)

Lactation Excretion in breast milk unknown/use caution

Use Treatment of pain and inflammation associated with cataract surgery

Available Dosage Forms

Suspension, ophthalmic:

Nevanac™: 0.1% (3 mL)

Dosing

Adult & Geriatric Pain, inflammation associated with cataract surgery: Ophthalmic: Instill 1 drop into affected eye(s) 3 times/day, beginning 1 day prior to surgery, the day of surgery, and through the first 2 weeks of the postoperative period

Pediatric Pain, inflammation associated with cataract surgery: Ophthalmic: Children ≥10 years: Refer to adult dosing.

Administration

Other

Ophthalmic: Shake well prior to use.

Monitoring and Teaching Issues

Patient Education Wash hands before instilling. Sit or lie down to instill. Open eye, look at the ceiling, and instill prescribed amount. Close eye and roll eye in all directions. Apply gentle pressure to inner corner of eye for 1-2 minutes after instillation. Do not wear soft contract lenses while using this medication.

Nesiritide (ni SIR i tide)

U.S. Brand Names Natrecor®

Index Terms B-type Natriuretic Peptide (Human); hBNP; Natriuretic Peptide

Generic Availability (U.S.) No

Pharmacologic Category Natriuretic Peptide, B-Type, Human; Vasodilator

Medication Safety Issues

High alert medication: The Institute for Safe Medication Practices (ISMP) includes this medication among its list of drugs which have a heightened risk of causing significant patient harm when used in error.

International issues:

Natrecor® may be confused with Nitrocor® which is a brand name for nitroglycerin in Chile and Italy

Pregnancy Risk Factor C

Lactation Excretion in breast milk unknown/use caution

Use Treatment of acutely decompensated heart failure (HF) with dyspnea at rest or with minimal activity

Mechanism of Action/Effect Binds to cell surface receptors in vasculature, resulting in smooth muscle cell relaxation. Has been shown to produce dose-dependent reductions in pulmonary capillary wedge pressure (PCWP) and systemic arterial pressure providing symptomatic improvements (dyspnea decreased) for several days.

Contraindications Hypersensitivity to natriuretic peptide or any component of the formulation; cardiogenic shock (when used as primary therapy); hypotension (systolic blood pressure <90 mm Hg)

Warnings/Precautions May cause hypotension; administer in clinical situations when blood pressure may be closely monitored. Use caution in patients systolic blood pressure <100 mm Hg (contraindicated if <90 mm Hg); more likely to experience hypotension. Effects may be additive with other agents capable of causing hypotension. Hypotensive effects may last for several hours.

Should not be used in patients with low cardiac filling pressures, or in patients with conditions which depend on venous return including significant valvular stenosis, restrictive or obstructive cardiomyopathy, constrictive pericarditis, and pericardial tamponade. May be associated with development of azotemia; use caution in patients with renal impairment or in patients where renal perfusion is dependent on renin-angiotensin-aldosterone system; avoid initiation at doses higher than recommended.

Monitor for allergic or anaphylactic reactions. Use caution with prolonged infusions; limited experience with infusions >48 hours.

Drug Interactions

Avoid Concomitant Use There are no known interactions where it is recommended to avoid concomitant use.

Decreased Effect There are no known significant interactions involving a decrease in effect.

Increased Effect/Toxicity

Nesiritide may increase the levels/effects of: Hypotensive Agents

Nutritional/Ethanol Interactions Herb/Nutraceutical: Avoid bayberry, blue cohosh, cayenne, ephedra, ginger, ginseng (American), kola, and licorice (may increase blood pressure). Avoid black cohosh, California poppy, coleus, golden seal, hawthorn, mistletoe, periwinkle, quinine, and shepherd's purse (may enhance decreased blood pressure).

Adverse Reactions Note: Frequencies cited below were recorded in VMAC trial at dosages similar to approved labeling. Higher frequencies have been observed in trials using higher dosages of nesiritide. The percentages marked with an asterisk (*) indicate frequency less than or equal to placebo or other standard therapy.

>10%:

Cardiovascular: Hypotension (total: 11%; symptomatic: 4% at recommended dose, up to 17% at higher doses)

Renal: Increased serum creatinine (28% with >0.5 mg/dL increase over baseline)

1% to 10%:

Cardiovascular: Ventricular tachycardia (3%)*, ventricular extrasystoles (3%)*, angina (2%)*, bradycardia (1%), tachycardia, atrial fibrillation, AV node conduction abnormalities

Central nervous system: Headache (8%)*, dizziness (3%), insomnia (2%)*, anxiety (3%), confusion, fever, paresthesia, somnolence, tremor

Dermatologic: Pruritus, rash

Gastrointestinal: Nausea (4%)*, abdominal pain (1%)*, vomiting (1%)*

Hematologic: Anemia

Local: Injection site reaction, catheter pain

Neuromuscular & skeletal: Back pain (4%), leg cramps

Ocular: Amblyopia

Respiratory: Apnea, cough increased, hemoptysis

Miscellaneous: Diaphoresis

Postmarketing and/or case reports: Hypersensitivity reactions (rare)

Pharmacodynamics/Kinetics

Onset of Action 15 minutes (60% of 3-hour effect achieved)

Duration of Action >60 minutes (up to several hours) for systolic blood pressure; hemodynamic effects persist longer than serum half-life would predict

Time to Peak 1 hour

Half-Life Elimination Initial (distribution) 2 minutes; Terminal: 18 minutes

Metabolism Proteolytic cleavage by vascular endopeptidases and proteolysis following binding to the membrane bound natriuretic peptide (NPR-C) and cellular internalization

Excretion Primarily eliminated by metabolism; also excreted in the urine

Available Dosage Forms

Injection, powder for reconstitution:

Natrecor®: 1.5 mg

Dosing

Adult & Geriatric

Acute decompensated heart failure: I.V.: Initial: 2 mcg/kg (bolus); followed by continuous infusion at 0.01 mcg/kg/minute. **Note:** Should not be initiated at a dosage higher than initial recommended dose. There is limited experience with increasing the dose >0.01 mcg/kg/minute; in one trial, a limited number of patients received higher doses that were increased no faster than every 3 hours by 0.005 mcg/kg/minute (preceded by a bolus of 1 mcg/kg), up to a maximum of 0.03 mcg/kg/minute. Increases beyond the initial infusion rate should be limited to selected patients and accompanied by close hemodynamic and renal function monitoring.

Patients experiencing hypotension during the infusion: Infusion dose should be reduced or discontinued. Other measures to support blood pressure should be initiated (eg, I.V. fluids, Trendelenburg position). May attempt to restart at a lower dose (reduce previous infusion dose by 30% and omit bolus).

Renal Impairment No adjustment required but use cautiously in patients with renal impairment or those patients who rely on the renin-angiotensin-aldosterone system for renal perfusion. Monitor renal function closely.

Hepatic Impairment No dosage adjustment recommended.

Administration

I.V. Do not administer through a heparin-coated catheter (concurrent administration of heparin via a separate catheter is acceptable, per manufacturer).

Stability

Reconstitution Reconstitute 1.5 mg vial with 5 mL of diluent removed from a preprefilled 250 mL plastic I.V. bag (compatible with D_5W, $D_5{}^1/_2NS$, $D_5{}^1/_4NS$, NS). Do not shake vial to dissolve (roll gently). Withdraw entire contents of vial and add to 250 mL I.V. bag. Invert several times to mix. Resultant concentration of solution is ~6 mcg/mL.

Storage Vials may be stored below 25°C (77°F); do not freeze. Protect from light. Following reconstitution, vials are stable at 2°C to 25°C (36°F to 77°F) for up to 24 hours. Use reconstituted solution within 24 hours.

Monitoring and Teaching Issues

Physical Assessment Blood pressure and cardiac function should be monitored before, at frequent intervals during, and for 24 hours following infusion (hemodynamic monitoring with larger doses). Assess renal function and monitor for hypersensitivity and hypotension on a regular basis throughout therapy.

Patient Education This medication can only be administered by infusion; you will be monitored closely during and following infusion. Report immediately any pain, burning, swelling at infusion site, or any signs of allergic reaction (eg, respiratory or swallowing difficulty, back pain, chest tightness, rash, hives, swelling of lips or mouth). Remain in bed until advised otherwise; call for assistance with turning or changing position. Report any chest pain, respiratory difficulty, persistent dizziness, or swelling of extremities.

Geriatric Considerations No specific data to date; elderly are liable to have hypotension, see Warnings/Precautions for blood pressure criteria. Elderly with reduced renal function should be monitored closely.

Pregnancy Considerations Adverse events were not observed in an animal reproduction study. Nesiritide is a recombinant B-type natriuretic peptide (rhBNP). BNP and NT-proBNP (which has been used as a marker of BNP), are endogenous peptides and NT-proBNP is measurable in the umbilical cord serum of normal pregnancies. Information related to the administration of nesiritide during pregnancy has not been located.

Additional Information The duration of symptomatic improvement with nesiritide following discontinuation of the infusion has been limited (generally lasting several days). Atrial natriuretic peptide, which is related to nesiritide, has been associated with increased vascular permeability. This has not been observed in clinical trials with nesiritide, but patients should be monitored for this effect.

Related Information

Compatibility of Drugs *on page* *1994*
Heart Failure (Systolic) *on page* *2040*

- ◆ **NESP** *see* Darbepoetin Alfa *on page* *463*
- ◆ **Neupogen®** *see* Filgrastim *on page* *760*
- ◆ **Neurontin®** *see* Gabapentin *on page* *843*
- ◆ **Neut®** *see* Sodium Bicarbonate *on page* *1658*
- ◆ **Neutra-Phos** *see* Potassium Phosphate and Sodium Phosphate *on page* *1486*
- ◆ **Neutra-Phos®-K [OTC] [DSC]** *see* Potassium Phosphate *on page* *1484*
- ◆ **Nevanac™** *see* Nepafenac *on page* *1299*

Nevirapine (ne VYE ra peen)

U.S. Brand Names Viramune®; Viramune® XR™

Index Terms NVP; Viramune® XR™

Generic Availability (U.S.) No

Pharmacologic Category Antiretroviral Agent, Reverse Transcriptase Inhibitor (Non-nucleoside)

Medication Safety Issues

Sound-alike/look-alike issues:

Nevirapine may be confused with nelfinavir

Viramune®, Viramune® XR™ may be confused with Viracept®

Medication Guide Available Yes

Pregnancy Risk Factor B

Lactation Enters breast milk/contraindicated

Use In combination therapy with other antiretroviral agents for the treatment of HIV-1

Mechanism of Action/Effect Blocks the RNA-dependent DNA polymerase activity

Contraindications Moderate-to-severe hepatic impairment (Child-Pugh class B or C); use in occupational or nonoccupational postexposure prophylaxis (PEP) regimens

Warnings/Precautions [U.S. Boxed Warning]: Severe hepatotoxic reactions may occur (fulminant and cholestatic hepatitis, hepatic necrosis) and, in some cases, have resulted in hepatic failure and death. The greatest risk of these reactions is within the initial 6 weeks of treatment. Patients with a history of chronic hepatitis (B or C) or increased baseline transaminase levels may be at increased risk of hepatotoxic reactions. Female gender and patients with increased CD4$^+$-cell counts may be at substantially greater risk of hepatic events (often associated with rash). Therapy in antiretroviral naive patients should not be started with elevated CD4$^+$-cell counts unless the benefit of therapy outweighs the risk of serious hepatotoxicity (adult/postpubertal females: CD4$^+$-cell counts >250 cells/mm^3; adult males: CD4$^+$-cell counts >400 cells/mm^3). Use with caution in patients with pre-existing dysfunction; monitor closely for drug-induced hepatotoxicity; contraindicated in patients with moderate-to-severe impairment (Child-Pugh class B or C).

[U.S. Boxed Warning]: Severe life-threatening skin reactions (eg, Stevens-Johnson syndrome, toxic epidermal necrolysis, hypersensitivity reactions with rash and organ dysfunction), including fatal cases, have occurred. The greatest risk of these reactions is within the initial 6 weeks of treatment; intensive monitoring is required during the initial 18 weeks of therapy to detect potentially life-threatening dermatologic, hypersensitivity, and hepatic reactions. Risk is greatest in African-Americans, Asian, or Hispanic race/ethnicity or in females. A 14-day lead-in dosing period with immediate release formulation must be initiated to decrease the incidence of adverse effects. The lead-in dosing can be extended up to 28 days if necessary, but an alternative regimen is necessary if >28 days is required. If a severe dermatologic or hypersensitivity reaction occurs, or if signs and symptoms of hepatitis occur, nevirapine should be permanently discontinued. These events may include a severe rash, or a rash associated with fever, blisters, oral lesions, conjunctivitis, facial edema, muscle or joint aches, transaminase elevations, general malaise, hepatitis, eosinophilia, granulocytopenia, lymphadenopathy, or renal dysfunction. Coadministration of prednisone during the first 6 weeks of therapy increases incidence and severity of rash; concomitant prednisone is not recommended to prevent rash.

May cause redistribution of fat (eg, buffalo hump, peripheral wasting with increased abdominal girth, cushingoid appearance). Patients may develop immune reconstitution syndrome resulting in the occurrence of an inflammatory response to an indolent or residual opportunistic infection; further evaluation and treatment may be required. Rhabdomyolysis has been observed in conjunction with skin and/or hepatic adverse events during postmarketing surveillance. Termination of therapy is warranted with evidence of severe skin or liver toxicity.

Use with caution in patients taking strong CYP3A4 inhibitors, moderate or strong CYP3A4 inducers and major CYP3A4 substrates (see Drug Interactions); consider alternative agents that avoid or lessen the potential for CYP-mediated interactions. Concurrent use of St John's wort or efavirenz is not recommended; may decrease the therapeutic efficacy (St John's wort) or increase adverse effects (efavirenz).

Nevirapine-based initial regimens should not be used in children <3 years of age if previously exposed to nevirapine during prevention of maternal-to-child transmission of HIV due to increased risk of resistance and treatment failure. Protease inhibitor-based initial regimens preferred in this population.

Due to rapid emergence of resistance, nevirapine should not be used as monotherapy or the only agent added to a failing regimen for the treatment of HIV. Consider alteration of antiretroviral therapies if disease progression occurs while patients are receiving nevirapine. Use care when timing discontinuation of regimens containing nevirapine; levels are sustained after levels of other medications decrease, leading to nevirapine resistance. Cross-resistance may be conferred to other non-nucleoside reverse transcriptase inhibitors (DHHS, 2011).

Drug Interactions

Metabolism/Transport Effects Substrate of CYP2B6 (minor), 2D6 (minor), 3A4 (major); **Inhibits** CYP1A2 (weak), 2D6 (weak), 3A4 (weak); **Induces** CYP2B6 (strong), 3A4 (strong)

Avoid Concomitant Use

Avoid concomitant use of Nevirapine with any of the following: Atazanavir; Dienogest; Dronedarone; Efavirenz; Etravirine; Everolimus; Lurasidone; Nilotinib; Nisoldipine; Pazopanib; Praziquantel; Ranolazine; Roflumilast; RomiDEPsin; St Johns Wort; Tolvaptan; Vandetanib

Decreased Effect

Nevirapine may decrease the levels/effects of: Atazanavir; Caspofungin; CYP2B6 Substrates; CYP3A4 Substrates; Dienogest; Dronedarone; Efavirenz; Etravirine; Everolimus; Exemestane; Fosamprenavir; Gefitinib; GuanFACINE; Imatinib; Indinavir; Ixabepilone; Lopinavir; Lurasidone; Maraviroc; Methadone; Nelfinavir; NIFEdipine; Nilotinib; Nisoldipine; Pazopanib; Praziquantel; Ranolazine; Rifabutin; Roflumilast; RomiDEPsin; Saquinavir; Saxagliptin; SORAfenib; Tadalafil; Tolvaptan; Ulipristal; Vandetanib; Voriconazole

The levels/effects of Nevirapine may be decreased by: CYP3A4 Inducers (Strong); Deferasirox; Peginterferon Alfa-2b; Rifabutin; Rifampin; St Johns Wort

Increased Effect/Toxicity

Nevirapine may increase the levels/effects of: Efavirenz; Etravirine; PACLitaxel; Rifabutin

The levels/effects of Nevirapine may be increased by: Atazanavir; Conivaptan; Efavirenz; Voriconazole

Nutritional/Ethanol Interactions Herb/Nutraceutical: Nevirapine serum concentration may be decreased by St John's wort; avoid concurrent use.

Adverse Reactions Note: Potentially life-threatening nevirapine-associated adverse effects may present with the following symptoms: Abrupt onset of flu-like symptoms, abdominal pain, jaundice, or fever with or without rash; may progress to hepatic failure with encephalopathy. Skin rash is present in ~50% of cases.

Percentages of adverse effects vary by clinical trial and may vary by formulation; incidences reported below are based on immediate release formulation:

>10%:

Dermatologic: Rash (grade 1/2: 13%; grade 3/4: 2%)

Hepatic: ALT >250 units/L (5% to 14%); symptomatic hepatic events (4%, range: up to 11%)

1% to 10%:

Central nervous system: Headache (1% to 4%), fatigue (≤5%)

Gastrointestinal: Nausea (<1% to 9%), abdominal pain (≤2%), diarrhea (≤2%)

Hematologic: Neutropenia (4%)

Hepatic: AST >250 units/L (4% to 8%)

Pharmacodynamics/Kinetics

Absorption >90%

Bioavailability 93% (immediate release tablet); ~75% (extended release tablet [relative to immediate release]); 91% (oral solution)

Time to Peak Serum: Immediate release: 4 hours; Extended release:~24 hours

Protein Binding Plasma: ~60%

Half-Life Elimination Decreases over 2- to 4-week time with chronic dosing due to autoinduction (ie, half-life = 45 hours initially and decreases to 25-30 hours)

Metabolism Extensively hepatic via CYP3A4 and CYP2B6 (hydroxylation to inactive compounds); may undergo enterohepatic recycling

Excretion Urine (~81%, primarily as metabolites, <3% as unchanged drug); feces (~10%)

Available Dosage Forms

Suspension, oral:

Viramune®: 50 mg/5 mL (240 mL)

Tablet, oral:

Viramune®: 200 mg

Tablet, extended release, oral:

Viramune® XR™: 400 mg

Dosing

Adult & Geriatric

HIV infection: Oral:

Note: Therapy in antiretroviral naive patients should not be initiated in patients with elevated CD4$^+$-cell counts unless the benefit of therapy outweighs the risk of serious hepatotoxicity (adult/postpubertal females: CD4$^+$-cell counts >250 cells/mm^3; adult males: CD4$^+$-cell counts >400 cells/mm^3).

Initial: Immediate release: 200 mg once daily for 14 days

Maintenance:

Immediate release: 200 mg twice daily (in combination with additional antiretroviral agents) if there is no rash or untoward effects during initial dosing period

Extended release: 400 mg once daily; maintenance therapy using the extended release must follow a 14-day initial dosing period (lead-in) using the immediate release formulation unless patient is already maintained on a nevirapine immediate release regimen

Note: If patient experiences a rash during the 14-day lead-in period, dose should not be increased until the rash has resolved. A lead-in period must always be done with immediate release formulation and regimen should not exceed 28 days; alternative treatment should be considered at that point. If a rash occurs within the first 18 weeks of therapy, immediately check serum transaminases. Discontinue if severe rash, rash with constitutional symptoms, or rash with elevated hepatic transaminases is noted. Coadministration of prednisone during the first 6 weeks of therapy increases incidence and severity of rash; concomitant prednisone is not recommended to prevent rash. Permanently discontinue if symptomatic hepatic events occur. If therapy with any formulation is interrupted for >7 days, restart with initial dose of immediate release formulation for 14 days.

Prevention of maternal-fetal HIV transmission (AIDS*info* perinatal guidelines; DHHS, 2011): Note: Nevirapine is used in combination with zidovudine (and possibly lamivudine) in select situations (eg, infants born to mothers with suboptimal viral suppression at delivery, infants born to mothers with only intrapartum therapy or no therapy, or infants born to mothers with known antiretroviral drug-resistant virus). Single-dose use in mother or neonate has not been associated with symptomatic hepatic events.

Mother: Immediate release: 200 mg as a single dose at onset of labor

Pediatric

HIV infection: Oral:

Note: If patient experiences a rash during the 14-day lead-in period, dose should not be increased until the rash has resolved. A lead-in period must always be done with immediate release formulation and regimen should not exceed 28 days; alternative treatment should be considered at that point. If a rash occurs within the first 18 weeks of therapy, immediately check serum transaminases. Discontinue if severe rash, rash with constitutional symptoms, or rash with elevated hepatic transaminases is noted. Coadministration of prednisone during the first 6 weeks of therapy increases incidence and severity of rash; concomitant prednisone is not recommended to prevent rash. Permanently discontinue if symptomatic hepatic events occur. If therapy with any formulation is interrupted for >7 days, restart with initial dose of immediate release formulation for 14 days.

Neonates ≥15 days, Infants, and Children:

Immediate release: 150 mg/m^2/dose once daily for first 14 days (maximum: 200 mg/day); increase dose to 150 mg/m^2/dose twice daily if no rash or untoward effects (maximum: 400 mg/day).

Extended release: Has not been evaluated in pediatric patients

AIDS*info* pediatric guidelines:

Note: Children <3 years of age: Nevirapine-based initial regimens should not be used in children previously exposed to nevirapine during prevention of maternal-to-child transmission of HIV

Neonates ≤14 days of age: Immediate release: Treatment dose not defined

Children <8 years: Immediate release: 200 mg/m^2/dose once daily for first 14 days (maximum dose: 200 mg); increase dose to 200 mg/m^2/dose twice daily if no rash or untoward effects (maximum: 400 mg/day)

Children ≥8 years: Immediate release: 120-150 mg/m^2/dose once daily for 14 days (maximum dose: 200 mg); increase dose to 120-150 mg/m^2/dose twice daily if no rash or untoward effects (maximum: 400 mg/day)

Adolescents: Immediate release: Refer to adult dosing.

Prevention of maternal-fetal HIV transmission (AIDS*info* perinatal guidelines; DHHS, 2011): Note: Nevirapine is used in combination with zidovudine (and possibly lamivudine) in select situations (eg, infants born to mothers with suboptimal viral suppression at delivery, infants born to mothers with only intrapartum therapy or no therapy, or infants born to mothers with known antiretroviral drug-resistant virus). Single-dose use in mother or neonate has not been associated with symptomatic hepatic events.

Neonate: Immediate release: 2 mg/kg as a single dose between birth and 72 hours if mother received intrapartum dose of nevirapine. If maternal dose was given ≤2 hours prior to delivery or not received, administer infant dose as soon as possible following birth (some experts consider giving a second dose at 48-72 hours of life).

Renal Impairment

Cl_{cr} ≥20 mL/minute: No adjustment required

Hemodialysis: Immediate release: An additional 200 mg dose is recommended following dialysis.

Hepatic Impairment Use is contraindicated with moderate-to-severe hepatic impairment (Child-Pugh Class B or C). Permanently discontinue if symptomatic hepatic events occur.

Administration

Oral May be administered with or without food. May be administered with an antacid or didanosine. Shake suspension gently prior to administration; the use of an oral dosing syringe is recommended, especially if the dose is ≤5 mL; if using a dosing cup, after administration, rinse cup with water and also administer rinse. Extended release tablets must be swallowed whole and not crushed, chewed, or divided.

Stability

Storage Store at 25°C (77°F); excursion permitted to 15°C to 30°C (59°F to 86°F).

Monitoring and Teaching Issues

Laboratory Monitoring Monitor CBC and viral load. Baseline liver function tests should be obtained prior to nevirapine's initiation. DHHS adult guidelines recommend serum transaminase monitoring every 2 weeks for the first 4 weeks of therapy, then monthly for the first 18 weeks, then frequently thereafter.. Patients receiving maintenance immediate release nevirapine who change to the extended release formulation should adhere to their regular monitoring schedule. AIDS*info* adult guidelines recommend serum transaminase monitoring every 2 weeks for the first 4 weeks of therapy, then monthly for 3 months, followed by every 3-4 months. AIDS*info* pediatric guidelines recommend serum transaminase monitoring every 2 weeks for the first 4 weeks of therapy, followed by every 4 months. Assess/evaluate AST/ALT immediately in any patients with a rash. Permanently discontinue if patient experiences severe rash, constitutional symptoms associated with rash, rash with elevated AST/ALT, or clinical hepatitis, Mild-to-moderate rash without AST/ALT elevation may continue treatment per discretion of prescriber. If mild-to-moderate urticarial rash, do not restart if treatment is interrupted.

Physical Assessment Use caution in presence of or history of hepatic disease. Patient response should be followed closely during 14-day lead-in dosing period to assess for hypersensitivity prior to increasing daily dose. Assess LFTs at baseline and frequently during therapy. Monitor patient regularly and frequently during initial 18 weeks of therapy to identify any symptoms of hypersensitivity (hepatic and or dermatologic reactions which may include severe rash, rash with fever, blisters, oral lesions, conjunctivitis, facial edema, muscle or joint aches, general malaise, jaundice, hepatitis, or renal dysfunction).

Patient Education You will be provided with an FDA-approved medication guide with your prescription; read this guide carefully. This is not a cure for HIV, nor has it been found to reduce transmission of HIV; use appropriate precautions to prevent spread to other persons. Shake suspension gently prior to use. Frequent blood tests may be required. If rash, blisters, or facial edema develops, stop medicine and contact prescriber immediately. Report any change in urinary pattern, dark urine or light stool, easy bleeding, unusual fatigue, flu-like symptoms, or abdominal pain.

Breast-Feeding Considerations In infants born to mothers who are HIV positive, HAART while breast-feeding may decrease postnatal infection. Infant prophylaxis with zidovudine in combination with nevirapine or nevirapine alone may also decrease the risk of HIV transmission to the infant. However, maternal or infant antiretroviral therapy does not completely eliminate the risk of postnatal HIV transmission. In addition, multiclass resistant virus has been detected in breast-feeding infants despite maternal therapy.

In the United States where formula is accessible, affordable, safe, and sustainable, complete avoidance of breast-feeding by HIV-infected women is recommended to decrease potential transmission of HIV.

Pregnancy Considerations Teratogenic effects were not observed in animal reproduction studies. Nevirapine crosses the placenta. No increased risk of overall birth defects has been observed following first trimester exposure according to data collected by the antiretroviral pregnancy registry. Pharmacokinetics are not altered during pregnancy and dose adjustment is not needed. The Perinatal HIV Guidelines Working Group recommends nevirapine as the NNRTI for use during pregnancy. Nevirapine may be initiated in pregnant women with a $CD4^+$ lymphocyte count <250/mm^3 or continued in women who are virologically suppressed and tolerating therapy once pregnancy is detected (regardless of $CD4^+$ lymphocyte count); however, do not initiate therapy in pregnant women with a $CD4^+$ lymphocyte count >250/mm^3 unless the benefit of therapy clearly outweighs the risk. Monitor for liver toxicity during first 18 weeks of therapy. In selected circumstances, nevirapine may also be used in HIV-infected women (regardless of $CD4^+$ lymphocyte count) who are in labor, but have had no prior antiretroviral therapy, in order to reduce the maternal-fetal transmission of HIV; intrapartum and postpartum zidovudine and lamivudine are also used to reduce nevirapine resistance.

Healthcare providers are encouraged to enroll pregnant women exposed to antiretroviral medications in the Antiretroviral Pregnancy Registry (1-800-258-4263 or www.APRegistry.com). Healthcare providers caring for HIV-infected women and their infants may contact the National Perinatal HIV Hotline (888-448-8765) for clinical consultation.

Additional Information Patients should never be taking more than one form (ie, immediate release or extended release) of nevirapine concomitantly. Potential compliance problems, frequency of administration, and adverse effects should be discussed with patients before initiating therapy to help prevent the emergence of resistance. Early virologic failure was observed with tenofovir and didanosine delayed release capsules, plus either efavirenz or nevirapine; use caution in treatment-naive patients with high baseline viral loads. Due to rapid emergence of resistance, nevirapine should not be used as monotherapy or as the only agent added to a failing regimen for the treatment of HIV. Use care when timing discontinuation of regimens containing nevirapine; levels of nevirapine are sustained after levels of other medications decrease, potentially leading to nevirapine resistance. Cross-resistance may be conferred to other non-nucleoside reverse transcriptase inhibitors.

- **NexAVAR®** *see* Sorafenib *on page* 1670
- **Nexiclon™ XR** *see* CloNIDine *on page* 408
- **NexIUM®** *see* Esomeprazole *on page* 667
- **NexIUM® I.V.** *see* Esomeprazole *on page* 667
- **Next Choice™** *see* Levonorgestrel *on page* 1097
- **Nexterone®** *see* Amiodarone *on page* 98
- **NFV** *see* Nelfinavir *on page* 1296

Niacin (NYE a sin)

U.S. Brand Names Niacin-Time® [OTC]; Niacor®; Niaspan®; Slo-Niacin® [OTC]

Index Terms Nicotinic Acid; Vitamin B_3

Generic Availability (U.S.) Yes

Pharmacologic Category Antilipemic Agent, Miscellaneous; Vitamin, Water Soluble

Medication Safety Issues

Sound-alike/look-alike issues:

Niacin may be confused with Minocin®, Niaspan®, Nispan®

Niaspan® may be confused with niacin

Nicobid® may be confused with Nitro-Bid®

Pregnancy Risk Factor A/C (dose exceeding RDA recommendation)

Lactation Enters breast milk/consider risk:benefit

Use Treatment of dyslipidemias (Fredrickson types IIa and IIb or primary hypercholesterolemia) as mono- or adjunctive therapy; to lower the risk of recurrent MI in patients with a history of MI and hyperlipidemia; to slow progression or promote regression of coronary artery disease; treatment of hypertriglyceridemia in patients at risk of pancreatitis

Unlabeled/Investigational Use Treatment of pellagra; dietary supplement

Mechanism of Action/Effect Component of two coenzymes which is necessary for tissue respiration, lipid metabolism, and glycogenolysis; inhibits the synthesis of very low density lipoproteins (VLDL) and low density lipoproteins (LDL); may also increase the rate of chylomicron triglyceride removal from plasma.

Contraindications Hypersensitivity to niacin, niacinamide, or any component of the formulation; active hepatic disease or significant or unexplained persistent elevations in hepatic transaminases; active peptic ulcer; arterial hemorrhage

Warnings/Precautions Use with caution in patients with unstable angina or MI, diabetes (may interfere with glucose control), renal disease, active gallbladder disease (can exacerbate), gout, or with anticoagulants (may slightly increase prothrombin time). Use with caution in patients with a past history of hepatic impairment and/or who consume substantial amounts of ethanol; contraindicated with active liver disease or unexplained persistent transaminase elevation. Rare cases of rhabdomyolysis have occurred during concomitant use with HMG-CoA reductase inhibitors. With concurrent use or if symptoms suggestive of myopathy occur, monitor creatine phosphokinase (CPK) and potassium; use with caution in patients with renal impairment, inadequately treated hypothyroidism, patients with diabetes or the elderly; risk for myopathy and rhabdomyolysis may be increased.

Immediate and extended or sustained release products are not interchangeable. Cases of severe hepatotoxicity have occurred when immediate release (crystalline) niacin products have been substituted with sustained-release (modified release, timed-release) niacin products at equivalent doses. Patients should be initiated with low doses (eg, 500 mg at bedtime) with titration to achieve desired response. Flushing and pruritus, common adverse effects of niacin, may be attenuated with a gradual increase in dose, and/or by taking aspirin (adults: 325 mg) or an NSAID 30-60 minutes before dosing. Compliance is enhanced with twice-daily dosing (extended-release product excluded). Prior to initiation, secondary causes for hypercholesterolemia (eg, poorly controlled diabetes mellitus, hypothyroidism) should be excluded; management with diet and other nonpharmacologic measures (eg, exercise or weight reduction) should be attempted prior to initiation. Use has not been evaluated in Fredrickson type I or III dyslipidemias.

Drug Interactions

Avoid Concomitant Use There are no known interactions where it is recommended to avoid concomitant use.

Decreased Effect

The levels/effects of Niacin may be decreased by: Bile Acid Sequestrants

Increased Effect/Toxicity

Niacin may increase the levels/effects of: HMG-CoA Reductase Inhibitors

Nutritional/Ethanol Interactions Ethanol: Avoid heavy use; avoid use around niacin dose.

Lab Interactions False elevations in some fluorometric determinations of plasma or urinary catecholamines; false-positive urine glucose (Benedict's reagent)

Adverse Reactions Frequency not defined.

Cardiovascular: Arrhythmias, atrial fibrillation, edema, flushing, hypotension, orthostasis, palpitation, syncope (rare), tachycardia

Central nervous system: Chills, dizziness, headache, insomnia, migraine, nervousness, pain

Dermatologic: Acanthosis nigricans, burning skin, dry skin, hyperpigmentation, maculopapular rash, pruritus, rash, skin discoloration, urticaria

Endocrine & metabolic: Glucose tolerance decreased, gout, phosphorous levels decreased, hyperuricemia

Gastrointestinal: Abdominal pain, amylase increased, diarrhea, dyspepsia, eructation, flatulence, nausea, peptic ulcers, vomiting

Hematologic: Platelet counts decreased

Hepatic: Hepatic necrosis (rare), hepatitis, jaundice, transaminases increased (dose-related), prothrombin time increased, total bilirubin increased

Neuromuscular & skeletal: CPK increased, leg cramps, myalgia, myasthenia, myopathy (with concurrent HMG-CoA reductase inhibitor), paresthesia, rhabdomyolysis (with concurrent HMG-CoA reductase inhibitor; rare), weakness

Ocular: Blurred vision, cystoid macular edema, toxic amblyopia

Respiratory: Cough, dyspnea

Miscellaneous: Diaphoresis, hypersensitivity reactions (rare; includes anaphylaxis, angioedema, laryngismus, vesiculobullous rash), LDH increased

Pharmacodynamics/Kinetics

Absorption Rapid and extensive (60% to 755)

Time to Peak Serum: Immediate release formulation: 30-60 minutes; extended release formulation: 4-5 hours

Half-Life Elimination 25-45 minutes

Metabolism Extensive first-pass effects; converted to nicotinamide adenine dinucleotide, nicotinuric acid, and other metabolites

Excretion Urine 60% to 88% (unchanged drug [up to 12% recovered after multiple dosing] and metabolites)

Available Dosage Forms

Caplet, timed release, oral: 500 mg

Capsule, oral: 50 mg, 250 mg

Capsule, extended release, oral: 250 mg, 500 mg

Capsule, timed release, oral: 250 mg, 400 mg, 500 mg

Tablet, oral: 50 mg, 100 mg, 250 mg, 500 mg

Niacor®: 500 mg

Tablet, controlled release, oral:

Slo-Niacin® [OTC]: 250 mg, 500 mg, 750 mg

Tablet, extended release, oral:

Niaspan®: 500 mg, 750 mg, 1000 mg

Tablet, timed release, oral: 250 mg, 500 mg, 750 mg, 1000 mg

Niacin-Time® [OTC]: 500 mg

Dosing

Adult & Geriatric Note: Formulations of niacin (regular release versus extended release) are not interchangeable.

Recommended daily allowances (National Academy of Sciences, 1998): Oral:

≥19 years: Female: 14 mg/day; Male: 16 mg/day

Pregnancy (all ages): 18 mg/day

Lactation (all ages): 17 mg/day

Dietary supplement (OTC labeling): Oral: 50 mg twice daily or 100 mg once daily. **Note:** Many over-the-counter formulations exist.

Hyperlipidemia: Oral:

Regular release formulation (Niacor®): Initial: 250 mg once daily (with evening meal); increase frequency and/or dose every 4-7 days to desired response or first-level therapeutic dose (1.5-2 g/day in 2-3 divided doses); after 2 months, may increase at 2- to 4-week intervals to 3 g/day in 3 divided doses (maximum dose: 6 g/day [NCEP recommends 4.5 g/day] in 3 divided doses). Usual daily dose after titration (NCEP, 2002): 1.5-3 g/day. **Note:** Many over-the-counter formulations exist.

Sustained release (or controlled release) formulations: **Note:** Several over-the-counter formulations exist. Usual daily dose after titration (NCEP, 2002): 1-2 g/day

Extended release formulation (Niaspan®): Initial: 500 mg at bedtime for 4 weeks, then 1 g at bedtime for 4 weeks; adjust dose to response and tolerance; may increase dose every 4 weeks by 500 mg/day to a maximum of 2 g/day. Usual daily dose after titration (NCEP, 2002): 1-2 g once daily

If additional LDL-lowering is necessary with lovastatin or simvastatin: Recommended initial lovastatin or simvastatin dose: 20 mg/day (maximum lovastatin or simvastatin dose: 40 mg/day); **Note:** Lovastatin prescribing information recommends a maximum dose of 20 mg/day with concurrent use of niacin (>1 g/day).

Pellagra (unlabeled use): Oral: 50-100 mg 3-4 times/day; maximum: 500 mg/day (some experts prefer niacinamide for treatment due to more favorable side effect profile)

Pediatric Note: Formulations of niacin (regular release versus extended release) are not interchangeable.

Adequate intake (National Academy of Sciences, 1998): Oral:

0-5 months: 2 mg/day
6-11 months: 3 mg/day

Recommended daily allowances (National Academy of Sciences, 1998): Oral:

1-3 years: 6 mg/day
4-8 years: 8 mg/day
9-13 years: 12 mg/day
14-18 years: Female: 14 mg/day; Male: 16 mg/day
≥19 years: Refer to adult dosing.

Pellagra (unlabeled use) Oral: 50-100 mg/dose 3 times/day (some experts prefer niacinamide for treatment due to more favorable side effect profile)

Renal Impairment No dosage adjustment recommended; use with caution.

Hepatic Impairment Contraindicated in patients with significant or unexplained hepatic dysfunction, active liver disease or unexplained persistent transaminase elevations.

Adjustment for Toxicity Hepatic toxicity: Transaminases rise ≥3 times ULN, either persistent or if symptoms of nausea, fever, and/or malaise occur: Discontinue therapy.

Administration

Oral Administer with food.

Niaspan®: Administer at bedtime. Tablet strengths are not interchangeable. When switching from immediate release tablet, initiate Niaspan® at lower dose and titrate. If therapy is interrupted for an extended period, dose should be retitrated. Long-acting forms should not be crushed, broken, or chewed. Do not substitute long-acting forms for immediate release ones.

Stability

Storage

Niaspan®: Store at room temperature of 20°C to 25°C (68°F to 77°F).

Niacor®: Store at controlled room temperature of 15°C to 30°C (59°F to 86°F).

Monitoring and Teaching Issues

Laboratory Monitoring Blood glucose (in diabetic patients); CPK and serum potassium (if on concurrent HMG-CoA reductase inhibitor); liver function tests pretreatment, every 6-12 weeks for first year, then periodically (approximately every 6 months), monitor liver function more frequently if history of transaminase elevation with prior use; lipid profile; platelets; PT (if on anticoagulants); uric acid (if predisposed to gout); phosphorus (if predisposed to hypophosphatemia)

Patient Education Take with food to reduce incidence of GI upset. Do not crush sustained release capsules. You may experience flushing, sensation of heat, or headache; these reactions may be decreased by increasing dose slowly or by taking aspirin 30-60 minutes prior to taking niacin. Avoid alcohol to minimize flushing. Taking at bedtime, after a low-fat snack, is also recommended. You may experience dizziness or lightheadedness. Report persistent GI disturbance or changes in color of urine or stool.

Dietary Considerations Should be taken with meal; low-fat meal if treating hyperlipidemia. Avoid hot drinks around the time of niacin dose.

Geriatric Considerations The definition of and, therefore, when to treat hyperlipidemia in the elderly is a controversial issue. The National Cholesterol Education Program recommends that all adults maintain a plasma cholesterol <160 mg/dL. Elderly with one additional risk factor, goal LDL would be <130 mg/dL. It is the authors' belief that pharmacologic treatment be reserved for those who are unable to obtain a desirable plasma cholesterol concentration by diet alone and for whom the benefits of treatment are believed to outweigh the potential adverse effects, drug interactions, and cost of treatment.

Breast-Feeding Considerations Niacin is excreted in human breast milk. Because lipid-lowering doses of niacin may cause serious adverse reactions in nursing infants, a decision should be made whether to discontinue nursing or discontinue the drug, taking into account the importance of the drug to the mother.

Pregnancy Considerations Animal reproduction studies have not been conducted. It is unknown whether or not niacin at lipid-lowering doses is harmful to the developing fetus. If a woman becomes pregnant while receiving niacin for primary hypercholesterolemia, niacin should be discontinued. If a woman becomes pregnant while receiving niacin for hypertriglyceridemia, the benefits and risks of continuing niacin should be assessed on an individual basis.

Related Information

Hyperlipidemia Management *on page* 2046

Niacin and Simvastatin (NYE a sin & sim va STAT in)

U.S. Brand Names Simcor®

Index Terms Simvastatin and Niacin

Generic Availability (U.S.) No

Pharmacologic Category Antilipemic Agent, HMG-CoA Reductase Inhibitor; Antilipemic Agent, Miscellaneous

Medication Safety Issues

International issue:

Simcor® is also a brand name for simvastatin in Indonesia.

Pregnancy Risk Factor X

Lactation Excretion in breast milk unknown/contraindicated

Use Reduce total cholesterol, LDL, Apo B, non-HDL, TG, and/or increase HDL in patients with primary hypercholesterolemia, mixed dyslipidemia, or hypertriglyceridemia in combination with standard cholesterol-lowering diet when simvastatin or niacin monotherapy is inadequate

Available Dosage Forms

Tablet, variable release, oral:

Simcor®: 500/20: Niacin 500 mg [extended release] and simvastatin 20 mg [immediate release]; 500/40: Niacin 500 mg [extended release] and simvastatin 40 mg [immediate release]; 750/20: Niacin 750 mg [extended release] and simvastatin 20 mg [immediate release]; 1000/20: Niacin 1000 mg [extended release] and simvastatin 20 mg [immediate release]; 1000/40: Niacin 1000 mg [extended release] and simvastatin 40 mg [immediate release]

Dosing

Adult Dosage forms are a fixed combination of niacin extended-release and simvastatin.

Dyslipidemia: Oral:

Initial dose:

Patients naïve to niacin therapy: Niacin 500 mg/simvastatin 20 mg once daily at bedtime; increase dose every 4 weeks as needed in increments of not more than 500 mg of niacin

Patients currently on immediate-release niacin products: Niacin 500 mg/simvastatin 20 mg once daily at bedtime; increase dose every 4 weeks as needed in increments of not more than 500 mg of niacin

Patients currently on simvastatin (20-40 mg/day): Niacin 500 mg/simvastatin 40 mg once daily at bedtime; increase dose every 4 weeks as needed in increments of not more than 500 mg of niacin

Maintenance dose: Niacin 1000-2000 mg/ simvastatin 20-40 mg once daily (maximum daily dose: niacin 2000 mg/simvastatin 40 mg)

Note: If therapy is interrupted for >7 days, reinstitution of therapy should begin with the lowest dose followed by retitration as tolerated. Not for use as initial therapy of dyslipidemias. May be substituted for equivalent dose of niacin extended-release, however, manufacturer does not recommend direct substitution with immediate-release preparations.

Dosage adjustment for simvastatin component with concomitant medications:

Cyclosporine, danazol, or gemfibrozil: Simvastatin dose should not exceed 10 mg/day. Therefore, use of niacin/simvastatin combination should not be used.

Amiodarone or verapamil: Simvastatin dose should not exceed 20 mg/day

Renal Impairment

Mild-to-moderate impairment: No dosage adjustment required; use caution.

Severe renal impairment: Use with extreme caution or avoid unless patient already tolerating simvastatin doses ≥10 mg.

Hepatic Impairment Contraindicated in active liver disease or unexplained persistent elevations of serum transaminases.

Adjustment for Toxicity Discontinue therapy if transaminases >3 times ULN persist or are accompanied by symptoms (nausea, fever, malaise).

Administration

Oral Tablets must be swallowed whole; do not crush or chew. Administer with a low-fat snack at bedtime.

Monitoring and Teaching Issues

Laboratory Monitoring Blood glucose (in patients with diabetes), CBC, LFTs, prothrombin time (surgical patients), and serum phosphorus (if predisposed to hypophosphatemia). Baseline CK levels, hepatic transaminase levels, and total cholesterol profile should be obtained prior to initiation of therapy. Repeat CK level with onset of unexplained muscle symptoms. Repeat hepatic transaminase levels every 12 weeks for first 6 months and periodically thereafter (approximately every 6 months).

Physical Assessment See individual agents.

Patient Education See individual agents.

Related Information

Hyperlipidemia Management *on page 2046*
Niacin *on page 1305*
Simvastatin *on page 1645*

◆ **Niacin-Time® [OTC]** *see* Niacin *on page 1305*
◆ **Niacor®** *see* Niacin *on page 1305*
◆ **Niaspan®** *see* Niacin *on page 1305*

NiCARdipine (nye KAR de peen)

U.S. Brand Names Cardene® I.V.; Cardene® SR

Index Terms Nicardipine Hydrochloride

Generic Availability (U.S.) Yes: Capsule, injection

Pharmacologic Category Calcium Channel Blocker; Calcium Channel Blocker, Dihydropyridine

Medication Safety Issues

Sound-alike/look-alike issues:

NiCARdipine may be confused with niacinamide, NIFEdipine, niMODipine
Cardene® may be confused with Cardizem®, Cardura®, codeine

International issues:

Cardene [U.S., Great Britain, Netherlands] may be confused with Cardem brand name for celiprolol [Spain]; Cardin brand name for simvastatin [Poland]

Significant differences exist between oral and I.V. dosing. Use caution when converting from one route of administration to another.

Pregnancy Risk Factor C

Lactation Enters breast milk

Use Chronic stable angina (immediate-release product only); management of hypertension (immediate and sustained release products); parenteral only for short-term use when oral treatment is not feasible

Unlabeled/Investigational Use Congestive heart failure, control of blood pressure in acute ischemic stroke and spontaneous intracranial hemorrhage, postoperative hypertension associated with carotid endarterectomy, perioperative hypertension, prevention of migraine headaches, subarachnoid hemorrhage associated cerebral vasospasm

Mechanism of Action/Effect Inhibits calcium ion from entering the "slow channels" or select voltage-sensitive areas of vascular smooth muscle and myocardium during depolarization, producing a relaxation of coronary vascular smooth muscle and coronary vasodilation; increases myocardial oxygen delivery in patients with vasospastic angina

Contraindications Hypersensitivity to nicardipine or any component of the formulation; advanced aortic stenosis

Warnings/Precautions Symptomatic hypotension with or without syncope can rarely occur; blood pressure must be lowered at a rate appropriate for the patient's clinical condition. Reflex tachycardia may occur resulting in angina and/or MI in patients with obstructive coronary disease especially in the absence of concurrent beta blockade. The most common side effect is peripheral edema (dose-dependent); occurs within 2-3 weeks of starting therapy. Use with caution in CAD (can cause increase in angina), HF (can worsen heart failure symptoms), aortic stenosis (may reduce coronary perfusion resulting in ischemia; use is contraindicated in patients with advanced aortic stenosis), and hypertrophic cardiomyopathy with outflow tract obstruction. To minimize infusion site reactions, peripheral infusion sites (for I.V. therapy) should be changed every 12 hours; use of small peripheral veins should be avoided. Titrate I.V. dose cautiously in patients with HF, renal or hepatic dysfunction. Use the I.V. form cautiously in patients with portal hypertension (can cause increase in hepatic pressure gradient). Initiate at the low end of the dosage range in the elderly. Concurrent use of fentanyl anesthesia may result in hypotension. Abrupt withdrawal may cause rebound angina in patients with CAD.

Drug Interactions

Metabolism/Transport Effects Substrate of CYP1A2 (minor), CYP2C9 (minor), CYP2D6 (minor), CYP2E1 (minor), CYP3A4 (major), P-glycoprotein; **Inhibits** CYP2C9 (strong), CYP2C19 (moderate), CYP2D6 (moderate), CYP3A4 (strong), P-glycoprotein

Avoid Concomitant Use

Avoid concomitant use of NiCARdipine with any of the following: Alfuzosin; Conivaptan; Dronedarone; Eplerenone; Everolimus; Halofantrine; Lurasidone; Nilotinib; Nisoldipine; Ranolazine; Rivaroxaban; RomiDEPsin; Salmeterol; Silodosin; Tamsulosin; Thioridazine; Tolvaptan; Topotecan; Toremifene

Decreased Effect

NiCARdipine may decrease the levels/effects of: Clopidogrel; Codeine; Prasugrel; QuiNIDine; TraMADol

The levels/effects of NiCARdipine may be decreased by: Barbiturates; Calcium Salts; CarBAMazepine; CYP3A4 Inducers (Strong); Deferasirox; Herbs (CYP3A4 Inducers); Herbs (Hypertensive Properties); Methylphenidate; Nafcillin; Peginterferon Alfa-2b; Rifamycin Derivatives; Yohimbine

Increased Effect/Toxicity

NiCARdipine may increase the levels/effects of: Alfuzosin; Almotriptan; Alosetron; Amifostine; Antihypertensives; Bortezomib; Brinzolamide; Calcium Channel Blockers (Nondihydropyridine); Ciclesonide; Colchicine; Conivaptan; Corticosteroids (Orally Inhaled); CYP2C19 Substrates; CYP2C9 Substrates (High risk); CYP2D6 Substrates; CYP3A4 Substrates; Dabigatran Etexilate; Dienogest; Dronedarone; Dutasteride; Eplerenone; Everolimus; FentaNYL; Fesoterodine; GuanFACINE; Halofantrine; Hypotensive Agents; Ixabepilone; Lumefantrine; Lurasidone; Magnesium Salts; Maraviroc; MethylPREDNISolone; Neuromuscular-Blocking Agents (Nondepolarizing); Nilotinib; Nisoldipine; Nitroprusside; Paricalcitol; Pazopanib; P-Glycoprotein Substrates; Phenytoin; Pimecrolimus; Ranolazine; RiTUXimab; Rivaroxaban; RomiDEPsin; Salmeterol; Saxagliptin; Silodosin; SORAfenib; Tacrolimus; Tacrolimus (Systemic); Tadalafil; Tamoxifen; Tamsulosin; Thioridazine; Tolvaptan; Topotecan; Toremifene; Vilazodone

The levels/effects of NiCARdipine may be increased by: Alpha1-Blockers; Antifungal Agents (Azole Derivatives, Systemic); Calcium Channel Blockers (Nondihydropyridine); CycloSPORINE; CycloSPORINE (Systemic); CYP3A4 Inhibitors (Moderate); CYP3A4 Inhibitors (Strong); Dasatinib; Diazoxide; Fluconazole; Grapefruit Juice; Herbs (Hypotensive Properties); Macrolide Antibiotics; Magnesium Salts; MAO Inhibitors; Pentoxifylline; P-Glycoprotein Inhibitors; Phosphodiesterase 5 Inhibitors; Prostacyclin Analogues; Protease Inhibitors

Nutritional/Ethanol Interactions

Ethanol: Avoid ethanol (may increase CNS depression).

Food: Nicardipine average peak concentrations may be decreased if taken with food. Serum concentrations/toxicity of nicardipine may be increased by grapefruit juice; avoid concurrent use.

Herb/Nutraceutical: St John's wort may decrease levels. Avoid bayberry, blue cohosh, cayenne, ephedra, ginger, ginseng (American), kola, licorice (may worsen hypertension). Avoid black cohosh, California poppy, coleus, golden seal, hawthorn, mistletoe, periwinkle, quinine, shepherd's purse (may have increased antihypertensive effect).

Adverse Reactions 1% to 10%:

Cardiovascular: Cardiovascular: Flushing (6% to 10%), peripheral edema (dose related; 6% to 8%), hypotension (I.V. 6%), increased angina (dose related; 6%), palpitation (3% to 4%), tachycardia (1% to 4%), vasodilation (1% to 5%), chest pain (I.V. 1%), ECG abnormal (I.V. 1%), extrasystoles (I.V. 1%), hemopericardium (I.V. 1%), hypertension (I.V. 1%), orthostasis (1%), supraventricular tachycardia (I.V. 1%), syncope (1%), ventricular extrasystoles (I.V. 1%), ventricular tachycardia (I.V. 1%)

Central nervous system: Headache (6% to 15%), dizziness (1% to 7%), hypoesthesia (1%), intracranial hemorrhage (1%) pain (1%), somnolence (1%)

Dermatologic: Rash (1%)

Endocrine & metabolic: Hypokalemia (I.V. 1%)

Gastrointestinal: Nausea (2% to 5%), vomiting (I.V. 5%), dyspepsia (oral 2%), abdominal pain (I.V. 1%), dry mouth (1%)

Genitourinary: Polyuria (1%)

Local: Injection site pain (I.V. 1%), injection site reaction (I.V. 1%)

Neuromuscular & skeletal: Weakness (1% to 6%), myalgia (1%), paresthesia (1%)

Renal: Hematuria (1%)

Respiratory: Dyspnea (1%)

Miscellaneous: Diaphoresis (1%)

Pharmacodynamics/Kinetics

Onset of Action Oral: 0.5-2 hours; I.V.: 10 minutes; Hypotension: ~20 minutes

Duration of Action I.V.: ≤8 hours; Oral: Immediate release capsules: ≤8 hours, Sustained release capsules: 8-12 hours

Absorption Oral: ~100%

Bioavailability 35%

Time to Peak Serum: Oral: Immediate release: 30-120 minutes; Sustained release: 60-240 minutes

Protein Binding >95%

Half-Life Elimination 2-4 hours

Metabolism Hepatic; CYP3A4 substrate (major); extensive first-pass effect (saturable)

Excretion Urine (49% to 60% as metabolites); feces (43% as metabolites)

Available Dosage Forms

Capsule, oral: 20 mg, 30 mg

Capsule, sustained release, oral:

Cardene® SR: 30 mg, 45 mg, 60 mg

Infusion, premixed iso-osmotic dextrose solution:

Cardene® I.V.: 20 mg (200 mL); 40 mg (200 mL)

Infusion, premixed iso-osmotic sodium chloride solution:

Cardene® I.V.: 20 mg (200 mL); 40 mg (200 mL)

Injection, solution: 2.5 mg/mL (10 mL)

Cardene® I.V.: 2.5 mg/mL (10 mL)

Dosing

Adult

Angina: Immediate release: Oral: 20 mg 3 times/day; usual range: 60-120 mg/day; increase dose at 3-day intervals

Hypertension: Oral:

Immediate release: Initial: 20 mg 3 times/day; usual: 20-40 mg 3 times/day (allow 3 days between dose increases)

Sustained release: Initial: 30 mg twice daily, titrate up to 60 mg twice daily

Note: The total daily dose of immediate-release product may not automatically be equivalent to the daily sustained-release dose; use caution in converting.

Acute hypertension: I.V.: Initial: Initial: 5 mg/hour increased by 2.5 mg/hour every 5 minutes (for rapid titration) to every 15 minutes (for gradual titration) up to a maximum of 15 mg/hour; rapidly titrated patients, consider reduction to 3 mg/hour after response is achieved. Monitor and titrate to lowest dose necessary to maintain stable blood pressure.

Arterial hypertension in acute ischemic stroke (unlabeled use [Adams, 2007; Jauch, 2010]): I.V.:

Patient otherwise eligible for reperfusion treatment (eg, alteplase): Blood pressure (BP): Systolic >185 mm Hg or diastolic >110 mm Hg: 5 mg/hour; titrate by 2.5 mg/hour at 5-15 minute intervals (maximum dose: 15 mg/hour). When goal BP obtained, reduce dose to 3 mg/hour. If BP does not decline and remains >185/110 mm Hg, alteplase should not be administered.

Management of BP during and after reperfusion treatment (eg, alteplase): BP: Systolic >230 mm Hg or diastolic >121-140 mm Hg: 5 mg/hour; titrate by 2.5 mg/hour at 5-minute intervals (maximum dose: 15 mg/hour). If hypertension is refractory, consider other I.V. antihypertensives (eg, nitroprusside).

Substitution for oral therapy (approximate equivalents):

20 mg every 8 hours oral, equivalent to 0.5 mg/hour I.V. infusion
30 mg every 8 hours oral, equivalent to 1.2 mg/hour I.V. infusion
40 mg every 8 hours oral, equivalent to 2.2 mg/hour I.V. infusion

Conversion to oral antihypertensive agent: Initiate oral antihypertensive at the same time that I.V. nicardipine is discontinued, if transitioning to oral nicardipine, start oral nicardipine 1 hour prior to I.V. discontinuation.

Geriatric Initiate at the low end of the dosage range. Specific guidelines for adjustment of nicardipine are not available, but careful monitoring is warranted and adjustment may be necessary.

Renal Impairment Oral: Titrate dose beginning with 20 mg 3 times/day (immediate release) or 30 mg twice daily (sustained release capsule). Specific guidelines for adjustment of nicardipine are not available, but careful monitoring is warranted and adjustment may be necessary.

Hepatic Impairment Oral: Starting dose: 20 mg twice daily (immediate release) with titration. Refer to **"Note"** in adult dosing. Specific guidelines for adjustment of nicardipine are not available, but careful monitoring is warranted and adjustment may be necessary.

Administration

Oral The total daily dose of immediate-release product may not automatically be equivalent to the daily sustained-release dose; use caution in converting. Do not chew or crush the sustained release formulation, swallow whole. Do not open or cut capsules.

I.V.

Vials must be diluted before use. Administer as a slow continuous infusion at a concentration of 0.1 mg/mL or 0.2 mg/mL. Concentrations of 0.5 mg/mL may be administered via a central line only.

Premixed bags: No further dilution needed. For single use only, discard any unused portion. Use only if solution is clear; the manufacturer recommends not to admix or run in the same line as other medications.

Stability

Reconstitution I.V.: Vial: Dilute 25 mg vial with 240 mL of compatible solution to provide a 250 mL total volume solution and a final concentration of 0.1 mg/mL.

Storage

I.V.:

Premixed bags: Store at controlled room temperature of 20°C to 25°C (68°F to 77°F). Protect from light and excessive heat. Do not freeze.

Vials: Store at controlled room temperature of 20°C to 25°C (68°F to 77°F). Protect from light. Diluted solution (0.1 mg/mL) is stable at room temperature for 24 hours in glass or PVC containers. Stability has also been demonstrated at room temperature at concentrations up to 0.5 mg/mL in PVC containers for 24 hours or in glass containers for up to 7 days (Baaske, 1996).

Oral (Cardene®, Cardene SR®): Store at 15°C to 30°C (59°F to 86°F). Protect from light. Freezing does not affect stability.

Monitoring and Teaching Issues

Physical Assessment Infusion site must be monitored closely to prevent extravasation; peripheral infusion sites should be changed every 12 hours. Evaluate cardiac status and blood pressure and monitor for rash, hypotension, bradycardia, confusion, and nausea when starting, adjusting dose, or discontinuing. Teach patient orthostatic precautions.

Patient Education This medication may be administered by intravenous infusion; report immediately any swelling, redness, burning, or pain at infusion site. Oral: Do not crush or chew sustained release forms; swallow whole. Take with nonfatty food. Avoid caffeine and alcohol. Consult prescriber before increasing exercise routine. May cause orthostatic hypotension, gum pain or swelling, dizziness, and constipation. Report chest pain or pressure, palpitations, severe constipation, swelling of extremities, or respiratory difficulty.

Dietary Considerations Avoid grapefruit juice.

Geriatric Considerations Elderly may experience a greater hypotensive response. Constipation may be more of a problem in the elderly. Calcium channel blockers are no more effective in the elderly than other therapies; however, they do not cause significant CNS effects which is an advantage over some antihypertensive agents.

Breast-Feeding Considerations Nicardipine is minimally excreted into breast milk. In one study, peak milk concentrations ranged from 1.9-18.8 mcg/mL following oral maternal doses of 40-150 mg/day. The estimated exposure to the breast-feeding infant was calculated to be 0.073% of the weight-adjusted maternal oral dose or 0.14% of the weight-adjusted maternal I.V. dose.

Pregnancy Considerations Adverse events were observed in some animal reproduction studies. Nicardipine crosses the placenta; changes in fetal heart rate have been observed following maternal use.

Related Information

Calcium Channel Blockers *on page* 1993

Hyperlipidemia Management *on page* 2046

◆ **Nicardipine Hydrochloride** *see* NiCARdipine *on page* 1309

◆ **NicoDerm® CQ® [OTC]** *see* Nicotine *on page* 1312

◆ **Nicorelief [OTC]** *see* Nicotine *on page* 1312

◆ **Nicorette® [OTC]** *see* Nicotine *on page* 1312

Nicotine (nik oh TEEN)

U.S. Brand Names Commit® [OTC]; NicoDerm® CQ® [OTC]; Nicorelief [OTC]; Nicorette® [OTC]; Nicotrol® Inhaler; Nicotrol® NS; Thrive™ [OTC]

Index Terms Habitrol; Nicotine Patch

Generic Availability (U.S.) Yes: Transdermal patch and gum

Pharmacologic Category Smoking Cessation Aid

Medication Safety Issues

Sound-alike/look-alike issues:

NicoDerm® may be confused with Nitroderm

Nicorette® may be confused with Nordette®

Transdermal patch may contain conducting metal (eg, aluminum); remove patch prior to MRI.

Pregnancy Risk Factor D (nasal)

Lactation Excretion in breast milk unknown/use caution

Use Treatment to aid smoking cessation for the relief of nicotine withdrawal symptoms (including nicotine craving)

Unlabeled/Investigational Use Management of ulcerative colitis (transdermal)

Available Dosage Forms

Gum, chewing, oral: 2 mg (20s, 40s, 50s, 100s, 108s, 110s); 4 mg (20s, 40s, 48s, 50s, 100s, 108s, 110s)

Nicorelief [OTC]: 2 mg (50s, 110s); 4 mg (50s, 110s)

Nicorette® [OTC]: 2 mg (40s, 48s, 50s, 100s, 108s, 110s, 168s, 170s, 192s, 200s, 216s); 4 mg (40s, 48s, 50s, 100s, 108s, 110s, 168s, 170s, 192s, 200s, 216s)

Thrive™ [OTC]: 2 mg (40s); 4 mg (40s)

Lozenge, oral:

Commit® [OTC]: 2 mg (48s, 72s); 4 mg (48s, 72s)

Nicorette® [OTC]: 4 mg (50s)

Oral inhalation system, for oral inhalation:

Nicotrol® Inhaler: 10 mg (10 mL)

Patch, transdermal: 7 mg/24 hours (7s, 14s, 30s); 14 mg/24 hours (7s, 14s, 30s); 21 mg/24 hours (7s, 14s, 30s)

NicoDerm® CQ® [OTC]: 7 mg/24 hours (14s); 14 mg/24 hours (14s); 21 mg/24 hours (7s, 14s)

Solution, intranasal:

Nicotrol® NS: 10 mg/mL (10 mL)

Dosing

Adult & Geriatric

Tobacco cessation (patients should be advised to completely stop smoking upon initiation of therapy):

Gum: Chew 1 piece of gum when urge to smoke, up to 24 pieces/day. Patients who smoke <25 cigarettes/day should start with 2-mg strength; patients smoking ≥25 cigarettes/day should start with the 4-mg strength. Use according to the following 12-week dosing schedule:

Weeks 1-6: Chew 1 piece of gum every 1-2 hours; to increase chances of quitting, chew at least 9 pieces/day during the first 6 weeks

Weeks 7-9: Chew 1 piece of gum every 2-4 hours

Weeks 10-12: Chew 1 piece of gum every 4-8 hours

Inhaler: Oral: Usually 6-16 cartridges per day; best effect was achieved by frequent continuous puffing (20 minutes); recommended duration of treatment is 3 months, after which patients may be weaned from the inhaler by gradual reduction of the daily dose over 6-12 weeks

Lozenge: Oral: Patients who smoke their first cigarette within 30 minutes of waking should use the 4-mg strength; otherwise the 2-mg strength is recommended. Use according to the following 12-week dosing schedule:

Weeks 1-6: One lozenge every 1-2 hours

Weeks 7-9: One lozenge every 2-4 hours

Weeks 10-12: One lozenge every 4-8 hours

Note: Use at least 9 lozenges/day during first 6 weeks to improve chances of quitting; do not use more than one lozenge at a time (maximum: 5 lozenges every 6 hours, 20 lozenges/day)

Spray: Nasal: 1-2 sprays/hour; do not exceed more than 5 doses (10 sprays) per hour [maximum: 40 doses/day (80 sprays); each dose (2 sprays) contains 1 mg of nicotine]

Transdermal patch: Topical: Apply new patch every 24 hours to nonhairy, clean, dry skin on the upper body or upper outer arm; each patch should be applied to a different site. **Note:** Adjustment may be required during initial treatment (move to higher dose if experiencing withdrawal symptoms; lower dose if side effects are experienced).

NicoDerm CQ®:

Patients smoking >10 cigarettes/day: Begin with step 1 (21 mg/day) for 6 weeks, **followed by** step 2 (14 mg/day) for 2 weeks; **finish with** step 3 (7 mg/day) for 2 weeks

Patients smoking ≤10 cigarettes/day: Begin with step 2 (14 mg/day) for 6 weeks, **followed by** step 3 (7 mg/day) for 2 weeks

Note: Patients who are receiving >600 mg/day of cimetidine: Decrease to the next lower patch size

Benefits of use of nicotine transdermal patches beyond 3 months have not been demonstrated

Administration

Oral

Gum: Should be chewed slowly to avoid jaw ache and to maximize benefit. Chew slowly until it tingles, then park gum between cheek and gum until tingle is gone; repeat process until most of tingle is gone (~30 minutes).

Lozenge: Should not be chewed or swallowed; allow to dissolve slowly (~20-30 minutes)

Inhalation

Nasal spray: Prime pump prior to first use (pump 6-8 times until fine spray appears) or if it has not been used for 24 hours (pump 1-2 times). Blow nose prior to use. Tilt head back slightly and insert tip of bottle into nostril. Breathe through mouth and spray once in each nostril. Do not sniff, swallow, or inhale through the nose during administration. After administration, wait 2-3 minutes before blowing nose.

Oral inhalant: Insert cartridge into inhaler and push hard until it pops into place. Replace mouthpiece and twist the top and bottom so that markings do not line up. Inhale deeply into the back of the throat or puff in short breaths. Nicotine in cartridge is used up after about 20 minutes of active puffing.

Topical Do not cut patch; causes rapid evaporation, rendering the patch useless.

Monitoring and Teaching Issues

Physical Assessment Monitor cardiac status and vital signs prior to, when beginning, and periodically during therapy.

Patient Education Do not smoke, chew tobacco, use snuff, nicotine gum, or any other form of nicotine.

Gum: Chew slowly for 30 minutes. Discard chewed gum away from access by children.

Lozenge: Allow to dissolve slowly in the mouth. Do not chew or swallow lozenge whole. Avoid food or drink 15 minutes prior to, during, or after lozenge.

Transdermal patch: Do not cut patches or wear more than one patch at a time. Remove backing from patch and press immediately on skin. Hold for 10 seconds. Apply to clean, dry skin in different site each day. Do not touch eyes; wash hands after application. You may experience vivid dreams and sleep disturbances, dizziness, lightheadedness, vomiting, or GI upset. Report persistent vomiting, diarrhea, chills, sweating, chest pain or palpitations, or burning or redness at application site. Remove patch while having MRI scan; can cause burns.

Spray: Blow nose gently before use. Use 1-2 sprays/hour; do not exceed 5 doses (10 sprays) per hour. Excessive use can result in severe (even life-threatening) reactions. You may experience temporary stinging or burning after spray.

◆ **Nicotine Patch** *see* Nicotine *on page* 1312
◆ **Nicotinic Acid** *see* Niacin *on page* 1305
◆ **Nicotrol® Inhaler** *see* Nicotine *on page* 1312
◆ **Nicotrol® NS** *see* Nicotine *on page* 1312
◆ **Nifediac CC®** *see* NIFEdipine *on page* 1313
◆ **Nifedical XL®** *see* NIFEdipine *on page* 1313

NIFEdipine (nye FED i peen)

U.S. Brand Names Adalat® CC; Afeditab® CR; Nifediac CC®; Nifedical XL®; Procardia XL®; Procardia®

Generic Availability (U.S.) Yes

Pharmacologic Category Calcium Channel Blocker; Calcium Channel Blocker, Dihydropyridine

Medication Safety Issues

Sound-alike/look-alike issues:

NIFEdipine may be confused with niCARdipine, niMODipine, nisoldipine

Procardia XL® may be confused with Cartia XT®

Beers Criteria medication: This drug may be inappropriate for use in geriatric patients (high severity risk).

International issues:
Depin [India] may be confused with Depen brand name for penicillamine [U.S.]; Depon brand name for acetaminophen [Greece]; Dipen brand name for diltiazem [Greece]
Nipin [Italy and Singapore] may be confused with Nipent brand name for pentostatin [U.S., Canada, and multiple international markets]

Pregnancy Risk Factor C

Lactation Enters breast milk/not recommended (AAP considers "compatible"; AAP 2001 update pending)

Use Management of chronic stable or vasospastic angina; treatment of hypertension (sustained release products only)

Unlabeled/Investigational Use Management of pulmonary hypertension, preterm labor, Raynaud's phenomenon

Mechanism of Action/Effect Inhibits calcium ion influx into vascular smooth muscle resulting in antianginal and antihypertensive effects.

Contraindications Hypersensitivity to nifedipine or any component of the formulation; concomitant use with strong CYP3A4 inducers (eg, rifampin); cardiogenic shock; immediate release preparation for treatment of urgent or emergent hypertension (Chobanian, 2003); acute MI (Antman, 2004)

Warnings/Precautions Symptomatic hypotension with or without syncope can rarely occur; blood pressure must be lowered at a rate appropriate for the patient's clinical condition. **The use of immediate release nifedipine (sublingually or orally) in hypertensive emergencies and urgencies is neither safe nor effective.** Serious adverse events (eg, death, cerebrovascular ischemia, syncope, stroke, acute myocardial infarction, and fetal distress) have been reported. **Immediate release nifedipine should not be used for acute blood pressure reduction.**

Blood pressure lowering should be done at a rate appropriate for the patient's condition. Rapid drops in blood pressure can lead to arterial insufficiency. Increased angina and/or MI have occurred with initiation or dosage titration of dihydropyridine calcium channel blockers; use with caution in patients with obstructive coronary disease especially in the absence of concurrent beta-blockade. Use with caution before major surgery. Cardiopulmonary bypass, intraoperative blood loss or vasodilating anesthesia may result in severe hypotension and/or increased fluid requirements. Consider withdrawing nifedipine (>36 hours) before surgery if possible.

The most common side effect is peripheral edema; occurs within 2-3 weeks of starting therapy. Reflex tachycardia may occur with use. Use with caution in HF or severe aortic stenosis (especially with concomitant beta-adrenergic blocker), severe left ventricular dysfunction, renal impairment, hypertrophic cardiomyopathy (especially obstructive), concomitant therapy with beta-blockers or digoxin, and edema. Use caution in patients with severe hepatic impairment. Clearance of nifedipine is reduced in cirrhotic patients leading to increased systemic exposure; monitor closely for adverse effects/toxicity and consider dose adjustments. Mild and transient elevations in liver function enzymes may be apparent within 8 weeks of therapy initiation. Abrupt withdrawal may cause rebound angina in patients with CAD. Short-acting nifedipine may be inappropriate for use in the elderly due to potential to cause hypotension and constipation (Beers Criteria). Immediate release formulations should not be used to manage essential hypertension, adequate studies to evaluate outcomes have not been conducted. Avoid use of extended release tablets (Procardia XL®) in patients with known stricture/narrowing of the GI tract.

Use with caution in patients taking CYP3A4 inhibitors; may result in increased nifedipine concentrations; monitor for adverse effects/toxicity and consider dose adjustments. Use with strong CYP3A4 inducers (eg, rifampin, rifabutin, phenobarbital, phenytoin, carbamazepine, St John's wort) is contraindicated due to reduced bioavailability and efficacy.

Drug Interactions

Metabolism/Transport Effects Substrate of CYP2D6 (minor), 3A4 (major); **Inhibits** CYP1A2 (moderate), 2C9 (weak), 2D6 (weak), 3A4 (weak)

Avoid Concomitant Use

Avoid concomitant use of NIFEdipine with any of the following: Grapefruit Juice

Decreased Effect

NIFEdipine may decrease the levels/effects of: Clopidogrel; QuiNIDine

The levels/effects of NIFEdipine may be decreased by: Barbiturates; Calcium Salts; CarBAMazepine; CYP3A4 Inducers (Strong); Deferasirox; Herbs (CYP3A4 Inducers); Herbs (Hypertensive Properties); Methylphenidate; Nafcillin; Peginterferon Alfa-2b; Rifamycin Derivatives; Yohimbine

Increased Effect/Toxicity

NIFEdipine may increase the levels/effects of: Amifostine; Antihypertensives; Calcium Channel Blockers (Nondihydropyridine); CYP1A2 Substrates; Hypotensive Agents; Magnesium Salts; Neuromuscular-Blocking Agents (Nondepolarizing); Nitroprusside; Phenytoin; RiTUXimab; Tacrolimus; Tacrolimus (Systemic); VinCRIStine

The levels/effects of NIFEdipine may be increased by: Alcohol (Ethyl); Alpha1-Blockers; Antifungal Agents (Azole Derivatives, Systemic); Calcium Channel Blockers (Nondihydropyridine); Cimetidine; Cisapride; Conivaptan; CycloSPORINE; CycloSPORINE (Systemic); CYP3A4 Inhibitors (Moderate); CYP3A4 Inhibitors (Strong); Dasatinib; Diazoxide; Fluconazole; Grapefruit Juice; Herbs (Hypotensive Properties); Macrolide Antibiotics; Magnesium Salts; MAO Inhibitors; Pentoxifylline; Phosphodiesterase 5 Inhibitors; Prostacyclin Analogues; Protease Inhibitors

Nutritional/Ethanol Interactions

Ethanol: Avoid ethanol (may increase CNS depression and may increase the effects of nifedipine). Monitor.

Food: Nifedipine serum levels may be decreased if taken with food. Food may decrease the rate but not the extent of absorption of Procardia XL®. Increased nifedipine concentrations resulting in therapeutic and vasodilator side effects, including severe hypotension and myocardial ischemia, may occur if nifedipine is taken by patients ingesting grapefruit.

Herb/Nutraceutical: St John's wort may decrease nifedipine levels (avoid use). Avoid use of bayberry, blue cohosh, cayenne, ephedra, ginger, ginseng (American), kola, licorice (may worsen hypertension). Avoid black cohosh, California poppy, coleus, golden seal, hawthorn, mistletoe, periwinkle, quinine, shepherd's purse (may have increased antihypertensive effect).

Adverse Reactions

>10%:

Cardiovascular: Flushing (10% to 25%; extended release products 3% to 4%), peripheral edema (dose related 7% to 30%)

Central nervous system: Dizziness/lightheadedness/giddiness (10% to 27%), headache (10% to 23%)

Gastrointestinal: Nausea/heartburn (10% to 11%)

≥1% to 10%:

Cardiovascular: Palpitation (≤2% to 7%), transient hypotension (dose related 5%), CHF (2%)

Central nervous system: Nervousness/mood changes (≤2% to 7%), fatigue (6%), shakiness (≤2%), jitteriness (≤2%), sleep disturbances (≤2%), difficulties in balance (≤2%), fever (≤2%), chills (≤2%)

Dermatologic: Dermatitis (≤2%), pruritus (≤2%), urticaria (≤2%)

Endocrine & metabolic: Sexual difficulties (≤2%)

Gastrointestinal: Diarrhea (≤2%), constipation (≤2%), cramps (≤2%), flatulence (≤2%), gingival hyperplasia (≤10%)

Neuromuscular & skeletal: Muscle cramps/tremor (≤2% to 8%), weakness (<3%), inflammation (≤2%), joint stiffness (≤2%)

Ocular: Blurred vision (≤2%)

Respiratory: Cough/wheezing (6%), nasal congestion/sore throat (≤2% to 6%), chest congestion (≤2%), dyspnea (≤2%)

Miscellaneous: Diaphoresis (≤2%)

Pharmacodynamics/Kinetics

Onset of Action Immediate release: ~20 minutes

Bioavailability Capsule: 40% to 77%; Sustained release: 65% to 89% relative to immediate release capsules; bioavailability increased with significant hepatic disease

Protein Binding Concentration dependent: 92% to 98%

Half-Life Elimination Adults: Healthy: 2-5 hours; Cirrhosis: 7 hours; Elderly: 7 hours (extended release tablet)

Metabolism Hepatic via CYP3A4 to inactive metabolites

Excretion Urine (60% to 80% as inactive metabolites); feces

Available Dosage Forms

Capsule, softgel, oral: 10 mg, 20 mg

Procardia®: 10 mg

Tablet, extended release, oral: 30 mg, 60 mg, 90 mg

Adalat® CC: 30 mg, 60 mg, 90 mg

Afeditab® CR: 30 mg, 60 mg

Nifediac CC®: 30 mg, 60 mg, 90 mg

Nifedical XL®: 30 mg, 60 mg

Procardia XL®: 30 mg, 60 mg, 90 mg

Dosing

Adult & Geriatric Dosage adjustments should occur at 7- to 14-day intervals, to allow for adequate assessment of new dose; when switching from immediate release to sustained release formulations, use same total daily dose.

Chronic stable or vasospastic angina: Oral:

Immediate release: Initial: 10 mg 3 times/day; usual dose: 10-20 mg 3 times/day; coronary artery spasm may require up to 20-30 mg 3-4 times/day; single doses >30 mg and total daily doses >120 mg are rarely needed; maximum: 180 mg/day; **Note:** Do not use for acute anginal episodes; may precipitate myocardial infarction

Extended release: Initial: 30 or 60 mg once daily; maximum: 120-180 mg/day

Hypertension: Oral: Extended release: Initial: 30 or 60 mg once daily; maximum: 90-120 mg/day

Pulmonary hypertension (unlabeled use; Galie, 2004): Oral: Extended release: Initial: 30 mg twice daily; may increase cautiously to 120-240 mg/day

Raynaud's phenomenon (unlabeled use; Wigley, 2002): Oral: Extended release: Dosage range: 30-120 mg once daily

Pediatric Hypertension (unlabeled use): Oral: Children 1-17 years: Extended release tablet: Initial: 0.25-0.5 mg/kg/day once daily or in 2 divided doses; maximum: 3 mg/kg/day up to 120 mg/day

Renal Impairment

Hemodialysis: Supplemental dose is not necessary.

Peritoneal dialysis effects: Supplemental dose is not necessary.

Hepatic Impairment Clearance of nifedipine is reduced in cirrhotic patients leading to increased systemic exposure; monitor closely for adverse effects/toxicity and consider dose adjustments.

Administration

Oral

Immediate release: In general, may be administered with or without food.

Extended release: Tablets should be swallowed whole; do not crush, split, or chew.

Adalat® CC, Afeditab® CR, Nifediac CC®: Administer on an empty stomach (per manufacturer). Other extended release products may not have this recommendation; consult product labeling.

Monitoring and Teaching Issues

Physical Assessment Use caution in presence of obstructive coronary disease (aortic stenosis), severe hepatic impairment, or heart failure. Monitor for hypotension, peripheral edema, and constipation when starting, adjusting dose, or discontinuing. Teach patient orthostatic precautions.

Patient Education Do not crush or chew sustained release forms; swallow whole. Avoid caffeine and alcohol. When used to manage angina, consult prescriber before increasing exercise routine. May cause dizziness, gum pain and swelling, difficulties in balance, fatigue, or constipation. Report chest pain or palpitations, swelling of extremities, respiratory difficulty, rash, or severe constipation.

Dietary Considerations Avoid grapefruit juice with all products.

Immediate release: Capsule is rapidly absorbed orally if it is administered without food, but may result in vasodilator side effects; if flushing is problematic, administration with low-fat meals may decrease. In general, can take with or without food.

Extended release: Adalat® CC, Afeditab® CR, Nifediac CC®: Take on an empty stomach (manufacturer recommendation). Other extended release products may not have this recommendation; consult product labeling.

Geriatric Considerations Elderly may experience a greater hypotensive response. Theoretically, constipation may be more of a problem in elderly patients. The half-life of nifedipine is extended in elderly patients (6.7 hours) as compared to younger subjects (3.8 hours).

This medication is considered to be potentially inappropriate in this patient population (Beers Criteria severity: High).

Pregnancy Considerations Adverse events were observed in animal reproduction studies. Nifedipine crosses the placenta. Use in pregnancy only when clearly needed and when the benefits outweigh the potential hazard to the fetus. Hypotension, IUGR reported. IUGR probably related to maternal hypertension. May be used for the treatment of preterm labor.

Additional Information When measuring smaller doses from the liquid-filled capsules, consider the following concentrations (for Procardia®) 10 mg capsule = 10 mg/0.34 mL; 20 mg capsule = 20 mg/0.45 mL; may be used preoperative to treat hypertensive urgency.

Considerable attention has been directed to potential increases in mortality and morbidity when short-acting nifedipine is used in treating hypertension. The rapid reduction in blood pressure may precipitate adverse cardiovascular events.

Short-acting nifedipine should not be used for acute anginal episodes since this may precipitate myocardial infarction. Extended-release formulations are preferred for the management of chronic or vasospastic angina (Poole-Wilson, 2004).

Equivalency of extended release formulation (Adalat® CC): The manufacturer states that it is acceptable to interchange two 30 mg tablets with one 60 mg tablet to effectively deliver a 60 mg dose. However, it is not recommended to substitute one 90 mg tablet with three 30 mg tablets, since the resulting C_{max} is 29% higher compared to giving the single 90 mg tablet.

Related Information

Calcium Channel Blockers *on page* 1993

◆ **Niftolid** *see* Flutamide *on page* 797

◆ **Nilandron®** *see* Nilutamide *on page* 1319

Nilotinib (nye LOE ti nib)

U.S. Brand Names Tasigna®

Index Terms AMN107; Nilotinib Hydrochloride Monohydrate

Generic Availability (U.S.) No

Pharmacologic Category Antineoplastic Agent, Tyrosine Kinase Inhibitor

Medication Safety Issues

Sound-alike/look-alike issues:

Nilotinib may be confused with dasatinib, imatinib, nilutamide, SUNItinib, vandetanib

High alert medication: This medication is in a class the Institute for Safe Medication Practices (ISMP) includes among its list of drug classes which have a heightened risk of causing significant patient harm when used in error.

Medication Guide Available Yes

Pregnancy Risk Factor D

Lactation Excretion in breast milk unknown/not recommended

Use Treatment of newly-diagnosed Philadelphia chromosome-positive chronic myelogenous leukemia (Ph+ CML) in chronic phase; treatment of chronic and accelerated phase Ph+ CML (refractory or intolerant to prior therapy, including imatinib)

Mechanism of Action/Effect Selective tyrosine kinase inhibitor that inhibits leukemic cell proliferation.

Contraindications Use in patients with hypokalemia, hypomagnesemia, or long QT syndrome

Warnings/Precautions [U.S. Boxed Warning]: May prolong the QT interval; sudden deaths have been reported. Use in patients with hypokalemia, hypomagnesemia, or long QT syndrome is contraindicated. Correct electrolyte imbalance prior to initiating therapy. Monitor ECG and QT_c (baseline, at 7 days, with dose change, and periodically). Avoid the use of QT-prolonging agents and strong CYP3A4 inhibitors. Concurrent use with other drugs which may prolong QT interval may increase the risk of potentially-fatal arrhythmias. Concurrent use with CYP3A4 inhibitors/inducers is not recommended; dosage reductions are recommended if concurrent use with CYP3A4 inhibitors cannot be avoided. Sudden deaths appear to be related to dose-dependent ventricular repolarization abnormalities. Prolonged QT interval may result in torsade de pointes, which may cause syncope, seizure, and/or death. Patients with uncontrolled or significant cardiovascular disease were excluded from studies.

[U.S. Boxed Warning]: Use with caution in patients with hepatic impairment; dosage reduction recommended. Nilotinib metabolism is primarily hepatic; carefully monitor for QT prolongation. May cause hepatotoxicity, including dose-limiting elevations in bilirubin, transaminases, and alkaline phosphatase; monitor liver function.

Reversible myelosuppression, including grades 3 and 4 thrombocytopenia, neutropenia, and anemia may occur; may require dose reductions and/or treatment delay. **[U.S. Boxed Warning]: Administer on an empty stomach, at least 1 hour before and 2 hours after food;** administration with food may prolong the QT_c. Use with caution in patients with a history of pancreatitis, may cause dose-limiting elevations of serum lipase and amylase; monitor. Consider alternative therapy or a dosage increase (with frequent monitoring) in patients with total gastrectomy. Capsules contain lactose; do not use with galactose intolerance, severe lactase deficiency, or glucose-galactose malabsorption syndromes. Safety and efficacy have not been established in children.

Drug Interactions

Metabolism/Transport Effects Substrate of CYP3A4 (major), P-glycoprotein (P-gp, ABCB1); **Inhibits** CYP3A4, 2C8, 2C9, 2D6, UGT1A1, P-glycoprotein (P-gp, ABCB1); **Induces** CYP2B6, 2C8, 2C9

Avoid Concomitant Use

Avoid concomitant use of Nilotinib with any of the following: Artemether; BCG; CYP3A4 Inducers (Strong); CYP3A4 Inhibitors (Strong); Dronedarone; Lumefantrine; Natalizumab; Pimecrolimus; Pimozide; QTc-Prolonging Agents; QuiNINE; Roflumilast; Silodosin; Tacrolimus (Topical); Tetrabenazine; Thioridazine; Topotecan; Toremifene; Vaccines (Live); Vandetanib; Ziprasidone

Decreased Effect

Nilotinib may decrease the levels/effects of: BCG; Cardiac Glycosides; Codeine; Sipuleucel-T; TraMADol; Vaccines (Inactivated); Vaccines (Live); Vitamin K Antagonists

The levels/effects of Nilotinib may be decreased by: CYP3A4 Inducers (Strong); Deferasirox; Echinacea; Herbs (CYP3A4 Inducers)

Increased Effect/Toxicity

Nilotinib may increase the levels/effects of: Carvedilol; Colchicine; CYP2C8 Substrates (High risk); CYP2C9 Substrates (High risk); CYP2D6 Substrates; Dabigatran Etexilate; Dronedarone; Everolimus; Fesoterodine; Leflunomide; Natalizumab; Nebivolol; P-Glycoprotein Substrates; Pimozide; QTc-Prolonging Agents; QuiNINE; Rivaroxaban; Silodosin; Tamoxifen; Tetrabenazine; Thioridazine; Topotecan; Toremifene; Vaccines (Live); Vandetanib; Vitamin K Antagonists; Ziprasidone

The levels/effects of Nilotinib may be increased by: Alfuzosin; Artemether; Chloroquine; Ciprofloxacin; Ciprofloxacin (Systemic); CYP3A4 Inhibitors (Moderate); CYP3A4 Inhibitors (Strong); Denosumab; Gadobutrol; Lumefantrine; Pimecrolimus; QuiNINE; Roflumilast; Tacrolimus (Topical); Trastuzumab

Nutritional/Ethanol Interactions

Food: Avoid grapefruit juice (may result in increased concentrations of nilotinib and potentiate QT prolongation).

Herb/Nutraceutical: Avoid St John's wort (may decrease nilotinib levels). Administration with grapefruit juice may result in increased concentrations of nilotinib and potentiate QT prolongation.

Adverse Reactions

>10%:

Cardiovascular: Peripheral edema (8% to 11%)

Central nervous system: Headache (21% to 31%), fatigue (16% to 28%), fever (10% to 24%)

Dermatologic: Rash (28% to 36%), pruritus (19% to 29%)

Endocrine & metabolic: Hyperglycemia (grades 3/4: 4% to 11%)

Gastrointestinal: Nausea (18% to 31%), diarrhea (14% to 22%), constipation (15% to 21%), vomiting (9% to 21%), lipase increased (grades 3/4: 7% to 17%), abdominal pain (11% to 15%)

Hematologic: Neutropenia (grades 3/4: 12% to 37%; median duration: 15 days), thrombocytopenia (grade 3/4: 10% to 37%; median duration: 22 days), anemia (grades 3/4: 4% to 23%)

Neuromuscular & skeletal: Arthralgia (15% to 18%), limb pain (9% to 16%), myalgia (14%), weakness (11% to 14%), muscle spasm (10% to 14%), bone pain (11% to 13%), back pain (10% to 12%)

Respiratory: Cough (12% to 17%), nasopharyngitis (11% to 19%), upper respiratory tract infection (≤13%), dyspnea (8% to 11%)

1% to 10%:

Cardiovascular: Angina, arrhythmia (including AV block, atrial fibrillation, bradycardia, cardiac flutter, and extrasystoles), chest pain, flushing, hypertension, palpitation, pericardial effusion, QT interval prolonged

Central nervous system: Depression, dizziness, dysphonia, hypoesthesia, insomnia, pain, vertigo
Dermatologic: Acne, alopecia, bruising, dry skin, dermatitis, eczema, erythema, folliculitis, hyperhidrosis, skin papilloma, urticaria
Endocrine & metabolic: Hypophosphatemia (grades 3/4: 5% to 10%), hypokalemia (grades 3/4: ≤5%), hyperkalemia (grades 3/4: 2% to 4%), hypocalcemia (grades 3/4: ≤4%), hyponatremia (grades 3/4: ≤3%), albumin decreased (grades 3/4: ≤1%), diabetes mellitus, hypercalcemia, hypercholesterolemia, hyperlipidemia, hyperphosphatemia, hypomagnesemia
Gastrointestinal: Abdominal discomfort, amylase increased, anorexia, dyspepsia, flatulence, pancreatitis
Genitourinary: Pollakuria
Hematologic: Lymphopenia, neutropenic fever, pancytopenia
Hepatic: Hyperbilirubinemia (grades 3/4: 4% to 10%), ALT increased (grades 3/4: 2% to 4%), alkaline phosphatase increased (grades 3/4: ≤3%), AST increased (grades 3/4: 1%), GGT increased
Neuromuscular & skeletal: Musculoskeletal pain, paresthesia
Ocular: Conjunctivitis, dry eye, eye hemorrhage, eyelid edema, periorbital edema, pruritus
Respiratory: Dyspnea (exertional), epistaxis, pleural effusion (≤1%), pneumonia
Miscellaneous: Night sweats

Pharmacodynamics/Kinetics

Bioavailability Increased 82% when administered 30 minutes after a high-fat meal

Time to Peak 3 hours

Protein Binding ~98%

Half-Life Elimination ~15-17 hour

Metabolism Hepatic; oxidation and hydroxylation, via CYP3A4 to primarily inactive metabolites

Excretion Feces (93%; 69% as parent drug)

Available Dosage Forms

Capsule, oral:
Tasigna®: 150 mg, 200 mg

Dosing

Adult & Geriatric

Ph+ CML, newly-diagnosed (chronic phase): Oral: 300 mg twice daily

Ph+ CML, resistant or intolerant (chronic or accelerated phase): Oral: 400 mg twice daily (continue treatment until disease progression or unacceptable toxicity)

Dosage adjustment for concomitant CYP3A4 inhibitors/inducers:

CYP3A4 inhibitors: The concomitant use of a strong CYP3A4 inhibitor with nilotinib is not recommended. If a strong CYP3A4 inhibitor is required, interruption of nilotinib treatment is recommended; if therapy cannot be interrupted and concurrent use can not be avoided, consider reducing the nilotinib dose to 300 mg once daily in patients with resistant or intolerant Ph+ CML or to 200 mg once daily in newly-diagnosed Ph+ CML, with careful monitoring, especially of the QT interval. When a strong CYP3A4 inhibitor is discontinued, allow a washout period prior to adjusting nilotinib dose upward.

CYP3A4 inducers: The concomitant use of a strong CYP3A4 inducer with nilotinib is not recommended.

Renal Impairment Not studied in patients with serum creatinine >1.5 times ULN, however, nilotinib and its metabolites have minimal renal excretion; dosage adjustments for renal dysfunction may not be needed.

Hepatic Impairment Note: Dosage adjustment for impairment at treatment initiation (if possible, consider alternative therapies first); recommendations vary by indication.

Newly-diagnosed Ph+ CML: Mild-to-severe impairment (Child-Pugh class A, B, or C): Initial: 200 mg twice daily; may increase to 300 mg twice daily based on patient tolerability

Resistant or intolerant Ph+ CML:
Mild-to-moderate impairment (Child-Pugh class A or B): Initial: 300 mg twice daily; may increase to 400 mg twice daily based on patient tolerability
Severe impairment (Child-Pugh class C): Initial: 200 mg twice daily; may increase to 300 mg twice daily and then further increased to 400 mg twice daily based on patient tolerability

For hepatotoxicity during treatment:
If bilirubin >3 times ULN (≥ grade 3): Withhold treatment, monitor bilirubin, resume treatment at 400 mg once daily when bilirubin returns to ≤1.5 times ULN (≤ grade 1)
If ALT or AST >5 times ULN (≥ grade 3): Withhold treatment, monitor transaminases, resume treatment at 400 mg once daily when ALT or AST returns to ≤2.5 times ULN (≤ grade 1)

Adjustment for Toxicity

Dosage adjustment for hematologic toxicity:
ANC <1000/mm^3 and/or platelets <50,000/mm^3: Withhold treatment, monitor blood counts
If ANC >1000/mm^3 and platelets >50,000/mm^3 within 2 weeks: Resume at prior dose
If ANC <1000/mm^3 and/or platelets <50,000/mm^3 for >2 weeks: Reduce dose to 400 mg once daily

Dosage adjustment for nonhematologic toxicity:
Amylase or lipase >2 times ULN (≥ grade 3): Withhold treatment, monitor serum amylase or lipase, resume treatment at 400 mg once daily when lipase or amylase returns to ≤1.5 times ULN (≤ grade 1)
Clinically-significant moderate or severe nonhematologic toxicity: Withhold treatment, upon resolution of toxicity, resume at 400 mg once daily; may escalate back to 300 mg or 400 mg twice daily (depending on indication) if clinically appropriate.

Dosage adjustment for QT prolongation: Note: Repeat ECG ~7 days after any dosage adjustment.

QT_c >480 msec: Withhold treatment, monitor and correct potassium and magnesium levels.

If QT_cF returns to <450 msec and to within 20 msec of baseline within 2 weeks: Resume at prior dose

If QT_cF returns to 450-480 msec for >2 weeks: Reduce dose to 400 mg once daily.

If QT_cF >480 msec after dosage reduction to 400 mg once daily, discontinue therapy.

Administration

Oral Administer twice daily doses ~12 hours apart. Swallow capsules whole with water. Administer on an empty stomach, at least 1 hour before or 2 hours after food.

Stability

Storage Store at 25°C (77°F); excursions permitted to 15°C to 30°C (59°F to 86°F).

Monitoring and Teaching Issues

Laboratory Monitoring CBC with differential (every 2 weeks for first 2 months, then monthly); electrolytes (including potassium and magnesium; baseline and periodic); lipid profile (periodic), hepatic function (ALT/AST, bilirubin, alkaline phosphatase; baseline and monthly or as clinically indicated); serum lipase (baseline and monthly or as clinically indicated)

Physical Assessment Assess for presence of hepatic impairment, history of pancreatitis, and galactose intolerance. Evaluate CBC, electrolytes, LFTs, and serum lipase at baseline and on a regular basis. Monitor for myelosuppression, cardiac changes, gastrointestinal disturbance, and hyperglycemia. Monitor pulmonary status.

Patient Education Take on an empty stomach, 1 hour before or 2 hours after a meal. Avoid grapefruit or grapefruit juice while taking this medication. Maintain adequate hydration unless instructed to restrict fluid intake. You may be required to have regularly scheduled laboratory tests while on this medication. You will be more susceptible to infection. You may experience diarrhea; constipation; insomnia or fatigue; nausea, vomiting, stomach pain, or dyspepsia; or unusual pain or weakness in joints, muscles, or bones. Report chest pain, rapid heart beat, or palpitations; swelling or unusual weight gain; unusual cough, respiratory difficulty, or wheezing; easy bruising; or unusual bleeding.

Dietary Considerations The bioavailability of nilotinib is increased with food. Take on an empty stomach, at least 1 hour before or 2 hours after food. Avoid grapefruit juice.

Breast-Feeding Considerations Due to the potential for serious adverse effects in the nursing infant, breast-feeding is not recommended.

Pregnancy Considerations Animal studies have demonstrated embryo-fetal toxicity and maternal toxicity. There are no adequate and well-controlled studies in pregnant women. Women of childbearing potential should be advised to use effective contraception during treatment.

Additional Information If clinically indicated, may be administered in combination with hematopoietic growth factors (eg, erythropoietin, filgrastim) and with hydroxyurea or anagrelide.

◆ **Nilotinib Hydrochloride Monohydrate** *see* Nilotinib *on page 1316*

Nilutamide (ni LOO ta mide)

U.S. Brand Names Nilandron®

Index Terms NSC-684588; RU-23908

Generic Availability (U.S.) No

Pharmacologic Category Antiandrogen; Antineoplastic Agent, Antiandrogen

Medication Safety Issues

Sound-alike/look-alike issues:

Nilutamide may be confused with nilotinib

Pregnancy Risk Factor C

Lactation Not indicated for use in women

Use Treatment of metastatic prostate cancer

Mechanism of Action/Effect Nonsteroidal antiandrogen that inhibits androgen uptake or inhibits binding of androgen in target tissues

Contraindications Hypersensitivity to nilutamide or any component of the formulation; severe hepatic impairment; severe respiratory insufficiency

Warnings/Precautions Hazardous agent - use appropriate precautions for handling and disposal. **[U.S. Boxed Warning]: Interstitial pneumonitis has been reported in 2% of patients exposed to nilutamide.** Patients typically experienced progressive exertional dyspnea, and possibly cough, chest pain and fever. X-rays showed interstitial or alveolo-interstitial changes. The suggestive signs of pneumonitis most often occurred within the first 3 months of nilutamide treatment.

Hepatitis or marked increases in liver enzymes leading to drug discontinuation occurred in 1% of nilutamide patients. Rare cases of elevated hepatic enzymes followed by death have been reported.

Thirteen percent to 57% of patients receiving nilutamide reported a delay in adaptation to the dark, ranging from seconds to a few minutes. This effect sometimes does not abate as drug treatment is continued. Caution patients who experience this effect about driving at night or through tunnels. This effect can be alleviated by wearing tinted glasses.

Drug Interactions

Metabolism/Transport Effects Substrate of CYP2C19 (major); **Inhibits** CYP2C19 (weak)

Avoid Concomitant Use There are no known interactions where it is recommended to avoid concomitant use.

Decreased Effect

The levels/effects of Nilutamide may be decreased by: CYP2C19 Inducers (Strong)

Increased Effect/Toxicity

The levels/effects of Nilutamide may be increased by: CYP2C19 Inhibitors (Moderate); CYP2C19 Inhibitors (Strong)

Nutritional/Ethanol Interactions

Ethanol: Avoid ethanol. Up to 5% of patients may experience a systemic reaction (flushing, hypotension, malaise) when combined with nilutamide.

Herb/Nutraceutical: St John's wort may decrease nilutamide levels.

Adverse Reactions

>10%:

- Central nervous system: Headache, insomnia
- Endocrine & metabolic: Hot flashes (30% to 67%), gynecomastia (10%)
- Gastrointestinal: Nausea (mild - 10% to 32%), abdominal pain (10%), constipation, anorexia
- Genitourinary: Testicular atrophy (16%), libido decreased
- Hepatic: Transaminases increased (8% to 13%; transient)
- Ocular: Impaired dark adaptation (13% to 57%), usually reversible with dose reduction, may require discontinuation of the drug in 1% to 2% of patients
- Respiratory: Dyspnea (11%)

1% to 10%:

- Cardiovascular: Chest pain, edema, heart failure, hypertension, syncope
- Central nervous system: Dizziness, drowsiness, fever, malaise, hypoesthesia, depression
- Dermatologic: Pruritus, alopecia, dry skin, rash
- Endocrine & metabolic: Disulfiram-like reaction (hot flashes, rash) (5%)
- Gastrointestinal: Vomiting, diarrhea, dyspepsia, GI hemorrhage, melena, weight loss, xerostomia
- Genitourinary: Hematuria, nocturia
- Hematologic: Anemia
- Hepatic: Hepatitis (1%)
- Neuromuscular & skeletal: Arthritis, paresthesia
- Ocular: Chromatopsia (9%), abnormal vision (6% to 7%), cataracts, photophobia
- Respiratory: Interstitial pneumonitis (2% - typically exertional dyspnea, cough, chest pain, and fever; most often occurring within the first 3 months of treatment); rhinitis
- Miscellaneous: Diaphoresis, flu-like syndrome

Pharmacodynamics/Kinetics

Absorption Rapid and complete

Protein Binding 72% to 85%

Half-Life Elimination Terminal: 23-87 hours; Metabolites: 35-137 hours

Metabolism Hepatic, forms active metabolites

Excretion Urine (up to 78% at 120 hours; <1% as unchanged drug); feces (1% to 7%)

Available Dosage Forms

Tablet, oral:

Nilandron®: 150 mg

Dosing

Adult & Geriatric Refer to individual protocols. **Prostate cancer:** Oral: 300 mg daily for 30 days starting the same day or day after surgical castration, then 150 mg/day

Administration

Oral Administer without regard to meals.

Stability

Storage Store at room temperature of 15°C to 30°C (59°F to 86°F). Protect from light.

Monitoring and Teaching Issues

Laboratory Monitoring Chest x-rays prior to and regularly during treatment. Measure serum hepatic enzyme levels at baseline and at regular intervals (3 months). If transaminases increase over 2-3 times the upper limit of normal, discontinue treatment. Perform appropriate laboratory testing at the first symptom/sign of liver injury (eg, jaundice, dark urine, fatigue, abdominal pain, or unexplained GI symptoms).

Physical Assessment Evaluate results of chest x-rays and laboratory tests at baseline and at regular 3-month intervals. Monitor for signs of interstitial pneumonitis (dyspnea, chest pain, cough, fever), hepatitis, or visual changes (impaired dark adaptation). Teach patient orthostatic precautions.

Patient Education Avoid alcohol while taking this medication; may cause severe adverse reaction. Periodic laboratory tests are necessary while taking this medication. May cause loss of light accommodation, dizziness, confusion, blurred vision, nausea, anorexia, hot flashes, gynecomastia, decreased libido, impotence, or sexual dysfunction (consult prescriber). Report any decreased respiratory function (eg, dyspnea, increased cough), unexplained fever, or difficulty or painful voiding or blood in urine.

Dietary Considerations May be taken without regard to meals.

Geriatric Considerations Your eyes may be slow to adapt to darkness; be careful when driving at night; tinted glasses may help.

Pregnancy Considerations Not indicated for use in women

◆ **Nimbex®** *see* Cisatracurium *on page* 382

NiMODipine (nye MOE di peen)

Generic Availability (U.S.) Yes

Pharmacologic Category Calcium Channel Blocker; Calcium Channel Blocker, Dihydropyridine

Medication Safety Issues

Sound-alike/look-alike issues:

NiMODipine may be confused with niCARdipine, NIFEdipine, nisoldipine

Administration issues: **For oral administration only.** For patients unable to swallow a capsule, the drug should be dispensed in an oral syringe (preferably amber in color) labeled **"WARNING: For ORAL use only"** or **"Not for I.V. use."** Nimodipine has inadvertently been administered I.V. when withdrawn from capsules into a syringe for subsequent nasogastric tube administration. Severe cardiovascular adverse events, including fatalities, have resulted. Employ precautions against such an event.

Pregnancy Risk Factor C

Lactation Enters breast milk/not recommended

Use Vasospasm following subarachnoid hemorrhage from ruptured intracranial aneurysms

Unlabeled/Investigational Use Prevention of migraines (inconsistent data)

Mechanism of Action/Effect Nimodipine shares the pharmacology of other calcium channel blockers; animal studies indicate that nimodipine has a greater effect on cerebral arterials than other arterials; inhibits calcium ion from entering the "slow channels" or select voltage sensitive areas of vascular smooth muscle and myocardium during depolarization

Contraindications Hypersensitivity to nimodipine or any component of the formulation

Warnings/Precautions Increased angina and/or MI has occurred with initiation or dosage titration of calcium channel blockers. The most common side effect is peripheral edema; occurs within 2-3 weeks of starting therapy. Reflex tachycardia may occur with use. Symptomatic hypotension with or without syncope can rarely occur; blood pressure must be lowered at a rate appropriate for the patient's clinical condition. Use caution in hepatic impairment. Intestinal pseudo-obstruction and ileus have been reported during the use of nimodipine. Use caution in patients with decreased GI motility of a history of bowel obstruction. Use caution when treating patients with hypertrophic cardiomyopathy.

[U.S. Boxed Warning]: Nimodipine has inadvertently been administered I.V. when withdrawn from capsules into a syringe for subsequent nasogastric administration. Severe cardiovascular adverse events, including fatalities, have resulted; precautions (eg, adequate labeling, use of oral syringes) should be employed against such an event.

Drug Interactions

Metabolism/Transport Effects Substrate of CYP3A4 (major)

Avoid Concomitant Use

Avoid concomitant use of NiMODipine with any of the following: Grapefruit Juice

Decreased Effect

NiMODipine may decrease the levels/effects of: Clopidogrel; QuiNIDine

The levels/effects of NiMODipine may be decreased by: Barbiturates; Calcium Salts; CarBAMazepine; CYP3A4 Inducers (Strong); Deferasirox; Herbs (CYP3A4 Inducers); Herbs (Hypertensive Properties); Methylphenidate; Nafcillin; Rifamycin Derivatives; Yohimbine

Increased Effect/Toxicity

NiMODipine may increase the levels/effects of: Amifostine; Antihypertensives; Calcium Channel Blockers (Nondihydropyridine); Hypotensive Agents; Magnesium Salts; Neuromuscular-Blocking Agents (Nondepolarizing); Nitroprusside; Phenytoin; RiTUXimab; Tacrolimus; Tacrolimus (Systemic)

The levels/effects of NiMODipine may be increased by: Alpha1-Blockers; Antifungal Agents (Azole Derivatives, Systemic); Calcium Channel Blockers (Nondihydropyridine); Cimetidine; Conivaptan; CycloSPORINE; CycloSPORINE (Systemic); CYP3A4 Inhibitors (Moderate); CYP3A4 Inhibitors (Strong); Dasatinib; Diazoxide; Fluconazole; Grapefruit Juice; Herbs (Hypotensive Properties); Macrolide Antibiotics; Magnesium Salts; MAO Inhibitors; Pentoxifylline; Phosphodiesterase 5 Inhibitors; Prostacyclin Analogues; Protease Inhibitors

Nutritional/Ethanol Interactions

Food: Nimodipine has shown a 1.5-fold increase in bioavailability when taken with grapefruit juice; avoid concurrent use.

Herb/Nutraceutical: St John's wort may decrease levels. Avoid dong quai if using for hypertension (has estrogenic activity). Avoid ephedra, yohimbe, ginseng (may worsen hypertension). Avoid garlic (may have increased antihypertensive effect).

Adverse Reactions 1% to 10%:

Cardiovascular: Reductions in systemic blood pressure (1% to 8%)

Central nervous system: Headache (1% to 4%)

Dermatologic: Rash (1% to 2%)

Gastrointestinal: Diarrhea (2% to 4%), abdominal discomfort (2%)

Pharmacodynamics/Kinetics

Bioavailability 13%

Time to Peak Serum: ~1 hour

Protein Binding >95%

Half-Life Elimination 1-2 hours; prolonged with renal impairment

Metabolism Extensively hepatic

Excretion Urine (50%) and feces (32%) within 4 days

Available Dosage Forms

Capsule, liquid filled, oral: 30 mg

Capsule, softgel, oral: 30 mg

Dosing

Adult & Geriatric Note: Capsules and contents are for oral/NG tube administration **ONLY.**

Subarachnoid hemorrhage: Oral: 60 mg every 4 hours for 21 days, start therapy within 96 hours after subarachnoid hemorrhage.

Renal Impairment Not removed by hemo- or peritoneal dialysis; supplemental dose is not necessary.

Hepatic Impairment Reduce dosage to 30 mg every 4 hours in patients with liver failure.

Administration

Oral For oral administration ONLY. Life-threatening adverse events have occurred when administered parenterally.

Nasogastric (NG) tube administration: If the capsules cannot be swallowed, the liquid may be removed by making a hole in each end of the capsule with an 18-gauge needle and extracting the contents into a syringe; transfer these contents into an oral syringe (amber-colored oral syringe preferred). It is strongly recommended that preparation be done in the pharmacy. Label oral syringe with **"WARNING: For ORAL use only"** or **"Not for I.V. use."** Follow with a flush of 30 mL NS.

Monitoring and Teaching Issues

Physical Assessment Assess blood pressure and cardiac status. Monitor for rash, hypotension, constipation, and peripheral edema when starting or adjusting dose and periodically during therapy.

Patient Education May cause orthostatic hypotension, headache, or constipation. Report chest pain, palpitations, severe constipation, ankle swelling, or respiratory difficulty.

Geriatric Considerations Elderly may experience a greater hypotensive response. Constipation may be more of a problem in the elderly. Studies in the treatment of Alzheimer's disease have not demonstrated clear clinical effect.

Pregnancy Considerations Use in pregnancy only when clearly needed and when the benefits outweigh the potential hazard to the fetus. Teratogenic and embryotoxic effects have been demonstrated in small animals. No well-controlled studies have been conducted in pregnant women.

Related Information

Calcium Channel Blockers *on page 1993*

◆ **Niravam™** *see* ALPRAZolam *on page 80*

Nisoldipine (nye SOL di peen)

U.S. Brand Names Sular®

Generic Availability (U.S.) Yes

Pharmacologic Category Calcium Channel Blocker; Calcium Channel Blocker, Dihydropyridine

Medication Safety Issues

Sound-alike/look-alike issues:

Nisoldipine may be confused with NIFEdipine, niMODipine

Pregnancy Risk Factor C

Lactation Excretion in breast milk unknown/not recommended

Use Management of hypertension, alone or in combination with other antihypertensive agents

Mechanism of Action/Effect As a dihydropyridine calcium channel blocker, structurally similar to nifedipine, nisoldipine impedes the movement of calcium ions into vascular smooth muscle and cardiac muscle. Dihydropyridines are potent vasodilators and are not as likely to suppress cardiac contractility and slow cardiac conduction as other calcium antagonists such as verapamil and diltiazem; nisoldipine is 5-10 times as potent a vasodilator as nifedipine.

Contraindications Hypersensitivity to nisoldipine, any component of the formulation, or other dihydropyridine calcium channel blockers

Warnings/Precautions With initiation or dosage titration of dihydropyridine calcium channel blockers, reflex tachycardia may occur resulting in angina and/or MI in patients with obstructive coronary disease especially in the absence of concurrent beta-blockade. Use with caution in patients with severe aortic stenosis, HF, and hypertrophic cardiomyopathy with outflow tract obstruction. Use with caution in hepatic impairment; lower starting dose required. The most common side effect is peripheral edema; occurs within 2-3 weeks of starting therapy. Symptomatic hypotension with or without syncope can rarely occur; blood pressure must be lowered at a rate appropriate for the patient's clinical condition. Some dosage forms contain tartrazine, which may cause allergic reactions in certain individuals (eg, aspirin hypersensitivity). Use with caution in patients >65 years of age; lower starting dose recommended.

Drug Interactions

Metabolism/Transport Effects Substrate of CYP3A4 (major); **Inhibits** CYP1A2 (weak), 3A4 (weak)

Avoid Concomitant Use

Avoid concomitant use of Nisoldipine with any of the following: CYP3A4 Inducers (Strong); CYP3A4 Inhibitors (Strong); Grapefruit Juice

Decreased Effect

Nisoldipine may decrease the levels/effects of: Clopidogrel

The levels/effects of Nisoldipine may be decreased by: Barbiturates; Calcium Salts; CarBAMazepine; CYP3A4 Inducers (Strong); Deferasirox; Herbs (CYP3A4 Inducers); Herbs (Hypertensive Properties); Methylphenidate; Nafcillin; Rifamycin Derivatives; Yohimbine

Increased Effect/Toxicity

Nisoldipine may increase the levels/effects of: Amifostine; Antihypertensives; Calcium Channel Blockers (Nondihydropyridine); Hypotensive Agents; Magnesium Salts; Neuromuscular-Blocking Agents (Nondepolarizing); Nitroprusside; Phenytoin; RiTUXimab; Tacrolimus; Tacrolimus (Systemic)

The levels/effects of Nisoldipine may be increased by: Alpha1-Blockers; Antifungal Agents (Azole Derivatives, Systemic); Calcium Channel Blockers (Nondihydropyridine); Cimetidine; CycloSPORINE; CycloSPORINE (Systemic); CYP3A4 Inhibitors (Moderate); CYP3A4 Inhibitors (Strong); Dasatinib; Diazoxide; Fluconazole; Grapefruit Juice; Herbs (Hypotensive Properties); Macrolide Antibiotics; Magnesium Salts; MAO Inhibitors; Pentoxifylline; Phosphodiesterase 5 Inhibitors; Prostacyclin Analogues; Protease Inhibitors

Nutritional/Ethanol Interactions

Food: Peak concentrations of nisoldipine may be significantly increased if taken with high-lipid foods; however, total exposure (AUC) may be reduced. Grapefruit juice has been shown to significantly increase the bioavailability of nisoldipine; avoid grapefruit products before and after dosing.

Herb/Nutraceutical: Avoid St John's wort (may decrease nisoldipine levels). Avoid bayberry, blue cohosh, cayenne, ephedra, ginger, ginseng (American), kola, licorice (may worsen hypertension). Avoid black cohosh, California poppy, coleus, golden seal, hawthorn, mistletoe, periwinkle, quinine, shepherd's purse (may have increased antihypertensive effect).

Adverse Reactions

>10%:

Cardiovascular: Peripheral edema (dose related; 7% to 29%)

Central nervous system: Headache (22%)

1% to 10%:

Cardiovascular: Vasodilation (4%), palpitation (3%), angina exacerbation (2%), chest pain (2%)

Central nervous system: Dizziness (3% to 10%)

Dermatologic: Rash (2%)

Gastrointestinal: Nausea (2%)

Respiratory: Pharyngitis (5%), sinusitis (3%)

Pharmacodynamics/Kinetics

Duration of Action >24 hours

Absorption Well absorbed. Peak concentrations significantly increased with high-lipid meals; however, AUC is reduced.

Bioavailability ~5%

Time to Peak 4-14 hours

Protein Binding >99%

Half-Life Elimination 9-18 hours

Metabolism Extensively hepatic; 1 active metabolite (10% of activity of parent); first-pass effect

Excretion Urine (60% to 80% as inactive metabolites); feces

Available Dosage Forms

Tablet, extended release, oral: 8.5 mg, 17 mg, 20 mg, 25.5 mg, 30 mg, 34 mg, 40 mg

Sular®: 8.5 mg, 17 mg, 25.5 mg, 34 mg

Dosing

Adult Hypertension: Oral:

Sular® (Geomatrix® delivery system): Oral: Initial: 17 mg once daily, then increase by 8.5 mg/week (or longer intervals) to attain adequate control of blood pressure

Usual dose range: 17-34 mg once daily; doses >34 mg once daily are not recommended

Nisoldipine extended-release tablet (original formulation): Initial: 20 mg once daily, then increase by 10 mg/week (or longer intervals) to attain adequate control of blood pressure

Usual dose range (JNC 7): 10-40 mg once daily; doses >60 mg once daily are not recommended

Conversion from nisoldipine extended-release (original formulation) to Sular® Geomatrix® delivery system:

Nisoldipine Extended Release Dosing Equivalency

Original Extended Release Formulation	Sular® Extended Release (Geomatrix® delivery system)
10 mg	8.5 mg
20 mg	17 mg
30 mg	25.5 mg
40 mg	34 mg

Geriatric Hypertension: Oral:

Sular® (Geomatrix® delivery system): Initial dose: 8.5 mg once daily; increase by 8.5 mg/week (or longer intervals) to attain adequate blood pressure control

Nisoldipine extended-release (original formulation): Initial dose: 10 mg once daily; increase by 10 mg/week (or longer intervals) to attain adequate blood pressure control.

Conversion from nisoldipine extended-release (original formulation) to Sular® Geomatrix® delivery system: Refer to adult dosing.

Hepatic Impairment

Sular® (Geomatrix® delivery system): An initial dose exceeding 8.5 mg once daily is not recommended for patients with hepatic impairment.

Nisoldipine extended-release (original formulation): An initial dose exceeding 10 mg once daily is not recommended for patients with hepatic impairment.

Administration

Oral Administer at the same time each day to ensure minimal fluctuation of serum levels. Avoid high-fat diet. Administer on an empty stomach (1 hour before or 2 hours after a meal). Swallow whole; do not crush, break, split, or chew.

Stability

Storage Store at controlled room temperature of 20°C to 25°C (68°F to 77°F). Protect from light; protect from moisture.

Monitoring and Teaching Issues

Physical Assessment Use caution in presence of severe aortic stenosis, HF, hypertrophic cardiomyopathy with outflow tract obstruction, or hepatic impairment. Assess cardiac status and blood pressure. Monitor for chest pain, dyspnea, edema, rash, and constipation when starting or adjusting dose and periodically during therapy. When discontinuing, taper dose gradually.

Patient Education Do not crush or chew tablets; swallow whole. Take on an empty stomach (1 hour before or 2 hours after a meal). This drug does not replace diet and other exercise recommendations of prescriber. May cause orthostatic hypotension, headache, dizziness, or constipation. Report weight gain or swelling of extremities, chest pain, palpitations, persistent dizziness, respiratory difficulty, rash, or fatigue.

Dietary Considerations Take on an empty stomach (1 hour before or 2 hours after a meal). Avoid grapefruit juice before and after dosing. Avoid grapefuit juice; avoid high-fat diet.

Geriatric Considerations Elderly have been found to have two- to threefold greater serum concentrations than younger adults. Therefore, begin therapy at lowest recommended doses. Elderly may experience a greater hypotensive response. Constipation may be more of a problem in the elderly. Calcium channel blockers are no more effective in the elderly than other therapies; however, they do not cause significant CNS effects which is an advantage over some antihypertensive agents.

Pregnancy Considerations Animal studies have demonstrated fetotoxic but not teratogenic effects. There are no adequate and well-controlled studies in pregnant women. Use during pregnancy only if potential benefit to the mother outweighs potential risk to the fetus.

Related Information

Calcium Channel Blockers *on page* 1993

◆ **Nitalapram** *see* Citalopram *on page* 386

Nitazoxanide (nye ta ZOX a nide)

U.S. Brand Names Alinia®

Index Terms NTZ

Generic Availability (U.S.) No

Pharmacologic Category Antiprotozoal

Pregnancy Risk Factor B

Lactation Excretion in breast milk unknown/use caution

Use Treatment of diarrhea caused by *Cryptosporidium parvum* or *Giardia lamblia*

Unlabeled/Investigational Use Alternative treatment for *Clostridium difficile*-associated diarrhea (CDAD)

Mechanism of Action/Effect Nitazoxanide is rapidly metabolized to the active metabolite tizoxanide *in vivo*. Nitazoxanide and its metabolite inhibit the growth of sporozoites and oocysts of *Cryptosporidium parvum* and trophozoites of *Giardia lamblia*.

Contraindications Hypersensitivity to nitazoxanide or any component of the formulation

Warnings/Precautions Use caution with renal or hepatic impairment. Safety and efficacy have not been established with HIV infection, immunodeficiency, or in children <1 year of age (suspension) and <12 years of age (tablet).

Drug Interactions

Avoid Concomitant Use There are no known interactions where it is recommended to avoid concomitant use.

Decreased Effect There are no known significant interactions involving a decrease in effect.

Increased Effect/Toxicity There are no known significant interactions involving an increase in effect.

Nutritional/Ethanol Interactions Food: Food increases AUC.

Adverse Reactions Rates of adverse effects were similar to those reported with placebo.

1% to 10%:

Central nervous system: Headache (1% to 3%)

Gastrointestinal: Abdominal pain (7% to 8%), diarrhea (2% to 4%), nausea (3%), vomiting (1%)

Pharmacodynamics/Kinetics

Bioavailability Relative bioavailability of suspension compared to tablet: 70%

Time to Peak Plasma: Tizoxanide and tizoxanide glucuronide: 1-4 hours

Protein Binding Tizoxanide: >99%

Metabolism Hepatic, to an active metabolite, tizoxanide. Tizoxanide undergoes conjugation to form tizoxanide glucuronide. Nitazoxanide is not detectable in the serum following oral administration.

Excretion Tizoxanide: Urine, bile, and feces; Tizoxanide glucuronide: Urine and bile

Available Dosage Forms

Powder for suspension, oral:
Alinia®: 100 mg/5 mL (60 mL)

Tablet, oral:
Alinia®: 500 mg

Dosing

Adult & Geriatric Diarrhea caused by *Cryptosporidium parvum* or *Giardia lamblia*: Oral: 500 mg every 12 hours for 3 days

***Clostridium difficile* -associated diarrhea (unlabeled use):** Oral: 500 mg every 12 hours for 10 days (Musher, 2009)

Pediatric Diarrhea caused by *Cryptosporidium parvum* or *Giardia lamblia*: Oral: **Note:** May consider increasing duration up to 14 days in HIV-exposed/-infected patients with crypotosporidiosis (CDC, 2009):

Children 1-3 years: 100 mg every 12 hours for 3 days; may consider increasing duration up to 14 days in HIV-exposed/-infected patients with crypotosporidiosis (CDC, 2009)

Children 4-11 years: 200 mg every 12 hours for 3 days; may consider increasing duration up to 14 days in HIV-exposed/-infected patients with crypotosporidiosis (CDC, 2009)

Children ≥12 years: Refer to adult dosing.

Renal Impairment Specific recommendations are not available; use with caution.

Hepatic Impairment Specific recommendations are not available; use with caution.

Administration

Oral Administer with food. Shake suspension well prior to administration.

Stability

Reconstitution For preparation at time of dispensing, add 48 mL incrementally to 60 mL bottle; shake vigorously. Resulting suspension is 20 mg/mL (100 mg per 5 mL).

Storage

Suspension: Prior to and following reconstitution, store at room temperature of 15°C to 30°C (59°F to 86°F). Following reconstitution, discard unused portion of suspension after 7 days.

Tablet: Store at room temperature.

Monitoring and Teaching Issues

Patient Education Administer with food. May cause headache, abdominal pain, diarrhea, or vomiting. If severe or persistent, contact prescriber.

Dietary Considerations Should be taken with food.

Pregnancy Considerations Teratogenic effects were not observed in animal studies. There are no adequate and well-controlled studies in pregnant women.

◆ **4'-Nitro-3'-Trifluoromethylisobutyrantide** *see* Flutamide *on page 797*

◆ **Nitro-Bid®** *see* Nitroglycerin *on page 1327*

◆ **Nitro-Dur®** *see* Nitroglycerin *on page 1327*

Nitrofurantoin (nye troe fyoor AN toyn)

U.S. Brand Names Furadantin®; Macrobid®; Macrodantin®

Generic Availability (U.S.) Yes: Excludes suspension

Pharmacologic Category Antibiotic, Miscellaneous

Medication Safety Issues

Sound alike/look alike issues:
Macrobid® may be confused with microK®, Nitro-Bid®
Nitrofurantoin may be confused with Neurontin®, nitroglycerin

Beers Criteria medication: This drug may be inappropriate for use in geriatric patients (high severity risk).

Pregnancy Risk Factor B (contraindicated at term)

Lactation Enters breast milk/not recommended (infants <1 month); AAP rates "compatible" (AAP 2001 update pending)

Use Prevention and treatment of urinary tract infections caused by susceptible strains of *E. coli, S. aureus, Enterococcus, Klebsiella,* and *Enterobacter*

Mechanism of Action/Effect Inhibits several bacterial enzyme systems including acetyl coenzyme A interfering with metabolism and possibly cell wall synthesis

Contraindications Hypersensitivity to nitrofurantoin or any component of the formulation; significant renal impairment (anuria, oliguria, significantly elevated serum creatinine, or Cl_{cr} <60 mL/minute); infants <1 month (due to the possibility of hemolytic anemia); pregnancy at term (38-42 weeks gestation), during labor and delivery, or when the onset of labor is imminent; use in patients with a history of cholestatic jaundice or hepatic impairment with previous nitrofurantoin therapy

Warnings/Precautions Use with caution in patients with G6PD deficiency (increased risk of hemolytic anemia). Therapeutic concentrations of nitrofurantoin are not attained in urine of patients with Cl_{cr} <60 mL/minute, therefore, use contraindicated in these patients. Use with caution if prolonged therapy is anticipated due to possible pulmonary toxicity. Acute, subacute, or chronic (usually after 6 months of therapy) pulmonary reactions (possibly fatal) have been observed in patients treated with nitrofurantoin; if these occur, discontinue therapy immediately; monitor closely for malaise, dyspnea, cough, fever, radiologic evidence of diffuse interstitial pneumonitis or fibrosis. Rare, but severe and sometimes fatal hepatic reactions (eg, cholestatic jaundice, hepatitis, hepatic necrosis) have been associated with nitrofurantoin (onset may be insidious); discontinue immediately if hepatitis occurs. Monitor liver function test periodically. Has been associated with peripheral neuropathy (rare); risk may be increased in patients with anemia, renal impairment, diabetes, vitamin B deficiency, debilitating disease, or electrolyte imbalance; use caution. Use in the elderly is not recommended due to potential for renal impairment; alternative agents preferred (Beers Criteria). Prolonged use may result in fungal or bacterial superinfection, including *C. difficile*-associated diarrhea (CDAD) and pseudomembranous colitis; CDAD has been observed >2 months postantibiotic treatment. Use is contraindicated in children <1 month of age (at increased risk for hemolytic anemia). Not indicated for the treatment of pyelonephritis or perinephric abscesses.

Drug Interactions

Avoid Concomitant Use

Avoid concomitant use of Nitrofurantoin with any of the following: BCG; Magnesium Trisilicate; Norfloxacin

Decreased Effect

Nitrofurantoin may decrease the levels/effects of: BCG; Norfloxacin; Typhoid Vaccine

The levels/effects of Nitrofurantoin may be decreased by: Magnesium Trisilicate

Increased Effect/Toxicity

The levels/effects of Nitrofurantoin may be increased by: Probenecid

Nutritional/Ethanol Interactions

Ethanol: Avoid ethanol (may increase CNS depression).

Food: Nitrofurantoin serum concentrations may be increased if taken with food.

Lab Interactions False-positive urine glucose (Benedict's and Fehling's methods); no false positives with enzymatic tests

Adverse Reactions Frequency not defined.

Cardiovascular: Cyanosis, ECG changes (nonspecific ST/T wave changes, bundle branch block)

Central nervous system: Bulging fontanels (infants), chills, confusion, depression, dizziness, drowsiness, fever, headache, malaise, pseudotumor cerebri, psychotic reaction, vertigo

Dermatologic: Alopecia, angioedema, erythema multiforme, exfoliative dermatitis, pruritus, rash (eczematous, erythematous, maculopapular), Stevens-Johnson syndrome, urticaria

Endocrine & metabolic: Hyperphosphatemia

Gastrointestinal: Abdominal pain, anorexia, *C. difficile* colitis, constipation, diarrhea, dyspepsia, flatulence, nausea, pancreatitis, pseudomembranous colitis, sialadenitis, vomiting

Genitourinary: Urine discoloration (brown)

Hematologic: Agranulocytosis, aplastic anemia, eosinophilia, glucose-6-phosphate dehydrogenase deficiency anemia, granulocytopenia, hemoglobin decreased, hemolytic anemia, leukopenia, megaloblastic anemia, thrombocytopenia

Hepatic: Hepatitis, hepatic necrosis, transaminases increased, jaundice (cholestatic)

Neuromuscular & skeletal: Arthralgia, myalgia, numbness, paresthesia, peripheral neuropathy, weakness

Ocular: Amblyopia, nystagmus, optic neuritis

Respiratory: Cough, dyspnea, pneumonitis, pulmonary fibrosis (with long-term use), pulmonary infiltration

Miscellaneous: Acute pulmonary reaction (symptoms include chills, chest pain, cough, dyspnea, fever, and eosinophilia), anaphylaxis, hypersensitivity (including acute pulmonary hypersensitivity), lupus-like syndrome, superinfections (eg, *Pseudomonas* or *Candida*)

Pharmacodynamics/Kinetics

Absorption Well absorbed; macrocrystalline is absorbed more slowly due to slower dissolution (causes less GI distress)

Bioavailability Increased with food

Protein Binding 60% to 90%

Half-Life Elimination 20-60 minutes; prolonged with renal impairment

Metabolism Body tissues (except plasma) metabolize 60% of drug to inactive metabolites

Excretion

Suspension: Urine (~40%) and feces (small amounts) as metabolites and unchanged drug

Macrocrystals: Urine (20% to 25% as unchanged drug)

Available Dosage Forms

Capsule, oral: 50 mg, 100 mg

Macrobid®: 100 mg

Macrodantin®: 25 mg, 50 mg, 100 mg

Suspension, oral:

Furadantin®: 25 mg/5 mL (230 mL)

Dosing

Adult

UTI treatment:

Furadantin®, Macrodantin®: Oral: 50-100 mg/dose every 6 hours; administer for 7 days or at least 3 days after obtaining sterile urine

Macrobid®: Oral: 100 mg twice daily for 7 days

UTI prophylaxis (Furadantin®, Macrodantin®): Oral: 50-100 mg/dose at bedtime

Geriatric Refer to adult dosing

Pediatric

UTI treatment:

Children >1 month (Furadantin®, Macrodantin®): Oral: 5-7 mg/kg/day in divided doses every 6 hours (maximum: 400 mg/day). Administer for 7 days or at least 3 days after obtaining sterile urine.

Children >12 years (Macrobid®): Oral: Refer to adult dosing.

UTI prophylaxis: Children >1 month (Furadantin®, Macrodantin®): Oral: 1-2 mg/kg/day in divided doses every 12-24 hours (maximum: 100 mg/day)

Renal Impairment

Cl_{cr} <60 mL/minute: Contraindicated

Contraindicated in hemo- and peritoneal dialysis and continuous arteriovenous or venovenous hemofiltration.

Administration

Oral Administer with meals to improve absorption and decrease adverse effects; suspension may be mixed with water, milk, fruit juice, or infant formula. Shake suspension well before use.

Stability

Storage Store at 20°C to 25°C (68°F to 77°F); excursions permitted to 15°C to 30°C (59°F to 86°F). Protect oral suspension from light.

Monitoring and Teaching Issues

Laboratory Monitoring CBC, periodic liver function, periodic renal function tests with long-term use; perform culture and sensitivity prior to initiating therapy

Physical Assessment Assess allergy history and renal status prior to beginning therapy.

Patient Education Take with food. Suspension may be mixed with water, milk, fruit juice, or infant formula. Shake suspension well before use. Maintain adequate hydration unless instructed to restrict fluid intake. May cause nausea, vomiting, or diarrhea. Report immediately any rash; swelling of face, tongue, mouth, or throat; or chest tightness. Report if condition being treated worsens or does not improve by the time prescription is completed.

Dietary Considerations Take with meals to improve absorption and decrease adverse effects.

Geriatric Considerations Because of nitrofurantoin's decreased efficacy in patients with a Cl_{cr} <60 mL/minute and its side effect profile, it is not an antibiotic of choice for acute or prophylactic treatment of urinary tract infections in the elderly. An increased rate of severe hepatic toxicity has been suggested by postmarketing reports.

This medication is considered to be potentially inappropriate in this patient population (Beers Criteria severity: High).

Breast-Feeding Considerations Minimal, if any, nitrofurantoin distributes to human milk. Use of nitrofurantoin during breast-feeding is not recommended by the manufacturer. Use with caution in patients at risk for G6PD deficiency or in newborns at risk for hyperbilirubinemia. Nondose-related effects could include modification of bowel flora.

Pregnancy Considerations Because adverse effects have not been observed in animals, nitrofurantoin is classified pregnancy category B. Nitrofurantoin crosses the placenta, but very little reaches the amniotic fluid. Most published experiences with nitrofurantoin use during pregnancy have failed to identify any increased obstetric or teratogenic risks. Isolated reports of a potential increased risk for cardiovascular defects and a case report of upper limb paralysis have not been replicated in other studies. Use of nitrofurantoin during pregnancy has been generally well tolerated with rare reports of maternal toxicity including severe pulmonary reactions or hematologic adverse effects. Nitrofurantoin is contraindicated in pregnant patients at term (38-42 weeks gestation), during labor and delivery, or when the onset of labor is imminent due to the possibility of hemolytic anemia in the neonate.

Nitroglycerin (nye troe GLI ser in)

U.S. Brand Names Minitran™; Nitro-Bid®; Nitro-Dur®; Nitro-Time®; Nitrolingual®; NitroMist®; Nitrostat®

Index Terms Glyceryl Trinitrate; Nitroglycerol; NTG; Tridil

Generic Availability (U.S.) Yes: Capsule, injection, patch, tablet

Pharmacologic Category Vasodilator

Medication Safety Issues

Sound-alike/look-alike issues:

Nitroglycerin may be confused with nitrofurantoin, nitroprusside

Nitro-Bid® may be confused with Macrobid®, Nicobid®

Nitroderm may be confused with NicoDerm®

Nitrol® may be confused with Nizoral®

Nitrostat® may be confused with Nilstat®, nystatin

Transdermal patch may contain conducting metal (eg, aluminum); remove patch prior to MRI.

International issues:

Nitrocor [Italy, Russia, and Venezuela] may be confused with Natrecor brand name for nesiritide [U.S., Canada, and multiple international markets] and Nutracort brand name for hydrocortisone in the [U.S. and multiple international markets]

Nitro-Dur [U.S., Canada, and multiple international markets] may be confused with Nitrocor [Italy, Russia, and Venezuela]

Pregnancy Risk Factor C

Lactation Excretion in breast milk unknown/use caution

Use Treatment or prevention of angina pectoris

Intravenous (I.V.) administration: Treatment or prevention of angina pectoris; acute decompensated heart failure (especially when associated with acute myocardial infarction); perioperative hypertension (especially during cardiovascular surgery); induction of intraoperative hypotension

Unlabeled/Investigational Use Short-term management of pulmonary hypertension (I.V.); esophageal spastic disorders

Mechanism of Action/Effect Relaxes smooth muscle, producing a vasodilator effect on the peripheral veins and arteries with more prominent effects on the veins. Primarily reduces cardiac oxygen demand by decreasing preload (left ventricular end-diastolic pressure); may modestly reduce afterload; dilates coronary arteries and improves collateral flow to ischemic regions

Contraindications Hypersensitivity to organic nitrates or any component of the formulation (includes adhesives for transdermal product); concurrent use with phosphodiesterase-5 (PDE-5) inhibitors (sildenafil, tadalafil, or vardenafil); increased intracranial pressure; severe anemia

Additional contraindications for I.V. product: Inadequate cerebral circulation; constrictive pericarditis; pericardial tamponade; restrictive cardiomyopathy

Note: According to the 2010 American Heart Association guidelines for the treatment of acute coronary syndromes, nitrates are considered contraindicated in the following conditions: Hypotension (SBP <90 mm Hg or ≥30 mm Hg below baseline), extreme bradycardia (<50 bpm), tachycardia in the absence of heart failure (>100 bpm), and right ventricular infarction (O'Connor, 2010).

Warnings/Precautions Severe hypotension can occur. Use with caution in volume depletion, moderate hypotension, and extreme caution with inferior wall MI and suspected right ventricular involvement. Use considered contraindicated in patients with severe hypotension (SBP <90 mm Hg or ≥30 mm Hg below baseline), extreme bradycardia (<50 bpm), and right ventricular MI (O'Connor, 2010).

Paradoxical bradycardia and increased angina pectoris can accompany hypotension. Orthostatic hypotension can also occur. Ethanol can accentuate this. Tolerance does develop to nitrates and appropriate dosing is needed to minimize this (drug-free interval). Avoid use of long-acting agents in acute MI or acute HF; cannot easily reverse effects. Nitrates may aggravate angina caused by hypertrophic cardiomyopathy. Nitroglycerin may precipitate or aggravate increased intracranial pressure and subsequently may worsen clinical outcomes in patients with neurologic injury (eg, intracranial hemorrhage, traumatic brain injury). Nitroglycerin transdermal patches may contain conducting metal (eg, aluminum); remove patch prior to MRI. Avoid concurrent use with PDE-5 inhibitors. When nitrate administration becomes medically necessary, may administer nitrates only if 24 hours have elapsed after use of sildenafil or vardenafil (48 hours after tadalafil use) (Trujillo, 2007).

Drug Interactions

Avoid Concomitant Use

Avoid concomitant use of Nitroglycerin with any of the following: Ergot Derivatives; Phosphodiesterase 5 Inhibitors

Decreased Effect

Nitroglycerin may decrease the levels/effects of: Alteplase; Heparin

The levels/effects of Nitroglycerin may be decreased by: Ergot Derivatives

Increased Effect/Toxicity

Nitroglycerin may increase the levels/effects of: Ergot Derivatives; Hypotensive Agents; Rosiglitazone

The levels/effects of Nitroglycerin may be increased by: Phosphodiesterase 5 Inhibitors

Nutritional/Ethanol Interactions

Ethanol: Avoid ethanol (may increase the hypotensive effects of nitroglycerin). Monitor.

Herb/Nutraceutical: Avoid bayberry, blue cohosh, cayenne, ephedra, ginger, ginseng (American), kola, licorice (may worsen hypertension). Avoid black cohosh, California poppy, coleus, golden seal, hawthorn, mistletoe, periwinkle, quinine, shepherd's purse (may cause hypotension).

Lab Interactions I.V. formulation: Due to propylene glycol content, triglyceride assays dependent on glycerol oxidase may be falsely elevated.

Adverse Reactions Frequency not defined.

Cardiovascular: Flushing, hypotension, peripheral edema, postural hypotension, syncope, tachycardia

Central nervous system: Headache (common), dizziness, lightheadedness

Gastrointestinal: Nausea, vomiting, xerostomia

Neuromuscular & skeletal: Paresthesia, weakness

Respiratory: Dyspnea, pharyngitis, rhinitis

Miscellaneous: Diaphoresis

Pharmacodynamics/Kinetics

Onset of Action Sublingual tablet: 1-3 minutes; Translingual spray: Similar to sublingual tablet; Sustained release: ~60 minutes; Topical: 15-30 minutes; Transdermal: ~30 minutes; I.V.: Immediate

Peak effect: Sublingual tablet: 5 minutes; Translingual spray: 4-10 minutes; Sustained release: 2.5-4 hours; Topical: ~60 minutes; Transdermal: 120 minutes; I.V.: Immediate

Duration of Action Sublingual tablet: At least 25 minutes; Translingual spray: Similar to sublingual tablet; Sustained release: 4-8 hours; Topical: 7 hours; Transdermal: 10-12 hours; I.V.: 3-5 minutes

Protein Binding 60%

Half-Life Elimination 1-4 minutes

Metabolism Extensive first-pass effect

Excretion Urine (as inactive metabolites)

Available Dosage Forms

Aerosol, translingual:

NitroMist®: 0.4 mg/spray (8.5 g)

Capsule, extended release, oral: 2.5 mg, 6.5 mg

Nitro-Time®: 2.5 mg, 6.5 mg, 9 mg

Capsule, sustained release, oral: 2.5 mg, 6.5 mg, 9 mg

Infusion, premixed in D_5W: 25 mg (250 mL); 50 mg (250 mL, 500 mL); 100 mg (250 mL)

Injection, solution: 5 mg/mL (5 mL, 10 mL)

Ointment, topical:

Nitro-Bid®: 2% (1 g, 30 g, 60 g)

Patch, transdermal: 0.1 mg/hr (30s); 0.2 mg/hr (30s); 0.4 mg/hr (30s); 0.6 mg/hr (30s)

Minitran™: 0.1 mg/hr (30s); 0.2 mg/hr (30s); 0.4 mg/hr (30s); 0.6 mg/hr (30s)

Nitro-Dur®: 0.1 mg/hr (30s); 0.2 mg/hr (30s); 0.3 mg/hr (30s); 0.4 mg/hr (30s); 0.6 mg/hr (30s); 0.8 mg/hr (30s)

Solution, translingual:

Nitrolingual®: 0.4 mg/spray (4.9 g, 12 g)

Tablet, sublingual:

Nitrostat®: 0.3 mg, 0.4 mg, 0.6 mg

Dosing

Adult & Geriatric Note: Hemodynamic and antianginal tolerance often develop within 24-48 hours of continuous nitrate administration. Nitrate-free interval (10-12 hours/day) is recommended to avoid tolerance development; gradually decrease dose in patients receiving NTG for prolonged period to avoid withdrawal reaction.

Angina/coronary artery disease:

Oral: 2.5-6.5 mg 3-4 times/day (maximum dose: 26 mg 4 times/day)

I.V.: 5 mcg/minute, increase by 5 mcg/minute every 3-5 minutes to 20 mcg/minute. If no response at 20 mcg/minute, may increase by 10-20 mcg/minute every 3-5 minutes (generally accepted maximum dose: 400 mcg/minute)

Topical ointment: 1/2" upon rising and 1/2" 6 hours later; if necessary, the dose may be doubled to 1" and subsequently doubled again to 2" if response is inadequate. Doses of 1/2" to 2" were used in clinical trials. Recommended maximum: 2 doses/day; include a nitrate free-interval ~10-12 hours/day.

Topical patch, transdermal: 0.2-0.4 mg/hour initially and titrate to doses of 0.4-0.8 mg/hour. Tolerance is minimized by using a patch-on period of 12-14 hours/day and patch-off period of 10-12 hours/day.

Sublingual: 0.3-0.6 mg every 5 minutes for maximum of 3 doses in 15 minutes; may also use prophylactically 5-10 minutes prior to activities which may provoke an attack.

Esophageal spastic disorders (unlabeled use): 0.3-0.6 mg

Translingual: 1-2 sprays onto or under tongue every 3-5 minutes for maximum of 3 doses in 15 minutes, may also be used prophylactically 5-10 minutes prior to activities which may provoke an angina attack

Administration

Oral

Oral (sustained release capsule): Swallow whole. Do not chew, break, or crush. Take with a full glass of water.

Sublingual: Do not crush sublingual product (tablet). Place under tongue and allow to dissolve.

Translingual spray: Do not shake container. Prior to initial use, the pump must be primed by spraying 5 times (Nitrolingual®) or 10 times (Nitromist®) into the air. Priming sprays should be directed away from patient and others. Release spray onto or under tongue. Close mouth after administration. Do not rinse the mouth for at least 5-10 minutes. The end of the pump should be covered by the fluid in the bottle. If pump is unused for 6 weeks, a single priming spray (Nitrolingual®) or 2 priming sprays (Nitromist®) should be completed.

I.V. Prepare in glass bottles, EXCEL® or PAB® containers. Adsorption occurs to soft plastic (eg, PVC); use administration sets intended for nitroglycerin.

Topical

Topical ointment: Wash hands prior to and after use. Application site should be clean, dry, and hair-free. Apply to chest or back with the applicator or dose-measuring paper. Spread in a thin layer over a 2.25 x 3.5 inch area. Do not rub into skin. Tape applicator into place.

Topical patch, transdermal: Application site should be clean, dry and hair-free. Remove patch after 12-14 hours. Rotate patch sites.

Stability

Reconstitution

Standard diluent: 50 mg/250 mL D_5W; 50 mg/500 mL D_5W.

Minimum volume: 100 mg/250 mL D_5W; concentration should not exceed 400 mcg/mL.

Storage

I.V. solution: Doses should be made in glass bottles, EXCEL® or PAB® containers. Adsorption occurs to soft plastic (eg, PVC). Nitroglycerin diluted in D_5W or NS in glass containers is physically and chemically stable for 48 hours at room temperature and 7 days under refrigeration. In D_5W or NS in EXCEL®/PAB® containers it is physically and chemically stable for 24 hours at room temperature. Premixed bottles are stable according to the manufacturer's expiration dating.

Store sublingual tablets and ointment in tightly closed containers at 20°C to 25°C (68°F to 77°F); slow release capsules at 20°C to 25°C (68°F to 77°F); translingual spray and transdermal patch at 15°C to 30°C (59°F to 86°F).

Monitoring and Teaching Issues

Physical Assessment Evaluate cardiac status and monitor for hypotension and GI disturbances. Teach patient importance of drug-free intervals.

Patient Education Keep medication in original container, tightly closed. If anginal chest pain is unresolved in 15 minutes, seek emergency medical help at once. Daily use may cause dizziness, headache, and GI disturbances. Report severe headache, persistent dizziness, loss of consciousness, or any rash.

Oral: Do not chew or swallow sublingual tablets; allow to dissolve under tongue. Sit down before using sublingual or buccal tablet or spray form. Do not chew or crush capsules; swallow with water.

Spray: Spray directly on mucous membranes; do not inhale.

Topical: Spread prescribed amount thinly on applicator; rotate application sites.

Transdermal: Place on hair-free area of skin and rotate sites (usually, patches will be removed for a period each day). Remove patch while having MRI scan; can cause burns.

Geriatric Considerations Caution should be used when using nitrate therapy in the elderly due to hypotension. Hypotension is enhanced in the elderly due to decreased baroreceptor response, decreased venous tone, and often hypovolemia (dehydration) or other hypotensive drugs.

Pregnancy Considerations Increased fetal mortality has been observed in animal studies using isosorbide mononitrate and isosorbide dinitrate at doses much higher than those used in humans. Toxic effects were not observed in animal studies following topical administration of nitroglycerin. There are no adequate and well-controlled studies in pregnant women.

Additional Information I.V. preparations contain alcohol and/or propylene glycol; may need to use nitrate-free interval (10-12 hours/day) to avoid tolerance development. Tolerance may possibly be reversed with acetylcysteine; gradually decrease dose in patients receiving NTG for prolonged period to avoid withdrawal reaction.

Concomitant use of sildenafil (Viagra®) or other phosphodiesterase-5 enzyme inhibitors (PDE-5) may precipitate acute hypotension, myocardial infarction, or death. Nitrates used in right ventricular infarction may induce acute hypotension. Nitrate use in severe pericardial effusion may reduce cardiac filling pressure and precipitate cardiac tamponade. In the management of heart failure, the combination of isosorbide dinitrate and hydralazine confers beneficial effects on disease progression and cardiac outcomes.

Related Information

Compatibility of Drugs *on page* 1994

Hyperlipidemia Management *on page* 2046

◆ **Nitroglycerol** *see* Nitroglycerin *on page* 1327

◆ **Nitrolingual®** *see* Nitroglycerin *on page* 1327

◆ **NitroMist®** *see* Nitroglycerin *on page* 1327

◆ **Nitropress®** *see* Nitroprusside *on page* 1330

Nitroprusside (nye troe PRUS ide)

U.S. Brand Names Nitropress®

Index Terms Nitroprusside Sodium; Sodium Nitroferricyanide; Sodium Nitroprusside

Generic Availability (U.S.) Yes

Pharmacologic Category Vasodilator

Medication Safety Issues

Sound-alike/look-alike issues:

Nitroprusside may be confused with nitroglycerin

High alert medication: The Institute for Safe Medication Practices (ISMP) includes this medication among its list of drugs which have a heightened risk of causing significant patient harm when used in error.

Pregnancy Risk Factor C

Lactation Excretion in breast milk unknown

Use Management of hypertensive crises; acute decompensated heart failure (HF); used for controlled hypotension to reduce bleeding during surgery

Mechanism of Action/Effect Causes peripheral vasodilation by direct action on venous and arteriolar smooth muscle, thus reducing peripheral resistance; will increase cardiac output by decreasing afterload; reduces aortal and left ventricular impedance

Contraindications Hypersensitivity to nitroprusside or any component of the formulation; treatment of compensatory hypertension (aortic coarctation, arteriovenous shunting); high output failure; congenital optic atrophy or tobacco amblyopia

Warnings/Precautions [U.S. Boxed Warning]: Continuous blood pressure monitoring is needed. Except when used briefly or at low (<2 mcg/kg/minute) infusion rates, nitroprusside gives rise to large cyanide quantities. Do not use the maximum dose for more than 10 minutes; if blood pressure not controlled then discontinue infusion. Monitor for cyanide toxicity via acid-base balance and venous oxygen concentration. Use with extreme caution in patients with elevated intracranial pressure (head trauma, cerebral hemorrhage), severe renal impairment, hepatic failure, hypothyroidism. Use the lowest end of the dosage range with renal impairment. Cyanide toxicity may occur in patients with decreased liver function. Thiocyanate toxicity occurs in patients with renal impairment or those on prolonged infusions. **[U.S. Boxed Warning]: Should not be administered by direct injection; must be further diluted with 5% dextrose in water.**

Drug Interactions

Avoid Concomitant Use There are no known interactions where it is recommended to avoid concomitant use.

Decreased Effect

The levels/effects of Nitroprusside may be decreased by: Herbs (Hypertensive Properties); Methylphenidate; Yohimbine

Increased Effect/Toxicity

Nitroprusside may increase the levels/effects of: Amifostine; Antihypertensives; Hypotensive Agents; RiTUXimab

The levels/effects of Nitroprusside may be increased by: Calcium Channel Blockers; Diazoxide; Herbs (Hypotensive Properties); MAO Inhibitors; Pentoxifylline; Phosphodiesterase 5 Inhibitors; Prostacyclin Analogues

Adverse Reactions Frequency not defined.

Cardiovascular: Excessive hypotensive response, palpitation, substernal distress
Central nervous system: Disorientation, psychosis, headache, restlessness
Endocrine & metabolic: Thyroid suppression (due to thiocyanate)
Gastrointestinal: Nausea, vomiting
Neuromuscular & skeletal: Hyper-reflexia (thiocyanate toxicity), muscle spasm, weakness
Ocular: Miosis (thiocyanate toxicity)
Otic: Tinnitus (thiocyanate toxicity)
Respiratory: Hypoxia
Miscellaneous: Diaphoresis

Pharmacodynamics/Kinetics

Onset of Action BP reduction <2 minutes

Duration of Action 1-10 minutes

Half-Life Elimination Parent drug: <10 minutes; Thiocyanate: 2.7-7 days

Metabolism Nitroprusside is converted to cyanide ions in the bloodstream; decomposes to prussic acid which in the presence of sulfur donor is converted to thiocyanate (hepatic and renal rhodanase systems)

Excretion Urine (as thiocyanate)

Available Dosage Forms

Injection, solution:

Nitropress®: 25 mg/mL (2 mL)

Dosing

Adult & Geriatric

Acute hypertension: I.V.: Initial: 0.3-0.5 mcg/kg/minute; increase in increments of 0.5 mcg/kg/minute, titrating to the desired hemodynamic effect or the appearance of headache or nausea; usual dose: 3 mcg/kg/minute; rarely need >4 mcg/kg/minute; maximum: 10 mcg/kg/minute. When >500 mcg/kg is administered by prolonged infusion of faster than 2 mcg/kg/minute, cyanide is generated faster than an unaided patient can handle.

Note: Administration requires the use of an infusion pump. Average dose: 5 mcg/kg/minute.

Pediatric

Pulmonary hypertension: I.V.: Children: Initial: 1 mcg/kg/minute by continuous I.V. infusion; increase in increments of 1 mcg/kg/minute at intervals of 20-60 minutes; titrating to the desired response; usual dose: 3 mcg/kg/minute, rarely need >4 mcg/kg/minute; maximum: 5 mcg/kg/minute.

Note: Administration requires the use of an infusion pump. Average dose: 5 mcg/kg/minute.

Renal Impairment Limit use; accumulation of thiocyanate may occur.

Hepatic Impairment Limit use; risk of cyanide toxicity.

Administration

I.V. I.V. infusion only, use only as an infusion with 5% dextrose in water. Infusion pump required. Not for direct injection.

Stability

Reconstitution Brownish solution is usable, discard if bluish in color. Nitroprusside sodium should be reconstituted freshly by diluting 50 mg in 250-1000 mL of D_5W.

Storage

Use only clear solutions; solutions of nitroprusside exhibit a color described as brownish, brown, brownish-pink, light orange, and straw. Solutions are highly sensitive to light. Exposure to light causes decomposition, resulting in a highly colored solution of orange, dark brown or blue. **A blue color indicates almost complete degradation and breakdown to cyanide.**

Solutions should be wrapped with aluminum foil or other opaque material to protect from light (do as soon as possible).

Stability of parenteral admixture at room temperature (25°C) and at refrigeration temperature (4°C) is 24 hours.

Monitoring and Teaching Issues

Physical Assessment Infusion site must be monitored closely to prevent extravasation. Continuous blood pressure monitoring is needed. Assess acid/base balance (metabolic acidosis is early sign of cyanide toxicity). Monitor for disorientation, hypoxia, and muscular twitching.

Patient Education This drug can only be given I.V. You will be monitored at all times during infusion. Promptly report any pain/burning at site of infusion.

Geriatric Considerations Elderly patients may have an increased sensitivity to nitroprusside possibly due to a decreased baroreceptor reflex, altered sensitivity to vasodilating effects or a resistance of cardiac adrenergic receptors to stimulation by catecholamines.

Related Information

Compatibility of Drugs *on page* *1994*

Hyperlipidemia Management *on page* *2046*

- **Nitroprusside Sodium** *see* Nitroprusside *on page* *1330*
- **Nitrostat®** *see* Nitroglycerin *on page* *1327*
- **Nitro-Time®** *see* Nitroglycerin *on page* *1327*

Nizatidine (ni ZA ti deen)

U.S. Brand Names Axid®; Axid® AR [OTC]

Generic Availability (U.S.) Yes: Excludes tablet

Pharmacologic Category Histamine H_2 Antagonist

Medication Safety Issues

Sound-alike/look-alike issues:

Axid® may be confused with Ansaid®

International issues:

Tazac [Australia] may be confused with Tazact brand name for piperacillin/tazobactam [India]; Tiazac brand name for diltiazem [U.S., Canada]

Pregnancy Risk Factor B

Lactation Enters breast milk/consider risk:benefit

Use Treatment and maintenance of duodenal ulcer; treatment of benign gastric ulcer; treatment of gastroesophageal reflux disease (GERD)

OTC labeling: Prevention of meal-induced heartburn, acid indigestion, and sour stomach

Unlabeled/Investigational Use Part of a multidrug regimen for *H. pylori* eradication to reduce the risk of duodenal ulcer recurrence

Available Dosage Forms

Capsule, oral: 150 mg, 300 mg

Solution, oral: 15 mg/mL (473 mL)

Axid®: 15 mg/mL (480 mL)

Tablet, oral:

Axid® AR [OTC]: 75 mg

Dosing

Adult & Geriatric

Duodenal ulcer: Oral:

Treatment of active ulcer: 300 mg at bedtime or 150 mg twice daily

Maintenance of healed ulcer: 150 mg/day at bedtime

Gastric ulcer: Oral: 150 mg twice daily or 300 mg at bedtime

GERD: Oral: 150 mg twice daily

Meal-induced heartburn, acid indigestion, and sour stomach (OTC labeling): Oral: 75 mg tablet [OTC] twice daily, 30-60 minutes prior to consuming food or beverages

Eradication of *Helicobacter pylori* (unlabeled use): Oral: 150 mg twice daily; requires combination therapy

Pediatric

GERD (unlabeled use): Oral:

Children <12 years: 10 mg/kg/day in divided doses given twice daily; may not be as effective in children <12 years

Children ≥12 years: Refer to adult dosing.

Meal-induced heartburn, acid indigestion and sour stomach: Oral: Children ≥12 years: Refer to adult dosing.

Renal Impairment

Active treatment:

Cl_{cr} 20-50 mL/minute: 150 mg/day

Cl_{cr} <20 mL/minute: 150 mg every other day

Maintenance treatment:

Cl_{cr} 20-50 mL/minute: 150 mg every other day

Cl_{cr} <20 mL/minute: 150 mg every 3 days

Monitoring and Teaching Issues

Patient Education May cause drowsiness. Report fever, sore throat, tarry stools, CNS changes, or muscle or joint pain.

- **Nizoral®** *see* Ketoconazole (Topical) *on page* *1039*
- **Nizoral® A-D [OTC]** *see* Ketoconazole (Topical) *on page* *1039*
- **N-Methylhydrazine** *see* Procarbazine *on page* *1510*
- **N-methylnaltrexone Bromide** *see* Methylnaltrexone *on page* *1202*
- **NN2211** *see* Liraglutide *on page* *1116*
- **No Doz® Maximum Strength [OTC]** *see* Caffeine *on page* *267*
- **Nolvadex** *see* Tamoxifen *on page* *1703*

- ◆ **Nora-BE®** *see* Norethindrone *on page* 1334
- ◆ **Noradrenaline** *see* Norepinephrine *on page* 1333
- ◆ **Noradrenaline Acid Tartrate** *see* Norepinephrine *on page* 1333
- ◆ **Norco®** *see* Hydrocodone and Acetaminophen *on page* 915
- ◆ **Norcuron** *see* Vecuronium *on page* 1852
- ◆ **Nordeoxyguanosine** *see* Ganciclovir (Systemic) *on page* 849
- ◆ **Nordette® 28** *see* Ethinyl Estradiol and Levonorgestrel *on page* 699
- ◆ **Norditropin®** *see* Somatropin *on page* 1664
- ◆ **Norditropin FlexPro®** *see* Somatropin *on page* 1664
- ◆ **Norditropin® NordiFlex®** *see* Somatropin *on page* 1664

Norepinephrine (nor ep i NEF rin)

U.S. Brand Names Levophed®

Index Terms Levarterenol Bitartrate; Noradrenaline; Noradrenaline Acid Tartrate; Norepinephrine Bitartrate

Generic Availability (U.S.) Yes

Pharmacologic Category Alpha/Beta Agonist

Medication Safety Issues

Sound-alike/look-alike issues:

Levophed® may be confused with levofloxacin

High alert medication: The Institute for Safe Medication Practices (ISMP) includes this medication among its list of drugs which have a heightened risk of causing significant patient harm when used in error.

Pregnancy Risk Factor C

Lactation Excretion in breast milk unknown

Use Treatment of shock which persists after adequate fluid volume replacement; severe hypotension

Mechanism of Action/Effect Stimulates $beta_1$-adrenergic receptors and alpha-adrenergic receptors causing increased contractility and heart rate as well as vasoconstriction, thereby increasing systemic blood pressure and coronary blood flow; clinically, alpha effects (vasoconstriction) are greater than beta effects (inotropic and chronotropic effects)

Contraindications Hypersensitivity to norepinephrine, bisulfites (contains metabisulfite), or any component of the formulation; hypotension from hypovolemia except as an emergency measure to maintain coronary and cerebral perfusion until volume could be replaced; mesenteric or peripheral vascular thrombosis unless it is a lifesaving procedure; during anesthesia with cyclopropane (not available in U.S.) or halothane (not available in U.S.) anesthesia (risk of ventricular arrhythmias)

Warnings/Precautions Assure adequate circulatory volume to minimize need for vasoconstrictors. Avoid hypertension; monitor blood pressure closely and adjust infusion rate. Use with extreme caution in patients taking MAO-Inhibitors. Avoid extravasation; infuse into a large vein if possible. Avoid infusion into leg veins. Watch I.V. site closely. **[U.S. Boxed Warning]: If extravasation occurs, infiltrate the area with diluted phentolamine (5-10 mg in 10-15 mL of saline) with a fine hypodermic needle. Phentolamine should be administered as soon as possible after extravasation is noted.** Product may contain sodium metasulfite.

Drug Interactions

Avoid Concomitant Use

Avoid concomitant use of Norepinephrine with any of the following: Inhalational Anesthetics; Iobenguane I 123

Decreased Effect

Norepinephrine may decrease the levels/effects of: Benzylpenicilloyl Polylysine; Iobenguane I 123

The levels/effects of Norepinephrine may be decreased by: Spironolactone

Increased Effect/Toxicity

Norepinephrine may increase the levels/effects of: Bromocriptine; Sympathomimetics

The levels/effects of Norepinephrine may be increased by: Antacids; Atomoxetine; Beta-Blockers; Cannabinoids; Carbonic Anhydrase Inhibitors; COMT Inhibitors; Inhalational Anesthetics; MAO Inhibitors; Serotonin/Norepinephrine Reuptake Inhibitors; Tricyclic Antidepressants

Adverse Reactions Frequency not defined.

Cardiovascular: Arrhythmias, bradycardia, peripheral (digital) ischemia
Central nervous system: Anxiety, headache (transient)
Local: Skin necrosis (with extravasation)
Respiratory: Dyspnea, respiratory difficulty

Pharmacodynamics/Kinetics

Onset of Action I.V.: Very rapid-acting

Duration of Action Vasopressor: 1-2 minutes

Metabolism Via catechol-o-methyltransferase (COMT) and monoamine oxidase (MAO)

Excretion Urine (84% to 96% as inactive metabolites)

Available Dosage Forms

Injection, solution: 1 mg/mL (4 mL)
Levophed®: 1 mg/mL (4 mL)

Dosing

Adult & Geriatric Administration requires the use of an infusion pump.

Note: Norepinephrine dosage is stated in terms of norepinephrine base.

Hypotension/shock: Continuous I.V. infusion:

Initial: 8-12 mcg/minute; titrate to desired response. Usual maintenance range: 2-4 mcg/minute; dosage range varies greatly depending on clinical situation. If patient remains hypotensive despite large doses, evaluate for occult hypovolemia and provide fluid resuscitation as appropriate.

ACLS dosing range (weight-based dosing): Post cardiac arrest care: Initial: 0.1-0.5 mcg/**kg**/minute (7-35 mcg/minute in a 70 kg patient); titrate to desired response (AHA, 2010)

Sepsis and septic shock (weight-based dosing): Range from clinical trials: 0.01-3 mcg/**kg**/minute (0.7-210 mcg/minute in a 70 kg patient) (Hollenberg, 2004)

Pediatric Administration requires the use of an infusion pump.

Note: Norepinephrine dosage is stated in terms of norepinephrine base.

Hypotension/shock: Continuous I.V. infusion: Initial: 0.05-0.1 mcg/kg/minute; titrate to desired effect; maximum dose: 2 mcg/kg/minute (Kliegman, 2007; AHA, 2010)

Administration

I.V. Administer as a continuous infusion with the use of an infusion pump. Dilute prior to use. Administration via central line recommended; may cause severe ischemic necrosis if extravasated. Do not administer sodium bicarbonate (or any alkaline solution) through an I.V. line containing norepinephrine; inactivation of norepinephrine may occur.

Stability

Reconstitution Dilute with D_5W, D_5NS, or NS; dilution in NS is not recommended by the manufacturer; however, stability in NS has been demonstrated (Tremblay, 2008).

Storage Readily oxidized. Protect from light. Do not use if brown coloration. Stability of parenteral admixture at room temperature (25°C) is 24 hours.

Monitoring and Teaching Issues

Physical Assessment Monitor blood pressure and cardiac status, CNS status, skin temperature, and color during and following infusion. Monitor fluid status. Assess infusion site frequently for extravasation. Blanching along vein pathway is a preliminary sign of extravasation.

Patient Education This drug is used in emergency situations. Patient information is based on patient condition.

Additional Information Norepinephrine dosage is stated in terms of norepinephrine base. Although the intravenous product vial designates the contents as norepinephrine bitartrate, the actual concentration shown is in terms of norepinephrine base 1 mg/mL.

Related Information

Compatibility of Drugs *on page 1994*

◆ **Norepinephrine Bitartrate** *see* Norepinephrine *on page 1333*

Norethindrone (nor ETH in drone)

U.S. Brand Names Aygestin®; Camila®; Errin®; Heather; Jolivette®; Nor-QD®; Nora-BE®; Ortho Micronor®

Index Terms Norethindrone Acetate; Norethisterone

Generic Availability (U.S.) Yes

Pharmacologic Category Contraceptive; Progestin

Medication Safety Issues

Sound-alike/look-alike issues:

Micronor® may be confused with miconazole, Micronase®

Pregnancy Risk Factor X

Lactation Enters breast milk/use caution

Use Treatment of amenorrhea; abnormal uterine bleeding; endometriosis; prevention of pregnancy

Available Dosage Forms

Tablet, oral: 0.35 mg, 5 mg

Aygestin®: 5 mg
Camila®: 0.35 mg
Errin®: 0.35 mg
Heather: 0.35 mg
Jolivette®: 0.35 mg
Nor-QD®: 0.35 mg
Nora-BE®: 0.35 mg
Ortho Micronor®: 0.35 mg

Dosing

Adult

Contraception (females): Oral: Progesterone only: Norethindrone 0.35 mg every day (no missed days)

Initial dose: Start on first day of menstrual period or the day after a miscarriage or abortion. If switching from a combined oral contraceptive, begin the day after finishing the last active combined tablet.

Missed dose: Take as soon as remembered. A back up method of contraception should be used for 48 hours if dose is taken ≥3 hours late.

Amenorrhea and abnormal uterine bleeding: Oral: Norethindrone acetate: 2.5-10 mg/day for 5-10 days during the second half of the menstrual cycle

Endometriosis: Oral: Norethindrone acetate: 5 mg/day for 14 days; increase at increments of 2.5 mg/day every 2 weeks to reach 15 mg/day; continue for 6-9 months or until breakthrough bleeding demands temporary termination

Pediatric Adolescents: Refer to adult dosing

Administration

Oral Administer at the same time each day. When used for the prevention of pregnancy, a back up method of contraception should be used for 48 hours if dose is missed or taken ≥3 hours late.

Monitoring and Teaching Issues

Physical Assessment Teach appropriate administration schedule. Schedule physical exam with reference to the breasts and pelvis, including a Papanicolaou smear. Exam may be deferred if appropriate; pregnancy should be ruled out prior to use. Monitor patient closely for loss of vision, sudden onset of proptosis, diplopia, migraine, blood pressure, signs and symptoms of thromboembolic disorders, signs or symptoms of depression, glycemic control in diabetics, and lipid profiles in patients being treated for hyperlipidemias. Adequate diagnostic measures, including endometrial sampling, if indicated, should be performed to rule out malignancy in all cases of undiagnosed abnormal vaginal bleeding. Emphasize need for regular breast self-exam and necessity of annual physical check-up with long-term use.

Patient Education Take according to prescribed schedule. Follow instructions for regular self-breast exam. You may experience dizziness or lightheadedness. Limit intake of caffeine. Avoid high-dose vitamin C. If you have diabetes, monitor blood glucose closely. You may experience photosensitivity, loss of hair (reversible), swelling of hands or feet, or weight gain or loss. Report sudden severe headache or vomiting; disturbances of vision or speech; sudden blindness; numbness or weakness in an extremity; chest pain; calf pain; respiratory difficulty; weight gain; depression or acute fatigue; or unusual bleeding, spotting, or changes in menstrual flow.

◆ **Norethindrone Acetate** *see* Norethindrone *on page* 1334

◆ **Norethindrone Acetate and Ethinyl Estradiol** *see* Ethinyl Estradiol and Norethindrone *on page* 701

◆ **Norethindrone and Estradiol** *see* Estradiol and Norethindrone *on page* 674

Norethindrone and Mestranol (nor eth IN drone & MES tra nole)

U.S. Brand Names Necon® 1/50; Norinyl® 1+50

Index Terms Mestranol and Norethindrone; Ortho Novum 1/50

Generic Availability (U.S.) Yes

Pharmacologic Category Contraceptive; Estrogen and Progestin Combination

Medication Safety Issues

Sound-alike/look-alike issues:

Norinyl® may be confused with Nardil®

Pregnancy Risk Factor X

Lactation Enters breast milk/not recommended

Use Prevention of pregnancy

Unlabeled/Investigational Use Treatment of hypermenorrhea (menorrhagia); pain associated with endometriosis; dysmenorrhea; dysfunctional uterine bleeding

Available Dosage Forms

Tablet, monophasic formulations:

Necon® 1/50: Norethindrone 1 mg and mestranol 0.05 mg [21 light blue tablets and 7 white inactive tablets] (28s)

Norinyl® 1+50: Norethindrone 1 mg and mestranol 0.05 mg [21 white tablets and 7 orange inactive tablets] (28s)

Dosing

Adult Female: Contraception: Oral:

Schedule 1 (Sunday starter): Dose begins on first Sunday after onset of menstruation; if the menstrual period starts on Sunday, take first tablet that very same day. **With a Sunday start, an additional method of contraception should be used until after the first 7 days of consecutive administration.**

For 21-tablet package: Dosage is 1 tablet daily for 21 consecutive days, followed by 7 days off of the medication; a new course begins on the 8th day after the last tablet is taken.

For 28-tablet package: Dosage is 1 tablet daily without interruption.

Schedule 2 (Day 1 starter): Dose starts on first day of menstrual cycle taking 1 tablet daily.

For 21-tablet package: Dosage is 1 tablet daily for 21 consecutive days, followed by 7 days off of the medication; a new course begins on the 8th day after the last tablet is taken.

For 28-tablet package: Dosage is 1 tablet daily without interruption.

Note: If all doses have been taken on schedule and one menstrual period is missed, continue dosing cycle. If two consecutive menstrual periods are missed, pregnancy test is required before new dosing cycle is started.

Missed doses: Monophasic formulations (refer to package insert for complete information):

One dose missed: Take as soon as remembered or take 2 tablets next day

Two consecutive doses missed in the first 2 weeks: Take 2 tablets as soon as remembered or 2 tablets next 2 days. **An additional method of contraception should be used for 7 days after missed dose.**

Two consecutive doses missed in week 3 or three consecutive doses missed at any time: **An additional method of contraception must be used for 7 days after a missed dose:**

Schedule 1 (Sunday starter): Continue dose of 1 tablet daily until Sunday, then discard the rest of the pack, and a new pack should be started that same day.

Schedule 2 (Day 1 starter): Current pack should be discarded, and a new pack should be started that same day.

Pediatric Female: Contraception: Oral: See adult dosing; not to be used prior to menarche.

Renal Impairment Specific guidelines not available; use with caution and monitor blood pressure closely. Consider other forms of contraception.

Hepatic Impairment Contraindicated in patients with hepatic impairment.

Administration

Oral Administer at the same time each day. Administer at bedtime to minimize occurrence of adverse effects.

Monitoring and Teaching Issues

Physical Assessment See individual agents.

Patient Education See individual agents.

Related Information

Norethindrone *on page* 1334

- **Norethisterone** *see* Norethindrone *on page* 1334
- **Norflex™** *see* Orphenadrine *on page* 1366
- **Norgestimate and Ethinyl Estradiol** *see* Ethinyl Estradiol and Norgestimate *on page* 704
- **Norinyl® 1+35** *see* Ethinyl Estradiol and Norethindrone *on page* 701
- **Norinyl® 1+50** *see* Norethindrone and Mestranol *on page* 1335
- **Normal Human Serum Albumin** *see* Albumin *on page* 57
- **Normal Serum Albumin (Human)** *see* Albumin *on page* 57
- **Norpramin®** *see* Desipramine *on page* 489
- **Nor-QD®** *see* Norethindrone *on page* 1334
- **Nortemp Children's [OTC]** *see* Acetaminophen *on page* 38
- **Nortrel® 0.5/35** *see* Ethinyl Estradiol and Norethindrone *on page* 701
- **Nortrel® 1/35** *see* Ethinyl Estradiol and Norethindrone *on page* 701
- **Nortrel® 7/7/7** *see* Ethinyl Estradiol and Norethindrone *on page* 701

Nortriptyline (nor TRIP ti leen)

U.S. Brand Names Pamelor®

Index Terms Nortriptyline Hydrochloride

Generic Availability (U.S.) Yes: Excludes solution

Pharmacologic Category Antidepressant, Tricyclic (Secondary Amine)

Medication Safety Issues

Sound-alike/look-alike issues:

Aventyl® HCl may be confused with Bentyl®

Nortriptyline may be confused with amitriptyline, desipramine, Norpramin®

Pamelor® may be confused with Demerol®, Dymelor®, Panlor® DC, Tambocor™

Medication Guide Available Yes

Lactation Enters breast milk/not recommended (AAP rates "of concern"; AAP 2001 update pending)

Use Treatment of symptoms of depression

Unlabeled/Investigational Use Chronic pain (including neuropathic pain), myofascial pain, burning mouth sydrome, anxiety disorders, attention-deficit/hyperactivity disorder (ADHD); enuresis; adjunctive therapy for smoking cessation

Available Dosage Forms

Capsule, oral: 10 mg, 25 mg, 50 mg, 75 mg

Pamelor®: 10 mg, 25 mg, 50 mg, 75 mg

Solution, oral: 10 mg/5 mL (473 mL, 480 mL)

Pamelor®: 10 mg/5 mL (480 mL)

Dosing

Adult

Depression: Oral: 25 mg 3-4 times/day up to 150 mg/day; doses may be given once daily.

Chronic urticaria, angioedema, nocturnal pruritus (unlabeled use): Oral: 75 mg/day

Myofascial pain, neuralgia, burning mouth syndrome (unlabeled uses): Initial: 10-25 mg at bedtime; dosage may be increased by 25 mg/day weekly, if tolerated; usual maintenance dose: 75 mg as a single bedtime dose or 2 divided doses

Smoking cessation (unlabeled use; Fiore, 2008): Oral: Initial: 25 mg/day; titrate dose to 75-100 mg/day 10-28 days prior to selected "quit" date; continue therapy for ≥12 weeks after "quit" day

Geriatric Initial: 30-50 mg/day, given as a single daily dose or in divided doses. **Note:** Nortriptyline is one of the best tolerated TCAs in the elderly)

Pediatric

Nocturnal enuresis (unlabeled use): Oral: 10-20 mg/day; titrate to a maximum of 40 mg/day

Depression (unlabeled use): Oral: 1-3 mg/kg/day

Hepatic Impairment Lower doses and slower titration are recommended dependent on individualization of dosage.

Monitoring and Teaching Issues

Physical Assessment Assess for suicidal tendencies before beginning therapy. Assess therapeutic effectiveness (mental status, mood, affect). Monitor for suicide ideation at beginning of therapy and periodically throughout. Taper dosage slowly when discontinuing. Caution patients with diabetes to monitor glucose levels closely; may increase or decrease serum glucose levels.

Patient Education Take once-a-day dose at bedtime. Do not increase dose or frequency; may take 2-3 weeks to achieve desired results. Avoid alcohol. Maintain adequate hydration unless instructed to restrict fluid intake. May cause drowsiness, lightheadedness, impaired coordination, dizziness, blurred vision, nausea, vomiting, loss of appetite, disturbed taste, constipation, urinary retention, postural hypotension, altered sexual drive or ability (reversible), or photosensitivity. Report chest pain, palpitations, or rapid heartbeat; persistent adverse CNS effects (eg, suicide ideation, nervousness, restlessness, insomnia, anxiety, excitation, headache, agitation, impaired coordination, changes in cognition); muscle cramping, weakness, tremors, or rigidity; blurred vision or eye pain; breast enlargement or swelling; yellowing of skin or eyes; or worsening of condition.

Related Information

Antidepressant Agents *on page 1982*
Peak and Trough Guidelines *on page 1958*
Pharmacotherapy of Urinary Incontinence *on page 2071*

◆ **Nortriptyline Hydrochloride** *see* Nortriptyline *on page 1336*
◆ **Norvasc®** *see* AmLODIPine *on page 104*
◆ **Norvir®** *see* Ritonavir *on page 1593*
◆ **Novantrone®** *see* Mitoxantrone *on page 1244*
◆ **Novarel®** *see* Chorionic Gonadotropin (Human) *on page 364*
◆ **Novel Erythropoiesis-Stimulating Protein** *see* Darbepoetin Alfa *on page 463*
◆ **NovoLIN® 70/30** *see* Insulin NPH and Insulin Regular *on page 993*
◆ **NovoLIN® N** *see* Insulin NPH *on page 992*
◆ **NovoLIN® R** *see* Insulin Regular *on page 994*
◆ **NovoLOG®** *see* Insulin Aspart *on page 981*
◆ **NovoLog 70/30** *see* Insulin Aspart Protamine and Insulin Aspart *on page 983*
◆ **NovoLOG® FlexPen®** *see* Insulin Aspart *on page 981*
◆ **NovoLOG® Mix 70/30** *see* Insulin Aspart Protamine and Insulin Aspart *on page 983*
◆ **NovoLOG® Mix 70/30 FlexPen®** *see* Insulin Aspart Protamine and Insulin Aspart *on page 983*
◆ **NovoLOG® Penfill®** *see* Insulin Aspart *on page 981*
◆ **NovoSeven® RT** *see* Factor VIIa (Recombinant) *on page 731*
◆ **Noxafil®** *see* Posaconazole *on page 1476*
◆ **NPH Insulin** *see* Insulin NPH *on page 992*
◆ **NPH Insulin and Regular Insulin** *see* Insulin NPH and Insulin Regular *on page 993*
◆ **NRP104** *see* Lisdexamfetamine *on page 1117*
◆ **NSC-750** *see* Busulfan *on page 257*
◆ **NSC-755** *see* Mercaptopurine *on page 1173*
◆ **NSC-13875** *see* Altretamine *on page 89*
◆ **NSC-15200** *see* Gallium Nitrate *on page 848*
◆ **NSC-71423** *see* Megestrol *on page 1158*
◆ **NSC-89199** *see* Estramustine *on page 675*
◆ **NSC-105014** *see* Cladribine *on page 389*
◆ **NSC-147834** *see* Flutamide *on page 797*
◆ **NSC-613795** *see* Sargramostim *on page 1624*
◆ **NSC-684588** *see* Nilutamide *on page 1319*
◆ **NSC-697732** *see* DAUNOrubicin Citrate (Liposomal) *on page 472*
◆ **NSC-714371** *see* Dalteparin *on page 459*
◆ **NTG** *see* Nitroglycerin *on page 1327*
◆ ***N*-trifluoroacetyladriamycin-14-valerate** *see* Valrubicin *on page 1836*
◆ **NTZ** *see* Nitazoxanide *on page 1324*
◆ **Nubain** *see* Nalbuphine *on page 1283*
◆ **Nucynta®** *see* Tapentadol *on page 1708*
◆ **Nuedexta™** *see* Dextromethorphan and Quinidine *on page 514*
◆ **NuLYTELY®** *see* Polyethylene Glycol-Electrolyte Solution *on page 1474*
◆ **Nuquin HP®** *see* Hydroquinone *on page 927*
◆ **Nutropin®** *see* Somatropin *on page 1664*
◆ **Nutropin AQ®** *see* Somatropin *on page 1664*

- ◆ **Nutropin AQ® NuSpin™** *see* Somatropin *on page 1664*
- ◆ **Nutropin AQ Pen®** *see* Somatropin *on page 1664*
- ◆ **Nuvigil®** *see* Armodafinil *on page 147*
- ◆ **NVP** *see* Nevirapine *on page 1301*
- ◆ **Nyamyc®** *see* Nystatin (Topical) *on page 1338*

Nystatin (Oral) (nye STAT in)

U.S. Brand Names Nystat-Rx [DSC]

Generic Availability (U.S.) Yes

Pharmacologic Category Antifungal Agent, Oral Nonabsorbed

Medication Safety Issues

Sound-alike/look-alike issues:

Nystatin may be confused with HMG-CoA reductase inhibitors (also known as "statins"; eg, atorvastatin, fluvastatin, lovastatin, pitavastatin, pravastatin, rosuvastatin, simvastatin), Nitrostat®

Pregnancy Risk Factor C

Lactation Excretion in breast milk unknown/use caution

Use Treatment of susceptible cutaneous, mucocutaneous, and oral cavity fungal infections normally caused by the *Candida* species

Available Dosage Forms

Powder, for prescription compounding: 50 million units (10 g); 150 million units (30 g); 500 million units (100 g)

Suspension, oral: 100,000 units/mL (5 mL, 60 mL, 473 mL)

Tablet, oral: 500,000 units

Dosing

Adult & Geriatric

Oral candidiasis: Suspension (swish and swallow): 400,000-600,000 units 4 times/day; swish in the mouth and retain for as long as possible (several minutes) before swallowing

Intestinal infections: Oral tablets: 500,000-1,000,000 units every 8 hours

Note: Powder for compounding: 1/8 teaspoon (500,000 units) to equal approximately 1/2 cup of water; give 4 times/day

Pediatric Oral candidiasis:

Suspension:

Premature infants: 100,000 units 4 times/day; paint suspension into recesses of the mouth

Infants: 200,000 units 4 times/day or 100,000 units to each side of mouth 4 times/day; paint suspension into recesses of the mouth

Children: 400,000-600,000 units 4 times/day; swish in the mouth and retain for as long as possible (several minutes) before swallowing

Powder for compounding: Children: Refer to adult dosing.

Administration

Oral Suspension: Shake well before using. Should be swished about the mouth and retained in the mouth for as long as possible (several minutes) before swallowing. For neonates and infants, paint nystatin suspension into recesses of the mouth.

Monitoring and Teaching Issues

Patient Education Maintain adequate hydration unless instructed to restrict fluid intake. Do not allow medication to come in contact with eyes. Report persistent nausea, vomiting, diarrhea, or if condition being treated worsens or does not improve.

Oral tablet: Swallow whole; do not crush or chew.

Oral suspension: Shake well before using. Remove dentures; clean mouth (do not replace dentures until after using medications). Swish suspension in mouth for several minutes before swallowing.

Nystatin (Topical) (nye STAT in)

U.S. Brand Names Nyamyc®; Nystop®; Pedi-Dri®

Generic Availability (U.S.) Yes

Pharmacologic Category Antifungal Agent, Topical; Antifungal Agent, Vaginal

Medication Safety Issues

Sound-alike/look-alike issues:

Nystatin may be confused with HMG-CoA reductase inhibitors (also known as "statins"; eg, atorvastatin, fluvastatin, lovastatin, pitavastatin, pravastatin, rosuvastatin, simvastatin), Nitrostat®

Pregnancy Risk Factor A (vaginal)/C (topical)

Lactation Excretion in breast milk unknown/not recommended

Use Treatment of susceptible cutaneous and mucocutaneous fungal infections normally caused by the *Candida* species

Available Dosage Forms

Cream, topical: 100,000 units/g (15 g, 30 g)

Ointment, topical: 100,000 units/g (15 g, 30 g)

Powder, topical: 100,000 units/g (15 g, 30 g, 60 g)

Nyamyc®: 100,000 units/g (15 g, 30 g, 60 g)

Nystop®: 100,000 units/g (15 g, 30 g, 60 g)

Pedi-Dri®: 100,000 units/g (56.7 g)

Tablet, vaginal: 100,000 units

Dosing

Adult & Geriatric

Mucocutaneous infections: Topical: Apply 2-3 times/day to affected areas; very moist topical lesions are treated best with powder.

Vaginal infections: Vaginal tablets: Insert 1 tablet/day at bedtime for 2 weeks. (May also be given orally.)

Pediatric Mucocutaneous infections: Children: Refer to adult dosing.

Monitoring and Teaching Issues

Physical Assessment Determine that cause of infection is fungal. Avoid skin contact when applying.

Patient Education Do not allow medication to come in contact with eyes. Report if condition being treated worsens or does not improve.

Topical: Wash and dry area before applying (do not reuse towels without washing, apply clean clothing after use). Report unresolved burning, redness, or swelling in treated areas.

Vaginal tablet: Wash hands before using. Lie down to insert high into vagina at bedtime.

Nystatin and Triamcinolone (nye STAT in & trye am SIN oh lone)

Index Terms Triamcinolone and Nystatin

Generic Availability (U.S.) Yes

Pharmacologic Category Antifungal Agent, Topical; Corticosteroid, Topical

Pregnancy Risk Factor C

Lactation Excretion in breast milk unknown

Use Treatment of cutaneous candidiasis

Available Dosage Forms

Cream: Nystatin 100,000 units and triamcinolone 0.1% (15 g, 30 g, 60 g)

Ointment: Nystatin 100,000 units and triamcinolone 0.1% (15 g, 30 g, 60 g)

Dosing

Adult & Geriatric Cutaneous *Candida*: Topical: Apply sparingly 2-4 times/day

Pediatric Refer to adult dosing.

Administration

Topical External use only; do not use on open wounds. Apply sparingly to occlusive dressings; should not be used in the presence of open or weeping lesions.

Monitoring and Teaching Issues

Physical Assessment See individual agents.

Patient Education See individual agents.

Related Information

Nystatin (Topical) *on page 1338*

Triamcinolone (Topical) *on page 1816*

◆ **Nystat-Rx [DSC]** *see* Nystatin (Oral) *on page 1338*

◆ **Nystop®** *see* Nystatin (Topical) *on page 1338*

◆ **Nytol® Quick Caps [OTC]** *see* DiphenhydrAMINE (Systemic) *on page 543*

◆ **Nytol® Quick Gels [OTC]** *see* DiphenhydrAMINE (Systemic) *on page 543*

◆ **OCBZ** *see* OXcarbazepine *on page 1375*

◆ **Ocella™** *see* Ethinyl Estradiol and Drospirenone *on page 696*

◆ **Octagam®** *see* Immune Globulin *on page 961*

Octreotide (ok TREE oh tide)

U.S. Brand Names SandoSTATIN LAR®; SandoSTATIN®

Index Terms Longastatin; Octreotide Acetate

Generic Availability (U.S.) Yes: Excludes depot formulation

Pharmacologic Category Antidiarrheal; Antidote; Somatostatin Analog

Medication Safety Issues

Sound-alike/look-alike issues:

SandoSTATIN® may be confused with SandIMMUNE®, SandoSTATIN LAR®, sargramostim, simvastatin

Pregnancy Risk Factor B

Lactation Excretion in breast milk unknown/use caution

Use Control of symptoms (diarrhea and flushing) in patients with metastatic carcinoid tumors; treatment of watery diarrhea associated with vasoactive intestinal peptide-secreting tumors (VIPomas); treatment of acromegaly

Unlabeled/Investigational Use Treatment of AIDS-associated diarrhea (including *Cryptosporidiosis*), chemotherapy-induced diarrhea, graft-versus-host disease (GVHD) associated diarrhea, postgastrectomy dumping syndrome; control of bleeding of esophageal varices; second-line treatment for thymic malignancies; Cushing's syndrome (ectopic); insulinomas; small bowel fistulas; islet cell tumors; Zollinger-Ellison syndrome; congenital hyperinsulinism; hypothalamic obesity; treatment of hypoglycemia secondary to sulfonylurea poisoning; treatment of malignant bowel obstruction

Available Dosage Forms

Injection, microspheres for suspension:
SandoSTATIN LAR®: 10 mg, 20 mg, 30 mg

Injection, solution: 0.2 mg/mL (5 mL); 0.5 mg/mL (1 mL); 1 mg/mL (5 mL)
SandoSTATIN®: 0.2 mg/mL (5 mL); 1 mg/mL (5 mL)

Injection, solution [preservative free]: 0.05 mg/mL (1 mL); 0.1 mg/mL (1 mL); 0.5 mg/mL (1 mL)
SandoSTATIN®: 0.05 mg/mL (1 mL); 0.1 mg/mL (1 mL); 0.5 mg/mL (1 mL)

Dosing

Adult

Acromegaly:

SubQ, I.V.: Initial: 50 mcg 3 times/day; titrate to achieve growth hormone levels <5 ng/mL or IGF-I (somatomedin C) levels <1.9 units/mL in males and <2.2 units/mL in females. Usual effective dose 100-200 mcg 3 times/day; range 300-1500 mcg/day. **Note:** Should be withdrawn yearly for a 4-week interval (8 weeks for depot injection) in patients who have received irradiation. Resume if levels increase and signs/symptoms recur.

I.M. depot injection: Patients must be stabilized on subcutaneous octreotide for at least 2 weeks before switching to the long-acting depot. Upon switch: 20 mg I.M. intragluteally every 4 weeks for 3 months, then the dose may be modified based upon response.

Dosage adjustment for acromegaly: After 3 months of depot injections, the dosage may be continued or modified as follows:

GH ≤1 ng/mL, IGF-1 normal, and symptoms controlled: Reduce octreotide depot to 10 mg I.M. every 4 weeks

GH ≤2.5 ng/mL, IGF-1 normal, and symptoms controlled: Maintain octreotide depot at 20 mg I.M. every 4 weeks

GH >2.5 ng/mL, IGF-1 elevated, and/or symptoms uncontrolled: Increase octreotide depot to 30 mg I.M. every 4 weeks

Note: Patients not adequately controlled at a dose of 30 mg may increase dose to 40 mg every 4 weeks. Dosages >40 mg are not recommended.

Carcinoid tumors:

Manufacturer labeling:

SubQ, I.V.: Initial 2 weeks: 100-600 mcg/day in 2-4 divided doses; usual range: 50-750 mcg/day (some patients may require up to 1500 mcg/day)

I.M. depot injection: Patients must be stabilized on subcutaneous octreotide for at least 2 weeks before switching to the long-acting depot. Upon switch: 20 mg I.M. intragluteally every 4 weeks for 2 months, then the dose may be modified based upon response.

NCCN guidelines (Neuroendocrine Tumor, v.2.2009):

SubQ: 150-250 mcg 3 times daily; dose and frequency may be increased if needed for symptom control

I.M. depot injection: 20-30 mg every 4 weeks; dose and frequency may be increased if needed for symptom control; SubQ octreotide may be used for breakthrough symptoms

Note: Patients should continue to receive their SubQ injections for the first 2 weeks at the same dose in order to maintain therapeutic levels (some patients may require 3-4 weeks of continued SubQ injections). Patients who experience periodic exacerbations of symptoms may require temporary SubQ injections in addition to depot injections (at their previous SubQ dosing regimen) until symptoms have resolved.

Dosage adjustment for carcinoid tumors: After 2 months of depot injections, the dosage may be continued or modified as follows:

Increase to 30 mg I.M. every 4 weeks if symptoms are inadequately controlled

Decrease to 10 mg I.M. every 4 weeks, for a trial period, if initially responsive to 20 mg dose

Dosage >30 mg is not recommended

VIPomas:

Manufacturer labeling:

SubQ, I.V.: Initial 2 weeks: 200-300 mcg/day in 2-4 divided doses; titrate dose based on response/tolerance. Range: 150-750 mcg/day (doses >450 mcg/day are rarely required)

I.M. depot injection: Patients must be stabilized on subcutaneous octreotide for at least 2 weeks before switching to the long-acting depot. Upon switch: 20 mg I.M. intragluteally every 4 weeks for 2 months, then the dose may be modified based upon response.

NCCN guidelines (Neuroendocrine Tumor, v.2.2009):

SubQ: 150-250 mcg 3 times daily; dose and frequency may be increased if needed for symptom control

I.M. depot injection: 20-30 mg every 4 weeks dose and frequency may be increased if needed for symptom control; SubQ octreotide may be used for breakthrough symptoms

Note: Patients receiving depot injection should continue to receive their SubQ injections for the first 2 weeks at the same dose in order to maintain therapeutic levels (some patients may require 3-4 weeks of continued SubQ injections). Patients who experience periodic exacerbations of symptoms may require temporary SubQ injections in addition to depot injections (at their previous SubQ dosing regimen) until symptoms have resolved.

Dosage adjustment for VIPomas: After 2 months of depot injections, the dosage may be continued or modified as follows:

Increase to 30 mg I.M. every 4 weeks if symptoms are inadequately controlled

Decrease to 10 mg I.M. every 4 weeks, for a trial period, if initially responsive to 20 mg dose

Dosage >30 mg is not recommended

Diarrhea (unlabeled use): I.V.: Initial: 50-100 mcg every 8 hours; increase by 100 mcg/dose at 48-hour intervals; maximum dose: 500 mcg every 8 hours

Diarrhea associated with chemotherapy (unlabeled use):

Low grade or uncomplicated: SubQ: 100-150 mcg every 8 hours (Benson, 2004; Kornblau, 2000)

Severe: Initial: SubQ: 100-150 mcg every 8 hours; may increase to 500-1500 mcg I.V. or SubQ every 8 hours (Kornblau, 2000)

Complicated: I.V., SubQ: Initial: 100-150 mcg 3 times daily or I.V. Infusion: 25-50 mcg/hour; may escalate to 500 mcg 3 times a day until controlled (Benson, 2004)

Diarrhea associated with GVHD (unlabeled use): I.V.: 500 mcg every 8 hours; discontinue within 24 hours of resolution; Maximum duration of therapy if diarrhea is not resolved: 7 days (Kornblau, 2000)

Esophageal varices bleeding (unlabeled use): I.V. bolus: 25-50 mcg followed by continuous I.V. infusion of 25-50 mcg/hour

Hypoglycemia in sulfonylurea poisoning (unlabeled use): SubQ is the preferred route of administration; repeat dosing, dose escalation, or initiation of a continuous infusion may be required in patients who experience recurrent hypoglycemia. Duration of treatment may exceed 24 hours. Optimal care decisions should be made based upon patient-specific details:

SubQ: 50-100 mcg; repeat in 6-12 hours as needed based upon blood glucose concentrations

I.V.: Doses up to 100-125 mcg/hour have been used successfully

Islet cell tumors (unlabeled use): SubQ: 150-250 mcg 3 times daily or I.M. (depot): 20-30 mg every 4 weeks dose and frequency may be increased if needed for symptom control; SubQ octreotide may be used for breakthrough symptoms (NCCN Neuroendocrine Tumor guidelines v.2.2009)

Malignant bowel obstruction (unlabeled use): SubQ: 150-300 mcg twice daily (Mercadante, 2007; NCCN Palliative Care guidelines v.1.2010)

Geriatric Refer to adult dosing. Elimination half-life is increased by 46% and clearance is decreased by 26%; dose adjustment may be required. Dosing should generally begin at the lower end of dosing range.

Pediatric Infants and Children:

Secretory diarrhea (unlabeled use): I.V., SubQ: Doses of 1-10 mcg/kg every 12 hours have been used in children beginning at the low end of the range and increasing by 0.3 mcg/kg/dose at 3-day intervals. Suppression of growth hormone (animal data) is of concern when used as long-term therapy.

Congenital hyperinsulinism (unlabeled use): SubQ: Doses of 3-40 mcg/kg/day have been used.

Hypoglycemia in sulfonylurea poisoning (unlabeled use): SubQ is the preferred route of administration; repeat dosing, dose escalation, or initiation of a continuous infusion may be required in patients who experience recurrent hypoglycemia. Duration of treatment may exceed 24 hours. Optimal care decisions should be made based upon patient-specific details: SubQ: 1-1.5 mcg/kg; repeat in 6-12 hours as needed based upon blood glucose concentrations

Renal Impairment

Nondialysis-dependent renal impairment: No dosage adjustment required

Dialysis-dependent renal impairment: Depot injection: Initial dose: 10 mg I.M. every 4 weeks; titrate based upon response (clearance is reduced by ~50%)

Hepatic Impairment Patients with established cirrhosis of the liver: Depot injection: Initial dose: 10 mg I.M. every 4 weeks; titrate based upon response.

Administration

I.M. Depot formulation: Administer I.M. intragluteal (avoid deltoid administration); alternate gluteal injection sites to avoid irritation. Do not administer Sandostatin LAR® intravenously or subcutaneously; must be administered immediately after mixing.

I.V. Regular injection only (not suspension): IVP should be administered undiluted over 3 minutes. IVPB should be administered over 15-30 minutes. Continuous I.V. infusion rates (unlabeled administration rate) have ranged from 25-50 mcg/hour for the treatment of esophageal variceal bleeding (unlabeled use); continuous I.V. infusion rates of 100-125 mcg/hour have been used for the treatment of sulfonylurea-induced hypoglycemia (unlabeled use).

Other SubQ: Regular injection formulation (not depot) can be administered SubQ. Use the concentration with smallest volume to deliver dose to reduce injection site pain. Rotate injection site; may bring to room temperature prior to injection.

Monitoring and Teaching Issues

Laboratory Monitoring

Acromegaly: Growth hormone, somatomedin C (IGF-1)

Carcinoid: 5-HIAA, plasma serotonin and plasma substance P

VIPomas: Vasoactive intestinal peptide

Chronic therapy: Thyroid function (baseline and periodic), vitamin B_{12} level, blood glucose, glycemic control and antidiabetic regimen (patients with diabetes mellitus), zinc level (patients with excessive fluid loss maintained on TPN)

Physical Assessment Use caution in presence of renal and/or hepatic impairment (dosage adjustment may be necessary). May effect response to insulin or sulfonylureas. Follow specific dosing directions when switching from SubQ to long-acting depot formulation. Evaluate therapeutic effectiveness according to use and adverse effects (eg, hyper-/hypoglycemia, hypothyroidism, cardiovascular changes, GI disturbances, CNS changes, dyspnea). Caution patients with diabetes to monitor serum glucose closely; may affect response to insulin or sulfonylureas. Teach patient appropriate injection technique and syringe/needle disposal.

Patient Education If self-administered, follow instructions for injection and syringe/needle disposal. Schedule injections between meals to decrease GI effects. Consult prescriber about appropriate diet. If you have diabetes, monitor serum glucose closely and notify prescriber of significant changes (this drug may alter the effects of insulin or sulfonylureas). May cause skin flushing, nausea, vomiting, dizziness, fatigue, drowsiness, or joint or muscle pain. Report unusual weight gain; swelling of extremities; respiratory difficulty; acute or persistent GI distress (eg, diarrhea, vomiting, constipation, abdominal pain); muscle weakness or tremors or loss of motor function; chest pain or palpitations; blurred vision; depression; or redness, swelling, burning, or pain at injection site.

◆ **Octreotide Acetate** *see* Octreotide *on page 1339*

◆ **Ocuflox®** *see* Ofloxacin (Ophthalmic) *on page 1343*

◆ **OcuNefrin™ [OTC]** *see* Phenylephrine (Ophthalmic) *on page 1452*

◆ **O-desmethylvenlafaxine** *see* Desvenlafaxine *on page 497*

◆ **ODV** *see* Desvenlafaxine *on page 497*

Ofatumumab (oh fa TOOM yoo mab)

U.S. Brand Names Arzerra™

Index Terms HuMax-CD20

Generic Availability (U.S.) No

Pharmacologic Category Antineoplastic Agent, Monoclonal Antibody; Monoclonal Antibody

Medication Safety Issues

Sound-alike/look-alike issues:

Ofatumumab may be confused with omalizumab

High alert medication: The Institute for Safe Medication Practices (ISMP) includes this medication among its list of drug classes which have a heightened risk of causing significant patient harm when used in error.

Pregnancy Risk Factor C

Lactation Excretion in breast milk unknown/use caution

Use Treatment of refractory chronic lymphocytic leukemia (CLL)

Available Dosage Forms

Injection, solution [preservative free]:

Arzerra™: 20 mg/mL (5 mL)

Dosing

Adult & Geriatric Note: Premedicate with acetaminophen, an antihistamine, and a corticosteroid 30-120 minutes prior to treatment (see Administration).

CLL: I.V. Initial dose: 300 mg week 1, followed 1 week later by 2000 mg once weekly for 7 doses (doses 2-8), followed 4 weeks later by 2000 mg once every 4 weeks for 4 doses (doses 9-12; for a total of 12 doses)

Renal Impairment When studied in patients with creatinine clearances ranging from 33-287 mL/minute, baseline creatinine clearance did not have a clinically relevant effect.

Adjustment for Toxicity Infusion reaction: Interrupt infusion for infusion reaction (any severity).

Grade 1 or 2 infusion reaction: Resume at one-half of the previous rate; may increase (see Administration) based on patient tolerance.

Grade 3: Resume infusion at 12 mL/hour; may increase (see Administration) based on patient tolerance.

Grade 4: Do not resume.

Administration

I.V. Do not administer I.V. push or as a bolus. Premedicate with acetaminophen, an antihistamine and a corticosteroid 30-120 minutes prior to administration. Administer with an in-line filter (supplied) and polyvinyl chloride (PVC) administration sets. Do not mix with or infuse with other medications. Flush line before and after infusion with NS. Begin infusion within 12 hours of preparation. The final concentration of dose 1 is 0.3 mg/mL and final concentration of doses 2-12 is 2 mg/mL.

Premedication: Premedicate with oral acetaminophen (1000 mg), an oral or I.V. antihistamine (eg, cetirizine 10 mg orally or equivalent), and an I.V. corticosteroid. Full dose corticosteroid is recommended for doses 1, 2, and 9; in the absence of infusion reaction ≥grade 3, may gradually reduce corticosteroid dose for doses 3-8; administer full or half corticosteroid dose with doses 10-12 if ≥grade 3 did not occur with dose 9.

Doses 1 and 2: Initiate infusion at 12 mL/hour for 30 minutes, if tolerated (no infusion reaction) increase to 25 mL/hour for 30 minutes, if tolerated, increase to 50 mL/hour for 30 minutes, if tolerated, increase to 100 mL/hour for 30 minutes, if tolerated, increase to 200 mL/hour for duration of infusion.

Doses 3-12: Initiate infusion at 25 mL/hour for 30 minutes, if tolerated (no infusion reaction) increase to 50 mL/hour for 30 minutes, if tolerated, increase to 100 mL/hour for 30 minutes, if tolerated, increase to 200 mL/hour for 30 minutes, if tolerated, increase to 400 mL/hour for remainder of infusion.

Monitoring and Teaching Issues

Laboratory Monitoring CBC with differential, hepatitis B screening (in patients at high-risk; prior to therapy initiation)

Physical Assessment Perform hepatitis B screening prior to prescribing therapy. Premedicate with acetaminophen, antihistamine, and a corticosteroid prior to administration. Patient must be monitored closely for infusion reactions; appropriate treatment for hypersensitivity reactions should be available. Evaluate patient response on a frequent basis throughout treatment; dosage adjustments may be necessary.

Patient Education You will be closely monitored during infusion. Report immediately any pain, burning, or swelling at infusion site; sudden chest pain or palpitations; difficulty breathing or swallowing; or chills. Between infusions, maintain adequate nutrition and hydration unless instructed to restrict fluid intake. You will need frequent laboratory tests during course of therapy. You will be more susceptible to infection. You may experience some nausea or vomiting. Report unresolved GI problems, persistent fever, chills, muscle pain, skin rash, unusual bleeding or bruising, signs of infection (mouth sores, sore throat, white plaques in mouth or perianal area, burning on urination), swelling of extremities, respiratory difficulty, chest pain, or palpitations.

◆ **Ofirmev™** *see* Acetaminophen *on page* 38

Ofloxacin (Ophthalmic) (oh FLOKS a sin)

U.S. Brand Names Ocuflox®

Generic Availability (U.S.) Yes

Pharmacologic Category Antibiotic, Ophthalmic; Antibiotic, Quinolone

Medication Safety Issues

Sound-alike/look-alike issues:

Ocuflox® may be confused with Occlusal®-HP, Ocufen®

Pregnancy Risk Factor C

Lactation Enters breast milk/not recommended (AAP rates "compatible"; AAP 2001 update pending)

Use Treatment of superficial ocular infections involving the conjunctiva or cornea due to strains of susceptible organisms

Available Dosage Forms

Solution, ophthalmic: 0.3% (5 mL, 10 mL)

Ocuflox®: 0.3% (5 mL)

Dosing

Adult

Conjunctivitis: Ophthalmic: Instill 1-2 drops in affected eye(s) every 2-4 hours for the first 2 days, then use 4 times/day for an additional 5 days.

Corneal ulcer: Ophthalmic: Instill 1-2 drops every 30 minutes while awake and every 4-6 hours after retiring for the first 2 days; beginning on day 3, instill 1-2 drops every hour while awake for 4-6 additional days; thereafter, 1-2 drops 4 times/day until clinical cure.

Pediatric

Conjunctivitis: Ophthalmic: Children ≥1 year: Refer to adult dosing.

Corneal ulcer: Ophthalmic: Children ≥1 year: Refer to adult dosing.

Administration

Other For ophthalmic use only; avoid touching tip of applicator to eye or other surfaces.

Monitoring and Teaching Issues

Patient Education Wash hands before instilling solution. Sit or lie down to instill. Open eye, look at ceiling, and instill prescribed amount of solution as directed. Close eye, roll eye in all directions, and apply gentle pressure to inner corner of eye. Do not touch tip of applicator or let tip of applicator touch eye (may cause eye infection, eye damage, or vision loss). Do not wear contact lenses during therapy. Temporary stinging, blurred vision, dry eyes, or a bad taste in your mouth may occur after installation. Report persistent pain, burning, excessive tearing, decreased visual acuity, swelling, itching, or worsening of condition.

Ofloxacin (Otic) (oh FLOKS a sin)

Index Terms Floxin Otic Singles

Generic Availability (U.S.) Yes

Pharmacologic Category Antibiotic, Quinolone

Medication Safety Issues

Sound-alike/look-alike issues:

Floxin® may be confused with Flexeril®

International issues:

Floxin: Brand name for ofloxacin [U.S., Canada], but also the brand name for flunarizine [Thailand], norfloxacin [South Africa], and perfloxacin [Philippines]

Floxin® [U.S., Canada] may be confused with Flexin brand name for diclofenac [Argentina], cyclobenzaprine [Chile], and orphenadrine [Israel]; Flogen brand name for naproxen [Mexico]; Fluoxin brand name for fluoxetine [Czech Republic]

Pregnancy Risk Factor C

Lactation Enters breast milk/not recommended (AAP rates "compatible"; AAP 2001 update pending)

Use Otitis externa, chronic suppurative otitis media, acute otitis media

Available Dosage Forms

Solution, otic: 0.3% (5 mL, 10 mL)

Dosing

Adult

Otitis media, chronic suppurative with perforated tympanic membranes: Otic: Instill 10 drops (or the contents of 2 single-dose containers) into affected ear twice daily for 14 days

Otitis externa: Otic: Instill 10 drops (or the contents of 2 single-dose containers) into affected ear(s) once daily for 7 days

Pediatric Not for systemic use.

Acute otitis media with tympanotomy tubes: Otic: Children 1-12 years: Instill 5 drops (or the contents of 1 single-dose container) into affected ear twice daily for 10 days.

Otitis externa: Otic:

Children 6 months to 13 years: Instill 5 drops (or the contents of 1 single-dose container) into affected ear(s) once daily for 7 days

Children ≥13 years: Refer to adult dosing.

Otitis media, chronic suppurative with perforated tympanic membranes: Otic: Children >12 years: Refer to adult dosing.

Administration

Other Prior to use, warm solution by holding container in hands for 1-2 minutes. Patient should lie down with affected ear upward and medication instilled. Pump tragus 4 times to ensure penetration of medication. Patient should remain in this position for 5 minutes.

Monitoring and Teaching Issues

Laboratory Monitoring Perform culture and sensitivity studies before initiating therapy. Monitor CBC, renal and hepatic function periodically if therapy is prolonged.

Patient Education Wash hands before and after applying drops. Warm solution by holding container in hands for a few minutes. Lie with affected ear up and instill prescribed number of drops into ear. Remain on side with ear up for 5 minutes.

◆ **Oforta™** *see* Fludarabine *on page* 776

◆ **9-OH-risperidone** *see* Paliperidone *on page* 1391

◆ **OKT3** *see* Muromonab-CD3 *on page* 1268

OLANZapine (oh LAN za peen)

U.S. Brand Names ZyPREXA®; ZyPREXA® IntraMuscular; ZyPREXA® Relprevv™; ZyPREXA® Zydis®

Index Terms LY170053; Olanzapine Pamoate; Zyprexa Zydis

Generic Availability (U.S.) No

Pharmacologic Category Antimanic Agent; Antipsychotic Agent, Atypical

Medication Safety Issues

Sound-alike/look-alike issues:

OLANZapine may be confused with olsalazine, QUEtiapine

ZyPREXA® may be confused with CeleXA®, Reprexain™, Zestril®, ZyrTEC®

ZyPREXA® Zydis® may be confused with Zelapar™

ZyPREXA® Relprevv™ may be confused with ZyPREXA® IntraMuscular

Medication Guide Available Yes

Prescribing and Access Restrictions As a requirement of the REMS program, only prescribers, healthcare facilities, and pharmacies registered with the Zyprexa® Relprevv™ Patient Care Program are able to prescribe, distribute, or dispense Zyprexa® Relprevv™ for patients who are enrolled in and meet all conditions of the program. Zyprexa® Relprevv™ must be administered at a registered healthcare facility. Prescribers will need to be recertified every 3 years. Contact the Zyprexa® Relprevv™ Patient Care Program at 1-877-772-9390.

Pregnancy Risk Factor C

Lactation Enters breast milk/not recommended

Use

Oral: Treatment of the manifestations of schizophrenia; treatment of acute or mixed mania episodes associated with bipolar I disorder (as monotherapy or in combination with lithium or valproate); maintenance treatment of bipolar disorder; in combination with fluoxetine for treatment-resistant or bipolar I depression

I.M., extended-release (Zyprexa® Relprevv™): Treatment of schizophrenia

I.M., short-acting (Zyprexa® IntraMuscular): Treatment of acute agitation associated with schizophrenia and bipolar I mania

Unlabeled/Investigational Use Treatment of psychosis/schizophrenia in children; chronic pain; prevention of chemotherapy-associated delayed nausea or vomiting; psychosis/agitation related to Alzheimer's dementia

Mechanism of Action/Effect The efficacy of olanzapine in schizophrenia and bipolar disorder is thought to be mediated through combined antagonism of dopamine and serotonin type 2 receptor sites.

Contraindications There are no contraindications listed in the manufacturer's labeling.

Canadian labeling: Hypersensitivity to olanzapine or any component of the formulation

Warnings/Precautions [U.S. Boxed Warning]: Elderly patients with dementia-related psychosis treated with antipsychotics are at an increased risk of death compared to placebo. Most deaths appeared to be either cardiovascular (eg, heart failure, sudden death) or infectious (eg, pneumonia) in nature. In addition, an increased incidence of cerebrovascular effects (eg, transient ischemic attack, stroke) has been reported in studies of placebo-controlled trials of olanzapine in elderly patients with dementia-related psychosis. Olanzapine is not approved for the treatment of dementia-related psychosis.

Moderate to highly sedating, use with caution in disorders where CNS depression is a feature; patients must be cautioned about performing tasks which require mental alertness (eg, operating machinery or driving). Use caution in patients with cardiac disease. Use with caution in Parkinson's disease, predisposition to seizures, or severe hepatic or renal disease. Life-threatening arrhythmias have occurred with therapeutic doses of some neuroleptics. May induce orthostatic hypotension; use caution with history of cardiovascular disease, hemodynamic instability, prior myocardial infarction, or ischemic heart disease. Increases in cholesterol and triglycerides have been noted. Use with caution in patients with pre-existing abnormal lipid profile. Esophageal dysmotility and aspiration have been associated with antipsychotic use; use with caution in patients at risk of aspiration pneumonia. May increase prolactin levels; clinical significance of hyperprolactinemia in patients with breast cancer or other prolactin-dependent tumors is unknown. Significant weight gain (>7% of baseline weight) may occur; monitor waist circumference and BMI. Impaired core body temperature regulation may occur; caution with strenuous exercise, heat exposure, dehydration, and concomitant medication possessing anticholinergic effects.

Leukopenia, neutropenia, and agranulocytosis (sometimes fatal) have been reported in clinical trials and postmarketing reports with antipsychotic use; presence of risk factors (eg, pre-existing low WBC or history of drug-induced leuko-/neutropenia) should prompt periodic blood count assessment. Discontinue therapy at first signs of blood dyscrasias or if absolute neutrophil count <1000/mm^3.

May cause anticholinergic effects; use with caution in patients with decreased gastrointestinal motility, urinary retention, BPH, xerostomia, or narrow-angle glaucoma. Relative to other neuroleptics, olanzapine has a moderate potency of cholinergic blockade. May cause extrapyramidal symptoms (EPS), although risk of these reactions is lower relative to other neuroleptics. Risk of dystonia (and probably other EPS) may be greater with increased doses, use of conventional antipsychotics, males, and younger patients. May be associated with neuroleptic malignant syndrome (NMS). May cause extreme and life-threatening hyperglycemia; use with caution in patients with diabetes or other disorders of glucose regulation; monitor. Olanzapine levels may be lower in patients who smoke; the manufacturer does not require dosage adjustments, although dosage adjustments may be considered. Use in adolescent patients ≥13 years of age may result in increased weight gain and sedation, as well as greater increases in LDL cholesterol, total cholesterol, triglycerides, prolactin, and liver transaminase levels when compared to adults. Adolescent patients should be maintained on the lowest dose necessary.

The possibility of a suicide attempt is inherent in psychotic illness or bipolar disorder; use caution in high-risk patients during initiation of therapy. Prescriptions should be written for the smallest quantity consistent with good patient care.

There are two Zyprexa® formulations for intramuscular injection: Zyprexa® Relprevv™ is an extended-release formulation and Zyprexa® Intramuscular is short-acting:

Extended-release I.M. injection (Zyprexa® Relprevv™): Monitor for post injection delirium/sedation syndrome; patients should be continuously watched (≥3 hours) for symptoms of olanzapine overdose. Only available through a restricted drug distribution program.

Short-acting I.M. injection (Zyprexa® IntraMuscular): Patients should remain recumbent if drowsy/dizzy until hypotension, bradycardia, and/or hypoventilation have been ruled out. Concurrent use of I.M./I.V. benzodiazepines is not recommended (fatalities have been reported, though causality not determined).

Drug Interactions

Metabolism/Transport Effects Substrate of CYP1A2 (major), 2D6 (minor); **Inhibits** CYP1A2 (weak), 2C9 (weak), 2C19 (weak), 2D6 (weak), 3A4 (weak)

Avoid Concomitant Use

Avoid concomitant use of OLANZapine with any of the following: Benzodiazepines; Metoclopramide

Decreased Effect

OLANZapine may decrease the levels/effects of: Amphetamines; Anti-Parkinson's Agents (Dopamine Agonist); Quinagolide

The levels/effects of OLANZapine may be decreased by: CYP1A2 Inducers (Strong); Lithium formulations; Peginterferon Alfa-2b

Increased Effect/Toxicity

OLANZapine may increase the levels/effects of: Alcohol (Ethyl); Anticholinergics; Benzodiazepines; CNS Depressants; Methotrimeprazine; Methylphenidate

The levels/effects of OLANZapine may be increased by: Acetylcholinesterase Inhibitors (Central); CYP1A2 Inhibitors (Moderate); CYP1A2 Inhibitors (Strong); Droperidol; FluvoxaMINE; LamoTRIgine; Lithium formulations; Methotrimeprazine; Methylphenidate; Metoclopramide; Pramlintide; Tetrabenazine

Nutritional/Ethanol Interactions

Ethanol: Avoid ethanol (may increase CNS depression).

Herb/Nutraceutical: Avoid dong quai, St John's wort (may also cause photosensitization). Avoid kava kava, gotu kola, valerian, St John's wort (may increase CNS depression).

Adverse Reactions

Oral: Unless otherwise noted, adverse events are reported for placebo-controlled trials in adult patients on monotherapy:

>10%:

Central nervous system: Somnolence (dose dependent; 20% to 39%; adolescents 39% to 48%), extrapyramidal symptoms (dose dependent; ≤32%), dizziness (11% to 18%), headache (adolescents 17%), fatigue (adolescents 3% to 14%), insomnia (12%)

Endocrine & metabolic: Prolactin increased (30%; adolescents 47%)

Gastrointestinal: Weight gain (5% to 6%, has been reported as high as 40%; adolescents 29% to 31%), appetite increased (3% to 6%; adolescents 17% to 29%), xerostomia (dose dependent; 3% to 22%), constipation (9% to 11%), dyspepsia (7% to 11%)

Hepatic: ALT increased ≥3 x ULN (adolescents 12%; adults 5%)

Neuromuscular & skeletal: Weakness (dose dependent; 8% to 20%)

Miscellaneous: Accidental injury (12%)

1% to 10%:

Cardiovascular: Chest pain, hypertension, peripheral edema, postural hypotension, tachycardia

Central nervous system: Fever, personality changes, restlessness (adolescents)

Dermatologic: Bruising

Endocrine & metabolic: Breast-related events ([adolescents] discharge, enlargement, galactorrhea, gynecomastia, lactation disorder); menstrual-related events (amenorrhea, hypomenorrhea, menstruation delayed, oligomenorrhea); sexual function-related events (anorgasmia, ejaculation delayed, erectile dysfunction, changes in libido, abnormal orgasm, sexual dysfunction)

Gastrointestinal: Abdominal pain (adolescents), diarrhea (adolescents), flatulence, nausea (dose dependent), vomiting

Genitourinary: Incontinence, UTI

Hepatic: Hepatic enzymes increased

Neuromuscular & skeletal: Abnormal gait, akathisia, articulation impairment, back pain, falling, hypertonia, joint/extremity pain, muscle stiffness (adolescents), tremor (dose dependent)

Ocular: Amblyopia

Respiratory: Cough, epistaxis (adolescents), pharyngitis, respiratory tract infection (adolescents), rhinitis, sinusitis (adolescents)

Injection: Unless otherwise noted, adverse events are reported for placebo-controlled trials in adult patients on extended-release I.M. injection (Zyprexa® Relprevv™). Also refer to adverse reactions noted with oral therapy.

>10%: Central nervous system: Headache (13 to 18%), sedation (8% to 13%)

1% to 10%:

Cardiovascular: Hypertension, hypotension (short-acting), postural hypotension (short-acting), QT prolongation

Central nervous system: Abnormal dreams, abnormal thinking, auditory hallucination, dizziness, dysarthria, extrapyramidal symptoms, fatigue, fever, pain, restlessness, somnolence

Dermatologic: Acne

Gastrointestinal: Abdominal pain, appetite increased, diarrhea, flatulence, nausea, vomiting, weight gain, xerostomia

Genitourinary: Vaginal discharge

Hepatic: Liver enzymes increased

Local: Injection site pain

Neuromuscular & skeletal: Arthralgia, back pain, muscle spasms, stiffness, tremor, weakness (short-acting)

Otic: Ear pain

Respiratory: Cough, nasal congestion, nasopharyngitis, pharyngolaryngeal pain, sneezing, upper respiratory tract infection

Miscellaneous: Toothache, tooth infection, viral infection

<1%, postmarketing, and/or case reports (limited to important or life-threatening): CPK increased, post-injection delirium/sedation syndrome, syncope (short-acting)

Pharmacodynamics/Kinetics

Absorption

Oral: Well absorbed; not affected by food; tablets and orally-disintegrating tablets are bioequivalent

Short-acting injection: Rapidly absorbed

Time to Peak Maximum plasma concentrations after I.M. administration are 5 times higher than maximum plasma concentrations produced by an oral dose.

Extended-release injection: ~7 days

Short-acting injection: 15-45 minutes

Oral: ~6 hours

Protein Binding Plasma: 93%, bound to albumin and alpha$_1$-glycoprotein

Half-Life Elimination 21-54 hours; approximately 1.5 times greater in elderly; Extended-release injection: ~30 days

Metabolism Highly metabolized via direct glucuronidation and cytochrome P450 mediated oxidation (CYP1A2, CYP2D6); 40% removed via first pass metabolism

Excretion Urine (57%, 7% as unchanged drug); feces (30%)

Clearance: 40% increase in olanzapine clearance in smokers; 30% decrease in females

Pharmacokinetic Note Tablets and orally-disintegrating tablets are bioequivalent.

Available Dosage Forms

Injection, powder for reconstitution:
ZyPREXA® IntraMuscular: 10 mg

Injection, powder for suspension, extended release:
ZyPREXA® Relprevv™: 210 mg, 300 mg, 405 mg

Tablet, oral:
ZyPREXA®: 2.5 mg, 5 mg, 7.5 mg, 10 mg, 15 mg, 20 mg

Tablet, orally disintegrating, oral:
ZyPREXA® Zydis®: 5 mg, 10 mg, 15 mg, 20 mg

Dosing

Adult & Geriatric

Schizophrenia:

Oral: Initial: 5-10 mg once daily (increase to 10 mg once daily within 5-7 days); thereafter, adjust by 5 mg/day at 1-week intervals, up to a recommended maximum of 20 mg/day. Maintenance: 10-20 mg once daily. Doses of 30-50 mg/day have been used; however, doses >10 mg/day have not demonstrated better efficacy, and safety and efficacy of doses >20 mg/day have not been evaluated.

Extended-release I.M. injection: **Note:** Establish tolerance to oral olanzapine prior to changing to extended-release I.M. injection. Maximum dose: 300 mg/2 weeks or 405 mg/4 weeks

Patients established on oral olanzapine 10 mg/day: Initial dose: 210 mg every 2 weeks for 4 doses or 405 mg every 4 weeks for 2 doses; Maintenance dose: 150 mg every 2 weeks or 300 mg every 4 weeks

Patients established on oral olanzapine 15 mg/day: Initial dose: 300 mg every 2 weeks for 4 doses; Maintenance dose: 210 mg every 2 weeks or 405 mg every 4 weeks

Patients established on oral olanzapine 20 mg/day: Initial and maintenance dose: 300 mg every 2 weeks

Acute mania associated with bipolar disorder: Oral:

Monotherapy: Initial: 10-15 mg once daily; increase by 5 mg/day at intervals of not less than 24 hours. Maintenance: 5-20 mg/day; recommended maximum dose: 20 mg/day.

Combination therapy (with lithium or valproate): Initial: 10 mg once daily; dosing range: 5-20 mg/day

Agitation (acute, associated with bipolar disorder or schizophrenia): Short-acting I.M. injection: Initial dose: 10 mg (a lower dose of 5-7.5 mg may be considered when clinical factors warrant); additional doses (up to 10 mg) may be considered; however, 2-4 hours should be allowed between doses to evaluate response (maximum total daily dose: 30 mg, per manufacturer's recommendation)

Depression:

Depression associated with bipolar disorder (in combination with fluoxetine): Oral: Initial: 5 mg in the evening; adjust as tolerated to usual range of 5-12.5 mg/day. See **"Note."**

Treatment-resistant depression (in combination with fluoxetine): Oral: Initial: 5 mg in the evening; adjust as tolerated to range of 5-20 mg/day. See **"Note."**

Note: When using individual components of fluoxetine with olanzapine rather than fixed dose combination product (Symbyax®), approximate dosage correspondence is as follows:

Olanzapine 2.5 mg + fluoxetine 20 mg = Symbyax® 3/25
Olanzapine 5 mg + fluoxetine 20 mg = Symbyax® 6/25
Olanzapine 12.5 mg + fluoxetine 20 mg = Symbyax® 12/25
Olanzapine 5 mg + fluoxetine 50 mg = Symbyax® 6/50
Olanzapine 12.5 mg + fluoxetine 50 mg = Symbyax® 12/50

Prevention of chemotherapy-associated delayed nausea or vomiting (unlabeled use; in combination with a corticosteroid and serotonin [$5HT_3$] antagonist): Oral: 10 mg once daily for 3-5 days, beginning on day 1 of chemotherapy **or** 5 mg once daily for 2 days before chemotherapy, followed by 10 mg once daily (beginning on the day of chemotherapy) for 3-8 days

Pediatric Schizophrenia/bipolar disorder: Adolescents ≥13 years: Oral: Initial: 2.5-5 mg once daily; adjust by 2.5-5 mg/day to target dose of 10 mg/day; dosing range: 2.5-20 mg/ day

Renal Impairment No dosage adjustment required. Not removed by dialysis.

Hepatic Impairment Dosage adjustment may be necessary; however, there are no specific recommendations. Monitor closely.

Administration

Oral

Tablet: May be administered without regard to meals.

Orally-disintegrating tablet: Remove from foil blister by peeling back (do not push tablet through the foil). Place tablet in mouth immediately upon removal. Tablet dissolves rapidly in saliva and may be swallowed with or without liquid. May be administered with or without food/meals.

I.M.

Short-acting I.M. injection: **For I.M. administration only**; do not administer injection intravenously or subcutaneously; inject slowly, deep into muscle. If dizziness and/or drowsiness are noted, patient should remain recumbent until examination indicates postural hypotension and/or bradycardia are not a problem.

Extended-release I.M. injection: **For I.M. gluteal injection only**; do not administer I.V. or subcutaneously. After needle insertion into muscle, aspirate to verify that no blood appears. Do not massage injection site. Use diluent, syringes, and needles provided in convenience kit; obtain a new kit if aspiration of blood occurs.

Stability

Reconstitution

Injection, extended-release: Dilute as directed to final concentration of 150 mg/mL. Shake vigorously to mix; will form yellow, opaque suspension. Following reconstitution, suspension may be stored at room temperature and used within 24 hours. Shake vigorously to resuspend prior to administration. Use immediately once suspension is in syringe. Suspension may be irritating to skin; wear gloves during reconstitution.

Injection, short-acting: Reconstitute 10 mg vial with 2.1 mL SWFI. Resulting solution is ~5 mg/mL. Use immediately (within 1 hour) following reconstitution. Discard any unused portion.

Storage

Injection, extended-release: Store at 20° to 25°C (68°F to 77°F); excursions permitted to 15°C to 30°C (59°F to 86°F).

Injection, short-acting: Store at 20° to 25°C (68°F to 77°F); excursions permitted to 15°C to 30°C (59°F to 86°F); do not freeze. Protect from light.

Tablet and orally-disintegrating tablet: Store at 20° to 25°C (68°F to 77°F); excursions permitted to 15°C to 30°C (59°F to 86°F). Protect from light and moisture.

Monitoring and Teaching Issues

Laboratory Monitoring Fasting lipid profile and fasting blood glucose/Hgb A_{1c} (prior to treatment, at 3 months, then annually); periodic assessment of hepatic transaminases (in patients with hepatic disease)

Physical Assessment Initiate at lower doses. Taper dosage slowly when discontinuing. Instruct patients with diabetes to monitor blood glucose levels closely; may cause hyperglycemia. Assess for extrapyramidal symptoms, suicide ideation, sedation, and CNS changes prior to treatment and periodically throughout. Monitor weight prior to initiating therapy and at least monthly. Consider titrating to a different antipsychotic agent for a weight gain ≥5% of initial weight. If Zyprexa® Relprevv™ is administered, monitor closely for at least 3 hours for symptoms of oversedation and/or delirium.

Patient Education It may take 2-3 weeks to achieve desired results. Avoid alcohol. Maintain adequate hydration. If you have diabetes, you may experience increased blood sugars; monitor closely. If you have glaucoma, periodic ophthalmic exams are recommended. You may experience excess drowsiness, restlessness, weakness, dizziness, or blurred vision; postural hypotension; constipation; heartburn; dry mouth; or weight gain. Report persistent CNS effects (eg, trembling fingers, altered gait or balance, excessive sedation, seizures, unusual movements, anxiety, abnormal thoughts, confusion, personality changes); suicide ideation; unresolved constipation or GI effects; vision changes; respiratory difficulty; unusual cough; or worsening of condition.

Orally-disintegrating tablet: Remove from foil blister by peeling back; do not push tablet through the foil. Place tablet in mouth immediately upon removal. Tablet dissolves rapidly in saliva and may be swallowed with or without liquid.

Dietary Considerations Tablets may be taken without regard to meals. Some products may contain phenylalanine.

Geriatric Considerations Elderly patients have an increased risk of adverse response to side effects or adverse reactions to antipsychotics. A higher incidence of falls has been reported in elderly patients, particularly in debilitated patients. Olanzapine half-life that was 1.5 times that of younger (<65 years of age) adults; therefore, lower initial doses are recommended. Olanzapine is not indicated in dementia-related psychosis.

Studies with patients ≥65 years of age with schizophrenia showed no difference in tolerability compared to younger adults. Studies in the elderly with dementia-related psychosis suggested a different tolerability compared to younger patients with schizophrenia. In light of significant risks and adverse effects in the elderly population (compared with limited data demonstrating efficacy in the treatment of dementia-related psychosis, aggression, and agitation), an extensive risk:benefit analysis should be performed prior to use. Therefore, use with caution and at lower recommended doses.

Breast-Feeding Considerations At steady-state concentrations, it is estimated that a breast-fed infant may be exposed to ~2% of the maternal dose.

Pregnancy Considerations No evidence of teratogenicity reported in animal studies. However, fetal toxicity and prolonged gestation have been observed. Antipsychotic use during the third trimester of pregnancy has a risk for abnormal muscle movements (extrapyramidal symptoms [EPS]) and withdrawal symptoms in newborns following delivery. Symptoms in the newborn may include agitation, feeding disorder, hypertonia, hypotonia, respiratory distress, somnolence, and tremor; these effects may be self-limiting or require hospitalization. There are no adequate and well-controlled studies in pregnant women. Healthcare providers are encouraged to enroll women 18-45 years of age exposed to olanzapine during pregnancy in the Atypical Antipsychotics Pregnancy Registry (1-866-961-2388).

Related Information

Antipsychotic Agents *on page 1986*

Olanzapine and Fluoxetine (oh LAN za peen & floo OKS e teen)

U.S. Brand Names Symbyax®

Index Terms Fluoxetine and Olanzapine; Olanzapine and Fluoxetine Hydrochloride

Generic Availability (U.S.) No

Pharmacologic Category Antidepressant, Selective Serotonin Reuptake Inhibitor; Antipsychotic Agent, Atypical

Medication Safety Issues

Sound-alike/look-alike issues:

Symbyax® may be confused with Cymbalta®

Medication Guide Available Yes

Pregnancy Risk Factor C

Lactation Enters breast milk/not recommended

Use Treatment of depressive episodes associated with bipolar I disorder; treatment-resistant depression (unresponsive to 2 trials of different antidepressants in the current episode)

Available Dosage Forms

Capsule:

Symbyax®:

3/25: Olanzapine 3 mg and fluoxetine 25 mg

6/25: Olanzapine 6 mg and fluoxetine 25 mg

6/50: Olanzapine 6 mg and fluoxetine 50 mg

12/25: Olanzapine 12 mg and fluoxetine 25 mg

12/50: Olanzapine 12 mg and fluoxetine 50 mg

Dosing

Adult Lower doses (olanzapine 3-6 mg/fluoxetine 25 mg) should be used in patients predisposed to hypotension, with hepatic impairment, with combined factors for reduced metabolism (females, the elderly, nonsmokers), or enhanced sensitivity to olanzapine; dose adjustments should be made with caution in this patient population.

Depression associated with bipolar I disorder: Initial: Olanzapine 6 mg/fluoxetine 25 mg once daily in the evening. Dosing range: Olanzapine 6-12 mg/fluoxetine 25-50 mg. Safety of daily doses of olanzapine >18 mg/fluoxetine >75 mg have not been evaluated.

Treatment-resistant depression: Initial: Olanzapine 6 mg/fluoxetine 25 mg once daily in the evening. Dosing range: Olanzapine 6-18 mg/fluoxetine 25-50 mg. Safety of daily doses of olanzapine >18 mg/fluoxetine >75 mg have not been evaluated.

Note: When using individual components of fluoxetine with olanzapine rather than fixed dose combination product (Symbyax®), approximate dosage correspondence is as follows:

Olanzapine 2.5 mg + fluoxetine 20 mg = Symbyax® 3/25

Olanzapine 5 mg + fluoxetine 20 mg = Symbyax® 6/25

Olanzapine 12.5 mg + fluoxetine 20 mg = Symbyax® 12/25

Olanzapine 5 mg + fluoxetine 50 mg = Symbyax® 6/50

Olanzapine 12.5 mg + fluoxetine 50 mg = Symbyax® 12/50

Geriatric Oral: Initial: Olanzapine 3-6 mg/fluoxetine 25 mg once daily in the evening; use caution adjusting dose (metabolism may be decreased). Safety and efficacy have not been established in patients >65 years of age.

Hepatic Impairment Initial: Olanzapine 3-6 mg/fluoxetine 25 mg once daily in the evening; use caution adjusting dose (metabolism may be decreased).

Administration

Oral Capsules should be taken once daily in the evening. May be taken without regard to meals.

Monitoring and Teaching Issues

Laboratory Monitoring CBC, lipid profile, fasting blood glucose/Hgb A_{1c}; BMI

Physical Assessment See individual agents.

Patient Education See individual agents.

Related Information

FLUoxetine *on page 789*

OLANZapine *on page 1344*

- **Olanzapine and Fluoxetine Hydrochloride** *see* Olanzapine and Fluoxetine *on page 1348*
- **Olanzapine Pamoate** *see* OLANZapine *on page 1344*
- **Oleptro™** *see* TraZODone *on page 1808*

Olmesartan (ole me SAR tan)

U.S. Brand Names Benicar®

Index Terms Olmesartan Medoxomil

Generic Availability (U.S.) No

Pharmacologic Category Angiotensin II Receptor Blocker

Medication Safety Issues

Sound-alike/look-alike issues:

Benicar® may be confused with Mevacor®

Pregnancy Risk Factor C (1st trimester); D (2nd and 3rd trimesters)

Lactation Excretion in breast milk unknown/not recommended

Use Treatment of hypertension with or without concurrent use of other antihypertensive agents

Mechanism of Action/Effect As a selective and competitive, nonpeptide angiotensin II receptor antagonist, olmesartan blocks the vasoconstrictor and aldosterone-secreting effects of angiotensin II. Olmesartan increases urinary flow rate and in addition to being natriuretic and kaliuretic, increases excretion of chloride, magnesium, uric acid, calcium, and phosphate.

Contraindications There are no contraindications listed in the manufacturer's labeling.

Warnings/Precautions [U.S. Boxed Warning]: Based on human data, drugs that act on the angiotensin system can cause injury and death to the developing fetus when used in the second and third trimesters. Angiotensin receptor blockers should be discontinued as soon as possible once pregnancy is detected. May cause hyperkalemia; avoid potassium supplementation unless specifically required by healthcare provider. Avoid use or use a smaller dose in patients who are volume depleted; correct depletion first. May be associated with deterioration of renal function and/or increases in serum creatinine, particularly in patients with low renal blood flow (eg, renal artery stenosis, heart failure) whose glomerular filtration rate (GFR) is dependent on efferent arteriolar vasoconstriction by angiotensin II. Use with caution in unstented unilateral/bilateral renal artery stenosis. When unstented bilateral renal artery stenosis is present, use is generally avoided due to the elevated risk of deterioration in renal function unless possible benefits outweigh risks. Use with caution with pre-existing renal insufficiency; significant aortic/mitral stenosis. Concurrent use of ACE inhibitors may increase the risk of clinically-significant adverse events (eg, renal dysfunction, hyperkalemia).

Drug Interactions

Metabolism/Transport Effects Substrate of SLCO1B1

Avoid Concomitant Use There are no known interactions where it is recommended to avoid concomitant use.

Decreased Effect

The levels/effects of Olmesartan may be decreased by: Herbs (Hypertensive Properties); Methylphenidate; Nonsteroidal Anti-Inflammatory Agents; Yohimbine

Increased Effect/Toxicity

Olmesartan may increase the levels/effects of: ACE Inhibitors; Amifostine; Antihypertensives; Hypotensive Agents; Lithium; Potassium-Sparing Diuretics; RiTUXimab

The levels/effects of Olmesartan may be increased by: Diazoxide; Eltrombopag; Eplerenone; Herbs (Hypotensive Properties); MAO Inhibitors; Pentoxifylline; Phosphodiesterase 5 Inhibitors; Potassium Salts; Prostacyclin Analogues; Tolvaptan; Trimethoprim

Nutritional/Ethanol Interactions

Food: Does not affect olmesartan bioavailability.

Herb/Nutraceutical: Avoid bayberry, blue cohosh, cayenne, ephedra, ginger, ginseng (American), kola, licorice (may worsen hypertension). Avoid black cohosh, California poppy, coleus, golden seal, hawthorn, mistletoe, periwinkle, quinine, shepherd's purse (may have increased antihypertensive effect).

Adverse Reactions 1% to 10%:

Central nervous system: Dizziness (3%), headache
Endocrine & metabolic: Hyperglycemia, hypertriglyceridemia
Gastrointestinal: Diarrhea
Neuromuscular & skeletal: Back pain, CPK increased
Renal: Hematuria
Respiratory: Bronchitis, pharyngitis, rhinitis, sinusitis
Miscellaneous: Flu-like syndrome

Pharmacodynamics/Kinetics

Bioavailability 26%

Time to Peak 1-2 hours

Protein Binding 99%

Half-Life Elimination Terminal: 13 hours

Metabolism Olmesartan medoxomil is hydrolyzed in the GI tract to active olmesartan. No further metabolism occurs.

Excretion All as unchanged drug: Feces (50% to 65%); urine (35% to 50%)

Available Dosage Forms

Tablet, oral:

Benicar®: 5 mg, 20 mg, 40 mg

Dosing

Adult Hypertension: Oral: Initial: Usual starting dose is 20 mg once daily; if initial response is inadequate, may be increased to 40 mg once daily after 2 weeks. May administer with other antihypertensive agents if blood pressure inadequately controlled with olmesartan. Consider lower starting dose in patients with possible depletion of intravascular volume (eg, patients receiving diuretics).

Geriatric No initial dosage adjustment necessary per labeling; however, may consider starting at 5-10 mg/day (due to concomitant disease or age changes).

Pediatric Hypertension: Children 6-16 years: Oral:

20 kg to <35 kg: Initial: 10 mg once daily; if initial response is inadequate, may be increased to 20 mg once daily after 2 weeks (maximum: 20 mg once daily)

≥35 kg: Initial: 20 mg once daily; if initial response is inadequate, may be increased to 40 mg once daily after 2 weeks (maximum: 40 mg once daily)

Renal Impairment No specific guidelines for dosage adjustment; patients undergoing hemodialysis have not been studied.

Hepatic Impairment No initial dosage adjustment necessary.

Administration

Oral May be administered with or without food.

Stability

Storage Store at 20°C to 25°C (68°F to 77°F).

Monitoring and Teaching Issues

Laboratory Monitoring Serum potassium

Physical Assessment Use caution in presence of volume depletion, renal insufficiency, or aortic/mitral stenosis. Evaluate blood pressure and monitor for tachycardia, hypotension, diarrhea, and bronchitis on a regular basis throughout therapy. Instruct patients with diabetes to monitor glucose levels closely (may cause hyperglycemia).

Patient Education Do not use potassium supplement or salt substitutes without consulting prescriber. May be taken with or without food. This drug does not eliminate the need for diet or exercise regimen as recommended by prescriber. If you have diabetes, check glucose levels closely (drug may alter glucose levels). May cause headache or dizziness, diarrhea, or back or joint pain. Report chest pain or palpitations, unrelieved headache, or flu-like symptoms or upper respiratory infection.

Dietary Considerations May be taken with or without food.

Geriatric Considerations No dosage adjustment is necessary when initiating angiotensin II receptor antagonists in the elderly. In clinical studies, no differences between younger adults and the elderly were demonstrated.

For age alone, consider hydration status to avoid hypotension; many elderly are volume depleted due to age-related blunting of the thirst reflex and diuretic use. May consider starting this medication at 5-10 mg once daily.

Pregnancy Considerations Medications which act on the renin-angiotensin system are reported to have the following fetal/neonatal effects: Hypotension, neonatal skull hypoplasia, anuria, renal failure, and death; oligohydramnios is also reported. These effects are reported to occur with exposure during the second and third trimesters. There are no adequate and well-controlled studies in pregnant women. **[U.S. Boxed Warning]: Based on human data, drugs that act on the angiotensin system can cause injury and death to the developing fetus when used in the second and third trimesters. Angiotensin receptor blockers should be discontinued as soon as possible once pregnancy is detected.**

Related Information

Angiotensin Agents *on page 1974*

◆ **Olmesartan and Amlodipine** *see* Amlodipine and Olmesartan *on page 108*

Olmesartan and Hydrochlorothiazide

(ole me SAR tan & hye droe klor oh THYE a zide)

U.S. Brand Names Benicar HCT®

Index Terms Hydrochlorothiazide and Olmesartan Medoxomil; Olmesartan Medoxomil and Hydrochlorothiazide

Generic Availability (U.S.) No

Pharmacologic Category Angiotensin II Receptor Blocker; Diuretic, Thiazide

Pregnancy Risk Factor C/D (2nd and 3rd trimesters)

Lactation Enters breast milk/contraindicated

Use Treatment of hypertension (not recommended for initial treatment)

Mechanism of Action/Effect Olmesartan blocks the vasoconstrictor and aldosterone-secreting effects of angiotensin II. Hydrochlorothiazide inhibits sodium reabsorption in the distal tubules causing increased excretion of sodium and water as well as potassium and hydrogen ions.

Contraindications Hypersensitivity to olmesartan, hydrochlorothiazide, or any component of the formulation; sulfonamide-derived drugs; anuria

Warnings/Precautions See individual agents.

Drug Interactions

Metabolism/Transport Effects Olmesartan: **Substrate** of SLCO1B1

Avoid Concomitant Use

Avoid concomitant use of Olmesartan and Hydrochlorothiazide with any of the following: Dofetilide

Decreased Effect

Olmesartan and Hydrochlorothiazide may decrease the levels/effects of: Antidiabetic Agents

The levels/effects of Olmesartan and Hydrochlorothiazide may be decreased by: Bile Acid Sequestrants; Herbs (Hypertensive Properties); Methylphenidate; Nonsteroidal Anti-Inflammatory Agents; Yohimbine

Increased Effect/Toxicity

Olmesartan and Hydrochlorothiazide may increase the levels/effects of: ACE Inhibitors; Allopurinol; Amifostine; Antihypertensives; Calcium Salts; CarBAMazepine; Dofetilide; Hypotensive Agents; Lithium; OXcarbazepine; Potassium-Sparing Diuretics; RiTUXimab; Topiramate; Toremifene; Vitamin D Analogs

The levels/effects of Olmesartan and Hydrochlorothiazide may be increased by: Alcohol (Ethyl); Analgesics (Opioid); Barbiturates; Corticosteroids (Orally Inhaled); Corticosteroids (Systemic); Eltrombopag; Eplerenone; Herbs (Hypotensive Properties); Licorice; MAO Inhibitors; Pentoxifylline; Phosphodiesterase 5 Inhibitors; Potassium Salts; Prostacyclin Analogues; Tolvaptan; Trimethoprim

Adverse Reactions Frequencies reported with combination product. See individual monographs for additional adverse effects reported with each agent.

Cardiovascular: Chest pain, peripheral edema

Central nervous system: Dizziness (9%), vertigo

Dermatologic: Rash

Endocrine & metabolic: Hyperuricemia (4%), hyperglycemia

Gastrointestinal: Nausea (3%), abdominal pain, dyspepsia, gastroenteritis, diarrhea

Genitourinary: Hematuria
Hepatic: Transaminases increased
Neuromuscular & skeletal: Back pain, arthritis, arthralgia, myalgia
Respiratory: Upper respiratory infection (7%), cough
Miscellaneous: CPK increased

Angioedema and rhabdomyolysis have been reported with angiotensin-receptor blockers. Severe dermatologic reactions, hypokalemia, and pancreatitis have been reported with hydrochlorothiazide.

Pharmacodynamics/Kinetics

Pharmacokinetic Note See individual agents.

Available Dosage Forms

Tablet:

Benicar HCT®: 20/12.5: Olmesartan 20 mg and hydrochlorothiazide 12.5 mg; 40/12.5: Olmesartan 40 mg and hydrochlorothiazide 12.5 mg; 40/25: Olmesartan 40 mg and hydrochlorothiazide 25 mg

Dosing

Adult & Geriatric

Hypertension: Oral: Dosage must be individualized; may be titrated at 2- to 4-week intervals.

Replacement therapy: May be substituted for titrated components.

Patients not controlled with single-agent therapy: Initiate by adding the lowest available dose of the alternative component (hydrochlorothiazide 12.5 mg or olmesartan 20 mg). Titrate to effect (maximum hydrochlorothiazide dose: 25 mg, maximum olmesartan dose: 40 mg).

Renal Impairment Not recommended in patients with Cl_{cr} <30 mL/minute.

Stability

Storage Store at 20°C to 25°C (68°F to 77°F).

Monitoring and Teaching Issues

Physical Assessment See individual agents.

Patient Education See individual agents.

Pregnancy Considerations The drug should be discontinued as soon as possible when pregnancy is detected. Drugs which act directly on renin-angiotensin can cause fetal and neonatal morbidity and death.

Related Information

Hydrochlorothiazide *on page 912*
Olmesartan *on page 1349*

◆ **Olmesartan Medoxomil** *see* Olmesartan *on page 1349*

◆ **Olmesartan Medoxomil and Hydrochlorothiazide** *see* Olmesartan and Hydrochlorothiazide *on page 1351*

Olopatadine (Nasal) (oh la PAT a deen)

U.S. Brand Names Patanase®

Index Terms Olopatadine Hydrochloride

Generic Availability (U.S.) No

Pharmacologic Category Histamine H_1 Antagonist; Histamine H_1 Antagonist, Second Generation; Piperidine Derivative

Pregnancy Risk Factor C

Lactation Excretion in breast milk unknown/use caution

Use Treatment of the symptoms of seasonal allergic rhinitis

Available Dosage Forms

Solution, intranasal:

Patanase®: 0.6% (30.5 g)

Dosing

Adult & Geriatric Seasonal allergic rhinitis: Intranasal: 2 sprays into each nostril twice daily

Pediatric Seasonal allergic rhinitis: Intranasal: Children ≥12 years: Refer to adult dosing.

Administration

Inhalation For intranasal use only. Before initial use of the nasal spray, the delivery system should be primed with 5 sprays or until a fine mist appears. If 7 or more days have elapsed since last use, the delivery system should be reprimed with 2 sprays or until a fine mist appears. Blow nose to clear nostrils. Keep head tilted downward when spraying. Insert applicator into nostril, keeping bottle upright, and close off the other nostril. Breathe in through nose. While inhaling, press pump to release spray. Alternate sprays between nostrils. After each use, wipe the spray tip with a clean tissue or cloth.

Monitoring and Teaching Issues

Physical Assessment Assess nasal mucosa periodically for ulceration.

Patient Education May cause drowsiness or bitter taste. Avoid alcohol use. Report ulcers or discomfort in nose.

Olopatadine (Ophthalmic) (oh la PAT a deen)

U.S. Brand Names Pataday™; Patanol®

Index Terms Olopatadine Hydrochloride

Generic Availability (U.S.) No

Pharmacologic Category Histamine H_1 Antagonist; Histamine H_1 Antagonist, Second Generation; Piperidine Derivative

Medication Safety Issues

Sound-alike/look-alike issues:

Patanol® may be confused with Platinol®

International issues:

Patanol [U.S., Canada, and multiple international markets] may be confused with Bétanol brand name for metipranolol [Monaco]

Pregnancy Risk Factor C

Lactation Excretion in breast milk unknown/use caution

Use Treatment of the signs and symptoms of allergic conjunctivitis

Available Dosage Forms

Solution, ophthalmic:

Pataday™: 0.2% (2.5 mL)

Patanol®: 0.1% (5 mL)

Dosing

Adult & Geriatric Allergic conjunctivitis: Ophthalmic:

Patanol®: Instill 1drop into affected eye(s) twice daily (allowing 6-8 hours between doses); results from an environmental study demonstrated that olopatadine was effective when dosed twice daily for up to 6 weeks

Pataday™: Instill 1 drop into affected eye(s) once daily

Pediatric Allergic conjunctivitis: Ophthalmic: Children ≥3 years: Refer to adult dosing.

Administration

Other For topical ophthalmic use only. After instilling drops, wait at least 10 minutes before inserting contact lenses. Do not insert contacts if eyes are red.

Monitoring and Teaching Issues

Patient Education For use in eyes only. Do not let tip of applicator touch eye; do not contaminate tip of applicator (may cause eye infection, eye damage, or vision loss). Do not wear contact lenses if eyes are red. Can cause cold-like symptoms and headache.

◆ **Olopatadine Hydrochloride** *see* Olopatadine (Nasal) *on page* 1352

◆ **Olopatadine Hydrochloride** *see* Olopatadine (Ophthalmic) *on page* 1352

Olsalazine (ole SAL a zeen)

U.S. Brand Names Dipentum®

Index Terms Olsalazine Sodium

Generic Availability (U.S.) No

Pharmacologic Category 5-Aminosalicylic Acid Derivative

Medication Safety Issues

Sound-alike/look-alike issues:

Olsalazine may be confused with OLANZapine

Dipentum® may be confused with Dilantin®

Pregnancy Risk Factor C

Lactation Enters breast milk/not recommended

Use Maintenance of remission of ulcerative colitis in patients intolerant to sulfasalazine

Available Dosage Forms

Capsule, oral:

Dipentum®: 250 mg

Dosing

Adult & Geriatric Ulcerative colitis: Oral: 1 g/day in 2 divided doses

Administration

Oral Administer with food in evenly divided doses.

Monitoring and Teaching Issues

Laboratory Monitoring CBC, hepatic function, renal function

Physical Assessment Assess allergy history before initiating therapy (salicylates, sulfasalazine, or mesalamine). Monitor for reduction of clinical signs of ulcerative colitis. Monitor for diarrhea.

Patient Education Take with meals, in evenly divided doses. May cause flu-like symptoms or muscle pain, diarrhea, nausea, or loss of appetite. Report persistent diarrhea or abdominal cramping, or skin rash or itching.

◆ **Olsalazine Sodium** *see* Olsalazine *on page* 1353

Omalizumab (oh mah lye ZOO mab)

U.S. Brand Names Xolair®

Index Terms rhuMAb-E25

Generic Availability (U.S.) No

Pharmacologic Category Monoclonal Antibody, Anti-Asthmatic

Medication Safety Issues

Sound-alike/look-alike issues:

Omalizumab may be confused with ofatumumab

Medication Guide Available Yes

Pregnancy Risk Factor B

Lactation Excretion in breast milk unknown/use caution

Use Treatment of moderate-to-severe, persistent allergic asthma not adequately controlled with inhaled corticosteroids

Mechanism of Action/Effect Blocks the binding of IgE to mast cells and basophils, decreasing the allergic response, corticosteroid usage, and asthma exacerbations.

Contraindications Hypersensitivity to omalizumab or any component of the formulation; acute bronchospasm, status asthmaticus

Warnings/Precautions **[U.S. Boxed Warning]: Anaphylaxis, including delayed-onset anaphylaxis, has been reported following administration; reactions usually occur within 2 hours of administration, but may occur up to 24 hours and in some cases >1 year after initiation of regular treatment.** Patients should receive treatment only under direct medical supervision and be observed for a minimum of 2 hours following administration; appropriate medications for the treatment of anaphylactic reactions should be available. Hypersensitivity reactions may occur following any dose, even during chronic therapy; discontinue therapy following any severe reaction.

For use in patients with a documented reactivity to a perennial aeroallergen and with symptoms uncontrolled using inhaled corticosteroids; not used to control acute asthma symptoms. Dosing is based on pretreatment IgE serum levels and body weight. IgE levels remain elevated up to 1 year following treatment, therefore, levels taken during treatment cannot be used as a dosage guide. Corticosteroid therapy should be tapered gradually, do not discontinue abruptly. Malignant neoplasms have been reported with use in short-term studies; impact of long-term use is not known. Use caution with and monitor patients at risk for parasitic (helminth) infections (risk of infection may be increased). Safety and efficacy in children <12 years of age have not been established.

Drug Interactions

Avoid Concomitant Use

Avoid concomitant use of Omalizumab with any of the following: BCG; Natalizumab; Pimecrolimus; Roflumilast; Tacrolimus (Topical); Vaccines (Live)

Decreased Effect

Omalizumab may decrease the levels/effects of: BCG; Sipuleucel-T; Vaccines (Inactivated); Vaccines (Live)

The levels/effects of Omalizumab may be decreased by: Echinacea

Increased Effect/Toxicity

Omalizumab may increase the levels/effects of: Leflunomide; Natalizumab; Vaccines (Live)

The levels/effects of Omalizumab may be increased by: Denosumab; Pimecrolimus; Roflumilast; Tacrolimus (Topical); Trastuzumab

Lab Interactions Total IgE levels are elevated for up to 1 year following treatment. Total serum IgE may be retested after interruption of therapy for 1 year or more.

Adverse Reactions

>10%:

Central nervous system: Headache (15%)

Local: Injection site reaction (45%; placebo 43%; severe 12%). Most reactions occurred within 1 hour, lasted <8 days, and decreased in frequency with additional dosing.

Respiratory: Upper respiratory tract infection (20%), sinusitis (16%), pharyngitis (11%)

Miscellaneous: Viral infection (23%)

1% to 10%:

Central nervous system: Pain (7%), fatigue (3%), dizziness (3%)

Dermatologic: Dermatitis (2%), pruritus (2%)

Neuromuscular & skeletal: Arthralgia (8%), leg pain (4%), arm pain (2%), fracture (2%)

Otic: Earache (2%)

Pharmacodynamics/Kinetics

Absorption Slow following SubQ injection

Bioavailability 62%

Time to Peak 7-8 days

Half-Life Elimination 26 days

Metabolism Hepatic; IgG degradation by reticuloendothelial system and endothelial cells

Excretion Primarily via hepatic degradation; intact IgG may be secreted in bile

Available Dosage Forms

Injection, powder for reconstitution:

Xolair®: 150 mg

Dosing

Adult & Geriatric Asthma: SubQ: Dose is based on pretreatment IgE serum levels and body weight. Dosing should not be adjusted based on IgE levels taken during treatment or <1 year following discontinuation of therapy; doses should be adjusted during treatment for significant changes in body weight.

IgE ≥30-100 int. units/mL:

30-90 kg: 150 mg every 4 weeks

>90-150 kg: 300 mg every 4 weeks

IgE >100-200 int. units/mL:

30-90 kg: 300 mg every 4 weeks

>90-150 kg: 225 mg every 2 weeks

IgE >200-300 int. units/mL:
30-60 kg: 300 mg every 4 weeks
>60-90 kg: 225 mg every 2 weeks
>90-150 kg: 300 mg every 2 weeks
IgE >300-400 int. units/mL:
30-70 kg: 225 mg every 2 weeks
>70-90 kg: 300 mg every 2 weeks
>90 kg: Do not administer dose
IgE >400-500 int. units/mL:
30-70 kg: 300 mg every 2 weeks
>70-90 kg: 375 mg every 2 weeks
>90 kg: Do not administer dose
IgE >500-600 int. units/mL:
30-60 kg: 300 mg every 2 weeks
>60-70 kg: 375 mg every 2 weeks
>70 kg: Do not administer dose
IgE >600-700 int. units/mL:
30-60 kg: 375 mg every 2 weeks
>60 kg: Do not administer dose

Pediatric Asthma: Children ≥12 years: SubQ: Refer to adult dosing.

Administration

Other For SubQ injection only; doses >150 mg should divided over more than one site. Injections may take 5-10 seconds to administer. Administer only under direct medical supervision and observe patient for a minimum of 2 hours following administration of any dose given.

Stability

Reconstitution Prepare using SWFI, USP only; add SWFI 1.4 mL to upright vial and swirl gently for 5-10 seconds every 5 minutes until dissolved; may take >20 minutes to dissolve completely. Resulting solution is 150 mg/1.2 mL. Do not use if powder takes >40 minutes to dissolve.

Storage Prior to reconstitution, store under refrigeration at 2°C to 8°C (36°F to 46°F); product may be shipped at room temperature. Following reconstitution, protect from direct sunlight. May be stored for up to 8 hours if refrigerated or 4 hours if stored at room temperature.

Monitoring and Teaching Issues

Laboratory Monitoring Anaphylactic/hypersensitivity reactions, baseline IgE; FEV_1, peak flow, and/or other pulmonary function tests

Physical Assessment For SubQ use only. Evaluate pulmonary function tests at baseline and as necessary with treatment. Anaphylactic reactions have been reported within 2-24 hours of initial dose; patient should be monitored for a minimum of 2 hours following injection and appropriate medications for the treatment of hypersensitivity reactions should be available. Monitor for hypersensitivity reaction, upper respiratory tract infection, viral infection, dermatitis, and arthralgia at beginning of and periodically during therapy.

Patient Education This medication is administered by injection and you will be closely monitored for some time following injection. Report immediately any sign of allergic response (redness, swelling, pain or itching at injection site; chest pain or tightness; difficulty breathing or swallowing; swelling of mouth or tongue; skin rash). If allergic response occurs, follow prescriber's directions for contacting emergency treatment immediately. May cause headache; dizziness; or joint, bone, or ear pain. Report unusual or increased respiratory difficulty, signs of infection, or skin rash.

Breast-Feeding Considerations IgG is excreted in human milk and excretion of omalizumab is expected. Effects to nursing infant are not known; use with caution.

Pregnancy Considerations Teratogenic effects were not observed in animal studies. There are no adequate and well-controlled studies in pregnant women. IgG molecules are known to cross the placenta; use during pregnancy only if clearly needed. A registry has been established to monitor outcomes of women exposed to omalizumab during pregnancy or within 8 weeks prior to pregnancy (866-496-5247).

◆ **Omega 3** *see* Omega-3-Acid Ethyl Esters *on page* *1355*

Omega-3-Acid Ethyl Esters (oh MEG a three AS id ETH il ES ters)

U.S. Brand Names Lovaza®

Index Terms Ethyl Esters of Omega-3 Fatty Acids; Fish Oil; Omega 3; P-OM3

Pharmacologic Category Antilipemic Agent, Miscellaneous

Medication Safety Issues

Sound-alike/look-alike issues:
Lovaza® may be confused with LORazepam
Omacor® may be confused with Amicar®

The Institute for Safe Medication Practices (ISMP) reported a case of a foam plastic cup dissolving after contact with the liquid contents from a Lovaza® capsule. ISMP is requesting the manufacturer to add warnings to its labeling and that healthcare providers add Lovaza® to their list of medications to not crush.

Pregnancy Risk Factor C

Lactation Excretion in breast milk unknown/use caution

Use Lovaza®: Adjunct to diet therapy in the treatment of hypertriglyceridemia (≥500 mg/dL)

Note: A number of OTC formulations containing omega-3 fatty acids are marketed as nutritional supplements; these do not have FDA-approved indications and may not contain the same amounts of the active ingredient.

Unlabeled/Investigational Use Lovaza®: Treatment of IgA nephropathy

Available Dosage Forms

Capsule, liquid gel, oral:

Lovaza®: 1 g

Dosing

Adult & Geriatric

Hypertriglyceridemia: Oral: 4 g/day as a single daily dose or in 2 divided doses.

Treatment of IgA nephropathy (unlabeled use): Oral: 4 g/day

Renal Impairment No dosage adjustment required.

Administration

Oral May be administered with or without food. Administer whole, do not crush.

Monitoring and Teaching Issues

Laboratory Monitoring Triglycerides and other lipids (LDL-C) should be monitored at baseline and periodically. Hepatic transaminase levels, particularly ALT, should be monitored periodically.

Physical Assessment Determine if patient is allergic to fish prior to prescribing. Encourage diet and exercise along with use of this medication.

Patient Education Do not use if allergic to fish. This medication should be used in addition to diet and exercise. Avoid alcohol use; significant use may increase triglycerides. You may experience flu-like syndrome, fever, burping, or an upset stomach.

Omeprazole (oh MEP ra zole)

U.S. Brand Names PriLOSEC OTC® [OTC]; PriLOSEC®

Index Terms Omeprazole Magnesium

Generic Availability (U.S.) Yes: Excludes granules for suspension

Pharmacologic Category Proton Pump Inhibitor; Substituted Benzimidazole

Medication Safety Issues

Sound-alike/look-alike issues:

Omeprazole may be confused with aripiprazole, fomepizole

PriLOSEC® may be confused with Plendil®, Prevacid®, predniSONE, prilocaine, Prinivil®, Proventil®, PROzac®

International issues:

Losec [multiple international markets] may be confused with Lasix, a brand name for furosemide [U.S., Canada, and multiple international markets]

Medral [Mexico] may be confused with Medrol brand name for methylprednisolone [U.S., Canada, and multiple international markets]

Norpramin: Brand name for omeprazole [Spain], but also the brand name for desipramine [U.S., Canada] and enalapril/hydrochlorothiazide [Portugal]

Pregnancy Risk Factor C

Lactation Enters breast milk/not recommended

Use Short-term (4-8 weeks) treatment of active duodenal ulcer disease or active benign gastric ulcer; treatment of heartburn and other symptoms associated with gastroesophageal reflux disease (GERD); short-term (4-8 weeks) treatment of endoscopically-diagnosed erosive esophagitis; maintenance healing of erosive esophagitis; long-term treatment of pathological hypersecretory conditions; as part of a multidrug regimen for *H. pylori* eradication to reduce the risk of duodenal ulcer recurrence

OTC labeling: Short-term treatment of frequent, uncomplicated heartburn occurring ≥2 days/week

Unlabeled/Investigational Use Healing NSAID-induced ulcers; prevention of NSAID-induced ulcer; stress-ulcer prophylaxis in the critically-ill

Mechanism of Action/Effect Proton pump inhibitor; suppresses gastric basal and stimulated acid secretion by inhibiting the parietal cell H+/K+ ATP pump

Contraindications Hypersensitivity to omeprazole, substituted benzimidazoles (eg, esomeprazole, lansoprazole), or any component of the formulation

Warnings/Precautions Use of proton pump inhibitors may increase the risk of gastrointestinal infections (eg, *Salmonella, Campylobacter*). Relief of symptoms does not preclude the presence of a gastric malignancy. Atrophic gastritis (by biopsy) has been noted with long-term omeprazole therapy. In long-term (2-year) studies in rats, omeprazole produced a dose-related increase in gastric carcinoid tumors. While available endoscopic evaluations and histologic examinations of biopsy specimens from human stomachs have not detected a risk from short-term exposure to omeprazole, further human data on the effect of sustained hypochlorhydria and hypergastrinemia are needed to rule out the possibility of an increased risk for the development of tumors in humans receiving long-term therapy. Proton pump inhibitors may diminish the therapeutic effect of clopidogrel thought to be due to reduced formation of the active metabolite of clopidogrel; an increase in the risk of cardiovascular events may occur. The manufacturer of clopidogrel recommends avoidance of concomitant administration of omeprazole even when scheduled 12 hours apart.

Increased incidence of osteoporosis-related bone fractures of the hip, spine, or wrist may occur with proton pump inhibitor therapy. Patients on high-dose (multiple daily doses)or long-term (≥1 year) therapy should be monitored. Use the lowest effective dose for the shortest duration of time, use vitamin D and calcium supplementation, and follow appropriate guidelines to reduce risk of fractures in patients at risk.

Decreased *H. pylori* eradication rates have been observed with short-term (≤7 days) combination therapy. The American College of Gastroenterology recommends 10-14 days of therapy (triple or quadruple) for eradication of *H. pylori* (Chey, 2007). Bioavailability may be increased in Asian populations and patients with hepatic dysfunction; consider dosage reductions, especially for maintenance healing of erosive esophagitis. Bioavailability may be increased in the elderly. When used for self-medication (OTC), do not use for >14 days.

Drug Interactions

Metabolism/Transport Effects Substrate of CYP2A6 (minor), 2C9 (minor), 2C19 (major), 2D6 (minor), 3A4 (major); **Inhibits** CYP1A2 (weak), 2C9 (moderate), 2C19 (moderate), 2D6 (weak), 3A4 (weak); **Induces** CYP1A2 (weak)

Avoid Concomitant Use

Avoid concomitant use of Omeprazole with any of the following: Clopidogrel; Delavirdine; Erlotinib; Nelfinavir; Posaconazole

Decreased Effect

Omeprazole may decrease the levels/effects of: Atazanavir; Bisphosphonate Derivatives; Cefditoren; Clopidogrel; CloZAPine; Dabigatran Etexilate; Dasatinib; Delavirdine; Erlotinib; Gefitinib; Indinavir; Iron Salts; Itraconazole; Ketoconazole; Ketoconazole (Systemic); Mesalamine; Mycophenolate; Nelfinavir; Posaconazole

The levels/effects of Omeprazole may be decreased by: CYP2C19 Inducers (Strong); Peginterferon Alfa-2b; Tipranavir

Increased Effect/Toxicity

Omeprazole may increase the levels/effects of: Amphetamines; Benzodiazepines (metabolized by oxidation); Carvedilol; Cilostazol; CloZAPine; CycloSPORINE; CycloSPORINE (Systemic); CYP2C19 Substrates; CYP2C9 Substrates (High risk); Dexmethylphenidate; Methotrexate; Methylphenidate; Phenytoin; Raltegravir; Saquinavir; Tacrolimus; Tacrolimus (Systemic); Vitamin K Antagonists; Voriconazole

The levels/effects of Omeprazole may be increased by: Conivaptan; Fluconazole; Ketoconazole; Ketoconazole (Systemic)

Nutritional/Ethanol Interactions

Ethanol: Avoid ethanol (may cause gastric mucosal irritation).
Food: Food delays absorption.

Adverse Reactions 1% to 10%:

Central nervous system: Headache (7%), dizziness (2%)
Dermatologic: Rash (2%)
Gastrointestinal: Abdominal pain (5%), diarrhea (4%), nausea (4%), vomiting (3%), flatulence (3%), acid regurgitation (2%), constipation (2%)
Neuromuscular & skeletal: Back pain (1%), weakness (1%)
Respiratory: Upper respiratory infection (2%), cough (1%)

Pharmacodynamics/Kinetics

Onset of Action Antisecretory: ~1 hour; Peak effect: Within 2 hours

Duration of Action Up to 72 hours; 50% of maximum effect at 24 hours; after stopping treatment, secretory activity gradually returns over 3-5 days

Absorption Rapid

Bioavailability Oral: ~30% to 40%; increased in Asian patients, elderly patients, and patients with hepatic dysfunction

Time to Peak Plasma: 0.5-3.5 hours

Protein Binding ~95%

Half-Life Elimination 0.5-1 hour; hepatic impairment: ~3 hours

Metabolism Hepatic via CYP2C19 primarily and (to a lesser extent) via 3A4 to hydroxy, desmethyl, and sulfone metabolites (all inactive); saturable first-pass effect

Excretion Urine (~77% as metabolites, very small amount as unchanged drug); feces

Available Dosage Forms

Capsule, delayed release, oral: 10 mg, 20 mg, 40 mg
PriLOSEC®: 10 mg, 20 mg, 40 mg

Granules for suspension, delayed release, enteric coated, oral:
PriLOSEC®: 2.5 mg/packet (30s); 10 mg/packet (30s)

Tablet, delayed release, oral: 20 mg, 40 mg
PriLOSEC OTC® [OTC]: 20 mg

Dosing

Adult & Geriatric

Active duodenal ulcer: Oral: 20 mg once daily for 4-8 weeks

Gastric ulcers: Oral: 40 mg once daily for 4-8 weeks

Symptomatic GERD (without esophageal lesions): Oral: 20 mg once daily for up to 4 weeks

Erosive esophagitis: Oral: 20 mg once daily for 4-8 weeks; maintenance of healing: 20 mg once daily for up to 12 months total therapy (including treatment period of 4-8 weeks)

***Helicobacter pylori* eradication:** Oral: Dose varies with regimen:

Manufacturer labeling: 40 mg once daily administered with clarithromycin 500 mg 3 times/day for 14 days **or** 20 mg twice daily administered with amoxicillin 1000 mg *and* clarithromycin 500 mg twice daily for 10 days. **Note:** Presence of ulcer at time of therapy initiation may necessitate an additional 14-18 days of omeprazole 20 mg/day (monotherapy) after completion of combination therapy.

American College of Gastroenterology guidelines (Chey, 2007):

Nonpenicillin allergy: 20 mg twice daily administered with amoxicillin 1000 mg *and* clarithromycin 500 mg twice daily for 10-14 days

Penicillin allergy: 20 mg twice daily administered with clarithromycin 500 mg *and* metronidazole 500 mg twice daily for 10-14 days **or** 20 mg once or twice daily administered with bismuth subsalicylate 525 mg *and* metronidazole 250 mg *plus* tetracycline 500 mg 4 times/day for 10-14 days

Pathological hypersecretory conditions: Oral: Initial: 60 mg once daily; doses up to 120 mg 3 times/day have been administered; administer daily doses >80 mg in divided doses

Stress-ulcer prophylaxis (ICU patients; unlabeled use): Oral: 40 mg once daily; periodically evaluate patient for continued need (Levy, 1997)

Frequent heartburn (OTC labeling): Oral: 20 mg once daily for 14 days; treatment may be repeated after 4 months if needed

Pediatric

GERD or other acid-related disorders: Oral: Children 1-16 years:

5 kg to <10 kg: 5 mg once daily

10 kg to <20 kg: 10 mg once daily

≥20 kg: 20 mg once daily

Renal Impairment No adjustment is necessary.

Hepatic Impairment Bioavailability is increased with chronic liver disease. Consider dosage adjustment, especially for maintenance of erosive esophagitis. Specific guidelines are not available.

Administration

Oral Best if administered before breakfast.

Capsule: Should be swallowed whole; do not chew or crush. Delayed release capsule may be opened and contents added to 1 tablespoon of applesauce (use immediately after adding to applesauce); mixture should not be chewed or warmed.

Oral suspension: Following reconstitution, the suspension should be left to thicken for 2-3 minutes and administered within 30 minutes. If any material remains after administration, add more water, stir, and administer immediately.

Tablet: Should be swallowed whole; do not crush or chew.

Other Nasogastric/orogastric (NG/OG) tube administration:

Capsule: When using capsules to extemporaneously prepare a solution for NG/OG administration, the manufacturers of Prilosec® recommend the use of an acidic juice for preparation and administration. Alternative methods have been described as follows:

NG/OG tube administration for the prevention of stress-related mucosal damage in ventilated, critically-ill patients:

Study 1 (Phillips, 1996): Pour the contents of one or two 20 mg omeprazole delayed release capsules (depending on the dose) into a syringe (after removing plunger); withdraw 10-20 mL of an 8.4% sodium bicarbonate solution into the syringe; allow 30 minutes for the enteric-coated omeprazole granules to break down. Shake the resulting milky substance prior to administration. Flush the NG tube with 5-10 mL of water and clamp for at least 1 hour.

Study 2 (Balaban, 1997): Open the omeprazole delayed release capsule (20 mg or 40 mg), then pour the intact granules into a container holding 30 mL of water. Pour one-third to one-half of the granules into a 30 mL syringe (with the plunger removed) attached to a nasogastric tube (NG). Replace the plunger with 1 cm of air between the granules and the plunger top while the plunger is depressed. Repeat this process until all the granules are flushed, then flush a final 15 mL of water through the tube.

Oral suspension: Following reconstitution in a catheter-tipped syringe, shake the suspension well and leave to thicken for 2-3 minutes. Administer within 30 minutes of reconstitution. Use an NG tube or gastric tube that is a size 6 French or larger; flush the syringe and tube with water.

Stability

Reconstitution Granules for oral suspension: For oral administration, empty the contents of the 2.5 mg packet into 5 mL of water (10 mg packet into 15 mL of water); stir. For NG administration, add 5 mL of water into a catheter-tipped syringe, and then add the contents of a 2.5 mg packet (15 mL water for the 10 mg packet); shake. **Note:** Regardless of the route of administration, the suspension should be left to thicken for 2-3 minutes prior to administration.

Storage

Capsules, tablets: Store at 15°C to 30°C (59°F to 86°F). Protect from light and moisture.

Granules for oral suspension: Store at 25°C (77°F); excursions permitted to 15°C to 30°C (59°F to 86°F).

Monitoring and Teaching Issues

Physical Assessment For patients at risk of osteoporosis-related fractures, optimize preventive measures and limit high-dose, prolonged therapy if possible.

Patient Education Take before eating. Do not crush or chew capsules. Delayed release capsule may be opened and contents added to applesauce. Avoid alcohol. You may experience anorexia; small frequent meals may help to maintain adequate nutrition. Report severe headache, unresolved severe diarrhea, or abdominal pain.

Dietary Considerations Should be taken on an empty stomach; best if taken before breakfast.

Geriatric Considerations In clinical trials, the incidence of side effects in the elderly is no different than that of younger adults (≤65 years) despite slight decrease in elimination and increase in bioavailability. Bioavailability may be increased in the elderly (≥65 years of age), however, dosage adjustments are not necessary.

An increased risk of fractures of the hip, spine, or wrist has been observed in epidemiologic studies with proton pump inhibitor (PPI) use, primarily in older adults ≥50 years of age. The greatest risk was seen in patients receiving high doses or on long-term therapy (≥1 year). Calcium and vitamin D supplementation and close monitoring are recommended to reduce the risk of fracture in high-risk patients.

Breast-Feeding Considerations Following administration of omeprazole 20 mg, peak concentrations detected in the breast milk were <7% of the maternal serum concentration.

Pregnancy Considerations Adverse events were observed in some animal reproduction studies. Based on data collected by the Teratogen Information System (TERIS), it was concluded that therapeutic doses used during pregnancy would be unlikely to pose a substantial teratogenic risk (quantity/quality of data: fair). Because the possibility of harm still exists, the manufacturer recommends use during pregnancy only if the potential benefit to the mother outweighs the possible risk to the fetus.

Related Information

Helicobacter pylori Treatment *on page 2045*

Omeprazole and Sodium Bicarbonate

(oh ME pray zol & SOW dee um bye KAR bun ate)

U.S. Brand Names Zegerid OTC™ [OTC]; Zegerid®

Index Terms Sodium Bicarbonate and Omeprazole

Generic Availability (U.S.) Yes: Capsule

Pharmacologic Category Proton Pump Inhibitor; Substituted Benzimidazole

Medication Safety Issues

Sound-alike/look-alike issues:

Zegerid® may be confused with Zestril®

Pregnancy Risk Factor C

Lactation Enters breast milk/not recommended

Use Short-term (4-8 weeks) treatment of active duodenal ulcer or active benign gastric ulcer; treatment of heartburn and other symptoms associated with gastroesophageal reflux disease (GERD); short-term (4-8 weeks) treatment of endoscopically-diagnosed erosive esophagitis; maintenance healing of erosive esophagitis; reduction of risk of upper gastrointestinal bleeding in critically-ill patients

OTC labeling: Short-term (2 weeks) treatment of frequent (2 days/week), uncomplicated heartburn

Available Dosage Forms

Capsule, oral: Omeprazole 20 mg [immediate release] and sodium bicarbonate 1100 mg; omeprazole 40 mg [immediate release] and sodium bicarbonate 1100 mg

Zegerid®: Omeprazole 20 mg [immediate release] and sodium bicarbonate 1100 mg

Zegerid®: Omeprazole 40 mg [immediate release] and sodium bicarbonate 1100 mg

Zegerid OTC™ [OTC]: Omeprazole 20 mg [immediate release] and sodium bicarbonate 1100 mg

Powder for oral suspension:

Zegerid®: Omeprazole 20 mg and sodium bicarbonate 1680 mg per packet

Zegerid®: Omeprazole 40 mg and sodium bicarbonate 1680 mg per packet

Dosing

Adult & Geriatric Note: Both strengths of Zegerid® capsule and powder for oral suspension have identical sodium bicarbonate content, respectively. Do not substitute two 20 mg capsules/packets for one 40 mg dose.

Active duodenal ulcer: Oral: 20 mg/day for 4-8 weeks

Gastric ulcers: Oral: 40 mg/day for 4-8 weeks

Heartburn (OTC labeling): Oral: 20 mg once daily for 14 days. Do not take for >14 days or more often than every 4 months, unless instructed by healthcare provider.

Symptomatic GERD: Oral: 20 mg/day for up to 4 weeks

Erosive esophagitis: Oral: 20 mg/day for 4-8 weeks; maintenance of healing: 20 mg/day for up to 12 months total therapy (including treatment period of 4-8 weeks)

Risk reduction of upper GI bleeding in critically-ill patients (Zegerid® powder for oral suspension): Oral:

Loading dose: Day 1: 40 mg every 6-8 hours for two doses

Maintenance dose: 40 mg/day for up to 14 days; therapy >14 days has not been evaluated

Renal Impairment No adjustment is necessary.

Hepatic Impairment Bioavailability is increased with chronic liver disease. Consider dosage adjustment, especially for maintenance of healing of erosive esophagitis. Specific guidelines are not available.

Administration

Oral Note: Both strengths of Zegerid® capsule and powder for oral suspension have identical sodium bicarbonate content, respectively. Do not substitute two 20 mg capsules/packets for one 40 mg dose.

Capsule: Should be swallowed whole with water (do not use other liquids); do not chew or crush. Capsules should **not** be opened, sprinkled on food, or administered via NG. Best if taken at least 1 hour before breakfast.

Powder for oral suspension: Administer 1 hour before a meal. Mix with 1-2 tablespoons of water; stir well and drink immediately. Rinse cup with water and drink. Do not use other liquids or sprinkle on food.

Other Nasogastric/orogastric tube: Powder for oral suspension: Mix well with 20 mL of water (do not use other liquids) and administer immediately; flush tube with an additional 20 mL of water. Suspend enteral feeding for 3 hours before and 1 hour after administering.

Monitoring and Teaching Issues

Physical Assessment See individual agents.

Patient Education See individual agents.

- **Omeprazole Magnesium** *see* Omeprazole *on page* 1356
- **Omnaris™** *see* Ciclesonide (Nasal) *on page* 368
- **Omnicef®** *see* Cefdinir *on page* 315
- **Omnipred™** *see* PrednisoLONE (Ophthalmic) *on page* 1500
- **Omnitrope®** *see* Somatropin *on page* 1664
- **Oncaspar®** *see* Pegaspargase *on page* 1421
- **Oncovin** *see* VinCRIStine *on page* 1865

Ondansetron (on DAN se tron)

U.S. Brand Names Zofran®; Zofran® ODT; Zuplenz®

Index Terms GR38032R; Ondansetron Hydrochloride; Zuplenz®

Generic Availability (U.S.) Yes: Excludes oral soluble film

Pharmacologic Category Antiemetic; Selective 5-HT_3 Receptor Antagonist

Medication Safety Issues

Sound-alike/look-alike issues:

Ondansetron may be confused with dolasetron, granisetron, palonosetron

Zofran® may be confused with Zantac®, Zosyn®

Pregnancy Risk Factor B

Lactation Excretion in breast milk unknown/use caution

Use Prevention of nausea and vomiting associated with moderately- to highly-emetogenic cancer chemotherapy; radiotherapy; prevention of postoperative nausea and vomiting (PONV); treatment of PONV if no prophylactic dose of ondansetron received

Unlabeled/Investigational Use Hyperemesis gravidarum; breakthrough treatment of nausea and vomiting associated with chemotherapy

Mechanism of Action/Effect Selective 5-HT_3 receptor antagonist, blocking serotonin, both peripherally on vagal nerve terminals and centrally in the chemoreceptor trigger zone

Contraindications Hypersensitivity to ondansetron, other selective 5-HT_3 antagonists, or any component of the formulation; concomitant use of apomorphine

Warnings/Precautions Ondansetron should be used on a scheduled basis, not on an "as needed" (PRN) basis, since data support the use of this drug only in the prevention of nausea and vomiting (due to antineoplastic therapy) and not in the rescue of nausea and vomiting. Ondansetron should only be used in the first 24-48 hours of chemotherapy. Data do not support any increased efficacy of ondansetron in delayed nausea and vomiting. Does not stimulate gastric or intestinal peristalsis; may mask progressive ileus and/or gastric distension. Use with caution in patients allergic to other 5-HT_3 receptor antagonists; cross-reactivity has been reported.

Use with caution in patients with congenital long QT syndrome or other risk factors for QT prolongation (eg, medications known to prolong QT interval, electrolyte abnormalities, and cumulative high-dose anthracycline therapy). 5-HT_3 antagonists have been associated with a number of dose-dependent increases in ECG intervals (eg, PR, QRS duration, QT/QT_c, JT), usually occurring 1-2 hours after I.V. administration. In general, these changes are not clinically relevant, however, when used in conjunction with other agents that prolong these intervals, arrhythmia may occur. When used with agents that prolong the QT interval (eg, Class I and III antiarrhythmics), clinically relevant QT interval prolongation may occur resulting in torsade de pointes. I.V. formulations of 5-HT_3 antagonists have more association with ECG interval changes, compared to oral formulations. Dose recommendations provided for patients with severe hepatic impairment (Child-Pugh class C); use with caution in mild-moderate hepatic impairment; clearance is decreased and half-life increased in hepatic impairment.

Orally-disintegrating tablets contain phenylalanine.

Drug Interactions

Metabolism/Transport Effects Substrate of CYP1A2 (minor), CYP2C9 (minor), CYP2D6 (minor), CYP2E1 (minor), CYP3A4 (major), P-glycoprotein; **Inhibits** CYP1A2 (weak), 2C9 (weak), 2D6 (weak)

Avoid Concomitant Use

Avoid concomitant use of Ondansetron with any of the following: Apomorphine

Decreased Effect

The levels/effects of Ondansetron may be decreased by: CYP3A4 Inducers (Strong); Deferasirox; Herbs (CYP3A4 Inducers); Peginterferon Alfa-2b; P-Glycoprotein Inducers; Rifamycin Derivatives

Increased Effect/Toxicity

Ondansetron may increase the levels/effects of: Apomorphine

The levels/effects of Ondansetron may be increased by: Conivaptan; P-Glycoprotein Inhibitors

Nutritional/Ethanol Interactions

Food: Tablet: Food slightly increases the extent of absorption.

Herb/Nutraceutical: St John's wort may decrease ondansetron levels.

Adverse Reactions Note: Percentages reported in adult patients.

>10%:

Central nervous system: Headache (9% to 27%), malaise/fatigue (9% to 13%)

Gastrointestinal: Constipation (6% to 11%)

1% to 10%:

Central nervous system: Drowsiness (8%), fever (2% to 8%), dizziness (4% to 7%), anxiety (6%), cold sensation (2%)

Dermatologic: Pruritus (2% to 5%), rash (1%)

Gastrointestinal: Diarrhea (2% to 7%)

Genitourinary: Gynecological disorder (7%), urinary retention (5%)

Hepatic: ALT increased (1% to 5%), AST increased (1% to 5%)

Local: Injection site reaction (4%; pain, redness, burning)

Neuromuscular & skeletal: Paresthesia (2%)

Respiratory: Hypoxia (9%)

Pharmacodynamics/Kinetics

Onset of Action ~30 minutes

Absorption Oral: Well absorbed from GI tract

Bioavailability Oral: 56% to 71% (some first pass metabolism); Rectal: 58% to 74%

Time to Peak Oral: ~2 hours; Oral soluble film: ~1 hour

Protein Binding Plasma: 70% to 76%

Half-Life Elimination Children <15 years: 2-7 hours; Adults: 3-6 hours

Mild-to-moderate hepatic impairment (Child-Pugh classes A and B): Adults: 12 hours

Severe hepatic impairment (Child-Pugh class C): Adults: 20 hours

Metabolism Extensively hepatic via hydroxylation, followed by glucuronide or sulfate conjugation; CYP1A2, CYP2D6, and CYP3A4 substrate, some demethylation occurs

Excretion Urine (44% to 60% as metabolites, ~5% as unchanged drug); feces (~25%)

Available Dosage Forms

Film, soluble, oral:

Zuplenz®: 4 mg (10s); 8 mg (10s)

Infusion, premixed in D_5W [preservative free]: 32 mg (50 mL)

Infusion, premixed in NS [preservative free]: 32 mg (50 mL)

Injection, solution: 2 mg/mL (2 mL, 20 mL)

Zofran®: 2 mg/mL (20 mL)

Injection, solution [preservative free]: 2 mg/mL (2 mL)

Solution, oral: 4 mg/5 mL (5 mL, 50 mL)

Zofran®: 4 mg/5 mL (50 mL)

Tablet, oral: 4 mg, 8 mg

Zofran®: 4 mg, 8 mg

Tablet, orally disintegrating, oral: 4 mg, 8 mg

Zofran® ODT: 4 mg, 8 mg

Dosing

Adult & Geriatric

Prevention of chemotherapy-induced emesis:

I.V.:

0.15 mg/kg 3 times/day beginning 30 minutes prior to chemotherapy **or**

0.45 mg/kg once daily **or**

8-10 mg 1-2 times/day **or**

24 mg or 32 mg once daily

Highly-emetogenic agents/single-day therapy: Oral: 24 mg given 30 minutes prior to the start of therapy

Moderately-emetogenic agents: Oral: 8 mg beginning 30 minutes before chemotherapy; repeat dose 8 hours after initial dose, then 8 mg every 12 hours for 1-2 days after chemotherapy completed

Radiation-induced emesis prophylaxis:

Total body irradiation: Oral: 8 mg 1-2 hours before each daily fraction of radiotherapy

Single high-dose fraction radiotherapy to abdomen: Oral: 8 mg 1-2 hours before irradiation, then 8 mg every 8 hours after first dose for 1-2 days after completion of radiotherapy

Daily fractionated radiotherapy to abdomen: Oral: 8 mg 1-2 hours before irradiation, then 8 mg 8 hours after first dose for each day of radiotherapy

Postoperative nausea and vomiting (PONV):

Oral: 16 mg given 1 hour prior to induction of anesthesia

I.M., I.V.: 4 mg as a single dose approximately 30 minutes before the end of anesthesia (see Note below) or as treatment if vomiting occurs after surgery (Gan, 2007).

Note: The manufacturer recommends administration immediately before induction of anesthesia; however, this has been shown not to be as effective as administration at the end of surgery (Sun, 1997). Repeat doses given in response to inadequate control of nausea/vomiting from preoperative doses are generally ineffective.

Treatment of hyperemesis gravidum (unlabeled use):

Oral: 8 mg every 12 hours

I.V.: 8 mg administered over 15 minutes every 12 hours or 1 mg/hour infused continuously for up to 24 hours

Pediatric Premixed injection not for use in children.

Prevention of chemotherapy-induced emesis: *I.V.:* Children 6 months to 18 years: 0.15 mg/kg/dose administered 30 minutes prior to chemotherapy, 4 and 8 hours after the first dose **or** 0.45 mg/kg/day as a single dose

Prevention of moderately-emetogenic chemotherapy-induced emesis: *Oral:*

4-11 years: 4 mg 30 minutes before chemotherapy; repeat 4 and 8 hours after initial dose, then 4 mg every 8 hours for 1-2 days after chemotherapy completed

≥12 years: Refer to adult dosing.

Prevention of postoperative nausea and vomiting (PONV): I.V.: Children 1 month to 12 years:

≤40 kg: 0.1 mg/kg as a single dose

>40 kg: 4 mg as a single dose

Renal Impairment No adjustment is necessary.

Hepatic Impairment Severe liver disease (Child-Pugh C): Maximum daily dose: 8 mg

Administration

Oral Oral dosage forms should be given 30 minutes prior to chemotherapy; 1-2 hours before radiotherapy; 1 hour prior to the induction of anesthesia.

Orally-disintegrating tablets: Do not remove from blister until needed. Peel backing off the blister, do not push tablet through. Using dry hands, place tablet on tongue and allow to dissolve. Swallow with saliva.

Oral soluble film: Do not remove from pouch until immediately before use. Using dry hands, place film on top of tongue and allow to dissolve (4-20 seconds). Swallow with or without liquid. If using more than one film, each film should be allowed to dissolve completely before administering the next film.

I.M. Should be given undiluted.

I.V.

IVPB: Dilute in 50 mL D_5W or NS. Infuse over 15-30 minutes; 24-hour continuous infusions have been reported, but are rarely used.

Chemotherapy-induced nausea and vomiting: Give first dose 30 minutes prior to beginning chemotherapy.

I.V. push: Prevention of postoperative nausea and vomiting: Single doses may be administered I.V. injection over 2-5 minutes as undiluted solution.

Stability

Reconstitution Prior to I.V. infusion, dilute in 50 mL D_5W or NS.

Storage

Oral soluble film: Store between 20°C and 25°C (68°F and 77°F). Store pouches in cartons; keep film in individual pouch until ready to use.

Oral solution: Store between 15°C and 30°C (59°F and 86°F). Protect from light.

Premixed bag: Store between 2°C and 30°C (36°F and 86°F). Protect from light.

Tablet: Store between 2°C and 30°C (36°F and 86°F).

Vial: Store between 2°C and 30°C (36°F and 86°F). Protect from light. Stable when mixed in D_5W or NS for 48 hours at room temperature.

Monitoring and Teaching Issues

Physical Assessment Assess allergy history (selective 5-HT_3 receptor antagonists) prior to administering. Use with caution in presence of, or potential for, cardiac conduction abnormalities (eg, QT prolongation, medication known to prolong QT interval, electrolyte abnormalities). Oral and I.V. doses have different schedules and should not be administered on "PRN" basis.

Patient Education This drug is given to prevent nausea and vomiting. If this medication is given by intravenous infusion you will be monitored during infusion. Report immediately any chest pain, respiratory difficulty, or pain or itching at infusion site. May cause headache, drowsiness, or dizziness. Report chest pain or palpitations, persistent headache, excessive drowsiness, fever, constipation, or diarrhea.

Orally-disintegrating tablets: Using dry hands, place tablet on tongue and allow to dissolve. Swallow with saliva.

Dietary Considerations Take without regard to meals. Some products may contain phenylalanine.

Geriatric Considerations Elderly have a slightly decreased hepatic clearance rate. This does not, however, require a dose adjustment.

Pregnancy Considerations Teratogenic effects were not observed in animal studies; however, there are no adequate and well-controlled studies in pregnant women. Use of ondansetron for the treatment of nausea and vomiting of pregnancy (NVP) has been evaluated. Additional studies are needed to determine safety to the fetus, particularly during the first trimester. Based on preliminary data, use is generally reserved for severe NVP (hyperemesis gravidarum) or when conventional treatments are not effective.

- **Ondansetron Hydrochloride** *see* Ondansetron *on page* 1360
- **Onsolis™** *see* FentaNYL *on page* 744
- **ONTAK®** *see* Denileukin Diftitox *on page* 484
- **Opana®** *see* Oxymorphone *on page* 1385
- **Opana® ER** *see* Oxymorphone *on page* 1385
- **OPC-13013** *see* Cilostazol *on page* 370
- **OPC-14597** *see* Aripiprazole *on page* 143
- **OPC-41061** *see* Tolvaptan *on page* 1785
- **o,p'-DDD** *see* Mitotane *on page* 1242
- **Opium and Belladonna** *see* Belladonna and Opium *on page* 194

Opium Tincture (OH pee um TING chur)

Index Terms Deodorized Tincture of Opium (error-prone synonym); DTO (error-prone abbreviation); Opium Tincture, Deodorized; Tincture of Opium

Generic Availability (U.S.) Yes

Pharmacologic Category Analgesic, Opioid; Antidiarrheal

Medication Safety Issues

Sound-alike/look-alike issues:

Opium tincture may be confused with camphorated tincture of opium (paregoric)

High alert medication: The Institute for Safe Medication Practices (ISMP) includes this medication among its list of drugs which have a heightened risk of causing significant patient harm when used in error.

Use care when prescribing opium tincture; opium tincture is 25 times more concentrated than paregoric, each undiluted mL of opium tincture contains the equivalent of morphine 10 mg/mL.

If opium tincture is used in neonates, a 25-fold dilution should be prepared (final concentration: 0.4 mg/mL morphine). Of note, paregoric (which contains the equivalent of morphine 0.4 mg/mL) is **not** recommended for use in neonates due to the high alcohol content (~45%) and the presence of other additives; as an alternative to the use of diluted opium tincture or paregoric, ISMP recommends using a diluted preservative free injectable morphine solution orally.

Although historically opium tincture is dosed as mL/kg, the preferred dosing units are **mg**/kg (Levine, 2001). ISMP suggests hospitals evaluate the need for this product at their institution.

DTO is an error-prone abbreviation and should never be used as an abbreviation for opium tincture (also known as *Deodorized* Tincture of Opium) due to potential for being mistaken as *Diluted* Tincture of Opium

Lactation Enters breast milk/use caution

Use Treatment of diarrhea in adults

Mechanism of Action/Effect Contains many narcotic alkaloids including morphine; its mechanism for gastric motility inhibition is primarily due to this morphine content; it results in a decrease in digestive secretions, an increase in GI muscle tone, and therefore a reduction in GI propulsion

Contraindications Hypersensitivity to opium, morphine sulfate, or any component of the formulation; diarrhea caused by poisoning prior to the toxic material being removed from the GI tract

Note: Manufacturer does not recommend use in children.

Warnings/Precautions May cause CNS depression, which may impair physical or mental abilities; patients must be cautioned about performing tasks which require mental alertness (eg, operating machinery or driving). Effects may be potentiated when used with other sedative drugs or ethanol. Opium shares the toxic potential of opiate agonists, and usual precautions of opiate agonist therapy should be observed; use with caution in patients with CNS depression or coma, morbid obesity, adrenal insufficiency, hepatic impairment, head trauma, GI hemorrhage, thyroid dysfunction, prostatic hyperplasia/urinary stricture, respiratory disease, or a history of drug abuse. Use with caution in patients with biliary tract dysfunction; acute pancreatitis may cause constriction of sphincter of Oddi. May cause hypotension; use with caution in patients with hypovolemia, cardiovascular disease (including acute MI), or with drugs which may exaggerate hypotensive effects (including phenothiazines or general anesthetics). May obscure diagnosis or clinical course of patients with acute abdominal conditions. Concurrent use of agonist/antagonist analgesics may precipitate withdrawal symptoms and/or reduced analgesic efficacy in patients following prolonged therapy with mu opioid agonists. Abrupt discontinuation following prolonged use may also lead to withdrawal symptoms. Use with caution in the elderly and debilitated patients; may be more sensitive to adverse effects. Some preparations contain sulfites which may cause allergic reactions. Infants <3 months of age are more susceptible to respiratory depression; if used, diluted doses are recommended and use with caution. Manufacturer does not recommend use in children.

Do not confuse opium tincture with paregoric; opium tincture is 25 times more potent than paregoric; opium shares the toxic potential of opiate agonists, usual precautions of opiate agonist therapy should be observed; opium may mask dehydration by producing fluid retention in the bowel; monitor patients with prolonged or severe diarrhea carefully; abrupt discontinuation after prolonged use may result in withdrawal symptoms.

Drug Interactions

Avoid Concomitant Use There are no known interactions where it is recommended to avoid concomitant use.

Decreased Effect

Opium Tincture may decrease the levels/effects of: Pegvisomant

The levels/effects of Opium Tincture may be decreased by: Ammonium Chloride; Mixed Agonist / Antagonist Opioids

Increased Effect/Toxicity

Opium Tincture may increase the levels/effects of: Alcohol (Ethyl); Alvimopan; CNS Depressants; Desmopressin; Selective Serotonin Reuptake Inhibitors; Thiazide Diuretics

The levels/effects of Opium Tincture may be increased by: Amphetamines; Antipsychotic Agents (Phenothiazines); Droperidol; Succinylcholine

Nutritional/Ethanol Interactions Ethanol: Avoid ethanol (may increase CNS depression).

Lab Interactions Increased aminotransferase [ALT/AST] (S)

Adverse Reactions Frequency not defined.

Cardiovascular: Palpitation, hypotension, bradycardia, peripheral vasodilation

Central nervous system: Drowsiness, dizziness, restlessness, headache, malaise, CNS depression, intracranial pressure increased, insomnia, mental depression

Gastrointestinal: Nausea, vomiting, constipation, anorexia, stomach cramps, biliary tract spasm

Genitourinary: Urination decreased, urinary tract spasm

Neuromuscular & skeletal: Weakness

Ocular: Miosis

Respiratory: Respiratory depression

Miscellaneous: Histamine release, physical and psychological dependence

Pharmacodynamics/Kinetics

Duration of Action 4-5 hours

Absorption Variable

Metabolism Hepatic

Excretion Urine

Controlled Substance C-II

Available Dosage Forms

Tincture, oral: Anhydrous morphine 10 mg/mL (120 mL, 480 mL)

Dosing

Adult & Geriatric Note: Opium tincture 10% contains morphine 10 mg/mL. Use caution in ordering, dispensing, and/or administering. The following doses are expressed in **mg** (milligram) dosing units of morphine.

Diarrhea: Oral: Usual: 6 **mg** of undiluted opium tincture (10 mg/mL) 4 times daily

Administration

Oral May administer with food to decrease GI upset.

Stability

Storage Store at 68° to 77°F (20° to 25°C). Protect from light.

Monitoring and Teaching Issues

Physical Assessment If being used to control diarrhea, monitor stools. Assess patient's physical and/or psychological dependence. For inpatients, implement safety measures to prevent falls. Discontinue slowly after prolonged use.

Patient Education May cause physical and/or psychological dependence. While using this medication, do not use alcohol and other prescription or OTC medications (especially sedatives, tranquilizers, antihistamines, or pain medications) without consulting prescriber. Maintain adequate hydration. May cause hypotension, dizziness, drowsiness, impaired coordination, blurred vision, or dry mouth. Report chest pain, slow or rapid heartbeat, dizziness, or persistent headache; confusion or respiratory difficulties; or severe constipation.

- **Opium Tincture, Deodorized** *see* Opium Tincture *on page* 1363
- **Oracea®** *see* Doxycycline *on page* 586
- **Oracit®** *see* Sodium Citrate and Citric Acid *on page* 1660
- **Oral Cholera Vaccine** *see* Travelers' Diarrhea and Cholera Vaccine *on page* 1806
- **Oralone®** *see* Triamcinolone (Topical) *on page* 1816
- **Oramorph® SR** *see* Morphine (Systemic) *on page* 1258
- **Oranyl [OTC]** *see* Pseudoephedrine *on page* 1529
- **Orap®** *see* Pimozide *on page* 1459
- **Orapred®** *see* PrednisoLONE (Systemic) *on page* 1497
- **Orapred ODT®** *see* PrednisoLONE (Systemic) *on page* 1497
- **OraVerse™** *see* Phentolamine *on page* 1448
- **Oraxyl™** *see* Doxycycline *on page* 586
- **Orbivan™** *see* Butalbital, Acetaminophen, and Caffeine *on page* 260
- **Orencia®** *see* Abatacept *on page* 33
- **Organidin® NR [OTC] [DSC]** *see* GuaiFENesin *on page* 890
- **ORG NC 45** *see* Vecuronium *on page* 1852

Orlistat (OR li stat)

U.S. Brand Names Alli™ [OTC]; Xenical®

Generic Availability (U.S.) No

Pharmacologic Category Lipase Inhibitor

Medication Safety Issues

Sound-alike/look-alike issues:

Xenical® may be confused with Xeloda®

Pregnancy Risk Factor B

Lactation Excretion in breast milk unknown/not recommended

Use Management of obesity, including weight loss and weight management, when used in conjunction with a reduced-calorie and low-fat diet; reduce the risk of weight regain after prior weight loss; indicated for obese patients with an initial body mass index (BMI) ≥30 kg/m^2 or ≥27 kg/m^2 in the presence of other risk factors (eg, diabetes, dyslipidemia, hypertension)

Mechanism of Action/Effect Inhibits gastric and pancreatic lipases, thus inhibiting the absorption of dietary fats (by 30% at doses of 120 mg 3 times/day)

Contraindications Hypersensitivity to orlistat or any component of the formulation; chronic malabsorption syndrome or cholestasis

Warnings/Precautions Prior to use other causes for obesity (eg, hypothyroidism) should be ruled out. Cases of severe liver injury (some fatal) with hepatocellular necrosis or acute hepatic failure have been reported (rare); liver transplantation has been required in some patients. Patients should be instructed to report any symptoms of hepatic dysfunction (eg, anorexia, pruritus, jaundice, dark urine, light colored stools, right upper quadrant pain); discontinue orlistat and obtain liver function test immediately if symptoms occur. Advise patients to adhere to dietary guidelines; if taken with a diet high in fat (>30% total daily calories from fat) gastrointestinal adverse events may increase. Distribute daily fat intake over 3 main meals. If taken with any 1 meal very high in fat, the possibility of gastrointestinal effects increases. Counsel patients to take a multivitamin supplement that contains fat-soluble vitamins ≥2 hours before or after orlistat administration to ensure adequate nutrition; orlistat has been shown to reduce the absorption of some fat-soluble vitamins and beta-carotene. Increased levels of urinary oxalate following treatment may occur in some patients; use with caution in patients with a history of hyperoxaluria or calcium oxalate nephrolithiasis. The potential exists for misuse in inappropriate patient populations (eg, patients with anorexia nervosa or bulimia) similar to any weight loss agent. In general, substantial weight loss may increase the risk of cholelithiasis. Safety and efficacy with >4 years of use have not been established.

Self-medication (OTC use): Prior to use, patients should contact their healthcare provider if they have ever had kidney stones, gall bladder disease, or pancreatitis. Patients taking medications for diabetes or thyroid disease, anticoagulants, or other weight-loss products should consult their healthcare provider or pharmacist. Patients who have had an organ transplant should not use orlistat. If severe and/or continuous abdominal pain, itching, yellowing of the eyes or skin, dark urine, or loss of appetite occurs, use should be discontinued and healthcare provider consulted.

Drug Interactions

Avoid Concomitant Use There are no known interactions where it is recommended to avoid concomitant use.

Decreased Effect

Orlistat may decrease the levels/effects of: Amiodarone; CycloSPORINE; CycloSPORINE (Systemic); Levothyroxine; Paricalcitol; Vitamin D Analogs; Vitamins (Fat Soluble)

Increased Effect/Toxicity

Orlistat may increase the levels/effects of: Warfarin

Nutritional/Ethanol Interactions Fat-soluble vitamins: Absorption of vitamins A, D, E, and K may be decreased by orlistat. A multivitamin containing the fat-soluble vitamins (A, D, E, and K) should be administered once daily at least 2 hours before or after orlistat.

Adverse Reactions Note: The frequency of most adverse reactions (especially gastrointestinal effects) decreases over time.

>10%:

Central nervous system: Headache (≤31%)

Gastrointestinal: Oily spotting (4% to 27%), abdominal pain/discomfort (≤26%), flatus with discharge (2% to 24%), fecal urgency (3% to 22%), fatty/oily stool (6% to 20%), oily evacuation (2% to 12%), defecation increased (3% to 11%)

Neuromuscular & skeletal: Back pain (≤14%)

Respiratory: Upper respiratory infection (26% to 38%)

Miscellaneous: Influenza (≤40%)

1% to 10%:

Cardiovascular: Pedal edema (≤3%)

Central nervous system: Fatigue (3% to 7%), anxiety (3% to 5%), sleep disorder (≤4%)

Dermatologic: Dry skin (≤2%)

Endocrine & metabolic: Menstrual irregularities (≤10%)

Gastrointestinal: Nausea (4% to 8%), fecal incontinence (2% to 8%), infectious diarrhea (≤5%), rectal pain/discomfort (3% to 5%), gingival disorder (2% to 4%), tooth disorder (3% to 4%)

Genitourinary: Urinary tract infection (6% to 8%), vaginitis (3% to 4%)

Neuromuscular & skeletal: Myalgia (≤4%)

Otic: Otitis (3% to 4%)

Respiratory: Lower respiratory infection (≤8%)

Pharmacodynamics/Kinetics

Onset of Action 24-48 hours

Duration of Action 48-72 hours

Absorption Minimal

Metabolism Metabolized within the gastrointestinal wall; forms inactive metabolites

Excretion Feces (~97%, 83% as unchanged drug); urine (<2%)

Available Dosage Forms

Capsule, oral:

Alli™ [OTC]: 60 mg

Xenical®: 120 mg

Dosing

Adult & Geriatric Obesity: Oral:

Xenical®: 120 mg 3 times/day with each main meal containing fat (during or up to 1 hour after the meal); omit dose if meal is occasionally missed or contains no fat.

Alli™: OTC labeling: 60 mg 3 times/day with each main meal containing fat

Pediatric Obesity (Xenical®): Children ≥12 years: Refer to adult dosing.

Administration

Oral Administer during or up to 1 hour after each main meal containing fat.

Stability

Storage Store at 25°C (77°F); excursions permitted to 15°C to 30°C (59°F to 86°F).

Monitoring and Teaching Issues

Laboratory Monitoring Serum glucose in patients with diabetes; thyroid function in patient with thyroid disease; liver function tests in patients exhibiting symptoms of hepatic dysfunction; cyclosporine levels closely if taking cyclosporine

Patient Education Maintain prescribed diet (ideally a low-fat diet; high-fat meals may result in GI distress), exercise regimen, and vitamin supplements as prescribed. You may experience dizziness, lightheadedness, or increased flatus and fecal urgency (this may lessen with continued use). Report persistent back, muscle, or joint pain; signs of respiratory tract infection or flu-like symptoms; skin rash or irritation; severe fatigue; fever; yellowing of skin or eyes; brown urine; abdominal pain; or persistent nausea or vomiting.

Dietary Considerations Multivitamin supplements that contain fat-soluble vitamins should be taken once daily at least 2 hours before or after the administration of orlistat (ie, bedtime). Gastrointestinal effects of orlistat may increase if taken with any one meal very high in fat. Distribute daily intake of carbohydrates, fat (~30% of daily calories), and protein over three main meals.

Pregnancy Considerations Teratogenic effects or embryotoxicity were not observed in animal studies. There are no adequate and well-controlled studies in pregnant women. Because animal reproductive studies are not always predictive of human response, orlistat is not recommended for use during pregnancy.

Related Information

Obesity Treatment Guidelines *on page 2064*

Orphenadrine (or FEN a dreen)

U.S. Brand Names Norflex™

Index Terms Orphenadrine Citrate

Generic Availability (U.S.) Yes

Pharmacologic Category Skeletal Muscle Relaxant

Medication Safety Issues

Sound-alike/look-alike issues:

Norflex™ may be confused with norfloxacin, Noroxin®

Beers Criteria medication: This drug may be inappropriate for use in geriatric patients (high severity risk).

International issues:

Flexin: Brand name for orphenadrine [Israel] but is also the brand name for cyclobenzaprine [Chile] and diclofenac [Argentina]

Flexin [Israel] may be confused with Floxin which is a brand name for flunarizine [Thailand], norfloxacin [South Africa], ofloxacin [U.S., Canada], and perfloxacin [Philippines]; Fluoxin brand name for fluoxetine [Czech Republic]

Pregnancy Risk Factor C

Lactation Excretion in breast milk unknown/use caution

Use Treatment of muscle spasm associated with acute painful musculoskeletal conditions

Available Dosage Forms

Injection, solution: 30 mg/mL (2 mL)

Norflex™: 30 mg/mL (2 mL)

Tablet, extended release, oral: 100 mg

Dosing

Adult Muscle spasms:

Oral: 100 mg twice daily

I.M., I.V.: 60 mg every 12 hours

Geriatric Use caution; generally not recommended for use in the elderly.

Administration

Oral Do not crush sustained release drug product.

Monitoring and Teaching Issues

Physical Assessment Do not discontinue abruptly if patient using chronically; taper dosage slowly.

Patient Education Do not chew or crush extended release tablets. Do not use alcohol. You may experience drowsiness, dizziness, or lightheadedness. Report excessive drowsiness.

◆ **Orphenadrine Citrate** *see* Orphenadrine *on page 1366*

◆ **Ortho Cept** *see* Ethinyl Estradiol and Desogestrel *on page 695*

◆ **Ortho-Cept®** *see* Ethinyl Estradiol and Desogestrel *on page 695*

◆ **Orthoclone OKT® 3 [DSC]** *see* Muromonab-CD3 *on page 1268*

◆ **Ortho Cyclen** *see* Ethinyl Estradiol and Norgestimate *on page 704*

◆ **Ortho-Cyclen®** *see* Ethinyl Estradiol and Norgestimate *on page 704*

◆ **Ortho Micronor®** *see* Norethindrone *on page 1334*

◆ **Ortho Novum** *see* Ethinyl Estradiol and Norethindrone *on page 701*

◆ **Ortho-Novum® 1/35** *see* Ethinyl Estradiol and Norethindrone *on page 701*

◆ **Ortho Novum 1/50** *see* Norethindrone and Mestranol *on page 1335*

◆ **Ortho-Novum® 7/7/7** *see* Ethinyl Estradiol and Norethindrone *on page 701*

◆ **Ortho,para-DDD** *see* Mitotane *on page 1242*

◆ **Ortho Tri Cyclen** *see* Ethinyl Estradiol and Norgestimate *on page 704*

◆ **Ortho Tri-Cyclen®** *see* Ethinyl Estradiol and Norgestimate *on page 704*

◆ **Ortho Tri-Cyclen® Lo** *see* Ethinyl Estradiol and Norgestimate *on page 704*

Oseltamivir (oh sel TAM i vir)

U.S. Brand Names Tamiflu®

Generic Availability (U.S.) No

Pharmacologic Category Antiviral Agent; Neuraminidase Inhibitor

Medication Safety Issues

Sound-alike/look-alike issues:

Tamiflu® may be confused with Thera-Flu®

Tamiflu® may be confused with Tambocor™

Dispensing issues:

Oseltamivir (Tamiflu®) oral suspension is packaged with an oral syringe. Healthcare providers dispensing this medication should be aware that the syringe is calibrated in 30 mg, 45 mg, and 60 mg graduations. **When the oral syringe is dispensed, instructions to the patient should be provided based on these units of measure (not mL or teaspoon). When dispensing the oral suspension for children <1 year of age, the oral syringe provided from the manufacturer should be removed and NOT provided to the caregiver.** Pharmacists and healthcare providers should instead supply an oral syringe capable of measuring mL doses. Patients should always be provided with a measuring device calibrated the same way as their labeled instructions.

Oseltamivir (Tamiflu®) 75 mg capsules can be compounded into a suspension when oseltamivir oral suspension is not commercially available. The commercially-available oral suspension concentration is 12 mg/mL; however, the extemporaneously prepared suspension concentration is 15 mg/mL. Prescriptions written in mL or teaspoons should specify the oral suspension concentration to be dispensed.

Pregnancy Risk Factor C

Lactation Enters breast milk/not recommended

Use Treatment of uncomplicated acute illness due to influenza (A or B) infection in children ≥1 year of age and adults who have been symptomatic for no more than 2 days; prophylaxis against influenza (A or B) infection in children ≥1 year of age and adults

The Advisory Committee on Immunization Practices (ACIP) recommends that **treatment** be considered for the following:

- Persons with severe, complicated or progressive illness
- Hospitalized persons
- Persons at higher risk for influenza complications:
  - Children <2 years of age (highest risk in children <6 months of age)
  - Adults ≥65 years of age
  - Persons with chronic disorders of the pulmonary (including asthma) or cardiovascular systems (except hypertension)
  - Persons with chronic metabolic diseases (including diabetes mellitus), hepatic disease, renal dysfunction, hematologic disorders (including sickle cell disease), or immunosuppression (including immunosuppression caused by medications or HIV)
  - Persons with neurologic/neuromuscular conditions (including conditions such as spinal cord injuries, seizure disorders, cerebral palsy, stroke, mental retardation, moderate to severe developmental delay, or muscular dystrophy) which may compromise respiratory function, the handling of respiratory secretions, or that can increase the risk of aspiration
  - Pregnant or postpartum women (≤2 weeks after delivery)
  - Persons <19 years of age on long-term aspirin therapy
  - American Indians and Alaskan Natives
  - Persons who are morbidly obese (BMI ≥40)
  - Residents of nursing homes or other chronic care facilities

- Use may also be considered for previously healthy, nonhigh-risk outpatients with confirmed or suspected influenza based on clinical judgment when treatment can be started within 48 hours of illness onset.

The ACIP recommends that **prophylaxis** be considered for the following:

- Postexposure prophylaxis may be considered for family or close contacts of suspected or confirmed cases, who are at higher risk of influenza complications, and who have not been vaccinated against the circulating strain at the time of the exposure.
- Postexposure prophylaxis may be considered for unvaccinated healthcare workers who had occupational exposure without protective equipment.
- Pre-exposure prophylaxis should only be used for persons at very high risk of influenza complications who cannot be otherwise protected at times of high risk for exposure.
- Prophylaxis should also be administered to all eligible residents of institutions that house patients at high risk when needed to control outbreaks.

The ACIP recommends that treatment and prophylaxis be given to children <1 year of age when indicated.

Mechanism of Action/Effect Thought to inhibit influenza virus by altering virus particle aggregation and release

Contraindications Hypersensitivity to oseltamivir or any component of the formulation

Warnings/Precautions Oseltamivir is not a substitute for the influenza virus vaccine. It has not been shown to prevent primary or concomitant bacterial infections that may occur with influenza virus. Use caution with renal impairment; dosage adjustment is required for creatinine clearance <30 mL/minute. Safety and efficacy for use in patients with chronic cardiac and/or kidney disease, severe hepatic impairment, or for treatment or prophylaxis in immunocompromised patients have not been established. Rare but severe hypersensitivity reactions (anaphylaxis, severe dermatologic reactions) have been associated with use. Rare occurrences of neuropsychiatric events (including confusion, delirium, hallucinations, and/or self-injury) have been reported from postmarketing surveillance (primarily in pediatric patients); direct causation is difficult to establish (influenza infection may also be associated with behavioral and neurologic changes). Monitor closely for signs of any unusual behavior.

Antiviral treatment should begin within 48 hours of symptom onset. However, the CDC recommends that treatment may still be beneficial and should be started in hospitalized patients with severe, complicated or progressive illness if >48 hours. Nonhospitalized persons who are not at high risk for developing severe or complicated illness and who have a mild disease are not likely to benefit if treatment is started >48 hours after symptom onset. Nonhospitalized persons who are already beginning to recover do not need treatment.

Drug Interactions

Avoid Concomitant Use There are no known interactions where it is recommended to avoid concomitant use.

Decreased Effect

Oseltamivir may decrease the levels/effects of: Influenza Virus Vaccine (Live/Attenuated)

Increased Effect/Toxicity

The levels/effects of Oseltamivir may be increased by: Probenecid

Adverse Reactions

>10%: Gastrointestinal: Vomiting (2% to 15%)

1% to 10%:

Gastrointestinal: Nausea (4% to 10%), abdominal pain (2% to 5%), diarrhea (1% to 3%)
Ocular: Conjunctivitis (1%)
Respiratory: Epistaxis (1%)

Pharmacodynamics/Kinetics

Absorption Well absorbed

Bioavailability 75% as oseltamivir carboxylate

Protein Binding Plasma: Oseltamivir carboxylate: 3%; Oseltamivir: 42%

Half-Life Elimination Oseltamivir: 1-3 hours; Oseltamivir carboxylate: 6-10 hours

Metabolism Hepatic (90%) to oseltamivir carboxylate; neither the parent drug nor active metabolite has any effect on the cytochrome P450 system

Excretion Urine (>90% as oseltamivir carboxylate); feces

Available Dosage Forms

Capsule:

Tamiflu®: 30 mg, 45 mg, 75 mg

Powder for oral suspension:

Tamiflu®: 12 mg/mL

Dosing

Adult & Geriatric

Influenza prophylaxis: Oral: 75 mg once daily; initiate prophylaxis within 48 hours of contact with an infected individual; duration of prophylaxis: 10 days. During community outbreaks, duration of protection lasts for length of dosing period; safety and efficacy have been demonstrated for use up to 6 weeks in immunocompetent patients and safety has been demonstrated for use up to 12 weeks in patients who are immunocompromised.

Prophylaxis (institutional outbreak, CDC 2011 recommendations): Continue for ≥2 weeks and until ~10 days after identification of illness onset in the last patient

Influenza treatment:

Treatment of influenza: Oral: 75 mg twice daily initiated within 48 hours of onset of symptoms; duration of treatment: 5 days

Note: Hospitalized patients with severe influenza infection may require longer (eg, ≥10 days) treatment courses. Some experts also recommend empirically doubling the treatment dose. Initiate as early as possible in any hospitalized patient with suspected/confirmed influenza (CDC, 2011); may be administered via naso- or orogastric tube in mechanically-ventilated patients (Taylor, 2008).

Pediatric

Influenza prophylaxis: Oral: Initiate prophylaxis within 48 hours of contact with an infected individual; duration of prophylaxis: 10 days:

Prophylaxis (institutional outbreak, CDC 2011 recommendations): Continue for ≥2 weeks and until ~10 days after identification of illness onset in the last patient

Children <1 year (unlabeled dosing, CDC 2011): **Note:** Prophylaxis is not recommended for infants <3 months of age unless clinically critical; weight-based dosing recommendations are not intended for premature neonates:

<12 months: 3 mg/kg/dose once daily

Alternate dosing based on age (use only if weight not available) (unlabeled dosing; AAP, 2010):

3-5 months: 20 mg once daily

6-11 months: 25 mg once daily

Children: 1-12 years: During community outbreaks, prophylaxis may be used for up to 6 weeks.

≤15 kg: 30 mg once daily

>15 kg to ≤23 kg: 45 mg once daily

>23 kg to ≤40 kg: 60 mg once daily

>40 kg: 75 mg once daily

Adolescents ≥13 years: Refer to adult dosing.

Influenza treatment: Oral: Initiate treatment within 48 hours of contact with an infected individual; duration of treatment: 5 days

Note: Hospitalized patients with severe influenza infection may require longer (eg, ≥10 days) treatment courses. Some experts also recommend empirically doubling the treatment dose. Doubling the dose in adult outpatients was not associated with increased adverse events. As no double dose studies have been published in children, use caution. Initiate as early as possible in any hospitalized patient with suspected/confirmed influenza (CDC, 2011); may be administered via naso- or orogastric tube in mechanically-ventilated patients (Taylor, 2008).

Treatment of influenza:

Children <1 year (unlabeled dosing, CDC 2011): **Note:** Weight-based dosing recommendations are not intended for premature neonates:

<12 months: 3 mg/kg/dose twice daily

Alternate dosing based on age (use only if weight not available) (unlabeled dosing; AAP, 2010):

<3 months: 12 mg twice daily

3-5 months: 20 mg twice daily

6-11 months: 25 mg twice daily

Children: 1-12 years:

≤15 kg: 30 mg twice daily

>15 kg to ≤23 kg: 45 mg twice daily

>23 kg to ≤40 kg: 60 mg twice daily

>40 kg: 75 mg twice daily

Adolescents ≥13 years: Refer to adult dosing.

Renal Impairment

Cl_{cr} 10-30 mL/minute: Adults:

Treatment: Reduce dose to 75 mg once daily for 5 days

High-dose treatment (unlabeled [eg, severely-ill hospitalized patients with 2009 H1N1 influenza]): Currently no data are available; consider 150 mg once daily

Prophylaxis: Administer 75 mg every other day or 30 mg once daily.

CAPD (unlabeled dose): Adults: 30 mg once weekly (Robson, 2006)

Hemodialysis:

Children >1 year (unlabeled dose; Schreuder, 2010):

≤15 kg: 7.5 mg after each hemodialysis session

>15 kg to ≤23 kg: 10 mg after each hemodialysis session

>23 kg to ≤40 kg: 15 mg after each hemodialysis session

>40 kg: 30 mg after each hemodialysis session

Adults (unlabeled dose; Robson, 2006): 30 mg after every other session

Hepatic Impairment

Mild-to-moderate impairment: No adjustment necessary

Severe impairment: Pharmacokinetics and safety have not been evaluated

Administration

Oral May be administered without regard to meals; take with food to improve tolerance. Capsules may be opened and mixed with sweetened liquid (eg, chocolate syrup).

Other Mechanically-ventilated critically-ill patients: May administer via naso- or orogastric (NG/OG) tube. For a 150 mg dose, dissolve powder from two 75 mg capsules in 20 mL of sterile water and inject down the NG/OG tube; follow with a 10 mL sterile water flush (Taylor, 2008).

Stability

Reconstitution Oral suspension: Reconstitute with 23 mL of water to a final concentration of 12 mg/mL (to make 25 mL total suspension).

Storage

Capsules: Store at 25°C (77°F); excursions permitted to 15°C to 30°C (59°F to 86°F).

Oral suspension: Store powder for suspension at 25°C (77°F); excursions permitted to 15°C to 30°C (59°F to 86°F). Once reconstituted, store suspension under refrigeration at 2°C to 8°C (36°F to 46°F); do not freeze. Use within 10 days of preparation if stored at room temperature or within 17 days of preparation if stored under refrigeration.

Monitoring and Teaching Issues

Laboratory Monitoring Critically-ill patients: Repeat rRT-PCR or viral culture may help to determine on-going viral replication

Physical Assessment Recommendations for antiviral susceptibility and effectiveness may change. Validate with the CDC recommendations for use prior to prescribing.

Patient Education This is not a substitute for the flu shot. Must be taken within 2 days of contact with an infected individual or onset of flu symptoms (eg, fever, cough, headache, fatigue, muscular weakness, and sore throat). You may experience nausea or vomiting. Report hallucinations or unusual behavior to your prescriber.

Dietary Considerations Take without regard to meals; take with food to improve tolerance.

Breast-Feeding Considerations Small amounts of oseltamivir and oseltamivir carboxylate have been detected in breast milk. Breast milk samples were obtained from a single patient (~9 months postpartum) over the course of 5 days of treatment. Using a maximum total milk concentration of oseltamivir (expressed as parent drug and metabolite) of 81.6 ng/mL, the estimated exposure to the breast-feeding infant would be ~0.5% of the weight-adjusted maternal dose (in a 60 kg woman). Breast-feeding is not recommended by the manufacturer. According to the CDC, breast-feeding while taking oseltamivir can be continued. The CDC recommends that women infected with the influenza virus follow general precautions (eg, frequent hand washing) to decrease viral transmission to the child. Mothers with influenza-like illnesses at delivery should consider avoiding close contact with the infant until they have received 48 hours of antiviral medication, fever has resolved, and cough and secretions can be controlled. These measures may help decrease (but not eliminate) the risk of transmitting influenza to the newborn. During this time, breast milk can be expressed and bottle-fed to the infant by another person who is well. Protective measures, such as wearing a face mask, changing into a clean gown or clothing, and strict hand hygiene should be continued by the mother for ≥7 days after the onset of symptoms or until symptom-free for 24 hours. Infant care should be performed by a noninfected person when possible (consult current CDC guidelines).

Pregnancy Considerations In animal reproduction studies, a dose-dependent increase in the rates of minor skeleton abnormalities was found in exposed offspring; therefore, the manufacturer classifies oseltamivir as pregnancy category C. The rate of each abnormality remained within the background rate of occurrence in the species studied. In an *in vitro* study, placental transfer of oseltamivir phosphate and its active metabolite oseltamivir carboxylate was found to be incomplete, resulting in minimal accumulation in the fetus. An increased risk of adverse neonatal outcomes has not been observed following maternal use of oseltamivir during pregnancy. Untreated influenza infection is associated with an increased risk of adverse events to the fetus and an increased risk of complications or death to the mother. Oseltamivir and zanamivir are currently recommended for the treatment or prophylaxis of influenza in pregnant women and women up to 2 weeks postpartum. Oseltamivir and zanamivir are currently recommended as an adjunct to vaccination and should not be used as a substitute for vaccination in pregnant women (consult current CDC guidelines).

Additional Information In clinical studies of the influenza virus, 1.3% of post-treatment isolates in adults and adolescents and 8.6% of isolates in children had decreased neuraminidase susceptibility *in vitro* to oseltamivir carboxylate.

The absence of symptoms does not rule out viral influenza infection and clinical judgment should guide the decision for therapy. Treatment should not be delayed while waiting for the results of diagnostic tests. Treatment should be considered for high-risk patients with symptoms despite a negative rapid influenza test when the illness cannot be contributed to another cause. Use of oseltamivir is not a substitute for vaccination (when available); susceptibility to influenza infection returns once therapy is discontinued.

- ◆ **OSI-774** *see* Erlotinib *on page* *652*
- ◆ **Osmitrol** *see* Mannitol *on page* *1146*
- ◆ **OTFC (Oral Transmucosal Fentanyl Citrate)** *see* FentaNYL *on page* *744*
- ◆ **Ovcon® 35** *see* Ethinyl Estradiol and Norethindrone *on page* *701*
- ◆ **Ovcon® 50** *see* Ethinyl Estradiol and Norethindrone *on page* *701*
- ◆ **Ovidrel®** *see* Chorionic Gonadotropin (Recombinant) *on page* *365*
- ◆ **Oxalatoplatin** *see* Oxaliplatin *on page* *1370*
- ◆ **Oxalatoplatinum** *see* Oxaliplatin *on page* *1370*

Oxaliplatin (ox AL i pla tin)

U.S. Brand Names Eloxatin®

Index Terms Diaminocyclohexane Oxalatoplatinum; L-OHP; Oxalatoplatin; Oxalatoplatinum

Generic Availability (U.S.) Yes

Pharmacologic Category Antineoplastic Agent, Alkylating Agent; Antineoplastic Agent, Platinum Analog

Medication Safety Issues

Sound-alike/look-alike issues:

Oxaliplatin may be confused with Aloxi®, carboplatin, cisplatin

High alert medication: The Institute for Safe Medication Practices (ISMP) includes this medication among its list of drug classes which have a heightened risk of causing significant patient harm when used in error.

Pregnancy Risk Factor D

Lactation Excretion in breast milk unknown/not recommended

Use Treatment of stage III colon cancer (adjuvant) and advanced colorectal cancer

Unlabeled/Investigational Use Treatment of esophageal cancer, gastric cancer, hepatobiliary cancer, non-Hodgkin's lymphoma, ovarian cancer, pancreatic cancer, testicular cancer

Mechanism of Action/Effect Oxaliplatin, a platinum derivative, is an alkylating agent. Following intracellular hydrolysis, the platinum compound binds to DNA forming cross-links which inhibit DNA replication and transcription, resulting in cell death. Cytotoxicity is cell-cycle nonspecific.

Contraindications Hypersensitivity to oxaliplatin, other platinum-containing compounds, or any component of the formulation

Canadian labeling: Additional contraindications (not in U.S. labeling): Pregnancy, breast-feeding; severe renal impairment (Cl_{cr} <30 mL/minute)

Warnings/Precautions Hazardous agent - use appropriate precautions for handling and disposal. **[U.S. Boxed Warning]: Anaphylactic/anaphylactoid reactions may occur within minutes of oxaliplatin administration; symptoms may be managed with epinephrine, corticosteroids, and antihistamines.** Grade 3 or 4 hypersensitivity has been observed. Allergic reactions may occur with any cycle and may include bronchospasm (rare), erythema, hypotension (rare), pruritus, rash, and/or urticaria.

Two different types of peripheral sensory neuropathy may occur: First, an acute (within first 2 days), reversible (resolves within 14 days), with primarily peripheral symptoms that are often exacerbated by cold (may include pharyngolaryngeal dysesthesia); may recur with subsequent doses; avoid mucositis prophylaxis with ice chips during oxaliplatin infusion. Secondly, a more persistent (>14 days) presentation that often interferes with daily activities (eg, writing, buttoning, swallowing), these symptoms may improve in some patients upon discontinuing treatment.

May cause pulmonary fibrosis; withhold treatment for unexplained pulmonary symptoms (eg, crackles, dyspnea, nonproductive cough, pulmonary infiltrates) until interstitial lung disease or pulmonary fibrosis are excluded. Hepatotoxicity (including rare cases of hepatitis and hepatic failure) has been reported. Liver biopsy has revealed peliosis, nodular regenerative hyperplasia, sinusoidal alterations, perisinusoidal fibrosis, and veno-occlusive lesions; the presence of hepatic vascular disorders (including veno-occlusive disease) should be considered, especially in individuals developing portal hypertension or who present with increased liver function tests. Use caution with renal dysfunction; increased toxicity may occur. When administered as sequential infusions, taxane derivatives (docetaxel, paclitaxel) should be administered before platinum derivatives (carboplatin, cisplatin, oxaliplatin) to limit myelosuppression and enhance efficacy. Concomitant use with 5-FU may increase risk for adverse hematologic or GI effects. Elderly patients are more sensitive to some adverse events including diarrhea, dehydration, hypokalemia, leukopenia, fatigue and syncope. Safety and efficacy in children have not been established.

Drug Interactions

Avoid Concomitant Use

Avoid concomitant use of Oxaliplatin with any of the following: BCG; Natalizumab; Pimecrolimus; Roflumilast; Tacrolimus (Topical); Vaccines (Live)

Decreased Effect

Oxaliplatin may decrease the levels/effects of: BCG; Cardiac Glycosides; Sipuleucel-T; Vaccines (Inactivated); Vaccines (Live); Vitamin K Antagonists

The levels/effects of Oxaliplatin may be decreased by: Echinacea

Increased Effect/Toxicity

Oxaliplatin may increase the levels/effects of: Leflunomide; Natalizumab; Taxane Derivatives; Topotecan; Vaccines (Live); Vitamin K Antagonists

The levels/effects of Oxaliplatin may be increased by: Denosumab; Pimecrolimus; Roflumilast; Tacrolimus (Topical); Trastuzumab

Adverse Reactions Percentages reported with monotherapy.

>10%:

Central nervous system: Fatigue (61%), fever (25%), pain (14%), headache (13%), insomnia (11%)

Gastrointestinal: Nausea (64%), diarrhea (46%), vomiting (37%), abdominal pain (31%), constipation (31%), anorexia (20%), stomatitis (14%)

Hematologic: Anemia (64%; grades 3/4: 1%), thrombocytopenia (30%; grades 3/4: 3%), leukopenia (13%)

Hepatic: AST increased (54%; grades 3/4: 4%), ALT increased (36%; grades 3/4: 1%), total bilirubin increased (13%; grades 3/4: 5%)

Neuromuscular & skeletal: Peripheral neuropathy (may be dose limiting; 76%; acute 65%; grades 3/4: 5%; persistent 43%; grades 3/4: 3%), back pain (11%)

Respiratory: Dyspnea (13%), cough (11%)

1% to 10%:

Cardiovascular: Edema (10%), chest pain (5%), peripheral edema (5%), flushing (3%), thromboembolism (2%)

Central nervous system: Dizziness (7%)

Dermatologic: Rash (5%), alopecia (3%), hand-foot syndrome (1%)

Endocrine & metabolic: Dehydration (5%), hypokalemia (3%)

Gastrointestinal: Dyspepsia (7%), taste perversion (5%), flatulence (3%), mucositis (2%), gastroesophageal reflux (1%), dysphagia (acute 1% to 2%)

Genitourinary: Dysuria (1%)

Hematologic: Neutropenia (7%)

Local: Injection site reaction (9%; redness/swelling/pain)

Neuromuscular & skeletal: Rigors (9%), arthralgia (7%)

Ocular: Abnormal lacrimation (1%)

Renal: Serum creatinine increased (5% to 10%)

Respiratory: URI (7%), rhinitis (6%), epistaxis (2%), pharyngitis (2%), pharyngolaryngeal dysesthesia (grades 3/4: 1% to 2%)

Miscellaneous: Allergic reactions (3%); hypersensitivity (includes urticaria, pruritus, facial flushing, shortness of breath, bronchospasm, diaphoresis, hypotension, syncope: grades 3/4: 2% to 3%); hiccup (2%)

Pharmacodynamics/Kinetics

Protein Binding >90% primarily albumin and gamma globulin (irreversible binding to platinum)

Half-Life Elimination Terminal: 391 hours

Metabolism Nonenzymatic (rapid and extensive), forms active and inactive derivatives

Excretion Urine (~54%); feces (~2%)

Available Dosage Forms

Injection, powder for reconstitution: 50 mg, 100 mg

Injection, solution: 5 mg/mL (10 mL, 20 mL)

Injection, solution [preservative free]:

Eloxatin®: 5 mg/mL (10 mL, 20 mL, 40 mL)

Dosing

Adult Details concerning dosing in combination regimens should also be consulted. Delay dosage in subsequent cycles until recovery of neutrophils ≥1.5 x 10^9/L and platelets ≥75 x 10^9/L.

Advanced colorectal cancer: I.V.: 85 mg/m^2 every 2 weeks until disease progression or unacceptable toxicity (in combination with fluorouracil/leucovorin)

Stage III colon cancer (adjuvant): I.V.: 85 mg/m^2 every 2 weeks for 12 cycles (in combination with fluorouracil/leucovorin)

Colon/colorectal cancer (unlabeled doses or combinations): I.V.: 85 mg/m^2/dose on days 1, 15, and 29 of an 8-week treatment cycle in combination with fluorouracil/leucovorin (Kuebler, 2007) **or** 85 mg/m^2 every 2 weeks in combination with fluorouracil/leucovorin/ irinotecan (Falcone, 2007) **or** 130 mg/m^2 every 3 weeks in combination with capecitabine (Cassidy, 2008)

Esophageal/gastric cancers (unlabeled use; as part of a combination chemotherapy regimen): I.V.: 85 mg/m^2 every 2 weeks (Al-Batran, 2008) **or** 130 mg/m^2 every 3 weeks (Cunningham, 2008)

or

Gastric cancer: 100 mg/m^2 every 2 weeks (Louvet, 2002)

Hepatobiliary cancer (unlabeled use; as part of a combination chemotherapy regimen): 100 mg/m^2 every 2 weeks (Andre, 2004) **or** 130 mg/m^2 every 3 weeks (Nehls, 2008)

Non-Hodgkin's lymphoma (unlabeled use; as part of a combination chemotherapy regimen): I.V.: 25 mg/m^2/day for 4 days every 4 weeks (Tsimberidou, 2008) **or** 100 mg/m^2 every 3 weeks (Lopez, 2008; Rodriguez, 2007) **or** 130 mg/m^2 every 3 weeks (Chau, 2001)

Ovarian cancer (unlabeled use): I.V.: 130 mg/m^2 every 3 weeks (Dieras, 2002; Piccart, 2000)

Pancreatic cancer (unlabeled use; as part of a combination chemotherapy regimen): I.V.: 85 mg/m^2 every 2 weeks (Conroy, 2005) **or** 100 mg/m^2 every 2 weeks (Louvet, 2005) **or** 110-130 mg/m^2 every 3 weeks (Xiong, 2008)

Testicular cancer (unlabeled use; in combination with gemcitabine): I.V.: 130 mg/m^2 every 3 weeks (Kollmannsberger, 2004; Pectasides, 2004)

Geriatric No dosing adjustment recommended.

Renal Impairment The FDA-approved labeling does not contain renal dosing adjustment guidelines. Oxaliplatin is primarily eliminated renally; in patients with Cl_{cr} <30 mL/minute, the AUC is increased ~190%. Oxaliplatin use has been studied in 25 patients with renal dysfunction; treatment was well-tolerated in patients with mild-to-moderate impairment (Cl_{cr} 20-59 mL/minute), suggesting that dose reduction is not necessary in this patient population (Takimoto, 2003). Patients with severe renal impairment (Cl_{cr} <20 mL/minute) have not been adequately studied; consider omitting dose or changing chemotherapy regimen if Cl_{cr} <20 mL/ minute.

Note: Canadian labeling: Use in patients with Cl_{cr} <30 mL/minute is contraindicated in Canadian labeling.

Hepatic Impairment Mild, moderate, or severe hepatic impairment: Dosage adjustment not necessary (Doroshow, 2003; Synold, 2007).

Adjustment for Toxicity Acute toxicities: Longer infusion times (up to 6 hours) may mitigate acute toxicities.

Neurosensory events:

Persistent (>7 days) grade 2 neurosensory events: Consider oxaliplatin dose reduction if symptoms do not resolve:

Adjuvant treatment of stage III colon cancer: Reduce dose to 75 mg/m^2

Advanced colorectal cancer: Reduce dose to 65 mg/m^2

Consider withholding oxaliplatin for grade 2 neuropathy lasting >7 days despite dose reduction.

Persistent grade 3 neurosensory events: Consider discontinuing oxaliplatin

Other toxicities (grade 3/4 gastrointestinal toxicity, grade 4 neutropenia, or grade 3/4 thrombocytopenia): After recovery from toxicity, oxaliplatin dose reductions are recommended:

Adjuvant treatment of stage III colon cancer: Reduce dose to 75 mg/m^2; delay next dose until neutrophils recover to ≥1500/mm^3 and platelets recover to ≥75,000/mm^3

Advanced colorectal cancer: Reduce dose to 65 mg/m^2; delay next dose until neutrophils recover to ≥1500/mm^3 and platelets recover to ≥75,000/mm^3

Administration

I.V. Administer as I.V. infusion over 2-6 hours. Flush infusion line with D_5W prior to administration of any concomitant medication. Patients should receive an antiemetic premedication regimen. Avoid mucositis prophylaxis with ice chips during oxaliplatin infusion (may exacerbate acute neurological symptoms).

Stability

Reconstitution Do not prepare using a chloride-containing solution such as NaCl due to rapid conversion to monochloroplatinum, dichloroplatinum, and diaquoplatinum; all highly reactive in sodium chloride (Takimoto, 2007). Use appropriate precautions for handling and disposal. Do not use needles or administration sets containing aluminum during preparation.

Aqueous solution: Dilution with D_5W (250 or 500 mL) is required prior to administration.

Lyophilized powder [CAN; not available in U.S.]: Use only water for injection or D_5W to reconstitute powder. To obtain final concentration of 5 mg/mL add 10 mL of diluent to 50 mg vial or 20 mL diluent to 100 mg vial. Gently swirl vial to dissolve powder. Dilution with D_5W (250 or 500 mL) is required prior to administration. Discard unused portion of vial.

Storage Store intact vials at room temperature of 25°C (77°F); excursions permitted to 15°C to 30°C (59°F to 86°F); do not freeze. Protect concentrated solution from light (store in original outer carton). According to the manufacturer, solutions diluted for infusion are stable up to 6 hours at room temperature of 20°C to 25°C (68°F to 77°F) or up to 24 hours under refrigeration at 2°C to 8°C (36°F to 46°F). Oxaliplatin solution diluted with D_5W to a final concentration of 0.7 mg/mL (polyolefin container) has been shown to retain >90% of its original concentration for up to 30 days when stored at room temperature or refrigerated; artificial light did not affect the concentration (Andre, 2007). As this study did not examine sterility, refrigeration would be preferred to limit microbial growth. Solutions diluted for infusion do not require protection from light.

Monitoring and Teaching Issues

Laboratory Monitoring CBC with differential, blood chemistries (including serum creatinine, ALT, AST, and bilirubin); INR and prothrombin time (in patients on oral anticoagulant therapy)

Physical Assessment Assess for use-related cautions prior to beginning therapy. Patient must be observed closely for anaphylactic-like reactions (can occur within minutes of administration; appropriate medications for the treatment of hypersensitivity reactions should be available). Monitor for pulmonary or hepatic toxicity, neuropathy (acute or persistent), GI disturbance, anemia, chest pain, and thromboembolism during and between each infusion.

Patient Education This medication can only be administered by infusion; you will be monitored closely during and following infusion. Report immediately any pain, burning, or swelling at infusion site or any signs of allergic reaction (eg, respiratory difficulty, difficulty swallowing, back pain, chest tightness, rash, hives, swelling of lips or mouth). It is important that you maintain adequate nutrition and hydration, unless instructed to restrict fluid intake. You may be more susceptible to infection. You may experience temporary numbness, pain, tingling, or loss of sensation in hands, feet, or throat (cold will exacerbate these effects; remain warm, cover skin before exposure to cold, and avoid cold drinks or the use of ice); if this condition persists or is severe contact prescriber. May cause fatigue, headache, insomnia, nausea, vomiting, loss of appetite, taste perversion, mouth sores, diarrhea, constipation, or loss of hair (reversible). Report chest pain or palpitations; swelling, pain, or hot areas in legs; unusual fatigue; unusual bruising or bleeding; cough, sore throat, or respiratory difficulty; or muscle cramps or twitching.

Breast-Feeding Considerations Due to the potential for serious adverse reactions in the nursing infant, breast-feeding is not recommended.

Pregnancy Considerations Decreased fetal weight, decreased ossification, and increased fetal deaths were observed in animal studies at one-tenth the equivalent human dose. There are no adequate and well-controlled studies in pregnant women. Women of childbearing potential should be advised to avoid pregnancy and use effective contraception during treatment.

Canadian labeling: Use in pregnant women is contraindicated in the Canadian labeling. Males should be advised not to father children during and for up to 6 months following therapy. May cause permanent infertility in males. Prior to initiating therapy, advise males desiring to father children, to seek counseling on sperm storage.

Additional Information Cold temperature may exacerbate acute neuropathy. Do not use ice for mucositis prophylaxis.

Oxaprozin (oks a PROE zin)

U.S. Brand Names Daypro®

Generic Availability (U.S.) Yes

Pharmacologic Category Nonsteroidal Anti-inflammatory Drug (NSAID), Oral

Medication Safety Issues

Sound-alike/look-alike issues:

Daypro® may be confused with Diupres®

Oxaprozin may be confused with oxazepam

Beers Criteria medication: This drug may be inappropriate for use in geriatric patients (high severity risk).

Medication Guide Available Yes

Pregnancy Risk Factor C

Lactation Excretion in breast milk unknown/not recommended

Use Acute and long-term use in the management of signs and symptoms of osteoarthritis and rheumatoid arthritis; juvenile idiopathic arthritis (JIA)

Available Dosage Forms

Caplet, oral:

Daypro®: 600 mg

Tablet, oral: 600 mg

Dosing

Adult & Geriatric

Osteoarthritis: Oral: 600-1200 mg once daily; patients should be titrated to lowest dose possible; patients with low body weight should start with 600 mg daily

Rheumatoid arthritis: Oral: 1200 mg once daily; a one-time loading dose of up to 1800 mg/day or 26 mg/kg (whichever is lower) may be given

Maximum doses:

Patient <50 kg: Maximum: 1200 mg/day

Patient >50 kg with normal renal/hepatic function and low risk of peptic ulcer: Maximum: 1800 mg or 26 mg/kg (whichever is lower) in divided doses

Pediatric

Juvenile idiopathic arthritis (JIA): Oral:

Note: Individualize to lowest effective dose.

Children 6-16 years:

22-31 kg: 600 mg once daily

32-54 kg: 900 mg once daily

≥55 kg: 1200 mg once daily

Renal Impairment In general, NSAIDs are not recommended for use in patients with advanced renal disease but the manufacturer of oxaprozin does provide some guidelines for adjustment in renal dysfunction.

Severe renal impairment or on dialysis: 600 mg once daily; may increase cautiously to 1200 mg/day with close monitoring.

Hepatic Impairment Use caution in patients with severe dysfunction.

Monitoring and Teaching Issues

Laboratory Monitoring CBC; hepatic, renal function

Physical Assessment Evaluate cardiac risk and potential for GI bleeding prior to prescribing this medication. Monitor blood pressure at the beginning of therapy and periodically during use. Schedule ophthalmic evaluations for patients who develop eye complaints during long-term NSAID therapy.

Patient Education Do not crush tablets. Take with food or milk to reduce GI distress. Do not use alcohol. You may experience drowsiness, dizziness, nervousness, anorexia, nausea, vomiting, or heartburn; GI bleeding, ulceration, or perforation can occur with or without pain. Discontinue medication and contact prescriber if persistent abdominal pain, cramping, or blood in stool occurs. Report vaginal bleeding; respiratory difficulty or unusual cough; chest pain, rapid heartbeat, or palpitations; bruising or bleeding (blood in urine, mouth, or vomitus); swollen extremities; skin rash or itching; or swelling of face, lips, tongue, or throat.

Related Information

Nonsalicylate / Nonsteroidal Anti-Inflammatory Agents *on page* 2002

Oxazepam (oks A ze pam)

U.S. Brand Names Serax®

Generic Availability (U.S.) Yes: Capsule

Pharmacologic Category Benzodiazepine

Medication Safety Issues

Sound-alike/look-alike issues:

Oxazepam may be confused with oxaprozin, quazepam

Serax® may be confused with Eurax®, Urex, ZyrTEC®

Beers Criteria medication: This drug may be inappropriate for use in geriatric patients (high severity risk).

International issues:

Murelax [Australia] may be confused with MiraLax brand name for polyethylene glycol 3350 [U.S.]

Use Treatment of anxiety; management of ethanol withdrawal

Unlabeled/Investigational Use Anticonvulsant in management of simple partial seizures; hypnotic

Controlled Substance C-IV

Available Dosage Forms

Capsule, oral: 10 mg, 15 mg, 30 mg
Serax®: 10 mg, 15 mg, 30 mg

Tablet, oral:
Serax®: 15 mg

Dosing

Adult

Anxiety: Oral: 10-30 mg 3-4 times/day
Ethanol withdrawal: Oral: 15-30 mg 3-4 times/day
Hypnotic: Oral: 15-30 mg

Geriatric Oral: Anxiety: 10 mg 2-3 times/day; increase gradually as needed to a total of 30-45 mg/day. Dose titration should be slow to evaluate sensitivity.

Renal Impairment Not dialyzable (0% to 5%)

Administration

Oral Administer orally in divided doses.

Monitoring and Teaching Issues

Physical Assessment Assess for history of addiction; long-term use can result in dependence, abuse, or tolerance; periodically evaluate need for continued use. For inpatient use, institute safety measures to prevent falls. Monitor for oversedation, dizziness, confusion, or ataxia which may impair physical and mental capabilities. Taper dosage slowly when discontinuing.

Patient Education Drug may cause physical and/or psychological dependence. Do not use alcohol. Maintain adequate hydration unless instructed to restrict fluid intake. You may experience drowsiness, lightheadedness, impaired coordination, dizziness, blurred vision, nausea, vomiting, dry mouth, or constipation. Report persistent CNS effects (eg, confusion, depression, suicide ideation, increased sedation, excitation, headache, agitation, insomnia or nightmares, dizziness, fatigue, impaired coordination, changes in personality, or changes in cognition) or worsening of condition.

Related Information

Benzodiazepines *on page 1988*

OXcarbazepine (ox car BAZ e peen)

U.S. Brand Names Trileptal®

Index Terms GP 47680; OCBZ

Generic Availability (U.S.) Yes

Pharmacologic Category Anticonvulsant, Miscellaneous

Medication Safety Issues

Sound-alike/look-alike issues:
OXcarbazepine may be confused with carBAMazepine
Trileptal® may be confused with TriLipix™

Medication Guide Available Yes

Pregnancy Risk Factor C

Lactation Enters breast milk/not recommended

Use Monotherapy or adjunctive therapy in the treatment of partial seizures in adults and children ≥4 years of age with epilepsy; adjunctive therapy in the treatment of partial seizures in children ≥2 years of age with epilepsy

Unlabeled/Investigational Use Bipolar disorder; treatment of neuropathic pain

Mechanism of Action/Effect Precise mechanism of action has not been determined. Believed to prevent the spread of seizures by decreasing propagation of synaptic impulses.

Contraindications Hypersensitivity to oxcarbazepine or any component of the formulation

Warnings/Precautions Antiepileptics are associated with an increased risk of suicidal behavior/thoughts with use (regardless of indication); patients should be monitored for signs/symptoms of depression, suicidal tendencies, and other unusual behavior changes during therapy and instructed to inform their healthcare provider immediately if symptoms occur.

Clinically-significant hyponatremia (sodium <125 mmol/L) can develop during oxcarbazepine use. Rare cases of anaphylaxis and angioedema have been reported, even after initial dosing; permanently discontinue should symptoms occur. Use caution in patients with previous hypersensitivity to carbamazepine (cross-sensitivity occurs in 25% to 30%). Potentially serious, sometimes fatal, dermatologic reactions (eg, Stevens-Johnson, toxic epidermal necrolysis) and multiorgan hypersensitivity reactions have been reported in adults and children; monitor for signs and symptoms of skin reactions and possible disparate manifestations associated with lymphatic, hepatic, renal, and/or hematologic organ systems; discontinuation and conversion to alternate therapy may be required. As with all antiepileptic drugs, oxcarbazepine should be withdrawn gradually to minimize the potential of increased seizure frequency. Use of oxcarbazepine has been associated with CNS-related adverse events, most significant of these were cognitive symptoms including psychomotor slowing, difficulty with concentration, speech or language problems, somnolence or fatigue, and coordination abnormalities, including ataxia and gait disturbances. Effects with other sedative drugs or ethanol may be potentiated. Single-dose studies show that half-life of the primary active metabolite is prolonged 3-4 fold and AUC is doubled in patients with Cl_{cr} <30 mL/minute; dose adjustment required in these patients. May reduce the efficacy of oral contraceptives (nonhormonal contraceptive measures are recommended).

Drug Interactions

Metabolism/Transport Effects Inhibits CYP2C19 (weak); **Induces** CYP3A4 (strong)

Avoid Concomitant Use

Avoid concomitant use of OXcarbazepine with any of the following: Dronedarone; Everolimus; Lurasidone; Nilotinib; Nisoldipine; Pazopanib; Praziquantel; Ranolazine; Roflumilast; RomiDEPsin; Selegiline; Tolvaptan; Vandetanib

Decreased Effect

OXcarbazepine may decrease the levels/effects of: Contraceptives (Estrogens); Contraceptives (Progestins); CYP3A4 Substrates; Dronedarone; Everolimus; Exemestane; Gefitinib; GuanFACINE; Imatinib; Ixabepilone; Lurasidone; Maraviroc; NIFEdipine; Nilotinib; Nisoldipine; Pazopanib; Praziquantel; Ranolazine; Roflumilast; RomiDEPsin; Saxagliptin; SORAfenib; Tadalafil; Tolvaptan; Ulipristal; Vandetanib

The levels/effects of OXcarbazepine may be decreased by: Divalproex; PHENobarbital; Phenytoin; Valproic Acid

Increased Effect/Toxicity

OXcarbazepine may increase the levels/effects of: Phenytoin; Selegiline

The levels/effects of OXcarbazepine may be increased by: Thiazide Diuretics

Nutritional/Ethanol Interactions

Ethanol: Avoid ethanol (may increase CNS depression).

Herb/Nutraceutical: St John's wort may decrease oxcarbazepine levels. Avoid evening primrose (seizure threshold decreased). Avoid valerian, St John's wort, kava kava, gotu kola.

Lab Interactions Thyroid function tests may depress serum T_4 without affecting T_3 levels or TSH.

Adverse Reactions As reported in adults with doses of up to 2400 mg/day (includes patients on monotherapy, adjunctive therapy, and those not previously on AEDs); incidence in children was similar.

>10%:

Central nervous system: Dizziness (22% to 49%), somnolence (20% to 36%), headache (13% to 32%), ataxia (5% to 31%), fatigue (12% to 15%), vertigo (6% to 15%)

Gastrointestinal: Vomiting (7% to 36%), nausea (15% to 29%), abdominal pain (10% to 13%)

Neuromuscular & skeletal: Abnormal gait (5% to 17%), tremor (3% to 16%)

Ocular: Diplopia (14% to 40%), nystagmus (7% to 26%), abnormal vision (4% to 14%)

1% to 10%:

Cardiovascular: Hypotension (1% to 2%), leg edema (1% to 2%)

Central nervous system: Nervousness (2% to 5%), amnesia (4%), abnormal thinking (2% to 4%), insomnia (2% to 4%), speech disorder (1% to 3%), EEG abnormalities (2%), abnormal feelings (1% to 2%), agitation (1% to 2%), confusion (1% to 2%)

Dermatologic: Rash (4%), acne (1% to 2%)

Endocrine & metabolic: Hyponatremia (1% to 3%)

Gastrointestinal: Diarrhea (5% to 7%), dyspepsia (5% to 6%), constipation (2% to 6%), gastritis (1% to 2%), weight gain (1% to 2%)

Neuromuscular & skeletal: Weakness (3% to 6%), back pain (4%), falling down (4%), abnormal coordination (1% to 4%), dysmetria (1% to 3%), sprains/strains (2%), muscle weakness (1% to 2%)

Ocular: Abnormal accommodation (2%)

Respiratory: Upper respiratory tract infection (7%), rhinitis (2% to 5%), chest infection (4%), epistaxis (4%), sinusitis (4%)

Pharmacodynamics/Kinetics

Absorption Complete; food has no affect on rate or extent

Bioavailability Decreased in children <8 years; increased in elderly >60 years

Time to Peak Serum (median): Tablets: 4.5 hours; oral suspension: 6 hours

Protein Binding Serum: MHD: 40%

Half-Life Elimination Parent drug: 2 hours; MHD: 9 hours; renal impairment (Cl_{cr} 30 mL/minute): MHD: 19 hours

Clearance of MHD is increased in younger children (~80% in children 2-4 years of age) and approaches that of adults by ~13 years of age

Metabolism Hepatic to 10-monohydroxy metabolite (MHD; active); MHD is further glucuronidated or oxidized to a 10,11-dihydroxy metabolite (DHD; inactive)

Excretion Urine (95%, <1% as unchanged oxcarbazepine, 27% as unchanged MHD, 49% as MHD glucuronides); feces (<4%)

Available Dosage Forms

Suspension, oral: 300 mg/5 mL (250 mL)

Trileptal®: 300 mg/5 mL (250 mL)

Tablet, oral: 150 mg, 300 mg, 600 mg

Trileptal®: 150 mg, 300 mg, 600 mg

Dosing

Adult & Geriatric

Adjunctive therapy, partial seizures (epilepsy): Oral: Initial: 300 mg twice daily; dosage may be increased by 600 mg/day at approximate weekly intervals. Recommended daily dose is 1200 mg/day in 2 divided doses. Although daily doses >1200 mg/day were somewhat more efficacious, most patients were unable to tolerate 2400 mg/day (due to CNS effects).

Conversion to monotherapy, partial seizures (epilepsy): Oral: Patients receiving concomitant antiepileptic drugs (AEDs): Initial: 300 mg twice daily while simultaneously reducing the dose of concomitant AEDs. Withdraw concomitant AEDs completely over 3-6 weeks, while increasing the oxcarbazine dose in increments of 600 mg/day at weekly intervals, reaching the maximum oxcarbazine dose (2400 mg/day) in about 2-4 weeks (lower doses have been effective in patients in whom monotherapy has been initiated).

Initiation of monotherapy, partial seizures (epilepsy): Oral: Patients not receiving prior AEDs: 300 mg twice daily (total dose 600 mg/day). Increase dose by 300 mg/day every third day to a dose of 1200 mg/day. Higher dosages (2400 mg/day) have been shown to be effective in patients converted to monotherapy from other AEDs.

Pediatric

Adjunctive treatment, partial seizures (epilepsy): Oral: Children 2-3 years:

Initial: 8-10 mg/kg/day (not to exceed 600 mg/day) given in a twice daily regimen.

Maintenance: The target maintenance dose should be achieved over 2 weeks, and depends on weight of the child:

<20 kg: 600 mg/day in 2 divided doses; consider initiating dose at 16-20 mg/kg/day; maximum maintenance dose should be achieved over 2-4 weeks and should not exceed 60 mg/kg/day

Adjunctive treatment, partial seizures (epilepsy): Oral: Children 4-16 years:

Initial: 8-10 mg/kg/day (not to exceed 600 mg/day) given in a twice daily regimen.

Maintenance: The target maintenance dose should be achieved over 2 weeks, and depends on weight of the child:

20-29 kg: 900 mg/day in 2 divided doses
29.1-39 kg: 1200 mg/day in 2 divided doses
>39 kg: 1800 mg/day in 2 divided doses

Conversion to monotherapy: Children 4-16 years: Oxcarbazepine 8-10 mg/kg/day in twice daily divided doses, while simultaneously initiating the reduction of the dose of the concomitant antiepileptic drug; the concomitant drug should be withdrawn over 3-6 weeks. Oxcarbazepine dose may be increased by a maximum of 10 mg/kg/day at weekly intervals. See below for recommended total daily dose by weight.

Initiation of monotherapy: Children 4-16 years: Oxcarbazepine should be initiated at 8-10 mg/kg/day in twice daily divided doses; doses may be titrated by 5 mg/kg/day every third day. See below for recommended total daily dose by weight.

Range of maintenance doses by weight during monotherapy:

20 kg: 600-900 mg/day
25-30 kg: 900-1200 mg/day
35-40 kg: 900-1500 mg/day
45 kg: 1200-1500 mg/day
50-55 kg: 1200-1800 mg/day
60-65 kg: 1200-2100 mg/day
70 kg: 1500-2100 mg/day

Renal Impairment Cl_{cr} <30 mL/minute: Therapy should be initiated at one-half the usual starting dose (300 mg/day in adults) and increased slowly to achieve the desired clinical response

Hepatic Impairment Adjustment not needed for mild-to-moderate impairment. No data in patients with severe impairment.

Administration

Oral Suspension: Prior to using for the first time, firmly insert the plastic adapter provided with the bottle. Cover adapter with child-resistant cap when not in use. Shake bottle for at least 10 seconds, remove child-resistant cap, and insert the oral dosing syringe provided to withdraw appropriate dose. Dose may be taken directly from oral syringe or may be mixed in a small glass of water immediately prior to swallowing. Rinse syringe with warm water after use and allow to dry thoroughly. Discard any unused portion after 7 weeks of first opening bottle.

Stability

Storage Store tablets and suspension at 25°C (77°F). Use suspension within 7 weeks of first opening container.

Monitoring and Teaching Issues

Laboratory Monitoring Serum sodium (particularly during first 3 months of therapy); additional serum sodium monitoring is recommended during maintenance treatment in patients receiving other medications known to decrease sodium levels, in patients with signs/symptoms of hyponatremia, and in patients with an increase in seizure frequency or severity.

Physical Assessment Assess complete allergy history (carbamazepine). Monitor therapeutic effectiveness (seizure activity, frequency, duration, type). Monitor for sedation, CNS changes, visual changes, and skin reactions. Dosage should be tapered when discontinuing to reduce risk of increased seizures. Teach patient safety and seizure precautions.

Patient Education While using the medication, do not use alcohol. Maintain adequate hydration unless instructed to restrict fluid intake. You may experience drowsiness, dizziness, blurred vision, nausea, or vomiting. Report CNS changes, increase in seizure frequency or severity, mentation changes, suicide ideation, depression, changes in cognition or memory, persistent fever, acute fatigue, weakness, insomnia, muscle cramping, weakness, abdominal pain, rash or skin irritations, unusual bruising or bleeding (mouth, urine, stool), or swelling of extremities.

Dietary Considerations May be taken without regard to meals.

Geriatric Considerations Studies in elderly volunteers (60-82 years of age) with both single dose (300 mg) and multiple doses (600 mg/day) reported maximum plasma concentrations and AUC as being 30% to 60% higher than younger volunteers (18-32 years of age). These results were due to differences in creatinine clearance between the two groups. Since elderly may have Cl_{cr} <30 mL/minute, dose reductions may be needed.

Breast-Feeding Considerations Oxcarbazepine and its active metabolite (MHD) are excreted in human breast milk. A milk-to-plasma concentration ratio of 0.5 was found for both. Because of the potential for serious adverse reactions to oxcarbazepine in nursing infants, a decision should be made whether to discontinue nursing or to discontinue the drug in nursing women.

Pregnancy Considerations Oxcarbazepine crosses the human placenta. Teratogenic effects have been observed in animal studies. There are no adequate and well-controlled studies in pregnant women; however, oxcarbazepine is structurally related to carbamazepine (teratogenic in humans); use during pregnancy only if the benefit to the mother outweighs the potential risk to the fetus. Nonhormonal forms of contraception should be used during therapy.

Patients exposed to oxcarbazepine during pregnancy are encouraged to enroll themselves into the AED Pregnancy Registry by calling 1-888-233-2334. Additional information is available at www.aedpregnancyregistry.org.

Related Information

Anticonvulsant Drugs of Choice *on page 1981*

◆ **Oxpentifylline** *see* Pentoxifylline *on page 1441*

◆ **Oxsoralen®** *see* Methoxsalen (Topical) *on page 1200*

Oxybutynin (oks i BYOO ti nin)

U.S. Brand Names Ditropan XL®; Gelnique™; Oxytrol®

Index Terms Ditropan; Oxybutynin Chloride

Generic Availability (U.S.) Yes: Excludes gel, transdermal patch

Pharmacologic Category Antispasmodic Agent, Urinary

Medication Safety Issues

Sound-alike/look-alike issues:

Oxybutynin may be confused with OxyCONTIN®

Ditropan may be confused with Detrol®, diazepam, Diprivan®, dithranol

Beers Criteria medication: This drug may be inappropriate for use in geriatric patients (high severity risk).

Transdermal patch may contain conducting metal (eg, aluminum); remove patch prior to MRI.

Pregnancy Risk Factor B

Lactation Excretion in breast milk unknown/use caution

Use Antispasmodic for neurogenic bladder (urgency, frequency, leakage, urge incontinence, dysuria); extended release formulation also indicated for treatment of symptoms associated with detrusor overactivity due to a neurological condition (eg, spina bifida)

Mechanism of Action/Effect Direct antispasmodic effect on smooth muscle, also inhibits the action of acetylcholine on smooth muscle (exhibits 1/5 the anticholinergic activity of atropine, but is 4-10 times the antispasmodic activity); does not block effects at skeletal muscle or at autonomic ganglia; increases bladder capacity, decreases uninhibited contractions, and delays desire to void, therefore, decreases urgency and frequency

Contraindications Hypersensitivity to oxybutynin or any component of the formulation; patients with or at risk for uncontrolled narrow-angle glaucoma, urinary retention, gastric retention or conditions with severely decreased GI motility

Warnings/Precautions Cases of angioedema have been reported with oral oxybutynin; some cases have occurred after a single dose. Discontinue immediately if develops. Use with caution in patients with bladder outflow obstruction, angle-closure glaucoma (treated), hyperthyroidism, reflux esophagitis (including concurrent therapy with oral bisphosphonates or drugs which may increase the risk of esophagitis), heart disease, hepatic or renal disease, prostatic hyperplasia, autonomic neuropathy, ulcerative colitis (may cause ileus and toxic megacolon), hypertension, hiatal hernia, myasthenia gravis, dementia, ulcerative colitis, or intestinal atony. May increase the risk of heat prostration. May cause anticholinergic effects (agitation, confusion, hallucinations, somnolence) which may require dose reduction or discontinuation of therapy. May cause CNS depression, which may impair physical or mental abilities; patients must be cautioned about performing tasks which require mental alertness (eg, operating machinery or driving).

This class of medication is poorly tolerated by the elderly due to anticholinergic effects, sedation, and weakness. Efficacy is questionable at dosages tolerated by elderly patients. Oxybutynin extended-release is considered an exception. (Beers Criteria).

The extended release formulation consists of drug within a nondeformable matrix; following drug release/absorption, the matrix/shell is expelled in the stool. The use of nondeformable products in patients with known stricture/narrowing of the GI tract has been associated with symptoms of obstruction. Transdermal patch may contain conducting metal (eg, aluminum); remove patch prior to MRI. When using the topical gel, cover treatment area with clothing after gel has dried to minimize transferring medication to others. Discontinue gel if skin irritation occurs. Gel contains ethanol; do not expose to open flame or smoking until gel has dried.

Drug Interactions

Metabolism/Transport Effects Substrate of CYP3A4 (minor); **Inhibits** CYP2C8 (weak), 2D6 (weak), 3A4 (weak)

Avoid Concomitant Use There are no known interactions where it is recommended to avoid concomitant use.

Decreased Effect

Oxybutynin may decrease the levels/effects of: Acetylcholinesterase Inhibitors (Central); Secretin

The levels/effects of Oxybutynin may be decreased by: Acetylcholinesterase Inhibitors (Central)

Increased Effect/Toxicity

Oxybutynin may increase the levels/effects of: AbobotulinumtoxinA; Anticholinergics; Cannabinoids; OnabotulinumtoxinA; Potassium Chloride; RimabotulinumtoxinB

The levels/effects of Oxybutynin may be increased by: Conivaptan; Pramlintide

Nutritional/Ethanol Interactions Ethanol: Use ethanol with caution (may increase CNS depression and toxicity). Watch for sedation.

Lab Interactions May suppress the wheal and flare reactions to skin test antigens.

Adverse Reactions

Oral:

>10%:

Central nervous system: Dizziness (4% to 17%), somnolence (2% to 14%)

Gastrointestinal: Xerostomia (29% to 71%; dose related), constipation (7% to 15%), nausea (2% to 12%)

5% to 10%:

Central nervous system: Headache (6% to 10%), pain (1% to 7%), nervousness (1% to 7%), insomnia (1% to 6%)

Gastrointestinal: Diarrhea (1% to 9%), dyspepsia (5% to 7%)

Genitourinary: Urinary hesitation (9%), urinary tract infection (5% to 7%), urinary retention (6%)

Neuromuscular & skeletal: Weakness (3% to 7%)

Ocular: Blurred vision (1% to 10%), dry eyes (3% to 6%)

Respiratory: Rhinitis (2% to 6%)

Topical gel:

1% to 10%:

Central nervous system: Dizziness (2% to 3%), fatigue (2%), headache (2%)

Dermatologic: Pruritus (1%)

Gastrointestinal: Xerostomia (7% to 8%), gastroenteritis (2%), constipation (1%)

Genitourinary: Urinary tract infection (7%)

Local: Application site reaction (5%; includes anesthesia, dermatitis, erythema, irritation, pain, papules, pruritus)

Respiratory: Nasopharyngitis (3%)

Transdermal:

>10%: Local: Application site reaction (17%), pruritus (14%)

1% to 10%:

Gastrointestinal: Xerostomia (4% to 10%), diarrhea (3%), constipation (3%)

Genitourinary: Dysuria (2%)

Local: Erythema (6% to 8%), vesicles (3%), rash (3%)

Ocular: Vision changes (3%)

Pharmacodynamics/Kinetics

Onset of Action Onset of action: Oral: 30-60 minutes; Peak effect: 3-6 hours

Duration of Action 6-10 hours (up to 24 hours for extended release oral formulation)

Absorption Oral: Rapid and well absorbed; Transdermal: High

Bioavailability Oral: ~6%

Time to Peak Serum: Oral: Immediate release: ~60 minutes; Extended release: 4-6 hours; Transdermal: 24-48 hours

Half-Life Elimination I.V.: ~2 hours (parent drug), 7-8 hours (metabolites); Oral: ~2-3 hours

Metabolism Hepatic via CYP3A4; Oral: High first-pass metabolism; forms active and inactive metabolites

Excretion Urine, as metabolites and unchanged drug (<0.1%)

Available Dosage Forms

Gel, topical:

Gelnique™: 10% (1 g)

Patch, transdermal:

Oxytrol®: 3.9 mg/24 hours (8s)

Syrup, oral: 5 mg/5 mL (5 mL, 473 mL, 480 mL)

Tablet, oral: 5 mg

Tablet, extended release, oral: 5 mg, 10 mg, 15 mg

Ditropan XL®: 5 mg, 10 mg, 15 mg

Dosing

Adult

Bladder spasms:

Oral:

Regular release: 5 mg 2-3 times/day up to maximum of 5 mg 4 times/day

Extended release: Initial: 5-10 mg once daily, adjust dose in 5 mg increments at weekly intervals; maximum: 30 mg daily

Topical gel: Apply contents of 1 sachet (100 mg/g) once daily

Transdermal: Apply one 3.9 mg/day patch twice weekly (every 3-4 days)

Note: Should be discontinued periodically to determine whether the patient can manage without the drug and to minimize resistance to the drug.

Geriatric

Oral: Regular release: Initial dose: 2.5 mg 2-3 times/day; increase as needed to 5 mg 2-3 times/day

Topical gel, transdermal patch: Refer to adult dosing. **Note:** Should be discontinued periodically to determine whether the patient can manage without the drug and to minimize resistance to the drug.

Pediatric

Bladder spasms: Oral: Children:

1-5 years (unlabeled use): 0.2 mg/kg/dose 2-4 times/day

>5 years: 5 mg twice daily, up to 5 mg 3 times/day maximum

>6 years: Extended release: 5 mg once daily; adjust dose in 5 mg increments; maximum dose: 20 mg/day

Administration

Oral Administer without regard to meals. Extended release tablets must be swallowed whole with liquid; do not crush, divide, or chew; take at approximately the same time each day.

Topical Topical gel: For topical use only. Apply to clean, dry, intact skin on abdomen, thighs, or upper arms/shoulders. Rotate site; do not apply to same site on consecutive days. Wash hands after use. Cover treated area with clothing after gel has dried to prevent transfer of medication to others. Do not bathe, shower, or swim until 1 hour after gel applied.

Other Transdermal: Apply to clean, dry skin on abdomen, hip, or buttock. Select a new site for each new system (avoid reapplication to same site within 7 days).

Stability

Storage

Immediate release: Store at controlled room temperature of 15°C to 30°C (59°F to 86°F). Protect syrup from light.

Extended release: Store at 25°C (77°F); excursions permitted to 15°C to 30°C (59°F to 86°F). Protect from moisture and humidity.

Gel sachet, transdermal patch: Store at 25°C (77°F); excursions permitted to 15°C to 30°C (59°F to 86°F). Protect from moisture and humidity. Keel gel away from open flame. Keep patch in sealed pouch. Throw away used sachets or patches where children and pets cannot reach.

Monitoring and Teaching Issues

Physical Assessment Assess voiding pattern, incontinent episodes, frequency, urgency, distention, and urinary retention prior to beginning therapy and periodically throughout.

Patient Education Swallow extended-release tablets whole; do not chew or crush. You may experience dizziness, lightheadedness, drowsiness, dry mouth or changes in appetite, constipation, decreased sexual ability (reversible with discontinuance of drug), or decreased sweating. Use alcohol with caution; may increase drowsiness. Report rapid heartbeat, palpitations, or chest pain; difficulty voiding; or vision changes.

Gel: Apply to dry, intact skin. Rotate application sites. Wash hands immediately after applying. Keep dry for 1 hour after application.

Dietary Considerations Food causes a slight delay in the absorption of the oral solution and bioavailability is increased by ~25%. Absorption of the extended release tablet is not affected by food. May be taken without regard to meals.

Geriatric Considerations Caution should be used in the elderly due to anticholinergic activity (eg, confusion, constipation, blurred vision, and tachycardia). Start with lower doses. Transdermal dosage form may have less potential for these effects. Oxybutynin may cause memory problems in the elderly. A study of 12 healthy volunteers with an average age of 69 showed cognitive decline while taking the drug (*J Am Geriatr Soc*, 1998, L46:8-13). Studies using transdermal dosage form did not reveal any differences in safety or efficacy between elderly and younger adults.

This medication is considered to be potentially inappropriate in this patient population (Beers Criteria severity: High).

Breast-Feeding Considerations Suppression of lactation has been reported.

Pregnancy Considerations Teratogenic effects were not observed in animal studies. There are no adequate and well-controlled studies in pregnant women; use during pregnancy only if clearly needed.

Related Information

Pharmacotherapy of Urinary Incontinence *on page* 2071

◆ **Oxybutynin Chloride** *see* Oxybutynin *on page* 1378

OxyCODONE (oks i KOE done)

U.S. Brand Names OxyCONTIN®; Roxicodone®

Index Terms Dihydrohydroxycodeinone; Oxycodone Hydrochloride

Generic Availability (U.S.) Yes: Excludes liquid, controlled release tablet

Pharmacologic Category Analgesic, Opioid

Medication Safety Issues

Sound-alike/look-alike issues:

OxyCODONE may be confused with HYDROcodone, OxyCONTIN®, oxymorphone

OxyCONTIN® may be confused with MS Contin®, oxybutynin, oxyCODONE

OxyFast® may be confused with Roxanol

Roxicodone® may be confused with Roxanol

High alert medication: The Institute for Safe Medication Practices (ISMP) includes this medication among its list of drug classes which have a heightened risk of causing significant patient harm when used in error.

International issues:

Supeudol® [Canada] may be confused with Supadol Mono which is a brand name for acetaminophen in Luxembourg

Medication Guide Available Yes

Prescribing and Access Restrictions As a requirement of the REMS program, healthcare providers who prescribe OxyContin® need to receive training on the proper use and potential risks of OxyContin®. For training, please refer to http://www.oxycontinrems.com. Prescribers will need retraining every 2 years or following any significant changes to the OxyContin® REMS program.

Pregnancy Risk Factor B

Lactation Enters breast milk/not recommended

Use Management of moderate-to-severe pain, normally used in combination with nonopioid analgesics

OxyContin® is indicated for around-the-clock management of moderate-to-severe pain when an analgesic is needed for an extended period of time.

Mechanism of Action/Effect Binds to opiate receptors in the CNS, causing inhibition of ascending pain pathways, altering the perception of and response to pain; produces generalized CNS depression

Contraindications Hypersensitivity to oxycodone or any component of the formulation; significant respiratory depression; hypercarbia; acute or severe bronchial asthma; paralytic ileus (known or suspected)

Warnings/Precautions May cause CNS depression, which may impair physical or mental abilities; patients must be cautioned about performing tasks which require mental alertness (eg, operating machinery or driving). Effects may be potentiated when used with other sedative drugs or ethanol. Use with caution in patients with hypersensitivity reactions to other phenanthrene derivative opioid agonists (morphine, hydrocodone, hydromorphone, levorphanol, oxymorphone), respiratory diseases including asthma, emphysema, or COPD. Use with caution in pancreatitis or biliary tract disease, acute alcoholism (including delirium tremens), morbid obesity, adrenocortical insufficiency, history of seizure disorders, CNS depression/coma, kyphoscoliosis (or other skeletal disorder which may alter respiratory function), hypothyroidism (including myxedema), prostatic hyperplasia, urethral stricture, and toxic psychosis. May obscure diagnosis or clinical course of patients with acute abdominal conditions.

Use with caution in the elderly, debilitated, and hepatic or renal function. Hemodynamic effects (hypotension, orthostasis) may be exaggerated in patients with hypovolemia, concurrent vasodilating drugs, or in patients with head injury. Respiratory depressant effects and capacity to elevate CSF pressure may be exaggerated in presence of head injury, other intracranial lesion, or pre-existing intracranial pressure.

[U.S. Boxed Warning]: Concomitant use with CYP3A4 inhibitors may result in increased effects and potentially fatal respiratory depression. Concurrent use of agonist/antagonist analgesics may precipitate withdrawal symptoms and/or reduced analgesic efficacy in patients following prolonged therapy with mu opioid agonists. Abrupt discontinuation following prolonged use may also lead to withdrawal symptoms. **[U.S. Boxed Warning]: Healthcare provider should be alert to problems of abuse, misuse, and diversion.** Tolerance or drug dependence may result from extended use. Patients should be assessed for risk of abuse or addition prior to therapy and all patients should be monitored for signs of misuse, abuse, and addiction.

Controlled-release formulations: [U.S. Boxed Warning]: OxyContin® is not intended for use as an "as needed" analgesic or for immediately-postoperative pain management (should be used postoperatively only if the patient has received it prior to surgery or if severe, persistent pain is anticipated). **[U.S. Boxed Warning]: Do NOT crush, break, or chew controlled-release tablets**; 60 mg and 80 mg strengths, a single dose >40 mg, or a total dose of >80 mg/day are for use only in opioid-tolerant patients.

Drug Interactions

Metabolism/Transport Effects Substrate of CYP2D6 (minor), 3A4 (major)

Avoid Concomitant Use There are no known interactions where it is recommended to avoid concomitant use.

Decreased Effect

OxyCODONE may decrease the levels/effects of: Pegvisomant

The levels/effects of OxyCODONE may be decreased by: Ammonium Chloride; CYP3A4 Inducers (Strong); Deferasirox; Mixed Agonist / Antagonist Opioids; Rifampin; St Johns Wort

Increased Effect/Toxicity

OxyCODONE may increase the levels/effects of: Alcohol (Ethyl); Alvimopan; CNS Depressants; Desmopressin; Selective Serotonin Reuptake Inhibitors; Thiazide Diuretics

The levels/effects of OxyCODONE may be increased by: Amphetamines; Antipsychotic Agents (Phenothiazines); Conivaptan; CYP3A4 Inhibitors (Moderate); CYP3A4 Inhibitors (Strong); Dasatinib; Droperidol; Succinylcholine; Voriconazole

Nutritional/Ethanol Interactions

Ethanol: Avoid ethanol (may increase CNS depression).

Herb/Nutraceutical: Avoid valerian, St John's wort, kava kava, gotu kola (may increase CNS depression).

Lab Interactions Some quinolones may produce a false-positive urine screening result for opiates using commercially-available immunoassay kits. This has been demonstrated most consistently for levofloxacin and ofloxacin, but other quinolones have shown cross-reactivity in certain assay kits. Confirmation of positive opiate screens by more specific methods should be considered.

Adverse Reactions Note: Percentages as reported with OxyContin®

>10%:

Central nervous system: Somnolence (23%), dizziness (13%)

Dermatologic: Pruritus (13%)

Gastrointestinal: Constipation (23%), nausea (23%), vomiting (12%)

1% to 10%:

Cardiovascular: Postural hypotension (1% to 5%)

Central nervous system: Headache (7%), abnormal dreams (1% to 5%), anxiety (1% to 5%), chills (1% to 5%), confusion (1% to 5%), dysphoria (1% to 5%), euphoria (1% to 5%), fever (1% to 5%), insomnia (1% to 5%), nervousness (1% to 5%), thought abnormalities (1% to 5%)

Dermatologic: Rash (1% to 5%)

Gastrointestinal: Xerostomia (6%), abdominal pain (1% to 5%), anorexia (1% to 5%), diarrhea (1% to 5%), dyspepsia (1% to 5%), gastritis (1% to 5%)

Neuromuscular & skeletal: Weakness (6%), twitching (1% to 5%)

Respiratory: Dyspnea (1% to 5%), hiccups (1% to 5%)

Miscellaneous: Diaphoresis (5%)

Pharmacodynamics/Kinetics

Onset of Action Pain relief: Immediate release: 10-15 minutes; Peak effect: Immediate release: 0.5-1 hour

Duration of Action Immediate release: 3-6 hours; Controlled release: ≤12 hours

Bioavailability Controlled release, immediate release: 60% to 87%

Time to Peak Plasma: Immediate release: 1.4-1.9 hours; Controlled release: 4-5 hours

Protein Binding ~45%

Half-Life Elimination Immediate release: 2-3 hours; Controlled release: ~5 hours

Metabolism Hepatically via CYP3A4 to noroxycodone (has weak analgesic), noroxymorphone, and alpha- and beta-noroxycodol. CYP2D6 mediated metabolism produces oxymorphone (has analgesic activity; low plasma concentrations), alpha- and beta-oxymorphol.

Excretion Urine (~19% as parent; >64% as metabolites)

Controlled Substance C-II

Available Dosage Forms

Capsule, oral: 5 mg

Solution, oral: 20 mg/mL (30 mL)

Tablet, oral: 5 mg, 15 mg, 30 mg

Roxicodone®: 5 mg, 15 mg, 30 mg

Tablet, controlled release, oral:

OxyCONTIN®: 10 mg, 15 mg, 20 mg, 30 mg, 40 mg, 60 mg, 80 mg

Dosing

Adult & Geriatric Management of pain: Oral:

Regular or immediate release formulations: Initial: 5-15 mg every 4-6 hours as needed; dosing range: 5-20 mg/dose (APS 6th edition). For severe chronic pain, administer on a regularly scheduled basis, every 4-6 hours, at the lowest dose that will achieve adequate analgesia.

Controlled release:

Opioid-naïve: 10 mg every 12 hours

Concurrent CNS depressants: Reduce usual dose by 1/3 to 1/2

Conversion from transdermal fentanyl: For each 25 mcg/hour transdermal dose, substitute 10 mg controlled release oxycodone every 12 hours; should be initiated 18 hours after the removal of the transdermal fentanyl patch

Currently on opioids: Use standard conversion chart to convert daily dose to oxycodone equivalent. Divide daily dose in 2 (for twice-daily dosing, usually every 12 hours) and round down to nearest dosage form.

Dose adjustment: Doses may be adjusted by changing the total daily dose (not by changing the dosing interval). Doses may be adjusted every 1-2 days and may be increased by 25% to 50%. Dose should be gradually tapered when no longer required in order to prevent withdrawal.

Note: 60 mg and 80 mg strengths, a single dose >40 mg, or a total dose of >80 mg/day are for use only in opioid-tolerant patients.

Multiplication factors for converting the daily dose of current oral opioid to the daily dose of oral oxycodone:

Current opioid mg/day dose x factor = Oxycodone mg/day dose

Codeine mg/day oral dose **x** 0.15 = Oxycodone mg/day dose

Hydrocodone mg/day oral dose **x** 0.9 = Oxycodone mg/day dose

Hydromorphone mg/day oral dose **x** 4 = Oxycodone mg/day dose

Levorphanol mg/day oral dose **x** 7.5 = Oxycodone mg/day dose

Meperidine mg/day oral dose **x** 0.1 = Oxycodone mg/day dose

Methadone mg/day oral dose **x** 1.5 = Oxycodone mg/day dose

Morphine mg/day oral dose **x** 0.5 = Oxycodone mg/day dose

Note: Divide the oxycodone mg/day dose into the appropriate dosing interval for the specific form being used.

Pediatric Management of pain (unlabeled use): Immediate release, initial dose: 0.1-0.2 mg/kg/dose (moderate pain) or 0.2 mg/kg/dose (severe pain) (APS 6th edition). For severe chronic pain, administer on a regularly scheduled basis, every 4-6 hours, at the lowest dose that will achieve adequate analgesia.

Renal Impairment Serum concentrations are increased ~50% in patients with Cl_{cr} <60 mL/minute; adjust dose based on clinical situation.

Hepatic Impairment Reduce dosage in patients with liver disease. Decrease the dose of controlled release tablets to 1/3 to 1/2 the usual starting dose; titrate carefully.

Administration

Oral Do not crush, break, or chew controlled release tablets. Controlled release tablets are not indicated for rectal administration; increased risk of adverse events due to better rectal absorption. Controlled release tablets should be administered one at a time and each followed with water immediately after placing in the mouth.

Appropriate laxatives should be administered to avoid the constipating side effects associated with use. Antiemetics may be needed for persistent nausea.

Stability

Storage Store at 25°C (77°F); excursions permitted between 15°C to 30°C (59°F to 86°F). Protect from light.

Monitoring and Teaching Issues

Physical Assessment Monitor for effectiveness of pain relief. Monitor CNS and respiratory status and degree of sedation at beginning of therapy and periodically thereafter. Assess patient's physical and/or psychological dependence. For inpatients, implement safety measures to prevent falls. Discontinue slowly after prolonged use.

Patient Education May cause physical and/or psychological dependence. Do not crush or chew controlled release tablets. While using this medication, do not use alcohol and other prescription or OTC medications (especially sedatives, tranquilizers, antihistamines, or pain medications) without consulting prescriber. Maintain adequate hydration, unless instructed to restrict fluid intake. May cause hypotension, dizziness, drowsiness, impaired coordination, or blurred vision; nausea, vomiting, or dry mouth; or constipation. The wax matrix from controlled release tablets may appear in stool. Report chest pain, slow or rapid heartbeat, dizziness, or persistent headache; confusion or respiratory difficulties; or severe constipation.

Dietary Considerations Instruct patient to avoid high-fat meals when taking some products (food has no effect on the reformulated OxyContin®).

Geriatric Considerations The elderly may be particularly susceptible to the CNS depressant and constipating effects of narcotics. Prophylactic use of a laxative should be considered. Serum levels at a given dose may also be increased relative to concentrations in younger patients.

Breast-Feeding Considerations Sedation and/or respiratory depression may occur in the infant; symptoms of opioid withdrawal may occur following the cessation of breast-feeding.

Pregnancy Considerations Adverse events were not observed in animal reproduction studies. Opioids cross the placenta; respiratory depression and withdrawal symptoms may occur in the neonate following use during pregnancy. Controlled release formulations should not be used immediately prior to or during labor.

Related Information

Opioid Analgesics *on page 2003*

Oxycodone and Acetaminophen (oks i KOE done & a seet a MIN oh fen)

U.S. Brand Names Endocet®; Percocet®; Primlev™; Roxicet™; Roxicet™ 5/500; Tylox®

Index Terms Acetaminophen and Oxycodone

Generic Availability (U.S.) Yes: Excludes caplet and solution

Pharmacologic Category Analgesic, Opioid

Medication Safety Issues

Sound-alike/look-alike issues:

Endocet® may be confused with Indocid®
Percocet® may be confused with Darvocet®, Fioricet®, Percodan®
Roxicet™ may be confused with Roxanol
Tylox® may be confused with Trimox®, Tylenol®, Wymox®, Xanax®

High alert medication: The Institute for Safe Medication Practices (ISMP) includes this medication among its list of drug classes which have a heightened risk of causing significant patient harm when used in error.

Duplicate therapy issues: This product contains acetaminophen, which may be a component of other combination products. Do not exceed the maximum recommended daily dose of acetaminophen.

Pregnancy Risk Factor C

Lactation Enters breast milk/use caution

Use Management of moderate-to-severe pain

Controlled Substance C-II

Available Dosage Forms

Caplet: Oxycodone 5 mg and acetaminophen 500 mg
Roxicet™ 5/500: Oxycodone 5 mg and acetaminophen 500 mg

Capsule: Oxycodone 5 mg and acetaminophen 500 mg
Tylox®: Oxycodone 5 mg and acetaminophen 500 mg

Solution, oral: Oxycodone 5 mg and acetaminophen 325 mg per 5 mL
Roxicet™: Oxycodone 5 mg and acetaminophen 325 mg per 5 mL
Tablet:
Generics:
Oxycodone 2.5 mg and acetaminophen 325 mg
Oxycodone 5 mg and acetaminophen 325 mg
Oxycodone 7.5 mg and acetaminophen 325 mg
Oxycodone 7.5 mg and acetaminophen 500 mg
Oxycodone 10 mg and acetaminophen 325 mg
Oxycodone 10 mg and acetaminophen 650 mg
Brands:
Endocet®:
5/325 [scored]: Oxycodone 5 mg and acetaminophen 325 mg
7.5/325: Oxycodone 7.5 mg and acetaminophen 325 mg
7.5/500: Oxycodone 7.5 mg and acetaminophen 500 mg
10/325: Oxycodone 10 mg and acetaminophen 325 mg
10/650: Oxycodone 10 mg and acetaminophen 650 mg
Percocet®:
2.5/325: Oxycodone 2.5 mg and acetaminophen 325 mg
5/325 [scored]: Oxycodone 5 mg and acetaminophen 325 mg
7.5/325: Oxycodone 7.5 mg and acetaminophen 325 mg
7.5/500: Oxycodone 7.5 mg and acetaminophen 500 mg
10/325: Oxycodone 10 mg and acetaminophen 325 mg
10/650: Oxycodone 10 mg and acetaminophen 650 mg
Primlev™:
5/300: Oxycodone 5 mg and acetaminophen 300 mg
7.5/300: Oxycodone 7.5 mg and acetaminophen 300 mg
10/300: Oxycodone 10 mg and acetaminophen 300 mg
Roxicet™ [scored]: Oxycodone 5 mg and acetaminophen 325 mg

Dosing

Adult

Note: Initial dose is based on the **oxycodone** content; however, the maximum daily dose is based on the **acetaminophen** content.

Management of pain: Doses should be given every 4-6 hours as needed and titrated to appropriate analgesic effects.

Maximum daily dose, based on acetaminophen content: Oral: 4 g/day.
Mild-to-moderate pain: Oral: Initial dose, **based on oxycodone content:** 2.5-5 mg
Severe pain: Oral: Initial dose, **based on oxycodone content:** 10-30 mg

Geriatric Doses should be titrated to appropriate analgesic effects: Oral: Initial dose, **based on oxycodone content:** 2.5-5 mg every 6 hours. Do not exceed 4 g/day of acetaminophen.

Pediatric

Note: Initial dose is based on the **oxycodone** content; however, the maximum daily dose is based on the **acetaminophen** content.

Management of pain: Doses should be given every 4-6 hours as needed and titrated to appropriate analgesic effects.

Mild-to-moderate pain: Oral: Initial dose, **based on oxycodone content:** 0.05-0.1 mg/kg/dose
Severe pain: Oral: Initial dose, **based on oxycodone content:** 0.3 mg/kg/dose

Maximum dose, based on acetaminophen content: Oral: Children <45 kg: 90 mg/kg/day; children >45 kg: 4 g/day

Hepatic Impairment Dose should be reduced in patients with severe liver disease.

Monitoring and Teaching Issues

Physical Assessment See individual agents.

Patient Education See individual agents.

Related Information

Acetaminophen *on page 38*
OxyCODONE *on page 1380*

Oxycodone and Ibuprofen (oks i KOE done & eye byoo PROE fen)

U.S. Brand Names Combunox™ [DSC]

Index Terms Ibuprofen and Oxycodone

Generic Availability (U.S.) Yes

Pharmacologic Category Analgesic, Opioid; Nonsteroidal Anti-inflammatory Drug (NSAID), Oral

Medication Safety Issues

High alert medication: The Institute for Safe Medication Practices (ISMP) includes this medication among its list of drug classes which have a heightened risk of causing significant patient harm when used in error.

Medication Guide Available Yes

Pregnancy Risk Factor C/D ≥30 weeks gestation

Lactation Enters breast milk/not recommended

Use Short-term (≤7 days) management of acute, moderate-to-severe pain

Controlled Substance C-II

Available Dosage Forms

Tablet: Oxycodone 5 mg and ibuprofen 400 mg

Dosing

Adult & Geriatric Pain: Oral: Take 1 tablet as needed (maximum: 4 tablets/24 hours); do not take for longer than 7 days

Administration

Oral Administer without regard to meals.

Monitoring and Teaching Issues

Laboratory Monitoring CBC, chemistry profile, occult blood loss; monitor renal function (urine output, serum BUN and creatinine)

Physical Assessment See individual agents.

Patient Education See individual agents.

◆ **Oxycodone Hydrochloride** *see* OxyCODONE *on page 1380*

◆ **OxyCONTIN®** *see* OxyCODONE *on page 1380*

Oxymorphone (oks i MOR fone)

U.S. Brand Names Opana®; Opana® ER

Index Terms Oxymorphone Hydrochloride

Generic Availability (U.S.) Yes: Tablet

Pharmacologic Category Analgesic, Opioid

Medication Safety Issues

Sound-alike/look-alike issues:

Oxymorphone may be confused with oxycodone, oxymetholone

High alert medication: The Institute for Safe Medication Practices (ISMP) includes this medication among its list of drug classes which have a heightened risk of causing significant patient harm when used in error.

Pregnancy Risk Factor C/D (prolonged use or high doses at term)

Lactation Excretion in breast milk unknown/use caution

Use

Parenteral: Management of moderate-to-severe pain

Oral, regular release: Management of moderate-to-severe pain

Oral, extended release: Management of moderate-to-severe pain in patients requiring around-the-clock opioid treatment for an extended period of time

Mechanism of Action/Effect Oxymorphone hydrochloride is a potent narcotic analgesic with uses similar to those of morphine. The drug is a semisynthetic derivative of morphine (phenanthrene derivative) and is closely related to hydromorphone chemically (Dilaudid®).

Contraindications Hypersensitivity to oxymorphone, other morphine analogs (phenanthrene derivatives), or any component of the formulation; paralytic ileus (known or suspected); increased intracranial pressure; moderate-to-severe hepatic impairment; severe respiratory depression (unless in monitored setting with resuscitative equipment); acute/severe bronchial asthma; hypercarbia; pregnancy (prolonged use or high doses at term).

Note: Injection formulation is also contraindicated in the treatment of upper airway obstruction and pulmonary edema due to a chemical respiratory irritant.

Warnings/Precautions An opioid-containing analgesic regimen should be tailored to each patient's needs and based upon the type of pain being treated (acute versus chronic), the route of administration, degree of tolerance for opioids (naive versus chronic user), age, weight, and medical condition. The optimal analgesic dose varies widely among patients. Doses should be titrated to pain relief/prevention.

May cause CNS depression, which may impair physical or mental abilities; patients must be cautioned about performing tasks which require mental alertness (eg, operating machinery or driving). Effects may be potentiated when used with other sedative drugs or ethanol. Use with caution in patients with hypersensitivity reactions to other phenanthrene-derivative opioid agonists (codeine, hydrocodone, hydromorphone, levorphanol, oxycodone). May cause respiratory depression. Use extreme caution in patients with COPD or other chronic respiratory conditions characterized by hypoxia, hypercapnia, or diminished respiratory reserve (myxedema, cor pulmonale, kyphoscoliosis, obstructive sleep apnea, severe obesity). Use with caution in patients (particularly elderly or debilitated) with impaired respiratory function, adrenal disease, morbid obesity, thyroid dysfunction, prostatic hyperplasia, or renal impairment. Use caution in mild hepatic dysfunction; use is contraindicated in moderate-to-severe hepatic impairment. Use only with extreme caution (if at all) in patients with head injury or increased intracranial pressure (ICP); potential to elevate ICP and/or blunt papillary response may be greatly exaggerated in these patients. Use with caution in biliary tract disease or acute pancreatitis (may cause constriction of sphincter of Oddi). May obscure diagnosis or clinical course of patients with acute abdominal conditions.

Oxymorphone shares the toxic potential of opiate agonists and usual precautions of opiate agonist therapy should be observed; may cause hypotension in patients with acute myocardial infarction, volume depletion, or concurrent drug therapy which may exaggerate vasodilation. The elderly may be particularly susceptible to adverse effects of narcotics.

[U.S. Boxed Warning]: Healthcare provider should be alert to problems of abuse, misuse, and diversion. Tolerance or drug dependence may result from extended use. Use caution in patients with a history of drug dependence or abuse. Abrupt discontinuation may precipitate withdrawal syndrome.

Extended release formulation:

[U.S. Boxed Warnings]: Opana® ER is an extended release oral formulation of oxymorphone and is not suitable for use as an "as needed" analgesic. Tablets should not be broken, chewed, dissolved, or crushed; tablets should be swallowed whole. Opana® ER is intended for use in long-term, continuous management of moderate-to-severe chronic pain. It is not indicated for use in the immediate postoperative period (12-24 hours). **[U.S. Boxed Warning]: The coingestion of ethanol or ethanol-containing medications with Opana® ER may result in accelerated release of drug from the dosage form, abruptly increasing plasma levels, which may have fatal consequences.**

Drug Interactions

Avoid Concomitant Use There are no known interactions where it is recommended to avoid concomitant use.

Decreased Effect

Oxymorphone may decrease the levels/effects of: Pegvisomant

The levels/effects of Oxymorphone may be decreased by: Ammonium Chloride; Mixed Agonist / Antagonist Opioids

Increased Effect/Toxicity

Oxymorphone may increase the levels/effects of: Alcohol (Ethyl); Alvimopan; CNS Depressants; Desmopressin; Selective Serotonin Reuptake Inhibitors; Thiazide Diuretics

The levels/effects of Oxymorphone may be increased by: Amphetamines; Antipsychotic Agents (Phenothiazines); Droperidol; Succinylcholine

Nutritional/Ethanol Interactions

Ethanol: Avoid ethanol (may increase CNS depression). Ethanol ingestion with extended-release tablets is specifically contraindicated due to possible accelerated release and potentially fatal overdose.

Food: When taken orally with a high-fat meal, peak concentration is 38% to 50% greater. Both immediate-release and extended-release tablets should be taken 1 hour before or 2 hours after eating.

Herb/Nutraceutical: Avoid valerian, St John's wort, kava kava, gotu kola (may increase CNS depression).

Lab Interactions Some quinolones may produce a false-positive urine screening result for opiates using commercially-available immunoassay kits. This has been demonstrated most consistently for levofloxacin and ofloxacin, but other quinolones have shown cross-reactivity in certain assay kits. Confirmation of positive opiate screens by more specific methods should be considered. May cause elevation in amylase (due to constriction of the sphincter of Oddi).

Adverse Reactions Frequency not defined.

Cardiovascular: Bradycardia, cardiac shock, flushing, hypotension, orthostatic hypotension, palpitation, peripheral vasodilation, shock, tachycardia

Central nervous system: Agitation, amnesia, anorexia, anxiety, CNS depression, coma, confusion, convulsion, dizziness, drowsiness, dysphoria, euphoria, fatigue, fever, hallucinations, headache, insomnia, intracranial pressure increased, malaise, mental depression, mental impairment, nervousness, restlessness, paradoxical CNS stimulation

Dermatologic: Pruritus, urticaria, rash

Endocrine & metabolic: Antidiuretic hormone release, weight loss

Gastrointestinal: Abdominal pain, appetite depression, biliary tract spasm, constipation, dehydration, dry mouth, dyspepsia, flatulence, nausea, paralytic ileus, stomach cramps, vomiting, xerostomia

Genitourinary: Urination decreased, urinary retention, urinary tract spasm

Local: Pain/reaction at injection site

Neuromuscular & skeletal: Weakness

Ocular: Blurred vision, diplopia, miosis

Renal: Oliguria

Respiratory: Apnea, bronchospasm, cyanosis, dyspnea, hypoventilation, laryngeal edema, laryngeal spasm, respiratory depression

Miscellaneous: Diaphoresis, histamine release, physical and psychological dependence

Pharmacodynamics/Kinetics

Onset of Action Parenteral: 5-10 minutes

Duration of Action Analgesic: Parenteral: 3-6 hours

Bioavailability Oral: 10%

Protein Binding 10% to 12%

Half-Life Elimination Oral: Immediate release: 7-9 hours; Extended release: 9-11 hours

Metabolism Hepatic via glucuronidation to active and inactive metabolites

Excretion Urine (<1% as unchanged drug); feces

Controlled Substance C-II

Available Dosage Forms

Injection, solution:

Opana®: 1 mg/mL (1 mL)

Tablet, oral: 5 mg, 10 mg

Opana®: 5 mg, 10 mg

Tablet, extended release, oral:

Opana® ER: 5 mg, 7.5 mg, 10 mg, 15 mg, 20 mg, 30 mg, 40 mg

Dosing

Adult Analgesia: **Note:** Dosage must be individualized.

I.M., SubQ: Initial: 1-1.5 mg; may repeat every 4-6 hours as needed

Labor analgesia: I.M.: 0.5-1 mg

I.V.: Initial: 0.5 mg

Oral:

Immediate release:

Opioid-naive: 10-20 mg every 4-6 hours as needed. Initial dosages as low as 5 mg may be considered in selected patients and/or patients with renal impairment. Dosage adjustment should be based on level of analgesia, side effects, and pain intensity. Initiation of therapy with initial dose >20 mg is **not** recommended.

Note: The American Pain Society recommends an initial dose of 5-10 mg for adult patients with severe pain.

Currently on stable dose of parenteral oxymorphone: ~10 times the daily parenteral requirement. The calculated amount should be divided and given in 4-6 equal doses.

Currently on other opioids: Use standard conversion chart to convert daily dose to oxymorphone equivalent. Generally start with 1/2 the calculated daily oxymorphone dosage and administered in divided doses every 4-6 hours.

Extended release (Opana® ER):

Opioid-naive: Initial: 5 mg every 12 hours. Supplemental doses of immediate-release oxymorphone may be used as "rescue" medication as dosage is titrated.

Note: Continued requirement for supplemental dosing may be used to titrate the dose of extended-release continuous therapy. Adjust therapy incrementally, by 5-10 mg every 12 hours at intervals of every 3-7 days. Ideally, basal dosage may be titrated to generally mild pain or no pain with the regular use of fewer than 2 supplemental doses per 24 hours.

Currently on stable dose of parenteral oxymorphone: Approximately 10 times the daily parenteral requirement. The calculated amount should be given in 2 divided doses (every 12 hours).

Currently on opioids: Use conversion chart (see **"Note"**) to convert daily dose to oxymorphone equivalent. Generally start with 1/2 the calculated daily oxymorphone dosage. Divide daily dose in 2 (for every 12-hour dosing) and round down to nearest dosage form.

Note: Per manufacturer, the following approximate oral dosages are equivalent to oxymorphone 10 mg:

Hydrocodone 20 mg
Oxycodone 20 mg
Methadone 20 mg
Morphine 30 mg

Conversion of stable dose of immediate-release oxymorphone to extended-release oxymorphone: Administer 1/2 of the daily dose of immediate-release oxymorphone (Opana®) as the extended-release formulation (Opana® ER) every 12 hours

Geriatric Refer to adult dosing. **Note:** Initiate dosing at the lower end of the dosage range.

Renal Impairment Cl_{cr} <50 mL/minute: Reduce initial dosage of oral formulations (bioavailability increased 57% to 65%). Begin therapy at lowest dose and titrate carefully.

Hepatic Impairment Generally, contraindicated for use in patients with moderate-to-severe liver disease. Initiate with lowest possible dose and titrate slowly in mild impairment.

Administration

Oral Administer immediate release and extended release tablets 1 hour before or 2 hours after eating. Opana® ER tablet should be swallowed; do not break, crush, or chew.

Stability

Storage Injection solution, tablet: Store at 15°C to 30°C (59°F to 86°F).

Monitoring and Teaching Issues

Physical Assessment If used to control diarrhea, monitor stools. Monitor for therapeutic effectiveness at beginning of therapy and periodically thereafter. Monitor blood pressure, CNS and respiratory status, and degree of sedation. Assess patient's physical and/or psychological dependence. For inpatients, implement safety measures to prevent falls. Discontinue slowly after prolonged use.

Patient Education May cause physical and/or psychological dependence. Do not break, chew, dissolve, or crush extended release tablets. Swallow whole. While using this medication, do not use alcohol and other prescription or OTC medications (especially sedatives, tranquilizers, antihistamines, or pain medications) without consulting prescriber. Maintain adequate hydration, unless instructed to restrict fluid intake. May cause hypotension, dizziness, drowsiness, impaired coordination, or blurred vision; nausea, vomiting, or dry mouth; or constipation. Report chest pain, slow or rapid heartbeat, dizziness, or persistent headache; confusion or respiratory difficulties; or severe constipation.

Dietary Considerations Immediate release and extended release tablets should be taken 1 hour before or 2 hours after eating.

Geriatric Considerations Elderly may be particularly susceptible to the CNS depressant and constipating effects of narcotics. Plasma levels of oxymorphone were about 40% higher in elderly patients as compared to younger patients.

Pregnancy Considerations Teratogenic effects were not observed in animal studies; however, decreased fetal weight, decreased litter size, increased stillbirths, and increased neonatal death were noted. Chronic opioid use during pregnancy may lead to a withdrawal syndrome in the neonate. Symptoms include irritability, hyperactivity, loss of sleep pattern, abnormal crying, tremor, vomiting, diarrhea, weight loss, or failure to gain weight. Opioid analgesics are considered pregnancy risk factor D if used for prolonged periods or in larger doses near term.

Related Information

Opioid Analgesics *on page 2003*

◆ **Oxymorphone Hydrochloride** *see* Oxymorphone *on page 1385*

Oxytocin (oks i TOE sin)

U.S. Brand Names Pitocin®

Index Terms Pit

Generic Availability (U.S.) Yes

Pharmacologic Category Oxytocic Agent

Medication Safety Issues

High alert medication: The Institute for Safe Medication Practices (ISMP) includes this medication among its list of drugs which have a heightened risk of causing significant patient harm when used in error.

Pregnancy Risk Factor X

Lactation Excretion in breast milk unknown/use caution

Use Induction of labor at term; control of postpartum bleeding; adjunctive therapy in management of abortion

Mechanism of Action/Effect Oxytocin stimulates uterine contraction by activating G-protein-coupled receptors that trigger increases in intracellular calcium levels in uterine myofibrils. Oxytocin also increases local prostaglandin production, further stimulating uterine contraction.

Contraindications Hypersensitivity to oxytocin or any component of the formulation; significant cephalopelvic disproportion; unfavorable fetal positions; fetal distress; hypertonic or hyperactive uterus; contraindicated vaginal delivery (invasive cervical cancer, active genital herpes, prolapse of the cord, cord presentation, total placenta previa, or vasa previa)

Warnings/Precautions Hazardous agent - use appropriate precautions for handling and disposal. **[U.S. Boxed Warning]: To be used for medical rather than elective induction of labor.** May produce antidiuretic effect (ie, water intoxication and excess uterine contractions). High doses or hypersensitivity to oxytocin may cause uterine hypertonicity, spasm, tetanic contraction, or rupture of the uterus. Severe water intoxication with convulsions, coma, and death is associated with a slow oxytocin infusion over 24 hours.

Drug Interactions

Avoid Concomitant Use There are no known interactions where it is recommended to avoid concomitant use.

Decreased Effect There are no known significant interactions involving a decrease in effect.

Increased Effect/Toxicity

The levels/effects of Oxytocin may be increased by: Dinoprostone; Misoprostol

Adverse Reactions Frequency not defined.

Fetus or neonate:

Cardiovascular: Arrhythmias (including premature ventricular contractions), bradycardia

Central nervous system: Brain or CNS damage (permanent), neonatal seizure

Hepatic: Neonatal jaundice

Ocular: Neonatal retinal hemorrhage

Miscellaneous: Fetal death, low Apgar score (5 minute)

Mother:

Cardiovascular: Arrhythmias, hypertensive episodes, premature ventricular contractions

Gastrointestinal: Nausea, vomiting

Genitourinary: Pelvic hematoma, postpartum hemorrhage, uterine hypertonicity, tetanic contraction of the uterus, uterine rupture, uterine spasm

Hematologic: Afibrinogenemia (fatal)

Miscellaneous: Anaphylactic reaction, subarachnoid hemorrhage

Pharmacodynamics/Kinetics

Onset of Action Uterine contractions: I.M.: 3-5 minutes; I.V.: ~1 minute

Duration of Action I.M.: 2-3 hour; I.V.: 1 hour

Half-Life Elimination 1-5 minutes

Metabolism Rapidly hepatic and via plasma (by oxytocinase) and to a smaller degree the mammary gland

Excretion Urine

Available Dosage Forms

Injection, solution: 10 units/mL (1 mL, 10 mL, 30 mL)

Pitocin®: 10 units/mL (1 mL, 10 mL)

Dosing

Adult Note: I.V. administration requires the use of an infusion pump.

Induction of labor: I.V.: 0.5-1 milliunits/minute; gradually increase dose in increments of 1-2 milliunits/minute until desired contraction pattern is established; dose may be decreased after desired frequency of contractions is reached and labor has progressed to 5-6 cm dilation. Infusion rates of 6 milliunits/minute provide oxytocin levels similar to those at spontaneous labor; rates >9-10 milliunits/minute are rarely required.

Postpartum bleeding:

I.M.: Total dose of 10 units after delivery

I.V.: 10-40 units by I.V. infusion in 1000 mL of intravenous fluid at a rate sufficient to control uterine atony

Adjunctive treatment of abortion: I.V.: 10-20 milliunits/minute; maximum total dose: 30 units/12 hours

Administration

I.V. Refer to Reconstitution for dilution information. An infusion pump is required for administration.

Stability

Reconstitution I.V.

Induction or stimulation of labor: Add oxytocin 10 units to NS or LR 1000 mL to yield a solution containing oxytocin 10 milliunits/mL. Rotate solution to mix.

Postpartum uterine bleeding: Add oxytocin 10-40 units to running I.V. infusion; maximum: 40 units/1000 mL.

Adjunctive management of abortion: Add oxytocin 10 units to 500 mL of a physiologic saline solution or D_5W.

Storage Store oxytocin at 2°C to 8°C (36°F to 46°F); do not freeze. Pitocin® may also be stored at 15°C to 25°C (59°F to 77°F) for up to 30 days.

Monitoring and Teaching Issues

Physical Assessment Monitor blood pressure, fluid intake and output, and labor closely if using oxytocin for induction; fetal monitoring is strongly recommended.

Breast-Feeding Considerations Endogenous levels of oxytocin naturally increase during breast-feeding.

Pregnancy Considerations [U.S. Boxed Warning]: To be used for medical rather than elective induction of labor. Reproduction studies have not been conducted. When used as indicated, teratogenic effects would not be expected. Nonteratogenic adverse reactions are reported in the neonate as well as the mother.

◆ **Oxytrol®** *see* Oxybutynin *on page* *1378*

◆ **Ozurdex®** *see* Dexamethasone (Ophthalmic) *on page* *503*

◆ **P-071** *see* Cetirizine *on page* *351*

◆ **Pacerone®** *see* Amiodarone *on page* *98*

Paclitaxel (pac li TAKS el)

Index Terms Taxol

Generic Availability (U.S.) Yes

Pharmacologic Category Antineoplastic Agent, Antimicrotubular; Antineoplastic Agent, Natural Source (Plant) Derivative; Antineoplastic Agent, Taxane Derivative

Medication Safety Issues

Sound-alike/look-alike issues:

PACLitaxel may be confused with DOCEtaxel, PARoxetine, Paxil®

PACLitaxel (conventional) may be confused with PACLitaxel (protein-bound)

Taxol® may be confused with Abraxane®, Paxil®, Taxotere®

High alert medication: This medication is in a class the Institute for Safe Medication Practices (ISMP) includes among its list of drug classes which have a heightened risk of causing significant patient harm when used in error.

Pregnancy Risk Factor D

Lactation Excretion in breast milk unknown/contraindicated

Use Treatment of breast, nonsmall cell lung, and ovarian cancers; treatment of AIDS-related Kaposi's sarcoma (KS)

Unlabeled/Investigational Use Treatment of bladder, cervical, small cell lung, and head and neck cancers; treatment of (unknown primary) adenocarcinoma

Available Dosage Forms

Injection, solution: 6 mg/mL (5 mL, 16.7 mL, 20 mL, 25 mL, 50 mL)

Dosing

Adult & Geriatric Note: Premedication with dexamethasone (20 mg orally or I.V. at 12 and 6 hours **or** 14 and 7 hours before the dose; reduce dexamethasone dose to 10 mg orally with advanced HIV disease), diphenhydramine (50 mg I.V. 30-60 minutes prior to the dose), and cimetidine, famotidine, or ranitidine (I.V. 30-60 minutes prior to the dose) is recommended.

Ovarian carcinoma:

I.V.: 135-175 mg/m^2 over 3 hours every 3 weeks **or**
135 mg/m^2 over 24 hours every 3 weeks **or**
50-80 mg/m^2 over 1-3 hours weekly **or**
1.4-4 mg/m^2/day continuous infusion for 14 days every 4 weeks

Intraperitoneal (unlabeled route): 60 mg/m^2 on day 8 of a 21-day treatment cycle for 6 cycles, in combination with I.V. paclitaxel and intraperitoneal cisplatin. **Note:** Administration of intraperitoneal paclitaxel should include the standard paclitaxel premedication regimen.

Metastatic breast cancer: I.V.: 175-250 mg/m^2 over 3 hours every 3 weeks **or**
50-80 mg/m^2 weekly **or**
1.4-4 mg/m^2/day continuous infusion for 14 days every 4 weeks

Nonsmall cell lung carcinoma: I.V.: 135 mg/m^2 over 24 hours every 3 weeks

AIDS-related Kaposi's sarcoma: I.V.: 135 mg/m^2 over 3 hours every 3 weeks **or** 100 mg/m^2 over 3 hours every 2 weeks

Renal Impairment There are no FDA-approved labeling guidelines for dosage adjustment in patients with renal impairment. Aronoff (2007) recommends no dosage adjustment necessary for adults with Cl_{cr} <50 mL/minute.

Hepatic Impairment Note: The FDA-approved labeling recommendations are based upon the patient's first course of therapy where the usual dose would be 135 mg/m^2 dose over 24 hours or the 175 mg/m^2 dose over 3 hours in patients with normal hepatic function. Dosage in subsequent courses should be based upon individual tolerance. Adjustments for other regimens are not available.

24-hour infusion:

Transaminases <2 times upper limit of normal (ULN) and bilirubin level ≤1.5 mg/dL: 135 mg/m^2

Transaminases 2-<10 times ULN and bilirubin level ≤1.5 mg/dL: 100 mg/m^2

Transaminases <10 times ULN and bilirubin level 1.6-7.5 mg/dL: 50 mg/m^2

Transaminases ≥10 times ULN or bilirubin level >7.5 mg/dL: Avoid use

3-hour infusion:

Transaminases <10 times ULN and bilirubin level ≤1.25 times ULN: 175 mg/m^2

Transaminases <10 times ULN and bilirubin level 1.26-2 times ULN: 135 mg/m^2

Transaminases <10 times ULN and bilirubin level 2.01-5 times ULN: 90 mg/m^2

Transaminases ≥10 times ULN or bilirubin level >5 times ULN: Avoid use

Adjustment for Toxicity

Dosage modification for toxicity (solid tumors, including ovary, breast, and lung carcinoma): Courses of paclitaxel should not be repeated until the neutrophil count is ≥1500 cells/mm^3 and the platelet count is ≥100,000 cells/mm^3; reduce dosage by 20% for patients experiencing severe peripheral neuropathy or severe neutropenia (neutrophil <500 cells/mm^3 for a week or longer)

Dosage modification for immunosuppression in advanced HIV disease: Paclitaxel should not be given to patients with HIV if the baseline or subsequent neutrophil count is <1000 cells/mm^3. Additional modifications include: Reduce dosage of dexamethasone in premedication to 10 mg orally; reduce dosage by 20% in patients experiencing severe peripheral neuropathy or severe neutropenia (neutrophil <500 cells/mm^3 for a week or longer); initiate concurrent hematopoietic growth factor (G-CSF) as clinically indicated

Administration

I.V. Infuse over 1-96 hours. When administered as sequential infusions, taxane derivatives should be administered before platinum derivatives (cisplatin, carboplatin) to limit myelosuppression and to enhance efficacy.

Premedication with dexamethasone (20 mg orally or I.V. at 12 and 6 hours **or** 14 and 7 hours before the dose; reduce to 10 mg with advanced HIV disease), diphenhydramine (50 mg I.V. 30-60 minutes prior to the dose), and cimetidine 300 mg, famotidine 20 mg, or ranitidine 50 mg (I.V. 30-60 minutes prior to the dose) is recommended.

Administer I.V. infusion over 1-24 hours; infuse through a 0.22 micron in-line filter and nonsorbing administration set.

Other Intraperitoneal: 1- to 2-hour infusion

Monitoring and Teaching Issues

Laboratory Monitoring CBC with differential and platelet count, liver and kidney function

Physical Assessment Paclitaxel (protein bound) is not interchangeable with paclitaxel (conventional). Assess patient carefully for cautious use indications and contraindications. Infusion site must be monitored closely to avoid extravasation. Monitor for hypersensitivity reaction, cardiovascular abnormalities, sensory neuropathy, myelosuppression, and GI irritation prior to, during, and between each infusion.

Patient Education This drug is only administered by intravenous infusion; you will be monitored closely during and following infusions. Immediately report burning, pain, or swelling at infusion site; unusual chest pain or tightness, rapid heartbeat, or palpitations; difficulty breathing; difficulty swallowing; or nausea or vomiting during infusion. You will be more susceptible to infection. It is important that you maintain adequate nutrition and fluid intake unless instructed to restrict fluid intake. May cause nausea, vomiting, sore mouth, loss of hair (will grow back after therapy), or diarrhea (if persistent, consult prescriber). Report chest pain, palpitations, or swelling of extremities; difficult breathing; pain or decreased sensation in extremities; unusual signs of weakness, fatigue, or lethargy; or persistent gastrointestinal disturbances.

◆ **Paclitaxel, Albumin-Bound** *see* Paclitaxel (Protein Bound) *on page 1390*

Paclitaxel (Protein Bound) (pac li TAKS el PROE teen bownd)

U.S. Brand Names Abraxane®

Index Terms ABI-007; Albumin-Bound Paclitaxel; Albumin-Stabilized Nanoparticle Paclitaxel; nab-Paclitaxel; Nanoparticle Albumin-Bound Paclitaxel; Paclitaxel, Albumin-Bound; Protein-Bound Paclitaxel

Generic Availability (U.S.) No

Pharmacologic Category Antineoplastic Agent, Antimicrotubular; Antineoplastic Agent, Natural Source (Plant) Derivative; Antineoplastic Agent, Taxane Derivative

Medication Safety Issues

Sound-alike/look-alike issues:

PACLitaxel may be confused with DOCEtaxel

PACLitaxel (protein bound) may be confused with PACLitaxel (conventional)

Abraxane® may be confused with Paxil®, Taxol®, Taxotere®

High alert medication: This medication is in a class the Institute for Safe Medication Practices (ISMP) includes among its list of drug classes which have a heightened risk of causing significant patient harm when used in error.

Pregnancy Risk Factor D

Lactation Excretion in breast milk unknown/not recommended

Use Treatment of refractory (metastatic) or relapsed (within 6 months of adjuvant therapy) breast cancer

Unlabeled/Investigational Use Treatment of advanced nonsmall cell lung cancer (NSCLC)

Available Dosage Forms

Injection, powder for reconstitution:

Abraxane®: 100 mg

Dosing

Adult & Geriatric

Breast cancer: I.V.: 260 mg/m^2 every 3 weeks

Breast cancer (weekly treatment; unlabeled schedule): I.V.: 100-150 mg/m^2 on days 1, 8, and 15 of a 28-day cycle (Gradishar, 2009)

NSCLC (unlabeled use): I.V.: 260 mg/m^2 every 3 weeks (Green, 2006) **or** 125 mg/m^2 on days 1, 8, and 15 of a 28-day cycle (Rizvi, 2008)

Renal Impairment Has not been studied; patients with serum creatinine >2 mg/dL were excluded from clinical trials.

Hepatic Impairment Every-3-week breast cancer regimen:

Mild impairment (AST <10 times ULN and bilirubin ≤1.25 times ULN): No adjustment required.

Moderate impairment (AST <10 times ULN and bilirubin 1.26-2 times ULN): Reduce dose to 200 mg/m^2.

Severe impairment:

AST <10 times ULN and bilirubin 2.01-5 times ULN: Reduce dose to 130 mg/m^2; may increase up to 200 mg/m^2 in subsequent cycles (based on individual tolerance).

AST >10 times ULN or bilirubin >5 times ULN: Use is not recommended.

Adjustment for Toxicity

Severe neutropenia (<500 cells/mm^3) ≥1 week: Reduce dose to 220 mg/m^2 for subsequent courses

Recurrent severe neutropenia: Reduce dose to 180 mg/m^2

Sensory neuropathy

Grade 1 or 2: Dosage adjustment generally not required

Grade 3: Hold treatment until resolved to grade 1 or 2, then resume with reduced dose for all subsequent cycles

Severe sensory neuropathy: Reduce dose to 220 mg/m^2 for subsequent courses

Recurrent severe sensory neuropathy: Reduce dose to 180 mg/m^2

Administration

I.V. Administer over 30 minutes. Do not use an in-line filter. Monitor infusion site; avoid extravasation. When given on a weekly (unlabeled) schedule, infusions were administered over ~30 minutes (Gradishar, 2009; Rizvi, 2008).

Monitoring and Teaching Issues

Laboratory Monitoring CBC, BP (during infusion); hepatic function

Physical Assessment Paclitaxel (protein bound) is not interchangeable with paclitaxel. Taxane derivatives should be administered before platinum derivatives to limit myelosuppression. Monitor for cardiovascular abnormalities, sensory neuropathy (numbness, tingling, burning pain), myelosuppression (anemia, opportunistic infection), and GI irritation (nausea, vomiting, mucositis, stomatitis) prior to, during, and between each infusion.

Patient Education This drug can only be administered by intravenous infusion; you will be monitored closely during and following infusions. Immediately report any burning, pain, or swelling at infusion site; any unusual chest pain or tightness, rapid heartbeat or palpitations; difficulty breathing; difficulty swallowing; or nausea or vomiting. You will be more susceptible to infection. It is important that you maintain adequate nutrition and fluid intake unless instructed to restrict fluid intake. May cause nausea, vomiting, mouth sores, diarrhea, or loss of hair (will grow back after therapy). Report chest pain, palpitations, swelling of extremities; difficult breathing; pain or decreased sensation in extremities; unusual sign of weakness, fatigue, lethargy, or persistent gastrointestinal disturbances (nausea, vomiting, diarrhea).

◆ **Pain Eze [OTC]** *see* Acetaminophen *on page 38*

◆ **Pain & Fever Children's [OTC]** *see* Acetaminophen *on page 38*

Paliperidone (pal ee PER i done)

U.S. Brand Names Invega®; Invega® Sustenna®

Index Terms 9-hydroxy-risperidone; 9-OH-risperidone; Paliperidone Palmitate

Generic Availability (U.S.) No

Pharmacologic Category Antipsychotic Agent, Atypical

Pregnancy Risk Factor C

Lactation Enters breast milk/not recommended

Use

Oral: Acute and maintenance treatment of schizophrenia; acute treatment of schizoaffective disorder (monotherapy or adjunctive therapy to mood stabilizers and/or antidepressants)

Injection: Acute and maintenance treatment of schizophrenia

Unlabeled/Investigational Use Psychosis/agitation related to Alzheimer's dementia

Mechanism of Action/Effect Paliperidone is the primary active metabolite of risperidone. Mixed central serotonergic and dopaminergic antagonism is thought to improve negative symptoms of psychoses and reduce the incidence of extrapyramidal side effects.

Contraindications Hypersensitivity to paliperidone, risperidone, or any component of the formulation

Warnings/Precautions [U.S. Boxed Warning]: Elderly patients with dementia-related psychosis treated with antipsychotics are at an increased risk of death compared to placebo. Most deaths appeared to be either cardiovascular (eg, heart failure, sudden death) or infectious (eg, pneumonia) in nature. In addition, an increased incidence of cerebrovascular adverse effects (eg, transient ischemic attack, cerebrovascular accidents) has been reported in studies of placebo-controlled trials of risperidone (paliperidone is the primary active metabolite of risperidone) in elderly patients with dementia-related psychosis. Paliperidone is not approved for the treatment of dementia-related psychosis.

Compared with risperidone, paliperidone is low to moderately sedating; use with caution in disorders where CNS depression is a feature. Use caution in patients with predisposition to seizures. Use with caution in renal dysfunction; dose reduction recommended. Esophageal dysmotility and aspiration have been associated with antipsychotic use; use with caution in patients at risk of aspiration pneumonia (eg, Alzheimer's disease).

Leukopenia, neutropenia, and agranulocytosis (sometimes fatal) have been reported in clinical trials and postmarketing reports with antipsychotic use; presence of risk factors (eg, pre-existing low WBC or history of drug-induced leuko-/neutropenia) should prompt periodic blood count assessment. Discontinue therapy at first signs of blood dyscrasias or if absolute neutrophil count <1000/mm^3.

Paliperidone is associated with increased prolactin levels; clinical significance of hyperprolactinemia in patients with breast cancer or other prolactin-dependent tumors is unknown. May alter temperature regulation. May mask toxicity of other drugs or conditions (eg intestinal obstruction, Reyes syndrome, brain tumor) due to antiemetic effects. Priapism has been reported rarely with use.

May cause orthostasis and syncope. Use with caution in patients with cardiovascular diseases (eg, heart failure, history of myocardial infarction or ischemia, cerebrovascular disease, conduction abnormalities). Use caution in patients receiving medications for hypertension (orthostatic effects may be exacerbated) or in patients with hypovolemia or dehydration. May alter cardiac conduction; life-threatening arrhythmias have occurred with therapeutic doses of neuroleptics. Avoid use in combination with QT_c-prolonging drugs. Avoid use in patients with congenital long QT syndrome and in patients with history of cardiac arrhythmia.

May cause extrapyramidal symptoms (EPS), including pseudoparkinsonism, acute dystonic reactions, akathisia, and tardive dyskinesia (risk of these reactions is low relative to other neuroleptics, and is dose dependent). Risk of dystonia (and probably other EPS) may be greater with increased doses, use of conventional antipsychotics, males, and younger patients. Risk of neuroleptic malignant syndrome (NMS) may be increased in patients with Parkinson's disease or Lewy body dementia; monitor for symptoms of confusion, obtundation, postural instability and extrapyramidal symptoms. May cause hyperglycemia; in some cases may be extreme and associated with ketoacidosis, hyperosmolar coma, or death. Use with caution in patients with diabetes (or risk factors) or other disorders of glucose regulation; monitor for worsening of glucose control. Significant weight gain has been observed with antipsychotic therapy; incidence varies with product. Monitor waist circumference and BMI. May cause lipid abnormalities (LDL and triglycerides increased; HDL decreased).

The possibility of a suicide attempt is inherent in psychotic illness or bipolar disorder; use caution in high-risk patients during initiation of therapy. Prescriptions should be written for the smallest quantity consistent with good patient care.

The tablet formulation consists of drug within a nonabsorbable shell that is expelled and may be visible in the stool. Use is not recommended in patients with pre-existing severe gastrointestinal narrowing disorders. Patients with upper GI tract alterations in transit time may have increased or decreased bioavailability of paliperidone. Do not use in patients unable to swallow the tablet whole.

Drug Interactions

Metabolism/Transport Effects Substrate of P-glycoprotein

Avoid Concomitant Use

Avoid concomitant use of Paliperidone with any of the following: Metoclopramide

Decreased Effect

Paliperidone may decrease the levels/effects of: Amphetamines; Anti-Parkinson's Agents (Dopamine Agonist); Quinagolide

The levels/effects of Paliperidone may be decreased by: CarBAMazepine; Lithium formulations; P-Glycoprotein Inducers

Increased Effect/Toxicity

Paliperidone may increase the levels/effects of: Alcohol (Ethyl); CNS Depressants; Methotrimeprazine; Methylphenidate

The levels/effects of Paliperidone may be increased by: Acetylcholinesterase Inhibitors (Central); Divalproex; Droperidol; Itraconazole; Lithium formulations; Methotrimeprazine; Methylphenidate; Metoclopramide; P-Glycoprotein Inhibitors; RisperiDONE; Tetrabenazine; Valproic Acid

Nutritional/Ethanol Interactions

Ethanol: Avoid ethanol (may increase CNS depression).

Herb/Nutraceutical: Avoid kava kava, gotu kola, valerian, St John's wort (may increase CNS depression).

Adverse Reactions Unless otherwise noted, frequency of adverse effects is reported for the oral/I.M. formulation in adults.

>10%:

Cardiovascular: Tachycardia (1% to 14%)

Central nervous system: EPS (≤26%; dose dependent), insomnia (10% to 15%), headache (6% to 15%), parkinsonism (3% to 14%; dose dependent), somnolence (adolescents 9% to 26%; adults 1% to 12%; dose dependent)

Neuromuscular & skeletal: Tremor (2% to 12%)

3% to 10%:

Cardiovascular: Orthostatic hypotension (1% to 4%; dose dependent), bundle branch block (≤3%)

Central nervous system: Agitation (4% to 10%), akathisia (adolescents 4% to 17%; adults 1% to 10%; dose dependent), anxiety (adolescents ≤9%; adults 3% to 8%), dizziness (1% to 6%), dystonia (1% to 5%; dose dependent), dysarthria (1% to 4%; dose dependent), fatigue (adolescents ≤4%), sleep disorder (≤3%), lethargy (adolescents ≤3%)

Endocrine & metabolic: Amenorrhea (adolescents ≤6%), galactorrhea (adolescents ≤4%), gynecomastia (adolescents ≤3%)

Gastrointestinal: Weight gain (1% to 9%; dose dependent), nausea (2% to 8%), dyspepsia (5% to 6%), vomiting (adolescents ≤11%; adults 2% to 5%), constipation (1% to 5%), salivation increased (adolescents ≤6%; adults ≤4%; dose dependent), appetite increased (2% to 3%), toothache (1% to 3%), abdominal pain (≤3%), diarrhea (≤3%), xerostomia (≤3%); tongue swelling (adolescents ≤3%), tongue paralysis (adolescents ≤3%)

Local: I.M. formulation: Injection site reaction (≤10%)

Neuromuscular & skeletal: Hyperkinesia (2% to 10% dose dependent), dyskinesia (1% to 9%), weakness (≤4%), myalgia (≤4% dose dependent), back pain (1% to 3%), extremity pain (≤3%)

Ocular: Blurred vision (adolescents ≤3%)

Respiratory: Nasopharyngitis (≤5%; dose dependent), upper respiratory tract infection (1% to 4%), cough (≤3%; dose dependent), rhinitis (1% to 3%; dose dependent)

Pharmacodynamics/Kinetics

Absorption I.M.: Slow release (begins on day 1 and continues up to 126 days)

Bioavailability 28%

Time to Peak Oral: ~24 hours; I.M.: 13 days

Protein Binding 74%

Half-Life Elimination

Oral: 23 hours; 24-51 hours with renal impairment (Cl_{cr} <80 mL/minute)

I.M. (following a single-dose administration): Range: 25-49 days

Metabolism Hepatic via CYP2D6 and 3A4 (limited role in elimination); minor metabolism (<10% each) via dealkylation, hydroxylation, dehydrogenation, and benzisoxazole scission

Excretion Urine (80%); feces (11%)

Available Dosage Forms

Injection, suspension, extended release:

Invega® Sustenna®: 39 mg/0.25 mL (0.25 mL); 78 mg/0.5 mL (0.5 mL); 117 mg/0.75 mL (0.75 mL); 156 mg/mL (1 mL); 234 mg/1.5 mL (1.5 mL)

Tablet, extended release, oral:

Invega®: 1.5 mg, 3 mg, 6 mg, 9 mg

Dosing

Adult

U.S. labeling:

Schizoaffective disorder, schizophrenia: Oral: Usual: 6 mg once daily in the morning; titration not required, though some may benefit from higher or lower doses. If exceeding 6 mg/day, increases of 3 mg/day are recommended no more frequently than every 4 days in schizoaffective disorder or every 5 days in schizophrenia, up to a maximum of 12 mg/day. Some patients may require only 3 mg/day.

Schizophrenia: I.M.: **Note:** Prior to initiation of I.M therapy, tolerability should be established with oral paliperidone or oral risperidone. Previous oral antipsychotics can be discontinued at the time of initiation of I.M. therapy. Dosing based on paliperidone palmitate.

Initiation of therapy:

Initial: 234 mg on treatment day 1 followed by 156 mg one week later. The second dose may be administered 2 days before or after the weekly timepoint.

Maintenance: Following the 1-week initiation regimen, begin a maintenance dose of 117 mg every month. Some patients may benefit from higher or lower monthly maintenance doses (monthly maintenance dosage range: 39-234 mg). The monthly maintenance dose may be administered 7 days before or after the monthly timepoint.

Conversion from oral paliperidone to I.M paliperidone: Initiate I.M. therapy as described using the one-week initiation regimen. Patients previously stabilized on oral doses can expect similar steady state exposure during maintenance treatment with I.M. therapy using the following conversion:

Oral extended release dose of 12 mg, then I.M. maintenance dose of 234 mg

Oral extended release dose of 6 mg, then I.M. maintenance dose of 117 mg

Oral extended release dose of 3 mg, then I.M. maintenance dose of 39-78 mg

Switching from other long-acting injectable antipsychotics to I.M. paliperidone: Initiate I.M. paliperidone in the place of the next scheduled injection and continue at monthly intervals. The one-week initiation regimen is not required in these patients.

Dosage adjustments: Adjustments may be made monthly (full effect from adjustments may not be seen for several months)

Missed doses:

If <6 weeks has elapsed since the last monthly injection: Administer the missed dose as soon as possible and continue therapy at monthly intervals.

If >6 weeks and ≤6 months has elapsed since the last monthly injection: Therapy may be resumed at same dose the patient was previously stabilized on, if the maintenance dose was <234 mg. If the dose was 234 mg, then administer a 156 mg dose as soon as possible, followed by a second dose of 156 mg one week later, then resume monthly maintenance dosing.

If >6 months has elapsed since last monthly maintenance injection: Therapy must be reinitiated following dosing recommendations for initiation of therapy.

Canadian labeling:

Schizophrenia: Oral: Usual: 6 mg once daily in the morning; titration not required, though some may benefit from higher or lower doses. If exceeding 6 mg/day, increases of 3 mg/day are recommended no more frequently than every 5 days in schizophrenia, up to a maximum of 12 mg/day. Some patients may require only 3 mg/day.

Schizophrenia: I.M.: **Note:** Prior to initiation of I.M therapy, tolerability should be established with oral paliperidone or oral risperidone. Previous oral antipsychotics can be discontinued at the time of initiation of I.M. therapy. Dosing based on paliperidone.

Initiation of therapy:

Initial: 150 mg on treatment day 1 followed by 100 mg one week later (day 8). The second dose may be administered 2 days before or after the weekly timepoint.

Maintenance: Following the 1-week initiation regimen, begin a maintenance dose of 75 mg every month. Some patients may benefit from higher or lower monthly maintenance doses (monthly maintenance dosage range: 25-150 mg). The monthly maintenance dose may be administered 7 days before or after the monthly timepoint.

Conversion from oral paliperidone to I.M paliperidone: Initiate I.M. therapy as described using the one-week initiation regimen. Patients previously stabilized on oral doses can expect similar steady state exposure during maintenance treatment with I.M. therapy using the following conversion:

Oral extended release dose of 12 mg, then I.M. maintenance dose of 150 mg

Oral extended release dose of 6 mg, then I.M. maintenance dose of 75 mg

Oral extended release dose of 3 mg, then I.M. maintenance dose of 25-50 mg

Switching from injectable risperidone (Risperdal® Consta®) to I.M. paliperidone:

Risperdal® Consta® dose of 25 mg every 2 weeks, then I.M. paliperidone maintenance dose of 50 mg

Risperdal® Consta® dose of 37.5 mg every 2 weeks, then I.M. paliperidone maintenance dose of 75 mg

Risperdal® Consta® dose of 50 mg every 2 weeks, then I.M. paliperidone maintenance dose of 100 mg

Switching from other long-acting injectable antipsychotics to I.M. paliperidone: Initiate I.M. paliperidone in the place of the next scheduled injection and continue at monthly intervals. The one-week initiation regimen is not required in these patients.

Dosage adjustments: Adjustments may be made monthly (full effect from adjustments may not be seen for several months)

Missed doses:

If <6 weeks has elapsed since the last monthly injection: Administer the missed dose as soon as possible and continue therapy at monthly intervals.

If >6 weeks and ≤6 months has elapsed since the last monthly injection: Therapy may be resumed at same dose (25-100 mg) the patient was previously stabilized on and then repeated one week later (day 8). Resume usual monthly maintenance dosing cycle thereafter. If the dose was 150 mg, administer a 100 mg dose as soon as possible and repeat one week later (day 8), then resume usual monthly maintenance dosing cycle 25-150 mg.

If >6 months has elapsed since last monthly maintenance injection: Therapy must be reinitiated following dosing recommendations for initiation of therapy.

Geriatric Refer to adult dosing. Additional monitoring of renal function and orthostatic blood pressure may be warranted.

Pediatric Schizophrenia: *U.S. labeling:* Adolescents 12-17 years: Oral: Initial: 3 mg once daily; titration not required (no known benefit from higher doses). If exceeding 3 mg/day, increases of 3 mg/day are recommended no more frequently than every 5 days.

Renal Impairment Clearance is decreased in renal impairment; adjust dose according to renal function:

Oral:

Mild impairment (Cl_{cr} 50-79 mL/minute): Initial dose: 3 mg once daily; maximum dose: 6 mg once daily

Moderate-to-severe impairment (Cl_{cr} 10-49 mL/minute): Initial dose: 1.5 mg once daily; maximum dose: 3 mg once daily

Severe impairment (Cl_{cr} <10 mL/minute): Use not recommended; not studied in this population

I.M., U.S. labeling:

Mild impairment (Cl_{cr} 50-79 mL/minute): Initiation of therapy: 156 mg on treatment day 1, followed by 117 mg one week later, followed by a maintenance dose of 78 mg every month

Moderate-to-severe impairment (Cl_{cr} <50 mL/minute): Use not recommended

I.M., Canadian labeling:

Mild impairment (Cl_{cr} 50-79 mL/minute): Initiation of therapy: 100 mg on treatment day 1, followed by 75 mg one week later followed by a maintenance dose of 50 mg every month

Moderate-to-severe impairment (Cl_{cr} <50 mL/minute): Use not recommended

Hepatic Impairment Oral, I.M.: No adjustment necessary for mild-to-moderate (Child-Pugh class A and B) impairment. Not studied in severe impairment.

Administration

Oral Administer in the morning without regard to meals. Extended release tablets should be swallowed whole with liquids; do not crush, chew, or divide.

I.M. Invega® Sustenna™ should be administered by I.M. route only as a single injection (do not divide); do not administer I.V. or subcutaneously. Avoid inadvertent injection into vasculature. Prior to injection, shake syringe for at least 10 seconds to ensure a homogenous suspension. The 2 initial injections should be administered in the deltoid muscle using a 1½ inch, 22-gauge needle for patients ≥90 kg, and a 1 inch, 23-gauge needle for patients <90 kg. The 2 initial deltoid intramuscular injections help attain therapeutic concentrations rapidly. Alternate deltoid injections (right and left deltoid muscle). The second dose may be administered 2 days before or after the weekly timepoint. Monthly maintenance doses can be administered in either the deltoid or gluteal muscle. Administer injections in the gluteal muscle using a 1½ inch, 22-gauge needle in the upper-outer quadrant of the gluteal area. Alternate gluteal injections (right and left gluteal muscle). The monthly maintenance dose may be administered 7 days before or after the monthly timepoint.

I.V. Do not administer I.V. or SubQ.

Stability

Storage Store at controlled room temperature of ≤25°C (77°F); excursions permitted to 15°C to 30°C (59°F to 86°F). Protect tablets from moisture.

Monitoring and Teaching Issues

Laboratory Monitoring Fasting lipid profile and fasting blood glucose/Hgb A_{1c} (prior to treatment, at 3 months, then annually), prolactin levels, CBC frequently during first few months of therapy in patients with pre-existing low WBC or a history of drug-induced leukopenia/neutropenia

Physical Assessment Assess for renal or cardiovascular disease, hypovolemia, and dehydration prior to treatment. Assess results of laboratory tests prior to treatment, at 3 months, and annually. Instruct patients with diabetes to monitor serum glucose closely; may seriously affect glucose control. Assess for suicide ideation, cardiovascular changes, extrapyramidal effects, and CNS changes.

Patient Education Do not chew, crush, or break tablet; swallow whole with liquids. It may take several weeks to achieve desired results. Avoid alcohol. Maintain adequate hydration. If you have diabetes, monitor blood sugars closely; may alter glucose control (notify prescriber of any change in glucose control). This medication comes in a nonabsorbable shell; after release of the drug, the shell is expelled and may be visible in stool (this is normal). May cause headache, dizziness, restlessness, anxiety, or blurred vision; orthostatic hypotension; or mild nausea, heartburn, abdominal pain, or sore mouth. Report immediately chest pain or rapid or irregular heart beat; muscle or bone pain, tremors, rigidity, or spasms; twitching of extremities or unusual movements; altered gait or loss of balance; CNS changes (persistent or unusual anxiety, nervousness, abnormal thought, confusion, fatigue, suicide ideation); or weight gain.

Dietary Considerations May be taken without regard to meals.

Geriatric Considerations Any changes in disease status in any organ system can result in behavior changes. Extrapyramidal syndrome symptoms occur less with this agent when total daily dose remains ≤6 mg as compared with phenothiazines and butyrophenone classes of antipsychotics.

In the treatment of agitated, demented, elderly patients, authors of meta-analysis of controlled trials of the response to the traditional antipsychotics (phenothiazines, butyrophenones) in controlling agitation have concluded that the use of neuroleptics results in a response rate of 18%. Clearly neuroleptic therapy for behavior control should be limited with frequent attempts to withdraw the agent given for behavior control. In light of significant risks and adverse effects in elderly population compared with limited data demonstrating efficacy in the treatment of dementia related psychosis, aggression, and agitation, an extensive risk:benefit analysis should be performed prior to use.

Pregnancy Considerations Animal studies with risperidone indicate an increase in fetal mortality. Antipsychotic use during the third trimester of pregnancy has a risk for abnormal muscle movements (extrapyramidal symptoms [EPS]) and withdrawal symptoms in newborns following delivery. Symptoms in the newborn may include agitation, feeding disorder, hypertonia, hypotonia, respiratory distress, somnolence, and tremor; these effects may be self-limiting or require hospitalization. There are no adequate and well-controlled studies in pregnant women. Reversible EPS symptoms were noted in neonates following maternal use of risperidone during the last trimester. Healthcare providers are encouraged to enroll women 18-45 years of age exposed to paliperidone during pregnancy in the Atypical Antipsychotics Pregnancy Registry (1-866-961-2388).

Additional Information Invega® is an extended release tablet based on the OROS® osmotic delivery system. Water from the GI tract enters through a semipermeable membrane coating the tablet, solubilizing the drug into a gelatinous form which, through hydrophilic expansion, is then expelled through laser-drilled holes in the coating.

Related Information

Antipsychotic Agents *on page 1986*

- **Paliperidone Palmitate** *see* Paliperidone *on page 1391*
- **Palmer's® Skin Success® Eventone® Fade Cream [OTC]** *see* Hydroquinone *on page 927*
- **Palmer's® Skin Success® Eventone® Fade Milk [OTC]** *see* Hydroquinone *on page 927*
- **Palmer's® Skin Success® Eventone® Ultra Fade Serum [OTC]** *see* Hydroquinone *on page 927*

Palonosetron (pal oh NOE se tron)

U.S. Brand Names Aloxi®

Index Terms Palonosetron Hydrochloride; RS-25259; RS-25259-197

Generic Availability (U.S.) No

Pharmacologic Category Antiemetic; Selective 5-HT_3 Receptor Antagonist

Medication Safety Issues

Sound-alike/look-alike issues:

Aloxi® may be confused with Eloxatin®, oxaliplatin

Palonosetron may be confused with dolasetron, granisetron, ondansetron

Pregnancy Risk Factor B

Lactation Excretion in breast milk unknown/not recommended

Use Prevention of chemotherapy-associated nausea and vomiting; indicated for prevention of acute (highly-emetogenic therapy) as well as acute and delayed (moderately-emetogenic therapy) nausea and vomiting; prevention of postoperative nausea and vomiting (PONV)

Mechanism of Action/Effect Selective 5-HT_3 receptor antagonist, blocking serotonin, both on vagal nerve terminals in the periphery and centrally in the chemoreceptor trigger zone

Contraindications Hypersensitivity to palonosetron or any component of the formulation

Warnings/Precautions Hypersensitivity has been observed rarely with I.V. palonosetron. Use caution in patients allergic to other 5-HT_3 receptor antagonists; cross-reactivity is possible. Some selective 5-HT_3 receptor antagonists have been associated with dose-dependent increases in ECG intervals (eg, PR, QRS duration, QT/QT_c, JT), usually occurring 1-2 hours after I.V. administration. In general, these changes are not clinically relevant, however, when these agents are used in conjunction with other agents that prolong these intervals, arrhythmia may occur. When used with agents that prolong the QT interval (eg, Class I and III antiarrhythmics), clinically relevant QT interval prolongation could result in torsade de pointes. A number of trials have shown that 5-HT_3 antagonists produce QT interval prolongation to variable degrees. Use with caution in patients at risk of QT prolongation and/or ventricular arrhythmia. Reduction in heart rate may also occur with the 5-HT_3 antagonists. Use with caution in patients with congenital long QT syndrome or other risk factors for QT prolongation (eg, medications known to prolong QT interval, electrolyte abnormalities, and cumulative high dose anthracycline therapy).

Not intended for treatment of nausea and vomiting or for chronic continuous therapy. **For chemotherapy, should be used on a scheduled basis, not on an "as needed" (PRN) basis,** since data support the use of this drug only in the prevention of nausea and vomiting (due to antineoplastic therapy) and not in the rescue of nausea and vomiting. For PONV, may use for low expectation of PONV if it is essential to avoid nausea and vomiting in the postoperative period; use is not recommended if there is little expectation of nausea and vomiting.

Drug Interactions

Metabolism/Transport Effects Substrate (minor) of CYP1A2, 2D6, 3A4

Avoid Concomitant Use

Avoid concomitant use of Palonosetron with any of the following: Apomorphine

Decreased Effect

The levels/effects of Palonosetron may be decreased by: Peginterferon Alfa-2b

Increased Effect/Toxicity

Palonosetron may increase the levels/effects of: Apomorphine

The levels/effects of Palonosetron may be increased by: Conivaptan

Adverse Reactions Adverse events may vary according to indication.

1% to 10%:

Cardiovascular: QT prolongation (chemotherapy-associated <1%; PONV 1% to 5%), bradycardia (chemotherapy-associated 1%; PONV 4%), hypotension (≤1%), sinus bradycardia (≤1%), tachycardia (nonsustained) (≤1%)

Central nervous system: Headache (chemotherapy-associated 5% to 9%; PONV 3%), anxiety (1%), dizziness (≤1%)

Dermatologic: Pruritus (≤1%)

Endocrine & metabolic: Hyperkalemia (1%)

Gastrointestinal: Constipation (2% to 5%), diarrhea (≤1%), flatulence (≤1%)

Genitourinary: Urinary retention (≤1%)

Hepatic: ALT increased (≤1%; transient), AST increased (≤1%; transient)

Neuromuscular & skeletal: Weakness (1%)

Pharmacodynamics/Kinetics

Protein Binding ~62%

Half-Life Elimination I.V.: Terminal: ~40 hours

Metabolism ~50% metabolized via CYP enzymes (and likely other pathways) to relatively inactive metabolites (N-oxide-palonosetron and 6-S-hydroxy-palonosetron); CYP1A2, 2D6, and 3A4 contribute to its metabolism

Excretion Urine (80% to 93%, 40% as unchanged drug); feces (5% to 8%)

Available Dosage Forms

Injection, solution:

Aloxi®: 0.05 mg/mL (1.5 mL, 5 mL)

Dosing

Adult

Chemotherapy-associated nausea and vomiting: I.V.: 0.25 mg 30 minutes prior to the start of chemotherapy administration

Breakthrough: Palonosetron has not been shown to be effective in terminating nausea or vomiting once it occurs and should not be used for this purpose.

PONV: I.V.: 0.075 mg immediately prior to anesthesia induction

Geriatric No dosage adjustment necessary.

Renal Impairment No dosage adjustment necessary.

Hepatic Impairment No dosage adjustment necessary.

Administration

I.V. Flush I.V. line with NS prior to and following administration.

Chemotherapy-associated nausea and vomiting: Infuse over 30 seconds, 30 minutes prior to the start of chemotherapy

PONV: Infuse over 10 seconds immediately prior to anesthesia induction

Stability

Storage Store intact vials at room temperature of 20°C to 25°C (68°F to 77°F); excursions permitted to 15°C to 30°C (59°F to 86°F); do not freeze. Protect from light. Solutions of 5 mcg/mL and 30 mcg/mL in NS, D_5W, $D_5{}^1/_2NS$, and D_5LR injection are stable for 48 hours at room temperature and 14 days under refrigeration (Trissel, 2004).

Monitoring and Teaching Issues

Physical Assessment Assess allergy history (selective 5-HT_3 receptor antagonists) prior to administering. Use with caution in presence of or potential for cardiac conduction abnormalities (eg, QT prolongation, medication known to prolong QT interval, electrolyte abnormalities). To be used on a scheduled basis for prevention of nausea and vomiting associated with moderately- to highly-emetogenic cancer chemotherapy and postoperative nausea and vomiting; not recommended for treatment of existing chemotherapy-induced emesis.

Patient Education This drug is given to prevent nausea and vomiting. If this medication is administered I.V., you will be monitored during infusion; report immediately any chest pain, respiratory difficulty, or pain or itching at infusion site. May cause headache, drowsiness, or dizziness. Report chest pain or palpitations, persistent headache, excessive drowsiness, fever, constipation, or diarrhea.

Breast-Feeding Considerations The extent to which palonosetron is excreted in breast milk, if at all, is unknown. Due to the potential for adverse effects in the nursing infant, breast-feeding is not recommended.

Pregnancy Considerations Teratogenic effects were not observed in animal studies. There are no adequate and well-controlled studies in pregnant women; use during pregnancy only if clearly needed.

◆ **Palonosetron Hydrochloride** *see* Palonosetron *on page 1396*

◆ **Pamelor®** *see* Nortriptyline *on page 1336*

Pamidronate (pa mi DROE nate)

U.S. Brand Names Aredia®

Index Terms Pamidronate Disodium

Generic Availability (U.S.) Yes

Pharmacologic Category Antidote; Bisphosphonate Derivative

Medication Safety Issues

Sound-alike/look-alike issues:

Aredia® may be confused with Adriamycin, Meridia®

Pamidronate may be confused with papaverine

International issues:

Linoten [Spain] may be confused with Loniten brand name for minoxidil [Canada and multiple international markets]

Pregnancy Risk Factor D

Lactation Excretion in breast milk unknown/use caution

Use Treatment of moderate or severe hypercalcemia associated with malignancy; treatment of osteolytic bone lesions associated with multiple myeloma or metastatic breast cancer; moderate-to-severe Paget's disease of bone

Unlabeled/Investigational Use Treatment of pediatric osteoporosis, treatment of osteogenesis imperfecta; treatment of symptomatic bone metastases of thyroid cancer; prevention of bone loss associated with androgen deprivation treatment in prostate cancer

Mechanism of Action/Effect A bisphosphonate which inhibits bone resorption via actions on osteoclasts or on osteoclast precursors. Does not appear to produce any significant effects on renal tubular calcium handling and is poorly absorbed following oral administration (high oral doses have been reported effective); therefore, I.V. therapy is preferred.

Contraindications Hypersensitivity to pamidronate, other bisphosphonates, or any component of the formulation

Warnings/Precautions Osteonecrosis of the jaw (ONJ) has been reported in patients receiving bisphosphonates. Risk factors include invasive dental procedures (eg, tooth extraction, dental implants, boney surgery); a diagnosis of cancer, with concomitant chemotherapy or corticosteroids; poor oral hygiene, ill-fitting dentures; and comorbid disorders (anemia, coagulopathy, infection, pre-existing dental disease). Most reported cases occurred after I.V. bisphosphonate therapy; however, cases have been reported following oral therapy. A dental exam and ▶

preventative dentistry should be performed prior to placing patients with risk factors on chronic bisphosphonate therapy. The manufacturer's labeling states that discontinuing bisphosphonates in patients requiring invasive dental procedures may reduce the risk of ONJ. However, other experts suggest that there is no evidence that discontinuing therapy reduces the risk of developing ONJ (Assael, 2009). The benefit/risk must be assessed by the treating physician and/or dentist/surgeon prior to any invasive dental procedure. Patients developing ONJ while on bisphosphonates should receive care by an oral surgeon.

Infrequently, severe (and occasionally debilitating) musculoskeletal (bone, joint, and/or muscle) pain have been reported during bisphosphonate treatment. The onset of pain ranged from a single day to several months. Consider discontinuing therapy in patients who experience severe symptoms; symptoms usually resolve upon discontinuation. Some patients experienced recurrence when rechallenged with same drug or another bisphosphonate; avoid use in patients with a history of these symptoms in association with bisphosphonate therapy.

Initial or single doses have been associated with renal deterioration, progressing to renal failure and dialysis. Withhold pamidronate treatment (until renal function returns to baseline) in patients with evidence of renal deterioration. Glomerulosclerosis (focal segmental) with or without nephrotic syndrome has also been reported. Longer infusion times (>2 hours) may reduce the risk for renal toxicity, especially in patients with pre-existing renal insufficiency. Single pamidronate doses should not exceed 90 mg. Patients with serum creatinine >3 mg/dL were not studied in clinical trials; limited data is available in patients with Cl_{cr} <30 mL/minute. Evaluate serum creatinine prior to each treatment. For the treatment of bone metastases, use is not recommended in patients with severe renal impairment; for renal impairment in indications other than bone metastases, use clinical judgment to determine if benefits outweigh potential risks.

Use has been associated with asymptomatic electrolyte abnormalities (including hypophosphatemia, hypokalemia, hypomagnesemia, and hypocalcemia). Rare cases of symptomatic hypocalcemia, including tetany have been reported. Patients with a history of thyroid surgery may have relative hypoparathyroidism; predisposing them to pamidronate-related hypocalcemia. Leukopenia has been observed with oral pamidronate and monitoring of white blood cell counts is suggested. Patients with pre-existing anemia, leukopenia, or thrombocytopenia should be closely monitored during the first 2 weeks of treatment.

According to the American Society of Clinical Oncology (ASCO) guidelines for bisphosphonates in multiple myeloma, treatment with pamidronate is not recommended for asymptomatic (smoldering) or indolent myeloma or with solitary plasmacytoma (Kyle, 2007). The National Comprehensive Cancer Network® (NCCN) multiple myeloma guidelines (v.2.2009) also do not recommend pamidronate use in stage 1 or smoldering disease, unless part of a clinical trial.

Adequate hydration is required during treatment (urine output ~2 L/day); avoid overhydration, especially in patients with heart failure. Vein irritation and thrombophlebitis may occur with infusions. Women of childbearing potential should be advised to use effective contraception and avoid becoming pregnant during therapy.

Drug Interactions

Avoid Concomitant Use There are no known interactions where it is recommended to avoid concomitant use.

Decreased Effect

The levels/effects of Pamidronate may be decreased by: Proton Pump Inhibitors

Increased Effect/Toxicity

Pamidronate may increase the levels/effects of: Phosphate Supplements

The levels/effects of Pamidronate may be increased by: Aminoglycosides; Nonsteroidal Anti-Inflammatory Agents; Thalidomide

Lab Interactions Bisphosphonates may interfere with diagnostic imaging agents such as technetium-99m-diphosphonate in bone scans.

Adverse Reactions Note: Actual percentages may vary by indication; treatment for multiple myeloma is associated with higher percentage.

>10%:

- Central nervous system: Fatigue (≤37%), fever (18% to 39%), headache (≤26%), insomnia (≤22%)
- Endocrine & metabolic: Hypophosphatemia (≤18%), hypokalemia (4% to 18%), hypomagnesemia (4% to 12%), hypocalcemia (≤12%)
- Gastrointestinal: Nausea (≤54%), vomiting (≤36%), anorexia (≤26%), abdominal pain (≤23%), dyspepsia (≤23%)
- Genitourinary: Urinary tract infection (≤19%)
- Hematologic: Anemia (≤43%), granulocytopenia (≤20%)
- Local: Infusion site reaction (≤18%; includes induration, pain, redness and swelling)
- Neuromuscular & skeletal: Weakness (≤22%), myalgia (≤26%), arthralgia (≤14%), osteonecrosis of the jaw (cancer patients: 1% to 11%)
- Renal: Serum creatinine increased (≤19%)
- Respiratory: Dyspnea (≤30%), cough (≤26%), upper respiratory tract infection (≤24%), sinusitis (≤16%), pleural effusion (≤11%)

1% to 10%:

- Cardiovascular: Atrial fibrillation (≤6%), hypertension (≤6%), syncope (≤6%), tachycardia (≤6%), atrial flutter (≤1%), cardiac failure (≤1%), edema (≤1%)
- Central nervous system: Somnolence (≤6%), psychosis (≤4%)
- Endocrine & metabolic: Hypothyroidism (≤6%)
- Gastrointestinal: Constipation (≤6%), gastrointestinal hemorrhage (≤6%), diarrhea (≤1%), stomatitis (≤1%)

Hematologic: Leukopenia (≤4%), neutropenia (≤1%), thrombocytopenia (≤1%)
Neuromuscular & skeletal: Back pain (≤5%), bone pain (≤5%)
Renal: Uremia (≤4%)
Respiratory: Rales (≤6%), rhinitis (≤6%)
Miscellaneous: Moniliasis (≤6%)

Pharmacodynamics/Kinetics

Onset of Action 24-48 hours; Peak effect: Maximum: 5-7 days

Absorption Poor; pharmacokinetic studies lacking

Half-Life Elimination 21-35 hours

Metabolism Not metabolized

Excretion Biphasic; urine (30% to 62% as unchanged drug; lower in patients with renal dysfunction) within 120 hours

Available Dosage Forms

Injection, powder for reconstitution: 30 mg, 90 mg
Aredia®: 30 mg, 90 mg

Injection, solution: 3 mg/mL (10 mL); 6 mg/mL (10 mL); 9 mg/mL (10 mL)

Injection, solution [preservative free]: 3 mg/mL (10 mL); 9 mg/mL (10 mL)

Dosing

Adult Dilute prior to administration and infuse intravenously slowly over at least 2 hours. Single doses should not exceed 90 mg.

Hypercalcemia of malignancy: I.V.:

Moderate cancer-related hypercalcemia (corrected serum calcium: 12-13.5 mg/dL): 60-90 mg, as a single dose over 2-24 hours

Severe cancer-related hypercalcemia (corrected serum calcium: >13.5 mg/dL): 90 mg, as a single dose over 2-24 hours

Repeat dosing: A period of 7 days should elapse before the use of second course; repeat infusions every 2-3 weeks have been suggested, however, could be administered every 2-3 months according to the degree and of severity of hypercalcemia and/or the type of malignancy.

Osteolytic bone lesions with multiple myeloma: 90 mg over 2-4 hours monthly or every 3-4 weeks

Osteolytic bone lesions with metastatic breast cancer: 90 mg over 2 hours repeated every 3-4 weeks

Paget's disease: 30 mg over 4 hours daily for 3 consecutive days

Prevention of androgen deprivation-induced osteoporosis (unlabeled use): 60 mg over 2 hours every 3 months (Smith, 2001) **or** 90 mg as a single dose over 3-4 hours (Diamond, 2001)

Geriatric Refer to adult dosing. Begin at lower end of adult dosing range.

Renal Impairment Safety and efficacy have not been established in patients with serum creatinine >5 mg/dL; studies are limited in multiple myeloma patients with serum creatinine ≥3 mg/dL

Manufacturer recommends the following guidelines:

Treatment of bone metastases: Use is not recommended in patients with severe renal impairment.

Renal impairment in indications other than bone metastases: Use clinical judgment to determine if benefits outweigh potential risks.

Multiple myeloma: American Society of Clinical Oncology (ASCO) guidelines (Kyle, 2007):

Severe renal impairment (serum creatinine >3 mg/dL **or** Cl_{cr} <30 mL/minute) and extensive bone disease: 90 mg over 4-6 hours. However, a reduced initial dose should be considered if renal impairment was pre-existing.

Albuminuria >500 mg/24 hours (unexplained): Withhold dose until returns to baseline, then recheck every 3-4 weeks; consider reinitiating at a dose not to exceed 90 mg every 4 weeks and with a longer infusion time of at least 4 hours

Dosing adjustment in renal toxicity: In patients with bone metastases, treatment should be withheld for deterioration in renal function (increase of serum creatinine ≥0.5 mg/dL in patients with normal baseline or ≥1.0 mg/dL in patients with abnormal baseline). Resumption of therapy may be considered when serum creatinine returns to within 10% of baseline.

Hepatic Impairment No adjustment required in patients with mild-to-moderate hepatic impairment; not studied in patients with severe hepatic impairment.

Administration

I.V. I.V. infusion over 2-24 hours. Longer infusion times (>2 hours) may reduce the risk for renal toxicity, especially in patients with pre-existing renal insufficiency. The manufacturer recommends infusing over 2-24 hours for hypercalcemia of malignancy; over 2 hours for osteolytic bone lesions with metastatic breast cancer; and over 4 hours for Paget's disease and for osteolytic bone lesions with multiple myeloma. The ASCO guidelines for bisphosphonate use in multiple myeloma recommend infusing pamidronate over at least 2 hours; if therapy is withheld due to renal toxicity, infuse over at least 4 hours upon reintroduction of treatment after renal recovery.

Stability

Reconstitution Powder for injection: Reconstitute by adding 10 mL of SWFI to each vial of lyophilized pamidronate disodium powder, the resulting solution will be 30 mg/10 mL or 90 mg/10 mL.

Pamidronate may be further diluted in 250-1000 mL of 0.45% or 0.9% sodium chloride or 5% dextrose. (The manufacturer recommends dilution in 1000 mL for hypercalcemia of malignancy, 500 mL for Paget's disease and bone metastases of myeloma, and 250 mL for bone metastases of breast cancer.)

Storage

Powder for reconstitution: Store below 30°C (86°F). The reconstituted solution is stable for 24 hours stored under refrigeration at 2°C to 8°C (36°F to 46°F).

Solution for injection: Store at 20°C to 25°C (68°F to 77°F).

Pamidronate solution for infusion is stable at room temperature for up to 24 hours.

Monitoring and Teaching Issues

Laboratory Monitoring Serum creatinine (prior to each treatment); serum electrolytes, including calcium, phosphate, magnesium, and potassium; CBC with differential; monitor for hypocalcemia for at least 2 weeks after therapy; patients with pre-existing anemia, leukopenia, or thrombocytopenia should be closely monitored during the first 2 weeks of treatment; monitor urine every 3-6 months for albuminuria in multiple myeloma patients

Physical Assessment Monitor for signs of hypocalcemia or renal failure. Monitor blood pressure at the beginning of therapy and periodically throughout. Teach patient lifestyle and dietary changes that will be beneficial.

Patient Education This medication can only be administered intravenously; report immediately any difficulty breathing, chest tightness, difficulty swallowing, redness, swelling, or pain at infusion site. You may experience nausea or vomiting, loss of appetite, abdominal pain, heartburn, recurrent bone pain, fever, headache, anxiety, insomnia, increased fatigue, or dizziness. Report palpitations or rapid heart beat, unusual muscle twitching or spasms, persistent diarrhea/constipation, persistent abdominal pain, unusual weight gain, decreased urine output, swelling of extremities, acute bone pain, or respiratory difficulty.

Dietary Considerations Multiple myeloma or metastatic bone lesions from solid tumors or Paget's disease: Take adequate daily calcium and vitamin D supplement

Geriatric Considerations Of the studies done with this drug, approximately 20% of the patients were ≥65 years of age with 15% ≥75 years. No differences were noted between elderly and younger adults. Dosing should be initiated with lowest recommended dose in elderly. Monitor serum electrolytes periodically since the elderly are often receiving diuretics which can result in decreases in serum calcium, potassium, and magnesium.

Pregnancy Considerations Pamidronate has been shown to cross the placenta and cause nonteratogenic embryo/fetal effects in animals. There are no adequate and well-controlled studies in pregnant women; manufacturer states pamidronate should not be used in pregnancy. Based on limited case reports, serum calcium levels in the newborn may be altered if pamidronate is administered during pregnancy. Bisphosphonates are incorporated into the bone matrix and gradually released over time. Theoretically, there may be a risk of fetal harm when pregnancy follows the completion of therapy. Women of childbearing potential should be advised to use effective contraception and avoid becoming pregnant during therapy.

◆ **Pamidronate Disodium** *see* Pamidronate *on page* 1397

◆ **p-Aminoclonidine** *see* Apraclonidine *on page* 139

◆ **Pamprin® Maximum Strength All Day Relief [OTC]** *see* Naproxen *on page* 1289

◆ **Pancrease® MT [DSC]** *see* Pancrelipase *on page* 1400

◆ **Pancreatic Enzymes** *see* Pancrelipase *on page* 1400

◆ **Pancreaze™** *see* Pancrelipase *on page* 1400

◆ **Pancrecarb MS® [DSC]** *see* Pancrelipase *on page* 1400

Pancrelipase (pan kre LYE pase)

U.S. Brand Names Creon®; Pancrease® MT [DSC]; Pancreaze™; Pancrecarb MS® [DSC]; Pancrelipase™; Ultrase® MT [DSC]; Ultrase® [DSC]; Viokase® [DSC]; Zenpep™

Index Terms Amylase, Lipase, and Protease; Lipancreatin; Lipase, Protease, and Amylase; Pancreatic Enzymes; Protease, Lipase, and Amylase

Generic Availability (U.S.) Yes

Pharmacologic Category Enzyme

Medication Safety Issues

Sound-alike/look-alike issues:

Pancrelipase may be confused with pancreatin

Medication Guide Available Yes

Pregnancy Risk Factor C

Lactation Excretion in breast milk unknown/use caution

Use Treatment of exocrine pancreatic insufficiency (EPI) due to conditions such as cystic fibrosis (Creon®, Pancreaze™, Zenpep™); chronic pancreatitis (Creon®); or pancreatectomy (Creon®)

Mechanism of Action/Effect Replaces endogenous pancreatic enzymes to assist in digestion of protein, starch, and fats

Contraindications There are no contraindications listed in the manufacturer's labeling.

Warnings/Precautions Fibrosing colonopathy advancing to colonic strictures have been reported with doses of lipase >6000 units/kg/meal over long periods of time in children <12 years of age. Patients taking doses of lipase >6000 units/kg/meal should be examined and the dose decreased. Doses of lipase >2500 units/kg/meal (or lipase >10,000 units/kg/day) should be used with caution and only with documentation of 3-day fecal fat measures. Crushing or chewing the contents of the capsules, or mixing the contents with foods outside of product labeling, may cause early release of the enzymes, causing irritation of the oral mucosa and/or loss of enzyme activity. When mixing the contents of capsules with food, the mixture should be swallowed immediately and followed with water or juice to ensure complete ingestion. Use caution in patients with gout, hyperuricemia, or renal impairment; products contain purines which may increase uric acid concentrations. Products are derived from porcine pancreatic glands. Severe, allergic reactions (rare) have been observed; use with caution in patients hypersensitive to pork proteins. Transmission of porcine viruses is theoretically a risk; however, testing and/or inactivation or removal of certain viruses, reduces the risk. There have been no cases of transmission of an infectious illness reported. Available brand products are **not** interchangeable.

Drug Interactions

Avoid Concomitant Use There are no known interactions where it is recommended to avoid concomitant use.

Decreased Effect

Pancrelipase may decrease the levels/effects of: Iron Salts

Increased Effect/Toxicity There are no known significant interactions involving an increase in effect.

Nutritional/Ethanol Interactions Food: Avoid placing contents of opened capsules on alkaline food; pancrelipase may impair absorption of oral iron.

Adverse Reactions The following adverse reactions were reported in a short-term safety studies; actual frequency varies with different products; adverse events, particularly gastrointestinal events, were often greater with placebo:

10%:

Central nervous system: Headache (6% to 15%)

Gastrointestinal: Abdominal pain (4% to 18%)

1% to 10%:

Central nervous system: Dizziness (6%)

Endocrine & metabolic: Diabetes mellitus exacerbation (4%), hyperglycemia (4%), hypoglycemia (4%)

Gastrointestinal: Flatulence (4% to 9%), early satiety (6%), weight loss (3% to 6%), upper abdominal pain (≤5%), diarrhea (≤4%), feces abnormal (≤4%)

Respiratory: Cough (6%), nasopharyngitis (4%)

Pharmacodynamics/Kinetics

Absorption None; acts locally in GI tract

Excretion Feces

Available Dosage Forms

Capsule, delayed release, enteric coated beads [porcine derived]:

Pancrelipase™: Lipase 5000 units, protease 17,000 units, amylase 27,000 units

Zenpep™: Lipase 5000 units, protease 17,000 units, amylase 27,000 units

Zenpep™: Lipase 10,000 units, protease 34,000 units, amylase 55,000 units

Zenpep™: Lipase 15,000 units, protease 51,000 units, amylase 82,000 units

Zenpep™: Lipase 20,000 units, protease 68,000 units, amylase 109,000 units

Capsule, delayed release, enteric coated microspheres [new formulation; porcine derived]:

Creon®: Lipase 6000 units, protease 19,000 units, and amylase 30,000 units

Creon®: Lipase 12000 units, protease 38,000 units, and amylase 60,000 units

Creon®: Lipase 24,000 units, protease 76,000 units, and amylase 120,000 units

Capsule, delayed release, enteric coated microtablets [porcine derived]:

Pancreaze™: Lipase 4200 units, protease 10,000 units, and amylase 17,500 units

Pancreaze™: Lipase 10,500 units, protease 25,000 units, and amylase 43,750 units

Pancreaze™: Lipase 16,800 units, protease 40,000 units, and amylase 70,000 units

Pancreaze™: Lipase 21,000 units, protease 37,000 units, and amylase 61,000 units

Capsule, enteric coated microspheres [porcine derived]:

Ultrase®: Lipase 4500 units, protease 25,000 units, and amylase 20,000 units

Dosing

Adult Note: Adjust dose based on body weight, clinical symptoms, and stool fat content. Allow several days between dose adjustments. Total daily dose reflects ~3 meals/day and 2-3 snacks/day, with half the mealtime dose given with a snack. Doses of lipase >2500 units/kg/meal (or lipase > 10,000 units/kg/day) should be used with caution and only with documentation of 3-day fecal fat measures. Doses of lipase >6000 units/kg/meal are associated with colonic stricture and should be decreased.

Pancreatic insufficiency: Oral: Initial: Lipase 500 units/kg/meal. Dosage range: Lipase 500-2500 units/kg/meal. Maximum dose: Lipase 10,000 units/kg/day **or** lipase 4000 units/g of fat per day

Pancreatic insufficiency due to chronic pancreatitis or pancreatectomy (Creon®): Oral: Lipase 72,000 units/meal while consuming ≥100 g of fat per day; alternatively, lower initial doses of lipase 500 units/kg/meal with individualized dosage titrations have also been used

Geriatric Refer to adult dosing.

Pediatric Note: Adjust dose based on body weight, clinical symptoms, and stool fat content. Allow several days between dose adjustments. Total daily dose reflects ~3 meals/day and 2-3 snacks/day, with half the mealtime dose given with a snack. Doses of lipase >2500 units/kg/meal (or lipase >10,000 units/kg/day) should be used with caution and only with documentation of 3-day fecal fat measures. Doses of lipase >6000 units/kg/meal are associated with colonic stricture and should be decreased.

Pancreatic insufficiency: Oral:

Children ≤1 year: Lipase 2000-4000 units per 120 mL of formula or breast milk

Children >1 and <4 years: Initial dose: Lipase 1000 units/kg/meal. Dosage range: Lipase 1000-2500 units/kg/meal. Maximum dose: Lipase 10,000 units/kg/day **or** lipase 4000 units/g of fat per day

Children ≥4 years: Refer to adult dosing.

Administration

Oral Administer with meals or snacks and swallow whole with a generous amount of liquid. Do not crush or chew; retention in the mouth before swallowing may cause mucosal irritation and stomatitis. If necessary, capsules may also be opened and contents added to a small amount of an acidic food (pH ≤4), such as applesauce. The food should be at room temperature and swallowed immediately after mixing. The contents of the capsule should not be crushed or chewed. Follow with water or juice to ensure complete ingestion and that no medication remains in the mouth.

Creon®: Capsules contain enteric coated spheres which are 0.71-1.6 mm in diameter

Pancreaze™: Capsules contain enteric coated microtablets which are ~2 mm in diameter

Zenpep™: Capsules contain enteric coated beads which are 1.8-2.5 mm in diameter

When administering to infants <1 year of age, do not mix with breast milk or infant formula. Open capsule and place the contents directly into the mouth or mix with a small amount of applesauce, commercially prepared pears, or bananas baby food. Administer immediately after mixing (or within 15 minutes of mixing using Pancreaze™). Follow with water or infant formula to ensure complete ingestion and that no medication remains in the mouth.

Stability

Storage

Creon®: Store at room temperature of 25°C (77°F); excursions permitted between 25°C to 40°C (77°F to 104°F) for ≤30 days. Protect from moisture, and discard if moisture conditions are >70%. Keep bottle tightly closed.

Pancreaze™: Store at ≤25°C (77°F). Protect from moisture; keep bottle tightly closed.

Zenpep™: Store at room temperature 20°C to 25°C (68°F to 77°F). Protect from moisture; keep bottle tightly closed after opening.

Monitoring and Teaching Issues

Physical Assessment Dosing and administration depend on purpose for use and formulation (available products are not interchangeable).

Patient Education Take right before or with foods, and swallow whole with a generous amount of liquid. Dairy products may have a high pH and should not be taken together with this medication. Do not crush or chew the contents of the capsules. Delayed-release capsules containing enteric-coated microspheres or microtablets may be opened and the contents sprinkled on soft food; do not chew. Report unusual rash, persistent GI upset, or respiratory difficulty.

Dietary Considerations Take with meals or snacks and swallow whole with a generous amount of liquid. Vitamin supplementation should be per current guidelines for patients with cystic fibrosis.

Geriatric Considerations No special considerations are necessary since drug is dosed to response; however, drug-induced diarrhea can result in unwanted side effects (eg, confusion, hypotension, lethargy, fluid and electrolyte loss).

Breast-Feeding Considerations Systemic absorption and concentration into the breast milk is unlikely, but unknown.

Pregnancy Considerations Reproduction studies have not been conducted. Nutrition should be optimized in pregnancy; in cystic fibrosis patients with malabsorption, pancreatic enzyme replacement is not considered to cause a risk to the pregnancy.

Additional Information Pancreatic enzyme replacement products (PEP) may **not** be used interchangeably; however, Pancrelipase™ lipase 5000 units strength manufactured by Eurand Pharmaceuticals and distributed by X-Gen Pharmaceuticals is an authorized generic which may be used interchangeably with the Zenpep™ lipase 5000 units product (manufactured by Eurand Pharmaceuticals).

◆ **Pancrelipase™** *see* Pancrelipase *on page 1400*

Pancuronium (pan kyoo ROE nee um)

Index Terms Pancuronium Bromide; Pavulon [DSC]

Generic Availability (U.S.) Yes

Pharmacologic Category Neuromuscular Blocker Agent, Nondepolarizing

Medication Safety Issues

Sound-alike/look-alike issues:

Pancuronium may be confused with pipecuronium

High alert medication: The Institute for Safe Medication Practices (ISMP) includes this medication among its list of drugs which have a heightened risk of causing significant patient harm when used in error.

United States Pharmacopeia (USP) 2006: The Interdisciplinary Safe Medication Use Expert Committee of the USP has recommended the following:

- Hospitals, clinics, and other practice sites should institute special safeguards in the storage, labeling, and use of these agents and should include these safeguards in staff orientation and competency training.
- Healthcare professionals should be on high alert (especially vigilant) whenever a neuromuscular-blocking agent (NMBA) is stocked, ordered, prepared, or administered.

Pregnancy Risk Factor C

Lactation Excretion in breast milk unknown/not recommended

Use Facilitation of endotracheal intubation and relaxation of skeletal muscles during surgery; facilitation of mechanical ventilation in ICU patients; does not relieve pain or produce sedation

Available Dosage Forms

Injection, solution: 1 mg/mL (10 mL)

Dosing

Adult & Geriatric Administer I.V.; dose to effect; doses will vary due to interpatient variability; use ideal body weight for obese patients

Neuromuscular blockade: Initial: 0.06-0.1 mg/kg or 0.05 mg/kg after initial dose of succinylcholine for intubation; maintenance dose: 0.01 mg/kg 60-100 minutes after initial dose and then 0.01 mg/kg every 25-60 minutes

Pretreatment/priming: 10% of intubating dose given 3-5 minutes before initial dose

Neuromuscular blockade in the ICU: 0.05-0.1 mg/kg bolus followed by 0.8-1.7 mcg/kg/minute once initial recovery from bolus observed or 0.1-0.2 mg/kg every 1-3 hours

Pediatric Infants >1 month and Children: Refer to adult dosing.

Renal Impairment Elimination half-life is doubled, plasma clearance is reduced, and rate of recovery is sometimes much slower.

Cl_{cr} 10-50 mL/minute: Administer 50% of normal dose.

Cl_{cr} <10 mL/minute: Do not use.

Hepatic Impairment Elimination half-life is doubled, plasma clearance is doubled, recovery time is prolonged, volume of distribution is increased (50%) and results in a slower onset, higher total dosage, and prolongation of neuromuscular blockade. Patients with liver disease may develop slow resistance to nondepolarizing muscle relaxant. Large doses may be required and problems may arise in antagonism.

Administration

I.V. May be administered undiluted by rapid I.V. injection.

Monitoring and Teaching Issues

Physical Assessment Dosage and rate of administration should be individualized and titrated to the desired effect, according to relevant clinical factors, premedication, concomitant medications, age, and general condition of the patient. Ventilatory support must be instituted and maintained until adequate respiratory muscle function and/or airway protection are assured. This drug is not an anesthetic or analgesic; pain must be treated with other agents. Continuous monitoring of vital signs, cardiac status, respiratory status, and degree of neuromuscular block (objective assessment with peripheral external nerve stimulator) is mandatory until full muscle tone has returned. Safety precautions must be maintained until full muscle tone has returned. It may take longer for return of muscle tone in obese or elderly patients or patients with renal or hepatic disease, myasthenia gravis, myopathy, other neuromuscular disease, dehydration, electrolyte imbalance, or severe acid/base imbalance.

Long-term use: Monitor level of neuromuscular blockade, skeletal muscle movement, and respiratory effort. Reposition patient and provide appropriate skin care, mouth care, and care of patient's eyes every 2-3 hours while sedated. Provide appropriate emotional and sensory support (auditory and environmental).

Patient Education Patient will usually be unconscious prior to administration. Reassurance of constant monitoring and emotional support to reduce fear and anxiety should precede and follow administration. Following return of muscle tone, do not attempt to change position or rise from bed without assistance.

◆ **Pancuronium Bromide** *see* Pancuronium *on page* 1402

◆ **Pandel®** *see* Hydrocortisone (Topical) *on page* 920

◆ **Panglobulin** *see* Immune Globulin *on page* 961

Panitumumab (pan i TOOM yoo mab)

U.S. Brand Names Vectibix®

Index Terms ABX-EGF; MOAB ABX-EGF; Monoclonal Antibody ABX-EGF; rHuMAb-EGFr

Generic Availability (U.S.) No

Pharmacologic Category Antineoplastic Agent, Monoclonal Antibody; Epidermal Growth Factor Receptor (EGFR) Inhibitor

Pregnancy Risk Factor C

Lactation Excretion in breast milk unknown/not recommended

Use Monotherapy in treatment of refractory metastatic colorectal cancer

Note: Subset analyses (retrospective) in metastatic colorectal cancer trials have not shown a benefit with EGFR inhibitor treatment in patients whose tumors have codon 12 or 13 *KRAS* mutations; use is not recommended in these patients.

Mechanism of Action/Effect Epidermal growth factor receptor (EGFR) inhibitor

Contraindications There are no contraindications listed in manufacturer's labeling.

Warnings/Precautions [U.S. Boxed Warning]: Dermatologic toxicities have been reported in ~90% of patients (severe in 12% of patients); may include dermatitis acneiform, pruritus, erythema, rash, skin exfoliation, paronychia, dry skin and skin fissures. Severe skin toxicities may be complicated by infection, sepsis, or abscesses. The median time to development of skin (or ocular) toxicity was 2 weeks, with resolution ~7 weeks after discontinuation. Withhold treatment (and monitor) for severe or life-threatening dermatologic toxicities; may require dose reduction or permanent discontinuation. The severity of dermatologic toxicity is predictive for response; grades 2-4 skin toxicity correlates with improved progression free survival and overall ▶

survival, compared to grade 1 skin toxicity (Peeters, 2009; Van Cutsem, 2007). Patients should minimize sunlight exposure; may exacerbate skin reactions. Gastric mucosal, ocular and nail toxicities have also been reported.

[U.S. Boxed Warning]: Severe infusion reactions (anaphylactic reaction, bronchospasm, fever, chills, and hypotension) have been reported in ~1% of patients. Discontinue infusion for severe reactions; permanently discontinue in patients with persistent severe infusion reactions. Appropriate medical support for the management of infusion reactions should be readily available. Mild-to-moderate infusion reactions are managed by slowing the infusion rate.

Pulmonary fibrosis has been reported (rarely); permanently discontinue treatment if interstitial lung disease, pneumonitis or lung infiltrates develop. Use caution with lung disease; patients with underlying lung disease were excluded from clinical trials. May cause diarrhea; the incidence and severity of chemotherapy-induced diarrhea and other toxicities (rash, electrolyte abnormalities, stomatitis) is increased with combination chemotherapy; acute renal failure resulting from severe diarrhea and dehydration has also been observed in patients receiving panitumumab with combination chemotherapy. In addition to increased toxicity, studies using panitumumab in combination with chemotherapy (with or without bevacizumab) resulted in decreased progression-free survival compared to regimens without panitumumab; therefore, panitumumab is not indicated for use in combination with chemotherapy. Electrolyte depletion may occur during treatment and after treatment is discontinued; monitor for hypomagnesemia and hypocalcemia during treatment and for at least 8 weeks after completion. Patients with colorectal cancer with tumors with a codon 12 or 13 *KRAS* mutation are unlikely to benefit from EGFR inhibitor therapy and should not receive panitumumab treatment. Safety and efficacy in children have not been established.

Drug Interactions

Avoid Concomitant Use There are no known interactions where it is recommended to avoid concomitant use.

Decreased Effect There are no known significant interactions involving a decrease in effect.

Increased Effect/Toxicity There are no known significant interactions involving an increase in effect.

Adverse Reactions

>10%:

Cardiovascular: Peripheral edema (12%)

Central nervous system: Fatigue (26%)

Dermatologic: Skin toxicity (90%; grades 3/4: 14% to 16%), erythema (65%; grades 3/4: 5%), acneiform rash (57%; grades 3/4: 7%), pruritus (57%; grades 3/4: 2%), exfoliation (25%; grades 3/4: 2%), paronychia (25%), rash (22%; grades 3/4: 1%), fissures (20%; grades 3/4: 1%), acne (13%; grades 3/4: 1%)

Endocrine & metabolic: Hypomagnesemia (38%; grades 3/4: 4%)

Gastrointestinal: Abdominal pain (25%), nausea (23%), diarrhea (21%; grades 3/4: 2%), constipation (21%), vomiting (19%)

Respiratory: Cough (14%)

1% to 10%:

Dermatologic: Dry skin (10%), nail disorder (other than paronychia: 9%)

Gastrointestinal: Stomatitis (7%), mucositis (6%)

Ocular: Eyelash growth (6%), conjunctivitis (4%), ocular hyperemia (3%), lacrimation increased (2%), eye/eye lid irritation (1%)

Miscellaneous: Antibody formation (≤5%), infusion reactions (3%; grades 3/4: 1%)

Pharmacodynamics/Kinetics

Half-Life Elimination ~7.5 days (range: 4-11 days)

Available Dosage Forms

Injection, solution [preservative free]:

Vectibix®: 20 mg/mL (5 mL, 20 mL)

Dosing

Adult & Geriatric Metastatic colorectal cancer: I.V.: 6 mg/kg every 2 weeks

Renal Impairment Has not been studied

Hepatic Impairment Has not been studied

Adjustment for Toxicity

Infusion reactions, mild-to-moderate (grade 1 or 2): Reduce the infusion rate by 50% for the duration of infusion

Infusion reactions, severe (grade 3 or 4): Immediately and permanently discontinue treatment

Dermatologic toxicity (≥grade 3, or intolerable): Withhold treatment; if skin toxicity does not improve to ≤grade 2 within 1 month, permanently discontinue. If skin toxicity improves to ≤grade 2 within 1 month (with patient missing ≤2 doses), resume treatment at 50% of the original dose. Dose may be increased in increments of 25% of the original dose (up to 6 mg/kg) if skin toxicities do not recur. For recurrent skin toxicity, permanently discontinue.

Administration

I.V. Doses ≤1000 mg, infuse over 1 hour; doses >1000 mg, infuse over 90 minutes; reduce infusion rate by 50% for mild-to-moderate infusion reactions (grades 1 and 2); discontinue for severe infusion reactions (grades 3 and 4). Administer through a low protein-binding 0.2 or 0.22 micrometer in-line filter. Flush with NS before and after infusion.

Stability

Reconstitution Dilute in 100-150 mL of normal saline to a final concentration of ≤10 mg/mL. Do not shake, invert gently to mix.

Storage Store unopened vials under refrigeration at 2°C to 8°C (36°F to 46°F). Do not freeze; do not shake; protect from light. Preparations in infusion containers are stable for 24 hours under refrigeration at 2°C to 8°C (36°F to 46°F) or for 6 hours at room temperature (do not freeze).

Monitoring and Teaching Issues

Laboratory Monitoring *KRAS* genotyping of tumor tissue. Monitor serum electrolytes, including magnesium and calcium (periodically during and for at least 8 weeks after therapy).

Physical Assessment Patient must be monitored closely during and following infusion for infusion reaction; appropriate medical support for the management of infusion reactions should be readily available. Monitor for severe skin reactions (may necessitate dose reduction), peripheral edema, and gastrointestinal upset (pain, nausea, diarrhea, constipation, vomiting) at each infusion and throughout therapy.

Patient Education This medication can only be administered by infusion; you will be closely monitored. Report immediately unusual back or abdominal pain; acute headache; difficulty breathing or chest tightness; difficulty swallowing; itching or rash; or redness, swelling, or pain at infusion site. Maintain adequate nutrition and hydration, unless instructed to restrict fluid intake. You may experience nausea, vomiting, diarrhea, or constipation. Report immediately any skin rash, redness, or infection; any unusual swelling of extremities or weight gain; unremitting abdominal pain, vomiting, diarrhea, or constipation; any changes in vision; or unusual infection (respiratory or wound).

Breast-Feeding Considerations Breast-feeding should be discontinued during treatment and for 2 months following the last dose.

Pregnancy Considerations Animal reproductive studies have demonstrated adverse fetal effects. Based on animal studies, panitumumab may disrupt normal menstrual cycles. There are no adequate and well-controlled studies in pregnant women. IgG is known to cross the placenta; therefore, it is possible the developing fetus may be exposed to panitumumab. Because panitumumab inhibits epidermal growth factor (EGF), a component of fetal development, adverse effects on pregnancy would be expected. Panitumumab should only be given to a pregnant woman if the potential benefit justifies the potential risk to the fetus. Women of childbearing potential should use effective contraception during and for 6 months after treatment. Women who become pregnant during panitumumab treatment are encouraged to enroll in Amgen's Pregnancy Surveillance Program (1-800-772-6436).

Additional Information Oncology Comment: The National Comprehensive Cancer Network® (NCCN) guidelines for colon cancer (v.2.2009) and the American Society of Clinical Oncology (ASCO) provisional clinical opinion (Allegra, 2009) recommend genotyping tumor tissue for *KRAS* mutation in all patients with metastatic colorectal cancer (genotyping may be done on archived specimens). Patients with known codon 12 or 13 *KRAS* gene mutations are unlikely to respond to EGFR inhibitors and should not receive panitumumab. Favorable progression-free survival and higher response rates have been demonstrated with panitumumab in patients with *KRAS* wild-type; patients with the *KRAS* mutation did not respond to panitumumab (Amado, 2008). Because EGFR testing in colorectal tumors does not correlate with response, the NCCN guidelines do not recommend routine EGFR testing in colorectal cancer. Severity of dermatologic toxicity associated with panitumumab is predictive for response; grades 2-4 skin toxicity correlates with improved progression free survival and overall survival, compared to patients with grade 1 skin toxicity (Van Cutsem, 2007). The association between dermatologic toxicity and progression free survival was not noted in patients with *KRAS* mutation (Peeters, 2009). The NCCN guidelines do not recommend the use of panitumumab after failure of cetuximab therapy.

◆ **Panretin®** *see* Alitretinoin *on page* 75

Pantoprazole (pan TOE pra zole)

U.S. Brand Names Protonix®

Generic Availability (U.S.) Yes: Delayed release tablet

Pharmacologic Category Proton Pump Inhibitor; Substituted Benzimidazole

Medication Safety Issues

Sound-alike/look-alike issues:

Pantoprazole may be confused with ARIPiprazole

Protonix® may be confused with Lotronex®, Lovenox®, protamine

Vials containing Protonix® I.V. for injection are not recommended for use with spiked I.V. system adaptors. Nurses and pharmacists have reported breakage of the glass vials during attempts to connect spiked I.V. system adaptors, which may potentially result in injury to healthcare professionals.

International issues:

Protonix [U.S., Canada] may be confused with Pretanix brand name for indapamide [Hungary]

Pregnancy Risk Factor B

Lactation Enters breast milk/not recommended

Use

Oral: Treatment and maintenance of healing of erosive esophagitis associated with GERD; reduction in relapse rates of daytime and nighttime heartburn symptoms in GERD; hypersecretory disorders associated with Zollinger-Ellison syndrome or other GI hypersecretory disorders

I.V.: Short-term treatment (7-10 days) of patients with gastroesophageal reflux disease (GERD) and a history of erosive esophagitis; hypersecretory disorders associated with Zollinger-Ellison syndrome or other neoplastic disorders

Unlabeled/Investigational Use Peptic ulcer disease, active ulcer bleeding (parenteral formulation); adjunct treatment with antibiotics for *Helicobacter pylori* eradication; stress-ulcer prophylaxis in the critically-ill

Mechanism of Action/Effect Suppresses gastric acid secretion by inhibiting the parietal cell H^+/K^+ ATP pump

Contraindications Hypersensitivity to pantoprazole, substituted benzamidazoles (eg, esomeprazole, lansoprazole, omeprazole, rabeprazole), or any component of the formulation

Canadian labeling: Additional contraindication (not in U.S. labeling): Concomitant use with atazanavir

Warnings/Precautions Use of proton pump inhibitors may increase the risk of gastrointestinal infections (eg, *Salmonella, Campylobacter*). Relief of symptoms does not preclude the presence of a gastric malignancy. Long-term pantoprazole therapy (especially in patients who were *H. pylori* positive) has caused biopsy-proven atrophic gastritis. No reports of enterochromaffin-like (ECL) cell carcinoids, dysplasia, or neoplasia such as those seen in rodent studies have occurred in humans. Not indicated for maintenance therapy; safety and efficacy for use beyond 16 weeks have not been established. Prolonged treatment (typically >3 years) may lead to vitamin B_{12} malabsorption and subsequent deficiency. Intravenous preparation contains edetate sodium (EDTA); use caution in patients who are at risk for zinc deficiency if other EDTA-containing solutions are coadministered. Decreased *H. pylori* eradication rates have been observed with short-term (≤7 days) combination therapy. The American College of Gastroenterology recommends 10-14 days of therapy (triple or quadruple) for eradication of *H. pylori* (Chey, 2007). Proton pump inhibitors may diminish the therapeutic effect of clopidogrel, thought to be due to reduced formation of the active metabolite of clopidogrel; an increase in the risk of cardiovascular events may occur. Of the PPIs, pantoprazole has the lowest degree of CYP2C19 inhibition and is preferred if concomitant use of a PPI is necessary.

Increased incidence of osteoporosis-related bone fractures of the hip, spine, or wrist may occur with proton pump inhibitor therapy. Patients on high-dose or long-term therapy should be monitored. Use the lowest effective dose for the shortest duration of time, use vitamin D and calcium supplementation, and follow appropriate guidelines to reduce risk of fractures in patients at risk.

Drug Interactions

Metabolism/Transport Effects Substrate of CYP2C9 (minor), 2C19 (major), 2D6 (minor), 3A4 (minor); **Inhibits** CYP2C9 (weak), 2C19 (moderate), ABCG2; **Induces** CYP1A2 (weak), 3A4 (weak)

Avoid Concomitant Use

Avoid concomitant use of Pantoprazole with any of the following: Delavirdine; Erlotinib; Nelfinavir; Posaconazole

Decreased Effect

Pantoprazole may decrease the levels/effects of: Atazanavir; Bisphosphonate Derivatives; Cefditoren; Clopidogrel; Dabigatran Etexilate; Dasatinib; Delavirdine; Erlotinib; Gefitinib; Indinavir; Iron Salts; Itraconazole; Ketoconazole; Ketoconazole (Systemic); Mesalamine; Mycophenolate; Nelfinavir; Posaconazole

The levels/effects of Pantoprazole may be decreased by: CYP2C19 Inducers (Strong); Peginterferon Alfa-2b; Tipranavir

Increased Effect/Toxicity

Pantoprazole may increase the levels/effects of: Amphetamines; CYP2C19 Substrates; Dexmethylphenidate; Methotrexate; Methylphenidate; Raltegravir; Saquinavir; Topotecan; Voriconazole

The levels/effects of Pantoprazole may be increased by: Conivaptan; Fluconazole; Ketoconazole; Ketoconazole (Systemic)

Nutritional/Ethanol Interactions

Ethanol: Avoid ethanol (may cause gastric mucosal irritation).

Herb/Nutraceutical: Prolonged treatment (typically >3 years) may lead to vitamin B_{12} malabsorption and subsequent deficiency.

Lab Interactions False-positive urine screening tests for tetrahydrocannabinol (THC) have been reported in patients receiving proton pump inhibitors, including pantoprazole.

Adverse Reactions ≥1%:

Cardiovascular: Chest pain

Central nervous system: Headache (2% to 9%), insomnia (≤1%), anxiety, dizziness, migraine, pain

Dermatologic: Rash (≤2%)

Endocrine & metabolic: Hyperglycemia (≤1%), hyperlipidemia

Gastrointestinal: Diarrhea (2% to 6%), flatulence (2% to 4%), abdominal pain (1% to 4%), nausea (≤2%), vomiting (≤2%), eructation (≤1%), constipation, dyspepsia, gastroenteritis, rectal disorder

Genitourinary: Urinary frequency, UTI

Hepatic: Liver function tests abnormal (≤2%)

Local: Injection site reaction (includes thrombophlebitis and abscess)

Neuromuscular & skeletal: Arthralgia, back pain, hypertonia, neck pain, weakness

Respiratory: Bronchitis, cough, dyspnea, pharyngitis, rhinitis, sinusitis, upper respiratory tract infection

Miscellaneous: Flu syndrome, infection

Pharmacodynamics/Kinetics

Absorption Rapid, well absorbed

Bioavailability 77%

Time to Peak Oral: 2.5 hours

Protein Binding 98%, primarily to albumin

Half-Life Elimination 1 hour; increased to 3.5-10 hours with CYP2C19 deficiency

Metabolism Extensively hepatic; CYP2C19 (demethylation), CYP3A4; no evidence that metabolites have pharmacologic activity

Excretion Urine (71%); feces (18%)

Available Dosage Forms

Granules for suspension, delayed release, enteric coated, oral:

Protonix®: 40 mg/packet (30s)

Injection, powder for reconstitution:

Protonix®: 40 mg

Tablet, delayed release, oral: 20 mg, 40 mg

Protonix®: 20 mg, 40 mg

Dosing

Adult & Geriatric

Erosive esophagitis associated with GERD:

Oral:

Treatment: 40 mg once daily for up to 8 weeks; an additional 8 weeks may be used in patients who have not healed after an 8-week course

Maintenance of healing: 40 mg once daily

Note: Lower doses (20 mg once daily) have been used successfully in mild GERD treatment and maintenance of healing

I.V.: 40 mg once daily for 7-10 days

Hypersecretory disorders (including Zollinger-Ellison):

Oral: Initial: 40 mg twice daily; adjust dose based on patient needs; doses up to 240 mg/day have been administered

I.V.: 80 mg twice daily; adjust dose based on acid output measurements; 160-240 mg/day in divided doses has been used for a limited period (up to 7 days)

Prevention of rebleeding in peptic ulcer bleed (unlabeled use): I.V.: 80 mg, followed by 8 mg/hour infusion for 72 hours. **Note:** A daily infusion of 40 mg does not raise gastric pH sufficiently to enhance coagulation in active GI bleeds.

***Helicobacter pylori* eradication (unlabeled use):** *Oral:* American College of Gastroenterology guidelines (Chey, 2007):

Nonpenicillin allergy: 40 mg twice daily administered with amoxicillin 1000 mg *and* clarithromycin 500 mg twice daily for 10-14 days

Penicillin allergy: 40 mg twice daily administered with clarithromycin 500 mg *and* metronidazole 500 mg twice daily for 10-14 days **or** 40 mg once or twice daily administered with bismuth subsalicylate 525 mg *and* metronidazole 250 mg *plus* tetracycline 500 mg 4 times/day for 10-14 days

Pediatric GERD, erosive esophagitis associated with GERD:

Oral:

Children <5 years: Dosage not established.

Children ≥5 years (unlabeled use): 20-40 mg once daily

I.V.: Dosage not established

Renal Impairment No adjustment is required. Pantoprazole is not removed by hemodialysis.

Hepatic Impairment No adjustment is required.

Administration

Oral

Tablet: Should be swallowed whole, do not crush or chew. Best if taken before breakfast.

Delayed-release oral suspension: Should only be administered in apple juice or applesauce and taken ~30 minutes before a meal. Do not administer with any other liquid (eg, water) or foods.

Oral administration in **applesauce**: Sprinkle intact granules on 1 tablespoon of applesauce and swallow within 10 minutes of preparation.

Oral administration in **apple juice**: Empty intact granules into 5 mL of apple juice (~1 teaspoonful), stir for 5 seconds, and swallow immediately after preparation. Rinse container once or twice with apple juice and swallow immediately.

Nasogastric tube administration: Separate the plunger from the barrel of a 60 mL catheter tip syringe and connect to a ≥16 French nasogastric tube. Holding the syringe attached to the tubing as high as possible, empty the contents of the packet into barrel of the syringe, add 10 mL of apple juice and gently tap/shake the barrel of the syringe to help empty the syringe. Add an additional 10 mL of apple juice and gently tap/shake the barrel to help rinse. Repeat rinse with at least 2-10 mL aliquots of apple juice. No granules should remain in the syringe.

I.V. Flush I.V. line before and after administration. In-line filter not required.

2-minute infusion: The volume of reconstituted solution (4 mg/mL) to be injected may be administered intravenously over at least 2 minutes.

15-minute infusion: Infuse over 15 minutes at a rate not to exceed 7 mL/minute (3 mg/minute).

Stability

Reconstitution Reconstitute with 10 mL NS (final concentration 4 mg/mL). Reconstituted solution may be given intravenously (over 2 minutes) or may be added to 100 mL D_5W, NS, or LR (for 15-minute infusion).

Storage

Oral: Store tablet and oral suspension at controlled room temperature of 20°C to 25°C (68°F to 77°F).

I.V.: Prior to reconstitution, store at controlled room temperature of 20°C to 25°C (68°F to 77°F). Protect from light. When reconstituted, solution is stable up to 96 hours at room temperature (Johnson, 2005). The preparation should be stored at 3°C to 5°C (37°F to 41°F) if it is stored beyond 48 hours to minimize discoloration. If further diluting in 100 mL of D_5W, LR, or NS, dilute within 6 hours of reconstitution. Diluted solution is stable at room temperature for up to 24 hours from the time of initial reconstitution; protection from light is not required.

Monitoring and Teaching Issues

Physical Assessment Assess other medications for effectiveness and interactions (cytochrome P450 enzyme substrate), especially those drugs in which absorption is determined by an acidic gastric pH.

Patient Education Take at similar time each day. Swallow tablet whole (do not crush or chew). Avoid alcohol. You may experience headache, vomiting, or diarrhea. Report persistent abdominal discomfort; chest pain; persistent headache; unresolved diarrhea; excessive fatigue; increased muscle, joint, or body pain; or changes in urinary pattern.

Dietary Considerations

Oral: May be taken with or without food; best if taken before breakfast.

I.V.: Due to EDTA in preparation, zinc supplementation may be needed in patients prone to zinc deficiency.

Geriatric Considerations Dosage adjustment not required.

Breast-Feeding Considerations Not recommended due to carcinogenicity in animal studies.

Pregnancy Considerations Teratogenic effects were not observed in animal studies. There are no adequate and well-controlled studies in pregnant women. Use in pregnancy only if clearly needed.

Related Information

Compatibility of Drugs *on page 1994*

Papillomavirus (Types 6, 11, 16, 18) Vaccine (Human, Recombinant)

(pap ih LO ma VYE rus typs six e LEV en SIX teen AYE teen vak SEEN YU man ree KOM be nant)

U.S. Brand Names Gardasil®

Index Terms HPV Vaccine; HPV4; Human Papillomavirus Vaccine; Papillomavirus Vaccine, Recombinant; Quadrivalent Human Papillomavirus Vaccine

Generic Availability (U.S.) No

Pharmacologic Category Vaccine, Inactivated (Viral)

Medication Safety Issues

Sound-alike/look-alike issues:

Papillomavirus vaccine types 6, 11, 16, 18 (Gardasil®) may be confused with Papillomavirus vaccine types 16, 18 (Cervarix®)

Pregnancy Risk Factor B

Lactation Excretion in breast milk unknown/use caution

Use

Females ≥9 years and ≤26 years of age: Prevention of cervical, vulvar, vaginal, and anal cancer caused by HPV types 16 and 18; genital warts caused by HPV types 6 and 11; cervical adenocarcinoma *in situ*, and vulvar, vaginal, cervical, or anal intraepithelial neoplasia caused by HPV types 6, 11, 16, 18

Males ≥9 years and ≤26 years of age: Prevention of genital warts caused by human papillomavirus (HPV) types 6 and 11; anal cancer caused by HPV types 16 and 18, and anal intraepithelial neoplasia caused by HPV types 6, 11, 16, and 18

Note: Canadian labeling: Approved for use in males ≥9 years of age and ≤17 years

The Advisory Committee on Immunization Practices (ACIP) recommends routine vaccination for females 11-12 years of age; catch-up vaccination is recommended for females 13-26 years of age; ACIP does not recommend routine use among males; however, eligible males 9-26 years of age may be vaccinated.

Unlabeled/Investigational Use Prevention of cervical, vulvar, and vaginal cancer caused by HPV types 16 and 18, genital warts caused by HPV types 6 and 11, cervical adenocarcinoma *in situ*, and vulvar, vaginal, or cervical intraepithelial neoplasia caused by HPV types 6, 11, 16, 18 in women 26-45 years of age

Available Dosage Forms

Injection, suspension [preservative free]:

Gardasil®: HPV 6 L1 protein 20 mcg, HPV 11 L1 protein 40 mcg, HPV 16 L1 protein 40 mcg, and HPV 18 L1 protein 20 mcg per 0.5 mL (0.5 mL)

Dosing

Adult Immunization regimen: I.M.: Children ≥9 years and Adults ≤26 years: 0.5 mL followed by 0.5 mL at 2 and 6 months after initial dose

CDC recommended immunization schedule: Administer first dose to females at age 11-12 years; begin series in females aged 13-26 years if not previously vaccinated. Minimum interval between first and second doses is 4 weeks; the minimum interval between first and third doses is 24 weeks. Inadequate doses or doses received following a shorter than recommended dosing interval should be repeated. The HPV vaccine series should be completed with the same product whenever possible. Currently, according to the CDC, HPV immunization may be given to eligible males to reduce their likelihood of acquiring genital warts; however, routine vaccination is not recommended (refer to current guidelines).

Pediatric Immunization regimen: Children ≥9 years: Refer to adult dosing.

Administration

I.M. Shake suspension well before use. Inject the entire dose I.M. into the deltoid region of the upper arm or higher anterolateral thigh area. Observe for syncope for 15 minutes following administration. If the vaccine series is interrupted and only one dose was given, administer the second dose as soon as possible and give the third dose ≥12 weeks later. If the vaccine series is interrupted and the first two doses were given, administer the third dose as soon as possible. The HPV vaccine series should be completed with the same product whenever possible.

For patients at risk of hemorrhage following intramuscular injection, the ACIP recommends "it should be administered intramuscularly if, in the opinion of the physician familiar with the patients bleeding risk, the vaccine can be administered by this route with reasonable safety. If the patient receives antihemophilia or other similar therapy, intramuscular vaccination can be scheduled shortly after such therapy is administered. A fine needle (23 gauge or smaller) can be used for the vaccination and firm pressure applied to the site (without rubbing) for at least 2 minutes. The patient should be instructed concerning the risk of hematoma from the injection." Patients on anticoagulant therapy should be considered to have the same bleeding risks and treated as those with clotting factor disorders (CDC, 2011).

Simultaneous administration of vaccines helps ensure the patients will be fully vaccinated by the appropriate age. Simultaneous administration of vaccines is defined as administering >1 vaccine on the same day at different anatomic sites. Separate vaccines should not be combined in the same syringe unless indicated by product specific labeling. Separate needles and syringes should be used for each injection. The ACIP prefers each dose of a specific vaccine in a series come from the same manufacturer when possible. Adolescents and adults should be vaccinated while seated or lying down. In general, preterm infants should be vaccinated at the same chronological age as full-term infants (CDC, 2011).

Antipyretics have not been shown to prevent febrile seizures. Antipyretics may be used to treat fever or discomfort following vaccination (CDC, 2011). One study reported that routine prophylactic administration of acetaminophen to prevent fever prior to vaccination decreased the immune response of some vaccines; the clinical significance of this reduction in immune response has not been established (Prymula, 2009).

Monitoring and Teaching Issues

Physical Assessment Assess for impaired immune responsiveness; may have reduced antibody response to immunizations. Treatment for anaphylactic/anaphylactoid reaction should be available during vaccine use; if there is a hypersensitivity response after receiving a dose of Gardasil®, patient should not receive further doses. All patients should be informed that the vaccine is not a treatment for active disease and is not a substitute for regular, routine cervical screening. All serious adverse reactions must be reported to the U.S. DHHS. Federal law also requires entry into the patient's medical record.

Patient Education This vaccine is not a treatment for active disease and does not substitute for regular, routine cervical cancer screening. Three doses will be required for effective immunity; consult prescriber for appropriate schedule of vaccinations. May cause fever, headache, or dizziness. May cause some redness, pain, or swelling at injection site; consult prescriber if excessive or persistent. Notify prescriber immediately of any allergic reaction (eg, difficulty breathing; rash; difficulty swallowing; or swelling of hands, feet, face, or lips).

Papillomavirus (Types 16, 18) Vaccine (Human, Recombinant)

(pap ih LO ma VYE rus typs SIX teen AYE teen vak SEEN YU man ree KOM be nant)

U.S. Brand Names Cervarix®

Index Terms Bivalent Human Papillomavirus Vaccine; GSK-580299; HPV 16/18 L1 VLP/AS04 VAC; HPV Vaccine; HPV2; Human Papillomavirus Vaccine; Papillomavirus Vaccine, Recombinant

Generic Availability (U.S.) No

Pharmacologic Category Vaccine, Inactivated (Viral)

Medication Safety Issues

Sound-alike/look-alike issues:

Papillomavirus vaccine types 16, 18 (Cervarix®) may be confused with Papillomavirus vaccine types 6, 11, 16, 18 (Gardasil®)

Cervarix® may be confused with Cerebyx®, Celebrex®

Pregnancy Risk Factor B

Lactation Excretion in breast milk unknown/use caution

Use Females 10 through 25 years of age: Prevention of cervical cancer, cervical adenocarcinoma *in situ*, and cervical intraepithelial neoplasia caused by human papillomavirus (HPV) types 16, 18

The Advisory Committee on Immunization Practices (ACIP) recommends routine vaccination for females 11-12 years of age; catch-up vaccination is recommended for females 13-25 years of age.

Available Dosage Forms

Injection, suspension [preservative free]:

Cervarix®: HPV 16 L1 protein 20 mcg and HPV 18 L1 protein 20 mcg per 0.5 mL (0.5 mL)

Dosing

Adult Immunization: I.M.: Females ≤25 years: 0.5 mL followed by 0.5 mL at 1 and 6 months after initial dose

CDC recommended immunization schedule: Administer first dose to females at age 11-12 years; begin series in females aged 13-25 years if not previously vaccinated. Minimum interval between first and second doses is 4 weeks; the minimum interval between first and third doses is 24 weeks. Inadequate doses or doses received following a shorter than recommended dosing interval should be repeated. The HPV vaccine series should be completed with the same product whenever possible.

Pediatric Immunization: I.M.: Females ≥10 years: 0.5 mL followed by 0.5 mL at 1 and 6 months after initial dose

CDC recommended immunization schedule: Administer first dose to females at age 11-12 years; begin series in females aged 13-25 years if not previously vaccinated. Minimum interval between first and second doses is 4 weeks; the minimum interval between first and third doses is 24 weeks. Inadequate doses or doses received following a shorter than recommended dosing interval should be repeated. The HPV vaccine series should be completed with the same product whenever possible.

Administration

I.M. Shake well prior to use. Do not use if discolored or if containing particulate matter, or if vial or syringe is cracked. Inject I.M. into the deltoid region of the upper arm. Do not administer I.V., SubQ, or intradermally.

For patients at risk of hemorrhage following intramuscular injection, the ACIP recommends "it should be administered intramuscularly if, in the opinion of the physician familiar with the patients bleeding risk, the vaccine can be administered by this route with reasonable safety. If the patient receives antihemophilia or other similar therapy, intramuscular vaccination can be scheduled shortly after such therapy is administered. A fine needle (23 gauge or smaller) can be used for the vaccination and firm pressure applied to the site (without rubbing) for at least 2 minutes. The patient should be instructed concerning the risk of hematoma from the injection." Patients on anticoagulant therapy should be considered to have the same bleeding risks and treated as those with clotting factor disorders (CDC, 2011).

Simultaneous administration of vaccines helps ensure the patients will be fully vaccinated by the appropriate age. Simultaneous administration of vaccines is defined as administering >1 vaccine on the same day at different anatomic sites. Separate vaccines should not be combined in the same syringe unless indicated by product specific labeling. Separate needles and syringes should be used for each injection. The ACIP prefers each dose of a specific vaccine in a series come from the same manufacturer when possible. Adolescents and adults should be vaccinated while seated or lying down. In general, preterm infants should be vaccinated at the same chronological age as full-term infants (CDC, 2011).

Antipyretics have not been shown to prevent febrile seizures. Antipyretics may be used to treat fever or discomfort following vaccination (CDC, 2011). One study reported that routine prophylactic administration of acetaminophen to prevent fever prior to vaccination decreased the immune response of some vaccines; the clinical significance of this reduction in immune response has not been established (Prymula, 2009).

Monitoring and Teaching Issues

Physical Assessment Have emergency treatment for anaphylactoid or hypersensitivity reaction available. Syncope following administration may occur. If latex sensitive, be advised that packaging may contain latex. Emphasize necessity to complete all 3 doses for maximum efficacy. All serious adverse reactions must be reported to the U.S. DHHS. Federal law also requires entry into the patient's medical record.

Patient Education This vaccine is not a substitute for routine cervical cancer screening. It is important for you to receive all 3 doses for maximum benefit. This medication does not protect against disease from HPV already exposed to through sexual activity. You may experience fatigue; headache; abdominal pain; nausea, vomiting, or diarrhea; flu-like symptoms; fever; muscle or joint pain; and redness and tenderness at injection site. Notify prescriber immediately of any allergic reaction (eg, difficulty breathing; rash; difficulty swallowing; or swelling of hands, feet, face, or lips).

◆ **Papillomavirus Vaccine, Recombinant** *see* Papillomavirus (Types 6, 11, 16, 18) Vaccine (Human, Recombinant) *on page 1408*

◆ **Papillomavirus Vaccine, Recombinant** *see* Papillomavirus (Types 16, 18) Vaccine (Human, Recombinant) *on page 1409*

◆ **Paracetamol** *see* Acetaminophen *on page 38*

◆ **Parafon Forte® DSC** *see* Chlorzoxazone *on page 362*

◆ **Paraplatin** *see* CARBOplatin *on page 295*

◆ **Parathyroid Hormone (1-34)** *see* Teriparatide *on page 1736*

◆ **Parcopa®** *see* Carbidopa and Levodopa *on page 291*

Paregoric (par e GOR ik)

Index Terms Camphorated Tincture of Opium (error-prone synonym)
Generic Availability (U.S.) Yes
Pharmacologic Category Analgesic, Opioid

Medication Safety Issues

Sound-alike/look-alike issues:

Camphorated tincture of opium is an error-prone synonym (mistaken as opium tincture)

Paregoric may be confused with Percogesic®

High alert medication: The Institute for Safe Medication Practices (ISMP) includes this medication among its list of drug classes which have a heightened risk of causing significant patient harm when used in error.

Use care when prescribing opium tincture; each mL contains the equivalent of morphine 10 mg; paregoric contains the equivalent of morphine 0.4 mg/mL

Pregnancy Risk Factor B/D (prolonged use or high doses)

Lactation Enters breast milk/use caution

Use Treatment of diarrhea or relief of pain; neonatal opiate withdrawal

Mechanism of Action/Effect Increases smooth muscle tone in GI tract, decreases motility and peristalsis, diminishes digestive secretions

Contraindications Hypersensitivity to opium or any component of the formulation; diarrhea caused by poisoning until the toxic material has been removed; pregnancy (prolonged use or high doses)

Warnings/Precautions May cause CNS depression, which may impair physical or mental abilities; patients must be cautioned about performing tasks which require mental alertness (eg, operating machinery or driving). Effects may be potentiated when used with other sedative drugs or ethanol. Use with caution in patients with respiratory, hepatic or renal dysfunction, adrenal insufficiency, morbid obesity, severe prostatic hyperplasia, urinary stricture, head trauma, thyroid dysfunction, seizure disorder, CNS depression/coma, or history of narcotic abuse. Use with caution in patients with biliary tract dysfunction; acute pancreatitis may cause constriction of sphincter of Oddi. May obscure diagnosis or clinical course of patients with acute abdominal conditions. Opium shares the toxic potential of opiate agonists, and usual precautions of opiate agonist therapy should be observed; some preparations contain sulfites which may cause allergic reactions; infants <3 months of age are more susceptible to respiratory depression, use with caution and generally in reduced doses in this age group; tolerance or drug dependence may result from extended use. Concurrent use of agonist/antagonist analgesics may precipitate withdrawal symptoms and/or reduced analgesic efficacy in patients following prolonged therapy with mu opioid agonists. Abrupt discontinuation following prolonged use may also lead to withdrawal symptoms. Use with caution in the elderly and debilitated patients; may be more sensitive to adverse effects.

Drug Interactions

Avoid Concomitant Use There are no known interactions where it is recommended to avoid concomitant use.

Decreased Effect

Paregoric may decrease the levels/effects of: Pegvisomant

The levels/effects of Paregoric may be decreased by: Ammonium Chloride; Mixed Agonist / Antagonist Opioids

Increased Effect/Toxicity

Paregoric may increase the levels/effects of: Alcohol (Ethyl); Alvimopan; CNS Depressants; Desmopressin; Selective Serotonin Reuptake Inhibitors; Thiazide Diuretics

The levels/effects of Paregoric may be increased by: Amphetamines; Antipsychotic Agents (Phenothiazines); Droperidol; Succinylcholine

Nutritional/Ethanol Interactions Ethanol: Avoid ethanol (may increase CNS depression).

Lab Interactions Increased aminotransferase [ALT/AST] (S)

Adverse Reactions Frequency not defined.

Cardiovascular: Hypotension, peripheral vasodilation

Central nervous system: Drowsiness, dizziness, insomnia, CNS depression, mental depression, increased intracranial pressure, restlessness, headache, malaise

Gastrointestinal: Constipation, anorexia, stomach cramps, nausea, vomiting, biliary tract spasm

Genitourinary: Ureteral spasms, decreased urination, urinary tract spasm

Hepatic: Increased liver function tests

Neuromuscular & skeletal: Weakness

Ocular: Miosis

Respiratory: Respiratory depression

Miscellaneous: Physical and psychological dependence, histamine release

Pharmacodynamics/Kinetics

Metabolism In terms of opium: Hepatic

Excretion In terms of opium: Urine (primarily as morphine glucuronide conjugates and unchanged drug - morphine, codeine, papaverine, etc)

Controlled Substance C-III

Available Dosage Forms

Liquid, oral: Morphine equivalent 2 mg/5 mL (473 mL)

Dosing

Adult & Geriatric Diarrhea: Oral: 5-10 mL 1-4 times/day

Pediatric

Neonatal opiate withdrawal: Oral: 3-6 drops every 3-6 hours as needed, or initially 0.2 mL every 3 hours; increase dosage by approximately 0.05 mL every 3 hours until withdrawal symptoms are controlled; it is rare to exceed 0.7 mL/dose. Stabilize withdrawal symptoms for 3-5 days, then gradually decrease dosage over a 2- to 4-week period.

Diarrhea: Oral: Children: 0.25-0.5 mL/kg 1-4 times/day

Stability

Storage Store in light-resistant, tightly-closed container.

Monitoring and Teaching Issues

Physical Assessment If used to control diarrhea, monitor stools. Monitor for excessive sedation, respiratory depression, or hypotension. For inpatients, implement safety measures (eg, side rails up, call light within reach, patient instructions to call for assistance). Assess patient's physical and/or psychological dependence. Discontinue slowly after prolonged use

Patient Education May cause dependence with prolonged or excessive use. Avoid alcohol or any other prescription and OTC medications that may cause sedation (eg, sleeping medications, some cough/cold remedies, antihistamines). You may experience drowsiness, dizziness, impaired judgment, or postural hypotension. You may experience nausea, loss of appetite, or constipation. Report unresolved nausea, vomiting, respiratory difficulty (shortness of breath or decreased respirations), chest pain, or palpitations.

Breast-Feeding Considerations Information regarding use while breast-feeding is based on experience with morphine. Probably safe with low doses and by administering dose after breast-feeding to further minimize exposure to the drug. Monitor the infant for possible side effects related to opiates.

Additional Information Contains morphine 0.4 mg/mL and alcohol 45%. Do **not** confuse this product with opium tincture which is 25 times **more** potent; each 5 mL of paregoric contains 2 mg morphine equivalent, 0.02 mL anise oil, 20 mg benzoic acid, 20 mg camphor, 0.2 mL glycerin and alcohol; final alcohol content 45%; paregoric also contains papaverine and noscapine; because all of these additives may be harmful to neonates, **a 25-fold dilution of opium tincture** is often preferred for treatment of neonatal abstinence syndrome (opiate withdrawal).

Paricalcitol (pah ri KAL si tole)

U.S. Brand Names Zemplar®

Generic Availability (U.S.) No

Pharmacologic Category Vitamin D Analog

Medication Safety Issues

Sound alike/look alike issues:

Paricalcitol may be confused with calcitriol

Pregnancy Risk Factor C

Lactation Excretion in breast milk unknown/not recommended

Use

I.V.: Prevention and treatment of secondary hyperparathyroidism associated with stage 5 chronic kidney disease (CKD)

Oral: Prevention and treatment of secondary hyperparathyroidism associated with stage 3 and 4 CKD and stage 5 CKD patients on hemodialysis or peritoneal dialysis

Mechanism of Action/Effect Vitamin D analog which suppresses parathyroid hormone release, improving calcium and phosphate homeostasis

Contraindications Hypersensitivity to paricalcitol or any component of the formulation; patients with evidence of vitamin D toxicity; hypercalcemia

Warnings/Precautions Excessive administration may lead to over suppression of PTH, hypercalcemia, hypercalciuria, hyperphosphatemia and adynamic bone disease. Acute hypercalcemia may increase risk of cardiac arrhythmias and seizures; use caution with cardiac glycosides as digitalis toxicity may be increased. Chronic hypercalcemia may lead to generalized vascular and other soft-tissue calcification. Phosphate and vitamin D (and its derivatives) should be withheld during therapy to avoid hypercalcemia. Risk of hypercalcemia may be increased by concomitant use of calcium-containing supplements and/or medications that increase serum calcium (eg, thiazide diuretics). Avoid regular administration to prevent aluminum overload and toxicity. Dialysate concentration of aluminum should be maintained at <10 mcg/L.

Drug Interactions

Metabolism/Transport Effects

Substrate of CYP3A4 (major)

Avoid Concomitant Use

Avoid concomitant use of Paricalcitol with any of the following: Aluminum Hydroxide; Sucralfate; Vitamin D Analogs

Decreased Effect

The levels/effects of Paricalcitol may be decreased by: Bile Acid Sequestrants; Mineral Oil; Orlistat

Increased Effect/Toxicity

Paricalcitol may increase the levels/effects of: Aluminum Hydroxide; Cardiac Glycosides; Digoxin; Sucralfate; Vitamin D Analogs

The levels/effects of Paricalcitol may be increased by: CYP3A4 Inhibitors (Strong); Thiazide Diuretics

Adverse Reactions

>10%:

Gastrointestinal: Nausea (5% to 13%), diarrhea (7% to 12%)

Miscellaneous: Infection (bacterial, fungal, viral: 3% to 15%)

2% to 10%:

Cardiovascular: Edema (7%), hypertension (7%), hypervolemia (5%), hypotension (5%), palpitation (3%), chest pain (3%), peripheral edema (3%), syncope (3%)

Central nervous system: Pain (8%), dizziness (5% to 7%), chills (5%), insomnia (5%), lightheadedness (5%), vertigo (5%), fever (3% to 5%), headache (3% to 5%), anxiety (3%), depression (3%)
Dermatologic: Rash (6%), bruising (3%), skin ulcer (3%)
Endocrine & metabolic: Dehydration (3%), hypoglycemia (3%)
Gastrointestinal: Vomiting (5% to 8%), GI bleeding (5%), constipation (4% to 5%), abdominal pain (4%), dyspepsia (3%), xerostomia (3%)
Genitourinary: Urinary tract infection (3%)
Neuromuscular & skeletal: Arthritis (5%), weakness (3% to 5%), back pain (4%), leg cramps (3%)
Renal: Uremia (3%)
Respiratory: Pneumonia (5%), rhinitis (5%), oropharyngeal pain (4%), bronchitis (3%), cough (3%), sinusitis (3%)
Miscellaneous: Allergic reaction (6%), flu-like syndrome (5%), peritonitis (5%), sepsis (5%)

Pharmacodynamics/Kinetics

Bioavailability Oral: 72% to 86% in healthy subjects

Time to Peak Plasma: 3 hours: Delayed by food

Protein Binding >99%

Half-Life Elimination

Healthy subjects: Oral: 4-6 hours; I.V.: 5-7 hours
Stage 3 and 4 CKD: Oral: 14-20 hours
Stage 5 CKD: Oral: 14-20 hours; I.V.: 14-15 hours

Metabolism Hydroxylation and glucuronidation via hepatic and nonhepatic enzymes, including CYP24, CYP3A4, UGT1A4; forms metabolites (at least one active)

Excretion Healthy subjects: Feces (oral: 70%; I.V.: 63%); urine (oral: 18%, I.V.: 19%)

Available Dosage Forms

Capsule, soft gelatin, oral:
Zemplar®: 1 mcg, 2 mcg, 4 mcg

Injection, solution:
Zemplar®: 2 mcg/mL (1 mL); 5 mcg/mL (1 mL, 2 mL)

Dosing

Adult & Geriatric Note: In stage 3 -5 CKD maintain Ca x P <55 mg^2/dL^2, reduce or interrupt dosing if recommended calcium phosphorus product (Ca x P) is exceeded or hypercalcemia is observed (K/DOQI Clinical Practice Guidelines, 2003).

Secondary hyperparathyroidism associated with chronic renal failure (stage 5 CKD):

I.V.: 0.04-0.1 mcg/kg (2.8-7 mcg) given as a bolus dose no more frequently than every other day at any time during dialysis; dose may be increased by 2-4 mcg every 2-4 weeks; doses as high as 0.24 mcg/kg (16.8 mcg) have been administered safely; the dose of paricalcitol should be adjusted based on serum intact PTH (iPTH) levels, as follows:
Same or increasing iPTH level: Increase paricalcitol dose
iPTH level decreased by <30%: Increase paricalcitol dose
iPTH level decreased by >30% and <60%: Maintain paricalcitol dose
iPTH level decrease by >60%: Decrease paricalcitol dose
iPTH level 1.5-3 times upper limit of normal: Maintain paricalcitol dose

Oral: Initial dose, in mcg, based on baseline iPTH level divided by 80. Administered 3 times weekly, no more frequently than every other day. **Note:** To reduce the risk of hypercalcemia initiate only after baseline serum calcium has been adjusted to ≤9.5 mg/dL.
Dose titration:
Titration dose (mcg) = Most recent iPTH level (pg/mL) divided by 80
Note: In situations where monitoring of iPTH, calcium, and phosphorus occurs less frequently than once per week, a more modest initial and dose titration rate may be warranted:
Modest titration dose (mcg) = Most recent iPTH level (pg/mL) divided by 100
Dosage adjustment for hypercalcemia or elevated Ca x P: Decrease calculated dose by 2-4 mcg. If further adjustment is required, dose should be reduced or interrupted until these parameters are normalized. If applicable, phosphate binder dosing may also be adjusted or withheld, or switch to a noncalcium-based phosphate binder

Secondary hyperparathyroidism associated with stage 3 and 4 CKD: Adults: Oral: Initial dose based on baseline serum iPTH:
iPTH ≤500 pg/mL: 1 mcg/day or 2 mcg 3 times/week
iPTH >500 pg/mL: 2 mcg/day or 4 mcg 3 times/week

Dosage adjustment based on iPTH level relative to baseline, adjust dose at 2-4 week intervals:
iPTH same or increased: Increase paricalcitol dose by 1 mcg/day or 2 mcg 3 times/week
iPTH decreased by <30%: Increase paricalcitol dose by 1 mcg/day or 2 mcg 3 times/week
iPTH decreased by ≥30% and ≤60%: Maintain paricalcitol dose
iPTH decreased by >60%: Decrease paricalcitol dose by 1 mcg/day* or 2 mcg 3 times/week
iPTH <60 pg/mL: Decrease paricalcitol dose by 1 mcg/day* or 2 mcg 3 times/week
*If patient is taking the lowest dose on a once-daily regimen, but further dose reduction is needed, decrease dose to 1 mcg 3 times/week. If further dose reduction is required, withhold drug as needed and restart at a lower dose. If applicable, calcium-phosphate binder dosing may also be adjusted or withheld, or switch to noncalcium-based binder.

Pediatric Secondary hyperparathyroidism associated with chronic renal failure (stage 5 CKD): I.V.: Children ≥5 years: Refer to adult dosing.

Renal Impairment Refer to adult dosing.

Hepatic Impairment
Mild-to-moderate hepatic impairment: No dosage adjustment required.
Severe hepatic impairment: Use has not been evaluated.

Administration

Oral May be administered with or without food. With the 3 times/week dosing schedule, doses should not be given more frequently than every other day.

I.V. Administered as a bolus dose at anytime during dialysis. Doses should not be administered more often than every other day.

Stability

Storage Store at 25°C (77°F); excursions permitted between 15°C to 30°C (59°F to 86°F).

Monitoring and Teaching Issues

Laboratory Monitoring

Serum calcium and phosphorus (closely monitor levels during dosage titration and after initiation of a strong CYP3A4 inhibitor):
- I.V.: Twice weekly during initial phase, then at least monthly once dose established
- Oral: At least every 2 weeks for 3 months or following dose adjustment, then monthly for 3 months, then every 3 months

Calcium phosphorus product (Ca x P): Maintain Ca x P <55 mg^2/dL^2 in stage 3-5 CKD
Serum or plasma intact PTH (iPTH):
- I.V.: Every 3 months
- Oral: At least every 2 weeks for 3 months or following dose adjustment, then monthly for 3 months, then every 3 months

Physical Assessment Instruct patient on dietary requirements.

Patient Education Adhere to diet as recommended (do not take any other vitamin D-related compounds while taking paricalcitol). You may experience nausea, vomiting, lightheadedness, or dizziness. Report gastric disturbances, bone pain, irritability, muscular twitching, or weakness.

Dietary Considerations May be taken with or without food. Some products may contain coconut or palm kernel oil.

Geriatric Considerations No specific dose changes necessary. Monitor closely. It may be advised to obtain baseline electrolytes, calcium, phosphorous, and digoxin serum concentrations, if applicable.

Pregnancy Considerations There are no adequate and well-controlled studies in pregnant women; use during pregnancy only if potential benefit to mother outweighs possible risk to fetus.

◆ **Pariprazole** *see* Rabeprazole *on page* 1544

◆ **Parlodel®** *see* Bromocriptine *on page* 231

◆ **Parlodel® SnapTabs®** *see* Bromocriptine *on page* 231

◆ **Parnate®** *see* Tranylcypromine *on page* 1803

PARoxetine (pa ROKS e teen)

U.S. Brand Names Paxil CR®; Paxil®; Pexeva®

Index Terms Paroxetine Hydrochloride; Paroxetine Mesylate

Generic Availability (U.S.) Yes: Excludes suspension, tablet (mesylate)

Pharmacologic Category Antidepressant, Selective Serotonin Reuptake Inhibitor

Medication Safety Issues

Sound-alike/look-alike issues:
- PARoxetine may be confused with FLUoxetine, PACLitaxel, piroxicam, pyridoxine
- Paxil® may be confused with Doxil®, paclitaxel, Plavix®, PROzac®, Taxol®

Medication Guide Available Yes

Pregnancy Risk Factor D

Lactation Enters breast milk/use caution (AAP rates "of concern"; AAP 2001 update pending)

Use Treatment of major depressive disorder (MDD); treatment of panic disorder with or without agoraphobia; obsessive-compulsive disorder (OCD); social anxiety disorder (social phobia); generalized anxiety disorder (GAD); post-traumatic stress disorder (PTSD); premenstrual dysphoric disorder (PMDD)

Unlabeled/Investigational Use May be useful in eating disorders, impulse control disorders, self-injurious behavior; vasomotor symptoms of menopause; treatment of depression and obsessive-compulsive disorder (OCD) in children; treatment of mild dementia-associated agitation in nonpsychotic patients

Mechanism of Action/Effect Paroxetine is a selective serotonin reuptake inhibitor, chemically unrelated to tricyclic, tetracyclic, or other antidepressants; presumably, the inhibition of serotonin reuptake from brain synapse stimulated serotonin activity in the brain

Contraindications Hypersensitivity to paroxetine or any component of the formulation; use with or within 14 days of MAO inhibitors; concurrent use with thioridazine or pimozide

Warnings/Precautions Hazardous agent - use appropriate precautions for handling and disposal. **[U.S. Boxed Warning]: Antidepressants increase the risk of suicidal thinking and behavior in children, adolescents, and young adults (18-24 years of age) with major depressive disorder (MDD) and other psychiatric disorders;** consider risk prior to prescribing. Short-term studies did not show an increased risk in patients >24 years of age and showed a decreased risk in patients ≥65 years. Closely monitor patients for clinical worsening, suicidality, or unusual changes in behavior, particularly during the initial 1-2 months of therapy or during periods of dosage adjustments (increases or decreases); the patient's family or caregiver should be instructed to closely observe the patient and communicate condition with healthcare provider. A medication guide concerning the use of antidepressants should be dispensed with each prescription. **Paroxetine is not FDA approved for use in children.**

The possibility of a suicide attempt is inherent in major depression and may persist until remission occurs. Patients treated with antidepressants (for any indication) should be observed for clinical worsening and suicidality, especially during the initial few months of a course of drug therapy, or at times of dose changes, either increases or decreases. Use caution in high-risk patients. Worsening depression and severe abrupt suicidality that are not part of the presenting symptoms may require discontinuation or modification of drug therapy. The patient's family or caregiver should be alerted to monitor patients for the emergence of suicidality and associated behaviors (such as agitation, irritability, hostility, impulsivity, and hypomania) and call healthcare provider.

May worsen psychosis in some patients or precipitate a shift to mania or hypomania in patients with bipolar disorder. Patients presenting with depressive symptoms should be screened for bipolar disorder. Monotherapy in patients with bipolar disorder should be avoided. **Paroxetine is not FDA approved for the treatment of bipolar depression.**

Serotonin syndrome and neuroleptic malignant syndrome (NMS)-like reactions have occurred with serotonin/norepinephrine reuptake inhibitors (SNRIs) and selective serotonin reuptake inhibitors (SSRIs) when used alone, and particularly when used in combination with serotonergic agents (eg, triptans) or antidopaminergic agents (eg, antipsychotics). Concurrent use with MAO inhibitors is contraindicated. May increase the risks associated with electroconvulsive therapy. Has a low potential to impair cognitive or motor performance - caution operating hazardous machinery or driving. Symptoms of agitation and/or restlessness may occur during initial few weeks of therapy. Low potential for sedation or anticholinergic effects relative to cyclic antidepressants.

Use caution in patients with a previous seizure disorder or condition predisposing to seizures such as brain damage, alcoholism, or concurrent therapy with other drugs which lower the seizure threshold. Use with caution in patients with hepatic dysfunction and in elderly patients. May cause hyponatremia/SIADH (elderly at increased risk); volume depletion (diuretics may increase risk). Use caution with concomitant use of NSAIDs, ASA, or other drugs that affect coagulation; the risk of bleeding may be potentiated. Use with caution in patients with renal insufficiency or other concurrent illness (due to limited experience); dose reduction recommended with severe renal impairment. May cause or exacerbate sexual dysfunction. Use caution in patients with narrow-angle glaucoma. Avoid use in the first trimester of pregnancy.

Upon discontinuation of paroxetine therapy, gradually taper dose and monitor for discontinuation symptoms (eg, dizziness, dysphoric mood, irritability, agitation, confusion, paresthesias). If intolerable symptoms occur following a decrease in dosage or upon discontinuation of therapy, then resuming the previous dose with a more gradual taper should be considered. Safety and efficacy in children have not been established.

Drug Interactions

Metabolism/Transport Effects **Substrate** of CYP2D6 (major); **Inhibits** CYP1A2 (weak), 2B6 (moderate), 2C9 (weak), 2C19 (weak), 2D6 (strong), 3A4 (weak)

Avoid Concomitant Use

Avoid concomitant use of PARoxetine with any of the following: Iobenguane I 123; MAO Inhibitors; Methylene Blue; Pimozide; Sibutramine; Tamoxifen; Thioridazine; Tryptophan

Decreased Effect

PARoxetine may decrease the levels/effects of: Aprepitant; Fosaprepitant; Iobenguane I 123

The levels/effects of PARoxetine may be decreased by: Aprepitant; CarBAMazepine; Cyproheptadine; Darunavir; Fosamprenavir; Fosaprepitant; Peginterferon Alfa-2b

Increased Effect/Toxicity

PARoxetine may increase the levels/effects of: Alcohol (Ethyl); Alpha-/Beta-Blockers; Anticoagulants; Antidepressants (Serotonin Reuptake Inhibitor/Antagonist); Antiplatelet Agents; Aspirin; Atomoxetine; Beta-Blockers; BusPIRone; CarBAMazepine; CloZAPine; CNS Depressants; Collagenase (Systemic); CYP2B6 Substrates; CYP2D6 Substrates; Desmopressin; Dextromethorphan; Drotrecogin Alfa; DULoxetine; Fesoterodine; Galantamine; Haloperidol; Ibritumomab; Lithium; Methadone; Methotrimeprazine; Methylene Blue; Mexiletine; NSAID (COX-2 Inhibitor); NSAID (Nonselective); Pimozide; Propafenone; RisperiDONE; Salicylates; Serotonin Modulators; Tamoxifen; Tetrabenazine; Thioridazine; Thrombolytic Agents; Tositumomab and Iodine I 131 Tositumomab; TraMADol; Tricyclic Antidepressants; Vitamin K Antagonists

The levels/effects of PARoxetine may be increased by: Analgesics (Opioid); Asenapine; BusPIRone; Cimetidine; CYP2D6 Inhibitors (Moderate); CYP2D6 Inhibitors (Strong); Dasatinib; Droperidol; Glucosamine; Herbs (Anticoagulant/Antiplatelet Properties); MAO Inhibitors; Methotrimeprazine; Metoclopramide; Omega-3-Acid Ethyl Esters; Pentosan Polysulfate Sodium; Pentoxifylline; Prostacyclin Analogues; Sibutramine; TraMADol; Tryptophan

Nutritional/Ethanol Interactions

Ethanol: Avoid ethanol (may increase CNS depression).

Food: Peak concentration is increased, but bioavailability is not significantly altered by food.

Herb/Nutraceutical: Avoid valerian, St John's wort, SAMe, kava kava.

Lab Interactions Increased LFTs

Adverse Reactions Frequency varies by dose and indication. Adverse reactions reported as a composite of all indications.

>10%:

Central nervous system: Somnolence (15% to 24%), insomnia (11% to 24%), headache (17% to 18%), dizziness (6% to 14%)

Endocrine & metabolic: Libido decreased (3% to 15%)

Gastrointestinal: Nausea (19% to 26%), xerostomia (9% to 18%), constipation (5% to 16%), diarrhea (9% to 12%)

Genitourinary: Ejaculatory disturbances (13% to 28%)

Neuromuscular & skeletal: Weakness (12% to 22%), tremor (4% to 11%)

Miscellaneous: Diaphoresis (5% to 14%)

1% to 10%:

Cardiovascular: Vasodilation (2% to 4%), chest pain (3%), palpitation (2% to 3%), hypertension (≥1%), tachycardia (≥1%)

Central nervous system: Nervousness (4% to 9%), anxiety (5%), agitation (3% to 5%), abnormal dreams (3% to 4%), concentration impaired (3% to 4%), yawning (2% to 4%), depersonalization (up to 3%), amnesia (2%), chills (2%), emotional lability (≥1%), vertigo (≥1%), confusion (1%)

Dermatologic: Rash (2% to 3%), pruritus (≥1%)

Endocrine & metabolic: Orgasmic disturbance (2% to 9%), dysmenorrhea (5%)

Gastrointestinal: Appetite decreased (5% to 9%), dyspepsia (2% to 5%), flatulence (4%), abdominal pain (4%), appetite increased (2% to 4%), vomiting (2% to 3%), taste perversion (2%), weight gain (≥1%)

Genitourinary: Genital disorder (male 10%; female 2% to 9%), impotence (2% to 9%), urinary frequency (2% to 3%), urinary tract infection (2%)

Neuromuscular & skeletal: Paresthesia (4%), myalgia (2% to 4%), back pain (3%), myoclonus (2% to 3%), myopathy (2%), myasthenia (1%), arthralgia (≥1%)

Ocular: Blurred vision (4%), abnormal vision (2% to 4%)

Otic: Tinnitus (≥1%)

Respiratory: Respiratory disorder (up to 7%), pharyngitis (4%), sinusitis (up to 4%), rhinitis (3%)

Miscellaneous: Infection (5% to 6%)

Pharmacodynamics/Kinetics

Onset of Action Depression: The onset of action is within a week, however, individual response varies greatly and full response may not be seen until 8-12 weeks after initiation of treatment.

Absorption Completely absorbed following oral administration

Time to Peak Immediate release: 5.2 hours; controlled release: 6-10 hours

Protein Binding 93% to 95%

Half-Life Elimination 21 hours (3-65 hours)

Metabolism Extensively hepatic via CYP2D6 enzymes; primary metabolites are formed via oxidation and methylation of parent drug, with subsequent glucuronide/sulfate conjugation; nonlinear pharmacokinetics (via 2D6 saturation) may be seen with higher doses and longer duration of therapy. Metabolites exhibit ~2% potency of parent compound. C_{min} concentrations are 70% to 80% greater in the elderly compared to nonelderly patients; clearance is also decreased.

Excretion Urine (64%, 2% as unchanged drug); feces (36% primarily via bile, <1% as unchanged drug)

Available Dosage Forms

Suspension, oral:

Paxil®: 10 mg/5 mL (250 mL)

Tablet, oral: 10 mg, 20 mg, 30 mg, 40 mg

Paxil®: 10 mg, 20 mg, 30 mg, 40 mg

Pexeva®: 10 mg, 20 mg, 30 mg, 40 mg

Tablet, controlled release, enteric coated, oral: 12.5 mg, 25 mg, 37.5 mg

Paxil CR®: 12.5 mg, 25 mg, 37.5 mg

Tablet, extended release, enteric coated, oral: 12.5 mg, 25 mg

Dosing

Adult

Major depressive disorder: Oral:

Paxil®, Pexeva®: Initial: 20 mg once daily, preferably in the morning; increase if needed by 10 mg/day increments at intervals of at least 1 week; maximum dose: 50 mg/day

Paxil CR®: Initial: 25 mg once daily; increase if needed by 12.5 mg/day increments at intervals of at least 1 week; maximum dose: 62.5 mg/day

Generalized anxiety disorder (Paxil®, Pexeva®): Oral: Initial: 20 mg once daily, preferably in the morning (if dose is increased, adjust in increments of 10 mg/day at 1-week intervals); doses of 20-50 mg/day were used in clinical trials, however, no greater benefit was seen with doses >20 mg.

Obsessive-compulsive disorder (Paxil®, Pexeva®): Oral: Initial: 20 mg once daily, preferably in the morning; increase if needed by 10 mg/day increments at intervals of at least 1 week; recommended dose: 40 mg/day; range: 20-60 mg/day; maximum dose: 60 mg/day

Panic disorder: Oral:

Paxil®, Pexeva®: Initial: 10 mg once daily, preferably in the morning; increase if needed by 10 mg/day increments at intervals of at least 1 week; recommended dose: 40 mg/day; range: 10-60 mg/day; maximum dose: 60 mg/day

Paxil CR®: Initial: 12.5 mg once daily; increase if needed by 12.5 mg/day at intervals of at least 1 week; maximum dose: 75 mg/day

Premenstrual dysphoric disorder (Paxil CR®): Oral: Initial: 12.5 mg once daily in the morning; may be increased to 25 mg/day; dosing changes should occur at intervals of at least 1 week. May be given daily throughout the menstrual cycle or limited to the luteal phase.

Post-traumatic stress disorder (Paxil®): Oral: Initial: 20 mg once daily, preferably in the morning; increase if needed by 10 mg/day increments at intervals of at least 1 week; range: 20-50 mg. Limited data suggest doses of 40 mg/day were not more efficacious than 20 mg/day.

Social anxiety disorder: Oral:

Paxil®: Initial: 20 mg once daily, preferably in the morning; recommended dose: 20 mg/day; range: 20-60 mg/day; doses >20 mg may not have additional benefit

Paxil CR®: Initial: 12.5 mg once daily, preferably in the morning; may be increased by 12.5 mg/day at intervals of at least 1 week; maximum dose: 37.5 mg/day

Menopause-associated vasomotor symptoms (unlabeled use, Paxil CR®): Oral: 12.5-25 mg/day

Note: Upon discontinuation of paroxetine therapy, gradually taper dose:

Paxil®, Pexeva®: 10 mg/day at weekly intervals; when 20 mg/day dose is reached, continue for 1 week before treatment is discontinued. Some patients may need to be titrated to 10 mg/day for 1 week before discontinuation.

Paxil CR®: Patients receiving 37.5 mg/day in clinical trials had their dose decreased by 12.5 mg/day to a dose of 25 mg/day and remained at a dose of 25 mg/day for 1 week before treatment was discontinued.

Geriatric

Major depressive disorder, obsessive compulsive disorder, panic attack, social anxiety disorder:

Paxil®, Pexeva®: Oral: Initial: 10 mg/day; increase if needed by 10 mg/day increments at intervals of at least 1 week; maximum dose: 40 mg/day

Paxil CR®: Initial: 12.5 mg/day; increase if needed by 12.5 mg/day increments at intervals of at least 1 week; maximum dose: 50 mg/day

Note: Upon discontinuation of paroxetine therapy, gradually taper dose:

Paxil®, Pexeva®: 10 mg/day at weekly intervals; when 20 mg/day dose is reached, continue for 1 week before treatment is discontinued. Some patients may need to be titrated to 10 mg/day for 1 week before discontinuation.

Paxil CR®: Patients receiving 37.5 mg/day in clinical trials had their dose decreased by 12.5 mg/day to a dose of 25 mg/day and remained at a dose of 25 mg/day for 1 week before treatment was discontinued.

Pediatric

Depression (unlabeled use; not recommended by FDA): Oral: Initial: 10 mg/day and adjusted upward on an individual basis to 20 mg/day

Obsessive-compulsive disorder (unlabeled use): Oral: Initial: 10 mg/day and titrate up as necessary to 60 mg/day

Self-injurious behavior (unlabeled use): Oral: 20 mg/day

Social anxiety disorder (unlabeled use): Oral: 2.5-15 mg/day

Renal Impairment

Cl_{cr} <30 mL/minute: Mean plasma concentrations ~4 times that seen in normal function.

Cl_{cr} 30-60 mL/minute: Plasma concentrations 2 times that seen in normal function.

Paxil®, Pexeva®: Adults: Initial: 10 mg/day; increase if needed by 10 mg/day increments at intervals of at least 1 week; maximum dose: 40 mg/day

Paxil CR®: Initial: 12.5 mg/day; increase if needed by 12.5 mg/day increments at intervals of at least 1 week; maximum dose: 50 mg/day

Hepatic Impairment In hepatic dysfunction, plasma concentration is 2 times that seen in normal function.

Paxil®, Pexeva®: Initial: 10 mg/day; increase if needed by 10 mg/day increments at intervals of at least 1 week; maximum dose: 40 mg/day

Paxil CR®: Initial: 12.5 mg/day; increase if needed by 12.5 mg/day increments at intervals of at least 1 week; maximum dose: 50 mg/day

Administration

Oral May be administered without regard to meals. Do not crush, break, or chew controlled release tablets.

Stability

Storage

Suspension: Store at ≤25°C (≤77°F).

Tablet: Store at 15°C to 30°C (59°F to 86°F).

Monitoring and Teaching Issues

Laboratory Monitoring Hepatic and renal function

Physical Assessment Monitor for clinical worsening and suicide ideation. Taper dosage slowly when discontinuing.

Patient Education It may take 2-3 weeks to achieve desired results. Take in the morning to reduce the incidence of insomnia (may be taken with or without food). Do not crush, break, or chew controlled release (Paxil CR®) tablets. Avoid alcohol. Maintain adequate hydration unless instructed to restrict fluid intake. You may experience drowsiness, dizziness, lightheadedness, nausea, vomiting, anorexia, dry mouth, or orthostatic hypotension. Report persistent insomnia or excessive daytime sedation; tremors or weakness; chest pain, palpitations, or rapid heartbeat; vision changes; abnormal bleeding; change in affect or thought processes or abnormal dreams; worsening of condition; or suicide ideation.

Dietary Considerations May be taken without regard to meals.

Geriatric Considerations Paroxetine is the most sedating and anticholinergic of the selective serotonin reuptake inhibitors. Paroxetine has been shown to be an equally effective antidepressant compared to nortriptyline in patients with ischemic heart disease. However, nortriptyline was associated with a significantly higher rate of adverse cardiac events (sustained increase in heart rate, sinus tachycardia, and asymptomatic increase in ventricular ectopy) compared to placebo. The elderly are more prone to SSRI/SNRI-induced hyponatremia.

Breast-Feeding Considerations Paroxetine is excreted in breast milk and concentrations in the hindmilk are higher than in foremilk. Paroxetine has not been detected in the serum of nursing infants and adverse events have not been reported. The manufacturer recommends that caution be exercised when administering paroxetine to nursing women.

The long-term effects on development and behavior have not been studied; therefore, one should prescribe paroxetine to a mother who is breast-feeding only when the benefits outweigh the potential risks.

Pregnancy Considerations Due to adverse events observed in human studies, paroxetine is classified as pregnancy category D. Paroxetine crosses the placenta. The risk of cardiovascular and other congenital malformations may be higher with paroxetine than with other antidepressants. Nonteratogenic effects in the newborn following SSRI exposure late in the third trimester include respiratory distress, cyanosis, apnea, seizures, temperature instability, feeding difficulty, vomiting, hypoglycemia, hypo- or hypertonia, hyper-reflexia, jitteriness, irritability, constant crying, and tremor. An increased risk of low birth weight, lower Apgar scores, and blunted behavioral response to pain for a prolonged period after delivery has also been reported. Exposure to SSRIs after the twentieth week of gestation has been associated with persistent pulmonary hypertension of the newborn (PPHN). Adverse effects may be due to toxic effects of the SSRI or drug withdrawal due to discontinuation. The long-term effects of *in utero* SSRI exposure on infant development and behavior are not known.

Due to pregnancy-induced physiologic changes, women who are pregnant may require increased doses of paroxetine to achieve euthymia. Women treated for major depression and who are euthymic prior to pregnancy are more likely to experience a relapse when medication is discontinued as compared to pregnant women who continue taking antidepressant medications. The ACOG recommends that therapy with SSRIs or SNRIs during pregnancy be individualized; treatment of depression during pregnancy should incorporate the clinical expertise of the mental health clinician, obstetrician, primary healthcare provider, and pediatrician. The ACOG also recommends that therapy with paroxetine be avoided during pregnancy if possible and that fetuses exposed in early pregnancy be assessed with a fetal echocardiography. If treatment during pregnancy is required, consider tapering therapy during the third trimester in order to prevent withdrawal symptoms in the infant. If this is done and the woman is considered to be at risk of relapse from her major depressive disorder, the medication can be restarted following delivery, although the dose should be readjusted to that required before pregnancy. Treatment algorithms have been developed by the ACOG and the APA for the management of depression in women prior to conception and during pregnancy (Yonkers, 2009).

Additional Information Paxil CR® incorporates a degradable polymeric matrix (Geomatrix™) to control dissolution rate over a period of 4-5 hours. An enteric coating delays the start of drug release until tablets have left the stomach.

Related Information

Antidepressant Agents *on page 1982*

- **Paroxetine Hydrochloride** *see* PARoxetine *on page 1414*
- **Paroxetine Mesylate** *see* PARoxetine *on page 1414*
- **Pataday™** *see* Olopatadine (Ophthalmic) *on page 1352*
- **Patanase®** *see* Olopatadine (Nasal) *on page 1352*
- **Patanol®** *see* Olopatadine (Ophthalmic) *on page 1352*
- **Pavulon [DSC]** *see* Pancuronium *on page 1402*
- **Paxil®** *see* PARoxetine *on page 1414*
- **Paxil CR®** *see* PARoxetine *on page 1414*

Pazopanib (paz OH pa nib)

U.S. Brand Names Votrient™

Index Terms GW786034; Pazopanib Hydrochloride

Generic Availability (U.S.) No

Pharmacologic Category Antineoplastic Agent, Tyrosine Kinase Inhibitor; Vascular Endothelial Growth Factor (VEGF) Inhibitor

Medication Safety Issues

Sound-alike/look-alike issues:

Pazopanib may be confused with SUNItinib, vandetanib
Votrient™ may be confused with vorinostat

High alert medication: This medication is in a class the Institute for Safe Medication Practices (ISMP) includes among its list of drug classes which have a heightened risk of causing significant patient harm when used in error.

Medication Guide Available Yes

Pregnancy Risk Factor D

Lactation Excretion in breast milk unknown/not recommended

Use Treatment of advanced renal cell cancer (RCC)

Mechanism of Action/Effect Tyrosine kinase (multikinase) inhibitor; inhibits angiogenesis

Contraindications There are no contraindications listed within the manufacturer's labeling.

Warnings/Precautions [U.S. Boxed Warning]: Severe and fatal hepatotoxicity (transaminase and bilirubin elevations) has been reported with use; monitor hepatic function; may require dosage interruption, reduction, or discontinuation. Transaminase elevations usually occur early in the treatment course. Safety has not been evaluated in patients with pre-existing severe hepatic impairment (bilirubin >3 times ULN with any ALT level) and is not recommended. Patients with total bilirubin ≤1.5 times ULN and ALT and AST ≤2 times ULN were included in clinical trials. Patients >60 years of age may be at higher risk for ALT >3 times ULN. Mild indirect (unconjugated) hyperbilirubinemia may occur in patients with Gilbert's syndrome; follow isolated ALT elevation dosage modification recommendations in patients with known Gilbert's syndrome, mild indirect bilirubin elevation and ALT >3 times ULN.

Arterial thrombotic events, including angina, transient ischemic attack, MI, and ischemic stroke were observed more frequently in the pazopanib group (versus placebo) in clinical trials; fatalities were observed. Use with caution in patients with a history of or an increased risk for these events. Use in patients with recent arteriothrombotic event (within 6 months) has not been studied and is not recommended. Hemorrhagic events (including fatal) have been reported; use is not recommended in patients with a history of hemoptysis, cerebral hemorrhage or clinically significant gastrointestinal hemorrhage within 6 months (these populations were excluded from clinical trials).

May cause and/or worsen hypertension; monitor; blood pressure should be controlled prior to treatment initiation; antihypertensive therapy should be used if needed. Hypertension usually occurs early in the treatment course. Dosage reduction may be necessary for persistent hypertension (despite antihypertensive therapy); discontinue for severe and persistent hypertension which is refractory to dose reduction and antihypertensive therapy. QT_c prolongation, including torsade de pointes, has been observed; use caution in patients with a history of QT_c prolongation, with medications known to prolong the QT interval, or with pre-existing cardiac disease. Obtain baseline and periodic 12-lead ECGs; correct electrolyte (potassium, calcium, and magnesium) abnormalities prior to and during treatment.

Gastrointestinal perforation and fistula (including fatal) have been reported; monitor for symptoms of gastrointestinal perforation and fistula. Proteinuria has been reported with use. Obtain baseline and periodic urinalysis. Discontinue for grade 4 proteinuria. Hypothyroidism has been reported with use; monitor thyroid function tests. Vascular endothelial growth factor (VEGF) receptor inhibitors are associated with impaired wound healing. Discontinue treatment at least 7 days prior to scheduled surgery; treatment reinitiation should be guided by clinical judgment. Discontinue if wound dehiscence occurs.

Patients with mild-to-moderate renal impairment (Cl_{cr} ≥30 mL/minute) were included in trials. There is no pharmacokinetic data in patients with severe renal impairment undergoing dialysis (peritoneal and hemodialysis); however, renal impairment is not expected to influence pazopanib pharmacokinetics or exposure. Avoid use with strong CYP3A4 inhibitors or inducers. If pazopanib must be administered concomitantly with a potent enzyme inhibitor, dose reductions are recommended. Use is not recommended in situations where the use of a strong CYP3A4 inducer is required. Pazopanib inhibits UGT1A1 and OATP1B1; pazopanib may increase concentration of drugs eliminated by UGT1A1 and OATP1B1. Concurrent use with other drugs which may prolong QT_c interval may increase the risk of potentially-fatal arrhythmias.

Drug Interactions

Metabolism/Transport Effects

Substrate of CYP3A4 (major), 1A2 (minor), 2C8 (minor); P-glycoprotein (P-gp, ABCB1); breast cancer resistance protein (BCRP, ABCG2); **Inhibits** CYP3A4 (weak), 2C8 (weak), 2D6 (weak); UGT1A1; OATP1B1

Avoid Concomitant Use

Avoid concomitant use of Pazopanib with any of the following: Artemether; BCG; CYP3A4 Inducers (Strong); Dronedarone; Grapefruit Juice; Lumefantrine; Natalizumab; Nilotinib; Pimecrolimus; Pimozide; QuiNINE; Roflumilast; Tacrolimus (Topical); Tetrabenazine; Thioridazine; Toremifene; Vaccines (Live); Vandetanib; Ziprasidone

Decreased Effect

Pazopanib may decrease the levels/effects of: BCG; Cardiac Glycosides; Sipuleucel-T; Vaccines (Inactivated); Vaccines (Live); Vitamin K Antagonists

The levels/effects of Pazopanib may be decreased by: CYP3A4 Inducers (Strong); Deferasirox; Echinacea; Herbs (CYP3A4 Inducers); P-Glycoprotein Inducers

Increased Effect/Toxicity

Pazopanib may increase the levels/effects of: Dronedarone; Leflunomide; Natalizumab; Pimozide; QTc-Prolonging Agents; QuiNINE; Tetrabenazine; Thioridazine; Toremifene; Vaccines (Live); Vandetanib; Vitamin K Antagonists; Ziprasidone

The levels/effects of Pazopanib may be increased by: Alfuzosin; Artemether; Chloroquine; Ciprofloxacin; Ciprofloxacin (Systemic); CYP3A4 Inhibitors (Moderate); CYP3A4 Inhibitors (Strong); Denosumab; Gadobutrol; Grapefruit Juice; Lapatinib; Lumefantrine; Nilotinib; P-Glycoprotein Inhibitors; Pimecrolimus; QuiNINE; Roflumilast; Tacrolimus (Topical); Trastuzumab

Nutritional/Ethanol Interactions

Food: Systemic exposure of pazopanib is increased when administered with food (AUC twofold higher with a meal). Avoid grapefruit juice (may increase the levels/effects of pazopanib).

Herb/Nutraceutical: Avoid St John's wort (may increase metabolism and decrease pazopanib concentrations).

Adverse Reactions

>10%:

Cardiovascular: Hypertension (40%; grade 3: 4%)

Central nervous system: Fatigue (19%)

Dermatologic: Hair color change (38%)

Endocrine & metabolic: Hyperglycemia (41%), hypophosphatemia (34%), hyponatremia (31%), hypomagnesemia (26%), hypoglycemia (17%)

Gastrointestinal: Diarrhea (52%; grade 3: 3%; grade 4: <1%), lipase increased (4% to 27%), nausea (26%), anorexia (22%), vomiting (21%), abdominal pain (11%)

Hematologic: Leukopenia (37%), neutropenia (34%; grade 3: 1%; grade 4: <1%), thrombocytopenia (32%; grades 3/4: <1%), lymphocytopenia (31%; grade 3: 4%; grade 4: <1%), hemorrhage (5% to 16%)

Hepatic: ALT increased (53%; grade 3: 10%; grade 4: 2%), AST increased (53%; grade 3: 7%; grade 4: <1%), bilirubin increased (36%; grade 3: 3%; grade 4: <1%)

Neuromuscular & skeletal: Weakness (14%)

1% to 10%:

Cardiovascular: Chest pain (5%), MI/ischemia (2%), facial edema (1%), QT prolongation (1%), transient ischemic event (1%)

Central nervous system: Headache (10%)

Dermatologic: Alopecia (8%), rash (8%), palmar-plantar erythrodysesthesia (6%), skin depigmentation (3%)

Endocrine & metabolic: Hypothyroidism (7%)

Gastrointestinal: Weight loss (9%), taste alteration (8%), dyspepsia (5%), rectal hemorrhage (1%)

Renal: Proteinuria (9%), hematuria (4%)

Respiratory: Epistaxis (2%), hemoptysis (2%)

Pharmacodynamics/Kinetics

Bioavailability Rate and extent of bioavailability are increased with food and increased if tablets are crushed (do not crush tablets)

Time to Peak Plasma: 2-4 hours

Protein Binding >99%

Half-Life Elimination ~31 hours

Metabolism Hepatic; primarily via CYP3A4, minor metabolism via CYP1A2 and CYP2C8

Excretion Feces (primarily); urine (<4%)

Available Dosage Forms

Tablet, oral:

Votrient™: 200 mg

Dosing

Adult & Geriatric RCC: Oral: 800 mg once daily.

Concomitant CYP3A4 inhibitors/inducers:

CYP3A4 inhibitors: Avoid concomitant strong CYP3A4 inhibitors (may increase pazopanib concentrations). If pazopanib must be administered concomitantly with a potent enzyme inhibitor, reduce pazopanib to 400 mg once daily with careful monitoring; further dosage reductions may be needed if adverse events occur.

CYP3A4 inducers: Avoid concomitant strong CYP3A4 inducers (may decrease pazopanib concentrations); use of pazopanib is not recommended in situations where the use of a strong CYP3A4 inducer is required.

Renal Impairment No adjustment required.

Hepatic Impairment

Pre-existing impairment:

Moderate: Reduce to 200 mg once daily (maximum tolerated dose in moderate hepatic impairment).

Severe (bilirubin >3 times ULN with any ALT level): Use is not recommended.

During treatment:

Isolated ALT elevations 3-8 times ULN: Continue treatment, monitor liver function weekly until ALT returns to grade 1 or baseline.

Isolated ALT elevations >8 times ULN: Interrupt treatment until ALT returns to grade 1 or baseline. If therapy benefit is greater than the risk of hepatotoxicity, may reinitiate treatment at ≤400 mg once daily (with liver function monitored weekly for 8 weeks); permanently discontinue if ALT >3 times ULN occur with reinitiation.

ALT >3 times ULN concurrently with bilirubin >2 times ULN: Permanently discontinue; monitor until resolution.

Gilbert's syndrome with mild indirect bilirubin elevation and ALT >3 times ULN: Refer to isolated ALT elevations dosage recommendations above.

Adjustment for Toxicity

Initial dosage reduction: Reduce to 400 mg once daily.

Further modification: Increase or decrease dose in 200 mg increments based on individual tolerance; maximum dose: 800 mg.

Proteinuria (grade 4), hypertension (severe, persistent, and refractory to antihypertensives and dose reduction), wound dehiscence: Discontinue treatment.

Administration

Oral Administer on an empty stomach, 1 hour before or 2 hours after a meal. Do not crush. If a dose is missed, do not take if <12 hours until the next dose.

Stability

Storage Store at room temperature of 25°C (77°F); excursions permitted between 15°C and 30°C (59°F and 86°F).

Monitoring and Teaching Issues

Laboratory Monitoring Monitor liver function tests at baseline and at least every 4 weeks for the first 4 months (more frequently if clinically indicated) and periodically thereafter; serum electrolytes (eg, calcium, magnesium, potassium); urinalysis (for proteinuria; baseline and periodic); thyroid function

Physical Assessment Monitor for hypertension, gastrointestinal perforation, diarrhea, hyper-/hypoglycemia, and cardiac changes; dose adjustments may be necessary.

Patient Education Take 1 hour before or 2 hours after food; do not crush. Avoid grapefruit juice. Maintain adequate nutrition and hydration, unless instructed to restrict fluid intake. May cause fatigue, rash or dry skin, loss of hair (may grow back when treatment is completed), nausea, or anorexia. Report persistent gastrointestinal changes, including diarrhea, abdominal pain, nausea, or vomiting; skin rash; dark-colored urine; chest pain or palpitations; difficulty breathing; unusual cough or fever; or signs of infection.

Dietary Considerations Take on an empty stomach, 1 hour before or 2 hours after a meal. Avoid grapefruit juice.

Breast-Feeding Considerations Due to the potential for serious adverse reaction in the nursing infant, breast-feeding is not recommended.

Pregnancy Considerations Adverse effects were observed in animal studies. There are no adequate and well-controlled studies in pregnant women. However, based on its mechanism of action, pazopanib would be expected to cause fetal harm if administered during pregnancy. Women of childbearing potential should avoid becoming pregnant during treatment.

Additional Information Oncology Comment: The National Comprehensive Cancer Network (NCCN) has added pazopanib to the kidney cancer guidelines (v.2.2010) as an option for first-line treatment in patients with either predominant clear cell histology or nonclear cell histology. Pazopanib may also be considered a subsequent treatment option for patients with predominant clear cell histology.

◆ **Pazopanib Hydrochloride** *see* Pazopanib *on page 1418*

◆ **PCA (error-prone abbreviation)** *see* Procainamide *on page 1508*

◆ **PCE®** *see* Erythromycin (Systemic) *on page 658*

◆ **PCEC** *see* Rabies Vaccine *on page 1546*

◆ **PCV** *see* Pneumococcal Conjugate Vaccine (7-Valent) *on page 1469*

◆ **PCV-7** *see* Pneumococcal Conjugate Vaccine (7-Valent) *on page 1469*

◆ **PCV-13** *see* Pneumococcal Conjugate Vaccine (13-Valent) *on page 1470*

◆ **PCV13-CRM(197)** *see* Pneumococcal Conjugate Vaccine (13-Valent) *on page 1470*

◆ **PDX** *see* Pralatrexate *on page 1487*

◆ **PediaCare® Children's Allergy [OTC]** *see* DiphenhydrAMINE (Systemic) *on page 543*

◆ **PediaCare® Children's Decongestant [OTC]** *see* Phenylephrine (Systemic) *on page 1449*

◆ **PediaCare® Children's NightTime Cough [OTC]** *see* DiphenhydrAMINE (Systemic) *on page 543*

◆ **Pediapred®** *see* PrednisoLONE (Systemic) *on page 1497*

◆ **Pediarix®** *see* Diphtheria, Tetanus Toxoids, Acellular Pertussis, Hepatitis B (Recombinant), and Poliovirus Vaccine *on page 555*

◆ **Pedi-Dri®** *see* Nystatin (Topical) *on page 1338*

◆ **PedvaxHIB®** *see* *Haemophilus* b Conjugate Vaccine *on page 893*

◆ **PEG-L-asparaginase** *see* Pegaspargase *on page 1421*

◆ **PEG-ASP** *see* Pegaspargase *on page 1421*

◆ **PEG-asparaginase** *see* Pegaspargase *on page 1421*

Pegaspargase (peg AS par jase)

U.S. Brand Names Oncaspar®

Index Terms L-asparaginase with Polyethylene Glycol; PEG-ASP; PEG-asparaginase; PEG-L-asparaginase; PEGLA; Polyethylene Glycol-L-asparaginase

Generic Availability (U.S.) No

Pharmacologic Category Antineoplastic Agent, Miscellaneous

Medication Safety Issues

Sound-alike/look-alike issues:

Oncaspar® may be confused with Elspar®

Pegaspargase may be confused with asparaginase

High alert medication: The Institute for Safe Medication Practices (ISMP) includes this medication among its list of drugs which have a heightened risk of causing significant patient harm when used in error.

Pregnancy Risk Factor C

Lactation Excretion in breast milk unknown/not recommended

Use Treatment of acute lymphocytic leukemia (ALL); treatment of ALL with previous hypersensitivity to native L-asparaginase

Mechanism of Action/Effect Pegaspargase is a modified version of asparaginase. Leukemic cells, especially lymphoblasts, require exogenous asparagine; normal cells can synthesize asparagine. Asparaginase contains L-asparaginase amidohydrolase type EC-2 which inhibits protein synthesis by deaminating asparagine to aspartic acid and ammonia in the plasma and extracellular fluid and therefore deprives tumor cells of the amino acid for protein synthesis. Asparaginase is cycle-specific for the G_1 phase of the cell cycle.

Contraindications History of serious allergic reactions to pegaspargase; history of any of the following with prior L-asparaginase treatment: pancreatitis, serious hemorrhagic events, serious thrombosis

Warnings/Precautions Hazardous agent - use appropriate precautions for handling and disposal. Serious allergic reactions may occur; discontinue in patients with serious allergic reaction. Observe patients for at least 1 hour after administration; immediate treatment for hypersensitivity reactions should be available during administration. Pegaspargase is indicated for use in patients who have had hypersensitivity reactions to native L-asparaginase; however, in one study, 32% of patients with a history of allergic reaction to *E. coli* asparaginase products also experienced allergic reaction to pegaspargase.

Serious thrombotic events, including sagittal sinus thrombosis may occur; discontinue with serious thrombotic event. Pancreatitis may occur; promptly evaluate patients with abdominal pain; discontinue if pancreatitis occurs during treatment. May cause glucose intolerance; irreversible in some cases; use with caution in patients with hyperglycemia, or diabetes. Coagulopathy has been reported; monitor coagulation parameters; severe or symptomatic coagulopathy may require treatment with fresh-frozen plasma; use with caution in patients with underlying coagulopathy. Reversible hepatotoxicity (hyperbilirubinemia and liver enzyme elevation) may occur; use with caution in patients with hepatic dysfunction or concomitant hepatotoxic medications. Use cautiously in patients with previous hematologic complications from asparaginase.

Drug Interactions

Avoid Concomitant Use

Avoid concomitant use of Pegaspargase with any of the following: BCG; Natalizumab; Pimecrolimus; Roflumilast; Tacrolimus (Topical); Vaccines (Live)

Decreased Effect

Pegaspargase may decrease the levels/effects of: BCG; Sipuleucel-T; Vaccines (Inactivated); Vaccines (Live)

The levels/effects of Pegaspargase may be decreased by: Echinacea; Pegloticase

Increased Effect/Toxicity

Pegaspargase may increase the levels/effects of: Leflunomide; Natalizumab; Vaccines (Live)

The levels/effects of Pegaspargase may be increased by: Denosumab; Pimecrolimus; Roflumilast; Tacrolimus (Topical); Trastuzumab

Adverse Reactions

>5%:

Cardiovascular: Edema
Central nervous system: Fever, malaise
Dermatologic: Rash
Gastrointestinal: Nausea, vomiting
Hematologic: Coagulopathy (7%; grades 3/4: 2%)
Hepatic: Transaminases increased (11%; grades 3/4: 3%)
Miscellaneous: Allergic reactions (including bronchospasm, chills, dyspnea, edema, erythema, hypotension, rash, swelling, urticaria; no prior asparaginase hypersensitivity: 1% to 10%; grades 3/4: 2%; prior asparaginase hypersensitivity: 32%; grades 3/4: 8%)

1% to 5%:

Cardiovascular: Hypotension, peripheral edema, tachycardia, thrombosis (4%)
Central nervous system: Chills, CNS thrombosis (2% to 4%; grades 3/4: 3%), CNS hemorrhage (2%), headache, seizure
Dermatologic: Lip edema, urticaria
Endocrine & metabolic: Hyperglycemia (3% to 5%; grades 3/4: ≤5%), hyperuricemia, hypoglycemia, hypoproteinemia
Gastrointestinal: Abdominal pain, anorexia, diarrhea, pancreatitis (1% to 2%; grades 3/4: 2%)
Hematologic: Anticoagulant effect decreased, disseminated intravascular coagulation (DIC), fibrinogen decreased, hemolytic anemia, leukopenia, pancytopenia, thrombocytopenia, thromboplastin increased, myelosuppression
Hepatic: Liver function tests abnormal (grades 3/4: 5%), hyperbilirubinemia (grades 3/4: 2%), jaundice
Local: Injection site hypersensitivity, pain or reaction
Neuromuscular & skeletal: Arthralgia, limb pain, myalgia, paresthesia
Respiratory: Dyspnea
Miscellaneous: Anaphylactic reactions, night sweats

Pharmacodynamics/Kinetics

Onset of Action Asparagine depletion: I.M.: Within 4 days

Duration of Action Asparagine depletion: I.M.: ~21 days; I.V. (in asparaginase naive adults): 2-4 weeks

Absorption I.M.: Slow

Time to Peak I.M.: 3-4 days

Half-Life Elimination I.M.: ~5.5-6 days; unaffected by age, renal or hepatic function; half-life decreased to 1.8-3.2 days in patients with previous hypersensitivity to native L-asparaginase; I.V.: Adults (asparaginase naive): 7 days

Metabolism Systemically degraded

Excretion Urine (trace amounts)

Available Dosage Forms

Injection, solution [preservative free]:
Oncaspar®: 750 int. units/mL (5 mL)

Dosing

Adult & Geriatric Details concerning dosing in combinations regimens should also be consulted.

Acute lymphoblastic leukemia (ALL): I.M., I.V.: 2500 units/m^2 (as part of a combination chemotherapy regimen), do not administer more frequently than every 14 days

Pediatric Details concerning dosing in combinations regimens should also be consulted.

Acute lymphoblastic leukemia: I.M., I.V.: Refer to adult dosing.

Renal Impairment Hemodialysis, peritoneal dialysis: Significant drug removal is unlikely based on physiochemical characteristics

Administration

I.M. Must only be administered as a deep intramuscular injection into a large muscle. Do not exceed 2 mL per injection site; use multiple injection sites for I.M. injection volume >2 mL.

I.V. Administer over 1-2 hours through a running I.V. infusion line; **do not administer I.V. push.**

Stability

Reconstitution I.V.: Dilute in 100 mL NS or D_5W.

Storage Refrigerate at 2°C to 8°C (36°F to 46°F); do not freeze. Do not use product if it is known to have been frozen. Do not use vial if stored at room temperature for >48 hours. Avoid excessive agitation; do not shake. Do not use if cloudy, discolored, or if precipitate is present. Solutions for infusion should be refrigerated immediately after aseptic preparation and administered within 24 hours of preparation [Data on file (Enzon Pharmaceuticals, 2009)].

Monitoring and Teaching Issues

Laboratory Monitoring CBC with differential, platelets, amylase, liver enzymes, fibrinogen, PT, PTT (coagulation parameters [baseline and periodic]), renal function tests, urine glucose, blood glucose

Physical Assessment Identify allergy with L-asparaginase before beginning therapy. Patient must be closely observed during and for at least 1 hour following administration; treatment for anaphylactic reactions should be available. Monitor for GI disturbance, thrombotic events, pancreatitis, depression of clotting factors, glucose intolerance, and hypotension.

Patient Education This drug is given by infusion or injection; report immediately any redness, swelling, burning, or pain at infusion/injection site or any signs of allergic reaction (eg, respiratory difficulty or swallowing, chest tightness, rash, hives, swelling of lips or mouth, palpitations or rapid heartbeat). Maintain adequate nutrition and hydration, unless instructed to restrict fluid intake. You may be more susceptible to infection. If you have diabetes, check your glucose levels closely and notify prescriber of significant changes; this medication can affect glucose control and diabetic medications may need to be adjusted. May cause nausea, vomiting, loss of appetite, mouth sores, dizziness, fatigue, drowsiness, syncope, or blurred vision. Report immediately any abdominal pain, unusual bruising or bleeding (nose bleeds, bleeding gums, black tarry stools, blood in urine or stool, pinpoint red spots on your skin), persistent nausea or vomiting, and edema (eg, swelling of extremities, sudden weight gain).

Breast-Feeding Considerations Due to the potential for serious adverse reactions in the nursing infant, breast-feeding is not recommended.

Pregnancy Considerations Reproduction studies have not been conducted with pegaspargase.

◆ **Pegasys®** *see* Peginterferon Alfa-2a *on page* 1423

Peginterferon Alfa-2a (peg in ter FEER on AL fa too aye)

U.S. Brand Names Pegasys®

Index Terms Interferon Alfa-2a (PEG Conjugate); Pegylated Interferon Alfa-2a

Generic Availability (U.S.) No

Pharmacologic Category Interferon

Medication Guide Available Yes

Pregnancy Risk Factor C / X in combination with ribavirin

Lactation Excretion in breast milk unknown/not recommended

Use Treatment of chronic hepatitis C (CHC), alone or in combination with ribavirin, in patients with compensated liver disease and not previously treated with alfa interferons (includes patients with histological evidence of cirrhosis [Child-Pugh class A] and patients with clinically-stable HIV disease); treatment of patients with HBeAg positive and HBeAg negative chronic hepatitis B with compensated liver disease and evidence of viral replication and liver inflammation

Mechanism of Action/Effect Alpha interferons are a family of proteins, produced by nucleated cells that have antiviral, antiproliferative, and immune-regulating activity. There are 16 known subtypes of alpha interferons. Interferons interact with cells through high affinity cell surface receptors. Following activation, multiple effects can be detected including induction of gene transcription. Inhibits cellular growth, alters the state of cellular differentiation, interferes with oncogene expression, alters cell surface antigen expression, increases phagocytic activity of macrophages, and augments cytotoxicity of lymphocytes for target cells.

Contraindications Hypersensitivity to polyethylene glycol (PEG), interferon alfa, or any component of the formulation; autoimmune hepatitis; decompensated liver disease in cirrhotic patients (Child-Pugh score >6); decompensated liver disease (Child-Pugh score ≥6, class B and C) in CHC coinfected with HIV; neonates and infants

Warnings/Precautions Hazardous agent: Use appropriate precautions for handling and disposal.

[U.S. Boxed Warning]: May cause or aggravate fatal or life-threatening autoimmune disorders, neuropsychiatric symptoms (including depression and/or suicidal thoughts/ behaviors), ischemic (including radiographic changes or worsening hepatic function) and/or infectious disorders; discontinue treatment for persistent severe or worsening symptoms.

Neuropsychiatric disorders: Severe psychiatric adverse effects (including depression, suicidal ideation, and suicide attempt) may occur. Avoid use in severe psychiatric disorders; use with extreme caution in patients with a history of depression. Patients who experience dizziness, confusion, somnolence or fatigue should use caution when performing tasks which require mental alertness (eg, operating machinery or driving).

Bone marrow suppression: May cause myelosuppression (including neutropenia, thrombocytopenia, lymphopenia, aplastic anemia). Use caution with baseline neutrophil count <1500/mm^3, platelet count <90,000/mm^3 or hemoglobin <10 g/dL. Discontinue therapy (at least temporarily) if ANC <500/mm^3 or platelet count <25,000/mm^3. Use with caution in patients with an increased risk for severe anemia (eg, spherocytosis, history of GI bleeding).

Hepatic disease: Hepatic decompensation and death have been associated with the use of alpha interferons including Pegasys®, in cirrhotic chronic hepatitis C patients; patients coinfected with HIV and receiving highly active antiretroviral therapy have shown an increased risk. Monitor hepatic function; discontinue if decompensation occurs (Child-Pugh score >6) in monoinfected patients and (Child-Pugh score ≥6, class B and C) in patients coinfected with HIV. In hepatitis B patients, flares (transient and potentially severe increases in serum ALT) may occur during or after treatment; more frequent monitoring of LFTs and a dose reduction are recommended. Discontinue if ALT elevation continues despite dose reduction or if increased bilirubin or hepatic decompensation occur.

Gastrointestinal disorders: Gastrointestinal hemorrhage, ulcerative and hemorrhagic/ischemic colitis have been observed with interferon alfa treatment; may be severe and/or life-threatening; discontinue if symptoms of colitis (eg, abdominal pain, bloody diarrhea, and/or fever) develop. Discontinue therapy if known or suspected pancreatitis develops.

Dermatologic disorders: Serious cutaneous reactions, including vesiculobullous eruptions, Stevens-Johnson syndrome and exfoliative dermatitis, have been reported (rarely) with use, with or without ribavirin therapy; discontinue with signs or symptoms of severe skin reactions.

Ophthalmic disease: Discontinue if new or worsening ophthalmologic disorders occur including retinal hemorrhages, cotton wool spots, and retinal artery or vein obstruction; visual exams are recommended in these instances, at the initiation of therapy, and periodically during therapy.

Pulmonary disorders: Dyspnea, pulmonary infiltrates, pneumonia, bronchiolitis obliterans, interstitial pneumonia, and sarcoidosis, resulting in potentially fatal respiratory failure may occur with treatment. Discontinue with unexplained pulmonary infiltrates or evidence of impaired pulmonary function. Use caution in patients with a history of pulmonary disease.

Endocrine disorders: Use with caution in patients with diabetes mellitus; hyper- or hypoglycemia have been reported which may require adjustments in medications. Use with caution in patients with pre-existing thyroid disease; thyroid disorders (hyper- or hypothyroidism) or exacerbations have been reported.

Severe acute hypersensitivity reactions have occurred rarely; prompt discontinuation is advised. Commonly associated with flu-like symptoms, including fever; rule out other causes/ infection with persistent or high fever. Serious and severe infections (bacterial, viral and fungal) have been reported with treatment. Use with caution in patients with renal dysfunction (Cl_{cr} <50 mL/minute); monitor for signs/symptoms of toxicity (dosage adjustment required if toxicity occurs). Use with caution in patients with pulmonary dysfunction, prior cardiovascular disease, or autoimmune disease. Use with caution in the elderly. Safety and efficacy have not been established in children. **Due to differences in dosage, patients should not change brands of interferon without the concurrence of their healthcare provider.** Safety and efficacy have not been established in patients who have failed other alpha interferon therapy, received organ transplants, been coinfected with HBV and HCV or HIV; or with HCV and HIV with a CD4+ cell count <100 cells/microL, or been treated for >48 weeks.

[U.S. Boxed Warning]: Combination treatment with ribavirin may cause birth defects and/ or fetal mortality (avoid pregnancy in females and female partners of male patients); hemolytic anemia (which may worsen cardiac disease), genotoxicity, mutagenicity, and may possibly be carcinogenic.

Drug Interactions

Metabolism/Transport Effects Inhibits CYP1A2 (weak)

Avoid Concomitant Use

Avoid concomitant use of Peginterferon Alfa-2a with any of the following: Telbivudine

Decreased Effect

The levels/effects of Peginterferon Alfa-2a may be decreased by: Pegloticase

Increased Effect/Toxicity

Peginterferon Alfa-2a may increase the levels/effects of: Aldesleukin; Methadone; Ribavirin; Telbivudine; Theophylline Derivatives; Zidovudine

Nutritional/Ethanol Interactions Ethanol: Avoid use in patients with hepatitis C virus.

Adverse Reactions Note: Percentages are reported for peginterferon alfa-2a in chronic hepatitis C (CHC) patients. Other percentages indicated as "with ribavirin" or "in HIV/CHC" are those which significantly exceed incidence reported for peginterferon monotherapy in CHC patients.

>10%:

Central nervous system: Headache (54%), fatigue (56%), pyrexia (37%; 41% with ribavirin; 54% in hepatitis B), insomnia (19%; 30% with ribavirin), depression (18%), dizziness (16%), irritability/anxiety/nervousness (19%; 33% with ribavirin), pain (11%)

Dermatologic: Alopecia (23%; 28% with ribavirin), pruritus (12%; 19% with ribavirin), dermatitis (16% with ribavirin)

Gastrointestinal: Nausea/vomiting (24%), anorexia (17%; 24% with ribavirin), diarrhea (16%), weight loss (16% in HIV/CHC), abdominal pain (15%)

Hematologic: Neutropenia (21%; 27% with ribavirin; 40% in HIV/CHC), lymphopenia (14% with ribavirin), anemia (11% with ribavirin; 14% in HIV/CHC)

Hepatic: ALT increases 5-10 x ULN during treatment (25% to 27% in hepatitis B); ALT increases >10 x ULN during treatment (12% to 18% in hepatitis B); ALT increases 5-10 x ULN after treatment (13% to 16% in hepatitis B); ALT increases >10 x ULN after treatment (7% to 12% in hepatitis B)

Local: Injection site reaction (22%)

Neuromuscular & skeletal: Weakness (56%; 65% with ribavirin), myalgia (37%), rigors (35%; 25% to 27% in hepatitis B), arthralgia (28%)

Respiratory: Dyspnea (13% with ribavirin)

1% to 10%:

Central nervous system: Concentration impaired (8%), memory impaired (5%), mood alteration (3%; 9% in HIV/CHC)

Dermatologic: Dermatitis (8%), rash (5%), dry skin (4%; 10% with ribavirin), eczema (1%; 5% with ribavirin)

Endocrine & metabolic: Hypothyroidism (3% to 4%), hyperthyroidism (≤1%)

Gastrointestinal: Xerostomia (6%), dyspepsia (<1%; 6% with ribavirin), weight loss (4%; 10% with ribavirin)

Hematologic: Thrombocytopenia (5%; 8% in HIV/CHC), lymphopenia (3%), anemia (2%)

Hepatic: Hepatic decompensation (2% in CHC/HIV)

Neuromuscular & skeletal: Back pain (9%)

Ocular: Blurred vision (4%)

Respiratory: Cough (4%; 10% with ribavirin), dyspnea (4%), exertional dyspnea (4% with ribavirin)

Miscellaneous: Diaphoresis (6%), bacterial infection (3%; 5% in HIV/CHC)

Pharmacodynamics/Kinetics

Time to Peak Serum: 72-96 hours

Half-Life Elimination Terminal: 50-160 hours; increased with renal dysfunction

Available Dosage Forms

Injection, solution:

Pegasys®: 180 mcg/mL (1 mL); 180 mcg/0.5 mL (0.5 mL)

Dosing

Adult & Geriatric

Chronic hepatitis C (monoinfection or coinfection with HIV): SubQ:

Monotherapy: 180 mcg once weekly for 48 weeks

Combination therapy with ribavirin: Recommended dosage: 180 mcg once/week with ribavirin (Copegus®)

Duration of therapy: Monoinfection (based on genotype):

Genotype 1,4: 48 weeks

Genotype 2,3: 24 weeks

Duration of therapy: Coinfection: 48 weeks

Note: *American Association for the Study of Liver Diseases (AASLD) guidelines recommendation:* Adults with chronic HCV infection (Ghany, 2009): Treatment of choice: Ribavirin plus **peginterferon**; clinical condition and ability of patient to tolerate therapy should be evaluated to determine length and/or likely benefit of therapy. Recommended treatment duration (AASLD guidelines): Genotypes 1,4: 48 weeks; Genotypes 2,3: 24 weeks; Coinfection with HIV: 48 weeks.

Chronic hepatitis B: SubQ: 180 mcg once weekly for 48 weeks

Renal Impairment

Cl_{cr} <50 mL/minute: Use caution; monitor for toxicity

End-stage renal disease requiring hemodialysis: 135 mcg/week; monitor for toxicity

Hepatic Impairment

HCV: ALT progressively rising above baseline: Decrease dose to 135 mcg/week. If ALT continues to rise or is accompanied by increased bilirubin or hepatic decompensation, discontinue therapy immediately.

HBV:

ALT >5 x ULN: Monitor LFTs more frequently; consider decreasing dose to 135 mcg/week or temporarily discontinuing (may resume after ALT flare subsides).

ALT >10 x ULN: Consider discontinuing.

Adjustment for Toxicity

Dose modifications for adverse events/toxicity:

For moderate-to-severe adverse reactions: Initial: 135 mcg/week; may need decreased to 90 mcg/week in some cases

Based on hematologic parameters:

ANC <750/mm^3: 135 mcg/week

ANC <500/mm^3: Suspend therapy until >1000/mm^3, then restart at 90 mcg/week; monitor ANC

Platelet count <50,000/mm^3: 90 mcg/week

Platelet count <25,000/mm^3: Discontinue therapy

Depression (severity based on DSM-IV criteria):

Mild depression: No dosage adjustment required; evaluate once weekly by visit/phone call. If depression remains stable, continue weekly visits. If depression improves, resume normal visit schedule

Moderate depression: Decrease interferon dose to 90-135 mcg once/week; evaluate once weekly with an office visit at least every other week. If depression remains stable, consider psychiatric evaluation and continue with reduced dosing. If symptoms improve and remain stable for 4 weeks, resume normal visit schedule; continue reduced dosing or return to normal dose.

Severe depression: Discontinue interferon permanently. Obtain immediate psychiatric consultation. Discontinue ribavirin if using concurrently.

Administration

Other SubQ: Administer in the abdomen or thigh. Rotate injection site. Do not use if solution contains particulate matter or is discolored. Discard unused solution. Administration should be done on the same day and at approximately the same time each week.

Stability

Storage Store in refrigerator at 2°C to 8°C (36°F to 46°F). Do not freeze or shake. Protect from light. The following stability information has also been reported:

Intact vial: May be stored at room temperature for up to 14 days (Cohen, 2007).

Prefilled syringe: May be stored at room temperature for up to 6 days (Cohen, 2007).

Monitoring and Teaching Issues

Laboratory Monitoring Clinical studies tested as follows: CBC (including hemoglobin, WBC, and platelets) and chemistries (including liver function tests and uric acid) measured at weeks 1, 2, 4, 6, and 8, and then every 4-6 weeks (more frequently if abnormal); TSH measured every 12 weeks

In addition, the following baseline values were used as entrance criteria:

Platelet count ≥90,000/mm^3 (as low as 75,000/mm^3 in patients with cirrhosis or transition to cirrhosis)

ANC ≥1500/mm^3

Serum creatinine <1.5 times ULN

TSH and T_4 within normal limits or adequately controlled

Serum HCV RNA levels (pretreatment, 12- and 24 weeks after therapy initiation, 24 weeks after completion of therapy). **Note:** Discontinuation of therapy may be considered after 12 weeks in patients with HCV (genotype 1) who fail to achieve an early virologic response (EVR) (defined as ≥2-log decrease in HCV RNA compared to pretreatment) or after 24 weeks with detectable HCV RNA. Treat patients with HCV (genotypes 2,3) for 24 weeks (if tolerated) and then evaluate HCV RNA levels (Ghany, 2009).

Prior to treatment, pregnancy screening should occur for women of childbearing age who are receiving treatment or who have male partners who are receiving treatment. In combination therapy with ribavirin, pregnancy tests should continue monthly up to 6 months after discontinuation of therapy.

Physical Assessment Evaluate for depression and other psychiatric symptoms before and during therapy. Patients may need baseline eye examination; patients with cardiac disease require baseline echocardiogram. Teach patient appropriate injection technique and syringe/ needle disposal.

Patient Education This medication must be given by injection; follow instructions for injection and syringe/needle disposal. Avoid alcohol. You will need laboratory tests and ophthalmic exams prior to and during therapy. May cause headache; insomnia; dizziness; loss of hair (will grow back after therapy); nausea or anorexia; diarrhea; weakness or fatigue; flu-like symptoms; or muscle, skeletal, or joint pain. Report any persistent nausea, vomiting, or abdominal pain; severe depression or suicide ideation; skin rash; pain, redness, or swelling at injection site; signs of infection; unusual bleeding or bruising; changes in vision; or chest pain, palpitations, or respiratory difficulty.

Dietary Considerations Avoid ethanol use in patients with hepatitis C virus.

Geriatric Considerations May require dosage reduction based upon renal dysfunction, but no established guidelines are available. Geriatric patients often have Cl_{cr} <50 mL/minute, as well as, many diseases that put them at risk for adverse effects with this agent. Calculation and measuring creatinine clearance must be done prior to initiating this drug.

Breast-Feeding Considerations Breast milk samples obtained from a lactating mother prior to and after administration of interferon alfa-2b showed that interferon alfa is present in breast milk and administration of the medication did not significantly affect endogenous levels. Breast-feeding is not linked to the spread of hepatitis C virus; however, if nipples are cracked or bleeding, breast-feeding is not recommended. Mothers co-infected with HIV are discouraged from breast-feeding to decrease potential transmission of HIV.

Pregnancy Considerations Reproduction studies with pegylated interferon alfa have not been conducted. Animal studies with nonpegylated interferon alfa-2b have demonstrated abortifacient effects. Disruption of the normal menstrual cycle was also observed in animal studies; therefore, the manufacturer recommends that reliable contraception is used in women of childbearing potential. Alfa interferon is endogenous to normal amniotic fluid. *In vitro* administration studies have reported that when administered to the mother, it does not cross the placenta. Case reports of use in pregnant women are limited. The Perinatal HIV Guidelines Working Group does not recommend that peginterferon-alfa be used during pregnancy. Peginterferon monotherapy should only be used in pregnancy when the potential benefit to the mother justifies the possible risk to the fetus. **[U.S. Boxed Warning]: Combination therapy with ribavirin may cause birth defects; avoid pregnancy in females and female partners of male patients;** combination therapy with ribavirin is contraindicated in pregnancy (refer to Ribavirin monograph); a pregnancy registry has been established for women inadvertently exposed to ribavirin while pregnant (800-593-2214).

◆ **PEGLA** *see* Pegaspargase *on page 1421*

Pegloticase (peg LOE ti kase)

U.S. Brand Names Krystexxa™

Index Terms PEG-Uricase; Pegylated Urate Oxidase; Polyethylene Glycol-Conjugated Uricase; Recombinant Urate Oxidase, Pegylated; Urate Oxidase, Pegylated

Generic Availability (U.S.) No

Pharmacologic Category Enzyme; Enzyme, Urate-Oxidase (Recombinant)

Medication Guide Available Yes

Pregnancy Risk Factor C

Lactation Excretion in breast milk unknown/not recommended

Use Treatment of chronic gout refractory to conventional therapy

Mechanism of Action/Effect Converts uric acid to allantoin (an inactive and water soluble metabolite of uric acid) which lowers serum uric acid concentrations; it does not inhibit the formation of uric acid

Contraindications Glucose-6-phosphate dehydrogenase (G6PD) deficiency

Warnings/Precautions **[U.S. Boxed Warning]: Anaphylaxis and infusion reactions have been reported during and after administration; patients should be closely monitored during infusion and for an appropriate period of time after the infusion. Therapy should be administered in a healthcare facility by skilled medical personnel prepared for the immediate treatment of anaphylaxis. All patients should be premedicated with antihistamines and corticosteroids.** Anaphylaxis may occur at any time during treatment (including the initial dose). **Reactions generally occur within 2 hours of administration; however, delayed hypersensitivity reactions have also been reported.** Infusion reactions are varied; symptoms range from chest pain, pruritus/urticaria, or dyspnea to a clinical presentation of anaphylaxis (eg, hemodynamic instability, perioral or lingual edema). If a less severe (non-anaphylactic) infusion reaction occurs, the infusion may be slowed, or stopped and restarted at a slower rate, at the physician's discretion. **Risk of an infusion reaction is increased in patients whose uric acid is >6 mg/dL; therefore, monitor serum uric acid concentrations prior to infusion and consider discontinuing treatment if concentrations exceed 6 mg/dL, particularly in the event of 2 consecutive concentrations >6 mg/dL.**

Therapy with antihyperuricemic agents commonly results in gout flare, particularly upon initiation due to rapid lowering of urate concentrations; gout flare-ups during treatment do not warrant discontinuation of therapy. Gout flare prophylaxis is recommended, using nonsteroidal anti-inflammatory agents (NSAID) or colchicines, unless contraindicated, beginning ≥1 week before initiation of pegloticase and continuing for at least 6 months. Exacerbation of heart failure has been observed in clinical trials; use caution in patients with pre-existing heart failure. Due to the risk for hemolysis and methemoglobinemia, pegloticase is contraindicated in patients with G6PD deficiency. Patients at higher risk for G6PD deficiency (eg, African, Mediterranean) should be screened prior to therapy. Therapy is not appropriate for the treatment of asymptomatic hyperuricemia. Potential for immunogenicity exists with the use of therapeutic proteins. Antipegloticase antibodies and antiPEG antibodies commonly occurred during clinical trials in pegloticase-treated patients. High antipegloticase antibody titers were associated with failure to maintain uric acid normalization and were also associated with a higher incidence of infusion reactions. Due to potential for immunogenicity, closely monitor patients who reinitiate therapy after discontinuing treatment for >4 weeks; patients may be at increased risk for anaphylaxis and infusion reactions.

Drug Interactions

Avoid Concomitant Use There are no known interactions where it is recommended to avoid concomitant use.

Decreased Effect

Pegloticase may decrease the levels/effects of: Certolizumab Pegol; Pegademase Bovine; Pegaptanib; Pegaspargase; Pegfilgrastim; Peginterferon Alfa-2a; Peginterferon Alfa-2b; Pegvisomant

Increased Effect/Toxicity There are no known significant interactions involving an increase in effect.

Adverse Reactions

>10%:

Dermatologic: Bruising (11%), urticaria (11%)

Gastrointestinal: Nausea (12%)

Miscellaneous: Antibody formation (antipegloticase antibodies: 92%; antiPEG antibodies: 42%), gout flare (74% within the first 3 months), infusion reactions (26%)

1% to 10%:

Cardiovascular: Chest pain (6% to 10%)

Dermatologic: Erythema (10%), pruritus (10%)

Gastrointestinal: Constipation (6%), vomiting (5%)

Respiratory: Dyspnea (7%), nasopharyngitis (7%)

Miscellaneous: Anaphylaxis (≤7%)

Frequency not defined: Anemia, diarrhea, headache, muscle spasms, nephrolithiasis

Pharmacodynamics/Kinetics

Onset of Action ~24 hours following the first dose, serum uric acid concentrations decreased

Duration of Action >300 hours (12.5 days)

Half-Life Elimination Median: ~14 days

Available Dosage Forms

Injection, solution:

Krystexxa™: Uricase protein 8 mg/mL (2 mL)

Dosing

Adult & Geriatric Refractory gout: I.V.: 8 mg every 2 weeks

Note: Premedicate with antihistamines and corticosteroids. Gout flare prophylaxis with either NSAIDs or colchicine is also recommended, beginning at least 1 week prior to initiation and continuing for at least 6 months.

Renal Impairment Creatinine clearance did not alter the pharmacokinetics; dosage adjustments are not needed.

Administration

I.V. Administer diluted solution by I.V. infusion over ≥120 minutes via gravity feed or an infusion pump or syringe-type pump. Do **not** administer by I.V. push or bolus. Administer in a healthcare setting by healthcare providers prepared to manage potential anaphylaxis. Monitor closely for infusion reactions during infusion and for an appropriate period of time after the infusion (anaphylaxis has been reported within 2 hours of the infusion). In the event or a less severe infusion reaction, infusion may be slowed, or stopped and restarted at a slower rate, based on the discretion of the physician.

Stability

Reconstitution To prepare solution for administration, withdraw 1 mL (8 mg) and add to a 250 mL bag of NS or ½NS; invert bag several times to mix thoroughly (do **not** shake). Do not use vial if particulate matter is present or if solution is discolored (solution should be a clear and colorless). After withdrawal, discard any unused portion of the product remaining in the vial.

Storage Prior to use, vials must be stored in the carton to protect from light and kept under refrigeration between 2°C to 8°C (36° to 46°F) at all times. Do **not** shake or freeze.

Diluted solution may be stored up to 4 hours at 2°C to 8°C (36°F to 46°F). Diluted solution is also stable for 4 hours at room temperature of 20°C to 25°C (68°F to 77°F); however, refrigeration is preferred. The diluted solution should be protected from light, not frozen, and used within 4 hours of dilution. Prior to administration, allow the diluted solution to reach room temperature; do not warm to room temperature using any form of artificial heating such as a microwave or warm water bath.

Monitoring and Teaching Issues

Breast-Feeding Considerations Due to the potential for serious adverse reactions in the nursing infant, breast-feeding is not recommended.

Pregnancy Considerations Adequate animal reproduction studies have not been conducted. There are no adequate and well-controlled studies in pregnant women. Use during pregnancy only if the benefit to the mother outweigh the potential risk to the fetus.

◆ **PEG-Uricase** *see* Pegloticase *on page 1427*

Pegvisomant (peg VI soe mant)

U.S. Brand Names Somavert®

Index Terms B2036-PEG

Generic Availability (U.S.) No

Pharmacologic Category Growth Hormone Receptor Antagonist

Pregnancy Risk Factor B

Lactation Excretion in breast milk unknown/use caution

Use Treatment of acromegaly in patients resistant to or unable to tolerate other therapies

Available Dosage Forms

Injection, powder for reconstitution:

Somavert®: 10 mg, 15 mg, 20 mg

Dosing

Adult & Geriatric Acromegaly: SubQ: Initial loading dose: 40 mg; maintenance dose: 10 mg once daily; doses may be adjusted by 5 mg increments in 4- to 6-week intervals based on IGF-I concentrations (maximum maintenance dose: 30 mg/day)

Hepatic Impairment

At initiation of therapy:

Normal liver function test (LFT): Initiate therapy; monitor LFT monthly for first 6 months, quarterly for next 6 months, then biannually the following year.

Baseline LFT elevated but ≤3 x ULN: May initiate therapy with monthly evaluation of LFT for 1 year then biannually the following year.

Baseline LFT >3 times ULN: Do not initiate treatment without comprehensive work-up to determine cause; monitor closely if treatment is started.

With ongoing therapy:

LFT ≥3 x but <5 x ULN without signs/symptoms of hepatitis, hepatic injury, or increase in total bilirubin: Continue treatment, but monitor LFT weekly for further increases; perform comprehensive hepatic work-up to rule out alternative cause of hepatic dysfunction

LFT ≥5 x ULN or transaminase ≥3 x ULN associated with any increase in total bilirubin: Discontinue immediately and perform comprehensive hepatic work-up. If LFTs return to normal, may cautiously consider restarting therapy with frequent LFT monitoring.

Signs or symptoms of hepatitis or hepatic injury: Discontinue therapy immediately and perform comprehensive hepatic work-up; discontinue permanently if liver injury is confirmed.

Administration

Other For SubQ administration only; to minimize the risk for lipohypertrophy, rotate injection site daily; may administer in upper arm, thigh, abdomen, or buttocks; do not rub injection site. The manufacturer recommends the initial dose be administered under the supervision of prescribing healthcare provider.

Monitoring and Teaching Issues

Laboratory Monitoring Serum glucose, serum IGF-I (every 4-6 weeks after initial dose and dosage change, every 6 months when normalized)

Liver function tests (ALT, AST, total bilirubin, and alkaline phosphatase levels):

Baseline:

Normal: Monthly for first 6 months, quarterly for next 6 months, biannually for the next year

Elevated, but ≤3 x ULN: Monitor monthly for at least 1 year, then biannually the next year

>3 x ULN: Withhold treatment; perform comprehensive liver function evaluation (rule out cholelithiasis or choledocholithiasis); if appropriate for treatment, closely monitor hepatic function and clinical status.

During therapy:

≥3 x but <5 x ULN without signs/symptoms of hepatitis, hepatic injury or increase in total bilirubin: monitor weekly for further increases; perform comprehensive hepatic work-up

≥5 x ULN or transaminase ≥3 x ULN associated with any increase in total bilirubin: Comprehensive hepatic work-up. If appropriate for treatment monitor closely

Physical Assessment First dose should be administered under supervision of prescriber.

Patient Education This medication may only be administered by injection. Report immediately any redness, swelling, or itching at injection site. May cause diarrhea, nausea, or allergic response (eg, chest pain, respiratory difficulty, skin rash).

- ◆ **Pegylated DOXOrubicin Liposomal** *see* DOXOrubicin (Liposomal) *on page* 582
- ◆ **Pegylated Interferon Alfa-2a** *see* Peginterferon Alfa-2a *on page* 1423
- ◆ **Pegylated Liposomal DOXOrubicin** *see* DOXOrubicin (Liposomal) *on page* 582
- ◆ **Pegylated Urate Oxidase** *see* Pegloticase *on page* 1427

Pemetrexed (pem e TREKS ed)

U.S. Brand Names Alimta®

Index Terms LY231514; Pemetrexed Disodium

Generic Availability (U.S.) No

Pharmacologic Category Antineoplastic Agent, Antimetabolite; Antineoplastic Agent, Antimetabolite (Antifolate)

Medication Safety Issues

Sound-alike/look-alike issues:

PEMEtrexed may be confused with methotrexate, PRALAtrexate

High alert medication: This medication is in a class the Institute for Safe Medication Practices (ISMP) includes among its list of drug classes which have a heightened risk of causing significant patient harm when used in error.

Pregnancy Risk Factor D

Lactation Excretion in breast milk unknown/not recommended

Use Treatment of unresectable malignant pleural mesothelioma (in combination with cisplatin); treatment of locally advanced or metastatic nonsquamous nonsmall cell lung cancer (NSCLC; as initial treatment in combination with cisplatin, as single-agent maintenance treatment after 4 cycles of initial platinum-based double therapy, and single-agent treatment after prior chemotherapy)

Unlabeled/Investigational Use Treatment of bladder cancer (metastatic), cervical cancer (recurrent or metastatic), ovarian cancer (recurrent or persistent), thymic malignancies; treatment of malignant pleural mesothelioma (either as a single agent or in combination with carboplatin)

Mechanism of Action/Effect Disrupts folate-dependent metabolic processes essential for cell replication.

Contraindications Severe hypersensitivity to pemetrexed or any component of the formulation

Canadian labeling (additional contraindications; not in U.S. labeling): Concomitant yellow fever vaccine

Warnings/Precautions Hazardous agent - use appropriate precautions for handling and disposal. Hypersensitivity (including anaphylaxis) has been reported with use. May cause bone marrow suppression (anemia, neutropenia, thrombocytopenia and/or pancytopenia); may require dose reductions in subsequent cycles. Prophylactic folic acid and vitamin B_{12} supplements are necessary to reduce hematologic and gastrointestinal toxicity and infection; initiate supplementation 1 week before the first dose of pemetrexed. Pretreatment with corticosteroids (dexamethasone or equivalent) reduces the incidence and severity of cutaneous reactions. Rarely, Stevens-Johnson syndrome and toxic epidermal necrolysis have been reported. Effects of third space fluid on drug disposition is unknown; consider draining effusion(s) prior to treatment. Use caution with hepatic dysfunction not due to metastases; may require dose adjustment. Interstitial pneumonitis with respiratory insufficiency has been observed with use; interrupt therapy and evaluate promptly with progressive dyspnea and cough.

The manufacturer does not recommend use in patients with Cl_{cr} <45 mL/minute. Decreased renal function results in increased toxicity. Use caution in patients receiving concurrent nephrotoxins; may result in delayed pemetrexed clearance. NSAIDs may reduce the clearance of pemetrexed; pemetrexed and ibuprofen (up to 1600 mg/day) may be administered in patients with Cl_{cr} ≥80 mL/minute; use with caution in patients with Cl_{cr} 45-79 mL/minute. Interruption of NSAID therapy may be necessary prior to, during, and immediately after pemetrexed therapy. Not indicated for use in patients with squamous cell NSCLC.

Drug Interactions

Avoid Concomitant Use

Avoid concomitant use of PEMEtrexed with any of the following: BCG; Natalizumab; Pimecrolimus; Roflumilast; Tacrolimus (Topical); Vaccines (Live)

Decreased Effect

PEMEtrexed may decrease the levels/effects of: BCG; Sipuleucel-T; Vaccines (Inactivated); Vaccines (Live)

The levels/effects of PEMEtrexed may be decreased by: Echinacea

Increased Effect/Toxicity

PEMEtrexed may increase the levels/effects of: Leflunomide; Natalizumab; Vaccines (Live)

The levels/effects of PEMEtrexed may be increased by: Denosumab; NSAID (Nonselective); Pimecrolimus; Roflumilast; Tacrolimus (Topical); Trastuzumab

Nutritional/Ethanol Interactions Lower ANC nadirs occur in patients with elevated baseline cystathionine or homocysteine concentrations. Levels of these substances can be reduced by folic acid and vitamin B_{12} supplementation.

Adverse Reactions Note: Reported for single-agent therapy in patients who received folate and B_{12} supplementation.

>10%:

Central nervous system: Fatigue (25% to 34%; dose-limiting)

Dermatologic: Rash/desquamation (10% to 14%)

Gastrointestinal: Nausea (19% to 31%), anorexia (19% to 22%), vomiting (9% to 16%), stomatitis (7% to 15%), diarrhea (5% to 13%)

Hematologic: Anemia (15% to 19%; grades 3/4: 3% to 4%), leukopenia (6% to 12%; grades 3/4: 2% to 4%), neutropenia (6% to 11%; grades 3/4: 3% to 5%; nadir: 8-10 days; recovery: 12-17 days; dose-limiting)

Respiratory: Pharyngitis (15%)

1% to 10%:

Cardiovascular: Edema (1% to 5%)

Central nervous system: Fever (1% to 8%)

Dermatologic: Pruritus (1% to 7%), alopecia (1% to 6%), erythema multiforme (≤5%)

Gastrointestinal: Constipation (1% to 6%), weight loss (1%), abdominal pain (≤5%)

Hematologic: Thrombocytopenia (1% to 8%; grades 3/4: 2%; dose-limiting), febrile neutropenia (grades 3/4: 2%)

Hepatic: ALT increased (8% to 10%; grades 3/4: ≤2%), AST increased (7% to 8%; grades 3/4: ≤1%)

Neuromuscular & skeletal: Sensory neuropathy (≤9%), motor neuropathy (≤5%)

Ocular: Conjunctivitis (≤5%), lacrimation increased (≤5%)

Renal: Creatinine increased/creatinine clearance decreased (1% to 5%)

Miscellaneous: Allergic reaction/hypersensitivity (≤5%), infection (≤5%), sepsis (1%)

Pharmacodynamics/Kinetics

Duration of Action V_{dss}: 16.1 L

Protein Binding ~73% to 81%

Half-Life Elimination Normal renal function: 3.5 hours; Cl_{cr} 40-59 mL/minute: 5.3-5.8 hours

Metabolism Minimal

Excretion Urine (70% to 90% as unchanged drug)

Available Dosage Forms

Injection, powder for reconstitution:

Alimta®: 100 mg, 500 mg

Dosing

Adult & Geriatric Details concerning dosing in combination regimens should also be consulted. **Note:** Start vitamin supplements 1 week before initial pemetrexed dose: Folic acid 350-1000 mcg/day orally (must be taken at least 5 out of 7 days prior to treatment initiation; continue daily during treatment and for 21 days after last pemetrexed dose) and vitamin B_{12} 1000 mcg I.M. during the week prior to treatment initiation and then every 3 cycles. Give dexamethasone 4 mg orally twice daily for 3 days, beginning the day before treatment to minimize cutaneous reactions. New treatment cycles should not begin unless ANC ≥1500/mm^3, platelets ≥100,000/mm^3, and Cl_{cr} ≥45 mL/minute.

Malignant pleural mesothelioma: I.V.: 500 mg/m^2 on day 1 of each 21-day cycle (in combination with cisplatin) **or** (unlabeled) in combination with carboplatin (Castagneto, 2008; Ceresoli, 2006) **or** (unlabeled) as single-agent therapy (Jassem, 2008; Taylor, 2008)

Nonsmall cell lung cancer: I.V:

Initial treatment: 500 mg/m^2 on day 1 of each 21-day cycle (in combination with cisplatin)

Maintenance or second-line treatment: 500 mg/m^2 on day 1 of each 21-day cycle (as a single-agent)

Bladder cancer (unlabeled use): I.V.: 500 mg/m^2 on day 1 of each 21-day cycle (Sweeney, 2006)

Renal Impairment

Cl_{cr} ≥45 mL/minute: No dosage adjustment required.

Cl_{cr} <45 mL/minute: No dosage adjustment guidelines are available; manufacturer recommends not using the drug.

Concomitant NSAID use with renal dysfunction:

Cl_{cr} 45 to 79 mL/minute and ibuprofen (up to 1600 mg/day): Use with caution.

Cl_{cr} 45 to 79 mL/minute and NSAIDs with short half-lives (eg, indomethacin, ketoprofen, ketorolac): Avoid for 2 days before, the day of, and for 2 days following a dose of pemetrexed.

Any creatinine clearance and NSAIDs with long half-lives (eg, nabumetone, naproxen, oxaprozin, piroxicam): Avoid for 5 days before, the day of, and 2 days following a dose of pemetrexed.

Hepatic Impairment Grade 3 (5.1-20 times ULN) **or** 4 (>20 times ULN) transaminase elevation: Reduce pemetrexed dose to 75% of previous dose (and cisplatin).

Adjustment for Toxicity

Toxicity: Discontinue if patient develops grade 3 or 4 toxicity after two dose reductions or immediately if grade 3 or 4 neurotoxicity develops

Hematologic toxicity: Upon recovery, reinitiate therapy

Nadir ANC <500/mm^3 and nadir platelets ≥50,000/mm^3: Reduce dose to 75% of previous dose of pemetrexed (and cisplatin)

Nadir platelets <50,000/mm^3 **without bleeding** (regardless of nadir ANC): Reduce dose to 75% of previous dose of pemetrexed (and cisplatin)

Nadir platelets <50,000/mm^3 **with bleeding** (regardless of nadir ANC): Reduce dose to 50% of previous dose of pemetrexed (and cisplatin)

Nonhematologic toxicity ≥grade 3 (excluding neurotoxicity): Withhold treatment until recovery to baseline; upon recovery, reinitiate therapy as follows:

Grade 3 or 4 toxicity (excluding mucositis): Reduce dose to 75% of previous dose of pemetrexed (and cisplatin)

Grade 3 or 4 diarrhea or any diarrhea requiring hospitalization: Reduce dose to 75% of previous dose of pemetrexed (and cisplatin)

Grade 3 or 4 mucositis: Reduce pemetrexed dose to 50% of previous dose (continue cisplatin at 100% of previous dose)

Neurotoxicity:

Grade 0-1: Continue pemetrexed at 100% of previous dose (and cisplatin)

Grade 2: Continue pemetrexed at 100% of previous dose; reduce cisplatin dose to 50% of previous dose

Administration

I.V. Infuse over 10 minutes.

Stability

Reconstitution Reconstitute with NS (preservative free); add 4.2 mL to the 100 mg vial and 20 mL to the 500 mg vial, resulting in a 25 mg/mL concentration. Gently swirl. Solution may be colorless to green-yellow. Further dilute in 100 mL NS for infusion; may also dilute in D_5W (Zhang, 2006), although the manufacturer recommends NS. Use appropriate precautions for handling and disposal.

Storage Store intact vials at room temperature of 25°C (77°F); excursions permitted to 15°C to 30°C (59°F to 86°F). Reconstituted solution in NS and infusion solutions (in D_5W or NS) are stable for 24 hours when refrigerated at 2°C to 8°C (36°F to 46°F) or stored at room temperature of 15°C to 30°C (59°F to 86°F). Concentrations at 25 mg/mL are stable in polypropylene syringes for 2 days at room temperature (23°C) (Zhang, 2005).

Monitoring and Teaching Issues

Laboratory Monitoring CBC with differential and platelets (before each dose; monitor for nadir and recovery); serum creatinine, BUN, total bilirubin, ALT, AST (periodic)

Physical Assessment See pre- and post-treatment medication requirements (eg, start oral folic acid and vitamin B_{12} [injection] 1 week before first dose). Corticosteroids may be used to reduce cutaneous reactions. Monitor for CNS changes, GI upset (nausea, vomiting, diarrhea, constipation), anemia, neuropathy, rash, and infection.

Patient Education This medication is only administered intravenously. Report immediately any burning, pain, itching, or redness at infusion site or any sudden feelings of anxiety, difficulty breathing, chest discomfort, or back pain. It is important that you maintain adequate nutrition and hydration, unless instructed to restrict fluid intake. Maintain regularly scheduled dietary supplements (vitamin B_{12} and folic acid) as prescribed. May cause severe nausea, vomiting, constipation, diarrhea, or mouth sores. Report immediately any chest pain, swelling of extremities, unusual weight gain, rash, tingling or loss of sensation in extremities, difficulty breathing, fever, chills, or unusual or persistent fatigue.

Dietary Considerations Initiate folic acid supplementation 1 week before first dose of pemetrexed, continue for full course of therapy, and for 21 days after last dose. Institute vitamin B_{12} 1 week before the first dose; administer every 9 weeks thereafter.

Breast-Feeding Considerations Due to the potential for serious adverse reactions in the nursing infant, breast-feeding is not recommended.

Pregnancy Considerations Adverse events were observed in animal reproduction studies. There are no adequate and well-controlled studies in pregnant women. Women of child-bearing potential should have a negative serum pregnancy test prior to treatment and should use effective contraceptive measures to avoid becoming pregnant during treatment. Irreversible infertility has been reported in males; prior to receiving treatment, males should be counseled on sperm storage. The Canadian labeling recommends that males receiving therapy use effective contraceptive measures and not father a child during, and for up to 6 months after therapy.

◆ **Pemetrexed Disodium** *see* Pemetrexed *on page 1429*

Penicillin G Benzathine (pen i SIL in jee BENZ a theen)

U.S. Brand Names Bicillin® L-A

Index Terms Benzathine Benzylpenicillin; Benzathine Penicillin G; Benzylpenicillin Benzathine

Generic Availability (U.S.) No

Pharmacologic Category Antibiotic, Penicillin

Medication Safety Issues

Sound-alike/look-alike issues:

Penicillin may be confused with penicillamine

Bicillin® may be confused with Wycillin®

Bicillin® C-R (penicillin G benzathine and penicillin G procaine) may be confused with Bicillin® L-A (penicillin G benzathine). Penicillin G benzathine is the only product currently approved for the treatment of syphilis. Administration of penicillin G benzathine and penicillin G procaine combination instead of Bicillin® L-A may result in inadequate treatment response.

Penicillin G benzathine may only be administered by deep intramuscular injection; intravenous administration of penicillin G benzathine has been associated with cardiopulmonary arrest and death.

Pregnancy Risk Factor B

Lactation Enters breast milk/use caution

Use Active against some gram-positive organisms, few gram-negative organisms such as *Neisseria gonorrhoeae*, and some anaerobes and spirochetes; used in the treatment of syphilis; used only for the treatment of mild to moderately-severe upper respiratory tract infections caused by organisms susceptible to low concentrations of penicillin G or for prophylaxis of infections caused by these organisms; primary and secondary prevention of rheumatic fever

Available Dosage Forms

Injection, suspension:

Bicillin® L-A: 600,000 units/mL (1 mL, 2 mL, 4 mL)

Dosing

Adult & Geriatric

Usual dosage range: I.M.: 1.2-2.4 million units as a single dose

Group A streptococcal upper respiratory infection: 1.2 million units as a single dose

Secondary prevention of glomerulonephritis: 1.2 million units every 4 weeks or 600,000 units twice monthly

Secondary prevention of rheumatic fever: 1.2 million units every 3-4 weeks or 600,000 units twice monthly

Syphilis (CDC, 2010):

Primary, Secondary, Early Latent (<1 year duration): 2.4 million units as a single dose in 2 injection sites

Late Latent, Latent with unknown duration: 2.4 million units in 2 injection sites once weekly for 3 doses

Neurosyphilis: Not indicated as single-drug therapy, but may be given once weekly for 3 weeks following I.V. treatment; refer to Penicillin G (Parenteral/Aqueous) monograph for dosing

Pediatric

Usual dosage range: I.M.: 25,000-50,000 units/kg as a single dose (maximum: 2.4 million units)

Congenital syphilis (asymptomatic): I.M.: Neonates >1200 g: 50,000 units/kg as a single dose

Group A streptococcal upper respiratory infection: I.M.: Infants and Children:

Primary prevention of rheumatic fever (Gerber, 2009): ≤27 kg: 600,000 units as a single dose; >27 kg: 1.2 million units as a single dose

Secondary prevention of rheumatic fever (Gerber, 2009): ≤27 kg: 600,000 units every 3-4 weeks; >27 kg: 1.2 million units every 3-4 weeks

Syphilis (CDC, 2010): I.M.:

Primary, Secondary, Early Latent (<1 year duration): Infants and Children: 50,000 units/kg as a single injection (maximum: 2.4 million units)

Late Latent, Latent with unknown duration: Children: 50,000 units/kg every week for 3 doses (maximum: 2.4 million units/dose)

Administration

I.M. Warm to room temperature before administration to lessen the pain associated with injection. Administer by deep I.M. injection in the upper outer quadrant of the buttock; in children <2 years of age, I.M. injections should be made into the midlateral muscle of the thigh, not the gluteal region. Do not inject near an artery or a nerve; permanent neurological damage or gangrene may result. When doses are repeated, rotate the injection site. **Do not administer I.V., intra-arterially, or SubQ.**

Monitoring and Teaching Issues

Laboratory Monitoring Perform culture and sensitivity before administering first dose.

Physical Assessment Assess results of culture and sensitivity tests and patient's allergy history prior to starting therapy. Use with caution in presence of impaired renal function or history of seizures. Monitor for hypersensitivity reactions and opportunistic infection.

Patient Education This drug can only be given by injection. Report immediately any redness, swelling, burning, or pain at injection site or any signs of allergic reaction (eg, respiratory difficulty or swallowing, chest tightness, rash, hives, swelling of lips or mouth). Maintain adequate hydration unless instructed to restrict fluid intake. If being treated for sexually-transmitted disease, partner will also need to be treated. May cause confusion or drowsiness. Report persistent adverse effects or signs of opportunistic infection (eg, fever, chills, diarrhea, unhealed sores, white plaques in mouth or vagina, purulent vaginal discharge).

Penicillin G (Parenteral/Aqueous) (pen i SIL in jee pa REN ter al AYE kwee us)

U.S. Brand Names Pfizerpen®

Index Terms Benzylpenicillin Potassium; Benzylpenicillin Sodium; Crystalline Penicillin; Penicillin G Potassium; Penicillin G Sodium

Generic Availability (U.S.) Yes

Pharmacologic Category Antibiotic, Penicillin

Medication Safety Issues

Sound-alike/look-alike issues:

Penicillin may be confused with penicillamine

Pregnancy Risk Factor B

Lactation Enters breast milk/compatible

Use Treatment of infections (including sepsis, pneumonia, pericarditis, endocarditis, meningitis, anthrax) caused by susceptible organisms; active against some gram-positive organisms, generally not *Staphylococcus aureus*; some gram-negative organisms such as *Neisseria gonorrhoeae*, and some anaerobes and spirochetes

Mechanism of Action/Effect Interferes with bacterial cell wall synthesis during active multiplication, causing cell wall death and resultant bactericidal activity against susceptible bacteria

Contraindications Hypersensitivity to penicillin or any component of the formulation

Warnings/Precautions Avoid intra-arterial administration or injection into or near major peripheral nerves or blood vessels since such injections may cause severe and/or permanent neurovascular damage; use with caution in patients with renal impairment (dosage reduction required), concomitant renal and hepatic impairment (further dosage adjustment may be required), pre-existing seizure disorders, or with a history of hypersensitivity to cephalosporins. Prolonged use may result in fungal or bacterial superinfection, including *C. difficile*-associated diarrhea (CDAD) and pseudomembranous colitis; CDAD has been observed >2 months postantibiotic treatment. Serious and occasionally severe or fatal hypersensitivity (anaphylactoid) reactions have been reported in patients on penicillin therapy, especially with a history of beta-lactam hypersensitivity, history of sensitivity to multiple allergens, or previous IgE-mediated reactions (eg, anaphylaxis, angioedema, urticaria). Use with caution in asthmatic patients. Extended duration of therapy or use associated with high serum concentrations may be associated with an increased risk for some adverse reactions. Neonates may have decreased renal clearance of penicillin and require frequent dosage adjustments depending on age. Product contains sodium and potassium; high doses of I.V. therapy may alter serum levels.

Drug Interactions

Avoid Concomitant Use

Avoid concomitant use of Penicillin G (Parenteral/Aqueous) with any of the following: BCG

Decreased Effect

Penicillin G (Parenteral/Aqueous) may decrease the levels/effects of: BCG; Mycophenolate; Typhoid Vaccine

The levels/effects of Penicillin G (Parenteral/Aqueous) may be decreased by: Fusidic Acid; Tetracycline Derivatives

Increased Effect/Toxicity

Penicillin G (Parenteral/Aqueous) may increase the levels/effects of: Methotrexate

The levels/effects of Penicillin G (Parenteral/Aqueous) may be increased by: Probenecid

Lab Interactions False-positive or negative urinary glucose determination using Clinitest®; positive Coombs' [direct]; false-positive urinary and/or serum proteins

Adverse Reactions Frequency not defined.

Central nervous system: Coma (high doses), hyper-reflexia (high doses), seizures (high doses)
Dermatologic: Contact dermatitis, rash
Endocrine & metabolic: Electrolyte imbalance (high doses)
Gastrointestinal: Pseudomembranous colitis
Hematologic: Neutropenia, positive Coombs' hemolytic anemia (rare, high doses)
Local: Injection site reaction, phlebitis, thrombophlebitis
Neuromuscular & skeletal: Myoclonus (high doses)
Renal: Acute interstitial nephritis (high doses), renal tubular damage (high doses)
Miscellaneous: Anaphylaxis, hypersensitivity reactions (immediate and delayed), Jarisch-Herxheimer reaction, serum sickness

Pharmacodynamics/Kinetics

Time to Peak Serum: I.M.: ~30 minutes; I.V.: ~1 hour

Protein Binding 65%

Half-Life Elimination

Neonates: <6 days old: 3.2-3.4 hours; 7-13 days old: 1.2-2.2 hours; >14 days old: 0.9-1.9 hours
Children and Adults: Normal renal function: 30-50 minutes
End-stage renal disease: 3.3-5.1 hours

Metabolism Hepatic (30%) to penicilloic acid

Excretion Urine (58% to 85% as unchanged drug)

Available Dosage Forms

Infusion, premixed iso-osmotic dextrose solution: 1 million units (50 mL); 2 million units (50 mL); 3 million units (50 mL)

Injection, powder for reconstitution: 5 million units, 20 million units
Pfizerpen®: 5 million units, 20 million units

Dosing

Adult & Geriatric

***Actinomyces* species:** I.V.: 10-20 million units/day divided every 4-6 hours for 4-6 weeks
Clostridium perfringens: I.V.: 24 million units/day divided every 4-6 hours with clindamycin
Corynebacterium diptheriae: I.V.: 2-3 million units/day in divided doses every 4-6 hours for 10-12 days
Erysipelas: I.V.: 1-2 million units every 4-6 hours
Erysipelothrix: I.V.: 2-4 million units every 4 hours
Fascial space infections: I.V.: 2-4 million units every 4-6 hours with metronidazole
Leptospirosis: I.V.: 1.5 million units every 6 hours for 7 days
Listeria: I.V.: 15-20 million units/day in divided doses every 4-6 hours for 2 weeks (meningitis) or 4 weeks (endocarditis)
Lyme disease (meningitis): I.V.: 20 million units/day in divided doses
Neurosyphilis: I.V.: 18-24 million units/day in divided doses every 4 hours (or by continuous infusion) for 10-14 days (CDC, 2006; CDC, 2009; CDC, 2010)
Streptococcus:
Brain abscess: I.V.: 18-24 million units/day in divided doses every 4 hours with metronidazole
Endocarditis or osteomyelitis: I.V.: 3-4 million units every 4 hours for at least 4 weeks
Pregnancy (prophylaxis GBS): I.V.: 5 million units x 1 dose, then 2.5 million units every 4 hours until delivery (ACOG, 2002; CDC, 2002)
Skin and soft tissue: I.V.: 3-4 million units every 4 hours for 10 days
Toxic shock: I.V.: 24 million units/day in divided doses with clindamycin
Streptococcal pneumonia: I.V.: 2-3 million units every 4 hours
Whipple's disease: I.V.: 2 million units every 4 hours for 2 weeks, followed by oral trimethoprim/sulfamethoxazole or doxycycline for 1 year
Relapse or CNS involvement: 4 million units every 4 hours for 4 weeks

Pediatric

Susceptible infections: I.M., I.V.:
Infants ≥1 month and Children: 100,000-400,000 units/kg/day in divided doses every 4-6 hours (maximum dose: 24 million units/day)
***Meningitis* (gonococcal):** I.V.: 250,000 units/kg/day in 4 divided doses
Moderate infections: I.M., I.V.: 100,000-250,000 units/kg/day in 4 divided doses
Neurosyphilis: I.V.: 200,000-300,000 units/kg/day divided every 4-6 hours for 10-14 days (maximum dose: 24 million units/day)
Severe infections: I.M., I.V.: 250,000-400,000 units/kg/day in divided doses every 4-6 hours (maximum dose: 24 million units/day)
Syphilis (congenital): I.V.:
Infants: 50,000 units/kg every 12 hours for first 7 days of life, then every 8 hours for a total of 10 days (CDC, 2010)
Children: 50,000 units/kg every 4-6 hours for 10 days (CDC, 2010)

Renal Impairment Dosage modification is required in patients with renal insufficiency.

Uremic patients with Cl_{cr} >10 mL/minute/1.73 m^2: Administer full loading dose followed by 1/2 of the loading dose given every 4-5 hours
Cl_{cr} <10 mL/minute/1.73 m^2: Administer full loading dose followed by 1/2 of the loading dose given every 8-10 hours

Administration

I.M. Administer I.M. by deep injection in the upper outer quadrant of the buttock. Administer injection around-the-clock to promote less variation in peak and trough levels. **Note:** The 20 million unit dosage form may be administered by continuous I.V. infusion only.

I.V. Usually administered by intermittent infusion. In some centers, large doses may be administered by continuous I.V. infusion. **Note:** The 20 million unit dosage form may by administered be continuous I.V. infusion only.

Intermittent I.V.: May be dissolved in small amounts of SWFI, NS, D_5W and administered peripherally as a 50,000-100,000 unit/mL solution. In fluid-restricted patients, 146,000 units/mL in SW results in a maximum recommended osmolality for peripheral infusion. Infuse over 15-30 minutes.

Continuous I.V. infusion: Determine the volume of fluid and rate of its administration required by the patient in a 24-hour period. Add the appropriate daily dosage of penicillin to this fluid. For example, if the daily dose is 10 million units and 2 L of fluid/day is required, add 5 million units to 1 L and adjust the rate of flow so the liter will be infused over 12 hours (83 mL/hour). Repeat steps (5 million units/L at 83 mL/hour) for the remaining 12 hours.

Stability

Reconstitution

Intermittent I.V.: 5 million unit vial: Add 8.2 mL for a final concentration of 500,000 units/mL; add 3.2 mL for a final concentration of 1,000,000 units/mL. Dilute further to 50,000-145,000 units/mL prior to infusion.

Continuous I.V. infusion: 20 million unit vial: Add 11.5 mL for a final concentration of 1,000,000 units/mL. Dilute further in 1-2 L of infusion solution and administer over a 24-hour period.

Storage

Penicillin G potassium powder for injection should be stored below 86°F (30°C). Following reconstitution, solution may be stored for up to 7 days under refrigeration. Premixed bags for infusion should be stored in the freezer (-20°C to -4°F); frozen bags may be thawed at room temperature or in refrigerator. Once thawed, solution is stable for 14 days if stored in refrigerator or for 24 hours when stored at room temperature. Do not refreeze once thawed.

Penicillin G sodium powder for injection should be stored at controlled room temperature. Reconstituted solution may be stored under refrigeration for up to 3 days.

Monitoring and Teaching Issues

Laboratory Monitoring Perform culture and sensitivity before administering first dose; periodic electrolyte, hepatic, renal, cardiac and hematologic function tests during prolonged/high-dose therapy

Physical Assessment Assess results of culture and sensitivity tests and patient's allergy history prior to starting therapy. Use with caution and monitor closely in presence of renal impairment or seizure disorder. Avoid intravascular or intra-arterial administration or injection into or near major peripheral nerves or blood vessels; may cause severe and/or permanent neurovascular damage. Monitor for hypersensitivity reactions, opportunistic infection (fever, chills, unhealed sores, white plaques in mouth or vagina, purulent vaginal discharge, fatigue), CNS changes, and thrombophlebitis.

Patient Education This drug can only be given by injection or infusion. Report immediately any redness, swelling, burning, or pain at infusion site or any signs of allergic reaction (eg, respiratory or swallowing difficulty, chest tightness, rash, hives, swelling of lips or mouth). Maintain adequate hydration unless instructed to restrict fluid intake. If being treated for sexually-transmitted disease, partner will also need to be treated. May cause confusion or drowsiness. Report signs of opportunistic infection (eg, fever, chills, diarrhea, unhealed sores, white plaques in mouth or vagina, purulent vaginal discharge).

Dietary Considerations Some products may contain potassium and/or sodium.

Geriatric Considerations Despite a reported prolonged half-life, it is usually not necessary to adjust the dose of penicillin G or VK in elderly to account for renal function changes with age, however, it is advised to calculate an estimated creatinine clearance and adjust dose accordingly.

Breast-Feeding Considerations Very small amounts of penicillin G transfer into breast milk. Peak milk concentrations occur at approximately 1 hour after an IM dose and are higher if multiple doses are given. The manufacturer recommends that caution be exercised when administering penicillin to nursing women. Nondose-related effects could include modification of bowel flora and allergic sensitization.

Pregnancy Considerations Adverse events have not been observed in animal studies; therefore, penicillin G is classified as pregnancy category B. Penicillin crosses the placenta and distributes into amniotic fluid. There is no evidence of adverse fetal effects after penicillin use during pregnancy in humans. Penicillin G is the drug of choice for treatment of syphilis during pregnancy and penicillin G (parenteral/aqueous) is the drug of choice for the prevention of early-onset Group B Streptococcal (GBS) disease in newborns.

Additional Information 1 million units is approximately equal to 625 mg.

Related Information

Antimicrobial Drugs of Choice *on page 2008*

◆ **Penicillin G Potassium** *see* Penicillin G (Parenteral/Aqueous) *on page 1433*

Penicillin G Procaine (pen i SIL in jee PROE kane)

Index Terms APPG; Aqueous Procaine Penicillin G; Procaine Benzylpenicillin; Procaine Penicillin G; Wycillin [DSC]

Generic Availability (U.S.) Yes

Pharmacologic Category Antibiotic, Penicillin

Medication Safety Issues

Sound-alike/look-alike issues:

Penicillin G procaine may be confused with penicillin V potassium

Wycillin® may be confused with Bicillin®

Pregnancy Risk Factor B

Lactation Enters breast milk/compatible

Use Treatment of moderately-severe infections due to *Treponema pallidum* and other penicillin G-sensitive microorganisms that are susceptible to low, but prolonged serum penicillin concentrations; anthrax due to *Bacillus anthracis* (postexposure) to reduce the incidence or progression of disease following exposure to aerolized *Bacillus anthracis*

Available Dosage Forms

Injection, suspension: 600,000 units/mL (1 mL, 2 mL)

Dosing

Adult & Geriatric

Anthrax:

Inhalational (postexposure prophylaxis): I.M.: 1,200,000 units every 12 hours

Note: Overall treatment duration should be 60 days. Available safety data suggest continued administration of penicillin G procaine for longer than 2 weeks may incur additional risk of adverse reactions. Clinicians may consider switching to effective alternative treatment for completion of therapy beyond 2 weeks.

Cutaneous (treatment): I.M.: 600,000-1,200,000 units/day; alternative therapy is recommended in severe cutaneous or other forms of anthrax infection

Endocarditis caused by susceptible viridans *Streptococcus* (when used in conjunction with an aminoglycoside): I.M.: 1.2 million units every 6 hours for 2-4 weeks

Gonorrhea (uncomplicated): 4.8 million units as a single dose divided in 2 sites given 30 minutes after probenecid 1 g orally

Neurosyphilis: I.M.: 2.4 million units/day with 500 mg probenecid by mouth 4 times/day for 10-14 days; **penicillin G aqueous I.V. is the preferred agent**

Whipple's disease: I.M.: 1.2 million units/day (with streptomycin) for 10-14 days, followed by oral trimethoprim/sulfamethoxazole or doxycycline for 1 year

Pediatric

Susceptible infections: I.M.: Infants and Children: 25,000-50,000 units/kg/day in divided doses 1-2 times/day; not to exceed 4.8 million units/24 hours

Anthrax, inhalational (postexposure prophylaxis): I.M.: 25,000 units/kg every 12 hours (maximum: 1,200,000 units every 12 hours).

Note: Overall treatment duration should be 60 days. Available safety data suggest continued administration of penicillin G procaine for longer than 2 weeks may incur additional risk for adverse reactions. Clinicians may consider switching to effective alternative treatment for completion of therapy beyond 2 weeks.

Syphilis (congenital): I.M.: 50,000 units/kg/day once daily for 10 days; if more than 1 day of therapy is missed, the entire course should be restarted

Renal Impairment

Cl_{cr} 10-30 mL/minute: Administer every 8-12 hours.

Cl_{cr} <10 mL/minute: Administer every 12-18 hours.

Moderately dialyzable (20% to 50%)

Administration

I.M. Procaine suspension is for deep I.M. injection only. Rotate the injection site. Do not inject in gluteal muscle in children <2 years of age. Avoid I.V., intravascular, or intra-arterial administration of penicillin G procaine since severe and/or permanent neurovascular damage may occur.

Monitoring and Teaching Issues

Laboratory Monitoring Periodic renal and hematologic function with prolonged therapy; WBC count; perform culture and sensitivity before administering first dose.

Physical Assessment Assess results of culture and sensitivity tests and patient's allergy history prior to starting therapy. Use with caution and monitor closely in presence of renal impairment or seizure disorder. Avoid intravascular or intra-arterial administration or injection into or near major peripheral nerves or blood vessels; may cause severe and/or permanent neurovascular damage. Monitor for hypersensitivity reactions and opportunistic infection (fever, chills, unhealed sores, white plaques in mouth or vagina, purulent vaginal discharge, fatigue), CNS changes, and thrombophlebitis.

Patient Education This drug can only be given by injection. Report immediately any redness, swelling, burning, or pain at injection site or any signs of allergic reaction (eg, respiratory or swallowing difficulty, chest tightness, rash, hives, swelling of lips or mouth). Maintain adequate hydration unless instructed to restrict fluid intake. If being treated for sexually-transmitted disease, partner will also need to be treated. May cause confusion or drowsiness. Report signs of opportunistic infection (eg, fever, chills, diarrhea, unhealed sores, white plaques in mouth or vagina, purulent vaginal discharge).

◆ **Penicillin G Sodium** *see* Penicillin G (Parenteral/Aqueous) *on page* 1433

Penicillin V Potassium (pen i SIL in vee poe TASS ee um)

Index Terms Pen VK; Phenoxymethyl Penicillin

Generic Availability (U.S.) Yes

Pharmacologic Category Antibiotic, Penicillin

Medication Safety Issues

Sound-alike/look-alike issues:

Penicillin V procaine may be confused with penicillin G potassium

Pregnancy Risk Factor B

Lactation Enters breast milk/compatible

Use Treatment of infections caused by susceptible organisms involving the respiratory tract, otitis media, sinusitis, skin, and urinary tract; prophylaxis in rheumatic fever

Mechanism of Action/Effect Inhibits bacterial cell wall synthesis by binding to one or more of the penicillin-binding proteins (PBPs); which in turn inhibits the final transpeptidation step of peptidoglycan synthesis in bacterial cell walls, thus inhibiting cell wall biosynthesis. Bacteria eventually lyse due to ongoing activity of cell wall autolytic enzymes (autolysins and murein hydrolases) while cell wall assembly is arrested.

Contraindications Hypersensitivity to penicillin or any component of the formulation

Warnings/Precautions Use with caution in patients with severe renal impairment (modify dosage) or history of seizures. Serious and occasionally severe or fatal hypersensitivity (anaphylactoid) reactions have been reported in patients on penicillin therapy, especially with a history of beta-lactam hypersensitivity, history of sensitivity to multiple allergens, or previous IgE-mediated reactions (eg, anaphylaxis, angioedema, urticaria). Use with caution in asthmatic patients. Extended duration of therapy or use associated with high serum concentrations may be associated with an increased risk for some adverse reactions. Prolonged use may result in fungal or bacterial superinfection, including *C. difficile*-associated diarrhea (CDAD) and pseudomembranous colitis; CDAD has been observed >2 months postantibiotic treatment.

Drug Interactions

Avoid Concomitant Use

Avoid concomitant use of Penicillin V Potassium with any of the following: BCG

Decreased Effect

Penicillin V Potassium may decrease the levels/effects of: BCG; Mycophenolate; Typhoid Vaccine

The levels/effects of Penicillin V Potassium may be decreased by: Fusidic Acid; Tetracycline Derivatives

Increased Effect/Toxicity

Penicillin V Potassium may increase the levels/effects of: Methotrexate

The levels/effects of Penicillin V Potassium may be increased by: Probenecid

Nutritional/Ethanol Interactions Food: Decreases drug absorption rate; decreases drug serum concentration.

Lab Interactions False-positive or negative urinary glucose determination using Clinitest®; positive Coombs' [direct]; false-positive urinary and/or serum proteins

Adverse Reactions >10%: Gastrointestinal: Mild diarrhea, vomiting, nausea, oral candidiasis

Pharmacodynamics/Kinetics

Absorption 60% to 73%

Time to Peak Serum: 0.5-1 hour

Protein Binding Plasma: 80%

Half-Life Elimination 30 minutes; prolonged with renal impairment

Excretion Urine (as unchanged drug and metabolites)

Available Dosage Forms

Powder for solution, oral: 125 mg/5 mL (100 mL, 200 mL); 250 mg/5 mL (100 mL, 200 mL)

Tablet, oral: 250 mg, 500 mg

Dosing

Adult & Geriatric

Actinomycosis:

Mild: 2-4 g/day in 4 divided doses for 8 weeks

Surgical: 2-4 g/day in 4 divided doses for 6-12 months (after I.V. penicillin G therapy of 4-6 weeks)

Erysipelas: 500 mg 4 times/day

Pharyngitis (streptococcal): 500 mg 3-4 times/day for 10 days

Prophylaxis of pneumococcal or recurrent rheumatic fever infections: 250 mg twice daily

Pediatric

Pharyngitis (streptococcal): 250 mg 2-3 times/day for 10 days

Prophylaxis of pneumococcal infections:

Children <5 years: 125 mg twice daily

Children ≥5 years: 250 mg twice daily

Prophylaxis of recurrent rheumatic fever:

Children <5 years: 125 mg twice daily

Children ≥5 years: 250 mg twice daily

Renal Impairment

Cl_{cr} 10-50 mL/minute: Administer every 8-12 hours.

Cl_{cr} <10 mL/minute: Administer every 12-16 hours.

Administration

Oral Administer around-the-clock to promote less variation in peak and trough serum levels. Take on an empty stomach 1 hour before or 2 hours after meals, to enhance absorption, take until gone, do not skip doses.

Stability

Storage Refrigerate suspension after reconstitution; discard after 14 days.

Monitoring and Teaching Issues

Laboratory Monitoring Periodic renal and hematologic function during prolonged therapy; perform culture and sensitivity before administering first dose.

Physical Assessment Assess results of culture and sensitivity tests and patient's allergy history prior to starting therapy. Use with caution in presence of renal impairment. Monitor for hypersensitivity reactions and opportunistic infection (fever, chills, unhealed sores, white plaques in mouth or vagina, purulent vaginal discharge, fatigue).

Patient Education Take at intervals around-the-clock, preferably on an empty stomach (1 hour before or 2 hours after a meal). Maintain adequate hydration unless instructed to restrict fluid intake. May cause nausea, vomiting, or diarrhea. Report signs of opportunistic infection (eg, fever, chills, diarrhea, unhealed sores, white plaques in mouth or vagina, purulent vaginal discharge) or signs of hypersensitivity reaction (rash, hives, itching, swelling of lips, tongue, mouth, or throat).

Dietary Considerations Take on an empty stomach 1 hour before or 2 hours after meals.

Geriatric Considerations Dosage adjustment in the elderly is usually not necessary.

Breast-Feeding Considerations Penicillins are excreted in breast milk. The manufacturer recommends that caution be exercised when administering penicillin to nursing women. Nondose-related effects could include modification of bowel flora and allergic sensitization.

Pregnancy Considerations Adverse events have not been observed in animal studies; therefore, penicillin V is classified as pregnancy category B. Penicillin crosses the placenta and distributes into amniotic fluid. There is no evidence of adverse fetal effects after penicillin use during pregnancy in humans. Due to pregnancy-induced physiologic changes, some pharmacokinetic parameters of penicillin V may be altered in the second and third trimester. Higher doses or increased dosing frequency may be required.

Additional Information 0.7 mEq of potassium per 250 mg penicillin V; 250 mg equals 400,000 units of penicillin

Related Information

Antimicrobial Drugs of Choice *on page 2008*

◆ **Penicilloyl-polylysine** *see* Benzylpenicilloyl Polylysine *on page 203*

◆ **Pennsaid®** *see* Diclofenac (Topical) *on page 522*

◆ **Pentacel®** *see* Diphtheria and Tetanus Toxoids, Acellular Pertussis, Poliovirus and *Haemophilus* b Conjugate Vaccine *on page 550*

◆ **Pentam® 300** *see* Pentamidine *on page 1438*

Pentamidine (pen TAM i deen)

U.S. Brand Names Nebupent®; Pentam® 300

Index Terms Pentamidine Isethionate

Generic Availability (U.S.) No

Pharmacologic Category Antibiotic, Miscellaneous; Antiprotozoal

Pregnancy Risk Factor C

Lactation Excretion in breast milk unknown/not recommended

Use Treatment and prevention of pneumonia caused by *Pneumocystis jiroveci* pneumonia (PCP)

Unlabeled/Investigational Use Treatment of African trypanosomiasis, cutaneous leishmaniasis, and amebic meningoencephalitis

Available Dosage Forms

Injection, powder for reconstitution:
Pentam® 300: 300 mg

Powder for solution, for nebulization [preservative free]:
Nebupent®: 300 mg

Dosing

Adult & Geriatric

PCP:

FDA-approved labeling:
Prevention: Inhalation: 300 mg every 4 weeks via Respirgard® II nebulizer
Treatment: I.M., I.V.: 4 mg/kg once daily for 14-21 days

CDC recommendation:
Prevention: Inhalation: 300 mg monthly via Respirgard® II nebulizer
Treatment: I.V.: 3-4 mg/kg once daily for 21 days

AIDSinfo guidelines (2009):
Prevention: Inhalation: 300 mg/dose monthly via Respirgard® II nebulizer
Treatment: I.V.: 4 mg/kg once daily, 3 mg/kg may be used by some clinicians

Cutaneous leishmaniasis (unlabeled use; CDC recommendation): I.M., I.V.: 2-3 mg/kg once daily or every second day for 4-7 doses

Trypanosomiasis (unlabeled use; CDC recommendation): I.M.: 4 mg/kg once daily for 7 days

Pediatric

PCP:

FDA-approved labeling: Children >4 months: Treatment: I.M., I.V.: 4 mg/kg once daily for 14-21 days

CDC recommendation:
Prevention (children ≥5 years): Inhalation: 300 mg/dose monthly via Respirgard® II nebulizer
Treatment: I.V.: 3-4 mg/kg once daily for 21 days

AIDSinfo guidelines (2009):

Prevention: Children ≥5 years: Inhalation: 300 mg/dose monthly via Respirgard® II nebulizer

Treatment: I.V.: 4 mg/kg once daily, if clinical improvement may change to atovaquone after 7-10 days

PCP prevention in pediatric oncology patients (age <5 years, intolerant to trimethoprim-sulfamethoxazole; unlabeled use): 4 mg/kg I.V. once monthly (Kim, 2008; Prasad, 2007)

Cutaneous leishmaniasis (unlabeled use; CDC recommendation): I.M., I.V.: 2-3 mg/kg once daily or every second day for 4-7 doses

Trypanosomiasis (unlabeled use; CDC recommendation): I.M.: 4 mg/kg once daily for 7 days

Renal Impairment I.V.: The FDA-approved labeling recommends that caution should be used in patients with renal impairment; however, no specific dosage adjustment guidelines are available. The following guidelines have been used by some clinicians (Aronoff, 2007):

Children:

Cl_{cr} >30 mL/minute: No adjustment required.

Cl_{cr} 10-30 mL/minute: Administer 4 mg/kg every 36 hours.

Cl_{cr} <10 mL/minute and peritoneal dialysis: Administer 4 mg/kg every 48 hours.

Hemodialysis: Administer 4 mg/kg every 48 hours, after dialysis on dialysis days.

Adults:

Cl_{cr} ≥10 mL/minute: No adjustment required.

Cl_{cr} <10 mL/minute: Administer 4 mg/kg every 24-36 hours.

Administration

I.M. Administer deep I.M. Do not use NS as a diluent.

I.V. Do not use NS as an initial diluent. Infuse slowly over 60-120 minutes. Avoid extravasation; assess catheter position before and during infusion.

Inhalation Deliver via Respirgard® II nebulizer until nebulizer is emptied (30-45 minutes). Use appropriate precautions to minimize exposure to healthcare personnel; refer to individual institutional policy.

Monitoring and Teaching Issues

Laboratory Monitoring Liver and renal function, blood glucose, serum potassium and calcium, CBC and platelets

Physical Assessment Assess patient for cautious use conditions and previous allergy history. I.V., I.M.: Patients should be lying down. Blood pressure, cardiac status, and respiratory function should be monitored closely during administration and several times thereafter until blood pressure is stable. Monitor for hypotension, rash, confusion, hallucinations, hypoglycemia, dyspnea, and cough. If self-administered, teach patient proper use of nebulizer.

Patient Education Inhalant drug must be prepared and used with a nebulizer exactly as directed and as often as prescribed. Frequent blood tests and blood pressure checks may be required while using this drug. PCP pneumonia may still occur despite use of this medication. Maintain adequate hydration unless instructed to restrict fluid intake. Avoid excessive alcohol (may exacerbate adverse effects). If you have diabetes, monitor glucose levels closely and frequently. May cause hypotension, metallic taste, nausea, vomiting, or anorexia. Report chest pain or irregular heartbeat; unusual confusion or hallucinations; rash; or unusual wheezing, coughing, or respiratory difficulty.

◆ **Pentamidine Isethionate** *see* Pentamidine *on page* 1438

◆ **Pentasa®** *see* Mesalamine *on page* 1177

◆ **Pentavalent Human-Bovine Reassortant Rotavirus Vaccine (PRV)** *see* Rotavirus Vaccine *on page* 1616

Pentazocine and Naloxone (pen TAZ oh seen & nal OKS one)

Index Terms Naloxone Hydrochloride and Pentazocine; Pentazocine Hydrochloride and Naloxone Hydrochloride; Talwin NX

Generic Availability (U.S.) Yes

Pharmacologic Category Analgesic, Opioid; Analgesic, Opioid Partial Agonist

Medication Safety Issues

High alert medication: The Institute for Safe Medication Practices (ISMP) includes this medication among its list of drug classes which have a heightened risk of causing significant patient harm when used in error.

Pregnancy Risk Factor C

Lactation Pentazocine enters breast milk/use caution

Use Relief of moderate-to-severe pain; indicated for oral use only

Controlled Substance C-IV

Available Dosage Forms

Tablet: Pentazocine 50 mg and naloxone 0.5 mg

Dosing

Adult Analgesia: Oral: Dose based on pentazocine component: 50 mg every 3-4 hours; may increase to 100 mg/dose if needed, but should not exceed 600 mg/day (maximum: 12 tablets/day)

Geriatric

Refer to adult dosing. Use with caution; may be more sensitive to analgesic and sedative effects; decrease initial dose when appropriate and monitor closely.

Pediatric Analgesia: Oral: Children ≥12 years: Refer to adult dosing.

Renal Impairment The FDA-approved labeling does not contain renal dosing adjustment guidelines for pentazocine; the following guidelines have been used by some clinicians (Aronoff, 2007):

Cl_{cr} 10-50 mL/minute: Administer 75% of normal dose.

Cl_{cr} <10 mL/minute: Administer 50% of normal dose.

Hepatic Impairment Use with caution.

Monitoring and Teaching Issues

Physical Assessment See individual agents.

Patient Education See individual agents.

Related Information

Naloxone *on page 1284*

◆ **Pentazocine Hydrochloride and Naloxone Hydrochloride** *see* Pentazocine and Naloxone *on page 1439*

Pentosan Polysulfate Sodium (PEN toe san pol i SUL fate SOW dee um)

U.S. Brand Names Elmiron®

Index Terms PPS

Generic Availability (U.S.) No

Pharmacologic Category Analgesic, Urinary

Medication Safety Issues

Sound-alike/look-alike issues:

Pentosan may be confused with pentostatin

Elmiron® may be confused with Imuran®

Pregnancy Risk Factor B

Lactation Excretion in breast milk unknown/use caution

Use Relief of bladder pain or discomfort due to interstitial cystitis

Contraindications Hypersensitivity to pentosan polysulfate sodium, related compounds (LMWHs or heparin), or any component of the formulation

Warnings/Precautions Pentosan polysulfate is a low-molecular weight heparin-like compound with anticoagulant and fibrinolytic effects, therefore, bleeding complications (such as ecchymosis, epistaxis, and gum bleeding) may occur. Patients with the following diseases should be carefully evaluated before initiating therapy: aneurysm, thrombocytopenia, hemophilia, gastrointestinal ulcerations, polyps, diverticula, or hepatic insufficiency. Patients undergoing invasive procedures or having signs or symptoms of underlying coagulopathies or other increased risk of bleeding (eg, receiving heparin, warfarin, thrombolytics, NSAIDs, or high dose aspirin) should be evaluated prior to use. Use with caution in patients with a history of heparin-induced thrombocytopenia. Safety and efficacy have not been established in children <16 years of age.

Drug Interactions

Avoid Concomitant Use There are no known interactions where it is recommended to avoid concomitant use.

Decreased Effect There are no known significant interactions involving a decrease in effect.

Increased Effect/Toxicity

Pentosan Polysulfate Sodium may increase the levels/effects of: Anticoagulants; Antiplatelet Agents

Adverse Reactions 1% to 10%:

Central nervous system: Headache (3%), dizziness (1%)

Dermatologic: Alopecia (4%), rash (3%)

Gastrointestinal: Rectal hemorrhage (6%), diarrhea (4%), nausea (4%), abdominal pain (2%), dyspepsia (2%)

Hepatic: Liver function test abnormalities (1%; dose related)

Pharmacodynamics/Kinetics

Absorption ~6%

Time to Peak Serum: 2 hours (range: 0.6-120 hours)

Half-Life Elimination 20-27 hours

Metabolism Hepatic and splenic via partial desulfation; partial depolymerization occurs in the renal parenchyma; saturable

Excretion Feces (58% to 84%, as unchanged drug); urine (6%, primarily as metabolites)

Available Dosage Forms

Capsule, oral:

Elmiron®: 100 mg

Dosing

Adult & Geriatric Interstitial cystitis: Oral: 100 mg 3 times/day taken with water 1 hour before or 2 hours after meals

Note: Patients should be evaluated at 3 months and may be continued an additional 3 months if there has been no improvement and if there are no therapy-limiting side effects. **The risks and benefits of continued use beyond 6 months in patients who have not responded is not yet known.**

Pediatric Children ≥16 years: Refer to adult dosing.

Administration

Oral Should be administered with water 1 hour before or 2 hours after meals.

Stability

Storage Store at room temperature of 15°C to 30°C (59°F to 86°F).

Monitoring and Teaching Issues

Dietary Considerations Should be taken with water 1 hour before or 2 hours after meals.

Pregnancy Considerations No adverse events were noted in animal reproduction studies; however, reversible limb bud abnormalities were noted during *in vitro* animal studies. There are no adequate and well-controlled studies in pregnant women. Use with caution and only if clearly needed during pregnancy. Based on limited data, pentosan polysulfate does not appear to cross the placenta.

Pentoxifylline (pen toks IF i lin)

U.S. Brand Names TRENtal®

Index Terms Oxpentifylline

Generic Availability (U.S.) Yes

Pharmacologic Category Blood Viscosity Reducer Agent

Medication Safety Issues

Sound-alike/look-alike issues:

Pentoxifylline may be confused with tamoxifen

TRENtal® may be confused with Bentyl®, TEGretol®, Trandate®

Pregnancy Risk Factor C

Lactation Enters breast milk/not recommended

Use Treatment of intermittent claudication on the basis of chronic occlusive arterial disease of the limbs; may improve function and symptoms, but not intended to replace more definitive therapy

Unlabeled/Investigational Use Venous leg ulcers (Jull, 2007)

Mechanism of Action/Effect Reduces blood viscosity improves tissue oxygenation through enhanced blood flow

Contraindications Hypersensitivity to pentoxifylline, xanthines (eg, caffeine, theophylline), or any component of the formulation; recent cerebral and/or retinal hemorrhage

Warnings/Precautions Use with caution in renal impairment; active metabolite may accumulate in renal impairment leading to increased risk of adverse effects. Use caution in the elderly and assess renal function before initiating. Safety and efficacy in pediatric patients have not been established.

Drug Interactions

Metabolism/Transport Effects Inhibits CYP1A2 (weak)

Avoid Concomitant Use

Avoid concomitant use of Pentoxifylline with any of the following: Ketorolac; Ketorolac (Systemic)

Decreased Effect There are no known significant interactions involving a decrease in effect.

Increased Effect/Toxicity

Pentoxifylline may increase the levels/effects of: Antihypertensives; Antiplatelet Agents; Heparin; Heparin (Low Molecular Weight); Theophylline Derivatives; Vitamin K Antagonists

The levels/effects of Pentoxifylline may be increased by: Cimetidine; Ciprofloxacin; Ciprofloxacin (Systemic); Ketorolac; Ketorolac (Systemic)

Nutritional/Ethanol Interactions Food: Food may decrease rate but not extent of absorption. Pentoxifylline peak serum levels may be decreased if taken with food.

Lab Interactions Decreased calcium (S), magnesium (S); false-positive theophylline levels

Adverse Reactions 1% to 10%: Gastrointestinal: Nausea (2%), vomiting (1%)

Pharmacodynamics/Kinetics

Absorption Well absorbed

Time to Peak Serum: 2-4 hours

Half-Life Elimination Parent drug: 24-48 minutes; Metabolites: 60-96 minutes

Metabolism Hepatic to 3-carboxybutyl (M-IV, inactive) and 3-carboxypropyl (M-V, active) and via erythrocytes to 5-hydroxyhexyl (M-I, active); extensive first-pass effect; M-I is further metabolized in the liver

Excretion Primarily urine (50% to 80% as M-V, 20% as other metabolites); feces (<4%)

Available Dosage Forms

Tablet, controlled release, oral:

TRENtal®: 400 mg

Tablet, extended release, oral: 400 mg

Dosing

Adult Peripheral vascular disease: Oral: 400 mg 3 times/day with meals; maximal therapeutic benefit may take 2-4 weeks to develop; recommended to maintain therapy for at least 8 weeks. May reduce to 400 mg twice daily if GI or CNS side effects occur.

Geriatric Refer to adult dosing. Dosage adjustment based on creatinine clearance can be considered (see Renal Impairment).

Renal Impairment Dosage adjustments are not required by manufacturer; however, consider dosing adjustments based on degree of renal impairment (Paap, 1996):

Moderate renal impairment (Cl_{cr} ~60 mL/minute): 400 mg twice daily

Severe renal impairment (Cl_{cr} ~20 mL/minute): 400 mg once daily; further reduction may be required; Paap suggests 200 mg once daily, but with current products (extended or controlled release; unscored) may require adaptation to 400 mg once every other day

Administration

Oral Tablets should be swallowed whole; do not chew, break, or crush. May be administered with food.

Stability

Storage Store between 15°C to 30°C (59°F to 86°F).

Monitoring and Teaching Issues

Physical Assessment Assess efficacy of therapy objectively.

Patient Education This may relieve pain of claudication, but additional therapy may be recommended. May cause dizziness, heartburn, nausea, or vomiting. Report chest pain; swelling of lips, mouth, or tongue; persistent headache; respiratory difficulty; rash; or unrelieved nausea or vomiting.

Dietary Considerations May be taken with meals.

Geriatric Considerations Pentoxifylline's value in the treatment of intermittent claudication is controversial. Walking distance improved statistically in some clinical trials, but the actual distance was minimal when applied to improving physical activity. Dose adjustment in moderate and severe kidney impairment has been recommended based on accumulation of two active metabolites. However, these doses have not been studied for clinical or safety outcomes.

Pregnancy Considerations Teratogenic effects were not observed in animal studies. There are no adequate and well-controlled studies in pregnant women.

- **Pen VK** *see* Penicillin V Potassium *on page 1436*
- **Pepcid®** *see* Famotidine *on page 733*
- **Pepcid® AC [OTC]** *see* Famotidine *on page 733*
- **Pepcid® AC Maximum Strength [OTC]** *see* Famotidine *on page 733*
- **Peptic Relief [OTC]** *see* Bismuth *on page 221*
- **Pepto-Bismol® [OTC]** *see* Bismuth *on page 221*
- **Pepto-Bismol® Maximum Strength [OTC]** *see* Bismuth *on page 221*
- **Pepto Relief [OTC]** *see* Bismuth *on page 221*
- **Percocet®** *see* Oxycodone and Acetaminophen *on page 1383*
- **Perforomist™** *see* Formoterol *on page 820*
- **Periactin** *see* Cyproheptadine *on page 443*

Perindopril Erbumine (per IN doe pril er BYOO meen)

U.S. Brand Names Aceon®

Generic Availability (U.S.) Yes

Pharmacologic Category Angiotensin-Converting Enzyme (ACE) Inhibitor

Pregnancy Risk Factor D

Lactation Excretion in breast milk unknown/use caution

Use Treatment of hypertension; reduction of cardiovascular mortality or nonfatal myocardial infarction in patients with stable coronary artery disease

Unlabeled/Investigational Use Treatment of heart failure; to delay the progression of nephropathy and reduce risks of cardiovascular events in hypertensive patients with type 1 or 2 diabetes mellitus

Mechanism of Action/Effect Perindopril is a prodrug for perindoprilat, which acts as a competitive inhibitor of angiotensin-converting enzyme (ACE); prevents conversion of angiotensin I to angiotensin II, a potent vasoconstrictor; results in lower levels of angiotensin II which, in turn, causes an increase in plasma renin activity and a reduction in aldosterone secretion

Contraindications Hypersensitivity to perindopril, any other ACE inhibitor, or any component of the formulation; angioedema related to previous treatment with an ACE inhibitor

Warnings/Precautions Anaphylactic reactions may occur rarely with ACE inhibitors. At any time during treatment (especially following first dose), angioedema may occur rarely with ACE inhibitors; it may involve the head and neck (potentially compromising airway) or the intestine (presenting with abdominal pain). African-Americans and patients with idiopathic or hereditary angioedema may be at an increased risk. Prolonged frequent monitoring may be required especially if tongue, glottis, or larynx are involved as they are associated with airway obstruction. Patients with a history of airway surgery may have a higher risk of airway obstruction. Aggressive early and appropriate management is critical. Use in patients with previous angioedema associated with ACE inhibitor therapy is contraindicated. Severe anaphylactoid reactions may be seen during hemodialysis (eg, CVVHD) with high-flux dialysis membranes (eg, AN69), and rarely, during low density lipoprotein apheresis with dextran sulfate cellulose. Rare cases of anaphylactoid reactions have been reported in patients undergoing sensitization treatment with hymenoptera (bee, wasp) venom while receiving ACE inhibitors.

Symptomatic hypotension with or without syncope can occur with ACE inhibitors (usually with the first several doses); effects are most often observed in volume-depleted patients; correct volume depletion prior to initiation; close monitoring of patient is required especially with initial dosing and dosing increases; blood pressure must be lowered at a rate appropriate for the patient's clinical condition. Initiation of therapy in patients with ischemic heart disease or cerebrovascular disease warrants close observation due to the potential consequences posed by falling blood pressure (eg, MI, stroke). Use with caution in hypertrophic cardiomyopathy with outflow tract obstruction, severe aortic stenosis, or before, during, or immediately after major surgery. **[U.S. Boxed Warning]: Based on human data, ACEIs can cause injury and death to the developing fetus when used in the second and third trimesters. ACEIs should be discontinued as soon as possible once pregnancy is detected.**

Hyperkalemia may occur with ACE inhibitors; risk factors include renal dysfunction, diabetes mellitus, concomitant use of potassium-sparing diuretics, potassium supplements, and/or potassium-containing salts. Use cautiously, if at all, with these agents and monitor potassium closely. Cough may occur with ACE inhibitors. Other causes of cough should be considered (eg, pulmonary congestion in patients with heart failure) and excluded prior to discontinuation.

May be associated with deterioration of renal function and/or increases in serum creatinine, particularly in patients with low renal blood flow (eg, renal artery stenosis, heart failure) whose glomerular filtration rate (GFR) is dependent on efferent arteriolar vasoconstriction by angiotensin II; deterioration may result in oliguria, acute renal failure, and progressive azotemia. Small increases in serum creatinine may occur following initiation; consider discontinuation only in patients with progressive and/or significant deterioration in renal function. Use with caution in patients with unstented unilateral/bilateral renal artery stenosis. When unstented bilateral renal artery stenosis is present, use is generally avoided due to the elevated risk of deterioration in renal function unless possible benefits outweigh risks. Concurrent use of angiotensin receptor blockers may increase the risk of clinically-significant adverse events (eg, renal dysfunction, hyperkalemia).

Rare toxicities associated with ACE inhibitors include cholestatic jaundice (which may progress to fulminant hepatic necrosis), agranulocytosis, neutropenia or leukopenia with myeloid hypoplasia. Patients with collagen vascular diseases (especially with concomitant renal impairment) or renal impairment alone may be at increased risk for hematologic toxicity; periodically monitor CBC with differential in these patients.

Drug Interactions

Avoid Concomitant Use There are no known interactions where it is recommended to avoid concomitant use.

Decreased Effect

The levels/effects of Perindopril Erbumine may be decreased by: Antacids; Aprotinin; Herbs (Hypertensive Properties); Methylphenidate; Nonsteroidal Anti-Inflammatory Agents; Salicylates; Yohimbine

Increased Effect/Toxicity

Perindopril Erbumine may increase the levels/effects of: Allopurinol; Amifostine; Antihypertensives; AzaTHIOprine; CycloSPORINE; CycloSPORINE (Systemic); Ferric Gluconate; Gold Sodium Thiomalate; Hypotensive Agents; Iron Dextran Complex; Lithium; RiTUXimab

The levels/effects of Perindopril Erbumine may be increased by: Angiotensin II Receptor Blockers; Diazoxide; DPP-IV Inhibitors; Eplerenone; Everolimus; Herbs (Hypotensive Properties); Loop Diuretics; MAO Inhibitors; Pentoxifylline; Phosphodiesterase 5 Inhibitors; Potassium Salts; Potassium-Sparing Diuretics; Prostacyclin Analogues; Sirolimus; Temsirolimus; Thiazide Diuretics; TiZANidine; Tolvaptan; Trimethoprim

Nutritional/Ethanol Interactions

Food: Perindopril active metabolite concentrations may be lowered if taken with food.

Herb/Nutraceutical: Avoid bayberry, blue cohosh, cayenne, ephedra, ginger, ginseng (American), kola, licorice (may worsen hypertension). Avoid black cohosh, California poppy, coleus, golden seal, hawthorn, mistletoe, periwinkle, quinine, shepherd's purse (may have increased antihypertensive effect).

Adverse Reactions

>10%:

Central nervous system: Headache (24%)

Respiratory: Cough (incidence is higher in women, 3:1) (12%)

1% to 10%:

Cardiovascular: Edema (4%), chest pain (2%), ECG abnormal (2%), palpitation (1%)

Central nervous system: Dizziness (8%, less than placebo), sleep disorders (3%), depression (2%), fever (2%), nervousness (1%), somnolence (1%)

Dermatologic: Rash (2%)

Endocrine & metabolic: Hyperkalemia (1%, less than placebo), triglycerides increased (1%), menstrual disorder (1%)

Gastrointestinal: Diarrhea (4%), abdominal pain (3%), nausea (2%), vomiting (2%), dyspepsia (2%), flatulence (1%)

Genitourinary: Urinary tract infection (3%), sexual dysfunction (male 1%)

Hepatic: ALT increased (2%)

Neuromuscular & skeletal: Weakness (8%), back pain (6%), lower extremity pain (5%), upper extremity pain (3%), hypertonia (3%), paresthesia (2%), joint pain (1%), myalgia (1%), arthritis (1%), neck pain (1%)

Renal: Proteinuria (2%)

Respiratory: Upper respiratory tract infection (9%), sinusitis (5%), rhinitis (5%), pharyngitis (3%)

Otic: Tinnitus (2%), ear infection (1%)

Miscellaneous: Viral infection (3%), seasonal allergy (2%)

Note: Some reactions occurred at an incidence >1% but ≤ placebo.

Additional adverse effects that have been reported with **ACE inhibitors** include agranulocytosis (especially in patients with renal impairment or collagen vascular disease), neutropenia, anemia, bullous pemphigoid, cardiac arrest, eosinophilic pneumonitis, exfoliative dermatitis, falls, hepatic failure, hyponatremia, jaundice, pancreatitis (acute), pancytopenia, pemphigus, psoriasis, thrombocytopenia; decreases in creatinine clearance in some elderly hypertensive patients or those with chronic renal failure, and worsening of renal function in patients with bilateral renal artery stenosis or hypovolemic patients (diuretic therapy). In addition, a syndrome which may include fever, myalgia, arthralgia, interstitial nephritis, vasculitis, rash, eosinophilia and positive ANA, and elevated ESR has been reported with ACE inhibitors.

Pharmacodynamics/Kinetics

Onset of Action Peak effect: 1-2 hours

Bioavailability Perindopril: 75%; Perindoprilat ~25% (~16% with food)

Time to Peak Chronic therapy: Perindopril: 1 hour; Perindoprilat: 3-7 hours (maximum perindoprilat serum levels are 2-3 times higher and T_{max} is shorter following chronic therapy); CHF: Perindoprilat: 6 hours

Protein Binding Perindopril: 60%; Perindoprilat: 10% to 20%

Half-Life Elimination Parent drug: 1.5-3 hours; Metabolite: Effective: 3-10 hours, Terminal: 30-120 hours

Metabolism Hydrolyzed hepatically to active metabolite, perindoprilat (~17% to 20% of a dose) and other inactive metabolites

Excretion Urine (75%, 4% to 12% as unchanged drug)

Available Dosage Forms

Tablet, oral: 2 mg, 4 mg, 8 mg

Aceon®: 2 mg, 4 mg, 8 mg

Dosing

Adult

Heart failure (unlabeled use): Oral: Initial: 2 mg once daily; increase at 1- to 2-week intervals; target dose: 8-16 mg once daily (ACC/AHA 2009 Heart Failure Guidelines)

Hypertension: Oral: Initial: 4 mg/day but may be titrated to response; usual range: 4-8 mg/day (may be given in 2 divided doses); increase at 1- to 2-week intervals (maximum: 16 mg/day)

Concomitant therapy with diuretics: To reduce the risk of hypotension, discontinue diuretic, if possible, 2-3 days prior to initiating perindopril. If unable to stop diuretic, initiate perindopril at 2-4 mg/day and monitor blood pressure closely for the first 2 weeks of therapy, and after any dose adjustment of perindopril or diuretic.

Stable coronary artery disease: Oral: Initial: 4 mg once daily for 2 weeks; increase as tolerated to 8 mg once daily.

Geriatric

Hypertension: >65 years of age: Initial: 4 mg/day; maintenance: 8 mg/day; experience with doses >8 mg/day is limited.

Stable coronary artery disease: >70 years of age: Initial: 2 mg/day for 1 week; increase as tolerated to 4 mg/day for 1 week; then increase as tolerated to 8 mg/day; experience with doses >8 mg/day is limited.

Renal Impairment

Cl_{cr} >30 mL/minute: Initial: 2 mg/day; maintenance dosing not to exceed 8 mg/day

Cl_{cr} <30 mL/minute: Safety and efficacy not established.

Hemodialysis: Perindopril and its metabolites are dialyzable

Hepatic Impairment No adjustment necessary.

Stability

Storage Store at room temperature of 20°C to 25°C (68°F to 77°F). Protect from moisture.

Monitoring and Teaching Issues

Laboratory Monitoring Serum creatinine and potassium; if patient has collagen vascular disease and/or renal impairment, periodically monitor CBC with differential

Physical Assessment Use with caution and monitor closely in presence of renal impairment, hypovolemia; collagen vascular diseases; valvular stenosis, hyperkalemia; or anesthesia. Monitor blood pressure closely (hypotension can occur, especially with first dose; angioedema can occur at any time during treatment, especially following first dose). Assess BP (standing and sitting), cardiac status, and fluid balance at beginning of therapy, when adjusting dose, and periodically throughout.

Patient Education Take first dose at bedtime. Do not take potassium supplements or salt substitutes containing potassium without consulting prescriber. This drug does not eliminate need for diet or exercise regimen as recommended by prescriber. May cause increased cough (if persistent or bothersome, contact prescriber), headache, postural hypotension, dizziness, nausea, vomiting, or diarrhea. Report chest pain, respiratory difficulty or persistent cough, painful muscles or joints, rash, or ringing in ears.

Geriatric Considerations Due to frequent decreases in glomerular filtration (also creatinine clearance) with aging, elderly patients may have exaggerated responses to ACE inhibitors; differences in clinical response due to hepatic changes are not observed. ACE inhibitors may be preferred agents in elderly patients with congestive heart failure and diabetes mellitus. Diabetic proteinuria is reduced and insulin sensitivity is enhanced. In general, the side effect profile is favorable in elderly and causes little or no CNS confusion; use lowest dose recommendations initially. Many elderly may be volume depleted due to diuretic use and/or blunted thirst reflex resulting in inadequate fluid intake.

Breast-Feeding Considerations It is not known if perindopril is excreted in human breast milk. The manufacturer recommends that caution be exercised when administering perindopril to nursing women.

Pregnancy Considerations Due to adverse events observed in humans, perindopril is considered pregnancy category D. Perindopril crosses the placenta. First trimester exposure to ACE inhibitors may cause major congenital malformations. An increased risk of cardiovascular and/or central nervous system malformations was observed in one study; however, an increased risk of teratogenic events was not observed in other studies. Second and third trimester use of an ACE inhibitor is associated with oligohydramnios. Oligohydramnios due to decreased fetal renal function may lead to fetal limb contractures, craniofacial deformation, and hypoplastic lung development. The use of ACE inhibitors during the second and third trimesters is also associated with anuria, hypotension, renal failure (reversible or irreversible), skull hypoplasia, and death in the fetus/neonate. Chronic maternal hypertension itself is also associated with adverse events in the fetus/infant. ACE inhibitors are not recommended during pregnancy to treat maternal hypertension or heart failure. Those who are planning a pregnancy should be considered for other medication options if an ACE inhibitor is currently prescribed or the ACE inhibitor should be discontinued as soon as possible once pregnancy is detected. The exposed fetus should be monitored for fetal growth, amniotic fluid volume, and organ formation. Infants exposed to an ACE inhibitor *in utero*, especially during the second and third trimester, should be monitored for hyperkalemia, hypotension, and oliguria.

[U.S. Boxed Warning]: Based on human data, ACE inhibitors can cause injury and death to the developing fetus. ACE inhibitors should be discontinued as soon as possible once pregnancy is detected.

Related Information

Angiotensin Agents *on page 1974*

Heart Failure (Systolic) *on page 2040*

◆ **Periostat®** *see* Doxycycline *on page 586*

Perphenazine (per FEN a zeen)

Generic Availability (U.S.) Yes

Pharmacologic Category Antiemetic; Antipsychotic Agent, Typical, Phenothiazine

Medication Safety Issues

Sound-alike/look-alike issues:

Trilafon® may be confused with Tri-Levlen®

Lactation Enters breast milk/not recommended (AAP rates "of concern"; AAP 2001 update pending)

Use Treatment of schizophrenia; severe nausea and vomiting

Unlabeled/Investigational Use Ethanol withdrawal; behavioral symptoms associated with dementia (elderly); Tourette's syndrome; Huntington's chorea; spasmodic torticollis; Reye's syndrome; psychosis; psychosis/agitation related to Alzheimer's dementia

Available Dosage Forms

Tablet, oral: 2 mg, 4 mg, 8 mg, 16 mg

Dosing

Adult

Schizophrenia/psychoses:

Nonhospitalized: Initial: 4-8 mg 3 times/day; reduce dose as soon as possible to minimum effective dosage (maximum: 64 mg/day)

Hospitalized: 8-16 mg 2-4 times/day (maximum: 64 mg/day)

Nausea/vomiting: Oral: 8-16 mg/day in divided doses up to 24 mg/day (maximum: 24 mg/day)

Geriatric Behavioral symptoms associated with dementia (unlabeled use): Oral: Initial: 2-4 mg 1-2 times/day; increase at 4- to 7-day intervals by 2-4 mg/day. Increase dose intervals (bid, tid, etc) as necessary to control behavior response or side effects. Maximum daily dose: 32 mg; gradual increase (titration) and bedtime administration may prevent some side effects or decrease their severity.

Renal Impairment Not dialyzable (0% to 5%)

Hepatic Impairment Dosage reductions should be considered in patients with liver disease although no specific guidelines are available.

Monitoring and Teaching Issues

Laboratory Monitoring Baseline liver and kidney function, CBC prior to and periodically during therapy, lipid profile, fasting blood glucose/Hgb A_{1c}; BMI

Physical Assessment Monitor ophthalmic screening at beginning of therapy and periodically throughout. Monitor blood pressure; can cause orthostatic hypotension. Initiate at lower doses and taper dosage slowly when discontinuing.

Patient Education It may take 2-3 weeks to achieve desired results. Avoid alcohol. Maintain adequate hydration unless instructed to restrict fluid intake. You may experience excess drowsiness, restlessness, dizziness, blurred vision, dry mouth, nausea, vomiting, constipation, postural hypotension, urinary retention, photosensitivity, or decreased perspiration. Report persistent CNS effects (eg, trembling fingers, altered gait or balance, excessive sedation, seizures, unusual movements, anxiety, confusion); chest pain, palpitations, or rapid heartbeat; severe dizziness; unresolved urinary retention; change in libido or ejaculatory difficulty; vision changes; skin rash or yellowing of skin; respiratory difficulty; or worsening of condition.

Related Information

Antipsychotic Agents *on page 1986*

◆ **Persantine®** *see* Dipyridamole *on page 556*

◆ **Pertussis, Acellular (Adsorbed)** *see* Diphtheria and Tetanus Toxoids, Acellular Pertussis, Poliovirus and *Haemophilus* b Conjugate Vaccine *on page 550*

◆ **Pethidine Hydrochloride** *see* Meperidine *on page 1172*

◆ **Pexeva®** *see* PARoxetine *on page 1414*

◆ **PFA** *see* Foscarnet *on page 828*

◆ **Pfizerpen®** *see* Penicillin G (Parenteral/Aqueous) *on page 1433*

◆ **PGE_1** *see* Alprostadil *on page 83*

◆ **PGE_2** *see* Dinoprostone *on page 540*

◆ **PGI_2** *see* Epoprostenol *on page* 643
◆ **PGX** *see* Epoprostenol *on page* 643
◆ **Phanasin® [OTC] [DSC]** *see* GuaiFENesin *on page* 890
◆ **Phanasin® Diabetic Choice® [OTC] [DSC]** *see* GuaiFENesin *on page* 890
◆ **Phenadoz®** *see* Promethazine *on page* 1517

Phenazopyridine (fen az oh PEER i deen)

U.S. Brand Names AZO Standard® Maximum Strength [OTC]; AZO Standard® [OTC]; Azo-Gesic™ [OTC]; Baridium [OTC]; Pyridium®; ReAzo [OTC]; UTI Relief® [OTC]

Index Terms Phenazopyridine Hydrochloride; Phenylazo Diamino Pyridine Hydrochloride

Generic Availability (U.S.) Yes

Pharmacologic Category Analgesic, Urinary

Medication Safety Issues

Sound-alike/look-alike issues:

Phenazopyridine may be confused with phenoxybenzamine

Pyridium® may be confused with Dyrenium®, Perdiem®, pyridoxine, pyrithione

Pregnancy Risk Factor B

Lactation Excretion in breast milk unknown

Use Symptomatic relief of urinary burning, itching, frequency, and urgency in association with urinary tract infection or following urologic procedures

Available Dosage Forms

Tablet, oral: 100 mg, 200 mg

AZO Standard® [OTC]: 95 mg

AZO Standard® Maximum Strength [OTC]: 97.5 mg

Azo-Gesic™ [OTC]: 95 mg

Baridium [OTC]: 97.2 mg

Pyridium®: 100 mg, 200 mg

ReAzo [OTC]: 95 mg

UTI Relief® [OTC]: 97.2 mg

Dosing

Adult & Geriatric Urinary analgesic: Oral: 100-200 mg 3 times/day after meals for 2 days when used concomitantly with an antibacterial agent

Pediatric Urinary analgesic: Oral: Children: 12 mg/kg/day in 3 divided doses administered after meals for 2 days

Renal Impairment

Cl_{cr} 50-80 mL/minute: Administer every 8-16 hours.

Cl_{cr} <50 mL/minute: Avoid use.

Administration

Oral Administer after meals.

Monitoring and Teaching Issues

Physical Assessment Instruct patients with diabetes to use serum glucose monitoring (phenazopyridine may interfere with certain urine testing reagents).

Patient Education May discolor urine (orange/yellow); this is normal, but will also stain fabric. If you have diabetes, use serum glucose tests; this medication may interfere with accuracy of urine testing. Report persistent headache, dizziness, or stomach cramping.

◆ **Phenazopyridine Hydrochloride** *see* Phenazopyridine *on page* 1446

Phenelzine (FEN el zeen)

U.S. Brand Names Nardil®

Index Terms Phenelzine Sulfate

Generic Availability (U.S.) No

Pharmacologic Category Antidepressant, Monoamine Oxidase Inhibitor

Medication Safety Issues

Sound-alike/look-alike issues:

Phenelzine may be confused with phenytoin

Nardil® may be confused with Norinyl®

Medication Guide Available Yes

Pregnancy Risk Factor C

Lactation Excretion in breast milk unknown/not recommended

Use Symptomatic treatment of atypical, nonendogenous, or neurotic depression

Unlabeled/Investigational Use Selective mutism

Available Dosage Forms

Tablet, oral:

Nardil®: 15 mg

Dosing

Adult Depression: Oral: 15 mg 3 times/day; may increase to 60-90 mg/day during early phase of treatment, then reduce dose for maintenance therapy slowly after maximum benefit is obtained. Takes 2-4 weeks for a significant response to occur.

Geriatric Oral: Initial: 7.5 mg/day; increase by 7.5-15 mg/day every 3-4 days as tolerated; usual therapeutic dose: 15-60 mg/day in 3-4 divided doses.

Pediatric Selective mutism (unlabeled use): Oral: 30-60 mg/day

Monitoring and Teaching Issues

Physical Assessment Assess other medications patient may be taking for effectiveness and interactions. Monitor therapeutic effectiveness and adverse reactions at beginning of therapy and periodically with long-term use. Monitor blood pressure. Observe for clinical worsening, suicidality, and unusual behavior changes, especially during the initial few months of therapy or during dosage changes. Taper dosage slowly when discontinuing; allow 3-4 weeks between discontinuing phenelzine and starting another antidepressant. Advise patients with diabetes to monitor serum glucose closely (phenelzine may lower glucose level). Assess knowledge/teach patient appropriate use, interventions to reduce side effects (including tyramine-free diet), and adverse symptoms to report.

Patient Education It may take 2-3 weeks to achieve desired results. Avoid alcohol. Avoid tyramine-containing foods. Maintain adequate hydration unless instructed to restrict fluid intake. You may experience postural hypotension, drowsiness, lightheadedness, dizziness, anorexia, dry mouth, constipation, or diarrhea. If you have diabetes, monitor serum glucose closely (Nardil® may effect glucose levels). Report persistent insomnia; chest pain, palpitations, irregular or rapid heartbeat, or swelling of extremities; muscle cramping, tremors, or altered gait; blurred vision or eye pain; yellowing of eyes or skin; pale stools/dark urine; suicide ideation; or worsening of condition.

Related Information

Antidepressant Agents *on page 1982*

◆ **Phenelzine Sulfate** *see* Phenelzine *on page 1446*

◆ **Phenergan®** *see* Promethazine *on page 1517*

PHENobarbital (fee noe BAR bi tal)

U.S. Brand Names Luminal® Sodium [DSC]

Index Terms Phenobarbital Sodium; Phenobarbitone; Phenylethylmalonylurea

Generic Availability (U.S.) Yes

Pharmacologic Category Anticonvulsant, Barbiturate; Barbiturate

Medication Safety Issues

Sound-alike/look-alike issues:

PHENobarbital may be confused with PENTobarbital, Phenergan®, phenytoin

Luminal® may be confused with Tuinal®

Pregnancy Risk Factor D

Lactation Enters breast milk/use caution (AAP recommends use "with caution"; AAP 2001 update pending)

Use Management of generalized tonic-clonic (grand mal), status epilepticus, and partial seizures; sedative/hypnotic

Unlabeled/Investigational Use Prevention and treatment of neonatal hyperbilirubinemia and lowering of bilirubin in chronic cholestasis; neonatal seizures

Controlled Substance C-IV

Available Dosage Forms

Elixir, oral: 20 mg/5 mL (5 mL, 7.5 mL, 15 mL)

Injection, solution: 65 mg/mL (1 mL); 130 mg/mL (1 mL)

Tablet, oral: 15 mg, 30 mg, 60 mg, 100 mg

Dosing

Adult

Sedation: Oral, I.M.: 30-120 mg/day in 2-3 divided doses

Hypnotic: Oral, I.M., I.V.: 100-320 mg at bedtime

Preoperative sedation: I.M.: 100-200 mg 1-1.5 hours before procedure

Anticonvulsant/status epilepticus:

Loading dose: I.V.: 10-20 mg/kg (maximum rate ≤60 mg/minute in patients ≥60 kg); may repeat dose in 20-minute intervals as needed (maximum total dose: 30 mg/kg)

Maintenance dose: Oral, I.V.: 1-3 mg/kg/day in divided doses or 50-100 mg 2-3 times/day

Sedative/hypnotic withdrawal (unlabeled use): Initial daily requirement is determined by substituting phenobarbital 30 mg for every 100 mg pentobarbital used during tolerance testing; then daily requirement is decreased by 10% of initial dose.

Geriatric Geriatric patients should be started at the lowest recommended dose. Refer to adult dosing.

Pediatric

Sedation: Oral: Children: 2 mg/kg 3 times/day

Hypnotic: I.M., I.V.: Children: 3-5 mg/kg at bedtime

Preoperative sedation: Oral, I.M., I.V.: Children: 1-3 mg/kg 1-1.5 hours before procedure

Anticonvulsant/status epilepticus (loading dose): I.V.: Infants and Children: 15-20 mg/kg (maximum: 1000 mg/dose, maximum rate ≤30 mg/minute in children <60 kg); may repeat dose after 15 minutes as needed (maximum total dose: 40 mg/kg)

Anticonvulsant maintenance dose: Oral, I.V.:

Infants: 5-8 mg/kg/day in 1-2 divided doses

Children:

1-5 years: 6-8 mg/kg/day in 1-2 divided doses

5-12 years: 4-6 mg/kg/day in 1-2 divided doses

>12 years: 1-3 mg/kg/day in divided doses or 50-100 mg 2-3 times/day

Renal Impairment

Cl_{cr} <10 mL/minute: Administer every 12-16 hours.

Moderately dialyzable (20% to 50%)

Hepatic Impairment Increased side effects may occur in severe liver disease. Monitor plasma levels and adjust dose accordingly.

Administration

I.M. Inject deep into muscle. Do not exceed 5 mL per injection site due to potential for tissue irritation.

I.V. Avoid rapid I.V. administration >60 mg/minute in adults and >30 mg/minute in children. Avoid extravasation. Intra-arterial injection is contraindicated. Avoid subcutaneous administration.

Monitoring and Teaching Issues

Laboratory Monitoring Phenobarbital serum concentrations, CBC, LFTs

Physical Assessment Assess for history of addiction or suicide ideation; long-term use can result in dependence, abuse, or tolerance; periodically evaluate need for continued use. **I.V.:** Monitor cardio/respiratory and CNS status; use safety precautions.

Patient Education I.V.: Patient instructions and information are determined by patient condition and therapeutic purpose. Oral: Drug may cause physical and/or psychological dependence. While using this medication, do not use alcohol and other prescription or OTC medications (especially pain medications, sedatives, antihistamines, or hypnotics) without consulting prescriber. Maintain adequate hydration unless instructed to restrict fluid intake. You may experience drowsiness, dizziness, blurred vision, nausea, vomiting, loss of appetite, or constipation. Report skin rash or irritation, CNS changes (confusion, depression, increased sedation, suicide ideation, excitation, headache, insomnia, or nightmares), respiratory difficulty or shortness of breath, changes in urinary pattern or menstrual pattern, muscle weakness or tremors, or difficulty swallowing or feeling of tightness in throat.

Related Information

Peak and Trough Guidelines *on page 1958*

◆ **Phenobarbital Sodium** *see* PHENobarbital *on page 1447*

◆ **Phenobarbitone** *see* PHENobarbital *on page 1447*

◆ **Phenoxymethyl Penicillin** *see* Penicillin V Potassium *on page 1436*

Phentolamine (fen TOLE a meen)

U.S. Brand Names OraVerse™

Index Terms Phentolamine Mesylate; Regitine [DSC]

Generic Availability (U.S.) Yes

Pharmacologic Category $Alpha_1$ Blocker

Medication Safety Issues

Sound-alike/look-alike issues:

Phentolamine may be confused with phentermine, Ventolin®

Pregnancy Risk Factor C

Lactation Excretion in breast milk unknown

Use Diagnosis of pheochromocytoma and treatment of hypertension associated with pheochromocytoma or other forms of hypertension caused by excess sympathomimetic amines; treatment of dermal necrosis after extravasation of drugs with alpha-adrenergic effects (ie, dopamine, epinephrine, norepinephrine, phenylephrine)

OraVerse™: Reversal of soft tissue anesthesia and the associated functional deficits resulting from a local dental anesthetic containing a vasoconstrictor

Unlabeled/Investigational Use Treatment of pralidoxime-induced hypertension

Available Dosage Forms

Injection, powder for reconstitution: 5 mg

Injection, solution [preservative free]:

OraVerse™: 0.4 mg/1.7 mL (1.7 mL)

Dosing

Adult & Geriatric

Treatment of alpha-adrenergic agonist drug extravasation: SubQ:

Infiltrate area with a small amount (eg, 1 mL) of solution (made by diluting 5-10 mg in 10 mL of NS) within 12 hours of extravasation; in general, do not exceed 0.1-0.2 mg/kg (5 mg total); typically doses of ≤5 mg are effective; a case using 50 mg for a large extravasation has been reported (Cooper, 1989).

If dose is effective, normal skin color should return to the blanched area within 1 hour.

Diagnosis of pheochromocytoma: I.M., I.V.: 5 mg

Surgery for pheochromocytoma: Hypertension: I.M., I.V.: 5 mg given 1-2 hours before procedure and repeated as needed every 2-4 hours

Hypertensive crisis: I.V.: 5-20 mg

Reversal of soft tissue (lip, tongue) anesthesia (OraVerse™): Infiltration or block technique: Submucosal oral injection: **Note:** Dose is based upon the number of cartridges of local anesthetic administered. Infiltration or block injection:

0.2 mg if one-half cartridge of anesthesia was administered

0.4 mg if 1 cartridge of anesthesia was administered

0.8 mg if 2 cartridges of anesthesia were administered

Treatment of pralidoxime-induced hypertension (unlabeled use): I.V.: 5 mg

Pediatric

Treatment of alpha-adrenergic agonist drug extravasation: SubQ: Infiltrate area with a small amount (eg, 1 mL) of solution (made by diluting 5-10 mg in 10 mL of NS) within 12 hours of extravasation; do not exceed 0.1-0.2 mg/kg (5 mg total)

Diagnosis of pheochromocytoma: I.M., I.V.: 0.05-0.1 mg/kg/dose, maximum single dose: 5 mg

Surgery for pheochromocytoma: Hypertension: I.M., I.V.: 0.05-0.1 mg/kg/dose given 1-2 hours before procedure; repeat as needed every 2-4 hours until hypertension is controlled; maximum single dose: 5 mg.

Treatment of pralidoxime-induced hypertension (unlabeled use): I.V.: 1 mg

Reversal of soft tissue (lip, tongue) anesthesia (OraVerse™): Infiltration or block technique: Submucosal oral injection:

Children: 15-30 kg: 0.2 mg maximum dose

Children >30 kg and <12 years: 0.4 mg maximum dose

Administration

I.V.

Vasoconstrictor (alpha-adrenergic agonist) extravasation: Infiltrate the area of extravasation with multiple small injections using only 27- or 30-gauge needles and changing the needle between each skin entry. Be careful not to cause so much swelling of the extremity or digit that a compartment syndrome occurs. If infiltration is severe, may also need to consult vascular surgeon.

Pheochromocytoma: Inject each 5 mg over 1 minute.

Monitoring and Teaching Issues

Physical Assessment When used to prevent tissue necrosis after extravasation, monitor effectiveness of treatment closely. Assess cardiac status.

Patient Education This medication can only be administered by infusion or by subQ injection. Assist patient with ambulation if used to manage pheochromocytoma. Report immediately any pain at infusion/injection site. May cause orthostatic hypotension. Report dizziness, rapid heartbeat, feelings of weakness, or nausea/vomiting.

Related Information

Hyperlipidemia Management *on page 2046*

◆ **Phentolamine Mesylate** *see* Phentolamine *on page 1448*

◆ **Phenylalanine Mustard** *see* Melphalan *on page 1162*

◆ **Phenylazo Diamino Pyridine Hydrochloride** *see* Phenazopyridine *on page 1446*

Phenylephrine (Systemic) (fen il EF rin)

U.S. Brand Names LuSonal™ [DSC]; Medi-First® Sinus Decongestant [OTC]; Medi-Phenyl [OTC]; PediaCare® Children's Decongestant [OTC]; Sudafed PE® Children's [OTC]; Sudafed PE® Congestion [OTC]; Sudafed PE™ Nasal Decongestant [OTC]; Sudogest™ PE [OTC]; Triaminic Thin Strips® Children's Cold with Stuffy Nose [OTC]

Index Terms Phenylephrine Hydrochloride

Generic Availability (U.S.) Yes: Excludes liquid, strips

Pharmacologic Category Alpha/Beta Agonist

Medication Safety Issues

Sound-alike/look-alike issues:

Neo-Synephrine® (phenylephrine) may be confused with Neo-Synephrine® (oxymetazoline)

Sudafed PE™ may be confused with Sudafed®

High alert medication: The Institute for Safe Medication Practices (ISMP) includes this medication among its list of drugs which have a heightened risk of causing significant patient harm when used in error.

Pregnancy Risk Factor C

Lactation Excretion in breast milk unknown/use caution

Use Treatment of hypotension, vascular failure in shock; as a vasoconstrictor in regional analgesia; supraventricular tachycardia (**Note:** Not for routine use in treatment of supraventricular tachycardias); as a decongestant [OTC]

Mechanism of Action/Effect Potent, direct-acting alpha-adrenergic agonist with virtually no beta-adrenergic activity; produces systemic arterial vasoconstriction

Contraindications Hypersensitivity to phenylephrine or any component of the formulation; hypertension; ventricular tachycardia

Oral: Use with or within 14 days of MAO inhibitor therapy

Warnings/Precautions Some products contain sulfites which may cause allergic reactions in susceptible individuals. Use with extreme caution in patients taking MAO inhibitors.

Intravenous: Use with caution in the elderly, patients with hyperthyroidism, bradycardia, partial heart block, myocardial disease, or severe CAD. Avoid or use with extreme caution in patients with heart failure or cardiogenic shock; increased systemic vascular resistance may significantly reduce cardiac output. Assure adequate circulatory volume to minimize need for vasoconstrictors. Avoid hypertension; monitor blood pressure closely and adjust infusion rate. Avoid extravasation; infuse into a large vein if possible. Avoid infusion into leg veins. Watch I.V. site closely. If extravasation occurs, infiltrate the area subcutaneously with diluted phentolamine (5-10 mg in 10 mL of saline) with a fine hypodermic needle. **Phentolamine should be administered as soon as possible after extravasation is noted. [U.S. Boxed Warning]: Should be administered by adequately trained individuals familiar with its use.**

Oral: Use caution with asthma, bowel obstruction/narrowing, hyperthyroidism, diabetes mellitus, cardiovascular disease, ischemic heart disease, increased intraocular pressure, prostatic hyperplasia or in the elderly. Notify healthcare provider if symptoms do not improve within 7 days or are accompanied by fever. Discontinue and contact healthcare provider if nervousness, dizziness, or sleeplessness occur.

Drug Interactions

Avoid Concomitant Use

Avoid concomitant use of Phenylephrine (Systemic) with any of the following: Iobenguane I 123; MAO Inhibitors

Decreased Effect

Phenylephrine (Systemic) may decrease the levels/effects of: Benzylpenicilloyl Polylysine; Iobenguane I 123

Increased Effect/Toxicity

Phenylephrine (Systemic) may increase the levels/effects of: Sympathomimetics

The levels/effects of Phenylephrine (Systemic) may be increased by: Atomoxetine; Cannabinoids; MAO Inhibitors; Tricyclic Antidepressants

Nutritional/Ethanol Interactions Herb/Nutraceutical: Avoid ephedra, yohimbe (may cause CNS stimulation).

Adverse Reactions Frequency not defined.

Injection:

Cardiovascular: Arrhythmia (rare), decreased cardiac output, hypertension, pallor, precordial pain or discomfort, reflex bradycardia, severe peripheral and visceral vasoconstriction

Central nervous system: Anxiety, dizziness, excitability, giddiness, headache, insomnia, nervousness, restlessness

Endocrine & metabolic: Metabolic acidosis

Gastrointestinal: Gastric irritation, nausea

Local: I.V.: Extravasation which may lead to necrosis and sloughing of surrounding tissue, blanching of skin

Neuromuscular & skeletal: Paresthesia, pilomotor response, tremor, weakness

Renal: Decreased renal perfusion, reduced urine output

Respiratory: Respiratory distress

Miscellaneous: Hypersensitivity reactions (including rash, urticaria, leukopenia, agranulocytosis, thrombocytopenia)

Oral: Central nervous system: Anxiety, dizziness, excitability, giddiness, headache, insomnia, nervousness, restlessness

Pharmacodynamics/Kinetics

Onset of Action

Blood pressure increase/vasoconstriction: I.M., SubQ: 10-15 minutes; I.V.: Immediate

Nasal decongestant: Oral: 15-30 minutes (Kollar, 2007)

Duration of Action

Blood pressure increase/vasoconstriction: I.M.: 1-2 hours; I.V.: ~15-20 minutes; SubQ: 50 minutes

Nasal decongestant: Oral: ≤4 hours (Kollar, 2007)

Absorption Oral: Rapid and complete (Kanfer, 1993)

Bioavailability Oral: ≤38% (Hengstmann, 1982; Kanfer, 1993)

Time to Peak Oral: 0.75-2 hours (Kanfer, 1993)

Half-Life Elimination Alpha phase: ~5 minutes; Terminal phase: 2-3 hours (Hengstmann, 1982; Kanfer, 1993)

Metabolism Hepatic via oxidative deamination (Oral: 24%; I.V.: 50%); Undergoes sulfation (Oral [mostly within gut wall]: 46%; I.V.: 8%) and some glucuronidation; forms inactive metabolites (Kanfer 1993)

Excretion Urine (mostly as inactive metabolites)

Available Dosage Forms

Injection, solution: 1% [10 mg/mL] (1 mL, 2 mL, 5 mL, 10 mL)

Liquid, oral:

PediaCare® Children's Decongestant [OTC]: 2.5 mg/5 mL (118 mL)

Sudafed PE® Children's [OTC]: 2.5 mg/5 mL (118 mL)

Strip, orally disintegrating, oral:

Triaminic Thin Strips® Children's Cold with Stuffy Nose [OTC]: 2.5 mg (14s)

Tablet, oral:

Medi-First® Sinus Decongestant [OTC]: 10 mg

Medi-Phenyl [OTC]: 5 mg

Sudafed PE® Congestion [OTC]: 10 mg

Sudafed PE™ Nasal Decongestant [OTC]: 10 mg

Sudogest™ PE [OTC]: 10 mg

Dosing

Adult & Geriatric

Hypotension/shock:

I.V. bolus: 0.1-0.5 mg/dose every 10-15 minutes as needed (initial dose should not exceed 0.5 mg)

I.V. infusion: Initial dose: 100-180 mcg/minute, **or alternatively**, 0.5 mcg/kg/minute; titrate to desired response. Dosing ranges between 0.4-9.1 mcg/kg/minute have been reported when treating septic shock (Gregory, 1991).

Nasal congestion: *Oral:* 10-20 mg every 4 hours as needed for ≤7 days

Paroxysmal supraventricular tachycardia (Note: Not recommended for routine use in treatment of supraventricular tachycardias): *I.V.:* 0.25-0.5 mg/dose over 20-30 seconds

Pediatric

Hypotension/shock:

I.V. bolus: 5-20 mcg/kg/dose every 10-15 minutes as needed

I.V. infusion: 0.1-0.5 mcg/kg/minute

Nasal congestion: *Oral:*

4 to <6 years: 2.5 mg every 4 hours as needed for ≤7 days

6 to <12 years: 5 mg every 4 hours as needed for ≤7 days

≥12 years: Refer to adult dosing.

Paroxysmal supraventricular tachycardia (Note: Not recommended for routine use in treatment of supraventricular tachycardias): *I.V.:* 5-10 mcg/kg/dose over 20-30 seconds

Stability

Reconstitution Solution for injection:

I.V. infusion: Usual concentration: 10 mg in 500 mL NS or D_5W. May also dilute 50 mg in 500 mL NS or 100 mg in 500 mL NS; both concentrations are stable for at least 14 days at room temperature of 25°C (77°F) (Gupta, 2004). Dilution of 1250 mg in 500 mL NS retained potency for at least 24 hours at 22°C (Weber, 1970).

I.V. injection: May dilute with SWFI to a concentration of 1 mg/mL.

Stability in syringes (Kiser, 2007): Concentration of 0.1 mg/mL in NS (polypropylene syringes) is stable for at least 30 days at -20°C (-4°F), 3°C to 5°C (37°F to 41°F), or 23°C to 25°C (73.4°F to 77°F).

Storage

Solution for injection: Store vials at controlled room temperature of 15°C to 25°C (59°F to 77°F). Protect from light. Do not use solution if brown or contains a precipitate.

Oral: Store at controlled room temperature of 15°C to 25°C (59°F to 77°F). Protect from light.

Monitoring and Teaching Issues

Physical Assessment Parenteral: Monitor arterial blood gases, vital signs, adverse reactions, and infusion site. If extravasation should occur, implement extravasation management immediately; can cause tissue sloughing.

Patient Education Oral: You may experience headache, trouble sleeping, nervousness, or dizziness.

Dietary Considerations Some products may contain phenylalanine and/or sodium.

Geriatric Considerations Elderly are more predisposed to the adverse effects of sympathomimetics since they frequently have cardiovascular disease and diabetes mellitus and are on multiple medications. Elderly patients should be counseled about their proper use of OTC products and in what disease states they should be avoided.

Breast-Feeding Considerations It is not known if phenylephrine is excreted into breast milk. The manufacturer recommends that caution be exercised when administering phenylephrine to nursing women.

Pregnancy Considerations Animal reproduction studies have not been conducted; therefore, the manufacturer classifies phenylephrine as pregnancy category C. Phenylephrine crosses the placenta at term. Maternal use of phenylephrine during the first trimester of pregnancy is not strongly associated with an increased risk of fetal malformations; maternal dose and duration of therapy were not reported in available publications. Phenylephrine is available over-the-counter (OTC) for the symptomatic relief of nasal congestion. Decongestants are not the preferred agents for the treatment of rhinitis during pregnancy. Oral phenylephrine should be avoided during the first trimester of pregnancy; short-term use (<3 days) of intranasal phenylephrine may be beneficial to some patients although its safety during pregnancy has not been studied. Phenylephrine injection is used at delivery for the prevention and/or treatment of maternal hypotension associated with spinal anesthesia in women undergoing cesarean section. Phenylephrine may be associated with a more favorable fetal acid base status than ephedrine; however, overall fetal outcomes appear to be similar. Nausea or vomiting may be less with phenylephrine than ephedrine but is also dependant upon blood pressure control. Phenylephrine may be preferred in the absence of maternal bradycardia.

Related Information

Vasoactive Agents, Intravenous *on page 2005*

Phenylephrine (Nasal) (fen il EF rin)

U.S. Brand Names 4 Way® Fast Acting [OTC]; 4 Way® Menthol [OTC]; Little Noses® Decongestant [OTC]; Neo-Synephrine® Extra Strength [OTC]; Neo-Synephrine® Mild Formula [OTC]; Neo-Synephrine® Regular Strength [OTC]; Rhinall® [OTC]; Vicks® Sinex® VapoSpray™ 4 Hour Decongestant [OTC]

Index Terms Phenylephrine Hydrochloride

Pharmacologic Category Alpha/Beta Agonist

Use For OTC use as symptomatic relief of nasal and nasopharyngeal mucosal congestion

Available Dosage Forms

Solution, intranasal:

4 Way® Fast Acting [OTC]: 1% (15 mL, 30 mL, 37 mL)

4 Way® Menthol [OTC]: 1% (15 mL, 30 mL)

Little Noses® Decongestant [OTC]: 0.125% (15 mL)

Neo-Synephrine® Extra Strength [OTC]: 1% (15 mL)

Neo-Synephrine® Mild Formula [OTC]: 0.25% (15 mL)

Neo-Synephrine® Regular Strength [OTC]: 0.5% (15 mL)

Rhinall® [OTC]: 0.25% (30 mL, 40 mL)

Vicks® Sinex® VapoSpray™ 4 Hour Decongestant [OTC]: 0.5% (15 mL)

Dosing

Adult & Geriatric Nasal congestion: Intranasal: 0.25% to 1% solution: Instill 2-3 sprays or 2-3 drops in each nostril every 4 hours as needed for ≤3 days

Pediatric Nasal congestion: Intranasal:

2-6 years: 0.125% solution: Instill 1 drop in each nostril every 2-4 hours as needed for ≤3 days

Little Noses® Decongestant: Instill 2-3 drops in each nostril every 4 hours as needed for ≤3 days

6-12 years: 0.25% solution: Instill 2-3 sprays in each nostril every 4 hours as needed for ≤3 days

>12 years: 0.25% to 0.5% solution: Instill 2-3 sprays or 2-3 drops in each nostril every 4 hours as needed for ≤3 days

Monitoring and Teaching Issues

Physical Assessment Ensure patient is not using chronically; may cause rebound congestion when discontinued.

Patient Education Do not use for more than 3 days in a row. Blow nose before use. Tilt head back and instill recommended dose of drops or spray. Do not blow nose for 5-10 minutes. You may experience transient stinging or burning. You may experience headache, trouble sleeping, nervousness, or dizziness.

Phenylephrine (Ophthalmic) (fen il EF rin)

U.S. Brand Names AK-Dilate™; Altafrin; Mydfrin®; Neofrin; OcuNefrin™ [OTC]

Index Terms Phenylephrine Hydrochloride

Generic Availability (U.S.) Yes

Pharmacologic Category Alpha/Beta Agonist; Ophthalmic Agent, Antiglaucoma; Ophthalmic Agent, Mydriatic

Medication Safety Issues

Sound-alike/look-alike issues:

Mydfrin® may be confused with Midrin®

Pregnancy Risk Factor C

Lactation Excretion in breast milk unknown/use caution

Use Used as a mydriatic in ophthalmic procedures and treatment of wide-angle glaucoma; OTC use as symptomatic relief of redness of the eye due to irritation

Available Dosage Forms

Solution, ophthalmic: 2.5% (2 mL, 3 mL, 5 mL, 15 mL)

AK-Dilate™: 2.5% (2 mL, 15 mL); 10% (5 mL)

Altafrin: 2.5% (15 mL); 10% (5 mL)

Mydfrin®: 2.5% (3 mL, 5 mL)

Neofrin: 2.5% (15 mL); 10% (5 mL)

OcuNefrin™ [OTC]: 0.12% (15 mL)

Dosing

Adult

Ocular procedures: Ophthalmic: Instill 1 drop of 2.5% or 10% solution; may repeat in 10-60 minutes as needed

Ophthalmic irritation (OTC formulation): Ophthalmic: Instill 1-2 drops 0.12% solution into affected eye up to 4 times/day; do not use for >72 hours

Geriatric

Ophthalmic preparations for pupil dilation: Instill 1 drop of 2.5% solution; may repeat in 1 hour if necessary

Other indications: Refer to adult dosing.

Pediatric Ocular procedures: Ophthalmic:

Infants <1 year: Instill 1 drop of 2.5% 15-30 minutes before procedures

Children ≥1 year: Refer to adult dosing.

Monitoring and Teaching Issues

Physical Assessment Systemic absorption from ophthalmic instillation is minimal, so there are no specific monitoring recommendations to identify adverse events.

Patient Education Do not let tip of applicator touch eye; do not contaminate tip of applicator (may cause eye infection, eye damage, or vision loss). Open eye, look at ceiling, and instill prescribed amount of solution. Close eye and roll eye in all directions, and apply gentle pressure to inner corner of eye for 1-2 minutes after instillation. Temporary stinging or blurred vision may occur. Report persistent pain, burning, double vision, or if condition worsens.

- **Phenylephrine and Diphenhydramine** *see* Diphenhydramine and Phenylephrine *on page 546*
- **Phenylephrine Hydrochloride** *see* Phenylephrine (Nasal) *on page 1451*
- **Phenylephrine Hydrochloride** *see* Phenylephrine (Ophthalmic) *on page 1452*
- **Phenylephrine Hydrochloride** *see* Phenylephrine (Systemic) *on page 1449*
- **Phenylephrine Hydrochloride and Diphenhydramine Hydrochloride** *see* Diphenhydramine and Phenylephrine *on page 546*
- **Phenylephrine Tannate and Diphenhydramine Tannate** *see* Diphenhydramine and Phenylephrine *on page 546*
- **Phenylethylmalonylurea** *see* PHENobarbital *on page 1447*
- **Phenytek®** *see* Phenytoin *on page 1453*

Phenytoin (FEN i toyn)

U.S. Brand Names Dilantin-125®; Dilantin®; Phenytek®

Index Terms Diphenylhydantoin; DPH; Phenytoin Sodium; Phenytoin Sodium, Extended; Phenytoin Sodium, Prompt

Generic Availability (U.S.) Yes: Excludes chewable tablet

Pharmacologic Category Anticonvulsant, Hydantoin

Medication Safety Issues

Sound-alike/look-alike issues:

Phenytoin may be confused with phenelzine, phentermine, PHENobarbital

Dilantin® may be confused with Dilaudid®, diltiazem, Dipentum®

High alert medication: The Institute for Safe Medication Practices (ISMP) includes this medication (I.V. formulation) among its list of drug classes which have a heightened risk of causing significant patient harm when used in error.

International issues:

Dilantin [U.S., Canada, and multiple international markets] may be confused with Dolantine brand name for pethidine [Belgium]

Medication Guide Available Yes

Pregnancy Risk Factor D

Lactation Enters breast milk/not recommended (AAP rates "compatible"; AAP 2001 update pending)

Use Management of generalized tonic-clonic (grand mal), complex partial seizures; prevention of seizures following head trauma/neurosurgery

Mechanism of Action/Effect Stabilizes neuronal membranes and decreases seizure activity by increasing efflux or decreasing influx of sodium ions across cell membranes in the motor cortex during generation of nerve impulses; prolongs effective refractory period and suppresses ventricular pacemaker automaticity, shortens action potential in the heart

Contraindications Hypersensitivity to phenytoin, other hydantoins, or any component of the formulation; pregnancy

Warnings/Precautions Antiepileptics are associated with an increased risk of suicidal behavior/thoughts with use (regardless of indication); patients should be monitored for signs/symptoms of depression, suicidal tendencies, and other unusual behavior changes during therapy and instructed to inform their healthcare provider immediately if symptoms occur.

[U.S. Boxed Warning]: Phenytoin must be administered slowly. Intravenous administration should not exceed 50 mg/minute in adult patients. In neonates, intravenous administration rate should not exceed 1-3 mg/kg/minute (most clinicians use a lower maximum rate of infusion in neonates of 0.5-1 mg/kg/minute). Hypotension may occur with rapid administration. I.V. form may cause skin necrosis at I.V. site; avoid I.V. administration in small veins; may increase frequency of petit mal seizures; use with caution in patients with porphyria; discontinue if rash or lymphadenopathy occurs; a spectrum of hematologic effects have been reported with use (eg, neutropenia, leukopenia, thrombocytopenia, pancytopenia, and anemias); use with caution in patients with hepatic dysfunction, sinus bradycardia, S-A block, or AV block; use with caution in elderly or debilitated patients, or in any condition associated with low serum albumin levels, which will increase the free fraction of phenytoin in the serum and, therefore, the pharmacologic response. Sedation, confusional states, or cerebellar dysfunction (loss of motor coordination) may occur at higher total serum concentrations, or at lower total serum concentrations when the free fraction of phenytoin is increased. Effects with other sedative drugs or ethanol may be potentiated. Abrupt withdrawal may precipitate status epilepticus. Severe reactions, including toxic epidermal necrolysis and Stevens-Johnson syndromes, although rarely reported, have resulted in fatalities; drug should be discontinued if there are any signs of rash. Patients of Asian descent with the variant *HLA-B*1502* may be at an increased risk of developing Stevens-Johnson syndrome and/or toxic epidermal necrolysis.

Drug Interactions

Metabolism/Transport Effects Substrate of CYP2C9 (major), 2C19 (major), 3A4 (minor); **Induces** CYP2B6 (strong), 2C8 (strong), 2C9 (strong), 2C19 (strong), 3A4 (strong)

Avoid Concomitant Use

Avoid concomitant use of Phenytoin with any of the following: Darunavir; Dronedarone; Etravirine; Everolimus; Lurasidone; Nilotinib; Pazopanib; Praziquantel; Ranolazine; Roflumilast; RomiDEPsin; Tolvaptan; Vandetanib

Decreased Effect

Phenytoin may decrease the levels/effects of: Acetaminophen; Amiodarone; Antifungal Agents (Azole Derivatives, Systemic); CarBAMazepine; Caspofungin; Chloramphenicol; CloZAPine; Contraceptives (Estrogens); Contraceptives (Progestins); CycloSPORINE; CycloSPORINE (Systemic); CYP2B6 Substrates; CYP2C19 Substrates; CYP2C8 Substrates (High risk); CYP2C9 Substrates (High risk); CYP3A4 Substrates; Darunavir; Deferasirox; Disopyramide; Divalproex; Doxycycline; Dronedarone; Efavirenz; Etoposide; Etoposide Phosphate; Etravirine; Everolimus; Exemestane; Felbamate; Flunarizine; Gefitinib; GuanFACINE; HMG-CoA Reductase Inhibitors; Imatinib; Irinotecan; Ixabepilone; Lacosamide; LamoTRIgine; Levodopa; Loop Diuretics; Lopinavir; Lurasidone; Maraviroc; Mebendazole; Meperidine; Methadone; MetroNIDAZOLE; MetroNIDAZOLE (Systemic); Metyrapone; Mexiletine; Nilotinib; OXcarbazepine; Pazopanib; Praziquantel; Primidone; QUEtiapine; QuiNIDine; Ranolazine; Ritonavir; Roflumilast; RomiDEPsin; Rufinamide; Saxagliptin; Sertraline; Sirolimus; SORAfenib; Tacrolimus; Tacrolimus (Systemic); Tadalafil; Temsirolimus; Teniposide; Theophylline Derivatives; Thyroid Products; Tipranavir; Tolvaptan; Topiramate; Treprostinil; Ulipristal; Valproic Acid; Vandetanib; Vecuronium; Zonisamide

The levels/effects of Phenytoin may be decreased by: Amphetamines; Antacids; CarBAMazepine; Ciprofloxacin; Ciprofloxacin (Systemic); CISplatin; Colesevelam; CYP2C19 Inducers (Strong); CYP2C9 Inducers (Highly Effective); Diazoxide; Divalproex; Folic Acid; Fosamprenavir; Ketorolac; Ketorolac (Systemic); Leucovorin Calcium-Levoleucovorin; Levomefolate; Lopinavir; Mefloquine; Methylfolate; Peginterferon Alfa-2b; Pyridoxine; Rifamycin Derivatives; Ritonavir; Theophylline Derivatives; Tipranavir; Valproic Acid; Vigabatrin

Increased Effect/Toxicity

Phenytoin may increase the levels/effects of: Alcohol (Ethyl); CNS Depressants; Fosamprenavir; Lithium; Methotrimeprazine; Vecuronium; Vitamin K Antagonists

The levels/effects of Phenytoin may be increased by: Allopurinol; Amiodarone; Antifungal Agents (Azole Derivatives, Systemic); Benzodiazepines; Calcium Channel Blockers; Capecitabine; CarBAMazepine; Carbonic Anhydrase Inhibitors; CeFAZolin; Chloramphenicol; Cimetidine; Conivaptan; CYP2C19 Inhibitors (Moderate); CYP2C19 Inhibitors (Strong); CYP2C9 Inhibitors (Moderate); CYP2C9 Inhibitors (Strong); Dexmethylphenidate; Disulfiram; Droperidol; Efavirenz; Felbamate; Floxuridine; Fluconazole; Fluorouracil; Fluorouracil (Systemic); Fluorouracil (Topical); FLUoxetine; FluvoxaMINE; Isoniazid; Methotrimeprazine; Methylphenidate; MetroNIDAZOLE; MetroNIDAZOLE (Systemic); OXcarbazepine; Proton Pump Inhibitors; Rufinamide; Sertraline; Sulfonamide Derivatives; Tacrolimus; Tacrolimus (Systemic); Ticlopidine; Topiramate; Trimethoprim; Vitamin K Antagonists

Nutritional/Ethanol Interactions

Ethanol:

Acute use: Avoid or limit ethanol (inhibits metabolism of phenytoin). Watch for sedation.

Chronic use: Avoid or limit ethanol (stimulates metabolism of phenytoin).

Food: Phenytoin serum concentrations may be altered if taken with food. If taken with enteral nutrition, phenytoin serum concentrations may be decreased. Tube feedings decrease bioavailability; hold tube feedings 1-2 hours before and 1-2 hours after phenytoin administration. May decrease calcium, folic acid, and vitamin D levels.

Herb/Nutraceutical: Avoid evening primrose (seizure threshold decreased). Avoid valerian, St John's wort, kava kava, gotu kola (may increase CNS depression).

Lab Interactions Increased glucose, alkaline phosphatase (S); decreased thyroxine (S), calcium (S)

Adverse Reactions I.V. effects: Hypotension, bradycardia, cardiac arrhythmia, cardiovascular collapse (especially with rapid I.V. use), venous irritation and pain, thrombophlebitis

Effects not related to plasma phenytoin concentrations: Hypertrichosis, gingival hypertrophy, thickening of facial features, carbohydrate intolerance, folic acid deficiency, peripheral neuropathy, vitamin D deficiency, osteomalacia, systemic lupus erythematosus

Concentration-related effects: Nystagmus, blurred vision, diplopia, ataxia, slurred speech, dizziness, drowsiness, lethargy, coma, rash, fever, nausea, vomiting, gum tenderness, confusion, mood changes, folic acid depletion, osteomalacia, hyperglycemia

Related to elevated concentrations:

>20 mcg/mL: Far lateral nystagmus

>30 mcg/mL: 45° lateral gaze nystagmus and ataxia

>40 mcg/mL: Decreased mentation

>100 mcg/mL: Death

Cardiovascular: Hypotension, bradycardia, cardiac arrhythmia, cardiovascular collapse

Central nervous system: Psychiatric changes, slurred speech, dizziness, drowsiness, headache, insomnia

Dermatologic: Rash

Gastrointestinal: Constipation, nausea, vomiting, gingival hyperplasia, enlargement of lips

Hematologic: Leukopenia, thrombocytopenia, agranulocytosis

Hepatic: Hepatitis

Local: Thrombophlebitis

Neuromuscular & skeletal: Tremor, peripheral neuropathy, paresthesia

Ocular: Diplopia, nystagmus, blurred vision

Rarely seen effects: Blood dyscrasias, coarsening of facial features, dyskinesias, hepatitis, hypertrichosis, lymphadenopathy, lymphoma, pseudolymphoma, SLE-like syndrome, Stevens-Johnson syndrome, toxic epidermal necrolysis, venous irritation and pain

Pharmacodynamics/Kinetics

Onset of Action I.V.: ~0.5-1 hour

Absorption Oral: Slow

Bioavailability Form dependent

Time to Peak Serum (form dependent): Oral: Extended-release capsule: 4-12 hours; Immediate release preparation: 2-3 hours

Protein Binding

Neonates: ≥80% (≤20% free)

Infants: ≥85% (≤15% free)

Adults: 90% to 95%

Others: Decreased protein binding

Disease states resulting in a decrease in serum albumin concentration: Burns, hepatic cirrhosis, nephrotic syndrome, pregnancy, cystic fibrosis

Disease states resulting in an apparent decrease in affinity of phenytoin for serum albumin: Renal failure, jaundice (severe), other drugs (displacers), hyperbilirubinemia (total bilirubin >15 mg/dL), Cl_{cr} <25 mL/minute (unbound fraction is increased two- to threefold in uremia)

Half-Life Elimination Oral: 22 hours (range: 7-42 hours)

Metabolism Follows dose-dependent capacity-limited (Michaelis-Menten) pharmacokinetics with increased V_{max} in infants >6 months of age and children versus adults; major metabolite (via oxidation), HPPA, undergoes enterohepatic recirculation

Excretion Urine (<5% as unchanged drug); as glucuronides

Clearance: Highly variable, dependent upon intrinsic hepatic function and dose administered; increased clearance and decreased serum concentrations with febrile illness

Available Dosage Forms

Capsule, extended release, oral: 100 mg, 200 mg, 300 mg

Dilantin®: 30 mg, 100 mg

Phenytek®: 200 mg, 300 mg

Injection, solution: 50 mg/mL (2 mL, 5 mL)

Suspension, oral: 100 mg/4 mL (4 mL); 125 mg/5 mL (120 mL, 237 mL, 240 mL)

Dilantin-125®: 125 mg/5 mL (240 mL)

Tablet, chewable, oral:

Dilantin®: 50 mg

Dosing

Adult & Geriatric Note: Phenytoin base (eg, oral suspension, chewable tablets) contains ~8% more drug than phenytoin sodium (~92 mg base is equivalent to 100 mg phenytoin sodium). Dosage adjustments and closer serum monitoring may be necessary when switching dosage forms.

Status epilepticus: I.V.: Loading dose: Manufacturer recommends 10-15 mg/kg, however, 15-20 mg/kg is generally recommended; maximum rate: 50 mg/minute

Anticonvulsant: Oral: Loading dose: 15-20 mg/kg; based on phenytoin serum concentrations and recent dosing history; administer oral loading dose in 3 divided doses given every 2-4 hours to decrease GI adverse effects and to ensure complete oral absorption; maintenance dose: 300 mg/day or 5-6 mg/kg/day in 3 divided doses or 1-2 divided doses using extended release (range: 200-1200 mg/day)

Dosage adjustment in obesity: Loading dose: Use adjusted body weight (ABW) correction based on a pharmacokinetic study of phenytoin loading doses in obese patients (Abernethy, 1985). The larger correction factor (ie, 1.33) is due to a doubling of V_d estimated in these obese patients.

ABW = [(Actual body weight – IBW) x 1.33] + IBW

Maximum loading dose: 2000 mg (Erstad, 2004)

Maintenance doses should be based on ideal body weight, conventional daily doses with adjustments based upon therapeutic drug monitoring and clinical effectiveness. (Abernethy, 1985; Erstad, 2002; Erstad, 2004)

Pediatric Note: Phenytoin base (eg, oral suspension, chewable tablets) contains ~8% more drug than phenytoin sodium (~92 mg base is equivalent to 100 mg phenytoin sodium). Dosage adjustments and closer serum monitoring may be necessary when switching dosage forms.

Status epilepticus: I.V.:

Infants and Children: Loading dose: 15-20 mg/kg in a single or divided dose; maintenance dose: Initial: 5 mg/kg/day in 2 divided doses, usual doses:

6 months to 3 years: 8-10 mg/kg/day

4-6 years: 7.5-9 mg/kg/day

7-9 years: 7-8 mg/kg/day

10-16 years: 6-7 mg/kg/day, some patients may require every 8 hours dosing

Anticonvulsant: Children: Oral: Refer to adult dosing.

Renal Impairment Phenytoin level in serum may be difficult to interpret in renal failure. Monitoring of free (unbound) concentrations or adjustment to allow interpretation is recommended.

Hepatic Impairment Safe in usual doses in mild liver disease; clearance may be substantially reduced in cirrhosis and plasma level monitoring with dose adjustment advisable. Free phenytoin levels should be monitored closely.

Administration

Oral Suspension: Shake well prior to use. Absorption is impaired when phenytoin suspension is given concurrently to patients who are receiving continuous nasogastric feedings. A method to resolve this interaction is to divide the daily dose of phenytoin and withhold the administration of nutritional supplements for 1-2 hours before and after each phenytoin dose.

I.M. Although approved for I.M. use, I.M. administration is not recommended due to erratic absorption and pain on injection. Fosphenytoin may be considered.

I.V. Vesicant. Fosphenytoin may be considered for loading in patients who are in status epilepticus, hemodynamically unstable or develop hypotension/bradycardia with I.V. administration of phenytoin. Phenytoin may be administered by IVP or IVPB administration. The maximum rate of I.V. administration is 50 mg/minute in adults. In neonates, the manufacturer recommends a maximum rate of 1-3 mg/kg/minute; however, a lower maximum rate of 0.5-1 mg/kg/minute is used clinically (Sankar, 2010; Shields, 1989). Highly sensitive patients (eg, elderly, patients with pre-existing cardiovascular conditions) should receive phenytoin more slowly (eg, 20 mg/minute).

Other SubQ administration is not recommended because of the possibility of local tissue damage (due to high pH).

Stability

Reconstitution I.V.: Further dilution of the solution for I.V. infusion is controversial and no consensus exists as to the optimal concentration and length of stability. Stability is concentration and pH dependent. Based on limited clinical consensus, NS or LR are recommended diluents; dilutions of 1-10 mg/mL have been used and should be administered as soon as possible after preparation (some recommend to discard if not used within 4 hours). Do not refrigerate.

Storage

Capsule, tablet: Store at controlled room temperature. Protect from light and moisture.

Oral suspension: Store at room temperature of 20°C to 25°C (68°F to 77°F); do not freeze. Protect from light.

Solution for injection: Store at room temperature of 15°C to 30°C (59°F to 86°F). Use only clear solutions free of precipitate and haziness; slightly yellow solutions may be used. Precipitation may occur if solution is refrigerated and may dissolve at room temperature.

Monitoring and Teaching Issues

Laboratory Monitoring Plasma phenytoin level, CBC, liver function. **Note:** If available, free phenytoin concentrations should be obtained in patients with renal impairment and/or hypoalbuminemia. If free phenytoin levels are unavailable, the adjusted total level is based upon equations in adult patients.

Physical Assessment When discontinuing oral formulation, taper dose gradually; abrupt discontinuance can cause exacerbation of seizures. **I.V.:** Monitor blood pressure. Infusion site should be monitored closely. Patient should be monitored closely for adverse/toxic results, including suicide ideation.

Patient Education Take preferably on an empty stomach. Do not crush, break, or chew extended release capsules. Shake liquid suspension well before using. Follow recommended diet, avoid alcohol, and maintain adequate hydration unless instructed to restrict fluid intake. May cause gum or mouth soreness, drowsiness, dizziness, nervousness, headache, nausea, or vomiting. Report chest pain, irregular heartbeat, or palpitations; slurred speech, unsteady gait, coordination difficulties, suicide ideation, or change in mentation; skin rash; unresolved nausea, vomiting, or constipation; swollen glands; swollen, sore, or bleeding gums; unusual bruising or bleeding; acute persistent fatigue; or vision changes.

Dietary Considerations

Folic acid: Phenytoin may decrease mucosal uptake of folic acid; to avoid folic acid deficiency and megaloblastic anemia, some clinicians recommend giving patients on anticonvulsants prophylactic doses of folic acid and cyanocobalamin. However, folate supplementation may increase seizures in some patients (dose dependent). Discuss with healthcare provider prior to using any supplements.

Calcium: Hypocalcemia has been reported in patients taking prolonged high-dose therapy with an anticonvulsant. Some clinicians have given an additional 4000 units/week of vitamin D (especially in those receiving poor nutrition and getting no sun exposure) to prevent hypocalcemia.

Vitamin D: Phenytoin interferes with vitamin D metabolism and osteomalacia may result; may need to supplement with vitamin D

Tube feedings: Tube feedings decrease phenytoin absorption. To avoid decreased serum levels with continuous NG feeds, hold feedings for 1-2 hours prior to and 1-2 hours after phenytoin administration, if possible. There is a variety of opinions on how to administer phenytoin with enteral feedings. Be **consistent** throughout therapy.

Injection may contain sodium.

Geriatric Considerations Elderly may have reduced hepatic clearance due to age decline in phase I metabolism. Elderly may have low albumin which will increase free fraction and, therefore, pharmacologic response. Monitor closely in those who are hypoalbuminemic. Free fraction measurements advised, also elderly may display a higher incidence of adverse effects (cardiovascular) when using the I.V. loading regimen; therefore, recommended to decrease loading I.V. dose to 25 mg/minute.

Breast-Feeding Considerations Phenytoin is excreted in breast milk; however, the amount to which the infant is exposed is considered small. The manufacturers of phenytoin do not recommend breast-feeding during therapy. Women should be counseled of the possible risks and benefits associated with breast-feeding while on phenytoin.

Pregnancy Considerations Phenytoin crosses the placenta. Congenital malformations (including a pattern of malformations termed the "fetal hydantoin syndrome" or "fetal anticonvulsant syndrome") have been reported in infants. Isolated cases of malignancies (including neuroblastoma) and coagulation defects in the neonate following delivery have also been reported. Epilepsy itself, the number of medications, genetic factors, or a combination of these probably influence the teratogenicity of anticonvulsant therapy.

Total plasma concentrations of phenytoin are decreased by 56% in the mother during pregnancy; unbound plasma (free) concentrations are decreased by 31%. Because protein binding is decreased, monitoring of unbound plasma concentrations is recommended. Concentrations should be monitored through the 8th week postpartum. The use of folic acid throughout pregnancy and vitamin K during the last month of pregnancy is recommended.

Patients exposed to phenytoin during pregnancy are encouraged to enroll themselves into the AED Pregnancy Registry by calling 1-888-233-2334. Additional information is available at www.aedpregnancyregistry.org.

Related Information

Anticonvulsant Drugs of Choice *on page 1981*

Peak and Trough Guidelines *on page 1958*

◆ **Phenytoin Sodium** *see* Phenytoin *on page 1453*

◆ **Phenytoin Sodium, Extended** *see* Phenytoin *on page 1453*

◆ **Phenytoin Sodium, Prompt** *see* Phenytoin *on page 1453*

◆ **Phos-NaK** *see* Potassium Phosphate and Sodium Phosphate *on page 1486*

◆ **Phospha 250™ Neutral** *see* Potassium Phosphate and Sodium Phosphate *on page 1486*

◆ **Phosphate, Potassium** *see* Potassium Phosphate *on page 1484*
◆ **Phosphonoformate** *see* Foscarnet *on page 828*
◆ **Phosphonoformic Acid** *see* Foscarnet *on page 828*
◆ **Phrenilin®** *see* Butalbital and Acetaminophen *on page 261*
◆ **Phrenilin® Forte** *see* Butalbital and Acetaminophen *on page 261*
◆ ***p*-Hydroxyampicillin** *see* Amoxicillin *on page 110*
◆ **Phylloquinone** *see* Phytonadione *on page 1457*
◆ **Phytomenadione** *see* Phytonadione *on page 1457*

Phytonadione (fye toe na DYE one)

U.S. Brand Names Mephyton®
Index Terms Methylphytyl Napthoquinone; Phylloquinone; Phytomenadione; Vitamin K_1
Generic Availability (U.S.) Yes
Pharmacologic Category Vitamin, Fat Soluble
Medication Safety Issues
Sound-alike/look-alike issues:
Mephyton® may be confused with melphalan, methadone
Pregnancy Risk Factor C
Lactation Enters breast milk/use caution (AAP rates "compatible"; AAP 2001 update pending)
Use Prevention and treatment of hypoprothrombinemia caused by coumarin derivative-induced or other drug-induced vitamin K deficiency, hypoprothrombinemia caused by malabsorption or inability to synthesize vitamin K; hemorrhagic disease of the newborn
Unlabeled/Investigational Use Treatment of hypoprothrombinemia caused by anticoagulant rodenticides
Mechanism of Action/Effect Promotes liver synthesis of clotting factors (II, VII, IX, X); however, the exact mechanism as to this stimulation is unknown. Menadiol is a water soluble form of vitamin K; phytonadione has a more rapid and prolonged effect than menadione; menadiol sodium diphosphate (K_4) is half as potent as menadione (K_3).
Contraindications Hypersensitivity to phytonadione or any component of the formulation
Warnings/Precautions [U.S. Boxed Warning]: Severe reactions resembling hypersensitivity (eg, anaphylaxis) reactions have occurred rarely during or immediately after I.V. administration. Allergic reactions have also occurred with I.M. and SubQ injections; oral administration is the safest. In obstructive jaundice or with biliary fistulas concurrent administration of bile salts is necessary. Manufacturers recommend the SubQ route over other parenteral routes. SubQ is less predictable when compared to the oral route. The American College of Chest Physicians recommends the I.V. route in patients with serious or life-threatening bleeding secondary to warfarin. The I.V. route should be restricted to emergency situations where oral phytonadione cannot be used. Efficacy is delayed regardless of route of administration; patient management may require other treatments in the interim. Administer a dose that will quickly lower the INR into a safe range without causing resistance to warfarin. High phytonadione doses may lead to warfarin resistance for at least one week. Use caution in newborns especially premature infants; hemolysis, jaundice and hyperbilirubinemia have been reported with larger than recommended doses. Some dosage forms contain benzyl alcohol which has been associated with "gasping syndrome" in premature infants. In liver disease, if initial doses do not reverse coagulopathy then higher doses are unlikely to have any effect. Ineffective in hereditary hypoprothrombinemia. Use caution with renal dysfunction (including premature infants). Injectable products may contain aluminum; may result in toxic levels following prolonged administration. Product may contain polysorbate 80.
Drug Interactions
Avoid Concomitant Use There are no known interactions where it is recommended to avoid concomitant use.
Decreased Effect
Phytonadione may decrease the levels/effects of: Vitamin K Antagonists

The levels/effects of Phytonadione may be decreased by: Mineral Oil; Orlistat
Increased Effect/Toxicity There are no known significant interactions involving an increase in effect.
Adverse Reactions Parenteral administration: Frequency not defined.
Cardiovascular: Cyanosis, flushing, hypotension
Central nervous system: Dizziness
Dermatologic: Scleroderma-like lesions
Endocrine & metabolic: Hyperbilirubinemia (newborn; greater than recommended doses)
Gastrointestinal: Abnormal taste
Local: Injection site reactions
Respiratory: Dyspnea
Miscellaneous: Anaphylactoid reactions, diaphoresis, hypersensitivity reactions
Pharmacodynamics/Kinetics
Onset of Action
Onset of action: Increased coagulation factors: Oral: 6-10 hours; I.V.: 1-2 hours
Peak effect: INR values return to normal: Oral: 24-48 hours; I.V.: 12-14 hours
Absorption Oral: From intestines in presence of bile; SubQ: Variable
Metabolism Rapidly hepatic
Excretion Urine and feces

Available Dosage Forms

Injection, aqueous colloidal: 1 mg/0.5 mL (0.5 mL); 10 mg/mL (1 mL)
Injection, aqueous colloidal [preservative free]: 1 mg/0.5 mL (0.5 mL)
Tablet, oral: 100 mcg
Mephyton®: 5 mg

Dosing

Adult & Geriatric Note: According to the manufacturer, SubQ is the preferred parenteral route; I.M. route should be avoided due to the risk of hematoma formation; I.V. route should be restricted for emergency use only. The American College of Chest Physicians recommends the I.V. route in patients with serious or life-threatening bleeding secondary to use of vitamin K antagonists.

Adequate intake: Males: 120 mcg/day; Females: 90 mcg/day

Hypoprothrombinemia due to drugs (other than coumarin derivatives) or factors limiting absorption or synthesis: Oral, SubQ, I.M., I.V.: Initial: 2.5-25 mg (rarely up to 50 mg)

Vitamin K deficiency (supratherapeutic INR) secondary to coumarin derivative (Ansell, 2008):

If INR above therapeutic range to <5 (no significant bleeding and rapid reversal unnecessary): Lower or hold next dose and monitor frequently; when INR approaches desired range, resume dosing with a lower dose.

If INR ≥5 and <9 (no significant bleeding): If no risk factors for bleeding exist, omit next 1 or 2 doses, monitor INR more frequently, and resume with an appropriately adjusted dose when INR in desired range.

Alternatively, if other risk factors for bleeding exist, omit next dose and administer vitamin K orally 1-2.5 mg; resume with an appropriately adjusted dose when INR in desired range.

If INR ≥5 and <9 (no significant bleeding and rapid reversal required for surgery): Administer vitamin K orally ≤5 mg and hold warfarin. Expect INR to be reduced within 24 hours; if INR still elevated, another 1-2 mg of vitamin K orally may be given.

If INR ≥9 (no significant bleeding): Hold warfarin, administer vitamin K orally 2.5-5 mg, expect INR to be reduced within 24-48 hours, monitor INR more frequently and give additional vitamin K at an appropriate dose if necessary. Resume warfarin at an appropriately adjusted dose when INR is in desired range.

If serious bleeding at any INR elevation: Hold warfarin, administer vitamin K 10 mg by slow I.V. infusion and supplement with FFP, PCC, or rFVIIa depending on the urgency of the situation; I.V. vitamin K may be repeated every 12 hours.

If life-threatening bleeding: Hold warfarin, give FFP, PCC, or rFVIIa supplemented with vitamin K 10 mg slow I.V. infusion; repeat if necessary, depending on INR.

Notes:

If mild-moderate INR elevation without major bleeding occurs, administer vitamin K orally instead of subcutaneously.

Use of high doses of vitamin K (eg, 10-15 mg) may cause warfarin resistance for ≥1 week. During this period of resistance, heparin or low molecular weight heparin may be given until INR responds.

FFP=fresh frozen plasma; PCC=prothrombin complex concentrate; rFVIIa=recombinant factor VIIa

Pediatric Note: According to the manufacturer, SubQ is the preferred parenteral route; I.M. route should be avoided due to the risk of hematoma formation; I.V. route should be restricted for emergency use only. The American College of Chest Physicians recommends the I.V. route in patients with serious or life-threatening bleeding secondary to use of vitamin K antagonists.

Adequate intake:

1-3 years: 30 mcg/day
4-8 years: 55 mcg/day
9-13 years: 60 mcg/day
14-18 years: 75 mcg/day

Hemorrhagic disease of the newborn:

Prophylaxis: I.M.: 0.5-1 mg within 1 hour of birth

Treatment: I.M., SubQ: 1 mg/dose/day; higher doses may be necessary if mother has been receiving oral anticoagulants

Administration

Oral The parenteral preparation has been administered orally to neonates.

I.V. Infuse slowly; rate of infusion should not exceed 1 mg/minute (3 mg/m^2/minute in children and infants). The injectable route should be used only if the oral route is not feasible or there is a greater urgency to reverse anticoagulation.

Stability

Reconstitution Dilute injection solution in preservative-free NS, D_5W, or D_5NS.

Storage

Injection: Store at 15°C to 30°C (59°F to 86°F). **Note:** Store Hospira product at 20°C to 25°C (68°F to 77°F).

Oral: Store tablets at 15°C to 30°C (59°F to 86°F). Protect from light.

Monitoring and Teaching Issues

Laboratory Monitoring PT, INR

Physical Assessment Note dosing specifics according to use. Assess degree of bleeding.

Patient Education Oral: Consult prescriber for recommended diet. Report bleeding gums; blood in urine, stool, or vomitus; unusual bruising or bleeding; or abdominal cramping.

Pregnancy Considerations Animal reproduction studies have not been conducted.

◆ **Pidorubicin** *see* Epirubicin *on page* 633

◆ **Pidorubicin Hydrochloride** *see* Epirubicin *on page* 633

Pimozide (PI moe zide)

U.S. Brand Names Orap®

Generic Availability (U.S.) No

Pharmacologic Category Antipsychotic Agent, Typical

Pregnancy Risk Factor C

Lactation Excretion in breast milk unknown/not recommended

Use Suppression of severe motor and phonic tics in patients with Tourette's disorder who have failed to respond satisfactorily to standard treatment

Unlabeled/Investigational Use Psychosis; reported use in individuals with delusions focused on physical symptoms (ie, preoccupation with parasitic infestation); Huntington's chorea

Available Dosage Forms

Tablet, oral:

Orap®: 1 mg, 2 mg

Dosing

Adult

Tourette's disorder: Oral: Initial: 1-2 mg/day, then increase dosage as needed every other day; range is usually 7-10 mg/day; maximum: 10 mg/day or 0.2 mg/kg/day (whichever is less)

Note: An ECG should be performed baseline and periodically thereafter, especially during dosage adjustment.

Geriatric Recommend initial dose of 1 mg/day; periodically attempt gradual reduction of dose to determine if tic persists; follow up for 1-2 weeks before concluding the tic is a persistent disease phenomenon and not a manifestation of drug withdrawal. **Note:** An ECG should be performed baseline and periodically thereafter, especially during dosage adjustment.

Pediatric

Tourette's disorder: Oral:

Children ≤12 years: Initial: 0.05 mg/kg preferably once at bedtime; may be increased every third day; usual range: 2-4 mg/day; do not exceed 10 mg/day (0.2 mg/kg/day); maximum dose: 10 mg/day or 0.2 mg/kg/day (whichever is less)

Children >12 years: Refer to adult dosing.

Note: An ECG should be performed baseline and periodically thereafter, especially during dosage adjustment.

Adjustment for Toxicity

ECG changes:

Children: QT_c prolongation >0.47 seconds or >25% above baseline: Decrease dose.

Adults: QT_c prolongation >0.52 seconds or >25% above baseline: Decrease dose.

NMS syndrome: Discontinue (monitor carefully if therapy is reinitiated).

Tardive dyskinesia signs/symptoms: Consider discontinuing.

Monitoring and Teaching Issues

Laboratory Monitoring Lipid profile, electrolytes, fasting blood glucose/Hgb A_{1c}; BMI

Physical Assessment Assess patient/caregiver knowledge of rationale for therapy and risks involved. Assess results of ophthalmic exam and blood pressure at beginning of therapy and periodically throughout. Conduct ECG at baseline and periodically during therapy (especially during dosage adjustment). Initiate at lower doses and decrease dosage slowly when discontinuing.

Patient Education It may take 2-3 weeks to achieve desired results. Avoid alcohol. Maintain adequate hydration unless instructed to restrict fluid intake. You may experience excess drowsiness, restlessness, dizziness, blurred vision, constipation, dry mouth, or anorexia. Report persistent CNS effects (eg, trembling fingers, altered gait or balance, excessive sedation, seizures, unusual muscle or facial movements, anxiety, abnormal thoughts, confusion, personality changes), unresolved constipation or GI effects, breast swelling (male and female) or decreased sexual ability, vision changes, respiratory difficulty, unusual cough or flu-like symptoms, or worsening of condition.

Related Information

Antipsychotic Agents *on page 1986*

Pindolol (PIN doe lole)

Generic Availability (U.S.) Yes

Pharmacologic Category Beta Blocker With Intrinsic Sympathomimetic Activity

Medication Safety Issues

Sound-alike/look-alike issues:

Pindolol may be confused with Parlodel®, Plendil®

Visken® may be confused with Visine®, Viskazide®

Pregnancy Risk Factor B

Lactation Enters breast milk/not recommended

Use Treatment of hypertension, alone or in combination with other agents

Unlabeled/Investigational Use Potential augmenting agent for antidepressants; ventricular arrhythmias/tachycardia, antipsychotic-induced akathisia, situational anxiety; aggressive behavior associated with dementia

Available Dosage Forms

Tablet, oral: 5 mg, 10 mg

Dosing

Adult

Hypertension: Oral: Initial: 5 mg twice daily, increase as necessary by 10 mg/day every 3-4 weeks (maximum daily dose: 60 mg); usual dose range (JNC 7): 10-40 mg twice daily.

Antidepressant augmentation (unlabeled use): Oral: 2.5 mg 3 times/day

Geriatric Oral: Initial: 5 mg once daily; increase as necessary by 5 mg/day every 3-4 weeks.

Renal Impairment Use with caution. Clearance significantly decreased in uremic patients. Dosage reduction may be necessary.

Hepatic Impairment Use with caution. Elimination half-life in cirrhotic patients may be 10 times as long compared to normal patients. Dosage reduction is necessary in severely impaired.

Administration

Oral May be administered without regard to meals.

Related Information

Beta-Blockers *on page* 1990

◆ **Pink Bismuth** *see* Bismuth *on page* 221

Pioglitazone (pye oh GLI ta zone)

U.S. Brand Names Actos®

Generic Availability (U.S.) No

Pharmacologic Category Antidiabetic Agent, Thiazolidinedione

Medication Safety Issues

Sound-alike/look-alike issues:

Actos® may be confused with Actidose®, Actonel®

International issues:

Tiazac: Brand name for piogitazone [Chile], but also the brand name for diltiazem [U.S, Canada]

Medication Guide Available Yes

Pregnancy Risk Factor C

Lactation Excretion in breast milk unknown/not recommended

Use

Type 2 diabetes mellitus (noninsulin dependent, NIDDM), monotherapy: Adjunct to diet and exercise, to improve glycemic control

Type 2 diabetes mellitus (noninsulin dependent, NIDDM), combination therapy with sulfonylurea, metformin, or insulin: When diet, exercise, and a single agent alone does not result in adequate glycemic control

Mechanism of Action/Effect Thiazolidinedione antidiabetic agent that lowers blood glucose by improving target cell response to insulin, without increasing pancreatic insulin secretion. It has a mechanism of action that is dependent on the presence of insulin for activity.

Contraindications Hypersensitivity to pioglitazone or any component of the formulation; NYHA Class III/IV heart failure (initiation of therapy)

Canadian labeling: Additional contraindications (not is U.S. labeling): Any stage of heart failure (eg, NYHA Class I, II, III, IV); serious hepatic impairment; pregnancy

Warnings/Precautions [U.S. Boxed Warning]: Thiazolidinediones, including pioglitazone, may cause or exacerbate heart failure; closely monitor for signs and symptoms of heart failure (eg, rapid weight gain, dyspnea, edema), particularly after initiation or dose increases. Not recommended for use in any patient with symptomatic heart failure. In the U.S., initiation of therapy is contraindicated in patients with NYHA class III or IV heart failure. If used in patients with NYHA class II (systolic heart failure), initiate at lowest dosage and monitor closely. In Canada, use in any stage of heart failure (NYHA I, II, III, IV) is contraindicated. Use with caution in patients with edema; may increase plasma volume and/or cause fluid retention. Dose reduction or discontinuation is recommended if heart failure suspected. Dose-related weight gain observed with use; mechanism unknown but likely associated with fluid retention and fat accumulation.

Should not be used in diabetic ketoacidosis. Mechanism requires the presence of insulin; therefore use in type 1 diabetes is not recommended. Use with caution in premenopausal, anovulatory women - may result in a resumption of ovulation, increasing the risk of pregnancy. Use with caution in patients with anemia (may reduce hemoglobin and hematocrit). Increased incidence of bone fractures in females treated with pioglitazone; majority of fractures occurred in the lower limb and distal upper limb.

Use with caution in patients with elevated transaminases (AST or ALT); do not initiate in patients with active liver disease of ALT >2.5 times the upper limit of normal at baseline. During therapy, if ALT >3 times the upper limit of normal, re-evaluate levels promptly and discontinue if elevation persists or if jaundice occurs at any time during use. Idiosyncratic hepatotoxicity has been reported with another thiazolidinedione agent (troglitazone); avoid use in patients who previously experienced jaundice during troglitazone therapy. Monitoring should include periodic determinations of liver function. Use caution with pre-existing macular edema or diabetic retinopathy. Postmarketing reports of new-onset or worsening diabetic macular edema with decreased visual acuity has been reported. Safety and efficacy have not been established in children.

Canadian labeling (not in U.S. labeling) states use with insulin **or** as part of triple therapy (pioglitazone in combination with a sulfonylurea and metformin) is not indicated.

Drug Interactions

Metabolism/Transport Effects Substrate of CYP2C8 (major), 3A4 (minor); **Inhibits** CYP2C8 (moderate), 2C9 (weak), 2C19 (weak) **Induces** CYP3A4 (weak)

Avoid Concomitant Use There are no known interactions where it is recommended to avoid concomitant use.

Decreased Effect

Pioglitazone may decrease the levels/effects of: Saxagliptin

The levels/effects of Pioglitazone may be decreased by: Bile Acid Sequestrants; Corticosteroids (Orally Inhaled); Corticosteroids (Systemic); CYP2C8 Inducers (Highly Effective); Luteinizing Hormone-Releasing Hormone Analogs; Rifampin; Somatropin; Thiazide Diuretics

Increased Effect/Toxicity

Pioglitazone may increase the levels/effects of: CYP2C8 Substrates (High risk); Hypoglycemic Agents

The levels/effects of Pioglitazone may be increased by: Conivaptan; CYP2C8 Inhibitors (Moderate); CYP2C8 Inhibitors (Strong); Deferasirox; Gemfibrozil; Herbs (Hypoglycemic Properties); Insulin; Pegvisomant; Pregabalin; Trimethoprim

Nutritional/Ethanol Interactions

Ethanol: Caution with ethanol (may cause hypoglycemia).

Food: Peak concentrations are delayed when administered with food, but the extent of absorption is not affected. Pioglitazone may be taken without regard to meals.

Herb/Nutraceutical: Caution with alfalfa, aloe, bilberry, bitter melon, burdock, celery, damiana, fenugreek, garcinia, garlic, ginger, ginseng (American), gymnema, marshmallow, and stinging nettle (may cause hypoglycemia).

Adverse Reactions

>10%:

Cardiovascular: Edema (5%; in combination trials with sulfonlyureas or insulin, the incidence of edema was as high as 15%)

Respiratory: Upper respiratory tract infection (13%)

1% to 10%:

Cardiovascular: Heart failure (requiring hospitalization; up to 6% in patients with prior macrovascular disease)

Central nervous system: Headache (9%), fatigue (4%)

Gastrointestinal: Tooth disorder (5%)

Hematologic: Anemia (≤2%)

Neuromuscular & skeletal: Myalgia (5%)

Respiratory: Sinusitis (6%), pharyngitis (5%)

Frequency not defined: HDL-cholesterol increased, hematocrit/hemoglobin decreased, hypoglycemia (in combination trials with sulfonylureas or insulin), serum triglycerides decreased, weight gain/loss

Pharmacodynamics/Kinetics

Onset of Action Delayed; Peak effect: Glucose control: Several weeks

Time to Peak ~2 hours; delayed with food

Protein Binding Pioglitazone >99% and active metabolites >98%; primarily to albumin

Half-Life Elimination Parent drug: 3-7 hours; Total: 16-24 hours

Metabolism Hepatic (99%) via CYP2C8 and 3A4 to both active and inactive metabolites

Excretion Urine (15% to 30%) and feces as metabolites

Available Dosage Forms

Tablet, oral:

Actos®: 15 mg, 30 mg, 45 mg

Dosing

Adult & Geriatric Type 2 diabetes: Oral:

Monotherapy: Initial: 15-30 mg once daily; if response is inadequate, the dosage may be increased in increments up to 45 mg once daily; maximum recommended dose: 45 mg once daily

Combination therapy:

Note: Maximum recommended dose: 45 mg/day

With sulfonylureas: Initial: 15-30 mg once daily; dose of sulfonylurea should be reduced if the patient reports hypoglycemia

With metformin: Initial: 15-30 mg once daily; it is unlikely that the dose of metformin will need to be reduced due to hypoglycemia

With insulin: Initial: 15-30 mg once daily; dose of insulin should be reduced by 10% to 25% if the patient reports hypoglycemia or if the plasma glucose falls to below 100 mg/dL.

Dosage adjustment in patients with CHF (NYHA Class II) in mono- or combination therapy: Oral: Initial: 15 mg once daily; may be increased after several months of treatment, with close attention to heart failure symptoms

Renal Impairment No adjustment is necessary.

Hepatic Impairment Clearance is significantly lower in hepatic impairment (Child-Pugh Grade B/C). Therapy should not be initiated if the patient exhibits active liver disease or increased transaminases (>2.5 times ULN) at baseline. During treatment if ALT levels elevate >3 times ULN, the test should be repeated as soon as possible. If ALT levels remain >3 times ULN or if the patient is jaundiced, therapy should be discontinued.

Administration

Oral May be administered without regard to meals.

Monitoring and Teaching Issues

Laboratory Monitoring Hemoglobin A_{1c}, serum glucose, liver enzymes prior to initiation and periodically during treatment (per clinician judgment); if the ALT is increased to >2.5 times ULN, liver function testing should be performed more frequently until the levels return to normal or pretreatment values. Patients with an elevation in ALT >3 times ULN should be rechecked as soon as possible. If the ALT levels remain >3 times ULN, therapy with pioglitazone should be discontinued.

Physical Assessment Monitor for signs of heart failure (weight gain, edema, dyspnea). Teach risks of hyperglycemia. Refer patient to a diabetic educator, if available.

Patient Education May be taken without regard to meals. Avoid or use caution with alcohol while taking this medication. If dose is missed, take as soon as possible. If dose is missed completely one day, do not double dose the next day. Follow dietary, exercise, and glucose monitoring instructions of prescriber (more frequent monitoring may be advised in periods of stress, trauma, surgery, increased exercise). Report respiratory infection, unusual weight gain, aggravation of hyper-/hypoglycemic condition, unusual swelling of extremities, shortness of breath, fatigue, yellowing of skin or eyes, dark urine, pale stool, nausea/vomiting, abdominal pain, or muscle pain.

Dietary Considerations Management of type 2 diabetes mellitus (noninsulin dependent, NIDDM) should include diet control. May be taken without regard to meals.

Geriatric Considerations No dosage adjustment is recommended in elderly patients. Intensive glucose control (Hb A_{1c} <6.5%) has been linked to increased all cause and cardiovascular mortality, hypoglycemia requiring assistance, and weight gain in adult type 2 diabetes. For elderly patients with diabetes who are relatively healthy, attaining target goals for aspirin use, blood pressure, lipids, smoking cessation, and diet and exercise may be more important than normalized glycemic control.

Breast-Feeding Considerations It is not known if pioglitazone is excreted in breast milk. Breast-feeding is not recommended by the manufacturer.

Pregnancy Considerations Pioglitazone is classified as pregnancy category C due to adverse effects observed in animal studies. The use of pioglitazone in pregnant women is limited to very few case reports where pregnancy occurred during treatment for polycystic ovarian syndrome (PCOS); details concerning fetal outcomes are limited. Thiazolidinediones may cause ovulation in anovulatory premenopausal women, increasing the risk of pregnancy; adequate contraception in premenopausal women is recommended. Maternal hyperglycemia can be associated with adverse effects in the fetus, including macrosomia, neonatal hyperglycemia, and hyperbilirubinemia; the risk of congenital malformations is increased when the Hb A_{1c} is above the normal range. Diabetes can also be associated with adverse effects in the mother. Poorly-treated diabetes may cause end-organ damage that may in turn negatively affect obstetric outcomes. Physiologic glucose levels should be maintained prior to and during pregnancy to decrease the risk of adverse events in the mother and the fetus. Until additional safety and efficacy data are obtained, the use of oral agents is generally not recommended as routine management of GDM or type 2 diabetes mellitus during pregnancy. Insulin is the drug of choice for the control of diabetes mellitus during pregnancy.

Related Information

Diabetes Mellitus Management, Adults *on page 2026*

Pioglitazone and Glimepiride (pye oh GLI ta zone & GLYE me pye ride)

U.S. Brand Names Duetact™

Index Terms Glimepiride and Pioglitazone; Glimepiride and Pioglitazone Hydrochloride

Generic Availability (U.S.) No

Pharmacologic Category Antidiabetic Agent, Sulfonylurea; Antidiabetic Agent, Thiazolidinedione; Hypoglycemic Agent, Oral

Medication Safety Issues

High alert medication: The Institute for Safe Medication Practices (ISMP) includes this medication among its list of drugs which have a heightened risk of causing significant patient harm when used in error.

Medication Guide Available Yes

Pregnancy Risk Factor C

Lactation Excretion in breast milk unknown/not recommended

Use Management of type 2 diabetes mellitus (noninsulin dependent, NIDDM) as an adjunct to diet and exercise

Available Dosage Forms

Tablet:

Duetact™: 30 mg/2 mg: Pioglitazone 30 mg and glimepiride 2 mg; 30 mg/4 mg: Pioglitazone 30 mg and glimepiride 4 mg

Dosing

Adult Type 2 diabetes mellitus: Oral: Initial dose should be based on current dose of pioglitazone and/or sulfonylurea.

Patients inadequately controlled on **glimepiride** alone: Initial dose: 30 mg/2 mg or 30 mg/4 mg once daily

Patients inadequately controlled on **pioglitazone** alone: Initial dose: 30 mg/2 mg once daily

Patients with systolic dysfunction (eg, NYHA Class I and II): Initiate only after patient has been safely titrated to 30 mg of pioglitazone. Initial dose: 30 mg/2 mg or 30 mg/4 mg once daily.

Note: No exact dosing relationship exists between glimepiride and other sulfonlyureas. Dosing should be limited to less than or equal to the maximum initial dose of glimepiride (2 mg). When converting patients from other sulfonylureas with longer half-lives (eg, chlorpropamide) to glimepiride, observe patient carefully for 1-2 weeks due to overlapping hypoglycemic effects.

Dosing adjustment: Dosage may be increased up to max dose and formulation strengths available; tablet should not be given more than once daily; see individual agents for frequency of adjustments. Dosage adjustments in patients with systolic dysfunction should be done carefully and patient monitored for symptoms of worsening heart failure.

Maximum dose: Pioglitazone 45 mg/glimepiride 8 mg daily

Geriatric Initial: Glimepiride 1 mg/day prior to initiating Duetact™; dose titration and maintenance dosing should be conservative to avoid hypoglycemia. Refer to adult dosing.

Renal Impairment Cl_{cr} <22 mL/minute: Initial dose should be 1 mg of glimepiride and dosage increments should be based on fasting blood glucose levels.

Hepatic Impairment Do not initiate treatment with active liver disease or ALT >2.5 times ULN. During treatment, if ALT levels elevate >3 times ULN, the test should be repeated as soon as possible. If ALT levels remain >3 times ULN or if the patient is jaundiced, Duetact™ should be discontinued.

Administration

Oral Administer once daily with the first main meal of the day. To avoid hypoglycemia, patients without oral intake may need to have the dose held.

Monitoring and Teaching Issues

Laboratory Monitoring Hemoglobin A_{1C}, serum glucose; liver enzymes and renal function prior to initiation and periodically during treatment

Note: If the ALT is increased to >2.5 times ULN, liver function testing should be performed more frequently until the levels return to normal or pretreatment values. If ALT levels elevate >3 times ULN, the test should be repeated as soon as possible. If ALT levels remain >3 times ULN or if the patient is jaundiced, therapy should be discontinued. Also monitor hemoglobin A_{1C}, serum glucose

Physical Assessment See individual agents.

Patient Education See individual agents.

Pioglitazone and Metformin (pye oh GLI ta zone & met FOR min)

U.S. Brand Names Actoplus Met®; Actoplus Met® XR

Index Terms Metformin Hydrochloride and Pioglitazone Hydrochloride

Generic Availability (U.S.) No

Pharmacologic Category Antidiabetic Agent, Biguanide; Antidiabetic Agent, Thiazolidinedione

Medication Guide Available Yes

Pregnancy Risk Factor C

Lactation

Metformin: Enters breast milk/not recommended

Pioglitazone: Excretion in breast milk unknown/not recommended

Use Management of type 2 diabetes mellitus (noninsulin dependent, NIDDM)

Mechanism of Action/Effect

Pioglitazone is a thiazolidinedione antidiabetic agent that lowers blood glucose by improving target cell response to insulin, without increasing pancreatic insulin secretion. It has a mechanism of action that is dependent on the presence of insulin for activity.

Metformin decreases hepatic glucose production, decreasing intestinal absorption of glucose, and improves insulin sensitivity (increases peripheral glucose uptake and utilization).

Contraindications Hypersensitivity to pioglitazone, metformin, or any component of the formulation; NYHA Class III/IV heart failure (initiation of therapy); renal disease or renal dysfunction (serum creatinine ≥1.5 mg/dL in males or ≥1.4 mg/dL in females, or abnormal creatinine clearance which may also result from conditions such as cardiovascular collapse, acute myocardial infarction, and septicemia); acute or chronic metabolic acidosis with or without coma (including diabetic ketoacidosis); concurrent iodinated radiocontrast adminstration (manufacturer recommends temporary discontinuation of metformin)

Warnings/Precautions [U.S. Boxed Warning]: Lactic acidosis is a rare, but potentially severe consequence of therapy with metformin. Lactic acidosis should be suspected in any patient with diabetes receiving metformin with evidence of acidosis but without evidence of ketoacidosis. Discontinue metformin in clinical situations predisposing to hypoxemia, including conditions such as cardiovascular collapse, respiratory failure, acute myocardial infarction, acute congestive heart failure, and septicemia.

Metformin is substantially excreted by the kidney. The risk of accumulation and lactic acidosis increases with the degree of impairment of renal function. Patients with renal function below the limit of normal for their age should not receive metformin. In elderly patients, renal function should be monitored regularly; should not be used in any patient ≥80 years of age unless normal renal function is confirmed. Use of concomitant medications that may affect renal function (ie, affect tubular secretion) may also affect metformin disposition. Metformin should be withheld in patients with dehydration and/or prerenal azotemia. Metformin therapy should be temporarily discontinued prior to or at the time of intravascular administration of iodinated contrast media (potential for acute alteration in renal function). Metformin should be withheld for 48 hours after the radiologic study and restarted only after renal function has been confirmed as normal.

[U.S. Boxed Warning]: Thiazolidinediones, including pioglitazone, may cause or exacerbate heart failure; closely monitor for signs and symptoms of heart failure (eg, rapid weight gain, dyspnea, edema), particularly after initiation or dose increases. Not recommended for use in any patient with symptomatic heart failure; initiation of therapy is contraindicated in patients with NYHA class III or IV heart failure. If used in patients with NYHA class II (systolic) heart failure, initiate at lowest dosage and monitor closely. In addition metformin should be used with caution in patients with heart failure requiring pharmacologic management, particularly in unstable or acute heart failure due to risk of lactic acidosis secondary to hypoperfusion. Use with caution in patients with edema; may increase plasma volume and/or cause fluid retention. Dose reduction or discontinuation is recommended if heart failure suspected. Dose-related weight gain observed with pioglitazone use; mechanism unknown but likely associated with fluid retention and fat accumulation.

Avoid metformin use in patients with impaired liver function due to potential for lactic acidosis. Use pioglitazone with caution in patients with elevated transaminases (AST or ALT); do not initiate in patients with active liver disease of ALT >2.5 times the upper limit of normal at baseline. During therapy, if ALT >3 times the upper limit of normal, reevaluate promptly and discontinue if elevation persists or if jaundice occurs at any time during use. Idiosyncratic hepatotoxicity has been reported with another thiazolidinedione agent (troglitazone); avoid use in patients who previously experienced jaundice during troglitazone therapy. Monitoring should include periodic determinations of liver function. Instruct patients to avoid excessive acute or chronic ethanol use; ethanol may potentiate metformin's effect on lactate metabolism.

Mechanism of pioglitazone requires the presence of insulin; therefore, use in type 1 diabetes (insulin dependent, IDDM) or diabetic ketoacidosis is not recommended. It may be necessary to discontinue metformin and administer insulin if the patient is exposed to stress (fever, trauma, infection, surgery). Increased incidence of bone fractures in females treated with pioglitazone; majority of fractures occurred in the lower limb and distal upper limb. Consider risk of fracture prior to initiation and during use. Pioglitazone may decrease hemoglobin/hematocrit; effects may be related to increased plasma volume. Metformin may impair vitamin B_{12} absorption; monitor for anemia. Use pioglitazone with caution in premenopausal, anovulatory women; may result in a resumption of ovulation, increasing the risk of pregnancy. Use pioglitazone with caution in patients with pre-existing macular edema or diabetic retinopathy; postmarketing events of new-onset or worsening diabetic macular edema with decreased visual acuity have been reported.

Drug Interactions

Metabolism/Transport Effects Pioglitazone: **Substrate** of CYP2C8 (major), 3A4 (minor); **Inhibits** CYP2C8 (moderate), 2C9 (weak), 2C19 (weak) **Induces** CYP3A4 (weak)

Avoid Concomitant Use There are no known interactions where it is recommended to avoid concomitant use.

Decreased Effect

Pioglitazone and Metformin may decrease the levels/effects of: Saxagliptin

The levels/effects of Pioglitazone and Metformin may be decreased by: Bile Acid Sequestrants; Corticosteroids (Orally Inhaled); Corticosteroids (Systemic); CYP2C8 Inducers (Highly Effective); Luteinizing Hormone-Releasing Hormone Analogs; Rifampin; Somatropin; Thiazide Diuretics

Increased Effect/Toxicity

Pioglitazone and Metformin may increase the levels/effects of: CYP2C8 Substrates (High risk); Hypoglycemic Agents

The levels/effects of Pioglitazone and Metformin may be increased by: Cephalexin; Cimetidine; Conivaptan; CYP2C8 Inhibitors (Moderate); CYP2C8 Inhibitors (Strong); Deferasirox; Gemfibrozil; Glycopyrrolate; Herbs (Hypoglycemic Properties); Insulin; Iodinated Contrast Agents; Pegvisomant; Pregabalin; Trimethoprim

Nutritional/Ethanol Interactions See individual agents.

Adverse Reactions Also see individual agents. Percentages of adverse effects as reported with the combination product.

>10%:

Cardiovascular: Edema (lower limb, 3% to 11%)
Respiratory: Upper respiratory infection (12% to 16%)

1% to 10%:

Central nervous system: Headache (2% to 6%), dizziness (5%)
Endocrine & metabolic: Weight gain (3% to 7%)
Gastrointestinal: Diarrhea (5% to 6%), nausea (4% to 6%)
Genitourinary: Urinary tract infection (5% to 6%)
Hematologic: Anemia (≤2%)
Respiratory: Sinusitis (4% to 5%)

Pharmacodynamics/Kinetics

Pharmacokinetic Note See individual agents.

Available Dosage Forms

Tablet, oral:

Actoplus Met®: 15/500: Pioglitazone 15 mg and metformin 500 mg; 15/850: Pioglitazone 15 mg and metformin 850 mg

Tablet, variable release, oral:

Actoplus Met® XR: 15/1000: Pioglitazone 15 mg and metformin 1000 mg; 30/1000: Pioglitazone 30 mg and metformin 1000 mg

Dosing

Adult Type 2 diabetes mellitus: Oral: Initial dose should be based on current dose of pioglitazone and/or metformin; metformin dose may be titrated every 1-2 weeks and pioglitazone dose may be titrated every 2-3 months as necessary to achieve goals

Immediate release tablet: **Note:** Daily doses higher than pioglitazone 15 mg plus metformin 850 mg should be divided. Initial: Pioglitazone 15 mg plus metformin 500 mg **or** pioglitazone 15 mg plus metformin 850 mg tablets once or twice daily. Maximum daily dose: Pioglitazone 45 mg/metformin 2550 mg

Variable release tablet: Pioglitazone 15 mg plus metformin 1000 mg tablet **or** pioglitazone 30 mg plus metformin 1000 mg tablet once daily with evening meal. Maximum daily dose: Pioglitazone 45 mg/metformin 2000 mg

Geriatric Refer to adult dosing. The initial and maintenance dosing should be conservative, due to the potential for decreased renal function (monitor). Generally, elderly patients should not be titrated to the maximum; do not use in patients ≥80 years of age unless normal renal function has been established.

Renal Impairment Do not use with renal disease or renal dysfunction (serum creatinine ≥1.5 mg/dL in males or ≥1.4 mg/dL in females or abnormal clearance).

Hepatic Impairment Do not initiate treatment with active liver disease or ALT >2.5 times ULN. During treatment, if ALT concentrations increase >3 times ULN, the test should be repeated as soon as possible. If ALT concentrations remain >3 times ULN or if the patient is jaundiced, therapy should be discontinued.

Administration

Oral

Immediate release formulation: Administer with meals.

Variable release formulation: Administer with the evening meal. Tablets should be swallowed whole; do not crush, split, or chew. Inactive tablet ingredients may be eliminated in the feces as a soft mass that resembles the orginal tablet.

Stability

Storage Store at 25°C (77°F); excursions permitted to 15°C to 30°C (59°F to 86°F). Protect from moisture and humidity

Monitoring and Teaching Issues

Laboratory Monitoring Hemoglobin A_{1c}, serum glucose; signs and symptoms of heart failure; liver enzymes prior to initiation and periodically during treatment (per clinician judgment). If the ALT is increased to >2.5 times ULN, liver function testing should be performed more frequently until the concentrations return to normal or pretreatment values. Patients with an elevation in ALT >3 times ULN should be rechecked as soon as possible. If the ALT concentrations remain >3 times ULN, therapy with pioglitazone should be discontinued. Initial and periodic monitoring of hematologic parameters (eg, hemoglobin/hematocrit and red blood cell indices) and renal function should performed. Check vitamin B_{12} and folate if anemia is present.

Physical Assessment See individual agents.

Patient Education See individual agents.

Dietary Considerations Immediate release tablets should be administered with meals. Variable release tablets should be administered with the evening meal. Avoid ethanol. Dietary modification based on ADA recommendations is a part of therapy. Monitor for signs and symptoms of vitamin B_{12} and/or folic acid deficiency; supplementation may be required.

Geriatric Considerations Intensive glucose control (Hb A_{1c} <6.5%) has been linked to increased all cause and cardiovascular mortality, hypoglycemia requiring assistance, and weight gain in adult type 2 diabetes. For elderly patients with diabetes who are relatively healthy, attaining target goals for aspirin use, blood pressure, lipids, smoking cessation, and diet and exercise may be more important than normalized glycemic control.

Breast-Feeding Considerations See individual agents.

Pregnancy Considerations Animal reproduction studies were not conducted with this combination; therefore, pioglitazone/metformin is classified as pregnancy category C. See individual agents.

◆ **Piperonyl Butoxide and Pyrethrins** *see* Pyrethrins and Piperonyl Butoxide *on page* 1530

Piroxicam (peer OKS i kam)

U.S. Brand Names Feldene®

Generic Availability (U.S.) Yes

Pharmacologic Category Nonsteroidal Anti-inflammatory Drug (NSAID), Oral

Medication Safety Issues

Sound-alike/look-alike issues:

Feldene® may be confused with FLUoxetine

Piroxicam may be confused with PARoxetine

International issues:

Flogene [Brazil] may be confused with Florone brand name for diflorasone [Germany, Greece]

Beers Criteria medication: This drug may be inappropriate for use in geriatric patients (high severity risk).

Medication Guide Available Yes

Pregnancy Risk Factor C

Lactation Enters breast milk/not recommended (AAP rates "compatible"; AAP 2001 update pending)

Use Symptomatic treatment of acute and chronic rheumatoid arthritis and osteoarthritis

Unlabeled/Investigational Use Ankylosing spondylitis

Available Dosage Forms

Capsule, oral: 10 mg, 20 mg

Feldene®: 10 mg, 20 mg

Dosing

Adult Inflammation, rheumatoid arthritis: Oral: 10-20 mg/day once daily; although associated with increase in GI adverse effects, doses >20 mg/day have been used (ie, 30-40 mg/day); maximum dose: 20 mg/day

Geriatric Refer to adult dosing. **Note:** Some clinicians have used 10 mg every other day to initiate therapy in the elderly to help avoid side effects and produce therapeutic effect at minimal dose. Maximum dose: 20 mg/day.

Pediatric Oral: Children (unlabeled use): 0.2-0.3 mg/kg/day once daily; maximum dose: 15 mg/day

Renal Impairment Not recommended in patients with advanced renal disease.

Hepatic Impairment Reduced dose is necessary.

Monitoring and Teaching Issues

Laboratory Monitoring Occult blood loss, hemoglobin, hematocrit, and periodic renal and hepatic function tests

Physical Assessment Evaluate cardiac risk and potential for GI bleeding prior to prescribing this medication. Monitor blood pressure at the beginning of therapy and periodically during use. Monitor for GI effects, hepatotoxicity, and ototoxicity at beginning of therapy and periodically throughout. Schedule ophthalmic evaluations for patients who develop eye complaints during long-term NSAID therapy. Advise patients with diabetes to use serum glucose testing.

Patient Education Take with food or milk to reduce GI distress. Do not use alcohol. You may experience drowsiness, dizziness, nervousness, anorexia, nausea, vomiting, flatulence, heartburn, or fluid retention; GI bleeding, ulceration, or perforation can occur with or without pain; discontinue medication and contact prescriber if persistent abdominal pain or cramping or blood in stool occurs. Report unusual swelling of extremities or unusual weight gain; breathlessness, respiratory difficulty, or unusual cough; chest pain, rapid heartbeat, or palpitations; bruising/bleeding; blood in urine, stool, mouth, or vomitus; unusual fatigue; skin rash; or ringing in ears.

Related Information

Nonsalicylate / Nonsteroidal Anti-Inflammatory Agents *on page 2002*

◆ ***p*-Isobutylhydratropic Acid** *see* Ibuprofen *on page 938*

◆ **Pit** *see* Oxytocin *on page 1388*

Pitavastatin (pi TA va sta tin)

U.S. Brand Names Livalo®

Index Terms Pitavastatin Calcium

Generic Availability (U.S.) No

Pharmacologic Category Antilipemic Agent, HMG-CoA Reductase Inhibitor

Medication Safety Issues

Sound-alike/look-alike issues:

Pitavastatin may be confused with atorvastatin, fluvastatin, lovastatin, nystatin, pravastatin, rosuvastatin, simvastatin

Pregnancy Risk Factor X

Lactation Excretion in breast milk unknown/contraindicated

Use Adjunct to dietary therapy to reduce elevations in total cholesterol (TC), LDL-C, apolipoprotein B (Apo B), and triglycerides (TG), and to increase low HDL-C in patients with primary hyperlipidemia and mixed dyslipidemia

Mechanism of Action/Effect Inhibitor of 3-hydroxy-3-methylglutaryl coenzyme A (HMG-CoA) reductase, the rate-limiting enzyme in cholesterol synthesis (reduces the production of mevalonic acid from HMG-CoA); this then results in a compensatory increase in the expression of LDL receptors on hepatocyte membranes and a stimulation of LDL catabolism

Contraindications Hypersensitivity to pitavastatin or any component of the formulation; active liver disease including unexplained persistent elevations of hepatic transaminases; concurrent use with cyclosporine; pregnancy; breast-feeding

Warnings/Precautions Secondary causes of hyperlipidemia should be ruled out prior to therapy. Pitavastatin has not been studied when the primary lipid abnormality is chylomicron elevation (Fredrickson types I and V) or in familial dysbetalipoproteinemia (Fredrickson type III). May cause hepatic dysfunction; in all patients, liver function must be monitored by periodic laboratory assessment. Use with caution in patients who consume large amounts of ethanol or have a history of liver disease; use is contraindicated in patients with active liver disease or unexplained persistent elevations of serum transaminases.

Myopathy and rhabdomyolysis with acute renal failure have occurred with use. Risk is dose related and is increased with concurrent use of lipid-lowering agents which may cause rhabdomyolysis (fibric acid derivatives or niacin at doses ≥1 g/day) or during concurrent use with erythromycin or protease inhibitors. Use caution in patients with renal impairment, inadequately treated hypothyroidism, and those taking other drugs associated with myopathy (eg, colchicine); these patients are predisposed to myopathy. Monitor closely if used with other drugs associated with myopathy. Weigh the risk versus benefit when combining any of these drugs with pitavastatin. Discontinue in any patient experiencing an acute or serious condition predisposing to renal failure secondary to rhabdomyolysis. Patients should be instructed to report unexplained muscle pain, tenderness, weakness, or brown urine. Concurrent use with cyclosporine is contraindicated. Ensure patient is on the lowest effective pitavastatin dose. Based upon current evidence, HMG-CoA reductase inhibitor therapy should be continued in the perioperative period unless risk outweighs cardioprotective benefit. Use with caution in elderly patients, as these patients are predisposed to myopathy.

Drug Interactions

Metabolism/Transport Effects Substrate of OATP1B1; (major) of UGT1A3 and UGT2B7; (minor) of CYP2C9, 2C8

Avoid Concomitant Use

Avoid concomitant use of Pitavastatin with any of the following: CycloSPORINE; CycloSPORINE (Systemic); Lopinavir; Red Yeast Rice; Ritonavir

Decreased Effect

The levels/effects of Pitavastatin may be decreased by: Antacids; Bosentan; Rifamycin Derivatives; St Johns Wort

Increased Effect/Toxicity

Pitavastatin may increase the levels/effects of: DAPTOmycin; Trabectedin; Vitamin K Antagonists

The levels/effects of Pitavastatin may be increased by: Atazanavir; Colchicine; CycloSPORINE; CycloSPORINE (Systemic); Danazol; Fenofibrate; Fenofibric Acid; Gemfibrozil; Grapefruit Juice; Lopinavir; Macrolide Antibiotics; Niacin; Niacinamide; Protease Inhibitors; Red Yeast Rice; Rifamycin Derivatives; Ritonavir; Sildenafil

Nutritional/Ethanol Interactions

Ethanol: Avoid excessive ethanol consumption (due to potential hepatic effects).

Food: Red yeast rice contains an estimated 2.4 mg lovastatin per 600 mg rice.

Adverse Reactions

2% to 10%:

Gastrointestinal: Constipation (2% to 4%), diarrhea (2% to 3%)

Neuromuscular & skeletal: Back pain (1% to 4%), myalgia (2% to 3%), pain in extremities (1% to 2%)

Additional class-related events or case reports (not necessarily reported with pitavastatin therapy): Cataracts, cirrhosis, dermatomyositis, eosinophilia, extraocular muscle movement impaired, fulminant hepatic necrosis, gynecomastia, hypersensitivity syndrome (symptoms may include anaphylaxis, angioedema, arthralgia, erythema multiforme, eosinophilia, hemolytic anemia, interstitial lung disease, lupus syndrome, photosensitivity, polymyalgia rheumatica, positive ANA, purpura, Stevens-Johnson syndrome, toxic epidermal necrolysis, urticaria, vasculitis), ophthalmoplegia, peripheral nerve palsy, rhabdomyolysis, renal failure (secondary to rhabdomyolysis), thyroid dysfunction, tremor, vertigo

Pharmacodynamics/Kinetics

Bioavailability 51%

Time to Peak ~1 hour

Protein Binding >99%

Half-Life Elimination ~12 hours

Metabolism Hepatic, via UGT1A3 and UGT 2B7; minimal metabolism via CYP2C9 and CYP2C8

Excretion Feces (79%); urine (15%)

Available Dosage Forms

Tablet, oral:

Livalo®: 1 mg, 2 mg, 4 mg

Dosing

Adult & Geriatric

Primary hyperlipidemia and mixed dyslipidemia: Oral: Initial: 2 mg once daily; may be increased to maximum 4 mg once daily

Note: Doses should be individualized according to the baseline LDL-cholesterol levels, the recommended goal of therapy, and patient response; adjustments should be made at intervals of 4 weeks.

Dosage adjustment with concomitant medications:

Erythromycin: Pitavastatin dose should not exceed 1 mg once daily

Rifampin: Pitavastatin dose should not exceed 2 mg once daily

Renal Impairment

Moderate renal impairment (Cl_{cr} 30-60 mL/minute/1.73 m^2) or end-stage renal disease receiving hemodialysis: Initial: 1 mg once daily; do not exceed 2 mg once daily

Severe renal impairment (Cl_{cr} <30 mL/minute/1.73 m^2) not receiving hemodialysis: Not recommended

Hepatic Impairment Contraindicated in active liver disease or in patients with unexplained persistent elevations of serum transaminases.

Administration

Oral May be administered with or without food; may take without regard to time of day.

Stability

Storage Store at controlled room temperature of 15°C to 30°C (59°F to 86°F). Protect from light.

Monitoring and Teaching Issues

Laboratory Monitoring Monitor total cholesterol, LDL, and HDL cholesterol within 4 weeks of treatment initiation or dose change; LFTs prior to initiation and 12 weeks after initiation or first dose or dose elevation, and periodically (semiannually) thereafter; baseline CPK (recheck CPK in any patient with symptoms suggestive of myopathy). Monitor LDL-C at intervals no less than 4 weeks.

Physical Assessment Use caution with history of hepatic disease. Assess risk potential for interactions with other prescriptions or herbal products patient may be taking that may increase risk of myopathy or rhabdomyolysis. Evaluate LFTs and lipid profile prior to treatment and at regular intervals. Teach proper diet and exercise program.

Patient Education Take with or without food. Follow prescribed diet and exercise regimen. You will have periodic blood tests to assess effectiveness. Avoid excessive alcohol. Report unusual muscle cramping or weakness, yellowing of skin or eyes, easy bruising or bleeding, or unusual fatigue.

Dietary Considerations May be taken with or without food; may take without regard to time of day. Red yeast rice contains an estimated 2.4 mg lovastatin per 600 mg rice.

Geriatric Considerations The definition of and, therefore, when to treat hyperlipidemia in the elderly is a controversial issue. The National Cholesterol Education Program recommends that all adults maintain a plasma cholesterol <160 mg/dL. Elderly patients with one additional risk factor, goal LDL would be <130 mg/dL. It is the authors' belief that pharmacologic treatment be reserved for those who are unable to obtain a desirable plasma cholesterol concentration by diet alone and for whom the benefits of treatment are believed to outweigh the potential adverse effects, drug interactions, and cost of treatment.

Pregnancy Considerations Cholesterol biosynthesis may be important in fetal development. Contraindicated in pregnancy. Administer to women of childbearing potential only when conception is highly unlikely and patients have been informed of potential hazards.

- ◆ **Pitavastatin Calcium** *see* Pitavastatin *on page* 1466
- ◆ **Pitocin®** *see* Oxytocin *on page* 1388
- ◆ **Pitressin®** *see* Vasopressin *on page* 1851
- ◆ **Plan B** *see* Levonorgestrel *on page* 1097
- ◆ **Plan B® One Step** *see* Levonorgestrel *on page* 1097
- ◆ **Plaquenil®** *see* Hydroxychloroquine *on page* 930
- ◆ **Plasbumin®-5** *see* Albumin *on page* 57
- ◆ **Plasbumin®-25** *see* Albumin *on page* 57
- ◆ **Platinol** *see* CISplatin *on page* 384
- ◆ **Platinol-AQ** *see* CISplatin *on page* 384
- ◆ **Plavix®** *see* Clopidogrel *on page* 413
- ◆ **Plendil** *see* Felodipine *on page* 738

Plerixafor (pler IX a fore)

U.S. Brand Names Mozobil™

Index Terms AMD3100; LM3100

Generic Availability (U.S.) No

Pharmacologic Category Hematopoietic Stem Cell Mobilizer

Pregnancy Risk Factor D

Lactation Excretion in breast milk unknown/not recommended

Use Mobilization of hematopoietic stem cells (HSC) for collection and subsequent autologous transplantation (in combination with filgrastim) in patients with non-Hodgkin's lymphoma (NHL) and multiple myeloma (MM)

Available Dosage Forms

Injection, solution [preservative free]:

Mozobil™: 20 mg/mL (1.2 mL)

Dosing

Adult & Geriatric Note: Dosing is based on actual body weight. Begin plerixafor after patient has received filgrastim 10 mcg/kg once daily for 4 days; plerixafor, filgrastim, and apheresis should be continued daily until sufficient cell collection up to a maximum of 4 days.

HSC mobilization: SubQ: 0.24 mg/kg once daily ~11 hours prior to apheresis for up to 4 consecutive days; maximum dose: 40 mg/day

Renal Impairment

Cl_{cr} >50 mL/minute: No adjustment required.

Cl_{cr} ≤50 mL/minute: 0.16 mg/kg; maximum dose: 27 mg/day.

Hemodialysis: Insufficient information for dosing recommendation

Administration

Other Administer subcutaneously, ~11 hours prior to initiation of apheresis. In some clinical trials, plerixafor administration began in the evening prior to apheresis. (filgrastim was begun on day 1, plerixafor initiated in the evening on day 4 and apheresis in the morning on day 5; with filgrastim, plerixafor and apheresis then continued daily until sufficient cell collection for autologous transplant.)

Monitoring and Teaching Issues

Laboratory Monitoring CBC with differential and platelets

Physical Assessment Teach patient appropriate injection techniques and syringe/needle disposal.

Patient Education This medication is administered via injection. Local injection site reactions, such as redness, inflammation, irritation, and itching, are not unusual. Contact prescriber if injection site reaction is severe. You may experience dizziness, nausea, diarrhea, gas, headache, muscle pain, problems sleeping, and fatigue. Report persistent abdominal pain to prescriber.

- ◆ **Pletal®** *see* Cilostazol *on page 370*
- ◆ **PMPA** *see* Tenofovir *on page 1728*
- ◆ **Pneumococcal 7-Valent Conjugate Vaccine** *see* Pneumococcal Conjugate Vaccine (7-Valent) *on page 1469*
- ◆ **Pneumococcal 13-Valent Conjugate Vaccine** *see* Pneumococcal Conjugate Vaccine (13-Valent) *on page 1470*

Pneumococcal Conjugate Vaccine (7-Valent)

(noo moe KOK al KON ju gate vak SEEN, seven vay lent)

U.S. Brand Names Prevnar®

Index Terms Diphtheria CRM_{197} Protein; PCV; PCV-7; PCV7; Pneumococcal 7-Valent Conjugate Vaccine

Generic Availability (U.S.) No

Pharmacologic Category Vaccine, Inactivated (Bacterial)

Medication Safety Issues

Sound-alike/look-alike issues:

Pneumococcal 7-Valent Conjugate Vaccine (Prevnar®) may be confused with Pneumococcal 13-Valent Conjugate Vaccine (Prevnar 13™) or with Pneumococcal 23-Valent Polysaccharide Vaccine (Pneumovax® 23)

Pregnancy Risk Factor C

Lactation

Excretion in breast milk unknown/not recommended

Use Note: In March 2010, the Advisory Committee on Immunization Practices (ACIP) released recommendations that pneumococcal 13-valent conjugate vaccine (PCV13; Prevnar 13™) replace pneumococcal 7-valent conjugate vaccine (PCV7; Prevnar®) for all doses for immunization of all children 2-59 months of age. Refer to the Pneumococcal Conjugate Vaccine (13-Valent) monograph for additional information.

Immunization of infants and toddlers against *Streptococcus pneumoniae* infection caused by serotypes included in the vaccine

Immunization of infants and toddlers against otitis media caused by serotypes included in the vaccine

The Advisory Committee on Immunization Practices (ACIP) recommends pneumococcal conjugate vaccine (PCV) for routine vaccination of all children 2-59 months and children 60-71 months with underlying medical conditions. PCV13 should be used to complete the vaccination of children who received ≥1 dose of PCV7.

Available Dosage Forms

Injection, suspension:

Prevnar®: 2 mcg of each capsular saccharide for serotypes 4, 9V, 14, 18C, 19F, and 23F, and 4 mcg of serotype 6B per 0.5 mL (0.5 mL)

Dosing

Adult & Geriatric Dosing established for infants and toddlers.

Pediatric Note: As of March 10, 2010, the Advisory Committee on Immunization Practices (ACIP) recommended that the use of pneumococcal 13-valent conjugate vaccine (PCV13; Prevnar 13™) replace all doses of pneumococcal 7-valent conjugate vaccine (PCV7; Prevnar®). The manufacturer, Wyeth Pharmaceuticals, intends to phase out the previous Prevnar® product. Refer to the Pneumococcal Conjugate Vaccine (13-Valent) monograph for transitioning from PCV7 to PCV13.

Immunization: Infants 2-6 months (manufacturer's labeling): I.M.: .5 mL at approximately 2-month intervals for 3 consecutive doses, followed by a fourth dose of 0.5 mL at 12-15 months of age; first dose may be given as young as 6 weeks of age, but is typically given at 2 months of age.

Administration

I.M. Shake well prior to use. Administer I.M. (deltoid muscle for toddlers and young children or lateral midthigh in infants). Do not inject I.V.; avoid intradermal route.

For patients at risk of hemorrhage following intramuscular injection, the ACIP recommends "it should be administered intramuscularly if, in the opinion of the physician familiar with the patients bleeding risk, the vaccine can be administered by this route with reasonable safety. If the patient receives antihemophilia or other similar therapy, intramuscular vaccination can be scheduled shortly after such therapy is administered. A fine needle (23 gauge or smaller) can be used for the vaccination and firm pressure applied to the site (without rubbing) for at least 2 minutes. The patient should be instructed concerning the risk of hematoma from the injection." Patients on anticoagulant therapy should be considered to have the same bleeding risks and treated as those with clotting factor disorders (CDC, 2011).

Antipyretics have not been shown to prevent febrile seizures. Antipyretics may be used to treat fever or discomfort following vaccination (CDC, 2011). One study reported that routine prophylactic administration of acetaminophen to prevent fever prior to vaccination decreased the immune response of some vaccines; the clinical significance of this reduction in immune response has not been established (Prymula, 2009).

Simultaneous administration of vaccines helps ensure the patients will be fully vaccinated by the appropriate age. Simultaneous administration of vaccines is defined as administering >1 vaccine on the same day at different anatomic sites. Separate vaccines should not be combined in the same syringe unless indicated by product specific labeling. Separate needles and syringes should be used for each injection. The ACIP prefers each dose of a specific vaccine in a series come from the same manufacturer when possible. Adolescents and adults should be vaccinated while seated or lying down. In general, preterm infants should be vaccinated at the same chronological age as full-term infants (CDC, 2011).

Monitoring and Teaching Issues

Physical Assessment Federal law requires entry into the patient's medical record.

Related Information

Immunization Recommendations *on page 1941*

Pneumococcal Conjugate Vaccine (13-Valent)

(noo moe KOK al KON ju gate vak SEEN, thur TEEN vay lent)

U.S. Brand Names Prevnar 13™

Index Terms Diphtheria CRM_{197} Protein; PCV-13; PCV13; PCV13-CRM(197); Pneumococcal 13-Valent Conjugate Vaccine

Generic Availability (U.S.) No

Pharmacologic Category Vaccine, Inactivated (Bacterial)

Medication Safety Issues

Sound-alike/look-alike issues:

Pneumococcal 13-Valent Conjugate Vaccine (Prevnar 13™) may be confused with Pneumococcal 7-Valent Conjugate Vaccine (Prevnar®) or with Pneumococcal 23-Valent Polysaccharide Vaccine (Pneumovax® 23)

Pregnancy Risk Factor C

Use

Immunization of infants and children against *Streptococcus pneumoniae* infection caused by serotypes included in the vaccine

Immunization of infants and children against otitis media caused by *Streptococcus pneumoniae* serotypes 4, 6B, 9V, 14, 18C, 19F, and 23F

The Advisory Committee on Immunization Practices (ACIP) recommends routine vaccination for the following:

All children age 2-59 months

Children 60-71 months with underlying medical conditions including: Cochlear implants, functional or anatomic asplenia (includes sickle cell disease and other hemoglobinopathies, congenital or acquired asplenia, or splenic dysfunction); immunocompromising conditions (includes HIV infection, congenital immunodeficiencies [excluding chronic granulomatous disease], chronic renal failure, nephrotic syndrome, diseases associated with immunosuppressive or radiation therapy, solid organ transplant); chronic illnesses (cardiac disease, cerebrospinal fluid leaks, diabetes mellitus, pulmonary disease [excluding asthma unless on high dose oral corticosteroids])

Children who received ≥1 dose of PCV7

Children 6-18 years of age at increased risk for invasive pneumococcal disease due to anatomic or functional asplenia (including sickle cell disease), HIV infection or other immunocompromising conditions, cochlear implant, or cerebrospinal fluid leaks (regardless of prior receipt of PCV7 or PPSV23). Routine use is not recommended for healthy children ≥5 years of age.

Available Dosage Forms

Injection, suspension:

Prevnar 13™: 2 mcg of each capsular saccharide for serotypes 1, 3, 4, 5, 6A, 7F, 9V, 14, 18C, 19A, 19F, and 23F, and 4 mcg of serotype 6B [bound to diphtheria CRM_{197} protein ~34 mcg] per 0.5 mL (0.5 mL)

Dosing

Adult & Geriatric Dosing established for Infants and Children.

Pediatric

Primary immunization: I.M.: *Infants and Children 6 weeks-59 months:* 0.5 mL/dose for a total of 4 doses. The first dose may be given as young as 6 weeks of age, but is typically given at 2 months of age. The 3 remaining doses are usually given at 4, 6, and 12-15 months of age. The recommended dosing interval is 4-8 weeks. The minimum interval between doses in children <1 year of age is 1 month. The minimum interval between the third and fourth dose is 2 months.

Previously unvaccinated Older Infants and Children: I.M.:

Children 7-11 months: 0.5 mL for a total of 3 doses; 2 doses at least 4 weeks apart, followed by a third dose after the 1-year birthday (12-15 months), separated from the second dose by at least 2 months

Children 12-23 months: 0.5 mL for a total of 2 doses, separated by at least 2 months

Healthy Children 24-59 months: 0.5 mL as a single dose

Children 24-71 months with an underlying medical condition: ACIP recommendations: 0.5 mL for a total of 2 doses, separated by 2 months

Previously vaccinated with PCV7 and/or PCV13, and with a lapse in vaccine administration (ACIP recommendations): I.M.:

Children 7-11 months: Previously received 1 or 2 doses: 0.5 mL dose at 7-11 months of age, followed by a second dose ≥2 months later at 12-15 months of age

Children 12-23 months:

Previously received 1 dose <12 months of age: 0.5 mL dose, followed by a second dose ≥2 months later

Previously received 1 dose at ≥12 months of age: 0.5 mL dose ≥2 months after the most recent dose

Previously received 2 or 3 doses before age 12 months: 0.5 mL dose ≥2 months after the most recent dose

Healthy Children 24-59 months with any incomplete schedule: 0.5 mL dose ≥ 2 months after the most recent dose

Children 24-71 months with an underlying medical condition:

Previously received <3 doses: 0.5 mL dose ≥2 months after the most recent dose, followed by a second dose ≥8 weeks later

Previously received 3 doses: 0.5 mL as a single dose ≥2 months after the most recent dose

Previously vaccinated with PCV7 and completed vaccination series of 4 doses (ACIP recommendations): I.M.:

Children 14-59 months: 0.5 mL as a single supplemental dose ≥2 months after the most recent dose

Children 24-71 months with an underlying medical condition: 0.5 mL as a single supplemental dose ≥2 months after the most recent dose of PCV7 or PPSV23

Previously vaccinated or not previously vaccinated with PCV7 or PPSV23 (ACIP recommendations): I.M.: *Children 6-18 years at high risk for invasive pneumococcal disease:* 0.5 mL as a single dose ≥2 months after the most recent dose

Administration

I.M. Shake well prior to use. Do not use if a homogenous white suspension does not form. Administer I.M. (deltoid muscle for toddlers and young children or lateral midthigh in infants). Do not inject I.V. or SubQ; avoid intradermal route. Concurrent administration of PCV13 and PPV23 has not been studied and is not recommended (CDC, 2010).

For patients at risk of hemorrhage following intramuscular injection, the ACIP recommends "it should be administered intramuscularly if, in the opinion of the physician familiar with the patients bleeding risk, the vaccine can be administered by this route with reasonable safety. If the patient receives antihemophilia or other similar therapy, intramuscular vaccination can be scheduled shortly after such therapy is administered. A fine needle (23 gauge or smaller) can be used for the vaccination and firm pressure applied to the site (without rubbing) for at least 2 minutes. The patient should be instructed concerning the risk of hematoma from the injection." Patients on anticoagulant therapy should be considered to have the same bleeding risks and treated as those with clotting factor disorders (CDC, 2011).

Antipyretics have not been shown to prevent febrile seizures. Antipyretics may be used to treat fever or discomfort following vaccination (CDC, 2011). One study reported that routine prophylactic administration of acetaminophen to prevent fever prior to vaccination decreased the immune response of some vaccines; the clinical significance of this reduction in immune response has not been established (Prymula, 2009).

Simultaneous administration of vaccines helps ensure the patients will be fully vaccinated by the appropriate age. Simultaneous administration of vaccines is defined as administering >1 vaccine on the same day at different anatomic sites. Separate vaccines should not be combined in the same syringe unless indicated by product specific labeling. Separate needles and syringes should be used for each injection. The ACIP prefers each dose of a specific vaccine in a series come from the same manufacturer when possible. Adolescents and adults should be vaccinated while seated or lying down. In general, preterm infants should be vaccinated at the same chronological age as full-term infants (CDC, 2011).

Monitoring and Teaching Issues

Physical Assessment Federal law requires entry into the patient's medical record.

Related Information

Immunization Recommendations *on page 1941*

Pneumococcal Polysaccharide Vaccine (Polyvalent)

(noo moe KOK al pol i SAK a ride vak SEEN, pol i VAY lent)

U.S. Brand Names Pneumovax® 23

Index Terms 23-Valent Pneumococcal Polysaccharide Vaccine; 23PS; PPSV; PPSV23; PPV23

Generic Availability (U.S.) No

Pharmacologic Category Vaccine, Inactivated (Bacterial)

Medication Safety Issues

Sound-alike/look-alike issues:

Pneumococcal 23-Valent Polysaccharide Vaccine (Pneumovax® 23) may be confused with Pneumococcal 7-Valent Conjugate Vaccine (Prevnar®) or with Pneumococcal 13-Valent Conjugate Vaccine (Prevnar 13™)

Pregnancy Risk Factor C

Lactation Excretion in breast milk unknown/use caution

Use Immunization against pneumococcal disease caused by serotypes included in the vaccine. Routine vaccination is recommended for persons ≥50 years of age and persons ≥2 years in certain situations.

The Advisory Committee on Immunization Practices (ACIP) recommends routine vaccination for the following:

All immunocompetent patients ≥65 years of age

Patients 2-18 years of age with certain high-risk condition(s):

- Chronic heart disease (particularly cyanotic congenital heart disease and cardiac failure)
- Chronic lung disease (including asthma if treated with high-dose oral corticosteroids)

Patients 2-64 years of age with certain high-risk condition(s):

- Diabetes mellitus
- Cochlear implants
- Cerebrospinal fluid leaks
- Functional or anatomic asplenia (including sickle cell disease and other hemoglobinopathies, splenic dysfunction, or splenectomy)
- Immunocompromising conditions including congenital immunodeficiency (includes B- or T-lymphocyte deficiency, complement deficiencies, and phagocytic disorders [excluding chronic granulomatous disease]); HIV infection; leukemia, lymphoma, Hodgkin's disease, multiple myeloma, generalized malignancy; chronic renal failure, nephrotic syndrome; patients requiring treatment with immunosuppressive therapy, including chemotherapy, long-term systemic corticosteroids, or radiation therapy; patients who have received a solid organ transplant

Patients 19-64 years of age with certain high-risk condition(s):

- Chronic heart disease (including heart failure and cardiomyopathy, and excluding hypertension)
- Chronic lung disease (including COPD, emphysema, and asthma)
- Persons who smoke cigarettes
- Alcoholism
- Chronic liver disease (including cirrhosis)

Routine vaccination is not recommended for Alaska Natives or American Indian persons unless they have underlying conditions which are indications for vaccination; in special situations, vaccination may be recommended when living in an area at increased risk of invasive pneumococcal disease.

Available Dosage Forms

Injection, solution:

Pneumovax® 23: 25 mcg each of 23 capsular polysaccharide isolates/0.5 mL (0.5 mL, 2.5 mL)

Dosing

Adult Immunization: I.M., SubQ: 0.5 mL

Revaccination: I.M., SubQ:

Immunocompetent individuals: Revaccination generally not recommended

Children ≥2 years and Adults at highest risk for pneumococcal disease: One revaccination ≥5 years after first dose of PPSV23. Patients at highest risk for infection include those with asplenia or immunocompromising conditions (eg, sickle cell anemia, HIV infection, leukemia, lymphoma, Hodgkin's disease, multiple myeloma, generalized malignancy, chronic renal failure, nephrotic syndrome, solid organ transplant, and patients on immunosuppressive therapy [including corticosteroids]) (CDC, September 3, 2010; CDC, December 10, 2010).

Geriatric

Primary immunization: I.M., SubQ: Refer to adult dosing.

Revaccination: I.M., SubQ: ≥65 years: One revaccination if ≥5 years after first dose of PPSV23 and if <65 years of age at the time of the initial vaccination (CDC, September 3, 2010).

Pediatric

Immunization: Children ≥2 years: I.M., SubQ: 0.5 mL

Children at increased risk of invasive pneumococcal disease: One dose of PPSV23 should be given at ≥2 years of age in children with underlying medical conditions. Immunization with PCV13 (or PCV7) should be completed prior to PPSV23 as recommended. The minimum interval between the last dose of PCV13 (or PCV7) and PPSV23 is 8 weeks (CDC, December 10, 2010).

Revaccination: Children ≥2 years: Refer to adult dosing.

Administration

I.M. Do not inject I.V.; avoid intradermal administration (may cause severe local reactions); administer SubQ or I.M. (deltoid muscle or lateral midthigh)

For patients at risk of hemorrhage following intramuscular injection, the ACIP recommends "it should be administered intramuscularly if, in the opinion of the physician familiar with the patients bleeding risk, the vaccine can be administered by this route with reasonable safety. If the patient receives antihemophilia or other similar therapy, intramuscular vaccination can be scheduled shortly after such therapy is administered. A fine needle (23 gauge or smaller) can be used for the vaccination and firm pressure applied to the site (without rubbing) for at least 2 minutes. The patient should be instructed concerning the risk of hematoma from the injection." Patients on anticoagulant therapy should be considered to have the same bleeding risks and treated as those with clotting factor disorders (CDC, 2011).

Antipyretics have not been shown to prevent febrile seizures. Antipyretics may be used to treat fever or discomfort following vaccination (CDC, 2011). One study reported that routine prophylactic administration of acetaminophen to prevent fever prior to vaccination decreased the immune response of some vaccines; the clinical significance of this reduction in immune response has not been established (Prymula, 2009).

Simultaneous administration of vaccines helps ensure the patients will be fully vaccinated by the appropriate age. Simultaneous administration of vaccines is defined as administering >1 vaccine on the same day at different anatomic sites. Separate vaccines should not be combined in the same syringe unless indicated by product specific labeling. Separate needles and syringes should be used for each injection. The ACIP prefers each dose of a specific vaccine in a series come from the same manufacturer when possible. Adolescents and adults should be vaccinated while seated or lying down. In general, preterm infants should be vaccinated at the same chronological age as full-term infants (CDC, 2011).

Other Do not inject I.V., avoid intradermal administration (may cause severe local reactions); administer SubQ or I.M. (deltoid muscle or lateral midthigh).

Monitoring and Teaching Issues

Physical Assessment Federal law requires entry into the patient's medical record.

Related Information

Immunization Recommendations *on page 1941*

- **Pneumovax® 23** *see* Pneumococcal Polysaccharide Vaccine (Polyvalent) *on page 1471*
- **PNU-140690E** *see* Tipranavir *on page 1771*
- **Podactin Cream [OTC]** *see* Miconazole (Topical) *on page 1224*
- **Poliovirus, Inactivated (IPV)** *see* Diphtheria and Tetanus Toxoids, Acellular Pertussis, and Poliovirus Vaccine *on page 548*
- **Poliovirus, Inactivated (IPV)** *see* Diphtheria and Tetanus Toxoids, Acellular Pertussis, Poliovirus and *Haemophilus* b Conjugate Vaccine *on page 550*

Poliovirus Vaccine (Inactivated) (POE lee oh VYE rus vak SEEN, in ak ti VAY ted)

U.S. Brand Names IPOL®

Index Terms Enhanced-potency Inactivated Poliovirus Vaccine; IPV; Salk Vaccine

Generic Availability (U.S.) No

Pharmacologic Category Vaccine, Inactivated (Viral)

Medication Safety Issues

Administration issues:

Poliovirus vaccine (inactivated) may be confused with tuberculin products. Medication errors have occurred when poliovirus vaccine (IPV) has been inadvertently administered instead of tuberculin skin tests (PPD). These products are refrigerated and often stored in close proximity to each other.

Pregnancy Risk Factor C

Lactation Excretion into breast milk unknown/use caution

Use Active immunization against poliomyelitis caused by poliovirus types 1, 2 and 3. **Note:** Combination products containing polio vaccine are also available and may be preferred in certain age groups if recipients are likely to be susceptible to the agents contained within each vaccine.

The Advisory Committee on Immunization Practices (ACIP) recommends routine vaccination for the following:

- All children (first dose given at 2 months of age)

Routine immunization of adults in the United States is generally not recommended. Adults with previous wild poliovirus disease, who have never been immunized, or those who are incompletely immunized may receive inactivated poliovirus vaccine if they fall into one of the following categories:

- Travelers to regions or countries where poliomyelitis is endemic or epidemic
- Healthcare workers in close contact with patients who may be excreting poliovirus
- Laboratory workers handling specimens that may contain poliovirus
- Members of communities or specific population groups with diseases caused by wild poliovirus
- Incompletely vaccinated or unvaccinated adults in a household or with other close contact with children receiving oral poliovirus (may be at increased risk of vaccine associated paralytic poliomyelitis)

Available Dosage Forms

Injection, suspension:

IPOL®: Type 1 poliovirus 40 D-antigen units, type 2 poliovirus 8 D-antigen units, and type 3 poliovirus 32 D-antigen units per 0.5 mL (0.5 mL, 5 mL)

Dosing

Adult & Geriatric Immunization: I.M., SubQ:

Previously unvaccinated: Two 0.5 mL doses administered at 1- to 2-month intervals, followed by a third dose 6-12 months later. If <3 months, but at least 2 months are available before protection is needed, 3 doses may be administered at least 1 month apart. If administration must be completed within 1-2 months, give 2 doses at least 1 month apart. If <1 month is available, give 1 dose.

Incompletely vaccinated: Adults with at least 1 previous dose of OPV, <3 doses of IPV, or a combination of OPV and IPV equaling <3 doses, administer at least one 0.5 mL dose of IPV. Additional doses to complete the series may be given if time permits.

Completely vaccinated and at increased risk of exposure: One 0.5 mL dose

Pediatric Immunization: I.M., SubQ:

Primary immunization: Administer three 0.5 mL doses, at 2, 4, and 6-18 months of age; do not administer more frequently than 4 weeks apart (preferably given more than 8 weeks apart).

Booster dose: 0.5 mL at 4-6 years of age; Minimum interval between booster and previous dose is 6 months. The final (booster) dose should be given at ≥4 years of age, regardless of the number of previous doses. If the final dose is not given at 4-6 years of age, it should be given as soon as feasible.

Note: Use of the minimum age and minimum intervals during the first 6 months of life should only be done when the vaccine recipient is at risk for imminent exposure to circulating poliovirus (shorter intervals and earlier start dates may lead to lower seroconversion).

Administration

I.M. Administer to midlateral aspect of the thigh in infants and small children. Administer in the deltoid area to adults or older children.

I.V. Do not administer I.V.

Other SubQ: Administer to midlateral aspect of the thigh in infants and small children. Administer in the deltoid area to adults or older children.

Simultaneous administration of vaccines helps ensure the patients will be fully vaccinated by the appropriate age. Simultaneous administration of vaccines is defined as administering >1 vaccine on the same day at different anatomic sites. The use of licensed combination vaccines is generally preferred over separate injections of the equivalent components. Separate vaccines should not be combined in the same syringe unless indicated by product specific labeling. Separate needles and syringes should be used for each injection. The ACIP prefers each dose of a specific vaccine in a series come from the same manufacturer when possible. Adolescents and adults should be vaccinated while seated or lying down. In general, preterm infants should be vaccinated at the same chronological age as full-term infants (CDC, 2011).

Antipyretics have not been shown to prevent febrile seizures. Antipyretics may be used to treat fever or discomfort following vaccination (CDC, 2011). One study reported that routine prophylactic administration of acetaminophen to prevent fever prior to vaccination decreased the immune response of some vaccines; the clinical significance of this reduction in immune response has not been established (Prymula, 2009).

Monitoring and Teaching Issues

Physical Assessment All serious adverse reactions must be reported to the U.S. DHHS. Federal law also requires entry into the patient's medical record.

Patient Education Inform healthcare provider if you have an allergy to neomycin, streptomycin, or polymyxin B. Contact healthcare provider immediately if you develop a high fever, unusual behavior, or a rash.

Related Information

Immunization Recommendations *on page* 1941

◆ **Polyethylene Glycol-L-asparaginase** *see* Pegaspargase *on page* 1421

◆ **Polyethylene Glycol-Conjugated Uricase** *see* Pegloticase *on page* 1427

Polyethylene Glycol-Electrolyte Solution

(pol i ETH i leen GLY kol ee LEK troe lite soe LOO shun)

U.S. Brand Names Colyte®; GaviLyte™-C; GaviLyte™-G; GaviLyte™-N; GoLYTELY®; MoviPrep®; NuLYTELY®; TriLyte®

Index Terms Electrolyte Lavage Solution

Generic Availability (U.S.) Yes

Pharmacologic Category Laxative, Osmotic

Medication Safety Issues

Sound-alike/look-alike issues:

GoLYTELY® may be confused with NuLYTELY®
NuLYTELY® may be confused with GoLYTELY®
TriLyte® may be confused with TriLipix™

Pregnancy Risk Factor C

Lactation Excretion in breast milk unknown/use caution

Use Bowel cleansing prior to GI examination

Unlabeled/Investigational Use Whole bowel irrigation (WBI) in the following toxic ingestions: Packets of illicit drugs (body packers, body stuffers), potentially toxic sustained-release or enteric-coated agents, substantial amounts of iron (AACT, 2004)

Available Dosage Forms

Powder, for solution, oral: PEG 3350 240 g, sodium sulfate 22.72 g, sodium bicarbonate 6.72 g, sodium chloride 5.84 g, and potassium 2.98 g; PEG 3350 236 g, sodium sulfate 22.74 g, sodium bicarbonate 6.74 g, sodium chloride 5.86 g, and potassium chloride 2.97 g; PEG 3350 240 g, sodium bicarbonate 5.72 g, sodium chloride 11.2 g, and potassium chloride 1.48 g

Colyte®: PEG 3350 240 g, sodium sulfate 22.72 g, sodium bicarbonate 6.72 g, sodium chloride 5.84 g, and potassium 2.98 g

GaviLyte™-C: PEG 3350 240 g, sodium sulfate 22.72 g, sodium bicarbonate 6.72 g, sodium chloride 5.84 g, and potassium chloride 2.98 g (4000 mL)

GaviLyte™-G: PEG 3350 236 g, sodium sulfate 22.74 g, sodium bicarbonate 6.74 g, sodium chloride 5.86 g, and potassium chloride 2.97 g (4000 mL)

GaviLyte™-N: PEG 3350 420 g, sodium bicarbonate 5.72 g, sodium chloride 11.2 g, and potassium chloride 1.48 g (4000 mL)

GoLYTELY®:

PEG 3350 236 g, sodium sulfate 22.74 g, sodium bicarbonate 6.74 g, sodium chloride 5.86 g, and potassium 2.97 g

PEG 3350 227.1 g, sodium sulfate 21.5 g, sodium bicarbonate 6.36 g, sodium chloride 5.53 g, and potassium 2.82 g per packet (1s)

MoviPrep®: Pouch A: PEG 3350 100g, sodium sulfate 7.5 g, sodium chloride 2.69 g, potassium chloride 1.015 g; Pouch B: Ascorbic acid 4.7 g, sodium ascorbate 5.9 g

NuLYTELY®: PEG 3350 420 g, sodium bicarbonate 5.72 g, sodium chloride 11.2 g, and potassium 1.48 g

TriLyte®: PEG 3350 420 g, sodium bicarbonate 5.72 g, sodium chloride 11.2 g, and potassium 1.48 g

Dosing

Adult & Geriatric

Bowel cleansing prior to GI exam:

Oral:

CoLyte®, GoLYTELY®, NuLYTELY®, TriLyte®: 240 mL (8 oz) every 10 minutes, until 4 L are consumed or the rectal effluent is clear; rapid drinking of each portion is preferred to drinking small amounts continuously. **Note:** The solution may be given via nasogastric tube to patients who are unwilling or unable to drink the solution.

MoviPrep®: Administer 2 L total with an additional 1 L of clear fluid prior to colonoscopy as follows:

Split dose: Evening before colonoscopy: 240 mL (8 oz) every 15 minutes until 1 L is consumed. Then drink 16 oz of clear liquid. On the morning of the colonoscopy, repeat process with second liter over 1 hour and then drink 16 oz of clear liquid at least 1 hour before the procedure.

Full dose: Evening before colonoscopy (~6 PM): 240 mL (8 oz every 15 minutes) until 1 L is consumed; 90 minutes later (~7:30 PM), repeat dose. Then drink 32 oz of clear liquid.

Nasogastric tube: 20-30 mL/minute (1.2-1.8 L/hour); the first bowel movement should occur ~1 hour after the start of administration.

Toxic ingestion (unlabeled use; AACT, 2004): *Nasogastric tube:* 1500-2000 mL/hour until rectal effluent is clear. **Note:** May take several hours for the rectal effluent to become clear. Duration may be extended if evidence of continued presence of toxins in GI tract (eg, radiographic evidence or ongoing elimination of toxins)

Pediatric

Bowel cleansing prior to GI exam: (CoLyte®, GoLYTELY®, NuLYTELY®, TriLyte®):

Oral: 25 mL/kg/hour (some studies have used up to 40 mL/kg/hour) for 4-10 hours until rectal effluent is clear (maximum total dose: 4 L)

Nasogastric tube: 25 mL/kg/hour until rectal effluent is clear

Toxic ingestion (unlabeled use; AACT, 2004): *Nasogastric tube:*

Children ≥9 months to 6 years: 500 mL/hour until rectal effluent is clear

Children 6-12 years: 1000 mL/hour until rectal effluent is clear

Adolescents: 1500-2000 mL/hour until rectal effluent is clear

Note: May take several hours for the rectal effluent to become clear. Duration may be extended if evidence of continued presence of toxins in GI tract (eg, radiographic evidence or ongoing elimination of toxins)

Administration

Oral Rapid drinking of each portion is preferred to drinking small amounts continuously. Do not add flavorings, unless provided by the manufacturer, as additional ingredients before use. Chilled solution often more palatable. Oral medications should not be administered within 1 hour of start of therapy.

Monitoring and Teaching Issues

Laboratory Monitoring Electrolytes, serum glucose, BUN, urine osmolality

Patient Education For bowel cleansing prior to GI exam, take every 10 minutes until recommended amount is consumed or the rectal effluent is clear. Rapid drinking of each portion is preferred to drinking small amounts continuously. The first bowel movement should occur approximately 1 hour after the start of administration. May cause abdominal bloating and distention before bowel starts to move. If severe discomfort or distention occurs, stop drinking temporarily or drink each portion at longer intervals until these symptoms disappear. Continue drinking until the watery stool is clear and free of solid matter.

Polyethylene Glycol-Electrolyte Solution and Bisacodyl

(pol i ETH i leen GLY kol ee LEK troe lite soe LOO shun & bis a KOE dil)

U.S. Brand Names HalfLytely® and Bisacodyl

Index Terms Bisacodyl and Polyethylene Glycol-Electrolyte Solution; Electrolyte Lavage Solution

Generic Availability (U.S.) No

Pharmacologic Category Laxative, Bowel Evacuant; Laxative, Stimulant

Medication Guide Available Yes

Pregnancy Risk Factor C

Lactation Excretion in breast milk unknown/use caution

Use Bowel cleansing prior to colonoscopy

Available Dosage Forms

Kit [each kit contains]:

HalfLytely® and Bisacodyl:

Powder for solution, oral (HalfLytely®): PEG 3350 210 g, sodium bicarbonate 2.86 g, sodium chloride 5.6 g, potassium chloride 0.74 g (2000 mL) [contains 4 flavor packs (each 1 g) cherry, lemon-lime, orange, pineapple flavors]

Tablet, delayed release (Bisacodyl): 5 mg (1s)

Dosing

Adult & Geriatric Bowel cleansing: Oral:

Bisacodyl: 5 mg as a single dose. After bowel movement or 6 hours (whichever occurs first), initiate polyethylene glycol-electrolyte solution

Polyethylene glycol-electrolyte solution: 8 ounces every 10 minutes until 2 L are consumed

Administration

Oral Administer bisacodyl tablet with water; do not chew or crush tablet. Do not take antacids within 1 hour of taking bisacodyl. Rapidly drinking the polyethylene glycol-electrolyte solution is preferred to drinking small amount continuously. If severe bloating, distention, or abdominal pain occurs, administration should be slowed or temporarily discontinued until symptoms resolve.

Monitoring and Teaching Issues

Laboratory Monitoring Electrolytes, renal function

Physical Assessment See individual agents.

Patient Education See individual agents.

◆ **Polyphenols** *see* Sinecatechins *on page* 1647

◆ **Polyphenon E** *see* Sinecatechins *on page* 1647

◆ **P-OM3** *see* Omega-3-Acid Ethyl Esters *on page* 1355

◆ **Portia®** *see* Ethinyl Estradiol and Levonorgestrel *on page* 699

Posaconazole (poe sa KON a zole)

U.S. Brand Names Noxafil®

Index Terms SCH 56592

Generic Availability (U.S.) No

Pharmacologic Category Antifungal Agent, Oral

Medication Safety Issues

Sound-alike/look-alike issues:

Noxafil® may be confused with minoxidil

International issues:

Noxafil [U.S. and multiple international markets] may be confused with Noxidil brand name for minoxidil [Thailand]

Pregnancy Risk Factor C

Lactation Excretion in breast milk unknown/not recommended

Use Prophylaxis of invasive *Aspergillus* and *Candida* infections in severely-immunocompromised patients [eg, hematopoietic stem cell transplant (HSCT) recipients with graft-versus-host disease (GVHD) or those with prolonged neutropenia secondary to chemotherapy for hematologic malignancies]; treatment of oropharyngeal candidiasis (including patients refractory to itraconazole and/or fluconazole)

Unlabeled/Investigational Use Salvage therapy of refractory or relapsed invasive fungal infections; mucormycosis; pulmonary infection (nonimmunosuppressed)

Mechanism of Action/Effect Interferes with fungal cytochrome P450 (latosterol-14α-demethylase) activity, decreasing ergosterol synthesis (principal sterol in fungal cell membrane) and inhibiting fungal cell membrane formation.

Contraindications Hypersensitivity to posaconazole, other azole antifungals, or any component of the formulation; coadministration of cisapride, ergot alkaloids, pimozide, quinidine, simvastatin, or sirolimus

Warnings/Precautions Hepatic dysfunction has occurred, ranging from reversible mild/moderate increases of ALT, AST, alkaline phosphatase, total bilirubin, and/or clinical hepatitis to severe reactions (cholestasis, hepatic failure including death). Consider discontinuation of therapy in patients who develop clinical evidence of liver disease that may be secondary to posaconazole. Use caution in patients with an increased risk of arrhythmia (long QT syndrome, concurrent QT_c-prolonging drugs, hypokalemia). Correct electrolyte abnormalities (eg, potassium, magnesium, and calcium) before initiating therapy. Concurrent use with cyclosporine or tacrolimus may significantly increase cyclosporine/tacrolimus concentrations and may result in rare serious adverse events (eg, nephrotoxicity, leukoencephalopathy, and death); dose reduction and close monitoring are recommended with initiation of posaconazole therapy. Concurrent use with midazolam may increase midazolam concentrations and potentiate midazolam-related adverse effects.

Use caution in hypersensitivity with other azole antifungal agents; cross-reaction may occur, but has not been established. Consider alternative therapy or closely monitor for breakthrough fungal infections in patients receiving drugs that decrease absorption or increase the metabolism of posaconazole or in any patient unable to eat or tolerate an oral liquid nutritional supplement. Use caution in severe renal impairment or GI disturbances; monitor for breakthrough fungal infections.

Drug Interactions

Metabolism/Transport Effects Inhibits CYP3A4 (strong)

Avoid Concomitant Use

Avoid concomitant use of Posaconazole with any of the following: Alfuzosin; Cisapride; Conivaptan; Dofetilide; Dronedarone; Efavirenz; Eplerenone; Ergot Derivatives; Everolimus; Halofantrine; Lurasidone; Nilotinib; Nisoldipine; Pimozide; Proton Pump Inhibitors; QuiNIDine; Ranolazine; Rivaroxaban; RomiDEPsin; Salmeterol; Silodosin; Sirolimus; Tamsulosin; Tolvaptan; Toremifene

Decreased Effect

Posaconazole may decrease the levels/effects of: Amphotericin B; Prasugrel; Saccharomyces boulardii

The levels/effects of Posaconazole may be decreased by: Didanosine; Efavirenz; Etravirine; Fosamprenavir; H2-Antagonists; Metoclopramide; Phenytoin; Proton Pump Inhibitors; Rifamycin Derivatives; Sucralfate

Increased Effect/Toxicity

Posaconazole may increase the levels/effects of: Alfentanil; Alfuzosin; Almotriptan; Alosetron; Antineoplastic Agents (Vinca Alkaloids); Aprepitant; Benzodiazepines (metabolized by oxidation); Bortezomib; Bosentan; Brinzolamide; BusPIRone; Busulfan; Calcium Channel Blockers; CarBAMazepine; Cardiac Glycosides; Ciclesonide; Cilostazol; Cinacalcet; Cisapride; Colchicine; Conivaptan; Corticosteroids (Orally Inhaled); Corticosteroids (Systemic); CycloSPORINE; CycloSPORINE (Systemic); CYP3A4 Substrates; Dienogest; DOCEtaxel; Dofetilide; Dronedarone; Dutasteride; Eletriptan; Eplerenone; Ergot Derivatives; Erlotinib; Eszopiclone; Etravirine; Everolimus; FentaNYL; Fesoterodine; Fosamprenavir; Fosaprepitant; Gefitinib; GlipiZIDE; GuanFACINE; Halofantrine; HMG-CoA Reductase Inhibitors; Imatinib; Irinotecan; Ixabepilone; Losartan; Lumefantrine; Lurasidone; Macrolide Antibiotics; Maraviroc; Methadone; MethylPREDNISolone; Nilotinib; Nisoldipine; Paricalcitol; Pazopanib; Phenytoin; Phosphodiesterase 5 Inhibitors; Pimecrolimus; Pimozide; Protease Inhibitors; QuiNIDine; Ramelteon; Ranolazine; Repaglinide; Rifamycin Derivatives; Rivaroxaban; RomiDEPsin; Salmeterol; Saxagliptin; Silodosin; Sirolimus; Solifenacin; SORAfenib; SUNItinib; Tacrolimus; Tacrolimus (Systemic); Tacrolimus (Topical); Tadalafil; Tamsulosin; Temsirolimus; Tolterodine; Tolvaptan; Toremifene; Vilazodone; Vitamin K Antagonists; Ziprasidone; Zolpidem

The levels/effects of Posaconazole may be increased by: Etravirine; Grapefruit Juice; Macrolide Antibiotics; Protease Inhibitors; Tacrolimus

Nutritional/Ethanol Interactions Food: Bioavailability increased ~3 times when posaconazole is administered with a nonfat meal or an oral liquid nutritional supplement; increased ~4 times when administered with a high-fat meal. Grapefruit juice may decrease the levels/effects of posaconazole; concurrent use should be avoided.

Adverse Reactions Note: Percentages reflect data from use in comparator trials with multiple concomitant conditions and medications; some adverse reactions may be due to underlying condition(s).

>10%:

- Cardiovascular: Hypertension (18%), edema (9% to 15%), hypotension (14%), tachycardia (12%)
- Central nervous system: Fever (6% to 45%), headache (8% to 28%), fatigue (3% to 17%), insomnia (1% to 17%), dizziness (11%), pain (1% to 11%)
- Endocrine & metabolic: Hypokalemia (≤30%), hypomagnesemia (18%), dehydration (1% to 11%), hyperglycemia (11%)
- Gastrointestinal: Diarrhea (10% to 42%), nausea (9% to 38%), vomiting (7% to 29%), abdominal pain (5% to 27%), constipation (21%), anorexia (2% to 19%), mucositis (17%), weight loss (1% to 14%), oral candidiasis (1% to 12%)
- Hematologic: Thrombocytopenia (29%), anemia (2% to 25%), neutropenia (4% to 23%), neutropenic fever (20%)
- Hepatic: ALT increased (6% to 17%)
- Neuromuscular & skeletal: Rigors (≤20%), musculoskeletal pain (16%), weakness (2% to 13%), arthralgia (11%)
- Respiratory: Cough (3% to 25%), dyspnea (1% to 20%), epistaxis (14%), pharyngitis (12%)
- Miscellaneous: Bacteremia (18%), herpes simplex (3% to 15%), CMV infection (14%)

1% to 10%:

- Central nervous system: Anxiety (9%)
- Endocrine & metabolic: Hypocalcemia (9%)
- Gastrointestinal: Dyspepsia (10%)
- Genitourinary: Vaginal hemorrhage (10%)
- Hepatic: Hyperbilirubinemia (7% to 10%), AST increased (3% to 4%), alkaline phosphatase increased (1% to 3%)
- Neuromuscular & skeletal: Back pain (10%)
- Respiratory: Pneumonia (3% to 10%), upper respiratory infection (7%)
- Miscellaneous: Diaphoresis (2% to 10%)

Pharmacodynamics/Kinetics

Absorption Coadministration with food, liquid nutritional supplements, and/or acidic carbonated beverages (eg, ginger ale) increases absorption; fasting states do not provide sufficient absorption to ensure adequate plasma concentrations.

Time to Peak ~3-5 hours

Protein Binding >98%; predominantly bound to albumin

Half-Life Elimination 35 hours (range: 20-66 hours)

Metabolism Not significantly metabolized; ~15% to 17% undergoes non-CYP-mediated metabolism, primarily via hepatic glucuronidation into metabolites

Excretion Feces 71% to 77% (~66% of the total dose as unchanged drug); urine 13% to 14% (<0.2% of the total dose as unchanged drug)

Available Dosage Forms

Suspension, oral:

Noxafil®: 40 mg/mL (123 mL)

Dosing

Adult & Geriatric

Aspergillosis, invasive: Oral:

Prophylaxis: 200 mg 3 times/day; duration of therapy is based is based on recovery from neutropenia or immunosuppression

Salvage treatment of refractory infection (unlabeled use): 200 mg 4 times/day initially; after disease stabilization may decrease frequency to 400 mg 2 times/day (Walsh, 2007). **Note:** Duration of therapy should be a minimum of 6-12 weeks or throughout period of immunosuppression (Walsh, 2008).

Candidal infections: Oral:

Prophylaxis: 200 mg 3 times/day; duration of therapy is based on recovery from neutropenia or immunosuppression

Treatment of oropharyngeal infection: Initial: 100 mg 2 times/day for 1 day; maintenance: 100 mg once daily for 13 days

Treatment of refractory oropharyngeal infection: 400 mg 2 times/day; duration of therapy is based on underlying disease and clinical response

Mucormycosis (unlabeled use): Oral: 800 mg/day in 2 or 4 divided doses; duration of therapy is based on response and risk of relapse due to immunosuppression (Greenburg, 2006)

Cryptococcal infections: Oral:

Pulmonary, nonimmunosuppressed (unlabeled use): 400 mg 2 times/day. **Note:** Fluconazole is considered first-line treatment (Perfect, 2010).

Salvage treatment of relapsed infection (unlabeled use): 400 mg 2 times/day (or 200 mg 4 times/day) for 10-12 weeks. **Note:** Salvage treatment should only be started after an appropriate course of an induction regimen (Perfect, 2010).

Pediatric

Aspergillosis, invasive: Oral: Children ≥13 years: Refer to adult dosing.

Candidal infections: Oral: Children ≥13 years: Refer to adult dosing.

Renal Impairment

Mild-to-moderate renal insufficiency (Cl_{cr} 20-80 mL/minute/1.73 m^2): No adjustment necessary

Severe renal insufficiency (Cl_{cr} <20 mL/minute/1.73 m^2): No adjustment necessary; however, monitor for breakthrough fungal infections due to variability in posaconazole exposure.

Hepatic Impairment

Mild-to-severe hepatic insufficiency (Child-Pugh classes A, B, and C): No adjustment necessary.

Clinical signs and symptoms of liver disease due to posaconazole: Consider discontinuing therapy.

Administration

Oral Shake well before use. Must be administered during or within 20 minutes following a full meal or an oral liquid nutritional supplement; alternatively, posaconazole may be administered with an acidic carbonated beverage (eg, ginger ale). In patients able to swallow, administer oral suspension using dosing spoon provided by the manufacturer; spoon should be rinsed clean with water after each use and before storage.

Stability

Storage Store at 25°C (77°F); excursions permitted to 15°C to 30°C (59°F to 86°F). Do not freeze.

Monitoring and Teaching Issues

Laboratory Monitoring Hepatic function (eg, AST/ALT, alkaline phosphatase and bilirubin) prior to initiation and during treatment; renal function; electrolyte disturbances (eg, calcium, magnesium, potassium); CBC

Physical Assessment Assess allergy history prior to beginning therapy. Use caution in presence of hepatic or renal dysfunction or risk of arrhythmia. Electrolyte abnormalities should be corrected prior to beginning therapy. Monitor for gastrointestinal disturbance, vision changes, hepatic toxicity, and CNS changes on a regular basis during therapy.

Patient Education Take preferably during or immediately after a full meal or liquid nutritional supplement (can alternatively be taken with an acidic carbonated beverage, such as ginger ale). Take full course of medication; fungal infections may take weeks or months of therapy. Maintain adequate hydration unless instructed to restrict fluid intake. You may experience nausea, vomiting, abdominal pain, loss of appetite, constipation, headache, dizziness, blurred vision, or insomnia. Report immediately chest pain or palpitations, unusual muscle pain or weakness, severe diarrhea or vomiting, urinary pattern changes, yellowing of skin or eyes, or changes in color of stool or urine.

Dietary Considerations Give during or within 20 minutes following a full meal or liquid nutritional supplement; alternatively, posaconazole may be administered with an acidic carbonated beverage (eg, ginger ale). Consider alternative antifungal therapy in patients with inadequate oral intake or severe diarrhea/vomiting; if alternative therapy is not an option, closely monitoring for breakthrough fungal infections. Adequate posaconazole absorption from GI tract and subsequent plasma concentrations are dependent on food for efficacy. Lower average plasma concentrations have been associated with an increased risk of treatment failure.

Geriatric Considerations Dosage adjustment not necessary.

Breast-Feeding Considerations Excretion in breast milk has not been investigated; use only if the benefit to the mother justifies potential risk to the fetus.

Pregnancy Considerations Posaconazole has been shown to be teratogenic in animal studies. There are no adequate and well-controlled studies in pregnant women. Use only if the benefit to the mother justifies potential risk to the fetus.

◆ **Posture® [OTC]** *see* Calcium Phosphate (Tribasic) *on page* *278*

Potassium Bicarbonate (poe TASS ee um bye KAR bun ate)

Generic Availability (U.S.) Yes

Pharmacologic Category Electrolyte Supplement, Oral

Pregnancy Risk Factor C

Use Potassium deficiency, hypokalemia

Available Dosage Forms

Tablet for solution, oral: Potassium 25 mEq

Dosing

Adult & Geriatric Hypokalemia: Oral: 25 mEq 2-4 times/day

Pediatric Hypokalemia: Oral: Children: 1-4 mEq/kg/day

Monitoring and Teaching Issues

Laboratory Monitoring Serum potassium, serum bicarbonate

Potassium Bicarbonate and Potassium Chloride
(poe TASS ee um bye KAR bun ate & poe TASS ee um KLOR ide)

Index Terms K-Lyte/Cl; Potassium Bicarbonate and Potassium Chloride (Effervescent)

Generic Availability (U.S.) Yes

Pharmacologic Category Electrolyte Supplement, Oral

Pregnancy Risk Factor C

Lactation Enters breast milk/compatible

Use Treatment or prevention of hypokalemia

Available Dosage Forms

Tablet for solution, oral [effervescent]: Potassium chloride 25 mEq

Dosing

Adult & Geriatric Hypokalemia: Oral:

Prevention: 16-24 mEq/day in 2-4 divided doses

Treatment: 40-100 mEq/day in 2-4 divided doses

Pediatric Oral: 1-4 mEq/kg/24 hours in divided doses as required to maintain normal serum potassium

Administration

Oral Administer with meals; solution should be sipped slowly, over 5-10 minutes

Monitoring and Teaching Issues

Laboratory Monitoring Serum potassium, serum bicarbonate

Physical Assessment See individual agents.

Patient Education See individual agents.

Related Information

Potassium Bicarbonate *on page* *1479*

Potassium Chloride *on page* *1480*

◆ **Potassium Bicarbonate and Potassium Chloride (Effervescent)** *see* Potassium Bicarbonate and Potassium Chloride *on page* *1479*

Potassium Bicarbonate and Potassium Citrate
(poe TASS ee um bye KAR bun ate & poe TASS ee um SIT rate)

U.S. Brand Names Effer-K®; Klor-Con®/EF

Index Terms Potassium Bicarbonate and Potassium Citrate (Effervescent)

Generic Availability (U.S.) Yes

Pharmacologic Category Electrolyte Supplement, Oral

Medication Safety Issues

Sound-alike/look-alike issues:

Klor-Con® may be confused with Klaron®

Pregnancy Risk Factor C

Use Treatment or prevention of hypokalemia

Available Dosage Forms

Tablet for solution, oral [effervescent]:

Effer-K®: Potassium 10 mEq; potassium 20 mEq; potassium 25 mEq

Klor-Con®/EF: Potassium 25 mEq

Dosing

Adult & Geriatric Hypokalemia: Oral:

Prevention: 16-24 mEq/day in 2-4 divided doses

Treatment: 40-100 mEq/day in 2-4 divided doses

Pediatric Hypokalemia: Oral: Children: 1-4 mEq/kg/24 hours in divided doses as required to maintain normal serum potassium

Monitoring and Teaching Issues

Laboratory Monitoring Serum potassium, serum bicarbonate

Physical Assessment See individual agents.

Patient Education See individual agents.

Related Information

Potassium Bicarbonate *on page* 1479

Potassium Citrate *on page* 1482

◆ **Potassium Bicarbonate and Potassium Citrate (Effervescent)** *see* Potassium Bicarbonate and Potassium Citrate *on page* 1479

Potassium Chloride (poe TASS ee um KLOR ide)

U.S. Brand Names Epiklor™; Epiklor™/25; K-Tab®; Kaon-CL® 10; Klor-Con®; Klor-Con® 10; Klor-Con® 8; Klor-Con® M10; Klor-Con® M15; Klor-Con® M20; Klor-Con®/25; microK®; microK® 10

Index Terms KCl; Kdur

Generic Availability (U.S.) Yes: Excludes powder for solution

Pharmacologic Category Electrolyte Supplement, Oral; Electrolyte Supplement, Parenteral

Medication Safety Issues

Sound-alike/look-alike issues:

Kaon-Cl-10® may be confused with kaolin

KCl may be confused with HCl

Klor-Con® may be confused with Klaron®

microK® may be confused with Macrobid®, Micronase®

High alert medication: The Institute for Safe Medication Practices (ISMP) includes this medication (I.V. formulation) among its list of drugs which have a heightened risk of causing significant patient harm when used in error.

Per JCAHO recommendations, concentrated electrolyte solutions should not be available in patient care areas.

Consider special storage requirements for intravenous potassium salts; I.V. potassium salts have been administered IVP in error, leading to fatal outcomes.

Pregnancy Risk Factor C

Lactation Enters breast milk/compatible

Use Treatment or prevention of hypokalemia

Contraindications Hypersensitivity to any component of the formulation; hyperkalemia. In addition, solid oral dosage forms are contraindicated in patients in whom there is a structural, pathological, and/or pharmacologic cause for delay or arrest in passage through the GI tract.

Warnings/Precautions Close monitoring of serum potassium concentrations is needed to avoid hyperkalemia. Use with caution in patients with renal impairment, cardiac disease, acid/base disorders, or potassium-altering conditions/disorders. Use with caution in digitalized patients or patients receiving concomitant medications or therapies that increase potassium (eg, ACEI, potassium-sparing diuretics, potassium containing salt substitutes). Do **NOT** administer undiluted or I.V. push; inappropriate parenteral administration may be fatal. Always administer potassium further diluted; refer to appropriate dilution and administration rate recommendations. Pain and phlebitis may occur during parenteral infusion requiring a decrease in infusion rate or potassium concentration. Avoid administering potassium diluted in dextrose solutions during initial therapy; potential for transient decreases in serum potassium due to intracellular shift of potassium from dextrose-stimulated insulin release. May cause GI upset (eg, nausea, vomiting, diarrhea, abdominal pain, discomfort) and lead to GI ulceration, bleeding, perforation, and/or obstruction. Oral liquid preparations (not solid) should be used in patients with esophageal compression or delayed gastric emptying.

Drug Interactions

Avoid Concomitant Use

Avoid concomitant use of Potassium Chloride with any of the following: Glycopyrrolate

Decreased Effect There are no known significant interactions involving a decrease in effect.

Increased Effect/Toxicity

Potassium Chloride may increase the levels/effects of: ACE Inhibitors; Angiotensin II Receptor Blockers; Potassium-Sparing Diuretics

The levels/effects of Potassium Chloride may be increased by: Anticholinergic Agents; Eplerenone; Glycopyrrolate

Adverse Reactions Frequency not defined.

Dermatologic: Rash

Endocrine & metabolic: Hyperkalemia

Gastrointestinal: Abdominal pain/discomfort, diarrhea, flatulence, GI bleeding (oral), GI obstruction (oral), GI perforation (oral), nausea, vomiting

Pharmacodynamics/Kinetics

Absorption Well absorbed from upper GI tract

Excretion Primarily urine; skin and feces (small amounts); most intestinal potassium reabsorbed

Available Dosage Forms

Capsule, extended release, microencapsulated, oral: 10 mEq
microK®: 8 mEq
microK® 10: 10 mEq

Infusion, premixed in ½ NS: 20 mEq (1000 mL)
Infusion, premixed in D_{10}¼ NS: 5 mEq (250 mL)
Infusion, premixed in D_5½ NS: 10 mEq (500 mL, 1000 mL); 20 mEq (1000 mL); 30 mEq (1000 mL); 40 mEq (1000 mL)
Infusion, premixed in D_5⅓ NS: 20 mEq (1000 mL)
Infusion, premixed in D_5¼ NS: 5 mEq (250 mL); 10 mEq (500 mL, 1000 mL); 20 mEq (1000 mL); 30 mEq (1000 mL); 40 mEq (1000 mL)
Infusion, premixed in D_5LR: 20 mEq (1000 mL)
Infusion, premixed in D_5NS: 20 mEq (1000 mL); 40 mEq (1000 mL)
Infusion, premixed in D_5W: 20 mEq (500 mL, 1000 mL); 40 mEq (1000 mL)
Infusion, premixed in NS: 20 mEq (1000 mL); 40 mEq (1000 mL)
Infusion, premixed in water for injection: 10 mEq (50 mL, 100 mL); 20 mEq (50 mL, 100 mL); 30 mEq (100 mL); 40 mEq (100 mL)
Injection, solution: 2 mEq/mL (5 mL, 10 mL, 15 mL, 20 mL, 30 mL, 250 mL, 500 mL)
Injection, solution [preservative free]: 2 mEq/mL (5 mL, 10 mL, 15 mL, 20 mL)

Powder for solution, oral:
Epiklor™: 20 mEq/packet (30s, 100s)
Epiklor™/25: 25 mEq/packet (30s, 100s)
Klor-Con®: 20 mEq/packet (30s, 100s)
Klor-Con®/25: 25 mEq/packet (30s, 100s)

Solution, oral: 20 mEq/15 mL (15 mL, 30 mL, 473 mL, 480 mL); 40 mEq/15 mL (15 mL, 473 mL)

Tablet, extended release, microencapsulated, oral: 8 mEq, 10 mEq, 20 mEq
Klor-Con® M10: 10 mEq
Klor-Con® M15: 15 mEq
Klor-Con® M20: 20 mEq

Tablet, extended release, wax matrix, oral: 8 mEq, 10 mEq
K-Tab®: 10 mEq
Kaon-CL® 10: 10 mEq
Klor-Con® 8: 8 mEq
Klor-Con® 10: 10 mEq

Dosing

Adult & Geriatric I.V. doses should be incorporated into the patient's maintenance I.V. fluids; intermittent I.V. potassium administration should be reserved for severe depletion situations in patients undergoing ECG monitoring. Doses expressed as mEq of potassium.

Normal daily requirements: *Oral, I.V.:* 40-80 mEq/day
Prevention of hypokalemia: *Oral:* 20-40 mEq/day in 1-2 divided doses
Treatment of hypokalemia:

Oral:

Asymptomatic, mild hypokalemia: Usual dosage range: 40-100 mEq/day divided in 2-5 doses; generally recommended to limit doses to 20-25 mEq/dose to avoid GI discomfort.

Mild-to-moderate hypokalemia: Some clinicians may administer up to 120-240 mEq/day divided in 3-4 doses; limit doses to 40-60 mEq/dose. If deficits are severe or ongoing losses are great, I.V. route should be considered.

I.V. intermittent infusion: Peripheral or central line: ≤10 mEq/hour; repeat as needed based on frequently obtained lab values; central line infusion and continuous ECG monitoring highly recommended for infusions >10 mEq/hour.

Potassium dosage/rate of infusion general guidelines (per product labeling): **Note:** High variability exists in dosing/infusion rate recommendations; therapy guided by patient condition and specific institutional guidelines.

Serum potassium >2.5 mEq/L: Maximum infusion rate: 10 mEq/hour; maximum concentration: 40 mEq/L; maximum 24-hour dose: 200 mEq

Serum potassium <2 mEq/L and symptomatic (excluding emergency treatment of cardiac arrest): Maximum infusion rate (central line only): 40 mEq/hour in presence of continuous ECG monitoring and frequent lab monitoring; In selected situations, patients may require up to 400 mEq/24 hours.

Pediatric I.V. doses should be incorporated into the patient's maintenance I.V. fluids; intermittent I.V. potassium administration should be reserved for severe depletion situations in patients undergoing ECG monitoring. Doses expressed as mEq of potassium.

Normal daily requirements: *Oral, I.V.:* 1-2 mEq/kg/day
Prevention of hypokalemia: *Oral:* 1-2 mEq/kg/day in 1-2 divided doses
Treatment of hypokalemia:

Oral: 1-2 mEq/kg initially, then as needed based on frequently obtained lab values. If deficits are severe or ongoing losses are great, I.V. route should be considered.

I.V. intermittent infusion: 0.5-1 mEq/kg/dose (maximum dose: 40 mEq). If infusion exceeds 0.5 mEq/kg/hour, physician should be at bedside and patient should have continuous ECG monitoring; repeat as needed based on frequently obtained lab values.

Administration

Oral Oral dosage forms should be taken with meals and a full glass of water or other liquid.

Capsule: MicroK®: Swallow whole, do not chew. Capsules may also be opened and contents sprinkled on a spoonful of applesauce or pudding and should be swallowed immediately without chewing. No more than 20 mEq should be given as a single dose.

Powder: Klor-Con®: Dissolve in 4-5 ounces of water or other beverage prior to administration.

Tablet:

K-Tab®, Kaon-Cl®, Klor-Con®: Swallow tablets whole; do not crush, chew, or suck on tablet. No more than 20 mEq should be given as a single dose.

Klor-Con® M: Tablet may also be broken in half and each half swallowed separately; the whole tablet may be dissolved in ~4 ounces of water (allow ~2 minutes to dissolve, stir well and drink immediately)

I.V. Potassium must be diluted prior to parenteral administration. Do not administer I.V. push. In general, the dose, concentration of infusion and rate of administration may be dependant on patient condition and specific institution policy. Some clinicians recommend that the maximum concentration for peripheral infusion is 10 mEq/100 mL and maximum rate of administration for peripheral infusion is 10 mEq/hour. ECG monitoring is recommended for peripheral or central infusions >10 mEq/hour in adults. Concentrations and rates of infusion may be greater with central line administration. Some clinicians recommend that the maximum concentration for central infusion is 20-40 mEq/100 mL and maximum rate of administration for central infusion is 40 mEq/hour.

Stability

Storage

Capsule: MicroK®: Store between 20°C to 25°C (68°F to 77°F).

Powder for oral solution: Klor-Con®: Store at room temperature of 15°C to 30°C (59°F to 86°F).

Solution for injection: Store at room temperature; do not freeze. Use only clear solutions. Use admixtures within 24 hours.

Tablet: K-Tab®: Store below 30°C (86°F).

Monitoring and Teaching Issues

Laboratory Monitoring Serum potassium, glucose, chloride

Patient Education Long-acting and wax matrix tablets should be swallowed whole; do not crush or chew. Powder must be dissolved in water before use. Liquid can be diluted or dissolved in water or juice. Take with food to avoid GI irritation and upset. Report abdominal pain, nausea, or vomiting.

Dietary Considerations Administer with plenty of fluid to decrease stomach irritation and discomfort. Some dietary sources of potassium include leafy green vegetables (eg, spinach, cabbage), tomatoes, cucumbers, zucchini, fruits (eg, apples, oranges, and bananas), root vegetables (eg, carrots, radishes), beans, and peas.

Geriatric Considerations Elderly may require less potassium than younger adults due to decreased renal function. For the elderly who do not respond to replacement therapy, check serum magnesium. Long-term use of diuretics may result in hypomagnesemic.

Breast-Feeding Considerations The normal content of potassium in human milk is ~13 mEq/L. Supplementation (that does not cause maternal hyperkalemia) would not be expected to affect normal levels.

Pregnancy Considerations Reproduction studies have not been conducted. Potassium supplementation (that does not cause maternal hyperkalemia) would not be expected to cause adverse fetal events.

Related Information

Compatibility of Drugs *on page* *1994*

Potassium Citrate (poe TASS ee um SIT rate)

U.S. Brand Names Urocit®-K

Generic Availability (U.S.) Yes

Pharmacologic Category Alkalinizing Agent, Oral

Medication Safety Issues

Sound-alike/look-alike issues:

Urocit®-K may be confused with Urised®

Pregnancy Risk Factor C

Lactation Excretion in breast milk unknown/use caution

Use Prevention of uric acid nephrolithiasis; prevention of calcium renal stones in patients with hypocitraturia; urinary alkalinizer when sodium citrate is contraindicated

Available Dosage Forms

Tablet, oral: 540 mg, 1080 mg

Urocit®-K: 540 mg, 1080 mg

Dosing

Adult & Geriatric Alkalinizer, bicarbonate precursor: Oral:

Mild-to-moderate hypocitraturia (>150 mg urinary citrate): 10 mEq 3 times daily; maximum dose: 100 mEq/day

Severe hypocitraturia (<150 mg/day urinary citrate): 20 mEq 3 times daily or 15 mEq 4 times daily; maximum dose: 100 mEq/day

Administration

Oral May be administered with meals. Swallow tablets whole with a full glass of water.

Monitoring and Teaching Issues

Laboratory Monitoring Serum electrolytes (potassium, chloride, sodium), serum creatinine, and CBC every 4 months; urinary citrate and/or urinary pH at initiation or dose change and every 4 months

Physical Assessment Assess kidney function prior to treatment. Monitor cardiac status and serum potassium prior to treatment and at regular intervals.

Patient Education Swallow tablet whole with full glass of water after meals (do not take on an empty stomach). Take any antacids 2 hours before or after potassium. Consult prescriber about advisability of increasing dietary potassium. Report unresolved nausea or vomiting, chest pain or palpitations, persistent abdominal pain, feelings of weakness, dizziness, acute muscle weakness, or cramping.

Potassium Iodide (poe TASS ee um EYE oh dide)

U.S. Brand Names iOSAT™ [OTC]; SSKI®; ThyroSafe™; Thyroshield™ [OTC]

Index Terms KI

Pharmacologic Category Antithyroid Agent; Expectorant

Medication Safety Issues

Sound-alike/look-alike issues:

Potassium iodide products, including saturated solution of potassium iodide (SSKI®) may be confused with potassium iodide and iodine (Strong Iodide Solution or Lugol's solution)

Pregnancy Risk Factor D

Lactation Enters breast milk/use caution (AAP rates "compatible"; AAP 2001 update pending)

Use Expectorant for the symptomatic treatment of chronic pulmonary diseases complicated by mucous; block thyroidal uptake of radioactive isotopes of iodine in a radiation emergency

Unlabeled/Investigational Use Lymphocutaneous and cutaneous sporotrichosis; reduce thyroid vascularity prior to thyroidectomy; management of thyrotoxic crisis; block thyroidal uptake of radioactive isotopes of iodine after therapeutic or diagnostic exposure to radioactive iodine

Available Dosage Forms

Solution, oral:

SSKI®: 1 g/mL (30 mL, 237 mL)

Thyroshield™ [OTC]: 65 mg/mL (30 mL)

Tablet, oral:

iOSAT™ [OTC]: 130 mg

ThyroSafe™: 65 mg

Dosing

Adult & Geriatric

RDA: 150 mcg (iodine)

Expectorant: Oral: *SSKI®:* 300-600 mg 3-4 times/day

Preoperative thyroidectomy (unlabeled use): Oral: 50-250 mg (1-5 drops SSKI®) 3 times/day; administer for 10 days before surgery

To reduce risk of thyroid cancer following nuclear accident (Iosat™, ThyroSafe™, ThyroShield™): Oral: Adults (including pregnant/lactating women): Oral: 130 mg once daily. **Note:** Dosing should continue until risk of exposure has passed or other measures have are implemented.

Thyroid gland protection during radiopharmaceutical use (unlabeled use): Oral: Tablet: 130 mg once daily or Solution (SSKI®): 4 drops 3 times/day. **Note:** Begin at 1-48 hours prior to exposure. Continue potassium iodide after radiopharmaceutical administration until risk of exposure has diminished (treatment duration and time of initiation is dependent on the radiopharmaceutical, consult specific protocol).

Thyrotoxic crisis (unlabeled use): Oral: 250 mg (5 drops SSKI®) every 6 hours (Nayak, 2006)

Sporotrichosis (cutaneous, lymphocutaneous; unlabeled use): Oral: Initial: 5 drops (SSKI®) 3 times/day; increase to 40-50 drops (SSKI®) 3 times/day as tolerated until 2-4 weeks after lesions have resolved (usual duration 3-6 months) (Kauffman, 2007)

Pediatric

Preoperative thyroidectomy (unlabeled use): Refer to adult dosing.

To reduce risk of thyroid cancer following nuclear accident (Iosat™, ThyroSafe™, ThyroShield™): Oral:

Neonates: 16.25 mg once daily

Children 1 month to 3 years: 32.5 mg once daily

Children 3-18 years: 65 mg once daily

Children >68 kg: Refer to adult dosing

Note: Dosing should continue until risk of exposure has passed or other measures are implemented.

Thyroid gland protection during radiopharmaceutical use (unlabeled use): Oral (Olivier, 2003; Giammarile, 2008):

Neonates: 16 mg once

Infants <5 kg: 16 mg once daily

Children 1 month to 3 years or 5-15 kg: 32 mg once daily

Children 3-13 years or 15-50 kg: 65 mg once daily

Children >13 years or >50 kg: 130 mg once daily

Note: Begin at 1-48 hours prior to exposure. Continue potassium iodide after radiopharmaceutical administration until risk of exposure has diminished (treatment duration and time of initiation is dependent on the radiopharmaceutical, consult specific protocol.

Thyrotoxic crisis (unlabeled use): Oral:
Infants: 100 mg (2 drops SSKI®) 4 times/day (Hassoun, 2008)
Children: Refer to adult dosing.

Administration

Oral SSKI®: Dilute in a glassful of water, fruit juice, or milk. Take with food to decrease gastric irritation.

Monitoring and Teaching Issues

Laboratory Monitoring Thyroid function

Patient Education SSKI®: Dilute in water, fruit juice, or milk and take with meals to reduce gastric irritation. May cause metallic taste, nausea, or vomiting; soreness of teeth, gums, or glands; fever, headache, or sore joints; or confusion or tiredness. Discontinue and report if you experience any swelling of lips, mouth, or tongue; difficulty swallowing; chest pain or irregular heartbeat; unusual muscle weakness; eye irritation or eyelid swelling; or skin rash.

Potassium Iodide and Iodine (poe TASS ee um EYE oh dide & EYE oh dine)

Index Terms Iodine and Potassium Iodide; Lugol's Solution; Strong Iodine Solution

Generic Availability (U.S.) Yes

Pharmacologic Category Antithyroid Agent

Medication Safety Issues

Sound-alike/look-alike issues:

Potassium iodide and iodine (Strong Iodide Solution or Lugol's solution) may be confused with potassium iodide products, including saturated solution of potassium iodide (SSKI®)

Pregnancy Risk Factor D (potassium iodide)

Lactation Enters breast milk/use caution (AAP rates "compatible"; AAP 2001 update pending)

Use Reduce thyroid vascularity prior to thyroidectomy and management of thyrotoxic crisis; block thyroidal uptake of radioactive isotopes of iodine in a radiation emergency or after therapeutic/diagnostic use of radioactive iodine; topical antiseptic

Available Dosage Forms

Solution, oral: Potassium iodide 100 mg/mL and iodine 50 mg/mL

Solution, topical: Potassium iodide 100 mg/mL and iodine 50 mg/mL (8 mL)

Dosing

Adult & Geriatric RDA: 150 mcg (iodine)

Preoperative thyroidectomy: Oral: 0.1-0.3 mL (3-5 drops) 3 times/day; administer for 10 days before surgery

Thyrotoxic crisis: Oral: 4-8 drops every 6-8 hours; begin administration ≥1 hour following the initial dose of either propylthiouracil or methimazole (Nayak, 2006)

Thyroid gland protection during radiopharmaceutical use: Oral: 1 drop/kg/day; (maximum: 40 drops/day or 20 drops twice daily) (Giammarile, 2008); alternatively, 20 drops 3 times/day has also been used (Bexxar® prescribing information, 2005)

Note: Initiate 1-48 hours prior to radiopharmaceutical exposure and continue after radiopharmaceutical administration until risk of exposure has diminished (treatment initiation time and duration is dependent on the radiopharmaceutical agent used, consult specific protocol or labeling.

Pediatric

Preoperative thyroidectomy: Refer to adult dosing.

Thyrotoxic crisis: Oral: 4-8 drops 3 times/day; begin therapy preferably 2 hours following the initial dose of propylthiouracil or alternatively, methimazole (Hassoun, 2008)

Monitoring and Teaching Issues

Physical Assessment See individual agents.

Patient Education See individual agents.

Potassium Phosphate (poe TASS ee um FOS fate)

U.S. Brand Names Neutra-Phos®-K [OTC] [DSC]

Index Terms Phosphate, Potassium

Generic Availability (U.S.) Yes: Injection

Pharmacologic Category Electrolyte Supplement, Parenteral

Medication Safety Issues

High alert medication: The Institute for Safe Medication Practices (ISMP) includes this medication (I.V. formulation) among its list of drugs which have a heightened risk of causing significant patient harm when used in error.

Per JCAHO recommendations, concentrated electrolyte solutions should not be available in patient care areas.

Consider special storage requirements for intravenous potassium salts; I.V. potassium salts have been administered IVP in error, leading to fatal outcomes.

Safe Prescribing: Because inorganic phosphate exists as monobasic and dibasic anions, with the mixture of valences dependent on pH, ordering by mEq amounts is unreliable and may lead to large dosing errors. In addition, I.V. phosphate is available in the sodium and potassium salt; therefore, the content of these cations must be considered when ordering phosphate. The most reliable method of ordering I.V. phosphate is by millimoles, then specifying the potassium or sodium salt. For example, an order for 15 mmol of phosphate as potassium phosphate in one liter of normal saline.

Pregnancy Risk Factor C

Use Treatment and prevention of hypophosphatemia; **Note:** The concomitant amount of potassium must be calculated into the total electrolyte content. For each 1 mmol of phosphate, ~1.5 mEq of potassium will be administered. Therefore, if ordering 30 mmol of potassium phosphate, the patient will receive ~45 mEq of potassium.

Contraindications Hyperphosphatemia, hyperkalemia, hypocalcemia, hypomagnesemia, renal failure (oral product)

Warnings/Precautions Close monitoring of serum potassium concentrations is needed to avoid hyperkalemia. Use with caution in patients with renal insufficiency, cardiac disease, metabolic alkalosis. Use with caution in digitalized patients and patients receiving concomitant potassium-altering therapies. Parenteral potassium may cause pain and phlebitis, requiring a decrease in infusion rate or potassium concentration. Solutions for injection may contain aluminum; toxic levels may occur following prolonged administration in premature neonates or patients with renal impairment.

Drug Interactions

Avoid Concomitant Use There are no known interactions where it is recommended to avoid concomitant use.

Decreased Effect There are no known significant interactions involving a decrease in effect.

Increased Effect/Toxicity

Potassium Phosphate may increase the levels/effects of: ACE Inhibitors; Angiotensin II Receptor Blockers; Potassium-Sparing Diuretics

The levels/effects of Potassium Phosphate may be increased by: Bisphosphonate Derivatives; Eplerenone

Nutritional/Ethanol Interactions Food: Avoid administering with oxalate (berries, nuts, chocolate, beans, celery, tomato) or phytate-containing foods (bran, whole wheat).

Adverse Reactions Frequency not defined.

Cardiovascular: Arrhythmia, bradycardia, chest pain, ECG changes, edema, heart block, hypotension

Central nervous system: Listlessness, mental confusion, tetany (with large doses of phosphate)

Endocrine & metabolic: Hyperkalemia

Gastrointestinal: Diarrhea, nausea, stomach pain, vomiting

Genitourinary: Urine output decreased

Local: Phlebitis

Neuromuscular & skeletal: Paralysis, paresthesia, weakness

Renal: Acute renal failure

Respiratory: Dyspnea

Available Dosage Forms

Injection, solution: Potassium 4.4 mEq and phosphorus 3 mmol per mL (5 mL, 15 mL, 50 mL)

Dosing

Adult & Geriatric Caution: The concomitant amount of potassium must be calculated into the total electrolyte content. For each 1 mmol of phosphate, ~1.5 mEq of potassium will be administered. Therefore, if ordering 30 mmol of potassium phosphate, the patient will receive ~45 mEq of potassium. With orders for I.V. phosphate, there is considerable confusion associated with the use of millimoles (mmol) versus milliequivalents (mEq) to express the phosphate requirement. The most reliable method of ordering I.V. phosphate is by millimoles, then specifying the potassium or sodium salt. Doses listed as mmol of phosphate.

Acute treatment of hypophosphatemia: I.V.: It is recommended that repletion of severe hypophosphatemia be done I.V. because large doses of oral phosphate may cause diarrhea and intestinal absorption may be unreliable. Intermittent I.V. infusion should be reserved for severe depletion situations; requires continuous cardiac monitoring. Guidelines differ based on degree of illness, need/use of TPN, and severity of hypophosphatemia. If potassium >4.0 mEq/L consider phosphate replacement strategy without potassium (eg, sodium phosphates). Obese patients and/or severe renal impairment were excluded from phosphate supplement trials. **Note:** 1 mmol phosphate = 31 mg phosphorus; 1 mg phosphorus = 0.032 mmol phosphate.

General replacement guidelines (Lentz, 1978):

Low dose: 0.08 mmol/kg over 6 hours; use if losses are recent and uncomplicated

Intermediate dose: 0.16-0.24 mmol/kg over 4-6 hours; use if serum phosphorus level 0.5-1 mg/dL (0.16-0.32 mmol/L)

Note: The initial dose may be increased by 25% to 50% if the patient is symptomatic secondary to hypophosphatemia and lowered by 25% to 50% if the patient is hypercalcemic.

Critically-ill adult trauma patients receiving concurrent TPN (Brown, 2006):

Low dose: 0.32 mmol/kg over 4-6 hours; use if serum phosphorus level 2.3-3 mg/dL (0.73-0.96 mmol/L)

Intermediate dose: 0.64 mmol/kg over 4-6 hours; use if serum phosphorus level 1.6-2.2 mg/dL (0.51-0.72 mmol/L)

High dose: 1 mmol/kg over 8-12 hours; use if serum phosphorus <1.5 mg/dL (<0.5 mmol/L)

Parenteral nutrition: I.V.: 10-15 mmol/1000 kcal (Hicks, 2001) **or** 20-40 mmol/24 hours (Mirtallo, 2004 [ASPEN guidelines])

Pediatric I.V. doses should be incorporated into the patient's maintenance I.V. fluids. Intermittent I.V. infusion should be reserved for severe depletion situations; requires continuous cardiac monitoring. It is difficult to determine total body phosphorus deficit; the following are empiric guidelines.

Note: Refer to notes under adult dosing

Pediatric I.V. phosphate repletion: Children: 0.25-0.5 mmol/kg **administer over 4-6 hours and repeat if symptomatic hypophosphatemia persists**; to assess the need for further phosphate administration, obtain serum inorganic phosphate after administration of the first dose and base further doses on serum levels and clinical status

Maintenance: *I.V. solutions:* Children: 0.5-2 mmol/kg/24 hours

Administration

I.V. Injection must be diluted in appropriate I.V. solution and volume prior to administration and administered over a minimum of 4 hours

Stability

Storage Store at room temperature; do not freeze. Use only clear solutions. Up to 10-15 mEq of calcium may be added per liter before precipitate may occur.

Stability of parenteral admixture at room temperature (25°C) is 24 hours.

Phosphate salts may precipitate when mixed with calcium salts. Solubility is improved in amino acid parenteral nutrition solutions. Check with a pharmacist to determine compatibility.

Monitoring and Teaching Issues

Laboratory Monitoring Serum potassium, phosphate, magnesium; after I.V. phosphate repletion, repeat serum phosphate level should be checked 2-4 hours later

Geriatric Considerations A complete drug history should be taken to rule out potential drug interactions since elderly frequently may be taking potassium and potassium-sparing diuretics or salicylates as antacids. Elderly may require less potassium than younger adults due to decreased renal function. Elderly who do not respond to replacement therapy, check serum magnesium. Long-term use of diuretics may result in hypomagnesemia. Monitor closely in elderly with Cl_{cr} <30 mL/minute.

Breast-Feeding Considerations Phosphorus, sodium, and potassium are normal constituents of human milk.

Pregnancy Considerations Reproduction studies have not been conducted with this product.

Related Information

Compatibility of Drugs *on page* 1994

Potassium Phosphate and Sodium Phosphate

(poe TASS ee um FOS fate & SOW dee um FOS fate)

U.S. Brand Names K-Phos® MF; K-Phos® Neutral; K-Phos® No. 2; Phos-NaK; Phospha 250™ Neutral; Uro-KP-Neutral®

Index Terms Neutra-Phos; Sodium Phosphate and Potassium Phosphate

Generic Availability (U.S.) Yes

Pharmacologic Category Electrolyte Supplement, Oral

Medication Safety Issues

Sound-alike/look-alike issues:

K-Phos® Neutral may be confused with Neutra-Phos-K®

Pregnancy Risk Factor C

Use Treatment of conditions associated with excessive renal phosphate loss or inadequate GI absorption of phosphate; to acidify the urine to lower calcium concentrations; to increase the antibacterial activity of methenamine; reduce odor and rash caused by ammonia in urine

Available Dosage Forms

Caplet:

Uro-KP-Neutral®: Dipotassium phosphate, disodium phosphate, and monobasic sodium phosphate

Powder, for oral solution:

Phos-NaK: Dibasic potassium phosphate, monobasic potassium phosphate, dibasic sodium phosphate, and monobasic sodium phosphate per packet (100s)

Tablet:

K-Phos® MF: Potassium phosphate 155 mg and sodium phosphate 350 mg

K-Phos® Neutral: Monobasic potassium phosphate 155 mg, dibasic sodium phosphate 852 mg, and monobasic sodium phosphate 130 mg

K-Phos® No. 2: Potassium phosphate 305 mg and sodium phosphate 700 mg

Phospha 250™ Neutral: Monobasic potassium phosphate 155 mg, dibasic sodium phosphate 852 mg, and monobasic sodium phosphate 130 mg

Dosing

Adult & Geriatric Phosphate supplement: Oral: Elemental phosphorus 250-500 mg 4 times/day after meals and at bedtime

Pediatric Phosphate supplement: Oral: Children ≥4 years: Elemental phosphorus 250 mg 4 times/day after meals and at bedtime

Administration

Oral Administer with food to reduce risk of diarrhea.

Caplet, tablet: Should be taken with a full glass of water.

Powder: Phos-NaK: Contents of 1 packet should be diluted in 75 mL water before administration. Following dilution of powder, solution may be chilled to increase palatability.

Monitoring and Teaching Issues

Laboratory Monitoring Serum potassium, phosphate

Physical Assessment See individual agents.

Patient Education See individual agents.

Related Information

Potassium Phosphate *on page 1484*

◆ **PPI-0903** *see* Ceftaroline Fosamil *on page 331*

◆ **PPI-0903M** *see* Ceftaroline Fosamil *on page 331*

◆ **PPL** *see* Benzylpenicilloyl Polylysine *on page 203*

◆ **PPS** *see* Pentosan Polysulfate Sodium *on page 1440*

◆ **PPSV** *see* Pneumococcal Polysaccharide Vaccine (Polyvalent) *on page 1471*

◆ **PPSV23** *see* Pneumococcal Polysaccharide Vaccine (Polyvalent) *on page 1471*

◆ **PPV23** *see* Pneumococcal Polysaccharide Vaccine (Polyvalent) *on page 1471*

Pralatrexate (pral a TREX ate)

U.S. Brand Names Folotyn®

Index Terms PDX

Generic Availability (U.S.) No

Pharmacologic Category Antineoplastic Agent, Antimetabolite (Antifolate)

Medication Safety Issues

Sound-alike/look-alike issues:

PRALAtrexate may be confused with methotrexate, PEMEtrexed, raltitrexed

Folotyn® may be confused with Focalin®

High alert medication: This medication is in a class the Institute for Safe Medication Practices (ISMP) includes among its list of drug classes which have a heightened risk of causing significant patient harm when used in error.

Pregnancy Risk Factor D

Lactation Excretion in breast milk unknown/not recommended

Use Treatment of relapsed or refractory peripheral T-cell lymphoma (PTCL)

Unlabeled/Investigational Use Treatment of relapsed or refractory cutaneous T-cell lymphoma (CTCL)

Mechanism of Action/Effect Antifolate analog; inhibits DNA, RNA, and protein synthesis by selectively entering cells expressing reduced folate carrier (RFC-1), is polyglutamylated by folylpolyglutamate synthetase (FPGS) and then competes for the DHFR-folate binding site to inhibit dihydrofolate reductase (DHFR)

Contraindications There are no contraindications listed within the manufacturer's labeling.

Warnings/Precautions Hazardous agent - use appropriate precautions for handling and disposal. May cause bone marrow suppression (thrombocytopenia, neutropenia and anemia); may require dosage modification. Mucositis, including stomatitis or mucosal inflammation of gastrointestinal and genitourinary tracts, may occur with treatment; may require dosage modification. Prophylactic folic acid and vitamin B_{12} supplements are necessary to reduce hematologic toxicity and treatment-related mucositis. Severe and potentially fatal dermatologic reactions, including skin exfoliation, ulceration, and toxic epidermal necrolysis (TEN) have been reported. Skin reaction may be progressive; severity may increase with continued treatment; may also involve skin and subcutaneous tissues which are affected by lymphoma; monitor all dermatologic reactions closely; withhold or discontinue treatment for severe dermatologic reaction.

Tumor lysis syndrome (TLS) has been reported in patients being treated for lymphoma; monitor closely, if TLS develops, treat for associated complications. Use with caution in patients with moderate-to-severe renal impairment (has not been studied in patients with renal impairment); monitor renal function and for systemic toxicity due to increased exposure. Concurrent use with drugs with substantial renal clearance (eg, NSAIDs, sulfamethoxazole/trimethoprim) may result in delayed pralatrexate clearance. Liver function test abnormalities have been observed with use; monitor liver function; persistent abnormalities may indicate hepatotoxicity and may require dosage modification.

Drug Interactions

Avoid Concomitant Use

Avoid concomitant use of PRALAtrexate with any of the following: BCG; Natalizumab; Pimecrolimus; Roflumilast; Tacrolimus (Topical); Vaccines (Live)

Decreased Effect

PRALAtrexate may decrease the levels/effects of: BCG; Cardiac Glycosides; Sapropterin; Sipuleucel-T; Vaccines (Inactivated); Vaccines (Live); Vitamin K Antagonists

The levels/effects of PRALAtrexate may be decreased by: Echinacea

Increased Effect/Toxicity

PRALAtrexate may increase the levels/effects of: Leflunomide; Natalizumab; Vaccines (Live); Vitamin K Antagonists

The levels/effects of PRALAtrexate may be increased by: Denosumab; Nonsteroidal Anti-Inflammatory Agents; Pimecrolimus; Probenecid; Roflumilast; Salicylates; Sulfamethoxazole; Tacrolimus (Topical); Trastuzumab; Trimethoprim

Adverse Reactions

>10%:

Cardiovascular: Edema (30%)

Central nervous system: Fatigue (36%), fever (32%)

Dermatologic: Rash (15%; grades 3/4: 0%), pruritus (14%; grade 3: 2%; grade 4: 0%)

Endocrine & metabolic: Hypokalemia (15%)

Gastrointestinal: Mucositis (70%; grade 3: 17%; grade 4: 4%), nausea (40%), constipation (33%), vomiting (25%), diarrhea (21%), anorexia (15%), abdominal pain (12%)
Hematologic: Thrombocytopenia (41%; grade 3: 14%; grade 4: 19%), anemia (34%; grade 4: 2%), neutropenia (24%; grade 3: 13%; grade 4: 7%), leukopenia (11%; grade 3: 3%; grade 4: 4%)
Hepatic: Transaminases increased (13%; grade 3: 5%; grade 4: 0%)
Neuromuscular & skeletal: Limb pain (12%), back pain (11%)
Respiratory: Cough (28%), epistaxis (26%), dyspnea (19%), pharyngolaryngeal pain (14%)
Miscellaneous: Night sweats (11%), infection

1% to 10%:
Cardiovascular: Tachycardia (10%)
Endocrine & metabolic: Dehydration (serious >3%)
Hematologic: Neutropenic fever (serious >3%)
Neuromuscular & skeletal: Weakness (10%)
Respiratory: Upper respiratory infection (10%)
Miscellaneous: Sepsis (serious >3%)

Pharmacodynamics/Kinetics

Protein Binding ~67%

Half-Life Elimination 12-18 hours

Excretion Urine (~34% as unchanged drug)

Available Dosage Forms

Injection, solution [preservative free]:
Folotyn®: 20 mg/mL (1 mL, 2 mL)

Dosing

Adult & Geriatric Note: Start vitamin supplements before initial pralatrexate dose: Folic acid 1-1.25 mg/day orally beginning within 10 days prior to initiating pralatrexate (continue during treatment and for 30 days after last pralatrexate dose) and vitamin B_{12} 1000 mcg I.M. within 10 weeks prior to treatment and every 8-10 weeks thereafter (after initial dose, B_{12} may be administered on the same day as pralatrexate).

Prior to administering any dose, mucositis should be ≤grade 1, platelets should be ≥100,000/mm^3 for the first dose and ≥50,000/mm^3 for subsequent doses, and absolute neutrophil count (ANC) should be ≥1000/mm^3.

Peripheral T-cell lymphoma (PTCL), relapsed or refractory: I.V.: 30 mg/m^2 once weekly for 6 weeks of a 7-week treatment cycle (continue until disease progression or unacceptable toxicity)

Cutaneous T-cell lymphoma (CTCL), relapsed or refractory (unlabeled use): I.V.: 15 mg/m^2 once weekly for 3 weeks of a 4-week treatment cycle (Horwitz, 2010)

Renal Impairment Moderate-to-severe renal impairment: Use with caution (has not been studied in patients with renal impairment). Monitor for possible systemic toxicity due to increased exposure.

Hepatic Impairment Patients with total bilirubin >1.5 mg/dL, AST or ALT >2.5 times the upper limit of normal (ULN), and ALT or AST >5 times ULN if documented hepatic lymphoma involvement were excluded from clinical trials. Persistent abnormalities may indicate hepatotoxicity requiring dosage modification; refer to dosage adjustment for nonhematologic (other than mucositis) toxicity for adjustment recommendations.

Adjustment for Toxicity Severe or intolerable adverse events may require dose omission, reduction or interruption. Do not make up omitted doses at the end of the cycle; do not re-escalate dose after a reduction due to toxicity.

Hematologic toxicity:

Platelets:
<50,000/mm^3 (for 1-week duration): Omit dose; continue at previous dose if platelets recover within 1 week
<50,000/mm^3 (for 2-week duration): Omit dose; decrease to 20 mg/m^2 if platelets recover within 2 weeks
<50,000/mm^3 (for 3-week duration): Discontinue treatment.

ANC:
500-1000/mm^3 without fever (for 1-week duration): Omit dose; continue at previous dose if ANC recovers within 1 week
500-1000/mm^3 with fever **or** ANC <500/mm^3 (for 1-week duration): Omit dose, give filgrastim or sargramostim support; continue at previous dose (with growth factor support) if ANC recovers within 1 week
500-1000/mm^3 with fever **or** ANC <500/mm^3 (recurrent or for 2-week duration): Omit dose and give filgrastim or sargramostim support; decrease to 20 mg/m^2 (with growth factor support) if ANC recovers within 2 weeks
500-1000/mm^3 with fever **or** ANC <500/mm^3 (second recurrence or for 3 week duration): Discontinue treatment.

Nonhematologic toxicity: Mucositis (on day of treatment):
Grade 2: Omit dose; continue at previous dose when recovers to ≤grade 1
Grade 3 or recurrent grade 2: Omit dose and decrease to 20 mg/m^2 when recovers to ≤grade 1
Grade 4: Discontinue treatment.

Nonhematologic toxicity (other than mucositis):
Grade 3: Omit dose; decrease to 20 mg/m^2 when recovers to ≤grade 2
Grade 4: Discontinue treatment.

Administration

I.V. Administer I.V. push over 3-5 minutes into the line of a free-flowing normal saline I.V.

Stability

Reconstitution Use appropriate precautions for handling (hazardous agent). Withdraw into syringe for administration; do not dilute (manufacturer recommends immediate use after placing in syringe). Discard unused portion in the vial.

Storage Store intact vials refrigerated at 2°C to 8°C (36°F to 46°F). Store in original carton to protect from light until use. Unopened vials (stored in the original carton) are stable for up to 72 hours at room temperature (discard after 72 hours).

Monitoring and Teaching Issues

Laboratory Monitoring CBC with differential (weekly), serum chemistries, including renal and liver function tests (prior to the first and fourth doses in each cycle)

Physical Assessment Use with caution and monitor in presence of renal or hepatic impairment (dosage adjustment may be necessary). Drugs with significant renal clearance may affect the levels/effects of pralatrexate. Monitor for mucositis, gastrointestinal disturbance, and renal or hepatic impairment.

Patient Education This drug is administered intravenously; report immediately any redness, swelling, pain, or burning at infusion/injection site. It is very important to maintain adequate nutrition and hydration, unless instructed to restrict fluid intake. You will be more susceptible to infection. May cause nausea, vomiting, fatigue or weakness, mouth sores, or limb or back pain. Report persistent or increasing gastrointestinal upset, mouth sores, rapid heartbeat or palpitations, black or tarry stools, fever, chills, unusual bleeding or bruising, shortness of breath, pain on urination, or change in urinary patterns.

Breast-Feeding Considerations Due to the potential for serious adverse reactions in the nursing infant, breast-feeding is not recommended.

Pregnancy Considerations Adverse effects were observed in animal studies. May cause fetal harm if administered to a pregnant woman.

Pramipexole (pra mi PEKS ole)

U.S. Brand Names Mirapex®; Mirapex® ER™

Index Terms Pramipexole Dihydrochloride Monohydrate

Generic Availability (U.S.) Yes: Excludes extended release tablet

Pharmacologic Category Anti-Parkinson's Agent, Dopamine Agonist

Medication Safety Issues

Sound-alike/look-alike issues:

Mirapex® may be confused with Hiprex®, Mifeprex®, MiraLax™

Pregnancy Risk Factor C

Lactation Excretion in breast milk unknown/not recommended

Use

Immediate release: Treatment of the signs and symptoms of idiopathic Parkinson's disease; treatment of moderate-to-severe primary Restless Legs Syndrome (RLS)

Extended release: Treatment of the signs and symptoms of idiopathic Parkinson's disease

Unlabeled/Investigational Use Treatment of depression; treatment of fibromyalgia

Mechanism of Action/Effect Pramipexole is a nonergot dopamine agonist with specificity for the D_2 subfamily dopamine receptor, and has also been shown to bind to D_3 and D_4 receptors. By binding to these receptors, it is thought that pramipexole can stimulate dopamine activity on the nerves of the striatum and substantia nigra.

Contraindications Hypersensitivity to pramipexole or any component of the formulation

Warnings/Precautions Caution should be taken in patients with renal insufficiency; dose adjustment necessary. May cause or exacerbate dyskinesias; use caution in patients with pre-existing dyskinesias. May cause orthostatic hypotension; Parkinson's disease patients appear to have an impaired capacity to respond to a postural challenge. Use with caution in patients at risk of hypotension or where transient hypotensive episodes would be poorly tolerated. Parkinson's patients being treated with dopaminergic agonists ordinarily require careful monitoring for signs and symptoms of postural hypotension, especially during dose escalation. May cause hallucinations.

Dopamine agonists have been associated with compulsive behaviors and/or loss of impulse control, which has manifested as pathological gambling, libido increases (hypersexuality), and/or binge eating. Causality has not been established, and controversy exists as to whether this phenomenon is related to the underlying disease, prior behaviors/addictions and/or drug therapy. Dose reduction or discontinuation of therapy has been reported to reverse these behaviors in some, but not all cases. Risk for melanoma development is increased in Parkinson's disease patients; drug causation or factors contributing to risk have not been established. Patients should be monitored closely and periodic skin examinations should be performed.

Taper gradually over a period of 1 week when discontinuing therapy; dopaminergic agents have been associated with a syndrome resembling neuroleptic malignant syndrome on abrupt withdrawal or significant dosage reduction after long-term use. Ergot-derived dopamine agonists have been associated with fibrotic complications (eg, retroperitoneal fibrosis, pleural thickening, and pulmonary infiltrates). Although pramipexole is not an ergot, there have been postmarketing reports of possible fibrotic complications with pramipexole; monitor closely for signs and symptoms of fibrosis.

Pramipexole has been associated with somnolence, particularly at higher dosages (>1.5 mg/day). In addition, patients have been reported to fall asleep during activities of daily living, including driving, while taking this medication. Whether these patients exhibited somnolence prior to these events is not clear. Patients should be advised of this issue and factors which may increase risk (sleep disorders, other sedating medications, or concomitant medications which increase pramipexole concentrations) and instructed to report daytime somnolence or sleepiness to the prescriber. Patients should use caution in performing activities which require alertness (driving or operating machinery), and to avoid other medications which may cause CNS depression, including ethanol. Use caution in the elderly as they may be more sensitive to these adverse drug reactions.

Pathologic degenerative changes were observed in the retinas of albino rats during studies with this agent, but were not observed in the retinas of albino mice or in other species. The significance of these data for humans remains uncertain. Augmentation (earlier onset of symptoms in the evening/afternoon, increase and/or spread of symptoms to other extremities) or rebound (shifting of symptoms to early morning hours) may occur in some RLS patients.

Drug Interactions

Avoid Concomitant Use There are no known interactions where it is recommended to avoid concomitant use.

Decreased Effect

Pramipexole may decrease the levels/effects of: Antipsychotics (Typical)

The levels/effects of Pramipexole may be decreased by: Antipsychotics (Atypical); Metoclopramide

Increased Effect/Toxicity

Pramipexole may increase the levels/effects of: Alcohol (Ethyl); CNS Depressants

The levels/effects of Pramipexole may be increased by: Antipsychotics (Typical); Cimetidine; MAO Inhibitors; Methylphenidate

Nutritional/Ethanol Interactions

Ethanol: Avoid ethanol (may increase CNS depression).

Food: Food intake does not affect the extent of drug absorption although the time to maximal plasma concentration is delayed when taken with a meal.

Herb/Nutraceutical: Avoid valerian, St John's wort, SAMe, kava kava (may increase risk of serotonin syndrome and/or excessive sedation).

Adverse Reactions

Parkinson's disease: Actual frequency may be dependent on dose and/or formulation:

>10%:

Cardiovascular: Postural hypotension (dose related; ≤53%)

Central nervous system: Somnolence (dose related; 9% to 36%), extrapyramidal syndrome (28%), insomnia (4% to 27%), dizziness (2% to 26%), hallucinations (5% to 17%), abnormal dreams (11%), headache (4% to 7%)

Gastrointestinal: Nausea (dose related; 11% to 28%), constipation (dose related; 6% to 14%)

Neuromuscular & skeletal: Dyskinesia (17% to 47%), weakness (1% to 14%)

1% to 10%:

Cardiovascular: Edema (2% to 8%), chest pain (3%)

Central nervous system: Confusion (4% to 10%), dystonia (2% to 8%), fatigue (6%), amnesia (dose related; 4% to 6%), sudden onset of sleep (3% to 6%), vertigo (2% to 4%), hypesthesia (3%), abnormal thinking (2% to 3%), akathisia (2% to 3%), malaise (2% to 3%), paranoia (2%), sleep disorder (1% to 3%), depression (≤2%), delusions (1%), fever (1%), myoclonus (1%)

Endocrine & metabolic: Libido decreased (1%)

Gastrointestinal: Xerostomia (4% to 7%), anorexia (1% to 5%), vomiting (4%), abdominal discomfort/pain (1% to 4%), dyspepsia (3%), appetite increased (2% to 3%), dysphagia (2%), weight loss (2%), salivary hypersecretion (≤2%), diarrhea (1% to 2%)

Genitourinary: Urinary frequency (6%), urinary tract infection (4%), impotence (2%), urinary incontinence (2%)

Neuromuscular & skeletal: Gait abnormalities (7%), hypertonia (7%), muscle spasm (3% to 5%), falls (4%), arthritis (3%), tremor (3%), back pain (2% to 3%), bursitis (2%), muscle twitching (2%), balance abnormalities (≤2%), CPK increased (1%), myasthenia (1%)

Ocular: Accommodation abnormalities (4%), vision abnormalities (3%), diplopia (1%)

Respiratory: Dyspnea (4%), cough (3%), rhinitis (3%), pneumonia (2%)

Restless legs syndrome: Actual frequency may be dependent on dose:

>10%:

Central nervous system: Headache (16%), insomnia (9% to 13%), abnormal dreams (1% to 8%), somnolence (6%)

Gastrointestinal: Nausea (11% to 27%), constipation (4%)

1% to 10%:

Central nervous system: Fatigue (3% to 9%)

Gastrointestinal: Diarrhea (1% to 7%), xerostomia (3%)

Neuromuscular & skeletal: Extremity pain (3% to 7%)

Respiratory: Nasal congestion (≤6%)

Miscellaneous: Influenza (1% to 7%)

Pharmacodynamics/Kinetics

Absorption Rapid

Bioavailability Immediate release: >90%; Extended release (as compared to immediate release): 100%

Time to Peak Serum: Immediate release: ~2 hours; Extended release: 6 hours

Protein Binding ~15%

Half-Life Elimination 8.5 hours; Elderly: 12 hours

Metabolism Negligible (<10%)

Excretion Urine (90% as unchanged drug)

Available Dosage Forms

Tablet, oral: 0.125 mg, 0.25 mg, 0.5 mg, 0.75 mg, 1 mg, 1.5 mg

Mirapex®: 0.125 mg, 0.25 mg, 0.5 mg, 0.75 mg, 1 mg, 1.5 mg

Tablet, extended release, oral:

Mirapex® ER™: 0.375 mg, 0.75 mg, 1.5 mg, 3 mg, 4.5 mg

Dosing

Adult & Geriatric

Parkinson's disease: Oral:

Immediate release formulation: Initial: 0.375 mg/day given in 3 divided doses; increase gradually every 5-7 days; range: 1.5-4.5 mg/day.

Extended release formulation (Mirapex® ER™): Initial: 0.375 mg once daily; increase gradually to 0.75 mg once daily. If necessary, may increase by 0.75 mg/dose not more frequently than every 5-7 days; maximum recommended dose 4.5 mg/day

Note: Converting from immediate release to extended release: May initiate extended release preparation the morning after the last immediate release evening tablet is taken. The total daily dose should remain the same.

Restless legs syndrome: Oral: Initial: 0.125 mg once daily 2-3 hours before bedtime. Dose may be doubled every 4-7 days up to 0.5 mg/day. Maximum dose: 0.5 mg/day (manufacturer's recommendation).

Note: Most patients require <0.5 mg/day, but higher doses have been used (2 mg/day). If augmentation occurs, dose earlier in the day.

Depression (unlabeled use): Initial: 0.25-0.375 mg/day given in 2-3 divided doses with a gradual titration; mean dose: 1.6-1.7 mg/day (Aiken, 2007; Goldberg, 2004)

Fibromyalgia (unlabeled use): Initial: 0.25 mg once daily at bedtime; may be increased weekly by 0.25 mg/day increments up to 4.5 mg/day (Holman, 2005)

Renal Impairment Use caution; renally-eliminated

Parkinson's disease: Immediate release formulation:

Cl_{cr} 35-59 mL/minute: Initial: 0.125 mg twice daily (maximum dose: 1.5 mg twice daily)

Cl_{cr} 15-34 mL/minute: Initial: 0.125 mg once daily (maximum dose: 1.5 mg once daily)

Cl_{cr} <15 mL/minute: Not adequately studied

Hemodialysis: Not adequately studied; a negligible amount of pramipexole is removed by dialysis

Parkinson's disease: Extended release formulation:

Cl_{cr} >50 mL/minute: Dosing adjustment not necessary

Cl_{cr} 30-50 mL/minute: Initial: 0.375 mg every other day; may increase to 0.375 mg once daily no sooner than 1 week after initiation. If necessary, may increase by 0.375 mg/dose not more frequently than every 7 days; maximum recommended dose: 2.25 mg/day

Cl_{cr} <30 mL/minute: Not recommended

Hemodialysis: Not recommended; a negligible amount of pramipexole is removed by dialysis

Restless legs syndrome: Immediate release formulation:

Cl_{cr} 20-60 mL/minute: Duration between titration should be increased to 14 days

Cl_{cr} <20 mL/minute: Not adequately studied

Administration

Oral Doses should be titrated gradually in all patients to avoid the onset of intolerable side effects. The dosage should be increased to achieve a maximum therapeutic effect, balanced against the side effects of dyskinesia, hallucinations, somnolence, and dry mouth. May be administered with or without food; may be administered with food to decrease nausea. Extended release tablets should be swallowed whole and not chewed, crushed, or divided.

Stability

Storage Store at 25°C (77°F); excursions permitted to 15°C to 30°C (59°F to 86°F). Protect from light and high humidity.

Monitoring and Teaching Issues

Physical Assessment Monitor blood pressure. Assess degree of somnolence. Taper dosage over one week when discontinuing.

Patient Education Avoid alcohol. May cause drowsiness and extreme sedation or somnolence, loss of impulse control (possibly manifested as pathological gambling, libido increases, and/or binge eating), postural hypotension, weakness, headache, nausea, abnormal dreams, dry mouth, nausea, hallucinations, new or increased occurrence of involuntary purposeless movements, constipation, or urinary frequency. Report to prescriber hallucinations, suicide ideation, changes in the appearance of skin moles or other unusual skin changes, or difficulty performing or controlling voluntary movements.

Dietary Considerations May be taken with or without food. May be taken with food to decrease nausea.

Breast-Feeding Considerations Prolactin secretion may be inhibited.

Pregnancy Considerations Early embryonic loss and postnatal growth inhibition were observed in animal studies. There are no adequate and well-controlled studies in pregnant women.

◆ **Pramipexole Dihydrochloride Monohydrate** *see* Pramipexole *on page* 1489

Pramlintide (PRAM lin tide)

U.S. Brand Names SymlinPen®; Symlin®

Index Terms Pramlintide Acetate

Generic Availability (U.S.) No

Pharmacologic Category Amylinomimetic; Antidiabetic Agent

Medication Safety Issues

High alert medication: The Institute for Safe Medication Practices (ISMP) includes this medication among its list of drug classes which have a heightened risk of causing significant patient harm when used in error.

Dosing: Use caution when drawing up doses from the vial (concentration 600 micrograms (mcg)/mL). Manufacturer recommended dosing ranges from 15 mcg to 120 mcg, which corresponds to injectable volumes of 0.025 mL to 0.2 mL. Patients and healthcare providers should exercise caution when administering this product to avoid inadvertent calculation of the dose based on "units," which could result in a sixfold overdose.

Medication Guide Available Yes

Pregnancy Risk Factor C

Lactation Excretion in breast milk unknown/use caution

Use

Adjunctive treatment with mealtime insulin in type 1 diabetes mellitus (insulin dependent, IDDM) patients who have failed to achieve desired glucose control despite optimal insulin therapy

Adjunctive treatment with mealtime insulin in type 2 diabetes mellitus (noninsulin dependent, NIDDM) patients who have failed to achieve desired glucose control despite optimal insulin therapy, with or without concurrent sulfonylurea and/or metformin

Mechanism of Action/Effect Human amylin analog which, in conjunction with insulin, reduces postprandial glucose

Contraindications Hypersensitivity to pramlintide or any component of the formulation; confirmed diagnosis of gastroparesis; hypoglycemia unawareness

Warnings/Precautions [U.S. Boxed Warning]: Coadministration with insulin may induce severe hypoglycemia (usually within 3 hours following administration); coadministration with insulin therapy is an approved indication but does require an initial dosage reduction of insulin and frequent pre and post blood glucose monitoring to reduce risk of severe hypoglycemia. Concurrent use of other glucose-lowering agents may increase risk of hypoglycemia. Avoid use in patients with poor compliance with their insulin regimen and/or blood glucose monitoring. Do not use in patients with Hb A_{1c} levels >9% or recent, recurrent episodes of hypoglycemia; obtain detailed history of glucose control (eg, Hb A_{1c}, incidence of hypoglycemia, glucose monitoring, and medication compliance) and body weight before initiating therapy. Use caution in patients with visual or dexterity impairment. Use caution when driving or operating heavy machinery until effects on blood sugar are known. Use caution with certain antihypertensive agents (eg, beta-adrenergic blockers) or neuropathic conditions which may mask signs/symptoms of hypoglycemia. Use caution in patients with history of nausea; avoid use in patients with conditions or concurrent medications likely to impair gastric motility (eg, anticholinergics); do not use in patients requiring medication(s) to stimulate gastric emptying.

Drug Interactions

Avoid Concomitant Use There are no known interactions where it is recommended to avoid concomitant use.

Decreased Effect There are no known significant interactions involving a decrease in effect.

Increased Effect/Toxicity

Pramlintide may increase the levels/effects of: Anticholinergics

Nutritional/Ethanol Interactions

Ethanol: Use caution with ethanol (may increase hypoglycemia).

Herb/Nutraceutical: Use caution with garlic, chromium, gymnema (may increase hypoglycemia).

Adverse Reactions

>10%:

Central nervous system: Headache (5% to 13%)
Gastrointestinal: Nausea (28% to 48%), vomiting (7% to 11%), anorexia (≤17%)
Endocrine & metabolic: Severe hypoglycemia (type 1 diabetes ≤17%)
Miscellaneous: Inflicted injury (8% to 14%)

1% to 10%:

Central nervous system: Fatigue (3% to 7%), dizziness (2% to 6%)
Endocrine & metabolic: Severe hypoglycemia (type 2 diabetes ≤8%)
Gastrointestinal: Abdominal pain (2% to 8%)
Respiratory: Pharyngitis (3% to 5%), cough (2% to 6%)
Neuromuscular & skeletal: Arthralgia (2% to 7%)
Miscellaneous: Allergic reaction (≤6%)

Pharmacodynamics/Kinetics

Duration of Action 3 hours

Bioavailability ~30% to 40%

Time to Peak 20 minutes

Protein Binding ~60%

Half-Life Elimination ~48 minutes

Metabolism Primarily renal to des-lys[1] pramlintide (active metabolite)

Excretion Primarily urine

Available Dosage Forms

Injection, solution:

SymlinPen®: 1000 mcg/mL (1.5 mL, 2.7 mL)
Symlin®: 600 mcg/mL (5 mL)

Dosing

Adult & Geriatric Note: When initiating pramlintide, reduce current insulin dose (including rapidly- and mixed-acting preparations) by 50% to avoid hypoglycemia. If pramlintide is discontinued for any reason, restart therapy with same initial titration protocol.

Type 1 diabetes mellitus (insulin dependent, IDDM): SubQ: Initial: 15 mcg immediately prior to meals; titrate in 15 mcg increments every 3 days (if no significant nausea occurs) to target dose of 30-60 mcg (consider discontinuation if intolerant of 30 mcg dose)

Type 2 diabetes mellitus (noninsulin dependent, NIDDM): SubQ: Initial: 60 mcg immediately prior to meals; after 3-7 days, increase to 120 mcg prior to meals if no significant nausea occurs (if nausea occurs at 120 mcg dose, reduce to 60 mcg)

Renal Impairment No dosage adjustment required; not evaluated in dialysis patients

Administration

Other Do not mix with other insulins; administer subcutaneously into abdominal or thigh areas at sites distinct from concomitant insulin injections (do not administer into arm due to variable absorption); rotate injection sites frequently. Allow solution to reach room temperature before administering; may reduce injection site reactions. For oral medications in which a rapid onset of action is desired, administer 1 hour before, or 2 hours after pramlintide, if possible. When using the pen-injector, do not transfer drug to a syringe; dosing errors could occur.

Stability

Storage Store unopened vials at 2°C to 8°C (36°F to 46°F); do not freeze. Opened vials may be kept refrigerated or at room temperature ≤30°C (≤86°F). Discard opened vial after 30 days. Protect from light.

Monitoring and Teaching Issues

Physical Assessment Monitor for hypoglycemia. Teach patient appropriate injection techniques and syringe/needle disposal.

Patient Education This medication is used to control diabetes; it is not a cure. It is imperative to follow other components of prescribed treatment (eg, diet and exercise regimen). This medication cannot be mixed with insulin. Use a different syringe for each medication. If you experience hypoglycemic reaction, contact prescriber immediately. Always carry quick source of sugar with you. Monitor glucose levels as directed by prescriber. You may experience nausea, headache, fatigue, or dizziness. Report unresolved nausea or vomiting and hypoglycemic reactions.

Dietary Considerations Dietary modification based on ADA recommendations is a part of therapy; pramlintide to be administered prior to major meals consisting of ≥250 Kcal or ≥30 g carbohydrates

Geriatric Considerations Patients must be able to adhere to their insulin regimen and self-monitor their blood glucose. In premarketing studies, the change in the Hb A_{1c} values and hypoglycemia frequencies did not differ by age. Monitor regimen closely.

Breast-Feeding Considerations It is not known if pramlintide is present in breast milk. The manufacturer recommends that pramlintide be used in nursing women only when the potential benefit to the mother outweighs the possible risk to the infant.

Pregnancy Considerations Due to adverse events observed in some animal studies, pramlintide is classified as pregnancy category C. Based on *in vitro* data, pramlintide has a low potential to cross the placenta. Maternal hyperglycemia can be associated with adverse effects in the fetus, including macrosomia, neonatal hyperglycemia, and hyperbilirubinemia; the risk of congenital malformations is increased when the Hb A_{1c} is above the normal range. Diabetes can also be associated with adverse effects in the mother. Poorly-treated diabetes may cause end-organ damage that may in turn negatively affect obstetric outcomes. Physiologic glucose levels should be maintained prior to and during pregnancy to decrease the risk of adverse events in the mother and the fetus. Until additional safety and efficacy data are obtained, the use of pramlintide is generally not recommended in the routine management of diabetes mellitus during pregnancy. Insulin is the drug of choice for the control of diabetes mellitus during pregnancy.

◆ **Pramlintide Acetate** *see* Pramlintide *on page* 1491

◆ **PrandiMet®** *see* Repaglinide and Metformin *on page* 1566

◆ **Prandin®** *see* Repaglinide *on page* 1564

Prasugrel (PRA soo grel)

U.S. Brand Names Effient®

Index Terms CS-747; LY-640315; Prasugrel Hydrochloride

Generic Availability (U.S.) No

Pharmacologic Category Antiplatelet Agent; Antiplatelet Agent, Thienopyridine

Medication Safety Issues

Sound-alike/look-alike issues:

Effient™ may be confused with EtheDent™

Prasugrel may be confused with pravastatin, propranolol

Medication Guide Available Yes

Pregnancy Risk Factor B

Lactation Excretion in breast milk unknown/consider risk:benefit

Use Reduces rate of thrombotic cardiovascular events (eg, stent thrombosis) in patients with unstable angina, non-ST-segment elevation MI, or ST-elevation MI (STEMI) managed with percutaneous coronary intervention (PCI)

Mechanism of Action/Effect Irreversibly blocks platelet activation and aggregation

Contraindications Active pathological bleeding such as peptic ulcer disease (PUD) or intracranial hemorrhage; history of transient ischemic attack (TIA) or stroke

Warnings/Precautions [U.S. Boxed Warning]: May cause significant or fatal bleeding. Use is contraindicated in patients with active pathological bleeding or history of TIA or stroke. Use with caution in patients who may be at risk of increased bleeding, including patients with active PUD, recent or recurrent GI bleeding, severe hepatic impairment, trauma, or surgery. Additional risk factors include body weight <60 kg, CABG or other surgical procedure, concomitant use of medications that increase risk of bleeding.

[U.S. Boxed Warning]: In patients ≥75 years of age, use is not recommended due to increased risk of fatal and intracranial bleeding and uncertain benefit; use may be considered in high-risk situations (eg, patients with diabetes or history of MI). **[U.S. Boxed Warning]: Discontinue ≥7 days before CABG;** increased risk of bleeding; do not initiate therapy in patients likely to undergo CABG.

If necessary, discontinue therapy for active bleeding, elective surgery, stroke, or TIA; reinitiate therapy as soon as possible unless patient suffers stroke or TIA where subsequent use is contraindicated. If possible, manage bleeding without discontinuing prasugrel. Use caution in concurrent treatment with oral anticoagulants (eg, warfarin), NSAIDs, or fibrinolytic agents; bleeding risk is increased. Use with caution in patients with severe liver impairment or end-stage renal disease (experience is limited). Cases of thrombotic thrombocytopenic purpura (usually occurring within the first 2 weeks of therapy), resulting in some fatalities, have been reported with other thienopyridines; urgent plasmapheresis is required. In patients <60 kg, consider lower maintenance dose.

Drug Interactions

Avoid Concomitant Use There are no known interactions where it is recommended to avoid concomitant use.

Decreased Effect

The levels/effects of Prasugrel may be decreased by: CYP3A4 Inhibitors (Strong); Nonsteroidal Anti-Inflammatory Agents; Ranitidine; Rifampin

Increased Effect/Toxicity

Prasugrel may increase the levels/effects of: Anticoagulants; Antiplatelet Agents; Collagenase (Systemic); Drotrecogin Alfa; Ibritumomab; Salicylates; Thrombolytic Agents; Tositumomab and Iodine I 131 Tositumomab

The levels/effects of Prasugrel may be increased by: Dasatinib; Glucosamine; Herbs (Anticoagulant/Antiplatelet Properties); Nonsteroidal Anti-Inflammatory Agents; Omega-3-Acid Ethyl Esters; Pentosan Polysulfate Sodium; Pentoxifylline; Prostacyclin Analogues

Adverse Reactions As with all drugs which may affect hemostasis, bleeding is associated with prasugrel. Hemorrhage may occur at virtually any site. Risk is dependent on multiple variables, including patient susceptibility and concurrent use of multiple agents which alter hemostasis.

2% to 10%:

Cardiovascular: Hypertension (8%), hypotension (4%), atrial fibrillation (3%), bradycardia (3%), noncardiac chest pain (3%), peripheral edema (3%)
Central nervous system: Headache (6%), dizziness (4%), fatigue (4%), fever (3%), extremity pain (3%)
Dermatologic: Rash (3%)
Endocrine & metabolic: Hypercholesterolemia/hyperlipidemia (7%)
Gastrointestinal: Nausea (5%), diarrhea (2%), gastrointestinal hemorrhage (2%)
Hematologic: Leukopenia (3%), anemia (2%)
Neuromuscular & skeletal: Back pain (5%)
Respiratory: Epistaxis (6%), dyspnea (5%), cough (4%)

Pharmacodynamics/Kinetics

Onset of Action Inhibition of platelet aggregation (IPA): Dose dependent: 60 mg loading dose: <30 minutes; median time to reach 20% IPA: 30 minutes (Brandt, 2007)

Peak effect: Time to maximal IPA: Dose-dependent: **Note:** Degree of IPA based on adenosine diphosphate (ADP) concentration used during light aggregometry: 60 mg loading dose: Occurs 4 hours post administration; mean IPA (ADP 5 µmol/L): 78.8%: mean IPA (ADP 20 µmol/L): 84.1%

Duration of Action Duration of effect: >3 days; platelet aggregation gradually returns to baseline values over 5-9 days after discontinuation; reflective of new platelet production

Absorption Rapid; ≥79%

Time to Peak Active metabolite: ~30 minutes (peak plasma levels begin to decrease at ~24 hours); with high-fat/high-calorie meal: 1.5 hours

Protein Binding Active metabolite: ~98%

Half-Life Elimination Half-life elimination: Active metabolite: ~7 hours (range 2-15 hours)

Metabolism Rapid intestinal and serum metabolism via esterase-mediated hydrolysis to a thiolactone (inactive), which is then converted, via CYP450-mediated (primarily CYP3A4 and CYP2B6) oxidation, to an active metabolite (R-138727)

Excretion Urine (~68% inactive metabolites); feces (27% inactive metabolites)

Available Dosage Forms

Tablet, oral:

Effient®: 5 mg, 10 mg

Dosing

Adult Acute coronary syndrome managed with PCI: Oral: Loading dose: 60 mg; Maintenance dose: 10 mg once daily (in combination with aspirin 81-325 mg/day). **Note:** In patients weighing <60 kg, the manufacturer suggests to consider decreasing maintenance dose to 5 mg once daily; however, prospective clinical trial data does not exist to support this recommendation and may place some patients at risk of thrombotic complications (eg, stent thrombosis); consider use of full dose while monitoring closely for bleeding complications or administration of an alternative agent (eg, clopidogrel). The 2009 ACCF/AHA/SCAI joint STEMI/PCI guidelines recommend prasugrel for at least 12 months in patients receiving either a bare metal stent (BMS) or drug eluting stent (DES); durations >15 months may be considered in patients with DES placement (Kushner, 2009).

Administration note: ST-elevation myocardial infarction (STEMI): Administer loading dose as soon as possible before **primary** percutaneous coronary intervention (PCI). If thrombolytic therapy has not been administered, once the coronary anatomy is known and **non-primary** PCI is planned, a loading dose of prasugrel should be given promptly and no later than 1 hour after PCI (Kushner, 2009).

Geriatric Refer to adult dosing. Patients ≥75 years: Use not recommended; may be considered in high-risk situations (eg, patients with diabetes or history of MI).

Renal Impairment No dosage adjustment necessary.

Hepatic Impairment No dosage adjustment necessary for mild-to-moderate hepatic impairment; use in severe hepatic impairment has not been evaluated.

Administration

Oral Administer without regard to meals.

Stability

Storage Store at 25°C (77°F); excursions permitted to 15°C to 30°C (59°F to 86°F).

Monitoring and Teaching Issues

Laboratory Monitoring Hemoglobin and hematocrit periodically

Physical Assessment Monitor for unusual bleeding. Monitor blood pressure at beginning of therapy and periodically throughout.

Patient Education It may take longer than usual to stop bleeding. You will be more prone to bruising and nosebleeds. Inform prescribers and dentists that you are taking this medication prior to scheduling any surgery or dental procedure. May cause headache, dizziness, nausea, or vomiting. Report immediately any unresolved bleeding that cannot be controlled, blood in urine or stool, blood in vomitus, coughing up blood, or acute, severe headache.

Dietary Considerations May be taken without regard to meals.

Geriatric Considerations See Warnings/Precautions. Not recommended for use in elderly 75 years or age and older due to risk of fatal intracranial bleeding and lack of certain benefit in this age group. Exceptions may be high risk patients (ie, diabetics or patients with a history of myocardial infarction).

Pregnancy Considerations There are no adequate and well-controlled studies in pregnant women. Use during pregnancy only if the benefits justify the risk to the fetus.

◆ **Prasugrel Hydrochloride** *see* Prasugrel *on page 1493*

◆ **Pravachol®** *see* Pravastatin *on page 1495*

Pravastatin (prav a STAT in)

U.S. Brand Names Pravachol®

Index Terms Pravastatin Sodium

Generic Availability (U.S.) Yes

Pharmacologic Category Antilipemic Agent, HMG-CoA Reductase Inhibitor

Medication Safety Issues

Sound-alike/look-alike issues:

Pravachol® may be confused with atorvastatin, Prevacid®, Prinivil®, propranolol

Pravastatin may be confused with nystatin, pitavastatin, prasugrel

Pregnancy Risk Factor X

Lactation Enters breast milk/contraindicated

Use Use with dietary therapy for the following:

Primary prevention of coronary events: In hypercholesterolemic patients without established coronary heart disease to reduce cardiovascular morbidity (myocardial infarction, coronary revascularization procedures) and mortality.

Secondary prevention of cardiovascular events in patients with established coronary heart disease: To slow the progression of coronary atherosclerosis; to reduce cardiovascular morbidity (myocardial infarction, coronary vascular procedures) and to reduce mortality; to reduce the risk of stroke and transient ischemic attacks

Hyperlipidemias: Reduce elevations in total cholesterol, LDL-C, apolipoprotein B, and triglycerides (elevations of 1 or more components are present in Fredrickson type IIa, IIb, III, and IV hyperlipidemias)

Heterozygous familial hypercholesterolemia (HeFH): In pediatric patients, 8-18 years of age, with HeFH having LDL-C ≥190 mg/dL **or** LDL ≥160 mg/dL with positive family history of premature cardiovascular disease (CVD) or 2 or more CVD risk factors in the pediatric patient

Mechanism of Action/Effect Pravastatin is a competitive inhibitor of 3-hydroxy-3-methylglutaryl coenzyme A (HMG-CoA) reductase, which is the rate-limiting enzyme involved in *de novo* cholesterol synthesis.

Contraindications Hypersensitivity to pravastatin or any component of the formulation; active liver disease; unexplained persistent elevations of serum transaminases; pregnancy; breast-feeding

Warnings/Precautions Secondary causes of hyperlipidemia should be ruled out prior to therapy. Liver function must be monitored by periodic laboratory assessment. Rhabdomyolysis with acute renal failure has occurred. Risk may be increased with concurrent use of other drugs which may cause rhabdomyolysis (including colchicine, gemfibrozil, fibric acid derivatives, or niacin at doses ≥1 g/day). Temporarily discontinue in any patient experiencing an acute or serious condition predisposing to renal failure secondary to rhabdomyolysis. Based upon current evidence, HMG-CoA reductase inhibitor therapy should be continued in the perioperative period unless risk outweighs cardioprotective benefit. Use with caution in patients with advanced age, these patients are predisposed to myopathy. Use caution in patients with previous liver disease or heavy ethanol use. Treatment in patients <8 years of age is not recommended.

Drug Interactions

Metabolism/Transport Effects **Substrate** of CYP3A4 (minor), P-glycoprotein, SLCO1B1; **Inhibits** CYP2C9 (weak), 2D6 (weak), 3A4 (weak)

Avoid Concomitant Use

Avoid concomitant use of Pravastatin with any of the following: Red Yeast Rice

Decreased Effect

The levels/effects of Pravastatin may be decreased by: Antacids; Bile Acid Sequestrants; Efavirenz; P-Glycoprotein Inducers; Phenytoin; Rifamycin Derivatives

Increased Effect/Toxicity

Pravastatin may increase the levels/effects of: DAPTOmycin; Trabectedin; Vitamin K Antagonists

The levels/effects of Pravastatin may be increased by: Antifungal Agents (Azole Derivatives, Systemic); Colchicine; Conivaptan; CycloSPORINE; CycloSPORINE (Systemic); Eltrombopag; Fenofibrate; Fenofibric Acid; Gemfibrozil; Niacin; Niacinamide; P-Glycoprotein Inhibitors; Protease Inhibitors; Red Yeast Rice; Rifamycin Derivatives

Nutritional/Ethanol Interactions

Ethanol: Consumption of large amounts of ethanol may increase the risk of liver damage with HMG-CoA reductase inhibitors.

Food: Red yeast rice contains an estimated 2.4 mg lovastatin per 600 mg rice.

Herb/Nutraceutical: St John's wort may decrease pravastatin levels.

Adverse Reactions As reported in short-term trials; safety and tolerability with long-term use were similar to placebo

1% to 10%:

- Cardiovascular: Chest pain (4%)
- Central nervous system: Headache (2% to 6%), fatigue (4%), dizziness (1% to 3%)
- Dermatologic: Rash (4%)
- Gastrointestinal: Nausea/vomiting (7%), diarrhea (6%), heartburn (3%)
- Hepatic: Transaminases increased (>3x normal on two occasions - 1%)
- Neuromuscular & skeletal: Myalgia (2%)
- Respiratory: Cough (3%)
- Miscellaneous: Influenza (2%)

Additional class-related events or case reports (not necessarily reported with pravastatin therapy): Angioedema, cataracts, depression, dyspnea, eosinophilia, erectile dysfunction, facial paresis, hypersensitivity reaction, impaired extraocular muscle movement, impotence, interstitial lung disease, leukopenia, malaise, memory loss, ophthalmoplegia, paresthesia, peripheral neuropathy, photosensitivity, psychic disturbance, skin discoloration, thrombocytopenia, thyroid dysfunction, toxic epidermal necrolysis, transaminases increased, vomiting

Pharmacodynamics/Kinetics

Onset of Action Several days; Peak effect: 4 weeks

Absorption Rapidly absorbed; average absorption 34%

Bioavailability 17%

Time to Peak Serum: 1-1.5 hours

Protein Binding 50%

Half-Life Elimination 77 hours (including all metabolites); pravastatin: ~2-3 hours (Pan, 1990); 3α-hydroxy-iso-pravastatin: ~1.5 hours (Gustavson, 2005)

Metabolism Hepatic multiple metabolites; primary metabolite is 3α-hydroxy-iso-pravastatin (2.5% to 10% activity of parent drug)

Excretion Feces (70%); urine (≤20%, 8% as unchanged drug)

Available Dosage Forms

Tablet, oral: 10 mg, 20 mg, 40 mg, 80 mg

Pravachol®: 10 mg, 20 mg, 40 mg, 80 mg

Dosing

Adult & Geriatric

Hyperlipidemias, primary prevention of coronary events, secondary prevention of cardiovascular events: Oral: Initial: 40 mg once daily; titrate dosage to response (usual range: 10-80 mg) (maximum dose: 80 mg once daily)

Dosage adjustment based on concomitant cyclosporine: Oral: Initial: 10 mg/day, titrate with caution (maximum dose: 20 mg/day)

Note: Doses should be individualized according to the baseline LDL-cholesterol levels, the recommended goal of therapy, and patient response; adjustments should be made at intervals of 4 weeks or more; doses may need adjusted based on concomitant medications

Pediatric

Heterozygous familial hypercholesterolemia (HeFH): Oral: Children:

8-13 years: 20 mg/day

14-18 years: 40 mg/day

Dosage adjustment based on concomitant cyclosporine: Refer to adult dosing.

Note: Doses should be individualized according to the baseline LDL-cholesterol levels, the recommended goal of therapy, and patient response; adjustments should be made at intervals of 4 weeks or more; doses may need adjusted based on concomitant medications

Renal Impairment Initial: 10 mg/day

Hepatic Impairment Initial: 10 mg/day

Administration

Oral May be administered without regard to meals.

Stability

Storage Store at 25°C (77°F); excursions permitted to 15°C to 30°C (59°F to 86°F). Protect from moisture and light.

Monitoring and Teaching Issues

Laboratory Monitoring Obtain baseline LFTs and total cholesterol profile; creatine phosphokinase due to possibility of myopathy. Repeat LFTs prior to elevation of dose. May be measured when clinically indicated and/or periodically thereafter; baseline CPK (recheck CPK in any patient with symptoms suggestive of myopathy). Monitor LDL-C at intervals no less than 4 weeks.

Physical Assessment Use caution with history of hepatic disease. Assess risk potential for interactions with other prescriptions or herbal products patient may be taking that may increase risk of myopathy or rhabdomyolysis. Evaluate LFTs and lipid profile prior to treatment and at regular intervals. Teach proper diet and exercise regimen.

Patient Education Take at same time each day, with or without food. Follow prescribed cholesterol-lowering diet and exercise regimen. Avoid excess alcohol. You will have periodic blood tests to assess effectiveness. Avoid excessive alcohol. Report unusual muscle cramping or weakness, yellowing of skin or eyes, easy bruising or bleeding, or unusual fatigue.

Dietary Considerations May be taken without regard to meals. Before initiation of therapy, patients should be placed on a standard cholesterol-lowering diet for 6 weeks and the diet should be continued during drug therapy. Red yeast rice contains an estimated 2.4 mg lovastatin per 600 mg rice.

Geriatric Considerations Effective and well tolerated in the elderly. No specific dosage recommendations. Clearance is reduced in elderly, resulting in an increase in AUC between 25% to 50%. However, substantial accumulation is not expected.

The definition of and, therefore, when to treat hyperlipidemia in elderly is a controversial issue. The National Cholesterol Education Program recommends that all adults maintain a plasma cholesterol <160 mg/dL. Elderly with one additional risk factor, goal LDL would be <130 mg/dL. It is the authors' belief that pharmacologic treatment be reserved for those who are unable to obtain a desirable plasma cholesterol concentration by diet alone and for whom the benefits of treatment are believed to outweigh the potential adverse effects, drug interactions, and cost of treatment.

Pregnancy Considerations Cholesterol biosynthesis may be important in fetal development. Contraindicated in pregnancy. Administer to women of childbearing potential only when conception is highly unlikely and patients have been informed of potential hazards.

Related Information

Hyperlipidemia Management *on page 2046*

◆ **Pravastatin Sodium** *see* Pravastatin *on page 1495*

◆ **Precose®** *see* Acarbose *on page 36*

◆ **Pred Forte®** *see* PrednisoLONE (Ophthalmic) *on page 1500*

◆ **Pred Mild®** *see* PrednisoLONE (Ophthalmic) *on page 1500*

PrednisoLONE (Systemic) (pred NISS oh lone)

U.S. Brand Names Millipred™; Orapred ODT®; Orapred®; Pediapred®; Prelone®; Veripred™ 20

Index Terms Prednisolone Sodium Phosphate

Generic Availability (U.S.) Yes: Excludes orally disintegrating tablet

Pharmacologic Category Corticosteroid, Systemic

Medication Safety Issues

Sound-alike/look-alike issues:

PrednisoLONE may be confused with predniSONE

Pediapred® may be confused with Pediazole®

Prelone® may be confused with Prozac®

Pregnancy Risk Factor C

Lactation Enters breast milk/use caution (AAP rates "compatible"; AAP 2001 update pending)

Use Treatment of endocrine disorders, rheumatic disorders, collagen diseases, allergic states, respiratory diseases, hematologic disorders, neoplastic diseases, edematous states, and gastrointestinal diseases; resolution of acute exacerbations of multiple sclerosis; management of fulminating or disseminated tuberculosis and trichinosis; acute or chronic solid organ rejection

Mechanism of Action/Effect Decreases inflammation by suppression of migration of polymorphonuclear leukocytes and reversal of increased capillary permeability; suppresses the immune system by reducing activity and volume of the lymphatic system

Contraindications Hypersensitivity to prednisolone or any component of the formulation; acute superficial herpes simplex keratitis; live or attenuated virus vaccines (with immunosuppressive doses of corticosteroids); systemic fungal infections; varicella

Warnings/Precautions May cause hypercorticism or suppression of hypothalamic-pituitary-adrenal (HPA) axis, particularly in younger children or in patients receiving high doses for prolonged periods. HPA axis suppression may lead to adrenal crisis. Withdrawal and discontinuation of a corticosteroid should be done slowly and carefully. Particular care is required when patients are transferred from systemic corticosteroids to inhaled products due to possible adrenal insufficiency or withdrawal from steroids, including an increase in allergic symptoms. Patients receiving >20 mg per day of prednisone (or equivalent) may be most susceptible. Fatalities have occurred due to adrenal insufficiency in asthmatic patients during and after transfer from systemic corticosteroids to aerosol steroids; aerosol steroids do **not** provide the systemic steroid needed to treat patients having trauma, surgery, or infections.

Acute myopathy has been reported with high dose corticosteroids, usually in patients with neuromuscular transmission disorders; may involve ocular and/or respiratory muscles; monitor creatine kinase; recovery may be delayed. Corticosteroid use may cause psychiatric disturbances, including depression, euphoria, insomnia, mood swings, and personality changes. Pre-existing psychiatric conditions may be exacerbated by corticosteroid use. Prolonged use of corticosteroids may also increase the incidence of secondary infection, mask acute infection (including fungal infections), prolong or exacerbate viral infections, or limit response to vaccines. Exposure to chickenpox should be avoided; corticosteroids should not be used to treat ocular herpes simplex. Corticosteroids should not be used for cerebral malaria or viral hepatitis. Close observation is required in patients with latent tuberculosis and/or TB reactivity; restrict use in active TB (only in conjunction with antituberculosis treatment). Prolonged use of corticosteroids may result in glaucoma; cataract formation may occur. Prolonged treatment with corticosteroids has been associated with the development of Kaposi's sarcoma (case reports); if noted, discontinuation of therapy should be considered.

Use with caution in patients with thyroid disease, hepatic impairment, renal impairment, cardiovascular disease, diabetes, glaucoma, cataracts, myasthenia gravis, patients at risk for osteoporosis, patients at risk for seizures, or GI diseases (diverticulitis, peptic ulcer, ulcerative colitis) due to perforation risk. Use caution following acute MI (corticosteroids have been associated with myocardial rupture). Because of the risk of adverse effects, systemic corticosteroids should be used cautiously in the elderly in the smallest possible effective dose for the shortest duration. Withdraw therapy with gradual tapering of dose. May affect growth velocity; growth should be routinely monitored in pediatric patients.

Drug Interactions

Metabolism/Transport Effects Substrate of CYP3A4 (minor); **Inhibits** CYP3A4 (weak)

Avoid Concomitant Use

Avoid concomitant use of PrednisoLONE (Systemic) with any of the following: Aldesleukin; BCG; Natalizumab; Pimecrolimus; Roflumilast; Tacrolimus (Topical)

Decreased Effect

PrednisoLONE (Systemic) may decrease the levels/effects of: Aldesleukin; Antidiabetic Agents; BCG; Calcitriol; Corticorelin; CycloSPORINE; CycloSPORINE (Systemic); Isoniazid; Salicylates; Sipuleucel-T; Vaccines (Inactivated)

The levels/effects of PrednisoLONE (Systemic) may be decreased by: Aminoglutethimide; Antacids; Barbiturates; Bile Acid Sequestrants; Echinacea; Mitotane; Primidone; Rifamycin Derivatives

Increased Effect/Toxicity

PrednisoLONE (Systemic) may increase the levels/effects of: Acetylcholinesterase Inhibitors; Amphotericin B; CycloSPORINE; CycloSPORINE (Systemic); Leflunomide; Loop Diuretics; Natalizumab; NSAID (COX-2 Inhibitor); NSAID (Nonselective); Thiazide Diuretics; Vaccines (Live); Warfarin

The levels/effects of PrednisoLONE (Systemic) may be increased by: Antifungal Agents (Azole Derivatives, Systemic); Aprepitant; Calcium Channel Blockers (Nondihydropyridine); Conivaptan; CycloSPORINE; CycloSPORINE (Systemic); Denosumab; Estrogen Derivatives; Fluconazole; Fosaprepitant; Macrolide Antibiotics; Neuromuscular-Blocking Agents (Nondepolarizing); Pimecrolimus; Quinolone Antibiotics; Roflumilast; Salicylates; Tacrolimus (Topical); Trastuzumab

Nutritional/Ethanol Interactions

Ethanol: Avoid ethanol (may increase gastric mucosal irritation).

Food: Prednisolone interferes with calcium absorption. Limit caffeine.

Herb/Nutraceutical: St John's wort may decrease prednisolone levels. Avoid cat's claw, echinacea (have immunostimulant properties).

Lab Interactions May respond to skin tests

Adverse Reactions Frequency not defined.

Cardiovascular: Cardiomyopathy, CHF, edema, facial edema, hypertension

Central nervous system: Headache, insomnia, malaise, nervousness, pseudotumor cerebri, psychic disorders, seizure, vertigo

Dermatologic: Bruising, facial erythema, hirsutism, petechiae, skin test reaction suppression, thin fragile skin, urticaria

Endocrine & metabolic: Carbohydrate tolerance decreased, Cushing's syndrome, diabetes mellitus, growth suppression, hyperglycemia, hypernatremia, hypokalemia, hypokalemic alkalosis, menstrual irregularities, negative nitrogen balance, pituitary adrenal axis suppression

Gastrointestinal: Abdominal distention, increased appetite, indigestion, nausea, pancreatitis, peptic ulcer, ulcerative esophagitis, weight gain

Hepatic: LFTs increased (usually reversible)

Neuromuscular & skeletal: Arthralgia, aseptic necrosis (humeral/femoral heads), fractures, muscle mass decreased, muscle weakness, osteoporosis, steroid myopathy, tendon rupture, weakness

Ocular: Cataracts, exophthalmus, eyelid edema, glaucoma, intraocular pressure increased, irritation

Respiratory: Epistaxis

Miscellaneous: Diaphoresis increased, impaired wound healing

Pharmacodynamics/Kinetics

Duration of Action 18-36 hours

Protein Binding Concentration dependent: 65% to 91%; decreased in elderly

Half-Life Elimination 3.6 hours; End-stage renal disease: 3-5 hours

Metabolism Primarily hepatic, but also metabolized in most tissues, to inactive compounds

Excretion Primarily urine (as glucuronides, sulfates, and unconjugated metabolites)

Available Dosage Forms

Solution, oral: 5 mg/5 mL (120 mL); 15 mg/5 mL (237 mL, 240 mL, 473 mL, 480 mL)
Millipred™: 10 mg/5 mL (237 mL)
Orapred®: 15 mg/5 mL (20 mL, 237 mL)
Pediapred®: 5 mg/5 mL (120 mL)
Veripred™ 20: 20 mg/5 mL (237 mL)

Syrup, oral: 15 mg/5 mL (240 mL, 480 mL)
Prelone®: 15 mg/5 mL (240 mL, 480 mL)

Tablet, orally disintegrating, oral:
Orapred ODT®: 10 mg, 15 mg, 30 mg

Dosing

Adult Dose depends upon condition being treated and response of patient. Oral dosage expressed in terms of prednisolone base. Consider alternate day therapy for long-term therapy. Discontinuation of long-term therapy requires gradual withdrawal by tapering the dose. Patients undergoing unusual stress while receiving corticosteroids, should receive increased doses prior to, during, and after the stressful situation.

Usual dose (range): Oral: 5-60 mg/day

Rheumatoid arthritis: Oral: Initial: 5-7.5 mg/day, adjust dose as necessary

Multiple sclerosis: Oral: 200 mg/day for 1 week followed by 80 mg every other day for 1 month

Dosing adjustment in hyperthyroidism: Prednisolone dose may need to be increased to achieve adequate therapeutic effects.

Geriatric Use lowest effective adult dose. Dose depends upon condition being treated and response of patient; alternate day dosing may be attempted in some disease states.

Pediatric Dose depends upon condition being treated and response of patient; dosage for infants and children should be based on severity of the disease and response of the patient rather than on strict adherence to dosage indicated by age, weight, or body surface area. Oral dosage expressed in terms of prednisolone base. Consider alternate day therapy for long-term therapy. Discontinuation of long-term therapy requires gradual withdrawal by tapering the dose. Patients undergoing unusual stress while receiving corticosteroids, should receive increased doses prior to, during, and after the stressful situation.

Acute asthma: Oral: 1-2 mg/kg/day in divided doses 1-2 times/day for 3-5 days

Anti-inflammatory or immunosuppressive dose: Oral: 0.1-2 mg/kg/day in divided doses 1-4 times/day

Nephrotic syndrome: Oral:

Initial (first 3 episodes): 2 mg/kg/day **or** 60 mg/m^2/day (maximum: 80 mg/day) in divided doses 3-4 times/day until urine is protein free for 3 consecutive days (maximum: 28 days); followed by 1-1.5 mg/kg/dose **or** 40 mg/m^2/dose given every other day for 4 weeks

Maintenance (for frequent relapses): 0.5-1 mg/kg/dose given every other day for 3-6 months

Dosing adjustment in hyperthyroidism: Refer to adult dosing.

Renal Impairment

Hemodialysis: Slightly dialyzable (5% to 20%); administer dose posthemodialysis

Peritoneal dialysis: Supplemental dose is not necessary

Administration

Oral Administer oral formulation with food or milk to decrease GI effects.

Orapred ODT®: Do not break or use partial tablet. Remove tablet from blister pack just prior to use. May swallow whole or allow to dissolve on tongue.

Stability

Storage

Millipred™: Store at 20°C to 25°C (68°F to 77°F).
Orapred ODT®: Store at 20°C to 25°C (68°F to 77°F) in blister pack. Protect from moisture.
Orapred®, Veripred™ 20: 2°C to 8°C (36°F to 46°F).
Pediapred®: 4°C to 25°C (39°F to 77°F); may be refrigerated.
Prelone®: 15°C to 30°C (59°F to 86°F).

Monitoring and Teaching Issues

Laboratory Monitoring Blood glucose, electrolytes

Physical Assessment Teach patients to report opportunistic infection and adrenal suppression. Instruct patients with diabetes to monitor serum glucose levels closely; corticosteroids can alter glycemic response. Dose may need to be increased if patient is experiencing higher than normal levels of stress. When discontinuing, taper dose and frequency slowly.

Patient Education Avoid alcohol. Prescriber may recommend increased dietary vitamins, minerals, or iron. If you have diabetes, monitor glucose levels closely (antidiabetic medication may need to be adjusted). Inform prescriber if you are experiencing greater-than-normal levels of stress (medication may need adjustment). This medication may cause GI upset (oral medication should be taken with meals to reduce GI upset). You may be more susceptible to infection. Report promptly excessive nervousness or sleep disturbances, any signs of infection (sore throat, unhealed injuries), excessive growth of body hair or loss of skin color, vision changes, weight gain, swelling of face or extremities, muscle weakness, change in color of stools (black or tarry) or persistent abdominal pain, or worsening of condition or failure to improve.

Dietary Considerations Should be taken after meals or with food or milk to decrease GI effects; increase dietary intake of pyridoxine, vitamin C, vitamin D, folate, calcium, and phosphorus.

Geriatric Considerations Useful in patients with inability to activate prednisone (liver disease). Because of the risk of adverse effects, systemic corticosteroids should be used cautiously in the elderly, in the smallest possible dose, and for the shortest possible time. For long-term use, monitor bone mineral density and institute fracture prevention strategies.

Breast-Feeding Considerations Prednisolone is excreted into breast milk with peak concentrations occurring ~1 hour after the maternal dose. The milk/plasma ratio was found to be 0.2 with doses ≥30 mg/day and 0.1 with doses <30 mg/day. Following a maternal dose of prednisolone 80 mg/day, a breast-feeding infant would ingest <0.1% of the dose.

Pregnancy Considerations Adverse events have been observed with corticosteroids in animal reproduction studies. Prednisolone crosses the placenta; prior to reaching the fetus, prednisolone is converted by placental enzymes to prednisone. As a result, the amount of prednisolone reaching the fetus is ~8-10 times lower than the maternal serum concentration (healthy women at term; similar results observed with preterm pregnancies complicated by HELLP syndrome). Some studies have shown an association between first trimester corticosteroid use and oral clefts; adverse events in the fetus/neonate have been noted in case reports following large doses of systemic corticosteroids during pregnancy. Women exposed to prednisolone during pregnancy for the treatment of an autoimmune disease may contact the OTIS Autoimmune Diseases Study at 877-311-8972.

Related Information

Corticosteroids *on page 1996*

PrednisoLONE (Ophthalmic) (pred NISS oh lone)

U.S. Brand Names Omnipred™; Pred Forte®; Pred Mild®

Index Terms Prednisolone Acetate, Ophthalmic; Prednisolone Sodium Phosphate, Ophthalmic

Generic Availability (U.S.) Yes

Pharmacologic Category Corticosteroid, Ophthalmic

Medication Safety Issues

Sound-alike/look-alike issues:

PrednisoLONE may be confused with predniSONE

Pregnancy Risk Factor C

Use Treatment of palpebral and bulbar conjunctivitis; corneal injury from chemical, radiation, thermal burns, or foreign body penetration; steroid-responsive inflammatory ophthalmic diseases

Available Dosage Forms

Solution, ophthalmic: 1% (5 mL, 10 mL, 15 mL)

Suspension, ophthalmic: 1% (5 mL, 10 mL, 15 mL)

Omnipred™: 1% (5 mL, 10 mL)

Pred Forte®: 1% (1 mL, 5 mL, 10 mL, 15 mL)

Pred Mild®: 0.12% (5 mL, 10 mL)

Dosing

Adult & Geriatric Conjunctivitis: Ophthalmic (suspension/solution): Instill 1-2 drops in the eye 2-4 times daily

Pediatric Conjunctivitis: Ophthalmic (suspension/solution): Children: Refer to adult dosing.

Monitoring and Teaching Issues

Patient Education For ophthalmic use only. Wash hands before using. Tilt head back and look upward. Put drops inside lower eyelid. Close eye and roll eyeball in all directions. Do not blink for 1/2 minute. Apply gentle pressure to inner corner of eye for 30 seconds. Do not use any other eye preparation for at least 5 minutes. Do not let tip of applicator touch eye; do not contaminate tip of applicator (may cause eye infection, eye damage, or vision loss). Wear sunglasses when in sunlight; you may be more sensitive to bright light. Inform prescriber if condition worsens or fails to improve or if you experience eye pain or disturbances of vision.

◆ **Prednisolone Acetate, Ophthalmic** *see* PrednisoLONE (Ophthalmic) *on page 1500*

◆ **Prednisolone Sodium Phosphate** *see* PrednisoLONE (Systemic) *on page 1497*

◆ **Prednisolone Sodium Phosphate, Ophthalmic** *see* PrednisoLONE (Ophthalmic) *on page 1500*

PredniSONE (PRED ni sone)

U.S. Brand Names PredniSONE Intensol™

Index Terms Deltacortisone; Deltadehydrocortisone

Generic Availability (U.S.) Yes

Pharmacologic Category Corticosteroid, Systemic

Medication Safety Issues

Sound-alike/look-alike issues:

PredniSONE may be confused with methylPREDNISolone, Pramosone®, prazosin, predniSOLONE, PriLOSEC®, primidone, promethazine

Lactation Enters breast milk/AAP rates "compatible" (AAP 2001 update pending)

Use Treatment of a variety of diseases, including:

Allergic states (including adjunctive treatment of anaphylaxis)
Autoimmune disorders (including systemic lupus erythematosus [SLE])
Collagen diseases
Dermatologic conditions/diseases
Edematous states (including nephrotic syndrome)
Endocrine disorders
Gastrointestinal diseases
Hematologic disorders (including idiopathic thrombocytopenia purpura [ITP])
Multiple sclerosis exacerbations
Neoplastic diseases
Ophthalmic diseases
Respiratory diseases (including acute asthma exacerbation)
Rheumatic disorders (including rheumatoid arthritis)
Trichinosis with neurologic or myocardial involvement
Tuberculous meningitis

Unlabeled/Investigational Use Adjunctive therapy for *Pneumocystis jiroveci* (formerly *carinni*) pneumonia (PCP); autoimmune hepatitis; adjunctive therapy for pain management in immunocompetent patients with herpes zoster; tuberculosis (severe, paradoxical reactions); Takayasu arteritis; giant cell arteritis

Mechanism of Action/Effect Decreases inflammation by suppression of migration of polymorphonuclear leukocytes and reversal of increased capillary permeability; suppresses the immune system by reducing activity and volume of the lymphatic system; suppresses adrenal function at high doses

Contraindications Hypersensitivity to any component of the formulation; systemic fungal infections; administration of live or live attenuated vaccines with immunosuppressive doses of prednisone

Warnings/Precautions May cause hypercorticism or suppression of hypothalamic-pituitary-adrenal (HPA) axis, particularly in younger children or in patients receiving high doses for prolonged periods. HPA axis suppression may lead to adrenal crisis. Withdrawal and discontinuation of a corticosteroid should be done slowly and carefully. Particular care is required when patients are transferred from systemic corticosteroids to inhaled products due to possible adrenal insufficiency or withdrawal from steroids, including an increase in allergic symptoms. Patients receiving >20 mg per day of prednisone (or equivalent) may be most susceptible. Fatalities have occurred due to adrenal insufficiency in asthmatic patients during and after transfer from systemic corticosteroids to aerosol steroids; aerosol steroids do **not** provide the systemic steroid needed to treat patients having trauma, surgery, or infections.

Acute myopathy has been reported with high dose corticosteroids, usually in patients with neuromuscular transmission disorders; may involve ocular and/or respiratory muscles; monitor creatine kinase; recovery may be delayed. Prolonged use of corticosteroids may increase the incidence of secondary infection, mask acute infection (including fungal infections), prolong or exacerbate viral infections, or limit response to vaccines. Exposure to chickenpox should be avoided. Corticosteroids should not be used to treat ocular herpes simplex or cerebral malaria. Close observation is required in patients with latent tuberculosis and/or TB reactivity; restrict use in active TB (only in conjunction with antituberculosis treatment). Prolonged treatment with corticosteroids has been associated with the development of Kaposi's sarcoma (case reports); if noted, discontinuation of therapy should be considered. Prolonged use may cause posterior subcapsular cataracts, glaucoma (with possible nerve damage) and may increase the risk for ocular infections. Corticosteroid use may cause psychiatric disturbances, including depression, euphoria, insomnia, mood swings, and personality changes. Pre-existing psychiatric conditions may be exacerbated by corticosteroid use.

Use with caution in patients with HF, diabetes, GI diseases (diverticulitis, peptic ulcer, ulcerative colitis; due to risk of perforation), hepatic impairment, myasthenia gravis, MI, patients with or who are at risk for osteoporosis, seizure disorders or thyroid disease. May affect growth velocity; growth should be routinely monitored in pediatric patients.

Prior to use, the dose and duration of treatment should be based on the risk versus benefit for each individual patient. In general, use the smallest effective dose for the shortest duration of time to minimize adverse events. A gradual tapering of dose may be required prior to discontinuing therapy.

Drug Interactions

Metabolism/Transport Effects Substrate of CYP3A4 (minor); **Induces** CYP2C19 (weak), 3A4 (weak)

Avoid Concomitant Use

Avoid concomitant use of PredniSONE with any of the following: Aldesleukin; BCG; Natalizumab; Pimecrolimus; Roflumilast; Tacrolimus (Topical)

Decreased Effect

PredniSONE may decrease the levels/effects of: Aldesleukin; Antidiabetic Agents; BCG; Calcitriol; Corticorelin; CycloSPORINE; CycloSPORINE (Systemic); Isoniazid; Salicylates; Sipuleucel-T; Vaccines (Inactivated)

The levels/effects of PredniSONE may be decreased by: Aminoglutethimide; Antacids; Barbiturates; Bile Acid Sequestrants; Echinacea; Mitotane; Primidone; Rifamycin Derivatives; Somatropin; Tesamorelin

Increased Effect/Toxicity

PredniSONE may increase the levels/effects of: Acetylcholinesterase Inhibitors; Amphotericin B; CycloSPORINE; CycloSPORINE (Systemic); Leflunomide; Loop Diuretics; Natalizumab; NSAID (COX-2 Inhibitor); NSAID (Nonselective); Thiazide Diuretics; Vaccines (Live); Warfarin

The levels/effects of PredniSONE may be increased by: Antifungal Agents (Azole Derivatives, Systemic); Aprepitant; Calcium Channel Blockers (Nondihydropyridine); Conivaptan; CycloSPORINE; CycloSPORINE (Systemic); Denosumab; Estrogen Derivatives; Fluconazole; Fosaprepitant; Macrolide Antibiotics; Neuromuscular-Blocking Agents (Nondepolarizing); Pimecrolimus; Quinolone Antibiotics; Ritonavir; Roflumilast; Salicylates; Tacrolimus (Topical); Trastuzumab

Nutritional/Ethanol Interactions

Ethanol: Avoid ethanol (may increase gastric mucosal irritation)

Food: Prednisone interferes with calcium absorption. Limit caffeine.

Herb/Nutraceutical: St John's wort may decrease prednisone levels. Avoid cat's claw, echinacea (have immunostimulant properties).

Lab Interactions Decreased response to skin tests

Adverse Reactions Frequency not defined.

Cardiovascular: Congestive heart failure (in susceptible patients), hypertension

Central nervous system: Emotional instability, headache, intracranial pressure increased (with papilledema), psychic derangements (including euphoria, insomnia, mood swings, personality changes, severe depression), seizure, vertigo

Dermatologic: Bruising, facial erythema, petechiae, thin fragile skin, urticaria, wound healing impaired

Endocrine & metabolic: Adrenocortical and pituitary unresponsiveness (in times of stress), carbohydrate intolerance, Cushing's syndrome, diabetes mellitus, fluid retention, growth suppression (in children), hypokalemic alkalosis, hypothyroidism enhanced, menstrual irregularities, negative nitrogen balance due to protein catabolism, potassium loss, sodium retention

Gastrointestinal: Abdominal distension, pancreatitis, peptic ulcer (with possible perforation and hemorrhage), ulcerative esophagitis

Hepatic: ALT increased, AST increased, alkaline phosphatase increased

Neuromuscular & skeletal: Aseptic necrosis of femoral and humeral heads, muscle mass loss, muscle weakness, osteoporosis, pathologic fracture of long bones, steroid myopathy, tendon rupture (particularly Achilles tendon), vertebral compression fractures

Ocular: Exophthalmos, glaucoma, intraocular pressure increased, posterior subcapsular cataracts

Miscellaneous: Allergic reactions, anaphylactic reactions, diaphoresis, hypersensitivity reactions, infections, Kaposi's sarcoma

Pharmacodynamics/Kinetics

Absorption 50% to 90% (may be altered in IBS or hyperthyroidism)

Protein Binding Concentration dependent: 65% to 91%

Half-Life Elimination Normal renal function: ~3.5 hours

Metabolism Hepatically converted from prednisone (inactive) to prednisolone (active); may be impaired with hepatic dysfunction

Excretion Urine (small portion)

Pharmacokinetic Note See Prednisolone (Systemic) monograph for complete information.

Available Dosage Forms

Solution, oral: 1 mg/mL (5 mL, 120 mL, 500 mL)

PredniSONE Intensol™: 5 mg/mL (30 mL)

Tablet, oral: 1 mg, 2.5 mg, 5 mg, 10 mg, 20 mg, 50 mg

Dosing

Adult General dosing range: Oral: Initial: 5-60 mg/day: **Note:** Dose depends upon condition being treated and response of patient; dosage for infants and children should be based on severity of the disease and response of the patient rather than on strict adherence to dosage indicated by age, weight, or body surface area. Consider alternate day therapy for long-term therapy. Discontinuation of long-term therapy requires gradual withdrawal by tapering the dose.

Prednisone taper (other regimens also available):

- Day 1: 30 mg divided as 10 mg before breakfast, 5 mg at lunch, 5 mg at dinner, 10 mg at bedtime
- Day 2: 5 mg at breakfast, 5 mg at lunch, 5 mg at dinner, 10 mg at bedtime
- Day 3: 5 mg 4 times/day (with meals and at bedtime)
- Day 4: 5 mg 3 times/day (breakfast, lunch, bedtime)
- Day 5: 5 mg 2 times/day (breakfast, bedtime)
- Day 6: 5 mg before breakfast

Indication-specific dosing:

Acute asthma (NIH guidelines, 2007): Oral: 40-60 mg per day for 3-10 days; administer as single or 2 divided doses

Anaphylaxis, adjunctive treatment (Lieberman, 2005): Oral: 0.5 mg/kg

Antineoplastic: Oral: Usual range: 10 mg/day to 100 mg/m²/day (depending on indication). **Note:** Details concerning dosing in combination regimens should also be consulted.

Autoimmune hepatitis (unlabeled use; Czaja, 2002): Oral: Initial treatment: 60 mg/day for 1 week, *followed by* 40 mg/day for 1 week, *then* 30 mg/day for 2 weeks, *then* 20 mg/day. Half this dose should be given when used in combination with azathioprine

Dermatomyositis/polymyositis: Oral: 1 mg/kg daily (range: 0.5-1.5 mg/kg/day), often in conjunction with steroid-sparing therapies; depending on response/tolerance, consider slow tapering after 2-8 weeks depending on response; taper regimens vary widely, but often involve 5-10 mg decrements per week and may require 6-12 months to reach a low once-daily or every-other-day dose to prevent disease flare (Briemberg, 2003; Hengstman, 2009; Iorizzo, 2008; Wiendl, 2008)

Giant cell arteritis (unlabeled use): Oral: Initial: 40-60 mg/day; typically requires 1-2 years of treatment, but may begin to taper after 2-3 months; alternative dosing of 30-40 mg/day has demonstrated similar efficacy (Hiratzka, 2010)

Herpes zoster (unlabeled use; Dworkin, 2007): Oral: 60 mg/day for 7 days, *followed by* 30 mg/day for 7 days, *then* 15 mg/day for 7 days

Idiopathic thrombocytopenia purpura (American Society of Hematology, 1997): Oral: 1-2 mg/kg/day

PCP pneumonia (AIDS*info* guidelines, 2008): Note: Begin within 72 hours of PCP therapy: 40 mg twice daily for 5 days, *followed by* 40 mg once daily for 5 days, *followed by* 20 mg once daily for 11 days or until antimicrobial regimen is completed

Rheumatoid arthritis (American College of Rheumatology, 2002): Oral: ≤10 mg/day

Systemic lupus erythematosus (American College of Rheumatology, 1999): Oral:
Mild SLE: ≤10 mg/day
Refractory or severe organ-threatening disease: 20-60 mg/day

Takayasu arteritis (unlabeled use): Oral: Initial: 40-60 mg/day; taper to lowest effective dose when ESR and CRP levels are normal; usual duration: 1-2 years (Hiratzka, 2010)

Thyrotoxicosis (type II amiodarone induced; unlabeled use): Oral: 30-40 mg/day for 7-14 days, gradually taper over 3 months

Tuberculosis, severe, paradoxical reactions (unlabeled use, AIDS*info* guidelines, 2008): Oral: 1 mg/kg/day, gradually reduce after 1-2 weeks

Geriatric Refer to adult dosing; use the lowest effective dose. Oral dose depends upon condition being treated and response of patient. Alternate day dosing may be attempted.

Pediatric

General dosing range: Oral: Refer to adult dosing. **Note:** Dose depends upon condition being treated and response of patient; dosage for infants and children should be based on severity of the disease and response of the patient rather than on strict adherence to dosage indicated by age, weight, or body surface area. Consider alternate day therapy for long-term therapy. Discontinuation of long-term therapy requires gradual withdrawal by tapering the dose.

Indication-specific dosing:

Acute asthma (NIH guidelines, 2007): Oral:
0-11 years 1-2 mg/kg/day for 3-10 days (maximum: 60 mg/day)
≥12 years: Refer to Adult dosing

Autoimmune hepatitis (unlabeled use; Czaja, 2002): Oral: Initial treatment: 2 mg/kg/day for 2 weeks (maximum: 60 mg/day), followed by a taper over 6-8 weeks to a dose of 0.1-0.2 mg/kg/day or 5 mg/day

Nephrotic syndrome (Pediatric Nephrology Panel recommendations [Hogg, 2000]): Oral: Initial: 2 mg/kg/day or 60 mg/m²/day given every day in 1-3 divided doses (maximum: 80 mg/day) until urine is protein free or for 4-6 weeks; followed by maintenance dose: 2 mg/kg/dose or 40 mg/m²/dose given every other day in the morning; gradually taper and discontinue after 4-6 weeks. **Note:** No definitive treatment guidelines exist. Dosing is dependant on institution protocols and individual response.

PCP pneumonia (AIDS*info* guidelines, 2008): Oral:
Children: 1 mg/kg twice daily for 5 days, *followed by* 0.5-1 mg/kg twice daily for 5 days, *followed by* 0.5 mg/kg once daily for 11-21 days
Adolescents: Refer to adult dosing.

Renal Impairment Hemodialysis effects: Supplemental dose is not necessary.

Administration

Oral Administer with food to decrease GI upset.

Monitoring and Teaching Issues

Laboratory Monitoring Blood glucose, electrolytes

Physical Assessment Teach patient to report opportunistic infection and adrenal suppression. Instruct patients with diabetes to monitor serum glucose levels closely; corticosteroids can alter glucose tolerance. Monitor growth with long-term use in pediatric patients. Dose may need to be increased if patient is experiencing higher than normal levels of stress. When discontinuing, taper dose and frequency slowly.

Patient Education Take with or after meals. Avoid alcohol. Maintain adequate nutrition; consult prescriber for possibility of special dietary recommendations. If you have diabetes, monitor serum glucose closely and notify prescriber of changes; this medication can alter glycemic response. Notify prescriber if you are experiencing higher than normal levels of stress; medication may need adjustment. Periodic ophthalmic examinations will be necessary. You will be susceptible to infection. You may experience insomnia or nervousness. Report weakness, change in menstrual pattern, vision changes, signs of hyperglycemia, signs of infection (eg, fever, chills, mouth sores, perianal itching, vaginal discharge), or worsening of condition.

Dietary Considerations Should be taken after meals or with food or milk; may require increased dietary intake of pyridoxine, vitamin C, vitamin D, folate, calcium, and phosphorus; may require decreased dietary intake of sodium

Geriatric Considerations Because of the risk of adverse effects, systemic corticosteroids should be used cautiously in the elderly, in the smallest possible dose, and for the shortest possible time.

Breast-Feeding Considerations Prednisone and its metabolite prednisolone are found in low concentrations in breast milk. Peak milk concentrations of both were found ~2 hours after the maternal dose in one case report. In a study which included 6 mother/infant pairs, adverse events were not observed in nursing infants (maternal prednisone dose not provided).

Pregnancy Considerations Adverse events have been observed with corticosteroids in animal reproduction studies. Prednisone and prednisolone cross the human placenta. In the mother, prednisone is converted to the active metabolite prednisolone by the liver. Prior to reaching the fetus, prednisolone is converted by placental enzymes back to prednisone. As a result, the level of prednisone remaining in the maternal serum and reaching the fetus are similar; however, the amount of prednisolone reaching the fetus is ~8-10 times lower than the maternal serum concentration (healthy women at term). Some studies have shown an association between first trimester prednisone use and oral clefts; adverse events in the fetus/neonate have been noted in case reports following large doses of systemic corticosteroids during pregnancy. Pregnant women exposed to prednisone for antirejection therapy following a transplant may contact the National Transplantation Pregnancy Registry (NTPR) at 215-955-4820. Women exposed to prednisone during pregnancy for the treatment of an autoimmune disease (eg, rheumatoid arthritis) may contact the OTIS Autoimmune Diseases Study at 877-311-8972.

Additional Information Tapering of corticosteroids after a short course of therapy (<7-10 days) is generally not required unless the disease/inflammatory process is slow to respond. Tapering after prolonged exposure is dependent upon the individual patient, duration of corticosteroid treatments, and size of steroid dose. Recovery of the HPA axis may require several months. Subtle but important HPA axis suppression may be present for as long as several months after a course of as few as 10-14 days duration. Testing of HPA axis (cosyntropin) may be required, and signs/symptoms of adrenal insufficiency should be monitored in patients with a history of use.

Related Information

Corticosteroids *on page 1996*

◆ **PredniSONE Intensol™** *see* PredniSONE *on page 1500*

Pregabalin (pre GAB a lin)

U.S. Brand Names Lyrica®

Index Terms CI-1008; S-(+)-3-isobutylgaba

Generic Availability (U.S.) No

Pharmacologic Category Analgesic, Miscellaneous; Anticonvulsant, Miscellaneous

Medication Safety Issues

Sound-alike/look-alike issues:

Lyrica® may be confused with Lopressor®

Medication Guide Available Yes

Pregnancy Risk Factor C

Lactation Excretion in breast milk unknown/not recommended

Use Management of pain associated with diabetic peripheral neuropathy; management of postherpetic neuralgia; adjunctive therapy for partial-onset seizure disorder in adults; management of fibromyalgia

Mechanism of Action/Effect Decreases symptoms of painful peripheral neuropathies and, as adjunctive therapy in partial seizures, decreases the frequency of seizures

Contraindications Hypersensitivity to pregabalin or any component of the formulation

Warnings/Precautions Antiepileptics are associated with an increased risk of suicidal behavior/thoughts with use (regardless of indication); patients should be monitored for signs/symptoms of depression, suicidal tendencies, and other unusual behavior changes during therapy and instructed to inform their healthcare provider immediately if symptoms occur.

Angioedema has been reported; may be life threatening; use with caution in patients with a history of angioedema episodes. Concurrent use with other drugs known to cause angioedema (eg, ACE inhibitors) may increase risk. Hypersensitivity reactions, including skin redness, blistering, hives, rash, dyspnea and wheezing have been reported; discontinue treatment of hypersensitivity occurs. May cause CNS depression and/or dizziness, which may impair physical or mental abilities. Patients must be cautioned about performing tasks which require mental alertness (eg, operating machinery or driving). Effects with other sedative drugs or ethanol may be potentiated. Visual disturbances (blurred vision, decreased acuity and visual field changes) have been associated with pregabalin therapy; patients should be instructed to notify their physician if these effects are noted.

Pregabalin has been associated with increases in CPK and rare cases of rhabdomyolysis. Patients should be instructed to notify their prescriber if unexplained muscle pain, tenderness, or weakness, particularly if fever and/or malaise are associated with these symptoms. Use may be associated with weight gain and peripheral edema; use caution in patients with congestive heart failure, hypertension, or diabetes. Effect on weight gain/edema may be additive to thiazolidinedione antidiabetic agent; particularly in patients with prior cardiovascular disease. May decrease platelet count or prolong PR interval.

Has been noted to be tumorigenic (increased incidence of hemangiosarcoma) in animal studies; significance of these findings in humans is unknown. Pregabalin has been associated with discontinuation symptoms following abrupt cessation, and increases in seizure frequency (when used as an antiepileptic) may occur. Should not be discontinued abruptly; dosage tapering over at least 1 week is recommended. Use caution in renal impairment; dosage adjustment required.

Drug Interactions

Avoid Concomitant Use There are no known interactions where it is recommended to avoid concomitant use.

Decreased Effect

The levels/effects of Pregabalin may be decreased by: Ketorolac; Ketorolac (Systemic); Mefloquine

Increased Effect/Toxicity

Pregabalin may increase the levels/effects of: Alcohol (Ethyl); Antidiabetic Agents (Thiazolidinedione); CNS Depressants; Methotrimeprazine

The levels/effects of Pregabalin may be increased by: Droperidol; Methotrimeprazine

Nutritional/Ethanol Interactions

Ethanol: Avoid ethanol (may increase CNS depression).

Herb/Nutraceutical: Avoid valerian, St John's wort, kava kava, gotu kola (may increase CNS depression).

Adverse Reactions Note: Frequency of adverse effects may be influenced by dose or concurrent therapy. In add-on trials in epilepsy, frequency of CNS and visual adverse effects were higher than those reported in pain management trials. Range noted below is inclusive of all trials.

>10%:

Cardiovascular: Peripheral edema (up to 16%)

Central nervous system: Dizziness (8% to 45%), somnolence (4% to 28%), ataxia (up to 20%), headache (up to 14%)

Gastrointestinal: Weight gain (up to 16%), xerostomia (1% to 15%)

Neuromuscular & skeletal: Tremor (up to 11%)

Ocular: Blurred vision (1% to 12%), diplopia (up to 12%)

Miscellaneous: Infection (up to 14%), accidental injury (2% to 11%)

1% to 10%:

Cardiovascular: Chest pain (up to 4%), edema (up to 6%)

Central nervous system: Neuropathy (up to 9%), thinking abnormal (up to 9%), fatigue (up to 8%), confusion (up to 7%), euphoria (up to 7%), speech disorder (up to 7%), attention disturbance (up to 6%), incoordination (up to 6%), amnesia (up to 6%), pain (up to 5%), memory impaired (up to 4%), vertigo (up to 4%), feeling abnormal (up to 3%), hypoesthesia (up to 3%), anxiety (up to 2%), depression (up to 2%), disorientation (up to 2%), lethargy (up to 2%), fever (≥1%), depersonalization (≥1%), hypertonia (≥1%), stupor (≥1%), nervousness (up to 1%)

Dermatologic: Facial edema (up to 3%), bruising (≥1%), pruritus (≥1%)

Endocrine & metabolic: Fluid retention (up to 3%), hypoglycemia (up to 3%), libido decreased (≥1%)

Gastrointestinal: Constipation (up to 10%), appetite increased (up to 7%), flatulence (up to 3%), vomiting (up to 3%), abdominal distension (up to 2%), abdominal pain (≥1%), gastroenteritis (≥1%)

Genitourinary: Incontinence (up to 2%), anorgasmia (≥1%), impotence (≥1%), urinary frequency (≥1%)

Hematologic: Thrombocytopenia (3%)

Neuromuscular & skeletal: Balance disorder (up to 9%), abnormal gait (up to 8%), weakness (up to 7%), arthralgia (up to 6%), twitching (up to 5%), back pain (up to 4%), muscle spasm (up to 4%), myoclonus (up to 4%), paresthesia (>2%), CPK increased (2%), leg cramps (≥1%), myalgia (≥1%), myasthenia (up to 1%)

Ocular: Visual abnormalities (up to 5%), visual field defect (≥2%), eye disorder (up to 2%), nystagmus (>2%), conjunctivitis (≥1%)

Otic: Otitis media (≥1%), tinnitus (≥1%)

Respiratory: Sinusitis (up to 7%), dyspnea (up to 3%), bronchitis (up to 3%), pharyngolaryngeal pain (up to 3%)

Miscellaneous: Flu-like syndrome (up to 2%), allergic reaction (≥1%)

Pharmacodynamics/Kinetics

Onset of Action Pain management: Effects may be noted as early as the first week of therapy

Bioavailability >90%

Time to Peak 1.5 hours (3 hours with food)

Protein Binding 0%

Half-Life Elimination 6.3 hours

Metabolism Negligible

Excretion Urine (90% as unchanged drug; minor metabolites)

Product Availability Lyrica® oral solution: FDA approved December 2009; anticipated availability is currently undetermined

Controlled Substance C-V

Available Dosage Forms

Capsule, oral:

Lyrica®: 25 mg, 50 mg, 75 mg, 100 mg, 150 mg, 200 mg, 225 mg, 300 mg

Dosing

Adult & Geriatric

Fibromyalgia: Oral: Initial: 150 mg/day in divided doses (75 mg 2 times/day); may be increased to 300 mg/day (150 mg 2 times/day) within 1 week based on tolerability and effect; may be further increased to 450 mg/day (225 mg 2 times/day). Maximum dose: 450 mg/day (dosages up to 600 mg/day were evaluated with no significant additional benefit and an increase in adverse effects)

Neuropathic pain (diabetes-associated): Oral: Initial: 150 mg/day in divided doses (50 mg 3 times/day); may be increased within 1 week based on tolerability and effect; maximum dose: 300 mg/day (dosages up to 600 mg/day were evaluated with no significant additional benefit and an increase in adverse effects)

Postherpetic neuralgia: Oral: Initial: 150 mg/day in divided doses (75 mg 2 times/day or 50 mg 3 times/day); may be increased to 300 mg/day within 1 week based on tolerability and effect; further titration (to 600 mg/day) after 2-4 weeks may be considered in patients who do not experience sufficient relief of pain provided they are able to tolerate pregabalin. Maximum dose: 600 mg/day

Partial onset seizures (adjunctive therapy): Oral: Initial: 150 mg per day in divided doses (75 mg 2 times/day or 50 mg 3 times/day); may be increased based on tolerability and effect (optimal titration schedule has not been defined). Maximum dose: 600 mg/day

Note: Discontinuing therapy: Pregabalin should not be abruptly discontinued; taper dosage over at least 1 week

Renal Impairment

Pregabalin Renal Impairment Dosing

Cl_{cr} (mL/minute)	Total Pregabalin Daily Dose (mg/day)				Dosing Frequency
≥60	150	300	450	600	2-3 divided doses
30-60	75	150	225	300	2-3 divided doses
15-30	25-50	75	100-150	150	1-2 divided doses
<15	25	25-50	50-75	75	Single daily dose

Posthemodialysis supplementary dosage (as a single additional dose):
25 mg/day schedule: Single supplementary dose of 25 mg **or** 50 mg
25-50 mg/day schedule: Single supplementary dose of 50 mg **or** 75 mg
50-75 mg/day schedule: Single supplementary dose of 75 mg **or** 100 mg
75 mg/day schedule: Single supplementary dose of 100 mg **or** 150 mg

Administration

Oral May be administered with or without food.

Stability

Storage Store at 15°C to 30°C (59°F to 86°F).

Monitoring and Teaching Issues

Laboratory Monitoring CPK

Physical Assessment Monitor weight. Assess for signs of fluid retention. Taper dosage over at least one week when discontinuing.

Patient Education Avoid alcohol; may increase drowsiness/CNS depression. Taper dosage slowly when discontinuing. Maintain adequate hydration unless instructed to restrict fluid intake by prescriber. May cause CNS depression and/or dizziness, headache, weight gain, or fluid retention. Report immediately any visual disturbances, suicide ideation, or depression. Report unexplained muscle pain, tenderness, or weakness, especially if accompanied by unexplained fever and malaise, dizziness, confusion or abnormal thinking, shortness of breath, weight gain, swelling of extremities, problems with coordination, tremor, facial swelling, excessively dry mouth, and excessive drowsiness.

Dietary Considerations May be taken with or without food.

Geriatric Considerations In clinical studies, no differences in safety and efficacy were noted between elderly. Since pregabalin is primarily excreted renally, dosage adjustment, based on Cl_{cr}, is necessary.

Pregnancy Considerations Increased incidence of fetal abnormalities, particularly skeletal malformations, were observed in animal studies. Male-mediated teratogenicity has been observed in animal studies; implications in humans are not defined. Impaired male and female fertility has been noted in animal studies. There are no adequate and well-controlled studies in pregnant women. Use only when potential benefit to the mother outweighs possible risk to the fetus.

Patients exposed to pregabalin during pregnancy are encouraged to enroll themselves into the AED Pregnancy Registry by calling 1-888-233-2334. Additional information is available at www.aedpregnancyregistry.org.

Related Information

Anticonvulsant Drugs of Choice *on page 1981*

- **Pregnenedione** *see* Progesterone *on page 1514*
- **Pregnyl®** *see* Chorionic Gonadotropin (Human) *on page 364*
- **Prelone®** *see* PrednisoLONE (Systemic) *on page 1497*
- **Premarin®** *see* Estrogens (Conjugated/Equine, Systemic) *on page 682*
- **Premarin®** *see* Estrogens (Conjugated/Equine, Topical) *on page 686*
- **Premjact®** *see* Lidocaine (Topical) *on page 1107*

- **Premphase®** *see* Estrogens (Conjugated/Equine) and Medroxyprogesterone *on page 686*
- **Prempro®** *see* Estrogens (Conjugated/Equine) and Medroxyprogesterone *on page 686*
- **Preparation H® Hydrocortisone [OTC]** *see* Hydrocortisone (Topical) *on page 920*
- **Pre-Pen®** *see* Benzylpenicilloyl Polylysine *on page 203*
- **Prepidil®** *see* Dinoprostone *on page 540*
- **Prevacid®** *see* Lansoprazole *on page 1061*
- **Prevacid® 24 HR [OTC]** *see* Lansoprazole *on page 1061*
- **Prevacid® SoluTab™** *see* Lansoprazole *on page 1061*
- **Prevalite®** *see* Cholestyramine Resin *on page 363*
- **Prevnar®** *see* Pneumococcal Conjugate Vaccine (7-Valent) *on page 1469*
- **Prevnar 13™** *see* Pneumococcal Conjugate Vaccine (13-Valent) *on page 1470*
- **Prevpac®** *see* Lansoprazole, Amoxicillin, and Clarithromycin *on page 1064*
- **Prezista®** *see* Darunavir *on page 469*
- **Prialt®** *see* Ziconotide *on page 1888*
- **PriLOSEC®** *see* Omeprazole *on page 1356*
- **PriLOSEC OTC® [OTC]** *see* Omeprazole *on page 1356*
- **Primaclone** *see* Primidone *on page 1507*
- **Primatene® Mist [OTC]** *see* EPINEPHrine (Systemic, Oral Inhalation) *on page 629*
- **Primaxin® I.M. [DSC]** *see* Imipenem and Cilastatin *on page 956*
- **Primaxin® I.V.** *see* Imipenem and Cilastatin *on page 956*

Primidone (PRI mi done)

U.S. Brand Names Mysoline®

Index Terms Desoxyphenobarbital; Primaclone

Generic Availability (U.S.) Yes

Pharmacologic Category Anticonvulsant, Miscellaneous; Barbiturate

Medication Safety Issues

Sound-alike/look-alike issues:

Primidone may be confused with predniSONE, primaquine, pyridoxine

Medication Guide Available Yes

Lactation Enters breast milk/not recommended (AAP recommends use "with caution"; AAP 2001 update pending)

Use Management of grand mal, psychomotor, and focal seizures

Unlabeled/Investigational Use Benign familial tremor (essential tremor)

Available Dosage Forms

Tablet, oral: 50 mg, 250 mg

Mysoline®: 50 mg, 250 mg

Dosing

Adult & Geriatric

Seizure disorders (grand mal, psychomotor, and focal): Oral: Days 1-3: 100-125 mg/day at bedtime; days 4-6: 100-125 twice daily; days 7-9: 100-125 mg 3 times daily; usual dose: 750-1500 mg/day in divided doses 3-4 times/day with maximum dosage of 2 g/day

Patients already receiving other anticonvulsants: Initial: 100-125 mg at bedtime; gradually increase to maintenance dose as other drug is gradually decreased, continue until desired level obtained or other drug completely withdrawn. If goal is monotherapy, conversion should be completed over ≥2 weeks.

Essential tremor (unlabeled use): Oral: Initial 12.5-25 mg/day at bedtime; titrate up to 250 mg/day in 1-2 divided doses; doses up to 750 mg/day may be beneficial

Pediatric Seizure disorders (grand mal, psychomotor, and focal): Oral:

Children <8 years: Initial: Days 1-3: 50 mg/day given at bedtime; days 4-6: 50 mg twice daily; days 7-9: 100 mg twice daily; usual dose: 375-750 mg/day in 3-4 divided doses (10-25 mg/kg/day)

Children ≥8 years: Refer to adult dosing.

Renal Impairment

Adults (Aronoff, 2007): **Note:** Avoid in renal failure if possible; due to active metabolites with long half-lives and complex kinetics:

Cl_{cr} ≥50 mL/minute: Administer every 12 hours

Cl_{cr} 10-50 mL/minute: Administer every 12-24 hours

Cl_{cr} <10 mL/minute: Administer every 24 hours

Hemodialysis: Administer dose postdialysis

Hepatic Impairment Increased side effects may occur in severe liver disease. Monitor plasma levels and adjust dose accordingly.

Monitoring and Teaching Issues

Laboratory Monitoring Serum primidone and phenobarbital concentration. Monitor CBC and sequential multiple analysis-12 (SMA-12) at 6-month intervals to compare with baseline obtained at start of therapy. Since elderly patients metabolize phenobarbital at a slower rate than younger adults, it is suggested to measure both primidone and phenobarbital levels together.

Physical Assessment Monitor for signs and symptoms of depression or suicide ideation. Taper dosage slowly when discontinuing. Teach patient safety and seizure precautions.

Patient Education While using this medication, do not use alcohol. Maintain adequate hydration unless instructed to restrict fluid intake. You may experience drowsiness, dizziness, blurred vision, nausea, vomiting, loss of appetite, or impotence (reversible). Wear identification of epileptic status and medications. Report behavioral or CNS changes (confusion, depression, increased sedation, excitation, headache, insomnia, or lethargy), suicide ideation, muscle weakness or tremors, unusual bruising or bleeding (mouth, urine, stool), or worsening of seizure activity or loss of seizure control.

Related Information

Peak and Trough Guidelines *on page 1958*

- **Primlev™** *see* Oxycodone and Acetaminophen *on page 1383*
- **Primsol®** *see* Trimethoprim *on page 1820*
- **Prinivil®** *see* Lisinopril *on page 1119*
- **Prinzide®** *see* Lisinopril and Hydrochlorothiazide *on page 1122*
- **Pristinamycin** *see* Quinupristin and Dalfopristin *on page 1543*
- **Pristiq®** *see* Desvenlafaxine *on page 497*
- **Privigen®** *see* Immune Globulin *on page 961*
- **ProAir® HFA** *see* Albuterol *on page 58*
- **ProAmatine® [DSC]** *see* Midodrine *on page 1228*

Probenecid (proe BEN e sid)

Index Terms Benemid [DSC]

Generic Availability (U.S.) Yes

Pharmacologic Category Uricosuric Agent

Medication Safety Issues

Sound-alike/look-alike issues:

Probenecid may be confused with Procanbid®

Lactation Excretion in breast milk unknown

Use Prevention of hyperuricemia associated with gout or gouty arthritis; prolongation and elevation of beta-lactam plasma levels

Available Dosage Forms

Tablet, oral: 500 mg

Dosing

Adult & Geriatric

Hyperuricemia with gout: Oral: 250 mg twice daily for 1 week; increase to 250-500 mg/day; may increase by 500 mg/month, if needed, to maximum of 2-3 g/day (dosages may be increased by 500 mg every 6 months if serum urate concentrations are controlled)

Prolong penicillin serum levels: Oral: 500 mg 4 times/day

Gonorrhea: CDC guidelines (alternative regimen): Probenecid 1 g orally with cefoxitin 2 g I.M.

Pelvic inflammatory disease: CDC guidelines: Cefoxitin 2 g I.M. plus probenecid 1 g orally as a single dose

Neurosyphilis: CDC guidelines (alternative regimen): Procaine penicillin 2.4 million units/day I.M. plus probenecid 500 mg orally 4 times/day; both administered for 10-14 days

Pediatric

Note: Contraindicated in children <2 years of age.

Prolong penicillin serum levels: Oral: Children 2-14 years: Initial: 25 mg/kg, then 40 mg/kg/day given 4 times/day (maximum: 500 mg/dose)

Treatment of gonorrhea: >45 kg: Refer to adult dosing.

Renal Impairment Cl_{cr} <30 mL/minute: Avoid use.

Administration

Oral Administer with food or antacids to minimize GI effects.

Monitoring and Teaching Issues

Laboratory Monitoring Uric acid, renal function, CBC

Patient Education May take 6-12 months to reduce gouty attacks (attacks may increase in frequency and severity for first few months of therapy). Take with food. If you have diabetes, use serum glucose monitoring. If you experience severe headache, contact prescriber for medication. You may experience dizziness, nausea, vomiting, headache, or loss of appetite. Report skin rash, signs of infection, blood in urine or painful urination, extreme tiredness or weakness, or easy bruising or bleeding.

- **Probenecid and Colchicine** *see* Colchicine and Probenecid *on page 426*

Procainamide (pro KANE a mide)

Index Terms PCA (error-prone abbreviation); Procainamide Hydrochloride; Procaine Amide Hydrochloride; Procanbid; Pronestyl

Generic Availability (U.S.) Yes

Pharmacologic Category Antiarrhythmic Agent, Class Ia

Medication Safety Issues

Sound-alike/look-alike issues:

Procanbid may be confused with probenecid, Procan SR®

Procan SR® may be confused with procanbid

Pronestyl may be confused with Ponstel®

High alert medication: The Institute for Safe Medication Practices (ISMP) includes this medication among its list of drugs which have a heightened risk of causing significant patient harm when used in error.

Procainamide hydrochloride is available in 10 mL vials of 100 mg/mL and in 2 mL vials with 500 mg/mL. Note that **BOTH** vials contain 1 gram of drug; confusing the strengths can lead to massive overdoses or underdoses.

PCA is an error-prone abbreviation (mistaken as patient controlled analgesia)

Pregnancy Risk Factor C

Lactation Enters breast milk/not recommended (AAP rates "compatible"; AAP 2001 update pending)

Use

Intravenous: Treatment of life-threatening ventricular arrhythmias

Oral (Canadian labeling; not available in U.S.): Treatment of supraventricular arrhythmias. **Note:** In the treatment of atrial fibrillation, use only when preferred treatment is ineffective or cannot be used. Use in paroxysmal atrial tachycardia when reflex stimulation or other measures are ineffective.

Unlabeled/Investigational Use

Paroxysmal supraventricular tachycardia (PSVT); prevent recurrence of ventricular tachycardia; symptomatic premature ventricular contractions

ACLS guidelines: I.V.: Treatment of the following arrhythmias in patients with preserved left ventricular function: Stable monomorphic VT; pre-excited atrial fibrillation; stable wide complex regular tachycardia (likely VT)

PALS guidelines: I.V.: Tachycardia with pulses and poor perfusion (probable SVT [unresponsive to vagal maneuvers and adenosine or synchronized cardioversion]; probable VT [unresponsive to synchronized cardioversion or adenosine])

Available Dosage Forms

Injection, solution: 100 mg/mL (10 mL); 500 mg/mL (2 mL)

Dosing

Adult Dose must be titrated to patient's response.

Antiarrhythmic:

I.M.: 50 mg/kg/day divided every 3-6 hours **or** 0.5-1 g every 4-8 hours (Koch-Weser, 1971)

I.V.:

Loading dose: 15-18 mg/kg administered as slow infusion over 25-30 minutes **or** 100 mg/dose at a rate not to exceed 50 mg/minute repeated every 5 minutes as needed to a total dose of 1 g.

Hemodynamically stable monomorphic VT or pre-excited atrial fibrillation (ACLS, 2010): Loading dose: Infuse 20-50 mg/minute **or** 100 mg every 5 minutes until arrhythmia controlled, hypotension occurs, QRS complex widens by 50% of its original width, or total of 17 mg/kg is given. Follow with a continuous infusion of 1-4 mg/minute. **Note:** Not recommended for use in ongoing ventricular fibrillation (VF) or pulseless ventricular tachycardia (VT) due to prolonged administration time and uncertain efficacy.

Maintenance dose: 1-4 mg/minute by continuous infusion. Maintenance infusions should be reduced by one-third in patients with moderate renal or cardiac impairment and by two-thirds in patients with severe renal or cardiac impairment.

Oral (not available in the U.S.; Canadian labeling): Sustained release formulation (Procan SR®): Maintenance: 50 mg/kg/24 hours given in divided doses every 6 hours

Suggested Procan SR® maintenance dose:

<55 kg: 500 mg every 6 hours

55-91 kg: 750 mg every 6 hours

>91 kg: 1000 mg every 6 hours

Geriatric Refer to adult dosing. Initiate doses at lower end of dosage range.

Pediatric Must be titrated to patient's response:

Arrhythmias:

I.M.: 20-30 mg/kg/day divided every 4-6 hours; maximum: 4 g/day

I.V.:

Load: 3-6 mg/kg/dose over 5 minutes not to exceed 100 mg/dose; may repeat every 5-10 minutes to maximum of 15 mg/kg/load

Maintenance as continuous I.V. infusion: 20-80 mcg/kg/minute; maximum: 2 g/24 hours

Possible VT (PALS, 2010): I.V.; I.O.: 15 mg/kg over 30-60 minutes

Renal Impairment

Oral:

Cl_{cr} 10-50 mL/minute: Administer every 6-12 hours.

Cl_{cr} <10 mL/minute: Administer every 8-24 hours.

I.V.:

Loading dose: Reduce dose to 12 mg/kg in severe renal impairment.

Maintenance infusion: Reduce dose by one-third in patients with mild renal impairment. Reduce dose by two-thirds in patients with severe renal impairment.

Dialysis:

Procainamide: Moderately hemodialyzable (20% to 50%): Monitor procainamide/N-acetyl-procainamide (NAPA) concentrations; supplementation may be necessary.

NAPA: Not dialyzable (0% to 5%)

Procainamide/NAPA: Not peritoneal dialyzable (0% to 5%)

Procainamide/NAPA: Replace according to blood concentration monitoring during continuous arteriovenous or venovenous hemofiltration.

Hepatic Impairment Reduce dose by 50%.

Administration

Oral Do **not** crush or chew sustained release drug products (not available in the U.S.).

I.V. Must dilute prior to I.V. administration. Loading dose: Maximum rate: 50 mg/minute

Monitoring and Teaching Issues

Laboratory Monitoring CBC with differential, platelet count; procainamide and NAPA blood concentrations in patients with hepatic impairment, renal failure, or receiving constant infusion >3 mg/minute for longer than 24 hours; ANA titers, serum creatinine, BUN

Physical Assessment I.V. requires use of infusion pump and continuous cardiac and hemodynamic monitoring. Monitor QT_c, QRS, and PR intervals.

Patient Education Oral: Avoid alcohol. You will need regular cardiac checkups and blood tests while taking this medication. You may experience dizziness, lightheadedness, visual changes, loss of appetite, headaches, or diarrhea (if persistent consult prescriber). Report chest pain, palpitation, or erratic heartbeat; increased weight or swelling of hands or feet; shortness of breath; acute diarrhea; or unusual fatigue and tiredness.

Related Information

Antiarrhythmic Drugs *on page 1978*

Peak and Trough Guidelines *on page 1958*

◆ **Procainamide Hydrochloride** *see* Procainamide *on page 1508*

◆ **Procaine Amide Hydrochloride** *see* Procainamide *on page 1508*

◆ **Procaine Benzylpenicillin** *see* Penicillin G Procaine *on page 1435*

◆ **Procaine Penicillin G** *see* Penicillin G Procaine *on page 1435*

◆ **Procanbid** *see* Procainamide *on page 1508*

Procarbazine (proe KAR ba zeen)

U.S. Brand Names Matulane®

Index Terms Benzmethyzin; N-Methylhydrazine; Procarbazine Hydrochloride

Generic Availability (U.S.) No

Pharmacologic Category Antineoplastic Agent, Alkylating Agent

Medication Safety Issues

Sound-alike/look-alike issues:

Procarbazine may be confused with dacarbazine

Matulane® may be confused with Materna®

High alert medication: The Institute for Safe Medication Practices (ISMP) includes this medication among its list of drugs which have a heightened risk of causing significant patient harm when used in error.

Pregnancy Risk Factor D

Lactation Excretion in breast milk unknown/not recommended

Use Treatment of Hodgkin's disease

Unlabeled/Investigational Use Treatment of non-Hodgkin's lymphoma, brain tumors

Mechanism of Action/Effect Mechanism of action is not clear, methylating of nucleic acids; inhibits DNA, RNA, and protein synthesis; may damage DNA directly and suppresses mitosis; metabolic activation required by host

Contraindications Hypersensitivity to procarbazine or any component of the formulation; pre-existing bone marrow aplasia; ethanol ingestion; pregnancy

Warnings/Precautions Hazardous agent - use appropriate precautions for handling and disposal. Use with caution in patients with pre-existing renal or hepatic impairment. Procarbazine possesses MAO inhibitor activity and has potential for severe drug and food interactions; follow MAO-I diet. Avoid ethanol consumption, may cause disulfiram-like reaction. May cause hemolysis and/or presence of Heinz inclusion bodies in erythrocytes. Bone marrow depression may occur 2-8 weeks after treatment initiation. Allow ≥1 month interval between radiation therapy or myelosuppressive chemotherapy and initiation of treatment. Withhold treatment for CNS toxicity, leukopenia (WBC <4000/mm^3), thrombocytopenia (platelets <100,000/mm^3), hypersensitivity, stomatitis, diarrhea, or hemorrhage. Procarbazine is a carcinogen which may cause acute leukemia. May cause infertility. **[U.S. Boxed Warning]: Should be administered under the supervision of an experienced cancer chemotherapy physician.**

Drug Interactions

Avoid Concomitant Use

Avoid concomitant use of Procarbazine with any of the following: Alpha-/Beta-Agonists (Indirect-Acting); Alpha1-Agonists; Alpha2-Agonists (Ophthalmic); Amphetamines; Anilidopiperidine Opioids; Atomoxetine; BCG; Bezafibrate; Buprenorphine; BuPROPion; BusPIRone; CarBAMazepine; Cyclobenzaprine; Dexmethylphenidate; Dextromethorphan; Diethylpropion; HYDROmorphone; Linezolid; Maprotiline; Meperidine; Methyldopa; Methylphenidate; Mirtazapine; Natalizumab; Pimecrolimus; Propoxyphene; Roflumilast; Selective Serotonin Reuptake Inhibitors; Serotonin 5-HT1D Receptor Agonists; Serotonin/Norepinephrine Reuptake

Inhibitors; Sibutramine; Tacrolimus (Topical); Tapentadol; Tetrabenazine; Tetrahydrozoline; Tetrahydrozoline (Nasal); Tricyclic Antidepressants; Tryptophan; Vaccines (Live)

Decreased Effect

Procarbazine may decrease the levels/effects of: BCG; Cardiac Glycosides; Sipuleucel-T; Vaccines (Inactivated); Vaccines (Live); Vitamin K Antagonists

The levels/effects of Procarbazine may be decreased by: Echinacea

Increased Effect/Toxicity

Procarbazine may increase the levels/effects of: Alpha-/Beta-Agonists (Direct-Acting); Alpha-/Beta-Agonists (Indirect-Acting); Alpha1-Agonists; Alpha2-Agonists (Ophthalmic); Amphetamines; Antihypertensives; Atomoxetine; Beta2-Agonists; Bezafibrate; BuPROPion; Dexmethylphenidate; Dextromethorphan; Diethylpropion; Doxapram; HYDROmorphone; Leflunomide; Linezolid; Lithium; Meperidine; Methadone; Methyldopa; Methylphenidate; Mirtazapine; Natalizumab; Orthostatic Hypotension Producing Agents; Reserpine; Selective Serotonin Reuptake Inhibitors; Serotonin 5-HT1D Receptor Agonists; Serotonin Modulators; Serotonin/Norepinephrine Reuptake Inhibitors; Tetrahydrozoline; Tetrahydrozoline (Nasal); Tricyclic Antidepressants; Vaccines (Live); Vitamin K Antagonists

The levels/effects of Procarbazine may be increased by: Altretamine; Anilidopiperidine Opioids; Buprenorphine; BusPIRone; CarBAMazepine; COMT Inhibitors; Cyclobenzaprine; Denosumab; Levodopa; MAO Inhibitors; Maprotiline; Pimecrolimus; Propoxyphene; Roflumilast; Sibutramine; Tacrolimus (Topical); Tapentadol; Tetrabenazine; TraMADol; Trastuzumab; Tryptophan

Nutritional/Ethanol Interactions

Ethanol: May enhance the adverse/toxic effects of procarbazine; concurrent use not recommended.

Food: Concurrent ingestion of foods rich in tyramine may cause sudden and severe high blood pressure (hypertensive crisis). Avoid tyramine-containing foods with MAO-Is. Food's freshness is also an important concern; improperly stored or spoiled food can create an environment where tyramine concentrations may increase.

Herb/Nutraceuticals: Avoid supplements containing caffeine, tyrosine, tryptophan, or phenylalanine. Ingestion of large quantities may increase the risk of severe side effects (eg, hypertensive reactions, serotonin syndrome).

Adverse Reactions Most frequencies not defined.

Cardiovascular: Edema, flushing, hypotension, syncope, tachycardia

Central nervous system: Apprehension, ataxia, chills, coma, confusion, depression, dizziness, drowsiness, fatigue, fever, hallucination, headache, insomnia, lethargy, nervousness, nightmares, pain, seizure, slurred speech

Dermatologic: Alopecia, dermatitis, hyperpigmentation, petechiae, pruritus, purpura, rash, urticaria

Endocrine & metabolic: Gynecomastia (in prepubertal and early pubertal males)

Hematologic: Eosinophilia; hemolysis (in patients with G6PD deficiency); hemolytic anemia; myelosuppression (leukopenia, anemia, thrombocytopenia); pancytopenia

Gastrointestinal: Abdominal pain, anorexia, constipation, diarrhea, dysphagia, hematemesis, melena; nausea and vomiting ([60% to 90%], increasing the dose in a stepwise fashion over several days may minimize); stomatitis, xerostomia

Genitourinary: Azoospermia (reported with combination chemotherapy), hematuria, nocturia, polyuria, reproductive dysfunction (>10%)

Hepatic: Hepatic dysfunction, jaundice

Neuromuscular & skeletal: Arthralgia, falling, foot drop, myalgia, neuropathy, paresthesia, reflex diminished, tremor, unsteadiness, weakness

Ocular: Diplopia, inability to focus, nystagmus, papilledema, photophobia, retinal hemorrhage

Otic: Hearing loss

Respiratory: Cough, epistaxis, hemoptysis, hoarseness, pleural effusion, pneumonitis, pulmonary toxicity (<1%)

Miscellaneous: Allergic reaction, diaphoresis, herpes, infection, secondary malignancies (2% to 15%; reported with combination therapy)

Pharmacodynamics/Kinetics

Absorption Rapid and complete

Time to Peak 1 hour

Half-Life Elimination 1 hour

Metabolism Hepatic and renal

Excretion Urine and respiratory tract (<5% as unchanged drug, 70% as metabolites)

Available Dosage Forms

Capsule, oral:

Matulane®: 50 mg

Dosing

Adult Refer to individual protocols.

Chemotherapy: Oral: Initial: 2-4 mg/kg/day in single or divided doses for 7 days then increase dose to 4-6 mg/kg/day until response is obtained or leukocyte count decreased <4000/mm^3 or the platelet count decreased <100,000/mm^3; maintenance: 1-2 mg/kg/day

Geriatric Refer to adult dosing; use with caution. Adjust for renal impairment.

Pediatric Refer to individual protocols. Manufacturer states that the dose is based on patient's ideal weight if the patient is obese or has abnormal fluid retention. Other studies suggest that ideal body weight may not be necessary. Oral (may be given as a single daily dose or in 2-3 divided doses): Children:

BMT aplastic anemia conditioning regimen (unlabeled use): 12.5 mg/kg/day every other day for 4 doses

Hodgkin's disease: MOPP/IC-MOPP regimens: 100 mg/m^2/day for 14 days and repeated every 4 weeks

Neuroblastoma and medulloblastoma (unlabeled use): Doses as high as 100-200 mg/m^2/ day once daily have been used.

Renal Impairment The FDA-approved labeling does not contain dosing adjustment guidelines; use with caution; may result in increased toxicity.

Hepatic Impairment The FDA-approved labeling does not contain dosing adjustment guidelines; use with caution; may result in increased toxicity. The following guidelines have been used by some clinicians:

Floyd, 2006:

Transaminases 1.6-6 times ULN: Administer 75% of dose

Transaminases >6 times ULN: Use clinical judgment

Serum bilirubin >5 mg/dL or transaminases >3 times ULN: Avoid use

King, 2001: Serum bilirubin >5 mg/dL or transaminases >180 units/L: Avoid use

Administration

Oral May be given as a single daily dose or in 2-3 divided doses.

Stability

Storage Protect from light.

Monitoring and Teaching Issues

Laboratory Monitoring CBC with differential, platelet and reticulocyte count, urinalysis, liver and renal function

Physical Assessment Assess potential for interactions with other pharmacological agents patient may be taking (eg, CNS depressants increase risk of adverse reactions). Emetic potential is high; antiemetic is generally required. Assess results of laboratory tests and patient response frequently (eg, neurotoxicity, nausea and vomiting, pneumonitis, arthralgia, paresthesia). Instruct patient about dietary and alcohol cautions (procarbazine has some MAO inhibitory effects, can result in life-threatening hypertension with tyramine; alcohol may cause disulfiram like reaction). Teach patient proper use, possible side effects/appropriate interventions, and adverse symptoms to report.

Patient Education Avoid alcohol; may cause acute disulfiram reaction (headache, respiratory difficulties, nausea, vomiting, sweating, thirst, hypotension, and flushing). Avoid tyramine-containing foods; could cause serious hypertensive effects. Maintain adequate hydration unless instructed to restrict fluid intake. You will be more sensitive to infection. May cause considerable nausea or vomiting, mental depression, nervousness, insomnia, nightmares, dizziness, confusion, lethargy, rash, hair loss or hyperpigmentation (reversible), loss of libido, sterility, or amenorrhea. Report persistent fever, chills, or sore throat; unusual bleeding, blood in urine, stool (black stool), or vomitus; unresolved depression; mania; hallucinations; nightmares; disorientation; seizures; chest pain or palpitations; respiratory difficulty; or vision changes.

Dietary Considerations Avoid tyramine-containing foods/beverages. Some examples include aged or matured cheese, air-dried or cured meats (including sausages and salamis), fava or broad bean pods, tap/draft beers, Marmite concentrate, sauerkraut, soy sauce and other soybean condiments.

Pregnancy Considerations Animal studies have demonstrated teratogenic effects. There are no adequate and well-controlled studies in pregnant women. There are, however, case reports of fetal malformations in the offspring of pregnant women exposed to procarbazine as part of a combination chemotherapy regimen. Women of childbearing potential should avoid becoming pregnant during treatment.

◆ **Procarbazine Hydrochloride** *see* Procarbazine *on page* 1510

◆ **Procardia®** *see* NIFEdipine *on page* 1313

◆ **Procardia XL®** *see* NIFEdipine *on page* 1313

◆ **ProCentra®** *see* Dextroamphetamine *on page* 509

◆ **Procetofene** *see* Fenofibrate *on page* 739

◆ **Prochieve® [DSC]** *see* Progesterone *on page* 1514

Prochlorperazine (proe klor PER a zeen)

U.S. Brand Names Compro®

Index Terms Chlormeprazine; Compazine; Prochlorperazine Edisylate; Prochlorperazine Maleate

Generic Availability (U.S.) Yes

Pharmacologic Category Antiemetic; Antipsychotic Agent, Typical, Phenothiazine

Medication Safety Issues

Sound-alike/look-alike issues:

Prochlorperazine may be confused with chlorproMAZINE

Compazine® may be confused with Copaxone®, Coumadin®

CPZ (occasional abbreviation for Compazine®) is an error-prone abbreviation (mistaken as chlorpromazine)

Lactation Excretion in breast milk unknown/use caution

Use Management of nausea and vomiting; psychotic disorders, including schizophrenia and anxiety

Unlabeled/Investigational Use Behavioral syndromes in dementia; psychosis/agitation related to Alzheimer's dementia

Available Dosage Forms

Injection, solution: 5 mg/mL (2 mL, 10 mL)

Suppository, rectal: 25 mg (12s)

Compro®: 25 mg (12s)

Tablet, oral: 5 mg, 10 mg

Dosing

Adult

Antiemetic:

Oral (tablet): 5-10 mg 3-4 times/day; usual maximum: 40 mg/day; larger doses may rarely be required

I.M. (deep): 5-10 mg every 3-4 hours; usual maximum: 40 mg/day

I.V.: 2.5-10 mg; maximum 10 mg/dose or 40 mg/day; may repeat dose every 3-4 hours as needed

Rectal: 25 mg twice daily

Surgical nausea/vomiting: Note: Should not exceed 40 mg/day

I.M.: 5-10 mg 1-2 hours before induction or to control symptoms during or after surgery; may repeat once if necessary

I.V. (administer slow IVP <5 mg/minute): 5-10 mg 15-30 minutes before induction or to control symptoms during or after surgery; may repeat once if necessary

Rectal (unlabeled use): 25 mg

Antipsychotic:

Oral: 5-10 mg 3-4 times/day; titrate dose slowly every 2-3 days; doses up to 150 mg/day may be required in some patients for treatment of severe disturbances

I.M.: Initial: 10-20 mg; if necessary repeat initial dose every 1-4 hours to gain control; more than 3-4 doses are rarely needed. If parenteral administration is still required; give 10-20 mg every 4-6 hours; change to oral as soon as possible.

Nonpsychotic anxiety: *Oral (tablet):* Usual dose: 15-20 mg/day in divided doses; do not give doses >20 mg/day or for longer than 12 weeks

Geriatric Dementia behavior (nonpsychotic, unlabeled use): Initial: 2.5-5 mg 1-2 times/day; increase dose at 4- to 7-day intervals by 2.5-5 mg/day. Increase dosing intervals (twice daily, 3 times/day, etc) as necessary to control response or side effects. Maximum daily dose should probably not exceed 75 mg in the elderly. Gradual increases (titration) may prevent some side effects or decrease their severity.

Pediatric Not recommended in children <10 kg or <2 years.

Antiemetic:

Oral, rectal: >9 kg: 0.4 mg/kg/24 hours in 3-4 divided doses; **or**

9-13 kg: 2.5 mg every 12-24 hours as needed; maximum: 7.5 mg/day

13.1-17 kg: 2.5 mg every 8-12 hours as needed; maximum: 10 mg/day

17.1-37 kg: 2.5 mg every 8 hours or 5 mg every 12 hours as needed; maximum: 15 mg/day

I.M.: 0.13 mg/kg/dose; change to oral as soon as possible

Antipsychotic: Children 2-12 years (not recommended in children <9 kg or <2 years):

Oral, rectal: 2.5 mg 2-3 times/day; do not give more than 10 mg the first day; increase dosage as needed to maximum daily dose of 20 mg for 2-5 years and 25 mg for 6-12 years

I.M.: 0.13 mg/kg/dose; change to oral as soon as possible

Administration

I.M. Inject by deep IM into outer quadrant of buttocks.

I.V. Administer slow I.V. at a rate not exceeding 5 mg/minute. To reduce the risk of hypotension, patients receiving I.V. prochlorperazine must remain lying down and be observed for at least 30 minutes following administration

Monitoring and Teaching Issues

Laboratory Monitoring Baseline liver and kidney function, CBC prior to and periodically during therapy, lipid profile, fasting blood glucose/Hgb A_{1c}; BMI

Physical Assessment For I.V., continuously monitor blood pressure and heart rate during administration. Monitor blood pressure and heart rate, fluid balance, and for dehydration. Monitor for seizures, especially with known seizure disorder. Monitor for excessive sedation, neuromuscular malignant syndrome, autonomic instability (eg, anticholinergic effects), and extrapyramidal symptoms.

Patient Education Avoid alcohol. You may experience appetite changes. Maintain adequate hydration unless instructed to restrict fluid intake. May cause dizziness, tremors, or visual disturbance (especially during early therapy). Do not change position rapidly(rise slowly). May cause photosensitivity reaction. Report immediately any changes in gait or muscular tremors. Report unresolved changes in voiding or elimination (constipation or diarrhea), acute dizziness or unresolved sedation, vision changes, palpitations, yellowing of skin or eyes, or changes in color of urine or stool (pink or red brown urine is expected).

Related Information

Compatibility of Drugs *on page 1994*

◆ **Prochlorperazine Edisylate** *see* Prochlorperazine *on page 1512*

◆ **Prochlorperazine Maleate** *see* Prochlorperazine *on page 1512*

◆ **Procrit®** *see* Epoetin Alfa *on page 638*

◆ **Proctocort®** *see* Hydrocortisone (Topical) *on page 920*

◆ **ProctoCream®-HC** *see* Hydrocortisone (Topical) *on page 920*

◆ **Proctofene** *see* Fenofibrate *on page 739*

◆ **Procto-Kit™ [DSC]** *see* Hydrocortisone (Topical) *on page 920*

◆ **Procto-Pak™** *see* Hydrocortisone (Topical) *on page 920*

- ◆ **Proctosol-HC®** *see* Hydrocortisone (Topical) *on page 920*
- ◆ **Proctozone-HC 2.5%™** *see* Hydrocortisone (Topical) *on page 920*

Progesterone (proe JES ter one)

U.S. Brand Names Crinone®; Endometrin®; First™-Progesterone VGS 100; First™-Progesterone VGS 200; First™-Progesterone VGS 25; First™-Progesterone VGS 400; First™-Progesterone VGS 50; Prochieve® [DSC]; Prometrium®

Index Terms Pregnenedione; Progestin

Generic Availability (U.S.) Yes: Injection, powder

Pharmacologic Category Progestin

Pregnancy Risk Factor B (Prometrium®, per manufacturer); none established for vaginal gel, vaginal tablet, or injection

Lactation Enters breast milk/use caution (AAP rates "compatible"; AAP 2001 update pending)

Use

Oral: Prevention of endometrial hyperplasia in nonhysterectomized, postmenopausal women who are receiving conjugated estrogen tablets; secondary amenorrhea

I.M.: Amenorrhea; abnormal uterine bleeding due to hormonal imbalance

Intravaginal gel: Part of assisted reproductive technology (ART) for infertile women with progesterone deficiency; secondary amenorrhea

Vaginal tablet: Part of ART for infertile women with progesterone deficiency

Mechanism of Action/Effect Natural steroid hormone that induces secretory changes in the endometrium, promotes mammary gland development, relaxes uterine smooth muscle, blocks follicular maturation and ovulation, and maintains pregnancy. When used as part of an ART program in the luteal phase, progesterone supports embryo implantation.

Contraindications Hypersensitivity to progesterone or any component of the formulation; undiagnosed abnormal vaginal bleeding; history of or current thrombophlebitis or venous thromboembolic disorders (including DVT, PE); history of, active or recent (within 1 year) arterial thromboembolic disease (eg, stroke, MI); history of or known or suspected carcinoma of the breast or genital organs; hepatic dysfunction or disease; missed abortion or ectopic pregnancy; diagnostic test for pregnancy; capsules are also contraindicated for use during pregnancy

Warnings/Precautions [U.S. Boxed Warning]: Progestins used in combination with estrogen should not be used to prevent cardiovascular disease. Use caution with cardiovascular disease or dysfunction. Progestins used in combination with estrogen may increase the risks of hypertension, myocardial infarction (MI), stroke, pulmonary emboli (PE), and deep vein thrombosis; incidence of these effects was shown to be significantly increased in postmenopausal women using CEE in combination with MPA. Similar risk should be assumed with other progestins.

[U.S. Boxed Warning]: The risk of dementia may be increased in postmenopausal women; progestins used in combination with estrogen should not be used to prevent dementia. Increased incidence was observed in women ≥65 years of age taking CEE alone or in combination with MPA.

[U.S. Boxed Warning]: An increased risk of invasive breast cancer was observed in postmenopausal women using conjugated equine estrogens (CEE) in combination with medroxyprogesterone acetate (MPA). An increase in abnormal mammograms has also been reported with estrogen and progestin therapy

Unopposed estrogens may increase the risk of endometrial carcinoma in postmenopausal women with an intact uterus. Risk appears to be associated with long-term use. The use of a progestin should be considered when administering estrogens to postmenopausal women with an intact uterus. Adequate diagnostic measures, including endometrial sampling (if indicated), should be performed to rule out malignancy in all cases of undiagnosed abnormal vaginal bleeding. Postmenopausal estrogen therapy and combined estrogen/progesterone therapy may increase the risk of ovarian cancer; however, the absolute risk to an individual woman is small. Although results from various studies are not consistent, risk does not appear to be significantly associated with the duration, route, or dose of therapy. In one study, the risk decreased after 2 years following discontinuation of therapy.

Discontinue pending examination in cases of sudden partial or complete vision loss, sudden onset of proptosis, diplopia, or migraine; discontinue permanently if papilledema or retinal vascular lesions are observed on examination. Use with caution in patients with diseases that may be exacerbated by fluid retention, including asthma, epilepsy, migraine, diabetes or renal dysfunction. Use caution with history of depression. Patients should be warned that progesterone might cause transient dizziness or drowsiness during initial therapy. Whenever possible, progestins in combination with estrogens should be discontinued at least 4-6 weeks prior to surgeries associated with an increased risk of thromboembolism or during periods of prolonged immobilization. Progestins used in combination with estrogen should be used for shortest duration possible consistent with treatment goals. Conduct periodic risk:benefit assessments.

Products may contain palm oil, peanut oil, sesame oil, or benzyl alcohol. Not for use prior to menarche.

Drug Interactions

Metabolism/Transport Effects Substrate of CYP1A2 (minor), 2A6 (minor), 2C9 (minor), 2C19 (major), 2D6 (minor), 3A4 (major); **Inhibits** CYP2C9 (weak), CYP2C19 (weak), CYP3A4 (weak), P-glycoprotein

Avoid Concomitant Use

Avoid concomitant use of Progesterone with any of the following: Silodosin; Topotecan

Decreased Effect

The levels/effects of Progesterone may be decreased by: Aminoglutethimide; CYP2C19 Inducers (Strong); CYP3A4 Inducers (Strong); Deferasirox; Herbs (CYP3A4 Inducers); Peginterferon Alfa-2b

Increased Effect/Toxicity

Progesterone may increase the levels/effects of: Colchicine; Dabigatran Etexilate; Everolimus; P-Glycoprotein Substrates; Rivaroxaban; Silodosin; Topotecan

The levels/effects of Progesterone may be increased by: Conivaptan; Herbs (Progestogenic Properties)

Nutritional/Ethanol Interactions

Food: Food increases oral bioavailability.

Herb/Nutraceutical: St John's wort may decrease progesterone levels. Herbs with progestogenic properties may enhance the adverse/toxic effects of progestin; example herbs include bloodroot, chasteberry, damiana, oregano, yucca.

Lab Interactions Thyroid function, metyrapone, liver function, coagulation tests, endocrine function tests

Adverse Reactions

Injection (I.M.):

Cardiovascular: Cerebral edema, cerebral thrombosis, edema
Central nervous system: Depression, fever, insomnia, somnolence
Dermatologic: Acne, allergic rash (rare), alopecia, hirsutism, pruritus, rash, urticaria
Endocrine & metabolic: Amenorrhea, breakthrough bleeding, breast tenderness, galactorrhea, menstrual flow changes, spotting
Gastrointestinal: Nausea, weight gain/loss
Genitourinary: Cervical erosion changes, cervical secretion changes
Hepatic: Cholestatic jaundice
Local: Injection site: Irritation, pain, redness
Ocular: Optic neuritis, retinal thrombosis
Respiratory: Pulmonary embolism
Miscellaneous: Anaphylactoid reactions

Oral capsule (percentages reported when used in combination with or cycled with conjugated estrogens):

>10%:

Central nervous system: Headache (16% to 31%), dizziness (15% to 24%), depression (19%)
Endocrine & metabolic: Breast tenderness (27%), breast pain (6% to 16%)
Gastrointestinal: Abdominal pain (10% to 20%), abdominal bloating (8% to 12%)
Genitourinary: Urinary problems (11%)
Neuromuscular & skeletal: Joint pain (20%), musculoskeletal pain (12%)
Miscellaneous: Viral infection (12%)

5% to 10%:

Cardiovascular: Chest pain (7%)
Central nervous system: Fatigue (8%), irritability (8%), worry (8%)
Gastrointestinal: Nausea/vomiting (8%), diarrhea (7% to 8%)
Genitourinary: Vaginal discharge (10%)
Respiratory: Cough (8%)

<5%: Breast biopsy, breast cancer, cholecystectomy, constipation

Vaginal gel (percentages reported with ART); also refer to oral capsule reactions listing for additional effects noted with progesterone:

>10%:

Central nervous system: Somnolence (27%), headache (13% to 17%), nervousness (16%), depression (11%)
Endocrine & metabolic: Breast enlargement (40%), breast pain (13%), libido decreased (11%)
Gastrointestinal: Constipation (27%), nausea (7% to 22%), cramps (15%), abdominal pain (12%)
Genitourinary: Perineal pain (17%), nocturia (13%)

5% to 10%:

Central nervous system: Pain (8%), dizziness (5%)
Gastrointestinal: Diarrhea (8%), bloating (7%), vomiting (5%)
Genitourinary: Vaginal discharge (7%), dyspareunia (6%), genital moniliasis (5%), genital pruritus (5%)
Neuromuscular & skeletal: Arthralgia (8%)

Vaginal tablet (percentages reported with ART); also refer to oral capsule reactions listing for additional effects noted with progesterone:

>10%:

Gastrointestinal: Abdominal pain (12%)
Miscellaneous: Post-oocyte retrieval pain (25% to 28%)

1% to 10%:

Central nervous system: Headache (3% to 4%), fatigue (2% to 3%)
Endocrine & metabolic: Ovarian hyperstimulation syndrome (7%)
Gastrointestinal: Nausea (7% to 8%), abdominal distension (4%), constipation (2% to 3%), vomiting (2% to 3%)
Genitourinary: Uterine spasm (3% to 4%), vaginal bleeding (3%), urinary tract infection (1% to 2%)

Pharmacodynamics/Kinetics

Absorption Vaginal gel: Prolonged; Absorption half-life: 25-50 hours

Time to Peak Oral: Within 3 hours; I.M.: ~8 hours; Vaginal tablet: ~17-24 hours

Protein Binding Albumin (50% to 54%) and cortisol-binding protein (43% to 48%)

Half-Life Elimination Vaginal gel: 5-20 minutes

Metabolism Hepatic

Excretion Urine, bile, feces

Available Dosage Forms

Capsule, oral:
Prometrium®: 100 mg, 200 mg

Gel, vaginal:
Crinone®: 4% (1.45 g); 8% (1.45 g)

Injection, oil: 50 mg/mL (10 mL)

Powder, for prescription compounding: USP: 100% (10 g, 25 g, 50 g, 100 g, 1000 g)

Suppository, vaginal:
First™-Progesterone VGS 25: 25 mg (30s)
First™-Progesterone VGS 50: 50 mg (30s)
First™-Progesterone VGS 100: 100 mg (30s)
First™-Progesterone VGS 200: 200 mg (30s)
First™-Progesterone VGS 400: 400 mg (30s)

Tablet, vaginal:
Endometrin®: 100 mg

Dosing

Adult & Geriatric Females:

Amenorrhea: I.M.: 5-10 mg/day for 6-8 consecutive days

Amenorrhea, secondary:

Intravaginal gel: 45 mg (4% gel) every other day for 6 doses; if response is inadequate, may increase to 90 mg (8% gel) at same schedule

Oral: 400 mg every evening for 10 days

ART in patients who require progesterone supplementation:

Intravaginal gel: 90 mg (8% gel) once daily. If pregnancy occurs, may continue treatment for 10-12 weeks.

Intravaginal tablet: 100 mg 2-3 times daily starting at oocyte retrieval and continuing for up to 10 weeks.

ART in patients with partial or complete ovarian failure:

Intravaginal gel: 90 mg (8% gel) twice daily. If pregnancy occurs, continue treatment for 10-12 weeks.

Endometrial hyperplasia prevention (in postmenopausal women with a uterus who are receiving daily conjugated estrogen tablets): Oral: 200 mg as a single daily dose every evening for 12 days sequentially per 28-day cycle

Functional uterine bleeding: I.M.: 5-10 mg/day for 6 doses

Administration

Oral Oral capsule: For patients who experience difficulty swallowing the capsules, taking with a full glass of water in the standing position may be beneficial.

I.M. Administer deep I.M. only

Other

Vaginal gel: (A small amount of gel will remain in the applicator following insertion): Administer into the vagina directly from sealed applicator. Remove applicator from wrapper; holding applicator by thickest end, shake down to move contents to thin end; while holding applicator by flat section of thick end, twist off tab; gently insert into vagina and squeeze thick end of applicator.

For use at altitudes above 2500 feet: Remove applicator from wrapper; hold applicator on both sides of bubble in the thick end; using a lancet, make a single puncture in the bubble to relieve air pressure; holding applicator by thickest end, shake down to move contents to thin end; while holding applicator by flat section of thick end, twist off tab; gently insert into vagina and squeeze thick end of applicator.

Vaginal tablet: Insert tablet in vagina using disposable applicator provided.

Stability

Storage Store at controlled room temperature. Protect capsules from excessive moisture.

Monitoring and Teaching Issues

Physical Assessment Assess blood pressure, mammogram, and results of Pap smears and pregnancy tests before beginning treatment and at least annually. Teach patient importance of annual physicals, Pap smears, and vision assessment.

Patient Education Inform prescriber if you are allergic to peanut or palm oil. Take at bedtime to minimize side effects. It is important that you have an annual physical assessment, Pap smear, and vision assessment while taking this medication and that you perform monthly self-breast exams. May cause temporary dizziness or drowsiness, headache, joint pain, nausea and/or vomiting, mood swings, or irritability. Report immediately warmth, swelling, or redness in calves; shortness of breath; chest pain; sudden loss or change in vision; breast mass; blurred vision; confusion; or depression.

Vaginal gel: A small amount of gel will remain in the applicator following insertion. Administer into the vagina directly from applicator.

Geriatric Considerations Not a progestin of choice in the elderly for hormonal cycling.

Pregnancy Considerations Adverse events were not observed following oral administration in animal reproduction studies. There is an increased risk of minor birth defects in children whose mothers take progesterones during the first 4 months of pregnancy. Hypospadias has been reported in male and mild masculinization of the external genitalia has been reported in female babies exposed during the first trimester. Cleft lip, cleft palate, congenital heart disease, patent ductus arteriosus, ventricular septal defect, intrauterine death, and spontaneous abortion have been noted in case reports following use of oral progesterone during pregnancy. High doses of progesterone would be expected to impair fertility. According to the American College of Obstetricians and Gynecologists, additional studies are needed to evaluate the use of progesterone to reduce the risk of preterm birth. If needed, use should be restricted to women with history of previous spontaneous abortion at <37 weeks. The vaginal gel and tablet are indicated for use in ART. The oral capsules are contraindicated for use during pregnancy.

- **Progestin** *see* Progesterone *on page 1514*
- **Prograf®** *see* Tacrolimus (Systemic) *on page 1695*
- **Proleukin®** *see* Aldesleukin *on page 62*
- **Prolia™** *see* Denosumab *on page 486*
- **Promacet** *see* Butalbital and Acetaminophen *on page 261*
- **Promacta®** *see* Eltrombopag *on page 610*

Promethazine (proe METH a zeen)

U.S. Brand Names Phenadoz®; Phenergan®; Promethegan™

Index Terms Promethazine Hydrochloride

Generic Availability (U.S.) Yes

Pharmacologic Category Antiemetic; Histamine H_1 Antagonist; Histamine H_1 Antagonist, First Generation; Phenothiazine Derivative

Medication Safety Issues

Sound-alike/look-alike issues:

Promethazine may be confused with chlorproMAZINE, predniSONE, promazine

Phenergan® may be confused with Phenaphen®, PHENobarbital, Phrenilin®, Theragran®

International issues:

Sominex: Brand name for promethazine in Great Britain, but also is a brand name for diphenhydrAMINE in the U.S.

High alert medication: The Institute for Safe Medication Practices (ISMP) includes this medication (I.V. formulation) among its list of drugs which have a heightened risk of causing significant patient harm when used in error.

Beers Criteria medication: This drug may be inappropriate for use in geriatric patients (high severity risk).

Administration issues:

To prevent or minimize tissue damage during I.V. administration, the Institute for Safe Medication Practices (ISMP) has the following recommendations:

Limit concentration available to the 25 mg/mL product
Consider limiting initial doses to 6.25-12.5 mg
Further dilute the 25 mg/mL strength into 10-20 mL NS
Administer through a large bore vein (not hand or wrist)
Administer via running I.V. line at port farthest from patient's vein
Consider administering over 10-15 minutes
Instruct patients to report immediately signs of pain or burning

Pregnancy Risk Factor C

Lactation Excretion in breast milk unknown/not recommended

Use Symptomatic treatment of various allergic conditions; antiemetic; motion sickness; sedative; adjunct to postoperative analgesia and anesthesia

Mechanism of Action/Effect Phenothiazine derivative; blocks postsynaptic mesolimbic dopaminergic receptors in the brain; exhibits a strong alpha-adrenergic blocking effect and depresses the release of hypothalamic and hypophyseal hormones; competes with histamine for the H_1-receptor; reduces stimuli to the brainstem reticular system

Contraindications Hypersensitivity to promethazine or any component of the formulation (cross-reactivity between phenothiazines may occur); coma; treatment of lower respiratory tract symptoms, including asthma; children <2 years of age; intra-arterial or subcutaneous administration

Warnings/Precautions [U.S. Boxed Warning]: Respiratory fatalities have been reported in children <2 years of age. Contraindicated in children <2 years of age. In children ≥2 years, use the lowest possible dose; other drugs with respiratory depressant effects should be avoided.

[U.S. Boxed Warning]: Promethazine injection can cause severe tissue injury (including gangrene) regardless of the route of administration. Tissue irritation and damage may result from perivascular extravasation, unintentional intra-arterial administration, and intraneuronal or perineuronal infiltration. In addition to gangrene, adverse events reported include tissue necrosis, abscesses, burning, pain, erythema, edema, paralysis, severe spasm of distal vessels, phlebitis, thrombophlebitis, venous thrombosis, sensory loss, paralysis, and palsies. Surgical intervention including fasciotomy, skin graft, and/or

amputation have been necessary in some cases. The preferred route of administration is by deep intramuscular (I.M.) injection. Subcutaneous administration is contraindicated. Discontinue intravenous injection immediately with onset of pain and evaluate for arterial injection or perivascular extravasation. Although there is no proven successful management of unintentional intra-arterial injection or perivascular extravasation, sympathetic block and heparinization have been used in the acute management of unintentional intra-arterial injection based on results from animal studies.

May be sedating; use with caution in disorders where CNS depression is a feature. May impair physical or mental abilities; patients must be cautioned about performing tasks which require mental alertness. Use with caution in hemodynamic instability; bone marrow suppression; subcortical brain damage; and in severe cardiac, hepatic or respiratory disease. Avoid use in Reye's syndrome. May lower seizure threshold; use caution in persons with seizure disorders or in persons using narcotics or local anesthetics which may also affect seizure threshold. May alter temperature regulation or mask toxicity of other drugs due to antiemetic effects. May alter cardiac conduction (life-threatening arrhythmias have occurred with therapeutic doses of phenothiazines). May cause orthostatic hypotension; use with caution in patients at risk of hypotension or where transient hypotensive episodes would be poorly tolerated (cardiovascular disease or cerebrovascular disease).

Phenothiazines may cause anticholinergic effects; therefore, they should be used with caution in patients with decreased gastrointestinal motility, GI or GU obstruction, urinary retention, BPH, xerostomia, or visual problems. Conditions which also may be exacerbated by cholinergic blockade include narrow-angle glaucoma (screening is recommended) and worsening of myasthenia gravis. Use with caution in Parkinson's disease. May cause extrapyramidal symptoms, including pseudoparkinsonism, acute dystonic reactions, akathisia, and tardive dyskinesia. May be associated with neuroleptic malignant syndrome (NMS). May cause photosensitivity. May be inappropriate for use in the elderly due to potent anticholinergic effects (Beers Criteria). Injection may contain sodium metabisulfite.

Drug Interactions

Metabolism/Transport Effects Substrate (major) of CYP2B6, 2D6; **Inhibits** CYP2D6 (weak)

Avoid Concomitant Use

Avoid concomitant use of Promethazine with any of the following: Metoclopramide; Sibutramine

Decreased Effect

Promethazine may decrease the levels/effects of: Acetylcholinesterase Inhibitors (Central)

The levels/effects of Promethazine may be decreased by: Acetylcholinesterase Inhibitors (Central); CYP2B6 Inducers (Strong); Peginterferon Alfa-2b

Increased Effect/Toxicity

Promethazine may increase the levels/effects of: Anticholinergics; Serotonin Modulators

The levels/effects of Promethazine may be increased by: CYP2B6 Inhibitors (Moderate); CYP2B6 Inhibitors (Strong); CYP2D6 Inhibitors (Moderate); CYP2D6 Inhibitors (Strong); Darunavir; MAO Inhibitors; Metoclopramide; Pramlintide; Quazepam; Sibutramine

Nutritional/Ethanol Interactions

Ethanol: Avoid ethanol (may increase CNS depression).

Herb/Nutraceutical: Avoid valerian, St John's wort, kava kava, gotu kola (may increase CNS depression).

Lab Interactions May interfere with urine detection of amphetamine/methamphetamine (false-positive); alters the flare response in intradermal allergen tests; hCG-based pregnancy tests may result in false-negatives or false-positives

Adverse Reactions Frequency not defined.

Cardiovascular: Bradycardia, hyper-/hypotension, nonspecific QT changes, postural hypotension, tachycardia,

Central nervous system: Agitation akathisia, catatonic states, confusion, delirium, disorientation, dizziness, drowsiness, dystonias, euphoria, excitation, extrapyramidal symptoms, faintness, fatigue, hallucinations, hysteria, insomnia, lassitude, pseudoparkinsonism, tardive dyskinesia, nervousness, neuroleptic malignant syndrome, nightmares, sedation, seizure, somnolence

Dermatologic: Angioneurotic edema, dermatitis, photosensitivity, skin pigmentation (slate gray), urticaria

Endocrine & metabolic: Amenorrhea, breast engorgement, gynecomastia, hyperglycemia, lactation

Gastrointestinal: Constipation, nausea, vomiting, xerostomia

Genitourinary: Ejaculatory disorder, impotence, urinary retention

Hematologic: Agranulocytosis, leukopenia, thrombocytopenia, thrombocytopenic purpura

Hepatic: Jaundice

Local: Abscess, distal vessel spasm, gangrene, injection site reactions (burning, edema, erythema, pain), palsies, paralysis, phlebitis, sensory loss, thrombophlebitis, tissue necrosis, venous thrombosis

Neuromuscular & skeletal: Incoordination, tremor

Ocular: Blurred vision, corneal and lenticular changes, diplopia, epithelial keratopathy, pigmentary retinopathy

Otic: Tinnitus

Respiratory: Apnea, asthma, nasal congestion, respiratory depression

Pharmacodynamics/Kinetics

Onset of Action Oral, I.M.: ~20 minutes; I.V.: ~5 minutes

Peak effect: C_{max}: ~9 ng/mL (suppository); ~19 ng/mL (syrup)

Duration of Action Usually 4-6 hours (up to 12 hours)

Absorption

I.M.: Bioavailability may be greater than with oral or rectal administration

Oral: Rapid and complete; large first pass effect limits systemic bioavailability

Time to Peak Maximum serum concentration: ~4.5 hours (syrup); ~7-9 hours (suppositories)

Protein Binding 93%

Half-Life Elimination 9-16 hours

Metabolism Hepatic; primarily oxidation; forms metabolites

Excretion Primarily urine and feces (as inactive metabolites)

Available Dosage Forms

Injection, solution: 25 mg/mL (1 mL); 50 mg/mL (1 mL)

Phenergan®: 25 mg/mL (1 mL); 50 mg/mL (1 mL)

Suppository, rectal: 12.5 mg (12s); 25 mg (12s)

Phenadoz®: 12.5 mg (12s); 25 mg (12s)

Promethegan™: 12.5 mg (12s); 25 mg (12s); 50 mg (12s)

Syrup, oral: 6.25 mg/5 mL (118 mL, 473 mL)

Tablet, oral: 12.5 mg, 25 mg, 50 mg

Dosing

Adult & Geriatric

Allergic conditions (including allergic reactions to blood or plasma):

Oral, rectal: 25 mg at bedtime **or** 12.5 mg before meals and at bedtime (range: 6.25-12.5 mg 3 times/day)

I.M., I.V.: 25 mg, may repeat in 2 hours when necessary; switch to oral route as soon as feasible

Antiemetic: Oral, I.M., I.V., rectal: 12.5-25 mg every 4-6 hours as needed

Motion sickness: Oral, rectal: 25 mg 30-60 minutes before departure, then every 12 hours as needed

Obstetrics (labor) analgesia adjunct: I.M., I.V.: Early labor: 50 mg; Established labor: 25-75 mg in combination with analgesic at reduced dosage; may repeat every 4 hours for up to 2 additional doses (maximum: 100 mg/day while in labor)

Pre-/postoperative analgesia/hypnotic adjunct: I.M., I.V.: 25-50 mg in combination with analgesic or hypnotic (at reduced dosage)

Sedation: Oral, I.M., I.V., rectal: 12.5-50 mg/dose

Pediatric

Allergic conditions: Children ≥2 years: Oral, rectal: 0.1 mg/kg/dose (maximum: 12.5 mg) every 6 hours during the day and 0.5 mg/kg/dose (maximum: 25 mg) at bedtime as needed

Antiemetic: Children ≥2 years: Oral, I.M., I.V., rectal: 0.25-1 mg/kg 4-6 times/day as needed (maximum: 25 mg/dose)

Motion sickness: Children ≥2 years: Oral, rectal: 0.5 mg/kg/dose 30 minutes to 1 hour before departure, then every 12 hours as needed (maximum dose: 25 mg twice daily)

Preoperative analgesia/hypnotic adjunct: Children ≥2 years: I.M., I.V.: 1.1 mg/kg in combination with an analgesic or hypnotic (at reduced dosage) and with an atropine-like agent (at appropriate dosage). **Note:** Promethazine dosage should not exceed half of suggested adult dosage.

Sedation: Children ≥2 years: Oral, I.M., I.V., rectal: 0.5-1 mg/kg/dose every 6 hours as needed (maximum: 50 mg/dose)

Administration

I.M. Preferred route of administration; administer into deep muscle

I.V. I.V. administration is **not** the preferred route; severe tissue damage may occur. Solution for injection should be administered in a maximum concentration of 25 mg/mL (more dilute solutions are recommended). Administer via running I.V. line at port farthest from patient's vein, or through a large bore vein (not hand or wrist). Consider administering over 10-15 minutes (maximum: 25 mg/minute). Discontinue immediately if burning or pain occurs with administration.

Other Not for SubQ or intra-arterial administration.

Stability

Storage

Injection: Prior to dilution, store at 20°C to 25°C (68°F to 77°F). Protect from light. Solutions in NS or D_5W are stable for 24 hours at room temperature.

Oral solution: Store at 15°C to 25°C (59°F to 77°F). Protect from light.

Suppositories: Store refrigerated at 2°C to 8°C (36°F to 46°F).

Tablets: Store at 20°C to 25°C (68°F to 77°F). Protect from light.

Monitoring and Teaching Issues

Physical Assessment Assess patient carefully for contraindications or cautions prior to beginning treatment. I.M. is the preferred route of administration. I.V.: Infusion site must be monitored closely; severe tissue damage may result. Not for SubQ or intra-arterial use. Monitor for sedation, bradycardia, akathisia, delirium, extrapyramidal symptoms, gastrointestinal upset, urinary retention, blurred vision, and respiratory depression. May be sedating and impair physical or mental abilities; use sedation safety measures to prevent falls (eg, side rails up, call light within reach).

Patient Education I.V.: Report immediately any pain or burning at infusion/injection site. Oral/suppository: Avoid alcohol; may increase CNS depression. May cause dizziness, drowsiness, blurred vision, orthostatic hypotension, photosensitivity, nausea, dry mouth, or appetite disturbances. Report unresolved nausea or diarrhea, palpitations, dizziness, excess/persistent sedation, changes in urination, sore throat, or respiratory difficulty.

Dietary Considerations Increase dietary intake of riboflavin.

Geriatric Considerations Because promethazine is a phenothiazine (and can, therefore, cause side effects such as extrapyramidal symptoms), it is not considered an antihistamine of choice in the elderly.

This medication is considered to be potentially inappropriate in this patient population (Beers Criteria severity: High).

Pregnancy Considerations Teratogenic effects were not observed in animal studies. There are no adequate and well-controlled studies in pregnant women. Crosses the placenta. Use during pregnancy only if benefits outweigh risk. May be used alone or as an adjunct to narcotic analgesics during labor.

Related Information

Compatibility of Drugs *on page 1994*

- **Promethazine Hydrochloride** *see* Promethazine *on page 1517*
- **Promethegan™** *see* Promethazine *on page 1517*
- **Prometrium®** *see* Progesterone *on page 1514*
- **Pronestyl** *see* Procainamide *on page 1508*
- **Pronto® Complete Lice Removal System [OTC]** *see* Pyrethrins and Piperonyl Butoxide *on page 1530*
- **Pronto® Plus Lice Killing Mousse Plus Vitamin E [OTC]** *see* Pyrethrins and Piperonyl Butoxide *on page 1530*
- **Pronto® Plus Lice Killing Mousse Shampoo Plus Natural Extracts and Oils [OTC]** *see* Pyrethrins and Piperonyl Butoxide *on page 1530*
- **Pronto® Plus Warm Oil Treatment and Conditioner [OTC]** *see* Pyrethrins and Piperonyl Butoxide *on page 1530*

Propafenone (pro PAF en one)

U.S. Brand Names Rythmol®; Rythmol® SR

Index Terms Propafenone Hydrochloride

Generic Availability (U.S.) Yes

Pharmacologic Category Antiarrhythmic Agent, Class Ic

Pregnancy Risk Factor C

Lactation Enters breast milk/use caution

Use Treatment of life-threatening ventricular arrhythmias

Rythmol® SR: Maintenance of normal sinus rhythm in patients with symptomatic atrial fibrillation

Unlabeled/Investigational Use Supraventricular tachycardias, including those patients with Wolff-Parkinson-White syndrome

Mechanism of Action/Effect Propafenone is a class 1c antiarrhythmic agent which possesses local anesthetic properties, blocks the fast inward sodium current, and slows the rate of increase of the action potential. Prolongs conduction and refractoriness in all areas of the myocardium, with a slightly more pronounced effect on intraventricular conduction; it prolongs effective refractory period, reduces spontaneous automaticity and exhibits some beta-blockade activity.

Contraindications Hypersensitivity to propafenone or any component of the formulation; sinoatrial, AV, and intraventricular disorders of impulse generation and/or conduction (except in patients with a functioning artificial pacemaker); sinus bradycardia; cardiogenic shock; uncompensated cardiac failure; hypotension; bronchospastic disorders; uncorrected electrolyte abnormalities; concurrent use of ritonavir (see Drug Interactions)

Warnings/Precautions Monitor for proarrhythmic events. May prolong QT_c interval; use caution with other QT_c-prolonging drugs. **[U.S. Boxed Warning]: In the Cardiac Arrhythmia Suppression Trial (CAST), recent (>6 days but <2 years ago) myocardial infarction patients with asymptomatic, non-life-threatening ventricular arrhythmias did not benefit and may have been harmed by attempts to suppress the arrhythmia with flecainide or encainide. An increased mortality or nonfatal cardiac arrest rate (7.7%) was seen in the active treatment group compared with patients in the placebo group (3%). The applicability of the CAST results to other populations is unknown. Antiarrhythmic agents should be reserved for patients with life-threatening ventricular arrhythmias.** Can cause or unmask a variety of conduction disturbances. May alter pacing and sensing thresholds of artificial pacemakers. Patients with bronchospastic disease should generally not receive this drug. Monitor for worsening HF if patient has underlying condition. Correct electrolyte disturbances, especially hypokalemia or hypomagnesemia, prior to use and throughout therapy. Administer cautiously in significant hepatic dysfunction. Use with caution in patients with myasthenia gravis; may exacerbate condition.

Drug Interactions

Metabolism/Transport Effects Substrate of CYP1A2 (minor), 2D6 (major), 3A4 (minor); **Inhibits** CYP1A2 (weak), 2D6 (weak)

Avoid Concomitant Use

Avoid concomitant use of Propafenone with any of the following: Artemether; Dronedarone; Lumefantrine; Nilotinib; Pimozide; QuiNINE; Ritonavir; Saquinavir; Tetrabenazine; Thioridazine; Tipranavir; Toremifene; Vandetanib; Ziprasidone

Decreased Effect

The levels/effects of Propafenone may be decreased by: Barbiturates; Etravirine; Peginterferon Alfa-2b; Rifamycin Derivatives

Increased Effect/Toxicity

Propafenone may increase the levels/effects of: Beta-Blockers; Cardiac Glycosides; Dronedarone; Pimozide; Propranolol; QTc-Prolonging Agents; QuiNINE; Tetrabenazine; Theophylline Derivatives; Thioridazine; Toremifene; Vandetanib; Venlafaxine; Vitamin K Antagonists; Ziprasidone

The levels/effects of Propafenone may be increased by: Alfuzosin; Artemether; Chloroquine; Cimetidine; Ciprofloxacin; Ciprofloxacin (Systemic); Conivaptan; CYP2D6 Inhibitors (Moderate); CYP2D6 Inhibitors (Strong); Darunavir; FLUoxetine; FluvoxaMINE; Gadobutrol; Lumefantrine; Nilotinib; PARoxetine; QuiNINE; Ritonavir; Saquinavir; Tipranavir

Nutritional/Ethanol Interactions

Food: Propafenone serum concentrations may be increased if taken with food.

Herb/Nutraceutical: St John's wort may decrease propafenone levels. Avoid ephedra (may worsen arrhythmia).

Adverse Reactions 1% to 10%:

Cardiovascular: New or worsened arrhythmia (proarrhythmic effect) (2% to 10%), angina (2% to 5%), CHF (1% to 4%), ventricular tachycardia (1% to 3%), palpitation (1% to 3%), AV block (first-degree) (1% to 3%), syncope (1% to 2%), increased QRS interval (1% to 2%), chest pain (1% to 2%), PVCs (1% to 2%), bradycardia (1% to 2%), edema (0% to 1%), bundle branch block (0% to 1%), atrial fibrillation (1%), hypotension (0% to 1%), intraventricular conduction delay (0% to 1%)

Central nervous system: Dizziness (4% to 15%), fatigue (2% to 6%), headache (2% to 5%), ataxia (0% to 2%), insomnia (0% to 2%), anxiety (1% to 2%), drowsiness (1%)

Dermatologic: Rash (1% to 3%)

Gastrointestinal: Nausea/vomiting (2% to 11%), unusual taste (3% to 23%), constipation (2% to 7%), dyspepsia (1% to 3%), diarrhea (1% to 3%), xerostomia (1% to 2%), anorexia (1% to 2%), abdominal pain (1% to 2%), flatulence (0% to 1%)

Neuromuscular & skeletal: Tremor (0% to 1%), arthralgia (0% to 1%), weakness (1% to 2%)

Ocular: Blurred vision (1% to 6%)

Respiratory: Dyspnea (2% to 5%)

Miscellaneous: Diaphoresis (1%)

Pharmacodynamics/Kinetics

Absorption Well absorbed

Bioavailability 150 mg: 3.4%; 300 mg: 10.6%

Time to Peak Serum: 3.5 hours

Protein Binding 85% to 95%

Half-Life Elimination Extensive metabolizers: 2-10 hours; Poor metabolizers: 10-32 hours

Metabolism Hepatic; two genetically determined metabolism groups exist (extensive and poor metabolizers); 10% of Caucasians are poor metabolizers. Exhibits nonlinear pharmacokinetics; when dose is increased from 300-900 mg/day, serum concentrations increase tenfold; this nonlinearity is thought to be due to saturable first-pass effect.

Available Dosage Forms

Capsule, extended release, oral: 225 mg, 325 mg, 425 mg

Rythmol® SR: 225 mg, 325 mg, 425 mg

Tablet, oral: 150 mg, 225 mg, 300 mg

Rythmol®: 150 mg, 225 mg

Dosing

Adult & Geriatric Note: Patients who exhibit significant widening of QRS complex or second- or third-degree AV block may need dose reduction.

Ventricular arrhythmias: Oral:

Immediate release tablet: Initial: 150 mg every 8 hours, increase at 3- to 4-day intervals up to 300 mg every 8 hours.

Extended release capsule: Initial: 225 mg every 12 hours; dosage increase may be made at a minimum of 5-day intervals; may increase to 325 mg every 12 hours; if further increase is necessary, may increase to 425 mg every 12 hours

Paroxysmal atrial fibrillation (unlabeled dose): Oral: *Immediate release:* Outpatient: "Pill-in-the-pocket" dose: 450 mg (weight <70 kg); 600 mg (weight ≥70 kg). May not repeat in ≤24 hours. **Note:** An initial inpatient conversion trial should have been successful before sending patient home on this approach. Patient must be taking an AV nodal-blocking agent (eg, beta-blocker, nondihydropyridine calcium channel blocker) prior to initiation of antiarrhythmic.

Hepatic Impairment Reduction is necessary; however, specific guidelines are not available.

Administration

Oral Capsules should be swallowed whole; do not crush or chew; may be taken without regard to meals.

Stability

Storage Store at 25°C (77°F); excursions permitted to 15°C to 30°C (59°F to 86°F).

Monitoring and Teaching Issues

Physical Assessment Evaluate for use cautions (eg, bronchospastic disorders, hepatic dysfunction, myasthenia gravis). Correct electrolyte abnormalities prior to and throughout use. Assess cardiac status when beginning therapy, titrating dosage, and on a regular basis; may cause new or worsened arrhythmias.

Patient Education You will need regular cardiac checkups. You may experience dizziness, drowsiness, insomnia, or blurred vision; abnormal taste, nausea, vomiting, or loss of appetite; headache; or muscle or joint pain. Report unusual weight gain, swelling of extremities, or respiratory difficulty. Report immediately or seek emergency help if you experience chest pain; palpitations; or increased, decreased, or erratic heartbeat.

Dietary Considerations Capsule: May be taken without regard to meals.

Geriatric Considerations Elderly may have age-related decreases in hepatic Phase I metabolism. Propafenone is dependent upon liver metabolism, therefore, monitor closely in the elderly and adjust dose more gradually during initial treatment. No differences in clearance noted with impaired renal function and, therefore, no adjustment for renal function in the elderly is necessary.

Pregnancy Considerations There are no adequate and well-controlled studies in pregnant women; use only if potential benefit to the mother justifies potential risk to the fetus.

Related Information

Antiarrhythmic Drugs *on page 1978*

- **Propafenone Hydrochloride** *see* Propafenone *on page 1520*
- **Propecia®** *see* Finasteride *on page 762*

Propoxyphene (proe POKS i feen)

U.S. Brand Names Darvon-N® [DSC]; Darvon® [DSC]

Index Terms Dextropropoxyphene; Propoxyphene Hydrochloride; Propoxyphene Napsylate

Generic Availability (U.S.) Yes: Capsule

Pharmacologic Category Analgesic, Opioid

Medication Safety Issues

Sound-alike/look-alike issues:

Propoxyphene may be confused with proparacaine
Darvon® may be confused with Devrom®, Diovan®
Darvon-N® may be confused with Darvocet-N®

High alert medication: The Institute for Safe Medication Practices (ISMP) includes this medication among its list of drug classes which have a heightened risk of causing significant patient harm when used in error.

Beers Criteria medication: This drug may be inappropriate for use in geriatric patients (low severity risk).

Medication Guide Available Yes

Pregnancy Risk Factor C

Lactation Enters breast milk/use caution (AAP rates "compatible"; AAP 2001 update pending)

Use Management of mild-to-moderate pain

Controlled Substance C-IV

Dosing

Adult Pain management: Oral:

Hydrochloride: 65 mg every 4 hours as needed; maximum: 390 mg/day
Napsylate: 100 mg every 4 hours as needed; maximum: 600 mg/day

Concurrent use with CYP3A4 inhibitors: Monitor closely; dosage adjustment may be necessary.

Discontinuation of therapy: In patients on prolonged therapy, gradually discontinue propoxyphene and acetaminophen by reducing dose by 25% to 50% daily and carefully monitor for signs/symptoms of withdrawal.

Geriatric Refer to adult dosing. Consider decreasing total daily dose.

Renal Impairment Serum concentrations of propoxyphene may be increased or elimination may be delayed. Use with caution; dosage reduction should be considered; however, no specific dosing recommendations are available.

Not dialyzable (8%)

Hepatic Impairment Serum concentrations of propoxyphene may be increased or elimination may be delayed. Use with caution; dosage reduction should be considered; however, no specific dosing recommendations are available.

Administration

Oral Food may decrease rate of absorption, but may slightly increase bioavailability.

Monitoring and Teaching Issues

Physical Assessment Assess for suicide ideation. Monitor respiratory and CNS status at beginning of therapy and periodically thereafter. Assess patient's physical and/or psychological dependence. Discontinue slowly after prolonged use

Patient Education Do not use alcohol, other prescription or OTC sedatives, tranquilizers, antihistamines, or pain medications without consulting prescriber. May cause dizziness, drowsiness, impaired judgment, vomiting, loss of appetite, or constipation. Report suicide ideation, unresolved nausea or vomiting, respiratory difficulty or shortness of breath, or unusual weakness.

Related Information

Opioid Analgesics *on page 2003*

- **Propoxyphene Hydrochloride** *see* Propoxyphene *on page 1522*
- **Propoxyphene Napsylate** *see* Propoxyphene *on page 1522*

Propranolol (proe PRAN oh lole)

U.S. Brand Names Inderal® LA; InnoPran XL®

Index Terms Propranolol Hydrochloride

Generic Availability (U.S.) Yes

Pharmacologic Category Antiarrhythmic Agent, Class II; Beta-Adrenergic Blocker, Nonselective

Medication Safety Issues

Sound-alike/look-alike issues:

Propranolol may be confused with prasugrel, Pravachol®, Propulsid®

Inderal® may be confused with Adderall®, Enduron®, Enduronyl®, Imdur®, Imuran®, Inderide®, Isordil®, Toradol®

Inderal® 40 may be confused with Enduronyl® Forte

High alert medication: The Institute for Safe Medication Practices (ISMP) includes this medication among its list of drugs which have a heightened risk of causing significant patient harm when used in error.

Significant differences exist between oral and I.V. dosing. Use caution when converting from one route of administration to another.

International issues:

Inderal [Canada and multiple international markets] and Inderal LA [U.S.] may be confused with Indiaral brand name for loperamide [France]

Pregnancy Risk Factor C

Lactation Enters breast milk/use caution (AAP rates "compatible"; AAP 2001 update pending)

Use Management of hypertension; angina pectoris; pheochromocytoma; essential tremor; supraventricular arrhythmias (such as atrial fibrillation and flutter, AV nodal re-entrant tachycardias), ventricular tachycardias (catecholamine-induced arrhythmias, digoxin toxicity); prevention of myocardial infarction; migraine headache prophylaxis; symptomatic treatment of hypertrophic subaortic stenosis (hypertrophic obstructive cardiomyopathy)

Unlabeled/Investigational Use Tremor due to Parkinson's disease; ethanol withdrawal; aggressive behavior (not recommended for dementia-associated aggression), anxiety, schizophrenia; antipsychotic-induced akathisia; primary and secondary prophylaxis of variceal hemorrhage; acute panic; thyrotoxicosis; tetralogy of Fallot (TOF) hypercyanotic spells

Mechanism of Action/Effect Nonselective beta-adrenergic blocker (class II antiarrhythmic); competitively blocks response to $beta_1$- and $beta_2$-adrenergic stimulation which results in decreases in heart rate, myocardial contractility, blood pressure, and myocardial oxygen demand; reduces portal pressure.

Contraindications Hypersensitivity to propranolol, beta-blockers, or any component of the formulation; uncompensated congestive heart failure (unless the failure is due to tachyarrhythmias being treated with propranolol), cardiogenic shock, severe sinus bradycardia or heart block greater than first-degree (except in patients with a functioning artificial pacemaker), severe hyperactive airway disease (asthma or COPD)

Warnings/Precautions Consider pre-existing conditions such as sick sinus syndrome before initiating. Administer cautiously in compensated heart failure and monitor for a worsening of the condition (efficacy of propranolol in HF has not been demonstrated). **[U.S. Boxed Warning]: Beta-blocker therapy should not be withdrawn abruptly (particularly in patients with CAD), but gradually tapered to avoid acute tachycardia, hypertension, and/or ischemia.** Use caution in patient with peripheral vascular disease (PVD). Use caution with concurrent use of beta-blockers and either verapamil or diltiazem; bradycardia or heart block can occur. Avoid concurrent I.V. use of both agents.

Use cautiously in patients with diabetes because it can mask prominent hypoglycemic symptoms. Use caution in hyperthyroidism since beta-blockade may mask signs of thyrotoxicosis. May alter thyroid-function tests. Use with caution in myasthenia gravis or psychiatric disease (may cause CNS depression). Use cautiously in renal and hepatic dysfunction; dosage adjustment required in hepatic impairment. Use care with anesthetic agents which decrease myocardial function. In general, patients with bronchospastic disease should not receive beta-blockers; if used at all, should be used cautiously with close monitoring. Adequate alpha-blockade is required prior to use of any beta-blocker for patients with untreated pheochromocytoma. May induce or exacerbate psoriasis. Use caution with history of severe anaphylaxis to allergens; patients taking beta-blockers may become more sensitive to repeated challenges. Treatment of anaphylaxis (eg, epinephrine) in patients taking beta-blockers may be ineffective or promote undesirable effects.

Drug Interactions

Metabolism/Transport Effects Substrate of CYP1A2 (major), 2C19 (minor), 2D6 (major), 3A4 (minor); **Inhibits** CYP1A2 (weak), CYP2D6 (weak), P-glycoprotein

Avoid Concomitant Use

Avoid concomitant use of Propranolol with any of the following: Methacholine; Topotecan

Decreased Effect

Propranolol may decrease the levels/effects of: Beta2-Agonists; Lacidipine; Theophylline Derivatives

The levels/effects of Propranolol may be decreased by: Alcohol (Ethyl); Barbiturates; Bile Acid Sequestrants; CYP1A2 Inducers (Strong); Herbs (Hypertensive Properties); Methylphenidate; Nonsteroidal Anti-Inflammatory Agents; Peginterferon Alfa-2b; Rifamycin Derivatives; Yohimbine

Increased Effect/Toxicity

Propranolol may increase the levels/effects of: Alpha-/Beta-Agonists (Direct-Acting); Alpha1-Blockers; Alpha2-Agonists; Amifostine; Antihypertensives; Antipsychotic Agents (Phenothiazines); Bupivacaine; Cardiac Glycosides; Colchicine; Dabigatran Etexilate; Everolimus; Fingolimod; Hypotensive Agents; Insulin; Lidocaine; Lidocaine (Systemic); Lidocaine (Topical); Mepivacaine; Methacholine; Midodrine; P-Glycoprotein Substrates; RiTUXimab; Rivaroxaban; Rizatriptan; Sulfonylureas; Topotecan; ZOLMitriptan

The levels/effects of Propranolol may be increased by: Acetylcholinesterase Inhibitors; Alcohol (Ethyl); Aminoquinolines (Antimalarial); Amiodarone; Anilidopiperidine Opioids; Antipsychotic Agents (Phenothiazines); Calcium Channel Blockers (Nondihydropyridine); Conivaptan; CYP1A2 Inhibitors (Moderate); CYP1A2 Inhibitors (Strong); CYP2D6 Inhibitors (Moderate); CYP2D6 Inhibitors (Strong); Darunavir; Diazoxide; Dipyridamole; Disopyramide; Dronedarone; FluvoxaMINE; Herbs (Hypotensive Properties); Lacidipine; MAO Inhibitors; Pentoxifylline; Phosphodiesterase 5 Inhibitors; Propafenone; Propoxyphene; Prostacyclin Analogues; QuiNIDine; Reserpine; Selective Serotonin Reuptake Inhibitors; Zileuton

Nutritional/Ethanol Interactions

Ethanol: Ethanol may increase or decrease plasma levels of propranolol. Reports are variable and have shown both enhanced as well as inhibited hepatic metabolism (of propranolol). Caution advised with consumption of alcohol and monitor for heart rate and/or blood pressure changes.

Food: Propranolol serum levels may be increased if taken with food. Protein-rich foods may increase bioavailability; a change in diet from high carbohydrate/low protein to low carbohydrate/high protein may result in increased oral clearance.

Cigarette: Smoking may decrease plasma levels of propranolol by increasing metabolism.

Herb/Nutraceutical: Avoid dong quai if using for hypertension (has estrogenic activity). Avoid bayberry, blue cohosh, cayenne, ephedra, ginger, ginseng (American), gotu kola, licorice, yohimbe (may worsen hypertension). Avoid black cohosh, california poppy, coleus, garlic, golden seal, hawthorn, mistletoe, periwinkle, quinine, shepherd's purse (have antihypertensive activity, may cause hypotension).

Lab Interactions Increased thyroxine (S)

Adverse Reactions Frequency not defined.

Cardiovascular: Angina, arterial insufficiency, AV conduction disturbance increased, bradycardia, cardiogenic shock, CHF, hypotension, impaired myocardial contractility, mesenteric arterial thrombosis (rare), Raynaud's syndrome, syncope

Central nervous system: Amnesia, catatonia, cognitive dysfunction, confusion, depression, dizziness, emotional lability, fatigue, hallucinations, hypersomnolence, insomnia, lethargy, lightheadedness, psychosis, vertigo, vivid dreams

Dermatologic: Alopecia, contact dermatitis, cutaneous ulcers, eczematous eruptions, erythema multiforme, exfoliative dermatitis, hyperkeratosis, nail changes, oculomucocutaneous reactions, pruritus, psoriasiform eruptions, rash, Stevens-Johnson syndrome, toxic epidermal necrolysis, ulcers, ulcerative lichenoid, urticaria

Endocrine & metabolic: Hyper-/hypoglycemia, hyperkalemia, hyperlipidemia

Gastrointestinal: Anorexia, cramping, constipation, diarrhea, ischemic colitis, nausea, stomach discomfort, vomiting

Genitourinary: Impotence, interstitial nephritis (rare), oliguria (rare), Peyronie's disease, proteinuria (rare)

Hematologic: Agranulocytosis, nonthrombocytopenic purpura, thrombocytopenia, thrombocytopenic purpura

Hepatic: Alkaline phosphatase increased, transaminases increased

Neuromuscular & skeletal: Arthropathy, carpal tunnel syndrome (rare), myotonus, paresthesia, polyarthritis, weakness

Ocular: Hyperemia of the conjunctiva, mydriasis, visual acuity decreased, visual disturbances, xerophthalmia

Renal: BUN increased

Respiratory: Bronchospasm, dyspnea, laryngospasm, pharyngitis, pulmonary edema, respiratory distress, wheezing

Miscellaneous: Anaphylactic/anaphylactoid allergic reaction, cold extremities, lupus-like syndrome (rare)

Pharmacodynamics/Kinetics

Onset of Action Beta-blockade: Oral: 1-2 hours

Duration of Action Immediate release: 6-12 hours; Extended-release formulations: ~24-27 hours

Absorption Oral: Rapid and complete

Bioavailability ~25% reaches systemic circulation due to high first-pass metabolism; protein-rich foods increase bioavailability by ~50%

Time to Peak Immediate release: 1-4 hours; Extended-release formulations: ~6-14 hours

Protein Binding Newborns: 68%; Adults: ~90% (S-isomer primarily to alpha$_1$-acid glycoprotein; R-isomer primarily to albumin)

Half-Life Elimination Neonates and Infants: Possible increased half-life; Children: 3.9-6.4 hours; Adults: Immediate release formulation: 3-6 hours; Extended-release formulations: 8-10 hours

Metabolism Hepatic via CYP2D6, and CYP1A2 to 4-hydroxypropranolol (active) and inactive compounds; extensive first-pass effect

Excretion Metabolites are excreted primarily in urine (96% to 99%); <1% excreted in urine as unchanged drug

Available Dosage Forms

Capsule, extended release, oral: 60 mg, 80 mg, 120 mg, 160 mg
InnoPran XL®: 80 mg, 120 mg

Capsule, sustained release, oral:
Inderal® LA: 60 mg, 80 mg, 120 mg, 160 mg

Injection, solution: 1 mg/mL (1 mL)

Injection, solution [preservative free]: 1 mg/mL (1 mL)

Solution, oral: 4 mg/mL (500 mL); 8 mg/mL (500 mL)

Tablet, oral: 10 mg, 20 mg, 40 mg, 60 mg, 80 mg

Dosing

Adult

Akathisia (unlabeled use): Oral: 30-120 mg/day in 2-3 divided doses

Essential tremor: Oral: 40 mg twice daily initially; maintenance doses: Usually 120-320 mg/day

Hypertension: Initial: Oral: 40 mg twice daily; increase dosage every 3-7 days; usual dose: 120-240 mg divided in 2-3 doses/day; maximum daily dose: 640 mg; usual dosage range (JNC 7): 40-160 mg/day in 2 divided doses

Extended release formulations:

Inderal® LA: Initial: 80 mg once daily; usual maintenance: 120-160 mg once daily; maximum daily dose: 640 mg; usual dosage range (JNC 7): 60-180 mg/day once daily

InnoPran XL®: Initial: 80 mg once daily at bedtime; if initial response is inadequate, may be increased at 2-3 week intervals to a maximum dose of 120 mg

Hypertrophic subaortic stenosis: Oral: 20-40 mg 3-4 times/day

Inderal® LA: 80-160 mg once daily

Migraine headache prophylaxis: Oral: Initial: 80 mg/day divided every 6-8 hours; increase by 20-40 mg/dose every 3-4 weeks to a maximum of 160-240 mg/day given in divided doses every 6-8 hours; if satisfactory response not achieved within 6 weeks of starting therapy, drug should be withdrawn gradually over several weeks

Inderal® LA: Initial: 80 mg once daily; effective dose range: 160-240 mg once daily

Pheochromocytoma: Oral: 30-60 mg/day in divided doses

Post-MI mortality reduction: Oral: 180-240 mg/day in 3-4 divided doses

Stable angina: Oral: 80-320 mg/day in doses divided 2-4 times/day

Inderal® LA: Initial: 80 mg once daily; maximum dose: 320 mg once daily

Tachyarrhythmias:

Oral: 10-30 mg/dose every 6-8 hours

I.V.: 1-3 mg/dose slow IVP; repeat every 2-5 minutes up to a total of 5 mg; titrate initial dose to desired response

or

0.5-1 mg over 1 minute; may repeat, if necessary, up to a total maximum dose of 0.1 mg/kg (ACLS guidelines, 2010)

Note: Once response achieved or maximum dose administered, additional doses should not be given for at least 4 hours.

Thyrotoxicosis (unlabeled use):

Oral: 10-40 mg/dose every 6 hours

I.V.: 1-3 mg/dose slow IVP as a single dose

Variceal hemorrhage prophylaxis (unlabeled use) (Garcia-Tsao, 2007): *Oral:*

Primary prophylaxis: Initial: 20 mg twice daily; adjust to maximal tolerated dose. **Note:** Risk factors for hemorrhage include Child-Pugh class B/C or variceal red wale markings on endoscopy.

Secondary prophylaxis: Initial: 20 mg twice daily; adjust to maximal tolerated dose

Geriatric

I.V.: Use caution; initiate at lower end of the dosing range.

Oral: Tachyarrhythmias: Initial: 10 mg twice daily; increase dosage every 3-7 days; usual dose range: 10-320 mg/day given in 1-2 divided doses. Refer to adult dosing for additional uses.

Pediatric

Hypertension (unlabeled use):

Oral: Initial: 0.5-1 mg/kg/day in divided doses every 6-12 hours; increase gradually every 5-7 days; maximum: 16 mg/kg/24 hours

Migraine headache prophylaxis (unlabeled use): Oral: Initial: 2-4 mg/kg/day **or**

≤35 kg: 10-20 mg 3 times/day

>35 kg: 20-40 mg 3 times/day

Tachyarrhythmias (unlabeled use):

Oral: Initial: 0.5-1 mg/kg/day in divided doses every 6-8 hours; titrate dosage upward every 3-7 days; usual dose: 2-6 mg/kg/day; higher doses may be needed; do not exceed 16 mg/kg/day or 60 mg/day

I.V.: 0.01-0.1 mg/kg/dose slow IVP over 10 minutes; maximum dose: 1 mg for infants; 3 mg for children

Thyrotoxicosis (unlabeled use): Oral:

2 mg/kg/day, divided every 6-8 hours, titrate to effective dose

Adolescents: Refer to adult dosing.

Hypercyanotic spells (TOF) (unlabeled use):

Oral: Palliation: Initial: 1 mg/kg/day every 6 hours; if ineffective, may increase dose after 1 week by 1 mg/kg/day to a maximum of 5 mg/kg/day, if patient becomes refractory, may increase slowly to a maximum of 10-15 mg/kg/day. Allow 24 hours between dosing changes.

I.V.: 0.01-0.2 mg/kg/dose infused over 10 minutes; maximum dose: 5 mg

Renal Impairment

Not dialyzable (0% to 5%); supplemental dose is not necessary.

Peritoneal dialysis effects: Supplemental dose is not necessary.

Hepatic Impairment Marked slowing of heart rate may occur in chronic liver disease with conventional doses; low initial dose and regular heart rate monitoring.

Administration

Oral Do not crush long-acting forms.

I.V. I.V. dose is much smaller than oral dose. When administered acutely for cardiac treatment, monitor ECG and blood pressure. May administer by rapid infusion (I.V. push) at a rate of 1 mg/minute or by slow infusion over ~30 minutes. Necessary monitoring for surgical patients who are unable to take oral beta-blockers (prolonged ileus) has not been defined. Some

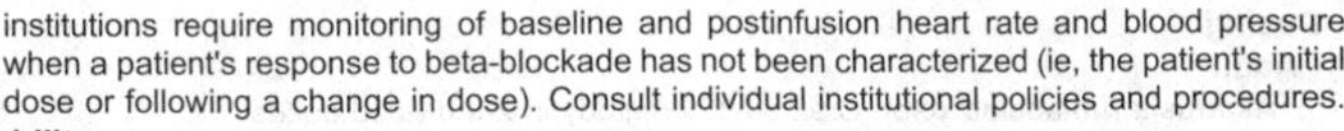

institutions require monitoring of baseline and postinfusion heart rate and blood pressure when a patient's response to beta-blockade has not been characterized (ie, the patient's initial dose or following a change in dose). Consult individual institutional policies and procedures.

Stability

Storage

Injection: Store at 20°C to 25°C (68°F to 77°F); protect from freezing or excessive heat. Once diluted, propranolol is stable for 24 hours at room temperature in D_5W or NS. Protect from light. Solution has a maximum stability at pH of 3 and decomposes rapidly in alkaline pH.

Capsule, tablet: Store at 20°C to 25°C (68°F to 77°F); protect from freezing or excessive heat. Protect from light and moisture.

Monitoring and Teaching Issues

Physical Assessment Assess potential for adverse interactions with cardiac medications, antihypertensives, antimalarials, antipsychotics, or antidiabetic agents. I.V. infusion usually requires hemodynamic monitoring; consult institution protocols. When discontinuing, drug must be tapered gradually over 2 weeks to avoid acute tachycardia, hypertension, and/or ischemia. Caution patients with diabetes to monitor blood glucose levels closely; beta-blockers can mask hypoglycemic symptoms.

Patient Education If administered by infusion, report immediately any pain, redness, or swelling at infusion site; palpitations or chest pain; dizziness; or difficulty breathing. **Oral:** If you have diabetes, monitor blood sugars carefully; beta-blockers may mask hypoglycemic symptoms. Do not crush or chew long-acting forms; swallow whole. You may experience orthostatic hypotension, dizziness, drowsiness, or blurred vision. May cause nausea, vomiting, or stomach discomfort. Report chest pain or palpitations; persistent dizziness or lethargy; any CNS symptoms (amnesia, change in cognition, confusion, depression, hallucinations, insomnia, vivid dreams); rash; difficulty breathing or wheezing; or weakness, pain, or loss of sensation in extremities.

Dietary Considerations Tablets (immediate release) should be taken on an empty stomach; capsules (extended release) may be taken with or without food, but should always be taken consistently (with food or on an empty stomach)

Geriatric Considerations Since bioavailability increased in about twofold in elderly patients, geriatrics may require lower maintenance doses. Also, as serum and tissue concentrations increase $beta_1$ selectivity diminishes. Beta-adrenergic blockade may result in less hemodynamic response than seen in younger adults due to alterations in the beta-adrenergic autonomic system. Studies indicate that despite decreased sensitivity to the chronotropic effects of beta-blockade with age, there appears to be an increased myocardial sensitivity to the negative inotropic effect during stress (ie, exercise). Controlled trials have shown the overall response rate for propranolol to be only 20% to 50% in elderly populations. Therefore, all beta-adrenergic blocking drugs may result in a decreased response as compared to younger adults. Due to propranolol's CNS penetration and nonselective action, it may not be the beta-blocker of choice for use in elderly.

Breast-Feeding Considerations Propranolol is excreted into breast milk with peak concentrations occurring ~2-3 hours after an oral dose. The inactive metabolites of propranolol have also been detected in breast milk. The manufacturer recommends that caution be exercised when administering propranolol to nursing women. Due to immature hepatic metabolism in newborns, breast-feeding infants should be monitored for adverse events.

Pregnancy Considerations Adverse events have been observed in some animal reproduction studies; therefore, the manufacturer classifies propranolol as pregnancy category C. Propranolol crosses the placenta and is measurable in the newborn serum following maternal use during pregnancy. In a cohort study, an increased risk of cardiovascular defects was observed following maternal use of beta-blockers during pregnancy. Intrauterine growth restriction (IUGR), small placentas, as well as fetal/neonatal bradycardia, hypoglycemia, and/or respiratory depression have been observed following *in utero* exposure to beta-blockers as a class. Adequate facilities for monitoring infants at birth should be available. Untreated chronic maternal hypertension and pre-eclampsia are also associated with adverse events in the fetus, infant, and mother. The peak maternal serum concentrations of propranolol and the active metabolite 4-hyrdoxypropranolol do not change during pregnancy; peak serum concentrations of naphthoxylactic acid are lower in the third trimester when compared to postpartum. Propranolol is recommended for use in the management of thyrotoxicosis in pregnancy. Propranolol has been evaluated for the treatment of hypertension in pregnancy, but other agents may be more appropriate for use. Propranolol has also been used in the management of hypertrophic obstructive cardiomyopathy in pregnancy and has been studied for use as an adjunctive agent in the management of dysfunctional labor (dystocia).

Related Information

Antiarrhythmic Drugs *on page 1978*

Beta-Blockers *on page 1990*

Propranolol and Hydrochlorothiazide

(proe PRAN oh lole & hye droe klor oh THYE a zide)

Index Terms Hydrochlorothiazide and Propranolol; Inderide

Generic Availability (U.S.) Yes

Pharmacologic Category Beta Blocker, Nonselective; Diuretic, Thiazide

Medication Safety Issues

Sound-alike/look-alike issues:

Inderide® may be confused with Inderal®

Pregnancy Risk Factor C

Lactation Enters breast milk/use caution

Use Management of hypertension

Available Dosage Forms

Tablet: Propranolol 40 mg and hydrochlorothiazide 25 mg; propranolol 80 mg and hydrochlorothiazide 25 mg

Dosing

Adult & Geriatric

Hypertension: Oral: Dose is individualized; typical dosages of **hydrochlorothiazide**: 12.5-50 mg/day; initial dose of **propranolol** 80 mg/day

Note: Daily dose of tablet form should be divided into 2 daily doses; may be used to maximum dosage of up to 160 mg of propranolol; higher dosages would result in higher than optimal thiazide dosages.

Monitoring and Teaching Issues

Physical Assessment See individual agents.

Patient Education See individual agents.

Related Information

Hydrochlorothiazide *on page 912*

Propranolol *on page 1522*

- **Propranolol Hydrochloride** *see* Propranolol *on page 1522*
- **Proprinal® [OTC]** *see* Ibuprofen *on page 938*
- **Propulsid®** *see* Cisapride *on page 381*
- **Propylene Glycol Diacetate, Acetic Acid, and Hydrocortisone** *see* Acetic Acid, Propylene Glycol Diacetate, and Hydrocortisone *on page 43*
- **2-Propylpentanoic Acid** *see* Valproic Acid *on page 1832*

Propylthiouracil (proe pil thye oh YOOR a sil)

Index Terms PTU (error-prone abbreviation)

Generic Availability (U.S.) Yes

Pharmacologic Category Antithyroid Agent; Thioamide

Medication Safety Issues

Sound-alike/look-alike issues:

Propylthiouracil may be confused with Purinethol®

PTU is an error-prone abbreviation (mistaken as mercaptopurine [Purinethol®; 6-MP])

Medication Guide Available Yes

Pregnancy Risk Factor D

Lactation Enters breast milk/AAP rates "compatible" (AAP 2001 update pending)

Use Adjunctive therapy in patients intolerant of methimazole to ameliorate hyperthyroidism symptoms in preparation for surgical treatment or radioactive iodine therapy; treatment of hyperthyroidism in patients intolerant of methimazole and not candidates for surgical/radiotherapy

Unlabeled/Investigational Use Management of thyrotoxic crisis

Available Dosage Forms

Tablet, oral: 50 mg

Dosing

Adult

Hyperthyroidism: Oral: Initial: 300 mg/day in 3 divided doses; 400 mg/day in patients with severe hyperthyroidism and/or very large goiters; an occasional patient will require 600-900 mg/day; usual maintenance: 100-150 mg/day

Thyrotoxic crisis/thyroid storm (unlabeled use): **Note:** Recommendations vary widely and have not been evaluated in comparative trials. Typical dosing is 800-1200 mg/day given as 200-300 mg every 4-6 hours; some clinicians advocate an initial loading dose of 600-1000 mg. After initial response, dose may be reduced gradually to a maintenance dosage (100-600 mg/day in divided doses) (Goldberg, 2003; Nayak, 2006).

Duration of therapy: Clinical improvement generally occurs in 1-3 months, after which dosage reduction may be employed (to prevent hypothyroidism), with discontinuation considered after 12-18 months of therapy. Thyroid function should be monitored every 2 months thereafter for 6 months until remission is confirmed, followed by annual evaluations (Cooper, 2005).

Pediatric

Hyperthyroidism: Oral: Children: Initial: 5-7 mg/kg/day **or** 150-200 mg/m²/day in divided doses every 8 hours **or**

6-10 years: 50-150 mg/day

>10 years: 150-300 mg/day

Note: Administer in equally divided doses every 8 hours. Adjust dosage to maintain T_3, T_4, and TSH levels in normal range; elevated T_3 may be sole indicator of inadequate treatment. Elevated TSH indicates excessive antithyroid treatment.

Renal Impairment Adjustment is not necessary.

Administration

Oral Administer at the same time in relation to meals each day, either always with meals or always between meals.

Monitoring and Teaching Issues

Laboratory Monitoring CBC with differential, prothrombin time, liver function tests (bilirubin, alkaline phosphatase, transaminases), and thyroid function tests (TSH, T_3, T_4) every 4-6 weeks until euthyroid; periodic blood counts are recommended for chronic therapy

Physical Assessment Monitor for rash, goiter, nausea, vomiting, leukopenia, agranulocytosis, anemia, jaundice, arthralgia, and CNS stimulation or depression.

Patient Education Take at the same time each day at around-the-clock intervals; take at the same time in relation to meals, either always with meals or always between meals. This drug may need to be taken for an extended period of time to achieve appropriate results and you may need periodic blood tests to assess effectiveness of therapy. May cause nausea or vomiting; constipation; or dizziness or drowsiness. Report rash, skin eruptions, or loss of hair; fever; unusual bleeding or bruising; unusual weight gain; unresolved headache or fever; yellowing of eyes or skin; changes in color of urine or feces; or joint or muscle pain or weakness.

- **2-Propylvaleric Acid** *see* Valproic Acid *on page 1832*
- **ProQuad®** *see* Measles, Mumps, Rubella, and Varicella Virus Vaccine *on page 1151*
- **Proquin® XR** *see* Ciprofloxacin (Systemic) *on page 375*
- **Proscar®** *see* Finasteride *on page 762*
- **Prostacyclin** *see* Epoprostenol *on page 643*
- **Prostaglandin E_1** *see* Alprostadil *on page 83*
- **Prostaglandin E_2** *see* Dinoprostone *on page 540*
- **Prostaglandin F_2** *see* Carboprost Tromethamine *on page 299*
- **Prostin E2®** *see* Dinoprostone *on page 540*
- **Prostin VR Pediatric®** *see* Alprostadil *on page 83*

Protamine Sulfate (PROE ta meen SUL fate)

Generic Availability (U.S.) Yes

Pharmacologic Category Antidote

Medication Safety Issues

Sound-alike/look-alike issues:

Protamine may be confused with ProAmatine®, Protonix®, Protopam®, Protropin®

Pregnancy Risk Factor C

Lactation Excretion in breast milk unknown

Use Treatment of heparin overdosage; neutralize heparin during surgery or dialysis procedures

Unlabeled/Investigational Use Treatment of low molecular weight heparin (LMWH) overdose

Available Dosage Forms

Injection, solution [preservative free]: 10 mg/mL (5 mL, 25 mL)

Dosing

Adult & Geriatric

Heparin neutralization: I.V.: Protamine dosage is determined by the dosage of heparin; 1 mg of protamine neutralizes 90 USP units of heparin (lung) and 115 USP units of heparin (intestinal); maximum dose: 50 mg

Heparin overdosage, following intravenous administration: I.V.: Since blood heparin concentrations decrease rapidly **after** administration, adjust the protamine dosage depending upon the duration of time since heparin administration as follows: See table.

Time Elapsed	Dose of Protamine (mg) to Neutralize 100 units of Heparin
Immediate	1-1.5
30-60 min	0.5-0.75
>2 h	0.25-0.375

Heparin overdosage, following SubQ injection: I.V.: 1-1.5 mg protamine per 100 units heparin; this may be done by a portion of the dose (eg, 25-50 mg) given slowly I.V. followed by the remaining portion as a continuous infusion over 8-16 hours (the expected absorption time of the SubQ heparin dose)

LMWH overdose (unlabeled use):

Enoxaparin: 1 mg protamine for each mg of enoxaparin; if PTT prolonged 2-4 hours after first dose, consider additional dose of 0.5 mg for each mg of enoxaparin.

Dalteparin or tinzaparin: 1 mg protamine for each 100 anti-Xa int. units of dalteparin or tinzaparin; if PTT prolonged 2-4 hours after first dose, consider additional dose of 0.5 mg for each 100 anti-Xa int. units of dalteparin or tinzaparin.

Note: Antifactor Xa activity never completely neutralized (maximum: ~60% to 75%). Excessive protamine doses may worsen bleeding potential.

Pediatric Refer to adult dosing.

Administration

I.V. For I.V. use only. Administer slow IVP (50 mg over 10 minutes). Rapid I.V. infusion causes hypotension. Reconstitute vial with 5 mL sterile water. Resulting solution equals 10 mg/mL. Inject without further dilution over 1-3 minutes; maximum of 50 mg in any 10-minute period.

Monitoring and Teaching Issues

Laboratory Monitoring Coagulation test, aPTT or ACT

Patient Education Report any respiratory difficulty, rash or flushing, feeling of warmth, tingling or numbness, dizziness, or disorientation.

◆ **Protease, Lipase, and Amylase** *see* Pancrelipase *on page 1400*

◆ **Protein C (Activated), Human, Recombinant** *see* Drotrecogin Alfa *on page 594*

◆ **Protein-Bound Paclitaxel** *see* Paclitaxel (Protein Bound) *on page 1390*

◆ **Protonix®** *see* Pantoprazole *on page 1405*

◆ **Protopic®** *see* Tacrolimus (Topical) *on page 1699*

◆ **Proventil® HFA** *see* Albuterol *on page 58*

◆ **Provera®** *see* MedroxyPROGESTERone *on page 1154*

◆ **Provigil®** *see* Modafinil *on page 1247*

◆ **PROzac®** *see* FLUoxetine *on page 789*

◆ **PROzac® Weekly™** *see* FLUoxetine *on page 789*

◆ **PRP-OMP** *see Haemophilus* b Conjugate Vaccine *on page 893*

◆ **PRP-T** *see Haemophilus* b Conjugate Vaccine *on page 893*

◆ **Prudoxin™** *see* Doxepin (Topical) *on page 578*

◆ **23PS** *see* Pneumococcal Polysaccharide Vaccine (Polyvalent) *on page 1471*

◆ **PS-341** *see* Bortezomib *on page 226*

Pseudoephedrine (soo doe e FED rin)

U.S. Brand Names Children's Nasal Decongestant [OTC]; Genaphed™ [OTC]; Oranyl [OTC]; Silfedrine Children's [OTC]; Sudafed® 12 Hour [OTC]; Sudafed® 24 Hour [OTC]; Sudafed® Children's [OTC]; Sudafed® Maximum Strength Nasal Decongestant [OTC]; Sudo-Tab® [OTC]; Sudogest 12 Hour [OTC]; SudoGest Children's [OTC]; SudoGest [OTC]

Index Terms *d*-Isoephedrine Hydrochloride; Pseudoephedrine Hydrochloride; Pseudoephedrine Sulfate; Sudafed

Generic Availability (U.S.) Yes: Excludes extended release products

Pharmacologic Category Alpha/Beta Agonist

Medication Safety Issues

Sound-alike/look-alike issues:

Sudafed® may be confused with sotalol, Sudafed PE™, Sufenta®

Lactation Enters breast milk (AAP rates "compatible"; AAP 2001 update pending)

Use Temporary symptomatic relief of nasal congestion due to common cold, upper respiratory allergies, and sinusitis; also promotes nasal or sinus drainage

Available Dosage Forms For available OTC formulations, consult specific product labeling.

Dosing

Adult Nasal congestion: General dosing guidelines: Oral: Immediate release: 60 mg every 4-6 hours; Extended release: 120 mg every 12 hours **or** 240 mg every 24 hours; maximum: 240 mg/24 hours

Geriatric Nasal congestion: Use caution in this population; initiate using immediate release formulation: 30-60 mg every 6 hours as needed

Pediatric Nasal congestion: General dosing guidelines: Oral:

Children:

4-5 years: 15 mg every 4-6 hours; maximum: 60 mg/24 hours

6-12 years: 30 mg every 4-6 hours; maximum: 120 mg/24 hours

>12 years: Refer to adult dosing.

Renal Impairment Consider reducing dose.

Administration

Oral Do not crush extended release drug product, swallow whole. May administer with or without food. Sudafed® 24 Hour tablet may not completely dissolve and appear in stool

Monitoring and Teaching Issues

Patient Education Do not chew or crush extended release forms. Maintain adequate hydration unless instructed to restrict fluid intake. You may experience nervousness, insomnia, dizziness, or drowsiness. Report persistent CNS changes (dizziness, tremor, or agitation), respiratory difficulty, chest pain, palpitations, rapid heartbeat; muscle tremor, or lack of improvement or worsening of condition.

Related Information

Pharmacotherapy of Urinary Incontinence *on page 2071*

◆ **Pseudoephedrine and Fexofenadine** *see* Fexofenadine and Pseudoephedrine *on page 759*

◆ **Pseudoephedrine and Loratadine** *see* Loratadine and Pseudoephedrine *on page 1129*

◆ **Pseudoephedrine Hydrochloride** *see* Pseudoephedrine *on page 1529*

◆ **Pseudoephedrine Sulfate** *see* Pseudoephedrine *on page 1529*

◆ **Pteroylglutamic Acid** *see* Folic Acid *on page 812*

◆ **PTG** *see* Teniposide *on page 1728*

◆ **PTU (error-prone abbreviation)** *see* Propylthiouracil *on page 1527*

◆ **Pulmicort Flexhaler®** *see* Budesonide (Systemic, Oral Inhalation) *on page 235*

◆ **Pulmicort Respules®** *see* Budesonide (Systemic, Oral Inhalation) *on page 235*

◆ **Pulmozyme®** *see* Dornase Alfa *on page 574*

◆ **Purified Chick Embryo Cell** *see* Rabies Vaccine *on page 1546*

◆ **Purinethol®** *see* Mercaptopurine *on page 1173*

Pyrazinamide (peer a ZIN a mide)

Index Terms Pyrazinoic Acid Amide

Generic Availability (U.S.) Yes

Pharmacologic Category Antitubercular Agent

Pregnancy Risk Factor C

Lactation Enters breast milk/use caution

Use Adjunctive treatment of tuberculosis in combination with other antituberculosis agents

Available Dosage Forms

Tablet, oral: 500 mg

Dosing

Adult Tuberculosis treatment: Oral: **Note:** Used as part of a multidrug regimen. Treatment regimens consist of an initial 2-month phase, followed by a continuation phase of 4 or 7 additional months; pyrazinamide is administered in the initial phase of treatment.

Suggested dosing based on lean body weight (Blumberg, 2003; CDC, 2003):

Daily therapy:

40-55 kg: 1000 mg
56-75 kg: 1500 mg
76-90 kg: 2000 mg (maximum dose regardless of weight)

Twice weekly directly observed therapy (DOT):

40-55 kg: 2000 mg
56-75 kg: 3000 mg
76-90 kg: 4000 mg (maximum dose regardless of weight)

Three times/week DOT:

40-55 kg: 1500 mg
56-75 kg: 2500 mg
76-90 kg: 3000 mg (maximum dose regardless of weight)

Pediatric Tuberculosis treatment: Oral: **Note:** Used as part of a multidrug regimen. Treatment regimens consist of an initial 2-month phase, followed by a continuation phase of 4 or 7 additional months; pyrazinamide is administered in the initial phase of treatment.

HIV negative (CDC, 2003):

Daily therapy: 15-30 mg/kg/day (maximum: 2 g/day)
Twice weekly directly observed therapy (DOT): 50 mg/kg/dose (maximum: 2 g/dose)

HIV-exposed/-infected: Daily therapy: 20-40 mg/kg/dose once daily (maximum: 2 g/day) (CDC, 2009)

Renal Impairment Adults: Cl_{cr} <30 mL/minute or receiving hemodialysis: Treatment of TB: 25-35 mg/kg/dose 3 times per week administered after dialysis (Blumberg, 2003; CDC, 2003)

Monitoring and Teaching Issues

Laboratory Monitoring Periodic liver function, serum uric acid, sputum culture, chest x-ray 2-3 months into treatment and at completion

Physical Assessment Assess patient history for use cautions and evaluate any history of alcohol intake prior to beginning treatment. Administer with at least one other effective agent for tuberculosis (other than rifampin). Evaluate results of chest x-ray regularly.

Patient Education You will need regular medical follow-up and laboratory tests while taking this medication. May cause nausea or loss of appetite. Report change in color of urine, pale stools, easy bruising or bleeding, blood in urine or difficulty urinating, yellowing of skin or eyes, extreme joint pain, unusual fever, or unresolved nausea or vomiting.

◆ **Pyrazinoic Acid Amide** *see* Pyrazinamide *on page 1530*

Pyrethrins and Piperonyl Butoxide (pye RE thrins & pi PER oh nil byo TOKS ide)

U.S. Brand Names A-200® Lice Treatment Kit [OTC]; A-200® Maximum Strength [OTC]; Licide® [OTC]; Pronto® Complete Lice Removal System [OTC]; Pronto® Plus Lice Killing Mousse Plus Vitamin E [OTC]; Pronto® Plus Lice Killing Mousse Shampoo Plus Natural Extracts and Oils [OTC]; Pronto® Plus Warm Oil Treatment and Conditioner [OTC]; RID® Maximum Strength [OTC]

Index Terms Piperonyl Butoxide and Pyrethrins

Generic Availability (U.S.) Yes: Shampoo

Pharmacologic Category Antiparasitic Agent, Topical; Pediculocide; Shampoo, Pediculocide

Pregnancy Risk Factor C

Use Treatment of *Pediculus humanus* infestations (head lice, body lice, pubic lice, and their eggs)

Available Dosage Forms

Kit:

A-200® Lice Treatment Kit [OTC]:
Shampoo: Pyrethrins 0.33% and piperonyl butoxide 4% (120 mL)
Solution: Permethrin 0.5% (180 mL)

Pronto® Complete Lice Removal System [OTC]:
Shampoo: Pyrethrins 0.33% and piperonyl butoxide 4% (60 mL)
Solution, topical: Benzalkonium chloride 0.1% (60 mL)

Oil, topical:
Pronto® Plus Warm Oil Treatment and Conditioner [OTC]: Pyrethrins 0.33% and piperonyl butoxide 4% (36 mL)

Shampoo: Pyrethrins 0.33% and piperonyl butoxide 4% (60 mL, 120 mL)
A-200® Maximum Strength [OTC]: Pyrethrins 0.33% and piperonyl butoxide 4% (60 mL, 120 mL)
Licide® [OTC], Pronto® Plus Lice Killing Mousse Shampoo Plus Vitamin E [OTC]: Pyrethrins 0.33% and piperonyl butoxide 4% (120 mL)
Pronto® Plus Lice Killing Mousse Shampoo Plus Natural Extracts and Oils [OTC]: Pyrethrins 0.33% and piperonyl butoxide 4% (60 mL)
Pronto® Plus Lice Killing Mousse Shampoo Plus Vitamin E [OTC]: Pyrethrins 0.33% and piperonyl butoxide 4% (120 mL)
RID® Maximum Strength [OTC]: Pyrethrins 0.33% and piperonyl butoxide 4% (60 mL, 120 mL, 180 mL, 240 mL)

Dosing

Adult & Geriatric Treatment of *Pediculus humanus* infestations: *Topical products:*
Apply enough solution to completely wet infested area, including hair
Allow to remain on area for 10 minutes
Wash and rinse with large amounts of warm water.
Use fine-toothed comb to remove lice and eggs from hair
Shampoo hair to restore body and luster
Treatment may be repeated if necessary once in a 24-hour period
Repeat treatment in 7-10 days to kill newly hatched lice
Note: Keep out of eyes when rinsing hair; protect eyes with a wash cloth or towel

Pediatric Head lice, body lice: Children: Refer to adult dosing.

Administration

Topical For external use only. Avoid touching eyes, mouth, or other mucous membranes.

◆ **Pyri-500 [OTC]** *see* Pyridoxine *on page* 1532
◆ **Pyridium®** *see* Phenazopyridine *on page* 1446

Pyridostigmine (peer id oh STIG meen)

U.S. Brand Names Mestinon®; Mestinon® Timespan®; Regonol®
Index Terms Pyridostigmine Bromide
Generic Availability (U.S.) Yes: Tablet
Pharmacologic Category Acetylcholinesterase Inhibitor
Medication Safety Issues
Sound-alike/look-alike issues:
Pyridostigmine may be confused with physostigmine
Mestinon® may be confused with Metatensin®
Regonol® may be confused with Reglan®, Renagel®
Pregnancy Risk Factor B
Lactation Enters breast milk/compatible
Use Symptomatic treatment of myasthenia gravis; antagonism of nondepolarizing neuromuscular blockers
Military use: Pretreatment for Soman nerve gas exposure
Available Dosage Forms
Injection, solution:
Regonol®: 5 mg/mL (2 mL)
Syrup, oral:
Mestinon®: 60 mg/5 mL (480 mL)
Tablet, oral: 60 mg
Mestinon®: 60 mg
Tablet, sustained release, oral:
Mestinon® Timespan®: 180 mg

Dosing

Adult & Geriatric

Myasthenia gravis:
Oral: Highly individualized dosing ranges: 60-1500 mg/day, usually 600 mg/day divided into 5-6 doses, spaced to provide maximum relief
Sustained release formulation: Highly individualized dosing ranges: 180-540 mg once or twice daily (doses separated by at least 6 hours); **Note:** Most clinicians reserve sustained release dosage form for bedtime dose only.
I.M. or slow I.V. push: To supplement oral dosage pre- and postoperatively during labor and postpartum, during myasthenic crisis, or when oral therapy is impractical): ~1/30th of oral dose; observe patient closely for cholinergic reactions
I.V. infusion: To supplement oral dosage pre- and postoperatively, during labor and postpartum, during myasthenic crisis, or when oral therapy is impractical): Initial: 2 mg/hour with gradual titration in increments of 0.5-1 mg/hour, up to a maximum rate of 4 mg/hour

Reversal of nondepolarizing muscle relaxants: *I.V.:* 0.1-0.25 mg/kg/dose; 10-20 mg is usually sufficient (full recovery usually occurs ≤15 minutes, but ≥30 minutes may be required).
Note: Atropine sulfate (0.6-1.2 mg) I.V. immediately prior to pyridostigmine to minimize side effects

Pretreatment for Soman nerve gas exposure (military use): *Oral:* 30 mg every 8 hours beginning several hours prior to exposure; discontinue at first sign of nerve agent exposure, then begin atropine and pralidoxime

Pediatric

Myasthenia gravis:

Oral: Children: 7 mg/kg/24 hours divided into 5-6 doses. Most clinicians reserve sustained release dosage form for bedtime dose only.

I.M., slow I.V. push: Children: 0.05-0.15 mg/kg/dose

Reversal of nondepolarizing muscle relaxants: I.V.: Children: Dosing range: 0.1-0.25 mg/kg/dose (full recovery usually occurs ≤15 minutes, but ≥30 minutes may be required).

Note: Atropine sulfate (0.6-1.2 mg) I.V. immediately prior to pyridostigmine to minimize side effects:

Renal Impairment Lower dosages may be required due to prolonged elimination; no specific recommendations have been published.

Administration

Oral Do **not** crush sustained release tablet.

Monitoring and Teaching Issues

Physical Assessment When used to reverse neuromuscular block (anesthesia or excessive acetylcholine), monitor patient safety until full return of neuromuscular functioning. Assess bladder and sphincter adequacy prior to treatment. Monitor for cholinergic crisis.

Patient Education This drug will not cure myasthenia gravis, but may help reduce symptoms. Take extended release tablets at bedtime; do not chew or crush extended release tablets. May cause dizziness, drowsiness, or hypotension; vomiting or loss of appetite; or diarrhea. Report persistent abdominal discomfort; significantly increased salivation, sweating, tearing, or urination; flushed skin; chest pain or palpitations; acute headache; unresolved diarrhea; excessive fatigue, insomnia, dizziness, or depression; increased muscle, joint, or body pain; vision changes or blurred vision; or shortness of breath or wheezing.

◆ **Pyridostigmine Bromide** *see* Pyridostigmine *on page 1531*

Pyridoxine (peer i DOKS een)

U.S. Brand Names Aminoxin® [OTC]; Pyri-500 [OTC]

Index Terms B6; B_6; Pyridoxine Hydrochloride; Vitamin B_6

Generic Availability (U.S.) Yes

Pharmacologic Category Vitamin, Water Soluble

Medication Safety Issues

Sound-alike/look-alike issues:

Pyridoxine may be confused with paroxetine, pralidoxime, Pyridium®

International issues:

Doxal® [Brazil] may be confused with Doxil® which is a brand name for doxorubicin in the U.S.

Doxal® [Brazil]: Brand name for doxycycline in Austria; brand name for pyridoxine/thiamine combination in Brazil; brand name for doxepin in Finland

Pregnancy Risk Factor A

Lactation Enters breast milk/compatible (AAP rates "compatible"; AAP 2001 update pending)

Use Prevention and treatment of vitamin B_6 deficiency, pyridoxine-dependent seizures in infants

Unlabeled/Investigational Use Treatment and prophylaxis of neurological toxicities (ie, seizures, coma) associated with isoniazid, hydrazine, and Gyromitrin-containing mushroom (false morel) overdose/toxicity

Available Dosage Forms

Capsule, oral: 50 mg, 250 mg

Aminoxin® [OTC]: 20 mg

Injection, solution: 100 mg/mL (1 mL)

Liquid, oral: 200 mg/5 mL (120 mL)

Tablet, oral: 25 mg, 50 mg, 100 mg, 250 mg, 500 mg

Tablet, sustained release, oral:

Pyri-500 [OTC]: 500 mg

Dosing

Adult & Geriatric

Recommended daily allowance (RDA):

Male: 1.7-2 mg

Female: 1.4-1.6 mg

Dietary deficiency: Oral: 10-20 mg/day for 3 weeks

Drug-induced neuritis (eg, isoniazid, hydralazine, penicillamine, cycloserine): Oral:

Treatment: 100-200 mg/24 hours

Prophylaxis: 25-100 mg/24 hours

Treatment of isoniazid-induced seizures and/or coma (unlabeled use): I.V.:

Acute ingestion of known amount: Initial: A total dose of pyridoxine equal to the amount of isoniazid ingested (maximum dose: 5 g); administer at a rate of 0.5-1 g/minute until seizures stop or the maximum initial dose has been administered; may repeat every 5-10 minutes as needed to control persistent seizure activity and/or CNS toxicity. If seizures stop prior to the administration of the calculated initial dose, infuse the remaining pyridoxine over 4-6 hours (Howland, 2006; Morrow, 2006).

Acute ingestion of unknown amount: Initial: 5 g; administer at a rate of 0.5-1 g/minute; may repeat every 5-10 minutes as needed to control persistent seizure activity and/or CNS toxicity (Howland, 2006; Morrow, 2006)

Prevention of isoniazid-induced seizures and/or coma (unlabeled use): I.V.: Asymptomatic patients who present within 2 hours of ingesting a potentially toxic amount of isoniazid should receive a prophylactic dose of pyridoxine (Boyer, 2006). Dosing recommendations are the same as for the treatment of symptomatic patients.

Treatment of acute hydrazine toxicity (unlabeled use): I.V.: A total dose of 25 mg/kg should be given over 15-30 minutes

Treatment of seizures from acute Gyromitrin-containing mushroom toxicity (unlabeled use; Diaz, 2005): I.V.: 25 mg/kg over 15-30 minutes; repeat dose as needed to control seizures

Pediatric

Recommended daily allowance (RDA):
1-3 years: 0.9 mg
4-6 years: 1.3 mg
7-10 years: 1.6 mg

Pyridoxine-dependent Infants:
Oral: 2-100 mg/day
I.M., I.V., SubQ: 10-100 mg

Dietary deficiency: Oral: 5-25 mg/24 hours for 3 weeks, then 1.5-2.5 mg/day in multiple vitamin product

Drug-induced neuritis (eg, isoniazid, hydralazine, penicillamine, cycloserine): Oral:
Treatment: 10-50 mg/24 hours
Prophylaxis: 1-2 mg/kg/24 hours

Treatment of isoniazid-induced seizures and/or coma (unlabeled use): I.V.:

Acute ingestion of known amount: Initial: A total dose of pyridoxine equal to the amount of isoniazid ingested (maximum dose: 70 mg/kg, up to 5 g); administer at a rate of 0.5-1 g/minute until seizures stop or the maximum initial dose has been administered; may repeat every 5-10 minutes as needed to control persistent seizure activity and/or CNS toxicity. If seizures stop prior to the administration of the calculated initial dose, infuse the remaining pyridoxine over 4-6 hours (Howland, 2006; Morrow, 2006).

Acute ingestion of unknown amount: Initial: 70 mg/kg (maximum dose: 5 g); administer at a rate of 0.5-1 g/minute; may repeat every 5-10 minutes as needed to control persistent seizure activity and/or CNS toxicity (Howland, 2006; Morrow, 2006; Santucci, 1999)

Prevention of isoniazid-induced seizures and/or coma (unlabeled use): Refer to adult dosing.

Treatment of seizures from acute Gyromitrin-containing mushroom toxicity (unlabeled use; Diaz, 2005): Refer to adult dosing.

Administration

I.M. Burning may occur at the injection site after I.M. or SubQ administration.

I.V. Seizures have occurred following I.V. administration of very large doses.

Isoniazid toxicity (unlabeled use): Initial doses should be administered at a rate of 0.5-1 g/minute. If the parenteral formulation is not available, anecdotal reports suggest that pyridoxine tablets may be crushed and made into a slurry and given at the same dose orally or via nasogastric (NG) tube (Boyer, 2006). Oral administration is not recommended for acutely poisoned patients with seizure activity.

Monitoring and Teaching Issues

Laboratory Monitoring For treatment of isoniazid, hydrazine, or Gyromitrin-containing mushroom toxicity: Anion gap, arterial blood gases, electrolytes

Physical Assessment Provide patient appropriate dietary instructions.

Patient Education Do not exceed recommended intake of dietary B_6. You may experience burning or pain at injection site; notify prescriber if this persists.

◆ **Pyridoxine Hydrochloride** *see* Pyridoxine *on page* 1532
◆ **Quadrivalent Human Papillomavirus Vaccine** *see* Papillomavirus (Types 6, 11, 16, 18) Vaccine (Human, Recombinant) *on page* 1408
◆ **Qualaquin®** *see* QuiNINE *on page* 1542
◆ **Quasense®** *see* Ethinyl Estradiol and Levonorgestrel *on page* 699
◆ **Quelicin®** *see* Succinylcholine *on page* 1683
◆ **Questran®** *see* Cholestyramine Resin *on page* 363
◆ **Questran® Light** *see* Cholestyramine Resin *on page* 363

QUEtiapine (kwe TYE a peen)

U.S. Brand Names SEROquel XR®; SEROquel®

Index Terms Quetiapine Fumarate

Generic Availability (U.S.) No

Pharmacologic Category Antipsychotic Agent, Atypical

Medication Safety Issues

Sound-alike/look-alike issues:
QUEtiapine may be confused with OLANZapine
SEROquel® may be confused with Serentil®, Serzone®, SINEquan®

Medication Guide Available Yes

Pregnancy Risk Factor C

Lactation Enters breast milk/use caution

Use Treatment of schizophrenia; treatment of acute manic or mixed episodes associated with bipolar I disorder (as monotherapy or in combination with lithium or divalproex); maintenance treatment of bipolar I disorder (in combination with lithium or divalproex); treatment of acute depressive episodes associated with bipolar disorder; adjunctive treatment of major depressive disorder

Unlabeled/Investigational Use Autism; delirium in the critically-ill patient; psychosis/agitation related to Alzheimer's dementia

Mechanism of Action/Effect Quetiapine is a dibenzothiazepine atypical antipsychotic. It has been proposed that this drug's antipsychotic activity is mediated through a combination of dopamine type 2 and serotonin type 2 antagonism.

Antagonism at receptors other than dopamine and 5-HT_2 with similar receptor affinities may explain some of the other effects of quetiapine. The drug's antagonism of histamine H_1-receptors may explain the somnolence observed. The drug's antagonism of adrenergic alpha$_1$-receptors may explain the orthostatic hypotension observed.

Contraindications There are no contraindications listed in manufacturers labeling.

Canadian labeling: Hypersensitivity to quetiapine or any component of the formulation

Warnings/Precautions [U.S. Boxed Warning]: Antidepressants increase the risk of suicidal thinking and behavior in children, adolescents, and young adults (18-24 years of age) with major depressive disorder (MDD) and other psychiatric disorders; consider risk prior to prescribing. Short-term studies did not show an increased risk in patients >24 years of age and showed a decreased risk in patients ≥65 years. Closely monitor all patients for clinical worsening, suicidality, or unusual changes in behavior; particularly during the initial 1-2 months of therapy or during periods of dosage adjustments (increased or decreases); the patient's family or caregiver should be instructed to closely observe the patient and communicate condition with healthcare provider. A medication guide concerning the use of antidepressants should be dispensed with each prescription.

[U.S. Boxed Warning]: Elderly patients with dementia-related psychosis treated with antipsychotics are at an increased risk of death compared to placebo. Most deaths appeared to be either cardiovascular (eg, heart failure, sudden death) or infectious (eg, pneumonia) in nature. Quetiapine is not approved for the treatment of dementia-related psychosis.

Leukopenia, neutropenia, and agranulocytosis (sometimes fatal) have been reported in clinical trials and postmarketing reports with antipsychotic use; presence of risk factors (eg, pre-existing low WBC or history of drug-induced leuko-/neutropenia) should prompt periodic blood count assessment. Discontinue therapy at first signs of blood dyscrasias or if absolute neutrophil count <1000/mm^3.

May be sedating, use with caution in disorders where CNS depression is a feature. Use with caution in Parkinson's disease. May induce orthostatic hypotension associated with dizziness, tachycardia, and, in some cases, syncope, especially during the initial dose titration period. Should be used with particular caution in patients with known cardiovascular disease (history of MI or ischemic heart disease, heart failure, or conduction abnormalities), cerebrovascular disease, or conditions that predispose to hypotension. Esophageal dysmotility and aspiration have been associated with antipsychotic use; use with caution in patients at risk of aspiration pneumonia (eg, Alzheimer's disease). Development of cataracts has been observed in animal studies; lens changes have been observed in humans during long-term treatment. Lens examination on initiation of therapy and every 6 months thereafter is recommended.

Due to anticholinergic effects, use with caution in patients with decreased gastrointestinal motility, urinary retention, BPH, xerostomia, visual problems, and narrow-angle glaucoma. Relative to other antipsychotics, quetiapine has a moderate potency of cholinergic blockade. May cause extrapyramidal symptoms (EPS), pseudoparkinsonism, and/or tardive dyskinesia. Risk of dystonia (and probably other EPS) may be greater with increased doses, use of conventional antipsychotics, males, and younger patients. Impaired core body temperature regulation may occur; caution with strenuous exercise, heat exposure, dehydration, and concomitant medication possessing anticholinergic effects. Neuroleptic malignant syndrome (NMS) is a potentially fatal symptom complex that has been reported in association with administration of antipsychotic drugs. Clinical manifestations of NMS are hyperpyrexia, muscle rigidity, altered mental status, and evidence of autonomic instability (irregular pulse or blood pressure, tachycardia, diaphoresis, and cardiac dysrhythmia). Management of NMS should include immediate discontinuation of antipsychotic drugs and other drugs not essential to concurrent therapy, intensive symptomatic treatment and medication monitoring, and treatment of any concomitant medical problems for which specific treatment are available.

Use caution in patients with a history of seizures. May cause decreases in total free thyroxine, elevations of liver enzymes, cholesterol levels, and/or triglyceride increases. Rare cases of priapism have been reported. May increase prolactin levels; clinical significance of hyperprolactinemia in patients with breast cancer or other prolactin-dependent tumors is unknown.

May cause hyperglycemia; in some cases may be extreme and associated with ketoacidosis, hyperosmolar coma, or death. Use with caution in patients with diabetes or other disorders of glucose regulation; monitor for worsening of glucose control. Significant weight gain has been observed with antipsychotic therapy; incidence varies with product. Monitor waist circumference and BMI. Patients using immediate release tablets may be switched to extended release tablets at the same total daily dose taken once daily. Dosage adjustments may be necessary based on response and tolerability. May cause withdrawal symptoms (rare) with abrupt cessation; gradually taper dose during discontinuation.

Drug Interactions

Metabolism/Transport Effects Substrate of CYP2D6 (minor), 3A4 (major)

Avoid Concomitant Use

Avoid concomitant use of QUEtiapine with any of the following: Artemether; Dronedarone; Lumefantrine; Metoclopramide; Nilotinib; Pimozide; QuiNINE; Tetrabenazine; Thioridazine; Toremifene; Vandetanib; Ziprasidone

Decreased Effect

QUEtiapine may decrease the levels/effects of: Amphetamines; Anti-Parkinson's Agents (Dopamine Agonist); Quinagolide

The levels/effects of QUEtiapine may be decreased by: CYP3A4 Inducers (Strong); Deferasirox; Herbs (CYP3A4 Inducers); Lithium formulations; Peginterferon Alfa-2b; Phenytoin

Increased Effect/Toxicity

QUEtiapine may increase the levels/effects of: Alcohol (Ethyl); Anticholinergics; CNS Depressants; Dronedarone; Methylphenidate; Pimozide; QTc-Prolonging Agents; QuiNINE; Tetrabenazine; Thioridazine; Toremifene; Vandetanib; Ziprasidone

The levels/effects of QUEtiapine may be increased by: Acetylcholinesterase Inhibitors (Central); Alfuzosin; Artemether; Chloroquine; Ciprofloxacin; Ciprofloxacin (Systemic); Conivaptan; CYP3A4 Inhibitors (Moderate); CYP3A4 Inhibitors (Strong); Gadobutrol; Lithium formulations; Lumefantrine; Methylphenidate; Metoclopramide; Nilotinib; Pramlintide; QuiNINE; Tetrabenazine

Nutritional/Ethanol Interactions

Ethanol: Avoid ethanol (may cause excessive impairment in cognition/motor function).

Food: In healthy volunteers, administration of quetiapine (immediate release) with food resulted in an increase in the peak serum concentration and AUC by 25% and 15%, respectively, compared to the fasting state. Administration of the extended release formulation with a high-fat meal (~800-1000 calories) resulted in an increase in peak serum concentration by 44% to 52% and AUC by 20% to 22% for the 50 mg and 300 mg tablets; administration with a light meal (≤300 calories) had no significant effect on the C_{max} or AUC.

Herb/Nutraceutical: St John's wort may decrease quetiapine levels. Avoid valerian, St John's wort, kava kava, gotu kola (may increase CNS depression).

Lab Interactions May interfere with urine detection of methadone (false-positives); may cause false-positive serum TCA screen

Adverse Reactions Actual frequency may be dependant upon dose and/or indication. Unless otherwise noted, frequency of adverse effects is reported for adult patients; spectrum and incidence of adverse effects similar in children (with significant exceptions noted).

>10%:

Cardiovascular: Diastolic blood pressure increased (children and adolescents, 41%), systolic blood pressure increased (children and adolescents, 15%)

Central nervous system: Somnolence (18% to 57%), headache (7% to 21%), agitation (5% to 20%), dizziness (1% to 18%), fatigue (3% to 14%), extrapyramidal symptoms (1% to 13%)

Endocrine & metabolic: Triglycerides increased (≥200 mg/dL, 8% to 22%), HDL cholesterol decreased (≤40 mg/dL, 6% to 19%), total cholesterol increased (≥240 mg/dL, 7% to 18%), LDL cholesterol increased (≥160 mg/dL, 4% to 17%), hyperglycemia (≥200 mg/dL post glucose challenge or fasting glucose ≥126 mg/dL, 2% to 12%)

Gastrointestinal: Xerostomia (9% to 44%), weight gain (dose related; 3% to 23%), appetite increased (2% to 12%), constipation (6% to 11%)

1% to 10%:

Cardiovascular: Orthostatic hypotension (2% to 7%; children and adolescents <1%), tachycardia (1% to 6%), syncope (<5%), palpitation (4%), peripheral edema (4%), hypotension (3%), hypertension (1% to 2%)

Central nervous system: Insomnia (9%), akathisia (≤8%), pain (1% to 7%), dystonia (≤6%), lethargy (1% to 5%), tardive dyskinesia (<5%), anxiety (2% to 4%), irritability (1% to 4%), parkinsonism (≤4%), abnormal dreams (2% to 3%), depression (1% to 3%), hypersomnia (1% to 3%), abnormal thinking (2%), ataxia (2%), attention disturbance (2%), coordination impaired (2%), disorientation (2%), hypoesthesia (2%), mental impairment (2%), migraine (2%), sluggishness (2%), vertigo (2%), confusion (1% to 2%), restlessness (1% to 2%), fever (1% to 2%), chills (1%)

Dermatologic: Rash (4%), hyperhidrosis (2%)

Endocrine & metabolic: Hyperprolactinemia (4%), libido decreased (≤2%), hypothyroidism (≤2%), female lactation (1%)

Gastrointestinal: Nausea (7% to 8%), abdominal pain (dose related; 4% to 7%), dyspepsia (dose related; 2% to 7%), vomiting (1% to 6%), drooling (<5%), gastroenteritis (2% to 4%), toothache (2% to 3%), appetite decreased (2%), dysphagia (2%), flatulence (2%), GERD (2%), anorexia (≥1%), abnormal taste (1%), abdominal distension (≤1%)

Genitourinary: Pollakiuria (2%), urinary tract infection (2%), impotence (1%)

Hematologic: Neutropenia (≤2%), leukopenia (≥1%), hemorrhage (1%)

Hepatic: Transaminases increased (1% to 6%), GGT increased (1%)

Neuromuscular & skeletal: Weakness (2% to 10%), tremor (2% to 8%), back pain (3% to 5%), dysarthria (1% to 5%), hypertonia (4%), twitching (4%), dyskinesia (≤4%), arthralgia (1% to 4%), paresthesia (3%), muscle spasm (1% to 3%), limb pain (2%), myalgia (2%), neck pain (2%), neck rigidity (1%)

Ocular: Blurred vision (1% to 4%), amblyopia (2% to 3%)

Otic: Ear pain (1% to 2%)

Respiratory: Pharyngitis (4% to 6%), nasal congestion (5%), rhinitis (3% to 4%), upper respiratory tract infection (2% to 3%), sinus congestion (2%), sinus headache (2%), sinusitis (2%), cough (3%), dyspnea (≥1%), dry throat (1%)

Miscellaneous: Diaphoresis (2%), restless legs syndrome (2%), flu-like syndrome (1% to 2%), lymphadenopathy (1%)

<1%, postmarketing, and/or case reports (limited to important or life-threatening): Acute renal failure, agranulocytosis, alkaline phosphatase increased, amnesia, anaphylactic reaction, anaphylaxis, anemia, angina, asthma, atrial arrhythmia, AV block, bradycardia, bundle branch block, cardiomyopathy, cataract formation, cerebral ischemia, cerebrovascular accident, HF, CPK increased, creatinine increased, dehydration, diabetes mellitus, dysuria, eosinophilia, epistaxis, exfoliative dermatitis, galactorrhea, hallucinations, hematemesis, hypoglycemia, hypothyroidism, hypersensitivity, hypokalemia, hyponatremia, intestinal obstruction, involuntary movements, leukocytosis, myocarditis, neuroleptic malignant syndrome, nightmares, pancreatitis, pneumonia, priapism, QRS duration increased, QT prolongation, rectal bleeding, rhabdomyolysis, seizure, SIADH, Stevens-Johnson syndrome, ST segment elevation, suicidal ideation, suicide attempt, thrombocytopenia, tinnitus, T-wave abnormal, T-wave inversion, urinary retention

Pharmacodynamics/Kinetics

Absorption Rapidly absorbed following oral administration

Bioavailability 100% (relative to oral solution)

Time to Peak Plasma: Immediate release: 1.5 hours; Extended release: 6 hours

Protein Binding Plasma: 83%

Half-Life Elimination

Mean: Terminal: Quetiapine: ~6 hours; Extended release: ~7 hours

Metabolite: N-desalkyl quetiapine: 9-12 hours

Metabolism Primarily hepatic; via CYP3A4; forms the metabolite N-desalkyl quetiapine (active) and two inactive metabolites

Excretion Urine (73% as metabolites, <1% of total dose as unchanged drug); feces (20%)

Available Dosage Forms

Tablet, oral:

SEROquel®: 25 mg, 50 mg, 100 mg, 200 mg, 300 mg, 400 mg

Tablet, extended release, oral:

SEROquel XR®: 50 mg, 150 mg, 200 mg, 300 mg, 400 mg

Dosing

Adult

Bipolar disorder: Oral:

Depression:

Immediate release tablet: Initial: 50 mg once daily the first day; increase to 100 mg once daily on day 2, further increasing by 100 mg/day each day until a target dose of 300 mg once daily is reached by day 4. Further increases up to 600 mg once daily by day 8 have been evaluated in clinical trials, but no additional antidepressant efficacy was noted.

Extended release tablet: Initial: 50 mg/day the first day; increase to 100 mg on day 2, further increasing by 100 mg/day each day until a target dose of 300 mg/day is reached by day 4.

Mania:

Immediate release tablet: Initial: 50 mg twice daily on day 1, increase dose in increments of 100 mg/day to 200 mg twice daily on day 4; may increase to a target dose of 800 mg/day by day 6 at increments ≤200 mg/day. Usual dosage range: 400-800 mg/day.

Extended release tablet: Initial: 300 mg on day 1; increase to 600 mg on day 2 and adjust dose to 400-800 mg once daily on day 3, depending on response and tolerance.

Maintenance therapy: Immediate release tablet: 200-400 mg twice daily with lithium or divalproex; **Note:** Average time of stabilization was 15 weeks in clinical trials.

Major depressive disorder (adjunct to antidepressants): Oral: Extended release tablet: Initial: 50 mg once daily; may be increased to 150 mg on day 3. Usual dosage range: 150-300 mg/day

Schizophrenia/psychoses: Oral:

Immediate release tablet: Initial: 25 mg twice daily; followed by increases in the total daily dose on the second and third day in increments of 25-50 mg divided 2-3 times/day, if tolerated, to a target dose of 300-400 mg/day in 2-3 divided doses by day 4. Make further adjustments as needed at intervals of at least 2 days in adjustments of 25-50 mg divided twice daily. Usual maintenance range: 300-800 mg/day.

Extended-release tablet: Initial: 300 mg once daily; increase in increments of up to 300 mg/day (in intervals of ≥1 day). Usual maintenance range: 400-800 mg/day.

Note: Dose reductions should be attempted periodically to establish lowest effective dose in patients with psychosis. Patients being restarted after 1 week of no drug need to be titrated as above.

ICU delirium: Oral: Initial: 50 mg twice daily; may increase as necessary on a daily basis in increments of 50 mg twice daily to a maximum dose of 400 mg/day (Devlin, 2010)

Geriatric Adults >65 years: 40% lower mean oral clearance of quetiapine in adults >65 years of age; higher plasma levels expected and, therefore, dosage adjustment may be needed; elderly patients usually require 50-200 mg/day of immediate release tablets or 50 mg/day of extended release tablets with a slower titration schedule. Increase immediate release dose by 25-50 mg/day or extended release dose by 50 mg/day to effective dose, based on clinical response and tolerability. If initiated with immediate release tablets, patient may transition to extended release formulation (at equivalent total daily dose) when effective dose has been reached. See "Note" in adult dosing.

Psychosis/agitation related to Alzheimer's dementia (unlabeled use): Initial: 12.5-50 mg/day; if necessary, gradually increase as tolerated not to exceed 200-300 mg/day (Rabins, 2007)

Pediatric Note: Total daily doses may also be divided into 3 doses per day.

Bipolar disorder: Children ≥10 years: Oral:

Mania: Immediate release tablet: Initial: 25 mg twice daily on day 1; increase to 50 mg twice daily on day 2, further increasing by 100 mg/day each day until a target dose of 400 mg/day is reached on day 5. May increase up to 600 mg/day at increments ≤100 mg/day; however, no additional benefit seen with 600 mg/day. Usual dosage range: 400-600 mg/day.

Maintenance therapy: Immediate release tablet: Continue therapy at lowest dose needed to maintain remission; periodically assess maintenance treatment needs.

Autism (unlabeled use): Children ≥10 years: Oral: 100-350 mg/day (1.6-5.2 mg/kg/day) (Martin, 1999)

Schizophrenia: Adolescents ≥13 years: Oral: Immediate release tablet: Initial: 25 mg twice daily on day 1; increase to 50 mg twice daily on day 2, further increasing by 100 mg/day each day until a target dose of 400 mg/day is reached on day 5. May increase up to 800 mg/day at increments ≤100 mg/day; however, no additional benefit seen with 800 mg/day. Usual dosage range: 400-800 mg/day; periodically assess maintenance treatment needs.

Renal Impairment No dosage adjustment required: 25% lower mean oral clearance of quetiapine than normal subjects; however, plasma concentrations similar to normal subjects receiving the same dose.

Hepatic Impairment Lower clearance in hepatic impairment (30%), may result in higher concentrations. Dosage adjustment may be required.

Immediate release tablet: Oral: Initial: 25 mg/day, increase dose by 25-50 mg/day to effective dose, based on clinical response and tolerability to patient. If initiated with immediate-release formulation, patient may transition to extended-release formulation (at equivalent total daily dose) when effective dose has been reached.

Extended release tablet Oral: Initial: 50 mg/day; increase dose by 50 mg/day to effective dose, based on clinical response and tolerability to patient.

Administration

Oral

Immediate release tablet: May be administered with or without food.

Extended release tablet: Administer without food or with a light meal (≤300 calories), preferably in the evening. Swallow tablet whole; do not break, crush, or chew.

Other Nasogastric/enteral tube (unlabeled route): Hold tube feeds for 30 minutes before administration; flush with 25 mL of sterile water. Crush dose using immediate-release formulation, mix in 10 mL water and administer via NG/enteral tube; follow with a 50 mL flush of sterile water (Devlin, 2010).

Stability

Storage Store at controlled room temperature of 25°C (77°F); excursions permitted to 15°C to 30°C (59°F to 86°F).

Monitoring and Teaching Issues

Laboratory Monitoring Fasting lipid profile and fasting blood glucose/Hgb A_{1c} (prior to treatment, at 3 months, then annually); CBC frequently during first few months of therapy in patients with pre-existing low WBC or a history of drug-induced leukopenia/neutropenia

Physical Assessment Assess mental status for depression and suicide ideation and observe for abnormal involuntary movements. Evaluate for cataracts before initiating treatment and every 6 months during chronic treatment. Monitor weight prior to initiating therapy and at least monthly. Consider titrating to a different antipsychotic agent for weight gain ≥5% of initial weight. Initiate at lower doses and taper dosage slowly when discontinuing.

Patient Education It may take 2-3 weeks to achieve desired results. Avoid alcohol. Maintain adequate hydration. If you have diabetes, you may experience increased blood sugars; monitor closely. Avoid overeating and/or dehydration. You may experience excess drowsiness, restlessness, dizziness, urinary retention, or blurred vision; mouth sores, dry mouth, or GI upset; weight gain; constipation; or postural hypotension. Report persistent CNS effects (eg, somnolence, agitation, insomnia), anormal involuntary movements, suicide ideation, severe dizziness, vision changes, respiratory difficulty, muscle stiffness, high fever, or worsening of condition.

Dietary Considerations Immediate-release tablet may be taken without regard to meals. Extended release tablet should be taken without food or with a light meal (≤300 calories).

Geriatric Considerations Any changes in disease status in any organ system can result in behavior changes.

Extrapyramidal syndrome symptoms occur less often than with traditional antipsychotics from the phenothiazine and butyrophenone classes. Many elderly patients receive antipsychotic medications for inappropriate nonpsychotic behavior. Before initiating antipsychotic medication, the clinician should investigate any possible reversible cause; any stress or stress from any disease can cause acute "confusion" or worsening of baseline nonpsychotic behavior. Most commonly acute changes in behavior are due to increases in drug dose or addition of new drug to regimen; fluid electrolyte loss; infections; and changes in environment.

In the treatment of agitated, demented elderly patients, authors of meta-analyses of controlled trials of the response to the traditional antipsychotics (eg, phenothiazines, butyrophenones) in controlling agitation, have concluded that the use of neuroleptics results in a response rate of 18%. Clearly neuroleptic therapy for behavior control should be limited with frequent attempts to withdraw the agent given for behavior control. In light of significant risks and adverse effects in elderly population compared with limited data demonstrating efficacy in the treatment of dementia related psychosis, aggression, and agitation, an extensive risk:benefit analysis should be performed prior to use.

Breast-Feeding Considerations Based on information from 8 mother/infant pairs, concentrations of quetiapine in breast milk have been reported as 0-170 µg/L. The estimated exposure to the breast-feeding infant would be up to 1 mg/kg/day (relative infant dose up to 0.43% based on a weight adjusted maternal dose of 400 mg/day).

Pregnancy Considerations Quetiapine was embryo and fetal toxic, but not teratogenic in animal reproduction studies. Congenital malformations have not been observed in humans (based on limited data). The long term effects of *in utero* exposure on infant development and behavior are not known. Antipsychotic use during the third trimester of pregnancy has a risk for abnormal muscle movements (extrapyramidal symptoms [EPS]) and withdrawal symptoms in newborns following delivery. Symptoms in the newborn may include agitation, feeding disorder, hypertonia, hypotonia, respiratory distress, somnolence, and tremor; these effects may be self-limiting or require hospitalization. Treatment algorithms have been developed by the ACOG and the APA for the management of depression in women prior to conception and during pregnancy. Healthcare providers are encouraged to enroll women 18-45 years of age exposed to quetiapine during pregnancy in the Atypical Antipsychotics Pregnancy Registry (1-866-961-2388).

Related Information

Antipsychotic Agents *on page 1986*

◆ **Quetiapine Fumarate** *see* QUEtiapine *on page 1533*

Quinapril (KWIN a pril)

U.S. Brand Names Accupril®

Index Terms Quinapril Hydrochloride

Generic Availability (U.S.) Yes

Pharmacologic Category Angiotensin-Converting Enzyme (ACE) Inhibitor

Medication Safety Issues

Sound-alike/look-alike issues:

Accupril® may be confused with Accolate®, Accutane®, AcipHex®, Monopril®

International issues:

Accupril [U.S., Canada] may be confused with Acepril which is a brand name for captopril [Great Britain]; enalapril [Hungary, Switzerland]; lisinopril [Malaysia]

Pregnancy Risk Factor C (1st trimester); D (2nd and 3rd trimesters)

Lactation Enters breast milk/use caution

Use Treatment of hypertension; treatment of heart failure

Unlabeled/Investigational Use Treatment of left ventricular dysfunction after myocardial infarction; pediatric hypertension; to delay the progression of nephropathy and reduce risks of cardiovascular events in hypertensive patients with type 1 or 2 diabetes mellitus

Mechanism of Action/Effect Competitive inhibitor of angiotensin-converting enzyme (ACE); prevents conversion of angiotensin I to angiotensin II, a potent vasoconstrictor; results in lower levels of angiotensin II which causes an increase in plasma renin activity and a reduction in aldosterone secretion

Contraindications Hypersensitivity to quinapril or any component of the formulation; angioedema related to previous treatment with an ACE inhibitor

Warnings/Precautions Anaphylactic reactions may occur rarely with ACE inhibitors. At any time during treatment (especially following first dose) angioedema may occur rarely with ACE inhibitors; it may involve the head and neck (potentially compromising airway) or the intestine (presenting with abdominal pain). African-Americans and patients with idiopathic or hereditary angioedema may be at an increased risk. Prolonged frequent monitoring may be required especially if tongue, glottis, or larynx are involved as they are associated with airway obstruction. Patients with a history of airway surgery may have a higher risk of airway obstruction. Aggressive early and appropriate management is critical. Use in patients with previous angioedema associated with ACE inhibitor therapy is contraindicated. Severe anaphylactoid reactions may be seen during hemodialysis (eg, CVVHD) with high-flux dialysis membranes (eg, AN69), and rarely, during low density lipoprotein apheresis with dextran sulfate cellulose. Rare cases of anaphylactoid reactions have been reported in patients undergoing sensitization treatment with hymenoptera (bee, wasp) venom while receiving ACE inhibitors.

Symptomatic hypotension with or without syncope can occur with ACE inhibitors (usually with the first several doses); effects are most often observed in volume-depleted patients; close monitoring of patient is required especially with initial dosing and dosing increases; blood pressure must be lowered at a rate appropriate for the patient's clinical condition. Initiation of therapy in patients with ischemic heart disease or cerebrovascular disease warrants close observation due to the potential consequences posed by falling blood pressure (eg, MI, stroke). Use with caution in hypertrophic cardiomyopathy with outflow tract obstruction, severe aortic stenosis, or before, during, or immediately after major surgery. **[U.S. Boxed Warning]: Based on human data, ACEIs can cause injury and death to the developing fetus when used in the second and third trimesters. ACEIs should be discontinued as soon as possible once pregnancy is detected.**

Hyperkalemia may occur with ACE inhibitors; risk factors include renal dysfunction, diabetes mellitus, concomitant use of potassium-sparing diuretics, potassium supplements, and/or potassium-containing salts. Use cautiously, if at all, with these agents and monitor potassium closely. Cough may occur with ACE inhibitors. Other causes of cough should be considered (eg, pulmonary congestion in patients with heart failure) and excluded prior to discontinuation.

May be associated with deterioration of renal function and/or increases in serum creatinine, particularly in patients with low renal blood flow (eg, renal artery stenosis, heart failure) whose glomerular filtration rate (GFR) is dependent on efferent arteriolar vasoconstriction by angiotensin II; deterioration may result in oliguria, acute renal failure, and progressive azotemia. Small increases in serum creatinine may occur following initiation; consider discontinuation only in patients with progressive and/or significant deterioration in renal function. Use with caution in patients with unstented unilateral/bilateral renal artery stenosis. When unstented bilateral renal artery stenosis is present, use is generally avoided due to the elevated risk of deterioration in renal function unless possible benefits outweigh risks. Concurrent use of angiotensin receptor blockers may increase the risk of clinically-significant adverse events (eg, renal dysfunction, hyperkalemia).

Rare toxicities associated with ACE inhibitors include cholestatic jaundice (which may progress to fulminant hepatic necrosis), agranulocytosis, neutropenia, or leukopenia with myeloid hypoplasia. Patients with collagen vascular diseases (especially with concomitant renal impairment) or renal impairment alone may be at increased risk for hematologic toxicity; periodically monitor CBC with differential in these patients.

Drug Interactions

Avoid Concomitant Use There are no known interactions where it is recommended to avoid concomitant use.

Decreased Effect

Quinapril may decrease the levels/effects of: Quinolone Antibiotics; Tetracycline Derivatives

The levels/effects of Quinapril may be decreased by: Antacids; Aprotinin; Herbs (Hypertensive Properties); Methylphenidate; Nonsteroidal Anti-Inflammatory Agents; Salicylates; Yohimbine

Increased Effect/Toxicity

Quinapril may increase the levels/effects of: Allopurinol; Amifostine; Antihypertensives; AzaTHIOprine; CycloSPORINE; CycloSPORINE (Systemic); Ferric Gluconate; Gold Sodium Thiomalate; Hypotensive Agents; Iron Dextran Complex; Lithium; RiTUXimab

The levels/effects of Quinapril may be increased by: Angiotensin II Receptor Blockers; Diazoxide; DPP-IV Inhibitors; Eplerenone; Everolimus; Herbs (Hypotensive Properties); Loop Diuretics; MAO Inhibitors; Pentoxifylline; Phosphodiesterase 5 Inhibitors; Potassium Salts; Potassium-Sparing Diuretics; Prostacyclin Analogues; Sirolimus; Temsirolimus; Thiazide Diuretics; TiZANidine; Tolvaptan; Trimethoprim

Nutritional/Ethanol Interactions Herb/Nutraceutical: Avoid bayberry, blue cohosh, cayenne, ephedra, ginger, ginseng (American), kola, licorice (may worsen hypertension). Avoid black cohosh, California poppy, coleus, golden seal, hawthorn, mistletoe, periwinkle, quinine, shepherd's purse (may have increased antihypertensive effect).

Adverse Reactions Note: Frequency ranges include data from hypertension and heart failure trials. Higher rates of adverse reactions have generally been noted in patients with CHF. However, the frequency of adverse effects associated with placebo is also increased in this population.

1% to 10%:

Cardiovascular: Hypotension (3%), chest pain (2%), first-dose hypotension (up to 3%)
Central nervous system: Dizziness (4% to 8%), headache (2% to 6%), fatigue (3%)
Dermatologic: Rash (1%)
Endocrine & metabolic: Hyperkalemia (2%)
Gastrointestinal: Vomiting/nausea (1% to 2%), diarrhea (2%)
Neuromuscular & skeletal: Myalgias (2% to 5%), back pain (1%)
Renal: BUN/serum creatinine increased (2%, transient elevations may occur with a higher frequency), worsening of renal function (in patients with bilateral renal artery stenosis or hypovolemia)
Respiratory: Upper respiratory symptoms, cough (2% to 4%; up to 13% in some studies), dyspnea (2%)

Pharmacodynamics/Kinetics

Onset of Action 1 hour

Duration of Action 24 hours

Absorption Quinapril: ≥60%

Time to Peak Serum: Quinapril: 1 hour; Quinaprilat: ~2 hours

Protein Binding Quinapril: 97%; Quinaprilat: 97%

Half-Life Elimination Quinapril: 0.8 hours; Quinaprilat: 3 hours; increases as Cl_{cr} decreases

Metabolism Rapidly hydrolyzed to quinaprilat, the active metabolite

Excretion Urine (50% to 60% primarily as quinaprilat)

Available Dosage Forms

Tablet, oral: 5 mg, 10 mg, 20 mg, 40 mg
Accupril®: 5 mg, 10 mg, 20 mg, 40 mg

Dosing

Adult

Heart failure: Oral: Initial: 5 mg once or twice daily, titrated at weekly intervals to 20-40 mg daily in 2 divided doses; target dose (heart failure): 20 mg twice daily (ACC/AHA 2009 Heart Failure Guidelines)

Hypertension: Oral: Initial: 10-20 mg once daily, adjust according to blood pressure response at peak and trough blood levels; initial dose may be reduced to 5 mg in patients receiving diuretic therapy if the diuretic is continued.

Usual dose range (JNC 7): 10-40 mg once daily

Geriatric Oral: Initial: 2.5-5 mg/day; increase dosage at increments of 2.5-5 mg at 1- to 2-week intervals; adjust for renal impairment.

Pediatric Hypertension (unlabeled use): Oral: Initial 5-10 mg once daily; maximum: 80 mg/day

Renal Impairment Lower initial doses should be used; after initial dose (if tolerated), administer initial dose twice daily; may be increased at weekly intervals to optimal response:

Heart failure: Oral: Initial:

Cl_{cr} >30 mL/minute: Administer 5 mg/day

Cl_{cr} 10-30 mL/minute: Administer 2.5 mg/day

Hypertension: Oral: Initial:

Cl_{cr} >60 mL/minute: Administer 10 mg/day

Cl_{cr} 30-60 mL/minute: Administer 5 mg/day

Cl_{cr} 10-30 mL/minute: Administer 2.5 mg/day

Hepatic Impairment In patients with alcoholic cirrhosis, hydrolysis of quinapril to quinaprilat is impaired; however, the subsequent elimination of quinaprilat is unaltered.

Stability

Reconstitution To prepare solution for oral administration, mix prior to administration and use within 10 minutes.

Storage Store at room temperature.

Monitoring and Teaching Issues

Laboratory Monitoring Serum creatinine and potassium; if patient has collagen vascular disease and/or renal impairment, periodically monitor CBC with differential

Physical Assessment Use caution in presence of renal impairment, hypovolemia, collagen vascular diseases, valvular stenosis, hyperkalemia, or before, during, or immediately after surgery. Assess potential for interactions with other pharmacological agents or herbal products that may impact fluid balance or cardiac status. Monitor first dose carefully (hypotension or angioedema can occur at any time during treatment, especially following first dose). Evaluate blood pressure and cardiac status. Monitor for hypovolemia, angioedema, and postural hypotension on a regular basis during therapy.

Patient Education Take first dose at bedtime or when sitting down (hypotension may occur). This drug does not eliminate need for diet or exercise regimen as recommended by prescriber. May cause increased cough (if persistent or bothersome, contact prescriber), postural hypotension, headache, dizziness, nausea, vomiting, or muscle or back pain. Immediately report swelling of face, mouth, lips, tongue, or throat; chest pain or respiratory difficulty; persistent cough; persistent pain in muscles, joints, or back; or skin rash.

Geriatric Considerations Due to frequent decreases in glomerular filtration (also creatinine clearance) with aging, elderly patients may have exaggerated responses to ACE inhibitors; differences in clinical response due to hepatic changes are not observed. ACE inhibitors may be preferred agents in elderly patients with CHF and diabetes mellitus. Diabetic proteinuria is reduced and insulin sensitivity is enhanced. In general, the side effect profile is favorable in elderly and causes little or no CNS confusion; use lowest dose recommendations initially. Adjust for renal function. Many elderly may be volume depleted due to diuretic use and/or blunted thirst reflex resulting in inadequate fluid intake.

Breast-Feeding Considerations Quinapril is excreted in breast milk. The manufacturer recommends that caution be exercised when administering quinapril to nursing women.

Pregnancy Considerations Due to adverse events observed in some animal studies, quinapril is considered pregnancy category C during the first trimester. Based on human data, quinapril is considered pregnancy category D if used during the second and third trimesters (per the manufacturer; however, one study suggests that fetal injury may occur at anytime during pregnancy). Quinapril crosses the placenta. First trimester exposure to ACE inhibitors may cause major congenital malformations. An increased risk of cardiovascular and/or central nervous system malformations was observed in one study; however, an increased risk of teratogenic events was not observed in other studies. Second and third trimester use of an ACE inhibitor is associated with oligohydramnios. Oligohydramnios due to decreased fetal renal function may lead to fetal limb contractures, craniofacial deformation, and hypoplastic lung development. The use of ACE inhibitors during the second and third trimesters is also associated with anuria, hypotension, renal failure (reversible or irreversible), skull hypoplasia, and death in the fetus/neonate. Chronic maternal hypertension itself is also associated with adverse events in the fetus/infant. ACE inhibitors are not recommended during pregnancy to treat maternal hypertension or heart failure. Those who are planning a pregnancy should be considered for other medication options if an ACE inhibitor is currently prescribed or the ACE inhibitor should be discontinued as soon as possible once pregnancy is detected. The exposed fetus should be monitored for fetal growth, amniotic fluid volume, and organ formation. Infants exposed to an ACE inhibitor *in utero*, especially during the second and third trimester, should be monitored for hyperkalemia, hypotension, and oliguria.

[U.S. Boxed Warning]: Based on human data, ACE inhibitors can cause injury and death to the developing fetus when used in the second and third trimesters. ACE inhibitors should be discontinued as soon as possible once pregnancy is detected.

Related Information

Angiotensin Agents *on page 1974*

Heart Failure (Systolic) *on page 2040*

Quinapril and Hydrochlorothiazide (KWIN a pril & hye droe klor oh THYE a zide)

U.S. Brand Names Accuretic®; Quinaretic

Index Terms Hydrochlorothiazide and Quinapril

Generic Availability (U.S.) Yes

Pharmacologic Category Angiotensin-Converting Enzyme (ACE) Inhibitor; Diuretic, Thiazide

Pregnancy Risk Factor C (1st trimester); D (2nd and 3rd trimesters)

Lactation Enters breast milk/use caution

Use Treatment of hypertension (not for initial therapy)

Available Dosage Forms

Tablet: 10/12.5: Quinapril 10 mg and hydrochlorothiazide 12.5 mg; 20/12.5: Quinapril 20 mg and hydrochlorothiazide 12.5 mg; 20/25: Quinapril 20 mg and hydrochlorothiazide 25 mg

Accuretic®, Quinaretic: 10/12.5: Quinapril 10 mg and hydrochlorothiazide 12.5 mg; 20/12.5: Quinapril 20 mg and hydrochlorothiazide 12.5 mg; 20/25: Quinapril 20 mg and hydrochlorothiazide 25 mg

Dosing

Adult

Hypertension: Oral:

Patients with inadequate response to quinapril monotherapy: Quinapril 10 mg/hydrochlorothiazide 12.5 mg **or** quinapril 20 mg/hydrochlorothiazide 12.5 mg once daily

Patients with adequate blood pressure control on hydrochlorothiazide 25 mg/day, but significant potassium loss: Quinapril 10 mg/hydrochlorothiazide 12.5 mg **or** quinapril 20 mg/hydrochlorothiazide 12.5 mg once daily

Note: Clinical trials of quinapril/hydrochlorothiazide combinations used quinapril doses of 2.5-40 mg/day and hydrochlorothiazide doses of 6.25-25 mg/day.

Geriatric If previous response to individual components is unknown, initial dose selection should be cautious, at the low end of adult dosage range; titration should occur at 1- to 2-week intervals.

Pediatric Safety and efficacy have not been established.

Renal Impairment Cl_{cr} <30 mL/minute/1.73 m^2 or serum creatinine ≥3 mg/dL: Use is not recommended.

Monitoring and Teaching Issues

Laboratory Monitoring BUN, serum creatinine, and electrolytes; if patient has collagen vascular disease and/or renal impairment, periodically monitor CBC with differential

Physical Assessment See individual agents.

Patient Education See individual agents.

Related Information

Hydrochlorothiazide *on page 912*

Quinapril *on page 1538*

◆ **Quinapril Hydrochloride** *see* Quinapril *on page 1538*

◆ **Quinaretic** *see* Quinapril and Hydrochlorothiazide *on page 1540*

QuiNIDine (KWIN i deen)

Index Terms Quinidine Gluconate; Quinidine Polygalacturonate; Quinidine Sulfate

Generic Availability (U.S.) Yes

Pharmacologic Category Antiarrhythmic Agent, Class Ia

Medication Safety Issues

Sound-alike/look-alike issues:

QuiNIDine may be confused with cloNIDine, quiNINE, Quinora®

High alert medication: The Institute for Safe Medication Practices (ISMP) includes this medication (I.V. formulation) among its list of drug classes which have a heightened risk of causing significant patient harm when used in error.

Pregnancy Risk Factor C

Lactation Enters breast milk/compatible

Use

Quinidine gluconate and sulfate salts: Conversion and prevention of relapse into atrial fibrillation and/or flutter; suppression of ventricular arrhythmias. **Note:** Due to proarrhythmic effects, use should be reserved for life-threatening arrhythmias. Moreover, the use of quinidine has largely been replaced by more effective/safer antiarrhythmic agents and/or nonpharmacologic therapies (eg, radiofrequency ablation).

Quinidine gluconate (I.V. formulation): Conversion of atrial fibrillation/flutter and ventricular tachycardia. **Note:** The use of I.V. quinidine gluconate for these indications has been replaced by more effective/safer antiarrhythmic agents (eg, amiodarone and procainamide).

Quinidine gluconate (I.V. formulation) and quinidine sulfate: Treatment of malaria (*Plasmodium falciparum*)

Unlabeled/Investigational Use Paroxysmal supraventricular tachycardia, paroxysmal AV junctional rhythm, and symptomatic atrial or ventricular premature contractions; short QT syndrome; Brugada syndrome

Available Dosage Forms

Injection, solution: 80 mg/mL (10 mL)

Tablet, oral: 200 mg, 300 mg

Tablet, extended release, oral: 300 mg, 324 mg

Dosing

Adult & Geriatric

Note: Dosage expressed in terms of the salt: 267 mg of quinidine gluconate = 275 mg of quinidine polygalacturonate = 200 mg of quinidine sulfate.

Antiarrhythmic: Oral:

Sulfate: 100-600 mg/dose every 4-6 hours; begin at 200 mg/dose and titrate to desired effect (maximum daily dose: 3-4 g)

Gluconate: 324-972 mg every 8-12 hours

Severe malaria, treatment: I.V. (quinidine gluconate): 10 mg/kg infused over 60-120 minutes followed by 0.02 mg/kg/minute continuous infusion for ≥24 hours; alternatively, may administer 24 mg/kg loading dose over 4 hours, followed by 12 mg/kg over 4 hours every 8 hours (beginning 8 hours after the loading dose); complete treatment with oral quinine once parasite density <1% and patient can receive oral medication; total duration of treatment (quinidine/quinine): 3 days (except in Southeast Asia or Oceania where treatment duration is 7 days); use in combination with doxycycline, tetracycline or clindamycin (CDC malaria guidelines, 2009). **Note:** Close monitoring, including telemetry, required.

Pediatric

Note: Dosage expressed in terms of the salt: 267 mg of quinidine gluconate = 200 mg of quinidine sulfate.

Antiarrhythmic: Oral (quinidine sulfate): 15-60 mg/kg/day in 4-5 divided doses or 6 mg/kg every 4-6 hours; usual 30 mg/kg/day or 900 mg/m²/day given in 5 daily doses

Severe malaria, treatment: Infants and Children: I.V. (quinidine gluconate): 10 mg/kg infused over 60-120 minutes followed by 0.02 mg/kg/minute continuous infusion for ≥24 hours; alternatively, may administer 24 mg/kg loading dose over 4 hours, followed by 12 mg/kg over 4 hours every 8 hours (beginning 8 hours after the loading dose); complete treatment with oral quinine once parasite density <1% and patient can receive oral medication; total duration of treatment (quinidine/quinine): 3 days (except in Southeast Asia or Oceania where treatment duration is 7 days); use in combination with doxycycline, tetracycline or clindamycin (CDC malaria guidelines, 2009). **Note:** Close monitoring, including telemetry, required.

Renal Impairment

Cl_{cr} <10 mL/minute: Administer 75% of normal dose.

Hemodialysis effects: Slightly hemodialyzable (5% to 20%); 200 mg supplemental dose posthemodialysis is recommended; not dialyzable (0% to 5%) by peritoneal dialysis.

Hepatic Impairment Larger loading dose may be indicated; reduce maintenance doses by 50% and monitor serum levels closely.

Administration

Oral Do not crush, chew, or break sustained release dosage forms. Give around-the-clock to promote less variation in peak and trough serum levels.

I.V. Give around-the-clock to promote less variation in peak and trough serum levels. Maximum I.V. infusion rate: 10 mg/minute. Minimize use of PVC tubing to enhance bioavailability.

Monitoring and Teaching Issues

Laboratory Monitoring Routine CBC, liver and renal function during long-term administration

Physical Assessment I.V. requires use of infusion pump and continuous cardiac and hemodynamic monitoring. Monitor cardiac functioning closely at beginning of therapy, when titrating dosage, and on a regular basis. Quinidine has a low TI and overdose may easily produce severe and life-threatening reactions.

Patient Education Take around-the-clock. Do not crush, chew, or break sustained release dosage forms. Do not take with grapefruit juice. You will need regular cardiac checkups and blood tests while taking this medication. You may experience dizziness, drowsiness, visual changes, abnormal taste, nausea, vomiting, loss of appetite, headaches, or diarrhea (if persistent consult prescriber). Report chest pain, palpitation, or erratic heartbeat; respiratory difficulty or wheezing; CNS changes (confusion, delirium, fever, consistent dizziness); skin rash; sense of fullness or ringing in ears; or vision changes.

Related Information

Antiarrhythmic Drugs *on page 1978*

Peak and Trough Guidelines *on page 1958*

◆ **Quinidine and Dextromethorphan** *see* Dextromethorphan and Quinidine *on page 514*

◆ **Quinidine Gluconate** *see* QuiNIDine *on page 1541*

◆ **Quinidine Polygalacturonate** *see* QuiNIDine *on page 1541*

◆ **Quinidine Sulfate** *see* QuiNIDine *on page 1541*

QuiNINE (KWYE nine)

U.S. Brand Names Qualaquin®

Index Terms Quinine Sulfate

Generic Availability (U.S.) No

Pharmacologic Category Antimalarial Agent

Medication Safety Issues

Sound-alike/look-alike issues:

QuiNINE may be confused with quiNIDine

Medication Guide Available Yes

Pregnancy Risk Factor C

Lactation Enters breast milk/use caution (AAP rate "compatible"; AAP 2001 update pending)

Use In conjunction with other antimalarial agents, treatment of uncomplicated chloroquine-resistant *P. falciparum* malaria

Unlabeled/Investigational Use Treatment of *Babesia microti* infection in conjunction with clindamycin; treatment of uncomplicated chloroquine-resistant *P. vivax* malaria (in conjunction with other antimalarial agents)

Available Dosage Forms

Capsule, oral:

Qualaquin®: 324 mg

Dosing

Adult & Geriatric Note: Actual duration of quinine treatment for malaria may be dependent upon the geographic region or pathogen. Dosage expressed in terms of the salt; 1 capsule Qualaquin® = 324 mg of quinine sulfate = 269 mg of base.

Treatment of uncomplicated chloroquine-resistant *P. falciparum* malaria (CDC guidelines): 648 mg every 8 hours for 3-7 days. Tetracycline, doxycycline, or clindamycin should also be given.

Treatment of uncomplicated chloroquine-resistant *P. vivax* malaria (unlabeled use; CDC guidelines): 648 mg every 8 hours for 3-7 days. Tetracycline or doxycycline plus primaquine should also be given.

Babesiosis (unlabeled use): 650 mg every 8 hours for 7-10 days with clindamycin

Pediatric Note: Actual duration of quinine treatment for malaria may be dependent upon the geographic region or pathogen. Dosage expressed in terms of the salt; 1 capsule Qualaquin® = 324 mg of quinine sulfate = 269 mg of base.

Treatment of uncomplicated chloroquine-resistant *P. falciparum* malaria (CDC guidelines): 30 mg/kg/day in divided doses every 8 hours for 3-7 days. Tetracycline, doxycycline, or clindamycin (consider risk versus benefit of using tetracycline or doxycycline in children <8 years) should also be given.

Treatment of uncomplicated chloroquine-resistant *P. vivax* malaria (unlabeled use; CDC guidelines): 30 mg/kg/day in divided doses every 8 hours for 3-7 days. Tetracycline or doxycycline (consider risk versus benefit of using tetracycline or doxycycline in children <8 years) plus primaquine should also be given.

Babesiosis (unlabeled use): 30 mg/kg/day divided every 8 hours for 7-10 days with clindamycin.

Renal Impairment

Cl_{cr} 10-50 mL/minute: Administer every 8-12 hours

Cl_{cr} <10 mL/minute: Administer every 24 hours

Severe chronic renal failure not on dialysis: Initial dose: 648 mg followed by 324 mg every 12 hours

Dialysis: Administer dose after dialysis. **Note:** Clearance of ~6.5% achieved with 1 hour of hemodialysis.

Not removed by hemo- or peritoneal dialysis; dose as for Cl_{cr} <10 mL/minute.

Continuous arteriovenous or hemodialysis: Dose as for Cl_{cr} 10-50 mL/minute.

Hepatic Impairment

Mild-to-moderate impairment: No dosing adjustment required; monitor closely.

Severe impairment (Child-Pugh class C): Data not available.

Administration

Oral Avoid use of aluminum- or magnesium-containing antacids because of drug absorption problems. Swallow dose whole to avoid bitter taste. May be administered with food.

Monitoring and Teaching Issues

Laboratory Monitoring Monitor CBC with platelet count, liver function tests, blood glucose, ophthalmologic examination

Physical Assessment Assess allergy history prior to beginning therapy. Use caution in presence of cardiac arrhythmias (quinine has quinidine-like activity) and myasthenia gravis.

Patient Education Take with 8 oz of water, with or without food. You will need to return for follow-up blood tests. May cause severe headache, nausea, vomiting, or diarrhea. Report any vision changes (blurring, night-blindness, double vision, etc) or ringing in ears. Seek emergency help for chest pain, respiratory difficulty, seizures, or bleeding.

◆ **Quinine Sulfate** *see* QuiNINE *on page 1542*

◆ **Quinol** *see* Hydroquinone *on page 927*

Quinupristin and Dalfopristin (kwi NYOO pris tin & dal FOE pris tin)

U.S. Brand Names Synercid®

Index Terms Dalfopristin and Quinupristin; Pristinamycin; RP-59500

Generic Availability (U.S.) No

Pharmacologic Category Antibiotic, Streptogramin

Pregnancy Risk Factor B

Lactation Excretion in breast milk unknown/use caution

Use Treatment of complicated skin and skin structure infections caused by methicillin-susceptible *Staphylococcus aureus* or *Streptococcus pyogenes*

Available Dosage Forms

Injection, powder for reconstitution:

Synercid®: 500 mg: Quinupristin 150 mg and dalfopristin 350 mg

Dosing

Adult & Geriatric Complicated skin and skin structure infection: I.V.: 7.5 mg/kg every 12 hours for at least 7 days

Pediatric Children ≥12 years: Refer to adult dosing.

Renal Impairment No adjustment is necessary in renal failure, hemodialysis, or peritoneal dialysis.

Hepatic Impairment Pharmacokinetic data suggest dosage adjustment may be necessary; however, specific recommendations have not been proposed.

Administration

I.V. Line should be flushed with 5% dextrose in water prior to and following administration. Infusion should be completed over 60 minutes (toxicity may be increased with shorter infusion). If severe venous irritation occurs following peripheral administration of quinupristin/dalfopristin diluted in 250 mL 5% dextrose in water, consideration should be given to increasing the infusion volume to 500 mL or 750 mL, changing the infusion site, or infusing by a peripherally-inserted central catheter (PICC) or a central venous catheter.

Monitoring and Teaching Issues

Laboratory Monitoring Culture and sensitivity

Physical Assessment Assess allergy history prior to starting treatment. Use caution in presence of hepatic or renal impairment. Infusion site must be closely monitored (may cause venous irritation). Monitor for arthralgia, headache, rash, hyperglycemia, opportunistic infection (fever, chills, sore throat, burning urination, fatigue), pseudomembranous colitis, hyperbilirubinemia, dyspnea, and ataxia.

Patient Education This drug can only be administered by intravenous infusion. Report immediately any pain, irritation, redness, burning, or swelling at infusion site. Report headache; rash; nausea; vomiting; diarrhea; pain; heat or swelling in muscle areas, especially in lower extremities; respiratory difficulty, tremors; or difficulty speaking.

Related Information

Antimicrobial Drugs of Choice *on page 2008*

◆ **QVAR®** *see* Beclomethasone (Oral Inhalation) *on page 192*

◆ **RabAvert®** *see* Rabies Vaccine *on page 1546*

Rabeprazole (ra BEP ra zole)

U.S. Brand Names AcipHex®

Index Terms Pariprazole

Generic Availability (U.S.) No

Pharmacologic Category Proton Pump Inhibitor; Substituted Benzimidazole

Medication Safety Issues

Sound-alike/look-alike issues:

AcipHex® may be confused with Acephen®, Accupril®, Aricept®, pHisoHex®

RABEprazole may be confused with ARIPiprazole, donepezil, lansoprazole, omeprazole, raloxifene

Pregnancy Risk Factor B

Lactation Excretion in breast milk unknown/not recommended

Use Short-term (4-8 weeks) treatment and maintenance of erosive or ulcerative gastroesophageal reflux disease (GERD); symptomatic GERD; short-term (up to 4 weeks) treatment of duodenal ulcers; long-term treatment of pathological hypersecretory conditions, including Zollinger-Ellison syndrome; *H. pylori* eradication (in combination therapy)

Canadian labeling: Additional uses (not in U.S. labeling): Treatment of nonerosive reflux disease (NERD); treatment of gastric ulcers

Unlabeled/Investigational Use Maintenance of duodenal ulcer

Mechanism of Action/Effect Prevents gastric acid secretion

Contraindications Hypersensitivity to rabeprazole, substituted benzimidazoles (ie, esomeprazole, lansoprazole, omeprazole, pantoprazole), or any component of the formulation

Warnings/Precautions Use of proton pump inhibitors may increase the risk of gastrointestinal infections (eg, *Salmonella, Campylobacter*). Use caution in severe hepatic impairment. Relief of symptoms with rabeprazole does not preclude the presence of a gastric malignancy. Decreased *H. pylori* eradication rates have been observed with short-term (≤7 days) combination therapy. The American College of Gastroenterology recommends 10-14 days of therapy (triple or quadruple) for eradication of *H. pylori* (Chey, 2007). Proton pump inhibitors may diminish the therapeutic effect of clopidogrel, thought to be due to reduced formation of the active metabolite of clopidogrel; an increase in the risk of cardiovascular events may occur. The manufacturer of clopidogrel recommends avoidance of concomitant administration of another PPI (ie, omeprazole); given the potency of CYP2C19 inhibitory activity, similar recommendations with rabeprazole would appear prudent. Increased incidence of osteoporosis-related bone fractures of the hip, spine, or wrist may occur with proton pump inhibitor therapy. Patients on high-dose (multiple daily doses) or long-term therapy (≥1 year) should be monitored. Use the lowest effective dose for the shortest duration of time, use vitamin D and calcium supplementation, and follow appropriate guidelines to reduce risk of fractures in patients at risk.

Drug Interactions

Metabolism/Transport Effects Substrate (major) of CYP2C19, 3A4; **Inhibits** CYP2C8 (moderate), 2C19 (moderate), 2D6 (weak), 3A4 (weak)

Avoid Concomitant Use

Avoid concomitant use of RABEprazole with any of the following: Delavirdine; Erlotinib; Nelfinavir; Posaconazole

Decreased Effect

RABEprazole may decrease the levels/effects of: Atazanavir; Bisphosphonate Derivatives; Cefditoren; Clopidogrel; Dabigatran Etexilate; Dasatinib; Delavirdine; Erlotinib; Gefitinib; Indinavir; Iron Salts; Itraconazole; Ketoconazole; Ketoconazole (Systemic); Mesalamine; Mycophenolate; Nelfinavir; Posaconazole

The levels/effects of RABEprazole may be decreased by: CYP2C19 Inducers (Strong); CYP3A4 Inducers (Strong); Deferasirox; Herbs (CYP3A4 Inducers); Tipranavir

Increased Effect/Toxicity

RABEprazole may increase the levels/effects of: Amphetamines; CYP2C19 Substrates; CYP2C8 Substrates (High risk); Dexmethylphenidate; Methotrexate; Methylphenidate; Raltegravir; Saquinavir; Tacrolimus; Tacrolimus (Systemic); Voriconazole

The levels/effects of RABEprazole may be increased by: Conivaptan; Fluconazole; Ketoconazole; Ketoconazole (Systemic)

Nutritional/Ethanol Interactions

Ethanol: Avoid ethanol (may cause gastric mucosal irritation).
Food: High-fat meals may delay absorption, but C_{max} and AUC are not altered.
Herb/Nutraceutical: St John's wort may increase the metabolism and thus decrease the levels/effects of rabeprazole.

Adverse Reactions 1% to 10%:

Central nervous system: Pain (3%), headache (2% to 5%)
Gastrointestinal: Diarrhea (3%), flatulence (3%), constipation (2%), nausea (2%)
Respiratory: Pharyngitis (3%)
Miscellaneous: Infection (2%)

Pharmacodynamics/Kinetics

Onset of Action Within 1 hour

Duration of Action 24 hours

Absorption Oral: Well absorbed within 1 hour

Bioavailability Oral: ~52%

Time to Peak Plasma: 2-5 hours

Protein Binding Serum: ~96%

Half-Life Elimination Dose dependent: 1-2 hours

Metabolism Hepatic via CYP3A and 2C19 to inactive metabolites

Excretion Urine (90% primarily as thioether carboxylic acid metabolites); remainder in feces

Available Dosage Forms

Tablet, delayed release, enteric coated, oral:
AcipHex®: 20 mg

Dosing

Adult & Geriatric

GERD, erosive/ulcerative: Oral: Treatment: 20 mg once daily for 4-8 weeks; if inadequate response, may repeat up to an additional 8 weeks; maintenance: 20 mg once daily
Canadian labeling: Oral: 20 mg once daily for 4 weeks; if inadequate response, may repeat for an additional 4 weeks (lack of symptom control after 4 weeks warrants further evaluation); maintenance: 10 mg once daily (maximum: 20 mg once daily)

GERD, symptomatic: Oral: Treatment: 20 mg once daily for 4 weeks; if inadequate response, may repeat for an additional 4 weeks
Canadian labeling: 10 mg once daily (maximum: 20 mg once daily) for 4 weeks; lack of symptom control after 4 weeks warrants further evaluation

Duodenal ulcer: Oral: 20 mg/day before breakfast for 4 weeks; additional therapy may be required for some patients

Gastric ulcers (*Canadian labeling*): Oral: 20 mg once daily up to 6 weeks; additional therapy may be required for some patients

***Helicobacter pylori* eradication:** Oral:
Manufacturer labeling: 20 mg twice daily administered with amoxicillin 1000 mg *and* clarithromycin 500 mg twice daily for 7 days
American College of Gastroenterology guidelines (Chey, 2007):
Nonpenicillin allergy: 20 mg twice daily administered with amoxicillin 1000 mg *and* clarithromycin 500 mg twice daily for 10-14 days
Penicillin allergy: 20 mg twice daily administered with clarithromycin 500 mg *and* metronidazole 500 mg twice daily for 10-14 days **or** 20 mg once or twice daily administered with bismuth subsalicylate 525 mg *and* metronidazole 250 mg *plus* tetracycline 500 mg 4 times/day for 10-14 days

Hypersecretory conditions: Oral: 60 mg once daily; dose may need to be adjusted as necessary. Doses as high as 100 mg once daily and 60 mg twice daily have been used, and continued as long as necessary (up to 1 year in some patients).

NERD (*Canadian labeling*): Oral: Treatment: 10 mg (maximum: 20 mg once daily) for 4 weeks; lack of symptom control after 4 weeks warrants further evaluation

Pediatric Short-term treatment of GERD: *U.S. labeling:* Children ≥12 years: 20 mg once daily for ≤8 weeks

Renal Impairment No dosage adjustment required.

Hepatic Impairment
Mild-to-moderate: Elimination decreased; no dosage adjustment required.
Severe: Use caution.

Administration

Oral May be administered without regard to meals; best if taken before breakfast. Do not crush, split, or chew tablet. May be administered with an antacid.

Stability

Storage Store at 25°C (77°F). Protect from moisture.

Monitoring and Teaching Issues

Physical Assessment Assess those medications requiring acid environment for absorption. Monitor reduction in symptoms.

Patient Education Swallow whole; do not crush, split, or chew. Follow recommended diet and activity instructions. Avoid alcohol. You may experience headache, diarrhea, or gas. Report persistent abdominal pain or headaches.

Dietary Considerations May be taken without regard to meals; best if taken before breakfast.

Geriatric Considerations No difference in efficacy or safety was noted in elderly subjects as compared to younger subjects. No dosage adjustment is necessary in the elderly.

An increased risk of fractures of the hip, spine, or wrist has been observed in epidemiologic studies with proton pump inhibitor (PPI) use, primarily in older adults ≥50 years of age. The greatest risk was seen in patients receiving high doses or on long-term therapy (≥1 year). Calcium and vitamin D supplementation and close monitoring are recommended to reduce the risk of fracture in high-risk patients.

Pregnancy Considerations Not shown to be teratogenic in animal studies, however, adequate and well-controlled studies have not been done in humans; use during pregnancy only if clearly needed

Related Information

Helicobacter pylori Treatment *on page 2045*

Rabies Vaccine (RAY beez vak SEEN)

U.S. Brand Names Imovax® Rabies; RabAvert®

Index Terms HDCV; Human Diploid Cell Cultures Rabies Vaccine; PCEC; Purified Chick Embryo Cell

Generic Availability (U.S.) No

Pharmacologic Category Vaccine, Inactivated (Viral)

Pregnancy Risk Factor C

Lactation Excretion in breast milk unknown

Use Pre-exposure and postexposure vaccination against rabies

The Advisory Committee on Immunization Practices (ACIP) recommends a primary course of prophylactic immunization (pre-exposure vaccination) for the following:

- Persons with continuous risk of infection, including rabies research laboratory and biologics production workers
- Persons with frequent risk of infection in areas where rabies is enzootic, including rabies diagnostic laboratory workers, cavers, veterinarians and their staff, and animal control and wildlife workers; persons who frequently handle bats
- Persons with infrequent risk of infection, including veterinarians and animal control staff with terrestrial animals in areas where rabies infection is rare, veterinary students, and travelers visiting areas where rabies is enzootic and immediate access to medical care and biologicals is limited

The ACIP recommends the use of postexposure vaccination for a particular person be assessed by the severity and likelihood versus the actual risk of acquiring rabies. Consideration should include the type of exposure, epidemiology of rabies in the area, species of the animal, circumstances of the incident, and the availability of the exposing animal for observation or rabies testing. Postexposure vaccination is used in both previously vaccinated and previously unvaccinated individuals.

Available Dosage Forms

Injection, powder for reconstitution [preservative free]:

Imovax® Rabies: ≥ 2.5 int. units

RabAvert®: ≥ 2.5 int. units

Dosing

Adult & Geriatric

Pre-exposure vaccination: I.M.: A total of 3 doses, 1 mL each, on days 0, 7, and 21-28. **Note:** Prolonging the interval between doses does not interfere with immunity achieved after the concluding dose of the basic series.

Postexposure vaccination: All postexposure treatment should begin with immediate cleansing of the wound with soap and water

Persons not previously immunized as above: I.M.: 5 doses (1 mL each) on days 0, 3, 7, 14, 28. In addition, patients should receive rabies immune globulin with the first dose (day 0). **Note:** A regimen of 4 doses (1 mL each) on days 0, 3, 7, 14 may be used in persons who are not immunosuppressed (ACIP recommendations, 2010).

Persons who have previously received postexposure prophylaxis with rabies vaccine, received a recommended I.M. pre-exposure series of rabies vaccine or have a previously documented rabies antibody titer considered adequate: I.M.: Two doses (1 mL each) on days 0 and 3; do not administer rabies immune globulin

Booster (for persons with continuous or frequent risk of infection): I.M.: 1 mL based on antibody titers

Pediatric Refer to adult dosing.

Administration

I.M. For I.M. administration only; this rabies vaccine product must not be administered intradermally; in adults and children, administer I.M. injections in the deltoid muscle, not the gluteal; for younger children, use the outer aspect of the thigh. Postexposure prophylaxis should begin with immediate cleansing of wounds with soap and water; if available, a virucidal agent (eg povidone-iodine solution) should be used to irrigate the wounds.

For patients at risk of hemorrhage following intramuscular injection, the ACIP recommends "it should be administered intramuscularly if, in the opinion of the physician familiar with the patients bleeding risk, the vaccine can be administered by this route with reasonable safety. If the patient receives antihemophilia or other similar therapy, intramuscular vaccination can be scheduled shortly after such therapy is administered. A fine needle (23 gauge or smaller) can be used for the vaccination and firm pressure applied to the site (without rubbing) for at least 2 minutes. The patient should be instructed concerning the risk of hematoma from the injection." Patients on anticoagulant therapy should be considered to have the same bleeding risks and treated as those with clotting factor disorders (CDC, 2011).

Simultaneous administration of vaccines helps ensure the patients will be fully vaccinated by the appropriate age. Simultaneous administration of vaccines is defined as administering >1 vaccine on the same day at different anatomic sites. The use of licensed combination vaccines is generally preferred over separate injections of the equivalent components. Separate vaccines should not be combined in the same syringe unless indicated by product specific labeling. Separate needles and syringes should be used for each injection. The ACIP prefers each dose of a specific vaccine in a series come from the same manufacturer when possible. Adolescents and adults should be vaccinated while seated or lying down. In general, preterm infants should be vaccinated at the same chronological age as full-term infants (CDC, 2011).

Antipyretics have not been shown to prevent febrile seizures. Antipyretics may be used to treat fever or discomfort following vaccination (CDC, 2011). One study reported that routine prophylactic administration of acetaminophen to prevent fever prior to vaccination decreased the immune response of some vaccines; the clinical significance of this reduction in immune response has not been established (Prymula, 2009).

Monitoring and Teaching Issues

Physical Assessment All serious adverse reactions must be reported to the U.S. DHHS. Federal law also requires entry into the patient's medical record.

Patient Education Common reactions include pain, irritation, swelling, and itching at the site of administration. Contact healthcare provider if you develop a high fever or signs of an allergic reaction.

Related Information

Immunization Recommendations *on page 1941*

- **Racemic Epinephrine** *see* EPINEPHrine (Systemic, Oral Inhalation) *on page 629*
- **Racepinephrine** *see* EPINEPHrine (Systemic, Oral Inhalation) *on page 629*
- **RAD001** *see* Everolimus *on page 720*
- **rAHF** *see* Antihemophilic Factor (Recombinant) *on page 133*
- **R-albuterol** *see* Levalbuterol *on page 1085*

Raloxifene (ral OKS i feen)

U.S. Brand Names Evista®

Index Terms Keoxifene Hydrochloride; Raloxifene Hydrochloride

Generic Availability (U.S.) No

Pharmacologic Category Selective Estrogen Receptor Modulator (SERM)

Medication Safety Issues

Sound-alike/look-alike issues:

Evista® may be confused with Avinza™, Eovist®

Medication Guide Available Yes

Pregnancy Risk Factor X

Lactation Excretion in breast milk unknown/contraindicated

Use Prevention and treatment of osteoporosis in postmenopausal women; risk reduction for invasive breast cancer in postmenopausal women with osteoporosis and in postmenopausal women with high risk for invasive breast cancer

Mechanism of Action/Effect A selective estrogen receptor modulator (SERM), meaning that it affects some of the same receptors that estrogen does, but not all, and in some instances, it antagonizes or blocks estrogen; it acts like estrogen to prevent bone loss and has the potential to block some estrogen effects in the breast uterine cancer tissues. Raloxifene decreases bone resorption, increasing bone mineral density and decreasing fracture incidence.

Contraindications History of or current venous thromboembolic disorders (including DVT, PE, and retinal vein thrombosis); pregnancy or women who could become pregnant; breast-feeding

Warnings/Precautions Hazardous agent - use appropriate precautions for handling and disposal. **[U.S. Boxed Warning]: May increase the risk for DVT or PE; use contraindicated in patients with history of or current venous thromboembolic disorders.** Use with caution in patients at high risk for venous thromboembolism; the risk for DVT and PE are higher in the first 4 months of treatment. Discontinue at least 72 hours prior to and during prolonged immobilization (postoperative recovery or prolonged bedrest). **[U.S. Boxed Warning]: The risk of death due to stroke may be increased in women with coronary heart disease or in**

women at risk for coronary events; use with caution in patients with cardiovascular disease. Not be used for the prevention of cardiovascular disease. Use caution with moderate-to-severe renal dysfunction, hepatic impairment, unexplained uterine bleeding, and in women with a history of elevated triglycerides in response to treatment with oral estrogens (or estrogen/progestin). Safety with concomitant estrogen therapy has not been established. Safety and efficacy in premenopausal women or men have not been established. Not indicated for treatment of invasive breast cancer, to reduce the risk of recurrence of invasive breast cancer or to reduce the risk of noninvasive breast cancer. The efficacy (for breast cancer risk reduction) in women with inherited BRCA1 and BRCA1 mutations has not been established.

Drug Interactions

Avoid Concomitant Use There are no known interactions where it is recommended to avoid concomitant use.

Decreased Effect

Raloxifene may decrease the levels/effects of: Levothyroxine

The levels/effects of Raloxifene may be decreased by: Bile Acid Sequestrants

Increased Effect/Toxicity There are no known significant interactions involving an increase in effect.

Nutritional/Ethanol Interactions Ethanol: Avoid ethanol (may increase risk of osteoporosis).

Adverse Reactions Note: Raloxifene has been associated with increased risk of thromboembolism (DVT, PE) and superficial thrombophlebitis; risk is similar to reported risk of HRT

>10%:
- Cardiovascular: Peripheral edema (3% to 14%)
- Endocrine & metabolic: Hot flashes (8% to 29%)
- Neuromuscular & skeletal: Arthralgia (11% to 16%), leg cramps/muscle spasm (6% to 12%)
- Miscellaneous: Flu syndrome (14% to 15%), infection (11%)

1% to 10%:
- Cardiovascular: Chest pain (3%), venous thromboembolism (1% to 2%)
- Central nervous system: Insomnia (6%)
- Dermatologic: Rash (6%)
- Endocrine & metabolic: Breast pain (4%)
- Gastrointestinal: Weight gain (9%), abdominal pain (7%), vomiting (5%), flatulence (2% to 3%), cholelithiasis (≤3%), gastroenteritis (≤3%)
- Genitourinary: Vaginal bleeding (6%), leukorrhea (3%), urinary tract disorder (3%), uterine disorder (3%), vaginal hemorrhage (3%), endometrial disorder (≤3%)
- Neuromuscular & skeletal: Myalgia (8%), tendon disorder (4%)
- Respiratory: Bronchitis (10%), sinusitis (10%), pharyngitis (8%), pneumonia (3%), laryngitis (≤2%)
- Miscellaneous: Diaphoresis (3%)

Pharmacodynamics/Kinetics

Onset of Action 8 weeks

Absorption Rapid; ~60%

Bioavailability ~2%

Protein Binding >95% to albumin and α-glycoprotein; does not bind to sex-hormone-binding globulin

Half-Life Elimination 28-33 hours

Metabolism Hepatic, extensive first-pass effect; metabolized to glucuronide conjugates

Excretion Primarily feces; urine (<0.2% as unchanged drug; <6% as glucuronide conjugates)

Available Dosage Forms

Tablet, oral:

Evista®: 60 mg

Dosing

Adult & Geriatric

Osteoporosis: Females: Oral: 60 mg once daily

Invasive breast cancer risk reduction: Female: Oral: 60 mg once daily for 5 years per ASCO guidelines (Visvanathan, 2009)

Renal Impairment Moderate-to-severe impairment: Use caution; safety and efficacy have not been established.

Hepatic Impairment Mild impairment (Child-Pugh class A): Plasma concentrations were higher and correlated with total bilirubin. Safety and efficacy in hepatic insufficiency have not been established.

Administration

Oral May be administered without regard to meals

Stability

Storage Store at controlled room temperature of 20°C to 25°C (68°F to 77°F); excursions permitted to 15°C to 30°C (59°F to 86°F).

Monitoring and Teaching Issues

Laboratory Monitoring Monitor lipid profile, bone mineral density (BMD)

Physical Assessment Evaluate lipid profile and BMD. Monitor for DVT, PE, chest pain, migraine, and rash on a regular basis during therapy.

Patient Education Avoid excessive use of alcohol (ethanol may increase risk of osteoporosis). May be taken at similar time each day without regard to meals. Additional vitamin and mineral supplements (vitamin D, calcium) may be recommended by your prescriber. May cause nausea, vomiting, diarrhea, or joint pain. Report immediately any pain, redness, warmth, or swelling in leg; sudden chest pain; respiratory difficulty; or sudden change in vision. Report acute migraine, weight gain, urinary infection, or vaginal burning or itching.

Dietary Considerations May be taken without regard to meals. Osteoporosis prevention or treatment: Ensure adequate calcium and vitamin D intake; postmenopausal women should consume ~1500 mg/day of elemental calcium and 400-800 int. units/day of vitamin D.

Geriatric Considerations No need to cycle with progesterone.

Pregnancy Considerations Animal studies have demonstrated teratogenicity and fetal loss. There are no adequate and well-controlled studies in pregnant women. Raloxifene should not be used by women who are or may become pregnant.

Additional Information The decrease in estrogen-related adverse effects with the selective estrogen-receptor modulators in general and raloxifene in particular should improve compliance and decrease the incidence of cardiovascular events and fractures while not increasing breast cancer.

Oncology Comment: The American Society of Clinical Oncology (ASCO) guidelines for breast cancer risk reduction (Visvanathan, 2009) recommend raloxifene (for 5 years) as an option to reduce the risk of ER-positive invasive breast cancer in postmenopausal women with a 5-year projected risk (based on NCI trial model) of ≥1.66%, or with lobular carcinoma *in situ*. Raloxifene should not be used in premenopausal women. Women with osteoporosis may use raloxifene beyond 5 years of treatment. According to the NCCN breast cancer risk reduction guidelines (v.2.2009), raloxifene is only recommended for postmenopausal women (≥35 years of age), and is equivalent to tamoxifen although, raloxifene has a better adverse event profile; however, tamoxifen is superior in reducing the risk on noninvasive breast cancer.

Related Information

Osteoporosis Management *on page 2067*

◆ **Raloxifene Hydrochloride** *see* Raloxifene *on page 1547*

Raltegravir (ral TEG ra vir)

U.S. Brand Names Isentress®

Index Terms MK-0518

Generic Availability (U.S.) No

Pharmacologic Category Antiretroviral Agent, Integrase Inhibitor

Pregnancy Risk Factor C

Lactation Excretion in breast milk unknown/contraindicated

Use Treatment of HIV-1 infection in combination with other antiretroviral agents

Mechanism of Action/Effect Inhibits the integration of viral DNA into host DNA, thereby blocking subsequent viral replication.

Contraindications There are no contraindications listed in the manufacturer's labeling.

Canadian labeling: Hypersensitivity to raltegravir or any other component of the formulation

Warnings/Precautions Patients may develop immune reconstitution syndrome resulting in the occurrence of an inflammatory response to an indolent or residual opportunistic infection; further evaluation and treatment may be required. Myopathy and rhabdomyolysis have been reported; use caution in patients with risk factors for CK elevations and/or skeletal muscle abnormalities. Use caution with medications known to induce (eg, rifampin) or inhibit (eg, atazanavir) UGT1A1 glucuronidation, as serum levels/therapeutic effects may be reduced or increased, respectively. Avoid use as a boosted PI replacement in antiretroviral experienced patients with documented resistance to nucleoside reverse transcriptase inhibitors.

Drug Interactions

Avoid Concomitant Use There are no known interactions where it is recommended to avoid concomitant use.

Decreased Effect

The levels/effects of Raltegravir may be decreased by: Efavirenz; Rifampin; Tipranavir

Increased Effect/Toxicity

The levels/effects of Raltegravir may be increased by: Proton Pump Inhibitors

Nutritional/Ethanol Interactions

Food: High-fat meal increased AUC by 19%, but raltegravir was administered without regard to meals in clinical trials.

Herb/Nutraceutical: Avoid St John's wort (may decrease the levels/effects of raltegravir).

Adverse Reactions

>10%: Endocrine & metabolic: Total cholesterol increased (grade 2: 16%; grade 3: 6%)

2% to 10%:

Cardiovascular: Hypertension (≤3%)

Central nervous system: Fatigue (<2% to 8%), dizziness (≤4%), insomnia (4%), headache (≥2%)

Dermatologic: Rash (≤5%), pruritus (≤3%), folliculitis (≤2%)

Endocrine & metabolic: LDL-cholesterol increased (grade 2: 9%; grade 3: 4%), glucose increased (126-250 mg/dL: 8%; 251-500 mg/dL: 2%), hypertriglyceridemia (grade 3: 4%)

Gastrointestinal: Abdominal pain (≤5%), lipase increased (1.6-3 x ULN: 4%), amylase increased (1.6-2 x ULN: 2%; 2.1-5 x ULN: 3%), gastroenteritis (≤3%), nausea (≥2%), constipation (≤2%)

Hepatic: AST increased (2.6-5 x ULN: 3% to 9%), hyperbilirubinemia (1.6-2.5 x ULN: 4% to 5%), ALT increased (5.1-10 x ULN: <1% to 3%), alkaline phosphatase increased (2.6-5 x ULN: <1% to 2%)

Neuromuscular & skeletal: Weakness (≥2%), creatine kinase increased (grade 4: 2%)

Renal: Creatinine increased (1.4-1.8 x ULN: 3%)

Respiratory: Nasopharyngitis (≤6%), cough (≤5%), influenza (≤3%)

Miscellaneous: Lymphadenopathy (≤3%), anogenital warts (≤2%)

Frequency <2% or not defined: Abnormal dreams, absolute neutrophil count decreased, acneiform dermatitis, allodynia, anemia, anxiety, appetite increased, arthralgia, back pain, cellulitis, central obesity, chest discomfort, chills, depression, diabetes mellitus, dry skin, dyspepsia, dyslipidemia, epistaxis, erectile dysfunction, erythema, extremity pain, facial wasting, flatulence, fever, gastritis, GERD, glossitis, gynecomastia, hepatitis, hepatomegaly, herpes simplex, herpes zoster, hyperhidrosis, hyperlactacidemia, hypersensitivity, insomnia, irritability, lipodystrophy, macrocytic anemia, maculopapular rash, MI, muscle atrophy, muscle spasms, myalgia, myopathy, myositis, nephrolithiasis, nephropathy, nephrotic syndrome, neuropathy, night sweats, nocturia, palpitation, paresthesia, platelets decreased, pollakiuria, prurigo, renal failure, renal tubular necrosis, rhabdomyolysis, somnolence, vertigo, ventricular extrasystoles, visual disturbance, vomiting, weight changes

Pharmacodynamics/Kinetics

Absorption AUC increased ~19% with high-fat meal

Time to Peak ~3 hours

Protein Binding ~83%

Half-Life Elimination ~9 hours

Metabolism Primarily hepatic glucuronidation mediated by UGT1A1

Excretion Feces (~51%, as unchanged drug); urine (~32%; 9% as unchanged drug)

Available Dosage Forms

Tablet, oral:

Isentress®: 400 mg

Dosing

Adult & Geriatric

HIV treatment: Oral: 400 mg twice daily. **Note:** Recommended as a first-line therapy with tenofovir/emtricitabine in antiretroviral naïve patients (Lennox, 2009; DHHS, 2011).

Dosage adjustment for rifampin coadministration: 800 mg twice daily

Pediatric HIV treatment: Adolescents ≥16 years: Refer to adult dosing.

Renal Impairment Severe renal impairment: No dosage adjustment required.

Hepatic Impairment

Mild-to-moderate hepatic impairment: No dosage adjustment required

Severe impairment: No data available

Administration

Oral May be administered without regard to meals.

Stability

Storage Store at room temperature of 20°C to 25°C (68°F to 77°F); excursions permitted to 15°C to 30°C (59°F to 86°F).

Monitoring and Teaching Issues

Laboratory Monitoring Viral load, CD4 count, lipid profile

Physical Assessment Evaluate CD4 count and viral load at baseline and periodically throughout; reduce cardiac risk factors.

Patient Education This drug will not cure HIV, nor has it been found to reduce the transmission of HIV; use appropriate precautions to prevent spread of the disease. This drug may be prescribed as one part of a multidrug combination; take exactly as directed for full course of therapy. If you miss a dose, take it as soon as you remember; do not double doses. You may be more susceptible to infection. May cause dizziness, headache, fatigue, nausea, vomiting, diarrhea, or itchy skin. Report signs of infection (unusual fever or chills, white plaques in mouth, vaginal itching or foul-smelling vaginal discharge, unusual cough, congestion, or unhealed wounds) or muscle pain, tenderness, or weakness.

Dietary Considerations May be taken without regard to meals.

Breast-Feeding Considerations In infants born to mothers who are HIV positive, HAART while breast-feeding may decrease postnatal infection. However, maternal or infant antiretroviral therapy does not completely eliminate the risk of postnatal HIV transmission. In addition, multiclass-resistant virus has been detected in breast-feeding infants despite maternal therapy.

In the United States where formula is accessible, affordable, safe, and sustainable, complete avoidance of breast-feeding by HIV-infected women is recommended to decrease potential transmission of HIV.

Pregnancy Considerations Animal studies revealed treatment-related increases in rib formation at 3-4 times human doses; no other embryo-/fetotoxic or teratogenic effects noted. There are no adequate and well-controlled studies in pregnant women and available data is insufficient to recommend use in pregnancy. An antiretroviral registry has been established to monitor maternal and fetal outcomes in women receiving antiretroviral drugs. Healthcare providers are encouraged to enroll pregnant women exposed to antiretroviral medications in the Antiretroviral Pregnancy Registry (1-800-258-4263 or www.APRegistry.com). Healthcare providers caring for HIV-infected women and their infants may contact the National Perinatal HIV Hotline (888-448-8765) for clinical consultation.

Ramelteon (ra MEL tee on)

U.S. Brand Names Rozerem™

Index Terms TAK-375

Generic Availability (U.S.) No

Pharmacologic Category Hypnotic, Nonbenzodiazepine

Medication Safety Issues
Sound-alike/look-alike issues:
Ramelteon may be confused with Remeron®
Rozerem® may be confused with Razadyne®, Remeron®

Medication Guide Available Yes

Pregnancy Risk Factor C

Lactation Excretion in breast milk unknown/use caution

Use Treatment of insomnia characterized by difficulty with sleep onset

Mechanism of Action/Effect Activates melatonin receptors within an area of the CNS controlling circadian rhythms and sleep-wake cycle.

Contraindications History of angioedema with previous ramelteon therapy (do not rechallenge); concurrent use with fluvoxamine

Warnings/Precautions Symptomatic treatment of insomnia should be initiated only after careful evaluation of potential causes of sleep disturbance. Failure of sleep disturbance to resolve after a reasonable period of treatment may indicate psychiatric and/or medical illness. Because of the rapid onset of action, administer immediately prior to bedtime or after the patient has gone to bed and is having difficulty falling asleep. Hypnotics/sedatives have been associated with abnormal thinking and behavior changes including decreased inhibition, aggression, bizarre behavior, agitation, hallucinations, and depersonalization. These changes may occur unpredictably and may indicate previously unrecognized psychiatric disorders; evaluate appropriately. Postmarketing studies have indicated that the use of hypnotic/sedative agents (including ramelteon) for sleep has been associated with hypersensitivity reactions including anaphylaxis as well as angioedema. Do not rechallenge patients who have developed angioedema with ramelteon therapy. An increased risk for hazardous sleep-related activities such as sleep-driving; cooking and eating food, and making phone calls while asleep have also been noted. Use caution with pre-existing depression or other psychiatric conditions. Caution when using with other CNS depressants; avoid engaging in hazardous activities or activities requiring mental alertness. Not recommended for use in patients with severe sleep apnea or COPD. Use caution with moderate hepatic impairment; not recommended in patients with severe impairment. May cause disturbances of hormonal regulation. Use caution when administered concomitantly with strong CYP1A2 inhibitors.

Drug Interactions

Metabolism/Transport Effects Substrate of CYP1A2 (major), CYP3A4 (minor), CYP2C family (minor)

Avoid Concomitant Use

Avoid concomitant use of Ramelteon with any of the following: FluvoxaMINE

Decreased Effect

The levels/effects of Ramelteon may be decreased by: Rifamycin Derivatives

Increased Effect/Toxicity

Ramelteon may increase the levels/effects of: Alcohol (Ethyl); CNS Depressants; Methotrimeprazine

The levels/effects of Ramelteon may be increased by: Antifungal Agents (Azole Derivatives, Systemic); Conivaptan; CYP1A2 Inhibitors (Moderate); CYP1A2 Inhibitors (Strong); Droperidol; Fluconazole; FluvoxaMINE; Methotrimeprazine

Nutritional/Ethanol Interactions
Ethanol: Avoid ethanol (may increase CNS depression).
Food: Taking with high-fat meal delays T_{max} and increases AUC (~31%).
Herb/Nutraceutical: Avoid valerian, St John's wort, kava kava, gotu kola (may increase CNS depression).

Adverse Reactions 1% to 10%:
Central nervous system: Dizziness (4% to 5%), somnolence (3% to 5%), fatigue (3% to 4%), insomnia worsened (3%), depression (2%)
Endocrine & metabolic: Serum cortisol decreased (1%)
Gastrointestinal: Nausea (3%), taste perversion (2%)
Neuromuscular & skeletal: Myalgia (2%), arthralgia (2%)
Respiratory: Upper respiratory infection (3%)
Miscellaneous: Influenza (1%)

Pharmacodynamics/Kinetics

Onset of Action 30 minutes

Absorption Rapid; high-fat meal delays T_{max} and increases AUC (~31%)

Bioavailability Absolute: 1.8%

Time to Peak Median: 0.5-1.5 hours

Protein Binding ~82%

Half-Life Elimination Ramelteon: 1-2.6 hours; M-II: 2-5 hours

Metabolism Extensive first-pass effect; oxidative metabolism primarily through CYP1A2 and to a lesser extent through CYP2C and CYP3A4; forms active metabolite (M-II)

Excretion Primarily as metabolites: Urine (84%); feces (4%)

Available Dosage Forms

Tablet, oral:
Rozerem™: 8 mg

Dosing

Adult & Geriatric Insomnia: Oral: One 8 mg tablet within 30 minutes of bedtime

Renal Impairment No dosage adjustment required

Hepatic Impairment No adjustment required for mild-to-moderate impairment; use caution. Not recommended with severe impairment.

Administration

Oral Do not administer with a high-fat meal. Swallow tablet whole; do not break.

Stability

Storage Store at 25°C (77°F); excursions permitted to 15°C to 30°C (59°F to 86°F). Protect from moisture.

Monitoring and Teaching Issues

Physical Assessment Monitor for CNS changes, abnormal thinking, and behavior changes.

Patient Education Take approximately 30 minutes before desiring to go to sleep. Avoid alcohol and other CNS depressants. You may experience dizziness, lightheadedness, or headache. Avoid meal high in fat prior to taking this medication. Report abnormal thinking or behavior; unusual swelling, especially on face or neck; or respiratory difficulty.

Dietary Considerations Do not take with high-fat meal.

Geriatric Considerations Although the C_{max} and AUC of ramelteon were increased in elderly patients, in clinical trials there were no significant differences in safety or efficacy between elderly and younger adult subjects.

Pregnancy Considerations Animal studies have demonstrated teratogenic effects. May cause disturbances of reproductive hormonal regulation (eg, disruption of menses or decreased libido). There are no adequate and well-controlled studies in pregnant women.

Ramipril (RA mi pril)

U.S. Brand Names Altace®

Generic Availability (U.S.) Yes: Capsule

Pharmacologic Category Angiotensin-Converting Enzyme (ACE) Inhibitor

Medication Safety Issues

Sound-alike/look-alike issues:

Ramipril may be confused with enalapril, Monopril®

Altace® may be confused with alteplase, Amaryl®, Amerge®, Artane®

International issues:

Altace [Canada] may be confused with Altace HCT brand name for ramipril/hydrochlorothiazide [Canada]

Pregnancy Risk Factor C (1st trimester); D (2nd and 3rd trimesters)

Lactation Excretion in breast milk unknown/not recommended

Use Treatment of hypertension, alone or in combination with thiazide diuretics; treatment of left ventricular dysfunction after MI; to reduce risk of MI, stroke, and death in patients at increased risk for these events

Unlabeled/Investigational Use Treatment of heart failure; to delay the progression of nephropathy and reduce risks of cardiovascular events in hypertensive patients with type 1 or 2 diabetes mellitus

Mechanism of Action/Effect Ramipril is an ACE inhibitor which prevents the formation of angiotensin II from angiotensin I and exhibits pharmacologic effects that are similar to captopril. Ramipril must undergo conversion in the liver to its biologically active metabolite, ramiprilat. The pharmacodynamic effects of ramipril result from the high-affinity, competitive, reversible binding of ramiprilat to angiotensin-converting enzyme thus preventing the formation of the potent vasoconstrictor angiotensin II.

Contraindications Hypersensitivity to ramipril or any component of the formulation; prior hypersensitivity (including angioedema) to ACE inhibitors

Warnings/Precautions Anaphylactic reactions may occur rarely with ACE inhibitors. At any time during treatment (especially following first dose) angioedema may occur rarely with ACE inhibitors; it may involve the head and neck (potentially compromising airway) or the intestine (presenting with abdominal pain). African-Americans and patients with idiopathic or hereditary angioedema may be at an increased risk. Prolonged frequent monitoring may be required especially if tongue, glottis, or larynx are involved as they are associated with airway obstruction. Patients with a history of airway surgery may have a higher risk of airway obstruction. Aggressive early and appropriate management is critical. Use in patients with previous angioedema associated with ACE inhibitor therapy is contraindicated. Severe anaphylactoid reactions may be seen during hemodialysis (eg, CVVHD) with high-flux dialysis membranes (eg, AN69), and rarely, during low density lipoprotein apheresis with dextran sulfate cellulose. Rare cases of anaphylactoid reactions have been reported in patients undergoing sensitization treatment with hymenoptera (bee, wasp) venom while receiving ACE inhibitors.

Symptomatic hypotension with or without syncope can occur with ACE inhibitors (usually with the first several doses); effects are most often observed in volume-depleted patients; close monitoring of patient is required especially with initial dosing and dosing increases; blood pressure must be lowered at a rate appropriate for the patient's clinical condition. Initiation of therapy in patients with ischemic heart disease or cerebrovascular disease warrants close observation due to the potential consequences posed by falling blood pressure (eg, MI, stroke). Use with caution in hypertrophic cardiomyopathy with outflow tract obstruction, severe aortic stenosis, or before, during, or immediately after major surgery. **[U.S. Boxed Warning]: Based on human data, ACEIs can cause injury and death to the developing fetus when used in the second and third trimesters. ACEIs should be discontinued as soon as possible once pregnancy is detected.**

Hyperkalemia may occur with ACE inhibitors; risk factors include renal dysfunction, diabetes mellitus, concomitant use of potassium-sparing diuretics, potassium supplements, and/or potassium containing salts. Use cautiously, if at all, with these agents and monitor potassium closely. Cough may occur with ACE inhibitors. Other causes of cough should be considered (eg, pulmonary congestion in patients with heart failure) and excluded prior to discontinuation.

May be associated with deterioration of renal function and/or increases in serum creatinine, particularly in patients with low renal blood flow (eg, renal artery stenosis, heart failure) whose glomerular filtration rate (GFR) is dependent on efferent arteriolar vasoconstriction by angiotensin II; deterioration may result in oliguria, acute renal failure, and progressive azotemia. Small increases in serum creatinine may occur following initiation; consider discontinuation only in patients with progressive and/or significant deterioration in renal function. Use with caution in patients with unstented unilateral/bilateral renal artery stenosis. When unstented bilateral renal artery stenosis is present, use is generally avoided due to the elevated risk of deterioration in renal function unless possible benefits outweigh risks. Concurrent use of angiotensin receptor blockers may increase the risk of clinically-significant adverse events (eg, renal dysfunction, hyperkalemia). Concurrent use with telmisartan is not recommended.

Rare toxicities associated with ACE inhibitors include cholestatic jaundice (which may progress to fulminant hepatic necrosis), agranulocytosis, neutropenia, or leukopenia with myeloid hypoplasia. Patients with collagen vascular diseases (especially with concomitant renal impairment) or renal impairment alone may be at increased risk for hematologic toxicity; periodically monitor CBC with differential in these patients.

Drug Interactions

Avoid Concomitant Use There are no known interactions where it is recommended to avoid concomitant use.

Decreased Effect

The levels/effects of Ramipril may be decreased by: Aprotinin; Herbs (Hypertensive Properties); Methylphenidate; Nonsteroidal Anti-Inflammatory Agents; Salicylates; Yohimbine

Increased Effect/Toxicity

Ramipril may increase the levels/effects of: Allopurinol; Amifostine; Antihypertensives; AzaTHIOprine; CycloSPORINE; CycloSPORINE (Systemic); Ferric Gluconate; Gold Sodium Thiomalate; Hypotensive Agents; Iron Dextran Complex; Lithium; RiTUXimab

The levels/effects of Ramipril may be increased by: Angiotensin II Receptor Blockers; Diazoxide; DPP-IV Inhibitors; Eplerenone; Everolimus; Herbs (Hypotensive Properties); Loop Diuretics; MAO Inhibitors; Pentoxifylline; Phosphodiesterase 5 Inhibitors; Potassium Salts; Potassium-Sparing Diuretics; Prostacyclin Analogues; Sirolimus; Telmisartan; Temsirolimus; Thiazide Diuretics; TiZANidine; Tolvaptan; Trimethoprim

Nutritional/Ethanol Interactions Herb/Nutraceutical: Avoid bayberry, blue cohosh, cayenne, ephedra, ginger, ginseng (American), kola, licorice (may worsen hypertension). Avoid black cohosh, California poppy, coleus, golden seal, hawthorn, mistletoe, periwinkle, quinine, shepherd's purse (may have increased antihypertensive effect).

Lab Interactions Positive Coombs' [direct]; may cause false-positive results in urine acetone determinations using sodium nitroprusside reagent

Adverse Reactions Note: Frequency ranges include data from hypertension and heart failure trials. Higher rates of adverse reactions have generally been noted in patients with CHF. However, the frequency of adverse effects associated with placebo is also increased in this population.

>10%: Respiratory: Cough increased (7% to 12%)

1% to 10%:

- Cardiovascular: Hypotension (11%), angina (up to 3%), postural hypotension (2%), syncope (up to 2%)
- Central nervous system: Headache (1% to 5%), dizziness (2% to 4%), fatigue (2%), vertigo (up to 2%)
- Endocrine & metabolic: Hyperkalemia (1% to 10%)
- Gastrointestinal: Nausea/vomiting (1% to 2%)
- Neuromuscular & skeletal: Chest pain (noncardiac) (1%)
- Renal: Renal dysfunction (1%), serum creatinine increased (1% to 2%), BUN increased (<1% to 3%); transient increases of creatinine and/or BUN may occur more frequently
- Respiratory: Cough (estimated 1% to 10%)

Worsening of renal function may occur in patients with bilateral renal artery stenosis or in hypovolemia. In addition, a syndrome which may include fever, myalgia, arthralgia, interstitial nephritis, vasculitis, rash, eosinophilia and positive ANA, and elevated ESR has been reported with ACE inhibitors. Risk of pancreatitis and agranulocytosis may be increased in patients with collagen vascular disease or renal impairment.

Pharmacodynamics/Kinetics

Onset of Action 1-2 hours

Duration of Action 24 hours

Absorption Well absorbed (50% to 60%)

Bioavailability Ramipril: 28%; Ramiprilat: 44%

Time to Peak Serum: Ramipril: ~1 hour; Ramiprilat: 2-4 hours

Protein Binding Ramipril: 73%; Ramiprilat: 56%

Half-Life Elimination Ramiprilat: Effective: 13-17 hours; Terminal: >50 hours

Metabolism Hepatic to the active form, ramiprilat

Excretion Urine (60%) and feces (40%) as parent drug and metabolites

Available Dosage Forms

Capsule, oral: 1.25 mg, 2.5 mg, 5 mg, 10 mg

Altace®: 1.25 mg, 2.5 mg, 5 mg, 10 mg

Dosing

Adult

Heart failure (unlabeled use): Initial: 1.25-2.5 mg once daily; target dose: 10 mg once daily (ACC/AHA 2009 Heart Failure Guidelines)

Hypertension: Oral: 2.5-5 mg once daily, maximum: 20 mg/day

LV dysfunction postmyocardial infarction: Oral: Initial: 2.5 mg twice daily titrated upward, if possible, to 5 mg twice daily

To reduce the risk of MI, stroke, and death from cardiovascular causes: Oral: Initial: 2.5 mg once daily for 1 week, then 5 mg once daily for the next 3 weeks, then increase as tolerated to 10 mg once daily (may be given as divided dose)

Note: The dose of any concomitant diuretic should be reduced. If the diuretic cannot be discontinued, initiate therapy with 1.25 mg. After the initial dose, the patient should be monitored carefully until blood pressure has stabilized.

Geriatric Refer to adult dosing. Adjust for renal function for elderly since glomerular filtration rates are decreased; may see exaggerated hypotensive effects if renal clearance is not considered.

Renal Impairment

Cl_{cr} <40 mL/minute: Administer 25% of normal dose.

Renal failure and heart failure: Administer 1.25 mg once daily, increasing to 1.25 mg twice daily up to 2.5 mg twice daily as tolerated.

Renal failure and hypertension: Administer 1.25 mg once daily, titrated upward as possible; maximum daily dose 5 mg.

Administration

Oral Capsule is usually swallowed whole, but contents may be mixed in water, apple juice, or applesauce.

Stability

Storage Store at controlled room temperature.

Monitoring and Teaching Issues

Laboratory Monitoring Serum creatinine and potassium; if patient has collagen vascular disease and/or renal impairment, periodically monitor CBC with differential

Physical Assessment Evaluate carefully for necessary use cautions. Assess potential for interactions with other pharmacological agents or herbal products that may impact fluid balance or cardiac status. Monitor first dose carefully. Assess blood pressure and cardiac status. Monitor for cough, renal dysfunction, nausea/vomiting, hypovolemia, angioedema, and postural hypotension on a regular basis during therapy.

Patient Education Take first dose at bedtime or when sitting down (hypotension may occur). This drug does not eliminate need for diet or exercise regimen as recommended by prescriber. May cause increased cough (if persistent or bothersome, contact prescriber), headache, postural hypotension, dizziness, nausea, or vomiting. Immediately report swelling of face, mouth, lips, tongue or throat; chest pain or irregular heartbeat. Report respiratory difficulty or persistent cough or persistent pain in muscles, joints, or back.

Geriatric Considerations Due to frequent decreases in glomerular filtration (also creatinine clearance) with aging, elderly patients may have exaggerated responses to ACE inhibitors; differences in clinical response due to hepatic changes are not observed. ACE inhibitors may be preferred agents in elderly patients with CHF and diabetes mellitus. Diabetic proteinuria is reduced and insulin sensitivity is enhanced. In general, the side effect profile is favorable in the elderly and causes little or no CNS confusion; use lowest dose recommendations initially. Many elderly may be volume depleted due to diuretic use and/or blunted thirst reflex resulting in inadequate fluid intake.

Breast-Feeding Considerations Ramipril and its metabolites were not detected in breast milk following a single oral dose of 10 mg. It is not known if multiple doses will produce detectable levels. Breast-feeding is not recommended by the manufacturer.

Pregnancy Considerations Due to adverse events observed in some animal studies, ramipril is considered pregnancy category C during the first trimester. Based on human data, ramipril is considered pregnancy category D if used during the second and third trimesters (per the manufacturer; however, one study suggests that fetal injury may occur at anytime during pregnancy). Ramipril crosses the placenta. First trimester exposure to ACE inhibitors may cause major congenital malformations. An increased risk of cardiovascular and/or central nervous system malformations was observed in one study; however, an increased risk of teratogenic events was not observed in other studies. Second and third trimester use of an ACE inhibitor is associated with oligohydramnios. Oligohydramnios due to decreased fetal renal function may lead to fetal limb contractures, craniofacial deformation, and hypoplastic lung development. The use of ACE inhibitors during the second and third trimesters is also associated with anuria, hypotension, renal failure (reversible or irreversible), skull hypoplasia, and death in the fetus/neonate. Chronic maternal hypertension itself is also associated with adverse events in the fetus/infant. ACE inhibitors are not recommended during pregnancy to treat maternal hypertension or heart failure. Those who are planning a pregnancy should be considered for other medication options if an ACE inhibitor is currently prescribed or the ACE inhibitor should be discontinued as soon as possible once pregnancy is detected. The exposed fetus should be monitored for fetal growth, amniotic fluid volume, and organ formation. Infants exposed to an ACE inhibitor *in utero*, especially during the second and third trimester, should be monitored for hyperkalemia, hypotension, and oliguria.

[U.S. Boxed Warning]: Based on human data, ACE inhibitors can cause injury and death to the developing fetus when used in the second and third trimesters. ACE inhibitors should be discontinued as soon as possible once pregnancy is detected.

Related Information

Angiotensin Agents *on page 1974*

Heart Failure (Systolic) *on page 2040*

◆ **Ranexa®** *see* Ranolazine *on page 1557*

◆ **Raniclor™** *see* Cefaclor *on page 310*

Ranitidine (ra NI ti deen)

U.S. Brand Names Zantac 150® [OTC]; Zantac 75® [OTC]; Zantac®; Zantac® EFFERdose®

Index Terms Ranitidine Hydrochloride

Generic Availability (U.S.) Yes: Excludes effervescent tablet, premixed infusion

Pharmacologic Category Histamine H_2 Antagonist

Medication Safety Issues

Sound-alike/look-alike issues:

Ranitidine may be confused with amantadine, rimantadine

Zantac® may be confused with Xanax®, Zarontin®, Zofran®, ZyrTEC®

International issues:

Antagon®: Brand name for astemizole in Mexico; brand name for ganirelix in the U.S.

Pregnancy Risk Factor B

Lactation Enters breast milk/use caution

Use

Zantac®: Short-term and maintenance therapy of duodenal ulcer, gastric ulcer, gastroesophageal reflux disease (GERD), active benign ulcer, erosive esophagitis, and pathological hypersecretory conditions; as part of a multidrug regimen for *H. pylori* eradication to reduce the risk of duodenal ulcer recurrence

Zantac 75® [OTC]: Relief of heartburn, acid indigestion, and sour stomach

Unlabeled/Investigational Use Recurrent postoperative ulcer, upper GI bleeding, prevention of acid-aspiration pneumonitis during surgery, and prevention of stress-induced ulcers

Mechanism of Action/Effect Competitive inhibition of histamine at H_2-receptors, gastric acid secretion, gastric volume and hydrogen ion concentration are reduced

Contraindications Hypersensitivity to ranitidine or any component of the formulation

Warnings/Precautions Ranitidine has been associated with confusional states (rare). Use with caution in patients with hepatic impairment; use with caution in renal impairment, dosage modification required. Avoid use in patients with history of acute porphyria (may precipitate attacks); long-term therapy may be associated with vitamin B_{12} deficiency. Symptoms of GI distress may be associated with a variety of conditions; symptomatic response to H_2 antagonists does not rule out the potential for significant pathology (eg, malignancy). EFFERdose® formulation contains phenylalanine.

Drug Interactions

Metabolism/Transport Effects Substrate of CYP1A2 (minor), CYP2C19 (minor), CYP2D6 (minor), P-glycoprotein; **Inhibits** CYP1A2 (weak), 2D6 (weak)

Avoid Concomitant Use

Avoid concomitant use of Ranitidine with any of the following: Delavirdine; Erlotinib

Decreased Effect

Ranitidine may decrease the levels/effects of: Atazanavir; Cefditoren; Cefpodoxime; Cefuroxime; Dasatinib; Delavirdine; Erlotinib; Fosamprenavir; Gefitinib; Indinavir; Iron Salts; Itraconazole; Ketoconazole; Ketoconazole (Systemic); Mesalamine; Nelfinavir; Posaconazole; Prasugrel

The levels/effects of Ranitidine may be decreased by: Peginterferon Alfa-2b; P-Glycoprotein Inducers

Increased Effect/Toxicity

Ranitidine may increase the levels/effects of: Dexmethylphenidate; Methylphenidate; Procainamide; Saquinavir; Sulfonylureas; Warfarin

The levels/effects of Ranitidine may be increased by: P-Glycoprotein Inhibitors

Nutritional/Ethanol Interactions

Ethanol: Avoid ethanol (may cause gastric mucosal irritation).

Food: Does not interfere with absorption of ranitidine.

Lab Interactions False-positive urine protein using Multistix®; gastric acid secretion test; skin test allergen extracts. May also interfere with urine detection of amphetamine/methamphetamine (false-positive).

Adverse Reactions Frequency not defined.

Cardiovascular: Asystole, atrioventricular block, bradycardia (with rapid I.V. administration), premature ventricular beats, tachycardia, vasculitis

Central nervous system: Agitation, dizziness, depression, hallucinations, headache, insomnia, malaise, mental confusion, somnolence, vertigo

Dermatologic: Alopecia, erythema multiforme, rash

Endocrine & metabolic: Prolactin levels increased

Gastrointestinal: Abdominal discomfort/pain, constipation, diarrhea, nausea, pancreatitis, vomiting

Hematologic: Acquired immune hemolytic anemia, acute porphyritic attack, agranulocytosis, aplastic anemia, granulocytopenia, leukopenia, pancytopenia, thrombocytopenia

Hepatic: Cholestatic hepatitis, hepatic failure, hepatitis, jaundice

Local: Transient pain, burning or itching at the injection site

Neuromuscular & skeletal: Arthralgia, involuntary motor disturbance, myalgia
Ocular: Blurred vision
Renal: Acute interstitial nephritis, serum creatinine increased
Respiratory: Pneumonia (causal relationship not established)
Miscellaneous: Anaphylaxis, angioneurotic edema, hypersensitivity reactions (eg, bronchospasm, fever, eosinophilia)

Pharmacodynamics/Kinetics

Absorption Oral: 50%

Bioavailability Oral: 48% to 50%; I.M.: 90% to 100%

Time to Peak Serum: Oral: 2-3 hours; I.M.: ≤15 minutes

Protein Binding 15%

Half-Life Elimination
Oral: Normal renal function: 2.5-3 hours; Cl_{cr} 25-35 mL/minute: 4.8 hours
I.V.: Normal renal function: 2-2.5 hours

Metabolism Hepatic to N-oxide, S-oxide, and N-desmethyl metabolites

Excretion Urine: Oral: 30%, I.V.: 70% (as unchanged drug); feces (as metabolites)

Available Dosage Forms

Capsule, oral: 150 mg, 300 mg
Infusion, premixed in 1/2 NS [preservative free]:
Zantac®: 50 mg (50 mL)
Injection, solution: 25 mg/mL (2 mL, 6 mL, 40 mL)
Zantac®: 25 mg/mL (2 mL, 6 mL, 40 mL)
Syrup, oral: 15 mg/mL (5 mL, 10 mL, 473 mL, 480 mL)
Zantac®: 15 mg/mL (480 mL)
Tablet, oral: 75 mg, 150 mg, 300 mg
Zantac 150® [OTC]: 150 mg
Zantac 75® [OTC]: 75 mg
Zantac®: 150 mg, 300 mg
Tablet for solution, oral:
Zantac® EFFERdose®: 25 mg

Dosing

Adult & Geriatric

Duodenal ulcer: Oral: Treatment: 150 mg twice daily, or 300 mg once daily after the evening meal or at bedtime; maintenance: 150 mg once daily at bedtime
Eradication of *Helicobacter pylori*: Oral: 150 mg twice daily; requires combination therapy
Pathological hypersecretory conditions:
Oral: 150 mg twice daily; adjust dose or frequency as clinically indicated; doses of up to 6 g/day have been used
I.V.: Continuous infusion for Zollinger-Ellison: Initial: 1 mg/kg/hour; measure gastric acid output at 4 hours, if >10 mEq or if patient is symptomatic, increase dose in increments of 0.5 mg/kg/hour; doses of up to 2.5 mg/kg/hour (or 220 mg/hour) have been used
Gastric ulcer, benign: *Oral:* 150 mg twice daily; maintenance: 150 mg once daily at bedtime
GERD: *Oral:* 150 mg twice daily
Erosive esophagitis: *Oral:* Treatment: 150 mg 4 times/day; maintenance: 150 mg twice daily
Prevention of heartburn: *Oral:* Zantac 75® [OTC]: 75 mg 30-60 minutes before eating food or drinking beverages which cause heartburn; maximum: 150 mg in 24 hours; do not use for more than 14 days
Patients not able to take oral medication:
I.M.: 50 mg every 6-8 hours
I.V.: Intermittent bolus or infusion: 50 mg every 6-8 hours
Continuous I.V. infusion: 6.25 mg/hour

Pediatric

Duodenal and gastric ulcer:
Oral: Children 1 month to 16 years:
Treatment: 4-8 mg/kg/day divided twice daily; maximum: 300 mg/day
Maintenance: 2-4 mg/kg/day once daily; maximum: 150 mg/day
I.V.: 2-4 mg/kg/day divided every 6-8 hours; maximum: 200 mg/day
GERD and erosive esophagitis: Children 1 month to 16 years:
Oral: 5-10 mg/kg/day divided twice daily; maximum: GERD: 300 mg/day, erosive esophagitis: 600 mg/day
I.V. (unlabeled): 2-4 mg/kg/day divided every 6-8 hours; maximum: 200 mg/day **or as an alternative**
Continuous infusion: Initial: 1 mg/kg/dose for one dose followed by infusion of 0.08-0.17 mg/kg/hour or 2-4 mg/kg/day
Prevention of heartburn: *Oral:* Children ≥12 years: Zantac 75® [OTC]: 75 mg 30-60 minutes before eating food or drinking beverages which cause heartburn; maximum: 150 mg/24 hours; do not use for more than 14 days

Renal Impairment Adults: Cl_{cr} <50 mL/minute:
Oral: 150 mg every 24 hours; adjust dose cautiously if needed
I.V.: 50 mg every 18-24 hours; adjust dose cautiously if needed
Hemodialysis: Adjust dosing schedule so that dose coincides with the end of hemodialysis.

Hepatic Impairment Patients with hepatic impairment may have minor changes in ranitidine half-life, distribution, clearance, and bioavailability; dosing adjustments are not necessary; monitor patient.

Administration

Oral EFFERdose®: Should not be chewed, swallowed whole, or dissolved on tongue: 25 mg tablet: Dissolve in at least 5 mL (1 teaspoonful) of water; wait until completely dissolved before administering

I.M. No dilution is needed

I.V.

I.V. push: Ranitidine (usually 50 mg) should be diluted to a total of 20 mL (or a concentration not exceeding 2.5 mg/mL) with NS or D_5W and administered over at least 5 minutes or a maximum rate of 10 mg/minute.

Intermittent I.V. infusion: Dilute to a maximum concentration of 0.5 mg/mL; administer over 15-20 minutes

Continuous I.V. infusion: Dilute to a maximum concentration of 2.5 mg/mL. Titrate dosage based on gastric pH.

Stability

Reconstitution Vials can be mixed with NS or D_5W.

Intermittent bolus injection, continuous infusion: Dilute to maximum of 2.5 mg/mL.

Intermittent infusion: Dilute to maximum of 0.5 mg/mL.

Storage

Injection: Vials: Store between 4°C to 25°C (39°F to 77°F); excursion permitted to 30°C (86°F). Protect from light. Solution is a clear, colorless to yellow solution; slight darkening does not affect potency. Vials mixed with NS or D_5W are stable for 48 hours at room temperature.

Premixed bag: Store between 2°C to 25°C (36°F to 77°F). Protect from light.

EFFERdose® formulations: Store between 2°C to 30°C (36°F to 86°F).

Syrup: Store between 4°C to 25°C (39°F to 77°F). Protect from light.

Tablets: Store in dry place, between 15°C to 30°C (59°F to 86°F). Protect from light.

Monitoring and Teaching Issues

Laboratory Monitoring AST, ALT, serum creatinine; when used to prevent stress-related GI bleeding, measure the intragastric pH and try to maintain pH >4; occult blood with GI bleeding; monitor renal function and adjust dosage as indicated.

Physical Assessment Use caution in presence of renal impairment; dosage adjustment may be necessary. Monitor for CNS changes (depression, hallucinations, confusion, malaise), rash, and GI disturbance.

Patient Education May take several days before you notice relief. Avoid excessive alcohol. May cause drowsiness, dizziness, or fatigue. Report immediately skin rash, CNS changes (mental confusion, hallucinations, somnolence), or unusual persistent weakness or lethargy.

Dietary Considerations Some products may contain phenylalanine and/or sodium. Oral dosage forms may be taken with or without food.

Geriatric Considerations Ulcer healing rates and incidence of adverse effects are similar in the elderly, when compared to younger patients; dosing adjustments not necessary based on age alone. Always adjust dose based upon creatinine clearance. Serum half-life is increased to 3-4 hours in elderly patients. H_2 blockers are the preferred drugs for treating PUD in the elderly due to cost and ease of administration. These agents are no less or more effective than any other therapy. The preferred agents, due to side effects and drug interaction profile and pharmacokinetics are ranitidine, famotidine, and nizatidine. Treatment for PUD in the elderly is recommended for 12 weeks since their lesions are larger; therefore, take longer to heal. This drug is substantially cleared renally, and elderly, having decreased renal function in general, should be monitored closely for adverse effects, especially CNS.

Breast-Feeding Considerations Ranitidine is excreted into breast milk. The manufacturer recommends that caution be exercised when administering ranitidine to nursing women. Peak milk concentrations of ranitidine occur ~5.5 hours after the dose (case report).

Pregnancy Considerations Adverse events were not observed in animal studies; therefore, ranitidine is classified as pregnancy category B. Ranitidine crosses the placenta. An increased risk of congenital malformations or adverse events in the newborn has generally not been observed following maternal use of ranitidine during pregnancy. Histamine H_2 antagonists have been evaluated for the treatment of gastroesophageal reflux disease (GERD) as well as gastric and duodenal ulcers during pregnancy. If needed, ranitidine is the agent of choice. Histamine H_2 antagonists may be used for aspiration prophylaxis prior to cesarean delivery.

Related Information

Compatibility of Drugs *on page* 1994

◆ **Ranitidine Hydrochloride** *see* Ranitidine *on page* 1555

Ranolazine (ra NOE la zeen)

U.S. Brand Names Ranexa®

Generic Availability (U.S.) No

Pharmacologic Category Cardiovascular Agent, Miscellaneous

Medication Safety Issues

Sound-alike/look-alike issues:

Ranexa® may be confused with Celexa®

Pregnancy Risk Factor C

Lactation Excretion in breast milk unknown/not recommended

Use Treatment of chronic angina

Mechanism of Action/Effect May increase myocardial relaxation during myocardial ischemia and improve energy supply during ischemia.

Contraindications Clinically significant hepatic impairment; concurrent strong CYP3A inhibitors; concurrent inducers of CYP3A

Warnings/Precautions Ranolazine does not relieve acute angina attacks. Has been shown to prolong QT interval in a dose/plasma concentration-related manner. Hepatically-impaired patients may have a more significant increase in QT interval. Use with caution in patients with mild (Child-Pugh class A) or moderate (Child-Pugh class B) hepatic impairment; use is contraindicated with clinically significant hepatic impairment. Use caution in patients ≥75 years of age; they may experience more adverse events. Use caution and monitor blood pressure in patients with renal dysfunction; has not been evaluated in patients requiring dialysis.

Ranolazine is a substrate for and a moderate inhibitor of P-glycoprotein. Inhibitors of P-glycoprotein may increase serum concentrations of ranolazine. Ranolazine may increase serum concentrations of substrates for P-glycoprotein (eg, digoxin). Ranolazine is primarily metabolized by CYP3A; use is contraindicated with inducers and strong inhibitors of CYP3A. Ranolazine has potential to prolong the QT-interval; use caution when administered concomitantly with QT-prolonging drugs. Use caution when administering ranolazine to patients with a history of malignant neoplasms or adenomatous polyps.

Drug Interactions

Metabolism/Transport Effects Substrate of CYP3A4 (major), CYP2D6 (minor), P-glycoprotein; **Inhibits** CYP3A4 (weak), CYP2D6 (moderate), P-glycoprotein

Avoid Concomitant Use

Avoid concomitant use of Ranolazine with any of the following: Antifungal Agents (Azole Derivatives, Systemic); Artemether; CYP3A4 Inducers (Strong); CYP3A4 Inhibitors (Strong); Dronedarone; Lumefantrine; Nilotinib; Pimozide; QuiNINE; Rifampin; Silodosin; Tetrabenazine; Thioridazine; Topotecan; Toremifene; Vandetanib; Ziprasidone

Decreased Effect

Ranolazine may decrease the levels/effects of: Codeine; TraMADol

The levels/effects of Ranolazine may be decreased by: CYP3A4 Inducers (Strong); Deferasirox; Herbs (CYP3A4 Inducers); Peginterferon Alfa-2b; P-Glycoprotein Inducers; Rifampin

Increased Effect/Toxicity

Ranolazine may increase the levels/effects of: Colchicine; CYP2D6 Substrates; Dabigatran Etexilate; Digoxin; Dronedarone; Everolimus; Fesoterodine; Nebivolol; P-Glycoprotein Substrates; Pimozide; QTc-Prolonging Agents; QuiNINE; Rivaroxaban; Silodosin; Simvastatin; Tacrolimus; Tacrolimus (Systemic); Tamoxifen; Tetrabenazine; Thioridazine; Topotecan; Toremifene; Vandetanib; Ziprasidone

The levels/effects of Ranolazine may be increased by: Alfuzosin; Antifungal Agents (Azole Derivatives, Systemic); Artemether; Calcium Channel Blockers (Nondihydropyridine); Chloroquine; Ciprofloxacin; Ciprofloxacin (Systemic); CYP3A4 Inhibitors (Moderate); CYP3A4 Inhibitors (Strong); Gadobutrol; Lumefantrine; Nilotinib; P-Glycoprotein Inhibitors; QuiNINE

Nutritional/Ethanol Interactions Food: Limit the use of grapefruit, grapefruit juice, or grapefruit-containing products; if use is significant and consistent, the dose of ranolazine should be limited to 500 mg twice daily.

Adverse Reactions

>10%:

Central nervous system: Dizziness (5% to 13%; dose related)

Gastrointestinal: Constipation (5% to 8%; 19% in the elderly)

>0.5% to 10%:

Cardiovascular: Syncope (≤3%), bradycardia (≤2%), hypotension (≤2%), orthostatic hypotension (≤2%), palpitation (≤2%), peripheral edema (≤2%), QT_c prolongation (>500 msec: ≤1%)

Central nervous system: Headache (3% to 6%), vertigo (≤2%)

Gastrointestinal: Nausea (4% to 9%), abdominal pain (≤2%), vomiting (≤2%), xerostomia (≤2%)

Hematologic: Hematocrit decreased (1%)

Otic: Tinnitus (≤2%)

Respiratory: Dyspnea (≤2%)

Pharmacodynamics/Kinetics

Absorption Highly variable; ranolazine is a substrate of P-glycoprotein; concurrent use of P-glycoprotein inhibitors may increase absorption

Bioavailability 35% to 55%

Time to Peak 2-5 hours

Protein Binding ~62%

Half-Life Elimination Terminal: 7 hours

Metabolism Hepatic via CYP3A (major) and 2D6 (minor); gut

Excretion Primarily urine (75% mostly as metabolites); feces (25% mostly as metabolites); in feces and urine, <5% to 7% excreted unchanged

Available Dosage Forms

Tablet, extended release, oral:

Ranexa®: 500 mg, 1000 mg

Dosing

Adult

Chronic angina: Oral: Initial: 500 mg twice daily; maximum recommended dose: 1000 mg twice daily

Dosage adjustment for ranolazine with concomitant medications:

Diltiazem, verapamil, and other moderate CYP3A inhibitors: Dose should not exceed 500 mg twice daily

P-glycoprotein inhibitors (eg, cyclosporine): Down-titrate ranolazine based on clinical response

Geriatric Refer to adult dosing. Select dose cautiously, starting at the lower end of the dosing range.

Renal Impairment Dosage adjustment recommendations have not been established. However, plasma ranolazine levels increased ~50% in patients with varying degrees of renal dysfunction. Patients with severe renal dysfunction had an increase in mean diastolic blood pressure of 10-15 mm Hg. Monitor blood pressure closely in these patients. Ranolazine has not been evaluated in patients requiring dialysis.

Hepatic Impairment Use with caution in patients with mild (Child-Pugh class A) and moderate (Child-Pugh class B) hepatic impairment. Use is contraindicated with clinically significant hepatic impairment.

Administration

Oral May be taken with or without meals. Swallow tablet whole; do not crush, break, or chew.

Stability

Storage Store at 25°C (77°F); excursions permitted to 15°C to 30°C (59°F to 86°F).

Monitoring and Teaching Issues

Laboratory Monitoring Baseline and follow up ECG to evaluate QT interval; correct and maintain serum potassium in normal limits

Physical Assessment Stress that this medication is not intended to treat an acute angina episode. Instruct patient in appropriate measures to take if an acute episode occurs.

Patient Education This medication is not intended to treat an acute angina episode. Follow instructions provided by prescriber for acute management. Swallow tablets whole; do not crush, break, or chew the tablets. You may experience dizziness or constipation. Report palpitations, dizziness, and chest pain that do not respond to recommended interventions.

Dietary Considerations May be taken without regard to meals. Limit the use of grapefuit juice.

Geriatric Considerations Elderly comprised 48% of study group participants. For those elderly, no overall difference in efficacy was observed between younger and older adults. There was, however, a higher incidence of adverse effects for those ≥75 years of age, resulting in drug discontinuations. The most common adverse effects were constipation (19%), nausea (6%), and dizziness (6%). Therefore, start dosing at lower end of dosing range recommended.

Breast-Feeding Considerations Due to the potential for serious adverse reactions in the nursing infant, breast-feeding is not recommended.

Pregnancy Considerations Adverse effects were observed in animal studies. There are no adequate and well-controlled studies in pregnant women.

◆ **Rapaflo®** *see* Silodosin *on page 1643*

◆ **Rapamune®** *see* Sirolimus *on page 1648*

◆ **Rapamycin** *see* Sirolimus *on page 1648*

Rasagiline (ra SA ji leen)

U.S. Brand Names Azilect®

Index Terms AGN 1135; Rasagiline Mesylate; TVP-1012

Generic Availability (U.S.) No

Pharmacologic Category Anti-Parkinson's Agent, MAO Type B Inhibitor

Medication Safety Issues

Sound-alike/look-alike issues:

Azilect® may be confused with Aricept®

Pregnancy Risk Factor C

Lactation Excretion in breast milk unknown/use caution

Use Treatment of idiopathic Parkinson's disease (initial monotherapy or as adjunct to levodopa)

Mechanism of Action/Effect Rasagiline selectively inhibits MAO-B which enhances brain dopamine levels, thus reducing symptomatic motor deficits.

Contraindications Concomitant use of cyclobenzaprine, dextromethorphan, methadone, propoxyphene, St John's wort, or tramadol; concomitant use of meperidine or an MAO inhibitor (including selective MAO-B inhibitors) within 14 days of rasagiline

Warnings/Precautions Hazardous agent - use appropriate precautions for handling and disposal.

Cardiovascular system: May cause orthostatic hypotension, particularly in combination with levodopa; use with caution in patients with hypotension or patients who would not tolerate transient hypotensive episodes (cardiovascular or cerebrovascular disease); orthostasis is usually most problematic during first 2 months of therapy and tends to abate thereafter. Due to the potential for hemodynamic instability, patients should not undergo elective surgery requiring general anesthesia and should avoid local anesthesia containing sympathomimetic vasoconstrictors within 14 days of discontinuing rasagiline. If surgery is required, benzodiazepines, mivacurium, fentanyl, morphine or codeine may be used cautiously. In patients taking recommended doses of rasagiline, dietary restriction of most tyramine-containing products is not necessary; however, certain foods (eg, aged cheeses) may contain high amounts

(>150 mg) of tyramine and could lead to hypertensive crisis. Avoid concomitant use with foods high in tyramine.

Central nervous system: Serotonin syndrome (SS)/neuroleptic malignant syndrome (NMS)-like reactions may occur rarely, particularly when used at doses exceeding recommendations or when used in combination with an antidepressant (eg, SSRI, SNRI, TCA). May cause hallucinations; signs of severe CNS toxicity (some fatal), including hyperpyrexia, hyperthermia, rigidity, altered mental status, seizure and coma have been reported with selective and nonselective MAO inhibitor use in combination with antidepressants. Do not use within 5 weeks of fluoxetine discontinuation; do not initiate tricyclic, SSRI, or SNRI therapy within 2 weeks of discontinuing rasagiline. Addition to levodopa therapy may result in exacerbation of dyskinesias, requiring a reduction in levodopa dosage.

Dermatologic: Risk of melanoma may be increased with rasagiline, although increased risk has been associated with Parkinson's disease itself; patients should have regular and frequent skin examinations.

Organ dysfunction: Use caution in mild hepatic impairment; dose reduction recommended. Do not use with moderate-to-severe hepatic impairment.

Drug Interactions

Metabolism/Transport Effects Substrate of CYP1A2 (major)

Avoid Concomitant Use

Avoid concomitant use of Rasagiline with any of the following: Alpha-/Beta-Agonists (Indirect-Acting); Alpha1-Agonists; Alpha2-Agonists (Ophthalmic); Amphetamines; Anilidopiperidine Opioids; Atomoxetine; Bezafibrate; Buprenorphine; BuPROPion; BusPIRone; CarBAMazepine; Cyclobenzaprine; Dexmethylphenidate; Dextromethorphan; Diethylpropion; HYDROmorphone; Linezolid; Maprotiline; Meperidine; Methyldopa; Methylphenidate; Mirtazapine; Propoxyphene; Selective Serotonin Reuptake Inhibitors; Serotonin 5-HT1D Receptor Agonists; Serotonin/Norepinephrine Reuptake Inhibitors; Sibutramine; Tapentadol; Tetrabenazine; Tetrahydrozoline; Tetrahydrozoline (Nasal); Tricyclic Antidepressants; Tryptophan

Decreased Effect

The levels/effects of Rasagiline may be decreased by: CYP1A2 Inducers (Strong)

Increased Effect/Toxicity

Rasagiline may increase the levels/effects of: Alpha-/Beta-Agonists (Direct-Acting); Alpha-/Beta-Agonists (Indirect-Acting); Alpha1-Agonists; Alpha2-Agonists (Ophthalmic); Amphetamines; Antihypertensives; Atomoxetine; Beta2-Agonists; Bezafibrate; BuPROPion; Dexmethylphenidate; Dextromethorphan; Diethylpropion; Doxapram; HYDROmorphone; Linezolid; Lithium; Meperidine; Methadone; Methyldopa; Methylphenidate; Mirtazapine; Orthostatic Hypotension Producing Agents; Reserpine; Selective Serotonin Reuptake Inhibitors; Serotonin 5-HT1D Receptor Agonists; Serotonin Modulators; Serotonin/Norepinephrine Reuptake Inhibitors; Tetrahydrozoline; Tetrahydrozoline (Nasal); Tricyclic Antidepressants

The levels/effects of Rasagiline may be increased by: Altretamine; Anilidopiperidine Opioids; Buprenorphine; BusPIRone; CarBAMazepine; COMT Inhibitors; Cyclobenzaprine; CYP1A2 Inhibitors (Moderate); CYP1A2 Inhibitors (Strong); Levodopa; MAO Inhibitors; Maprotiline; Propoxyphene; Sibutramine; Tapentadol; Tetrabenazine; TraMADol; Tryptophan

Nutritional/Ethanol Interactions

Ethanol: Avoid ethanol.

Food: Concurrent ingestion of foods rich in tyramine may cause sudden and severe high blood pressure (hypertensive crisis). Avoid foods (such as aged cheeses) containing high amounts (>150 mg) of tyramine.

Herb/Nutraceutical: Avoid valerian, St John's wort, SAMe, kava kava (may increase risk of serotonin syndrome and/or excessive sedation); Avoid supplements containing caffeine, tyrosine, tryptophan, or phenylalanine. Ingestion of large quantities may increase the risk of severe side effects (eg, hypertensive reactions, serotonin syndrome).

Adverse Reactions Unless otherwise noted, the following adverse reactions are as reported for monotherapy. Spectrum of adverse events was generally similar with adjunctive (levodopa) therapy, though the incidence tended to be higher.

>10%:

Cardiovascular: Postural hypotension (6% to 13% adjunct therapy, dose dependent)
Central nervous system: Dyskinesia (18% adjunct therapy), headache (14%)
Gastrointestinal: Nausea (10% to 12% adjunct therapy)

1% to 10%:

Cardiovascular: Angina, bundle branch block, chest pain, syncope
Central nervous system: Depression (5%), hallucinations (4% to 5% adjunct therapy), fever (3%), malaise (2%), vertigo (2%), anxiety, dizziness
Dermatologic: Bruising (2%), alopecia, skin carcinoma, vesiculobullous rash
Endocrine & metabolic: Impotence, libido decreased
Gastrointestinal: Constipation (4% to 9% adjunct therapy), weight loss (2% to 9% adjunct therapy; dose dependent), dyspepsia (7%), xerostomia (2% to 6% adjunct therapy; dose dependent), gastroenteritis (3%), anorexia, diarrhea, gastrointestinal hemorrhage, vomiting
Genitourinary: Hematuria, urinary incontinence
Hematologic: Leukopenia
Hepatic: Liver function tests increased
Neuromuscular & skeletal: Arthralgia (7%), neck pain (2%), arthritis (2%), paresthesia (2%), abnormal gait, hyperkinesias, hypertonia, neuropathy, tremor, weakness
Ocular: Conjunctivitis (3%)
Renal: Albuminuria
Respiratory: Rhinitis (3%), asthma, cough increased
Miscellaneous: Fall (5%), flu-like syndrome (5%), allergic reaction

Pharmacodynamics/Kinetics

Onset of Action Therapeutic: Within 1 hour

Duration of Action ~1 week (irreversible inhibition); may require ~14-40 days for complete restoration of (brain) MAO-B activity

Absorption Rapid

Bioavailability ~36%

Time to Peak ~1 hour

Protein Binding 88% to 94%,primarily to albumin

Half-Life Elimination ~1.3-3 hours (no correlation with biologic effect due to irreversible inhibition)

Metabolism Hepatic N-dealkylation and/or hydroxylation via CYP1A2 to multiple inactive metabolites (nonamphetamine derivatives)

Excretion Urine (62%, <1% of total dose as unchanged drug); feces (7%)

Available Dosage Forms

Tablet, oral:

Azilect®: 0.5 mg, 1 mg

Dosing

Adult & Geriatric Parkinson's disease: Oral:

Monotherapy: 1 mg once daily

Adjunctive therapy with levodopa: Initial: 0.5 mg once daily; may increase to 1 mg once daily based on response and tolerability

Note: When added to existing levodopa therapy, a dose reduction of levodopa may be required to avoid exacerbation of dyskinesias; typical dose reductions of ~9% to 13% were employed in clinical trials.

Dose reduction with concomitant ciprofloxacin or other CYP1A2 inhibitors: 0.5 mg once daily

Renal Impairment

Mild-to-moderate impairment: No adjustment necessary.

Severe impairment: Not studied.

Hepatic Impairment

Mild impairment (Child-Pugh ≤6): 0.5 mg once daily

Moderate-to-severe impairment: Not recommended.

Administration

Oral Administer without regard to meals.

Stability

Storage Store at 25°C (77°F); excursions permitted to 15°C to 30°C (59°F to 86°F).

Monitoring and Teaching Issues

Physical Assessment Assess effectiveness and interactions of other medications patient may be taking. Monitor therapeutic effectiveness according to rationale for therapy and adverse reactions at beginning of therapy and periodically throughout therapy. Monitor blood pressure. Be alert to thoughts of suicide. Patient should be cautioned against eating foods high in tyramine. Assess knowledge/teach patient appropriate use, interventions to reduce side effects, and adverse symptoms to report.

Patient Education May be prescribed in conjunction with levodopa/carbidopa. Therapeutic effects may take several weeks or months to achieve and you may need frequent monitoring during first weeks of therapy. Take with meals if GI upset occurs. Take at the same time each day. Avoid tyramine-containing foods during treatment and for two weeks after the medication had been stopped. Maintain adequate hydration unless instructed to restrict fluid intake. Do not use alcohol. You may experience drowsiness, dizziness, confusion, vision changes, orthostatic hypotension, constipation, runny nose or flu-like symptoms, nausea, vomiting, loss of appetite, or stomach discomfort. You are at an increased risk of melanoma. Have skin monitored by a qualified professional. Report any skin changes or suspicious areas. Report unresolved constipation or vomiting; chest pain, palpitations, irregular heartbeat; CNS changes (hallucination, loss of memory, seizures, acute headache, nervousness, suicide ideation, etc); painful or difficult urination; increased muscle spasticity, rigidity, or involuntary movements; skin rash; or significant worsening of condition.

Dietary Considerations May be taken without regard to meals. Avoid products containing high amounts of tyramine (>150 mg), such as aged cheeses (eg, Stilton cheese). Restriction of tyramine-containing products with lower amounts (<150 mg) of tyramine is not necessary in patients taking recommended doses. Some examples of tyramine-containing products include aged or matured cheese, air-dried or cured meats (including sausages and salamis), fava or broad bean pods, tap/draft beers, Marmite concentrate, sauerkraut, soy sauce and other soybean condiments. Food's freshness is also an important concern; improperly stored or spoiled food can create an environment where tyramine concentrations may increase.

Geriatric Considerations In clinical trials, no significant differences in the safety profile were seen between elderly and younger adults.

Breast-Feeding Considerations Animal studies have shown rasagiline is capable of inhibiting prolactin secretion.

Pregnancy Considerations Animal studies have documented decreased offspring survival and birth weight. An increased incidence of teratogenic effects, embryo-fetal deaths, and cardiovascular abnormalities were also noted with rasagiline in combination with levodopa/carbidopa. There are no adequate and well-controlled studies in pregnant women.

Additional Information When adding rasagiline to levodopa/carbidopa, the dose of the latter can usually be decreased. Studies are investigating the use of rasagiline in early Parkinson's disease to slow the progression of the disease.

◆ **Rasagiline Mesylate** *see* Rasagiline *on page 1559*

Rasburicase (ras BYOOR i kayse)

U.S. Brand Names Elitek™

Index Terms Recombinant Urate Oxidase; Urate Oxidase

Generic Availability (U.S.) No

Pharmacologic Category Enzyme; Enzyme, Urate-Oxidase (Recombinant)

Pregnancy Risk Factor C

Lactation Excretion in breast milk unknown/not recommended

Use Initial management of uric acid levels in patients with leukemia, lymphoma, and solid tumor malignancies receiving chemotherapy expected to result in tumor lysis and elevation of plasma uric acid

Mechanism of Action/Effect Converts uric acid to allantoin (an inactive and soluble metabolite of uric acid); it does not inhibit the formation of uric acid.

Contraindications History of anaphylaxis or severe hypersensitivity to rasburicase or any component of the formulation; history of hemolytic reaction or methemoglobinemia associated with rasburicase; glucose-6-phosphatase dehydrogenase (G6PD) deficiency

Warnings/Precautions [U.S. Boxed Warning]: Severe hypersensitivity reactions (including anaphylaxis) have been reported; immediately and permanently discontinue in patients developing serious hypersensitivity reaction; reactions may occur at any time during treatment, including the initial dose. Signs and symptoms of hypersensitivity may include bronshospasm, chest pain/tightness, dyspnea, hypotension, hypoxia, shock, or urticaria. **[U.S. Boxed Warning]: Due to the risk for hemolysis (<1%), rasburicase is contraindicated in patients with G6PD deficiency; discontinue immediately and permanently in any patient developing hemolysis. Patients at higher risk for G6PD deficiency (eg, African, Mediterranean, or Southeast Asian descent) should be screened prior to therapy;** severe hemolytic reactions occurred within 2-4 days of rasburicase initiation. **[U.S. Boxed Warning]: Methemoglobinemia has been reported (<1%). Discontinue immediately and permanently in any patient developing methemoglobinemia;** initiate appropriate treatment (eg, transfusion, methylene blue) if methemoglobinemia occurs.

[U.S. Boxed Warning]: Enzymatic degradation of uric acid in blood samples will occur if left at room temperature, which may interfere with serum uric acid measurements; specific guidelines for the collection of plasma uric acid samples must be followed, including collection in pre-chilled tubes with heparin anticoagulant, immediate ice water bath immersion and assay within 4 hours. Patients at risk for tumor lysis syndrome should receive appropriate I.V. hydration as part of uric acid management; however, alkalinization (with sodium bicarbonate) concurrently with rasburicase is not recommended (Coiffier, 2008). Rasburicase is immunogenic and can elicit an antibody response; administration of more than one course is not recommended.

Drug Interactions

Avoid Concomitant Use There are no known interactions where it is recommended to avoid concomitant use.

Decreased Effect There are no known significant interactions involving a decrease in effect.

Increased Effect/Toxicity There are no known significant interactions involving an increase in effect.

Lab Interactions Specific handling procedures must be followed to prevent the degradation of uric acid in plasma samples. Blood must be collected in prechilled tubes containing heparin anticoagulant. Samples must then be **immediately** immersed in an ice water bath. Prepare samples by centrifugation in a precooled centrifuge (4°C). Samples must be kept in ice water bath and analyzed within 4 hours of collection.

Adverse Reactions

>10%:

Cardiovascular: Peripheral edema (≤50%), fluid overload (≤12%)

Central nervous system: Fever (46%; serious: 5%), headache (26%), anxiety (≤24%)

Dermatologic: Rash (13%; serious: 1%)

Endocrine & metabolic: Hypophosphatemia (≤17%)

Gastrointestinal: Vomiting (50%), nausea (27%), abdominal pain (20%), constipation (20%), diarrhea (20%), mucositis (15%; serious: 2%)

Hepatic: Hyperbilirubinemia (≤16%), ALT increased (≤11%)

Respiratory: Pharyngolaryngeal pain (≤14%)

Miscellaneous: Antibody formation (healthy volunteers: 61% to 64%; patients with malignancies: 11%), sepsis (≤12%; serious: 3% to 5%)

1% to 10%:

Cardiovascular: Ischemic coronary disorder, supraventricular arrhythmia

Endocrine & metabolic: Hyperphosphatemia (≤10%)

Gastrointestinal: Abdominal/gastrointestinal infection

Hematologic: Neutropenic fever (serious: 4%), neutropenia (serious: 2%)

Respiratory: Respiratory distress (serious: 3%), pulmonary hemorrhage, respiratory failure

Miscellaneous: Hypersensitivity (≤4%)

Pharmacodynamics/Kinetics

Onset of Action Uric acid levels decrease within 4 hours of initial administration

Half-Life Elimination ~16-23 hours

Available Dosage Forms

Injection, powder for reconstitution:

Elitek™: 1.5 mg, 7.5 mg

Dosing

Adult Hyperuricemia associated with malignancy: I.V.: 0.2 mg/kg once daily for up to 5 days (manufacturer-recommended dose) **or**

Alternate dosing (unlabeled; Coiffier, 2008): 0.05-0.2 mg/kg once daily for 1-7 days (average of 2-3 days) with the duration of treatment dependant on plasma uric acid levels and clinical judgment (patients with significant tumor burden may require an increase to twice daily); the following dose levels are recommended based on risk of tumor lysis syndrome (TLS):

High risk: 0.2 mg/kg once daily (duration is based on plasma uric acid levels)

Intermediate risk: 0.15 mg/kg once daily (duration is based on plasma uric acid levels)

Low risk: 0.1 mg/kg once daily (duration is based on clinical judgment); a dose of 0.05 mg/kg was used effectively in one trial

Single-dose rasburicase (unlabeled use; based on limited data): 0.15 mg/kg (Campara, 2009; Liu, 2005) **or** 3-7.5 mg as a single dose (Hutcherson, 2006; McDonnell, 2006; Reeves, 2008; Trifilio, 2006); repeat doses (1.5-6 mg) may be needed based on serum uric acid levels

Geriatric Refer to adult dosing.

Pediatric Hyperuricemia associated with malignancy: I.V.: 0.2 mg/kg once daily for up to 5 days (manufacturer-recommended dose) **or**

Alternate dosing (unlabeled; Coiffier, 2008): 0.05-0.2 mg/kg once daily for 1-7 days (average of 2-3 days) with the duration of treatment dependant on plasma uric acid levels and clinical judgment (patients with significant tumor burden may require an increase to twice daily); the following dose levels are recommended based on risk of tumor lysis syndrome (TLS):

High risk: 0.2 mg/kg once daily (duration is based on plasma uric acid levels)

Intermediate risk: 0.15 mg/kg once daily (duration is based on plasma uric acid levels); may consider managing initially with a single dose

Low risk: 0.1 mg/kg once daily (duration is based on clinical judgment); a dose of 0.05 mg/kg was used effectively in one trial

Single-dose rasburicase (unlabeled use; based on limited data): 0.15 mg/kg; additional doses may be needed based on serum uric acid levels (Liu, 2005)

Administration

I.V. I.V. infusion over 30 minutes; do **not** administer as a bolus infusion. Do **not** filter during infusion. If not possible to administer through a separate line, I.V. line should be flushed with at least 15 mL saline prior to and following rasburicase infusion. May begin chemotherapy 4 hours after the initiation of rasburicase (Coiffier, 2008).

Stability

Reconstitution Reconstitute with provided diluent (use 1 mL diluent for the 1.5 mg vial and 5 mL diluent for the 7.5 mg vial). Mix by gently swirling; do **not** shake or vortex. Discard if discolored or containing particulate matter. Total dose should be further diluted in NS to a final volume of 50 mL.

Storage Prior to reconstitution, store with diluent at 2°C to 8°C (36°F to 46°F); do not freeze. Protect from light. Reconstituted and final solution may be stored up to 24 hours at 2°C to 8°C (36°F to 46°F). Discard unused product.

Monitoring and Teaching Issues

Laboratory Monitoring Plasma uric acid levels (4 hours after rasburicase administration, then every 6-8 hours until TLS resolution), CBC, G6PD deficiency screening (in patients at high risk for deficiency)

Physical Assessment Evaluate carefully for use-related cautions prior to instituting therapy. Patient must be observed closely for hypersensitivity reaction.

Patient Education This medication can only be administered by infusion; you will be monitored closely during and following infusion. Report immediately any swelling or any signs of allergic reaction (eg, respiratory difficulty or swallowing, back pain, chest tightness, rash, hives, swelling of lips or mouth). Report severe headache, persistent gastrointestinal upset (nausea, vomiting, or abdominal pain), respiratory difficulty, or swelling of extremities.

Breast-Feeding Considerations Due to the potential for serious adverse reactions in the nursing infant, breast-feeding should be discontinued during treatment.

Pregnancy Considerations Adverse effects were observed in animal studies. There are no adequate and well-controlled studies in pregnant women. Use during pregnancy only if the benefit to the mother outweighs the potential risk to the fetus.

- **Razadyne®** *see* Galantamine *on page 847*
- **Razadyne® ER** *see* Galantamine *on page 847*
- **ReAzo [OTC]** *see* Phenazopyridine *on page 1446*
- **Rebetol®** *see* Ribavirin *on page 1571*
- **Rebif®** *see* Interferon Beta-1a *on page 1003*
- **Reclast®** *see* Zoledronic Acid *on page 1899*
- **Reclipsen®** *see* Ethinyl Estradiol and Desogestrel *on page 695*
- **Recombinant Desulfatohirudin** *see* Desirudin *on page 490*
- **Recombinant Hirudin** *see* Desirudin *on page 490*
- **Recombinant Hirudin** *see* Lepirudin *on page 1075*
- **Recombinant Human Deoxyribonuclease** *see* Dornase Alfa *on page 574*
- **Recombinant Human Interleukin-2** *see* Aldesleukin *on page 62*
- **Recombinant Human Luteinizing Hormone** *see* Lutropin Alfa *on page 1142*
- **Recombinant Human Parathyroid Hormone (1-34)** *see* Teriparatide *on page 1736*
- **Recombinant Plasminogen Activator** *see* Reteplase *on page 1567*

◆ **Recombinant Urate Oxidase** *see* Rasburicase *on page 1562*
◆ **Recombinant Urate Oxidase, Pegylated** *see* Pegloticase *on page 1427*
◆ **Recombinate** *see* Antihemophilic Factor (Recombinant) *on page 133*
◆ **Recombivax HB®** *see* Hepatitis B Vaccine (Recombinant) *on page 905*
◆ **Recort [OTC]** *see* Hydrocortisone (Topical) *on page 920*
◆ **Refenesen™ [OTC]** *see* GuaiFENesin *on page 890*
◆ **Refenesen™ 400 [OTC]** *see* GuaiFENesin *on page 890*
◆ **Refissa™** *see* Tretinoin (Topical) *on page 1811*
◆ **Refludan®** *see* Lepirudin *on page 1075*
◆ **Regenecare®** *see* Lidocaine (Topical) *on page 1107*
◆ **Regenecare® HA [OTC]** *see* Lidocaine (Topical) *on page 1107*
◆ **Regitine [DSC]** *see* Phentolamine *on page 1448*
◆ **Reglan®** *see* Metoclopramide *on page 1213*
◆ **Regonol®** *see* Pyridostigmine *on page 1531*
◆ **Regular Insulin** *see* Insulin Regular *on page 994*
◆ **Relafen** *see* Nabumetone *on page 1275*
◆ **Relenza®** *see* Zanamivir *on page 1885*
◆ **Relistor®** *see* Methylnaltrexone *on page 1202*
◆ **Relpax®** *see* Eletriptan *on page 608*
◆ **Remeron®** *see* Mirtazapine *on page 1239*
◆ **Remeron SolTab®** *see* Mirtazapine *on page 1239*
◆ **Remicade®** *see* InFLIXimab *on page 973*
◆ **Remodulin®** *see* Treprostinil *on page 1809*
◆ **Renagel®** *see* Sevelamer *on page 1637*
◆ **Renova®** *see* Tretinoin (Topical) *on page 1811*
◆ **Renvela®** *see* Sevelamer *on page 1637*

Repaglinide (re PAG li nide)

U.S. Brand Names Prandin®

Generic Availability (U.S.) No

Pharmacologic Category Antidiabetic Agent, Meglitinide Derivative

Medication Safety Issues

Sound-alike/look-alike issues:

Prandin® may be confused with Avandia®

High alert medication: The Institute for Safe Medication Practices (ISMP) includes this medication among its list of drug classes which have a heightened risk of causing significant patient harm when used in error.

Pregnancy Risk Factor C

Lactation Excretion in breast milk unknown/not recommended

Use Management of type 2 diabetes mellitus (noninsulin dependent, NIDDM) as an adjunct to diet and exercise; may be used in combination with metformin or thiazolidinediones

Mechanism of Action/Effect Nonsulfonylurea hypoglycemic agent of the meglitinide class (the nonsulfonylurea moiety of glyburide) used in the management of type 2 diabetes mellitus; stimulates insulin release from the pancreatic beta cells. Repaglinide-induced insulin release is glucose-dependent.

Contraindications Hypersensitivity to repaglinide or any component of the formulation; diabetic ketoacidosis, with or without coma; type 1 diabetes (insulin dependent, IDDM); concurrent gemfibrozil therapy

Warnings/Precautions Use with caution in patients with hepatic impairment. Use caution in severe renal dysfunction, elderly, malnourished, or patients with adrenal/pituitary dysfunction; may be more susceptible to glucose-lowering effects. May cause hypoglycemia; appropriate patient selection, dosage, and patient education are important to avoid hypoglycemic episodes. It may be necessary to discontinue repaglinide and administer insulin if the patient is exposed to stress (fever, trauma, infection, surgery). Theoretically, repaglinide may increase cardiovascular events as observed in some studies using sulfonylureas, but there are no long-term studies assessing this concern. Not indicated for use in combination with NPH insulin as there have been case reports of myocardial ischemia; further evaluation required to assess the safety of this combination.

Drug Interactions

Metabolism/Transport Effects Substrate of CYP2C8 (major), CYP3A4 (major), SLCO1B1

Avoid Concomitant Use

Avoid concomitant use of Repaglinide with any of the following: Gemfibrozil

Decreased Effect

The levels/effects of Repaglinide may be decreased by: Corticosteroids (Orally Inhaled); Corticosteroids (Systemic); CYP2C8 Inducers (Highly Effective); CYP3A4 Inducers (Strong); Deferasirox; Herbs (CYP3A4 Inducers); Luteinizing Hormone-Releasing Hormone Analogs; Rifamycin Derivatives; Somatropin; Thiazide Diuretics

Increased Effect/Toxicity

Repaglinide may increase the levels/effects of: Hypoglycemic Agents

The levels/effects of Repaglinide may be increased by: Antifungal Agents (Azole Derivatives, Systemic); Conivaptan; CycloSPORINE; CycloSPORINE (Systemic); CYP2C8 Inhibitors (Moderate); CYP2C8 Inhibitors (Strong); CYP3A4 Inhibitors (Moderate); CYP3A4 Inhibitors (Strong); Dasatinib; Deferasirox; Eltrombopag; Gemfibrozil; Herbs (Hypoglycemic Properties); Macrolide Antibiotics; Pegvisomant; Trimethoprim

Nutritional/Ethanol Interactions

Ethanol: Avoid ethanol; may increase risk of hypoglycemia.

Food: When given with food, the AUC of repaglinide is decreased.

Herb/Nutraceutical: Avoid alfalfa, aloe, bilberry, bitter melon, burdock, celery, damiana, fenugreek, garcinia, garlic, ginger, ginseng (American), gymnema, marshmallow, and stinging nettle (may enhance the hypoglycemic effects of antidiabetic agents). St John's wort may decrease the levels/effect of repaglinide.

Adverse Reactions

>10%:

Central nervous system: Headache (9% to 11%)

Endocrine & metabolic: Hypoglycemia (16% to 31%)

Respiratory: Upper respiratory tract infection (10% to 16%)

1% to 10%:

Cardiovascular: Ischemia (4%), chest pain (2% to 3%)

Gastrointestinal: Diarrhea (4% to 5%), constipation (2% to 3%), tooth disorder (≤2%)

Genitourinary: Urinary tract infection (2% to 3%)

Neuromuscular & skeletal: Back pain (5% to 6%), arthralgia (3% to 6%)

Respiratory: Sinusitis (3% to 6%), bronchitis (2% to 6%)

Miscellaneous: Allergy (1% to 2%)

Pharmacodynamics/Kinetics

Onset of Action Single dose: Increased insulin levels: ~15-60 minutes

Duration of Action 4-6 hours

Absorption Rapid and complete

Bioavailability ~56%

Time to Peak Plasma: ~1 hour

Protein Binding Plasma: >98% to albumin

Half-Life Elimination ~1 hour

Metabolism Hepatic via CYP3A4 and CYP2C8 isoenzymes and glucuronidation to inactive metabolites

Excretion Feces (~90%, <2% as unchanged drug); Urine (~8%, 0.1% as unchanged drug)

Available Dosage Forms

Tablet, oral:

Prandin®: 0.5 mg, 1 mg, 2 mg

Dosing

Adult & Geriatric

Type 2 diabetes: Oral:

Patients not previously treated or whose Hb A_{1c} is <8%: Initial: 0.5 mg before each meal

Patients previously treated with blood glucose-lowering agents whose Hb A_{1c} is ≥8%: Initial: 1 or 2 mg before each meal.

Dose adjustment: Determine dosing adjustments by blood glucose response, usually fasting blood glucose. Double the preprandial dose up to 4 mg until satisfactory blood glucose response is achieved. At least 1 week should elapse to assess response after each dose adjustment.

Dose range: 0.5-4 mg taken with meals. Repaglinide may be dosed preprandially 2, 3, or 4 times/day in response to changes in the patient's meal pattern. Maximum recommended daily dose: 16 mg.

Patients receiving other oral hypoglycemic agents: When repaglinide is used to replace therapy with other oral hypoglycemic agents, it may be started the day after the final dose is given. Observe patients carefully for hypoglycemia because of potential overlapping of drug effects. When transferred from longer half-life sulfonylureas (eg, chlorpropamide), close monitoring may be indicated for up to ≥1 week.

Note: Combination therapy: If repaglinide monotherapy does not result in adequate glycemic control, metformin or a thiazolidinedione may be added. Or, if metformin or thiazolidinedione therapy does not provide adequate control, repaglinide may be added. The starting dose and dose adjustments for combination therapy are the same as repaglinide monotherapy. Carefully adjust the dose of each drug to determine the minimal dose required to achieve the desired pharmacologic effect. Failure to do so could result in an increase in the incidence of hypoglycemic episodes. Use appropriate monitoring of FPG and Hb A_{1c} measurements to ensure that the patient is not subjected to excessive drug exposure or increased probability of secondary drug failure. If glucose is not achieved after a suitable trial of combination therapy, consider discontinuing these drugs and using insulin.

Renal Impairment

Cl_{cr} 40-80 mL/minute (mild-to-moderate renal dysfunction): Initial dosage adjustment does not appear to be necessary.

Cl_{cr} 20-40 mL/minute (severe renal impairment): Initial: 0.5 mg with meals; titrate carefully.

Cl_{cr} <20 mL/minute: Not studied.

Hemodialysis: Not studied

Hepatic Impairment Use conservative initial and maintenance doses. Use longer intervals between dosage adjustments.

Administration

Oral Administer 15 minutes before meals; however, time may vary from immediately preceding a meal to as long as 30 minutes before a meal. If the patient misses a meal or is unable to take anything by mouth, repaglinide should not be administered to avoid hypoglycemia. Patients consuming extra meals should be instructed to add a dose for the extra meal.

Stability

Storage Do not store above 25°C (77°F). Protect from moisture.

Monitoring and Teaching Issues

Laboratory Monitoring Fasting blood glucose (periodically) and glycosylated hemoglobin (Hb A_{1c}) levels (every 3 months)

Physical Assessment Instruct patient to treat signs of hypoglycemia and report instances to health care provider.

Patient Education Take 3-4 times a day 15-30 minutes prior to a meal. If you skip a meal, skip a dose for that meal. Follow dietary and lifestyle directions of prescriber or diabetic educator. Avoid alcohol. You will be instructed in signs of hyper-/hypoglycemia by prescriber or diabetic educator; be alert for adverse hypoglycemia (lightheadedness, tachycardia or palpitations, sweaty palms or profuse perspiration, yawning, tingling of lips and tongue, seizures, or change in sensorium) and follow prescriber's instructions for intervention. May cause headache or mild GI effects during first weeks of therapy (nausea, vomiting, diarrhea, constipation, heartburn); if these do not diminish, consult prescriber for approved medication. Report chest pain, respiratory difficulty or symptoms of upper respiratory infection, urinary tract infection (burning or itching on urination), or muscle or back pain.

Dietary Considerations Take repaglinide 15-30 minutes before meals. Individualized medical nutrition therapy (MNT) based on ADA recommendations is an integral part of therapy. May cause hypoglycemia. Must be able to recognize symptoms of hypoglycemia (palpitations, tachycardia, sweaty palms, diaphoresis, lightheadedness).

Geriatric Considerations Repaglinide has not been studied exclusively in the elderly; information from the manufacturer states that no differences in its effectiveness or adverse effects had been identified between persons younger than and older than 65 years of age. How "tightly" a geriatric patient's blood glucose should be controlled is controversial; however, a fasting blood glucose <150 mg/dL is now an acceptable endpoint. Such a decision should be based on the patient's functional status, how well he/she recognizes hypoglycemic or hyperglycemic symptoms, and how to respond to them and their other disease states. Intensive glucose control (Hb A_{1c} <6.5%) has been linked to increased all cause and cardiovascular mortality, hypoglycemia requiring assistance, and weight gain in adult type 2 diabetes. For elderly patients with diabetes who are relatively healthy, attaining target goals for aspirin use, blood pressure, lipids, smoking cessation, and diet and exercise may be more important than normalized glycemic control.

Breast-Feeding Considerations It is not known if repaglinide is excreted in breast milk. Breast-feeding is not recommended by the manufacturer.

Pregnancy Considerations Adverse events have been observed in some animal studies; therefore, repaglinide is classified as pregnancy category C. Information describing the effects of repaglinide on pregnancy outcomes is limited. Maternal hyperglycemia can be associated with adverse effects in the fetus, including macrosomia, neonatal hyperglycemia, and hyperbilirubinemia; the risk of congenital malformations is increased when the Hb A_{1c} is above the normal range. Diabetes can also be associated with adverse effects in the mother. Poorly-treated diabetes may cause end-organ damage that may in turn negatively affect obstetric outcomes. Physiologic glucose levels should be maintained prior to and during pregnancy to decrease the risk of adverse events in the mother and the fetus. Until additional safety and efficacy data are obtained, the use of oral agents is generally not recommended as routine management of GDM or type 2 diabetes mellitus during pregnancy. Insulin is the drug of choice for the control of diabetes mellitus during pregnancy.

Related Information

Diabetes Mellitus Management, Adults *on page 2026*

Repaglinide and Metformin (re PAG li nide & met FOR min)

U.S. Brand Names PrandiMet®

Index Terms Metformin and Repaglinide; Repaglinide and Metformin Hydrochloride

Generic Availability (U.S.) No

Pharmacologic Category Antidiabetic Agent, Biguanide; Antidiabetic Agent, Meglitinide Derivative; Hypoglycemic Agent, Oral

Medication Safety Issues

Sound-alike/look-alike issues:

PrandiMet® may be confused with Avandamet®, Prandin®

High alert medication: The Institute for Safe Medication Practices (ISMP) includes this medication among its list of drug classes which have a heightened risk of causing significant patient harm when used in error.

Pregnancy Risk Factor C

Lactation

Metformin: Enters breast milk/not recommended

Repaglinide: Excretion in breast milk unknown/not recommended

Use Management of type 2 diabetes mellitus (noninsulin dependent, NIDDM), as an adjunct to diet and exercise, in patients currently receiving or not adequately controlled on metformin and/or a meglitinide

Available Dosage Forms

Tablet:

PrandiMet®: 1/500: Repaglinide 1 mg and metformin hydrochloride 500 mg; 2/500: Repaglinide 2 mg and metformin hydrochloride 500 mg

Dosing

Adult & Geriatric Type 2 diabetes mellitus: Oral: **Note:** Daily doses should be divided and given 2-3 times daily with meals (maximum single dose: 4 mg/dose [repaglinide], 1000 mg/dose [metformin]; maximum daily dose: 10 mg/day [repaglinide], 2500 mg/day [metformin])

Patients currently taking repaglinide and metformin: Initial doses should be based on (but not exceeding) the patient's current doses of repaglinide and metformin; titrate as needed to the maximum daily dose to achieve targeted glycemic control

Patients inadequately controlled on metformin alone: Initial dose: repaglinide 1 mg/ metformin 500 mg twice daily with meals. Titrate slowly to reduce the risk of repaglinide-induced hypoglycemia.

Patients inadequately controlled on a meglitinide alone: Initial dose: metformin 500 mg twice daily plus repaglinide at a dose similar to (but not exceeding) the patient's current dose. Titrate slowly to reduce the risk of metformin-induced gastrointestinal adverse effects.

Renal Impairment Do not use in renal impairment; metformin use is contraindicated in patients with renal impairment (serum creatinine ≥1.5 mg/dL in males or ≥1.4 mg/dL in females).

Hepatic Impairment Avoid use in patients with impaired liver function.

Administration

Oral Administer 15-30 minutes before meals to avoid risk of hypoglycemia/GI upset; if a meal skipped or patient is unable to take anything by mouth, do not administer dose.

Monitoring and Teaching Issues

Laboratory Monitoring Regular assessment of fasting blood glucose, postprandial blood glucose, and hemoglobin A_{1c}; initial and periodic monitoring of hematologic parameters (eg, hemoglobin/hematocrit, red blood cell indices) and renal function should be performed at least annually. Evaluation of vitamin B_{12} and folate should be performed if anemia is present.

Physical Assessment See individual agents.

Patient Education See individual agents.

Related Information

Diabetes Mellitus Management, Adults *on page 2026*

MetFORMIN *on page 1182*

Repaglinide *on page 1564*

- **Repaglinide and Metformin Hydrochloride** *see* Repaglinide and Metformin *on page 1566*
- **Repan®** *see* Butalbital, Acetaminophen, and Caffeine *on page 260*
- **Reprexain™** *see* Hydrocodone and Ibuprofen *on page 916*
- **Repronex®** *see* Menotropins *on page 1170*
- **Requip®** *see* Ropinirole *on page 1606*
- **Requip® XL™** *see* Ropinirole *on page 1606*
- **Rescriptor®** *see* Delavirdine *on page 482*
- **Respa®-BR [DSC]** *see* Brompheniramine *on page 234*
- **Restasis®** *see* CycloSPORINE (Ophthalmic) *on page 442*
- **Restoril™** *see* Temazepam *on page 1720*
- **Retavase®** *see* Reteplase *on page 1567*

Reteplase (RE ta plase)

U.S. Brand Names Retavase®

Index Terms r-PA; Recombinant Plasminogen Activator

Generic Availability (U.S.) No

Pharmacologic Category Thrombolytic Agent

Medication Safety Issues

High alert medication: The Institute for Safe Medication Practices (ISMP) includes this medication (I.V.) among its list of drugs which have a heightened risk of causing significant patient harm when used in error.

Pregnancy Risk Factor C

Lactation Excretion in breast milk unknown/use caution

Use Management of ST-elevation myocardial infarction (STEMI); improvement of ventricular function; reduction of the incidence of CHF and the reduction of mortality following AMI

Recommended criteria for treatment: STEMI: Chest pain ≥20 minutes duration, onset of chest pain within 12 hours of treatment (or within prior 12-24 hours in patients with continuing ischemic symptoms), and ST-segment elevation >0.1 mV in at least two contiguous precordial leads or two adjacent limb leads on ECG or new or presumably new left bundle branch block (LBBB)

Mechanism of Action/Effect Reteplase initiates local fibrinolysis by binding to fibrin in a thrombus (clot) and converting entrapped plasminogen to plasmin. Dissolution of thrombus occluding a coronary artery restores perfusion to ischemic myocardium. Reteplase is manufactured by recombinant DNA technology using *E. coli*.

Contraindications Hypersensitivity to reteplase or any component of the formulation; active internal bleeding; history of cerebrovascular accident; recent intracranial or intraspinal surgery or trauma; intracranial neoplasm, arteriovenous malformations, or aneurysm; known bleeding diathesis; severe uncontrolled hypertension

Warnings/Precautions Concurrent heparin anticoagulation can contribute to bleeding; careful attention to all potential bleeding sites. I.M. injections and nonessential handling of the patient should be avoided. Venipunctures should be performed carefully and only when necessary. If arterial puncture is necessary, use an upper extremity vessel that can be manually compressed. If serious bleeding occurs then the infusion of anistreplase and heparin should be stopped.

For the following conditions the risk of bleeding is higher with use of reteplase and should be weighed against the benefits of therapy: recent major surgery (eg, CABG, obstetrical delivery, organ biopsy, previous puncture of noncompressible vessels), cerebrovascular disease, recent gastrointestinal or genitourinary bleeding, recent trauma including CPR, hypertension (systolic BP >180 mm Hg and/or diastolic BP >110 mm Hg), high likelihood of left heart thrombus (eg, mitral stenosis with atrial fibrillation), acute pericarditis, subacute bacterial endocarditis, hemostatic defects including ones caused by severe renal or hepatic dysfunction, significant hepatic dysfunction, pregnancy, diabetic hemorrhagic retinopathy or other hemorrhagic ophthalmic conditions, septic thrombophlebitis or occluded AV cannula at seriously infected site, advanced age (eg, >75 years), patients receiving oral anticoagulants, any other condition in which bleeding constitutes a significant hazard or would be particularly difficult to manage because of location.

Coronary thrombolysis may result in reperfusion arrhythmias. Follow standard MI management. Rare anaphylactic reactions can occur. Safety and efficacy in pediatric patients have not been established.

Drug Interactions

Avoid Concomitant Use There are no known interactions where it is recommended to avoid concomitant use.

Decreased Effect

The levels/effects of Reteplase may be decreased by: Aprotinin

Increased Effect/Toxicity

Reteplase may increase the levels/effects of: Anticoagulants; Drotrecogin Alfa

The levels/effects of Reteplase may be increased by: Antiplatelet Agents; Herbs (Anticoagulant/Antiplatelet Properties); Nonsteroidal Anti-Inflammatory Agents; Salicylates

Adverse Reactions Bleeding is the most frequent adverse effect associated with reteplase. Heparin and aspirin have been administered concurrently with reteplase in clinical trials. The incidence of adverse events is a reflection of these combined therapies, and are comparable with comparison thrombolytics.

>10%: Local: Injection site bleeding (4.6% to 48.6%)

1% to 10%:

- Gastrointestinal: Bleeding (1.8% to 9.0%)
- Genitourinary: Bleeding (0.9% to 9.5%)
- Hematologic: Anemia (0.9% to 2.6%)

Other adverse effects noted are frequently associated with MI (and therefore may or may not be attributable to Retavase®) and include arrhythmia, hypotension, cardiogenic shock, pulmonary edema, cardiac arrest, reinfarction, pericarditis, tamponade, thrombosis, and embolism.

Pharmacodynamics/Kinetics

Onset of Action Thrombolysis: 30-90 minutes

Half-Life Elimination 13-16 minutes

Excretion Feces and urine

Clearance: Plasma: 250-450 mL/minute

Available Dosage Forms

Injection, powder for reconstitution [preservative free]:

Retavase®: 10.4 units

Dosing

Adult & Geriatric

STEMI: I.V.: 10 units I.V. over 2 minutes, followed by a second dose 30 minutes later of 10 units I.V. over 2 minutes; withhold second dose if serious bleeding or anaphylaxis occurs.

Note: All patients should receive 162-325 mg of chewable nonenteric coated aspirin as soon as possible and then daily. Administer concurrently with heparin 60 units/kg bolus (maximum: 4000 units) followed by continuous infusion of 12 units/kg/hour (maximum: 1000 units/hour) and adjust to aPTT target of 50-70 seconds (or 1.5-2 times the upper limit of control).

Pediatric Not recommended

Administration

I.V. Infuse over 2 minutes.

Stability

Reconstitution Reteplase should be reconstituted using the diluent, syringe, needle, and dispensing pin provided with each kit.

Storage Dosage kits should be stored at 2°C to 25°C (36°F to 77°F) and remain sealed until use in order to protect from light.

Monitoring and Teaching Issues

Laboratory Monitoring CBC, PTT, signs and symptoms of bleeding, ECG monitoring

Physical Assessment Use caution when there is significant risk of bleeding. Patient should be closely monitored for bleeding during and following treatment. Monitor infusion site, neurological status (eg, intracranial hemorrhage), vital signs, and ECG. Bleeding precautions should be maintained; avoid I.M. injections, venipunctures (unless absolutely necessary), and nonessential handling of the patient. If arterial puncture is necessary, use an upper extremity vessel that can be manually compressed.

Patient Education This medication can only be administered by infusion; you will be monitored closely during and after treatment. You will have a tendency to bleed easily; use caution to prevent injury. Follow instructions for strict bedrest to reduce the risk of injury. If bleeding occurs, report immediately and apply pressure to bleeding spot until bleeding stops completely. Report unusual pain (acute headache, joint pain, chest pain); unusual bruising or bleeding; blood in urine, stool, or vomitus; bleeding gums; vision changes; or change in mentation.

Geriatric Considerations No specific changes in use in the elderly are necessary.

- ◆ **Retin-A®** *see* Tretinoin (Topical) *on page 1811*
- ◆ **Retin-A Micro®** *see* Tretinoin (Topical) *on page 1811*
- ◆ **Retinoic Acid** *see* Tretinoin (Topical) *on page 1811*
- ◆ **Retrovir®** *see* Zidovudine *on page 1890*
- ◆ **Revatio®** *see* Sildenafil *on page 1641*
- ◆ **ReVia®** *see* Naltrexone *on page 1286*
- ◆ **Revlimid®** *see* Lenalidomide *on page 1071*
- ◆ **Revolade®** *see* Eltrombopag *on page 610*
- ◆ **Revonto™** *see* Dantrolene *on page 462*
- ◆ **rFSH-alpha** *see* Follitropin Alfa *on page 813*
- ◆ **rFSH-beta** *see* Follitropin Beta *on page 815*
- ◆ **rFVIIa** *see* Factor VIIa (Recombinant) *on page 731*
- ◆ **rhAPC** *see* Drotrecogin Alfa *on page 594*
- ◆ **r-hCG** *see* Chorionic Gonadotropin (Recombinant) *on page 365*
- ◆ **rhDNase** *see* Dornase Alfa *on page 574*
- ◆ **Rheumatrex®** *see* Methotrexate *on page 1193*
- ◆ **rhFSH-alpha** *see* Follitropin Alfa *on page 813*
- ◆ **rhFSH-beta** *see* Follitropin Beta *on page 815*
- ◆ **RhIG** *see* $Rh_o(D)$ Immune Globulin *on page 1569*
- ◆ **Rhinall® [OTC]** *see* Phenylephrine (Nasal) *on page 1451*
- ◆ **Rhinocort Aqua®** *see* Budesonide (Nasal) *on page 238*
- ◆ **r-Hirudin** *see* Desirudin *on page 490*
- ◆ **r-hLH** *see* Lutropin Alfa *on page 1142*
- ◆ **Rho(D) Immune Globulin (Human)** *see* $Rh_o(D)$ Immune Globulin *on page 1569*

$Rh_o(D)$ Immune Globulin (ar aych oh (dee) i MYUN GLOB yoo lin)

U.S. Brand Names HyperRHO™ S/D Full Dose; HyperRHO™ S/D Mini-Dose; MICRhoGAM® UF Plus; RhoGAM® UF Plus; Rhophylac®; WinRho® SDF

Index Terms RhIG; Rho(D) Immune Globulin (Human); RhoIGIV; RhoIVIM

Generic Availability (U.S.) No

Pharmacologic Category Blood Product Derivative; Immune Globulin

Pregnancy Risk Factor C

Lactation Does not enter breast milk

Use

Suppression of Rh isoimmunization: Use in the following situations when an $Rh_o(D)$-negative individual is exposed to $Rh_o(D)$-positive blood: During delivery of an $Rh_o(D)$-positive infant; abortion; amniocentesis; chorionic villus sampling; ruptured tubal pregnancy; abdominal trauma; hydatidiform mole; transplacental hemorrhage. Used when the mother is $Rh_o(D)$-negative, the father of the child is either $Rh_o(D)$-positive or $Rh_o(D)$-unknown, or the baby is either $Rh_o(D)$-positive or $Rh_o(D)$-unknown.

Transfusion: Suppression of Rh isoimmunization in $Rh_o(D)$-negative individuals transfused with $Rh_o(D)$ antigen-positive RBCs or blood components containing $Rh_o(D)$ antigen-positive RBCs

Treatment of idiopathic thrombocytopenic purpura (ITP): Used intravenously in the following nonsplenectomized $Rh_o(D)$-positive individuals: Children with acute or chronic ITP, adults with chronic ITP, and children and adults with ITP secondary to HIV infection

Available Dosage Forms

Injection, solution [preservative free]:

HyperRHO™ S/D Full Dose: ≥300 mcg/mL (1 mL)

HyperRHO™ S/D Mini-Dose: ≥50 mcg/0.17 mL (0.17 mL)

MICRhoGAM® UF Plus: ~50 mcg/0.75 mL (0.75 mL)

RhoGAM® UF Plus: ~300 mcg/0.75 mL (0.75 mL)

Rhophylac®: ≥300 mcg/2 mL (2 mL)

WinRho® SDF: 300 mcg/~1.3 mL (1.3 mL); 3000 mcg/~13 mL (13 mL); 500 mcg/~2.2 mL (2.2 mL); 1000 mcg/~4.4 mL (4.4 mL)

Dosing

Adult

ITP:

Rhophylac®: I.V.: 50 mcg/kg

WinRho® SDF: I.V.:

Initial: 50 mcg/kg as a single injection, or can be given as a divided dose on separate days.

If hemoglobin is <10 g/dL: Dose should be reduced to 25-40 mcg/kg

Subsequent dosing: 25-60 mcg/kg can be used if required to increase platelet count

Maintenance dosing if patient **did respond** to initial dosing: 25-60 mcg/kg based on platelet count and hemoglobin concentration

Maintenance dosing if patient **did not respond** to initial dosing:

Hemoglobin <8 g/dL: Alternative treatment should be used

Hemoglobin 8-10 g/dL: Redose between 25-40 mcg/kg

Hemoglobin >10 g/dL: Redose between 50-60 mcg/kg

Rh_o (D) suppression: Note: One "full dose" (300 mcg) provides enough antibody to prevent Rh sensitization if the volume of RBC entering the circulation is ≤15 mL. When >15 mL is suspected, a fetal red cell count should be performed to determine the appropriate dose.

Pregnancy:

Antepartum prophylaxis: In general, dose is given at 28 weeks. If given early in pregnancy, administer every 12 weeks to ensure adequate levels of passively acquired anti-Rh

HyperRHO™ S/D Full Dose, RhoGAM®: I.M.: 300 mcg

Rhophylac®, WinRho® SDF: I.M., I.V.: 300 mcg

Postpartum prophylaxis: In general, dose is administered as soon as possible after delivery, preferably within 72 hours. Can be given up to 28 days following delivery

HyperRHO™ S/D Full Dose, RhoGAM®: I.M.: 300 mcg

Rhophylac®: I.M., I.V.: 300 mcg

WinRho® SDF: I.M., I.V.: 120 mcg

Threatened abortion, any time during pregnancy (with continuation of pregnancy):

HyperRHO™ S/D Full Dose, RhoGAM®: I.M.: 300 mcg; administer as soon as possible

Rhophylac®, WinRho® SDF: I.M./I.V.: 300 mcg; administer as soon as possible

Abortion, miscarriage, termination of ectopic pregnancy:

RhoGAM®: I.M.: ≥13 weeks gestation: 300 mcg.

HyperRHO™ S/D Mini Dose, MICRhoGAM®: <13 weeks gestation: I.M.: 50 mcg

Rhophylac®: I.M., I.V.: 300 mcg

WinRho® SDF: I.M., I.V.: After 34 weeks gestation: 120 mcg; administer immediately or within 72 hours

Amniocentesis, chorionic villus sampling:

HyperRHO™ S/D Full Dose, RhoGAM®: I.M.: At 15-18 weeks gestation or during the 3rd trimester: 300 mcg. If dose is given between 13-18 weeks, repeat at 26-28 weeks and within 72 hours of delivery.

Rhophylac®: I.M., I.V.: 300 mcg

WinRho® SDF: I.M., I.V.:

Before 34 weeks gestation: 300 mcg; administer immediately, repeat dose every 12 weeks during pregnancy

After 34 weeks gestation: 120 mcg, administered immediately or within 72 hours

Excessive fetomaternal hemorrhage (>15 mL): Rhophylac®: I.M., I.V.: 300 mcg within 72 hours plus 20 mcg/mL fetal RBCs in excess of 15 mL if excess transplacental bleeding is quantified **or** 300 mcg/dose if bleeding cannot be quantified

Abdominal trauma, manipulation:

HyperRHO™ S/D Full Dose, RhoGAM®: I.M.: 2nd or 3rd trimester: 300 mcg. If dose is given between 13-18 weeks, repeat at 26-28 weeks and within 72 hours of delivery.

Rhophylac®: I.M., I.V.: 300 mcg within 72 hours

WinRho® SDF: I.M., I.V.: After 34 weeks gestation: 120 mcg; administer immediately or within 72 hours

Transfusion:

HyperRHO™ S/D Full Dose, RhoGAM®: I.M.: Multiply the volume of Rh positive whole blood administered by the hematocrit of the donor unit to equal the volume of RBCs transfused. The volume of RBCs is then divided by 15 mL, providing the number of 300 mcg doses (vials/syringes) to administer. If the dose calculated results in a fraction, round up to the next higher whole 300 mcg dose (vial/syringe).

WinRho® SDF: Administer within 72 hours after exposure of incompatible blood transfusions or massive fetal hemorrhage.

I.V.: Calculate dose as follows; administer 600 mcg every 8 hours until the total dose is administered:

Exposure to Rh_o(D) positive whole blood: 9 mcg/mL blood

Exposure to Rh_o(D) positive red blood cells: 18 mcg/mL cells

I.M.: Calculate dose as follows; administer 1200 mcg every 12 hours until the total dose is administered:

Exposure to Rh_o(D) positive whole blood: 12 mcg/mL blood

Exposure to Rh_o(D) positive red blood cells: 24 mcg/mL cells

Rhophylac®: I.M., I.V.:20 mcg per 2 mL transfused blood or 1 mL erythrocyte concentrate

Geriatric Refer to adult dosing. Patients >65 years of age with a concurrent comorbid condition (eg, infection, malignancy, autoimmune disorders) may be at increased risk of developing acute hemolytic reactions. Fatal outcomes associated with IVH have occurred most frequently in those >65 years. Careful consideration should be used when selecting dosage for elderly patients due to a higher probability of decreased hepatic, renal, or cardiac function; consider starting at lower doses.

Pediatric ITP, transfusion: Rhophylac®, WinRho® SDF: Refer to adult dosing.

Renal Impairment I.V. infusion: Use caution; may require infusion rate reduction or discontinuation.

Administration

I.M. Administer into the deltoid muscle of the upper arm or anterolateral aspect of the upper thigh. Avoid gluteal region due to risk of sciatic nerve injury. If large doses (>5 mL) are needed, administration in divided doses at different sites is recommended. **Note:** Do not administer I.M. Rh_o(D) immune globulin for ITP.

I.V.

WinRho® SDF: Infuse over at least 3-5 minutes; do not administer with other medications

Rhophylac®: ITP: Infuse at 2 mL per 15-60 seconds

Monitoring and Teaching Issues

Laboratory Monitoring

Patients with suspected IVH: CBC, haptoglobin, plasma hemoglobin, urine dipstick, BUN, serum creatinine, liver function tests, DIC-specific tests (D-dimer, fibrin degradation products [FDP] or fibrin split products [FSP]) for differential diagnosis. In patients at increased risk of developing acute renal failure, periodically monitor renal function and urine output. Clinical response may be determined by monitoring platelets, red blood cell (RBC) counts, hemoglobin, and reticulocyte levels.

ITP: Check blood type, CBC, reticulocyte count, DAT, urine dipstick before initiating treatment with WinRho® SDF, repeat urine dipstick at 2 and 4 hours after administration and prior to end of the 8-hour monitoring period.

Physical Assessment Monitor blood pressure; may cause hyper-/hypotension. Be alert to the possibility of allergic reactions, including anaphylaxis. Assess for signs and symptoms of intravascular hemolysis (IVH) in patients with ITP, anemia, renal insufficiency, back pain, shaking, chills, discolored urine, or hematuria; observe patient for side effects for 8 hours following administration.

Patient Education Do not have live virus vaccinations within 6 months of receiving this medication. This medication can only be administered by injection or infusion; report immediately any difficulty breathing; rapid heartbeat; chills; back rash; pain; redness, swelling, or pain at injection site; discolored urine or blood in the urine; decreased urine output; sudden weight gain; or swelling of extremities. You may experience headache, sleepiness, or dizziness.

- ◆ **RhoGAM® UF Plus** *see* Rh_o(D) Immune Globulin *on page* 1569
- ◆ **RhoIGIV** *see* Rh_o(D) Immune Globulin *on page* 1569
- ◆ **RhoIVIM** *see* Rh_o(D) Immune Globulin *on page* 1569
- ◆ **Rhophylac®** *see* Rh_o(D) Immune Globulin *on page* 1569
- ◆ **rhPTH(1-34)** *see* Teriparatide *on page* 1736
- ◆ ***r*HuEPO-α** *see* Epoetin Alfa *on page* 638
- ◆ **rhuGM-CSF** *see* Sargramostim *on page* 1624
- ◆ **rhuMAb-E25** *see* Omalizumab *on page* 1353
- ◆ **rHuMAb-EGFr** *see* Panitumumab *on page* 1403
- ◆ **rhuMAb HER2** *see* Trastuzumab *on page* 1804
- ◆ **rhuMAb-VEGF** *see* Bevacizumab *on page* 211
- ◆ **RibaPak™ [DSC]** *see* Ribavirin *on page* 1571
- ◆ **Ribasphere®** *see* Ribavirin *on page* 1571
- ◆ **Ribasphere® RibaPak®** *see* Ribavirin *on page* 1571

Ribavirin (rye ba VYE rin)

U.S. Brand Names Copegus®; Rebetol®; RibaPak™ [DSC]; Ribasphere®; Ribasphere® RibaPak®; Virazole®

Index Terms RTCA; Tribavirin

Generic Availability (U.S.) Yes: Capsule, tablet

Pharmacologic Category Antiviral Agent

Medication Safety Issues

Sound-alike/look-alike issues:

Ribavirin may be confused with riboflavin, rifampin, Robaxin®

Medication Guide Available Yes

Pregnancy Risk Factor X

Lactation Excretion in breast milk unknown/not recommended

Use

Inhalation: Treatment of patients with respiratory syncytial virus (RSV) infections; specially indicated for treatment of severe lower respiratory tract RSV infections in patients with an underlying compromising condition (prematurity, bronchopulmonary dysplasia and other chronic lung conditions, congenital heart disease, immunodeficiency, immunosuppression), and recent transplant recipients

Oral capsule:

In combination with interferon alfa-2b (Intron® A) injection for the treatment of chronic hepatitis C in patients with compensated liver disease who have relapsed after alpha interferon therapy or were previously untreated with alpha interferons

In combination with peginterferon alfa-2b (PEG-Intron®) injection for the treatment of chronic hepatitis C in patients with compensated liver disease who were previously untreated with alpha interferons

Oral solution: In combination with interferon alfa 2b (Intron® A) injection for the treatment of chronic hepatitis C in patients with compensated liver disease who were previously untreated with alpha interferons or patients who have relapsed after alpha interferon therapy

Oral tablet: In combination with peginterferon alfa-2a (Pegasys®) injection for the treatment of chronic hepatitis C in patients with compensated liver disease who were previously untreated with alpha interferons (includes patients with histological evidence of cirrhosis [Child-Pugh class A] and patients with clinically-stable HIV disease)

Unlabeled/Investigational Use Used in other viral infections including influenza A and B and adenovirus

Mechanism of Action/Effect Inhibits viral protein synthesis

Contraindications Hypersensitivity to ribavirin or any component of the formulation; women of childbearing age who will not use contraception reliably; pregnancy

Additional contraindications for oral formulation: Male partners of pregnant women; hemoglobinopathies (eg, thalassemia major, sickle cell anemia); patients with autoimmune hepatitis; ribavirin tablets are contraindicated in patients with hepatic decompensation (Child-Pugh class B and C); concomitant use of didanosine

Refer to individual monographs for Interferon Alfa-2b (Intron® A) and Peginterferon Alfa-2a (Pegasys®) for additional contraindication information.

Warnings/Precautions Oral: **[U.S. Boxed Warning]: Significant teratogenic effects have been observed in all animal studies.** A negative pregnancy test is required before initiation and monthly thereafter. Avoid pregnancy in female patients and female partners of male patients, during therapy, and for at least 6 months after treatment; two forms of contraception should be used. Safety and efficacy have not been established in patients who have failed other alfa interferon therapy, received organ transplants, or been coinfected with hepatitis B or HIV (Copegus® may be used in HIV coinfected patients unless CD4+ cell count is <100 cells/microL). Oral products should not be used for HIV infection, adenovirus, RSV, or influenza infections.

[U.S. Boxed Warning]: Monotherapy not effective for chronic hepatitis C infection. Severe psychiatric events have occurred including depression and suicidal behavior during combination therapy. Avoid use in patients with a psychiatric history; discontinue if severe psychiatric symptoms occur. Acute hypersensitivity reactions (eg, anaphylaxis, angioedema, bronchoconstriction, and urticaria) have been observed (rarely) with ribavirin and alfa interferon combination therapy. Severe cutaneous reactions, including Stevens-Johnson syndrome and exfoliative dermatitis have been reported (rarely) with ribavirin and alfa interferon combination therapy; discontinue with signs or symptoms of severe skin reactions. Use with caution in patients with renal impairment; avoid use in patients with Cl_{cr} <50 mL/minute. Elderly patients are more susceptible to adverse effects; use caution.

[U.S. Boxed Warning]: Hemolytic anemia is the primary toxicity of oral therapy; usually occurring within 1-2 weeks of therapy initiation; observed in ~10% to 13% of patients when alfa interferons were combined with ribavirin. Assess cardiac disease before initiation. Anemia may worsen underlying cardiac disease; avoid use in patients with significant/unstable cardiac disease. If deterioration in cardiovascular status occurs, discontinue therapy. Patients with renal dysfunction and/or those >50 years of age should be carefully assessed for development of anemia. Pancytopenia and bone marrow suppression have been reported with the combination of ribavirin, interferon, and azathioprine. Use caution in pulmonary disease; pulmonary symptoms have been associated with administration. Discontinue therapy if evidence of hepatic decompensation (Child-Pugh score ≥6) is observed. Use caution in patients with sarcoidosis (exacerbation reported). Dental and periodontal disorders have been reported with ribavirin and interferon therapy; patients should be instructed to brush teeth twice daily and have regular dental exams. Serious ophthalmologic disorders have occurred with combination therapy. All patients require an eye exam at baseline; those with pre-existing ophthalmologic disorders (eg, diabetic or hypertensive retinopathy) require periodic follow up. In combination with peginterferon alfa-2b, ribavirin may cause a reduction in growth velocity in pediatric patients during treatment and for about 6 months post-treatment.

Inhalation: **[U.S. Boxed Warning]: Use with caution in patients requiring assisted ventilation because precipitation of the drug in the respiratory equipment may interfere with safe and effective patient ventilation; sudden deterioration of respiratory function has been observed;** monitor carefully in patients with COPD and asthma for deterioration of respiratory function. Ribavirin is potentially mutagenic, tumor-promoting, and gonadotoxic. Although anemia has not been reported with inhalation therapy, consider monitoring for anemia 1-2 weeks post-treatment. Pregnant healthcare workers may consider unnecessary occupational exposure; ribavirin has been detected in healthcare workers' urine. Healthcare professionals or family members who are pregnant (or may become pregnant) should be counseled about potential risks of exposure and counseled about risk reduction strategies. Hazardous agent - use appropriate precautions for handling and disposal.

Drug Interactions

Avoid Concomitant Use

Avoid concomitant use of Ribavirin with any of the following: Didanosine

Decreased Effect

Ribavirin may decrease the levels/effects of: Influenza Virus Vaccine (Live/Attenuated)

Increased Effect/Toxicity

Ribavirin may increase the levels/effects of: AzaTHIOprine; Didanosine; Reverse Transcriptase Inhibitors (Nucleoside)

The levels/effects of Ribavirin may be increased by: Interferons (Alfa); Zidovudine

Nutritional/Ethanol Interactions Food: Oral: High-fat meal increases the AUC and C_{max}.

Adverse Reactions

Inhalation:

1% to 10%:

Central nervous system: Fatigue, headache, insomnia
Gastrointestinal: Nausea, anorexia
Hematologic: Anemia

<1%: Hypotension, cardiac arrest, digitalis toxicity, conjunctivitis, mild bronchospasm, worsening of respiratory function, apnea

Note: Incidence of adverse effects (approximate) in healthcare workers: Headache (51%); conjunctivitis (32%); rhinitis, nausea, rash, dizziness, pharyngitis, and lacrimation (10% to 20%); bronchospasm and/or chest pain (case reports in individuals with underlying airway disease)

Oral (all adverse reactions are documented while receiving combination therapy with alfa interferons; percentages as reported in adults); asterisked (*) percentages are those similar to interferon therapy alone:

>10%:

Central nervous system: Fatigue (60% to 70%)*, headache (43% to 66%)*, fever (32% to 55%)*, insomnia (26% to 41%), depression (20% to 36%)*, irritability (23% to 33%), dizziness (14% to 26%), impaired concentration (10% to 21%)*, emotional lability (7% to 12%)*

Dermatologic: Alopecia (27% to 36%), pruritus (13% to 29%), rash (5% to 28%), dry skin (10% to 24%), dermatitis (≤16%)

Endocrine and metabolic: Hyperuricemia (33% to 38%)

Gastrointestinal: Nausea (25% to 47%), anorexia (21% to 32%), weight decrease (10% to 29%), vomiting (9% to 25%)*, diarrhea (10% to 22%), dyspepsia (6% to 16%), abdominal pain (8% to 13%), xerostomia (≤12%), RUQ pain (≤12%)

Hematologic: Leukopenia (6% to 45%), neutropenia (8% to 42%; grade 4: 2% to 11%; 40% with HIV coinfection), hemoglobin decreased (11% to 35%), anemia (11% to 17%), thrombocytopenia (<1% to 15%), lymphopenia (12% to 14%), hemolytic anemia (10% to 13%)

Hepatic: Bilirubin increase (10% to 32%)

Neuromuscular & skeletal: Myalgia (40% to 64%)*, rigors (25% to 48%), arthralgia (22% to 34%)*, musculoskeletal pain (19% to 28%)

Respiratory: Dyspnea (13% to 26%), cough (7% to 23%), pharyngitis (≤13%), sinusitis (≤12%)*

Miscellaneous: Flu-like syndrome (13% to 18%)*, viral infection (≤12%), diaphoresis (≤11%)

1% to 10%:

Cardiovascular: Chest pain (5% to 9%)*, flushing (≤4%)

Central nervous system: Pain (≤10%), mood alteration (≤6%; 9% with HIV coinfection), agitation (5% to 8%), nervousness (6%)*, memory impairment (≤6%), malaise (≤6%), suicidal ideation (adolescents: 2%; adults: 1%)

Dermatologic: Eczema (4% to 5%)

Endocrine & metabolic: Menstrual disorder (≤7%), hypothyroidism (≤5%)

Gastrointestinal: Taste perversion (4% to 9%), constipation (5%)

Hepatic: Hepatomegaly (4%), transaminases increased (1% to 3%), hepatic decompensation (2% with HIV coinfection)

Neuromuscular & skeletal: Weakness (9% to 10%), back pain (5%)

Ocular: Blurred vision (≤6%), conjunctivitis (≤5%)

Respiratory: Rhinitis (≤8%), exertional dyspnea (≤7%)

Miscellaneous: Fungal infection (≤6%), bacterial infection (3% to 5%)

Note: Incidence of anorexia, headache, fever, suicidal ideation, and vomiting are higher in children.

Pharmacodynamics/Kinetics

Absorption Inhalation: Systemic; dependent upon respiratory factors and method of drug delivery; maximal absorption occurs with the use of aerosol generator via endotracheal tube; highest concentrations in respiratory tract and erythrocytes

Bioavailability Oral: 64%

Time to Peak Serum: Inhalation: At end of inhalation period; Oral capsule: Multiple doses: 3 hours; Tablet: 2 hours

Protein Binding Oral: None

Half-Life Elimination Plasma:

Children: Inhalation: 6.5-11 hours

Adults: Oral:

Capsule, single dose (Rebetol®, Ribasphere®): 24 hours in healthy adults, 44 hours with chronic hepatitis C infection (increases to ~298 hours at steady state)

Tablet, single dose (Copegus®): ~120-170 hours

Metabolism Hepatically and intracellularly (forms active metabolites); may be necessary for drug action

Excretion Inhalation: Urine (40% as unchanged drug and metabolites); Oral capsule: Urine (61%), feces (12%)

Available Dosage Forms

Capsule, oral: 200 mg

Rebetol®: 200 mg

Ribasphere®: 200 mg

Combination package, oral:

Ribasphere® RibaPak®: Tablet: 400 mg (7s) [medium blue tablets] and Tablet: 600 mg (7s) [dark blue tablets] (14s, 56s)

Powder for solution, for nebulization:

Virazole®: 6 g

Solution, oral:

Rebetol®: 40 mg/mL (100 mL)

Tablet, oral: 200 mg

Copegus®: 200 mg

Ribasphere®: 200 mg, 400 mg, 600 mg

Ribasphere® RibaPak®: 400 mg, 600 mg

Dosing

Adult & Geriatric

Chronic hepatitis C (in combination with peginterferon alfa-2a): Oral: Tablet (Copegus®):

Monoinfection, genotype 1,4:

<75 kg: 1000 mg/day, in 2 divided doses for 48 weeks

≥75 kg: 1200 mg/day, in 2 divided doses for 48 weeks

Monoinfection, genotype 2,3: 800 mg/day, in 2 divided doses for 24 weeks

Coinfection with HIV: 800 mg/day in 2 divided doses for 48 weeks (regardless of genotype)

Chronic hepatitis C (in combination with interferon alfa-2b): Oral: Capsule (Rebetol®, Ribasphere®):

≤75 kg: 400 mg in the morning, then 600 mg in the evening

>75 kg: 600 mg in the morning, then 600 mg in the evening

Chronic hepatitis C (in combination with peginterferon alfa-2b): Oral: Capsule (Rebetol®, Ribasphere®): 400 mg twice daily

Note: *American Association for the Study of Liver Diseases (AASLD) guidelines recommendation:* Adults with chronic HCV infection (Ghany, 2009): Treatment of choice: Ribavirin plus **peginterferon**; clinical condition and ability of patient to tolerate therapy should be evaluated to determine length and/or likely benefit of therapy. Recommended treatment duration (AASLD guidelines): Genotypes 1,4: 48 weeks; Genotypes 2,3: 24 weeks; Coinfection with HIV: 48 weeks.

Pediatric

RSV infection: Infants and Children: Aerosol inhalation: Use with Viratek® small particle aerosol generator (SPAG-2): A concentration of 20 mg/mL (6 g reconstituted with 300 mL of sterile water without preservatives) administered for 12-18 hours/day for 3 days, up to 7 days in length.

Chronic hepatitis C (in combination with interferon alfa-2b): Oral solution should be used in children 3-5 years of age, children ≤25 kg, or those unable to swallow capsules. Recommended therapy duration (manufacturer labeling): Genotype 1: 48 weeks; genotypes 2,3: 24 weeks

Capsule/oral solution: Children ≥3 years: 15 mg/kg/day in 2 divided doses.

Capsule dosing recommendations:

25-36 kg: 400 mg/day (200 mg morning and evening)

37-49 kg: 600 mg/day (200 mg in the morning and 400 mg in the evening)

50-61 kg: 800 mg/day (400 mg in the morning and evening)

>61 kg: Refer to adult dosing.

Note: *American Association for the Study of Liver Diseases (AASLD) guidelines recommendation:* Children 2-17 years with chronic HCV infection (Ghany, 2009): Treatment of choice: Ribavirin 15 mg/kg daily in combination with SubQ peginterferon alfa-2b 60 mcg/m^2 once weekly for 48 weeks

Renal Impairment Cl_{cr} <50 mL/minute: Oral route is not recommended.

Hepatic Impairment Hepatic decompensation (Child-Pugh class B and C): Use of ribavirin tablets is contraindicated.

Adjustment for Toxicity Oral: Capsule, solution, tablet:

Patient **without** cardiac history:

Hemoglobin <10 g/dL:

Children: Decrease dose to 7.5 mg/kg/day

Adults: Decrease dose to 600 mg/day

Hemoglobin <8.5 g/dL: Children and Adults: Permanently discontinue treatment

Patient **with** cardiac history:

Hemoglobin has decreased ≥2 g/dL during any 4-week period of treatment:

Children: Decrease dose to 7.5 mg/kg/day

Adults: Decrease dose to 600 mg/day

Hemoglobin <12 g/dL after 4 weeks of reduced dose: Children and Adults: Permanently discontinue treatment

Administration

Oral Administer concurrently with interferon alfa injection. Capsule should not be opened, crushed, chewed, or broken. Capsules are not for use in children <5 years of age. Use oral solution for children 3-5 years, those ≤25 kg, or those who cannot swallow capsules.

Capsule, in combination with interferon alfa-2b: May be administered with or without food, but always in a consistent manner in regard to food intake.

Capsule, in combination with peginterferon alfa-2b: Administer with food.

Solution, in combination with interferon alfa-2b: May be administered with or without food, but always in a consistent manner in regard to food intake.

Tablet: Should be administered with food.

Inhalation Ribavirin should be administered in well-ventilated rooms (at least 6 air changes/hour). In mechanically-ventilated patients, ribavirin can potentially be deposited in the ventilator delivery system depending on temperature, humidity, and electrostatic forces; this deposition can lead to malfunction or obstruction of the expiratory valve, resulting in inadvertently high positive end-expiratory pressures. The use of one-way valves in the inspiratory lines, a breathing circuit filter in the expiratory line, and frequent monitoring and filter replacement have been effective in preventing these problems. Solutions in SPAG-2 unit should be discarded at least every 24 hours and when the liquid level is low before adding newly reconstituted solution. Should not be mixed with other aerosolized medication.

Stability

Reconstitution Inhalation: Do not use any water containing an antimicrobial agent to reconstitute drug. Reconstituted solution is stable for 24 hours at room temperature.

Storage

Inhalation: Store vials in a dry place at 15°C to 30°C (59°F to 86°F).

Oral: Store at controlled room temperature of 25°C (77°F). Solution may also be refrigerated at 2°C to 8°C (36°F to 46°F).

Monitoring and Teaching Issues

Laboratory Monitoring

Inhalation: Respiratory function, hemoglobin, reticulocyte count, CBC with differential, I & O

Oral: Clinical studies tested as follows: CBC (including hemoglobin, WBC, and platelets) and chemistries (including liver function tests and uric acid) measured at weeks 1, 2, 4, 6, and 8, and then every 4 weeks; TSH measured every 12 weeks

Baseline values used in clinical trials:

Platelet count ≥90,000/mm^3 (75,000/mm^3 for cirrhosis or 70,000/mm^3 for coinfection with HIV)

ANC ≥1500/mm^3

Hemoglobin ≥12 g/dL for women and ≥13 g/dL for men (11 g/dL for HIV coinfected women and 12 g/dL for HIV coinfected men)

TSH and T_4 within normal limits or adequately controlled

CD4$^+$ cell count ≥200 cells/microL or CD4$^+$ cell count 100-200 cells/microL and HIV-1 RNA <5000 copies/mL for coinfection with HIV

Serum HCV RNA (pretreatment, week 12 and week 24, and 24 weeks after completion of therapy). **Note:** Discontinuation of therapy may be considered after 12 weeks in patients with HCV (genotypes 1,4) who fail to achieve an early virologic response (EVR) (defined as ≥2-log decrease in HCV RNA compared to pretreatment) or after 24 weeks with detectable HCV RNA. Treat patients with HCV (genotypes 2,3) for 24 weeks (if tolerated) and then evaluate HCV RNA levels (Ghany, 2009).

Pretreatment and monthly pregnancy test up to 6 months following discontinuation of therapy for women of childbearing age; pretreatment ECG in patients with pre-existing cardiac disease; dental exams

Physical Assessment Note specific cautions for healthcare professionals' exposure risks with inhalation formulation. Evaluate patient health status and history for contraindications and use cautions prior to beginning therapy. Evaluate weight on a regular basis throughout therapy. Monitor for headache; fatigue; irritability; impaired concentration; nausea, vomiting, or anorexia; anemia; or deterioration of hepatic, respiratory, or cardiac status on a regular basis.

Patient Education For oral administration, take capsules with food and solution with or without food. Do not allow pregnant women or women of childbearing age to come in any contact with this medication. If prescribed in conjunction with other medications, maintain schedule as directed. Maintain adequate hydration, unless instructed to restrict fluid intake. You will need regular blood tests while taking this drug. You may experience increased susceptibility to infection. May cause dental or periodontal disorders. You may be required to have regular ophthalmic exams during therapy. May cause confusion, dizziness, insomnia, impaired concentration, emotional liability, headache, nausea, vomiting, anorexia, extreme fatigue, diarrhea, loss of hair (reversible), or dermatitis. Report chest pain or palpitations; unusual cough or difficulty breathing; rash; signs of infection (fever, chills, unusual bleeding or bruising, infection, or unhealed sores or white plaques in mouth); tingling, weakness, or pain in extremities; CNS changes (suicide ideation, fatigue, insomnia, irritability, depression, impaired concentration); or changes in vision.

Dietary Considerations When used in combination with interferon alfa-2b, capsules and solution may be taken with or without food, but always in a consistent manner in regard to food intake (ie, always take with food or always take on an empty stomach). When used in combination with peginterferon alfa-2b, capsules should be taken with food. Tablets should be taken with food.

Geriatric Considerations No specific recommendations are necessary in the elderly; however, in patients with creatinine clearance <50 mL/minute, the oral route not recommended. Many elderly will fall into this category.

Pregnancy Considerations [U.S. Boxed Warning]: Significant teratogenic effects have been observed in all animal studies at ~0.01 times the maximum recommended daily human dose. Use is contraindicated in pregnancy. Negative pregnancy test is required before initiation and monthly thereafter. Avoid pregnancy in female patients and female partners of male patients during therapy by using two effective forms of contraception; continue contraceptive measures for at least 6 months after completion of therapy. If patient or female partner becomes pregnant during treatment, she should be counseled about potential risks of exposure. If pregnancy occurs during use or within 6 months after treatment, report to the ribavirin pregnancy registry (800-593-2214).

◆ **RID® Maximum Strength [OTC]** *see* Pyrethrins and Piperonyl Butoxide *on page* 1530

Rifabutin (rif a BYOO tin)

U.S. Brand Names Mycobutin®

Index Terms Ansamycin

Generic Availability (U.S.) No

Pharmacologic Category Antibiotic, Miscellaneous; Antitubercular Agent

Medication Safety Issues

Sound-alike/look-alike issues:

Rifabutin may be confused with rifampin

Pregnancy Risk Factor B

Lactation Excretion in breast milk unknown/not recommended

Use Prevention of disseminated *Mycobacterium avium* complex (MAC) in patients with advanced HIV infection

Unlabeled/Investigational Use Utilized in multidrug regimens for treatment of MAC; alternative to rifampin as prophylaxis for latent tuberculosis infection (LTBI) or part of multidrug regimen for treatment active tuberculosis infection

Mechanism of Action/Effect Inhibits DNA-dependent RNA polymerase at the beta subunit which prevents chain initiation

Contraindications Hypersensitivity to rifabutin, any other rifamycins, or any component of the formulation

Warnings/Precautions Rifabutin must not be administered for MAC prophylaxis to patients with active tuberculosis since its use may lead to the development of tuberculosis that is resistant to both rifabutin and rifampin. May be associated with neutropenia and/or thrombocytopenia (rarely). Dosage reduction recommended in severe impairment (Cl_{cr} <30 mL/minute). Prolonged use may result in fungal or bacterial superinfection, including *C. difficile*-associated diarrhea (CDAD) and pseudomembranous colitis; CDAD has been observed >2 months postantibiotic treatment. May cause brown/orange discoloration of urine, feces, saliva, sweat, tears, and skin. Remove soft contact lenses during therapy since permanent staining may occur.

Drug Interactions

Metabolism/Transport Effects Substrate of CYP3A4 (major); **Induces** CYP3A4 (strong)

Avoid Concomitant Use

Avoid concomitant use of Rifabutin with any of the following: BCG; Dronedarone; Everolimus; Lurasidone; Mycophenolate; Nilotinib; Pazopanib; Praziquantel; Ranolazine; Roflumilast; RomiDEPsin; Tolvaptan; Vandetanib; Voriconazole

Decreased Effect

Rifabutin may decrease the levels/effects of: Alfentanil; Amiodarone; Angiotensin II Receptor Blockers; Antiemetics (5HT3 Antagonists); Antifungal Agents (Azole Derivatives, Systemic); Aprepitant; Atovaquone; Barbiturates; BCG; Benzodiazepines (metabolized by oxidation); BusPIRone; Calcium Channel Blockers; Contraceptives (Estrogens); Contraceptives (Progestins); Corticosteroids (Systemic); CycloSPORINE; CycloSPORINE (Systemic); CYP3A4 Substrates; Dapsone; Dapsone (Systemic); Delavirdine; Disopyramide; Dronedarone; Efavirenz; Etravirine; Everolimus; Exemestane; FentaNYL; Fluconazole; Gefitinib; GuanFACINE; HMG-CoA Reductase Inhibitors; Imatinib; Indinavir; Ixabepilone; Lurasidone; Maraviroc; Morphine (Systemic); Morphine Sulfate; Mycophenolate; Nelfinavir; Nevirapine; Nilotinib; Pazopanib; Phenytoin; Praziquantel; Propafenone; QuiNIDine; Ramelteon; Ranolazine; Repaglinide; Roflumilast; RomiDEPsin; Saxagliptin; SORAfenib; SUNItinib; Tacrolimus; Tacrolimus (Systemic); Tadalafil; Tamoxifen; Temsirolimus; Terbinafine (Systemic); Tolvaptan; Typhoid Vaccine; Ulipristal; Vandetanib; Vitamin K Antagonists; Voriconazole; Zaleplon; Zolpidem

The levels/effects of Rifabutin may be decreased by: CYP3A4 Inducers (Strong); Deferasirox; Efavirenz; Herbs (CYP3A4 Inducers); Nevirapine

Increased Effect/Toxicity

Rifabutin may increase the levels/effects of: Clopidogrel; Darunavir; Fosamprenavir; HMG-CoA Reductase Inhibitors; Isoniazid; Lopinavir

The levels/effects of Rifabutin may be increased by: Antifungal Agents (Azole Derivatives, Systemic); Atazanavir; Conivaptan; Darunavir; Delavirdine; Fluconazole; Fosamprenavir; Indinavir; Lopinavir; Macrolide Antibiotics; Nelfinavir; Nevirapine; Ritonavir; Saquinavir; Tipranavir; Voriconazole

Nutritional/Ethanol Interactions Food: High-fat meal may decrease the rate but not the extent of absorption.

Adverse Reactions

>10%:

Dermatologic: Rash (11%)

Genitourinary: Discoloration of urine (30%)

Hematologic: Neutropenia (25%), leukopenia (17%)

1% to 10%:

Central nervous system: Headache (3%), fever (2%)

Gastrointestinal: Nausea (3% to 6%), abdominal pain (4%), dyspepsia (3%), eructation (3%), taste perversion (3%), vomiting (3%), flatulence (2%)

Hematologic: Thrombocytopenia (5%)

Hepatic: ALT increased (7% to 9%; incidence less than placebo), AST increased (7% to 9%; incidence less than placebo)
Neuromuscular & skeletal: Myalgia (2%)

Pharmacodynamics/Kinetics

Absorption Readily, 53%

Bioavailability Absolute: HIV: 20%

Time to Peak Serum: 2-4 hours

Protein Binding 85%

Half-Life Elimination Terminal: 45 hours (range: 16-69 hours)

Metabolism To 5 metabolites; predominantly 25-O-desacetyl-rifabutin (antimicrobial activity equivalent to parent drug; serum AUC 10% of parent drug) and 31-hydroxy-rifabutin (serum AUC 7% of parent drug)

Excretion Urine (53% as metabolites); feces (30%)

Available Dosage Forms

Capsule, oral:
Mycobutin®: 150 mg

Dosing

Adult & Geriatric

Disseminated MAC in advanced HIV infection: Oral:
Prophylaxis: 300 mg once daily or 150 mg twice daily to reduce gastrointestinal upset
Treatment (unlabeled use; AIDSinfo guidelines): 300 mg once daily as an optional add-on to primary therapy of clarithromycin and ethambutol

Tuberculosis (unlabeled use as alternative to rifampin; AIDS *info* guidelines): Oral:
Prophylaxis of LTBI: 300 mg once daily for 4 months
Treatment of active TB: 300 mg once daily or intermittently 2-3 times weekly as part of multidrug regimen

Dosage adjustment for concurrent nelfinavir, amprenavir, indinavir: Reduce rifabutin dose to 150 mg/day; no change in dose if administered twice weekly

Dosage adjustment for concurrent efavirenz (no concomitant protease inhibitor): Increase rifabutin dose to 450-600 mg daily, or 600 mg 3 times/week

Pediatric

Prophylaxis for recurrence of *Mycobacterium avium* complex (MAC) in HIV-exposed/-infected patients (unlabeled use; CDC, 2009): Oral: Infants and Children: 5 mg/kg (maximum dose: 300 mg) once daily as an optional add-on to primary therapy of clarithromycin and ethambutol

Prophylaxis for first episode of MAC in HIV-exposed/-infected patients (unlabeled use; CDC, 2009): Oral: Children ≥6 years: 300 mg once daily

Treatment of active TB (as alternative to rifampin) in HIV-exposed/-infected patients (unlabeled use; CDC, 2009): Oral: Infants and Children: 10-20 mg/kg (maximum dose: 300 mg) once daily or intermittently 2-3 times weekly

Treatment of severe MAC in HIV-exposed/-infected patients (unlabeled use; CDC, 2009): Oral: Infants and Children: 10-20 mg/kg (maximum dose: 300 mg) once daily, in addition to primary therapy of clarithromycin and ethambutol

Adolescents: Refer to adult dosing.

Renal Impairment Cl_{cr} <30 mL/minute: Reduce dose by 50%

Administration

Oral May be taken with meals to minimize nausea or vomiting.

Stability

Storage Store at 25°C (77°F); excursions permitted to 15°C to 30°C (59°F to 86°F).

Monitoring and Teaching Issues

Laboratory Monitoring Periodic liver function, CBC with differential, platelet count

Physical Assessment Monitor for anemia, neutropenia, GI disturbance, and rash.

Patient Education Will discolor urine, stool, saliva, tears, sweat, and other body fluids a red-brown color; this is normal. Stains on clothing or contact lenses are permanent. May cause headache, vomiting, loss of appetite, or taste perversion. Report skin rash, persistent vomiting or diarrhea, or persistent muscle pain.

Dietary Considerations May be taken with meals.

Geriatric Considerations No specific recommendations for the elderly.

◆ **Rifadin®** *see* Rifampin *on page* 1577

◆ **Rifamate®** *see* Rifampin and Isoniazid *on page* 1580

◆ **Rifampicin** *see* Rifampin *on page* 1577

Rifampin (rif AM pin)

U.S. Brand Names Rifadin®

Index Terms Rifampicin

Generic Availability (U.S.) Yes

Pharmacologic Category Antibiotic, Miscellaneous; Antitubercular Agent

Medication Safety Issues

Sound-alike/look-alike issues:
Rifadin® may be confused with Rifater®, Ritalin®
Rifampin may be confused with ribavirin, rifabutin, Rifamate®, rifapentine, rifaximin

Pregnancy Risk Factor C

Lactation Enters breast milk/not recommended (AAP rates "compatible"; AAP 2001 update pending)

Use Management of active tuberculosis in combination with other agents; elimination of meningococci from the nasopharynx in asymptomatic carriers

Unlabeled/Investigational Use Prophylaxis of *Haemophilus influenzae* type b infection; *Legionella* pneumonia; used in combination with other anti-infectives in the treatment of staphylococcal infections; treatment of *M. leprae* infections

Mechanism of Action/Effect Inhibits bacterial RNA synthesis by binding to the beta subunit of DNA-dependent RNA polymerase, blocking RNA transcription

Contraindications Hypersensitivity to rifampin, any rifamycins, or any component of the formulation; concurrent use of amprenavir, saquinavir/ritonavir (possibly other protease inhibitors)

Warnings/Precautions Use with caution and modify dosage in patients with liver impairment; observe for hyperbilirubinemia; discontinue therapy if this in conjunction with clinical symptoms or any signs of significant hepatocellular damage develop. Use with caution in patients receiving concurrent medications associated with hepatotoxicity. Use with caution in patients with a history of alcoholism (even if ethanol consumption is discontinued during therapy). Since rifampin since rifampin has enzyme-inducing properties, porphyria exacerbation is possible; use with caution in patients with porphyria; do not use for meningococcal disease, only for short-term treatment of asymptomatic carrier states

Regimens of >600 mg once or twice weekly have been associated with a high incidence of adverse reactions including a flu-like syndrome, hypersensitivity, thrombocytopenia, leukopenia, and anemia. Urine, feces, saliva, sweat, tears, and CSF may be discolored to red/orange; remove soft contact lenses during therapy since permanent staining may occur. Do not administer I.V. form via I.M. or SubQ routes; restart infusion at another site if extravasation occurs. Prolonged use may result in fungal or bacterial superinfection, including *C. difficile*-associated diarrhea (CDAD) and pseudomembranous colitis; CDAD has been observed >2 months postantibiotic treatment. Monitor for compliance in patients on intermittent therapy.

Drug Interactions

Metabolism/Transport Effects Substrate of P-glycoprotein, SLCO1B1; **Induces** CYP1A2 (strong), CYP2A6 (strong), CYP2B6 (strong), CYP2C8 (strong), CYP2C9 (strong), CYP2C19 (strong), CYP3A4 (strong), P-glycoprotein

Avoid Concomitant Use

Avoid concomitant use of Rifampin with any of the following: Atazanavir; BCG; Dabigatran Etexilate; Darunavir; Dronedarone; Etravirine; Everolimus; Fosamprenavir; Indinavir; Lopinavir; Lurasidone; Mycophenolate; Nelfinavir; Nilotinib; Pazopanib; Praziquantel; QuiNINE; Ranolazine; Ritonavir; Roflumilast; RomiDEPsin; Saquinavir; Tipranavir; Tolvaptan; Vandetanib; Voriconazole

Decreased Effect

Rifampin may decrease the levels/effects of: Alfentanil; Amiodarone; Angiotensin II Receptor Blockers; Antidiabetic Agents (Thiazolidinedione); Antiemetics (5HT3 Antagonists); Antifungal Agents (Azole Derivatives, Systemic); Aprepitant; Atazanavir; Atovaquone; Barbiturates; BCG; Bendamustine; Benzodiazepines (metabolized by oxidation); Beta-Blockers; BusPIRone; Calcium Channel Blockers; Caspofungin; Chloramphenicol; Contraceptives (Estrogens); Contraceptives (Progestins); Corticosteroids (Systemic); CycloSPORINE; CycloSPORINE (Systemic); CYP1A2 Substrates; CYP2A6 Substrates; CYP2B6 Substrates; CYP2C19 Substrates; CYP2C8 Substrates (High risk); CYP2C9 Substrates (High risk); CYP3A4 Substrates; Dabigatran Etexilate; Dapsone; Dapsone (Systemic); Darunavir; Deferasirox; Delavirdine; Disopyramide; Divalproex; Dronedarone; Efavirenz; Erlotinib; Etravirine; Everolimus; Exemestane; FentaNYL; Fexofenadine; Fluconazole; Fosamprenavir; Fosaprepitant; Gefitinib; GuanFACINE; HMG-CoA Reductase Inhibitors; Imatinib; Indinavir; Ixabepilone; LamoTRIgine; Lopinavir; Lurasidone; Maraviroc; Methadone; Morphine (Systemic); Morphine Sulfate; Mycophenolate; Nelfinavir; Nevirapine; Nilotinib; OxyCODONE; Pazopanib; P-Glycoprotein Substrates; Phenytoin; Prasugrel; Praziquantel; Propafenone; QuiNIDine; QuiNINE; Raltegravir; Ramelteon; Ranolazine; Repaglinide; Ritonavir; Roflumilast; RomiDEPsin; Saquinavir; Saxagliptin; Sirolimus; SORAfenib; Sulfonylureas; SUNItinib; Tacrolimus; Tacrolimus (Systemic); Tadalafil; Tamoxifen; Temsirolimus; Terbinafine; Terbinafine (Systemic); Thyroid Products; Tipranavir; Tolvaptan; Treprostinil; Typhoid Vaccine; Ulipristal; Valproic Acid; Vandetanib; Vitamin K Antagonists; Voriconazole; Zaleplon; Zidovudine; Zolpidem

The levels/effects of Rifampin may be decreased by: P-Glycoprotein Inducers

Increased Effect/Toxicity

Rifampin may increase the levels/effects of: Clopidogrel; Gadoxetate; HMG-CoA Reductase Inhibitors; Isoniazid; Leflunomide; Lopinavir; Saquinavir

The levels/effects of Rifampin may be increased by: Antifungal Agents (Azole Derivatives, Systemic); Delavirdine; Eltrombopag; Fluconazole; Macrolide Antibiotics; P-Glycoprotein Inhibitors; Pyrazinamide; Voriconazole

Nutritional/Ethanol Interactions

Ethanol: Avoid ethanol (may increase risk of hepatotoxicity).

Food: Food decreases the extent of absorption; rifampin concentrations may be decreased if taken with food.

Herb/Nutraceutical: St John's wort may decrease rifampin levels.

Lab Interactions May interfere with urine detection of opiates (false-positive); positive Coombs' reaction [direct], rifampin inhibits standard assay's ability to measure serum folate and B_{12}; transient increase in LFTs and decreased biliary excretion of contrast media

Adverse Reactions

Frequency not defined:

Cardiovascular: Edema, flushing

Central nervous system: Ataxia, behavioral changes, concentration impaired, confusion, dizziness, drowsiness, fatigue, fever, headache, numbness, psychosis

Dermatologic: Pemphigoid reaction, pruritus, urticaria

Endocrine & metabolic: Adrenal insufficiency, menstrual disorders

Hematologic: Agranulocytosis (rare), DIC, eosinophilia, hemoglobin decreased, hemolysis, hemolytic anemia, leukopenia, thrombocytopenia (especially with high-dose therapy)

Hepatic: Hepatitis (rare), jaundice

Neuromuscular & skeletal: Myalgia, osteomalacia, weakness

Ocular: Exudative conjunctivitis, visual changes

Renal: Acute renal failure, BUN increased, hemoglobinuria, hematuria, interstitial nephritis, uric acid increased

Miscellaneous: Flu-like syndrome

1% to 10%:

Dermatologic: Rash (1% to 5%)

Gastrointestinal (1% to 2%): Anorexia, cramps, diarrhea, epigastric distress, flatulence, heartburn, nausea, pseudomembranous colitis, pancreatitis, vomiting

Hepatic: LFTs increased (up to 14%)

Pharmacodynamics/Kinetics

Duration of Action ≤24 hours

Absorption Oral: Well absorbed; food may delay or slightly reduce peak

Time to Peak Serum: Oral: 2-4 hours

Protein Binding 80%

Half-Life Elimination 3-4 hours, prolonged with hepatic impairment; End-stage renal disease: 1.8-11 hours

Metabolism Hepatic; undergoes enterohepatic recirculation

Excretion Feces (60% to 65%) and urine (~30%) as unchanged drug

Available Dosage Forms

Capsule, oral: 150 mg, 300 mg

Rifadin®: 150 mg, 300 mg

Injection, powder for reconstitution: 600 mg

Rifadin®: 600 mg

Dosing

Adult & Geriatric

Tuberculosis, active: Oral, I.V.: **Note:** A four-drug regimen (isoniazid, rifampin, pyrazinamide, and ethambutol) is preferred for the initial, empiric treatment of TB. When the drug susceptibility results are available, the regimen should be altered as appropriate.

Daily therapy: 10 mg/kg/day (maximum: 600 mg/day)

Twice weekly directly observed therapy (DOT): 10 mg/kg (maximum: 600 mg); 3 times/ week: 10 mg/kg (maximum: 600 mg)

Tuberculosis, latent infection (LTBI): As an alternative to isoniazid: Oral, I.V.: 10 mg/kg/day (maximum: 600 mg/day) for 4 months. **Note:** Combination with pyrazinamide should not generally be offered (*MMWR*, Aug 8, 2003).

Endocarditis, prosthetic valve due to MRSA (unlabeled use): Oral, I.V.: 300 mg every 8 hours for at least 6 weeks (combine with vancomycin for the entire duration of therapy and gentamicin for the first 2 weeks) (Liu, 2011)

***H. influenzae* prophylaxis (unlabeled use):** Oral, I.V.: 600 mg every 24 hours for 4 days

Leprosy (unlabeled use): Oral, I.V.:

Multibacillary: 600 mg once monthly for 24 months in combination with ofloxacin and minocycline

Paucibacillary: 600 mg once monthly for 6 months in combination with dapsone

Single lesion: 600 mg as a single dose in combination with ofloxacin 400 mg and minocycline 100 mg

Meningococcal meningitis prophylaxis (unlabeled use): Oral, I.V.: 600 mg every 12 hours for 2 days

Meningitis *(Pneumococcus* or *Staphylococcus)* (unlabeled use): Oral, I.V.: 600 mg once daily

Nasal carriers of *Staphylococcus aureus* (unlabeled use): Oral, I.V.: 600 mg/day for 5-10 days; **Note: Must use in combination with at least one other systemic antistaphylococcal antibiotic.** Not recommended as first-line drug for decolonization; evidence is weak for use in patients with recurrent infections (Liu, 2011).

Nontuberculous mycobacterium *(M. kansasii)* (unlabeled use): Oral, I.V.: 10 mg/kg/day (maximum: 600 mg/day) for duration to include 12 months of culture-negative sputum; typically used in combination with ethambutol and isoniazid

***Staphylococcus aureus* infections, adjunctive therapy (unlabeled use):** Oral, I.V.: 600 mg once daily or 300-450 mg every 12 hours with other antibiotics. **Note:** Must be used in combination with another antistaphylococcal antibiotic to avoid rapid development of resistance (Liu, 2011).

Pediatric

Tuberculosis, active: Oral, I.V.:

Infants and Children <12 years:

Daily therapy: 10-20 mg/kg/day usually as a single dose (maximum: 600 mg/day)

Twice weekly directly observed therapy (DOT): 10-20 mg/kg (maximum: 600 mg)

See "Note" in adult dosing.

Tuberculosis, latent infection (LTBI): As an alternative to isoniazid: Children: 10-20 mg/kg/ day (maximum: 600 mg/day) for 6 months

***H. influenzae* prophylaxis (unlabeled use):** Oral, I.V.: Infants and Children: 20 mg/kg/day every 24 hours for 4 days, not to exceed 600 mg/dose

Meningococcal prophylaxis (unlabeled use): Oral:

<1 month: 10 mg/kg/day in divided doses every 12 hours for 2 days

Infants and Children: 20 mg/kg/day in divided doses every 12 hours for 2 days (maximum: 600 mg/dose)

Nasal carriers of *Staphylococcus aureus* (unlabeled use): Oral, I.V.: 15 mg/kg/day divided every 12 hours for 5-10 days; **Note: Must use in combination with at least one other systemic antistaphylococcal antibiotic.** Not recommended as first-line drug for decolonization; evidence is weak for use in patients with recurrent infections (Liu, 2011).

Renal Impairment Plasma rifampin concentrations are not significantly affected by hemodialysis or peritoneal dialysis.

Hepatic Impairment Dose reductions are necessary to reduce hepatotoxicity.

Administration

Oral Administer on an empty stomach with a glass of water (ie, 1 hour prior to, or 2 hours after meals or antacids) to increase total absorption (food may delay and reduce the amount of rifampin absorbed). The compounded oral suspension must be shaken well before using. May mix contents of capsule with applesauce or jelly.

I.M. Do not administer I.M. or SubQ

I.V. Administer I.V. preparation by slow I.V. infusion over 30 minutes to 3 hours at a final concentration not to exceed 6 mg/mL.

Stability

Reconstitution Reconstitute powder for injection with SWFI. Prior to injection, dilute in appropriate volume of compatible diluent (eg, 100 mL D_5W).

Storage Rifampin powder is reddish brown. Intact vials should be stored at room temperature and protected from excessive heat and light. Reconstituted vials are stable for 24 hours at room temperature.

Stability of parenteral admixture at room temperature (25°C) is 4 hours for D_5W and 24 hours for NS.

Monitoring and Teaching Issues

Laboratory Monitoring Periodic monitoring of liver function (AST, ALT), CBC, sputum culture, chest x-ray 2-3 months into treatment

Physical Assessment Concurrent use with rifampin may decrease levels/effects of multiple other drugs; analyze complete medical regimen. Infusion site must be monitored to prevent extravasation. Assess results of chest x-ray. Monitor for hypersensitivity reactions, hepatotoxicity, CNS changes, hematologic changes, visual disturbances, and gastrointestinal upset on a regular basis during therapy. Monitor patient compliance with treatment regimen.

Patient Education Rifampin may be prescribed in conjunction with other antibiotics; maintain dosing schedule as directed. Take rifampin on an empty stomach, 1 hour before or 2 hours after meals. Keep appointments for scheduled laboratory tests and chest x-rays. This medication will discolor urine, stool, saliva, tears, sweat, and other body fluids a red-brown color. Stains on contact lenses and clothing are permanent. Report persistent vomiting, diarrhea, rash, fever, chills, flu-like symptoms, or unusual bruising or bleeding.

Dietary Considerations Rifampin should be taken on an empty stomach.

Geriatric Considerations Rifampin, in combination with isoniazid, is the foundation of tuberculosis treatment. Since most older patients acquired their *Mycobacterium tuberculosis* infection before effective chemotherapy was available, either a 9-month regimen of isoniazid and rifampin or a 6-month regimen of isoniazid and rifampin with pyrazinamide (the first 2 months) should be effective.

Breast-Feeding Considerations The manufacturer does not recommend breast-feeding due to tumorigenicity observed in animal studies; however, the CDC does not consider rifampin a contraindication to breast-feeding.

Pregnancy Considerations Teratogenic effects have been reported in animal studies. Rifampin crosses the human placenta. Due to the risk of tuberculosis to the fetus, treatment is recommended when the probability of maternal disease is moderate to high. Postnatal hemorrhages have been reported in the infant and mother with isoniazid administration during the last few weeks of pregnancy.

Related Information

Antimicrobial Drugs of Choice *on page 2008*

Prophylaxis for Patients Exposed to Common Communicable Diseases *on page 2073*

Rifampin and Isoniazid (rif AM pin & eye soe NYE a zid)

U.S. Brand Names IsonaRif™; Rifamate®

Index Terms Isoniazid and Rifampin

Generic Availability (U.S.) Yes

Pharmacologic Category Antibiotic, Miscellaneous

Medication Safety Issues

Sound-alike/look-alike issues:

Rifamate® may be confused with rifampin

Pregnancy Risk Factor C

Lactation Enters breast milk/compatible

Use Management of active tuberculosis; see individual agents for additional information

Available Dosage Forms

Capsule:

IsonaRif™, Rifamate®: 300/150: Rifampin 300 mg and isoniazid 150 mg

Dosing

Adult Tuberculosis: Oral: 2 capsules/day

Geriatric Refer to dosing in individual monographs.

Monitoring and Teaching Issues

Physical Assessment See individual agents.

Patient Education See individual agents.

Related Information

Isoniazid *on page 1024*

Rifampin *on page 1577*

◆ **rIFN beta-1a** *see* Interferon Beta-1a *on page 1003*

◆ **rIFN beta-1b** *see* Interferon Beta-1b *on page 1005*

Rilonacept (ri LON a sept)

U.S. Brand Names Arcalyst™

Generic Availability (U.S.) No

Pharmacologic Category Interleukin-1 Inhibitor

Pregnancy Risk Factor C

Lactation Excretion in breast milk unknown/use caution

Use Orphan drug: Treatment of cryopyrin-associated periodic syndromes (CAPS) including familial cold autoinflammatory syndrome (FCAS) and Muckle-Wells syndrome (MWS)

Mechanism of Action/Effect Rilonacept reduces inflammation by binding to IL-1β and preventing interaction with cell surface receptors in patients with Cryopyrin-associated periodic syndromes (CAPS).

Contraindications There are no contraindications listed in the manufacturer's labeling.

Warnings/Precautions May cause rare hypersensitivity, anaphylaxis, or anaphylactoid reactions; medications for the treatment of hypersensitivity reactions should be available for immediate use. Caution should be exercised when considering use in patients with a history of new/recurrent infections, with conditions that predispose them to infections, or with latent or localized infections. Therapy should not be initiated in patients with active or chronic infections. Use may impair defenses against malignancies; impact on the development and course of malignancies is not fully defined. Use may increase total cholesterol, HDL, LDL, and triglycerides; periodic assessment of lipid profile should occur. Tumor necrosis factor (TNF)-blocking agents should not be used in combination with rilonacept; risk of serious infection is increased. Immunizations should be up to date including pneumococcal and influenza vaccines before initiating therapy. Live vaccines should not be given concurrently. Administration of inactivated (killed) vaccines while on therapy may not be effective. Use with caution in the elderly due to the potential higher risk for infections. Safety and efficacy has not been established in patients <12 years of age.

Drug Interactions

Avoid Concomitant Use

Avoid concomitant use of Rilonacept with any of the following: Anti-TNF Agents; BCG; Canakinumab; Natalizumab; Pimecrolimus; Roflumilast; Tacrolimus (Topical); Vaccines (Live)

Decreased Effect

Rilonacept may decrease the levels/effects of: BCG; Sipuleucel-T; Vaccines (Inactivated); Vaccines (Live)

The levels/effects of Rilonacept may be decreased by: Echinacea

Increased Effect/Toxicity

Rilonacept may increase the levels/effects of: Canakinumab; Leflunomide; Natalizumab; Vaccines (Live)

The levels/effects of Rilonacept may be increased by: Anti-TNF Agents; Denosumab; Pimecrolimus; Roflumilast; Tacrolimus (Topical); Trastuzumab

Adverse Reactions

>10%:

Local: Injection site reactions (48%; majority mild-moderate; typically lasting 1-2 days; characterized by erythema, bruising, dermatitis, inflammation, pain, pruritus, swelling, urticaria, vesicles, warmth, and hemorrhage)

Respiratory: Upper respiratory tract infection (26%)

Miscellaneous: Infection (48% during winter months; 18% during summer months), antibody formation to rilonacept (35%)

1% to 10%:

Central nervous system: Hypoesthesia (9%)

Respiratory: Cough (9%), sinusitis (9%)

Pharmacodynamics/Kinetics

Onset of Action Steady state reached by 6 weeks

Available Dosage Forms

Injection, powder for reconstitution:

Arcalyst™: 220 mg

Dosing

Adult & Geriatric Cryopyrin-associated periodic syndromes: SubQ: Loading dose 320 mg given as 2 separate injections (160 mg each) on the same day at 2 different sites, followed a week later by 160 mg, then once weekly. **Note:** Do not administer more frequently than once weekly.

Pediatric Cryopyrin-associated periodic syndromes: Children ≥12 years: SubQ: Loading dose 4.4 mg/kg (maximum dose: 320 mg) given as 1-2 separate injections (maximum: 2 mL/injection) on the same day, followed by 2.2 mg/kg (maximum dose: 160 mg) once weekly. **Note:** Do not administer more frequently than once weekly.

Administration

Other SubQ: Rotate injection sites (thigh, abdomen, upper arm); injections should never be made at sites that are bruised, red, tender, or hard

Stability

Reconstitution Reconstitute rilonacept 220 mg powder for injection with SWFI 2.3 mL; do not use bacteriostatic water containing benzyl alcohol or parabens. After reconstituting with SWFI, gently shake the vial for 1 minute, then allow solution to sit for 1 minute. Each reconstituted vial allows for withdrawal of 2 mL (160 mg) for SubQ administration.

Storage Store powder in refrigerator at 2°C to 8°C (36°F to 46°F); do not freeze. Do not shake. Protect from light. After reconstitution, may be stored at controlled room temperature. Protect from light. Use within 3 hours of reconstitution.

Monitoring and Teaching Issues

Laboratory Monitoring CBC with differential, lipid profile, C-reactive protein (CRP), serum amyloid A

Physical Assessment Evaluate for signs and symptoms of infection. This drug should not be used when active or chronic infections are present. Immunization should be given prior to initiating therapy. Teach patient appropriate injection techniques and syringe/needle disposal.

Patient Education You may experience redness, pain, itching, or swelling at the site of injection. This typically lasts 1-2 days. Do not receive any immunizations unless approved by prescriber. You may be susceptible to infections. Report signs of infection immediately.

Breast-Feeding Considerations It is unknown whether or not rilonacept is excreted in human breast milk. Use with caution in breast-feeding.

Pregnancy Considerations Animal studies have demonstrated teratogenic effects and fetal loss. There are no adequate and well-controlled studies in pregnant women. Use during pregnancy only if potential benefit to the mother outweighs potential risk to the fetus.

◆ **Rilutek®** *see* Riluzole *on page 1582*

Riluzole (RIL yoo zole)

U.S. Brand Names Rilutek®

Index Terms 2-Amino-6-Trifluoromethoxy-benzothiazole; RP-54274

Generic Availability (U.S.) No

Pharmacologic Category Glutamate Inhibitor

Pregnancy Risk Factor C

Lactation Excretion in breast milk unknown/not recommended

Use Treatment of amyotrophic lateral sclerosis (ALS); riluzole can extend survival or time to tracheostomy

Mechanism of Action/Effect Mechanism of action is not known. Pharmacologic properties include inhibitory effect on glutamate release, inactivation of voltage-dependent sodium channels; and ability to interfere with intracellular events that follow transmitter binding at excitatory amino acid receptors

Contraindications Severe hypersensitivity reactions to riluzole or any component of the formulation

Warnings/Precautions Among 4000 patients given riluzole for ALS, there were 3 cases of marked neutropenia (ANC <500/mm^3), all seen within the first 2 months of treatment. Interstitial lung disease (primarily hypersensitivity pneumonitis) has occurred, requires prompt evaluation and possible discontinuation. Use with caution in patients with concomitant renal insufficiency. Use with caution in patients with current evidence or history of abnormal liver function; do not administer if baseline liver function tests are elevated. May cause elevations in transaminases (usually transient). May cause elevations in transaminases (usually transient) within first 3 months of therapy; discontinue if ALT levels are ≥5 times upper limit of normal or if jaundice develops. The elderly or female patients may have decreased clearance of riluzole; use with caution. May cause dizziness or somnolence; caution should be used performing tasks which require alertness (operating machinery or driving).

Drug Interactions

Metabolism/Transport Effects Substrate of CYP1A2 (major)

Avoid Concomitant Use There are no known interactions where it is recommended to avoid concomitant use.

Decreased Effect

The levels/effects of Riluzole may be decreased by: CYP1A2 Inducers (Strong)

Increased Effect/Toxicity There are no known significant interactions involving an increase in effect.

Nutritional/Ethanol Interactions

Ethanol: Avoid ethanol (due to CNS depression and possible risk of liver toxicity).

Food: A high-fat meal decreases absorption of riluzole (decreasing AUC by 20% and peak blood levels by 45%). Charbroiled food may increase riluzole elimination.

Adverse Reactions

>10%:

Gastrointestinal: Nausea (16%)

Neuromuscular & skeletal: Weakness (19%)

1% to 10%:

Cardiovascular: Hypertension (5%), peripheral edema (3%), tachycardia (3%)

Central nervous system: Dizziness (4%), somnolence (2%), vertigo (2%), malaise (1%)

Dermatologic: Pruritus (4%), eczema (2%), exfoliative dermatitis (1%)

Gastrointestinal: Abdominal pain (5%), vomiting (4%), flatulence (3%), oral moniliasis (1%), stomatitis (1%), tooth disorder (1%)

Genitourinary: Urinary tract infection (3%), dysuria (1%)

Hepatic: Liver function tests increased (8% >3 x ULN; 2% >5 x ULN)

Neuromuscular & skeletal: Arthralgia (4%), paresthesia (circumoral; 2%), tremor (1%)

Respiratory: Lung function decreased (10%), cough increased (3%)

Pharmacodynamics/Kinetics

Absorption ~90%; high-fat meal decreases AUC by 20% and peak blood levels by 45%

Bioavailability Oral: Absolute: ~60%

Protein Binding Plasma: 96%, primarily to albumin and lipoproteins

Half-Life Elimination 12 hours

Metabolism Extensively hepatic to six major and a number of minor metabolites via CYP1A2 dependent hydroxylation and glucuronidation

Excretion Urine (90%; 85% as metabolites, 2% as unchanged drug) and feces (5%) within 7 days

Available Dosage Forms

Tablet, oral:

Rilutek®: 50 mg

Dosing

Adult & Geriatric

ALS treatment: Oral: 50 mg every 12 hours; no increased benefit can be expected from higher daily doses, but adverse events are increased.

Dosage adjustment in smoking: Cigarette smoking is known to induce CYP1A2; patients who smoke cigarettes would be expected to eliminate riluzole faster. There is no information, however, on the effect of, or need for, dosage adjustment in these patients.

Renal Impairment No specific dosage adjustments recommended by manufacturer; use caution.

Hepatic Impairment No specific dosage adjustments recommended by manufacturer; use caution.

Administration

Oral Administer at the same time each day, at least 1 hour before or 2 hours after a meal.

Stability

Storage Store at 20°C to 25°C (68°F to 77°F). Protect from bright light.

Monitoring and Teaching Issues

Laboratory Monitoring Monitor serum aminotransferases (including ALT levels) before and during therapy. Evaluate serum ALT levels every month during the first 3 months of therapy, every 3 months during the remainder of the first year, and periodically thereafter. Evaluate ALT levels more frequently in patients who develop elevations. Maximum increases in serum ALT usually occurred within 3 months after the start of therapy and were usually transient when <5 times ULN. Discontinue therapy if ALT levels are ≥ 5 times upper limit of normal or if jaundice develops.

In trials, if ALT levels were <5 times ULN, treatment continued and ALT levels usually returned to below 2 times ULN within 2-6 months. Treatment in studies was discontinued, however, if ALT levels exceed 5 times ULN, so that there is no experience with continued treatment of ALS patients once ALT values exceed 5 times ULN.

Physical Assessment Monitor for decreased liver function at beginning of therapy and periodically throughout.

Patient Education This drug will not cure or stop disease, but it may slow progression. Take at the same time each day, preferably on an empty stomach, 1 hour before or 2 hours after meals. Avoid alcohol. You may experience increased spasticity, dizziness, sleepiness, nausea, vomiting, or anorexia. Report fever; severe vomiting, diarrhea, or constipation; change in color of urine or stool; yellowing of skin or eyes; acute back pain or muscle pain; or worsening of condition.

Dietary Considerations Take at least 1 hour before or 2 hours after a meal.

Geriatric Considerations In clinical trials, no difference was demonstrated between elderly and younger adults. However, renal and hepatic changes with age can be expected to result in higher serum concentrations of the parent drug and its metabolites.

Pregnancy Considerations Impaired fertility, decreased implantation, increased intrauterine death, and adverse effects on offspring growth and viability were observed in animal studies. There are no adequate or well-controlled studies in pregnant women.

Rimantadine (ri MAN ta deen)

U.S. Brand Names Flumadine®

Index Terms Rimantadine Hydrochloride

Generic Availability (U.S.) Yes

Pharmacologic Category Antiviral Agent; Antiviral Agent, Adamantane

Medication Safety Issues

Sound-alike/look-alike issues:

Rimantadine may be confused with amantadine, ranitidine, Rimactane®

Flumadine® may be confused with fludarabine, flunisolide, flutamide

Pregnancy Risk Factor C

Lactation Excretion in breast milk unknown/ not recommended

Use Prophylaxis (adults and children >1 year of age) and treatment (adults) of influenza A viral infection (per manufacturer labeling; also refer to current ACIP guidelines for recommendations during current flu season)

Note: In certain circumstances, the ACIP recommends use of rimantadine in combination with oseltamivir for the treatment or prophylaxis of influenza A infection when resistance to oseltamivir is suspected.

Mechanism of Action/Effect Exerts its inhibitory effect on three antigenic subtypes of influenza A virus (H1N1, H2N2, H3N2) early in the viral replicative cycle, possibly inhibiting the uncoating process; it has no activity against influenza B virus and is two- to eightfold more active than amantadine

Contraindications Hypersensitivity to drugs of the adamantine class, including rimantadine and amantadine, or any component of the formulation

Warnings/Precautions Use with caution in patients with renal and hepatic dysfunction; avoid use, if possible, in patients with uncontrolled psychosis or severe psychoneurosis. An increase in seizure incidence may occur in patients with seizure disorders; discontinue drug if seizures occur; resistance may develop during treatment; viruses exhibit cross-resistance between amantadine and rimantadine. Due to increased resistance, the ACIP has recommended that rimantadine and amantadine no longer be used for the treatment or prophylaxis of influenza A in the United States until susceptibility has been re-established; consult current guidelines. Rimantadine is not effective in the prevention or treatment of influenza B virus infections. The elderly are at higher risk for CNS (eg, dizziness, headache, weakness) and gastrointestinal (eg, nausea/vomiting, abdominal pain) adverse events; dosage adjustment is recommended in elderly patients >65 years of age.

Drug Interactions

Avoid Concomitant Use There are no known interactions where it is recommended to avoid concomitant use.

Decreased Effect

Rimantadine may decrease the levels/effects of: Influenza Virus Vaccine (Live/Attenuated)

Increased Effect/Toxicity

The levels/effects of Rimantadine may be increased by: MAO Inhibitors

Nutritional/Ethanol Interactions Food: Food does not affect rate or extent of absorption

Adverse Reactions 1% to 10%:

Central nervous system: Insomnia (2% to 3%), concentration impaired (≤2%), dizziness (1% to 2%), nervousness (1% to 2%), fatigue (1%), headache (1%)

Gastrointestinal: Nausea (3%), anorexia (2%), vomiting (2%), xerostomia (2%), abdominal pain (1%)

Neuromuscular & skeletal: Weakness (1%)

Pharmacodynamics/Kinetics

Onset of Action Antiviral activity: No data exist establishing a correlation between plasma concentration and antiviral effect

Time to Peak 6 hours

Protein Binding ~40%, primarily to albumin

Half-Life Elimination 25.4 hours; prolonged with elderly, severe liver and severe renal impairment

Metabolism Extensively hepatic

Excretion Urine (<25% as unchanged drug)

Clearance: Hemodialysis does not contribute to clearance

Available Dosage Forms

Tablet, oral: 100 mg

Flumadine®: 100 mg

Dosing

Adult

Prophylaxis of influenza A: Oral: 100 mg twice daily

Note: Prophylaxis (institutional outbreak): In order to control outbreaks in institutions, if influenza A virus subtyping is unavailable and oseltamivir resistant viruses are circulating, rimantadine may be used in combination with oseltamivir if zanamivir cannot be used. Treatment should continue for ≥2 weeks and until ~10 days after illness onset in the last patient (CDC, 2011; Harper 2009).

Treatment of influenza A: Oral: 100 mg twice daily

Geriatric Prophylaxis or treatment of influenza A: Oral: 100 mg daily in the elderly (≥65 years), including elderly nursing home patients.

Pediatric

Prophylaxis of influenza A: Oral:

Children:

1-9 years: 5 mg/kg/day in 1-2 divided doses; maximum: 150 mg/day

≥10 years and <40 kg: 5 mg/kg/day in 2 divided doses (CDC, 2011)

≥10 years and ≥40 kg: Refer to adult dosing.

Prophylaxis (institutional outbreak): Refer to adult dosing.

Treatment of influenza A: Oral: Children ≥17 years: Refer to adult dosing.

Renal Impairment

Cl_{cr} ≥30 mL/minute: Dose adjustment not required.

Cl_{cr} <30 mL/minute: 100 mg daily

Hepatic Impairment Severe dysfunction: 100 mg daily

Administration

Oral Initiation of rimantadine within 48 hours of the onset of influenza A illness halves the duration of illness and significantly reduces the duration of viral shedding and increased peripheral airways resistance. Continue therapy for 5-7 days after symptoms begin; discontinue as soon as clinically warranted to reduce the emergence of antiviral drug resistant viruses

Stability

Storage Store at 25°C (77°F); excursions permitted to 15°C to 30°C (59°F to 86°F).

Monitoring and Teaching Issues

Physical Assessment Recommendations for antiviral susceptibility and effectiveness may change. Validate with the CDC recommendations for use prior to prescribing. Use caution with hepatic or renal impairment, seizure disorders, uncontrolled psychoses, or severe psychoneurosis. Monitor for hypotension, CNS changes (confusion, anxiety, agitation), gastrointestinal upset, and anticholinergic effects (dry mouth, urinary retention, mydriases).

Patient Education May cause dizziness, insomnia, fatigue, nervousness, or gastrointestinal upset. Report rash, palpitations, severe nausea or vomiting, or persistent CNS changes (eg, confusion, insomnia, anxiety, restlessness, irritability, hallucinations).

Geriatric Considerations Refer to current CDC guidelines for appropriate use. Adverse CNS and GI effects occur frequently if dosage is not adjusted. Monitor GI effects in the elderly or patients with renal or hepatic impairment. Dosing must be individualized (100 mg 1-2 times/day). It is recommended that nursing home patients receive 100 mg/day.

Breast-Feeding Considerations Do not use in nursing mothers due to potential adverse effect in infants. The CDC recommends that women infected with the influenza virus follow general precautions (eg, frequent hand washing) to decrease viral transmission to the child. Mothers with influenza-like illnesses at delivery should consider avoiding close contact with the infant until they have received 48 hours of antiviral medication, fever has resolved, and cough and secretions can be controlled. These measures may help decrease (but not eliminate) the risk of transmitting influenza to the newborn during breast-feeding. During this time, breast milk can be expressed and bottle-fed to the infant by another person who is not infected. Protective measures, such as wearing a face mask, changing into a clean gown or clothing, and strict hand hygiene should be continued by the mother for ≥7 days after the onset of symptoms or until symptom-free for 24 hours. Infant care should be performed by a noninfected person when possible (consult current CDC guidelines).

Pregnancy Considerations Animal data suggest embryotoxicity, maternal toxicity, and offspring mortality at doses 7-11 times the recommended human dose. There are no adequate and well-controlled studies in pregnant women.

Influenza infection may be more severe in pregnant women. Untreated influenza infection is associated with an increased risk of adverse events to the fetus and an increased risk of complications or death to the mother. Oseltamivir and zanamivir are currently recommended for the treatment or prophylaxis influenza in pregnant women and women up to 2 weeks postpartum. Appropriate antiviral agents are currently recommended as an adjunct to vaccination and should not be used as a substitute for vaccination in pregnant women (consult current CDC guidelines).

Healthcare providers are encouraged to refer women exposed to influenza vaccine, or who have taken an antiviral medication during pregnancy to the Vaccines and Medications in Pregnancy Surveillance System (VAMPSS) by contacting The Organization of Teratology Information Specialists (OTIS) at (877) 311-8972.

◆ **Rimantadine Hydrochloride** *see* Rimantadine *on page 1583*

◆ **Riomet®** *see* MetFORMIN *on page 1182*

Risedronate (ris ED roe nate)

U.S. Brand Names Actonel®; Atelvia™

Index Terms Risedronate Sodium

Generic Availability (U.S.) No

Pharmacologic Category Bisphosphonate Derivative

Medication Safety Issues

Sound-alike/look-alike issues:

Actonel® may be confused with Actos®

Risedronate may be confused with alendronate

Medication Guide Available Yes

Pregnancy Risk Factor C

Lactation Excretion in breast milk unknown/not recommended

Use

Actonel®: Treatment of Paget's disease of the bone; treatment and prevention of glucocorticoid-induced osteoporosis; treatment and prevention of osteoporosis in postmenopausal women; treatment of osteoporosis in men

Atelvia™: Treatment of osteoporosis in postmenopausal women

Mechanism of Action/Effect A bisphosphonate which inhibits bone resorption via actions on osteoclasts or on osteoclast precursors; decreases the rate of bone resorption, leading to an indirect increase in bone mineral density. In Paget's disease, characterized by disordered resorption and formation of bone, inhibition of resorption leads to an indirect decrease in bone formation; but the newly-formed bone has a more normal architecture.

Contraindications Hypersensitivity to risedronate, bisphosphonates, or any component of the formulation; hypocalcemia; inability to stand or sit upright for at least 30 minutes; abnormalities of the esophagus which delay esophageal emptying, such as stricture or achalasia

Warnings/Precautions Bisphosphonates may cause upper gastrointestinal disorders such as dysphagia, esophagitis, esophageal ulcer, and gastric ulcer; risk increases in patients unable to comply with dosing instructions. Use with caution in patients with dysphagia, esophageal disease, gastritis, duodenitis, or ulcers (may worsen underlying condition). Discontinue if new or worsening symptoms occur. Use caution in patients with renal impairment (not recommended in patients with a Cl_{cr} <30 mL/minute). Hypocalcemia must be corrected before therapy initiation with risedronate. Ensure adequate calcium and vitamin D intake, especially for patients with Paget's disease in whom the pretreatment rate of bone turnover may be greatly elevated.

Bisphosphonate therapy has been associated with osteonecrosis, primarily of the jaw. Risk factors for osteonecrosis of the jaw (ONJ) include invasive dental procedures (eg, tooth extraction, dental implants, boney surgery); a diagnosis of cancer, with concomitant chemotherapy or corticosteroids; poor oral hygiene, ill-fitting dentures; and comorbid disorders (anemia, coagulopathy, infection, pre-existing dental disease). Most reported cases occurred after I.V. bisphosphonate therapy; however, cases have been reported following oral therapy. A dental exam and preventative dentistry should be performed prior to placing patients with risk factors on chronic bisphosphonate therapy. The manufacturer's labeling states that discontinuing bisphosphonates in patients requiring invasive dental procedures may reduce the risk of ONJ. However, other experts suggest that there is no evidence that discontinuing therapy reduces the risk of developing ONJ (Assael, 2009). The benefit/risk must be assessed by the treating physician and/or dentist/surgeon prior to any invasive dental procedure. Patients developing ONJ while on bisphosphonates should receive care by an oral surgeon.

Atypical femur fractures have been reported in patients receiving bisphosphonates for treatment/prevention of osteoporosis. The fractures include subtrochanteric femur (bone just below the hip joint) and diaphyseal femur (long segment of the thigh bone). Some patients experience prodromal pain weeks or months before the fracture occurs. It is unclear if bisphosphonate therapy is the cause for these fractures, although the majority have been reported in patients taking bisphosphonates. Patients receiving long-term (>3-5 years) therapy may be at an increased risk. Discontinue bisphosphonate therapy in patients who develop a femoral shaft fracture.

Infrequently, severe (and occasionally debilitating) bone, joint, and/or muscle pain have been reported during bisphosphonate treatment. The onset of pain ranged from a single day to several months. Consider discontinuing therapy in patients who experience severe symptoms; symptoms usually resolve upon discontinuation. Some patients experienced recurrence when rechallenged with same drug or another bisphosphonate; avoid use in patients with a history of these symptoms in association with bisphosphonate therapy.

When using for glucocorticoid-induced osteoporosis, evaluate sex steroid hormonal status prior to treatment initiation; consider appropriate hormone replacement if necessary. Not approved for use in pediatric patients with osteogenesis imperfecta due to lack of efficacy in reducing the risk of fracture.

Drug Interactions

Avoid Concomitant Use There are no known interactions where it is recommended to avoid concomitant use.

Decreased Effect

The levels/effects of Risedronate may be decreased by: Antacids; Calcium Salts; Iron Salts; Magnesium Salts; Proton Pump Inhibitors

Increased Effect/Toxicity

Risedronate may increase the levels/effects of: Phosphate Supplements

The levels/effects of Risedronate may be increased by: Aminoglycosides; Nonsteroidal Anti-Inflammatory Agents

Nutritional/Ethanol Interactions

Ethanol: Avoid ethanol (may increase risk of osteoporosis).

Food: Food reduces absorption (similar to other bisphosphonates); mean oral bioavailability is decreased when given with food.

Lab Interactions Bisphosphonates may interfere with diagnostic imaging agents such as technetium-99m-diphosphonate in bone scans.

Adverse Reactions Frequency may vary with product, dose, and indication.

>10%:

Cardiovascular: Hypertension (11%)
Central nervous system: Headache (3% to 18%)
Dermatologic: Rash (8% to 12%)
Endocrine & metabolic: Serum PTH levels increased (transient; <30%)
Gastrointestinal: Diarrhea (5% to 20%), nausea (4% to 13%), constipation (3% to 13%), abdominal pain (2% to 12%), dyspepsia (4% to 11%)
Genitourinary: Urinary tract infection (11%)
Neuromuscular & skeletal: Arthralgia (7% to 33%), back pain (6% to 28%)
Miscellaneous: Infection (≤31%)

1% to 10%:

Cardiovascular: Peripheral edema (8%), chest pain (5% to 7%), arrhythmia (2%)

Central nervous system: Depression (7%), dizziness (3% to 7%)

Endocrine & metabolic: Hypocalcemia (≤5%), hypophosphatemia (<3%)

Gastrointestinal: Vomiting (2% to 5%), gastritis (3%), duodenitis (≤1%), glossitis (≤1%)

Genitourinary: Prostatic hyperplasia (5%; benign), nephrolithiasis (3%)

Neuromuscular & skeletal: Joint disorder (7%), myalgia (2% to 7%), neck pain (5%), muscle spasm (1% to 2%)

Ocular: Cataract (7%)

Respiratory: Bronchitis (3% to 10%), pharyngitis (6%), rhinitis (6%), dyspnea (4%)

Miscellaneous: Flu-like syndrome (10%), acute phase reaction (≤8%; includes fever, influenza-like illness)

Pharmacodynamics/Kinetics

Onset of Action May require weeks

Absorption Rapid

Bioavailability Poor, ~0.54% to 0.75%

Time to Peak Serum: 1-3 hours

Protein Binding ~24%

Half-Life Elimination Initial: 1.5 hours; Terminal: 480-561 hours

Metabolism None

Excretion Urine (up to 85%); feces (as unabsorbed drug)

Available Dosage Forms

Tablet, oral:

Actonel®: 5 mg, 30 mg, 35 mg, 150 mg

Tablet, delayed release, oral:

Atelvia™: 35 mg

Dosing

Adult & Geriatric Note: Patients should receive supplemental calcium and vitamin D if dietary intake is inadequate.

Paget's disease of bone: Oral: *Immediate release tablet:* 30 mg once daily for 2 months

Note: Retreatment may be considered (following post-treatment observation of at least 2 months) if relapse occurs, or if treatment fails to normalize serum alkaline phosphatase. For retreatment, the dose and duration of therapy are the same as for initial treatment. No data are available on more than one course of retreatment.

Osteoporosis (postmenopausal): Oral:

Immediate release tablet: Prevention and treatment: 5 mg once daily **or** 35 mg once weekly **or** 150 mg once a month

Delayed release tablet: Treatment: 35 mg once weekly

Osteoporosis (male) treatment: Oral: *Immediate release tablet:* 35 mg once weekly

Osteoporosis (glucocorticoid-induced) prevention and treatment: Oral: *Immediate release tablet:* 5 mg once daily

Renal Impairment

Cl_{cr} ≥30 mL/minute: No adjustment required

Cl_{cr} <30 mL/minute: Use is not recommended

Hepatic Impairment No studies performed in hepatic impairment; no dosage adjustment necessary due to lack of hepatic metabolism.

Administration

Oral Note: Avoid administration of oral calcium supplements, antacids, magnesium supplements/laxatives, and iron preparations within 30 minutes of risedronate administration.

Immediate release tablet: Risedronate immediate release tablets must be taken on an empty stomach with a full glass (6-8 oz) of **plain water** (not mineral water) at least 30 minutes before any food, drink, or other medications orally to avoid interference with absorption. Patient must remain sitting upright or standing for at least 30 minutes after taking (to reduce esophageal irritation). Tablet should be swallowed whole; do not crush or chew.

Delayed release tablet: Risedronate delayed release tablets must be taken with at least 4 oz of **plain water** (not mineral water) immediately **after** breakfast. Patient must remain sitting upright or standing for at least 30 minutes after taking (to reduce esophageal irritation). Tablet should be swallowed whole; do not cut, split, crush, or chew.

Stability

Storage Store at room temperature of 20°C to 25°C (68°F to 77°F).

Monitoring and Teaching Issues

Laboratory Monitoring

Osteoporosis: Serum calcium and 25(OH)D; consider measuring biochemical markers of bone turnover

Paget's disease: Alkaline phosphatase, serum calcium and 25(OH)D

Physical Assessment Assess history for any previous adverse response to bisphosphonates and ability to comply with administration instructions. Use caution with renal impairment. Correct any hypocalcemia prior to beginning treatment. Patients at risk for osteonecrosis of the jaw (eg, chemotherapy, corticosteroids, poor oral hygiene) should have dental exams; necessary preventive dentistry should be done before beginning bisphosphonate therapy. Monitor for immediate or long-term musculoskeletal pain. Teach patient specific administration directions. Instruct patient in lifestyle and dietary changes.

Patient Education Stay in upright sitting or standing position for 30 minutes following administration to reduce potential for esophageal irritation. Take immediate release tablets with a full glass (6-8 oz) of water on an empty stomach at least 30 minutes before eating or taking anything else. Take delayed release tablets with at least 4 ounces of water immediately after breakfast. Do not cut, crush, or chew tablets. Certain dental procedures should be avoided if possible while you are taking this medication. You may experience temporary nausea or vomiting, diarrhea, or bone pain. Report persistent muscle or bone pain; leg cramps; muscle twitching; unusual fever; seizures; difficulty breathing; rash; bloody stool; or pain in mouth, jaws, or teeth.

Dietary Considerations Ensure adequate calcium and vitamin D intake. Take immediate release tablet with at least 6 oz of **plain water** (not mineral water) ≥30 minutes before the first food or drink of the day other than water. Take delayed release tablet with at least 4 ounces of **plain water** immediately **after** breakfast.

Geriatric Considerations No dosage adjustment required if Cl_{cr} ≥30 mL/minute. Since elderly often receive diuretics, evaluate electrolyte status periodically due to the drug class (bisphosphonates). Ensure that immobilized patients remain sitting upright for at least 30 minutes after swallowing tablet. The elderly are frequently treated long-term for osteoporosis and patients should be advised to report any lower extremity pain that cannot be explained or lasts for more than a week.

Breast-Feeding Considerations The manufacturer recommends discontinuing nursing or discontinuing risedronate.

Pregnancy Considerations Teratogenic and nonteratogenic embryo/fetal effects have been reported in animal studies. There are no adequate and well-controlled studies in pregnant women. Bisphosphonates are incorporated into the bone matrix and gradually released over time. Theoretically, there may be a risk of fetal harm when pregnancy follows the completion of therapy. Based on limited case reports with pamidronate, serum calcium levels in the newborn may be altered if administered during pregnancy.

Related Information

Osteoporosis Management *on page* 2067

◆ **Risedronate Sodium** *see* Risedronate *on page* 1585

◆ **RisperDAL®** *see* Risperidone *on page* 1588

◆ **Risperdal M-Tab** *see* Risperidone *on page* 1588

◆ **RisperDAL® M-Tab®** *see* Risperidone *on page* 1588

◆ **RisperDAL® Consta®** *see* Risperidone *on page* 1588

Risperidone (ris PER i done)

U.S. Brand Names RisperDAL®; RisperDAL® Consta®; RisperDAL® M-Tab®

Index Terms Risperdal M-Tab

Generic Availability (U.S.) Yes: Excludes injection

Pharmacologic Category Antimanic Agent; Antipsychotic Agent, Atypical

Medication Safety Issues

Sound-alike/look-alike issues:

RisperiDONE may be confused with reserpine, rOPINIRole

RisperDAL® may be confused with lisinopril, reserpine, Restoril™

Pregnancy Risk Factor C

Lactation Enters breast milk/not recommended

Use

Oral: Treatment of schizophrenia; treatment of acute mania or mixed episodes associated with bipolar I disorder (as monotherapy in children or adults, or in combination with lithium or valproate in adults); treatment of irritability/aggression associated with autistic disorder

Injection: Treatment of schizophrenia; maintenance treatment of bipolar I disorder in adults as monotherapy or in combination with lithium or valproate

Unlabeled/Investigational Use Treatment of Tourette's syndrome; treatment of pervasive developmental disorder; psychosis/agitation related to Alzheimer's dementia; post-traumatic stress disorder (PTSD)

Mechanism of Action/Effect Risperidone is a benzisoxazole atypical antipsychotic with affinity for dopamine and serotonin. Results in improvement of psychotic symptoms and reduction of extrapyramidal side effects.

Contraindications Hypersensitivity to risperidone or any component of the formulation

Warnings/Precautions Hazardous agent - use appropriate precautions for handling and disposal. **[U.S. Boxed Warning]: Elderly patients with dementia-related psychosis treated with antipsychotics are at an increased risk of death compared to placebo.** Most deaths appeared to be either cardiovascular (eg, heart failure, sudden death) or infectious (eg, pneumonia) in nature. In addition, an increased incidence of cerebrovascular effects (eg, transient ischemic attack, cerebrovascular accidents) has been reported in studies of placebo-controlled trials of risperidone in elderly patients with dementia-related psychosis. Risperidone is not approved for the treatment of dementia-related psychosis.

Leukopenia, neutropenia, and agranulocytosis (sometimes fatal) have been reported in clinical trials and postmarketing reports with antipsychotic use; presence of risk factors (eg, pre-existing low WBC or history of drug-induced leuko-/neutropenia) should prompt periodic blood count assessment. Discontinue therapy at first signs of blood dyscrasias or if absolute neutrophil count <1000/mm^3.

Low to moderately sedating, use with caution in disorders where CNS depression is a feature. Use with caution in Parkinson's disease. Caution in patients with predisposition to seizures. Use with caution in renal or hepatic dysfunction; dose reduction recommended. Esophageal dysmotility and aspiration have been associated with antipsychotic use; use with caution in patients at risk of aspiration pneumonia (ie, Alzheimer's disease). Use is associated with increased prolactin levels; clinical significance of hyperprolactinemia in patients with breast cancer or other prolactin-dependent tumors is unknown. May alter temperature regulation. May mask toxicity of other drugs or conditions (eg intestinal obstruction, Reyes syndrome, brain tumor) due to antiemetic effects. Neutropenia has been reported with antipsychotic use, including fatal cases of agranulocytosis. Pre-existing myelosuppression (disease or drug-induced) increases risk and these patients should have frequent CBC monitoring; decreased blood counts in absence of other causative factors should prompt discontinuation of therapy.

Use with caution in patients with cardiovascular diseases (eg, heart failure, history of myocardial infarction or ischemia, cerebrovascular disease, conduction abnormalities). May cause orthostatic hypotension; use with caution in patients at risk of this effect (eg, concurrent medication use which may predispose to hypotension/bradycardia or presence of hypovolemia) or in those who would not tolerate transient hypotensive episodes. May alter cardiac conduction (low risk relative to other neuroleptics); life-threatening arrhythmias have occurred with therapeutic doses of neuroleptics.

May cause anticholinergic effects (confusion, agitation, constipation, xerostomia, blurred vision, urinary retention); therefore, they should be used with caution in patients with decreased gastrointestinal motility, urinary retention, BPH, xerostomia, or visual problems (including narrow-angle glaucoma). Relative to other neuroleptics, risperidone has a low potency of cholinergic blockade.

May cause extrapyramidal symptoms (EPS), including pseudoparkinsonism, acute dystonic reactions, akathisia, and tardive dyskinesia (risk of these reactions is low relative to other neuroleptics, and is dose dependent). Risk of dystonia (and probably other EPS) may be greater with increased doses, use of conventional antipsychotics, males, and younger patients. Risk of neuroleptic malignant syndrome (NMS) may be increased in patients with Parkinson's disease or Lewy body dementia; monitor for symptoms of confusion, obtundation, postural instability and extrapyramidal symptoms. May cause hyperglycemia; in some cases may be extreme and associated with ketoacidosis, hyperosmolar coma, or death. Use with caution in patients with diabetes or other disorders of glucose regulation; monitor for worsening of glucose control. Significant weight gain has been observed with antipsychotic therapy; incidence varies with product. Monitor waist circumference and BMI. Rare cases of priapism have been reported.

The possibility of a suicide attempt is inherent in psychotic illness or bipolar disorder; use caution in high-risk patients during initiation of therapy. Prescriptions should be written for the smallest quantity consistent with good patient care. Long-term effects on growth or sexual maturation have not been evaluated. Vehicle used in injectable (polylactide-co-glycolide microspheres) has rarely been associated with retinal artery occlusion in patients with abnormal arteriovenous anastomosis.

Drug Interactions

Metabolism/Transport Effects Substrate of CYP2D6 (major), 3A4 (minor); **Inhibits** CYP2D6 (weak), 3A4 (weak)

Avoid Concomitant Use

Avoid concomitant use of RisperiDONE with any of the following: Artemether; Dronedarone; Lumefantrine; Metoclopramide; Nilotinib; Pimozide; QuiNINE; Tetrabenazine; Thioridazine; Toremifene; Vandetanib; Ziprasidone

Decreased Effect

RisperiDONE may decrease the levels/effects of: Amphetamines; Anti-Parkinson's Agents (Dopamine Agonist); Quinagolide

The levels/effects of RisperiDONE may be decreased by: CarBAMazepine; Lithium formulations; Peginterferon Alfa-2b

Increased Effect/Toxicity

RisperiDONE may increase the levels/effects of: Alcohol (Ethyl); Anticholinergics; CNS Depressants; Dronedarone; Methylphenidate; Paliperidone; Pimozide; QTc-Prolonging Agents; QuiNINE; Tetrabenazine; Thioridazine; Toremifene; Vandetanib; Ziprasidone

The levels/effects of RisperiDONE may be increased by: Acetylcholinesterase Inhibitors (Central); Alfuzosin; Artemether; Chloroquine; Ciprofloxacin; Ciprofloxacin (Systemic); Conivaptan; CYP2D6 Inhibitors (Moderate); CYP2D6 Inhibitors (Strong); Darunavir; Divalproex; Gadobutrol; Lithium formulations; Lumefantrine; Methylphenidate; Metoclopramide; Nilotinib; Pramlintide; QuiNINE; Selective Serotonin Reuptake Inhibitors; Tetrabenazine; Valproic Acid; Verapamil

Nutritional/Ethanol Interactions

Ethanol: May increase CNS depression; monitor for increased effects with coadministration. Caution patients about effects.

Herb/Nutraceutical: Avoid kava kava, gotu kola, valerian, St John's wort (may increase CNS depression).

Adverse Reactions The frequency of adverse effects is reported as absolute percentages and is not based upon net frequencies as compared to placebo. Actual frequency may be dependant upon dose and/or indication. Events are reported from placebo-controlled studies and not with combination therapy. Unless otherwise noted, frequency of adverse effects is reported for the oral formulation in adults.

>10%:

Central nervous system: Somnolence (children 12% to 67%; adults 5% to 14%; I.M. injection 5% to 6%), fatigue (children 18% to 42%; adults 1% to 3%), headache (I.M. injection 15% to 21%), fever (children 20%; adults 1% to 2%), dystonia (children 9% to 18%; adults 5% to 11%), anxiety (children ≤16%; adults 2% to 16%), dizziness (children 7% to 16%; adults 4% to 10%), Parkinsonism (children 2% to 16%; adults 12% to 20%)

Dermatologic: Rash (children ≤11%; adults 2% to 4%)
Gastrointestinal: Appetite increased (children 4% to 49%), vomiting (children 10% to 25%), salivation increased (children ≤22%; adults 1% to 3%), constipation (children 21%; adults 8% to 9%), abdominal pain (children 15% to 18%; adults 3% to 4%), nausea (children 8% to 16%; adults 4% to 9%), dyspepsia (children 5% to 16%; adults 4% to 10%), xerostomia (children 13%; adults ≤4%)
Genitourinary: Urinary incontinence (children 5% to 22%; adults <2%)
Neuromuscular & skeletal: Tremor (adults 6%; children 10% to 12%)
Respiratory: Rhinitis (children 13% to 36%; adults 7% to 11%), upper respiratory infection (children 34%; adults 2% to 3%), cough (children 34%; adults 3%)

1% to 10%:
Cardiovascular: Tachycardia (children ≤7%; adults 1% to 5%), hypertension (I.M. injection 3%), chest pain (1% to 3%), creatine phosphokinase increased (≤2%), postural hypotension (≤2%), arrhythmia (≤1%), edema (≤1%), hypotension (≤1%), syncope (≤1%)
Central nervous system: Akathisia (children ≤10%; adults 5% to 9%), automatism (children 7%), confusion (children 5%)
Dermatologic: Seborrhea (up to 2%), acne (1%)
Endocrine & metabolic: Lactation nonpuerperal (children 2% to 5%; adults 1%), ejaculation failure (≤1%)
Gastrointestinal: Diarrhea (children 7% to 8%; adults ≤3%), anorexia (children 8%; adults ≤2%;), weight gain (children 5%; adults ≤1%), toothache (I.M. injection 1% to 3%)
Genitourinary: Urinary tract infection (≤3%)
Hematologic: Neutropenia (I.M. injection <2%), anemia (I.M. injection <2%; oral ≤1%)
Hepatic: Transaminases increased (I.M. injection ≥1%; oral 1%)
Neuromuscular & skeletal: Dyskinesia (children 7%; adults 1%), arthralgia (2% to 3%), back pain (2% to 3%), myalgia (≤2%), weakness (1%)
Ocular: Abnormal vision (children 4% to 7%; adults 1% to 3%), blurred vision (I.M. injection 2% to 3%)
Otic: Earache (1%)
Respiratory: Dyspnea (children 2% to 5%; adults 2%), epistaxis (≤2%)

Pharmacodynamics/Kinetics

Absorption

Oral: Rapid and well absorbed; food does not affect rate or extent
Injection: <1% absorbed initially; main release occurs at ~3 weeks and is maintained from 4-6 weeks

Bioavailability Oral: 70%; Tablet (relative to solution): 94%; orally-disintegrating tablets and oral solution are bioequivalent to tablets

Time to Peak Plasma: Oral: Risperidone: Within 1 hour; 9-hydroxyrisperidone: Extensive metabolizers: 3 hours; Poor metabolizers: 17 hours

Protein Binding Plasma: Risperidone 90%; 9-hydroxyrisperidone: 77%

Half-Life Elimination Active moiety (risperidone and its active metabolite 9-hydroxyrisperidone)
Oral: 20 hours (mean)
Extensive metabolizers: Risperidone: 3 hours; 9-hydroxyrisperidone: 21 hours
Poor metabolizers: Risperidone: 20 hours; 9-hydroxyrisperidone: 30 hours
Injection: 3-6 days; related to microsphere erosion and subsequent absorption of risperidone

Metabolism Extensively hepatic via CYP2D6 to 9-hydroxyrisperidone (similar pharmacological activity as risperidone); *N*-dealkylation is a second minor pathway

Excretion Urine (70%); feces (14%)

Available Dosage Forms

Injection, microspheres for reconstitution, extended release:
RisperDAL® Consta®: 12.5 mg, 25 mg, 37.5 mg, 50 mg
Solution, oral: 1 mg/mL (30 mL)
RisperDAL®: 1 mg/mL (30 mL)
Tablet, oral: 0.25 mg, 0.5 mg, 1 mg, 2 mg, 3 mg, 4 mg
RisperDAL®: 0.25 mg, 0.5 mg, 1 mg, 2 mg, 3 mg, 4 mg
Tablet, orally disintegrating, oral: 0.25 mg, 0.5 mg, 1 mg, 2 mg, 3 mg, 4 mg
RisperDAL® M-Tab®: 0.5 mg, 1 mg, 2 mg, 3 mg, 4 mg

Dosing

Adult Note: When reinitiating treatment after discontinuation, the initial titration schedule should be followed.

Bipolar mania: *Oral:* Recommended starting dose: 2-3 mg once daily; if needed, adjust dose by 1 mg/day in intervals ≥24 hours; dosing range: 1-6 mg/day.
Maintenance: No dosing recommendation available for treatment >3 weeks duration

Bipolar I maintenance: *I.M. (Risperdal® Consta®):* 25 mg every 2 weeks; if unresponsive, some may benefit from larger doses (37.5-50 mg); maximum dose: 50 mg every 2 weeks. Dosage adjustments should not be made more frequently than every 4 weeks. A lower initial dose of 12.5 mg may be appropriate in some patients (eg, demonstrated poor tolerability to other psychotropic medications).

Note: Oral risperidone (or other antipsychotic) should be administered with the initial injection of Risperdal® Consta® and continued for 3 weeks (then discontinued) to maintain adequate therapeutic plasma concentrations prior to main release phase of risperidone from injection site. When switching from depot administration to a short-acting formulation, administer short-acting agent in place of the next regularly-scheduled depot injection.

Schizophrenia:
Oral: Initial: 2 mg/day in 1-2 divided doses; may be increased by 1-2 mg/day at intervals ≥24 hours to a recommended dosage range of 4-8 mg/day; may be given as a single daily dose once maintenance dose is achieved; daily dosages >6 mg do not appear to confer any

additional benefit, and the incidence of extrapyramidal symptoms is higher than with lower doses. Further dose adjustments should be made in increments/decrements of 1-2 mg/day on a weekly basis. Dose range studied in clinical trials: 4-16 mg/day. Maintenance: Recommended dosage range: 2-8 mg/day

I.M. (Risperdal® Consta®): Initial: 25 mg every 2 weeks; if unresponsive, some may benefit from larger doses (37.5-50 mg); maximum dose: 50 mg every 2 weeks. Dosage adjustments should not be made more frequently than every 4 weeks. A lower initial dose of 12.5 mg may be appropriate in some patients (eg, demonstrated poor tolerability to other psychotropic medications).

Note: Oral risperidone (or other antipsychotic) should be administered with the initial injection of Risperdal® Consta® and continued for 3 weeks (then discontinued) to maintain adequate therapeutic plasma concentrations prior to main release phase of risperidone from injection site. When switching from depot administration to a short-acting formulation, administer short-acting agent in place of the next regularly-scheduled depot injection.

Post-traumatic stress disorder (PTSD) (unlabeled use): *Oral:* 0.5-8 mg/day (Bandelow, 2008; Benedek, 2009)

Tourette's syndrome (unlabeled use): *Oral:* Initial: 0.25 mg once daily for 2 days, then 0.25 mg twice daily for 3 days, then 0.5 mg twice daily for 2 days; titrate slowly thereafter in increments/decrements ≤0.5 mg twice daily and at intervals ≥3 days; maximum dose: 6 mg/day (Dion, 2002)

Geriatric

Oral: Initial: 0.5 mg twice daily; titration should progress slowly in increments of no more than 0.5 mg twice daily; increases to dosages >1.5 mg twice daily should occur at intervals of ≥1 week.

Note: Additional monitoring of renal function and orthostatic blood pressure may be warranted. If once-a-day dosing in the elderly or debilitated patient is considered, a twice daily regimen should be used to titrate to the target dose, and this dose should be maintained for 2-3 days prior to attempts to switch to a once-daily regimen.

Psychosis/agitation related to Alzheimer's dementia (unlabeled use): Initial: 0.25-1 mg/day; if necessary, gradually increase as tolerated not to exceed 1.5-2 mg/day; doses >1 mg/day are associated with higher rates of extrapyramidal symptoms (Rabins, 2007)

I.M. (Risperdal® Consta®): 25 mg every 2 weeks; a lower initial dose of 12.5 mg may be appropriate in some patients.

Note: Oral risperidone (or other antipsychotic) should be administered with the initial injection of Risperdal® Consta® and continued for 3 weeks (then discontinued) to maintain adequate therapeutic plasma concentrations prior to main release phase of risperidone from injection site. When switching from depot administration to a short-acting formulation, administer short-acting agent in place of the next regularly-scheduled depot injection.

Pediatric Note: When reinitiating treatment after discontinuation, the initial titration schedule should be followed.

Autism: Children ≥5 years and Adolescents: *Oral:*

<15 kg: Use with caution; specific dosing recommendations not available

<20 kg: Initial: 0.25 mg/day; may increase dose to 0.5 mg/day after ≥4 days, maintain dose for ≥14 days. In patients not achieving sufficient clinical response, may increase dose by 0.25 mg/day in ≥2-week intervals. Therapeutic effect reached plateau at 1 mg/day in clinical trials. Following clinical response, consider gradually lowering dose. May be administered once daily or in divided doses twice daily.

≥20 kg: Initial: 0.5 mg/day; may increase dose to 1 mg/day after ≥4 days, maintain dose for ≥14 days. In patients not achieving sufficient clinical response, may increase dose by 0.5 mg/day in ≥2-week intervals. Therapeutic effect reached plateau at 2.5 mg/day (3 mg/day in children >45 kg) in clinical trials. Following clinical response, consider gradually lowering dose. May be administered once daily or in divided doses twice daily.

Bipolar mania: Children and Adolescents 10-17 years: *Oral:* Initial: 0.5 mg once daily; dose may be adjusted in increments of 0.5-1 mg/day at intervals ≥24 hours to a dose of 2.5 mg/day. Doses ranging from 0.5-6 mg/day have been evaluated, however doses >2.5 mg/day do not confer additional benefit and are associated with increased adverse events.

Maintenance: No dosing recommendation available for treatment >3 weeks duration

Pervasive developmental disorder (unlabeled use): Children and Adolescents: *Oral:*

Initial: 0.25 mg twice daily; titrate up 0.25 mg/day every 5-7 days; optimal dose range: 0.75-1.5 mg/day (Fisman, 1996)

or

Initial: 0.5 mg at bedtime; titrate up 0.5 mg/day every 7 days in a morning and bedtime dosing regimen; dose range: 1-4 mg/day (McDougal, 1997)

Schizophrenia: Adolescents 13-17 years: *Oral:* Initial: 0.5 mg once daily; dose may be adjusted in increments of 0.5-1 mg/day at intervals ≥24 hours to a dose of 3 mg/day. Doses ranging from 1-6 mg/day have been evaluated, however, doses >3 mg/day do not confer additional benefit and are associated with increased adverse events.

Tourette's syndrome (unlabeled use): Adolescents: *Oral:* Refer to adult dosing.

Renal Impairment

Oral: Starting dose of 0.5 mg twice daily; titration should progress slowly in increments of no more than 0.5 mg twice daily; increases to dosages >1.5 mg twice daily should occur at intervals of ≥1 week. Clearance of the active moiety is decreased by 60% in patients with moderate-to-severe renal disease compared to healthy subjects.

I.M.: Initiate with **oral** dosing (0.5 mg twice daily for 1 week then 2 mg/day for 1 week); if tolerated, begin 25 mg **I.M.** every 2 weeks; continue oral dosing for 3 weeks after the first I.M. injection. An initial I.M. dose of 12.5 mg may also be considered.

Hepatic Impairment

Oral: Starting dose of 0.5 mg twice daily; titration should progress slowly in increments of no more than 0.5 mg twice daily; increases to dosages >1.5 mg twice daily should occur at intervals of ≥1 week. The mean free fraction of risperidone in plasma was increased by 35% in patients with hepatic impairment compared to healthy subjects.

I.M.: Initiate with **oral** dosing (0.5 mg twice daily for 1 week then 2 mg/day for 1 week); if tolerated, begin 25 mg **I.M.** every 2 weeks; continue oral dosing for 3 weeks after the first I.M. injection. An initial I.M. dose of 12.5 mg may also be considered.

Administration

Oral

Oral: May be administered without regard to meals.

Oral solution can be administered directly from the provided pipette or may be mixed with water, coffee, orange juice, or low-fat milk, but is **not compatible** with cola or tea.

In children or adolescents experiencing somnolence, half the daily dose may be administered twice daily **or** the once-daily dose may be administered at bedtime.

Risperdal® M-Tab® should not be removed from blister pack until administered. Using dry hands, place immediately on tongue. Tablet will dissolve within seconds, and may be swallowed with or without liquid. Do not split or chew.

I.M. Risperdal® Consta® should be administered I.M. into either the deltoid muscle or the upper outer quadrant of the gluteal area. Avoid inadvertent injection into vasculature. Injection should alternate between the two arms or buttocks. Do not combine two different dosage strengths into one single administration. Do not substitute any components of the dose-pack; administer with needle provided (1-inch needle for deltoid administration or 2-inch needle for gluteal administration).

Stability

Reconstitution Risperdal® Consta®: Bring to room temperature prior to reconstitution. Reconstitute with provided diluent only. Shake vigorously to mix; will form thick, milky suspension. Following reconstitution, store at room temperature and use within 6 hours. Suspension settles in ~2 minutes; shake vigorously to resuspend prior to administration.

Storage

Injection: Risperdal® Consta®: Store in refrigerator at 2°C to 8°C (36°F to 46°F) and protect from light. May be stored at room temperature of 25°C (77°F) for up to 7 days prior to administration. Following reconstitution, store at room temperature and use within 6 hours. Suspension settles in ~2 minutes; shake vigorously to resuspend prior to administration.

Oral solution, tablet: Store at 15°C to 25°C (59°F to 77°F). Protect from light and moisture. Keep orally-disintegrating tablets sealed in foil pouch until ready to use. Do not freeze solution.

Monitoring and Teaching Issues

Laboratory Monitoring Fasting lipid profile and fasting blood glucose/Hgb A_{1c} (prior to treatment, at 3 months, then annually); CBC

Physical Assessment Monitor results of periodic ophthalmic exams. Monitor weight prior to treatment and at least monthly. Be alert to the potential for suicide ideation and orthostatic hypotension, especially during the titration phase. Initiate at lower doses and titrate to target dose. Taper dosage slowly when discontinuing.

Patient Education It may take several weeks to achieve desired results. Dilute solution with water, milk, or orange juice; do not dilute with beverages containing tannin or pectinate (eg, colas, tea). Avoid alcohol. Maintain adequate hydration. If you have diabetes, you may experience increased blood sugars; monitor closely. You may experience excess sedation, drowsiness, restlessness, dizziness, or blurred vision; dry mouth, nausea, or GI upset; postural hypotension; or urinary retention (void before taking medication). Report persistent CNS effects (eg, trembling fingers, altered gait or balance, excessive sedation, seizures, unusual muscle or skeletal movements, anxiety, abnormal thoughts [especially suicide ideation], confusion, personality changes); chest pain, palpitations, irregular or rapid heartbeat, or severe dizziness; signs of infection or fever; altered menstrual pattern or sexual dysfunction; pain or difficulty on urination; vision changes; skin rash or yellowing of skin; respiratory difficulty; or worsening of condition.

Dietary Considerations May be taken without regard to meals. Some products may contain phenylalanine.

Geriatric Considerations Any changes in disease status in any organ system can result in behavior changes.

Extrapyramidal syndrome symptoms occur less with this agent when total daily dose remains <6 mg as compared with phenothiazines and butyrophenone classes of antipsychotics. Many elderly patients receive antipsychotic medications for inappropriate nonpsychotic behavior. Before initiating antipsychotic medication, the clinician should investigate any possible reversible cause; any stress or stress from any disease can cause acute "confusion" or worsening of baseline nonpsychotic behavior. Most commonly acute changes in behavior are due to increases in drug dose or addition of new drug to regimen; fluid electrolyte loss; infections; and changes in environment.

In the treatment of agitated, demented, elderly patients, authors of meta-analysis of controlled trials of the response to the traditional antipsychotics (phenothiazines, butyrophenones) in controlling agitation have concluded that the use of neuroleptics results in a response rate of 18%. Clearly neuroleptic therapy for behavior control should be limited with frequent attempts to withdraw the agent given for behavior control. In light of significant risks and adverse effects in elderly population compared with limited data demonstrating efficacy in the treatment of dementia related psychosis, aggression, and agitation, an extensive risk:benefit analysis should be performed prior to use.

Breast-Feeding Considerations Risperidone and its metabolite are excreted in breast milk; it is recommended that women not breast-feed during therapy or for 12 weeks after the last injection if using Risperdal® Consta®.

Pregnancy Considerations Animal studies indicate an increase in fetal mortality. Reversible EPS symptoms were noted in neonates following use of risperidone during the last trimester. Agenesis of the corpus callosum has also been noted in one case report of an infant exposed *in utero*. Antipsychotic use during the third trimester of pregnancy has a risk for abnormal muscle movements (extrapyramidal symptoms [EPS]) and withdrawal symptoms in newborns following delivery. Symptoms in the newborn may include agitation, feeding disorder, hypertonia, hypotonia, respiratory distress, somnolence, and tremor; these effects may be self-limiting or require hospitalization. There are no adequate and well-controlled studies in pregnant women. When using Risperdal® Consta®, patients should notify healthcare provider if they become or intend to become pregnant during therapy or within 12 weeks of last injection. Risperidone may cause hyperprolactinemia, which may decrease reproductive function in both males and females. Healthcare providers are encouraged to enroll women 18-45 years of age exposed to risperidone during pregnancy in the Atypical Antipsychotics Pregnancy Registry (1-866-961-2388).

Additional Information Risperdal® Consta® is an injectable formulation of risperidone using the extended release Medisorb® drug-delivery system; small polymeric microspheres degrade slowly, releasing the medication at a controlled rate.

Related Information

Antipsychotic Agents *on page 1986*

- **Ritalin®** *see* Methylphenidate *on page 1204*
- **Ritalin LA®** *see* Methylphenidate *on page 1204*
- **Ritalin-SR®** *see* Methylphenidate *on page 1204*

Ritonavir (ri TOE na veer)

U.S. Brand Names Norvir®

Generic Availability (U.S.) No

Pharmacologic Category Antiretroviral Agent, Protease Inhibitor

Medication Safety Issues

Sound-alike/look-alike issues:

Ritonavir may be confused with Retrovir®

Norvir® may be confused with Norvasc®

Pregnancy Risk Factor B

Lactation Excretion in breast milk unknown/not recommended

Use Treatment of HIV infection; should always be used as part of a multidrug regimen (at least three antiretroviral agents); may be used as a pharmacokinetic "booster" for other protease inhibitors

Mechanism of Action/Effect Blocks the site of HIV-1 protease activity, resulting in the formation of immature, noninfectious viral particles.

Contraindications Hypersensitivity to ritonavir or any component of the formulation; concurrent alfuzosin, amiodarone, bepridil, cisapride, dihydroergotamine, ergonovine, ergotamine, flecainide, lovastatin, methylergonovine, midazolam (oral), pimozide, propafenone, quinidine, sildenafil (when used for the treatment of pulmonary arterial hypertension [eg, Revatio®]), simvastatin, St John's wort, triazolam, and voriconazole (when ritonavir ≥800 mg/day)

Warnings/Precautions [U.S. Boxed Warning]: Ritonavir may interact with many medications, resulting in potentially serious and/or life-threatening adverse events. Use with caution in patients taking strong CYP3A4 inhibitors, moderate or strong CYP3A4 inducers and major CYP3A4 substrates (see Drug Interactions); consider alternative agents that avoid or lessen the potential for CYP-mediated interactions. Concomitant use with fluticasone, salmeterol, or high-dose or long-term use of meperidine is not recommended. Do not coadminister colchicine in patient with renal or hepatic impairment

Pancreatitis has been observed; use with caution in patients with increased triglycerides; monitor serum lipase and amylase and for gastrointestinal symptoms. Increases in total cholesterol and triglycerides have been reported; screening should be done prior to therapy and periodically throughout treatment.

Protease inhibitors have been associated with a variety of hypersensitivity events (some severe), including rash, anaphylaxis (rare), angioedema, bronchospasm, erythema multiforme, and/or Stevens-Johnson syndrome (rare). It is generally recommended to discontinue treatment if severe rash or moderate symptoms accompanied by other systemic symptoms occur. Use with caution in patients with cardiomyopathy, ischemic heart disease, pre-existing conduction abnormalities, or structural heart disease; may be at increased risk of conduction abnormalities (eg, second- or third-degree AV block). Ritonavir has been associated with AV block due to prolongation of PR interval; use caution with drugs that prolong the PR interval. Use with caution in patients with hemophilia A or B; increased bleeding during protease inhibitor therapy has been reported. Changes in glucose tolerance, hyperglycemia, exacerbation of diabetes, DKA, and new-onset diabetes mellitus have been reported in patients receiving protease inhibitors. May be associated with fat redistribution (buffalo hump, increased abdominal girth, breast engorgement, facial atrophy, and dyslipidemia). Immune reconstitution syndrome may develop resulting in the occurrence of an inflammatory response to an indolent or residual opportunistic infection; further evaluation and treatment may be required. May cause hepatitis or exacerbate pre-existing hepatic dysfunction; use with caution in patients with hepatitis B or C and in hepatic disease. Norvir® tablets are **not** bioequivalent to Norvir®

capsules. Gastrointestinal side effects (eg, nausea, vomiting, abdominal pain, diarrhea) or paresthesias may be more common when patients are switching from the capsule to the tablet formulation due to a higher C_{max} (26% increase) observed with the tablet formulation compared to the capsule. These side effects should decrease as therapy is continued. Safety and efficacy have not been established in children <1 month of age.

Drug Interactions

Metabolism/Transport Effects Substrate of CYP1A2 (minor), CYP2B6 (minor), CYP2D6 (major), CYP3A4 (major), P-glycoprotein; **Inhibits** CYP2C8 (strong), CYP2C9 (weak), CYP2C19 (weak), CYP2D6 (strong), CYP2E1 (weak), CYP3A4 (strong), P-glycoprotein; **Induces** CYP1A2 (weak), 2C8 (weak), 2C9 (weak), 3A4 (weak)

Avoid Concomitant Use

Avoid concomitant use of Ritonavir with any of the following: Alfuzosin; Amiodarone; Cisapride; Conivaptan; Disulfiram; Dronedarone; Eplerenone; Ergot Derivatives; Etravirine; Everolimus; Flecainide; Fluticasone (Nasal); Halofantrine; Lovastatin; Lurasidone; Midazolam; Nilotinib; Nisoldipine; Pimozide; Pitavastatin; Propafenone; QuiNIDine; Ranolazine; Rifampin; Rivaroxaban; RomiDEPsin; Salmeterol; Silodosin; Simvastatin; St Johns Wort; Tamoxifen; Tamsulosin; Thioridazine; Tolvaptan; Topotecan; Toremifene; Triazolam; Voriconazole

Decreased Effect

Ritonavir may decrease the levels/effects of: Abacavir; Atovaquone; BuPROPion; Clarithromycin; Codeine; Contraceptives (Estrogens); Deferasirox; Delavirdine; Divalproex; Etravirine; LamoTRIgine; Meperidine; Methadone; Phenytoin; Prasugrel; Theophylline Derivatives; TraMADol; Valproic Acid; Voriconazole; Warfarin; Zidovudine

The levels/effects of Ritonavir may be decreased by: Antacids; CarBAMazepine; Contraceptives (Estrogens); CYP3A4 Inducers (Strong); Efavirenz; Garlic; Peginterferon Alfa-2b; P-Glycoprotein Inducers; Phenytoin; Rifampin; St Johns Wort; Tenofovir

Increased Effect/Toxicity

Ritonavir may increase the levels/effects of: Alfuzosin; Almotriptan; Alosetron; ALPRAZolam; Amiodarone; Antifungal Agents (Azole Derivatives, Systemic); Atomoxetine; Bortezomib; Bosentan; Brinzolamide; Calcium Channel Blockers (Dihydropyridine); Calcium Channel Blockers (Nondihydropyridine); CarBAMazepine; Ciclesonide; Cisapride; Clarithromycin; Clorazepate; Colchicine; Conivaptan; Corticosteroids (Orally Inhaled); CycloSPORINE; CycloSPORINE (Systemic); CYP2C8 Substrates (High risk); CYP2D6 Substrates; CYP3A4 Substrates; Dabigatran Etexilate; Diazepam; Dienogest; Digoxin; Dronabinol; Dronedarone; Dutasteride; Enfuvirtide; Eplerenone; Ergot Derivatives; Estazolam; Everolimus; FentaNYL; Fesoterodine; Flecainide; Flurazepam; Fluticasone (Nasal); Fusidic Acid; GuanFACINE; Halofantrine; HMG-CoA Reductase Inhibitors; Ixabepilone; Lovastatin; Lumefantrine; Lurasidone; Maraviroc; Meperidine; MethylPREDNISolone; Midazolam; Nebivolol; Nefazodone; Nilotinib; Nisoldipine; Paricalcitol; Pazopanib; P-Glycoprotein Substrates; Pimecrolimus; Pimozide; Pitavastatin; PrednisoLONE; PredniSONE; Propafenone; Protease Inhibitors; QuiNIDine; Ranolazine; Rifabutin; Rivaroxaban; RomiDEPsin; Salmeterol; Saxagliptin; Sildenafil; Silodosin; Simvastatin; Sirolimus; SORAfenib; Tacrolimus; Tacrolimus (Systemic); Tacrolimus (Topical); Tadalafil; Tamoxifen; Tamsulosin; Temsirolimus; Tenofovir; Tetrabenazine; Thioridazine; Tolvaptan; Topotecan; Toremifene; TraZODone; Treprostinil; Triazolam; Tricyclic Antidepressants; Vardenafil; Vilazodone; VinBLAStine; VinCRIStine

The levels/effects of Ritonavir may be increased by: Antifungal Agents (Azole Derivatives, Systemic); Clarithromycin; CycloSPORINE; CycloSPORINE (Systemic); Delavirdine; Disulfiram; Efavirenz; Enfuvirtide; Fusidic Acid; MetroNIDAZOLE (Topical); P-Glycoprotein Inhibitors

Nutritional/Ethanol Interactions

Food: Food enhances absorption.

Herb/Nutraceutical: St John's wort may decrease ritonavir serum levels. Avoid use.

Adverse Reactions Percentages as reported for combined experiences in both treatment-naive and experienced adults:

>10%:

- Endocrine & metabolic: Hypercholesterolemia (>240 mg/dL: 37% to 45%), triglycerides increased (>800 mg/dL: 17% to 34%; >1500 mg/dL: 1% to 13%)
- Gastrointestinal: Nausea (26% to 30%), diarrhea (15% to 23%), vomiting (14% to 17%), taste perversion (7% to 11%)
- Hepatic: GGT increased (5% to 20%)
- Neuromuscular & skeletal: Weakness (10% to 15%), creatine phosphokinase increased (9% to 12%)

2% to 10%:

- Cardiovascular: Vasodilation (2%), syncope (1% to 2%)
- Central nervous system: Headache (6% to 7%), fever (1% to 5%), dizziness (3% to 4%), insomnia (2% to 3%), somnolence (2% to 3%), depression (2%), anxiety (up to 2%), malaise (1% to 2%)
- Dermatologic: Rash (up to 4%)
- Endocrine & metabolic: Uric acid increased (up to 4%)
- Gastrointestinal: Abdominal pain (6% to 8%), anorexia (2% to 8%), dyspepsia (up to 6%), local throat irritation (2% to 3%), flatulence (1% to 2%)
- Hepatic: Transaminases increased (6% to 10%)
- Neuromuscular & skeletal: Paresthesia (3% to 7%), arthralgia (up to 2%), myalgia (2%)
- Respiratory: Pharyngitis (≤1% to 3%)
- Miscellaneous: Diaphoresis (2% to 3%)

Pharmacodynamics/Kinetics

Absorption Variable; increased with food; In the fed state, mean C_{max} of the tablet formulation increased by 26% compared to the capsule.

Time to Peak Oral solution: 2 hours (fasted); 4 hours (nonfasted)

Protein Binding 98% to 99%

Half-Life Elimination 3-5 hours

Metabolism Hepatic via CYP3A4 and 2D6; five metabolites, low concentration of an active metabolite (M-2) achieved in plasma (oxidative)

Excretion Urine (~11%, ~4% as unchanged drug); feces (~86%, ~34% as unchanged drug)

Available Dosage Forms

Capsule, soft gelatin, oral:

Norvir®: 100 mg

Solution, oral:

Norvir®: 80 mg/mL (240 mL)

Tablet, oral:

Norvir®: 100 mg

Dosing

Adult & Geriatric Note: Norvir® tablets are **not** bioequivalent to Norvir® capsules. Gastrointestinal side effects or paresthesias may be more common initially when patients are switching from the capsule to the tablet formulation.

Treatment of HIV infection (not recommended as the primary protease inhibitor in any regimen [DHHS, 2011]): Oral: 600 mg twice daily; dose escalation tends to avoid nausea that many patients experience upon initiation of full dosing. Escalate the dose as follows: 300 mg twice daily for 1 day, 400 mg twice daily for 2 days, 500 mg twice daily for 1 day, then increase by 100 mg twice daily every 2-3 days to recommended dosage of 600 mg twice daily

Pharmacokinetic "booster" in combination with other protease inhibitors: 100-400 mg/day

Note: Recommended as the "booster" component in the following regimens in treatment-naive patients: Atazanavir and tenofovir/emtricitabine, or darunavir and tenofovir/emtricitabine (DHHS, 2011). In patients without evidence of PI resistance, once daily booster-dosing of 100 mg ritonavir may be preferred to 200 mg/day due to less gastrointestinal and metabolic adverse events. Refer to individual protease inhibitor monographs; specific dosage recommendations often require adjustment of both agents.

Dosage adjustments for concomitant therapy: Oral:

Coadministration with bosentan:

Coadministration of bosentan in patients currently receiving ritonavir: For patients receiving ritonavir for at least 10 days, begin with bosentan 62.5 mg once daily or every other day based on tolerability

Coadministration of ritonavir in patients currently receiving bosentan: Discontinue bosentan 36 hours prior to the initiation of ritonavir. After at least 10 days of ritonavir, resume bosentan 62.5 mg once daily or every other day based on tolerability.

Coadministration with colchicine:

Familial Mediterranean fever (FMF): Maximum colchicine dose: 0.6 mg/day (0.3 mg twice daily)

Gout prophylaxis:

If original colchicine dose is 0.6 mg twice daily, adjust dose to 0.3 mg once daily

If original colchicine dose is 0.6 mg once daily, adjust dose to 0.3 mg every other day

Gout flare treatment: Initial: Colchicine 0.6 mg, followed in 1 hour by a single dose of 0.3 mg; do not repeat for at least 3 days

Coadministration with phosphodiesterase-5 enzyme (PDE-5) inhibitor:

Pulmonary arterial hypertension: Ritonavir coadministered with tadalafil:

Patient receiving ritonavir for at least 1 week: Initiate tadalafil at 20 mg once daily; increase to 40 mg once daily based on individual tolerability

Patient receiving tadalafil when initiating ritonavir: Stop tadalafil at least 24 hours prior to starting ritonavir. After at least 1 week following the initiation of ritonavir, resume tadalafil at 20 mg once daily; increase to 40 mg once daily based on individual tolerability.

Erectile dysfunction: Ritonavir coadministered with:

Sildenafil (Viagra®): Maximum sildenafil dose: 25 mg in a 48-hour period

Tadalafil (Cialis®): Maximum tadalafil dose: 10 mg in a 72-hour period

Vardenafil: Maximum vardenafil dose: 2.5 mg in a 72-hour period

Pediatric Note: Norvir® tablets are **not** bioequivalent to Norvir® capsules. Gastrointestinal side effects or paresthesias may be more common initially when patients are switching from the capsule to the tablet formulation.

HIV infection: Oral: Children >1 month: 350-400 mg/m^2 twice daily (maximum dose: 600 mg twice daily). Initiate dose at 250 mg/m^2 twice daily; titrate dose upward every 2-3 days by 50 mg/m^2 twice daily.

Hepatic Impairment No adjustment required in mild or moderate impairment; however, careful monitoring is required in moderate hepatic impairment (levels may be decreased); caution advised with severe impairment (no data available).

Administration

Oral Administer capsules or oral solution with or without food (DHHS, 2011). Food improves tolerability. Liquid formulations usually have an unpleasant taste. Consider mixing it with chocolate milk or a liquid nutritional supplement. Whenever possible, administer oral solution with calibrated dosing syringe. Shake liquid well before use. Tablets should be administered with food and swallowed whole; do not chew, break, or crush.

Stability

Storage

Capsule: Store under refrigeration at 2°C to 8°C (36°F to 46°F); may be left out at room temperature of <25°C (<77°F) if used within 30 days. Protect from light. Avoid exposure to excessive heat.

Solution: Store at room temperature at 20°C to 25°C (68°F to 77°F); do not refrigerate. Avoid exposure to excessive heat.

Tablet: Store at room temperature at 20°C to 25°C (68°F to 77°F); excursions permitted to 15°C to 30°C (59°F to 86°F); avoid exposure to excessive heat. Exposure to high humidity outside of the original container (or a USP equivalent container) for >2 weeks is not recommended.

Monitoring and Teaching Issues

Laboratory Monitoring Triglycerides, cholesterol, LFTs, CBC, CPK, uric acid, viral load, CD4 count, glucose, serum amylase and lipase

Physical Assessment Assess CD4 count and hepatic function at regular intervals during therapy. Monitor for gastrointestinal disturbance (nausea, vomiting, diarrhea) that can lead to dehydration and weight loss, hyperlipidemia and redistribution of body fat, rash, CNS effects (malaise, insomnia, abnormal thinking), and electrolyte imbalance. Caution patients to monitor glucose levels closely; protease inhibitors may cause hyperglycemia or new-onset diabetes. Teach patient proper timing of multiple medications. Instruct patient on glucose testing (protease inhibitors may cause hyperglycemia; exacerbation or new-onset diabetes).

Patient Education This is not a cure for HIV, nor has it been found to reduce transmission of HIV; use appropriate precautions to prevent spread to other persons. Take with meals. Mix liquid formulation with chocolate milk or liquid nutritional supplement. Maintain adequate hydration, unless instructed to restrict fluid intake. Frequent blood tests may be required. You may be advised to check your glucose levels (this drug can cause exacerbation or new-onset diabetes). May cause body changes due to redistribution of body fat, facial atrophy, or breast enlargement (normal effects of drug). May cause dizziness, insomnia, abnormal thinking, nausea, vomiting, taste perversion, muscle weakness, or headache. Inform prescriber if you experience muscle numbness or tingling; unresolved persistent vomiting, diarrhea, or abdominal pain; respiratory difficulty or chest pain; unusual skin rash; or change in color of stool or urine.

Dietary Considerations Should be taken with food. Oral solution contains 43% ethanol by volume.

Breast-Feeding Considerations In infants born to mothers who are HIV positive, HAART while breast-feeding may decrease postnatal infection. However, maternal or infant antiretroviral therapy does not completely eliminate the risk of postnatal HIV transmission. In addition, multiclass-resistant virus has been detected in breast-feeding infants despite maternal therapy.

In the United States where formula is accessible, affordable, safe, and sustainable, complete avoidance of breast-feeding by HIV-infected women is recommended to decrease potential transmission of HIV.

Pregnancy Considerations Ritonavir crosses the placenta in minimal amounts; no increased risk of overall birth defects has been observed following 1st trimester exposure according to data collected by the antiretroviral pregnancy registry. Early studies have shown lower plasma levels during pregnancy compared to postpartum. If needed during pregnancy, use in combination with another PI to boost levels of second PI. Pregnancy and protease inhibitors are both associated with an increased risk of hyperglycemia. Glucose levels should be closely monitored. The Perinatal HIV Guidelines Working Group considers ritonavir to be an alternative PI for use during pregnancy. Healthcare providers are encouraged to enroll pregnant women exposed to antiretroviral medications in the Antiretroviral Pregnancy Registry (1-800-258-4263 or www.APRegistry.com). Healthcare providers caring for HIV-infected women and their infants may contact the National Perinatal HIV Hotline (888-448-8765) for clinical consultation.

Additional Information Potential compliance problems, frequency of administration and adverse effects should be discussed with patients before initiating therapy to help prevent the emergence of resistance.

Tipranavir with "boosted" ritonavir is not a recommended regimen due to inferior virilogic efficacy; do not use (DHHS, 2011).

◆ **Ritonavir and Lopinavir** *see* Lopinavir and Ritonavir *on page 1127*

◆ **Rituxan®** *see* RITUXimab *on page 1596*

RITUXimab (ri TUK si mab)

U.S. Brand Names Rituxan®

Index Terms Anti-CD20 Monoclonal Antibody; C2B8 Monoclonal Antibody; IDEC-C2B8

Generic Availability (U.S.) No

Pharmacologic Category Antineoplastic Agent, Monoclonal Antibody; Monoclonal Antibody

Medication Safety Issues

Sound-alike/look-alike issues:

Rituxan® may be confused with Remicade®

RiTUXimab may be confused with bevacizumab, inFLIXimab

High alert medication: The medication is in a class the Institute for Safe Medication Practices (ISMP) includes among its list of drug classes which have a heightened risk of causing significant patient harm when used in error.

The rituximab dose for rheumatoid arthritis is a flat dose (1000 mg) and is not based on body surface area (BSA).

Medication Guide Available Yes

Pregnancy Risk Factor C

Lactation Excretion in breast milk unknown/not recommended

Use

Treatment of CD20-positive non-Hodgkin's lymphomas (NHL):

- Relapsed or refractory, low-grade or follicular B-cell NHL (as a single agent)
- Follicular B-cell NHL, previously untreated (in combination with first-line chemotherapy, and as single-agent maintenance therapy if response to first-line rituximab with chemotherapy)
- Nonprogressing, low-grade B-cell NHL (as a single agent after first-line CVP treatment)
- Diffuse large B-cell NHL, previously untreated (in combination with CHOP chemotherapy [or other anthracycline-based regimen])

Treatment of CD20-positive chronic lymphocytic leukemia (CLL) (in combination with fludarabine and cyclophosphamide)

Treatment of moderately- to severely-active rheumatoid arthritis (in combination with methotrexate) in adult patients with inadequate response to one or more TNF antagonists

Treatment of Wegener's granulomatosis (WG) (in combination with glucocorticoids)

Treatment of microscopic polyangiitis (MPA) (in combination with glucocorticoids)

Unlabeled/Investigational Use Treatment of Burkitt's lymphoma, central nervous system lymphoma, Hodgkin's lymphoma (lymphocyte predominant); mucosal associated lymphoid tissue (MALT) lymphoma (gastric and nongastric), splenic marginal zone lymphoma; Waldenström's macroglobulinemia (WM); post-transplant lymphoproliferative disorder (PTLD); autoimmune hemolytic anemia (AIHA) in children; chronic immune thrombocytopenic purpura (ITP); refractory pemphigus vulgaris; treatment of steroid-refractory chronic graft-versus-host disease (GVHD)

Mechanism of Action/Effect Binds to the CD20 antigen on B-lymphocytes and recruits immune effector functions to mediate B-cell lysis *in vitro*. The antibody induces cell death in the DHL-4 human B-cell lymphoma line.

Contraindications There are no contraindications listed in the FDA-approved manufacturer's labeling.

Canadian labeling (not in U.S. labeling): Type 1 hypersensitivity or anaphylactic reaction to murine proteins, Chinese Hamster Ovary (CHO) cell proteins, or any component of the formulation; patients who have or have had progressive multifocal leukoencephalopathy (PML)

Warnings/Precautions [U.S. Boxed Warning]: Severe (occasionally fatal) infusion-related reactions have been reported, usually with the first infusion; fatalities have been reported within 24 hours of infusion; monitor closely during infusion; discontinue with grades 3 or 4 infusion reactions. Reactions usually occur within 30-120 minutes and may include hypotension, angioedema, bronchospasm, hypoxia, urticaria, and in more severe cases pulmonary infiltrates, acute respiratory distress syndrome, myocardial infarction, ventricular fibrillation, cardiogenic shock and/or anaphylaxis. Risk factors associated with fatal outcomes include chronic lymphocytic leukemia, female gender, mantle cell lymphoma, or pulmonary infiltrates. Closely monitor patients with a history of prior cardiopulmonary reactions or with pre-existing cardiac or pulmonary conditions and patients with high numbers of circulating malignant cells (>25,000/mm^3). Prior to infusion, premedicate patients with acetaminophen and an antihistamine (and methylprednisolone for patients with RA). Discontinue infusion for severe reactions; treatment is symptomatic. Medications for the treatment of hypersensitivity reactions (eg, bronchodilators, epinephrine, antihistamines, corticosteroids) should be available for immediate use. Discontinue infusion for serious or life-threatening cardiac arrhythmias; subsequent doses should include cardiac monitoring during and after the infusion. Mild-to-moderate infusion-related reactions (eg, chills, fever, rigors) occur frequently and are typically managed through slowing or interrupting the infusion. Infusion may be resumed at a 50% infusion rate reduction upon resolution of symptoms. Due to the potential for hypotension, consider withholding antihypertensives 12 hours prior to treatment.

[U.S. Boxed Warning]: Progressive multifocal leukoencephalopathy (PML) due to JC virus infection has been reported with rituximab use; may be fatal. Cases were reported in patients with hematologic malignancies receiving rituximab either with combination chemotherapy, or with hematopoietic stem cell transplant. Cases were also reported in patients receiving rituximab for autoimmune diseases who had received prior or concurrent immunosuppressant therapy. Onset may be delayed, although most cases were diagnosed within 12 months of the last rituximab dose. A retrospective analysis of patients (n=57) diagnosed with PML following rituximab therapy, found a median of 16 months (following rituximab initiation), 5.5 months (following last rituximab dose), and 6 rituximab doses preceded PML diagnosis. Clinical findings included confusion/disorientation, motor weakness/hemiparesis, altered vision/speech, and poor motor coordination with symptoms progressing over weeks to months (Carson, 2009). Promptly evaluate any patient presenting with neurological changes; consider neurology consultation, brain MRI and lumbar puncture for suspected PML. Discontinue rituximab in patients who develop PML; consider reduction/discontinuation of concurrent chemotherapy or immunosuppressants. Avoid use if severe active infection is present. Serious and potentially fatal bacterial, fungal, and either new or reactivated viral infections may occur during treatment, and up to 1 year after completing rituximab. Associated new or reactivated viral infections have included cytomegalovirus, herpes simplex virus, parvovirus B19, varicella zoster virus, West Nile virus, and hepatitis B and C. Rarely, reactivation of hepatitis B (with fulminant hepatitis, hepatic failure, and death) has been reported in association with rituximab;

median time to hepatitis diagnosis was ~4 months after initiation of therapy and 1 month following last dose; screen high-risk patients prior to therapy initiation. initiation; monitor for several months following completion of therapy. Discontinue rituximab (and concomitant chemotherapy) in patients who develop viral hepatitis and initiate antiviral therapy. Discontinue rituximab in patients who develop other serious infections and initiate appropriate anti-infective treatment.

[U.S. Boxed Warning]: Tumor lysis syndrome leading to acute renal failure requiring dialysis may occur 12-24 hours following the first dose when used as a single agent in the treatment of NHL. Hyperkalemia, hypocalcemia, hyperuricemia, and/or hyperphosphatemia may occur. Administer prophylaxis (allopurinol, hydration) in patients at high risk (high numbers of circulating malignant cells ≥25,000/mm^3 or high tumor burden). May cause fatal renal toxicity in patients with hematologic malignancies. Patients who received combination therapy with cisplatin and rituximab for NHL experienced renal toxicity during clinical trials; this combination is not an approved treatment regimen. Monitor for signs of renal failure; discontinue rituximab with increasing serum creatinine or oliguria. Correct electrolyte abnormalities; monitor hydration status.

[U.S. Boxed Warning]: Severe and sometimes fatal mucocutaneous reactions (lichenoid dermatitis, paraneoplastic pemphigus, Stevens-Johnson syndrome, toxic epidermal necrolysis and vesiculobullous dermatitis) have been reported, occurring from 1-13 weeks following exposure. Discontinue in patients experiencing severe mucocutaneous skin reactions; the safety of re-exposure following mucocutaneous reactions has not been evaluated. Use caution with pre-existing cardiac or pulmonary disease, or prior cardiopulmonary events. Rheumatoid arthritis patients are at increased risk for cardiovascular events; monitor closely during and after each infusion. Elderly patients are at higher risk for cardiac (supraventricular arrhythmia) and pulmonary adverse events (pneumonia, pneumonitis). Abdominal pain, bowel obstruction, and perforation (rarely fatal) have been reported with an average onset of symptoms of ~6 days (range: 1-77 days); complaints of abdominal pain should be evaluated, especially if early in the treatment course. Live vaccines should not be given concurrently with rituximab; there is no data available concerning secondary transmission of live vaccines with or following rituximab treatment. RA patients should be brought up to date with nonlive immunizations (following current guidelines) at least 4 weeks before initiating therapy; evaluate risks of therapy delay versus benefit (of nonlive vaccines) for NHL patients. Safety and efficacy of rituximab in combination with biologic agents or disease-modifying antirheumatic drugs (DMARD) other than methotrexate have not been established. Rituximab is not recommended for use in RA patients who have not had prior inadequate response to TNF antagonists. Safety and efficacy of retreatment for RA have not been established. The safety of concomitant immunosuppressants other than corticosteroids has not been evaluated in patients with Wegener's granulomatosis (WG) or microscopic polyangiitis (MPA) after rituximab-induced B-cell depletion. There are only limited data on subsequent courses of rituximab for WG or MPA; safety and efficacy of retreatment has not been established.

Drug Interactions

Avoid Concomitant Use

Avoid concomitant use of RiTUXimab with any of the following: BCG; Belimumab; Certolizumab Pegol; Natalizumab; Pimecrolimus; Roflumilast; Tacrolimus (Topical); Vaccines (Live)

Decreased Effect

RiTUXimab may decrease the levels/effects of: BCG; Sipuleucel-T; Vaccines (Inactivated); Vaccines (Live)

The levels/effects of RiTUXimab may be decreased by: Echinacea

Increased Effect/Toxicity

RiTUXimab may increase the levels/effects of: Belimumab; Certolizumab Pegol; Hypoglycemic Agents; Leflunomide; Natalizumab; Vaccines (Live)

The levels/effects of RiTUXimab may be increased by: Abciximab; Antihypertensives; Denosumab; Herbs (Hypoglycemic Properties); Pimecrolimus; Roflumilast; Tacrolimus (Topical); Trastuzumab

Nutritional/Ethanol Interactions Herb/Nutraceutical: Avoid echinacea (may diminish the therapeutic effect of immunosuppressants). Avoid hypoglycemic herbs, including alfalfa, aloe, bilberry, bitter melon, burdock, celery, damiana, fenugreek, garcinia, garlic, ginger, ginseng (American), gymnema, marshmallow, and stinging nettle (may enhance the hypoglycemic effect of rituximab).

Adverse Reactions Note: Patients treated with rituximab for rheumatoid arthritis (RA) may experience fewer adverse reactions.

>10%:

Cardiovascular: Peripheral edema (8% to 16%), hypertension (6% to 12%)

Central nervous system: Fever (5% to 53%), fatigue (13% to 39%), chills (3% to 33%), headache (17% to 19%), insomnia (≤14%), pain (12%)

Dermatologic: Rash (10% to 17%; grades 3/4: 1%), pruritus (5% to 17%), angioedema (11%; grades 3/4: 1%)

Gastrointestinal: Nausea (8% to 23%), diarrhea (10% to 17%), abdominal pain (2% to 14%), weight gain (11%)

Hematologic: Cytopenias (grades 3/4: ≤48%; may be prolonged), lymphopenia (48%; grades 3/4: 40%; median duration 14 days), anemia (8% to 35%; grades 3/4: 3%), leukopenia (NHL: 14%; grades 3/4: 4%; CLL: grades 3/4: 23%; WG/MPA: 10%), neutropenia (NHL: 14%; grades 3/4: 4% to 6%; median duration 13 days; CLL: grades 3/4: 30% to 49%), neutropenic fever (CLL: grades 3/4: 9% to 15%), thrombocytopenia (12%; grades 3/4: 2% to 11%)

Hepatic: ALT increased (≤13%)

Neuromuscular & skeletal: Neuropathy (≤30%), weakness (2% to 26%), muscle spasm (≤17%), arthralgia (6% to 13%)
Respiratory: Cough (13%), rhinitis (3% to 12%), epistaxis (≤11%)
Miscellaneous: Infusion-related reactions (lymphoma: first dose 77%; decreases with subsequent infusions; may include angioedema, bronchospasm, chills, dizziness, fever, headache, hyper-/hypotension, myalgia, nausea, pruritus, rash, rigors, urticaria, and vomiting; reactions reported are lower [first infusion: 32%] in RA; CLL: 59%; grades 3/4: 7% to 9%; WG/MPA: 12%); infection (19% to 62%; grades 3/4: 4%; bacterial: 19%; viral 10%; fungal: 1%), human antichimeric antibody (HACA) positive (1% to 23%), night sweats (15%)

1% to 10%:
Cardiovascular: Hypotension (10%; grades 3/4: 2%), flushing (5%)
Central nervous system: Dizziness (10%), anxiety (2% to 5%), migraine (RA: 2%)
Dermatologic: Urticaria (2% to 8%)
Endocrine & metabolic: Hyperglycemia (9%)
Gastrointestinal: Vomiting (10%), dyspepsia (RA: 3%)
Neuromuscular & skeletal: Back pain (10%), myalgia (10%), paresthesia (2%)
Respiratory: Dyspnea (≤10%), throat irritation (2% to 9%), bronchospasm (8%), dyspnea (7%), upper respiratory tract infection (RA: 7%), sinusitis (6%)
Miscellaneous: LDH increased (7%)

Pharmacodynamics/Kinetics

Duration of Action Detectable in serum 3-6 months after completion of treatment; B-cell recovery begins ~6 months following completion of treatment; median B-cell levels return to normal by 12 months following completion of treatment

Absorption I.V.: Immediate and results in a rapid and sustained depletion of circulating and tissue-based B cells

Half-Life Elimination
CLL: Median terminal half-life: 32 days (range: 14-62 days)
NHL: Median terminal half-life: 22 days (range: 6-52 days)
RA: Mean terminal half-life: 18 days (range: 5-78 days)
WG/MPA: 23 days (range: 9-49 days)

Excretion Uncertain; may undergo phagocytosis and catabolism in the reticuloendothelial system (RES)

Available Dosage Forms

Injection, solution [preservative free]:
Rituxan®: 10 mg/mL (10 mL, 50 mL)

Dosing

Adult & Geriatric Note: Details concerning dosing in combination regimens should also be consulted. Pretreatment with acetaminophen and an antihistamine is recommended for all indications. For oncology uses, a uricostatic agent (eg, allopurinol) and aggressive hydration is recommended for patients at risk for tumor lysis syndrome (high tumor burden or lymphocytes >25,000/mm^3). In patients with CLL, *Pneumocystis jiroveci* pneumonia (PCP) and antiherpetic viral prophylaxis is recommended during treatment (and for up to 12 months following treatment). In patients with WG and MPA, PCP prophylaxis is recommended during and for 6 months after rituximab treatment. For patients with RA, premedication with methylprednisolone 100 mg I.V. (or equivalent) is recommended 30 minutes prior to each dose.

Chronic lymphocytic leukemia (CLL): I.V. infusion: 375 mg/m^2 on the day prior to fludarabine/cyclophosphamide in cycle 1, then 500 mg/m^2 on day 1 (every 28 days) of cycles 2-6

Non-Hodgkin's lymphoma (NHL; relapsed/refractory, low-grade or follicular CD20-positive, B-cell): I.V. infusion: 375 mg/m^2 once weekly for 4 or 8 doses
Retreatment following disease progression: 375 mg/m^2 once weekly for 4 doses

NHL (diffuse large B-cell): I.V. infusion: 375 mg/m^2 given on day 1 of each chemotherapy cycle for up to 8 doses

NHL (follicular, CD20-positive, B-cell, previously untreated): I.V. infusion: 375 mg/m^2 given on day 1 of each chemotherapy cycle for up to 8 doses
Maintenance therapy (as a single agent, in patients with partial or complete response to rituximab plus chemotherapy; begin 8 weeks after completion of combination chemotherapy): I.V. infusion: 375 mg/m^2 every 8 weeks for 12 doses

NHL (nonprogressing, low-grade, CD20-positive, B-cell, after first line CVP): I.V. infusion: 375 mg/m^2 once weekly for 4 doses every 6 months for up to 4 cycles (initiate after 6-8 cycles of chemotherapy are completed)

NHL: Combination therapy with ibritumomab: I.V. infusion: 250 mg/m^2 I.V. day 1; repeat in 7-9 days with ibritumomab

Canadian labeling: **NHL, low grade or follicular:** I.V. infusion:
Initial: 375 mg/m^2 once weekly for 4 doses (as a single agent) **or** 375 mg/m^2 on day 1 of each 21-day cycle for 8 cycles (in combination with CVP chemotherapy)
Maintenance (responding to induction therapy): 375 mg/m^2 every 3 months until disease progression or up to a maximum of 2 years

Rheumatoid arthritis: I.V. infusion: 1000 mg on days 1 and 15 in combination with methotrexate; subsequent courses may be administered every 24 weeks (based on clinical evaluation), if necessary may be repeated no sooner than every 16 weeks

Wegener's granulomatosis (WG): I.V. infusion: 375 mg/m^2 once weekly for 4 doses (in combination with methylprednisolone I.V. for 1-3 days followed by daily prednisone)

Microscopic polyangiitis (MPA): I.V. infusion: 375 mg/m^2 once weekly for 4 doses (in combination with methylprednisolone I.V. for 1-3 days followed by daily prednisone)

Chronic graft-versus-host disease (GVHD), refractory (unlabeled use): I.V. infusion: 375 mg/m^2 once weekly for 4 doses (Cutler, 2006)

Chronic immune thrombocytopenic purpura (ITP; unlabeled use): I.V. infusion: 375 mg/m^2 once weekly for 4 doses (Arnold, 2007; Godeau, 2008)

Hodgkin's lymphoma (unlabeled use): I.V. infusion: 375 mg/m^2 once weekly for 4 weeks (Ekstrand, 2003; Schulz, 2008)

Pemphigus vulgaris, refractory (unlabeled use): I.V. infusion: 375 mg/m^2 once weekly of weeks 1, 2, and 3 of a 4-week cycle, repeat for 1 additional cycle, then 1 dose per month for 4 months (total of 10 doses in 6 months) (Ahmed, 2006)

Post-transplant lymphoproliferative disorder (unlabeled use): I.V. infusion: 375 mg/m^2 once weekly for 4 doses (Choquet, 2006)

Waldenström's macroglobulinemia (unlabeled use): I.V. infusion: 375 mg/m^2 once weekly for 4 weeks (Dimopoulos, 2002)

Pediatric Note: Pretreatment with acetaminophen and an antihistamine is recommended.

Autoimmune hemolytic anemia (AIHA; unlabeled use): I.V. infusion: 375 mg/m^2 once weekly for 2-4 doses (Zecca, 2003)

Chronic immune thrombocytopenic purpura (ITP; unlabeled use): I.V. infusion: 375 mg/m^2 once weekly for 4 doses (Parodi, 2009; Wang, 2005)

Administration

I.V. Do **not** administer I.V. push or bolus.

Initial infusion: Start rate of 50 mg/hour; if there is no reaction, increase the rate by 50 mg/hour increments every 30 minutes, to a maximum rate of 400 mg/hour.

Subsequent infusions: If patient did not tolerate initial infusion follow initial infusion guidelines. If patient tolerated initial infusion, start at 100 mg/hour; if there is no reaction, increase the rate by 100 mg/hour increments every 30 minutes, to a maximum rate of 400 mg/hour.

Note: If a reaction occurs, slow or stop the infusion. If the reaction abates, restart infusion at 50% of the previous rate.

In patients with NHL who are receiving a corticosteroid as part of their combination chemotherapy regimen and after tolerance has been established at the recommended infusion rate in cycle 1, a rapid infusion rate has been used beginning with cycle 2. The daily corticosteroid, acetaminophen, and diphenhydramine are administered prior to treatment, then the rituximab dose is administered over 90 minutes, with 20% of the dose administered in the first 30 minutes and the remaining 80% is given over 60 minutes (Sehn, 2007).

Stability

Reconstitution Withdraw necessary amount of rituximab and dilute to a final concentration of 1-4 mg/mL with 0.9% sodium chloride or 5% dextrose in water. Gently invert the bag to mix the solution. Do not shake.

Storage Store vials under refrigeration at 2°C to 8°C (36°F to 46°F); do not freeze. Do not shake. Protect vials from direct sunlight. Solutions for infusion are stable at 2°C to 8°C (36°F to 46°F) for 24 hours and at room temperature for an additional 24 hours.

Monitoring and Teaching Issues

Laboratory Monitoring CBC with differential and platelets (obtain at weekly to monthly intervals and more frequently in patients with cytopenias, or at 2-4 month intervals in rheumatoid arthritis patients, WG and MPA), peripheral CD20+ cells. Patients with elevated HAMA/HACA titers may have an allergic reaction when treated with rituximab or other antibodies from a mouse genetic source.

Physical Assessment Patient must be monitored closely during and following each infusion; severe infusion reactions can occur. Pretreatment with acetaminophen and diphenhydramine is recommended (corticosteroid when used to treat RA). Emergency equipment and medications (epinephrine, antihistamines, corticosteroids) should be immediately available during infusion. In the event of severe infusion reaction, infusion should be stopped and patient assessed. Monitor patient closely for abdominal pain (bowel obstruction and perforation), hyper-/hypotension, CNS changes, hyper-/hypoglycemia, and rash after each dose and following discontinuation of therapy. Bowel obstruction and perforation can occur early in therapy; acute tumor lysis syndrome leading to acute renal failure can occur 12-24 hours after first dose; severe mucocutaneous reactions can occur from 1-13 weeks following treatment; and new or reactivated serious viral infection may occur up to one year following discontinuation of therapy.

Patient Education This medication is only administered by infusion. You may experience a reaction during the infusion of this medication, including high fever, chills, respiratory difficulty, or congestion. You will be closely monitored and comfort measures provided. Maintain adequate hydration during entire course of therapy, unless instructed to restrict fluid intake. You will be susceptible to infection. If you have diabetes, monitor glucose levels closely; this medication may impact glucose control. May cause dizziness, trembling, nausea, vomiting, loss of appetite, diarrhea, or bone or muscle pain. Report immediately any unusual abdominal pain; skin rash or redness; persistent dizziness; swelling of extremities; unusual weight gain; respiratory difficulty; chest pain or tightness; symptoms of respiratory infection (wheezing, bronchospasms, or difficulty breathing); unresolved GI disturbance (nausea, vomiting); opportunistic infection (sore or irritated throat, unusual and persistent fatigue, chills, fever, unhealed sores, white plaques in mouth or genital area, unusual bruising or bleeding); CNS changes (confusion, agitation, insomnia); pain, tingling, or loss of sensation in extremities; or loss of coordination.

Breast-Feeding Considerations It is not known if rituximab is excreted in human milk. However, human IgG is excreted in breast milk, and therefore, rituximab may also be excreted in milk. The manufacturer recommends discontinuing breast-feeding until circulating levels of rituximab are no longer detectable.

Pregnancy Considerations Animal studies have demonstrated adverse effects including decreased (reversible) B-cells and immunosuppression. IgG molecules are known to cross the placenta (rituximab is an engineered IgG molecule) and rituximab has been detected in the serum of infants exposed in utero. B-Cell lymphocytopenia lasting <6 months may occur in exposed infants. Retrospective case reports of inadvertent pregnancy during rituximab treatment (often combined with concomitant teratogenic therapies) describe premature births, and infant hematologic abnormalities and infections; no specific pattern of birth defects has been observed (limited data). Effective contraception should be used during and for 12 months following treatment. Healthcare providers are encouraged to enroll women with rheumatoid arthritis exposed to rituximab during pregnancy in the OTIS AutoImmune Diseases Study by contacting the Organization of Teratology Information Specialists (877-311-8972).

Rivastigmine (ri va STIG meen)

U.S. Brand Names Exelon®

Index Terms ENA 713; Rivastigmine Tartrate; SDZ ENA 713

Generic Availability (U.S.) Yes: Capsule

Pharmacologic Category Acetylcholinesterase Inhibitor (Central)

Pregnancy Risk Factor B

Lactation Excretion in breast milk unknown/use caution

Use Treatment of mild-to-moderate dementia associated with Alzheimer's disease or Parkinson's disease

Unlabeled/Investigational Use Severe dementia associated with Alzheimer's disease; Lewy body dementia

Mechanism of Action/Effect A deficiency of cortical acetylcholine is thought to account for some of the symptoms of Alzheimer's disease and the dementia of Parkinson's disease; rivastigmine increases acetylcholine in the central nervous system through reversible inhibition of its hydrolysis by cholinesterase

Contraindications Hypersensitivity to rivastigmine, other carbamate derivatives (eg, neostigmine, pyridostigmine, physostigmine), or any component of the formulation

Warnings/Precautions Significant nausea, vomiting, anorexia, and weight loss are associated with use; occurs more frequently in women and during the titration phase. Nausea and/or vomiting may be severe, particularly at doses higher than recommended. Monitor weight during therapy. Therapy should be initiated at lowest dose and titrated; if treatment is interrupted for more than several days, reinstate at the lowest daily dose. Cholinesterase inhibitors may have vagotonic effects which may cause bradycardia and/or heart block with or without a history of cardiac disease. Alzheimer's treatment guidelines consider bradycardia to be a relative contraindication for use of centrally-active cholinesterase inhibitors. Post-market cases of overdose (including a few fatalities) have been reported in association with medication errors/improper use of rivastigmine transdermal patches. No more than 1 patch should be applied daily and existing patch must be removed prior to applying new patch.

Use caution in patients with a history of peptic ulcer disease or concurrent NSAID use. Use caution in patients undergoing anesthesia who will receive succinylcholine-type muscle relaxation, patients with sick-sinus syndrome, bradycardia or supraventricular conduction conditions, urinary obstruction, seizure disorders, or pulmonary conditions such as asthma or COPD. Use caution in patients with low body weight (<50 kg) due to increased risk of adverse reactions.

Drug Interactions

Avoid Concomitant Use There are no known interactions where it is recommended to avoid concomitant use.

Decreased Effect

Rivastigmine may decrease the levels/effects of: Anticholinergics; Neuromuscular-Blocking Agents (Nondepolarizing)

The levels/effects of Rivastigmine may be decreased by: Anticholinergics

Increased Effect/Toxicity

Rivastigmine may increase the levels/effects of: Antipsychotics; Beta-Blockers; Cholinergic Agonists; Succinylcholine

The levels/effects of Rivastigmine may be increased by: Corticosteroids (Systemic)

Nutritional/Ethanol Interactions

Smoking: Nicotine increases the clearance of rivastigmine by 23%.

Ethanol: Avoid ethanol (due to risk of sedation; may increase GI irritation).

Food: Food delays absorption by 90 minutes, lowers C_{max} by 30% and increases AUC by 30%.

Herb/Nutraceutical: Avoid ginkgo biloba (may increase cholinergic effects).

Adverse Reactions Note: Many concentration-related effects are reported at a lower frequency by transdermal route.

>10%:

Central nervous system: Dizziness (2% to 21%), headache (3% to 17%)

Gastrointestinal: Nausea (7% to 47%), vomiting (6% to 31%), diarrhea (5% to 19%), anorexia (3% to 17%), abdominal pain (1% to 13%)

1% to 10%:

Cardiovascular: Syncope (3%), hypertension (3%)

Central nervous system: Fatigue (2% to 9%), insomnia (1% to 9%), confusion (8%), depression (4% to 6%), anxiety (2% to 5%), malaise (5%), somnolence (4% to 5%), hallucinations (4%), aggressiveness (3%), parkinsonism symptoms worsening (2% to 3%), vertigo (≤2%)

Gastrointestinal: Dyspepsia (9%), constipation (5%), flatulence (4%), weight loss (3% to 8%), eructation (2%), dehydration (2%)

Genitourinary: Urinary tract infection (1% to 7%)

Neuromuscular & skeletal: Weakness (2% to 6%), tremor (1%; up to 10% in Parkinson's patients)
Respiratory: Rhinitis (4%)
Miscellaneous: Diaphoresis (4%), flu-like syndrome (3%)

Pharmacodynamics/Kinetics

Duration of Action Anticholinesterase activity (CSF): ~10 hours (6 mg oral dose)

Absorption Oral: Fasting: Rapid and complete within 1 hour

Bioavailability Oral: 36% to 40%

Time to Peak Oral: 1 hour; Transdermal patch: 10-16 hours following first dose

Protein Binding 40%

Half-Life Elimination Oral: 1.5 hours; Transdermal patch: 3 hours (after removal)

Metabolism Extensively via cholinesterase-mediated hydrolysis in the brain; metabolite undergoes N-demethylation and/or sulfate conjugation hepatically; minimal CYP involvement; linear kinetics at 3 mg twice daily, but nonlinear at higher doses

Excretion Urine (97% as metabolites); feces (0.4%)

Available Dosage Forms

Capsule, oral: 1.5 mg, 3 mg, 4.5 mg, 6 mg
Exelon®: 1.5 mg, 3 mg, 4.5 mg, 6 mg

Patch, transdermal:
Exelon®: 4.6 mg/24 hours (30s); 9.5 mg/24 hours (30s)

Solution, oral:
Exelon®: 2 mg/mL (120 mL)

Dosing

Adult Note: Exelon® oral solution and capsules are bioequivalent.

Mild-to-moderate Alzheimer's dementia:

Oral: Initial: 1.5 mg twice daily; may increase by 3 mg/day (1.5 mg/dose) every 2 weeks based on tolerability (maximum recommended dose: 6 mg twice daily)

Note: If GI adverse events occur, discontinue treatment for several doses then restart at the same or next lower dosage level; antiemetics have been used to control GI symptoms. If treatment is interrupted for longer than several days, restart the treatment at the lowest dose and titrate as previously described.

Transdermal patch: Initial: 4.6 mg/24 hours; if well tolerated, may be increased (after at least 4 weeks) to 9.5 mg/24 hours (recommended effective dose). Maintenance: 9.5 mg/24 hours (maximum dose: 9.5 mg/24 hours).

Note: If intolerance is noted (nausea, vomiting), patch should be removed and treatment interrupted for several days and restarted at the same or lower dosage. If interrupted for more than several days, reinitiate at lowest dosage and increase to maintenance dose after 4 weeks.

Conversion from oral therapy: If oral daily dose <6 mg, switch to 4.6 mg/24 hours patch; if oral daily dose 6-12 mg, switch to 9.5 mg/24 hours patch. Apply patch on the next day following last oral dose.

Mild-to-moderate Parkinson's-related dementia:

Oral: Initial: 1.5 mg twice daily; may increase by 3 mg/day (1.5 mg/dose) every 4 weeks based on tolerability (maximum recommended dose: 6 mg twice daily)

Transdermal patch: See transdermal dosing for Alzheimer's dementia.

Geriatric Following oral administration, clearance is significantly lower in patients >60 years of age, but dosage adjustments are not recommended. Age was not associated with exposure in patients treated transdermally. Titrate dose to individual's tolerance. Refer to adult dosing.

Renal Impairment Dosage adjustments are not recommended; however, titrate the dose to the individual's tolerance.

Hepatic Impairment Clearance is significantly reduced in mild to moderately impaired patients. Although dosage adjustments are not recommended, use lowest possible dose and titrate according to individual's tolerance. Consider intervals of >2 weeks between dosage adjustments.

Administration

Oral Should be administered with meals (breakfast or dinner). Capsule should be swallowed whole. Liquid form is available for patients who cannot swallow capsules (can be swallowed directly from syringe or mixed with water, soda, or cold fruit juice). Stir well and drink within 4 hours of mixing.

Topical Transdermal patch: Apply transdermal patch to upper or lower back (alternatively, may apply to upper arm or chest). Avoid reapplication to same spot of skin for 14 days (may rotate sections of back, for example). Do not apply to red, irritated, or broken skin. Avoid areas of recent application of lotion or powder. After removal, fold patch to press adhesive surfaces together, and discard. Avoid eye contact; wash hands after handling patch. Replace patch every 24 hours. Avoid exposing the patch to external sources of heat (eg, sauna, excessive light) for prolonged periods of time. No more than 1 patch should be applied daily and existing patch must be removed prior to applying new patch.

Stability

Storage

Oral: Store at 15°C to 30°C (59°F to 86°F); do not freeze. Store solution in an upright position.
Transdermal patch: Store at 15°C to 30°C (59°F to 86°F). Patches should be kept in sealed pouch until use.

Monitoring and Teaching Issues

Physical Assessment Assess bladder and sphincter adequacy prior to treatment. Monitor weight prior to treatment and regularly throughout. Assess cognitive function at periodic intervals.

Patient Education This drug is not a cure for Alzheimer's disease, but it may reduce the symptoms. Swallow capsule whole with meals (do not crush or chew). Liquid can be swallowed directly from syringe or mixed with water, soda, or cold fruit juice; stir well and drink within 4 hours of mixing. Apply transdermal patch to skin free from redness or irritation. Rotate sites; do not apply to same site within 14 days. No more than 1 patch should be applied daily and existing patch must be removed prior to applying new patch. Avoid alcohol. May cause dizziness, drowsiness, or postural hypotension; vomiting or loss of appetite; diarrhea; constipation; or urinary frequency. Report persistent abdominal discomfort, diarrhea, or constipation; significantly increased salivation, sweating, tearing, or urination; chest pain or palpitations; acute headache; CNS changes (eg, excessive fatigue, agitation, insomnia, dizziness, confusion, aggressiveness, depression); increased muscle, joint, or body pain; vision changes or blurred vision; shortness of breath, coughing, or wheezing; or skin rash.

Dietary Considerations Capsules should be taken with meals.

Geriatric Considerations Titrate dose to tolerance.

Pregnancy Considerations Teratogenic effects were not observed in animal studies. There are no adequate and well-controlled studies in pregnant women. Should be used only if the benefit outweighs the potential risk to the fetus.

◆ **Rivastigmine Tartrate** *see* Rivastigmine *on page 1601*

Rizatriptan (rye za TRIP tan)

U.S. Brand Names Maxalt-MLT®; Maxalt®

Index Terms MK462

Generic Availability (U.S.) No

Pharmacologic Category Antimigraine Agent; Serotonin 5-$HT_{1B,\ 1D}$ Receptor Agonist

Pregnancy Risk Factor C

Lactation Excretion in breast milk unknown/use caution

Use Acute treatment of migraine with or without aura

Mechanism of Action/Effect Selective agonist for serotonin receptor in cranial arteries; causes vasoconstriction and relief of migraine

Contraindications Hypersensitivity to rizatriptan or any component of the formulation; documented ischemic heart disease or Prinzmetal's angina; uncontrolled hypertension; basilar or hemiplegic migraine; during or within 2 weeks of MAO inhibitors; during or within 24 hours of treatment with another 5-HT_1 agonist, or an ergot-containing or ergot-type medication (eg, methysergide, dihydroergotamine)

Warnings/Precautions Only indicated for treatment of acute migraine; if a patient does not respond to the first dose, the diagnosis of migraine should be reconsidered. Coronary artery vasospasm, transient ischemia, myocardial infarction, ventricular tachycardia/fibrillation, cardiac arrest, and death have been reported with 5-HT_1 agonist administration. Patients who experience sensations of chest pain/pressure/tightness or symptoms suggestive of angina following dosing should be evaluated for coronary artery disease or Prinzmetal's angina before receiving additional doses. Should not be given to patients who have risk factors for CAD (eg, hypertension, hypercholesterolemia, smoker, obesity, diabetes, strong family history of CAD, menopause, male >40 years of age) without adequate cardiac evaluation. Patients with suspected CAD should have cardiovascular evaluation to rule out CAD before considering use; if cardiovascular evaluation "is satisfactory," first dose should be given in the healthcare provider's office. Periodic evaluation of cardiovascular status should be done in all patients. Significant elevation in blood pressure, including hypertensive crisis, has also been reported on rare occasions in patients with and without a history of hypertension. Cerebral/subarachnoid hemorrhage, stroke, peripheral vascular ischemia, and colonic ischemia have been reported with 5-HT_1 agonist administration.

Use with caution in elderly or patients with hepatic or renal impairment (including dialysis patients). Symptoms of agitation, confusion, hallucinations, hyper-reflexia, myoclonus, shivering, and tachycardia may occur with concomitant proserotonergic drugs (eg, SSRIs/SNRIs or triptans) or agents which reduce rizatriptan's metabolism. Concurrent use of serotonin precursors (eg, tryptophan) is not recommended. Maxalt-MLT® tablets contain phenylalanine.

Drug Interactions

Avoid Concomitant Use

Avoid concomitant use of Rizatriptan with any of the following: Ergot Derivatives; MAO Inhibitors; Sibutramine

Decreased Effect There are no known significant interactions involving a decrease in effect.

Increased Effect/Toxicity

Rizatriptan may increase the levels/effects of: Ergot Derivatives; Serotonin Modulators

The levels/effects of Rizatriptan may be increased by: Ergot Derivatives; MAO Inhibitors; Propranolol; Sibutramine

Nutritional/Ethanol Interactions Food: Food delays absorption.

Adverse Reactions 1% to 10%:

Cardiovascular: Systolic/diastolic blood pressure increases (5-10 mm Hg), chest pain (5%), palpitation

Central nervous system: Dizziness, drowsiness, fatigue (13% to 30%, dose related)

Dermatologic: Skin flushing

Endocrine & metabolic: Mild increase in growth hormone, hot flashes

Gastrointestinal: Abdominal pain, dry mouth (<5%), nausea

Respiratory: Dyspnea

Pharmacodynamics/Kinetics

Onset of Action ~30 minutes

Duration of Action 14-16 hours

Bioavailability 40% to 50%

Time to Peak 1-1.5 hours

Protein Binding 14%

Half-Life Elimination 2-3 hours

Metabolism Via monoamine oxidase-A; first-pass effect

Excretion Urine (82%, 8% to 16% as unchanged drug); feces (12%)

Available Dosage Forms

Tablet, oral:

Maxalt®: 5 mg, 10 mg

Tablet, orally disintegrating, oral:

Maxalt-MLT®: 5 mg, 10 mg

Dosing

Adult & Geriatric Note: In patients with risk factors for coronary artery disease, following adequate evaluation to establish the absence of coronary artery disease, the initial dose should be administered in a setting where response may be evaluated (physician's office or similarly staffed setting). ECG monitoring may be considered.

Migraine: Oral: 5-10 mg, repeat after 2 hours if significant relief is not attained; maximum: 30 mg in a 24-hour period (use 5 mg dose in patients receiving propranolol with a maximum of 15 mg in 24 hours)

Note: For orally-disintegrating tablets (Maxalt-MLT®): Patient should be instructed to place tablet on tongue and allow to dissolve. Dissolved tablet will be swallowed with saliva.

Stability

Storage Store in blister pack until administration.

Monitoring and Teaching Issues

Laboratory Monitoring Consider monitoring vital signs and ECG with first dose in patients with unrecognized coronary disease, such as patients with significant hypertension, hypercholesterolemia, obese patients, patients with diabetes, smokers with other risk factors or strong family history of coronary artery disease

Physical Assessment For use only with clear diagnosis of migraine. Cardiovascular status should be evaluated prior to initiating medication and periodically thereafter. Monitor for drowsiness, nausea/vomiting, chest pain, and palpitations.

Patient Education This drug is to be used to reduce your migraine, not to prevent or reduce the number of attacks. For orally-disintegrating tablets (Maxalt-MLT®), do not open blister pack before using. Open with dry hands, place on tongue, and allow to dissolve (dissolved tablet will be swallowed with saliva). Do not crush, break, or chew. If first dose brings relief, second dose may be taken anytime after 2 hours if migraine returns. Do not take more than two doses without consulting prescriber. May cause dizziness, drowsiness, dry mouth, skin flushing or hot flashes, mild abdominal discomfort, nausea, or vomiting. Report immediately any chest pain, palpitations, or irregular heartbeat; severe dizziness, acute headache, stiff or painful neck or facial swelling; muscle weakness or pain; changes in mental acuity; blurred vision or eye pain; or excessive perspiration or urination.

Dietary Considerations Some products may contain phenylalanine.

Geriatric Considerations Since the elderly often have cardiovascular disease, careful evaluation of the use of 5-HT agonists is needed to avoid complications with the use of these agents. The pharmacokinetic disposition of these agents is similar to that seen in younger adults.

Pregnancy Considerations There are no adequate and well-controlled studies using rizatriptan in pregnant women. Use only if potential benefit to the mother outweighs the potential risk to the fetus. A pregnancy registry has been established to monitor outcomes of women exposed to rizatriptan during pregnancy (800-986-8999). In some animal studies, administration was associated with decreased weight gain, developmental toxicity and increased mortality in the offspring. Teratogenic effects were not observed.

Related Information

Antimigraine Drugs: 5-HT_1 Receptor Agonists *on page 1985*

◆ **rLFN-α2** *see* Interferon Alfa-2b *on page 1000*

◆ **R-modafinil** *see* Armodafinil *on page 147*

◆ **Robafen [OTC]** *see* GuaiFENesin *on page 890*

◆ **Robafen AC** *see* Guaifenesin and Codeine *on page 891*

◆ **Robaxin®** *see* Methocarbamol *on page 1193*

◆ **Robaxin®-750** *see* Methocarbamol *on page 1193*

◆ **Robinul®** *see* Glycopyrrolate *on page 881*

◆ **Robinul® Forte** *see* Glycopyrrolate *on page 881*

◆ **Robitussin AC** *see* Guaifenesin and Codeine *on page 891*

◆ **Robitussin® Chest Congestion [OTC] [DSC]** *see* GuaiFENesin *on page 890*

◆ **Robitussin® Children's Cough & Cold Long-Acting [OTC]** *see* Dextromethorphan and Chlorpheniramine *on page 513*

◆ **Robitussin® Cough & Cold Long-Acting [OTC]** *see* Dextromethorphan and Chlorpheniramine *on page 513*

- **Robitussin® Night Time Cough & Cold [OTC]** *see* Diphenhydramine and Phenylephrine *on page 546*
- **Rocaltrol®** *see* Calcitriol *on page 271*
- **Rocephin®** *see* CefTRIAXone *on page 336*

Roflumilast (roe FLUE mi last)

Index Terms Daliresp™

Generic Availability (U.S.) No

Pharmacologic Category Phosphodiesterase-4 Enzyme Inhibitor

Use Adjunct to bronchodilator therapy in the maintenance treatment of severe chronic obstructive pulmonary disease (COPD) associated with chronic bronchitis

Mechanism of Action/Effect Roflumilast and its active metabolite selectively inhibit phosphodiesterase-4 (PDE4) leading to an accumulation of cyclic AMP (cAMP) within inflammatory and structural cells important in the development of COPD. Inflammation, pulmonary remodeling, and mucociliary malfunction are decreased.

Contraindications Hypersensitivity to roflumilast or any component of the formulation; moderate or severe hepatic impairment (Child-Pugh class B or C)

Warnings/Precautions Not indicated for relieving acute bronchospasms or for use as monotherapy of COPD; use only as adjunctive therapy to bronchodilator therapy. Avoid and/or discontinue use in patients with cancer (excluding basal cell carcinoma) and patients with congestive heart failure (NYHA III/IV). Neuropsychiatric effects (eg, anxiety, depression) have been reported with use; rarely, suicidal behavior/ ideation and completed suicide were reported. Avoid use in patients with a history of depression with suicidal behavior/ideations; instruct patients/caregivers to report psychiatric symptoms and consider discontinuation of therapy in such patients. Avoid and/or discontinue use in patients with a severe acute infection, severe immunosuppression, or those receiving immunosuppressive therapy (excludes short-term systemic corticosteroid use for COPD exacerbation). Systemic exposure may be increased in patients with mild hepatic impairment; use in moderate-to-severe impairment is contraindicated.

May cause diarrhea (sometimes severe) and/or weight loss; diarrhea usually observed within 4 weeks and weight loss within 6 months of initiating therapy. Instruct patients to monitor weight regularly. Avoid initiation of therapy or discontinue therapy with unexplained/pronounced weight loss. Hypersensitivity may occur following administration; monitor for signs/symptoms of hypersensitivity. Safety and efficacy not established in patients <18 years of age.

Drug Interactions

Avoid Concomitant Use

Avoid concomitant use of Roflumilast with any of the following: CYP3A4 Inducers (Strong); Immunosuppressants; Rifampin

Decreased Effect

The levels/effects of Roflumilast may be decreased by: CYP3A4 Inducers (Strong); Deferasirox; Herbs (CYP3A4 Inducers); Rifampin

Increased Effect/Toxicity

Roflumilast may increase the levels/effects of: Immunosuppressants

The levels/effects of Roflumilast may be increased by: Cimetidine; Conivaptan; FluvoxaMINE

Nutritional/Ethanol Interactions Food: Food delays roflumilast T_{max} by 1 hour and reduces its C_{max} ~40%, but does not affect total PDE4 inhibition (tPDE4i); C_{max} and T_{max} of roflumilast N-oxide (active metabolite) are unaffected by food.

Adverse Reactions

>10%: Gastrointestinal: Diarrhea (12%)

1% to 10%:

Cardiovascular: Supraventricular arrhythmia (1%)

Central nervous system: Headache (5%), dizziness (3%), insomnia (3%), anxiety (1%), depression (1%), fatigue (1%)

Gastrointestinal: Weight loss (7%), nausea (5%), abdominal pain (4%), appetite decreased (3%), gastritis (1%), vomiting (1%)

Neuromuscular & skeletal: Back pain (3%), muscle spasms (2%), tremor (2%)

Pharmacodynamics/Kinetics

Bioavailability ~80%

Time to Peak ~1 hour (delayed by food); N-oxide metabolite: ~8 hours

Protein Binding 99%; N-oxide metabolite: 97%

Half-Life Elimination 17 hours; N-oxide metabolite: 30 hours

Metabolism Hepatic via CYP3A4 and CYP1A2 to active N-oxide metabolite; also undergoes conjugation

Excretion Urine (~70% as unchanged drug)

Product Availability

Daliresp™: FDA approved March 2011; availability expected in second quarter 2011.

Daliresp™ is an oral selective phosphodiesterase-4 inhibitor approved to reduce the risk of COPD exacerbations in patients with severe COPD secondary to chronic bronchitis with a history of exacerbations.

Dosing

Adult & Geriatric COPD: Oral: 500 mcg once daily

Renal Impairment No dosage adjustment is required.

Hepatic Impairment
Mild impairment: No dosage adjustment is required.
Moderate-to-severe impairment (Child-Pugh class B or C): Use is contraindicated.

Administration

Oral Administer without regards to meals.

Stability

Storage Store at 15°C to 30°C (59°F to 86°F).

Monitoring and Teaching Issues

Dietary Considerations May be given with or without food.

Breast-Feeding Considerations Roflumilast and/or its metabolites are excreted into the breast milk of lactating rats. Excretion into human breast milk is likely. Avoid use while breast-feeding.

Pregnancy Considerations Animal studies have demonstrated reproductive toxicity (incomplete ossification, post-implantive losses) at doses greater than the human recommended dose. There are no adequate and well controlled studies in pregnant women. Avoid use during pregnancy.

◆ **Romazicon®** *see* Flumazenil *on page* 782

Ropinirole (roe PIN i role)

U.S. Brand Names Requip®; Requip® XL™

Index Terms Ropinirole Hydrochloride

Generic Availability (U.S.) Yes: Excludes combination package, extended-release tablets

Pharmacologic Category Anti-Parkinson's Agent, Dopamine Agonist

Medication Safety Issues
Sound-alike/look-alike issues:
Requip® may be confused with Reglan®
ROPINIRole may be confused with RisperDAL®, risperiDONE, ropivacaine

Pregnancy Risk Factor C

Lactation Excretion in breast milk unknown/not recommended

Use Treatment of idiopathic Parkinson's disease; in patients with early Parkinson's disease who were not receiving concomitant levodopa therapy as well as in patients with advanced disease on concomitant levodopa; treatment of moderate-to-severe primary Restless Legs Syndrome (RLS)

Contraindications Hypersensitivity to ropinirole or any component of the formulation

Warnings/Precautions Syncope, sometimes associated with bradycardia, was observed in association with ropinirole in both early Parkinson's disease (without levodopa) patients and advanced Parkinson's disease (with levodopa) patients. Dopamine agonists appear to impair the systemic regulation of blood pressure resulting in postural hypotension, especially during dose escalation. Parkinson's disease patients appear to have an impaired capacity to respond to a postural challenge; use with caution in patients at risk of hypotension (ie, those receiving antihypertensive or antiarrhythmic drugs) or where transient hypotensive episodes would be poorly tolerated (cardiovascular disease or cerebrovascular disease). Parkinson's patients being treated with dopaminergic agonists ordinarily require careful monitoring for signs and symptoms of postural hypotension, especially during dose escalation, and should be informed of this risk.

May cause hallucinations (dose dependent); risk may be increased in the elderly. Use with caution in patients with pre-existing dyskinesia, hepatic or severe renal dysfunction (use in patients with severe renal impairment and who are not undergoing regular hemodialysis is not recommended in the Canadian labeling). Avoid use in patients with a major psychotic disorder; may exacerbate psychosis.

Patients treated with ropinirole have reported falling asleep while engaging in activities of daily living; this has been reported to occur without significant warning signs. Monitor for daytime somnolence or pre-existing sleep disorder; caution with concomitant sedating medication; discontinue if significant daytime sleepiness or episodes of falling asleep occur. Patients must be cautioned about performing tasks which require mental alertness (eg, operating machinery or driving). Use with caution in patients receiving other CNS depressants or psychoactive agents. Effects with other sedative drugs or ethanol may be potentiated.

Dopamine agonists have been associated with compulsive behaviors and/or loss of impulse control, which has manifested as pathological gambling, libido increases (hypersexuality), and/or binge eating. Causality has not been established, and controversy exists as to whether this phenomenon is related to the underlying disease, prior behaviors/addictions and/or drug therapy. Dose reduction or discontinuation of therapy has been reported to reverse these behaviors in some, but not all cases. Risk for melanoma development is increased in Parkinson's disease patients; drug causation or factors contributing to risk have not been established. Patients should be monitored closely and periodic skin examinations should be performed.

Some patients treated for RLS may experience worsening of symptoms in the early morning hours (rebound) or an increase and/or spread of daytime symptoms (augmentation); clinical management of these phenomena has not been evaluated in controlled clinical trials. Pathologic degenerative changes were observed in the retinas of albino rats during studies with this agent, but were not observed in the retinas of albino mice or in other species. The significance of these data for humans remains uncertain.

Other dopaminergic agents have been associated with a syndrome resembling neuroleptic malignant syndrome on withdrawal or significant dosage reduction after long-term use. Risk of fibrotic complications (eg, pleural effusion/fibrosis, interstitial lung disease) and melanoma has been reported in patients receiving ropinirole; drug causation has not been established.

Drug Interactions

Metabolism/Transport Effects Substrate of CYP1A2 (major), 3A4 (minor); **Inhibits** CYP1A2 (weak)

Avoid Concomitant Use There are no known interactions where it is recommended to avoid concomitant use.

Decreased Effect

ROPINIRole may decrease the levels/effects of: Antipsychotics (Typical)

The levels/effects of ROPINIRole may be decreased by: Antipsychotics (Atypical); CYP1A2 Inducers (Strong); Metoclopramide

Increased Effect/Toxicity

The levels/effects of ROPINIRole may be increased by: Antipsychotics (Typical); Ciprofloxacin; Ciprofloxacin (Systemic); Conivaptan; CYP1A2 Inhibitors (Moderate); CYP1A2 Inhibitors (Strong); Estrogen Derivatives; MAO Inhibitors; Methylphenidate

Nutritional/Ethanol Interactions

Ethanol: Avoid ethanol (may increase CNS depression).

Herb/Nutraceutical: Avoid kava kava, gotu kola, valerian, St John's wort (may increase CNS depression).

Adverse Reactions

Data inclusive of trials in early Parkinson's disease (without levodopa) and Restless Legs Syndrome:

>10%:

- Cardiovascular: Syncope (1% to 12%)
- Central nervous system: Somnolence (11% to 40%), dizziness (6% to 40%), fatigue (8% to 11%)
- Gastrointestinal: Nausea (immediate release: 40% to 60%; extended release: 19%), vomiting (11% to 12%)
- Miscellaneous: Viral infection (11%)

1% to 10%:

- Cardiovascular: Dependent/leg edema (2% to 7%), orthostasis (1% to 6%), hypertension (5%), chest pain (4%), flushing (3%), palpitation (3%), peripheral ischemia (2% to 3%), atrial fibrillation (2%), extrasystoles (2%), hypotension (2%), tachycardia (2%)
- Central nervous system: Pain (3% to 8%), headache (extended release: 6%), confusion (5%), hallucinations (up to 5%; dose related), hypoesthesia (4%), amnesia (3%), malaise (3%), yawning (3%), concentration impaired (2%), vertigo (2%)
- Dermatologic: Hyperhidrosis (3%)
- Gastrointestinal: Dyspepsia (4% to 10%), abdominal pain (3% to 7%), constipation (≥5%), xerostomia (3% to 5%), diarrhea (5%), anorexia (4%), flatulence (3%)
- Genitourinary: Urinary tract infection (5%), impotence (3%)
- Hepatic: Alkaline phosphatase increased (3%)
- Neuromuscular & skeletal: Weakness (6%), arthralgia (4%), muscle cramps (3%), paresthesia (3%), hyperkinesia (2%)
- Ocular: Abnormal vision (6%), xerophthalmia (2%)
- Respiratory: Pharyngitis (6% to 9%), rhinitis (4%), sinusitis (4%), bronchitis (3%), dyspnea (3%), influenza (3%), cough (3%), nasal congestion (2%)
- Miscellaneous: Diaphoresis increased (3% to 6%)

Advanced Parkinson's disease (with levodopa):

>10%:

- Central nervous system: Dizziness (immediate release: 26%; extended-release: 8%), somnolence (immediate release: 20%, extended release: 7%), headache (17%)
- Gastrointestinal: Nausea (immediate release: 30%; extended-release: 11%)
- Neuromuscular & skeletal: Dyskinesias (immediate release: 34%; extended-release: 13%; dose related)

1% to 10%:

- Cardiovascular: Hypotension (2% to 5%; including orthostatic), peripheral edema (4%), syncope (3%), hypertension (3%; dose related)
- Central nervous system: Hallucinations (7% to 10%; dose related), confusion (9%), anxiety (2% to 6%), amnesia (5%), nervousness (5%), pain (5%), vertigo (4%), abnormal dreaming (3%), paresis (3%), aggravated parkinsonism, insomnia
- Gastrointestinal: Abdominal pain (6% to 9%), vomiting (7%), constipation (4% to 6%), diarrhea (3% to 5%), xerostomia (2% to 5%), dysphagia (2%), flatulence (2%), salivation increased (2%), weight loss (2%)
- Genitourinary: Urinary tract infection (6%), pyuria (2%), urinary incontinence (2%)
- Hematologic: Anemia (2%)
- Neuromuscular & skeletal: Falls (2% to 10%; dose related), arthralgia (7%), tremor (6%), hypokinesia (5%), paresthesia (5%), arthritis (3%), back pain (3%)
- Ocular: Diplopia (2%)
- Respiratory: Upper respiratory tract infection (9%), dyspnea (3%)
- Miscellaneous: Injury, diaphoresis increased (7%), viral infection, increased drug level (7%)

Other adverse effects (all phase 2/3 trials for Parkinson's disease and Restless Leg Syndrome): ≥1%: Asthma, BUN increased, depression, gastroenteritis, gastrointestinal reflux, irritability, migraine, muscle spasm, myalgia, neck pain, neuralgia, osteoarthritis, pharyngolaryngeal pain, rash, rigors, sleep disorder, tendonitis

Pharmacodynamics/Kinetics

Absorption Not affected by food

Bioavailability Absolute: 45% to 55%

Time to Peak Immediate release: ~1-2 hours; Extended release: 6-10 hours; T_{max} increased by 2.5-3 hours when drug taken with food

Protein Binding 40%

Half-Life Elimination ~6 hours

Metabolism Extensively hepatic via CYP1A2 to inactive metabolites; first-pass effect

Excretion Urine (<10% as unchanged drug, 60% as metabolites); Clearance: Reduced by 15% to 30% in patients >65 years of age

Available Dosage Forms

Tablet, oral: 0.25 mg, 0.5 mg, 1 mg, 2 mg, 3 mg, 4 mg, 5 mg

Requip®: 0.25 mg, 0.5 mg, 1 mg, 2 mg, 3 mg, 4 mg, 5 mg

Tablet, extended release, oral:

Requip® XL™: 2 mg, 4 mg, 6 mg, 8 mg, 12 mg

Dosing

Adult

Parkinson's disease: Oral:

Immediate release tablet: The dosage should be increased to achieve a maximum therapeutic effect, balanced against the principal side effects of nausea, dizziness, somnolence and dyskinesia. Recommended starting dose is 0.25 mg 3 times/day; based on individual patient response, the dosage should be titrated with weekly increments as described below:

- Week 1: 0.25 mg 3 times/day; total daily dose: 0.75 mg
- Week 2: 0.5 mg 3 times/day; total daily dose: 1.5 mg
- Week 3: 0.75 mg 3 times/day; total daily dose: 2.25 mg
- Week 4: 1 mg 3 times/day; total daily dose: 3 mg

Note: After week 4, if necessary, daily dosage may be increased by 1.5 mg/day on a weekly basis up to a dose of 9 mg/day, and then by up to 3 mg/day weekly to a total of 24 mg/day

Parkinson's disease discontinuation taper: Ropinirole should be gradually tapered over 7 days as follows: reduce frequency of administration from 3 times daily to twice daily for 4 days, then reduce to once daily for remaining 3 days.

Extended release tablet: Initial: 2 mg once daily for 1-2 weeks, followed by increases of 2 mg/day at weekly or longer intervals based on therapeutic response and tolerability (maximum: 24 mg/day); **Note:** When discontinuing gradually taper over 7 days.

Restless legs syndrome: Oral: Immediate release tablets: Initial: 0.25 mg once daily 1-3 hours before bedtime. Dose may be increased after 2 days to 0.5 mg daily, and after 7 days to 1 mg daily. Dose may be further titrated upward in 0.5 mg increments every week until reaching a daily dose of 3 mg during week 6. If symptoms persist or reappear, the daily dose may be increased to a maximum of 4 mg beginning week 7.

Note: Doses up to 4 mg per day may be discontinued without tapering.

Converting from ropinirole immediate release tablets to ropinirole extended-release tablets: Choose a once daily extended-release dose that most closely matches current immediate-release daily dose.

Geriatric Clearance is reduced; however, no dosage adjustment necessary. Titrate dose to clinical response. Refer to adult dosing.

Renal Impairment

Moderate renal impairment (Cl_{cr} 30-50 mL/minute): No adjustment needed

Severe renal impairment (Cl_{cr} <30 mL/minute): Use with caution; has not been studied in this patient population. **Note:** The Canadian labeling recommends to avoid use in patients with severe renal impairment and who are not undergoing regular hemodialysis.

Hemodialysis: Canadian labeling (not in U.S. labeling): Initial: 0.25 mg 3 times daily; may titrate dose upward based on tolerability and efficacy (maximum dose: 18 mg/day); post-dialysis supplemental doses are not required

Hepatic Impairment Titrate with caution; has not been studied.

Administration

Oral May be administered without regard to meals; taking with food may reduce nausea. Swallow extended-release tablet whole; do not crush, split, or chew.

Stability

Storage Store at controlled room temperature of 20°C to 25°C (68°F to 77°F). Protect from light.

Monitoring and Teaching Issues

Physical Assessment Monitor blood pressure periodically. Monitor for CNS depression/ somnolence.

Patient Education Take without regard to food. Avoid alcohol. May cause dizziness; sudden, overwhelming sleepiness; postural hypotension; loss of impulse control (possibly manifested as pathological gambling, libido increases, and/or binge eating); nausea; vomiting; lack of appetite; or mouth sores. Report unusual and persistent sleepiness, chest pain or palpitations, CNS changes (confusion, hallucinations, amnesia, abnormal dreaming, insomnia), suicide ideation, skeletal weakness or increased random tremors or movements, gait changes or difficulty walking, signs of urinary tract or respiratory infection (pain or burning on urination, pus or blood in urine, or unusual cough and chest tightness), changes in the appearance of skin moles, or other unusual skin changes.

Dietary Considerations May be taken without regard to meals; taking with food may reduce nausea.

Geriatric Considerations Since the dose is titrated to clinical response, no specific dosage adjustment is necessary in the elderly.

Breast-Feeding Considerations Ropinirole inhibits prolactin secretion in humans and may potentially inhibit lactation. It is not known if ropinirole is excreted into breast milk. Due to the potential for serious adverse reactions, a decision should be made whether to discontinue nursing or discontinue the drug, taking into account the importance of the drug to the mother.

Pregnancy Considerations Teratogenic effects have been observed in animal studies. There are no adequate and well-controlled studies in pregnant women; use only if potential benefit outweighs the risk to the fetus.

Additional Information If therapy with a drug known to be a potent inhibitor of CYP1A2 is stopped or started during treatment with ropinirole, adjustment of ropinirole dose may be required. Ropinirole binds to melanin-containing tissues (ie, eyes, skin) in pigmented rats. After a single dose, long-term retention of drug was demonstrated, with a half-life in the eye of 20 days; not known if ropinirole accumulates in these tissues over time.

◆ **Ropinirole Hydrochloride** *see* Ropinirole *on page 1606*

Rosiglitazone (roh si GLI ta zone)

U.S. Brand Names Avandia®

Generic Availability (U.S.) No

Pharmacologic Category Antidiabetic Agent, Thiazolidinedione

Medication Safety Issues

Sound-alike/look-alike issues:

Avandia® may be confused with Avalide®, Coumadin®, Prandin®

International issues:

Avandia [U.S., Canada, and multiple international markets] may be confused with Avanza brand name for mirtazapine [Australia]

Medication Guide Available Yes

Prescribing and Access Restrictions Health Canada requires written informed consent for new and current patients receiving rosiglitazone.

Pregnancy Risk Factor C

Lactation Excretion in breast milk unknown/not recommended

Use Type 2 diabetes mellitus (noninsulin dependent, NIDDM):

Monotherapy: Improve glycemic control as an adjunct to diet and exercise

Note: Canadian labeling approves use as monotherapy only when metformin is contraindicated or not tolerated.

Combination therapy: **Note:** Use when diet, exercise, and a single agent do not result in adequate glycemic control.

U.S. labeling: In combination with a sulfonylurea, metformin, or sulfonylurea plus metformin

Canadian labeling: In combination with metformin; in combination with a sulfonylurea only when metformin use is contraindicated or not tolerated

Mechanism of Action/Effect Thiazolidinedione antidiabetic agent that lowers blood glucose by improving target cell response to insulin, without increasing pancreatic insulin secretion. It has a mechanism of action that is dependent on the presence of insulin for activity.

Contraindications NYHA Class III/IV heart failure (initiation of therapy)

Canadian labeling: Hypersensitivity to rosiglitazone or any component of the formulation; any stage of heart failure (eg, NYHA Class I, II, III, IV); serious hepatic impairment; pregnancy

Warnings/Precautions [U.S. Boxed Warning]: Thiazolidinediones, including rosiglitazone, may cause or exacerbate congestive heart failure; closely monitor for signs/symptoms of congestive heart failure (eg, rapid weight gain, dyspnea, edema), particularly after initiation or dose increases. Not recommended for use in any patient with symptomatic heart failure. In the U.S., initiation of therapy is contraindicated in patients with NYHA class III or IV heart failure; in Canada use is contraindicated in patients with any stage of heart failure (NYHA Class I, II, III, IV). Use with caution in patients with edema; may increase plasma volume and/or cause fluid retention, leading to heart failure. Dose-related weight gain observed with use; mechanism unknown but likely associated with fluid retention and fat accumulation. Use may also be associated with an increased risk of angina and MI. Use caution in patients at risk for cardiovascular events and monitor closely. Discontinue if any deterioration in cardiac status occurs.

Should not be used in diabetic ketoacidosis. Mechanism requires the presence of insulin; therefore, use in type 1 diabetes (insulin dependent, IDDM) is not recommended. Combination therapy with other hypoglycemic agents may increase risk for hypoglycemic events; dose reduction with the concomitant agent may be warranted. Concomitant use with nitrates is not recommended due to increased risk of myocardial ischemia. Avoid use with insulin due to an increased risk of edema, congestive heart failure, and myocardial ischemic events.

Use with caution in patients with elevated transaminases (AST or ALT); do not initiate in patients with active liver disease or ALT >2.5 times ULN at baseline; evaluate patients with ALT ≤2.5 times ULN at baseline or during therapy for cause of enzyme elevation; during therapy, if ALT >3 times ULN, reevaluate levels promptly and discontinue if elevation persists or if jaundice occurs at any time during use. Idiosyncratic hepatotoxicity has been reported with another thiazolidinedione agent (troglitazone); avoid use in patients who previously experienced jaundice during troglitazone therapy. Monitoring should include periodic determinations of liver function. Increased incidence of bone fractures in females treated with rosiglitazone observed during analysis of long-term trial; majority of fractures occurred in the upper arm, hand, and foot ▶

(differing from the hip or spine fractures usually associated with postmenopausal osteoporosis). May decrease hemoglobin/hematocrit and/or WBC count (slight); effects may be related to increased plasma volume and/or dose related; use with caution in patients with anemia.

Rosiglitazone has been associated with new onset and/or worsening of macular edema in patients with diabetes. Rosiglitazone should be used with caution in patients with a pre-existing macular edema or diabetic retinopathy. Discontinuation of rosiglitazone should be considered in any patient who reports visual deterioration. In addition, ophthalmological consultation should be initiated in these patients. Use with caution in premenopausal, anovulatory women; may result in resumption of ovulation, increasing the risk of pregnancy. Safety and efficacy in pediatric patients have not been established.

Additional Canadian warnings (not included in U.S. labeling): If glycemic control is inadequate, rosiglitazone may be added to metformin or a sulfonylurea (if metformin use is contraindicated or not tolerated); use of triple therapy (rosiglitazone in combination with both metformin and a sulfonylurea) is not indicated due to increased risks of heart failure and fluid retention.

Drug Interactions

Metabolism/Transport Effects Substrate of CYP2C8 (major), 2C9 (minor); **Inhibits** CYP2C8 (moderate), 2C9 (weak), 2C19 (weak)

Avoid Concomitant Use There are no known interactions where it is recommended to avoid concomitant use.

Decreased Effect

The levels/effects of Rosiglitazone may be decreased by: Bile Acid Sequestrants; Corticosteroids (Orally Inhaled); Corticosteroids (Systemic); CYP2C8 Inducers (Highly Effective); Luteinizing Hormone-Releasing Hormone Analogs; Rifampin; Somatropin; Thiazide Diuretics

Increased Effect/Toxicity

Rosiglitazone may increase the levels/effects of: CYP2C8 Substrates (High risk); Hypoglycemic Agents

The levels/effects of Rosiglitazone may be increased by: CYP2C8 Inhibitors (Moderate); CYP2C8 Inhibitors (Strong); Deferasirox; Gemfibrozil; Herbs (Hypoglycemic Properties); Insulin; Pegvisomant; Pregabalin; Trimethoprim; Vasodilators (Organic Nitrates)

Nutritional/Ethanol Interactions

Ethanol: Avoid ethanol (may cause hypoglycemia).

Food: Peak concentrations are lower by 28% and delayed when administered with food, but these effects are not believed to be clinically significant.

Herb/Nutraceutical: Avoid alfalfa, aloe, bilberry, bitter melon, burdock, celery, damiana, fenugreek, garcinia, garlic, ginger, ginseng (American), gymnema, marshmallow, stinging nettle (may cause hypoglycemia).

Adverse Reactions Note: The rate of certain adverse reactions (eg, anemia, edema, hypoglycemia) may be higher with some combination therapies.

>10%: Endocrine & metabolic: HDL-cholesterol increased, LDL-cholesterol increased, total cholesterol increased, weight gain

1% to 10%:

Cardiovascular: Edema (5%), hypertension (4%); heart failure/CHF (up to 2% to 3% in patients receiving insulin; incidence likely higher in patients with pre-existing HF; myocardial ischemia (3%; incidence likely higher in patients with preexisting CAD)

Central nervous system: Headache (6%)

Endocrine & metabolic: Hypoglycemia (1% to 3%; combination therapy with insulin: 12% to 14%)

Gastrointestinal: Diarrhea (3%)

Hematologic: Anemia (2%)

Neuromuscular & skeletal: Fractures (up to 9%; incidence greater in females; usually upper arm, hand, or foot), arthralgia (5%), back pain (4% to 5%)

Respiratory: Upper respiratory tract infection (4% to 10%), nasopharyngitis (6%)

Miscellaneous: Injury (8%)

Pharmacodynamics/Kinetics

Onset of Action Delayed; Maximum effect: Up to 12 weeks

Bioavailability 99%

Time to Peak 1 hour; delayed with food

Protein Binding 99.8%; primarily albumin

Half-Life Elimination 3-4 hours

Metabolism Hepatic (99%) via CYP2C8; minor metabolism via CYP2C9

Excretion Urine (~64%) and feces (~23%) as metabolites

Available Dosage Forms

Tablet, oral:

Avandia®: 2 mg, 4 mg, 8 mg

Dosing

Adult & Geriatric Type 2 diabetes: Oral: **Note:** All patients should be initiated at the lowest recommended dose.

Monotherapy: Initial: 4 mg daily as a single daily dose or in divided doses twice daily. If response is inadequate after 8-12 weeks of treatment, the dosage may be increased to 8 mg daily as a single daily dose or in divided doses twice daily. In clinical trials, the 4 mg twice-daily regimen resulted in the greatest reduction in fasting plasma glucose and Hb A_{1c}.

Combination therapy: When adding rosiglitazone to existing therapy, continue current dose(s) of previous agents:

U.S. labeling: With sulfonylureas or metformin (or sulfonylurea plus metformin): Initial: 4 mg daily as a single daily dose or in divided doses twice daily. If response is inadequate after

8-12 weeks of treatment, the dosage may be increased to 8 mg daily as a single daily dose or in divided doses twice daily. Reduce dose of sulfonylurea if hypoglycemia occurs. It is unlikely that the dose of metformin will need to be reduced due to hypoglycemia.

Canadian labeling:

With metformin: Initial: 4 mg daily as a single daily dose or in divided doses twice daily. If response is inadequate after 8-12 weeks of treatment, the dosage may be increased to 8 mg daily as a single daily dose or in divided doses twice daily.

With a sulfonylurea: 4 mg daily as a single daily dose or in divided doses twice daily. Dose should not exceed 4 mg daily when using in combination with a sulfonylurea. Reduce dose of sulfonylurea if hypoglycemia occurs.

Renal Impairment No adjustment is necessary.

Hepatic Impairment Clearance is significantly lower in hepatic impairment. Therapy should not be initiated if the patient exhibits active liver disease or increased transaminases (ALT >2.5 times the upper limit of normal) at baseline.

Administration

Oral May be administered without regard to meals.

Stability

Storage Store at 15°C to 30°C (59°F to 86°F). Protect from light.

Monitoring and Teaching Issues

Laboratory Monitoring Hemoglobin A_{1c}, serum glucose; liver enzymes (prior to initiation of therapy, then periodically thereafter). Evaluate patients with ALT ≤2.5 times ULN at baseline or during therapy for cause of enzyme elevation. Patients with an elevation in ALT >3 times ULN should be rechecked as soon as possible. If the ALT levels remain >3 times ULN, therapy with rosiglitazone should be discontinued.

Physical Assessment Assess for signs of fluid retention and heart failure. Monitor weight. Monitor response to therapy closely until response is stable. Teach risks of hyperglycemia, its symptoms, treatment, and predisposing conditions. Refer patient to a diabetic educator, if possible.

Patient Education May be taken without regard to meals. If dose is missed at the usual meal, take it with next meal. Do not double dose if daily dose is missed completely. Monitor serum glucose as recommended by prescriber. More frequent monitoring is required during periods of stress, trauma, surgery, pregnancy, increased activity, or exercise. Avoid alcohol. Report chest pain, rapid heartbeat or palpitations, abdominal pain, fever, rash, hypoglycemia reactions, yellowing of skin or eyes, dark urine or light stool, unusual fatigue, or nausea/vomiting. Report unusually rapid weight gain; swelling of ankles, legs, or abdomen; or weakness or shortness of breath.

Dietary Considerations Management of type 2 diabetes mellitus (noninsulin dependent, NIDDM) should include diet control. May be taken without regard to meals.

Geriatric Considerations No dosage adjustment required. Due to the increased incidence of fractures in the hand, upper arm, and foot, rosiglitazone's benefits should be weighed against its risks in patients with a history of fractures, low bone mineral density, or falling. Intensive glucose control (Hb A_{1c} <6.5%) has been linked to increased all cause and cardiovascular mortality, hypoglycemia requiring assistance, and weight gain in adult type 2 diabetes. For elderly patients with diabetes who are relatively healthy, attaining target goals for aspirin use, blood pressure, lipids, smoking cessation, and diet and exercise may be more important than normalized glycemic control.

Breast-Feeding Considerations It is not known if rosiglitazone is excreted in breast milk. Breast-feeding is not recommended by the manufacturer.

Pregnancy Considerations Rosiglitazone is classified as pregnancy category C due to adverse effects observed in initial animal studies. Rosiglitazone has been found to cross the placenta during the first trimester of pregnancy. Inadvertent use early in pregnancy has not shown adverse fetal effects although in the majority of cases, the medication was stopped as soon as pregnancy was detected. Thiazolidinediones may cause ovulation in anovulatory premenopausal women, increasing the risk of pregnancy; adequate contraception in premenopausal women is recommended. Maternal hyperglycemia can be associated with adverse effects in the fetus, including macrosomia, neonatal hyperglycemia, and hyperbilirubinemia; the risk of congenital malformations is increased when the Hb A_{1c} is above the normal range. Diabetes can also be associated with adverse effects in the mother. Poorly-treated diabetes may cause end-organ damage that may in turn negatively affect obstetric outcomes. Physiologic glucose levels should be maintained prior to and during pregnancy to decrease the risk of adverse events in the mother and the fetus. Until additional safety and efficacy data are obtained, the use of oral agents is generally not recommended as routine management of GDM or type 2 diabetes mellitus during pregnancy. Insulin is the drug of choice for the control of diabetes mellitus during pregnancy.

Related Information

Diabetes Mellitus Management, Adults *on page* 2026

Rosiglitazone and Glimepiride (roh si GLI ta zone & GLYE me pye ride)

U.S. Brand Names Avandaryl®

Index Terms Glimepiride and Rosiglitazone Maleate

Generic Availability (U.S.) No

Pharmacologic Category Antidiabetic Agent, Sulfonylurea; Antidiabetic Agent, Thiazolidinedione

Medication Safety Issues

High alert medication: The Institute for Safe Medication Practices (ISMP) includes this medication among its list of drugs which have a heightened risk of causing significant patient harm when used in error.

Medication Guide Available Yes

Prescribing and Access Restrictions Health Canada requires written informed consent for new and current patients receiving rosiglitazone

Pregnancy Risk Factor C

Lactation Excretion in breast milk unknown/not recommended

Use Management of type 2 diabetes mellitus (noninsulin dependent, NIDDM) as an adjunct to diet and exercise

Available Dosage Forms

Tablet:

Avandaryl®: 4 mg/1 mg: Rosiglitazone 4 mg and glimepiride 1 mg; 4 mg/2 mg: Rosiglitazone 4 mg and glimepiride 2 mg; 4 mg/4 mg: Rosiglitazone 4 mg and glimepiride 4 mg; 8 mg/2 mg: Rosiglitazone 8 mg and glimepiride 2 mg; 8 mg/4 mg: Rosiglitazone 8 mg and glimepiride 4 mg

Dosing

Adult Type 2 diabetes mellitus: Oral: Initial: Rosiglitazone 4 mg and glimepiride 1 mg once daily **or** rosiglitazone 4 mg and glimepiride 2 mg once daily (for patients previously treated with sulfonylurea or thiazolidinedione monotherapy)

Patients switching from combination rosiglitazone and glimepiride as separate tablets: Use current dose.

Titration:

Dose adjustment in patients previously on sulfonylurea monotherapy: May take 2 weeks to observe decreased blood glucose and 2-3 months to see full effects of rosiglitazone component. If not adequately controlled after 8-12 weeks, increase daily dose of rosiglitazone component.

Dose adjustment in patients previously on thiazolidinedione monotherapy: If not adequately controlled after 1-2 weeks, increase daily dose of glimepiride component in ≤2 mg increments in 1-2 week intervals.

Maximum dose:

U.S. labeling: Rosiglitazone 8 mg and glimepiride 4 mg once daily

Canadian labeling: Rosiglitazone 4 mg and glimepiride 4 mg once daily

Geriatric Rosiglitazone 4 mg and glimepiride 1 mg once daily. Carefully titrate dose.

Renal Impairment Rosiglitazone 4 mg and glimepiride 1 mg once daily. Carefully titrate dose.

Hepatic Impairment Rosiglitazone 4 mg and glimepiride 1 mg once daily. Carefully titrate dose.

ALT ≤2.5 times ULN: Use with caution.

ALT >2.5 times ULN: Do not initiate therapy.

ALT >3 times ULN or jaundice: Discontinue.

Administration

Oral Should be administered with the first meal of the day.

Monitoring and Teaching Issues

Laboratory Monitoring Hemoglobin A_{1c}, fasting serum glucose; liver enzymes (prior to initiation of therapy, then periodically thereafter). Evaluate patients with ALT ≤2.5 times ULN at baseline or during therapy for cause of enzyme elevation. Patients with an elevation in ALT >3 times ULN should be rechecked as soon as possible. If the ALT levels remain >3 times ULN, therapy should be discontinued.

Physical Assessment See individual agents.

Patient Education See individual agents.

Related Information

Glimepiride *on page 870*

Rosiglitazone *on page 1609*

Rosiglitazone and Metformin (roh si GLI ta zone & met FOR min)

U.S. Brand Names Avandamet®

Index Terms Metformin and Rosiglitazone; Metformin Hydrochloride and Rosiglitazone Maleate; Rosiglitazone Maleate and Metformin Hydrochloride

Generic Availability (U.S.) No

Pharmacologic Category Antidiabetic Agent, Biguanide; Antidiabetic Agent, Thiazolidinedione

Medication Safety Issues

Sound-alike/look-alike issues:

Avandamet® may be confused with Anzemet®

Medication Guide Available Yes

Prescribing and Access Restrictions

Health Canada requires written informed consent for new and current patients receiving rosiglitazone.

Pregnancy Risk Factor C

Lactation

Rosiglitazone: Excretion in breast milk unknown/not recommended

Metformin: Enters breast milk/not recommended

Use Management of type 2 diabetes mellitus (noninsulin dependent, NIDDM) as an adjunct to diet and exercise in patients where dual rosiglitazone and metformin therapy is appropriate

Available Dosage Forms

Tablet:

Avandamet®: 2/500: Rosiglitazone 2 mg and metformin 500 mg; 4/500: Rosiglitazone 4 mg and metformin 500 mg; 2/1000: Rosiglitazone 2 mg and metformin 1000 mg; 4/1000: Rosiglitazone 4 mg and metformin 1000 mg

Dosing

Adult Type 2 diabetes mellitus: Oral:

First-line therapy (drug-naive patients): Initial: Rosiglitazone 2 mg and metformin 500 mg once or twice daily; may increase by 2 mg/500 mg per day after 4 weeks to a maximum of 8 mg/2000 mg per day.

Second-line therapy:

Patients inadequately controlled on metformin alone: Initial dose: Rosiglitazone 4 mg/day plus current dose of metformin

Patients inadequately controlled on rosiglitazone alone: Initial dose: Metformin 1000 mg/day plus current dose of rosiglitazone

Note: When switching from combination rosiglitazone and metformin as separate tablets: Use current dose

Dose adjustment: Doses may be increased as increments of rosiglitazone 4 mg and/or metformin 500 mg, up to the maximum dose; doses should be titrated gradually.

After a change in the metformin dosage, titration can be done after 1-2 weeks

After a change in the rosiglitazone dosage, titration can be done after 8-12 weeks

Maximum dose: Rosiglitazone 8 mg/metformin 2000 mg daily

Geriatric The initial and maintenance dosing should be conservative, due to the potential for decreased renal function (monitor). Generally, elderly patients should not be titrated to the maximum. Do not use in patients ≥80 years unless normal renal function has been established.

Renal Impairment Do not use with renal disease or renal dysfunction (serum creatinine ≥1.5 mg/dL in males or ≥1.4 mg/dL in females or abnormal clearance).

Hepatic Impairment Do not initiate therapy with active liver disease or ALT >2.5 times the upper limit of normal.

Administration

Oral Administer with meals. Patients who are NPO may need to have their dose held to avoid hypoglycemia.

Monitoring and Teaching Issues

Laboratory Monitoring See individual components listed in Related Information.

Physical Assessment See individual agents.

Patient Education See individual agents.

Related Information

MetFORMIN *on page 1182*

Rosiglitazone *on page 1609*

◆ **Rosiglitazone Maleate and Metformin Hydrochloride** *see* Rosiglitazone and Metformin *on page 1612*

Rosuvastatin (roe soo va STAT in)

U.S. Brand Names Crestor®

Index Terms Rosuvastatin Calcium

Generic Availability (U.S.) No

Pharmacologic Category Antilipemic Agent, HMG-CoA Reductase Inhibitor

Medication Safety Issues

Sound-alike/look-alike issues:

Rosuvastatin may be confused with atorvastatin, nystatin, pitavastatin

Pregnancy Risk Factor X

Lactation Excretion in breast milk unknown/contraindicated

Use

Treatment of dyslipidemias:

Used with dietary therapy for hyperlipidemias to reduce elevations in total cholesterol (TC), LDL-C, apolipoprotein B, nonHDL-C, and triglycerides (TG) in patients with primary hypercholesterolemia (elevations of 1 or more components are present in Fredrickson type IIa, IIb, and IV hyperlipidemias); increase HDL-C; treatment of primary dysbetalipoproteinemia (Fredrickson type III hyperlipidemia); treatment of homozygous familial hypercholesterolemia (FH); to slow progression of atherosclerosis as an adjunct to diet to lower TC and LDL-C

Heterozygous familial hypercholesterolemia (HeFH): In adolescent patients (10-17 years of age, females >1 year postmenarche) with HeFH having LDL-C >190 mg/dL or LDL >160 mg/dL with positive family history of premature cardiovascular disease (CVD), or ≥2 other CVD risk factors.

Primary prevention of cardiovascular disease: To reduce the risk of stroke, myocardial infarction, or arterial revascularization procedures in patients without clinically evident coronary heart disease or lipid abnormalities but with all of the following: 1) an increased risk of cardiovascular disease based on age ≥50 years old in men and ≥60 years old in women, 2) hsCRP ≥2 mg/L, and 3) the presence of at least one additional cardiovascular disease risk factor such as hypertension, low HDL-C, smoking, or a family history of premature coronary heart disease.

Secondary prevention of cardiovascular disease: To slow progression of atherosclerosis

Mechanism of Action/Effect Inhibitor of 3-hydroxy-3-methylglutaryl coenzyme A (HMG-CoA) reductase, the rate limiting enzyme in cholesterol synthesis (reduces the production of mevalonic acid from HMG-CoA); lowers TC, LDL-C, TG and improves HDL:LDL ratio

Contraindications Hypersensitivity to rosuvastatin or any component of the formulation; active liver disease; unexplained persistent elevations of serum transaminases (>3 times ULN); pregnancy; breast-feeding

Canadian labeling: Additional contraindications (not in U.S. labeling): Concomitant administration of cyclosporine; use of 40 mg dose in Asian patients, patients with predisposing risk factors for myopathy/rhabdomyolysis (eg, hereditary muscle disorders, history of myotoxicity with other HMC-CoA reductase inhibitors, concomitant use with fibrates or niacin, severe hepatic impairment, severe renal impairment [Cl_{cr} <30 mL/minute/1.73 m^2], hypothyroidism, alcohol abuse)

Warnings/Precautions Secondary causes of hyperlipidemia should be ruled out prior to therapy. Rosuvastatin has not been studied when the primary lipid abnormality is chylomicron elevation (Fredrickson types I and V). Liver function must be monitored by periodic laboratory assessment. Use with caution in patients who consume large amounts of ethanol or have a history of liver disease. Use is contraindicated with active liver disease or unexplained transaminase elevations; may cause hepatic dysfunction. Rhabdomyolysis with acute renal failure has occurred. Hematuria (microscopic) and proteinuria have been observed; more commonly reported in patients receiving rosuvastatin 40 mg daily. Typically, transient and not associated with a decrease in renal function. Consider dosage reduction if unexplained hematuria and proteinuria persists. Discontinue in any patient in which CPK levels are markedly elevated (>10 times ULN) or if myopathy is suspected/diagnosed. An increased incidence of rosuvastatin-associated myopathy has been reported during concomitant therapy with fibric acid derivatives, niacin, cyclosporine, and lopinavir/ritonavir, and in certain subgroups of the Asian population; dosage adjustment should be considered for patients of Asian descent. The Canadian labeling contraindicates concomitant use of rosuvastatin with cyclosporine and the use of rosuvastatin 40 mg/day in Asian patients and/or patients receiving fibrates or niacin. Use with caution with concurrent protease inhibitor/ritonavir combinations. Atazanavir/ritonavir and lopinavir/ritonavir significantly increase rosuvastatin serum concentration; limit dose of rosuvastatin to 10 mg/day. Monitor closely if used with other drugs associated with myopathy (eg, colchicine). Risk is also elevated at higher dosages of rosuvastatin. Patients should be instructed to report unexplained muscle pain, tenderness, or weakness, particularly if associated with fever and/or malaise. Use caution in patients predisposed to myopathy (eg, renal failure, advanced age, inadequately treated hypothyroidism). Temporarily withhold in patients experiencing an acute or serious condition predisposing to renal failure secondary to rhabdomyolysis (sepsis, hypotension, major surgery, trauma, severe metabolic or endocrine or electrolyte disorders, uncontrolled seizures). Based upon current evidence, HMG-CoA reductase inhibitor therapy should be continued in the perioperative period unless risk outweighs cardioprotective benefit. In the JUPITER study, small increases in hemoglobin (Hb) A1c (mean HbA1c increased by ~0.1%) and physician-reported diabetes was significantly higher in the rosuvastatin group compared to placebo (Ridker, 2008). Overall, evidence supporting an association with diabetes risk is lacking. Because the clear benefits on cardiovascular disease risk outweigh any potential detrimental effects on glucose metabolism, the use of HMG-CoA reductase inhibitors in patients with diabetes continues to be recommended (ADA, 2011).

Drug Interactions

Metabolism/Transport Effects Substrate (minor) of CYP2C9, CYP3A4, SLCO1B1

Avoid Concomitant Use

Avoid concomitant use of Rosuvastatin with any of the following: Red Yeast Rice

Decreased Effect

The levels/effects of Rosuvastatin may be decreased by: Antacids

Increased Effect/Toxicity

Rosuvastatin may increase the levels/effects of: DAPTOmycin; Trabectedin; Vitamin K Antagonists

The levels/effects of Rosuvastatin may be increased by: Amiodarone; Colchicine; Conivaptan; CycloSPORINE; CycloSPORINE (Systemic); Eltrombopag; Fenofibrate; Fenofibric Acid; Gemfibrozil; Niacin; Niacinamide; Protease Inhibitors; Red Yeast Rice

Nutritional/Ethanol Interactions

Ethanol: Avoid excessive ethanol consumption (due to potential hepatic effects).

Food: Red yeast rice contains an estimated 2.4 mg lovastatin per 600 mg rice.

Adverse Reactions

>10%: Neuromuscular & skeletal: Myalgia (3% to 13%)

2% to 10%:

Central nervous system: Headache (6%), dizziness (4%)

Gastrointestinal: Nausea (3%), abdominal pain (2%), constipation (2%)

Hepatic: ALT increased (2%; >3 times ULN)

Neuromuscular & skeletal: Arthralgia (4% to 10%), CPK increased (3%; >10 x ULN: Children 3%), weakness (3%)

Adverse reactions reported with other HMG-CoA reductase inhibitors (not necessarily reported with rosuvastatin therapy) include a hypersensitivity syndrome (symptoms may include anaphylaxis, angioedema, arthralgia, erythema multiforme, eosinophilia, hemolytic anemia, interstitial lung disease, lupus syndrome, photosensitivity, polymyalgia rheumatica, positive ANA, purpura, Stevens-Johnson syndrome, toxic epidermal necrolysis, urticaria, vasculitis)

Pharmacodynamics/Kinetics

Onset of Action Within 1 week; maximal at 4 weeks

Bioavailability 20% (high first-pass extraction by liver)

Time to Peak Plasma: 3-5 hours

Protein Binding 88%

Half-Life Elimination 19 hours

Metabolism Hepatic (10%), via CYP2C9 (1 active metabolite identified: N-desmethyl rosuvastatin, one-sixth to one-half the HMG-CoA reductase activity of the parent compound)

Excretion Feces (90%), primarily as unchanged drug

Pharmacokinetic Note Asian patients have been noted to have increased bioavailability.

Available Dosage Forms

Tablet, oral:

Crestor®: 5 mg, 10 mg, 20 mg, 40 mg

Dosing

Adult & Geriatric Note: Doses should be individualized according to the baseline LDL-cholesterol levels, the recommended goal of therapy, and patient response; adjustments should be made at intervals of 4 weeks or more.

Hyperlipidemia, mixed dyslipidemia, hypertriglyceridemia, primary dysbetalipoproteinemia, slowing progression of atherosclerosis: Oral:

Initial dose:

General dosing: 10 mg once daily; 20 mg once daily may be used in patients with severe hyperlipidemia (LDL >190 mg/dL) and aggressive lipid targets

Conservative dosing: Patients requiring less aggressive treatment or predisposed to myopathy (including patients of Asian descent): 5 mg once daily

Titration: After 2 weeks, may be increased by 5-10 mg once daily; dosing range: 5-40 mg/day (maximum dose: 40 mg once daily)

Note: The 40 mg dose should be reserved for patients who have not achieved goal cholesterol levels on a dose of 20 mg/day, including patients switched from another HMG-CoA reductase inhibitor.

Homozygous familial hypercholesterolemia (FH): Oral: Initial: 20 mg once daily (maximum dose: 40 mg/day)

Dosage adjustment with concomitant medications: Oral:

U.S. labeling:

Cyclosporine: Rosuvastatin dose should not exceed 5 mg/day

Gemfibrozil: Avoid concurrent use; if unable to avoid concurrent use, rosuvastatin dose should not exceed 10 mg/day

Atazanavir/ritonavir or lopinavir/ritonavir: Rosuvastatin dose should not exceed 10 mg/day

Canadian labeling:

Cyclosporine: Concomitant use is contraindicated

Gemfibrozil: Rosuvastatin dose should not exceed 20 mg/day

Dosage adjustment for hematuria and/or persistent, unexplained proteinuria while on 40 mg/day: Reduce dose and evaluate causes.

Pediatric Note: Doses should be individualized according to the baseline LDL-cholesterol levels, the recommended goal of therapy, and patient response; adjustments should be made at intervals of 4 weeks or more.

Heterozygous familial hypercholesterolemia (HeFH):

U.S. labeling: Children 10-17 years (females >1 year postmenarche): Oral: 5-20 mg once daily; maximum: 20 mg/day

Dosage adjustment for rosuvastatin with concomitant cyclosporine, atazanavir/ritonavir or lopinavir/ritonavir: Refer to drug-specific dosing in adult dosing section.

Canadian labeling: Oral: 5-10 mg once daily; maximum: 10 mg/day

Renal Impairment

Mild-to-moderate impairment: No dosage adjustment required.

Cl_{cr} <30 mL/minute/1.73 m^2: Initial: 5 mg/day; do not exceed 10 mg once daily

Hepatic Impairment

U.S. labeling: Active hepatic disease, including unexplained persistent transaminase elevations: Use is contraindicated.

Canadian labeling:

Active hepatic disease or unexplained persistent transaminase >3 x ULN: Use is contraindicated.

Mild-to-moderate impairment: No dosage adjustment required.

Severe impairment: Initial: 5 mg/day; do not exceed 20 mg once daily.

Administration

Oral May be administered with or without food. May be taken at any time of the day.

Stability

Storage Store between 20°C and 25°C (68°F to 77°F). Protect from moisture.

Monitoring and Teaching Issues

Laboratory Monitoring Total cholesterol, LDL, and HDL cholesterol within 2-4 weeks of treatment initiation or dose change; liver function tests should be determined at baseline (prior to initiation), 3 months following initiation, 3 months after any increase in dose, and periodically thereafter (eg, semiannually); baseline CPK (recheck CPK in any patient with symptoms suggestive of myopathy). Monitor LDL-C at intervals no less than 4 weeks.

Physical Assessment Use caution with history of hepatic or renal disease. Assess risk potential for interactions with other prescriptions or herbal products patient may be taking that may increase risk of myopathy or rhabdomyolysis. Assess LFTs or cholesterol profile prior to treatment and at regular intervals. Teach proper diet and exercise regimen.

Patient Education Take at same time each day, with or without food. Follow prescribed cholesterol-lowering diet and exercise regimen. You will have periodic blood tests to assess effectiveness. Avoid excessive alcohol. Report unusual muscle cramping or weakness, yellowing of skin or eyes, easy bruising or bleeding, or unusual fatigue.

Dietary Considerations May be taken with or without food. Red yeast rice contains an estimated 2.4 mg lovastatin per 600 mg rice.

Geriatric Considerations Effective and well tolerated in the elderly. The definition of and, therefore, when to treat hyperlipidemia in geriatrics is a controversial issue. The National Cholesterol Education Program recommends that all adults maintain a plasma cholesterol <160 mg/dL. Elderly with one additional risk factor, goal LDL would be <130 mg/dL. It is the authors' belief that pharmacologic treatment be reserved for those who are unable to obtain a desirable plasma cholesterol concentration by diet alone and for whom the benefits of treatment are believed to outweigh the potential adverse effects, drug interactions, and cost of treatment.

Pregnancy Considerations Cholesterol biosynthesis may be important in fetal development. Contraindicated in pregnancy. Administer to women of childbearing potential only when conception is highly unlikely and patients have been informed of potential hazards.

Related Information

Hyperlipidemia Management *on page 2046*

◆ **Rosuvastatin Calcium** *see* Rosuvastatin *on page 1613*

◆ **Rotarix®** *see* Rotavirus Vaccine *on page 1616*

◆ **RotaTeq®** *see* Rotavirus Vaccine *on page 1616*

Rotavirus Vaccine (ROE ta vye rus vak SEEN)

U.S. Brand Names Rotarix®; RotaTeq®

Index Terms Human Rotavirus Vaccine, Attenuated (HRV); Pentavalent Human-Bovine Reassortant Rotavirus Vaccine (PRV); Rotavirus Vaccine, Pentavalent; RV1 (Rotarix®); RV5 (RotaTeq®)

Generic Availability (U.S.) No

Pharmacologic Category Vaccine, Live (Viral)

Pregnancy Risk Factor C

Use Prevention of rotavirus gastroenteritis in infants and children

The Advisory Committee on Immunization Practices (ACIP) recommends routine vaccination of all infants.

Available Dosage Forms

Powder, for suspension, oral [preservative free; human derived]:

Rotarix®: G1P[8] ≥10^6 infectious units per 1 mL [oral applicator contains natural latex/natural rubber]

Suspension, oral [preservative free]:

RotaTeq®: G1 ≥2.2 10^6 infectious units, G2 ≥2.8 10^6 infectious units, G3 ≥2.2 10^6 infectious units, G4 ≥2 10^6 infectious units, and P1 [8] ≥2.3 10^6 infectious units per 2 mL (2 mL)

Dosing

Pediatric Prevention of rotavirus gastroenteritis: Oral:

Manufacturer's labeling:

Infants 6-24 weeks of age: Rotarix®: A total of two 1 mL doses, the first dose given at 6 weeks of age. The first and second dose should be separated by ≥4 weeks. The 2-dose series should be completed by 24 weeks of age.

Infants 6-32 weeks: RotaTeq®: A total of three 2 mL doses given at 2-, 4-, and 6 months of age; the first given at 6-12 weeks of age, followed by subsequent doses at 4- to 10-week intervals. Administer all doses by 32 weeks of age.

ACIP recommendations: The first dose can be given at 6-14 weeks of age. The series should not be started in infants ≥15 weeks. The final dose in the series should be administered by 8 months 0 days of age. The minimum interval between doses is 4 weeks. RotaTeq® should be given in 3 doses administered at 2-, 4-, and 6 months of age. Rotarix® should be given in 2 doses administered at 2- and 4 months of age. For infants inadvertently administered rotavirus vaccine at ≥15 weeks of age, the vaccine series may be completed according to schedule. The ACIP recommendations for vaccination recommend completing the vaccine series with the same product whenever possible. If continuing with same product will cause vaccination to be deferred, or if product used previously is unknown, vaccination should be completed with the product available. If RotaTeq® was used in any previous doses, or if the specific product used was unknown, a total of 3 doses should be given. Infants who have had rotavirus gastroenteritis before getting the full course of vaccine should still initiate or complete the recommended schedule; initial infection provides only partial immunity.

Administration

Oral

Rotarix®: Using oral applicator, administer contents into infant's inner cheek. Dispose of applicator and vaccine vial in biologic waste container.

RotaTeq®: Gently squeeze dose from ready-to-use dosing tube into infant's inner cheek. After use, dispose of the empty tube and cap in a biologic waste container.

Note: A single dose of the rotavirus vaccine should not be readministered to an infant who regurgitates, spits out, or vomits the vaccine during administration. Any remaining dose(s) should be administered on schedule (CDC, 2009).

Simultaneous administration of vaccines helps ensure the patients will be fully vaccinated by the appropriate age. Simultaneous administration of vaccines is defined as administering >1 vaccine on the same day at different anatomic sites. Separate vaccines should not be combined in the same syringe unless indicated by product specific labeling. The ACIP prefers each dose of a specific vaccine in a series come from the same manufacturer when possible. In general, preterm infants should be vaccinated at the same chronological age as full-term infants (CDC, 2011).

Antipyretics have not been shown to prevent febrile seizures. Antipyretics may be used to treat fever or discomfort following vaccination (CDC, 2011). One study reported that routine prophylactic administration of acetaminophen to prevent fever prior to vaccination decreased the immune response of some vaccines; the clinical significance of this reduction in immune response has not been established (Prymula, 2009).

Monitoring and Teaching Issues

Physical Assessment Have treatment for anaphylactoid or hypersensitivity reaction available. If latex sensitive, be advised that packaging may contain latex. Consider deferring administration in patients with moderate or severe acute illness; may administer to patients with mild acute illness (with or without fever). Federal law requires entry into the patient's medical record.

Patient Education May experience fever, irritability, diarrhea, vomiting, and otitis media. Acetaminophen may be helpful. Notify prescriber if symptoms persist.

Related Information

Immunization Recommendations *on page 1941*

- ◆ **Rotavirus Vaccine, Pentavalent** *see* Rotavirus Vaccine *on page 1616*
- ◆ **Rowasa®** *see* Mesalamine *on page 1177*
- ◆ **Roxanol** *see* Morphine (Systemic) *on page 1258*
- ◆ **Roxicet™** *see* Oxycodone and Acetaminophen *on page 1383*
- ◆ **Roxicet™ 5/500** *see* Oxycodone and Acetaminophen *on page 1383*
- ◆ **Roxicodone®** *see* OxyCODONE *on page 1380*
- ◆ **Rozerem™** *see* Ramelteon *on page 1550*
- ◆ **RP-6976** *see* Docetaxel *on page 563*
- ◆ **RP-54274** *see* Riluzole *on page 1582*
- ◆ **RP-59500** *see* Quinupristin and Dalfopristin *on page 1543*
- ◆ **r-PA** *see* Reteplase *on page 1567*
- ◆ **RPR-116258A** *see* Cabazitaxel *on page 264*
- ◆ **(R,R)-Formoterol L-Tartrate** *see* Arformoterol *on page 141*
- ◆ **RS-25259** *see* Palonosetron *on page 1396*
- ◆ **RS-25259-197** *see* Palonosetron *on page 1396*
- ◆ **RTCA** *see* Ribavirin *on page 1571*
- ◆ **RU 0211** *see* Lubiprostone *on page 1139*
- ◆ **RU-486** *see* Mifepristone *on page 1229*
- ◆ **RU-23908** *see* Nilutamide *on page 1319*
- ◆ **RU-38486** *see* Mifepristone *on page 1229*
- ◆ **Rubella, Measles and Mumps Vaccines** *see* Measles, Mumps, and Rubella Virus Vaccine *on page 1150*
- ◆ **Rubella, Varicella, Measles, and Mumps Vaccine** *see* Measles, Mumps, Rubella, and Varicella Virus Vaccine *on page 1151*
- ◆ **Rubidomycin Hydrochloride** *see* DAUNOrubicin Hydrochloride *on page 474*
- ◆ **RUF 331** *see* Rufinamide *on page 1617*

Rufinamide (roo FIN a mide)

U.S. Brand Names Banzel®

Index Terms CGP 33101; E 2080; RUF 331; Xilep

Generic Availability (U.S.) No

Pharmacologic Category Anticonvulsant, Triazole Derivative

Medication Guide Available Yes

Pregnancy Risk Factor C

Lactation Excretion in breast milk unknown/not recommended

Use Adjunctive therapy in the treatment of generalized seizures of Lennox-Gastaut syndrome

Available Dosage Forms

Suspension, oral:

Banzel®: 40 mg/mL (460 mL)

Tablet, oral:

Banzel®: 200 mg, 400 mg

Dosing

Adult & Geriatric Lennox-Gastaut (adjunctive): Oral: Initial: 400-800 mg/day in 2 equally divided doses; increase dose by 400-800 mg/day every other day to a target dose of 3200 mg/day in 2 equally divided doses

Dosage adjustment for concomitant medications: Valproate: Initial rufinamide dose should be <400 mg/day

Pediatric Lennox-Gastaut (adjunctive): Children ≥4 years: Oral: Initial: 10 mg/kg/day in 2 equally divided doses; increase dose by ~10 mg/kg every other day to a target dose of 45 mg/kg/day **or** 3200 mg/day (whichever is lower) in 2 equally divided doses

Dosage adjustment for concomitant medications: Valproate: Initial rufinamide dose should be <10 mg/kg/day

Renal Impairment

Cl_{cr} <30 mL/minute: No dosage adjustment needed.

Hemodialysis: No specific guidelines available; consider dosage adjustment for loss of drug.

Hepatic Impairment

Mild-to-moderate impairment: Use caution.

Severe impairment: Use in severe impairment has not been studied and is not recommended.

Administration

Oral Administer with food. Tablets may be swallowed whole, split in half, or crushed. Oral suspension should be administered using the provided adapter and oral syringe; shake well before every administration.

Monitoring and Teaching Issues

Laboratory Monitoring Serum levels of concurrent anticonvulsants

Physical Assessment Monitor for signs and symptoms of suicide ideation (eg, anxiety, depression, unusual mood or behavior changes).

Patient Education Take with food. Avoid alcohol. You may experience drowsiness or dizziness. May cause headache, fatigue, nausea, or vomiting. Report suicide ideation, depression, rash (especially if accompanied by fever), problems with vision, tremors, or problems with gait.

- ◆ **RV1 (Rotarix®)** *see* Rotavirus Vaccine *on page* 1616
- ◆ **RV5 (RotaTeq®)** *see* Rotavirus Vaccine *on page* 1616
- ◆ **Rybix™ ODT** *see* TraMADol *on page* 1797
- ◆ **Rythmol®** *see* Propafenone *on page* 1520
- ◆ **Rythmol® SR** *see* Propafenone *on page* 1520
- ◆ **Ryzolt™** *see* TraMADol *on page* 1797
- ◆ **S2® [OTC]** *see* EPINEPHrine (Systemic, Oral Inhalation) *on page* 629
- ◆ **S-(+)-3-isobutylgaba** *see* Pregabalin *on page* 1504
- ◆ **S-4661** *see* Doripenem *on page* 573
- ◆ **Safyral™** *see* Ethinyl Estradiol, Drospirenone, and Levomefolate *on page* 706
- ◆ **SAHA** *see* Vorinostat *on page* 1875
- ◆ **Saizen®** *see* Somatropin *on page* 1664
- ◆ **Salbutamol** *see* Albuterol *on page* 58
- ◆ **Salbutamol and Ipratropium** *see* Ipratropium and Albuterol *on page* 1011
- ◆ **Salbutamol Sulphate** *see* Albuterol *on page* 58
- ◆ **Salicylazosulfapyridine** *see* Sulfasalazine *on page* 1688
- ◆ **Salk Vaccine** *see* Poliovirus Vaccine (Inactivated) *on page* 1473

Salmeterol (sal ME te role)

U.S. Brand Names Serevent® Diskus®

Index Terms Salmeterol Xinafoate

Generic Availability (U.S.) No

Pharmacologic Category $Beta_2$-Adrenergic Agonist; $Beta_2$-Adrenergic Agonist, Long-Acting

Medication Safety Issues

Sound-alike/look-alike issues:

Salmeterol may be confused with Salbutamol, Solu-Medrol®

Serevent® may be confused with Atrovent®, Combivent®, Serentil®, sertraline, Sinemet®, Spiriva®, Zoloft®

Medication Guide Available Yes

Pregnancy Risk Factor C

Lactation Enters breast milk/use caution

Use Maintenance treatment of asthma and prevention of bronchospasm (as concomitant therapy) in patients with reversible obstructive airway disease, including patients with symptoms of nocturnal asthma; prevention of exercise-induced bronchospasm (monotherapy may be indicated in patients without persistent asthma); maintenance treatment of bronchospasm associated with COPD

Mechanism of Action/Effect Relaxes bronchial smooth muscle by selective action on $beta_2$-receptors with little effect on heart rate; salmeterol acts locally in the lung.

Contraindications Hypersensitivity to salmeterol or any component of the formulation (milk proteins); monotherapy in the treatment of asthma (ie, use without a concomitant long-term asthma control medication, such as an inhaled corticosteroid); status asthmaticus or other acute episodes of asthma or COPD

Warnings/Precautions

Asthma treatment: [U.S. Boxed Warning]: Long-acting beta$_2$-agonists (LABAs) increase the risk of asthma-related deaths. Salmeterol should only be used in asthma patients as adjuvant therapy in patients who are currently receiving but are not adequately controlled on a long-term asthma control medication (ie, an inhaled corticosteroid). Monotherapy with an LABA is contraindicated in the treatment of asthma. In a large, randomized, placebo-controlled U.S. clinical trial (SMART, 2006), salmeterol was associated with an increase in asthma-related deaths (when added to usual asthma therapy); risk is considered a class effect among all LABAs. Data are not available to determine if the addition of an inhaled corticosteroid lessens this increased risk of death associated with LABA use. Assess patients at regular intervals once asthma control is maintained on combination therapy to determine if step-down therapy is appropriate and the LABA can be discontinued (without loss of asthma control), and the patient can be maintained on an inhaled corticosteroid. LABAs are not appropriate in patients whose asthma is adequately controlled on low- or medium-dose inhaled corticosteroids. Do **not** use for acute bronchospasm. Short-acting beta$_2$-agonist (eg, albuterol) should be used for acute symptoms and symptoms occurring between treatments. Do **not** initiate in patients with significantly worsening or acutely deteriorating asthma; reports of severe (sometimes fatal) respiratory events have been reported when salmeterol has been initiated in this situation. Corticosteroids should not be stopped or reduced when salmeterol is initiated. During initiation, watch for signs of worsening asthma. Patients must be instructed to use short-acting beta$_2$-agonists (eg, albuterol) for acute asthmatic or COPD symptoms and to seek medical attention in cases where acute symptoms are not relieved or a previous level of response is diminished. The need to increase frequency of use of short-acting beta$_2$-agonist may indicate deterioration of asthma, and treatment must not be delayed. Because LABAs may disguise poorly controlled persistent asthma, frequent or chronic use of LABAs for exercise-induced bronchospasm is discouraged by the NIH Asthma Guidelines (NIH, 2007). Salmeterol should not be used more than twice daily; do not use with other long-acting beta$_2$-agonists. **[U.S. Boxed Warning]: LABAs may increase the risk of asthma-related hospitalization in pediatric and adolescent patients.** In general, a combination product containing a LABA and an inhaled corticosteroid is preferred in patients <18 years of age to ensure compliance.

COPD treatment: Appropriate use: Do **not** use for acute episodes of COPD. Do **not** initiate in patients with significantly worsening or acutely deteriorating COPD. Data are not available to determine if LABA use increases the risk of death in patients with COPD.

Concurrent diseases: Use caution in patients with cardiovascular disease (eg, arrhythmia, hypertension, or HF), seizure disorders, diabetes, hyperthyroidism, hepatic impairment, or hypokalemia. Beta-agonists may cause elevation in blood pressure, heart rate, CNS stimulation/excitation, increased risk of arrhythmia, increase serum glucose, or decrease serum potassium.

Adverse events: Immediate hypersensitivity reactions (urticaria, angioedema, rash, bronchospasm) have been reported. There have been reports of laryngeal spasm, irritation, swelling (stridor, choking) with use. Salmeterol should not be used more than twice daily; do not exceed recommended dose; do not use with other long-acting beta$_2$-agonists; serious adverse events have been associated with excessive use of inhaled sympathomimetics. Rarely, paradoxical bronchospasm may occur with use of inhaled bronchodilating agents; this should be distinguished from inadequate response. Use with strong CYP3A4 inhibitors (see Drug Interactions) is not recommended due to potential for an increased risk of cardiovascular events. Powder for oral inhalation contains lactose; very rare anaphylactic reactions have been reported in patients with severe milk protein allergy.

Drug Interactions

Metabolism/Transport Effects Substrate of CYP3A4 (major)

Avoid Concomitant Use

Avoid concomitant use of Salmeterol with any of the following: CYP3A4 Inhibitors (Strong); Iobenguane I 123

Decreased Effect

Salmeterol may decrease the levels/effects of: Iobenguane I 123

The levels/effects of Salmeterol may be decreased by: Alpha-/Beta-Blockers; Beta-Blockers (Beta1 Selective); Beta-Blockers (Nonselective); Betahistine

Increased Effect/Toxicity

Salmeterol may increase the levels/effects of: Loop Diuretics; Sympathomimetics

The levels/effects of Salmeterol may be increased by: Atomoxetine; Cannabinoids; CYP3A4 Inhibitors (Moderate); CYP3A4 Inhibitors (Strong); MAO Inhibitors; Tricyclic Antidepressants

Adverse Reactions

>10%:

- Central nervous system: Headache (13% to 17%)
- Neuromuscular & skeletal: Pain (1% to 12%)

1% to 10%:

- Cardiovascular: Hypertension (4%), edema (1% to 3%), pallor
- Central nervous system: Dizziness (4%), sleep disturbance (1% to 3%), fever (1% to 3%), anxiety (1% to 3%), migraine (1% to 3%)
- Dermatologic: Rash (1% to 4%), contact dermatitis (1% to 3%), eczema (1% to 3%), urticaria (3%), photodermatitis (1% to 2%)

Endocrine & metabolic: Hyperglycemia (1% to 3%)
Gastrointestinal: Throat irritation (7%), nausea (1% to 3%), dyspepsia (1% to 3%), dental pain (1% to 3%), gastrointestinal infection (1% to 3%), oropharyngeal candidiasis (1% to 3%), xerostomia (1% to 3%)
Hepatic: Liver enzymes increased
Neuromuscular & skeletal: Muscular cramps/spasm (3%), articular rheumatism (1% to 3%), arthralgia (1% to 3%), joint pain (1% to 3%), muscular stiffness (1% to 3%), paresthesia (1% to 3%), rigidity (1% to 3%)
Ocular: Keratitis/conjunctivitis (1% to 3%)
Respiratory: Nasal congestion (4% to 9%), tracheitis/bronchitis (7%), pharyngitis (≤6%), cough (5%), influenza (5%), viral respiratory tract infection (5%), sinusitis (4% to 5%), rhinitis (4% to 5%), asthma (3% to 4%)

Pharmacodynamics/Kinetics

Onset of Action Asthma: 30-48 minutes, COPD: 2 hours; Peak effect: Asthma: 3 hours, COPD: 2-5 hours

Duration of Action 12 hours

Absorption Systemic: Inhalation: Undetectable to poor

Time to Peak Serum: ~20 minutes

Protein Binding 96%

Half-Life Elimination 5.5 hours

Metabolism Hepatic; hydroxylated via CYP3A4

Excretion Feces (60%); urine (25%)

Available Dosage Forms

Powder, for oral inhalation:
Serevent® Diskus®: 50 mcg (28s, 60s)

Dosing

Adult & Geriatric

Asthma, maintenance and prevention: Inhalation, powder (50 mcg/inhalation): One inhalation twice daily (~12 hours apart); maximum: 1 inhalation twice daily. **Note:** For asthma control, long acting beta$_2$-agonists (LABAs) should be used in combination with inhaled corticosteroids and not as monotherapy.

Exercise-induced asthma, prevention: Inhalation, powder (50 mcg/inhalation): One inhalation at least 30 minutes prior to exercise; additional doses should not be used for 12 hours; should not be used in individuals already receiving salmeterol twice daily. **Note:** Because LABAs may disguise poorly controlled persistent asthma, frequent or chronic use of LABAs for exercise-induced bronchospasm is discouraged by the NIH Asthma Guidelines (NIH, 2007).

COPD maintenance: Inhalation, powder (50 mcg/inhalation): One inhalation twice daily (~12 hours apart); maximum: 1 inhalation twice daily

Pediatric Asthma (maintenance/prevention) and exercise-induced asthma (prevention): Inhalation, powder (50 mcg/inhalation): Children ≥4 years: Refer to adult dosing.

Hepatic Impairment No dosage adjustment required; manufacturer suggests close monitoring of patients with hepatic impairment.

Administration

Inhalation Not to be used for the relief of acute attacks. Not for use with a spacer device. Administer with Diskus® in a level, horizontal position. Do not wash mouthpiece; Diskus® should be kept dry.

Stability

Storage Inhalation powder (Serevent® Diskus®): Store at controlled room temperature 20°C to 25°C (68°F to 77°F) in a dry place away from direct heat or sunlight. Stable for 6 weeks after removal from foil pouch.

Monitoring and Teaching Issues

Laboratory Monitoring FEV$_1$, peak flow, and/or other pulmonary function tests

Physical Assessment Not for use to relieve acute asthmatic attacks. Evaluate for increased use of short-acting beta$_2$-agonist inhalers; may be marker of a deteriorating asthma condition. For inpatient care, monitor vital signs and lung sounds prior to and periodically during therapy.

Patient Education This medication is not to be used as a rescue treatment for acute asthmatic symptoms. You may experience headache, nervousness, dizziness, fatigue, dry mouth, or stomach upset. Report immediately any swelling of face, tongue, or throat; rash; or difficulty swallowing or choking. Report unresolved GI upset; dizziness or fatigue; vision changes; chest pain, rapid heartbeat, or palpitations; insomnia; nervousness or hyperactivity; or muscle cramping or tremors.

Dietary Considerations Some products may contain lactose; very rare anaphylactic reactions have been reported in patients with severe milk protein allergy.

Geriatric Considerations Geriatric patients were included in four clinical studies of salmeterol; no apparent differences in efficacy and safety were noted in geriatric patients compared to younger adults. Because salmeterol is only to be used for prevention of bronchospasm, patients also need a short-acting beta-agonist to treat acute attacks. Elderly patients should be carefully counseled about which inhaler to use and the proper scheduling of doses.

Pregnancy Considerations Animal studies have demonstrated (dose-dependent) teratogenicity. There are no adequate and well-controlled studies in pregnant women. Beta-agonists may interfere with uterine contractility if administered during labor. Use only if clearly needed.

◆ **Salmeterol and Fluticasone** *see* Fluticasone and Salmeterol *on page 804*
◆ **Salmeterol Xinafoate** *see* Salmeterol *on page 1618*
◆ **Salt Poor Albumin** *see* Albumin *on page 57*

◆ **Sal-Tropine™** *see* Atropine *on page 172*
◆ **Samsca™** *see* Tolvaptan *on page 1785*
◆ **Sancuso®** *see* Granisetron *on page 887*
◆ **SandIMMUNE®** *see* CycloSPORINE (Systemic) *on page 437*
◆ **SandoSTATIN®** *see* Octreotide *on page 1339*
◆ **SandoSTATIN LAR®** *see* Octreotide *on page 1339*
◆ **Saphris®** *see* Asenapine *on page 150*

Saquinavir (sa KWIN a veer)

U.S. Brand Names Invirase®

Index Terms Saquinavir Mesylate

Generic Availability (U.S.) No

Pharmacologic Category Antiretroviral Agent, Protease Inhibitor

Medication Safety Issues

Sound-alike/look-alike issues:

Saquinavir may be confused with SINEquan®

Medication Guide Available Yes

Pregnancy Risk Factor B

Lactation Excretion in breast milk unknown/contraindicated

Use Treatment of HIV infection; used in combination with at least two other antiretroviral agents

Mechanism of Action/Effect Blocks the site of HIV-1 protease activity, resulting in the formation of immature, noninfectious viral particles.

Contraindications Hypersensitivity to saquinavir or any component of the formulation; congenital or acquired QT prolongation, refractory hypokalemia or hypomagnesemia, concomitant use of other medications that both increase saquinavir plasma concentrations and prolong the QT interval; complete AV block (without implanted ventricular pacemaker) or patients at high risk of complete AV block; severe hepatic impairment; coadministration of saquinavir/ritonavir with alfuzosin, amiodarone, bepridil, cisapride, dofetilide, ergot derivatives, flecainide, lidocaine (systemic), lovastatin, midazolam (oral), pimozide, propafenone, quinidine, rifampin, sildenafil (when used for pulmonary artery hypertension [eg, Revatio®]),simvastatin, trazodone, or triazolam

Warnings/Precautions Use caution in patients with hepatic insufficiency. May exacerbate preexisting hepatic dysfunction; use with caution in patients with hepatitis B or C and in cirrhosis. May be associated with fat redistribution (buffalo hump, increased abdominal girth, breast engorgement, facial atrophy). Use caution in hemophilia. May increase cholesterol and/or triglycerides. Changes in glucose tolerance, hyperglycemia, exacerbation of diabetes, DKA, and new-onset diabetes mellitus have been reported in patients receiving protease inhibitors.

Altered cardiac conduction: Saquinavir/ritonavir prolongs the QT interval, potentially leading to torsade de pointes, and prolongs the PR interval, potentially leading to heart block. An ECG should be performed for all patients prior to starting saquinavir/ritonavir therapy; do not initiate therapy in patients with a baseline QT interval >450 msec. If baseline QT interval <450 msec, may initiate therapy but a subsequent ECG is recommended after ~3-4 days of therapy. If subsequent QT interval is >480 msec or is prolonged over baseline by >20 msec, therapy should be discontinued. Patients who may be at increased risk for QT- or PR-interval prolongation include those with heart failure, bradyarrhythmias, hepatic impairment, electrolyte abnormalities, ischemic heart disease, cardiomyopathy, structural heart disease, or those with pre-existing cardiac conduction abnormalities; ECG monitoring is recommended for these patients.

Use with caution in patients taking strong CYP3A4 inhibitors, moderate or strong CYP3A4 inducers and major CYP3A4 substrates (see Drug Interactions); consider alternative agents that avoid or lessen the potential for CYP-mediated interactions. St John's wort, lovastatin, and simvastatin should not be used concurrently with saquinavir/ritonavir. A listing of medications that should not be used is available with each bottle and patients should be provided with this information. Do not coadminister colchicine in patient with renal or hepatic impairment; avoid concurrent use with salmeterol. Patients may develop immune reconstitution syndrome resulting in the occurrence of an inflammatory response to an indolent or residual opportunistic infection; further evaluation and treatment may be required. Invirase® may be used only if combined with ritonavir. Safety and efficacy have not been established in children ≤16 years of age.

Drug Interactions

Metabolism/Transport Effects Substrate of CYP2D6 (minor), CYP3A4 (major), P-glycoprotein; **Inhibits** CYP2C9 (weak), CYP2C19 (weak), CYP2D6 (weak), CYP3A4 (moderate), P-glycoprotein

Avoid Concomitant Use

Avoid concomitant use of Saquinavir with any of the following: Alfuzosin; Amiodarone; Artemether; Bepridil [Off Market]; Cisapride; Conivaptan; Darunavir; Dofetilide; Dronedarone; Eplerenone; Ergot Derivatives; Everolimus; Flecainide; Halofantrine; Lidocaine (Systemic); Lovastatin; Lumefantrine; Lurasidone; Midazolam; Nilotinib; Nisoldipine; Pimozide; Propafenone; QuiNIDine; QuiNINE; Ranolazine; Rifampin; Rivaroxaban; RomiDEPsin; Salmeterol; Silodosin; Simvastatin; St Johns Wort; Tamsulosin; Tetrabenazine; Thioridazine; Tolvaptan; Topotecan; Toremifene; TraZODone; Triazolam; Vandetanib; Ziprasidone

Decreased Effect

Saquinavir may decrease the levels/effects of: Abacavir; Clarithromycin; Contraceptives (Estrogens); Darunavir; Delavirdine; Divalproex; Etravirine; Meperidine; Methadone; Prasugrel; Theophylline Derivatives; Valproic Acid; Zidovudine

The levels/effects of Saquinavir may be decreased by: Antacids; CarBAMazepine; Contraceptives (Estrogens); CYP3A4 Inducers (Strong); Deferasirox; Efavirenz; Garlic; Nevirapine; Peginterferon Alfa-2b; P-Glycoprotein Inducers; Rifampin; St Johns Wort

Increased Effect/Toxicity

Saquinavir may increase the levels/effects of: Alfuzosin; Almotriptan; Alosetron; ALPRAZolam; Amiodarone; Antifungal Agents (Azole Derivatives, Systemic); Bepridil [Off Market]; Bortezomib; Brinzolamide; Calcium Channel Blockers (Dihydropyridine); Calcium Channel Blockers (Nondihydropyridine); CarBAMazepine; Ciclesonide; Cisapride; Clarithromycin; Clorazepate; Colchicine; Conivaptan; Corticosteroids (Orally Inhaled); CycloSPORINE; CycloSPORINE (Systemic); CYP3A4 Substrates; Dabigatran Etexilate; Diazepam; Dienogest; Digoxin; Dofetilide; Dronedarone; Dutasteride; Enfuvirtide; Eplerenone; Ergot Derivatives; Everolimus; FentaNYL; Fesoterodine; Flecainide; Flurazepam; Fusidic Acid; GuanFACINE; Halofantrine; HMG-CoA Reductase Inhibitors; Ixabepilone; Lidocaine (Systemic); Lovastatin; Lumefantrine; Lurasidone; Maraviroc; Meperidine; MethylPREDNISolone; Midazolam; Nefazodone; Nilotinib; Nisoldipine; Paricalcitol; Pazopanib; P-Glycoprotein Substrates; Pimecrolimus; Pimozide; Propafenone; Protease Inhibitors; QTc-Prolonging Agents; QuiNIDine; QuiNINE; Ranolazine; Rifabutin; Rivaroxaban; RomiDEPsin; Salmeterol; Saxagliptin; Sildenafil; Silodosin; Simvastatin; Sirolimus; SORAfenib; Tacrolimus; Tacrolimus (Systemic); Tacrolimus (Topical); Tadalafil; Tamsulosin; Temsirolimus; Tetrabenazine; Thioridazine; Tolvaptan; Topotecan; Toremifene; TraZODone; Triazolam; Tricyclic Antidepressants; Vandetanib; Vardenafil; Vilazodone; Warfarin; Ziprasidone

The levels/effects of Saquinavir may be increased by: Alfuzosin; Antifungal Agents (Azole Derivatives, Systemic); Artemether; Bepridil [Off Market]; Chloroquine; Ciprofloxacin; Ciprofloxacin (Systemic); Clarithromycin; CycloSPORINE; CycloSPORINE (Systemic); Delavirdine; Efavirenz; Enfuvirtide; Etravirine; Fusidic Acid; Gadobutrol; H2-Antagonists; Lumefantrine; Nilotinib; P-Glycoprotein Inhibitors; Proton Pump Inhibitors; QuiNINE; Rifampin

Nutritional/Ethanol Interactions

Food: A high-fat meal maximizes bioavailability. Saquinavir levels may increase if taken with grapefruit juice.

Herb/Nutraceutical: Saquinavir serum concentrations may be decreased by St John's wort; avoid concurrent use. Garlic capsules may decrease saquinavir serum concentrations; avoid use if saquinavir is the only protease inhibitor.

Adverse Reactions

Incidence data shown for saquinavir soft gel capsule formulation (no longer available) in combination with ritonavir.

10%: Gastrointestinal: Nausea (11%)

1% to 10%:

Cardiovascular: Chest pain

Central nervous system: Fatigue (6%), fever (3%), anxiety, depression, headache, insomnia, pain

Dermatologic: Pruritus (3%), rash (3%), dry lips/skin (2%), eczema (2%), verruca

Endocrine & metabolic: Lipodystrophy (5%), hyperglycemia (3%), hypoglycemia, hyperkalemia, libido disorder, serum amylase increased

Gastrointestinal: Diarrhea (8%), vomiting (7%), abdominal pain (6%), constipation (2%), abdominal discomfort, appetite decreased, buccal mucosa ulceration, dyspepsia, flatulence, taste alteration

Hepatic: AST increased, ALT increased, bilirubin increased

Neuromuscular & skeletal: Back pain (2%), CPK increased, paresthesia, weakness

Renal: Creatinine kinase increased

Respiratory: Pneumonia (5%), bronchitis (3%), sinusitis (3%)

Miscellaneous: Influenza (3%)

Incidence not currently defined (limited to significant reactions; reported for hard or soft gel capsule with/without ritonavir)

Cardiovascular: Cyanosis, heart valve disorder (including murmur), hyper-/hypotension, peripheral vasoconstriction, prolonged QT interval, prolonged PR interval, syncope, thrombophlebitis

Central nervous system: Agitation, amnesia, ataxia, confusion, hallucination, hyper-/hyporeflexia, myelopolyradiculoneuritis, neuropathies, poliomyelitis, progressive multifocal encephalopathy, psychosis, seizures, somnolence, speech disorder, suicide attempt

Dermatologic: Alopecia, bullous eruption, dermatitis, erythema, maculopapular rash, photosensitivity, Stevens-Johnson syndrome, skin ulceration, urticaria

Endocrine & metabolic: Dehydration, diabetes, electrolyte changes, TSH increased

Gastrointestinal: Ascites, colic, dysphagia, esophagitis, bloody stools, gastritis, intestinal obstruction, hemorrhage (rectal), pancreatitis, stomatitis

Genitourinary: impotence, prostate enlarged, hematuria, UTI

Hematologic; Acute myeloblastic leukemia, anemia (including hemolytic), leukopenia, neutropenia, pancytopenia, splenomegaly, thrombocytopenia

Hepatic: Alkaline phosphatase increased, GGT increased, hepatitis, hepatomegaly, hepatosplenomegaly, jaundice, liver disease exacerbation

Neuromuscular & skeletal: Arthritis, LDH increased

Ocular: Blepharitis, visual disturbance

Otic: Otitis, hearing decreased, tinnitus
Renal: Nephrolithiasis, renal calculus
Respiratory: Dyspnea, hemoptysis, pharyngitis, upper respiratory tract infection
Miscellaneous: Infections (bacterial, fungal, viral)

Pharmacodynamics/Kinetics

Absorption Poor; increased with high fat meal; Fortovase® has improved absorption over Invirase®

Bioavailability Invirase®: ~4%

Protein Binding Plasma: ~98%

Metabolism Extensively hepatic via CYP3A4; extensive first-pass effect

Excretion Feces (81% to 88%), urine (1% to 3%) within 5 days

Available Dosage Forms

Capsule, oral:
Invirase®: 200 mg

Tablet, oral:
Invirase®: 500 mg

Dosing

Adult Note: ECG should be done prior to starting therapy; do not initiate therapy if pretreatment QT interval >450 msec. Saquinavir should not be used in "unboosted regimens."

HIV infection: Oral: 1000 mg (five 200 mg capsules or two 500 mg tablets) twice daily given in combination with ritonavir 100 mg twice daily. This combination should be given together and within 2 hours after a full meal in combination with a nucleoside analog.

Dosage adjustments when administered in combination therapy: Saquinavir: 1000 mg twice daily administered with lopinavir 400 mg/ritonavir 100 mg (Kaletra™) twice daily; no additional ritonavir is necessary

Dosage adjustments for concomitant therapy: Oral:

Coadministration with bosentan:

Coadministration of bosentan in patients currently receiving saquinavir/ritonavir: For patients receiving saquinavir/ritonavir for at least 10 days, begin with bosentan 62.5 mg once daily or every other day based on tolerability

Coadministration of saquinavir/ritonavir in patients currently receiving bosentan: Discontinue bosentan 36 hours prior to the initiation of saquinavir/ritonavir. After at least 10 days of saquinavir/ritonavir, resume bosentan 62.5 mg once daily or every other day based on tolerability.

Coadministration with colchicine:

Familial Mediterranean fever (FMF): Maximum colchicine dose: 0.6 mg/day (0.3 mg twice daily)

Gout prophylaxis:
If original colchicine dose is 0.6 mg twice daily, adjust dose to 0.3 mg once daily
If original colchicine dose is 0.6 mg once daily, adjust dose to 0.3 mg every other day

Gout flare treatment: Initial: Colchicine 0.6 mg, followed in 1 hour by a single dose of 0.3 mg; do not repeat for at least 3 days

Coadministration with phosphodiesterase-5 enzyme (PDE-5) inhibitor:

Pulmonary arterial hypertension: Saquinavir/ritonavir coadministered with tadalafil:
Patient receiving saquinavir/ritonavir for at least 1 week: Initiate tadalafil at 20 mg once daily; increase to 40 mg once daily based on individual tolerability
Patient receiving tadalafil when initiating saquinavir/ritonavir: Stop tadalafil at least 24 hours prior to starting saquinavir/ritonavir. After at least 1 week following the initiation of saquinavir/ritonavir, resume tadalafil at 20 mg once daily; increase to 40 mg once daily based on individual tolerability.

Erectile dysfunction: Saquinavir/ritonavir coadministered with:
Sildenafil: Maximum sildenafil dose: 25 mg in a 48-hour period
Tadalafil: Maximum tadalafil dose: 10 mg in a 72-hour period
Vardenafil: Maximum vardenafil dose: 2.5 mg in a 72-hour period

Geriatric Clinical studies did not include sufficient numbers of patients ≥65 years of age. Use caution due to increased frequency of organ dysfunction.

Pediatric

HIV infection: Oral: Children >16 years: Refer to adult dosing.

Administration

Oral Administer within 2 hours after a full meal. When used with ritonavir, saquinavir and ritonavir should be administered at the same time.

Stability

Storage Invirase®: Store at room temperature.

Monitoring and Teaching Issues

Laboratory Monitoring Serum potassium and magnesium levels, triglycerides and cholesterol (prior to initiation and periodically during therapy); viral load, CD4 count; glucose

Physical Assessment Assess CD4 count and hepatic function. Monitor for gastrointestinal disturbance (nausea, vomiting, diarrhea) that can lead to dehydration and weight loss, hyperlipidemia and redistribution of body fat, rash, CNS effects (malaise, insomnia, abnormal thinking), and electrolyte imbalance at regular intervals during therapy. Caution patients to monitor glucose levels closely; protease inhibitors may cause hyperglycemia or new-onset diabetes. Teach patient proper timing of multiple medications.

Patient Education This is not a cure for HIV, nor has it been found to reduce transmission of HIV; use appropriate precautions to prevent spread to other persons. Maintain adequate hydration unless instructed to restrict fluid intake. Frequent blood tests may be required. You may be advised to check your glucose levels (this drug can cause exacerbation or new-onset diabetes). May cause body changes due to redistribution of body fat, facial atrophy, or breast enlargement (normal effects of drug). May cause dizziness, insomnia, abnormal thinking, nausea, vomiting, taste perversion, muscle weakness, headache, or insomnia. Inform prescriber if you experience muscle numbness or tingling; unresolved persistent vomiting, diarrhea, or abdominal pain; respiratory difficulty or chest pain; unusual skin rash; or change in color of stool or urine.

Dietary Considerations Take within 2 hours of a meal. Invirase® capsules contain lactose (not expected to induce symptoms of intolerance).

Breast-Feeding Considerations In infants born to mothers who are HIV positive, HAART while breast-feeding may decrease postnatal infection. However, maternal or infant antiretroviral therapy does not completely eliminate the risk of postnatal HIV transmission. In addition, multiclass-resistant virus has been detected in breast-feeding infants despite maternal therapy.

In the United States where formula is accessible, affordable, safe, and sustainable, complete avoidance of breast-feeding by HIV-infected women is recommended to decrease potential transmission of HIV.

Pregnancy Considerations Adverse events were not observed in animal studies and saquinavir crosses the human placenta in minimal amounts. Based on limited data, Invirase® 1000 mg (capsules and tablets) administered twice daily with ritonavir 100 mg twice daily provide adequate levels in pregnant women. The Perinatal HIV Guidelines Working Group considers Invirase® capsules and ritonavir to be an alternative combination for use during pregnancy. Pregnancy and protease inhibitors are both associated with an increased risk of hyperglycemia. Glucose levels should be closely monitored. Healthcare providers are encouraged to enroll pregnant women exposed to antiretroviral medications in the Antiretroviral Pregnancy Registry (1-800-258-4263 or www.APRegistry.com). Healthcare providers caring for HIV-infected women and their infants may contact the National Perinatal HIV Hotline (888-448-8765) for clinical consultation.

◆ **Saquinavir Mesylate** *see* Saquinavir *on page* 1621

◆ **Sarafem®** *see* FLUoxetine *on page* 789

Sargramostim (sar GRAM oh stim)

U.S. Brand Names Leukine®

Index Terms GM-CSF; Granulocyte-Macrophage Colony Stimulating Factor; NSC-613795; rhuGM-CSF

Generic Availability (U.S.) No

Pharmacologic Category Colony Stimulating Factor

Medication Safety Issues

Sound-alike/look-alike issues:

Leukine® may be confused with Leukeran®, leucovorin

Pregnancy Risk Factor C

Lactation Excretion in breast milk unknown/use caution

Use

Acute myelogenous leukemia (AML) following induction chemotherapy in older adults (≥55 years of age) to shorten time to neutrophil recovery and to reduce the incidence of severe and life-threatening infections and infections resulting in death

Bone marrow transplant (allogeneic or autologous) failure or engraftment delay

Myeloid reconstitution after allogeneic bone marrow transplantation

Myeloid reconstitution after autologous bone marrow transplantation: Non-Hodgkin's lymphoma (NHL), acute lymphoblastic leukemia (ALL), Hodgkin's lymphoma

Peripheral stem cell transplantation: Mobilization and myeloid reconstitution following autologous peripheral stem cell transplantation

Mechanism of Action/Effect Stimulates proliferation, differentiation and functional activity of neutrophils, eosinophils, monocytes, and macrophages.

Contraindications Hypersensitivity to sargramostim, yeast-derived products, or any component of the formulation; concurrent (24 hours preceding/following) myelosuppressive chemotherapy or radiation therapy; patients with excessive (≥10%) leukemic myeloid blasts in bone marrow or peripheral blood

Warnings/Precautions Simultaneous administration, or administration 24 hours preceding/following cytotoxic chemotherapy or radiotherapy is not recommended. Use with caution in patients with pre-existing cardiac problems or HF; supraventricular arrhythmias have been reported in patients with history of arrhythmias. Edema, capillary leak syndrome, pleural and/or pericardial effusion have been reported; use with caution in patients with pre-existing fluid retention; may worsen. Use with caution in patients with hepatic or renal impairment; monitor hepatic and/or renal function in patients with history of hepatic or renal dysfunction. Elevations in bilirubin, transaminases, and serum creatinine have been observed with use. Dyspnea may occur; monitor respiratory symptoms during and following infusion; use with caution in patients with hypoxia or pulmonary infiltrates.

With rapid increase in blood counts (ANC >20,000/mm^3, WBC >50,000/mm^3, or platelets >500,000/mm^3); decrease dose by 50% or discontinue drug (counts will fall to normal within 3-7 days after discontinuing drug). May potentially act as a growth factor for any tumor type, particularly myeloid malignancies; caution should be exercised when using in any malignancy with myeloid characteristics; tumors of nonhematopoietic origin may have surface receptors for sargramostim. Discontinue use if disease progression occurs during treatment.

There is a "first-dose effect" (refer to Adverse Reactions for details) which is seen (rarely) with the first dose of a cycle and does not usually occur with subsequent doses within that cycle. Anaphylaxis or other serious allergic reactions have been reported; discontinue immediately if occur. Solution contains benzyl alcohol; do not use in premature infants or neonates.

Drug Interactions

Avoid Concomitant Use There are no known interactions where it is recommended to avoid concomitant use.

Decreased Effect There are no known significant interactions involving a decrease in effect.

Increased Effect/Toxicity

Sargramostim may increase the levels/effects of: Bleomycin

Lab Interactions May interfere with bone imaging studies; increased hematopoietic activity of the bone marrow may appear as transient positive bone imaging changes

Adverse Reactions

>10%:

Cardiovascular: Hypertension (34%), pericardial effusion (4% to 25%), edema (13% to 25%), chest pain (15%), peripheral edema (11%), tachycardia (11%)

Central nervous system: Fever (81%), malaise (57%), headache (26%), chills (25%), anxiety (11%), insomnia (11%)

Dermatologic: Rash (44%), pruritus (23%)

Endocrine & metabolic: Hyperglycemia (25%), hypercholesterolemia (17%), hypomagnesemia (15%)

Gastrointestinal: Diarrhea (≤89%), nausea (58% to 70%), vomiting (46% to 70%), abdominal pain (38%), weight loss (37%), anorexia (13%), hematemesis (13%), dysphagia (11%), gastrointestinal hemorrhage (11%)

Genitourinary: Urinary tract disorder (14%)

Hepatic: Hyperbilirubinemia (30%)

Neuromuscular & skeletal: Weakness (66%), bone pain (21%), arthralgia (11% to 21%) myalgia (18%)

Ocular: Eye hemorrhage (11%)

Renal: BUN increased (23%), serum creatinine increased (15%)

Respiratory: Pharyngitis (23%), epistaxis (17%), dyspnea (15%)

1% to 10%: Respiratory: Pleural effusion (1%)

Pharmacodynamics/Kinetics

Onset of Action Increase in WBC: 7-14 days

Duration of Action WBCs return to baseline within 1 week of discontinuing drug

Time to Peak Serum: SubQ: 1-3 hours

Half-Life Elimination I.V.: 60 minutes; SubQ: 2.7 hours

Available Dosage Forms

Injection, powder for reconstitution:

Leukine®: 250 mcg

Injection, solution:

Leukine®: 500 mcg/mL (1 mL)

Dosing

Adult & Geriatric

I.V. infusion over ≥2 hours or SubQ: **Rounding the dose to the nearest vial size enhances patient convenience and reduces costs without clinical detrement.**

Myeloid reconstitution after allogeneic or autologous bone marrow transplant: I.V.: 250 mcg/m²/day (over 2 hours), begin 2-4 hours after the marrow infusion and ≥24 hours after chemotherapy or radiotherapy, when the post marrow infusion ANC is <500 cells/mm³, and continue until ANC >1500 cells/mm³ for 3 consecutive days

If a severe adverse reaction occurs, reduce the dose by 50% or temporarily discontinue until the reaction abates

If blast cells appear or progression of the underlying disease occurs, discontinue treatment

If ANC >20,000 cells/mm³, interrupt treatment or reduce the dose by 50%

Neutrophil recovery following chemotherapy in AML: I.V.: 250 mcg/m²/day (over 4 hours) starting approximately on day 11 or 4 days following the completion of induction chemotherapy, if day 10 bone marrow is hypoplastic with <5% blasts

If a second cycle of chemotherapy is necessary, administer ~4 days after the completion of chemotherapy if the bone marrow is hypoplastic with <5% blasts

Continue sargramostim until ANC is >1500 cells/mm³ for 3 consecutive days or a maximum of 42 days

Discontinue sargramostim immediately if leukemic regrowth occurs

If a severe adverse reaction occurs, reduce the dose by 50% or temporarily discontinue the dose until the reaction abates

If ANC >20,000 cells/mm³, interrupt treatment or reduce the dose by 50%

Mobilization of peripheral blood progenitor cells: I.V., SubQ: 250 mcg/m²/day I.V. over 24 hours or SubQ once daily

Continue the same dose through the period of PBPC collection

The optimal schedule for PBPC collection has not been established (usually begun by day 5 and performed daily until protocol specified targets are achieved)

If WBC >50,000 cells/mm³, reduce the dose by 50%

If adequate numbers of progenitor cells are not collected, consider other mobilization therapy

Postperipheral blood progenitor cell transplantation: I.V., SubQ: 250 mcg/m²/day I.V. over 24 hours or SubQ once daily beginning immediately following infusion of progenitor cells and continuing until ANC is >1500 cells/mm³ for 3 consecutive days is attained

BMT failure or engraftment delay: I.V.: 250 mcg/m²/day over 2 hours for 14 days

May be repeated after 7 days off therapy if engraftment has not occurred

If engraftment still has not occurred, a third course of 500 mcg/m²/day for 14 days may be tried after another 7 days off therapy; if there is still no improvement, it is unlikely that further dose escalation will be beneficial

If a severe adverse reaction occurs, reduce the dose by 50% or temporarily discontinue the dose until the reaction abates

If blast cells appear or disease progression occurs, discontinue treatment

If ANC >20,000 cells/mm³, interrupt treatment or reduce the dose by 50%

Pediatric Dosage not established in children (unlabeled use). Refer to adult dosing.

Administration

I.V. Can premedicate with analgesics and antipyretics (eg, acetaminophen) to control adverse events (eg, fever, chills, myalgia, etc); control bone pain with non-narcotic analgesics I.V. infusion should be over 2-24 hours; incompatible with dextrose-containing solutions. An in-line membrane filter should **NOT** be used for intravenous administration.

Other Administer by SubQ (undiluted). Do not shake solution. When administering GM-CSF subcutaneously, rotate injection sites.

Stability

Reconstitution

Powder for injection: May be reconstituted with preservative free SWFI or bacteriostatic water for injection (with benzyl alcohol 0.9%). Gently swirl to reconstitute; do not shake.

Sargramostim may also be further diluted in 25-50 mL NS to a concentration ≥10 mcg/mL for I.V. infusion administration.

If the final concentration of sargramostim is <10 mcg/mL, 1 mg of human albumin/1 mL of NS (eg, 1 mL of 5% human albumin/50 mL of NS) should be added.

Storage Store at 2°C to 8°C (36°F to 46°F); do not freeze. Do not shake.

Solution for injection: May be stored for up to 20 days at 2°C to 8°C (36°F to 46°F) once the vial has been entered. Discard remaining solution after 20 days.

Powder for injection: Preparations made with SWFI should be administered as soon as possible, and discarded within 6 hours of reconstitution. Preparations made with bacteriostatic water may be stored for up to 20 days at 2°C to 8°C (36°F to 46°F).

I.V. infusion administration: Preparations diluted with NS are stable for 48 hours at room temperature and refrigeration.

Monitoring and Teaching Issues

Laboratory Monitoring CBC with differential twice weekly during therapy, renal/liver function tests at least biweekly during therapy (in patients displaying renal or hepatic dysfunction prior to initiation of treatment)

Physical Assessment Use with caution in presence of pre-existing cardiac problems or hepatic, renal, or pulmonary impairment. Patient must be monitored closely during and following infusion for respiratory symptoms and "first-dose effect" (hypotension, tachycardia, flushing, and syncope with the first dose of a cycle). Premedication may be used to control adverse events. Monitor for respiratory symptoms, fluid balance (I and O), rash, hypotension, tachycardia, GI disturbance (diarrhea, stomatitis, mucositis), myalgia, and bone pain.

Patient Education This medication can only be administered by infusion or injection. Report immediately any redness, swelling, pain, or burning at infusion/injection site; difficulty breathing; or chest pain. You will require frequent blood tests during treatment. You may experience bone, joint, or muscle pain; nausea, vomiting, or loss of appetite; hair loss (reversible); diarrhea; headache; dizziness; or insomnia. At any time during treatment, report chest pain or palpitations, signs or symptoms of edema (eg, swollen extremities, difficulty breathing, rapid weight gain), onset of severe headache, acute back or chest pain, muscular tremors, or seizure activity.

Pregnancy Considerations Clinical effects to the fetus: Animal reproduction studies have not been conducted. It is not known whether sargramostim can cause fetal harm when administered to a pregnant woman or can affect reproductive capability. Sargramostim should be given to a pregnant woman only if clearly needed.

Additional Information Reimbursement Hotline (Leukine®): 1-800-321-4669

◆ **Savella®** *see* Milnacipran *on page* 1233

Saxagliptin and Metformin (sax a GLIP tin & met FOR min)

U.S. Brand Names Kombiglyze™ XR

Index Terms Metformin and Saxagliptin; Metformin Hydrochloride and Saxagliptin; Saxagliptin and Metformin Hydrochloride

Pharmacologic Category Antidiabetic Agent, Biguanide; Antidiabetic Agent, Dipeptidyl Peptidase IV (DPP-IV) Inhibitor

Medication Safety Issues

Sound-alike/look-alike issues:

Saxagliptin and Metformin may be confused with sitaGLIPtin and Metformin

Pregnancy Risk Factor B

Lactation

Saxagliptin: Excretion in breast milk unknown/use caution

Metformin: Enters breast milk/not recommended

Use Management of type 2 diabetes mellitus (noninsulin dependent, NIDDM) as an adjunct to diet and exercise when treatment with both saxagliptin and metformin is appropriate

Available Dosage Forms

Tablet, variable release, oral:

Kombiglyze™ XR 2.5/1000: Saxagliptin 2.5 mg [immediate release] and metformin hydrochloride 1000 mg [extended release]; 5/500: Saxagliptin 5 mg [immediate release] and metformin hydrochloride 500 mg [extended release]; 5/1000: Saxagliptin 5 mg [immediate release] and metformin hydrochloride 1000 mg [extended release]

Dosing

Adult Note: Patients receiving concomitant insulin secretagogues (eg, sulfonylureas) may require dosage adjustments of these agents.

Type 2 diabetes mellitus: Oral: Initial doses should be based on current dose of saxagliptin and metformin; daily doses should be given once daily with the evening meal. Maximum: Saxagliptin 5 mg/metformin 2000 mg daily

Patients inadequately controlled on metformin alone: Initial dose: Saxagliptin 2.5-5 mg/day plus current dose of metformin. **Note:** Patients who require saxagliptin 2.5 mg (eg, dose adjusted for concomitant use of strong CYP3A4/5 inhibitors) and metformin >1000 mg should not be switched to the combination product.

Patients inadequately controlled on saxagliptin alone: Initial dose: Metformin 500 mg/day plus saxagliptin 5 mg/day. **Note:** Metformin-naïve patients currently receiving saxagliptin 2.5 mg daily (eg, dose adjusted for concomitant use of strong CYP3A4/5 inhibitors) should not be switched to the combination product.

Concomitant use with strong CYP3A4/5 inhibitors: Maximum: Saxagliptin 2.5 mg/metformin 1000 mg daily

Geriatric Refer to adult dosing. The initial and maintenance dosing should be conservative, due to the potential for decreased renal function (monitor). Do not use in patients ≥80 years of age unless normal renal function has been established.

Renal Impairment Do not use in patients with renal disease or renal dysfunction (serum creatinine ≥1.5 mg/dL [≥136 μmol/L] in males or ≥1.4 mg/dL [≥124 μmol/L] in females or abnormal clearance).

Hepatic Impairment Avoid metformin; liver disease is a risk factor for the development of lactic acidosis during metformin therapy.

Administration

Oral Administer once daily with the evening meal. Swallow whole; do not crush, cut, or chew tablets.

Monitoring and Teaching Issues

Laboratory Monitoring Plasma glucose; Hb A_{1c}; hematologic parameters (eg, hemoglobin/hematocrit and red blood cell indices); hepatic function; renal function (prior to initiation of therapy then annually or more frequent if necessary); vitamin B_{12} (periodically with long-term treatment) and folate (if megaloblastic anemia is suspected)

Physical Assessment See individual agents.

Patient Education See individual agents.

◆ **Saxagliptin and Metformin Hydrochloride** *see* Saxagliptin and Metformin *on page 1626*

◆ **SB-265805** *see* Gemifloxacin *on page 861*

◆ **SB-497115** *see* Eltrombopag *on page 610*

◆ **SB-497115-GR** *see* Eltrombopag *on page 610*

◆ **SC 33428** *see* IDArubicin *on page 945*

◆ **Scalpana [OTC]** *see* Hydrocortisone (Topical) *on page 920*

◆ **SCH 13521** *see* Flutamide *on page 797*

◆ **SCH 52365** *see* Temozolomide *on page 1721*

◆ **SCH 56592** *see* Posaconazole *on page 1476*

◆ **SCIG** *see* Immune Globulin *on page 961*

◆ **S-Citalopram** *see* Escitalopram *on page 662*

◆ **Scopace™** *see* Scopolamine (Systemic) *on page 1627*

Scopolamine (Systemic) (skoe POL a mee)

U.S. Brand Names Scopace™; Transderm Scōp®

Index Terms Hyoscine Butylbromide; Scopolamine Base; Scopolamine Butylbromide; Scopolamine Hydrobromide

Generic Availability (U.S.) Yes: Injection

Pharmacologic Category Anticholinergic Agent

Medication Safety Issues Transdermal patch may contain conducting metal (eg, aluminum); remove patch prior to MRI.

Pregnancy Risk Factor C

Lactation Enters breast milk/use caution (AAP rates "compatible"; AAP 2001 update pending)

Use

Scopolamine base: Transdermal: Prevention of nausea/vomiting associated with motion sickness and recovery from anesthesia and surgery

Scopolamine hydrobromide:

Injection: Preoperative medication to produce amnesia, sedation, tranquilization, antiemetic effects, and decrease salivary and respiratory secretions

Oral: Symptomatic treatment of postencephalitic parkinsonism and paralysis agitans; in spastic states; inhibits excessive motility and hypertonus of the gastrointestinal tract in such conditions as the irritable colon syndrome, mild dysentery, diverticulitis, pylorospasm, and cardiospasm

Scopolamine butylbromide [not available in the U.S.]: Oral/injection: Treatment of smooth muscle spasm of the genitourinary or gastrointestinal tract; injection may also be used to prior to radiological/diagnostic procedures to prevent spasm

Mechanism of Action/Effect Blocks the action of acetylcholine at parasympathetic sites in smooth muscle, secretory glands and the CNS; increases cardiac output, dries secretions, antagonizes histamine and serotonin

Contraindications Hypersensitivity to scopolamine, other belladonna alkaloids, or any component of the formulation; narrow-angle glaucoma; acute hemorrhage; paralytic ileus; tachycardia secondary to cardiac insufficiency; myasthenia gravis

Tablet formulations are also contraindicated in patients with prostatic hyperplasia, pyloric obstruction, or patients with an idiosyncrasy to anticholinergic drugs.

Injectable formulations are also contraindicated in patients with chronic lung disease (repeated administration).

Warnings/Precautions Use with caution in patients with coronary artery disease, tachyarrhythmias, heart failure, or hypertension; evaluate tachycardia prior to administration. Use with caution with hepatic or renal impairment; adverse CNS effects occur more often in these patients. Use injectable and transdermal products with caution in patients with prostatic hyperplasia (nonobstructive) or urinary retention; oral products are contraindicated. Discontinue if patient reports unusual visual disturbances or pain within the eye. Use caution in hiatal hernia, reflux esophagitis, and ulcerative colitis. Use with caution in patients with a history of seizure or psychosis; may exacerbate these conditions. Patients with idiosyncratic reaction to anticholinergics, including scopolamine, may experience disorientation, delirium and/or marked somnolence; may be accompanied by dilated pupils, rapid pulse and xerostomia. May cause CNS depression, which may impair physical or mental abilities; patients must be cautioned about performing tasks which require mental alertness (eg, operating machinery or driving).

Transdermal patch may contain conducting metal (eg, aluminum); remove patch prior to MRI. Scopolamine (hyoscine) hydrobromide should not be interchanged with scopolamine butylbromide formulations; dosages are not equivalent.

Use with caution in infants and children since they may be more susceptible to adverse effects of scopolamine. Safety and efficacy have not been established for the use of transdermal and oral scopolamine in children.

Drug Interactions

Avoid Concomitant Use There are no known interactions where it is recommended to avoid concomitant use.

Decreased Effect

Scopolamine (Systemic) may decrease the levels/effects of: Acetylcholinesterase Inhibitors (Central); Secretin

The levels/effects of Scopolamine (Systemic) may be decreased by: Acetylcholinesterase Inhibitors (Central)

Increased Effect/Toxicity

Scopolamine (Systemic) may increase the levels/effects of: AbobotulinumtoxinA; Alcohol (Ethyl); Anticholinergics; Cannabinoids; CNS Depressants; Methotrimeprazine; OnabotulinumtoxinA; Potassium Chloride; RimabotulinumtoxinB

The levels/effects of Scopolamine (Systemic) may be increased by: Droperidol; Methotrimeprazine; Pramlintide

Nutritional/Ethanol Interactions Ethanol: Avoid ethanol (may increase CNS depression).

Lab Interactions Interferes with gastric secretion test

Adverse Reactions Frequency not defined.

Cardiovascular: Orthostatic hypotension, ventricular fibrillation, tachycardia, palpitation
Central nervous system: Confusion, drowsiness, headache, loss of memory, ataxia, fatigue
Dermatologic: Dry skin, photosensitivity increased, rash
Endocrine & metabolic: Decreased flow of breast milk
Gastrointestinal: Constipation, xerostomia, dry throat, dysphagia, bloated feeling, nausea, vomiting
Genitourinary: Dysuria
Local: Irritation at injection site
Neuromuscular & skeletal: Weakness
Ocular: Increased intraocular pain, blurred vision
Respiratory: Dry nose
Miscellaneous: Diaphoresis decreased

Pharmacodynamics/Kinetics

Onset of Action Oral, I.M.: 0.5-1 hour; I.V.: 10 minutes

Peak effect: 20-60 minutes; may take 3-7 days for full recovery; transdermal: 24 hours

Duration of Action Oral, I.M.: 4-6 hours; I.V.: 2 hours

Absorption Tertiary salts (hydrobromide) are well absorbed; quaternary salts (butylbromide) are poorly absorbed (local concentrations in the GI tract following oral dosing may be high)

Half-Life Elimination Hyoscine-N-butylbromide: 4.8 hours; Scopolamine: 9.5 hours

Metabolism Hepatic

Excretion Urine (<10%, as parent drug and metabolites)

Available Dosage Forms

Injection, solution: 0.4 mg/mL (1 mL)

Patch, transdermal:

Transderm Scōp®: 1.5 mg (4s, 10s, 24s)

Tablet, soluble, oral:

Scopace™: 0.4 mg

Dosing

Adult & Geriatric Note: Scopolamine (hyoscine) hydrobromide should not be interchanged with scopolamine butylbromide formulations. Dosages are not equivalent.

Scopolamine base:

Preoperative: Transdermal patch: Apply 1 patch to hairless area behind ear the night before surgery or 1 hour prior to cesarean section (apply no sooner than 1 hour before surgery to minimize newborn exposure); remove 24 hours after surgery

Motion sickness: Transdermal patch: Apply 1 patch behind the ear at least 4 hours prior to exposure and every 3 days as needed; effective if applied as soon as 2-3 hours before anticipated need, best if 12 hours before

Scopolamine hydrobromide:

Antiemetic: SubQ: 0.6-1 mg

Preoperative: I.M., I.V., SubQ: 0.3-0.65 mg

Sedation, tranquilization: I.M., I.V., SubQ: 0.6 mg 3-4 times/day

Parkinsonism, spasticity, motion sickness: Oral: 0.4-0.8 mg. May repeat every 8-12 hours as needed; the dosage may be cautiously increased in parkinsonism and spastic states. For motion sickness, administration at least 1 hour before exposure is recommended.

Scopolamine butylbromide: *Gastrointestinal/genitourinary spasm* (Buscopan® [CAN]; not available in the U.S.):

Oral: 10-20 mg daily (1-2 tablets); maximum: 6 tablets/day

I.M., I.V., SubQ: 10-20 mg; maximum: 100 mg/day. Intramuscular injections should be administered 10-15 minutes prior to radiological/diagnostic procedures

Pediatric Scopolamine hydrobromide:

Antiemetic: SubQ: 0.006 mg/kg

Preoperative: I.M., I.V., SubQ:

Children 6 months to 3 years: 0.1-0.15 mg

Children 3-6 years: 0.2-0.3 mg

Administration

I.V.

Hydrobromide: Inject over 2-3 minutes

Butylbromide:

I.V.: Inject at a rate of 1 mL/minute

I.M.: Intramuscular injections should be administered 10-15 minutes prior to radiological/diagnostic procedures.

Topical Transdermal: Topical patch is programmed to deliver 1 mg over 3 days. Once applied, do not remove the patch for 3 full days. Apply to hairless area of skin behind the ear. Wash hands before and after applying the disc to avoid drug contact with eyes.

Stability

Storage

Injection: Store at room temperature of 15°C to 30°C (58°F to 86°F). Protect from light.

Hydrobromide injection: Avoid acid solutions, hydrolysis occurs at pH <3.

Butylbromide injection: Stable in D_5W, NS, $D_{10}W$, and LR for up to 8 hours.

Tablet: Store at room temperature of 15°C to 30°C (58°F to 86°F).

Transdermal system: Store at 20°C to 25°C (68°F to 77°F).

Monitoring and Teaching Issues

Physical Assessment When used preoperatively, safety precautions should be observed and patient should be advised about blurred vision.

Patient Education May cause drowsiness, confusion, impaired judgment, vision changes, dry mouth, nausea, vomiting, orthostatic hypotension, constipation, increased sensitivity to heat and decreased perspiration, or decreased milk if breast-feeding. Report hot, dry, flushed skin; blurred vision or vision changes; difficulty swallowing; chest pain, palpitations, or rapid heartbeat; painful or difficult urination; increased confusion, depression, or loss of memory; rapid or difficult respirations; muscle weakness or tremors; or eye pain.

Transdermal: Apply patch behind ear the day before traveling. Wash hands before and after applying and avoid contact with the eyes. Do not remove for 3 days. Patch may contain metal; remove prior to MRI; can cause burns.

Geriatric Considerations Anticholinergic agents are not well tolerated in the elderly and their use should be avoided when possible.

Pregnancy Considerations Teratogenic effects were not observed in animal studies; embryotoxic events were observed in some studies. Scopolamine crosses the placenta; may cause respiratory depression and/or neonatal hemorrhage when used during pregnancy. Transdermal scopolamine has been used as an adjunct to epidural anesthesia for cesarean delivery without adverse CNS effects on the newborn. Except when used prior to cesarean section, use during pregnancy only if the benefit to the mother outweighs the potential risk to the fetus.

◆ **Scopolamine Base** *see* Scopolamine (Systemic) *on page* 1627

◆ **Scopolamine Butylbromide** *see* Scopolamine (Systemic) *on page* 1627

◆ **Scopolamine Hydrobromide** *see* Scopolamine (Systemic) *on page* 1627

- **Scot-Tussin® DM Maximum Strength [OTC]** *see* Dextromethorphan and Chlorpheniramine *on page 513*
- **Scot-Tussin® Expectorant [OTC]** *see* GuaiFENesin *on page 890*
- **SDX-105** *see* Bendamustine *on page 198*
- **SDZ ENA 713** *see* Rivastigmine *on page 1601*
- **Seasonale®** *see* Ethinyl Estradiol and Levonorgestrel *on page 699*
- **Seasonique®** *see* Ethinyl Estradiol and Levonorgestrel *on page 699*
- **Secura® Antifungal Extra Thick [OTC]** *see* Miconazole (Topical) *on page 1224*
- **Secura® Antifungal Greaseless [OTC]** *see* Miconazole (Topical) *on page 1224*
- **Sedapap®** *see* Butalbital and Acetaminophen *on page 261*

Selegiline (se LE ji leen)

U.S. Brand Names Eldepryl®; Emsam®; Zelapar™

Index Terms Deprenyl; L-Deprenyl; Selegiline Hydrochloride

Generic Availability (U.S.) Yes: Capsule, tablet

Pharmacologic Category Anti-Parkinson's Agent, MAO Type B Inhibitor; Antidepressant, Monoamine Oxidase Inhibitor

Medication Safety Issues

Sound-alike/look-alike issues:

Selegiline may be confused with Salagen®, Serentil®, sertraline, Serzone®, Stelazine®

Eldepryl® may be confused with Elavil®, enalapril

Zelapar™ may be confused with zaleplon, Zemplar®, ZyPREXA® Zydis®

Medication Guide Available Yes

Pregnancy Risk Factor C

Lactation Excretion in breast milk unknown/use caution

Use Adjunct in the management of parkinsonian patients in which levodopa/carbidopa therapy is deteriorating (oral products); treatment of major depressive disorder (transdermal product)

Unlabeled/Investigational Use Early Parkinson's disease; attention-deficit/hyperactivity disorder (ADHD); negative symptoms of schizophrenia; extrapyramidal symptoms

Mechanism of Action/Effect At lower oral doses (capsule/tablet ≤10 mg/day; orally disintegrating tablet <2.5 mg/day), selegiline is a selective monoamine oxidase (MAO) type B inhibitor, which increases dopaminergic synaptic activity thus reducing symptoms of Parkinsonism. At higher oral doses or administered transdermally in recommended doses, selegiline nonselectively inhibits both MAO-B and MAO-A which blocks catabolism of other centrally-active biogenic amine neurotransmitters leading to improved mood

Contraindications Hypersensitivity to selegiline or any component of the formulation; concomitant use of meperidine

Orally disintegrating tablet: Additional contraindications: Concomitant use of dextromethorphan, methadone, propoxyphene, tramadol, oral selegiline, other MAO inhibitors

Transdermal: Additional contraindications: Pheochromocytoma; concomitant use of bupropion, selective or dual serotonin reuptake inhibitors (including SSRIs and SNRIs), tricyclic antidepressants, buspirone, tramadol, propoxyphene, methadone, dextromethorphan, St. John's wort, mirtazapine, cyclobenzaprine, oral selegiline and other MAO inhibitors; carbamazepine, and oxcarbazepine; elective surgery requiring general anesthesia, local anesthesia containing sympathomimetic vasoconstrictors; sympathomimetics (and related compounds); foods high in tyramine content; supplements containing tyrosine, phenylalanine, tryptophan, or caffeine

Warnings/Precautions

Oral: MAO-B selective inhibition should not pose a problem with tyramine-containing products as long as the typical oral doses are employed, however, rare reactions have been reported. Increased risk of nonselective MAO inhibition occurs with oral capsule/tablet doses >10 mg/day or orally disintegrating tablet doses >2.5 mg/day. Use of oral selegiline with tricyclic antidepressants and SSRIs has also been associated with rare reactions and should generally be avoided. Addition to levodopa therapy may result in exacerbation of levodopa adverse effects, requiring a reduction in levodopa dosage. Dopaminergic agents used for Parkinson's disease or restless legs syndrome have been associated with compulsive behaviors and/or loss of impulse control, which has manifested as pathological gambling, libido increases (hypersexuality), and/or binge eating. Causality has not been established, and controversy exists as to whether this phenomenon is related to the underlying disease, prior behaviors/addictions and/or drug therapy. Dose reduction or discontinuation of therapy has been reported to reverse these behaviors in some, but not all cases. Risk for melanoma development is increased in Parkinson's disease patients; drug causation or factors contributing to risk have not been established. Patients should be monitored closely and periodic skin examinations should be performed.

Transdermal: Nonselective MAO inhibition occurs with transdermal delivery and is necessary for antidepressant efficacy. Hypertensive crisis as a result of ingesting tyramine-rich foods is always a concern with nonselective MAO inhibition. Although transdermal delivery minimizes inhibition of MAO-A in the gut, there is limited data with higher transdermal doses; dietary restrictions are recommended with doses >6 mg/24 hours.

Transdermal patch: May contain conducting metal (eg, aluminum); remove patch prior to MRI.

Transdermal: **[U.S. Boxed Warning]: Antidepressants increase the risk of suicidal thinking and behavior in children, adolescents, and young adults (18-24 years of age) with major depressive disorder (MDD) and other psychiatric disorders;** consider risk prior to prescribing. Short-term studies did not show an increased risk in patients >24 years of age and showed a decreased risk in patients ≥65 years. Closely monitor patients for worsening of depression, suicidality and/or associated behaviors, particularly during the initial 1-2 months of therapy or during periods of dosage adjustments (increases or decreases); the patient's family or caregiver should be instructed to closely observe the patient and communicate condition with healthcare provider. A medication guide concerning the use of antidepressants should be dispensed with each prescription. **Transdermal selegiline is not FDA approved for use in children <12 years of age.**

Transdermal: The possibility of a suicide attempt is inherit in major depression and may persist until remission occurs. Patients treated with antidepressants (for any indication) should be observed for clinical worsening and suicidality, especially during the initial few months of a course of drug therapy, or at times of dose changes, either increases or decreases. Use caution in high-risk patients. Worsening depression and severe abrupt suicidality that are not part of the presenting symptoms may require discontinuation or modification of drug therapy. Use caution in high-risk patients during initiation of therapy. The patient's family or caregiver should be alerted to monitor patients for the emergence of suicidality and associated behaviors (such as agitation, irritability, hostility, and hypomania) and call healthcare provider.

Transdermal selegiline may worsen psychosis in some patients or precipitate a shift to mania or hypomania in patients with bipolar disorder. Monotherapy in patients with bipolar disorder should be avoided. Patients presenting with depressive symptoms should be screened for bipolar disorder. **Selegiline is not FDA approved for the treatment of bipolar depression.**

Drug Interactions

Metabolism/Transport Effects Substrate of CYP1A2 (minor), 2A6 (minor), 2B6 (major), 2C8 (minor), 2C19 (minor), 2D6 (minor), 3A4 (minor); **Inhibits** CYP1A2 (weak), 2A6 (weak), 2C9 (weak), 2C19 (weak), 2D6 (weak), 2E1 (weak), 3A4 (weak)

Avoid Concomitant Use

Avoid concomitant use of Selegiline with any of the following: Alpha-/Beta-Agonists (Indirect-Acting); Alpha1-Agonists; Alpha2-Agonists (Ophthalmic); Amphetamines; Anilidopiperidine Opioids; Atomoxetine; Bezafibrate; Buprenorphine; BuPROPion; BusPIRone; CarBAMazepine; Cyclobenzaprine; Dexmethylphenidate; Dextromethorphan; Diethylpropion; HYDROmorphone; Linezolid; Maprotiline; Meperidine; Methyldopa; Methylphenidate; Mirtazapine; OXcarbazepine; Propoxyphene; Selective Serotonin Reuptake Inhibitors; Serotonin 5-HT1D Receptor Agonists; Serotonin/Norepinephrine Reuptake Inhibitors; Sibutramine; Tapentadol; Tetrabenazine; Tetrahydrozoline; Tetrahydrozoline (Nasal); Tricyclic Antidepressants; Tryptophan

Decreased Effect

The levels/effects of Selegiline may be decreased by: CYP2B6 Inducers (Strong); Peginterferon Alfa-2b

Increased Effect/Toxicity

Selegiline may increase the levels/effects of: Alpha-/Beta-Agonists (Direct-Acting); Alpha-/Beta-Agonists (Indirect-Acting); Alpha1-Agonists; Alpha2-Agonists (Ophthalmic); Amphetamines; Antihypertensives; Atomoxetine; Beta2-Agonists; Bezafibrate; BuPROPion; Dexmethylphenidate; Dextromethorphan; Diethylpropion; Doxapram; HYDROmorphone; Linezolid; Lithium; Meperidine; Methadone; Methyldopa; Methylphenidate; Mirtazapine; Orthostatic Hypotension Producing Agents; Reserpine; Selective Serotonin Reuptake Inhibitors; Serotonin 5-HT1D Receptor Agonists; Serotonin Modulators; Serotonin/Norepinephrine Reuptake Inhibitors; Tetrahydrozoline; Tetrahydrozoline (Nasal); Tricyclic Antidepressants

The levels/effects of Selegiline may be increased by: Altretamine; Anilidopiperidine Opioids; Buprenorphine; BusPIRone; CarBAMazepine; COMT Inhibitors; Conivaptan; Contraceptives (Estrogens); Contraceptives (Progestins); Cyclobenzaprine; CYP2B6 Inhibitors (Moderate); CYP2B6 Inhibitors (Strong); Levodopa; MAO Inhibitors; Maprotiline; OXcarbazepine; Propoxyphene; Quazepam; Sibutramine; Tapentadol; Tetrabenazine; TraMADol; Tryptophan

Nutritional/Ethanol Interactions

Ethanol: Avoid ethanol (based on CNS depressant effects and potential tyramine content)

Food: Concurrent ingestion of foods rich in tyramine may cause sudden and severe high blood pressure (hypertensive crisis). Avoid tyramine-containing foods with MAO-Is.

Herb/Nutraceuticals: Avoid valerian, St John's wort, SAMe, kava kava. Avoid supplements containing caffeine, tryptophan, or phenylalanine. Ingestion of large quantities may increase the risk of severe side effects (eg, hypertensive reactions, serotonin syndrome).

Lab Interactions May interfere with urine detection of amphetamine/methamphetamine (false-positive).

Adverse Reactions Unless otherwise noted, the percentage of adverse events is reported for the transdermal patch (**Note:** ODT = orally disintegrating tablet, Oral = capsule/tablet)

>10%:

- Central nervous system: Headache (18%; ODT 7%; oral 2%), insomnia (12%; ODT 7%), dizziness (ODT 11%; oral 7%)
- Gastrointestinal: Nausea (ODT 11%; oral 10%)
- Local: Application site reaction (24%)

1% to 10%:

- Cardiovascular: Hypotension (including postural 3% to 10%), chest pain (≥1%; ODT 2%), hypertension (≥1%), peripheral edema (≥1%)
- Central nervous system: Pain (ODT 8%), hallucinations (ODT 4%; oral 3%), confusion (ODT 4%; oral 3%), headache (ODT 7%; oral 2%), ataxia (ODT 3%), somnolence (ODT 3%), agitation (≥1%), amnesia (≥1%), paresthesia (≥1%), thinking abnormal (≥1%), depression (<1%; ODT 2%)
- Dermatologic: Rash (4%), ecchymosis (ODT 2%), bruising (≥1%), pruritus (≥1%), acne (≥1%)
- Endocrine & metabolic: Weight loss (5%), hypokalemia (ODT 2%), sexual side effects (≤1%)

Gastrointestinal: Diarrhea (9%; ODT 2%), xerostomia (8%; ODT 4%), stomatitis (ODT 5%), abdominal pain (oral 4%), dyspepsia (4%; ODT 5%), constipation (≥1%; ODT 4%), flatulence (≥1%; ODT 2%), anorexia (≥1%), gastroenteritis (≥1%), taste perversion (≥1%; ODT 2%), vomiting (≥1%; ODT 3%), tooth disorder (ODT 2%), dysphagia (ODT 2%)
Genitourinary: Dysmenorrhea (≥1%), metrorrhagia (≥1%), UTI (≥1%), urinary frequency (≥1%)
Neuromuscular & skeletal: Dyskinesia (ODT 6%), back pain (ODT 5%), ataxia (<1%; ODT 3%), leg cramps (ODT 3%), myalgia (≥1%; ODT 3%), neck pain (≥1%), tremor (<1%; ODT 3%)
Otic: Tinnitus (≥1%)
Respiratory: Rhinitis (ODT 7%), pharyngitis (3%; ODT 4%), sinusitis (3%), cough (≥1%), bronchitis (≥1%), dyspnea (<1%; ODT 3%)
Miscellaneous: Diaphoresis (≥1%)

Pharmacodynamics/Kinetics

Onset of Action Therapeutic: Oral: Within 1 hour

Duration of Action Oral: 24-72 hours

Absorption
Orally disintegrating tablet: Rapid; greater bioavailability than capsule/tablet
Transdermal: 25% to 30% (of total selegiline content) over 24 hours

Protein Binding Protein binding: ~90%

Half-Life Elimination 18-25 hours

Metabolism Hepatic, primarily via CYP2B6 to active (N-desmethylselegiline, amphetamine, methamphetamine) and inactive metabolites

Excretion Urine (primarily metabolites); feces

Available Dosage Forms

Capsule, oral: 5 mg
Eldepryl®: 5 mg

Patch, transdermal:
Emsam®: 6 mg/24 hours (30s); 9 mg/24 hours (30s); 12 mg/24 hours (30s)

Tablet, oral: 5 mg

Tablet, orally disintegrating, oral:
Zelapar™: 1.25 mg

Dosing

Adult

Parkinson's disease:
Capsule/tablet: 5 mg twice daily with breakfast and lunch or 10 mg in the morning
Orally disintegrating tablet (Zelapar™): Initial 1.25 mg daily for at least 6 weeks; may increase to 2.5 mg daily based on clinical response (maximum: 2.5 mg daily)

Depression: Transdermal (Emsam®): Initial: 6 mg/24 hours once daily; may titrate based on clinical response in increments of 3 mg/day every 2 weeks up to a maximum of 12 mg/24 hours

Geriatric

Parkinson's disease:
Capsule/tablet: Initial: 5 mg in the morning; may increase to a total of 10 mg/day.
Orally disintegrating tablet (Zelapar™): Initial 1.25 mg daily for at least 6 weeks; may increase to 2.5 mg daily based on clinical response (maximum: 2.5 mg daily)

Depression: Transdermal (Emsam®): 6 mg/24 hours

Pediatric ADHD (unlabeled use): Children and Adolescents: Oral: 5-15 mg/day

Renal Impairment No adjustment necessary.

Hepatic Impairment No adjustment necessary in mild-moderate hepatic impairment.

Administration

Oral Orally disintegrating tablet (Zelapar™): Take in morning before breakfast; place on top of tongue and allow to dissolve. Avoid food or liquid 5 minutes before and after administration.

Topical Transdermal (Emsam®): Apply to clean, dry, intact skin to the upper torso (below the neck and above the waist), upper thigh, or outer surface of the upper arm. Avoid exposure of application site to external heat source, which may increase the amount of drug absorbed. Apply at the same time each day and rotate application sites. Wash hands with soap and water after handling. Avoid touching the sticky side of the patch.

Stability

Storage
Capsule, tablet: Store at controlled room temperature 15°C to 30°C (59°F to 86°F).
Orally-disintegrating tablet: Store at controlled room temperature 15°C to 30°C (59°F to 86°F). Use within 3 months of opening pouch and immediately after opening individual blister.
Transdermal: Store at 20°C to 25°C (68°F to 77°F).

Monitoring and Teaching Issues

Physical Assessment Assess effectiveness and interactions of other medications patient may be taking. Monitor therapeutic effectiveness according to rationale for therapy and adverse reactions at beginning of therapy and periodically throughout therapy. Monitor blood pressure. Be alert to thoughts of suicide. Patient should be cautioned against eating foods high in tyramine. Assess knowledge/teach patient appropriate use, interventions to reduce side effects, and adverse symptoms to report. Discontinue at least 10 days prior to elective surgery. Taper dose when discontinuing.

Patient Education May be prescribed in conjunction with levodopa/carbidopa. Therapeutic effects may take several weeks or months to achieve and you may need frequent monitoring during first weeks of therapy. Take oral capsule/tablet with meals if GI upset occurs. Do not take food or liquid for 5 minutes before or after administering orally disintegrating tablets. Do not swallow orally disintegrating tablet; allow to dissolve on tongue. Take at the same time each day. Avoid tyramine-containing foods (low potential for reaction) with oral products. Maintain adequate hydration unless instructed to restrict fluid intake. Do not use alcohol. You may experience drowsiness, dizziness, confusion, vision changes, orthostatic hypotension, constipation, runny nose or flu-like symptoms, nausea, vomiting, loss of appetite, or stomach discomfort. Report unresolved constipation or vomiting; chest pain, palpitations, irregular heartbeat; CNS changes (hallucination, loss of memory, seizures, acute headache, nervousness, suicide ideation); painful or difficult urination; stiff neck; increased muscle spasticity, rigidity, or involuntary movements; changes in the appearance of skin moles, skin rash, or other unusual skin changes; or significant worsening of condition.

Dietary Considerations Avoid tyramine-containing foods/beverages. Some examples include aged or matured cheese, air-dried or cured meats (including sausages and salamis), fava or broad bean pods, tap/draft beers, Marmite concentrate, sauerkraut, soy sauce and other soybean condiments. Food's freshness is also an important concern; improperly stored or spoiled food can create an environment where tyramine concentrations may increase.

Emsam® 9 mg/24 hours or 12 mg/24 hours: Avoid tyramine-rich foods or beverages beginning the first day of treatment or for 2 weeks after discontinuation or dose reduction to 6 mg/24 hours.

Zelapar™: Do not take with food or liquid.

Some products may contain phenylalanine.

Geriatric Considerations Do not use capsule/tablet at doses >10 mg/day or orally disintegrating tablet at doses >2.5 mg/day because of the risks associated with nonselective inhibition of MAO.

Orally-disintegrating tablets: In clinical trials, adverse effects were seen more frequently in the elderly compared to younger adults. This is particularly of concern for hypertension, orthostatic hypotension, dizziness, and somnolence. If using the orally disintegrating tablets, administer at the lowest dose and monitor for side effects.

Pregnancy Considerations Teratogenic and adverse behavioral events were noted in animal studies. There are no adequate and well-controlled studies in pregnant women.

Additional Information When adding selegiline to levodopa/carbidopa, the dose of the latter can usually be decreased.

Related Information

Antidepressant Agents *on page 1982*

- **Selegiline Hydrochloride** *see* Selegiline *on page 1630*
- **Selfemra® [DSC]** *see* FLUoxetine *on page 789*
- **Selzentry™** *see* Maraviroc *on page 1147*
- **Sensipar®** *see* Cinacalcet *on page 373*
- **Sensorcaine®** *see* Bupivacaine *on page 244*
- **Sensorcaine®-MPF** *see* Bupivacaine *on page 244*
- **Sensorcaine®-MPF Spinal** *see* Bupivacaine *on page 244*
- **Septra® [DSC]** *see* Sulfamethoxazole and Trimethoprim *on page 1686*
- **Septra® DS** *see* Sulfamethoxazole and Trimethoprim *on page 1686*
- **Serax®** *see* Oxazepam *on page 1374*
- **Serevent® Diskus®** *see* Salmeterol *on page 1618*
- **Serophene®** *see* ClomiPHENE *on page 402*
- **SEROquel®** *see* QUEtiapine *on page 1533*
- **SEROquel XR®** *see* QUEtiapine *on page 1533*
- **Serostim®** *see* Somatropin *on page 1664*

Sertraline (SER tra leen)

U.S. Brand Names Zoloft®

Index Terms Sertraline Hydrochloride

Generic Availability (U.S.) Yes

Pharmacologic Category Antidepressant, Selective Serotonin Reuptake Inhibitor

Medication Safety Issues

Sound-alike/look-alike issues:

Sertraline may be confused with selegiline, Serentil®, Serevent®, Soriatane®

Zoloft® may be confused with Zocor®

Medication Guide Available Yes

Pregnancy Risk Factor C

Lactation Enters breast milk/use caution (AAP rates "of concern"; AAP 2001 update pending)

Use Treatment of major depression; obsessive-compulsive disorder (OCD); panic disorder; post-traumatic stress disorder (PTSD); premenstrual dysphoric disorder (PMDD); social anxiety disorder

Unlabeled/Investigational Use Eating disorders; generalized anxiety disorder (GAD); impulse control disorders; treatment of mild dementia-associated agitation in nonpsychotic patients

Mechanism of Action/Effect Antidepressant with selective inhibitory effects on presynaptic serotonin (5-HT) reuptake and only very weak effects on norepinephrine and dopamine neuronal uptake

Contraindications Hypersensitivity to sertraline or any component of the formulation; use of MAO inhibitors within 14 days; concurrent use of pimozide; concurrent use of sertraline oral concentrate with disulfiram

Warnings/Precautions [U.S. Boxed Warning]: Antidepressants increase the risk of suicidal thinking and behavior in children, adolescents, and young adults (18-24 years of age) with major depressive disorder (MDD) and other psychiatric disorders; consider risk prior to prescribing. Short-term studies did not show an increased risk in patients >24 years of age and showed a decreased risk in patients ≥65 years. Closely monitor patients for clinical worsening, suicidality, or unusual changes in behavior, particularly during the initial 1-2 months of therapy or during periods of dosage adjustments (increases or decreases); the patient's family or caregiver should be instructed to closely observe the patient and communicate condition with healthcare provider. A medication guide concerning the use of antidepressants should be dispensed with each prescription. **Sertraline is not FDA approved for use in children with major depressive disorder (MDD). However, it is approved for the treatment of obsessive-compulsive disorder (OCD) in children ≥6 years of age.**

The possibility of a suicide attempt is inherent in major depression and may persist until remission occurs. Use caution in high-risk patients. Worsening depression and severe abrupt suicidality that are not part of the presenting symptoms may require discontinuation or modification of drug therapy. The patient's family or caregiver should be alerted to monitor patients for the emergence of suicidality and associated behaviors (such as agitation, irritability, hostility, impulsivity, and hypomania) and call healthcare provider.

May worsen psychosis in some patients or precipitate a shift to mania or hypomania in patients with bipolar disorder. Patients presenting with depressive symptoms should be screened for bipolar disorder. Monotherapy in patients with bipolar disorder should be avoided. **Sertraline is not FDA approved for the treatment of bipolar depression.**

Serotonin syndrome and neuroleptic malignant syndrome (NMS)-like reactions have occurred with serotonin/norepinephrine reuptake inhibitors (SNRIs) and selective serotonin reuptake inhibitors (SSRIs) when used alone, and particularly when used in combination with serotonergic agents (eg, triptans) or antidopaminergic agents (eg, antipsychotics). Concurrent use with MAO inhibitors is contraindicated. Has a very low potential to impair cognitive or motor performance. However, caution patients regarding activities requiring alertness until response to sertraline is known. Does not appear to potentiate the effects of alcohol, however, ethanol use is not advised.

Use caution in patients with a previous seizure disorder or condition predisposing to seizures such as brain damage, alcoholism, or concurrent therapy with other drugs which lower the seizure threshold. May increase the risks associated with electroconvulsive therapy. Use with caution in patients with hepatic or renal dysfunction and in elderly patients. May cause hyponatremia/SIADH (elderly at increased risk); volume depletion (diuretics may increase risk). Use with caution in patients with renal insufficiency or other concurrent illness (due to limited experience). Sertraline acts as a mild uricosuric; use with caution in patients at risk of uric acid nephropathy. Use caution with concomitant use of NSAIDs, ASA, or other drugs that affect coagulation; the risk of bleeding may be potentiated. Use with caution in patients where weight loss is undesirable. May cause or exacerbate sexual dysfunction.

Use oral concentrate formulation with caution in patients with latex sensitivity; dropper dispenser contains dry natural rubber. Monitor growth in pediatric patients. Discontinuation symptoms (eg, dysphoric mood, irritability, agitation, confusion, anxiety, insomnia, hypomania) may occur upon abrupt discontinuation. Taper dose when discontinuing therapy.

Drug Interactions

Metabolism/Transport Effects Substrate of CYP2B6 (minor), 2C9 (minor), 2C19 (major), 2D6 (major), 3A4 (minor); **Inhibits** CYP1A2 (weak), 2B6 (moderate), 2C8 (weak), 2C9 (weak), 2C19 (moderate), 2D6 (moderate), 3A4 (moderate)

Avoid Concomitant Use

Avoid concomitant use of Sertraline with any of the following: Clopidogrel; Disulfiram; Iobenguane I 123; MAO Inhibitors; Methylene Blue; Pimozide; Sibutramine; Thioridazine; Tolvaptan; Tryptophan

Decreased Effect

Sertraline may decrease the levels/effects of: Clopidogrel; Iobenguane I 123

The levels/effects of Sertraline may be decreased by: CarBAMazepine; Cyproheptadine; Darunavir; Efavirenz; Peginterferon Alfa-2b; Phenytoin

Increased Effect/Toxicity

Sertraline may increase the levels/effects of: Alcohol (Ethyl); Alpha-/Beta-Blockers; Anticoagulants; Antidepressants (Serotonin Reuptake Inhibitor/Antagonist); Antiplatelet Agents; Aspirin; Beta-Blockers; BusPIRone; CarBAMazepine; CloZAPine; CNS Depressants; Colchicine; Collagenase (Systemic); CYP2B6 Substrates; CYP2C19 Substrates; CYP2D6 Substrates; CYP3A4 Substrates; Desmopressin; Dextromethorphan; Drotrecogin Alfa; Eplerenone; Everolimus; Fesoterodine; Galantamine; Halofantrine; Haloperidol; Ibritumomab; Lithium; Lurasidone; Methadone; Methotrimeprazine; Methylene Blue; NSAID (COX-2 Inhibitor); NSAID (Nonselective); Phenytoin; Pimecrolimus; Pimozide; Ranolazine; RisperiDONE; Salicylates; Salmeterol; Saxagliptin; Serotonin Modulators; Tamoxifen; Thioridazine; Thrombolytic Agents; Tolvaptan; Tositumomab and Iodine I 131 Tositumomab; TraMADol; Tricyclic Antidepressants; Vitamin K Antagonists

The levels/effects of Sertraline may be increased by: Analgesics (Opioid); BusPIRone; Cimetidine; Conivaptan; CYP2D6 Inhibitors (Moderate); CYP2D6 Inhibitors (Strong); Dasatinib; Disulfiram; Droperidol; Glucosamine; Herbs (Anticoagulant/Antiplatelet Properties);

Macrolide Antibiotics; MAO Inhibitors; Methotrimeprazine; Metoclopramide; Omega-3-Acid Ethyl Esters; Pentosan Polysulfate Sodium; Pentoxifylline; Prostacyclin Analogues; Sibutramine; TraMADol; Tryptophan

Nutritional/Ethanol Interactions

Ethanol: Avoid ethanol (may increase CNS depression).

Food: Sertraline average peak serum levels may be increased if taken with food.

Herb/Nutraceutical: Avoid valerian, St John's wort, kava kava, gotu kola (may increase CNS depression).

Lab Interactions

Increased (minor) serum triglycerides, LFTs; decreased serum uric acid; may interfere with urine detection of benzodiazepines (false-positive)

Adverse Reactions

>10%:

Central nervous system: Dizziness, fatigue, headache, insomnia, somnolence
Endocrine & metabolic: Libido decreased
Gastrointestinal: Anorexia, diarrhea, nausea, xerostomia
Genitourinary: Ejaculatory disturbances
Neuromuscular & skeletal: Tremors
Miscellaneous: Diaphoresis

1% to 10%:

Cardiovascular: Chest pain, palpitation
Central nervous system: Agitation, anxiety, hypoesthesia, malaise, nervousness, pain
Dermatologic: Rash
Endocrine & metabolic: Impotence
Gastrointestinal: Appetite increased, constipation, dyspepsia, flatulence, vomiting, weight gain
Neuromuscular & skeletal: Back pain, hypertonia, myalgia, paresthesia, weakness
Ocular: Visual difficulty, abnormal vision
Otic: Tinnitus
Respiratory: Rhinitis
Miscellaneous: Yawning

Additional adverse reactions reported in pediatric patients (frequency >2%): Aggressiveness, epistaxis, hyperkinesia, purpura, sinusitis, urinary incontinence

Pharmacodynamics/Kinetics

Onset of Action Depression: The onset of action is within a week, however, individual response varies greatly and full response may not be seen until 8-12 weeks after initiation of treatment.

Absorption Slow

Bioavailability Bioavailability of tablets and solution are equivalent

Time to Peak Plasma: Sertraline: 4.5-8.4 hours

Protein Binding 98%

Half-Life Elimination Sertraline: 26 hours; N-desmethylsertraline: 66 hours (range: 62-104 hours)

Metabolism Hepatic; may involve CYP2C19 and CYP2D6; extensive first pass metabolism; forms metabolite N-desmethylsertraline

Excretion Urine and feces

Available Dosage Forms

Solution, oral: 20 mg/mL (60 mL)
Zoloft®: 20 mg/mL (60 mL)

Tablet, oral: 25 mg, 50 mg, 100 mg
Zoloft®: 25 mg, 50 mg, 100 mg

Dosing

Adult

Depression/obsessive-compulsive disorder: Oral: Initial: 50 mg/day

Note: May increase daily dose, at intervals of not less than 1 week, to a maximum of 200 mg/day. If somnolence is noted, give at bedtime.

Panic disorder, post-traumatic stress disorder, social anxiety disorder: Oral: Initial: 25 mg once daily; increased after 1 week to 50 mg once daily; maximum dose: 200 mg/day

Premenstrual dysphoric disorder: 50 mg/day either daily throughout menstrual cycle **or** limited to the luteal phase of menstrual cycle, depending on physician assessment. Patients not responding to 50 mg/day may benefit from dose increases (50 mg increments per menstrual cycle) up to 150 mg/day when dosing throughout menstrual cycle **or** up to 100 mg day when dosing during luteal phase only. If a 100 mg/day dose has been established with luteal phase dosing, a 50 mg/day titration step for 3 days should be utilized at the beginning of each luteal phase dosing period.

Geriatric Oral: Initial: 25 mg/day in the morning; increase by 25 mg/day increments every 2-3 days if tolerated to 50-100 mg/day; additional increases may be necessary; maximum: 200 mg/day. **Note:** Patients with Alzheimer's dementia-related depression may require a lower starting dosage of 12.5 mg/day, with titration intervals of 1-2 weeks, up to 150-200 mg/day maximum.

Pediatric

Obsessive-compulsive disorder: Oral: Children:

6-12 years: Initial: 25 mg once daily
13-17 years: Initial: 50 mg once daily

May increase daily dose, at intervals of not less than 1 week, to a maximum: 200 mg/day. If somnolence is noted, give at bedtime.

Renal Impairment Multiple-dose pharmacokinetics are unaffected by renal impairment.

Hemodialysis effect: Not removed by hemodialysis

Hepatic Impairment Sertraline is extensively metabolized by the liver. Caution should be used in patients with hepatic impairment. A lower dose or less frequent dosing should be used.

Administration

Oral Oral concentrate: Must be diluted before use. Immediately before administration, use the dropper provided to measure the required amount of concentrate; mix with 4 ounces (1/2 cup) of water, ginger ale, lemon/lime soda, lemonade, or orange juice **only**. Do not mix with any other liquids than these. The dose should be taken immediately after mixing; do not mix in advance. A slight haze may appear after mixing; this is normal. **Note:** Use with caution in patients with latex sensitivity; dropper dispenser contains dry natural rubber.

Stability

Storage Tablets and oral solution should be stored at controlled room temperature of 15°C to 30°C (59°F to 86°F).

Monitoring and Teaching Issues

Physical Assessment Assess mental status for worsening of depression, suicide ideation, anxiety, social functioning, mania, or panic attack (especially during initiation of therapy and when dosage is changed). Taper dosage slowly when discontinuing. Pediatric patients: Monitor growth pattern.

Patient Education It may take 2-3 weeks to achieve desired results. Take in the morning to reduce the incidence of insomnia. Avoid alcohol. Maintain adequate hydration unless instructed to restrict fluid intake. You may experience drowsiness, dizziness, lightheadedness, nausea, vomiting, anorexia, dry mouth, postural hypotension, urinary pattern changes, or male sexual dysfunction (reversible). Report persistent insomnia or daytime sedation, agitation, nervousness, fatigue; muscle cramping, tremors, or weakness; chest pain, palpitations, or swelling of extremities; vision changes; ringing in ears; skin rash or irritation; suicide ideation; or worsening of condition.

Geriatric Considerations Sertraline's favorable side effect profile makes it a useful alternative to the traditional tricyclic antidepressants; its potential stimulation effect and anorexia may be bothersome. Has the shortest half-life of the currently marketed serotonin-reuptake inhibitors. Data from a clinical trial comparing fluoxetine to tricyclics suggest that fluoxetine is significantly less effective than nortriptyline in hospitalized elderly patients with unipolar major affective disorder, especially those with melancholia and concurrent cardiovascular diseases. The elderly are more prone to SSRI/SNRI-induced hyponatremia.

Breast-Feeding Considerations Sertraline and desmethylsertraline are excreted in breast milk. Infants exposed to sertraline while breast-feeding generally receive a low relative dose and serum concentrations are not detectable in most infants. Adverse reactions have not been reported in nursing infants. Sertraline concentrations in the hindmilk are higher than in foremilk. If the benefits of the mother receiving the sertraline and breast-feeding outweigh the risks, the mother may consider pumping and discarding breast milk with the feeding 7-9 hours after the daily dose to decrease sertraline exposure to the infant. The long-term effects on development and behavior have not been studied. The manufacturer recommends that caution be exercised when administering sertraline to nursing women.

Pregnancy Considerations Due to adverse effects observed in animal studies, sertraline is classified as pregnancy category C. Sertraline crosses the human placenta. Nonteratogenic effects in the newborn following SSRI exposure late in the third trimester include respiratory distress, cyanosis, apnea, seizures, temperature instability, feeding difficulty, vomiting, hypoglycemia, hypo- or hypertonia, hyper-reflexia, jitteriness, irritability, constant crying, and tremor. An increased risk of low birth weight, lower Apgar scores, and blunted behavioral response to pain for a prolonged period after delivery has also been reported. Exposure to SSRIs after the twentieth week of gestation has been associated with persistent pulmonary hypertension of the newborn (PPHN). Adverse effects may be due to toxic effects of the SSRI or drug discontinuation. The long-term effects of *in utero* SSRI exposure on infant development and behavior are not known.

Due to pregnancy-induced physiologic changes, women who are pregnant may require increased doses of sertraline to achieve euthymia. Women treated for major depression and who are euthymic prior to pregnancy are more likely to experience a relapse when medication is discontinued as compared to pregnant women who continue taking antidepressant medications. The ACOG recommends that therapy with SSRIs or SNRIs during pregnancy be individualized; treatment of depression during pregnancy should incorporate the clinical expertise of the mental health clinician, obstetrician, primary healthcare provider, and pediatrician. If treatment during pregnancy is required, consider tapering therapy during the third trimester in order to prevent withdrawal symptoms in the infant. If this is done and the woman is considered to be at risk of relapse from her major depressive disorder, the medication can be restarted following delivery, although the dose should be readjusted to that required before pregnancy. Treatment algorithms have been developed by the ACOG and the APA for the management of depression in women prior to conception and during pregnancy (Yonkers, 2009).

Additional Information Buspirone (15-60 mg/day) may be useful in treatment of sexual dysfunction during treatment with a selective serotonin reuptake inhibitor. May exacerbate tics in Tourette's syndrome.

Related Information

Antidepressant Agents *on page* 1982

◆ **Sertraline Hydrochloride** *see* Sertraline *on page* 1633

◆ **Serzone** *see* Nefazodone *on page* 1296

Sevelamer (se VEL a mer)

U.S. Brand Names Renagel®; Renvela®

Index Terms Sevelamer Carbonate; Sevelamer Hydrochloride

Generic Availability (U.S.) No

Pharmacologic Category Phosphate Binder

Medication Safety Issues

Sound-alike/look-alike issues:

Renagel® may be confused with Reglan®, Regonol®, Renal Caps, Renvela®

Renvela® may be confused with Reglan®, Regonol®, Renagel®, Renal Caps

Sevelamer may be confused with Savella™

International issues:

Renagel [U.S., Canada, and multiple international markets] may be confused with Remegel brand name for aluminium hydroxide and magnesium carbonate [Netherlands] and for calcium carbonate [Hungary, Great Britain and Ireland] and with Remegel Wind Relief brand name for calcium carbonate and simethicone [Great Britain]

Pregnancy Risk Factor C

Lactation Excretion in breast milk unknown/use caution (not absorbed systemically but may alter maternal nutrition)

Use Reduction or control of serum phosphorous in patients with chronic kidney disease on hemodialysis

Mechanism of Action/Effect Sevelamer (a polymeric compound) binds phosphate within the intestinal lumen, limiting absorption and decreasing serum phosphate concentrations without altering calcium, aluminum, or bicarbonate concentrations.

Contraindications Hypophosphatemia; bowel obstruction

Warnings/Precautions Use with caution in patients with gastrointestinal disorders including dysphagia, swallowing disorders, severe gastrointestinal motility disorders (including constipation), or major gastrointestinal surgery. May cause reductions in vitamin D, E, K, and folic acid absorption. May bind to some drugs in the gastrointestinal tract and decrease their absorption; when changes in absorption of oral medications may have significant clinical consequences (such as antiarrhythmic and antiseizure medications), these medications should be taken at least 1 hour before or 3 hours after a dose of sevelamer. Tablets should not be taken apart or chewed; broken or crushed tablets will rapidly expand in water/saliva and may be a choking hazard.

Drug Interactions

Avoid Concomitant Use There are no known interactions where it is recommended to avoid concomitant use.

Decreased Effect

Sevelamer may decrease the levels/effects of: Calcitriol; Levothyroxine; Mycophenolate; Quinolone Antibiotics

Increased Effect/Toxicity There are no known significant interactions involving an increase in effect.

Adverse Reactions Note: A decreased incidence of gastrointestinal adverse events was observed in a clinical trial of sevelamer carbonate compared to sevelamer hydrochloride.

>10%:

Dermatologic: Pruritus (13%)

Gastrointestinal: Vomiting (22%), nausea (7% to 20%), diarrhea (4% to 19%), dyspepsia (5% to 16%)

Neuromuscular & skeletal: Limb pain (13%), arthralgia (12%)

Respiratory: Nasopharyngitis (14%), bronchitis (11%)

1% to 10%:

Cardiovascular: Hypertension (10%)

Central nervous system: Headache (9%), pyrexia (5%)

Endocrine & metabolic: Hypercalcemia (5% to 7%)

Gastrointestinal: Abdominal pain (9%), flatulence (4% to 8%), constipation (2% to 8%)

Neuromuscular & skeletal: Back pain (4%)

Respiratory: Dyspnea (10%), cough (7%), upper respiratory tract infection (5%)

Miscellaneous: Peritonitis (peritoneal dialysis: 8%)

Pharmacodynamics/Kinetics

Absorption Not systemically absorbed

Excretion Feces

Available Dosage Forms

Powder for suspension, oral:

Renvela®: 0.8 g/packet (90s); 2.4 g/packet (90s)

Tablet, oral:

Renagel®: 400 mg, 800 mg

Renvela®: 800 mg

Dosing

Adult & Geriatric Note: The dosing of sevelamer carbonate and sevelamer hydrochloride are expected to be similar, when switching from one product to another, the same dose (on a mg per mg basis) should be utilized.

Control of serum phosphorous: Oral:

Patients not taking a phosphate binder: 800-1600 mg 3 times/day with meals; the initial dose may be based on serum phosphorous levels:

>5.5 mg/dL to <7.5 mg/dL: 800 mg 3 times/day

≥7.5 mg/dL to <9.0 mg/dL: 1200-1600 mg 3 times/day

≥9.0 mg/dL: 1600 mg 3 times/day

Maintenance dose adjustment based on serum phosphorous concentration (goal range of 3.5-5.5 mg/dL; maximum dose studied was equivalent to 13 g/day [sevelamer hydrochloride] or 14 g/day [sevelamer carbonate]):

>5.5 mg/dL: Increase by 400-800 mg per meal at 2-week intervals

3.5-5.5 mg/dL: Maintain current dose

<3.5 mg/dL: Decrease by 400-800 mg per meal

Dosage adjustment when switching between phosphate binder products: 667 mg of calcium acetate is equivalent to 800 mg sevelamer (carbonate or hydrochloride)

Pediatric Control of serum phosphorous (unlabeled use): Oral: Sevelamer hydrochloride: Doses of 121-163 mg/kg/day divided 3 times/day given with meals have been used in small studies. Doses should be rounded to nearest tablet size.

Maintenance dose adjustment based on serum phosphorous concentration (based on age).

Administration

Oral Must be administered with meals.

Powder for oral suspension: Mix powder with water prior to administration. The 0.8 g packet should be mixed with 30 mL of water and the 2.4 g packet should be mixed with 60 mL of water (multiple packets may be mixed together using the appropriate amount of water). Stir vigorously to suspend mixture just prior to drinking; powder does not dissolve. Drink within 30 minutes of preparing or resuspend just prior to drinking.

Tablets: Swallow whole; do not crush, chew, or break

Stability

Storage Store at controlled room temperature of 25°C (77°F); excursions permitted to 15°C to 30°C (59°F to 86°F). Protect from moisture.

Monitoring and Teaching Issues

Laboratory Monitoring Serum chemistries, including phosphorus, calcium, bicarbonate, chloride

Physical Assessment Monitor blood pressure; calcium (phosphate) product.

Patient Education Take with meals. Do not break or chew tablets. You may experience headache, dizziness, nausea, vomiting, heartburn, diarrhea, itching, or mild neuromuscular pain or stiffness.

Dietary Considerations Take with meals. Reduced levels of folic acid, and vitamins D, E, and K may occur; most hemodialysis patients in clinical trials received vitamin supplementation.

Geriatric Considerations No specific dose changes needed for the elderly. Since electrolyte changes (ie, phosphorus, calcium) can have dramatic effects in the elderly, monitor closely.

Breast-Feeding Considerations It is not known whether sevelamer is excreted in human milk. Because sevelamer may cause a reduction in the absorption of some vitamins, it should be used with caution in nursing women.

Pregnancy Considerations Animal studies have shown reduced or irregular ossification of fetal bones. Because sevelamer may cause a reduction in the absorption of some vitamins, it should be used with caution in pregnant women.

◆ **Sevelamer Carbonate** *see* Sevelamer *on page* 1637

◆ **Sevelamer Hydrochloride** *see* Sevelamer *on page* 1637

◆ **sfRowasa™** *see* Mesalamine *on page* 1177

◆ **Shingles Vaccine** *see* Zoster Vaccine *on page* 1910

◆ **Shohl's Solution (Modified)** *see* Sodium Citrate and Citric Acid *on page* 1660

Sibutramine (si BYOO tra meen)

U.S. Brand Names Meridia® [DSC]

Index Terms Sibutramine Hydrochloride Monohydrate

Generic Availability (U.S.) No

Pharmacologic Category Anorexiant; Sympathomimetic

Medication Safety Issues

Sound-alike/look-alike issues:

Meridia® may be confused with Aredia®

Medication Guide Available Yes

Pregnancy Risk Factor C

Lactation Excretion in breast milk unknown/not recommended

Use Management of obesity in patients with an initial body mass index (BMI) ≥30 kg/m^2 or ≥27 kg/m^2 in the presence of other risk factors (eg, diabetes, hyperlipidemia, hypertension)

Mechanism of Action/Effect Sibutramine blocks the neuronal uptake of norepinephrine, serotonin, and (to a lesser extent) dopamine

Contraindications Hypersensitivity to sibutramine or any component of the formulation; patients >65 years of age; during or within 2 weeks of MAO inhibitors or concomitant centrally-acting appetite suppressants; anorexia nervosa, bulimia nervosa; poorly-controlled or uncontrolled hypertension; history of coronary artery disease, heart failure (HF), arrhythmia, stroke, tachycardia, TIA, or peripheral arterial disease

Warnings/Precautions Pharmacotherapy for weight loss is recommended only for obese patients with a body mass index ≥30 kg/m^2, or ≥27 kg/m^2 in the presence of other risk factors, such as hypertension, diabetes, and/or dyslipidemia or a high waist circumference; therapy should be used in conjunction with a comprehensive weight management program. Rule out organic causes of obesity (eg, untreated hypothyroidism) prior to use. Discontinue or reevaluate therapy/dose if significant weight loss has not occurred (eg, <4 pounds within the first 4 weeks of treatment).

The use of some anorexigens has been associated with the development of valvular heart disease. Avoid use in patients with known serious structural cardiac abnormalities, cardiomyopathy, serious heart rhythm abnormalities, or other serious cardiac problems that could increase the risk of sudden death that these conditions alone carry.

May cause increase in blood pressure or pulse rate. For patients experiencing a sustained increase in blood pressure or pulse, dose reduction or discontinuation should be considered. Caution should be used in patients with controlled hypertension; use is contraindicated in patients with poorly-controlled or uncontrolled hypertension. Use of sibutramine in patients with CVD increased the risk of cardiovascular events in one clinical trial. Use is contraindicated in patients with a history of coronary artery disease, HF, tachycardia, arrhythmia, stroke or TIA, or peripheral arterial disease.

Primary pulmonary hypertension (PPH), a rare and frequently fatal disease of the lungs, has been found to occur with increased frequency in patients receiving some anorexigens. Although not reported in clinical trials, it is possible that sibutramine may share this potential, and patients should be monitored closely.

Use with caution in mild-moderate renal impairment or hepatic dysfunction, seizure disorder, gallstones, narrow-angle glaucoma, and elderly patients; not for use in patients with severe renal or hepatic impairment. Use caution with diabetes; antidiabetic agent requirements may be altered with anorexigens and concomitant dietary restrictions. Serotonin syndrome and neuroleptic malignant syndrome (NMS)-like reactions have occurred with serotonin/norepinephrine reuptake inhibitors (SNRIs) and selective serotonin reuptake inhibitors (SSRIs), including sibutramine, when used alone and particularly when used in combination with serotonergic agents (eg, triptans) or antidopaminergic agents (eg, antipsychotics). Avoid concurrent use with other serotonergic agents, due to the risk of developing serotonin syndrome. Rare cases of bleeding have been reported; use caution in patients with bleeding disorders. Stimulants may unmask tics in individuals with coexisting Tourette's syndrome. Rare reports of depression, mania, psychosis, suicide, and suicidal ideation have been documented; use caution and monitor closely in patients with history of psychiatric symptoms. May impair the ability to engage in potentially hazardous activities.

Drug Interactions

Metabolism/Transport Effects **Substrate** of CYP3A4 (major)

Avoid Concomitant Use

Avoid concomitant use of Sibutramine with any of the following: Iobenguane I 123; Serotonin Modulators

Decreased Effect

Sibutramine may decrease the levels/effects of: Iobenguane I 123

Increased Effect/Toxicity

Sibutramine may increase the levels/effects of: Ergot Derivatives; Serotonin Modulators; Sympathomimetics

The levels/effects of Sibutramine may be increased by: Atomoxetine; Cannabinoids; Conivaptan; CYP3A4 Inhibitors (Moderate); CYP3A4 Inhibitors (Strong); Dasatinib

Nutritional/Ethanol Interactions

Ethanol: Avoid excess ethanol ingestion.

Food: Administration with a standard breakfast reduced the peak concentrations of the active metabolites, M1 and M2 (27% and 32%, respectively) and delayed the time to peak by ~3 hours; AUC and was not significantly altered.

Herb/Nutraceutical: St John's wort and SAMe may decrease sibutramine levels.

Adverse Reactions

>10%:

Central nervous system: Headache (30%), insomnia (11%)

Gastrointestinal: Xerostomia (17%), anorexia (13%), constipation (12%)

1% to 10%:

Cardiovascular: Tachycardia (3%), vasodilation (2%), hypertension (2%), palpitation (2%), chest pain (2%), peripheral edema (≥1%)

Central nervous system: Dizziness (7%), nervousness (5%), anxiety (5%), depression (4%), CNS stimulation (2%), migraine (2%), somnolence (2%), emotional lability (1%), agitation (≥1%), fever (≥1%), thinking abnormal (≥1%)

Dermatologic: Rash (4%), pruritus (≥1%)

Endocrine & metabolic: Dysmenorrhea (4%)

Gastrointestinal: Appetite increased (9%), nausea (6%), abdominal pain (5%), dyspepsia (5%), gastritis (2%), taste perversion (2%), vomiting (2%), diarrhea (≥1%), flatulence (≥1%), gastroenteritis (≥1%), tooth disorder (≥1%)

Hepatic: Abnormal LFTs (2%)

Neuromuscular & skeletal: Back pain (8%), weakness (6%), arthralgia (6%), neck pain (2%), myalgia (2%), paresthesia (2%), tenosynovitis (1%), arthritis (≥1%), hypertonia (≥1%), leg cramps (≥1%)

Ocular: Amblyopia (≥1%)

Otic: Ear disorder (2%)

Respiratory: Pharyngitis (10%), rhinitis (10%), sinusitis (5%), cough (4%), bronchitis (≥1%), dyspnea (≥1%)

Miscellaneous: Flu-like syndrome (8%), diaphoresis (3%), allergic reactions (2%), thirst (2%)

Pharmacodynamics/Kinetics

Absorption 77%; rapid

Time to Peak Sibutramine: 1.2 hours; Metabolites (M_1 and M_2): 3-4 hours

Protein Binding Plasma: Parent drug and metabolites: >94%

Half-Life Elimination Sibutramine: 1 hour; Metabolites: M_1: 14 hours; M_2: 16 hours

Metabolism Hepatic; undergoes first-pass metabolism via CYP3A4; forms two primary metabolites (M_1 and M_2; active)

Excretion Primarily urine (77% as inactive metabolites); feces

Controlled Substance C-IV

Available Dosage Forms

Capsule, oral:

Meridia®: 5 mg, 10 mg, 15 mg

Dosing

Adult Obesity: Oral:

Initial: 10 mg once daily; may increase to 15 mg once daily after 4 weeks as needed and tolerated (maximum daily dose: 15 mg); may be used for up to 2 years, per manufacturer labeling

Maintenance: 5-15 mg once daily

Geriatric Contraindicated in patients >65 years of age

Pediatric Children ≥16 years: Refer to adult dosing.

Renal Impairment

Mild-to-moderate renal impairment: Use with caution.

Severe renal impairment (CL_{cr} ≤30 mL/minute): Use not recommended in this patient population (including patients on dialysis)

Hepatic Impairment

Mild-to-moderate hepatic impairment: No adjustment necessary

Severe hepatic impairment: Use not recommended

Administration

Oral May administer without regard to meals.

Stability

Storage Store at 25°C (77°F); excursions permitted to 15°C to 30°C (59°F to 86°F).

Monitoring and Teaching Issues

Physical Assessment Monitor vital signs, weight, and adverse reactions at start of therapy, when changing dosage, and at regular intervals during therapy.

Patient Education May be taken with meals (do not take at bedtime). Avoid caffeine. You may experience restlessness, dizziness, sleepiness, insomnia, nausea, vomiting, constipation, diarrhea, or altered menstrual periods (reversible when drug is discontinued). Report chest pain, palpitations, or irregular heartbeat; excessive nervousness, excitation, or sleepiness; back pain, muscle weakness, or tremors; CNS changes (acute headache, aggressiveness, restlessness, excitation, sleep disturbances); menstrual pattern changes; rash; blurred vision; runny nose, sinusitis, cough, or respiratory difficulty.

Dietary Considerations Most effective when combined with a low calorie diet and behavior modification counseling. May be taken without regard to meals.

Breast-Feeding Considerations Weight loss therapy is generally not recommended for lactating women. Weight loss programs which include physical activity and nutrition components should be discussed at the 6-week postpartum visit.

Pregnancy Considerations Teratogenic effects were not observed in animal studies except at doses also causing maternal toxicity. Weight loss therapy is generally not recommended for pregnant women. Obese and overweight women should be encouraged to participate in weight reduction programs prior to attempting pregnancy; weight gain during pregnancy should be determined by their prepregnancy BMI and current guidelines. Women of child-bearing potential should be instructed to use effective contraception while taking sibutramine.

Additional Information Physicians should carefully evaluate patients for history of drug abuse and follow such patients closely, observing them for signs of misuse or abuse (eg, development of tolerance, excessive increases of doses, drug seeking behavior).

Related Information

Obesity Treatment Guidelines *on page* 2064

◆ **Sibutramine Hydrochloride Monohydrate** *see* Sibutramine *on page* 1638

◆ **Siladryl Allergy [OTC]** *see* DiphenhydrAMINE (Systemic) *on page* 543

◆ **Silapap Children's [OTC]** *see* Acetaminophen *on page* 38

◆ **Silapap Infant's [OTC]** *see* Acetaminophen *on page* 38

Sildenafil (sil DEN a fil)

U.S. Brand Names Revatio®; Viagra®

Index Terms Sildenafil Citrate; UK92480

Generic Availability (U.S.) No

Pharmacologic Category Phosphodiesterase-5 Enzyme Inhibitor

Medication Safety Issues

Sound-alike/look-alike issues:

Revatio® may be confused with ReVia®, Revonto™

Sildenafil may be confused with silodosin, tadalafil, vardenafil

Viagra® may be confused with Allegra®, Vaniqa®

Pregnancy Risk Factor B

Lactation Excretion in breast milk unknown/use caution

Use

Revatio®: Treatment of pulmonary arterial hypertension (WHO Group I) to improve exercise ability and delay clinical worsening

Viagra®: Treatment of erectile dysfunction (ED)

Unlabeled/Investigational Use Pulmonary arterial hypertension in children

Mechanism of Action/Effect Sildenafil enhances the effect of nitric oxide by inhibiting phosphodiesterase type 5 (PDE-5), resulting in smooth muscle relaxation. In erectile dysfunction, smooth muscle relaxation results in the inflow of blood into the corpus cavernosum with sexual stimulation. In pulmonary hypertension, smooth muscle relaxation results in pulmonary vasculature; vasodilation reducing pulmonary pressure.

Contraindications Hypersensitivity to sildenafil or any component of the formulation; concurrent use (regularly/intermittently) of organic nitrates in any form (eg, nitroglycerin, isosorbide dinitrate); concurrent use with a protease inhibitor regimen when sildenafil used for pulmonary artery hypertension (eg, Revatio®)

Warnings/Precautions Decreases in blood pressure may occur due to vasodilator effects; use with caution in patients with left ventricular outflow obstruction (aortic stenosis or hypertrophic obstructive cardiomyopathy); may be more sensitive to hypotensive actions. Concurrent use with alpha-adrenergic antagonist therapy or substantial ethanol consumption may cause symptomatic hypotension; patients should be hemodynamically stable prior to initiating therapy at the lowest possible dose. Use with caution in patients with hypotension (<90/50 mm Hg); uncontrolled hypertension (>170/110 mm Hg); life-threatening arrhythmias, stroke or MI within the last 6 months; cardiac failure or coronary artery disease causing unstable angina; safety and efficacy have not been studied in these patients. There is a degree of cardiac risk associated with sexual activity; therefore, physicians should consider the cardiovascular status of their patients prior to initiating any treatment for erectile dysfunction. If pulmonary edema occurs when treating pulmonary arterial hypertension, consider the possibility of pulmonary veno-occlusive disease (PVOD); continued use is not recommended in patient with PVOD.

Sildenafil should be used with caution in patients with anatomical deformation of the penis (angulation, cavernosal fibrosis, or Peyronie's disease) and in patients who have conditions which may predispose them to priapism (sickle cell anemia, multiple myeloma, leukemia). All patients should be instructed to seek medical attention if erection persists >4 hours.

Vision loss may occur rarely and be a sign of nonarteritic anterior ischemic optic neuropathy (NAION). Risk may be increased with history of vision loss. Other risk factors for NAION include low cup-to-disc ratio ("crowded disc"), coronary artery disease, diabetes, hypertension, hyperlipidemia, smoking, and age >50 years. May cause dose-related impairment of color discrimination. Use caution in patients with retinitis pigmentosa; a minority have genetic disorders of retinal phosphodiesterases (no safety information available). Sudden decrease or loss of hearing has been reported rarely; hearing changes may be accompanied by tinnitus and dizziness. A direct relationship between therapy and vision or hearing loss has not been determined.

The potential underlying causes of erectile dysfunction should be evaluated prior to treatment. The safety and efficacy of sildenafil with other treatments for erectile dysfunction have not been established; use is not recommended. Efficacy with concurrent bosentan therapy has not been evaluated; use with caution. Use with caution in patients taking strong CYP3A4 inhibitors or alpha-blockers. Concomitant use with all forms of nitrates is contraindicated. If nitrate administration is medically necessary, it is not known when nitrates can be safely administered following the use of sildenafil (per manufacturer); the ACC/AHA 2007 guidelines supports administration of nitrates only if 24 hours have elapsed.

Avoid abrupt discontinuation, especially if used as monotherapy in PAH as exacerbation may occur. Use caution in patients with bleeding disorders or with active peptic ulcer disease; safety and efficacy have not been established. Efficacy has not be established for treatment of pulmonary hypertension associated with sickle cell disease. Use with caution in the elderly, or patients with renal or hepatic dysfunction; dose adjustment may be needed.

Drug Interactions

Metabolism/Transport Effects Substrate of CYP2C9 (minor), 3A4 (major); **Inhibits** CYP1A2 (weak), 2C9 (weak), 2C19 (weak), 2D6 (weak), 2E1 (weak), 3A4 (weak)

Avoid Concomitant Use

Avoid concomitant use of Sildenafil with any of the following: Amyl Nitrite; Phosphodiesterase 5 Inhibitors; Vasodilators (Organic Nitrates)

Decreased Effect

The levels/effects of Sildenafil may be decreased by: Bosentan; CYP3A4 Inducers (Strong); Deferasirox; Etravirine; Herbs (CYP3A4 Inducers); Peginterferon Alfa-2b

Increased Effect/Toxicity

Sildenafil may increase the levels/effects of: Alpha1-Blockers; Amyl Nitrite; Antihypertensives; Bosentan; HMG-CoA Reductase Inhibitors; Phosphodiesterase 5 Inhibitors; Vasodilators (Organic Nitrates)

The levels/effects of Sildenafil may be increased by: Antifungal Agents (Azole Derivatives, Systemic); Conivaptan; CYP3A4 Inhibitors (Moderate); CYP3A4 Inhibitors (Strong); Dasatinib; Macrolide Antibiotics; Protease Inhibitors; Sapropterin

Nutritional/Ethanol Interactions

Food: Amount and rate of absorption of sildenafil is reduced when taken with a high-fat meal. Serum concentrations/toxicity may be increased with grapefruit juice; avoid concurrent use.

Herb/Nutraceutical: St John's wort may decrease sildenafil levels.

Adverse Reactions Based upon normal doses for either indication or route. (Adverse effects such as flushing, diarrhea, myalgia, and visual disturbances may be increased with doses >100 mg/24 hours.)

>10%:

Central nervous system: Headache (16% to 46%)
Gastrointestinal: Dyspepsia (7% to 17%; dose related)

2% to 10%:

Cardiovascular: Flushing (10%)
Central nervous system: Insomnia (≤7%), pyrexia (6%), dizziness (2%)
Dermatologic: Erythema (6%), rash (2%)
Gastrointestinal: Diarrhea (3% to 9%), gastritis (≤3%)
Genitourinary: Urinary tract infection (3%)
Hepatic: LFTs increased
Neuromuscular & skeletal: Myalgia (≤7%), paresthesia (≤3%)
Ocular: Abnormal vision (color changes, blurred vision, or increased sensitivity to light 3% to 11%; dose related)
Respiratory: Epistaxis (9% to 13%), dyspnea exacerbated (≤7%), nasal congestion (4%), rhinitis (4%), sinusitis (3%)

Pharmacodynamics/Kinetics

Onset of Action ~60 minutes

Duration of Action 2-4 hours

Absorption Rapid; slower with a high-fat meal

Bioavailability 40% (25% to 63%)

Time to Peak 30-120 minutes; delayed by 60 minutes with a high-fat meal

Protein Binding Plasma: ~96%

Half-Life Elimination ~4 hours; the elderly and those with severe renal impairment have reduced clearance of sildenafil and its active N-desmethyl metabolite

Metabolism Hepatic via CYP3A4 (major) and CYP2C9 (minor route); forms N-desmethyl metabolite (active)

Excretion Feces (~80%); urine (~13%)

Available Dosage Forms

Injection, solution:
Revatio®: 0.8 mg/mL (12.5 mL)

Tablet, oral:
Revatio®: 20 mg
Viagra®: 25 mg, 50 mg, 100 mg

Dosing

Adult

Erectile dysfunction (Viagra®): Oral: Usual dose: 50 mg once daily 1 hour (range: 30 minutes to 4 hours) before sexual activity; dosing range: 25-100 mg once daily.

Pulmonary arterial hypertension (Revatio®):

I.V.: 10 mg 3 times/day

Oral: 20 mg 3 times/day, taken 4-6 hours apart. **Note:** A delay in clinical worsening was observed in a short-term trial in which most patients achieved a target dose of 80 mg 3 times daily (unlabeled dose). The patients had an incremental dosage escalation while on a stable epoprostenol regimen (Simonneau, 2008).

Dosage considerations for patients stable on alpha-blockers: Viagra®: Initial: 25 mg

Dosage adjustment for concomitant use of potent CYP34A inhibitors:

Revatio®:
Erythromycin: No dosage adjustment
Itraconazole, ketoconazole: Not recommended

Viagra®:
Erythromycin, itraconazole, ketoconazole: Starting dose of 25 mg should be considered
Protease inhibitors: Maximum sildenafil dose: 25 mg every 48 hours

Geriatric Elderly >65 years: Use with caution.
Revatio®: Refer to adult dosing.
Viagra®: Starting dose of 25 mg should be considered.

Pediatric Pulmonary arterial hypertension (unlabeled use): Oral: Children ≥1 month: 0.25-2 mg/kg/dose every 4-6 hours. Most reports used 0.5 mg/kg/dose and titrated up to 2 mg/kg/dose

Renal Impairment

Revatio®: Dose adjustment not necessary

Viagra®: Cl_{cr} <30 mL/minute: Starting dose of 25 mg should be considered.

Hepatic Impairment

Revatio®: Child-Pugh class A and B: Dose adjustment not necessary; not studied in severe impairment (Child-Pugh class C).

Viagra®: Child-Pugh class A and B: Starting dose of 25 mg should be considered; not studied in severe impairment (Child-Pugh class C).

Administration

Oral

Revatio®: Administer tablets without regard to meals at least 4-6 hours apart.

Viagra®: Administer orally 30 minutes to 4 hours before sexual activity.

I.V. Revatio®: Administer injection as an I.V. bolus.

Stability

Storage Store at controlled room temperature of 25°C (77°F); excursions permitted to 15°C to 30°C (59°F to 86°F).

Monitoring and Teaching Issues

Patient Education Sildenafil provides no protection against sexually-transmitted diseases, including HIV. You may experience headache, flushing, or abnormal vision (color changes, blurred or increased sensitivity to light). Report immediately acute allergic reactions, chest pain or palpitations, persistent dizziness, signs of urinary tract infection, skin rash, respiratory difficulty, change in vision, change in hearing or ringing in the ears, or genital swelling. If erection lasts longer than 4 hours, contact prescriber immediately; permanent damage to the penis can occur. If taking for pulmonary arterial hypertension, do not discontinue abruptly.

Dietary Considerations Avoid grapefruit juice.

Geriatric Considerations Since the elderly often have concomitant diseases, many of which may contraindicate the use of sildenafil, a thorough knowledge of diseases and medications used must be assessed. Adjust dose for renal/hepatic function.

Pregnancy Considerations Teratogenic effects were not observed in animal studies. There are no adequate and well-controlled studies in pregnant women. Less than 0.001% appears in the semen.

Additional Information Sildenafil is ~10 times more selective for PDE-5 as compared to PDE6. This enzyme is found in the retina and is involved in phototransduction. At higher plasma levels, interference with PDE6 is believed to be the basis for changes in color vision noted in some patients.

◆ **Sildenafil Citrate** *see* Sildenafil *on page* 1641

◆ **Silenor®** *see* Doxepin (Systemic) *on page* 577

◆ **Silfedrine Children's [OTC]** *see* Pseudoephedrine *on page* 1529

Silodosin (SI lo doe sin)

U.S. Brand Names Rapaflo®

Index Terms KMD 3213

Generic Availability (U.S.) No

Pharmacologic Category $Alpha_1$ Blocker

Medication Safety Issues

Sound-alike/look-alike issues:

Rapaflo™ may be confused with Rapamune®, Raptiva®

Silodosin may be confused with sildenafil

Pregnancy Risk Factor B

Use Treatment of signs and symptoms of benign prostatic hyperplasia (BPH)

Mechanism of Action/Effect Selectively antagonizes $alpha_{1A}$-adrenoreceptors in the prostate (and bladder) which mediate the dynamic component of urine flow obstruction by regulating smooth muscle tone of the bladder neck and prostate. When given to patients with BPH, blockade of alpha-receptors leads to relaxation of these muscles, resulting in an improvement in urine flow rate and symptoms. Alpha-blockade does not influence the static component of urinary obstruction, which is related to tissue proliferation.

Contraindications Concurrent use with strong CYP3A4 inhibitors (eg, clarithromycin, itraconazole, ketoconazole, ritonavir); severe renal impairment (Cl_{cr} <30 mL/minute); severe hepatic impairment (Child-Pugh class C)

Warnings/Precautions Not intended for use as an antihypertensive drug. May cause significant orthostatic hypotension and syncope, especially with first dose; anticipate a similar effect if therapy is interrupted for a few days, if dosage is rapidly increased, or if another antihypertensive drug (particularly vasodilators) or a PDE-5 inhibitor (eg, sildenafil, tadalafil, vardenafil) is introduced. "First-dose" orthostatic hypotension may occur 4-8 hours after dosing; may be dose related. Patients should be cautioned about performing hazardous tasks when starting new therapy or adjusting dosage upward. Rule out prostatic carcinoma before beginning therapy with silodosin. Intraoperative floppy iris syndrome has been observed in cataract surgery patients who were on or were previously treated with $alpha_1$-blockers; causality has not been established and there appears to be no benefit in discontinuing alpha-blocker therapy prior to surgery. Use with caution in patients with mild-to-moderate hepatic impairment; contraindicated with severe impairment; not studied. Use with caution in patients with moderate renal impairment; dosage adjustment recommended. Contraindicated in patients with severe impairment (Cl_{cr} <30 mL/minute). Not indicated for use in women or children.

Drug Interactions

Metabolism/Transport Effects Substrate of CYP3A4, UGT2B7, P-glycoprotein

Avoid Concomitant Use

Avoid concomitant use of Silodosin with any of the following: Alpha1-Blockers; CYP3A4 Inhibitors (Strong); P-Glycoprotein Inhibitors

Decreased Effect

The levels/effects of Silodosin may be decreased by: CYP3A4 Inducers (Strong); Deferasirox; Herbs (CYP3A4 Inducers); P-Glycoprotein Inducers

Increased Effect/Toxicity

Silodosin may increase the levels/effects of: Alpha1-Blockers; Calcium Channel Blockers

The levels/effects of Silodosin may be increased by: Beta-Blockers; CYP3A4 Inhibitors (Moderate); CYP3A4 Inhibitors (Strong); Dasatinib; MAO Inhibitors; P-Glycoprotein Inhibitors; Phosphodiesterase 5 Inhibitors

Nutritional/Ethanol Interactions

Food: AUC decrease by 4% to 49% and C_{max} decreased by ~18% to 43% with moderate calorie/fat meal.

Herb/Nutraceutical: Avoid St. John's wort (may decrease the levels/effects of silodosin). Avoid herbs with hypotensive properties (black cohosh, California poppy, coleus, golden seal, hawthorn, mistletoe, periwinkle, quinine, Shepherd's purse); may enhance the hypotensive effect of silodosin. Avoid saw palmetto (due to limited experience with this combination).

Adverse Reactions

>10%: Miscellaneous: Retrograde ejaculation (28%)

1% to 10%:

Cardiovascular: Orthostatic hypotension (3%)

Central nervous system: Dizziness (3%), headache (2%), insomnia (1% to 2%)

Gastrointestinal: Diarrhea (3%), abdominal pain (1% to 2%)

Genitourinary: PSA increased (1% to 2%)

Neuromuscular & skeletal: Weakness (1% to 2%)

Respiratory: Nasal congestion (2%), nasopharyngitis (2%), rhinorrhea (1% to 2%), sinusitis (1% to 2%)

Pharmacodynamics/Kinetics

Bioavailability ~32%

Time to Peak ~3 hours

Protein Binding ~97%

Half-Life Elimination Healthy volunteers: Silodosin: 5-21 hours; KMD-3213G: ~24 hours

Metabolism Extensive, via CYP3A4, glucuronidation, and alcohol and aldehyde dehydrogenase pathways; KMD-3213G (active *in vitro*) and KMD-3293 (not significant) metabolites formed

Excretion Feces (55%); urine (34%)

Available Dosage Forms

Capsule, oral:

Rapaflo®: 4 mg, 8 mg

Dosing

Adult & Geriatric BPH: Oral: 8 mg once daily with a meal

Renal Impairment

Cl_{cr} >50 mL/minute: No adjustment needed.

Cl_{cr} 30-50 mL/minute: 4 mg once daily.

Cl_{cr} <30 mL/minute: Use is contraindicated.

Hepatic Impairment

Mild-to-moderate impairment (Child-Pugh classes A and B): No adjustment needed.

Severe impairment (Child-Pugh class C): Use is contraindicated.

Administration

Oral Administer once daily with a meal.

Stability

Storage Store at room temperature of 25°C (77°F); excursions permitted to 15°C to 30°C (59°F to 86°F). Protect from light. Protect from moisture.

Monitoring and Teaching Issues

Physical Assessment Not intended for use as an antihypertensive. Use with caution in presence of hepatic or renal impairment; dosing adjustment may be necessary. Assess potential for interactions or toxicity with other antihypertensives or drugs that may increase hypotensive effect. Assess symptomatic relief of BPH regularly. Monitor for orthostatic hypotension and syncope when beginning therapy, if therapy is interrupted, or if dose is increased (may be dose related). When discontinuing, dose should be tapered and blood pressure monitored closely. Teach patient about possible side effects, including orthostatic hypotension.

Patient Education Take at the same time each day with a meal. May cause postural hypotension, especially if taken with antihypertensive medications. May cause retrograde ejaculation (consult prescriber).

Dietary Considerations Take with a meal.

Geriatric Considerations See Renal Impairment. In clinical studies, older men had a higher incidence of orthostatic hypotension when using silodosin.

Pregnancy Considerations Teratogenic effects were not observed in animal studies; however, silodosin is not approved for use in women.

◆ **Silphen [OTC]** *see* DiphenhydrAMINE (Systemic) *on page* 543

- **Siltussin DAS [OTC] [DSC]** *see* GuaiFENesin *on page 890*
- **Siltussin SA [OTC]** *see* GuaiFENesin *on page 890*
- **Simcor®** *see* Niacin and Simvastatin *on page 1308*
- **Simply Sleep® [OTC]** *see* DiphenhydrAMINE (Systemic) *on page 543*
- **Simponi™** *see* Golimumab *on page 883*
- **Simulect®** *see* Basiliximab *on page 189*

Simvastatin (sim va STAT in)

U.S. Brand Names Zocor®

Generic Availability (U.S.) Yes

Pharmacologic Category Antilipemic Agent, HMG-CoA Reductase Inhibitor

Medication Safety Issues

Sound-alike/look-alike issues:

Simvastatin may be confused with atorvastatin, nystatin, pitavastatin

Zocor® may be confused with Cozaar®, Lipitor®, Yocon®, Zoloft®, ZyrTEC®

International issues:

Cardin [Poland] may be confused with Cardem brand name for celiprolol [Spain]; Cardene brand name for nicardipine [U.S., Great Britain, Netherlands]

Pregnancy Risk Factor X

Lactation Excretion in breast milk unknown/contraindicated

Use Used with dietary therapy for the following:

Secondary prevention of cardiovascular events in hypercholesterolemic patients with established coronary heart disease (CHD) or at high risk for CHD: To reduce cardiovascular morbidity (myocardial infarction, coronary/noncoronary revascularization procedures) and mortality; to reduce the risk of stroke

Hyperlipidemias: To reduce elevations in total cholesterol (total-C), LDL-C, apolipoprotein B, triglycerides, and VLDL-C, and to increase HDL-C in patients with primary hypercholesterolemia (elevations of 1 or more components are present in Fredrickson type IIa, IIb, III, and IV hyperlipidemias); treatment of homozygous familial hypercholesterolemia

Heterozygous familial hypercholesterolemia (HeFH): In adolescent patients (10-17 years of age, females >1 year postmenarche) with HeFH having LDL-C ≥190 mg/dL **or** LDL-C ≥160 mg/dL with positive family history of premature cardiovascular disease (CVD), or 2 or more CVD risk factors in the adolescent patient

Mechanism of Action/Effect Simvastatin is a derivative of lovastatin that acts by competitively inhibiting 3-hydroxy-3-methylglutaryl-coenzyme A (HMG-CoA) reductase, the enzyme that catalyzes the rate-limiting step in cholesterol biosynthesis; lowers total and LDL-cholesterol with increase in HDL

Contraindications Hypersensitivity to simvastatin or any component of the formulation; active liver disease; unexplained persistent elevations of serum transaminases; pregnancy; breast-feeding

Warnings/Precautions Secondary causes of hyperlipidemia should be ruled out prior to therapy. Liver function must be monitored by laboratory assessment. Rhabdomyolysis with acute renal failure has occurred. Risk is dose-related and is increased with high doses (80 mg) or concurrent use of lipid-lowering agents which may cause rhabdomyolysis (gemfibrozil, other fibric acid derivatives, or niacin at doses ≥1 g/day), during concurrent use with danazol or moderate-to-strong CYP3A4 inhibitors (including amiodarone, cyclosporine, grapefruit juice in large quantities, or verapamil). Avoid concurrent use of strong CYP3A4 inhibitors (eg, itraconazole, ketoconazole, erythromycin, clarithromycin, telithromycin, nefazodone, and HIV protease inhibitors). Monitor closely if used with other drugs associated with myopathy (eg, colchicine). Weigh the risk versus benefit when combining any of these drugs with simvastatin. Do not initiate simvastatin-containing treatment in a patient with pre-existing therapy of cyclosporine or danazol, unless the patient has previously demonstrated tolerance to ≥5 mg/day simvastatin. Temporarily discontinue in any patient experiencing an acute or serious major medical or surgical condition which may increase the risk of rhabdomyolysis. Discontinue temporarily for elective surgical procedures. Based upon current evidence, HMG-CoA reductase inhibitor therapy should be continued in the perioperative period unless risk outweighs cardioprotective benefit. Use caution in patients with renal insufficiency. Use with caution in patients with advanced age, these patients are predisposed to myopathy. Use with caution in patients who consume large amounts of ethanol or have a history of liver disease. Use is contraindicated with active liver disease and with unexplained transaminase elevations. Concomitant use of high-dose simvastatin (80 mg) and niacin ≥1 g/day may increase risk of myopathy in Chinese patients.

Drug Interactions

Metabolism/Transport Effects Substrate of CYP3A4 (major), SLCO1B1; **Inhibits** CYP2C8 (weak), 2C9 (weak), 2D6 (weak)

Avoid Concomitant Use

Avoid concomitant use of Simvastatin with any of the following: Protease Inhibitors; Red Yeast Rice

Decreased Effect

The levels/effects of Simvastatin may be decreased by: Antacids; Bosentan; CYP3A4 Inducers (Strong); Deferasirox; Efavirenz; Etravirine; Phenytoin; Rifamycin Derivatives; St Johns Wort

Increased Effect/Toxicity

Simvastatin may increase the levels/effects of: DAPTOmycin; Diltiazem; Trabectedin; Vitamin K Antagonists

The levels/effects of Simvastatin may be increased by: Amiodarone; Antifungal Agents (Azole Derivatives, Systemic); Colchicine; Conivaptan; CycloSPORINE; CycloSPORINE (Systemic); CYP3A4 Inhibitors (Moderate); CYP3A4 Inhibitors (Strong); Danazol; Dasatinib; Diltiazem; Dronedarone; Eltrombopag; Fenofibrate; Fenofibric Acid; Fluconazole; Fusidic Acid; Gemfibrozil; Grapefruit Juice; Green Tea; Imatinib; Macrolide Antibiotics; Nefazodone; Niacin; Niacinamide; Protease Inhibitors; QuiNINE; Ranolazine; Red Yeast Rice; Rifamycin Derivatives; Sildenafil; Verapamil

Nutritional/Ethanol Interactions

Ethanol: Avoid excessive ethanol consumption (due to potential hepatic effects).

Food: Simvastatin serum concentration may be increased when taken with grapefruit juice; avoid concurrent intake of large quantities (>1 quart/day). Red yeast rice contains an estimated 2.4 mg lovastatin per 600 mg rice.

Herb/Nutraceutical: St John's wort may decrease simvastatin levels.

Adverse Reactions

1% to 10%:

Cardiovascular: Atrial fibrillation (6%; placebo 5%), edema (3%; placebo 2%)
Central nervous system: Headache (3% to 7%), vertigo (5%)
Dermatologic: Eczema (5%)
Gastrointestinal: Abdominal pain (7%), constipation (2% to 7%), gastritis (5%), nausea (5%)
Hepatic: Transaminases increased (>3 x ULN; 1%)
Neuromuscular & skeletal: CPK increased (>3 x normal; 5%), myalgia (4%)
Respiratory: Upper respiratory infections (9%), bronchitis (7%)

Additional class-related events or case reports (not necessarily reported with simvastatin therapy): Alteration in taste, anorexia, anxiety, bilirubin increased, cataracts, cholestatic jaundice, cirrhosis, decreased libido, depression, erectile dysfunction/impotence, facial paresis, fatty liver, fulminant hepatic necrosis, gynecomastia, hepatoma, hyperbilirubinemia, impaired extraocular muscle movement, increased CPK (>10 x normal), interstitial lung disease, ophthalmoplegia, peripheral nerve palsy, psychic disturbance, renal failure (secondary to rhabdomyolysis), thyroid dysfunction, tremor, vertigo

Pharmacodynamics/Kinetics

Onset of Action >3 days; Peak effect: 2 weeks

Absorption 85%

Bioavailability <5%

Time to Peak 1.3-2.4 hours

Protein Binding ~95%

Half-Life Elimination Unknown

Metabolism Hepatic via CYP3A4; extensive first-pass effect

Excretion Feces (60%); urine (13%)

Available Dosage Forms

Tablet, oral: 5 mg, 10 mg, 20 mg, 40 mg, 80 mg
Zocor®: 5 mg, 10 mg, 20 mg, 40 mg, 80 mg

Dosing

Adult Note: Doses should be individualized according to the baseline LDL-cholesterol levels, the recommended goal of therapy, and the patient's response; adjustments should be made at intervals of 4 weeks or more; doses may need adjusted based on concomitant medications

Homozygous familial hypercholesterolemia: Oral: 40 mg once daily in the evening **or** 80 mg/day (given in 3 divided doses as 20 mg, 20 mg, and 40 mg evening dose)

Prevention of cardiovascular events, hyperlipidemias: Oral: 20-40 mg once daily in the evening; range: 5-80 mg/day

Patients requiring only moderate reduction of LDL-cholesterol: May be started at 10 mg once daily in the evening

Patients requiring reduction of >45% in low-density lipoprotein (LDL) cholesterol: May be started at 40 mg once daily in the evening

Patients with CHD or at high risk for CHD: Dosing should be started at 40 mg once daily in the evening; simvastatin should be started simultaneously with diet therapy.

Dosage adjustment for simvastatin with concomitant medications:

Cyclosporine or danazol: Initial: 5 mg, should **not** exceed 10 mg/day
Gemfibrozil: Dose should **not** exceed 10 mg/day
Amiodarone or verapamil: Dose should **not** exceed 20 mg/day
Diltiazem: Simvastatin dose should **not** exceed 40 mg/day

Dosage adjustment in Chinese patients on niacin doses ≥1 g/day: Because of an increased risk of myopathy, do not administer simvastatin 80 mg concurrently.

Geriatric Oral: Initial: Maximum reductions in LDL-cholesterol may be achieved with daily dose ≤20 mg.

Pediatric HeFH: Oral: Children 10-17 years (females >1 year postmenarche): 10 mg once daily in the evening; range: 10-40 mg/day (maximum: 40 mg/day)

Dosage adjustment with concomitant medications: With concomitant amiodarone, cyclosporine, danazol, diltiazem, gemfibrozil, or verapamil: Refer to adult dosing.

Note: Doses should be individualized according to the baseline LDL-cholesterol levels, the recommended goal of therapy, and the patient's response; adjustments should be made at intervals of 4 weeks or more; doses may need adjusted based on concomitant medications

Renal Impairment Because simvastatin does not undergo significant renal excretion, modification of dose should not be necessary in patients with mild-to-moderate renal insufficiency.

Severe renal impairment: Cl_{cr} <10 mL/minute: Initial: 5 mg/day with close monitoring.

Administration

Oral May be administered without regard to meals. Administer in the evening for maximal efficacy.

Stability

Storage Tablets should be stored in tightly-closed containers at temperatures between 5°C to 30°C (41°F to 86°F).

Monitoring and Teaching Issues

Laboratory Monitoring Creatine phosphokinase levels due to possibility of myopathy; serum cholesterol (total and fractionated); baseline CPK (recheck CPK in any patient with symptoms suggestive of myopathy)

Obtain liver function tests prior to initiation, dose, and thereafter when clinically indicated. Patients titrated to the 80 mg dose should be tested prior to initiation and 3 months after initiating the 80 mg dose. Thereafter, periodic monitoring (ie, semiannually) is recommended for the first year of treatment. Patients with elevated transaminase levels should have a second (confirmatory) test and frequent monitoring until values normalize. Discontinue if increase in ALT/AST is persistently >3 times ULN. Monitor LDL-C at intervals no less than 4 weeks.

Physical Assessment Monitor closely in presence of impaired liver function. Assess risk potential for interactions with other prescriptions or herbal products patient may be taking that may increase risk of myopathy or rhabdomyolysis. Assess LFTs and cholesterol profile prior to treatment and at regular intervals. Evaluate possible reduction in lipid levels. Teach proper diet and exercise regimen.

Patient Education Take at same time each day, in the evening, with or without food. Follow prescribed cholesterol-lowering diet and exercise regimen. Avoid excessive grapefruit juice (>1 quart/day) and alcohol. You will have periodic blood tests to assess effectiveness. Report unusual muscle cramping or weakness, yellowing of skin or eyes, easy bruising or bleeding, or unusual fatigue.

Dietary Considerations May be taken without regard to meals. Red yeast rice contains an estimated 2.4 mg lovastatin per 600 mg rice.

Geriatric Considerations Effective and well tolerated in the elderly. The definition of and, therefore, when to treat hyperlipidemia in the elderly is a controversial issue. The National Cholesterol Education Program recommends that all adults maintain a plasma cholesterol <160 mg/dL. In elderly with one additional risk factor, goal LDL would be <130 mg/dL. It is the authors' belief that pharmacologic treatment be reserved for those who are unable to obtain a desirable plasma cholesterol concentration by diet alone and for whom the benefits of treatment are believed to outweigh the potential adverse effects, drug interactions, and cost of treatment.

Breast-Feeding Considerations Excretion in breast milk is unknown, but would be expected; other medications in this class are excreted in human milk. Breast-feeding is contraindicated.

Pregnancy Considerations Cholesterol biosynthesis may be important in fetal development. Contraindicated in pregnancy. Administer to women of childbearing potential only when conception is highly unlikely and patients have been informed of potential hazards. If pregnancy occurs during treatment, discontinue simvastatin immediately.

Related Information

Hyperlipidemia Management *on page 2046*

◆ **Simvastatin and Ezetimibe** *see* Ezetimibe and Simvastatin *on page 729*

◆ **Simvastatin and Niacin** *see* Niacin and Simvastatin *on page 1308*

Sinecatechins (sin e KAT e kins)

U.S. Brand Names Veregen™

Index Terms Catechins; Green Tea Extract; Kunecatechins; Polyphenols; Polyphenon E

Generic Availability (U.S.) No

Pharmacologic Category Immunomodulator, Topical; Topical Skin Product

Pregnancy Risk Factor C

Lactation Excretion in breast milk unknown/use caution

Use Treatment of external genital and perianal warts secondary to *Condylomata acuminata*

Mechanism of Action/Effect Unknown; possibly related to antioxidant effects

Contraindications There are no contraindications listed in the manufacturer's labeling.

Warnings/Precautions Sinecatechins has not been evaluated from the treatment of urethral, intravaginal, cervical, rectal, or intra-anal human papilloma viral disease and is not recommended for these conditions. Women should continue to undergo regular gynecological examination, including monitoring and screening for cervical dysplasia. Local skin reactions are common, if possible, continue treatment; severe reactions may require treatment interruption or discontinuation. Women may be at a greater risk for severe local reactions (eg, erosion/ulceration, burning, itching, pain). Avoid exposure of treated area to sun and/or UV-light. Avoid application of the product to open wounds may increase the risk of severe local reactions. Ointment is for topical use only; not intended for internal use. Treatment should continue until all warts have cleared or for 16 weeks, whichever is shorter; the safety and efficacy of treatment >16 weeks has not been established. The safety and efficacy of the use of sinecatechins has not been established in pediatric and immunosuppressed patients.

Drug Interactions

Avoid Concomitant Use There are no known interactions where it is recommended to avoid concomitant use.

Decreased Effect There are no known significant interactions involving a decrease in effect.

Increased Effect/Toxicity There are no known significant interactions involving an increase in effect.

Adverse Reactions

>10%:

Dermatologic: Erythema (70%), pruritus (69%), edema (45%), vesicular rash (20%)

Local: Burning (67%), pain/discomfort (56%), erosion/ulceration (49%), induration (35%)

1% to 10%:

Dermatologic: Desquamation (5%), rash (1%), scar formation (1%)

Local: Discharge (3%), lymphadenitis (3%), bleeding (2%), reaction (2%), irritation (1%)

Miscellaneous: Phimosis (uncircumcised males; 3%), hypersensitivity (2%)

Available Dosage Forms

Ointment, topical:

Veregen™: 15% (15 g)

Dosing

Adult *Condylomata acuminata:* Topical: Apply a thin layer (~0.5 cm strand) 3 times/day to all external genital and perianal warts until all warts have been cleared (maximum duration: 16 weeks)

Renal Impairment No adjustment required.

Hepatic Impairment No adjustment required.

Administration

Topical Wash hands before and after application; apply with fingers, leaving a thin layer of ointment; do not wash ointment off affected area after application. Discontinue treatment if the severity of local skin reactions becomes unacceptable. Do not apply internally; do not apply to open wounds; do not apply occlusive dressing. Sexual contact should be avoided while ointment is on skin. For females requiring tampon use during treatment, tampon should be inserted prior to application of ointment to prevent accidental application of ointment into the vagina. May stain clothing or bedding.

Stability

Storage Store at 2°C to 8°C (36°F to 46°F) until dispensed; after dispensing, patient may store under refrigeration or up to 25°C (77°F). Do not freeze.

Monitoring and Teaching Issues

Patient Education Apply thin layer of medication; do not wash off. Wash your hands immediately after application. Avoid contact with eyes, nostrils, or mouth. Women using tampons should insert the tampon prior to application so as not to introduce the ointment into the vagina. Avoid exposure to sunlight. Do not apply to open wounds, vagina, or anal area. Avoid sexual contact. Genital warts are sexually transmitted; you may infect your partner. Wash off the ointment before use of a condom or diaphragm; ointment may weaken these forms of birth control. Avoid use of occlusive dressing. You may experience redness, swelling, or itching at the site of application. Report development of open sores or severe reactions.

Pregnancy Considerations Teratogenic effects were not observed in animal studies. There are no adequate and well-controlled studies in pregnant women; use only if possible benefit outweighs potential risk to the fetus. Sinecatechins ointment may weaken condoms and diaphragms.

Additional Information Sinecatechins ointment represents the first botanical drug product to be approved by the FDA. The product contains an extract of dried green tea leaves. The active ingredient(s) are not known; however, sinecatechins is a mixture of catechins (85% to 95% by weight) with the major component being (-)-Epigallocatechin gallate (EGCg). Approximately 2.5% of the mixture contains gallic acid, caffeine, and theobromine.

- ◆ **Sinemet®** *see* Carbidopa and Levodopa *on page* 291
- ◆ **Sinemet® CR** *see* Carbidopa and Levodopa *on page* 291
- ◆ **Singulair®** *see* Montelukast *on page* 1256
- ◆ **Sirdalud®** *see* TiZANidine *on page* 1775

Sirolimus (sir OH li mus)

U.S. Brand Names Rapamune®

Index Terms Rapamycin

Generic Availability (U.S.) No

Pharmacologic Category Immunosuppressant Agent; mTOR Kinase Inhibitor

Medication Safety Issues

Sound-alike/look-alike issues:

Rapamune® may be confused with Rapaflo™

Sirolimus may be confused with everolimus, tacrolimus, temsirolimus

Medication Guide Available Yes

Pregnancy Risk Factor C

Lactation Excretion in breast milk unknown/not recommended

Use Prophylaxis of organ rejection in patients receiving renal transplants

Unlabeled/Investigational Use Prophylaxis of organ rejection in heart transplant recipients; prevention acute graft-versus-host disease (GVHD) in allogeneic stem cell transplantation; treatment of refractory acute or chronic GVHD; treatment of soft tissue sarcoma (chordoma, angiomyolipoma, or lymphangioleiomyomatosis)

Mechanism of Action/Effect Sirolimus inhibits T-lymphocyte activation and proliferation in response to antigenic and cytokine stimulation and inhibits antibody production (mechanism differs from other immunosuppressants) to inhibit acute rejection of allografts and prolongs graft survival. Sirolimus binds to FKBP-12, an intracellular protein, to form an immunosuppressive complex which inhibits the regulatory kinase, mTOR (mammalian target of rapamycin), which suppresses cytokine mediated T-cell proliferation, halting progression from the G1 to the S phase of the cell cycle.

Contraindications Hypersensitivity to sirolimus or any component of the formulation

Warnings/Precautions Hazardous agent - use appropriate precautions for handling and disposal. **[U.S. Boxed Warning]: Immunosuppressive agents, including sirolimus, increase the risk of infection and may be associated with the development of lymphoma.** Immune suppression may also increase the risk of opportunistic infections (including activation of latent viral infections including BK virus-associated nephropathy), fatal infections, and sepsis. Prophylactic treatment for *Pneumocystis jiroveci* pneumonia (PCP) should be administered for 1 year post-transplant; prophylaxis for cytomegalovirus (CMV) should be taken for 3 months post-transplant in patients at risk for CMV. Progressive multifocal leukoencephalopathy (PML), an opportunistic CNS infection caused by reactivation of the JC virus, has been reported in patients receiving immunosuppressive therapy, including sirolimus. Clinical findings of PML include apathy, ataxia, cognitive deficiency, confusion, and hemiparesis; promptly evaluate any patient presenting with neurological changes; consider decreasing the degree of immunosuppression with consideration to the risk of organ rejection in transplant patients.

[U.S. Boxed Warning]: Sirolimus is not recommended for use in liver or lung transplantation. Bronchial anastomotic dehiscence cases have been reported in lung transplant patients when sirolimus was used as part of an immunosuppressive regimen; most of these reactions were fatal. Studies indicate an association with an increase risk of hepatic artery thrombosis (HAT), graft failure, and increased mortality (with evidence of infection) in liver transplant patients when sirolimus is used in combination with cyclosporine and/or tacrolimus. Most cases of HAT occurred within 30 days of transplant.

In renal transplant patients, *de novo* use without cyclosporine has been associated with higher rates of acute rejection. Sirolimus should be used in combination with cyclosporine (and corticosteroids) initially. Cyclosporine may be withdrawn in low-to-moderate immunologic risk patients after 2-4 months, in conjunction with an increase in sirolimus dosage. In high immunologic risk patients, use in combination with cyclosporine and corticosteroids is recommended for the first year. Safety and efficacy of combination therapy with cyclosporine in high immunologic risk patients has not been studied beyond 12 months of treatment; adjustment of immunosuppressive therapy beyond 12 months should be considered based on clinical judgement. Monitor renal function closely when combined with cyclosporine; consider dosage adjustment or discontinue in patients with increasing serum creatinine.

May increase serum creatinine and decrease GFR. Use caution when used concurrently with medications which may alter renal function. May delay recovery of renal function in patients with delayed allograft function. Increased urinary protein excretion has been observed when converting renal transplant patients from calcineurin inhibitors to sirolimus during maintenance therapy. A higher level of proteinuria prior to sirolimus conversion correlates with a higher degree of proteinuria after conversion. In some patients, proteinuria may reach nephrotic levels; nephrotic syndrome (new onset) has been reported. Increased risk of BK viral-associated nephropathy which may impair renal function and cause graft loss; consider decreasing immunosuppressive burden if evidence of deteriorating renal function.

Use caution with hepatic impairment; a reduction in the maintenance dose is recommended. Has been associated with an increased risk of fluid accumulation and lymphocele; peripheral edema, lymphedema, ascites, and pleural and pericardial effusions (including significant effusions and tamponade) were reported; use with caution in patients in whom fluid accumulation may be poorly tolerated, such as in cardiovascular disease (heart failure or hypertension) and pulmonary disease. Cases of interstitial lung disease (eg, pneumonitis, bronchiolitis obliterans organizing pneumonia [BOOP], pulmonary fibrosis) have been observed; risk may be increased with higher trough levels. Avoid concurrent use of strong CYP3A4 and/or P-glycoprotein (P-gp) inhibitors (eg, clarithromycin, erythromycin, telithromycin, itraconazole, ketoconazole, voriconazole) and strong inducers of CYP3A4 and/or P-gp (eg, rifampin, rifabutin). Concurrent use with a calcineurin inhibitor (cyclosporine, tacrolimus) may increase the risk of calcineurin inhibitor-induced hemolytic uremic syndrome/thrombotic thrombocytopenic purpura/thrombotic microangiopathy (HUS/TTP/TMA).

Hypersensitivity reactions, including anaphylactic/anaphylactoid reactions, angioedema, exfoliative dermatitis, and hypersensitivity vasculitis have been reported. Concurrent use with other drugs known to cause angioedema (eg, ACE inhibitors) may increase risk. Immunosuppressant therapy is associated with an increased risk of skin cancer; limit sun and ultraviolet light exposure; use appropriate sun protection. May increase serum lipids (cholesterol and triglycerides); use with caution in patients with hyperlipidemia. May be associated with wound dehiscence and impaired healing; use caution in the perioperative period. Patients with a body mass index (BMI) >30 kg/m^2 are at increased risk for abnormal wound healing.

Sirolimus tablets and oral solution are not bioequivalent, due to differences in absorption. Clinical equivalence was seen using 2 mg tablet and 2 mg solution. It is not known if higher doses are also clinically equivalent. Monitor sirolimus levels if changes in dosage forms are ▶

made. **[U.S. Boxed Warning]: Should only be used by physicians experienced in immunosuppressive therapy and management of transplant patients. Adequate laboratory and supportive medical resources must be readily available.** Sirolimus concentrations are dependant on the assay method (eg, chromatographic and immunoassay) used; assay methods are not interchangeable. Variations in methods to determine sirolimus whole blood concentrations, as well as interlaboratory variations, may result in improper dosage adjustments, which may lead to subtherapeutic or toxic levels. Determine the assay method used to assure consistency (or accommodations if changes occur), and for monitoring purposes, be aware of alterations to assay method or reference range. The manufacturer recommends high performance liquid chromatography (HPLC) as the reference standard to determine sirolimus trough concentrations.

Drug Interactions

Metabolism/Transport Effects Substrate of CYP3A4 (major), P-glycoprotein; **Inhibits** CYP3A4 (weak)

Avoid Concomitant Use

Avoid concomitant use of Sirolimus with any of the following: BCG; Natalizumab; Pimecrolimus; Posaconazole; Roflumilast; Tacrolimus (Systemic); Tacrolimus (Topical); Vaccines (Live); Voriconazole

Decreased Effect

Sirolimus may decrease the levels/effects of: BCG; Sipuleucel-T; Tacrolimus; Tacrolimus (Systemic); Vaccines (Inactivated); Vaccines (Live)

The levels/effects of Sirolimus may be decreased by: CYP3A4 Inducers (Strong); Deferasirox; Echinacea; Efavirenz; Herbs (CYP3A4 Inducers); P-Glycoprotein Inducers; Phenytoin; Rifampin

Increased Effect/Toxicity

Sirolimus may increase the levels/effects of: ACE Inhibitors; CycloSPORINE; CycloSPORINE (Systemic); Hypoglycemic Agents; Leflunomide; Natalizumab; Tacrolimus; Tacrolimus (Systemic); Tacrolimus (Topical); Vaccines (Live)

The levels/effects of Sirolimus may be increased by: Conivaptan; CycloSPORINE; CycloSPORINE (Systemic); CYP3A4 Inhibitors (Moderate); CYP3A4 Inhibitors (Strong); Dasatinib; Denosumab; Fluconazole; Herbs (Hypoglycemic Properties); Itraconazole; Ketoconazole; Ketoconazole (Systemic); Macrolide Antibiotics; P-Glycoprotein Inhibitors; Pimecrolimus; Posaconazole; Protease Inhibitors; Roflumilast; Tacrolimus; Tacrolimus (Systemic); Tacrolimus (Topical); Trastuzumab; Voriconazole

Nutritional/Ethanol Interactions

Food: Avoid grapefruit juice; may decrease clearance of sirolimus. Ingestion with high-fat meals decreases peak concentrations but increases AUC by 23% to 35%. Sirolimus should be taken consistently (either with or without food) to minimize variability.

Herb/Nutraceutical: St John's wort may decrease sirolimus levels; avoid concurrent use. Avoid cat's claw, echinacea (have immunostimulant properties; consider therapy modifications). Herbs with hypoglycemic properties may increase the risk of sirolimus-induced hypoglycemia; includes alfalfa, aloe, bilberry, bitter melon, burdock, celery, damiana, fenugreek, garcinia, garlic, ginger, ginseng (American), gymnema, marshmallow, stinging nettle.

Adverse Reactions Incidence of many adverse effects is dose related.

>20%:

Cardiovascular: Peripheral edema (54% to 58%), hypertension (45% to 49%), edema (18% to 20%)

Central nervous system: Headache (34%), pain (20% to 33%), insomnia (13% to 22%)

Dermatologic: Acne (22%)

Endocrine & metabolic: Hypertriglyceridemia (45% to 57%), hypercholesterolemia (43% to 46%)

Gastrointestinal: Constipation (36% to 38%), abdominal pain (29% to 36%), diarrhea (25% to 36%), nausea (25% to 31%)

Genitourinary: Urinary tract infection (26% to 33%)

Hematologic: Anemia (23% to 33%), thrombocytopenia (14% to 30%)

Neuromuscular & skeletal: Arthralgia (25% to 31%)

Renal: Serum creatinine increased (39% to 40%)

3% to 20%:

Cardiovascular: Atrial fibrillation, CHF, DVT, facial edema, hypervolemia, hypotension, palpitation, peripheral vascular disorder, postural hypotension, syncope, tachycardia, thrombosis, vasodilation

Central nervous system: Anxiety, chills, confusion, depression, dizziness, emotional lability, hypoesthesia, malaise, neuropathy, somnolence

Dermatologic: Rash (10% to 20%), skin carcinoma (up to 3%; includes basal cell carcinoma, squamous cell carcinoma, melanoma), cellulitis, dermal ulcer, dermatitis (fungal), ecchymosis, hirsutism, pruritus, skin hypertrophy, wound healing abnormal

Endocrine & metabolic: Acidosis, Cushing's syndrome, dehydration, diabetes mellitus, glycosuria, hypercalcemia, hyperglycemia, hyperphosphatemia, hypocalcemia, hypoglycemia, hypokalemia, hypomagnesemia, hyponatremia

Gastrointestinal: Abdomen enlarged, anorexia, dysphagia, eructation, esophagitis, flatulence, gastritis, gastroenteritis, gingival hyperplasia, gingivitis, ileus, mouth ulceration, oral moniliasis, stomatitis, weight loss

Genitourinary: Impotence, pelvic pain, scrotal edema, testis disorder

Hematologic: Hemolytic-uremic syndrome, hemorrhage, leukopenia, leukocytosis, polycythemia, TTP

Hepatic: Abnormal liver function tests, alkaline phosphatase increased, LDH increased

Local: Thrombophlebitis

Neuromuscular & skeletal: Arthrosis, bone necrosis, CPK increased, hyper-/hypotonia, leg cramps, myalgia, osteoporosis, paresthesia, tetany

Ocular: Abnormal vision, cataract, conjunctivitis

Otic: Ear pain, otitis media, tinnitus

Renal: Albuminuria, bladder pain, BUN increased, dysuria, hematuria, hydronephrosis, kidney pain, nephropathy (toxic), nocturia, oliguria, pyelonephritis, pyuria, tubular necrosis, urinary frequency, urinary incontinence, urinary retention

Respiratory: Asthma, atelectasis, bronchitis, cough, epistaxis, hypoxia, lung edema, pleural effusion, pneumonia, pulmonary embolism, rhinitis, sinusitis

Miscellaneous: Lymphoproliferative disease/lymphoma (1% to 3%), abscess, diaphoresis, flu-like syndrome, hernia, herpesvirus infection, infection (including opportunistic), lymphadenopathy, lymphocele, peritonitis, sepsis

Pharmacodynamics/Kinetics

Absorption Rapid

Bioavailability Oral solution: 14%; Oral tablet: 18%

Time to Peak Oral solution: 1-3 hours; Tablet: 1-6 hours

Protein Binding ~92%, primarily to albumin

Half-Life Elimination Half-life elimination: Mean: 62 hours (range; 46-78 hours); extended in hepatic impairment (Child-Pugh class A or B) to 113 hours

Metabolism Extensive; in intestinal wall via P-glycoprotein and hepatic via CYP3A4; to 7 major metabolites

Excretion Feces (91% via P-glycoprotein-mediated efflux into gut lumen); urine (2%)

Available Dosage Forms

Solution, oral:

Rapamune®: 1 mg/mL (60 mL)

Tablet, oral:

Rapamune®: 0.5 mg, 1 mg, 2 mg

Dosing

Adult & Geriatric

Low-to-moderate immunologic risk renal transplant patients: Oral:

<40 kg: Loading dose: 3 mg/m^2 on day 1, followed by maintenance dosing of 1 mg/m^2 once daily

≥40 kg: Loading dose: 6 mg on day 1; maintenance: 2 mg once daily

High immunologic risk renal transplant patients: Oral: Loading dose: Up to 15 mg on day 1; maintenance: 5 mg/day; obtain trough concentration between days 5-7 and adjust accordingly. Continue concurrent cyclosporine/sirolimus therapy for 1 year following transplantation. Further adjustment of the regimen must be based on clinical status.

Dosage adjustment: Sirolimus dosages should be adjusted to maintain trough concentrations within desired range based on risk and concomitant therapy. Maximum daily dose: 40 mg. Dosage should be adjusted at intervals of 7-14 days to account for the long half-life of sirolimus. In general, dose proportionality may be assumed. New sirolimus dose **equals** current dose **multiplied by** (target concentration **divided by** current concentration). **Note:** If large dose increase is required, consider loading dose calculated as:

Loading dose **equals** (new maintenance dose **minus** current maintenance dose) **multiplied by** 3

Maximum dose in 1 day: 40 mg; if required dose is >40 mg (due to loading dose), divide loading dose over 2 days. Whole blood concentrations should not be used as the sole basis for dosage adjustment (monitor clinical signs/symptoms, tissue biopsy, and laboratory parameters).

Maintenance therapy after withdrawal of cyclosporine: Cyclosporine withdrawal is not recommended in high immunological risk patients. Following 2-4 months of combined therapy, withdrawal of cyclosporine may be considered in low-to-moderate immunologic risk patients. Cyclosporine should be discontinued over 4-8 weeks, and a necessary increase in the dosage of sirolimus (up to fourfold) should be anticipated due to removal of metabolic inhibition by cyclosporine and to maintain adequate immunosuppressive effects. Dose-adjusted trough target concentrations are typically 16-24 ng/mL for the first year post-transplant and 12-20 ng/mL thereafter (measured by chromatographic methodology).

GVHD prophylaxis (unlabeled use): Oral: 12 mg loading dose on day -3, followed by 4 mg daily (target trough level: 3-12 ng/mL); taper off after 6-9 months (Armand, 2008; Cutler, 2007)

Treatment of refractory acute GVHD (unlabeled use): Oral: 4-5 mg/m^2 for 14 days (no loading dose) (Benito, 2001)

Treatment of chronic GVHD (unlabeled use): Oral: 6 mg loading dose, followed by 2 mg daily (target trough level: 7-12 ng/mL) for 6-9 months (Couriel, 2005)

Pediatric

Immunosuppression: Children ≥13 years: Oral: Refer to adult dosing.

Renal Impairment No dosage adjustment (in loading or maintenance dose) is necessary in renal impairment. However, adjustment of regimen (including discontinuation of therapy) should be considered when used concurrently with cyclosporine and elevated or increasing serum creatinine is noted.

Hepatic Impairment

Loading dose: No adjustment required

Maintenance dose:

Mild-to-moderate hepatic impairment: reduce maintenance dose by ~33%.

Severe hepatic impairment: reduce maintenance dose by ~50%.

Administration

Oral Initial dose should be administered as soon as possible after transplant. Sirolimus should be taken 4 hours after oral cyclosporine (Neoral® or Gengraf®). Should be administered consistently (with or without food).

Solution: Mix (by stirring vigorously) with at least 2 ounces of water or orange juice. No other liquids should be used for dilution. Patient should drink diluted solution immediately. The cup should then be refilled with an additional 4 ounces of water or orange juice, stirred vigorously, and the patient should drink the contents at once.

Tablet: Do not crush, split, or chew.

Stability

Storage

Oral solution: Store under refrigeration, 2°C to 8°C (36°F to 46°F). Protect from light. A slight haze may develop in refrigerated solutions, but the quality of the product is not affected. After opening, solution should be used in 1 month. If necessary, may be stored at temperatures up to 25°C (77°F) for ≤15 days after opening. Product may be stored in amber syringe for a maximum of 24 hours (at room temperature or refrigerated). Discard syringe after single use. Solution should be used immediately following dilution.

Tablet: Store at room temperature of 20°C to 25°C (68°F to 77°F). Protect from light.

Monitoring and Teaching Issues

Laboratory Monitoring Monitor LFTs and CBC during treatment. Monitor sirolimus levels in all patients (especially in pediatric patients, patients ≥13 years of age weighing <40 kg, patients with hepatic impairment, or on concurrent potent inhibitors or inducers of CYP3A4 or P-gp, and/or if cyclosporine dosing is markedly reduced or discontinued), and when changing dosage forms of sirolimus. Also monitor serum cholesterol and triglycerides, serum creatinine, and urinary protein. Serum drug concentrations should be determined 3-4 days after loading doses and 7-14 days after dosage adjustments; however, these concentrations should not be used as the sole basis for dosage adjustment, especially during withdrawal of cyclosporine (monitor clinical signs/symptoms, tissue biopsy, and laboratory parameters). **Note:** Concentrations and ranges are dependent on and will vary with assay methodology (chromatographic or immunoassay); assay methods are not interchangeable.

Physical Assessment Assess lipid profiles; evaluate the need for medication intervention. Monitor blood pressure, weight, and renal function. Assess for signs of fluid retention and infection.

Patient Education Do not mix sirolimus solution with anything other than water or orange juice. Do not crush, split, or chew tablets. May be taken with or without food, but should be taken consistently with regard to food (always on an empty stomach or always with food). Maintain adequate hydration, unless instructed to restrict fluid intake. You will be susceptible to infection. If you have diabetes, monitor glucose levels closely (drug may alter glucose levels). Limit exposure to sunlight by wearing protective clothing or sunscreen. You may experience nausea, vomiting, loss of appetite, constipation, diarrhea, rash, acne, tremor, weight gain, or muscle or back pain. Inform prescriber of unresolved GI problems; respiratory difficulty, cough, or infection; persistent fever; skin rash or irritation; headache, insomnia, anxiety, confusion, or emotional lability; unusual bleeding; changes in voiding pattern or burning, itching, or pain on urination; persistent bone, joint, or muscle cramping, pain or weakness; numbness or tingling of extremities; chest pain, palpitations, or swelling of extremities; weight gain; or hearing or vision changes.

Dietary Considerations Take consistently (with or without food) to minimize variability of absorption.

Breast-Feeding Considerations Due to the potential for adverse reactions in the breast-fed infant, including possible immunosuppression, breast-feeding is not recommended.

Pregnancy Considerations Animal studies have demonstrated embryotoxicity and fetotoxicity, as evidenced by increased mortality, reduced fetal weights and delayed ossification. There are no adequate and well-controlled studies in pregnant women. Effective contraception must be initiated before therapy with sirolimus and continued for 12 weeks after discontinuation.

The National Transplantation Pregnancy Registry (NTPR, Temple University) is a registry for pregnant women taking immunosuppressants following any solid organ transplant. The NTPR encourages reporting of all immunosuppressant exposures during pregnancy in transplant recipients at 877-955-6877.

Additional Information Sirolimus tablets and oral solution are not bioequivalent, due to differences in absorption. Clinical equivalence was seen using 2 mg tablet and 2 mg solution. It is not known if higher doses are also clinically equivalent. Monitor sirolimus levels if changes in dosage forms are made.

Sirolimus solution may cause irritation if administered undiluted.

High-risk renal transplant patients are defined (per the manufacturer's labeling) as African-American transplant recipients and/or repeat renal transplant recipients who lost a previous allograft based on an immunologic process and/or patients with high PRA (panel-reactive antibodies; peak PRA level >80%). Individual transplant centers may have differences in their definitions. For example, some centers would consider a PRA >50% to be at higher risk of rejection.

SitaGLIPtin (sit a GLIP tin)

U.S. Brand Names Januvia®

Index Terms MK-0431; Sitagliptin Phosphate

Generic Availability (U.S.) No

Pharmacologic Category Antidiabetic Agent, Dipeptidyl Peptidase IV (DPP-IV) Inhibitor

Medication Safety Issues

Sound-alike/look-alike issues:

Januvia® may be confused with Enjuvia™, Janumet®, Jantoven™

SitaGLIPtin may be confused with saxagliptin, SUMAtriptan

Medication Guide Available Yes

Pregnancy Risk Factor B

Lactation Excretion in breast milk unknown/use caution

Use Management of type 2 diabetes mellitus (noninsulin dependent, NIDDM) as an adjunct to diet and exercise as monotherapy or in combination therapy with other antidiabetic agents

Mechanism of Action/Effect Sitagliptin inhibits dipeptidyl peptidase IV (DPP-IV) enzyme resulting in prolonged active incretin levels. Incretin hormones (eg, glucagon-like peptide-1 [GLP-1] and glucose-dependent insulinotropic polypeptide [GIP]) regulate glucose homeostasis by increasing insulin synthesis and release from pancreatic beta cells and decreasing glucagon secretion from pancreatic alpha cells. Decreased glucagon secretion results in decreased hepatic glucose production. Under normal physiologic circumstances, incretin hormones are released by the intestine throughout the day and levels are increased in response to a meal; incretin hormones are rapidly inactivated by the DPP-IV enzyme.

Contraindications Serious hypersensitivity (eg, anaphylaxis, angioedema) to sitagliptan or any component of the formulation

Warnings/Precautions Avoid use in type 1 diabetes mellitus (insulin dependent, IDDM) and diabetic ketoacidosis (DKA) due to lack of efficacy in these populations. Use caution when used in conjunction with insulin or insulin secretagogues; risk of hypoglycemia is increased. Monitor blood glucose closely; dosage adjustments of insulin or insulin secretagogues may be necessary. Use with caution in patients with moderate-to-severe renal dysfunction and end-stage renal disease (ESRD) requiring hemodialysis or peritoneal dialysis; dosing adjustment required. Safety and efficacy have not been established in severe hepatic dysfunction.

Rare hypersensitivity reactions, including anaphylaxis, angioedema, and/or severe dermatologic reactions (such as Stevens-Johnson syndrome), have been reported in postmarketing surveillance; discontinue if signs/symptoms of hypersensitivity reactions occur. Cases of acute pancreatitis (including hemorrhagic and necrotizing with some fatalities) have been reported with use; monitor for signs/symptoms of pancreatitis. Discontinue use immediately if pancreatitis is suspected and initiate appropriate management. Use with caution in patients with a history of pancreatitis (not known if this population is at greater risk).

Clinical trials included only a limited number of patients with heart failure (HF). No specific recommendations regarding this population are provided in the approved U.S. labeling (Canadian labeling recommends against use in this population). Diabetes self-management education (DSME) is essential to maximize the effectiveness of therapy.

Drug Interactions

Metabolism/Transport Effects **Substrate** of CYP2C8 (minor), CYP3A4 (minor), P-glycoprotein

Avoid Concomitant Use There are no known interactions where it is recommended to avoid concomitant use.

Decreased Effect

The levels/effects of SitaGLIPtin may be decreased by: Corticosteroids (Orally Inhaled); Corticosteroids (Systemic); Luteinizing Hormone-Releasing Hormone Analogs; P-Glycoprotein Inducers; Somatropin; Thiazide Diuretics

Increased Effect/Toxicity

SitaGLIPtin may increase the levels/effects of: ACE Inhibitors; Digoxin; Hypoglycemic Agents

The levels/effects of SitaGLIPtin may be increased by: Herbs (Hypoglycemic Properties); Pegvisomant; P-Glycoprotein Inhibitors

Adverse Reactions As reported with monotherapy: 1% to 10%:

Cardiovascular: Peripheral edema (2%)

Endocrine & metabolic: Hypoglycemia (1%)

Gastrointestinal: Diarrhea (4%), constipation (3%), nausea (2%)

Neuromuscular & skeletal: Osteoarthritis (1%)

Respiratory: Nasopharyngitis (5%), pharyngitis (1%), upper respiratory tract infection (viral; 1%)

Pharmacodynamics/Kinetics

Absorption Rapid

Bioavailability ~87%

Time to Peak 1-4 hours

Protein Binding 38%

Half-Life Elimination 12 hours

Metabolism Not extensively metabolized; minor metabolism via CYP3A4 and 2C8 to metabolites (inactive) suggested by *in vitro* studies

Excretion Urine 87% (79% as unchanged drug, 16% as metabolites); feces 13%

Available Dosage Forms

Tablet, oral:

Januvia®: 25 mg, 50 mg, 100 mg

Dosing

Adult Type 2 diabetes: Oral: 100 mg once daily

Concomitant use with insulin and/or insulin secretagogues (eg, sulfonylureas): Reduced dose of insulin and/or insulin secretagogues may be needed.

Renal Impairment

Cl_{cr} ≥50 mL/minute: No adjustment required

Cl_{cr} ≥30 to <50 mL/minute: 50 mg once daily

S_{cr}: Males: >1.7 to ≤3.0 mg/dL; Females: >1.5 to ≤2.5 mg/dL: 50 mg once daily

Cl_{cr}<30 mL/minute: 25 mg once daily

S_{cr}: Males: >3.0 mg/dL; Females: >2.5 mg/dL: 25 mg once daily

ESRD requiring hemodialysis or peritoneal dialysis: 25 mg once daily; administered without regard to timing of hemodialysis

Hepatic Impairment

Mild-to-moderate impairment (Child-Pugh score 7-9): No dosage adjustment required

Severe impairment (Child-Pugh score >9): Not studied

Administration

Oral May be administered with or without food.

Stability

Storage Store at 20°C to 25°C (68°F to 77°F); excursions permitted to 15°C to 30°C (59°F to 86°F).

Monitoring and Teaching Issues

Laboratory Monitoring Hb A_{1C}, serum glucose; renal function prior to initiation and periodically during treatment

Physical Assessment With insulin or sulfonylureas, the risk of hypoglycemia may be increased and dosage adjustments may be necessary. Assess renal function prior to treatment and throughout. Monitor for hypersensitivity reactions and development of pancreatitis. Refer patient to diabetic educator for diabetic education if necessary.

Patient Education This medication will not cure diabetes and may be prescribed in conjunction with another antidiabetic medication. Do not chew or crush tablets. May be taken with or without food. It is important to follow dietary and lifestyle recommendations and glucose monitoring instructions of prescriber or diabetic educator. You will be instructed in signs of hyper-/hypoglycemia; always carry a source of glucose with you in event of hypoglycemia. You may experience mild headache, upper respiratory infection, stuffy or runny nose, sore throat, diarrhea, or constipation when beginning treatment. Notify prescriber of any persistent abdominal pain, anorexia, nausea, or vomiting; or signs of hypersensitivity reaction (swelling of face, lips, or mouth; severe skin rash or eruption; difficulty breathing).

Dietary Considerations May be taken with or without food. Individualized medical nutrition therapy (MNT) based on ADA recommendations is an integral part of therapy.

Geriatric Considerations Sitagliptin has not been studied exclusively in the elderly. The manufacturer reports that 725 out of 3884 patients in clinical trials were >65 years (only 61 were age 75 years and older), with no difference in safety or efficacy compared to younger patients. How "tightly" a geriatric patient's blood glucose should be controlled is controversial; however, a fasting blood sugar of <150 mg/dL is now an acceptable endpoint. Such a decision should be based on the patient's functional and cognitive status, how well they recognize hypoglycemic or hyperglycemic symptoms, and how to respond to them and their other disease states. Intensive glucose control (Hb A_{1c} <6.5%) has been linked to increased all cause and cardiovascular mortality, hypoglycemia requiring assistance, and weight gain in adult type 2 diabetes. For elderly patients with diabetes who are relatively healthy, attaining target goals for aspirin use, blood pressure, lipids, smoking cessation, and diet and exercise may be more important than normalized glycemic control.

Breast-Feeding Considerations It is not known if sitagliptin is excreted in breast milk. The manufacturer recommends that caution be used if administered to breast-feeding women.

Pregnancy Considerations Adverse events have not been observed in animal reproduction studies; therefore, sitagliptan is classified as pregnancy category B. There are no adequate and well controlled studies in pregnant women. Maternal hyperglycemia can be associated with adverse effects in the fetus, including macrosomia, neonatal hyperglycemia, and hyperbilirubinemia; the risk of congenital malformations is increased when the Hb A_{1c} is above the normal range. Diabetes can also be associated with adverse effects in the mother. Poorly-treated diabetes may cause end-organ damage that may in turn negatively affect obstetric outcomes. Physiologic glucose levels should be maintained prior to and during pregnancy to decrease the risk of adverse events in the mother and the fetus. Until additional safety and efficacy data are obtained, the use of oral agents is generally not recommended as routine management of GDM or type 2 diabetes mellitus during pregnancy. Insulin is the drug of choice for the control of diabetes mellitus during pregnancy. Health professionals are encouraged to report any prenatal exposure to sitagliptin by contacting Merck's pregnancy registry (1-800-986-8999).

Related Information

Diabetes Mellitus Management, Adults *on page 2026*

Sitagliptin and Metformin (sit a GLIP tin & met FOR min)

U.S. Brand Names Janumet®

Index Terms Metformin and Sitagliptin; Sitagliptin Phosphate and Metformin Hydrochloride

Generic Availability (U.S.) No

Pharmacologic Category Antidiabetic Agent, Biguanide; Antidiabetic Agent, Dipeptidyl Peptidase IV (DPP-IV) Inhibitor; Hypoglycemic Agent, Oral

Medication Safety Issues

Sound-alike/look-alike issues:

Janumet® may be confused with Jantoven™, Januvia®

Medication Guide Available Yes

Pregnancy Risk Factor B

Lactation

Sitagliptin: Excretion in breast milk unknown/use caution

Metformin: Enters breast milk

Use Management of type 2 diabetes mellitus (noninsulin dependent, NIDDM) as an adjunct to diet and exercise in patients not adequately controlled on metformin or sitagliptin monotherapy

Contraindications Hypersensitivity to sitagliptin, metformin, or any component of the formulation; renal disease or renal dysfunction (serum creatinine ≥1.5 mg/dL [≥136 µmol/L] in males or ≥1.4 mg/dL [≥124 µmol/L] in females), or abnormal creatinine clearance which may also result from conditions such as cardiovascular collapse, acute myocardial infarction, and septicemia); acute or chronic metabolic acidosis including diabetic ketoacidosis (with or without coma).

Canadian labeling: Additional contraindications (not in U.S. labeling): Unstable and/or insulin-dependent (type 1) diabetes mellitus (IDDM); history of lactic acidosis, regardless of precipitating factors; acute or chronic excessive alcohol intake; severe hepatic disease; cardiovascular collapse and disease states associated with hypoxemia (eg, cardiorespiratory insufficiency) which are often associated with hyperlactacidemia; use during stress conditions (eg, severe infection, trauma, surgery) and the recovery phase thereafter; severe dehydration; breast-feeding; pregnancy

Warnings/Precautions Rare hypersensitivity reactions, including anaphylaxis, angioedema and/or severe dermatologic reactions (such as Stevens-Johnson syndrome), have been reported in postmarketing surveillance; discontinue if signs/symptoms of hypersensitivity reactions occur. Events have generally been noted within the first 3 months of therapy, and may occur with the initial dose. **[U.S. Boxed Warning]: Lactic acidosis is a rare, but potentially severe consequence of therapy with metformin.** Lactic acidosis should be suspected in any patient with diabetes receiving metformin with evidence of acidosis but without evidence of ketoacidosis. Discontinue metformin in clinical situations predisposing to hypoxemia, including conditions such as cardiovascular collapse, respiratory failure, acute myocardial infarction, acute heart failure, and septicemia. Not indicated for use in patients with insulin-dependent diabetes mellitus (IDDM) (type 1). Use caution in patients with heart failure requiring pharmacologic management, particularly in patients with unstable of acute heart failure; risk of lactic acidosis may be increased secondary to hypoperfusion. The Canadian labeling recommends avoiding use in patients with heart failure. Avoid use in patients with impaired liver function due to potential for lactic acidosis. Patients should be instructed to avoid excessive acute or chronic ethanol use; ethanol may potentiate metformin's effect on lactate metabolism. Cases of acute pancreatitis (including hemorrhagic and necrotizing with some fatalities) have been reported with use of sitagliptin. Monitor for signs/symptoms of pancreatitis; discontinue use immediately if pancreatitis is suspected and initiate appropriate management. Use with caution in patients with a history of pancreatitis as it is not known if this population is at greater risk.

Sitagliptin and metformin are substantially excreted by the kidney; patients with renal function below the limit of normal for their age should not receive therapy. In elderly patients, renal function should be monitored regularly; should not be used in any patient ≥80 years of age unless normal renal function is confirmed. The risk of accumulation and lactic acidosis increases with the degree of impairment of renal function. Use of concomitant medications that may affect renal function (eg, affect tubular secretion) may also affect metformin disposition. Metformin should be withheld in patients with dehydration and/or prerenal azotemia. Metformin therapy should be temporarily discontinued prior to or at the time of intravascular administration of iodinated contrast media (potential for acute alteration in renal function). Metformin should be withheld for 48 hours after the radiologic study and restarted only after renal function has been confirmed as normal. Therapy should be suspended for any surgical procedures (resume only after normal intake resumed and normal renal function is verified). It may be necessary to discontinue metformin and administer insulin if the patient is exposed to stress (fever, trauma, infection, surgery). May impair vitamin B_{12} absorption; very rarely associated with anemia. Rapid reversal of vitamin B_{12} deficiency may be observed with discontinuation of therapy or supplementation; monitor vitamin B_{12} serum concentrations periodically with long-term therapy. Use with caution in conjunction with insulin or insulin secretagogues (eg, sulfonylureas); risk of hypoglycemia is increased. Monitor blood glucose closely; dosage adjustments of insulin or the secretagogue may be necessary.

Drug Interactions

Metabolism/Transport Effects Sitagliptin: **Substrate** of CYP2C8 (minor), CYP3A4 (minor), P-glycoprotein

Avoid Concomitant Use There are no known interactions where it is recommended to avoid concomitant use.

Decreased Effect

The levels/effects of Sitagliptin and Metformin may be decreased by: Corticosteroids (Orally Inhaled); Corticosteroids (Systemic); Luteinizing Hormone-Releasing Hormone Analogs; P-Glycoprotein Inducers; Somatropin; Thiazide Diuretics

Increased Effect/Toxicity

Sitagliptin and Metformin may increase the levels/effects of: ACE Inhibitors; Digoxin; Hypoglycemic Agents

The levels/effects of Sitagliptin and Metformin may be increased by: Cephalexin; Cimetidine; Glycopyrrolate; Herbs (Hypoglycemic Properties); Iodinated Contrast Agents; Pegvisomant; P-Glycoprotein Inhibitors

Nutritional/Ethanol Interactions Ethanol: Excessive ethanol intake (acute or chronic) should be avoided due to increased risks for metformin accumulation and lactic acidosis.

Adverse Reactions See individual agents.

Pharmacodynamics/Kinetics

Pharmacokinetic Note See individual agents.

Available Dosage Forms

Tablet, oral:

Janumet®: 50/500: Sitagliptin 50 mg and metformin 500 mg; 50/1000: Sitagliptin 50 mg and metformin 1000 mg

Dosing

Adult Note: Patients receiving concomitant insulin and/or insulin secretagogues (eg, sulfonylureas) may require dosage adjustments of these agents.

Type 2 diabetes mellitus: Oral: Initial doses should be based on current dose of sitagliptin and metformin; daily doses should be divided and given twice daily with meals. Maximum: Sitagliptin 100 mg/metformin 2000 mg daily

Patients inadequately controlled on metformin alone: Initial dose: Sitagliptin 100 mg/day plus current dose of metformin. **Note:** The U.S. labeling recommends that patients currently receiving metformin 850 mg twice daily receive an initial dose of sitagliptin 50 mg and metformin 1000 mg twice daily

Patients inadequately controlled on sitagliptin alone: Initial dose: Metformin 1000 mg/day plus sitagliptin 100 mg/day. **Note:** Patients currently receiving a renally adjusted dose of sitagliptin should not be switched to combination product.

Dosing adjustment: Metformin component may be gradually increased up to the maximum dose. Maximum dose: Sitagliptin 100 mg/metformin 2000 mg daily

Geriatric Refer to adult dosing. The initial and maintenance dosing should be conservative, due to the potential for decreased renal function (monitor). Do not use in patients ≥80 years of age unless normal renal function has been established.

Renal Impairment Do not use with renal disease or renal dysfunction (serum creatinine ≥1.5 mg/dL [≥136 µmol/L] in males or ≥1.4 mg/dL [≥124 µmol/L] in females or abnormal clearance).

Hepatic Impairment Avoid metformin; liver disease is a risk factor for the development of lactic acidosis during metformin therapy.

Administration

Oral Administer with meals, at the same time each day.

Stability

Storage Store at 20°C to 25°C (68°F to 77°F); excursions permitted to 15°C to 30°C (59°F to 86°F).

Monitoring and Teaching Issues

Laboratory Monitoring Hb A_{1c} and serum glucose, hematologic parameters (eg, hemoglobin/hematocrit, red blood cell indices); hepatic function, renal function (prior to initiation of therapy then annually or more frequent if necessary); vitamin B_{12} (periodically with long-term treatment) and folate (if megaloblastic anemia is suspected)

Physical Assessment See individual agents.

Patient Education See individual agents.

Dietary Considerations Should be taken with meals (to decrease GI upset). Take at the same time each day. Individualized medical nutrition therapy (MNT) based on ADA recommendations is an integral part of therapy. Monitor for signs and symptoms of vitamin B_{12} and/or folic acid deficiency; supplementation may be required.

Geriatric Considerations Sitagliptin has not been studied exclusively in the elderly. The manufacturer reports that 725 out of 3884 patients in clinical trials were >65 years of age (only 61 were ≥75 years), with no difference in safety or efficacy compared to younger patients. Limited data suggest that metformin's total body clearance may be decreased and AUC and half-life increased in elderly patients; presumably due to decreased renal clearance. Metformin has been well tolerated by the elderly but lower doses and frequent monitoring are recommended. In one study of elderly subjects, its effects could not be distinguished from tolbutamide, except for weight loss. The initial and maintenance dosing should be conservative, due to the potential for decreased renal function. Generally, elderly patients should not be titrated to the maximum dose of metformin. Do not use in patients ≥80 years of age unless normal renal function has been established. How "tightly" an elderly patient's blood glucose should be controlled is controversial; however, a fasting blood sugar of <150 mg/dL is now an acceptable endpoint. Such a decision should be based on the patient's functional and cognitive status, how well they recognize hypoglycemic or hyperglycemic symptoms, and how to respond to them and their other disease states. Intensive glucose control (Hb A_{1c} <6.5%) has been linked to increased all cause and cardiovascular mortality, hypoglycemia requiring assistance, and weight gain in adult type 2 diabetes. For elderly patients with diabetes who are relatively healthy, attaining target goals for aspirin use, blood pressure, lipids, smoking cessation, and diet and exercise may be more important than normalized glycemic control.

Breast-Feeding Considerations See individual agents.

Pregnancy Considerations

Reproduction studies have not been conducted with this combination. Adverse events were not observed in animal studies of the individual agents; therefore, sitagliptin/metformin is classified as pregnancy category B. See individual agents. Health professionals are encouraged to report any prenatal exposure to Janumet® by contacting Merck's pregnancy registry (1-800-986-8999).

Related Information

Diabetes Mellitus Management, Adults *on page 2026*

◆ **Sitagliptin Phosphate** *see* SitaGLIPtin *on page 1652*

◆ **Sitagliptin Phosphate and Metformin Hydrochloride** *see* Sitagliptin and Metformin *on page 1654*

Sitaxsentan (sye TACKS en tan)

Index Terms Sitaxsentan; Sitaxsentan Sodium

Generic Availability (U.S.) No

Pharmacologic Category Endothelin Antagonist; Vasodilator

Lactation Excretion into breast milk unknown/contraindicated

Use Treatment of primary pulmonary arterial hypertension (PAH) or pulmonary hypertension secondary to connective tissue disease, in World Health Organization (WHO) class III patients unresponsive to conventional therapy; treatment of PAH in WHO class II patients who are unresponsive to conventional therapy and have no alternative treatment options

Product Availability Not available in U.S.

Dosing

Adult & Geriatric Pulmonary arterial hypertension: Oral: 100 mg once daily. (**Note:** Doses above 100 mg/day are not recommended; higher doses have not been shown to provide additional benefit and may increase risk of hepatic toxicity).

Renal Impairment No adjustment required.

Adjustment for Toxicity Dosage modifications based on transaminase elevation:

AST/ALT >3 but ≤8 times ULN: Confirm with additional test; if confirmed, interrupt treatment. Monitor transaminase levels at least every 2 weeks until levels are <3 times ULN. Reinitiate treatment as appropriate with return to pretreatment values and with more frequent checks of transaminase levels (3 days after restarting therapy and every 2 weeks thereafter).

AST/ALT >8 times ULN: Stop treatment and do not reintroduce.

Note: If any elevation, regardless of degree, is accompanied by clinical symptoms of hepatic injury (unusual fatigue, nausea, vomiting, abdominal pain, fever, or jaundice) or a serum bilirubin >2 times ULN, treatment should be stopped and not reintroduced.

Administration

Oral Administer with or without food.

Monitoring and Teaching Issues

Laboratory Monitoring Serum transaminase (AST and ALT) and bilirubin should be determined prior to the initiation of therapy and at monthly intervals thereafter. Monitor for clinical signs and symptoms of liver injury (eg, abdominal pain, fatigue, fever, jaundice, nausea, vomiting). Interrupt therapy if transaminases >3 times ULN and ≤8 times ULN. Monitor levels every 2 weeks until they are <3 times ULN. Therapy may be resumed with more frequent monitoring of levels. Discontinue therapy with transaminase levels >8 times ULN and in patients with elevated transaminases with accompanying symptoms of hepatic injury, or bilirubin >2 times ULN.

Hemoglobin and hematocrit should be measured at baseline, 1 month, 3 months, and every 3 months thereafter (levels generally stabilize within 4 weeks from the initiation of therapy). Obtain baseline blood pressure and initiate therapy with caution with SBP <85 mm Hg. A woman of childbearing potential must have a negative pregnancy test prior to the initiation of therapy and monthly thereafter.

Physical Assessment Monitor blood pressure at the beginning of therapy and periodically thereafter. Teach patient the need for careful contraception.

Patient Education May cause headache, nausea, nasal congestion, nose bleeds, or peripheral edema. Report increase in shortness of breath, weight gain, unusual fatigue, jaundice, nausea, vomiting, abdominal pain, or fever.

◆ **Sitaxsentan** *see* Sitaxsentan *on page 1657*
◆ **Sitaxsentan Sodium** *see* Sitaxsentan *on page 1657*
◆ **Skelaxin®** *see* Metaxalone *on page 1181*
◆ **Skelid®** *see* Tiludronate *on page 1762*
◆ **SKF 104864** *see* Topotecan *on page 1790*
◆ **SKF 104864-A** *see* Topotecan *on page 1790*
◆ **Sleep-ettes D [OTC]** *see* DiphenhydrAMINE (Systemic) *on page 543*
◆ **Sleepinal® [OTC]** *see* DiphenhydrAMINE (Systemic) *on page 543*
◆ **Sleep-Tabs [OTC]** *see* DiphenhydrAMINE (Systemic) *on page 543*
◆ **S-leucovorin** *see* LEVOleucovorin *on page 1096*
◆ **6S-leucovorin** *see* LEVOleucovorin *on page 1096*
◆ **Slo-Niacin® [OTC]** *see* Niacin *on page 1305*
◆ **Slow FE® [OTC]** *see* Ferrous Sulfate *on page 754*
◆ **Slow-Mag® [OTC]** *see* Magnesium Chloride *on page 1143*
◆ **SM-13496** *see* Lurasidone *on page 1140*
◆ **SMX-TMP** *see* Sulfamethoxazole and Trimethoprim *on page 1686*
◆ **SMZ-TMP** *see* Sulfamethoxazole and Trimethoprim *on page 1686*
◆ **(+)-(*S*)-*N*-Methyl-γ-(1-naphthyloxy)-2-thiophenepropylamine Hydrochloride** *see* DULoxetine *on page 596*
◆ **Sodium 2-Mercaptoethane Sulfonate** *see* Mesna *on page 1180*
◆ **Sodium Acid Carbonate** *see* Sodium Bicarbonate *on page 1658*

◆ **Sodium Benzoate and Caffeine** *see* Caffeine *on page* 267

Sodium Bicarbonate (SOW dee um bye KAR bun ate)

U.S. Brand Names Brioschi® [OTC]; Neut®

Index Terms Baking Soda; $NaHCO_3$; Sodium Acid Carbonate; Sodium Hydrogen Carbonate

Generic Availability (U.S.) Yes: Excludes granules

Pharmacologic Category Alkalinizing Agent; Antacid; Electrolyte Supplement, Oral; Electrolyte Supplement, Parenteral

Pregnancy Risk Factor C

Lactation Enters breast milk/compatible

Use Management of metabolic acidosis; gastric hyperacidity; as an alkalinization agent for the urine; treatment of hyperkalemia; management of overdose of certain drugs, including tricyclic antidepressants and aspirin

Unlabeled/Investigational Use Prevention of contrast-induced nephropathy (CIN)

Mechanism of Action/Effect Dissociates to provide bicarbonate ion which neutralizes hydrogen ion concentration and raises blood and urinary pH

Contraindications Alkalosis, hypernatremia, severe pulmonary edema, hypocalcemia, unknown abdominal pain

Warnings/Precautions Rapid administration in neonates and children <2 years of age has led to hypernatremia, decreased CSF pressure and intracranial hemorrhage. **Use of I.V. $NaHCO_3$ should be reserved for documented metabolic acidosis and for hyperkalemia-induced cardiac arrest.** Routine use in cardiac arrest is not recommended. Avoid extravasation, tissue necrosis can occur due to the hypertonicity of $NaHCO_3$. May cause sodium retention especially if renal function is impaired; not to be used in treatment of peptic ulcer; use with caution in patients with HF, edema, cirrhosis, or renal failure. Not the antacid of choice for the elderly because of sodium content and potential for systemic alkalosis.

Drug Interactions

Avoid Concomitant Use There are no known interactions where it is recommended to avoid concomitant use.

Decreased Effect

Sodium Bicarbonate may decrease the levels/effects of: ACE Inhibitors; Anticonvulsants (Hydantoin); Antipsychotic Agents (Phenothiazines); Atazanavir; Bisacodyl; Cefditoren; Cefpodoxime; Cefuroxime; Chloroquine; Corticosteroids (Oral); Dabigatran Etexilate; Dasatinib; Delavirdine; Erlotinib; Flecainide; HMG-CoA Reductase Inhibitors; Iron Salts; Isoniazid; Itraconazole; Ketoconazole; Ketoconazole (Systemic); Lithium; Mesalamine; Methenamine; Penicillamine; Phosphate Supplements; Protease Inhibitors; Tetracycline Derivatives; Trientine

Increased Effect/Toxicity

Sodium Bicarbonate may increase the levels/effects of: Alpha-/Beta-Agonists; Amphetamines; Calcium Polystyrene Sulfonate; Dexmethylphenidate; Flecainide; Memantine; Methylphenidate; QuiNIDine; QuiNINE

Nutritional/Ethanol Interactions Herb/Nutraceutical: Concurrent doses with iron may decrease iron absorption.

Adverse Reactions Frequency not defined.

Cardiovascular: Cerebral hemorrhage, CHF (aggravated), edema

Central nervous system: Tetany

Gastrointestinal: Belching, flatulence (with oral), gastric distension

Endocrine & metabolic: Hypernatremia, hyperosmolality, hypocalcemia, hypokalemia, increased affinity of hemoglobin for oxygen-reduced pH in myocardial tissue necrosis when extravasated, intracranial acidosis, metabolic alkalosis, milk-alkali syndrome (especially with renal dysfunction)

Respiratory: Pulmonary edema

Pharmacodynamics/Kinetics

Onset of Action Oral: Rapid; I.V.: 15 minutes

Duration of Action Oral: 8-10 minutes; I.V.: 1-2 hours

Absorption Oral: Well absorbed

Excretion Urine (<1%)

Available Dosage Forms

Granules for solution, oral:

Brioschi® [OTC]: 2.69 g/capful (120 g, 240 g); 2.69 g/packet (12s)

Injection, solution: 4.2% (10 mL); 7.5% (50 mL); 8.4% (10 mL, 50 mL, 250 mL, 500 mL)

Neut®: 4% (5 mL)

Injection, solution [preservative free]: 4.2% (5 mL, 10 mL); 7.5% (50 mL); 8.4% (10 mL, 50 mL)

Powder, oral: USP: 100% (120 g, 454 g, 480 g)

Tablet, oral: 325 mg, 650 mg

Dosing

Adult & Geriatric

Cardiac arrest (ACLS, 2010): I.V.: Initial: 1 mEq/kg/dose; repeat doses should be guided by arterial blood gases

Routine use of $NaHCO_3$ is not recommended. May be considered in the setting of prolonged cardiac arrest only after adequate alveolar ventilation has been established and effective cardiac compressions. **Note:** In some cardiac arrest situations (eg, metabolic acidosis, hyperkalemia, or tricyclic antidepressant overdose), sodium bicarbonate may be beneficial.

Metabolic acidosis: I.V.: Dosage should be based on the following formula if blood gases and pH measurements are available:

HCO_3^-(mEq) = 0.2 x weight (kg) x base deficit (mEq/L)

Administer 1/2 dose initially, then remaining 1/2 dose over the next 24 hours; monitor pH, serum HCO_3^-, and clinical status

Note: If acid-base status is not available: 2-5 mEq/kg I.V. infusion over 4-8 hours; subsequent doses should be based on patient's acid-base status

Hyperkalemia (ACLS, 2010): I.V.: 50 mEq over 5 minutes (as appropriate, consider methods of enhancing potassium removal/excretion)

Chronic renal failure: Oral: Initiate when plasma HCO_3^- <15 mEq/L Start with 20-36 mEq/day in divided doses, titrate to bicarbonate level of 18-20 mEq/L

Renal tubular acidosis: Oral:

Distal: 0.5-2 mEq/kg/day in 4-5 divided doses

Proximal: Initial: 5-10 mEq/kg/day; maintenance: Increase as required to maintain serum bicarbonate in the normal range

Urine alkalinization: Oral: Initial: 48 mEq (4 g), then 12-24 mEq (1-2 g) every 4 hours; dose should be titrated to desired urinary pH; doses up to 16 g/day (200 mEq) in patients <60 years and 8 g (100 mEq) in patients >60 years

Antacid: Oral: 325 mg to 2 g 1-4 times/day

Prevention of contrast-induced nephropathy (unlabeled use): I.V. infusion: 154 mEq/L sodium bicarbonate in D_5W solution: 3 mL/kg/hour for 1 hour immediately before contrast injection, then 1mL/kg/hour during contrast exposure and for 6 hours after procedure

To prepare solution, remove 154 mL from 1000 mL bag of D_5W; replace with 154 mL of 8.4% sodium bicarbonate; resultant concentration is 154 mEq/L (Merten, 2004); more practically, institutions may remove 150 mL from 1000 mL bag of D_5W and replace with 150 mL of 8.4% sodium bicarbonate; resultant concentration is 150 mEq/L

Pediatric

Cardiac arrest (PALS, 2010): I.V., I.O.: Infants and Children: 1 mEq/kg/dose; repeat doses should be guided by arterial blood gases; neonates and children <2 years of age should receive 4.2% (0.5 mEq/mL) solution. **Note:** If I.O. route is used for administration and is subsequently used to obtain blood samples for acid-base analysis, results will be inaccurate.

Routine use of $NaHCO_3$ is not recommended. May be considered in the setting of prolonged cardiac arrest only after adequate alveolar ventilation has been established and effective cardiac compressions. **Note:** In some cardiac arrest situations (eg, metabolic acidosis, hyperkalemia, or tricyclic antidepressant overdose), sodium bicarbonate may be beneficial.

Metabolic acidosis: I.V.: Infants and Children: Dosage should be based on the following formula if blood gases and pH measurements are available:

HCO_3^- (mEq) = 0.3 x weight (kg) x base deficit (mEq/L)

Administer 1/2 dose initially, then remaining 1/2 dose over the next 24 hours; monitor pH, serum HCO_3^-, and clinical status

Note: If acid-base status is not available: Dose for older Children: 2-5 mEq/kg I.V. infusion over 4-8 hours; subsequent doses should be based on patient's acid-base status.

Chronic renal failure: Oral: Children: Initiate when plasma HCO_3^- <15 mEq/L: 1-3 mEq/kg/day

Renal tubular acidosis, distal: Oral: Children: 2-3 mEq/kg/day

Renal tubular acidosis, proximal: Children: Initial: 5-10 mEq/kg/day; maintenance: Increase as required to maintain serum bicarbonate in the normal range

Urine alkalinization: Oral: Children: 1-10 mEq (84-840 mg)/kg/day in divided doses every 4-6 hours; dose should be titrated to desired urinary pH.

Administration

Oral Oral product should be administered 1-3 hours after meals.

Stability

Reconstitution Prevention of contrast-induced nephropathy (unlabeled use): Remove 154 mL from 1000 mL bag of D_5W; replace with 154 mL of 8.4% sodium bicarbonate; resultant concentration is 154 mEq/L (Merten, 2004); more practically, institutions may remove 150 mL from 1000 mL bag of D_5W and replace with 150 mL of 8.4% sodium bicarbonate; resultant concentration is 150 mEq/L

Storage Store injection at room temperature. Protect from heat and from freezing. Use only clear solutions.

Monitoring and Teaching Issues

Physical Assessment I.V.: Monitor infusion site (if extravasation occurs, elevate extravasation site and apply warm compresses). Monitor for signs of fluid retention.

Patient Education Do not use for chronic gastric acidity. Chew tablets thoroughly and follow with a full glass of water, preferably on an empty stomach (2 hours before or after food). Report CNS effects (eg, irritability, confusion), muscle rigidity or tremors, swelling of feet or ankles, respiratory difficulty, chest pain or palpitations, respiratory changes, or tarry stools.

Dietary Considerations Some products may contain sodium. Oral product should be taken 1-3 hours after meals.

Geriatric Considerations Not the antacid of choice for the elderly because of sodium content and potential for systemic alkalosis (see maximum daily dose under Dosing).

Related Information

Compatibility of Drugs *on page 1994*

◆ **Sodium Bicarbonate and Omeprazole** *see* Omeprazole and Sodium Bicarbonate *on page 1359*

Sodium Citrate and Citric Acid (SOW dee um SIT rate & SI trik AS id)

U.S. Brand Names Cytra-2; Oracit®; Shohl's Solution (Modified)

Index Terms Bicitra; Citric Acid and Sodium Citrate; Modified Shohl's Solution

Generic Availability (U.S.) Yes

Pharmacologic Category Alkalinizing Agent, Oral

Medication Safety Issues

Sound-alike/look-alike issues:

Bicitra may be confused with Polycitra®

Pregnancy Risk Factor Not established

Lactation Excretion in breast milk unknown/compatible

Use Treatment of metabolic acidosis; alkalinizing agent in conditions where long-term maintenance of an alkaline urine is desirable

Available Dosage Forms Contains sodium 1 mEq/mL and is equivalent to bicarbonate 1 mEq/mL

Solution, oral: Sodium citrate 500 mg and citric acid 334 mg per 5 mL

Cytra-2: Sodium citrate 500 mg and citric acid 334 mg per 5 mL

Oracit®: Sodium citrate 490 mg and citric acid 640 mg per 5 mL

Shohl's Solution (Modified): Sodium citrate 500 mg and citric acid 300 mg er 5 mL

Dosing

Adult & Geriatric Systemic alkalization: Oral: 10-30 mL with water after meals and at bedtime

Pediatric Systemic alkalization: Oral: Infants and Children: 2-3 mEq/kg/day in divided doses 3-4 times/day **or** 5-15 mL with water after meals and at bedtime

Administration

Oral Administer after meals. Dilute with 30-90 mL of water to enhance taste. Chilling solution prior to dosing helps to enhance palatability.

Monitoring and Teaching Issues

Physical Assessment Assess kidney function prior to treatment. Monitor cardiac status and serum potassium prior to treatment and at regular intervals.

Patient Education Take after meals. Dilute with 1-3 oz of water and follow with additional water; chilling solution prior to taking will help to improve taste. You may experience diarrhea or nausea and vomiting; if severe, contact prescriber. Report CNS changes (eg, irritability, tremors, confusion), swelling of feet or ankles, respiratory difficulty or palpitations, abdominal pain, or tarry stools.

◆ **Sodium Edecrin®** *see* Ethacrynic Acid *on page* 692

◆ **Sodium Hydrogen Carbonate** *see* Sodium Bicarbonate *on page* 1658

◆ **Sodium Nafcillin** *see* Nafcillin *on page* 1282

◆ **Sodium Nitroferricyanide** *see* Nitroprusside *on page* 1330

◆ **Sodium Nitroprusside** *see* Nitroprusside *on page* 1330

◆ **Sodium Phosphate and Potassium Phosphate** *see* Potassium Phosphate and Sodium Phosphate *on page* 1486

Sodium Polystyrene Sulfonate (SOW dee um pol ee STYE reen SUL fon ate)

U.S. Brand Names Kalexate; Kayexalate®; Kionex®; SPS®

Generic Availability (U.S.) No

Pharmacologic Category Antidote

Medication Safety Issues

Sound-alike/look-alike issues:

Kayexalate® may be confused with Kaopectate®

Sodium polystyrene sulfonate may be confused with calcium polystyrene sulfonate

Always prescribe either one-time doses or as a specific number of doses (eg, 15 g q6h x 2 doses). Scheduled doses with no dosage limit could be given for days leading to dangerous hypokalemia.

International issues:

Kionex [U.S.] may be confused with Kinex brand name for biperiden [Mexico]

Pregnancy Risk Factor C

Lactation Excretion in breast milk unknown/use caution

Use Treatment of hyperkalemia

Mechanism of Action/Effect Removes potassium by exchanging sodium ions for potassium ions in the intestine (especially the large intestine) before the resin is passed from the body

Contraindications Hypersensitivity to sodium polystyrene sulfonate or any component of the formulation; hypokalemia; obstructive bowel disease; neonates with reduced gut motility (postoperatively or drug-induced); oral administration in neonates

Additional contraindications: Sodium polystyrene sulfonate suspension (**with** sorbitol): Rectal administration in neonates (particularly in premature infants); any postoperative patient until normal bowel function resumes

Warnings/Precautions Intestinal necrosis (including fatalities) and other serious gastrointestinal events (eg, bleeding, ischemic colitis, perforation) have been reported, especially when administered with sorbitol. Increased risk may be associated with a history of intestinal disease or surgery, hypovolemia, prematurity, and renal insufficiency or failure; use with sorbitol is not recommended. Avoid use in any postoperative patient until normal bowel function resumes or in patients at risk for constipation or impaction; discontinue use if constipation occurs. Oral or rectal administration of sorbitol-containing sodium polystyrene sulfonate suspensions is contraindicated in neonates (particularly with prematurity). Use with caution in patients with severe HF, hypertension, or edema; sodium load may exacerbate condition. Effective lowering of serum potassium from sodium polystyrene sulfonate may take hours to days after administration; consider alternative measures (eg, dialysis) or concomitant therapy (eg, I.V. sodium bicarbonate) in situations where rapid correction of severe hyperkalemia is required. Severe hypokalemia may occur; frequent monitoring of serum potassium is recommended within each 24-hour period; ECG monitoring may be appropriate in select patients. In addition to serum potassium-lowering effects, cation-exchange resins may also affect other cation concentrations possibly resulting in decreased serum magnesium and calcium. Large oral doses may cause fecal impaction (especially in elderly).

Concomitant administration of oral sodium polystyrene sulfonate with nonabsorbable cation-donating antacids or laxatives (eg, magnesium hydroxide) may result in systemic alkalosis and may diminish ability to reduce serum potassium concentrations; use with such agents is not recommended. In addition, intestinal obstruction has been reported with concomitant administration of aluminum hydroxide due to concretion formation. Enema will reduce the serum potassium faster than oral administration, but the oral route will result in a greater reduction over several hours. Oral administration in neonates and use in neonates with reduced gut motility (postoperatively or drug-induced) is contraindicated. Oral or rectal administration of sorbitol-containing sodium polystyrene sulfonate suspensions in neonates (particularly with prematurity) is also contraindicated due to propylene glycol content and risk of intestinal necrosis and digestive hemorrhage. Use sodium polystyrene sulfonate (**without** sorbitol) with caution in premature or low-birth-weight infants. Use with caution in children when administering rectally; excessive dosage or inadequate dilution may result in fecal impaction.

Drug Interactions

Avoid Concomitant Use

Avoid concomitant use of Sodium Polystyrene Sulfonate with any of the following: Laxatives; Sorbitol

Decreased Effect

Sodium Polystyrene Sulfonate may decrease the levels/effects of: Lithium; Thyroid Products

Increased Effect/Toxicity

Sodium Polystyrene Sulfonate may increase the levels/effects of: Aluminum Hydroxide; Digoxin

The levels/effects of Sodium Polystyrene Sulfonate may be increased by: Antacids; Laxatives; Sorbitol

Adverse Reactions Frequency not defined.

Endocrine & metabolic: Hypernatremia, hypocalcemia, hypokalemia, hypomagnesemia, sodium retention

Gastrointestinal: Anorexia, constipation, diarrhea, fecal impaction, intestinal necrosis (rare), intestinal obstruction (due to concretions in association with aluminum hydroxide), nausea, vomiting

Pharmacodynamics/Kinetics

Onset of Action 2-24 hours

Absorption None

Excretion Completely feces (primarily as potassium polystyrene sulfonate)

Available Dosage Forms

Powder for suspension, oral/rectal: (454 g)

Kalexate: (454 g)

Kayexalate®: (454 g)

Kionex®: (454 g)

Suspension, oral/rectal:

Kionex®: 15 g/60 mL (60 mL, 480 mL)

SPS®: 15 g/60 mL (60 mL, 120 mL, 473 mL)

Dosing

Adult & Geriatric Hyperkalemia:

Oral: 15 g 1-4 times/day

Rectal: 30-50 g every 6 hours

Pediatric Hyperkalemia:

Oral: Children: 1 g/kg/dose every 6 hours

Rectal: Children: 1 g/kg/dose every 2-6 hours (in small children and infants, employ lower doses by using the practical exchange ratio of 1 mEq K^+/g of resin as the basis for calculation)

Administration

Oral Shake suspension well prior to administration. Administer orally (or via NG tube) as a suspension. **Do not mix in orange juice.** Chilling the oral mixture will increase palatability. Powder for suspension: For each 1 g of the powdered resin, add 3-4 mL of water or syrup (amount of fluid usually ranges from 20-100 mL)

Other Rectal: Enema route is less effective than oral administration. Administer cleansing enema first. Each dose of the powder for suspension should be suspended in 100 mL of aqueous vehicle and administered as a warm emulsion (body temperature). The commercially available suspension should also be warmed to body temperature. During administration, the solution should be agitated gently. Retain enema in colon for at least 30-60 minutes and for several hours, if possible. Once retention time is complete, irrigate colon with a nonsodium-containing solution to remove resin.

Stability

Storage Store at 25°C (77°F); excursions permitted to 15°C to 30°C (59°F to 86°F). Store repackaged product in refrigerator and use within 14 days. Freshly prepared suspensions should be used within 24 hours. Do not heat resin suspension.

Monitoring and Teaching Issues

Laboratory Monitoring Serum electrolytes (potassium, sodium, calcium, magnesium)

Physical Assessment Monitor ECG until potassium levels are normal. Monitor bowel function; can cause constipation and/or fecal impaction.

Patient Education You will be monitored for effects of this medication and frequent blood tests may be necessary. Oral: Mix well with a full glass of a chilled liquid (not orange juice or any other juice containing potassium). Avoid use of antacids, laxatives, or preparations containing sorbitol while taking this medication. You may experience nausea, vomiting, or constipation. Report persistent constipation, abdominal pain, or GI distress; chest pain or rapid heartbeat; or mental confusion or muscle weakness.

Dietary Considerations Do **not** mix in orange juice or in any fruit juice known to contain potassium. Some products may contain sodium.

Geriatric Considerations Large doses in the elderly may cause fecal impaction and intestinal obstruction.

Pregnancy Considerations Animal reproductive studies have not been conducted. There are no adequate and well-controlled studies in pregnant women. Use during pregnancy only if benefits outweigh the risks.

Additional Information 1 g of resin binds approximately 1 mEq of potassium

Historically, sorbitol was often recommended as a cathartic agent to be administered with sodium polystyrene sulfonate (SPS) to prevent SPS-induced fecal impaction. However, SPS, particularly when used with sorbitol, has been associated with cases of intestinal necrosis and other serious GI adverse events. Due to the concern that sorbitol may increase the risk of intestinal necrosis, concomitant use of sorbitol is no longer recommended.

Sodium polystyrene sulfonate is commercially available in a liquid suspension containing 33% sorbitol (~20 grams sorbitol per 60 mL suspension).

- **Solaraze®** *see* Diclofenac (Topical) *on page* *522*
- **Solarcaine® cool aloe Burn Relief [OTC]** *see* Lidocaine (Topical) *on page* *1107*
- **Solia® [DSC]** *see* Ethinyl Estradiol and Desogestrel *on page* *695*

Solifenacin (sol i FEN a sin)

U.S. Brand Names VESIcare®

Index Terms Solifenacin Succinate; YM905

Generic Availability (U.S.) No

Pharmacologic Category Anticholinergic Agent

Medication Safety Issues

Sound-alike/look-alike issues:

VESIcare® may be confused with Vesinoid®,Visicol®

Pregnancy Risk Factor C

Lactation Excretion in breast milk unknown/not recommended

Use Treatment of overactive bladder with symptoms of urinary frequency, urgency, or urge incontinence

Mechanism of Action/Effect Inhibits muscarinic receptors resulting in decreased urinary bladder contraction, increased residual urine volume, and decreased detrusor muscle pressure.

Contraindications Hypersensitivity to solifenacin or any component of the formulation; urinary retention; gastric retention; uncontrolled narrow-angle glaucoma.

Warnings/Precautions Cases of angioedema involving the face, lips, tongue, and/or larynx have been reported. Immediately discontinue if tongue, hypopharynx, or larynx are involved. May cause drowsiness and/or blurred vision, which may impair physical or mental abilities; patients must be cautioned about performing tasks which require mental alertness (eg, operating machinery or driving). Heat prostration may occur in the presence of increased environmental temperature; use caution in hot weather and/or exercise. Use with caution in patients with bladder outflow obstruction, gastrointestinal obstructive disorders, and decreased gastrointestinal motility. Use with caution in patients with a known history of QT prolongation or other risk factors for QT prolongation (eg, concomitant use of medications known to prolong QT interval and/or electrolyte abnormalities); the risk for QT prolongation is dose-related. Use with caution in patients with controlled (treated) narrow-angle glaucoma; use is contraindicated with uncontrolled narrow-angle glaucoma. Dosage adjustment is required for patients with severe renal impairment (Cl_{cr} <30 mL/minute) or moderate (Child-Pugh class B) hepatic impairment; use is not recommended with severe hepatic impairment (Child-Pugh class C). Patients on potent CYP3A4 inhibitors require the lower dose of solifenacin.

Drug Interactions

Metabolism/Transport Effects Substrate of CYP3A4 (major)

Avoid Concomitant Use There are no known interactions where it is recommended to avoid concomitant use.

Decreased Effect

Solifenacin may decrease the levels/effects of: Acetylcholinesterase Inhibitors (Central); Secretin

The levels/effects of Solifenacin may be decreased by: Acetylcholinesterase Inhibitors (Central); CYP3A4 Inducers (Strong); Deferasirox; Herbs (CYP3A4 Inducers)

Increased Effect/Toxicity

Solifenacin may increase the levels/effects of: AbobotulinumtoxinA; Anticholinergics; Cannabinoids; OnabotulinumtoxinA; Potassium Chloride; RimabotulinumtoxinB

The levels/effects of Solifenacin may be increased by: Antifungal Agents (Azole Derivatives, Systemic); Conivaptan; CYP3A4 Inhibitors (Moderate); CYP3A4 Inhibitors (Strong); Dasatinib; Pramlintide

Nutritional/Ethanol Interactions

Food: Grapefruit juice may increase the serum level effects of solifenacin.

Herb/Nutraceutical: St John's wort (*Hypericum*) may decrease the levels/effects of solifenacin.

Adverse Reactions

>10%: Gastrointestinal: Xerostomia (11% to 28%; dose-related), constipation (5% to 13%; dose-related)

1% to 10%:

- Cardiovascular: Edema (≤1%), hypertension (≤1%)
- Central nervous system: Headache (3% to 6%), fatigue (1% to 2%), depression (≤1%)
- Gastrointestinal: Dyspepsia (1% to 4%), nausea (2% to 3%), upper abdominal pain (1% to 2%)
- Genitourinary: Urinary tract infection (3% to 5%), urinary retention (≤1%)
- Ocular: Blurred vision (4% to 5%), dry eyes (≤2%)
- Respiratory: Cough (≤1%)
- Miscellaneous: Influenza (≤2%)

Pharmacodynamics/Kinetics

Bioavailability ~90%

Time to Peak Plasma: 3-8 hours

Protein Binding ~98% bound primarily to alpha$_1$-acid glycoprotein

Half-Life Elimination 45-68 hours following chronic dosing; prolonged in severe renal (Cl_{cr} <30 mL/minute) or moderate hepatic (Child-Pugh class B) impairment

Metabolism Extensively hepatic; via N-oxidation and 4 R-hydroxylation, forms 1 active and 3 inactive metabolites; primary pathway for elimination is via CYP3A4

Excretion Urine 69% (<15% as unchanged drug); feces 23%

Available Dosage Forms

Tablet, oral:

VESIcare®: 5 mg, 10 mg

Dosing

Adult Overactive bladder: Oral: 5 mg once daily; if tolerated, may increase to 10 mg once daily

Dosage adjustment with concomitant CYP3A4 inhibitors: Maximum solifenacin dose: 5 mg/day

Geriatric Base dosing on renal/hepatic function.

Renal Impairment Use with caution in reduced renal function; Cl_{cr} <30 mL/minute: Maximum dose: 5 mg/day

Hepatic Impairment Use with caution in reduced hepatic function:

Moderate (Child-Pugh class B): Maximum dose: 5 mg/day

Severe (Child-Pugh class C): Use is not recommended

Administration

Oral Swallow tablet whole; administer with liquids; may be administered without regard to meals.

Stability

Storage Store at controlled room temperature of 25°C (77°F); excursions permitted to 15°C to 30°C (59°F to 86°F).

Monitoring and Teaching Issues

Laboratory Monitoring Creatinine clearance (prior to treatment for dosing adjustment); liver function tests

Physical Assessment Monitor urination pattern.

Patient Education Maintain adequate hydration unless instructed to restrict fluid intake by prescriber. This medication may cause dry mouth. You may be more susceptible to heat prostration due to decreased ability to sweat. Use caution in hot weather. You may experience constipation, nausea, vomiting, blurred vision, and dry eyes. Report difficulty, pain, or burning on urination.

Dietary Considerations May be taken without regard to meals.

Geriatric Considerations In patients with Cl_{cr} <30 mL/minute, doses >5 mg/day are not recommended. Similar safety and effectiveness were observed in elderly and younger patients.

Pregnancy Considerations Decreased fetal weight, increased incidence of cleft palate, and delayed physical development were observed in some animal studies. There are no adequate or well-controlled studies in pregnant women. Use during pregnancy only if the benefit to the mother outweighs the potential risk to the fetus.

Related Information

Pharmacotherapy of Urinary Incontinence *on page 2071*

◆ **Solifenacin Succinate** *see* Solifenacin *on page 1662*
◆ **Soliris®** *see* Eculizumab *on page 601*
◆ **Solodyn®** *see* Minocycline *on page 1236*
◆ **Solu-CORTEF®** *see* Hydrocortisone (Systemic) *on page 917*
◆ **Solumedrol** *see* MethylPREDNISolone *on page 1208*
◆ **Solu-MEDROL®** *see* MethylPREDNISolone *on page 1208*
◆ **Soma®** *see* Carisoprodol *on page 300*
◆ **Soma® Compound** *see* Carisoprodol and Aspirin *on page 301*

Somatropin (soe ma TROE pin)

U.S. Brand Names Genotropin Miniquick®; Genotropin®; Humatrope®; Norditropin FlexPro®; Norditropin®; Norditropin® NordiFlex®; Nutropin AQ Pen®; Nutropin AQ®; Nutropin AQ® NuSpin™; Nutropin®; Omnitrope®; Saizen®; Serostim®; Tev-Tropin®; Zorbtive®

Index Terms Growth Hormone, Human; hGH; Human Growth Hormone

Generic Availability (U.S.) No

Pharmacologic Category Growth Hormone

Medication Safety Issues

Sound-alike/look-alike issues:

Humatrope® may be confused with homatropine
Somatrem may be confused with somatropin
Somatropin may be confused with homatropine, somatrem, sumatriptan

Pregnancy Risk Factor B/C (depending upon manufacturer)

Lactation Excretion in breast milk unknown/use caution

Use

Children:

Treatment of growth failure due to inadequate endogenous growth hormone secretion (Genotropin®, Humatrope®, Norditropin®, Nutropin®, Nutropin AQ®, Omnitrope®, Saizen®, Tev-Tropin®)

Treatment of short stature associated with Turner syndrome (Genotropin®, Humatrope®, Norditropin®, Nutropin®, Nutropin AQ®)

Treatment of Prader-Willi syndrome (Genotropin®, Omnitrope®)

Treatment of growth failure associated with chronic renal insufficiency (CRI) up until the time of renal transplantation (Nutropin®, Nutropin AQ®)

Treatment of growth failure in children born small for gestational age who fail to manifest catch-up growth by 2 years of age (Genotropin®, Omnitrope®) or by 2-4 years of age (Humatrope®, Norditropin®)

Treatment of idiopathic short stature (nongrowth hormone-deficient short stature) defined by height standard deviation score (SDS) ≤-2.25 and growth rate not likely to attain normal adult height (Genotropin®, Humatrope®, Nutropin®, Nutropin AQ®, Omnitrope®)

Treatment of short stature or growth failure associated with short stature homeobox gene (SHOX) deficiency (Humatrope®)

Treatment of short stature associated with Noonan syndrome (Norditropin®)

Adults:

HIV patients with wasting or cachexia with concomitant antiviral therapy (Serostim®)

Replacement of endogenous growth hormone in patients with adult growth hormone deficiency who meet both of the following criteria (Genotropin®, Humatrope®, Norditropin®, Nutropin®, Nutropin AQ®, Omnitrope®, Saizen®):

Biochemical diagnosis of adult growth hormone deficiency by means of a subnormal response to a standard growth hormone stimulation test (peak growth hormone ≤5 mcg/L). Confirmatory testing may not be required in patients with congenital/genetic growth hormone deficiency or multiple pituitary hormone deficiencies due to organic diseases.

and

Adult-onset: Patients who have adult growth hormone deficiency whether alone or with multiple hormone deficiencies (hypopituitarism) as a result of pituitary disease, hypothalamic disease, surgery, radiation therapy, or trauma

or

Childhood-onset: Patients who were growth hormone deficient during childhood, confirmed as an adult before replacement therapy is initiated

Treatment of short-bowel syndrome (Zorbtive®)

Unlabeled/Investigational Use Investigational: Pediatric HIV patients with wasting/cachexia (Serostim®); HIV-associated adipose redistribution syndrome (HARS) (Serostim®)

Mechanism of Action/Effect Human growth hormone assists in growth of linear bone, skeletal muscle, and organs; stimulates erythropoietin which increases red blood cell mass; exerts both insulin-like and diabetogenic effects; enhances transmucosal transport of water, electrolytes, and nutrients across the gut

Contraindications Hypersensitivity to growth hormone or any component of the formulation; growth promotion in pediatric patients with closed epiphyses; progression or recurrence of any underlying intracranial lesion or actively growing intracranial tumor; acute critical illness due to complications following open heart or abdominal surgery; multiple accidental trauma or acute respiratory failure; evidence of active malignancy; active proliferative or severe nonproliferative diabetic retinopathy; use in patients with Prader-Willi syndrome **without** growth hormone deficiency (except Genotropin®) or in patients with Prader-Willi syndrome **with** growth hormone deficiency who are severely obese, have a history of upper airway obstruction or sleep apnea, or have severe respiratory impairment

Warnings/Precautions Initiation of somatropin is contraindicated with acute critical illness due to complications following open heart or abdominal surgery, multiple accidental trauma, or acute respiratory failure; mortality may be increased. The safety of continuing somatropin in patients who develop these illnesses during therapy has not been established; use with caution. Use in contraindicated with active malignancy; monitor patients with pre-existing tumors or growth failure secondary to an intracranial lesion for recurrence or progression of underlying disease; discontinue therapy with evidence of recurrence. An increased risk of second neoplasm has been reported in childhood cancer survivors treated with somatropin; the most common second neoplasms were meningiomas in patients treated with radiation to the head for their first neoplasm. Monitor patients for any malignant transformation of skin lesions.

Somatropin may decrease insulin sensitivity; use with caution in patients with diabetes or with risk factors for impaired glucose tolerance. Adjustment of antidiabetic medications may be necessary. Pancreatitis has been rarely reported; incidence in children (especially girls) with Turner syndrome may be greater than adults. Monitor for hypersensitivity reactions. Patients with hypoadrenalism may require increased dosages of glucocorticoids (especially cortisone acetate and prednisone) due to somatropin-mediated inhibition of 11 beta-hydroxysteroid dehydrogenase type 1; undiagnosed central hypoadrenalism may be unmasked. Excessive glucocorticoid therapy may inhibit the growth promoting effects of somatropin in children; monitor and adjust glucocorticoids carefully. Untreated/undiagnosed hypothyroidism may decrease response to therapy; monitor thyroid function test periodically and initiate/adjust thyroid replacement therapy as needed. Closely monitor other hormonal replacement treatments in patients with hypopituitarism. Obese patients may experience an increased incidence of adverse events when using a weight-based dosing regimen. Intracranial hypertension (IH) with headache, nausea, papilledema, visual changes, and/or vomiting has been reported with somatropin; funduscopic examination prior to initiation of therapy and periodically thereafter is recommended. Treatment should be discontinued in patients who develop papilledema; resuming treatment at a lower dose may be considered once IH-associated signs and symptoms have resolved. Patients with Turner syndrome, chronic renal failure and Prader-Willi syndrome may be at increased risk for IH. Progression of scoliosis may occur in children experiencing rapid growth. Patients with growth hormone deficiency may develop slipped capital epiphyses more frequently, evaluate any child with new onset of a limp or with complaints of hip or knee pain. Patients with Turner syndrome are at increased risk for otitis media and other ear/hearing disorders, cardiovascular disorders (including stroke, aortic aneurysm, hypertension), and thyroid disease, monitor carefully. Fluid retention may occur frequently in adults during use; manifestations of fluid retention (eg, edema, arthralgia, myalgia, nerve compression syndromes/paresthesias) are generally transient and dose dependent. Products may contain benzyl alcohol or m-cresol. When administering to newborns, reconstitute with sterile water or saline for injection. Not for I.V. injection.

Fatalities have been reported in pediatric patients with Prader-Willi syndrome following the use of growth hormone. The reported fatalities occurred in patients with one or more risk factors, including severe obesity, sleep apnea, respiratory impairment, or unidentified respiratory infection; male patients with one or more of these factors may be at greater risk. Treatment interruption is recommended in patients who show signs of upper airway obstruction, including the onset of, or increased, snoring. In addition, evaluation of and/or monitoring for sleep apnea and respiratory infections are recommended.

Patients with HIV infection should be maintained on antiretroviral therapy to prevent the potential increase in viral replication.

Elderly patients may be more sensitive to the actions of somatropin; consider lower starting doses. Safety and efficacy have not been established for the treatment of Noonan syndrome in children with significant cardiac disease. Children with epiphyseal closure who are treated for adult GHD need reassessment of therapy and dose. Administration site rotation is necessary to prevent tissue atrophy.

Drug Interactions

Avoid Concomitant Use There are no known interactions where it is recommended to avoid concomitant use.

Decreased Effect

Somatropin may decrease the levels/effects of: Antidiabetic Agents; Cortisone; PredniSONE

The levels/effects of Somatropin may be decreased by: Estrogen Derivatives

Increased Effect/Toxicity There are no known significant interactions involving an increase in effect.

Adverse Reactions

Growth hormone deficiency: Adverse reactions reported with growth hormone deficiency vary greatly by age. Generally, percentages are less in pediatric patients than adults, and many of the reactions reported in adults are dose related. Percentages reported also vary by product. Below is a listing by age group; events reported more commonly overall are noted with an asterisk (*).

Children: Antibodies development, arthralgia, benign intracranial hypertension, edema, eosinophilia, glycosuria, Hb A_{1c} increased, headache, hematoma, hematuria, hyperglycemia (mild), hypertriglyceridemia, hypoglycemia, hypothyroidism, injection site reaction, intracranial tumor, leg pain, lipoatrophy, leukemia, meningioma, muscle pain, papilledema, pseudotumor cerebri, psoriasis exacerbation, rash, scoliosis progression, seizure, slipped capital femoral epiphysis, weakness

Adults: Acne, ALT increased, AST increased, arthralgia*, back pain, bronchitis, carpal tunnel syndrome, chest pain, cough, depression, diabetes mellitus (type 2), diaphoresis, dizziness, edema*, fatigue, flu-like syndrome*, gastritis, glucose intolerance, glucosuria, headache*, hyperglycemia (mild), hypertension, hypoesthesia, hypothyroidism, infection, insomnia, insulin resistance, joint disorder, leg edema, muscle pain, myalgia*, nausea, pain in extremities, paresthesia*, peripheral edema*, pharyngitis, retinopathy, rhinitis, skeletal pain*, stiffness in extremities, surgical procedure, upper respiratory tract infection, weakness

Additional/postmarketing reactions observed with growth hormone deficiency: Gynecomastia, increased growth of pre-existing nevi, pancreatitis

HARS: Serostim®: Limited to >10%: Edema (peripheral) (19% to 45%), arthralgia (28% to 37%), pain (extremity) (5% to 19%), hypoesthesia (9% to 15%), headache (4% to 14%), blood glucose increased (4% to 14%), paresthesia (11% to 13%), myalgia (3% to 13%)

Idiopathic short stature: Percentages reported using Humatrope® versus placebo: Myalgia (24%), scoliosis (19%), otitis media (16%), arthralgia (11%), arthrosis (11%), hyperlipidemia (8%), gynecomastia (5%), hip pain (3%), hypertension (3%). Additional adverse reactions listed as reported using other products from ISS NCGS Cohort (frequencies <1%): Aggressiveness, benign intracranial hypertension, diabetes, edema, hair loss, headache, injection site reaction

Prader-Willi syndrome: Genotropin® (frequency not defined): Aggressiveness, arthralgia, edema, hair loss, headache, benign intracranial hypertension, myalgia; fatalities associated with use in this population have been reported

Turner syndrome: Percentages reported using Humatrope® compared to untreated patients. Additional adverse reactions reported from other products, frequency not specified: Surgical procedures (45%), otitis media (43%), ear disorders (18%), joint pain, respiratory illness, urinary tract infection

HIV patients with wasting or cachexia: Serostim® (limited to ≥5%): Musculoskeletal disorders (arthralgia, arthrosis, myalgia: 78%), peripheral edema (26%), headache (13%), nausea (9%), paresthesia (8%), edema (6%), gynecomastia (6%), hypoesthesia (5%)

Short-bowel syndrome: Zorbtive® (limited to >10%): Peripheral edema (69% to 81%), facial edema (44% to 50%), arthralgia (31% to 44%), nausea (13% to 31%), injection site pain (up to 31%), flatulence (25%), injection site reaction (19% to 25%), abdominal pain (13% to 25%), vomiting (19%), pain (6% to 19%), chest pain (up to 19%), dehydration (up to 19%), infection (up to 19%), rhinitis (up to 19%), hearing symptoms (13%), dizziness (6% to 13%), rash (6% to 13%), diaphoresis (up to 13%), generalized edema (up to 13%), malaise (up to 13%), moniliasis (up to 13%), myalgia (up to 13%)

SHOX deficiency: Humatrope®: Arthralgia (11%), gynecomastia (8%), excessive cutaneous nevi (7%), scoliosis (4%)

Small for gestational age: Genotropin®, Humatrope® (frequency not defined): Mild, transient hyperglycemia; benign intracranial hypertension (rare); central precocious puberty; jaw prominence (rare); aggravation of pre-existing scoliosis (rare); injection site reactions; progression of pigmented nevi; carpal tunnel syndrome (rare) diabetes mellitus (rare); otitis media; headache; slipped capital femoral epiphysis

Pharmacodynamics/Kinetics

Duration of Action Maintains supraphysiologic levels for 18-20 hours

Absorption I.M., SubQ: Well absorbed

Bioavailability SubQ: ~70% to 90%; **Note:** Variable; product-dependent

Half-Life Elimination Preparation and route of administration dependent; SubQ: ~2-4 hours

Metabolism Hepatic and renal (~90%)

Excretion Urine (small amount)

Available Dosage Forms

Injection, powder for reconstitution:

Genotropin Miniquick®: 0.2 mg, 0.4 mg, 0.6 mg, 0.8 mg, 1 mg, 1.2 mg, 1.4 mg, 1.6 mg, 1.8 mg, 2 mg
Genotropin®: 5.8 mg, 13.8 mg
Humatrope®: 5 mg, 6 mg, 12 mg, 24 mg
Nutropin®: 5 mg, 10 mg
Omnitrope®: 5.8 mg
Saizen®: 5 mg, 8.8 mg
Serostim®: 4 mg, 5 mg, 6 mg
Tev-Tropin®: 5 mg
Zorbtive®: 8.8 mg

Injection, solution:

Norditropin FlexPro®: 5 mg/1.5 mL (1.5 mL); 10 mg/1.5 mL (1.5 mL); 15 mg/1.5 mL (1.5 mL)
Norditropin®: 5 mg/1.5 mL (1.5 mL); 15 mg/1.5 mL (1.5 mL)
Norditropin® NordiFlex®: 5 mg/1.5 mL (1.5 mL); 10 mg/1.5 mL (1.5 mL); 30 mg/3 mL (3 mL)
Nutropin AQ Pen®: 10 mg/2 mL (2 mL); 20 mg/2 mL (2 mL)
Nutropin AQ®: 10 mg/2 mL (2 mL)
Nutropin AQ® NuSpin™: 5 mg/2 mL (2 mL); 10 mg/2 mL (2 mL); 20 mg/2 mL (2 mL)
Omnitrope®: 5 mg/1.5 mL (1.5 mL); 10 mg/1.5 mL (1.5 mL)

Dosing

Adult

Growth hormone deficiency: Adjust dose based on individual requirements: To minimize adverse events in older or overweight patients, reduced dosages may be necessary. During therapy, dosage should be decreased if required by the occurrence of side effects or excessive IGF-I levels.

Weight-based dosing:

Norditropin®: SubQ: Initial dose ≤0.004 mg/kg/day; after 6 weeks of therapy, may increase dose up to 0.016 mg/kg/day

Nutropin®, Nutropin® AQ: SubQ: ≤0.006 mg/kg/day; dose may be increased up to a maximum of 0.025 mg/kg/day in patients <35 years of age, or up to a maximum of 0.0125 mg/kg/day in patients ≥35 years of age

Humatrope®: SubQ: ≤0.006 mg/kg/day; dose may be increased up to a maximum of 0.0125 mg/kg/day

Genotropin®, Omnitrope®: SubQ: Weekly dosage: ≤0.04 mg/kg divided into equal doses 6-7 days per week; dose may be increased at 4- to 8-week intervals to a maximum of 0.08 mg/kg/week

Saizen®: SubQ: ≤0.005 mg/kg/day; dose may be increased to not more than 0.01 mg/kg/day after 4 weeks

Nonweight-based dosing: SubQ: Initial: 0.2 mg/day (range: 0.15-0.3 mg/day); may increase every 1-2 months by 0.1-0.2 mg/day based on response and/or serum IGF-I levels

Dosage adjustment with estrogen supplementation (growth hormone deficiency): Larger doses of somatropin may be needed for women taking oral estrogen replacement products; dosing not affected by topical products

HARS (unlabeled use): Serostim®: SubQ: Induction: 4 mg once daily at bedtime for 12 weeks; Maintenance: 2 mg or 4 mg every other day at bedtime for 12-24 weeks. **Note:** Every-other-day dosing during induction has also been studied. Although a greater response was seen with daily dosing, it was associated with an increased incidence of adverse events.

HIV patients with wasting or cachexia:

Serostim®: SubQ: 0.1 mg/kg once daily at bedtime (maximum: 6 mg/day). Alternately, patients at risk for side effects may be started at 0.1 mg/kg every other day. Patients who continue to lose weight after 12 weeks should be re-evaluated for opportunistic infections or other clinical events; rotate injection sites to avoid lipodystrophy Adjust dose if needed to manage side effects.

Daily dose based on body weight:

<35 kg: 0.1 mg/kg
35-45 kg: 4 mg
45-55 kg: 5 mg
>55 kg: 6 mg

Short-bowel syndrome: *Zorbtive®:* SubQ: 0.1 mg/kg once daily for 4 weeks (maximum: 8 mg/day)

Fluid retention (moderate) or arthralgias: Treat symptomatically or reduce dose by 50%

Severe toxicity: Discontinue therapy for up to 5 days; when symptoms resolve, restart at 50% of dose. If severe toxicity recurs or does not disappear within 5 days after discontinuation, permanently discontinue treatment.

Geriatric Patients ≥65 years of age may be more sensitive to the action of growth hormone and more prone to adverse effects; in general, dosing should be cautious, beginning at low end of dosing range.

Pediatric

Growth hormone deficiency:

Genotropin®, Omnitrope®: SubQ: Weekly dosage: 0.16-0.24 mg/kg divided into equal doses 6-7 days per week

Humatrope®: SubQ: Weekly dosage: 0.18-0.3 mg/kg divided into equal doses 6-7 days per week

Norditropin®: SubQ: 0.024-0.034 mg/kg/day, 6-7 days per week

Nutropin®, Nutropin® AQ: SubQ: Weekly dosage: 0.3 mg/kg divided into equal daily doses; pubertal patients: ≤0.7 mg/kg divided into equal daily doses

Tev-Tropin®: SubQ: Up to 0.1 mg/kg administered 3 days per week

Saizen®: I.M., SubQ: Weekly dosage: 0.18 mg/kg divided into equal daily doses **or** as 0.06 mg/kg/dose administered 3 days per week **or** as 0.03 mg/kg/dose administered 6 days per week

Note: Therapy should be discontinued when patient has reached satisfactory adult height, when epiphyses have fused, or when the patient ceases to respond. Growth of 5 cm/year or more is expected, if growth rate does not exceed 2.5 cm in a 6-month period, double the dose for the next 6 months; if there is still no satisfactory response, discontinue therapy

Chronic renal insufficiency (CRI): *Nutropin®, Nutropin® AQ:* SubQ: Weekly dosage: 0.35 mg/kg divided into daily injections; continue until the time of renal transplantation

Dosage recommendations in patients treated for CRI who require dialysis:

Hemodialysis: Administer dose at night prior to bedtime or at least 3-4 hours after hemodialysis to prevent hematoma formation from heparin

CCPD: Administer dose in the morning following dialysis

CAPD: Administer dose in the evening at the time of overnight exchange

Turner syndrome:

Genotropin®: SubQ: Weekly dosage: 0.33 mg/kg divided into equal doses 6-7 days per week

Humatrope®: SubQ: Weekly dosage: 0.375 mg/kg divided into equal doses 6-7 days per week

Norditropin®: SubQ: Up to 0.067 mg/kg/day

Nutropin®, Nutropin® AQ: SubQ: Weekly dosage: ≤0.375 mg/kg divided into equal doses 3-7 days per week

Prader-Willi syndrome: *Genotropin®, Omnitrope®:* SubQ: Weekly dosage: 0.24 mg/kg divided into equal doses 6-7 days per week

Small for gestational age:

Genotropin®, Omnitrope®: SubQ: Weekly dosage: 0.48 mg/kg divided into equal doses 6-7 days per week

Humatrope®: SubQ: Weekly dosage: 0.47 mg/kg divided into equal doses 6-7 days per week

Norditropin®: SubQ: Up to 0.067 mg/kg/day

Alternate dosing (small for gestational age): In older/early pubertal children or children with very short stature, consider initiating therapy at higher doses (0.067 mg/kg/day) and then consider reducing the dose (0.033 mg/kg/day) if substantial catch-up growth observed. In younger children (<4 years) with less severe short stature, consider initiating therapy with lower doses (0.033 mg/kg/day) and then titrating the dose upwards as needed.

Idiopathic short stature:

Genotropin®, Omnitrope®: SubQ: Weekly dosage: 0.47 mg/kg divided into equal doses 6-7 days per week

Humatrope®: SubQ: Weekly dosage: 0.37 mg/kg divided into equal doses 6-7 days per week

Nutropin®, Nutropin AQ®: SubQ: Weekly dosage: Up to 0.3 mg/kg divided into equal daily doses

SHOX deficiency: *Humatrope®:* SubQ: Weekly dosage: 0.35 mg/kg divided into equal doses 6-7 days per week

HIV patients with wasting or cachexia (unlabeled use): *Serostim®:* SubQ: Limited data; doses of 0.04 mg/kg/day were reported in five children, 6-17 years of age; doses of 0.07 mg/kg/day were reported in six children, 8-14 years of age

Noonan syndrome: *Norditropin®:* SubQ: Up to 0.066 mg/kg/day

Renal Impairment Reports indicate patients with chronic renal failure tend to have decreased clearance; specific dosing suggestions not available

Hepatic Impairment Clearance may be reduced in patients with severe hepatic dysfunction; specific dosing suggestions are not available.

Administration

I.M. Not all products are approved for I.M. administration. Rotate administration sites to avoid tissue atrophy.

Other Do not shake; administer SubQ or I.M. (not all products are approved for I.M. administration). Rotate administration sites to avoid tissue atrophy. When administering to newborns, do not reconstitute with a diluent that contains benzyl alcohol; sterile water for injection may be used as an alternative. Norditropin® cartridge must be administered using the corresponding color-coded NordiPen® injection pen. Solution in the Omnitrope® cartridges must be administered using the Omnitrope® pen; when installing a new cartridge, prime pen prior to first use. When administering Tev-Tropin®, SubQ injections of solutions >1 mL not recommended.

Stability

Reconstitution

Genotropin®: Reconstitute with diluent provided.

Genotropin MiniQuick®: Reconstitute with diluent provided. Consult the instructions provided with the reconstitution device.

Humatrope®:

Cartridge: Consult HumatroPen™ User Guide for complete instructions for reconstitution. **Dilute with solution provided with cartridges ONLY; do not use diluent provided with vials.**

Vial: 5 mg: Reconstitute with 1.5-5 mL diluent provided. Swirl gently; do not shake.

Nutropin®: Vial:

5 mg: Reconstitute with 1-5 mL bacteriostatic water for injection. Swirl gently, do not shake.

10 mg: Reconstitute with 1-10 mL bacteriostatic water for injection. Swirl gently, do not shake.

Omnitrope® powder: Reconstitute with provided diluent. Swirl gently; do not shake.

Saizen®: Vial:

5 mg: Reconstitute with 1-3 mL bacteriostatic water for injection or sterile water for injection. Gently swirl; do not shake.

8.8 mg: Reconstitute with 2-3 mL bacteriostatic water for injection or sterile water for injection. Gently swirl; do not shake.

Serostim®: Vial: Reconstitute with 0.5-1 mL sterile water for injection.

Tev-Tropin®: Reconstitute with 1-5 mL of diluent provided. Gently swirl; do not shake. May use preservative-free NS for use in newborns.

Zorbtive®: 8.8 mg vial: Reconstitute with 1-2 mL bacteriostatic water for injection. Swirl gently.

Storage

Genotropin®: Store at 2°C to 8°C (36°F to 46°F); do not freeze. Protect from light. Following reconstitution of 5.8 mg and 13.8 mg cartridge, store under refrigeration and use within 21 days.

Genotropin® Miniquick®: Store in refrigerator prior to dispensing, but may be stored ≤25°C (77°F) for up to 3 months after dispensing. Once reconstituted, solution must be refrigerated and used within 24 hours. Discard unused portion.

Humatrope®:

Vial: Before and after reconstitution, store at 2°C to 8°C (36°F to 46°F); do not freeze. When reconstituted with provided diluent or bacteriostatic water for injection, use within 14 days. When reconstituted with sterile water for injection, use within 24 hours and discard unused portion.

Cartridge: Before and after reconstitution, store at 2°C to 8°C (36°F to 46°F); do not freeze. Following reconstitution with provided diluent, stable for 28 days under refrigeration.

Norditropin®: Store at 2°C to 8°C (36°F to 46°F); do not freeze. Avoid direct light.

Cartridge: When refrigerated, must be used within 4 weeks once inserted into pen. Orange cartridges (5 mg/1.5 mL) may also be stored up to 3 weeks at ≤25°C (77°F).

Prefilled pen: When refrigerated, must be used within 4 weeks after initial injection. Orange and blue prefilled pens may also be stored up to 3 weeks at ≤25°C (77°F).

Nutropin®: Before and after reconstitution, store at 2°C to 8°C (36°F to 46°F); do not freeze.

Nutropin® vial: Use reconstituted vials within 14 days. When reconstituted with sterile water for injection, use immediately and discard unused portion.

Nutropin® AQ formulations: Use within 28 days following initial use.

Omnitrope®:

Powder for injection: Prior to reconstitution, store under refrigeration at 2°C to 8°C (36°F to 46°F); do not freeze. Protect from light. Reconstitute with provided diluent. Swirl gently; do not shake. Following reconstitution with the provided diluents, the 5.8 mg vial may be stored under refrigeration for up to 3 weeks. Store vial in carton to protect from light.

Solution: Prior to use, store under refrigeration at 2°C to 8°C (36°F to 46°F). Once the cartridge is loaded into the pen delivery system, store under refrigeration for up to 21 days after first use.

Saizen®: Prior to reconstitution, store at room temperature 15°C to 30°C (59°F to 86°F). Following reconstitution with bacteriostatic water for injection, reconstituted solution should be refrigerated and used within 14 days. When reconstituted with sterile water for injection, use immediately and discard unused portion. The Saizen® easy click cartridge, when reconstituted with the provided bacteriostatic water, should be stored under refrigeration and used within 21 days.

Serostim®: Prior to reconstitution, store at room temperature 15°C to 30°C (59°F to 86°F). When reconstituted with sterile water for injection, use immediately and discard unused portion.

Tev-Tropin®: Prior to reconstitution, store at 2°C to 8°C (36°F to 46°F). Following reconstitution with bacteriostatic NS, solution should be refrigerated and used within 14 days. Some cloudiness may occur; do not use if cloudiness persists after warming to room temperature.

Zorbtive®: Store unopened vials and diluent at room temperature of 15°C to 30°C (59°F to 86°F). Store reconstituted vial under refrigeration at 2°C to 8°C (36°F to 46°F) for up to 14 days; do not freeze.

Monitoring and Teaching Issues

Laboratory Monitoring Periodic thyroid function tests, periodical urine testing for glucose, somatomedin C (IGF-I) levels; serum phosphorus, alkaline phosphatase and parathyroid hormone. If growth deceleration is observed in children treated for growth hormone deficiency, and not due to other causes, evaluate for presence of antibody formation. Periodic blood glucose monitoring; strict blood glucose monitoring in patients with diabetes. **Note:** Practice guidelines recommend monitoring for efficacy and adverse effects every 1-2 months during dose titration and semiannually, thereafter (TES, 2006).

Physical Assessment Perform funduscopic examinations at initiation of therapy and periodically during treatment. Instruct patients with diabetes to monitor glucose levels closely (may induce insulin intolerance). Instruct patient in proper use if self-administered (storage, reconstitution, injection techniques, and syringe/needle disposal). Pediatrics: Monitor growth curve; annually determine bone age.

Patient Education This drug can only be administered by injection. If self-administered, you will be instructed by prescriber on proper storage, reconstitution, injection technique, and syringe/needle disposal. Report immediately pain, redness, burning, drainage, or swelling at injection site. If you have diabetes, monitor glucose levels closely. Report immediately swelling of extremities, headache, nausea or vomiting, any rash, sudden change in vision, increased urination, thirst, or weight loss.

Dietary Considerations

Prader-Willi syndrome: All patients should have effective weight control (use is contraindicated in severely-obese patients).

Short-bowel syndrome: Intravenous parenteral nutrition requirements may need reassessment as gastrointestinal absorption improves.

Pregnancy Considerations Teratogenic effects were not observed in animal studies. Reproduction studies have not been conducted with all agents. During normal pregnancy, maternal production of endogenous growth hormone decreases as placental growth hormone production increases. Data with somatropin use during pregnancy is limited.

◆ **Somavert®** *see* Pegvisomant *on page 1428*

◆ **Sominex® [OTC]** *see* DiphenhydrAMINE (Systemic) *on page 543*

◆ **Sominex® Maximum Strength [OTC]** *see* DiphenhydrAMINE (Systemic) *on page* 543
◆ **Somnote®** *see* Chloral Hydrate *on page* 356
◆ **Sonata®** *see* Zaleplon *on page* 1883

Sorafenib (sor AF e nib)

U.S. Brand Names NexAVAR®

Index Terms BAY 43-9006; Sorafenib Tosylate

Generic Availability (U.S.) No

Pharmacologic Category Antineoplastic Agent, Tyrosine Kinase Inhibitor; Vascular Endothelial Growth Factor (VEGF) Inhibitor

Medication Safety Issues

Sound-alike/look-alike issues:

NexAVAR® may be confused with NexIUM®

SORAfenib may be confused with gefitinib, imatinib, SUNItinib, vandetanib

High alert medication: This medication is in a class the Institute for Safe Medication Practices (ISMP) includes among its list of drug classes which have a heightened risk of causing significant patient harm when used in error.

Pregnancy Risk Factor D

Lactation Excretion in breast milk unknown/not recommended

Use Treatment of advanced renal cell cancer (RCC); treatment of unresectable hepatocellular cancer (HCC)

Unlabeled/Investigational Use Treatment of advanced thyroid cancer, recurrent or metastatic angiosarcoma, resistant gastrointestinal stromal tumor (GIST)

Mechanism of Action/Effect Prevents tumor growth by inhibiting both tumor cell proliferation and tumor angiogenesis through kinase inhibition

Contraindications Hypersensitivity to sorafenib or any component of the formulation; use in combination with carboplatin and paclitaxel in patients with squamous cell lung cancer

Warnings/Precautions Hazardous agent - use appropriate precautions for handling and disposal. May cause hypertension (generally mild-to-moderate), especially in the first 6 weeks of treatment; monitor; use caution in patients with underlying or poorly-controlled hypertension; consider discontinuing (temporary or permanent) in patients who develop severe or persistent hypertension. May cause cardiac ischemia or infarction; consider discontinuing (temporarily or permanently) in patients who develop these; use in patients with unstable coronary artery disease or recent myocardial infarction has not been studied. Use with caution in patients with cardiovascular disease. Serious bleeding events may occur; monitor PT/INR in patients on warfarin therapy. May complicate wound healing; temporarily withhold treatment for patients undergoing major surgical procedures. Gastrointestinal perforation has been reported (rare); monitor patients for signs/symptoms (abdominal pain, constipation, or vomiting); discontinue treatment if gastrointestinal perforation occurs. Avoid concurrent use (if possible) with strong CYP3A4 inducers (eg, carbamazepine, dexamethasone, phenobarbital, phenytoin, rifampin, St John's wort); may decrease sorafenib levels/effects. Use caution when administering sorafenib with compounds that are metabolized predominantly via UGT1A1 (eg, irinotecan). Use in combination with carboplatin and paclitaxel in patients with squamous cell lung cancer is contraindicated.

Hand-foot skin reaction and rash are the most common adverse events and typically appear within the first 6 weeks of treatment; usually managed with topical treatment, treatment delays, and/or dose reductions. The risk for hand-foot syndrome increased with cumulative doses of sorafenib. The incidence of hand-foot syndrome is also increased in patients treated with sorafenib plus bevacizumab in comparison to those treated with sorafenib monotherapy. Sorafenib levels may be lower in HCC patients with mild-to-moderate hepatic impairment (Child-Pugh classes A and B); has not been studied in patients with severe hepatic impairment. Use with extreme caution in patients with HCC with elevated bilirubin levels. The optimal dose in non-HCC patients with hepatic impairment has not been established. In a small study of Asian patients with advanced HCC, sorafenib demonstrated efficacy with adequate tolerability in a hepatitis B-endemic area (Yau, 2009). Monitor fluid balance and electrolytes in patients at risk of renal dysfunction.

Drug Interactions

Metabolism/Transport Effects Substrate of CYP3A4 (minor); **Inhibits** CYP2B6 (moderate), 2C8 (strong), 2C9 (moderate)

Avoid Concomitant Use

Avoid concomitant use of SORAfenib with any of the following: BCG; CARBOplatin; Natalizumab; PACLitaxel; Pimecrolimus; Roflumilast; Tacrolimus (Topical); Vaccines (Live)

Decreased Effect

SORAfenib may decrease the levels/effects of: BCG; Cardiac Glycosides; Dacarbazine; Fluorouracil; Fluorouracil (Systemic); Fluorouracil (Topical); Sipuleucel-T; Vaccines (Inactivated); Vaccines (Live); Vitamin K Antagonists

The levels/effects of SORAfenib may be decreased by: CYP3A4 Inducers (Strong); Echinacea; Herbs (CYP3A4 Inducers); Neomycin

Increased Effect/Toxicity

SORAfenib may increase the levels/effects of: Acetaminophen; CARBOplatin; Carvedilol; CYP2B6 Substrates; CYP2C8 Substrates (High risk); CYP2C9 Substrates (High risk); DOCEtaxel; DOXOrubicin; Fluorouracil; Fluorouracil (Systemic); Fluorouracil (Topical); Irinotecan; Leflunomide; Natalizumab; PACLitaxel; Treprostinil; Vaccines (Live); Vitamin K Antagonists; Warfarin

The levels/effects of SORAfenib may be increased by: Acetaminophen; Bevacizumab; CYP3A4 Inhibitors (Strong); Denosumab; Pimecrolimus; Roflumilast; Tacrolimus (Topical); Trastuzumab

Nutritional/Ethanol Interactions

Food: Bioavailability is decreased 29% with a high-fat meal (bioavailability is similar to fasting state when administered with a moderate-fat meal).

Herb/Nutraceutical: Avoid St John's wort (may decrease the levels/effects of sorafenib).

Adverse Reactions

>10%:

Cardiovascular: Hypertension (9% to 17%; grade 3: 3% to 4%; grade 4: <1%; onset: ~3 weeks)

Central nervous system: Fatigue (37% to 46%), sensory neuropathy (≤13%), pain (11%)

Dermatologic: Rash/desquamation (19% to 40%; grade 3: ≤1%), hand-foot syndrome (21% to 30%; grade 3: 6% to 8%), alopecia (14% to 27%), pruritus (14% to 19%), dry skin (10% to 11%), erythema

Endocrine & metabolic: Hypoalbuminemia (≤59%), hypophosphatemia (35% to 45%; grade 3: 11% to 13%; grade 4: <1%)

Gastrointestinal: Diarrhea (43% to 55%; grade 3: 2% to 10%; grade 4: <1%), lipase increased (40% to 41% [usually transient]), amylase increased (30% to 34% [usually transient]), abdominal pain (11% to 31%), weight loss (10% to 30%), anorexia (16% to 29%), nausea (23% to 24%), vomiting (15% to 16%), constipation (14% to 15%)

Hematologic: Lymphopenia (23% to 47%; grades 3/4: ≤13%), thrombocytopenia (12% to 46%; grades 3/4: 1% to 4%), INR increased (≤42%), neutropenia (≤18%; grades 3/4: ≤5%), hemorrhage (15% to 18%; grade 3: 2% to 3%; grade 4: ≤2%), leukopenia

Hepatic: Liver dysfunction (≤11%; grade 3: 2%; grade 4: 1%)

Neuromuscular & skeletal: Muscle pain, weakness

Respiratory: Dyspnea (≤14%), cough (≤13%)

1% to 10%:

Cardiovascular: Cardiac ischemia/infarction (≤3%), heart failure (2%; congestive), flushing

Central nervous system: Headache (≤10%), depression, fever

Dermatologic: Acne, exfoliative dermatitis

Gastrointestinal: Appetite decreased, dyspepsia, dysphagia, esophageal varices bleeding (2%), glossodynia, mucositis, stomatitis, xerostomia

Genitourinary: Erectile dysfunction

Hematologic: Anemia

Hepatic: Transaminases increased (transient)

Neuromuscular & skeletal: Joint pain (≤10%), arthralgia, myalgia

Renal: Renal failure

Respiratory: Hoarseness

Miscellaneous: Flu-like syndrome

Pharmacodynamics/Kinetics

Bioavailability 38% to 49%; reduced when administered with a high-fat meal

Time to Peak ~3 hours

Protein Binding 99.5%

Half-Life Elimination 25-48 hours

Metabolism Hepatic, via CYP3A4 (primarily oxidated to the pyridine N-oxide; active, minor) and UGT1A9 (glucuronidation)

Excretion Feces (77%, 51% of dose as unchanged drug); urine (19%, as metabolites)

Available Dosage Forms

Tablet, oral:

NexAVAR®: 200 mg

Dosing

Adult & Geriatric

Advanced renal cell carcinoma: Oral: 400 mg twice daily; continue until no longer clinically benefiting or until unacceptable toxicity

Hepatocellular cancer: Oral: 400 mg twice daily; continue until no longer clinically benefiting or until unacceptable toxicity

Angiosarcoma (unlabeled use): Oral: 400 mg twice daily (Maki, 2009)

GIST (unlabeled use): Oral: 400 mg twice daily (Wiebe, 2008)

Thyroid cancer (unlabeled use): Oral: 400 mg twice daily (Gupta-Abramson, 2008)

Dosage adjustment for concomitant CYP3A4 inducers: Avoid the concomitant use of a strong CYP3A4 inducer (eg, carbamazepine, dexamethasone, phenobarbital, phenytoin, rifampin, St. John's wort) with sorafenib. If concomitant use of a strong CYP3A4 inducer cannot be avoided, the sorafenib dose may need to be increased, with careful monitoring. When the strong CYP3A4 inducer is discontinued, reduce sorafenib to the indicated dose.

Renal Impairment

FDA-approved labeling: No adjustment is required for mild, moderate, or severe renal impairment (not dependant on dialysis); has not been studied in dialysis patients.

Safety and pharmacokinetics were studied in varying degrees of renal dysfunction with the following empiric dose levels recommended based on patient tolerance (Miller, 2009):

Mild renal dysfunction (Cl_{cr} 40-59 mL/minute): 400 mg twice daily

Moderate renal dysfunction (Cl_{cr} 20-39 mL/minute): 200 mg twice daily
Severe renal dysfunction (Cl_{cr} <20 mL/minute): Data inadequate to define dose
Hemodialysis (any Cl_{cr}): 200 mg once daily

Hepatic Impairment

FDA-approved labeling: No adjustment is required for mild (Child-Pugh class A) to moderate (Child-Pugh class B) hepatic impairment; not studied in severe hepatic impairment (Child-Pugh class C). Use with extreme caution in patients with HCC with elevated bilirubin levels.

Safety and pharmacokinetics were studied in varying degrees of hepatic dysfunction with the following empiric dose levels recommended based on patient tolerance (Miller, 2009):

Mild hepatic dysfunction (bilirubin >1 to ≤1.5 times ULN and/or AST >ULN): 400 mg twice daily
Moderate hepatic dysfunction (bilirubin >1.5 to ≤3 times ULN; any AST): 200 mg twice daily
Severe hepatic dysfunction:
Bilirubin >3-10 x ULN (any AST): 200 mg every 3 days was **not** tolerated
Albumin <2.5 g/dL (any bilirubin and any AST): 200 mg once daily

Adjustment for Toxicity Temporary interruption and/or dosage reduction may be necessary for management of adverse drug reactions. The dose may be reduced to 400 mg once daily and then further reduced to 400 mg every other day.

Dose modification for severe/persistent hypertension (despite antihypertensive therapy) or cardiac ischemia/infarction: Consider temporarily or permanently discontinuing treatment.

Dose modification for gastrointestinal perforation: Permanently discontinue treatment.

Dose modification for hemorrhage requiring medical intervention: Consider permanently discontinuing treatment.

Dose modification for skin toxicity:

Grade 1 (numbness, dysesthesia, paresthesia, tingling, painless swelling, erythema, or discomfort of the hands or feet which do not disrupt normal activities): Continue sorafenib and consider symptomatic treatment with topical therapy.

Grade 2 (painful erythema and swelling of the hands or feet and/or discomfort affecting normal activities):

1st occurrence: Continue sorafenib and consider symptomatic treatment with topical therapy. **Note:** If no improvement within 7 days, see dosing for 2nd or 3rd occurrence.
2nd or 3rd occurrence: Hold treatment until resolves to grade 0-1; resume treatment with dose reduced by one dose level (400 mg daily or 400 mg every other day)
4th occurrence: Discontinue treatment

Grade 3 (moist desquamation, ulceration, blistering, or severe pain of the hands or feet or severe discomfort that prevents working or performing daily activities):

1st or 2nd occurrence: Hold treatment until resolves to grade 0-1; resume treatment with dose reduced by one dose level (400 mg daily or 400 mg every other day)
3rd occurrence: Discontinue treatment

Administration

Oral Administer with water on an empty stomach (1 hour before or 2 hours after eating). Swallow tablet whole.

Stability

Storage Store at room temperature of 25°C (77°F); excursions permitted to 15°C and 30°C (59°F and 86°F). Protect from moisture.

Monitoring and Teaching Issues

Laboratory Monitoring CBC with differential, electrolytes, phosphorus, lipase and amylase levels; monitor fluid balance (and electrolytes) in patients at risk for renal dysfunction

Physical Assessment Evaluate for hypertension, cardiac artery disease, or recent MI prior to prescribing therapy. Monitor for gastrointestinal perforation (abdominal pain, constipation, vomiting), diarrhea, fatigue, rash, or hand-foot syndrome; dosing adjustments may be necessary.

Patient Education Take on an empty stomach 1 hour before or 2 hours after eating. You may need periodic laboratory tests while taking this medication. Maintain adequate hydration unless instructed to restrict fluid intake. You may experience loss of appetite, nausea, vomiting, diarrhea, or hair loss (may grow back when treatment is discontinued). Report immediately persistent or acute headache, dizziness, or vision changes (monitor blood pressure if recommended by prescriber); chest pain or palpitations; or unusual bleeding. Report unusual skin rash; hand and foot syndrome (redness, tenderness, dryness, peeling, numbness, or tingling of the palms and soles); persistent gastrointestinal upset (diarrhea, constipation, abdominal pain); unusual or persistent cough; bone, joint, or muscle weakness or pain or loss of sensation; or flu-like symptoms.

Dietary Considerations Take without food (1 hour before or 2 hours after eating).

Geriatric Considerations No difference in efficacy or safety was observed between older and younger patients, but only 4% of patients studied were >75 years of age.

Breast-Feeding Considerations Due to the potential for serious adverse effects in the nursing infant, breast-feeding is not recommended.

Pregnancy Considerations Animal studies have demonstrated teratogenicity and fetal loss. There are no adequate and well-controlled studies in pregnant women. Because sorafenib inhibits angiogenesis, a critical component of fetal development, adverse effects on pregnancy would be expected. Women of childbearing potential should be advised to avoid pregnancy. Men and women should use effective birth control during treatment and for at least 2 weeks after treatment is discontinued.

Additional Information Hand-foot skin reaction (HFSR) management (Lacouture, 2008): The following treatments may be used in addition to the recommended dosage modifications. Prior to treatment initiation, a pedicure is recommended to remove hyperkeratotic areas/calluses, which may predispose to HFSR; avoid vigorous exercise/activities which may stress hands or feet. During therapy, patients should reduce exposure to hot water (may exacerbate hand-foot symptoms); avoid constrictive footwear and excessive skin friction. Patients may also wear thick cotton gloves or socks and should wear shoes with padded insoles. Grade 1 HFSR may be relieved with moisturizing creams, cotton gloves and socks (at night) and/or keratolytic creams such as urea (20% to 40%) or salicylic acid (6%). Apply topical steroid (eg, clobetasol ointment) twice daily to erythematous areas of Grade 2 HFSR; topical anesthetics (eg, lidocaine 2%) and then systemic analgesics (if appropriate) may be used for pain control. Resolution of acute erythema may result in keratotic areas which may be softened with keratolytic agents.

◆ **Sorafenib Tosylate** *see* Sorafenib *on page 1670*

Sorbitol (SOR bi tole)

Generic Availability (U.S.) Yes

Pharmacologic Category Genitourinary Irrigant; Laxative, Osmotic

Pregnancy Risk Factor C

Lactation Excretion in breast milk unknown

Use Genitourinary irrigant in transurethral prostatic resection or other transurethral resection or other transurethral surgical procedures; diuretic; humectant; sweetening agent; hyperosmotic laxative; facilitate the passage of sodium polystyrene sulfonate through the intestinal tract

Available Dosage Forms

Solution, genitourinary irrigation [preservative free]: 3% (3000 mL, 5000 mL); 3.3% (2000 mL, 4000 mL)

Solution, oral: 70% (30 mL, 473 mL, 480 mL, 3840 mL)

Dosing

Adult & Geriatric

Hyperosmotic laxative (as single dose, at infrequent intervals):

Oral: 30-150 mL (as 70% solution)

Rectal enema: 120 mL as 25% to 30% solution

Adjunct to sodium polystyrene sulfonate: 15 mL as 70% solution orally until diarrhea occurs (10-20 mL/2 hours) or 20-100 mL as an oral vehicle for the sodium polystyrene sulfonate resin

When administered with charcoal:

Oral: 4.3 mL/kg of 70% sorbitol with 1 g/kg of activated charcoal every 4 hours until first stool containing charcoal is passed

Transurethral surgical procedures: Irrigation: Topical: 3% to 3.3% as transurethral surgical procedure irrigation

Pediatric

Hyperosmotic laxative (as single dose, at infrequent intervals):

Children 2-11 years:

Oral: 2 mL/kg (as 70% solution)

Rectal enema: 30-60 mL as 25% to 30% solution

Children >12 years: Oral, Rectal enema: Refer to adult dosing.

When administered with charcoal: Oral: Children: 4.3 mL/kg of 35% sorbitol with 1 g/kg of activated charcoal

Monitoring and Teaching Issues

Laboratory Monitoring Electrolytes

Physical Assessment When used as cathartic, determine cause of constipation before use.

◆ **Sorine®** *see* Sotalol *on page 1673*

Sotalol (SOE ta lole)

U.S. Brand Names Betapace AF®; Betapace®; Sorine®

Index Terms Sotalol Hydrochloride

Generic Availability (U.S.) Yes

Pharmacologic Category Antiarrhythmic Agent, Class II; Antiarrhythmic Agent, Class III; Beta-Adrenergic Blocker, Nonselective

Medication Safety Issues

Sound-alike/look-alike issues:

Sotalol may be confused with Stadol®, Sudafed®

Betapace® may be confused with Betapace AF®

Betapace AF® may be confused with Betapace®

Pregnancy Risk Factor B

Lactation Enters breast milk/consider risk:benefit (AAP rates "compatible"; AAP 2001 update pending)

Use Treatment of documented ventricular arrhythmias (ie, sustained ventricular tachycardia), that in the judgment of the physician are life-threatening; maintenance of normal sinus rhythm in patients with symptomatic atrial fibrillation and atrial flutter who are currently in sinus rhythm. Manufacturer states substitutions should not be made for Betapace AF® since Betapace AF® is distributed with a patient package insert specific for atrial fibrillation/flutter.

Injection: Substitution for oral sotalol in those who are unable to take sotalol orally

Unlabeled/Investigational Use Fetal tachycardia

Injection: Hemodynamically stable monomorphic ventricular tachycardia (ACLS, 2010)

Mechanism of Action/Effect

Beta-blocker which contains both beta-adrenoreceptor-blocking (Vaughan Williams Class II) and cardiac action potential duration prolongation (Vaughan Williams Class III) properties

Class II effects: Increased sinus cycle length, slowed heart rate, decreased AV nodal conduction, and increased AV nodal refractoriness

Class III effects: Prolongation of the atrial and ventricular monophasic action potentials, and effective refractory prolongation of atrial muscle, ventricular muscle, and atrioventricular accessory pathways in both the antegrade and retrograde directions

Sotalol is a racemic mixture of *d*- and *l*-sotalol; both isomers have similar Class III antiarrhythmic effects while the *l*-isomer is responsible for virtually all of the beta-blocking activity

Sotalol has both $beta_1$- and $beta_2$-receptor blocking activity. The beta-blocking effect of sotalol is a noncardioselective [half maximal at about 80 mg/day and maximal at doses of 320-640 mg/day]. Significant beta-blockade occurs at oral doses as low as 25 mg/day.

Significant Class III effects are seen only at oral doses ≥160 mg/day.

Contraindications Hypersensitivity to sotalol or any component of the formulation; bronchial asthma; sinus bradycardia; second- or third-degree AV block (unless a functioning pacemaker is present); congenital or acquired long QT syndromes; cardiogenic shock; uncontrolled heart failure

Additional contraindications: Betapace AF® and the injectable formulation: Baseline QT_c interval >450 msec; bronchospastic conditions; Cl_{cr} <40 mL/minute; serum potassium <4 mEq/L; sick sinus syndrome

Warnings/Precautions [U.S. Boxed Warning] Manufacturer recommends initiation (or reinitiation) and doses increased in a hospital setting with continuous monitoring and staff familiar with the recognition and treatment of life-threatening arrhythmias. Some experts will initiate therapy on an outpatient basis in a patient without heart disease or bradycardia, who has a baseline uncorrected QT interval <450 msec, and normal serum potassium and magnesium levels; close ECG monitoring during this time is necessary. ACC/AHA guidelines for management of atrial fibrillation also recommend that for outpatient initiation the patient not have risk factors predisposing to drug-induced ventricular proarrhythmia (Fuster, 2006). Dosage should be adjusted gradually with 3 days between dosing increments to achieve steady-state concentrations, and to allow time to monitor QT intervals. **[U.S. Boxed Warning]: Adjust dosing interval based on creatinine clearance to decrease risk of proarrhythmia; QT interval prolongation is directly related to sotalol concentration.** Creatinine clearance must be calculated with dose initiation and dose increases. Use cautiously in the renally-impaired (dosage adjustment required). Betapace AF® and the injectable formulation are contraindicated in patients with Cl_{cr} <40 mL/minute.

[U.S. Boxed Warning]: Sotalol injection: Sotalol can cause life-threatening ventricular tachycardia associated with QT interval prolongation (ie, torsade de pointes). Do not initiate if baseline QT_c interval is >450 msec. If QT_c exceeds 500 msec during therapy, reduce the dose, prolong the infusion duration, or discontinue use. If while on oral sotalol therapy baseline QT_c interval is >500 msec, use I.V. sotalol with particular caution; serious consideration should be given to reducing the dose or discontinuing I.V. sotalol when QT_c exceeds 520 msec. QT_c prolongation is directly related to the concentration of sotalol; reduced creatinine clearance, female gender, and large doses increase the risk of QT_c prolongation and subsequent torsade de pointes. Monitor and adjust dose to prevent QT_c prolongation. Concurrent use with other QT_c-prolonging drugs (including Class I and Class III antiarrhythmics) and use within 3 months of discontinuing amiodarone is generally not recommended. To reduce the chance of excessive QT_c-prolongation, withhold QT_c-prolonging drugs for at least 3 half-lives (or 3 months for amiodarone) before initiating sotalol.

Correct electrolyte imbalances before initiating (especially hypokalemia and hypomagnesemia). Consider pre-existing conditions such as sick sinus syndrome before initiating. Conduction abnormalities can occur particularly sinus bradycardia. Use cautiously within the first 2 weeks post-MI especially in patients with markedly impaired ventricular function (experience limited). Administer cautiously in compensated heart failure and monitor for a worsening of the condition. Use caution in patients with peripheral vascular disease (can aggravate arterial insufficiency). Beta-blocker therapy should not be withdrawn abruptly (particularly in patients with CAD), but gradually tapered to avoid acute tachycardia, hypertension, and/or ischemia; abrupt discontinuation may exacerbate symptoms of hyperthyroidism and may also induce thyroid storm. Use caution with concurrent use of verapamil or diltiazem; bradycardia or heart block can occur. Use cautiously in diabetics because it can mask prominent hypoglycemic symptoms. Use with caution in patients with bronchospastic disease, myasthenia gravis or psychiatric disease. Use care with anesthetic agents which decrease myocardial function. Adequate alpha-blockade is required prior to use of any beta-blocker for patients with untreated pheochromocytoma. Beta-blockade may mask signs of hyperthyroidism (eg, tachycardia). Use caution with history of severe anaphylaxis to allergens; patients taking beta-blockers may become more sensitive to repeated challenges. Treatment of anaphylaxis (eg, epinephrine) in patients taking beta-blockers may be ineffective or promote undesirable effects.

[U.S. Boxed Warning]: Betapace® should not be substituted for Betapace® AF; Betapace® AF is distributed with an educational insert specifically for patients with atrial fibrillation/flutter.

Drug Interactions

Avoid Concomitant Use

Avoid concomitant use of Sotalol with any of the following: Artemether; Dronedarone; Lumefantrine; Methacholine; Nilotinib; Pimozide; QuiNINE; Tetrabenazine; Thioridazine; Toremifene; Vandetanib; Ziprasidone

Decreased Effect

Sotalol may decrease the levels/effects of: Beta2-Agonists; Theophylline Derivatives

The levels/effects of Sotalol may be decreased by: Barbiturates; Herbs (Hypertensive Properties); Methylphenidate; Nonsteroidal Anti-Inflammatory Agents; Rifamycin Derivatives; Yohimbine

Increased Effect/Toxicity

Sotalol may increase the levels/effects of: Alpha-/Beta-Agonists (Direct-Acting); Alpha1-Blockers; Alpha2-Agonists; Amifostine; Antihypertensives; Antipsychotic Agents (Phenothiazines); Bupivacaine; Cardiac Glycosides; Dronedarone; Fingolimod; Hypotensive Agents; Insulin; Lidocaine; Lidocaine (Systemic); Lidocaine (Topical); Mepivacaine; Methacholine; Midodrine; Pimozide; QTc-Prolonging Agents; QuiNINE; RiTUXimab; Sulfonylureas; Tetrabenazine; Thioridazine; Toremifene; Vandetanib; Ziprasidone

The levels/effects of Sotalol may be increased by: Acetylcholinesterase Inhibitors; Alfuzosin; Aminoquinolines (Antimalarial); Amiodarone; Anilidopiperidine Opioids; Antipsychotic Agents (Phenothiazines); Artemether; Calcium Channel Blockers (Nondihydropyridine); Chloroquine; Ciprofloxacin; Ciprofloxacin (Systemic); Diazoxide; Dipyridamole; Disopyramide; Dronedarone; Eribulin; Fingolimod; Gadobutrol; Herbs (Hypotensive Properties); Lumefantrine; MAO Inhibitors; Nilotinib; Pentoxifylline; Phosphodiesterase 5 Inhibitors; Propafenone; Propoxyphene; Prostacyclin Analogues; QuiNIDine; QuiNINE; Reserpine

Nutritional/Ethanol Interactions

Food: Sotalol peak serum concentrations may be decreased if taken with food.

Herb/Nutraceutical: Avoid ephedra (may worsen arrhythmia).

Adverse Reactions Note: No clinical experience with I.V. sotalol; however, since exposure is similar between I.V. and oral sotalol, adverse reactions are expected to be similar.

>10%:

Cardiovascular: Bradycardia (13% to 16%), chest pain (3% to 16%), palpitation (14%)

Central nervous system: Fatigue (20%), dizziness (20%), lightheadedness (12%)

Neuromuscular & skeletal: Weakness (13%)

Respiratory: Dyspnea (21%)

1% to 10%:

Cardiovascular: Edema (8%), abnormal ECG (7%), hypotension (6%), proarrhythmia (5%), syncope (5%), CHF (5%), torsade de pointes (dose related; 1% to 4%), peripheral vascular disorders (3%), ventricular tachycardia worsened (1%), QT_c interval prolongation (dose related)

Central nervous system: Headache (8%), sleep problems (8%), mental confusion (6%), anxiety (4%), depression (4%)

Dermatologic: Itching/rash (5%)

Endocrine & metabolic: Sexual ability decreased (3%)

Gastrointestinal: Nausea/vomiting (10%), diarrhea (7%), stomach discomfort (3% to 6%), flatulence (2%)

Genitourinary: Impotence (2%)

Hematologic: Bleeding (2%)

Neuromuscular & skeletal: Extremity pain (7%), paresthesia (4%), back pain (3%)

Ocular: Visual problems (5%)

Respiratory: Upper respiratory problems (5% to 8%), asthma (2%)

Pharmacodynamics/Kinetics

Onset of Action Oral: Rapid, 1-2 hours; when administered I.V. for ongoing VT over 5 minutes, onset of action is ~5-10 minutes (Ho, 1994)

Duration of Action 8-16 hours

Absorption Oral: Decreased 20% to 30% by meals compared to fasting

Bioavailability Oral: 90% to 100%

Time to Peak Serum: Oral: 2.5-4 hours

Protein Binding None

Half-Life Elimination 12 hours; Children: 9.5 hours; terminal half-life decreases with age <2 years (time to steady state may be ≥1 week in neonates); increases with renal dysfunction

Metabolism None

Excretion Urine (as unchanged drug)

Available Dosage Forms

Injection, solution [preservative free]: 15 mg/mL (10 mL)

Tablet, oral: 80 mg, 120 mg, 160 mg, 240 mg

Betapace AF®: 80 mg, 120 mg, 160 mg

Betapace®: 80 mg, 120 mg, 160 mg, 240 mg

Sorine®: 80 mg, 120 mg, 160 mg, 240 mg

Dosing

Adult & Geriatric Baseline QT_c interval and creatinine clearance must be determined prior to initiation. Sotalol should be initiated and doses increased in a hospital with facilities for cardiac rhythm monitoring and assessment. Proarrhythmic events can occur after initiation of therapy and with each upward dosage adjustment.

Conversion from oral sotalol to I.V. sotalol:

80 mg oral equivalent to 75 mg I.V.

120 mg oral equivalent to 112.5 mg I.V.

160 mg oral equivalent to 150 mg I.V.

Ventricular arrhythmias:

I.V.: **Note:** The effects of the initial I.V. dose must be monitored and the dose titrated either upward or downward, if needed, based on clinical effect, QT_c interval, or adverse reactions.

Substitution for oral sotalol: Initial dose: 75 mg infused over 5 hours twice daily

Dose adjustment: If the frequency of relapse does not reduce and excessive QT_c prolongation does not occur, may increase to 112.5 mg twice daily. For ventricular arrhythmias, may increase dose every 3 days in increments of 75 mg/day.

Dose range: Usual therapeutic dose: 75-150 mg twice daily; maximum dose: 300 mg twice daily.

Hemodynamically stable monomorphic VT, ongoing (unlabeled use): 1.5 mg/kg over 5 minutes (ACLS, 2010); **Note:** Clinical trial employed standard dose of 100 mg (Ho, 1994).

Oral (Betapace®, Sorine®):

Initial: 80 mg twice daily; dose may be increased gradually to 240-320 mg/day; allow 3 days between dosing increments (to attain steady-state plasma concentrations and to allow monitoring of QT_c intervals).

Usual range: Most patients respond to 160-320 mg/day in 2-3 divided doses.

Maximum: Some patients, with life-threatening refractory ventricular arrhythmias, may require doses as high as 480-640 mg/day; prescribed ONLY when the potential benefit outweighs the increased of adverse events.

Atrial fibrillation or atrial flutter:

I.V.: **Note:** The effects of the initial I.V. dose must be monitored and the dose titrated either upward or downward, if needed, based on clinical effect, QT_c interval, or adverse reactions.

Substitution for oral sotalol: Initial dose: 75 mg infused over 5 hours twice daily

Dose adjustment: If the frequency of relapse does not reduce and excessive QT_c prolongation does not occur, may increase to 112.5 mg twice daily. For ventricular arrhythmias, may increase dose every 3 days in increments of 75 mg/day.

Dose range: Usual therapeutic dose: 112.5 mg twice daily; maximum dose: 150 mg twice daily

Oral (Betapace AF®): Initial: 80 mg twice daily. If the frequency of relapse does not reduce and excessive QT_c prolongation does not occur after 3 days, the dose may be increased to 120 mg twice daily; may further increase to 160 mg twice daily if response is inadequate and QT_c prolongation is not excessive.

Pediatric Baseline QT_c interval and creatinine clearance must be determined prior to initiation. Sotalol should be initiated and doses increased in a hospital with facilities for cardiac rhythm monitoring and assessment. Proarrhythmic events can occur after initiation of therapy and with each upward dosage adjustment.

Note: The safety and efficacy of sotalol in children have not been established

Supraventricular arrhythmias: Oral: **Note:** Dosing per manufacturer, based on pediatric pharmacokinetic data; wait at least 36 hours between dosage adjustments to allow monitoring of QT_c intervals

Children ≤2 years: Dosage should be adjusted (decreased) by plotting of the child's age on a logarithmic scale; see graph or refer to manufacturer's package labeling.

Sotalol Age Factor Nomogram for Patients ≤2 Years of Age

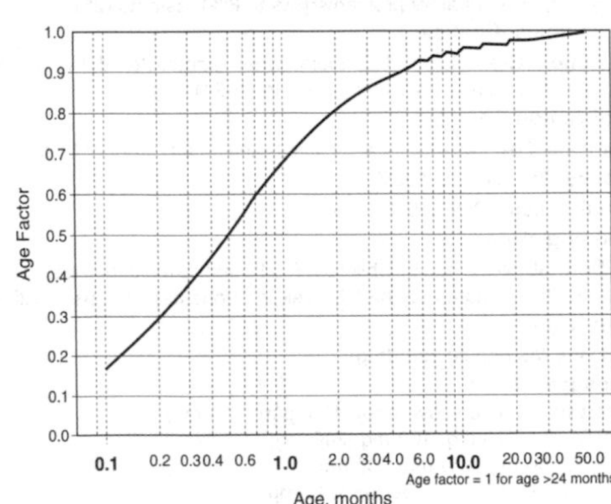

Adapted from U.S. Food and Drug Administration.
http://www.fda.gov/cder/foi/label/2001/2115s3lbl.PDF

Children >2 years: Initial: 90 mg/m²/day in 3 divided doses; may be incrementally increased to a maximum of 180 mg/m²/day

Renal Impairment Adults: Impaired renal function can increase the terminal half-life, resulting in increased drug accumulation. Sotalol (Betapace AF®, injectable formulation) is contraindicated per the manufacturers for treatment of atrial fibrillation/flutter in patients with a Cl_{cr} <40 mL/minute.

Ventricular arrhythmias (Betapace®, Sorine®):

Cl_{cr} >60 mL/minute: Administer every 12 hours.

Cl_{cr} 30-60 mL/minute: Administer every 24 hours.

Cl_{cr} 10-29 mL/minute: Administer every 36-48 hours.

Cl_{cr} <10 mL/minute: Individualize dose.

Atrial fibrillation/flutter (Betapace AF®):

Cl_{cr} >60 mL/minute: Administer every 12 hours.

Cl_{cr} 40-60 mL/minute: Administer every 24 hours.

Cl_{cr} <40 mL/minute: Use is contraindicated.

Note: The manufacturer of the injectable formulation recommends adjustment similar to that used for Betapace AF®. However, the injectable formulation may be used for either indication.

Dialysis: Hemodialysis would be expected to reduce sotalol plasma concentrations because sotalol is not bound to plasma proteins and does not undergo extensive metabolism. Administer dose postdialysis or administer supplemental 80 mg dose. Peritoneal dialysis does not remove sotalol; supplemental dose is not necessary.

Adjustment for Toxicity

QT_c ≥500 msec during initiation period:

Betapace AF®: Reduce dose or discontinue sotalol

Injectable formulation: Reduce dose, decrease infusion rate, or discontinue sotalol

QT_c ≥520 msec (or JT interval ≥430 msec if the QRS >100 msec) during maintenance therapy (Betapace AF®, injectable formulation): Reduce dose and carefully monitor QT_c until <520 msec. If QT_c interval ≥520 msec on the lowest maintenance dose, discontinue sotalol.

QT_c ≥550 msec (Betapace®, Sorine®): Reduce dose or discontinue sotalol.

Administration

Oral Administer without regard to meals.

I.V.

Substitution for oral: Administer over 5 hours.

Hemodynamically stable monomorphic VT: Administer I.V. push over 5 minutes; use with caution due to increased risk of adverse events (eg, bradycardia, hypotension, torsade de pointes) (ACLS, 2010)

Stability

Storage Store at 25°C (77°F); excursions permitted to 15°C to 30°C (59°F to 86°F). To prepare sotalol infusion, see manufacturer's prescribing information.

Monitoring and Teaching Issues

Laboratory Monitoring Serum creatinine, magnesium, potassium

Physicai Assessment Assess blood pressure and heart rate prior to and following first dose and with any change in dosage. Consider cardiac monitoring to observe for QT changes and arrhythmias, especially if giving I.V. Assess cardiac and pulmonary status. Advise patients with diabetes to monitor glucose levels closely (beta-blockers may alter glucose tolerance). Do not discontinue abruptly; dose should be tapered gradually. Teach patient hypotension precautions.

Patient Education Take pulse daily (prior to medication) and follow prescriber's instruction about holding of medication. If you have diabetes, monitor serum sugar closely; drug may alter glucose tolerance or mask signs of hypoglycemia. May cause fatigue, dizziness, lightheadedness, postural hypotension, alteration in sexual performance (reversible), nausea, vomiting, or diarrhea. Report immediately any chest pain, palpitations, irregular heartbeat; swelling of extremities, weight gain, respiratory difficulty, new cough, or unusual fatigue; persistent nausea, vomiting, or diarrhea; or unusual muscle weakness.

Dietary Considerations May be taken without regard to meals.

Geriatric Considerations Since elderly frequently have Cl_{cr} <60 mL/minute, attention to dose, creatinine clearance, and monitoring is important. Make dosage adjustments at 3-day intervals or after 5-6 doses at any dosage.

Breast-Feeding Considerations Sotalol is excreted into breast milk in concentrations higher than those found in the maternal serum. Although adverse events in nursing infants have not been observed in case reports, close monitoring for bradycardia, hypotension, respiratory distress, and hypoglycemia is advised. According to the manufacturer, the decision to continue or discontinue breast-feeding during therapy should take into account the risk of exposure to the infant and the benefits of treatment to the mother.

Pregnancy Considerations Adverse events were not observed in the initial animal reproduction studies; therefore, the manufacturer classifies sotalol as pregnancy category B. Sotalol crosses the placenta and is found in amniotic fluid. In a cohort study, an increased risk of cardiovascular defects was observed following maternal use of beta-blockers during pregnancy. Intrauterine growth restriction (IUGR), small placentas, as well as fetal/neonatal bradycardia, hypoglycemia, and/or respiratory depression have been observed following *in utero* exposure to beta-blockers as a class. Adequate facilities for monitoring infants at birth should be available. Untreated chronic maternal hypertension and pre-eclampsia are also associated with adverse events in the fetus, infant, and mother; however, sotalol is currently not recommended for the initial treatment of hypertension in pregnancy. Because sotalol crosses the placenta in concentrations similar to the maternal serum, it has been used for the treatment of fetal atrial flutter or fetal supraventricular tachycardia without hydrops. The clearance of sotalol is increased during the third trimester of pregnancy, but other pharmacokinetic parameters do not significantly differ from nonpregnant values.

Additional Information Pharmacokinetics in children are more relevant for BSA than age.

Related Information

Antiarrhythmic Drugs *on page 1978*

Beta-Blockers *on page 1990*

- ◆ **Sotalol Hydrochloride** *see* Sotalol *on page 1673*
- ◆ **Sotret®** *see* Isotretinoin *on page 1030*
- ◆ **SPA** *see* Albumin *on page 57*
- ◆ **SPD417** *see* CarBAMazepine *on page 287*
- ◆ **Spectracef®** *see* Cefditoren *on page 317*
- ◆ **SPI 0211** *see* Lubiprostone *on page 1139*
- ◆ **Spiriva® HandiHaler®** *see* Tiotropium *on page 1769*

Spironolactone (speer on oh LAK tone)

U.S. Brand Names Aldactone®

Generic Availability (U.S.) Yes

Pharmacologic Category Diuretic, Potassium-Sparing; Selective Aldosterone Blocker

Medication Safety Issues

Sound-alike/look-alike issues:

Aldactone® may be confused with Aldactazide®

International issues:

Aldactone: Brand name for spironolactone [U.S., Canada], but also the brand name for potassium canrenoate [Austria, Czech Republic, Germany, Hungary, Poland]

Pregnancy Risk Factor C

Lactation Enters breast milk/not recommended (AAP rates "compatible"; AAP 2001 update pending)

Use Management of edema associated with excessive aldosterone excretion; hypertension; primary hyperaldosteronism; hypokalemia; cirrhosis of liver accompanied by edema or ascites; nephritic syndrome; severe heart failure (NYHA class III-IV) to increase survival and reduce hospitalization when added to standard therapy

Unlabeled/Investigational Use Female acne (adjunctive therapy); hirsutism; hypertension (pediatric); diuretic (pediatric)

Mechanism of Action/Effect Competes with aldosterone for receptor sites in the distal renal tubules, increasing sodium chloride and water excretion while conserving potassium and hydrogen ions; may block the effect of aldosterone on arteriolar smooth muscle as well

Contraindications Anuria; acute renal insufficiency; significant impairment of renal excretory function; hyperkalemia

Warnings/Precautions Monitor serum potassium closely in patients being treated for heart failure. Avoid potassium supplements, potassium-containing salt substitutes, a diet rich in potassium, or other drugs that can cause hyperkalemia. Excess amounts can lead to profound diuresis with fluid and electrolyte loss; close medical supervision and dose evaluation are required. Watch for and correct electrolyte disturbances; adjust dose to avoid dehydration. In cirrhosis, avoid electrolyte and acid/base imbalances that might lead to hepatic encephalopathy. Gynecomastia is related to dose and duration of therapy. Discontinue use prior to adrenal vein catheterization. When evaluating a heart failure patient for spironolactone treatment, creatinine should be ≤2.5 mg/dL in men or ≤2 mg/dL in women and potassium <5 mEq/L. Discontinue or interrupt therapy if serum potassium >5 mEq/L or serum creatinine >4 mg/dL. **[U.S. Boxed Warning]: Shown to be a tumorigen in chronic toxicity animal studies. Avoid unnecessary use.**

Drug Interactions

Avoid Concomitant Use

Avoid concomitant use of Spironolactone with any of the following: Tacrolimus

Decreased Effect

Spironolactone may decrease the levels/effects of: Alpha-/Beta-Agonists; Cardiac Glycosides; Mitotane; QuiNIDine

The levels/effects of Spironolactone may be decreased by: Herbs (Hypertensive Properties); Methylphenidate; Nonsteroidal Anti-Inflammatory Agents; Yohimbine

Increased Effect/Toxicity

Spironolactone may increase the levels/effects of: ACE Inhibitors; Amifostine; Ammonium Chloride; Antihypertensives; Cardiac Glycosides; Digoxin; Hypotensive Agents; Neuromuscular-Blocking Agents (Nondepolarizing); RiTUXimab; Tacrolimus

The levels/effects of Spironolactone may be increased by: Angiotensin II Receptor Blockers; Diazoxide; Drospirenone; Eplerenone; Herbs (Hypotensive Properties); MAO Inhibitors; Nonsteroidal Anti-Inflammatory Agents; Pentoxifylline; Phosphodiesterase 5 Inhibitors; Potassium Salts; Prostacyclin Analogues; Tolvaptan

Nutritional/Ethanol Interactions

Ethanol: Increases risk of orthostasis.

Food: Food increases absorption.

Herb/Nutraceutical: Avoid natural licorice (due to mineralocorticoid activity)

Lab Interactions May cause false elevation in serum digoxin concentrations measured by RIA.

Adverse Reactions Frequency not always defined.

Cardiovascular: Vasculitis

Central nervous system: Ataxia, confusion, drowsiness, drug fever, fatigue, headache, lethargy

Dermatologic: Eosinophilia, maculopapular or erythematous cutaneous eruptions, urticaria
Endocrine & metabolic: Gynecomastia (men 9%), breast pain (men 2%), hyperkalemia (serious; 2%), dehydration, hyperchloremic metabolic acidosis in decompensated hepatic cirrhosis, hyponatremia, impotence, irregular menses, amenorrhea, postmenopausal bleeding
Gastrointestinal: Anorexia, cramps, diarrhea, gastritis, nausea, ulceration, vomiting, xerostomia
Hematologic: Agranulocytosis
Hepatic: Cholestatic/hepatocellular toxicity
Renal: BUN increased, renal dysfunction, renal failure
Miscellaneous: Anaphylactic reaction, breast cancer, deepening of the voice

Pharmacodynamics/Kinetics

Duration of Action 2-3 days

Time to Peak Serum: 3-4 hours (primarily as the active metabolite)

Protein Binding 91% to 98%

Half-Life Elimination Spironolactone: 78-84 minutes; Canrenone: 10-23 hours; 7-alpha-spirolactone: 7-20 hours

Metabolism Hepatic to multiple metabolites, including active metabolites canrenone and 7-alpha-spirolactone

Excretion Urine and feces

Available Dosage Forms

Tablet, oral: 25 mg, 50 mg, 100 mg
Aldactone®: 25 mg, 50 mg, 100 mg

Dosing

Adult To reduce delay in onset of effect, a loading dose of 2 or 3 times the daily dose may be administered on the first day of therapy.

Edema: Oral: 25-200 mg/day in 1-2 divided doses
Hypokalemia: Oral: 25-100 mg daily
Hypertension (JNC 7): Oral: 25-50 mg/day in 1-2 divided doses
Diagnosis of primary aldosteronism: Oral: Long test: 400 mg daily for 3-4 weeks; short test: 400 mg daily for 4 days; maintenance until surgical correction: 100-400 mg/day in 1-2 divided doses
Heart failure, severe (NYHA class III-IV; with ACE inhibitor and a loop diuretic ± digoxin): 12.5-25 mg/day; maximum daily dose: 50 mg. If 25 mg once daily not tolerated, reduce to 25 mg every other day was the lowest maintenance dose possible.
Note: If potassium >5 mEq/L or serum creatinine >4 mg/dL, discontinue or interrupt therapy.
Acne in women (unlabeled use): Oral: 25-200 mg once daily
Hirsutism in women (unlabeled use): Oral: 50-200 mg/day in 1-2 divided doses

Geriatric Oral: Indication specific: Initial: 25-50 mg/day in 1-2 divided doses; increase by 25-50 mg every 5 days as needed. Adjust for renal impairment.

Pediatric Administration with food increases absorption. To reduce delay in onset of effect, a loading dose of 2 or 3 times the daily dose may be administered on the first day of therapy.

Edema, hypertension (unlabeled use): Oral: Children 1-17 years: Initial: 1 mg/kg/day divided every 12-24 hours (maximum dose: 3.3 mg/kg/day, up to 100 mg/day)
Diagnosis of primary aldosteronism (unlabeled use): Oral: 125-375 mg/m^2/day in divided doses

Renal Impairment Heart failure:
Cl_{cr} 31-50 mL/minute: Decrease initial dose to 12.5 mg once daily.
Cl_{cr} <30 mL/minute: Not recommended.

Stability

Storage Store below 25°C (77°F).

Monitoring and Teaching Issues

Laboratory Monitoring Serum electrolytes (potassium, sodium), renal function
HF: Potassium levels and renal function should be checked in 3 days and 1 week after initiation or increase in dose, then every 2-4 weeks for 3 months, then quarterly for a year, then every 6 months thereafter.

Physical Assessment Diuretic effect may be delayed 2-3 days. Assess serum electrolytes on a regular basis. Assess fluid status and monitor for CNS changes (drowsiness, headache, confusion), rash, gynecomastia, dehydration, and hyperkalemia during therapy.

Patient Education Take with meals. Avoid any potassium supplements (vitamin/mineral products), potassium-containing salt substitutes, natural licorice, or extra dietary intake of potassium. Weigh yourself weekly and report weight loss. May cause dizziness, drowsiness, confusion, headache, nausea, vomiting, dry mouth, or gynecomastia. Report mental confusion; clumsiness; persistent fatigue, chills, numbness, or muscle weakness in hands, feet, or face; acute persistent diarrhea; chest pain, rapid heartbeat, or palpitations; excessive thirst; respiratory difficulty; breast tenderness or increased body hair in females; breast enlargement; or inability to achieve erection in males.

Dietary Considerations Should be taken with food to decrease gastrointestinal irritation and to increase absorption. Excessive potassium intake (eg, salt substitutes, low-salt foods, bananas, nuts) should be avoided.

Geriatric Considerations When used in combination with ACE inhibitors, monitor patient for hyperkalemia.

Breast-Feeding Considerations The active metabolite of spironolactone has been found in breast milk. Effects to humans are not known; however, this metabolite was found to be carcinogenic in rats. The manufacturer recommends discontinuing spironolactone or using an alternative method of feeding.

Pregnancy Considerations Teratogenic effects were not observed in animal studies; however, doses used were less than or equal to equivalent doses in humans. The antiandrogen effects of spironolactone have been shown to cause feminization of the male fetus in animal studies. Two case reports did not demonstrate this effect in humans however, the authors caution that adequate data is lacking. Use of diuretics during normal pregnancies is not appropriate; use may be considered when edema is due to pathologic causes (as in the nonpregnant patient); monitor.

Additional Information Maximum diuretic effect may be delayed 2-3 days and maximum hypertensive effects may be delayed 2-3 weeks.

Related Information

Heart Failure (Systolic) *on page 2040*

- **Spironolactone and Hydrochlorothiazide** *see* Hydrochlorothiazide and Spironolactone *on page 914*
- **SPM 927** *see* Lacosamide *on page 1051*
- **Sporanox®** *see* Itraconazole *on page 1034*
- **SPP100** *see* Aliskiren *on page 71*
- **Sprintec®** *see* Ethinyl Estradiol and Norgestimate *on page 704*
- **SPS®** *see* Sodium Polystyrene Sulfonate *on page 1660*
- **SR33589** *see* Dronedarone *on page 591*
- **Sronyx®** *see* Ethinyl Estradiol and Levonorgestrel *on page 699*
- **SS734** *see* Besifloxacin *on page 204*
- **SSKI®** *see* Potassium Iodide *on page 1483*
- **Stadol** *see* Butorphanol *on page 263*
- **Stagesic™** *see* Hydrocodone and Acetaminophen *on page 915*
- **Stalevo®** *see* Levodopa, Carbidopa, and Entacapone *on page 1091*
- **Starlix®** *see* Nateglinide *on page 1293*

Stavudine (STAV yoo deen)

U.S. Brand Names Zerit®

Index Terms d4T

Generic Availability (U.S.) Yes: Capsule

Pharmacologic Category Antiretroviral Agent, Reverse Transcriptase Inhibitor (Nucleoside)

Medication Safety Issues

Sound-alike/look-alike issues:

Zerit® may be confused with Zestril®, Ziac®, ZyrTEC®

Medication Guide Available Yes

Pregnancy Risk Factor C

Lactation Excretion in breast milk unknown/contraindicated

Use Treatment of HIV infection in combination with other antiretroviral agents

Mechanism of Action/Effect Inhibits reverse transcriptase of the human immunodeficiency virus (HIV)

Contraindications Hypersensitivity to stavudine or any component of the formulation

Warnings/Precautions Use with caution in patients who demonstrate previous hypersensitivity to zidovudine, didanosine, zalcitabine, pre-existing bone marrow suppression, renal insufficiency (dosage adjustment recommended), hepatic impairment, or peripheral neuropathy. Peripheral neuropathy may be a treatment-limiting side effect; consider permanent discontinuation. Zidovudine should not be used in combination with stavudine. **[U.S. Boxed Warning]: Lactic acidosis and severe hepatomegaly with steatosis have been reported with stavudine use, including fatal cases;** combination therapy with didanosine may increase risk; use with caution in patients with risk factors for liver disease (although acidosis has occurred in patients without known risk factors, risk may be increased with female gender, obesity, pregnancy, or prolonged exposure). Suspend treatment in any patient who develops clinical or laboratory findings suggestive of lactic acidosis or hepatotoxicity. Severe motor weakness (resembling Guillain-Barré syndrome) has been reported (including fatal cases, usually in association with lactic acidosis); manufacturer recommends discontinuation if motor weakness develops (with or without lactic acidosis). May cause redistribution of fat (eg, buffalo hump, peripheral wasting with increased abdominal girth, cushingoid appearance). Patients may develop immune reconstitution syndrome resulting in the occurrence of an inflammatory response to an indolent or residual opportunistic infection; further evaluation and treatment may be required. **[U.S. Boxed Warning]: Pancreatitis (including some fatal cases) has occurred during combination therapy with didanosine.** Suspend stavudine and didanosine combination therapy, and any other agents toxic to the pancreas, in patients with suspected pancreatitis. If pancreatitis diagnosis confirmed, use extreme caution if reinitiating stavudine; monitor closely and do not use didanosine in regimen. Use with caution in combination with interferon alfa with or without ribavirin in HIV/HBV coinfected patients; monitor closely for hepatic decompensation, anemia, or neutropenia; dose reduction or discontinuation of interferon and/or ribavirin may be required if toxicity evident. Combination therapy with didanosine or hydroxyurea may increase risk of hepatotoxicity, pancreatitis, or severe peripheral neuropathy; avoid stavudine and hydroxyurea combination.

Drug Interactions

Avoid Concomitant Use

Avoid concomitant use of Stavudine with any of the following: Hydroxyurea; Zidovudine

Decreased Effect

The levels/effects of Stavudine may be decreased by: DOXOrubicin; DOXOrubicin (Liposomal); Zidovudine

Increased Effect/Toxicity

Stavudine may increase the levels/effects of: Didanosine; Hydroxyurea

The levels/effects of Stavudine may be increased by: Hydroxyurea; Ribavirin

Adverse Reactions Adverse reactions reported below represent experience with combination therapy with other nucleoside analogues and protease inhibitors.

>10%:

Central nervous system: Headache (25% to 46%)

Dermatologic: Rash (18% to 30%)

Gastrointestinal: Nausea (43% to 53%; less than comparator group), vomiting (18% to 30%; less than comparator group), diarrhea (34% to 45%)

Hepatic: Hyperbilirubinemia (65% to 68%; grade 3/4: 7% to 16%), AST increased (42% to 53%; grade 3/4: 5% to 7%), ALT increased (40% to 50%; grade 3/4: 6% to 8%), GGT increased (15% to 28%; grade 3/4: 2% to 5%)

Neuromuscular & skeletal: Peripheral neuropathy (8% to 21%)

Miscellaneous: Amylase increased (21% to 31%; grade 3/4: 4% to 8%), lipase increased (~27%; grade 3/4: 5% to 6%)

Pharmacodynamics/Kinetics

Bioavailability Children: 76.9%; Adults: 86.4%

Time to Peak Serum: 1 hour

Half-Life Elimination HIV-infected Children: 0.96 hours, HIV-infected Adults: 1.6 hours

Metabolism Undergoes intracellular phosphorylation to an active metabolite (stavudine triphosphate)

Excretion Urine 95% (74% as unchanged drug); feces 3% (62% as unchanged drug)

Available Dosage Forms

Capsule, oral: 15 mg, 20 mg, 30 mg, 40 mg

Zerit®: 15 mg, 20 mg, 30 mg, 40 mg

Powder for solution, oral:

Zerit®: 1 mg/mL (200 mL)

Dosing

Adult HIV infection (in combination with other antiretrovirals): Oral:

<60 kg: 30 mg every 12 hours

≥60 kg: 40 mg every 12 hours

Geriatric Older patients should be closely monitored for signs and symptoms of peripheral neuropathy. Dosage should be carefully adjusted to renal function.

Pediatric HIV infection: Oral:

Newborns (Birth to 13 days): 0.5 mg/kg every 12 hours

Children:

≥14 days and <30 kg: 1 mg/kg every 12 hours

≥30 kg: Refer to adult dosing.

Renal Impairment

Children: Specific recommendations not available. Reduction in dose or increase in dosing interval should be considered.

Adults:

Cl_{cr} >50 mL/minute:

<60 kg: 30 mg every 12 hours

≥60 kg: 40 mg every 12 hours

Cl_{cr} 26-50 mL/minute:

<60 kg: 15 mg every 12 hours

≥60 kg: 20 mg every 12 hours

Cl_{cr} 10-25 mL/minute, hemodialysis (administer dose after hemodialysis on day of dialysis):

<60 kg: 15 mg every 24 hours

≥60 kg: 20 mg every 24 hours

Administration

Oral May be administered without regard to meals. Oral solution should be shaken vigorously prior to use.

Stability

Reconstitution Reconstitute powder for oral suspension with 202 mL of purified water as specified on the bottle. Shake vigorously until suspended. Final suspension will be 1 mg/mL (200 mL).

Storage Capsules and powder for reconstitution may be stored at controlled room temperature of 25°C (77°F). Reconstituted oral solution should be stored in refrigerator at 2°C to 8°C (36°F to 46°F) and is stable for 30 days.

Monitoring and Teaching Issues

Laboratory Monitoring Liver function, renal function tests, viral load

Physical Assessment Assess closely for any previous allergy history prior to beginning treatment. Patient must be monitored frequently during therapy for peripheral neuropathy, lactic acidosis, hepatomegaly, and motor weakness; may require suspension of therapy. Assess decrease in infections, progression of disease, and viral load periodically during therapy. Teach patient proper timing of multiple medications.

Patient Education This drug will not cure HIV, nor has it been found to reduce transmission of HIV; use appropriate precautions to prevent spread to other persons. This drug is prescribed as one part of a multidrug combination; take exactly as directed, for full course of therapy. Maintain adequate hydration unless advised by prescriber to restrict fluids. Frequent blood tests may be required. May cause dizziness, weakness, nausea, or vomiting. Report immediately any tingling, pain, or loss of sensation in hands or feet; alterations in urinary pattern; swelling of extremities; or weight gain. If you are instructed to stop the medication, do not restart without specific instruction by your prescriber.

Dietary Considerations May be taken without regard to meals. Some products may contain sucrose.

Breast-Feeding Considerations In infants born to mothers who are HIV positive, HAART while breast-feeding may decrease postnatal infection. However, maternal or infant antiretroviral therapy does not completely eliminate the risk of postnatal HIV transmission. In addition, multiclass resistant virus has been detected in breast-feeding infants despite maternal therapy.

In the United States where formula is accessible, affordable, safe, and sustainable, complete avoidance of breast-feeding by HIV-infected women is recommended to decrease potential transmission of HIV.

Pregnancy Considerations Adverse events were observed in some animal reproduction studies. No increased risk of overall birth defects has been observed following first trimester exposure according to data collected by the antiretroviral pregnancy registry. Cases of lactic acidosis/hepatic steatosis syndrome related to mitochondrial toxicity have been reported in pregnant women receiving nucleoside analogues. It is not known if pregnancy itself potentiates this known side effect; however, women may be at increased risk of lactic acidosis and liver damage. In addition, these adverse events are similar to other rare but life-threatening syndromes which occur during pregnancy (eg, HELLP syndrome). Combination treatment with didanosine may also contribute to the risk of lactic acidosis, and should be considered only if benefit outweighs risk. Hepatic enzymes and electrolytes should be monitored frequently during the third trimester of pregnancy and clinicians should watch for early signs of the syndrome. Pharmacokinetics of stavudine are not significantly altered during pregnancy; dose adjustments are not needed. There are no adequate and well-controlled studies in pregnant women; however, the Perinatal HIV Guidelines Working Group considers stavudine to be an alternative NRTI in dual nucleoside combination regimens; use with didanosine only if no alternatives are available; do not use with zidovudine.

Healthcare providers are encouraged to enroll pregnant women exposed to antiretroviral medications in the Antiretroviral Pregnancy Registry (1-800-258-4263 or www.APRegistry.com). Healthcare providers caring for HIV-infected women and their infants may contact the National Perinatal HIV Hotline (888-448-8765) for clinical consultation.

Additional Information Potential compliance problems, frequency of administration and adverse effects should be discussed with patients before initiating therapy to help prevent the emergence of resistance.

◆ **Stavzor™** *see* Valproic Acid *on page 1832*

◆ **Staxyn™** *see* Vardenafil *on page 1846*

◆ **STI-571** *see* Imatinib *on page 951*

◆ **Stimate®** *see* Desmopressin *on page 493*

◆ **St Joseph® Adult Aspirin [OTC]** *see* Aspirin *on page 155*

◆ **Strattera®** *see* Atomoxetine *on page 164*

Streptozocin (strep toe ZOE sin)

U.S. Brand Names Zanosar®

Generic Availability (U.S.) No

Pharmacologic Category Antineoplastic Agent, Alkylating Agent

Medication Safety Issues

Sound-alike/look-alike issues:

Streptozocin may be confused with streptomycin

High alert medication: The Institute for Safe Medication Practices (ISMP) includes this medication among its list of drugs which have a heightened risk of causing significant patient harm when used in error.

Pregnancy Risk Factor D

Lactation Enters breast milk/contraindicated

Use Treatment of metastatic islet cell carcinoma of the pancreas

Unlabeled/Investigational Use Treatment of adrenal tumors

Available Dosage Forms

Injection, powder for reconstitution:

Zanosar®: 1 g

Dosing

Adult & Geriatric Antineoplastic: Refer to individual protocols.

Single agent therapy: I.V.: 1-1.5 g/m^2 weekly for 6 weeks followed by a 4-week rest period

Combination therapy: I.V.: 0.5-1 g/m^2 for 5 consecutive days followed by a 4- to 6-week rest period

Pediatric Refer to adult dosing.

Renal Impairment The FDA-approved labeling does not contain dosing adjustments; however, it is recommended to use clinical judgment weighing benefit vs risk of renal toxicity in patients with pre-existing renal impairment. The following dosing adjustments have been used by some clinicians (Aronoff, 2007): Adults:

Cl_{cr} 10-50 mL/minute: Administer 75% of dose

Cl_{cr} <10 mL/minute: Administer 50% of dose

Hepatic Impairment There are no specific guidelines on dosage adjustment in patients with hepatic impairment. Streptozocin is rapidly hepatically metabolized; dose should be decreased in patients with severe liver disease.

Administration

I.V. Administer as short (30-60 minutes) or 6-hour infusion; may be given by rapid I.V. push

Monitoring and Teaching Issues

Laboratory Monitoring Liver function tests, CBC, renal function tests (BUN, serum creatinine) at baseline and weekly during therapy

Physical Assessment Antiemetic should be administered prior to therapy (emetic potential 100%). Infusion site should be monitored closely to prevent extravasation. Monitor for nephrotoxicity/renal dysfunction (I & O, hematuria, edema, BUN), hepatotoxicity (jaundice, fatigue, LFTs), hypoglycemia, and diarrhea (dehydration) on a regular basis. Caution patients with diabetes to monitor glucose levels closely (may precipitate hypoglycemia).

Patient Education This drug can only be given I.V.; report immediately any redness, swelling, pain, or burning at infusion site. Maintain adequate hydration unless instructed to restrict fluid intake. You will be more sensitive to infection. If you have diabetes, monitor glucose levels closely; may cause hypoglycemia. May cause nausea and vomiting; nervousness, dizziness, confusion, or lethargy; or loss of body hair (reversible when treatment is finished). Report unusual back pain, change in urinary pattern; persistent fever, chills, or sore throat; unusual bleeding; blood in urine, vomitus, or stool; chest pain, palpitations, or respiratory difficulty; or swelling of feet or lower legs.

◆ **Striant®** *see* Testosterone *on page 1739*

◆ **Strong Iodine Solution** *see* Potassium Iodide and Iodine *on page 1484*

◆ **Suberoylanilide Hydroxamic Acid** *see* Vorinostat *on page 1875*

◆ **Sublimaze® [DSC]** *see* FentaNYL *on page 744*

◆ **Suboxone®** *see* Buprenorphine and Naloxone *on page 249*

◆ **Subutex®** *see* Buprenorphine *on page 246*

Succinylcholine (suks in il KOE leen)

U.S. Brand Names Anectine®; Quelicin®

Index Terms Succinylcholine Chloride; Suxamethonium Chloride

Generic Availability (U.S.) No

Pharmacologic Category Neuromuscular Blocker Agent, Depolarizing

Medication Safety Issues

International issues:

Quelicin [U.S., Brazil, Canada, Indonesia] may be confused with Keflin, a brand name for cefalotin [Argentina, Brazil, Mexico, Netherlands, Norway]

High alert medication: The Institute for Safe Medication Practices (ISMP) includes this medication among its list of drugs which have a heightened risk of causing significant patient harm when used in error.

United States Pharmacopeia (USP) 2006: The Interdisciplinary Safe Medication Use Expert Committee of the USP has recommended the following:

- Hospitals, clinics, and other practice sites should institute special safeguards in the storage, labeling, and use of these agents and should include these safeguards in staff orientation and competency training.
- Healthcare professionals should be on high alert (especially vigilant) whenever a neuromuscular-blocking agent (NMBA) is stocked, ordered, prepared, or administered.

Pregnancy Risk Factor C

Lactation Excretion in breast milk unknown/use caution

Use To facilitate both rapid sequence and routine endotracheal intubation and to relax skeletal muscles during surgery; to reduce the intensity of muscle contractions of pharmacologically- or electrically-induced convulsions; does not relieve pain or produce sedation

Available Dosage Forms

Injection, solution:

Anectine®: 20 mg/mL (10 mL)

Quelicin®: 20 mg/mL (10 mL)

Injection, solution [preservative free]:

Quelicin®: 100 mg/mL (10 mL)

Dosing

Adult & Geriatric Neuromuscular blockade: I.M., I.V.: Dose to effect; doses will vary due to interpatient variability; use total body weight for obese patients (Bentley, 1982; Brunette, 2004; Rose, 2000)

I.M.: Up to 3-4 mg/kg, total dose should not exceed 150 mg

I.V.: Initial:

Short surgical procedures: 0.6 mg/kg (range 0.3-1.1 mg/kg)

Long surgical procedures:

Continuous infusion: 2.5-4.3 mg/minute; adjust dose based on response

Intermittent: Initial: 0.3-1.1 mg/kg; maintenance: 0.04-0.07 mg/kg/dose as required

Note: Initial dose of succinylcholine must be increased when nondepolarizing agent pretreatment used because of the antagonism between succinylcholine and nondepolarizing neuromuscular-blocking agents.

Dose adjustment with reduced plasma cholinesterase activity: Administer a test dose of 5-10 mg to evaluate sensitivity, or cautiously administer 1 mg/mL by slow I.V. infusion to produce neuromuscular blockade

Pediatric Neuromuscular blockade: I.M., I.V.: Dose to effect; doses will vary due to interpatient variability; use total body weight for obese patients (Bentley, 1982; Brunette, 2004; Rose, 2000)

I.M.: Children: Refer to adult dosing.

I.V.: Children: **Note:** Because of the risk of malignant hyperthermia, use of continuous infusions is not recommended in infants and children

Smaller Children: Intermittent: Initial: 2 mg/kg/dose one time; maintenance: 0.3-0.6 mg/kg/dose every 5-10 minutes as needed

Older Children and Adolescents: Intermittent: Initial: 1 mg/kg/dose one time; maintenance: 0.3-0.6 mg/kg every 5-10 minutes as needed

Note: Initial dose of succinylcholine must be increased when nondepolarizing agent pretreatment used because of the antagonism between succinylcholine and nondepolarizing neuromuscular-blocking agents.

Hepatic Impairment Dose should be reduced in patients with severe liver disease.

Administration

I.M. I.M. injections should be made deeply, preferably high into deltoid muscle. Use only when I.V. access is not available.

I.V. May be given by rapid I.V. injection without further dilution.

Monitoring and Teaching Issues

Laboratory Monitoring Serum potassium and calcium

Physical Assessment Dosage and rate of administration should be individualized and titrated to the desired effect, according to relevant clinical factors, premedication, concomitant medications, age, and general condition of patient. Ventilatory support must be instituted and maintained until adequate respiratory muscle function and/or airway protection are assured. This drug is not an anesthetic or analgesic; pain must be treated with appropriate agents. Continuous monitoring of vital signs, cardiac status, respiratory status, and degree of neuromuscular block (objective assessment with external nerve stimulator) is mandatory during infusion and until full muscle tone has returned. Safety precautions regarding ventilation must be maintained until full muscle tone has returned.

Patient Education Patient will usually be unconscious prior to administration. Reassurance of constant monitoring and emotional support to reduce fear and anxiety should precede and follow administration. Following return of muscle tone, do not attempt to change position or rise from bed without assistance. Report immediately any skin rash or hives, pounding heartbeat, respiratory difficulty, or muscle tremors.

◆ **Succinylcholine Chloride** *see* Succinylcholine *on page* 1683

Sucralfate (soo KRAL fate)

U.S. Brand Names Carafate®

Index Terms Aluminum Sucrose Sulfate, Basic

Generic Availability (U.S.) Yes

Pharmacologic Category Gastrointestinal Agent, Miscellaneous

Medication Safety Issues

Sound-alike/look-alike issues:

Sucralfate may be confused with salsalate

Carafate® may be confused with Cafergot®

Pregnancy Risk Factor B

Lactation Excretion in breast milk unknown/use caution

Use Short-term (≤8 weeks) management of duodenal ulcers; maintenance therapy for duodenal ulcers

Unlabeled/Investigational Use Gastric ulcers; suspension may be used topically for treatment of stomatitis due to cancer chemotherapy and other causes of esophageal and gastric erosions; GERD, esophagitis; treatment of NSAID mucosal damage; prevention of stress ulcers; postsclerotherapy for esophageal variceal bleeding

Available Dosage Forms

Suspension, oral: 1 g/10 mL (10 mL)

Carafate®: 1 g/10 mL (420 mL)

Tablet, oral: 1 g

Carafate®: 1 g

Dosing

Adult & Geriatric

Stress ulcer prophylaxis (unlabeled use): Oral: 1 g 4 times/day

Stress ulcer treatment (unlabeled use): Oral: 1 g every 4 hours

Treatment of duodenal ulcer: Oral:

Initial treatment: 1 g 4 times/day, 1 hour before meals or food and at bedtime for 4-8 weeks, or alternatively 2 g twice daily; treatment is recommended for 4-8 weeks in adults

Maintenance/prophylaxis of duodenal ulcer: 1 g twice daily

Stomatitis (unlabeled use): Oral: 10 mL (1 g/10 mL suspension); swish and spit or swish and swallow 4 times/day.

Pediatric Doses of 40-80 mg/kg/day divided every 6 hours have been used

Stomatitis (unlabeled use): Oral: Children: 5-10 mL (1 g/10 mL suspension), swish and spit or swish and swallow 4 times/day

Renal Impairment Aluminum salt is minimally absorbed (<5%), however, may accumulate in renal failure.

Administration

Oral Tablet may be broken or dissolved in water before ingestion. Administer with water on an empty stomach.

Monitoring and Teaching Issues

Physical Assessment Use caution in presence of renal failure. Teach patient proper timing of other medications. May cause constipation.

Patient Education Take recommended dose with water on an empty stomach, 1 hour before or 2 hours after meals. Take any other medications at least 2 hours before taking sucralfate. May cause constipation. If constipation persists, consult prescriber for stool softener.

- ◆ **Sudafed** *see* Pseudoephedrine *on page 1529*
- ◆ **Sudafed® 12 Hour [OTC]** *see* Pseudoephedrine *on page 1529*
- ◆ **Sudafed® 24 Hour [OTC]** *see* Pseudoephedrine *on page 1529*
- ◆ **Sudafed® Children's [OTC]** *see* Pseudoephedrine *on page 1529*
- ◆ **Sudafed® Maximum Strength Nasal Decongestant [OTC]** *see* Pseudoephedrine *on page 1529*
- ◆ **Sudafed PE® Children's [OTC]** *see* Phenylephrine (Systemic) *on page 1449*
- ◆ **Sudafed PE® Congestion [OTC]** *see* Phenylephrine (Systemic) *on page 1449*
- ◆ **Sudafed PE™ Nasal Decongestant [OTC]** *see* Phenylephrine (Systemic) *on page 1449*
- ◆ **SudoGest [OTC]** *see* Pseudoephedrine *on page 1529*
- ◆ **Sudogest 12 Hour [OTC]** *see* Pseudoephedrine *on page 1529*
- ◆ **SudoGest Children's [OTC]** *see* Pseudoephedrine *on page 1529*
- ◆ **Sudogest™ PE [OTC]** *see* Phenylephrine (Systemic) *on page 1449*
- ◆ **Sudo-Tab® [OTC]** *see* Pseudoephedrine *on page 1529*
- ◆ **Sular®** *see* Nisoldipine *on page 1322*
- ◆ **Sulbactam and Ampicillin** *see* Ampicillin and Sulbactam *on page 127*

SulfADIAZINE (sul fa DYE a zeen)

Generic Availability (U.S.) Yes

Pharmacologic Category Antibiotic, Sulfonamide Derivative

Medication Safety Issues

Sound-alike/look-alike issues:

SulfADIAZINE may be confused with sulfaSALAzine

Pregnancy Risk Factor C

Lactation Enters breast milk/contraindicated

Use Treatment of urinary tract infections and nocardiosis; adjunctive treatment in toxoplasmosis; uncomplicated attack of malaria

Unlabeled/Investigational Use Rheumatic fever prophylaxis

Available Dosage Forms

Tablet, oral: 500 mg

Dosing

Adult & Geriatric

Toxoplasmosis: Oral: 2-6 g/day divided every 6 hours in conjunction with pyrimethamine 50-75 mg/day and with supplemental leucovorin calcium

Asymptomatic meningococcal carriers: 1 g twice daily for 2 days

Nocardiosis: 4-8 g/day for a minimum of 6 weeks

Prevention of recurrent attacks of rheumatic fever (unlabeled use): 1 g/day

Pediatric

Congenital toxoplasmosis: Oral:

Newborns and Children <2 months: 100 mg/kg/day divided every 6 hours in conjunction with pyrimethamine 1 mg/kg/day once daily and supplemental leucovorin calcium 5 mg every 3 days for 6 months

Children >2 months: 25-50 mg/kg/dose 4 times/day

Toxoplasmosis: Oral: Children >2 months: Loading dose: 75 mg/kg; maintenance dose: 120-150 mg/kg/day, maximum dose: 6 g/day; divided every 4-6 hours in conjunction with pyrimethamine 2 mg/kg/day divided every 12 hours for 3 days followed by 1 mg/kg/day once daily with supplemental leucovorin calcium

Secondary prophylaxis of toxoplasmosis in HIV-exposed/-positive patients (unlabeled use: CDC, 2009): Oral: Infants and Children: 85-120 mg/kg/day divided every 6-12 hours (maximum: 4 g/day) plus pyrimethamine and leucovorin calcium

Prevention of recurrent attacks of rheumatic fever (unlabeled use): Oral: <30 kg: 0.5 g/day; >30 kg: 1 g/day

Administration

Oral Tablets may be crushed to prepare oral suspension of the drug in water or with a sucrose-containing solution. Aqueous suspension with concentrations of 100 mg/mL should be stored in the refrigerator and used within 7 days. Administer around-the-clock to promote less variation in peak and trough serum levels.

Monitoring and Teaching Issues

Laboratory Monitoring Perform culture and sensitivity prior to initiating therapy.

Physical Assessment Assess for allergy history prior to starting therapy (sulfonamides). Monitor for rash, photosensitivity, gastrointestinal disturbance (nausea, vomiting, anorexia), anemia, jaundice, and hematuria.

Patient Education Inform prescriber of any allergies you have. Take as directed at regular intervals around-the-clock. Take on an empty stomach, 1 hour before or 2 hours after meals with full glass of water. Avoid large quantities of vitamin C. Maintain adequate hydration to prevent kidney damage, unless instructed to restrict fluid intake. May cause dizziness, headache, photosensitivity, nausea, vomiting, or loss of appetite. Report skin rash, persistent nausea, vomiting, diarrhea, opportunistic infection (sore throat, fever, vaginal itching or discharge, unusual bruising or bleeding, fatigue), blood in urine or change in urinary pattern, persistent headache, abdominal pain, or respiratory difficulty.

Sulfamethoxazole and Trimethoprim

(sul fa meth OKS a zole & trye METH oh prim)

U.S. Brand Names Bactrim™; Bactrim™ DS; Septra® DS; Septra® [DSC]; Sulfatrim®

Index Terms Co-Trimoxazole; SMX-TMP; SMZ-TMP; Sulfatrim; TMP-SMX; TMP-SMZ; Trimethoprim and Sulfamethoxazole

Generic Availability (U.S.) Yes

Pharmacologic Category Antibiotic, Miscellaneous; Antibiotic, Sulfonamide Derivative

Medication Safety Issues

Sound-alike/look-alike issues:

Bactrim™ may be confused with bacitracin, Bactine®, Bactroban®
Co-trimoxazole may be confused with clotrimazole
Septra® may be confused with Ceptaz®, Sectral®
Septra® DS may be confused with Semprex®-D

Pregnancy Risk Factor C

Lactation Enters breast milk/contraindicated (AAP rates "compatible"; AAP 2001 update pending)

Use

Oral treatment of urinary tract infections due to *E. coli*, *Klebsiella* and *Enterobacter* sp, *M. morganii*, *P. mirabilis* and *P. vulgaris*; acute otitis media in children; acute exacerbations of chronic bronchitis in adults due to susceptible strains of *H. influenzae* or *S. pneumoniae*; treatment and prophylaxis of *Pneumocystis jiroveci* pneumonitis (PCP); traveler's diarrhea due to enterotoxigenic *E. coli*; treatment of enteritis caused by *Shigella flexneri* or *Shigella sonnei*

I.V. treatment of severe or complicated infections when oral therapy is not feasible, for documented PCP, empiric treatment of PCP in immune compromised patients; treatment of documented or suspected shigellosis, typhoid fever, *Nocardia asteroides* infection, or other infections caused by susceptible bacteria

Unlabeled/Investigational Use Cholera and *Salmonella*-type infections and nocardiosis; chronic prostatitis; as prophylaxis in neutropenic patients with *P. jiroveci* infections, in leukemia patients, and in patients following renal transplantation, to decrease incidence of PCP; treatment of *Cyclospora* infection, typhoid fever, *Nocardia asteroides* infection; prophylaxis against urinary tract infection; alternative treatment for MRSA infections

Available Dosage Forms The 5:1 ratio (SMX:TMP) remains constant in all dosage forms.

Injection, solution: Sulfamethoxazole 80 mg and trimethoprim 16 mg per mL (5 mL, 10 mL, 30 mL)

Suspension, oral: Sulfamethoxazole 200 mg and trimethoprim 40 mg per 5 mL
Sulfatrim®: Sulfamethoxazole 200 mg and trimethoprim 40 mg per 5 mL

Tablet: Sulfamethoxazole 400 mg and trimethoprim 80 mg
Bactrim™: Sulfamethoxazole 400 mg and trimethoprim 80 mg

Tablet, double-strength: Sulfamethoxazole 800 mg and trimethoprim 160 mg
Bactrim™ DS, Septra® DS: Sulfamethoxazole 800 mg and trimethoprim 160 mg

Dosing

Adult & Geriatric Dosage recommendations are based on the trimethoprim component. double-strength tablets are equivalent to sulfamethoxazole 800 mg and trimethoprim 160 mg.

General dosing guidelines:

Oral: 1-2 double-strength tablets (sulfamethoxazole 800 mg; trimethoprim 160 mg) every 12-24 hours

I.V.: 8-20 mg TMP/kg/day divided every 6-12 hours

Chronic bronchitis (acute): Oral: One double-strength tablet every 12 hours for 10-14 days

Cyclosporiasis (unlabeled use): Oral, I.V.: 160 mg TMP twice daily for 7-10 days. **Note:** AIDS patients: Oral: One double-strength tablet 2-4 times/day for 10 days, then 1 double-strength tablet 3 times/week for 10 weeks (Pape, 1994; Verdier, 2000).

Granuloma inguinale (donovanosis) (unlabeled use): Oral: One double-strength tablet every 12 hours for at least 3 weeks and until lesions have healed (CDC, 2010)

Meningitis (bacterial): I.V.: 10-20 mg TMP/kg/day in divided doses every 6-12 hours

Nocardia (unlabeled use): Oral, I.V.:

Cutaneous infections: 5-10 mg TMP/kg/day in 2-4 divided doses

Severe infections (pulmonary/cerebral): 15 mg TMP/kg/day in 2-4 divided doses for 3-4 weeks, then 10 mg TMP/kg/day in 2-4 divided doses. Treatment duration is controversial; an average of 7 months has been reported.

Note: Therapy for severe infection may be initiated I.V. and converted to oral therapy (frequently converted to approximate dosages of oral solid dosage forms: 2 DS tablets every 8-12 hours). Although not widely available, sulfonamide levels should be considered in patients with questionable absorption, at risk for dose-related toxicity, or those with poor therapeutic response.

Osteomyelitis due to MRSA (unlabeled use): Oral, I.V.: 3.5-4 mg TMP/kg/dose every 8-12 hours for a minimum of 8 weeks with rifampin 600 mg once daily (Liu, 2011)

***Pneumocystis jirovecii*:**

Prophylaxis: Oral: One double-strength tablet daily or 3 times/week

Treatment: Oral, I.V.: 15-20 mg TMP/kg/day in 3-4 divided doses

Sepsis: I.V.: 20 TMP/kg/day divided every 6 hours

Septic arthritis due to MRSA (unlabeled use): Oral, I.V.: 3.5-4 mg TMP/kg/dose every 8-12 hours for 3-4 weeks (some experts combine with rifampin) (Liu, 2011)

Shigellosis:

Oral: One double-strength tablet every 12 hours for 5 days

I.V.: 8-10 mg TMP/kg/day in divided doses every 6, 8, or 12 hours for up to 5 days

Skin/soft tissue infection due to community-acquired MRSA (unlabeled use): Oral: 1-2 double-strength tablets every 12 hours for 5-10 days (Liu, 2011); **Note:** If beta-hemolytic *Streptococcus* spp are also suspected, a beta-lactam antibiotic should be added to the regimen (Liu, 2011)

Stenotrophomonas maltophilia **(ventilator-associated pneumonia):** I.V.: Most clinicians have utilized 12-15 mg TMP/kg/day for the treatment of VAP caused by *Stenotrophomonas maltophilia*. Higher doses (up to 20 mg TMP/kg/day) have been mentioned for treatment of severe infection in patients with normal renal function (Vartivarian, 1989; Looney, 2009; Wood, 2010)

Travelers' diarrhea: Oral: One double-strength tablet every 12 hours for 5 days

Urinary tract infection:

Oral: One double-strength tablet every 12 hours

Duration of therapy: Uncomplicated: 3-5 days; Complicated: 7-10 days

Pyelonephritis: 14 days

Prostatitis: Acute: 2 weeks; Chronic: 2-3 months

I.V.: 8-10 mg TMP/kg/day in divided doses every 6, 8, or 12 hours for up to 14 days with severe infections

Pediatric Recommendations are based on the trimethoprim component.

General dosing guidelines: Children >2 months:

Mild-to-moderate infections: Oral: 8-12 mg TMP/kg/day in divided doses every 12 hours

Serious infection:

Oral: 20 mg TMP/kg/day in divided doses every 6 hours

I.V.: 8-12 mg TMP/kg/day in divided doses every 6 hours

Acute otitis media: Oral: 8 mg TMP/kg/day in divided doses every 12 hours for 10 days. **Note:** Recommended by the American Academy of Pediatrics as an alternative agent in penicillin allergic patients at a dose of 6-10mg TMP/kg/day (AOM guidelines, 2004).

Cyclosporiasis (unlabeled use): Oral, I.V.: 5 mg TMP/kg twice daily for 7-10 days

***Pneumocystis*:**

Treatment: Oral, I.V.: 15-20 mg TMP/kg/day in divided doses every 6-8 hours for 21 days

Prophylaxis: Oral: 150 mg TMP/m^2/day in divided doses every 12 hours and administered for 3 days/week on consecutive or alternate days; an alternative dosing regimen allows for same dose to be administered in 2 divided doses daily (maximum: trimethoprim 320 mg and sulfamethoxazole 1600 mg daily) (CDC, 2009)

Shigellosis:

Oral: 8 mg TMP/kg/day in divided doses every 12 hours for 5 days

I.V.: 8-10 mg TMP/kg/day in divided doses every 6, 8, or 12 hours for up to 5 days

Skin/soft tissue infection due to community-acquired MRSA (unlabeled use): Oral: 4-6 mg TMP/kg/dose every 12 hours for 5-10 days (Liu, 2011); **Note:** If beta-hemolytic *Streptococcus* spp are also suspected, a beta-lactam antibiotic should be added to the regimen (Liu, 2011)

Toxoplasmosis primary prophylaxis (HIV-exposed/infected): Oral: 150 mg TMP/m^2/day in 2 divided doses (CDC, 2009)

Urinary tract infection:

Treatment:

Oral: 6-12 mg TMP/kg/day in divided doses every 12 hours

I.V.: 8-10 mg TMP/kg/day in divided doses every 6, 8, or 12 hours for up to 14 days with serious infections

Prophylaxis: Oral: 2 mg TMP/kg/dose daily or 5 mg TMP/kg/dose twice weekly

Renal Impairment Oral, I.V.:

Manufacturer's recommendation: Children and Adults:

Cl_{cr} 15-30 mL/minute: Administer 50% of recommended dose

Cl_{cr} <15 mL/minute: Use is not recommended

Alternate recommendations:

Cl_{cr} 15-30 mL/minute:

Treatment: Administer full daily dose (divided every 12 hours) for 24-48 hours, then decrease daily dose by 50% and administer every 24 hours (**Note:** For serious infections including *Pneumocystis jiroveci* pneumonia (PCP), full daily dose is given in divided doses every 6-8 hours for 2 days, followed by reduction to 50% daily dose divided every 12 hours) (Nahata, 1995).

PCP prophylaxis: One-half single-strength tablet (40 mg trimethoprim) daily **or** 1 single-strength tablet (80 mg trimethoprim) daily or 3 times weekly (Masur, 2002).

Cl_{cr} <15 mL/minute:

Treatment: Administer full daily dose every 48 hours (Nahata, 1995)

PCP prophylaxis: One-half single-strength tablet (40 mg trimethoprim) daily **or** 1 single-strength tablet (80 mg trimethoprim) 3 times weekly (Masur, 2002). While the guidelines do acknowledge the alternative of giving 1 single-strength tablet daily, this may be inadvisable in the uremic/ESRD patient.

Hemodialysis:

Treatment: Full daily dose before dialysis and 50% dose after dialysis (Nahata, 1995)

Children: GFR <10 mL/minute/1.73 m^2: Not recommended, but if required 5-10 mg TMP/kg every 24 hours (Arnoff, 2007)

PCP prophylaxis: One single-strength tablet (80 mg trimethoprim) after each dialysis session (Masur, 2002)

CAPD:

Use Cl_{cr} <15 mL/minute dosing recommendations. Not significantly removed by CAPD; supplemental dosing is not required (Aronoff, 2007):

Exit-site and tunnel infections: Oral: One single-strength tablet daily (Li, 2010)

Peritonitis: Oral: One double-strength tablet twice daily (Li, 2010)

Children: GFR <10 mL/minute/1.73 m^2: Not recommended, but if required 5-10 mg TMP/kg every 24 hours. Intraperitoneal: Loading dose: TMP-SMX 320/1600 mg/L; Maintenance: TMP-SMX 80/400 mg/L (Arnoff, 2007; Warady, 2000)

CRRT: 2.5-10 mg TMP/kg/dose every 12 hours (Heintz, 2009)

Administration

Oral Administer without regard to meals. Administer with at least 8 ounces of water.

I.V. Infuse over 60-90 minutes, must dilute well before giving (ie, 1:15 to 1:25, which equates to 5 mL of drug solution diluted in 75-125 mL base solution).

Monitoring and Teaching Issues

Laboratory Monitoring Perform culture and sensitivity testing prior to initiating therapy; CBC, serum potassium, creatinine, BUN

Physical Assessment See individual agents.

Patient Education See individual agents.

Related Information

Antimicrobial Drugs of Choice *on page 2008*

I.V. to Oral Conversion *on page 1956*

Trimethoprim *on page 1820*

Sulfasalazine (sul fa SAL a zeen)

U.S. Brand Names Azulfidine EN-tabs®; Azulfidine®

Index Terms Salicylazosulfapyridine

Generic Availability (U.S.) Yes

Pharmacologic Category 5-Aminosalicylic Acid Derivative

Medication Safety Issues

Sound-alike/look-alike issues:

SulfaSALAzine may be confused with salsalate, sulfADIAZINE, sulfiSOXAZOLE

Azulfidine® may be confused with Augmentin®, azaTHIOprine

Pregnancy Risk Factor B

Lactation Enters breast milk/use caution (AAP recommends use "with caution"; AAP 2001 update pending)

Use Treatment of mild-to-moderate ulcerative colitis or as adjunctive therapy in severe ulcerative colitis; enteric coated tablets are also used for rheumatoid arthritis (including juvenile idiopathic arthritis [JIA]) in patients who inadequately respond to analgesics and NSAIDs

Unlabeled/Investigational Use Ankylosing spondylitis, Crohn's disease, psoriasis, psoriatic arthritis

Available Dosage Forms

Tablet, oral: 500 mg

Azulfidine®: 500 mg

Tablet, delayed release, enteric coated, oral: 500 mg

Azulfidine EN-tabs®: 500 mg

Dosing

Adult & Geriatric

Ulcerative colitis: Oral:

Initial: 3-4 g/day in evenly divided doses at ≤8-hour intervals. **Note:** American College of Gastroenterology guideline recommendations: Titrate to 4-6 g/day in 4 divided doses (Kornbluth, 2010).

Maintenance dose: 2 g/day in evenly divided doses at ≤8-hour intervals; may initiate therapy with 1-2 g/day to reduce GI intolerance

Rheumatoid arthritis: Oral (enteric coated tablet): Initial: 0.5-1 g/day; increase weekly to maintenance dose of 2 g/day in 2 divided doses; maximum: 3 g/day (if response to 2 g/day is inadequate after 12 weeks of treatment)

Pediatric

Ulcerative colitis: Oral: Children ≥6 years: Initial: 40-60 mg/kg/day in 3-6 divided doses; maintenance dose: 30 mg/kg/day in 4 divided doses

Juvenile idiopathic arthritis (JIA): Oral (enteric coated tablet): Children ≥6 years: 30-50 mg/kg/day in 2 divided doses; Initial: Begin with 1/4 to 1/3 of expected maintenance dose; increase weekly; maximum: 2 g/day typically

Renal Impairment Use not recommended; weigh risk vs benefit.

Hepatic Impairment Use not recommended; weigh risk vs benefit.

Administration

Oral GI intolerance is common during the first few days of therapy (give with meals). Do not crush enteric coated tablets.

Monitoring and Teaching Issues

Laboratory Monitoring CBC with differential and liver function tests (prior to therapy, then every other week for first 3 months of therapy, followed by every month for the second 3 months, then once every 3 months thereafter); periodic urinalysis and renal function tests

Physical Assessment Assess for use-related cautions and allergy history prior to starting therapy (sulfa drugs, salicylates). Monitor for blood dyscrasias, photosensitivity, gastrointestinal disturbance, anemia, jaundice, hematuria, or CNS changes.

Patient Education Take with food, at regular intervals. Do not crush, chew, or dissolve coated tablets. Maintain adequate hydration to prevent kidney damage, unless instructed to restrict fluid intake. May cause dizziness, headache, nausea, vomiting, or loss of appetite. Report rash; persistent nausea, vomiting, diarrhea, or GI pain; opportunistic infection (sore throat, fever, vaginal itching or discharge, unusual bruising or bleeding, fatigue); blood in urine or change in urinary pattern; swelling of face, lips, or tongue; or tightness in chest, bad cough, or blue skin color.

◆ **Sulfatrim** *see* Sulfamethoxazole and Trimethoprim *on page 1686*

◆ **Sulfatrim®** *see* Sulfamethoxazole and Trimethoprim *on page 1686*

Sulindac (SUL in dak)

U.S. Brand Names Clinoril®

Generic Availability (U.S.) Yes

Pharmacologic Category Nonsteroidal Anti-inflammatory Drug (NSAID), Oral

Medication Safety Issues

Sound-alike/look-alike issues:

Clinoril® may be confused with Cleocin®, Clozaril®

Medication Guide Available Yes

Pregnancy Risk Factor C

Lactation Excretion in breast milk unknown/not recommended

Use Management of inflammatory diseases including osteoarthritis, rheumatoid arthritis, acute gouty arthritis, ankylosing spondylitis, acute painful shoulder (bursitis/tendonitis)

Unlabeled/Investigational Use Management of preterm labor

Mechanism of Action/Effect Reversibly inhibits cyclooxygenase-1 and 2 (COX-1 and 2) enzymes, which results in decreased formation of prostaglandin precursors; has antipyretic, analgesic, and anti-inflammatory properties

Contraindications Hypersensitivity or allergic-type reactions to sulindac, aspirin, other NSAIDs, or any component of the formulation; perioperative pain in the setting of coronary artery bypass graft (CABG) surgery

Warnings/Precautions [U.S. Boxed Warning]: NSAIDs are associated with an increased risk of adverse cardiovascular thrombotic events, including MI and stroke. Use caution with fluid retention. Avoid use in heart failure. Concurrent administration of ibuprofen, and potentially other nonselective NSAIDs, may interfere with aspirin's cardioprotective effect. May cause new-onset hypertension or worsening of existing hypertension. NSAID use may compromise existing renal function; dose-dependent decreases in prostaglandin synthesis may result from NSAID use, reducing renal blood flow which may cause renal decompensation. NSAID use may increase the risk for hyperkalemia. Patients with impaired renal function, dehydration, heart failure, liver dysfunction, those taking diuretics, and ACE inhibitors, and the elderly are at greater risk of renal toxicity and hyperkalemia. Rehydrate patient before starting therapy; monitor renal function closely. Not recommended for use in patients with advanced renal disease. Long-term NSAID use may result in renal papillary necrosis. Use caution in patients with renal lithiasis; sulindac metabolites have been reported as components of renal stones. Maintain adequate hydration in patients with a history of renal stones. Use with caution in patients with decreased hepatic function. May require dosage adjustment in hepatic dysfunction; sulfide and sulfone metabolites may accumulate. The elderly are at increased risk for adverse effects. **[U.S. Boxed Warning]: Use is contraindicated for treatment of perioperative pain in the setting of coronary artery bypass graft (CABG) surgery.** Risk of MI and stroke may be increased with use following CABG surgery.

[U.S. Boxed Warning]: NSAIDs may increase risk of gastrointestinal irritation, inflammation, ulceration, bleeding, and perforation. Use the lowest effective dose for the shortest duration of time, consistent with individual patient goals, to reduce risk of cardiovascular or GI adverse events. When used concomitantly with ≤325 mg of aspirin, a substantial increase in the risk of gastrointestinal complications (eg, ulcer) occurs; concomitant gastroprotective therapy (eg, proton pump inhibitors) is recommended (Bhatt, 2008). Pancreatitis has been reported; discontinue with suspected pancreatitis.

NSAIDS may cause drowsiness, dizziness, blurred vision and other neurologic effects which may impair physical or mental abilities; patients must be cautioned about performing tasks which require mental alertness (eg, operating machinery or driving). Discontinue use with blurred or diminished vision and perform ophthalmologic exam. Monitor vision with long-term therapy.

Platelet adhesion and aggregation may be decreased, may prolong bleeding time; patients with coagulation disorders or who are receiving anticoagulants should be monitored closely. Anemia may occur; patients on long-term NSAID therapy should be monitored for anemia. Rarely, NSAID use may cause severe blood dyscrasias (eg, agranulocytosis, aplastic anemia, thrombocytopenia). NSAIDs may cause serious skin adverse events including exfoliative dermatitis, Stevens-Johnson syndrome (SJS) and toxic epidermal necrolysis (TEN); discontinue use at first sign of skin rash or hypersensitivity. Anaphylactoid reactions may occur. Do not use in patients who experience bronchospasm, asthma, rhinitis, or urticaria with NSAID or aspirin therapy. Use caution in other forms of asthma. May increase the risk of aseptic meningitis, especially in patients with systemic lupus erythematosus (SLE) and mixed connective tissue disorders.

Withhold for at least 4-6 half-lives prior to surgical or dental procedures.

Drug Interactions

Avoid Concomitant Use

Avoid concomitant use of Sulindac with any of the following: Ketorolac; Ketorolac (Systemic)

Decreased Effect

Sulindac may decrease the levels/effects of: ACE Inhibitors; Angiotensin II Receptor Blockers; Antiplatelet Agents; Beta-Blockers; Eplerenone; HydrALAZINE; Loop Diuretics; Potassium-Sparing Diuretics; Salicylates; Thiazide Diuretics

The levels/effects of Sulindac may be decreased by: Bile Acid Sequestrants; Nonsteroidal Anti-Inflammatory Agents; Salicylates

Increased Effect/Toxicity

Sulindac may increase the levels/effects of: Aminoglycosides; Anticoagulants; Antiplatelet Agents; Bisphosphonate Derivatives; Collagenase (Systemic); CycloSPORINE; CycloSPORINE (Systemic); Desmopressin; Digoxin; Drotrecogin Alfa; Eplerenone; Haloperidol; Ibritumomab; Methotrexate; Nonsteroidal Anti-Inflammatory Agents; PEMEtrexed; Potassium-Sparing Diuretics; PRALAtrexate; Quinolone Antibiotics; Salicylates; Thrombolytic Agents; Tositumomab and Iodine I 131 Tositumomab; Vancomycin; Vitamin K Antagonists

The levels/effects of Sulindac may be increased by: Antidepressants (Tricyclic, Tertiary Amine); Corticosteroids (Systemic); Dasatinib; Dimethyl Sulfoxide; Glucosamine; Herbs (Anticoagulant/Antiplatelet Properties); Ketorolac; Ketorolac (Systemic); Nonsteroidal Anti-Inflammatory Agents; Omega-3-Acid Ethyl Esters; Pentosan Polysulfate Sodium; Pentoxifylline; Probenecid; Prostacyclin Analogues; Selective Serotonin Reuptake Inhibitors; Serotonin/Norepinephrine Reuptake Inhibitors; Treprostinil

Nutritional/Ethanol Interactions

Ethanol: Avoid ethanol (may enhance gastric mucosal irritation).

Herb/Nutraceutical: Avoid alfalfa, anise, bilberry, bladderwrack, bromelain, cat's claw, celery, chamomile, coleus, cordyceps, dong quai, evening primrose, fenugreek, feverfew, garlic, ginger, ginkgo biloba, ginseng (American, Panax, Siberian), grapeseed, green tea, guggul, horse chestnut seed, horseradish, licorice, prickly ash, red clover, reishi, SAMe (S-adenosylmethionine), sweet clover, turmeric, white willow (all have additional antiplatelet activity).

Lab Interactions Increased chloride (S), sodium (S), bleeding time

Adverse Reactions 1% to 10%:

Cardiovascular: Edema (1% to 3%)

Central nervous system: Dizziness (3% to 9%), headache (3% to 9%), nervousness (1% to 3%)

Dermatologic: Rash (3% to 9%), pruritus (1% to 3%)

Gastrointestinal: GI pain (10%), constipation (3% to 9%), diarrhea (3% to 9%), dyspepsia (3% to 9%), nausea (3% to 9%), abdominal cramps (1% to 3%), anorexia (1% to 3%), flatulence (1% to 3%), vomiting (1% to 3%)

Otic: Tinnitus (1% to 3%)

Pharmacodynamics/Kinetics

Absorption 90%

Time to Peak Sulindac: 3-4 hours; Sulfide and sulfone metabolites: 5-6 hours

Protein Binding Sulindac: 93%, sulfone metabolite: 95%, sulfide metabolite: 98%; primarily to albumin

Half-Life Elimination Sulindac: ~8 hours; Sulfide metabolite: ~16 hours

Metabolism Hepatic; prodrug metabolized to sulfide metabolite (active) for therapeutic effects and to sulfone metabolites (inactive); parent and inactive sulfone metabolite undergo extensive enterohepatic recirculation

Excretion Urine (~50%, primarily as inactive metabolites, <1% as active metabolite); feces (~25%, primarily as metabolites)

Available Dosage Forms

Tablet, oral: 150 mg, 200 mg

Clinoril®: 200 mg

Dosing

Adult & Geriatric Note: Maximum daily dose: 400 mg

Osteoarthritis, rheumatoid arthritis, ankylosing spondylitis: 150 mg twice daily

Acute painful shoulder (bursitis/tendonitis): 200 mg twice daily; usual treatment: 7-14 days

Acute gouty arthritis: 200 mg twice daily; usual treatment: 7 days

Pediatric Dose not established

Renal Impairment Not recommended with advanced renal impairment; if required, decrease dose and monitor closely.

Hepatic Impairment Dose reduction is necessary; discontinue if abnormal liver function tests occur.

Administration

Oral Should be administered with food or milk.

Stability

Storage Store at room temperature of 15°C to 30°C (59°F to 86°F).

Monitoring and Teaching Issues

Laboratory Monitoring Liver enzymes, BUN, serum creatinine, CBC, platelets

Physical Assessment Evaluate cardiac risk and potential for GI bleeding prior to prescribing this medication. Monitor blood pressure at the beginning of therapy and periodically during use. Monitor for GI bleeding, hepatotoxicity, and ototoxicity at beginning of therapy and periodically throughout. Schedule ophthalmic evaluations for patients who are taking NSAIDs for long periods of time.

Patient Education Take with food or milk to reduce GI distress. Do not use alcohol. Regularly scheduled ophthalmic exams are advised with long-term use of NSAIDs. You may experience dizziness, nervousness, headache, nausea, vomiting, heartburn, or constipation; GI bleeding, ulceration, or perforation can occur with or without pain; discontinue medication and contact prescriber if persistent abdominal pain, cramping, or blood in stool occurs. Report respiratory difficulty; chest pain; bruising or bleeding; blood in urine, stool, mouth, or vomitus; unusual fatigue; skin rash; or ringing in ears.

Dietary Considerations Drug may cause GI upset, bleeding, ulceration, perforation; take with food or milk to minimize GI upset.

Geriatric Considerations Elderly are a high-risk population for adverse effects from NSAIDs. As much as 60% of the elderly who develop GI complications can develop peptic ulceration and/or hemorrhage asymptomatically. The concomitant use of H_2 blockers and sucralfate is not effective as prophylaxis with the exception of NSAID-induced duodenal ulcers which may be prevented by the use of ranitidine. Misoprostol and proton pump inhibitors are the only agents proven to help prevent the development of NSAID-induced ulcers. Also, concomitant disease and drug use contribute to the risk for GI adverse effects. Use lowest effective dose for shortest period possible. Consider renal function decline with age. Use of NSAIDs can compromise existing renal function especially when Cl_{cr} is ≤30 mL/minute. Tinnitus may be a difficult and unreliable indication of toxicity due to age-related hearing loss or eighth cranial nerve damage. CNS adverse effects such as confusion, agitation, and hallucination are generally seen in overdose or high-dose situations, but the elderly may demonstrate these adverse effects at lower doses than younger adults.

Breast-Feeding Considerations It is not known if sulindac is excreted into breast milk. Breast-feeding is not recommended by the manufacturer.

Pregnancy Considerations Adverse events were not observed in the initial animal reproduction studies; therefore, the manufacturer classifies sulindac as pregnancy category C. Sulindac and the sulfide metabolite have been found to cross the placenta. NSAID exposure during the first trimester is not strongly associated with congenital malformations; however, cardiovascular anomalies and cleft palate have been observed following NSAID exposure in some studies. The use of an NSAID in the first trimester may be associated with an increased risk of miscarriage. Nonteratogenic effects have been observed following NSAID administration during the third trimester including myocardial degenerative changes, prenatal constriction of the ductus arteriosus, failure of the ductus arteriosus to close postnatally, and fetal tricuspid regurgitation; renal dysfunction or failure, oligohydramnios; gastrointestinal bleeding or perforation, increased risk of necrotizing enterocolitis; intracranial bleeding, platelet dysfunction with resultant bleeding; or pulmonary hypertension. Because they may cause premature closure of the ductus arteriosus, use of NSAIDs late in pregnancy should be avoided (use after 31-32 weeks gestation is not recommended by some clinicians). Sulindac has been used in the management of preterm labor. The chronic use of NSAIDs in women of reproductive age may be associated with infertility that is reversible upon discontinuation of the medication. A registry is available for pregnant women exposed to autoimmune medications including sulindac. For additional information contact the Organization of Teratology Information Specialists, OTIS Autoimmune Diseases Study, at (877) 311-8972.

Related Information

Nonsalicylate / Nonsteroidal Anti-Inflammatory Agents *on page 2002*

SUMAtriptan (soo ma TRIP tan)

U.S. Brand Names Alsuma™; Imitrex®; Sumavel™ DosePro™

Index Terms Sumatriptan Succinate

Generic Availability (U.S.) Yes

Pharmacologic Category Antimigraine Agent; Serotonin 5-$HT_{1B, 1D}$ Receptor Agonist

Medication Safety Issues

Sound-alike/look-alike issues:

SUMAtriptan may be confused with saxagliptin, sitaGLIPtin, somatropin, ZOLMitriptan

Pregnancy Risk Factor C

Lactation Enters breast milk/use caution (AAP rates "compatible"; AAP 2001 update pending)

Use

Intranasal, Oral, SubQ: Acute treatment of migraine with or without aura

SubQ: Acute treatment of cluster headache episodes

Mechanism of Action/Effect Selective agonist for serotonin receptor in cranial arteries; causes vasoconstriction and relief of migraine

Contraindications Hypersensitivity to sumatriptan or any component of the formulation; patients with ischemic heart disease or signs or symptoms of ischemic heart disease (including Prinzmetal's angina, angina pectoris, myocardial infarction, silent myocardial ischemia); cerebrovascular syndromes (including strokes, transient ischemic attacks); peripheral vascular disease (including ischemic bowel disease); uncontrolled hypertension; use within 24 hours of ergotamine derivatives; use within 24 hours of another 5-HT_1 agonist; concurrent administration or within 2 weeks of discontinuing an MAO type A inhibitors (oral and nasal sumatriptan only; see Warnings/Precautions); management of hemiplegic or basilar migraine; severe hepatic impairment (oral and nasal sumatriptan, and injectable Imitrex® only); not for I.V. administration

Warnings/Precautions Sumatriptan is only indicated for the acute treatment of migraine or cluster headache; not indicated for migraine prophylaxis, or for the treatment of hemiplegic or basilar migraine. If a patient does not respond to the first dose, the diagnosis of migraine or cluster headache should be reconsidered; rule out underlying neurologic disease in patients with atypical headache and in patients with no prior history of migraine or cluster headache. Cardiac events (coronary artery vasospasm, transient ischemia, myocardial infarction, ventricular tachycardia/fibrillation, cardiac arrest and death), cerebral/subarachnoid hemorrhage, and stroke have been reported with 5-HT_1 agonist administration. Do not give to patients with risk factors for CAD until a cardiovascular evaluation has been performed; if evaluation is satisfactory, the healthcare provider should administer the first dose and cardiovascular status should be periodically evaluated.

Significant elevation in blood pressure, including hypertensive crisis, has also been reported on rare occasions in patients with and without a history of hypertension; use is contraindicated in patients with uncontrolled hypertension. Vasospasm-related reactions have been reported other than coronary artery vasospasm. Peripheral vascular ischemia and colonic ischemia with abdominal pain and bloody diarrhea have occurred. Transient and permanent blindness and significant partial vision loss have been very rarely reported. Use with caution in patients with a history of seizure disorder or in patients with a lowered seizure threshold. Use the oral formulation with caution in patients with hepatic impairment. Presystemic clearance of orally administered sumatriptan is reduced in hepatic impairment, leading to increased plasma concentrations; dosage reduction of the oral product is recommended. Non-oral routes of administration (nasal, subcutaneous formulations) do not undergo similar hepatic first-pass metabolism and are not expected to result in significantly altered pharmacokinetics in patients with hepatic impairment. Use of the oral, nasal, or Imitrex® injectable is contraindicated in severe hepatic impairment.

Symptoms of agitation, confusion, hallucinations, hyper-reflexia, myoclonus, shivering, and tachycardia (serotonin syndrome) may occur with concomitant proserotonergic drugs (ie, SSRIs/SNRIs or triptans) or agents which reduce sumatriptan's metabolism. Concurrent use of serotonin precursors (eg, tryptophan) is not recommended. Concurrent use with an MAO inhibitor may result in increased sumatriptan concentrations and increased risk for dose-related adverse effects (eg, serotonin syndrome); use with oral or nasal sumatriptan is contraindicated. Although generally not recommended, if concomitant use with injectable sumatriptan is deemed necessary, careful monitoring and appropriate dosage adjustments are required. I.V. administration is contraindicated due to the potential to cause coronary vasospasm. Not recommended for use in elderly patients; older adults are at a higher risk for coronary artery disease and may be more likely to have reduced hepatic function.

Drug Interactions

Avoid Concomitant Use

Avoid concomitant use of SUMAtriptan with any of the following: Ergot Derivatives; MAO Inhibitors; Sibutramine

Decreased Effect There are no known significant interactions involving a decrease in effect.

Increased Effect/Toxicity

SUMAtriptan may increase the levels/effects of: Ergot Derivatives; Serotonin Modulators

The levels/effects of SUMAtriptan may be increased by: Ergot Derivatives; MAO Inhibitors; Sibutramine

Adverse Reactions

Injection:

>10%:

Central nervous system: Dizziness (12%), warm/hot sensation (11%)

Local: Injection site reaction (≤86%; includes bleeding, bruising, edema, and erythema)

Neuromuscular & skeletal: Paresthesia (5% to 14%)

1% to 10%:

Cardiovascular: Chest discomfort/tightness/pressure (2% to 5%)

Central nervous system: Burning sensation (7%), feeling of heaviness (7%), flushing (7%), pressure sensation (7%), feeling of tightness (5%), drowsiness (3%), feeling strange (2%), headache (2%), tight feeling in head (2%), anxiety (1%), cold sensation (1%), malaise/fatigue (1%)

Gastrointestinal: Nausea/vomiting (4%), abdominal discomfort (1%), dysphagia (1%)

Neuromuscular & skeletal: Neck pain/stiffness (5%), numbness (5%), weakness (5%), jaw discomfort (2%), myalgia (2%), muscle cramps (1%)

Ocular: Vision alterations (1%)

Respiratory: Throat discomfort (3%), nasal disorder/discomfort (2%), bronchospasm (1%)

Miscellaneous: Diaphoresis (2%)

Nasal spray:

>10%: Gastrointestinal: Bad taste (13% to 24%), nausea (11% to 13%), vomiting (11% to 13%)

1% to 10%:

Central nervous system: Dizziness (1% to 2%)

Respiratory: Nasal disorder/discomfort (2% to 4%), throat discomfort (1% to 2%)

Tablet:

1% to 10%:

Cardiovascular: Chest pain/tightness/heaviness/pressure (1% to 2%), palpitation (1%), syncope (1%)

Central nervous system: Burning (1%), dizziness (>1%), drowsiness (>1%), malaise/fatigue (2% to 3%), headache (>1%), nonspecified pain (1% to 2%, placebo 1%), vertigo (<1% to 2%), migraine (>1%), sleepiness (>1%)

Gastrointestinal: Diarrhea (1%), nausea (>1%), vomiting (>1%), hyposalivation (>1%)

Genitourinary: Hematuria (1%)

Hematologic: Hemolytic anemia (1%)

Neuromuscular & skeletal: Neck, throat, and jaw pain/tightness/pressure (2% to 3%), paresthesia (3% to 5%), myalgia (1%), numbness (1%)

Otic: Ear hemorrhage (1%), hearing loss (1%), sensitivity to noise (1%), tinnitus (1%)

Respiratory: Allergic rhinitis (1%), dyspnea (1%), nasal inflammation (1%), nose/throat hemorrhage (1%), sinusitis (1%), upper respiratory inflammation (1%)

Miscellaneous: Hypersensitivity reactions (1%), nonspecified pressure/tightness/heaviness (1% to 3%, placebo 2%); warm/cold sensation (2% to 3%, placebo 2%)

Pharmacodynamics/Kinetics

Onset of Action Oral: ~30 minutes; Nasal: ~15-30 minutes; SubQ: ~10 minutes

Bioavailability Nasal: 17% (compared to SubQ); Oral: 15%; SubQ: 97% ± 16%

Time to Peak Oral: 2-2.5 hours; SubQ: 12 minutes (range: 4-20 minutes)

Protein Binding 14% to 21%

Half-Life Elimination ~2-2.5 hours

Metabolism Hepatic, primarily via MAO-A isoenzyme; extensive first-pass metabolism following oral administration

Excretion

Nasal spray: Urine (42% of total dose as indole acetic acid metabolite; 3% of total dose as unchanged drug)

Oral: Urine (~60% of total dose, mostly as indole acetic acid metabolite; 3% of total dose as unchanged drug); feces (~40%)

SubQ: Urine (38% of total dose as indole acetic acid metabolite; 22% of total dose as unchanged drug)

Available Dosage Forms

Injection, solution: 4 mg/0.5 mL (0.5 mL); 6 mg/0.5 mL (0.5 mL)

Alsuma™: 6 mg/0.5 mL (0.5 mL)

Imitrex®: 4 mg/0.5 mL (0.5 mL); 6 mg/0.5 mL (0.5 mL)

Sumavel™ DosePro™: 6 mg/0.5 mL (0.5 mL)

Solution, intranasal: 5 mg/0.1 mL (6s); 20 mg/0.1 mL (6s)

Imitrex®: 5 mg/0.1 mL (6s); 20 mg/0.1 mL (6s)

Tablet, oral: 25 mg, 50 mg, 100 mg

Imitrex®: 25 mg, 50 mg, 100 mg

Dosing

Adult

Migraine:

Oral: A single dose of 25 mg, 50 mg, or 100 mg (taken with fluids). If a satisfactory response has not been obtained at 2 hours, a second dose may be administered. Results from clinical trials show that initial doses of 50 mg and 100 mg are more effective than doses of 25 mg, and that 100 mg doses do not provide a greater effect than 50 mg and may have increased incidence of side effects. Although doses of up to 300 mg/day have been studied, the total daily dose should not exceed 200 mg. The safety of treating an average of >4 headaches in a 30-day period have not been established.

Intranasal: A single dose of 5 mg, 10 mg, or 20 mg administered in one nostril. A 10 mg dose may be achieved by administering a single 5 mg dose in each nostril. If headache returns, the dose may be repeated once after 2 hours, not to exceed a total daily dose of 40 mg. In clinical trials, a greater number of patients responded to initial doses of 20 mg versus 5 or 10 mg. The safety of treating an average of >4 headaches in a 30-day period has not been established.

SubQ: Initial: Up to 6 mg; may repeat if needed ≥1 hour after initial dose (maximum: Two 6 mg injections per 24-hour period). However, controlled clinical trials have failed to document a benefit with administration of a second 6 mg dose in nonresponders.

Cluster headache: SubQ: Initial: Up to 6 mg; may repeat if needed ≥1 hour after initial dose (maximum: Two 6-mg injections per 24-hour period)

Geriatric Not recommended due to increased potential for adverse effects.

Renal Impairment Dosage adjustment is not necessary.

Hepatic Impairment

Mild-to-moderate hepatic impairment:

Oral: Bioavailability of oral sumatriptan is increased with liver disease. If treatment is needed, do not exceed single doses of 50 mg.

Nasal spray: Has not been studied in patients with hepatic impairment, however, because the spray does not undergo first-pass metabolism, levels would not be expected to be altered.

Subcutaneous: Has been studied and pharmacokinetics were not altered in patients with hepatic impairment compared to healthy patients.

Severe hepatic impairment: Oral, nasal, and subcutaneous (limited to Imitrex® injection, per prescribing information) formulations are contraindicated with severe hepatic impairment.

Administration

Oral Should be administered as soon as symptoms appear.

I.V. Do **not** administer I.V.; may cause coronary vasospasm.

Other

SubQ: Not for I.M. or I.V. use. Needle penetrates 1/4 inch of skin; use in areas of the body with adequate skin and subcutaneous thickness. Alsuma™ is a prefilled single-use autoinjector device.

Needleless administration (Sumavel™ DosePro™): Administer to the abdomen (>2 inches from the navel) or thigh; not for I.M. or I.V. administration. Do not administer to other areas of the body (eg, arm). Device is for single use only, discard after use; do not use if the tip of the device is tilted or broken.

Stability

Storage

Alsuma™: Store at 25°C (77°F); excursions permitted between 15°C and 30°C (59°F and 86°F); do not refrigerate. Protect from light.

Imitrex® injectable, tablet, nasal spray: Store at 2°C to 30°C (36°F to 86°F). Protect from light.

Sumavel™ DosePro™: Store at 20°C to 25°C (68°F to 77°F); excursions permitted between 15°C and 30°C (59°F and 86°F); do not freeze.

Monitoring and Teaching Issues

Physical Assessment For use only with a clear diagnosis of acute migraine or cluster headaches (not for prophylaxis). Cardiovascular status should be evaluated prior to initiating medication and periodically thereafter. Evaluate carefully for use-related cautions (eg, history of, current, or risk factors for coronary heart disease; hepatic impairment; or seizure history). Monitor for hypertension, cardiac event, cerebrovascular event, dizziness, tingling, drowsiness, myalgia, vision alternation, nausea, and vomiting. With SubQ, teach patient appropriate injection technique and syringe/needle disposal.

Patient Education Take at first sign of migraine attack. This drug is to be used to reduce your migraine, not to prevent or reduce the number of attacks. If using injection formulation, follow instructions for injection and disposal of needle and syringe. May cause dizziness, fatigue, drowsiness, vision alterations, nausea, or vomiting. Report immediately any chest tightness, pain, or pressure; respiratory difficulty; acute headache, pressure, or tight feeling in head; muscle weakness, pain, cramping, or numbness; abdominal pain; or blood in stool.

Geriatric Considerations Use cautiously in the elderly, particularly since many elderly have cardiovascular disease which would put them at risk for cardiovascular adverse effects. Safety and efficacy in the elderly (>65 years) have not been established. Pharmacokinetic disposition is, however, similar to that in young adults.

Breast-Feeding Considerations The amount of sumatriptan an infant would be exposed to following breast-feeding is considered to be small (although the mean milk-to-plasma ratio is ~4.9, weight adjusted doses estimates suggest breast-fed infants receive 3.5% of a maternal dose). Expressing and discarding the milk for 8-12 hours after a single dose is suggested to reduce the amount present even further. The half-life of sumatriptan in breast milk is 2.22 hours.

Pregnancy Considerations There are no adequate and well-controlled studies using sumatriptan in pregnant women. Use only if potential benefit to the mother outweighs the potential risk to the fetus. A pregnancy registry has been established to monitor outcomes of women exposed to sumatriptan during pregnancy (800-336-2176). Preliminary data from the registry do not suggest a greater risk of birth defects than the general population and so far a specific pattern of malformations has not been identified. However, sample sizes are small and studies are ongoing. In some (but not all) animal studies, administration was associated with embryolethality, fetal malformations and pup mortality.

Related Information

Antimigraine Drugs: 5-HT_1 Receptor Agonists *on page* 1985

Sumatriptan and Naproxen (soo ma TRIP tan & na PROKS en)

U.S. Brand Names Treximet™

Index Terms Naproxen and Sumatriptan; Naproxen Sodium and Sumatriptan; Naproxen Sodium and Sumatriptan Succinate; Sumatriptan Succinate and Naproxen; Sumatriptan Succinate and Naproxen Sodium

Generic Availability (U.S.) No

Pharmacologic Category Antimigraine Agent; Nonsteroidal Anti-inflammatory Drug (NSAID), Oral; Serotonin 5-$HT_{1B, 1D}$ Receptor Agonist

Medication Safety Issues

Sound-alike/look-alike issues:

Naproxen may be confused with Natacyn®, Nebcin®, neomycin, niacin
SUMAtriptan may be confused with somatropin, ZOLMitriptan
Treximet™ may be confused with Trexall™

Medication Guide Available Yes

Pregnancy Risk Factor C

Lactation Enters breast milk/not recommended

Use Acute treatment of migraine with or without aura

Available Dosage Forms

Tablet:

Treximet™ 85/500: Sumatriptan 85 mg and naproxen sodium 500 mg

Dosing

Adult & Geriatric Migraine: Oral: 1 tablet (sumatriptan 85 mg and naproxen 500 mg). If a satisfactory response has not been obtained at 2 hours, a second dose may be administered (maximum: 2 tablets/24 hours). **Note:** The safety of treating an average of >5 migraine headaches in a 30-day period has not been established.

Renal Impairment

Cl_{cr} ≥30 mL/minute Dosage adjustment not necessary.
Cl_{cr} <30 mL/minute: Use not recommended.

Hepatic Impairment Mild-to-severe impairment: Use is contraindicated by the manufacturer.

Administration

Oral May be administered with or without food. Swallow tablet whole; tablet should not be divided, crushed, or chewed.

Monitoring and Teaching Issues

Laboratory Monitoring Occult blood loss; periodic liver function test, CBC, BUN, serum creatinine

Physical Assessment See individual agents.

Patient Education See individual agents.

- **Sumatriptan Succinate** *see* SUMAtriptan *on page 1691*
- **Sumatriptan Succinate and Naproxen** *see* Sumatriptan and Naproxen *on page 1694*
- **Sumatriptan Succinate and Naproxen Sodium** *see* Sumatriptan and Naproxen *on page 1694*
- **Sumavel™ DosePro™** *see* SUMAtriptan *on page 1691*
- **Suprax®** *see* Cefixime *on page 320*
- **Surmontil®** *see* Trimipramine *on page 1822*
- **Sustiva®** *see* Efavirenz *on page 604*
- **Suxamethonium Chloride** *see* Succinylcholine *on page 1683*
- **Symbicort®** *see* Budesonide and Formoterol *on page 239*
- **Symbyax®** *see* Olanzapine and Fluoxetine *on page 1348*
- **Symlin®** *see* Pramlintide *on page 1491*
- **SymlinPen®** *see* Pramlintide *on page 1491*
- **Symmetrel** *see* Amantadine *on page 91*
- **Synalgos®-DC** *see* Dihydrocodeine, Aspirin, and Caffeine *on page 535*
- **Synarel®** *see* Nafarelin *on page 1280*
- **Synercid®** *see* Quinupristin and Dalfopristin *on page 1543*
- **Synthroid®** *see* Levothyroxine *on page 1101*
- **T_4** *see* Levothyroxine *on page 1101*
- **T-20** *see* Enfuvirtide *on page 621*
- **T-91825** *see* Ceftaroline Fosamil *on page 331*
- **Tabloid®** *see* Thioguanine *on page 1752*
- **Taclonex®** *see* Calcipotriene and Betamethasone *on page 268*
- **Taclonex Scalp®** *see* Calcipotriene and Betamethasone *on page 268*

Tacrolimus (Systemic) (ta KROE li mus)

U.S. Brand Names Prograf®

Index Terms FK506

Generic Availability (U.S.) Yes: Capsule

Pharmacologic Category Calcineurin Inhibitor; Immunosuppressant Agent

Medication Safety Issues

Sound-alike/look-alike issues:

Prograf® may be confused with Gengraf®, PROzac®
Tacrolimus may be confused with everolimus, pimecrolimus, sirolimus, temsirolimus

Medication Guide Available Yes

Pregnancy Risk Factor C

Lactation Enters breast milk/not recommended

Use Prevention of organ rejection in heart, kidney, or liver transplant recipients

Unlabeled/Investigational Use Prevention of organ rejection in lung, small bowel transplant recipients; prevention and treatment of graft-versus-host disease (GVHD) in allogenic hematopoietic stem cell transplantation

Mechanism of Action/Effect Suppresses cellular immunity (inhibits T-lymphocyte activation)

Contraindications Hypersensitivity to tacrolimus or any component of the formulation

Warnings/Precautions Hazardous agent - use appropriate precautions for handling and disposal. **[U.S. Boxed Warning]: Increased susceptibility to infection and the possible development of lymphoma may result from immunosuppression with tacrolimus.** The risk of developing other malignancies may also be increased. Insulin-dependent post-transplant diabetes mellitus (PTDM) has been reported including in patients without pretransplant history of diabetes mellitus; risk increases in African-American and Hispanic kidney transplant patients. Posterior reversible encephalopathy syndrome (PRES) may occur with therapy; symptoms are reversible with dose reduction or discontinuation of immunosuppressant therapy; stabilize blood pressure and reduce dose with suspected or confirmed diagnosis. Nephrotoxicity has has been reported, especially with higher doses; to avoid excess nephrotoxicity do not administer simultaneously with other nephrotoxic drugs (eg sirolimus, cyclosporine). Neurotoxicity may occur especially when used in high doses; tremor headache, coma and delirium have been reported and are associated with serum concentrations. Seizures may also occur. Monitoring of serum concentrations (trough for oral therapy) is essential to prevent organ rejection and reduce drug-related toxicity. Variable absorption is seen in bone marrow transplantation relative to total body radiation and/or methotrexate use. A period of ≥24 hours should elapse between discontinuation of cyclosporine and the initiation of tacrolimus. Delay initiation further with persistently elevated tacrolimus/cyclosporine levels. Use caution in renal or hepatic dysfunction, dosing adjustments may be required. Delay initiation if postoperative oliguria occurs. Use may be associated with the development of hypertension (common); hyperkalemia has been reported; avoid use of potassium-sparing diuretics. Myocardial hypertrophy has been reported (rare). Each mL of injection contains polyoxyl 60 hydrogenated castor oil (HCO-60) (200 mg) and dehydrated alcohol USP 80% v/v. Anaphylaxis has been reported with the injection, use should be reserved for those patients not able to take oral medications. **[U.S. Boxed Warning]: Should be administered under the supervision of a physician experienced in immunosuppressive therapy and organ transplantation in a facility appropriate for monitoring and managing therapy.**

Drug Interactions

Metabolism/Transport Effects **Substrate** of CYP3A4 (major), P-glycoprotein; **Inhibits** CYP3A4 (weak), P-glycoprotein

Avoid Concomitant Use

Avoid concomitant use of Tacrolimus (Systemic) with any of the following: Artemether; BCG; CycloSPORINE (Systemic); Dronedarone; Grapefruit Juice; Lumefantrine; Natalizumab; Nilotinib; Pimecrolimus; Pimozide; QuiNINE; Roflumilast; Silodosin; Sirolimus; Tacrolimus (Topical); Temsirolimus; Tetrabenazine; Thioridazine; Topotecan; Toremifene; Vaccines (Live); Vandetanib; Ziprasidone

Decreased Effect

Tacrolimus (Systemic) may decrease the levels/effects of: BCG; Sipuleucel-T; Vaccines (Inactivated); Vaccines (Live)

The levels/effects of Tacrolimus (Systemic) may be decreased by: Caspofungin; Cinacalcet; CYP3A4 Inducers (Strong); Deferasirox; Echinacea; Efavirenz; P-Glycoprotein Inducers; Phenytoin; Rifamycin Derivatives; Sirolimus; St Johns Wort; Temsirolimus

Increased Effect/Toxicity

Tacrolimus (Systemic) may increase the levels/effects of: Colchicine; CycloSPORINE (Systemic); Dabigatran Etexilate; Dronedarone; Everolimus; Leflunomide; Natalizumab; P-Glycoprotein Substrates; Phenytoin; Pimozide; QTc-Prolonging Agents; QuiNINE; Rivaroxaban; Silodosin; Sirolimus; Temsirolimus; Tetrabenazine; Thioridazine; Topotecan; Toremifene; Vaccines (Live); Vandetanib; Ziprasidone

The levels/effects of Tacrolimus (Systemic) may be increased by: Alfuzosin; Antidepressants (Serotonin Reuptake Inhibitor/Antagonist); Artemether; Calcium Channel Blockers (Dihydropyridine); Calcium Channel Blockers (Nondihydropyridine); Chloroquine; Ciprofloxacin; Ciprofloxacin (Systemic); Clotrimazole; Clotrimazole (Oral); Conivaptan; CycloSPORINE (Systemic); CYP3A4 Inhibitors (Moderate); CYP3A4 Inhibitors (Strong); Denosumab; Fluconazole; Gadobutrol; Grapefruit Juice; Itraconazole; Ketoconazole; Ketoconazole (Systemic); Lumefantrine; Macrolide Antibiotics; MetroNIDAZOLE; MetroNIDAZOLE (Systemic); Nilotinib; P-Glycoprotein Inhibitors; Pimecrolimus; Posaconazole; Protease Inhibitors; Proton Pump Inhibitors; QuiNINE; Ranolazine; Roflumilast; Sirolimus; Tacrolimus (Topical); Temsirolimus; Trastuzumab; Voriconazole

Nutritional/Ethanol Interactions

Food: Decreases rate and extent of absorption. High-fat meals have most pronounced effect (37% decrease in AUC, 77% decrease in C_{max}). Grapefruit juice, CYP3A4 inhibitor, may increase serum level and/or toxicity of tacrolimus; avoid concurrent use.

Herb/Nutraceutical: St John's wort: May reduce tacrolimus serum concentrations (avoid concurrent use).

Adverse Reactions As reported for kidney, liver, and heart transplantation:

≥15%:

Cardiovascular: Hypertension (13% to 62%), edema (peripheral 11% to 36%), chest pain (19%), edema (18%), pericardial effusion (heart transplant 15%)

Central nervous system: Headache (25% to 64%), insomnia (30% to 64%), pain (24% to 63%), fever (19% to 48%), postprocedural pain (kidney transplant 29%), dizziness (19%)

Dermatologic: Pruritus (15% to 36%), rash (10% to 24%)
Endocrine & metabolic: Hypophosphatemia (28% to 49%), hypomagnesemia (16% to 48%), hyperglycemia (21% to 47%), hyperkalemia (8% to 45%), hyperlipemia (10% to 31%), hypokalemia (13% to 29%), diabetes mellitus (24% to 26%)
Gastrointestinal: Diarrhea (24% to 72%), abdominal pain (29% to 59%), nausea (32% to 46%), constipation (23% to 36%), anorexia (7% to 34%), vomiting (14% to 29%), dyspepsia (18% to 28%)
Genitourinary: Urinary tract infection (16% to 34%)
Hematologic: Anemia (5% to 50%), leukopenia (13% to 48%), leukocytosis (8% to 32%), thrombocytopenia (14% to 24%)
Hepatic: Liver function tests abnormal (6% to 36%), ascites (7% to 27%)
Local: Incision site complication (kidney transplant 28%)
Neuromuscular & skeletal: Tremor (34% to 56%; heart transplant 15%), weakness (11% to 52%), paresthesia (17% to 40%), back pain (17% to 30%), arthralgia (25%)
Renal: Abnormal kidney function (36% to 56%), creatinine increased (23% to 45%), BUN increased (12% to 30%), oliguria (18% to 19%)
Respiratory: Atelectasis (5% to 28%), pleural effusion (30% to 36%), dyspnea (5% to 29%), cough increased (18%), bronchitis (17%)
Miscellaneous: Infection (24% to 45%), CMV infection (32%), graft dysfunction (kidney transplant 24%)

<15%:

Cardiovascular: Abnormal ECG (QRS or ST segment abnormal), arrhythmia, atrial fibrillation, atrial flutter, bradycardia, cardiopulmonary failure, deep thrombophlebitis, heart failure, heart rate decreased, hemorrhage, hemorrhagic stroke, hypervolemia, hypotension, peripheral vascular disorder, phlebitis, postural hypotension, syncope, tachycardia, thrombosis, vasodilation, ventricular fibrillation
Central nervous system: Abnormal dreams, abnormal thinking, agitation, amnesia, anxiety, chills, confusion, depression, emotional lability, encephalopathy, flaccid paralysis, hallucinations, mood elevated, nervousness, psychosis, quadriparesis, seizure, somnolence
Dermatologic: Acne, alopecia, bruising, cellulitis, exfoliative dermatitis, fungal dermatitis, hirsutism, photosensitivity reaction, skin discoloration, skin disorder, skin neoplasm, skin ulcer, wound healing impaired
Endocrine & metabolic: Acidosis, alkalosis, bicarbonate decreased, Cushing's syndrome, dehydration, gout, hypercholesterolemia, hyper-/hypocalcemia, hyperphosphatemia, hyperuricemia, hypoproteinemia, serum iron decreased
Gastrointestinal: Appetite increased, cramps, duodenitis, dysphagia, enlarged abdomen, esophagitis (including ulcerative), flatulence, gastritis, gastroesophagitis, GI perforation/hemorrhage, ileus, oral moniliasis, pancreatic pseudocyst, rectal disorder, stomatitis, weight gain
Genitourinary: Bladder spasm, cystitis, dysuria, nocturia, urge incontinence, urinary frequency, urinary incontinence, urinary retention, vaginitis
Hematologic: Coagulation disorder, decreased prothrombin, hypochromic anemia, polycythemia
Hepatic: Alkaline phosphatase increased, bilirubinemia, cholangitis, cholestatic jaundice, GGT increased, hepatitis (including granulomatous), jaundice, LDH increased, liver damage
Local: Phlebitis
Neuromuscular & skeletal: Hypertonia, incoordination, joint disorder, leg cramps, myalgia, myasthenia, myoclonus, nerve compression, neuropathy, osteoporosis
Ocular: Abnormal vision, amblyopia
Otic: Ear pain, otitis media, tinnitus
Renal: Acute renal failure, albuminuria, BK nephropathy, hematuria, hydronephrosis, renal tubular necrosis, toxic nephropathy
Respiratory: Asthma, lung disorder, pharyngitis, pneumonia, pneumothorax, pulmonary edema, respiratory disorder, rhinitis, sinusitis, voice alteration
Miscellaneous: Abscess, abnormal healing, allergic reaction, crying, diaphoresis, flu-like syndrome, generalized spasm, hernia, herpes simplex, peritonitis, sepsis, writing impaired

Pharmacodynamics/Kinetics

Absorption Better in resected patients with a closed stoma; unlike cyclosporine, clamping of the T-tube in liver transplant patients does not alter trough concentrations or AUC; Oral: Incomplete and variable; the rate and extent of absorption is affected by food and may be most pronounced with a high-fat meal

Bioavailability Oral: Children: 7% to 55%, Adults: 7% to 32%; Absolute: Unknown

Time to Peak 0.5-6 hours

Protein Binding 99% primarily to albumin and alpha$_1$-acid glycoprotein glycoprotein

Half-Life Elimination Variable, 23-46 hours in healthy volunteers; 2.1-36 hours in transplant patients

Metabolism Extensively hepatic via CYP3A4 to eight possible metabolites (major metabolite, 31-demethyl tacrolimus, shows same activity as tacrolimus *in vitro*)

Excretion Feces (~93%); urine (<2% as unchanged drug)

Available Dosage Forms

Capsule, oral: 0.5 mg, 1 mg, 5 mg
Prograf®: 0.5 mg, 1 mg, 5 mg

Injection, solution:
Prograf®: 5 mg/mL (1 mL)

Dosing

Adult & Geriatric

Prevention of organ rejection in transplant recipients: Note: The initial dose of tacrolimus should begin no sooner than 6 hours post-transplant; adjunctive therapy with corticosteroids is recommended early post-transplant. I.V. route should only be used in patients not able to take oral medications and continued only until oral medication can be tolerated; anaphylaxis has been reported with I.V. administration. If switching from I.V. to oral, the oral dose should be started 8-12 hours after stopping the infusion.

Liver transplant:

Oral: Initial dose: 0.1-0.15 mg/kg/day in 2 divided doses, given every 12 hours

I.V.: Initial dose: 0.03-0.05 mg/kg/day as a continuous infusion

Heart transplant: Use in combination with azathioprine or mycophenolate mofetil is recommended.

Oral: Initial dose: 0.075 mg/kg/day in 2 divided doses, given every 12 hours

I.V.: Initial dose: 0.01 mg/kg/day as a continuous infusion

Kidney transplant: Use in combination with azathioprine or mycophenolate mofetil is recommended.

Oral: Initial dose: 0.2 mg/kg/day in combination with azathioprine **or** 0.1 mg/kg/day in combination with mycophenolate mofetil. Administer in 2 divided doses, given every 12 hours; initial dose may be given within 24 hours of transplant, but should be delayed until renal function has recovered; African-American patients may require larger doses to maintain trough concentration

I.V.: Initial dose: 0.03-0.05 mg/kg/day as a continuous infusion

Prevention of graft-versus-host disease (unlabeled use):

Oral: Convert from I.V. to oral dose (1:4 ratio): Multiply total daily I.V. dose times 4 and administer in 2 divided oral doses per day, every 12 hours (Uberti, 1999).

I.V.: Initial: 0.03 mg/kg/day (based on lean body weight) as continuous infusion. Treatment should begin at least 24 hours prior to stem cell infusion and continued only until oral medication can be tolerated (Przepiorka, 1999)

Treatment of graft-versus-host disease (unlabeled use): *I.V.:* Initial: 0.03 mg/kg/day (based on lean body weight) as continuous infusion (Furlong, 2000; Przepiorka, 1999)

Pediatric

Liver transplant:

Oral: Initial dose: 0.15-0.20 mg/kg/day in 2 divided doses, given every 12 hours

I.V.: Initial dose: 0.03-0.05 mg/kg/day as a continuous infusion.

Note: The initial dose of tacrolimus should begin no sooner than 6 hours post-transplant; adjunctive therapy with corticosteroids is recommended early post-transplant. I.V. route should only be used in patients not able to take oral medications and continued only until oral medication can be tolerated; anaphylaxis has been reported with I.V. administration. If switching from I.V. to oral, the oral dose should be started 8-12 hours after stopping the infusion. Patients without pre-existing renal or hepatic dysfunction have required (and tolerated) higher doses than adults to achieve similar blood concentrations. It is recommended that therapy be initiated at ***high end*** of the recommended adult I.V. and oral dosing ranges; dosage adjustments may be required.

Prevention of graft-vs-host disease (unlabeled use):

Oral: Convert from I.V. to oral dose (1:4 ratio): Multiply total daily I.V. dose times 4 and administer in 2 divided oral doses per day, every 12 hours (Yanik, 2000)

I.V.: Initial: 0.03 mg/kg/day (based on lean body weight) as continuous infusion. Treatment should begin at least 24 hours prior to stem cell infusion and continued only until oral medication can be tolerated (Yanik, 2000)

Renal Impairment Evidence suggests that lower doses should be used; patients should receive doses at the lowest value of the recommended I.V. and oral dosing ranges; further reductions in dose below these ranges may be required.

Tacrolimus therapy should usually be delayed up to 48 hours or longer in patients with postoperative oliguria.

Hemodialysis: Not removed by hemodialysis; supplemental dose is not necessary.

Peritoneal dialysis: Significant drug removal is unlikely based on physiochemical characteristics.

Hepatic Impairment Use of tacrolimus in liver transplant recipients experiencing post-transplant hepatic impairment may be associated with increased risk of developing renal insufficiency related to high whole blood levels of tacrolimus. The presence of moderate-to-severe hepatic dysfunction (serum bilirubin >2 mg/dL; Child-Pugh score ≥10) appears to affect the metabolism of tacrolimus. The half-life of the drug was prolonged and the clearance reduced after I.V. administration. The bioavailability of tacrolimus was also increased after oral administration. The higher plasma concentrations as determined by ELISA, in patients with severe hepatic dysfunction are probably due to the accumulation of metabolites of lower activity. These patients should be monitored closely and dosage adjustments should be considered. Some evidence indicates that lower doses could be used in these patients.

Administration

Oral Administer on an empty stomach; be consistent with timing and composition of meals if GI intolerance occurs and administration with food becomes necessary (per manufacturer). If dosed once daily (not common), administer in the morning. If dosed twice daily, doses should be 12 hours apart. If the morning and evening doses differ, the larger dose (differences are never >0.5-1 mg) should be given in the morning. If dosed 3 times/day, separate doses by 8 hours.

I.V. If I.V. administration is necessary, administer by continuous infusion only. Do not use PVC tubing when administering diluted solutions. Tacrolimus is usually intended to be administered as a continuous infusion over 24 hours.

Stability

Reconstitution Dilute with 5% dextrose injection or 0.9% sodium chloride injection to a final concentration between 0.004 mg/mL and 0.02 mg/mL.

Storage

Injection: Prior to dilution, store at 5°C to 25°C (41°F to 77°F). Following dilution, stable for 24 hours in D_5W or NS in glass or polyethylene containers.

Capsules: Store at room temperature of 25°C (77°F); excursions permitted to 15°C to 30°C (59°F to 86°F).

Monitoring and Teaching Issues

Laboratory Monitoring Renal function, hepatic function, serum electrolytes (especially potassium), glucose. Since pharmacokinetics show great inter- and intrapatient variability over time, monitoring of serum concentrations (trough for oral therapy) has proven helpful to prevent organ rejection and reduce drug-related toxicity. Measure 3 times/week for first few weeks, then gradually decrease frequency as patient stabilizes.

Tacrolimus serum levels may be falsely elevated in infected liver transplant patients due to interference from β-galactosidase antibodies.

Physical Assessment Monitor blood pressure frequently. Patients with diabetes should be advised to monitor glucose levels closely (this medication may alter glucose levels). Monitor for signs of opportunistic infection.

Patient Education Take on an empty stomach. Maintain adequate hydration during entire course of therapy, unless instructed to restrict fluid intake. You will be susceptible to infection. If you have diabetes, monitor glucose levels closely (drug may alter glucose levels). You may experience nausea, vomiting, or diarrhea. Report chest pain, severe headache, respiratory difficulty, unresolved GI effects, fatigue, chills, fever, unhealed sores, white plaques in mouth, pain on urination or change in urinary patterns, or rash.

Dietary Considerations Capsule: Take on an empty stomach; be consistent with timing and composition of meals if GI intolerance occurs and administration with food becomes necessary (per manufacturer). Avoid grapefruit juice.

Breast-Feeding Considerations Concentrations of tacrolimus in breast milk are lower than that of the maternal serum. The low bioavailability of tacrolimus following oral absorption may also decrease the amount of exposure to a nursing infant.

Pregnancy Considerations Adverse events were observed in animal reproduction studies. Tacrolimus crosses the human placenta and is measurable in the cord blood, amniotic fluid, and newborn serum. Tacrolimus concentrations in the placenta may be higher than the maternal serum. No consistent pattern of congenital anomalies has been observed. Transient neonatal hyperkalemia and renal dysfunction have been reported.

The National Transplantation Pregnancy Registry (NTPR, Temple University) is a registry for pregnant women taking immunosuppressants following any solid organ transplant. The NTPR encourages reporting of all immunosuppressant exposures during pregnancy in transplant recipients at 877-955-6877.

Tacrolimus (Topical) (ta KROE li mus)

U.S. Brand Names Protopic®

Generic Availability (U.S.) No

Pharmacologic Category Calcineurin Inhibitor; Topical Skin Product

Medication Safety Issues

Sound-alike/look-alike issues:

Tacrolimus may be confused with everolimus, pimecrolimus, sirolimus, temsirolimus

Medication Guide Available Yes

Pregnancy Risk Factor C

Lactation Enters breast milk/not recommended

Use Moderate-to-severe atopic dermatitis in immunocompetent patients not responsive to conventional therapy or when conventional therapy is not appropriate

Canadian labeling: Additional use (not in U.S. labeling): Maintenance therapy to prevent flares and extend flare-free intervals in patients with moderate-to-severe atopic dermatitis who are responsive to initial therapy and experiencing ≥5 flares per year

Available Dosage Forms

Ointment, topical:

Protopic®: 0.03% (30 g, 60 g, 100 g); 0.1% (30 g, 60 g, 100 g)

Dosing

Adult & Geriatric Atopic dermatitis (moderate-to-severe): Topical:

Treatment: Apply thin layer of 0.03% or 0.1% ointment to affected area twice daily; rub in gently and completely. Discontinue use when symptoms have cleared. If no improvement within 6 weeks, patients should be re-examined to confirm diagnosis.

Maintenance therapy (Canadian labeling; not in U.S. labeling): Apply one application (thin layer of 0.03% or 0.1% ointment) to areas usually affected twice a week, allowing 2-3 days between applications (eg, one application on Monday and Thursday). Reevaluate after 12 months. Safety of maintenance therapy >12 months has not been established.

Note: Patients experiencing flares should resume twice daily treatment.

Pediatric Moderate-to-severe atopic dermatitis: Topical:

Treatment:

Children ≥2-15 years: Apply thin layer of 0.03% ointment to affected area twice daily; rub in gently and completely. Discontinue use when symptoms have cleared. If no improvement within 6 weeks, patients should be re-examined to confirm diagnosis.

Children >15 years: Refer to adult dosing.

Maintenance therapy (Canadian labeling; not in U.S. labeling):

Children ≥2-15 years: Apply one application (thin layer of 0.03% ointment) to areas usually affected twice a week, allowing 2-3 days between applications (eg, one application on Monday and Thursday). Reevaluate after 12 months. Safety of maintenance therapy >12 months has not been established.

Children >15 years: Refer to adult dosing.

Note: Patients experiencing flares should resume twice daily treatment.

Administration

Topical Do not use with occlusive dressings. Burning at the application site is most common in first few days; improves as atopic dermatitis improves. Limit application to involved areas. Continue as long as signs and symptoms persist; discontinue if resolution occurs; re-evaluate if symptoms persist >6 weeks.

Monitoring and Teaching Issues

Physical Assessment Monitor for signs of opportunistic infection.

Patient Education Before applying, wash area gently and thoroughly. Apply in thin film to affected area. Do not cover skin with bandages. Wash hands only if not treating skin on the hands. Protect skin from sunlight or exposure to UV light.

Tadalafil (tah DA la fil)

U.S. Brand Names Adcirca®; Cialis®

Index Terms GF196960

Generic Availability (U.S.) No

Pharmacologic Category Phosphodiesterase-5 Enzyme Inhibitor

Medication Safety Issues

Sound-alike/look-alike issues:

Tadalafil may be confused with sildenafil, vardenafil

Adcirca® may be confused with Advair® Diskus®, Advair® HFA, Advicor®

Pregnancy Risk Factor B

Lactation Excretion in breast milk unknown/use caution

Use

Adcirca®: Treatment of pulmonary arterial hypertension (PAH) (WHO Group I) to improve exercise ability

Cialis®: Treatment of erectile dysfunction (ED)

Mechanism of Action/Effect

Erectile dysfunction: Tadalafil enhances the effect of nitric oxide (NO) by inhibiting phosphodiesterase type 5 (PDE-5), which is responsible for degradation of cGMP in the corpus cavernosum; when sexual stimulation causes local release of NO, inhibition of PDE-5 by tadalafil causes increased levels of cGMP in the corpus cavernosum, resulting in smooth muscle relaxation and inflow of blood to the corpus cavernosum. At recommended doses, it has no effect in the absence of sexual stimulation.

PAH: Inhibits phosphodiesterase type 5 (PDE-5) in smooth muscle of pulmonary vasculature where PDE-5 is responsible for the degradation of cyclic guanosine monophosphate (cGMP). Increased cGMP concentration results in pulmonary vasculature relaxation; vasodilation in the pulmonary bed and the systemic circulation (to a lesser degree) may occur.

Contraindications Known serious hypersensitivity to tadalafil; concurrent use (regularly/intermittently) of organic nitrates in any form (eg, nitroglycerin, isosorbide dinitrate)

Warnings/Precautions There is a degree of cardiac risk associated with sexual activity; therefore, physicians should consider the cardiovascular status of their patients prior to initiation. Use for erectile dysfunction is not recommended in patients with hypotension (<90/50 mm Hg), uncontrolled hypertension (>170/100 mm Hg), NYHA class II-IV heart failure within the last 6 months, uncontrolled arrhythmias, stroke within the last 6 months, MI within the last 3 months, unstable angina or angina during sexual intercourse; safety and efficacy have not been evaluated in these patients. Safety and efficacy in PAH have not been evaluated in patients with clinically significant aortic and/or mitral valve disease, life-threatening arrhythmias, hypotension (<90/50 mm Hg), uncontrolled hypertension, significant left ventricular dysfunction, pericardial constriction, restrictive or congestive cardiomyopathy, symptomatic coronary artery disease. Use caution in patients with left ventricular outflow obstruction (eg, aortic stenosis, hypertrophic obstructive cardiomyopathy); may be more sensitive to vasodilator effects.

Patients experiencing anginal chest pain after tadalafil administration should seek immediate medical attention. Concomitant use (regularly/intermittently) with all forms of nitrates is contraindicated. When used for either erectile dysfunction or PAH and nitrate administration is medically necessary following use, at least 48 hours should elapse after the tadalafil dose and nitrate administration. When used for PAH, per the manufacturer, nitrate may be administered within 48 hours of tadalafil. For both situations, administration of nitrates should only be done under close medical supervision with hemodynamic monitoring.

Concurrent use with alpha-adrenergic antagonist therapy or substantial alcohol consumption may cause symptomatic hypotension; patients should be hemodynamically stable prior to initiating tadalafil therapy at the lowest possible dose. When used for erectile dysfunction, use caution in patients receiving strong CYP3A4 inhibitors. When used for PAH, avoid use in patients taking strong CYP3A4 inducers/inhibitors. Use in patients receiving or about to receive ritonavir requires dosage adjustment or interruption of therapy, respectively. Pulmonary vasodilators may exacerbate the cardiovascular status in patients with pulmonary veno-occlusive disease (PVOD); use is not recommended. In patients with unrecognized PVOD, signs of pulmonary edema should prompt investigation into this diagnosis. Use with caution in patients with mild-to-moderate hepatic impairment; dosage adjustment/limitation is needed. Use is not recommended in patients with severe hepatic impairment or cirrhosis. Use with caution in patients with renal impairment; dosage adjustment/limitation is needed. Safety and efficacy with other tadalafil brands or other PDE-5 inhibitors (ie, sildenafil and vardenafil) have not been established. Patients should be informed not to take with other tadalafil brands or other PDE-5 inhibitors. Use caution in patients with bleeding disorders or peptic ulcer disease due to effect on platelets (bleeding).

When used to treat erectile dysfunction, potential underlying causes of erectile dysfunction should be evaluated prior to treatment. Use with caution in patients with anatomical deformation of the penis (angulation, cavernosal fibrosis, or Peyronie's disease), or who have conditions which may predispose them to priapism (sickle cell anemia, multiple myeloma, leukemia). Instruct patients to seek immediate medical attention if erection persists >4 hours. Safety and efficacy with other tadalafil brands or other PDE-5 inhibitors (ie, sildenafil and vardenafil) have not been established. Patients should be informed not to take with other tadalafil brands or other PDE-5 inhibitors. The safety and efficacy of tadalafil with other treatments for erectile dysfunction have not been studied and are, therefore, not recommended as combination therapy.

Rare cases of nonarteritic anterior ischemic optic neuropathy (NAION) have been reported; risk may be increased with history of vision loss or NAION in one eye. Other risk factors for NAION include heart disease, diabetes, hypertension, smoking, age >50 years, or history of certain eye problems. Sudden decrease or loss of hearing has been reported rarely; hearing changes may be accompanied by tinnitus and dizziness. A direct relationship between therapy and vision or hearing loss has not been determined. Instruct patients to seek medical assistance for sudden loss of vision in one or both eyes, sudden decrease in hearing, or sudden loss of hearing.

Patients with genetic retinal disorders (eg, retinitis pigmentosa) were not evaluated in clinical trials; use is not recommended. Use with caution in the elderly.

Drug Interactions

Metabolism/Transport Effects Substrate of CYP3A4 (major)

Avoid Concomitant Use

Avoid concomitant use of Tadalafil with any of the following: Amyl Nitrite; Phosphodiesterase 5 Inhibitors; Vasodilators (Organic Nitrates)

Decreased Effect

The levels/effects of Tadalafil may be decreased by: Bosentan; CYP3A4 Inducers (Strong); Etravirine

Increased Effect/Toxicity

Tadalafil may increase the levels/effects of: Alpha1-Blockers; Amyl Nitrite; Antihypertensives; Bosentan; Phosphodiesterase 5 Inhibitors; Vasodilators (Organic Nitrates)

The levels/effects of Tadalafil may be increased by: Antifungal Agents (Azole Derivatives, Systemic); CYP3A4 Inhibitors (Moderate); CYP3A4 Inhibitors (Strong); Dasatinib; Macrolide Antibiotics; Ritonavir; Sapropterin

Nutritional/Ethanol Interactions

Ethanol: Substantial consumption of ethanol may increase the risk of hypotension and orthostasis. Lower ethanol consumption has not been associated with significant changes in blood pressure or increase in orthostatic symptoms.

Food: Rate and extent of absorption are not affected by food. Grapefruit juice may increase serum levels/toxicity of tadalafil. Use tadalafil with caution in patients who regularly consume grapefruit juice. In general, use of grapefruit juice should be limited or avoided; the manufacturer does not give specific recommendations.

Herb/Nutraceutical: St John's wort: Use caution with concomitant use.

Adverse Reactions Based upon usual doses for either indication. For erectile dysfunction, similar adverse events are reported with once-daily versus intermittent dosing, but are generally lower than with doses used intermittently.

>10%:

Cardiovascular: Flushing (1% to 13%; dose related)

Central nervous system: Headache (3% to 42%; dose related)

Gastrointestinal: Dyspepsia (1% to 13%), nausea (10% to 11%)

Neuromuscular & skeletal: Myalgia (1% to 14%; dose related), back pain (2% to 12%), extremity pain (1% to 11%)

Respiratory: Respiratory tract infection (3% to 13%), nasopharyngitis (2% to 13%)

2% to 10%:

Cardiovascular: Hypertension (1% to 3%)

Gastrointestinal: Gastroenteritis (viral; 3% to 5%), GERD (1% to 3%), abdominal pain (1% to 2%), diarrhea (1% to 2%)

Genitourinary: Urinary tract infection (≤2%)

Respiratory: Nasal congestion (≤9%), cough (2% to 4%), bronchitis (≤2%)

Miscellaneous: Flu-like syndrome (2% to 5%)

Pharmacodynamics/Kinetics

Onset of Action Within 1 hour

Peak effect: Pulmonary artery vasodilation: 75-90 minutes (Ghofrani, 2004)

Duration of Action Erectile dysfunction: Up to 36 hours

Time to Peak Plasma: ~2-4 hours (range: 30 minutes to 8 hours)

Protein Binding 94%

Half-Life Elimination 15-17.5 hours; Pulmonary hypertension (not receiving bosentan): 35 hours

Metabolism Hepatic, via CYP3A4 to metabolites (inactive)

Excretion Feces (~61%, predominantly as metabolites); urine (~36%, predominantly as metabolites)

Available Dosage Forms

Tablet, oral:

Adcirca®: 20 mg

Cialis®: 2.5 mg, 5 mg, 10 mg, 20 mg

Dosing

Adult

Erectile dysfunction (Cialis®): Oral:

As-needed dosing: 10 mg at least 30 minutes prior to anticipated sexual activity (dosing range: 5-20 mg); to be given as one single dose and not given more than once daily. **Note:** Erectile function may be improved for up to 36 hours following a single dose; adjust dose.

Once-daily dosing: 2.5 mg once daily (dosing range: 2.5-5 mg/day) to be given at approximately the same time daily without regard to timing of sexual activity

Dosing adjustment with concomitant medications:

Alpha$_1$-blockers: If stabilized on either alpha-blockers or tadalafil therapy, initiate new therapy with the other agent at the lowest possible dose.

Protease inhibitors: Maximum tadalafil dose: 10 mg in a 72-hour period

Other CYP3A4 inhibitors: Dose reduction of tadalafil is recommended with strong CYP3A4 inhibitors. When used on an as-needed basis, the dose of tadalafil should not exceed 10 mg, and tadalafil should not be taken more frequently than once every 72 hours. When used on a once-daily basis, the dose of tadalafil should not exceed 2.5 mg. Examples of such inhibitors include clarithromycin, conivaptan, delavirdine, diclofenac, imatinib, isoniazid, itraconazole, ketoconazole, miconazole, nefazodone, nicardipine, propofol, quinidine, and telithromycin.

Pulmonary arterial hypertension (Adcirca®): Oral: 40 mg once daily

Dosing adjustment with concomitant medications:

Coadministration with protease inhibitor regimen:

Concurrent use with atazanavir/ritonavir, darunavir/ritonavir, fosamprenavir, ritonavir, saquinavir/ritonavir, tipranavir/ritonavir:

Coadministration of tadalafil in patients currently receiving one of these protease inhibitor regimens for at least 1 week: Initiate tadalafil at 20 mg once daily; increase to 40 mg once daily based on individual tolerability.

Coadministration of one of these protease inhibitor regimens in patients currently receiving tadalafil: Discontinue tadalafil at least 24 hours prior to the initiation of the protease inhibitor regimen. After at least 1 week of the protease inhibitor regimen, resume tadalafil at 20 mg once daily; increase to 40 mg once daily based on individual tolerability.

Concurrent use with indinavir or nelfinavir:

Patient receiving indinavir/nelfinavir when initiating tadalafil: Initiate tadalafil at 20 mg once daily; increase to 40 mg once daily based on individual tolerability

Patient receiving tadalafil when initiating indinavir/nelfinavir: Adjust tadalafil to 20 mg once daily; increase to 40 mg once daily based on individual tolerability

Other potent CYP3A4 inhibitors: Avoid concurrent use when tadalafil used for PAH. Examples of such inhibitors include clarithromycin, conivaptan, delavirdine, diclofenac, imatinib, isoniazid, itraconazole, ketoconazole, miconazole, nefazodone, nicardipine, propofol, quinidine, and telithromycin.

Potent CYP3A4 inducers (eg, rifampin): Avoid concurrent use when tadalafil used for PAH.

Geriatric Refer to adult dosing. No dose adjustment for patients >65 years of age in the absence of renal or hepatic impairment.

Renal Impairment

Erectile dysfunction (Cialis®):

As-needed use:

Cl_{cr} ≥51 mL/minute: Dosage adjustment not required.

Cl_{cr} 31-50 mL/minute: Initial: 5 mg once daily; maximum: 10 mg (not to be given more frequently than every 48 hours).

Cl_{cr} <30 mL/minute and on hemodialysis: Maximum: 5 mg (not to be given more frequently than every 72 hours).

Once-daily use:

Cl_{cr} ≥31 mL/minute: Dose adjustment not required.

Cl_{cr} <30 mL/minute and on hemodialysis: Use not recommended.

Pulmonary arterial hypertension (Adcirca®):

Cl_{cr} 31-80 mL/minute: Initial: 20 mg once daily; increase to 40 mg once daily based on individual tolerability.

Cl_{cr} <30 mL/minute and on hemodialysis: Avoid use due to increased tadalafil exposure, limited clinical experience, and lack of ability to influence clearance by dialysis.

Hepatic Impairment

Erectile dysfunction (Cialis®):

As-needed use:

Mild-to-moderate hepatic impairment (Child-Pugh class A or B): Use with caution; dose should not exceed 10 mg once daily.

Severe hepatic impairment (Child-Pugh class C): Use is not recommended.

Once-daily use:

Mild-to-moderate hepatic impairment (Child-Pugh class A or B): Use with caution.

Severe hepatic impairment (Child-Pugh class C): Use is not recommended.

Pulmonary arterial hypertension (Adcirca®):

Mild-to-moderate hepatic impairment (Child-Pugh class A or B): Use with caution; consider initial dose of 20 mg once daily.

Severe hepatic impairment (Child-Pugh class C): Avoid use; has not been studied in patients with severe hepatic cirrhosis.

Administration

Oral May be administered with or without food.

Adcirca®: Administer daily dose all at once; dividing doses throughout the day is not advised.

Cialis®: When used on an as-needed basis, should be taken at least 30 minutes prior to sexual activity. When used on a once-daily basis, should be taken at the same time each day, without regard to timing of sexual activity.

Stability

Storage Store at 25°C (77°F); excursions permitted to 15°C to 30°C (59°F to 86°F).

Monitoring and Teaching Issues

Patient Education Avoid substantial consumption of alcohol. This drug provides no protection against sexually-transmitted diseases, including HIV. You may experience headache, fatigue, dizziness, blurred vision, or back or limb pain. Report immediately chest pain, palpitations, respiratory difficulty, unusual dizziness, change in vision, change in hearing or ringing in the ears, signs of urinary tract infection, skin rash, genital swelling or priapism, or erection lasting >4 hours.

Dietary Considerations May be taken with or without food.

Geriatric Considerations No significant differences in pharmacokinetics were seen in elderly men versus younger men. Dosing should be adjusted for renal function. Since older adults often have concomitant diseases, many of which may be contraindicated with the use of tadalafil, prescriber should complete a thorough review of diseases and medications prior to prescribing tadalafil.

Pregnancy Considerations Teratogenic events were not reported in animal reproduction studies. Postnatal development and pup survival was decreased at some doses. There are no adequate and well-controlled studies in pregnant women. Less than 0.0005% is found in the semen of healthy males.

- **Tagamet HB 200® [OTC]** *see* Cimetidine *on page* 372
- **TAK-375** *see* Ramelteon *on page* 1550
- **TAK-390MR** *see* Dexlansoprazole *on page* 504
- **TAK-599** *see* Ceftaroline Fosamil *on page* 331
- **Talwin NX** *see* Pentazocine and Naloxone *on page* 1439
- **Tambocor™** *see* Flecainide *on page* 766
- **Tamiflu®** *see* Oseltamivir *on page* 1367

Tamoxifen (ta MOKS i fen)

Index Terms ICI-46474; Nolvadex; Tamoxifen Citras; Tamoxifen Citrate

Generic Availability (U.S.) Yes

Pharmacologic Category Antineoplastic Agent, Estrogen Receptor Antagonist; Selective Estrogen Receptor Modulator (SERM)

Medication Safety Issues

Sound-alike/look-alike issues:

Tamoxifen may be confused with pentoxifylline, Tambocor™, tamsulosin, temazepam

Medication Guide Available Yes

Pregnancy Risk Factor D

Lactation Excretion in breast milk unknown/not recommended

Use Treatment of metastatic (female and male) breast cancer; adjuvant treatment of breast cancer after primary treatment with surgery and radiation; reduce risk of invasive breast cancer in women with ductal carcinoma *in situ* (DCIS) after surgery and radiation; reduce the incidence of breast cancer in women at high risk

Unlabeled/Investigational Use Treatment of mastalgia, gynecomastia, ovarian cancer, endometrial cancer, uterine sarcoma, and desmoid tumors; risk reduction in women with Paget's disease of the breast (with DCIS or without associated cancer); induction of ovulation; treatment of precocious puberty in females, secondary to McCune-Albright syndrome

Mechanism of Action/Effect Competitively binds to estrogen receptors on tumors and other tissue targets, producing a nuclear complex that decreases DNA synthesis and inhibits estrogen effects; nonsteroidal agent with potent antiestrogenic properties which compete with estrogen for binding sites in breast and other tissues; cells accumulate in the G_0 and G_1 phases; therefore, tamoxifen is cytostatic rather than cytocidal.

Contraindications Hypersensitivity to tamoxifen or any component of the formulation; concurrent warfarin therapy or history of deep vein thrombosis or pulmonary embolism (when tamoxifen is used for cancer risk reduction in women at high-risk for breast cancer and in women with DCIS)

Warnings/Precautions Hazardous agent - use appropriate precautions for handling and disposal. **[U.S. Boxed Warning]: Serious and life-threatening events (including stroke, pulmonary emboli, and uterine malignancy) have occurred at an incidence greater than placebo during use for breast cancer risk reduction in women at high-risk for breast cancer and in women with DCIS;** these events are rare, but require consideration in risk: benefit evaluation. An increased incidence of thromboembolic events, including DVT and pulmonary embolism, has been associated with use for breast cancer; risk is increased with concomitant chemotherapy; use with caution in individuals with a history of thromboembolic events. Thrombocytopenia and/or leukopenia may occur; neutropenia and pancytopenia have been reported rarely. Although the relationship to tamoxifen therapy is uncertain, rare hemorrhagic episodes have occurred in patients with significant thrombocytopenia. Use with caution in patients with hyperlipidemias; infrequent postmarketing cases of hyperlipidemias have been reported. Decreased visual acuity, retinal vein thrombosis, retinopathy, corneal changes, color perception changes, and increased incidence of cataracts (and the need for cataract surgery), have been reported. Hypercalcemia has occurred in patients with bone metastasis, usually within a few weeks of therapy initiation; institute appropriate hypercalcemia management; discontinue if severe. Local disease flare and increased bone and tumor pain may occur in patients with metastatic breast cancer; may be associated with (good) tumor response.

Tamoxifen is associated with a high potential for drug interactions, including CYP- and Pgp-mediated interactions. Decreased efficacy and an increased risk of breast cancer recurrence has been reported with concurrent moderate or strong CYP2D6 inhibitors (Aubert, 2009; Dezentje, 2009). Concomitant use with select SSRIs may result in decreased tamoxifen efficacy. Strong CYP2D6 inhibitors (eg, fluoxetine, paroxetine) and moderate CYP2D6 inhibitors (eg, sertraline) are reported to interfere with transformation to the active metabolite endoxifen. Weak CYP2D6 inhibitors (eg, venlafaxine, citalopram) have minimal effect on the conversion to endoxifen (Jin, 2005; NCCN Breast Cancer Risk Reduction Guidelines v.2.2010); escitalopram is also a weak CYP2D6 inhibitor. Lower plasma concentrations of endoxifen (active metabolite) have been observed in patients associated with reduced CYP2D6 activity (Jin, 2005) and may be associated with reduced efficacy. In a retrospective analysis of breast cancer patients taking tamoxifen and SSRIs, concomitant use of paroxetine and tamoxifen was associated with an increased risk of death due to breast cancer (Kelly, 2010).

Tamoxifen use may be associated with changes in bone mineral density (BMD) and the effects may be dependent upon menstrual status. In postmenopausal women, tamoxifen use is associated with a protective effect on bone mineral density (BMD), preventing loss of BMD which lasts over the 5-year treatment period. In premenopausal women, a decline (from baseline) in BMD mineral density has been observed in women who continued to menstruate; may be associated with an increased risk of fractures. Liver abnormalities such as cholestasis, fatty liver, hepatitis, and hepatic necrosis have occurred. Hepatocellular carcinomas have been reported in some studies; relationship to treatment is unclear. Tamoxifen is associated with an increased incidence of uterine or endometrial cancers. Endometrial hyperplasia, polyps, endometriosis, uterine fibroids, and ovarian cysts have occurred. Monitor and promptly evaluate any report of abnormal vaginal bleeding. Amenorrhea and menstrual irregularities have been reported with tamoxifen use.

Drug Interactions

Metabolism/Transport Effects **Substrate** of CYP2A6 (minor), 2B6 (minor), 2C9 (major), 2D6 (major), 2E1 (minor), 3A4 (major); **Inhibits** CYP2B6 (weak), 2C8 (moderate), 2C9 (weak), 3A4 (weak), p-glycoprotein

Avoid Concomitant Use

Avoid concomitant use of Tamoxifen with any of the following: CYP2D6 Inhibitors (Strong); Silodosin; Topotecan; Vitamin K Antagonists

Decreased Effect

Tamoxifen may decrease the levels/effects of: Anastrozole; Letrozole

The levels/effects of Tamoxifen may be decreased by: Aminoglutethimide; CYP2C9 Inducers (Highly Effective); CYP3A4 Inducers (Strong); Deferasirox; Herbs (CYP3A4 Inducers); Peginterferon Alfa-2b; Rifamycin Derivatives

Increased Effect/Toxicity

Tamoxifen may increase the levels/effects of: Colchicine; CYP2C8 Substrates (High risk); Dabigatran Etexilate; Everolimus; P-Glycoprotein Substrates; Rivaroxaban; Silodosin; Topotecan; Vitamin K Antagonists

The levels/effects of Tamoxifen may be increased by: Conivaptan; CYP2C9 Inhibitors (Moderate); CYP2C9 Inhibitors (Strong); CYP2D6 Inhibitors (Moderate); CYP2D6 Inhibitors (Strong); CYP3A4 Inhibitors (Moderate); CYP3A4 Inhibitors (Strong); Darunavir; Dasatinib

Nutritional/Ethanol Interactions

Food: Avoid grapefruit juice (may decrease the metabolism of tamoxifen).

Herb/Nutraceutical: Avoid black cohosh, dong quai in estrogen-dependent tumors. Avoid St John's wort (may decrease levels/effects of tamoxifen).

Lab Interactions T_4 elevations (which may be explained by increases in thyroid-binding globulin) have been reported; not accompanied by clinical hyperthyroidism

Adverse Reactions

>10%:

Cardiovascular: Vasodilation (41%), flushing (33%), hypertension (11%), peripheral edema (11%)

Central nervous system: Mood changes (12% to 18%), pain (3% to 16%), depression (2% to 12%)
Dermatologic: Skin changes (6% to 19%), rash (13%)
Endocrine & metabolic: Hot flashes (3% to 80%), fluid retention (32%), altered menses (13% to 25%), amenorrhea (16%)
Gastrointestinal: Nausea (5% to 26%), weight loss (23%), vomiting (12%)
Genitourinary: Vaginal discharge (13% to 55%), vaginal bleeding (2% to 23%)
Neuromuscular & skeletal: Weakness (18%), arthritis (14%), arthralgia (11%)
Respiratory: Pharyngitis (14%)
Miscellaneous: Lymphedema (11%)

1% to 10%:
Cardiovascular: Chest pain (5%), venous thrombotic events (5%), edema (4%), cardiovascular ischemia (3%), angina (2%), deep venous thrombus (≤2%), MI (1%)
Central nervous system: Insomnia (9%), dizziness (8%), headache (8%), anxiety (6%), fatigue (4%)
Dermatologic: Alopecia (≤5%)
Endocrine & metabolic: Oligomenorrhea (9%), breast pain (6%), menstrual disorder (6%), breast neoplasm (5%), hypercholesterolemia (4%)
Gastrointestinal: Abdominal pain (9%), weight gain (9%), constipation (4% to 8%), diarrhea (7%), dyspepsia (6%), throat irritation (oral solution 5%), abdominal cramps (1%), anorexia (1%)
Genitourinary: Urinary tract infection (10%), leukorrhea (9%), vaginal hemorrhage (6%), vaginitis (5%), vulvovaginitis (5%), ovarian cyst (3%)
Hematologic: Thrombocytopenia (≤10%), anemia (5%)
Hepatic: AST increased (5%), serum bilirubin increased (2%)
Neuromuscular & skeletal: Back pain (10%), bone pain (6% to 10%), osteoporosis (7%), fracture (7%), arthrosis (5%), joint disorder (5%), myalgia (5%), paresthesia (5%), musculoskeletal pain (3%)
Ocular: Cataract (7%)
Renal: Serum creatinine increased (≤2%)
Respiratory: Cough (4% to 9%), dyspnea (8%), bronchitis (5%), sinusitis (5%)
Miscellaneous: Infection/sepsis (≤9%), diaphoresis (6%), flu-like syndrome (6%), cyst (5%), neoplasm (5%), allergic reaction (3%)

Pharmacodynamics/Kinetics

Absorption Well absorbed

Time to Peak Serum: ~5 hours

Protein Binding 99%

Half-Life Elimination Tamoxifen: ~5-7 days; N-desmethyl tamoxifen: ~14 days

Metabolism Hepatic; via CYP2D6 to 4-hydroxytamoxifen and via CYP3A4/5 to N-desmethyl-tamoxifen. Each is then further metabolized into endoxifen (4-hydroxy-tamoxifen via CYP3A4/5 and N-desmethyl-tamoxifen via CYP2D6); both 4-hydroxy-tamoxifen and endoxifen are 30- to 100-fold more potent than tamoxifen

Excretion Feces (26% to 51%); urine (9% to 13%)

Available Dosage Forms

Tablet, oral: 10 mg, 20 mg

Dosing

Adult & Geriatric Note: For the treatment of breast cancer, patients receiving both tamoxifen and chemotherapy, should receive treatment sequentially, with tamoxifen following completion of chemotherapy.

Breast cancer treatment:

Adjuvant therapy (females): 20 mg once daily for 5 years

Metastatic (males and females): 20-40 mg/day (doses >20 mg should be given in 2 divided doses). **Note:** Although the FDA-approved labeling recommends dosing up to 40 mg/day, clinical benefit has not been demonstrated with doses above 20 mg/day (Bratherton, 1984).

Premenopausal women: Duration of treatment is 5 years (NCCN Breast Cancer guidelines v.1.2011)

Postmenopausal women: Duration of tamoxifen treatment is 2-3 years followed by an aromatase inhibitor (AI) to complete 5 years; if contraindications or intolerant to AI, may take tamoxifen for the full 5 years **or** extended therapy: 4.5-6 years of tamoxifen followed by 5 years of an AI (NCCN Breast Cancer guidelines v.1.2011)

DCIS (females), to reduce the risk for invasive breast cancer: 20 mg once daily for 5 years

Breast cancer risk reduction (pre- and postmenopausal high-risk females): 20 mg once daily for 5 years

Induction of ovulation (unlabeled use): 20 mg once daily (range: 20-80 mg once daily) for 5 days (Steiner, 2005)

Paget's disease of the breast (risk reduction; with DCIS or without associated cancer): 20 mg once daily for 5 years (NCCN Breast Cancer Guidelines, v.1.2011)

Dosage adjustment for DVT, pulmonary embolism, cerebrovascular accident, or prolonged immobilization: Discontinue tamoxifen (NCCN Breast Cancer Risk Reduction Guidelines, v.2.2010)

Pediatric Females: Precocious puberty and McCune-Albright syndrome (unlabeled use): Oral: A dose of 20 mg/day has been reported in patients 2-10 years of age; safety and efficacy have not been established for treatment of longer than 1 year duration (Eugster, 2003)

Administration

Oral Administer with or without food.

Stability

Storage Store at room temperature of 20°C to 25°C (68°F to 77°F). Protect from light.

Monitoring and Teaching Issues

Laboratory Monitoring CBC with platelets, serum calcium, LFTs; triglycerides and cholesterol (in patients with pre-existing hyperlipidemias); INR and PT (in patients on vitamin K antagonists)

Physical Assessment Evaluate for use-related precautions prior to beginning therapy. Monitor for thromboembolism, flushing, fluid retention, hot flashes, vaginal bleeding or discharge, constipation, rash, or mood changes. Teach patient importance of periodic ophthalmic evaluations and annual gynecological exams and mammograms with long-term use.

Patient Education It is important to maintain adequate nutrition and hydration, unless instructed to restrict fluid intake. You should schedule an annual ophthalmic examination, gynecological exam, and mammogram if this medication is used long-term. You may experience hot flashes, hair loss, or loss of libido (these will subside when treatment is completed). May cause nausea, vomiting, loss of appetite, photosensitivity, or hot flashes. Notify prescriber if menstrual irregularities, vaginal bleeding, or intolerable hot flashes occur. Report unusual bleeding or bruising, severe weakness or unusual fatigue, CNS changes (depression, mood changes), persistent bone changes, swelling or pain in calves, respiratory difficulty, or vision changes.

Dietary Considerations May be taken with or without food. Avoid grapefruit and grapefruit juice.

Geriatric Considerations Studies have shown tamoxifen to be effective in the treatment of primary breast cancer in elderly women. Comparative studies with other antineoplastic agents in elderly women with breast cancer had more favorable survival rates with tamoxifen. Initiation of hormone therapy rather than chemotherapy is justified for elderly patients with metastatic breast cancer who are responsive. Reduction of mortality and recurrence was greater in those studies that used tamoxifen for ≥2 years than those that use it for <2 years.

Breast-Feeding Considerations It is not known if tamoxifen is excreted in breast milk, however, it has been shown to inhibit lactation. Due to the potential for adverse reactions, women taking tamoxifen should not breast-feed.

Pregnancy Considerations Animal studies have demonstrated fetal adverse effects and fetal loss. There have been reports of vaginal bleeding, birth defects and fetal loss in pregnant women. Tamoxifen use during pregnancy may have a potential long term risk to the fetus of a DES-like syndrome. For sexually-active women of childbearing age, initiate during menstruation (negative β-hCG immediately prior to initiation in women with irregular cycles). Tamoxifen may induce ovulation. Barrier or nonhormonal contraceptives are recommended. Pregnancy should be avoided during treatment and for 2 months after treatment has been discontinued.

Additional Information Estrogen receptor status may predict if adjuvant treatment with tamoxifen is of benefit. In metastatic breast cancer, patients with estrogen receptor positive tumors are more likely to benefit from tamoxifen treatment. With tamoxifen use to reduce the incidence of breast cancer in high risk-women, high risk is defined as women ≥35 years of age with a 5 year NCI Gail model predicted risk of breast cancer ≥1.67%.

Oncology Comment: The American Society of Clinical Oncology (ASCO) guidelines for adjuvant endocrine therapy in postmenopausal women with HR-positive breast cancer (Burstein, 2010) recommend considering aromatase inhibitor (AI) therapy at some point in the treatment course (primary, sequentially, or extended). Optimal duration at this time is not known; however, treatment with an AI should not exceed 5 years in primary and extended therapies, and 2-3 years if followed by tamoxifen in sequential therapy (total of 5 years). If initial therapy with AI has been discontinued before the 5 years, consideration should be taken to receive tamoxifen for a total of 5 years. The optimal time to switch to an AI is also not known; but data supports switching after 2-3 years of tamoxifen (sequential) or after 5 years of tamoxifen (extended). If patient becomes intolerant or has poor adherence, consideration should be made to switch to another AI or initiate tamoxifen.

The adjuvant endocrine therapy of choice is tamoxifen for men with breast cancer and for pre- or perimenopausal women at diagnosis. CYP2D6 genotyping is not recommended, however, due to the potential for drug-drug interactions use caution and consider avoiding concomitant therapy with tamoxifen and known CYP2D6 inhibitors.

◆ **Tamoxifen Citras** *see* Tamoxifen *on page 1703*

◆ **Tamoxifen Citrate** *see* Tamoxifen *on page 1703*

Tamsulosin (tam SOO loe sin)

U.S. Brand Names Flomax®

Index Terms Tamsulosin Hydrochloride

Generic Availability (U.S.) Yes

Pharmacologic Category Alpha$_1$ Blocker

Medication Safety Issues

Sound-alike/look-alike issues:

Flomax® may be confused with Flonase®, Flovent®, Foltx®, Fosamax®

Tamsulosin may be confused with tacrolimus, tamoxifen, terazosin

International issues:

Flomax [U.S., Canada, and multiple international markets] may be confused with Flomox brand name for cefcapene [Japan] and Volmax brand name for salbutamol [multiple international markets]

Flomax: Brand name for tamsulosin [U.S., Canada, and multiple international markets], but also the brand name for morniflumate [Italy]

Pregnancy Risk Factor B

Use Treatment of signs and symptoms of benign prostatic hyperplasia (BPH)

Unlabeled/Investigational Use Symptomatic treatment of bladder outlet obstruction or dysfunction

Mechanism of Action/Effect Antagonizes alpha$_{1A}$-adrenoreceptors in the prostate which mediate the dynamic component of urine flow obstruction by regulating smooth muscle tone of the bladder neck and prostate. When given to patients with BPH, blockade of alpha-receptors leads to relaxation of these muscles, resulting in an improvement in urine flow rate and symptoms. Alpha-blockade does not influence the static component of urinary obstruction, which is related to tissue proliferation.

Contraindications Hypersensitivity to tamsulosin or any component of the formulation

Warnings/Precautions Not intended for use as an antihypertensive drug. May cause significant orthostatic hypotension and syncope, especially with first dose; anticipate a similar effect if therapy is interrupted for a few days, if dosage is rapidly increased, or if another antihypertensive drug (particularly vasodilators) or a PDE-5 inhibitor (eg, sildenafil, tadalafil, vardenafil) is introduced. "First-dose" orthostatic hypotension may occur 4-8 hours after dosing; may be dose related. Patients should be cautioned about performing hazardous tasks when starting new therapy or adjusting dosage upward. Discontinue if symptoms of angina occur or worsen. Rule out prostatic carcinoma before beginning therapy with tamsulosin. Intraoperative floppy iris syndrome has been observed in cataract surgery patients who were on or were previously treated with alpha$_1$-blockers; causality has not been established and there appears to be no benefit in discontinuing alpha-blocker therapy prior to surgery; instruct patients to inform ophthalmologist of tamsulosin use when considering eye surgery. Priapism has been associated with use (rarely). Rarely, patients with a sulfa allergy have also developed an allergic reaction to tamsulosin; avoid use when previous reaction has been severe. Not indicated for use in women.

Drug Interactions

Metabolism/Transport Effects Substrate (major) of CYP2D6, 3A4

Avoid Concomitant Use

Avoid concomitant use of Tamsulosin with any of the following: Alpha1-Blockers; CYP3A4 Inhibitors (Strong)

Decreased Effect

The levels/effects of Tamsulosin may be decreased by: CYP3A4 Inducers (Strong); Deferasirox; Herbs (CYP3A4 Inducers); Peginterferon Alfa-2b

Increased Effect/Toxicity

Tamsulosin may increase the levels/effects of: Alpha1-Blockers; Calcium Channel Blockers

The levels/effects of Tamsulosin may be increased by: Beta-Blockers; CYP2D6 Inhibitors (Moderate); CYP2D6 Inhibitors (Strong); CYP3A4 Inhibitors (Moderate); CYP3A4 Inhibitors (Strong); Dasatinib; MAO Inhibitors; Phosphodiesterase 5 Inhibitors

Nutritional/Ethanol Interactions

Food: Fasting increases bioavailability by 30% and peak concentration 40% to 70%.

Herb/Nutraceutical: St John's wort: May decrease the levels/effects of tamsulosin. Avoid herbs with hypotensive properties (black cohosh, California poppy, coleus, golden seal, hawthorn, mistletoe, periwinkle, quinine, Shepherd's purse); may enhance the hypotensive effect of tamsulosin. Avoid saw palmetto (due to limited experience with this combination).

Adverse Reactions

>10%:

Cardiovascular: Orthostatic hypotension (6 % to 19%)
Central nervous system: Headache (19% to 21%), dizziness (15% to 17%)
Genitourinary: Abnormal ejaculation (8% to 18%)
Respiratory: Rhinitis (13% to 18%)
Miscellaneous: Infection (9% to 11%)

1% to 10%:

Cardiovascular: Chest pain (4%)
Central nervous system: Somnolence (3% to 4%), insomnia (1% to 2%), vertigo (≤1%)
Endocrine & metabolic: Libido decreased (1% to 2%)
Gastrointestinal: Diarrhea (4% to 6%), nausea (3% to 4%), gum pain, toothache
Neuromuscular & skeletal: Weakness (8% to 9%), back pain (7% to 8%)
Ocular: Blurred vision (≤2%)
Respiratory: Pharyngitis (5% to 6%), cough (3% to 5%), sinusitis (2% to 4%)

Pharmacodynamics/Kinetics

Absorption >90%

Bioavailability Fasting: 30% increase

Time to Peak Fasting: 4-5 hours; With food: 6-7 hours

Steady-state: By the fifth day of once daily dosing

Protein Binding 94% to 99%, primarily to alpha$_1$ acid glycoprotein (AAG)

Half-Life Elimination Healthy volunteers: 9-13 hours; Target population: 14-15 hours

Metabolism Hepatic (extensive) via CYP3A4 and 2D6; metabolites undergo extensive conjugation to glucuronide or sulfate

Excretion Urine (76%, <10% as unchanged drug); feces (21%)

Available Dosage Forms

Capsule, oral: 0.4 mg

Flomax®: 0.4 mg

Tablet, oral: 0.4 mg

Dosing

Adult & Geriatric

BPH: Oral: 0.4 mg once daily ~30 minutes after the same meal each day; dose may be increased after 2-4 weeks to 0.8 mg once daily in patients who fail to respond. If therapy is interrupted for several days, restart with 0.4 mg once daily.

Bladder outlet obstruction (unlabeled use): Oral: 0.4 mg once daily ~30 minutes after the same meal each day

Renal Impairment

Cl_{cr} ≥10 mL/minute: No adjustment needed.

Cl_{cr} <10 mL/minute: Not studied.

Hepatic Impairment

Mild-to-moderate impairment: No adjustment needed

Severe impairment: Not studied

Administration

Oral Administer 30 minutes after the same meal each day. Capsules should be swallowed whole; do not crush, chew, or open.

Stability

Storage Store at room temperature of 25°C (77°F); excursions permitted to 15°C to 30°C (59°F to 86°F).

Monitoring and Teaching Issues

Physical Assessment Not for use as an antihypertensive. Assess potential for interactions with pharmacological agents that may increase risk of hypotension. Monitor for improved urine flow. Monitor for "first dose" orthostatic hypotension, headache, or gastrointestinal disturbance (nausea, vomiting) at beginning of therapy and on a regular basis. When discontinuing, dose should be tapered and blood pressure monitored closely.

Patient Education May cause dizziness with first doses, postural hypotension, ejaculatory disturbance (reversible, may resolve with continued use of drug), headache, or rhinitis. Report palpitations or rapid heartbeat, dizziness, muscle weakness, fatigue, blurred vision, or headache.

Dietary Considerations Take once daily, 30 minutes after the same meal each day.

Geriatric Considerations Metabolism of tamsulosin may be slower, and older patients may be more sensitive to the orthostatic hypotension caused by this medication. A 40% higher exposure (AUC) is anticipated in patients between 55 and 75 years of age as compared to younger subjects (20-32 years).

Pregnancy Considerations Teratogenic effects were not observed in animal studies, however, tamsulosin is not approved for use in women.

Related Information

Pharmacotherapy of Urinary Incontinence *on page 2071*

◆ **Tamsulosin and Dutasteride** *see* Dutasteride and Tamsulosin *on page 600*

◆ **Tamsulosin Hydrochloride** *see* Tamsulosin *on page 1706*

◆ **Tamsulosin Hydrochloride and Dutasteride** *see* Dutasteride and Tamsulosin *on page 600*

◆ **TanaCof-XR [DSC]** *see* Brompheniramine *on page 234*

◆ **TAP-144** *see* Leuprolide *on page 1082*

◆ **Tapazole®** *see* Methimazole *on page 1192*

Tapentadol (ta PEN ta dol)

U.S. Brand Names Nucynta®

Index Terms CG5503; Tapentadol Hydrochloride

Generic Availability (U.S.) No

Pharmacologic Category Analgesic, Opioid

Medication Safety Issues

Sound-alike/look-alike issues:

Tapentadol may be confused with traMADol

Medication Guide Available Yes

Pregnancy Risk Factor C

Lactation Excretion in breast milk unknown/not recommended

Use Relief of moderate-to-severe acute pain

Mechanism of Action/Effect Binds to μ-opiate receptors in the CNS causing inhibition of ascending pain pathways, altering the perception of and response to pain; also inhibits the reuptake of norepinephrine, which also modifies the ascending pain pathway

Contraindications Impaired pulmonary function (severe respiratory depression, acute or severe asthma or hypercapnia) in unmonitored settings or in absence of resuscitative equipment or ventilatory support; paralytic ileus; use of MAO inhibitors within 14 days

Warnings/Precautions Use with caution in patients with respiratory disease or respiratory compromise (eg, asthma, chronic obstructive pulmonary disease [COPD], cor pulmonale, sleep apnea, severe obesity, kyphoscoliosis, hypoxia, hypercapnia); critical respiratory depression may occur, even at therapeutic dosages. May cause CNS depression, which may impair physical or mental abilities; patients must be cautioned about performing tasks which require mental alertness (eg, operating machinery or driving). Use with caution in patients with CNS depression or coma. Effects may be potentiated when used with other sedative drugs or ethanol.

Serotonin syndrome (SS) may occur with serotonin/norepinephrine reuptake inhibitors (SNRIs), including tapentadol. Signs of SS may include agitation, tachycardia, hyperthermia, nausea, and vomiting. Avoid use with serotonergic agents such as TCAs, triptans, venlafaxine, trazodone, lithium, sibutramine, meperidine, dextromethorphan, St John's wort, SNRIs, and SSRIs; concomitant use has been associated with the development of serotonin syndrome. Contraindicated with MAO inhibitor use within 14 days.

Use caution in patients with biliary tract dysfunction or acute pancreatitis; opioids may cause spasm of the sphincter of Oddi. Opioid use may obscure diagnosis or clinical course of patients with acute abdominal conditions. Use with extreme caution in patients with head injury, intracranial lesions, or elevated intracranial pressure (ICP); exaggerated elevation of ICP may occur. Serum concentrations are increased in hepatic impairment; use with caution in patients with moderate hepatic impairment (dosage adjustment required). Not recommended for use in severe hepatic impairment (not studied). Use with caution in patients with mild-to-moderate renal impairment (no dosage adjustment recommended). Not recommended for use in severe renal impairment (not studied). Use caution in patients with a history of seizures or conditions predisposing patients to seizures; patients with a history of seizures were excluded in clinical trials of tapentadol. Tramadol, an analgesic with similar pharmacologic properties to tapentadol, has been associated with seizures, particularly in patients with predisposing factors.

Approved for acute pain (not approved for chronic use); prolonged use increases risk of abuse, addiction, and withdrawal symptoms. An opioid-containing regimen should be tailored to each patient's needs with respect to degree of tolerance for opioids (naïve versus chronic user), age, weight, and medical condition. Healthcare provider should be alert to problems of abuse, misuse, and diversion. Abrupt discontinuation may lead to withdrawal symptoms. Symptoms may be decreased by tapering prior to discontinuation. Use opioids with caution in elderly; consider decreasing initial dose. Use caution in debilitated patients; there is a greater potential for critical respiratory depression, even at therapeutic dosages.

Drug Interactions

Avoid Concomitant Use

Avoid concomitant use of Tapentadol with any of the following: MAO Inhibitors; Sibutramine

Decreased Effect

Tapentadol may decrease the levels/effects of: Pegvisomant

The levels/effects of Tapentadol may be decreased by: Ammonium Chloride; Mixed Agonist / Antagonist Opioids; Peginterferon Alfa-2b

Increased Effect/Toxicity

Tapentadol may increase the levels/effects of: Alcohol (Ethyl); Alvimopan; CNS Depressants; Desmopressin; MAO Inhibitors; Selective Serotonin Reuptake Inhibitors; Serotonin Modulators; Thiazide Diuretics

The levels/effects of Tapentadol may be increased by: Amphetamines; Antipsychotic Agents (Phenothiazines); Droperidol; Sibutramine; Succinylcholine

Nutritional/Ethanol Interactions

Ethanol: Avoid ethanol (may increase CNS depression).

Food: When administered after a high fat/calorie meal, the AUC and C_{max} increased by 25% and 16%, respectively; may administer without regard to meals.

Herb/Nutraceutical: Avoid St John's wort (may increase CNS depression and risk of serotonin syndrome).

Adverse Reactions

>10%:

Central nervous system: Dizziness (24%), somnolence (15%)

Gastrointestinal: Nausea (30%), vomiting (18%)

1% to 10%:

Central nervous system: Fatigue (3%), insomnia (2%), anxiety (1%), confusion (1%), dreams abnormal (1%), lethargy (1%)

Dermatologic: Pruritus (3% to 5%), hyperhidrosis (3%), rash (1%)

Endocrine & metabolic: Hot flushes (1%)

Gastrointestinal: Constipation (8%), xerostomia (4%), appetite decreased (2%), dyspepsia (2%)

Genitourinary: Urinary tract infection (1%)

Neuromuscular & skeletal: Arthralgia (1%), tremor (1%)

Respiratory: Nasopharyngitis (1%), upper respiratory tract infection (1%)

Pharmacodynamics/Kinetics

Absorption Rapid and complete

Bioavailability ~32%

Time to Peak Plasma: 1.25 hours

Protein Binding ~20%

Half-Life Elimination ~4 hours

Metabolism Extensive metabolism, including first pass metabolism; metabolized primarily via phase 2 glucuronidation to glucuronides (major metabolite: tapentadol-O-glucuronide); minimal phase 1 oxidative metabolism; also metabolized to a lesser degree by CYP2C9, CYP2C19, and CYP2D6; all metabolites pharmacologically inactive

Excretion Urine (99%: 70% conjugated metabolites; 3% unchanged drug)

Controlled Substance C-II

Available Dosage Forms

Tablet, oral:

Nucynta®: 50 mg, 75 mg, 100 mg

Dosing

Adult Dose and dosage intervals should be individualized according to pain severity with respect to patient's previous experience with similar opioid analgesics.

Acute moderate-severe pain: Oral: Day 1: 50-100 mg every 4-6 hours as needed; may administer a second dose ≥1 hour after the initial dose (maximum dose on first day: 700 mg/day); Day 2 and subsequent dosing: 50-100 mg every 4-6 hours as needed (maximum: 600 mg/day)

Geriatric Initial: Consider initiating at lower range of dosing. Refer to adult dosing.

Renal Impairment

Mild-moderate renal impairment: No adjustment necessary.

Severe renal impairment: Not recommended (not studied).

Hepatic Impairment

Mild hepatic impairment: No adjustment necessary.

Moderate hepatic impairment: Initial: 50 mg every 8 hours or longer (maximum: 3 doses/24 hours). Further treatment for maintenance of analgesia may be achieved by either shortening or lengthening the dosing interval.

Severe hepatic impairment: Not recommended (not studied).

Administration

Oral Administer with or without food.

Stability

Storage Store at room temperature up to 25°C (77°F); excursions permitted to 15°C to 30°C (59°F to 86°F). Protect from moisture.

Monitoring and Teaching Issues

Physical Assessment Monitor respiratory and CNS status. Assess patient's physical and/or psychological dependence. For inpatients, implement safety measures to prevent falls. Discontinue slowly after prolonged use.

Patient Education May cause physical and/or psychological dependence. While using this medication, do not use alcohol and other prescription or OTC medications (especially sedatives, tranquilizers, antihistamines, or pain medications) without consulting prescriber. Maintain adequate hydration, unless instructed to restrict fluid intake. May cause itching, hypotension, dizziness, drowsiness, impaired coordination, or blurred vision; loss of appetite, dry mouth, nausea, or vomiting; or constipation. Report dizziness, changes in mental status, skin rash, or shortness of breath.

Dietary Considerations May be taken without regard to meals.

Geriatric Considerations In clinical studies, patients ≥65 years had a higher incidence of constipation as compared to younger patients. See Dosing: Geriatric.

Breast-Feeding Considerations Limited information available on the excretion of tapentadol in human milk; however, data suggests it may be excreted in human milk. The possibility of sedation or respiratory depression in the nursing infant should be considered.

Pregnancy Considerations Embryo-fetal toxicity, including malformations, was observed in animal studies only at doses that were maternally toxic. There are no adequate and well-controlled studies in pregnant women. Not recommended for use during labor and delivery. Neonates exposed to tapentadol in utero should be monitored for respiratory depression.

- **Tapentadol Hydrochloride** *see* Tapentadol *on page 1708*
- **Tarceva®** *see* Erlotinib *on page 652*
- **Targretin®** *see* Bexarotene (Systemic) *on page 215*
- **Targretin®** *see* Bexarotene (Topical) *on page 217*
- **Tarka®** *see* Trandolapril and Verapamil *on page 1802*
- **Tasigna®** *see* Nilotinib *on page 1316*
- **Tasmar®** *see* Tolcapone *on page 1781*
- **Tavist® ND Allergy [OTC]** *see* Loratadine *on page 1128*
- **Taxol** *see* Paclitaxel *on page 1389*
- **Taxotere®** *see* Docetaxel *on page 563*

Tazarotene (taz AR oh teen)

U.S. Brand Names Avage®; Tazorac®

Generic Availability (U.S.) No

Pharmacologic Category Acne Products; Keratolytic Agent; Topical Skin Product, Acne

Pregnancy Risk Factor X

Lactation Excretion in breast milk unknown/use caution

Use Topical treatment of facial acne vulgaris; topical treatment of stable plaque psoriasis; mitigation (palliation) of facial skin wrinkling, facial mottled hyper-/hypopigmentation, and benign facial lentigines

Contraindications Hypersensitivity to tazarotene, other retinoids or vitamin A derivatives (isotretinoin, tretinoin, etretinate), or any component of the formulation; use in women of childbearing potential who are unable to comply with birth control requirements; pregnancy (negative pregnancy test required)

Warnings/Precautions Women of childbearing potential must use adequate contraceptive measures because of potential teratogenicity. Treatment can increase skin sensitivity to weather extremes of wind or cold. Also, concomitant topical medications (eg, medicated or abrasive soaps, cleansers, or cosmetics with a strong drying effect) should be used with caution due to increased skin irritation. May cause photosensitivity; exposure to sunlight should be avoided unless deemed medically necessary, and in such cases, exposure should be minimized (including use of sunscreens/protective clothing) during use of tazarotene. Risk may be increased by concurrent therapy with known photosensitizers (thiazides, tetracyclines, fluoroquinolones, phenothiazines, sulfonamides). For external use only; avoid contact with eyes, eyelids, and mouth. Not for use on eczematous, broken, or sunburned skin; not for treatment of lentigo maligna. Avoid application over extensive areas; specifically, safety and efficacy of gel applied over >20% of BSA have not been established.

Drug Interactions

Avoid Concomitant Use There are no known interactions where it is recommended to avoid concomitant use.

Decreased Effect There are no known significant interactions involving a decrease in effect.

Increased Effect/Toxicity There are no known significant interactions involving an increase in effect.

Adverse Reactions Percentage of incidence varies with formulation and/or strength:

>10%: Dermatologic: Burning/stinging, desquamation, dry skin, erythema, irritation, pruritus, skin pain, worsening of psoriasis

1% to 10%:

Cardiovascular: Peripheral edema

Dermatologic: Cheilitis, contact dermatitis, discoloration, eczema, fissuring, inflammation, localized bleeding, rash

Endocrine & metabolic: Hypertriglyceridemia

Frequency not defined: Dermatologic: Photosensitization

Pharmacodynamics/Kinetics

Duration of Action Therapeutic: Psoriasis: Effects have been observed for up to 3 months after a 3-month course of topical treatment

Absorption Minimal following cutaneous application (≤6% of dose)

Protein Binding >99%

Half-Life Elimination 18 hours

Metabolism Prodrug, rapidly metabolized via esterases to an active metabolite (tazarotenic acid) following topical application and systemic absorption; tazarotenic acid undergoes further hepatic metabolism

Excretion Urine and feces (as metabolites)

Available Dosage Forms

Cream, topical:

Avage®: 0.1% (30 g)

Tazorac®: 0.05% (30 g, 60 g); 0.1% (30 g, 60 g)

Gel, topical:

Tazorac®: 0.05% (30 g, 100 g); 0.1% (30 g, 100 g)

Dosing

Adult & Geriatric Note: In patients experiencing excessive pruritus, burning, skin redness, or peeling, discontinue until integrity of the skin is restored, or reduce dosing to an interval the patient is able to tolerate.

Acne: Topical: Tazorac® cream/gel 0.1%: Apply a thin film (2 mg/cm^2) to affected area once daily.

Palliation of fine facial wrinkles, facial mottled hyper-/hypopigmentation, benign facial lentigines: Topical: Avage™: Apply a pea-sized amount once daily.

Psoriasis: Topical: Tazorac® cream/gel: Initial: 0.05%: Apply once daily to psoriatic lesions using enough (2 mg/cm^2) to cover only the lesion with a thin film. May increase strength to 0.1% if tolerated and necessary.

Pediatric Note: In patients experiencing excessive pruritus, burning, skin redness, or peeling, discontinue until integrity of the skin is restored, or reduce dosing to an interval the patient is able to tolerate.

Acne: Children ≥12 years: Refer to adult dosing.

Psoriasis: Children ≥12 years: Topical: Tazorac® gel: Initial: 0.05%: Apply once daily to psoriatic lesions using enough (2 mg/cm^2) to cover only the lesion with a thin film to no more than 20% of body surface area. May increase strength to 0.1% if tolerated and necessary.

Palliation of fine facial wrinkles, facial mottled hyper-/hypopigmentation, benign facial lentigines: Children ≥17 years: Topical: Avage™: Refer to adult dosing.

Administration

Topical Do not apply to eczematous or sunburned skin; avoid eyes and mouth

Acne: Apply in evening after gently cleansing and drying face; apply enough to cover entire affected area.

Palliation of fine facial wrinkles, facial mottled hyper-/hypopigmentation, benign facial lentigines: Apply to clean dry face at bedtime; lightly cover entire face including eyelids if desired. Emollients or moisturizers may be applied before or after; if applied before tazarotene, ensure cream or lotion has absorbed into the skin and has dried completely.

Psoriasis: Apply in evening. If a bath or shower is taken prior to application, dry the skin before applying. If emollients are used, apply them at least 1 hour prior to application. Unaffected skin may be more susceptible to irritation, avoid application to these areas.

Stability

Storage Store at 25°C (77°F).

Monitoring and Teaching Issues

Physical Assessment Assess for accumulated photosensitivity.

Patient Education This medication is for external use only; avoid using near eyes or mouth. Severe skin reactions may occur. Avoid any other skin products (including cosmetics or personal products that may contain medications, alcohols, or irritants) that are not approved by your prescriber. May cause photosensitivity, which will cause severe rash or burning (use sunblock SPF 15 or higher, wear protective clothing and eyewear, and avoid direct sunlight, sunlamps, or tanning beds). Report redness or discoloration, irritation, burning, stinging, excessive dryness, or worsening of condition.

Application: Wash affected area gently and completely dry before applying medication. Apply a thin layer to cover affected area. Wash off any medication that gets on unaffected skin areas and wash hands thoroughly after application.

Geriatric Considerations No differences in safety or efficacy were seen when the cream formulation was administered to patients >65 years of age; may experience increased sensitivity. Increased incidence of adverse effects and lower treatment success rates were observed with the gel formulation in the treatment of psoriasis.

Pregnancy Considerations May cause fetal harm if administered to a pregnant woman. A negative pregnancy test should be obtained within 2 weeks prior to treatment; treatment should begin during a normal menstrual period.

- **Tazicef®** *see* Ceftazidime *on page* 332
- **Tazorac®** *see* Tazarotene *on page* 1710
- **Taztia XT®** *see* Diltiazem *on page* 536
- **3TC** *see* LamiVUDine *on page* 1054
- **3TC, Abacavir, and Zidovudine** *see* Abacavir, Lamivudine, and Zidovudine *on page* 32
- **T-Cell Growth Factor** *see* Aldesleukin *on page* 62
- **TCGF** *see* Aldesleukin *on page* 62
- **TCN** *see* Tetracycline *on page* 1744
- **Tdap** *see* Diphtheria and Tetanus Toxoids, and Acellular Pertussis Vaccine *on page* 552
- **TDF** *see* Tenofovir *on page* 1728
- **Teflaro™** *see* Ceftaroline Fosamil *on page* 331

Tegaserod (teg a SER od)

U.S. Brand Names Zelnorm®

Index Terms HTF919; Tegaserod Maleate

Generic Availability (U.S.) No

Pharmacologic Category Serotonin 5-HT_4 Receptor Agonist

Prescribing and Access Restrictions Available in U.S. under an emergency investigational new drug (IND) process. Emergency situations are defined as immediately life-threatening or requiring hospitalization. Physicians with patients who may qualify can contact the FDA's Division of Drug Information via email (druginfo@fda.hhs.gov). The FDA may either deny the request or authorize shipment of Zelnorm® by Novartis. Additional information can be found at http://www.fda.gov/Drugs/DrugSafety/PostmarketDrugSafetyInformationforPatientsandProviders/ucm103223.htm.

Pregnancy Risk Factor B

Lactation Excretion in breast milk unknown/not recommended

Use Emergency treatment of irritable bowel syndrome with constipation (IBS-C) and chronic idiopathic constipation (CIC) in women (<55 years of age) in which no alternative therapy exists

Mechanism of Action/Effect Normalizes impaired motility by stimulating peristalsis and decreasing transit time in the gastrointestinal tract.

Contraindications Per product labeling: Hypersensitivity to tegaserod or any component of the formulation; severe renal impairment; moderate or severe hepatic impairment; history of bowel obstruction, symptomatic gallbladder disease, suspected sphincter of Oddi dysfunction, or abdominal adhesions. Treatment should not be started in patients with diarrhea or in those who experience diarrhea frequently.

Exclusion criteria under the emergency-IND process: Unstable angina, history of MI or stroke, hypertension, hyperlipidemia, diabetes, age ≥55 years, smoking, obesity, depression, anxiety, or suicidal ideation.

Warnings/Precautions Serious cardiovascular events (eg, MI, stroke, unstable angina) may occur; patients should seek emergency care following any sign and symptom suggestive of a serious cardiac event. Use under the emergency IND process will not be permitted in patients with unstable angina, a history of MI or stroke, cigarette smoking, hypertension, hyperlipidemia, obesity, or diabetes. In addition, use will not be permitted in patients with depression, anxiety, or with any signs of suicidal ideation or behavior. Use has been associated with rare intestinal ischemic events. Discontinue immediately with new or sudden worsening abdominal pain or rectal bleeding. Diarrhea may occur after the start of treatment, most cases reported as a single episode within the first week of therapy, and may resolve with continued dosing. However, serious consequences of diarrhea (hypovolemia, syncope) have been reported. Patients should be warned to contact healthcare provider immediately if they develop severe diarrhea, or diarrhea with severe cramping, abdominal pain, or dizziness. Use caution with mild hepatic impairment; not recommended with moderate or severe impairment. Potential benefits should be weighed against potential risks in patients eligible for emergency-IND use. Safety and efficacy have not been established in males with IBS. Use in elderly women (≥55 years of age) is contraindicated.

Drug Interactions

Avoid Concomitant Use There are no known interactions where it is recommended to avoid concomitant use.

Decreased Effect There are no known significant interactions involving a decrease in effect.

Increased Effect/Toxicity There are no known significant interactions involving an increase in effect.

Nutritional/Ethanol Interactions Food: Bioavailability is decreased by 40% to 65% and C_{max} is decreased by 20% to 40% when taken with food. T_{max} is prolonged from 1 hour up to 2 hours when taken following a meal, but decreased to 0.7 hours when taken 30 minutes before a meal.

Adverse Reactions

>10%:

Central nervous system: Headache (15%)
Gastrointestinal: Abdominal pain (12%)

1% to 10%:

Central nervous system: Dizziness (4%), migraine (2%)
Gastrointestinal: Diarrhea (9%; severe <1%), nausea (8%), flatulence (6%)
Neuromuscular & skeletal: Back pain (5%), arthropathy (2%), leg pain (1%)

Pharmacodynamics/Kinetics

Bioavailability Fasting: 10%

Time to Peak 1 hour

Protein Binding 98% primarily to α_1-acid glycoprotein

Half-Life Elimination I.V.: 11 ± 5 hours

Metabolism GI: Hydrolysis in the stomach; Hepatic: oxidation, conjugation, and glucuronidation; metabolite (negligible activity); significant first-pass effect

Excretion Feces (~66% as unchanged drug); urine (~33% as metabolites)

Available Dosage Forms

Tablet, oral:
Zelnorm®: 2 mg, 6 mg

Dosing

Adult

IBS with constipation: Females <55 years of age: Oral: 6 mg twice daily, before meals, for 4-6 weeks; may consider continuing treatment for an additional 4-6 weeks in patients who respond initially

Chronic idiopathic constipation: Females <55 years of age: Oral: 6 mg twice daily, before meals; the need for continued therapy should be reassessed periodically

Geriatric Use in elderly women (≥55 years of age) is contraindicated.

Renal Impairment C_{max} and AUC of the inactive metabolite are increased with renal impairment.

Mild-to-moderate impairment: No dosage adjustment recommended
Severe impairment: Use is contraindicated

Hepatic Impairment C_{max} and AUC of tegaserod are increased with hepatic impairment.

Mild impairment: No dosage adjustment recommended; however, use caution
Moderate-to-severe impairment: Use is contraindicated

Administration

Oral Administer 30 minutes before meals.

Stability

Storage Store at controlled room temperature of 15°C to 30°C (59°F to 86°F). Protect from moisture.

Monitoring and Teaching Issues

Physical Assessment For emergency use only under FDA emergency investigational new drug process. Monitor for cardiac event, clinically-significant diarrhea (hypovolemia, hypotension, syncope), and ischemic colitis (rectal bleeding, bloody diarrhea, abdominal pain) frequently when beginning therapy and at regular intervals during treatment.

Patient Education Take on an empty stomach, 30 minutes before meals. Effectiveness of treatment will need to be evaluated by prescriber; maintain contact/appointment schedule as directed. May cause headache, dizziness, nausea, flatulence, or diarrhea. Stop taking Zelnorm® and contact prescriber immediately with any new or sudden worsening abdominal pain or rectal bleeding, or severe or bloody diarrhea. Seek emergency medical care immediately if you experience severe chest pain, shortness of breath, dizziness, sudden onset of weakness, or difficulty walking or talking.

Dietary Considerations Take on an empty stomach, 30 minutes before meals.

Geriatric Considerations No dosing adjustment is required.

Pregnancy Considerations Safety and efficacy have not been established in pregnant women. Use during pregnancy only if clearly needed.

- **Tegaserod Maleate** *see* Tegaserod *on page* 1712
- **TEGretol®** *see* CarBAMazepine *on page* 287
- **TEGretol®-XR** *see* CarBAMazepine *on page* 287
- **TEI-6720** *see* Febuxostat *on page* 737
- **Tekamlo™** *see* Aliskiren and Amlodipine *on page* 73
- **Tekturna®** *see* Aliskiren *on page* 71
- **Tekturna HCT®** *see* Aliskiren and Hydrochlorothiazide *on page* 74

Telbivudine (tel BI vyoo deen)

U.S. Brand Names Tyzeka®

Index Terms L-Deoxythymidine; LdT

Generic Availability (U.S.) No

Pharmacologic Category Antiretroviral Agent, Reverse Transcriptase Inhibitor (Nucleoside)

Medication Guide Available Yes

Pregnancy Risk Factor B

Lactation Excretion in breast milk unknown/not recommended

Use Treatment of chronic hepatitis B with evidence of viral replication and either persistent transaminase elevations or histologically-active disease

Mechanism of Action/Effect Telbivudine, a synthetic thymidine nucleoside analogue (L-enantiomer of thymidine), is intracellularly phosphorylated to the active triphosphate form, which competes with the natural substrate, thymidine 5'-triphosphate, to inhibit hepatitis B viral DNA polymerase; enzyme inhibition blocks reverse transcriptase activity thereby reducing viral DNA replication.

Contraindications There are no contraindications in the manufacturers labeling.

Warnings/Precautions [U.S. Boxed Warnings]: Cases of lactic acidosis and severe hepatomegaly with steatosis, some fatal, have been reported with the use of nucleoside analogues. Severe, acute exacerbation of hepatitis B may occur upon discontinuation. Monitor liver function several months after stopping treatment; reinitiation of antihepatitis B therapy may be required. Myopathy (eg, unexplained muscle aches and/or muscle weakness in conjunction with increases serum creatine kinase) has been reported with telbivudine initiation after several weeks to months; therapy should be interrupted if myopathy suspected and discontinued if diagnosed. Patients taking concomitant medications associated with myopathy should be monitored closely. Concomitant use with peginterferon alfa-2a has been associated with an increased risk of peripheral neuropathy; interrupt therapy for suspected peripheral neuropathy and discontinue if confirmed. Use caution in patients with renal impairment or patients receiving concomitant therapy which may reduce renal function; dosage adjustment required (Cl_{cr} <50 mL/minute). Monitor renal function before and during treatment in liver transplant patients receiving concurrent therapy of cyclosporine or tacrolimus; telbivudine may need to be adjusted. Safety and efficacy in liver transplant patients have not been established.

Not recommended as first-line therapy of chronic HBV due to high rate of resistance; use may be appropriate in short-term treatment of acute HBV (Lok, 2009). Cross-resistance among other antivirals for hepatitis B may occur; use caution in patients failing previous therapy with lamivudine. Telbivudine does not exhibit any clinically-relevant activity against human immunodeficiency virus (HIV type 1). Safety and efficacy have not been studied in patients coinfected with HIV, hepatitis C virus (HCV), or hepatitis D virus (HDV).

Drug Interactions

Avoid Concomitant Use

Avoid concomitant use of Telbivudine with any of the following: Interferon Alfa-2b; Peginterferon Alfa-2a; Peginterferon Alfa-2b

Decreased Effect There are no known significant interactions involving a decrease in effect.

Increased Effect/Toxicity

The levels/effects of Telbivudine may be increased by: Interferon Alfa-2b; Peginterferon Alfa-2a; Peginterferon Alfa-2b

Nutritional/Ethanol Interactions

Ethanol: Should be avoided in hepatitis B infection due to potential hepatic toxicity.

Food: Does not have a significant effect on telbivudine absorption.

Adverse Reactions

>10%:

Central nervous system: Fatigue (13%), headache (10%)

Neuromuscular & skeletal: CPK increased (79%; grades 3/4: 13%)

1% to 10%:

Central nervous system: Dizziness (4%), fever (4%), insomnia (3%)

Dermatologic: Rash (4%), pruritus (2%)

Endocrine & metabolic: Lipase increased (grades 3/4: 2%)

Gastrointestinal: Abdominal pain (3% to 6%), diarrhea (6%), nausea (5%), abdominal distension (3%), dyspepsia (3%)

Hematologic: Neutropenia (grades 3/4: 2%)

Hepatic: ALT increased (grades 3/4: 5% to 7%), AST increased (grades 3/4: 6%)

Neuromuscular & skeletal: Arthralgia (4%), back pain (4%), myalgia (3%)

Respiratory: Cough (6%), pharyngolaryngeal pain (5%)

Pharmacodynamics/Kinetics

Time to Peak 1-4 hours

Protein Binding ~3%

Half-Life Elimination Terminal: 40-49 hours

Metabolism No metabolites detected

Excretion Urine (as unchanged drug)

Product Availability Tyzeka® oral solution: FDA approved April 2009; anticipated availability is currently undetermined

Available Dosage Forms

Tablet, oral:

Tyzeka®: 600 mg

Dosing

Adult Chronic hepatitis B: Oral: 600 mg once daily.

Treatment duration (AASLD practice guidelines):

Hepatitis Be antigen (HBeAg) positive chronic hepatitis: Treat ≥1 year until HBeAg seroconversion and undetectable serum HBV DNA; continue therapy for ≥6 months after HBeAg seroconversion.

HBeAg negative chronic hepatitis: Treat >1 year until hepatitis B surface antigen (HBsAg) clearance.

Note: Patients achieving <2 log decrease in serum HBV DNA after at least 6 months of therapy should either receive additional treatment or be switched to an alternative therapy (Lok, 2009).

Pediatric Chronic hepatitis B: Oral: Adolescents ≥16 years: Refer to adult dosing.

Renal Impairment

Cl_{cr} 30-49 mL/minute: 600 mg every 48 hours

Cl_{cr} <30 mL/minute (not requiring dialysis): 600 mg every 72 hours

End-stage renal disease: 600 mg every 96 hours

Hemodialysis: Administer after dialysis session

Hepatic Impairment No adjustment necessary.

Administration

Oral May be administered without regard to food.

Stability

Storage Store at 25°C (77°F); excursions permitted to 15°C to 30°C (59°F to 86°F).

Monitoring and Teaching Issues

Laboratory Monitoring LFTs (eg, AST and ALT) periodically during therapy and for several months following discontinuation of therapy; renal function prior to initiation and periodically during treatment; serum creatine kinase; HBV DNA (every 3-6 months during therapy); HBeAg and anti-HBe

Physical Assessment Use caution in presence of impaired renal function. Assess suppression of HBV DNA on a regular basis throughout therapy. Monitor for peripheral neuropathy or myopathy (may be necessary to discontinue drug), gastrointestinal effects (pain or vomiting), or upper respiratory infection. Patients should be assessed for several months following discontinuation of therapy for possible clinical exacerbations.

Patient Education This medication does not stop you from spreading HBV to others; consult prescriber about safe sex practices and do not share needles or personal items that may have blood or body fluids on them. Take as directed with or without food. Avoid alcohol (may increase potential for liver damage). Maintain adequate hydration unless instructed to restrict fluid intake. Frequent blood tests may be required. May cause dizziness, fatigue, headache, muscle pain, or rash. Report immediately any signs of lactic acidosis (eg, persistent lethargy or fatigue, unusual muscle pain or weakness, cold feeling [especially in arms and legs], rapid or irregular heart beat, or difficulty breathing); liver toxicity (eg, yellowing of eyes or skin, pale stool and dark urine); or upper respiratory infection.

Dietary Considerations May be taken without regard to food.

Geriatric Considerations Insufficient clinical data in elderly to determine differences between aged patients and younger patients. Since elderly often have Cl_{cr} <50 mL/minute, dosage should be determined accordingly.

Pregnancy Considerations Teratogenic effects have not been observed in animal studies. There are no adequate and well-controlled studies in pregnant women. Health professionals are encouraged to contact the antiretroviral pregnancy registry to monitor outcomes of pregnant women exposed to antiretroviral medications (1-800-258-4263).

Telithromycin (tel ith roe MYE sin)

U.S. Brand Names Ketek®

Index Terms HMR 3647

Generic Availability (U.S.) No

Pharmacologic Category Antibiotic, Ketolide

Medication Safety Issues

Sound-alike/look-alike issues:

Telithromycin may be confused with telavancin

Medication Guide Available Yes

Pregnancy Risk Factor C

Lactation Excretion in breast milk unknown/use caution

Use Treatment of community-acquired pneumonia (mild-to-moderate) caused by susceptible strains of *Streptococcus pneumoniae* (including multidrug-resistant isolates), *Haemophilus influenzae*, *Chlamydophila pneumoniae*, *Moraxella catarrhalis*, and *Mycoplasma pneumoniae*

Mechanism of Action/Effect Inhibits bacterial protein synthesis by binding to two sites on the 50S ribosomal subunit.

Contraindications Hypersensitivity to telithromycin, macrolide antibiotics, or any component of the formulation; myasthenia gravis; history of hepatitis and/or jaundice associated with telithromycin or other macrolide antibiotic use; concurrent use of cisapride or pimozide

Warnings/Precautions Acute hepatic failure and severe liver injury, including hepatitis and hepatic necrosis (leading to some fatalities) have been reported, in some cases after only a few doses; if signs/symptoms of hepatitis or liver damage occur, discontinue therapy and initiate liver function tests. **[U.S. Boxed Warning]: Life-threatening (including fatal) respiratory failure has occurred in patients with myasthenia gravis;** use in these patients is contraindicated. May prolong QT_c interval, leading to a risk of ventricular arrhythmias; closely-related antibiotics have been associated with malignant ventricular arrhythmias and torsade de pointes. Avoid in patients with prolongation of QTc interval due to congenital causes, history of long QT syndrome, uncorrected electrolyte disturbances (hypokalemia or hypomagnesemia), significant bradycardia (<50 bpm), or concurrent therapy with QT_c-prolonging drugs (eg, class Ia and class III antiarrhythmics). Avoid use in patients with a prior history of confirmed cardiogenic syncope or ventricular arrhythmias while receiving macrolide antibiotics or other QT_c-prolonging drugs. May cause severe visual disturbances (eg, changes in accommodation ability, diplopia, blurred vision). May cause loss of consciousness (possibly vagal-related); caution patients that these events may interfere with ability to operate machinery or drive, and to use caution until effects are known. Use caution in renal impairment; severe impairment (Cl_{cr} <30 mL/minute) requires dosage adjustment. Pseudomembranous colitis has been reported. Safety and efficacy not established in pediatric patients <13 years of age per Canadian approved labeling and <18 years of age per U.S. approved labeling.

Drug Interactions

Metabolism/Transport Effects **Substrate** of CYP1A2 (minor), 3A4 (major); **Inhibits** CYP2D6 (weak), 3A4 (strong)

Avoid Concomitant Use

Avoid concomitant use of Telithromycin with any of the following: Alfuzosin; Artemether; BCG; Cisapride; Conivaptan; Disopyramide; Dronedarone; Eplerenone; Everolimus; Halofantrine; Lumefantrine; Lurasidone; Nilotinib; Nisoldipine; Pimozide; QuiNINE; Ranolazine; Rivaroxaban; RomiDEPsin; Salmeterol; Silodosin; Tamsulosin; Tetrabenazine; Thioridazine; Tolvaptan; Toremifene; Vandetanib; Ziprasidone

Decreased Effect

Telithromycin may decrease the levels/effects of: BCG; Clopidogrel; Prasugrel; Typhoid Vaccine

The levels/effects of Telithromycin may be decreased by: CYP3A4 Inducers (Strong); Deferasirox; Etravirine; Herbs (CYP3A4 Inducers)

Increased Effect/Toxicity

Telithromycin may increase the levels/effects of: Alfentanil; Alfuzosin; Almotriptan; Alosetron; Antifungal Agents (Azole Derivatives, Systemic); Antineoplastic Agents (Vinca Alkaloids); Benzodiazepines (metabolized by oxidation); Bortezomib; Brinzolamide; BusPIRone; Calcium Channel Blockers; CarBAMazepine; Cardiac Glycosides; Ciclesonide; Cilostazol; Cisapride; CloZAPine; Colchicine; Conivaptan; Corticosteroids (Orally Inhaled); Corticosteroids (Systemic); CycloSPORINE; CycloSPORINE (Systemic); CYP3A4 Substrates; Dienogest; Disopyramide; Dronedarone; Dutasteride; Eletriptan; Eplerenone; Ergot Derivatives; Everolimus; FentaNYL; Fesoterodine; GuanFACINE; Halofantrine; HMG-CoA Reductase Inhibitors; Ixabepilone; Lumefantrine; Lurasidone; Maraviroc; MethylPREDNISolone; Nilotinib; Nisoldipine; Paricalcitol; Pazopanib; Phosphodiesterase 5 Inhibitors; Pimecrolimus; Pimozide; QTc-Prolonging Agents; QuiNIDine; QuiNINE; Ranolazine; Repaglinide; Rifamycin Derivatives; Rivaroxaban; RomiDEPsin; Salmeterol; Saxagliptin; Selective Serotonin Reuptake Inhibitors; Silodosin; Sirolimus; SORAfenib; Tacrolimus; Tacrolimus (Systemic); Tacrolimus (Topical); Tadalafil; Tamsulosin; Temsirolimus; Tetrabenazine; Thioridazine; Tolvaptan; Toremifene; Vandetanib; Verapamil; Vilazodone; Vitamin K Antagonists; Ziprasidone; Zopiclone

The levels/effects of Telithromycin may be increased by: Alfuzosin; Antifungal Agents (Azole Derivatives, Systemic); Artemether; Chloroquine; Ciprofloxacin; Ciprofloxacin (Systemic); CYP3A4 Inhibitors (Moderate); CYP3A4 Inhibitors (Strong); Gadobutrol; Lumefantrine; Nilotinib; QuiNINE

Nutritional/Ethanol Interactions Herb/nutraceutical: St John's wort: May decrease the levels/effects of telithromycin.

Adverse Reactions

>10%: Gastrointestinal: Diarrhea (10% to 11%)

2% to 10%:

Central nervous system: Headache (2% to 6%), dizziness (3% to 4%)

Gastrointestinal: Nausea (7% to 8%), vomiting (2% to 3%), loose stools (2%), dysgeusia (2%)

≥0.2% to <2%:

Central nervous system: Fatigue, insomnia, somnolence, vertigo

Dermatologic: Rash

Gastrointestinal: Abdominal distension, abdominal pain, anorexia, constipation, dyspepsia, flatulence, gastritis, gastroenteritis, GI upset, glossitis, stomatitis, watery stools, xerostomia

Genitourinary: Vaginal candidiasis

Hematologic: Platelets increased

Hepatic: Transaminases increased

Ocular: Blurred vision, accommodation delayed, diplopia

Miscellaneous: Candidiasis, diaphoresis increased

Pharmacodynamics/Kinetics

Absorption Rapid

Bioavailability 57% (significant first-pass metabolism)

Time to Peak Plasma: 1 hour

Protein Binding 60% to 70%; primarily to albumin

Half-Life Elimination 10 hours

Metabolism Hepatic, via CYP3A4 (50%) and non-CYP-mediated pathways

Excretion Urine (13% unchanged drug, remainder as metabolites); feces (7%)

Available Dosage Forms

Tablet, oral:

Ketek®: 300 mg, 400 mg

Dosing

Adult & Geriatric

Community-acquired pneumonia: Oral: 800 mg once daily for 7-10 days

Pediatric Tonsillitis/pharyngitis (unlabeled use; Canadian indication): Children ≥13 years: Oral: Refer to adult dosing.

Renal Impairment

Cl_{cr} <30 mL/minute, including dialysis:

U.S. product labeling: 600 mg once daily; when renal impairment is accompanied by hepatic impairment, reduce dosage to 400 mg once daily

Canadian product labeling: Reduce dose to 400 mg once daily

Hemodialysis: Administer following dialysis

Hepatic Impairment No adjustment recommended, unless concurrent severe renal impairment is present.

Administration

Oral May be administered with or without food.

Stability

Storage Store at 15°C to 30°C (59°F to 86°F).

Monitoring and Teaching Issues

Laboratory Monitoring Culture and sensitivity; liver function tests

Physical Assessment Assess culture and sensitivity report and previous experience with telithromycin or macrolide antibiotics prior to therapy. Assess patient for contraindications (history of hepatic dysfunction, myasthenia gravis, history of prolonged QT interval). Assess results of LFTs. Monitor for hepatic necrosis or failure, gastrointestinal disturbance (nausea, vomiting, diarrhea), CNS (vertigo, insomnia), rash, opportunistic infection, and QT prolongation during therapy. Teach patient to report any signs of jaundice or hepatic impairment.

Patient Education Take with or without food. May cause headache, dizziness, insomnia, blurred vision, difficulty focusing, nausea, vomiting, loss of appetite, diarrhea, or watery stools (consult prescriber if persistent). If you experience visual difficulties, loss of consciousness (fainting), dark urine, pale stool, or yellowing of skin or eyes, contact prescriber immediately before taking another dose. Report chest pain, palpitations, or irregular heart beat; flushing or facial swelling; CNS disturbance (dizziness, headache, anxiety, abnormal dreams, tremor); unusual muscle weakness; skin rash; or vaginal itching, burning, or discharge.

Dietary Considerations May be taken with or without food.

Geriatric Considerations Bioavailability (57%) equivalent in persons ≥65 years compared to younger adults; although a 1.4- to 2-fold increase in AUC found in older adults. No dosage adjustment required.

Breast-Feeding Considerations It is not known if telithromycin is excreted in breast milk. The manufacturer recommends caution if using telithromycin in a breast-feeding woman.

Pregnancy Considerations Because adverse effects were observed in some animal studies, telithromycin is classified pregnancy category C. There are no adequate and well-controlled studies of telithromycin in pregnant women.

Telmisartan (tel mi SAR tan)

U.S. Brand Names Micardis®

Generic Availability (U.S.) No

Pharmacologic Category Angiotensin II Receptor Blocker

Pregnancy Risk Factor C (1st trimester); D (2nd and 3rd trimesters)

Lactation Excretion in breast milk unknown/not recommended

Use Treatment of hypertension (may be used alone or in combination with other antihypertensive agents); cardiovascular risk reduction in patients ≥55 years of age unable to take ACE inhibitors and who are at high risk of major cardiovascular events (eg, MI, stroke, death)

Mechanism of Action/Effect Telmisartan, a nonpeptide angiotensin receptor antagonist, binds to the AT1 angiotensin II receptor thereby blocking the vasoconstriction and the aldosterone secreting effects of angiotensin II.

Contraindications There are no contraindications listed in manufacturer's labeling.

Canadian labeling: Hypersensitivity to telmisartan or any component of the formulation; second and third trimesters of pregnancy; breast-feeding; fructose intolerance

Warnings/Precautions [U.S. Boxed Warning]: Based on human data, drugs that act on the angiotensin system can cause injury and death to the developing fetus when used in the second and third trimesters. Angiotensin receptor blockers should be discontinued as soon as possible once pregnancy is detected. May cause hyperkalemia; avoid potassium supplementation unless specifically required by healthcare provider. Avoid use or use a smaller dose in patients who are volume depleted; correct depletion first. May be associated with deterioration of renal function and/or increases in serum creatinine, particularly in patients with low renal blood flow (eg, renal artery stenosis, heart failure) whose glomerular filtration rate (GFR) is dependent on efferent arteriolar vasoconstriction by angiotensin II. Use with caution in unstented unilateral/bilateral renal artery stenosis. When unstented bilateral renal artery stenosis is present, use is generally avoided due to the elevated risk of deterioration in renal function unless possible benefits outweigh risks. Use with caution with pre-existing renal insufficiency; significant aortic/mitral stenosis. Concurrent use of ACE inhibitors may increase the risk of clinically-significant adverse events (eg, renal dysfunction, hyperkalemia). Concurrent use with ramipril is not recommended. Use with caution in patients who have biliary obstructive disorders or hepatic dysfunction. Product contains sorbitol. The Canadian labeling (not in U.S. labeling) contraindicates use in fructose intolerant patients.

Drug Interactions

Metabolism/Transport Effects Inhibits CYP2C19 (weak)

Avoid Concomitant Use There are no known interactions where it is recommended to avoid concomitant use.

Decreased Effect

The levels/effects of Telmisartan may be decreased by: Herbs (Hypertensive Properties); Methylphenidate; Nonsteroidal Anti-Inflammatory Agents; Yohimbine

Increased Effect/Toxicity

Telmisartan may increase the levels/effects of: ACE Inhibitors; Amifostine; Antihypertensives; Cardiac Glycosides; Hypotensive Agents; Lithium; Potassium-Sparing Diuretics; Ramipril; RiTUXimab

The levels/effects of Telmisartan may be increased by: Diazoxide; Eplerenone; Herbs (Hypotensive Properties); MAO Inhibitors; Pentoxifylline; Phosphodiesterase 5 Inhibitors; Potassium Salts; Prostacyclin Analogues; Tolvaptan; Trimethoprim

Nutritional/Ethanol Interactions Herb/Nutraceutical: Avoid herbs with hypertensive properties (bayberry, blue cohosh, cayenne, ephedra, ginger, ginseng [American], kola, licorice); may diminish the antihypertensive effect of telmisartan. Avoid herbs with hypotensive properties (black cohosh, California poppy, coleus, golden seal, hawthorn, mistletoe, periwinkle, quinine, shepherd's purse); may enhance the hypotensive effect of telmisartan.

Adverse Reactions May be associated with worsening of renal function in patients dependent on renin-angiotensin-aldosterone system.

1% to 10%:

Cardiovascular: Intermittent claudication (7%; placebo 6%), chest pain (≥1%), hypertension (≥1%), peripheral edema (≥1%)

Central nervous system: Dizziness (≥1%), fatigue (≥1%), headache (≥1%), pain (≥1%)

Dermatologic: Skin ulcer (3%; placebo 2%)

Gastrointestinal: Diarrhea (3%), abdominal pain (≥1%), dyspepsia (≥1%), nausea (≥1%)

Genitourinary: Urinary tract infection (≥1%)

Neuromuscular & skeletal: Back pain (3%), myalgia (≥1%)

Respiratory: Upper respiratory infection (7%), sinusitis (3%), cough (≥1%), pharyngitis (1%)

Pharmacodynamics/Kinetics

Onset of Action 1-2 hours; Peak effect: 0.5-1 hours

Duration of Action Up to 24 hours

Bioavailability Dose dependent: 42% to 58%; Hepatic impairment: Approaches 100%

Time to Peak Plasma: 0.5-1 hours

Protein Binding >99.5%; primarily to albumin and alpha$_1$-acid glycoprotein

Half-Life Elimination Terminal: 24 hours

Metabolism Hepatic via conjugation to inactive metabolites; not metabolized via CYP

Excretion Feces (97%)

Clearance: Total body: 800 mL/minute

Pharmacokinetic Note Orally active, not a prodrug.

Available Dosage Forms

Tablet, oral:

Micardis®: 20 mg, 40 mg, 80 mg

Dosing

Adult

Hypertension: Oral: Initial: 40 mg once daily; usual maintenance dose range: 20-80 mg/day. Patients with volume depletion should be initiated on the lower dosage with close supervision.

Cardiovascular risk reduction: Oral: Initial: 80 mg once daily. **Note:** It is unknown whether doses <80 mg/day are associated with a reduction in risk of cardiovascular morbidity or mortality.

Geriatric

Hypertension: Oral: Initial: 20 mg/day; usual maintenance dose range: 20-80 mg/day

Cardiovascular risk reduction: Oral: Initial 80 mg once daily

Renal Impairment No adjustment required; hemodialysis patients are more susceptible to orthostatic hypotension

Hepatic Impairment Initiate therapy with low dose; titrate slowly and monitor closely.

Canadian labeling: Recommended initial dose: 40 mg/day

Administration

Oral May be administered without regard to meals.

Stability

Storage Store at 25°C (77°F); excursions between 15°C to 30°C (59°F to 86°F) permitted. Protect from moisture and do not remove from blister pack until immediately before use.

Monitoring and Teaching Issues

Laboratory Monitoring Electrolytes, serum creatinine, BUN

Physical Assessment Assess potential for interactions with other pharmacological agents and herbal products (eg, increased risk of hypercalcemia or increased hypotensive effects). Monitor for hypotension, diarrhea, URI, and cough on a regular basis during therapy. Teach patient need for regular blood pressure monitoring.

Patient Education Monitor blood pressure on a regular basis at same time of day, as advised by prescriber. This drug does not eliminate need for diet or exercise regimen as recommended by prescriber. May cause dizziness, fainting, lightheadedness, or postural hypotension. Report unusual weight gain and swelling of ankles, hands, face, lips, throat, or tongue; persistent fatigue; dry cough or respiratory difficulty; palpitations or chest pain; CNS changes; GI disturbances; muscle or bone pain, cramping, or tremors; change in urinary pattern; or changes in hearing or vision.

Dietary Considerations May be taken without regard to meals. Product contains sorbitol.

Geriatric Considerations No initial dose adjustment is required. There appear to be no significant differences in response between the elderly and younger adults (limited data available). Monitor closely during initiation phase. Many elderly may be volume depleted due to diuretics and/or blunted thirst reflex resulting in inadequate fluid intake.

Pregnancy Considerations Medications which act on the renin-angiotensin system are reported to have the following fetal/neonatal effects: Hypotension, neonatal skull hypoplasia, anuria, renal failure, and death; oligohydramnios is also reported. These effects are reported to occur with exposure during the second and third trimesters. There are no adequate and well-controlled studies in pregnant women. **[U.S. Boxed Warning]: Based on human data, drugs that act on the angiotensin system can cause injury and death to the developing fetus when used in the second and third trimesters. Angiotensin receptor blockers should be discontinued as soon as possible once pregnancy is detected.**

Related Information

Angiotensin Agents *on page 1974*

Telmisartan and Amlodipine (tel mi SAR tan & am LOE di peen)

U.S. Brand Names Twynsta®

Index Terms Amlodipine and Telmisartan; Amlodipine Besylate and Telmisartan

Generic Availability (U.S.) No

Pharmacologic Category Angiotensin II Receptor Blocker; Calcium Channel Blocker; Calcium Channel Blocker, Dihydropyridine

Pregnancy Risk Factor C (1st trimester); D (2nd and 3rd trimesters)

Lactation Excretion in breast milk unknown/not recommended

Use Treatment of hypertension, including initial treatment in patients who will require multiple antihypertensives for adequate control

Available Dosage Forms

Tablet, oral:

Twynsta® 40/5: Telmisartan 40 mg and amlodipine 5 mg; Twynsta® 40/10: telmisartan 40 mg and amlodipine 10 mg; Twynsta® 80/5: telmisartan 80 mg and amlodipine 5 mg; Twynsta® 80/10: telmisartan 80 mg and amlodipine10 mg

Dosing

Adult Dose is individualized; combination product may be substituted for individual components in patients currently maintained on both agents separately or in patients not adequately controlled with monotherapy (using one of the agents or an agent within the same antihypertensive class). May also be used as initial therapy in patients who are likely to need >1 antihypertensive to control blood pressure.

Hypertension: Oral:

Initial therapy (antihypertensive naive): Telmisartan 40 mg/amlodipine 5 mg once daily; dose may be increased after 2 weeks of therapy. Patients requiring larger blood pressure reductions may be started on telmisartan 80 mg/amlodipine 5 mg once daily. Maximum recommended dose: Telmisartan 80 mg/day, amlodipine 10 mg/day

Add-on/replacement therapy: Telmisartan 40-80 mg and amlodipine 5-10 mg once daily depending upon previous doses, current control, and goals of therapy; dose may be titrated after 2 weeks of therapy. Maximum recommended dose: Telmisartan 80 mg/day; amlodipine 10 mg/day

Geriatric Initial therapy is not recommended in patients ≥75 years. Amlodipine therapy should be initiated at 2.5 mg once daily and slowly titrated up. The appropriate combination form is not available.

Renal Impairment

Mild-to-moderate impairment: No adjustment necessary.

Severe impairment: Titrate slowly.

Hepatic Impairment Initial therapy is not recommended. Initiate amlodipine therapy at 2.5 mg once daily and titrate slowly. The appropriate combination form is not available.

Administration

Oral May be administered without regard to meals.

Monitoring and Teaching Issues

Laboratory Monitoring Baseline and periodic electrolyte panels (especially serum potassium); renal function; hepatic function

Physical Assessment See individual agents.

Patient Education See individual agents.

Related Information

AmLODIPine *on page 104*

Telmisartan *on page 1717*

Telmisartan and Hydrochlorothiazide

(tel mi SAR tan & hye droe klor oh THYE a zide)

U.S. Brand Names Micardis® HCT

Index Terms Hydrochlorothiazide and Telmisartan

Generic Availability (U.S.) No

Pharmacologic Category Angiotensin II Receptor Blocker; Diuretic, Thiazide

Pregnancy Risk Factor C (1st trimester); D (2nd and 3rd trimesters)

Lactation Enters breast milk/not recommended

Use Treatment of hypertension; combination product should not be used for initial therapy

Available Dosage Forms

Tablet, oral:

Micardis® HCT: 40/12.5: Telmisartan 40 mg and hydrochlorothiazide 12.5 mg; 80/12.5: Telmisartan 80 mg and hydrochlorothiazide 12.5 mg; 80/25: Telmisartan 80 mg and hydrochlorothiazide 25 mg

Dosing

Adult Hypertension: Oral: Replacement therapy: Combination product can be substituted for individual titrated agents. Initiation of combination therapy when monotherapy has failed to achieve desired effects:

Patients currently on telmisartan: Initial dose if blood pressure is not currently controlled on monotherapy of 80 mg telmisartan: Telmisartan 80 mg/hydrochlorothiazide 12.5 mg once daily; may titrate up to telmisartan 160 mg/hydrochlorothiazide 25 mg if needed.

Patients currently on hydrochlorothiazide: Initial dose if blood pressure is not currently controlled on monotherapy of 25 mg once daily: Telmisartan 80 mg/hydrochlorothiazide 12.5 mg once daily or telmisartan 80 mg/hydrochlorothiazide 25 mg once daily; may titrate up to telmisartan 160 mg/hydrochlorothiazide 25 mg if blood pressure remains uncontrolled after 2-4 weeks of therapy. Patients who develop hypokalemia while on hydrochlorothiazide 25 mg may be switched to telmisartan 80 mg/hydrochlorothiazide 12.5 mg.

Geriatric Refer to adult dosing. Monitor renal function.

Renal Impairment

Cl_{cr} >30 mL/minute: No dosage adjustment necessary.

Cl_{cr} ≤30 mL/minute: Not recommended.

Hepatic Impairment

Mild-to-moderate hepatic impairment or biliary obstructive disorders: Initial: Telmisartan 40 mg/hydrochlorothiazide 12.5 mg.

Severe hepatic impairment: Not recommended.

Administration

Oral May be administered without regard to meals.

Monitoring and Teaching Issues

Laboratory Monitoring Electrolytes, serum creatinine, BUN

Physical Assessment See individual agents.

Patient Education See individual agents.

Related Information

Hydrochlorothiazide *on page* 912

Telmisartan *on page* 1717

Temazepam (te MAZ e pam)

U.S. Brand Names Restoril™

Generic Availability (U.S.) Yes

Pharmacologic Category Hypnotic, Benzodiazepine

Medication Safety Issues

Sound-alike/look-alike issues:

Temazepam may be confused with flurazepam, LORazepam, tamoxifen

Restoril™ may be confused with, RisperDAL®, Vistaril®, Zestril®

Beers Criteria medication: This drug may be inappropriate for use in geriatric patients (high severity risk).

Medication Guide Available Yes

Pregnancy Risk Factor X

Lactation Enters breast milk/use caution (AAP rates "of concern"; AAP 2001 update pending)

Use Short-term treatment of insomnia

Unlabeled/Investigational Use Treatment of anxiety

Controlled Substance C-IV

Available Dosage Forms

Capsule, oral: 7.5 mg, 15 mg, 22.5 mg, 30 mg

Restoril™: 7.5 mg, 15 mg, 22.5 mg, 30 mg

Dosing

Adult Insomnia: Oral: Usual dose: 15-30 mg at bedtime; some patients may respond to 7.5 mg in transient insomnia

Geriatric Initial: 7.5 mg in elderly or debilitated patients at bedtime

Monitoring and Teaching Issues

Physical Assessment For short-term use. Assess for history of addiction; long-term use can result in dependence, abuse, or tolerance. For inpatient use, institute safety measures to prevent falls. For outpatients, monitor for CNS depression at beginning of therapy and periodically throughout.

Patient Education Drug may cause physical and/or psychological dependence. May take with food to decrease GI upset. While using this medication, do not use alcohol. Maintain adequate hydration unless instructed to restrict fluid intake. You may experience drowsiness, dizziness, lightheadedness, blurred vision, dry mouth, or GI discomfort. Report CNS changes (confusion, depression, increased sedation, excitation, headache, abnormal thinking, insomnia, or nightmares, memory impairment, impaired coordination), respiratory difficulty, persistent dizziness, alterations in normal gait, vision changes, or ineffectiveness of medication.

Related Information

Benzodiazepines *on page 1988*

◆ **Temodar®** *see* Temozolomide *on page 1721*

Temozolomide (te moe ZOE loe mide)

U.S. Brand Names Temodar®

Index Terms SCH 52365; TMZ

Generic Availability (U.S.) No

Pharmacologic Category Antineoplastic Agent, Alkylating Agent (Triazene)

Medication Safety Issues

Sound-alike/look-alike issues:

Temodar® may be confused with Tambocor®

Temozolomide may be confused with temsirolimus

High alert medication: This medication is in a class the Institute for Safe Medication Practices (ISMP) includes among its list of drug classes which have a heightened risk of causing significant patient harm when used in error.

Pregnancy Risk Factor D

Lactation Excretion in breast milk unknown/not recommended

Use Treatment of newly-diagnosed glioblastoma multiforme (initially in combination with radiotherapy, then as maintenance treatment); treatment of refractory anaplastic astrocytoma

Canadian labeling (not an approved indication in the U.S.): Treatment of recurrent or progressive glioblastoma multiforme

Unlabeled/Investigational Use Treatment of recurrent glioblastoma multiforme, low-grade astrocytoma, low-grade oligodendroglioma, anaplastic oligodendroglioma, metastatic CNS lesions, refractory primary CNS lymphoma, advanced or metastatic melanoma, cutaneous T-cell lymphomas (mycosis fungoides [MF] and Sézary syndrome [SS]), advanced neuroendocrine tumors (carcinoid or islet cell), Ewing's sarcoma (recurrent or progressive), soft tissue sarcomas (extremity/retroperitoneal/intra-abdominal or hemangiopericytoma/solitary fibrous tumor), treatment of pediatric neuroblastoma

Available Dosage Forms

Capsule, oral:

Temodar®: 5 mg, 20 mg, 100 mg, 140 mg, 180 mg, 250 mg

Injection, powder for reconstitution:

Temodar®: 100 mg

Dosing

Adult

Anaplastic astrocytoma (refractory): Oral, I.V.: Initial dose: 150 mg/m^2/day for 5 days; repeat every 28 days. Subsequent doses of 100-200 mg/m^2/day for 5 days per treatment cycle; based upon hematologic tolerance.

Dosage modification for toxicity:

ANC <1000/mm^3 or platelets <50,000/mm^3 on day 22 or day 29 (day 1 of next cycle): Postpone therapy until ANC >1500/mm^3 and platelets >100,000/mm^3; reduce dose by 50 mg/m^2/day for subsequent cycle

ANC 1000-1500/mm^3 or platelets 50,000-100,000/mm^3 on day 22 or day 29 (day 1 of next cycle): Postpone therapy until ANC >1500/mm^3 and platelets >100,000/mm^3; maintain initial dose

ANC ≥1500/mm^3 and platelets ≥100,000/mm^3 on day 22 or day 29 (day 1 of next cycle): Increase dose to or maintain dose at 200 mg/m^2/day for 5 days for subsequent cycle

Glioblastoma multiforme (newly diagnosed, high-grade glioma): Oral, I.V.:

Concomitant phase: 75 mg/m^2/day for 42 days with focal radiotherapy (60Gy administered in 30 fractions). **Note:** PCP prophylaxis is required during concomitant phase and should continue in patients who develop lymphocytopenia until lymphocyte recovery to ≤ grade 1. Obtain weekly CBC.

Continue at 75 mg/m^2/day throughout the 42-day concomitant phase (up to 49 days) as long as ANC ≥1500/mm^3, platelet count ≥100,000/mm^3, and nonhematologic toxicity ≤ grade 1 (excludes alopecia, nausea/vomiting)

Dosage modification for toxicity:

ANC ≥500/mm^3 but <1500/mm^3 **or** platelet count ≥10,000/mm^3 but <100,000/mm^3 **or** grade 2 nonhematologic toxicity (excludes alopecia, nausea/vomiting): Interrupt therapy

ANC <500/mm^3 **or** platelet count <10,000/mm^3 **or** grade 3/4 nonhematologic toxicity (excludes alopecia, nausea/vomiting): Discontinue therapy

Maintenance phase (consists of 6 treatment cycles): Begin 4 weeks after concomitant phase completion. **Note:** Each subsequent cycle is 28 days (consisting of 5 days of drug treatment followed by 23 days without treatment). Draw CBC within 48 hours of day 22; hold next cycle and do weekly CBC until ANC >1500/mm^3 and platelet count >100,000/mm^3; dosing modification should be based on lowest blood counts and worst nonhematologic toxicity during the previous cycle.

Cycle 1: 150 mg/m^2/day for 5 days; repeat every 28 days

Cycles 2-6: May increase to 200 mg/m^2/day for 5 days every 28 days (if ANC ≥1500/mm^3, platelets ≥100,000/mm^3 and nonhematologic toxicities for cycle 1 are ≤ grade 2 [excludes alopecia, nausea/vomiting]); **Note:** If dose was not escalated at the onset of cycle 2, do not increase for cycles 3-6)

Dosage modification (during maintenance phase) for toxicity:

ANC <1000/mm^3, platelet count <50,000/mm^3, or grade 3 nonhematologic toxicity (excludes for alopecia, nausea/vomiting) during previous cycle: Decrease dose by 1 dose level (by 50 mg/m^2/day for 5 days), unless dose has already been lowered to 100 mg/m^2/day, then discontinue therapy.

If dose reduction <100 mg/m^2/day is required or grade 4 nonhematologic toxicity (excludes for alopecia, nausea/vomiting), or if the same grade 3 nonhematologic toxicity occurs after dose reduction: Discontinue therapy

Glioblastoma multiforme (recurrent glioma): *Canadian labeling (unlabeled use in the U.S.):* 200 mg/m^2/day for 5 days every 28 days; if previously treated with chemotherapy, initiate at 150 mg/m^2/day for 5 days every 28 days and increase to 200 mg/m^2/day for 5 days every 28 days with cycle 2 if no hematologic toxicity (Brada, 2001; Yung, 2000)

Ewing's sarcoma, recurrent or progressive (unlabeled use): Oral: 100 mg/m^2/dose days 1-5 every 21 days (in combination with irinotecan) (Casey, 2009)

Melanoma, advanced or metastatic (unlabeled use): Oral: 200 mg/m^2/day for 5 days every 28 days (for up to 12 cycles). For subsequent cycles reduce dose to 75% of the original dose for grade 3/4 hematologic toxicity and reduce the dose to 50% of the original dose for grade 3/4 nonhematologic toxicity (Middleton, 2000).

Neuroendocrine tumors, advanced (unlabeled use): Oral: 150 mg/m^2/day for 7 days every 14 days in combination with thalidomide (Kulke, 2006)

Primary CNS lymphoma, refractory (unlabeled use): Oral: 150 mg/m^2/day for 5 days every 28 days, initially in combination with rituximab, followed by temozolomide monotherapy: 150 mg/m^2/day for 5 days every 28 days (Wong, 2004) **or** 150 mg/m^2/day for 7 days every 14 days, initially in combination with rituximab, followed by temozolomide monotherapy: 150 mg/m^2/day for 5 days every 28 days (Enting, 2004)

Soft tissue sarcoma (unlabeled use): Oral: 75 mg/m^2/day for 6 weeks (Garcia del Muro, 2005)

Geriatric Refer to adult dosing. **Note:** Patients ≥70 years of age in the anaplastic astrocytoma study had a higher incidence of grade 4 neutropenia and thrombocytopenia in the first cycle of therapy than patients <70 years of age.

Pediatric

Ewing's sarcoma, recurrent or progressive (unlabeled use): Oral: Refer to adult dosing.

Neuroblastoma, relapsed or refractory (unlabeled use): Oral: 100 mg/m^2/dose days 1-5 days every 21 days (in combination with irinotecan) for up to 6 cycles (Bagatell, 2011)

Renal Impairment Oral:

Cl_{cr} ≥36 mL/minute/m^2: No effect on temozolomide clearance was demonstrated.

Severe renal impairment (Cl_{cr} <36 mL/minute/m^2): Use with caution.

Dialysis patients: Use has not been studied.

Hepatic Impairment Severe hepatic impairment: Use with caution.

Administration

Oral Swallow capsules whole with a glass of water. Absorption is affected by food. Administer consistently either with food or without food (was administered in studies under fasting and nonfasting conditions). May administer on an empty stomach or at bedtime to reduce nausea and vomiting. Standard antiemetics may be administered if needed. Do not repeat dose if vomiting occurs after dose is administered; wait until the next scheduled dose. Do not open or chew capsules; avoid contact with skin if capsules are accidentally opened or damaged.

I.V. Infuse over 90 minutes. Flush line before and after administration. May be administered through the same I.V. line as sodium chloride 0.9%; do not administer other medications through the same I.V. line.

Monitoring and Teaching Issues

Laboratory Monitoring CBC with differential and platelets (prior to each cycle; weekly during glioma concomitant phase treatment; at or within 48 hours of day 22 and weekly until ANC >1500/mm^3 for glioma maintenance and astrocytoma treatment)

Physical Assessment Monitor for CNS effects, gastrointestinal disturbance, myelosuppression, opportunistic infection, vision disturbance, and cough on a regular basis; dosage adjustments may be necessary for toxicity.

Patient Education If administered I.V., report immediately any swelling, pain, or burning at infusion site. May cause headache, dizziness, confusion, fatigue, anxiety, insomnia, impaired coordination, nausea, vomiting, loss of appetite, constipation, or diarrhea. Report chest pain or palpitations; acute headache; unusual swelling of legs or feet; visual disturbances; unresolved GI problems; itching or burning on urination or vaginal discharge; acute joint, back, bone, or muscle pain or unusual weakness; difficulty breathing; cough; or signs of respiratory infection.

Oral: Take always with food or always without food; taking at bedtime may reduce nausea or vomiting. Swallow whole with 8 ounces of water. Do not open, crush, or chew capsules; if capsule is accidentally broken, do not inhale powder (wash hands thoroughly if powder gets on skin).

Temsirolimus (tem sir OH li mus)

U.S. Brand Names Torisel®

Index Terms CCI-779

Generic Availability (U.S.) No

Pharmacologic Category Antineoplastic Agent, mTOR Kinase Inhibitor

Medication Safety Issues

Sound-alike/look-alike issues:

Temsirolimus may be confused with everolimus, sirolimus, tacrolimus, temozolomide, tesamorelin

High alert medication: This medication is in a class the Institute for Safe Medication Practices (ISMP) includes among its list of drug classes which have a heightened risk of causing significant patient harm when used in error.

Temsirolimus requires a two-step dilution process prior to administration. Dilute initially to 10 mg/mL (with provided diluent), then further dilute for infusion in 250 mL sodium chloride 0.9%. Errors have occurred due to improper preparation.

Temsirolimus, for the treatment of advanced renal cell cancer, is a flat dose (25 mg) and is not based on body surface area (BSA).

Pregnancy Risk Factor D

Lactation Excretion in breast milk unknown/not recommended

Use Treatment of advanced renal cell cancer (RCC)

Mechanism of Action/Effect Targeted inhibitor of mTOR (rapamycin kinase), which regulates tumor cell growth and angiogenesis

Contraindications Bilirubin >1.5 times the upper limit of normal (ULN)

Canadian labeling: Additional contraindications (not in U.S. labeling): History of anaphylaxis after exposure to temsirolimus, sirolimus, or any component of the formulation

Warnings/Precautions Hazardous agent - use appropriate precautions for handling and disposal.

Hypersensitivity/infusion reactions (eg, anaphylaxis, apnea, dyspnea, flushing, loss of consciousness, hypotension, and/or chest pain) have been reported. Infusion reaction may occur with initial or subsequent infusions. Premedicate with an antihistamine (H_1 antagonist) prior to infusion; monitor during infusion; interrupt infusion for hypersensitivity reaction and observe patient for 30-60 minutes. With discretion, treatment may be resumed at a slower infusion rate; administer an H_1 antagonist (if not given as premedication) and/or an H_2 antagonist 30 minutes prior to resuming infusion. Use with caution in patients with hypersensitivity temsirolimus, sirolimus (a metabolite), or polysorbate 80. Angioneurotic edema has been reported; concurrent use with other drugs known to cause angioedema (eg, ACE inhibitors) may increase risk.

Temsirolimus is predominantly cleared by the liver; use with caution and reduce dose in patients with mild hepatic impairment (bilirubin >1-1.5 x ULN or AST >ULN with bilirubin ≤ULN). Use is contraindicated in patients with moderate-to-severe hepatic impairment (bilirubin >1.5 x ULN).

Avoid concomitant use with strong CYP3A4 inhibitors and strong CYP3A4 inducers (see Drug Interactions); consider alternative agents that avoid or lessen the potential for CYP-mediated interactions. Patients should not be immunized with live, viral vaccines during or shortly after treatment and should avoid close contact with recently vaccinated (live vaccine) individuals. Patients who are receiving anticoagulant therapy or those with CNS tumors/metastases may be at increased risk for developing intracerebral bleeding. Combination therapy with temsirolimus and sunitinib has resulted in dose-limiting toxicities, including grade 3 or 4 rash, gout, and/or cellulitis.

Increases in serum glucose commonly occur during treatment; initiation or alteration of insulin and/or oral hypoglycemic therapy may be required; monitor serum glucose before and during treatment; use with caution in patients with diabetes. Use with caution in patients with hyperlipidemia; may increase serum lipids (cholesterol and triglycerides); initiation or dosage adjustment of of antihyperlipidemic agents may be required. Treatment may result in immunosuppression, may increase risk of opportunistic infections and/or sepsis. Interstitial lung disease (ILD), sometimes fatal, has been reported; symptoms include dyspnea, cough, hypoxia, and/or fever, although asymptomatic cases may present; promptly evaluate worsening respiratory symptoms; may require corticosteroids, antibiotic therapy, or treatment discontinuation. Cases of bowel perforation (fatal) have occurred (usually presenting with abdominal pain, bloody stools, diarrhea, fever, or metabolic acidosis); promptly evaluate any new or worsening abdominal pain or bloody stools. Temsirolimus may be associated with impaired wound healing; use caution in the perioperative period. Cases of acute renal failure with rapid progression have been reported (unrelated to disease progression), including cases unresponsive to dialysis.

Drug Interactions

Metabolism/Transport Effects **Substrate** of CYP3A4 (major), P-glycoprotein; **Inhibits** CYP3A4 (weak), 2D6 (weak)

Avoid Concomitant Use

Avoid concomitant use of Temsirolimus with any of the following: BCG; Natalizumab; Pimecrolimus; Roflumilast; SUNItinib; Tacrolimus; Tacrolimus (Systemic); Tacrolimus (Topical); Vaccines (Live)

Decreased Effect

Temsirolimus may decrease the levels/effects of: BCG; Sipuleucel-T; Tacrolimus; Tacrolimus (Systemic); Vaccines (Inactivated); Vaccines (Live)

The levels/effects of Temsirolimus may be decreased by: CarBAMazepine; CYP3A4 Inducers (Strong); Deferasirox; Echinacea; Herbs (CYP3A4 Inducers); P-Glycoprotein Inducers; Phenytoin; Rifamycin Derivatives

Increased Effect/Toxicity

Temsirolimus may increase the levels/effects of: ACE Inhibitors; CycloSPORINE; CycloSPORINE (Systemic); Hypoglycemic Agents; Leflunomide; Natalizumab; SUNItinib; Tacrolimus; Tacrolimus (Systemic); Tacrolimus (Topical); Vaccines (Live)

The levels/effects of Temsirolimus may be increased by: Conivaptan; CYP3A4 Inhibitors (Moderate); CYP3A4 Inhibitors (Strong); Dasatinib; Denosumab; Fluconazole; Herbs (Hypoglycemic Properties); Itraconazole; Ketoconazole; Ketoconazole (Systemic); Macrolide Antibiotics; P-Glycoprotein Inhibitors; Pimecrolimus; Posaconazole; Protease Inhibitors; Roflumilast; Tacrolimus; Tacrolimus (Systemic); Tacrolimus (Topical); Trastuzumab

Nutritional/Ethanol Interactions Herb/Nutraceutical: St John's wort may decrease sirolimus (the active metabolite of temsirolimus) levels; avoid concurrent use. Herbs with hypoglycemic properties may increase the risk of temsirolimus-induced hypoglycemia; includes alfalfa, aloe, bilberry, bitter melon, burdock, celery, damiana, fenugreek, garcinia, garlic, ginger, ginseng (American), gymnema, marshmallow, stinging nettle. Avoid grapefruit and grapefruit juice (may increase the levels/effects of sirolimus).

Adverse Reactions

>10%:

Cardiovascular: Edema (35%), peripheral edema (27%), chest pain (16%)
Central nervous system: Pain (28%), fever (24%), headache (15%), insomnia (12%)
Dermatologic: Rash (47%), pruritus (19%), nail disorder/thinning (14%), dry skin (11%)
Endocrine & metabolic: Hyperglycemia (26% to 89%; grades 3/4: 16%), hypercholesterolemia (24% to 87%; grades 3/4: 2%), hypertriglyceridemia (83%; grades 3/4: 44%), hypophosphatemia (49%; grades 3/4: 18%), hyperlipidemia (27%), hypokalemia (21%; grades 3/4: 5%)
Gastrointestinal: Mucositis (41%), nausea (37%), anorexia (32%), diarrhea (27%), abdominal pain (21%), constipation (20%), stomatitis (20%), taste disturbance (20%), vomiting (19%), weight loss (19%)
Genitourinary: Urinary tract infection (15%)
Hematologic: Anemia (45% to 94%; grades 3/4: 20%), lymphopenia (53%; grades 3/4: 16%), thrombocytopenia (14% to 40%; grades 3/4: 1%; dose-limiting toxicity), leukopenia (6% to 32%; grades 3/4: 1%), neutropenia (7% to 19%; grades 3/4: 3% to 5%)
Hepatic: Alkaline phosphatase increased (68%; grades 3/4: 3%), AST increased (8% to 38%; grades 3/4: 1% to 2%)
Neuromuscular & skeletal: Weakness (51%), back pain (20%), arthralgia (18%)
Renal: Creatinine increased (14% to 57%; grades 3/4: 3%)
Respiratory: Dyspnea (28%), cough (26%), epistaxis (12%), pharyngitis (12%)
Miscellaneous: Infection (20% to 27%; includes abscess, bronchitis, cellulitis, herpes simplex, herpes zoster)

1% to 10%:

Cardiovascular: Hypertension (7%), venous thromboembolism (2%, includes DVT and PE), thrombophlebitis (1%)
Central nervous system: Chills (8%), depression (4%)
Dermatologic: Acne (10%), wound healing impaired (1%)
Gastrointestinal: Bowel perforation (fatal: 1%)
Hepatic: Hyperbilirubinemia (8%; grades 3/4: 1%)
Neuromuscular & skeletal: Myalgia (8%)
Ocular: Conjunctivitis (7%)
Respiratory: Rhinitis (10%), pneumonia (8%), upper respiratory tract infection (7%), interstitial lung disease (2%)
Miscellaneous: Allergic/hypersensitivity/infusion reaction (9%; includes anaphylaxis, apnea, chest pain, dyspnea, flushing, hypotension, loss of consciousness)

Pharmacodynamics/Kinetics

Time to Peak Temsirolimus: At end of infusion; Sirolimus: 0.5-2 hours after temsirolimus infusion

Half-Life Elimination Temsirolimus: ~17 hours; Sirolimus: ~55 hours

Metabolism Hepatic; via CYP3A4 to sirolimus (primary active metabolite) and 4 minor metabolites

Excretion Feces (78%); urine (<5%)

Available Dosage Forms

Injection, solution:

Torisel®: 25 mg/mL (1.2 mL)

Dosing

Adult & Geriatric Note: For infusion reaction prophylaxis, premedicate with an H_1 antagonist (eg, diphenhydramine 25-50 mg I.V.) 30 minutes prior to infusion.

RCC: I.V.: 25 mg once weekly; continue until disease progression or unacceptable toxicity

Dosage adjustment for concomitant CYP3A4 inhibitors/inducers:

CYP3A4 inhibitors: Avoid concomitant administration with strong CYP3A4 inhibitors (eg, clarithromycin, itraconazole, ketoconazole, nefazodone, protease inhibitors, telithromycin, voriconazole); if concomitant administration with a strong CYP3A4 inhibitor cannot be avoided, consider a dose reduction to 12.5 mg/week. When a strong CYP3A4 inhibitor is discontinued; allow ~1 week to elapse prior to adjusting the temsirolimus upward to the dose used prior to initiation of the CYP3A4 inhibitor.

CYP3A4 inducers: Avoid concomitant administration with strong CYP3A4 inducers (eg, carbamazepine, dexamethasone, phenobarbital, phenytoin, rifampin, St John's wort); if concomitant administration with a strong CYP3A4 inducer cannot be avoided, consider adjusting temsirolimus dose up to 50 mg/week. If the strong CYP3A4 enzyme inducer is discontinued, reduce the temsirolimus to the dose used prior to initiation of the CYP3A4 inducer.

Renal Impairment Not studied in renal dysfunction; however, due to the minimal renal elimination (<5%), dosage adjustment for renal dysfunction is not recommended.

Hemodialysis: Has not been studied in hemodialysis patients.

Hepatic Impairment

Mild hepatic impairment (bilirubin >1-1.5 x ULN or AST >ULN with bilirubin ≤ULN): Reduce dose to 15 mg once weekly.

Moderate-to-severe hepatic impairment (bilirubin >1.5 x ULN): Use is contraindicated.

Adjustment for Toxicity

Hematologic toxicity: ANC <1000/mm^3 or platelets <75,000/mm^3: Withhold treatment until resolves and reinitiate treatment with a 5 mg/week dose reduction; minimum dose: 15 mg/week if adjustment for toxicity is needed.

Nonhematologic toxicity: Any toxicity ≥grade 3: Withhold treatment until resolves to ≤grade 2; reinitiate treatment with a 5 mg/week dose reduction; minimum dose: 15 mg/week if adjustment for toxicity is needed.

Infusion/hypersensitivity reaction: Interrupt infusion and observe for 30-60 minutes; treatment may be resumed with discretion at a slower infusion rate (up to 60 minutes); administer an H1 antagonist (if not given as premedication) and/or an H_2 antagonist 30 minutes prior to resuming infusion.

Administration

I.V. Infuse over 30-60 minutes via an infusion pump (preferred). Use non-DEHP containing administration tubing. Administer through an inline polyethersulfone filter ≤5 micron. Premedicate with an H_1 antagonist (eg, diphenhydramine 25-50 mg I.V. 30 minutes prior to infusion. Monitor during infusion; interrupt infusion for hypersensitivity/infusion reaction; monitor for 30-60 minutes; may reinitiate at a reduced infusion rate (over 60 minutes) with discretion, 30 minutes after administration of a histamine H_1 antagonist and/or a histamine H_2 antagonist (eg, famotidine or ranitidine). Administration should be completed within 6 hours of admixture.

Stability

Reconstitution Preparation requires a two-step dilution process. Vials should initially be diluted with 1.8 mL of provided diluent to a concentration of 10 mg/mL (vial contains overfill). Mix by inverting vial. After allowing air bubbles to subside, further dilute in 250 mL of NS in a non-DEHP/non-PVC container (glass, polyolefin, or polypropylene). Avoid excessive shaking (may result in foaming). Use appropriate precautions for handling and disposal.

Storage Store intact vials under refrigeration at 2°C to 8°C (36°F to 46°F). Diluted solution in the vial (10 mg/mL) is stable for 24 hours at room temperature. Solutions diluted for infusion (in normal saline) must be infused within 6 hours of preparation. Protect from light during storage, preparation, and handling.

Monitoring and Teaching Issues

Laboratory Monitoring CBC with differential and platelets (weekly), serum chemistries including glucose (baseline and every other week), serum cholesterol and triglycerides (baseline and periodic), liver function (baseline and periodic), renal function tests (baseline and periodic)

Physical Assessment Premedicate with antihistamine prior to infusion. Patient must be monitored closely for anaphylaxis, dyspnea, flushing, and chest pain during and following each infusion; medication/equipment for treating reactions should be readily available. Monitor for hypersensitivity, altered glucose control, opportunistic infection or impaired wound healing, interstitial lung disease, bowel perforations, and renal failure at each infusion and throughout therapy; discontinuation may be necessary.

Patient Education This medication can only be administered by infusion; you will be closely monitored during infusion. Report immediately unusual back or abdominal pain; acute headache; difficulty breathing or chest pain; difficulty swallowing; itching or rash; or redness, swelling, or pain at infusion site. Maintain adequate nutrition and hydration between treatments, unless instructed to restrict fluid intake. You will be required to have regularly scheduled laboratory tests while on this medication. You will be more susceptible to infection. If you have diabetes, you will be instructed to check your glucose levels closely and notify prescriber of significant changes, excessive thirst, or frequency of urination. This medication can affect glucose control and diabetic medications may need to be adjusted. You may experience headache, insomnia, loss of appetite, nausea, dry mouth, taste changes, rash, or dry skin. Report immediately changes in respiratory status (difficulty breathing, dyspnea, unusual cough, or fever), abdominal pain or blood in stool, signs or symptoms of any urinary tract infection (difficulty urinating, burning on urination, or perineal itching), or unusual infection or delayed wound healing.

Breast-Feeding Considerations Due to the potential for serious adverse reactions in the nursing infant, breast-feeding is not recommended.

Pregnancy Considerations Embryotoxicity and fetotoxicity (as evidenced by increased mortality, reduced fetal weights, and delayed ossification) occurred in animal studies at oral doses lower than the usual human dose. There are no adequate and well-controlled studies in pregnant women. Women of childbearing potential should be advised to avoid pregnancy. Men and women should use effective birth control during temsirolimus treatment, and continue for 3 months after temsirolimus discontinuation.

Tenecteplase (ten EK te plase)

U.S. Brand Names TNKase®

Generic Availability (U.S.) No

Pharmacologic Category Thrombolytic Agent

Medication Safety Issues

Sound-alike/look-alike issues:

TNKase® may be confused with Activase®, t-PA

TNK (occasional abbreviation for TNKase®) is an error-prone abbreviation (mistaken as TPA)

High alert medication: The Institute for Safe Medication Practices (ISMP) includes this medication (I.V.) among its list of drugs which have a heightened risk of causing significant patient harm when used in error.

Pregnancy Risk Factor C

Lactation Use caution

Use Thrombolytic agent used in the management of ST-elevation myocardial infarction (STEMI) for the lysis of thrombi in the coronary vasculature to restore perfusion and reduce mortality.

Recommended criteria for treatment: STEMI: Chest pain ≥20 minutes duration, onset of chest pain within 12 hours of treatment (or within prior 12-24 hours in patients with continuing ischemic symptoms), and S-T segment elevation >0.1 mV in at least two contiguous precordial leads or two adjacent limb leads on ECG or new or presumably new left bundle branch block (LBBB)

Unlabeled/Investigational Use Acute MI - combination regimen of tenecteplase (unlabeled dose), abciximab, and heparin (unlabeled dose)

Mechanism of Action/Effect Initiates fibrinolysis by binding to fibrin and converting plasminogen to plasmin.

Contraindications Hypersensitivity to tenecteplase or any component of the formulation; active internal bleeding; history of stroke; intracranial/intraspinal surgery or trauma within 2 months; intracranial neoplasm; arteriovenous malformation or aneurysm; bleeding diathesis; severe uncontrolled hypertension

Warnings/Precautions Stop antiplatelet agents and heparin if serious bleeding occurs. Avoid I.M. injections and nonessential handling of the patient for a few hours after administration. Monitor for bleeding complications. Venipunctures should be performed carefully and only when necessary. If arterial puncture is necessary, then use an upper extremity that can be easily compressed manually. For the following conditions, the risk of bleeding is higher with use of tenecteplase and should be weighed against the benefits: Recent major surgery, cerebrovascular disease, recent GI or GU bleed, recent trauma, uncontrolled hypertension (systolic BP ≥180 mm Hg and/or diastolic BP ≥110 mm Hg), suspected left heart thrombus, acute pericarditis, subacute bacterial endocarditis, hemostatic defects, severe hepatic dysfunction, pregnancy, hemorrhagic diabetic retinopathy or other hemorrhagic ophthalmic conditions, septic thrombophlebitis or occluded arteriovenous cannula at seriously infected site, advanced age (see Dosing: Geriatric), anticoagulants, recent administration of GP IIb/IIIa inhibitors. Coronary thrombolysis may result in reperfusion arrhythmias. Caution with readministration of tenecteplase. Safety and efficacy have not been established in pediatric patients. Cholesterol embolism has rarely been reported.

Drug Interactions

Avoid Concomitant Use There are no known interactions where it is recommended to avoid concomitant use.

Decreased Effect

The levels/effects of Tenecteplase may be decreased by: Aprotinin

Increased Effect/Toxicity

Tenecteplase may increase the levels/effects of: Anticoagulants; Drotrecogin Alfa

The levels/effects of Tenecteplase may be increased by: Antiplatelet Agents; Herbs (Anticoagulant/Antiplatelet Properties); Nonsteroidal Anti-Inflammatory Agents; Salicylates

Adverse Reactions As with all drugs which may affect hemostasis, bleeding is the major adverse effect associated with tenecteplase. Hemorrhage may occur at virtually any site. Risk is dependent on multiple variables, including the dosage administered, concurrent use of multiple agents which alter hemostasis, and patient predisposition. Rapid lysis of coronary artery thrombi by thrombolytic agents may be associated with reperfusion-related arterial and/or ventricular arrhythmia. The incidence of stroke and bleeding increase in patients >65 years.

>10%:

- Hematologic: Bleeding (22% minor: ASSENT-2 trial)
- Local: Hematoma (12% minor)

1% to 10%:

- Central nervous system: Stroke (2%)
- Gastrointestinal: GI hemorrhage (1% major, 2% minor), epistaxis (2% minor)
- Genitourinary: GU bleeding (4% minor)
- Hematologic: Bleeding (5% major: ASSENT-2 trial)
- Local: Bleeding at catheter puncture site (4% minor), hematoma (2% major)
- Respiratory: Pharyngeal bleeding (3% minor)

Additional cardiovascular events associated with use in MI: Cardiogenic shock, arrhythmia, AV block, pulmonary edema, heart failure, cardiac arrest, recurrent myocardial ischemia, myocardial reinfarction, myocardial rupture, cardiac tamponade, pericarditis, pericardial effusion, mitral regurgitation, thrombosis, embolism, electromechanical dissociation, hypotension, fever, nausea, vomiting

Pharmacodynamics/Kinetics

Half-Life Elimination 90-130 minutes

Metabolism Primarily hepatic

Excretion Clearance: Plasma: 99-119 mL/minute

Available Dosage Forms

Injection, powder for reconstitution:
TNKase®: 50 mg

Dosing

Adult

STEMI: I.V.: The recommended total dose should not exceed 50 mg and is based on weight. Administer as a bolus over 5 seconds:
<60 kg: 30 mg dose
≥60 to <70 kg: 35 mg
≥70 to <80 kg: 40 mg
≥80 to <90 kg: 45 mg
≥90 kg: 50 mg

Note: All patients should receive 162-325 mg of chewable nonenteric coated aspirin as soon as possible and then daily. Administer concurrently with heparin 60 units/kg bolus (maximum: 4000 units) followed by continuous infusion of 12 units/kg/hour (maximum: 1000 units/hour) and adjust to aPTT target of 50-70 seconds (or 1.5-2 times the upper limit of control).

Combination regimen (unlabeled): Half-dose tenecteplase (15-25 mg based on weight) and abciximab 0.25 mg/kg bolus then 0.125 mcg/kg/minute (maximum: 10 mcg/minute) for 12 hours with heparin dosing as follows: Concurrent bolus of 40 units/kg (maximum: 3000 units), then 7 units/kg/hour (maximum: 800 units/hour) as continuous infusion. Adjust to aPTT target of 50-70 seconds.

Note: The 2004 ACC/AHA guidelines for the management of patients with STEMI suggests that abciximab and half-dose reteplase or tenecteplase may be considered for prevention of reinfarction in patients with anterior MI, who are <75 years of age and have no risk factors for bleeding. However, more recently the American College of Chest Physicians recommends against the combination of half-dose reteplase or tenecteplase and standard-dose abciximab (with low dose unfractionated heparin) in any patient with STEMI due to the lack of mortality benefit and the risk of major bleeding (Goodman, 2008).

Geriatric Refer to adult dosing. Although dosage adjustments are not recommended, the elderly have a higher incidence of morbidity and mortality with the use of tenecteplase. The 30-day mortality in the ASSENT-2 trial was 2.5% for patients younger than 65 years, 8.5% for patients between 65 and 74 years, and 16.2% for patients 75 years and older. The intracranial hemorrhage rate was 0.4% for patient younger than 65 years, 1.6% for patients between 65 and 74 years, and 1.7% for patients 75 years and older. The risks and benefits of use should be weighted carefully in the elderly.

Renal Impairment No adjustment is necessary.

Hepatic Impairment Severe hepatic failure is a relative contraindication. Recommendations were not made for mild-to-moderate hepatic impairment.

Administration

I.V. Tenecteplase should be reconstituted using the supplied 10 mL syringe with TwinPak™ Dual Cannula Device and 10 mL SWFI. Do not shake when reconstituting. Slight foaming is normal; will dissipate if left standing for several minutes. Any unused solution should be discarded. The reconstituted solution is 5 mg/mL. Dextrose-containing lines must be flushed with a saline solution before and after administration. Check frequently for signs of bleeding. Avoid I.M. injections and nonessential handling of patient.

Stability

Reconstitution Tenecteplase should be reconstituted using the supplied 10 mL syringe with TwinPak™ Dual Cannula Device and 10 mL sterile water for injection.

Storage Store at room temperature not to exceed 30°C (86°F) or under refrigeration 2°C to 8°C (36°F to 46°F). If reconstituted and not used immediately, store in refrigerator and use within 8 hours.

Monitoring and Teaching Issues

Laboratory Monitoring CBC, PTT, signs and symptoms of bleeding, ECG monitoring

Physical Assessment Patient should be closely monitored for bleeding during and following treatment. Monitor infusion site, neurological status (eg, intracranial hemorrhage), vital signs, and ECG (reperfusion arrhythmias). Arrhythmias may occur; treatment should be immediately available. Bedrest and bleeding precautions should be maintained; avoid I.M. injections, venipuncture (unless absolutely necessary), and nonessential handling of the patient. If arterial puncture is necessary, an upper extremity vessel that can be manually compressed should be used.

Patient Education This medication is only administered by infusion; you will be monitored closely during and after treatment. Immediately report burning, pain, redness, swelling, or oozing at infusion site. Following infusion you will have a tendency to bleed easily; use caution to prevent injury and follow instructions for strict bedrest to reduce the risk of injury. If bleeding does occur, report immediately and apply pressure to bleeding spot until bleeding stops completely. Report unusual pain (acute headache, joint pain, chest pain); unusual bruising or bleeding; blood in urine, stool, or vomitus; bleeding gums; vision changes; or respiratory difficulty.

Pregnancy Considerations Administer to pregnant women only if the potential benefits justify the risk to the fetus.

Teniposide (ten i POE side)

U.S. Brand Names Vumon®
Index Terms EPT; PTG; VM-26
Generic Availability (U.S.) No
Pharmacologic Category Antineoplastic Agent, Podophyllotoxin Derivative
Medication Safety Issues
Sound-alike/look-alike issues:
Teniposide may be confused with etoposide

High alert medication: This medication is in a class the Institute for Safe Medication Practices (ISMP) includes among its list of drug classes which have a heightened risk of causing significant patient harm when used in error.

Pregnancy Risk Factor D
Lactation Excretion in breast milk unknown/not recommended
Use Treatment of refractory childhood acute lymphoblastic leukemia (ALL) in combination with other chemotherapy
Unlabeled/Investigational Use Treatment of refractory acute lymphoblastic leukemia (ALL) in adults
Available Dosage Forms
Injection, solution:
Vumon®: 10 mg/mL (5 mL)
Dosing
Adult Note: Patients with Down syndrome and leukemia may be more sensitive to the myelosuppressive effects; administer the first course at half the usual dose and adjust dose in subsequent cycles upward based on degree of toxicities (myelosuppression and mucositis) in the previous course(s).
Acute lymphoblastic leukemia (ALL) consolidation treatment (unlabeled use; combination chemotherapy): I.V.: 165 mg/m^2/dose days 1, 4, 8, and 11 of alternating consolidation cycles (Linker, 1991)
Pediatric Note: Patients with Down syndrome and leukemia may be more sensitive to the myelosuppressive effects; administer the first course at half the usual dose and adjust dose in subsequent cycles upward based on degree of toxicities (myelosuppression and mucositis) in the previous course(s).

Acute lymphoblastic leukemia (ALL; combination chemotherapy): I.V.: 165 mg/m^2 twice weekly for 8-9 doses **or** 250 mg/m^2 weekly for 4-8 weeks **or** (unlabeled dosing) 165 mg/m^2/dose days 1 and 2 of weeks 3, 13, and 23 (Lauer, 2001)

Renal Impairment Data is insufficient, but dose adjustments may be necessary in patient with significant renal impairment.

Hepatic Impairment Data is insufficient, but dose adjustments may be necessary in patient with significant hepatic impairment.

Administration
I.V. Must be administered slowly (over at least 30-60 minutes); do not administer by rapid I.V. injection. Administer through non-DEHP-containing administration sets. Incompatible with heparin; flush infusion line with D_5W or NS before and after infusion. Precipitation may occur at any concentration; administer as soon as possible after preparation; inspect solution prior to administration. Observe patient continuously for at least the first 60 minutes of infusion, observe frequently thereafter. Stop infusion for signs of anaphylaxis (may require treatment with epinephrine, corticosteroids, antihistamines, pressors, or volume expanders); discontinue for clinically significant hypotension during infusion; if infusion is restarted after being withheld for hypotension, reinitiate at a slower infusion rate.
Monitoring and Teaching Issues
Laboratory Monitoring CBC, platelet count, renal and hepatic function tests
Physical Assessment Premedication with corticosteroids and antiemetic. Infusion site should be closely monitored to prevent extravasation. Patient should be monitored closely during infusion for hypersensitivity reactions (chills, fever, tachycardia, dyspnea, hypotension, anaphylaxis); immediate treatment for anaphylaxis should be available during infusion. Monitor for mucositis, diarrhea, myelosuppression, and leucopenia prior to each infusion and throughout therapy.
Patient Education This medication can only be administered by infusion; you will be monitored closely during and following infusion. Report immediately any pain, burning, or swelling at infusion site or any signs of allergic reaction (eg, respiratory difficulty, difficulty swallowing, back pain, chest tightness, rash, hives, swelling of lips or mouth). Maintain adequate nutrition and hydration, unless instructed to restrict fluid intake. You will be more susceptible to infection. May cause nausea, vomiting, diarrhea (consult prescriber if acute or persistent), or loss of hair (reversible). Report unusual bleeding or bruising, persistent fever or chills, sore throat, sores in mouth or vagina, or respiratory difficulty.

Tenofovir (te NOE fo veer)

U.S. Brand Names Viread®
Index Terms PMPA; TDF; Tenofovir Disoproxil Fumarate
Generic Availability (U.S.) No
Pharmacologic Category Antiretroviral Agent, Reverse Transcriptase Inhibitor (Nucleotide)
Pregnancy Risk Factor B

Lactation Excretion in breast milk unknown/contraindicated

Use Management of HIV infections in combination with at least two other antiretroviral agents; treatment of chronic hepatitis B virus (HBV) in patients with compensated or decompensated liver disease

Mechanism of Action/Effect Tenofovir blocks replication of HIV virus by inhibiting the reverse transcriptase enzyme. It is chemically similar to adenosine 5'-monophosphate (a nucleotide), which is required to form DNA. Tenofovir inhibits replication of HBV by inhibiting HBV polymerase.

Contraindications There are no contraindications listed within the FDA-approved labeling.

Warnings/Precautions [U.S Boxed Warning]: Lactic acidosis and severe hepatomegaly with steatosis have been reported with tenofovir and other nucleoside analogues, including fatal cases; use with caution in patients with risk factors for liver disease (risk may be increased in obese patients or prolonged exposure) and suspend treatment in any patient who develops clinical or laboratory findings suggestive of lactic acidosis (transaminase elevation may/may not accompany hepatomegaly and steatosis). May cause redistribution of fat (eg, buffalo hump, peripheral wasting with increased abdominal girth, cushingoid appearance). Immune reconstitution syndrome may develop resulting in the occurrence of an inflammatory response to an indolent or residual opportunistic infection; further evaluation and treatment may be required. Use caution in hepatic impairment; no dosage adjustment is required; limited studies indicate the pharmacokinetics of tenofovir are not altered in hepatic dysfunction. Limited data supporting treatment of chronic hepatitis B in patients with decompensated liver disease; observe for increased adverse reactions, including renal dysfunction.

May cause osteomalacia; increased biochemical markers of bone metabolism, serum parathyroid hormone levels, and 1,25 vitamin D levels have been noted with tenofovir use. A 5% to 7% loss of bone mineral density (BMD) has been reported in some patients. BMD monitoring should be considered in patients with a history of bone fracture or risk factors for osteopenia or bone loss. Bone effects in tenofovir-treated HIV adolescents were similar to adults; long-term bone health and fracture risk unknown.

Do not use as monotherapy in treatment of HIV. Treatment of HIV in patients with unrecognized/untreated HBV may lead to rapid HBV resistance. Patients should be tested for presence of chronic hepatitis B infection prior to initiation of therapy.

Use caution in renal impairment. Calculate creatinine clearance prior to initiation of therapy and monitor renal function (including recalculation of creatinine clearance and serum phosphorus) during therapy. Dosage adjustment required in patients with Cl_{cr} <50 mL/minute. May cause acute renal failure or Fanconi syndrome; use caution with other nephrotoxic agents (especially those which compete for active tubular secretion), patients with low body weight, or concurrent medications which increase tenofovir levels. Use caution in the elderly; dosage adjustment based on renal function may be required.

[U.S. Boxed Warning]: If treating HBV, acute exacerbation of hepatitis B may occur upon discontinuation. Monitor liver function closely for several months after discontinuing treatment; reinitiation of antihepatitis B therapy may be required. Treatment of HBV in patients with unrecognized/untreated HIV may lead to HIV resistance; patients should be tested for presence of HIV infection prior to initiating therapy. Do not use as monotherapy in treatment of HIV. Treatment of HIV in patients with unrecognized/untreated HBV may lead to rapid HBV resistance. Patients should be tested for presence of chronic hepatitis B prior to initiation of therapy. Use with caution in patients taking strong CYP3A4 inhibitors, moderate or strong CYP3A4 inducers and major CYP3A4 substrates (see Drug Interactions); consider alternative agents that avoid or lessen the potential for CYP-mediated interactions. Do not use concurrently with adefovir or tenofovir combination products.

Drug Interactions

Metabolism/Transport Effects Inhibits CYP1A2 (weak)

Avoid Concomitant Use

Avoid concomitant use of Tenofovir with any of the following: Didanosine

Decreased Effect

Tenofovir may decrease the levels/effects of: Atazanavir; Didanosine; Protease Inhibitors

The levels/effects of Tenofovir may be decreased by: Adefovir

Increased Effect/Toxicity

Tenofovir may increase the levels/effects of: Adefovir; Didanosine; Ganciclovir-Valganciclovir

The levels/effects of Tenofovir may be increased by: Acyclovir-Valacyclovir; Atazanavir; Ganciclovir-Valganciclovir; Lopinavir; Protease Inhibitors

Nutritional/Ethanol Interactions Food: Fatty meals may increase the bioavailability of tenofovir. Tenofovir may be taken with or without food.

Adverse Reactions Frequencies listed are treatment-emergent adverse effects noted at higher frequency than in the placebo group or comparator group. Only adverse events from treatment-naive studies which varied significantly were noted (eg, rash event). Patients treated for chronic hepatitis B had similar reactions and frequencies.

>10%:

Central nervous system: Insomnia (3% to 4%; decompensated liver disease 18%), pain (7% to 13%), dizziness (3%; treatment naive 8%; decompensated liver disease 13%), depression (4% to 8%; treatment naive 9% to 11%), fever (2% to 4%; treatment naive 8%; decompensated liver disease 11%)

Dermatologic: Rash event (includes maculopapular, pustular, or vesiculobullous rash, pruritus or urticaria 5% to 7%; treatment naive 18%)

Endocrine & metabolic: Triglycerides increased (grades 3/4: 11%; treatment naive 4%)

Gastrointestinal: Abdominal pain (4% to 7%; decompensated liver disease 22%), nausea (8% to 11%; decompensated liver disease 20%), diarrhea (11% to 16%), vomiting (4% to 7%; decompensated liver disease 13%)

Neuromuscular & skeletal: Creatine kinase increased (9% to 12%), weakness (7% to 11%)

1% to 10%:

Cardiovascular: Chest pain (3%)

Central nervous system: Fatigue (9%), headache (5% to 8%), anxiety (6%)

Endocrine & metabolic: Hyperglycemia (grades 3/4: 3%)

Gastrointestinal: Serum amylase increased (grades 3/4: 4% to 7%; treatment naive 8% to 9%), anorexia (3% to 4%), dyspepsia (3% to 4%), flatulence (3% to 4%), weight loss (2% to 4%)

Genitourinary: Hematuria (grades 3/4: 3% to 7%)

Hematologic: Neutropenia (1% to 3%)

Hepatic: Transaminases increased (2% to 5%), alkaline phosphatase increased (1%)

Neuromuscular & skeletal: Back pain (3% to 4%; treatment naive 9%), peripheral neuropathy (3% to 5%), myalgia (3% to 4%)

Renal: Serum creatinine increased (decompensated liver disease 9%), renal failure (decompensated liver disease 7%), glycosuria (grades 3/4: 3%)

Respiratory: Upper respiratory tract infection (8%), sinusitis (8%), nasopharyngitis (5%), pneumonia (2% to 3%; treatment naive 5%)

Miscellaneous: Diaphoresis (3%)

Pharmacodynamics/Kinetics

Bioavailability Fasting: ~25%; increases ~40% with high-fat meal

Time to Peak Serum: Fasting: 36-84 minutes; With food: 96-144 minutes

Protein Binding <7% to serum proteins

Half-Life Elimination ~17 hours

Metabolism Tenofovir disoproxil fumarate (TDF) is converted intracellularly by hydrolysis (by non-CYP enzymes) to tenofovir, then phosphorylated to the active tenofovir diphosphate

Excretion Urine (70% to 80%) via filtration and active secretion, primarily as unchanged tenofovir

Available Dosage Forms

Tablet, oral:

Viread®: 300 mg

Dosing

Adult & Geriatric

HIV infection: Oral: 300 mg once daily (in combination with other antiretrovirals)

Hepatitis B infection: Oral: 300 mg once daily

Note: Tenofovir is recommended for first-line treatment of HBV (Lok, 2009). Concurrent use with adefovir and/or tenofovir combination products should be avoided.

Treatment duration (AASLD practice guidelines, 2009):

Note: Patients achieving <2 log decrease in serum HBV DNA after at least 6 months of therapy should either receive additional treatment or be switched to an alternative therapy (Lok, 2009).

Hepatitis Be antigen (HBeAg) positive chronic hepatitis: Treat ≥1 year until HBeAg seroconversion and undetectable serum HBV DNA; continue therapy for ≥6 months after HBeAg seroconversion

HBeAg negative chronic hepatitis: Treat >1 year until hepatitis B surface antigen (HBsAg) clearance

Decompensated liver disease: Lifelong treatment is recommended

Pediatric HIV infection: Oral: Children ≥ 12 years and ≥35 kg: 300 mg once daily

Renal Impairment Adults:

Cl_{cr} ≥50 mL/minute: No adjustment necessary.

Cl_{cr} 30-49 mL/minute: 300 mg every 48 hours

Cl_{cr} 10-29 mL/minute: 300 mg every 72-96 hours

Cl_{cr} <10 mL/minute without hemodialysis: No recommendation available.

Hemodialysis: 300 mg following dialysis every 7 days or after a total of ~12 hours of dialysis (usually once weekly assuming 3 dialysis sessions lasting about 4 hours each)

Hepatic Impairment No dosage adjustment required.

Administration

Oral May be administered without regard to meals.

Stability

Storage Store at 25°C (77°F); excursions permitted to 15°C to 30°C (59°F to 86°F).

Monitoring and Teaching Issues

Laboratory Monitoring

Patients with HIV: CBC with differential, reticulocyte count, creatine kinase, CD4 count, HIV RNA plasma levels, renal and hepatic function tests, bone density (long-term), serum phosphorus; testing for HBV is recommended prior to the initiation of antiretroviral therapy

Patients with HBV: HIV status (prior to initiation of therapy); bone density (long-term), serum phosphorus; serum creatinine (prior to initiation and as clinically indicated therapy; HBV DNA (every 3-6 months during therapy); HBeAg and anti-HBe; LFTs every 3 months during therapy and for several months following discontinuation of tenofovir

Patients with HIV and HBV coinfection should be monitored for several months following tenofovir discontinuation.

Physical Assessment Assess closely for any previous allergy history prior to beginning treatment. Monitor for lactic acidosis osteomalacia, gastrointestinal disturbance, neutropenia, myalgia, and peripheral neuropathy on a regular basis. Teach patient drugs that should not be used concurrently.

Patient Education This drug will not cure HIV, nor has it been found to reduce transmission of HIV; use appropriate precautions to prevent spread to other people. When used to treat HIV, this drug will be prescribed as one part of a multidrug combination; take exactly as directed for full course of therapy. Maintain adequate hydration, unless advised by prescriber to restrict fluids. You may be susceptible to infection. Frequent blood tests may be required with prolonged therapy. May cause dizziness, headache, nausea, or vomiting. Report immediately any tingling, pain, or loss of sensation in toes, feet, muscles, or joints; swollen glands; alterations in urinary pattern; swelling of extremities; weight gain or loss; unusual weakness; or signs of opportunistic infection (burning on urination, perineal itching, white plaques in mouth, unhealed sores, persistent sore throat or cough). If you are instructed to stop the medication; do not restart without specific instruction by your prescriber.

Dietary Considerations May be taken without regard to meals. Consider calcium and vitamin D supplementation in patients with history of bone fracture or osteopenia.

Breast-Feeding Considerations In infants born to mothers who are HIV positive, HAART while breast-feeding may decrease postnatal infection. However, maternal or infant antiretroviral therapy does not completely eliminate the risk of postnatal HIV transmission. In addition, multiclass resistant virus has been detected in breast-feeding infants despite maternal therapy.

In the United States where formula is accessible, affordable, safe, and sustainable, complete avoidance of breast-feeding by HIV-infected women is recommended to decrease potential transmission of HIV.

Pregnancy Considerations Animal studies have shown decreased fetal growth and reduced fetal bone porosity. Clinical studies in children have shown bone demineralization with chronic use. Tenofovir crosses the human placenta. No increased risk of overall birth defects has been observed following first trimester exposure according to data collected by the antiretroviral pregnancy registry. Limited data indicate decreased maternal bioavailability during the third trimester. Due to the potential for bone effects and limited data in pregnancy, use in pregnancy only in special circumstances (eg, coinfection with hepatitis B) after considering use of other alternatives. Cases of lactic acidosis/hepatic steatosis syndrome related to mitochondrial toxicity have been reported in pregnant women receiving nucleoside analogues. It is not known if pregnancy itself potentiates this known side effect; however, women may be at increased risk of lactic acidosis and liver damage. In addition, these adverse events are similar to other rare but life-threatening syndromes which occur during pregnancy (eg HELLP syndrome). Hepatic enzymes and electrolytes should be monitored frequently during the third trimester of pregnancy in women receiving nucleoside analogues and clinicians should watch for early signs of the syndrome. Renal function should also be monitored. Use caution with hepatitis B coinfection; hepatitis B flare may occur if tenofovir is discontinued postpartum.

Healthcare providers are encouraged to enroll pregnant women exposed to antiretroviral medications in the Antiretroviral Pregnancy Registry (1-800-258-4263 or www.APRegistry.com). Healthcare providers caring for HIV-infected women and their infants may contact the National Perinatal HIV Hotline (888-448-8765) for clinical consultation.

Additional Information Approval was based on two clinical trials involving patients who were previously treated with antiretrovirals with continued evidence of HIV replication despite therapy. The risk:benefit ratio for untreated patients has not been established (studies currently ongoing), however, patients who received tenofovir showed significant decreases in HIV replication as compared to continuation of standard therapy.

A high rate of early virologic nonresponse was observed when abacavir, lamivudine, and tenofovir were used as the initial regimen in treatment-naive patients. A high rate of early virologic nonresponse was also observed when didanosine, lamivudine, and tenofovir were used as the initial regimen in treatment-naive patients. Use of either of these combinations is not recommended; patients currently on either of these regimens should be closely monitored for modification of therapy. Early virologic failure was also observed with tenofovir and didanosine delayed release capsules, plus either efavirenz or nevirapine; use caution in treatment-naive patients with high baseline viral loads.

- **Tenofovir and Emtricitabine** *see* Emtricitabine and Tenofovir *on page* 615
- **Tenofovir Disoproxil Fumarate** *see* Tenofovir *on page* 1728
- **Tenofovir Disoproxil Fumarate, Efavirenz, and Emtricitabine** *see* Efavirenz, Emtricitabine, and Tenofovir *on page* 606
- **Tenoretic®** *see* Atenolol and Chlorthalidone *on page* 164
- **Tenormin®** *see* Atenolol *on page* 161
- **Terazol® 3** *see* Terconazole *on page* 1735
- **Terazol® 7** *see* Terconazole *on page* 1735

Terazosin (ter AY zoe sin)

Index Terms Hytrin

Generic Availability (U.S.) Yes

Pharmacologic Category $Alpha_1$ Blocker

Pregnancy Risk Factor C

Lactation Excretion in breast milk unknown/use caution

Use Management of mild-to-moderate hypertension; alone or in combination with other agents such as diuretics or beta-blockers; benign prostate hyperplasia (BPH)

Unlabeled/Investigational Use Pediatric hypertension

Mechanism of Action/Effect Alpha$_1$-specific blocking agent with minimal alpha$_2$ effects; this allows peripheral postsynaptic blockade, with the resultant decrease in arterial tone, while preserving the negative feedback loop which is mediated by the peripheral presynaptic alpha$_2$-receptors; terazosin relaxes the smooth muscle of the bladder neck, thus reducing bladder outlet obstruction

Contraindications Hypersensitivity to terazosin or any component of the formulation

Warnings/Precautions Can cause significant orthostatic hypotension and syncope, especially with first dose; anticipate a similar effect if therapy is interrupted for a few days, if dosage is rapidly increased, or if another antihypertensive drug (particularly vasodilators) or a PDE-5 inhibitor is introduced. Discontinue if symptoms of angina occur or worsen. Patients should be cautioned about performing hazardous tasks when starting new therapy or adjusting dosage upward. Prostate cancer should be ruled out before starting for BPH. Intraoperative floppy iris syndrome has been observed in cataract surgery patients who were on or were previously treated with alpha$_1$-blockers. Causality has not been established and there appears to be no benefit in discontinuing alpha-blocker therapy prior to surgery. Priapism has been associated with use (rarely).

Drug Interactions

Avoid Concomitant Use

Avoid concomitant use of Terazosin with any of the following: Alpha1-Blockers

Decreased Effect

The levels/effects of Terazosin may be decreased by: Herbs (Hypertensive Properties); Methylphenidate; Yohimbine

Increased Effect/Toxicity

Terazosin may increase the levels/effects of: Alpha1-Blockers; Amifostine; Antihypertensives; Calcium Channel Blockers; Hypotensive Agents; RiTUXimab

The levels/effects of Terazosin may be increased by: Beta-Blockers; Diazoxide; Herbs (Hypotensive Properties); MAO Inhibitors; Pentoxifylline; Phosphodiesterase 5 Inhibitors; Prostacyclin Analogues

Nutritional/Ethanol Interactions Herb/Nutraceutical: Avoid dong quai if using for hypertension (has estrogenic activity). Avoid ephedra, yohimbe, ginseng (may worsen hypertension). Avoid saw palmetto. Avoid garlic (may have increased antihypertensive effect).

Adverse Reactions

>10%:

Central nervous system: Dizziness (9% to 19%)

Neuromuscular & skeletal: Muscle weakness (7% to 11%)

1% to 10%:

Cardiovascular: Peripheral edema (1% to 6%), orthostatic hypotension (1% to 4%), palpitation (≤4%), tachycardia (≤2%), syncope (≤1%

Central nervous system: Somnolence (4% to 5%), vertigo (1%)

Gastrointestinal: Nausea (2% to 4%)

Genitourinary: Impotence (≤2%), libido decreased (≤1%)

Neuromuscular & skeletal: Extremity pain (≤4%), paresthesia (≤3%), back pain (≤2%)

Ocular: Blurred vision (≤2%)

Respiratory: Nasal congestion (2% to 6%), dyspnea (2% to 3%), sinusitis (≤3%)

Pharmacodynamics/Kinetics

Onset of Action 1-2 hours

Absorption Rapid and complete

Time to Peak Serum: ~1 hour

Protein Binding 90% to 95%

Half-Life Elimination ~12 hours

Metabolism Hepatic; minimal first-pass

Excretion Feces (~60%, ~20% as unchanged drug); urine (~40%, ~10% as unchanged drug)

Available Dosage Forms

Capsule, oral: 1 mg, 2 mg, 5 mg, 10 mg

Dosing

Adult & Geriatric

Hypertension: Oral: Initial: 1 mg at bedtime; slowly increase dose to achieve desired blood pressure, up to 20 mg/day; usual dose range (JNC 7): 1-20 mg once daily

Benign prostatic hyperplasia: Oral: Initial: 1 mg at bedtime; thereafter, titrate upwards, if needed, over several weeks, balancing therapeutic benefit with terazosin-induced postural hypotension; most patients require 10 mg day; if no response after 4-6 weeks of 10 mg/day, may increase to 20 mg/day

Concurrent use with a diuretic or other antihypertensive agent (especially verapamil): Dosage reduction may be needed when adding.

Concurrent use with PDE-5 inhibitors: Initiate PDE-5 inhibitor therapy at the lowest dose due to additive orthostatic and blood pressure lowering effects.

Note: If drug is discontinued for greater than several days, consider beginning with initial dose and retitrate as needed; dosage may be given on a twice daily regimen if response is diminished at 24 hours and hypotension is observed at 2-4 hours following a dose.

Pediatric Hypertension (unlabeled use): Oral: Initial: 1 mg once daily; gradually increase dose as necessary, up to maximum of 20 mg/day

Administration

Oral Administered without regard to meals at the same time each day.

Stability

Storage Store below 30°C (86°F).

Monitoring and Teaching Issues

Physical Assessment Assess blood pressure and monitor for hypotension, dizziness, somnolence, and impotence at beginning of therapy and on a regular basis. When discontinuing, dose should be tapered and blood pressure monitored closely.

Patient Education Take at the same time each day. Follow recommended diet and exercise program. May cause drowsiness, dizziness, postural hypotension, nausea, or sexual dysfunction (reversible, may resolve with continued use). Report altered CNS status (eg, fatigue, lethargy, confusion, nervousness); sudden weight gain; unusual or persistent swelling of ankles, feet, or extremities; palpitations or rapid heartbeat; respiratory difficulty; or muscle weakness.

Dietary Considerations May be taken without regard to meals at the same time each day.

Geriatric Considerations Adverse reactions such as dry mouth and urinary problems can be particularly bothersome in the elderly.

Pregnancy Considerations Teratogenic effects have not been observed in animal studies. Decreased fetal weight and increased risk of fetal mortality were noted in some animal reproduction studies. There are no adequate and well-controlled studies in pregnant women. Use only if benefit outweighs risk.

Related Information

Pharmacotherapy of Urinary Incontinence *on page 2071*

Terbinafine (Systemic) (TER bin a feen)

U.S. Brand Names LamISIL®

Index Terms Terbinafine Hydrochloride

Generic Availability (U.S.) Yes: Tablet

Pharmacologic Category Antifungal Agent, Oral

Medication Safety Issues

Sound-alike/look-alike issues:

Terbinafine may be confused with terbutaline

LamISIL® may be confused with LaMICtal®, Lomotil®

Pregnancy Risk Factor B

Lactation Enters breast milk/not recommended

Use Active against most strains of *Trichophyton mentagrophytes*, *Trichophyton rubrum*; may be effective for infections of *Microsporum gypseum* and *M. nanum*, *Trichophyton verrucosum*, *Epidermophyton floccosum*, *Candida albicans*, and *Scopulariopsis brevicaulis*

Onychomycosis of the toenail or fingernail due to susceptible dermatophytes; treatment of tinea capitis

Mechanism of Action/Effect Synthetic allylamine derivative which inhibits squalene epoxidase, a key enzyme in sterol biosynthesis in fungi. This results in a deficiency in ergosterol within the fungal cell wall and results in fungal cell death.

Contraindications Hypersensitivity to terbinafine or any component of the formulation

Warnings/Precautions While rare, the following complications have been reported and may require discontinuation of therapy: Changes in the ocular lens and retina, pancytopenia, neutropenia, Stevens-Johnson syndrome, toxic epidermal necrolysis. Precipitation or exacerbation of cutaneous or systemic lupus erythematosus has been observed; discontinue if signs and/or symptoms develop. Rare cases of hepatic failure, including fatal cases, have been reported following treatment of onychomycosis. Not recommended for use in patients with active or chronic liver disease. Discontinue if symptoms or signs of hepatobiliary dysfunction or cholestatic hepatitis develop. Products are not recommended for use with pre-existing liver or renal disease (Cl_{cr} ≤50 mL/minute). Use caution in patients sensitive to allylamine antifungals (eg, naftifine, butenafine); cross sensitivity to terbinafine may exist.

Drug Interactions

Metabolism/Transport Effects Substrate (minor) of 1A2, 2C9, 2C19, 3A4; **Inhibits** CYP2D6 (strong); **Induces** CYP3A4 (weak)

Avoid Concomitant Use

Avoid concomitant use of Terbinafine (Systemic) with any of the following: Tamoxifen; Thioridazine

Decreased Effect

Terbinafine (Systemic) may decrease the levels/effects of: Codeine; CycloSPORINE; Saccharomyces boulardii; Saxagliptin; TraMADol

The levels/effects of Terbinafine (Systemic) may be decreased by: Rifamycin Derivatives

Increased Effect/Toxicity

Terbinafine (Systemic) may increase the levels/effects of: Atomoxetine; CYP2D6 Substrates; Fesoterodine; Nebivolol; Tamoxifen; Tetrabenazine; Thioridazine; Tricyclic Antidepressants

The levels/effects of Terbinafine (Systemic) may be increased by: Conivaptan

Adverse Reactions Adverse events listed for tablets unless otherwise specified. Granules were studied in patients 4-12 years of age.

>10%: Central nervous system: Headache (13%; granules 7%)

1% to 10%:

Central nervous system: Fever (granules 7%)

Dermatologic: Rash (6%; granules 2%), pruritus (3%; granules 1%), urticaria (1%)

Gastrointestinal: Diarrhea (6%; granules 3%), vomiting (granules 5%), dyspepsia (4%), nausea (3%; granules 2%), taste disturbance (3%), abdominal pain (2%; granules 2% to 4%), toothache (granules 1%)

Hepatic: Liver enzyme abnormalities (3%)

Respiratory: Nasopharyngitis (granules 10%), cough (granules 6%), nasal congestion (granules 2%), pharyngeal pain (granules 2%), rhinorrhea (granules 2%)

Pharmacodynamics/Kinetics

Absorption Children and Adults: >70%

Bioavailability 40%; Children 36% to 64%

Time to Peak Plasma: Children and Adults: 1-2 hours

Protein Binding Children and Adults: Plasma: >99%

Half-Life Elimination Terminal half-life: 200-400 hours; very slow release of drug from skin and adipose tissues occurs; effective half-life: ~36 hours; Children 27-31 hours

Metabolism Hepatic; no active metabolites; first-pass effect (40%); little effect on CYP

Excretion Urine (70% to 75%; Children 70%)

Available Dosage Forms

Granules, oral:

LamISIL®: 125 mg/packet (14s, 42s); 187.5 mg/packet (14s, 42s)

Tablet, oral: 250 mg

LamISIL®: 250 mg

Dosing

Adult & Geriatric

Superficial mycoses (onychomycosis): Oral:

Fingernail: 250 mg daily for up to 6 weeks; may be given in 2 divided doses

Toenail: 250 mg daily for 12 weeks; may be given in 2 divided doses

Systemic mycosis (unlabeled use): Oral: 250-500 mg/day for up to 16 months

Pediatric

Tinea capitis: Oral: Granules: Children ≥4 years:

<25 kg: 125 mg once daily for 6 weeks

25-35 kg: 187.5 mg once daily for 6 weeks

>35 kg: 250 mg once daily for 6 weeks

Onychomycosis (unlabeled use): Oral: Tablet: Children:

10-20 kg: 62.5 mg once daily for 6 weeks (fingernails) **or** 12 weeks (toenails)

20-40 kg: 125 mg once daily for 6 weeks (fingernails) **or** 12 weeks (toenails)

>40 kg: 250 mg once daily for 6 weeks (fingernails) **or** 12 weeks (toenails)

Renal Impairment Cl_{cr} <50 mL/minute: Oral administration is not recommended; clearance is decreased by ~50%.

Hepatic Impairment Hepatic cirrhosis: Oral administration is not recommended; clearance is decreased by ~50%.

Administration

Oral Tablets may be administered without regard to meals. Granules should be sprinkled on a spoonful of nonacidic food (eg, mashed potatoes); swallow granules without chewing.

Stability

Storage

Granules: Store at controlled room temperature of 15°C to 30°C (59°F to 86°F).

Tablet: Store below 25°C (77°F). Protect from light.

Monitoring and Teaching Issues

Laboratory Monitoring AST/ALT prior to initiation, repeat if used >6 weeks; CBC

Physical Assessment Use with caution in presence of hepatic or renal impairment.

Patient Education Take at same time of day, with or without regard to meals. Granules may be sprinkled on a spoonful of nonacidic food; swallow granules without chewing. It is important to take full prescription, even if symptoms appear resolved; may take several months for full treatment (inadequate treatment may result in reinfection). May cause altered taste (normal); nausea, vomiting, or abdominal pain; or diarrhea. Report unusual fatigue; persistent gastrointestinal upset; nasal congestion, runny nose, sore throat, or unusual cough; skin rash or blistering; or dark urine/pale stool.

Geriatric Considerations No specific information on use in the elderly is available; however, since many elderly will have creatinine clearances <50 mL/minute, this drug is not a drug of choice for elderly with onychomycosis.

Breast-Feeding Considerations Terbinafine is found in breast milk following oral administration. The milk/plasma ratio is 7:1.

Pregnancy Considerations Adverse events were not observed in animal reproduction studies. Avoid use in pregnancy since treatment of onychomycosis is postponable.

Additional Information Due to potential toxicity, the manufacturer recommends confirmation of diagnosis testing of nail specimens prior to treatment of onychomycosis. Patients should not be considered therapeutic failures until they have been symptom-free for 2-4 weeks off following a course of treatment; GI complaints usually subside with continued administration.

A meta-analysis of efficacy studies for toenail infections revealed that weighted average mycological cure rates for continuous therapy were 36.7% (griseofulvin), 54.7% (itraconazole), and 77% (terbinafine). Cure rate for 4-month pulse therapy for itraconazole and terbinafine were 73.3% and 80%. Additionally, the final outcome measure of final costs per cured infections for continuous therapy was significantly lower for terbinafine.

◆ **Terbinafine Hydrochloride** *see* Terbinafine (Systemic) *on page* 1733

Terbutaline (ter BYOO ta leen)

Index Terms Brethaire [DSC]; Brethine; Bricanyl [DSC]
Generic Availability (U.S.) Yes
Pharmacologic Category $Beta_2$-Adrenergic Agonist
Medication Safety Issues
Sound-alike/look-alike issues:
Brethine may be confused with Methergine®
Terbutaline may be confused with terbinafine, TOLBUTamide
Terbutaline and methylergonovine parenteral dosage forms look similar. Due to their contrasting indications, use care when administering these agents.
Pregnancy Risk Factor B
Lactation Enters breast milk/compatible
Use Bronchodilator in reversible airway obstruction and bronchial asthma
Unlabeled/Investigational Use Injection: Tocolytic agent (short-term [≤72 hours] prevention or management of preterm labor
Available Dosage Forms
Injection, solution: 1 mg/mL (1 mL)
Tablet, oral: 2.5 mg, 5 mg
Dosing
Adult & Geriatric
Asthma or bronchoconstriction:
Oral: 5 mg/dose every 6 hours 3 times/day; if side effects occur, reduce dose to 2.5 mg every 6 hours; not to exceed 15 mg in 24 hours.
SubQ: 0.25 mg/dose; may repeat in 15-30 minutes (maximum: 0.5 mg/4-hour period)
Bronchospasm (acute): *Inhalation* (Bricanyl® [CAN] MDI: 500 mcg/puff, *not labeled for use in the U.S.*): One puff as needed; may repeat with 1 inhalation (after 5 minutes); more than 6 inhalations should not be necessary in any 24 hour period. **Note:** If a previously effective dosage regimen fails to provide the usual relief, or the effects of a dose last for >3 hours, medical advice should be sought immediately; this is a sign of seriously worsening asthma that requires reassessment of therapy.
Premature labor (acute; short-term [≤72 hours] tocolysis; unlabeled use):
I.V.: 2.5-5 mcg/minute; increased gradually every 20-30 minutes by 2.5-5 mcg/minute; effective maximum dosages from 17.5-30 mcg/minute have been used with caution. Duration of infusion is at least 12 hours (Travis, 1993).
SubQ: 0.25 mg every 20 minutes to 3 hours; hold for pulse >120 beats per minute. Terbutaline has not been approved for and should not be used for prolonged tocolysis (beyond 48-72 hours) (ACOG, 2003)
Pediatric
Asthma or bronchoconstriction:
Oral: Children:
<12 years: Initial: 0.05 mg/kg/dose 3 times/day, increased gradually as required; maximum: 0.15 mg/kg/dose 3-4 times/day or a total of 5 mg/24 hours
12-15 years: 2.5 mg every 6 hours 3 times/day; not to exceed 7.5 mg in 24 hours
>15 years: 5 mg/dose every 6 hours 3 times/day; if side effects occur, reduce dose to 2.5 mg every 6 hours; not to exceed 15 mg in 24 hours
SubQ: Children:
<12 years: 0.005-0.01 mg/kg/dose to a maximum of 0.3 mg/dose; may repeat in 15-20 minutes
≥12 years: Refer to adult dosing.
Bronchospasm (acute): *Inhalation:* Bricanyl® [CAN] MDI: 500 mcg/puff, *not labeled for use in the U.S.*): Children ≥6 years: Refer to adult dosing.
Renal Impairment
Cl_{cr} 10-50 mL/minute: Administer 50% of normal dose.
Cl_{cr} <10 mL/minute: Avoid use.
Administration
Oral Administer around-the-clock to promote less variation in peak and trough serum levels.
I.V. Use infusion pump.
Monitoring and Teaching Issues
Laboratory Monitoring FEV_1, peak flow, and/or other pulmonary function tests; serum potassium, serum glucose (in selected patients)
Tocolysis: Frequent glucose and potassium during the infusion
Physical Assessment Respiratory use: For inpatient care, monitor vital signs and lung sounds prior to and periodically during therapy. **Preterm labor use: Inpatient:** Monitor maternal vital signs; respiratory, fluid, cardiac, and electrolyte status; frequency, duration, and intensity of contractions; and fetal heart rate.
Patient Education You may experience nervousness, dizziness, fatigue, dry mouth, and stomach upset. Report unresolved GI upset; dizziness or fatigue; vision changes; sudden weight gain; swelling of extremities; chest pain, rapid heartbeat, or palpitations; insomnia, nervousness, or hyperactivity; muscle cramping, tremors, or pain; or rash.

Terconazole (ter KONE a zole)

U.S. Brand Names Terazol® 3; Terazol® 7; Zazole™ [DSC]
Index Terms Triaconazole

Generic Availability (U.S.) Yes

Pharmacologic Category Antifungal Agent, Vaginal

Medication Safety Issues

Sound-alike/look-alike issues:

Terconazole may be confused with tioconazole

International issues:

Terazol [U.S., Canada] may be confused with Theradol brand name for tramadol [Netherlands]

Pregnancy Risk Factor C

Lactation Excretion in breast milk unknown/not recommended

Use Local treatment of vulvovaginal candidiasis

Available Dosage Forms

Cream, vaginal: 0.4% (45 g); 0.8% (20 g)

Terazol® 7: 0.4% (45 g)

Terazol® 3: 0.8% (20 g)

Suppository, vaginal: 80 mg (3s)

Terazol® 3: 80 mg (3s)

Dosing

Adult & Geriatric Vulvovaginal candidiasis: Intravaginal:

Terazol® 3, Zazole™ (0.8%) vaginal cream: Insert 1 applicatorful intravaginally at bedtime for 3 consecutive days.

Terazol® 7, Zazole™ (0.4%) vaginal cream: Insert 1 applicatorful intravaginally at bedtime for 7 consecutive days.

Terazol® 3 vaginal suppository: Insert 1 suppository intravaginally at bedtime for 3 consecutive days.

Monitoring and Teaching Issues

Patient Education Sexual partner may experience irritation; best to refrain from intercourse during period of treatment. Suppositories may cause breakdown of rubber/latex products such as diaphragms; avoid concurrent use. Report persistent vaginal burning, itching, irritation, or rash.

Teriparatide (ter i PAR a tide)

U.S. Brand Names Forteo®

Index Terms Parathyroid Hormone (1-34); Recombinant Human Parathyroid Hormone (1-34); rhPTH(1-34)

Generic Availability (U.S.) No

Pharmacologic Category Parathyroid Hormone Analog

Medication Guide Available Yes

Pregnancy Risk Factor C

Lactation Excretion in breast milk unknown/not recommended

Use Treatment of osteoporosis in postmenopausal women at high risk of fracture; treatment of primary or hypogonadal osteoporosis in men at high risk of fracture; treatment of glucocorticoid-induced osteoporosis in men and women at high risk for fracture

Mechanism of Action/Effect An analog of parathyroid hormone, teriparatide stimulates osteoblast function, increases gastrointestinal calcium absorption, and increases renal tubular reabsorption of calcium. Treatment with teriparatide increases bone mineral density, bone mass, and strength. In postmenopausal women, it has been shown to decrease osteoporosis-related fractures.

Contraindications Hypersensitivity to teriparatide or any component of the formulation

Warnings/Precautions **[U.S. Boxed Warning]: In animal studies, teriparatide has been associated with an increase in osteosarcoma;** risk was dependent on both dose and duration. Avoid use in patients with an increased risk of osteosarcoma (including Paget's disease, prior radiation, unexplained elevation of alkaline phosphatase, or in patients with open epiphyses). Do not use in patients with a history of skeletal metastases, hyperparathyroidism, or pre-existing hypercalcemia. Not for use in patients with metabolic bone disease other than osteoporosis. Use caution in patients with active or recent urolithiasis. Use caution in patients at risk of orthostasis (including concurrent antihypertensive therapy), or in patients who may not tolerate transient hypotension (cardiovascular or cerebrovascular disease). Use caution in patients with cardiac, renal or hepatic impairment (limited data available concerning safety and efficacy). Use of teriparatide for longer than 2 years is not recommended. Not approved for use in pediatric patients.

Drug Interactions

Avoid Concomitant Use There are no known interactions where it is recommended to avoid concomitant use.

Decreased Effect There are no known significant interactions involving a decrease in effect.

Increased Effect/Toxicity There are no known significant interactions involving an increase in effect.

Nutritional/Ethanol Interactions

Ethanol: Excessive intake may increase risk of osteoporosis.

Herb/Nutraceutical: Ensure adequate calcium and vitamin D intake.

Lab Interactions Transiently increases serum calcium; maximal effect 4-6 hours postdose; generally returns to baseline ~16 hours postdose

Adverse Reactions

>10%: Endocrine & metabolic: Hypercalcemia (transient increases noted 4-6 hours postdose [women 11%; men 6%])

1% to 10%:

Cardiovascular: Orthostatic hypotension (5%; transient), chest pain (3%), syncope (3%)

Central nervous system: Dizziness (8%), insomnia (4% to 5%), anxiety (≤4%), depression (4%), vertigo (4%)

Dermatologic: Rash (5%)

Endocrine & metabolic: Hyperuricemia (3%)

Gastrointestinal: Nausea (9% to 14%), gastritis (≤7%), dyspepsia (5%), vomiting (3%), tooth disorder (2%)

Neuromuscular & skeletal: Arthralgia (10%), weakness (9%), leg cramps (3%)

Respiratory: Rhinitis (10%), pharyngitis (6%), dyspnea (4% to 6%), pneumonia (4% to 6%)

Miscellaneous: Antibodies to teriparatide (3% of women in long-term treatment; hypersensitivity reactions or decreased efficacy were not associated in preclinical trials), herpes zoster (≤3%)

Pharmacodynamics/Kinetics

Bioavailability 95%

Time to Peak Serum: ~30 minutes

Half-Life Elimination I.V.: 5 minutes; SubQ: ~1 hour

Metabolism Hepatic (nonspecific proteolysis)

Excretion Urine (as metabolites)

Available Dosage Forms

Injection, solution:

Forteo®: 250 mcg/mL (2.4 mL)

Dosing

Adult & Geriatric Osteoporosis: SubQ: 20 mcg once daily; **Note:** Initial administration should occur under circumstances in which the patient may sit or lie down, in the event of orthostasis.

Renal Impairment No dosage adjustment required. Bioavailability and half-life increase with Cl_{cr} <30 mL/minute.

Administration

Other Administer by subcutaneous injection into the thigh or abdominal wall. Initial administration should occur under circumstances in which the patient may sit or lie down, in the event of orthostasis.

Stability

Storage Store at 2°C to 8°C (36°F to 46°F); do not freeze. Protect from light. Discard pen 28 days after first injection. Do not use if solution is cloudy, colored, or contains solid particles.

Monitoring and Teaching Issues

Laboratory Monitoring Serum calcium, serum phosphorus

Physical Assessment Initial administration should occur where patient may sit or lie down, in the event of orthostasis. Assess calcium and phosphorus levels prior to and periodically during therapy. Monitor for chest pain, hypotension, nausea, vomiting, arthralgia, leg cramps, and dyspnea at beginning of and regular intervals during therapy. Teach patient proper administration and disposal and proper diet with adequate calcium and vitamin D.

Patient Education Rotate injection sites in thigh or abdominal wall. Sit when administering to reduce possibility of falling or injury. Avoid excess alcohol (may increase risk of osteoporosis) and follow dietary instructions of prescriber. May cause dizziness; nausea, vomiting, or upset stomach; or muscle or skeletal pain, weakness, or cramping. Report chest pain or palpitations or respiratory difficulty.

Geriatric Considerations No age-related differences in pharmacokinetics have been seen. In studies, no significant difference was seen in either efficacy or adverse effects between older patients and younger patients. Teriparatide should be considered as a last resort in patents who cannot tolerate or have not responded to other treatments for osteoporosis.

Breast-Feeding Considerations Indicated for use in postmenopausal women. Studies have not been conducted to determine excretion in breast milk. Not recommended for use in breast-feeding women.

Pregnancy Considerations Adverse events were observed in animal studies; the effect on human fetal development has not been studied. Teriparatide is not indicated for use in pregnant or premenopausal women.

Additional Information Teriparatide was formerly marketed as a diagnostic agent (Perithar™); that agent was withdrawn from the market in 1997. Teriparatide (Forteo®) is manufactured through recombinant DNA technology using a strain of *E. coli*.

Patients are encouraged to enroll in the Forteo® Patient Registry which is designed to monitor the potential risk of osteosarcoma and teriparatide treatment. Enrollment information may be found at www.forteoregistry.rti.org or by calling 1-866-382-6813.

Tesamorelin (tes a moe REL in)

U.S. Brand Names Egrifta™

Index Terms Tesamorelin Acetate; TH9507

Pharmacologic Category Growth Hormone Releasing Factor

Medication Safety Issues

Sound-alike/look-alike issues:

Tesamorelin may be confused with temsirolimus

Prescribing and Access Restrictions In order to prescribe Egrifta™, healthcare providers must call the Axis Center at 1-877-714-2947. Egrifta™ is only available through specialty pharmacy distribution.

Pregnancy Risk Factor X

Lactation Excretion in breast milk unknown/not recommended

Use Reduction of excess abdominal fat in HIV-infected patients with lipodystrophy

Mechanism of Action/Effect Tesamorelin stimulates the release of growth hormone which promotes the reduction of total fat mass.

Contraindications Hypersensitivity to tesamorelin, mannitol, or any component of the formulation; disruption of hypothalamic-pituitary-axis due to hypophysectomy, hypopituitarism, pituitary tumor/surgery, head irradiation or head trauma; active malignancy (newly diagnosed or recurrent); pregnancy

Warnings/Precautions Hypersensitivity reactions (eg, pruritus, erythema, flushing, urticaria, rash) may occur. If hypersensitivity is suspected; discontinue and instruct patient to seek immediate medical attention. Tesamorelin use may result in peripheral edema manifested by increased skin turgor and musculoskeletal discomfort. Injection site reactions (including erythema, pruritus, pain, irritation, and bruising) may occur; incidence decreases with treatment continued beyond 26 weeks; rotating the site of injection to different areas of the abdomen may reduce incidence of reactions. Tesamorelin may increase risk of development of diabetes due to glucose intolerance; evaluate glucose status prior to treatment initiation; monitor periodically for glucose metabolism changes. Patients with diabetes should be monitored for the development or worsening of retinopathy due to increased IGF-1 levels.

HIV-positive patients are at an increased risk for development of malignancies. Due to increased IGF-1 levels, use may be associated with a reactivation of malignancies in patients with a history of malignancies. Use is contraindicated in patients with active malignancies; treatment for malignancy should be completed prior to initiation of tesamorelin. IGF-1 levels should be monitored during treatment; consider discontinuing with persistent IGF-1 elevations. Growth hormone is associated with an increased risk of mortality in patients with acute critical illness due to complications following open heart surgery, abdominal surgery, trauma, or acute respiratory failure; consider discontinuing in critically ill patients. Should not be used in children due to risk of excess growth (gigantism) when epiphyses are open and is not indicated for weight loss management in non-HIV infected patients

Drug Interactions

Avoid Concomitant Use There are no known interactions where it is recommended to avoid concomitant use.

Decreased Effect

Tesamorelin may decrease the levels/effects of: Cortisone; PredniSONE

Increased Effect/Toxicity There are no known significant interactions involving an increase in effect.

Adverse Reactions Note: The incidence of adverse reactions generally decreases with treatment continued beyond 26 weeks.

10%:

Local: Injection site reactions (6% to 25%; includes erythema [1% to 9%], pruritus [2% to 8%], pain [4%], irritation [3%], hemorrhage [2%], swelling [2%], urticaria [2%], rash [1%])

Neuromuscular & skeletal: Arthralgia (13%)

1% to 10%:

Cardiovascular: Peripheral edema (2% to 6%), hypertension (1% to 2%), chest pain (1%), palpitation (1%)

Central nervous system: Hypoesthesia (2% to 4%), depression (2%), pain (2%), insomnia (1%)

Dermatologic: Rash (4%), pruritus (1% to 2%), urticaria (1%)

Endocrine & metabolic: Hb A_{1c} increased (5%), hot flush (1%), hyperglycemia

Gastrointestinal: Nausea (4%), vomiting (2% to 3%), dyspepsia (2%), abdominal pain (1%)

Neuromuscular & skeletal: Pain in extremity (3% to 6%), myalgia (1% to 6%), paresthesia (2% to 5%), carpal tunnel syndrome (2%), creatine phosphokinase increased (2%), muscle stiffness (2%), musculoskeletal pain (2%), joint stiffness (2%), peripheral neuropathy (2%), joint swelling (1%), muscle spasm (1%), muscle strain (1%)

Miscellaneous: Hypersensitivity reactions (1% to 4%), night sweats (1%)

Pharmacodynamics/Kinetics

Bioavailability SubQ: Healthy adults: <4%

Time to Peak 9 minutes

Half-Life Elimination Healthy adults: 26 minutes; HIV-infected patients: 38 minutes

Available Dosage Forms

Injection, powder for reconstitution:

Egrifta™: 1 mg

Dosing

Adult & Geriatric HIV-associated lipodystrophy: SubQ: 2 mg once daily

Adjustment for Toxicity Discontinue if symptoms of hypersensitivity occur.

Administration

Other SubQ: The abdomen is the preferred site of administration; site should be rotated within the abdomen. Avoid injection into scar tissue, bruises, or the navel. The reconstituted solution should be visually inspected for particulate matter and discoloration; do not administer if solution is not clear, colorless and free of particulate matter. **Note:** Syringes and needles are single-use only and should not be shared between patients.

Stability

Reconstitution Use reconstituted solution immediately after prepared.

Storage Store refrigerated at 2°C to 8°C (36°F to 46°F). Protect from light and store in original container until time of use. Store diluent, (sterile water for injection USP), syringes, and needles at room temperature at 20°C to 25°C (68°F to 77°F). Do not refrigerate or freeze reconstituted solution. Discard if not used immediately.

Monitoring and Teaching Issues

Laboratory Monitoring Serum IGF-1 levels should be monitored at baseline and during therapy due to the potential increased risk of malignancy from sustained elevation of IGF-1 levels.

Breast-Feeding Considerations In the United States where formula is accessible, affordable, safe, and sustainable, complete avoidance of breast-feeding by HIV-infected women is recommended to decrease potential transmission of HIV.

Pregnancy Considerations Adverse effects were noted in animal reproduction studies. During pregnancy, there is an increased deposition of visceral adipose tissue due to metabolic and hormonal changes. Tesamorelin decreases the deposition of visceral fat and could potentially cause harm to the unborn fetus. Therefore, use during pregnancy is contraindicated.

◆ **Tesamorelin Acetate** *see* Tesamorelin *on page* 1737

◆ **TESPA** *see* Thiotepa *on page* 1754

◆ **Tessalon®** *see* Benzonatate *on page* 201

◆ **Tessalon Perles** *see* Benzonatate *on page* 201

◆ **Testim®** *see* Testosterone *on page* 1739

◆ **Testopel®** *see* Testosterone *on page* 1739

Testosterone (tes TOS ter one)

U.S. Brand Names Androderm®; AndroGel®; Axiron®; Delatestryl®; Depo®-Testosterone; First®-Testosterone; First®-Testosterone MC; Fortesta™; Striant®; Testim®; Testopel®

Index Terms Axiron®; Testosterone Cypionate; Testosterone Enanthate

Generic Availability (U.S.) Yes: Injection, powder

Pharmacologic Category Androgen

Medication Safety Issues

Sound-alike/look-alike issues:

Testosterone may be confused with testolactone

Testoderm® may be confused with Estraderm®

Transdermal patch may contain conducting metal (eg, aluminum); remove patch prior to MRI.

Medication Guide Available Yes

Pregnancy Risk Factor X

Lactation Enters breast milk/contraindicated

Use

Injection: Androgen replacement therapy in the treatment of delayed male puberty; male hypogonadism (primary or hypogonadotropic); inoperable metastatic female breast cancer (enanthate only)

Pellet: Androgen replacement therapy in the treatment of delayed male puberty; male hypogonadism (primary or hypogonadotropic)

Buccal system, topical gel, topical solution, transdermal system: Male hypogonadism (primary or hypogonadotropic)

Capsule (not available in U.S.): Conditions associated with a deficiency or absence of endogenous testosterone

Unlabeled/Investigational Use Androgen deficiency in men with AIDS wasting; postmenopausal women (short-term use in select cases)

Mechanism of Action/Effect Principal endogenous androgen responsible for promoting the growth and development of the male sex organs and maintaining secondary sex characteristics in androgen-deficient males

Contraindications Hypersensitivity to testosterone or any component of the formulation; males with known or suspected carcinoma of the breast or prostate; specific products are contraindicated in women

Depo®-Testosterone: Also contraindicated in serious hepatic, renal, or cardiac disease

Warnings/Precautions When used to treat delayed male puberty, perform radiographic examination of the hand and wrist every 6 months to determine the rate of bone maturation. May cause hypercalcemia in patients with prolonged immobilization or cancer. May accelerate bone maturation without producing compensating gain in linear growth. Has both androgenic and anabolic activity, the anabolic action may enhance hypoglycemia. May alter serum cholesterol; use caution with history of MI or coronary artery disease. Use caution in elderly patients or patients with other demographic factors which may increase the risk of prostatic carcinoma; careful monitoring is required. Urethral obstruction may develop in patients with BPH; treatment should be discontinued if this should occur (use lower dose if restarted). Withhold treatment pending urological evaluation in patients with palpable prostate nodule or induration, PSA >4 ng/mL, or PSA >3 ng/mL in men at high risk of prostate cancer (Bhasin 2010). Use with caution in patients with conditions influenced by edema (eg, cardiovascular disease, migraine, seizure disorder, renal or hepatic impairment) or medications that enhance edema formation (eg, corticosteroids); testosterone may cause fluid retention. May cause gynecomastia. Large doses may suppress spermatogenesis. During treatment for metastatic breast cancer, women should be monitored for signs of virilization; discontinue if mild virilization is present to prevent irreversible symptoms.

Prolonged use of high doses of androgens has been associated with serious hepatic effects (peliosis hepatis, hepatic neoplasms, cholestatic hepatitis, jaundice). May potentiate sleep apnea in some male patients (obesity or chronic lung disease). May increase hematocrit requiring dose adjustment or discontinuation; monitor.

[U.S. Boxed Warning]: Virilization in children has been reported following contact with unwashed or unclothed application sites of men using topical testosterone. Patients should strictly adhere to instructions for use in order to prevent secondary exposure. Virilization of female sexual partners has also been reported with male use of topical testosterone. Symptoms of virilization generally regress following removal of exposure; however, in some children, enlarged genitalia and bone age did not fully return to age appropriate normal. Signs of inappropriate virilization in women or children following secondary exposure to topical testosterone should be brought to the attention of a healthcare provider. Axiron® and Fortesta™ are not interchangeable with other topical testosterone products. Transdermal patch may contain conducting metal (eg, aluminum); remove patch prior to MRI. Gels and buccal system have not been evaluated in males <18 years of age; safety and efficacy of injection have not been established in males <12 years of age. Some testosterone products may be chemically synthesized from soy. Some products may contain benzyl alcohol. Use of Axiron® in males with BMI >35 kg/m^2 has not been established.

Drug Interactions

Metabolism/Transport Effects Substrate (minor) of CYP2B6, 2C9, 2C19, 3A4; **Inhibits** CYP3A4 (weak)

Avoid Concomitant Use There are no known interactions where it is recommended to avoid concomitant use.

Decreased Effect There are no known significant interactions involving a decrease in effect.

Increased Effect/Toxicity

Testosterone may increase the levels/effects of: CycloSPORINE; CycloSPORINE (Systemic); Vitamin K Antagonists

The levels/effects of Testosterone may be increased by: Conivaptan

Nutritional/Ethanol Interactions Herb/Nutraceutical: St John's wort may decrease testosterone levels.

Lab Interactions Testosterone may decrease thyroxine-binding globulin, resulting in decreased total T_4; free thyroid hormone levels are not changed.

Adverse Reactions Frequency not always defined.

Cardiovascular: Deep venous thrombosis, edema, hypertension, vasodilation

Central nervous system: Abnormal dreams, aggressive behavior, anger, amnesia, anxiety, blood pressure decreased, depression, dizziness, emotional lability, excitation, headache, hostility, insomnia, malaise, memory loss, mood swings, nervousness, seizure, sleep apnea, sleeplessness

Dermatologic: Acne, alopecia, dry skin, folliculitis, hair discoloration, hirsutism (increase in pubic hair growth), pruritus, rash, seborrhea

Endocrine & metabolic: Breast pain/soreness, gonadotropin secretion decreased, growth acceleration, gynecomastia, hot flashes, hypercalcemia, hyperchloremia, hypercholesterolemia, hyper-/hypoglycemia, hyper-/hypokalemia, hyperlipidemia, hypernatremia, inorganic phosphate retention, libido changes, menstrual problems (including amenorrhea), virilism, water retention

Gastrointestinal: Appetite increased, diarrhea, GI bleeding, GI irritation, nausea, taste disorder, vomiting, weight gain

Following buccal administration (most common): Bitter taste, gum edema, gum or mouth irritation, gum pain, gum tenderness, taste perversion

Genitourinary: Bladder irritability, impotence, oligospermia, penile erections (spontaneous), priapism, prostatic carcinoma, prostatic hyperplasia, PSA increased, testicular atrophy, urination impaired

Hepatic: Bilirubin increased, cholestatic hepatitis, cholestatic jaundice, hepatic dysfunction, hepatic necrosis, hepatocellular neoplasms, liver function test changes, peliosis hepatis

Hematologic: Anemia, bleeding, hematocrit/hemoglobin increased, leukopenia, polycythemia, suppression of clotting factors

Local: Application site reaction (gel, solution), injection site inflammation/pain

Transdermal system: Pruritus at application site (37%), burn-like blisters under system (12%), erythema at application site (7%), vesicles at application site (6%), allergic contact dermatitis to system (4%), burning at application site (3%), induration at application site (3%)

Neuromuscular & skeletal: Hyperkinesias, paresthesia, weakness

Ocular: Lacrimation increased

Renal: Creatinine increased

Respiratory: Dyspnea, nasopharyngitis

Miscellaneous: Anaphylactoid reactions, diaphoresis, hypersensitivity reactions, smell disorder

Pharmacodynamics/Kinetics

Duration of Action Route and ester dependent; I.M.: Cypionate and enanthate esters have longest duration, ≤2-4 weeks; gel: 24-48 hours

Absorption Transdermal gel: ~10% of applied dose

Protein Binding 98% bound to sex hormone-binding globulin (40%) and albumin

Half-Life Elimination Variable: 10-100 minutes

Metabolism Hepatic; forms metabolites, including dihydrotestosterone (DHT) and estradiol (both active)

Excretion Urine (90%); feces (6%)

Controlled Substance C-III

Available Dosage Forms

Cream, topical:
First®-Testosterone MC: 2% (60 g)

Gel, topical:
AndroGel®: 1% [5 g gel/packet] (30s); 1% [2.5 g gel/packet] (30s); 1% [1.25 g gel/actuation] (75 g)
Fortesta™: 10 mg/actuation (60 g)
Testim®: 1% [5 g gel/tube] (30s)

Implant, subcutaneous:
Testopel®: 75 mg (10s, 24s, 100s)

Injection, oil: 100 mg/mL (10 mL); 200 mg/mL (1 mL, 5 mL, 10 mL)
Delatestryl®: 200 mg/mL (5 mL)
Depo®-Testosterone: 100 mg/mL (10 mL); 200 mg/mL (1 mL, 10 mL)

Mucoadhesive, for buccal application:
Striant®: 30 mg (60s)

Ointment, topical:
First®-Testosterone: 2% (60 g)

Patch, transdermal:
Androderm®: 2.5 mg/24 hours (60s); 5 mg/24 hours (30s)

Powder, for prescription compounding: USP: 100% (5 g, 25 g)

Solution, topical:
Axiron®: 30 mg/actuation (110 mL)

Dosing

Adult & Geriatric

Conditions associated with a deficiency or absence of endogenous testosterone: *Oral capsule (Andriol®; not available in U.S.):* Initial: 120-160 mg/day in 2 divided doses for 2-3 weeks; adjust according to individual response; usual maintenance dose: 40-120 mg/day (in divided doses)

Inoperable metastatic breast cancer (females): *I.M. (testosterone enanthate):* 200-400 mg every 2-4 weeks

Hypogonadism or hypogonadotropic hypogonadism (males):
I.M. (testosterone enanthate or testosterone cypionate): 50-400 mg every 2-4 weeks (FDA-approved dosing range); 75-100 mg/week or 150-200 mg every 2 weeks (Bhasin, 2010)
Pellet (for subcutaneous implantation): 150-450 mg every 3-6 months
Topical:
Buccal: 30 mg twice daily (every 12 hours) applied to the gum region above the incisor tooth
Transdermal system: Androderm®: Primary hypogonadism or hypogonadotropic hypogonadism: Initial: Apply 5 mg/day once nightly; dosing range: 2.5-7.5 mg/day; in nonvirilized patients, dose may be initiated at 2.5 mg/day. Apply to clean, dry, intact skin. **Do not apply to the scrotum.**
Gel: Apply to clean, dry, intact skin. **Do not apply testosterone gel to the genitals.**
AndroGel®, Testim®: 5 g (to deliver 50 mg of testosterone with 5 mg systemically absorbed) applied once daily (preferably in the morning) to clean, dry, intact skin of the shoulder and upper arms. AndroGel® may also be applied to the abdomen. Dosage may be increased to a maximum of 10 g (100 mg).
Dose adjustment based on testosterone levels:
Less than normal range: Increase dose from 5 g to 7.5 g to 10 g
Greater than normal range: Decrease dose. Discontinue if consistently above normal at 5 g/day
Fortesta™: 40 mg once daily in the morning. Apply to the thighs. Dosing range: 10-70 mg/day
Dose adjustment based on serum testosterone levels:
≥2500 ng/dL: Decrease dose by 20 mg/day
≥1250 to <2500 ng/dL: Decrease dose by 10 mg/day
≥500 and <1250 ng/dL: Maintain current dose
<500 ng/dL: Increase by 10 mg/day
Solution (Axiron®): 60 mg once daily. (Dosage range 30-120 mg/day). Apply to the axilla at the same time each morning; do not apply to other parts of the body. Apply to clean, dry, intact skin. **Do not apply testosterone solution to the genitals.**
Dose adjustment based on serum testosterone levels:
>1050 ng/dL: Decrease 60 mg/day dose to 30 mg/day; if levels >1050 ng/dL persist after dose reduction discontinue therapy
<300 ng/dL: Increase 60 mg/day dose to 90 mg/day, or increase 90 mg/day dose to 120 mg/day

Delayed puberty (males):
I.M. (testosterone enanthate): 50-200 mg every 2-4 weeks for a limited duration
Pellet (for subcutaneous implantation): 150-450 mg every 3-6 months

Pediatric

Delayed puberty (adolescent males):
I.M. (testosterone enanthate): Refer to adult dosing.
Pellet (for subcutaneous implantation): Refer to adult dosing.

Hypogonadism or hypogonadotropic hypogonadism (adolescent males):
I.M. (testosterone enanthate or testosterone cypionate): Refer to adult dosing.
Pellet (for subcutaneous implantation): Refer to adult dosing.

Hypogonadism or hypogonadotropic hypogonadism (males ≥ 15 years of age): *Transdermal system (Androderm®):* Refer to adult dosing.

Renal Impairment Use with caution; may enhance edema formation.

Hepatic Impairment Use with caution; may enhance edema formation.

Administration

Oral

Oral, buccal application (Striant®): One mucoadhesive for buccal application (buccal system) should be applied to a comfortable area above the incisor tooth. Apply flat side of system to gum. Rotate to alternate sides of mouth with each application. Hold buccal system firmly in place for 30 seconds to ensure adhesion. The buccal system should adhere to gum for 12 hours. If the buccal system falls out, replace with a new system. If the system falls out within 4 hours of next dose, the new buccal system should remain in place until the time of the following scheduled dose. System will soften and mold to shape of gum as it absorbs moisture from mouth. Do not chew or swallow the buccal system. The buccal system will not dissolve; gently remove by sliding downwards from gum; avoid scratching gum.

Oral, capsule (Andriol®; not available in the U.S.): Should be administered with meals. Should be swallowed whole; do not crush or chew.

I.M. Warm injection to room temperature and shaking vial will help redissolve crystals that have formed after storage. Administer by deep I.M. injection into the upper outer quadrant of the gluteus maximus.

Other

Transdermal patch (Androderm®): Apply patch to clean, dry area of skin on the back, abdomen, upper arms, or thigh. Do not apply to bony areas or parts of the body that are subject to prolonged pressure while sleeping or sitting. **Do not apply to the scrotum.** Following patch removal, mild skin irritation may be treated with OTC hydrocortisone cream. A small amount of triamcinolone acetonide 0.1% cream may be applied under the system to decrease irritation; do not use ointment. Patch should be applied nightly. Rotate administration sites, allowing 7 days between applying to the same site.

Topical gel and solution: Apply to clean, dry, intact skin. Application sites should be allowed to dry for a few minutes prior to dressing. Hands should be washed with soap and water after application. **Do not apply testosterone gel or solution to the genitals.** Alcohol-based gels and solutions are flammable; avoid fire or smoking until dry. Testosterone may be transferred to another person following skin-to-skin contact with the application site. Strict adherence to application instructions is needed in order to decrease secondary exposure. Thoroughly wash hands after application and cover application site with clothing (ie, shirt) once gel or solution has dried, or clean application site thoroughly with soap and water prior to contact in order to minimize transfer. In addition to skin-to-skin contact, secondary exposure has also been reported following exposure to secondary items (eg, towel, shirt, sheets). If secondary exposure occurs, the other person should thoroughly wash the skin with soap and water as soon as possible.

AndroGel®, Testim®: Apply (preferably in the morning) to clean, dry, intact skin of the shoulder and upper arms. AndroGel® may also be applied to the abdomen; do not apply Testim® to the abdomen. Area of application should be limited to what will be covered by a short sleeve t-shirt. Apply at the same time each day. Upon opening the packet(s), the entire contents should be squeezed into the palm of the hand and immediately applied to the application site(s). Alternatively, a portion may be squeezed onto palm of hand and applied, repeating the process until entire packet has been applied. Application site should not be washed for ≥2 hours following application of Testim®.

AndroGel® multidose pump: Prime pump 3 times (and discard this portion of product) prior to initial use. Each actuation delivers 1.25 g of gel (4 actuations = 5 g; 6 actuations = 7.5 g; 8 actuations = 10 g); each actuation may be applied individually or all at the same time.

Axiron®: Apply using the applicator to the axilla at the same time each morning. Do not apply to other parts of the body (eg, abdomen, genitals, shoulders, upper arms). Avoid washing the site or swimming for 2 hours after application. Prior to first use, prime the applicator pump by depressing it 3 times (discard this portion of the product). After priming, position the nozzle over the applicator cup and depress pump fully one time; ensure liquid enters cup. Each pump actuation delivers testosterone 30 mg. No more than 30 mg (one pump) should be added to the cup at one time. The total dose should be divided between axilla (example, 30 mg/day: apply to one axilla only; 60 mg/day: apply 30 mg to each axilla; 90 mg/day: apply 30 mg to each axilla, allow to dry, then apply an additional 30 mg to one axilla; etc). To apply dose, keep applicator upright and wipe into the axilla; if solution runs or drips, use cup to wipe. Do not rub into skin with fingers or hand. If more than one 30 mg dose is needed, repeat process. Apply roll-on or stick antiperspirants or deodorants prior to testosterone. Once application site is dry, cover with clothing. After use, rinse applicator under running water and pat dry with a tissue. The application site and dose of this product are not interchangeable with other topical testosterone products.

Fortesta™: Apply to skin of front and inner thighs. Do not apply to other parts of the body. Use one finger to rub gel evenly onto skin of each thigh. Avoid showering, washing the site, or swimming for 2 hours after application. Prior to first dose, prime the pump by holding canister upright and fully depressing the pump 8 times (discard this portion of the product). Each pump actuation delivers testosterone 10 mg. The total dose should be divided between thighs (example, 10 mg/day: apply 10 mg to one thigh only; 20 mg/day: apply 10 mg to each thigh; 30 mg/day: apply 20 mg to one thigh and 10 mg to the other thigh; etc). Once application site is dry, cover with clothing. The application site and dose of this product are not interchangeable with other topical testosterone products.

Stability

Storage

Androderm®: Store at room temperature. Do not store outside of pouch. Excessive heat may cause system to burst.

AndroGel®, Axiron®, Delatestryl®, Striant®, Testim®: Store at room temperature.

Depo® Testosterone: Store at room temperature. Protect from light.

Fortesta™: Store at room temperature; do not freeze

Testopel®: Store in a cool location.

Monitoring and Teaching Issues

Laboratory Monitoring Periodic liver function tests, cholesterol, hemoglobin and hematocrit (prior to therapy, at 3-6 months, then annually); radiologic examination of wrist and hand every 6 months (when using in prepubertal children). Withhold initial treatment with hematocrit >54%, hyperviscosity, untreated obstructive sleep apnea, or uncontrolled severe heart failure. Monitor urine and serum calcium and signs of virilization in women treated for breast cancer. Serum glucose (may be decreased by testosterone, monitor patients with diabetes). Evaluate males for response to treatment and adverse events 3-6 months after initiation and then annually.

Bone mineral density: Monitor after 1-2 years of therapy in hypogonadal men with osteoporosis or low trauma fracture (Bhasin, 2010)

PSA: In men >40 years of age with baseline PSA >0.6 ng/mL, PSA and prostate exam (prior to therapy, at 3-6 months, then as based on current guidelines). Withhold treatment pending urological evaluation in patients with palpable prostate nodule or induration or PSA >4 ng/mL or if PSA >3 ng/mL in men at high risk of prostate cancer (Bhasin, 2010).

Do not treat with severe untreated BPH with IPSS symptom score >19.

Serum testosterone: Monitor 3-6 months after initiating treatment, then annually.

Injection: Measure midway between injections. Adjust dose or frequency if testosterone concentration is <400 ng/dL or >700 ng/dL (Bhasin, 2010).

AndroGel®, Testim®: Morning serum testosterone levels ~14 days after start of therapy

Androderm®: Morning serum testosterone levels following application the previous evening

Axiron®: Serum testosterone levels can be measured 2-8 hours after application and after 14 days of starting therapy or dose adjustments

Fortesta™: Serum testosterone levels can be measured 2 hours after application and after 14 and 35 days of starting therapy or dose adjustments

Striant®: Application area of gums; total serum testosterone 4-12 weeks after initiating treatment, prior to morning dose

Testopel®: Measure at the end of the dosing interval (Bhasin, 2010)

Physical Assessment Caution patients with diabetes; may cause hypoglycemic reaction. Teach patient to protect others from accidental exposure.

Patient Education For topical application (patch or gel), use precautions to avoid accidental skin-to-skin exposure with others. If using self-administered injections, follow prescriber's instructions for injection procedure and disposal of syringes/needles. If you have diabetes, monitor serum glucose closely and notify prescriber of changes; this medication may alter hypoglycemic requirements. You may experience acne, growth of body hair, loss of libido, impotence, menstrual irregularity (usually reversible), nausea, taste disorder, or vomiting. Report changes in menstrual pattern; enlarged or painful breasts; deepening of voice or unusual growth of body hair; persistent or spontaneous penile erection; fluid retention (swelling of ankles, feet, or hands; respiratory difficulty; sudden weight gain); unresolved changes in CNS (nervousness, chills, insomnia, depression, aggressiveness); altered urinary patterns; change in color of urine or stool; yellowing of eyes or skin; unusual bruising or bleeding; blood in urine or stool; difficulty sleeping or sleep apnea; or skin irritation, redness, burning, or swelling at application site or injection site.

Dietary Considerations Testosterone USP may be synthesized from soy. Food and beverages have not been found to interfere with buccal system; ensure system is in place following eating, drinking, or brushing teeth.

Geriatric Considerations Elderly males treated with androgens may be at increased risk of developing prostatic hyperplasia and prostatic carcinoma. Increase in libido may occur.

Breast-Feeding Considerations High levels of endogenous maternal testosterone, such as those caused by certain ovarian cysts, suppress milk production. Maternal serum testosterone levels generally fall following pregnancy and return to normal once breast-feeding is stopped. The amount of testosterone present in breast milk or the effect to the nursing infant following maternal supplementation is not known. Some products are contraindicated while breast-feeding. Females who are nursing should avoid skin-to-skin contact to areas where testosterone has been applied topically on another person.

Pregnancy Considerations Testosterone may cause adverse effects, including masculinization of the female fetus, if used during pregnancy. Females who are or may become pregnant should also avoid skin-to-skin contact to areas where testosterone has been applied topically on another person.

- **Testosterone Cypionate** *see* Testosterone *on page* 1739
- **Testosterone Enanthate** *see* Testosterone *on page* 1739
- **Testred®** *see* MethylTESTOSTERone *on page* 1212
- **Tetanus Toxoid** *see* Diphtheria and Tetanus Toxoids, Acellular Pertussis, Poliovirus and *Haemophilus* b Conjugate Vaccine *on page* 550
- **Tetanus Toxoid, Reduced Diphtheria Toxoid, and Acellular Pertussis, Adsorbed** *see* Diphtheria and Tetanus Toxoids, and Acellular Pertussis Vaccine *on page* 552

Tetrabenazine (tet ra BEN a zeen)

U.S. Brand Names Xenazine®

Pharmacologic Category Central Monoamine-Depleting Agent

Medication Guide Available Yes

Prescribing and Access Restrictions Xenazine® is available only through specialty pharmacies. For more information regarding the procurement of Xenazine®, healthcare providers, patients, and caregivers may contact the Xenazine® Information Center (XIC) at 1-888-882-6013 or at:

Healthcare providers: http://www.xenazineusa.com/HCP/PrescribingXenazine/Default.aspx

Patients and caregivers: http://www.xenazineusa.com/AboutXenazine/Getting-Your-Prescription.aspx

Pregnancy Risk Factor C

Lactation Excretion in breast milk unknown/not recommended

Use Treatment of chorea associated with Huntington's disease

Canadian labeling: Treatment of hyperkinetic movement disorders, including Huntington's chorea, hemiballismus, senile chorea, Tourette syndrome, and tardive dyskinesia

Available Dosage Forms

Tablet, oral:

Xenazine®: 12.5 mg, 25 mg

Dosing

Adult Dose should be individualized; titrate slowly

Chorea associated with Huntington's disease: Oral:

Initial: 12.5 mg once daily, may increase to 12.5 mg twice daily after 1 week

Maintenance: May be increased by 12.5 mg/day at weekly intervals; doses >37.5 mg/day should be divided into 3 doses (maximum single dose: 25 mg)

Patients requiring doses >50 mg/day: Genotype for CYP2D6:

Extensive/intermediate metabolizers: Maximum: 100 mg/day; 37.5 mg/dose

Poor metabolizers: Maximum: 50 mg/day; 25 mg/dose

Concomitant use with strong CYP2D6 inhibitors (eg, fluoxetine, paroxetine, quinidine): Dose of tetrabenazine should be reduced by 50% in patients receiving strong CYP2D6 inhibitors, follow dosing for poor CYP2D6 metabolizers. Use caution when adding a CYP2D6 inhibitor to patients already taking tetrabenazine.

Note: If treatment is interrupted for >5 days, retitration is recommended. If treatment is interrupted for <5 days resume at previous maintenance dose.

Canadian labeling: Hyperkinetic movement disorders: Initial: 12.5 mg twice daily (may be given 3 times/day); may be increased by 12.5 mg/day every 3-5 days; should be titrated slowly to maximal tolerated and effective dose (dose is individualized)

Usual maximum tolerated dosage: 25 mg 3 times/day; maximum recommended dose: 200 mg/day

Note: If there is no improvement at the maximum tolerated dose after 7 days, improvement is unlikely; discontinuation should be considered.

Geriatric Canadian labeling: Elderly and/or debilitated patients: Consider initiation at lower doses; must be titrated slowly to individualize dosage.

Hepatic Impairment Use is contraindicated.

Adjustment for Toxicity For toxicity/adverse reaction, including akathisia, restlessness, parkinsonism, insomnia, depression, suicidality, anxiety, sedation (intolerable): Suspend upward dosage titration and reduce dose; consider discontinuing if adverse reaction does not resolve (may be discontinued without tapering).

Administration

Oral May administer without regard to meals.

Monitoring and Teaching Issues

Physical Assessment Evaluate closely for presence or history of depression or other psychiatric disorders, hepatic impairment, cardiac abnormalities, or recent use of MAO inhibitors. Dosing should be individualized and titrated slowly. Monitor psychiatric status and for CNS changes at beginning of therapy, with any dose change, and at frequent intervals during therapy.

Patient Education May cause dizziness, headache, sedation, nausea, or vomiting. Report immediately any signs of CNS changes (mood changes, increased irritability or anxiety, depression, suicide ideation) or difficulty breathing.

Tetracycline (tet ra SYE kleen)

Index Terms Achromycin; TCN; Tetracycline Hydrochloride

Generic Availability (U.S.) Yes: Capsule

Pharmacologic Category Antibiotic, Tetracycline Derivative

Medication Safety Issues

Sound-alike/look-alike issues:

Tetracycline may be confused with tetradecyl sulfate

Achromycin may be confused with actinomycin, Adriamycin PFS®

Pregnancy Risk Factor D

Lactation Enters breast milk/not recommended (AAP rates "compatible"; AAP 2001 update pending)

Use Treatment of susceptible bacterial infections of both gram-positive and gram-negative organisms; also infections due to *Mycoplasma*, *Chlamydia*, and *Rickettsia*; indicated for acne, exacerbations of chronic bronchitis, and treatment of gonorrhea and syphilis in patients who are allergic to penicillin; as part of a multidrug regimen for *H. pylori* eradication to reduce the risk of duodenal ulcer recurrence

Mechanism of Action/Effect Inhibits protein synthesis of susceptible bacteria; bacteriostatic, causes cell death.

Contraindications Hypersensitivity to tetracycline or any component of the formulation; do not administer to children ≤8 years of age; pregnancy

Warnings/Precautions Use with caution in patients with renal or hepatic impairment (eg, elderly); dosage modification required in patients with renal impairment since it may increase BUN as an antianabolic agent. Hepatotoxicity has been reported rarely; risk may be increased in patients with pre-existing hepatic or renal impairment. Pseudotumor cerebri has been reported with tetracycline use (usually resolves with discontinuation); outdated drug can cause nephropathy; use protective measure to avoid photosensitivity. Prolonged use may result in fungal or bacterial superinfection, including *C. difficile*-associated diarrhea (CDAD) and pseudomembranous colitis; CDAD has been observed >2 months postantibiotic treatment. May cause tissue hyperpigmentation, enamel hypoplasia, or permanent tooth discoloration; use of tetracyclines should be avoided during tooth development (children ≤8 years of age) unless other drugs are not likely to be effective or are contraindicated. However, recommended in treatment of anthrax exposure. Do not use during pregnancy. In addition to affecting tooth development, tetracycline use has been associated with retardation of skeletal development and reduced bone growth.

Drug Interactions

Metabolism/Transport Effects Substrate of CYP3A4 (major); **Inhibits** CYP3A4 (moderate)

Avoid Concomitant Use

Avoid concomitant use of Tetracycline with any of the following: BCG; Retinoic Acid Derivatives; Tolvaptan

Decreased Effect

Tetracycline may decrease the levels/effects of: Atovaquone; BCG; Penicillins; Typhoid Vaccine

The levels/effects of Tetracycline may be decreased by: Antacids; Bile Acid Sequestrants; Bismuth; Bismuth Subsalicylate; CYP3A4 Inducers (Strong); Deferasirox; Herbs (CYP3A4 Inducers); Iron Salts; Magnesium Salts; Quinapril; Sucralfate; Zinc Salts

Increased Effect/Toxicity

Tetracycline may increase the levels/effects of: Colchicine; CYP3A4 Substrates; Eplerenone; Everolimus; FentaNYL; Halofantrine; Lurasidone; Neuromuscular-Blocking Agents; Pimecrolimus; Ranolazine; Retinoic Acid Derivatives; Salmeterol; Saxagliptin; Tolvaptan; Vilazodone; Vitamin K Antagonists

The levels/effects of Tetracycline may be increased by: Conivaptan

Nutritional/Ethanol Interactions

Food: Serum concentrations may be decreased if taken with dairy products.

Herb/Nutraceutical: Avoid dong quai, St John's wort (may also cause photosensitization)

Lab Interactions False-negative urine glucose with Clinistix®

Adverse Reactions Frequency not defined.

Cardiovascular: Pericarditis

Central nervous system: Intracranial pressure increased, bulging fontanels in infants, pseudotumor cerebri, paresthesia

Dermatologic: Photosensitivity, pruritus, pigmentation of nails, exfoliative dermatitis

Endocrine & metabolic: Diabetes insipidus syndrome

Gastrointestinal: Discoloration of teeth and enamel hypoplasia (young children), nausea, diarrhea, vomiting, esophagitis, anorexia, abdominal cramps, antibiotic-associated pseudomembranous colitis, staphylococcal enterocolitis, pancreatitis

Hematologic: Thrombophlebitis

Hepatic: Hepatotoxicity

Renal: Acute renal failure, azotemia, renal damage

Miscellaneous: Superinfection, anaphylaxis, hypersensitivity reactions, candidal superinfection

Pharmacodynamics/Kinetics

Absorption Oral: 75%

Time to Peak Serum: Oral: 2-4 hours

Protein Binding ~65%

Half-Life Elimination Normal renal function: 8-11 hours; End-stage renal disease: 57-108 hours

Excretion Urine (60% as unchanged drug); feces (as active form)

Available Dosage Forms

Capsule, oral: 250 mg, 500 mg

Dosing

Adult & Geriatric

Usual dosage range: Oral: 250-500 mg every 6 hours

Acne: Oral: 250-500 twice daily

Chronic bronchitis, acute exacerbation: Oral: 500 mg 4 times/day

Erlichiosis: Oral: 500 mg 4 times/day for 7-14 days

Peptic ulcer disease: Eradication of *Helicobacter pylori*: Oral: 500 mg 2-4 times/day depending on regimen; requires combination therapy with at least one other antibiotic and an acid-suppressing agent (proton pump inhibitor or H_2 blocker)

Periodontitis: Oral: 250 mg every 6 hours until improvement (usually 10 days)

Vibrio cholerae: Oral: 500 mg 4 times/day for 3 days

Pediatric Usual dosage range: Children >8 years: Oral: 25-50 mg/kg/day in divided doses every 6 hours

Renal Impairment
Cl_{cr} 50-80 mL/minute: Administer every 8-12 hours.
Cl_{cr} 10-50 mL/minute: Administer every 12-24 hours.
Cl_{cr} <10 mL/minute: Administer every 24 hours.
Slightly dialyzable (5% to 20%) via hemo- and peritoneal dialysis or via continuous arterio-venous or venovenous hemofiltration; supplemental dose is not necessary.

Hepatic Impairment Use caution; no dosing adjustment required

Administration

Oral Oral should be given on an empty stomach (ie, 1 hour prior to, or 2 hours after meals) to increase total absorption. Administer at least 1-2 hours prior to, or 4 hours after antacid because aluminum and magnesium cations may chelate with tetracycline and reduce its total absorption. Administer around-the-clock to promote less variation in peak and trough serum levels.

Stability

Storage Outdated tetracyclines have caused a Fanconi-like syndrome (nausea, vomiting, acidosis, proteinuria, glycosuria, aminoaciduria, polydipsia, polyuria, hypokalemia). Protect oral dosage forms from light.

Monitoring and Teaching Issues

Laboratory Monitoring Renal, hepatic, and hematologic function; WBC. Perform culture and sensitivity studies prior to initiating therapy to determine the causative organism and its susceptibility to tetracycline.

Physical Assessment Assess results of culture and sensitivity tests and patient's allergy history prior to beginning therapy. Monitor for nausea, diarrhea, pericarditis, photosensitivity, rash, opportunistic infection, and hypersensitivity.

Patient Education Preferable to take on an empty stomach, 1 hour before or 2 hours after meals. Avoid antacids, iron, or dairy products within 2 hours of taking tetracycline. You may experience photosensitivity, dizziness, lightheadedness, or nausea/vomiting. Report rash or intense itching, yellowing of skin or eyes, fever or chills, blackened stool, vaginal itching or discharge, foul-smelling stools, excessive thirst or urination, acute headache, unresolved or persistent diarrhea, respiratory difficulty, if condition does not improve, or worsening of condition.

Dietary Considerations Take on an empty stomach (ie, 1 hour prior to, or 2 hours after meals). Take at least 1-2 hours prior to, or 4 hours after antacid.

Geriatric Considerations The role of tetracycline has decreased because of the emergence of resistant organisms. Doxycycline is the tetracycline of choice when one is indicated because of its better GI absorption, less interactions with divalent cations, longer half-life, and the fact that the majority is cleared by nonrenal mechanisms.

Breast-Feeding Considerations Tetracyclines are excreted in breast milk. Tetracycline binds to calcium. The calcium in the maternal milk will decrease the amount of tetracycline absorbed by the breast-feeding infant. Nondose-related effects could include modification of bowel flora.

Pregnancy Considerations Tetracyclines cross the placenta, enter fetal circulation, and may cause permanent discoloration of teeth if used during the second or third trimester. Maternal hepatic toxicity has been associated with the use of tetracycline during pregnancy, especially in patients with azotemia or pyelonephritis. Because use during pregnancy may cause fetal harm, tetracycline is classified as pregnancy category D.

Related Information

Antimicrobial Drugs of Choice *on page* 2008
Helicobacter pylori Treatment *on page* 2045

◆ **Tetracycline Hydrochloride** *see* Tetracycline *on page* 1744
◆ **Tetrahydrocannabinol** *see* Dronabinol *on page* 590
◆ **Teveten®** *see* Eprosartan *on page* 646
◆ **Teveten® HCT** *see* Eprosartan and Hydrochlorothiazide *on page* 648
◆ **Tev-Tropin®** *see* Somatropin *on page* 1664
◆ **Texacort®** *see* Hydrocortisone (Topical) *on page* 920
◆ **TG** *see* Thioguanine *on page* 1752
◆ **6-TG (error-prone abbreviation)** *see* Thioguanine *on page* 1752
◆ **TH9507** *see* Tesamorelin *on page* 1737

Thalidomide (tha LI doe mide)

U.S. Brand Names Thalomid®

Generic Availability (U.S.) No

Pharmacologic Category Angiogenesis Inhibitor; Immunomodulator, Systemic; Tumor Necrosis Factor (TNF) Blocking Agent

Medication Safety Issues

Sound-alike/look-alike issues:
Thalidomide may be confused with flutamide, lenalidomide
Thalomid® may be confused with thiamine

High alert medication: This medication is in a class the Institute for Safe Medication Practices (ISMP) includes among its list of drugs which have a heightened risk of causing significant patient harm when used in error.

International issues:

Thalomid [U.S., Canada] may be confused with Thilomide brand name for lodoxamide [Greece, Turkey]

Medication Guide Available Yes

Prescribing and Access Restrictions U.S.: As a requirement of the REMS program, access to this medication is restricted. Thalidomide is approved for marketing only under a special distribution program. This program, called the "System for Thalidomide Education and Prescribing Safety" (STEPS® 1-888-423-5436), has been approved by the FDA. Prescribers and pharmacists must be registered with the program. No more than a 4-week supply should be dispensed. Blister packs should be dispensed intact (do not repackage capsules). Prescriptions must be filled within 7 days. Subsequent prescriptions may be filled only if fewer than 7 days of therapy remain on the previous prescription. A new prescription is required for further dispensing (a telephone prescription may not be accepted.) Pregnancy testing is required for females of childbearing potential.

Canada: Access to thalidomide is restricted through a controlled distribution program called RevAid®. Only physicians and pharmacists enrolled in this program are authorized to prescribe or dispense thalidomide. Patients must be enrolled in the program by their physicians. Further information is available by calling 1-888-738-2431.

Pregnancy Risk Factor X

Lactation Excretion in breast milk unknown/not recommended

Use Treatment of newly-diagnosed multiple myeloma; treatment and maintenance of cutaneous manifestations of erythema nodosum leprosum (ENL)

Unlabeled/Investigational Use Treatment of refractory Crohn's disease; treatment of chronic graft-versus-host disease (GVHD) in hematopoietic stem cell transplantation; AIDS-related aphthous stomatitis; Waldenström's macroglobulinemia; maintenance therapy of multiple myeloma (following autologous stem cell transplant)

Available Dosage Forms

Capsule, oral:

Thalomid®: 50 mg, 100 mg, 150 mg, 200 mg

Dosing

Adult & Geriatric

Cutaneous ENL: Oral: Initial: 100-300 mg once daily

Adjustments to initial dose:

Patients weighing <50 kg: Initiate at lower end of the dosing range

Severe cutaneous reaction or patients previously requiring high dose may be initiated at 400 mg/day; doses may be divided, but taken 1 hour after meals

Duration and tapering/maintenance:

Maintenance: Dosing should continue until active reaction subsides (usually at least 2 weeks), then tapered in 50 mg decrements every 2-4 weeks

Patients who flare during tapering or with a history of requiring prolonged maintenance should be maintained on the minimum dosage necessary to control the reaction. Efforts to taper should be repeated every 3-6 months, in decrements of 50 mg every 2-4 weeks.

Multiple myeloma: Oral: **Note:** Details concerning dosing for multiple myeloma with combination regimens should also be consulted.

200 mg once daily at bedtime (in combination with dexamethasone 40 mg daily on days 1-4, 9-12, and 17-20 of a 28-day treatment cycle)

In combination with melphalan and prednisone (unlabeled combination in U.S.): 200-400 mg once daily (Facon, 2007) **or** 100 mg once daily (Palumbo, 2008)

Canadian labeling: Adults ≥65 years: 200 mg once daily (in combination with melphalan and prednisone)

AIDS-related aphthous stomatitis (unlabeled use): Oral: 200 mg once daily at bedtime for up to 8 weeks, if no response, then 200 mg twice daily for 4 weeks (Jacobson, 1997)

Chronic graft-versus-host disease (refractory), treatment (unlabeled second-line use; optimum dose not determined): Oral: Initial: 100 mg at bedtime, with dose escalation up to 400 mg/day in 3-4 divided doses (Wolff, 2010) **or** Initial: 50-100 mg 3 times/day; maximum dose: 600-1200 mg/day (Kulkarni, 2003) **or** 200 mg 4 times/day (dose adjusted to goal thalidomide concentration of ≥5 mcg/mL 2 hours postdose) (Vogelsang, 1992) **or** 100-300 mg 4 times/day (Parker, 1995)

Crohn's disease, refractory (unlabeled use): Oral: 50-100 mg/day at bedtime (Vasiliauskas, 1999) **or** 200-300 mg/day at bedtime (Ehrenpreis, 1999)

Multiple myeloma, maintenance (following autologous stem cell transplant; unlabeled use): Oral: 200 mg/day starting 3-6 months after transplant; continue until disease progression or unacceptable toxicity (Brinker, 2006) **or** 100 mg/day starting 42-60 days following transplant; increase to 200 mg/day after 2 weeks if tolerated; continue for up to 12 months (in combination with prednisolone) (Spencer, 2009)

Waldenström's macroglobulinemia (unlabeled use): Oral: 200 mg/day for up to 52 weeks (in combination with rituximab) (Treon, 2008)

Pediatric Cutaneous ENL: Children ≥12 years: Oral: Refer to adult dosing.

Chronic graft-versus-host disease (refractory), treatment (unlabeled second-line use; limited data): Children ≥3 years: Oral: 3 mg/kg 4 times/day (dose adjusted to goal thalidomide concentration of ≥5 mcg/mL 2 hours postdose) (Vogelsang, 1992) **or** Initial: 3-6 mg/kg/day in 2-4 divided doses; target dose 12 mg/kg/day; Maximum daily dose: 800 mg (Rovelli, 1998)

Adjustment for Toxicity

ANC ≤750/mm^3: Withhold treatment if clinically appropriate

Multiple myeloma:

U.S. labeling: Constipation, oversedation, peripheral neuropathy: Temporarily withhold or continue with a reduced dose

Canadian labeling:

ANC <1500/mm^3: Withhold melphalan and prednisone for 1 week; resume melphalan and prednisone after 1 week if ANC >1500/mm^3 **or** if ANC 1000-1500/mm^3 reduce melphalan dose by 50% **or** if ANC <1000/mm^3 adjust chemotherapy dose based on clinical status of patient.

Constipation, oversedation: Temporarily withhold thalidomide treatment or continue with a reduced dose

Peripheral neuropathy, Grade 1 (paresthesia, weakness and/or loss of reflexes) without loss of function): Evaluate patient and consider dose reduction with worsening of symptoms; symptom improvement may not follow dose reduction, however.

Peripheral neuropathy, Grade 2 (interferes with function but not with daily activities), Grade 3 (interferes with daily activities), or Grade 4 (disabling neuropathy): Discontinue thalidomide treatment

Thromboembolic events: Withhold therapy and initiate standard anticoagulant treatment; may resume thalidomide therapy at original dose following stabilization of patient and resolution of thromboembolic event; maintain anticoagulant treatment for duration of thalidomide therapy

Administration

Oral Administer orally with water, preferably at bedtime once daily on an empty stomach, at least 1 hour after the evening meal. Doses >400 mg/day may be given in 2-3 divided doses. For missed doses, if <12 hours patient may receive dose; if >12 hours wait till next dose due.

Avoid extensive handling of capsules; capsules should remain in blister pack until ingestion. If exposed to the powder content from broken capsules or body fluids from patients receiving thalidomide, the exposed area should be washed with soap and water.

Monitoring and Teaching Issues

Laboratory Monitoring Pregnancy testing (sensitivity of at least 50 mIU/mL) is required within 24 hours prior to initiation of therapy, weekly during the first 4 weeks, then every 4 weeks in women with regular menstrual cycles or every 2 weeks in women with irregular menstrual cycles. In HIV-seropositive patients; monitor viral load after 1 and 3 months, then every 3 months. CBC with differential, platelets. Consider monitoring of sensory nerve application potential amplitudes at baseline and every 6 months to detect asymptomatic neuropathy.

Physical Assessment Patient must be capable of complying with STEPS® program. Instruct patient on risks of pregnancy, appropriate contraceptive measures, and necessity for frequent pregnancy testing (schedule pregnancy testing at time of dispensing and give patient schedule in writing). Monitor for signs of fluid retention, weight gain, and hypotension. Monitor closely for signs of neuropathy, neutropenia, and CNS depression.

Patient Education You will be given oral and written instructions about the necessity of using two methods of contraception and the necessity of keeping return visits for pregnancy testing. Do not donate blood while taking this medicine. Male patients should not donate sperm. Avoid extensive handling of capsules; capsules should remain in blister pack until ingestion. If exposed to the powder content from broken capsules or body fluids from patients receiving thalidomide, the exposed area should be washed with soap and water. Avoid alcohol. You may experience postural hypotension, sleepiness, dizziness, fatigue, fever, headaches, lack of concentration, nausea or vomiting or loss of appetite, constipation or diarrhea, oral thrush (frequent mouth care is necessary), or sexual dysfunction (reversible). Report any of the above if persistent or severe. Report chest pain or palpitations or swelling of extremities; respiratory difficulty; back, neck, muscle pain, muscle weakness, or stiffness; numbness or pain in extremities; significant weight loss or gain; skin rash or eruptions; or increased nervousness, anxiety, confusion, or insomnia.

◆ **Thalitone®** *see* Chlorthalidone *on page 361*

◆ **Thalomid®** *see* Thalidomide *on page 1746*

◆ **THC** *see* Dronabinol *on page 590*

◆ **Theo-24®** *see* Theophylline *on page 1748*

◆ **Theochron™** *see* Theophylline *on page 1748*

Theophylline (thee OFF i lin)

U.S. Brand Names Elixophyllin® Elixir; Theo-24®; Theochron™

Index Terms Theophylline Anhydrous

Generic Availability (U.S.) Yes: Extended release tablet, infusion, solution

Pharmacologic Category Theophylline Derivative

Pregnancy Risk Factor C

Lactation Enters breast milk/compatible (AAP rates "compatible"; AAP 2001 update pending)

Use Treatment of symptoms and reversible airway obstruction due to chronic asthma, or other chronic lung diseases; apnea of prematurity

Note: The Global Initiative for Asthma Guidelines (2009) and the National Heart, Lung and Blood Institute Guidelines (2007) do not recommend oral theophylline as a long-term control medication for asthma in children ≤5 years of age; use has been shown to be effective as an add-on (but not preferred) agent in older children and adults with severe asthma treated with inhaled or oral glucocorticoids. The guidelines do not recommend theophylline for the treatment of exacerbations of asthma.

The Global Initiative for Chronic Obstructive Lung Disease Guidelines (2009) suggest that while higher doses of slow release formulations of theophylline have been proven to be effective for use in COPD, it is not a preferred agent due to its potential for toxicity.

Available Dosage Forms

Capsule, extended release, oral:
Theo-24®: 100 mg, 200 mg, 300 mg, 400 mg

Infusion, premixed in D_5W: 400 mg (100 mL, 250 mL, 500 mL, 1000 mL); 800 mg (250 mL, 500 mL, 1000 mL)

Solution, oral: 80 mg/15 mL (15 mL)
Elixophyllin® Elixir: 80 mg/15 mL (473 mL)

Tablet, extended release, oral: 100 mg, 200 mg, 300 mg, 400 mg, 450 mg, 600 mg
Theochron™: 100 mg, 200 mg, 300 mg, 450 mg

Dosing

Adult Doses should be individualized based on steady-state serum concentrations and ideal body weight.

Acute symptoms: Loading dose: Oral, I.V.:

Asthma exacerbations: While theophylline may be considered for relief of asthma symptoms, the role of treating exacerbations is not supported by current practice.

COPD treatment: Theophylline is currently considered second-line intravenous therapy in the emergency department or hospital setting when there is inadequate or insufficient response to short acting bronchodilators (Global Initiative for COPD Guidelines, 2009).

If no theophylline received within the previous 24 hours: 4.6 mg/kg loading dose (~5.8 mg/kg hydrous aminophylline) I.V. or 5 mg/kg orally. Loading dose intended to achieve a serum level of approximately 10 mcg/mL; loading doses should be given intravenously (preferred) or with a rapidly absorbed oral product (not an extended-release product). **Note:** On the average, for every 1 mg/kg theophylline given, blood levels will rise 2 mcg/mL.

If theophylline has been administered in the previous 24 hours: A loading dose is not recommended without obtaining a serum theophylline concentration. The loading dose should be calculated as follows:

Dose = (desired serum theophylline concentration - measured serum theophylline concentration) (V_d)

Acute symptoms: Maintenance dose: I.V.: **Note:** To achieve a target concentration of 10 mcg/mL unless otherwise noted. Lower initial doses may be required in patients with reduced theophylline clearance. Dosage should be adjusted according to serum level measurements during the first 12- to 24-hour period.

Adults 16-60 years (otherwise healthy, nonsmokers): 0.4 mg/kg/hour; maximum 900 mg/day unless serum levels indicate need for larger dose

Adults >60 years: 0.3 mg/kg/hour; maximum 400 mg/day unless serum levels indicate need for larger dose

Treatment of chronic conditions: With newer guidelines suggesting lower therapeutic theophylline ranges, it is unlikely that doses larger than >10 mg/kg/day will be required in children ≥1 year of age.

Oral solution: Initial dose: 300 mg/day administered in divided doses every 6-8 hours; Maintenance: 400-600 mg/day (maximum: 600 mg/day)

Oral extended release formulations: Initial dose: 300-400 mg once daily; Maintenance: 400-600 mg once daily (maximum: 600 mg/day)

Dosage adjustment after serum theophylline measurement: Asthma: Within normal limits: Adults: 5-15 mcg/mL: Maintain dosage if tolerated. Recheck serum theophylline concentration at 24-hour intervals (for acute I.V. dosing) or at 6- to 12-month intervals (for oral dosing). Finer adjustments in dosage may be needed for some patients. If levels ≥15 mcg/mL, consider 10% dose reduction to improve safety margin.

Note: Recheck serum theophylline levels after 3 days when using oral dosing, or after 12 hours (children) or 24 hours (adults) when dosing intravenously. Patients maintained with oral therapy may be reassessed at 6- to 12-month intervals.

Geriatric

Acute symptoms: Adults >60 years:

Loading dose: Oral, I.V.: Refer to adult dosing.

Maintenance dose: I.V.: 0.3 mg/kg/hour; maximum 400 mg/day unless serum levels indicate need for larger dose

Chronic conditions: Oral: Adults >60 years: Do not exceed a dose of 400 mg/day

Cardiac decompensation, cor pulmonale, hepatic dysfunction, sepsis with multiorgan failure, shock: Refer to adult dosing.

Pediatric Doses should be individualized based on steady-state serum concentrations and ideal body weight.

Acute symptoms: Loading dose: Oral, I.V.: Asthma exacerbations: While theophylline may be considered for relief of asthma symptoms, the role of treating exacerbations is not supported by current practice.

If no theophylline received within the previous 24 hours: 4.6 mg/kg loading dose (~5.8 mg/kg hydrous aminophylline) I.V. or 5 mg/kg orally. Loading dose intended to achieve a serum level of approximately 10 mcg/mL; loading doses should be given intravenously (preferred) or with a rapidly absorbed oral product (not an extended-release product). **Note:** On the average, for every 1 mg/kg theophylline given, blood levels will rise 2 mcg/mL.

If theophylline has been administered in the previous 24 hours: A loading dose is not recommended without obtaining a serum theophylline concentration. The loading dose should be calculated as follows:

Dose = (desired serum theophylline concentration - measured serum theophylline concentration) (V_d)

Acute symptoms: Maintenance dose: I.V.: **Note:** To achieve a target concentration of 10 mcg/mL unless otherwise noted. Lower initial doses may be required in patients with reduced theophylline clearance. Dosage should be adjusted according to serum level measurements during the first 12- to 24-hour period.

Neonates ≤24 days: 1 mg/kg every 12 hours to achieve a target concentration of 7.5 mcg/mL for apnea of prematurity

Neonates >24 days: 1.5 mg/kg every 12 hours to achieve a target concentration of 7.5 mcg/mL for apnea of prematurity

Infants 6-52 weeks: mg/kg/hour = (0.008) (age in weeks) + 0.21

Children 1-9 years: 0.8 mg/kg/hour

Children 9-12 years: 0.7 mg/kg/hour

Adolescents 12-16 years (cigarette or marijuana smokers): 0.7 mg/kg/hour

Adolescents 12-16 years (nonsmokers): 0.5 mg/kg/hour; maximum 900 mg/day unless serum levels indicate need for larger dose

Treatment of chronic conditions: With newer guidelines suggesting lower therapeutic theophylline ranges, it is unlikely that doses larger than >10 mg/kg/day will be required in children ≥1 year of age.

Oral solution:

Infants <1 year: **Note:** Doses should be adjusted to maintain the peak steady state serum concentrations. The time to reach steady state will vary based on age and the presence of risk factors which may affect theophylline clearance.

Premature Neonates <24 days postnatal age: 1 mg/kg/dose every 12 hours

Premature Neonates ≥24 days postnatal age: 1.5 mg/kg/dose every 12 hours

Full-term Infants and Infants <26 weeks: Total daily dose (mg)= [(0.2 x age in weeks) +5] x (weight in kg); divide dose into 3 equal amounts and administer at 8-hour intervals

Full-term Infants and Infants ≥26 weeks and <52 weeks: Total daily dose (mg) = [(0.2 x age in weeks) +5] x (weight in kg); divide dose into 4 equal amounts and administer at 6-hour intervals

Children ≥1 year and <45 kg: Initial dose: 10-14 mg/kg/day (maximum 300 mg/day) administered in divided doses every 4-6 hours; Maintenance: Up to 20 mg/kg/day (maximum: 600 mg/day)

Children >45 kg: Refer to adult dosing.

Oral extended release formulations:

Children ≥1 year and <45 kg: Initial: 10-14 mg/kg once daily (maximum 300 mg/day); Maintenance up to 20 mg/kg/day (maximum: 600 mg/day)

Children >45 kg: Refer to adult dosing.

Dosage adjustment after serum theophylline measurement: Asthma: Within normal limits: Children: 5-10 mcg/mL: Maintain dosage if tolerated. Recheck serum theophylline concentration at 24-hour intervals (for acute I.V. dosing) or at 6- to 12-month intervals (for oral dosing). Finer adjustments in dosage may be needed for some patients. If levels ≥15 mcg/mL, consider 10% dose reduction to improve safety margin.

Note: Recheck serum theophylline levels after 3 days when using oral dosing, or after 12 hours (children) or 24 hours (adults) when dosing intravenously. Patients maintained with oral therapy may be reassessed at 6- to 12-month intervals.

Administration

Oral Long-acting preparations should be taken with a full glass of water, swallowed whole, or cut in half if scored. Do **not** crush. Extended release capsule forms may be opened and the contents sprinkled on soft foods; do **not** chew beads.

I.V. Administer loading dose over 30 minutes; follow with a continuous infusion as appropriate.

Monitoring and Teaching Issues

Laboratory Monitoring Arterial or capillary blood gases (if applicable)

Theophylline levels: Serum theophylline levels should be monitored prior to making dose increases; in the presence of signs or symptoms of toxicity; or when a new illness, worsening of a present illness, or medication changes occur that may change theophylline clearance

I.V. loading dose: Measure serum concentrations 30 minutes after the end of an I.V. loading dose

I.V. infusion: Measure serum concentrations one half-life after starting a continuous infusion, then every 12-24 hours

Physical Assessment Monitor effectiveness of therapy (respiratory rate, lung sounds, characteristics of cough and sputum). For inpatient care, monitor vital signs prior to and periodically during therapy.

Patient Education Preferable to take on empty stomach, 1 hour before or 2 hours after meals, with a full glass of water. Do not chew of crush sustained release forms; capsules may be opened and contents sprinkled on soft food (do not chew beads). Avoid dietary stimulants (eg, caffeine, tea, colas, or chocolate). You may experience nausea, vomiting, or loss of appetite.

Report acute insomnia or restlessness, chest pain or rapid heartbeat, emotional lability or agitation, muscle tremors or cramping, acute headache, persistent and repetitive vomiting, abdominal pain and cramping, blackened stool, or worsening of respiratory condition.

Related Information

Peak and Trough Guidelines *on page 1958*

◆ **Theophylline Anhydrous** *see* Theophylline *on page 1748*

◆ **Theraflu® Thin Strips® Multi Symptom [OTC]** *see* DiphenhydrAMINE (Systemic) *on page 543*

◆ **Thiamazole** *see* Methimazole *on page 1192*

◆ **Thiamin** *see* Thiamine *on page 1751*

Thiamine (THYE a min)

Index Terms Aneurine Hydrochloride; Thiamin; Thiamine Hydrochloride; Thiaminium Chloride Hydrochloride; Vitamin B_1

Generic Availability (U.S.) Yes

Pharmacologic Category Vitamin, Water Soluble

Medication Safety Issues

Sound-alike/look-alike issues:

Thiamine may be confused with Tenormin®, Thalomid®, Thorazine®

International issues:

Doxal® [Brazil] may be confused with Doxil® which is a brand name for doxorubicin in the U.S.

Doxal® [Brazil]: Brand name for doxycycline in Austria; brand name for pyridoxine/thiamine combination in Brazil; brand name for doxepin in Finland

Pregnancy Risk Factor A

Lactation Enters breast milk/use caution (AAP rates "compatible"; AAP 2001 update pending)

Use Treatment of thiamine deficiency including beriberi, Wernicke's encephalopathy, Korsakoff's syndrome, neuritis associated with pregnancy, or in alcoholic patients; dietary supplement

Available Dosage Forms

Injection, solution: 100 mg/mL (2 mL)

Tablet, oral: 50 mg, 100 mg, 250 mg, 500 mg

Dosing

Adult & Geriatric

Recommended daily intake:

≥19 years: Female: 1.1 mg; Male: 1.2 mg

Pregnancy, lactation: 1.4 mg

Parenteral nutrition supplementation: 6 mg/day; may be increased to 25-50 mg/day with history of alcohol abuse

Thiamine deficiency (beriberi): 5-30 mg/dose I.M. or I.V. 3 times/day (if critically ill); then orally 5-30 mg/day in single or divided doses 3 times/day for 1 month

Alcohol withdrawal syndrome: 100 mg/day I.M. or I.V. for several days, followed by 50-100 mg/day orally

Wernicke's encephalopathy: Treatment (manufacturer labeling): Initial: 100 mg I.V., then 50-100 mg/day I.M. or I.V. until consuming a regular, balanced diet. However, larger doses may be required based on failure of lower doses to produce clinical improvement in some patients.

Alternate dosage: The Royal College of Physicians (U.K.) has recommended the use of higher doses of thiamine (in combination with other B vitamins, ascorbic acid, potassium, phosphate, and magnesium) for the management of Wernicke's encephalopathy (Thomson, 2002):

Prophylaxis: 250 mg I.V. once daily for 3-5 days

Treatment: Initial: 500 mg I.V. 3 times/day for 3 days. If response to thiamine after 3 days, continue with 250 mg I.M. or I.V. once daily for an additional 5 days or until clinical improvement.

Pediatric

Adequate Intake:

0-6 months: 0.2 mg/day

7-12 months: 0.3 mg/day

Recommended daily intake:

1-3 years: 0.5 mg

4-8 years: 0.6 mg

9-13 years: 0.9 mg

14-18 years: Female: 1 mg; Male: 1.2 mg

≥19 years: Refer to adult dosing.

Parenteral nutrition supplementation: Infants: 1.2 mg/day

Thiamine deficiency (beriberi): Children: 10-25 mg/dose I.M. or I.V. daily (if critically ill), or 10-50 mg/dose orally every day for 2 weeks, then 5-10 mg/dose orally daily for 1 month

Administration

I.M. Parenteral form may be administered I.M.

I.V. Parenteral form may be administered by I.V. injection. Various rates of administration have been reported. Local injection reactions may be minimized by slow administration (~30 minutes) into larger, more proximal veins. Thiamine should be administered prior to parenteral glucose solutions to prevent precipitation of acute symptoms of thiamine deficiency in the poorly nourished.

Monitoring and Teaching Issues

Physical Assessment If self-administered, teach patient appropriate injection technique and needle disposal. Provide patient appropriate dietary instruction. Be alert to the potential for hypersensitivity reaction, especially if given I.V.

Patient Education Follow dietary instructions. Report shortness of breath, itching, or rash.

◆ **Thiamine Hydrochloride** *see* Thiamine *on page 1751*

◆ **Thiaminium Chloride Hydrochloride** *see* Thiamine *on page 1751*

Thioguanine (thye oh GWAH neen)

U.S. Brand Names Tabloid®

Index Terms 2-Amino-6-Mercaptopurine; 6-TG (error-prone abbreviation); 6-Thioguanine (error-prone abbreviation); TG; Tioguanine

Generic Availability (U.S.) No

Pharmacologic Category Antineoplastic Agent, Antimetabolite (Purine Analog)

Medication Safety Issues

Sound-alike/look-alike issues:

Thioguanine may be confused with thiotepa

International issues:

Lanvis [Canada and multiple international markets] may be confused with Lantus brand name for insulin glargine [U.S., Canada, and multiple international markets]

High alert medication: This medication is in a class the Institute for Safe Medication Practices (ISMP) includes among its list of drugs which have a heightened risk of causing significant patient harm when used in error.

6-thioguanine and 6-TG are error-prone abbreviations (associated with sixfold overdoses of thioguanine)

Pregnancy Risk Factor D

Lactation Excretion in breast milk unknown/not recommended

Use Treatment of acute myelogenous (nonlymphocytic) leukemia (AML)

Unlabeled/Investigational Use Treatment of pediatric acute lymphoblastic leukemia (ALL)

Mechanism of Action/Effect Purine analog that is incorporated into DNA and RNA resulting in the blockage of synthesis and metabolism of purine nucleotides

Contraindications Prior resistance to thioguanine (or mercaptopurine)

Canadian labeling: Additional contraindications (not in US labeling): Hypersensitivity to thioguanine or any component of the formulation

Warnings/Precautions Hazardous agent - use appropriate precautions for handling and disposal.

Not recommended for maintenance therapy or long-term continuous treatment; long-term continuous therapy or maintenance treatment is associated with a high risk for hepatotoxicity, hepatic veno-occlusive disease (VOD), or portal hypertension; monitor liver function carefully for liver toxicity and discontinue in patients with evidence of hepatic VOD (eg, hyperbilirubinemia, hepatomegaly [tender], and weight gain due to ascites and fluid retention) or portal hypertension (eg, splenomegaly, thrombocytopenia, esophageal varices); hepatotoxicity with or without transaminase elevations may occur; pathologic findings of hepatotoxicity include hepatoportal sclerosis, nodular regenerative hyperplasia, peliosis hepatitis, and periportal fibrosis.

Myelosuppression (anemia, leukopenia, and/or thrombocytopenia) is a common dose-related toxicity (may be delayed); monitor for infection (due to leukopenia) or bleeding(due to thrombocytopenia); withhold treatment with abnormally significant drop in blood counts. Patients with genetic enzyme deficiency of thiopurine methyltransferase (TPMT) or who are receiving drugs which inhibit this enzyme (mesalazine, olsalazine, sulfasalazine) may be highly sensitive to myelosuppressive effects and may require substantial dose reductions.

Hyperuricemia occurs commonly with treatment; institute adequate hydration and prophylactic allopurinol. Thioguanine is potentially carcinogenic. Cross resistance with mercaptopurine generally occurs. Avoid vaccination with live vaccines during treatment.

Drug Interactions

Avoid Concomitant Use

Avoid concomitant use of Thioguanine with any of the following: BCG; Natalizumab; Pimecrolimus; Roflumilast; Tacrolimus (Topical); Vaccines (Live)

Decreased Effect

Thioguanine may decrease the levels/effects of: BCG; Sipuleucel-T; Vaccines (Inactivated); Vaccines (Live)

The levels/effects of Thioguanine may be decreased by: Echinacea

Increased Effect/Toxicity

Thioguanine may increase the levels/effects of: Leflunomide; Natalizumab; Vaccines (Live)

The levels/effects of Thioguanine may be increased by: 5-ASA Derivatives; Denosumab; Pimecrolimus; Roflumilast; Tacrolimus (Topical); Trastuzumab

Nutritional/Ethanol Interactions Ethanol: Avoid; may increase the risk for hepatotoxicity.

Adverse Reactions Frequency not defined.

Endocrine & metabolic: Fluid retention, hyperuricemia (common)

Gastrointestinal: Anorexia, intestinal necrosis, intestinal perforation, nausea, splenomegaly, stomatitis, vomiting, weight gain

Hematologic: Anemia (may be delayed), bleeding, granulocytopenia, leukopenia (common; may be delayed), marrow hypoplasia, pancytopenia, thrombocytopenia (common; may be delayed)

Hepatic: Ascites, esophageal varices, hepatic necrosis (centrilobular), hepatic veno-occlusive disease (VOD), hepatitis, hepatomegaly [tender], hepatoportal sclerosis, hepatotoxicity, hyperbilirubinemia, jaundice, LFTs increased, nodular regenerative hyperplasia, peliosis hepatitis, periportal fibrosis, portal hypertension

Miscellaneous: Infection

Pharmacodynamics/Kinetics

Absorption ~30% (range: 14% to 46%; highly variable)

Time to Peak Serum: Within 8 hours; predominantly metabolite(s)

Half-Life Elimination Terminal: 5-9 hours

Metabolism Hepatic; rapidly and extensively via thiopurine methyltransferase (TPMT) to 2-amino-6-methylthioguanine (MTG; active) and inactive compounds

Available Dosage Forms

Tablet, oral:

Tabloid®: 40 mg

Dosing

Pediatric Pediatric ALL (unlabeled use; combination therapy): Oral: Delayed intensification treatment phase: 60 mg/m^2/day for 14 days (Lange, 2002; Nachman, 1998)

Renal Impairment Children: No adjustment required (Aronoff, 2007).

Hepatic Impairment Deterioration in transaminases, alkaline phosphatase or bilirubin, toxic hepatitis, biliary stasis, clinical jaundice, evidence of hepatic VOD, or evidence of portal hypertension: Discontinue treatment.

Administration

Oral For oral use; total daily dose can be given at one time.

Stability

Storage Store tablet at room temperature at 15°C to 25°C (59°F to 77°F). Protect from moisture.

Monitoring and Teaching Issues

Laboratory Monitoring CBC with differential and platelet count; liver function tests (weekly when beginning therapy then monthly, more frequently in patients with liver disease or concurrent hepatotoxic drugs); serum uric acid, renal function; some laboratories offer testing for TPMT deficiency

Physical Assessment Use caution with hepatic impairment. Monitor for myelosuppression, nausea, vomiting, anorexia, malaise, and hepatotoxicity weekly when beginning therapy, then monthly. Teach patient necessity for contraception and importance of adequate hydration.

Patient Education Maintain adequate hydration, unless instructed to restrict fluid intake. You may be required to have regularly scheduled laboratory testing to evaluate response to this medication. May cause nausea, vomiting, loss of appetite, weakness or lethargy, or mouth sores. You will be more susceptible to infection. Report signs or symptoms of infection (eg, fever, chills, sore throat, burning urination, fatigue); bleeding or easy bruising; dark urine, light-colored stool, or yellowing of skin or eyes; unresolved mouth sores, nausea, or vomiting; weight gain; or swelling of abdomen.

Breast-Feeding Considerations Due to the potential for serious adverse reactions in the nursing infant, the manufacturer recommends to discontinue breast-feeding during therapy.

Pregnancy Considerations Animal studies have demonstrated adverse effects. There are no adequate and well-controlled studies in pregnant women. May cause fetal harm if administered during pregnancy. Women of childbearing potential should avoid becoming pregnant during treatment.

◆ **6-Thioguanine (error-prone abbreviation)** *see* Thioguanine *on page 1752*

◆ **Thiophosphoramide** *see* Thiotepa *on page 1754*

◆ **Thioplex** *see* Thiotepa *on page 1754*

Thioridazine (thye oh RID a zeen)

Index Terms Thioridazine Hydrochloride

Generic Availability (U.S.) Yes

Pharmacologic Category Antipsychotic Agent, Typical, Phenothiazine

Medication Safety Issues

Sound-alike/look-alike issues:

Thioridazine may be confused with thiothixene, Thorazine®

Mellaril® may be confused with Elavil®, Mebaral®

Beers Criteria medication: This drug may be inappropriate for use in geriatric patients (high severity risk).

Pregnancy Risk Factor C

Use Management of schizophrenic patients who fail to respond adequately to treatment with other antipsychotic drugs, either because of insufficient effectiveness or the inability to achieve an effective dose due to intolerable adverse effects from those medications

Unlabeled/Investigational Use Behavior problems (children); severe psychoses (children); schizophrenia/psychoses (children); depressive disorders/dementia (children and adults); behavioral symptoms associated with dementia (elderly); psychosis/agitation related to Alzheimer's dementia

Available Dosage Forms

Tablet, oral: 10 mg, 25 mg, 50 mg, 100 mg

Dosing

Adult

Schizophrenia/psychosis: Oral: Initial: 50-100 mg 3 times/day with gradual increments as needed and tolerated; maximum: 800 mg/day in 2-4 divided doses

Depressive disorders, dementia (unlabeled use): Oral: Initial: 25 mg 3 times/day; maintenance dose: 20-200 mg/day

Geriatric Behavioral symptoms associated with dementia (unlabeled use): Oral: Initial: 10-25 mg 1-2 times/day; increase at 4- to 7-day intervals by 10-25 mg/day; increase dose intervals (once daily, twice daily, etc) as necessary to control response or side effects. Maximum daily dose: 400 mg; gradual increases (titration) may prevent some side effects or decrease their severity.

Pediatric

Schizophrenia/psychosis (unlabeled use): Oral:

Children >2-12 years: Range: 0.5-3 mg/kg/day in 2-3 divided doses; usual: 1 mg/kg/day; maximum: 3 mg/kg/day

Children >12 years: Refer to adult dosing.

Behavior problems (unlabeled use): Oral:

Children >2-12 years: Initial: 10 mg 2-3 times/day, increase gradually.

Children >12 years: Refer to adult dosing.

Severe psychoses (unlabeled use): Oral:

Children >2-12 years: Initial: 25 mg 2-3 times/day, increase gradually.

Children >12 years: Refer to adult dosing.

Renal Impairment Not dialyzable (0% to 5%)

Administration

Oral Do not take antacid within 2 hours of taking drug.

Monitoring and Teaching Issues

Laboratory Monitoring Baseline ECG; serum potassium, lipid profile, fasting blood glucose and Hgb A_{1c}; BMI; do not initiate if QT_c >450 msec

Physical Assessment Review ophthalmic exam at beginning of therapy and periodically throughout. Monitor for CNS depression/level of sedation. Avoid skin contact with liquid medication; may cause contact dermatitis (wash immediately with warm, soapy water). Initiate at lower doses and taper dosage slowly when discontinuing.

Patient Education May be taken with food. Avoid alcohol. Maintain adequate hydration unless instructed to restrict fluid intake. You may experience excess drowsiness, lightheadedness, dizziness, blurred vision, nausea, vomiting, dry mouth, constipation, urinary retention, ejaculatory dysfunction (reversible), decreased perspiration, or photosensitivity. Report persistent CNS effects (eg, trembling fingers, altered gait or balance, excessive sedation, seizures, unusual movements, anxiety, confusion); chest pain, palpitations, or rapid heartbeat; severe dizziness; unresolved urinary retention; altered menstrual pattern; change in libido; swelling or pain in breasts (male or female); vision changes; skin rash or changes in color of skin (gray-blue); or worsening of condition.

Related Information

Antipsychotic Agents *on page 1986*

◆ **Thioridazine Hydrochloride** *see* Thioridazine *on page 1753*

Thiotepa (thye oh TEP a)

Index Terms TESPA; Thiophosphoramide; Thioplex; Triethylenethiophosphoramide; TSPA

Generic Availability (U.S.) Yes

Pharmacologic Category Antineoplastic Agent, Alkylating Agent

Medication Safety Issues

Sound-alike/look-alike issues:

Thiotepa may be confused with thioguanine

High alert medication: This medication is in a class the Institute for Safe Medication Practices (ISMP) includes among its list of drugs which have a heightened risk of causing significant patient harm when used in error.

Intrathecal medication safety: The American Society of Clinical Oncology (ASCO)/Oncology Nursing Society (ONS) chemotherapy administration safety standards (Jacobson, 2009) encourage the following safety measures for intrathecal chemotherapy:

- Intrathecal medication should not be prepared during the preparation of any other agents
- After preparation, store in an isolated location or container clearly marked with a label identifying as "intrathecal" use only
- Delivery to the patient should only be with other medications intended for administration into the central nervous system

Pregnancy Risk Factor D

Lactation Excretion in breast milk unknown/not recommended

Use Treatment of superficial papillary bladder cancer; palliative treatment of adenocarcinoma of breast or ovary; controlling intracavitary effusions caused by metastatic tumors

Unlabeled/Investigational Use Intrathecal treatment of leptomeningeal metastases

Mechanism of Action/Effect Alkylating agent that reacts with DNA phosphate groups to produce cross-linking of DNA strands leading to inhibition of DNA, RNA, and protein synthesis; mechanism of action has not been explored as thoroughly as the other alkylating agents, it is presumed that the aziridine rings open and react as nitrogen mustard; reactivity is enhanced at a lower pH

Contraindications Hypersensitivity to thiotepa or any component of the formulation

Note: May be contraindicated in certain circumstances of hepatic, renal, and/or bone marrow failure; evaluate on an individual basis as lower dose treatment (with close monitoring) may still be appropriate if the potential benefit outweighs the risks

Warnings/Precautions Hazardous agent - use appropriate precautions for handling and disposal. Myelosuppression is common; monitor for infection or bleeding. Myelosuppression has also been reported with intravesicular administration (due to systemic absorption). Potentially teratogenic, mutagenic, and carcinogenic; myelodysplastic syndrome and acute myeloid leukemia (AML) have been reported. Reduce dosage and use extreme caution in patients with hepatic, renal, or bone marrow damage. Use may be contraindicated with impairment/damage and should be limited to cases where benefit outweighs risk.

When used for intrathecal administration, should not be prepared during the preparation of any other agents; after preparation, store intrathecal medications in an isolated location or container clearly marked with a label identifying as "intrathecal" use only; delivery of intrathecal medications to the patient should only be with other medications intended for administration into the central nervous system (Jacobson, 2009).

Drug Interactions

Metabolism/Transport Effects Inhibits CYP2B6 (strong)

Avoid Concomitant Use

Avoid concomitant use of Thiotepa with any of the following: BCG; Natalizumab; Pimecrolimus; Roflumilast; Tacrolimus (Topical); Vaccines (Live)

Decreased Effect

Thiotepa may decrease the levels/effects of: BCG; Sipuleucel-T; Vaccines (Inactivated); Vaccines (Live)

The levels/effects of Thiotepa may be decreased by: Echinacea

Increased Effect/Toxicity

Thiotepa may increase the levels/effects of: CYP2B6 Substrates; Leflunomide; Natalizumab; Vaccines (Live)

The levels/effects of Thiotepa may be increased by: Denosumab; Pimecrolimus; Roflumilast; Tacrolimus (Topical); Trastuzumab

Nutritional/Ethanol Interactions

Ethanol: Avoid ethanol (due to GI irritation).

Herb/Nutraceutical: Avoid black cohosh, dong quai in estrogen-dependent tumors.

Adverse Reactions Frequency not defined.

Central nervous system: Chills, dizziness, fatigue, fever, headache

Dermatologic: Alopecia, contact dermatitis, depigmentation (with topical treatment), dermatitis, rash, urticaria

Endocrine & metabolic: Amenorrhea, spermatogenesis inhibition

Gastrointestinal: Abdominal pain, anorexia, nausea, vomiting

Genitourinary: Dysuria, urinary retention

Hematologic: Anemia, bleeding, leukopenia, thrombocytopenia

Local: Injection site pain

Neuromuscular & skeletal: Weakness

Ocular: Blurred vision, conjunctivitis

Renal: Hematuria

Respiratory: Asthma, epistaxis, laryngeal edema, wheezing

Miscellaneous: Allergic reaction, anaphylactic shock, infection

Pharmacodynamics/Kinetics

Absorption Intracavitary instillation: Unreliable (10% to 100%) through bladder mucosa

Half-Life Elimination Terminal: Dose-dependent clearance: ~2 hours

Metabolism Extensively hepatic; major metabolite (active): TEPA

Excretion Urine (as metabolites and unchanged drug)

Available Dosage Forms

Injection, powder for reconstitution: 15 mg

Dosing

Adult & Geriatric

Bladder cancer: Intravesical: 60 mg in 30-60 mL NS retained for 2 hours once weekly for 4 weeks

Ovarian, breast cancer: I.V.: 0.3-0.4 mg/kg by rapid I.V. administration every 1-4 weeks

Effusions: Intracavitary: 0.6-0.8 mg/kg

Leptomeningeal metastases (unlabeled use): Intrathecal: 10 mg twice a week for 4 weeks, then (if CSF cytology is negative) weekly for 4 weeks, then monthly for 4 doses (NCCN CNS cancer guidelines v.1.2010)

HSCT for CNS malignancy (unlabeled use; combination chemotherapy): I.V.: 250 mg/m^2/day for 3 days beginning 9 days prior to transplant (Soussain, 2008) **or** 150 mg/m^2/dose every 12 hours for 6 doses, followed by stem cell reinfusion 96 hours after completion of thiotepa (Abrey, 2006)

Pediatric HSCT for CNS malignancy (unlabeled use; combination chemotherapy): 300 mg/m²/day for 3 days beginning 8 days prior to transplant (Gilheeney, 2010) **or** 300 mg/m²/day for 3 days beginning 5 days prior to transplant (Dunkel, 2010; Grodman, 2009)

Renal Impairment Use with extreme caution, reduced dose may be warranted. Use may be contraindicated with existing renal impairment and should be limited to cases where benefit outweighs risk.

Hepatic Impairment Use with extreme caution, reduced dose may be warranted. Use may be contraindicated with existing hepatic impairment and should be limited to cases where benefit outweighs risk.

Adjustment for Toxicity I.V.: **Note:** Use may be contraindicated with pre-existing marrow damage and should be limited to cases where benefit outweighs risk.

WBC ≤3000/mm³: Discontinue treatment

Platelets ≤150,000/mm³: Discontinue treatment

Administration

I.V. Administer as a rapid injection. Infusion times may be longer for high-dose (unlabeled use) treatment; refer to specific protocols.

Other Intravesical instillation: Instill directly into the bladder and retain for 2 hours; patient should be repositioned every 15-30 minutes for maximal exposure.

Stability

Reconstitution Use appropriate precautions for handling and disposal. Reconstitute each 15 mg vial with 1.5 mL SWFI to a concentration of 10 mg/mL. Solutions for I.V. use should be further diluted in 0.9% sodium chloride injection prior to infusion. Filter through a 0.22 micron filter (polysulfone membrane [eg, Sterile Aerodisc®] or triton-free cellulose mixed ester [eg, Millex®-GS]) prior to administration; do not use solutions which precipitate or remain opaque after filtering. Solutions for intravesicular administration should be diluted in 30-60 mL NS. Solutions for intrathecal administration should be diluted to a concentration of 1-5 mg/mL in preservative-free NS. Intrathecal medications should not be prepared during the preparation of any other agents.

Storage Store intact vials under refrigeration (2°C to 8°C). Protect from light. Reconstituted solutions (10 mg/mL) are stable for up to 28 days under refrigeration (4°C to 8°C) or 7 days at room temperature (25°C), although the manufacturer recommends use within 8 hours when reconstituted solutions are stored under refrigeration. Solutions further diluted (for I.V. use) in NS to 1 mg/mL are stable for 24 hours and to 3 mg/mL are stable for 48 hours at room temperature, although the manufacturer recommends immediate use. After preparation, store intrathecal medications in an isolated location or container clearly marked with a label identifying as "intrathecal" use only.

Monitoring and Teaching Issues

Laboratory Monitoring CBC with differential and platelet count (monitor weekly during treatment and for at least 3 weeks after treatment); renal and liver function tests; uric acid, urinalysis

Physical Assessment Use caution in presence of hepatic or renal impairment or compromised bone marrow reserve; dosing adjustment may be warranted. Evaluate results of laboratory tests regularly during treatment and for at least 3 weeks following treatment. Monitor for myelosuppression, leukopenia, dysuria, bleeding, and infection. Teach patient importance of adequate hydration.

Patient Education Do not take any aspirin or aspirin-containing products during therapy unless approved by prescriber. If administered by infusion, report immediately any redness, pain, swelling, or burning at infusion site. You will require regular blood tests to assess response to therapy. Maintain adequate hydration to prevent kidney damage, unless instructed to restrict fluid intake. You may have increased sensitivity to infection. May cause mild nausea, vomiting, or loss of appetite; rash; hair loss; or change in skin color (usually reversible after discontinuing treatment). Report any changes in urinary pattern or blood in your urine, unusual bleeding or bruising, persistent fever or chills, sore throat, sores in mouth or vagina, blackened stool, unusual or persistent weakness, difficulty swallowing, or respiratory difficulty.

Breast-Feeding Considerations Due to the potential for serious adverse reactions in the nursing infant, breast-feeding is not recommended.

Pregnancy Considerations Animal studies have demonstrated teratogenicity and fetal loss. There are no adequate and well-controlled studies in pregnant women. May cause harm if administered during pregnancy. Effective contraception is recommended for men and women of childbearing potential.

Thiothixene (thye oh THIKS een)

U.S. Brand Names Navane®

Index Terms Tiotixene

Generic Availability (U.S.) Yes

Pharmacologic Category Antipsychotic Agent, Typical

Medication Safety Issues

Sound-alike/look-alike issues:

Thiothixene may be confused with FLUoxetine, thioridazine

Navane® may be confused with Norvasc®, Nubain®

Use Management of schizophrenia

Unlabeled/Investigational Use Psychotic disorders (children); rapid tranquilization of the agitated patient (children); nonpsychotic patient, dementia behavior (elderly); psychosis/agitation related to Alzheimer's dementia

Available Dosage Forms

Capsule, oral: 1 mg, 2 mg, 5 mg, 10 mg

Navane®: 2 mg, 10 mg, 20 mg

Dosing

Adult

Mild-to-moderate psychosis: Oral: 2 mg 3 times/day, up to 20-30 mg/day; more severe psychosis: Initial: 5 mg 2 times/day, may increase gradually, if necessary; maximum: 60 mg/day

Rapid tranquilization of the agitated patient (administered every 30-60 minutes): Oral: 5-10 mg; average total dose for tranquilization: 15-30 mg

Geriatric Nonpsychotic patient, dementia behavior (unlabeled use): Initial: 1-2 mg 1-2 times/day; increase dose at 4- to 7-day intervals by 1-2 mg/day. Increase dosing intervals (bid, tid, etc) as necessary to control response or side effects; maximum daily dose: 30 mg. Gradual increases in dose may prevent some side effects or decrease their severity.

Pediatric

Children <12 years (unlabeled use): Oral: 0.25 mg/kg/24 hours in divided doses (dose not well established; use not recommended)

Children >12 years (unlabeled use): Mild-to-moderate psychosis: Refer to adult dosing.

Renal Impairment Not dialyzable (0% to 5%)

Monitoring and Teaching Issues

Laboratory Monitoring Lipid profile, fasting blood glucose/Hgb A_{1c}; BMI

Physical Assessment Review ophthalmic exam at beginning of therapy and periodically throughout. Initiate at lower doses and taper dosage slowly when discontinuing.

Patient Education Capsules may be taken with food. Avoid alcohol. Maintain adequate hydration unless instructed to restrict fluid intake. You may experience excess drowsiness, lightheadedness, dizziness, blurred vision, nausea, vomiting, constipation, postural hypotension, urinary retention, ejaculatory dysfunction (reversible), decreased perspiration, or photosensitivity. Report persistent CNS effects (eg, trembling fingers, altered gait or balance, excessive sedation, seizures, unusual movements, anxiety, abnormal thoughts, confusion, personality changes); chest pain, palpitations, or rapid heartbeat; severe dizziness; unresolved urinary retention or changes in urinary pattern; altered menstrual pattern; change in libido; swelling or pain in breasts (male or female); vision changes; skin rash, irritation, or changes in color of skin (gray-blue); or worsening of condition.

Related Information

Antipsychotic Agents *on page 1986*

- **Thorazine** *see* ChlorproMAZINE *on page 360*
- **Thrive™ [OTC]** *see* Nicotine *on page 1312*
- **Thymocyte Stimulating Factor** *see* Aldesleukin *on page 62*

Thyroid, Desiccated (THYE roid DES i kay tid)

U.S. Brand Names Armour® Thyroid; Nature-Throid™; Westhroid™

Index Terms Desiccated Thyroid; Thyroid Extract; Thyroid USP

Generic Availability (U.S.) Yes

Pharmacologic Category Thyroid Product

Medication Safety Issues

Beers Criteria medication: This drug may be inappropriate for use in geriatric patients (high severity risk).

Pregnancy Risk Factor A

Lactation Enters breast milk/compatible

Use Replacement or supplemental therapy in hypothyroidism; pituitary TSH suppressants (thyroid nodules, thyroiditis, multinodular goiter, thyroid cancer), thyrotoxicosis, diagnostic suppression tests

Available Dosage Forms

Tablet, oral:

Armour® Thyroid: 15 mg, 30 mg, 60 mg, 90 mg, 120 mg, 180 mg, 240 mg, 300 mg

Nature-Throid™: 16.25 mg, 32.5 mg, 65 mg, 130 mg, 195 mg

Westhroid™: 32.5 mg, 65 mg, 130 mg

Dosing

Adult Hypothyroidism: Oral: Initial: 15-30 mg; increase with 15 mg increments every 2-4 weeks; use 15 mg in patients with cardiovascular disease or myxedema. Maintenance dose: Usually 60-120 mg/day; monitor TSH and clinical symptoms.

Note: Thyroid cancer requires larger amounts than replacement therapy.

Geriatric Not recommended for use in the elderly.

Pediatric Hypothyroidism: Oral: See table.

Recommended Pediatric Dosage for Congenital Hypothyroidism

Age	Daily Dose (mg)	Daily Dose/kg (mg)
0-6 mo	15-30	4.8-6
6-12 mo	30-45	3.6-4.8
1-5 y	45-60	3-3.6
6-12 y	60-90	2.4-3
>12 y	>90	1.2-1.8

Administration

Oral Administer on an empty stomach.

Monitoring and Teaching Issues

Laboratory Monitoring Monitor T_4 and TSH. TSH is the most reliable guide for evaluating adequacy of thyroid replacement dosage. TSH may be elevated during the first few months of thyroid replacement despite patients being clinically euthyroid. In cases where T_4 remains low and TSH is within normal limits, an evaluation of "free" (unbound) T_4 is needed to evaluate further increase in dosage.

Physical Assessment Monitor for hyperthyroidism (weight loss, nervousness, sweating, tachycardia, insomnia, heat intolerance, palpitations, vomiting, psychosis, fever, seizures, angina, arrhythmias). Caution patients with diabetes to monitor glucose levels closely (may increase need for oral hypoglycemics or insulin).

Patient Education Thyroid replacement therapy is generally for life. Take in the morning before breakfast. Do not take antacids or iron preparations within 8 hours of thyroid medication. If you have diabetes, monitor glucose levels closely (may increase need for oral hypoglycemics or insulin). Report chest pain, rapid heart rate, palpitations, heat intolerance, excessive sweating, increased nervousness, agitation, or lethargy.

◆ **Thyroid Extract** *see* Thyroid, Desiccated *on page* *1757*

◆ **Thyroid USP** *see* Thyroid, Desiccated *on page* *1757*

◆ **ThyroSafe™** *see* Potassium Iodide *on page* *1483*

◆ **Thyroshield™ [OTC]** *see* Potassium Iodide *on page* *1483*

TiaGABine (tye AG a been)

U.S. Brand Names Gabitril®

Index Terms Tiagabine Hydrochloride

Generic Availability (U.S.) No

Pharmacologic Category Anticonvulsant, Miscellaneous

Medication Safety Issues

Sound-alike/look-alike issues:

TiaGABine may be confused with tiZANidine

Medication Guide Available Yes

Pregnancy Risk Factor C

Lactation Enters breast milk/not recommended

Use Adjunctive therapy in adults and children ≥12 years of age in the treatment of partial seizures

Mechanism of Action/Effect The exact mechanism by which tiagabine exerts antiseizure activity is not definitively known; however, *in vitro* experiments demonstrate that it enhances the activity of gamma aminobutyric acid (GABA), the major neuroinhibitory transmitter in the nervous system; it is thought that binding to the GABA uptake carrier inhibits the uptake of GABA into presynaptic neurons, allowing an increased amount of GABA to be available to postsynaptic neurons; based on *in vitro* studies, tiagabine does not inhibit the uptake of dopamine, norepinephrine, serotonin, glutamate, or choline

Contraindications Hypersensitivity to tiagabine or any component of the formulation

Warnings/Precautions Antiepileptics are associated with an increased risk of suicidal behavior/thoughts with use (regardless of indication); patients should be monitored for signs/symptoms of depression, suicidal tendencies, and other unusual behavior changes during therapy and instructed to inform their healthcare provider immediately if symptoms occur. New-onset seizures and status epilepticus have been associated with tiagabine use when taken for unlabeled indications. Often these seizures have occurred shortly after the initiation of treatment or shortly after a dosage increase. Seizures have also occurred with very low doses or after several months of therapy. In most cases, patients were using concomitant medications (eg, antidepressants, antipsychotics, stimulants, narcotics). In these instances, the discontinuation of tiagabine, followed by an evaluation for an underlying seizure disorder, is suggested. Use for unapproved indications, however, has not been proven to be safe or effective and is not recommended. When tiagabine is used as an adjunct in partial seizures (an FDA-approved indication), it should not be abruptly discontinued because of the possibility of increasing seizure frequency, unless safety concerns require a more rapid withdrawal. Rarely, nonconvulsive status epilepticus has been reported following abrupt discontinuation or dosage reduction.

Use with caution in patients with hepatic impairment. Experience in patients not receiving enzyme-inducing drugs has been limited; caution should be used in treating any patient who is not receiving one of these medications (decreased dose and slower titration may be required). Weakness, sedation, and confusion may occur with tiagabine use. Patients must be cautioned about performing tasks which require mental alertness (eg, operating machinery or driving). Effects with other sedative drugs or ethanol may be potentiated. May cause serious rash, including Stevens-Johnson syndrome.

Drug Interactions

Metabolism/Transport Effects Substrate of 3A4 (major)

Avoid Concomitant Use There are no known interactions where it is recommended to avoid concomitant use.

Decreased Effect

The levels/effects of TiaGABine may be decreased by: CYP3A4 Inducers (Strong); Deferasirox; Herbs (CYP3A4 Inducers); Ketorolac; Ketorolac (Systemic); Mefloquine

Increased Effect/Toxicity

TiaGABine may increase the levels/effects of: Alcohol (Ethyl); CNS Depressants; Methotrimeprazine

The levels/effects of TiaGABine may be increased by: Conivaptan; CYP3A4 Inhibitors (Moderate); CYP3A4 Inhibitors (Strong); Dasatinib; Droperidol; Methotrimeprazine

Nutritional/Ethanol Interactions

Ethanol: Avoid ethanol (may increase CNS depression).

Food: Food reduces the rate but not the extent of absorption.

Herb/Nutraceutical: St John's wort may decrease tiagabine levels. Avoid valerian, St John's wort, kava kava, gotu kola (may increase CNS depression).

Adverse Reactions

>10%:

Central nervous system: Concentration decreased, dizziness, nervousness, somnolence

Gastrointestinal: Nausea

Neuromuscular & skeletal: Weakness, tremor

1% to 10%:

Cardiovascular: Chest pain, edema, hypertension, palpitation, peripheral edema, syncope, tachycardia, vasodilation

Central nervous system: Agitation, ataxia, chills, confusion, difficulty with memory, confusion, depersonalization, depression, euphoria, hallucination, hostility, insomnia, malaise, migraine, paranoid reaction, personality disorder, speech disorder

Dermatologic: Alopecia, bruising, dry skin, pruritus, rash

Gastrointestinal: Abdominal pain, diarrhea, gingivitis, increased appetite, mouth ulceration, stomatitis, vomiting, weight gain/loss

Neuromuscular & skeletal: Abnormal gait, arthralgia, dysarthria, hyper-/hypokinesia, hyper-/hypotonia, myasthenia, myalgia, myoclonus, neck pain, paresthesia, reflexes decreased, stupor, twitching, vertigo

Ocular: Abnormal vision, amblyopia, nystagmus

Otic: Ear pain, hearing impairment, otitis media, tinnitus

Respiratory: Bronchitis, cough, dyspnea, epistaxis, pneumonia

Miscellaneous: Allergic reaction, cyst, diaphoresis, flu-like syndrome, lymphadenopathy

Pharmacodynamics/Kinetics

Absorption Rapid (45 minutes); prolonged with food

Bioavailability Oral: Absolute: 90%

Time to Peak Plasma: 45 minutes

Protein Binding 96%, primarily to albumin and α_1-acid glycoprotein

Half-Life Elimination 2-5 hours when administered with enzyme inducers; 7-9 hours when administered without enzyme inducers

Metabolism Hepatic via CYP (primarily 3A4)

Excretion Feces (63%); urine (25%); 2% as unchanged drug; primarily as metabolites

Available Dosage Forms

Tablet, oral:

Gabitril®: 2 mg, 4 mg, 12 mg, 16 mg

Dosing

Adult & Geriatric Partial seizures (adjunct): Oral:

Patients receiving enzyme-inducing AED regimens: 4 mg once daily for 1 week; may increase by 4-8 mg weekly to response or up to 56 mg daily in 2-4 divided doses; usual maintenance: 32-56 mg/day

Patients **not** receiving enzyme-inducing AED regimens: The estimated plasma concentrations of tiagabine in patients not taking enzyme-inducing medications is twice that of patients receiving enzyme-inducing AEDs. Lower doses are required; slower titration may be necessary.

Pediatric Partial seizures: Oral:

Patients receiving enzyme-inducing AED regimens: Children 12-18 years: 4 mg once daily for 1 week; may increase to 8 mg daily in 2 divided doses for 1 week; then may increase by 4-8 mg weekly to response or up to 32 mg daily in 2-4 divided doses

Patients **not** receiving enzyme-inducing AED regimens: Refer to adult dosing.

Monitoring and Teaching Issues

Laboratory Monitoring A therapeutic range for tiagabine has not been established. Monitor complete blood counts, renal function tests, liver function tests, and routine blood chemistry.

Physical Assessment Monitor therapeutic effectiveness (seizure activity, type, duration) at beginning of therapy and throughout. Taper dosage slowly when discontinuing. Teach patient seizure safety precautions.

Patient Education While using this medication, do not use alcohol. Maintain adequate hydration unless instructed to restrict fluid intake. You may experience drowsiness, dizziness, disturbed concentration, blurred vision, nausea, vomiting, or loss of appetite. Wear identification of epileptic status and medications. Report behavioral or CNS changes, suicide ideation, or depression; skin rash; muscle cramping, weakness, tremors, changes in gait; vision difficulties; persistent GI distress (cramping, pain, vomiting); chest pain, irregular heartbeat, or palpitations; cough or respiratory difficulty; or worsening of seizure activity or loss of seizure control.

Dietary Considerations Take with food.

Geriatric Considerations No special recommendations are made for the elderly; dose according to response.

Pregnancy Considerations Patients exposed to tiagabine during pregnancy are encouraged to enroll themselves into the AED Pregnancy Registry by calling 1-888-233-2334. Additional information is available at www.aedpregnancyregistry.org.

Additional Information Animal studies suggest that tiagabine may bind to retina and uvea; however, no treatment-related ophthalmoscopic changes were seen long-term; periodic monitoring may be considered.

◆ **Tiagabine Hydrochloride** *see* TiaGABine *on page 1758*

◆ **Tiazac®** *see* Diltiazem *on page 536*

Ticarcillin and Clavulanate Potassium

(tye kar SIL in & klav yoo LAN ate poe TASS ee um)

U.S. Brand Names Timentin®

Index Terms Ticarcillin and Clavulanic Acid

Generic Availability (U.S.) No

Pharmacologic Category Antibiotic, Penicillin

Pregnancy Risk Factor B

Lactation Enters breast milk/use caution

Use Treatment of lower respiratory tract, urinary tract, skin and skin structures, bone and joint, gynecologic (endometritis) and intra-abdominal (peritonitis) infections, and septicemia caused by susceptible organisms. Clavulanate expands activity of ticarcillin to include beta-lactamase producing strains of *S. aureus*, *H. influenzae*, *Bacteroides* species, and some other gram-negative bacilli

Available Dosage Forms

Infusion [premixed, frozen]:

Timentin®: Ticarcillin 3 g and clavulanic acid 0.1 g (100 mL)

Injection, powder for reconstitution:

Timentin®: Ticarcillin 3 g and clavulanic acid 0.1 g (3.1 g, 31 g)

Dosing

Adult Note: Timentin® (ticarcillin/clavulanate) is a combination product; each 3.1 g dosage form contains 3 g ticarcillin disodium and 0.1 g clavulanic acid.

Systemic infections: I.V.: 3.1 g (ticarcillin 3 g plus clavulanic acid 0.1 g) every 4-6 hours (maximum: 24 g of ticarcillin component/day)

Amnionitis, cholangitis, diverticulitis, endometritis, epididymo-orchitis, mastoiditis, orbital cellulitis, peritonitis, pneumonia (aspiration): I.V.: 3.1 g every 6 hours

Intra-abdominal infection, complicated, community-acquired, mild-to-moderate: I.V.: 3.1 g every 6 hours for 4-7 days (provided source controlled)

Liver abscess, parafascial space infections, septic thrombophlebitis: I.V.: 3.1 g every 4 hours

***Pseudomonas* infections:** I.V.: 3.1 g every 4 hours

Urinary tract infections: I.V.: 3.1 g every 6-8 hours

Geriatric I.V.: 3.1 g every 4-6 hours; adjust for renal function.

Pediatric Note: Timentin® (ticarcillin/clavulanate) is a combination product; each 3.1 g dosage form contains 3 g ticarcillin disodium and 0.1 g clavulanic acid.

Systemic infections:

Children <60 kg: 200-300 mg of ticarcillin component/kg/day in divided doses every 4-6 hours

Children ≥60 kg: 3.1 g (ticarcillin 3 g plus clavulanic acid 0.1 g) every 4-6 hours; maximum: 24 g of ticarcillin component/day

Bite wounds (animal): 200 mg of ticarcillin component/kg/day in divided doses

Neutropenic fever: 75 mg of ticarcillin component/kg every 6 hours (maximum: 3.1 g/dose)

Pneumonia (nosocomial): 300 mg of ticarcillin component/kg/day in 4 divided doses (maximum: 18-24 g of ticarcillin component/day)

Renal Impairment

Loading dose: I.V.: 3.1 g one dose, followed by maintenance dose based on creatinine clearance:

Cl_{cr} 30-60 mL/minute: Administer 2 g of ticarcillin component every 4 hours or 3.1 g every 8 hours

Cl_{cr} 10-30 mL/minute: Administer 2 g of ticarcillin component every 8 hours or 3.1 g every 12 hours

Cl_{cr} <10 mL/minute: Administer 2 g of ticarcillin component every 12 hours

Cl_{cr} <10 mL/minute with concomitant hepatic dysfunction: 2 g of ticarcillin component every 24 hours

Moderately dialyzable (20% to 50%)

Continuous ambulatory peritoneal dialysis: 3.1 g every 12 hours

Hemodialysis: 2 g of ticarcillin component every 12 hours; supplemented with 3.1 g after each dialysis

Continuous renal replacement therapy (CRRT): Drug clearance is highly dependent on the method of renal replacement, filter type, and flow rate. Appropriate dosing requires close monitoring of pharmacologic response, signs of adverse reactions due to drug accumulation, as well as drug levels in relation to target trough (if appropriate). The following are general recommendations only (based on dialysate flow/ultrafiltration rates of 1 L/hour) and should not supersede clinical judgment:

CVVH: 2 g every 6-8 hours

CVVHD/CVVHDF: 3.1 g every 6 hours

Note: Do not administer in intervals exceeding every 8 hours. Clavulanate component is hepatically eliminated; extending the dosing interval beyond 8 hours may result in loss of beta-lactamase inhibition.

Hepatic Impairment With concomitant renal dysfunction (Cl_{cr} <10 mL/minute): 2 g of ticarcillin component every 24 hours.

Administration

I.V. Infuse over 30 minutes.

Some penicillins (eg, carbenicillin, ticarcillin, and piperacillin) have been shown to inactivate aminoglycosides *in vitro*. This has been observed to a greater extent with tobramycin and gentamicin, while amikacin has shown greater stability against inactivation. Concurrent use of these agents may pose a risk of reduced antibacterial efficacy *in vivo*, particularly in the setting of profound renal impairment. However, definitive clinical evidence is lacking. If combination penicillin/aminoglycoside therapy is desired in a patient with renal dysfunction, separation of doses (if feasible), and routine monitoring of aminoglycoside levels, CBC, and clinical response should be considered.

Monitoring and Teaching Issues

Laboratory Monitoring Serum electrolytes, bleeding time, and periodic tests of renal, hepatic, and hematologic function; perform culture and sensitivity before administering first dose.

◆ **Ticarcillin and Clavulanic Acid** *see* Ticarcillin and Clavulanate Potassium *on page 1760*

◆ **Tigan®** *see* Trimethobenzamide *on page 1819*

Tigecycline (tye ge SYE kleen)

U.S. Brand Names Tygacil®

Index Terms GAR-936

Generic Availability (U.S.) No

Pharmacologic Category Antibiotic, Glycylcycline

Pregnancy Risk Factor D

Lactation Excretion in breast milk unknown/use caution

Use Treatment of complicated skin and skin structure infections caused by susceptible organisms, including methicillin-resistant *Staphylococcus aureus* and vancomycin-sensitive *Enterococcus faecalis*; complicated intra-abdominal infections (cIAI); community-acquired pneumonia

Available Dosage Forms

Injection, powder for reconstitution:

Tygacil®: 50 mg

Dosing

Adult & Geriatric Note: Duration of therapy dependant on severity/site of infection and clinical status and response to therapy.

Pneumonia, community-acquired: I.V.: Initial: 100 mg as a single dose; Maintenance dose: 50 mg every 12 hours for 7-14 days

Intra-abdominal infections, complicated (cIAI): I.V.: Initial: 100 mg as a single dose; Maintenance dose: 50 mg every 12 hours for 5-14 days; **Note:** 2010 IDSA guidelines recommend a treatment duration of 4-7 days (provided source controlled) for community-acquired, mild-to-moderate IAI

Skin/skin structure infections, complicated: I.V.: Initial: 100 mg as a single dose; Maintenance dose: 50 mg every 12 hours for 5-14 days

Renal Impairment No dosage adjustment required in renal impairment or in patients undergoing hemodialysis.

Hepatic Impairment

Mild-to-moderate hepatic impairment (Child-Pugh classes A and B): No dosage adjustment required.

Severe hepatic impairment (Child-Pugh class C): Initial: 100 mg single dose; Maintenance: 25 mg every 12 hours.

Administration

I.V. Infuse over 30-60 minutes through dedicated line or via Y-site

Monitoring and Teaching Issues

Physical Assessment Assess results of culture and sensitivity tests and patient's allergy history (tetracyclines) prior to beginning therapy. Use caution in presence of hepatic impairment; dosage adjustment may be necessary. May cause life-threatening anaphylaxis/anaphylactoid reactions. Monitor for nausea, vomiting, diarrhea, headache, rash, anemia, dyspnea, and opportunistic infection.

Patient Education This medication is only administered intravenously. Report immediately any burning, pain, or swelling at infusion site; difficulty breathing or swallowing; chest pain; or chills. Report gastrointestinal upset (nausea, vomiting, diarrhea, constipation, stomach pain), headache or dizziness, changes in respirations, increased sweating, or rash.

◆ **Tikosyn®** *see* Dofetilide *on page* 565

◆ **Tilia™ Fe** *see* Ethinyl Estradiol and Norethindrone *on page* 701

Tiludronate (tye LOO droe nate)

U.S. Brand Names Skelid®

Index Terms Tiludronate Disodium

Generic Availability (U.S.) No

Pharmacologic Category Bisphosphonate Derivative

Pregnancy Risk Factor C

Lactation Excretion in breast milk unknown/use caution

Use Treatment of Paget's disease of the bone (osteitis deformans) in patients who have a level of serum alkaline phosphatase (SAP) at least twice the upper limit of normal, or who are symptomatic, or who are at risk for future complications of their disease

Mechanism of Action/Effect A bisphosphonate which inhibits osteoclast activity, reducing enzymatic and transport processes that lead to resorption of bone. At least two possible mechanisms may be involved: detachment of osteoclasts from the bone surface (due to inhibition of protein-tyrosine-phosphatase) and inhibition of the osteoclastic proton pump, required to alter local pH to solubilize ions and bone matrix during resorption.

Contraindications Hypersensitivity to tiludronate, bisphosphonates, or any component of the formulation; inability to stand or sit upright for at least 30 minutes

Warnings/Precautions Not recommended in patients with severe renal impairment (Cl_{cr} <30 mL/minute). Use with caution in patients with active upper GI problems (eg, dysphagia, symptomatic esophageal diseases, gastritis, duodenitis, ulcers); discontinue use if new or worsening symptoms develop.

Osteonecrosis of the jaw (ONJ) has been reported in patients receiving bisphosphonates. Risk factors include invasive dental procedures (eg, tooth extraction, dental implants, boney surgery); a diagnosis of cancer, with concomitant chemotherapy or corticosteroids; poor oral hygiene, ill-fitting dentures; and comorbid disorders (anemia, coagulopathy, infection, preexisting dental disease). Most reported cases occurred after I.V. bisphosphonate therapy; however, cases have been reported following oral therapy. A dental exam and preventative dentistry should be performed prior to placing patients with risk factors on chronic bisphosphonate therapy. The manufacturer's labeling states that discontinuing bisphosphonates in patients requiring invasive dental procedures may reduce the risk of ONJ. However, other experts suggest that there is no evidence that discontinuing therapy reduces the risk of developing ONJ (Assael, 2009). The benefit/risk must be assessed by the treating physician and/or dentist/surgeon prior to any invasive dental procedure. Patients developing ONJ while on bisphosphonates should receive care by an oral surgeon.

Infrequently, severe (and occasionally debilitating) bone, joint, and/or muscle pain have been reported during bisphosphonate treatment. The onset of pain ranged from a single day to several months. Consider discontinuing therapy in patients who experience severe symptoms; symptoms usually resolve upon discontinuation. Some patients experienced recurrence when rechallenged with same drug or another bisphosphonate; avoid use in patients with a history of these symptoms in association with bisphosphonate therapy.

Drug Interactions

Avoid Concomitant Use There are no known interactions where it is recommended to avoid concomitant use.

Decreased Effect

The levels/effects of Tiludronate may be decreased by: Antacids; Aspirin; Calcium Salts; Iron Salts; Magnesium Salts; Proton Pump Inhibitors

Increased Effect/Toxicity

Tiludronate may increase the levels/effects of: Phosphate Supplements

The levels/effects of Tiludronate may be increased by: Aminoglycosides; Indomethacin; Nonsteroidal Anti-Inflammatory Agents

Nutritional/Ethanol Interactions Food: In single-dose studies, the bioavailability of tiludronate was reduced by 90% when an oral dose was administered with, or 2 hours after, a standard breakfast compared to the same dose administered after an overnight fast and 4 hours before a standard breakfast.

Lab Interactions Bisphosphonates may interfere with diagnostic imaging agents such as technetium-99m-diphosphonate in bone scans.

Adverse Reactions 1% to 10%:

Cardiovascular: Chest pain (3%), edema (3%), peripheral edema (3%), flushing, hypertension, syncope

Central nervous system: Anxiety, fatigue, insomnia, nervousness, somnolence, vertigo

Dermatologic: Rash (3%), skin disorder (3%), pruritus
Endocrine & metabolic: Hyperparathyroidism (3%)
Gastrointestinal: Nausea (9%), diarrhea (9%), dyspepsia (5%), vomiting (4%), flatulence (3%), tooth disorder (3%), abdominal pain, anorexia, constipation, gastritis, xerostomia
Genitourinary: Urinary tract infection
Neuromuscular & skeletal: Paresthesia (4%), arthrosis (3%), fractures, muscle spasm, weakness
Ocular: Cataract (3%), conjunctivitis (3%), glaucoma (3%)
Respiratory: Rhinitis (5%), sinusitis (5%), pharyngitis (3%), bronchitis
Miscellaneous: Accidental injury (4%), infection (3%), diaphoresis

Pharmacodynamics/Kinetics

Onset of Action Delayed, may require several weeks

Absorption Rapid

Bioavailability ~6% (range: 2% to 11%); reduced by 90% when given with food

Time to Peak Plasma: Within 2 hours

Protein Binding ~90%, primarily to albumin

Half-Life Elimination Healthy volunteers: Single dose: 50 hours; Cl_{cr} 11-18 mL/minute: 205 hours; Pagetic patients: Repeated dosing: 150 hours

Metabolism Little, if any

Excretion Urine (~60%, as tiludronic acid within 13 days)

Available Dosage Forms

Tablet, oral:
Skelid®: 200 mg

Dosing

Adult & Geriatric Paget's disease: Oral: 400 mg (2 tablets of tiludronic acid) daily for a period of 3 months

Renal Impairment Tiludronate is excreted renally. It is not recommended for use in patients with severe renal impairment (Cl_{cr} <30 mL/minute) and is not removed by dialysis.

Administration

Oral Administer as a single oral dose, take with 6-8 oz of plain water. Should not be taken with beverages containing minerals (eg, mineral water), food, or with other medications (may reduce absorption). Do not take within 2 hours of food. Take calcium or mineral supplements at least 2 hours before or after tiludronate. Take aluminum- or magnesium-containing antacids at least 2 hours after taking tiludronate. Patients should be instructed to stay upright (not to lie down) for at least 30 minutes and until after first food of the day (to reduce esophageal irritation).

Stability

Storage Store at 25°C (77°F); excursions permitted to 15°C to 30°C (59°F to 86°F). Do not remove tablets from foil strips until they are to be used.

Monitoring and Teaching Issues

Laboratory Monitoring Alkaline phosphatase, serum calcium and 25(OH)D

Physical Assessment Assess history for any previous adverse response to bisphosphonates. Use caution with renal impairment. Monitor blood pressure at the beginning of therapy and periodically during use. Patients at risk for osteonecrosis of the jaw (eg, chemotherapy, corticosteroids, poor oral hygiene) should have dental exams; necessary preventive dentistry should be done before beginning bisphosphonate therapy. Teach patient appropriate administration of medication (eg, timing with food, supplements, and other medications. Instruct patient in lifestyle and dietary changes that will have a beneficial impact on Paget's disease.

Patient Education In order to be effective, this medication must be taken with a full glass of water (6-8 oz) at least 2 hours before or 2 hours after food. Do not take aspirin, antacids, or vitamin-mineral supplements containing calcium, magnesium, or aluminum within 2 hours of this medication. Consult prescriber to determine recommended lifestyle changes (eg, decreased smoking, decreased alcohol intake, dietary supplements). Certain dental procedures should be avoided if possible while you are taking this medication. Notify prescriber at once if experiencing any difficulty swallowing, pain when swallowing, or severe or persistent heartburn. You may experience mild/temporary skin rash, abdominal pain, or constipation. Report persistent muscle or bone pain or pain in the mouth, jaw, or teeth.

Dietary Considerations Do not take within 2 hours of food. Ensure adequate intake of vitamin D and calcium supplements during treatment.

Geriatric Considerations No dose adjustment necessary.

Pregnancy Considerations Teratogenic and nonteratogenic embryo/fetal effects have been reported in animal studies. There are no adequate and well-controlled studies in pregnant women. Bisphosphonates are incorporated into the bone matrix and gradually released over time. Theoretically, there may be a risk of fetal harm when pregnancy follows the completion of therapy. Based on limited case reports with pamidronate, serum calcium levels in the newborn may be altered if bisphosphonates are administered during pregnancy.

◆ **Tiludronate Disodium** *see* Tiludronate *on page 1762*

◆ **Timentin®** *see* Ticarcillin and Clavulanate Potassium *on page 1760*

Timolol (Ophthalmic) (TIM oh lol)

U.S. Brand Names Betimol®; Istalol®; Timolol GFS; Timoptic-XE®; Timoptic®; Timoptic® in OcuDose®

Index Terms Timolol Hemihydrate; Timolol Maleate

Generic Availability (U.S.) Yes: Excludes solution as maleate (preservative free), solution as hemihydrate

Pharmacologic Category Beta-Adrenergic Blocker, Nonselective; Ophthalmic Agent, Antiglaucoma

Medication Safety Issues

Sound-alike/look-alike issues:

Timolol may be confused with atenolol, Tylenol®

Timoptic® may be confused with Betoptic® S, Talacen, Viroptic®

Bottle cap color change:

Timoptic®: Both the 0.25% and 0.5% strengths are now packaged in bottles with yellow caps; previously, the color of the cap on the product corresponded to different strengths.

International issues:

Betimol [U.S., Finland] may be confused with Betanol brand name for metipranolol [Monaco]

Pregnancy Risk Factor C

Lactation Enters breast milk/ consider risk:benefit (AAP rates "compatible"; AAP 2001 update pending)

Use Treatment of elevated intraocular pressure such as glaucoma or ocular hypertension

Available Dosage Forms

Gel forming solution, ophthalmic: 0.25% (5 mL); 0.5% (5 mL)

Timolol GFS: 0.25% (5 mL); 0.5% (5 mL)

Timoptic-XE®: 0.25% (5 mL); 0.5% (5 mL)

Solution, ophthalmic: 0.25% (5 mL, 10 mL, 15 mL); 0.5% (5 mL, 10 mL, 15 mL)

Betimol®: 0.25% (5 mL); 0.5% (5 mL, 10 mL, 15 mL)

Istalol®: 0.5% (2.5 mL, 5 mL)

Timoptic®: 0.25% (5 mL); 0.5% (5 mL, 10 mL)

Solution, ophthalmic [preservative free]:

Timoptic® in OcuDose®: 0.25% (0.2 mL); 0.5% (0.2 mL)

Dosing

Adult & Geriatric Glaucoma: Ophthalmic:

Solution: Initial: 0.25% solution, instill 1 drop twice daily into affected eye(s); increase to 0.5% solution if response not adequate; decrease to 1 drop/day if controlled; do not exceed 1 drop twice daily of 0.5% solution.

Istalol®: Instill 1 drop (0.5% solution) once daily in the morning.

Gel-forming solution (Timolol GFS, Timoptic-XE®): Instill 1 drop (either 0.25% or 0.5%) once daily

Pediatric Glaucoma: Ophthalmic:

Solution: Initial: Instill 1 drop (0.25% solution) into affected eye(s) twice daily; increase to 0.5% solution if response not adequate; decrease to 1 drop/day if controlled; do not exceed 1 drop twice daily of 0.5% solution

Gel-forming solution (Timolol GFS, Timoptic-XE®): Instill 1 drop (either 0.25% or 0.5% solution) once daily

Administration

Other Ophthalmic: Administer other topically-applied ophthalmic medications at least 10 minutes before Timoptic-XE®; wash hands before use; invert closed bottle and shake once before use; remove cap carefully so that tip does not touch anything; hold bottle between thumb and index finger; use index finger of other hand to pull down the lower eyelid to form a pocket for the eye drop and tilt head back; place the dispenser tip close to the eye and gently squeeze the bottle to administer 1 drop; remove pressure after a single drop has been released; **do not allow the dispenser tip to touch the eye**; replace cap and store bottle in an upright position in a clean area; do **not** enlarge hole of dispenser; do **not** wash tip with water, soap, or any other cleaner. Some solutions contain benzalkonium chloride; wait at least 10 minutes after instilling solution before inserting soft contact lenses.

Monitoring and Teaching Issues

Patient Education Wash hands before using. Do not let tip of applicator touch eye; do not contaminate tip of applicator (may cause eye infection, eye damage, or vision loss). Tilt head back and look upward. Gently pull down lower lid and put drop(s) inside lower eyelid at inner corner. Close eye and roll eyeball in all directions. Do not blink for 1/2 minute. Apply gentle pressure to inner corner of eye for 30 seconds. Wipe away excess from skin around eye. Do not use any other eye preparation for at least 10 minutes. Temporary stinging or blurred vision may occur. Remove contact lenses prior to administration. Lenses may be reinserted 15 minutes following administration. Report persistent eye pain, irritation, double vision, vision changes, slow heart rate, dizziness, worsening of condition, or lack of improvement.

- ◆ **Timolol GFS** *see* Timolol (Ophthalmic) *on page 1763*
- ◆ **Timolol Hemihydrate** *see* Timolol (Ophthalmic) *on page 1763*
- ◆ **Timolol Maleate** *see* Timolol (Ophthalmic) *on page 1763*
- ◆ **Timoptic®** *see* Timolol (Ophthalmic) *on page 1763*
- ◆ **Timoptic® in OcuDose®** *see* Timolol (Ophthalmic) *on page 1763*
- ◆ **Timoptic-XE®** *see* Timolol (Ophthalmic) *on page 1763*
- ◆ **Tincture of Opium** *see* Opium Tincture *on page 1363*
- ◆ **Tindamax®** *see* Tinidazole *on page 1765*
- ◆ **Ting® Spray Powder [OTC]** *see* Miconazole (Topical) *on page 1224*

Tinidazole (tye NI da zole)

U.S. Brand Names Tindamax®

Generic Availability (U.S.) No

Pharmacologic Category Amebicide; Antibiotic, Miscellaneous; Antiprotozoal, Nitroimidazole

Pregnancy Risk Factor C

Lactation Enters breast milk/contraindicated (AAP rates "of concern"; AAP 2001 update pending)

Use Treatment of trichomoniasis caused by *T. vaginalis*; treatment of giardiasis caused by *G. duodenalis* (*G. lamblia*); treatment of intestinal amebiasis and amebic liver abscess caused by *E. histolytica*; treatment of bacterial vaginosis caused by *Bacteroides* spp, *Gardnerella vaginalis*, and *Prevotella* spp in nonpregnant females

Mechanism of Action/Effect After diffusing into the organism, it is proposed that tinidazole causes cytotoxicity by damaging DNA and preventing further DNA synthesis.

Contraindications Hypersensitivity to tinidazole, nitroimidazole derivatives (including metronidazole), or any component of the formulation; pregnancy (1st trimester); breast-feeding

Warnings/Precautions Use caution with CNS diseases; seizures and peripheral neuropathy have been reported with tinidazole and other nitroimidazole derivatives. **[U.S. Boxed Warning]: Carcinogenicity has been observed with another nitroimidazole derivative (metronidazole) in animal studies;** use should be reserved for approved indications only. Use caution with current or history of blood dyscrasias or hepatic impairment. When used for amebiasis, not indicated for the treatment of asymptomatic cyst passage. Prolonged use may result in fungal or bacterial superinfection, including *C. difficile*-associated diarrhea (CDAD), pseudomembranous colitis, and/or vaginal candidiasis. CDAD has been observed >2 months postantibiotic treatment. Safety and efficacy have not been established in children ≤3 years of age.

Drug Interactions

Metabolism/Transport Effects Substrate of CYP3A4 (major), 2B6 (minor)

Avoid Concomitant Use There are no known interactions where it is recommended to avoid concomitant use.

Decreased Effect Specific interaction studies have not been conducted. Refer to Metronidazole (Systemic) monograph on page 1220.

Increased Effect/Toxicity Specific interaction studies have not been conducted. Refer to Metronidazole (Systemic) monograph on page 1220.

Nutritional/Ethanol Interactions

Ethanol: The manufacturer recommends to avoid all ethanol or any ethanol-containing drugs (may cause disulfiram-like reaction characterized by flushing, headache, nausea, vomiting, sweating or tachycardia) during and for at least 3 days after completion of treatment.

Food: Peak antibiotic serum concentration lowered and delayed, but total drug absorbed not affected.

Lab Interactions May interfere with AST, ALT, triglycerides, glucose, and LDH testing

Adverse Reactions

1% to 10%:

Central nervous system: Fatigue/malaise (1% to 2%), dizziness (≤1%), headache (≤1%)

Endocrine & metabolic: Menorrhagia (>2%)

Gastrointestinal: Metallic/bitter taste (4% to 6%), nausea (3% to 5%), anorexia (2% to 3%), appetite decreased (>2%), flatulence (>2%), dyspepsia/cramps/epigastric discomfort (1% to 2%), vomiting (1% to 2%), constipation (≤1%)

Genitourinary: *Candida* vaginitis (5%), painful urination (>2%), pelvic pain (>2%), urine abnormality (>2%), vaginal odor (>2%), vulvovaginal discomfort (>2%)

Neuromuscular & skeletal: Weakness (1% to 2%)

Renal: Urinary tract infection (>2%)

Respiratory: Upper respiratory tract infection (>2%)

Frequency not defined:

Cardiovascular: Flushing, palpitation

Central nervous system: Ataxia, coma (rare), confusion (rare), depression (rare), drowsiness, fever, giddiness, insomnia, seizure, vertigo

Dermatologic: Angioedema, pruritus, rash, urticaria

Gastrointestinal: Abdominal pain, diarrhea, furry tongue (rare), oral candidiasis, salivation, stomatitis, thirst, tongue discoloration, xerostomia

Genitourinary: Urine darkened, vaginal discharge increased

Hematologic: Leukopenia (transient), neutropenia (transient), thrombocytopenia (reversible; rare)

Hepatic: Transaminases increased

Neuromuscular & skeletal: Arthralgia, arthritis, myalgia, peripheral neuropathy (transient, includes numbness and paresthesia)

Respiratory: Bronchospasm (rare), dyspnea (rare), pharyngitis (rare)

Miscellaneous: Burning sensation, *Candida* overgrowth, diaphoresis

Pharmacodynamics/Kinetics

Absorption Rapid and complete

Time to Peak 1.6 hours

Protein Binding 12%

Half-Life Elimination 13 hours

Metabolism Hepatic via CYP3A4 (primarily); undergoes oxidation, hydroxylation and conjugation; forms a metabolite

Excretion Urine (20% to 25%); feces (12%)

Available Dosage Forms

Tablet, oral:

Tindamax®: 250 mg, 500 mg

Dosing

Adult & Geriatric

Amebiasis, intestinal: Oral: 2 g/day for 3 days

Amebiasis, liver abscess: Oral: 2 g/day for 3-5 days

Bacterial vaginosis: 2 g/day for 2 days or 1 g/day for 5 days

Giardiasis: Oral: 2 g as a single dose

Trichomoniasis: Oral: 2 g as a single dose; sexual partners should be treated at the same time

Urethritis (unlabeled use): Oral: 2 g as a single dose with azithromycin (CDC, 2010)

Pediatric

Amebiasis, intestinal: Oral: Children >3 years: 50 mg/kg/day for 3 days (maximum dose: 2 g/day)

Amebiasis, liver abscess: Oral: Children >3 years: 50 mg/kg/day for 3-5 days (maximum dose: 2 g/day)

Giardiasis: Oral: Children >3 years: 50 mg/kg as a single dose (maximum dose: 2 g)

Renal Impairment Adjustment not necessary. An additional dose equal to $1/2$ the usual dose, should be administered at the end of hemodialysis if tinidazole is administered on a day hemodialysis occurs.

Hepatic Impairment Specific recommendations are not available; use with caution.

Administration

Oral Administer with food.

Stability

Storage Store at controlled room temperature of 15°C to 30°C (59°F to 86°F). Protect from light.

Monitoring and Teaching Issues

Patient Education Avoid all alcohol while taking this medication and for 3 days following completion; may cause unpleasant reaction (flushing, nausea, vomiting, sweating, headache, rapid heart beat). Refrain from sexual intercourse or use contraceptive if being treated for trichomoniasis. May cause headache, drowsiness or dizziness; mild gastrointestinal disturbance (nausea, vomiting, constipation, diarrhea, metallic/bitter taste, abdominal discomfort). Report severe fatigue or weakness, chest pain or palpitations, swelling of lips or mouth, or lack of improvement or worsening of condition.

Dietary Considerations Take with food. The manufacturer recommends that ethanol be avoided during treatment and for 3 days after therapy is complete.

Breast-Feeding Considerations Tinidazole is excreted into breast milk in concentrations similar to those in the maternal serum and can be detected for up to 72 hours after administration. Tinidazole is contraindicated in nursing mothers unless breast-feeding is interrupted during therapy and for 3 days after the last dose.

Pregnancy Considerations Adverse events have been observed in some animal reproduction studies; therefore, the manufacturer classifies tinidazole as pregnancy category C. Carcinogenicity studies have not been completed with tinidazole; however, metronidazole has a similar chemical structure and has caused carcinogenic effects in rats and mice. Tinidazole crosses the human placenta and enters the fetal circulation. Use of tinidazole is contraindicated during the first trimester of pregnancy.

Tinzaparin (tin ZA pa rin)

U.S. Brand Names Innohep®

Index Terms Tinzaparin Sodium

Generic Availability (U.S.) No

Pharmacologic Category Low Molecular Weight Heparin

Medication Safety Issues

High alert medication: The Institute for Safe Medication Practices (ISMP) includes this medication among its list of drug classes which have a heightened risk of causing significant patient harm when used in error.

2009 National Patient Safety Goals: The Joint Commission (TJC) requires healthcare organizations that provide anticoagulant therapy to have a process in place to reduce the risk of anticoagulant-associated patient harm. Patients receiving anticoagulants should receive individualized care through a defined process that includes standardized ordering, dispensing, administration, monitoring and education. This does not apply to routine short-term use of anticoagulants for prevention of venous thromboembolism when the expectation is that the patient's laboratory values will remain within or close to normal values (NPSG.03.05.01).

Pregnancy Risk Factor B

Lactation Excretion in breast milk unknown/use caution

Use Treatment of acute symptomatic deep vein thrombosis, with or without pulmonary embolism, in conjunction with warfarin sodium

Unlabeled/Investigational Use Prophylaxis of deep vein thrombosis following hip or knee replacement surgery, and general surgery

Mechanism of Action/Effect Standard heparin consists of components with molecular weights ranging from 4000-30,000 daltons with a mean of 16,000 daltons. Heparin acts as an anticoagulant by enhancing the inhibition rate of clotting proteases by antithrombin III, impairing normal hemostasis and inhibition of factor Xa. Low molecular weight heparins have a small effect on the activated partial thromboplastin time and strongly inhibit factor Xa. The primary inhibitory activity of tinzaparin is through antithrombin. Tinzaparin is derived from porcine heparin that undergoes controlled enzymatic depolymerization. The average molecular weight of tinzaparin ranges between 5500 and 7500 daltons which is distributed as <2000 daltons (<10%), 2000-8000 daltons (60% to 72%), and >8000 daltons (22% to 36%). The anti-Xa activity is approximately 100 int. units/mg.

Contraindications Hypersensitivity to tinzaparin sodium, heparin, or any component of the formulation; active major bleeding; heparin-induced thrombocytopenia (current or history of)

Warnings/Precautions **[U.S. Boxed Warning]: Spinal or epidural hematomas, including subsequent paralysis, may occur with recent or anticipated neuraxial anesthesia (epidural or spinal) or spinal puncture in patients anticoagulated with LMWH or heparinoids.** Consider risk versus benefit prior to spinal procedures; risk is increased by the use of concomitant agents which may alter hemostasis, the use of indwelling epidural catheters for analgesia, a history of spinal deformity or spinal surgery, as well as traumatic or repeated epidural or spinal punctures. Patient should be observed closely for signs and symptoms of neurological impairment. Not to be used interchangeably (unit for unit) with heparin or any other low molecular weight heparins.

Monitor patient closely for signs or symptoms of bleeding. Certain patients are at increased risk of bleeding. Risk factors include bacterial endocarditis; congenital or acquired bleeding disorders; active ulcerative or angiodysplastic GI diseases; severe uncontrolled hypertension; history of hemorrhagic stroke; use shortly after brain, spinal, or ophthalmologic surgery; patients treated concomitantly with platelet inhibitors; recent GI bleeding; thrombocytopenia or platelet defects; severe liver disease; hypertensive or diabetic retinopathy; or in patients undergoing invasive procedures. Monitor platelet count closely. Rare cases of thrombocytopenia have occurred. Manufacturer recommends discontinuation of therapy if platelets are <100,000/mm^3. Rare cases of thrombocytopenia with thrombosis have occurred.

Reduced tinzaparin clearance was observed in patients with moderate-to-severe renal impairment; use with caution or avoid use in patients with renal insufficiency. The 2008 *Chest* guidelines recommend that patients with Cl_{cr} <30 mL/minute be treated with unfractionated heparin instead of LMWH (Hirsh, 2008). Use with caution in the elderly (delayed elimination may occur). Use in patients ≥70 years of age with renal insufficiency (Cl_{cr} ≤30 mL/minute or ≥75 years of age and Cl_{cr} ≤60 mL/minute) has been associated with an increased risk of death compared to use of unfractionated heparin; consider alternative treatments in these patients.

Heparin can cause hyperkalemia by suppressing aldosterone production; similar reactions could occur with LMWHs. Monitor for hyperkalemia which most commonly occurs in patients with risk factors for the development of hyperkalemia (eg, renal dysfunction, concomitant use of potassium-sparing diuretics or potassium supplements, hematoma in body tissues). For subcutaneous use only; do not administer intramuscularly or intravenously. Clinical experience is limited in patients with BMI >40 kg/m^2. Derived from porcine intestinal mucosa. Contains benzyl alcohol and sodium metabisulfite.

Drug Interactions

Avoid Concomitant Use There are no known interactions where it is recommended to avoid concomitant use.

Decreased Effect There are no known significant interactions involving a decrease in effect.

Increased Effect/Toxicity

Tinzaparin may increase the levels/effects of: Anticoagulants; Collagenase (Systemic); Drotrecogin Alfa; Ibritumomab; Tositumomab and Iodine I 131 Tositumomab

The levels/effects of Tinzaparin may be increased by: 5-ASA Derivatives; Antiplatelet Agents; Dasatinib; Herbs (Anticoagulant/Antiplatelet Properties); Nonsteroidal Anti-Inflammatory Agents; Pentosan Polysulfate Sodium; Pentoxifylline; Prostacyclin Analogues; Salicylates; Thrombolytic Agents

Adverse Reactions As with all anticoagulants, bleeding is the major adverse effect of tinzaparin. Hemorrhage may occur at virtually any site. Risk is dependent on multiple variables.

>10%:
- Hepatic: ALT increased (13%)
- Local: Injection site hematoma (16%)

1% to 10%:
- Cardiovascular: Angina pectoris, chest pain (2%), hyper-/hypotension, tachycardia
- Central nervous system: Confusion, dizziness, fever (2%), headache (2%), insomnia, pain (2%)
- Dermatologic: Bullous eruption, pruritus, rash (1%), skin disorder
- Gastrointestinal: Constipation (1%), dyspepsia, flatulence, nausea (2%), nonspecified gastrointestinal disorder, vomiting (1%)
- Genitourinary: Dysuria, urinary retention, urinary tract infection (4%)
- Hematologic: Anemia, hematoma, hemorrhage (2%), thrombocytopenia (1%)
- Hepatic: AST increased (9%)
- Local: Thrombophlebitis (deep)
- Neuromuscular & skeletal: Back pain (2%)
- Renal: Hematuria (1%)
- Respiratory: Dyspnea (1%), epistaxis (2%), pneumonia, pulmonary embolism (2%), respiratory disorder
- Miscellaneous: Impaired healing, infection, unclassified reactions

Pharmacodynamics/Kinetics

Onset of Action 2-3 hours

Bioavailability 87%

Time to Peak 4-5 hours

Half-Life Elimination 3-4 hours

Metabolism Partially metabolized by desulphation and depolymerization

Excretion Urine

Available Dosage Forms

Injection, solution:

Innohep®: 20,000 anti-Xa int. units/mL (2 mL)

Dosing

Adult

DVT (with or without PE) treatment: SubQ: 175 anti-Xa int. units/kg once daily. The 2008 *Chest* guidelines recommend starting warfarin on the first treatment day and continuing tinzaparin until INR is between 2 and 3 (usually 5-7 days). Administer tinzaparin for at least 5 days and until INR ≥2 for at least 24 hours (Hirsh, 2008).

Note: To calculate the volume of solution to administer per treatment dose: Volume to be administered (mL) = patient weight (kg) x 0.00875 mL/kg (may be rounded off to the nearest 0.05 mL)

DVT prophylaxis (unlabeled use): SubQ:

Hip replacement surgery: 75 anti-Xa int. units/kg once daily, with initial dose given 18-24 hours after surgery for up to 14 days **or** 4500 anti-Xa int. units once daily, with initial dose given 12 hours prior to surgery and continued for up to 15 days (Hull, 1993; Planes, 1999)

Knee replacement surgery: 75 anti-Xa int. units/kg once daily, with initial dose given 18-24 hours after surgery and continued for up to 14 days (Hull, 1993)

General surgery: 3500 anti-Xa int. units once daily, with initial dose given 2 hours prior to surgery and continued for 7-10 days (Leizorovicz, 1991)

Dosing adjustment in obesity: Weight based dosing (175 anti-Xa int. units/kg once daily) provided in product labeling for patients up to 162 kg. Limited clinical experience in patients with a BMI >40 kg/m^2.

Geriatric Refer to adult dosing. Increased sensitivity to tinzaparin in elderly patients may be possible due to a decline in renal function. Increased all-cause mortality noted in patients ≥70 years of age with Cl_{cr} ≤30 mL/minute or ≥75 years of age and Cl_{cr} ≤60 mL/minute; consider alternative treatments in these patients.

Renal Impairment

Cl_{cr} ≤50 mL/minute: Use with caution; clearance is decreased.

Cl_{cr} <30 mL/minute: Per manufacturer's labeling, use with caution. The 2008 *Chest* guidelines recommend avoiding use (in patients requiring therapeutic anticoagulation); if used, consider monitoring anti-Xa levels (Hirsh, 2008).

Hepatic Impairment No adjustment necessary.

Administration

Other Patient should be lying down or sitting. Administer by deep SubQ injection, alternating between the left and right anterolateral and left and right posterolateral abdominal wall. Vary site daily. The entire needle should be introduced into the skin fold formed by the thumb and forefinger. Hold the skin fold until injection is complete. To minimize bruising, do not rub the injection site.

Stability

Storage Store at 15°C to 30°C (59°F to 86°F).

Monitoring and Teaching Issues

Laboratory Monitoring CBC including platelet count and hematocrit or hemoglobin, and stool for occult blood; the monitoring of PT and/or PTT is not of clinical value. Patients receiving both warfarin and tinzaparin should have their INR drawn just prior to the next scheduled dose of tinzaparin.

According to 2008 *Chest* guidelines, routine monitoring of anti-Xa levels is generally not recommended; however, anti-Xa levels may be beneficial in certain patients (eg, obese patients, patients with severe renal insufficiency receiving therapeutic doses, and possibly pregnant women receiving therapeutic doses; Hirsh, 2008)

Physical Assessment Use caution in the presence of renal insufficiency, advanced age, or increased risk of bleeding. Monitor for bleeding, rash, and confusion regularly throughout therapy. Observe and teach bleeding precautions. If self-administered, teach patient appropriate injection technique and syringe/needle disposal.

Patient Education This drug can only be administered I.V.; if self-administered, inject exactly as directed and follow instructions for syringe disposal. Report excessive bruising, swelling, or redness at injection site. You may have a tendency to bleed easily while taking this drug. Report immediately any unusual bleeding or bruising (eg, mouth, nose, blood in urine or stool), severe headache or confusion, dizziness, or skin rash.

Geriatric Considerations No significant differences in safety or response were seen when used in patients ≥65 years of age. However, increased sensitivity to tinzaparin in elderly patients may be possible due to a decline in renal function. Results from the Innohep in Renal Insufficiency Study (IRIS) study showed an increased in all-cause mortality in elderly patients receiving tinzaparin compared to unfractionated heparin for treatment of DVT and/or PE. The at-risk population has defined as patients ≥70 years of age with Cl_{cr} ≤30 mL/minute or ≥75 years of age and Cl_{cr} ≤60 mL/minute.

Pregnancy Considerations Teratogenic events were not observed in animal studies. Tinzaparin does not cross the human placenta. A pharmacokinetic study in pregnant women found no dose adjustment was needed during pregnancy. Pregnancy may increase the risk of thromboembolism; risk may be further increased with certain pre-existing conditions. As with all anticoagulants, bleeding is the major adverse effect of tinzaparin. Vaginal bleeding was reported in ~10% of pregnant patients during tinzaparin therapy. Contains benzyl alcohol; use with caution in pregnant women.

◆ **Tinzaparin Sodium** *see* Tinzaparin *on page 1766*

Tioconazole (tye oh KONE a zole)

U.S. Brand Names 1-Day™ [OTC]; Vagistat®-1 [OTC]

Generic Availability (U.S.) No

Pharmacologic Category Antifungal Agent, Vaginal

Medication Safety Issues

Sound-alike/look-alike issues:

Tioconazole may be confused with terconazole

Pregnancy Risk Factor C

Lactation Excretion in breast milk unknown/not recommended

Use Local treatment of vulvovaginal candidiasis

Available Dosage Forms For available OTC formulations, consult specific product labeling.

Dosing

Adult & Geriatric Vulvovaginal candidiasis: Vaginal: Insert 1 applicatorful in vagina, just prior to bedtime, as a single dose

Monitoring and Teaching Issues

Patient Education Consult with prescriber if treating a vaginal yeast infection for the first time. Insert high into the vagina. Refrain from intercourse during treatment. May interact with condoms and vaginal contraceptive diaphragms (ie, weaken latex); do not rely on these products for 3 days following treatment. Do not use tampons, douches, spermicides, or other vaginal products during treatment. Although product is used for a single day, relief from symptoms usually takes longer than 1 day. Report persistent (>3 days) vaginal burning, irritation, or discharge.

◆ **Tioguanine** *see* Thioguanine *on page 1752*

◆ **Tiotixene** *see* Thiothixene *on page 1756*

Tiotropium (ty oh TRO pee um)

U.S. Brand Names Spiriva® HandiHaler®

Index Terms Tiotropium Bromide Monohydrate

Generic Availability (U.S.) No

Pharmacologic Category Anticholinergic Agent

Medication Safety Issues

Sound-alike/look-alike issues:

Spiriva® may be confused with Inspra™, Serevent®

Tiotropium may be confused with ipratropium

Spiriva® capsules for inhalation are for administration via HandiHaler® device and are **not** for oral use

Pregnancy Risk Factor C

Lactation Excretion in breast milk unknown/use caution

Use Maintenance treatment of bronchospasm associated with COPD (including bronchitis and emphysema); reduction of COPD exacerbations

Mechanism of Action/Effect Blocks the action of acetylcholine at parasympathetic sites in bronchial smooth muscle causing bronchodilation

Contraindications Hypersensitivity to tiotropium or ipratropium, or any component of the formulation (contains lactose)

Warnings/Precautions Rarely, paradoxical bronchospasm may occur with use of inhaled bronchodilating agents; discontinue use and consider other therapy if bronchospasm occurs.

Not indicated for the initial (rescue) treatment of acute episodes of bronchospasm. Use with caution in patients with myasthenia gravis, narrow-angle glaucoma, prostatic hyperplasia, moderate-severe renal impairment (Cl_{cr} ≤50 mL/minute), or bladder neck obstruction; avoid inadvertent instillation of powder into the eyes. Immediate hypersensitivity reactions may occur; discontinue immediately if signs/symptoms occur. Use with caution in patients with a history of hypersensitivity to atropine.

The contents of Spiriva® capsules are for inhalation only via the HandiHaler® device. There have been reports of incorrect administration (swallowing of the capsules). Capsule for oral inhalation contains lactose; use with caution in patients with severe milk protein allergy.

Drug Interactions

Metabolism/Transport Effects Substrate (minor) of CYP2D6, 3A4

Avoid Concomitant Use There are no known interactions where it is recommended to avoid concomitant use.

Decreased Effect

Tiotropium may decrease the levels/effects of: Acetylcholinesterase Inhibitors (Central); Secretin

The levels/effects of Tiotropium may be decreased by: Acetylcholinesterase Inhibitors (Central); Peginterferon Alfa-2b

Increased Effect/Toxicity

Tiotropium may increase the levels/effects of: AbobotulinumtoxinA; Anticholinergics; Cannabinoids; OnabotulinumtoxinA; Potassium Chloride; RimabotulinumtoxinB

The levels/effects of Tiotropium may be increased by: Conivaptan; Pramlintide

Adverse Reactions

>10%:

Gastrointestinal: Xerostomia (5% to 16%)

Respiratory: Upper respiratory tract infection (41%), pharyngitis (9% to 13%), sinusitis (7% to 11%)

1% to 10%:

Cardiovascular: Chest pain (1% to 7%), edema (dependent, 5%)

Central nervous system: Headache (6%), insomnia (4%), depression (1% to 4%), dysphonia (1% to 3%)

Dermatologic: Rash (4%)

Endocrine & metabolic: Hypercholesterolemia (1% to 3%), hyperglycemia (1% to 3%)

Gastrointestinal: Dyspepsia (6%), abdominal pain (5%), constipation (4% to 5%), vomiting (4%), gastroesophageal reflux (1% to 3%), stomatitis (including ulcerative; 1% to 3%)

Genitourinary: Urinary tract infection (7%)

Neuromuscular & skeletal: Arthralgia (4%), myalgia (4%), arthritis (≥3%), leg pain (1% to 3%), paresthesia (1% to 3%), skeletal pain (1% to 3%)

Ocular: Cataract (1% to 3%)

Respiratory: Rhinitis (6%), epistaxis (4%), cough (≥3%), laryngitis (1% to 3%)

Miscellaneous: Infection (4%), moniliasis (4%), flu-like syndrome (≥3%), allergic reaction (1% to 3%), herpes zoster (1% to 3%)

Pharmacodynamics/Kinetics

Absorption Poorly absorbed from GI tract, systemic absorption may occur from lung.

Bioavailability Following inhalation: 19.5%; oral solution: 2% to 3%

Time to Peak Plasma: 5 minutes (following inhalation)

Protein Binding 72%

Half-Life Elimination 5-6 days

Metabolism Hepatic (minimal), via CYP2D6 and CYP3A4

Excretion Urine (14% of an inhaled dose); feces (primarily nonabsorbed drug)

Available Dosage Forms

Powder, for oral inhalation:

Spiriva® HandiHaler®: 18 mcg/capsule (5s, 30s, 90s)

Dosing

Adult & Geriatric COPD: Oral inhalation: Contents of 1 capsule (18 mcg) inhaled once daily using HandiHaler® device. **Note:** To ensure drug delivery the contents of each capsule should be inhaled twice.

Renal Impairment Plasma concentrations may increase in renal impairment. Use caution in moderate-to-severe impairment (Cl_{cr} ≤50 mL/minute); although no dosage adjustment is required, monitor closely.

Administration

Oral For oral inhalation only. Capsule should not be swallowed.

Inhalation Administer once daily at the same time each day. Remove capsule from foil blister immediately before use. Capsule should not be swallowed. Place capsule in the capsule-chamber in the base of the HandiHaler® Inhaler. Must only use the HandiHaler® Inhaler. Close mouthpiece until a click is heard, leaving dustcap open. Exhale fully. Do not exhale into inhaler. Tilt head slightly back and inhale (rapidly, steadily and deeply); the capsule vibration may be heard within the device. Hold breath as long as possible. If any powder remains in capsule, exhale and inhale again. Repeat until capsule is empty. Throw away empty capsule; do not leave in inhaler. Do not use a spacer with the HandiHaler® Inhaler. Do not use HandiHaler® device for other medications. Always keep capsules and inhaler dry.

Delivery of dose: Instruct patient to place mouthpiece gently between teeth, closing lips around inhaler. Instruct patient to inhale deeply and hold breath for 5-10 seconds. The amount of drug delivered is small, and the individual will not sense the medication as it is inhaled. Remove mouthpiece prior to exhalation. Patient should not breathe out through the mouthpiece.

Stability

Storage Store at 25°C (77°F); excursions permitted to 15°C to 30°C (59°F to 86°F). Avoid excessive temperatures and moisture. Do not store capsules in HandiHaler® device. Capsules should be stored in the blister pack and only removed immediately before use. Once protective foil is peeled back and/or removed the capsule should be used immediately; if capsule is not used immediately it should be discarded.

Monitoring and Teaching Issues

Laboratory Monitoring FEV_1, peak flow (or other pulmonary function studies)

Physical Assessment Assess results of pulmonary tests prior to and periodically during therapy.

Patient Education Use inhaler and medication as instructed - once daily, at same time each day. Do not use as an acute "rescue" bronchodilator. Capsules are not to be swallowed. May cause nausea or vomiting, dry mouth, hyperglycemia (if you have diabetes, monitor serum glucose closely), or muscle or skeletal pain. Report swelling of face, mouth, or tongue; skin rash; chest pain or palpitations; persistent gastrointestinal effects; muscle or skeletal pain or weakness; change in vision; numbness or weakness of extremities; slurred speech; or respiratory changes, sore throat, or flu-like symptoms.

Administration of HandiHaler® Inhaler: Remove capsule from blister pack immediately before using. Place capsule in capsule chamber in the base of inhaler. Close mouthpiece until a click is heard, leaving dustcap open. Exhale fully (do not exhale into inhaler). Place mouthpiece gently between teeth, closing lips around inhaler. Tilt head back slightly and inhale once rapidly, steadily, and deeply (the capsule vibration may be heard within the inhaler, but you will not sense the medication as it is inhaled.) Hold breath as long as possible. Remove inhaler from mouth before exhaling. If any powder remains in capsule, repeat inhalation again. Throw away empty capsule. Do not store capsule in inhaler and always keep inhaler and capsules dry.

Geriatric Considerations Assess patient's ability to use the HandiHaler®. In elderly patients, renal clearance of tiotropium was decreased and plasma concentrations were increased, due to decreased renal function. In clinical trials, the incidence of constipation, UTIs and xerostomia increased with age. No dosage adjustments are recommended due to age or renal function. However, the manufacturer recommends monitoring patients with moderate-to-severe renal impairment.

Pregnancy Considerations Adverse events (fetal loss, decreased birth weights, delayed sexual maturation) were observed in some animal studies. There are no adequate and well-controlled studies in pregnant women. Use only when expected benefit to mother outweighs potential risk to the fetus.

◆ **Tiotropium Bromide Monohydrate** *see* Tiotropium *on page 1769*

Tipranavir (tip RA na veer)

U.S. Brand Names Aptivus®

Index Terms PNU-140690E; TPV

Generic Availability (U.S.) No

Pharmacologic Category Antiretroviral Agent, Protease Inhibitor

Pregnancy Risk Factor C

Lactation Excretion in breast milk unknown/contraindicated

Use Treatment of HIV-1 infections in combination with ritonavir and other antiretroviral agents; limited to highly treatment-experienced or multiprotease inhibitor-resistant patients.

Mechanism of Action/Effect Blocks the site of HIV-1 protease activity, resulting in the formation of immature, noninfectious viral particles.

Contraindications Concurrent therapy of tipranavir/ritonavir with alfuzosin, amiodarone, bepridil, cisapride, ergot derivatives (eg, dihydroergotamine, ergonovine, ergotamine, methylergonovine), flecainide, lovastatin, midazolam (oral), pimozide, propafenone, quinidine, rifampin, sildenafil (for pulmonary arterial hypertension [eg, Revatio®]), simvastatin, St John's wort, and triazolam; moderate-to-severe hepatic impairment (Child-Pugh class B or C)

Warnings/Precautions Coadministration with ritonavir is required. **[U.S. Boxed Warning]: In combination with ritonavir, may cause hepatitis (including fatalities) and/or exacerbate pre-existing hepatic dysfunction (causal relationship not established); patients with chronic hepatitis B or C are at increased risk.** Monitor patients closely; discontinue use if signs or symptoms of toxicity occur or if asymptomatic AST/ALT elevations >10 times upper limit of normal or AST/ALT elevations >5-10 times upper limit of normal concurrently with total bilirubin >2.5 times the upper limit of normal occur. Use with caution in patients with mild hepatic impairment; contraindicated in moderate-to-severe impairment. May be associated with fat redistribution (buffalo hump, increased abdominal girth, breast engorgement, facial atrophy). Use caution in hemophilia. May increase cholesterol and/or triglycerides; hypertriglyceridemia may increase risk of pancreatitis. May cause hyperglycemia. Use with caution in patients with sulfonamide allergy. Protease inhibitors have been associated with a variety of hypersensitivity events (some severe), including rash, anaphylaxis (rare), angioedema, bronchospasm, erythema multiforme, and/or Stevens-Johnson syndrome (rare). It is generally recommended to discontinue treatment if severe rash or moderate symptoms accompanied by other systemic symptoms occur. Immune reconstitution syndrome, including inflammatory responses to indolent infections, has been associated with antiretroviral therapy; additional evaluation and treatment may be required.

[U.S. Boxed Warning]: Tipranavir in combination with ritonavir has been associated with rare reports of fatal and nonfatal intracranial hemorrhage; causal relationship not established. Events often occurred in patients with medical conditions (eg, CNS lesions, head trauma, recent neurosurgery, coagulopathy, alcohol abuse) or concurrent therapy which may have influenced these events. Tipranavir may inhibit platelet aggregation. Use with caution in patients who may be at risk for increased bleeding (trauma, surgery or other medical conditions) or in patients receiving concurrent medications which may increase the risk of bleeding, including antiplatelet agents and anticoagulants.

Use with caution in patients taking strong CYP3A4 inhibitors and moderate CYP3A4 inducers. Concomitant use with selected major CYP3A4 substrates and strong CYP3A4 inducers is contraindicated (see Drug Interactions); consider alternative agents that avoid or lessen the potential for CYP-mediated interactions. Do not coadminister colchicine in patient with renal or ▶

hepatic impairment; avoid concurrent use with salmeterol. Coadministration with anticoagulants or antiplatelet agents may increase the risk of bleeding. Women receiving estrogen (as hormonal contraception or replacement therapy) have an increased incidence of rash. Alternative forms of contraception may be needed. Do not coadminister with etravirine. Oral solution formulation contains vitamin E; additional vitamin E supplements should be avoided. Safety and efficacy have not been established in children <2 years of age.

Drug Interactions

Metabolism/Transport Effects Substrate of CYP3A4 (major); **Induces** P-glycoprotein

Avoid Concomitant Use

Avoid concomitant use of Tipranavir with any of the following: Alfuzosin; Amiodarone; Bepridil [Off Market]; Cisapride; Dabigatran Etexilate; Ergot Derivatives; Etravirine; Flecainide; Lovastatin; Midazolam; Pimozide; Propafenone; QuiNIDine; Rifampin; Simvastatin; St Johns Wort; Tamoxifen; Thioridazine; Triazolam

Decreased Effect

Tipranavir may decrease the levels/effects of: Abacavir; Clarithromycin; Codeine; Contraceptives (Estrogens); Dabigatran Etexilate; Delavirdine; Didanosine; Divalproex; Estrogen Derivatives; Etravirine; Meperidine; Methadone; P-Glycoprotein Substrates; PHENobarbital; Phenytoin; Proton Pump Inhibitors; Raltegravir; Theophylline Derivatives; TraMADol; Valproic Acid; Zidovudine

The levels/effects of Tipranavir may be decreased by: Antacids; CarBAMazepine; Contraceptives (Estrogens); CYP3A4 Inducers (Strong); Deferasirox; Efavirenz; Garlic; PHENobarbital; Phenytoin; Rifampin; St Johns Wort; Tenofovir

Increased Effect/Toxicity Note: Listed interactions include interactions resulting from coadministration with ritonavir. Refer to Ritonavir monograph on page 1593 for additional interaction concerns. The serum concentrations of tipranavir may be increased by ritonavir. This combination is recommended to enhance the effect ("boost") tipranavir.

Tipranavir/ritonavir may increase the levels/effects of CYP3A4 substrates. Tipranavir/ritonavir may increase the toxicity of benzodiazepines; concurrent use of midazolam and triazolam is specifically contraindicated. Tipranavir may increase serum concentrations of cisapride, increasing the risk of malignant arrhythmias; use is contraindicated. Toxicity of pimozide is significantly increased by tipranavir/ritonavir; concurrent use is contraindicated. Tipranavir/ritonavir may increase serum concentrations/toxicity of several antiarrhythmic agents; contraindicated with amiodarone, flecainide, propafenone, and quinidine (use extreme caution with lidocaine). Tipranavir/ritonavir may also increase serum concentrations/effects of calcium channel blockers and immunosuppressants (cyclosporine, sirolimus, tacrolimus).

Serum concentrations of HMG-CoA reductase inhibitors (atorvastatin, cerivastatin, lovastatin, simvastatin) may be increased by tipranavir/ritonavir, increasing the risk of myopathy/rhabdomyolysis. Lovastatin and simvastatin are not recommended. Use lowest possible dose of atorvastatin. Fluvastatin and pravastatin may be safer alternatives. Serum concentrations of rifabutin may be increased by tipranavir/ritonavir; dosage adjustment of rifabutin is required.

The toxicity of ergot alkaloids (dihydroergotamine, ergotamine, ergonovine, methylergonovine) is increased by tipranavir; concurrent use is contraindicated. Effects of hypoglycemic agents may be altered by tipranavir/ritonavir. Concurrent therapy with tipranavir may increase serum concentrations of normeperidine, and decrease serum concentrations of meperidine. The serum concentrations of sildenafil, tadalafil, and vardenafil may be increased by tipranavir/ritonavir; dose adjustment and limitations related to ritonavir coadministration must be recognized.

Concurrent use of disulfiram with tipranavir oral solution is contraindicated due to risk of adverse reaction (due to alcohol content of formulation). Clarithromycin may increase serum concentrations of tipranavir. Tipranavir/ritonavir may increase serum concentrations of clarithromycin. Use with caution and adjust dose of clarithromycin during concurrent therapy in renally impaired patients.

Nutritional/Ethanol Interactions

Ethanol: Capsules contain dehydrated alcohol 7% w/w (0.1 g per capsule)

Herb/Nutraceutical: St Johns wort may decrease the levels/effects of tipranavir/ritonavir; concurrent use is contraindicated. Vitamin E (high dose) may increase the risk of bleeding.

Adverse Reactions

>10%:

- Dermatologic: Rash (children 21%; adults 3% to 10%)
- Endocrine & metabolic: Hypertriglyceridemia (>400 mg/dL: 61%), hypercholesterolemia (>300 mg/dL: 22%)
- Gastrointestinal: Diarrhea (15%)
- Hepatic: Transaminases increased (>2.5 x ULN: 26% to 32%; grade 3/4: 10% to 20%)
- Neuromuscular & skeletal: CPK increased (grade 3/4: children 11%)

2% to 10%:

- Central nervous system: Fever (6% to 8%), fatigue (6%), headache (5%)
- Endocrine & metabolic: Dehydration (2%)
- Gastrointestinal: Nausea (5% to 9%), amylase increased (grade 3: 6% to 8%), vomiting (6%), abdominal pain (4%), diarrhea (children 4%), weight loss (3%)
- Hematologic: Bleeding (children 8%), WBC decreased (grades 3: 5%), anemia (3%), neutropenia (2%)
- Hepatic: ALT increased (2%, grades 3/4: 10%), AST increased (grades 3/4: 6%), GGT increased (2%)
- Neuromuscular & skeletal: Myalgia (2%)
- Respiratory: Cough (children 6%), dyspnea (2%), epistaxis (children 4%)

Pharmacodynamics/Kinetics

Absorption Incomplete (percentage not established)

Bioavailability Not established

Time to Peak 3 hours

Protein Binding >99% (albumin, alpha$_1$-acid glycoprotein)

Half-Life Elimination Children 2-<6 years of age: ~8 hours, 6-<12 years of age: ~7 hours, 12-18 years: ~5 hours; Adults: 6 hours

Metabolism Hepatic, via CYP3A4 (minimal when coadministered with ritonavir)

Excretion Feces (82%); urine (4%); primarily as unchanged drug (when coadministered with ritonavir)

Available Dosage Forms

Capsule, soft gelatin, oral:

Aptivus®: 250 mg

Solution, oral:

Aptivus®: 100 mg/mL (95 mL)

Dosing

Adult & Geriatric HIV infection: Oral: 500 mg twice daily; **Note:** Coadministration with ritonavir (200 mg twice daily) is required.

Dosage adjustments for concomitant therapy: Oral:

Coadministration with bosentan:

Coadministration of bosentan in patients currently receiving tipranavir/ritonavir: For patients receiving tipranavir/ritonavir for at least 10 days, begin with bosentan 62.5 mg once daily or every other day based on tolerability

Coadministration of tipranavir/ritonavir in patients currently receiving bosentan: Discontinue bosentan 36 hours prior to the initiation of tipranavir/ritonavir. After at least 10 days of tipranavir/ritonavir, resume bosentan 62.5 mg once daily or every other day based on tolerability.

Coadministration with colchicine:

Familial Mediterranean fever (FMF): Maximum colchicine dose: 0.6 mg/day (0.3 mg twice daily)

Gout prophylaxis:

If original colchicine dose is 0.6 mg twice daily, adjust dose to 0.3 mg once daily

If original colchicine dose is 0.6 mg once daily, adjust dose to 0.3 mg every other day

Gout flare treatment: Initial: Colchicine 0.6 mg, followed in 1 hour by a single dose of 0.3 mg; do not repeat for at least 3 days

Coadministration with phosphodiesterase-5 enzyme (PDE-5) inhibitor:

Pulmonary arterial hypertension: Tipranavir/ritonavir coadministered with tadalafil:

Patient receiving tipranavir/ritonavir for at least 1 week: Initiate tadalafil at 20 mg once daily; increase to 40 mg once daily based on individual tolerability

Patient receiving tadalafil when initiating tipranavir/ritonavir: Stop tadalafil at least 24 hours prior to starting tipranavir/ritonavir. After at least 1 week following the initiation of tipranavir/ritonavir, resume tadalafil at 20 mg once daily; increase to 40 mg once daily based on individual tolerability.

Erectile dysfunction: Tipranavir/ritonavir coadministered with:

Sildenafil (Viagra®): Maximum sildenafil dose: 25 mg in a 48-hour period

Tadalafil (Cialis®): Maximum tadalafil dose: 10 mg in a 72-hour period

Vardenafil: Maximum vardenafil dose: 2.5 mg in a 72-hour period

Pediatric HIV infection: Children ≥2 years: Oral: 14 mg/kg or 375 mg/m^2 (maximum: 500 mg/dose) twice daily. **Note:** Coadministration with ritonavir (6 mg/kg or 150 mg/m^2 [maximum: 200 mg/dose] twice daily) is required.

If intolerance or toxicity develops and virus is not resistant to multiple protease inhibitors: May decrease dose to 12 mg/kg or 290 mg/m^2 twice daily. **Note:** Coadministration with ritonavir (5 mg/kg or 115 mg/m^2 twice daily) is required.

Renal Impairment No adjustment required.

Hepatic Impairment

Mild impairment (Child-Pugh class A): No adjustment required.

Moderate-to-severe impairment (Child-Pugh class B or C): Concurrent use is contraindicated.

Administration

Oral Coadministration with ritonavir is required. Administer with ritonavir capsules or solution without regard to meals; administer with ritonavir tablets with meals.

Stability

Storage

Capsule: Prior to opening bottle, store under refrigeration at 2°C to 8°C (36°F to 46°F). After bottle is opened, may be stored at controlled room temperature of 25°C (77°F) for up to 60 days.

Oral solution: Store at 15°C to 30°C (59°F to 86°F). After bottle is open, use within 60 days. Do not refrigerate or freeze oral solution.

Monitoring and Teaching Issues

Laboratory Monitoring Viral load, CD4, serum glucose, liver function tests, bilirubin

Physical Assessment Assess CD4 count and hepatic function. Monitor for gastrointestinal disturbance (nausea, vomiting, diarrhea) that can lead to dehydration and weight loss, hyperlipidemia, redistribution of body fat, rash, and electrolyte imbalance. Caution patients to monitor glucose levels closely; may alter effects of hypoglycemic agents or cause hyperglycemia. Teach patient proper timing of multiple medications.

Patient Education This is not a cure for HIV, nor has it been found to reduce transmission of HIV; use appropriate precautions to prevent spread to other persons. Maintain adequate hydration, unless instructed to restrict fluid intake. Frequent blood tests may be required. You may be advised to check your glucose levels; this drug can cause exacerbation or new-onset diabetes. May cause body changes due to redistribution of body fat, facial atrophy, or breast enlargement (normal effects of drug). May cause dizziness, insomnia, abnormal thinking, nausea, vomiting, taste perversion, muscle weakness, headache, or insomnia. Inform prescriber if you experience muscle numbness or tingling; unresolved persistent vomiting, diarrhea, or abdominal pain; respiratory difficulty or chest pain; unusual skin rash; or change in color of stool or urine.

Dietary Considerations Capsule contains dehydrated ethanol. Oral solution formulation contains vitamin E; additional vitamin E supplements should be avoided.

Breast-Feeding Considerations In infants born to mothers who are HIV positive, HAART while breast-feeding may decrease postnatal infection. However, maternal or infant antiretroviral therapy does not completely eliminate the risk of postnatal HIV transmission. In addition, multiclass-resistant virus has been detected in breast-feeding infants despite maternal therapy.

In the United States where formula is accessible, affordable, safe, and sustainable, complete avoidance of breast-feeding by HIV-infected women is recommended to decrease potential transmission of HIV.

Pregnancy Considerations Teratogenic effects were not observed in animal reproduction studies; fetotoxity was observed with some doses. It is not known if tipranavir crosses the human placenta. Pregnancy and protease inhibitors are both associated with an increased risk of hyperglycemia. Glucose levels should be closely monitored. Women receiving estrogen (as hormonal contraception or replacement therapy) have an increased incidence of rash. Alternative forms of contraception may be needed. The Perinatal HIV Guidelines Working Group notes there is insufficient data to recommend use during pregnancy; however, if used, tipranavir must be given with low-dose ritonavir boosting. Healthcare providers are encouraged to enroll pregnant women exposed to antiretroviral medications in the Antiretroviral Pregnancy Registry (1-800-258-4263 or www.APRegistry.com). Healthcare providers caring for HIV-infected women and their infants may contact the National Perinatal HIV Hotline (888-448-8765) for clinical consultation.

Tirofiban (tye roe FYE ban)

U.S. Brand Names Aggrastat®

Index Terms MK383; Tirofiban Hydrochloride

Generic Availability (U.S.) No

Pharmacologic Category Antiplatelet Agent, Glycoprotein IIb/IIIa Inhibitor

Medication Safety Issues

Sound-alike/look-alike issues:

Aggrastat® may be confused with Aggrenox®, argatroban

High alert medication: The Institute for Safe Medication Practices (ISMP) includes this medication among its list of drugs which have a heightened risk of causing significant patient harm when used in error.

Pregnancy Risk Factor B

Lactation Excretion in breast milk unknown/contraindicated

Use Treatment of acute coronary syndrome (ie, unstable angina/non-ST-elevation myocardial infarction [UA/NSTEMI]) in combination with heparin

Unlabeled/Investigational Use To support PCI during ST-elevation myocardial infarction (STEMI) (administered at the time of primary PCI)

Mechanism of Action/Effect A reversible antagonist of fibrinogen binding to the GP IIb/IIIa receptor, the major platelet surface receptor involved in platelet aggregation. Platelet aggregation inhibition is reversible following cessation of the infusion.

Contraindications Hypersensitivity to tirofiban or any component of the formulation; active internal bleeding or a history of bleeding diathesis within the previous 30 days; history of intracranial hemorrhage, intracranial neoplasm, arteriovenous malformation, or aneurysm; history of thrombocytopenia following prior exposure; history of CVA within 30 days or any history of hemorrhagic stroke; major surgical procedure or severe physical trauma within the previous month; history, symptoms, or findings suggestive of aortic dissection; severe hypertension (systolic BP >180 mm Hg and/or diastolic BP >110 mm Hg); concomitant use of another parenteral GP IIb/IIIa inhibitor; acute pericarditis

Warnings/Precautions Bleeding is the most common complication encountered during this therapy; most major bleeding occurs at the arterial access site for cardiac catheterization. Caution in patients with platelets <150,000/mm^3; patients with hemorrhagic retinopathy; chronic dialysis patients; when used in combination with other drugs impacting on coagulation. Prior to pulling the sheath, heparin should be discontinued for 3-4 hours and ACT <180 seconds or aPTT <45 seconds. Use standard compression techniques after sheath removal. Watch the site closely afterwards for further bleeding. Sheath hemostasis should be achieved at least 4 hours before hospital discharge. Other trauma and vascular punctures should be minimized. Avoid obtaining vascular access through a noncompressible site (eg, subclavian or jugular vein). Patients with severe renal insufficiency require dosage reduction.

Drug Interactions

Avoid Concomitant Use There are no known interactions where it is recommended to avoid concomitant use.

Decreased Effect

The levels/effects of Tirofiban may be decreased by: Nonsteroidal Anti-Inflammatory Agents

Increased Effect/Toxicity

Tirofiban may increase the levels/effects of: Anticoagulants; Antiplatelet Agents; Collagenase (Systemic); Drotrecogin Alfa; Ibritumomab; Salicylates; Thrombolytic Agents; Tositumomab and Iodine I 131 Tositumomab

The levels/effects of Tirofiban may be increased by: Dasatinib; Glucosamine; Herbs (Anticoagulant/Antiplatelet Properties); Nonsteroidal Anti-Inflammatory Agents; Omega-3-Acid Ethyl Esters; Pentosan Polysulfate Sodium; Pentoxifylline; Prostacyclin Analogues

Adverse Reactions Bleeding is the major drug-related adverse effect. Patients received background treatment with aspirin and heparin. Major bleeding was reported in 1.4% to 2.2%; minor bleeding in 10.5% to 12%; transfusion was required in 4% to 4.3%.

>1% (nonbleeding adverse events):

Cardiovascular: Coronary artery dissection (5%), bradycardia (4%), edema (2%)

Central nervous system: Dizziness (3%), vasovagal reaction (2%), fever (>1%), headache (>1%)

Gastrointestinal: Nausea (>1%)

Genitourinary: Pelvic pain (6%)

Hematologic: Thrombocytopenia: <90,000/mm^3 (1.5%), <50,000/mm^3 (0.3%)

Neuromuscular & skeletal: Leg pain (3%)

Miscellaneous: Diaphoresis (2%)

Pharmacodynamics/Kinetics

Half-Life Elimination 2 hours

Metabolism Minimally hepatic

Excretion Urine (65%) and feces (25%) primarily as unchanged drug

Clearance: Elderly: Reduced by 19% to 26%

Available Dosage Forms

Infusion, premixed in NS [preservative free]:

Aggrastat®: 50 mcg/mL (250 mL)

Dosing

Adult & Geriatric

Unstable angina/non-ST-elevation myocardial infarction (UA/NSTEMI): I.V.: Initial rate of 0.4 mcg/kg/minute for 30 minutes and then continued at 0.1 mcg/kg/minute. Dosing should be continued through angiography and for 12-24 hours after angioplasty or atherectomy.

ST-elevation myocardial infarction (STEMI) undergoing percutaneous coronary intervention (PCI) (unlabeled use): Loading dose: 25 mcg/kg over 3 minutes at the time of PCI; Maintenance infusion: 0.15 mcg/kg/minute continued for up to 18 hours (Kushner, 2009)

Renal Impairment Cl_{cr} <30 mL/minute: Reduce dose to 50% of normal rate.

Administration

I.V. For unstable angina/non-ST-elevation MI (UA/NSTEMI), infuse loading dose over 30 minutes, followed by continuous infusion. When used during percutaneous coronary intervention (PCI), may administer loading dose over 3 minutes, followed by continuous infusion. Tirofiban injection must be diluted to a concentration of 50 mcg/mL (premixed solution does not require dilution). Unused solution should be discarded.

Stability

Storage Store at 25°C (77°F); do not freeze. Protect from light during storage.

Monitoring and Teaching Issues

Laboratory Monitoring Platelet count, persistent reductions <90,000/mm^3 may require interruption or discontinuation of infusion. Hemoglobin and hematocrit should be monitored prior to treatment, within 6 hours following loading infusion, and at least daily thereafter during therapy. Platelet count may need to be monitored earlier in patients who received prior glycoprotein IIb/IIa antagonists. Because tirofiban requires concurrent heparin therapy, aPTT levels should also be followed.

Physical Assessment Monitor vital signs prior to, during, and after therapy. Assess infusion insertion site during and after therapy. Monitor closely for bleeding and teach bleeding precautions.

Patient Education This medication can only be administered I.V. You will have a tendency to bleed easily during administration of this medication. If bleeding occurs, apply pressure to bleeding spot until bleeding stops completely. Report unusual bruising or bleeding (eg, blood in urine, stool, or vomitus; bleeding gums; vaginal bleeding; nosebleeds); unusual and persistent fever; dizziness or vision changes; back, leg, or pelvic pain; or persistent nausea or vomiting.

Geriatric Considerations Elderly patients receiving tirofiban with heparin or heparin alone had a higher incidence of bleeding in clinical trials. Caution must be used when using other drugs affecting hemostasis, which are commonly used in elderly.

◆ **Tirofiban Hydrochloride** *see* Tirofiban *on page 1774*

◆ **Tirosint®** *see* Levothyroxine *on page 1101*

TiZANidine (tye ZAN i deen)

U.S. Brand Names Zanaflex Capsules®; Zanaflex®

Index Terms Sirdalud®

Generic Availability (U.S.) Yes: Tablet

Pharmacologic Category Alpha$_2$-Adrenergic Agonist

Medication Safety Issues

Sound-alike/look-alike issues:

TiZANidine may be confused with tiaGABine

Zanaflex® may be confused with Xiaflex™

Zanaflex® capsules and Zanaflex® tablets (or generic tizanidine tablets) are not interchangeable

Pregnancy Risk Factor C

Lactation Excretion in breast milk unknown/not recommended

Use Skeletal muscle relaxant used for treatment of muscle spasticity

Unlabeled/Investigational Use Tension headaches, low back pain, and trigeminal neuralgia

Mechanism of Action/Effect Acts within CNS at the level of the spinal cord to reduce excitation of motor neurons, resulting in muscle relaxation

Contraindications Hypersensitivity to tizanidine or any component of the formulation; concomitant therapy with ciprofloxacin or fluvoxamine (potent CYP1A2 inhibitors)

Warnings/Precautions Significant hypotension (possibly with bradycardia or orthostatic hypotension) and sedation may occur; use caution in patients with cardiac disease or those at risk for severe hypotensive or sedative effects. Avoid concomitant administration with CYP1A2 inhibitors; increased tizanidine levels/effects (severe hypotension and sedation) may occur. These effects may also be increased with concomitant administration with other CNS depressants and/or antihypertensives; use caution. Elderly patients are at risk due to decreased clearance, particulary in elderly patients with renal insufficiency (Cl_{cr} <25 mL/minute) compared to healthy elderly subjects; this may lead to an increased risk of adverse effects and/or a longer duration of effects. Use caution in any patient with renal impairment; reduced initial doses recommended in patient with Cl_{cr} <25 mL/minute. Use with extreme caution or avoid in hepatic impairment due to extensive hepatic metabolism and potential hepatotoxicity; AST/ALT elevations (≥2 times baseline) and rarely hepatic failure have occurred; monitoring recommended.

Use has been associated with visual hallucinations or delusions, generally in first 6 weeks of therapy; use caution in patients with psychiatric disorders. Withdrawal resulting in rebound hypertension, tachycardia, and hypertonia may occur upon discontinuation; doses should be decreased slowly, particularly in patients receiving high doses for prolonged periods. Pharmacokinetics and bioequivalence between capsules and tablets altered by nonfasting vs fasting conditions. Limited data exists for chronic use of single doses >8 mg and multiple doses >24 mg/day.

Drug Interactions

Metabolism/Transport Effects Substrate of CYP1A2 (major)

Avoid Concomitant Use

Avoid concomitant use of TiZANidine with any of the following: Ciprofloxacin; Ciprofloxacin (Systemic); FluvoxaMINE; Iobenguane I 123

Decreased Effect

TiZANidine may decrease the levels/effects of: Iobenguane I 123

The levels/effects of TiZANidine may be decreased by: Antidepressants (Alpha2-Antagonist); Serotonin/Norepinephrine Reuptake Inhibitors; Tricyclic Antidepressants

Increased Effect/Toxicity

TiZANidine may increase the levels/effects of: ACE Inhibitors; Alcohol (Ethyl); CNS Depressants; Hypotensive Agents; Lisinopril; Methotrimeprazine

The levels/effects of TiZANidine may be increased by: Beta-Blockers; Ciprofloxacin; Ciprofloxacin (Systemic); Contraceptives (Estrogens); CYP1A2 Inhibitors (Moderate); CYP1A2 Inhibitors (Strong); Droperidol; FluvoxaMINE; MAO Inhibitors; Methotrimeprazine

Nutritional/Ethanol Interactions

Ethanol: Avoid ethanol (may increase CNS depression).

Food: The tablet and capsule dosage forms are not bioequivalent when administered with food. Food increases both the time to peak concentration and the extent of absorption for both the tablet and capsule. However, maximal concentrations of tizanidine achieved when administered with food were increased by 30% for the tablet, but decreased by 20% for the capsule. Under fed conditions, the capsule is approximately 80% bioavailable relative to the tablet.

Herb/Nutraceutical: Avoid valerian, St John's wort, kava kava, gotu kola (may increase CNS depression). Avoid black cohosh, California poppy, coleus, golden seal, hawthorn, mistletoe, periwinkle, quinine, shepherd's purse (may increase hypotensive effects).

Adverse Reactions Frequency percentages below reported during multiple-dose studies, unless specified otherwise.

>10%:

Cardiovascular: Hypotension (single-dose study with doses ≥8 mg: 16% to 33%)

Central nervous system: Somnolence (48%), dizziness (16%)

Gastrointestinal: Xerostomia (49%)

Neuromuscular & skeletal: Weakness (41%)

1% to 10%:

Cardiovascular: Bradycardia (single-dose study with doses ≥8 mg: 2% to 10%)

Central nervous system: Nervousness (3%), speech disorder (3%), visual hallucinations/delusions (3%; generally occurring in first 6 weeks of therapy), anxiety (1%), depression (1%), fever (1%)

Dermatologic: Rash (1%), skin ulcer (1%)

Gastrointestinal: Constipation (4%), vomiting (3%), abdominal pain (1%), diarrhea (1%), dyspepsia (1%)

Genitourinary: UTI (10%), urinary frequency (3%)
Hepatic: Liver enzymes increased (3% to 5%)
Neuromuscular & skeletal: Dyskinesia (3%), back pain (1%), myasthenia (1%), paresthesia (1%)
Ocular: Blurred vision (3%)
Respiratory: Pharyngitis (3%), rhinitis (3%)
Miscellaneous: Infection (6%), flu-like syndrome (3%), diaphoresis (1%)

Pharmacodynamics/Kinetics

Duration of Action 3-6 hours

Absorption Tablets and capsules are bioequivalent under fasting conditions, but not under nonfasting conditions.

Tablets administered with food: Peak plasma concentration is increased by ~30%; time to peak increased by 25 minutes; extent of absorption increased by ~30%.

Capsules administered with food: Peak plasma concentration decreased by 20%; time to peak increased by 2-3 hours; extent of absorption increased by ~10%.

Capsules opened and sprinkled on applesauce are not bioequivalent to administration of intact capsules under fasting conditions. Peak plasma concentration and AUC are increased by 15% to 20%.

Bioavailability ~40% (extensive first-pass metabolism)

Time to Peak

Fasting state: Capsule, tablet: 1 hour
Fed state: Capsule: 3-4 hours, Tablet: 1.5 hours

Protein Binding ~30%

Half-Life Elimination 2.5 hours

Metabolism Extensively hepatic

Excretion Urine (60%); feces (20%)

Available Dosage Forms

Capsule, oral:
Zanaflex Capsules®: 2 mg, 4 mg, 6 mg

Tablet, oral: 2 mg, 4 mg
Zanaflex®: 4 mg

Dosing

Adult Spasticity: Usual initial dose: 4 mg, may increase by 2-4 mg as needed for satisfactory reduction of muscle tone every 6-8 hours to a maximum of 3 doses in any 24 hour period
Range: 2-4 mg 3 times/day
Maximum: 36 mg/day

Geriatric No specific dosing guidelines exist; clearance is decreased; dose cautiously.

Renal Impairment Cl_{cr} <25 mL/minute: Use with caution; clearance reduced >50%. During initial dose titration, use reduced doses. If higher doses necessary, increase dose instead of increasing dosing frequency.

Hepatic Impairment Avoid use in hepatic impairment; if used, lowest possible dose should be used initially with close monitoring for adverse effects (eg, hypotension).

Administration

Oral Capsules may be opened and contents sprinkled on food; however, extent of absorption is increased up to 20% relative to administration of the capsule under fasted conditions.

Monitoring and Teaching Issues

Laboratory Monitoring Monitor liver function (aminotransferases) at baseline, 1, 3, 6 months and periodically thereafter; renal function

Physical Assessment May cause hypotension; monitor blood pressure periodically. Do not discontinue medication abruptly; can cause hypertension and tachycardia.

Patient Education If you miss a dose, take the missed dose as soon as possible if it is within an hour or so of the regular time. If not within an hour or so, skip the missed dose and go back to your regular dosing schedule. Do not double doses. Avoid alcohol. May cause dizziness, nervousness, insomnia, daytime drowsiness, postural hypotension, nausea, vomiting, dry mouth, mouth sores, or upset stomach. Report persistent dizziness or GI symptoms, chest pain or palpitations, CNS disturbances (delusions, confusion), muscle weakness or tremors, rash, or respiratory difficulty.

Dietary Considerations Administration with food compared to administration in the fasting state results in clinically-significant differences in absorption and other pharmacokinetic parameters. Patients should be consistent and should not switch administration of the tablets or the capsules between the fasting and nonfasting state. In addition, switching between the capsules and the tablets in the fed state will also result in significant differences. Opening capsule contents to sprinkle on applesauce compared to swallowing intact capsules whole will also result in significant absorption differences. Patients should be consistent with regards to administration.

Geriatric Considerations Since elderly commonly have renal function of Cl_{cr} <30 mL/minute, creatinine clearance should be estimated before dosing this medication. Low doses should be started initially because of the possibility of CNS effects.

◆ **TMC-114** *see* Darunavir *on page* 469
◆ **TMC125** *see* Etravirine *on page* 718
◆ **TMP** *see* Trimethoprim *on page* 1820
◆ **TMP-SMX** *see* Sulfamethoxazole and Trimethoprim *on page* 1686
◆ **TMP-SMZ** *see* Sulfamethoxazole and Trimethoprim *on page* 1686
◆ **TMX-67** *see* Febuxostat *on page* 737

◆ **TMZ** *see* Temozolomide *on page* 1721

◆ **TNKase®** *see* Tenecteplase *on page* 1726

◆ **TOBI®** *see* Tobramycin (Systemic, Oral Inhalation) *on page* 1778

Tobramycin (Systemic, Oral Inhalation) (toe bra MYE sin)

U.S. Brand Names TOBI®

Index Terms Tobramycin Sulfate

Generic Availability (U.S.) Yes: Excludes solution for nebulization

Pharmacologic Category Antibiotic, Aminoglycoside

Medication Safety Issues

Sound-alike/look-alike issues:

Tobramycin may be confused with Trobicin®, vancomycin

Nebcin® may be confused with Inapsine®, Naprosyn®, Nubain®

High alert medication: The Institute for Safe Medication Practices (ISMP) includes this medication (intrathecal administration) among its list of drug classes which have a heightened risk of causing significant patient harm when used in error.

Pregnancy Risk Factor D

Lactation Enters breast milk/not recommended

Use Treatment of documented or suspected infections caused by susceptible gram-negative bacilli, including *Pseudomonas aeruginosa*. Tobramycin solution for inhalation is indicated for the management of cystic fibrosis patients (>6 years of age) with *Pseudomonas aeruginosa*.

Mechanism of Action/Effect Interferes with bacterial protein synthesis, resulting in a defective bacteriocidal cell membrane

Contraindications Hypersensitivity to tobramycin, other aminoglycosides, or any component of the formulation; pregnancy

Warnings/Precautions [U.S. Boxed Warning]: Aminoglycosides may cause neurotoxicity and/or nephrotoxicity; usual risk factors include pre-existing renal impairment, concomitant neuro-/nephrotoxic medications, advanced age, and dehydration. Ototoxicity may be directly proportional to the amount of drug given and the duration of treatment; tinnitus or vertigo are indications of vestibular injury and impending hearing loss; renal damage is usually reversible. May cause neuromuscular blockade and respiratory paralysis, especially when given soon after anesthesia or muscle relaxants.

Not intended for long-term therapy due to toxic hazards associated with extended administration; use caution in pre-existing renal insufficiency, vestibular or cochlear impairment, myasthenia gravis, hypocalcemia, and conditions which depress neuromuscular transmission. Dosage modification required in patients with impaired renal function. Prolonged use may result in fungal or bacterial superinfection, including *C. difficile*-associated diarrhea (CDAD) and pseudomembranous colitis; CDAD has been observed >2 months postantibiotic treatment. Solution may contain sodium metabisulfate; use caution in patients with sulfite allergy.

Drug Interactions

Avoid Concomitant Use

Avoid concomitant use of Tobramycin (Systemic, Oral Inhalation) with any of the following: BCG; Gallium Nitrate

Decreased Effect

Tobramycin (Systemic, Oral Inhalation) may decrease the levels/effects of: BCG; Typhoid Vaccine

The levels/effects of Tobramycin (Systemic, Oral Inhalation) may be decreased by: Penicillins

Increased Effect/Toxicity

Tobramycin (Systemic, Oral Inhalation) may increase the levels/effects of: AbobotulinumtoxinA; Bisphosphonate Derivatives; CARBOplatin; Colistimethate; CycloSPORINE; CycloSPORINE (Systemic); Gallium Nitrate; Neuromuscular-Blocking Agents; OnabotulinumtoxinA; RimabotulinumtoxinB

The levels/effects of Tobramycin (Systemic, Oral Inhalation) may be increased by: Amphotericin B; Capreomycin; CISplatin; Loop Diuretics; Nonsteroidal Anti-Inflammatory Agents; Vancomycin

Lab Interactions Some penicillin derivatives may accelerate the degradation of aminoglycosides *in vitro*, leading to a potential underestimation of aminoglycoside serum concentration.

Adverse Reactions

Injection: Frequency not defined:

Central nervous system: Confusion, disorientation, dizziness, fever, headache, lethargy, vertigo

Dermatologic: Exfoliative dermatitis, itching, rash, urticaria

Endocrine & metabolic: Serum calcium, magnesium, potassium, and/or sodium decreased

Gastrointestinal: Diarrhea, nausea, vomiting

Hematologic: Anemia, eosinophilia, granulocytopenia, leukocytosis, leukopenia, thrombocytopenia

Hepatic: ALT increased, AST increased, bilirubin increased, LDH increased

Local: Pain at the injection site

Otic: Hearing loss, tinnitus, ototoxicity (auditory), ototoxicity (vestibular), roaring in the ears

Renal: BUN increased, cylindruria, serum creatinine increased, oliguria, proteinuria

Inhalation:

>10%:

Gastrointestinal: Sputum discoloration (21%)

Respiratory: Voice alteration (13%)

1% to 10%:

Central nervous system: Malaise (6%)

Otic: Tinnitus (3%)

Pharmacodynamics/Kinetics

Absorption

Oral: Poorly absorbed

I.M.: Rapid and complete

Inhalation: Peak serum concentrations are ~1 mcg/mL following a 300 mg dose

Time to Peak Serum: I.M.: 30-60 minutes; I.V.: ~30 minutes

Protein Binding <30%

Half-Life Elimination

Neonates: ≤1200 g: 11 hours; >1200 g: 2-9 hours

Adults: 2-3 hours; directly dependent upon glomerular filtration rate

Adults with impaired renal function: 5-70 hours

Excretion Normal renal function: Urine (~90% to 95%) within 24 hours

Available Dosage Forms

Infusion, premixed in NS: 60 mg (50 mL); 80 mg (100 mL)

Injection, powder for reconstitution: 1.2 g

Injection, solution: 10 mg/mL (2 mL, 8 mL); 40 mg/mL (2 mL, 30 mL, 50 mL)

Solution, for nebulization [preservative free]:

TOBI®: 300 mg/5 mL (56s)

Dosing

Adult Note: Individualization is **critical** because of the low therapeutic index.

Use of ideal body weight (IBW) for determining the mg/kg/dose appears to be more accurate than dosing on the basis of total body weight (TBW). In morbid obesity, dosage requirement may best be estimated using a dosing weight of IBW + 0.4 (TBW - IBW).

Initial and periodic plasma drug levels (eg, peak and trough with conventional dosing) should be determined, particularly in critically-ill patients with serious infections or in disease states known to significantly alter aminoglycoside pharmacokinetics (eg, cystic fibrosis, burns, or major surgery).

Severe life-threatening infections: I.M., I.V.:

Conventional: 1-2.5 mg/kg/dose every 8-12 hours; to ensure adequate peak concentrations early in therapy, higher initial dosage may be considered in selected patients when extracellular water is increased (edema, septic shock, postsurgical, and/or trauma)

Once-daily: 4-7 mg/kg/dose once daily; some clinicians recommend this approach for all patients with normal renal function; this dose is at least as efficacious with similar, if not less, toxicity than conventional dosing.

Brucellosis: I.M., I.V.: 240 mg (I.M.) daily or 5 mg/kg (I.V.) daily for 7 days; either regimen recommended in combination with doxycycline

Cholangitis: I.M., I.V.: 4-6 mg/kg once daily with ampicillin

CNS shunt infection: Intrathecal (unlabeled route): 5-20 mg/day (Tunkel, 2004)

Cystic fibrosis: Inhalation (TOBI®): 300 mg every 12 hours (do not administer doses <6 hours apart); administer in repeated cycles of 28 days on drug followed by 28 days off drug.

Diverticulitis, complicated: I.M., I.V.: 1.5-2 mg/kg every 8 hours (with ampicillin and metronidazole)

Infective endocarditis or synergy (for gram-positive infections): I.M., I.V.: 1 mg/kg every 8 hours (with ampicillin)

Meningitis *(Enterococcus or Pseudomonas aeruginosa)*: I.V.: 5 mg/kg/day in divided doses every 8 hours (administered with another bacteriocidal drug)

Pelvic inflammatory disease: I.M., I.V.: Loading dose: 2 mg/kg, then 1.5 mg/kg every 8 hours **or** 4.5 mg/kg once daily

Plague *(Yersinia pestis)*: I.M., I.V.: Treatment: 5 mg/kg/day, followed by postexposure prophylaxis with doxycycline

Pneumonia, hospital- or ventilator-associated: I.M., I.V.: 7 mg/kg/day (with antipseudomonal beta-lactam or carbapenem)

Prophylaxis against endocarditis (dental, oral, upper respiratory procedures, GI/GU procedures): I.M., I.V.: 1.5 mg/kg with ampicillin (50 mg/kg) 30 minutes prior to procedure. **Note:** AHA guidelines now recommend prophylaxis only in patients undergoing invasive procedures and in whom underlying cardiac conditions may predispose to a higher risk of adverse outcomes should infection occur. As of April 2007, routine prophylaxis no longer recommended by the AHA.

Tularemia: I.M., I.V.: 5 mg/kg/day divided every 8 hours for 1-2 weeks

Urinary tract infection: I.M., I.V.: 1.5 mg/kg/dose every 8 hours

Geriatric Dosage should be based on an estimate of ideal body weight.

I.M., I.V.: 1.5-5 mg/kg/day in 1-2 divided doses

I.V.: Once daily or extended interval: 5-7 mg/kg/dose given every 24, 36, or 48 hours based on creatinine clearance

Pediatric Individualization is **critical** because of the low therapeutic index

Use of ideal body weight (IBW) for determining the mg/kg/dose appears to be more accurate than dosing on the basis of total body weight (TBW). In morbid obesity, dosage requirement may best be estimated using a dosing weight of IBW + 0.4 (TBW - IBW).

Usual dosage range: I.M., I.V.:
Infants and Children <5 years: 2.5 mg/kg/dose every 8 hours
Children >5 years: 2-2.5 mg/kg/dose every 8 hours

CNS shunt infection: Intrathecal (unlabeled route): Refer to adult dosing.

Cystic fibrosis:
I.M., I.V.: 2.5-3.3 mg/kg every 6-8 hours. **Note:** Some patients may require larger or more frequent doses if serum levels document the need (eg, cystic fibrosis or febrile granulocytopenic patients).
Inhalation: TOBI®: Children ≥6 years: Refer to adult dosing.

Meningitis: Neonates: I.M., I.V.:
0-7 days: <2000 g: 2.5 mg/kg every 18-24 hours; >2000 g: 2.5 mg/kg every 12 hours
8-28 days: <2000 g: 2.5 mg/kg every 8-12 hours; >2000 g: 2.5 mg/kg every 8 hours

Renal Impairment I.M., I.V.:

Conventional dosing:
Cl_{cr} ≥60 mL/minute: Administer every 8 hours.
Cl_{cr} 40-60 mL/minute: Administer every 12 hours.
Cl_{cr} 20-40 mL/minute: Administer every 24 hours.
Cl_{cr} 10-20 mL/minute: Administer every 48 hours.
Cl_{cr} <10 mL/minute: Administer every 72 hours.

High-dose therapy: Interval may be extended (eg, every 48 hours) in patients with moderate renal impairment (Cl_{cr} 30-59 mL/minute) and/or adjusted based on serum level determinations.

Dialyzable; 30% removal of aminoglycosides occurs during 4 hours of HD - administer dose after dialysis and follow levels.

Continuous arteriovenous or venovenous hemofiltration: Dose as for Cl_{cr} of 10-40 mL/minute and follow levels.

Administration via CAPD fluid:
Gram-negative infection: 4-8 mg/L (4-8 mcg/mL) of CAPD fluid
Gram-positive infection (ie, synergy): 3-4 mg/L (3-4 mcg/mL) of CAPD fluid

Administration IVPB/I.M.: Dose as for Cl_{cr} <10 mL/minute and follow levels.

Hepatic Impairment Monitor plasma concentrations.

Administration

I.V. Infuse over 30-60 minutes.

Some penicillins (eg, carbenicillin, ticarcillin, and piperacillin) have been shown to inactivate aminoglycosides *in vitro*. This has been observed to a greater extent with tobramycin and gentamicin, while amikacin has shown greater stability against inactivation. Concurrent use of these agents may pose a risk of reduced antibacterial efficacy *in vivo*, particularly in the setting of profound renal impairment. However, definitive clinical evidence is lacking. If combination penicillin/aminoglycoside therapy is desired in a patient with renal dysfunction, separation of doses (if feasible), and routine monitoring of aminoglycoside levels, CBC, and clinical response should be considered.

Inhalation TOBI®: To be inhaled over ~15 minutes using a handheld nebulizer (PARI-LC PLUS™). If multiple different nebulizer treatments are required, administer bronchodilator first, followed by chest physiotherapy, any other nebulized medications, and then TOBI® last. Do not mix with other nebulizer medications.

Stability

Reconstitution Dilute in 50-100 mL NS, D_5W for I.V. infusion.

Storage

Injection: Stable at room temperature both as the clear, colorless solution and as the dry powder. Reconstituted solutions remain stable for 24 hours at room temperature and 96 hours when refrigerated.

Solution, for inhalation (TOBI®): Store under refrigeration at 2°C to 8°C (36°F to 46°F). May be stored in foil pouch at room temperature of 25°C (77°F) for up to 28 days. Avoid intense light. Solution may darken over time; however, do not use if cloudy or contains particles.

Monitoring and Teaching Issues

Laboratory Monitoring Urinalysis, BUN, serum creatinine, plasma tobramycin levels (as appropriate to dosing method). Peak levels are drawn 30 minutes after the end of a 30-minute infusion or 1 hour after initiation of infusion or I.M. injection. The trough is drawn just before the next dose. Levels are typically obtained after the third dose in conventional dosing. Perform culture and sensitivity studies prior to initiating therapy to determine the causative organism and its susceptibility to tobramycin. Some penicillin derivatives may accelerate the degradation of aminoglycosides.

Physical Assessment Assess patient's hearing level before, during, and following therapy. Monitor for ototoxicity and nephrotoxicity at beginning of therapy and throughout.

Patient Education Maintain adequate hydration unless instructed to restrict fluid intake. Report decreased urine output, swelling of extremities, respiratory difficulty, vaginal itching or discharge, rash, diarrhea, oral thrush, dizziness, change in hearing acuity or ringing in ears, or worsening of condition.

Dietary Considerations May require supplementation of calcium, magnesium, potassium.

Geriatric Considerations The aminoglycosides are an important therapeutic intervention for susceptible organisms and as empiric therapy in seriously ill patients. Their use is not without risk of toxicity; however, these risks can be minimized if initial dosing is adjusted for estimated renal function and appropriate monitoring is performed. High dose, once daily aminoglycosides have been advocated as an alternative to traditional dosing regimens. Once daily or extended interval dosing is as effective and may be safer than traditional dosing. Interval must be adjusted for renal function.

Breast-Feeding Considerations Tobramycin is excreted into breast milk and breast-feeding is not recommended by the manufacturer; however, tobramycin is not well absorbed when taken orally. This limited oral absorption may minimize exposure to the nursing infant. Nondose-related effects could include modification of bowel flora.

Pregnancy Considerations [U.S. Boxed Warning]: Aminoglycosides may cause fetal harm if administered to a pregnant woman. There are several reports of total irreversible bilateral congenital deafness in children whose mothers received another aminoglycoside (streptomycin) during pregnancy; therefore, tobramycin is classified as pregnancy category D. Tobramycin crosses the placenta and produces detectable serum levels in the fetus. Although serious side effects to the fetus have not been reported following maternal use of tobramycin, a potential for harm exists.

Due to pregnancy-induced physiologic changes, some pharmacokinetic parameters of tobramycin may be altered. Pregnant women have an average-to-larger volume of distribution which may result in lower serum peak levels than for the same dose in nonpregnant women. Serum half-life is also shorter.

Additional Information Once-daily dosing: Higher peak serum drug concentration to MIC ratios, demonstrated aminoglycoside postantibiotic effect, decreased renal cortex drug uptake, and improved cost-time efficiency are supportive reasons for the use of once daily dosing regimens for aminoglycosides. Current research indicates these regimens to be as effective for non-life-threatening infections, with no higher incidence of nephrotoxicity, than those requiring multiple daily doses. Doses are determined by calculating the entire day's dose via usual multiple dose calculation techniques and administering this quantity as a single dose. Doses are then adjusted to maintain mean serum concentrations above the MIC(s) of the causative organism(s). (Example: 2.5-5 mg/kg as a single dose; expected Cp_{max}: 10-20 mcg/mL and Cp_{min}: <1 mcg/mL). Further research is needed for universal recommendation in all patient populations and gram-negative disease; exceptions may include those with known high clearance (eg, children, patients with cystic fibrosis, or burns who may require shorter dosage intervals) and patients with renal function impairment for whom longer than conventional dosage intervals are usually required.

Related Information

Antimicrobial Drugs of Choice *on page 2008*
Peak and Trough Guidelines *on page 1958*

◆ **Tobramycin and Loteprednol Etabonate** *see* Loteprednol and Tobramycin *on page 1137*
◆ **Tobramycin Sulfate** *see* Tobramycin (Systemic, Oral Inhalation) *on page 1778*
◆ **Tofranil®** *see* Imipramine *on page 958*
◆ **Tofranil-PM®** *see* Imipramine *on page 958*

Tolcapone (TOLE ka pone)

U.S. Brand Names Tasmar®

Generic Availability (U.S.) No

Pharmacologic Category Anti-Parkinson's Agent, COMT Inhibitor

Prescribing and Access Restrictions A patient signed consent form acknowledging the risks of hepatic injury should be obtained by the treating physician.

Pregnancy Risk Factor C

Lactation Excretion in breast milk unknown/not recommended

Use Adjunct to levodopa and carbidopa for the treatment of signs and symptoms of idiopathic Parkinson's disease in patients with motor fluctuations not responsive to other therapies

Mechanism of Action/Effect Tolcapone is a selective and reversible inhibitor of catechol-o-methyltransferase (COMT) which leads to more sustained blood levels of levodopa.

Contraindications Hypersensitivity to tolcapone or any component of the formulation; history of liver disease or tolcapone-induced hepatocellular injury; nontraumatic rhabdomyolysis or hyperpyrexia and confusion

Warnings/Precautions [U.S. Boxed Warning]: Due to reports of fatal liver injury associated with use of this drug, the manufacturer is advising that tolcapone be reserved for patients who are experiencing inadequate symptom control or who are not appropriate candidates for other available treatments. Patients must provide written consent acknowledging the risks of hepatic injury. Liver disease should be excluded prior to initiation; laboratory monitoring is recommended. Discontinue if signs and/or symptoms of hepatic injury are noted (eg, transaminases >2 times upper limit of normal) or if clinical improvement is not evident after 3 weeks of therapy. Use with caution in patients with pre-existing dyskinesias; exacerbation of pre-existing dyskinesia and severe rhabdomyolysis has been reported. Levodopa dosage reduction may be required, particularly in patients with levodopa dosages >600 mg daily or with moderate-to-severe dyskinesia prior to initiation.

May cause orthostatic hypotension and syncope; Parkinson's disease patients appear to have an impaired capacity to respond to a postural challenge; use with caution in patients at risk of hypotension (such as those receiving antihypertensive drugs) or where transient hypotensive episodes would be poorly tolerated (cardiovascular disease or cerebrovascular disease). Parkinson's patients being treated with dopaminergic agonists ordinarily require careful monitoring for signs and symptoms of postural hypotension, especially during dose escalation, and should be informed of this risk. May cause hallucinations, which may improve with reduction in levodopa therapy. Use with caution in patients with lower gastrointestinal disease or an increased risk of dehydration; tolcapone has been associated with delayed development of diarrhea (onset after 2-12 weeks).

Tolcapone, in conjunction with other drug therapy that alters brain biogenic amine concentrations (eg, MAO inhibitors, SSRIs), has been associated with a syndrome resembling neuroleptic malignant syndrome (hyperpyrexia and confusion - some fatal) on abrupt withdrawal or dosage reduction. Concomitant use of tolcapone and nonselective MAO inhibitors should be avoided. Selegiline is a selective MAO type B inhibitor (when given orally at ≤10 mg/day) and can be taken with tolcapone. Dopaminergic agents have been associated with compulsive behaviors and/or loss of impulse control, which has manifested as pathological gambling, libido increases (hypersexuality), and/or binge eating. Causality has not been established, and controversy exists as to whether this phenomenon is related to the underlying disease, prior behaviors/addictions and/or drug therapy. Dose reduction or discontinuation of therapy has been reported to reverse these behaviors in some, but not all cases. Risk for melanoma development is increased in Parkinson's disease patients; drug causation or factors contributing to risk have not been established. Patients should be monitored closely and periodic skin examinations should be performed. Dopaminergic agents from the ergot class have also been associated with fibrotic complications, such as retroperitoneal fibrosis, pulmonary infiltrates or effusion and pleural thickening. It is unknown whether non-ergot, pro-dopaminergic agents like tolcapone confer this risk. Use caution in patients with hepatic impairment or severe renal impairment.

Drug Interactions

Metabolism/Transport Effects Inhibits CYP2C9 (weak)

Avoid Concomitant Use There are no known interactions where it is recommended to avoid concomitant use.

Decreased Effect There are no known significant interactions involving a decrease in effect.

Increased Effect/Toxicity

Tolcapone may increase the levels/effects of: Alcohol (Ethyl); CNS Depressants; COMT Substrates; MAO Inhibitors; Methotrimeprazine

The levels/effects of Tolcapone may be increased by: Droperidol; MAO Inhibitors; Methotrimeprazine

Nutritional/Ethanol Interactions

Ethanol: Avoid ethanol (may increase CNS depression).

Food: Tolcapone, taken with food within 1 hour before or 2 hours after the dose, decreases bioavailability by 10% to 20%.

Avoid valerian, St John's wort, kava kava, gotu kola (may increase CNS depression).

Adverse Reactions

>10%:

Cardiovascular: Orthostatic hypotension (17%)

Central nervous system: Somnolence (14% to 32%), sleep disorder (24% to 25%), hallucinations (8% to 24%), excessive dreaming (16% to 21%), dizziness (6% to 13%), headache (10% to 11%), confusion (10% to 11%)

Gastrointestinal: Nausea (28% to 50%), diarrhea (16% to 34%; approximately 3% to 4% severe), anorexia (19% to 23%)

Neuromuscular & skeletal: Dyskinesia (42% to 51%), dystonia (19% to 22%), muscle cramps (17% to 18%)

1% to 10%:

Cardiovascular: Syncope (4% to 5%), chest pain (1% to 3%), hypotension (2%), palpitation

Central nervous system: Fatigue (3% to 7%), loss of balance (2% to 3%), agitation (1%), euphoria (1%), hyperactivity (1%), malaise (1%), panic reaction (1%), irritability (1%), mental deficiency (1%), fever (1%), depression, hypoesthesia, tremor, speech disorder, vertigo, emotional lability, hyperkinesia

Dermatologic: Alopecia (1%), bleeding (1%), tumor (1%), rash

Gastrointestinal: Vomiting (8% to 10%), constipation (6% to 8%), xerostomia (5% to 6%), abdominal pain (5% to 6%), dyspepsia (3% to 4%), flatulence (2% to 4%), tooth disorder

Genitourinary: UTI (5%), hematuria (4% to 5%), urine discoloration (2% to 3%), urination disorder (1% to 2%), uterine tumor (1%), incontinence, impotence

Hepatic: Transaminases increased (1% to 3%; 3 times ULN, usually with first 6 months of therapy)

Neuromuscular & skeletal: Paresthesia (1% to 3%), hyper-/hypokinesia (1% to 3%), arthritis (1% to 2%), neck pain (2%), stiffness (2%), myalgia, rhabdomyolysis

Ocular: Cataract (1%), eye inflammation (1%)

Otic: Tinnitus

Respiratory: Upper respiratory infection (5% to 7%), dyspnea (3%), sinus congestion (1% to 2%), bronchitis, pharyngitis

Miscellaneous: Diaphoresis (4% to 7%), influenza (3% to 4%), burning (1% to 2%), flank pain, injury, infection

Pharmacodynamics/Kinetics

Absorption Rapid

Bioavailability 65%

Time to Peak ~2 hours

Protein Binding >99.0%

Half-Life Elimination 2-3 hours

Metabolism Hepatic, via glucuronidation, to inactive metabolite (>99%)

Excretion Urine (60% as metabolites; 0.5% as unchanged drug); feces (40%)

Available Dosage Forms

Tablet, oral:

Tasmar®: 100 mg

Dosing

Adult & Geriatric Note: If clinical improvement is not observed after 3 weeks of therapy (regardless of dose), tolcapone treatment should be discontinued.

Parkinson's Disease: Oral: Initial: 100 mg 3 times/day; may increase as tolerated to 200 mg 3 times/day. **Note:** Levodopa dose may need to be decreased upon initiation of tolcapone (average reduction in clinical trials was 30%). As many as 70% of patients receiving levodopa doses >600 mg daily required levodopa dosage reduction in clinical trials. Patients with moderate-to-severe dyskinesia prior to initiation are also more likely to require dosage reduction.

Renal Impairment No adjustment necessary for mild-moderate impairment. Use caution with severe impairment; no safety information available in patients with Cl_{cr} <25 mL/minute.

Hepatic Impairment Do not use. Discontinue immediately if signs/symptoms of hepatic impairment develop.

Administration

Oral May be administered without regard to meals. In clinical studies, the first dose of the day was administered with carbidopa/levodopa, and the subsequent doses were administered 6 hours and 12 hours later.

Stability

Storage Store at 20°C to 25°C (68°F to 77°F).

Monitoring and Teaching Issues

Laboratory Monitoring Liver enzymes at baseline and then every 2-4 weeks for the first 6 months of therapy; thereafter, periodic monitoring should be conducted as deemed clinically relevant. If the dose is increased to 200 mg 3 times/day, reinitiate LFT monitoring every 2-4 weeks for 6 months, and then resume periodic monitoring. Discontinue therapy if the ALT or AST exceeds 2 times the upper limit of normal or if the clinical signs and symptoms suggest the onset of liver failure.

Physical Assessment Assess therapeutic effectiveness (eg, mental status and involuntary movements). Monitor for CNS depression. Monitor blood pressure.

Patient Education May be prescribed in conjunction with levodopa/carbidopa. Therapeutic effects may take several weeks or months to achieve and you may need frequent monitoring during first weeks of therapy. Best to take 2 hours before or after a meal; however, may be taken with meals if GI upset occurs. Take at the same time each day. Maintain adequate hydration unless instructed to restrict fluid intake. Do not use alcohol and prescription or OTC sedatives or CNS depressants without consulting prescriber. Urine or perspiration may appear darker. You may experience drowsiness, dizziness, confusion, vision changes, orthostatic hypotension, increased susceptibility to heat stroke, decreased perspiration, constipation, dry skin or nasal passages, nausea, vomiting, loss of appetite, or stomach discomfort. Report unresolved constipation or vomiting; chest pain or irregular heartbeat; respiratory difficulty; acute headache or dizziness; CNS changes (hallucination, loss of memory, nervousness, etc); painful or difficult urination; unusual muscle cramping or pain; yellowing of skin or eyes; easy bruising or bleeding; dry, colored stools; abdominal pain or blood in stool; increased muscle spasticity, rigidity, or involuntary movements; skin rash, persistent itching, changes in the appearance of skin moles, or other unusual skin changes; or significant worsening of condition.

Dietary Considerations May be taken without regard to meals.

Geriatric Considerations No specific data in elderly patients, but based on the pharmacokinetic profile, no dosage adjustment appears necessary.

Pregnancy Considerations Tolcapone may be teratogenic based on animal studies. There are no adequate and well-controlled studies in pregnant women. Use only if benefit outweighs risk.

Tolterodine (tole TER oh deen)

U.S. Brand Names Detrol®; Detrol® LA

Index Terms Tolterodine Tartrate

Generic Availability (U.S.) No

Pharmacologic Category Anticholinergic Agent

Medication Safety Issues

Sound-alike/look-alike issues:

Tolterodine may be confused with fesoterodine

Detrol® may be confused with Ditropan

Pregnancy Risk Factor C

Lactation Excretion in breast milk unknown/not recommended

Use Treatment of patients with an overactive bladder with symptoms of urinary frequency, urgency, or urge incontinence

Mechanism of Action/Effect Antagonizes muscarinic receptors of the urinary bladder resulting in decreased bladder pressure and contraction.

Contraindications Hypersensitivity to tolterodine or any component of the formulation; urinary retention; gastric retention; uncontrolled narrow-angle glaucoma

Warnings/Precautions May cause drowsiness and/or blurred vision, which may impair physical or mental abilities; patients must be cautioned about performing tasks which require mental alertness (eg, operating machinery or driving). Use with caution in patients with bladder flow obstruction, may increase the risk of urinary retention. Use with caution in patients with gastrointestinal obstructive disorders (ie, pyloric stenosis), may increase the risk of gastric retention. Use with caution in patients with myasthenia gravis and controlled (treated) narrow-angle glaucoma; metabolized in the liver and excreted in the urine and feces, dosage adjustment is required for patients with renal or hepatic impairment. Tolterodine has been associated with QT_c prolongation at high (supratherapeutic) doses. The manufacturer recommends caution in patients with congenital prolonged QT or in patients receiving concurrent therapy with QT_c-prolonging drugs (class Ia or III antiarrhythmics). However, the mean change in QT_c even at supratherapeutic dosages was less than 15 msec. Individuals who are CYP2D6 poor metabolizers or in the presence of inhibitors of CYP2D6 and CYP3A4 may be more likely to exhibit prolongation. Dosage adjustment is recommended in patients receiving CYP3A4 inhibitors (a lower dose of tolterodine is recommended).

Drug Interactions

Metabolism/Transport Effects Substrate of CYP2C9 (minor), 2C19 (minor), 2D6 (major), 3A4 (major)

Avoid Concomitant Use There are no known interactions where it is recommended to avoid concomitant use.

Decreased Effect

Tolterodine may decrease the levels/effects of: Acetylcholinesterase Inhibitors (Central); Secretin

The levels/effects of Tolterodine may be decreased by: Acetylcholinesterase Inhibitors (Central); CYP3A4 Inducers (Strong); Deferasirox; Herbs (CYP3A4 Inducers); Peginterferon Alfa-2b

Increased Effect/Toxicity

Tolterodine may increase the levels/effects of: AbobotulinumtoxinA; Anticholinergics; Cannabinoids; OnabotulinumtoxinA; Potassium Chloride; RimabotulinumtoxinB; Warfarin

The levels/effects of Tolterodine may be increased by: Antifungal Agents (Azole Derivatives, Systemic); Conivaptan; CYP2D6 Inhibitors (Moderate); CYP2D6 Inhibitors (Strong); CYP3A4 Inhibitors (Moderate); CYP3A4 Inhibitors (Strong); Darunavir; Dasatinib; Fluconazole; Pramlintide; VinBLAStine

Nutritional/Ethanol Interactions

Food: Increases bioavailability (~53% increase) of tolterodine tablets (dose adjustment not necessary); does not affect the pharmacokinetics of tolterodine extended release capsules. As a CYP3A4 inhibitor, grapefruit juice may increase the serum level and/or toxicity of tolterodine, but unlikely secondary to high oral bioavailability.

Herb/Nutraceutical: St John's wort (*Hypericum*) appears to induce CYP3A enzymes.

Adverse Reactions As reported with immediate release tablet, unless otherwise specified

>10%: Gastrointestinal: Dry mouth (35%; extended release capsules 23%)

1% to 10%:

Cardiovascular: Chest pain (2%)

Central nervous system: Headache (7%; extended release capsules 6%), somnolence (3%; extended release capsules 3%), fatigue (4%; extended release capsules 2%), dizziness (5%; extended release capsules 2%), anxiety (extended release capsules 1%)

Dermatologic: Dry skin (1%)

Gastrointestinal: Abdominal pain (5%; extended release capsules 4%), constipation (7%; extended release capsules 6%), dyspepsia (4%; extended release capsules 3%), diarrhea (4%), weight gain (1%)

Genitourinary: Dysuria (2%; extended release capsules 1%)

Neuromuscular & skeletal: Arthralgia (2%)

Ocular: Abnormal vision (2%; extended release capsules 1%), dry eyes (3%; extended release capsules 3%)

Respiratory: Bronchitis (2%), sinusitis (extended release capsules 2%)

Miscellaneous: Flu-like syndrome (3%), infection (1%)

Pharmacodynamics/Kinetics

Absorption Immediate release tablet: Rapid; ≥77%

Bioavailability Immediate release tablet: Increased 53% with food

Time to Peak Immediate release tablet: 1-2 hours; Extended release tablet: 2-6 hours

Protein Binding >96% (primarily to $alpha_1$-acid glycoprotein)

Half-Life Elimination

Immediate release tablet: Extensive metabolizers: ~2 hours; Poor metabolizers: ~10 hours

Extended release capsule: Extensive metabolizers: ~7 hours; Poor metabolizers: ~18 hours

Metabolism Extensively hepatic, primarily via CYP2D6 to 5-hydroxymethyltolterodine (active) and 3A4 usually (minor pathway). In patients with a genetic deficiency of CYP2D6, metabolism via 3A4 predominates.

Excretion Urine (77%); feces (17%); primarily as metabolites (<1% unchanged drug) of which the active 5-hydroxymethyl metabolite accounts for 5% to 14% (<1% in poor metabolizers); as unchanged drug (<1%; <2.5% in poor metabolizers)

Available Dosage Forms

Capsule, extended release, oral:

Detrol® LA: 2 mg, 4 mg

Tablet, oral:

Detrol®: 1 mg, 2 mg

Dosing

Adult & Geriatric Treatment of overactive bladder: Oral:

Immediate release tablet: 2 mg twice daily; the dose may be lowered to 1 mg twice daily based on individual response and tolerability

Dosing adjustment in patients concurrently taking CYP3A4 inhibitors: 1 mg twice daily

Extended release capsule: 4 mg once a day; dose may be lowered to 2 mg daily based on individual response and tolerability

Dosing adjustment in patients concurrently taking CYP3A4 inhibitors: 2 mg daily

Renal Impairment Use with caution (studies conducted in patients with Cl_{cr} 10-30 mL/minute):

Immediate release tablet: 1 mg twice daily

Extended release capsule: 2 mg daily

Hepatic Impairment

Immediate release tablet: 1 mg twice daily

Extended release capsule: 2 mg daily

Administration

Oral Extended release capsule: Swallow whole; do not crush, chew, or open

Stability

Storage Store at 25°C (77°F); excursions permitted to 15°C to 30°C (59°F to 86°F). Protect from light.

Monitoring and Teaching Issues

Laboratory Monitoring Renal function (BUN, creatinine); hepatic function

Patient Education Take as directed. Do not break, crush, or chew extended release medication. May cause headache, dry mouth, dizziness, nervousness, sleepiness, abdominal discomfort, diarrhea, constipation, nausea, or vomiting. Report back pain, muscle spasms, alteration in gait, or numbness of extremities; unresolved or persistent constipation, diarrhea, or vomiting; or symptoms of upper respiratory infection or flu. Report immediately any chest pain or palpitations, difficulty urinating, or pain on urination.

Geriatric Considerations No difference in safety has been noted between elderly and younger patients, therefore, no dosage adjustment is recommended.

Pregnancy Considerations Teratogenic effects were observed in some animal studies. There are no adequate and well-controlled studies in pregnant women. Use during pregnancy only if the potential benefit to the mother outweighs the possible risk to the fetus.

Related Information

Pharmacotherapy of Urinary Incontinence *on page* 2071

◆ **Tolterodine Tartrate** *see* Tolterodine *on page* 1783

Tolvaptan (tol VAP tan)

U.S. Brand Names Samsca™

Index Terms OPC-41061

Generic Availability (U.S.) No

Pharmacologic Category Vasopressin Antagonist

Medication Guide Available Yes

Pregnancy Risk Factor C

Lactation Excretion in breast milk unknown/use caution

Use Treatment of clinically significant hypervolemic or euvolemic hyponatremia (associated with heart failure, cirrhosis or SIADH) with either a serum sodium <125 mEq/L or less marked hyponatremia that is symptomatic and resistant to fluid restriction

Mechanism of Action/Effect Tolvaptan blocks the antidiuretic action of arginine vasopressin in the kidney, leading to the excretion of free water without loss of serum sodium.

Contraindications Hypovolemic hyponatremia; urgent need to raise serum sodium acutely; use in patients unable to sense or appropriately respond to thirst; anuria; concurrent use with strong CYP3A inhibitors (eg, ketoconazole, itraconazole, ritonavir, indinavir, nelfinavir, saquinavir, nefazodone, telithromycin, clarithromycin)

Warnings/Precautions [U.S. Boxed Warning]: Tolvaptan should be initiated and reinitiated in patients only in a hospital where serum sodium can be closely monitored. Too rapid correction of hyponatremia (ie, >12 mEq/L/24 hours) can cause osmotic demyelination resulting in dysarthria, mutism, dysphagia, lethargy, affective changes, spastic quadriparesis, seizures, coma, and death. In susceptible patients (including those with severe malnutrition, alcoholism, or advanced liver disease), slower rates of correction may be advisable. Patients with SIADH or very low baseline serum sodium concentrations may be at greater risk of overly-rapid correction.

Interrupt or discontinue therapy in patients who develop medically significant signs or symptoms of hypovolemia. Patients should ingest fluids in response to thirst. Gastrointestinal bleeding can occur in patients with cirrhosis; use only if the need to treat outweighs the risk. Reductions in extracellular fluid volumes may cause hyperkalemia. Patients with a pretreatment serum potassium >5 mEq/L should be monitored after initiation of therapy.

Use in patients with creatinine clearance <10 mL/minute has not been studied. Do not use in anuric patients. Use with hypertonic saline is not recommended. Use contraindicated in patients taking strong CYP3A inhibitors; avoid use in patients taking moderate CYP3A4 inhibitors. If possible, avoid use with CYP3A4 inducers; if administered with CYP3A4 inducers, dose increases may be necessary. Dose reductions may be necessary if administered with P-gp inhibitors. Consider alternative agents that avoid or lessen the potential for CYP- or P-gp mediated interactions. Patients receiving medications known to increase potassium should be monitored for hyperkalemia.

Monitor closely for rate of serum sodium increase and neurological status; rapid serum sodium correction (>12 mEq/L/24 hours) can lead to permanent neurological damage. Discontinue use if rate of serum sodium increase is undesirable; fluid restriction during the first 24 hours of sodium correction can increase the risk of overly-rapid correction and should generally be avoided; not intended for urgent correction of serum sodium to prevent or treat serious neurologic symptoms; it has not been demonstrated that raising serum sodium with tolvaptan provides a symptomatic benefit.

Drug Interactions

Metabolism/Transport Effects Substrate of P-glycoprotein

Avoid Concomitant Use

Avoid concomitant use of Tolvaptan with any of the following: CYP3A4 Inducers (Strong); CYP3A4 Inhibitors (Moderate); CYP3A4 Inhibitors (Strong); Sodium Chloride

Decreased Effect

The levels/effects of Tolvaptan may be decreased by: CYP3A4 Inducers (Strong); Deferasirox; Herbs (CYP3A4 Inducers); P-Glycoprotein Inducers

Increased Effect/Toxicity

Tolvaptan may increase the levels/effects of: ACE Inhibitors; Angiotensin II Receptor Blockers; Digoxin; Potassium-Sparing Diuretics

The levels/effects of Tolvaptan may be increased by: CYP3A4 Inhibitors (Moderate); CYP3A4 Inhibitors (Strong); Dasatinib; P-Glycoprotein Inhibitors; Sodium Chloride

Nutritional/Ethanol Interactions

Food: Tolvaptan exposure may be doubled when taken with grapefruit juice.
Herb/Nutraceutical: St John's wort may decrease tolvaptan serum concentrations.

Adverse Reactions

>10%:
- Gastrointestinal: Nausea (21%), xerostomia (7% to 13%)
- Renal: Pollakiuria (4% to 11%), polyuria (4% to 11%)
- Miscellaneous: Thirst (12% to 16%)

2% to 10%:
- Central nervous system: Pyrexia (4%)
- Endocrine & metabolic: Hyperglycemia (6%)
- Gastrointestinal: Constipation (7%), anorexia (4%)
- Neuromuscular & skeletal: Weakness (9%)

Pharmacodynamics/Kinetics

Onset of Action 2-4 hour; Peak effect: 4-8 hours

Duration of Action 60% peak serum sodium elevation is retained at 24 hours; urinary excretion of free water is no longer elevated

Bioavailability ~40%

Time to Peak Plasma: 2-4 hours

Protein Binding 99%

Half-Life Elimination 5-12 hours; dominant half-life <12 hours

Metabolism Hepatic via CYP3A4

Excretion Feces

Available Dosage Forms

Tablet, oral:
Samsca™: 15 mg, 30 mg

Dosing

Adult & Geriatric Hyponatremia: Oral: Initial: 15 mg once daily; after at least 24 hours, may increase to 30 mg once daily to a maximum of 60 mg once daily titrating at 24-hour intervals to desired serum sodium concentration.

Administration

Oral Treatment should be initiated or reinitiated in a hospital. May be administered without regards to meals.

Stability

Storage Store at 25°C (77°F); excursions permitted between 15°C and 30°C (59°F and 86°F).

Monitoring and Teaching Issues

Laboratory Monitoring Serum sodium concentration, rate of serum sodium increase, serum potassium concentration (if >5 mEq/L prior to administration or receiving medications known to elevate serum potassium)

Physical Assessment Therapy should be initiated (or reinitiated) in hospital with appropriate laboratory and neurological monitoring. Evaluate serum sodium and neurological status at beginning of therapy and on a regular basis throughout. Teach patient importance of adequate fluid intake.

Patient Education May be taken with or without food. Do not drink grapefruit juice while being treated; may cause dangerous increase in levels of tolvaptan. Follow directions for fluid intake. Report vomiting or diarrhea or if you cannot drink normally, dizziness, unusual weakness, or change in thinking.

Dietary Considerations May be taken without regards to meals. Avoid grapefruit juice.

Pregnancy Considerations Animal studies indicate reduced fetal weight, delayed ossification, increased abortions, fetal death, microphthalmia, open eyelids, cleft palate, brachymelia, and skeletal malformations. There are no adequate and well-controlled studies in pregnant women. Use only if benefit outweighs risk.

◆ **Tomoxetine** *see* Atomoxetine *on page 164*

◆ **Topamax®** *see* Topiramate *on page 1787*

◆ **TopCare® Junior Strength [OTC]** *see* Ibuprofen *on page 938*

◆ **Topicaine® [OTC]** *see* Lidocaine (Topical) *on page 1107*

Topiramate (toe PYRE a mate)

U.S. Brand Names Topamax®

Generic Availability (U.S.) Yes

Pharmacologic Category Anticonvulsant, Miscellaneous

Medication Safety Issues

Sound-alike/look-alike issues:

Topamax® may be confused with Sporanox®, Tegretol®, Tegretol®-XR, Toprol-XL®

Medication Guide Available Yes

Pregnancy Risk Factor D

Lactation Enters breast milk/use caution

Use Monotherapy or adjunctive therapy for partial onset seizures and primary generalized tonic-clonic seizures; adjunctive treatment of seizures associated with Lennox-Gastaut syndrome; prophylaxis of migraine headache

Unlabeled/Investigational Use Infantile spasms, neuropathic pain; prophylaxis of cluster headache

Mechanism of Action/Effect Anticonvulsant activity may be due to a combination of potential mechanisms: Blocks neuronal voltage-dependent sodium channels, enhances GABA(A) activity, antagonizes AMPA/kainate glutamate receptors, and weakly inhibits carbonic anhydrase.

Contraindications There are no contraindications listed in the manufacturers' labeling.

Canadian labeling (not in U.S. labeling): Hypersensitivity to topiramate or any component of the formulation or container; pregnancy and women in childbearing years not using effective contraception (migraine prophylaxis only)

Warnings/Precautions Antiepileptics are associated with an increased risk of suicidal behavior/thoughts with use (regardless of indication); patients should be monitored for signs/symptoms of depression, suicidal tendencies, and other unusual behavior changes during therapy and instructed to inform their healthcare provider immediately if symptoms occur. Use with caution in patients with hepatic, respiratory, or renal impairment. Topiramate may decrease serum bicarbonate concentrations (up to 67% of patients); treatment-emergent metabolic acidosis is less common. Risk may be increased in patients with a predisposing condition (organ dysfunction, ketogenic diet, or concurrent treatment with other drugs which may cause acidosis). Metabolic acidosis may occur at dosages as low as 50 mg/day. Monitor serum bicarbonate as well as potential complications of chronic acidosis (nephrolithiasis, osteomalacia, and reduced growth rates in children). Kidney stones have been reported in both children and adults; the risk of kidney stones is about 2-4 times that of the untreated population; the risk of this event may be reduced by increasing fluid intake.

Cognitive dysfunction, psychiatric disturbances (mood disorders), and sedation (somnolence or fatigue) may occur with topiramate use; incidence may be related to rapid titration and higher doses. Patients must be cautioned about performing tasks which require mental alertness (eg, operating machinery or driving). Topiramate may also cause paresthesia, dizziness, and ataxia. Topiramate has been associated with acute myopia and secondary angle-closure glaucoma in adults and children, typically within 1 month of initiation; discontinue in patients with acute onset of decreased visual acuity or ocular pain. Hyperammonemia with or without encephalopathy may occur with or without concomitant valproate administration; valproic acid dose-dependency was observed in limited pediatric studies; use with caution in patients with inborn errors of metabolism or decreased hepatic mitochondrial activity. Topiramate may be associated (rarely) with severe oligohydrosis and hyperthermia, most frequently in children; use caution and monitor closely during strenuous exercise, during exposure to high environmental temperature, or in patients receiving receiving other carbonic anhydrase inhibitors and drugs with anticholinergic activity. Concurrent use of topiramate and hydrochlorothiazide may increase the risk for hypokalemia; monitor potassium closely.

Avoid abrupt withdrawal of topiramate therapy, it should be withdrawn/tapered slowly to minimize the potential of increased seizure frequency. Doses were also gradually withdrawn in migraine prophylaxis studies. Effects with other sedative drugs or ethanol may be potentiated. Safety and efficacy have not been established in children <2 years of age for adjunctive treatment of seizures and <10 years of age for monotherapy treatment of seizures. In pediatric patients, weight loss may occur most often early in therapy; in clinical trials of at least 1 year, the majority of patients with weight loss had a resumption of weight gain within the study period. Safety and efficacy have not been established in children for migraine prophylaxis.

Drug Interactions

Metabolism/Transport Effects Inhibits CYP2C19 (weak); **Induces** CYP3A4 (weak)

Avoid Concomitant Use There are no known interactions where it is recommended to avoid concomitant use.

Decreased Effect

Topiramate may decrease the levels/effects of: Contraceptives (Estrogens); Contraceptives (Progestins); Saxagliptin

The levels/effects of Topiramate may be decreased by: CarBAMazepine; Ketorolac; Ketorolac (Systemic); Mefloquine; Phenytoin

Increased Effect/Toxicity

Topiramate may increase the levels/effects of: Alcohol (Ethyl); CNS Depressants; Divalproex; Lithium; Methotrimeprazine; Phenytoin; Valproic Acid

The levels/effects of Topiramate may be increased by: Droperidol; Methotrimeprazine; Thiazide Diuretics

Nutritional/Ethanol Interactions

Ethanol: Avoid ethanol (may increase CNS depression).

Food: Ketogenic diet may increase the possibility of acidosis and/or kidney stones.

Herb/Nutraceutical: Avoid evening primrose (seizure threshold decreased).

Adverse Reactions Adverse events are reported for placebo-controlled trials of adjunctive therapy in adult and pediatric patients. Unless otherwise noted, the percentages refer to incidence in epilepsy trials. **Note:** A wide range of dosages were studied; incidence of adverse events was frequently lower in the pediatric population studied.

>10%:

Central nervous system: Somnolence (15% to 29%), dizziness (4% to 25%; dose dependent), fatigue (9% to 16%; dose-dependent), nervousness (9% to 18%), ataxia (6% to 16%), psychomotor slowing (3% to 13%; dose dependent), speech problems (2% to 13%), memory difficulties (2% to 12%), behavior problems (children 11%), confusion (4% to 11%)

Endocrine & metabolic: Serum bicarbonate decreased (dose related: 7% to 67%; marked reductions [to <17 mEq/L] 1% to 11%)

Gastrointestinal: Anorexia (4% to 24%; dose dependent), nausea (6% to 10%; migraine trial: 9% to 14%)

Neuromuscular & skeletal: Paresthesia (1% to 11%; migraine trial: 35% to 51%)

Ocular: Abnormal vision (2% to 13%)

Respiratory: Upper respiratory infection (migraine trial: 12% to 14%)

Miscellaneous: Injury (14%)

1% to 10%:

Cardiovascular: Chest pain (2% to 4%), edema (2%), hypertension (1% to 2%), bradycardia (1%), pallor (1%), syncope (1%)

Central nervous system: Difficulty concentrating (5% to 10%), aggressive reactions (2% to 9%), depression (5% to 9%; dose dependent, insomnia (4% to 8%), mood problems (≤6%), abnormal coordination (4%), agitation (3%), cognitive problems (3%), emotional lability (3%), anxiety (2% to 3%; dose dependent), hypoesthesia (2%; migraine trial: 6% to 8%), stupor (2%), vertigo (2%), fever (migraine trial: 1% to 2%), apathy (1%), hallucination (1%), neurosis (1%), psychosis (1%), seizure (1%), suicide attempt (1%)

Dermatologic: Pruritus (migraine trial: 2% to 4%), skin disorder (2% to 3%), alopecia (2%), dermatitis (2%), hypertrichosis (2%), rash erythematous (1% to 2%), eczema (1%), seborrhea (1%), skin discoloration (1%)

Endocrine & metabolic: Breast pain (4%), hot flashes (1% to 2%), libido decreased (<1% to 2%), menstrual irregularities (1% to 2%), hypoglycemia (1%), metabolic acidosis (hyperchloremia, nonanion gap)

Gastrointestinal: Weight loss (4% to 9%), dyspepsia (2% to 7%), abdominal pain (5% to 6%), salivation increased (6%), constipation (4% to 5%), gastroenteritis (2% to 3%), vomiting (migraine trial: 1% to 3%), diarrhea (2%; migraine trial: 9% to 11%), dysgeusia (2%; migraine trial: 8% to 15%), xerostomia (2%), loss of taste (migraine trial: ≤2%), appetite increased (1%), dysphagia (1%), fecal incontinence (1%), flatulence (1%), GERD (1%), gingivitis (1%), glossitis (1%), gum hyperplasia (1%), weight gain (1%)

Genitourinary: Incontinence (2% to 4%), UTI (2%), premature ejaculation (migraine trial: ≤3%), cystitis (2%), leukorrhea (2%), impotence (1%), nocturia (1%)

Hematologic: Purpura (8%), leukopenia (2%), anemia (1%), hematoma (1%), prothrombin time increased (1%), thrombocytopenia (1%)

Neuromuscular & skeletal: Tremor (3% to 9%), gait abnormal (3% to 8%), arthralgia (migraine trial: 1% to 7%), weakness (6%), hyperkinesia (5%), back pain (1% to 5%), involuntary muscle contractions (2%; migraine trial: 2% to 4%), leg cramps (2%), leg pain (2%), myalgia (2%), hyporeflexia (2%), rigors (1%), skeletal pain (1%)

Ocular: Diplopia (1% to 10%), nystagmus (10%), conjunctivitis (1%), lacrimation abnormal (1%), myopia (1%)

Otic: Hearing decreased (2%), tinnitus (2%), otitis media (migraine trial: 1% to 2%)

Renal: Hematuria (2%), renal calculus (migraine trial ≤2%)

Respiratory: Rhinitis (4% to 7%), pharyngitis (6%), sinusitis (5%; migraine trial: 6% to 10%), pneumonia (5%), epistaxis (2% to 4%), cough (migraine trial: 2% to 4%), bronchitis (migraine trial: 3%), dyspnea (migraine trial: 1% to 3%)

Miscellaneous: Viral infection (2% to 7%: migraine trial: 3% to 4%), flu-like syndrome (3%), allergy (2%), infection (2%), thirst (2%), body odor (1%), diaphoresis (1%), moniliasis (1%)

Pharmacodynamics/Kinetics

Absorption Good, rapid; unaffected by food

Bioavailability ~80%

Time to Peak Serum: ~1-4 hours

Protein Binding 15% to 41% (inversely related to plasma concentrations)

Half-Life Elimination Mean: Adults: Normal renal function: 21 hours; shorter in pediatric patients; clearance is 50% higher in pediatric patients; Elderly: ~24 hours

Metabolism Hepatic via P450

Excretion Urine (~70% to 80% as unchanged drug)

Dialyzable: Significantly hemodialyzed; dialysis clearance: 120 mL/minute (4-6 times higher than in adults with normal renal function); supplemental doses may be required

Available Dosage Forms

Capsule, sprinkle, oral: 15 mg, 25 mg

Topamax®: 15 mg, 25 mg

Tablet, oral: 25 mg, 50 mg, 100 mg, 200 mg

Topamax®: 25 mg, 50 mg, 100 mg, 200 mg

Dosing

Adult Note: Do not abruptly discontinue therapy; taper dosage gradually to prevent rebound effects. (In clinical trials, adult doses were withdrawn by decreasing in weekly intervals of 50-100 mg/day gradually over 2-8 weeks for seizure treatment, and by decreasing in weekly intervals by 25-50 mg/day for migraine prophylaxis.)

Epilepsy, monotherapy:

Partial onset seizure and primary generalized tonic-clonic seizures: Oral: Initial: 25 mg twice daily; may increase weekly by 50 mg/day up to 100 mg twice daily (week 4 dose); thereafter, may further increase weekly by 100 mg/day up to the recommended maximum of 200 mg twice daily

Canadian labeling: Oral: Initial: 25 mg once daily (in evening); may increase to 25 mg twice daily in weeks 2 or 3 and up to 50 mg twice daily by weeks 3 or 4; may further increase weekly in increments of 50 mg/day up to recommended maximum of 200 mg twice daily

Epilepsy, adjunctive therapy:

Partial onset seizures: Oral: Initial: 25 mg once or twice daily for 1 week; may increase weekly by 25-50 mg/day until response; usual maintenance dose: 100-200 mg twice daily. Doses >1600 mg/day have not been studied

Primary generalized tonic-clonic seizures: Oral: Use initial dose as listed above for partial onset seizures, but use slower initial titration rate; titrate upwards to recommended dose by the end of 8 weeks; usual maintenance dose: 200 mg twice daily. Doses >1600 mg/day have not been studied.

Canadian labeling: Oral: Initial: 25 mg once or twice daily; may increase weekly by 50 mg/day up to the recommended dose of 100-200 mg twice daily (maximum recommended dose: 800 mg/day; doses >400 mg/day have shown no additional benefit)

Migraine prophylaxis:Oral: Initial: 25 mg once daily (in evening); may increase weekly by 25 mg/day up to the recommended dose of 100 mg/day given in 2 divided doses. Doses >100 mg/day have shown no additional benefit.

Cluster headache prophylaxis (unlabeled use): Oral: Initial: 25 mg/day, titrated at weekly intervals in 25 mg increments, up to 200 mg/day (Pascual, 2007)

Neuropathic pain (unlabeled use): Oral: Initial: 25 mg/day, titrated at weekly intervals in 25-50 mg increments to target dose of 400 mg daily in 2 divided doses (Raskin, 2004; Thienel, 2004)

Geriatric Most older adults have creatinine clearances <70 mL/minute/1.73 m^2; obtain a serum creatinine and calculate creatinine clearance prior to initiation of therapy. An initial dose of 25 mg/day may be recommended, followed by incremental increases of 25 mg at weekly intervals until an effective dose is reached; refer to adult dosing for titration schedule.

Pediatric Note: Do not abruptly discontinue therapy; taper dosage gradually to prevent rebound effects.

Epilepsy monotherapy:

Partial onset seizure and primary generalized tonic-clonic seizure: Children ≥10 years: Oral: Refer to adult dosing.

Canadian labeling: Children ≥6 years: Refer to adult dosing.

Epilepsy, adjunctive therapy:

Partial onset seizure or seizure associated with Lennox-Gastaut syndrome:

Children 2-16 years: Oral: Initial: 25 mg (1-3 mg/kg/day) once daily (in evening); may increase every 1-2 weeks in increments of 1-3 mg/kg/day up to the recommended maximum of 5-9 mg/kg/day in 2 divided doses

Adolescents ≥17 years: Refer to adult dosing.

Primary generalized tonic-clonic seizure:

Children 2-16 years: Oral: Use initial dose listed above for partial onset seizures, but use slower initial titration rate; titrate to the recommended maintenance dose of 6 mg/kg/day by the end of 8 weeks

Adolescents ≥17 years: Refer to adult dosing.

Canadian labeling:

Children 2-16 years: Oral: Initial: 25 mg (1-3 mg/kg/day) once daily (in evening); may increase every 1-2 weeks in increments of 1-3 mg/kg/day up to the recommended maximum of 5-9 mg/kg/day in 2 divided doses

Adolescents ≥17 years: Refer to adult dosing.

Renal Impairment Cl_{cr} <70 mL/minute/1.73 m^2: Administer 50% dose and titrate more slowly.

Hemodialysis: Supplemental dose may be needed during hemodialysis

Hepatic Impairment Clearance may be reduced; however the manufacturer's labeling provides no specific dosing recommendations.

Administration

Oral May be administered without regard to meals

Capsule sprinkles: May be swallowed whole or opened to sprinkle the contents on a small amount (~1 teaspoon) of soft food (drug/food mixture should not be chewed; swallow immediately).

Tablet: Because of bitter taste, tablets should not be broken or chewed.

Stability

Storage Store at room temperature of 15°C to 30°C (59°F to 86°F). Protect from moisture.

Monitoring and Teaching Issues

Laboratory Monitoring Recommended monitoring includes serum bicarbonate (baseline and periodically during treatment) and serum creatinine. Ammonia level in patients with unexplained lethargy, vomiting, or mental status changes.

Physical Assessment Monitor therapeutic effectiveness (seizure activity, type, duration) at beginning of therapy and throughout. Taper dosage slowly when discontinuing. May cause weight loss; monitor weight periodically. Teach patient seizure safety precautions.

Patient Education While using this medication, do not use alcohol. Maintain adequate hydration, unless instructed to restrict fluid intake, to prevent the development of kidney stones and dehydration. You may be at risk for decreased sweating and increased body temperature, especially in hot weather. You may experience drowsiness, dizziness, disturbed concentration, memory changes, blurred vision, mouth sores, nausea, vomiting, or loss of appetite. Wear identification of epileptic status and medications. Report behavioral or CNS changes, suicide ideation, depression, skin rash, muscle cramping, numbness in extremities, weakness, tremors, changes in gait, chest pain, irregular heartbeat, palpitations, hearing loss, cough, respiratory difficulty, or worsening of seizure activity or loss of seizure control. Seek immediate medical evaluation if you experience sudden vision changes, periorbital pain, flank pain, or blood in urine.

Geriatric Considerations This drug may not be a drug of choice in the elderly until all other therapies for seizures have been exhausted. Follow the recommended titration schedule and adjust time intervals to meet patient's needs. Since most elderly will have a Cl_{cr} <70 mL/minute, it is important to either measure or estimate by calculation the Cl_{cr} prior to initiating therapy.

Breast-Feeding Considerations Based on limited data, topiramate was found in breast milk. Infant plasma concentrations of topiramate have been reported as 10% to 20% of the maternal plasma concentration.

Pregnancy Considerations Topiramate was found to be teratogenic in animal studies. Based on limited data, topiramate was found to cross the placenta. An increase risk of oral clefts (cleft lip and/or palate) has been observed following first trimester exposure. Data, from the North American Antiepileptic Drug (NAAED) Pregnancy Registry, reported that the prevalence of oral clefts was 1.4% for infants exposed to topiramate during the first trimester of pregnancy, versus 0.38% to 0.55% for infants exposed to other antiepileptic drugs and 0.07% with no exposure. Hypospadias and other congenital anomalies have also been reported. Although not evaluated during pregnancy, metabolic acidosis may be induced by topiramate. In general, metabolic acidosis during pregnancy may result in adverse effects and fetal death. Maternal serum concentrations may decrease during the second and third trimesters of pregnancy therefore therapeutic drug monitoring should be considered in pregnant women who require therapy.

Patients exposed to topiramate during pregnancy are encouraged to enroll themselves into the AED Pregnancy Registry by calling 1-888-233-2334. Additional information is available at www.aedpregnancyregistry.org.

Additional Information May be associated with weight loss in some patients

Related Information

Anticonvulsant Drugs of Choice *on page* 1981

◆ **Toposar®** *see* Etoposide *on page* 712

Topotecan (toe poe TEE kan)

U.S. Brand Names Hycamtin®

Index Terms Hycamptamine; SKF 104864; SKF 104864-A; Topotecan Hydrochloride

Generic Availability (U.S.) Yes: Injection

Pharmacologic Category Antineoplastic Agent, Camptothecin; Antineoplastic Agent, Natural Source (Plant) Derivative; Antineoplastic Agent, Topoisomerase I Inhibitor

Medication Safety Issues

Sound-alike/look-alike issues:

Hycamtin® may be confused with Hycomine®, Mycamine®

High alert medication: This medication is in a class the Institute for Safe Medication Practices (ISMP) includes among its list of drug classes which have a heightened risk of causing significant patient harm when used in error.

Pregnancy Risk Factor D

Lactation Excretion in breast milk unknown/contraindicated

Use Treatment of metastatic ovarian cancer, relapsed or refractory small cell lung cancer, recurrent or resistant cervical cancer (in combination with cisplatin)

Unlabeled/Investigational Use Treatment of nonsmall cell lung cancer, sarcoma (pediatrics), neuroblastoma (pediatrics), refractory solid tumors (pediatrics)

Mechanism of Action/Effect Binds to topoisomerase I and stabilizes the cleavable complex so that religation of the cleaved DNA strand cannot occur. This results in the accumulation of cleavable complexes and single-strand DNA breaks. Topotecan acts in S phase of the cell cycle.

Contraindications Hypersensitivity to topotecan or any component of the formulation; severe bone marrow depression; pregnancy; breast-feeding

Canadian labeling: Additional contraindications (not in U.S. labeling): Severe renal impairment (Cl_{cr} <20 mL/minute)

Warnings/Precautions Hazardous agent - use appropriate precautions for handling and disposal. The dose-limiting toxicity is bone marrow suppression (primarily neutropenia; may also cause thrombocytopenia and anemia); monitor bone marrow function. Neutropenia is not cumulative overtime. **[U.S. Boxed Warning]: Should only administer to patients with adequate bone marrow reserves, baseline neutrophils at least 1500 cells/mm^3** and platelet counts at least 100,000/mm^3. In a clinical study comparing I.V. to oral topotecan, G-CSF support was administered in a higher percentage of patients receiving oral topotecan. Topotecan-induced neutropenia may lead to neutropenic colitis; should be considered in patients presenting with neutropenia, fever and abdominal pain. Diarrhea has been reported with oral topotecan; may be severe; incidence may be higher in the elderly; educate patients on proper management. Use caution in renal impairment; may require dose adjustment. Interstitial lung disease (ILD) (with fatalities) has been reported; discontinue use in patients with confirmed ILD; risk factors for ILD include a history of ILD, pulmonary fibrosis, lung cancer, thoracic radiation, and the use of colony-stimulating factors or medication with pulmonary toxicity. Diarrhea has been reported with oral topotecan; may be severe; incidence may be higher in the elderly; educate patients on proper management. Use caution in renal impairment; may require dose adjustment (use in severe renal impairment is contraindicated in the Canadian labeling).

Drug Interactions

Avoid Concomitant Use

Avoid concomitant use of Topotecan with any of the following: BCG; Natalizumab; P-Glycoprotein Inhibitors; Pimecrolimus; Roflumilast; Tacrolimus (Topical); Vaccines (Live)

Decreased Effect

Topotecan may decrease the levels/effects of: BCG; Sipuleucel-T; Vaccines (Inactivated); Vaccines (Live)

The levels/effects of Topotecan may be decreased by: Echinacea

Increased Effect/Toxicity

Topotecan may increase the levels/effects of: Leflunomide; Natalizumab; Vaccines (Live)

The levels/effects of Topotecan may be increased by: BCRP/ABCG2 Inhibitors; Denosumab; Filgrastim; P-Glycoprotein Inhibitors; Pimecrolimus; Platinum Derivatives; Roflumilast; Tacrolimus (Topical); Trastuzumab

Nutritional/Ethanol Interactions Ethanol: Avoid ethanol (due to GI irritation).

Lab Interactions None known

Adverse Reactions

>10%:

Central nervous system: Fatigue (11% to 29%), fever (5% to 28%), pain (23%), headache (18%)

Dermatologic: Alopecia (10% to 49%), rash (16%)

Gastrointestinal: Nausea (27% to 64%), vomiting (19% to 45%), diarrhea (14% to 32%; Oral: grade 3: 4%; grade 4: ≤1%; onset: 9 days), constipation (29%), abdominal pain (22%), anorexia (7% to 19%), stomatitis (18%)

Hematologic: Neutropenia (83% to 97%; grade 4: 32% to 80%; nadir 8-11 days; duration: 7 days; recovery <21 days), leukopenia (86% to 97%; grade 4: 15% to 32%), anemia (89% to 98%; grade 4: 7% to 10%), thrombocytopenia (69% to 81%; grade 4: 6% to 29%; duration: 3 days), neutropenic fever/sepsis (2% to 28%)

Neuromuscular & skeletal: Weakness (3% to 25%)

Respiratory: Dyspnea (22%), cough (15%)

1% to 10%:

Hepatic: Liver enzymes increased (transient; 8%)

Neuromuscular & skeletal: Paresthesia (7%)

Miscellaneous: Sepsis (grades 3/4: 5%)

Pharmacodynamics/Kinetics

Absorption Oral: Rapid

Bioavailability Oral: ~40%

Time to Peak Oral 1-2 hours; delayed with high-fat meal (1.5-4 hours)

Protein Binding ~35%

Half-Life Elimination I.V.: 2-3 hours; renal impairment: 5 hours; Oral: 3-6 hours

Metabolism Undergoes a rapid, pH-dependent hydrolysis of the lactone ring to yield a relatively inactive hydroxy acid in plasma; metabolized in the liver to N-demethylated metabolite

Excretion

I.V.: Urine (51%; 3% as N-desmethyl topotecan); feces (18%; 2% as N-desmethyl topotecan)

Oral: Urine (20%; 2% as N-desmethyl topotecan); feces (33%; <2% as N-desmethyl topotecan)

Available Dosage Forms

Capsule, oral:

Hycamtin®: 0.25 mg, 1 mg

Injection, powder for reconstitution: 4 mg

Hycamtin®: 4 mg

Injection, solution: 1 mg/mL (4 mL)

Dosing

Adult & Geriatric Refer to individual protocols: **Note:** Baseline neutrophil count should be >1500/mm^3; retreatment neutrophil count should be >1000/mm^3; baseline and retreatment platelet count should be >100,000/mm^3; (also, for oral topotecan, retreatment hemoglobin should be ≥9 g/dL):

Small cell lung cancer:

IVPB: 1.5 mg/m^2/day for 5 days; repeated every 21 days

Oral: 2.3 mg/m^2/day for 5 days; repeated every 21 days (round dose to the nearest 0.25 mg); if patient vomits after dose is administered, do not give a replacement dose.

Metastatic ovarian cancer:

IVPB: 1.5 mg/m^2/day for 5 days; repeated every 21 days

I.V. continuous infusion (unlabeled dose): 0.2-0.7 mg/m^2/day for 7-21 days

Cervical cancer: IVPB: 0.75 mg/m^2/day for 3 days (followed by cisplatin 50 mg/m^2 on day 1 only, [with hydration]); repeated every 21 days

Renal Impairment

Manufacturer's labeling recommends the following dosage adjustment:

I.V.:

Cl_{cr} ≥40 mL/minute: No dosage adjustment required

Cl_{cr} 20-39 mL/minute: Reduce to 0.75 mg/m^2/dose

Cl_{cr} <20 mL/minute: Insufficient data available for dosing recommendation (contraindicated in the Canadian labeling)

Note: For topotecan in combination with cisplatin for cervical cancer, do not initiate treatment in patients with serum creatinine >1.5 mg/dL; consider discontinuing treatment in patients with serum creatinine >1.5 mg/dL in subsequent cycles.

Oral:

Cl_{cr} 30-49 mL/minute: Reduce dose to 1.8 mg/m^2/day

Cl_{cr} <30 mL/minute: Insufficient data available for dosing recommendation

The following guidelines have been used by some clinicians:

Aronoff, 2007: *I.V.:*

Children:

Cl_{cr} 30-50 mL/minute: Administer 75% of dose

Cl_{cr} 10-29 mL/minute: Administer 50% of dose or reduce by 0.75 mg/m^2/dose

Cl_{cr} <10 mL/minute: Administer 25% of dose

Hemodialysis: 0.75 mg/m^2

Continuous renal replacement therapy (CRRT): Administer 50% of dose or reduce by 0.75 mg/m^2/dose

Adults:

Cl_{cr} >50 mL/minute: Administer 75% of dose

Cl_{cr} 10-50 mL/minute: Administer 50% of dose

Cl_{cr} <10 mL/minute: Administer 25% of dose

Hemodialysis: Avoid use

Continuous ambulatory peritoneal dialysis (CAPD): Avoid use

Continuous renal replacement therapy (CRRT): 0.75 mg/m^2

Kintzel, 1995:

Cl_{cr} 46-60 mL/minute: Administer 80% of dose

Cl_{cr} 31-45 mL/minute: Administer 75% of dose

Cl_{cr} <30 mL/minute: Administer 70% of dose

Hepatic Impairment Manufacturer's labeling recommends the following:

I.V.: Bilirubin 1.5-10 mg/dL: No adjustment necessary.

Oral: Bilirubin >1.5 mg/dL: No adjustment necessary.

Adjustment for Toxicity

I.V.:

Ovarian and small cell lung cancer: Dosage adjustment for hematological effects: Severe neutropenia or platelet count <25,000/mm^3: Reduce dose to 1.25 mg/m^2/day for subsequent cycles (may consider G-CSF support [beginning on day 6] prior to instituting dose reduction for neutropenia). **Note:** The Canadian labeling states that the dose may be further reduced to 1 mg/m^2/day if necessary.

Cervical cancer: Severe febrile neutropenia (ANC <1000/mm^3 with temperature of 38°C) or platelet count <10,000/mm^3: Reduce topotecan to 0.6 mg/m^2/day for subsequent cycles (may consider C-CSF support [beginning on day 4] prior to instituting dose reduction for neutropenic fever.

For neutropenic fever despite G-CSF use, reduce dose to 0.45 mg/m^2/day for subsequent cycles). **Note:** Cisplatin may also require dose adjustment.

Oral:

Small cell lung cancer: Severe neutropenia (neutrophils <500/mm^3 associated with fever or infection or lasting >7 days) or prolonged neutropenia (neutrophils ≥500/mm^3 to ≤1000/mm^3 lasting beyond day 21) or platelets <25,000/mm^3 or grades 3/4 diarrhea: Reduce dose to 1.9 mg/m^2/day for subsequent cycles (may consider same dosage reduction for grade 2 diarrhea if clinically indicated).

Administration

Oral Administer without regard to meals. Swallow whole; do not crush, chew, or divide capsule. If vomiting occurs after dose, do not take replacement dose.

I.V. Administer IVPB over 30 minutes or by 24-hour continuous infusion (unlabeled administration rate). For combination chemotherapy with cisplatin, administer pretreatment hydration.

Stability

Reconstitution Reconstitute lyophilized powder with 4 mL SWFI. Further dilute in 50-100 mL D_5W or NS for infusion.

Storage

I.V.:

Solution for injection: Store intact vials at 2°C to 8°C (36°F to 45°F). Protect from light. Single-use vials should be discarded after initial vial entry; solutions for infusion are stable for 24 hours at room temperature after diluted.

Lyophilized powder: Store intact vials at room temperature of 20°C to 25°C (68°F to 77°F). Protect from light. Reconstituted solution is stable for up to 28 days at room temperature of 20°C to 25°C (68°F to 77°F). Solutions further diluted for infusion are stable for 24 hours at room temperature or up to 7 days under refrigeration.

Oral: Store at 2°C to 8°C (36°F to 46°F). Protect from light.

Monitoring and Teaching Issues

Laboratory Monitoring CBC with differential and platelet count, renal function tests, bilirubin

Physical Assessment Evaluate renal function (I & O, edema) and monitor for signs of myelosuppression, gastrointestinal disturbance (nausea, vomiting, diarrhea, pain), and dyspnea prior to each infusion and on a regular basis with oral formulation.

Patient Education If this drug is administered by intravenous infusion, report immediately any burning, pain, redness, or swelling at infusion site; sudden chest pain; difficulty breathing or swallowing; or chills. Oral form may be taken with or without food. Swallow whole; do not crush, chew, or divide capsule. If vomiting occurs after dose, do not take replacement dose; take next dose at scheduled time. Maintain adequate hydration (3-4 L/day of fluids) unless instructed to restrict fluid intake during therapy. Maintain good oral hygiene. You will be more susceptible to infection. May cause nausea, vomiting, diarrhea, or hair loss (will regrow after treatment is completed). Report unresolved diarrhea, nausea, vomiting, or unusual abdominal pain; alterations in urinary pattern (increased or decreased); opportunistic infection (fever, chills, unusual bruising or bleeding, fatigue, purulent vaginal discharge, unhealed mouth sores); chest pain; respiratory difficulty; or unexplained weakness or fatigue.

Dietary Considerations May be taken without regard to meals.

Breast-Feeding Considerations Breast-feeding should be discontinued in women who are receiving topotecan.

Pregnancy Considerations Animal studies found reduced fetal body weight, eye, brain, skull, and vertebrae malformations. May cause fetal harm in pregnant women. Use during pregnancy is contraindicated.

◆ **Topotecan Hydrochloride** *see* Topotecan *on page 1790*

◆ **Toprol-XL®** *see* Metoprolol *on page 1217*

◆ **Toradol** *see* Ketorolac (Systemic) *on page 1043*

Toremifene (tore EM i feen)

U.S. Brand Names Fareston®

Index Terms FC1157a; Toremifene Citrate

Generic Availability (U.S.) No

Pharmacologic Category Antineoplastic Agent, Estrogen Receptor Antagonist; Selective Estrogen Receptor Modulator (SERM)

Pregnancy Risk Factor D

Lactation Excretion in breast milk unknown/not recommended

Use Treatment of metastatic breast cancer in postmenopausal women with estrogen receptor positive or estrogen receptor status unknown

Unlabeled/Investigational Use Treatment of soft tissue sarcoma (desmoid tumors)

Mechanism of Action/Effect Nonsteroidal agent that competitively binds to estrogen receptors on tumors and other tissue targets (including breast and other tissues), producing a nuclear complex that decreases DNA synthesis and inhibits estrogen effects (also has estrogenic effects). Cells accumulate in the G_0 and G_1 phases; therefore, toremifene is cytostatic rather than cytocidal.

Contraindications Hypersensitivity to toremifene or any component of the formulation; long QT syndrome (congenital or acquired QT prolongation), uncorrected hypokalemia, uncorrected hypomagnesemia

Warnings/Precautions Hazardous agent - use appropriate precautions for handling and disposal.

[U.S. Boxed Warning]: May prolong the QT interval; QT_c prolongation is dose-dependent and concentration dependant. Torsade de pointes, syncope, seizure and/or sudden death may occur. Use is contraindicated in patients with congenital or acquired long QT syndrome, uncorrected hypokalemia, or uncorrected hypomagnesemia. Avoid use with other medications known to prolong the QT interval and with strong CYP3A4 inhibitors. Use with caution in patients with heart failure, hepatic impairment, or electrolyte abnormalities. Monitor electrolytes; correct hypokalemia and hypomagnesemia prior to treatment. Obtain ECG at baseline and as clinically indicated in patients at risk for QT prolongation

Hypercalcemia and tumor flare have been reported during the first weeks of treatment in some breast cancer patients with bone metastases; monitor closely for hypocalcemia. Institute appropriate measures if hypercalcemia occurs, and if severe, discontinue treatment. Tumor flare consists of diffuse musculoskeletal pain and erythema with initial increased size of tumor lesions that later regress; is often accompanied by hypercalcemia. Tumor flare does not imply treatment failure or represent tumor progression. Drugs that decrease renal calcium excretion (eg, thiazide diuretics) may increase the risk of hypercalcemia in patients receiving toremifene. Leukopenia and thrombocytopenia have been reported rarely; monitor leukocyte and platelet ▶

counts. Endometrial hyperplasia has been reported; some patients have developed endometrial cancer, although a role of toremifene in endometrial cancer development has not been established. Avoid long-term use in patients with pre-existing endometrial hyperplasia. Use with caution in patients with hepatic failure. Avoid use in patients with a history of thromboembolic disease.

Drug Interactions

Metabolism/Transport Effects Substrate of CYP1A2 (minor), 3A4 (major)

Avoid Concomitant Use

Avoid concomitant use of Toremifene with any of the following: Artemether; CYP3A4 Inhibitors (Strong); Dronedarone; Lumefantrine; Nilotinib; Pimozide; QTc-Prolonging Agents; QuiNINE; Tetrabenazine; Thioridazine; Vandetanib; Ziprasidone

Decreased Effect

The levels/effects of Toremifene may be decreased by: CYP3A4 Inducers (Strong); Deferasirox; Herbs (CYP3A4 Inducers)

Increased Effect/Toxicity

Toremifene may increase the levels/effects of: Dronedarone; Pimozide; QTc-Prolonging Agents; QuiNINE; Tetrabenazine; Thioridazine; Vandetanib; Vitamin K Antagonists; Ziprasidone

The levels/effects of Toremifene may be increased by: Alfuzosin; Artemether; Chloroquine; Ciprofloxacin; Ciprofloxacin (Systemic); CYP3A4 Inhibitors (Strong); Gadobutrol; Lumefantrine; Nilotinib; QTc-Prolonging Agents; QuiNINE; Thiazide Diuretics

Nutritional/Ethanol Interactions

Food: Avoid grapefruit juice (may increase toremifene levels).
Herb/Nutraceutical: Avoid St John's wort (may decrease toremifene levels).

Adverse Reactions

>10%:

Endocrine & metabolic: Hot flashes (35%)
Gastrointestinal: Nausea (14%)
Genitourinary: Vaginal discharge (13%)
Hepatic: Alkaline phosphatase increased (8% to 19%), AST increased (5% to 19%)
Miscellaneous: Diaphoresis (20%)

1% to 10%:

Cardiovascular: Edema (5%), arrhythmia (≤2%), CVA/TIA (≤2%), thrombosis (≤2%), cardiac failure (≤1%), MI (≤1%)
Central nervous system: Dizziness (9%)
Endocrine & metabolic: Hypercalcemia (≤3%)
Gastrointestinal: Vomiting (4%)
Genitourinary: Vaginal bleeding (2%)
Hepatic: Bilirubin increased (1% to 2%)
Local: Thrombophlebitis (≤2%)
Ocular: Cataracts (≤10%), xerophthalmia (≤9%), visual field abnormal (≤4%), corneal keratopathy (≤2%), glaucoma (≤2%), vision abnormal/diplopia (≤2%)
Respiratory: Pulmonary embolism (≤2%)

Pharmacodynamics/Kinetics

Absorption Well absorbed

Bioavailability Not affected by food

Time to Peak Serum: ≤3 hours

Protein Binding Plasma: >99.5%, primarily to albumin

Half-Life Elimination Toremifene: ~5 days; N-demethyltoremifene: 6 days

Metabolism Extensively hepatic, principally by CYP3A4 to N-demethyltoremifene (a weak antiestrogen)

Excretion Primarily feces; urine (10%) during a 1-week period

Available Dosage Forms

Tablet, oral:
Fareston®: 60 mg

Dosing

Adult & Geriatric Metastatic breast cancer (postmenopausal): Oral: 60 mg once daily, continue until disease progression

Administration

Oral Administer orally, as a single daily dose, with or without food.

Stability

Storage Store at 25°C (77°F); excursions permitted to 15°C to 30°C (59°F to 86°F); protect from heat. Protect from light.

Monitoring and Teaching Issues

Laboratory Monitoring CBC with differential, electrolytes (calcium, magnesium, and potassium), hepatic function. In patients with bone metastases, monitor closely for hypercalcemia during the first few weeks of treatment.

Physical Assessment Monitor for thromboembolism, MI, edema, hypercalcemia, endometriosis, nausea, vomiting, and vision changes.

Patient Education Take without regard to food. You may experience an initial "flare" of this disease (eg, increased bone pain and hot flashes), which will subside with continued use. May cause nausea, vomiting, loss of appetite, or dizziness. Report vomiting that occurs immediately after taking medication; chest pain, palpitations, or swollen extremities; vaginal bleeding, hot flashes, or excessive perspiration; chest pain, unusual coughing, or respiratory difficulty; or any vision changes or dry eyes.

Dietary Considerations May be taken with or without food. Avoid grapefruit juice.

Geriatric Considerations No specific information concerning elderly patients.

Pregnancy Considerations Animal studies have demonstrated embryotoxicity and fetal adverse effects. There are no adequate and well-controlled studies in pregnant women. Only approved for use in postmenopausal women. May cause fetal harm if administered during pregnancy.

◆ **Toremifene Citrate** *see* Toremifene *on page 1793*

◆ **Torisel®** *see* Temsirolimus *on page 1723*

Torsemide (TORE se mide)

U.S. Brand Names Demadex®

Generic Availability (U.S.) Yes

Pharmacologic Category Diuretic, Loop

Medication Safety Issues

Sound-alike/look-alike issues:

Torsemide may be confused with furosemide

Demadex® may be confused with Denorex®

Pregnancy Risk Factor B

Lactation Excretion in breast milk unknown/use caution

Use Management of edema associated with heart failure and hepatic or renal disease (including chronic renal failure); treatment of hypertension

Mechanism of Action/Effect Inhibits reabsorption of sodium and chloride in the ascending loop of Henle and distal renal tubule, interfering with the chloride-binding cotransport system, thus causing increased excretion of water, sodium, chloride, magnesium, and calcium; does not alter GFR, renal plasma flow, or acid-base balance

Contraindications Hypersensitivity to torsemide, any component of the formulation, or any sulfonylurea; anuria

Warnings/Precautions Loop diuretics are potent diuretics; excess amounts can lead to profound diuresis with fluid and electrolyte loss; close medical supervision and dose evaluation are required. Potassium supplementation and/or use of potassium-sparing diuretics may be necessary to prevent hypokalemia. Use with caution in patients with cirrhosis; avoid sudden changes in fluid and electrolyte balance and acid/base status which may lead to hepatic encephalopathy. Administration with an aldosterone antagonist or potassium-sparing diuretic may provide additional diuretic efficacy and maintain normokalemia. Coadministration of antihypertensives may increase the risk of hypotension.

Monitor fluid status and renal function in an attempt to prevent oliguria, azotemia, and reversible increases in BUN and creatinine; close medical supervision of aggressive diuresis required. Ototoxicity has been demonstrated following oral administration of torsemide and following rapid I.V. administration of other loop diuretics. Other possible risk factors may include use in renal impairment, excessive doses, and concurrent use of other ototoxins (eg, aminoglycosides).

Chemical similarities are present among sulfonamides, sulfonylureas, carbonic anhydrase inhibitors, thiazides, and loop diuretics (except ethacrynic acid). Use in patients with sulfonylurea allergy is specifically contraindicated in product labeling; a risk of cross-reaction exists in patients with allergy to any of these compounds; avoid use when previous reaction has been severe. Discontinue if signs of hypersensitivity are noted.

Drug Interactions

Metabolism/Transport Effects Substrate of CYP2C8 (minor), CYP2C9 (major), SLCO1B1; **Inhibits** CYP2C19 (weak)

Avoid Concomitant Use There are no known interactions where it is recommended to avoid concomitant use.

Decreased Effect

Torsemide may decrease the levels/effects of: Lithium; Neuromuscular-Blocking Agents

The levels/effects of Torsemide may be decreased by: Bile Acid Sequestrants; CYP2C9 Inducers (Highly Effective); Herbs (Hypertensive Properties); Methylphenidate; Nonsteroidal Anti-Inflammatory Agents; Peginterferon Alfa-2b; Phenytoin; Probenecid; Salicylates; Yohimbine

Increased Effect/Toxicity

Torsemide may increase the levels/effects of: ACE Inhibitors; Allopurinol; Amifostine; Aminoglycosides; Antihypertensives; CISplatin; Dofetilide; Hypotensive Agents; Lithium; Neuromuscular-Blocking Agents; RiTUXimab; Salicylates; Warfarin

The levels/effects of Torsemide may be increased by: Beta2-Agonists; Corticosteroids (Orally Inhaled); Corticosteroids (Systemic); CYP2C9 Inhibitors (Moderate); CYP2C9 Inhibitors (Strong); Diazoxide; Eltrombopag; Herbs (Hypotensive Properties); Licorice; MAO Inhibitors; Pentoxifylline; Phosphodiesterase 5 Inhibitors; Probenecid; Prostacyclin Analogues

Nutritional/Ethanol Interactions Herb/Nutraceutical: Avoid herbs with *hypertensive* properties (bayberry, blue cohosh, cayenne, ephedra, ginger, ginseng [American], kola, licorice); may diminish the antihypertensive effect of torsemide. Avoid herbs with *hypotensive* properties (black cohosh, California poppy, coleus, golden seal, hawthorn, mistletoe, periwinkle, quinine, shepherd's purse); may enhance the hypotensive effect of torsemide.

Adverse Reactions

1% to 10%:

Cardiovascular: ECG abnormality (2%), chest pain (1%)

Central nervous system: Nervousness (1%)

Gastrointestinal: Constipation (2%), diarrhea (2%), dyspepsia (2%), nausea (2%), sore throat (2%)

Genitourinary: Excessive urination (7%)

Neuromuscular & skeletal: Arthralgia (2%), myalgia (2%), weakness (2%)

Respiratory: Rhinitis (3%), cough (2%)

Pharmacodynamics/Kinetics

Onset of Action Diuresis: Oral: Within 1 hour; Peak effect: Diuresis: Oral: 1-2 hours; Antihypertensive: Oral: 4-6 weeks (up to 12 weeks)

Duration of Action Diuresis: Oral: ~6-8 hours

Absorption Oral: Rapid

Bioavailability ~80%

Time to Peak Plasma: Oral: 1 hour; delayed ~30 minutes when administered with food

Protein Binding Plasma: >99%

Half-Life Elimination ~3.5 hours; Cirrhosis: 7-8 hours

Metabolism Hepatic (~80%) via CYP

Excretion Urine (~20% as unchanged drug)

Available Dosage Forms

Injection, solution: 10 mg/mL (2 mL, 5 mL)

Tablet, oral: 5 mg, 10 mg, 20 mg, 100 mg

Demadex®: 5 mg, 10 mg, 20 mg, 100 mg

Dosing

Adult & Geriatric Note: I.V. and oral dosing are equivalent.

Edema:

Chronic renal failure: Oral, I.V.: Initial: 20 mg once daily; may increase gradually by doubling dose until the desired diuretic response is obtained (maximum recommended daily dose: 200 mg)

Heart failure:

Oral: Initial: 10-20 mg once daily; may increase gradually by doubling dose until the desired diuretic response is obtained. **Note:** ACC/AHA 2009 guidelines for heart failure maximum daily dose: 200 mg (Hunt, 2009)

I.V.: Initial: 10-20 mg; may repeat every 2 hours with double the dose as needed. **Note:** ACC/AHA 2009 guidelines for heart failure recommend maximum single dose: 100-200 mg (Hunt, 2009)

Continuous I.V. infusion (unlabeled dose): Initial: 20 mg I.V. load, then 5-20 mg/hour (Hunt, 2009)

Hepatic cirrhosis: Oral: Initial: 5-10 mg once daily; may increase gradually by doubling dose until the desired diuretic response is obtained (maximum recommended single dose: 40 mg). **Note:** Administer with an aldosterone antagonist or a potassium-sparing diuretic.

Hypertension: Oral: Initial: 5 mg once daily; may increase to 10 mg once daily after 4-6 weeks if adequate antihypertensive response is not apparent; if still not effective, an additional antihypertensive agent may be added. Usual dosage range (JNC 7): 2.5-10 mg once daily. **Note:** Thiazide-type diuretics are preferred in the treatment of hypertension (Chobanian, 2003)

Administration

Oral Administer without regard to meals; patients may be switched from the I.V. form to the oral (and vice-versa) with no change in dose.

I.V. Administer over ≥2 minutes; reserve I.V. administration for situations which require rapid onset of action.

Stability

Storage

I.V.: Store at 15°C to 30°C (59°F to 86°F). If torsemide is to be administered via continuous infusion, stability has been demonstrated through 24 hours at room temperature in plastic containers for the following fluids and concentrations:

200 mg torsemide (10 mg/mL) added to 250 mL D_5W, 250 mL NS or 500 mL 0.45% sodium chloride

50 mg torsemide (10 mg/mL) added to 500 mL D_5W, 500 mL NS, or 500 mL 0.45% sodium chloride

Tablets: Store at 15°C to 30°C (59°F to 86°F).

Monitoring and Teaching Issues

Laboratory Monitoring Renal function, electrolytes

Physical Assessment Assess for allergy to sulfonylurea before beginning therapy. Monitor for dehydration, electrolyte imbalance, and postural hypotension on a regular basis during therapy.

Patient Education Take with food or milk (to reduce GI distress), early in the day. If taken twice daily, take last dose in early afternoon in order to avoid sleep disturbance and achieve maximum therapeutic effect. Include potassium-rich foods in daily diet. Do not take potassium supplements without consulting prescriber. Weigh yourself each day when beginning therapy and weekly on long-term therapy; report unusual or unanticipated weight gain or loss. May cause transient drowsiness, blurred vision, dizziness, or constipation. Report unusual weight gain or loss, swelling of ankles and hands, persistent fatigue, weakness, fatigue, dizziness, vomiting, cramps, change in hearing, or chest pain or palpitations.

Dietary Considerations May be taken without regard to meals; however, food slows the rate and reduces the extent of absorption and may reduce diuretic efficacy (Bard, 2004). May require increased intake of potassium-rich foods.

Geriatric Considerations Loop diuretics are potent diuretics, excess amounts can lead to profound diuresis with fluid and electrolyte loss. Close medical supervision and dose evaluation is required, particularly in elderly.

Pregnancy Considerations A decrease in fetal weight, an increase in fetal resorption, and delayed fetal ossification has occurred in animal studies.

Additional Information 10-20 mg torsemide is approximately equivalent to furosemide 40 mg or bumetanide 1 mg.

Related Information

Heart Failure (Systolic) *on page 2040*

◆ **Totect®** *see* Dexrazoxane *on page 508*

◆ **Toviaz™** *see* Fesoterodine *on page 757*

◆ **tPA** *see* Alteplase *on page 86*

◆ **TPV** *see* Tipranavir *on page 1771*

TraMADol (TRA ma dole)

U.S. Brand Names Rybix™ ODT; Ryzolt™; Ultram®; Ultram® ER

Index Terms Tramadol Hydrochloride

Generic Availability (U.S.) Yes: Excludes orally disintegrating tablet

Pharmacologic Category Analgesic, Opioid

Medication Safety Issues

Sound-alike/look-alike issues:

TraMADol may be confused with tapentadol, Toradol®, Trandate®, traZODone, Voltaren®

Ultram® may be confused with Ultane®, Ultracet®, Voltaren®

International issues:

Theradol [Netherlands] may be confused with Foradil brand name for formoterol [U.S., Canada, and multiple international markets], Terazol brand name for terconazole [U.S. and Canada], and Toradol brand name for ketorolac [Canada and multiple international markets]

Trexol [Mexico] may be confused with Trexall brand name for methotrexate [U.S.]; Truxal brand name for chlorprothixene [multiple international markets]

Pregnancy Risk Factor C

Lactation Enters breast milk/not recommended

Use Relief of moderate to moderately-severe pain

Extended release formulations are indicated for patients requiring around-the-clock management of moderate to moderately-severe pain for an extended period of time

Mechanism of Action/Effect Tramadol and its active metabolite (M1) binds to μ-opiate receptors in the CNS causing inhibition of ascending pain pathways, altering the perception of and response to pain; also inhibits the reuptake of norepinephrine and serotonin, which also modifies the ascending pain pathway

Contraindications Hypersensitivity to tramadol, opioids, or any component of the formulation; opioid-dependent patients; acute intoxication with alcohol, hypnotics, centrally-acting analgesics, opioids, or psychotropic drugs

Additional contraindications for Ryzolt™: Severe/acute bronchial asthma, hypercapnia, or significant respiratory depression in the absence of appropriately monitored setting and/or resuscitative equipment

Canadian product labeling:

Tramadol is contraindicated during or within 14 days following MAO inhibitor therapy

Extended release formulations (Ralivia™ ER [CAN], Tridural™[CAN], and Zytram® XL [CAN]): Additional contraindications: Severe (Cl_{cr} <30 mL/minute) renal dysfunction, severe (Child-Pugh class C) hepatic dysfunction

Warnings/Precautions Rare but serious anaphylactoid reactions (including fatalities) often following initial dosing have been reported. Pruritus, hives, bronchospasm, angioedema, toxic epidermal necrolysis (TEN) and Stevens-Johnson syndrome also have been reported with use. Previous anaphylactoid reactions to opioids may increase risks for similar reactions to tramadol. Caution patients to swallow extended release tablets whole. Rapid release and absorption of tramadol from extended release tablets that are broken, crushed, or chewed may lead to a potentially lethal overdose. May cause CNS depression, which may impair physical or mental abilities; patients must be cautioned about performing tasks which require mental alertness (eg, operating machinery or driving). May cause CNS depression and/or respiratory depression, particularly when combined with other CNS depressants. Use with caution and reduce dosage when administered to patients receiving other CNS depressants. An increased risk of seizures may occur in patients receiving serotonin reuptake inhibitors (SSRIs or anorectics), tricyclic antidepressants or other cyclic compounds (including cyclobenzaprine, promethazine), neuroleptics, drugs which may lower seizure threshold, or drugs which impair metabolism of tramadol (ie, CYP2D6 and 3A4 inhibitors). Patients with a history of seizures, or with a risk of seizures (head trauma, metabolic disorders, CNS infection, or malignancy, or during ethanol/drug withdrawal) are also at increased risk. Avoid use, if possible, with serotonergic agents such as TCAs, MAO inhibitors (use with extreme caution; contraindicated in Canadian product labeling), triptans, venlafaxine, trazodone, lithium, sibutramine, meperidine, dextromethorphan,

St John's wort, SNRIs, and SSRIs; use caution with drugs which impair metabolism of tramadol (ie, CYP2D6 and 3A4 inhibitors); concomitant may increase the risk of serotonin syndrome.

Elderly (particularly >75 years of age), debilitated patients and patients with chronic respiratory disorders may be at greater risk of adverse events. Use with caution in patients with increased intracranial pressure or head injury. Avoid use in patients who are suicidal or addiction prone; use with caution in patients taking tranquilizers and/or antidepressants, or those with an emotional disturbance including depression. Healthcare provider should be alert to problems of abuse, misuse, and diversion. Use caution in heavy alcohol users. Use caution in treatment of acute abdominal conditions; may mask pain. Use tramadol with caution and reduce dosage in patients with liver disease or renal dysfunction. Avoid using extended release tablets in severe hepatic impairment. Do not use Ryzolt™ in any degree of hepatic impairment. Tolerance or drug dependence may result from extended use (withdrawal symptoms have been reported); abrupt discontinuation should be avoided. Tapering of dose at the time of discontinuation limits the risk of withdrawal symptoms. Some products may contain phenylalanine.

Drug Interactions

Metabolism/Transport Effects Substrate of CYP2D6 (major), 3A4 (major)

Avoid Concomitant Use

Avoid concomitant use of TraMADol with any of the following: Sibutramine

Decreased Effect

TraMADol may decrease the levels/effects of: Pegvisomant

The levels/effects of TraMADol may be decreased by: Ammonium Chloride; CYP2D6 Inhibitors (Moderate); CYP2D6 Inhibitors (Strong); CYP3A4 Inducers (Strong); Deferasirox; Mixed Agonist / Antagonist Opioids

Increased Effect/Toxicity

TraMADol may increase the levels/effects of: Alcohol (Ethyl); Alvimopan; CNS Depressants; Desmopressin; MAO Inhibitors; Selective Serotonin Reuptake Inhibitors; Serotonin Modulators; Thiazide Diuretics; Vitamin K Antagonists

The levels/effects of TraMADol may be increased by: Amphetamines; Antipsychotic Agents (Phenothiazines); Conivaptan; CYP3A4 Inhibitors (Moderate); CYP3A4 Inhibitors (Strong); Dasatinib; Droperidol; Selective Serotonin Reuptake Inhibitors; Sibutramine; Succinylcholine; Tricyclic Antidepressants

Nutritional/Ethanol Interactions

Ethanol: Avoid ethanol (may increase CNS depression).

Food:

Immediate release: Does not affect the rate or extent of absorption.

Extended release: Reduced C_{max} and AUC and T_{max} occurred 3 hours earlier when taken with a high-fat meal.

Ryzolt™: Increased C_{max}; no effect on AUC.

Herb/Nutraceutical: Avoid valerian, St John's wort, kava kava, gotu kola (may increase CNS depression).

Lab Interactions May interfere with urine detection of PCP (false-positive).

Adverse Reactions

>10%:

Cardiovascular: Flushing (8% to 16%)

Central nervous system: Dizziness (10% to 33%), headache (4% to 32%), somnolence (7% to 25%), insomnia (2% to 11%)

Dermatologic: Pruritus (5% to 12%)

Gastrointestinal: Constipation (10% to 46%), nausea (15% to 40%), vomiting (5% to 17%), dyspepsia (1% to 13%)

Neuromuscular & skeletal: Weakness (4% to 12%)

1% to 10%:

Cardiovascular: Postural hypotension (2% to 5%), chest pain (1% to <5%), vasodilation (1% to <5%)

Central nervous system: Anxiety (1% to <5%), confusion (1% to <5%), coordination impaired (1% to <5%), depression (1% to <5%), euphoria (1% to <5%), hypoesthesia (1% to <5%), lethargy (1% to <5%), nervousness (1% to <5%), pain (1% to <5%), pyrexia (1% to <5%), restlessness (1% to <5%), malaise (<1% to <5%), fatigue (2%), vertigo (2%)

Dermatologic: Dermatitis (1% to <5%), rash (1% to <5%)

Endocrine & metabolic: Hot flashes (2% to 9%), menopausal symptoms (1% to <5%)

Gastrointestinal: Diarrhea (5% to 10%), xerostomia (3% to 10%), anorexia (1% to <6%), abdominal pain (1% to <5%), appetite decreased (1% to <5%), weight loss (1% to <5%), flatulence (<1% to <5%)

Genitourinary: Urinary tract infection (1% to <5%), urinary frequency (<1% to <5%), urinary retention (<1% to <5%)

Neuromuscular & skeletal: Arthralgia (1% to <5%), back pain (1% to <5%), hypertonia (1% to <5%), rigors (1% to <5%), paresthesia (1% to <5%), tremor (1% to <5%), creatine phosphokinase increased (1% to <5%)

Ocular: Blurred vision (1% to <5%), miosis (1% to <5%)

Respiratory: Bronchitis (1% to <5%), congestion (nasal/sinus) (1% to <5%), cough (1% to <5%), dyspnea (1% to <5%), nasopharyngitis (1% to <5%), rhinorrhea (1% to <5%), sinusitis (1% to <5%), sneezing (1% to <5%), sore throat (1% to <5%), upper respiratory infection (1% to <5%)

Miscellaneous: Diaphoresis (2% to 9%), flu-like syndrome (1% to < 5%), shivering (<1% to <5%)

A withdrawal syndrome may occur with abrupt discontinuation; includes anxiety, diarrhea, hallucinations (rare), nausea, pain, piloerection, rigors, sweating, and tremor. Uncommon discontinuation symptoms may include severe anxiety, panic attacks, or paresthesia.

Pharmacodynamics/Kinetics

Onset of Action Immediate release: ~1 hour

Duration of Action 9 hours

Absorption Immediate release formulation: Rapid and complete; Extended release formulation: Delayed

Bioavailability Immediate release: 75%; Extended release: Ultram® ER: 85% to 90% (as compared to immediate release), Zytram® XL, Tridural™: 70%; Ryzolt™: ~95% (as compared to immediate release)

Time to Peak Immediate release: ~2 hours; Extended release: Ultram® ER: ~12 hours, Ryzolt™, Tridural™: ~4 hours

Protein Binding Plasma: 20%

Half-Life Elimination Tramadol: ~6-8 hours; Active metabolite: 7-9 hours, prolonged in elderly, hepatic, or renal impairment; Zytram® XL: ~16 hours; Ralivia™ ER, Ryzolt™, Tridural™: ~5-9 hours

Metabolism Extensively hepatic via demethylation (mediated by CYP3A4 and CYP2B6), glucuronidation, and sulfation; has pharmacologically active metabolite formed by CYP2D6 (M1; O-desmethyl tramadol)

Excretion Urine (30% as unchanged drug; 60% as metabolites)

Available Dosage Forms

Tablet, oral: 50 mg

Ultram®: 50 mg

Tablet, extended release, oral: 100 mg, 200 mg

Ryzolt™: 100 mg, 200 mg, 300 mg

Ultram® ER: 100 mg, 200 mg, 300 mg

Tablet, orally disintegrating, oral:

Rybix™ ODT: 50 mg

Dosing

Adult Moderate-to-severe pain: Oral:

Immediate release formulation: 50-100 mg every 4-6 hours (not to exceed 400 mg/day)

For patients not requiring rapid onset of effect, tolerability may be improved by starting dose at 25 mg/day and titrating dose by 25 mg every 3 days, until reaching 25 mg 4 times/day. The total daily dose may then be increased by 50 mg every 3 days as tolerated, to reach dose of 50 mg 4 times/day. After titration, 50-100 mg may be given every 4-6 hours as needed up to a maximum 400 mg/day.

Extended release formulation:

Ultram® ER:

Patients not currently on immediate-release: 100 mg once daily; titrate every 5 days (maximum: 300 mg/day)

Patients currently on immediate-release: Calculate 24-hour immediate release total dose and initiate total extended release daily dose (round dose to the next lowest 100 mg increment); titrate (maximum: 300 mg/day)

Ralivia™ ER (Canadian labeling, not available in U.S.): 100 mg once daily; titrate every 5 days as needed based on clinical response and severity of pain (maximum: 300 mg/day)

Ryzolt™:

Patients not currently on immediate-release: 100 mg once daily; titrate every 2-3 days by 100 mg/day increments; usual daily dose: 200-300 mg/day (maximum: 300 mg/day)

Patients currently on immediate-release: Calculate 24 hour immediate release total dose and initiate total extended release daily dose (round dose to the next lowest 100 mg increment); titrate (maximum: 300 mg/day)

Tridural™ (Canadian labeling, not available in U.S.): 100 mg once daily; titrate by 100 mg/day every 2 days as needed based on clinical response and severity of pain (maximum: 300 mg/day)

Zytram® XL (Canadian labeling, not available in U.S.): 150 mg once daily; if pain relief is not achieved may titrate by increasing dosage incrementally, with sufficient time to evaluate effect of increased dosage; generally not more often than every 7 days (maximum: 400 mg/day)

Geriatric Elderly >65 years: Oral: Use caution and initiate at the lower end of the dosing range. Refer to adult dosing.

Immediate release: Elderly >75 years: Do not exceed 300 mg/day; see dosing adjustments for renal and hepatic impairment.

Extended release formulation: Elderly >75 years: Use with great caution; see dosing for adults, renal, and hepatic impairment.

Pediatric Moderate-to-severe pain: Oral:

Children 7-16 years (unlabeled use): 1-2 mg/kg/dose every 4-6 hours; maximum: 400 mg/day

Children ≥17 years: Refer to adult dosing.

Renal Impairment

Immediate release: Cl_{cr} <30 mL/minute: Administer 50-100 mg dose every 12 hours (maximum: 200 mg/day).

Extended release: Should not be used in patients with Cl_{cr} <30 mL/minute.

Hepatic Impairment

Immediate release: Cirrhosis: Recommended dose: 50 mg every 12 hours.

Extended release: Should not be used in patients with severe (Child-Pugh class C) hepatic dysfunction; Ryzolt™ should not be used in any degree of hepatic impairment

Administration

Oral

Extended release tablet: Swallow whole; do not crush, chew, or split. Administer without regard to meals, but consistently administering with or without meals.

Orally-disintegrating tablet: Remove from foil blister by peeling back (do not push tablet through the foil). Place tablet on tongue and allow to dissolve (may take ~1 minute); water is not needed, but may be administered with water. Do not chew, break, or split tablet.

Stability

Storage Store at 25°C (77°F); excursions permitted to 15°C to 30°C (59°F to 86°F).

Monitoring and Teaching Issues

Physical Assessment Assess patient's physical and/or psychological dependence. Discontinue slowly after prolonged use.

Patient Education Extended release tablet must be swallowed whole; do not break, chew, or crush. May cause physical and/or psychological dependence. While using this medication, do not use alcohol and other prescription or OTC medications (especially pain medications, sedatives, antihistamines, or cough preparations) without consulting prescriber. Maintain adequate hydration, unless instructed to restrict fluid intake. You may experience headache, drowsiness, dizziness, dry mouth, or blurred vision; nausea, vomiting, or loss of appetite; insomnia; or constipation. Report severe unresolved constipation, respiratory difficulty or shortness of breath, excessive sedation or increased insomnia and restlessness, rash or hives, seizures, muscle weakness or tremors, or chest pain or palpitations.

Dietary Considerations May be taken without regard to meals. Ultram® ER: Be consistent; always give with food or always give on an empty stomach. Some products may contain phenylalanine.

Geriatric Considerations One study in the elderly found that tramadol 50 mg was similar in efficacy as acetaminophen 300 mg with codeine 30 mg. In Ultram® ER trials, elderly patients experienced more adverse effects than younger adults, particularly constipation, fatigue, weakness, postural hypotension, and dyspepsia. For this reason, the extended release formulation should probably be avoided in the elderly, or only used with great caution.

Breast-Feeding Considerations Sixteen hours following a single 100 mg I.V. dose, the amount of tramadol found in breast milk was 0.1% of the maternal dose. Use is not recommended by the manufacturer for postdelivery analgesia in nursing mothers.

Pregnancy Considerations Adverse events were observed in animal studies. Tramadol has been shown to cross the human placenta when administered during labor. Postmarketing reports following tramadol use during pregnancy include neonatal seizures, withdrawal syndrome, fetal death, and stillbirth. Not recommended for use during labor and delivery.

◆ **Tramadol Hydrochloride** *see* TraMADol *on page* *1797*

◆ **Trandate®** *see* Labetalol *on page* *1048*

Trandolapril (tran DOE la pril)

U.S. Brand Names Mavik®

Generic Availability (U.S.) Yes

Pharmacologic Category Angiotensin-Converting Enzyme (ACE) Inhibitor

Pregnancy Risk Factor C (1st trimester); D (2nd and 3rd trimesters)

Lactation Excretion in breast milk unknown/not recommended

Use Treatment of hypertension alone or in combination with other antihypertensive agents; treatment of heart failure (HF) or left ventricular (LV) dysfunction after myocardial infarction (MI)

Unlabeled/Investigational Use To delay the progression of nephropathy and reduce risks of cardiovascular events in hypertensive patients with type 1 or 2 diabetes mellitus

Mechanism of Action/Effect Competitive inhibitor of angiotensin-converting enzyme (ACE); prevents conversion of angiotensin I to angiotensin II, a potent vasoconstrictor; results in lower levels of angiotensin II which causes an increase in plasma renin activity and a reduction in aldosterone secretion

Contraindications Hypersensitivity to trandolapril or any component of the formulation; history of angioedema related to previous treatment with an ACE inhibitor

Warnings/Precautions Anaphylactic reactions may occur rarely with ACE inhibitors. At any time during treatment (especially following first dose) angioedema may occur rarely with ACE inhibitors; it may involve the head and neck (potentially compromising the airway) or the intestine (presenting with abdominal pain). African-Americans and patients with idiopathic or hereditary angioedema may be at an increased risk. Prolonged frequent monitoring may be required especially if tongue, glottis, or larynx are involved as they are associated with airway obstruction. Patients with a history of airway surgery may have a higher risk of airway obstruction. Aggressive early and appropriate management is critical. Use in patients with previous angioedema associated with ACE inhibitor therapy is contraindicated. Severe anaphylactoid reactions may be seen during hemodialysis (eg, CVVHD) with high-flux dialysis membranes (eg, AN69). Rare cases of anaphylactoid reactions have been reported in patients undergoing sensitization treatment with hymenoptera (bee, wasp) venom while receiving ACE inhibitors.

Symptomatic hypotension with or without syncope can occur with ACE inhibitors (usually with the first several doses); effects are most often observed in volume-depleted patients; correct volume depletion prior to initiation; close monitoring of patient is required especially with initial dosing and dosing increases; blood pressure must be lowered at a rate appropriate for the patient's clinical condition. Initiation of therapy in patients with ischemic heart disease or cerebrovascular disease warrants close observation due to the potential consequences posed by falling blood pressure (eg, MI, stroke). Use with caution in hypertrophic cardiomyopathy with outflow tract obstruction, severe aortic stenosis, or before, during, or immediately after major surgery. **[U.S. Boxed Warning]: Based on human data, ACEIs can cause injury and death to the developing fetus when used in the second and third trimesters. ACEIs should be discontinued as soon as possible once pregnancy is detected.**

Hyperkalemia may occur with ACE inhibitors; risk factors include renal dysfunction, diabetes mellitus, concomitant use of potassium-sparing diuretics, potassium supplements, and/or potassium-containing salts. Use cautiously, if at all, with these agents and monitor potassium closely. Cough may occur with ACE inhibitors. Other causes of cough should be considered (eg, pulmonary congestion in patients with heart failure) and excluded prior to discontinuation.

Dosage adjustment needed in severe renal dysfunction (Cl_{cr} <30 mL/minute) or hepatic cirrhosis. May be associated with deterioration of renal function and/or increases in serum creatinine, particularly in patients with low renal blood flow (eg, renal artery stenosis, heart failure) whose glomerular filtration rate (GFR) is dependent on efferent arteriolar vasoconstriction by angiotensin II; deterioration may result in oliguria, acute renal failure, and progressive azotemia. Small increases in serum creatinine may occur following initiation; consider discontinuation only in patients with progressive and/or significant deterioration in renal function. Use with caution in patients with unstented unilateral/bilateral renal artery stenosis. When unstented bilateral renal artery stenosis is present, use is generally avoided due to the elevated risk of deterioration in renal function unless possible benefits outweigh risks. Concurrent use of angiotensin receptor blockers may increase the risk of clinically-significant adverse events (eg, renal dysfunction, hyperkalemia).

Rare toxicities associated with ACE inhibitors include cholestatic jaundice (which may progress to fulminant hepatic necrosis), agranulocytosis, neutropenia, or leukopenia with myeloid hypoplasia. Patients with collagen vascular diseases (especially with concomitant renal impairment) or renal impairment alone may be at increased risk for hematologic toxicity; periodically monitor CBC with differential in these patients.

Drug Interactions

Avoid Concomitant Use There are no known interactions where it is recommended to avoid concomitant use.

Decreased Effect

The levels/effects of Trandolapril may be decreased by: Antacids; Aprotinin; Herbs (Hypertensive Properties); Methylphenidate; Nonsteroidal Anti-Inflammatory Agents; Salicylates; Yohimbine

Increased Effect/Toxicity

Trandolapril may increase the levels/effects of: Allopurinol; Amifostine; Antihypertensives; AzaTHIOprine; CycloSPORINE; CycloSPORINE (Systemic); Ferric Gluconate; Gold Sodium Thiomalate; Hypotensive Agents; Iron Dextran Complex; Lithium; RiTUXimab

The levels/effects of Trandolapril may be increased by: Angiotensin II Receptor Blockers; Diazoxide; DPP-IV Inhibitors; Eplerenone; Everolimus; Herbs (Hypotensive Properties); Loop Diuretics; MAO Inhibitors; Pentoxifylline; Phosphodiesterase 5 Inhibitors; Potassium Salts; Potassium-Sparing Diuretics; Prostacyclin Analogues; Sirolimus; Temsirolimus; Thiazide Diuretics; TiZANidine; Tolvaptan; Trimethoprim

Nutritional/Ethanol Interactions Herb/Nutraceutical: Avoid bayberry, blue cohosh, cayenne, ephedra, ginger, ginseng (American), kola, licorice (may worsen hypertension). Avoid black cohosh, California poppy, coleus, golden seal, hawthorn, mistletoe, periwinkle, quinine, shepherd's purse (may have increased antihypertensive effect).

Adverse Reactions Note: Frequency ranges include data from hypertension and heart failure trials. Higher rates of adverse reactions have generally been noted in patients with CHF. However, the frequency of adverse effects associated with placebo is also increased in this population.

>1%:

Cardiovascular: Hypotension (<1% to 11%), syncope (6%), bradycardia (<1% to 5%), intermittent claudication (4%)

Central nervous system: Dizziness (1% to 23%)

Endocrine & metabolic: Uric acid increased (15%), hyperkalemia (5%), hypocalcemia (5%)

Gastrointestinal: Diarrhea (1%)

Neuromuscular & skeletal: Myalgia (5%)

Renal: BUN increased (9%), serum creatinine increased (1% to 5%)

Respiratory: Cough (2% to 35%)

Worsening of renal function may occur in patients with bilateral renal artery stenosis or hypovolemia. In addition, a syndrome which may include fever, myalgia, arthralgia, interstitial nephritis, vasculitis, rash, eosinophilia and positive ANA, and elevated ESR has been reported with ACE inhibitors. Eosinophilic pneumonitis has also been reported with other ACE inhibitors.

Pharmacodynamics/Kinetics

Onset of Action 1-2 hours; Peak effect: Reduction in blood pressure: 6 hours

Duration of Action Prolonged; 72 hours after single dose

Absorption Rapid

Bioavailability Trandolapril: 10%; Trandolaprilat: 70%

Time to Peak Parent: 1 hour; Active metabolite trandolaprilat: 4-10 hours

Protein Binding Trandolapril: ~80%; Trandolaprilat: 65% to 94% (concentration dependent)

Half-Life Elimination

Trandolapril: 6 hours; Trandolaprilat: Effective: 22.5 hours

Metabolism Hepatically hydrolyzed to active metabolite, trandolaprilat

Excretion Urine (33%); feces (66%)

Clearance: Reduce dose in renal failure; creatinine clearances ≤30 mL/minute result in accumulation of active metabolite

Available Dosage Forms

Tablet, oral: 1 mg, 2 mg, 4 mg

Mavik®: 1 mg, 2 mg, 4 mg

Dosing

Adult & Geriatric

Hypertension: Initial dose in patients not receiving a diuretic: Oral: 1 mg once daily (2 mg/day in black patients). Adjust dosage at intervals of ≥1 week according to blood pressure response; most patients require 2-4 mg/day. There is little experience with doses >8 mg/day. Patients inadequately treated with once daily dosing at 4 mg may be treated with twice daily dosing. If blood pressure is not adequately controlled with trandolapril monotherapy, a diuretic may be added.

Usual dose range (JNC 7): 1-4 mg once daily

Post-MI heart failure or LV dysfunction: Oral: Initial: 1 mg once daily; titrate (as tolerated) towards target dose of 4 mg/day. If 4 mg dose is not tolerated, patients may continue therapy with the greatest tolerated dose.

Renal Impairment Cl_{cr} <30 mL/minute: Recommended starting dose: 0.5 mg once daily.

Hepatic Impairment Cirrhosis: Recommended starting dose: 0.5 mg once daily.

Stability

Storage Store at controlled room temperature of 20°C to 25°C (68°F to 77°F).

Monitoring and Teaching Issues

Laboratory Monitoring Serum creatinine and potassium; if patient has collagen vascular disease and/or renal impairment, periodically monitor CBC with differential

Physical Assessment Assess potential for interactions with other pharmacological agents or herbal products that may impact fluid balance or cardiac status. Monitor for hypovolemia, angioedema, and postural hypotension with first doses and on a regular basis during therapy.

Patient Education Take first dose at bedtime. This drug does not eliminate need for diet or exercise regimen as recommended by prescriber. May cause dizziness, fainting, lightheadedness, postural hypotension, or diarrhea. Report immediately any swelling of face, mouth, lips, tongue or throat; or respiratory difficulty. Report chest pain or palpitations, swelling of extremities, skin rash, or unusual cough.

Geriatric Considerations Due to frequent decreases in glomerular filtration (also creatinine clearance) with aging, elderly patients may have exaggerated responses to ACE inhibitors; differences in clinical response due to hepatic changes are not observed. ACE inhibitors may be preferred agents in elderly patients with CHF and diabetes mellitus. Diabetic proteinuria is reduced and insulin sensitivity is enhanced. In general, the side effect profile is favorable in the elderly and causes little or no CNS confusion; use lowest dose recommendations initially. Adjust for renal function. Many elderly may be volume depleted due to diuretic use and/or blunted thirst reflex resulting in inadequate fluid intake.

Breast-Feeding Considerations It is not known if trandolapril is excreted in breast milk. Breast-feeding is not recommended by the manufacturer.

Pregnancy Considerations Due to adverse events observed in some animal studies, trandolapril is considered pregnancy category C during the first trimester. Based on human data, trandolapril is considered pregnancy category D if used during the second and third trimesters (per the manufacturer; however, one study suggests that fetal injury may occur at anytime during pregnancy). First trimester exposure to ACE inhibitors may cause major congenital malformations. An increased risk of cardiovascular and/or central nervous system malformations was observed in one study; however, an increased risk of teratogenic events was not observed in other studies. Second and third trimester use of an ACE inhibitor is associated with oligohydramnios. Oligohydramnios due to decreased fetal renal function may lead to fetal limb contractures, craniofacial deformation, and hypoplastic lung development. The use of ACE inhibitors during the second and third trimesters is also associated with anuria, hypotension, renal failure (reversible or irreversible), skull hypoplasia, and death in the fetus/neonate. Chronic maternal hypertension itself is also associated with adverse events in the fetus/infant. ACE inhibitors are not recommended during pregnancy to treat maternal hypertension or heart failure. Those who are planning a pregnancy should be considered for other medication options if an ACE inhibitor is currently prescribed or the ACE inhibitor should be discontinued as soon as possible once pregnancy is detected. The exposed fetus should be monitored for fetal growth, amniotic fluid volume, and organ formation. Infants exposed to an ACE inhibitor *in utero*, especially during the second and third trimester, should be monitored for hyperkalemia, hypotension, and oliguria.

[U.S. Boxed Warning]: Based on human data, ACE inhibitors can cause injury and death to the developing fetus when used in the second and third trimesters. ACE inhibitors should be discontinued as soon as possible once pregnancy is detected.

Related Information

Angiotensin Agents *on page 1974*

Heart Failure (Systolic) *on page 2040*

Trandolapril and Verapamil (tran DOE la pril & ver AP a mil)

U.S. Brand Names Tarka®

Index Terms Verapamil and Trandolapril

Generic Availability (U.S.) Yes

Pharmacologic Category Angiotensin-Converting Enzyme (ACE) Inhibitor; Calcium Channel Blocker

Pregnancy Risk Factor C/D (2nd and 3rd trimesters)

Lactation Enters breast milk/contraindicated

Use Treatment of hypertension; however, not indicated for initial treatment of hypertension

Available Dosage Forms

Tablet, variable release: Trandolapril 2 mg [immediate release] and verapamil 180 mg [sustained release]; Trandolapril 2 mg [immediate release] and verapamil 240 mg [sustained release]; Trandolapril 4 mg [immediate release] and verapamil 240 mg [sustained release]

Tarka®:

1/240: Trandolapril 1 mg [immediate release] and verapamil 240 mg [sustained release]
2/180: Trandolapril 2 mg [immediate release] and verapamil 180 mg [sustained release]
2/240: Trandolapril 2 mg [immediate release] and verapamil 240 mg [sustained release]
4/240: Trandolapril 4 mg [immediate release] and verapamil 240 mg [sustained release]

Dosing

Adult Hypertension: Oral: Individualize dose. Patients receiving trandolapril (up to 8 mg) and verapamil (up to 240 mg) in separate tablets may wish to receive Tarka® at equivalent dosages once daily.

Geriatric Refer to dosing in individual monographs.

Renal Impairment Usual regimen need not be adjusted unless patient's creatinine clearance is <30 mL/minute. Titration of individual components must be done prior to switching to combination product

Hepatic Impairment Has not been evaluated in hepatic impairment. Verapamil is hepatically metabolized, adjustment of dosage in hepatic impairment is recommended.

Monitoring and Teaching Issues

Laboratory Monitoring Serum creatinine and potassium; if patient has collagen vascular disease and/or renal impairment, periodically monitor CBC with differential

Physical Assessment See individual agents.

Patient Education See individual agents.

Related Information

Trandolapril *on page 1800*
Verapamil *on page 1858*

◆ **Transamine Sulphate** *see* Tranylcypromine *on page 1803*
◆ **Transderm Scōp®** *see* Scopolamine (Systemic) *on page 1627*
◆ ***trans*-Retinoic Acid** *see* Tretinoin (Topical) *on page 1811*
◆ **Tranxene T-Tab** *see* Clorazepate *on page 415*
◆ **Tranxene® T-Tab®** *see* Clorazepate *on page 415*

Tranylcypromine (tran il SIP roe meen)

U.S. Brand Names Parnate®

Index Terms Transamine Sulphate; Tranylcypromine Sulfate

Generic Availability (U.S.) No

Pharmacologic Category Antidepressant, Monoamine Oxidase Inhibitor

Medication Guide Available Yes

Lactation Enters breast milk/not recommended

Use Treatment of major depressive episode without melancholia

Available Dosage Forms

Tablet, oral: 10 mg

Parnate®: 10 mg

Dosing

Adult & Geriatric Depression: Oral: Usual effective dose: 30 mg/day in divided doses; if symptoms don't improve after 2 weeks, increase by 10 mg increments at 1- to 3-week intervals; maximum: 60 mg/day

Transitioning from another MAO inhibitor or dibenzazepine derivative (eg, TCAs, carbamazepine, cyclobenzaprine) to tranylcypromine therapy: Allow at least 1 medication-free week, then initiate tranylcypromine at 50% of usual starting dose for at least 1 week.

Monitoring and Teaching Issues

Laboratory Monitoring Blood glucose

Physical Assessment Evaluate need for continued therapy on a regular basis. Monitor blood pressure. Monitor for CNS depression. Observe for clinical worsening, suicidality, or unusual behavior changes, especially during the initial few months of therapy or during dosage changes. Taper dosage slowly when discontinuing.

Patient Education It may take 2-3 weeks to achieve desired results. Take in the morning to reduce the incidence of insomnia. Avoid alcohol, caffeine, and other prescription or OTC medications not approved by prescriber. Avoid tyramine-containing foods; see prescriber for complete list of foods to be avoided. Maintain adequate hydration unless instructed to restrict fluid intake. If you have diabetes, monitor blood glucose closely at the beginning of therapy. May cause hypoglycemia. You may experience drowsiness, dizziness, blurred vision, anorexia, dry mouth, constipation, diarrhea, orthostatic hypotension, or altered sexual ability (reversible). Report persistent excessive sedation; muscle cramping, tremors, weakness, or change in gait; chest pain, palpitations, rapid heartbeat, or swelling of extremities; vision changes; suicide ideation; or worsening of condition.

Related Information

Antidepressant Agents *on page 1982*

◆ **Tranylcypromine Sulfate** *see* Tranylcypromine *on page 1803*

Trastuzumab (tras TU zoo mab)

U.S. Brand Names Herceptin®

Index Terms anti-c-erB-2; anti-ERB-2; MOAB HER2; rhuMAb HER2

Generic Availability (U.S.) No

Pharmacologic Category Antineoplastic Agent, Monoclonal Antibody; Monoclonal Antibody

Medication Safety Issues

High alert medication: This medication is in a class the Institute for Safe Medication Practices (ISMP) includes among its list of drug classes which have a heightened risk of causing significant patient harm when used in error.

Pregnancy Risk Factor D

Lactation Excretion in breast milk unknown/not recommended

Use Treatment (adjuvant) of HER-2 overexpressing breast cancer; treatment of HER-2 overexpressing metastatic breast cancer; treatment of HER-2 overexpressing metastatic gastric or gastroesophageal junction adenocarcinoma (in patients who have not received prior treatment)

Mechanism of Action/Effect Trastuzumab is a monoclonal antibody which binds to the extracellular domain of the human epidermal growth factor receptor 2 protein (HER-2). It mediates antibody-dependent cellular cytotoxicity by inhibiting proliferation of cells which overexpress HER-2 protein.

Contraindications There are no contraindications listed within the manufacturer's labeling.

Canadian labeling: Hypersensitivity to trastuzumab, Chinese hamster ovary (CHO) cell proteins, or any component of the formulation

Warnings/Precautions Hazardous agent - use appropriate precautions for handling and disposal. **[U.S. Boxed Warning]: Trastuzumab is associated with symptomatic and asymptomatic reductions in left ventricular ejection fraction (LVEF) and heart failure (HF); the incidence is highest in patients receiving trastuzumab with an anthracycline-containing chemotherapy regimen. Evaluate LVEF in all patients prior to and during treatment; discontinue for cardiomyopathy.** Extreme caution should be used in patients with pre-existing cardiac disease or dysfunction. Prior or concurrent exposure to anthracyclines or radiation therapy significantly increases the risk of cardiomyopathy; other potential risk factors include advanced age, high or low body mass index, smoking, diabetes, and hyper/hypothyroidism. Discontinuation should be strongly considered in patients who develop a clinically significant reduction in LVEF during therapy; treatment with HF medications (eg, ACE inhibitors, beta-blockers) should be initiated. Withhold treatment for ≥16% decrease from pretreatment levels or LVEF below normal limits and ≥10% decrease from baseline (see Dosing Adjustment for Cardiotoxicity). Cardiomyopathy due to trastuzumab is generally reversible over a period of 1-3 months after discontinuation. Trastuzumab is also associated with arrhythmias, hypertension, mural thrombus formation, stroke, and even cardiac death.

[U.S. Boxed Warning]: Serious adverse events, including hypersensitivity reaction (anaphylaxis), infusion reactions (including fatalities), and pulmonary events (including acute respiratory distress syndrome [ARDS]) have been associated with trastuzumab. Discontinue for anaphylaxis, angioedema, ARDS or interstitial pneumonitis. Most of these events occur with the first infusion; pulmonary events may occur during or within 24 hours of the first infusion; delayed reactions have occurred. Interrupt infusion for dyspnea or significant hypotension; monitor until symptoms resolve. Infusion reactions may consist of fever and chills, and may also include nausea, vomiting, pain, headache dizziness, dyspnea, hypotension, rash and weakness. Retreatment of patients who experienced severe hypersensitivity reactions has been attempted (with premedication). Some patients tolerated retreatment, while others experienced a second severe reaction. When used in combination with myelosuppressive chemotherapy, trastuzumab may increase the incidence of neutropenia (moderate-to-severe) and febrile neutropenia; the incidence of anemia may be higher when trastuzumab is added to chemotherapy. Rare cases of nephrotic syndrome with evidence of glomerulopathy have been reported, with an onset of 4-18 months from trastuzumab initiation; complications may include volume overload and HF. The incidence of renal impairment was increased in metastatic gastric cancer patients when trastuzumab is added to chemotherapy.

May cause serious pulmonary toxicity (dyspnea, hypoxia, interstitial pneumonitis, pulmonary infiltrates, pleural effusion, noncardiogenic pulmonary edema, pulmonary insufficiency, acute respiratory distress syndrome, and/or pulmonary fibrosis); use caution in patients with pre-existing pulmonary disease or patients with extensive pulmonary tumor involvement. **[U.S. Boxed Warning]: Trastuzumab exposure during pregnancy may result in oligohydramnios and oligohydramnios sequence (pulmonary hypoplasia, skeletal malformations and neonatal death).** Effective contraception is recommended during and for 6 months after treatment for women of childbearing potential.

Drug Interactions

Avoid Concomitant Use

Avoid concomitant use of Trastuzumab with any of the following: Belimumab

Decreased Effect

Trastuzumab may decrease the levels/effects of: PACLitaxel

Increased Effect/Toxicity

Trastuzumab may increase the levels/effects of: Antineoplastic Agents (Anthracycline); Belimumab; Immunosuppressants

The levels/effects of Trastuzumab may be increased by: Abciximab; PACLitaxel

Adverse Reactions Note: Percentages reported with single-agent therapy.

>10%:

Cardiovascular: LVEF decreased (4% to 22%)

Central nervous system: Pain (47%), fever (6% to 36%), chills (5% to 32%), headache (10% to 26%), insomnia (14%), dizziness (4% to 13%)

Dermatologic: Rash (4% to 18%)

Gastrointestinal: Nausea (6% to 33%), diarrhea (7% to 25%), vomiting (4% to 23%), abdominal pain (2% to 22%), anorexia (14%)

Neuromuscular & skeletal: Weakness (4% to 42%), back pain (5% to 22%)

Respiratory: Cough (5% to 26%), dyspnea (3% to 22%), rhinitis (2% to 14%), pharyngitis (12%)

Miscellaneous: Infusion reaction (21% to 40%, chills and fever most common; severe: 1%), infection (20%)

1% to 10%:

Cardiovascular: Peripheral edema (5% to 10%), edema (8%), HF (2% to 7%; severe: <1%), tachycardia (5%), hypertension (4%), arrhythmia (3%), palpitation (3%)

Central nervous system: Depression (6%)

Dermatologic: Acne (2%), nail disorder (2%), pruritus (2%)

Gastrointestinal: Constipation (2%), dyspepsia (2%)

Genitourinary: Urinary tract infection (3% to 5%)

Hematologic: Anemia (4%), leukopenia (3%)

Neuromuscular & skeletal: Paresthesia (2% to 9%), bone pain (3% to 7%), arthralgia (6% to 8%), myalgia (4%), muscle spasm (3%), peripheral neuritis (2%), neuropathy (1%)

Respiratory: Sinusitis (2% to 9%), nasopharyngitis (8%), upper respiratory infection (3%), epistaxis (2%), pharyngolaryngeal pain (2%)

Miscellaneous: Flu-like syndrome (2% to 10%), accidental injury (6%), influenza (4%), allergic reaction (3%), herpes simplex (2%)

Pharmacodynamics/Kinetics

Half-Life Elimination Weekly dosing: Mean: 6 days (range: 1-32 days); every 3 week regimen: Mean: 16 days (range: 11-23 days)

Available Dosage Forms

Injection, powder for reconstitution:

Herceptin®: 440 mg

Dosing

Adult & Geriatric Details concerning dosing in combination regimens should also be consulted.

Note: Missed dose recommendation (Canadian labeling, 2010): If a dose is missed by ≤1 week, the usual maintenance dose (based on patient's schedule) should be administered as soon as possible (do not wait until the next planned cycle); if a dose is missed by >1 week, then a loading dose (4 mg/kg if patient receives trastuzumab weekly; 8 mg/kg if on an every-3-week schedule) should be administered, followed by the usual maintenance dose and schedule.

Breast cancer, adjuvant treatment: I.V. infusion:

With concurrent paclitaxel or docetaxel:

Initial loading dose: 4 mg/kg infused over 90 minutes

Maintenance dose: 2 mg/kg infused over 30 minutes weekly for total of 12 weeks, followed 1 week later (when concurrent chemotherapy completed) by 6 mg/kg infused over 30-90 minutes every 3 weeks for total therapy duration of 52 weeks

With concurrent docetaxel/carboplatin:

Initial loading dose: 4 mg/kg infused over 90 minutes

Maintenance dose: 2 mg/kg infused over 30 minutes weekly for total of 18 weeks, followed 1 week later (when concurrent chemotherapy completed) by 6 mg/kg infused over 30-90 minutes every 3 weeks for total therapy duration of 52 weeks

Following completion of anthracycline-based chemotherapy:

Initial loading dose: 8 mg/kg infused over 90 minutes

Maintenance dose: 6 mg/kg infused over 30-90 minutes every 3 weeks for total therapy duration of 52 weeks

Breast cancer, metastatic (either as a single agent or in combination with paclitaxel): I.V. infusion:

Initial loading dose: 4 mg/kg infused over 90 minutes

Maintenance dose: 2 mg/kg infused over 30 minutes weekly until disease progression

Gastric cancer, metastatic (in combination with cisplatin and either capecitabine or fluorouracil for 6 cycles followed by trastuzumab monotherapy; Bang, 2010; Van Cutsem, 2009): I.V. infusion:

Initial loading dose: 8 mg/kg infused over 90 minutes

Maintenance dose: 6 mg/kg infused over 30-90 minutes every 3 weeks until disease progression

Renal Impairment Data suggest that the disposition of trastuzumab is not altered based on serum creatinine (up to 2 mg/dL)

Adjustment for Toxicity

Cardiotoxicity: LVEF ≥16% decrease from baseline within normal limits or LVEF below normal limits and ≥10% decrease from baseline: Withhold treatment for at least 4 weeks and repeat LVEF every 4 weeks. May resume trastuzumab treatment if LVEF returns to normal limits within 4-8 weeks and remains at ≤15% decrease from baseline value. Discontinue permanently for persistent (>8 weeks) LVEF decline or for >3 incidents of treatment interruptions for cardiomyopathy.

Infusion-related events:

Mild-moderate infusion reactions: Decrease infusion rate.

Dyspnea, clinically significant hypotension: Interrupt infusion.

Severe or life-threatening infusion reactions: Discontinue.

Administration

I.V. Administered by I.V. infusion; loading doses are infused over 90 minutes; maintenance doses may be infused over 30 minutes if tolerated. Do not administer with D_5W. **Do not administer I.V. push or by rapid bolus.** Treatment with acetaminophen, diphenhydramine, and/or meperidine is usually effective for managing infusion-related events.

Stability

Reconstitution Reconstitute each vial with 20 mL of bacteriostatic sterile water for injection to a concentration of 21 mg/mL. Swirl gently; do not shake. Allow vial to rest for ~5 minutes. If the patient has a known hypersensitivity to benzyl alcohol, trastuzumab may be reconstituted with sterile water for injection without preservatives, which must be used immediately. Further dilute the appropriate volume for the trastuzumab dose in 250 mL NS prior to administration. Gently invert bag to mix.

Storage Prior to reconstitution, store intact vials under refrigeration at 2°C to 8°C (36°F to 46°F). Following reconstitution with bacteriostatic SWFI, the solution in the vial is stable refrigerated for 28 days from the date of reconstitution; do not freeze. Solutions reconstituted with sterile water for injection without preservatives must be used immediately. The solution diluted in 250 mL NS for infusion is stable for 24 hours refrigerated; do not freeze.

Monitoring and Teaching Issues

Physical Assessment Assess for signs of infusion reaction during infusion. If patient is pregnant, monitor amniotic fluid volume. Evaluate cardiac and respiratory function and vital signs. Monitor for arrhythmias, difficulty breathing, peripheral edema, and sudden weight gain.

Patient Education This medication can only be administered by infusion. Report immediately any respiratory difficulty, chills, fever, headache, backache, nausea, or vomiting. You will be susceptible to infection. You may experience dizziness, weakness, nausea, vomiting, diarrhea, headache, or back or joint pain. Report persistent GI effects; sore throat, runny nose, or respiratory difficulty; chest pain, irregular heartbeat, palpitations, swelling of extremities, or unusual weight gain; muscle or joint weakness, numbness, or pain; skin rash or irritation; itching or pain on urination; unhealed sores, white plaques in mouth or genital area, or unusual bruising or bleeding.

Breast-Feeding Considerations It is not known whether trastuzumab is secreted in human milk. Because many immunoglobulins are secreted in milk, and the potential for serious adverse reactions in the nursing infant exists, patients should discontinue nursing during treatment; the extended half-life should be considered for decisions regarding breast-feeding after therapy completion.

Pregnancy Considerations Reproductive studies in cynomolgus monkeys showed no evidence of impaired fertility or fetal harm. Trastuzumab inhibits HER2 protein, which has a role in embryonic development. There are no adequate and well-controlled studies in pregnant women. Effective contraception is recommended during and for 6 months after treatment for women of childbearing potential. **[U.S. Boxed Warning]: Trastuzumab exposure during pregnancy may result in oligohydramnios and oligohydramnios sequence (pulmonary hypoplasia, skeletal malformations and neonatal death).** Oligohydramnios (reversible in some cases) has been reported with trastuzumab use alone or with combination chemotherapy. If trastuzumab exposure occurs during pregnancy, monitor for oligohydramnios. Women exposed to trastuzumab during pregnancy are encouraged to enroll in MotHER (the Herceptin Pregnancy Registry; 1-800-690-6720).

The National Comprehensive Cancer Network (NCCN) breast cancer guidelines (v.3.2010) consider pregnancy a contraindication to trastuzumab treatment and recommend administering trastuzumab (if indicated) in the postpartum period.

◆ **Trav-L-Tabs® [OTC]** *see* Meclizine *on page 1153*

◆ **Travatan® [DSC]** *see* Travoprost *on page 1807*

◆ **Travatan Z®** *see* Travoprost *on page 1807*

Travelers' Diarrhea and Cholera Vaccine

(TRAV uh lerz dahy uh REE uh & KOL er uh vak SEEN)

Index Terms *Vibrio cholera* and Enterotoxigenic *Escherichia coli Vaccine*; Cholera and Traveler's Diarrhea Vaccine; Cholera Vaccine; Enterotoxigenic *Escherichia coli* and *Vibrio cholera* Vaccine; Oral Cholera Vaccine; Traveller's Diarrhea Vaccine and Cholera

Pharmacologic Category Vaccine

Use Protection against travelers' diarrhea and/or cholera in adults and children ≥2 years of age who will be visiting areas where there is a risk of contracting travelers' diarrhea caused by enterotoxigenic *E. coli* (ETEC) or cholera caused by *V. cholerae* O1 (classical and El Tor biotypes; Inaba and Ogawa serotypes)

Product Availability Not available in U.S.

Dosing

Adult & Geriatric

Cholera: Oral:

Primary immunization: 2 doses given at intervals of ≥1 week and completed at least 1 week prior to trip to endemic/epidemic areas; restart treatment if interval between doses >6 weeks

Booster:

2-5 years **since last dose**: 1 booster dose

>5 years **since last dose**: Repeat primary immunization schedule

ETEC: Oral:

Primary immunization: 2 doses given at intervals of ≥1 week and completed at least 1 week prior to trip to endemic/epidemic areas; restart treatment if interval between doses >6 weeks

Booster:

3 months to 5 years **since last dose**: 1 booster dose

>5 years **since last dose**: Repeat primary immunization schedule

Pediatric

Cholera: Oral:

Primary immunization:

Children 2-6 years: 3 doses given at intervals of ≥1 week and completed at least 1 week prior to trip to endemic/epidemic areas; restart treatment if interval between doses >6 weeks

Children >6 years: Refer to adult dosing.

Booster:

Children 2-6 years:

6 months to 5 years **since last dose**: 1 booster dose

>5 years **since last dose**: Repeat primary immunization schedule

Children >6 years: Refer to adult dosing.

ETEC: Oral: Children ≥2 years: Refer to adult dosing.

Administration

Oral For oral use only; do no administer I.M., I.V., or SubQ. Oral administration of other medications, vaccines, and consumption of food should be avoided 1 hour before and 1 hour following vaccine administration.

Administration with other vaccines (manufacturer recommendations): *Typhoid vaccine, oral:* Separate by at least 8 hours

Acetaminophen may be used when needed to provide comfort; however, routine prophylactic administration of acetaminophen to prevent fever due to vaccine use is not recommended. There is evidence of a decreased immune response to some vaccines associated with acetaminophen administration; the clinical significance of this reduction in immune response has not been established.

Monitoring and Teaching Issues

Physical Assessment Assess any previous exposure to cholera vaccine prior to treatment. Instruct patient about safe eating and drinking practice. All serious adverse reactions must be reported to the U.S. DHHS. Federal law also requires entry into the patient's medical record. Instruct patient about anaphylactic treatment that should be available during use.

Patient Education Emergency treatment for anaphylactic reaction should be available during use. Granules must be dissolved in a glass with water (do not use juice, milk, or other beverages). Contact healthcare provider if you develop severe belly pain, diarrhea, or rash. May cause mild transient abdominal pain or diarrhea.

◆ **Traveller's Diarrhea Vaccine and Cholera** *see* Travelers' Diarrhea and Cholera Vaccine *on page 1806*

Travoprost (TRA voe prost)

U.S. Brand Names Travatan Z®; Travatan® [DSC]

Generic Availability (U.S.) No

Pharmacologic Category Ophthalmic Agent, Antiglaucoma; Prostaglandin, Ophthalmic

Medication Safety Issues

Sound-alike/look-alike issues:

Travatan® may be confused with Xalatan®

Pregnancy Risk Factor C

Lactation Excretion in breast milk unknown/use caution

Use Reduction of elevated intraocular pressure in patients with open-angle glaucoma or ocular hypertension who are intolerant of the other IOP-lowering medications or insufficiently responsive (failed to achieve target IOP determined after multiple measurements over time) to another IOP-lowering medication

Available Dosage Forms

Solution, ophthalmic:

Travatan Z®: 0.004% (2.5 mL, 5 mL)

Dosing

Adult & Geriatric Glaucoma (open angle) or ocular hypertension: Ophthalmic: Instill 1 drop into affected eye(s) once daily in the evening; do not exceed once-daily dosing (may decrease IOP-lowering effect). If used with other topical ophthalmic agents, separate administration by at least 5 minutes.

Administration

Other May be used with other eye drops to lower intraocular pressure. If using more than one ophthalmic product, wait at least 5 minutes in between application of each medication. Travatan®: Remove contact lenses prior to administration and wait 15 minutes before reinserting.

Monitoring and Teaching Issues

Patient Education For use in eyes only. Wash hands before instilling. Sit or lie down to instill. Open eye, look at ceiling, and instill prescribed amount of solution. Apply gentle pressure to inner corner of eye. Do not let tip of applicator touch eye; do not contaminate tip of applicator (may cause eye infection, eye damage, or vision loss). May cause permanent changes in eye color, eyelid, and eyelashes. May also increase the length and/or number of eyelashes. Changes may occur slowly (months to years). May be used with other eye drops to lower intraocular pressure. If using more than one eye drop medicine, wait at least 5 minutes in between application of each medication. Notify prescriber if conjunctivitis or eyelid reactions occur with use of this product.

TraZODone (TRAZ oh done)

U.S. Brand Names Oleptro™

Index Terms Desyrel; Trazodone Hydrochloride

Generic Availability (U.S.) Yes: Excludes extended release tablet

Pharmacologic Category Antidepressant, Serotonin Reuptake Inhibitor/Antagonist

Medication Safety Issues

Sound-alike/look-alike issues:

Desyrel may be confused with Demerol®, Delsym®, Zestril®

TraZODone may be confused with traMADol, ziprasidone

International issues:

Desyrel [Canada, Turkey] may be confused with Deseril brand name for methysergide [Australia, Belgium, Great Britain, Netherlands]

Medication Guide Available Yes

Pregnancy Risk Factor C

Lactation Enters breast milk/use caution (AAP rates "of concern"; AAP 2001 update pending)

Use Treatment of major depressive disorder

Unlabeled/Investigational Use Potential augmenting agent for antidepressants, hypnotic

Available Dosage Forms

Tablet, oral: 50 mg, 100 mg, 150 mg, 300 mg

Tablet, extended release, oral:

Oleptro™: 150 mg, 300 mg

Dosing

Adult

Depression: Oral: Initial: 150 mg/day in 3 divided doses (may increase by 50 mg/day every 3-7 days); maximum dose: 600 mg/day

Extended release formulation: Initial: 150 mg once daily at bedtime (may increase by 75 mg/day every 3 days); maximum dose: 375 mg/day; once adequate response obtained, gradually reduce with adjustment based on therapeutic response

Note: Therapeutic effects may take up to 6 weeks. Therapy is normally maintained for 6-12 months after optimum response is reached to prevent recurrence of depression.

Sedation/hypnotic (unlabeled use): Oral: 25-50 mg at bedtime (often in combination with daytime SSRIs). May increase up to 200 mg at bedtime.

Geriatric

Immediate release: Oral: 25-50 mg at bedtime with 25-50 mg/day dose increase every 3 days for inpatients and weekly for outpatients, if tolerated; usual dose: 75-150 mg/day

Extended release: Refer to adult dosing. Use with caution in the elderly; clinical experience is limited.

Pediatric

Depression (unlabeled use):

Children 6-12 years: Initial: 1.5-2 mg/kg/day in divided doses; increase gradually every 3-4 days as needed; maximum: 6 mg/kg/day in 3 divided doses

Adolescents: Initial: 25-50 mg/day; increase to 100-150 mg/day in divided doses

Administration

Oral

Immediate release tablet: Dosing after meals may decrease lightheadedness and postural hypotension

Extended release tablet: Take on an empty stomach; swallow whole or as a half tablet without food. Tablet may be broken along the score line, but do not crush or chew.

Monitoring and Teaching Issues

Laboratory Monitoring Baseline liver function prior to and periodically during therapy

Physical Assessment Initiate at lower doses and taper dosage slowly when discontinuing.

Patient Education It may take 2-4 weeks to achieve desired results. Take immediate release tablet after meals. Extended release tablet should be taken on an empty stomach. Avoid excessive alcohol. Maintain adequate hydration unless instructed to restrict fluid intake. You may experience drowsiness, lightheadedness, dizziness, postural hypotension, nausea, dry mouth, constipation, or diarrhea. Report persistent dizziness or headache; muscle cramping, tremors, or altered gait; blurred vision or eye pain; chest pain or irregular heartbeat; suicide ideation; or worsening of condition. Report prolonged or inappropriate erections.

Related Information

Antidepressant Agents *on page 1982*

- **Trazodone Hydrochloride** *see* TraZODone *on page 1808*
- **Treanda®** *see* Bendamustine *on page 198*
- **Trelstar®** *see* Triptorelin *on page 1824*
- **TRENtal®** *see* Pentoxifylline *on page 1441*

Treprostinil (tre PROST in il)

U.S. Brand Names Remodulin®; Tyvaso™

Index Terms Treprostinil Sodium

Generic Availability (U.S.) No

Pharmacologic Category Prostacyclin; Prostaglandin; Vasodilator

Pregnancy Risk Factor B

Lactation Excretion in breast milk unknown/use caution

Use

Injection: Treatment of pulmonary arterial hypertension (PAH) in patients with NYHA Class II-IV symptoms to decrease exercise-associated symptoms; to diminish clinical deterioration when transitioning from epoprostenol (I.V.)

Inhalation: Treatment of pulmonary arterial hypertension (PAH) in patients with NYHA Class III symptoms to increase walk distance. **Note:** Nearly all controlled clinical trial experience has been with concomitant bosentan or sildenafil.

Mechanism of Action/Effect Treprostinil is a direct vasodilator of both pulmonary and systemic arterial vascular beds.

Contraindications There are no contraindications listed in the FDA-approved labeling.

Warnings/Precautions May produce symptomatic hypotension; use with caution in patients with low systemic arterial blood pressure. Abrupt withdrawal/large dosage reductions may worsen symptoms of PAH. I.V./SubQ: If infusion is restarted within a few hours of discontinuation, the same dose rate may be used. Interruptions for longer periods may require retitration. Regardless of administration route (inhalation, I.V., or SubQ), treatment interruptions should be avoided. Immediate access to medication, back-up inhalation device, or pump and infusion sets is essential to prevent treatment interruptions. Chronic continuous I.V. infusion of treprostinil via a chronic indwelling central venous catheter has been associated with serious blood stream infections. This method of administration should be reserved for patients who are intolerant of the SubQ route or in whom the benefit outweighs the potential risks. Treprostinil should only be used by clinicians experienced in the treatment of PAH. Prior to initiation, patients should be carefully evaluated for ability to administer treprostinil, either as an I.V./SubQ infusion or inhalation, and care for the infusion system/inhalation device. Initiation of infusion must occur in a setting where adequate personnel and equipment necessary for hemodynamic monitoring and emergency treatment is available. Use with caution in patients with hepatic impairment; dose reduction is recommended for the initial dose (I.V./SubQ) in patients with mild-to-moderate hepatic insufficiency; titrate dose slowly in patients with hepatic insufficiency; has not been studied in severe hepatic impairment. Has not been studied in renal impairment; use with caution in renal impairment; titrate dose slowly in patients with renal insufficiency. Use with caution in patients ≥65 years of age. Inhalation: Safety and efficacy have not been established in patients with underlying pulmonary disease (eg, asthma, COPD). Patients with acute pulmonary infections should be monitored closely for exacerbation or reduced efficacy. Treprostinil inhibits platelet aggregation, increasing the risk of bleeding; use with caution in patients receiving concurrent anticoagulant/antiplatelet therapy. Safety and efficacy have not been established in children ≤16 years of age (I.V., SubQ) or <18 years of age (inhalation).

Drug Interactions

Avoid Concomitant Use There are no known interactions where it is recommended to avoid concomitant use.

Decreased Effect

The levels/effects of Treprostinil may be decreased by: CYP2C8 Inducers (Highly Effective)

Increased Effect/Toxicity

Treprostinil may increase the levels/effects of: Anticoagulants; Antihypertensives; Antiplatelet Agents; Nonsteroidal Anti-Inflammatory Agents; Salicylates

The levels/effects of Treprostinil may be increased by: CYP2C8 Inhibitors (Strong)

Adverse Reactions

>10%:

Cardiovascular: Flushing (inhalation: 15%), vasodilation (11%)

Central nervous system: Headache (27% to 41%)

Dermatologic: Rash (14%)

Gastrointestinal: Diarrhea (25%), nausea (19% to 22%)

Local: Infusion site pain (SubQ: 85%; may improve after several months of therapy); infusion site reaction (SubQ: 83%)

Neuromuscular & skeletal: Jaw pain (13%)

Respiratory: Cough (inhalation: 54%), throat irritation/pharyngolaryngeal pain (inhalation: 25%)

1% to 10%:

Cardiovascular: Edema (9%), syncope (inhalation: 6%), hypotension (4%), epistaxis (inhalation), wheezing (inhalation)

Central nervous system: Dizziness (9%)

Dermatologic: Pruritus (8%)
Respiratory: Pneumonia (inhalation: 4%), hemoptysis (inhalation: 2%)

Pharmacodynamics/Kinetics

Absorption SubQ: Rapidly and completely

Bioavailability Inhalation: 64% to 72% (dose-dependent); SubQ: 100%

Protein Binding 91%

Half-Life Elimination Terminal: ~4 hours

Metabolism Hepatic (primarily by CYP2C8); forms 5 inactive metabolites (HU1-HU5)

Excretion Urine (79%; 4% as unchanged drug, 64% as metabolites); feces (13%)

Available Dosage Forms

Injection, solution:
Remodulin®: 1 mg/mL (20 mL); 2.5 mg/mL (20 mL); 5 mg/mL (20 mL); 10 mg/mL (20 mL)

Solution, for oral inhalation:
Tyvaso™: 0.6 mg/mL (2.9 mL)

Dosing

Adult & Geriatric

Pulmonary arterial hypertension (PAH):

Inhalation: **Note:** Prior to initiation, patients should be carefully evaluated for ability to administer treprostinil and care for the inhalation system and accessories required for administration. Immediate access to a back-up inhalation device, accessories, and medication is essential to prevent treatment interruptions.

Initial: 18 mcg (or 3 inhalations) every 4 hours 4 times/day; if 3 inhalations are not tolerated, reduce to 1-2 inhalations, then increase to 3 inhalations as tolerated

Maintenance: If tolerated, increase dose by an additional 3 inhalations at approximately 1- to 2-week intervals; maximum dose: 54 mcg (or 9 inhalations) 4 times/day

SubQ (preferred) or I.V. infusion: **Note:** Prior to initiation, patients should be carefully evaluated for ability to administer treprostinil and care for the infusion system outside of inpatient setting. Immediate access to a back-up pump, infusion sets, and medication is essential to prevent treatment interruptions.

Initial: New to prostacyclin therapy: 1.25 ng/kg/minute continuous; if dose cannot be tolerated due to systemic effects, reduce to 0.625 ng/kg/minute. Increase at rate not >1.25 ng/kg/minute per week for first 4 weeks, and not >2.5 ng/kg/minute per week for remainder of therapy. Limited experience with doses >40 ng/kg/minute. **Note:** Dose must be carefully and individually titrated (symptom improvement with minimal adverse effects). Avoid abrupt withdrawal. If infusion is restarted within a few hours of discontinuation, the same dose rate may be used. Interruptions for longer periods may require retitration.

Transitioning from epoprostenol (see table): SubQ (preferred) or I.V. infusion: **Note:** Transition should occur in a hospital setting to follow response (eg, walking distance, sign/symptoms of disease progression). May take 24-48 hours to transition. Transition is accomplished by initiating the infusion of treprostinil, and increasing it while simultaneously reducing the dose of intravenous epoprostenol. During transition, increases in PAH symptoms should be first treated with an increase in treprostinil dose. Occurrence of prostacyclin associated side effects should be treated by decreasing the dose of epoprostenol.

Transitioning From I.V. Epoprostenol to SubQ (Preferred) or I.V. Treprostinil

Step	Epoprostenol Dose	Treprostinil Dose
1	Maintain current dose	Initiate at 10% initial epoprostenol dose
2	Decrease to 80% initial dose	Increase to 30% initial epoprostenol dose
3	Decrease to 60% initial dose	Increase to 50% initial epoprostenol dose
4	Decrease to 40% initial dose	Increase to 70% initial epoprostenol dose
5	Decrease to 20% initial dose	Increase to 90% initial epoprostenol dose
6	Decrease to 5% initial dose	Increase to 110% initial epoprostenol dose
7	Discontinue epoprostenol	Maintain current dose plus additional 5% to 10% as needed

Pediatric

Inhalation: Dosage not established.
I.V./SubQ: Limited experience in patients <16 years of age.

Renal Impairment Titrate slowly in patients with renal impairment.

Hepatic Impairment

Mild-to-moderate: Use with caution and titrate slowly in patients with hepatic impairment
I.V./SubQ: Initial: 0.625 ng/kg/minute (ideal body weight)
Severe: Has not been studied in patients with severe hepatic impairment

Administration

I.V. Avoid abrupt withdrawal (including interruptions in delivery) or rapid large dosage reductions. Immediate access to a back-up pump, infusion sets, and medication is essential to prevent treatment interruptions.

I.V. infusion: I.V. use is recommended when SubQ infusion is not tolerated or when the benefit outweighs the potential risks of an indwelling central venous catheter. Solution must be diluted in SWFI or NS prior to use and administered by continuous infusion using a central indwelling catheter and infusion pump. Peripheral infusion may be used temporarily until central line is established. Avoid abrupt withdrawal (including interruptions in delivery) or rapid large dosage reductions. Immediate access to back up pump, infusion sets and medication is essential to prevent treatment interruptions.

Other Avoid abrupt withdrawal (including interruptions in delivery) or rapid large dosage reductions. Immediate access to medication, a back-up inhalation device, or pump and infusion sets is essential to prevent treatment interruptions.

Inhalation: Do not mix with other medications. For inhalation only via the Tyvaso™ Inhalation System; consists of the Optineb-ir Model ON-100/7 (an ultrasonic, pulsed-delivery device) and accessories. Prior to the first treatment session of each day, transfer the entire contents of one ampule into the medicine chamber; one ampule contains sufficient volume of medication for all 4 treatment sessions in a single day. Between each session, the device should be capped and stored upright with the remaining medication inside. At the end of each day, the medicine chamber and any remaining medication must be discarded. Avoid contact of solution with eyes or skin; wash hands after handling.

SubQ infusion (preferred): Administer undiluted via continuous SubQ infusion using an appropriately-designed infusion pump. Avoid abrupt withdrawal (including interruptions in delivery) or rapid large dosage reductions. Immediate access to back up pump, infusion sets and medication is essential to prevent treatment interruptions. Infusion site reactions may be helped by moving the infusion site every 3 days, local application of topical hot and cold packs, topical or oral analgesics. Injection site pain and erythema may improve after several months of therapy.

Stability

Reconstitution Injection solution: For SubQ infusion, **product should not be diluted prior to use**. For I.V. infusion, dilute in SWFI, NS, or Flolan® sterile diluent to a final volume of either 50 mL or 100 mL (dependent on system reservoir and calculated dose).

Storage

Injection solution: Store vials at 15°C to 30°C (59°F to 86°F). Contents of a vial should not be used past 30 days after initial needle access into the vial. Stability for up to 48 hours has been shown for concentrations as low as 4000 ng/mL. Solutions diluted for infusion may be used for up to 48 hours at 37°C.

Solution for inhalation: Store ampules in foil packs at 25°C (77°F); excursions permitted to 15°C to 30°C (59°F to 89°F). Protect from light. Once foil pack is opened, ampules should be used within 7 days. Following transfer of solution to inhalation device, solution should remain in device for no more than 24 hours; discard unused portion.

Monitoring and Teaching Issues

Physical Assessment Initiation of therapy must be performed in a setting with necessary continuous pulmonary and hemodynamic arterial monitoring and emergency care. Chronic therapy may be needed; patient's ability to prepare and administer the medication should be carefully assessed. Evaluate effectiveness of therapy (improved pulmonary function and quality of life). Instruct patient/caregiver to monitor vital signs on regular basis.

Patient Education Therapy will probably be long-term. You will be taught how to store and prepare medication and how to care for and monitor the equipment; follow these directions completely. Notify contact person immediately with any problems or questions with equipment. You will be required to monitor your blood pressure and heart rate at regular intervals. You may experience mild headache, nervousness, dizziness, nausea, vomiting, diarrhea, or muscular pain. Report immediately any signs or symptoms of increased dizziness, acute or severe headache, increased difficulty breathing, fever or chills, unusual bleeding or bruising, or chest pain or palpitations. If administering through an I.V., notify healthcare provider if site is increasingly painful, red, or has pus forming.

Pregnancy Considerations Some skeletal malformations and maternal toxicity noted in animal studies. There are no adequate and well-controlled studies in pregnant women. Use with caution and only if clearly needed.

Related Information

Heart Failure (Systolic) *on page 2040*

◆ **Treprostinil Sodium** *see* Treprostinil *on page 1809*

◆ **Tretin-X™** *see* Tretinoin (Topical) *on page 1811*

◆ **Tretinoin and Clindamycin** *see* Clindamycin and Tretinoin *on page 401*

Tretinoin (Topical) (TRET i noyn TOP i kal)

U.S. Brand Names Atralin™; Avita®; Refissa™; Renova®; Retin-A Micro®; Retin-A®; Tretin-X™

Index Terms *trans*-Retinoic Acid; Retinoic Acid; Vitamin A Acid

Generic Availability (U.S.) Yes

Pharmacologic Category Acne Products; Retinoic Acid Derivative; Topical Skin Product, Acne

Medication Safety Issues

Sound-alike/look-alike issues:

Tretinoin may be confused with ISOtretinoin, Tenormin®, triamcinolone, trientine

International issues:

Renova [U.S., Canada] may be confused with Remov brand name for nimesulide [Italy]

Pregnancy Risk Factor C

Lactation Enters breast milk/compatible

Use Treatment of acne vulgaris; photodamaged skin; palliation of fine wrinkles, mottled hyperpigmentation, and tactile roughness of facial skin as part of a comprehensive skin care and sun avoidance program

Unlabeled/Investigational Use Some skin cancers

Available Dosage Forms

Cream, topical: 0.025% (20 g, 45 g); 0.05% (20 g, 45 g); 0.1% (20 g, 45 g)
Avita®: 0.025% (20 g, 45 g)
Refissa™: 0.05% (40 g)
Renova®: 0.02% (40 g, 44 g, 60 g)
Retin-A®: 0.025% (20 g, 45 g); 0.05% (20 g, 45 g); 0.1% (20 g, 45 g)
Tretin-X™: 0.025% (35 g); 0.0375% (35 g); 0.05% (35 g); 0.1% (35 g)

Gel, topical: 0.01% (15 g, 45 g); 0.025% (15 g, 45 g)
Atralin™: 0.05% (45 g)
Avita®: 0.025% (20 g, 45 g)
Retin-A Micro®: 0.04% (20 g, 45 g, 50 g); 0.1% (20 g, 45 g, 50 g)
Retin-A®: 0.01% (15 g, 45 g); 0.025% (15 g, 45 g)
Tretin-X™: 0.01% (35 g); 0.025% (35 g)

Dosing

Adult

Acne vulgaris: Topical: Begin therapy with a weaker formulation of tretinoin (0.025% cream, 0.04% microsphere gel, or 0.01% gel) and increase the concentration as tolerated; apply once daily to acne lesions before retiring or on alternate days; if stinging or irritation develop, decrease frequency of application

Palliation of fine wrinkles, mottled hyperpigmentation, and tactile roughness of facial skin: Topical: Pea-sized amount of the 0.02% or 0.05% cream applied to entire face once daily in the evening

Geriatric Use of the 0.02% cream in patients 65-71 years of age showed similar improvement in fine wrinkles as seen in patients <65 years. Safety and efficacy of the 0.02% cream have not been established in patients >71 years of age. Safety and efficacy of the 0.05% cream have not been established in patients >50 years of age.

Pediatric Children >12 years: Acne vulgaris: Topical: Refer to adult dosing.

Administration

Topical Palliation of fine wrinkles, mottled hyperpigmentation, and tactile roughness of facial skin: Cream: Prior to application, gently wash face with a mild soap. Pat dry. Wait 20-30 minutes to apply cream. Avoid eyes, ears, nostrils, and mouth.

Monitoring and Teaching Issues

Patient Education For once-daily use, do not overuse. Thoroughly wash hands before applying. Wash area to be treated at least 30 minutes before applying. Do not wash face more frequently than 2-3 times a day. Do not apply to areas near your mouth, eyes, corners of your nose, or open sores. Avoid using topical preparations that contain alcohol or harsh chemicals during treatment. It may take several weeks before the full benefit of the medication is seen. You may experience increased sensitivity to sunlight; protect skin with sunblock (minimum SPF 15), wear protective clothing, and avoid direct sunlight. Stop treatment and inform prescriber if rash, skin irritation, redness, scaling, or excessive dryness occurs. When used for hyperpigmentation and tactile redness of facial skin, wrinkles will not be eliminated. Must be used in combination with a comprehensive skin care program.

◆ **Trexall™** *see* Methotrexate *on page 1193*

◆ **Treximet™** *see* Sumatriptan and Naproxen *on page 1694*

◆ **Triaconazole** *see* Terconazole *on page 1735*

Triamcinolone (Systemic) (trye am SIN oh lone)

U.S. Brand Names Aristospan®; Kenalog®-10; Kenalog®-40

Index Terms Triamcinolone Acetonide, Parenteral; Triamcinolone Hexacetonide

Generic Availability (U.S.) No

Pharmacologic Category Corticosteroid, Systemic

Medication Safety Issues

Sound-alike/look-alike issues:

Kenalog® may be confused with Ketalar®

TAC (occasional abbreviation for triamcinolone) is an error-prone abbreviation (mistaken as tetracaine-adrenaline-cocaine)

Pregnancy Risk Factor C

Lactation Excretion in breast milk unknown/use caution

Use

Intra-articular (soft tissue): Acute gouty arthritis, acute/subacute bursitis, acute tenosynovitis, epicondylitis, rheumatoid arthritis, synovitis of osteoarthritis

Intralesional: Alopecia areata, discoid lupus erythematosus, keloids, granuloma annulare lesions (localized hypertrophic, infiltrated, or inflammatory), lichen planus plaques, lichen simplex chronicus plaques, psoriatic plaques, necrobiosis lipoidica diabeticorum, cystic tumors of aponeurosis or tendon (ganglia)

Systemic: Adrenocortical insufficiency, dermatologic diseases, endocrine disorders, gastrointestinal diseases, hematologic and neoplastic disorders, nervous system disorders, nephrotic syndrome, rheumatic disorders, allergic states, respiratory diseases, systemic lupus erythematosus (SLE), and other diseases requiring anti-inflammatory or immunosuppressive effects

Mechanism of Action/Effect Decreases inflammation by suppression of migration of polymorphonuclear leukocytes and reversal of increased capillary permeability; suppresses the immune system by reducing activity and volume of the lymphatic system; suppresses adrenal function at high doses

Contraindications Hypersensitivity to triamcinolone or any component of the formulation; systemic fungal infections; cerebral malaria; idiopathic thrombocytopenic purpura (I.M. injection)

Warnings/Precautions May cause hypercorticism or suppression of hypothalamic-pituitary-adrenal (HPA) axis, particularly in younger children or in patients receiving high doses for prolonged periods. HPA axis suppression may lead to adrenal crisis. Withdrawal and discontinuation of a corticosteroid should be done slowly and carefully.

Acute myopathy has been reported with high-dose corticosteroids, usually in patients with neuromuscular transmission disorders; may involve ocular and/or respiratory muscles; monitor creatine kinase; recovery may be delayed. Corticosteroid use may cause psychiatric disturbances, including depression, euphoria, insomnia, mood swings, and personality changes. Pre-existing psychiatric conditions may be exacerbated by corticosteroid use. Prolonged use of corticosteroids may also increase the incidence of secondary infection, mask acute infection (including fungal infections), prolong or exacerbate viral infections, or limit response to vaccines. Exposure to chickenpox should be avoided; corticosteroids should not be used to treat ocular herpes simplex. Corticosteroids should not be used for cerebral malaria or viral hepatitis. Close observation is required in patients with latent tuberculosis and/or TB reactivity; restrict use in active TB (only in conjunction with antituberculosis treatment). Use with caution in patients with threadworm infection; may cause serious hyperinfection. Prolonged treatment with corticosteroids has been associated with the development of Kaposi's sarcoma (case reports); if noted, discontinuation of therapy should be considered. Avoid use in head injury patients.

Use with caution in patients with thyroid disease, hepatic impairment, renal impairment, cardiovascular disease, diabetes, myasthenia gravis, patients at risk for osteoporosis, patients at risk for seizures, or GI diseases (diverticulitis, peptic ulcer, ulcerative colitis) due to perforation risk. Avoid use in head injury patients. Use caution following acute MI (corticosteroids have been associated with myocardial rupture). Because of the risk of adverse effects, systemic corticosteroids should be used cautiously in the elderly in the smallest possible effective dose for the shortest duration. Patients should not be immunized with live, viral vaccines while receiving immunosuppressive doses of corticosteroids. The ability to respond to dead viral vaccines is unknown.

Withdraw therapy with gradual tapering of dose. There have been reports of systemic corticosteroid withdrawal symptoms (eg, joint/muscle pain, lassitude, depression) when withdrawing oral inhalation therapy. Injection suspension contains benzyl alcohol; benzyl alcohol has been associated with the "gasping syndrome" in neonates and low-birth-weight infants.

Drug Interactions

Avoid Concomitant Use

Avoid concomitant use of Triamcinolone (Systemic) with any of the following: Aldesleukin; BCG; Natalizumab; Pimecrolimus; Roflumilast; Tacrolimus (Topical)

Decreased Effect

Triamcinolone (Systemic) may decrease the levels/effects of: Aldesleukin; Antidiabetic Agents; BCG; Calcitriol; Corticorelin; Isoniazid; Salicylates; Sipuleucel-T; Vaccines (Inactivated)

The levels/effects of Triamcinolone (Systemic) may be decreased by: Aminoglutethimide; Barbiturates; Echinacea; Mitotane; Primidone; Rifamycin Derivatives

Increased Effect/Toxicity

Triamcinolone (Systemic) may increase the levels/effects of: Acetylcholinesterase Inhibitors; Amphotericin B; Leflunomide; Loop Diuretics; Natalizumab; NSAID (COX-2 Inhibitor); NSAID (Nonselective); Thiazide Diuretics; Vaccines (Live); Warfarin

The levels/effects of Triamcinolone (Systemic) may be increased by: Antifungal Agents (Azole Derivatives, Systemic); Aprepitant; Calcium Channel Blockers (Nondihydropyridine); Denosumab; Estrogen Derivatives; Fluconazole; Fosaprepitant; Macrolide Antibiotics; Neuromuscular-Blocking Agents (Nondepolarizing); Pimecrolimus; Quinolone Antibiotics; Roflumilast; Salicylates; Tacrolimus (Topical); Trastuzumab

Adverse Reactions Frequency not defined; reactions reported with corticosteroid therapy in general:

Cardiovascular: Arrhythmia, bradycardia, cardiac arrest, cardiac enlargement, CHF, circulatory collapse, edema, hypertension, hypertrophic cardiomyopathy (premature infants), myocardial rupture (following recent MI), syncope, tachycardia, thromboembolism, vasculitis

Central nervous system: Arachnoiditis (I.T.), depression, emotional instability, euphoria, headache, insomnia, intracranial pressure increased, malaise, meningitis (I.T.), mood changes, neuritis, neuropathy, personality change, pseudotumor cerebri (with discontinuation), seizure, vertigo
Dermatologic: Abscess (sterile), acne, allergic dermatitis, angioedema, atrophy (cutaneous/subcutaneous), bruising, dry skin, erythema, hair thinning, hirsutism, hyper-/hypopigmentation, hypertrichosis, impaired wound healing, lupus erythematosus-like lesions, petechiae, purpura, rash, skin test suppression, striae, thin skin
Endocrine & metabolic: Carbohydrate intolerance, Cushingoid state, diabetes mellitus, fluid retention, glucose intolerance, growth suppression (children), hypokalemia, hypokalemic alkalosis, menstrual irregularities, negative nitrogen balance, sodium retention, sperm motility altered
Gastrointestinal: Abdominal distention, appetite increased, GI hemorrhage, GI perforation, nausea, pancreatitis, peptic ulcer, ulcerative esophagitis, weight gain
Hepatic: Hepatomegaly, liver function tests increased
Local: Thrombophlebitis
Neuromuscular & skeletal: Aseptic necrosis of femoral and humeral heads, calcinosis, Charcot-like arthropathy, fractures, joint tissue damage, muscle mass loss, myopathy, osteoporosis, parasthesia, tendon rupture, vertebral compression fractures, weakness
Ocular: Cataracts, exophthalmos, glaucoma, ocular pressure increased, papilledema
Renal: Glycosuria
Respiratory: Pulmonary edema
Miscellaneous: Abnormal fat deposits, anaphylactoid reaction, anaphylaxis, diaphoresis, hiccups, infection, moon face

Pharmacodynamics/Kinetics

Time to Peak I.M.: 8-10 hours
Protein Binding ~68%
Half-Life Elimination Biologic: 18-36 hours
Excretion Urine (~40%); feces (~60%)

Available Dosage Forms

Injection, suspension:
Aristospan®: 5 mg/mL (5 mL); 20 mg/mL (1 mL, 5 mL)
Kenalog®-10: 10 mg/mL (5 mL)
Kenalog®-40: 40 mg/mL (1 mL, 5 mL, 10 mL)

Dosing

Adult & Geriatric The lowest possible dose should be used to control the condition; when dose reduction is possible, the dose should be reduced gradually.

Dermatoses (steroid-responsive, including contact/atopic dermatitis): Injection:
Acetonide: Intradermal: Initial: 1 mg
Hexacetonide: Intralesional, sublesional: Up to 0.5 mg/square inch of affected skin; range: 2-48 mg/day

Hay fever/pollen asthma: I.M.: 40-100 mg as a single injection/season

Multiple sclerosis (acute exacerbation): I.M.: 160 mg daily for 1 week, followed by 64 mg every other day for 1 month

Rheumatic or arthritic disorders:
Intra-articular (or similar injection as designated):
Acetonide: Intra-articular, intrabursal, tendon sheaths: Initial: Smaller joints: 2.5-5 mg, larger joints: 5-15 mg; may require up to 10 mg for small joints and up to 40 mg for large joints; maximum dose/treatment (several joints at one time): 20-80 mg
Hexacetonide: Intra-articular: Average dose: 2-20 mg; smaller joints: 2-6 mg; larger joints: 10-20 mg. Frequency of injection into a single joint is every 3-4 weeks as necessary; to avoid possible joint destruction use as infrequently as possible.
I.M.: Acetonide: Range: 2.5-100 mg/day; Initial: 60 mg
See table.

Triamcinolone Dosing

	Acetonide	Hexacetonide
Intrasynovial	5-40 mg	
Intralesional	1-30 mg (usually 1 mg per injection site); 10 mg/mL suspension usually used	Up to 0.5 mg/sq inch affected area
Sublesional	1-30 mg	
Systemic I.M.	2.5-60 mg/dose (usual adult dose: 60 mg; may repeat with 20-100 mg dose when symptoms recur)	
Intra-articular	2.5-40 mg	2-20 mg average
large joints	5-15 mg	10-20 mg
small joints	2.5-5 mg	2-6 mg
Tendon sheaths	2.5-10 mg	
Intradermal	1 mg/site	

Pediatric Rheumatic conditions: *I.M. (acetonide):* Range: 2.5-100 mg/day
Children: Initial: 0.11-1.6 mg/kg/day in 3-4 divided doses
Children 6-12 years: Initial: 40 mg
Children ≥12 years: Refer to adult dosing.

Administration

I.M. Inject I.M. dose deep in large muscle mass, avoid deltoid.

Other Avoid subcutaneous administration.

Stability

Reconstitution Hexacetonide injectable suspension: Avoid diluents containing parabens, phenol, or other preservatives (may cause flocculation). Suspension for intralesional use may be diluted with D_5NS, D_{10}NS, NS, or SWFI to a 1:1, 1:2, or 1:4 concentration. Solutions for intra-articular use, may be diluted with lidocaine 1% or 2%.

Storage Injection, suspension:
Acetonide injectable suspension: Kenalog®: Store at 20°C to 25°C (68°F to 77°F); avoid freezing. Protect from light.
Hexacetonide injectable suspension: Store at 20°C to 25°C (68°F to 77°F); avoid freezing. Protect from light. Diluted suspension stable up to 1 week.

Monitoring and Teaching Issues

Physical Assessment Patients with diabetes should monitor glucose levels closely (corticosteroids may alter glucose levels). When used for >10-14 days, do not discontinue abruptly; decrease dosage incrementally.

Patient Education Avoid alcohol. If you have diabetes, monitor glucose levels closely (antidiabetic medication may need to be adjusted). Inform prescriber if you are experiencing greater than normal levels of stress (medication may need adjustment). You may be more susceptible to infection. Report promptly excessive nervousness or sleep disturbances, any signs of infection (sore throat, unhealed injuries), excessive growth of body hair or loss of skin color, vision changes, weight gain, swelling of face or extremities, muscle weakness, change in color of stools (black or tarry) or persistent abdominal pain, or worsening of condition or failure to improve.

Dietary Considerations Ensure adequate intake of calcium and vitamins (or consider supplementation) in patients on medium-to-high doses of systemic corticosteroids.

Geriatric Considerations Because of the risk of adverse effects, corticosteroids should be used cautiously in the elderly, in the smallest possible dose, and for the shortest possible time.

Breast-Feeding Considerations Corticosteroids are excreted in human milk; information specific to triamcinolone has not been located.

Pregnancy Considerations Triamcinolone was shown to be teratogenic in animal reproduction studies. Some studies have shown an association between first trimester corticosteroid use and oral clefts; adverse events in the fetus/neonate have been noted in case reports following large doses of systemic corticosteroids during pregnancy.

Related Information

Asthma *on page 2015*
Corticosteroids *on page 1996*

Triamcinolone (Nasal) (trye am SIN oh lone)

U.S. Brand Names Nasacort® AQ

Index Terms Triamcinolone acetonide

Generic Availability (U.S.) No

Pharmacologic Category Corticosteroid, Nasal

Medication Safety Issues

Sound-alike/look-alike issues:
Nasacort® may be confused with NasalCrom®

TAC (occasional abbreviation for triamcinolone) is an error-prone abbreviation (mistaken as tetracaine-adrenaline-cocaine)

Pregnancy Risk Factor C

Lactation Excretion in breast milk unknown/use caution

Use Management of seasonal and perennial allergic rhinitis

Available Dosage Forms

Suspension, intranasal:
Nasacort® AQ: 55 mcg/inhalation (16.5 g)

Dosing

Adult & Geriatric Allergic rhinitis (perennial or seasonal):

Nasal spray: 220 mcg/day as 2 sprays in each nostril once daily; once symptoms controlled reduce to 110 mcg/day

Nasal inhaler: Initial: 220 mcg/day as 2 sprays in each nostril once daily; may increase dose to 440 mcg/day (given once daily or divided and given 2 or 4 times/day)

Pediatric Allergic rhinitis (perennial or seasonal):

Nasal spray:
Children 2-5 years: 110 mcg/day as 1 spray in each nostril once daily (maximum: 110 mcg/day)
Children 6-11 years: Initial: 110 mcg/day as 1 spray in each nostril once daily; may increase to 220 mcg/day as 2 sprays in each nostril if response not adequate; once symptoms controlled may reduce to 110 mcg/day
Children ≥12 years: Refer to adult dosing.

Nasal inhaler:
Children 6-11 years: Initial: 220 mcg/day as 2 sprays in each nostril once daily
Children ≥12 years: Refer to adult dosing.

Administration

Inhalation Shake well prior to use. Gently blow nose to clear nostrils.

Nasacort® AQ: Prime prior to first use, by shaking contents well and releasing 5 sprays into the air. If product is not used for more than 2 weeks, reprime with 1 spray.

Monitoring and Teaching Issues

Patient Education Do not use if you have a nasal infection, nasal injury, or recent nasal surgery. Report unusual cough or spasm; persistent nasal bleeding, burning, or irritation; or worsening of condition.

Triamcinolone (Topical) (trye am SIN oh lone)

U.S. Brand Names Kenalog®; Oralone®; Triderm®; Zytopic™

Generic Availability (U.S.) Yes: Excludes aerosol

Pharmacologic Category Corticosteroid, Topical

Medication Safety Issues

Sound-alike/look-alike issues:
Kenalog® may be confused with Ketalar®

TAC (occasional abbreviation for triamcinolone) is an error-prone abbreviation (mistaken as tetracaine-adrenaline-cocaine)

Pregnancy Risk Factor C

Lactation Excretion in breast milk unknown/use caution

Use

Oral topical: Adjunctive treatment and temporary relief of symptoms associated with oral inflammatory lesions and ulcerative lesions resulting from trauma

Topical: Inflammatory dermatoses responsive to steroids

Available Dosage Forms

Aerosol, topical:
Kenalog®: 0.2 mg/2-second spray (63 g)

Cream, topical: 0.025% (15 g, 80 g, 454 g); 0.1% (15 g, 30 g, 80 g, 454 g, 2240 g, 2270 g); 0.5% (15 g)
Triderm®: 0.1% (30 g, 85 g)
Zytopic™: 0.1% (85 g)

Lotion, topical: 0.025% (60 mL); 0.1% (60 mL)

Ointment, topical: 0.025% (15 g, 80 g, 454 g); 0.05% (430 g); 0.1% (15 g, 80 g, 454 g); 0.5% (15 g)

Paste, oral: 0.1% (5 g)

Paste, oral, topical: 0.1% (5 g)
Oralone®: 0.1% (5 g)

Dosing

Adult & Geriatric

Dermatoses (steroid-responsive, including contact/atopic dermatitis): Topical:
Cream, Ointment:
0.025%: Apply thin film to affected areas 2-4 times/day
0.1% or 0.5%: Apply thin film to affected areas 2-3 times/day
Spray: Apply to affected area 3-4 times/day

Oral inflammatory lesions/ulcers: Oral topical: Press a small dab (about 1/4 inch) to the lesion until a thin film develops; a larger quantity may be required for coverage of some lesions. For optimal results, use only enough to coat the lesion with a thin film; do not rub in.

Administration

Topical

Oral topical: Apply small dab to lesion until a thin film develops; do not rub in. Apply at bedtime or after meals if applications are needed throughout the day.

Topical:

Ointment: Apply a thin film sparingly. Do not use on open skin or wounds. Do not occlude area unless directed; if using occluding dressing, monitor for infection.

Spray: Avoid eyes and do not inhale if spraying near face. Occlusive dressing may be used if instructed; monitor for infection.

Monitoring and Teaching Issues

Patient Education Report promptly any signs of infection. For external use only. Not for eyes or mucous membranes or open wounds. Apply in very thin layer. Avoid prolonged or excessive use around sensitive tissues, genital, or rectal areas. Inform prescriber if condition worsens (swelling, redness, irritation, pain, open sores) or fails to improve.

Related Information

Corticosteroids *on page 1996*

◆ **Triamcinolone acetonide** *see* Triamcinolone (Nasal) *on page 1815*
◆ **Triamcinolone Acetonide, Parenteral** *see* Triamcinolone (Systemic) *on page 1812*
◆ **Triamcinolone and Nystatin** *see* Nystatin and Triamcinolone *on page 1339*
◆ **Triamcinolone Hexacetonide** *see* Triamcinolone (Systemic) *on page 1812*
◆ **Triaminic™ Children's Fever Reducer Pain Reliever [OTC]** *see* Acetaminophen *on page 38*

◆ **Triaminic® Children's Night Time Cold & Cough [OTC]** *see* Diphenhydramine and Phenylephrine *on page 546*

◆ **Triaminic® Children's Softchews® Cough & Runny Nose [OTC]** *see* Dextromethorphan and Chlorpheniramine *on page 513*

◆ **Triaminic® Children's Thin Strips® Night Time Cold & Cough [OTC]** *see* Diphenhydramine and Phenylephrine *on page 546*

◆ **Triaminic Thin Strips® Children's Cold with Stuffy Nose [OTC]** *see* Phenylephrine (Systemic) *on page 1449*

◆ **Triaminic Thin Strips® Children's Cough & Runny Nose [OTC]** *see* DiphenhydrAMINE (Systemic) *on page 543*

◆ **Triamterene and Hydrochlorothiazide** *see* Hydrochlorothiazide and Triamterene *on page 914*

Triazolam (trye AY zoe lam)

U.S. Brand Names Halcion®

Generic Availability (U.S.) Yes

Pharmacologic Category Hypnotic, Benzodiazepine

Medication Safety Issues

Sound-alike/look-alike issues:

Triazolam may be confused with alPRAZolam

Halcion® may be confused with halcinonide, Haldol®

Beers Criteria medication: This drug may be inappropriate for use in geriatric patients (high severity risk).

Medication Guide Available Yes

Pregnancy Risk Factor X

Lactation Excretion in breast milk unknown/not recommended

Use Short-term treatment of insomnia

Controlled Substance C-IV

Available Dosage Forms

Tablet, oral: 0.125 mg, 0.25 mg

Halcion®: 0.25 mg

Dosing

Adult Note: Onset of action is rapid, patient should be in bed when taking medication.

Insomnia (short-term): Oral: 0.125-0.25 mg at bedtime (maximum dose: 0.5 mg/day)

Dental (preprocedure): Oral: 0.25 mg taken the evening before oral surgery; or 0.25 mg 1 hour before procedure

Geriatric Oral: Insomnia (short-term use): Initial: 0.125 mg at bedtime; maximum dose: 0.25 mg/day

Hepatic Impairment Reduce dose or avoid use in cirrhosis.

Administration

Oral May take with food. Tablet may be crushed or swallowed whole. Onset of action is rapid, patient should be in bed when taking medication.

Monitoring and Teaching Issues

Physical Assessment Assess for history of addiction; long-term use can result in dependence, abuse, or tolerance; periodically evaluate need for continued use. For inpatient use, institute safety measures to prevent falls. Monitor for CNS depression. Taper dosage slowly when discontinuing.

Patient Education Drug may cause physical and/or psychological dependence. Do not use alcohol. Avoid grapefruit juice. Maintain adequate hydration unless instructed to restrict fluid intake. You may experience drowsiness, lightheadedness, impaired coordination, dizziness, blurred vision, nausea, vomiting, dry mouth, constipation, or photosensitivity. Report persistent CNS effects (eg, memory impairment; confusion; depression; increased sedation; excitation; headache; agitation; insomnia or nightmares; dizziness; fatigue; impaired coordination; changes in personality, behavior, or cognition) or worsening of condition.

Related Information

Benzodiazepines *on page 1988*

◆ **Tribavirin** *see* Ribavirin *on page 1571*

◆ **Tri-Buffered Aspirin [OTC]** *see* Aspirin *on page 155*

◆ **Tricalcium Phosphate** *see* Calcium Phosphate (Tribasic) *on page 278*

◆ **Trichloroacetaldehyde Monohydrate** *see* Chloral Hydrate *on page 356*

◆ **TriCor®** *see* Fenofibrate *on page 739*

◆ **Tricosal** *see* Choline Magnesium Trisalicylate *on page 363*

◆ **Triderm®** *see* Triamcinolone (Topical) *on page 1816*

◆ **Tridil** *see* Nitroglycerin *on page 1327*

◆ **Triethylenethiophosphoramide** *see* Thiotepa *on page 1754*

◆ **Triglide®** *see* Fenofibrate *on page 739*

Trihexyphenidyl (trye heks ee FEN i dil)

Index Terms Artane; Benzhexol Hydrochloride; Trihexyphenidyl Hydrochloride

Generic Availability (U.S.) Yes

Pharmacologic Category Anti-Parkinson's Agent, Anticholinergic; Anticholinergic Agent

Medication Safety Issues

Sound-alike/look-alike issues:

Trihexyphenidyl may be confused with trifluoperazine

Lactation Excretion in breast milk unknown/use caution

Use Adjunctive treatment of Parkinson's disease; treatment of drug-induced extrapyramidal symptoms

Mechanism of Action/Effect Exerts a direct inhibitory effect on the parasympathetic nervous system. It also has a relaxing effect on smooth musculature; exerted both directly on the muscle itself and indirectly through parasympathetic nervous system (inhibitory effect)

Contraindications There are no contraindications listed within the manufacturer's labeling.

Warnings/Precautions Use with caution in hot weather or during exercise, especially when administered concomitantly with other atropine-like drugs to chronically-ill patients, alcoholics, patients with CNS disease, or persons doing manual labor in a hot environment. Use with caution in patients with cardiovascular disease (including hypertension), glaucoma, prostatic hyperplasia or any tendency toward urinary retention, liver or kidney disorders, and obstructive disease of the GI tract. May exacerbate mental symptoms when used to treat extrapyramidal symptoms. When given in large doses or to susceptible patients, may cause weakness. May impair physical or mental abilities; patients must be cautioned about performing tasks which require mental alertness (eg, operating machinery or driving). Does not improve symptoms of tardive dyskinesias. Elderly patients require strict dosage regulation.

Drug Interactions

Avoid Concomitant Use There are no known interactions where it is recommended to avoid concomitant use.

Decreased Effect

Trihexyphenidyl may decrease the levels/effects of: Acetylcholinesterase Inhibitors (Central); Secretin

The levels/effects of Trihexyphenidyl may be decreased by: Acetylcholinesterase Inhibitors (Central)

Increased Effect/Toxicity

Trihexyphenidyl may increase the levels/effects of: AbobotulinumtoxinA; Anticholinergics; Cannabinoids; OnabotulinumtoxinA; Potassium Chloride; RimabotulinumtoxinB

The levels/effects of Trihexyphenidyl may be increased by: Pramlintide

Nutritional/Ethanol Interactions Ethanol: Avoid ethanol (may increase CNS depression).

Adverse Reactions Frequency not defined.

Cardiovascular: Tachycardia

Central nervous system: Agitation, confusion, delusions, dizziness, drowsiness, euphoria, hallucinations, headache, nervousness, paranoia, psychiatric disturbances

Dermatologic: Rash

Gastrointestinal: Constipation, dilatation of colon, ileus, nausea, parotitis, vomiting, xerostomia

Genitourinary: Urinary retention

Neuromuscular & skeletal: Weakness

Ocular: Blurred vision, glaucoma, intraocular pressure increased, mydriasis

Pharmacodynamics/Kinetics

Time to Peak Serum: 1.3 hours

Half-Life Elimination 33 hours

Metabolism Hydroxylation of the alicyclic groups

Excretion Urine and bile

Available Dosage Forms

Elixir, oral: 2 mg/5 mL (473 mL)

Tablet, oral: 2 mg, 5 mg

Dosing

Adult

Parkinson's disease: Oral: Initial: 1 mg/day, increase by 2 mg increments at intervals of 3-5 days; usual dose: 6-10 mg/day in 3-4 divided doses; doses of 12-15 mg/day may be required

Drug-induced EPS: Oral: Initial: 1 mg/day; increase as necessary to usual range: 5-15 mg/day in 3-4 divided doses

Use in combination with levodopa: Usual range: 3-6 mg/day in divided doses

Geriatric Parkinson's disease: Refer to adult dosing. **Note:** Conservative initial doses and gradual titration is especially important in patients >60 years of age.

Administration

Oral May be administered before or after meals; tolerated best if given in 3 daily doses and with food. High doses (>10 mg/day) may be divided into 4 doses, at meal times and at bedtime.

Stability

Storage Store at 20°C to 25°C (68°F to 77°F).

Monitoring and Teaching Issues

Physical Assessment Monitor renal function. Monitor for anticholinergic syndrome. Intraocular pressure monitoring and gonioscopic evaluations should be performed periodically.

Patient Education Take with meals if GI upset occurs. Maintain adequate hydration unless instructed to restrict fluid intake; void before taking medication. Do not use alcohol. You may experience drowsiness, confusion, vision changes, increased susceptibility to heat stroke, decreased perspiration, constipation, or dry skin or nasal passages. Report unresolved constipation, chest pain or palpitations, respiratory difficulty, CNS changes (hallucination, loss of memory, nervousness, etc), painful or difficult urination, increased muscle spasticity or rigidity, skin rash, or significant worsening of condition.

Dietary Considerations May be taken before or after meals; tolerated best if given with food.

Geriatric Considerations Anticholinergic agents are generally not well tolerated in the elderly (eg, confusion, constipation, urinary retention) and their use should be avoided when possible. In elderly, anticholinergic agents should not be used as prophylaxis against extrapyramidal symptoms.

Breast-Feeding Considerations Anticholinergic agents may suppress lactation.

Additional Information Incidence and severity of side effects are dose related. Patients may be switched to sustained-action capsules when stabilized on conventional dosage forms.

- ◆ **Trihexyphenidyl Hydrochloride** *see* Trihexyphenidyl *on page 1818*
- ◆ **TriHIBit® [DSC]** *see* Diphtheria and Tetanus Toxoids, Acellular Pertussis and *Haemophilus influenzae* b Conjugate Vaccine *on page 548*
- ◆ **Tri-Legest™ Fe** *see* Ethinyl Estradiol and Norethindrone *on page 701*
- ◆ **Trileptal®** *see* OXcarbazepine *on page 1375*
- ◆ **TriLipix®** *see* Fenofibric Acid *on page 742*
- ◆ **Trilisate** *see* Choline Magnesium Trisalicylate *on page 363*
- ◆ **TriLyte®** *see* Polyethylene Glycol-Electrolyte Solution *on page 1474*

Trimethobenzamide (trye meth oh BEN za mide)

U.S. Brand Names Tigan®

Index Terms Trimethobenzamide Hydrochloride

Generic Availability (U.S.) Yes

Pharmacologic Category Antiemetic

Medication Safety Issues

Sound-alike/look-alike issues:

Tigan® may be confused with Tiazac®, Ticar®, Ticlid®

Trimethobenzamide may be confused with metoclopramide, trimethoprim

Beers Criteria medication: This drug may be inappropriate for use in geriatric patients (high severity risk).

Lactation Excretion in breast milk unknown

Use Treatment of postoperative nausea and vomiting; treatment of nausea associated with gastroenteritis

Mechanism of Action/Effect Acts centrally to inhibit the medullary chemoreceptor trigger zone by blocking emetic impulses to the vomiting center

Contraindications Hypersensitivity to trimethobenzamide or any component of the formulation; injection contraindicated in children

Warnings/Precautions May mask emesis due to Reye's syndrome or mimic CNS effects of Reye's syndrome in patients with emesis of other etiologies. Antiemetic effects may mask toxicity of other drugs or conditions (eg, intestinal obstruction). May cause drowsiness; patient should avoid tasks requiring alertness (eg, driving, operating machinery). May cause extrapyramidal symptoms (EPS) which may be confused with CNS symptoms of primary disease responsible for emesis. May be inappropriate for use in the elderly due to the risk of EPS adverse effects combined with lower efficacy, as compared to other antiemetics (Beers Criteria). Risk of CNS adverse effects (eg, coma, EPS, seizure) may be increased in patients with acute febrile illness, dehydration, electrolyte imbalance, encephalitis, or gastroenteritis; use caution. Allergic-type skin reactions have been reported with use; discontinue with signs of sensitization. Trimethobenzamide clearance is predominantly renal; dosage reductions may be recommended in patient with renal impairment. Use capsule formulation with caution in children; antiemetics are not recommended for uncomplicated vomiting in children, limit antiemetic use to prolonged vomiting of known etiology. Use of injection is contraindicated in children.

Drug Interactions

Avoid Concomitant Use There are no known interactions where it is recommended to avoid concomitant use.

Decreased Effect

Trimethobenzamide may decrease the levels/effects of: Acetylcholinesterase Inhibitors (Central); Secretin

The levels/effects of Trimethobenzamide may be decreased by: Acetylcholinesterase Inhibitors (Central)

Increased Effect/Toxicity

Trimethobenzamide may increase the levels/effects of: AbobotulinumtoxinA; Anticholinergics; Cannabinoids; OnabotulinumtoxinA; Potassium Chloride; RimabotulinumtoxinB

The levels/effects of Trimethobenzamide may be increased by: Pramlintide

Nutritional/Ethanol Interactions Ethanol: Concomitant use should be avoided (sedative effects may be additive).

Adverse Reactions Frequency not defined.

Cardiovascular: Hypotension (I.V. administration)

Central nervous system: Coma, depression, disorientation, dizziness, drowsiness, EPS, headache, Parkinson-like symptoms, seizure

Dermatologic: Allergic-type skin reactions

Gastrointestinal: Diarrhea

Hematologic: Blood dyscrasias

Hepatic: Jaundice

Local: Injection site burning, pain, redness, stinging, or swelling

Neuromuscular & skeletal: Muscle cramps, opisthotonos

Ocular: Blurred vision

Miscellaneous: Hypersensitivity reactions

Pharmacodynamics/Kinetics

Onset of Action Antiemetic: Oral: 10-40 minutes; I.M.: 15-35 minutes

Duration of Action 3-4 hours

Bioavailability Oral: 60% to 100%

Time to Peak Oral: ~45 minutes; I.M.: ~30 minutes

Half-Life Elimination 7-9 hours

Metabolism Via oxidation, forms metabolite trimethobenzamide N-oxide

Excretion Urine (30% to 50%, as unchanged drug)

Available Dosage Forms

Capsule, oral: 300 mg

Tigan®: 300 mg

Injection, solution:

Tigan®: 100 mg/mL (20 mL)

Injection, solution [preservative free]:

Tigan®: 100 mg/mL (2 mL)

Dosing

Adult

Nausea, vomiting:

Oral: 300 mg 3-4 times/day

I.M.: 200 mg 3-4 times/day

Postoperative nausea and vomiting (PONV): I.M.: 200 mg, followed 1 hour later by a second 200 mg dose

Geriatric Refer to adult dosing. Consider dosage reduction or increasing dosing interval in elderly patients with renal impairment (specific adjustment guidelines are not provided in the manufacturer's labeling).

Pediatric Nausea, vomiting: Children >40 kg: Oral: Refer to adult dosing. (Injection is contraindicated in children.)

Renal Impairment Cl_{cr} ≤70 mL/minute: Consider dosage reduction or increasing dosing interval (specific adjustment guidelines are not provided in the manufacturer's labeling)

Administration

Oral Capsule: Administer capsule orally without regard to meals.

I.M. Injection: Administer I.M. only. Inject deep into upper outer quadrant of gluteal muscle.

I.V. Injection: Not for I.V. administration.

Stability

Storage Store capsules and injection solution at room temperature of 25°C (77°F); excursions permitted to 15°C to 30°C (59°F to 86°F).

Monitoring and Teaching Issues

Laboratory Monitoring Renal function (at baseline)

Physical Assessment Monitor for hypovolemia, angioedema, and postural hypotension. If self-administered injection, teach patient appropriate injection technique and syringe disposal.

Patient Education If using injection formulation, follow directions for injection and disposal of syringe. May cause drowsiness, blurred vision, or diarrhea. Report chest pain or palpitations, persistent dizziness or blurred vision, or CNS changes (disorientation, depression, confusion).

Geriatric Considerations No specific data for use in the elderly have been established; as with any drug which has EPS adverse effects and possibility of confusion, caution should be used when administering to elderly.

This medication is considered to be potentially inappropriate in this patient population (Beers Criteria severity: High).

Pregnancy Considerations Teratogenic effects were not observed in animal studies. Safety and efficacy have not been established in pregnant patients. Trimethobenzamide has been used to treat nausea and vomiting of pregnancy.

◆ **Trimethobenzamide Hydrochloride** *see* Trimethobenzamide *on page* 1819

Trimethoprim (trye METH oh prim)

U.S. Brand Names Primsol®

Index Terms TMP

Generic Availability (U.S.) Yes: Tablet

Pharmacologic Category Antibiotic, Miscellaneous

Medication Safety Issues

Sound-alike/look-alike issues:

Trimethoprim may be confused with trimethaphan

Pregnancy Risk Factor C

Lactation Enters breast milk/use caution

Use Treatment of urinary tract infections due to susceptible strains of *E. coli*, *P. mirabilis*, *K. pneumoniae*, *Enterobacter* sp and coagulase-negative *Staphylococcus* including *S. saprophyticus*; acute otitis media in children; acute exacerbations of chronic bronchitis in adults; in combination with other agents for treatment of toxoplasmosis, *Pneumocystis jiroveci*; treatment of superficial ocular infections involving the conjunctiva and cornea

Mechanism of Action/Effect Inhibits folic acid reduction to tetrahydrofolate, and thereby inhibits microbial growth

Contraindications Hypersensitivity to trimethoprim or any component of the formulation; megaloblastic anemia due to folate deficiency

Warnings/Precautions Use with caution in patients with impaired renal or hepatic function or with possible folate deficiency. Prolonged use may result in fungal or bacterial superinfection, including *C. difficile*-associated diarrhea (CDAD) and pseudomembranous colitis; CDAD has been observed >2 months postantibiotic treatment.

Drug Interactions

Metabolism/Transport Effects Substrate (major) of CYP2C9, 3A4; **Inhibits** CYP2C8 (moderate), 2C9 (moderate)

Avoid Concomitant Use

Avoid concomitant use of Trimethoprim with any of the following: BCG; Dofetilide

Decreased Effect

Trimethoprim may decrease the levels/effects of: BCG; Typhoid Vaccine

The levels/effects of Trimethoprim may be decreased by: CYP2C9 Inducers (Highly Effective); CYP3A4 Inducers (Strong); Deferasirox; Herbs (CYP3A4 Inducers); Leucovorin Calcium-Levoleucovorin; Peginterferon Alfa-2b

Increased Effect/Toxicity

Trimethoprim may increase the levels/effects of: ACE Inhibitors; Amantadine; Angiotensin II Receptor Blockers; Antidiabetic Agents (Thiazolidinedione); AzaTHIOprine; Carvedilol; CYP2C8 Substrates (High risk); CYP2C9 Substrates (High risk); Dapsone; Dapsone (Systemic); Dapsone (Topical); Dofetilide; LamiVUDine; Memantine; Methotrexate; Phenytoin; PRALAtrexate; Procainamide; Repaglinide

The levels/effects of Trimethoprim may be increased by: Amantadine; Conivaptan; CYP2C9 Inhibitors (Moderate); CYP2C9 Inhibitors (Strong); Dapsone; Dapsone (Systemic); Memantine

Adverse Reactions Frequency not defined.

Central nervous system: Aseptic meningitis (rare), fever

Dermatologic: Maculopapular rash (3% to 7% at 200 mg/day; incidence higher with larger daily doses), erythema multiforme (rare), exfoliative dermatitis (rare), pruritus (common), phototoxic skin eruptions, Stevens-Johnson syndrome (rare), toxic epidermal necrolysis (rare)

Endocrine & metabolic: Hyperkalemia, hyponatremia

Gastrointestinal: Epigastric distress, glossitis, nausea, vomiting

Hematologic: Leukopenia, megaloblastic anemia, methemoglobinemia, neutropenia, thrombocytopenia

Hepatic: Cholestatic jaundice (rare), liver enzymes increased

Renal: BUN and creatinine increased

Miscellaneous: Anaphylaxis, hypersensitivity reactions

Pharmacodynamics/Kinetics

Absorption Readily and extensive

Time to Peak Serum: 1-4 hours

Protein Binding 42% to 46%

Half-Life Elimination 8-14 hours; prolonged with renal impairment

Metabolism Partially hepatic

Excretion Urine (60% to 80%) as unchanged drug

Available Dosage Forms

Solution, oral:

Primsol®: 50 mg (base)/5 mL (473 mL)

Tablet, oral: 100 mg

Dosing

Adult & Geriatric Susceptible infections: Oral: 100 mg every 12 hours or 200 mg every 24 hours for 10 days; longer treatment periods may be necessary for prostatitis (ie, 4-16 weeks); in the treatment of *Pneumocystis jiroveci* pneumonia; dose may be as high as 15-20 mg/kg/day in 3-4 divided doses

Pediatric Oral: Children (>2 months or age): 4 mg/kg/day in divided doses every 12 hours

Renal Impairment

Cl_{cr} 15-30 mL/minute: Administer 100 mg every 18 hours or 50 mg every 12 hours.

Cl_{cr} <15 mL/minute: Administer 100 mg every 24 hours or avoid use.

Moderately dialyzable (20% to 50%)

Administration

Oral Administer with milk or food.

Stability

Storage Protect the 200 mg tablet from light.

Monitoring and Teaching Issues

Laboratory Monitoring Periodic CBC and serum potassium during long-term therapy. Perform culture and sensitivity prior to initiating therapy.

Physical Assessment Perform culture and sensitivity tests prior to initiating therapy.

Patient Education Maintain adequate hydration unless instructed to restrict fluid intake. May cause nausea, vomiting, or GI upset. Report skin rash, redness, or irritation; feelings of acute fatigue or weakness; or unusual bleeding or bruising.

Dietary Considerations May cause folic acid deficiency, supplements may be needed. Should be taken with milk or food.

Geriatric Considerations Trimethoprim is often used in combination with sulfamethoxazole; it can be used alone in patients who are allergic to sulfonamides; adjust dose for renal function (see Pharmacodynamics/Kinetics and Dosing).

Breast-Feeding Considerations Trimethoprim is excreted in breast milk. The manufacturer recommends caution while using trimethoprim in a breast-feeding woman because trimethoprim may interfere with folic acid metabolism. Nondose-related effects could include modification of bowel flora. Also see the sulfamethoxazole/trimethoprim monograph for additional information.

Pregnancy Considerations Because adverse effects have been observed in animals, trimethoprim is classified pregnancy category C. Trimethoprim crosses the placenta and can be detected in the fetal serum and amniotic fluid. Due to trimethoprim's potential effect on folic acid metabolism, TMP should only be used during pregnancy if the benefit justifies the potential risk. The use of dihydrofolate reductase inhibitors, including trimethoprim, during pregnancy may increase the risk of congenital anomalies including cardiovascular defects, oral clefts, urinary tract anomalies, and neural tube defects. Folic acid supplementation may decrease this risk. The majority of studies evaluating the effects of trimethoprim administration in pregnancy have been conducted with sulfamethoxazole/trimethoprim. Trimethoprim in combination with sulfamethoxazole is used in pregnancy for various indications (see the sulfamethoxazole/trimethoprim monograph for details).

◆ **Trimethoprim and Sulfamethoxazole** *see* Sulfamethoxazole and Trimethoprim *on page 1686*

Trimipramine (trye MI pra meen)

U.S. Brand Names Surmontil®

Index Terms Trimipramine Maleate

Generic Availability (U.S.) No

Pharmacologic Category Antidepressant, Tricyclic (Tertiary Amine)

Medication Safety Issues

Sound-alike/look-alike issues:

Trimipramine may be confused with triamterene, trimeprazine

Medication Guide Available Yes

Pregnancy Risk Factor C

Lactation Enters breast milk/contraindicated

Use Treatment of depression

Mechanism of Action/Effect Increases the synaptic concentration of serotonin and/or norepinephrine in the central nervous system by inhibition of their reuptake by the presynaptic neuronal membrane

Contraindications Hypersensitivity to trimipramine, any component of the formulation, or other dibenzodiazepines; use of MAO inhibitors within 14 days; use in a patient during the acute recovery phase of MI

Warnings/Precautions **[U.S. Boxed Warning]: Antidepressants increase the risk of suicidal thinking and behavior in children, adolescents, and young adults (18-24 years of age) with major depressive disorder (MDD) and other psychiatric disorders;** consider risk prior to prescribing. Short-term studies did not show an increased risk in patients >24 years of age and showed a decreased risk in patients ≥65 years. Closely monitor for clinical worsening, suicidality, or unusual changes in behavior; the patient's family or caregiver should be instructed to closely observe the patient and communicate condition with healthcare provider. A medication guide should be dispensed with each prescription. **Trimipramine is not FDA approved for use in children.**

The possibility of a suicide attempt is inherent in major depression and may persist until remission occurs. Monitor for worsening of depression or suicidality, especially during initiation of therapy (generally first 1-2 months) or with dose increases or decreases. Use caution in high-risk patients. Worsening depression and severe abrupt suicidality that are not part of the presenting symptoms may require discontinuation or modification of drug therapy. The patient's family or caregiver should be alerted to monitor patients for the emergence of suicidality and associated behaviors (such as agitation, irritability, hostility, impulsivity, and hypomania) and call healthcare provider.

May worsen psychosis in some patients or precipitate a shift to mania or hypomania in patients with bipolar disorder. Patients presenting with depressive symptoms should be screened for bipolar disorder. Monotherapy in patients with bipolar disorder should be avoided. **Trimipramine is not FDA approved for the treatment of bipolar depression.**

The degree of sedation, anticholinergic effects, orthostasis, and conduction abnormalities are high relative to other antidepressants. Trimipramine often causes drowsiness/sedation, resulting in impaired performance of tasks requiring alertness (eg, operating machinery or driving).

Sedative effects may be additive with other CNS depressants and/or ethanol. Use with caution in patients with a history of cardiovascular disease (including previous MI, stroke, tachycardia, or conduction abnormalities). Use with caution in patients with urinary retention, benign prostatic hyperplasia, narrow-angle glaucoma, xerostomia, visual problems, constipation, or a history of bowel obstruction.

May alter glucose control - use with caution in patients with diabetes. Consider discontinuing, when possible, prior to elective surgery. Therapy should not be abruptly discontinued in patients receiving high doses for prolonged periods. May lower seizure threshold - use caution in patients with a previous seizure disorder or condition predisposing to seizures such as brain damage, alcoholism, or concurrent therapy with other drugs which lower the seizure threshold. May increase the risks associated with electroconvulsive therapy. Use with caution in hyperthyroid patients or those receiving thyroid supplementation. Use with caution in patients with hepatic or renal dysfunction and in elderly patients.

Drug Interactions

Metabolism/Transport Effects Substrate (major) of CYP2C19, 2D6, 3A4

Avoid Concomitant Use

Avoid concomitant use of Trimipramine with any of the following: Artemether; Dronedarone; Iobenguane I 123; Lumefantrine; MAO Inhibitors; Methylene Blue; Nilotinib; Pimozide; QuiNINE; Sibutramine; Tetrabenazine; Thioridazine; Toremifene; Vandetanib; Ziprasidone

Decreased Effect

Trimipramine may decrease the levels/effects of: Acetylcholinesterase Inhibitors (Central); Alpha2-Agonists; Iobenguane I 123

The levels/effects of Trimipramine may be decreased by: Acetylcholinesterase Inhibitors (Central); Barbiturates; CarBAMazepine; CYP2C19 Inducers (Strong); CYP3A4 Inducers (Strong); Deferasirox; Peginterferon Alfa-2b; St Johns Wort

Increased Effect/Toxicity

Trimipramine may increase the levels/effects of: Alcohol (Ethyl); Alpha-/Beta-Agonists (Direct-Acting); Alpha1-Agonists; Amphetamines; Anticholinergics; Aspirin; Beta2-Agonists; CNS Depressants; Desmopressin; Dronedarone; Methylene Blue; NSAID (COX-2 Inhibitor); NSAID (Nonselective); Pimozide; QTc-Prolonging Agents; QuiNIDine; QuiNINE; Serotonin Modulators; Sulfonylureas; Tetrabenazine; Thioridazine; Toremifene; TraMADol; Vandetanib; Vitamin K Antagonists; Yohimbine; Ziprasidone

The levels/effects of Trimipramine may be increased by: Alfuzosin; Altretamine; Artemether; BuPROPion; Chloroquine; Cimetidine; Cinacalcet; Ciprofloxacin; Ciprofloxacin (Systemic); Conivaptan; CYP2C19 Inhibitors (Moderate); CYP2C19 Inhibitors (Strong); CYP2D6 Inhibitors (Moderate); CYP2D6 Inhibitors (Strong); CYP3A4 Inhibitors (Moderate); CYP3A4 Inhibitors (Strong); Dexmethylphenidate; Divalproex; DULoxetine; Gadobutrol; Lithium; Lumefantrine; MAO Inhibitors; Methylphenidate; Metoclopramide; Nilotinib; Pramlintide; Propoxyphene; Protease Inhibitors; QuiNIDine; QuiNINE; Selective Serotonin Reuptake Inhibitors; Sibutramine; Terbinafine; Terbinafine (Systemic); Valproic Acid

Nutritional/Ethanol Interactions

Ethanol: Avoid ethanol (may increase CNS depression).

Food: Grapefruit juice may inhibit the metabolism of some TCAs and clinical toxicity may result.

Herb/Nutraceutical: Avoid valerian, St John's wort, SAMe, kava kava (may increase risk of serotonin syndrome and/or excessive sedation).

Lab Interactions Increased glucose

Adverse Reactions Frequency not defined.

Cardiovascular: Arrhythmias, facial edema, flushing, heart block, hyper-/hypotension, MI, palpitation, stroke, tachycardia

Central nervous system: Agitation, anxiety, confusion, delusions, disorientation, dizziness, drowsiness, EEG abnormalities, exacerbation of psychosis, fatigue, hallucinations, headache, hypomania, insomnia, nightmares, restlessness, seizure

Dermatologic: Alopecia, itching, petechiae, photosensitivity, rash, urticaria

Endocrine & metabolic: Breast enlargement, galactorrhea, gynecomastia, hyper-/hypoglycemia, libido (changes in), parotid swelling, syndrome of inappropriate ADH secretion (SIADH)

Gastrointestinal: Abdominal cramps, anorexia, black tongue, constipation, diarrhea, epigastric distress, nausea, paralytic ileus, stomatitis, tongue edema, unpleasant taste, tongue edema, vomiting, weight gain/loss, xerostomia

Genitourinary: Delayed/difficult urination, impotence, polyuria, testicular edema, urinary retention

Hematologic: Agranulocytosis, eosinophilia, purpura, thrombocytopenia

Hepatic: Cholestatic jaundice, liver enzymes increased

Neuromuscular & skeletal: Ataxia, extrapyramidal symptoms, incoordination, numbness, paresthesia, peripheral neuropathy, tingling, tremor, weakness

Ocular: Blurred vision, disturbances in accommodation, mydriasis

Otic: Tinnitus

Miscellaneous: Diaphoresis, withdrawal syndrome

Pharmacodynamics/Kinetics

Bioavailability 18% to 63%

Protein Binding 95%; free drug: 3% to 7%

Half-Life Elimination 16-40 hours

Metabolism Hepatic; significant first-pass effect

Excretion Urine

Available Dosage Forms

Capsule, oral:

Surmontil®: 25 mg, 50 mg, 100 mg

Dosing

Adult Depression: Oral:

Outpatients: Initial: 75 mg/day in divided doses; may increase to 150 mg/day; Maintenance: 50-150 mg/day as a single bedtime dose; maximum: 200 mg/day

Inpatients: Initial: 100 mg /day in divided doses; may increase to 200 mg/day; if no improvement after 2-3 weeks, dose may be increased to 250-300 mg/day

Geriatric Oral: 50 mg/day; gradually increase dose to 100 mg/day

Pediatric Depression: Adolescents: Oral: Initial: 50 mg/day; gradually increase dose to 100 mg/day; Maintenance: Lowest effective dose at bedtime

Stability

Storage Solutions stable at a pH of 4-5. Turns yellowish or reddish on exposure to light. Slight discoloration does not affect potency; marked discoloration is associated with loss of potency. Capsules stable for 3 years following date of manufacture.

Monitoring and Teaching Issues

Physical Assessment Monitor for CNS depression, thoughts of suicide. Taper dosage slowly when discontinuing.

Patient Education It may take 2-3 weeks to achieve desired results. Take at bedtime. Avoid alcohol. Maintain adequate hydration unless instructed to restrict fluid intake. You may experience drowsiness, lightheadedness, dizziness, blurred vision, nausea, altered taste, dry mouth, constipation, diarrhea, increased appetite, postural hypotension, urinary retention, or sexual dysfunction (reversible). Report persistent CNS effects (eg, insomnia, restlessness, fatigue, anxiety, impaired cognitive function, seizures, suicide ideation); muscle cramping or tremors; chest pain, palpitations, rapid heartbeat, swelling of extremities, or severe dizziness; unresolved urinary retention; vision changes or eye pain; yellowing of eyes or skin; pale stools/dark urine; suicide ideation; or worsening of condition.

Geriatric Considerations Similar to doxepin in its side effect profile; has not been well studied in the elderly; very anticholinergic and, therefore, not considered a drug of first choice in the elderly when selecting an antidepressant. Data from a clinical trial comparing fluoxetine to tricyclics suggest that fluoxetine is significantly less effective than nortriptyline in hospitalized elderly patients with unipolar major affective disorder, especially those with melancholia and concurrent cardiovascular diseases.

Additional Information May cause alterations in bleeding time.

Related Information

Antidepressant Agents *on page 1982*

◆ **Trimipramine Maleate** *see* Trimipramine *on page 1822*

◆ **TriNessa®** *see* Ethinyl Estradiol and Norgestimate *on page 704*

◆ **Tri-Norinyl®** *see* Ethinyl Estradiol and Norethindrone *on page 701*

◆ **Tripedia® [DSC]** *see* Diphtheria and Tetanus Toxoids, and Acellular Pertussis Vaccine *on page 552*

Triptorelin (trip toe REL in)

U.S. Brand Names Trelstar®

Index Terms AY-25650; CL-118,532; D-Trp(6)-LHRH; Detryptoreline; Triptorelin Pamoate; Tryptoreline

Generic Availability (U.S.) No

Pharmacologic Category Gonadotropin Releasing Hormone Agonist

Pregnancy Risk Factor X

Lactation Excretion in breast milk unknown/not recommended

Use Palliative treatment of advanced prostate cancer

Unlabeled/Investigational Use Treatment of endometriosis, *in vitro* fertilization, precocious puberty, uterine sarcoma

Mechanism of Action/Effect Causes suppression of ovarian and testicular steroidogenesis due to decreased levels of LH and FSH with subsequent decrease in testosterone (male) and estrogen (female) levels. After chronic and continuous administration, usually 2-4 weeks after initiation, a sustained decrease in LH and FSH secretion occurs.

Contraindications Hypersensitivity to triptorelin or any component of the formulation, other GnRH agonists or GnRH; pregnancy

Warnings/Precautions Hazardous agent - use appropriate precautions for handling and disposal. Transient increases in testosterone can lead to worsening symptoms (bone pain, hematuria, bladder outlet obstruction, neuropathy, spinal cord compression) of prostate cancer during the first few weeks of therapy. Androgen-deprivation therapy may increase the risk for cardiovascular disease (Levine, 2010). Hyperglycemia has been reported with androgen deprivation therapy (in prostate cancer) and may manifest as diabetes or worsening of pre-existing diabetes; monitor blood glucose and/or Hb A_{1c}. Cases of spinal cord compression have been reported with GnRH agonists. Closely observe (during the first 2 weeks of treatment) patients with metastatic vertebral lesions or urinary tract obstruction. Hypersensitivity reactions including angioedema, anaphylaxis and anaphylactic shock have rarely occurred; discontinue if severe reaction occurs. Rare cases of pituitary apoplexy (frequently secondary to pituitary adenoma) have been observed with leuprolide administration (onset from 1 hour to usually <2 weeks); may present as sudden headache, vomiting, visual or mental status changes, and infrequently cardiovascular collapse; immediate medical attention required.

Drug Interactions

Avoid Concomitant Use There are no known interactions where it is recommended to avoid concomitant use.

Decreased Effect

Triptorelin may decrease the levels/effects of: Antidiabetic Agents

Increased Effect/Toxicity There are no known significant interactions involving an increase in effect.

Lab Interactions Pituitary-gonadal function may be suppressed with chronic administration and for up to 8 weeks after triptorelin therapy has been discontinued.

Adverse Reactions As reported with all strengths; frequency of effect may vary by strength:

>10%:

Endocrine & metabolic: Hot flashes (59% to 73%), glucose increased, testosterone levels increased (peak: days 2-4; decline to low levels by weeks 3-4)

Hematologic: Hemoglobin decreased, RBC count decreased

Hepatic: Alkaline phosphatase increased (2% to >10%), ALT increased, AST increased

Neuromuscular & skeletal: Skeletal pain (12% to 13%)

Renal: BUN increased

1% to 10%:

Cardiovascular: Leg edema (6%), hypertension (1% to 4%), chest pain (2%), edema (2%), peripheral edema (≤1%)

Central nervous system: Headache (2% to 7%), pain (2% to 3%), dizziness (1% to 3%), fatigue (2%), insomnia (1% to 2%), emotional lability (1%)

Dermatologic: Rash (2%), pruritus (1%)

Endocrine & metabolic: Breast pain (2%), gynecomastia (2%), libido decreased (2%)

Gastrointestinal: Nausea (3%), anorexia (2%), constipation (2%), dyspepsia (2%), vomiting (2%), abdominal pain (1%), diarrhea (1%)

Genitourinary: Erectile dysfunction (10%), testicular atrophy (8%), impotence (2% to 7%), dysuria (5%), urinary retention (≤1%), urinary tract infection (≤1%)

Hematologic: Anemia (1%)

Local: Injection site pain (4%)

Neuromuscular & skeletal: Leg pain (2% to 5%), back pain (1% to 3%), leg cramps (2%), arthralgia (1% to 2%), extremity pain (1%), myalgia (1%), weakness (1%)

Ocular: Conjunctivitis (1%), eye pain (1%)

Respiratory: Cough (2%), dyspnea (1%), pharyngitis (1%)

Pharmacodynamics/Kinetics

Time to Peak 1-3 hours

Protein Binding None

Half-Life Elimination 2.8 ± 1.2 hours

Moderate-to-severe renal impairment: 6.5-7.7 hours

Hepatic impairment: 7.6 hours

Metabolism Unknown; unlikely to involve CYP; no known metabolites

Excretion Urine (42% as intact peptide); hepatic

Available Dosage Forms

Injection, powder for reconstitution:

Trelstar®: 3.75 mg, 11.25 mg, 22.5 mg

Dosing

Adult & Geriatric Advanced prostate carcinoma: I.M.:

3.75 mg once every 4 weeks **or**

11.25 mg once every 12 weeks **or**

22.5 mg once every 24 weeks

Administration

I.M. Administer by I.M. injection into the buttock; alternate injection sites. Administer immediately after reconstitution.

Stability

Reconstitution Reconstitute with 2 mL sterile water for injection. Shake well to obtain a uniform suspension. Solution will appear milky. Administer immediately after reconstitution.

MIXJECT® System: Follow manufacturer's instructions for mixing prior to use.

Storage Store at 20°C to 25°C (68°F to 77°F). Do not freeze MIXJECT® system.

Monitoring and Teaching Issues

Laboratory Monitoring Serum testosterone levels, prostate-specific antigen

Physical Assessment Hypersensitivity reactions, including angioedema, anaphylaxis, and anaphylactic shock, have rarely occurred; discontinue if severe reaction occurs. Be alert to the potential onset of spinal cord compression, diabetes, and/or cardiovascular disease.

Patient Education This medication can only be administered by injection. If you have diabetes, monitor blood sugar closely; may alter blood glucose levels. Report swelling, pain, or burning at injection site. May cause disease flare (increased bone pain), blood in urine, urinary retention during early treatment (usually resolves within 1 week), impotence, or hot flashes. Report any persistent adverse GI upset; chest pain, rapid heartbeat, or palpations; numbness in extremities; acute headache; or alterations in urinary pattern. Report immediately sudden headache, severe vomiting, visual or mental status change, and cardiovascular collapse.

Geriatric Considerations No dosage adjustments are needed in the elderly. Monitoring for bone density changes, serum lipid, hemoglobin A_{1c}, blood pressure, and serum calcium changes is recommended.

Pregnancy Considerations Contraindicated in women who are or may become pregnant. Hormonal changes induced by triptorelin may increase the risk of pregnancy loss or fetal harm.

- **Triptorelin Pamoate** *see* Triptorelin *on page 1824*
- **Trisenox®** *see* Arsenic Trioxide *on page 149*
- **Tri-Sprintec®** *see* Ethinyl Estradiol and Norgestimate *on page 704*
- **Trivalent Inactivated Influenza Vaccine (TIV)** *see* Influenza Virus Vaccine (Inactivated) *on page 978*
- **Trivora®** *see* Ethinyl Estradiol and Levonorgestrel *on page 699*
- **Trizivir®** *see* Abacavir, Lamivudine, and Zidovudine *on page 32*
- **Trusopt®** *see* Dorzolamide *on page 574*
- **Truvada®** *see* Emtricitabine and Tenofovir *on page 615*
- **Tryptoreline** *see* Triptorelin *on page 1824*
- **TSPA** *see* Thiotepa *on page 1754*
- **Tucks® Anti-Itch [OTC] [DSC]** *see* Hydrocortisone (Topical) *on page 920*
- **Tusso-C™** *see* Guaifenesin and Codeine *on page 891*
- **TVP-1012** *see* Rasagiline *on page 1559*
- **Twelve Resin-K [OTC]** *see* Cyanocobalamin *on page 431*
- **Twilite® [OTC]** *see* DiphenhydrAMINE (Systemic) *on page 543*
- **Twinject®** *see* EPINEPHrine (Systemic, Oral Inhalation) *on page 629*
- **Twinrix®** *see* Hepatitis A and Hepatitis B Recombinant Vaccine *on page 903*
- **Twynsta®** *see* Telmisartan and Amlodipine *on page 1719*
- **Tygacil®** *see* Tigecycline *on page 1761*
- **Tykerb®** *see* Lapatinib *on page 1064*
- **Tylenol® [OTC]** *see* Acetaminophen *on page 38*
- **Tylenol #2** *see* Acetaminophen and Codeine *on page 41*
- **Tylenol #3** *see* Acetaminophen and Codeine *on page 41*
- **Tylenol® 8 Hour [OTC]** *see* Acetaminophen *on page 38*
- **Tylenol® Arthritis Pain Extended Relief [OTC]** *see* Acetaminophen *on page 38*
- **Tylenol® Children's [OTC]** *see* Acetaminophen *on page 38*
- **Tylenol® Children's Meltaways [OTC]** *see* Acetaminophen *on page 38*
- **Tylenol Codeine** *see* Acetaminophen and Codeine *on page 41*
- **Tylenol® Extra Strength [OTC]** *see* Acetaminophen *on page 38*
- **Tylenol® Infant's Concentrated [OTC]** *see* Acetaminophen *on page 38*
- **Tylenol® Jr. Meltaways [OTC]** *see* Acetaminophen *on page 38*
- **Tylenol® with Codeine No. 3** *see* Acetaminophen and Codeine *on page 41*
- **Tylenol® with Codeine No. 4** *see* Acetaminophen and Codeine *on page 41*
- **Tylox®** *see* Oxycodone and Acetaminophen *on page 1383*
- **Tysabri®** *see* Natalizumab *on page 1292*
- **Tyvaso™** *see* Treprostinil *on page 1809*
- **Tyzeka®** *see* Telbivudine *on page 1714*
- **U-90152S** *see* Delavirdine *on page 482*
- **UCB-P071** *see* Cetirizine *on page 351*
- **U-Cort™** *see* Hydrocortisone (Topical) *on page 920*
- **UK-88,525** *see* Darifenacin *on page 467*
- **UK-427,857** *see* Maraviroc *on page 1147*
- **UK92480** *see* Sildenafil *on page 1641*
- **UK109496** *see* Voriconazole *on page 1871*

Ulipristal (ue li PRIS tal)

U.S. Brand Names ella®

Index Terms CDB-2914; Ulipristal Acetate

Generic Availability (U.S.) No

Pharmacologic Category Contraceptive; Progestin Receptor Modulator

Medication Safety Issues

Sound-alike/look-alike issues:

Ulipristal may be confused with ursodiol

Pregnancy Risk Factor X

Lactation Excretion unknown/not recommended

Use Emergency contraception following unprotected intercourse or possible contraceptive failure

Available Dosage Forms

Tablet, oral:

ella®: 30 mg

Dosing

Adult Emergency contraception: Oral: One tablet (30 mg) within 120 hours (5 days) of unprotected intercourse or contraceptive failure

Geriatric Not indicated for use in postmenopausal women.

Pediatric Not for use prior to menarche.

Administration

Oral Administer with or without food at anytime during menstrual cycle. If vomiting occurs within 3 hours of administration, consider repeating dose.

Monitoring and Teaching Issues

Laboratory Monitoring Evaluate for pregnancy or ectopic pregnancy if menses is delayed for ≥1 week following emergency contraception, or if lower abdominal pain (3-5 weeks after administration) or persistent irregular bleeding develops.

- ◆ **Ulipristal Acetate** *see* Ulipristal *on page* 1826
- ◆ **Uloric®** *see* Febuxostat *on page* 737
- ◆ **Ultram®** *see* TraMADol *on page* 1797
- ◆ **Ultram® ER** *see* TraMADol *on page* 1797
- ◆ **Ultraprin [OTC]** *see* Ibuprofen *on page* 938
- ◆ **Ultrase® [DSC]** *see* Pancrelipase *on page* 1400
- ◆ **Ultrase® MT [DSC]** *see* Pancrelipase *on page* 1400
- ◆ **Unasyn®** *see* Ampicillin and Sulbactam *on page* 127
- ◆ **Unburn® [OTC]** *see* Lidocaine (Topical) *on page* 1107
- ◆ **Uniretic®** *see* Moexipril and Hydrochlorothiazide *on page* 1252
- ◆ **Unisom® SleepGels® Maximum Strength [OTC]** *see* DiphenhydrAMINE (Systemic) *on page* 543
- ◆ **Unisom® SleepMelts™ [OTC]** *see* DiphenhydrAMINE (Systemic) *on page* 543
- ◆ **Unithroid®** *see* Levothyroxine *on page* 1101
- ◆ **Univasc®** *see* Moexipril *on page* 1249
- ◆ **Urate Oxidase** *see* Rasburicase *on page* 1562
- ◆ **Urate Oxidase, Pegylated** *see* Pegloticase *on page* 1427
- ◆ **Urecholine®** *see* Bethanechol *on page* 210
- ◆ **Urocit®-K** *see* Potassium Citrate *on page* 1482
- ◆ **Uro-KP-Neutral®** *see* Potassium Phosphate and Sodium Phosphate *on page* 1486
- ◆ **Uroxatral®** *see* Alfuzosin *on page* 69
- ◆ **Urso 250®** *see* Ursodiol *on page* 1827
- ◆ **Ursodeoxycholic Acid** *see* Ursodiol *on page* 1827

Ursodiol (ur soe DYE ol)

U.S. Brand Names Actigall®; Urso 250®; Urso Forte®

Index Terms Ursodeoxycholic Acid

Generic Availability (U.S.) Yes

Pharmacologic Category Gallstone Dissolution Agent

Medication Safety Issues

Sound-alike/look-alike issues:

Ursodiol may be confused with ulipristal

Pregnancy Risk Factor B

Lactation Excretion in breast milk unknown/use caution

Use

Actigall®: Gallbladder stone dissolution; prevention of gallstones in obese patients experiencing rapid weight loss

Urso®, Urso Forte®: Primary biliary cirrhosis

Available Dosage Forms

Capsule, oral: 300 mg

Actigall®: 300 mg

Tablet, oral: 250 mg, 500 mg

Urso 250®: 250 mg

Urso Forte®: 500 mg

Dosing

Adult & Geriatric

Gallstone dissolution (Actigall®): Oral: 8-10 mg/kg/day in 2-3 divided doses; use beyond 24 months is not established

Gallstone prevention (Actigall®): Oral: 300 mg twice daily

Primary biliary cirrhosis (Urso®, Urso Forte®): Oral: 13-15 mg/kg/day in 2-4 divided doses (with food)

Administration

Oral Do not administer with aluminum-based antacids. If aluminum-based antacids are needed, administer 2 hours after ursodiol. Urso Forte® can be split into halves for appropriate dosage; do not chew. Urso® and Urso Forte® should be taken with food.

Monitoring and Teaching Issues

Laboratory Monitoring

Gallstone disease: ALT, AST, ALP; sonogram may be required

Hepatic disease: Monitor hepatic function tests frequently

Patient Education Take with food. Drug will need to be taken for 1-3 months after stone is dissolved; stones may recur. Report any persistent nausea, vomiting, abdominal pain, or yellowing of skin or eyes.

◆ **Urso Forte®** *see* Ursodiol *on page 1827*

◆ **UTI Relief® [OTC]** *see* Phenazopyridine *on page 1446*

◆ **Vagistat®-1 [OTC]** *see* Tioconazole *on page 1769*

ValACYclovir (val ay SYE kloe veer)

U.S. Brand Names Valtrex®

Index Terms Valacyclovir Hydrochloride

Generic Availability (U.S.) Yes

Pharmacologic Category Antiviral Agent; Antiviral Agent, Oral

Medication Safety Issues

Sound-alike/look-alike issues:

Valtrex® may be confused with Keflex®, Valcyte®, Zovirax®

ValACYclovir may be confused with acyclovir, valGANciclovir, vancomycin

Pregnancy Risk Factor B

Lactation Enters breast milk/use caution

Use Treatment of herpes zoster (shingles) in immunocompetent patients; treatment of first-episode and recurrent genital herpes; suppression of recurrent genital herpes and reduction of heterosexual transmission of genital herpes in immunocompetent patients; suppression of genital herpes in HIV-infected individuals; treatment of herpes labialis (cold sores); chickenpox in immunocompetent children

Unlabeled/Investigational Use Prophylaxis of cancer-related HSV, VZV, and CMV infections; treatment of cancer-related HSV, VZV infection

Mechanism of Action/Effect Valacyclovir is rapidly converted to acyclovir before it exerts its antiviral activity against HSV-1, HSV-2, or VZV. Inhibits viral DNA synthesis and replication.

Contraindications Hypersensitivity to valacyclovir, acyclovir, or any component of the formulation

Warnings/Precautions Thrombotic thrombocytopenic purpura/hemolytic uremic syndrome has occurred in immunocompromised patients (at doses of 8 g/day). Safety and efficacy have not been established for treatment/suppression of recurrent genital herpes or disseminated herpes in patients with profound immunosuppression (eg, advanced HIV with CD4 <100 cells/mm^3). CNS adverse effects (including agitation, hallucinations, confusion, delirium, seizures, and encephalopathy) have been reported. Use caution in patients with renal impairment, the elderly, and/or those receiving nephrotoxic agents. Acute renal failure has been observed in patients with renal dysfunction; dose adjustment may be required. Decreased precipitation in renal tubules may occur leading to urinary precipitation; adequately hydrate patient. For cold sores, treatment should begin at with earliest symptom (tingling, itching, burning). For genital herpes, treatment should begin as soon as possible after the first signs and symptoms (within 72 hours of onset of first diagnosis or within 24 hours of onset of recurrent episodes). For herpes zoster, treatment should begin within 72 hours of onset of rash. For chickenpox, treatment should begin with earliest sign or symptom. Use with caution in the elderly; CNS effects have been reported. Safety and efficacy have not been established in patients <2 years of age.

Drug Interactions

Avoid Concomitant Use

Avoid concomitant use of ValACYclovir with any of the following: Zoster Vaccine

Decreased Effect

ValACYclovir may decrease the levels/effects of: Zoster Vaccine

Increased Effect/Toxicity

ValACYclovir may increase the levels/effects of: Mycophenolate; Tenofovir; Zidovudine

The levels/effects of ValACYclovir may be increased by: Mycophenolate

Adverse Reactions

>10%:

Central nervous system: Headache (13% to 38%)

Gastrointestinal: Nausea (5% to 15%), abdominal pain (1% to 11%)

Hematologic: Neutropenia (≤18%)

Hepatic: ALT increased (≤14%), AST increased (2% to 16%)

Respiratory: Nasopharyngitis (≤16%)

1% to 10%:

Central nervous system: Fatigue (≤8%), depression (≤7%), fever (children 4%), dizziness (2% to 4%)

Dermatologic: Rash (≤8%)

Endocrine: Dysmenorrhea (≤1% to 8%), dehydration (children 2%)

Gastrointestinal: Vomiting (<1% to 6%), diarrhea (children 5%; adults <1%)

Hematologic: Thrombocytopenia (≤3%)

Hepatic: Alkaline phosphatase increased (≤4%)

Neuromuscular & skeletal: Arthralgia (<1 to 6%)
Respiratory: Rhinorrhea (children 2%)
Miscellaneous: Herpes simplex (children 2%)

Pharmacodynamics/Kinetics

Absorption Rapid

Bioavailability ~55% once converted to acyclovir

Protein Binding ~14% to 18%

Half-Life Elimination Normal renal function: Adults: 2.5-3.3 hours (acyclovir), ~30 minutes (valacyclovir); End-stage renal disease: 14-20 hours (acyclovir); During hemodialysis: 4 hours

Metabolism Hepatic; valacyclovir is rapidly and nearly completely converted to acyclovir and L-valine by first-pass effect; acyclovir is hepatically metabolized to a very small extent by aldehyde oxidase and by alcohol and aldehyde dehydrogenase (inactive metabolites)

Excretion Urine, primarily as acyclovir (89%); **Note:** Following oral administration of radiolabeled valacyclovir, 46% of the label is eliminated in the feces (corresponding to nonabsorbed drug), while 47% of the radiolabel is eliminated in the urine.

Available Dosage Forms

Caplet, oral: 500 mg, 1 g
Valtrex®: 500 mg, 1 g

Tablet, oral: 500 mg, 1 g

Dosing

Adult & Geriatric

CMV prophylaxis in allogeneic HSCT recipients (unlabeled use): 2 g 4 times/day
Herpes labialis (cold sores): Oral: 2 g twice daily for 1 day (separate doses by ~12 hours)
Herpes zoster (shingles): Oral: 1 g 3 times/day for 7 days
HSV, VZV in cancer patients (unlabeled use):
Prophylaxis: 500 mg 2-3 times/day
Treatment: 1 g 3 times/day
Genital herpes: Oral:
Initial episode: 1 g twice daily for 10 days
Recurrent episode: 500 mg twice daily for 3 days
Reduction of transmission: 500 mg once daily (source partner)
Suppressive therapy:
Immunocompetent patients: 1000 mg once daily (500 mg once daily in patients with <9 recurrences per year)
HIV-infected patients (CD4 ≥100 cells/mm^3): 500 mg twice daily

Pediatric

Chickenpox: Children 2 to <18 years: 20 mg/kg/dose 3 times/day for 5 days (maximum: 1 g 3 times/day)
Herpes labialis (cold sores): Children ≥12 years: Refer to adult dosing.

Renal Impairment

Herpes zoster: Adults:
Cl_{cr} 30-49 mL/minute: 1 g every 12 hours
Cl_{cr} 10-29 mL/minute: 1 g every 24 hours
Cl_{cr} <10 mL/minute: 500 mg every 24 hours
Genital herpes: Adults:
Initial episode:
Cl_{cr} 10-29 mL/minute: 1 g every 24 hours
Cl_{cr} <10 mL/minute: 500 mg every 24 hours
Recurrent episode: Cl_{cr} <29 mL/minute: 500 mg every 24 hours
Suppressive therapy: Cl_{cr} <29 mL/minute:
For usual dose of 1 g every 24 hours, decrease dose to 500 mg every 24 hours
For usual dose of 500 mg every 24 hours, decrease dose to 500 mg every 48 hours
HIV-infected patients: 500 mg every 24 hours
Herpes labialis: Adolescents and Adults:
Cl_{cr} 30-49 mL/minute: 1 g every 12 hours for 2 doses
Cl_{cr} 10-29 mL/minute: 500 mg every 12 hours for 2 doses
Cl_{cr} <10 mL/minute: 500 mg as a single dose
Hemodialysis: Dialyzable (~33% removed during 4-hour session); administer dose post-dialysis
Chronic ambulatory peritoneal dialysis/continuous arteriovenous hemofiltration dialysis: Pharmacokinetic parameters are similar to those in patients with ESRD; supplemental dose not needed following dialysis

Hepatic Impairment No adjustment required.

Administration

Oral If GI upset occurs, administer with meals.

Stability

Storage Store at 15°C to 25°C (59°F to 77°F).

Monitoring and Teaching Issues

Laboratory Monitoring Urinalysis, BUN, serum creatinine, liver enzymes, and CBC

Physical Assessment Monitor for CNS changes (dizziness, depression), nausea, vomiting, dysmenorrhea, and arthralgia. Teach patient appropriate timing of treatment.

Patient Education This medication is not a cure for genital herpes; it is not known if it will prevent transmission to others. Use appropriate precautions to prevent spread to other persons. Begin use at first sign of herpes. Maintain adequate hydration, unless instructed to restrict fluid intake. May cause headache, dizziness, nausea, vomiting, or abdominal pain. Immediately report difficulty swallowing or breathing, rash, or hives.

Dietary Considerations May be taken with or without food.

Geriatric Considerations More convenient dosing and increased bioavailability, without increasing side effects, make valacyclovir a favorable choice compared to acyclovir. Has been shown to accelerate resolution of postherpetic pain. Adjust dose for renal impairment.

Breast-Feeding Considerations Peak concentrations in breast milk range from 0.5-2.3 times the corresponding maternal acyclovir serum concentration. This is expected to provide a nursing infant with a dose of acyclovir equivalent to ~0.6 mg/kg/day following ingestion of valacyclovir 500 mg twice daily by the mother. Use with caution while breast-feeding.

Pregnancy Considerations Teratogenic events were not observed in animal studies. Data from a pregnancy registry has shown no increased rate of birth defects than that of the general population; however, the registry is small and use during pregnancy is only warranted if the potential benefit to the mother justifies the risk of the fetus.

◆ **Valacyclovir Hydrochloride** *see* ValACYclovir *on page 1828*

◆ **Valcyte®** *see* ValGANCIclovir *on page 1830*

◆ **23-Valent Pneumococcal Polysaccharide Vaccine** *see* Pneumococcal Polysaccharide Vaccine (Polyvalent) *on page 1471*

ValGANCIclovir (val gan SYE kloh veer)

U.S. Brand Names Valcyte®

Index Terms Valganciclovir Hydrochloride

Generic Availability (U.S.) No

Pharmacologic Category Antiviral Agent

Medication Safety Issues

Sound-alike/look-alike issues:

Valcyte® may be confused with Valium®, Valtrex®

ValGANciclovir may be confused with valACYclovir

Pregnancy Risk Factor C

Lactation Excretion in breast milk unknown/not recommended

Use Treatment of cytomegalovirus (CMV) retinitis in patients with acquired immunodeficiency syndrome (AIDS); prevention of CMV disease in high-risk patients (donor CMV positive/ recipient CMV negative) undergoing kidney, heart, or kidney/pancreas transplantation

Mechanism of Action/Effect Valganciclovir is a prodrug of ganciclovir, and is rapidly metabolized in the body to form ganciclovir. Ganciclovir inhibits the formation of viral DNA within infected cells, blocking reproduction of the virus.

Contraindications Hypersensitivity to valganciclovir, ganciclovir, or any component of the formulation

Warnings/Precautions Hazardous agent - use appropriate precautions for handling and disposal. **[U.S. Boxed Warning]: May cause dose- or therapy-limiting granulocytopenia, anemia, and/or thrombocytopenia;** do not use in patients with an absolute neutrophil count <500/mm^3, platelet count <25,000/mm^3, or hemoglobin <8 g/dL. Uuse with caution in patients with impaired renal function (dose adjustment required). Acute renal failure (ARF) may occur; ensure adequate hydration and use with caution in patients receiving concomitant nephrotoxic agents. Elderly patients with or without pre-existing renal impairment may develop ARF; use with caution and adjust dose as needed. **[U.S. Boxed Warning]: Ganciclovir may be teratogenic, carcinogenic, and cause aspermatogenesis.** Due to its teratogenic potential, contraceptive precautions for female and male patients need to be followed during and for at least 90 days after therapy with the drug. Fertility may be temporarily or permanently impaired in males and females. Due to differences in bioavailability, valganciclovir tablets cannot be substituted for ganciclovir capsules on a one-to-one basis. The preferred dosage form for pediatric patients is the oral solution; however, valganciclovir tablets may used so long as the calculated dose is within 10% of the available tablet strength (450 mg). Not indicated for use in liver transplant patients (higher incidence of tissue-invasive CMV relative to oral ganciclovir was observed in trials). Use of valganciclovir for the treatment of congenital CMV disease has not been evaluated.

Drug Interactions

Avoid Concomitant Use

Avoid concomitant use of ValGANciclovir with any of the following: Imipenem

Decreased Effect There are no known significant interactions involving a decrease in effect.

Increased Effect/Toxicity

ValGANciclovir may increase the levels/effects of: Imipenem; Mycophenolate; Reverse Transcriptase Inhibitors (Nucleoside); Tenofovir

The levels/effects of ValGANciclovir may be increased by: Mycophenolate; Probenecid; Tenofovir

Nutritional/Ethanol Interactions Food: Coadministration with a high-fat meal increased AUC by 30%.

Adverse Reactions

>10%:

Cardiovascular: Hypertension (12% to 18%)

Central nervous system: Fever (9% to 31%), headache (6% to 22%), insomnia (6% to 20%)

Gastrointestinal: Diarrhea (16% to 41%), nausea (8% to 30%), vomiting (3% to 21%), abdominal pain (15%), constipation

Hematologic: Anemia (≤31%), thrombocytopenia (≤22%), neutropenia (3% to 19%)

Neuromuscular & skeletal: Tremor (12% to 28%)

Ocular: Retinal detachment (15%)

Renal: Serum creatinine increased (S_{cr} >1.5-2.5 mg/dL: 12% to 50%; S_{cr} >2.5: 3% to 17%)

Respiratory: Cough, upper respiratory tract infection

5% to 10%: Central nervous system: Peripheral neuropathy (9%), paresthesia (8%)

<5%:

Cardiovascular: Edema, hypotension, peripheral edema

Central nervous system: Agitation, confusion, depression, dizziness, fatigue, hallucination, pain, psychosis, seizure

Dermatologic: Acne, dermatitis, pruritus

Endocrine & metabolic: Dehydration, hyperglycemia, hyper-/hypokalemia, hypocalcemia, hypomagnesemia, hypophosphatemia

Gastrointestinal: Abdominal distention/pain, appetite (decreased), dyspepsia

Genitourinary: Urinary tract infection

Hematologic: Aplastic anemia, bleeding (potentially life-threatening due to thrombocytopenia), bone marrow depression, pancytopenia

Hepatic: Ascites

Neuromuscular & skeletal: Arthralgia, back pain, limb pain, muscle cramps, weakness

Renal: Creatinine clearance (decreased), dysuria, renal impairment

Respiratory: Dyspnea, nasopharyngitis, pharyngitis, pleural effusion, rhinorrhea

Miscellaneous: Allergic reaction, local and systemic infection (including sepsis)

Pharmacodynamics/Kinetics

Absorption Well absorbed; high-fat meal increases AUC by 30%

Bioavailability With food: 60%

Time to Peak Ganciclovir: 1-3 hours

Protein Binding Ganciclovir: 1% to 2%

Half-Life Elimination Ganciclovir: 4.08 hours, prolonged with renal impairment; Severe renal impairment: Up to 68 hours

Metabolism Converted to ganciclovir by intestinal mucosal cells and hepatocytes

Excretion Urine (primarily as ganciclovir)

Available Dosage Forms

Powder for solution, oral:

Valcyte®: 50 mg/mL (100 mL)

Tablet, oral:

Valcyte®: 450 mg

Dosing

Adult & Geriatric

CMV retinitis: Oral:

Induction (active retinitis): 900 mg twice daily for 21 days

Maintenance: Following induction treatment, or for patients with inactive CMV retinitis who require maintenance therapy: 900 mg once daily

Prevention of CMV disease following transplantation: 900 mg once daily beginning within 10 days of transplantation; continue therapy until 100 days (heart or kidney-pancreas transplant) or 200 days (kidney transplant) post-transplantation

Pediatric

Prevention of CMV disease following kidney or heart transplantation: Oral:

Children 4 months to 16 years: Dose (mg) = 7 x body surface area x creatinine clearance* once daily beginning within 10 days of transplantation; continue therapy until 100 days post-transplantation. Doses should be rounded to the nearest 25 mg increment; maximum dose: 900 mg/day

*Cl_{cr} (mL/minute/1.73 m^2) = [k x Height (cm)] divided by serum creatinine (mg/dL)

Note: If the calculated Cl_{cr} is >150 mL/minute/1.73 m^2, then a maximum value of 150 mL/minute/1.73 m^2 should be used to calculate the dose.

Note: Calculated using *modified* Schwartz formula where k is as follows:

Patients <2 years: k = 0.45

Girls 2-16 years: k = 0.55

Boys 2 to <13 years: k = 0.55

Boys 13-16 years: k = 0.7

Children >16 years: Refer to adult dosing.

Renal Impairment

Children 4 months to 16 years: No additional dosage adjustments required; calculation for all patients adjusts for renal function.

Children >16 years and Adults:

Induction dose:

Cl_{cr} 40-59 mL/minute: 450 mg twice daily

Cl_{cr} 25-39 mL/minute: 450 mg once daily

Cl_{cr} 10-24 mL/minute: 450 mg every 2 days

Maintenance dose:

Cl_{cr} 40-59 mL/minute: 450 mg once daily

Cl_{cr} 25-39 mL/minute: 450 mg every 2 days

Cl_{cr} 10-24 mL/minute: 450 mg twice weekly

Note: Valganciclovir is not recommended in patients receiving hemodialysis. For patients on hemodialysis (Cl_{cr} <10 mL/minute), it is recommended that ganciclovir be used (dose adjusted as specified for ganciclovir).

Hepatic Impairment Use has not been studied.

Administration

Oral Valganciclovir should be taken with meals. The preferred dosage form for pediatric patients is the oral solution; however, valganciclovir tablets may used so long as the calculated dose is within 10% of the available tablet strength (450 mg).

Due to the carcinogenic and mutagenic potential, avoid direct contact with broken or crushed tablets, powder for oral solution, and oral solution. Consideration should be given to handling and disposal according to guidelines issued for antineoplastic drugs. However, there is no consensus on the need for these precautions.

Stability

Reconstitution Oral solution: Prior to dispensing, prepare the oral solution by adding 91 mL of purified water to the bottle; shake well. Discard any unused medication after 49 days. A reconstituted 100 mL bottle will only provide 88 mL of solution for administration.

Storage

Oral solution: Store dry powder at 25°C (77°F); excursions permitted to 15°C to 30°C (59°F to 86°F). Store oral solution under refrigeration at 2°C to 8°C (36°F to 46°F); do not freeze. Discard any unused medication after 49 days.

Tablet: Store at 25°C (77°F); excursions permitted to 15°C to 30°C (59°F to 86°F).

Monitoring and Teaching Issues

Laboratory Monitoring Retinal exam (at least every 4-6 weeks), CBC, platelet counts, serum creatinine

Physical Assessment Use caution with renal impairment. Monitor for peripheral neuropathy, neutropenia, anemia, nephrotoxicity, vomiting, and bloody diarrhea on a regular basis during therapy.

Patient Education This medication is not a cure for CMV retinitis. You will need frequent and regular laboratory tests and ophthalmic exams while taking this medication. Maintain adequate hydration, unless instructed to restrict fluid intake. May cause headache, insomnia, nausea, vomiting, diarrhea, or photosensitivity. Report fever, chills, unusual bleeding or bruising, infection or unhealed sores, white plaques in mouth or vaginal discharge, CNS disturbances (eg, hallucinations, confusion, nightmares), or weakness or loss of feeling in nerves or muscles.

Dietary Considerations Should be taken with meals.

Breast-Feeding Considerations HIV-infected mothers are discouraged from breast-feeding to decrease the potential transmission of HIV.

Pregnancy Considerations Valganciclovir is converted to ganciclovir and shares its reproductive toxicity. **[U.S. Boxed Warning]: Ganciclovir may be teratogenic and cause aspermatogenesis.** Based on animal data, temporary or permanent impairment of fertility may occur in males and females. Ganciclovir is also teratogenic in animals. Females should use effective contraception during treatment and for 30 days after; males should use barrier contraception during treatment and for 90 days after.

◆ **Valganciclovir Hydrochloride** *see* ValGANCIclovir *on page 1830*

◆ **Valium®** *see* Diazepam *on page 514*

◆ **Valorin [OTC]** *see* Acetaminophen *on page 38*

◆ **Valorin Extra [OTC]** *see* Acetaminophen *on page 38*

◆ **Valproate Semisodium** *see* Divalproex *on page 557*

◆ **Valproate Semisodium** *see* Valproic Acid *on page 1832*

◆ **Valproate Sodium** *see* Valproic Acid *on page 1832*

Valproic Acid (val PROE ik AS id)

U.S. Brand Names Depacon®; Depakene®; Stavzor™

Index Terms 2-Propylpentanoic Acid; 2-Propylvaleric Acid; Dipropylacetic Acid; DPA; Valproate Semisodium; Valproate Sodium

Generic Availability (U.S.) Yes: Excludes delayed release capsule

Pharmacologic Category Anticonvulsant, Miscellaneous; Antimanic Agent; Histone Deacetylase Inhibitor

Medication Safety Issues

Sound-alike/look-alike issues:

Depakene® may be confused with Depakote®

Valproate sodium may be confused with vecuronium

Pregnancy Risk Factor D

Lactation Enters breast milk/not recommended (AAP considers "compatible"; AAP 2001 update pending)

Use Monotherapy and adjunctive therapy in the treatment of patients with complex partial seizures; monotherapy and adjunctive therapy of simple and complex absence seizures; adjunctive therapy in patients with multiple seizure types that include absence seizures

Stavzor™: Mania associated with bipolar disorder; migraine prophylaxis

Unlabeled/Investigational Use Status epilepticus

Mechanism of Action/Effect Causes increased availability of gamma-aminobutyric acid (GABA), an inhibitory neurotransmitter, to brain neurons or may enhance the action of GABA or mimic its action at postsynaptic receptor sites

Contraindications Hypersensitivity to valproic acid, derivatives, or any component of the formulation; hepatic disease or significant impairment; urea cycle disorders

Warnings/Precautions **[U.S. Boxed Warning]: Hepatic failure resulting in fatalities has occurred in patients; children <2 years of age are at considerable risk.** Other risk factors include organic brain disease, mental retardation with severe seizure disorders, congenital metabolic disorders, and patients on multiple anticonvulsants. Hepatotoxicity has usually been reported within 6 months of therapy initiation. Monitor patients closely for appearance of malaise, weakness, facial edema, anorexia, jaundice, and vomiting; discontinue immediately with signs/symptom of significant or suspected impairment. Liver function tests should be performed at baseline and at regular intervals after initiation of therapy, especially within the first 6 months. Hepatic dysfunction may progress despite discontinuing treatment. Should only be used as monotherapy in children <2 years of age and patients at high risk for hepatotoxicity. Contraindicated with severe impairment.

[U.S. Boxed Warning]: Cases of life-threatening pancreatitis, occurring at the start of therapy or following years of use, have been reported in adults and children. Some cases have been hemorrhagic with rapid progression of initial symptoms to death. Promptly evaluate symptoms of abdominal pain, nausea, vomiting, and/or anorexia; should generally be discontinued if pancreatitis is diagnosed.

[U.S. Boxed Warning]: May cause teratogenic effects such as neural tube defects (eg, spina bifida). Use in women of childbearing potential requires that benefits of use in mother be weighed against the potential risk to fetus, especially when used for conditions not associated with permanent injury or risk of death (eg, migraine).

May cause severe thrombocytopenia, inhibition of platelet aggregation, and bleeding. Tremors may indicate overdosage; use with caution in patients receiving other anticonvulsants. Hypersensitivity reactions affecting multiple organs have been reported in association with valproic acid use; may include dermatologic and/or hematologic changes (eosinophilia, neutropenia, thrombocytopenia) or symptoms of organ dysfunction.

Hyperammonemia and/or encephalopathy, sometimes fatal, have been reported following the initiation of valproic acid therapy and may be present with normal transaminase levels. Ammonia levels should be measured in patients who develop unexplained lethargy and vomiting, changes in mental status, or in patients who present with hypothermia (unintentional drop in core body temperature to <35°C/95°F). Discontinue therapy if ammonia levels are increased and evaluate for possible urea cycle disorder (UCD); contraindicated in patients with UCD. Evaluation of UCD should be considered for the following patients prior to the start of therapy: History of unexplained encephalopathy or coma; encephalopathy associated with protein load; pregnancy or postpartum encephalopathy; unexplained mental retardation; history of elevated plasma ammonia or glutamine; history of cyclical vomiting and lethargy; episodic extreme irritability, ataxia; low BUN or protein avoidance; family history of UCD or unexplained infant deaths (particularly male); or signs or symptoms of UCD (hyperammonemia, encephalopathy, respiratory alkalosis). Hypothermia has been reported with valproic acid therapy; may or may not be associated with hyperammonemia; may also occur with concomitant topiramate therapy.

In vitro studies have suggested valproic acid stimulates the replication of HIV and CMV viruses under experimental conditions. The clinical consequence of this is unknown, but should be considered when monitoring affected patients.

Antiepileptics are associated with an increased risk of suicidal behavior/thoughts with use (regardless of indication); patients should be monitored for signs/symptoms of depression, suicidal tendencies, and other unusual behavior changes during therapy and instructed to inform their healthcare provider immediately if symptoms occur.

Use of Depacon® injection is not recommended for post-traumatic seizure prophylaxis following acute head trauma. Anticonvulsants should not be discontinued abruptly because of the possibility of increasing seizure frequency; valproic acid should be withdrawn gradually to minimize the potential of increased seizure frequency, unless safety concerns require a more rapid withdrawal. Concomitant use with carbapenem antibiotics may reduce valproic acid levels to subtherapeutic levels; monitor levels frequently and consider alternate therapy if levels drop significantly or lack of seizure control occurs. Concomitant use with clonazepam may induce absence status. Patients treated for bipolar disorder should be monitored closely for clinical worsening or suicidality; prescriptions should be written for the smallest quantity consistent with good patient care.

CNS depression may occur with valproic acid use. Patients must be cautioned about performing tasks which require mental alertness (operating machinery or driving). Effects with other sedative drugs or ethanol may be potentiated. Use with caution in the elderly.

Drug Interactions

Metabolism/Transport Effects For valproic acid: **Substrate** (minor) of CYP2A6, 2B6, 2C9, 2C19, 2E1; **Inhibits** CYP2C9 (weak), 2C19 (weak), 2D6 (weak), 3A4 (weak); **Induces** CYP2A6 (weak)

Avoid Concomitant Use There are no known interactions where it is recommended to avoid concomitant use.

Decreased Effect

Valproic Acid may decrease the levels/effects of: CarBAMazepine; OXcarbazepine; Phenytoin

The levels/effects of Valproic Acid may be decreased by: Barbiturates; CarBAMazepine; Carbapenems; Ethosuximide; Methylfolate; Phenytoin; Primidone; Protease Inhibitors; Rifampin

Increased Effect/Toxicity

Valproic Acid may increase the levels/effects of: Barbiturates; Ethosuximide; LamoTRIgine; LORazepam; Paliperidone; Primidone; RisperiDONE; Rufinamide; Temozolomide; Tricyclic Antidepressants; Vorinostat; Zidovudine

The levels/effects of Valproic Acid may be increased by: ChlorproMAZINE; Felbamate; GuanFACINE; Salicylates; Topiramate

Nutritional/Ethanol Interactions

Ethanol: Avoid ethanol (may increase CNS depression).

Food: Food may delay but does not affect the extent of absorption. Valproic acid serum concentrations may be decreased if taken with food. Milk has no effect on absorption.

Herb/Nutraceutical: Avoid evening primrose (seizure threshold decreased).

Lab Interactions Valproic acid may cause abnormalities in liver function tests; false-positive result for urine ketones

Adverse Reactions

>10%:

Central nervous system: Headache (≤31%), somnolence (≤30%), dizziness (12% to 25%), insomnia (>1% to 15%), nervousness (>1% to 11%), pain (1% to 11%)

Dermatologic: Alopecia (>1% to 24%)

Gastrointestinal: Nausea (15% to 48%), vomiting (7% to 27%), diarrhea (7% to 23%), abdominal pain (7% to 23%), dyspepsia (7% to 23%), anorexia (>1% to 12%)

Hematologic: Thrombocytopenia (1% to 24%; dose related)

Neuromuscular & skeletal: Tremor (≤57%), weakness (6% to 27%)

Ocular: Diplopia (>1% to 16%), amblyopia/blurred vision (≤12%)

Miscellaneous: Infection (≤20%), flu-like syndrome (12%)

1% to 10%:

Cardiovascular: Peripheral edema (>1% to 8%), chest pain (>1% to <5%), edema (>1% to <5%), facial edema (>1% to <5%), hypertension (>1% to <5%), hypotension (>1% to <5%), palpitation (>1% to <5%), postural hypotension (>1% to <5%), tachycardia (>1% to <5%), vasodilation (>1% to <5%), arrhythmia

Central nervous system: Ataxia (>1% to 8%), amnesia (>1% to 7%), emotional lability (>1% to 6%), fever (>1% to 6%), abnormal thinking (≤6%), depression (>1% to 5%), abnormal dreams (>1% to <5%), agitation (>1% to <5%), anxiety (>1% to <5%), catatonia (>1% to <5%), chills (>1% to <5%), confusion (>1% to <5%), coordination abnormal (>1% to <5%), hallucination (>1% to <5%), malaise (>1% to <5%), personality disorder (>1% to <5%), speech disorder (>1% to <5%), tardive dyskinesia (>1% to <5%), vertigo (>1% to <5%), euphoria (1%), hypoesthesia (1%)

Dermatologic: Rash (>1% to 6%), bruising (>1% to 5%), discoid lupus erythematosus (>1% to <5%), dry skin (>1% to <5%), furunculosis (>1% to <5%), petechia (>1% to <5%), pruritus (>1% to <5), seborrhea (>1% to <5%)

Endocrine & metabolic: Amenorrhea (>1% to <5%), dysmenorrhea (>1% to <5%), metrorrhagia (>1% to <5%), hypoproteinemia

Gastrointestinal: Weight gain (4% to 9%), weight loss (6%), appetite increased (≤6%), constipation (>1% to 5%), xerostomia (>1% to 5%), eructation (>1% to <5%), fecal incontinence (>1% to <5%), flatulence (>1% to <5%), gastroenteritis (>1% to <5%), glossitis (>1% to <5%), hematemesis (>1% to <5%), pancreatitis (>1% to <5%), periodontal abscess (>1% to <5%), stomatitis (>1% to <5%), taste perversion (>1% to <5%), dysphagia, gum hemorrhage, mouth ulceration

Genitourinary: Cystitis (>1% to 5%), dysuria (>1% to 5%), urinary frequency (>1% to <5%), urinary incontinence (>1% to <5%), vaginal hemorrhage (>1% to 5%), vaginitis (>1% to <5%)

Hepatic: ALT increased (>1% to <5%), AST increased (>1% to <5%)

Local: Injection site pain (3%), injection site reaction (2%), injection site inflammation (1%)

Neuromuscular & skeletal: Back pain (≤8%), abnormal gait (>1% to <5%), arthralgia (>1% to <5%), arthrosis (>1% to <5%), dysarthria (>1% to <5%), hypertonia (>1% to <5%), hypokinesia (>1% to <5%), leg cramps (>1% to <5%), myalgia (>1% to <5%), myasthenia (>1% to <5%), neck pain (>1% to <5%), neck rigidity (>1% to <5%), paresthesia (>1% to <5%), reflex increased (>1% to <5%), twitching (>1% to <5%)

Ocular: Nystagmus (1% to 8%), dry eyes (>1% to 5%), eye pain (>1% to 5%), abnormal vision (>1% to <5%), conjunctivitis (>1% to <5%)

Otic: Tinnitus (1% to 7%), ear pain (>1% to 5%), deafness (>1% to <5%), otitis media (>1% to <5%)

Respiratory: Pharyngitis (2% to 8%), bronchitis (5%), rhinitis (>1% to 5%), dyspnea (1% to 5%), cough (>1% to <5%), epistaxis (>1% to <5%), pneumonia (>1% to <5%), sinusitis (>1% to <5%)

Miscellaneous: Diaphoresis (1%), hiccups

Pharmacodynamics/Kinetics

Time to Peak Serum: Stavzor™: 2 hours

Protein Binding Dose dependent: 80% to 90%; decreased in the elderly and with hepatic or renal dysfunction

Half-Life Elimination Increased in neonates and with liver disease; Children >2 months: 7-13 hours; Adults: 9-16 hours

Metabolism Extensively hepatic via glucuronide conjugation and mitochondrial beta-oxidation. The relationship between dose and total valproate concentration is nonlinear; concentration does not increase proportionally with the dose, but increases to a lesser extent due to saturable plasma protein binding. The kinetics of unbound drug are linear.

Excretion Urine (30% to 50% as glucuronide conjugate, 3% as unchanged drug)

Available Dosage Forms

Capsule, softgel, oral: 250 mg

Depakene®: 250 mg

Capsule, softgel, delayed release, oral:

Stavzor™: 125 mg, 250 mg, 500 mg

Injection, solution [preservative free]: 100 mg/mL (5 mL)
Depacon®: 100 mg/mL (5 mL)
Solution, oral: 250 mg/5 mL (473 mL, 480 mL)
Syrup, oral: 250 mg/5 mL (5 mL, 10 mL, 473 mL, 480 mL)
Depakene®: 250 mg/5 mL (473 mL)

Dosing

Adult

Seizures: Administer doses >250 mg/day in divided doses.

Oral:

Simple and complex absence seizure: Initial: 15 mg/kg/day; increase by 5-10 mg/kg/day at weekly intervals until therapeutic levels are achieved; maximum: 60 mg/kg/day.

Complex partial seizure: Initial: 10-15 mg/kg/day; increase by 5-10 mg/kg/day at weekly intervals until therapeutic levels are achieved; maximum: 60 mg/kg/day.

Note: Regular release and delayed release formulations are usually given in 2-4 divided doses/day

I.V.: Administer as a 60-minute infusion (≤20 mg/minute) with the same frequency as oral products; switch patient to oral products as soon as possible. Rapid infusions ≤45 mg/kg over 5-10 minutes (1.5-6 mg/kg/minute) were generally well tolerated in clinical trials.

Rectal (unlabeled): Dilute syrup 1:1 with water for use as a retention enema; loading dose: 17-20 mg/kg one time; maintenance: 10-15 mg/kg/dose every 8 hours

Status epilepticus (unlabeled use):

Loading dose: I.V.: 15-45 mg/kg administered at ≤ 6 mg/kg/minute

Maintenance dose: I.V. infusion: 1-4 mg/kg/hour; titrate dose as needed based upon patient response and evaluation of drug-drug interactions

Mania (Stavzor™): *Oral:* Initial: 750 mg/day in divided doses; dose should be adjusted as rapidly as possible to desired clinical effect; maximum recommended dosage: 60 mg/kg/day

Migraine prophylaxis (Stavzor™): *Oral:* 250 mg twice daily; adjust dose based on patient response, up to 1000 mg/day

Geriatric Initiate at lower doses; dose escalation should be managed more slowly (in persons of advanced age). Refer to adult dosing.

Pediatric

Seizures:

Oral, I.V.:

Simple and complex absence seizures: Refer to adult dosing. Larger maintenance doses may be required in younger children.

Complex partial seizures: Children ≥10 years: Refer to adult dosing. Larger maintenance doses may be required in younger children.

Rectal (unlabeled): Refer to adult dosing.

Migraine prophylaxis: *Oral:* Children ≥12 years: Refer to adult dosing.

Renal Impairment A 27% reduction in clearance of unbound valproate is seen in patients with Cl_{cr} <10 mL/minute. Hemodialysis reduces valproate concentrations by 20%, therefore, no dose adjustment is needed in patients with renal failure. Protein binding is reduced, monitoring only total valproate concentrations may be misleading.

Hepatic Impairment Dosage reduction is required. Clearance is decreased with liver impairment. Hepatic disease is also associated with decreased albumin concentrations and 2- to 2.6-fold increase in the unbound fraction. Free concentrations of valproate may be elevated while total concentrations appear normal. Use is contraindicated in severe impairment.

Administration

Oral Depakene® capsule, Stavzor™: Swallow whole; do not chew.

I.V. Depacon®: Following dilution to final concentration, administer over 60 minutes at a rate ≤20 mg/minute. Alternatively, single doses up to 45 mg/kg have been administered as a rapid infusion over 5-10 minutes (1.5-6 mg/kg/minute).

Stability

Reconstitution Depacon®: Injection should be diluted in 50 mL of a compatible diluent.

Storage

Depakene® solution: Store below 30°C (86°F).
Stavzor™: Store at controlled room temperature of 25°C (77°F).
Depakene® capsule: Store at controlled room temperature of 15°C to 25°C (59°F to 77°F).
Depacon®: Store vial at room temperature of 15°C to 30°C (59°F to 86°F). Stable in D_5W, NS, and LR for at least 24 hours when stored in glass or PVC.

Monitoring and Teaching Issues

Laboratory Monitoring Liver enzymes (at baseline and during therapy), CBC with platelets (baseline and periodic intervals), PT/PTT (especially prior to surgery), serum ammonia (with symptoms of lethargy, mental status change), serum valproate levels

Physical Assessment I.V.: Monitor therapeutic effectiveness (type of seizure activity, and duration). Monitor vital signs; neurological, cardiac, and respiratory status. Monitor for signs and symptoms of hepatic failure (malaise, weakness, facial edema, anorexia, jaundice, and vomiting), especially when used in children <2 years of age. Monitor for signs and symptoms of pancreatitis (abdominal pain, nausea, vomiting, and/or anorexia). Taper dosage slowly when discontinuing. Teach patient seizure safety precautions. Some adverse reactions, including hepatic failure and thrombocytopenia, can occur 3 days to 6 months after beginning therapy.

Patient Education Oral: Do not crush or chew capsule or enteric-coated pill. While using this medication, do not use alcohol. Maintain adequate hydration unless instructed to restrict fluid intake. You may experience nervousness, decreased appetite, insomnia, headache, sleepiness, dizziness, visual changes, and hair loss. Report suicide ideation or depression; alterations in menstrual cycle; abdominal cramps, unresolved diarrhea, vomiting, or constipation; skin rash; tremors; unusual bruising or bleeding; blood in urine, stool, or vomitus; malaise; weakness; facial swelling; yellowing of skin or eyes; persistent abdominal pain; excessive sedation; change in mental status; extreme lethargy; or restlessness.

Dietary Considerations Valproic acid may cause GI upset; take with large amount of water or food to decrease GI upset. May need to split doses to avoid GI upset. Valproate sodium oral solution will generate valproic acid in carbonated beverages and may cause mouth and throat irritation; do not mix valproate sodium oral solution with carbonated beverages.

Geriatric Considerations Although there is little data in elderly for the use of valproic acid in the treatment of seizures, there are a number of studies which demonstrate its benefit in the treatment of agitation and dementia and other psychiatric disorders. It is important that the clinician understand that serum concentrations do not correlate with behavior response; likewise, it is imperative to monitor LFTs and CBC during the first 6 months of therapy. See Warnings/Precautions and Laboratory Monitoring.

Elimination is decreased in elderly. Studies of older adults with dementia show a high incidence of somnolence (which is usually transient); cognitive side effects generally minimal. In some patients, this was associated with weight loss. Starting doses should be lower and increased slowly, with careful monitoring of nutritional intake and dehydration. Safety and efficacy for use in patients >65 years of age have not been studied for migraine prophylaxis.

Breast-Feeding Considerations Breast milk concentrations of valproic acid have been reported as 1% to 10% of maternal concentration. The weight-adjusted dose to the infant has been calculated to be ~4%.

Pregnancy Considerations [U.S. Boxed Warning]: May cause teratogenic effects such as neural tube defects (eg, spina bifida). Teratogenic effects have been reported in animals and humans. Valproic acid crosses the placenta. Neural tube, cardiac, facial (characteristic pattern of dysmorphic facial features), skeletal, multiple other defects reported. Epilepsy itself, number of medications, genetic factors, or a combination of these probably influence the teratogenicity of anticonvulsant therapy. Information from the North American Antiepileptic Drug Pregnancy Registry notes a fourfold increase in congenital malformations with exposure to valproic acid monotherapy during the 1st trimester of pregnancy when compared to monotherapy with other antiepileptic drugs (AED). The risk of neural tube defects is ~1% to 2% (general population risk estimated to be 0.14% to 0.2%). The effect of folic acid supplementation to decrease this risk is unknown, however, folic acid supplementation is recommended for all women contemplating pregnancy. An information sheet describing the teratogenic potential is available from the manufacturer.

Nonteratogenic effects have also been reported. Afibrinogenemia leading to fatal hemorrhage and hepatotoxicity have been noted in case reports of infants following *in utero* exposure to valproic acid. Developmental delay, autism and/or autism spectrum disorder have also been reported. Use in women of childbearing potential requires that benefits of use in mother be weighed against the potential risk to fetus, especially when used for conditions not associated with permanent injury or risk of death (eg, migraine).

Patients exposed to valproic acid during pregnancy are encouraged to enroll themselves into the AED Pregnancy Registry by calling 1-888-233-2334. Additional information is available at www.aedpregnancyregistry.org.

Related Information

Anticonvulsant Drugs of Choice *on page* 1981

◆ **Valproic Acid Derivative** *see* Divalproex *on page* 557

Valrubicin (val ROO bi sin)

U.S. Brand Names Valstar®

Index Terms *N*-trifluoroacetyladriamycin-14-valerate; AD32

Generic Availability (U.S.) No

Pharmacologic Category Antineoplastic Agent, Anthracycline

Medication Safety Issues

Sound-alike/look-alike issues:

Valrubicin may be confused with DAUNOrubicin, DOXOrubicin, epirubicin, IDArubicin

Valstar® may be confused with valsartan

High alert medication: The Institute for Safe Medication Practices (ISMP) includes this medication among its list of drug classes which have a heightened risk of causing significant patient harm when used in error.

Pregnancy Risk Factor C

Lactation Excretion in breast milk unknown/not recommended

Use Intravesical therapy of BCG-refractory bladder carcinoma *in situ*

Mechanism of Action/Effect Blocks function of DNA topoisomerase II; inhibits DNA synthesis, causes extensive chromosomal damage, and arrests cell development; unlike other anthracyclines, does not appear to intercalate DNA; readily penetrates cells.

Contraindications Hypersensitivity to anthracyclines, polyoxyl castor oil (Cremophor® EL), or any component of the formulation; concurrent urinary tract infection; small bladder capacity (unable to tolerate a 75 mL instillation)

Warnings/Precautions Hazardous agent - use appropriate precautions for handling and disposal. Delay valrubicin therapy for at least 2 weeks after transurethral resection and/or fulguration. Do not administer if mucosal integrity of bladder has been compromised or bladder perforation is present; evaluate bladder status prior to instillation. Use aseptic technique to prevent urinary tract infection or traumatizing urinary mucosa. Although clamping of the urinary catheter after administration is not recommended, use caution and appropriate medical supervision if performed. Irritable bladder symptoms may occur during instillation and retention, and for a brief time after voiding. Use caution in patients with severe irritable bladder symptoms. Red-tinged urine is typical for the first 24 hours after instillation. Prolonged symptoms or discoloration should prompt contact with the physician.

Contains polyoxyl castor oil (Cremophor® EL) which is associated with hypersensitivity reactions; use is contraindicated in patients with hypersensitivity to polyoxyl castor oil. Delaying cystectomy during treatment may lead to metastatic bladder cancer; reconsider cystectomy if complete response to treatment does not occur within 3 months.

Drug Interactions

Avoid Concomitant Use

Avoid concomitant use of Valrubicin with any of the following: BCG; Natalizumab; Pimecrolimus; Roflumilast; Tacrolimus (Topical); Vaccines (Live)

Decreased Effect

Valrubicin may decrease the levels/effects of: BCG; Cardiac Glycosides; Sipuleucel-T; Vaccines (Inactivated); Vaccines (Live)

The levels/effects of Valrubicin may be decreased by: Cardiac Glycosides; Echinacea

Increased Effect/Toxicity

Valrubicin may increase the levels/effects of: Leflunomide; Natalizumab; Vaccines (Live)

The levels/effects of Valrubicin may be increased by: Bevacizumab; Denosumab; Pimecrolimus; Roflumilast; Tacrolimus (Topical); Taxane Derivatives; Trastuzumab

Adverse Reactions **Note:** In general, local adverse reactions occur during or shortly after instillation and resolve within 1-7 days.

>10%: Genitourinary: Bladder irritation (88%), urinary frequency (61%), urinary urgency (57%), dysuria (56%), bladder spasm (31%), hematuria (29%; gross: 1%), bladder pain (28%), urinary incontinence (22%), cystitis (15%), urinary tract infection (15%), urine red-tinged

1% to 10%:

Cardiovascular: Chest pain (3%), vasodilation (2%), peripheral edema (1%)
Central nervous system: Headache (4%), malaise (4%), dizziness (3%), fever (2%)
Dermatologic: Rash (3%)
Endocrine & metabolic: Hyperglycemia (1%)
Gastrointestinal: Abdominal pain (5%), nausea (5%), diarrhea (3%), vomiting (2%), flatulence (1%)
Genitourinary: Nocturia (7%), burning symptoms (5%), urinary retention (4%), urethral pain (3%), pelvic pain (1%), hematuria (microscopic) (3%)
Hematologic: Anemia (2%)
Neuromuscular & skeletal: Weakness (4%), back pain (3%), myalgia (1%)
Respiratory: Pneumonia (1%)

Pharmacodynamics/Kinetics

Absorption Intravesical: Penetrates into bladder wall; negligible systemic absorption (dependant on bladder wall condition; trauma to mucosa may increase absorption, bladder wall perforation may significantly increase absorption and systemic myelotoxicity).

Metabolism Negligible after intravesical instillation and 2-hour retention

Excretion Urine (post 2-hour retention): 98.6% as intact drug; 0.4% as *N*-trifluoroacetyladriamycin)

Available Dosage Forms

Injection, solution [preservative free]:

Valstar®: 40 mg/mL (5 mL)

Dosing

Adult & Geriatric Bladder cancer: Intravesical: 800 mg once weekly (retain for 2 hours) for 6 weeks

Adjustment for Toxicity In clinical trials (Steinberg, 2000), treatment was delayed for 1 week for the following adverse events: Grade 3 dysuria (not controlled with phenazopyridine), frequency/urgency lasting >24 hours, grade 2 gross hematuria (without clots) lasting >48 hours, grade 3 hematuria (with clots) lasting >48 hours. For local toxicities <grade 4 (eg, dysuria [not controlled with phenazopyridine] or severe bladder spasm), anticholinergic therapy (systemic or topical) or topical anesthesia was administered prior to subsequent instillations.

Administration

Other Intravesicular bladder instillation: Insert urinary catheter, empty bladder prior to instillation, slowly by gravity flow, instill 800 mg/75 mL (in 0.9% sodium chloride injection), remove catheter. Retain in the bladder for 2 hours, then void. Administer through non-PVC tubing due to the polyoxyl castor oil (Cremophor® EL) diluent. Maintain adequate hydration following treatment.

Stability

Reconstitution Allow vials to warm to room temperature (without heating) prior to use. A waxy precipitate (due to polyoxyl castor oil) may form at temperatures <4°C, warm vial in the hand until solution is clear (do not use vial if particulate still present). Use appropriate precautions for handling and disposal. Dilute 800 mg (20 mL) with 55 mL NS (total volume of 75 mL). Use non-PVC containers (glass, polyolefin, or polypropylene) and administration sets to avoid leaching of DEHP plasticizers. Stable for 12 hours at room temperature when diluted in 0.9% sodium chloride. Do not mix with other drugs.

Storage Store unopened vials under refrigeration at 2°C to 8°C (36°F to 48°F). Stable for 12 hours at room temperature when diluted in 0.9% sodium chloride.

Monitoring and Teaching Issues

Laboratory Monitoring Cystoscopy, biopsy, and urine cytology every 3 months for recurrence or progression

Physical Assessment Use caution to prevent inadvertent exposure to this medication. Assess patient response during and following instillation (genitourinary [frequency, urgency, incontinence, dysuria, bladder spasm or pain, hematuria, urinary tract infection], rash, nausea, vomiting, myalgia, hyperglycemia).

Patient Education This medication will be instilled into your bladder through a catheter. After the catheter is withdrawn, you should not void for two hours (if possible); after 2 hours you should void. It is important that you maintain adequate hydration, unless instructed to restrict fluid intake. If you have diabetes, monitor glucose levels closely (may cause hyperglycemia). Your urine will be red-tinged for the next 24 hours; report promptly if this continues for a longer period. May cause altered urination patterns (increased or decreased frequency or incontinence), bladder pain, pain on urination, or pelvic pain; report if these persist. May cause dizziness, fatigue, nausea, vomiting, or taste disturbance. Report chest pain or palpitations; persistent dizziness; swelling of extremities; persistent nausea, vomiting, diarrhea, or abdominal pain; muscle weakness, pain, or tremors; unusual cough; or respiratory difficulty.

Breast-Feeding Considerations Due to the potential for serious adverse reactions in the nursing infant, breast-feeding should be discontinued prior to initiation of therapy.

Pregnancy Considerations Embryotoxicity and teratogenic effects were observed in animal studies. There are no adequate and well-controlled studies in pregnant women. All patients of reproductive age should use an effective method of contraception during the treatment period.

Valsartan (val SAR tan)

U.S. Brand Names Diovan®

Generic Availability (U.S.) No

Pharmacologic Category Angiotensin II Receptor Blocker

Medication Safety Issues

Sound-alike/look-alike issues:

Valsartan may be confused with losartan, Valstar™, Valturna®

Diovan® may be confused with Darvon®, Dioval®, Zyban®

International issues:

Diovan [U.S., Canada, and multiple international markets] may be confused with Dianben, a brand name for metformin [Spain]

Pregnancy Risk Factor D

Lactation Excretion in breast milk unknown/not recommended

Use Alone or in combination with other antihypertensive agents in the treatment of essential hypertension; reduction of cardiovascular mortality in patients with left ventricular dysfunction postmyocardial infarction; treatment of heart failure (NYHA Class II-IV)

Mechanism of Action/Effect Valsartan produces direct antagonism of the angiotensin II (AT2) receptors. Valsartan blocks the vasoconstrictor and aldosterone-secreting effects of angiotensin II. It displaces angiotensin II from the AT1 receptor and produces its blood pressure-lowering effects by antagonizing AT1-induced vasoconstriction, aldosterone release, catecholamine release, arginine vasopressin release, water intake, and hypertrophic responses. This action results in more efficient blockade of the cardiovascular effects of angiotensin II and fewer side effects than the ACE inhibitors.

Contraindications

There are no contraindications listed in manufacturer's labeling.

Canadian labeling: Hypersensitivity to valsartan or any component of the formulation

Warnings/Precautions [U.S. Boxed Warning]: Based on human data, drugs that act on the angiotensin system can cause injury and death to the developing fetus when used in the second and third trimesters. Angiotensin receptor blockers should be discontinued as soon as possible once pregnancy is detected. May cause hyperkalemia; avoid potassium supplementation unless specifically required by healthcare provider. During the initiation of therapy, hypotension may occur, particularly in patients with heart failure or post-MI patients. Use extreme caution with concurrent administration of potassium-sparing diuretics or potassium supplements, in patients with mild-to-moderate hepatic dysfunction (adjust dose), in those who may be sodium/water depleted (eg, on high-dose diuretics), and in the elderly; correct depletion first.

Use caution with unstented unilateral/bilateral renal artery stenosis. When unstented bilateral renal artery stenosis is present, use is generally avoided due to the elevated risk of deterioration in renal function unless possible benefits outweigh risks. Use with caution with preexisting renal insufficiency; significant aortic/mitral stenosis. May be associated with deterioration of renal function and/or increases in serum creatinine, particularly in patients with low renal blood flow (eg, renal artery stenosis, heart failure) whose glomerular filtration rate (GFR) is dependent on efferent arteriolar vasoconstriction by angiotensin II. Use caution in patients with severe renal impairment or significant hepatic dysfunction. Monitor renal function closely in patients with severe heart failure; changes in renal function should be anticipated and dosage adjustments of valsartan or concomitant medications may be needed. Concurrent use of ACE inhibitors may increase the risk of clinically-significant adverse events (eg, renal dysfunction, hyperkalemia). In Canada, use is not approved in patients <18 years of age.

Drug Interactions

Metabolism/Transport Effects Substrate of SLCO1B1; **Inhibits** CYP2C9 (weak)

Avoid Concomitant Use There are no known interactions where it is recommended to avoid concomitant use.

Decreased Effect

The levels/effects of Valsartan may be decreased by: Herbs (Hypertensive Properties); Methylphenidate; Nonsteroidal Anti-Inflammatory Agents; Yohimbine

Increased Effect/Toxicity

Valsartan may increase the levels/effects of: ACE Inhibitors; Amifostine; Antihypertensives; Hypotensive Agents; Lithium; Potassium-Sparing Diuretics; RiTUXimab

The levels/effects of Valsartan may be increased by: Diazoxide; Eltrombopag; Eplerenone; Herbs (Hypotensive Properties); MAO Inhibitors; Pentoxifylline; Phosphodiesterase 5 Inhibitors; Potassium Salts; Prostacyclin Analogues; Tolvaptan; Trimethoprim

Nutritional/Ethanol Interactions

Food: Decreases the peak plasma concentration and extent of absorption by 50% and 40%, respectively.

Herb/Nutraceutical: Avoid bayberry, blue cohosh, cayenne, ephedra, ginger, ginseng (American), kola, licorice (may worsen hypertension). Avoid black cohosh, California poppy, coleus, golden seal, hawthorn, mistletoe, periwinkle, quinine, shepherd's purse (may have increased antihypertensive effect).

Adverse Reactions

>10%:

Central nervous system: Dizziness (heart failure trials 17%)

Renal: BUN increased >50% (heart failure trials 17%)

1% to 10%:

Cardiovascular: Hypotension (heart failure trials 7%; MI trial 1%), postural hypotension (heart failure trials 2%), syncope (up to >1%)

Central nervous system: Dizziness (hypertension trial 2% to 8%), fatigue (heart failure trials 3%; hypertension trial 2%), postural dizziness (heart failure trials 2%), headache (heart failure trials >1%), vertigo (up to >1%)

Endocrine & metabolic: Serum potassium increased by >20% (4% to 10%), hyperkalemia (heart failure trials 2%)

Gastrointestinal: Diarrhea (heart failure trials 5%), abdominal pain (2%), nausea (heart failure trials >1%), upper abdominal pain (heart failure trials >1%)

Hematologic: Neutropenia (2%)

Neuromuscular & skeletal: Arthralgia (heart failure trials 3%), back pain (up to 3%)

Ocular: Blurred vision (heart failure trials >1%)

Renal: Creatinine doubled (MI trial 4%), creatinine increased >50% (heart failure trials 4%), renal dysfunction (up to >1%)

Respiratory: Cough (1% to 3%)

Miscellaneous: Viral infection (3%)

Pharmacodynamics/Kinetics

Onset of Action ~2 hours

Duration of Action 24 hours

Bioavailability Tablet: 25% (range: 10% to 35%); suspension: ~40% (~1.6 times more than tablet)

Time to Peak Serum: 2-4 hours

Protein Binding 95%, primarily albumin

Half-Life Elimination ~6 hours

Metabolism To inactive metabolite

Excretion Feces (83%) and urine (13%) as unchanged drug

Available Dosage Forms

Tablet, oral:

Diovan®: 40 mg, 80 mg, 160 mg, 320 mg

Dosing

Adult & Geriatric

Hypertension: Initial: 80 mg or 160 mg once daily (in patients who are not volume depleted); dose may be increased to achieve desired effect; maximum recommended dose: 320 mg/day

Heart failure: Initial: 40 mg twice daily; titrate dose to 80-160 mg twice daily, as tolerated; maximum daily dose: 320 mg

Left ventricular dysfunction after MI: Initial: 20 mg twice daily; titrate dose to target of 160 mg twice daily as tolerated; may initiate ≥12 hours following MI

Pediatric Hypertension: Oral: Children 6-16 years: Initial: 1.3 mg/kg once daily (maximum: 40 mg/day); dose may be increased to achieve desired effect; doses >2.7 mg/kg (maximum: 160 mg) have not been studied.

Renal Impairment

Children: Use is not recommended if Cl_{cr} <30 mL/minute.

Adults: No dosage adjustment necessary if Cl_{cr} >10 mL/minute.

Dialysis: Not significantly removed.

Hepatic Impairment In mild-to-moderate liver disease no adjustment is needed. Use caution in patients with liver disease. Patients with mild-to-moderate chronic disease have twice the exposure as healthy volunteers.

Administration

Oral Administer with or without food.

Stability

Storage Store at 25°C (77°F); excursions permitted to 15°C to 30°C (59°F to 86°F). Protect from moisture.

Monitoring and Teaching Issues

Laboratory Monitoring Baseline and periodic electrolyte panels, renal and liver function, urinalysis; in CHF, serum potassium during dose escalation and periodically thereafter

Physical Assessment Assess effectiveness and interactions with other pharmacological agents and herbal products (eg, concurrent use of potassium supplements, ACE inhibitors, potassium-sparing diuretics may increase risk of hyperkalemia). Monitor for changes in renal function, dizziness, cough, headache, nausea, hypotension, and hyperkalemia.

Patient Education This drug does not eliminate need for diet or exercise regimen as recommended by prescriber. May cause dizziness, lightheadedness, postural hypotension, or diarrhea. Report changes in urinary pattern, swelling of extremities, unusual back ache, chest pain or palpitations, unrelenting headache, or unusual cough.

Dietary Considerations Avoid salt substitutes which contain potassium. May be taken with or without food.

Geriatric Considerations No dosage adjustment is necessary when initiating angiotensin II receptor antagonists in the elderly. In clinical studies, no differences between younger adults and elderly were demonstrated. Many elderly may be volume depleted due to diuretic use and/or blunted thirst reflex resulting in inadequate fluid intake.

Breast-Feeding Considerations It is not known if valsartan is found in breast milk; the manufacturer recommends discontinuing the drug or discontinuing nursing based on the importance of the drug to the mother.

Pregnancy Considerations Medications which act on the renin-angiotensin system are reported to have the following fetal/neonatal effects: Hypotension, neonatal skull hypoplasia, anuria, renal failure, and death; oligohydramnios is also reported. These effects are reported to occur with exposure during the second and third trimesters. **[U.S. Boxed Warning]: Based on human data, drugs that act on the angiotensin system can cause injury and death to the developing fetus when used in the second and third trimesters. Angiotensin receptor blockers should be discontinued as soon as possible once pregnancy is detected.**

Additional Information Valsartan may have an advantage over losartan due to minimal metabolism requirements and consequent use in mild-to-moderate hepatic impairment.

Related Information

Angiotensin Agents *on page 1974*

Heart Failure (Systolic) *on page 2040*

◆ **Valsartan and Aliskiren** *see* Aliskiren and Valsartan *on page 75*

◆ **Valsartan and Amlodipine** *see* Amlodipine and Valsartan *on page 108*

Valsartan and Hydrochlorothiazide (val SAR tan & hye droe klor oh THYE a zide)

U.S. Brand Names Diovan HCT®

Index Terms Hydrochlorothiazide and Valsartan

Generic Availability (U.S.) No

Pharmacologic Category Angiotensin II Receptor Blocker; Diuretic, Thiazide

Medication Safety Issues

Sound-alike/look-alike issues:

Diovan® may be confused with Darvon®, Dioval®, Zyban®

Pregnancy Risk Factor D

Lactation Enters breast milk/not recommended

Use Treatment of hypertension

Mechanism of Action/Effect Valsartan produces direct antagonism of the angiotensin II (AT2) receptors. Valsartan blocks the vasoconstrictor and aldosterone-secreting effects of angiotensin II. It displaces angiotensin II from the AT1 receptor and produces its blood pressure-lowering effects by antagonizing AT1-induced vasoconstriction, aldosterone release, catecholamine release, arginine vasopressin release, water intake, and hypertrophic responses. This action results in more efficient blockade of the cardiovascular effects of angiotensin II and fewer side effects than the ACE inhibitors.

Hydrochlorothiazide inhibits sodium reabsorption in the distal tubules causing increased excretion of sodium and water as well as potassium and hydrogen ions

Contraindications Hypersensitivity to valsartan, hydrochlorothiazide, sulfonamide-derived drugs, or any component of the formulation; anuria

Warnings/Precautions See individual agents.

Drug Interactions

Metabolism/Transport Effects Valsartan: **Substrate** of SLCO1B1; **Inhibits** CYP2C9 (weak)

Avoid Concomitant Use

Avoid concomitant use of Valsartan and Hydrochlorothiazide with any of the following: Dofetilide

Decreased Effect

Valsartan and Hydrochlorothiazide may decrease the levels/effects of: Antidiabetic Agents

The levels/effects of Valsartan and Hydrochlorothiazide may be decreased by: Bile Acid Sequestrants; Herbs (Hypertensive Properties); Methylphenidate; Nonsteroidal Anti-Inflammatory Agents; Yohimbine

Increased Effect/Toxicity

Valsartan and Hydrochlorothiazide may increase the levels/effects of: ACE Inhibitors; Allopurinol; Amifostine; Antihypertensives; Calcium Salts; CarBAMazepine; Dofetilide; Hypotensive Agents; Lithium; OXcarbazepine; Potassium-Sparing Diuretics; RiTUXimab; Topiramate; Toremifene; Vitamin D Analogs

The levels/effects of Valsartan and Hydrochlorothiazide may be increased by: Alcohol (Ethyl); Analgesics (Opioid); Barbiturates; Corticosteroids (Orally Inhaled); Corticosteroids (Systemic); Eltrombopag; Eplerenone; Herbs (Hypotensive Properties); Licorice; MAO Inhibitors; Pentoxifylline; Phosphodiesterase 5 Inhibitors; Potassium Salts; Prostacyclin Analogues; Tolvaptan; Trimethoprim

Adverse Reactions Percentages reported with combination product; other reactions have been reported (see individual agents for additional information)

>10%: Renal: BUN increased (15%)

1% to 10%:

Cardiovascular: Hypotension (1%)

Central nervous system: Dizziness (6%; dose related)

Endocrine & metabolic: Hypokalemia (3%)

Renal: Creatinine increased (2%)

Respiratory: Nasopharyngitis (2%)

Pharmacodynamics/Kinetics

Pharmacokinetic Note See individual agents.

Available Dosage Forms

Tablet:

Diovan HCT®: 80 mg/12.5 mg: Valsartan 80 mg and hydrochlorothiazide 12.5 mg; 160 mg/12.5 mg: Valsartan 160 mg and hydrochlorothiazide 12.5 mg; 160 mg/25 mg: Valsartan 160 mg and hydrochlorothiazide 25 mg; 320 mg/12.5 mg: Valsartan 320 mg and hydrochlorothiazide 12.5 mg; 320 mg/25 mg: Valsartan 320 mg and hydrochlorothiazide 25 mg

Dosing

Adult & Geriatric Note: Dose is individualized; combination product may be used as initial therapy or substituted for individual components in patients currently maintained on both agents separately or in patients not adequately controlled with monotherapy (using one of the agents or an agent within same antihypertensive class).

Hypertension: Oral:

Initial therapy: Valsartan 160 mg and hydrochlorothiazide 12.5 mg once daily; dose may be titrated after 1-2 weeks of therapy. Maximum recommended daily doses: Valsartan 320 mg; hydrochlorothiazide 25 mg.

Add-on/replacement therapy: Valsartan 80-160 mg and hydrochlorothiazide 12.5-25 mg once daily; dose may be titrated after 3-4 weeks of therapy. Maximum recommended daily dose: Valsartan 320 mg; hydrochlorothiazide 25 mg.

Renal Impairment

Cl_{cr} >30 mL/minute: No adjustment needed

Cl_{cr} ≤30 mL/minute: Use of combination not recommended. Contraindicated in patients with anuria.

Hepatic Impairment Use with caution; initiate at lower dose and titrate slowly.

Administration

Oral Administer with or without food.

Stability

Storage Store at controlled room temperature of 25°C (77°F); excursions permitted to 15°C to 30°C (59°F to 86°F). Protect from moisture.

Monitoring and Teaching Issues

Physical Assessment See individual agents.

Patient Education See individual agents.

Dietary Considerations Avoid salt substitutes which contain potassium. May be taken with or without food.

Breast-Feeding Considerations Excretion of valsartan in breast milk is not known and use during nursing is not recommended; hydrochlorothiazide is excreted in breast milk

Pregnancy Considerations Medications which act on the renin-angiotensin system are reported to have the following fetal/neonatal effects: Hypotension, neonatal skull hypoplasia, anuria, renal failure, and death; oligohydramnios is also reported. These effects are reported to occur with exposure during the 2nd and 3rd trimesters. Valsartan should be discontinued as soon as possible after pregnancy is detected. Hydrochlorothiazide crosses the placenta; adverse (but not teratogenic) effects have been reported in the fetus.

Related Information

Hydrochlorothiazide *on page 912*

Valsartan *on page 1838*

◆ **Valsartan, Hydrochlorothiazide, and Amlodipine** *see* Amlodipine, Valsartan, and Hydrochlorothiazide *on page 109*

◆ **Valstar®** *see* Valrubicin *on page 1836*

◆ **Valtrex®** *see* ValACYclovir *on page 1828*

- ◆ **Valturna®** *see* Aliskiren and Valsartan *on page 75*
- ◆ **Vancenase** *see* Beclomethasone (Oral Inhalation) *on page 192*
- ◆ **Vancocin®** *see* Vancomycin *on page 1842*

Vancomycin (van koe MYE sin)

U.S. Brand Names Vancocin®
Index Terms Vancomycin Hydrochloride
Generic Availability (U.S.) Yes: Excludes capsule
Pharmacologic Category Glycopeptide
Medication Safety Issues
Sound-alike/look-alike issues:
I.V. vancomycin may be confused with Invanz®
Vancomycin may be confused with clindamycin, gentamicin, tobramycin, valACYclovir, vecuronium, Vibramycin®

High alert medication: The Institute for Safe Medication Practices (ISMP) includes this medication (intrathecal administration) among its list of drug classes which have a heightened risk of causing significant patient harm when used in error.

Pregnancy Risk Factor B (oral); C (injection)
Lactation Enters breast milk/not recommended
Use Treatment of patients with infections caused by staphylococcal species and streptococcal species; used orally for staphylococcal enterocolitis or for antibiotic-associated pseudomembranous colitis produced by *C. difficile*
Unlabeled/Investigational Use Bacterial endophthalmitis; treatment of infections caused by gram-positive organisms in patients who have serious allergies to beta-lactam agents; treatment of beta-lactam resistant gram-positive infections
Mechanism of Action/Effect Inhibits bacterial cell wall synthesis
Contraindications Hypersensitivity to vancomycin or any component of the formulation; avoid in patients with previous severe hearing loss
Warnings/Precautions May cause nephrotoxicity although limited data suggest direct causal relationship; usual risk factors include pre-existing renal impairment, concomitant nephrotoxic medications, advanced age, and dehydration. If multiple sequential (≥2) serum creatinine concentrations demonstrate an increase of 0.5 mg/dL or ≥50% increase from baseline (whichever is greater) in the absence of an alternative explanation, the patient should be identified as having vancomycin-induced nephrotoxicity (Rybak, 2009). Discontinue treatment if signs of nephrotoxicity occur; renal damage is usually reversible. May cause neurotoxicity; usual risk factors include pre-existing renal impairment, concomitant neuro-/nephrotoxic medications, advanced age, and dehydration. Ototoxicity, although rarely associated with monotherapy, is proportional to the amount of drug given and the duration of treatment. Tinnitus or vertigo may be indications of vestibular injury and impending bilateral irreversible damage. Discontinue treatment if signs of ototoxicity occur. Prolonged therapy (>1 week) or total doses exceeding 25 g may increase the risk of neutropenia; prompt reversal of neutropenia is expected after discontinuation of therapy. Prolonged use may result in fungal or bacterial superinfection, including *C. difficile*-associated diarrhea (CDAD) and pseudomembranous colitis; CDAD has been observed >2 months postantibiotic treatment. Use with caution in patients with renal impairment or those receiving other nephrotoxic or ototoxic drugs; dosage modification required in patients with impaired renal function (especially elderly). Rapid I.V. administration may result in hypotension, flushing, erythema, urticaria, and/or pruritus. Oral vancomycin is only indicated for the treatment of pseudomembranous colitis due to *C. difficile* and enterocolitis due to *S. aureus* and is not effective for systemic infections; parenteral vancomycin is not effective for the treatment of colitis due to *C. difficile* and enterocolitis due to *S. aureus*. **Note:** The Infectious Disease Society of America (IDSA) recommends the use of oral metronidazole for initial treatment of mild-to-moderate *C. difficile* infection and the use of oral vancomycin for initial treatment of severe *C. difficile* infection (Cohen, 2010).

Drug Interactions

Avoid Concomitant Use

Avoid concomitant use of Vancomycin with any of the following: BCG; Gallium Nitrate

Decreased Effect

Vancomycin may decrease the levels/effects of: BCG; Typhoid Vaccine

Increased Effect/Toxicity

Vancomycin may increase the levels/effects of: Aminoglycosides; Colistimethate; Gallium Nitrate; Neuromuscular-Blocking Agents

The levels/effects of Vancomycin may be increased by: Nonsteroidal Anti-Inflammatory Agents

Adverse Reactions
Oral:
>10%: Gastrointestinal: Bitter taste, nausea, vomiting
1% to 10%:
Central nervous system: Chills, drug fever
Hematologic: Eosinophilia
Parenteral:
>10%:
Cardiovascular: Hypotension accompanied by flushing
Dermatologic: Erythematous rash on face and upper body (red neck or red man syndrome - infusion rate related)

1% to 10%:

Central nervous system: Chills, drug fever

Dermatologic: Rash

Hematologic: Eosinophilia, reversible neutropenia

Local: Phlebitis

Pharmacodynamics/Kinetics

Absorption Oral: Poor; I.M.: Erratic; Intraperitoneal: ~38%

Time to Peak Serum: I.V.: Immediately after completion of infusion

Protein Binding ~50%

Half-Life Elimination Biphasic: Terminal:

Newborns: 6-10 hours

Infants and Children 3 months to 4 years: 4 hours

Children >3 years: 2.2-3 hours

Adults: 5-11 hours; significantly prolonged with renal impairment

End-stage renal disease: 200-250 hours

Excretion I.V.: Urine (80% to 90% as unchanged drug); Oral: Primarily feces

Available Dosage Forms

Capsule, oral:

Vancocin®: 125 mg, 250 mg

Infusion, premixed iso-osmotic dextrose solution: 500 mg (100 mL); 750 mg (150 mL); 1 g (200 mL)

Injection, powder for reconstitution: 500 mg, 750 mg, 1 g, 5 g, 10 g

Dosing

Adult & Geriatric

Usual dosage range: Initial intravenous dosing should be based on actual body weight; subsequent dosing adjusted based on serum trough vancomycin concentrations.

I.V.: 2-3 g/day (or 30-60 mg/kg/day) in divided doses every 8-12 hours (Rybak, 2009); **Note:** Dose requires adjustment in renal impairment

Oral: 500-2000 mg/day in divided doses every 6 hours

Indication-specific dosing:

Catheter-related infections: Antibiotic lock technique (Mermel, 2009): 2 mg/mL ± 10 units heparin/mL **or** 2.5 mg/mL ± 2500 **or** 5000 units heparin/mL **or** 5 mg/mL ± 5000 units heparin/mL (preferred regimen); instill into catheter port with a volume sufficient to fill the catheter (2-5 mL). **Note:** May use SWFI/NS or D_5W as diluents. Do not mix with any other solutions. Dwell times generally should not exceed 48 hours before renewal of lock solution. Remove lock solution prior to catheter use, then replace.

C. difficile **-associated diarrhea (CDAD):** Oral:

Manufacturer recommendations: 500-2000 mg/day in 3-4 divided doses for 7-10 days (usual dose: 125-500 mg every 6 hours)

IDSA guideline recommendations: Severe infection: 125 mg 4 times/day for 10-14 days; Severe, complicated infection: 500 mg 4 times/day with or without concurrent I.V. metronidazole. May consider vancomycin retention enema (in patients with complete ileus) (Cohen, 2010).

Complicated infections in seriously-ill patients: I.V.: Loading dose: 25-30 mg/kg (based on actual body weight) may be used to rapidly achieve target concentration; then 15-20 mg/kg/dose every 8-12 hours (Rybak, 2009)

Enterocolitis *(S. aureus):* Oral: 500-2000 mg/day in 3-4 divided doses for 7-10 days (usual dose: 125-500 mg every 6 hours)

Endophthalmitis (unlabeled use): Intravitreal: Usual dose: 1 mg/0.1 mL NS instilled into vitreum; may repeat administration if necessary in 3-4 days, usually in combination with ceftazidime or an aminoglycoside. **Note:** Some clinicians have recommended using a lower dose of 0.2 mg/0.1 mL, based on concerns for retinotoxicity.

Hospital-acquired pneumonia (HAP): I.V.: 15-20 mg/kg/dose every 8-12 hours (American Thoracic Society [ATS], 2005 guidelines; Rybak, 2009)

Meningitis:

I.V.: 30-60 mg/kg/day in divided doses every 8-12 hours (Rybak, 2009) **or** 500-750 mg every 6 hours (with third-generation cephalosporin for PCN-resistant *Streptococcus pneumoniae*)

Intrathecal, intraventricular (unlabeled route): 5-20 mg/day

MRSA infections: I.V.:

Bacteremia (Liu, 2011): 15-20 mg/kg/dose every 8-12 hours for 2-6 weeks depending on severity

Brain abscess, subdural empyema, spinal epidural abscess (Liu, 2011): 15-20 mg/kg/dose every 8-12 hours for 4-6 weeks (some experts combine with rifampin)

Complicated skin and skin structure infections (Liu, 2011): 15-20 mg/kg/dose every 8-12 hours for 7-14 days

Endocarditis, native valve (Liu, 2011): 15-20 mg/kg/dose every 8-12 hours for 6 weeks

Endocarditis, prosthetic valve (Liu, 2011): 15-20 mg/kg/dose every 8-12 hours for at least 6 weeks (combine with rifampin for the entire duration of therapy and gentamicin for the first 2 weeks)

Meningitis (Liu, 2011): 15-20 mg/kg/dose every 8-12 hours for 2 weeks (some experts combine with rifampin)

Osteomyelitis (Liu, 2011): 15-20 mg/kg/dose every 8-12 hours for a minimum of 8 weeks (some experts combine with rifampin)

Pneumonia (Liu, 2011): 15-20 mg/kg/dose every 8-12 hours for 7-21 days depending on severity

Septic arthritis (Liu, 2011): 15-20 mg/kg/dose every 8-12 hours for 3-4 weeks

Septic thrombosis of cavernous or dural venous sinus (Liu, 2011): 15-20 mg/kg/dose every 8-12 hours for 4-6 weeks (some experts combine with rifampin)

Prophylaxis against infective endocarditis:

Dental, oral, or upper respiratory tract surgery: 1 g 1 hour before surgery. **Note:** AHA guidelines now recommend prophylaxis only in patients undergoing invasive procedures and in whom underlying cardiac conditions may predispose to a higher risk of adverse outcomes should infection occur

GI/GU procedure: 1 g plus 1.5 mg/kg gentamicin 1 hour prior to surgery. **Note:** As of April 2007, routine prophylaxis no longer recommended by the AHA.

Susceptible (MIC ≤1 mcg/mL; Rybak, 2009) gram-positive infections: 15-20 mg/kg/dose (usual: 750-1500 mg) every 8-12 hours. **Note:** If MIC ≥2 mcg/mL, alternative therapies are recommended.

Pediatric

Usual dosage range: Infants >1 month and Children: I.V.: 10-15 mg/kg every 6 hours

Indication-specific dosing:

***C. difficile* -associated diarrhea (CDAD):** Infants >1 month and Children: Oral: 40 mg/kg/day in 3-4 divided doses added to fluids for 7-10 days (maximum: 2000 mg/day)

Enterocolitis (S. aureus): Infants >1 months and Children: Oral: 40 mg/kg/day in 3-4 divided doses added to fluids for 7-10 days (maximum: 2000 mg/day)

Meningitis: Infants >1 month and Children:

I.V.: 15 mg/kg every 6 hours (Tunkel, 2004)

Intrathecal, intraventricular (unlabeled route): 5-20 mg/day (Tunkel, 2004)

MRSA infections: I.V.:

Bacteremia (Liu, 2011): Children: 15 mg/kg/dose every 6 hours for 2-6 weeks depending on severity

Brain abscess, subdural empyema, spinal epidural abscess (Liu, 2011): Children: 15 mg/kg/dose every 6 hours for 4-6 weeks (some experts combine with rifampin)

Complicated skin and skin structure infections (Liu, 2011): Children: 15 mg/kg/dose every 6 hours for 7-14 days

Endocarditis, native valve (Liu, 2011): Children: 15 mg/kg/dose every 6 hours for 6 weeks

Endocarditis, prosthetic valve (Liu, 2011): Children: 15 mg/kg/dose every 6 hours for at least 6 weeks

Meningitis (Liu, 2011): Children: 15 mg/kg/dose every 6 hours for 2 weeks (some experts combine with rifampin)

Osteomyelitis (Liu, 2011): Children: 15 mg/kg/dose every 6 hours for 4-6 weeks

Pneumonia (Liu, 2011): Children: 15 mg/kg/dose every 6 hours for 7-21 days depending on severity

Septic arthritis (Liu, 2011): Children: 15 mg/kg/dose every 6 hours for minimum of 3-4 weeks

Septic thrombosis of cavernous or dural venous sinus (Liu, 2011): Children: 15 mg/kg/dose every 6 hours for 4-6 weeks (some experts combine with rifampin)

Prophylaxis against infective endocarditis: Children:

Dental, oral, or upper respiratory tract surgery: 20 mg/kg/dose administered 1 hour prior to the procedure. **Note:** American Heart Association (AHA) guidelines recommend prophylaxis only in patients undergoing invasive procedures and in whom underlying cardiac conditions may predispose to a higher risk of adverse outcomes should infection occur.

GI/GU procedure: 20 mg/kg (plus gentamicin 1.5 mg/kg) administered 1 hour prior to surgery. **Note:** Routine prophylaxis no longer recommended by the AHA.

Susceptible (MIC ≤1 mcg/mL; Rybak, 2009) gram-positive infections: Infants >1 month and Children: 10 mg/kg every 6 hours (manufacturer recommendations) **or** 15 mg/kg every 6 hours (Liu, 2011). **Note:** If MIC ≥2 mcg/mL, alternative therapies are recommended.

Renal Impairment Vancomycin levels should be monitored in patients with any renal impairment:

Cl_{cr} >50 mL/minute: Start with 15-20 mg/kg/dose (usual: 750-1500 mg) every 8-12 hours

Cl_{cr} 20-49 mL/minute: Start with 15-20 mg/kg/dose (usual: 750-1500 mg) every 24 hours

Cl_{cr} <20 mL/minute: Will need longer intervals; determine by serum concentration monitoring

Note: In the critically-ill patient with renal insufficiency, the initial loading dose (25-30 mg/kg) should not be reduced. However, subsequent dosage adjustments should be made based on renal function and trough serum concentrations.

Dialysis: Variable, depending on method; poorly dialyzable by conventional hemodialysis (0% to 5%). Use of high-flux membranes and continuous renal replacement therapy (CRRT) increases vancomycin clearance, and generally requires replacement dosing.

Hemodialysis (HD): Following loading dose of 15-20 mg/kg, give 500 mg to 1 g after each dialysis session, depending on factors such as HD membrane type and flow rate; monitor levels closely.

Continuous ambulatory peritoneal dialysis (CAPD):

Administration via CAPD fluid: 15-30 mg/L (15-30 mcg/mL) of CAPD fluid

Systemic: 1 g loading dose, followed by 500 mg to 1 g every 48-72 hours with close monitoring of levels

Continuous renal replacement therapy (CRRT): Removal of vancomycin is highly dependent on the method of replacement, filter type, and flow rate. Appropriate dosing requires close monitoring of levels in relation to target trough. The following are general recommendations only (Heintz, 2009; Trotman, 2005), and require consideration of the aforementioned parameters.

CVVH: Following loading dose of 15-25 mg/kg, give 1 g every 48 hours **or** 10-15 mg/kg every 24-48 hours

CVVHD or CVVHDF: Following loading dose of 15-25 mg/kg, give 1 g every 24 hours **or** 10-15 mg/kg every 24 hours (for CVVHD) **or** 7.5-10 mg/kg every 12 hours (CVVHDF)

Administration

Oral May be administered with food. If patient cannot swallow capsules, the powder for injection (not premixed solution) may be diluted in 30 mL of water for oral administration; flavoring may be added to improve taste. The unflavored, diluted solution may also be administered via nasogastric tube.

I.M. Do not administer I.M.

I.V. Administer vancomycin with a final concentration not to exceed 5 mg/mL by I.V. intermittent infusion over at least 60 minutes (recommended infusion period of ≥30 minutes for every 500 mg administered).

Red man syndrome may occur if the infusion is too rapid. It is not an allergic reaction, but may be characterized by hypotension and/or a maculopapular rash appearing on the face, neck, trunk, and/or upper extremities. If this should occur, slow the infusion rate to over 1½ to 2 hours and increase the dilution volume. Reactions are often treated with antihistamines and steroids.

Extravasation treatment: Monitor I.V. site closely; extravasation will cause serious injury with possible necrosis and tissue sloughing. Rotate infusion site frequently.

Other Vancomycin is available as a powder for injection and may be diluted to 1-5 mg/mL concentration in preservative-free 0.9% sodium chloride for intrathecal administration. May be administered by intravitreal injection (unlabeled use).

Stability

Reconstitution Reconstitute vials with 20 mL of SWFI for each 1 g of vancomycin (10 mL/500 mg vial; 20 mL/1 g vial; 100 mL/5 g vial; 200 mL/10 g vial). The reconstituted solution must be further diluted with at least 100 mL of a compatible diluent per 500 mg of vancomycin prior to parenteral administration.

Intrathecal: Vancomycin is available as a powder for injection and may be diluted to 1-5 mg/mL concentration in preservative free 0.9% sodium chloride for administration into the CSF.

Storage Reconstituted 500 mg and 1 g vials are stable for at either room temperature or under refrigeration for 14 days. **Note:** Vials contain no bacteriostatic agent. Solutions diluted for administration in either D_5W or NS are stable under refrigeration for 14 days or at room temperature for 7 days.

Monitoring and Teaching Issues

Laboratory Monitoring Perform culture and susceptibility studies prior to first dose. Periodic renal function, urinalysis; WBC; serum trough vancomycin concentrations in select patients (eg, aggressive dosing, unstable renal function, concurrent nephrotoxins, prolonged courses). Obtain drug levels after the third or fourth dose unless otherwise directed. Troughs are the most accurate and practical method for monitoring and should be obtained just before the next dose (approximately after the fourth dose).

Physical Assessment Assess results of culture and sensitivity tests and patient's allergy history prior to first dose. Use caution with renal impairment or previous hearing loss. Premedication with antihistamines may prevent or minimize "red man" reaction. Infusion site must be monitored closely to prevent extravasation. Monitor for hypotension, rash, neutropenia, nausea, vomiting, and auditory changes on a regular basis during therapy.

Patient Education If administered by infusion, report immediately any chills; pain, swelling, or redness at infusion site; or respiratory difficulty. May cause nausea, vomiting, or GI upset. Report rash or hives, chills or fever, persistent GI disturbances, opportunistic infection (sore throat, chills, fever, burning, itching on urination, vaginal discharge, white plaques in mouth), respiratory difficulty, any change in urine output, chest pain or palpitations, changes in hearing or feeling of fullness in ears, or worsening of condition.

Dietary Considerations May be taken with food.

Geriatric Considerations As a result of age-related changes in renal function and volume of distribution, accumulation and toxicity are a risk in the elderly. Careful monitoring and dosing adjustment is necessary.

Breast-Feeding Considerations Small amounts of vancomycin are excreted in human milk and use during breast-feeding is not recommended by the manufacturer. If given orally to the mother, the minimal systemic absorption of the dose would limit the amount available to pass into the milk. If given intravenously, the small amount that distributes to the milk would not be expected to cause systemic toxicity due to the lack of GI absorption. Nondose-related effects could include modification of bowel flora.

Pregnancy Considerations Adverse effects have not been observed in animal studies and there are no controlled studies in pregnant women; however, oral vancomycin is not systemically absorbed. Therefore, I.V. vancomycin has been classified pregnancy category C and oral vancomycin has been classified pregnancy category B. Vancomycin crosses the placenta. *In vivo* studies and human case reports have documented placental transfer of vancomycin in the second and third trimesters of pregnancy resulting in therapeutic fetal concentrations. Vancomycin has not caused adverse fetal effects, including hearing loss or nephrotoxicity, when administered during pregnancy. A case report has been published of a vancomycin dose rapidly administered over 3 minutes leading to maternal hypotension and fetal bradycardia.

The pharmacokinetics of vancomycin may be altered during pregnancy and pregnant patients may need a higher dose of vancomycin. Maternal half-life is unchanged, but the volume of distribution and the total plasma clearance are increased. Individualization of therapy through serum concentration monitoring may be warranted. Vancomycin is recommended for use in pregnant women for prevention of early-onset group B streptococcal (GBS) disease in newborns.

Additional Information Because of its long half-life, vancomycin should be dosed on an every 8- to 12-hour basis. Monitoring of trough serum concentrations is advisable in certain situations. "Red man syndrome", characterized by skin rash and hypotension, is not an allergic reaction but rather is associated with too rapid infusion of the drug. To alleviate or prevent the reaction, infuse vancomycin at a rate of ≥30 minutes for each 500 mg of drug being administered (eg, 1 g over ≥60 minutes); 1.5 g over ≥90 minutes.

Related Information

Antimicrobial Drugs of Choice *on page 2008*
Compatibility of Drugs *on page 1994*
Peak and Trough Guidelines *on page 1958*

◆ **Vancomycin Hydrochloride** *see* Vancomycin *on page 1842*
◆ **Vanos™** *see* Fluocinonide *on page 786*
◆ **Vantin** *see* Cefpodoxime *on page 328*
◆ **VAQTA®** *see* Hepatitis A Vaccine *on page 904*
◆ **VAR** *see* Varicella Virus Vaccine *on page 1850*

Vardenafil (var DEN a fil)

U.S. Brand Names Levitra®; Staxyn™

Index Terms Vardenafil Hydrochloride

Generic Availability (U.S.) No

Pharmacologic Category Phosphodiesterase-5 Enzyme Inhibitor

Medication Safety Issues

Sound-alike/look-alike issues:

Vardenafil may be confused with sildenafil, tadalafil
Levitra® may be confused with Kaletra®, Lexiva®

Pregnancy Risk Factor B

Lactation Excretion in breast milk unknown/not indicated for use in women.

Use Treatment of erectile dysfunction (ED)

Mechanism of Action/Effect Vardenafil enhances the effect of nitric oxide by inhibiting phosphodiesterase type 5 (PDE-5), resulting in smooth muscle relaxation and inflow of blood into the corpus cavernosum with sexual stimulation.

Contraindications Hypersensitivity to vardenafil or any component of the formulation; concurrent (regular or intermittent) use of organic nitrates in any form (eg, nitroglycerin, isosorbide dinitrate)

Warnings/Precautions There is a degree of cardiac risk associated with sexual activity; therefore, physicians may wish to consider the patient's cardiovascular status prior to initiating any treatment for erectile dysfunction. Use caution in patients with anatomical deformation of the penis (angulation, cavernosal fibrosis, or Peyronie's disease) and in patients who have conditions which may predispose them to priapism (sickle cell anemia, multiple myeloma, leukemia). Instruct patients to seek immediate medical attention if erection persists >4 hours.

Use is not recommended in patients with hypotension (<90/50 mm Hg); uncontrolled hypertension (>170/100 mm Hg); unstable angina or angina during intercourse; life-threatening arrhythmias, stroke, or MI within the last 6 months; cardiac failure or coronary artery disease causing unstable angina. Safety and efficacy have not been studied in these patients. Use caution in patients with left ventricular outflow obstruction (eg, aortic stenosis). Use caution with alpha-blockers, effective CYP3A4 inhibitors, the elderly, or those with hepatic impairment (Child-Pugh class B); dosage adjustment is needed.

Rare cases of nonarteritic ischemic optic neuropathy (NAION) have been reported; risk may be increased with history of vision loss. Other risk factors for NAION include heart disease, diabetes, hypertension, smoking, age >50 years, or history of certain eye problems. Sudden decrease or loss of hearing has been reported rarely; hearing changes may be accompanied by tinnitus and dizziness.

Safety and efficacy have not been studied in patients with the following conditions, therefore, use in these patients is not recommended at this time: Congenital QT prolongation, patients taking medications known to prolong the QT interval (avoid use in patients taking Class Ia or III antiarrhythmics); severe hepatic impairment (Child-Pugh class C); end-stage renal disease requiring dialysis; retinitis pigmentosa or other degenerative retinal disorders. The safety and efficacy of vardenafil with other treatments for erectile dysfunction have not been studied and are not recommended as combination therapy. Concomitant use with all forms of nitrates is contraindicated. If nitrate administration is medically necessary, it is not known when nitrates can be safely administered following the use of vardenafil; the ACC/AHA 2007 guidelines support administration of nitrates only if 24 hours have elapsed. Potential underlying causes of erectile dysfunction should be evaluated prior to treatment. Some products may contain phylalanine. Some products may contain sorbitol; do not use in patients with fructose intolerance.

Drug Interactions

Metabolism/Transport Effects Substrate of CYP2C (minor), 3A4 (major)

Avoid Concomitant Use

Avoid concomitant use of Vardenafil with any of the following: Amyl Nitrite; Phosphodiesterase 5 Inhibitors; Vasodilators (Organic Nitrates)

Decreased Effect

The levels/effects of Vardenafil may be decreased by: Bosentan; Etravirine

Increased Effect/Toxicity

Vardenafil may increase the levels/effects of: Alpha1-Blockers; Amyl Nitrite; Antihypertensives; Bosentan; Phosphodiesterase 5 Inhibitors; Vasodilators (Organic Nitrates)

The levels/effects of Vardenafil may be increased by: Antifungal Agents (Azole Derivatives, Systemic); Conivaptan; CYP3A4 Inhibitors (Moderate); CYP3A4 Inhibitors (Strong); Dasatinib; Macrolide Antibiotics; Protease Inhibitors; Sapropterin

Nutritional/Ethanol Interactions Food: High-fat meals decrease maximum serum concentration 18% to 50%. Serum concentrations/toxicity may be increased with grapefruit juice; avoid concurrent use.

Adverse Reactions

>10%:

Cardiovascular: Flushing (8% to 11%)
Central nervous system: Headache (14% to 15%)

2% to 10%:

Central nervous system: Dizziness (2%)
Gastrointestinal: Dyspepsia (3% to 4%), nausea (2%)
Neuromuscular & skeletal: Back pain (2%), CPK increased (2%)
Respiratory: Rhinitis (9%), nasal congestion (3%), sinusitis (3%)
Miscellaneous: Flu-like syndrome (3%)

Pharmacodynamics/Kinetics

Onset of Action ~60 minutes

Absorption Rapid

Bioavailability ~15%; Film-coated tablet: Elderly (≥65 years): AUC increased by 52%; Hepatic impairment (moderate, Child-Pugh class B): AUC increased by 160%; Oral disintegrating tablet: Elderly (≥65 years): AUC increased by 21% more compared to film-coated tablet. When administered with water, AUC decreases by 29%.

Time to Peak Plasma: 0.5-2 hours

Protein Binding ~95% (parent drug and metabolite)

Half-Life Elimination Terminal: Vardenafil and metabolite: 3-6 hours

Metabolism Hepatic via CYP3A4 (major), CYP2C and 3A5 (minor); forms metabolite (active)

Excretion Feces (~91% to 95% as metabolites); urine (~2% to 6%)

Product Availability

Staxyn™: FDA approved June 2010; availability expected near the end of 2010
Staxyn™ orally disintegrating tablets are indicated for the treatment of erectile dysfunction.

Available Dosage Forms

Tablet, oral:
Levitra®: 2.5 mg, 5 mg, 10 mg, 20 mg

Dosing

Adult Note: Oral disintegrating tablets should not be used interchangeably with film-coated tablets; patients requiring a dose other than 10 mg should use the film-coated tablets.

Erectile dysfunction: Oral:

Film-coated tablet (Levitra®): 10 mg 60 minutes prior to sexual activity; dosing range: 5-20 mg; to be given as one single dose and not given more than once daily

Oral disintegrating tablet (Staxyn™): 10 mg 60 minutes prior to sexual activity; maximum: 10 mg/day

Dosing adjustment with concomitant medications:

Alpha-blocker (dose should be stable at time of vardenafil initiation):

Film-coated tablet (Levitra®): Initial vardenafil dose: 5 mg/24 hours; if an alpha-blocker is added to vardenafil therapy, it should be initiated at the smallest possible dose and titrated carefully.

Oral disintegrating tablet (Staxyn™): Do not use to initiate therapy. Initial therapy should be with film-coated tablets at lower doses. Patients who have previously used film-coated tablets may be switched to oral disintegrating tablets as recommended by healthcare provider.

Film-coated tablet (Levitra®):

Atazanavir: Maximum vardenafil dose: 2.5 mg/24 hours
Clarithromycin: Maximum vardenafil dose: 2.5 mg/24 hours
Darunavir: Maximum vardenafil dose: 2.5 mg/72 hours
Erythromycin: Maximum vardenafil dose: 5 mg/24 hours
Fosamprenavir: Maximum vardenafil dose: 2.5 mg/24 hours
Fosamprenavir/ritonavir: Maximum vardenafil dose: 2.5 mg/72 hours
Indinavir: Maximum vardenafil dose: 2.5 mg/24 hours
Itraconazole:
200 mg/day: Maximum vardenafil dose: 5 mg/24 hours
400 mg/day: Maximum vardenafil dose: 2.5 mg/24 hours
Ketoconazole:
200 mg/day: Maximum vardenafil dose: 5 mg/24 hours
400 mg/day: Maximum vardenafil dose: 2.5 mg/24 hours
Lopinavir/ritonavir: Maximum vardenafil dose: 2.5 mg/72 hours

Nelfinavir: Maximum vardenafil dose: 2.5 mg/24 hours
Ritonavir: Maximum vardenafil dose: 2.5 mg/72 hours
Saquinavir: Maximum vardenafil dose: 2.5 mg/24 hours
Tipranavir: Maximum vardenafil dose: 2.5 mg/72 hours

Oral disintegrating tablet (Staxyn™): Concurrent use not recommended with potent or moderate CYP3A4 inhibitors (atazanavir, clarithromycin, erythromycin, indinavir, itraconazole, ketoconazole, ritonavir, saquinavir)

Geriatric Erectile dysfunction: Elderly ≥65 years: Oral: Initial: 5 mg 60 minutes prior to sexual activity; to be given as one single dose and not given more than once daily.

Renal Impairment Dose adjustment not needed for mild, moderate, or severe impairment; use not recommended in patients on hemodialysis.

Hepatic Impairment

Child-Pugh class A: No adjustment required

Child-Pugh class B:

Film-coated tablet (Levitra®): Initial: 5 mg 60 minutes prior to sexual activity (maximum dose: 10 mg); to be given as one single dose and not given more than once daily

Oral disintegrating tablet (Staxyn™): Use not recommended

Child-Pugh class C: Has not been studied; use is not recommended by the manufacturer

Administration

Oral May be administered with or without food, 60 minutes prior to sexual activity.

Oral disintegrating tablet should not be removed from blister pack until administered. Using dry hands, place immediately on tongue. Tablet will dissolve within seconds; do not take with liquid. Do not crush, split, or chew.

Stability

Storage Store at controlled room temperature of 25°C (77°F); excursions permitted to 15°C to 25°C (59°F to 86°F). Keep oral disintegrating tablets sealed in blisterpack until ready to use.

Monitoring and Teaching Issues

Patient Education Use 60 minutes prior to sexual activity. Avoid taking with high-fat meals. This medication does not provide protection against sexually-transmitted diseases, including HIV. You may experience headache, flushing, or blurred vision. Report immediately chest pain, acute head pain, respiratory difficulty, change in vision (seeing a blue tinge to objects or having difficulty telling the difference between the colors blue and green), change in hearing or ringing in the ears, allergic response (eg, chills, fever, respiratory difficulty, rash), genital swelling, or erection lasting >4 hours.

Dietary Considerations May take with or without food. Avoid grapefruit juice. Some products may contain phenylalanine. Some products may contain sorbitol; do not use in patients with fructose intolerance.

Geriatric Considerations In adults ≥65 years of age, vardenafil plasma concentrations were higher than younger males (mean C_{max} was 34% higher), therefore, initial dose should be lower than the usual adult dose. Since the elderly often have concomitant diseases, many of which may be contraindicated with the use of vardenafil, a thorough knowledge of disease and medications must be accessed.

Pregnancy Considerations Teratogenic effects were not observed in animal studies; however, vardenafil is not indicated for use in women. No effects on sperm motility or morphology were observed in healthy males.

◆ **Vardenafil Hydrochloride** *see* Vardenafil *on page* 1846

Varenicline (var e NI kleen)

U.S. Brand Names Chantix®

Index Terms Varenicline Tartrate

Generic Availability (U.S.) No

Pharmacologic Category Partial Nicotine Agonist; Smoking Cessation Aid

Medication Guide Available Yes

Pregnancy Risk Factor C

Lactation Excretion in breast milk unknown/not recommended

Use Treatment to aid in smoking cessation

Mechanism of Action/Effect Decreases nicotine dependence, craving, and withdrawal

Contraindications Known history of serious hypersensitivity or skin reactions to varenicline

Warnings/Precautions **[U.S. Boxed Warning]: Serious neuropsychiatric events (including depression, suicidal thoughts, and suicide) have been reported with use;** some cases may have been complicated by symptoms of nicotine withdrawal following smoking cessation. Smoking cessation (with or without treatment) is associated with nicotine withdrawal symptoms and the exacerbation of underlying psychiatric illness; however, some of the behavioral disturbances were reported in treated patients who continued to smoke. Neuropsychiatric symptoms (eg, mood disturbances, psychosis, hostility) have occurred in patients with and without pre-existing psychiatric disease; many cases resolved following therapy discontinuation although in some cases, symptoms persisted. Monitor all patients for behavioral changes and psychiatric symptoms (eg, agitation, depression, suicidal behavior, suicidal ideation); inform patients to discontinue treatment and contact their healthcare provider immediately if they experience any behavioral and/or mood changes. **[U.S. Boxed Warning]: Before prescribing, the risks of serious neuropsychiatric events must be weighed against the immediate and long term benefits of smoking abstinence for each patient.**

Hypersensitivity reactions (including angioedema) and rare cases of serious skin reactions (including Stevens-Johnson syndrome and erythema multiforme) have been reported. Patients should be instructed to discontinue use and contact healthcare provider if signs/symptoms occur. Dose-dependent nausea may occur; both transient and persistent nausea has been reported. Dosage reduction may be considered for intolerable nausea. May cause sedation, which may impair physical or mental abilities; patients must be cautioned about performing tasks which require mental alertness (eg, operating machinery or driving).

Use caution in renal dysfunction; dosage adjustment required. Safety and efficacy of varenicline with other smoking cessation therapies have not been established; increased adverse events when used concurrently with nicotine replacement therapy.

Drug Interactions

Avoid Concomitant Use There are no known interactions where it is recommended to avoid concomitant use.

Decreased Effect There are no known significant interactions involving a decrease in effect.

Increased Effect/Toxicity There are no known significant interactions involving an increase in effect.

Adverse Reactions

>10%:

Central nervous system: Insomnia (18% to 19%), headache (15% to 19%), abnormal dreams (9% to 13%)

Gastrointestinal: Nausea (16% to 40%; dose related)

1% to 10%:

Central nervous system: Malaise (≤7%), sleep disorder (≤5%), somnolence (3%), nightmares (1% to 2%), lethargy (1% to 2%)

Dermatologic: Rash (≤3%)

Gastrointestinal: Flatulence (6% to 9%), constipation (5% to 8%), abnormal taste (5% to 8%), abdominal pain (≤7%), xerostomia (≤6%), dyspepsia (5%), vomiting (≤5%), appetite increased (3% to 4%), anorexia (≤2%), gastroesophageal reflux (1%)

Respiratory: Upper respiratory tract disorder (5% to 7%), dyspnea (≤2%), rhinorrhea (≤1%)

Pharmacodynamics/Kinetics

Absorption Well absorbed; unaffected by food

Time to Peak Plasma: ~3-4 hours

Protein Binding ≤20%

Half-Life Elimination ~24 hours

Metabolism Minimal (<10% of clearance is through metabolism)

Excretion Urine (92% as unchanged drug)

Available Dosage Forms

Combination package, oral:

Chantix®: Tablet: 0.5 mg (11s) [white tablets] and Tablet: 1 mg (42s) [light blue tablets]

Tablet, oral:

Chantix®: 0.5 mg, 1 mg

Dosing

Adult & Geriatric Smoking cessation: Oral:

Initial:

Days 1-3: 0.5 mg once daily

Days 4-7: 0.5 mg twice daily

Maintenance (≥ Day 8): 1 mg twice daily

Note: Start 1 week before target quit date. Patients who cannot tolerate adverse events may require temporary (or permanent) reduction in dose. If patient successfully quits smoking at the end of the 12 weeks, may continue for another 12 weeks to help maintain success. If not successful in first 12 weeks, then stop medication and reassess factors contributing to failure.

Renal Impairment

Cl_{cr} ≥30 mL/minute: No adjustment required

Cl_{cr} <30 mL/minute: Initiate: 0.5 mg once daily; maximum dose: 0.5 mg twice daily

Hemodialysis: Maximum dose: 0.5 mg once daily

Hepatic Impairment Dosage adjustment not required

Adjustment for Toxicity Lower dose for a period of time, then may increase dose again or remain on lower dose.

Administration

Oral Administer with food and a full glass of water.

Stability

Storage Store at 25°C (77°F); excursions permitted to 15°C to 30°C (59°F to 86°F).

Monitoring and Teaching Issues

Physical Assessment Provide educational materials and counseling to support an attempt at quitting smoking. Carefully instruct patient in appropriate titration of doses. Monitor for behavioral and emotional changes, such as hostility, agitation, and suicide ideation. Monitor other medications patient is taking for potential need for dose adjustment after quitting smoking.

Patient Education Start medication 1 week prior to quit date designated. Take after eating, with a full glass of water. You may experience nausea, vomiting, constipation, headaches, problems sleeping, or unusual dreams. Report depression, suicide ideation, or emotional/behavioral changes to prescriber.

Dietary Considerations Should be given with food and a full glass of water to decrease gastric upset.

Geriatric Considerations Dosage adjustment for renal function may be necessary. Although studies to date do not demonstrate any significant pharmacokinetic differences between elderly (65-75 years of age) and younger adults.

Pregnancy Considerations Teratogenic effects were not observed in animal studies; however, decreased fertility, decreased fetal weight, and increased auditory startle response were observed in the offspring. There are no adequate or well-controlled studies in pregnant women. Use only if benefit outweighs the potential risk to fetus.

Additional Information In all studies, patients received an educational booklet on smoking cessation and received up to 10 minutes of counseling at each weekly visit. Dosing started 1 week before target quit date. Successful cessation of smoking may alter pharmacokinetic properties of other medications (eg, theophylline, warfarin, insulin).

◆ **Varenicline Tartrate** *see* Varenicline *on page 1848*

◆ **Varicella, Measles, Mumps, and Rubella Vaccine** *see* Measles, Mumps, Rubella, and Varicella Virus Vaccine *on page 1151*

Varicella Virus Vaccine (var i SEL a VYE rus vak SEEN)

U.S. Brand Names Varivax®

Index Terms Chickenpox Vaccine; VAR; Varicella-Zoster Virus (VZV) Vaccine (Varicella); VZV Vaccine (Varicella)

Generic Availability (U.S.) No

Pharmacologic Category Vaccine, Live (Viral)

Medication Safety Issues

Sound-alike/look-alike issues:

Varicella virus vaccine has been given in error (instead of the indicated varicella immune globulin) to pregnant women exposed to varicella.

Both varicella vaccine and zoster vaccine are live, attenuated strains of varicella-zoster virus. Their indications, dosing, and composition are distinct. Varicella is indicated in children to prevent chickenpox, while zoster vaccine is indicated in older individuals to prevent reactivation of the virus which causes shingles. Zoster vaccine is **not** a substitute for varicella vaccine and should not be used in children.

Pregnancy Risk Factor C

Lactation Excretion in breast milk unknown/use caution

Use Immunization against varicella in children ≥12 months of age and adults

The ACIP recommends vaccination for all children, adolescents, and adults who do not have evidence of immunity. Vaccination is especially important for:

- Persons with close contact to those at high risk for severe disease
- Persons living or working in environments where transmission is likely (teachers, child-care workers, residents and staff of institutional settings)
- Persons in environments where transmission has been reported
- Nonpregnant women of childbearing age
- Adolescents and adults in households with children
- International travelers

Postexposure prophylaxis: Vaccination within 3 days (possibly 5 days) after exposure to rash is effective in preventing illness or modifying severity of disease

Available Dosage Forms

Injection, powder for reconstitution [preservative free]:

Varivax®: 1350 PFU

Dosing

Adult & Geriatric Varicella immunization: SubQ: 2 doses of 0.5 mL separated by 4-8 weeks.

Note: The ACIP recommends that all children and adults who received only 1 dose of vaccine receive a second dose (CDC, 2007).

Pediatric

Children 12 months to 12 years: Varicella immunization: SubQ: 0.5 mL; a second dose may be administered ≥3 months later

Note: The ACIP recommends the routine childhood vaccination be 2 doses, with the first dose administered at 12-15 months of age. School age children should receive the second dose at 4-6 years of age, but it may be administered earlier provided ≥3 months have elapsed after the first dose. All children and adolescents who received only 1 dose of vaccine should receive a second dose (CDC, 2007).

Children ≥13 years: Varicella immunization: Refer to adult dosing.

Administration

I.M. SubQ administration is recommended; however, doses inadvertently given I.M. have resulted in similar seroconversion.

I.V. Do not administer I.V.

Other For SubQ injection only; inject in the outer aspect of upper arm. Administer immediately following reconstitution.

Simultaneous administration of vaccines helps ensure the patients will be fully vaccinated by the appropriate age. Simultaneous administration of vaccines is defined as administering >1 vaccine on the same day at different anatomic sites. The use of licensed combination vaccines is generally preferred over separate injections of the equivalent components. Separate vaccines should not be combined in the same syringe unless indicated by product specific labeling. Separate needles and syringes should be used for each injection. The ACIP prefers each dose of a specific vaccine in a series come from the same manufacturer when possible. Adolescents and adults should be vaccinated while seated or lying down. In general, preterm infants should be vaccinated at the same chronological age as full-term infants (CDC, 2011).

Antipyretics have not been shown to prevent febrile seizures. Antipyretics may be used to treat fever or discomfort following vaccination (CDC, 2011). One study reported that routine prophylactic administration of acetaminophen to prevent fever prior to vaccination decreased the immune response of some vaccines; the clinical significance of this reduction in immune response has not been established (Prymula, 2009).

Monitoring and Teaching Issues

Physical Assessment Federal law requires entry into the patient's medical record.

Related Information

Immunization Recommendations *on page 1941*

◆ **Varicella-Zoster Virus (VZV) Vaccine (Varicella)** *see* Varicella Virus Vaccine *on page 1850*

◆ **Varicella-Zoster (VZV) Vaccine (Zoster)** *see* Zoster Vaccine *on page 1910*

◆ **Varivax®** *see* Varicella Virus Vaccine *on page 1850*

◆ **Vaseretic®** *see* Enalapril and Hydrochlorothiazide *on page 620*

Vasopressin (vay soe PRES in)

U.S. Brand Names Pitressin®

Index Terms 8-Arginine Vasopressin; ADH; Antidiuretic Hormone; AVP

Generic Availability (U.S.) Yes

Pharmacologic Category Antidiuretic Hormone Analog; Hormone, Posterior Pituitary

Medication Safety Issues

Use care when prescribing and/or administering vasopressin solutions. Close attention should be given to concentration of solution, route of administration, dose, and rate of administration (units/minute, units/kg/minute, units/kg/hour).

Pregnancy Risk Factor C

Lactation Enters breast milk/use caution

Use Treatment of central diabetes insipidus; differential diagnosis of diabetes insipidus

Unlabeled/Investigational Use ACLS guidelines: Pulseless arrest (ventricular tachycardia [VT]/ventricular fibrillation [VF], asystole/pulseless electrical activity [PEA]); cardiac arrest secondary to anaphylaxis (unresponsive to epinephrine)

Adjunct in the treatment of GI hemorrhage and esophageal varices; adjunct in the treatment of vasodilatory shock (septic shock); donor management in brain-dead patients (hormone replacement therapy)

Available Dosage Forms

Injection, solution: 20 units/mL (0.5 mL, 1 mL, 10 mL)

Pitressin®: 20 units/mL (1 mL)

Dosing

Adult & Geriatric

Central diabetes insipidus: Note: Dosage is highly variable; titrated based on serum and urine sodium and osmolality in addition to fluid balance and urine output. Use of vasopressin is impractical for chronic therapy.

I.M., SubQ: 5-10 units 2-4 times/day as needed

Continuous I.V. infusion (unlabeled route): Continuous infusion has not been formally evaluated in the post-neurosurgical adult. However, some convert I.M./SubQ requirement to an hourly continuous I.V. infusion rate.

Central diabetes insipidus, post-traumatic (unlabeled use): *I.V.:* Initial: 2.5 units/hour; titrate to adequately reduce urine output (Levitt, 1984)

Donor management in brain-dead patients (hormone replacement therapy) (unlabeled use): *I.V.:* Initial: 1 unit bolus followed by 0.5-4 units/hour (Rosendale, 2003; UNOS Critical Pathway, 2002)

Variceal hemorrhage (unlabeled use): *Continuous I.V. infusion:* Dilute in NS or D_5W to 0.1-1 unit/mL. **Note:** Other therapies may be preferred.

[AASLD guidelines, 2007]: *Continuous I.V. infusion:* Initial: 0.2-0.4 units/minute, may titrate dose as needed to a maximum dose of 0.8 units/minute; maximum duration: 24 hours at highest effective dose continuously (to reduce incidence of adverse effects). Patient should also receive I.V. nitroglycerin concurrently to prevent myocardial ischemic complications. Monitor closely for signs/symptoms of ischemia (myocardial, peripheral, bowel).

Pulseless arrest (unlabeled use) [ACLS, 2010]: I.V., I.O.: 40 units; may give 1 dose to replace first or second dose of epinephrine. I.V./I.O. drug administration is preferred, but if no access, may give endotracheally. ACLS guidelines do not recommend a specific endotracheal dose; however, may be given endotracheally using the same I.V. dose (ACLS, 2010; Wenzel, 1997).

Vasodilatory shock/septic shock (unlabeled use): *I.V.:* 0.01-0.04 units/minute for the treatment of septic shock. **Note:** Recommended as a second-line vasopressor in addition to norepinephrine (Dellinger, 2008). Doses >0.04 units/minute may have more cardiovascular side effects. Most case reports have used 0.04 units/minute continuous infusion as a fixed dose.

Pediatric

Central diabetes insipidus: Note: Dosage is highly variable; titrated based on serum and urine sodium and osmolality in addition to fluid balance and urine output. Use of vasopressin is impractical for chronic therapy.

I.M., SubQ: 2.5-10 units 2-4 times/day as needed

Continuous I.V. infusion (unlabeled route): Initial: 0.0005 units/kg/hour; increase dose by 0.0005 units/kg/hour increments every 5-10 minutes as needed to adequately reduce urine output (maximum dose: 0.01 unit/kg/hour) (Wise-Faberowski, 2004). **Note:** Although clinical trial titrated every 5-10 minutes, a reduced frequency of titration (eg, every 30 minutes) may be more appropriate given the half-life of vasopressin.

GI hemorrhage (unlabeled use): *Continuous I.V. infusion:* Dilute in NS or D_5W to 0.1-1 unit/mL. **Note:** Other therapies may be preferred.

Initial I.V. bolus: 0.3 units/kg (maximum: 20 units) may be given

Continuous I.V. infusion: 0.001-0.01 units/kg/minute; titrate dose as needed; maximum: 0.01 unit/kg/minute; if bleeding controlled for 12-24 hours, then taper off over 24-36 hours

Hepatic Impairment Some patients respond to much lower doses with cirrhosis.

Administration

I.V. Usual concentration: 100 units in 500 mL D_5W. **Note:** In one clinical trial with lower dosing (eg, 0.0005 units/kg/hour) in pediatric patients, a more dilute solution (eg, 20 units in 500 mL D_5W) was employed (Wise-Faberowski, 2004).

Vasodilatory shock: Administration through a central catheter is recommended.

Topical Topical administration on nasal mucosa: Administer injectable vasopressin on cotton plugs, as nasal spray, or by dropper. Should not be inhaled.

Other Endotracheal: If no I.V./I.O. access may give endotracheally. ACLS guidelines do not recommend a specific endotracheal dose; however, may be given endotracheally using the same I.V. dose (ACLS, 2010; Wenzel, 1997). Mix with 5-10 mL of water or normal saline, and administer down the endotracheal tube.

Monitoring and Teaching Issues

Laboratory Monitoring Serum and urine sodium, urine specific gravity, urine and serum osmolality

Physical Assessment Evaluate patient history closely for use cautions. I.V. requires use of infusion pump and close monitoring to prevent extravasation (may cause severe necrosis and gangrene). Monitor cardiac status, blood pressure, CNS status, fluid balance, and for signs or symptoms of water intoxication or intranasal irritation.

Patient Education This drug will usually be administered by infusion or injection and you will be closely monitored. Report immediately any chest pain or palpitations; difficulty breathing; abdominal cramping; or redness, swelling, pain, or burning at infusion/injection site. May cause dizziness or drowsiness. Report persistent nausea, vomiting, or abdominal cramps; tremor, acute headache, or dizziness; chest pain or irregular heartbeat; respiratory difficulty or excessive perspiration; or CNS changes (confusion, drowsiness).

◆ **Vasotec®** *see* Enalapril *on page 616*

◆ **Vectibix®** *see* Panitumumab *on page 1403*

◆ **Vectical™** *see* Calcitriol *on page 271*

Vecuronium (vek ue ROE nee um)

Index Terms Norcuron; ORG NC 45

Generic Availability (U.S.) Yes

Pharmacologic Category Neuromuscular Blocker Agent, Nondepolarizing

Medication Safety Issues

Sound-alike/look-alike issues:

Vecuronium may be confused with valproate sodium, vancomycin

Norcuron® may be confused with Narcan®

High alert medication: The Institute for Safe Medication Practices (ISMP) includes this medication among its list of drugs which have a heightened risk of causing significant patient harm when used in error.

United States Pharmacopeia (USP) 2006: The Interdisciplinary Safe Medication Use Expert Committee of the USP has recommended the following:

- Hospitals, clinics, and other practice sites should institute special safeguards in the storage, labeling, and use of these agents and should include these safeguards in staff orientation and competency training.
- Healthcare professionals should be on high alert (especially vigilant) whenever a neuromuscular-blocking agent (NMBA) is stocked, ordered, prepared, or administered.

Pregnancy Risk Factor C

Lactation Excretion in breast milk unknown/use caution

Use To facilitate endotracheal intubation and to relax skeletal muscles during surgery; to facilitate mechanical ventilation in ICU patients; does not relieve pain or produce sedation

Mechanism of Action/Effect Blocks acetylcholine from binding to receptors on motor endplate inhibiting depolarization

Contraindications Hypersensitivity to vecuronium or any component of the formulation

Warnings/Precautions Ventilation must be supported during neuromuscular blockade. Vecuronium does not relieve pain or produce sedation; use should include appropriate anesthesia, pain control, and sedation. In patients requiring long-term administration, use of a peripheral nerve stimulator to monitor drug effects is strongly recommended. Additional doses of vecuronium or any other neuromuscular-blocking agent should be avoided unless nerve stimulation response suggests inadequate neuromuscular blockade. Certain clinical conditions may result in potentiation or antagonism of neuromuscular blockade:

Antagonism: Alkalosis, hypercalcemia, demyelinating lesions, peripheral neuropathies, denervation, immobilization, infection, and muscle trauma

Potentiation: Electrolyte abnormalities, severe hyponatremia, severe hypocalcemia, severe hypokalemia, hypermagnesemia, cachexia, neuromuscular diseases, acidosis, Eaton-Lambert syndrome, and myasthenia gravis

Resistance may occur in burn patients (>30% of body) for period of 5-70 days postinjury. Hypothermia may prolong the duration of action. Use with caution in patients with hepatic impairment; clinical duration may be prolonged. Use with caution in patients who are anephric; clinical duration may be prolonged. Use with caution in patients who have underlying respiratory disease. Some patients may experience delayed recovery of neuromuscular function after administration (especially after prolonged use). Other factors associated with delayed recovery should be considered (eg, corticosteroid use, disease-related conditions). Cross-sensitivity with other neuromuscular-blocking agents may occur; use extreme caution in patients with previous anaphylactic reactions. Use caution in the elderly. Children 1-10 years of age may require slightly higher initial doses and slightly more frequent supplementation. **[U.S. Boxed Warning]: Should be administered by adequately trained individuals familiar with its use.** Some dosage forms may contain benzyl alcohol which has been associated with "gasping syndrome" in neonates.

Drug Interactions

Avoid Concomitant Use

Avoid concomitant use of Vecuronium with any of the following: QuiNINE

Decreased Effect

The levels/effects of Vecuronium may be decreased by: Acetylcholinesterase Inhibitors; CarBAMazepine; Loop Diuretics; Phenytoin

Increased Effect/Toxicity

Vecuronium may increase the levels/effects of: Cardiac Glycosides; Corticosteroids (Systemic); OnabotulinumtoxinA; RimabotulinumtoxinB

The levels/effects of Vecuronium may be increased by: AbobotulinumtoxinA; Aminoglycosides; Calcium Channel Blockers; Capreomycin; Colistimethate; Inhalational Anesthetics; Ketorolac; Ketorolac (Systemic); Lincosamide Antibiotics; Lithium; Loop Diuretics; Magnesium Salts; Phenytoin; Polymyxin B; Procainamide; QuiNIDine; QuiNINE; Spironolactone; Tetracycline Derivatives; Vancomycin

Pharmacodynamics/Kinetics

Onset of Action Good intubation conditions: Within 2.5-3 minutes; Maximum neuromuscular blockade: Within 3-5 minutes

Duration of Action Under balanced anesthesia (time to recovery to 25% of control): 25-40 minutes; recovery 95% complete ~45-65 minutes after injection of intubating dose

Protein Binding 60% to 80%

Half-Life Elimination Healthy surgical patients and renal failure patients undergoing transplant surgery: 65-75 minutes; Late pregnancy: 35-40 minutes

Metabolism Active metabolite: 3-desacetyl vecuronium (1/2 the activity of parent drug)

Excretion Primarily feces (40% to 75%); urine (30% as unchanged drug and metabolites)

Available Dosage Forms

Injection, powder for reconstitution: 10 mg, 20 mg

Dosing

Adult & Geriatric Dose to effect; doses will vary due to interpatient variability.

Surgical relaxation: I.V. (do not administer I.M.): **Note:** For obese (≥130% of IBW) adult patients, may use ideal body weight (IBW) (Erstad, 2004; Schwartz, 1992; Weinstein, 1988); onset time may be slightly delayed using IBW.

Tracheal intubation: I.V.: Initial: 0.08-0.1 mg/kg. **Note:** If intubation is performed using succinylcholine (not preferred agent in pediatric patients), the initial dose of vecuronium may be reduced to 0.04-0.06 mg/kg with inhalation anesthesia and 0.05-0.06 mg/kg with balanced anesthesia. Inhaled anesthetic agents prolong the duration of action of vecuronium.

Pretreatment/priming: Adults: 10% of intubating dose given 3-5 minutes before intubating dose

Maintenance for continued surgical relaxation: Intermittent dosing (see **"Note"** below): 0.01-0.015 mg/kg administered at 25% recovery of control T_1 or continuous infusion: Initial: 1 mcg/kg/minute only after early evidence of spontaneous recovery of neuromuscular function. Infusion rates range: 0.8-1.2 mcg/kg/minute.

Note: Use lower end of the dosing range when anesthesia is maintained with an inhaled anesthetic agent, with the redosing interval guided by monitoring with a peripheral nerve stimulator.

ICU paralysis (eg, facilitate mechanical ventilation) in selected adequately sedated patients (Darrah, 1989; Murray, 2002; Rudis, 1997): I.V.: Initial bolus dose: 0.08-0.1 mg/kg, then a continuous I.V. infusion of 0.8-1.7 mcg/kg/minute; monitor depth of blockade every 1-2 hours initially until stable dose, then every 8-12 hours. Usual maintenance infusion dose range: 0.8-1.2 mcg/kg/minute.

Dosage adjustment (Rudis, 1996; Rudis, 1997): Adjust rate of administration in increments of 0.3 mcg/kg/minute or by 50% reductions of previous dose according to peripheral nerve stimulation response (eg, train-of-four [TOF] count) or desired clinical response as long as TOF count >1/4 is present. If no response on TOF, discontinue infusion and reinitiate when TOF count ≥1/4 occurs.

Note: When possible, minimize depth and duration of paralysis. Stopping the infusion daily for some time until forced to restart based on patient condition is recommended to reduce post-paralytic complications (eg, acute quadriplegic myopathy syndrome [AQMS]) (Murray, 2002, Segredo, 1992).

Intermittent bolus dosing (Hunter, 1985): 0.1-0.2 mg/kg/dose; may be repeated when TOF count >1/4

Control of refractory shivering in adequately sedated patients during therapeutic hypothermia after cardiac arrest (unlabeled use; Bernard, 2002; Nolan, 2003; Polderman, 2009): I.V.: 8-12 mg; redose as needed to control shivering. **Note:** Duration of action prolonged in patients undergoing induced hypothermia. May also mask seizure activity.

Pediatric Dose to effect; doses will vary due to interpatient variability.

Surgical relaxation: Tracheal intubation: I.V. (do not administer I.M.): Children ≥1 year: Refer to adult dosing. **Note:** Children 1-10 years may require slightly higher initial doses and more frequent supplementation.

ICU paralysis (eg, facilitate mechanical ventilation) in selected adequately sedated patients (unlabeled; Martin, 1999): I.V.: Initial bolus dose: 0.1-0.15 mg/kg, then a continuous I.V. infusion of 1-2.5 mcg/kg/minute; monitor depth of blockade using train-of-four (TOF) every 2-3 hours initially until stable dose, then every 8-12 hours

Intermittent bolus dosing (Eldadah, 1989): 0.1 mg/kg every 1 hour as needed when TOF count ≥1/4

Renal Impairment In general, patients with renal impairment do not experience clinically significant prolongation of neuromuscular blockade with vecuronium; however, in patients who are anephric, the clinical duration may be prolonged.

Hepatic Impairment Dose reductions are necessary in patients with liver disease.

Administration

I.V. Concentration of 1 mg/mL may be administered by rapid I.V. injection. May further dilute reconstituted vial to 0.1-0.2 mg/mL in a compatible solution for I.V. infusion. Concentration of 1 mg/mL may be used for I.V. infusion in fluid-restricted patients.

Stability

Reconstitution Reconstitute with compatible solution for injection to final concentration of 1 mg/mL.

Storage Store intact vials of powder for injection at room temperature 20°C to 25°C (68°F to 77°F). Vials reconstituted with bacteriostatic water for injection (BWFI) may be stored for 5 days under refrigeration or at room temperature. Vials reconstituted with other compatible diluents (nonbacteriostatic) should be stored under refrigeration and used within 24 hours.

Monitoring and Teaching Issues

Physical Assessment Dosage and rate of administration should be individualized and titrated to the desired effect, according to relevant clinical factors, premedication, concomitant medications, age, and general condition of patient. Ventilatory support must be instituted and maintained until adequate respiratory muscle function and/or airway protection are assured. This drug is not an anesthetic or analgesic; pain must be treated with other agents. Continuous monitoring of vital signs, cardiac status, respiratory status, and degree of neuromuscular block (objective assessment with peripheral external nerve stimulator) is mandatory during infusion and until full muscle tone has returned. Safety precautions must be maintained until full muscle tone has returned. It may take longer for return of muscle tone in obese or elderly patients or patients with renal or hepatic disease, myasthenia gravis, myopathy, other neuromuscular disease, dehydration, electrolyte imbalance, or severe acid/base imbalance.

Long-term use: Monitor level of neuromuscular blockade, skeletal muscle movement, and respiratory effort. Reposition patient and provide appropriate skin care, mouth care, and care of patient's eyes every 2-3 hours while sedated. Provide appropriate emotional and sensory support (auditory and environmental).

Patient Education Patient will usually be unconscious prior to administration. Reassurance of constant monitoring and emotional support to reduce fear and anxiety should precede and follow administration. Following return of muscle tone, do not attempt to change position or rise from bed without assistance.

Pregnancy Considerations There are no adequate and well-controlled studies in pregnant women. Use in cesarean section has been reported. Umbilical venous concentrations were 11% of maternal. Use only if the potential benefit justifies the potential risk to the fetus.

Additional Information Vecuronium is classified as an intermediate-duration neuromuscular-blocking agent. It produces minimal, if any, histamine release; does not relieve pain or produce sedation. It may produce cumulative effect on duration of blockade.

◆ **Velban** *see* VinBLAStine *on page* 1862

◆ **Velcade®** *see* Bortezomib *on page* 226

◆ **Veletri®** *see* Epoprostenol *on page* 643

◆ **Velivet™** *see* Ethinyl Estradiol and Desogestrel *on page* 695

◆ **Veltin™** *see* Clindamycin and Tretinoin *on page* 401

◆ **Veltin™** *see* Clindamycin and Tretinoin *on page* 401

Venlafaxine (ven la FAX een)

U.S. Brand Names Effexor XR®; Effexor®

Generic Availability (U.S.) Yes

Pharmacologic Category Antidepressant, Serotonin/Norepinephrine Reuptake Inhibitor

Medication Safety Issues

Sound-alike/look-alike issues:

Effexor® may be confused with Effexor XR®

Medication Guide Available Yes

Pregnancy Risk Factor C

Lactation Enters breast milk/not recommended

Use Treatment of major depressive disorder, generalized anxiety disorder (GAD), social anxiety disorder (social phobia), panic disorder

Unlabeled/Investigational Use Obsessive-compulsive disorder (OCD); hot flashes; neuropathic pain; attention-deficit/hyperactivity disorder (ADHD); post-traumatic stress disorder (PTSD)

Mechanism of Action/Effect Venlafaxine and its active metabolite, o-desmethylvenlafaxine (ODV), inhibit the reuptake of both norepinephrine and serotonin (SNRI); improves symptoms of depression.

Contraindications Hypersensitivity to venlafaxine or any component of the formulation; use of MAO inhibitors within 14 days; should not initiate MAO inhibitor within 7 days of discontinuing venlafaxine

Warnings/Precautions [U.S. Boxed Warning]: Antidepressants increase the risk of suicidal thinking and behavior in children, adolescents, and young adults (18-24 years of age) with major depressive disorder (MDD) and other psychiatric disorders; consider risk prior to prescribing. Short-term studies did not show an increased risk in patients >24 years of age and showed a decreased risk in patients ≥65 years. Closely monitor for clinical worsening, suicidality, or unusual changes in behavior; the patient's family or caregiver should be instructed to closely observe the patient and communicate condition with healthcare provider. Reduced growth rate has been observed with venlafaxine therapy in children. A medication guide should be dispensed with each prescription. **Venlafaxine is not FDA approved for use in children.**

The possibility of a suicide attempt is inherent in major depression and may persist until remission occurs. Monitor for worsening of depression or suicidality, especially during initiation of therapy (generally first 1-2 months) or with dose increases or decreases. Use caution in high-risk patients. Worsening depression and severe abrupt suicidality that are not part of the presenting symptoms may require discontinuation or modification of drug therapy. The patient's family or caregiver should be alerted to monitor patients for the emergence of suicidality and associated behaviors (such as agitation, irritability, hostility, impulsivity, and hypomania) and call healthcare provider.

May worsen psychosis in some patients or precipitate a shift to mania or hypomania in patients with bipolar disorder. Patients presenting with depressive symptoms should be screened for bipolar disorder. Monotherapy in patients with bipolar disorder should be avoided. **Venlafaxine is not FDA approved for the treatment of bipolar depression.**

Serotonin syndrome and neuroleptic malignant syndrome (NMS)-like reactions have occurred with serotonin/norepinephrine reuptake inhibitors (SNRIs) and selective serotonin reuptake inhibitors (SSRIs) when used alone, and particularly when used in combination with serotonergic agents (eg, triptans) or antidopaminergic agents (eg, antipsychotics). Concurrent use with MAO inhibitors is contraindicated. May cause sustained increase in blood pressure or tachycardia; dose related and increases are generally modest (12-15 mm Hg diastolic). Control pre-existing hypertension prior to initiation of venlafaxine. Use caution in patients with recent history of MI, unstable heart disease, or hyperthyroidism; may cause increase in anxiety, nervousness, insomnia; may cause weight loss (use with caution in patients where weight loss is undesirable); may cause increases in serum cholesterol. Use caution with hepatic or renal impairment; dosage adjustments recommended. May cause hyponatremia/SIADH (elderly at increased risk); volume depletion (diuretics may increase risk).

May impair platelet aggregation resulting in increased risk of bleeding events, particularly if used concomitantly with aspirin or NSAIDs. Bleeding related to SSRI or SNRI use has been reported to range from relatively minor bruising and epistaxis to life-threatening hemorrhage. Interstitial lung disease and eosinophilic pneumonia have been rarely reported; may present as progressive dyspnea, cough, and/or chest pain. Prompt evaluation and possible discontinuation of therapy may be necessary. Venlafaxine may increase the risks associated with electroconvulsive therapy. Use cautiously in patients with a history of seizures. The risks of cognitive or motor impairment, as well as the potential for anticholinergic effects are very low. May cause or exacerbate sexual dysfunction.

Abrupt discontinuation or dosage reduction after extended (≥6 weeks) therapy may lead to agitation, dysphoria, nervousness, anxiety, and other symptoms. When discontinuing therapy, dosage should be tapered gradually over at least a 2-week period. If intolerable symptoms occur following a decrease in dosage or upon discontinuation of therapy, then resuming the previous dose with a more gradual taper should be considered. Use caution in patients with increased intraocular pressure or at risk of acute narrow-angle glaucoma.

Drug Interactions

Metabolism/Transport Effects Substrate of CYP2C9 (minor), 2C19 (minor), 2D6 (major), 3A4 (major); **Inhibits** CYP2B6 (weak), 2D6 (weak), 3A4 (weak)

Avoid Concomitant Use

Avoid concomitant use of Venlafaxine with any of the following: Iobenguane I 123; MAO Inhibitors; Methylene Blue; Sibutramine

Decreased Effect

Venlafaxine may decrease the levels/effects of: Alpha2-Agonists; Indinavir; Iobenguane I 123

The levels/effects of Venlafaxine may be decreased by: CYP3A4 Inducers (Strong); Deferasirox; Peginterferon Alfa-2b

Increased Effect/Toxicity

Venlafaxine may increase the levels/effects of: Alcohol (Ethyl); Alpha-/Beta-Agonists; Aspirin; CNS Depressants; Methotrimeprazine; Methylene Blue; NSAID (Nonselective); Serotonin Modulators; TraZODone; Vitamin K Antagonists

The levels/effects of Venlafaxine may be increased by: Conivaptan; CYP2D6 Inhibitors (Moderate); CYP2D6 Inhibitors (Strong); CYP3A4 Inhibitors (Moderate); CYP3A4 Inhibitors (Strong); Darunavir; Dasatinib; Droperidol; MAO Inhibitors; Methotrimeprazine; Metoclopramide; Propafenone; Sibutramine; Voriconazole

Nutritional/Ethanol Interactions

Ethanol: Avoid ethanol (may increase CNS effects).

Herb/Nutraceutical: Avoid valerian, St John's wort, SAMe, kava kava, tryptophan (may increase risk of serotonin syndrome and/or excessive sedation).

Lab Interactions May interfere with urine detection of PCP (false-positive).

Adverse Reactions Note: Actual frequency may be dependant upon formulation and/or indication

>10%:

Central nervous system: Headache (25% to 38%), somnolence (12% to 26%), dizziness (11% to 24%), insomnia (15% to 24%), nervousness (6% to 21%), anxiety (2% to 11%),

Gastrointestinal: Nausea (21% to 58%), xerostomia (12% to 22%), anorexia (8% to 17%), constipation (8% to 15%)

Genitourinary: Abnormal ejaculation/orgasm (2% to 19%)

Neuromuscular & skeletal: Weakness (8% to 19%)

Miscellaneous: Diaphoresis (7% to 19%)

1% to 10%:

Cardiovascular: Vasodilation (2% to 6%), hypertension (dose related; 3% in patients receiving <100 mg/day, up to 13% in patients receiving >300 mg/day), palpitation (3%), tachycardia (2%), chest pain (2%), postural hypotension (1%), edema

Central nervous system: Yawning (3% to 8%), abnormal dreams (3% to 7%), chills (2% to 7%), agitation (2% to 5%), confusion (2%), abnormal thinking (2%), depersonalization (1%), depression (1% to 3%), fever, migraine, amnesia, hypoesthesia, vertigo

Dermatologic: Rash (3%), pruritus (1%), bruising

Endocrine & metabolic: Libido decreased (2% to 8%), hypercholesterolemia (5%), triglycerides increased

Gastrointestinal: Abdominal pain (8%), diarrhea (8%), vomiting (3% to 8%), dyspepsia (5% to 7%), weight loss (1% to 6%), flatulence (3% to 4%), taste perversion (2%), appetite increased, belching, weight gain

Genitourinary: Impotence (4% to 6%), urinary frequency (3%), urination impaired (2%), urinary retention (1%), metrorrhagia, prostatic disorder, vaginitis

Neuromuscular & skeletal: Tremor (1% to 10%), hypertonia (3%), paresthesia (2% to 3%), twitching (1% to 3%), arthralgia, neck pain, trismus

Ocular: Accommodation abnormal (6% to 9%), abnormal or blurred vision (4% to 6%), mydriasis (2%)

Otic: Tinnitus (2%)

Renal: Albuminuria

Respiratory: Pharyngitis (7%), sinusitis (2%), bronchitis, cough increased, dyspnea

Miscellaneous: Infection (6%), flu-like syndrome (2%), trauma (2%)

Pharmacodynamics/Kinetics

Absorption Oral: ≥92%; food has no significant effect on absorption or formation of active metabolite

Bioavailability Oral: ~45%

Time to Peak

Immediate release: Venlafaxine: 2 hours, ODV: 3 hours

Extended release: Venlafaxine: 5.5 hours, ODV: 9 hours

Protein Binding Venlafaxine 27% ± 2%, ODV 30% ± 12%

Half-Life Elimination Venlafaxine: 5 ± 2 hours; ODV: 11 ± 2 hours; prolonged with cirrhosis (venlafaxine: ~30%, ODV: ~60%), renal impairment (venlafaxine: ~50%, ODV: ~40%), and during dialysis (venlafaxine: ~180%, ODV: ~142%)

Metabolism Hepatic via CYP2D6 to active metabolite, O-desmethylvenlafaxine (ODV); other metabolites include N-desmethylvenlafaxine and N,O-didesmethylvenlafaxine

Excretion Urine (~87%; 5% of total dose as unchanged drug; 29% of total dose as unconjugated ODV; 26% of total dose as conjugated ODV; 27% of total dose as minor inactive metabolites)

Available Dosage Forms

Capsule, extended release, oral: 37.5 mg, 75 mg, 150 mg

Effexor XR®: 37.5 mg, 75 mg, 150 mg

Tablet, oral: 25 mg, 37.5 mg, 50 mg, 75 mg, 100 mg

Effexor®: 50 mg

Tablet, extended release, oral: 37.5 mg, 75 mg, 150 mg, 225 mg

Dosing

Adult

Depression: Oral:

Immediate-release tablets: Initial: 75 mg/day, administered in 2 or 3 divided doses; may increase in ≤75 mg/day increments at intervals of ≥4 days as tolerated (maximum daily dose: 225-375 mg)

Extended-release capsules or tablets: Initial: 37.5-75 mg once daily; in patients who are initiated at 37.5 mg once daily, may increase to 75 mg once daily after 4-7 days; dose may then be increased by ≤75 mg/day increments at intervals of ≥4 days as tolerated (maximum daily dose: 225 mg)

Generalized anxiety disorder: Oral: *Extended-release capsules:* Initial: 37.5-75 mg once daily; in patients who are initiated at 37.5 mg once daily, may increase to 75 mg once daily after 4-7 days; may then be increased by ≤75 mg/day increments at intervals of ≥4 days as tolerated (maximum daily dose: 225 mg)

Panic disorder: Oral: *Extended-release capsules:* Initial: 37.5 mg once daily for 1 week; may increase to 75 mg once daily after 7 days, may then be increased by ≤75 mg/day increments at intervals of ≥7 days (maximum daily dose: 225 mg).

Social anxiety disorder: Oral: *Extended-release capsules or tablets:* 75 mg once daily (maximum daily dose: 75 mg); no evidence that doses >75 mg/day offer any additional benefit

Obsessive-compulsive disorder (unlabeled use): Oral: Titrate to usual dosage range of 150-300 mg/day; however, doses up to 375 mg/day have been used; response may be seen in 4 weeks (Phelps, 2005)

Neuropathic pain (unlabeled use): Oral: Dosages evaluated varied considerably based on etiology of chronic pain, but efficacy has been shown for many conditions in the range of 75-225 mg/day; onset of relief may occur in 1-2 weeks, or take up to 6 weeks for full benefit (Grothe, 2004).

Hot flashes (unlabeled use): Oral: Doses of 37.5-75 mg/day have demonstrated significant improvement of vasomotor symptoms after 4-8 weeks of treatment; in one study, doses >75 mg/day offered no additional benefit (Evans, 2005; Loprinzi, 2000); however, higher doses (225 mg/day) may be beneficial in patients with perimenopausal depression.

Attention-deficit disorder (unlabeled use): Oral: Initial: Doses vary between 18.75 to 75 mg/day; may increase after 4 weeks to 150 mg/day; if tolerated, doses up to 225 mg/day have been used (Maidment, 2003)

Post-traumatic stress disorder (PTSD) (unlabeled use): Oral: *Extended release formulation:* 37.5-300 mg/day (Bandelow, 2008; Benedek, 2009)

Note: When discontinuing this medication after more than 1 week of treatment, it is generally recommended that the dose be tapered. If venlafaxine is used for 6 weeks or longer, the dose should be tapered over 2 weeks when discontinuing its use.

Geriatric Refer to adult dosing. No specific recommendations for elderly, but may be best to start lower at 25-50 mg twice daily and increase as tolerated by 25 mg/dose. Extended-release formulation: 37.5 mg once daily, increase by 37.5 mg every 4-7 days as tolerated

Alzheimer's dementia-related depression (unlabeled use; Rabins, 2007):

Immediate-release tablets: Initial: 25 mg/day; may increase at weekly intervals to maximum of 375 mg/day in divided doses

Extended-release capsules: Initial: 37.5 mg/day; may increase at weekly intervals to maximum of 225 mg/day

Pediatric Attention-deficit/hyperactivity disorder (unlabeled use; Olvera, 1996): Children and Adolescents: Oral: Initial: 12.5 mg/day

Children <40 kg: Increase by 12.5 mg/week to maximum of 50 mg/day in 2 divided doses

Children ≥40 kg: Increase by 25 mg/week to maximum of 75 mg/day in 3 divided doses.

Mean dose: 60 mg or 1.4 mg/kg administered in 2-3 divided doses

Renal Impairment

GFR: 10-70 mL/minute: Reduce total daily dose by 25% to 50%

Hemodialysis: Reduce total daily dose by 50%

Hepatic Impairment Mild-to-moderate hepatic impairment: Reduce total daily dose by 50%; further reductions may be necessary in some patients

Administration

Oral Administer with food.

Extended-release formulations: Swallow capsule or tablet whole; do not crush or chew. Contents of capsule may be sprinkled on a spoonful of applesauce and swallowed immediately without chewing; followed with a glass of water to ensure complete swallowing of the pellets.

Stability

Storage Store at controlled room temperature of 20°C to 25°C (68°F to 77°F).

Monitoring and Teaching Issues

Laboratory Monitoring Cholesterol

Physical Assessment Monitor blood pressure and weight/height at beginning of therapy and periodically throughout. Observe for clinical worsening, suicide ideation, or unusual behavior changes, especially during the initial few months of therapy or during dosage changes. Taper dosage when discontinuing.

Patient Education It may take 2-3 weeks to achieve desired results. Take with food. Extended release capsules should be swallowed whole; do not crush or chew. Alternatively, contents may be emptied onto a spoonful of applesauce and swallowed without chewing. Avoid alcohol. Maintain adequate hydration unless instructed to restrict fluid intake. You may experience excess drowsiness or insomnia, lightheadedness, dizziness, blurred vision, headache, nausea, vomiting, anorexia, altered taste, dry mouth, constipation, diarrhea, postural hypotension, urinary retention, or sexual dysfunction (reversible). Report persistent CNS effects (eg, insomnia, restlessness, fatigue, anxiety, abnormal thoughts, suicide ideation, confusion, personality changes, impaired cognitive function), muscle cramping or tremors, chest pain, palpitations, rapid heartbeat, swelling of extremities, severe dizziness, unresolved urinary retention, vision changes or eye pain, hearing changes or ringing in ears, skin rash or irritation, or worsening of condition.

Dietary Considerations Should be taken with food.

Geriatric Considerations Venlafaxine's low anticholinergic activity, minimal sedation, and hypotension properties makes this a valuable antidepressant in treating elderly with depression or anxiety disorders. No dose adjustment is necessary for age alone; adjust dose for renal function in the elderly. The elderly are more prone to SSRI/SNRI-induced hyponatremia.

Breast-Feeding Considerations Venlafaxine and ODV are found in human milk. Low concentrations of ODV have been found in the serum of nursing infants whose mothers are taking venlafaxine; venlafaxine has also been detected in some infants. Adverse events have not been observed; however, it is recommended to monitor the infant for adverse events if the decision to breast-feed has been made. The long-term effects on neurobehavior have not been studied, thus one should prescribe venlafaxine to a mother who is breast-feeding only when the benefits outweigh the potential risks. The manufacturer does not recommend breast-feeding during therapy.

Pregnancy Considerations Venlafaxine is classified as pregnancy category C due to adverse effects observed in animal studies. Venlafaxine and its active metabolite ODV cross the human placenta. Neonatal seizures and neonatal abstinence syndrome have been noted in case reports following maternal use of venlafaxine during pregnancy. Nonteratogenic effects in the newborn following SSRI/SNRI exposure late in the third trimester include respiratory distress, cyanosis, apnea, seizures, temperature instability, feeding difficulty, vomiting, hypoglycemia, hyper- or hypotonia, hyper-reflexia, jitteriness, irritability, constant crying, and tremor. The long-term effects on neurobehavior have not been studied.

Due to pregnancy-induced physiologic changes, some pharmacokinetic parameters of venlafaxine may be altered. Women should be monitored for decreased efficacy. Women treated for major depression and who are euthymic prior to pregnancy are more likely to experience a relapse when medication is discontinued as compared to pregnant women who continue taking antidepressant medications. The ACOG recommends that therapy with SSRIs or SNRIs during pregnancy be individualized; treatment of depression during pregnancy should incorporate the clinical expertise of the mental health clinician, obstetrician, primary healthcare provider, and pediatrician. If treatment during pregnancy is required, consider tapering therapy during the third trimester in order to prevent withdrawal symptoms in the infant. If this is done and the woman is considered to be at risk of relapse from her major depressive disorder, the medication can be restarted following delivery, although the dose should be readjusted to that required before pregnancy. Treatment algorithms have been developed by the ACOG and the APA for the management of depression in women prior to conception and during pregnancy (Yonkers, 2009).

Related Information

Antidepressant Agents *on page 1982*

◆ **Venofer®** *see* Iron Sucrose *on page 1022*
◆ **Ventolin® HFA** *see* Albuterol *on page 58*
◆ **VePesid** *see* Etoposide *on page 712*
◆ **Veramyst®** *see* Fluticasone (Nasal) *on page 802*

Verapamil (ver AP a mil)

U.S. Brand Names Calan®; Calan® SR; Covera-HS®; Isoptin® SR; Verelan®; Verelan® PM

Index Terms Iproveratril Hydrochloride; Verapamil Hydrochloride

Generic Availability (U.S.) Yes: Excludes caplet (sustained release) and tablet (extended release, controlled onset)

Pharmacologic Category Antiarrhythmic Agent, Class IV; Calcium Channel Blocker; Calcium Channel Blocker, Nondihydropyridine

Medication Safety Issues

Sound-alike/look-alike issues:

Calan® may be confused with Colace®, diltiazem
Covera-HS® may be confused with Provera®
Isoptin® may be confused with Isopto® Tears
Verelan® may be confused with Virilon®, Voltaren®

High alert medication: The Institute for Safe Medication Practices (ISMP) includes this medication (I.V. formulation) among its list of drug classes which have a heightened risk of causing significant patient harm when used in error.

Significant differences exist between oral and I.V. dosing. Use caution when converting from one route of administration to another.

International issues:

Dilacor [Brazil] may be confused with Dilacor XR brand name for diltiazem [U.S.]

Pregnancy Risk Factor C

Lactation Enters breast milk/not recommended (AAP considers "compatible"; AAP 2001 update pending)

Use

Oral: Treatment of hypertension; angina pectoris (vasospastic, chronic stable, unstable) (Calan®, Covera-HS®); supraventricular tachyarrhythmia (PSVT, atrial fibrillation/flutter [rate control])

I.V.: Supraventricular tachyarrhythmia (PSVT, atrial fibrillation/flutter [rate control])

Unlabeled/Investigational Use Migraine; hypertrophic cardiomyopathy; bipolar disorder (manic manifestations)

Mechanism of Action/Effect Produces relaxation of coronary vascular smooth muscle and coronary vasodilation. Increases myocardial oxygen delivery in patients with vasospastic (Prinzmetal's) angina. Slows automaticity and conduction of AV node.

Contraindications Hypersensitivity to verapamil or any component of the formulation; severe left ventricular dysfunction; hypotension (systolic pressure <90 mm Hg) or cardiogenic shock; sick sinus syndrome (except in patients with a functioning artificial ventricular pacemaker); second- or third-degree AV block (except in patients with a functioning artificial ventricular pacemaker); atrial flutter or fibrillation and an accessory bypass tract (Wolff-Parkinson-White [WPW] syndrome, Lown-Ganong-Levine syndrome)

I.V.: Additional contraindications include concurrent use of I.V. beta-blocking agents; ventricular tachycardia

Warnings/Precautions Avoid use in heart failure; can exacerbate condition; use is contraindicated in severe left ventricular dysfunction. Symptomatic hypotension with or without syncope can rarely occur; blood pressure must be lowered at a rate appropriate for the patient's clinical condition. Rare increases in hepatic enzymes can be observed. Can cause first-degree AV block or sinus bradycardia; use is contraindicated in patients with sick sinus syndrome, second- or third-degree AV block (except in patients with a functioning artificial pacemaker), or an accessory bypass tract (eg, WPW syndrome). Other conduction abnormalities are rare. Considered contraindicated in patients with wide complex tachycardias unless known to be supraventricular in origin; severe hypotension likely to occur upon administration (ACLS, 2010). Use caution when using verapamil together with a beta-blocker. Administration of I.V. verapamil and an I.V. beta-blocker within a few hours of each other may result in asystole and should be avoided; simultaneous administration is contraindicated. Use with other agents known to reduce SA node function and/or AV nodal conduction (eg, digoxin) or reduce sympathetic outflow (eg, clonidine) may increase the risk of serious bradycardia. Verapamil significantly increases digoxin serum concentrations; adjust digoxin dose. Use with caution in patients with hypertrophic cardiomyopathy with outflow tract obstruction (especially those with resting outflow obstruction and severe limiting symptoms); may be used in patients who cannot tolerate beta-blockade.

Decreased neuromuscular transmission has been reported with verapamil; use with caution in patients with attenuated neuromuscular transmission (Duchenne's muscular dystrophy, myasthenia gravis); dosage reduction may be required. Use with caution in renal impairment; monitor hemodynamics and possibly ECG if severe impairment, particularly if concomitant hepatic impairment. Use with caution in patients with hepatic impairment; dosage reduction may be required; monitor hemodynamics and possibly ECG if severe impairment. May prolong recovery from nondepolarizing neuromuscular-blocking agents. Use Covera-HS® (extended-release delivery system) with caution in patients with severe GI narrowing. In patients with extremely short GI transit times (eg, <7 hours), dosage adjustment may be required; inadequate pharmacokinetic data. I.V. use for SVT for is not recommended in infants; use with caution in children as myocardial depression/hypotension may occur.

Drug Interactions

Metabolism/Transport Effects Substrate of CYP1A2 (minor), CYP2B6 (minor), CYP2C9 (minor), CYP2C18 (minor), CYP2E1 (minor), CYP3A4 (major), P-glycoprotein; **Inhibits** CYP1A2 (weak), CYP2C9 (weak), CYP2D6 (weak), CYP3A4 (moderate), P-glycoprotein

Avoid Concomitant Use

Avoid concomitant use of Verapamil with any of the following: Disopyramide; Dofetilide; Tolvaptan; Topotecan

Decreased Effect

Verapamil may decrease the levels/effects of: Clopidogrel

The levels/effects of Verapamil may be decreased by: Barbiturates; Calcium Salts; CarBAMazepine; CYP3A4 Inducers (Strong); Deferasirox; Herbs (CYP3A4 Inducers); Herbs (Hypertensive Properties); Methylphenidate; Nafcillin; P-Glycoprotein Inducers; Rifamycin Derivatives; Yohimbine

Increased Effect/Toxicity

Verapamil may increase the levels/effects of: Alcohol (Ethyl); Aliskiren; Amifostine; Amiodarone; Antihypertensives; Atorvastatin; Benzodiazepines (metabolized by oxidation); Beta-Blockers; BusPIRone; Calcium Channel Blockers (Dihydropyridine); CarBAMazepine; Cardiac Glycosides; Colchicine; Corticosteroids (Systemic); CycloSPORINE; CycloSPORINE (Systemic); CYP3A4 Substrates; Dabigatran Etexilate; Disopyramide; Dofetilide; Dronedarone; Eletriptan; Eplerenone; Everolimus; Fexofenadine; Fingolimod; Flecainide; Halofantrine; Hypotensive Agents; Lithium; Lovastatin; Lurasidone; Magnesium Salts; Midodrine; Neuromuscular-Blocking Agents (Nondepolarizing); Nitroprusside; P-Glycoprotein Substrates; Phenytoin; Pimecrolimus; QuiNIDine; Ranolazine; Red Yeast Rice; RisperiDONE; RiTUXimab; Rivaroxaban; Salicylates; Salmeterol; Saxagliptin; Simvastatin; Tacrolimus; Tacrolimus (Systemic); Tacrolimus (Topical); Tolvaptan; Topotecan; Vilazodone

The levels/effects of Verapamil may be increased by: Alpha1-Blockers; Anilidopiperidine Opioids; Antifungal Agents (Azole Derivatives, Systemic); Atorvastatin; Calcium Channel Blockers (Dihydropyridine); Cimetidine; Conivaptan; CycloSPORINE; CycloSPORINE (Systemic); CYP3A4 Inhibitors (Moderate); CYP3A4 Inhibitors (Strong); Dasatinib; Diazoxide;

Dronedarone; Fluconazole; Grapefruit Juice; Herbs (Hypotensive Properties); Macrolide Antibiotics; Magnesium Salts; MAO Inhibitors; Pentoxifylline; P-Glycoprotein Inhibitors; Phosphodiesterase 5 Inhibitors; Prostacyclin Analogues; Protease Inhibitors; QuiNIDine; Telithromycin

Nutritional/Ethanol Interactions

Ethanol: Avoid or limit ethanol (may increase ethanol levels).

Food: Grapefruit juice may increase the serum concentration of verapamil; use with caution and monitor for increased verapamil effects.

Herb/Nutraceutical: St John's wort may decrease levels. Avoid herbs with hypertensive properties (bayberry, blue cohosh, cayenne, ephedra, ginger, ginseng [American], kola, licorice); may diminish the antihypertensive effect of verapamil. Avoid herbs with hypotensive properties (black cohosh, California poppy, coleus, golden seal, hawthorn, mistletoe, periwinkle, quinine, shepherd's purse); may enhance the hypotensive effect of verapamil.

Lab Interactions May interfere with urine detection of methadone (false-positive).

Adverse Reactions

>10%:

Central nervous system: Headache (1% to 12%)

Gastrointestinal: Gingival hyperplasia (≤19%), constipation (7% to 12%)

1% to 10%:

Cardiovascular: Peripheral edema (1% to 4%), hypotension (3%), CHF/pulmonary edema (2%), AV block (1% to 2%), bradycardia (HR <50 bpm: 1%), flushing (1%)

Central nervous system: Fatigue (2% to 5%), dizziness (1% to 5%), lethargy (3%), pain (2%), sleep disturbance (1%)

Dermatologic: Rash (1% to 2%)

Gastrointestinal: Dyspepsia (3%), nausea (1% to 3%), diarrhea (2%)

Hepatic: Liver enzymes increased (1%)

Neuromuscular & skeletal: Myalgia (1%), paresthesia (1%)

Respiratory: Dyspnea (1%)

Miscellaneous: Flu-like syndrome (4%)

Pharmacodynamics/Kinetics

Onset of Action Oral (immediate release tablets): Peak effect: 1-2 hours; I.V.: Peak effect: 1-5 minutes

Duration of Action Oral: Immediate release tablets: 6-8 hours; I.V.: 10-20 minutes

Absorption Well absorbed

Bioavailability Oral: 20% to 35%

Time to Peak Serum: Oral:

Immediate release: 1-2 hours

Extended release (Covera-HS®, Verelan PM®): ~11 hours, drug release delayed ~4-5 hours

Sustained release: 5.21 hours (Calan® SR, Isoptin® SR); 7-9 hours (Verelan®)

Protein Binding ~90%

Half-Life Elimination Infants: 4.4-6.9 hours; Adults: Single dose: 3-7 hours, Multiple doses: 4.5-12 hours; severe hepatic impairment: 14-16 hours

Metabolism Hepatic (extensive first-pass effect) via multiple CYP isoenzymes; primary metabolite is norverapamil (20% pharmacologic activity of verapamil)

Excretion Urine (70% as metabolites, 3% to 4% as unchanged drug); feces (16%)

Available Dosage Forms

Caplet, sustained release, oral:

Calan® SR: 120 mg, 180 mg, 240 mg

Capsule, extended release, oral: 120 mg, 180 mg, 240 mg

Capsule, extended release, controlled onset, oral: 100 mg, 200 mg, 300 mg

Verelan® PM: 100 mg, 200 mg, 300 mg

Capsule, sustained release, oral: 120 mg, 180 mg, 240 mg, 360 mg

Verelan®: 120 mg, 180 mg, 240 mg, 360 mg

Injection, solution: 2.5 mg/mL (2 mL, 4 mL)

Tablet, oral: 40 mg, 80 mg, 120 mg

Calan®: 80 mg, 120 mg

Tablet, extended release, oral: 120 mg, 180 mg, 240 mg

Tablet, extended release, controlled onset, oral:

Covera-HS®: 180 mg, 240 mg

Tablet, sustained release, oral: 240 mg

Isoptin® SR: 120 mg, 180 mg, 240 mg

Dosing

Adult

Angina: Oral: **Note:** When switching from immediate-release to extended/sustained release formulations, the total daily dose remains the same unless formulation strength does not allow for equal conversion.

Immediate release: Initial: 80-120 mg 3 times/day (elderly or small stature: 40 mg 3 times/day); Usual dose range (Gibbons, 2002): 80-160 mg 3 times/day

Extended release (Covera-HS®): Initial: 180 mg once daily at bedtime; if inadequate response, may increase dose at weekly intervals to 240 mg once daily, then 360 mg once daily, then 480 mg once daily; maximum dose: 480 mg/day

Chronic atrial fibrillation (rate-control), PSVT prophylaxis: Oral: Immediate release: 240-480 mg/day in 3-4 divided doses; Usual dose range (Fuster, 2006): 120-360 mg/day in divided doses

Hypertension: Oral: **Note:** When switching from immediate-release to extended/sustained release formulations, the total daily dose remains the same unless formulation strength does not allow for equal conversion.

Immediate release: 80 mg 3 times/day; usual dose range (JNC 7): 80-320 mg/day in 2 divided doses

Sustained release: Usual dose range (JNC 7): 120-480 mg/day in 1-2 divided doses; **Note:** There is no evidence of additional benefit with doses >360 mg/day.

Calan® SR, Isoptin® SR: Initial: 180 mg once daily in the morning (elderly or small stature: 120 mg/day); if inadequate response, may increase dose at weekly intervals to 240 mg once daily, then 180 mg twice daily (or 240 mg in the morning followed by 120 mg in the evening); maximum dose: 240 mg twice daily.

Verelan®: Initial: 180 mg once daily in the morning (elderly or small stature: 120 mg/day); if inadequate response, may increase dose at weekly intervals to 240 mg once daily, then 360 mg once daily, then 480 mg once daily; maximum dose: 480 mg/day

Extended release: Usual dose range (JNC 7): 120-360 mg once daily (once-daily dosing is recommended at bedtime)

Covera-HS®: Initial: 180 mg once daily at bedtime; if inadequate response, may increase dose at weekly intervals to 240 mg once daily, then 360 mg once daily, then 480 mg once daily; maximum dose: 480 mg/day

Verelan® PM: Initial: 200 mg once daily at bedtime (elderly or small stature: 100 mg/day); if inadequate response, may increase dose at weekly intervals to 300 mg once daily, then 400 mg once daily; maximum dose: 400 mg/day

SVT (ACLS, 2010): I.V.: 2.5-5 mg over 2 minutes; second dose of 5-10 mg (~0.15 mg/kg) may be given 15-30 minutes after the initial dose if patient tolerates, but does not respond to initial dose; maximum total dose: 20-30 mg

Geriatric

Immediate release: Oral: 120-480 mg/24 hours divided 2-4 times/day

Extended release (Verelan PM®): Oral: Initial: 100 mg once daily at bedtime

Sustained release: Oral: 120 mg/day; adjust dose after 24 hours by increases of 120 mg/day. When switching from immediate release forms, total daily dose may remain the same. Controlled onset: initiate therapy with 180 mg in the evening; titrate upward as needed to obtain desired response and avoiding adverse effects.

Pediatric SVT: Note: Verapamil is no longer included in the Pediatric Advanced Life Support (PALS) tachyarrhythmia algorithm.

Children: 1-15 years: I.V.: 0.1-0.3 mg/kg/dose over 2 minutes; maximum: 5 mg/dose, may repeat dose in 30 minutes if inadequate response; maximum for second dose: 10 mg

Renal Impairment Manufacturer recommends caution and additional ECG monitoring in patients with renal insufficiency. The manufacturer of Verelan PM® recommends an initial dose of 100 mg/day at bedtime. **Note:** A multiple dose study in adults suggests reduced renal clearance of verapamil and its metabolite (norverapamil) with advanced renal failure (Storstein, 1984). Additionally, several clinical papers report adverse effects of verapamil in patients with chronic renal failure receiving recommended doses of verapamil (Pritza, 1991; Váquez, 1996). In contrast, a number of single dose studies show no difference in verapamil (or norverapamil metabolite) disposition between chronic renal failure and control patients (Beyerlein, 1990; Hanyok, 1988; Mooy, 1985; Zachariah, 1991).

Dialysis: Not removed by hemodialysis (Mooy, 1985); supplemental dose is not necessary.

Hepatic Impairment In cirrhosis, reduce dose to 20% and 50% of normal for oral and intravenous administration, respectively, and monitor ECG (Somogyi, 1981). The manufacturer of Verelan PM® recommends an initial adult dose of 100 mg/day at bedtime. The manufacturers of Calan®, Calan® SR, Covera-HS®, Isoptin® SR, and Verelan® recommend giving 30% of the normal dose to patients with severe hepatic impairment.

Administration

Oral Do not crush or chew sustained or extended release products.

Calan® SR, Isoptin® SR: Administer with food.

Verelan®, Verelan® PM: Capsules may be opened and the contents sprinkled on 1 tablespoonful of applesauce, then swallowed immediately without chewing. Do not subdivide contents of capsules.

I.V. Administer over 2 minutes (over 3 minutes in older patients [ACLS, 2010])

Stability

Storage Store at controlled room temperature of 15°C to 30°C (59°F to 86°F). Protect from light.

Monitoring and Teaching Issues

Laboratory Monitoring Periodic liver function tests

Physical Assessment I.V. requires use of infusion pump and continuous cardiac and hemodynamic monitoring. Monitor gums for gingival hyperplasia. Encourage good oral hygiene. Refer to dentist if indicated.

Patient Education Oral: Do not crush or chew sustained or extended release forms. Avoid grapefruit juice; avoid (or limit) alcohol and caffeine. Maintain good oral hygiene to avoid gum disease. You may experience dizziness or lightheadedness, nausea, vomiting, constipation, or diarrhea. Report chest pain, palpitations, or irregular heartbeat; unusual cough, respiratory difficulty, or swelling of extremities (feet/ankles); muscle tremors or weakness; confusion or acute lethargy; or skin irritation or rash. **Pregnancy precaution:** Inform prescriber if you are or intend to become pregnant.

Dietary Considerations Calan® SR and Isoptin® SR products may be taken with food or milk, other formulations may be administered without regard to meals; sprinkling contents of Verelan® or Verelan® PM capsule onto applesauce does not affect oral absorption.

Geriatric Considerations Elderly may experience a greater hypotensive response. Constipation may be more of a problem in the elderly. Calcium channel blockers are no more effective in the elderly than other therapies; however, they do not cause significant CNS effects which is an advantage over some antihypertensive agents. Generic verapamil products which are bioequivalent in young adults may not be bioequivalent in the elderly; use generics cautiously.

Breast-Feeding Considerations Crosses into breast milk; manufacturer recommends to discontinue breast-feeding while taking verapamil.

Pregnancy Considerations In some animal reproduction studies verapamil has been shown to cause fetal harm; adverse maternal effects were also observed. Verapamil crosses the placenta. Although verapamil is not considered a major human teratogen, use during pregnancy may cause adverse fetal effects (bradycardia, heart block, hypotension).

Related Information

Antiarrhythmic Drugs *on page 1978*
Calcium Channel Blockers *on page 1993*

- ◆ **Verapamil and Trandolapril** *see* Trandolapril and Verapamil *on page 1802*
- ◆ **Verapamil Hydrochloride** *see* Verapamil *on page 1858*
- ◆ **Veregen™** *see* Sinecatechins *on page 1647*
- ◆ **Verelan®** *see* Verapamil *on page 1858*
- ◆ **Verelan® PM** *see* Verapamil *on page 1858*
- ◆ **Veripred™ 20** *see* PrednisoLONE (Systemic) *on page 1497*
- ◆ **Vermox** *see* Mebendazole *on page 1152*
- ◆ **Versed** *see* Midazolam *on page 1225*
- ◆ **VESIcare®** *see* Solifenacin *on page 1662*
- ◆ **VFEND®** *see* Voriconazole *on page 1871*
- ◆ **Viagra®** *see* Sildenafil *on page 1641*
- ◆ **Vibramycin®** *see* Doxycycline *on page 586*
- ◆ ***Vibrio cholera* and Enterotoxigenic *Escherichia coli* Vaccine** *see* Travelers' Diarrhea and Cholera Vaccine *on page 1806*
- ◆ **Vicks® Casero™ Chest Congestion Relief [OTC]** *see* GuaiFENesin *on page 890*
- ◆ **Vicks® DayQuil® Mucus Control [OTC]** *see* GuaiFENesin *on page 890*
- ◆ **Vicks® Sinex® VapoSpray™ 4 Hour Decongestant [OTC]** *see* Phenylephrine (Nasal) *on page 1451*
- ◆ **Vicodin®** *see* Hydrocodone and Acetaminophen *on page 915*
- ◆ **Vicodin® ES** *see* Hydrocodone and Acetaminophen *on page 915*
- ◆ **Vicodin® HP** *see* Hydrocodone and Acetaminophen *on page 915*
- ◆ **Vicoprofen®** *see* Hydrocodone and Ibuprofen *on page 916*
- ◆ **Victoza®** *see* Liraglutide *on page 1116*
- ◆ **Vidaza®** *see* AzaCITIDine *on page 175*
- ◆ **Videx®** *see* Didanosine *on page 524*
- ◆ **Videx® EC** *see* Didanosine *on page 524*
- ◆ **Vigamox®** *see* Moxifloxacin (Ophthalmic) *on page 1267*
- ◆ **Vimovo™** *see* Naproxen and Esomeprazole *on page 1290*
- ◆ **Vimpat®** *see* Lacosamide *on page 1051*

VinBLAStine (vin BLAS teen)

Index Terms Velban; Vinblastine Sulfate; Vincaleukoblastine; VLB

Generic Availability (U.S.) Yes

Pharmacologic Category Antineoplastic Agent, Natural Source (Plant) Derivative; Antineoplastic Agent, Vinca Alkaloid

Medication Safety Issues

Sound-alike/look-alike issues:

VinBLAStine may be confused with vinCRIStine, vinorelbine

High alert medication: The Institute for Safe Medication Practices (ISMP) includes this medication among its list of drug classes which have a heightened risk of causing significant patient harm when used in error.

Note: Must be dispensed in overwrap which bears the statement **"Do not remove covering until the moment of injection. Fatal if given intrathecally. For I.V. use only."** Syringes should be labeled: **"Fatal if given intrathecally. For I.V. use only."**

Pregnancy Risk Factor D

Lactation Excretion in breast milk unknown/not recommended

Use Treatment of Hodgkin's and non-Hodgkin's lymphoma; testicular cancer; breast cancer; mycosis fungoides; Kaposi's sarcoma; histiocytosis (Letterer-Siwe disease); choriocarcinoma

Unlabeled/Investigational Use Treatment of bladder cancer, melanoma, nonsmall cell lung cancer (NSCLC), ovarian cancer, soft tissue sarcoma (desmoid tumors)

Mechanism of Action/Effect Vinblastine arrests cell cycle growth in metaphase. Also inhibits RNA synthesis and amino acid metabolism resulting in inhibition of metabolic pathways and cell growth.

Contraindications Significant granulocytopenia; presence of bacterial infection; I.T. administration is contraindicated (may result in death)

Warnings/Precautions Hazardous agent - use appropriate precautions for handling and disposal. **[U.S. Boxed Warning]: For I.V. use only. Intrathecal administration may result in death.** Must be dispensed in overwrap which bears the statement **"Do not remove covering until the moment of injection. Fatal if given intrathecally. For I.V. use only." [U.S. Boxed Warning]: Vinblastine is a moderate vesicant; avoid extravasation. Individuals administering should be experienced in vinblastine administration;** assure proper needle or catheter placement prior to administration. Leukopenia is common; granulocytopenia may be severe with higher doses. Leukopenia may be more pronounced in cachectic patients and patients with skin ulceration. Thrombocytopenia and anemia may occur rarely.

Use with caution in patients with hepatic impairment; toxicity may be increased; may require dosage modification. Neurotoxicity is rare at clinical doses; may occur with high doses (symptoms are similar to vincristine toxicity, including peripheral neuropathy, loss of deep tendon reflexes, headache, weakness, urinary retention, and GI symptoms). May rarely cause disabling neurotoxicity (usually reversible). Itraconazole may decrease the metabolism of vinblastine via CYP3A4 inhibition and may increase the effects of vinblastine via P-glycoprotein effects; severe myelosuppression and neurotoxicity may occur. Acute shortness of breath and severe bronchospasm have been reported, most often in association with concurrent administration of mitomycin; may occur within minutes to several hours following vinblastine administration or up to 14 days following mitomycin administration; use caution in patients with pre-existing pulmonary disease. Use with caution in patients with ischemic heart disease. **[U.S. Boxed Warning]: Should be administered under the supervision of an experienced cancer chemotherapy physician.** Some dosage forms may contain benzyl alcohol which has been associated with "gasping syndrome" in neonates.

Drug Interactions

Metabolism/Transport Effects **Substrate** of CYP2D6 (minor), CYP3A4 (major), P-glycoprotein; **Inhibits** CYP2D6 (weak), CYP3A4 (weak); **Induces** P-glycoprotein

Avoid Concomitant Use

Avoid concomitant use of VinBLAStine with any of the following: BCG; Dabigatran Etexilate; Natalizumab; Pimecrolimus; Roflumilast; Tacrolimus (Topical); Vaccines (Live)

Decreased Effect

VinBLAStine may decrease the levels/effects of: BCG; Dabigatran Etexilate; P-Glycoprotein Substrates; Sipuleucel-T; Vaccines (Inactivated); Vaccines (Live)

The levels/effects of VinBLAStine may be decreased by: CYP3A4 Inducers (Strong); Deferasirox; Echinacea; Herbs (CYP3A4 Inducers); Peginterferon Alfa-2b; P-Glycoprotein Inducers

Increased Effect/Toxicity

VinBLAStine may increase the levels/effects of: Leflunomide; MitoMYcin; Natalizumab; Tolterodine; Vaccines (Live)

The levels/effects of VinBLAStine may be increased by: Conivaptan; CYP3A4 Inhibitors (Moderate); CYP3A4 Inhibitors (Strong); Dasatinib; Denosumab; Itraconazole; Lopinavir; Macrolide Antibiotics; MAO Inhibitors; P-Glycoprotein Inhibitors; Pimecrolimus; Posaconazole; Ritonavir; Roflumilast; Tacrolimus (Topical); Trastuzumab; Voriconazole

Nutritional/Ethanol Interactions Herb/Nutraceutical: Avoid St John's wort (may decrease vinblastine levels). Avoid black cohosh, dong quai in estrogen-dependent tumors.

Adverse Reactions Frequency not defined.

Common:

Cardiovascular: Hypertension
Central nervous system: Malaise
Dermatologic: Alopecia
Gastrointestinal: Constipation
Hematologic: Myelosuppression, leukopenia/granulocytopenia (nadir: 5-10 days; recovery: 7-14 days; dose-limiting toxicity)
Neuromuscular & skeletal: Bone pain, jaw pain, tumor pain

Less common:

Cardiovascular: Angina, cerebrovascular accident, coronary ischemia, ECG abnormalities, MI, Raynaud's phenomenon
Central nervous system: Depression, dizziness, headache, neurotoxicity (duration: >24 hours), seizure, vertigo
Dermatologic: Dermatitis, photosensitivity (rare), rash, skin blistering
Endocrine & metabolic: Aspermia, hyperuricemia, SIADH
Gastrointestinal: Abdominal pain, anorexia, diarrhea, gastrointestinal bleeding, hemorrhagic enterocolitis, ileus, metallic taste, nausea (mild), paralytic ileus, rectal bleeding, stomatitis, vomiting (mild)
Genitourinary: Urinary retention
Hematologic: Anemia, thrombocytopenia (recovery within a few days)
Local: Cellulitis (with extravasation), irritation, phlebitis (with extravasation), radiation recall
Neuromuscular & skeletal: Deep tendon reflex loss, myalgia, paresthesia, peripheral neuritis, weakness
Ocular: Nystagmus
Otic: Auditory damage, deafness, vestibular damage
Respiratory: Bronchospasm, dyspnea, pharyngitis

Pharmacodynamics/Kinetics

Protein Binding 99%

Half-Life Elimination Biphasic: Initial: 4 minutes; Terminal: 25 hours

Metabolism Hepatic to active metabolite

Excretion Feces (95%); urine (<1% as unchanged drug)

Available Dosage Forms

Injection, powder for reconstitution: 10 mg

Injection, solution: 1 mg/mL (10 mL)

Dosing

Adult & Geriatric Details concerning dosing in combination regimens should also be consulted. **Note:** Frequency and duration of therapy may vary by indication, concomitant combination chemotherapy and hematologic response. **For I.V. use only.**

Antineoplastic (typical dosages): I.V.: Initial: 3.7 mg/m^2; adjust dose every 7 days (based on white blood cell response) up to 5.5 mg/m^2 (second dose); 7.4 mg/m^2 (third dose); 9.25 mg/m^2 (fourth dose); and 11.1 mg/m^2 (fifth dose); do not administer more frequently than every 7 days.

Usual range: 5.5-7.4 mg/m^2 every 7 days; Maximum dose: 18.5 mg/m^2; dosage adjustment goal is to reduce white blood cell count to ~3000/mm^3

Indication-specific dosing:

Hodgkin's disease: Usual dose: 6 mg/m^2 every 2 weeks (as part of a combination chemotherapy regimen) (Bartlett, 1995; Horning, 2002)

Testicular cancer: Usual dose: 0.11 mg/kg daily for 2 days every 3 weeks (as part of a combination chemotherapy regimen) (Loehrer, 1998) **or** 6 mg/m^2/day for 2 days every 3-4 weeks (as part of a combination chemotherapy regimen) (Clemm, 1986)

Bladder cancer (unlabeled use): Usual dose: 3 mg/m^2 every 7 days for 3 out of 4 weeks (as part of combination chemotherapy) (Sternberg, 2001) **or** 3 mg/m^2 days 2, 15, and 22 of a 28-day treatment cycle (as part of a combination chemotherapy regimen) (von der Maase, 2000)

Melanoma (unlabeled used): 2 mg/m^2 days 1-4 and 22-25 of a 6-week treatment cycle (as part of a combination chemotherapy regimen) (Eton, 2002)

Nonsmall cell lung cancer (unlabeled use): 4 mg/m^2 days 1, 8, 15, 22, and 29, then every 2 weeks (as part of combination chemotherapy) (Arriagada, 2004)

Ovarian cancer (unlabeled use): 0.11 mg/kg daily for 2 days every 3 weeks (as part of a combination chemotherapy regimen) (Loehrer, 1998)

Pediatric Details concerning dosing in combination regimens should also be consulted. **Note:** Frequency and duration of therapy may vary by indication, concomitant combination chemotherapy and hematologic response. **For I.V. use only.**

Hodgkin's disease: I.V.: Initial dose: 6 mg/m^2; do not administer more frequently than every 7 days

Letterer-Siwe disease: I.V.: Initial dose: 6.5 mg/m^2; do not administer more frequently than every 7 days

Testicular cancer: I.V.: Initial dose: 3 mg/m^2; do not administer more frequently than every 7 days

Renal Impairment According to FDA-approved labeling, no adjustment is necessary in patients with renal impairment.

Hepatic Impairment

The FDA-approved labeling recommends the following guidelines: Serum bilirubin >3 mg/dL: Administer 50% of dose

The following guidelines have been used by some clinicians:

Serum bilirubin >3.1 or transaminases >3 times ULN: Avoid use (Floyd, 2006) **or**

Serum bilirubin 1.5-3 mg/dL or AST 60-180 units: Administer 50% of dose

Serum bilirubin 3-5 mg/dL: Administer 25% of dose

Serum bilirubin >5 mg/dL or AST >180 units: Avoid use

Administration

I.V. Vesicant. **Fatal if given intrathecally.** For I.V. administration only, usually as a slow (2-3 minutes) push, or a bolus (5-15 minutes) infusion; the manufacturer recommends an undiluted 1-minute infusion to prevent venous irritation/extravasation. Prolonged administration times and/or increased administration volumes may the risk of vein irritation and extravasation. Assure proper needle or catheter placement prior to administration.

Stability

Reconstitution Reconstitute lyophilized powder to a concentration of 1 mg/mL with NS or bacteriostatic NS. For infusion, may dilute in 50 mL NS or D_5W; dilution in larger volumes (≥100 mL) of I.V. fluids is not recommended. Use appropriate precautions for handling and disposal.

Storage Note: Must be dispensed in overwrap which bears the statement "Do not remove covering until the moment of injection. Fatal if given intrathecally. For I.V. use only." Syringes should be labeled: "Fatal if given intrathecally. For I.V. use only."

Store intact vials under refrigeration at 2°C to 8°C (36°F to 46°F). Protect from light. Solutions reconstituted in bacteriostatic NS are stable for 28 days under refrigeration.

Monitoring and Teaching Issues

Laboratory Monitoring CBC with differential and platelet count, serum uric acid, hepatic function

Physical Assessment Use caution with impaired liver function. Premedication with antiemetic is advisable. Infusion site must be monitored closely to prevent extravasation (vesicant will cause tissue damage and necrosis). Assess renal function. Monitor for SIADH, bone marrow suppression, leukopenia, hypertension, gastrointestinal disturbance, myalgia, depression, and paresthesia throughout therapy.

Patient Education This medication can only be administered by infusion; report immediately any redness, swelling, burning, or pain at infusion site; sudden difficulty breathing; swelling; chest pain; or chills. Maintain adequate nutrition and hydration, unless instructed to restrict fluid intake. You will be more susceptible to infection. May cause hair loss (will grow back after therapy), nausea or vomiting (request antiemetic), photosensitivity, feelings of extreme weakness or lethargy, or mouth sores. Report persistent constipation or abdominal pain, numbness or tingling in fingers or toes, weakness or pain in muscles or jaw, signs of infection (eg, fever, chills, sore throat, burning urination, fatigue), unusual bleeding (eg, tarry stools, easy bruising, blood in stool, urine, or mouth), unresolved mouth sores, skin rash or itching, or respiratory difficulty.

Breast-Feeding Considerations Due to the potential for serious adverse reactions in the nursing infant, breast-feeding is not recommended.

Pregnancy Considerations Animal studies have demonstrated resorption and teratogenic effects. There are no adequate and well-controlled studies in pregnant women. Women of childbearing potential should avoid becoming pregnant during vinblastine treatment. Aspermia has been reported in males who have received treatment with vinblastine.

◆ **Vinblastine Sulfate** *see* VinBLAStine *on page 1862*
◆ **Vincaleukoblastine** *see* VinBLAStine *on page 1862*
◆ **Vincasar PFS®** *see* VinCRIStine *on page 1865*

VinCRIStine (vin KRIS teen)

U.S. Brand Names Vincasar PFS®

Index Terms Leurocristine Sulfate; Oncovin; Vincristine Sulfate

Generic Availability (U.S.) Yes

Pharmacologic Category Antineoplastic Agent, Natural Source (Plant) Derivative; Antineoplastic Agent, Vinca Alkaloid

Medication Safety Issues

Sound-alike/look-alike issues:

VinCRIStine may be confused with vinBLAStine, vinorelbine
Oncovin® may be confused with Ancobon®

High alert medication: This medication is in a class the Institute for Safe Medication Practices (ISMP) includes among its list of drugs which have a heightened risk of causing significant patient harm when used in error.

Administration safety measures: For I.V. use only. Fatal if administered by other routes. To prevent fatal inadvertent intrathecal injection, it is recommended that vincristine doses be dispensed in a small minibag. Vincristine should **NOT** be prepared during the preparation of any intrathecal medications. After preparation, store vincristine in a location **away** from the separate storage location recommended for intrathecal medications. Vincristine should **NOT** be delivered to the patient at the same time with any medications intended for central nervous system administration.

Pregnancy Risk Factor D

Lactation Excretion in breast milk unknown/not recommended

Use Treatment of acute lymphocytic leukemia (ALL), Hodgkin's lymphoma, non-Hodgkin's lymphomas, Wilms' tumor, neuroblastoma, rhabdomyosarcoma

Unlabeled/Investigational Use Treatment of multiple myeloma, chronic lymphocytic leukemia (CLL), brain tumors, small cell lung cancer, ovarian germ cell tumors

Mechanism of Action/Effect Binds to microtubular protein of the mitotic spindle causing metaphase arrest; cell-cycle phase specific in the M and S phases

Contraindications Patients with demyelinating form of Charcot-Marie-Tooth syndrome

Warnings/Precautions Hazardous agent - use appropriate precautions for handling and disposal; avoid eye contamination.

[U.S. Boxed Warning]: For I.V. administration only; intrathecal administration has uniformly caused severe neurologic damage and/or death; vincristine should never be administered by this route. Vincristine should **NOT** be prepared during the preparation of any intrathecal medications. After preparation, store vincristine in a location **away** from the separate storage location recommended for intrathecal medications. Vincristine should **NOT** be delivered to the patient with any medications intended for central nervous system administration.

[U.S. Boxed Warning]: Vincristine is a vesicant; avoid extravasation. (Individuals administering should be experienced in vincristine administration.) Check for proper needle placement; if extravasation occurs, discontinue vincristine infusion and initiate appropriate extravasation management.

Neurotoxicity, including alterations in mental status such as depression, confusion, or insomnia may occur; neurologic effects are dose-limiting (may require dosage reduction) and may be additive with those of other neurotoxic agents and spinal cord irradiation. Use with caution in patients with pre-existing neuromuscular disease and/or with concomitant neurotoxic agents. Constipation, paralytic ileus, intestinal necrosis and/or perforation may occur; constipation may present as upper colon impaction with an empty rectum (may require flat film of abdomen for diagnosis); generally responds to high enemas and laxatives. All patients should be on a prophylactic bowel management regimen.

Use with caution in patients receiving concurrent therapy which alters CYP3A4 activity, may require therapy alterations. Acute shortness of breath and severe bronchospasm have been reported with vinca alkaloids, usually when used in combination with mitomycin-C. Onset may be several minutes to hours after vincristine administration and up to 2 weeks after mitomycin-C. Progressive dyspnea may occur. Permanently discontinue vincristine in this situation.

Use with caution in patients with hepatic impairment; dosage modification required. May be associated with hepatic veno-occlusive disease (VOD), increased risk in children <3 years of age; use with caution in hepatobiliary dysfunction. Monitor for signs or symptoms of hepatic VOD, including bilirubin >1.4 mg/dL, unexplained weight gain, ascites, hepatomegaly, or unexplained right upper quadrant pain (Arndt, 2004). Acute uric acid nephropathy has been reported with vincristine. Use with caution in the elderly.

Drug Interactions

Metabolism/Transport Effects Substrate of CYP3A4 (major), P-glycoprotein; **Inhibits** CYP3A4 (weak)

Avoid Concomitant Use

Avoid concomitant use of VinCRIStine with any of the following: BCG; Natalizumab; Pimecrolimus; Roflumilast; Tacrolimus (Topical); Vaccines (Live)

Decreased Effect

VinCRIStine may decrease the levels/effects of: BCG; Cardiac Glycosides; Sipuleucel-T; Vaccines (Inactivated); Vaccines (Live); Vitamin K Antagonists

The levels/effects of VinCRIStine may be decreased by: CYP3A4 Inducers (Strong); Deferasirox; Echinacea; Herbs (CYP3A4 Inducers); P-Glycoprotein Inducers

Increased Effect/Toxicity

VinCRIStine may increase the levels/effects of: Leflunomide; MitoMYcin; Natalizumab; Vaccines (Live); Vitamin K Antagonists

The levels/effects of VinCRIStine may be increased by: Conivaptan; CYP3A4 Inhibitors (Moderate); CYP3A4 Inhibitors (Strong); Dasatinib; Denosumab; Itraconazole; Lopinavir; Macrolide Antibiotics; MAO Inhibitors; NIFEdipine; P-Glycoprotein Inhibitors; Pimecrolimus; Posaconazole; Ritonavir; Roflumilast; Tacrolimus (Topical); Teniposide; Trastuzumab; Voriconazole

Nutritional/Ethanol Interactions Herb/Nutraceutical: St John's wort may decrease vincristine levels.

Adverse Reactions Frequency not defined.

Cardiovascular: Edema, hyper-/hypotension

Central nervous system: Ataxia, coma, cranial nerve dysfunction (auditory damage, extraocular muscle impairment, laryngeal muscle impairment, paralysis, paresis, vestibular damage, vocal cord paralysis), dizziness, fever, headache, neurotoxicity, neuropathic pain (common), seizure, vertigo

Dermatologic toxicity: Alopecia (common), rash

Endocrine & metabolic: Hyperuricemia, parotid pain, SIADH (rare)

Gastrointestinal: Abdominal cramps, abdominal pain, anorexia, constipation (common), diarrhea, intestinal necrosis, intestinal perforation, nausea, oral ulcers, paralytic ileus, vomiting, weight loss

Genitourinary: Bladder atony, dysuria, polyuria, urinary retention

Hematologic: Anemia (mild), leukopenia (mild), thrombocytopenia (mild)

Hepatic: Hepatic veno-occlusive disease (VOD)

Local: Phlebitis, tissue irritation/necrosis (if infiltrated)

Neuromuscular & skeletal: Back pain, bone pain, deep tendon reflex loss, difficulty walking, foot drop, gait changes, jaw pain, limb pain, motor difficulties, muscle wasting, myalgia, paralysis, paresthesia, peripheral neuropathy (common), sensorimotor dysfunction, sensory loss

Ocular: Cortical blindness (transient), nystagmus, optic atrophy with blindness

Otic: Deafness

Renal: Acute uric acid nephropathy

Respiratory: Bronchospasm, dyspnea, pharyngeal pain

Miscellaneous: Allergic reactions (rare), anaphylaxis (rare), hypersensitivity (rare)

Pharmacodynamics/Kinetics

Half-Life Elimination Terminal: 85 hours (range: 19-155 hours)

Metabolism Extensively hepatic, via CYP3A4

Excretion Feces (~80%); urine (10% to 20%; <1% as unchanged drug)

Available Dosage Forms

Injection, solution [preservative free]: 1 mg/mL (1 mL, 2 mL)

Vincasar PFS®: 1 mg/mL (1 mL, 2 mL)

Dosing

Adult & Geriatric Note: Doses may be capped at a maximum of 2 mg/dose; refer to individual protocol.

Doses in the manufacturer's FDA-approved labeling: I.V.: 1.4 mg/m^2/dose; frequency may vary based on protocol

Additional dosing in combination therapy; indication-specific and/or unlabeled dosing:

ALL: I.V.:

Hyper-CVAD regimen: 2 mg/dose days 4 and 11 during odd-numbered cycles (cycles 1, 3, 5, 7) of an 8-cycle phase, followed by maintenance treatment (if needed) of 2 mg monthly for 2 years (Kantarjian, 2004)

Larson (CALBG 8811) regimen: Induction phase: 2 mg/dose days 1, 8, 15, and 22 (4-week treatment cycle); Early intensification phase: 2 mg/dose days 15, and 22 (4-week treatment cycle, repeat once); Late intensification phase: 2 mg/dose days 1, 8, 15 (8-week treatment cycle); Maintenance phase: 2 mg/dose day 1 every 4 weeks until 24 months from diagnosis (Larson, 1995)

Brain tumors: I.V.: PCV regimen: 1.4 mg/m^2/dose (maximum dose: 2 mg) on days 8 and 29 of a 6-week treatment cycle for a total of 6 cycles (van de Bent, 2006) **or** 1.4 mg/m^2/dose (no maximum dose) on days 8 and 29 of a 6-week treatment cycle for up to 4 cycles (Cairncross, 2006)

Hodgkin's lymphoma: I.V.:

BEACOPP regimen: 1.4 mg/m^2/dose (maximum dose: 2 mg) on day 8 of a 21-day treatment cycle (Diehl, 2003)

Stanford-V regimen: 1.4 mg/m^2/dose (maximum dose: 2 mg) in weeks 2, 4, 6, 8, 10, and 12 (Horning, 2000; Horning, 2002)

Non-Hodgkin's lymphoma: I.V.:

CHOP regimen: 1.4 mg/m^2/dose (maximum dose: 2 mg) on day 1 of a 21-day treatment cycle for 8 cycles (Coiffier, 2002)

CVP regimen: 1.4 mg/m^2/dose (maximum dose: 2 mg) on day 1 of a 21-day treatment cycle for 8 cycles (Marcus, 2005)

EPOCH regimen: 0.4 mg/m^2/day continuous infusion for 4 days (over 96 hours) (total 1.6 mg/m^2/cycle; dose not usually capped) of a 21-day treatment cycle (Wilson, 2002)

Multiple myeloma (unlabeled use):

DVD regimen: 1.4 mg/m^2/dose (maximum dose: 2 mg) on day 1 of a 28-day treatment cycle (Rifkin, 2006)

VAD regimen: 0.4 mg/day continuous infusion for 4 days (over 96 hours) (total 1.6 mg/cycle) of a 28-day treatment cycle (Rifkin, 2006)

Ovarian cancer (unlabeled use): I.V.: VAC regimen: 1.5 mg/m^2/dose (maximum dose: 2 mg) weekly for 8-12 weeks (Slayton, 1985)

Small cell lung cancer (unlabeled use): I.V.: CAV regimen: 1.4 mg/m^2/dose day 1 of a 21-day treatment cycle (Hong, 1989) **or** 2 mg/dose on day 1 of a 21-day treatment cycle (von Pawel, 1999)

Pediatric Note: Doses may be capped at a maximum of 2 mg/dose; refer to individual protocol.

Doses in the manufacturer's FDA-approved labeling: I.V.:

Children ≤10 kg: 0.05 mg/kg/dose once weekly

Children >10 kg: 1.5-2 mg/m^2/dose; frequency may vary based on protocol

Additional dosing in combination therapy; indication-specific and/or unlabeled dosing:

ALL: I.V.: Induction phase: 1.5 mg/m^2/dose days 0, 7, 14, and 21; Consolidation phase: 1.5 mg/m^2/dose days 0, 28, and 56; Delayed intensification phase: 1.5 mg/m^2/dose days 0, 7, and 14; Maintenance phase: 1.5 mg/m^2/dose days 0, 28, and 56 (Bostrom, 2003) **or** Induction phase: 1.5 mg/m^2/dose days 0, 7, 14, and 21; Consolidation phase: 1.5 mg/m^2/dose days 0, 28, and 56; Interim maintenance phases: 1.5 mg/m^2/dose days 0 and 28; Delayed intensification phase: 1.5 mg/m^2/dose days 0, 7, and 14; Maintenance phase: 1.5 mg/m^2/dose every 4 weeks (Avramis, 2002)

Ewing's sarcoma: I.V.: 2 mg/m^2/dose (maximum dose: 2 mg) on day 1 of a 21-day cycle, administer either every cycle or during odd-numbered cycles (Grier, 2003) **or** 0.67 mg/m^2/day continuous infusion days 1, 2, and 3 (total 2 mg/m^2/cycle; maximum dose/cycle: 2 mg) during cycles 1, 2, 3, and 6 (Kolb, 2003)

Hodgkin's lymphoma: I.V.: BEACOPP regimen: 2 mg/m^2/dose (maximum dose: 2 mg) on day 7 of a 21-day treatment cycle (Kelly, 2002)

Rhabdomyosarcoma: I.V.:

VA regimen: 1.5 mg/m^2/dose (maximum dose: 2 mg) weeks 1-8, weeks 13-20, and weeks 25-32 (Crist, 2001)

VAC regimen: 1.5 mg/m^2/dose (maximum dose: 2 mg) weeks 0-12, week 16, weeks 20-25; Continuation therapy: Weeks 29-34, and weeks 38-43 (Crist, 2001)

Wilms' tumor: I.V.:

Children <1 year: 0.75 mg/m^2/dose weekly for 10-11 weeks, then every 3 weeks for 15 additional weeks (total 25-26 weeks) (Pritchard, 1995)

Children ≥1 year: 1.5 mg/m^2/dose weekly for 10-11 weeks, then every 3 weeks for 15 additional weeks (total 25-26 weeks) (Pritchard, 1995)

or

Children ≤30 kg: 0.05 mg/kg/dose (maximum dose: 2 mg) weeks 1, 2, 4, 5, 6, 7, 8, 10, and 11, followed by 0.067 mg/kg/dose (maximum dose: 2 mg) weeks 12, 13, 18, and 24 (Green, 2007)

Children >30 kg: 1.5 mg/m^2/dose (maximum dose: 2 mg) weeks 1, 2, 4, 5, 6, 7, 8, 10, and 11, followed by 2 mg/m^2/dose (maximum dose: 2 mg) weeks 12, 13, 18, and 24 (Green, 2007)

Renal Impairment No adjustment is necessary in patients with renal impairment.

Hepatic Impairment

The FDA-approved labeling recommends the following guidelines: Serum bilirubin >3 mg/dL: Administer 50% of normal dose

The following guidelines have been used by some clinicians:

Serum bilirubin 1.5-3 mg/dL or AST 60-180 units: Administer 50% of dose

Serum bilirubin 3-5 mg/dL: Administer 25% of dose

Serum bilirubin >5 mg/dL or AST >180 units: Avoid use

Floyd, 2006: Serum bilirubin 1.5-3 mg/dL or transaminases 2-3 times ULN or alkaline phosphatase increased: Administer 50% of dose

Administration

I.V. Vesicant; avoid extravasation. **For I.V. administration only. FATAL IF GIVEN INTRATHECALLY.** Vincristine should **NOT** be delivered to the patient at the same time with any medications intended for central nervous system administration.

Usually administered as short 5-10 minute infusion (preferred); may also be administered as a slow (1 minute) push or by a 24-hour continuous infusions (depending on the protocol)

Stability

Reconstitution Use appropriate precautions for handling and disposal. Solutions for I.V. infusion may be mixed in NS or D_5W. **Note:** In order to prevent inadvertent intrathecal administration the World Health Organization (WHO) and the Institute for Safe Medical Practices (ISMP) recommend dispensing vincristine in a minibag (rather than a syringe). Vincristine should **NOT** be prepared during the preparation of any intrathecal medications. If dispensing vincristine in a syringe, it must be packaged in the manufacturer-provided overwrap which bears the statement **"Do not remove covering until the moment of injection. For intravenous use only. Fatal if given intrathecally."**

Storage Store intact vials under refrigeration. May be stable for up to 30 days at room temperature. Protect from light.

I.V. solution: Diluted in 25-50 mL NS or D_5W, stable for 7 days under refrigeration, or 2 days at room temperature. In ambulatory pumps, solution is stable for 7 days at room temperature. After preparation, store vincristine in a location away from the separate storage location recommended for intrathecal medications.

Monitoring and Teaching Issues

Laboratory Monitoring Serum electrolytes (sodium), hepatic function, CBC, serum uric acid

Physical Assessment Use caution with impaired liver function or pre-existing neuromuscular disease. Premedication with antiemetic is advisable. Infusion site must be monitored closely to prevent extravasation (vesicant will cause tissue damage and necrosis). May cause severe constipation, paralytic ileus, intestinal obstruction, necrosis, and/or perforation; prophylactic bowel management regimen may be advisable. Assess CNS status (motor difficulties, seizure, depression), neuromuscular status (myalgia, peripheral neuropathy, cramping), and photophobia throughout therapy.

Patient Education This medication can only be administered by infusion; report immediately any redness, swelling, burning, or pain at infusion site. Maintain adequate nutrition and hydration, unless instructed to restrict fluid intake. You will be more susceptible to infection. May cause postural hypotension, hair loss (will grow back after therapy), nausea or vomiting (request antiemetic if persistent), photosensitivity, feelings of extreme weakness or lethargy, or mouth sores. Report persistent gastrointestinal changes (eg, constipation, abdominal cramps, bloating); numbness, tingling, or pain in legs, fingers, or toes; signs of infection (eg, fever, chills, sore throat, burning urination, fatigue); unusual bleeding (eg, tarry stools, easy bruising, blood in stool, urine, or mouth); unresolved mouth sores; skin rash or itching; or respiratory difficulty.

Breast-Feeding Considerations Due to the potential for serious adverse reactions in the nursing infant, breast-feeding is not recommended.

Pregnancy Considerations Animal studies have demonstrated teratogenicity and fetal loss. There are no adequate and well-controlled studies in pregnant women. May cause fetal harm if administered during pregnancy. Women of childbearing potential should avoid becoming pregnant during treatment.

◆ **Vincristine Sulfate** *see* VinCRIStine *on page* 1865

Vinorelbine (vi NOR el been)

U.S. Brand Names Navelbine®

Index Terms Dihydroxydeoxynorvinkaleukoblastine; Vinorelbine Tartrate

Generic Availability (U.S.) Yes

Pharmacologic Category Antineoplastic Agent, Natural Source (Plant) Derivative; Antineoplastic Agent, Vinca Alkaloid

Medication Safety Issues

Sound-alike/look-alike issues:

Vinorelbine may be confused with vinBLAStine, vinCRIStine

High alert medication: This medication is in a class the Institute for Safe Medication Practices (ISMP) includes among its list of drug classes which have a heightened risk of causing significant patient harm when used in error.

Administration safety measures: Vinorelbine is intended **for I.V. use only**: Inadvertent intrathecal administration of other vinca alkaloids has resulted in death. Syringes containing vinorelbine should be labeled **"For I.V. use only. Fatal if given intrathecally."** Vinorelbine should **NOT** be prepared during the preparation of any intrathecal medications. After preparation, store vinorelbine in a location **away** from the separate storage location recommended for intrathecal medications.

Pregnancy Risk Factor D

Lactation Excretion in breast milk unknown/not recommended

Use Treatment of nonsmall cell lung cancer (NSCLC)

Unlabeled/Investigational Use Treatment of breast cancer (metastatic), cervical cancer, ovarian cancer, malignant pleural mesothelioma, and soft tissue sarcoma

Mechanism of Action/Effect Mitotic inhibition that causes metaphase arrest in neoplastic cells

Contraindications Pretreatment granulocyte counts <1000/mm^3

Warnings/Precautions Hazardous agent - use appropriate precautions for handling and disposal. **[U.S. Boxed Warning]: For I.V. use only; do not administer intrathecally;** intrathecal administration may result in death. **[U.S. Boxed Warning]: Avoid extravasation;** infiltration may cause irritation, thrombophlebitis and/or local tissue necrosis. **[U.S. Boxed Warning]: Severe granulocytopenia may occur with treatment;** granulocytopenia is a dose-limiting toxicity; granulocyte counts should be ≥1000/mm^3 prior to treatment initiation; monitor closely for infections and/or fever; may require dosage adjustment. The incidence of granulocytopenia is significantly higher when given in combination with cisplatin when compared to single-agent vinorelbine. Use with caution in patients with compromised marrow reserve due to prior chemotherapy therapy or prior radiation therapy.

Fatal cases of interstitial pulmonary changes and ARDS have been reported (with single-agent therapy); promptly evaluate changes in baseline pulmonary symptoms or any new onset pulmonary symptoms. Acute shortness of breath and severe bronchospasm have been reported rarely; usually associated with the concurrent administration of mitomycin.

Vinorelbine should **NOT** be prepared during the preparation of any intrathecal medications. After preparation, store vinorelbine in a location **away** from the separate storage location recommended for intrathecal medications. Dosage modification required in patients with impaired hepatic function and neurotoxicity; use with caution. May cause new onset or worsening of pre-existing neuropathy; use with caution in patients with neuropathy. May cause severe constipation (grade 3-4), paralytic ileus, intestinal obstruction, necrosis, and/or perforation. May have radiosensitizing effects with prior or concurrent radiation therapy; radiation recall reactions may occur in patients who have received prior radiation therapy. Avoid eye contamination (exposure may cause severe irritation). **[U.S. Boxed Warning]: Should be administered under the supervision of an experienced cancer chemotherapy physician.**

Drug Interactions

Metabolism/Transport Effects Substrate of CYP2D6 (minor), 3A4 (major); **Inhibits** CYP2D6 (weak), 3A4 (weak)

Avoid Concomitant Use

Avoid concomitant use of Vinorelbine with any of the following: BCG; Natalizumab; Pimecrolimus; Roflumilast; Tacrolimus (Topical); Vaccines (Live)

Decreased Effect

Vinorelbine may decrease the levels/effects of: BCG; Sipuleucel-T; Vaccines (Inactivated); Vaccines (Live)

The levels/effects of Vinorelbine may be decreased by: CYP3A4 Inducers (Strong); Deferasirox; Echinacea; Herbs (CYP3A4 Inducers); Peginterferon Alfa-2b

Increased Effect/Toxicity

Vinorelbine may increase the levels/effects of: Leflunomide; MitoMYcin; Natalizumab; Vaccines (Live)

The levels/effects of Vinorelbine may be increased by: CISplatin; Conivaptan; CYP3A4 Inhibitors (Moderate); CYP3A4 Inhibitors (Strong); Dasatinib; Denosumab; Gefitinib; Itraconazole; Macrolide Antibiotics; PACLitaxel; PACLitaxel (Protein Bound); Pimecrolimus; Posaconazole; Roflumilast; Tacrolimus (Topical); Trastuzumab; Voriconazole

Nutritional/Ethanol Interactions Herb/Nutraceutical: Avoid St John's wort (may decrease vinorelbine levels).

Adverse Reactions Note: Reported with single-agent therapy.

>10%:

Central nervous system: Fatigue (27%)

Dermatologic: Alopecia (12% to 30%)

Gastrointestinal: Nausea (31% to 44%; grade 3: 1% to 2%), constipation (35%; grade 3: 3%), vomiting (20% to 31%; grade 3: 1% to 2%), diarrhea (12% to 17%)

Hematologic: Leukopenia (83% to 92%; grade 4: 6% to 15%), granulocytopenia (90%; grade 4: 36%; nadir: 7-10 days; recovery 14-21 days; dose-limiting), neutropenia (85%; grade 4: 28%), anemia (83%; grades 3/4: 9%)

Hepatic: AST increased (67%; grade 3: 5%; grade 4: 1%), total bilirubin increased (5% to 13%; grade 3: 4%; grade 4: 3%)

Local: Injection site reaction (22% to 28%; includes erythema, vein discoloration), injection site pain (16%)

Neuromuscular & skeletal: Weakness (36%), peripheral neuropathy (25%; grade 3: 1%; grade 4: <1%)

Renal: Creatinine increased (13%)

1% to 10%:

Cardiovascular: Chest pain (5%)

Dermatologic: Rash (<5%)

Gastrointestinal: Paralytic ileus (1%)

Hematologic: Neutropenic fever/sepsis (8%; grade 4: 4%), thrombocytopenia (3% to 5%; grades 3/4: 1%)

Local: Phlebitis (7% to 10%)

Neuromuscular & skeletal: Loss of deep tendon reflexes (<5%), myalgia (<5%), arthralgia (<5%), jaw pain (<5%)

Otic: Ototoxicity (≤1%)

Respiratory: Dyspnea (7%)

Pharmacodynamics/Kinetics

Absorption Unreliable; must be given I.V.

Bioavailability Oral (not approved in the U. S.): 26% to 45%

Protein Binding 80% to 91%

Half-Life Elimination Triphasic: Terminal: 28-44 hours

Metabolism Extensively hepatic, via CYP3A4, to two metabolites, deacetylvinorelbine (active) and vinorelbine N-oxide

Excretion Feces (46%); urine (18%, 10% to 12% as unchanged drug)

Clearance: Plasma: Mean: 0.97-1.26 L/hour/kg

Available Dosage Forms

Injection, solution [preservative free]: 10 mg/mL (1 mL, 5 mL)

Navelbine®: 10 mg/mL (1 mL, 5 mL)

Dosing

Adult & Geriatric Details concerning dosing in combination regimens should also be consulted.

Nonsmall cell lung cancer: I.V.:

Single-agent therapy: 30 mg/m²/dose every 7 days

Combination therapy with cisplatin: 25-30 mg/m²/dose every 7 days (in combination with cisplatin)

Breast cancer (unlabeled use): I.V.: 25 mg/m²/dose every 7 days (Zelek, 2001)

Cervical cancer (unlabeled use): I.V.: 30 mg/m²/dose days 1 and 8 of a 21-day treatment cycle (Muggia, 2004; Muggia, 2005)

Malignant pleural mesothelioma (unlabeled use): I.V.: 30 mg/m²/dose (maximum dose: 60 mg) every 7 days for 6 weeks (Stebbing, 2009) **or** 30 mg/m²/dose (maximum dose: 60 mg) every 7 days for 6 weeks, off 2 weeks, then repeat cycle (Muers, 2008)

Ovarian cancer (unlabeled use): I.V.: 25 mg/m²/dose every 7 days (Bajetta, 1996) **or** 30 mg/m²/dose days 1 and 8 of a 21-day treatment cycle (Rothenberg, 2004)

Soft tissue sarcoma (unlabeled use; in combination with gemcitabine): I.V.: 25 mg/m²/dose days 1 and 8 of a 21-day treatment cycle (Dileo, 2007)

Renal Impairment No adjustment is necessary.

Hepatic Impairment

Note: In patients with concurrent hematologic toxicity and hepatic impairment, administer the lower of the doses determined from the adjustment recommendations.

The FDA-approved labeling guidelines are as follows: Vinorelbine should be administered with caution in patients with hepatic insufficiency. In patients who develop hyperbilirubinemia during treatment with vinorelbine, the dose should be adjusted for total bilirubin as follows:

Serum bilirubin ≤2 mg/dL: Administer 100% of dose

Serum bilirubin 2.1-3 mg/dL: Administer 50% of dose

Serum bilirubin >3 mg/dL: Administer 25% of dose

Adjustment for Toxicity

Note: In patients with concurrent hematologic toxicity and hepatic impairment, administer the lower of the doses determined from the adjustment recommendations.

Dosage adjustment in hematological toxicity (based on granulocyte counts):

Granulocytes ≥1500 cells/mm³ on day of treatment: Administer 100% of starting dose.

Granulocytes 1000-1499 cells/mm³ on day of treatment: Administer 50% of starting dose.

Granulocytes <1000 cells/mm³ on day of treatment: Do not administer. Repeat granulocyte count in 1 week. If 3 consecutive doses are held because granulocyte count is <1000 cells/mm³, discontinue vinorelbine.

Adjustment: For patients who, during treatment, have experienced fever or sepsis while granulocytopenic or had 2 consecutive weekly doses held due to granulocytopenia, subsequent doses of vinorelbine should be:

75% of starting dose for granulocytes ≥1500 cells/mm³

37.5% of starting dose for granulocytes 1000-1499 cells/mm³

Dosage adjustment for neurotoxicity: Neurotoxicity ≥grade 2: Discontinue treatment

Administration

I.V. FATAL IF GIVEN INTRATHECALLY. Administer as a direct intravenous push or rapid bolus, over 6-10 minutes (up to 30 minutes). Longer infusions may increase the risk of pain and phlebitis. Intravenous doses should be followed by at least 75-125 mL of saline or D_5W to reduce the incidence of phlebitis and inflammation. Assure proper needle or catheter position prior to administration.

Stability

Reconstitution Dilute in D_5W or NS to a final concentration of 1.5-3 mg/mL (for syringe) or 0.5-2 mg/mL (for I.V. bag). Vinorelbine should **NOT** be prepared during the preparation of any intrathecal medications.

Storage Store intact vials under refrigeration at 2°C to 8°C (36°F to 46°F); do not freeze. Protect from light. Intact vials are stable at room temperature of 25°C (77°F) for up to 72 hours. Dilutions in D_5W or NS are stable for 24 hours at room temperature. After preparation, store vinorelbine in a location **away** from the separate storage location recommended for intrathecal medications.

Monitoring and Teaching Issues

Laboratory Monitoring CBC with differential and platelet count, hepatic function

Physical Assessment For intravenous use only. Use caution with hepatic impairment, neurotoxicity, or compromised marrow reserve. Premedication with antiemetic is advisable. May cause severe constipation, paralytic ileus, intestinal obstruction, necrosis, and/or perforation; prophylactic bowel management regimen may be advisable. Infusion site must be monitored closely to prevent extravasation; may cause tissue damage and necrosis. Monitor for peripheral neuropathy. Assess pulmonary status and liver function prior to each infusion and throughout therapy.

Patient Education This medication can only be administered by infusion; report immediately any redness, swelling, burning, or pain at infusion site. Maintain adequate hydration and nutrition. You will be more susceptible to infection. May cause hair loss (will grow back after therapy), nausea or vomiting (request antiemetic if persistent), feelings of weakness or lethargy, or mouth sores. Report persistent constipation or abdominal pain; numbness or tingling in fingers or toes; weakness, numbness, or pain in muscles or extremities; signs of infection (eg, fever, chills, sore throat, burning urination, fatigue); unusual bleeding (eg, tarry stools; easy bruising; blood in stool, urine, or mouth); unresolved mouth sores; skin rash or itching; or respiratory difficulty.

Breast-Feeding Considerations Due to the potential for serious adverse reactions in the nursing infant, breast-feeding is not recommended.

Pregnancy Considerations Animal studies have demonstrated embryotoxicity, fetotoxicity, decreased fetal weight, and delayed ossification. There are no adequate and well-controlled studies in pregnant women. Women of childbearing potential should avoid becoming pregnant during vinorelbine treatment.

- **Vinorelbine Tartrate** *see* Vinorelbine *on page 1868*
- **Viokase® [DSC]** *see* Pancrelipase *on page 1400*
- **Viosterol** *see* Ergocalciferol *on page 650*
- **Viracept®** *see* Nelfinavir *on page 1296*
- **Viramune®** *see* Nevirapine *on page 1301*
- **Viramune® XR™** *see* Nevirapine *on page 1301*
- **Viramune® XR™** *see* Nevirapine *on page 1301*
- **Virazole®** *see* Ribavirin *on page 1571*
- **Viread®** *see* Tenofovir *on page 1728*
- **Viscous Lidocaine** *see* Lidocaine (Topical) *on page 1107*
- **Vistaril®** *see* HydrOXYzine *on page 934*
- **Vistide®** *see* Cidofovir *on page 368*
- **Vitamin A Acid** *see* Tretinoin (Topical) *on page 1811*
- **Vitamin B_1** *see* Thiamine *on page 1751*
- **Vitamin B_3** *see* Niacin *on page 1305*
- **Vitamin B_6** *see* Pyridoxine *on page 1532*
- **Vitamin B_{12}** *see* Cyanocobalamin *on page 431*
- **Vitamin B_{12a}** *see* Hydroxocobalamin *on page 928*
- **Vitamin D2** *see* Ergocalciferol *on page 650*
- **Vitamin K_1** *see* Phytonadione *on page 1457*
- **Vivaglobin® [DSC]** *see* Immune Globulin *on page 961*
- **Vivarin® [OTC]** *see* Caffeine *on page 267*
- **Vivelle-Dot®** *see* Estradiol (Systemic) *on page 670*
- **Vivitrol®** *see* Naltrexone *on page 1286*
- **VLB** *see* VinBLAStine *on page 1862*
- **VM-26** *see* Teniposide *on page 1728*
- **Voltaren® Gel** *see* Diclofenac (Topical) *on page 522*
- **Voltaren®-XR** *see* Diclofenac (Systemic) *on page 518*
- **von Willebrand Factor/Factor VIII Complex** *see* Antihemophilic Factor/von Willebrand Factor Complex (Human) *on page 134*

Voriconazole (vor i KOE na zole)

U.S. Brand Names VFEND®

Index Terms UK109496

Generic Availability (U.S.) Yes: Tablet

Pharmacologic Category Antifungal Agent, Oral; Antifungal Agent, Parenteral

Pregnancy Risk Factor D

Lactation Excretion in breast milk unknown/not recommended

Use Treatment of invasive aspergillosis; treatment of esophageal candidiasis; treatment of candidemia (in non-neutropenic patients); treatment of disseminated *Candida* infections of the skin and viscera; treatment of serious fungal infections caused by *Scedosporium apiospermum* and *Fusarium* spp (including *Fusarium solani*) in patients intolerant of, or refractory to, other therapy

Unlabeled/Investigational Use Fungal infection prophylaxis in intermediate or high risk neutropenic cancer patients with myelodysplastic syndrome (MDS) or acute myelogenous leukemia (AML), neutropenic allogeneic hematopoietic stem cell recipients, and patients with significant graft-versus-host disease; empiric antifungal therapy (second-line) for persistent neutropenic fever

Mechanism of Action/Effect Interferes with fungal cytochrome P450 activity (selectively inhibits 14-alpha-lanosterol demethylation), decreasing ergosterol synthesis (principal sterol in fungal cell membrane) and inhibiting fungal cell membrane formation.

Contraindications Hypersensitivity to voriconazole or any component of the formulation (cross-reaction with other azole antifungal agents may occur but has not been established, use caution); coadministration of CYP3A4 substrates which may lead to QT_c prolongation (cisapride, pimozide, or quinidine); coadministration with barbiturates (long acting), carbamazepine, efavirenz (with standard [eg, not adjusted] voriconazole and efavirenz doses), ergot derivatives, rifampin, rifabutin, ritonavir (≥800 mg/day), sirolimus, St John's wort

Warnings/Precautions Visual changes, including blurred vision, changes in visual acuity, color perception, and photophobia, are commonly associated with treatment; postmarketing cases of optic neuritis and papilledema (lasting >1 month) have also been reported. Patients should be warned to avoid tasks which depend on vision, including operating machinery or driving. Changes are reversible on discontinuation following brief exposure/treatment regimens (≤28 days).

Serious hepatic reactions (including hepatitis, cholestasis, and fulminant hepatic failure) have occurred during treatment, primarily in patients with serious concomitant medical conditions. However, hepatotoxicity has occurred in patients with no identifiable risk factors. Use caution in patients with pre-existing hepatic impairment (dose adjustment or discontinuation may be required).

Voriconazole tablets contain lactose; avoid administration in hereditary galactose intolerance, Lapp lactase deficiency, or glucose-galactose malabsorption. Suspension contains sucrose; use caution with fructose intolerance, sucrose-isomaltase deficiency, or glucose-galactose malabsorption. Avoid/limit use of intravenous formulation in patients with renal impairment; intravenous formulation contains excipient cyclodextrin (sulfobutyl ether beta-cyclodextrin), which may accumulate in renal insufficiency. Acute renal failure has been observed in severely ill patients; use with caution in patients receiving concomitant nephrotoxic medications. Anaphylactoid-type infusion-related reactions may occur with intravenous dosing. Consider discontinuation of infusion if reaction is severe.

Use caution in patients taking strong cytochrome P450 inducers, CYP2C9 inhibitors, and major 3A4 substrates (see Drug Interactions); consider alternative agents that avoid or lessen the potential for CYP-mediated interactions. QT interval prolongation has been associated with voriconazole use; rare cases of arrhythmia (including torsade de pointes), cardiac arrest, and sudden death have been reported, usually in seriously ill patients with comorbidities and/or risk factors (eg, prior cardiotoxic chemotherapy, cardiomyopathy, electrolyte imbalance, or concomitant QT_c-prolonging drugs). Use with caution in these patient populations; correct electrolyte abnormalities (eg, hypokalemia, hypomagnesemia, hypocalcemia) prior to initiating therapy. Do not infuse concomitantly with blood products or short-term concentrated electrolyte solutions, even if the two infusions are running in separate intravenous lines (or cannulas).

Rare cases of malignancy (melanoma, squamous cell carcinoma) have been reported in patients (mostly immunocompromised) with prior onset of severe photosensitivity reactions and exposure to long-term voriconazole therapy. Other serious exfoliative cutaneous reactions, including Stevens-Johnson syndrome, have also been reported. Patient should avoid strong, direct exposure to sunlight; may cause photosensitivity, especially with long-term use. Discontinue use in patients who develop an exfoliative cutaneous reaction or a skin lesion consistent with squamous cell carcinoma or melanoma. Periodic total body skin examinations should be performed, particularly with prolonged use.

Monitor pancreatic function in patients (children and adults) at risk for acute pancreatitis (eg, recent chemotherapy or hematopoietic stem cell transplantation); there have been postmarketing reports of pancreatitis in children.

Drug Interactions

Metabolism/Transport Effects Substrate of CYP2C9 (major), 2C19 (major), 3A4 (minor); **Inhibits** CYP2C9 (moderate), 2C19 (weak), 3A4 (moderate)

Avoid Concomitant Use

Avoid concomitant use of Voriconazole with any of the following: Alfuzosin; Artemether; Barbiturates; CarBAMazepine; Cisapride; Conivaptan; Darunavir; Dofetilide; Dronedarone; Eplerenone; Ergot Derivatives; Everolimus; Halofantrine; Lopinavir; Lumefantrine; Lurasidone; Nilotinib; Nisoldipine; Pimozide; QuiNIDine; QuiNINE; Ranolazine; Rifamycin Derivatives; Ritonavir; Rivaroxaban; RomiDEPsin; Salmeterol; Silodosin; Sirolimus; St Johns Wort; Tamsulosin; Tetrabenazine; Thioridazine; Tolvaptan; Toremifene; Vandetanib; Ziprasidone

Decreased Effect

Voriconazole may decrease the levels/effects of: Amphotericin B; Prasugrel; Saccharomyces boulardii

The levels/effects of Voriconazole may be decreased by: Barbiturates; CarBAMazepine; CYP2C19 Inducers (Strong); CYP2C9 Inducers (Highly Effective); Darunavir; Didanosine; Etravirine; Lopinavir; Peginterferon Alfa-2b; Phenytoin; Reverse Transcriptase Inhibitors (Non-Nucleoside); Rifamycin Derivatives; Ritonavir; St Johns Wort; Sucralfate

Increased Effect/Toxicity

Voriconazole may increase the levels/effects of: Alfentanil; Alfuzosin; Almotriptan; Alosetron; Antineoplastic Agents (Vinca Alkaloids); Aprepitant; Benzodiazepines (metabolized by oxidation); Bortezomib; Bosentan; Brinzolamide; BusPIRone; Busulfan; Calcium Channel Blockers; CarBAMazepine; Carvedilol; Ciclesonide; Cilostazol; Cinacalcet; Cisapride; Colchicine; Conivaptan; Contraceptives (Estrogens); Contraceptives (Progestins); Corticosteroids (Orally Inhaled); Corticosteroids (Systemic); CycloSPORINE; CycloSPORINE (Systemic); CYP2C9 Substrates (High risk); CYP3A4 Substrates; Diclofenac; Diclofenac (Systemic); Diclofenac (Topical); Dienogest; DOCEtaxel; Dofetilide; Dronedarone; Dutasteride; Eletriptan; Eplerenone; Ergot Derivatives; Erlotinib; Eszopiclone; Etravirine; Everolimus; FentaNYL; Fesoterodine; Fosaprepitant; Gefitinib; GuanFACINE; Halofantrine; HMG-CoA Reductase Inhibitors;

Ibuprofen; Imatinib; Irinotecan; Ixabepilone; Losartan; Lumefantrine; Lurasidone; Macrolide Antibiotics; Maraviroc; Meloxicam; Methadone; MethylPREDNISolone; Nilotinib; Nisoldipine; OxyCODONE; Paricalcitol; Pazopanib; Phenytoin; Phosphodiesterase 5 Inhibitors; Pimecrolimus; Pimozide; Protease Inhibitors; QTc-Prolonging Agents; QuiNIDine; QuiNINE; Ramelteon; Ranolazine; Repaglinide; Reverse Transcriptase Inhibitors (Non-Nucleoside); Rifamycin Derivatives; Rivaroxaban; RomiDEPsin; Salmeterol; Saxagliptin; Silodosin; Sirolimus; Solifenacin; SORAfenib; Sulfonylureas; SUNItinib; Tacrolimus; Tacrolimus (Systemic); Tacrolimus (Topical); Tadalafil; Tamsulosin; Tetrabenazine; Thioridazine; Tolterodine; Tolvaptan; Toremifene; Vandetanib; Venlafaxine; Vilazodone; Vitamin K Antagonists; Ziprasidone; Zolpidem

The levels/effects of Voriconazole may be increased by: Alfuzosin; Artemether; Chloramphenicol; Chloroquine; Ciprofloxacin; Ciprofloxacin (Systemic); Contraceptives (Estrogens); Contraceptives (Progestins); CYP2C19 Inhibitors (Moderate); CYP2C19 Inhibitors (Strong); CYP2C9 Inhibitors (Moderate); CYP2C9 Inhibitors (Strong); Etravirine; Gadobutrol; Grapefruit Juice; Lumefantrine; Macrolide Antibiotics; Nilotinib; Protease Inhibitors; Proton Pump Inhibitors; QuiNINE

Nutritional/Ethanol Interactions

Food: May decrease voriconazole absorption. Oral voriconazole should be taken 1 hour before or 1 hour after a meal. Avoid grapefruit juice (may decrease voriconazole levels).

Herb/Nutraceutical: St John's wort may decrease voriconazole levels; concurrent use with voriconazole is contraindicated.

Adverse Reactions

>10%:

- Central nervous system: Hallucinations (4% to 12%; auditory and/or visual and likely serum concentration-dependent)
- Ocular: Visual changes (dose related; photophobia, color changes, increased or decreased visual acuity, or blurred vision occur in ~21%)
- Renal: Creatinine increased (1% to 21%)

2% to 10%:

- Cardiovascular: Tachycardia (≤2%)
- Central nervous system: Fever (≤6%), chills (≤4%), headache (≤3%)
- Dermatologic: Rash (≤7%)
- Endocrine & metabolic: Hypokalemia (≤2%)
- Gastrointestinal: Nausea (1% to 5%), vomiting (1% to 4%)
- Hepatic: Alkaline phosphatase increased (4% to 5%), AST increased (2% to 4%), ALT increased (2% to 3%), cholestatic jaundice (1% to 2%)
- Ocular: Photophobia (2% to 3%)

Pharmacodynamics/Kinetics

Absorption Well absorbed after oral administration; administration of crushed tablets is considered bioequivalent to whole tablets

Bioavailability 96%

Time to Peak Oral: 1-2 hours; 0.5 hours (crushed tablet)

Protein Binding 58%

Half-Life Elimination Variable, dose dependent

Metabolism Hepatic, via CYP2C19 (major pathway) and CYP2C9 and CYP3A4 (less significant); saturable (may demonstrate nonlinearity)

Excretion Urine (as inactive metabolites; <2% as unchanged drug)

Available Dosage Forms

Injection, powder for reconstitution:
VFEND®: 200 mg

Powder for suspension, oral:
VFEND®: 40 mg/mL (70 mL)

Tablet, oral: 50 mg, 200 mg
VFEND®: 50 mg, 200 mg

Dosing

Adult & Geriatric

Aspergillosis, invasive, including disseminated and extrapulmonary infection: Duration of therapy should be a minimum of 6-12 weeks or throughout period of immunosuppression (Walsh, 2008):

I.V.: Initial: Loading dose: 6 mg/kg every 12 hours for 2 doses; followed by maintenance dose of 4 mg/kg every 12 hours

Oral: Maintenance dose:

Manufacturer's recommendations:

Patients <40 kg: 100 mg every 12 hours; maximum: 300 mg/day
Patients ≥40 kg: 200 mg every 12 hours; maximum: 600 mg/day

IDSA recommendations (Walsh, 2008): May consider oral therapy in place of I.V. with dosing of 4 mg/kg (rounded up to convenient tablet dosage form) every 12 hours; however, I.V. administration is preferred in serious infections since comparative efficacy with the oral formulation has not been established.

Scedosporiosis, fusariosis:

I.V.: Initial: Loading dose: 6 mg/kg every 12 hours for 2 doses; followed by maintenance dose of 4 mg/kg every 12 hours

Oral: Maintenance dose:

Patients <40 kg: 100 mg every 12 hours; maximum 300 mg/day
Patients ≥40 kg: 200 mg every 12 hours; maximum: 600 mg/day

Candidemia and other deep tissue *Candida* infections: Treatment should continue for a minimum of 14 days following resolution of symptoms or following last positive culture, whichever is longer.

I.V.: Initial: Loading dose 6 mg/kg every 12 hours for 2 doses; followed by maintenance dose of 3-4 mg/kg every 12 hours

Oral:

Manufacturer's recommendations: Maintenance dose:

Patients <40 kg: 100 mg every 12 hours; maximum: 300 mg/day

Patients ≥40 kg: 200 mg every 12 hours; maximum: 600 mg/day

IDSA recommendations (Pappas, 2009): Initial: Loading dose: 400 mg every 12 hours for 2 doses; followed by 200 mg every 12 hours

Endophthalmitis, fungal (unlabeled use; Pappas, 2009): I.V.: 6 mg/kg every 12 hours for 2 doses, then 3-4 mg/kg every 12 hours

Esophageal candidiasis: Oral: Treatment should continue for a minimum of 14 days, and for at least 7 days following resolution of symptoms:

Patients <40 kg: 100 mg every 12 hours; maximum: 300 mg/day

Patients ≥40 kg: 200 mg every 12 hours; maximum: 600 mg/day

Dosage adjustment in patients unable to tolerate treatment:

I.V.: Dose may be reduced to 3 mg/kg every 12 hours

Oral: Dose may be reduced in 50 mg decrements to a minimum dosage of 200 mg every 12 hours in patients weighing ≥40 kg (100 mg every 12 hours in patients <40 kg)

Dosage adjustment in patients receiving concomitant CYP450 enzyme inducers or substrates:

Cyclosporine: Reduce cyclosporine dose by one-half and monitor closely; upon discontinuation of voriconazole, monitor cyclosporine concentrations and escalate the cyclosporine dose as needed

Efavirenz: Oral: Increase maintenance dose of voriconazole to 400 mg every 12 hours and reduce efavirenz dose to 300 mg once daily; upon discontinuation of voriconazole, return to the initial dose of efavirenz

Omeprazole: Reduce omeprazole dose by one-half in patients maintained on ≥40 mg/day of omeprazole

Phenytoin:

I.V.: Increase voriconazole maintenance dosage to 5 mg/kg every 12 hours

Oral: Increase voriconazole dose to 400 mg every 12 hours in patients ≥40 kg (200 mg every 12 hours in patients <40 kg)

Tacrolimus: Reduce tacrolimus dose by one-third and monitor closely; upon discontinuation of voriconazole, monitor tacrolimus concentrations and escalate the tacrolimus dose as needed.

Pediatric

Aspergillosis, invasive including disseminated and extrapulmonary infection in HIV-exposed/-positive patients: (unlabeled; CDC, 2009): Infants and Children:

Oral: Loading dose: 8 mg/kg/dose (maximum: 400 mg/dose) every 12 hours for 2 doses on day 1, followed by maintenance dose of 7 mg/kg/dose (maximum: 200 mg/dose) every 12 hours for ≥12 weeks

I.V.: Loading dose: 6-8 mg/kg/dose (maximum: 400 mg/dose) every 12 hours for 2 doses on day 1, followed by maintenance dose of 7 mg/kg/dose (maximum: 200 mg/dose) every 12 hours for ≥12 weeks

Children ≥12 years: Refer to adult dosing.

Renal Impairment In patients with Cl_{cr} <50 mL/minute, accumulation of the intravenous vehicle (cyclodextrin) occurs. After initial I.V. loading dose, oral voriconazole should be administered to these patients, unless an assessment of the benefit:risk to the patient justifies the use of I.V. voriconazole. Monitor serum creatinine and change to oral voriconazole therapy when possible.

Hemodialysis: Oral dosage adjustment not required; I.V. dosing not recommended since cyclodextrin vehicle is cleared at half the rate of voriconazole and may accumulate

Hepatic Impairment

Mild-to-moderate hepatic dysfunction (Child-Pugh class A and B): Following standard loading dose, reduce maintenance dosage by 50%

Severe hepatic impairment: Should only be used if benefit outweighs risk; monitor closely for toxicity

Administration

Oral Administer 1 hour before or 1 hour after a meal.

I.V. Infuse over 1-2 hours (rate not to exceed 3 mg/kg/hour). Do not infuse concomitantly into same line or cannula with other drug infusions, including TPN.

Stability

Reconstitution

Powder for injection: Reconstitute 200 mg vial with 19 mL of sterile water for injection (use of automated syringe is not recommended). Resultant solution (20 mL) has a concentration of 10 mg/mL. Prior to infusion, must dilute to 0.5-5 mg/mL with NS, LR, D_5WLR, $D_5W^1/_2NS$, D_5W, D_5W with KCl 20 mEq, $^1/_2NS$, or D_5WNS. Do not dilute with 4.2% sodium bicarbonate infusion.

Powder for oral suspension: Add 46 mL of water to the bottle to make 40 mg/mL suspension. Discard unused portion after 14 days.

Storage

Powder for injection: Store at 15°C to 30°C (59°F to 86°F). Reconstituted solutions are stable for up to 24 hours under refrigeration at 2°C to 8°C (36°F to 46°F).

Powder for oral suspension: Store at 2°C to 8°C (36°F to 46°F). Reconstituted oral suspension may be stored at 15°C to 30°C (59°F to 86°F).

Tablets: Store at 15°C to 30°C (59°F to 86°F).

Monitoring and Teaching Issues

Laboratory Monitoring Hepatic function at initiation and during course of treatment; renal function; serum electrolytes (particularly calcium, magnesium and potassium) prior to therapy initiation; may consider obtaining voriconazole trough level in patients failing therapy or exhibiting signs of toxicity; pancreatic function (in patients at risk for acute pancreatitis)

Physical Assessment Evaluate hepatic function, renal function, and allergy history prior to beginning therapy. Monitor for vision changes (photophobia, changed visual acuity, blurred vision), hepatic toxicity (increased liver enzymes, jaundice), tachycardia, and dermatologic reactions (can be severe; periodic total body examinations should be performed with long-term use).

Patient Education Maintain adequate hydration unless instructed to restrict fluid intake. Avoid direct exposure to strong sunlight. You may experience headache, dizziness, blurred vision, photophobia, changes in visual acuity (vision changes are reversible shortly after treatment is completed or discontinued), nausea, vomiting, or abdominal pain. Report immediately any change in vision. Report unusual tiredness, flu-like feelings, skin rash or itching, dark urine, light colored stool, yellowing of skin or eyes, fever, chest pain, or rapid heartbeat.

I.V.: You will be monitored during intravenous administration; report immediately any pain, swelling, or redness at infusion site; difficulty breathing or swallowing; back pain; or itching.

Oral: Preferable to take on empty stomach 1 hour before or 1 hour after a meal.

Dietary Considerations Oral: Should be taken 1 hour before or 1 hour after a meal. Voriconazole tablets contain lactose; avoid administration in hereditary galactose intolerance, Lapp lactase deficiency, or glucose-galactose malabsorption. Suspension contains sucrose; use caution with fructose intolerance, sucrose-isomaltase deficiency, or glucose-galactose malabsorption.

Geriatric Considerations The manufacturer reports that median voriconazole plasma concentrations were increased in patients 65 years and older compared to those 65 years and younger. The recommendation that a dose adjustment is not needed for the elderly was based on a similar safety profile between young and older patients.

Breast-Feeding Considerations Excretion in breast milk has not been investigated; avoid breast-feeding until additional data are available.

Pregnancy Considerations Voriconazole can cause fetal harm when administered to a pregnant woman. Voriconazole was teratogenic and embryotoxic in animal studies, and lowered plasma estradiol in animal models. Women of childbearing potential should use effective contraception during treatment. Should be used in pregnant woman only if benefit to mother justifies potential risk to the fetus.

Vorinostat (vor IN oh stat)

U.S. Brand Names Zolinza™

Index Terms SAHA; Suberoylanilide Hydroxamic Acid

Generic Availability (U.S.) No

Pharmacologic Category Antineoplastic Agent, Histone Deacetylase Inhibitor

Medication Safety Issues

Sound-alike/look-alike issues:

Vorinostat may be confused with Votrient™

High alert medication: The Institute for Safe Medication Practices (ISMP) includes this medication among its list of drug classes which have a heightened risk of causing significant patient harm when used in error.

Pregnancy Risk Factor D

Lactation Excretion in breast milk unknown/not recommended

Use Treatment of progressive, persistent, or recurrent cutaneous T-cell lymphoma (CTCL)

Mechanism of Action/Effect Histone deacetylase inhibitor; causes termination of cell growth leading to cell death

Contraindications There are no contraindications listed within the FDA-approved manufacturer's labeling.

Canadian labeling: Hypersensitivity to vorinostat or any component of the formulation; severe hepatic impairment (total bilirubin ≥3 times ULN)

Warnings/Precautions Hazardous agent - use appropriate precautions for handling and disposal. Pulmonary embolism and deep vein thrombosis (DVT) have been reported; monitor. Use caution in patients with a history of thrombotic events. Dose-related thrombocytopenia and/or anemia may occur; may require dosage adjustments or discontinuation. QT_c prolongation has been observed; baseline and periodic ECGs were done in clinical trials (Duvic, 2007; Olsen, 2007). Correct electrolyte abnormalities prior to treatment and monitor and correct potassium, calcium, and magnesium levels during therapy. Use caution in patients with a history of QT_c prolongation or with medications known to prolong the QT interval. May cause hyperglycemia; monitor and use with caution in diabetics; may require diet and/or therapy modifications. Nausea, vomiting, and diarrhea may occur; antiemetics and antidiarrheals may be required; control pre-existing nausea and vomiting prior to treatment initiation; replace fluids and electrolytes to avoid dehydration. May cause dizziness or fatigue; caution patients about performing tasks which require mental alertness (eg, operating machinery or driving). Use with caution in patients with hepatic impairment (elimination is predominantly hepatic); in the Canadian labeling, use is not recommended in patients with moderate hepatic impairment (total bilirubin 1.5-3 times ULN) and is contraindicated in patients with severe hepatic impairment (total bilirubin >3 times ULN).

Drug Interactions

Avoid Concomitant Use

Avoid concomitant use of Vorinostat with any of the following: Artemether; Dronedarone; Lumefantrine; Nilotinib; Pimozide; QuiNINE; Tetrabenazine; Thioridazine; Toremifene; Vandetanib; Ziprasidone

Decreased Effect There are no known significant interactions involving a decrease in effect.

Increased Effect/Toxicity

Vorinostat may increase the levels/effects of: Dronedarone; Pimozide; QTc-Prolonging Agents; QuiNINE; Tetrabenazine; Thioridazine; Toremifene; Vandetanib; Vitamin K Antagonists; Ziprasidone

The levels/effects of Vorinostat may be increased by: Alfuzosin; Artemether; Chloroquine; Ciprofloxacin; Ciprofloxacin (Systemic); Divalproex; Gadobutrol; Lumefantrine; Nilotinib; QuiNINE; Valproic Acid

Adverse Reactions

>10%:

Cardiovascular: Peripheral edema (13%)

Central nervous system: Fatigue (52%), chills (16%), dizziness (15%), headache (12%), fever (11%)

Dermatologic: Alopecia (19%), pruritus (12%)

Endocrine & metabolic: Hyperglycemia (8% to 69%; grade 3: 5%), dehydration (1% to 16%)

Gastrointestinal: Diarrhea (52%), nausea (41%), taste alteration (28%), anorexia (24%), weight loss (21%), xerostomia (16%), constipation (15%), vomiting (15%), appetite decreased (14%)

Hematologic: Thrombocytopenia (26%; grades 3/4: 6%), anemia (14%; grades 3/4: 2%)

Neuromuscular & skeletal: Muscle spasm (20%)

Renal: Proteinuria (51%), creatinine increased (16% to 47%)

Respiratory: Cough (11%), upper respiratory infection (11%)

1% to 10%:

Cardiovascular: QT_c prolongation (3% to 4%)

Dermatologic: Squamous cell carcinoma (4%)

Respiratory: Pulmonary embolism (5%)

Pharmacodynamics/Kinetics

Bioavailability Fasting: ~43%

Time to Peak Plasma: With high-fat meal: ~4 hours (range: 2-10 hours)

Protein Binding ~71%

Half-Life Elimination ~2 hours

Metabolism Glucuronidated and hydrolyzed (followed by beta-oxidation) to inactive metabolites

Excretion Urine: 52% (<1% as unchanged drug, ~52% as inactive metabolites)

Available Dosage Forms

Capsule, oral:

Zolinza™: 100 mg

Dosing

Adult & Geriatric Cutaneous T-cell lymphoma: Oral: 400 mg once daily (continue until disease progression or unacceptable toxicity)

In clinical trials, treatment was withheld for grade 4 anemia or thrombocytopenia or other grade 3 or 4 drug related toxicity, until resolved to ≤ grade 1. Therapy was reinitiated with dose modification (Olsen, 2007).

Renal Impairment Not studied, however, based on the minimal renal elimination, adjustment not required.

Hepatic Impairment Not studied; use caution based on predominant hepatic metabolism.

Canadian labeling (not in the FDA-approved labeling):

Moderate hepatic impairment (total bilirubin 1.5-3 times ULN): Use is not recommended.

Severe hepatic impairment (total bilirubin >3 times ULN): Use is contraindicated.

Adjustment for Toxicity Intolerance: Reduce dose to 300 mg once daily; may further reduce to 300 mg daily for 5 consecutive days per week

In clinical trials, **dose reductions** were instituted for the following adverse events: Increased serum creatinine, decreased appetite, hypokalemia, leukopenia, nausea, neutropenia, thrombocytopenia, and vomiting. Vorinostat was **discontinued** for the following adverse events: Anemia, angioneurotic edema, weakness, chest pain, exfoliative dermatitis, DVT, ischemic stroke, lethargy, pulmonary embolism, and spinal cord injury.

Administration

Oral Administer with food. Do not open, crush, or chew capsules. Maintain adequate hydration (≥2 L/day fluids) during treatment.

Stability

Storage Store at 20°C to 25°C (68°F to 77°F); excursions permitted to 15°C to 30°C (59°F to 86°F).

Monitoring and Teaching Issues

Laboratory Monitoring CBC with differential and serum chemistries, including calcium, magnesium, potassium, glucose and creatinine (baseline, then every 2 weeks for 2 months, then monthly)

Physical Assessment Use with caution in presence of hepatic impairment. Electrolyte abnormalities should be corrected prior to treatment. Caution patients with diabetes to monitor serum glucose closely. Teach patient correct use and proper handling of capsules.

Patient Education Take with food. Do not open, chew, or crush capsules. If capsule is accidentally opened or crushed, do not touch the capsules or powder. If powder gets on your skin, wash well with water. If you have diabetes, you should monitor your glucose levels closely and report immediately if your blood sugar is higher than normal. Maintain adequate nutrition and hydration, unless instructed to restrict fluid intake. You may experience dry mouth, taste changes, diarrhea, nausea, vomiting, loss of hair (may grow back after treatment is discontinued), dizziness, or headache. Report persistent diarrhea; chest pain or palpitations; upper respiratory infection or difficulty breathing; muscle pain, tremors, weakness, or spasms; swelling in foot, ankle, or leg; or rash or itching.

Dietary Considerations Take with food.

Breast-Feeding Considerations Due to the potential for serious adverse reactions in the nursing infant, breast-feeding is not recommended.

Pregnancy Considerations Animal studies have demonstrated adverse fetal effects, including fetal loss, decreased fetal weight, and skeletal malformation. There are no adequate and well-controlled studies in pregnant women. Inform patient of potential hazard if used during pregnancy or if pregnancy occurs during treatment.

- ◆ **VoSol® HC** *see* Acetic Acid, Propylene Glycol Diacetate, and Hydrocortisone *on page 43*
- ◆ **VoSpire ER®** *see* Albuterol *on page 58*
- ◆ **Votrient™** *see* Pazopanib *on page 1418*
- ◆ **VP-16** *see* Etoposide *on page 712*
- ◆ **VP-16-213** *see* Etoposide *on page 712*
- ◆ **Vumon®** *see* Teniposide *on page 1728*
- ◆ **VWF/FVIII Concentrate** *see* Antihemophilic Factor/von Willebrand Factor Complex (Human) *on page 134*
- ◆ **VWF:RCo** *see* Antihemophilic Factor/von Willebrand Factor Complex (Human) *on page 134*
- ◆ **vWF:RCof** *see* Antihemophilic Factor/von Willebrand Factor Complex (Human) *on page 134*
- ◆ **Vytorin®** *see* Ezetimibe and Simvastatin *on page 729*
- ◆ **Vyvanse®** *see* Lisdexamfetamine *on page 1117*
- ◆ **VZV Vaccine (Varicella)** *see* Varicella Virus Vaccine *on page 1850*
- ◆ **VZV Vaccine (Zoster)** *see* Zoster Vaccine *on page 1910*

Warfarin (WAR far in)

U.S. Brand Names Coumadin®; Jantoven®

Index Terms Warfarin Sodium

Generic Availability (U.S.) Yes: Tablet

Pharmacologic Category Anticoagulant, Coumarin Derivative; Vitamin K Antagonist

Medication Safety Issues

Sound-alike/look-alike issues:

Coumadin® may be confused with Avandia®, Cardura®, Compazine®, Kemadrin®

Jantoven® may be confused with Janumet®, Januvia®

High alert medication: The Institute for Safe Medication Practices (ISMP) includes this medication among its list of drugs which have a heightened risk of causing significant patient harm when used in error.

2009 National Patient Safety Goals: The Joint Commission on Accreditation of Healthcare Organizations requires healthcare organizations that provide anticoagulant therapy to have a process in place to reduce the risk of anticoagulant-associated patient harm. Patients receiving anticoagulants should receive individualized care through a defined process that includes standardized ordering, dispensing, administration, monitoring and education. This does not apply to routine short-term use of anticoagulants for prevention of venous thromboembolism when the expectation is that the patient's laboratory values will remain within or close to normal values (NPSG.03.05.01).

Medication Guide Available Yes

Pregnancy Risk Factor X

Lactation Does not enter breast milk (AAP rates "compatible"; AAP 2001 update pending)

Use Prophylaxis and treatment of thromboembolic disorders (eg, venous, pulmonary) and embolic complications arising from atrial fibrillation or cardiac valve replacement; adjunct to reduce risk of systemic embolism (eg, recurrent MI, stroke) after myocardial infarction

Unlabeled/Investigational Use Prevention of recurrent transient ischemic attacks

Mechanism of Action/Effect Interferes with hepatic synthesis of vitamin K-dependent coagulation factors (II, VII, IX, X)

Contraindications Hypersensitivity to warfarin or any component of the formulation; hemorrhagic tendencies (eg, patients bleeding from the GI, respiratory, or GU tract; aneurysm; cerebrovascular hemorrhage; following spinal puncture and other diagnostic or therapeutic procedures with potential for significant bleeding; history of bleeding diathesis); recent or potential surgery of the eye or CNS; major regional lumbar block anesthesia or surgery resulting in large, open surfaces; blood dyscrasias; severe uncontrolled or malignant hypertension; pericarditis or pericardial effusion; subacute bacterial endocarditis; history of warfarin-induced necrosis; an unreliable, noncompliant patient; alcoholism; patient who has a history of falls or is a significant fall risk; unsupervised senile or psychotic patient; eclampsia/pre-eclampsia, threatened abortion, pregnancy

Warnings/Precautions Hazardous agent - use appropriate precautions for handling and disposal. Use care in the selection of patients appropriate for this treatment. Ensure patient cooperation especially from the alcoholic, illicit drug user, demented, or psychotic patient; ability to comply with routine laboratory monitoring is essential. Use with caution in trauma, acute infection, moderate-severe renal insufficiency, prolonged dietary insufficiencies, moderate-severe hypertension, polycythemia vera, vasculitis, open wound, active TB, any disruption in normal GI flora, history of PUD, anaphylactic disorders, indwelling catheters, severe diabetes, thyroid disease, and menstruating and postpartum women. Use with caution in protein C deficiency. Use with caution in patients with heparin-induced thrombocytopenia and DVT. Warfarin monotherapy is contraindicated in the initial treatment of active HIT. Reduced liver function, regardless of etiology, may impair synthesis of coagulation factors leading to increased warfarin sensitivity.

[U.S. Boxed Warning]: May cause major or fatal bleeding. Risk factors for bleeding include high intensity anticoagulation (INR >4), age (>65 years), variable INRs, history of GI bleeding, hypertension, cerebrovascular disease, serious heart disease, anemia, malignancy, trauma, renal insufficiency, drug-drug interactions, long duration of therapy, or known genetic deficiency in CYP2C9 activity. Patient must be instructed to report bleeding, accidents, or falls. Unrecognized bleeding sites (eg, colon cancer) may be uncovered by anticoagulation. Patient must also report any new or discontinued medications, herbal or alternative products used, or significant changes in smoking or dietary habits. Necrosis or gangrene of the skin and other tissue can occur, usually in conjunction with protein C or S deficiency. "Purple toes syndrome," due to cholesterol microembolization, may rarely occur. Women may be at risk of developing ovarian hemorrhage at the time of ovulation. The elderly may be more sensitive to anticoagulant therapy. Safety and efficacy have not been established in children; monitor closely.

Presence of the CYP2C9*2 or *3 allele and/or polymorphism of the vitamin K oxidoreductase (VKORC1) gene may increase the risk of bleeding. Lower doses may be required in these patients; genetic testing may help determine appropriate dosing.

Drug Interactions

Metabolism/Transport Effects Substrate of CYP1A2 (minor), 2C9 (major), 2C19 (minor), 3A4 (minor); **Inhibits** CYP2C9 (moderate), 2C19 (weak)

Avoid Concomitant Use

Avoid concomitant use of Warfarin with any of the following: Tamoxifen

Decreased Effect

The levels/effects of Warfarin may be decreased by: Aminoglutethimide; Antineoplastic Agents; Antithyroid Agents; Aprepitant; AzaTHIOprine; Barbiturates; Bile Acid Sequestrants; Bosentan; CarBAMazepine; Coenzyme Q-10; Contraceptives (Estrogens); Contraceptives (Progestins); CYP2C9 Inducers (Highly Effective); Darunavir; Dicloxacillin; Efavirenz; Fosaprepitant; Ginseng (American); Glutethimide; Green Tea; Griseofulvin; Lopinavir; Mercaptopurine; Nafcillin; Nelfinavir; Peginterferon Alfa-2b; Phytonadione; Rifamycin Derivatives; Ritonavir; St Johns Wort; Sucralfate

Increased Effect/Toxicity

Warfarin may increase the levels/effects of: Anticoagulants; Collagenase (Systemic); Drotrecogin Alfa; Ethotoin; Phenytoin

The levels/effects of Warfarin may be increased by: Acetaminophen; Allopurinol; Amiodarone; Androgens; Antineoplastic Agents; Antiplatelet Agents; Atazanavir; Bicalutamide; Capecitabine; Cephalosporins; Chloral Hydrate; Chloramphenicol; Cimetidine; Clopidogrel; Corticosteroids (Systemic); Cranberry; CYP2C9 Inhibitors (Moderate); CYP2C9 Inhibitors (Strong); Desvenlafaxine; Dexmethylphenidate; Disulfiram; Dronedarone; Efavirenz; Erythromycin (Ophthalmic); Esomeprazole; Ethacrynic Acid; Ethotoin; Etoposide; Exenatide; Fenofibrate; Fenofibric Acid; Fenugreek; Fibric Acid Derivatives; Fluconazole; Fluorouracil; Fluorouracil (Systemic); Fluorouracil (Topical); Fosamprenavir; Gefitinib; Ginkgo Biloba; Glucagon; Green Tea; Herbs (Anticoagulant/Antiplatelet Properties); HMG-CoA Reductase Inhibitors; Ifosfamide; Imatinib; Itraconazole; Ivermectin; Ketoconazole; Ketoconazole (Systemic); Lansoprazole; Leflunomide; Macrolide Antibiotics; Methylphenidate; MetroNIDAZOLE; MetroNIDAZOLE (Systemic); Miconazole (Oral); Miconazole (Topical); Milnacipran; Mirtazapine; Nelfinavir; NSAID (COX-2 Inhibitor); NSAID (Nonselective); Omega-3-Acid Ethyl Esters; Omeprazole; Orlistat; Pentosan Polysulfate Sodium; Pentoxifylline; Phenytoin; Posaconazole; Propafenone; Propoxyphene; Prostacyclin Analogues; QuiNIDine; Quinolone Antibiotics; Ranitidine; Salicylates; Saquinavir; Selective Serotonin Reuptake Inhibitors; Sitaxentan; SORAfenib; Sulfinpyrazone [Off Market]; Sulfonamide Derivatives; Tamoxifen; Tetracycline Derivatives; Thrombolytic Agents; Thyroid Products; Tigecycline; Tolterodine; Toremifene; Torsemide; TraMADol; Tricyclic Antidepressants; Venlafaxine; Vitamin E; Voriconazole; Vorinostat; Zafirlukast; Zileuton

Nutritional/Ethanol Interactions

Ethanol: Avoid ethanol. Acute ethanol ingestion (binge drinking) decreases the metabolism of warfarin and increases PT/INR. Chronic daily ethanol use increases the metabolism of warfarin and decreases PT/INR.

Food: The anticoagulant effects of warfarin may be decreased if taken with foods rich in vitamin K. Vitamin E may increase warfarin effect. Cranberry juice may increase warfarin effect.

Herb/Nutraceutical: Cranberry, fenugreek, ginkgo biloba, glucosamine, may enhance bleeding or increase warfarin's effect. Ginseng (American), coenzyme Q_{10}, and St John's wort may decrease warfarin levels and effects. Avoid alfalfa, anise, bilberry, bladderwrack, bromelain, cat's claw, celery, chamomile, coleus, cordyceps, dong quai, evening primrose oil, fenugreek, feverfew, garlic, ginger, ginkgo biloba, ginseng (American), ginseng (Panax), ginseng (Siberian), grapeseed, green tea, guggul, horse chestnut seed, horseradish, licorice, omega-3-acids, prickly ash, red clover, reishi, SAMe (s-adenosylmethionine), sweet clover, turmeric, and white willow (all have additional antiplatelet activity).

Adverse Reactions Bleeding is the major adverse effect of warfarin. Hemorrhage may occur at virtually any site. Risk is dependent on multiple variables, including the intensity of anticoagulation and patient susceptibility.

Cardiovascular: Angina, chest pain, edema, hemorrhagic shock, hypotension, pallor, syncope, vasculitis

Central nervous system: Coma, dizziness, fatigue, fever, headache, lethargy, malaise, pain, stroke

Dermatologic: Alopecia, bullous eruptions, dermatitis, rash, pruritus, urticaria

Gastrointestinal: Abdominal cramps, abdominal pain, anorexia, diarrhea, flatulence, gastrointestinal bleeding, mouth ulcers, nausea, taste disturbance, vomiting

Genitourinary: Hematuria, priapism

Hematologic: Agranulocytosis, anemia, leukopenia, retroperitoneal hematoma, unrecognized bleeding sites (eg, colon cancer) may be uncovered by anticoagulation

Hepatic: Cholestatic jaundice, hepatic injury, hepatitis, transaminases increased

Neuromuscular & skeletal: Joint pain, muscle pain, osteoporosis (potential association with long-term use), paralysis, paresthesia, weakness

Respiratory: Dyspnea, tracheobronchial calcification

Miscellaneous: Anaphylactic reaction, cold intolerance, hypersensitivity/allergic reactions, skin necrosis, gangrene, "purple toes" syndrome

Pharmacodynamics/Kinetics

Onset of Action Anticoagulation: Oral: 24-72 hours; Peak effect: Full therapeutic effect: 5-7 days; INR may increase in 36-72 hours

Duration of Action 2-5 days

Absorption Oral: Rapid, complete

Time to Peak Oral: ~4 hours

Protein Binding 99%

Half-Life Elimination 20-60 hours; Mean: 40 hours; highly variable among individuals

Metabolism Hepatic, primarily via CYP2C9; minor pathways include CYP2C8, 2C18, 2C19, 1A2, and 3A4

Genomic variants: Approximately 37% reduced clearance of S-warfarin in patients heterozygous for 2C9 (*1/*2 or *1/*3), and ~70% reduced in patients homozygous for reduced function alleles (*2/*2, *2/*3, or *3/*3)

Excretion Urine (92%), primarily as metabolites)

Available Dosage Forms

Injection, powder for reconstitution:

Coumadin®: 5 mg

Tablet, oral: 1 mg, 2 mg, 2.5 mg, 3 mg, 4 mg, 5 mg, 6 mg, 7.5 mg, 10 mg

Coumadin®: 1 mg, 2 mg, 2.5 mg, 3 mg, 4 mg, 5 mg, 6 mg, 7.5 mg, 10 mg

Jantoven®: 1 mg, 2 mg, 2.5 mg, 3 mg, 4 mg, 5 mg, 6 mg, 7.5 mg, 10 mg

Dosing

Adult Note: Labeling identifies genetic factors which may increase patient sensitivity to warfarin. Specifically, genetic variations in the proteins CYP2C9 and VKORC1, responsible for warfarin's primary metabolism and pharmacodynamic activity, respectively, have been identified as predisposing factors associated with decreased dose requirement and increased bleeding risk. Genotyping tests are available, and may provide important guidance on initiation of anticoagulant therapy.

Prevention/treatment of thrombosis/embolism:

I.V. (administer as a slow bolus injection): 2-5 mg/day

Oral: Initial dosing must be individualized. Consider the patient (hepatic function, cardiac function, age, nutritional status, concurrent therapy, risk of bleeding) in addition to prior dose response (if available) and the clinical situation. Start 2-5 mg daily for 2 days **or** 5-10 mg daily for 1-2 days (Ansell, 2008). Adjust dose according to INR results; usual maintenance dose ranges from 2-10 mg daily (individual patients may require loading and maintenance doses outside these general guidelines).

Note: Lower starting doses may be required for patients with hepatic impairment, poor nutrition, CHF, elderly, high risk of bleeding, or patients who are debilitated, or those with reduced function genomic variants of the catabolic enzymes CYP2C9 (*2 or *3 alleles) or VKORC1 (-1639 polymorphism); see table. Higher initial doses may be reasonable in selected patients (ie, receiving enzyme-inducing agents and with low risk of bleeding).

Range[1] of Expected Therapeutic Maintenance Dose Based on CYP2C9[2] and VKORC1[3] Genotypes

VKORC1	CYP2C9					
	*1/*1	*1/*2	*1/*3	*2/*2	*2/*3	*3/*3
GG	5-7 mg	5-7 mg	3-4 mg	3-4 mg	3-4 mg	0.5-2 mg
AG	5-7 mg	3-4 mg	3-4 mg	3-4 mg	0.5-2 mg	0.5-2 mg
AA	3-4 mg	3-4 mg	0.5-2 mg	0.5-2 mg	0.5-2 mg	0.5-2 mg

Note: Must also take into account other patient related factors when determining initial dose (eg, age, body weight, concomitant medications, comorbidities).

[1]Ranges derived from multiple published clinical studies.

[2]Patients with CYP2C9 *1/*3, *2/*2, *2/*3, and *3/*3 alleles may take up to 4 weeks to achieve maximum INR with a given dose regimen.

[3]VKORC1 -1639G>A (rs 9923231) variant is used in this table; other VKORC1 variants may also be important determinants of dose.

Geriatric Oral: Initial dose ≤5 mg. Usual maintenance dose: 2-5 mg/day. The elderly tend to require lower dosages to produce a therapeutic level of anticoagulation (due to changes in the pattern of warfarin metabolism).

Pediatric Prevention/treatment of thrombosis: Oral: Infants and Children (unlabeled use): Initial loading dose (if baseline INR is 1-1.3): 0.2 mg/kg (maximum: 10 mg/dose); adjust dose based on INR (reported ranges to maintain INR of 2-3: 0.09-0.33 mg/kg/day). Infants <12 months of age may require doses at or near the high end of this range; consistent anti-coagulation may be difficult to maintain in children <5 years of age.

Renal Impairment No adjustment required, however, patients with renal failure have an increased risk of bleeding complications. Monitor closely.

Hepatic Impairment Monitor effect at usual doses. The response to oral anticoagulants may be markedly enhanced in obstructive jaundice, hepatitis, and cirrhosis. INR should be closely monitored.

Administration

Oral Administer with or without food. Take at the same time each day.

I.V. Administer as a slow bolus injection over 1-2 minutes. Avoid all I.M. injections.

Stability

Reconstitution Reconstitute with 2.7 mL of sterile water (yields 2 mg/mL solution).

Storage

Injection: Prior to reconstitution, store at 15°C to 30°C (59°F to 86°F). Following reconstitution with 2.7 mL of sterile water (yields 2 mg/mL solution), stable for 4 hours at 15°C to 30°C (59°F to 86°F). Protect from light.

Tablet: Store at 15°C to 30°C (59°F to 86°F). Protect from light.

Monitoring and Teaching Issues

Laboratory Monitoring Prothrombin time (desirable range usually 1.5-2 times the control), hematocrit, INR (desirable range usually 2-3 with standard therapy, 2.5-3.5 with high-dose therapy); consider genotyping of CYP2C9 and VKORC1 prior to initiation of therapy, if available

Physical Assessment Use caution with any condition that increases risk of bleeding or that may impact patient ability to comply with therapeutic regimen (eg, dietary vitamin K or C deficiency, hypertension, open wounds, TB, PUD, diabetes, thyroid or renal disease, recent surgery) or any condition that may impact patient's ability to comply with therapeutic regimen (eg, unreliable patient, alcoholism, history of falls or significant fall risk, unsupervised senile or psychotic patient). Assess potential for interactions with other prescriptions, OTC medications, or herbal products patient may be taking that may affect coagulation or platelet aggregation. Monitor for bleeding from any site, rash, urticaria, gastrointestinal upset, abdominal pain, diarrhea, or hypersensitivity reaction.

Patient Education If dose is missed, take as soon as possible; do not double dose. Laboratory tests will be required. Follow prescriber's recommended diet and activity. Avoid excessive alcohol. Do not make major changes in your dietary intake of vitamin K (green vegetables). You will have a tendency to bleed easily while taking this drug. Report unusual bleeding or bruising, skin rash or irritation, unusual fever, persistent nausea or GI upset, pain in joints or back, swelling or pain at injection site, or unhealed wounds.

Dietary Considerations Foods high in vitamin K (eg, beef liver, pork liver, green tea, and leafy green vegetables) inhibit anticoagulant effect. Do not change dietary habits once stabilized on warfarin therapy. A balanced diet with a consistent intake of vitamin K is essential. Avoid large amounts of alfalfa, asparagus, broccoli, Brussels sprouts, cabbage, cauliflower, green teas, kale, lettuce, spinach, turnip greens, and watercress; decreased efficacy of warfarin. It is recommended that the diet contain a CONSISTENT vitamin K content of 70-140 mcg/day. Check with healthcare provider before changing diet.

Geriatric Considerations Before committing an elderly patient to long-term anticoagulation therapy, the risk for bleeding complications secondary to falls, drug interactions, living situation, and cognitive status should be considered. A risk of bleeding complications has been associated with increased age.

Breast-Feeding Considerations Breast-feeding women may be treated with warfarin. Based on limited data, warfarin does not pass into breast milk; however, prolonged PT may occur in some infants (product labeling). Women who are breast-feeding should be carefully monitored to avoid excessive anticoagulation. ACCP guidelines recommend continuation of warfarin in lactating women who wish to breast-feed their infants (Bates, 2008). Warfarin was not detected in breast milk in 2 reports of warfarin exposure during breast-feeding in 9 infants.

Evaluation of coagulation tests and vitamin K status of breast-feeding infant is considered prudent (product labeling).

Pregnancy Considerations Warfarin crosses the placenta; concentrations in the fetal plasma are similar to maternal values. Teratogenic effects have been reported following first trimester exposure and may include coumarin embryopathy (nasal hypoplasia and/or stippled epiphyses; limb hypoplasia may also be present). Adverse events to the fetus have also been observed following second and third trimester exposure and may include CNS abnormalities (including ventral midline dysplasia, dorsal midline dysplasia). Use is contraindicated during pregnancy (or in women of reproductive potential), threatened abortion, eclampsia, or preeclampsia. Frequent pregnancy tests are recommended for women who are planning to become pregnant and adjusted dose heparin or low molecular weight heparin should be substituted as soon as pregnancy is confirmed. In pregnant women with high-risk mechanical heart valves, the benefits of warfarin therapy should be discussed with the risks of available treatments; when possible avoid warfain use during the first trimester and close to delivery.

Additional Information Prospective genotyping is available, and may provide important guidance on initiation of anticoagulant therapy. Commercial testing with PGxPredict™: WARFARIN is available from PGxHealth™ (Division of Clinical Data, Inc, New Haven, CT). The test genotypes patients for presence of the CYP2C9*2 or *3 alleles and the VKORC1 -1639G>A polymorphism. The results of the test allow patients to be phenotyped as extensive, intermediate, or poor metabolizers (CYP2C9) and as low, intermediate, or high warfarin sensitivity (VKORC1). Ordering information is available at 888-592-7327 or warfarininfo@pgxhealth.com.

Related Information

Peak and Trough Guidelines *on page 1958*

- **Xyntha™** *see* Antihemophilic Factor (Recombinant) *on page* *133*
- **Xyzal®** *see* Levocetirizine *on page* *1091*
- **Yasmin®** *see* Ethinyl Estradiol and Drospirenone *on page* *696*
- **Yaz®** *see* Ethinyl Estradiol and Drospirenone *on page* *696*
- **YM905** *see* Solifenacin *on page* *1662*
- **Z4942** *see* Ifosfamide *on page* *947*

Zafirlukast (za FIR loo kast)

U.S. Brand Names Accolate®

Index Terms ICI-204,219

Generic Availability (U.S.) Yes

Pharmacologic Category Leukotriene-Receptor Antagonist

Medication Safety Issues

Sound-alike/look-alike issues:

Accolate® may be confused with Accupril®, Accutane®, Aclovate®

Pregnancy Risk Factor B

Lactation Enters breast milk/contraindicated

Use Prophylaxis and chronic treatment of asthma in adults and children ≥5 years of age

Mechanism of Action/Effect Leukotrienes are inflammatory mediators of asthma. Zafirlukast blocks leukotriene receptors and is able to reduce bronchoconstriction and inflammatory cell infiltration.

Contraindications Hypersensitivity to zafirlukast or any component of the formulation

Warnings/Precautions Zafirlukast is not FDA approved for use in the reversal of bronchospasm in acute asthma attacks, including status asthmaticus. Therapy with zafirlukast can be continued during acute exacerbations of asthma.

Hepatic adverse events (including hepatitis, hyperbilirubinemia, and hepatic failure) have been reported; female patients may be at greater risk. Discontinue immediately if liver dysfunction is suspected. Periodic testing of liver function may be considered (early detection is generally believed to improve the likelihood of recovery). If hepatic dysfunction is suspected (due to clinical signs/symptoms), liver function tests should be measured immediately. Do not resume or restart if hepatic function studies are consistent with dysfunction. Use caution in patients with alcoholic cirrhosis; clearance is reduced. Postmarketing reports of behavioral changes (ie, depression, insomnia) have been noted. Monitor INR closely with concomitant warfarin use. Rare cases of eosinophilic vasculitis (Churg-Strauss) have been reported in patients receiving zafirlukast (usually, but not always, associated with reduction in concurrent steroid dosage). No causal relationship established. Monitor for eosinophilic vasculitis, rash, pulmonary symptoms, cardiac symptoms, or neuropathy.

An increased proportion of zafirlukast patients >55 years of age reported infections as compared to placebo-treated patients. These infections were mostly mild or moderate in intensity and predominantly affected the respiratory tract. Infections occurred equally in both sexes, were dose-proportional to total milligrams of zafirlukast exposure, and were associated with coadministration of inhaled corticosteroids.

Drug Interactions

Metabolism/Transport Effects **Substrate** of CYP2C9 (major); **Inhibits** CYP1A2 (weak), 2C8 (weak), 2C9 (moderate), 2C19 (weak), 2D6 (weak), 3A4 (weak)

Avoid Concomitant Use There are no known interactions where it is recommended to avoid concomitant use.

Decreased Effect

The levels/effects of Zafirlukast may be decreased by: CYP2C9 Inducers (Highly Effective); Erythromycin; Erythromycin (Systemic); Peginterferon Alfa-2b; Theophylline Derivatives

Increased Effect/Toxicity

Zafirlukast may increase the levels/effects of: Carvedilol; CYP2C9 Substrates (High risk); Theophylline Derivatives; Vitamin K Antagonists

The levels/effects of Zafirlukast may be increased by: CYP2C9 Inhibitors (Moderate); CYP2C9 Inhibitors (Strong)

Nutritional/Ethanol Interactions Food: Decreases bioavailability of zafirlukast by 40%.

Adverse Reactions

>10%: Central nervous system: Headache (13%)

1% to 10%:

Central nervous system: Dizziness (2%), pain (2%), fever (2%)

Gastrointestinal: Nausea (3%), diarrhea (3%), abdominal pain (2%), vomiting (2%), dyspepsia (1%)

Hepatic: ALT increased (2%)

Neuromuscular & skeletal: Back pain (2%), myalgia (2%), weakness (2%)

Miscellaneous: Infection (4%)

Pharmacodynamics/Kinetics

Bioavailability Reduced 40% with food

Time to Peak Serum: 3 hours

Protein Binding >99%, primarily to albumin

Half-Life Elimination 10 hours

Metabolism Extensively hepatic via CYP2C9

Excretion Urine (10%); feces

Available Dosage Forms

Tablet, oral: 10 mg, 20 mg

Accolate®: 10 mg, 20 mg

Dosing

Adult & Geriatric Asthma: Oral: 20 mg twice daily

Pediatric Asthma: Oral:

Children 5-11 years: 10 mg twice daily. Safety and effectiveness have not been established in children <5 years of age.

Children ≥12 years: Refer to adult dosing.

Renal Impairment Dosage adjustment not required.

Hepatic Impairment Clearance of zafirlukast is reduced with a greater C_{max} and AUC of 50% to 60% in patients with alcoholic cirrhosis.

Administration

Oral Administer 1 hour before or 2 hours after meals.

Stability

Storage Store tablets at controlled room temperature of 20°C to 25°C (68°F to 77°F). Protect from light and moisture; dispense in original airtight container.

Monitoring and Teaching Issues

Laboratory Monitoring Monitor for improvements in air flow; periodic monitoring of LFTs may be considered (not proved to prevent serious injury, but early detection may enhance recovery)

Physical Assessment Not for use in acute asthma attack. Monitor for liver dysfunction.

Patient Education Do not use during acute bronchospasm. Take regularly as prescribed, even during symptom-free periods. This medication should be taken on an empty stomach, 1 hour before or 2 hours after meals. Do not stop taking other antiasthmatic medications unless instructed by prescriber. You may experience headache, drowsiness, dizziness, blurred vision, gastric upset, nausea, or vomiting. Report persistent CNS or GI symptoms; muscle or back pain; weakness, fever, or chills; yellowing of skin or eyes; dark urine or pale stool; or skin rash. Contact prescriber immediately if experiencing right upper abdominal pain; nausea; fatigue; itching; flu-like symptoms; swelling of the eyes, face, neck, or throat; anorexia; or worsening of condition.

Dietary Considerations Should be taken on an empty stomach (1 hour before or 2 hours after meals).

Geriatric Considerations The mean dose (mg/kg) normalized AUC and C_{max} increase and plasma clearance decreases with increasing age. In patients >65 years of age, there is a two- to threefold greater C_{max} and AUC compared to younger adults. Some studies have demonstrated slightly higher adverse effect reports in elderly compared to younger adults: Headache (4.7%), diarrhea and nausea (1.8%), and pharyngitis (1.3%). No changes in dose recommended for elderly.

Breast-Feeding Considerations The manufacturer does not recommend breast-feeding due to tumorigenicity observed in animal studies.

Pregnancy Considerations There are no adequate and well-controlled trials in pregnant women. Teratogenic effects not observed in animal studies; fetal defects were observed when administered in maternally toxic doses.

Zaleplon (ZAL e plon)

U.S. Brand Names Sonata®

Generic Availability (U.S.) Yes

Pharmacologic Category Hypnotic, Nonbenzodiazepine

Medication Safety Issues

Sound-alike/look-alike issues:

Sonata® may be confused with Soriatane®

Zaleplon may be confused with zolpidem

Medication Guide Available Yes

Pregnancy Risk Factor C

Lactation Enters breast milk/not recommended

Use Short-term (7-10 days) treatment of insomnia (has been demonstrated to be effective for up to 5 weeks in controlled trial)

Mechanism of Action/Effect Zaleplon is unrelated to benzodiazepines, barbiturates, or other hypnotics. However, it interacts with the benzodiazepine GABA receptor complex. Nonclinical studies have shown that it binds selectively to the brain omega-1 receptor situated on the alpha subunit of the GABA-A receptor complex.

Contraindications Hypersensitivity to zaleplon or any component of the formulation

Warnings/Precautions Symptomatic treatment of insomnia should be initiated only after careful evaluation of potential causes of sleep disturbance. Failure of sleep disturbance to resolve after 7-10 days may indicate psychiatric and/or medical illness.

Use with caution in patients with depression, particularly if suicidal risk may be present. Use with caution in patients with a history of drug dependence. Abrupt discontinuance may lead to withdrawal symptoms. Hypnotics/sedatives have been associated with abnormal thinking and behavior changes including decreased inhibition, aggression, bizarre behavior, agitation, hallucinations, and depersonalization. These changes may occur unpredictably and may indicate previously unrecognized psychiatric disorders; evaluate appropriately. May impair physical and mental capabilities. Patients must be cautioned about performing tasks which require mental alertness (operating machinery or driving). Amnesia can occur. Use with caution in patients receiving other CNS depressants or psychoactive medications. Effects with other sedative drugs or ethanol may be potentiated. Postmarketing studies have indicated that the use of hypnotic/sedative agents for sleep has been associated with hypersensitivity reactions including anaphylaxis as well as angioedema. An increased risk for hazardous sleep-related activities such as sleep-driving, cooking and eating food, and making phone calls while asleep have been noted.

Use with caution in the elderly, those with compromised respiratory function, or hepatic impairment (dosage adjustment recommended in mild-to-moderate hepatic impairment; avoid use in severe impairment). Because of the rapid onset of action, zaleplon should be administered immediately prior to bedtime or after the patient has gone to bed and is having difficulty falling asleep. Capsules contain tartrazine (FDC yellow #5); avoid in patients with sensitivity (caution in patients with asthma).

Drug Interactions

Metabolism/Transport Effects Substrate of CYP3A4 (minor)

Avoid Concomitant Use There are no known interactions where it is recommended to avoid concomitant use.

Decreased Effect

The levels/effects of Zaleplon may be decreased by: Flumazenil; Rifamycin Derivatives

Increased Effect/Toxicity

Zaleplon may increase the levels/effects of: Alcohol (Ethyl); CNS Depressants; Methotrimeprazine

The levels/effects of Zaleplon may be increased by: Cimetidine; Conivaptan; Droperidol; Methotrimeprazine

Nutritional/Ethanol Interactions

Ethanol: Avoid ethanol (may increase CNS depression).

Food: High fat meal prolonged absorption; delayed T_{max} by 2 hours, and reduced C_{max} by 35%.

Herb/Nutraceutical: St John's wort may decrease zaleplon levels. Avoid valerian, St John's wort, kava kava, gotu kola (may increase CNS depression).

Adverse Reactions

>10%: Central nervous system: Headache (30% to 42%)

1% to 10%:

Cardiovascular: Chest pain (≥1%), peripheral edema (≤1%)

Central nervous system: Dizziness (7% to 9%), somnolence (5% to 6%), amnesia (2% to 4%), depersonalization (<1% to 2%), hypoesthesia (<1% to 2%), malaise (<1% to 2%), abnormal thinking (≥1%), anxiety (≥1%), depression (≥1%), fever (≥1%), migraine (≥1%), nervousness (≥1%), confusion (≤1%), hallucination (≤1%), vertigo (≤1%)

Dermatologic: Pruritus (≥1%), rash (≥1%), photosensitivity reaction (≤1%)

Endocrine & metabolic: Dysmenorrhea (3% to 4%)

Gastrointestinal: Nausea (6% to 8%), abdominal pain (6%), anorexia (<1% to 2%), constipation (≥1%), dyspepsia (≥1%), taste perversion (≥1%), xerostomia (≥1%), colitis (up to 1%)

Neuromuscular & skeletal: Weakness (5% to 7%), paresthesia (3%), tremor (2%), arthralgia (≥1%), arthritis (≥1%), back pain (≥1%), myalgia (≥1%), hypertonia (1%)

Ocular: Eye pain (3% to 4%), abnormal vision (<1% to 2%), conjunctivitis (≥1%)

Otic: Hyperacusis (1% to 2%), ear pain (≤1%)

Respiratory: Bronchitis (≥1%), epistaxis (≤1%)

Miscellaneous: Parosmia (<1% to 2%)

Pharmacodynamics/Kinetics

Onset of Action Rapid

Duration of Action 6-8 hours

Absorption Rapid and almost complete; high-fat meal delays absorption

Bioavailability ~30%

Time to Peak Serum: 1 hour

Protein Binding ~45% to 75%

Half-Life Elimination 1 hour

Metabolism Extensive, primarily via aldehyde oxidase to form 5-oxo-zaleplon and, to a lesser extent, by CYP3A4 to desethylzaleplon; all metabolites are pharmacologically inactive

Excretion Urine (~70% primarily metabolites, <1% as unchanged drug); feces (~17%)

Clearance: Plasma: Oral: 3 L/hour/kg

Controlled Substance C-IV

Available Dosage Forms

Capsule, oral: 5 mg, 10 mg

Sonata®: 5 mg, 10 mg

Dosing

Adult Insomnia (short-term use): Oral: 10 mg at bedtime (range: 5-20 mg)

Geriatric Reduce dose to 5 mg at bedtime; recommended maximum: 10 mg/day

Renal Impairment No adjustment for mild-to-moderate renal impairment; use in severe renal impairment has not been adequately studied.

Hepatic Impairment Mild-to-moderate impairment: 5 mg; not recommended for use in patients with severe hepatic impairment.

Administration

Oral Administer immediately before bedtime or when the patient is in bed and cannot fall asleep.

Stability

Storage Store at controlled room temperature of 20°C to 25°C (68°F to 77°F). Protect from light.

Monitoring and Teaching Issues

Physical Assessment Evaluate etiology of insomnia; failure of sleep disturbance to resolve after 7-10 days may indicate psychiatric and/or medical illness. Evaluate risk for suicide and assess for history of addiction (long-term use may result in dependence, abuse, or tolerance). Prescription quantities should not exceed a 1 month supply; periodically evaluate need for continued use. For inpatient use, institute safety measures to prevent falls.

Patient Education Take immediately before bedtime, or when you cannot fall asleep. May be habit forming. Avoid alcohol. You may experience drowsiness, dizziness, or lightheadedness. Discontinue drug and report any severe CNS disturbances (hallucinations, anxiety, persistent sleepiness or lethargy, impaired coordination, amnesia); skin rash; vision changes; respiratory difficulty; or unusual swelling, especially on face or neck.

Dietary Considerations Avoid taking with or after a heavy, high-fat meal; reduces absorption.

Geriatric Considerations In clinical trials, elderly responded to the 5 mg dose with decreased sleep latency. As with all hypnotics, assess underlying cause of insomnia.

Pregnancy Considerations Not recommended for use during pregnancy

Additional Information Prescription quantities should not exceed a 1-month supply.

◆ **Zamicet™** *see* Hydrocodone and Acetaminophen *on page 915*

◆ **Zanaflex®** *see* TiZANidine *on page 1775*

◆ **Zanaflex Capsules®** *see* TiZANidine *on page 1775*

Zanamivir (za NA mi veer)

U.S. Brand Names Relenza®

Generic Availability (U.S.) No

Pharmacologic Category Antiviral Agent; Neuraminidase Inhibitor

Medication Safety Issues

Sound-alike/look-alike issues:

Relenza® may be confused with Albenza®, Aplenzin™

Prescribing and Access Restrictions Zanamivir *aqueous solution* intended for nebulization or intravenous (I.V.) administration is **not** currently approved for use. Data on safety and efficacy via these routes of administration are limited. However, limited supplies of zanamivir aqueous solution may be made available through the Zanamivir Compassionate Use Program for qualifying patients for the treatment of serious influenza illness. For information, contact the GlaxoSmithKline Clinical Support Help Desk at 1-866-341-9160 or gskclinicalsupportHD@gsk.-com.

Pregnancy Risk Factor C

Lactation Excretion in breast milk unknown/use caution

Use Treatment of uncomplicated acute illness due to influenza virus A and B in patients who have been symptomatic for no more than 2 days; prophylaxis against influenza virus A and B

The Advisory Committee on Immunization Practices (ACIP) recommends that **treatment** be considered for the following:

- Persons with severe, complicated or progressive illness
- Hospitalized persons
- Persons at higher risk for influenza complications:
  - Children <2 years of age (highest risk in children <6 months of age)
  - Adults ≥65 years of age
  - Persons with chronic disorders of the pulmonary (including asthma) or cardiovascular systems (except hypertension)
  - Persons with chronic metabolic diseases (including diabetes mellitus), hepatic disease, renal dysfunction, hematologic disorders (including sickle cell disease), or immunosuppression (including immunosuppression caused by medications or HIV)
  - Persons with neurologic/neuromuscular conditions (including conditions such as spinal cord injuries, seizure disorders, cerebral palsy, stroke, mental retardation, moderate to severe developmental delay, or muscular dystrophy) which may compromise respiratory function, the handling of respiratory secretions, or that can increase the risk of aspiration
  - Pregnant or postpartum women (≤2 weeks after delivery)
  - Persons <19 years of age on long-term aspirin therapy
  - American Indians and Alaskan Natives
  - Persons who are morbidly obese (BMI ≥40)
  - Residents of nursing homes or other chronic care facilities
- Use may also be considered for previously healthy, nonhigh-risk outpatients with confirmed or suspected influenza based on clinical judgment when treatment can be started within 48 hours of illness onset.

The ACIP recommends that **prophylaxis** be considered for the following:

- Postexposure prophylaxis may be considered for family or close contacts of suspected or confirmed cases, who are at higher risk of influenza complications, and who have not been vaccinated against the circulating strain at the time of the exposure.
- Postexposure prophylaxis may be considered for unvaccinated healthcare workers who had occupational exposure without protective equipment.

- Pre-exposure prophylaxis should only be used for persons at very high risk of influenza complications who cannot be otherwise protected at times of high risk for exposure.
- Prophylaxis should also be administered to all eligible residents of institutions that house patients at high risk when needed to control outbreaks.

Mechanism of Action/Effect Zanamivir inhibits influenza virus neuraminidase enzymes, potentially altering virus particle aggregation and release.

Contraindications Hypersensitivity to zanamivir or any component of the formulation

Warnings/Precautions Allergic-like reactions, including anaphylaxis, oropharyngeal edema, and serious skin rashes have been reported. Rare occurrences of neuropsychiatric events (including confusion, delirium, hallucinations, and/or self-injury) have been reported from postmarketing surveillance; direct causation is difficult to establish (influenza infection may also be associated with behavioral and neurologic changes). Patients must be instructed in the use of the delivery system. Antiviral treatment should begin within 48 hours of symptom onset. However, the CDC recommends that treatment may still be beneficial and should be started in hospitalized patients with severe, complicated or progressive illness if >48 hours. Nonhospitalized persons who are not at high risk for developing severe or complicated illness and who have a mild disease are not likely to benefit if treatment is started >48 hours after symptom onset. Nonhospitalized persons who are already beginning to recover do not need treatment. Effectiveness has not been established in patients with significant underlying medical conditions or for prophylaxis of influenza in nursing home patients (per manufacturer). The CDC recommends zanamivir to be used to control institutional outbreaks of influenza when circulating strains are suspected of being resistant to oseltamivir (refer to current guidelines). Not recommended for use in patients with underlying respiratory disease, such as asthma or COPD, due to lack of efficacy and risk of serious adverse effects. Bronchospasm, decreased lung function, and other serious adverse reactions, including those with fatal outcomes, have been reported in patients with and without airway disease; discontinue with bronchospasm or signs of decreased lung function. For a patient with an underlying airway disease where a medical decision has been made to use zanamivir, a fast-acting bronchodilator should be made available, and used prior to each dose. Not a substitute for annual flu vaccination; has not been shown to reduce risk of transmission of influenza to others. Consider primary or concomitant bacterial infections. Powder for oral inhalation contains lactose. The inhalation powder should only be administered via inhalation using the provided Diskhaler® delivery device. The commercially available formulation is **not** intended to be solubilized or administered via any nebulizer/mechanical ventilator; inappropriate administration has resulted in death. Safety and efficacy of repeated courses or use with hepatic impairment or severe renal impairment have not been established. Indicated for children ≥5 years of age (for influenza prophylaxis) and children ≥7 years of age (for influenza treatment); children ages 5-6 years may have inadequate inhalation (via Diskhaler®) for the treatment of influenza.

Drug Interactions

Avoid Concomitant Use There are no known interactions where it is recommended to avoid concomitant use.

Decreased Effect

Zanamivir may decrease the levels/effects of: Influenza Virus Vaccine (Live/Attenuated)

Increased Effect/Toxicity There are no known significant interactions involving an increase in effect.

Adverse Reactions Most adverse reactions occurred at a frequency which was less than or equal to the control (lactose vehicle).

>10%:

Central nervous system: Headache (prophylaxis 13% to 24%; treatment 2%)

Gastrointestinal: Throat/tonsil discomfort/pain (prophylaxis 8% to 19%)

Respiratory: Nasal signs and symptoms (prophylaxis 12% to 20%; treatment 2%), cough (prophylaxis 7% to 17%; treatment ≤2%)

Miscellaneous: Viral infection (prophylaxis 3% to 13%)

1% to 10%:

Central nervous system: Fever/chills (prophylaxis 5% to 9%; treatment <1.5%), fatigue (prophylaxis 5% to 8%; treatment <1.5%), malaise (prophylaxis 5% to 8%; treatment <1.5%), dizziness (treatment 1% to 2%)

Dermatologic: Urticaria (treatment <1.5%)

Gastrointestinal: Anorexia/appetite decreased (prophylaxis 2% to 4%), appetite increased (prophylaxis 2% to 4%), nausea (prophylaxis 1% to 2%; treatment ≤3%), diarrhea (prophylaxis 2%; treatment 2% to 3%), vomiting (prophylaxis 1% to 2%; treatment 1% to 2%), abdominal pain (treatment <1.5%)

Neuromuscular & skeletal: Muscle pain (prophylaxis 3% to 8%), musculoskeletal pain (prophylaxis 6%), arthralgia/articular rheumatism (prophylaxis 2%), arthralgia (treatment <1.5%), myalgia (treatment <1.5%)

Respiratory: Infection (ear/nose/throat; prophylaxis 2%; treatment 1% to 5%), sinusitis (treatment 3%), bronchitis (treatment 2%), nasal inflammation (prophylaxis 1%)

Pharmacodynamics/Kinetics

Absorption Inhalation: Systemic: ~4% to 17%

Time to Peak 1-2 hours

Protein Binding Plasma: <10%

Half-Life Elimination Serum: 2.5-5.1 hours; Mild-to-moderate renal impairment: 4.7 hours; Severe renal impairment: 18.5 hours

Metabolism None

Excretion Urine (as unchanged drug); feces (unabsorbed drug)

Available Dosage Forms

Powder, for oral inhalation:

Relenza®: 5 mg/blister (20s)

Dosing

Adult & Geriatric Influenza virus A and B:

Prophylaxis: Oral inhalation:

Household setting: Two inhalations (10 mg) once daily for 10 days. Begin within 36 hours following onset of signs or symptoms of index case.

Institutional outbreak, CDC 2011 recommendations: Continue for ≥2 weeks and until ~10 days after identification of illness onset in the last patient. Zanamivir is to be used to control institutional outbreaks of influenza when circulating strains are suspected of being resistant to oseltamivir.

Community outbreak: Two inhalations (10 mg) once daily for 28 days. Begin within 5 days of outbreak.

Treatment: Oral inhalation: Two inhalations (10 mg total) twice daily for 5 days. Doses on first day should be separated by at least 2 hours; on subsequent days, doses should be spaced by ~12 hours. Begin within 2 days of signs or symptoms. Longer treatment may be considered for patients who remain severely ill after 5 days.

Pediatric Influenza virus A and B:

Prophylaxis: Oral inhalation:

Household setting: Children ≥5 years: Refer to adult dosing.

Institutional outbreak: Children ≥5 years: Refer to adult dosing.

Community outbreak: Adolescents: Refer to adult dosing.

Treatment: Oral inhalation: Children ≥7 years: Refer to adult dosing.

Renal Impairment Adjustment not necessary following a 5-day course of treatment due to low systemic absorption; however the potential for drug accumulation should be considered.

Administration

Inhalation Must be used with Diskhaler® delivery device. The foil blister disk containing zanamivir inhalation powder should not be manipulated, solubilized, or administered via a nebulizer. Patients who are scheduled to use an inhaled bronchodilator should use their bronchodilator prior to zanamivir. With the exception of the initial dose when used for treatment, administer at the same time each day.

Stability

Storage Store at 25°C (77°F); excursions permitted to 15°C to 30°C (59°F to 86°F). Do not puncture blister until taking a dose using the Diskhaler®.

Monitoring and Teaching Issues

Physical Assessment Recommendations for antiviral susceptibility and effectiveness may change. Validate with the CDC recommendations for use prior to prescribing. Therapy for treatment must be started within 48 hours of first influenza symptoms. Monitor for change in behavior.

Patient Education This is not a substitute for the influenza vaccine. If you have asthma or COPD you may be at risk for bronchospasm; see prescriber for appropriate bronchodilator before using zanamivir. Stop using this medication and contact your prescriber if you experience shortness of breath, increased wheezing, or other signs of bronchospasm. You may experience dizziness, headache, sore throat, or nasal congestion. Report unresolved diarrhea, vomiting, or nausea; fever or muscle pain; or change in behavior, including hallucinations, confusion, delirium, or seizures.

Geriatric Considerations A recent study demonstrated that most elderly were unable to use an inhaler device effectively.

Breast-Feeding Considerations It is not known if zanamivir is found in human milk and the manufacturer recommends that caution be exercised when administering zanamivir to nursing women. According to the CDC, breast-feeding while taking zanamivir can be continued. The CDC recommends that women infected with the influenza virus follow general precautions (eg, frequent hand washing) to decrease viral transmission to the child. Mothers with influenza-like illnesses at delivery should consider avoiding close contact with the infant until they have received 48 hours of antiviral medication, fever has resolved, and cough and secretions can be controlled. These measures may help decrease (but not eliminate) the risk of transmitting influenza to the newborn. During this time, breast milk can be expressed and bottle-fed to the infant by another person who is well. Protective measures, such as wearing a face mask, changing into a clean gown or clothing, and strict hand hygiene should be continued by the mother for ≥7 days after the onset of symptoms or until symptom-free for 24 hours. Infant care should be performed by a noninfected person when possible (consult current CDC guidelines).

Pregnancy Considerations Adverse events were not observed in animal reproduction studies; therefore, the manufacturer classifies zanamivir as pregnancy category C. Influenza infection may be more severe in pregnant women. Untreated influenza infection is associated with an increased risk of adverse events to the fetus and an increased risk of complications or death to the mother. Oseltamivir and zanamivir are currently recommended for the treatment or prophylaxis of influenza in pregnant women and women up to 2 weeks postpartum. Oseltamivir and zanamivir are currently recommended as an adjunct to vaccination and should not be used as a substitute for vaccination in pregnant women (consult current CDC guidelines).

Additional Information Majority of patients included in clinical trials were infected with influenza A, however, a number of patients with influenza B infections were also enrolled. Patients with lower temperature or less severe symptoms appeared to derive less benefit from therapy. No consistent treatment benefit was demonstrated in patients with chronic underlying medical conditions.

The absence of symptoms does not rule out viral influenza infection and clinical judgment should guide the decision for therapy. Treatment should not be delayed while waiting for the results of diagnostic tests. Treatment should be considered for high-risk patients with symptoms despite a negative rapid influenza test when the illness cannot be contributed to another cause. Use of zanamivir is not a substitute for vaccination (when available); susceptibility to influenza infection returns once therapy is discontinued.

- ◆ **Zanosar®** *see* Streptozocin *on page 1682*
- ◆ **Zantac®** *see* Ranitidine *on page 1555*
- ◆ **Zantac 75® [OTC]** *see* Ranitidine *on page 1555*
- ◆ **Zantac 150® [OTC]** *see* Ranitidine *on page 1555*
- ◆ **Zantac® EFFERdose®** *see* Ranitidine *on page 1555*
- ◆ **Zarah®** *see* Ethinyl Estradiol and Drospirenone *on page 696*
- ◆ **Zaroxolyn®** *see* Metolazone *on page 1215*
- ◆ **Zazole™ [DSC]** *see* Terconazole *on page 1735*
- ◆ **ZD1033** *see* Anastrozole *on page 128*
- ◆ **ZD1839** *see* Gefitinib *on page 853*
- ◆ **ZD9238** *see* Fulvestrant *on page 838*
- ◆ **ZDV** *see* Zidovudine *on page 1890*
- ◆ **ZDV, Abacavir, and Lamivudine** *see* Abacavir, Lamivudine, and Zidovudine *on page 32*
- ◆ **ZDX** *see* Goserelin *on page 885*
- ◆ **Zeasorb®-AF [OTC]** *see* Miconazole (Topical) *on page 1224*
- ◆ **Zebeta®** *see* Bisoprolol *on page 222*
- ◆ **Zebutal®** *see* Butalbital, Acetaminophen, and Caffeine *on page 260*
- ◆ **Zegerid®** *see* Omeprazole and Sodium Bicarbonate *on page 1359*
- ◆ **Zegerid OTC™ [OTC]** *see* Omeprazole and Sodium Bicarbonate *on page 1359*
- ◆ **Zelapar™** *see* Selegiline *on page 1630*
- ◆ **Zeldox** *see* Ziprasidone *on page 1896*
- ◆ **Zelnorm®** *see* Tegaserod *on page 1712*
- ◆ **Zemplar®** *see* Paricalcitol *on page 1412*
- ◆ **Zenapax® [DSC]** *see* Daclizumab *on page 453*
- ◆ **Zenchent™** *see* Ethinyl Estradiol and Norethindrone *on page 701*
- ◆ **Zenpep™** *see* Pancrelipase *on page 1400*
- ◆ **Zeosa™** *see* Ethinyl Estradiol and Norethindrone *on page 701*
- ◆ **Zerit®** *see* Stavudine *on page 1680*
- ◆ **Zestoretic®** *see* Lisinopril and Hydrochlorothiazide *on page 1122*
- ◆ **Zestril®** *see* Lisinopril *on page 1119*
- ◆ **Zetia®** *see* Ezetimibe *on page 728*
- ◆ **Ziac®** *see* Bisoprolol and Hydrochlorothiazide *on page 223*
- ◆ **Ziagen®** *see* Abacavir *on page 30*
- ◆ **Ziana™** *see* Clindamycin and Tretinoin *on page 401*

Ziconotide (zi KOE no tide)

U.S. Brand Names Prialt®

Generic Availability (U.S.) No

Pharmacologic Category Analgesic, Nonopioid; Calcium Channel Blocker, N-Type

Medication Safety Issues

High alert medication: The Institute for Safe Medication Practices (ISMP) includes this medication among its list of drugs which have a heightened risk of causing significant patient harm when used in error.

Pregnancy Risk Factor C

Lactation Excretion in breast milk unknown/not recommended

Use Management of severe chronic pain in patients requiring intrathecal (I.T.) therapy and who are intolerant or refractory to other therapies

Mechanism of Action/Effect Ziconotide selectively binds to N-type voltage-sensitive calcium channels located on the nociceptive afferent nerves of the dorsal horn in the spinal cord. This binding is thought to block N-type calcium channels, leading to a blockade of excitatory neurotransmitter release and reducing sensitivity to painful stimuli.

Contraindications Hypersensitivity to ziconotide or any component of the formulation; history of psychosis; I.V. administration

I.T. administration is contraindicated in patients with infection at the injection site, uncontrolled bleeding, or spinal canal obstruction that impairs CSF circulation

Warnings/Precautions [U.S Boxed Warning]: Severe psychiatric symptoms and neurological impairment have been reported; interrupt or discontinue therapy if cognitive impairment, hallucinations, mood changes, or changes in consciousness occur. May cause or worsen depression and/or risk of suicide. Cognitive impairment may appear gradually during treatment and is generally reversible after discontinuation (may take up to 2 weeks for cognitive effects to reverse). Use caution in the elderly; may experience a higher incidence of confusion. Patients should be instructed to use caution in performing tasks which require alertness (eg, operating machinery or driving). May have additive effects with opiates or other CNS-depressant medications; may potentiate opioid-induced decreased GI motility; does not interact with opioid receptors or potentiate opiate-induced respiratory depression. Will not prevent or relieve symptoms associated with opiate withdrawal and opiates should not be abruptly discontinued. Unlike opioids, ziconotide therapy can be interrupted abruptly or discontinued without evidence of withdrawal.

Meningitis may occur with use of I.T. pumps; monitor for signs and symptoms of meningitis; treatment of meningitis may require removal of system and discontinuation of intrathecal therapy. Elevated serum creatine kinase can occur, particularly during the first 2 months of therapy; consider dose reduction or discontinuing if combined with new neuromuscular symptoms (myalgias, myasthenia, muscle cramps, weakness) or reduction in physical activity. Safety and efficacy have not been established with renal or hepatic dysfunction, or in pediatric patients. Should not be used in combination with intrathecal opiates.

Drug Interactions

Avoid Concomitant Use There are no known interactions where it is recommended to avoid concomitant use.

Decreased Effect There are no known significant interactions involving a decrease in effect.

Increased Effect/Toxicity

Ziconotide may increase the levels/effects of: Alcohol (Ethyl); CNS Depressants; Methotrimeprazine

The levels/effects of Ziconotide may be increased by: Droperidol; Methotrimeprazine

Nutritional/Ethanol Interactions Ethanol: Avoid ethanol (may increase CNS adverse effects).

Adverse Reactions

>10%:

Central nervous system: Dizziness (46%), confusion (15% to 33%), memory impairment (7% to 22%), somnolence (17%), ataxia (14%), speech disorder (14%), headache (13%), aphasia (12%), hallucination (12%; including auditory and visual)

Gastrointestinal: Nausea (40%), diarrhea (18%), vomiting (16%)

Neuromuscular & skeletal: Creatine kinase increased (40%; ≥3 times ULN: 11%), weakness (18%), gait disturbances (14%)

Ocular: Blurred vision (12%)

2% to 10%:

Cardiovascular: Hypotension, peripheral edema, postural hypotension

Central nervous system: Abnormal thinking (8%), amnesia (8%), anxiety (8%), vertigo (7%), insomnia (6%), fever (5%), paranoid reaction (3%), delirium (2%), hostility (2%), stupor (2%), agitation, attention disturbance, balance impaired, burning sensation, coordination abnormal, depression, disorientation, fatigue, fever, hypoesthesia, irritability, lethargy, mental impairment, mood disorder, nervousness, pain, sedation

Dermatologic: Pruritus (7%)

Gastrointestinal: Anorexia (6%), taste perversion (5%), abdominal pain, appetite decreased, constipation, xerostomia

Genitourinary: Urinary retention (9%), dysuria, urinary hesitance

Neuromuscular & skeletal: Dysarthria (7%), paresthesia (7%), rigors (7%), tremor (7%), muscle spasm (6%), limb pain (5%), areflexia, muscle cramp, muscle weakness, myalgia

Ocular: Nystagmus (8%), diplopia, visual disturbance

Respiratory: Sinusitis (5%)

Miscellaneous: Diaphoresis (5%)

Pharmacodynamics/Kinetics

Protein Binding ~50%

Half-Life Elimination I.V.: 1-1.6 hours (plasma); I.T.: 2.9-6.5 hours (CSF)

Metabolism Metabolized via endopeptidases and exopeptidases present on multiple organs including kidney, liver, lung; degraded to peptide fragments and free amino acids

Excretion I.V.: Urine (<1%)

Available Dosage Forms

Injection, solution [preservative free]:

Prialt®: 25 mcg/mL (20 mL); 100 mcg/mL (1 mL, 5 mL)

Dosing

Adult Chronic pain: I.T.: Initial dose: ≤2.4 mcg/day (0.1 mcg/hour)

Dose may be titrated by ≤2.4 mcg/day (0.1 mcg/hour) at intervals ≤2-3 times/week to a maximum dose of 19.2 mcg/day (0.8 mcg/hour) by day 21; average dose at day 21: 6.9 mcg/day (0.29 mcg/hour). A faster titration should be used only if the urgent need for analgesia outweighs the possible risk to patient safety.

Geriatric Refer to adult dosing. Use with caution.

Adjustment for Toxicity

Cognitive impairment: Reduce dose or discontinue. Effects are generally reversible within 3-15 days of discontinuation.

Reduced level of consciousness: Discontinue until event resolves.

CK elevation with neuromuscular symptoms: Consider dose reduction or discontinuation.

Administration

I.V. Not for I.V. administration

Other Not for I.V. administration. **For I.T. administration only** using Medtronic SynchroMed® EL, SynchroMed® II Infusion System, or CADD-Micro® ambulatory infusion pump.

Medtronic SynchroMed® EL or SynchroMed® II Infusion Systems:

Naive pump priming (first time use with ziconotide): Use 2 mL of undiluted ziconotide 25 mcg/mL solution to rinse the internal surfaces of the pump; repeat twice for a total of 3 rinses

Initial pump fill: Use only undiluted 25 mcg/mL solution and fill pump after priming. Following the initial fill only, adsorption on internal device surfaces will occur, requiring the use of the undiluted solution and refill within 14 days.

Pump refills: Contents should be emptied prior to refill. Subsequent pump refills should occur at least every 40 days if using diluted solution or at least every 84 days if using undiluted solution.

CADD-Micro® ambulatory infusion pump: Refer to manufacturers' manual for initial fill and refill instructions

pH: 4-5

Stability

Reconstitution Preservative free NS should be used when dilution is needed.

CADD-Micro® ambulatory infusion pump: Initial fill: Dilute to final concentration of 5 mcg/mL.

Medtronic SynchroMed® EL or SynchroMed® II infusion system: Prior to initial fill, rinse internal pump surfaces with 2 mL ziconotide (25 mcg/mL), repeat twice. Only the 25 mcg/mL concentration (undiluted) should be used for initial pump fill.

Storage Prior to use, store vials at 2°C to 8°C (36°F to 46°F). Once diluted, may be stored at 2°C to 8°C (36°F to 46°F) for 24 hours; refrigerate during transit. Do not freeze. Protect from light.

When using the Medtronic SynchroMed® EL or SynchroMed® II Infusion System, solutions expire as follows:

25 mcg/mL: Undiluted:

Initial fill: Use within 14 days.

Refill: Use within 84 days.

100 mcg/mL:

Undiluted: Refill: Use within 84 days.

Diluted: Refill: Use within 40 days.

Monitoring and Teaching Issues

Laboratory Monitoring CPK (every other week for first month, then monthly)

Physical Assessment This medication is given intrathecally via pump. Monitor for changes in behavior, cognitive impairment, hallucinations, or changes in mood or consciousness.

Patient Education Do not use alcohol. You may experience dizziness, sleepiness, or lightheadedness; nausea or vomiting; constipation; diarrhea; or loss of appetite. Report chest pain, swelling of extremities, muscle weakness and poor coordination, hallucinations, confusion, or extreme weakness.

Geriatric Considerations Manufacturer reports that in all trials there was a higher incidence of confusion in the elderly compared to younger adults.

Breast-Feeding Considerations The manufacturer recommends discontinuing breast-feeding or discontinuing ziconotide.

Pregnancy Considerations Teratogenic effects were not observed in animal studies, but increased postimplantation pup loss was reported. Maternal toxicity was also noted. There are no adequate and well-controlled studies in pregnant women.

Zidovudine (zye DOE vyoo deen)

U.S. Brand Names Retrovir®

Index Terms Azidothymidine; AZT (error-prone abbreviation); Compound S; ZDV

Generic Availability (U.S.) Yes: Capsule, syrup, tablet

Pharmacologic Category Antiretroviral Agent, Reverse Transcriptase Inhibitor (Nucleoside)

Medication Safety Issues

Sound-alike/look-alike issues:

Azidothymidine may be confused with azaTHIOprine, aztreonam

Retrovir® may be confused with acyclovir, ritonavir

AZT is an error-prone abbreviation (mistaken as azathioprine, aztreonam)

Pregnancy Risk Factor C

Lactation Enters breast milk/contraindicated

Use Treatment of HIV infection in combination with at least two other antiretroviral agents; prevention of maternal/fetal HIV transmission as monotherapy

Unlabeled/Investigational Use Postexposure prophylaxis for HIV exposure as part of a multidrug regimen

Mechanism of Action/Effect Zidovudine is a thymidine analog which interferes with the HIV virus that results in inhibition of viral replication.

Contraindications Life-threatening hypersensitivity to zidovudine or any component of the formulation

Warnings/Precautions Hazardous agent - use appropriate precautions for handling and disposal. **[U.S. Boxed Warning]: Often associated with hematologic toxicity including granulocytopenia, severe anemia requiring transfusions, or (rarely) pancytopenia.** Use with caution in patients with bone marrow compromise (granulocytes <1000 cells/mm^3 or hemoglobin <9.5 mg/dL); dosage adjustment may be required in patients who develop anemia or neutropenia. **[U.S. Boxed Warning]: Lactic acidosis and severe hepatomegaly with**

steatosis have been reported, including fatal cases; use with caution in patients with risk factors for liver disease (risk may be increased in obese patients or prolonged exposure) and suspend treatment with zidovudine in any patient who develops clinical or laboratory findings suggestive of lactic acidosis (transaminase elevation may/may not accompany hepatomegaly and steatosis). Use caution in combination with interferon alfa with or without ribavirin in HIV/HBV coinfected patients; monitor closely for hepatic decompensation, anemia, or neutropenia; dose reduction or discontinuation of interferon and/or ribavirin may be required if toxicity evident. **[U.S. Boxed Warning]: Prolonged use has been associated with symptomatic myopathy and myositis.** May cause redistribution of fat (eg, buffalo hump, peripheral wasting with increased abdominal girth, cushingoid appearance). Immune reconstitution syndrome may develop resulting in the occurrence of an inflammatory response to an indolent or residual opportunistic infection; further evaluation and treatment may be required. Reduce dose in patients with severe renal impairment. Do not administer with combination products that contain zidovudine as one of their components (eg, COMBIVIR® [lamivudine and zidovudine] or TRIZIVIR® [abacavir sulfate, lamivudine, and zidovudine]).

Drug Interactions

Metabolism/Transport Effects Substrate (minor) of CYP2A6, 2C9, 2C19, 3A4

Avoid Concomitant Use

Avoid concomitant use of Zidovudine with any of the following: Stavudine

Decreased Effect

Zidovudine may decrease the levels/effects of: Stavudine

The levels/effects of Zidovudine may be decreased by: Clarithromycin; DOXOrubicin; DOXOrubicin (Liposomal); Protease Inhibitors; Rifamycin Derivatives

Increased Effect/Toxicity

Zidovudine may increase the levels/effects of: Ribavirin

The levels/effects of Zidovudine may be increased by: Acyclovir-Valacyclovir; Clarithromycin; Conivaptan; Divalproex; DOXOrubicin; DOXOrubicin (Liposomal); Fluconazole; Ganciclovir-Valganciclovir; Interferons; Methadone; Probenecid; Ribavirin; Valproic Acid

Adverse Reactions As reported in adult patients with asymptomatic HIV infection. Frequency and severity may increase with advanced disease.

>10%:

Central nervous system: Headache (63%), malaise (53%)
Gastrointestinal: Nausea (51%), anorexia (20%), vomiting (17%)

1% to 10%:

Gastrointestinal: Constipation (6%)
Hematologic: Granulocytopenia (2%; onset 6-8 weeks), anemia (1%; onset 2-4 weeks)
Hepatic: Transaminases increased (1% to 3%)
Neuromuscular & skeletal: Weakness (9%)

Frequency not defined:

Cardiovascular: Cardiomyopathy, chest pain, syncope, vasculitis
Central nervous system: Anxiety, chills, confusion, depression, dizziness, fatigue, insomnia, loss of mental acuity, mania, seizure, somnolence, vertigo
Dermatologic: Pruritus, rash, skin/nail pigmentation changes, Stevens-Johnson syndrome, toxic epidermal necrolysis, urticaria
Endocrine & metabolic: Body fat redistribution, gynecomastia
Gastrointestinal: Abdominal cramps, abdominal pain, dyspepsia, dysphagia, flatulence, mouth ulcer, oral mucosa pigmentation, pancreatitis, taste perversion
Genitourinary: Urinary frequency, urinary hesitancy
Hematologic: Aplastic anemia, hemolytic anemia, leukopenia, lymphadenopathy, pancytopenia with marrow hypoplasia, pure red cell aplasia
Hepatic: Hepatitis, hepatomegaly with steatosis, hyperbilirubinemia, jaundice, lactic acidosis
Neuromuscular & skeletal: Arthralgia, back pain, CPK increased, LDH increased, musculoskeletal pain, myalgia, neuropathy, muscle spasm, myopathy, myositis, paresthesia, rhabdomyolysis, tremor
Ocular: Amblyopia, macular edema, photophobia
Otic: Hearing loss
Respiratory: Cough, dyspnea, rhinitis, sinusitis
Miscellaneous: Allergic reactions, anaphylaxis, angioedema, diaphoresis, flu-like syndrome, immune reconstitution syndrome

Pharmacodynamics/Kinetics

Bioavailability 54% to 74%

Time to Peak Serum: 30-90 minutes

Protein Binding 25% to 38%

Half-Life Elimination Terminal: 0.5-3 hours

Metabolism Hepatic via glucuronidation to inactive metabolites; extensive first-pass effect

Excretion

Oral: Urine (72% to 74% as metabolites, 14% to 18% as unchanged drug)
I.V.: Urine (45% to 60% as metabolites, 18% to 29% as unchanged drug)

Available Dosage Forms

Capsule, oral: 100 mg
Retrovir®: 100 mg

Injection, solution [preservative free]:
Retrovir®: 10 mg/mL (20 mL)

Syrup, oral: 50 mg/5 mL (240 mL)
Retrovir®: 50 mg/5 mL (240s)

Tablet, oral: 300 mg
Retrovir®: 300 mg

Dosing

Adult & Geriatric

Prevention of maternal-fetal HIV transmission: Maternal (per AIDS*info* guidelines): Begin oral therapy with usual recommended dose as soon as possible in women who require treatment for their own health (including use during the first trimester); may delay therapy until after 10-12 weeks gestation (but no later than 28 weeks gestation) in women who are using antiretroviral medications solely for the prevention of perinatal transmission. Dose adjustment is not required for pregnant women. Change to I.V. dosing during labor.

Note: Consider use of zidovudine in combination with nevirapine (and possibly lamivudine) in select situations (eg, infants born to mothers with suboptimal viral suppression at delivery, infants born to mothers with only intrapartum therapy or no therapy, or infants born to mothers with known antiretroviral drug-resistant virus) (AIDS*info* guidelines).

During labor and delivery, administer zidovudine I.V. at 2 mg/kg as loading dose followed by a continuous I.V. infusion of 1 mg/kg/hour until the umbilical cord is clamped. For scheduled cesarean delivery, begin I.V. zidovudine 3 hours before surgery.

HIV infection:

Oral: 300 mg twice daily or 200 mg 3 times/day

I.V.: 1 mg/kg/dose administered every 4 hours around-the-clock (5-6 doses/day)

Prevention of HIV following needlesticks (unlabeled use): Oral: 200 mg 3 times/day plus lamivudine 150 mg twice daily; a protease inhibitor (eg, indinavir) may be added for high risk exposures; begin therapy within 2 hours of exposure if possible

Note: Patients should receive I.V. therapy only until oral therapy can be administered

Pediatric

Prevention of maternal-fetal HIV transmission (in neonates): Note: Consider use of zidovudine in combination with nevirapine (and possibly lamivudine) in select situations (eg, infants born to mothers with suboptimal viral suppression at delivery, infants born to mothers with only intrapartum therapy or no therapy, or infants born to mothers with known antiretroviral drug-resistant virus) (AIDS*info* guidelines).

Note: Dosing should begin 6-12 hours after birth and continue for the first 6 weeks of life.

Oral:

Full-term infants: 2 mg/kg/dose every 6 hours

Infants ≥30 weeks and <35 weeks gestation at birth: 2 mg/kg/dose every 12 hours; at 2 weeks of age, advance to 2 mg/kg/dose every 8 hours

Infants <30 weeks gestation at birth: 2 mg/kg/dose every 12 hours; at 4 weeks of age, advance to 2 mg/kg/dose every 8 hours

Alternate dosing for infants >35 weeks gestation (for use in low resource settings; may also be considered for use in higher resource settings if simplicity in dosing/administration is important):

Infants <2.5 kg at birth: 10 mg twice daily

Infants >2.5 kg at birth: 15 mg twice daily

I.V. (infants unable to receive oral dosing):

Full term: 1.5 mg/kg/dose every 6 hours

Infants ≥30 weeks and <35 weeks gestation at birth: 1.5 mg/kg/dose every 12 hours; at 2 weeks of age, advance to 1.5 mg/kg/dose every 8 hours

Infants <30 weeks gestation at birth: 1.5 mg/kg/dose every 12 hours; at 4 weeks of age, advance to 1.5 mg/kg/dose every 8 hours

Treatment of HIV infection:

Children 4 weeks to <18 years:

Oral: Dose should be calculated by body weight (in kg) or body surface area and should not exceed the recommended adult dose. **Note:** Doses calculated by body weight may not be the same as those calculated by body surface area.

Dosing based on body surface area: 240 mg/m^2 every 12 hours (maximum: 300 mg every 12 hours) **or** 160 mg/m^2/dose every 8 hours (maximum: 200 mg every 8 hours)

Dosing based on weight (**Note:** 3 times daily dose is approved but rarely used in clinical practice):

4 to <9 kg: 12 mg/kg/dose twice daily **or** 8 mg/kg/dose 3 times/day

≥9 to <30 kg: 9 mg/kg/dose twice daily **or** 6 mg/kg/dose 3 times/day

≥30 kg: 300 mg twice daily **or** 200 mg 3 times/day

Children 6 weeks to <12 years:

I.V. continuous infusion: 20 mg/m^2/hour

I.V. intermittent infusion: 120 mg/m^2/dose every 6 hours

Children ≥12 years: *I.V. intermittent infusion:* 1 mg/kg/dose every 4 hours around-the-clock

Renal Impairment

Cl_{cr} <15 mL/minute including hemo-/peritoneal dialysis: 100 mg (oral) or 1 mg/kg (I.V.) every 6-8 hours

Continuous arteriovenous or venovenous hemodiafiltration: Administer 100 mg every 8 hours

Hepatic Impairment Insufficient data to make dosing recommendation.

Adjustment for Toxicity Consider dose interruption for significant anemia (hemoglobin <7.5 g/dL or >25% reduction from baseline) and/or neutropenia (granulocyte count <750 cells/mm^3 or >50% reduction from baseline) until evidence of recovery. Anemia associated with chronic zidovudine may warrant dose reduction.

Administration

Oral Administer around-the-clock to promote less variation in peak and trough serum levels. Oral zidovudine may be administered without regard to meals.

I.M. Do not give I.M.

I.V. Avoid rapid infusion or bolus injection

Neonates: Infuse over 30 minutes

Adults: Infuse loading dose over 1 hour, followed by continuous infusion

Stability

Reconstitution Solution for injection should be diluted with D_5W to a concentration ≤4 mg/mL. Attempt to administer diluted solution within 8 hours if stored at room temperature or 24 hours if refrigerated to minimize potential for microbial-contaminated solutions ≥≥(vials are single-use and do not contain preservative).

Storage

I.V.: Store undiluted vials at 15°C to 25°C (59°F to 77°F). Protect from light. When diluted, solution is physically and chemically stable for 24 hours at room temperature and 48 hours if refrigerated.

Tablets, capsules, syrup: Store at 15°C to 25°C (59°F to 77°F). Protect capsules from moisture.

Monitoring and Teaching Issues

Laboratory Monitoring Monitor CBC and platelet count at least every 2 weeks, liver function tests, MCV, serum creatinine kinase, CD4 cell count, viral load

Physical Assessment Assess closely for any previous allergy history prior to beginning treatment. Use caution in presence of bone marrow compromise or renal impairment; dose reduction may be necessary. Assess CD4 count and viral load, CBC and platelet count, and LFTs. Monitor for lactic acidosis (elevated transaminases), anemia, neutropenia, hepatic decompensation, gastrointestinal disturbance (nausea, vomiting, diarrhea), myalgia, and peripheral neuropathy. Teach patient proper timing of multiple medications.

Patient Education This drug will not cure HIV, nor has it been found to reduce transmission of HIV; use appropriate precautions to prevent spread to other persons. This drug is prescribed as one part of a multidrug combination; take exactly as directed for full course of therapy. Maintain adequate hydration unless advised by prescriber to restrict fluids. Avoid alcohol. Frequent blood tests may be required. May cause body changes due to redistribution of body fat, facial atrophy, or breast enlargement (normal effects of drug). May cause headache, dizziness, weakness, nausea, vomiting, mouth sores, constipation, CNS changes (anxiety, chills, confusion, depression, loss of mental acuity, or seizures - contact prescriber), or back or muscle pain. Report excessive fatigue, easy bruising or bleeding, change in urinary pattern, dark urine or light stool, chest pain or palpitations, rash or skin sores, muscle or bone pain, or tremor. Stop drug and report immediately symptoms of hypersensitivity/allergic reaction (eg, swelling of lips, face, mouth, or throat; rash; difficulty breathing or chest tightness; excessive sweating; numbness or loss of sensation). Do not restart without specific instruction by your prescriber.

Dietary Considerations May be taken without regard to meals.

Breast-Feeding Considerations In infants born to mothers who are HIV positive, HAART while breast-feeding may decrease postnatal infection. Infant prophylaxis with zidovudine in combination with nevirapine or nevirapine alone may also decrease the risk of HIV transmission to the infant. However, maternal or infant antiretroviral therapy does not completely eliminate the risk of postnatal HIV transmission. In addition, multiclass resistant virus has been detected in breast-feeding infants despite maternal therapy.

In the United States where formula is accessible, affordable, safe, and sustainable, complete avoidance of breast-feeding by HIV-infected women is recommended to decrease potential transmission of HIV.

Pregnancy Considerations Adverse events have been observed in some animal reproduction studies. Zidovudine crosses the placenta and the placenta also metabolizes zidovudine to the active metabolite. No increased risk of overall birth defects has been observed following first trimester exposure according to data collected by the antiretroviral pregnancy registry. The pharmacokinetics of zidovudine are not significantly altered in pregnancy and dosing adjustment is not needed. The Perinatal HIV Guidelines Working Group considers zidovudine the preferred NRTI for use in combination regimens during pregnancy. The use of zidovudine reduces the maternal-fetal transmission of HIV by ~70% and should be used for antenatal therapy unless there is severe toxicity, concurrent stavudine use, documented resistance, or the mother is already on a fully suppressive regimen. In HIV-infected mothers not previously on antiretroviral therapy, and who do not need therapy for their own health, treatment may be delayed until after 10-12 weeks gestation (but no later than 28 weeks gestation). Intrapartum zidovudine is recommended for all women regardless of their antepartum regimen. Cases of lactic acidosis/hepatic steatosis syndrome related to mitochondrial toxicity have been reported in pregnant women receiving nucleoside analogues. It is not known if pregnancy itself potentiates this known side effect; however, women may be at increased risk of lactic acidosis and liver damage. In addition, these adverse events are similar to other rare but life-threatening syndromes which occur during pregnancy (eg HELLP syndrome). Hepatic enzymes and electrolytes should be monitored frequently during the third trimester of pregnancy in women receiving nucleoside analogues and clinicians should watch for early signs of the syndrome. Women in labor with an unknown HIV status should have a rapid HIV test. If the test is positive, begin I.V. zidovudine therapy. (If a postpartum confirmatory test is negative, zidovudine therapy in the infant can be stopped).

Healthcare providers are encouraged to enroll pregnant women exposed to antiretroviral medications in the Antiretroviral Pregnancy Registry (1-800-258-4263 or www.APRegistry.com). Healthcare providers caring for HIV-infected women and their infants may contact the National Perinatal HIV Hotline (888-448-8765) for clinical consultation.

Other Issues Anemia occurs usually after 4-6 weeks of therapy. Dose adjustments and/or transfusions may be required.

Additional Information Potential compliance problems, frequency of administration, and adverse effects should be discussed with patients before initiating therapy to help prevent the emergence of resistance.

◆ **Zidovudine, Abacavir, and Lamivudine** *see* Abacavir, Lamivudine, and Zidovudine *on page 32*

Zidovudine and Lamivudine (zye DOE vyoo deen & la MI vyoo deen)

U.S. Brand Names Combivir®

Index Terms AZT + 3TC (error-prone abbreviation); Lamivudine and Zidovudine

Generic Availability (U.S.) No

Pharmacologic Category Antiretroviral Agent, Reverse Transcriptase Inhibitor (Nucleoside)

Medication Safety Issues

Sound-alike/look-alike issues:

Combivir® may be confused with Combivent®, Epivir®

AZT is an error-prone abbreviation (mistaken as azaTHIOprine, aztreonam)

Pregnancy Risk Factor C

Lactation See individual agents.

Use Treatment of HIV infection when therapy is warranted based on clinical and/or immunological evidence of disease progression

Available Dosage Forms

Tablet:

Combivir®: Zidovudine 300 mg and lamivudine 150 mg [scored]

Dosing

Adult Treatment of HIV infection: Oral: 1 tablet twice daily. Because this is a fixed-dose combination product, avoid use in patients requiring dosage reduction including children <30 kg, renally-impaired patients with a creatinine clearance ≤50 mL/minute, hepatic impairment, or those patients experiencing dose-limiting adverse effects.

Pediatric Adolescents ≥30 kg: Refer to adult dosing.

Monitoring and Teaching Issues

Laboratory Monitoring Amylase, bilirubin; monitor CBC with differential and platelet count at least every 2 weeks, liver function tests (including signs/symptoms of hepatomegaly), MCV, serum creatinine kinase, viral load, and CD4 count; blood lactate levels and signs of acidosis

Physical Assessment See individual agents.

Patient Education See individual agents.

Related Information

LamiVUDine *on page 1054*

Zidovudine *on page 1890*

Zileuton (zye LOO ton)

U.S. Brand Names Zyflo CR®; Zyflo®

Generic Availability (U.S.) No

Pharmacologic Category 5-Lipoxygenase Inhibitor

Pregnancy Risk Factor C

Lactation Excretion in breast milk unknown/not recommended

Use Prophylaxis and chronic treatment of asthma

Mechanism of Action/Effect Inhibits leukotriene formation which contributes to inflammation, edema, mucous secretion, and bronchoconstriction in the airway of the asthmatic.

Contraindications Hypersensitivity to zileuton or any component of the formulation; active liver disease or transaminase elevations ≥3 times ULN

Warnings/Precautions Not appropriate or indicated for the reversal of bronchospasm in acute asthma attacks, including status asthmaticus; therapy may be continued during acute asthma exacerbations. Hepatic adverse effects have been reported (elevated transaminase levels); females >65 years and patients with pre-existing elevated transaminases may be at greater risk. Serum ALT should be monitored. Discontinue zileuton and follow transaminases until normal if patients develop clinical signs/symptoms of liver dysfunction or with transaminase levels >5 times ULN (use caution with history of liver disease and/or in those patients who consume substantial quantities of ethanol). Postmarketing reports of behavioral changes and sleep disorders have been noted.

Drug Interactions

Metabolism/Transport Effects Substrate (minor) of CYP1A2, 2C9, 3A4; **Inhibits** CYP1A2 (moderate)

Avoid Concomitant Use There are no known interactions where it is recommended to avoid concomitant use.

Decreased Effect There are no known significant interactions involving a decrease in effect.

Increased Effect/Toxicity

Zileuton may increase the levels/effects of: Propranolol; Theophylline; Warfarin

The levels/effects of Zileuton may be increased by: Conivaptan

Nutritional/Ethanol Interactions

Ethanol: Avoid ethanol (may increase CNS depression; may increase risk of hepatic toxicity).

Food: Zyflo CR®: Improved absorption when administered with food.

Herb/Nutraceutical: St John's wort may decrease zileuton levels.

Adverse Reactions

>10%: Central nervous system: Headache (23% to 25%)

1% to 10%:

Cardiovascular: Chest pain

Central nervous system: Pain (8%), dizziness, fever, insomnia, malaise, nervousness, somnolence

Dermatologic: Pruritus, rash

Gastrointestinal: Dyspepsia (8%), diarrhea (5%), nausea (5% to 6%), abdominal pain (5%), constipation, flatulence, vomiting

Genitourinary: Urinary tract infection, vaginitis

Hematologic: Leukopenia (1% to 3%)

Hepatic: ALT increased (≥3 x ULN: 2% to 5%), hepatotoxicity

Neuromuscular & skeletal: Myalgia (7%), weakness (4%), arthralgia, hypertonia, neck pain/rigidity

Ocular: Conjunctivitis

Respiratory: Upper respiratory tract infection (9%), sinusitis (7%), pharyngolaryngeal pain (5%)

Miscellaneous: Hypersensitivity reactions, lymphadenopathy

Pharmacodynamics/Kinetics

Time to Peak Immediate release: 1.7 hours

Protein Binding 93%, primarily albumin

Half-Life Elimination ~3 hours

Metabolism Hepatic and gastrointestinal; zileuton and N-dehydroxylated metabolite can be metabolized via CYP1A2, 2C9, and 3A4

Excretion Urine (~95% primarily as metabolites); feces (~2%)

Available Dosage Forms

Tablet, oral:

Zyflo®: 600 mg [scored]

Tablet, extended release, oral:

Zyflo CR®: 600 mg

Dosing

Adult & Geriatric Asthma: Oral:

Immediate release: 600 mg 4 times/day

Extended release: 1200 mg twice daily

Pediatric Asthma: Oral: Children ≥12 years: Refer to adult dosing.

Renal Impairment Adjustment not necessary in renal dysfunction or with hemodialysis.

Hepatic Impairment Contraindicated with hepatic dysfunction.

Administration

Oral

Immediate release: Administer without regard to meals.

Extended release: Do not crush, cut, or chew tablet; administer within 1 hour after morning and evening meals.

Stability

Storage Store tablets at 20°C to 25°C (68°F to 77°F). Protect from light.

Monitoring and Teaching Issues

Laboratory Monitoring Hepatic transaminases (prior to initiation and during therapy), specifically monitor serum ALT (prior to initiation, once-a-month for the first 3 months, every 2-3 months for the remainder of the first year, and periodically thereafter for patients receiving long-term therapy)

Physical Assessment Not for use to relieve acute asthmatic attacks. Monitor for improvement in number of asthma attacks.

Patient Education This medication is not for an acute asthmatic attack. Do not stop other asthma medication. Avoid alcohol. You may experience mild headache, belly pain, nausea, vomiting, or diarrhea. Report skin rash; flu-like symptoms; severe nausea, vomiting, or diarrhea; inability to eat; itching; jaundice or dark urine; or worsening of asthmatic condition.

Dietary Considerations

Immediate release: Take without regard to meals.

Extended release: Take with food.

Geriatric Considerations No differences in the pharmacokinetics found between younger adults and elderly; no dosage adjustments necessary. However, monitor liver effects closely as with any patient regardless of age.

Breast-Feeding Considerations Due to the potential tumorigenicity of zileuton in animal studies, the manufacturer does not recommend breast-feeding.

Pregnancy Considerations In developmental studies, reduced body weight and increased skeletal variations were observed in rats. There are no adequate and well-controlled studies in pregnant women.

◆ **Zinacef®** *see* Cefuroxime *on page 340*

◆ **Zinecard®** *see* Dexrazoxane *on page 508*

Ziprasidone (zi PRAS i done)

U.S. Brand Names Geodon®

Index Terms Zeldox; Ziprasidone Hydrochloride; Ziprasidone Mesylate

Generic Availability (U.S.) No

Pharmacologic Category Antipsychotic Agent, Atypical

Medication Safety Issues

Sound-alike/look-alike issues:

Ziprasidone may be confused with TraZODone

Pregnancy Risk Factor C

Lactation Excretion in breast milk unknown/not recommended

Use Treatment of schizophrenia; treatment of acute manic or mixed episodes associated with bipolar disorder with or without psychosis; maintenance treatment of bipolar disorder as an adjunct to lithium or valproate; acute agitation in patients with schizophrenia

Unlabeled/Investigational Use Tourette's syndrome; psychosis/agitation related to Alzheimer's dementia

Mechanism of Action/Effect Ziprasidone is a benzylisothiazolylpiperazine antipsychotic which blocks a number of CNS receptors, including dopamine, serotonin, alpha$_1$ adrenergic, and histamine receptors. Also inhibits reuptake of serotonin and epinephrine. Results in improvement in positive and negative symptoms of schizophrenia.

Contraindications Hypersensitivity to ziprasidone or any component of the formulation; history of (or current) prolonged QT; congenital long QT syndrome; recent myocardial infarction; uncompensated heart failure; concurrent use of other QT_c-prolonging agents including arsenic trioxide, chlorpromazine, class Ia antiarrhythmics (eg, disopyramide, quinidine, procainamide), class III antiarrhythmics (eg, amiodarone, dofetilide, ibutilide, sotalol), dolasetron, droperidol, gatifloxacin, levomethadyl, mefloquine, mesoridazine, moxifloxacin, pentamidine, pimozide, probucol, tacrolimus, and thioridazine

Warnings/Precautions [U.S. Boxed Warning]: Elderly patients with dementia-related behavioral disorders treated with antipsychotics are at an increased risk of death compared to placebo. Most deaths appeared to be either cardiovascular (eg, heart failure, sudden death) or infectious (eg, pneumonia) in nature. Ziprasidone is not approved for the treatment of dementia-related psychosis.

May result in QT_c prolongation (dose related), which has been associated with the development of malignant ventricular arrhythmias (torsade de pointes) and sudden death. Note contraindications related to this effect. Observed prolongation was greater than with other atypical antipsychotic agents (risperidone, olanzapine, quetiapine), but less than with thioridazine. Correct electrolyte disturbances, especially hypokalemia or hypomagnesemia, prior to use and throughout therapy. Use caution in patients with bradycardia. Discontinue in patients found to have persistent QT_c intervals >500 msec. Patients with symptoms of dizziness, palpitations, or syncope should receive further cardiac evaluation. May cause orthostatic hypotension. Use is contraindicated in patients with recent acute myocardial infarction (MI), QT prolongation, or uncompensated heart failure. Avoid use in patients with a history of cardiac arrhythmias; use with caution in patients with history of MI or unstable heart disease.

Leukopenia, neutropenia, and agranulocytosis (sometimes fatal) have been reported in clinical trials and postmarketing reports with antipsychotic use; presence of risk factors (eg, pre-existing low WBC or history of drug-induced leuko-/neutropenia) should prompt periodic blood count assessment. Discontinue therapy at first signs of blood dyscrasias or if absolute neutrophil count <1000/mm^3.

May cause extrapyramidal symptoms (EPS). Risk of dystonia (and probably other EPS) may be greater with increased doses, use of conventional antipsychotics, males, and younger patients. Impaired core body temperature regulation may occur; caution with strenuous exercise, heat exposure, dehydration, and concomitant medication possessing anticholinergic effects; not reported in premarketing trials of ziprasidone. Antipsychotic use may also be associated with neuroleptic malignant syndrome (NMS). Use with caution in patients at risk of seizures.

Atypical antipsychotics have been associated with development of hyperglycemia. There is limited documentation with ziprasidone and specific risk associated with this agent is not known. Use caution in patients with diabetes or other disorders of glucose regulation; monitor for worsening of glucose control. May increase prolactin levels; clinical significance of hyperprolactinemia in patients with breast cancer or other prolactin-dependent tumors is unknown.

Cognitive and/or motor impairment (sedation) is common with ziprasidone. Use with caution in disorders where CNS depression is a feature. Use with caution in Parkinson's disease. Antipsychotic use has been associated with esophageal dysmotility and aspiration; use with caution in patients at risk of pneumonia (ie, Alzheimer's disease). Use caution in hepatic impairment. Ziprasidone has been associated with a fairly high incidence of rash (5%). Significant weight gain has been observed with antipsychotic therapy; incidence varies with product. Monitor waist circumference and BMI. Rare cases of priapism have been reported. Use the intramuscular formulation with caution in patients with renal impairment; formulation contains cyclodextrin, an excipient which may accumulate in renal insufficiency.

The possibility of a suicide attempt is inherent in psychotic illness or bipolar disorder; use caution in high-risk patients during initiation of therapy. Prescriptions should be written for the smallest quantity consistent with good patient care.

Drug Interactions

Metabolism/Transport Effects Substrate (minor) of CYP1A2, 3A4; **Inhibits** CYP2D6 (weak), 3A4 (weak)

Avoid Concomitant Use

Avoid concomitant use of Ziprasidone with any of the following: Artemether; Dronedarone; Lumefantrine; Metoclopramide; Nilotinib; Pimozide; QTc-Prolonging Agents; QuiNINE; Tetrabenazine; Thioridazine; Toremifene; Vandetanib

Decreased Effect

Ziprasidone may decrease the levels/effects of: Amphetamines; Anti-Parkinson's Agents (Dopamine Agonist); Quinagolide

The levels/effects of Ziprasidone may be decreased by: CarBAMazepine; Lithium formulations

Increased Effect/Toxicity

Ziprasidone may increase the levels/effects of: Alcohol (Ethyl); CNS Depressants; Dronedarone; Methylphenidate; Pimozide; QTc-Prolonging Agents; QuiNINE; Tetrabenazine; Thioridazine; Toremifene; Vandetanib

The levels/effects of Ziprasidone may be increased by: Acetylcholinesterase Inhibitors (Central); Alfuzosin; Antifungal Agents (Azole Derivatives, Systemic); Artemether; Chloroquine; Ciprofloxacin; Ciprofloxacin (Systemic); Conivaptan; Gadobutrol; Lithium formulations; Lumefantrine; Methylphenidate; Metoclopramide; Nilotinib; QTc-Prolonging Agents; QuiNINE; Tetrabenazine

Nutritional/Ethanol Interactions

Ethanol: Avoid ethanol (may increase CNS depression).

Food: Administration with food increases serum levels twofold. Grapefruit juice may increase serum concentration of ziprasidone.

Herb/Nutraceutical: St John's wort may decrease serum levels of ziprasidone, due to a potential effect on CYP3A4. This has not been specifically studied. Avoid kava kava, chamomile (may increase CNS depression).

Lab Interactions Increased cholesterol, triglycerides, eosinophils

Adverse Reactions Note: Although minor QT_c prolongation (mean: 10 msec at 160 mg/day) may occur more frequently (incidence not specified), clinically-relevant prolongation (>500 msec) was rare (0.06%) and less than placebo (0.23%).

>10%:

Central nervous system: Extrapyramidal symptoms (2% to 31%), somnolence (8% to 31%), headache (3% to 18%), dizziness (3% to 16%)

Gastrointestinal: Nausea (4% to 12%)

1% to 10%:

Cardiovascular: Postural hypotension (5%), chest pain (3%), hypertension (2% to 3%), tachycardia (2%), bradycardia (≤2%), facial edema (1%), vasodilation (≤1%), orthostatic hypotension

Central nervous system: Akathisia (2% to 10%), anxiety (2% to 5%), insomnia (3%), agitation (2%), speech disorder (2%), personality disorder (2%), akinesia (≥1%), amnesia (≥1%), ataxia (≥1%), confusion (≥1%), coordination abnormal (≥1%), delirium (≥1%), dystonia (≥1%), hostility (≥1%), oculogyric crisis (≥1%), vertigo (≥1%), chills (1%), fever (1%), hypothermia (1%), psychosis (1%)

Dermatologic: Rash (4% to 5%), fungal dermatitis (2%)

Endocrine & metabolic: Dysmenorrhea (2%)

Gastrointestinal: Weight gain (6% to 10%), constipation (2% to 9%), dyspepsia (1% to 8%), diarrhea (3% to 5%), vomiting (3% to 5%), xerostomia (1% to 5%), salivation increased (4%), tongue edema (≤3%), anorexia (2%), abdominal pain (≤2%), dysphagia (≤2%), rectal hemorrhage (≤2%), buccoglossal syndrome (≥1%), tooth disorder (1%)

Genitourinary: Priapism (1%)

Local: Injection site pain (7% to 9%)

Neuromuscular & skeletal: Weakness (2% to 6%), hypoesthesia (2%), myalgia (2%), paresthesia (2%), abnormal gait (≥1%), choreoathetosis (≥1%), dysarthria (≥1%), dyskinesia (≥1%), hyper-/hypokinesia (≥1%), hypotonia (≥1%), neuropathy (≥1%), tremor (≥1%), twitching (≥1%), back pain (1%), cogwheel rigidity (1%), hypertonia (1%)

Ocular: Vision abnormal (3% to 6%), diplopia (≥1%)

Respiratory: Infection (8%), rhinitis (1% to 4%), cough (3%), pharyngitis (3%), dyspnea (2%)

Miscellaneous: Diaphoresis (2%), furunculosis (2%), withdrawal syndrome (≥1%), flank pain (1%), flu-like syndrome (1%), photosensitivity reaction (1%),

Pharmacodynamics/Kinetics

Absorption Well absorbed

Bioavailability Oral (with food): 60% (up to twofold increase with food); I.M.: 100%

Time to Peak Oral: 6-8 hours; I.M.: ≤60 minutes

Protein Binding >99%, primarily to albumin and $alpha_1$-acid glycoprotein

Half-Life Elimination 2-7 hours

Metabolism Extensively hepatic, primarily via aldehyde oxidase; less than 1/3 of total metabolism via CYP3A4 and CYP1A2 (minor)

Excretion Feces (~66%; <4% of total dose as unchanged drug); urine (~20%; <1% of total dose as unchanged drug)

Available Dosage Forms

Capsule, oral:

Geodon®: 20 mg, 40 mg, 60 mg, 80 mg

Injection, powder for reconstitution:

Geodon®: 20 mg

Dosing

Adult

Bipolar mania (acute): Oral: Initial: 40 mg twice daily

Adjustment: May increase to 60 mg or 80 mg twice daily on second day of treatment; average dose 40-80 mg twice daily.

Bipolar disorder (maintenance; as adjunct to lithium or valproate): Oral: Continue ziprasidone dose at which the patient was initially stabilized; usual dosage range: 40-80 mg twice daily

Schizophrenia: Oral: Initial: 20 mg twice daily

Adjustment: Increases (if indicated) should be made no more frequently than every 2 days; ordinarily patients should be observed for improvement over several weeks before adjusting the dose.

Maintenance: Range: 20-100 mg twice daily; however, dosages >80 mg twice daily are generally not recommended.

Acute agitation (schizophrenia): I.M.: 10 mg every 2 hours **or** 20 mg every 4 hours (maximum: 40 mg/day). Oral therapy should replace I.M. administration as soon as possible.

Geriatric No dosage adjustment is recommended; consider initiating at a low end of the dosage range, with slower titration.

Pediatric

Tourette's syndrome (unlabeled use): Children and adolescents: Oral: 5-40 mg/day

Renal Impairment

Oral: No dosage adjustment is recommended

I.M.: Cyclodextrin, an excipient in the I.M. formulation, is cleared by renal filtration; use with caution.

Ziprasidone is not removed by hemodialysis.

Hepatic Impairment No adjustment necessary.

Administration

Oral Administer with food.

I.M. Injection: For I.M. administration only.

Stability

Reconstitution Each vial should be reconstituted with 1.2 mL SWFI. Shake vigorously; will form a pale, pink solution containing 20 mg/mL ziprasidone.

Storage

Capsule: Store at 25°C (77°F); excursion permitted to 15°C to 30°C (59°F to 86°F).

Vials for injection: Store at 25°C (77°F); excursion permitted to 15°C to 30°C (59°F to 86°F). Protect from light. Following reconstitution, injection may be stored at room temperature up to 24 hours or under refrigeration for up to 7 days. Protect from light.

Monitoring and Teaching Issues

Laboratory Monitoring Serum potassium and magnesium; fasting lipid profile and fasting blood glucose, Hgb A_{1c} (prior to treatment, at 3 months, then annually).

Physical Assessment Assess seizure risk (seizure history, ethanol use, head trauma, brain damage, or current therapy with medications that reduce seizure threshold) and cardiac status (bradycardia, QT prolongation) prior to treatment. Monitor weight prior to initiating therapy and at least monthly. Consider titrating to a different antipsychotic agent for a weight gain ≥5% of initial weight.

Patient Education It may take 2-3 weeks to achieve desired results. Avoid alcohol. Maintain adequate hydration. If you have diabetes, you may experience increased blood sugars; monitor closely. You may experience drowsiness, lightheadedness, impaired coordination, dizziness, or blurred vision; dry mouth, nausea, or GI upset; postural hypotension; urinary retention; or constipation. Report persistent CNS effects (eg, trembling, altered gait or balance, excessive sedation, seizures, unusual muscle or skeletal movements, excessive anxiety, hallucinations, nightmares, suicide ideation, confusion), swelling or pain in breasts (male or female), altered menstrual pattern, sexual dysfunction, alteration in urinary pattern, vision changes, rash, respiratory difficulty, or chest pain or palpitations.

Dietary Considerations Take with food.

Geriatric Considerations Extrapyramidal syndrome symptoms occur less with this agent than phenothiazine and butyrophenone classes of antipsychotics.

Many elderly patients receive antipsychotic medications for inappropriate nonpsychotic behavior. Before initiating antipsychotic medication, the clinician should investigate any possible reversible cause; any stress or stress from any disease can cause acute "confusion" or worsening of baseline nonpsychotic behavior. Most commonly, acute changes in behavior are due to increases in drug dose or addition of a new drug to regimen, fluid electrolyte loss, infection, and changes in environment. Any changes in disease status and any organ system can result in behavior changes.

In the treatment of agitated, demented, elderly patients, authors of meta-analysis of controlled trials of the response to the traditional antipsychotics (phenothiazines, butyrophenones) in controlling agitation have concluded that the use of neuroleptics results in a response rate of 18%. Clearly, neuroleptic therapy for behavior control should be limited with frequent attempts to withdraw the agent given for behavior control. In light of significant risks and adverse effects in elderly population compared with limited data demonstrating efficacy in the treatment of dementia related psychosis, aggression, and agitation, an extensive risk:benefit analysis should be performed prior to use.

Since diabetes is prevalent in elderly, monitor closely when using this agent in this population.

Pregnancy Considerations Developmental toxicity demonstrated in animals. Antipsychotic use during the third trimester of pregnancy has a risk for abnormal muscle movements (extrapyramidal symptoms [EPS]) and withdrawal symptoms in newborns following delivery. Symptoms in the newborn may include agitation, feeding disorder, hypertonia, hypotonia, respiratory distress, somnolence, and tremor; these effects may be self-limiting or require hospitalization. There are no adequate and well-controlled studies in pregnant women. Use only if potential benefit justifies risk to the fetus. Healthcare providers are encouraged to enroll women 18-45 years of age exposed to ziprasidone during pregnancy in the Atypical Antipsychotics Pregnancy Registry (1-866-961-2388).

Additional Information The increased potential to prolong QT_c, as compared to other available antipsychotic agents, should be considered in the evaluation of available alternatives.

Related Information

Antipsychotic Agents *on page 1986*

- **Ziprasidone Hydrochloride** *see* Ziprasidone *on page 1896*
- **Ziprasidone Mesylate** *see* Ziprasidone *on page 1896*
- **Zipsor™** *see* Diclofenac (Systemic) *on page 518*
- **Zithromax®** *see* Azithromycin (Systemic) *on page 181*
- **Zithromax TRI-PAK™** *see* Azithromycin (Systemic) *on page 181*
- **Zithromax® TRI-PAK™** *see* Azithromycin (Systemic) *on page 181*
- **Zithromax Z-PAK®** *see* Azithromycin (Systemic) *on page 181*
- **Zithromax® Z-PAK®** *see* Azithromycin (Systemic) *on page 181*
- **Zmax®** *see* Azithromycin (Systemic) *on page 181*
- **Zocor®** *see* Simvastatin *on page 1645*
- **Zofran®** *see* Ondansetron *on page 1360*
- **Zofran® ODT** *see* Ondansetron *on page 1360*
- **Zol 446** *see* Zoledronic Acid *on page 1899*
- **Zoladex®** *see* Goserelin *on page 885*
- **Zoledronate** *see* Zoledronic Acid *on page 1899*

Zoledronic Acid (zoe le DRON ik AS id)

U.S. Brand Names Reclast®; Zometa®

Index Terms CGP-42446; Zol 446; Zoledronate

Generic Availability (U.S.) No

Pharmacologic Category Antidote; Bisphosphonate Derivative

Medication Safety Issues

Sound-alike/look-alike issues:

Zometa® may be confused with Zofran®, Zoladex®

Duplicate therapy issues:

Reclast® and Aclasta® contain zoledronic acid, which is the same ingredient contained in Zometa®; patients receiving Zometa® should not be treated with Reclast® or Aclasta®

Medication Guide Available Yes

Pregnancy Risk Factor D

Lactation Excretion in breast milk unknown/not recommended

Use

Oncology-related uses: Treatment of hypercalcemia of malignancy (albumin-corrected serum calcium >12 mg/dL); treatment of multiple myeloma; treatment of bone metastases of solid tumors

Nononcology uses: Treatment of Paget's disease of bone; treatment of osteoporosis in postmenopausal women (to reduce the incidence of fractures or to reduce the incidence of new clinical fractures in patients with low-trauma hip fracture); prevention of osteoporosis in postmenopausal women, treatment of osteoporosis in men (to increase bone mass); treatment and prevention of glucocorticoid-induced osteoporosis (in patients initiating or continuing prednisone ≥7.5 mg/day [or equivalent] and expected to remain on glucocorticoids for at least 12 months)

Unlabeled/Investigational Use Prevention of bone loss associated with aromatase inhibitor therapy in postmenopausal women with breast cancer; prevention of bone loss associated with androgen deprivation therapy in prostate cancer

Mechanism of Action/Effect A bisphosphonate which inhibits bone resorption via actions on osteoclasts or on osteoclast precursors; inhibits osteoclastic activity and skeletal calcium release induced by tumors. Decreases serum calcium and phosphorus, and increases their elimination. In osteoporosis, zoledronic acid inhibits osteoclast-mediated resorption, therefore reducing bone turnover.

Contraindications Hypersensitivity to zoledronic acid, other bisphosphonates, or any component of the formulation; hypocalcemia (Reclast®)

Canadian labeling: Aclasta® is also contraindicated with uncorrected hypocalcemia at the time of infusion and in pregnancy and breast-feeding.

Warnings/Precautions Osteonecrosis of the jaw (ONJ) has been reported in patients receiving bisphosphonates. Risk factors include invasive dental procedures (eg, tooth extraction, dental implants, boney surgery); a diagnosis of cancer, with concomitant chemotherapy or corticosteroids; poor oral hygiene, ill-fitting dentures; and comorbid disorders (anemia, coagulopathy, infection, pre-existing dental disease). Most reported cases occurred after I.V. bisphosphonate therapy; however, cases have been reported following oral therapy. A dental exam and preventative dentistry should be performed prior to placing patients with risk factors on chronic bisphosphonate therapy. The manufacturer's labeling states that discontinuing bisphosphonates in patients requiring invasive dental procedures may reduce the risk of ONJ. However, other experts suggest that there is no evidence that discontinuing therapy reduces the risk of developing ONJ (Assael, 2009). The benefit/risk must be assessed by the treating physician and/or dentist/surgeon prior to any invasive dental procedure. Patients developing ONJ while on bisphosphonates should receive care by an oral surgeon.

Atypical femur fractures have been reported in patients receiving bisphosphonates for treatment/prevention of osteoporosis. The fractures include subtrochanteric femur (bone just below the hip joint) and diaphyseal femur (long segment of the thigh bone). Some patients experience prodromal pain weeks or months before the fracture occurs. It is unclear if bisphosphonate therapy is the cause for these fractures, although the majority have been reported in patients taking bisphosphonates. Patients receiving long-term (>3-5 years) therapy may be at an increased risk. Discontinue bisphosphonate therapy in patients who develop a femoral shaft fracture.

Infrequently, severe (and occasionally debilitating) musculoskeletal (bone, joint, and/or muscle) pain have been reported during bisphosphonate treatment. The onset of pain ranged from a single day to several months. Consider discontinuing therapy in patients who experience severe symptoms; symptoms usually resolve upon discontinuation. Some patients experienced recurrence when rechallenged with same drug or another bisphosphonate; avoid use in patients with a history of these symptoms in association with bisphosphonate therapy.

May cause hypocalcemia in patients with Paget's disease, in whom the pretreatment rate of bone turnover may be greatly elevated. Hypocalcemia must be corrected before initiation of therapy in patients with Paget's disease and osteoporosis. Ensure adequate calcium and vitamin D intake during therapy. Use caution in patients with disturbances of calcium and mineral metabolism (eg, hypoparathyroidism, thyroid surgery, malabsorption syndromes).

Reclast®: Use is not recommended in patients with Cl_{cr} <35 mL/minute.

Zometa®: Use caution in mild-to-moderate renal dysfunction; dosage adjustment required. In cancer patients, renal toxicity has been reported with doses >4 mg or infusions administered over 15 minutes. Risk factors for renal deterioration include pre-existing renal insufficiency and repeated doses of zoledronic acid and other bisphosphonates. Dehydration and the use of other nephrotoxic drugs which may contribute to renal deterioration should be identified and managed. Use is not recommended in patients with severe renal impairment (serum creatinine >3 mg/dL or Cl_{cr} <30 mL/minute) and bone metastases (limited data); use in patients with hypercalcemia of malignancy and severe renal impairment (serum creatinine >4.5 mg/dL for hypercalcemia of malignancy) should only be done if the benefits outweigh the risks. Renal function should be assessed prior to treatment; if decreased after treatment, additional treatments should be withheld until renal function returns to within 10% of baseline. Diuretics should not be used before correcting hypovolemia. Renal deterioration, resulting in renal failure and dialysis has occurred in patients treated with zoledronic acid after single and multiple infusions at recommended doses of 4 mg over 15 minutes.

Aclasta® [CAN; not available in U.S.]: Use is not recommended in patients with Cl_{cr} <30 mL/minute.

According to the American Society of Clinical Oncology (ASCO) guidelines for bisphosphonates in multiple myeloma, treatment with zoledronic acid is not recommended for asymptomatic (smoldering) or indolent myeloma or with solitary plasmacytoma (Kyle, 2007). The National Comprehensive Cancer Network® (NCCN) multiple myeloma guidelines (v.2.2009) also do not recommend zoledronic acid use in stage 1 or smoldering disease, unless part of a clinical trial.

Adequate hydration is required during treatment (urine output ~2 L/day); avoid overhydration, especially in patients with heart failure. Pre-existing renal compromise, severe dehydration, and concurrent use with diuretics or other nephrotoxic drugs may increase the risk for renal impairment. Single and multiple infusions in patients with both normal and impaired renal function have been associated with renal deterioration, resulting in renal failure and dialysis (rare). Use caution in patients with aspirin-sensitive asthma (may cause bronchoconstriction) and the elderly. Women of childbearing age should be advised against becoming pregnant. Not approved for use in children.

Drug Interactions

Avoid Concomitant Use There are no known interactions where it is recommended to avoid concomitant use.

Decreased Effect

The levels/effects of Zoledronic Acid may be decreased by: Proton Pump Inhibitors

Increased Effect/Toxicity

Zoledronic Acid may increase the levels/effects of: Phosphate Supplements

The levels/effects of Zoledronic Acid may be increased by: Aminoglycosides; Nonsteroidal Anti-Inflammatory Agents; Thalidomide

Lab Interactions Bisphosphonates may interfere with diagnostic imaging agents such as technetium-99m-diphosphonate in bone scans.

Adverse Reactions Note: An acute reaction (eg, arthralgia, fever, flu-like symptoms, myalgia) may occur within the first 3 days following infusion in up to 44% of patients; usually resolves within 3-4 days of onset, although may take up to 14 days to resolve. The incidence may be decreased with acetaminophen (prior to infusion and for 72 hours postinfusion).

Zometa®:

>10%:

Cardiovascular: Leg edema (5% to 21%), hypotension (11%)

Central nervous system: Fatigue (39%), fever (32% to 44%), headache (5% to 19%), dizziness (18%), insomnia (15% to 16%), anxiety (11% to 14%), depression (14%), agitation (13%), confusion (7% to 13%), hypoesthesia (12%)

Dermatologic: Alopecia (12%), dermatitis (11%)

Endocrine & metabolic: Dehydration (5% to 14%), hypophosphatemia (12% to 13%), hypokalemia (12%), hypomagnesemia (11%)

Gastrointestinal: Nausea (29% to 46%), vomiting (14% to 32%), constipation (27% to 31%), diarrhea (17% to 24%), anorexia (9% to 22%), abdominal pain (14% to 16%), weight loss (16%), appetite decreased (13%)

Genitourinary: Urinary tract infection (12% to 14%)

Hematologic: Anemia (22% to 33%), neutropenia (12%)

Neuromuscular & skeletal: Bone pain (55%), weakness (5% to 24%), myalgia (23%), arthralgia (5% to 21%), back pain (15%), paresthesia (15%), limb pain (14%), skeletal pain (12%), rigors (11%)

Renal: Renal deterioration (8% to 17%; up to 40% in patients with abnormal baseline creatinine)

Respiratory: Dyspnea (22% to 27%), cough (12% to 22%)

Miscellaneous: Cancer progression (16%), moniliasis (12%)

1% to 10%:

Cardiovascular: Chest pain (5% to 10%)

Central nervous system: Somnolence (5% to 10%)

Endocrine & metabolic: Hypocalcemia (5% to 10%; grades 3/4: ≤1%), hypermagnesemia (2%)

Gastrointestinal: Dysphagia (5% to 10%), dyspepsia (10%), mucositis (5% to 10%), stomatitis (8%), sore throat (8%)

Hematologic: Granulocytopenia (5% to 10%), pancytopenia (5% to 10%), thrombocytopenia (5% to 10%)

Renal: Serum creatinine increased (grades 3/4: ≤2%)

Respiratory: Pleural effusion, upper respiratory tract infection (10%)

Miscellaneous: Infection (nonspecific; 5% to 10%), metastases (5% to 10%)

Reclast®:

>10%:

Cardiovascular: Hypertension (5% to 13%)

Central nervous system: Pain (2% to 24%), fever (9% to 22%), headache (4% to 20%), chills (2% to 18%), fatigue (2% to 18%)

Endocrine & metabolic: Hypocalcemia (≤3%; Paget's disease 21%)

Gastrointestinal: Nausea (5% to 18%)

Neuromuscular & skeletal: Arthralgia (9% to 27%), myalgia (5% to 23%), back pain (4% to 18%), limb pain (3% to 16%), musculoskeletal pain (≤12%)

Miscellaneous: Acute phase reaction (4% to 25%), flu-like syndrome (1% to 11%)

1% to 10%:

Cardiovascular: Chest pain (1% to 8%), peripheral edema (3% to 6%), atrial fibrillation (1% to 3%), palpitation (≤3%)

Central nervous system: Dizziness (2% to 9%), malaise (1% to 7%), hypoesthesia (≤6%), lethargy (3% to 5%), vertigo (1% to 4%), hyperthermia (≤2%)

Dermatologic: Rash (2% to 3%), hyperhidrosis (≤3%)

Gastrointestinal: Abdominal pain (1% to 9%), diarrhea (5% to 8%), vomiting (2% to 8%), constipation (6% to 7%), dyspepsia (2% to 7%), abdominal discomfort/distension (1% to 2%), anorexia (1% to 2%)

Neuromuscular & skeletal: Bone pain (3% to 9%), arthritis (2% to 9%), rigors (8%), shoulder pain (≤7%), neck pain (1% to 7%), weakness (2% to 6%), muscle spasm (2% to 6%), stiffness (1% to 5%), jaw pain (2% to 4%), joint swelling (≤3%), paresthesia (2%)

Ocular: Eye pain (≤2%)

Renal: Serum creatinine increased (2%)

Respiratory: Dyspnea (5% to 7%)

Miscellaneous: C-reactive protein increased (≤5%)

Pharmacodynamics/Kinetics

Protein Binding 28% to 53%

Half-Life Elimination Triphasic; Terminal: 146 hours

Excretion Urine (39% ± 16% as unchanged drug) within 24 hours; feces (<3%)

Available Dosage Forms

Infusion, solution, premixed:

Reclast®: 5 mg (100 mL)

Injection, solution:

Zometa®: 4 mg/5 mL (5 mL)

Dosing

Adult & Geriatric Note: Acetaminophen administration after the infusion may reduce symptoms of acute-phase reactions. Patients treated for multiple myeloma, osteoporosis, and Paget's disease should receive a daily calcium supplement and multivitamin containing vitamin D (if dietary intake is inadequate).

Hypercalcemia of malignancy (albumin-corrected serum calcium ≥12 mg/dL) (Zometa®): I.V.: 4 mg (maximum) given as a single dose. Wait at least 7 days before considering retreatment. Dosage adjustment may be needed in patients with decreased renal function following treatment.

Multiple myeloma or metastatic bone lesions from solid tumors (Zometa®): I.V.: 4 mg every 3-4 weeks

Osteoporosis, glucocorticoid-induced, treatment and prevention (Reclast®, Aclasta® [CAN]): 5 mg infused over at least 15 minutes once a year

Osteoporosis, prevention (Reclast®): 5 mg infused over at least 15 minutes every 2 years

Osteoporosis, treatment (Reclast®, Aclasta® [CAN]): 5 mg infused over at least 15 minutes once a year

Paget's disease: I.V.: 5 mg infused over at least 15 minutes. **Note:** Data concerning retreatment is not available; retreatment may be considered for relapse if appropriate, for inadequate response, or in patients who are symptomatic.

Prevention of aromatase inhibitor-induced bone loss in breast cancer (unlabeled use): 4 mg every 6 months (Brufsky, 2007)

Prevention of androgen deprivation-induced bone loss in nonmetastatic prostate cancer (unlabeled use): 4 mg every 3 months for 1 year (Smith, 2003) or 4 mg every 12 months (Michaelson, 2007)

Renal Impairment

Reclast®:

Cl_{cr} ≥35 mL/minute: No adjustment required.
Cl_{cr} <35 mL/minute: Use is not recommended.

Zometa®: Multiple myeloma and bone metastases (at treatment initiation):

Cl_{cr} >60 mL/minute: 4 mg
Cl_{cr} 50-60 mL/minute: 3.5 mg
Cl_{cr} 40-49 mL/minute: 3.3 mg
Cl_{cr} 30-39 mL/minute: 3 mg
Cl_{cr} <30 mL/minute: Not recommended.

Zometa®: Hypercalcemia of malignancy (at treatment initiation):

Mild-to-moderate impairment: No adjustment necessary.
Severe impairment (serum creatinine >4.5 mg/dL): Evaluate risk versus benefit.

Aclasta® [CAN]:

Cl_{cr} ≥30 mL/minute: No adjustment required.
Cl_{cr} <30 mL/minute: Use is not recommended.

Renal toxicity (during treatment):

Hypercalcemia of malignancy: Evidence of renal deterioration: Evaluate risk versus benefit.

Multiple myeloma and bone metastases: Evidence of renal deterioration: Withhold dose until renal function returns to within 10% of baseline: renal deterioration defined as follows:

Normal baseline creatinine: Increase of 0.5 mg/dL
Abnormal baseline creatinine: Increase of 1 mg/dL

Reinitiate dose at the same dose administered prior to treatment interruption.

Multiple myeloma: Albuminuria >500 mg/24 hours (unexplained): Withhold dose until return to baseline, then re-evaluate every 3-4 weeks; consider reinitiating with a longer infusion time of at least 30 minutes (Kyle, 2007).

Hepatic Impairment Specific guidelines are not available.

Administration

I.V. Infuse over 15-30 minutes; do not infuse over <15 minutes. Infuse in a line separate from other medications. Patients should be appropriately hydrated prior to treatment.

Reclast®, Zometa®: If refrigerated, allow to reach room temperature prior to administration. Acetaminophen or ibuprofen after administration may reduce the incidence of acute reaction (eg, arthralgia, fever, flu-like symptoms, myalgia).

Stability

Reconstitution Zometa®: Dilute solution for injection in 100 mL NS or D_5W prior to administration.

Storage

Aclasta® [CAN]: Store at room temperature of 15°C to 30°C (59°F to 86°F).

Reclast®: Store at room temperature of 25°C (77°F); excursions permitted to 15°C to 30°C (59°F to 86°F). After opening, stable for 24 hours at 2°C to 8°C (36°F to 46°F).

Zometa®: Store vials at 25°C (77°F); excursions permitted to 15°C to 30°C (59°F to 86°F). Solutions for infusion which are not used immediately after preparation should be refrigerated at 2°C to 8°C (36°F to 46°F). Infusion of solution must be completed within 24 hours of preparation.

Monitoring and Teaching Issues

Laboratory Monitoring

Aclasta® [CAN], Reclast®: Serum creatinine prior to each dose

Osteoporosis: Bone mineral density as measured by central dual-energy x-ray absorptiometry (DXA) of the hip or spine (prior to initiation of therapy and at least every 2 years; after 6-12 months of combined glucocorticoid and zoledronic acid treatment); serum calcium and 25(OH)D; may consider monitoring biochemical markers of bone turnover

Paget's disease: Alkaline phosphatase, serum calcium and 25(OH)D

Zometa®: Serum creatinine prior to each dose; serum electrolytes, phosphate, magnesium, and hemoglobin/hematocrit should be evaluated regularly. Monitor serum calcium to assess response and avoid overtreatment. In patients with multiple myeloma, monitor urine every 3-6 months for albuminuria.

Physical Assessment Assess for use-related cautions (according to formulation and purpose for use) prior to beginning therapy. Patients at risk for osteonecrosis (eg, chemotherapy, corticosteroids, poor oral hygiene) should have dental exams and necessary preventive dentistry should be done before beginning bisphosphonate therapy. Teach patient need for adequate hydration.

Patient Education This medication is only administered by infusion or injection; report immediately any burning, redness, or pain at infusion/injection site. Maintain adequate hydration, unless instructed to restrict fluid intake. Certain dental procedures should be avoided if possible while you are taking this medication; consult prescriber. You may experience a brief reaction (3-14 days), including fever, flu-like symptoms, or muscle pain. You may experience nausea, vomiting, loss of appetite, headache, dizziness, insomnia, or confusion. Report difficulty breathing; chest pain or swelling of extremities; persistent CNS changes (fatigue, depression, insomnia, agitation, confusion); acute or persistent bone, joint, or muscle pain; changes in elimination pattern (urine or stool); skin rash; or burning or itching on urination.

Dietary Considerations

Multiple myeloma or metastatic bone lesions from solid tumors: Take daily calcium supplement (500 mg) and daily multivitamin (with 400 int. units vitamin D).

Osteoporosis: Ensure adequate calcium and vitamin D supplementation; general requirements are calcium 1200 mg/day and vitamin D 800-1000 int. units/day.

Paget's disease: Take calcium 1500 mg/day and vitamin D 800 units/day, particularly during the first 2 weeks after administration.

Geriatric Considerations This drug requires adequate hydration and adjustments for creatinine clearance for its use. Elderly are often volume depleted secondary to drugs and a blunted thirst reflex. See disease related concerns in Dosing: Renal Impairment. The elderly are frequently treated long-term for osteoporosis and patients should be advised to report any lower extremity pain that cannot be explained or lasts for more than a week.

Breast-Feeding Considerations Because it binds to bone long term, zoledronic acid use is not recommended in nursing women.

Pregnancy Considerations Animal studies resulted in embryotoxicity and losses. Zoledronic acid should not be used during pregnancy; may cause fetal harm if administered to a pregnant woman. Bisphosphonates are incorporated into the bone matrix and gradually released over time. Theoretically, there may be a risk of fetal harm when pregnancy follows the completion of therapy. Based on limited case reports with pamidronate, serum calcium levels in the newborn may be altered if administered during pregnancy.

Related Information

Osteoporosis Management *on page 2067*

◆ **Zolinza™** *see* Vorinostat *on page 1875*

Zolmitriptan (zohl mi TRIP tan)

U.S. Brand Names Zomig-ZMT®; Zomig®

Index Terms 311C90

Generic Availability (U.S.) No

Pharmacologic Category Antimigraine Agent; Serotonin 5-HT$_{1B,\ 1D}$ Receptor Agonist

Medication Safety Issues

Sound-alike/look-alike issues:

ZOLMitriptan may be confused with SUMAtriptan

Pregnancy Risk Factor C

Lactation Excretion in breast milk unknown/use caution

Use Acute treatment of migraine with or without aura

Mechanism of Action/Effect Selective agonist for serotonin receptor in cranial arteries; causes vasoconstriction and relief of migraine

Contraindications Hypersensitivity to zolmitriptan or any component of the formulation; ischemic heart disease or vasospastic coronary artery disease, including Prinzmetal's angina; signs or symptoms of ischemic heart disease; uncontrolled hypertension; symptomatic Wolff-Parkinson-White syndrome or arrhythmias associated with other cardiac accessory conduction pathway disorders; use with ergotamine derivatives (within 24 hours of); use within 24 hours of another 5-HT$_1$ agonist; concurrent administration or within 2 weeks of discontinuing an MAO inhibitor; management of hemiplegic or basilar migraine

Nasal spray: Additional contraindications with nasal spray: Cerebrovascular syndromes (eg, stroke, TIA); peripheral vascular disease (including ischemic bowel disease)

Warnings/Precautions Zolmitriptan is indicated only in patient populations with a clear diagnosis of migraine. Not for prophylactic treatment of migraine headaches. Cardiac events (coronary artery vasospasm, transient ischemia, myocardial infarction, ventricular tachycardia/fibrillation, cardiac arrest, and death) have been reported with 5-HT$_1$ agonist administration. Should not be given to patients who have risk factors for CAD (eg, hypertension, hypercholesterolemia, smoker, obesity, diabetes, strong family history of CAD, menopause, male >40 years of age) without adequate cardiac evaluation. Patients with suspected CAD should have cardiovascular evaluation to rule out CAD before considering zolmitriptan's use; if cardiovascular evaluation negative, first dose would be safest if given in the healthcare provider's office. ▶

Periodic evaluation of those without cardiovascular disease, but with continued risk factors, should be done. Significant elevation in blood pressure, including hypertensive crisis, has also been reported on rare occasions in patients with and without a history of hypertension. Vasospasm-related reactions have been reported other than coronary artery vasospasm. Peripheral vascular ischemia and colonic ischemia with abdominal pain and bloody diarrhea have occurred. Cerebral/subarachnoid hemorrhage and stroke have been reported with 5-HT_1 agonist administration; nasal spray contraindicated in patients with cerebrovascular syndromes. Rarely, partial vision loss and blindness (transient and permanent) have been reported with 5-HT_1 agonists. Use with caution in patients with hepatic impairment. Zomig-ZMT™ tablets contain phenylalanine. Symptoms of agitation, confusion, hallucinations, hyper-reflexia, myoclonus, shivering, and tachycardia (serotonin syndrome) may occur with concomitant proserotonergic drugs (eg, SSRIs/SNRIs or triptans) or agents which reduce zolmitriptan's metabolism. Concurrent use of serotonin precursors (eg, tryptophan) is not recommended.

Drug Interactions

Metabolism/Transport Effects Substrate of CYP1A2 (minor)

Avoid Concomitant Use

Avoid concomitant use of ZOLMitriptan with any of the following: Ergot Derivatives; MAO Inhibitors; Sibutramine

Decreased Effect There are no known significant interactions involving a decrease in effect.

Increased Effect/Toxicity

ZOLMitriptan may increase the levels/effects of: Ergot Derivatives; Serotonin Modulators

The levels/effects of ZOLMitriptan may be increased by: Cimetidine; Ergot Derivatives; MAO Inhibitors; Propranolol; Sibutramine

Nutritional/Ethanol Interactions Ethanol: Limit use (may have additive CNS toxicity).

Lab Interactions No interferences have been identified

Adverse Reactions Percentages noted from oral preparations.

1% to 10%:

Cardiovascular: Chest pain (2% to 4%), palpitation (up to 2%)

Central nervous system: Dizziness (6% to 10%), somnolence (5% to 8%), pain (2% to 3%), vertigo (≤2%)

Gastrointestinal: Nausea (4% to 9%), xerostomia (3% to 5%), dyspepsia (1% to 3%), dysphagia (≤2%)

Neuromuscular & skeletal: Paresthesia (5% to 9%), weakness (3% to 9%), warm/cold sensation (5% to 7%), hypoesthesia (1% to 2%), myalgia (1% to 2%), myasthenia (up to 2%)

Miscellaneous: Neck/throat/jaw pain (4% to 10%), diaphoresis (up to 3%), allergic reaction (up to 1%)

Pharmacodynamics/Kinetics

Onset of Action 0.5-1 hour

Absorption Well absorbed

Bioavailability 40%

Time to Peak Serum: Tablet: 1.5 hours; Orally-disintegrating tablet and nasal spray: 3 hours

Protein Binding 25%

Half-Life Elimination 2.8-3.7 hours

Metabolism Converted to an active N-desmethyl metabolite (2-6 times more potent than zolmitriptan)

Excretion Urine (~60% to 65% total dose); feces (30% to 40%)

Available Dosage Forms

Solution, intranasal:

Zomig®: 5 mg/0.1 mL (0.1 mL)

Tablet, oral:

Zomig®: 2.5 mg, 5 mg

Tablet, orally disintegrating, oral:

Zomig-ZMT®: 2.5 mg, 5 mg

Dosing

Adult

Migraine headache:

Oral:

Tablet: Initial: ≤2.5 mg at the onset of migraine headache; may break 2.5 mg tablet in half

Orally-disintegrating tablet: Initial: 2.5 mg at the onset of migraine headache

Nasal spray: Initial: 1 spray (5 mg) at the onset of migraine headache

Note: Use the lowest possible dose to minimize adverse events. If the headache returns, the dose may be repeated after 2 hours; do not exceed 10 mg within a 24-hour period. Controlled trials have not established the effectiveness of a second dose if the initial one was ineffective.

Geriatric Refer to adult dosing. No dosage adjustment needed, but elderly patients are more likely to have underlying cardiovascular disease and should have careful evaluation of cardiovascular system before prescribing.

Renal Impairment No dosage adjustment recommended. There is a 25% reduction in zolmitriptan's clearance in patients with severe renal impairment (Cl_{cr} 5-25 mL/minute).

Hepatic Impairment Administer with caution in patients with liver disease, generally using doses <2.5 mg (doses <5 mg can only be achieved using oral tablets). Patients with moderate-to-severe hepatic impairment may have decreased clearance of zolmitriptan, and significant elevation in blood pressure was observed in some patients.

Administration

Oral Administer as soon as migraine headache starts. Tablets may be broken. Orally-disintegrating tablets: Must be taken whole; do not break, crush or chew. Place on tongue and allow to dissolve. Administration with liquid is not required

Other Nasal spray: Administer as soon as migraine headache starts. Blow nose gently prior to use. After removing protective cap, instill device into nostril. Block opposite nostril; breathe in gently through nose while pressing plunger of spray device. One dose (5 mg) is equal to 1 spray in 1 nostril.

Stability

Storage Store at 20°C to 25°C (68°F to 77°F). Protect from light and moisture.

Monitoring and Teaching Issues

Physical Assessment For use only with a clear diagnosis of migraine headaches. Cardiovascular status should be evaluated prior to initiating medication and periodically thereafter. Use caution in presence of cardiovascular risk factors and hepatic impairment. Monitor for chest pain, nausea, dizziness, paresthesia, myalgia, and pain.

Patient Education This drug is to be used to reduce your migraine, not to prevent or reduce the number of attacks. Remove orally-disintegrating tablet from blister package just before using, place on tongue, and allow to dissolve. Do not crush, break, or chew. Regular tablet may be broken in half for use. Do not remove protective cap from nasal spray until ready to use. If first dose brings relief, second dose may be taken anytime after 2 hours if migraine returns. If you have no relief with first dose, do not take a second dose without consulting prescriber. Do not exceed 10 mg in 24 hours. May cause dizziness, drowsiness, or dry mouth. Report immediately any chest pain, heart throbbing, or tightness in throat; swelling of eyelids, face, or lips; skin rash or hives; easy bruising; blood in urine, stool, or vomitus; pain or itching with urination; or pain, warmth, or numbness in extremities.

Dietary Considerations Some products may contain phenylalanine.

Geriatric Considerations No dosage adjustment needed, but elderly patients are more likely to have underlying cardiovascular disease and should have careful evaluation of the cardiovascular system before prescribing.

Pregnancy Considerations There are no adequate and well-controlled studies using zolmitriptan in pregnant women. Use only if potential benefit to the mother outweighs the potential risk to the fetus. In animal studies, administration was associated with embryolethality, fetal abnormalities, and pup mortality.

Additional Information Not recommended if the patient has risk factors for heart disease (high blood pressure, high cholesterol, obesity, diabetes, smoking, strong family history of heart disease, postmenopausal woman, or a male >40 years of age).

This agent is intended to relieve migraine, but not to prevent or reduce the number of attacks. Use only to treat an actual migraine attack.

Related Information

Antimigraine Drugs: 5-HT_1 Receptor Agonists *on page 1985*

◆ **Zoloft®** *see* Sertraline *on page 1633*

Zolpidem (zole PI dem)

U.S. Brand Names Ambien CR®; Ambien®; Edluar™; Zolpimist®

Index Terms Zolpidem Tartrate

Generic Availability (U.S.) Yes: Excludes oral spray, sublingual tablet

Pharmacologic Category Hypnotic, Nonbenzodiazepine

Medication Safety Issues

Sound-alike/look-alike issues:

Ambien® may be confused with Abilify®, Ativan®, Ambi 10®

Zolpidem may be confused with lorazepam, zaleplon

International issues:

Ambien® may be confused with Ambyen which is a brand name for amiodarone in Great Britain

Medication Guide Available Yes

Pregnancy Risk Factor C

Lactation Enters breast milk/use caution (AAP rates "compatible"; AAP 2001 update pending)

Use

Ambien®, Edluar™, Zolpimist®: Short-term treatment of insomnia (with difficulty of sleep onset)

Ambien CR®: Treatment of insomnia (with difficulty of sleep onset and/or sleep maintenance)

Mechanism of Action/Effect Zolpidem is structurally dissimilar to benzodiazepines but enhances the activity of γ-aminobutyric acid (GABA) resulting in increased sedation. Zolpidem exhibits minimal anxiolytic, myorelaxant, and anticonvulsant properties.

Contraindications Hypersensitivity to zolpidem or any component of the formulation

Warnings/Precautions Should be used only after evaluation of potential causes of sleep disturbance. Failure of sleep disturbance to resolve after 7-10 days may indicate psychiatric or medical illness. Hypnotics/sedatives have been associated with abnormal thinking and behavior changes including decreased inhibition, aggression, bizarre behavior, agitation, hallucinations, and depersonalization. These changes may occur unpredictably and may indicate previously unrecognized psychiatric disorders; evaluate appropriately. Sedative/hypnotics may produce withdrawal symptoms following abrupt discontinuation. Use with caution in patients with depression; worsening of depression, including suicide or suicidal ideation has been reported with the use of hypnotics. Intentional overdose may be an issue in this ▶

population. The minimum dose that will effectively treat the individual patient should be used. Prescriptions should be written for the smallest quantity consistent with good patient care. Causes CNS depression, which may impair physical and mental capabilities. Zolpidem should only be administered when the patient is able to stay in bed a full night (7-8 hours) before being active again. Effects with other sedative drugs or ethanol may be potentiated.

Use caution in patients with myasthenia gravis. Avoid use in patients with sleep apnea or a history of sedative-hypnotic abuse. Postmarketing studies have indicated that the use of hypnotic/sedative agents for sleep has been associated with hypersensitivity reactions including anaphylaxis as well as angioedema. An increased risk for hazardous sleep-related activities such as sleep-driving; cooking and eating food, and making phone calls while asleep have also been noted; amnesia may also occur. Discontinue treatment in patients who report any sleep-related episodes.

Use caution with respiratory disease. Use caution with hepatic impairment; dose adjustment required. Because of the rapid onset of action, administer immediately prior to bedtime or after the patient has gone to bed and is having difficulty falling asleep.

Use caution in the elderly; dose adjustment recommended. Closely monitor elderly or debilitated patients for impaired cognitive or motor performance. When studied for the unapproved use of insomnia associated with ADHD in children, a higher incidence (~7%) of hallucinations was reported. In addition, sleep latency did not decrease compared to placebo. Zolpidem is **not** FDA-approved for use in pediatric patients.

Drug Interactions

Metabolism/Transport Effects Substrate of CYP1A2 (minor), 2C9 (minor), 2C19 (minor), 2D6 (minor), 3A4 (major)

Avoid Concomitant Use There are no known interactions where it is recommended to avoid concomitant use.

Decreased Effect

The levels/effects of Zolpidem may be decreased by: CarBAMazepine; CYP3A4 Inducers (Strong); Deferasirox; Flumazenil; Herbs (CYP3A4 Inducers); Peginterferon Alfa-2b; Rifamycin Derivatives

Increased Effect/Toxicity

Zolpidem may increase the levels/effects of: Alcohol (Ethyl); CarBAMazepine; CNS Depressants; Methotrimeprazine

The levels/effects of Zolpidem may be increased by: Antifungal Agents (Azole Derivatives, Systemic); Conivaptan; CYP3A4 Inhibitors (Moderate); CYP3A4 Inhibitors (Strong); Dasatinib; Droperidol; Methotrimeprazine

Nutritional/Ethanol Interactions

Ethanol: May enhance the adverse/toxic effects of zolpidem; avoid use.

Food: Maximum plasma concentration and bioavailability are decreased with food; time to peak plasma concentration is increased; half-life remains unchanged. Grapefruit juice may decrease the metabolism of zolpidem.

Herb/Nutraceutical: St John's wort may decrease the levels/effects of zolpidem; avoid concomitant use. In addition, concomitant use of valerian, kava kava, and gotu kola should be avoided due to the risk of increased CNS depression.

Lab Interactions Increased aminotransferase [ALT/AST], bilirubin (S); decreased RAI uptake

Adverse Reactions Actual frequency may be dosage form, dose, and/or age dependent

>10%: Central nervous system: Headache (7% to 19%), somnolence (6% to 15%), dizziness (1% to 12%)

1% to 10%:

Cardiovascular: Blood pressure increased, chest discomfort/pain, palpitation

Central nervous system: Abnormal dreams, anxiety, apathy, amnesia, ataxia, attention disturbance, body temperature increased, burning sensation, confusion, depersonalization, depression, disinhibition, disorientation, drowsiness, drugged feeling, euphoria, fatigue, fever, hallucinations, hypoesthesia, insomnia, lethargy, lightheadedness, memory disorder, mood swings, sleep disorder, stress

Dermatologic: Rash, urticaria, wrinkling

Endocrine & metabolic: Menorrhagia

Gastrointestinal: Abdominal discomfort, abdominal pain, abdominal tenderness, appetite disorder, constipation, diarrhea, dyspepsia, flatulence, gastroenteritis, gastroesophageal reflux, hiccup, nausea, vomiting, xerostomia

Genitourinary: Urinary tract infection, vulvovaginal dryness

Neuromuscular & skeletal: Arthralgia, back pain, balance disorder, involuntary muscle contractions, myalgia, neck pain, paresthesia, psychomotor retardation, tremor, weakness

Ocular: Asthenopia, blurred vision, depth perception altered, diplopia, red eye, visual disturbance

Otic: Labyrinthitis, tinnitus, vertigo

Renal: Dysuria

Respiratory: Pharyngitis, sinusitis, throat irritation, upper respiratory tract infection

Miscellaneous: Allergy, binge eating, flu-like syndrome

Pharmacodynamics/Kinetics

Onset of Action Immediate release: 30 minutes

Duration of Action Immediate release: 6-8 hours

Absorption Rapid

Bioavailability 70%

Time to Peak
Immediate release: 1.6 hours; 2.2 hours with food
Extended release: 1.5 hours; 4 hours with food
Spray: ~0.9 hours
Sublingual: ~1.4 hours; ~1.8 hours with food

Protein Binding ~93%

Half-Life Elimination
Immediate release, Extended release: ~2.5 hours (range 1.4-4.5 hours); Cirrhosis: Up to 9.9 hours; Elderly: Prolonged up to 32%
Spray: ~3 hours (range: 1.7-8.4)
Sublingual: ~3 hours (range: 1.6-6.7 hours)

Metabolism Hepatic methylation and hydroxylation via CYP3A4 (~60%), CYP2C9 (~22%), CYP1A2 (~14%), CYP2D6 (~3%), and CYP2C19 (~3%) to three inactive metabolites

Excretion Urine (48% to 67%, primarily as metabolites); feces (29% to 42%, primarily as metabolites)

Controlled Substance C-IV

Available Dosage Forms

Solution, oral:
Zolpimist®: 5 mg/actuation (8.2 g)

Tablet, oral: 5 mg, 10 mg
Ambien®: 5 mg, 10 mg

Tablet, sublingual:
Edluar™: 5 mg, 10 mg

Tablet, extended release, oral: 6.25 mg
Ambien CR®: 6.25 mg, 12.5 mg

Dosing

Adult Insomnia: Oral:
Immediate release tablet, spray, sublingual tablet: 10 mg immediately before bedtime; maximum dose: 10 mg
Extended release tablet: 12.5 mg immediately before bedtime

Geriatric
Immediate release tablet, spray, sublingual tablet: 5 mg immediately before bedtime
Extended release tablet: 6.25 mg immediately before bedtime

Renal Impairment Dose adjustment not required; monitor closely.
Not dialyzable

Hepatic Impairment
Immediate release tablet, spray, sublingual tablet: 5 mg
Extended release tablet: 6.25 mg

Administration

Oral Ingest immediately before bedtime due to rapid onset of action.
Ambien CR® tablets should be swallowed whole; do not divide, crush, or chew.
Edluar™ sublingual tablets should be placed under the tongue and allowed to disintegrate; do not swallow or administer with water.
Zolpimist® oral spray should be sprayed directly into the mouth over the tongue. Prior to initial use, pump should be primed by spraying 5 times. If pump is not used for at least 14 days, re-prime pump with 1 spray.

Stability

Storage
Ambien®, Edluar™: Store at 20°C to 25°C (68°F to 77°F). Protect sublingual tablets from light and moisture.
Ambien CR®: Store at 15°C to 25°C (59°F to 77°F); limited excursions permitted up to 30°C (86°F).
Zolpimist®: Store at 25°C (77°F); do not freeze. Avoid prolonged exposure to temperatures >30°C (86°F).

Monitoring and Teaching Issues

Physical Assessment For short-term use. Assess for history of addiction; long-term use can result in dependence, abuse, or tolerance; periodically evaluate need for continued use. Monitor for CNS depression. For inpatient use, institute safety measures to prevent falls.

Patient Education Take immediately before going to bed. Only use this medication if you can get a full night's sleep (at least 7-8 hours). Drug may cause physical and/or psychological dependence. While using this medication, do not use alcohol. Avoid grapefruit or grapefruit juice when taking this medication. You may experience drowsiness, dizziness, blurred vision, nausea, or diarrhea. Report CNS changes (confusion, memory problems, depression, excitation, headache, abnormal thinking or behavior, nightmares); muscle pain or weakness; respiratory difficulty; unusual swelling, especially on face or neck; chest pain or palpitations; or ineffectiveness of medication. Report episodes of "sleep driving" or other complex behaviors, such as driving a vehicle, preparing food, or other activities which you have no memory of performing.

Dietary Considerations For faster sleep onset, do not administer with (or immediately after) a meal.

Geriatric Considerations In doses >5 mg, there was subjective evidence of impaired sleep on the first post-treatment night. There have been few reports of increased hypotension and/or falls in the elderly with this drug. Can be considered a drug of choice in the elderly when a hypnotic is indicated. With Ambien CR®, the adverse event profile of 6.25 mg in elderly patients was similar to the 12.5 mg dose in younger adults. Until there is more experience with this dosage form, use with caution in the elderly.

Pregnancy Considerations Teratogenic effects were not observed in animal studies. Adverse effects were noted in animal reproductive studies at doses 20-100 times the maximum recommended human dose. Severe neonatal respiratory depression has been reported when zolpidem was used at the end of pregnancy, especially when used concurrently with other CNS depressants. Studies of prenatal exposure to zolpidem have not been conducted in children. Children born of mothers taking sedative/hypnotics may be at risk for withdrawal; neonatal flaccidity has been reported in infants following maternal use of sedative/hypnotics during pregnancy. Use during pregnancy only if the benefits justify the risk to the fetus.

Additional Information Causes fewer disturbances in sleep stages as compared to benzodiazepines. Time spent in sleep stages 3 and 4 are maintained; zolpidem decreases sleep latency; should not be prescribed in quantities exceeding a 1-month supply.

- **Zolpidem Tartrate** *see* Zolpidem *on page 1905*
- **Zolpimist®** *see* Zolpidem *on page 1905*
- **Zolvit™** *see* Hydrocodone and Acetaminophen *on page 915*
- **Zometa®** *see* Zoledronic Acid *on page 1899*
- **Zomig®** *see* Zolmitriptan *on page 1903*
- **Zomig-ZMT®** *see* Zolmitriptan *on page 1903*
- **Zonalon®** *see* Doxepin (Topical) *on page 578*
- **Zonatuss™** *see* Benzonatate *on page 201*
- **Zonegran®** *see* Zonisamide *on page 1908*

Zonisamide (zoe NIS a mide)

U.S. Brand Names Zonegran®

Generic Availability (U.S.) Yes

Pharmacologic Category Anticonvulsant, Miscellaneous

Medication Safety Issues

Sound-alike/look-alike issues:

Zonegran® may be confused with SINEquan®

Zonisamide may be confused with lacosamide

Medication Guide Available Yes

Pregnancy Risk Factor C

Lactation Excreted into breast milk /not recommended

Use Adjunct treatment of partial seizures in children >16 years of age and adults with epilepsy

Unlabeled/Investigational Use Bipolar disorder

Mechanism of Action/Effect The exact mechanism of action is not known. May stabilize neuronal membranes and suppress neuronal hypersynchronization through action at sodium and calcium channels. Does not affect GABA activity.

Contraindications Hypersensitivity to zonisamide, sulfonamides, or any component of the formulation

Warnings/Precautions Hazardous agent - use appropriate precautions for handling and disposal. Rare, but potentially fatal sulfonamide reactions have occurred following the use of zonisamide. These reactions include Stevens-Johnson syndrome, fulminant hepatic necrosis, agranulocytosis, aplastic anemia, and toxic epidermal necrolysis, usually appearing within 2-16 weeks of drug initiation. Discontinue zonisamide if rash develops. Chemical similarities are present among sulfonamides, sulfonylureas, carbonic anhydrase inhibitors, thiazides, and loop diuretics (except ethacrynic acid). Use in patients with sulfonamide allergy is specifically contraindicated in product labeling, however, a risk of cross-reaction exists in patients with allergy to any of these compounds; avoid use when previous reaction has been severe. Use may be associated with the development of metabolic acidosis (generally dose-dependent) in certain patients; predisposing conditions/therapies include renal disease, severe respiratory disease, diarrhea, surgery, ketogenic diet, and other medications. Pediatric patients may also be at an increased risk for and may have more severe metabolic acidosis. Serum bicarbonate should be monitored in all patients prior to and during use; if metabolic acidosis occurs, consider decreasing the dose or tapering the dose to discontinue. If use continued despite acidosis, alkali treatment should be considered. Untreated metabolic acidosis may increase the risk of developing nephrolithiasis, nephrocalcinosis, osteomalacia (or rickets in children), or osteoporosis; pediatric patients may also have decreased growth rates.

Pooled analysis of trials involving various antiepileptics (regardless of indication) showed an increased risk of suicidal thoughts/behavior (incidence rate: 0.43% treated patients compared to 0.24% of patients receiving placebo); risk observed as early as 1 week after initiation and continued through duration of trials (most trials ≤24 weeks). Monitor all patients for notable changes in behavior that might indicate suicidal thoughts or depression; notify healthcare provider immediately if symptoms occur.

Discontinue zonisamide in patients who develop acute renal failure or a significant sustained increase in creatinine/BUN concentration. Kidney stones have been reported. Do not use in patients with renal impairment (GFR <50 mL/minute); use with caution in patients with hepatic impairment.

Significant CNS effects include psychiatric symptoms, psychomotor slowing, and fatigue or somnolence. Fatigue and somnolence occur within the first month of treatment, most commonly at doses of 300-500 mg/day. Effects with other sedative drugs or ethanol may be potentiated.

May cause sedation, which may impair physical or mental abilities; patients must be cautioned about performing tasks which require mental alertness (eg, operating machinery or driving). Abrupt withdrawal may precipitate seizures; discontinue or reduce doses gradually.

Safety and efficacy in children <16 years of age has not been established. Decreased sweating (oligohydrosis) and hyperthermia requiring hospitalization have been reported in children. Pediatric patients may also be at an increased risk and may have more severe metabolic acidosis.

Drug Interactions

Metabolism/Transport Effects Substrate of CYP2C19 (minor), 3A4 (major)

Avoid Concomitant Use There are no known interactions where it is recommended to avoid concomitant use.

Decreased Effect

The levels/effects of Zonisamide may be decreased by: CYP3A4 Inducers (Strong); Deferasirox; Herbs (CYP3A4 Inducers); Ketorolac; Ketorolac (Systemic); Mefloquine; PHENobarbital; Phenytoin

Increased Effect/Toxicity

Zonisamide may increase the levels/effects of: Alcohol (Ethyl); CNS Depressants; Methotrimeprazine

The levels/effects of Zonisamide may be increased by: Conivaptan; CYP3A4 Inhibitors (Moderate); CYP3A4 Inhibitors (Strong); Dasatinib; Droperidol; Methotrimeprazine

Nutritional/Ethanol Interactions

Ethanol: Avoid ethanol (may increase CNS depression).

Food: Food delays time to maximum concentration, but does not affect bioavailability.

Adverse Reactions Adjunctive therapy: Frequencies noted in patients receiving other anticonvulsants:

>10%:

Central nervous system: Somnolence (17%), dizziness (13%)

Gastrointestinal: Anorexia (13%)

1% to 10%:

Central nervous system: Headache (10%), agitation/irritability (9%), fatigue (8%), tiredness (7%), ataxia (6%), confusion (6%), concentration decreased (6%), memory impairment (6%), depression (6%), insomnia (6%), speech disorders (5%), mental slowing (4%), anxiety (3%), nervousness (2%), schizophrenic/schizophreniform behavior (2%), difficulty in verbal expression (2%), status epilepticus (1%), convulsion (1%), hyperesthesia (1%), incoordination (1%)

Dermatologic: Rash (3%), bruising (2%), pruritus (1%)

Gastrointestinal: Nausea (9%), abdominal pain (6%), diarrhea (5%), dyspepsia (3%), weight loss (3%), constipation (2%), taste perversion (2%), xerostomia (2%), vomiting (1%)

Neuromuscular & skeletal: Paresthesia (4%), abnormal gait (1%), tremor (1%), weakness (1%)

Ocular: Diplopia (6%), nystagmus (4%), amblyopia (1%)

Otic: Tinnitus (1%)

Respiratory: Rhinitis (2%), pharyngitis (1%), increased cough (1%)

Miscellaneous: Flu-like syndrome (4%) accidental injury (1%)

Pharmacodynamics/Kinetics

Time to Peak 2-6 hours

Protein Binding 40%

Half-Life Elimination Plasma: ~63 hours

Metabolism Hepatic via CYP3A4; forms N-acetyl zonisamide and 2-sulfamoylacetyl phenol (SMAP)

Excretion Urine (62%, 35% as unchanged drug, 65% as metabolites); feces (3%)

Available Dosage Forms

Capsule, oral: 25 mg, 50 mg, 100 mg

Zonegran®: 25 mg, 100 mg

Dosing

Adult

Adjunctive treatment of partial seizures: Oral: Initial: 100 mg/day. Dose may be increased to 200 mg/day after 2 weeks. Further dosage increases to 300 mg and 400 mg/day can then be made with a minimum of 2 weeks between adjustments, in order to reach steady state at each dosage level. Doses of up to 600 mg/day have been studied, however, there is no evidence of increased response with doses >400 mg/day.

Mania (unlabeled use): Oral: Initial: 100-200 mg/day; maximum: 600 mg/day (Kanba, 1994)

Geriatric Data from clinical trials is insufficient for patients older than 65. Begin dosing at the low end of the dosing range.

Pediatric Children >16 years: Refer to adult dosing.

Renal Impairment Slower titration and frequent monitoring are indicated in patients with renal disease. Use is not recommended in patients with GFR <50 mL/minute. Marked renal impairment (Cl_{cr} <20 mL/minute) was associated with a 35% increase in AUC.

Hepatic Impairment Slower titration and frequent monitoring are indicated.

Administration

Oral Capsules should be swallowed whole. Dose may be administered once or twice daily. Doses of 300 mg/day and higher are associated with increased side effects. Steady-state levels are reached in 14 days.

Stability

Storage Store at controlled room temperature 25°C (77°F). Protect from moisture and light.

Monitoring and Teaching Issues

Laboratory Monitoring Metabolic profile, specifically BUN, serum creatinine; serum bicarbonate (prior to initiation and periodically during therapy)

Physical Assessment Observe and teach seizure precautions.

Patient Education Take at the same time each day, with or without food. Do not chew, crush, or open capsules; swallow whole. Maintain adequate hydration unless instructed to restrict fluid intake. While using this medication, avoid alcohol. Wear/carry identification of epileptic status and medications. You may experience drowsiness, dizziness, blurred vision, nausea, vomiting, constipation, dry mouth, or loss of appetite. Report CNS changes (changes in speech patterns, mentation changes, suicide ideation, depression, changes in cognition or memory, unusual thought patterns, coordination difficulties, or excessive drowsiness); extreme fatigue, loss of appetite, or hyperventilation; respiratory difficulty or tightening of the throat; swelling of mouth, lips, or tongue; muscle cramping, weakness, or pain; rash or skin irritations; unusual bruising or bleeding (mouth, urine, stool); fever, sore throat, or sores in your mouth; swelling of extremities; sudden back pain, pain on urination, or dark/bloody urine (signs of kidney stones); or change in seizure type or frequency.

Dietary Considerations May be taken without regard to meals.

Geriatric Considerations Consider the CNS effects commonly experienced in the first month of therapy.

Breast-Feeding Considerations Zonisamide is excreted into breast milk in concentrations similar to those in the maternal plasma and has been detected in the plasma of a nursing infant. According to the manufacturer, the decision to continue or discontinue breast-feeding during therapy should take into account the risk of exposure to the infant and the benefits of treatment to the mother.

Pregnancy Considerations Teratogenic effects were observed in animal reproduction studies; therefore, zonisamide is classified as pregnancy category C. Zonisamide crosses the placenta and can be detected in the newborn following delivery. Although adverse fetal events have been reported, the risk of teratogenic effects following maternal use of zonisamide in not clearly defined. Other agents may be preferred until additional data is available. Newborns should be monitored for transient metabolic acidosis after birth. Zonisamide clearance may increase in the second trimester of pregnancy, requiring dosage adjustment. Women of childbearing potential are advised to use effective contraception during therapy.

Patients exposed to zonisamide during pregnancy are encouraged to enroll themselves into the AED Pregnancy Registry by calling 1-888-233-2334. Additional information is available at http://www.aedpregnancyregistry.org.

Related Information

Anticonvulsant Drugs of Choice *on page 1981*

◆ **Zorbtive®** *see* Somatropin *on page 1664*

◆ **ZORprin® [DSC]** *see* Aspirin *on page 155*

◆ **Zortress®** *see* Everolimus *on page 720*

◆ **ZOS** *see* Zoster Vaccine *on page 1910*

◆ **Zostavax®** *see* Zoster Vaccine *on page 1910*

Zoster Vaccine (ZOS ter vak SEEN)

U.S. Brand Names Zostavax®

Index Terms Shingles Vaccine; Varicella-Zoster (VZV) Vaccine (Zoster); VZV Vaccine (Zoster); ZOS

Generic Availability (U.S.) No

Pharmacologic Category Vaccine, Live (Viral)

Medication Safety Issues

Both varicella vaccine and zoster vaccine are live, attenuated strains of varicella-zoster virus. Their indications, dosing, and composition are distinct. Varicella vaccine is indicated for the prevention of chickenpox, while zoster vaccine is indicated in older individuals to prevent reactivation of the virus which causes shingles. Zoster vaccine is **not** a substitute for varicella vaccine and should not be used in children.

Lactation Excretion in breast milk unknown/use caution

Use Prevention of herpes zoster (shingles) in patients ≥50 years of age

The Advisory Committee on Immunization Practices (ACIP) recommends routine vaccination of all patients ≥60 years of age, including:

- Patients who report a previous episode of zoster.
- Patients with chronic medical conditions (eg, chronic renal failure, diabetes mellitus, rheumatoid arthritis, chronic pulmonary disease) unless those conditions are contraindications.
- Residents of nursing homes and other long-term care facilities ≥60 years of age, without contraindications.

Available Dosage Forms

Injection, powder for reconstitution [preservative free]:

Zostavax®: 19,400 PFU

Dosing

Adult & Geriatric Shingles: Adults ≥50 years: SubQ: 0.65 mL administered as a single dose; there are no data to support readministration of the vaccine

Renal Impairment No adjustment required.

Administration

I.M. Not for I.M. administration

I.V. Not for I.V. administration

Other Inject immediately after reconstitution. Inject SubQ into the deltoid region of the upper arm, if possible. In persons anticipating immunosuppression, give at least 14 days to 1 month prior to starting immunosuppressant.

Administration with chronic use of acyclovir, famciclovir, or valacyclovir: Discontinue ≥24 hours before administration of zoster vaccine. Do not use for ≥14 days after vaccination.

Simultaneous administration of vaccines helps ensure the patients will be fully vaccinated by the appropriate age. Simultaneous administration of vaccines is defined as administering >1 vaccine on the same day at different anatomic sites. Separate vaccines should not be combined in the same syringe unless indicated by product specific labeling. Separate needles and syringes should be used for each injection. The ACIP prefers each dose of a specific vaccine in a series come from the same manufacturer when possible. Adolescents and adults should be vaccinated while seated or lying down (CDC, 2011).

Antipyretics have not been shown to prevent febrile seizures. Antipyretics may be used to treat fever or discomfort following vaccination (CDC, 2011). One study reported that routine prophylactic administration of acetaminophen to prevent fever prior to vaccination decreased the immune response of some vaccines; the clinical significance of this reduction in immune response has not been established (Prymula, 2009).

Monitoring and Teaching Issues

Physical Assessment This is not a substitute for varicella vaccine. Not for use in patients <50 years of age or in the treatment of active zoster outbreak. Assess patient history for contraindications prior to treatment. Deferring treatment should be considered in presence of acute illness or fever >101.3°F. Treatment for anaphylactic/anaphylactoid reaction should be immediately available. Federal law requires entry into the patient's medical record.

Patient Education This vaccine is not a treatment for shingles, but may help prevent the occurrence of shingles or reduce the pain if shingles develops despite the vaccination. Avoid other vaccinations for 2 months following this vaccine unless approved by prescriber. Avoid close and/or prolonged contact with highly susceptible individuals (newborns, pregnant women, immunocompromised persons) for six weeks following vaccination; there is a rare risk of transmitting the vaccine virus to those who have not had chickenpox. Notify prescriber immediately of any acute reaction to vaccination (eg, difficulty breathing, chest pain, acute headache, rash, or difficulty swallowing). May cause mild fever and some irritation or swelling at injection site; consult prescriber if excessive or persisting. Federal law requires entry into the patient's medical record.

Related Information

Immunization Recommendations *on page 1941*

- **Zovia®** *see* Ethinyl Estradiol and Ethynodiol Diacetate *on page 698*
- **Zovirax®** *see* Acyclovir (Systemic) *on page 44*
- **Zovirax®** *see* Acyclovir (Topical) *on page 48*
- **Z-Pak** *see* Azithromycin (Systemic) *on page 181*
- **Zuplenz®** *see* Ondansetron *on page 1360*
- **Zuplenz®** *see* Ondansetron *on page 1360*
- **Zyban®** *see* BuPROPion *on page 252*
- **Zyclara™** *see* Imiquimod *on page 959*
- **Zydone®** *see* Hydrocodone and Acetaminophen *on page 915*
- **Zyflo®** *see* Zileuton *on page 1894*
- **Zyflo CR®** *see* Zileuton *on page 1894*
- **Zylet®** *see* Loteprednol and Tobramycin *on page 1137*
- **Zyloprim®** *see* Allopurinol *on page 76*
- **Zymar® [DSC]** *see* Gatifloxacin *on page 852*
- **Zymaxid™** *see* Gatifloxacin *on page 852*
- **ZyPREXA®** *see* OLANZapine *on page 1344*
- **ZyPREXA® IntraMuscular** *see* OLANZapine *on page 1344*
- **ZyPREXA® Relprevv™** *see* OLANZapine *on page 1344*
- **Zyprexa Zydis** *see* OLANZapine *on page 1344*
- **ZyPREXA® Zydis®** *see* OLANZapine *on page 1344*
- **ZyrTEC® Allergy [OTC]** *see* Cetirizine *on page 351*
- **ZyrTEC® Children's Allergy [OTC]** *see* Cetirizine *on page 351*
- **ZyrTEC® Children's Hives Relief [OTC]** *see* Cetirizine *on page 351*
- **Zytopic™** *see* Triamcinolone (Topical) *on page 1816*
- **Zyvox®** *see* Linezolid *on page 1112*

PHARMACOLOGIC CATEGORY INDEX

APPENDIX TABLE OF CONTENTS

DIAGNOSTICS AND SURGICAL AIDS

Agent	Use
Arginine (R-Gene® 10)	Pituitary function test (growth hormone)
Atopiclair® (multiple ingredients)	Manage and relieve symptoms of dermatoses, including atopic dermatitis and allergic contact dermatitis; helps to relieve dry, waxy skin by maintaining a moist skin environment
Candida albicans (Monilia) (Candin®)	Screen for the detection of nonresponsiveness to antigens in immunocompromised individuals
Cellulose (oxidized regenerated) (Surgicel®)	Hemostatic; temporary packing for the control of capillary, venous, or small arterial hemorrhage
Chondroitin sulfate – sodium hyaluronate (DisCoVisc®; Viscoat®)	Ophthalmic surgical aid in the anterior segment during cataract extraction and intraocular lens implantation
Collagen hemostat (Avitene®; EndoAvitene®; Helistat®; Helitene®; Instat™; SyringeAvitene™)	Adjunct to hemostasis when control of bleeding by ligature is ineffective or impractical
Corticorelin (Acthrel®)	Diagnostic test used in adrenocorticotropic hormone (ACTH)-dependent Cushing's syndrome to differentiate between pituitary and ectopic production of ACTH
Corticotropin (H.P. Acthar® Gel)	Acute exacerbations of multiple sclerosis; diagnostic aid in adrenocortical insufficiency, severe muscle weakness in myasthenia gravis Cosyntropin is preferred over corticotropin for diagnostic test of adrenocortical insufficiency (cosyntropin is less allergenic and test is shorter in duration)
Cosyntropin (Cortrosyn®)	Diagnostic test to differentiate primary adrenal from secondary (pituitary) adrenocortical insufficiency
Cyclopentolate (AK-Pentolate™; Cyclogyl®; Cylate™)	Diagnostic procedures requiring mydriasis and cycloplegia
Cyclopentolate and phenylephrine (Cyclomydril®)	Induce mydriasis greater than that produced with cyclopentolate HCl alone
Fluorescein (AK-Fluor®; Angiofluor™; Angiofluor™ Lite; Fluorescite®; Fluorets®; Ful-Glo®)	Injection: Diagnostic aid in ophthalmic angiography and angioscopy Topical: To stain the anterior segment of the eye for procedures (such as fitting contact lenses), disclosing corneal injury, and in applanation tonometry
Fluorescein and benoxinate (EyeFlur; Fluress®; Flurox™)	For use in ophthalmic procedures when a topical disclosing agent is needed along with an anesthetic
Gelatin, absorbable (Gelfilm®; Gelfoam®)	Adjunct to provide hemostasis in surgery; used in open prostatic surgery
Hydroxyamphetamine and tropicamide (Paremyd®)	Short-term pupil dilation for diagnostic procedures and exams
Hydroxypropyl methylcellulose (Cellugel®; GenTeal® Mild; GenTeal®; Gonak™; Goniosoft™; Isopto® Tears; Tearisol®; Tears Again® MC)	Relief of burning and minor irritation due to dry eyes; diagnostic agent in gonioscopic examination
Indocyanine green (IC-Green™)	Determine hepatic function, cardiac output, and liver blood flow; ophthalmic angiography
Isosulfan Blue (Lymphazurin™)	Adjunct to lymphography for visualization of the lymphatic system; sentinel node identification
Methacholine (Provocholine®)	Diagnosis of bronchial airway hyperactivity
Metyrapone (Metopirone®)	Diagnostic test for hypothalamic-pituitary ACTH function
MimyX® (multiple ingredients)	Manage and relieve the symptoms of dermatoses, including atopic dermatitis, allergic contact dermatitis, and radiation dermatitis; used to maintain a moist wound and skin environment; restores the natural components of the stratum corneum; re-establishes barrier function of the outer layers of the epidermis

Agent	Use
Perflutren Protein Type A (Optison™)	Opacification of left ventricular chamber and improvement of delineation of the left ventricular endocardial border in patients with suboptimal echocardiograms
Proparacaine (Alcaine®; Ophthetic®; Parcaine™)	Anesthesia for tonometry, gonioscopy; suture removal from cornea; removal of corneal foreign body; cataract extraction, glaucoma surgery; short operative procedure involving the cornea and conjunctiva
Proparacaine and fluorescein (Flucaine®)	Anesthesia for tonometry, gonioscopy; suture removal from cornea; removal of corneal foreign body; cataract extraction, glaucoma surgery
Regadenoson (Lexiscan®)	Radionuclide myocardial perfusion imaging (MPI) in patients unable to undergo adequate exercise stress testing
Secretin (ChiRhoStim™)	Secretin-stimulation testing to aid in diagnosis of pancreatic exocrine dysfunction; diagnosis of gastrinoma (Zollinger-Ellison syndrome); facilitation of endoscopic retrograde cholangiopancreatography (ERCP) visualization
Sincalide (Kinevac®)	Postevacuation cholecystography; gallbladder bile sampling; stimulate pancreatic secretion for analysis; accelerate the transit of barium through the small bowel
Thrombin (topical) (Evithrom™; Recothrom™; Thrombi-Gel®; Thrombi-Pad®; Thrombin-JMI®)	Hemostasis whenever minor bleeding from capillaries and small venules is accessible Thrombi-Gel®; Thrombi-Pad®: Temporary control as trauma dressing for moderate-to-severe bleeding wounds; control of surface bleeding from vascular access sites and percutaneous catheter/tubes
Thyrotropin Alfa (Thyrogen®)	As an adjunctive diagnostic tool for serum thyroglobulin (Tg) testing; adjunctive treatment for radioiodine ablation of thyroid tissue remnants after total or near-total thyroidectomy in patients with well-differentiated thyroid cancer without evidence of metastatic disease Potential clinical uses include: Patients with an undetectable Tg on thyroid hormone suppressive therapy to exclude the diagnosis of residual or recurrent thyroid cancer, patients requiring serum Tg testing and radioiodine imaging who are unwilling to undergo thyroid hormone withdrawal testing and whose treating physician believes that use of a less sensitive test is justified, patients who are either unable to mount an adequate endogenous TSH response to thyroid hormone withdrawal or in whom withdrawal is medically contraindicated, and patients without evidence of metastatic disease to ablate thyroid remnants (in combination with radioiodine [I^{131}]) following near-total thyroidectomy.
Trichophyton skin test	Assess cell-mediated immunity
Tropicamide (Mydral™; Mydriacyl®; Tropicacyl®)	Short-acting mydriatic used in diagnostic procedures, as well as preoperatively and postoperatively; treatment of some cases of acute iritis, iridocyclitis, and keratitis

HERBAL AND NUTRITIONAL PRODUCTS

HERBS AND COMMON NATURAL AGENTS

The authors have chosen to include this list of natural products and proposed medical claims. However, due to limited scientific investigation to support these claims, this list is not intended to imply that these claims have been scientifically proven.

Proposed Treatments

Herb	Treatment
Agrimony	Digestive disorders
Alfalfa	High cholesterol; menopause
Allspice	General health
Aloe vera	Healing agent; minor bites and stings; constipation
Alpha-lipoic acid	Glaucoma; neuropathies
Androstenedione	Increased strength and muscle mass
Anise (seed)	Prevent gas
Astragalus	Enhance energy reserves; immune system modulation; adjunctive treatment for cancer
Barberry (bark)	Halitosis
Bayberry (bark)	Relieve and prevent varicose veins
Bay (leaf)	Relieves cramps
Bee pollen	Renewal of enzymes, hormones, vitamins, amino acids, and others
Bergamot	Calming effect
Bifidobacterium bifidum (bifidus)	Gastrointestinal microflora recolonization (anaerobic)
Bilberry (leaf)	Increases night vision; reduces eye fatigue; antioxidant; circulation
Birch (bark)	Urinary problems; used for rheumatism
Blackberry (leaf)	Diarrhea
Black cohosh	Relieves menstrual cramps; menopause
Blueberry (leaf)	Diarrhea
Blue cohosh	Regulate menstrual flow
Blue flag	Skin diseases and constipation
Boldo (leaf)	Stimulates digestion; gallstones
Boneset	Colds and flu
Bromelain	Digestive enzyme
Buchu (leaf)	Diuretic
Buckthorn (bark)	Expels worms; laxative
Burdock (leaf and root)	Eczema
Butternut	Works well for constipation
Calendula	Mending and healing of cuts or wounds topically; burns
Capsicum (cayenne)	Normalizes blood pressure; circulation; arthritis; neuralgia pain
Caraway (seed)	Aids digestion
Cascara sagrada	Remedies for chronic constipation
Catnip	Calming effect in children
Cat's claw	Asthma; cancer
Celery	Blood pressure; diuretic
Centaury	Stimulates the salivary gland
Chamomile	Headache; colic; minor bites and stings; anxiety/tension

Proposed Treatments *(continued)*

Herb	Treatment
Chaste tree	Acne; menopause
Chickweed	Rich in vitamin C and minerals (calcium, magnesium, and potassium); diuretic; thyroid stimulant
Chicory (root)	Effective in disorders of the kidneys, liver, and urinary canal
Chondroitin	Osteoarthritis
Cinnamon (bark)	Prevents infection and indigestion; helps break down fats during digestion
Cleavers	Kidney and bladder disorders; useful in obstructions of the urinary organ
Cloves	General medicinal
Coenzyme Q_{10}	Cardiovascular disorders (angina, heart failure, hypertension)
Coriander (seed)	Stomach tonic
Cranberry	Urinary tract health; bladder infections; cystitis
Cubeb (berry)	Chronic bladder trouble; increases flow of urine
Damiana (leaf)	Sexual impotency
Dandelion (leaf)	Diuretic; appetite stimulation; liver conditions
Dandelion (root)	Detoxify poisons in the liver; beneficial in lowering blood pressure
Dehydroepiandrosterone (DHEA)	Improvement in energy, muscle mass, mood, memory
Devil's claw	Arthritis; back pain
Dill weed	Digestive health
Dong quai (root)	Menopause and PMS symptoms; anemia
Echinacea (root)	Colds and viruses; immune modulating
Eucalyptus (leaf)	Mucolytic
Elder	Antiviral; boils and skin ulcers; cough
Elecampane (root)	Cough with mucus
Evening primrose	Arthritis; diabetes; eczema
Eyebright (*Euphrasia officinalis*)	Eye-related inflammatory conditions
Fennel (seed)	Remedies for gas and acid stomach
Fenugreek (seed)	Allergies; coughs; digestion; emphysema; headaches; migraines; intestinal inflammation; ulcers; lungs; mucous membranes; and sore throat
Feverfew	Migraines
Fish oil	Hypercholesterolemia; cardiovascular health
Flax seed	Cardiovascular health
Garlic (bulb)	Lowers blood cholesterol; anti-infective; protective against cancer
Gentian	Digestive health
Ginger (root)	Antiemetic; arthritis
Ginkgo biloba	Improves blood circulation to the brain; dementia; impotence
Ginseng, Siberian (root)	Resistance against stress; slows the aging process; fatigue
Glucosamine	Osteoarthritis
Goldenseal	Digestive disorders
Gota kola	"Memory herb"; nerve tonic; wound healing
Gravelroot (queen of the meadow)	Remedy for stones in the kidney and bladder
Green tea	Antioxidant
Hawthorn	Cardiotonic; hypertension; circulatory problems
Hibiscus (flower)	Diuretic
Hops (flower)	Insomnia; used to decrease the desire for alcohol
Horehound	Acute or chronic sore throat and coughs

Proposed Treatments *(continued)*

Herb	Treatment
Horsetail (shavegrass)	Rich in minerals, especially silica; used to develop strong fingernails and hair, good for split ends; diuretic
Hydrangea (root)	Backaches
Juniper (berry)	Diuretic; arthritis; bladder infections; cystitis
Kava (root)	Calm nervousness; anxiety; pain
Kelp	High contents of natural plant iodine, for proper function of the thyroid; high levels of natural calcium, potassium, and magnesium
Lactobacillus acidophilus	Gastrointestinal microflora recolonization (anaerobic)
Lavender (oil)	Wound healing; decrease scarring (topical)
Lecithin	Break up cholesterol; prevent arteriosclerosis
Licorice (root)	Expectorant; used in peptic ulceration; adrenal exhaustion; canker sores
Lobelia	Cough
Ma huang (ephedra)	Asthma
Malva (flower)	Soothes inflammation in the mouth and throat; helpful for earaches
Marjoram	Beneficial for a sour stomach or loss of appetite
Marshmallow (leaf)	Demulcent
Milk thistle	Liver detoxifier; antioxidant; diuretic
Motherwort	Hypertension; regulate blood circulation
Mugwort	Used for rheumatism and gout
Mullein (leaf)	High in iron, magnesium, and potassium; sinuses; relieves swollen joints; soothing bronchial tissue
Mustard (seed)	General medicinal
Myrrh (gum)	Removes bad breath; sinus problems
Nettle (leaf)	Dandruff; antihistaminic qualities; allergies; asthma; hay fever
Nettle (root)	Used in benign prostatic hyperplasia (BPH); arthritis
Nutmeg	Gas
Oregano (leaf)	Settles the stomach after meals; helps treat colds
Oregon grape (root)	Gallbladder problems
Papaya (leaf)	Digestive stimulant; contains the enzyme papain
Paprika (sweet)	Stimulates the appetite and gastric secretions
Passion (flower)	Mild sedative
Pau d'arco	Protects immune system; antifungal
Peppermint (leaf)	Excellent for headaches; digestive stimulation; indigestion; colic
Poppy seed blue	Excellent in the making of breads and desserts
Prickly ash (bark)	Increases circulation
Psyllium (seed)	Lubricant to the intestinal tract
Red clover	Phytoestrogenic properties
Red raspberry (leaf)	Decreases menstrual bleeding; childbirth; diarrhea
Red yeast rice	Lowers cholesterol levels
Rhubarb (root)	Powerful laxative
Rose hips	High content of vitamin C
SAMe (S-adenosyl methionine)	Depression
Sassafras oil	Mild counterirritant on skin (eg, insect bites)
Saw palmetto (berry)	Benign prostatic hyperplasia (BPH)
Schisandra	Increasing the body's ability to adapt to stresses from chemical, physical, psychological, and environmental sources
Scullcap	Anxiety and tension
Seawrack (bladderwrack)	Combat obesity; contains iodine

Proposed Treatments *(continued)*

Herb	Treatment
Senna (leaf)	Laxative
Shepherd's purse	Female reproductive health
Sheep sorrel	Diuretic
Slippery elm (bark)	Normalize bowel movement; beneficial for hemorrhoids and constipation
Solomon's seal (root)	Poultice for bruises
Spikenard	Skin ailments such as acne, pimples, blackheads, rashes, and general skin problems
Star anise	Promotes appetite and relieves flatulence
St John's wort	Depression; neuralgia pain
Summer savory (leaf)	Diarrhea, upset stomach, and sore throat
Tea tree oil	Antifungal, antibacterial; dental and oral health (mouthwash); burns, cuts, scrapes, insect bites, dandruff; acne
Thyme (leaf)	Ulcers (peptic); cough; antifungal
Tumeric	Arthritis; liver detoxifier
Uva-ursi (leaf)	Diuretic; used in urinary tract health; bladder infections; cystitis
Valerian (root)	Insomnia; anxiety and tension; neuralgia pain
Vanadium	Diabetes mellitus
Vervain	Remedy for fevers
White oak (bark)	Strong astringent
White willow	Arthritis; back pain; migraines
Wild alum (root)	Powerful astringent; used as rinse for sores in mouth and bleeding gums
Wild cherry	Cough suppressant
Wild Oregon grape (root)	Chronic skin disease
Wild yam (root)	Menopause
Wintergreen (leaf)	Valuable for colic and gas in the bowels
Witch hazel (bark and leaf)	Hemorrhoids
Wormwood	Antiparasitic
Yarrow (root)	Fevers; hemorrhoid
Yellow dock (root)	Good in all skin problems
Yerba santa	Bronchial congestion
Yohimbe	Natural aphrodisiac
Yucca (root)	Reduces inflammation of the joints

IMMUNIZATION ADMINISTRATION RECOMMENDATIONS

The following tables are taken from the General Recommendations on Immunization, 2011:

- Guidelines for Spacing of Live and Inactivated Antigens
- Guidelines for Administering Antibody-Containing Products and Vaccines
- Recommended Intervals Between Administration of Antibody-Containing Products and Measles- or Varicella-Containing Vaccine, by Product and Indication for Vaccination
- Vaccination of persons with Primary and Secondary Immunodeficiencies
- Needle length and Injection Site of I.M. injections

Guidelines for Spacing of Live and Inactivated Antigens

Antigen Combination	Recommended Minimum Interval Between Doses
Two or more inactivated[1]	May be administered simultaneously or at any interval between doses
Inactivated and live	May be administered simultaneously or at any interval between doses
Two or more live injectable[2]	28 days minimum interval, if not administered simultaneously

[1]Certain experts suggest a 28-day interval between tetanus toxoid, reduced diphtheria toxoid, and reduced acellular pertussis (Tdap) vaccine and tetravalent meningococcal conjugate vaccine if they are not administered simultaneously.

[2]Live oral vaccines (eg, Ty21a typhoid vaccine and rotavirus vaccine) may be administered simultaneously or at any interval before or after inactivated or live injectable vaccines.

Adapted from American Academy of Pediatrics, Pertussis. In: Pickering LK, Baker CJ, Kimberlin DW, Long SS, eds, Red Book: 2009 Report of the Committee on Infectious Diseases, 28th ed, Elk Grove Village, IL: American Academy of Pediatrics, 2009, 22.

Guidelines for Administering Antibody-Containing Products[1] and Vaccines

Simultaneous Administration (during the same office visit)

Products Administered	Recommended Minimum Interval Between Doses
Antibody-containing products and inactivated antigen	Can be administered simultaneously at different anatomic sites or at any time interval between doses.
Antibody-containing products and live antigen	Should **not** be administered simultaneously.[2] If simultaneous administration of measles-containing vaccine or varicella vaccine is unavoidable, administer at different sites and revaccinate or test for seroconversion after the recommended interval.

Nonsimultaneous Administration

Products Administered: Administered first	Products Administered: Administered second	Recommended Minimum Interval Between Doses
Antibody-containing products	Inactivated antigen	No interval necessary
Inactivated antigen	Antibody-containing products	No interval necessary
Antibody-containing products	Live antigen	Dose-related[2,3]
Live antigen	Antibody-containing products	2 weeks[2]

[1]Blood products containing substantial amounts of immune globulin include intramuscular and intravenous immune globulin, specific hyperimmune globulin (eg, hepatitis B immune globulin, tetanus immune globulin, varicella zoster immune globulin, and rabies immune globulin), whole blood, packed red blood cells, plasma, and platelet products.

[2]Yellow fever vaccine; rotavirus vaccine; oral Ty21a typhoid vaccine; live-attenuated influenza vaccine; and zoster vaccine are exceptions to these recommendations. These live-attenuated vaccines can be administered at any time before, after, or simultaneously with an antibody-containing product.

[3]The duration of interference of antibody-containing products with the immune response to the measles component of measles-containing vaccine, and possibly varicella vaccine, is dose-related.

Recommended Intervals Between Administration of Antibody-Containing Products and Measles- or Varicella-Containing Vaccine, by Product and Indication for Vaccination

Product / Indication	Dose (mg IgG/kg) and Route[1]	Recommended Interval Before Measles- or Varicella-Containing Vaccine[2] Administration (mo)
Tetanus IG	I.M.: 250 units (10 mg IgG/kg)	3
Hepatitis A IG		
Contact prophylaxis	I.M.: 0.02 mL/kg (3.3 mg IgG/kg)	3
International travel	I.M.: 0.06 mL/kg (10 mg IgG/kg)	3
Hepatitis B IG	I.M.: 0.06 mL/kg (10 mg IgG/kg)	3
Rabies IG	I.M.: 20 int. units/kg (22 mg IgG/kg)	4
Varicella IG	I.M.: 125 units/10 kg (60-200 mg IgG/kg) (maximum: 625 units)	5
Measles prophylaxis IG		
Standard (ie, nonimmunocompromised) contact	I.M.: 0.25 mL/kg (40 mg IgG/kg)	5
Immunocompromised contact	I.M.: 0.50 mL/kg (80 mg IgG/kg)	6
Blood transfusion		
Red blood cells (RBCs), washed	I.V.: 10 mL/kg (negligible IgG/kg)	None
RBCs, adenine-saline added	I.V.: 10 mL/kg (10 mg IgG/kg)	3
Packed RBCs (hematocrit 65%)[3]	I.V.: 10 mL/kg (60 mg IgG/kg)	6
Whole blood cells (hematocrit 35% to 50%)[3]	I.V.: 10 mL/kg (80-100 mg IgG/kg)	6
Plasma/platelet products	I.V.: 10 mL/kg (160 mg IgG/kg)	7
Cytomegalovirus intravenous immune globulin (IGIV)	150 mg/kg maximum	6
IGIV		
Replacement therapy for immune deficiencies[4]	I.V.: 300-400 mg/kg[4]	8
Immune thrombocytopenic purpura treatment	I.V.: 400 mg/kg	8
Postexposure varicella prophylaxis[5]	I.V.: 400 mg/kg	8
Immune thrombocytopenic purpura treatment	I.V.: 1000 mg/kg	10
Kawasaki disease	I.V.: 2 g/kg	11
Monoclonal antibody to respiratory syncytial virus F protein (Synagis® [Medimmune])[6]	I.M.: 15 mg/kg	None

HIV = human immunodeficiency virus; IG = immune globulin; IgG = immune globulin G; IGIV = intravenous immune globulin; mg IgG/kg = milligrams of immune globulin G per kilogram of body weight; I.M. = intramuscular; I.V. = intravenous; RBCs = red blood cells

[1]This table is not intended for determining the correct indications and dosages for using antibody-containing products. Unvaccinated persons might not be fully protected against measles during the entire recommended interval, and additional doses of IG or measles vaccine might be indicated after measles exposure. Concentrations of measles antibody in an IG preparation can vary by manufacturer's lot. Rates of antibody clearance after receipt of an IG preparation also might vary. Recommended intervals are extrapolated from an estimated half-life of 30 days for passively acquired antibody and an observed interference with the immune response to measles vaccine for 5 months after a dose of 80 mg IgG/kg.

[2]Does not include zoster vaccine. Zoster vaccine may be given with antibody-containing blood products.

[3]Assumes a serum IgG concentration of 16 mg/mL.

[4]Measles and varicella vaccinations are recommended for children with asymptomatic or mildly symptomatic HIV infection but are contraindicated for persons with severe immunosuppression from HIV or any other immunosuppressive disorder.

[5]The investigational product VariZIG™, similar to licensed varicella-zoster IG (VZIG), is a purified human IG preparation made from plasma containing high levels of anti-varicella antibodies (IgG). The interval between VariZIG™ and varicella vaccine (Var or MMRV) is 5 months.

[6]Contains antibody only to respiratory syncytial virus.

Vaccination of Persons With Primary and Secondary Immunodeficiencies

Category	Specific Immunodeficiency	Contraindicated Vaccines[1]	Risk-Specific Recommended Vaccines[1]	Effectiveness and Comments
Primary				
B-lymphocyte (humoral)	Severe antibody deficiencies (eg, X-linked agammaglobulinemia and common variable immunodeficiency)	Oral poliovirus (OPV)[2] Smallpox Live-attenuated influenza vaccine (LAIV) BCG Ty21a (live oral typhoid) Yellow fever	Pneumococcal Consider measles and varicella vaccination	The effectiveness of any vaccine is uncertain if it depends only on the humoral response (eg, PPSV or MPSV4) IGIV interferes with the immune response to measles vaccine and possibly varicella vaccine.
	Less severe antibody deficiencies (eg, selective IgA deficiency and IgG subclass deficiency)	OPV[2] BCG Yellow Fever Other live-vaccines appear to be safe	Pneumococcal	All vaccines likely effective; immune response may be attenuated.
T-lymphocyte (cell-mediated and humoral)	Complete defects (eg, severe combined immunodeficiency [SCID] disease, complete DiGeorge syndrome)	All live vaccines[3,4,5]	Pneumococcal	Vaccines might be ineffective.
	Partial defects (eg, most patients with DiGeorge syndrome, Wiskott-Aldrich syndrome, ataxia- telangiectasia)	All live vaccines[3,4,5]	Pneumococcal Meningococcal Hib (if not administered in infancy)	Effectiveness of any vaccine depends on degree of immune suppression.
Complement	Persistent complement, properdin, or factor B deficiency	None	Pneumococcal Meningococcal	All routine vaccines likely effective.
Phagocytic function	Chronic granulomatous disease, leukocyte adhesion defect, and myeloperoxidase deficiency	Live bacterial vaccines[3]	Pneumococcal[6]	All inactivated vaccines safe and likely effective. Live viral vaccines likely safe and effective.

Vaccination of Persons With Primary and Secondary Immunodeficiencies *continued*

Category	Specific Immunodeficiency	Contraindicated Vaccines[1]	Risk-Specific Recommended Vaccines[1]	Effectiveness and Comments
Secondary				
	HIV/AIDS	OPV[2] Smallpox BCG LAIV Withhold MMR and varicella in severely immunocompromised persons Yellow fever vaccine might have a contraindication or a precaution depending on clinical parameters of immune function[9]	Pneumococcal Consider Hib (if not administered in infancy) and meningococcal vaccination.	MMR, varicella, rotavirus, and all inactivated vaccines, including inactivated influenza, might be effective.[7]
	Malignant neoplasm, transplantation, immunosuppressive or radiation therapy	Live viral and bacterial, depending on immune status[3,4]	Pneumococcal	Effectiveness of any vaccine depends on degree of immune suppression.
	Asplenia	None	Pneumococcal Meningococcal Hib (if not administered in infancy)	All routine vaccines likely effective.
	Chronic renal disease	LAIV	Pneumococcal Hepatitis B[8]	All routine vaccines likely effective.

AIDS = acquired immunodeficiency syndrome; BCG = bacille Calmette-Guerin; Hib = *Haemophilus influenzae* type b; HIV = human immunodeficiency virus; IG = immunoglobulin; IGIV = immune globulin intravenous; LAIV = live, attenuated influenza vaccine; MMR = measles, mumps, and rubella; MPSV4 = quadrivalent meningococcal polysaccharide vaccine; OPV = oral poliovirus vaccine (live); PPSV = pneumococcal polysaccharide vaccine; TIV = trivalent inactivated influenza vaccine

[1]Other vaccines that are universally or routinely recommended should be administered if not contraindicated.

[2]OPV is no longer available in the United States.

[3]Live bacterial vaccines: BCG and oral Ty21a *Salmonella typhi* vaccine.

[4]Live viral vaccines: MMR, MMRV, OPV, LAIV, yellow fever, zoster, rotavirus, varicella, and vaccinia (smallpox). Smallpox vaccine is not recommended for children or the general public.

[5]Regarding T-lymphocyte immunodeficiency as a contraindication for rotavirus vaccine, data exist only for severe combined immunodeficiency.

[6]Pneumococcal vaccine is not indicated for children with chronic granulomatous disease beyond age-based universal recommendations for PCV. Children with chronic granulomatous disease are not at increased risk for pneumococcal disease.

[7]HIV-infected children should receive IG after exposure to measles, and may receive varicella and measles vaccine if $CD4^+$ lymphocyte count is ≥15%.

[8]Indicated based on the risk from dialysis-based bloodborne transmission.

[9]Symptomatic HIV infection or $CD4^+$ T-lymphocyte count of <200/mm^3 or <15% of total lymphocytes for children aged <6 years is a containdication to yellow fever vaccine administration. Asymptomatic HIV infection with $CD4^+$ T-lymphocyte count of 200-499/mm^3 for persons aged ≥6 years or 15% to 24% of total lymphocytes for children aged <6 years is a precaution for yellow fever vaccine administration. Details of yellow fever vaccine recommendations are available from CDC. (CDC. Yellow fever vaccine: recommendations of the Advisory Committee on Immunization Practices [ACIP]. MMWR 2010, 59[No. RR-7])

Adapted from American Academy of Pediatrics. Passive Immunization. In: Pickering LK, Baker CJ, Kimberline DW, Long SS, eds, Red Book: 2009 Report of the Committee on Infectious Diseases, 28th ed, Elk Grove Village, IL: American Academy of Pediatrics, 2009, 74-5.

Needle Length and Injection Site of I.M. for Children Aged ≤18 years (by age) and Adults Aged ≥19 years (by sex and weight)

Age Group	Needle Length	Injection Site
Children (birth to 18 y)		
Neonates[1]	5/8" (16 mm)[2]	Anterolateral thigh
Infant 1-12 mo	1" (25 mm)	Anterolateral thigh
Toddler 1-2 y	1-1 1/4" (25-32 mm)	Anterolateral thigh[3]
	5/8[2]-1" (16-25 mm)	Deltoid muscle of the arm
Children 3-18 y	5/8[2]-1" (16-25 mm)	Deltoid muscle of the arm[3]
	1-1 1/4" (25-32 mm)	Anterolateral thigh
Adults ≥19 y		
Men and women <60 kg (130 lb)	1" (25 mm)[4]	Deltoid muscle of the arm
Men and women 60-70 kg (130-152 lb)	1" (25 mm)	
Men 70-118 kg (152-260 lb)	1-1 1/2" (25-38 mm)	
Women 70-90 kg (152-200 lb)		
Men >118 kg (260 lb)	1 1/2" (38 mm)	
Women >90 kg (200 lb)		

I.M. = intramuscular

[1]First 28 days of life.

[2]If skin is stretched tightly and subcutaneous tissues are not bunched.

[3]Preferred site.

[4]Some experts recommend a 5/8" needle for men and women who weigh <60 kg.

Adapted from Poland GA, Borrud A, Jacobsen RM, et al, "Determination of Deltoid Fat Pad Thickness: Implications for Needle Length in Adult Immunization," *JAMA*, 1997, 277:1709-11.

RECOMMENDATIONS FOR TRAVELERS

The Centers for Disease Control and Prevention (CDC) also provides guidance to assist travelers and their healthcare providers in deciding the vaccines, medications, and other measures necessary to prevent illness and injury during international travel. Information can be found on the following website: http://wwwnc.cdc.gov/travel/

Reference:

Centers for Disease Control, "Recommendations of the Advisory Committee on Immunization Practices (ACIP): General Recommendations on Immunization," *MMWR Recomm Rep*, 2011, 60 (2):1-61.

IMMUNIZATION RECOMMENDATIONS

Recommended Immunization Schedule for Persons Aged 0 Through 6 Years—United States • 2011

For those who fall behind or start late, see the catch-up schedule

Vaccine ▼ Age ▶	Birth	1 month	2 months	4 months	6 months	12 months	15 months	18 months	19–23 months	2–3 years	4–6 years
Hepatitis B[1]	HepB	HepB			HepB						
Rotavirus[2]			RV	RV	RV[2]						
Diphtheria, Tetanus, Pertussis[3]			DTaP	DTaP	DTaP	see footnote[3]	DTaP				DTaP
Haemophilus influenzae type b[4]			Hib	Hib	Hib[4]	Hib					
Pneumococcal[5]			PCV	PCV	PCV	PCV				PPSV	
Inactivated Poliovirus[6]			IPV	IPV	IPV						IPV
Influenza[7]					Influenza (Yearly)						
Measles, Mumps, Rubella[8]						MMR		see footnote[8]			MMR
Varicella[9]						Varicella		see footnote[9]			Varicella
Hepatitis A[10]						HepA (2 doses)				HepA Series	
Meningococcal[11]										MCV4	

Range of recommended ages for all children

Range of recommended ages for certain high-risk groups

This schedule includes recommendations in effect as of December 21, 2010. Any dose not administered at the recommended age should be administered at a subsequent visit, when indicated and feasible. The use of a combination vaccine generally is preferred over separate injections of its equivalent component vaccines. Considerations should include provider assessment, patient preference, and the potential for adverse events. Providers should consult the relevant Advisory Committee on Immunization Practices statement for detailed recommendations: **http://www.cdc.gov/vaccines/pubs/acip-list.htm**. Clinically significant adverse events that follow immunization should be reported to the Vaccine Adverse Event Reporting System (VAERS) at http://www.vaers.hhs.gov or by telephone, **800-822-7967**.

Footnotes to Recommended Immunization Schedule for Ages 0-6 Years

[1]**Hepatitis B vaccine (HepB).** *(Minimum age: birth)*

At birth:

- Administer monovalent HepB to all newborns before hospital discharge.
- If mother is hepatitis B surface antigen (HB_sAg)-positive, administer HepB and 0.5 mL of hepatitis B immune globulin (HBIG) within 12 hours of birth.
- If mother's HB_sAg status is unknown, administer HepB within 12 hours of birth. Determine mother's HB_sAg status as soon as possible and, if HB_sAg-positive, administer HBIG (no later than age 1 week).

Doses following the birth dose:

- The second dose should be administered at age 1 or 2 months. Monovalent HepB should be used for doses administered before age 6 weeks.
- Infants born to HB_sAg-positive mothers should be tested for HB_sAg and antibody to HB_sAg 1-2 months after completion of at least 3 doses of the HepB series, at age 9-18 months (generally at the next well-child visit).
- Administration of 4 doses of HepB to infants is permissible when combination vaccine containing HepB is administered after the birth dose.
- Infants who did not receive a birth dose should receive 3 doses of HepB on a schedule of 0, 1, and 6 months.
- The final (3rd or 4th) dose in the HepB series should be administered no earlier than age 24 weeks.

[2]**Rotavirus vaccine (RV).** *(Minimum age: 6 weeks)*

- Administer the first dose at age 6-14 weeks (maximum age: 14 weeks 6 days). Vaccination should not be initiated for infants aged 15 weeks 0 days or older.
- The maximum age for the final dose in the series is 8 months 0 days.
- If Rotarix® is administered at ages 2 and 4 months, a dose at 6 months is not indicated.

[3]**Diphtheria and tetanus toxoids and acellular pertussis vaccine (DTaP).** *(Minimum age: 6 weeks)*

- The fourth dose may be administered as early as age 12 months, provided at least 6 months have elapsed since the third dose.

[4]***Haemophilus influenzae* type b conjugate vaccine (Hib).** *(Minimum age: 6 weeks)*
- If PRP-OMP (PedvaxHIB® or ComVax® [HepB-Hib]) is administered at ages 2 and 4 months, a dose at age 6 months is not indicated.
- Hiberix® should not be used for doses at ages 2, 4, or 6 months for the primary series but can be used as the final dose in children aged 12 months through 4 years.

[5]**Pneumococcal vaccine.** *(Minimum age: 6 weeks for pneumococcal conjugate vaccine [PCV]; 2 years for pneumococcal polysaccharide vaccine [PPSV])*
- PCV is recommended for all children aged <5 years. Administer 1 dose of PCV to all healthy children aged 24-59 months who are not completely vaccinated for their age.
- A PCV series begun with 7-valent PCV (PCV7) should be completed with 13-valent PCV (PCV13).
- A single supplemental dose of PCV13 is recommended for all children aged 14-59 months who have received an age-appropriate series of PCV7.
- A single supplemental dose of PCV13 is recommended for all children aged 60-71 months with underlying medical conditions who have received an age-appropriate series of PCV7.
- The supplemental dose of PCV13 should be administered at least 8 weeks after the previous dose of PCV7. See *MMWR* 2010:59(No. RR-11).
- Administer PPSV at least 8 weeks after last dose of PCV to children aged ≥2 years with certain underlying medical conditions, including a cochlear implant.

[6]**Inactivated poliovirus vaccine (IPV).** *(Minimum age: 6 weeks)*
- If 4 or more doses are administered prior to age 4 years an additional dose should be administered at age 4-6 years.
- The final dose in the series should be administered on or after the fourth birthday and at least 6 months following the previous dose.

[7]**Influenza vaccine (seasonal).** *(Minimum age: 6 months for trivalent inactivated influenza vaccine [TIV]; 2 years for live, attenuated influenza vaccine [LAIV])*
- For healthy children aged ≥2 years (ie, those who do not have underlying medical conditions that predispose them to influenza complications), either LAIV or TIV may be used, except LAIV should not be given to children aged 2-4 years who have had wheezing in the past 12 months.
- Administer 2 doses (separated by at least 4 weeks) to children aged 6 months through 8 years who are receiving seasonal influenza vaccine for the first time or who were vaccinated for the first time during the previous influenza season but only received 1 dose.
- Children aged 6 months through 8 years who received no doses of monovalent 2009 H1N1 vaccine should receive 2 doses of 2010–2011 seasonal influenza vaccine. See *MMWR* 2010;59(No. RR-8):33–34.

[8]**Measles, mumps, and rubella vaccine (MMR).** *(Minimum age: 12 months)*
- The second dose may be administered before age 4 years, provided at least 4 weeks have elapsed since the first dose.

[9]**Varicella vaccine.** *(Minimum age: 12 months)*
- The second dose may be administered before age 4 years, provided at least 3 months have elapsed since the first dose.
- For children aged 12 months through 12 years the recommended minimum interval between doses is 3 months. However, if the second dose was administered at least 4 weeks after the first dose, it can be accepted as valid.

[10]**Hepatitis A vaccine (HepA).** *(Minimum age: 12 months)*
- Administer 2 doses at least 6 months apart.
- HepA is recommended for children aged older than 23 months who live in areas where vaccination programs target older children, who are at increased risk for infection, or for whom immunity against hepatitis A is desired.

[11]**Meningococcal conjugate vaccine, quadrivalent (MCV4).** *(Minimum age: 2 years)*
- Administer 2 doses of MCV4 at least 8 weeks apart to children aged 2-10 years with persistent complement component deficiency and anatomic or functional asplenia, and 1 dose every 5 years thereafter.
- Persons with human immunodeficiency virus (HIV) infection who are vaccinated with MCV4 should receive 2 doses at least 8 weeks apart.
- Administer 1 dose of MCV4 to children aged 2-10 years who travel to countries with highly endemic or epidemic disease and during outbreaks caused by a vaccine serogroup.
- Administer MCV4 to children at continued risk for meningococcal disease who were previously vaccinated with MCV4 or meningococcal polysaccharide vaccine after 3 years if the first dose was administered at age 2-6 years.

The recommended immunization schedules for persons aged 0-18 years are approved by the Advisory Committee on Immunization Practices (**http://www.cdc.gov/vaccines/recs/acip**), the American Academy of Pediatrics (**http://www.aap.org**), and the American Academy of Family Physicians (**http://www.aafp.org**).

Recommended Immunization Schedule for Persons Aged 7 Through 18 Years—United States • 2011

For those who fall behind or start late, see the schedule below and the catch-up schedule

Vaccine ▼ Age ▶	7–10 years	11–12 years	13–18 years
Tetanus, Diphtheria, Pertussis[1]		Tdap	Tdap
Human Papillomavirus[2]	*see footnote*[2]	HPV (3 doses)(females)	HPV series
Meningococcal[3]	MCV4	MCV4	MCV4
Influenza[4]		Influenza (Yearly)	
Pneumococcal[5]		Pneumococcal	
Hepatitis A[6]		HepA Series	
Hepatitis B[7]		Hep B Series	
Inactivated Poliovirus[8]		IPV Series	
Measles, Mumps, Rubella[9]		MMR Series	
Varicella[10]		Varicella Series	

Range of recommended ages for all children

Range of recommended ages for catch-up immunization

Range of recommended ages for certain high-risk groups

This schedule includes recommendations in effect as of December 21, 2010. Any dose not administered at the recommended age should be administered at a subsequent visit, when indicated and feasible. The use of a combination vaccine generally is preferred over separate injections of its equivalent component vaccines. Considerations should include provider assessment, patient preference, and the potential for adverse events. Providers should consult the relevant Advisory Committee on Immunization Practices statement for detailed recommendations: **http://www.cdc.gov/vaccines/pubs/acip-list.htm**. Clinically significant adverse events that follow immunization should be reported to the Vaccine Adverse Event Reporting System (VAERS) at **http://www.vaers.hhs.gov** or by telephone, **800-822-7967**.

Footnotes to Recommended Immunization Schedule for Ages 7-18 Years

[1]**Tetanus and diphtheria toxoids and acellular pertussis vaccine (Tdap).** *(Minimum age: 10 years for Boostrix® and 11 years for Adacel®)*

- Persons aged 11-18 years who have not received Tdap should receive a dose followed by Td booster doses every 10 years thereafter.
- Persons aged 7 through 10 years who are not fully immunized against pertussis (including those never vaccinated or with unknown pertussis vaccination status) should receive a single dose of Tdap. Refer to the catch-up schedule if additional doses of tetanus and diphtheria toxoid–containing vaccine are needed.
- Tdap can be administered regardless of the interval since the last tetanus and diphtheria toxoid–containing vaccine.

[2]**Human papillomavirus vaccine (HPV).** *(Minimum age: 9 years)*

- Quadrivalent HPV vaccine (HPV4) or bivalent HPV vaccine (HPV2) is recommended for the prevention of cervical precancers and cancers in females.
- HPV4 is recommended for prevention of cervical precancers, cancers, and genital warts in females.
- HPV4 may be administered in a 3-dose series to males aged 9-18 years to reduce their likelihood of genital warts.
- Administer the second dose 1-2 months after the first dose and the third dose 6 months after the first dose (at least 24 weeks after the first dose).

[3]**Meningococcal conjugate vaccine, quadrivalent (MCV4).** *(Minimum age: 2 years)*

- Administer MCV4 at age 11-12 years with a booster dose at age 16 years.
- Administer 1 dose at age 13-18 years if not previously vaccinated.
- Persons who received their first dose at age 13-15 years should receive a booster dose at age 16-18 years.
- Administer 1 dose to previously unvaccinated college freshmen living in a dormitory.
- Administer 2 doses at least 8 weeks apart to children aged 2-10 years with persistent complement component deficiency and anatomic or functional asplenia, and 1 dose every 5 years thereafter.
- Persons with HIV infection who are vaccinated with MCV4 should receive 2 doses at least 8 weeks apart.
- Administer 1 dose of MCV4 to children aged 2-10 years who travel to countries with highly endemic or epidemic disease and during outbreaks caused by a vaccine serogroup.
- Administer MCV4 to children at continued risk for meningococcal disease who were previously vaccinated with MCV4 or meningococcal polysaccharide vaccine after 3 years (if first dose administered at age 2-6 years) or after 5 years (if first dose administered at age 7 years or older).

[4]Influenza vaccine (seasonal).

- For healthy nonpregnant persons aged 7-18 years (ie, those who do not have underlying medical conditions that predispose them to influenza complications), either LAIV or TIV may be used.
- Administer 2 doses (separated by at least 4 weeks) to children aged 6 months through 8 years who are receiving seasonal influenza vaccine for the first time or who were vaccinated for the first time during the previous influenza season but only received 1 dose.
- Children 6 months through 8 years of age who received no doses of monovalent 2009 H1N1 vaccine should receive 2 doses of 2010-2011 seasonal influenza vaccine. See *MMWR* 2010;59(No. RR-8):33–34.

[5]Pneumococcal vaccines.

- A single dose of 13-valent pneumococcal conjugate vaccine (PCV13) may be administered to children aged 6-18 years who have functional or anatomic asplenia, HIV infection or other immunocompromising condition, cochlear implant or CSF leak. See *MMWR* 2010;59(No. RR-11).
- The dose of PCV13 should be administered at least 8 weeks after the previous dose of PCV7.
- Administer pneumococcal polysaccharide vaccine at least 8 weeks after the last dose of PCV to children aged 2 years or older with certain underlying medical conditions, including a cochlear implant. A single revaccination should be administered after 5 years to children with functional or anatomic asplenia or an immunocompromising condition.

[6]Hepatitis A vaccine (HepA).

- Administer 2 doses at least 6 months apart.
- HepA is recommended for children >23 months who live in areas where vaccination programs target older children, who are at increased risk of infection, or for whom immunity against hepatitis A is desired.

[7]Hepatitis B vaccine (HepB).

- Administer the 3-dose series to those not previously vaccinated. For those with incomplete vaccination, follow the catch-up schedule.
- A 2-dose series (separated by at least 4 months) of adult formulation Recombivax HB® is licensed for children aged 11-15 years.

[8]Inactivated poliovirus vaccine (IPV).

- The final dose in the series should be administered on or after the fourth birthday and at least 6 months following the previous dose.
- If both OPV and IPV were administered as part of a series, a total of 4 doses should be administered, regardless of the child's current age.

[9]Measles, mumps, and rubella vaccine (MMR).

- The minimum interval between the 2 doses of MMR is 4 weeks.

[10]Varicella vaccine.

- For persons aged 7-18 years without evidence of immunity [see *MMWR*, 2007, 56(RR-4)], administer 2 doses if not previously vaccinated or the second dose if only 1 dose has been administered.
- For persons aged 7-12 years, the recommended minimum interval between doses is 3 months. However, if the second dose was administered at least 4 weeks after the first dose, it can be accepted as valid.
- For persons aged ≥13 years, the minimum interval between doses is 4 weeks.

The recommended immunization schedules for persons age 0-18 years are approved by the Advisory Committee on Immunization Practices (**http://www.cdc.gov/vaccines/recs/acip**), the American Academy of Pediatrics (**http://www.aap.org**), and the American Academy of Family Physicians (**http://www.aafp.org**).

Catch-up Immunization Schedule for Persons Aged 4 Months - 18 Years Who Start Late or Who Are >1 Month Behind - United States, 2011

The table below provides catch-up schedules and minimum intervals between doses for children whose vaccinations have been delayed. A vaccine series does not need to be restarted, regardless of the time that has elapsed between doses. Use the section appropriate for the child's age.

Vaccine	Minimum Age for Dose 1	Minimum Interval Between Doses			
		Dose 1 to Dose 2	Dose 2 to Dose 3	Dose 3 to Dose 4	Dose 4 to Dose 5
Catch-up Schedule for Persons Age 4 Months – 6 Years					
Hepatitis B[1]	Birth	**4 weeks**	**8 weeks** (and ≥16 weeks after 1st dose)		
Rotavirus[2]	6 wk	**4 weeks**	**4 weeks**[2]		
Diphtheria, tetanus, pertussis[3]	6 wk	**4 weeks**	**4 weeks**	**6 months**	**6 months**[3]

(continued)

Vaccine	Minimum Age for Dose 1	Minimum Interval Between Doses			
		Dose 1 to Dose 2	Dose 2 to Dose 3	Dose 3 to Dose 4	Dose 4 to Dose 5
Haemophilus influenzae type b[4]	6 wk	**4 weeks** if 1st dose administered at age <12 months **8 weeks (as final dose)** if 1st dose administered at age 12-14 months **No further doses needed** if 1st dose administered at age ≥15 months	**4 weeks**[4] if current age <12 months **8 weeks (as final dose)**[4] if current age ≥12 months and 1st dose is administered at age <12 months and 2nd dose administered at age <15 months **No further doses needed** if previous dose administered at age ≥15 months	**8 weeks (as final dose)** This dose only necessary for children age 12-59 months who received 3 doses before age 12 months	
Pneumococcal[5]	6 wk	**4 weeks** if 1st dose administered at age <12 months **8 weeks (as final dose for healthy children)** if 1st dose administered at age ≥12 months or current age 24-59 months **No further doses needed** for healthy children if 1st dose administered at age ≥24 months	**4 weeks** if current age <12 months **8 weeks (as final dose for healthy children)** if current age ≥12 months **No further doses needed** for healthy children if previous dose administered at age ≥24 months	**8 weeks (as final dose)** This dose only necessary for children age 12-59 months who received 3 doses before age 12 months or for high-risk children who received 3 doses at any age	
Inactivated poliovirus[6]	6 wk	**4 weeks**	**4 weeks**	**6 months**[6]	
Measles, mumps, rubella[7]	12 mo	**4 weeks**			
Varicella[8]	12 mo	**3 months**			
Hepatitits A[9]	12 mo	**6 months**			
Catch-up Schedule for Persons Age 7-18 Years					
Tetanus, diphtheria/ tetanus, diphtheria, pertussis[10]	7 y	**4 weeks**	**4 weeks** if 1st dose administered at age <12 months **6 months** if 1st dose administered at age ≥12 months	**6 months** if 1st dose administered at age <12 months	
Human papillomavirus[11]	9 y	**Routine dosing intervals are recommended**[11]			
Hepatitis A[9]	12 mo	**6 months**			
Hepatitis B[1]	Birth	**4 weeks**	**8 weeks** (and ≥16 weeks after 1st dose)		
Inactivated poliovirus[6]	6 wk	**4 weeks**	**4 weeks**[6]	**6 months**[6]	
Measles, mumps, rubella[7]	12 mo	**4 weeks**			
Varicella[8]	12 mo	**3 months** if the person is age <13 years **4 weeks** if the person is age ≥13 years			

Footnotes to Catch-up Immunization Schedule Table

[1]**Hepatitis B vaccine (HepB).**
- Administer the 3-dose series to those not previously vaccinated.
- The minimum age for the third dose of HepB is 24 weeks.
- A 2-dose series (separated by at least 4 months) of adult formulation Recombivax HB® is licensed for children aged 11-15 years.

[2]**Rotavirus vaccine (RV).**
- The maximum age for the first dose is 14 weeks 6 days. Vaccination should not be initiated for infants aged ≥15 weeks 0 days.
- The maximum age for the final dose in the series is 8 months 0 days.
- If Rotarix® was administered for the first and second doses, a third dose is not indicated.

[3]**Diphtheria and tetanus toxoids and acellular pertussis vaccine (DTaP).**
- The fifth dose is not necessary if the fourth dose was administered at age ≥4 years.

[4]***Haemophilus influenzae* type b conjugate (Hib).**
- 1 dose of Hib vaccine should be considered for unvaccinated persons aged 5 years or older who have sickle cell disease, leukemia, or HIV infection, or who have had a splenectomy.
- If the first 2 doses were PRP-OMP (PedvaxHIB® or ComVax®), and administered at age ≤11 months, the third (and final) dose should be administered at age 12-15 months and ≥8 weeks after the second dose.
- If first dose administered at age 7-11 months, administer second dose ≥4 weeks later and a final dose at age 12-15 months.

[5]**Pneumococcal vaccine.**
- Administer 1 dose of 13-valent pneumococcal conjugate vaccine (PCV13) to all healthy children aged 24-59 months with any incomplete PCV schedule (PCV7 or PCV13).
- For children aged 24-71 months with underlying medical conditions, administer 1 dose of PCV13 if 3 doses of PCV were received previously or administer 2 doses of PCV13 ≥8 weeks apart if <3 doses of PCV were received previously.
- A single dose of PCV13 is recommended for certain children with underlying medical conditions through 18 years of age. See age-specific schedules for details.
- Administer pneumococcal polysaccharide vaccine (PPSV) to children aged ≥2 years with certain underlying medical conditions, including a cochlear implant, at ≥8 weeks after the last dose of PCV. A single revaccination should be administered after 5 years to children with functional or anatomic asplenia or an immunocompromising condition. See *MMWR* 2010;59(No. RR-11).

[6]**Inactivated poliovirus vaccine (IPV).**
- The final dose in the series should be administered on or after the fourth birthday and ≥6 months following the previous dose.
- A fourth dose is not necessary if the third dose was administered at age ≥4 years and ≥6 months following the previous dose.
- In the first 6 months of life, minimum age and minimum intervals are only recommended if the person is at risk for imminent exposure to circulating poliovirus (ie, travel to a polio-endemic region or during an outbreak).

[7]**Measles, mumps, and rubella vaccine (MMR).**
- Administer the second dose routinely at age 4-6 years. The minimum interval between the 2 doses of MMR is 4 weeks.

[8]**Varicella vaccine.**
- Administer the second dose routinely at age 4-6 years.
- If the second dose was administered at least 4 weeks after the first dose, it can be accepted as valid.

[9]**Hepatitis A vaccine (HepA).**
- HepA is recommended for children aged >23 months who live in areas where vaccination programs target older children, who are at increased risk for infection, or for whom immunity against hepatitis A is desired.

[10]**Tetanus and diphtheria toxoids (Td) and tetanus and diphtheria toxoids and acellular pertussis vaccine (Tdap).**
- Doses of DTaP are counted as part of the Td/Tdap series.
- Tdap should be substituted for a single dose of Td in the catch-up series for children aged 7-10 years or as a booster for children aged 11-18 years; use Td for other doses.

[11]**Human papillomavirus vaccine (HPV).**
- Administer the series to females at age 13-18 years if not previously vaccinated or have not completed the vaccine series.
- Quadrivalent HPV vaccine (HPV4) may be administered in a 3-dose series to males aged 9-18 years to reduce their likelihood of genital warts.
- Use recommended routine dosing intervals for series catch-up (ie, the second and third doses should be administered at 1-2 and 6 months after the first dose). The minimum interval between the first and second doses is 4 weeks. The minimum interval between the second and third doses is 12 weeks, and the third dose should be administered ≥24 weeks after the first dose.

Information about reporting reactions after immunization is available online at **http://www.vaers.hhs.gov** or by telephone, 800-822-7967. Suspected cases of vaccine-preventable diseases should be reported to the state or local health department. Additional information, including precautions and contraindications for immunization, is available from the National Center for Immunization and Respiratory Diseases at **http://www.cdc.gov/vaccines** or telephone, **800-CDC-INFO** (800-232-4636).

Recommended adult immunization schedule, by vaccine and age group—United States, 2011

VACCINE ▼ / AGE GROUP ▶	19–26 years	27–49 years	50–59 years	60–64 years	≥65 years
Influenza[1,*]	1 dose annually				
Tetanus, diphtheria, pertussis (Td/Tdap)[2,*]	Substitute 1-time dose of Tdap for Td booster; then boost with Td every 10 years				Td booster every 10 years
Varicella[3,*]	2 doses				
Human papillomavirus (HPV)[4,*]	3 doses (females)				
Zoster[5]				1 dose	
Measles, mumps, rubella (MMR)[6,*]	1 or 2 doses		1 dose		
Pneumococcal (polysaccharide)[7,8]	1 or 2 doses				1 dose
Meningococcal[9,*]	1 or more doses				
Hepatitis A[10,*]	2 doses				
Hepatitis B[11,*]	3 doses				

*Covered by the Vaccine Injury Compensation Program

For all persons in this category who meet the age requirements and who lack evidence of immunity (e.g., lack documentation of vaccination or have no evidence of previous infection)

Recommended if some other risk factor is present (e.g., based on medical, occupational, lifestyle, or other indications)

No recommendation

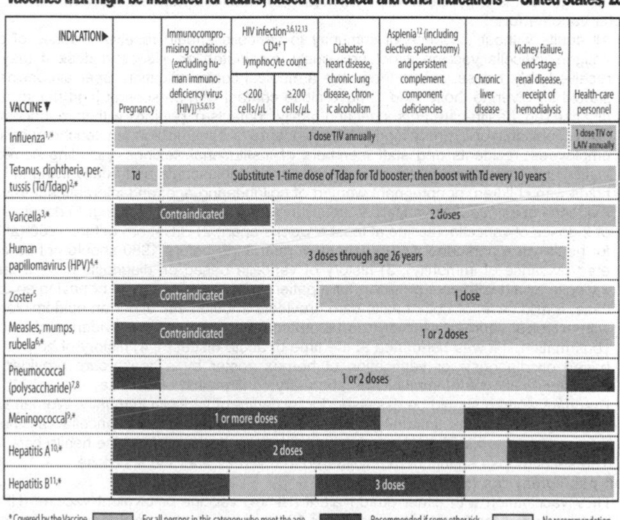

Vaccines that might be indicated for adults, based on medical and other indications—United States, 2011

VACCINE ▼ / INDICATION ▶	Pregnancy	Immunocompromising conditions (excluding human immunodeficiency virus [HIV])[3,5,6,13]	HIV infection[3,6,12,13] CD4+ T lymphocyte count: <200 cells/μL	HIV infection CD4+ T lymphocyte count: ≥200 cells/μL	Diabetes, heart disease, chronic lung disease, chronic alcoholism	Asplenia[12] (including elective splenectomy) and persistent complement component deficiencies	Chronic liver disease	Kidney failure, end-stage renal disease, receipt of hemodialysis	Health-care personnel
Influenza[1,*]	1 dose TIV annually								1 dose TIV or LAIV annually
Tetanus, diphtheria, pertussis (Td/Tdap)[2,*]	Td	Substitute 1-time dose of Tdap for Td booster; then boost with Td every 10 years							
Varicella[3,*]	Contraindicated			2 doses					
Human papillomavirus (HPV)[4,*]		3 doses through age 26 years							
Zoster[5]	Contraindicated				1 dose				
Measles, mumps, rubella[6,*]	Contraindicated			1 or 2 doses					
Pneumococcal (polysaccharide)[7,8]		1 or 2 doses							
Meningococcal[9,*]	1 or more doses								
Hepatitis A[10,*]	2 doses								
Hepatitis B[11,*]				3 doses					

*Covered by the Vaccine Injury Compensation Program

For all persons in this category who meet the age requirements and who lack evidence of immunity (e.g., lack documentation of vaccination or have no evidence of previous infection)

Recommended if some other risk factor is present (e.g., on the basis of medical, occupational, lifestyle, or other indications)

No recommendation

Footnotes to Recommended Adult Immunization Schedule

[1]Influenza vaccination.

- Annual vaccination against influenza is recommended for all persons aged 6 months and older, including all adults. Healthy, nonpregnant adults aged less than 50 years without high-risk medical conditions can receive either intranasally administered live, attenuated influenza vaccine (FluMist®), or inactivated vaccine. Other persons should receive the inactivated vaccine. Adults aged 65 years and older can receive the standard influenza vaccine or the high-dose (Fluzone®) influenza vaccine. Additional information about influenza vaccination is available at http://www.cdc.gov/vaccines/vpd-vac/flu/default.htm.

[2]Tetanus, diphtheria, and acellular pertussis (Td/Tdap) vaccination.

- Administer a one-time dose of Tdap to adults aged less than 65 years who have not received Tdap previously or for whom vaccine status is unknown to replace one of the 10-year Td boosters, and as soon as feasible to all 1) postpartum women, 2) close contacts of infants younger than age 12 months (eg, grandparents and child-care providers), and 3) health-care personnel with direct patient contact. Adults aged 65 years and older who have not previously received Tdap and who have close contact with an infant aged less than 12 months also should be vaccinated. Other adults aged 65 years and older may receive Tdap. Tdap can be administered regardless of interval since the most recent tetanus or diphtheria-containing vaccine.
- Adults with uncertain or incomplete history of completing a 3-dose primary vaccination series with Td-containing vaccines should begin or complete a primary vaccination series. For unvaccinated adults, administer the first 2 doses at least 4 weeks apart and the third dose 6–12 months after the second. If incompletely vaccinated (ie, less than 3 doses), administer remaining doses. Substitute a one-time dose of Tdap for one of the doses of Td, either in the primary series or for the routine booster, whichever comes first.
- If a woman is pregnant and received the most recent Td vaccination 10 or more years previously, administer Td during the second or third trimester. If the woman received the most recent Td vaccination less than 10 years previously, administer Tdap during the immediate postpartum period. At the clinician's discretion, Td may be deferred during pregnancy and Tdap substituted in the immediate postpartum period, or Tdap may be administered instead of Td to a pregnant woman after an informed discussion with the woman.
- The ACIP statement for recommendations for administering Td as prophylaxis in wound management is available at http://www.cdc.gov/vaccines/pubs/acip-list.htm.

[3]Varicella vaccination.

- All adults without evidence of immunity to varicella should receive 2 doses of single-antigen varicella vaccine if not previously vaccinated or a second dose if they have received only 1 dose, unless they have a medical contraindication. Special consideration should be given to those who 1) have close contact with persons at high risk for severe disease (eg, health-care personnel and family contacts of persons with immunocompromising conditions) or 2) are at high risk for exposure or transmission (eg, teachers; child-care employees; residents and staff members of institutional settings, including correctional institutions; college students; military personnel; adolescents and adults living in households with children; nonpregnant women of childbearing age; and international travelers).
- Evidence of immunity to varicella in adults includes any of the following: 1) documentation of 2 doses of varicella vaccine at least 4 weeks apart; 2) U.S.-born before 1980 (although for health-care personnel and pregnant women, birth before 1980 should not be considered evidence of immunity); 3) history of varicella based on diagnosis or verification of varicella by a health-care provider (for a patient reporting a history of or having an atypical case, a mild case, or both, health-care providers should seek either an epidemiologic link with a typical varicella case or to a laboratory-confirmed case or evidence of laboratory confirmation, if it was performed at the time of acute disease); 4) history of herpes zoster based on diagnosis or verification of herpes zoster by a health-care provider; or 5) laboratory evidence of immunity or laboratory confirmation of disease.
- Pregnant women should be assessed for evidence of varicella immunity. Women who do not have evidence of immunity should receive the first dose of varicella vaccine upon completion or termination of pregnancy and before discharge from the health-care facility. The second dose should be administered 4–8 weeks after the first dose.

[4]Human papillomavirus (HPV) vaccination.

- HPV vaccination with either quadrivalent (HPV4) vaccine or bivalent vaccine (HPV2) is recommended for females at age 11 or 12 years and catch-up vaccination for females aged 13-26 years.
- Ideally, vaccine should be administered before potential exposure to HPV through sexual activity; however, females who are sexually active should still be vaccinated consistent with age-based recommendations. Sexually active females who have not been infected with any of the four HPV vaccine types (types 6, 11, 16, and 18, all of which HPV4 prevents) or any of the two HPV vaccine types (types 16 and 18, both of which HPV2 prevents) receive the full benefit of the vaccination. Vaccination is less beneficial for females who have already been infected with one or more of the HPV vaccine types. HPV4 or HPV2 can be administered to persons with a history of genital warts, abnormal Papanicolaou test, or positive HPV DNA test, because these conditions are not evidence of previous infection with all vaccine HPV types.
- HPV4 may be administered to males aged 9-26 years to reduce their likelihood of genital warts. HPV4 would be most effective when administered before exposure to HPV through sexual contact.

- A complete series for either HPV4 or HPV2 consists of 3 doses. The second dose should be administered 1–2 months after the first dose; the third dose should be administered 6 months after the first dose.
- Although HPV vaccination is not specifically recommended for persons with the medical indications described in Figure 2, "Vaccines that might be indicated for adults based on medical and other indications," it may be administered to these persons because the HPV vaccine is not a live-virus vaccine. However, the immune response and vaccine efficacy might be less for persons with the medical indications described in Figure 2 than in persons who do not have the medical indications described or who are immunocompetent.

[5]Herpes zoster vaccination.

- A single dose of zoster vaccine is recommended for adults aged 60 years and older regardless of whether they report a previous episode of herpes zoster. Persons with chronic medical conditions may be vaccinated unless their condition constitutes a contra-indication.

[6]Measles, mumps, rubella (MMR) vaccination.

- Adults born before 1957 generally are considered immune to measles and mumps. All adults born in 1957 or later should have documentation of 1 or more doses of MMR vaccine unless they have a medical contraindication to the vaccine, laboratory evidence of immunity to each of the three diseases, or documentation of provider-diagnosed measles or mumps disease. For rubella, documentation of provider-diagnosed disease is not considered acceptable evidence of immunity.
- *Measles component:* A second dose of MMR vaccine, administered a minimum of 28 days after the first dose, is recommended for adults who 1) have been recently exposed to measles or are in an outbreak setting; 2) are students in postsecondary educational institutions; 3) work in a health-care facility; or 4) plan to travel internationally. Persons who received inactivated (killed) measles vaccine or measles vaccine of unknown type during 1963–1967 should be revaccinated with 2 doses of MMR vaccine.
- *Mumps component:* A second dose of MMR vaccine, administered a minimum of 28 days after the first dose, is recommended for adults who 1) live in a community experiencing a mumps outbreak and are in an affected age group; 2) are students in postsecondary educational institutions; 3) work in a health-care facility; or 4) plan to travel internationally. Persons vaccinated before 1979 with either killed mumps vaccine or mumps vaccine of unknown type who are at high risk for mumps infection (eg, persons who are working in a health-care facility) should be revaccinated with 2 doses of MMR vaccine.
- *Rubella component:* For women of childbearing age, regardless of birth year, rubella immunity should be determined. If there is no evidence of immunity, women who are not pregnant should be vaccinated. Pregnant women who do not have evidence of immunity should receive MMR vaccine upon completion or termination of pregnancy and before discharge from the health-care facility.
- *Health-care personnel born before 1957:* For unvaccinated health-care personnel born before 1957 who lack laboratory evidence of measles, mumps, and/or rubella immunity or laboratory confirmation of disease, health-care facilities should 1) consider routinely vaccinating personnel with 2 doses of MMR vaccine at the appropriate interval (for measles and mumps) and 1 dose of MMR vaccine (for rubella), and 2) recommend 2 doses of MMR vaccine at the appropriate interval during an outbreak of measles or mumps, and 1 dose during an outbreak of rubella. Complete information about evidence of immunity is available at http://www.cdc.gov/vaccines/recs/provisional/default.htm.

[7]Pneumococcal polysaccharide (PPSV) vaccination.

- Vaccinate all persons with the following indications:
  - *Medical:* Chronic lung disease (including asthma); chronic cardiovascular diseases; diabetes mellitus; chronic liver diseases; cirrhosis; chronic alcoholism; functional or anatomic asplenia (eg, sickle cell disease or splenectomy [if elective splenectomy is planned, vaccinate at least 2 weeks before surgery]); immunocompromising conditions (including chronic renal failure or nephrotic syndrome); and cochlear implants and cerebrospinal fluid leaks. Vaccinate as close to HIV diagnosis as possible.
  - *Other:* Residents of nursing homes or long-term care facilities and persons who smoke cigarettes. Routine use of PPSV is not recommended for American Indians/Alaska Natives or persons aged less than 65 years unless they have underlying medical conditions that are PPSV indications. However, public health authorities may consider recommending PPSV for American Indians/Alaska Natives and persons aged 50-64 years who are living in areas where the risk for invasive pneumococcal disease is increased.

[8]Revaccination with PPSV.

- One-time revaccination after 5 years is recommended for persons aged 19-64 years with chronic renal failure or nephrotic syndrome; functional or anatomic asplenia (eg, sickle cell disease or splenectomy); and for persons with immunocompromising conditions. For persons aged 65 years and older, one-time revaccination is recommended if they were vaccinated 5 or more years previously and were aged less than 65 years at the time of primary vaccination.

[9]Meningococcal vaccination.

- Meningococcal vaccine should be administered to persons with the following indications:
  - *Medical:* A 2-dose series of meningococcal conjugate vaccine is recommended for adults with anatomic or functional asplenia, or persistent complement component deficiencies. Adults with HIV infection who are vaccinated should also receive a routine 2-dose series. The 2 doses should be administered at 0 and 2 months.

- *Other:* A single dose of meningococcal vaccine is recommended for unvaccinated first-year college students living in dormitories; microbiologists routinely exposed to isolates of *Neisseria meningitidis*; military recruits; and persons who travel to or live in countries in which meningococcal disease is hyperendemic or epidemic (eg, the "meningitis belt" of sub-Saharan Africa during the dry season [December through June]), particularly if their contact with local populations will be prolonged. Vaccination is required by the government of Saudi Arabia for all travelers to Mecca during the annual Hajj.

- Meningococcal conjugate vaccine, quadrivalent (MCV4) is preferred for adults with any of the preceding indications who are aged 55 years and younger; meningococcal polysaccharide vaccine (MPSV4) is preferred for adults aged 56 years and older. Revaccination with MCV4 every 5 years is recommended for adults previously vaccinated with MCV4 or MPSV4 who remain at increased risk for infection (eg, adults with anatomic or functional asplenia, or persistent complement component deficiencies).

[10]Hepatitis A vaccination.

- Vaccinate persons with any of the following indications and any person seeking protection from hepatitis A virus (HAV) infection:
  - *Behavioral:* Men who have sex with men and persons who use injection drugs.
  - *Occupational:* Persons working with HAV-infected primates or with HAV in a research laboratory setting.
  - *Medical:* Persons with chronic liver disease and persons who receive clotting factor concentrates.
  - *Other:* Persons traveling to or working in countries that have high or intermediate endemicity of hepatitis A (a list of countries is available at http://wwwn.cdc.gov/travel/contentdiseases.aspx).
- Unvaccinated persons who anticipate close personal contact (eg, household or regular babysitting) with an international adoptee during the first 60 days after arrival in the United States from a country with high or intermediate endemicity should be vaccinated. The first dose of the 2-dose hepatitis A vaccine series should be administered as soon as adoption is planned, ideally 2 or more weeks before the arrival of the adoptee.
- Single-antigen vaccine formulations should be administered in a 2-dose schedule at either 0 and 6–12 months (Havrix®), or 0 and 6–18 months (VAQTA®). If the combined hepatitis A and hepatitis B vaccine (Twinrix®) is used, administer 3 doses at 0, 1, and 6 months; alternatively, a 4-dose schedule may be used, administered on days 0, 7, and 21–30, followed by a booster dose at month 12.

[11]Hepatitis B vaccination.

- Vaccinate persons with any of the following indications and any person seeking protection from hepatitis B virus (HBV) infection:
  - *Behavioral:* Sexually active persons who are not in a long-term, mutually monogamous relationship (eg, persons with more than one sex partner during the previous 6 months); persons seeking evaluation or treatment for a sexually transmitted disease (STD); current or recent injection-drug users; and men who have sex with men.
  - *Occupational:* Health-care personnel and public-safety workers who are exposed to blood or other potentially infectious body fluids.
  - *Medical:* Persons with end-stage renal disease, including patients receiving hemodialysis; persons with HIV infection; and persons with chronic liver disease.
  - *Other:* Household contacts and sex partners of persons with chronic HBV infection; clients and staff members of institutions for persons with developmental disabilities; and international travelers to countries with high or intermediate prevalence of chronic HBV infection (a list of countries is available at http://wwwn.cdc.gov/travel/contentdiseases.aspx).
- Hepatitis B vaccination is recommended for all adults in the following settings: STD treatment facilities; HIV testing and treatment facilities; facilities providing drug-abuse treatment and prevention services; health-care settings targeting services to injection-drug users or men who have sex with men; correctional facilities; end-stage renal disease programs and facilities for chronic hemodialysis patients; and institutions and nonresidential day-care facilities for persons with developmental disabilities.
- Administer missing doses to complete a 3-dose series of hepatitis B vaccine to those persons not vaccinated or not completely vaccinated. The second dose should be administered 1 month after the first dose; the third dose should be given at least 2 months after the second dose (and at least 4 months after the first dose). If the combined hepatitis A and hepatitis B vaccine (Twinrix®) is used, administer 3 doses at 0, 1, and 6 months; alternatively, a 4-dose Twinrix® schedule, administered on days 0, 7, and 21-30, followed by a booster dose at month 12 may be used.
- Adult patients receiving hemodialysis or with other immunocompromising conditions should receive 1 dose of 40 µg/mL (Recombivax HB®) administered on a 3-dose schedule or 2 doses of 20 µg/mL (Engerix-B®) administered simultaneously on a 4-dose schedule at 0, 1, 2, and 6 months.

[12]Selected conditions for which *Haemophilus influenzae* type b (Hib) vaccine may be used.

- 1 dose of Hib vaccine should be considered for persons who have sickle cell disease, leukemia, or HIV infection, or who have had a splenectomy, if they have not previously received Hib vaccine.

[13]Immunocompromising conditions.

- Inactivated vaccines generally are acceptable (eg, pneumococcal, meningococcal, influenza [inactivated influenza vaccine]) and live vaccines generally are avoided in persons with immune deficiencies or immunocompromising conditions. Information on specific conditions is available at http://www.cdc.gov/vaccines/pubs/acip-list.htm.

Reference

"Recommended Adult Immunization Schedule - United States, 2011," *MMWR*, 2011, 60(4):Q1-4.

These schedules indicate the recommended age groups and medical indications for which administration of currently licensed vaccines is commonly indicated for adults ages 19 years and older, as of January 1, 2011. For all vaccines being recommended on the adult immunization schedule: a vaccine series does not need to be restarted, regardless of the time that has elapsed between doses. Licensed combination vaccines may be used whenever any components of the combination are indicated and when the vaccine's other components are not contraindicated. For detailed recommendations on all vaccines, including those used primarily for travelers or that are issued during the year, consult the manufacturers' package inserts and the complete statements from the Advisory Committee on Immunization Practices (http:// www.cdc.gov/vaccines/pubs/acip-list.htm).

Report all clinically significant postvaccination reactions to the Vaccine Adverse Event Reporting System (VAERS). Reporting forms and instructions on filing a VAERS report are available at http://www.vaers.hhs.gov or by telephone, 800-822-7967.

Information on how to file a Vaccine Injury Compensation Program claim is available at http:// www.hrsa.gov/vaccinecompensation or by telephone, 800-338-2382. Information about filing a claim for vaccine injury is available through the U.S. Court of Federal Claims, 717 Madison Place, N.W., Washington, D.C. 20005; telephone, 202-357-6400.

Additional information about the vaccines in this schedule, extent of available data, and contraindications for vaccination also is available at http://www.cdc.gov/vaccines or from the CDC-INFO Contact Center at 800-CDC-INFO (800-232-4636) in English and Spanish, 24 hours a day, 7 days a week.

Use of trade names and commercial sources is for identification only and does not imply endorsement by the U.S. Department of Health and Human Services.

The recommendations in this schedule were approved by ACIP, the American Academy of Family Physicians, the American College of Obstetricians and Gynecologists, and the American College of Physicians.

VACCINE INJURY TABLE

The Vaccine Injury Table makes it easier for some people to get compensation. The table lists and explains injuries/conditions that are presumed to be caused by vaccines. It also lists time periods in which the first symptom of these injuries/conditions must occur after receiving the vaccine. If the first symptom of these injuries/conditions occurs within the listed time periods, it is presumed that the vaccine was the cause of the injury or condition unless another cause is found. For example, if the patient received the tetanus vaccines and had a severe allergic reaction (anaphylaxis) within 4 hours after receiving the vaccine, then it is presumed that the tetanus vaccine caused the injury if no other cause is found.

If the injury/condition is not on the table or if the injury/condition did not occur within the time period on the table, it must be proven that the vaccine caused the injury/condition. Such proof must be based on medical records or opinion, which may include expert witness testimony.

Vaccine Injury Table[1]

Vaccine		Adverse Event	Time Interval
Tetanus toxoid-containing vaccines (eg, DTaP, Tdap, DTP-Hib, DT, Td, TT)	A.	Anaphylaxis or anaphylactic shock	0-4 hours
	B.	Brachial neuritis	2-28 days
	C.	Any acute complication or sequela (including death) of above events	Not applicable
Pertussis antigen-containing vaccines (eg, DTaP, Tdap, DTP, P, DTP-Hib)	A.	Anaphylaxis or anaphylactic shock	0-4 hours
	B.	Encephalopathy (or encephalitis)	0-72 hours
	C.	Any acute complication or sequela (including death) of above events	Not applicable
Measles, mumps, and rubella virus-containing vaccines in any combination (eg, MMR, MR, M, R)	A.	Anaphylaxis or anaphylactic shock	0-4 hours
	B.	Encephalopathy (or encephalitis)	5-15 days
	C.	Any acute complication or sequela (including death) of above events	Not applicable
Rubella virus-containing vaccines (eg, MMR, MR, R)	A.	Chronic arthritis	7-42 days
	B.	Any acute complication or sequela (including death) of above events	Not applicable
Measles virus-containing vaccines (eg, MMR, MR, M)	A.	Thrombocytopenic purpura	7-30 days
	B.	Vaccine-strain measles viral infection in an immunodeficient recipient	0-6 months
	C.	Any acute complication or sequela (including death) of above events	Not applicable

Vaccine Injury Table[1] *(continued)*

Vaccine		Adverse Event	Time Interval
Polio live virus-containing vaccines (OPV)	A.	Paralytic polio	
	•	In a nonimmunodeficient recipient	0-30 days
	•	In an immunodeficient recipient	0-6 months
	•	In a vaccine associated community case	Not applicable
	B.	Vaccine-strain polio viral infection	
	•	In a nonimmunodeficient recipient	0-30 days
	•	In an immunodeficient recipient	0-6 months
	•	In a vaccine associated community case	Not applicable
	C.	Any acute complication or sequela (including death) of above events	Not applicable
Polio inactivated-virus containing vaccines (eg, IPV)	A.	Anaphylaxis or anaphylactic shock	0-4 hours
	B.	Any acute complication or sequela (including death) of above events	Not applicable
Hepatitis B antigen-containing vaccines	A.	Anaphylaxis or anaphylactic shock	0-4 hours
	B.	Any acute complication or sequela (including death) of above events	Not applicable
Hemophilus influenzae (type b polysaccharide conjugate vaccines)	A.	No condition specified for compensation	Not applicable
Varicella vaccine	A.	No condition specified for compensation	Not applicable
Rotavirus vaccine	A.	No condition specified for compensation	Not applicable
Pneumococcal conjugate vaccines	A.	No condition specified for compensation	Not applicable
Any new vaccine recommended by the Centers for Disease Control and Prevention for routine administration to children, after publication by Secretary, HHS of a notice of coverage[2,3]	A.	No condition specified for compensation	Not applicable

[1]Effective date: November 10, 2008.

[2]As of **December 1, 2004**, hepatitis A vaccines have been added to the Vaccine Injury Table under this category. As of **July 1, 2005**, trivalent influenza vaccines have been added to the table under this category. Trivalent influenza vaccines are given annually during the flu season either by needle and syringe or in a nasal spray. All influenza vaccines routinely administered in the U.S. are trivalent vaccines covered under this category. See Federal Register Notice: April 12, 2005.

[3]As of February 1, 2007, meningococcal (conjugate and polysaccharide) and human papillomavirus (HPV) vaccines have been added to the table under this category.

See *News* on the VICP website for more information. Available at: http://www.hrsa.gov/vaccinecompensation.

APOTHECARY / METRIC EQUIVALENTS

Approximate Liquid Measures

Basic equivalent: 1 fluid ounce = 30 mL

Examples:

1 gallon	=	3800 mL	1 gallon	=	128 fluid ounces
1 quart	=	960 mL	1 quart	=	32 fluid ounces
1 pint	=	480 mL	1 pint	=	16 fluid ounces
8 fluid oz	=	240 mL	15 minims	=	1 mL
4 fluid oz	=	120 mL	10 minims	=	0.6 mL

Approximate Household Equivalents

1 teaspoonful	=	5 mL	1 tablespoonful	=	15 mL

Weights

Basic equivalents:

1 oz	=	30 g	15 gr	=	1 g

Examples:

4 oz	=	120 g	1 gr	=	60 mg
2 oz	=	60 g	1/100 gr	=	600 mcg
10 gr	=	600 mg	1/150 gr	=	400 mcg
7 1/2 gr	=	500 mg	1/200 gr	=	300 mcg
16 oz	=	1 lb			

Metric Conversions

Basic equivalents:

1 g	=	1000 mg	1 mg	=	1000 mcg

Examples:

5 g	=	5000 mg	5 mg	=	5000 mcg
0.5 g	=	500 mg	0.5 mg	=	500 mcg
0.05 g	=	50 mg	0.05 mg	=	50 mcg

Exact Equivalents

1 g	=	15.43 gr	0.1 mg	=	1/600 gr
1 mL	=	16.23 minims	0.12 mg	=	1/500 gr
1 minim	=	0.06 mL	0.15 mg	=	1/400 gr
1 gr	=	64.8 mg	0.2 mg	=	1/300 gr
1 pint (pt)	=	473.2 mL	0.3 mg	=	1/200 gr
1 oz	=	28.35 g	0.4 mg	=	1/150 gr
1 lb	=	453.6 g	0.5 mg	=	1/120 gr
1 kg	=	2.2 lb	0.6 mg	=	1/100 gr
1 qt	=	946.4 mL	0.8 mg	=	1/80 gr
			1 mg	=	1/65 gr

Solids[1]

1/4 grain	=	15 mg	1 1/2 grains	=	90 mg
1/2 grain	=	30 mg	5 grains	=	300 mg
1 grain	=	60 mg	10 grains	=	600 mg

[1]Use exact equivalents for compounding and calculations requiring a high degree of accuracy.

AVERAGE WEIGHTS AND SURFACE AREAS

Average Height, Weight, and Surface Area by Age and Gender

Age	Girls			Boys		
	Height (cm)	Weight (kg)	BSA (m^2)	Height (cm)	Weight (kg)	BSA (m^2)
Birth	49.5	3.4	0.22	50	3.6	0.22
3 mo	59	5.6	0.3	61	6	0.32
6 mo	65	7.2	0.36	67	7.9	0.38
9 mo	70	8.3	0.4	72	9.3	0.43
12 mo	74.5	9.5	0.44	75.5	10.3	0.46
15 mo	77	10.3	0.47	79	11.1	0.49
18 mo	80	11	0.49	82	11.7	0.52
21 mo	83	11.6	0.52	85	12.2	0.54
2 y	86	12	0.54	87.5	12.6	0.55
2.5 y	91	13	0.57	92	13.5	0.59
3 y	94.5	13.8	0.6	96	14.3	0.62
3.5 y	97	15	0.64	98	15	0.64
4 y	101	16	0.67	102	16	0.67
4.5 y	104	17	0.7	105	17	0.7
5 y	107.5	18	0.73	109	18.5	0.75
6 y	115	20	0.80	115	21	0.82
7 y	121.5	23	0.88	122	23	0.88
8 y	127.5	25.5	0.95	127.5	26	0.96
9 y	133	29	1.04	133.5	28.5	1.03
10 y	138	33	1.12	138.5	32	1.1
11 y	144	37	1.22	143.5	36	1.2
12 y	151	41.5	1.32	149	40.5	1.29
13 y	157	46	1.42	156	45.5	1.4
14 y	160.5	49.5	1.49	163.5	51	1.52
15 y	162	52	1.53	170	56	1.63
16 y	162.5	54	1.56	173.5	61	1.71
17 y	163	55	1.58	175	64.5	1.77
Adult[1]	163.5	58	1.62	177	83.5	2.03

Data extracted from the CDC growth charts based on the 50th percentile height and weight for a given age.[2]

Body surfaced area calculation[3]: Square root of [(Ht x Wt) / 3600]

[1]McDowell MA, Fryar CD, Hirsch R, et al, "Anthropometric Reference Data for Children and Adults: U.S. Population, 1999-2002," *Adv Data*, 2005, (361):1-5.

[2]Centers for Disease Control and Prevention, "2000 CDC Growth Charts: United States," Available at: http://www.cdc.gov/growthcharts/. Accessed November 16, 2007.

[3]Mosteller RD, "Simplified Calculation of Body-Surface Area," *N Engl J Med*, 1987, 317(17):1098.

BODY SURFACE AREA OF ADULTS AND CHILDREN

Calculating Body Surface Area in Children

In a child of average size, find weight and corresponding surface area on the boxed scale to the left; or, use the nomogram to the right. Lay a straightedge on the correct height and weight points for the child, then read the intersecting point on the surface area scale.

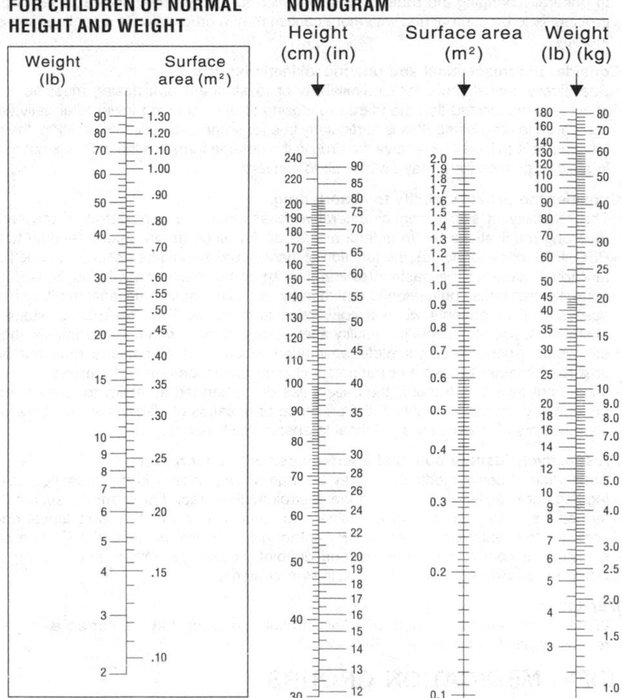

BODY SURFACE AREA FORMULA (Adult and Pediatric)

$$\text{BSA (m}^2) = \sqrt{\frac{\text{Ht (in)} \times \text{Wt (lb)}}{3131}} \quad \text{or, in metric: BSA (m}^2) = \sqrt{\frac{\text{Ht (cm)} \times \text{Wt (kg)}}{3600}}$$

References

Lam TK and Leung DT, "More on Simplified Calculation of Body Surface Area," *N Engl J Med*, 1988, 318(17):1130 (Letter).

Mosteller RD, "Simplified Calculation of Body Surface Area", *N Engl J Med*, 1987, 317(17):1098 (Letter).

IDEAL BODY WEIGHT CALCULATION

Adults (18 years and older) (IBW is in kg)

IBW (male) = 50 + (2.3 x height in inches over 5 feet)

IBW (female) = 45.5 + (2.3 x height in inches over 5 feet)

Children (IBW is in kg; height is in cm)

a. 1-18 years

IBW = ((height)^2 x 1.65) / 1000

b. 5 feet and taller

IBW (male) = 39 + (2.27 x height in inches over 5 feet)

IBW (female) = 42.2 + (2.27 x height in inches over 5 feet)

I.V. TO ORAL CONVERSION

1. **Consider drug class and indication. Conversion is acceptable only if the risk and benefit evaluation justifies conversion. Conversion should never be made only because of drug costs. The cost of failed therapy is much higher.**

   Assuming access is available, intravenous dosing rapidly produces effective serum concentrations, suitable when this benefit outweighs the risk of venous irritation/trauma, infection, and cost. Conversion from I.V. to oral is often dependent on the patient's specific clinical situation. As the clinical situation improves, oral administration may be acceptable. In general, changing the route of administration for a drug treating the patient's primary problem is to be approached with more caution than a drug which is a continuation of prior therapy.

2. **Consider pharmaceutical and pharmacokinetic issues.**
   Specifically, adjustments for bioavailability or to standard oral dosing must be made. It should be recognized that standard oral dosing is often a much lower total daily dose as compared to oral dosing (this is particularly true for some antibiotics. In addition, the patient must be able to ingest or receive the drug in the dosage form available. Drugs not available in a liquid dosage form may be difficult to convert.

3. **Consider the patient's ability to absorb drug.**
   The reliability of swallowing or enteral access should be considered. If the patient is receiving medications by an enteral access device such as an enteral feeding tube (eg, PEG, PEJ, or nasogastric), the function of these tubes should be assured. In addition, the functional status of the gastrointestinal tract must be evaluated. Obviously, NPO status normally precludes conversion to oral therapy. However, gastrointestinal motility should be assessed in all patients when a conversion is planned. The presence or suspicion of obstruction, use of multiple promotility agents, or problems with nausea/emesis should be assessed. Agents with complete absorption in ambulatory patients may not be well absorbed in acute illness. For patients receiving continuous enteral feedings, conversion should not be attempted until the patient has demonstrated an ability to tolerate feedings up to their goal rate. In addition, the presence or absence of diarrhea should be assessed as indicators of the patient's potential to absorb medications.

4. **Prospectively identify potential interferences with absorption.**
   Absorption of some medications may be dramatically altered in the presence of enteral feedings or specific electrolytes in the gastrointestinal tract. For example, sucralfate may reduce the absorption of fluoroquinolones to ineffective levels. In this instance, one may consider the replacement with an H_2 antagonist to eliminate potential interferences or selection of comparable nonquinolone antibiotic coverage. Other drug binding agents include bile acid sequestrants and activated charcoal.

5. **Monitoring**
   With any change in the route of administration, consider that a recurrence may require reconsideration of the route.

SPECIFIC MEDICATION GROUPS

Antibiotics

May be readily converted to oral therapy in most situations. Most institutions encourage evaluation of an initial response (3- to 5-day period) prior to oral therapy. In most cases, a lack of clinical improvement over the evaluation period or a recent change in the status should delay prompting to oral therapy.

I.V. Agent	Usual I.V. Dose	Oral Agent (if different)	Common Oral Dose
Ampicillin	1 g q6h	Amoxicillin	500 mg q6h[1]
Ampicillin/ sulbactam	1.5-3 g q6h	Amoxicillin/ clavulanate	500 mg q8h or 875 mg q12h
Azithromycin	500 mg qd		250 mg qd
Cefazolin	1 g q8h	Cephalexin	500 mg q6h
Cefuroxime	750 mg q8h	Cefuroxime axetil	250-500 mg q12h[1,2]
Ciprofloxacin	400-600 mg q12h		500-750 mg q12h
Clindamycin	300-600 mg q8h		300-450 mg orally q6h
Co-trimoxazole	7.5-20 mg/kg		Equivalent # tablets (divide q6h or q12h)
Doxycycline	100 mg q12h		100 mg q12h
Erythromycin	500-1000 mg q6h		500 mg q6h
Fluconazole	100 mg qd		100 mg qd
Gatifloxacin	200-400 mg q24h		200-400 mg q24h

(continued)

I.V. Agent	Usual I.V. Dose	Oral Agent (if different)	Common Oral Dose
Levofloxacin	500 mg q24h		500 mg q24h
Metronidazole	500 mg q8-12h		500 mg q8h or 250 mg q6h
Ofloxacin	200-400 mg q12h		200-400 mg q12h
Trovafloxacin	100-200 mg qd		100-200 mg qd

[1]Oral dose represents dose reduction.

[2]Poor oral absorption.

Others

- H_2 antagonists – generally converted 1:1 to equivalent dose and scheduled orally.
- Methylprednisolone – may be converted to oral prednisone (each 4 mg methylprednisolone = 5 mg prednisone).
- Aminophylline – must be calculated based on infusion rate. However, a simple conversion calculation is possible: Dose in mg/h x 10 = dose of sustained release product to be given every 12 hours (ie, a typical infusion of 30 mg/h = 300 mg of sustained release theophylline q12h or 150 mg q6h of nonsustained release product.

PEAK AND TROUGH GUIDELINES

Drug	When to Sample	Therapeutic Levels*	Usual Half-Life	Steady State (Ideal Sampling Time)	Potentially Toxic Levels*
Antibiotics					
Gentamicin Tobramycin	30 min after 30 min infusion Trough: <0.5 h before next dose	Peak: 4-10 mcg/mL Trough: <2.0 mcg/mL	2 h	15 h	Peak: >12 mcg/mL Trough: >2 mcg/mL
Amikacin		Peak: 20-35 mcg/mL Trough: <8 mcg/mL			Peak: >35 mcg/mL Trough: >8 mcg/mL
Vancomycin	Peak: 1 h after 1 h infusion Trough: <0.5 h before next dose	Peak: 30-40 mcg/mL Trough: ≥10-20 mcg/mL depending upon severity/type of infection	6-8 h	24 h	Peak: >80 mcg/mL
Anticonvulsants					
Carbamazepine	Trough: Just before next oral dose In combination with other anticonvulsants	4-12 mcg/mL 4-8 mcg/mL	15-20 h	7-12 d	>12 mcg/mL
Ethosuximide	Trough: Just before next oral dose	40-100 mcg/mL	30-60 h	10-13 d	>100 mcg/mL
Phenobarbital	Trough: Just before next dose	15-40 mcg/mL	40-120 h	20 d	>40 mcg/mL
Phenytoin Free phenytoin	Trough: Just before next dose Draw at same time as total level.	10-20 mcg/mL 1-2 mcg/mL	Concentration dependent	5-14 d	>20 mcg/mL
Primidone	Trough: Just before next dose (**Note:** Primidone is metabolized to phenobarb, order levels separately.)	5-12 mcg/mL	10-12 h	5 d	>12 mcg/mL
Valproic acid	Trough: Just before next dose	Seizures: 50-100 mcg/mL Mania: 85-125 mcg/mL	5-20 h	4 d	>150 mcg/mL
Bronchodilators					
Aminophylline (I.V.)	18-24 h after starting or changing a maintenance dose; given as a constant infusion	5-15 mcg/mL	Nonsmoking adult: 8 h Children and smoking adults: 4 h	2 d	>20 mcg/mL
Theophylline (P.O.)	Peak levels: Not recommended Trough level: Just before next dose				

Drug	When to Sample	Therapeutic Levels*	Usual Half-Life	Steady State (Ideal Sampling Time)	Potentially Toxic Levels*
Cardiovascular Agents					
Digoxin	Trough: Just before next dose (levels drawn earlier than 6 h after a dose will be artificially elevated)	0.5-2 ng/mL	36 h	5 d	>2 ng/mL
Lidocaine	Steady-state levels are usually achieved after 6-12 h	1.2-5.0 mcg/mL	1.5 h	5-10 h	>6 mcg/mL
Procainamide	Trough: Just before next oral dose I.V.: 6-12 h after infusion started Combined procainamide plus NAPA	4-10 mcg/mL NAPA: 6-10 h 5-30 mcg/mL	Procain: 2.7-5 h >30 (NAPA + procain)	20 h	>10 mcg/mL
Quinidine	Trough: Just before next oral dose	2-5 mcg/mL	6 h	24 h	>10 mcg/mL
Warfarin	Same time of day each draw	See Warfarin monograph.	42 h	5-7 d	See Warfarin monograph.
Other Agents					
Amitriptyline plus nortriptyline	Trough: Just before next dose	120-250 ng/mL		4-80 d	
Cyclosporine		Months post-transplant: Plasma: 50-150 ng/mL Whole blood: 150-450 ng/mL		Variable	
Desipramine		50-300 ng/mL	12-54 h	3-11 d	
Imipramine plus desipramine		150-300 ng/mL	9-24 h	2-5 d	
Lithium		0.6-1.2 mEq/mL (acute)	18-20 h	2-7 d	>1.5 mEq/mL
Nortriptyline		50-140 ng/mL		4-19 d	

*Due to methodology differences, reference ranges may vary from laboratory to laboratory; check with the laboratory service used for their appropriate levels.

POUNDS / KILOGRAMS CONVERSION

1 pound = 0.45359 kilograms
1 kilogram = 2.2 pounds

lb	=	kg	lb	=	kg	lb	=	kg
1		0.45	70		31.75	140		63.50
5		2.27	75		34.02	145		65.77
10		4.54	80		36.29	150		68.04
15		6.80	85		38.56	155		70.31
20		9.07	90		40.82	160		72.58
25		11.34	95		43.09	165		74.84
30		13.61	100		45.36	170		77.11
35		15.88	105		47.63	175		79.38
40		18.14	110		49.90	180		81.65
45		20.41	115		52.16	185		83.92
50		22.68	120		54.43	190		86.18
55		24.95	125		56.70	195		88.45
60		27.22	130		58.91	200		90.72
65		29.48	135		61.24			

TEMPERATURE CONVERSION

Celsius to Fahrenheit = (°C x 9/5) + 32 = °F
Fahrenheit to Celsius = (°F - 32) x 5/9 = °C

°C	=	°F	°C	=	°F	°C	=	°F
100.0		212.0	39.0		102.2	36.8		98.2
50.0		122.0	38.8		101.8	36.6		97.9
41.0		105.8	38.6		101.5	36.4		97.5
40.8		105.4	38.4		101.1	36.2		97.2
40.6		105.1	38.2		100.8	36.0		96.8
40.4		104.7	38.0		100.4	35.8		96.4
40.2		104.4	37.8		100.1	35.6		96.1
40.0		104.0	37.6		99.7	35.4		95.7
39.8		103.6	37.4		99.3	35.2		95.4
39.6		103.3	37.2		99.0	35.0		95.0
39.4		102.9	37.0		98.6	0		32.0
39.2		102.6						

REFERENCE VALUES FOR CHILDREN

CHEMISTRY		Normal Values
Albumin	0-1 y	2-4 g/dL
	1 y to adult	3.5-5.5 g/dL
Ammonia	Newborns	90-150 mcg/dL
	Children	40-120 mcg/dL
	Adults	18-54 mcg/dL
Amylase	Newborns	0-60 units/L
	Adults	30-110 units/L
Bilirubin, conjugated, direct	Newborns	<1.5 mg/dL
	1 mo to adult	0-0.5 mg/dL
Bilirubin, total	0-3 d	2-10 mg/dL
	1 mo to adult	0-1.5 mg/dL
Bilirubin, unconjugated, indirect		0.6-10.5 mg/dL
Calcium	Newborns	7-12 mg/dL
	0-2 y	8.8-11.2 mg/dL
	2 y to adult	9-11 mg/dL
Calcium, ionized, whole blood		4.4-5.4 mg/dL
Carbon dioxide, total		23-33 mEq/L
Chloride		95-105 mEq/L
Cholesterol	Newborns	45-170 mg/dL
	0-1 y	65-175 mg/dL
	1-20 y	120-230 mg/dL
Creatinine	0-1 y	≤0.6 mg/dL
	1 y to adult	0.5-1.5 mg/dL
Glucose	Newborns	30-90 mg/dL
	0-2 y	60-105 mg/dL
	Children to Adults	70-110 mg/dL
Iron		
	Newborns	110-270 mcg/dL
	Infants	30-70 mcg/dL
	Children	55-120 mcg/dL
	Adults	70-180 mcg/dL
Iron binding	Newborns	59-175 mcg/dL
	Infants	100-400 mcg/dL
	Adults	250-400 mcg/dL
Lactic acid, lactate		2-20 mg/dL
Lead, whole blood		<10 mcg/dL
Lipase		
	Children	20-140 units/L
	Adults	0-190 units/L
Magnesium		1.5-2.5 mEq/L
Osmolality, serum		275-296 mOsm/kg
Osmolality, urine		50-1400 mOsm/kg
Phosphorus	Newborns	4.2-9 mg/dL
	6 wk to 19 mo	3.8-6.7 mg/dL
	19 mo to 3 y	2.9-5.9 mg/dL
	3-15 y	3.6-5.6 mg/dL

CHEMISTRY (continued)		Normal Values
	>15 y	2.5-5 mg/dL
Potassium, plasma	Newborns	4.5-7.2 mEq/L
	2 d to 3 mo	4-6.2 mEq/L
	3 mo to 1 y	3.7-5.6 mEq/L
	1-16 y	3.5-5 mEq/L
Protein, total	0-2 y	4.2-7.4 g/dL
	>2 y	6-8 g/dL
Sodium		136-145 mEq/L
Triglycerides	Infants	0-171 mg/dL
	Children	20-130 mg/dL
	Adults	30-200 mg/dL
Urea nitrogen, blood	0-2 y	4-15 mg/dL
	2 y to Adult	5-20 mg/dL
Uric acid	Male	3-7 mg/dL
	Female	2-6 mg/dL
ENZYMES		
Alanine aminotransferase (ALT)	0-2 mo	8-78 units/L
	>2 mo	8-36 units/L
Alkaline phosphatase (ALKP)	Newborns	60-130 units/L
	0-16 y	85-400 units/L
	>16 y	30-115 units/L
Aspartate aminotransferase (AST)	Infants	18-74 units/L
	Children	15-46 units/L
	Adults	5-35 units/L
Creatine kinase (CK)	Infants	20-200 units/L
	Children	10-90 units/L
	Adult male	0-206 units/L
	Adult female	0-175 units/L
Lactate dehydrogenase (LDH)	Newborns	290-501 units/L
	1 mo to 2 y	110-144 units/L
	>16 y	60-170 units/L

Blood Gases

	Arterial	Capillary	Venous
pH	7.35-7.45	7.35-7.45	7.32-7.42
pCO_2 (mm Hg)	35-45	35-45	38-52
pO_2 (mm Hg)	70-100	60-80	24-48
HCO_3 (mEq/L)	19-25	19-25	19-25
TCO_2 (mEq/L)	19-29	19-29	23-33
O_2 saturation (%)	90-95	90-95	40-70
Base excess (mEq/L)	-5 to +5	-5 to +5	-5 to +5

Thyroid Function Tests

T_4 (thyroxine)	1-7 d	10.1-20.9 mcg/dL
	8-14 d	9.8-16.6 mcg/dL
	1 mo to 1 y	5.5-16 mcg/dL
	>1 y	4-12 mcg/dL
FTI	1-3 d	9.3-26.6
	1-4 wk	7.6-20.8
	1-4 mo	7.4-17.9
	4-12 mo	5.1-14.5
	1-6 y	5.7-13.3
	>6 y	4.8-14
T_3 by RIA	Newborns	100-470 ng/dL
	1-5 y	100-260 ng/dL
	5-10 y	90-240 ng/dL
	10 y to Adult	70-210 ng/dL
T_3 uptake		35%-45%
TSH	Cord	3-22 μIU/mL
	1-3 d	<40 μIU/mL
	3-7 d	<25 μIU/mL
	>7 d	0-10 μIU/mL

REFERENCE VALUES FOR ADULTS

CHEMISTRY

Test	Values	Remarks
Serum / Plasma		
Acetone	Negative	
Albumin	3.2-5 g/dL	
Alcohol, ethyl	Negative	
Aldolase	1.2-7.6 IU/L	
Ammonia	20-70 mcg/dL	Specimen to be placed on ice as soon as collected.
Amylase	30-110 units/L	
Bilirubin, direct	0-0.3 mg/dL	
Bilirubin, total	0.1-1.2 mg/dL	
Calcium	8.6-10.3 mg/dL	
Calcium, ionized	2.24-2.46 mEq/L	
Chloride	95-108 mEq/L	
Cholesterol, total	≤200 mg/dL	Fasted blood required – normal value affected by dietary habits. This reference range is for a general adult population.
HDL cholesterol	40-60 mg/dL	Fasted blood required – normal value affected by dietary habits.
LDL cholesterol	<160 mg/dL	If triglyceride is >400 mg/dL, LDL cannot be calculated accurately (Friedewald equation). Target LDL-C depends on patient's risk factors.
CO_2	23-30 mEq/L	
Creatine kinase (CK) isoenzymes		
CK-BB	0%	
CK-MB (cardiac)	0%-3.9%	
CK-MM (muscle)	96%-100%	
CK-MB levels must be both ≥4% and 10 IU/L to meet diagnostic criteria for CK-MB positive result consistent with myocardial injury.		
Creatine phosphokinase (CPK)	8-150 IU/L	
Creatinine	0.5-1.4 mg/dL	
Ferritin	13-300 ng/mL	
Folate	3.6-20 ng/dL	
GGT (gamma-glutamyltranspeptidase)		
male	11-63 IU/L	
female	8-35 IU/L	
GLDH	To be determined	
Glucose (preprandial)	<115 mg/dL	Goals different for diabetics.
Glucose, fasting	60-110 mg/dL	Goals different for diabetics.
Glucose, nonfasting (2-h postprandial)	<120 mg/dL	Goals different for diabetics.
Hemoglobin A_{1c}	<8	
Hemoglobin, plasma free	<2.5 mg/100 mL	
Hemoglobin, total glycosolated (Hb A_1)	4%-8%	
Iron	65-150 mcg/dL	
Iron binding capacity, total (TIBC)	250-420 mcg/dL	
Lactic acid	0.7-2.1 mEq/L	Specimen to be kept on ice and sent to lab as soon as possible.
Lactate dehydrogenase (LDH)	56-194 IU/L	

CHEMISTRY *(continued)*

Test	Values	Remarks
Lactate dehydrogenase (LDH) isoenzymes		
LD_1	20%-34%	
LD_2	29%-41%	
LD_3	15%-25%	
LD_4	1%-12%	
LD_5	1%-15%	
Flipped LD_1/LD_2 ratios (>1 may be consistent with myocardial injury) particularly when considered in combination with a recent CK-MB positive result.		
Lipase	23-208 units/L	
Magnesium	1.6-2.5 mg/dL	Increased by slight hemolysis.
Osmolality	289-308 mOsm/kg	
Phosphatase, alkaline		
adults 25-60 y	33-131 IU/L	
adults ≥61 y	51-153 IU/L	
infancy-adolescence	Values range up to 3-5 times higher than adults	
Phosphate, inorganic	2.8-4.2 mg/dL	
Potassium	3.5-5.2 mEq/L	Increased by slight hemolysis.
Prealbumin	>15 mg/dL	
Protein, total	6.5-7.9 g/dL	
AST	<35 IU/L (20-48)	
ALT (10-35)	<35 IU/L	
Sodium	134-149 mEq/L	
Thyroid stimulating hormone (TSH)		
adults ≤20 y	0.7-6.4 mIU/L	
21-54 y	0.4-4.2 mIU/L	
55-87 y	0.5-8.9 mIU/L	
Transferrin	>200 mg/dL	
Triglycerides	45-155 mg/dL	Fasted blood required.
Troponin I	<1.5 ng/mL	
Urea nitrogen (BUN)	7-20 mg/dL	
Uric acid		
male	2-8 mg/dL	
female	2-7.5 mg/dL	
Cerebrospinal Fluid		
Glucose	50-70 mg/dL	
Protein	15-45 mg/dL	CSF obtained by lumbar puncture.
Note: Bloody specimen gives erroneously high value due to contamination with blood proteins		
Urine (24-hour specimen is required for all these tests unless specified)		
Amylase	32-641 units/L	The value is in units/L and **not** calculated for total volume.
Amylase, fluid (random samples)		Interpretation of value left for physician, depends on the nature of fluid.
Calcium	Depends upon dietary intake	
Creatine		
male	150 mg/24 h	Higher value on children and during pregnancy.
female	250 mg/24 h	
Creatinine	1000-2000 mg/24 h	

CHEMISTRY *(continued)*

Test	Values	Remarks
Creatinine clearance (endogenous)		
male	85-125 mL/min	A blood sample must accompany urine specimen.
female	75-115 mL/min	
Glucose	1 g/24 h	
5-hydroxyindoleacetic acid	2-8 mg/24 h	
Iron	0.15 mg/24 h	Acid washed container required.
Magnesium	146-209 mg/24 h	
Osmolality	500-800 mOsm/kg	With normal fluid intake.
Oxalate	10-40 mg/24 h	
Phosphate	400-1300 mg/24 h	
Potassium	25-120 mEq/24 h	Varies with diet; the interpretation of urine electrolytes and osmolality should be left for the physician.
Sodium	40-220 mEq/24 h	
Porphobilinogen, qualitative	Negative	
Porphyrins, qualitative	Negative	
Proteins	0.05-0.1 g/24 h	
Salicylate	Negative	
Urea clearance	60-95 mL/min	A blood sample must accompany specimen.
Urea N	10-40 g/24 h	Dependent on protein intake.
Uric acid	250-750 mg/24 h	Dependent on diet and therapy.
Urobilinogen	0.5-3.5 mg/24 h	For qualitative determination on random urine, send sample to urinalysis section in Hematology Lab.
Xylose absorption test		
children	16%-33% of ingested xylose	
Feces		
Fat, 3-day collection	<5 g/d	Value depends on fat intake of 100 g/d for 3 days preceding and during collection.
Gastric Acidity		
Acidity, total, 12 h	10-60 mEq/L	Titrated at pH 7.

Blood Gases

	Arterial	Capillary	Venous
pH	7.35-7.45	7.35-7.45	7.32-7.42
pCO_2 (mm Hg)	35-45	35-45	38-52
pO_2 (mm Hg)	70-100	60-80	24-48
HCO_3 (mEq/L)	19-25	19-25	19-25
TCO_2 (mEq/L)	19-29	19-29	23-33
O_2 saturation (%)	90-95	90-95	40-70
Base excess (mEq/L)	-5 to +5	-5 to +5	-5 to +5

HEMATOLOGY

Complete Blood Count

Age	Hgb (g/dL)	Hct (%)	RBC (mill/mm^3)	RDW
0-3 d	15.0-20.0	45-61	4.0-5.9	<18
1-2 wk	12.5-18.5	39-57	3.6-5.5	<17
1-6 mo	10.0-13.0	29-42	3.1-4.3	<16.5
7 mo to 2 y	10.5-13.0	33-38	3.7-4.9	<16
2-5 y	11.5-13.0	34-39	3.9-5.0	<15
5-8 y	11.5-14.5	35-42	4.0-4.9	<15
13-18 y	12.0-15.2	36-47	4.5-5.1	<14.5
Adult male	13.5-16.5	41-50	4.5-5.5	<14.5
Adult female	12.0-15.0	36-44	4.0-4.9	<14.5

Age	MCV (fL)	MCH (pg)	MCHC (%)	Plts (x 10^3/mm^3)
0-3 d	95-115	31-37	29-37	250-450
1-2 wk	86-110	28-36	28-38	250-450
1-6 mo	74-96	25-35	30-36	300-700
7 mo to 2 y	70-84	23-30	31-37	250-600
2-5 y	75-87	24-30	31-37	250-550
5-8 y	77-95	25-33	31-37	250-550
13-18 y	78-96	25-35	31-37	150-450
Adult male	80-100	26-34	31-37	150-450
Adult female	80-100	26-34	31-37	150-450

WBC and Differential

Age	WBC (x 10^3/mm^3)	Segs	Bands	Lymphs	Monos
0-3 d	9.0-35.0	32-62	<18	19-29	5-7
1-2 wk	5.0-20.0	14-34	<14	36-45	6-10
1-6 mo	6.0-17.5	13-33	<12	41-71	4-7
7 mo to 2 y	6.0-17.0	15-35	<11	45-76	3-6
2-5 y	5.5-15.5	23-45	<11	35-65	3-6
5-8 y	5.0-14.5	32-54	<11	28-48	3-6
13-18 y	4.5-13.0	34-64	<11	25-45	3-6
Adults	4.5-11.0	35-66	<11	24-44	3-6

Age	Eosinophils	Basophils	Atypical Lymphs	No. of NRBCs
0-3 d	0-2	0-1	0-8	0-2
1-2 wk	0-2	0-1	0-8	0
1-6 mo	0-3	0-1	0-8	0
7 mo to 2 y	0-3	0-1	0-8	0
2-5 y	0-3	0-1	0-8	0
5-8 y	0-3	0-1	0-8	0
13-18 y	0-3	0-1	0-8	0
Adults	0-3	0-1	0-8	0

Segs = segmented neutrophils.

Bands = band neutrophils.

Lymphs = lymphocytes.

Monos = monocytes.

Erythrocyte Sedimentation Rates and Reticulocyte Counts

Sedimentation rate, Westergren	Children	0-20 mm/h
	Adult male	0-15 mm/h
	Adult female	0-20 mm/h
Sedimentation rate, Wintrobe	Children	0-13 mm/h
	Adult male	0-10 mm/h
	Adult female	0-15 mm/h
Reticulocyte count	Newborns	2%-6%
	1-6 mo	0%-2.8%
	Adults	0.5%-1.5%

RENAL FUNCTION ESTIMATION IN ADULT PATIENTS

Evaluation of a patient's renal function often includes the use of equations to estimate glomerular filtration rate (GFR) (eg, estimated GFR [eGFR] creatinine clearance [Cl_{Cr}]) using an endogenous filtration marker (eg, serum creatinine) and other patient variables. For example, the Cockcroft-Gault equation estimates renal function by calculating Cl_{Cr} and is typically used to steer medication dosing. Equations which calculate eGFR are primarily used to categorize chronic kidney disease (CKD) staging. The rate of creatinine clearance does not always accurately represent GFR; creatinine may be cleared by other renal mechanisms in addition to glomerular filtration and serum creatinine concentrations may be affected by non-renal factors (eg, age, gender, race, body habitus, illness, diet). In addition, these equations were developed based on studies in limited populations and may either over- or underestimate the renal function of a specific patient.

Nevertheless, most clinicians estimate renal function using Cl_{Cr} as an indicator of actual renal function for the purpose of adjusting medication doses. Utilization of eGFR for renal medication dosing may overestimate renal function by up to 40% which may result in supratherapeutic medication doses (Hermsen, 2009). These equations should only be used in the clinical context of patient-specific factors noted during the physical exam/work-up. Decisions regarding drug therapy and doses must be made on clinical judgment.

RENAL FUNCTION ESTIMATION EQUATIONS

Commonly used equations include the Cockcroft-Gault, Jelliffe, four-variable Modification of Diet in Renal Disease (MDRD), and six-variable MDRD (aka, MDRD extended). All of these equations were originally developed using a serum creatinine assay measured by the alkaline picrate-based (Jaffe) method. Many substances, including proteins, can interfere with the accuracy of this assay and overestimate serum creatinine concentration. The National Kidney Foundation and The National Kidney Disease Education Program (NDKEP) advocate for a universal creatinine assay, in order to ensure an accurate estimate of renal function in patients. As a result, a more specific enzymatic assay with an isotope dilution mass spectrometry (IDMS)-traceable international standard has been developed. Compared to the older methods, IDMS-traceable assays may report lower serum creatinine values and may, therefore, overestimate renal function when used in the original equations (eg, Cockcroft-Gault, Jelliffe, original MDRD). Updated four-variable MDRD and six-variable MDRD equations based on serum creatinine measured by the IDMS-traceable method has been proposed for adults (Levey, 2006); the Cockcroft-Gault and Jelliffe equations have not been re-expressed and may overestimate renal function when used with a serum creatinine measured by the IDMS-traceable method. Clinicians should be aware of the serum creatinine assay used by their institution and the ramifications the assay may have on the equations used for renal function estimation.

Regardless of the serum creatinine assay used, the following factors may contribute to an inaccurate estimation of renal function (Stevens, 2006):

- Increased creatinine generation (may underestimate renal function):
  - Black or African American patients
  - Muscular body habitus
  - Ingestion of cooked meats
- Decreased creatinine generation (may overestimate renal function):
  - Increased age
  - Female patients
  - Hispanic patients
  - Asian patients
  - Amputees
  - Malnutrition, inflammation, or deconditioning (eg, cancer, severe cardiovascular disease, hospitalized patients)
  - Neuromuscular disease
  - Vegetarian diet
- Rapidly changing serum creatinine (either up or down): In patients with rapidly rising serum creatinines (ie, increasing by >0.5-0.7 mg/dL/day), it is best to assume that the patient's renal function is severely impaired

Use extreme caution when estimating renal function in the following patient populations:

- Low body weight (actual body weight < ideal body weight)
- Liver transplant
- Elderly (>90 years old)
- Dehydration
- Recent kidney transplantation (serum creatinine values may decrease rapidly and can lead to renal function underestimation; conversely, delayed graft function may be present)

Note: In most situations, the use of the patient's ideal body weight (IBW) is recommended for estimating renal function, except when the patient's actual body weight (ABW) is less than ideal. Use of actual body weight (ABW) in obese patients (and possibly patients with ascites) may significantly overestimate renal function. Some clinicians prefer to use an adjusted body weight in such cases [eg, IBW + 0.4 (ABW - IBW)]; the adjustment factor may vary based on practitioner and/or institutional preference.

Alkaline picrate-based (Jaffe) methods

Note: These equations have not been updated for use with serum creatinine methods traceable to IDMS. Use with IDMS-traceable serum creatinine methods may overestimate renal function; use with caution.

Method 1: MDRD equation:

$eGFR = 186 \times (Creatinine)^{-1.545} \times (Age)^{-0.203} \times (Gender) \times (Race)$
where:
eGFR = estimated GFR; calculated in mL/minute/1.73 m^2
Creatinine is input in mg/dL
Age is input in years
Gender: Females: Gender = 0.762; Males: Gender = 1
Race: Black: Race = 1.18; White or other: Race = 1

Method 2: MDRD Extended equation:

$eGFR = 170 \times (Creatinine)^{-0.999} \times (Age)^{-0.176} \times (SUN)^{-0.170} \times (Albumin)^{0.318} \times (Gender) \times (Race)$
where:
eGFR = estimated GFR; calculated in mL/minute/1.73 m^2
Creatinine is input in mg/dL
Age is input in years
SUN = Serum Urea Nitrogen; input in mg/dL
Albumin = Serum Albumin; input in g/dL
Gender: Females: Gender = 0.762; Males: Gender = 1
Race: Black: Race = 1.18; White or other: Race = 1

Method 3: Cockroft-Gault equation[1]

Males: $Cl_{Cr} = [(140 - Age) \times Weight] / (72 \times Creatinine)$
Females: $Cl_{Cr} = \{[(140 - Age) \times Weight] / (72 \times Creatinine)\} \times 0.85$
where:
Cl_{Cr} = creatinine clearance; calculated in mL/minute
Age is input in years
Weight is input in kg
Creatinine is input in mg/dL

Method 4: Jelliffe equation

Males: $Cl_{Cr} = \{98 - [0.8 \times (Age - 20)]\} / (Creatinine)$
Females: Cl_{Cr} = Use above equation, then multiply result by 0.9
where:
Cl_{Cr} = creatinine clearance; calculated in mL/minute/1.73m^2
Age is input in years
Creatinine is input in mg/dL

IDMS-traceable methods

Method 1: MDRD equation[2]:

$eGFR = 175 \times (Creatinine)^{-1.154} \times (Age)^{-0.203} \times (Gender) \times (Race)$
where:
eGFR = estimated GFR; calculated in mL/minute/1.73 m^2
Creatinine is input in mg/dL
Age is input in years
Gender: Females: Gender = 0.762; Males: Gender = 1
Race: Black: Race = 1.18; White or other: Race = 1

Method 2: MDRD Extended equation:

$eGFR = 161.5 \times (Creatinine)^{-0.999} \times (Age)^{-0.176} \times (SUN)^{-0.170} \times (Albumin)^{0.318} \times (Gender) \times (Race)$
where:
eGFR = estimated GFR; calculated in mL/minute/1.73 m^2
Creatinine is input in mg/dL
Age is input in years
SUN = Serum Urea Nitrogen; input in mg/dL
Albumin = Serum Albumin; input in g/dL
Gender: Females: Gender = 0.762; Males: Gender = 1
Race: Black: Race = 1.18; White or other: Race = 1

FOOTNOTES

[1]Equation typically used for adjusting medication doses
[2]Preferred equation for CKD staging National Kidney Disease Foundation Program

REFERENCES

Cockcroft DW and Gault MH, "Prediction of Creatinine Clearance From Serum Creatinine," *Nephron*, 1976, 16(1):31-41.

Dowling TC, Matzke GR, Murphy JE, et al, "Evaluation of Renal Drug Dosing: Prescribing Information and Clinical Pharmacist Approaches," *Pharmacotherapy*, 2010, 30(8):776-86.

Hermsen ED, Maiefski M, Florescu MC, et al, "Comparison of the Modification of Diet in Renal Disease and Cockcroft-Gault Equations for Dosing Antimicrobials," *Pharmacotherapy*, 2009, 29(6):649-55.

Jelliffe RW, "Letter: Creatinine Clearance: Bedside Estimate," *Ann Intern Med*, 1973, 79(4):604-5.

Levey AS, Bosch JP, Lewis JB, et al, "A More Accurate Method to Estimate Glomerular Filtration Rate From Serum Creatinine: A New Prediction Equation. Modification of Diet in Renal Disease Study Group," *Ann Intern Med*, 1999, 16;130(6):461–70.

Levey AS, Coresh J, Greene T, et al, "Using Standardized Serum Creatinine Values in the Modification of Diet in Renal Disease Study Equation for Estimating Glomerular Filtration Rate," *Ann Intern Med*, 2006, 145(4):247-54.

National Kidney Disease Education Program, "GFR Calculators." Available at: http://www.nkdep.nih.gov/professionals/gfr_calculators. Last accessed: January 20, 2011.

Stevens LA, Coresh J, Greene T, et al, "Assessing Kidney Function - Measured and Estimated Glomerular Filtration Rate," *N Engl J Med*, 2006, 354(23):2473-83.

RENAL FUNCTION ESTIMATION IN PEDIATRIC PATIENTS

Evaluation of a patient's renal function often includes the use of equations to estimate glomerular filtration rate (GFR) (eg, estimated GFR [eGFR] creatinine clearance [Cl_{Cr}]) using an endogenous filtration marker (eg, serum creatinine) and other patient variables. For example, the Schwartz equation estimates renal function by calculating eGFR and is typically used to steer medication dosing or categorize chronic kidney disease (CKD) staging. The rate of creatinine clearance does not always accurately represent GFR; creatinine may be cleared by other renal mechanisms in addition to glomerular filtration and serum creatinine concentrations may be affected by non-renal factors (eg, age, gender, race, body habitus, illness, diet). In addition, these equations were developed based on studies in limited populations and may either over- or underestimate the renal function of a specific patient.

Nevertheless, most clinicians use an eGFR or Cl_{Cr} as an indicator of renal function in pediatric patients for the purposes of adjusting medication doses. These equations should only be used in the clinical context of patient-specific factors noted during the physical exam/work-up. **Decisions regarding drug therapy and doses must be made on clinical judgment.**

RENAL FUNCTION ESTIMATION EQUATIONS

Commonly used equations include the Schwartz and Traub-Johnson equations. Both equations were originally developed using a serum creatinine assay measured by the alkaline picrate-based (Jaffe) method. Many substances, including proteins, can interfere with the accuracy of this assay and overestimate serum creatinine concentration. The National Kidney Foundation and The National Kidney Disease Education Program advocate for a universal creatinine assay, in order to ensure an accurate estimate of GFR in patients. As a result, a more specific enzymatic assay with an isotope dilution mass spectrometry (IDMS)-traceable international standard has been developed. Compared to the older methods, IDMS-traceable assays may report lower serum creatinine values and may, therefore, overestimate renal function when used in the original equations. An updated Schwartz equation (eg, Bedside Schwartz) based on serum creatinine measured by the IDMS-traceable method has been proposed for pediatrics (Schwartz, 2009); the Traub-Johnson equation has not been re-expressed. The original Schwartz and Traub-Johnson equations may overestimate renal function when used with a serum creatinine measured by the IDMS-traceable method. Clinicians should be aware of the serum creatinine assay used by their institution and the ramifications the assay may have on the equations used for renal function estimation.

Regardless of the serum creatinine assay used, the following factors may contribute to an inaccurate estimation of renal function (Stevens, 2006):

- Increased creatinine generation (may underestimate renal function):
  - Black or African American patients
  - Muscular body habitus
  - Ingestion of cooked meats
- Decreased creatinine generation (may overestimate renal function):
  - Increased age
  - Female patients
  - Asian patients
  - Amputees
  - Malnutrition, inflammation, or deconditioning (eg, cancer, severe cardiovascular disease, hospitalized patients)
  - Neuromuscular disease
  - Vegetarian diet
- Rapidly changing serum creatinine (either up or down):
  - In patients with rapidly rising serum creatinines (ie, increasing by >0.5-0.7 mg/dL/day), it is best to assume that the patient's renal function is severely impaired

Use extreme caution when estimating renal function in the following patient populations:

- Low body weight (actual body weight < ideal body weight)
- Liver transplant
- Prematurity (especially very low birth weight)
- Dehydration
- Recent kidney transplantation (serum creatinine values may decrease rapidly and can lead to renal function underestimation; conversely, delayed graft function may be present)

Alkaline picrate-based (Jaffe) methods

Note: These equations have not been updated for use with serum creatinine methods traceable to IDMS. Use with IDMS-traceable serum creatinine methods may overestimate renal function; use with caution.

Method 1: Schwartz equation

Note: This equation may not provide an accurate estimation of creatinine clearance for infants <6 months of age or for patients with severe starvation or muscle wasting.

eGFR = (k X Height) / Creatinine

where:

eGFR = estimated GFR; calculated in mL/minute/1.73 m^2

Height (length) is input in cm

k = constant of proportionality that is age-specific

<1 year preterm: 0.33

<1 year full-term: 0.45

1-12 years: 0.55

>12 years female: 0.55

>12 years male: 0.7

Creatinine is input in mg/dL

Method 2: Traub-Johnson equation

Note: This equation is for use in ages 1-18 years.

Cl_{Cr} = (0.48 X Height) / Creatinine

where:

Cl_{Cr} = estimated creatinine clearance; calculated in mL/minute/1.73 m^2

Height (length) is input in cm

Creatinine = Sr_{Cr} input in mg/dL

IDMS-traceable method: Bedside Schwartz[1]

Note: This equation is for use in ages 1-16 years.

eGFR = (0.413 X Height) / Creatinine

where:

eGFR = estimated GFR; calculated in mL/minute/1.73 m^2

Height (length) is input in cm

Creatinine = Sr_{Cr} input in mg/dL

FOOTNOTES

[1]National Kidney Disease Foundation Program preferred equation

REFERENCES

Dowling TC, Matzke GR, Murphy JE, et al, "Evaluation of Renal Drug Dosing: Prescribing Information and Clinical Pharmacist Approaches," *Pharmacotherapy*, 2010, 30(8):776-86.

Myers GL, Miller WG, Coresh J, et al, "Recommendations for Improving Serum Creatinine Measurement: A Report From the Laboratory Working Group of the National Kidney Disease Education Program," *Clin Chem*, 2006, 52(1):5-18.

National Kidney Disease Education Program, "GFR Calculators." Available at: http://www.nkdep.nih.gov/professionals/gfr_calculators. Last accessed: January 20, 2011.

Pottel H, Mottaghy FM, Zaman Z, et al, "On the Relationship Between Glomerular Filtration Rate and Serum Creatinine in Children," *Pediatr Nephrol*, 2010, 25(5):927-34.

Schwartz GJ, Brion LP, and Spitzer A, "The Use of Plasma Creatinine Concentration for Estimating Glomerular Filtration Rate in Infants, Children, and Adolescents," *Pediatr Clin North Am*, 1987, 34 (3):571-90.

Schwartz GJ, Haycock GB, Edelmann CM Jr, et al, "A Simple Estimate of Glomerular Filtration Rate in Children Derived From Body Length and Plasma Creatinine," *Pediatrics*, 1976, 58(2):259-63.

Schwartz GJ, Muñoz A, Schneider MF, et al, "New Equations to Estimate GFR in Children With CKD," *J Am Soc Nephrol*, 2009, 20(3):629-37.

Staples A, LeBlond R, Watkins S, et al, "Validation of the Revised Schwartz Estimating Equation in a Predominantly Non-CKD Population," *Pediatr Nephrol*, 2010, 25(11):2321-6.

Stevens LA, Coresh J, Greene T, et al, "Assessing Kidney Function - Measured and Estimated Glomerular Filtration Rate," *N Engl J Med*, 2006, 354(23):2473-83.

Traub SL and Johnson CE, "Comparison of Methods of Estimating Creatinine Clearance in Children," *Am J Hosp Pharm*, 1980, 37(2):195-201.

ANGIOTENSIN AGENTS

Comparison of Indications and Adult Dosages

Drug	Hypertension	HF	Renal Dysfunction	Dialyzable	Strengths (mg)
ACE Inhibitors					
Benazepril (Lotensin®)	10-40 mg/day	Not FDA-approved	Cl_{cr} <30 mL/min: 5 mg/day initially Maximum: 40 mg/day	Yes	Tablets 5, 10, 20, 40
Captopril (Capoten® [DSC])	25-100 mg/day bid-tid	6.25-100 mg tid Maximum: 450 mg/day	Cl_{cr} 10-50 mL/min: 75% of usual dose Cl_{cr} <10 mL/min: 50% of usual dose	Yes	Tablets 12.5, 25, 50, 100
Cilazapril (Inhibace®) **Note:** Not available in U.S.	2.5-10 mg/day	0.5-2.5 mg/day	Cl_{cr} 10-40 mL/min: Initial: 0.5 mg/day (0.25-0.5 mg/day for HF) (maximum: 2.5 mg/day) Cl_{cr} <10 mL/minute: 0.25-0.5 mg once or twice weekly	Yes	Tablets 1, 2.5, 5
Enalapril (Vasotec®)	2.5-40 mg/day qd-bid	2.5-20 mg bid Maximum: 20 mg bid	Cl_{cr} 30-80 mL/min: 5 mg/day initially Cl_{cr} <30 mL/min: 2.5 mg/day initially	Yes	Tablets 2.5, 5, 10, 20
Enalaprilat[1]	0.625 mg, 1.25 mg, 2.5 mg q6h Maximum: 5 mg q6h	Not FDA-approved	Cl_{cr} <30 mL/min: 0.625 mg q6h	Yes	1.25 mg/mL (1 mL, 2 mL vials)
Fosinopril (Monopril®)	10-40 mg/day	10-40 mg/day	No dosage reduction necessary	Not well dialyzed	Tablets 10, 20, 40
Lisinopril (Prinivil®, Zestril®)	10-40 mg/day Maximum: 40 mg/day	5-40 mg/day	Cl_{cr} 10-30 mL/min: 5 mg/day initially Cl_{cr} <10 mL/min: 2.5 mg/day initially	Yes	Tablets 2.5, 5, 10, 20, 30, 40
Moexipril (Univasc®)	7.5-30 mg/day qd-bid Maximum: 30 mg/day	LV dysfunction (post-MI): 7.5-30 mg/day	Cl_{cr} <40 mL/min: 3.75 mg/day initially Maximum: 15 mg/day	Unknown	Tablets 7.5, 15
Perindopril (Aceon®)	4-8 mg/day	4-8 mg/day Maximum: 16 mg/day	Cl_{cr} 30-60 mL/min: 2 mg/day Cl_{cr} 15-29 mL/min: 2 mg qod Cl_{cr} <15 mL/min: 2 mg on dialysis days	Yes	Tablets 2, 4, 8
Quinapril (Accupril®)	10-40 mg/day qd-bid	5-20 mg bid	Cl_{cr} 30-60 mL/min: 5 mg/day initially Cl_{cr} <10-30 mL/min: 2.5 mg/day initially	Not well dialyzed	Tablets 5, 10, 20, 40
Ramipril (Altace®)	2.5-20 mg/day qd-bid	2.5-10 mg/day	Cl_{cr} <40 mL/min: 25% of normal dose	Unknown	Capsules 1.25, 2.5, 5, 10
Trandolapril (Mavik®)	1-4 mg/day Maximum: 8 mg/day qd-bid	LV dysfunction (post-MI): 1-4 mg/day	Cl_{cr} <30 mL/min: 0.5 mg/day initially	No	Tablets 1, 2, 4

Comparison of Indications and Adult Dosages *continued*

Drug	Hypertension	HF	Renal Dysfunction	Dialyzable	Strengths (mg)
Angiotensin II Receptor Blockers					
Azilsartan (Edarbi™)	40-80 mg/day	Not FDA-approved	No dosage adjustment necessary	Unknown	Tablets 40, 80
Candesartan (Atacand®)	8-32 mg/day	Target: 32 mg once daily	No dosage adjustment necessary	No	Tablets 4, 8, 16, 32
Eprosartan (Teveten®)	400-800 mg/day qd-bid	Not FDA-approved	No dosage adjustment necessary	Unknown	Tablets 400, 600
Irbesartan (Avapro®)	150-300 mg/day	Not FDA-approved	No dosage reduction necessary	No	Tablets 75, 150, 300
Losartan (Cozaar®)	25-100 mg qd or bid	Not FDA-approved	No dosage adjustment necessary	No	Tablets 25, 50, 100
Olmesartan (Benicar®)	20-40 mg/day	Not FDA-approved	No dosage adjustment necessary	Unknown	Tablets 5, 20, 40
Telmisartan (Micardis®)	20-80 mg/day	Not FDA-approved	No dosage reduction necessary	No	Tablets 20, 40, 80
Valsartan (Diovan®)	80-320 mg/day	Target: 160 mg bid	Decrease dose only if Cl_{cr} <10 mL/minute	No	Tablets 40, 80, 160, 320
Renin Inhibitors					
Aliskiren (Tekturna®)	150-300 mg once daily	Not FDA-approved	No dosage adjustment necessary in mild-to-moderate impairment; not adequately studied in severe impairment	Unknown	Tablets 150, 300

Dosage is based on 70 kg adult with normal hepatic and renal function.

[1]Enalaprilat is the only available ACE inhibitor in a parenteral formulation.

ACE Inhibitors: Comparative Pharmacokinetics

Drug	Prodrug	Absorption (%)	Serum $t_{1/2}$ (h) Normal Renal Function	Serum Protein Binding (%)	Elimination	Onset of BP Lowering Action (h)	Peak BP Lowering Effects (h)	Duration of BP Lowering Effects (h)
Benazepril	Yes	37		~97	Renal (32%), biliary (~12%)	1	2-4	24
Benazeprilat			10-11 (effective)	~95%				
Captopril	No	60-75 (fasting)	1.9 (elimination)	25-30	Renal	0.25-0.5	1-1.5	~6
Enalapril	Yes	55-75	2	50-60	Renal (60%-80%), fecal	1	4-6	12-24
Enalaprilat			11 (effective)			0.25	1-4	~6
Fosinopril		36			Renal (~50%), biliary (~50%)	1		24
Fosinoprilat			12 (effective)	>99				
Lisinopril	No	25	11-12	25	Renal	1	6	24
Moexipril	Yes		1	90	Fecal (53%), renal (8%)		1-2	>24
Moexiprilat			2-10	50				
Perindopril	Yes		1.5-3	60	Renal		3-7	
Perindoprilat			3-10 (effective)	10-20				
Quinapril	Yes	>60	0.8	97	Renal (~60%) as metabolite, fecal	1	2-4	24
Quinaprilat			2					
Ramipril	Yes	50-60	1-2	73	Renal (60%), fecal (40%)	1-2	3-6	24
Ramiprilat			13-17 (effective)	56				
Trandolapril	Yes		6	80	Renal (33%), fecal (66%)	1-2	6	≥24
Trandolaprilat			10	65-94				

Angiotensin II Receptor Blockers and Renin Inhibitors: Comparative Pharmacokinetics

Drug	Prodrug	Time to Peak	Bioavailability	Food "Area-Under-the-Curve"	Elimination Half-Life	Elimination Altered in Renal Dysfunction	Precautions in Severe Renal Dysfunction	Elimination Altered in Hepatic Dysfunction	Precautions in Hepatic Dysfunction	Protein Binding
Angiotensin II Receptor Blockers										
Azilsartan (Edarbi™)	Yes	1.5-3 h	60%	No effect	11 h	No	Yes	No	No	>99%
Candesartan (Atacand®)	Yes[1]	3-4 h	15%	No effect	9 h	Yes[2]	Yes	No	Yes	>99%
Eprosartan (Teveten®)	No	1-2 h	13%	No effect	5-9 h	No	Yes	No	Yes	98%
Irbesartan (Avapro®)	No	1.5-2 h	60%-80%	No effect	11-15 h	No	Yes	No	No	90%
Losartan (Cozaar®)	Yes[3]	1 h / 3-4 h[3]	33%	9%-10%	1.5-2 h / 6-9 h[3]	No	Yes	Yes	Yes	~99%
Olmesartan (Benicar®)	Yes	1-2 h	26%	No effect	13 h	Yes	Yes	Yes	No	99%
Telmisartan (Micardis®)	No	0.5-1 h	42%-58%	9.6%-20%	24 h	No	Yes	Yes	Yes	>99.5%
Valsartan (Diovan®)	No	2-4 h	25%	9%-40%	6 h	No	Yes	Yes	Yes	95%
Renin Inhibitors										
Aliskiren (Tekturna®)	No	1-3 h	~3%	85% (high-fat meal)	16-32 h	Yes[4]	Yes	No	No	?

[1]Candesartan cilexetil: Active metabolite candesartan.

[2]Dosage adjustments are not necessary.

[3]Losartan: Active metabolite E-3174.

[4]No initial dosage adjustment in mild-to-moderate impairment.

ANTIARRHYTHMIC DRUGS

Vaughan Williams Classification of Antiarrhythmic Drugs Based on Cardiac Effects

Class	Drug(s)	Conduction Velocity[1]	Refractory Period	Automaticity
I				
Ia	Disopyramide Procainamide Quinidine	↓	↑	↓
Ib	Lidocaine Mexiletine	0/↓	↓	↓
Ic	Flecainide Propafenone[2]	↓↓	0	↓
II	Beta-blockers	0	0	↓
III	Amiodarone Dofetilide Ibutilide Sotalol[2]	0	↑↑	0
IV	Diltiazem Verapamil[3]	↓	↑	↓
Miscellaneous	Dronedarone[4]	↓	↑	↓

[1]Variables for normal tissue models in ventricular tissue.

[2]Also has type II, beta-blocking action.

[3]Variables for SA and AV nodal tissue only.

[4]Dronedarone has effects of all V-W classes similar to amiodarone; yet to be classified

Expected Electrocardiographic Changes of Antiarrhythmic Agents

Class	Drug(s)	PR Interval	QRS Duration	QT Interval
I				
Ia	Disopyramide Procainamide Quinidine	0/↑	↑	↑
Ib	Lidocaine Mexiletine	0	0	0
Ic	Flecainide	↑	↑	↑
	Propafenone	↑	↑	0
II	Beta-blockers	↑	0	0
III	Amiodarone	↑	0/↑	↑
	Dofetilide	0	0	↑↑
	Ibutilide	0	0	↑↑
	Sotalol	↑	0	↑
IV	Diltiazem Verapamil	↑↑	0	0
Miscellaneous	Dronedarone	↑	0	↑

Vaughan Williams Classification, Indications, and Adverse Effects of Antiarrhythmic Agents

Class	Drug(s)	Primary Uses	Route of Administration	Adverse Effects
I				
Ia	Disopyramide	AF, VT	P.O.	Anticholinergic effects, CHF
	Procainamide	AF, VT, WPW	P.O. (not available in U.S.)/I.V.	GI, CNS, lupus, fever, hematological, anticholinergic effects
	Quinidine	AF, PSVT, VT, WPW	P.O./I.V.	Hypotension, GI, thrombocytopenia, cinchonism
Ib	Lidocaine	VT, VF, PVC	I.V.	CNS, GI
	Mexiletine	VT	P.O.	GI, CNS
Ic	Flecainide	AF, PSVT, VT	P.O.	CHF, GI, CNS, blurred vision
	Propafenone	AF, PSVT, VT	P.O.	GI, blurred vision, dizziness

Vaughan Williams Classification, Indications, and Adverse Effects of Antiarrhythmic Agents *(continued)*

Class	Drug(s)	Primary Uses	Route of Administration	Adverse Effects
II	Esmolol	VT, SVT	I.V.	CHF, CNS, lupus-like syndrome, hypotension, bradycardia, bronchospasm
	Propranolol	SVT, VT, PVC	P.O./I.V.	CHF, bradycardia, hypotension, CNS, fatigue
III	Amiodarone	AF, SVT, VF, VT	P.O./I.V.	CNS, GI, thyroid, pulmonary fibrosis, liver, corneal deposits
	Dofetilide	AF	P.O.	Headache, dizziness, VT, torsade de pointes
	Ibutilide	AF	I.V.	Torsade de pointes, hypotension, bundle branch block, AV block
	Sotalol	AF, VT	P.O./I.V.	Bradycardia, hypotension, CHF, CNS, fatigue, torsade de pointes
IV	Diltiazem	AF, PSVT	P.O./I.V.	Hypotension, CHF, bradycardia
	Verapamil	AF, PSVT	P.O./I.V.	Hypotension, CHF, bradycardia, vertigo, constipation
Miscellaneous	Adenosine	SVT, PSVT	I.V.	Flushing, dizziness, bradycardia, syncope
	Digoxin	AF, PSVT	P.O./I.V.	GI, CNS, arrhythmias
	Dronedarone	AF	P.O.	Bradycardia, diarrhea, nausea
	Magnesium	VT, VF	I.V.	Hypotension, CNS, hypothermia, myocardial depression

AF = atrial fibrillation; PSVT = paroxysmal supraventricular tachycardia; VT = ventricular tachycardia; WPW = Wolf-Parkinson-White arrhythmias; VF = ventricular fibrillation; SVT = supraventricular tachycardia.

Comparative Pharmacokinetic Properties of Antiarrhythmic Agents

Class	Drug(s)	Bioavailability (%)	Primary Route of Elimination	Volume of Distribution (L/kg)	Protein Binding (%)	Half-Life	Therapeutic Range (mcg/mL)
I							
Ia	Disopyramide	60-83	Hepatic/renal	0.8-2	20-60	4-10 h	2-6
	Procainamide	80-90[1]	Hepatic/renal	2	15-20	PA: 2.5-5 h NAPA: 6-8 h	PA: 4-10 NAPA: 15-25
	Quinidine	70-80	Hepatic	2-3	80-90	6-8 h	2-6
Ib	Lidocaine	NA	Hepatic	1-2	60-80	Initial: 7-30 min Terminal: 90-120 min	1.5-5
	Mexiletine	80-95	Hepatic	5-7	50-60	10-14 h	0.8-2
Ic	Flecainide	85-90	Hepatic/renal	5-13	40-50	7-22 h	0.3-2.5
	Propafenone	3-11	Hepatic	2-5	85-95	PM: 10-32 h EM: 2-10 h	—
II	Esmolol	Refer to Beta-Blocker Comparison Chart					
	Propranolol	Refer to Beta-Blocker Comparison Chart					
III	Amiodarone	35-65	Hepatic	18-148	95-97	26-107 d	1-2.5[2]
	Dofetilide	>90%	Renal	3	60-70	10 h	—
	Ibutilide	NA	Hepatic	11	40	2-12 h	—
	Sotalol	90-100	Renal	1.2-2.4	Negligible	12-15 h	—
IV	Diltiazem	40	Hepatic	3-13	70-80	3-5 h	—
	Verapamil	20-35	Hepatic	4	90	2-12 h	—
Miscellaneous	Adenosine	NA	—	—	—	<10 sec	—
	Digoxin	70-80	Renal	6-7	30	38-48 h	0.8-2 ng/mL[3]
	Dronedarone	4-15	Hepatic	~20	>98	13-19 h	—

DEA = desethylamiodarone; EM = extensive metabolizers; PA = procainamide; PM = poor metabolizers; NAPA = N-acetylprocainamide

[1]Oral formulation not available in the U.S.

[2]The active metabolite, desethylamiodarone (DEA) equates to levels of the parent compound. Poor correlation exists between level and therapeutic or toxic effects of amiodarone.

[3]Higher end of range may be necessary to control ventricular response; monitor closely for digoxin toxicity. Therapeutic range for patients with heart failure without atrial arrhythmia is 0.5-0.8 ng/mL

ANTICONVULSANT DRUGS OF CHOICE

Seizure Type	First Line Therapy	Alternatives
Partial (including secondary generalization)	Carbamazepine, lamotrigine, levetiracetam, or oxcarbazepine	Divalproex, gabapentin, lacosamide, phenytoin, pregabalin, topiramate, valproic acid, or zonisamide
Generalized tonic-clonic	Divalproex, lamotrigine, or valproic acid	Carbamazepine, levetiracetam, oxcarbazepine, phenytoin, topiramate, or zonisamide
Childhood absence epilepsy	Divalproex, ethosuximide (only if no generalized seizures), lamotrigine, or valproic acid	Clonazepam, levetiracetam, or zonisamide
Atypical absence, myoclonic, or atonic	Divalproex, lamotrigine, levetiracetam, or valproic acid	Clonazepam, felbamate, topiramate, or zonisamide

Note: Table includes non-FDA approved indications.

References

"Drugs for Epilepsy," *Treat Guidel Med Lett*, 2008, 6(70):37-46.

Glauser T, Ben-Menachem E, Bourgeois B, et al, "ILAE Treatment Guidelines: Evidence-Based Analysis of Antiepileptic Drug Efficacy and Effectiveness as Initial Monotherapy for Epileptic Seizures and Syndromes," *Epilepsia*, 2006, 47(7):1094-120.

ANTIDEPRESSANT AGENTS

Comparison of Usual Adult Dosage, Mechanism of Action, and Adverse Effects

Drug	Initial Adult Dose	Usual Adult Dosage (mg/d)	Dosage Forms	Adverse Effects						Comments
				ACH	Drowsiness	Orthostatic Hypotension	Conduction Abnormalities	GI Distress	Weight Gain	
Tricyclic Antidepressants and Related Compounds[1]										
Amitriptyline	25-75 mg qhs	100-300	T	4+	4+	3+	3+	1+	4+	Also used in chronic pain, migraine, and as a hypnotic; contraindicated with cisapride
Amoxapine	50 mg bid	100-400	T	2+	2+	2+	2+	0	2+	May cause extrapyramidal symptom (EPS)
ClomiPRAMINE[2] (Anafranil®)	25-75 mg qhs	100-250	C	4+	4+	2+	3+	1+	4+	Only approved for OCD
Desipramine (Norpramin®)	25-75 mg qhs	100-300	T	1+	2+	2+	2+	0	1+	Blood levels useful for therapeutic monitoring
Doxepin	25-75 mg qhs	100-300	C, L	3+	4+	2+	2+	0	4+	
Imipramine (Tofranil®, Tofranil-PM®)	25-75 mg qhs	100-300	T, C	3+	3+	4+	3+	1+	4+	Blood levels useful for therapeutic monitoring
Maprotiline	25-75 mg qhs	100-225	T	2+	3+	2+	2+	0	2+	
Nortriptyline (Pamelor®)	25-50 mg qhs	50-150	C, L	2+	2+	1+	2+	0	1+	Blood levels useful for therapeutic monitoring
Protriptyline (Vivactil®)	15 mg qAM	15-60	T	2+	1+	2+	3+	1+	1+	
Trimipramine (Surmontil®)	25-75 mg qhs	100-300	C	4+	4+	3+	3+	0	4+	
Selective Serotonin Reuptake Inhibitors[3]										
Citalopram (Celexa®)	20 mg qAM	20-60	T, L	0	0	0	0	3+[4]	1+	
Escitalopram (Lexapro®)	10 mg qAM	10-20	T, L	0	0	0	0	3+	1+	S-enantiomer of citalopram
FLUoxetine (Prozac®, Prozac® Weekly™, Sarafem®, Selfemra®)	10-20 mg qAM	20-80	C, CDR, L, T	0	0	0	0	3+[4]	1+	CYP2B6 and 2D6 inhibitor
Fluvoxamine[2] (Luvox® CR)	50 mg qhs	100-300	T, CXR	0	0	0	0	3+[4]	1+	Contraindicated with pimozide, thioridazine, mesoridazine, CYP1A2, 2B6, 2C19, and 3A4 inhibitors
PARoxetine (Paxil®, Paxil CR®, Pexeva®)	10-20 mg qAM	20-50	T, CXR, L	1+	1+	0	0	3+[4]	2+	CYP2B6 and 2D6 inhibitor
Sertraline (Zoloft®)	25-50 mg qAM	50-200	T, L	0	0	0	0	3+[4]	1+	CYP2B6 and 2C19 inhibitor
Vilazodone (Viibryd™)	10 mg qAM	10-40	T	0	0	0	0	3+	0	CYP2C8, 2C19, and 2D6 inhibitor; also is a 5-HT_{1A} partial agonist

Comparison of Usual Adult Dosage, Mechanism of Action, and Adverse Effects *continued*

Drug	Initial Adult Dose	Usual Adult Dosage (mg/d)	Dosage Forms	Adverse Effects						Comments
				ACH	Drowsiness	Orthostatic Hypotension	Conduction Abnormalities	GI Distress	Weight Gain	
Dopamine-Reuptake Blocking Compounds										
BuPROPion (Aplenzin™, Buproban®, Budeprion SR®, Budeprion XL®, Wellbutrin®, Wellbutrin SR®, Wellbutrin XL®, Zyban®)	100 mg bid-tid IR[5] 150 mg qAM-bid SR[6]	300-450	T, TSR, TXR	0	0	0	1+/0	1+	0	Contraindicated with seizures, bulimia, and anorexia; low incidence of sexual dysfunction IR: A 6-h interval between doses preferred SR: An 8-h interval between doses preferred XL: Administer once daily
Serotonin / Norepinephrine Reuptake Inhibitors[7]										
Desvenlafaxine (Pristiq®)	50 mg/d	50-100	TXR	0	1+	1+	0	3+[4]	0	Active metabolite of venlafaxine
DULoxetine (Cymbalta®)	40-60 mg/d	40-60	CDR	1+	1+	0	1+	3+	0	Also indicated for GAD, management of pain associated with diabetic neuropathy, and management of fibromyalgia
Milnacipran[8] (Savella™)	12.5 mg/d	100-200	T	2+	1+	0	1+	3+	0	Only indicated for fibromyalgia
Venlafaxine (Effexor®, Effexor XR®)	25 mg bid-tid IR 37.5 mg qd XR	75-375 IR 75-225 XR	T, TXR, CXR	1+	1+	0	1+	3+[4]	0	High-dose may be useful to treat refractory depression; frequency of hypertension increases with dosage >225 mg/d
5-HT_2 Receptor Antagonist Properties										
Nefazodone	100 mg bid	300-600	T	1+	1+	2+	1+	1+	0	Contraindicated with carbamazepine, pimozide, astemizole, cisapride, and terfenadine; caution with triazolam and alprazolam; low incidence of sexual dysfunction
TraZODone	50 mg tid	150-600	T	0	4+	3+	1+	1+	2+	
Noradrenergic Antagonist										
Mirtazapine (Remeron®, Remeron SolTab®)	15 mg qhs	15-45	T, TOD	1+	3+	1+	1+	0	3+	Dose >15 mg/d less sedating, low incidence of sexual dysfunction

Comparison of Usual Adult Dosage, Mechanism of Action, and Adverse Effects *continued*

Drug	Initial Adult Dose	Usual Adult Dosage (mg/d)	Dosage Forms	Adverse Effects						Comments
				ACH	Drowsiness	Orthostatic Hypotension	Conduction Abnormalities	GI Distress	Weight Gain	
Monoamine Oxidase Inhibitors										
Isocarboxazid (Marplan®)	10 mg tid	10-30	T	2+	2+	2+	1+	1+	2+	Diet must be low in tyramine; contraindicated with sympathomimetics and other antidepressants
Phenelzine (Nardil®)	15 mg tid	15-90	T	2+	2+	2+	0	1+	3+	
Tranylcypromine (Parnate®)	10 mg bid	10-60	T	2+	1+	2+	1+	1+	2+	
Selegiline (EmSam®)	6 mg/d	6-12	Transdermal	2+	1+	2+	0	1+	0	Low tyramine diet not required for 6 mg/d dosage

ACH = anticholinergic effects (dry mouth, blurred vision, urinary retention, constipation); 0 - 4+ = absent or rare - relatively common. T = tablet, TSR = tablet, sustained release, TXR - tablet, extended release, TOD = tablet, orally disintegrating, L = liquid, C = capsule, CDR = capsule, delayed release, CXR = capsule, extended release; IR = immediate release, SR = sustained release, XR = extended release.

[1]**Important note:** A 1-week supply taken all at once in a patient receiving the maximum dose can be fatal.

[2]Not approved by FDA for depression. Approved for OCD.

[3]Flat dose response curve, headache, nausea, and sexual dysfunction are common side effects for SSRIs.

[4]Nausea is usually mild and transient.

[5]IR: 100 mg bid, may be increased to 100 mg tid no sooner than 3 days after beginning therapy.

[6]SR: 150 mg qAM, may be increased to 150 mg bid as early as day 4 of dosing. To minimize seizure risk, do not exceed SR 200 mg/dose.

[7]Do not use with sibutramine; relatively safe in overdose.

[8]Milnacipran is only approved for fibromyalgia.

ANTIMIGRAINE DRUGS: 5-HT_1 RECEPTOR AGONISTS

Pharmacokinetic Differences

Pharmacokinetic Parameter	Almotriptan (Axert®)	Eletriptan (Relpax®)	Frovatriptan (Frova®)	Naratriptan (Amerge®)	Rizatriptan (Maxalt®, Maxalt-MLT®)		Sumatriptan (Imitrex®)			Zolmitriptan (Zomig®, Zomig-ZMT®)		
	Oral (6.25-12.5 mg)	Tablets	Oral	Oral	Tablets	Disintegrating Tablets	SubQ (6 mg)	Oral (100 mg)	Nasal (20 mg)	Oral (5 mg)	Disintegrat-ing Tablets (5 mg)	Nasal (5 mg)
Onset	<60 min	<2 h	<2 h	1-2 h	~30 min	~30 min	10 min	~30 min	15-30 min	0.5-1 h	0.5-1 h	0.5-1 h
Duration	Short	Short	Long	Long	Short	Short	Short	Short	Short	Short		
Time to peak serum concentration (h)	1-3	1.5-2	2-4	2-3	1-1.5	1-1.5	4-20 min	2-2.5	1	1.5	3	3
Average bioavailability (%)	70	50	20-30	70	45	45	97	15	17	40	40	40
Volume of distribution (L)	180-200	138	210-280	170	110-140	110-140	170	170	NA	—	402	NA
Half-life (h)	3-4	4	26	6	2-3	2-3	2	2-2.5[1]	2	2.8-3.74	2.8-3.7	2.8-3.7
Fraction excreted unchanged in urine (%)	40	—	<10	50	12	12	22	3	3	8	8	—

[1]With extended dosing, the half-life extends to 7 hours.

ANTIPSYCHOTIC AGENTS

Antipsychotic Agent	Dosage Forms	I.M./P.O. Potency	Equiv. Dosages (approx) (mg/d)	Usual Adult Daily Maint. Dose (mg)	Sedation (Incidence)	Extrapyramidal Side Effects	Anticholinergic Side Effects	Orthostatic Hypotension	Comments
ARIPiprazole (Abilify®)	Solution; tablet; tablet, orally disintegrating; injection		7.5	10-30	Low	Low	Very low	Very low	Low weight gain; activating
Asenapine (Saphris®)	Tablet, sublingual			10-20	Moderate	Low	Very low	Low / moderate	Low weight gain; activating
ChlorproMAZINE	Injection; tablet	4:1	100	200-1000	High	Moderate	Moderate	Moderate / high	
CloZAPine (Clozaril®, FazaClo®)	Tablet; tablet, orally disintegrating		100	75-900	High	Very low	High	High	~1% incidence of agranulocytosis; weekly-biweekly CBC required; potential for weight gain, lipid abnormalities, and diabetes
FluPHENAZine	Solution, concentrate; injection; tablet	2:1	2	0.5-20	Low	High	Low	Low	
	Injection, long-acting			12.5-25*					
Haloperidol (Haldol®)	Solution, concentrate; injection; tablet	2:1	2	0.5-20	Low	High	Low	Low	
(Haldol® Decanoate)	Injection, long-acting			50-200*					
Iloperidone (Fanapt™)	Tablet			12-24	Low	Low	Very low	Low / moderate	
Loxapine (Loxitane®)	Capsule		10	25-250	Moderate	Moderate	Low	Low	
Lurasidone (Latuda®)	Tablet			40-80	Moderate	Low/Moderate	Low	Low	Contraindicated with strong CYP3A4 inducers and inhibitors. Take with food.
OLANZapine (Zyprexa®)	Injection; tablet; tablet, orally disintegrating		5	5-20	Moderate / high	Low	Moderate	Moderate	Potential for weight gain, lipid abnormalities, diabetes
(Zyprexa® Relprew™)	Injection, long-acting			210-405*					

continued

Antipsychotic Agent	Dosage Forms	I.M./P.O. Potency	Equiv. Dosages (approx) (mg/d)	Usual Adult Daily Maint. Dose (mg)	Sedation (Incidence)	Extrapyramidal Side Effects	Anticholinergic Side Effects	Orthostatic Hypotension	Comments
Paliperidone (Invega®)	Tablet, extended release			3-12	Low / moderate	Low	Very low	Moderate	Active metabolite of risperidone
(Invega® Sustenna®)	Injection, long-acting			39-234*					
Perphenazine	Tablet		10	16-64	Low	Moderate	Low	Low	
Pimozide (Orap®)	Tablet		2	1-10	Moderate	High	Moderate	Low	Contraindicated with CYP3A inhibitors
QUEtiapine (Seroquel®, Seroquel XR®)	Tablet; tablet, extended release		75	50-800	Moderate / high	Very low	Moderate	Moderate	Moderate weight gain; potential for lipid abnormalities; diabetes
RisperiDONE (Risperdal®)	Solution; tablet; tablet, orally disintegrating		2	0.5-6	Low / moderate	Low	Very low	Moderate	Low to moderate weight gain; potential for diabetes
(Risperdal® Consta®)	Injection, long-acting			25-50*					
Thioridazine	Tablet		100	200-800	High	Low	High	Moderate / high	May cause irreversible retinitis pigmentosa at doses >800 mg/d; prolongs QTc; use only in treatment of refractory illness
Thiothixene (Navane®)	Capsule	4:1	4	5-40	Low	High	Low	Low / moderate	
Trifluoperazine	Tablet		5	2-40	Low	High	Low	Low	
Ziprasidone (Geodon®)	Capsule; injection, powder	2:1	60	40-160	Low / moderate	Low	Very low	Low / moderate	Low weight gain; contraindicated with QTc-prolonging agents. Take with food.

* Administered every 2 or 4 weeks; consult drug monograph for specific dosage details

Woods SW, "Chlorpromazine Equivalent Doses for the Newer Atypical Antipsychotics," *J Clin Psychiatry*, 2003, 64(6):663-7.

BENZODIAZEPINES

Agent	FDA-Approved Indication	Dosage Forms	Relative Potency (mg)	Peak Blood Levels (oral) (h)	Protein Binding (%)	Volume of Distribution (L/kg)	Major Active Metabolite	Onset	Metabolism	Half-Life (parent) (h)	Half-Life[1] (metabolite) (h)	Elimination	Usual Initial Oral Dose	Adult Oral Dosage Range
Anxiolytic														
Alprazolam (Xanax XR®; Xanax®)	Anxiety, anxiety associated with depression, panic disorder treatment	Sol, tab	0.5	IR: 1-2 XR: 9	80	0.9-1.2	No	Intermediate	Hepatic via CYP3A4	12-15	—	Urine	0.25-0.5 tid	0.75-4 mg/d
Chlordiazepoxide (Librium®)	Anxiety, EtOH withdrawal, adjunct to anesthesia (I.V.)	Cap, powd for inj	10	2-4	90-98	0.3	Yes	Intermediate	Hepatic via CYP3A4	5-30	24-96	Urine	5-25 mg tid-qid	15-100 mg/d
Diazepam (Diastat®, Valium®)	Anxiety, EtOH withdrawal, adjunct to anesthesia (I.V.), anxiety/amnesiac during cardioversion (I.V.), anxiety/amnesia in endoscopic procedures, convulsions/status epilepticus (I.V.), adjunct in epilepsy (rectal gel), skeletal muscle spasms	Gel, inj, sol, tab	5	0.5-2	98	1.1	Yes	Rapid	Hepatic via 2C19 and 3A4	20-80	50-100	Urine	2-10 mg bid-qid	4-40 mg/d
Lorazepam (Ativan®)[2]	Anxiety, anxiety associated with depression, adjunct to anesthesia (I.V.), convulsions/status epilepticus (I.V.)	Inj, sol, tab	1	1-6	88-92	1.3	No	Intermediate	Hepatic	10-20	—	Urine and feces (minimal)	0.5-2 mg tid-qid	2-4 mg/d
Oxazepam (Serax®)	Anxiety, anxiety associated with depression, EtOH withdrawal	Cap, tab	15-30	2-4	86-99	0.6-2	No	Slow	Hepatic via glucoronide conjugation	5-20	—	Urine as unchanged (50%) and glucoronide	10-30 mg tid-qid	30-120 mg/d
Sedative / Hypnotic														
Estazolam	Insomnia	Tab	0.3	2	93	—	No	Slow	Hepatic via CYP3A4	10-24	—	Urine	1 mg qhs	1-2 mg
Flurazepam (Dalmane®)	Insomnia	Cap	5	0.5-2	97	—	Yes	Rapid	Hepatic via CYP3A4	Not significant	40-114	Urine	15 mg qhs	15-60 mg
Quazepam (Doral®)	Insomnia	Tab	5	2	95	5	Yes	Intermediate	Hepatic via CYP3A4	25-41	28-114	Urine	15 mg qhs	7.5-15 mg
Temazepam (Restoril™)	Insomnia	Cap	5	2-3	96	1.4	No	Slow	Hepatic via CYP2B6, 2C8/9, 2C19, 3A4	10-40	—	Urine as inactive metabolites	15-30 mg qhs	15-30 mg

Agent	FDA-Approved Indication	Dosage Forms	Relative Potency (mg)	Peak Blood Levels (oral) (h)	Protein Binding (%)	Volume of Distribution (L/kg)	Major Active Metabolite	Onset	Metabolism	Half-Life (parent) (h)	Half-Life[1] (metabolite) (h)	Elimination	Usual Initial Oral Dose	Adult Oral Dosage Range
Triazolam (Halcion®)	Insomnia	Tab	0.1	1	89-94	0.8-1.3	No	Intermediate	Hepatic via CYP3A4	2.3	—	Urine as unchanged drug and metabolites	0.125-0.25 qhs	0.125-0.25 mg
Miscellaneous														
Clonazepam (Klonopin®)	Adjunct in Lennox-Gastuat syndrome, akinetic seizures, myoclonic seizures, adjunct in absence seizures, panic disorder treatment	Tab	0.25-0.5	1-2	86	1.8-4	No	Intermediate	Hepatic via glucoronide and sulfate conjugation	18-50	—	Urine as glucoronide or sulfate conjugate	0.5 mg tid	1.5-20 mg/d
Clorazepate (Tranxene® T-Tab®)	Anxiety, EtOH withdrawal, adjunct in partial seizures	Cap, tab	7.5	1-2	80-95	—	Yes	Rapid	Decarboxylated in acidic stomach prior to absorption and hepatic via CYP3A4	Not significant	50-100	Urine	7.5-15 mg bid-qid	15-60 mg
Midazolam	Adjunct to anesthesia, anxiety/amnesiac during cardioversion, anxiety/amnesia in endoscopic procedures	Inj	NA	0.4-0.7[3]	95	0.8-6.6	Yes	Rapid	Hepatic via CYP3A4	2-5 h	12 h	Urine	NA	NA

IR = immediate release; XR = extended release; NA = not available.

Rapid = 15 minutes or less; intermediate = 15-30 minutes; slow = 30-60 minutes.

[1]Significant metabolite.

[2]Reliable bioavailability when given I.M.

[3]I.V. only.

BETA-BLOCKERS

Agent	Adrenergic Receptor Blocking Activity	Intrinsic Sympathomimetic Activity (ISA)	Lipid Solubility	Protein Bound (%)	Half-Life (h)	Bioavailability (%)	Primary Site of Metabolism	Primary (Secondary) Route of Elimination	Indications	Usual Dosage
Acebutolol (Sectral®)	$beta_1$	Yes	Low	15-25	3-4	40 7-fold[1]	Hepatic	Feces (renal)	Hypertension, arrhythmias	P.O.: 400-1200 mg/d
Atenolol (Tenormin®)	$beta_1$	No	Low	<5-10	6-9	50-60 4-fold[1]	Hepatic (limited)	Feces (renal)	Hypertension, angina pectoris, acute MI	P.O.: 50-200 mg/d I.V.: Acute MI: 5 mg x 2 doses
Betaxolol (Kerlone®)	$beta_1$	No	Low	50-55	14-22	84-94	Hepatic	Renal	Hypertension	P.O.: 5-20 mg/d
Bisoprolol (Zebeta®)	$beta_1$	No	Low	26-33	9-12	80	Hepatic	Renal	Hypertension, heart failure	P.O.: HF: 2.5-10 mg/d HTN: 2.5-20 mg/d
Carvedilol (Coreg®, Coreg CR®)	$alpha_1$ $beta_1$ $beta_2$	No	ND	98	7-10	25-35	Hepatic	Feces	Hypertension, heart failure (mild to severe)	P.O.: 3.125-25 mg twice daily
Esmolol (Brevibloc)	$beta_1$	No	Low	55	0.15	NA 5-fold[1]	Red blood cell esterase	Renal	Supraventricular tachycardia, sinus tachycardia, atrial fibrillation/flutter, hypertension	I.V. infusion: 25-300 mcg/kg/min
Labetalol (Trandate®)	$alpha_1$ $beta_1$ $beta_2$	No	Moderate	50	5.5-8	18-30 10-fold[1]	Hepatic	Renal	Hypertension	P.O.: 200-2400 mg/d I.V.: 20-80 mg at 10-min intervals up to a maximum of 300 mg **or** continuous infusion of 2-6 mg/min

Agent	Adrenergic Receptor Blocking Activity	Intrinsic Sympathomimetic Activity (ISA)	Lipid Solubility	Protein Bound (%)	Half-Life (h)	Bioavailability (%)	Primary Site of Metabolism	Primary (Secondary) Route of Elimination	Indications	Usual Dosage
Metoprolol (Lopressor®, Toprol-XL®)	$beta_1$	No	Moderate	10-12	3-7	50 7- to 10-fold[1] (Toprol XL®: 77)	Hepatic	Renal	Hypertension, angina pectoris, acute MI, heart failure (mild to moderate; XL formulation only), atrial tachyarrhythmias (rate control)	P.O.: 100-450 mg/d HF: (Toprol-XL®): 12.5-200 mg/d I.V.: Acute MI: 5 mg q2 min x 3 doses AF (rate control): 2.5-5 mg q2-5 min (max total dose: 15 mg over 0-15 min)
Nadolol (Corgard®)	$beta_1$ $beta_2$	No	Low	25-30	20-24	30 5- to 8-fold[1]	None	Renal	Hypertension, angina pectoris	P.O.: 40-320 mg/d
Nebivolol (Bystolic®)	$beta_1$	No	High	98	10-32	12-96	Hepatic	Renal (feces)	Hypertension	P.O.: 5-40 mg/d
Penbutolol (Levatol®)	$beta_1$ $beta_2$	Yes	High	80-98	5	~100	Hepatic	Renal	Hypertension	P.O.: 20-80 mg/d
Pindolol	$beta_1$ $beta_2$	Yes	Moderate	57	3-4	90 2- to 2.5-fold[1]	Hepatic	Renal (feces)	Hypertension	P.O.: 20-60 mg/d
Propranolol (Inderal®, various)	$beta_1$ $beta_2$	No	High	90	3-5	25 2- to 3-fold[1]	Hepatic	Renal	Hypertension, angina pectoris, arrhythmias, prophylaxis (post-MI)	P.O.: 40-480 mg/d I.V.: Tachyarrhythmias: 1-3 mg q2-5 min (max: 5 mg)
Propranolol long-acting (Inderal-LA®, InnoPran XL™)	$beta_1$ $beta_2$	No	High	90	9-18	25 2- to 3-fold[1]	Hepatic	Renal	Hypertrophic cardiomyopathy with outflow tract obstruction, prophylaxis (post-MI)	P.O.: 180-240 mg/d

continued

Agent	Adrenergic Receptor Blocking Activity	Intrinsic Sympathomimetic Activity (ISA)	Lipid Solubility	Protein Bound (%)	Half-Life (h)	Bioavailability (%)	Primary Site of Metabolism	Primary (Secondary) Route of Elimination	Indications	Usual Dosage
Sotalol (Betapace®, Betapace AF®, Sorine®)	$beta_1$ $beta_2$	No	Low	0	12	90-100	None	Renal	Atrial and ventricular tachyarrhythmias	P.O. 160-320 mg/d
Timolol (Blocadren®)	$beta_1$ $beta_2$	No	Low to moderate	<10	4	75 7-fold[1]	Hepatic	Renal	Hypertension, prophylaxis (post-MI)	P.O.: 20-60 mg/d

Dosage is based on 70 kg adult with normal hepatic and renal function.

Note: All $beta_1$-selective agents will inhibit $beta_2$ receptors at higher doses.

[1]Interpatient variations in plasma levels.

CALCIUM CHANNEL BLOCKERS

Comparative Pharmacokinetics

Agent	Bioavailability (%)	Protein Binding (%)	Onset of BP Effect (min)	Duration of BP Effect (h)	Half-Life (h)	Volume of Distribution	Route of Metabolism	Route of Excretion
Dihydropyridines								
Amlodipine (Norvasc®)	64-90	93-98	30-50	24	30-50	21 L/kg	Hepatic; inactive metabolites	Urine; 10% as parent
Clevidipine (Cleviprex™)		>99.5	2-4	5-15 min	1-15 min	0.17 L/kg	Blood and extravascular tissue esterases	Urine (63% to 74%; as metabolites); feces (7% to 22%)
Felodipine (Plendil)	20	>99	2-5 h	24	11-16	10 L/kg	Hepatic; CYP3A4 substrate (major); inactive metabolites; extensive first pass	Urine (70%; as metabolites); feces 10%
Isradipine (DynaCirc CR®)	15-24	95	20	>12	8	3 L/kg	Hepatic; CYP3A4 substrate (major); inactive metabolites; extensive first pass	Urine as metabolites
Nicardipine (Cardene®)	35	>95	30	≤8	2-4		Hepatic; CYP3A4 substrate (major); saturable first pass	Urine (60%; as metabolites); feces 35%
Nifedipine (Procardia®)	40-77	92-98	Within 20		2-5		Hepatic; CYP3A4 substrate (major); inactive metabolites	Urine as metabolites
Nimodipine (Nimotop®)	13	>95	ND	4-6	1-2		Hepatic; CYP3A4 substrate (major); metabolites inactive or less active than parent; extensive first pass	Urine (50%; as metabolites); feces 32%
Nisoldipine (Sular®)	5	>99	ND	6-12	7-12		Hepatic; CYP3A4 substrate (major); 1 active metabolite (10% of parent); extensive first pass	Urine as metabolites
Phenylalkylamines								
Verapamil (Calan®, Verelan®)	20-35	90	30	6-8	4.5-12		Hepatic; CYP3A4 substrate (major); 1 active metabolite (20% of parent); extensive first pass	Urine (70%; 3%-4% as unchanged drug); feces 16%
Benzothiazepines								
Diltiazem (Cardizem®)	~40	70-80	30-60	6-8	3-4.5	3-13 L/kg	Hepatic; CYP3A4 substrate (major); 1 major metabolite (20%-50% of parent); extensive first pass	Urine as metabolites

COMPATIBILITY OF DRUGS

Drug Compatibility Guide

KEY
C = Compatible
X = Incompatible
Ø = Conflicting Reports
Blank = No information

	azithromycin	butorphanol	calcium gluconate	cefazolin	ciprofloxacin	cisatracurium	clindamycin	dobutamine	dopamine	drotrecogin alfa	fentanyl	fluconazole	furosemide	heparin	lansoprazole	levofloxacin	lorazepam	magnesium
azithromycin	■				X		X				X		X			X		
butorphanol		■				C									X			
calcium gluconate			■		C	C					C	X		C	X			
cefazolin				■		Ø					C	C		C	X			C
ciprofloxacin	X		C		■	C		C	C	X			X	X	X		C	X
cisatracurium		C	C	Ø	C	■	C	C	C	C	C	C	Ø	Ø			C	C
clindamycin	X					C	■			X	C	X		C	X	C		C
dobutamine					C	C		■		X	C	C		Ø	X	C		
dopamine					C	C			■	X	C	C		C	X	C		
drotrecogin alfa					X	C	X	X	X	■		C	X	X		X		X
fentanyl	X		C	C		C	C	C	C		■		C	C	C	C	C	
fluconazole			X	C		C	X	C	C	C		■	X	C	C		C	
furosemide	X				X	Ø				X	C	X	■	C	X	X	C	
heparin			C	C	X	Ø	C	Ø	C	X	C	C	C	■	C	X	C	C
lansoprazole		X	X	X	X		X	X	X		C	C	X	C	■	X	X	X
levofloxacin	X						C	C	C	X	C		X	X	X	■	C	
lorazepam					C	C					C	C	C	C	X	C	■	
magnesium				C	X	C	C			X				C	X			■
methylprednisolone					X	Ø								Ø	X			
metronidazole					C	C			Ø	X	C	C		C	X	C	C	C
midazolam			C	C	C	C	C	Ø	C	X	C	C	X	C	X			
morphine	X			C		C	C		C			C	X	C	X	C		C
nesiritide								C	C		C		X	X				
nitroglycerin						C				C	C	C	X	Ø	X	X		
nitroprusside						Ø				X				C		X		
norepinephrine						C			C	X				C				
pantoprazole			X	X	X		X	Ø	X		X	X	X	X		X	X	Ø
piperacillin & tazobactam																		
potassium chloride	X		C		C	C			C	C	C		C		X		C	C
potassium phosphate					X					X					X			
prochlorperazine			Ø			C						C		C	X			
promethazine					C	C						C	X	C	X			
propofol		C	C	C	C		C	C	C		Ø	C	C	C			Ø	C
ranitidine				C	C	C		C	C	X		C		C	X		C	
sodium bicarbonate					Ø	Ø					C			C	X	C		
vancomycin				Ø		C				X	C	C		Ø	X	C	C	C

Note: Because the compatibility of two or more drugs in solution depends on several variables such as the solution itself, drug concentration and the method of mixing (bottle, syringe, or Y-site), this table is intended to be used solely as a guide to general drug compatibilities. Before mixing any drugs, the healthcare professional should ascertain if a potential incompatibility exists by referring to an appropriate information source.

Drug Compatibility Guide

KEY
C = Compatible
X = Incompatible
Ø = Conflicting Reports
Blank = No information

	methylprednisolone	metronidazole	midazolam	morphine	nesiritide	nitroglycerin	nitroprusside	norepinephrine	pantoprazole	piperacillin & tazobactam	potassium chloride	potassium phosphate	prochlorperazine	promethazine	propofol	ranitidine	sodium bicarbonate	vancomycin
azithromycin				X							X							
butorphanol															C			
calcium gluconate			C						X		C		Ø		C			
cefazolin			C	C					X						C	C		Ø
ciprofloxacin	X	C	C						X		C	X		C	C	C	Ø	
cisatracurium	Ø	C	C	C		C	Ø	C			C		C	C		C	Ø	C
clindamycin			C	C					X						C			
dobutamine			Ø		C				Ø						C	C		
dopamine		Ø	C	C	C			C	X		C				C	C		
drotrecogin alfa		X	X			C	X	X			C	X				X		X
fentanyl		C	C		C	C			X		C				Ø		C	C
fluconazole		C	C	C		C			X				C	C	C	C		C
furosemide			X	X	X	X			X		C			X	C			
heparin	Ø	C	C	C	X	Ø	C	C	X				C	C	C	C	C	Ø
lansoprazole	X	X	X	X		X					X	X	X	X		X	X	X
levofloxacin		C		C		X	X		X								C	C
lorazepam		C							X		C				Ø	C		C
magnesium		C		C					Ø		C				C			C
methylprednisolone	■	C	X	C					X		X				X			
metronidazole	C	■	C	C					X									
midazolam	X	C	■	C		C	C	C	X		Ø				C	C	X	C
morphine	C	C	C	■	C		C	C	X		C				C			C
nesiritide				C	■	C	C	C										
nitroglycerin			C		C	■			X						C	C		
nitroprusside			C	C	C		■		X									
norepinephrine			C	C	C			■	X		C				C			
pantoprazole	X	X	X	X		X	X	X	■	X	C	X	X		X	X	X	C
piperacillin & tazobactam									X	■								
potassium chloride	X		Ø	C				C	C		■		C	C	C		C	
potassium phosphate									X			■						
prochlorperazine									X		C		■		C			
promethazine											C			■				
propofol	X		X	C		C		C	X		C		C		■	C	C	C
ranitidine			C			C			X						C	■		
sodium bicarbonate			X						X		C				C		■	
vancomycin			C	C					C						C			■

Chart created using the King Guide to Parental Admixtures, available through Lexi-Drugs Online www.lexi.com.

CORTICOSTEROIDS

Corticosteroids, Systemic Equivalencies

Glucocorticoid	Approximate Equivalent Dose (mg)	Routes of Administration	Relative Anti-inflammatory Potency	Relative Mineralocorticoid Potency	Protein Binding (%)	Half-life Plasma (min)
Short-Acting						
Cortisone	25	P.O., I.M.	0.8	0.8	90	30
Hydrocortisone	20	I.M., I.V.	1	1	90	90
Intermediate-Acting						
Methylprednisolone[1]	4	P.O., I.M., I.V.	5	0	—	180
Prednisolone	5	P.O., I.M., I.V., intra-articular, intradermal, soft tissue injection	4	0.8	90-95	200
Prednisone	5	P.O.	4	0.8	70	60
Triamcinolone[1]	4	I.M., intra-articular, intradermal, intrasynovial, soft tissue injection	5	0	—	300
Long-Acting						
Betamethasone	0.75	P.O., I.M., intra-articular, intradermal, intrasynovial, soft tissue injection	25	0	64	100-300
Dexamethasone	0.75	P.O., I.M., I.V., intra-articular, intradermal, soft tissue injection	25-30	0	—	100-300
Mineralocorticoids						
Fludrocortisone	—	P.O.	10	125	42	200

[1]May contain propylene glycol as an excipient in injectable forms.

Reference

Asare K, "Diagnosis and Treatment of Adrenal Insufficiency in the Critically Ill Patient," *Pharmacotherapy*, 2007, 27(11):1512-28.

GUIDELINES FOR SELECTION AND USE OF TOPICAL CORTICOSTEROIDS

The quantity prescribed and the frequency of refills should be monitored to reduce the risk of adrenal suppression. In general, short courses of high-potency agents are preferable to prolonged use of low potency. After control is achieved, control should be maintained with a low potency preparation.

1. Low-to-medium potency agents are usually effective for treating thin, acute, inflammatory skin lesions; whereas, high or super-potent agents are often required for treating chronic, hyperkeratotic, or lichenified lesions.
2. Since the stratum corneum is thin on the face and intertriginous areas, low-potency agents are preferred but a higher potency agent may be used for 2 weeks.
3. Because the palms and soles have a thick stratum corneum, high or super-potent agents are frequently required.
4. Low potency agents are preferred for infants and the elderly. Infants have a high body surface area to weight ratio; elderly patients have thin, fragile skin.
5. The vehicle in which the topical corticosteroid is formulated influences the absorption and potency of the drug. Ointment bases are preferred for thick, lichenified lesions; they enhance penetration of the drug. Creams are preferred for acute and subacute dermatoses; they may be used on moist skin areas or intertriginous areas. Solutions, gels, and sprays are preferred for the scalp or for areas where a nonoil-based vehicle is needed.
6. In general, super-potent agents should not be used for longer than 2-3 weeks unless the lesion is limited to a small body area. Medium-to-high potency agents usually cause only rare adverse effects when treatment is limited to 3 months or less, and use on the face and intertriginous areas are avoided. If long-term treatment is needed, intermittent vs continued treatment is recommended.
7. Most preparations are applied once or twice daily. More frequent application may be necessary for the palms or soles because the preparation is easily removed by normal activity and penetration is poor due to a thick stratum corneum. Every-other-day or week-end-only application may be effective for treating some chronic conditions.

Corticosteroids, Topical

	Steroid	Dosage Form
	Very High Potency	
0.05%	Betamethasone dipropionate, augmented	Cream, gel, lotion, ointment
0.05%	Clobetasol propionate	Cream, foam, gel, lotion, ointment, shampoo, spray
0.05%	Diflorasone diacetate	Ointment
0.05%	Halobetasol propionate	Cream, ointment
	High Potency	
0.1%	Amcinonide	Cream, ointment, lotion
0.05%	Betamethasone dipropionate, augmented	Cream
0.05%	Betamethasone dipropionate	Cream, ointment
0.1%	Betamethasone valerate	Ointment
0.05%	Desoximetasone	Gel
0.25%	Desoximetasone	Cream, ointment
0.05%	Diflorasone diacetate	Cream, ointment
0.05%	Fluocinonide	Cream, ointment, gel
0.1%	Halcinonide	Cream, ointment
0.5%	Triamcinolone acetonide	Cream, spray
	Intermediate Potency	
0.05%	Betamethasone dipropionate	Lotion
0.1%	Betamethasone valerate	Cream
0.1%	Clocortolone pivalate	Cream
0.05%	Desoximetasone	Cream
0.025%	Fluocinolone acetonide	Cream, ointment
0.05%	Flurandrenolide	Cream, ointment, lotion, tape
0.005%	Fluticasone propionate	Ointment
0.05%	Fluticasone propionate	Cream, lotion
0.1%	Hydrocortisone butyrate[1]	Ointment, solution
0.2%	Hydrocortisone valerate[1]	Cream, ointment

Corticosteroids, Topical *(continued)*

	Steroid	Dosage Form
0.1%	Mometasone furoate[1]	Cream, ointment, lotion
0.1%	Prednicarbate	Cream, ointment
0.025%	Triamcinolone acetonide	Cream, ointment, lotion
0.1%	Triamcinolone acetonide	Cream, ointment, lotion
	Low Potency	
0.05%	Alclometasone dipropionate[1]	Cream, ointment
0.05%	Desonide	Cream, ointment
0.01%	Fluocinolone acetonide	Cream, solution
0.5%	Hydrocortisone[1]	Cream, ointment, lotion
0.5%	Hydrocortisone acetate[1]	Cream, ointment
1%	Hydrocortisone acetate[1]	Cream, ointment
1%	Hydrocortisone[1]	Cream, ointment, lotion, solution
2.5%	Hydrocortisone[1]	Cream, ointment, lotion

[1]Not fluorinated.

INTRAVENOUS IMMUNE GLOBULIN

Brand Name	FDA-Approved Indications	Labeled Contraindications	IgA Content	Half-Life	pH	Osmolarity / Osmolality	Recommended Infusion Rates	Additional Comments
Carimune® NF	Primary immunodeficiency; ITP	IgA deficiency with IgA antibody; severe systemic reaction to human immune globulins	720 mcg/mL	3 weeks	6.4-6.8	3% solution in NS: 498 mOsmol/kg 6% solution in NS: 690 mOsmol/kg 9% solution in NS: 882 mOsmol/kg 12% solution in NS: 1074 mOsmol/kg 3% solution in D_5W: 444 mOsmol/kg 6% solution in D_5W: 636 mOsmol/kg 9% solution in D_5W: 828 mOsmol/kg 12% solution in D_5W: 1020 mOsmol/kg 3% solution in SWFI: 192 mOsmol/kg 6% solution in SWFI: 384 mOsmol/kg 9% solution in SWFI: 576 mOsmol/kg 12% solution in SWFI: 768 mOsmol/kg	Initial (3% solution): 0.5-1 mL/min Maximum (3% solution): 2 mg/kg/min	Contains sucrose
Flebogamma®	Primary immunodeficiency	selective IgA deficiency; hyperprolimia (Privigen); hypersensitvity to immune globulin	<50 mcg/mL	30-32 days	5-6	240-370 mOsmol/L	Initial (5% solution): 0.01 mL/kg/min (0.5 mg/kg/min) Maximum (5% solution): 0.1 mL/kg/min (5 mg/kg/min) Maximum in patients with renal dysfunction (5% solution): 0.06 mL/kg/min (3 mg/kg/min)	Contains sorbitol

continued

Brand Name	FDA-Approved Indications	Labeled Contraindications	IgA Content	Half-Life	pH	Osmolarity / Osmolality	Recommended Infusion Rates	Additional Comments
Flebogamma® DIF	Primary immunodeficiency	IgA deficiency with IgA antibody; history of anaphylaxis with immune globulin	<50 mcg/mL	30-32 days	5-6	240-370 mOsmol/L	Initial (5% solution): 0.01 mL/kg/min (0.5 mg/kg/min) Maximum (5% solution): 0.1 mL/kg/min (5 mg/kg/min) Maximum in patients with renal dysfunction (5% solution): 0.06 mL/kg/min (3 mg/kg/min)	Contains sorbitol
Gammagard® Liquid	Primary immunodeficiency	IgA deficiency, history of anaphylaxis with immune globulin	37 mcg/mL	35 days	4.6-5.1	240-300 mOsmol/kg	Initial (10% solution): 0.5 mL/kg/h (0.8 mg/kg/min) Maximum (10% solution): 5 mL/kg/h (8.9 mg/kg/min); <2 mL/kg/h (3.3 mg/kg/min) in patients at risk for renal impairment or thrombosis	
Gammagard S/D®	Primary immunodeficiency, ITP, CLL, Kawasaki syndrome	IgA deficiency	≤1 mcg/mL	~23-53 days	6.4-7.2		Initial (5% solution): 0.5 mL/kg/h Maximum (5% solution): 4 mL/kg/h Maximum concentration for infusion: 10%	Contains glucose
Gamunex®	Primary immunodeficiency, ITP, chronic inflammatory demyelinating polyneuropathy (CIDP)	IgA deficiency with IgA antibody; history of anaphylaxis with immune globulin	46 mcg/mL	35 days	4-4.5	258 mOsmol/kg	Initial (10% solution): 0.01 mL/kg/min Maximum (10% solution): 0.08 mL/kg/min Maximum concentration for infusion: 10%	

Brand Name	FDA-Approved Indications	Labeled Contraindications	IgA Content	Half-Life	pH	Osmolarity / Osmolality	Recommended Infusion Rates	Additional Comments
Octagam®	Primary immunodeficiency	IgA deficiency with IgA antibody	≤200 mcg/mL	Immuno-deficiency: 40 days	5.1-6.0	310-380 mOsmol/kg	Initial: 30 mg/kg/h (0.01 mL/kg/min) Maximum: <200 mg/kg/h (<0.07 mL/kg/min) Maximum concentration for infusion: 5%	Contains maltose
Privigen®	Primary immunodeficiency, ITP	IgA deficiency; history of anaphylaxis with immune globulin; hyperprolinemia	≤25 mcg/mL	~37 days	4.6-5	240-440 mOsmol/kg	Initial: 0.5 mg/kg/min (0.005 mL/kg/min) Maximum primary immunodeficiency: 8 mg/kg/min (0.08 mL/kg/min; ITP: 4 mg/kg/min (0.04 mL/kg/min) Maximum concentration for solution: 10%	L-proline

Carimune® NF prescribing information, ZLB Behring LLC, Kankakee, IL, January 2005.

Flebogamma® 5% prescribing information, Grifols Biologicals, Inc, Los Angeles, CA, December 2009.

Gammagard Liquid prescribing information, Baxter Healthcare Corporation, Westlake Village, CA, April 2005.

Gammagard S/D prescribing information, Baxter Healthcare Corporation, Westlake Village, CA, March 2007.

Gamunex® prescribing information, Talecris Biotherapeutics, Inc, Research Triangle Park, NC, September 2008.

Octagam® prescribing information, Octapharma USA, Inc, Centreville, VA, March 2007.

Privigen® prescribing information, CSL Behring, King of Prussia, PA, July 2007.

NONSALICYLATE / NONSTEROIDAL ANTI-INFLAMMATORY AGENTS

Name	Plasma Half-Life (h)	Time to Peak[1] (h)	Usual Duration (h)	Maximum Recommended Daily Dose (mg)	Considerations
Celecoxib (Celebrex®)	11	~3	12	400	Selective COX-2 inhibitor
Choline magnesium trisalicylate	2-30	2	8-24	4500	Nonacetylated salicylates: limited antiplatelet effects
Diclofenac potassium immediate release (Cataflam®)	~2	1	8	200 day 1; 150 thereafter	Less GI distress, less CNS depression
Diclofenac sodium delayed release (Voltaren®-XR)	~2	5	8-12	200	Less GI distress, less CNS depression
Diflunisal	8-12	2-3	8-12	1500	
Etodolac	5-8	1-2	6-8	1000	Less GI distress
Fenoprofen (Nalfon®)	2.5-3	~2	4-6	3200	Increased nephrotoxicity, increased antiplatelet activity
Flurbiprofen (Ansaid®)	5.7	1.5	6-12	300	Increased GI distress
Ibuprofen (Motrin®, Advil®)	2-4	1-2	4-6	3200	Less GI distress, moderately increased nephrotoxicity
Indomethacin (Indocin®)	4.5	2	4-6	200	Increased nephrotoxicity, GI distress, and CNS depression
Indomethacin SR, (Indocin® SR)	4.5-6	2-4	6-12	150	
Ketoprofen	2-4	0.5-2	4-6	300	
Ketoprofen, extended release	~3-7.5	6-7	–	200	
Ketorolac (Toradol®)	2-6	1	6-8	P.O.: 40[2] I.M.: 120	Increased nephrotoxicity and GI distress
Meclofenamate (Meclomen®)	0.8-2.1	0.5-1.5	2-4	400	Less hepatic injury, increased GI distress
Mefenamic acid (Ponstel®)	~2	2-4	≤6	1500	
Meloxicam (Mobic®)	15-20	4-5	>24	15	
Nabumetone (Relafen®)	24	2.5-4	>24	2000	Less GI distress
Naproxen (Aleve®, Naprosyn®)	12-17	1-4	≤7	1500	Less GI distress
Naproxen sodium (Anaprox®)	12-17	1-4	≤7	1375	
Oxaprozin (Daypro™)	40-50	2-4	>24	1800	Less GI distress
Piroxicam (Feldene®)	50	P.O.: 3-5	24	20	Less hepatic injury
Salsalate	7-8	2	8-24	3000	Nonacetylated salicylates: limited antiplatelet effects
Sulindac (Clinoril®)	8 (16)[3]	3-4	12	400	
Tolmetin	5	0.5-1	6-8	1800	

Dosage is based on a 70 kg adult with normal hepatic and renal function.

[1]Food decreases the rate of absorption and may delay the time to peak levels.

[2]150 mg on the first day.

[3]Half-life of active sulfide metabolite.

OPIOID ANALGESICS

This table serves as a general guide to opioid conversion. Utilization of a direct conversion without a detailed patients and medication assessment is not recommended and may result in over- or underdosing. Chronic administration may alter pharmacokinetics and change parenteral:oral ratio.

Opioid Analgesics – Initial Oral Dosing Commonly Used for Severe Pain

Drug	Equianalgesic Dose (mg)		Initial Oral Dose	
	Oral[1]	Parenteral[2]	Children[3] (mg/kg)	Adults (mg)
Buprenorphine	—	0.4	—	—
Butorphanol	—	2	—	—
Fentanyl	—	0.1	—	—
Hydromorphone	7.5	1.5	0.06	2-4
Levorphanol	Acute: 4 Chronic: 1	Acute: 2 Chronic: 1	0.04	2-4
Meperidine[4]	300	75	Not recommended	
Methadone[5]	See Guidelines for Conversion to Oral Methadone in Adults	Variable	0.2	5-10
Morphine	30	10	0.3	15-30
Nalbuphine	—	10	—	—
Pentazocine	50	30	—	—
Oxycodone	15-30	—	0.2	10-20
Oxymorphone	10	1	—	5-10

Guidelines for Conversion to Oral Methadone in Adults[5]

Oral Morphine Dose or Equivalent (mg/day)	Oral Morphine:Oral Methadone (Conversion Ratio)
<90	4:1
90-300	8:1
>300	12:1

[1]Elderly: Starting dose should be lower for this population group.

[2]Standard parenteral doses (I.M.) for acute pain in adults; can be used to convert doses for I.V. infusions and repeated small I.V. boluses. For single I.V. boluses, use half the I.M. dose.

[3]The pharmacokinetics of opioids in children and infants >6 months old are similar to adults but infants <6 months old, especially premature or physically compromised ones, are at risk of apnea.

[4]Not recommended for routine use.

[5]Conversion of higher doses may be guided by the following (consult a pain or palliative care specialist if unfamiliar with methadone prescribing): As the total daily chronic dose of morphine increases, the equianalgesic dose ratio (morphine:methadone) changes (American Pain Society, 2008). Total daily dose should be divided by 3; delivered every 8 hours. Methadone is significantly more potent with repetitive dosing (due to its active metabolite). Begin methadone at lower doses and gradually titrate. Applicability to pediatric patients is unknown.

References

National Cancer Institute, "Pain (PDQ®)," Last Modified 5/7/09. Available at http://www.cancer.gov/cancertopics/pdq/supportivecare/pain/HealthProfessional/page1.

National Comprehensive Cancer Network® (NCCN), "Clinical Practice Guidelines in Oncology™: Adult Cancer Pain," Version 1, 2009. Available at http://www.nccn.org/professionals/physician_gls/PDF/pain.pdf.

Patanwala AE, Duby J, Waters D, et al, "Opioid Conversions in Acute Care," *Ann Pharmacother*, 2007, 41(2):255-66.

Principles of Analgesic Use in the Treatment of Acute Pain and Cancer Pain, 6th ed, Glenview, IL: American Pain Society, 2008.

THIAZOLIDINEDIONES

Lipid Effects

Parameter	Pioglitazone (Actos®)	Rosiglitazone (Avandia®)
LDL	↑ up to 7%	↑ up to 18.6%
HDL	↑ up to 13%	↑ up to 18.5%
Total cholesterol	No significant change	↑
Total cholesterol/HDL ratio	↓	↓
LDL/HDL ratio	Slightly ↓	No change
Triglycerides	↓ up to 26%	Variable effects

Thiazolidinedione Pharmacokinetics

Parameter	Pioglitazone (Actos®)	Rosiglitazone (Avandia®)
Absorption	Food slightly delays but does not alter the extent of absorption	Absolute bioavailability is 99% Food ↓ C_{max} and delays T_{max}, but not change in AUC
T_{max}	2 h	1 h
Distribution	0.63 L	17.6 L
Plasma protein binding	>99% to serum albumin	99.8% to serum albumin
Metabolism	Extensive liver metabolism by hydroxylation and oxidation. Some metabolites are pharmacologically active. CYP2C8 and CYP3A4 metabolism	Extensive liver metabolism via N-demethylation and hydroxylation with no unchanged drug excreted in the urine CYP2C8 and some CYP2C9 metabolism
Excretion	Urine (15% to 30%) and feces	Urine (64%) and feces (23%)
Half-life	Pioglitazone: 3-7 h Pioglitazone and metabolites: 16-24 h	3-4 h
Effect of hemodialysis	Not removed	Not removed

VASOACTIVE AGENTS, INTRAVENOUS

Drug	Dose	Hemodynamic Effects				
		HR	MAP	PAOP	CI	SVR
Dopamine	1-3 mcg/kg/min	↑	0	↓	0/↑	0/↓
	3-10 mcg/kg/min	↑	↑	0	↑	0
	>10-20 mcg/kg/min	↑↑	↑↑	0	↑	↑
Epinephrine	0.01-0.05 mcg/kg/min	↑	↑	0/↓	↑↑	0/↓
	>0.05 mcg/kg/min	↑↑	↑↑	↑	↑↑	↑↑
Norepinephrine	0.02-3 mcg/kg/min	0/↑	↑↑↑	↑↑	0/↓/↑	↑↑↑
Phenylephrine	0.5-9 mcg/kg/min	0/↓	↑	↑	0/↓/↑	↑↑↑
Vasopressin	0.04 units/min	0/↓	↑↑	↑	0/↓	↑↑
Dobutamine	2-10 mcg/kg/min	0/↑	↑	↓	↑	0/↓
	>10-20 mcg/kg/min	↑↑	↓/↑	↓	↑↑	↓
Milrinone	0.375-0.75 mcg/kg/min	↑↑	0/↓/↑	↓	↑	↓↓
Nesiritide	2 mcg/kg bolus	0	↓	↓	0/↑	↓
	0.01-0.03 mcg/kg/min					
Nitroglycerin	0.1-2 mcg/kg/min	0/↑	0/↓	↓	0/↑	↓
Nitroprusside	0.25-10 mcg/kg/min	0/↑↑	0/↓↓	↓	↑/↑↑	↓/↓↓

HR = heart rate; MAP = mean arterial pressure; PAOP = pulmonary artery occlusion pressure; CI = cardiac index; SVR = systemic vascular resistance.

↑ = increase; ↓ = decrease; 0 = no change.

Drug	Dose	Receptor Activity						
		α_1	α_2	β_1	β_2	DA_1	V_1	V_2
Dobutamine	2-10 mcg/kg/min	+	0	+++	++	0	0	0
	>10-20 mcg/kg/min	++	0	++++	+++	0	0	0
Dopamine	1-3 mcg/kg/min	0	0	+	0	++++	0	0
	3-10 mcg/kg/min	0/+	0	++++	++	++++	0	0
	>10-20 mcg/kg/min	+++	0	++++	+	0	0	0
Epinephrine	0.01-0.05 mcg/kg/min	++	++	++++	+++	0	0	0
	>0.05 mcg/kg/min	++++	++++	+++	+	0	0	0
Norepinephrine	0.02-3 mcg/kg/min	++++	++	++	0	0	0	0
Phenylephrine	0.5-9 mcg/kg/min	++++	+	0	0	0	0	0
Vasopressin	0.04 units/min	0	0	0	0	0	+++	+

Activity ranges from no activity (0) or maximal activity (++++).

DA = dopaminergic; V = vasopressin

SELECTED READINGS

Biaggioni I and Robertson D, "Adrenoceptor Agonists & Sympathomimetic Drugs," *Basic and Clinical Pharmacology*, 11th ed, Katzung BG, Masters SB, and Trevor AJ, eds, Stamford, CT: McGraw-Hill, 2009, 127-148.

Hollenberg SM, Ahrens TS, Annane D, et al, "Practice Parameters for Hemodynamic Support of Sepsis in Adult Patients: 2004 Update," *Crit Care Med*, 2004, 32(9):1928-48.

Hollenberg SM, "Vasopressor Support in Septic Shock," *Chest*, 2007, 132(5):1678-87.

MacLaren R, Rudis MI, and Dasta JF, "Use of Vasopressors and Inotropes in the Pharmacotherapy of Shock," *Pharmacotherapy: A Pathophysiologic Approach*, 7th ed, Dipiro JT, Talbert RL, Yee GC, et al, eds, Stamford, CT: McGraw-Hill, 2008, 417-39.

CYTOCHROME P450 ENZYMES: SUBSTRATES, INHIBITORS, AND INDUCERS

INTRODUCTION

Most drugs are eliminated from the body, at least in part, by being chemically altered to less lipid-soluble products (ie, metabolized), and thus are more likely to be excreted via the kidneys or the bile. Phase I metabolism includes drug hydrolysis, oxidation, and reduction, and results in drugs that are more polar in their chemical structure, while Phase II metabolism involves the attachment of an additional molecule onto the drug (or partially metabolized drug) in order to create an inactive and/or more water soluble compound. Phase II processes include (primarily) glucuronidation, sulfation, glutathione conjugation, acetylation, and methylation.

Virtually any of the Phase I and II enzymes can be inhibited by some xenobiotic or drug. Some of the Phase I and II enzymes can be induced. Inhibition of the activity of metabolic enzymes will result in increased concentrations of the substrate (drug), whereas induction of the activity of metabolic enzymes will result in decreased concentrations of the substrate. For example, the well-documented enzyme-inducing effects of phenobarbital may include a combination of Phase I and II enzymes. Phase II glucuronidation may be increased via induced UDP-glucuronosyltransferase (UGT) activity, whereas Phase I oxidation may be increased via induced cytochrome P450 (CYP) activity. However, for most drugs, the primary route of metabolism (and the primary focus of drug-drug interaction) is Phase I oxidation.

CYP enzymes may be responsible for the metabolism (at least partial metabolism) of approximately 75% of all drugs, with the CYP3A subfamily responsible for nearly half of this activity. Found throughout plant, animal, and bacterial species, CYP enzymes represent a superfamily of xenobiotic metabolizing proteins. There have been several hundred CYP enzymes identified in nature, each of which has been assigned to a family (1, 2, 3, etc), subfamily (A, B, C, etc), and given a specific enzyme number (1, 2, 3, etc) according to the similarity in amino acid sequence that it shares with other enzymes. Of these many enzymes, only a few are found in humans, and even fewer appear to be involved in the metabolism of xenobiotics (eg, drugs). The key human enzyme subfamilies include CYP1A, CYP2A, CYP2B, CYP2C, CYP2D, CYP2E, and CYP3A. However, the number of distinct isozymes (eg, CYP2C9) found to be functionally active in humans, as well as, the number of genetically variant forms of these isozymes (eg, CYP2C9*2) in individuals continues to expand.

CYP enzymes are found in the endoplasmic reticulum of cells in a variety of human tissues (eg, skin, kidneys, brain, lungs), but their predominant sites of concentration and activity are the liver and intestine. Though the abundance of CYP enzymes throughout the body is relatively equally distributed among the various subfamilies, the relative contribution to drug metabolism is (in decreasing order of magnitude) CYP3A4 (nearly 50%), CYP2D6 (nearly 25%), CYP2C8/9 (nearly 15%), then CYP1A2, CYP2C19, CYP2A6, and CYP2E1. Owing to their potential for numerous drug-drug interactions, those drugs that are identified in preclinical studies as substrates of CYP3A enzymes are often given a lower priority for continued research and development in favor of drugs that appear to be less affected by (or less likely to affect) this enzyme subfamily.

Each enzyme subfamily possesses unique selectivity toward potential substrates. For example, CYP1A2 preferentially binds medium-sized, planar, lipophilic molecules, while CYP2D6 preferentially binds molecules that possess a basic nitrogen atom. Some CYP subfamilies exhibit polymorphism (ie, genetic variation that results in a modified enzyme with small changes in amino acid sequences that may manifest differing catalytic properties). The best described polymorphisms involve CYP2C9, CYP2C19, and CYP2D6. Individuals possessing "wild type" genes exhibit normal functioning CYP capacity. Others, however, possess genetic variants that leave the person with a subnormal level of catalytic potential (so called "poor metabolizers"). Poor metabolizers would be more likely to experience toxicity from drugs metabolized by the affected enzymes (or less effects if the enzyme is responsible for converting a prodrug to it's active form as in the case of codeine). The percentage of people classified as poor metabolizers varies by enzyme and population group. As an example, approximately 7% of Caucasians and only about 1% of Asians appear to be CYP2D6 poor metabolizers.

CYP enzymes can be both inhibited and induced by other drugs, leading to increased or decreased serum concentrations (along with the associated effects), respectively. Induction occurs when a drug causes an increase in the amount of smooth endoplasmic reticulum, secondary to increasing the amount of the affected CYP enzymes in the tissues. This "revving up" of the CYP enzyme system may take several days to reach peak activity, and likewise, may take several days, even months, to return to normal following discontinuation of the inducing agent.

CYP inhibition occurs via several potential mechanisms. Most commonly, a CYP inhibitor competitively (and reversibly) binds to the active site on the enzyme, thus preventing the substrate from binding to the same site, and preventing the substrate from being metabolized. The affinity of an inhibitor for an enzyme may be expressed by an inhibition constant (Ki) or IC50 (defined as the concentration of the inhibitor required to cause 50% inhibition under a given set of conditions). In addition to reversible competition for an enzyme site, drugs may inhibit enzyme activity by binding to sites on the enzyme other than that to which the substrate would bind, and thereby cause a change in the functionality or physical structure of the enzyme. A drug may also bind to the enzyme in an irreversible (ie, "suicide") fashion. In such a case, it is not the concentration of drug at the enzyme site that is important (constantly binding and releasing), but the number of molecules available for binding (once bound, always bound).

Although an inhibitor or inducer may be known to affect a variety of CYP subfamilies, it may only inhibit one or two in a clinically important fashion. Likewise, although a substrate is known to be at least partially metabolized by a variety of CYP enzymes, only one or two enzymes may contribute significantly enough to its overall metabolism to warrant concern when used with potential inducers or inhibitors. Therefore, when attempting to predict the level of risk of using two drugs that may affect each other via altered CYP function, it is important to identify the relative effectiveness of the inhibiting/inducing drug on the CYP subfamilies that significantly contribute to the metabolism of the substrate. The contribution of a specific CYP pathway to substrate metabolism should be considered not only in light of other known CYP pathways, but also other nonoxidative pathways for substrate metabolism (eg, glucuronidation) and transporter proteins (eg, P-glycoprotein) that may affect the presentation of a substrate to a metabolic pathway.

Selected Readings

Bjornsson TD, Callaghan JT, Einolf HJ, et al, "The Conduct of *in vitro* and *in vivo* Drug-Drug Interaction Studies: A PhRMA Perspective," *J Clin Pharmacol*, 2003, 43(5):443-69.

Drug-Drug Interactions, Rodrigues AD, ed, New York, NY: Marcel Dekker, Inc, 2002.

Levy RH, Thummel KE, Trager WF, et al, eds, *Metabolic Drug Interactions*, Philadelphia, PA: Lippincott Williams & Wilkins, 2000.

Michalets EL, "Update: Clinically Significant Cytochrome P-450 Drug Interactions," *Pharmacotherapy*, 1998, 18(1):84-112.

Thummel KE and Wilkinson GR, " *In vitro* and *in vivo* Drug Interactions Involving Human CYP3A," *Annu Rev Pharmacol Toxicol*, 1998, 38:389-430.

Zhang Y and Benet LZ, "The Gut as a Barrier to Drug Absorption: Combined Role of Cytochrome P450 3A and P-Glycoprotein," *Clin Pharmacokinet*, 2001, 40(3):159-68.

Selected Websites

http://www.imm.ki.se/CYPalleles
http://medicine.iupui.edu/flockhart
http://www.fda.gov/Drugs/DevelopmentApprovalProcess/DevelopmentResources/DrugInteraction-sLabeling/ucm080499.htm

ANTIMICROBIAL DRUGS OF CHOICE

Empirical treatment of some common infecting organisms is listed below. These recommendations are based on results of susceptibility studies, clinical trials, and the opinions of *Medical Letter* consultants. The site and severity of the infection, pharmacokinetic characteristics of antibiotics, local resistance patterns, potential drug interactions, and specific patient factors should be taken into account in choosing an appropriate regimen.

Infecting Organism	Drug of First Choice	Alternative Drugs
GRAM-POSITIVE COCCI		
**Enterococcus* spp.[1]		
endocarditis or other severe infection	Penicillin G or ampicillin + gentamicin or streptomycin[2]	Vancomycin + gentamicin or streptomycin[2]; linezolid[3]; daptomycin[4]; quinupristin/dalfopristin[5]
uncomplicated urinary tract infection	Ampicillin or amoxicillin	Nitrofurantoin; a fluoroquinolone[6]; fosfomycin
**Staphylococcus aureus* or *epidermidis*		
methicillin-susceptible	A penicillinase-resistant penicillin[7]	A cephalosporin[8,9]; vancomycin; imipenem or meropenem; clindamycin; linezolid[3]; daptomycin[4]; a fluoroquinolone[6]
methicillin-resistant[10]	Vancomycin ± gentamicin ± rifampin	Linezolid[3]; daptomycin[4]; tigecycline[11]; a fluoroquinolone[6]; trimethoprim/sulfamethoxazole; quinupristin/dalfopristin; a doxycycline[11]
Streptococcus pyogenes (group A[12]) and groups C and G	Penicillin G or V[13]	Clindamycin; erythromycin; a cephalosporin[8,9]; vancomycin; clarithromycin[14]; azithromycin; linezolid[3]; daptomycin[4]
Streptococcus, group B	Penicillin G or ampicillin	A cephalosporin[8,9]; vancomycin; daptomycin[4]; erythromycin
**Streptococcus*, viridans group[1]	Penicillin G ± gentamicin	A cephalosporin[8,9]; vancomycin
Streptococcus bovis	Penicillin G	A cephalosporin[8,9]; vancomycin
Streptococcus, anaerobic or *Peptostreptococcus*	Penicillin G	Clindamycin; a cephalosporin[8,9]; vancomycin
**Streptococcus pneumoniae*[15] (pneumococcus)		
penicillin-susceptible (MIC <0.1 mcg/mL)	Penicillin G or V[13]; amoxicillin	A cephalosporin[8,9]; erythromycin; azithromycin; clarithromycin[14]; levofloxacin, gemifloxacin, or moxifloxacin[6]; meropenem, imipenem, or ertapenem; trimethoprim/sulfamethoxazole; clindamycin; a tetracycline[11]; vancomycin
penicillin-intermediate resistance (MIC 0.1-1 mcg/mL)	Penicillin G I.V. (12 million units/day for adults); ceftriaxone or cefotaxime	Levofloxacin, gemifloxacin, or moxifloxacin[6]; vancomycin; clindamycin
penicillin-high level resistance (MIC ≥2 mcg/mL)	**Meningitis:** Vancomycin + ceftriaxone or cefotaxime, ± rifampin	
	Other Infections: Vancomycin + ceftriaxone or cefotaxime; levofloxacin, gemifloxacin, or moxifloxacin[6]	Linezolid[3]; quinupristin/dalfopristin
GRAM-NEGATIVE COCCI		
Moraxella (Branhamella) catarrhalis	Cefuroxime[8]; a fluoroquinolone[6]	Trimethoprim/sulfamethoxazole; amoxicillin/clavulanate; erythromycin; clarithromycin[14]; azithromycin; doxycycline[11]; cefotaxime[8]; ceftizoxime[8]; ceftriaxone[8]; cefpodoxime[8]
**Neisseria gonorrhoeae* (gonococcus)[16]	Ceftriaxone[8]	Cefixime[8]; cefotaxime[8]; penicillin G

Infecting Organism	Drug of First Choice	Alternative Drugs
Neisseria meningitidis[17] (meningococcus)	Penicillin G	Cefotaxime[8]; ceftizoxime[8]; ceftriaxone[8]; chloramphenicol[18]; a sulfonamide[19]; a fluoroquinolone[6]
GRAM-POSITIVE BACILLI		
**Bacillus anthracis*[20] (anthrax)	Ciprofloxacin[6]; a tetracycline[11]	Penicillin G; amoxicillin; erythromycin; imipenem; clindamycin; levofloxacin[6]
Bacillus cereus, subtilis	Vancomycin	Imipenem or meropenem; clindamycin
Clostridium perfringens[21]	Penicillin G; clindamycin	Metronidazole; imipenem, meropenem, or ertapenem; chloramphenicol[18]
Clostridium tetani[22]	Metronidazole	Penicillin G; a doxycycline[11]
Clostridium difficile[23]	Metronidazole (oral)	Vancomycin (oral)
Corynebacterium diphtheriae[24]	Erythromycin	Penicillin G
Corynebacterium, jeikeium	Vancomycin	Penicillin G + gentamicin; erythromycin
**Erysipelothrix rhusiopathiae*	Penicillin G	Erythromycin; a cephalosporin[8,9]; a fluoroquinolone[6]
Listeria monocytogenes	Ampicillin ± gentamicin	Trimethoprim/sulfamethoxazole
ENTERIC GRAM-NEGATIVE BACILLI		
**Campylobacter fetus*	A third-generation cephalosporin[9]; gentamicin	Ampicillin; imipenem or meropenem
**Campylobacter jejuni*	Erythromycin or azithromycin	A fluoroquinolone[6]; a tetracycline[11]; gentamicin
**Citrobacter freundi*	Imipenem or meropenem[25]	A fluoroquinolone[6]; ertapenem; amikacin; doxycycline[11]; trimethoprim/sulfamethoxazole; cefotaxime[8,25], ceftizoxime[8,25], ceftriaxone[8,25], cefepime[8,25] or ceftazidime[8,25]
**Enterobacter* spp.	Imipenem or meropenem[25]; cefepime[8,25]	Gentamicin, tobramycin or amikacin; trimethoprim/sulfamethoxazole; ciprofloxacin[6]; ticarcillin/clavulanate[26] or piperacillin/tazobactam[26]; aztreonam[25]; cefotaxime, ceftizoxime, ceftriaxone, or ceftazidime[8,25]; tigecycline[11]
**Escherichia coli*[27]	Cefotaxime, ceftriaxone, cefepime, or ceftazidime[8,25]	Ampicillin ± gentamicin, tobramycin, or amikacin; gentamicin, tobramycin, or amikacin; amoxicillin/clavulanate; ticarcillin/clavulanate[26]; piperacillin/tazobactam[26]; ampicillin/sulbactam[25]; trimethoprim/sulfamethoxazole; imipenem, meropenem, or ertapenem[25]; aztreonam[25]; a fluoroquinolone[6]; another cephalosporin[8,9]; tigecycline[11]
**Klebsiella pneumoniae*[27]	Cefotaxime, ceftriaxone, cefepime, or ceftazidime[8,25]	Imipenem, meropenem, or ertapenem[25]; gentamicin, tobramycin, or amikacin; amoxicillin/clavulanate; ticarcillin/clavulanate[26]; piperacillin/tazobactam[26]; ampicillin/sulbactam[25]; trimethoprim/sulfamethoxazole; aztreonam[25]; a fluoroquinolone[6]; another cephalosporin[8,9]; tigecycline[11]
**Proteus mirabilis*[27]	Ampicillin[28]	A cephalosporin[8,9,25]; ticarcillin/clavulanate or piperacillin/tazobactam[26]; gentamicin, tobramycin, or amikacin; trimethoprim/sulfamethoxazole; imipenem, meropenem, or ertapenem[25]; aztreonam[25]; a fluoroquinolone[6]; chloramphenicol[18]
**Proteus*, indole-positive (including *Providencia rettgeri, Morganella morganii*, and *Proteus vulgaris*)	Cefotaxime, ceftriaxone, cefepime, or ceftazidime[8,25]	Imipenem, meropenem, or ertapenem[25]; gentamicin, tobramycin, or amikacin; amoxicillin/clavulanate; ticarcillin/clavulanate[26]; piperacillin/tazobactam[26]; ampicillin/sulbactam[25]; aztreonam[25]; trimethoprim/sulfamethoxazole; a fluoroquinolone[6]

(continued)

Infecting Organism	Drug of First Choice	Alternative Drugs
**Providencia stuartii*	Cefotaxime, ceftriaxone, cefepime, or ceftazidime[8,25]	Imipenem, meropenem, or ertapenem[25]; ticarcillin/clavulanate[26]; piperacillin/tazobactam[26]; gentamicin, tobramycin, or amikacin; aztreonam[25]; trimethoprim/sulfamethoxazole; a fluoroquinolone[6]
**Salmonella typhi* (typhoid fever)[29]	A fluoroquinolone[6] or ceftriaxone[8]	Chloramphenicol[18]; trimethoprim/sulfamethoxazole; ampicillin; amoxicillin; azithromycin[30]
*Other *Salmonella* spp.[31]	Cefotaxime[8] or ceftriaxone[8] or a fluoroquinolone[6]	Ampicillin or amoxicillin; trimethoprim/sulfamethoxazole; chloramphenicol[18]
**Serratia* spp.	Imipenem or meropenem[25]	Gentamicin or amikacin; cefotaxime, ceftizoxime, ceftriaxone, cefepime, or ceftazidime[8,25]; aztreonam[25]; trimethoprim/sulfamethoxazole; a fluoroquinolone[6]
**Shigella* spp.	A fluoroquinolone[6]	Azithromycin; trimethoprim/sulfamethoxazole; ampicillin; ceftriaxone[8]
**Yersinia enterocolitica*	Trimethoprim/sulfamethoxazole	A fluoroquinolone[6]; gentamicin, tobramycin, or amikacin; cefotaxime[8]
OTHER GRAM-NEGATIVE BACILLI		
**Acinetobacter*	Imipenem or meropenem[25]	An aminoglycoside; ciprofloxacin[6]; trimethoprim/sulfamethoxazole; ticarcillin/clavulanate[26] or piperacillin/tazobactam[26]; ceftazidime[25]; doxycycline[11]; sulbactam[32]; colistin[18]
**Aeromonas*	Trimethoprim/sulfamethoxazole	Gentamicin or tobramycin; imipenem; a fluoroquinolone[6]
**Bacteroides*	Metronidazole	Imipenem, meropenem, or ertapenem; amoxicillin/clavulanate; ticarcillin/clavulanate; piperacillin/tazobactam or ampicillin/sulbactam; chloramphenicol[18]
Bartonella henselae or *quintana* (bacillary angiomatosis, trench fever)	Erythromycin	Azithromycin; doxycycline[11]
Bartonella henselae[33] (cat scratch bacillus)	Azithromycin	Erythromycin; ciprofloxacin[6]; trimethoprim/sulfamethoxazole; gentamicin; rifampin
Bordetella pertussis (whooping cough)	Azithromycin; erythromycin; clarithromycin[14]	Trimethoprim/sulfamethoxazole
**Brucella* spp.	A tetracycline[11] + rifampin	A tetracycline[11] + streptomycin or gentamicin; chloramphenicol[18] ± streptomycin; trimethoprim/sulfamethoxazole ± gentamicin; ciprofloxacin[6] + rifampin
**Burkholderia cepacia*	Trimethoprim/sulfamethoxazole	Ceftazidime[8]; chloramphenicol[18]; imipenem
Burkholderia (Pseudomonas) mallei (glanders)	Streptomycin + a tetracycline[11]	Streptomycin + chloramphenicol[18]; imipenem
**Burkholderia (Pseudomonas) pseudomallei* (melioidosis)	Imipenem; ceftazidime[8]	Meropenem; chloramphenicol[18] + doxycycline[11] + trimethoprim/sulfamethoxazole; amoxicillin/clavulanate
Calymmatobacterium granulomatis (granuloma inguinale)	Trimethoprim/sulfamethoxazole	Doxycycline[11] or ciprofloxacin[6] ± gentamicin
Capnocytophaga canimorsus[34]	Penicillin G	Cefotaxime, ceftizoxime, or ceftriaxone[8]; imipenem or meropenem; vancomycin; a fluoroquinolone[6]; clindamycin
**Eikenella corrodens*	Ampicillin	Erythromycin; azithromycin; clarithromycin[14]; doxycycline[11]; amoxicillin/clavulanate; ampicillin/sulbactam; ceftriaxone[8]
**Francisella tularensis* (tularemia)[35]	Gentamicin (or streptomycin) + a tetracycline[11]	Chloramphenicol[18]; ciprofloxacin[6]
**Fusobacterium*	Penicillin G; metronidazole	Clindamycin; cefoxitin[8]; chloramphenicol[18]

Infecting Organism	Drug of First Choice	Alternative Drugs
Gardnerella vaginalis (bacterial vaginosis)	Oral metronidazole[36]	Topical clindamycin or metronidazole; oral clindamycin
**Haemophilus ducreyi* (chancroid)	Azithromycin or ceftriaxone	Ciprofloxacin[6] or erythromycin
**Haemophilus influenzae*		
meningitis, epiglottitis, arthritis, and other serious infections	Cefotaxime or ceftriaxone[8]	Cefuroxime[8] (not for meningitis); chloramphenicol[18]; meropenem
upper respiratory infections and bronchitis	Trimethoprim/ sulfamethoxazole	Cefuroxime[8]; amoxicillin/clavulanate; cefuroxime axetil[8]; cefpodoxime[8]; cefaclor[8]; cefotaxime[8]; ceftizoxime[8]; ceftriaxone[8]; cefixime[8]; doxycycline[11]; clarithromycin[14]; azithromycin; a fluoroquinolone[6]; ampicillin or amoxicillin
**Helicobacter pylori*[37]	Proton pump inhibitor[38] + clarithromycin[14] + either amoxicillin or metronidazole	Bismuth subsalicylate + metronidazole + tetracycline HCl[11] + either a proton pump inhibitor[38] or H_2-blocker[38]
Legionella species	Azithromycin or a fluoroquinolone[6] ± rifampin	Doxycycline[11] ± rifampin; trimethoprim/sulfamethoxazole; erythromycin
Leptotrichia buccalis	Penicillin G	Doxycycline[11]; clindamycin; erythromycin
Pasteurella multocida	Penicillin G	Doxycycline[11]; a second- or third-generation cephalosporin[8,9]; amoxicillin/clavulanate; ampicillin/ sulbactam
**Pseudomonas aeruginosa*		
urinary tract infection	Ciprofloxacin[6]	Levofloxacin[6]; piperacillin/ tazobactam; ceftazidime[8]; cefepime[8]; imipenem or meropenem; aztreonam; tobramycin; gentamicin or amikacin
other infections	Piperacillin/ tazobactam or ticarcillin/clavulanate, **plus/minus** tobramycin, gentamicin, or amikacin[39]	Ceftazidime[8]; ciprofloxacin[6]; imipenem or meropenem; aztreonam; cefepime[8] **plus/minus** tobramycin, gentamicin, or amikacin
Spirillum minus (rat bite fever)	Penicillin G	Doxycycline[11]; streptomycin[18]
**Stenotrophomonas maltophilia*	Trimethoprim/ sulfamethoxazole	Ticarcillin/clavulanate[26]; minocycline[11]; a fluoroquinolone[6]; tigecycline[11]
Streptobacillus moniliformis (rat bite fever, Haverhill fever)	Penicillin G	Doxycycline[11]; streptomycin[18]
Vibrio cholerae (cholera)[40]	A tetracycline[11]	A fluoroquinolone[6]; trimethoprim/ sulfamethoxazole
Vibrio vulnificus	A tetracycline[11]	Cefotaxime[8]; ciprofloxacin[14]
Yersinia pestis (plague)	Streptomycin ± a tetracycline[11]	Chloramphenicol[18]; gentamicin; trimethoprim/sulfamethoxazole; ciprofloxacin[14]
MYCOBACTERIA		
**Mycobacterium tuberculosis*[41]	Isoniazid + rifampin + pyrazinamide ± ethambutol or streptomycin[18]	A fluoroquinolone[6]; cycloserine[18]; capreomycin[18] or kanamycin[18] or amikacin[18]; ethionamide[18]; para-aminosalicylic acid[18]
**Mycobacterium kansasii*[41]	Isoniazid + rifampin ± ethambutol or streptomycin[18]	Clarithromycin[14] or azithromycin; ethionamide[18]; cycloserine[18]
**Mycobacterium avium* complex		
treatment	Clarithromycin[14] or azithromycin + ethambutol ± rifabutin	Ciprofloxacin[6]; amikacin[18]
prophylaxis	Clarithromycin[14] or azithromycin ± rifabutin	
**Mycobacterium fortuitum/ chelonae*[41] complex	Amikacin + clarithromycin[14]	Cefoxitin[8]; rifampin; a sulfonamide; doxycycline[11]; ethambutol; linezolid[3]

(continued)

Infecting Organism	Drug of First Choice	Alternative Drugs
Mycobacterium marinum (balnei)[42]	Minocycline[11]	Trimethoprim/sulfamethoxazole; rifampin; clarithromycin[14]; doxycycline[11]
Mycobacterium leprae (leprosy)	Dapsone + rifampin ± clofazimine	Minocycline[11]; ofloxacin[6]; clarithromycin[14]
ACTINOMYCETES		
Actinomyces israelii (actinomycosis)	Penicillin G	Doxycycline[11]; erythromycin; clindamycin
Nocardia	Trimethoprim/ sulfamethoxazole	Sulfisoxazole; amikacin[18]; a tetracycline[11]; ceftriaxone; imipenem or meropenem; cycloserine[18]; linezolid[3]
**Rhodococcus equi*	Vancomycin ± a fluoroquinolone,[6] rifampin, imipenem, or meropenem; amikacin	Erythromycin
Tropheryma whippelii[43] (Whipple's disease)	Trimethoprim/ sulfamethoxazole	Penicillin G; a tetracycline[11]; ceftriaxone
CHLAMYDIAE		
Chlamydia trachomatis		
trachoma	Azithromycin	Doxycycline[11]; a sulfonamide (topical plus oral)
inclusion conjunctivitis	Erythromycin (oral or I.V.)	A sulfonamide
pneumonia	Erythromycin	A sulfonamide
urethritis, cervicitis	Azithromycin or doxycycline[11]	Erythromycin; ofloxacin[6]; amoxicillin
lymphogranuloma venereum	A tetracycline[11]	Erythromycin
Chlamydophilia (formerly *Chlamydia*) *pneumoniae*	Erythromycin; a tetracycline[11]; clarithromycin[14] or azithromycin	A fluoroquinolone[6]
Chlamydophilia (formerly *Chlamydia*) *psittaci* (psittacosis, ornithosis)	A tetracycline[11]	Chloramphenicol[18]
EHRLICHIA		
Anaplasma phagocytophilum (formerly *Ehrlichia phagocytophila*)	Doxycycline[11]	Rifampin
Ehrlichia chaffeensis	Doxycycline[11]	Chloramphenicol[18]
Ehrlichia ewingii	Doxycycline[11]	
MYCOPLASMA		
Mycoplasma pneumoniae	Erythromycin; a tetracycline[11]; clarithromycin[14] or azithromycin	A fluoroquinolone[6]
Ureaplasma urealyticum	Azithromycin	Erythromycin; a tetracycline[11]; clarithromycin[14]; ofloxacin[6]
RICKETTSIOSES		
Rickettsia rickettsii (Rocky Mountain spotted fever)	Doxycycline[11]	A fluoroquinolone[6]; chloramphenicol[18]
Rickettsia typhi (endemic typhus – murine)	Doxycycline[11]	A fluoroquinolone[6]; chloramphenicol[18]
Rickettsia prowazekii (epidemic typhus – louse-borne)	Doxycycline[11]	A fluoroquinolone[6]; chloramphenicol[18]
Orientia tsutsugamushi (scrub typhus)	Doxycycline[11]	A fluoroquinolone[6]; chloramphenicol[18]
Coxiella burnetii (Q fever)	Doxycycline[11]	A fluoroquinolone[6]; chloramphenicol[18]
SPIROCHETES		
Borrelia burgdorferi (Lyme disease)[44]	Doxycycline[11]; amoxicillin; cefuroxime axetil[8]	Ceftriaxone[8]; cefotaxime[8]; penicillin G; azithromycin; clarithromycin[14]
Borrelia recurrentis (relapsing fever)	A tetracycline[11]	Penicillin G; erythromycin

Infecting Organism	Drug of First Choice	Alternative Drugs
Leptospira	Penicillin G	Doxycycline[11]; ceftriaxone[8,45]
Treponema pallidum (syphilis)	Penicillin G[13]	Doxycycline[11]; ceftriaxone[8]
Treponema pertenue (yaws)	Penicillin G	Doxycycline[11]

***Resistance may be a problem; susceptibility tests should be used to guide therapy.**

[1]Disk sensitivity testing may not provide adequate information; beta-lactamase assays, "E" tests, and dilution tests for susceptibility should be used in serious infections.

[2]Aminoglycoside resistance is increasingly common among enterococci; treatment options include ampicillin 2 g I.V. every 4 hours, continuous infusion of ampicillin, a combination of ampicillin plus a fluoroquinolone, or a combination of ampicillin, imipenem, and vancomycin.

[3]Reversible bone marrow suppression has occurred, especially with therapy for more than 2 weeks. Linezolid is an MAO inhibitor and can interact with serotonergic and adrenergic drugs and with tyramine-containing foods (Taylor JJ, Wilson JW, and Estes LL, "Linezolid and Serotonergic Drug Interactions: A Retrospective Survey," *Clin Infect Dis*, 2006, 43(2):180-7).

[4]Daptomycin should not be used to treat pneumonia.

[5]Quinupristin/dalfopristin is not active against *Enterococcus faecalis*.

[6]Among the fluoroquinolones, levofloxacin, gemifloxacin, and moxifloxacin have excellent *in vitro* activity against *S. pneumoniae*, including penicillin- and cephalosporin-resistant strains. Levofloxacin, gemifloxacin, and moxifloxacin also have good activity against many strains of *S. aureus*, but resistance has become frequent among methicillin-resistant strains. Gemifloxacin is associated with a high rate of rash; other fluoroquinolones are preferred. Ciprofloxacin has the greatest activity against *Pseudomonas aeruginosa*. For urinary tract infections, norfloxacin can be used. For tuberculosis, levofloxacin, ofloxacin, ciprofloxacin, or moxifloxacin could be used ("Drugs for Tuberculosis," *Treat Guidel Med Lett*, 2007, 5(55):15-22). Ciprofloxacin, ofloxacin, levofloxacin, and moxifloxacin are available for I.V. use. None of these agents is recommended for use in children or pregnant women.

[7]For oral use against staphylococci, cloxacillin or dicloxacillin is preferred; for severe infections, a parenteral formulation (nafcillin or oxacillin) should be used. Ampicillin, amoxicillin, carbenicillin, ticarcillin, and piperacillin are not effective against penicillinase-producing staphylococci. The combinations of clavulanate with amoxicillin or ticarcillin, sulbactam with ampicillin, and tazobactam with piperacillin may be active against these organisms.

[8]Cephalosporins have been used as alternatives to penicillins in patients allergic to penicillins, but such patients may also have allergic reactions to cephalosporins.

[9]For parenteral treatment of staphylococcal or nonenterococcal streptococcal infections, a first-generation cephalosporin such as cefazolin can be used. For oral therapy, cephalexin or cephradine can be used. The second-generation cephalosporins cefamandole, cefprozil, cefuroxime, cefotetan, cefoxitin, and loracarbef are more active than the first-generation drugs against gram-negative bacteria. Cefotetan and cefamandole are no longer available. Cefuroxime is active against ampicillin-resistant strains of *H. influenzae*. Cefoxitin is the most active of the cephalosporins against *B. fragilis*. The third-generation cephalosporins cefotaxime, cefoperazone, ceftizoxime, ceftriaxone, and ceftazidime, and the fourth-generation cefepime have greater activity than the second-generation drugs against enteric gram-negative bacilli. Ceftazidime has poor activity against many gram-positive cocci and anaerobes, and ceftizoxime has poor activity against penicillin-resistant *S. pneumoniae*. Cefepime has *in vitro* activity against gram-positive cocci similar to cefotaxime and ceftriaxone and somewhat greater activity against enteric gram-negative bacilli. The activity of cefepime against *P. aeruginosa* is similar to that of ceftazidime. Cefixime, cefpodoxime, cefdinir, ceftibuten, and cefditoren are oral cephalosporins with more activity than second-generation cephalosporins against facultative gram-negative bacilli; they have no useful activity against anaerobes or *P. aeruginosa*, and cefixime and ceftibuten have no useful activity against staphylococci. With the exception of cefoperazone (which can cause bleeding), ceftazidime, and cefepime, the activity of all currently available cephalosporins against *P. aeruginosa* is poor or inconsistent.

[10]Many strains of coagulase-positive and coagulase-negative staphylococci are resistant to penicillinase-resistant penicillins; these strains are also resistant to cephalosporins and carbapenems and are often resistant to fluoroquinolones, trimethoprim/sulfamethoxazole, and clindamycin. Community-acquired MRSA often is susceptible to clindamycin and trimethoprim/sulfamethoxazole.

[11]Tetracyclines and tigecycline, a derivative of minocycline, are generally not recommended for pregnant women or children less than 8 years old.

[12]For serious soft-tissue infection due to group A streptococci, clindamycin may be more effective than penicillin. Group A streptococci may, however, be resistant to clindamycin; therefore, some *Medical Letter* consultants suggest using both clindamycin and penicillin, with or without I.V. immune globulin, to treat serious soft-tissue infections. Surgical debridement is usually needed for necrotizing soft tissue infections due to group A streptococci. Group A streptococci may also be resistant to erythromycin, azithromycin, and clarithromycin.

[13]Penicillin V (or amoxicillin) is preferred for oral treatment of infections caused by nonpenicillinase-producing streptococci. For initial therapy of severe infections, penicillin G, administered parenterally, is the first choice. For somewhat longer action in less severe infections due to group A streptococci, pneumococci, or *Treponema pallidum*, procaine penicillin G, an I.M. formulation, can be given once or twice daily, but is seldom used now. Benzathine penicillin G, a slowly absorbed preparation, is usually given in a single monthly injection for prophylaxis of rheumatic fever, once for treatment of group A streptococcal pharyngitis and once or more for treatment of syphilis.

[14]Not recommended for use in pregnancy.

[15]Some strains of *S. pneumoniae* are resistant to erythromycin, clindamycin, trimethoprim/sulfamethoxazole, clarithromycin, azithromycin, and chloramphenicol, and resistance to the newer fluoroquinolones is rare but increasing. Nearly all strains tested so far are susceptible to linezolid and quinupristin/dalfopristin *in vitro*.

[16]Patients with gonorrhea should be treated presumptively for coinfection with *C. trachomatis* with azithromycin or doxycycline. Fluoroquinolones are no longer recommended for treatment (Centers for

Disease Control and Prevention [CDC], "Update to CDC's Sexually Transmitted Diseases Treatment Guidelines, 2006: Fluoroquinolones No Longer Recommended for Treatment of Gonococcal Infections," *MMWR Morb Mortal Wkly Rep*, 2007, 56(14):332-6).

[17]Rare strains of *N. meningitidis* are resistant or relatively resistant to penicillin. A fluoroquinolone or rifampin is recommended for prophylaxis after close contact with infected patients.

[18]Because of the possibility of serious adverse effects, this drug should be used only for severe infections when less hazardous drugs are ineffective.

[19]Sulfonamide-resistant strains are frequent in the U.S; sulfonamides should be used only when susceptibility is established by susceptibility tests.

[20]For postexposure prophylaxis, ciprofloxacin for 4 weeks if given with vaccination, and 60 days if not given with vaccination, might prevent disease; if the strain is susceptible, doxycycline is an alternative (Bartlett JG, Inglesby TV Jr, and Borio L, "Management of Anthrax," *Clin Infect Dis*, 2002, 35(7):851-8).

[21]Debridement is primary. Large doses of penicillin G are required. Hyperbaric oxygen therapy may be a useful adjunct to surgical debridement in management of the spreading, necrotizing type of infection.

[22]For prophylaxis, a tetanus toxoid booster and, for some patients, tetanus immune globulin (human) are required.

[23]In order to decrease the emergence of vancomycin-resistant enterococci in hospitals and to reduce costs, most clinicians now recommend use of metronidazole first in treatment of patients with *C. difficile* associated diarrhea, with oral vancomycin used only for seriously ill patients, or those who do not respond to metronidazole. Patients who are unable to take oral medications can be treated with I.V. metronidazole.

[24]Antitoxin is primary; antimicrobials are used only to halt further toxin production and to prevent the carrier state.

[25]In severely ill patients, most *Medical Letter* consultants would add gentamicin, tobramycin, or amikacin.

[26]In severely ill patients, most *Medical Letter* consultants would add gentamicin, tobramycin, or amikacin (but see footnote 39).

[27]For an acute, uncomplicated urinary tract infection, before the infecting organism is known, the drug of first choice is trimethoprim/sulfamethoxazole. Antibacterial treatment of gastroenteritis due to *E. coli* O157:H7 may increase toxin release and risk of hemolytic uremic syndrome and is not recommended (Centers for Disease Control and Prevention [CDC], "Ongoing Multistate Outbreak of Escherichia coli Serotype O157:H7 Infections Associated With Consumption of Fresh Spinach–United States, September 2006," *MMWR Morb Mortal Wkly Rep*, 2006, 55(38):1045-6).

[28]Large doses (≥6 g/day) are usually necessary for systemic infections. In severely ill patients, some *Medical Letter* consultants would add gentamicin, tobramycin, or amikacin.

[29]A fluoroquinolone or amoxicillin is the drug of choice for *S. typhi* carriers (Parry CM, Hien TT, Dougan G, "Typhoid Fever," *N Engl J Med*, 2002, 347(22):1770-82).

[30]Frenck RW Jr, Nakhla I, Sultan Y, et al, "Azithromycin Versus Ceftriaxone for the Treatment of Uncomplicated Typhoid Fever in Children," *Clin Infect Dis*, 2000, 31(5):1134-8.

[31]Most cases of *Salmonella* gastroenteritis subside spontaneously without antimicrobial therapy. Immunosuppressed patients, young children, and the elderly may benefit the most from antibacterials.

[32]Sulbactam may be useful to treat multidrug resistant *Acinetobacter*. It is only available in combination with ampicillin as Unasyn®. *Medical Letter* consultants recommend 3 g I.V. every 4 hours.

[33]Role of antibiotics is not clear (Conrad DA, "Treatment of Cat-Scratch Disease," *Curr Opin Pediatr*, 2001, 13(1):56-9).

[34]Pers C, Gahrn-Hansen B, Frederiksen W, et al, "*Capnocytophaga canimorsus* Septicemia in Denmark, 1982-1995: Review of 39 Cases," *Clin Infect Dis*, 1996, 23(1):71-5.

[35]For postexposure prophylaxis, doxycycline or ciprofloxacin begun during the incubation period and continued for 14 days might prevent disease ("Drugs and Vaccines for Biological Weapons," *Med Lett Drugs Ther*, 2001, 43(1115):87-9).

[36]Metronidazole is effective for bacterial vaginosis even though it is not usually active *in vitro* against *Gardnerella*.

[37]Eradication of *H. pylori* with various antibacterial combinations, given concurrently with a proton pump inhibitor or H_2-blocker, has led to rapid healing of active peptic ulcers and low recurrence rates.

[38]Proton pump inhibitors available in the U.S. are omeprazole (Prilosec® and others), lansoprazole (Prevacid®), pantoprazole (Protonix®), esomeprazole (Nexium®), and rabeprazole (Aciphex®). Available H_2-blockers include cimetidine (Tagamet® and others), famotidine (Pepcid® and others), nizatidine (Axid® and others), and ranitidine (Zantac® and others).

[39]Neither gentamicin, tobramycin, netilmicin, or amikacin should be mixed in the same bottle with carbenicillin, ticarcillin, mezlocillin, or piperacillin for I.V. administration. When used in high doses or in patients with renal impairment, these penicillins may inactivate the aminoglycosides.

[40]Antibiotic therapy is an adjunct to and not a substitute for prompt fluid and electrolyte replacement.

[41]Multidrug regimens are necessary for successful treatment. Drugs listed as alternatives are substitutions for primary regimens and are meant to be used in combination. For additional treatment recommendations for tuberculosis, see "Drugs for Tuberculosis," *Treat Guidel Med Lett*, 2007, 5 (55):15-22.

[42]Most infections are self-limited without drug treatment.

[43]Fenollar F, Puéchal X, and Raoult D, "Whipple's Disease," *N Engl J Med*, 2007, 356(1):55-66.

[44]For treatment of erythema migrans, uncomplicated facial nerve palsy, mild cardiac disease, and arthritis, oral therapy is satisfactory; for other neurologic or more serious cardiac disease, parenteral therapy with ceftriaxone, cefotaxime, or penicillin G is recommended. For recurrent arthritis after an oral regimen, another course of oral therapy or a parenteral drug may be given ("Treatment of Lyme Disease," *Med Lett Drugs Ther*, 2005, 47(1209):41-3).

[45]Vinetz JM, "A Mountain Out of a Molehill: Do We Treat Acute Leptospirosis, and if so, With What?" *Clin Infect Dis*, 2003, 36(12):1514-5; Panaphut T, Domrongkitchaiporn S, Vibhagool A, et al, "Ceftriaxone Compared With Sodium Penicillin G for Treatment of Severe Leptospirosis," *Clin Infect Dis*, 2003, 36(12):1507-13.

ASTHMA

MANAGEMENT OF ASTHMA IN ADULTS AND CHILDREN

Goals of Asthma Treatment

- Prevent chronic and troublesome symptoms: Minimal or no chronic symptoms day or night
- No limitations on activities; no school/work missed
- Minimal use of inhaled short-acting beta$_2$-agonist (≤2 days/week, <1 canister/month) (not including prevention of exercise induced asthma)
- Minimal or no adverse effects from medications
- Maintain (near) normal pulmonary function
- Prevent recurrent exacerbations (ie, trips to emergency department or hospitalizations)

All Patients

- Short-acting bronchodilator: **Inhaled beta$_2$ -agonists** as needed for symptoms.
- Intensity of treatment will depend on severity of exacerbation; see "Management of Asthma Exacerbations".
- Use of short-acting inhaled beta$_2$-agonists on a daily basis, or increasing use, indicates the need to initiate or titrate long-term control therapy.

Education

- Teach self-management.
- Teach about controlling environmental factors (avoidance of allergens or other factors that contribute to asthma severity).
- Review administration technique and compliance with patient.
- Use a written action plan to help educate.

Stepwise Approach for Managing Asthma in Adults and Children ≥12 Years of Age

Symptoms	Lung Function	Daily Medications
	STEP 6: Severe Asthma	
Day: Throughout the day Night: Often 7 times/week SABA use: Several times/day	FEV_1 <60% predicted FEV_1/FVC reduced 5%	**Preferred:** High dose ICS plus LABA plus oral corticosteroid AND Consider: Omalizumab (in those with allergies)[1]
	STEP 5: Severe Asthma	
Day: Throughout the day Night: Often 7 times/week SABA use: Several times/day	FEV_1 <60% predicted FEV_1/FVC reduced 5%	**Preferred:** High dose ICS plus LABA AND Consider: Omalizumab (in those with allergies)[1]
	STEP 4: Severe Asthma	
Day: Throughout the day Night: Often 7 times/week SABA use: Several times/day	FEV_1 <60% predicted FEV_1/FVC reduced 5%	**Preferred:** Medium dose ICS plus LABA **Alternatives[2]:** Medium dose ICS plus either LTRA, theophylline, or zileuton[3]
	STEP 3: Moderate Asthma	
Day: Daily Night: >1 night/week (not nightly) SABA use: Daily	FEV_1 >60%, <80% predicted FEV_1/FVC reduced 5%	**Preferred:** Low dose ICS plus LABA OR Medium dose ICS **Alternatives[2]:** Low dose ICS plus either LTRA, theophylline, or zileuton[3]
	STEP 2: Mild Asthma	
Day: >2 days/week (not daily) Night: 3-4 times/month SABA use: >2 days/week, no more than once per day (not daily)	FEV_1 <80% FEV_1/FVC normal	**Preferred:** Low dose ICS **Alternatives[2]:** LTRA, nedocromil, or theophylline
	STEP 1: Intermittent Asthma	
Day: ≤2 days/week Night: ≤2 nights/month SABA use: ≤2 days/week	FEV_1 normal between exacerbations FEV_1 >80% predicted FEV_1/FVC normal	Preferred: SABA as needed

Note: Treatment options within each step are listed in alphabetical order.

Steps 2-4: Consider subcutaneous allergen immunotherapy for patients with allergic asthma.[1]

Consult with asthma specialist if Step 4 or higher care is needed.

FEV_1 = forced expiratory volume in 1 second; FVC = forced vital capacity; ICS = inhaled corticosteroid; LABA = long-acting inhaled beta$_2$-agonist; SABA = short-acting inhaled beta$_2$-agonist; LTRA = leukotriene receptor antagonist.

[1]When using immunotherapy or omalizumab, clinicians should be prepared to identify and treat anaphylaxis in the event it occurs.

[2]If alternative treatment is used and response is inadequate, discontinue it and use preferred treatment before stepping up.

[3]Zileuton is less desirable alternative due to limited studies and need to monitor liver function.

Notes:

- **The stepwise approach presents general guidelines to assist clinical decision making; it is not intended to be a specific prescription. Asthma is highly variable; clinicians should tailor specific medication plans to the needs and circumstances of individual patients.**
- Gain control as quickly as possible; then decrease treatment to the least medication necessary to maintain control.
- A rescue course of systemic corticosteroids may be needed at any time and at any step.
- Some patients with intermittent asthma experience severe and life-threatening exacerbations separated by long periods of normal lung function and no symptoms. This may be especially common with exacerbations provoked by respiratory infections.
- At each step, patient education, environmental control, management of comorbidities emphasized.
- Antibiotics are not recommended for treatment of acute asthma exacerbations except where there is evidence or suspicion of bacterial infection.
- Consultation with an asthma specialist is recommended for moderate or severe persistent asthma.
- Peak flow monitoring for patients with moderate-severe persistent asthma and patients who have a history of severe exacerbations should be considered.

MANAGEMENT OF ASTHMA IN INFANTS AND YOUNG CHILDREN (<12 YEARS OF AGE)

Stepwise Approach for Managing Asthma in Children 0-4 Years of Age

Symptoms	Daily Medications[1]
STEP 6: Severe Asthma	
Day: Throughout the day Night: >1 time/week SABA use: Several times/day	**Preferred:** High dose ICS plus either LABA or montelukast Oral systemic corticosteroids
STEP 5: Severe Asthma	
Day: Throughout the day Night: >1 time/week SABA use: Daily	**Preferred:** High dose ICS plus either LABA or montelukast
STEP 4: Moderate Asthma	
Day: Daily Night: 3-4 times/month SABA use: Daily	**Preferred:** Medium dose ICS plus either LABA or montelukast
STEP 3: Moderate Asthma	
Day: Daily Night: 3-4 times/month SABA use: Daily	**Preferred:** Medium dose ICS
STEP 2: Mild Asthma	
Day: >2 days/week (not daily) Night: 1-2 times/month SABA use: >2 days/week, no more than once per day (not daily)	**Preferred:** Low dose ICS **Alternative**[2]: Montelukast
STEP 1: Intermittent Asthma	
Day: ≤2 days/week Night: No symptoms SABA use: ≤2 days/week	SABA as needed

Consult with asthma specialist if Step 3 or higher care is needed.

FEV_1 = forced expiratory volume in 1 second; FVC = forced vital capacity; ICS = inhaled corticosteroid; LABA = long-acting inhaled $beta_2$-agonist; SABA = short-acting inhaled $beta_2$-agonist.

[1]Studies on children 0-4 years old are limited. Many recommendations are based on expert opinion and extrapolation from studies of older children.

[2]If alternative treatment is used and response is inadequate, discontinue it and use preferred treatment before stepping up.

Stepwise Approach for Managing Asthma in Children 5-11 Years

Symptoms	Lung Function	Daily Medications
STEP 6: Severe Asthma		
Day: Throughout the day Night: Often 7 times/week SABA use: Several times/day	FEV_1 <60% predicted FEV_1/FVC <75%	**Preferred:** High dose ICS plus LABA plus oral corticosteroid **Alternative**[1]**:** High dose ICS plus either LTRA or theophylline[2] plus oral systemic corticosteroid
STEP 5: Severe Asthma		
Day: Throughout the day Night: Often 7 times/week SABA use: Several times/day	FEV_1 <60% predicted FEV_1/FVC <75%	**Preferred:** High dose ICS plus LABA **Alternative**[1]**:** High dose ICS plus either LTRA or theophylline[2]
STEP 4: Severe Asthma		
Day: Throughout the day Night: Often 7 times/week SABA use: Several times/day	FEV_1 <60% predicted FEV_1/FVC <75%	**Preferred:** Medium dose ICS plus LABA **Alternative**[1]**:** Medium dose ICS plus either LTRA or theophylline[2]
STEP 3: Moderate Asthma		
Day: Daily Night: >1 time/week (not nightly) SABA use: Daily	FEV_1 60% to 80% predicted FEV_1/FVC 75% to 80%	**Preferred:** Low dose ICS plus either LABA, LTRA, or theophylline[2] OR Medium dose ICS
STEP 2: Mild Asthma		
Day: >2 days/week (not daily) Night: 3-4 times/month SABA use: >2 days/week, no more than once per day (not daily)	FEV_1 ≥80% predicted FEV_1/FVC >80%	**Preferred:** Low dose ICS **Alternatives**[1]**:** LTRA, nedocromil, or theophylline[2]
STEP 1: Intermittent Asthma		
Day: ≤2 days/week Night: ≤2 times/month SABA use: ≤2 days/week	FEV_1 normal between exacerbations FEV_1 >80% predicted FEV_1/FVC >85%	SABA as needed

Steps 2-4: Consider subcutaneous allergen immunotherapy for patients with allergic asthma.[3]

Consult with asthma specialist if Step 4 or higher care is needed.

FEV_1 = forced expiratory volume in 1 second; FVC = forced vital capacity; ICS = inhaled corticosteroid; LABA = long-acting inhaled $beta_2$-agonist; SABA = short-acting inhaled $beta_2$-agonist; LTRA = leukotriene receptor antagonist.

[1]If alternative treatment is used and response is inadequate, discontinue it and use preferred treatment before stepping up.

[2]Theophylline is a less desirable alternative due monitoring required.

[3]When using immunotherapy, clinicians should be prepared to identify and treat anaphylaxis in the event it occurs.

Management of Asthma Exacerbations: Home Treatment

Assess Severity

- **Patients at high risk for a fatal attack require immediate medical attention after initial treatment.**
- Symptoms and signs suggestive of a more serious exacerbation such as marked breathlessness, inability to speak more than short phrases, use of accessory muscles, or drowsiness should result in initial treatment while immediately consulting with a clinician.
- If available, measure PEF—values of 50% to 79% predicted or personal best indicate the need for quick-relief mediation. Depending on the response to treatment, contact with a clinician may also be indicated. Values below 50% indicate the need for immediate medical care.

↓

Initial Treatment

- Inhaled SABA: Up to two treatments 20 minutes apart of 2–6 puffs by metered-dose inhaler (MDI) or nebulizer treatments.
- Note: Medication delivery is highly variable. Children and individuals who have exacerbations of lesser severity may need fewer puffs than suggested above.

↓

Good Response

No wheezing or dyspnea (assess tachypnea in young children).

PEF ≥80% predicted or personal best.

- Contact clinician for followup instructions and further management.
- May continue inhaled SABA every 3–4 hours for 24–48 hours.
- Consider short course of oral systemic corticosteroids.

Incomplete Response

Persistent wheezing and dyspnea (tachypnea).

PEF 50% to 79% predicted or personal best.

- Add oral systemic corticosteroid.
- Continue inhaled SABA.
- Contact clinician urgently (this day) for further instruction.

Poor Response

Marked wheezing and dyspnea.

PEF <50% predicted or personal best.

- Add oral systemic corticosteroid
- Repeat inhaled SABA immediately.
- If distress is severe and nonresponsive to initial treatment:
  - Call your doctor AND
  - **PROCEED TO EMERGENCY DEPARTMENT**;
  - Consider calling 911 (ambulance transport).

↓

- To emergency department.

MDI: Metered-dose inhaler; PEF: Peak expiratory flow; SABA: Short-acting beta$_2$-agonist (quick relief inhaler)

Management of Asthma Exacerbations: Emergency Department and Hospital-Based Care

Initial Assessment
Brief history, physical examination (auscultation, use of accessory muscles, heart rate, respiratory rate), PEF or FEV_1, oxygen saturation, and other tests as indicated

FEV_1 or PEF ≥40% (Mild-to-Moderate)
- Oxygen to achieve SaO_2 ≥90%
- Inhaled SABA by nebulizer or MDI with valved holding chamber, up to 3 doses in first hour
- Oral systemic corticosteroids if no immediate response or if patient recently took oral systemic corticosteroids

FEV_1 or PEF <40% (Severe)
- Oxygen to achieve SaO_2 ≥90%
- High-dose inhaled SABA plus ipratropium by nebulizer or MDI plus valved holding chamber, every 20 minutes or continuously for 1 hour
- Oral systemic corticosteroids

Impending or Actual Respiratory Arrest
- Intubation and mechanical ventilation with 100% oxygen
- Nebulized SABA and ipratropium
- I.V. corticosteroids
- Consider adjunct therapies

→ **Admit to Hospital Intensive Care** (see box)

Repeat Assessment
Symptoms, physical examination, PEF, O_2 saturation, other tests as needed

Moderate Exacerbation
FEV_1 or PEF 40% to 69% predicted/personal best
Physical exam: Moderate symptoms
- Inhaled SABA every 60 minutes
- Oral systemic corticosteroid
- Continue treatment 1-3 hours, provided there is improvement; make admit decision in <4 hours

Severe Exacerbation
FEV_1 or PEF <40% predicted/personal best
Physical exam: Severe symptoms at rest, accessory muscle use, chest retraction
History: High-risk patient
No improvement after initial treatment
- Oxygen
- Nebulized SABA plus iparopium, hourly or continuous
- Oral systemic corticosteroids
- Concider adjunct therapies

Good Response
- FEV_1 or PEF ≥70%
- Response sustained 60 minutes after last treatment
- No distress
- Physical exam: Normal

Incomplete Response
- FEV_1 or PEF 40% to 69%
- Mild-to-moderate symtoms

Individualized decision re: Hospitalization (see text)

Poor Response
- FEV_1 or PEF <40%
- PCO_2 ≥42 mm Hg
- Physical exam: Symptoms severe, drowsiness, confusion

Discharge Home
- Continue treatment with inhaled SABA.
- Continue course of oral systemic corticosteroid.
- Consider initiation of an ICS
- Patient Education
  - Review medications, including inhaler technique.
  - Review/initiate action plan.
  - Recommend close medical follow-up.

Admit to Hospital Ward
- Oxygen
- Inhaled SABA
- Systemic (oral or intravenous) corticosteroid
- Consider adjunct therapies
- Monitor vital signs, FEV_1 or PEF, SaO_2

Admit to Hospital Intensive Care
- Oxygen
- Inhaled SABA hourly or continuously
- Intravenous corticosteroid
- Consider adjunct therapies
- Possible intubation and mechanical ventilation

Improve (Hospital Ward → Discharge Home)

Improve (Intensive Care → Hospital Ward)

Discharge Home
- Continue treatment with inhaled SABAs.
- Continue course of oral systemic corticosteroid.
- Continue on ICS. For those not on long-term control therapy, consider initiation of an ICS.
- Patient education (eg, review medications, including inhaler technique and, whenever possible, environmental control measures; review/initiate action plan; recommend close medical follow-up).
- Before discharge, schedule follow-up appointment with primary care provider and/or asthma specialist in 1-4 weeks.

FEV_1 = forced expiratory volume in 1 second; ICS = inhaled corticosteroid; MDI = metered dose inhaler; PCO_2 = partial pressure carbon dioxide; PEF = peak expiratory flow; SABA = short-acting $beta_2$-agonist; SaO_2 = oxygen saturation

ESTIMATED COMPARATIVE DAILY DOSAGES FOR INHALED CORTICOSTEROIDS

Children ≥12 Years of Age and Adults

Drug	Low Daily Dose	Medium Daily Dose	High Daily Dose
Beclomethasone HFA 40 mcg/puff 80 mcg/puff	80-240 mcg	>240-480 mcg	>480 mcg
Budesonide DPI 90 mcg/puff 180 mcg/puff 200 mcg/puff	180-600 mcg	>600-1200 mcg	>1200 mcg
Flunisolide 250 mcg/puff	500-1000 mcg	>1000-2000 mcg	>2000 mcg
Flunisolide HFA 80 mcg/puff	320 mcg	>320-640 mcg	>640 mcg
Fluticasone HFA 44 mcg/puff 110 mcg/puff 220 mcg/puff	88-264 mcg	>264-440 mcg	>440 mcg
Mometasone DPI 220 mcg/puff	220 mcg	440 mcg	>440 mcg

DPI = dry powder inhaler; HFA = hydrofluoroalkane.

Children <12 Years of Age

Drug	Low Daily Dose	Medium Daily Dose	High Daily Dose
Beclomethasone HFA 40 mcg/puff 80 mcg/puff	0-4 years: NA 5-11 years: 80-160 mcg	0-4 years: NA 5-11 years: >160-320 mcg	0-4 years: NA 5-11 years: >320 mcg
Budesonide DPI 90 mcg/puff 180 mcg/puff 200 mcg/puff	0-4 years: NA 5-11 years: 180-400 mcg	0-4 years: NA 5-11 years: >400-800 mcg	0-4 years: NA 5-11 years: >800 mcg
Budesonide nebulized 0.25 mg/2 mL 0.5 mg/2 mL	0-4 years: 0.25-0.5 mg 5-11 years: 0.5 mg	0-4 years: >0.5-1 mg 5-11 years: 1 mg	0-4 years: >1 mg 5-11 years: 2 mg
Flunisolide 250 mcg/puff	0-4 years: NA 5-11 years: 500-750 mcg	0-4 years: NA 5-11 years: 1000-1250 mcg	0-4 years: NA 5-11 years: >1250 mcg
Flunisolide HFA 80 mcg/puff	0-4 years: NA 5-11 years: 160 mcg	0-4 years: NA 5-11 years: 320 mcg	0-4 years: NA 5-11 years: ≥640 mcg
Fluticasone HFA 44 mcg/puff 110 mcg/puff 220 mcg/puff	0-4 years: 176 mcg 5-11 years: 88-176 mcg	0-11 years: >176-352 mcg	0-11 years: >352 mcg
Fluticasone DPI 50 mcg/puff 100 mcg/puff 250 mcg/puff	0-4 years: NA 5-11 years: 100-200 mcg	0-4 years: NA 5-11 years: >200-400 mcg	0-4 years: NA 5-11 years: >400 mcg
Mometasone	NA	NA	NA

DPI = dry powder inhaler; HFA = hydrofluoroalkane.

NA = not approved for use in this age group or no data available.

Reference

Expert Panel Report 3, "Guidelines for the Diagnosis and Management of Asthma," *Clinical Practice Guidelines*, National Institutes of Health, National Heart, Lung, and Blood Institute, NIH Publication No. 08-4051, prepublication 2007. Available at http://www.nhlbi.nih.gov/guidelines/asthma/asthgdln.-htm.

COMMUNITY-ACQUIRED PNEUMONIA IN ADULTS

Alternative methods exist to facilitate the objective rating of disease severity in community-acquired pneumonia patients in order to guide appropriate site of care and aggressiveness of treatment. The first option, the Pneumonia Severity Index (PSI) was derived from the Pneumonia Patient Outcomes Research Team (PORT). This is a well-validated instrument which stratifies patients based on risk of mortality; however, calculation of the patient's score requires assessment of 19 variables. The second method is referred to as the "Confusion, Uremia, Respiratory rate, Blood pressure, and age >65 years (CURB-65)" score. This system has fewer variables to evaluate and focuses more on assessment of disease severity, but is less well validated. In either case, these measures should not be used in exclusion to appropriate clinical judgement.

PNEUMONIA SEVERITY INDEX (PSI)

The initial site of treatment should be based on a 3-step process:

1. Assessment of pre-existing conditions that compromise safety of home care
2. Calculation of the Pneumonia Severity Index with recommendation for home care for risk classes I, II, and III, and
3. Clinical judgment

Algorithm

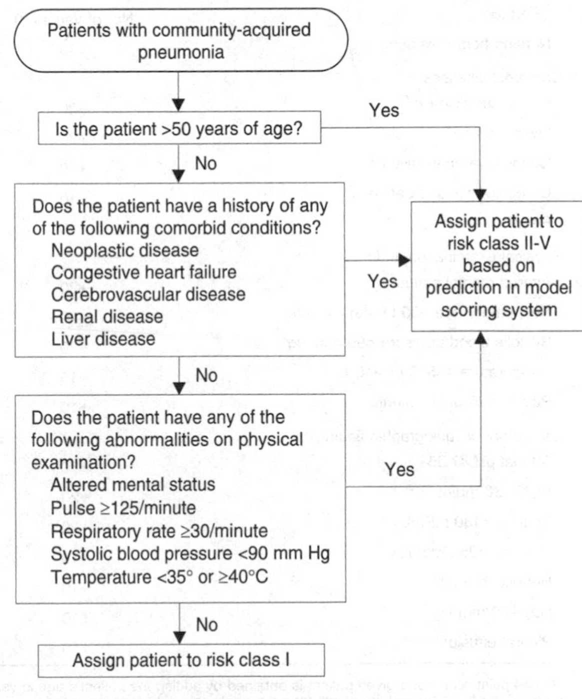

Stratification of Risk Score

Risk	Risk Class	Based on
Low	I	Algorithm
	II	≤70 total points
	III	71-90 total points
Moderate	IV	91-130 total points
High	V	>130 total points

Risk-Class Mortality Rates for Patients With Pneumonia

Risk Class	No. of Points	Validation Cohort: No. of Patients	Mortality (%)	Recommended Site of Care
I	No predictors	3034	0.1	Outpatient
II	≤70	5778	0.6	Outpatient
III	71-90	6790	2.8	Outpatient or brief inpatient
IV	91-130	13,104	8.2	Inpatient
V	>130	9333	29.2	Inpatient

Scoring System: Assignment to Risk Classes II-V

Patient Characteristic	Points Assigned[1]
Demographic factors	
Age	
Male	No. of years
Female	No. of years -10
Nursing home resident	+10
Comorbid illnesses	
Neoplastic disease[2]	+30
Liver disease[3]	+20
Congestive heart failure[4]	+10
Cerebrovascular disease[5]	+10
Renal disease[6]	+10
Physical examination findings	
Altered mental status[7]	+20
Respiratory rate >30 breaths/minute	+20
Systolic blood pressure <90 mm Hg	+20
Temperature <35°C or >40°C	+15
Pulse >125 beats/minute	+10
Laboratory or radiographic findings	
Arterial pH <7.35	+30
BUN >30 mg/dL	+20
Sodium <130 mEq/L	+20
Glucose >250 mg/dL	+10
Hematocrit <30%	+10
pO_2 <60 mm Hg[8]	+10
Pleural effusion	+10

[1]A total point score for a given patient is obtained by adding the patient's age in years (age -10, for females) and the points for each applicable patient characteristic.

[2]Any cancer, except basal or squamous cell cancer of the skin, that was active at the time of presentation or diagnosed within 1 year of presentation.

[3]A clinical or histologic diagnosis of cirrhosis or other form of chronic liver disease such as chronic active hepatitis.

[4]Systolic or diastolic ventricular dysfunction documented by history and physical examination, as well as chest radiography, echocardiography, Muga scanning, or left ventriculography.

[5]A clinical diagnosis of stroke, transient ischemic attack, or stroke documented by MRI or computed axial tomography.

[6]A history of chronic renal disease or abnormal blood urea nitrogen (BUN) and creatinine values documented in the medical record.

[7]Disorientation (to person, place, or time; not known to be chronic), stupor, or coma.

[8]In the Pneumonia Patient Outcome Research Team cohort study, an oxygen saturation value <90% on pulse oximetry or intubation before admission was also considered abnormal.

CONFUSION, UREMIA, RESPIRATORY RATE, BLOOD PRESSURE, AND AGE >65 YEARS (CURB-65)

Risk factors:

1. Presence of confusion (based on specific tests or noted disorientation to people, place, or time)
2. Blood urea nitrogen (BUN) of >7mmol/L (20 mg/dL)
3. Respiratory rate >30 breaths/minute
4. Systolic blood pressure <90 mmHg or diastolic <60 mmHg
5. Age >65 years

Number of Risk Factors	30-Day Mortality Risk (%)
0	0.7
1	2.1
2	9.2
3	14.5
4	40
5	57

Scoring:

0-1 risk factors: Treat as outpatient.

2 risk factors: Treat as inpatient.

3-5 risk factors: Treat as inpatient; likely requires more aggressive management, possibly ICU.

Epidemiological Conditions Related to Specific Pathogens in Patients With Selected Community-Acquired Pneumonia

Condition	Commonly Encountered Pathogens
Alcoholism	*Streptococcus pneumoniae*, anaerobes
COPD and/or smoker	*S. pneumoniae, Haemophilus influenzae, Moraxella catarrhalis, Legionella* species
Nursing home residency	*S. pneumoniae*, gram-negative bacilli, *H. influenzae, Staphylococcus aureus*, anaerobes, *Chlamydia pneumoniae*
Poor dental hygiene	Anaerobes
Epidemic Legionnaires' disease	*Legionella* species
Exposure to bats or soil enriched with bird droppings	*Histoplasma capsulatum*
Exposure to birds	*Chlamydia psittaci*
Exposure to rabbits	*Francisella tularensis*
HIV infection (early stage)	*S. pneumoniae, H. influenzae, Mycobacterium tuberculosis*
HIV infection (late stage)	Above plus *P. carinii, Cryptococcus, Histoplasma* species
Travel to southwestern United States	*Coccidioides* species
Exposure to farm animals or parturient cats	*Coxiella burnetii* (Q fever)
Influenza active in community	Influenza, *S. pneumoniae, S. aureus, Streptococcus pyogenes, H. influenzae*
Suspected large-volume aspiration	Anaerobes (chemical pneumonitis, obstruction)
Structural disease of the lung (bronchiectasis, cystic fibrosis, etc)	*Pseudomonas aeruginosa, Burkholderia (Pseudomonas) cepacia, S. aureus*
Injection drug use	*S. aureus*, anaerobes, *M. tuberculosis, S. pneumoniae*
Airway obstruction	Anaerobes, *S. pneumoniae, H. influenzae, S. aureus*

COPD = chronic obstructive pulmonary disease.

Initial Empiric Therapy for Suspected Bacterial Community-Acquired Pneumonia (CAP) in Immunocompetent Adults

Patient Variable	Preferred Treatment Options
Outpatient	
Previously healthy	
No recent antibiotic therapy or risk for DRSP	A macrolide[1] or doxycycline
Comorbidities[2]; recent antibiotic therapy[3]; risk factors for DRSP[4]	A respiratory fluoroquinolone[5] alone, or an advanced macrolide[6] plus high-dose amoxicillin,[7] high-dose amoxicillin-clavulanate,[8] cefpodoxime, ceftriaxone, or cefuroxime.
Suspected aspiration with infection	Amoxicillin-clavulanate or clindamycin
Influenza with bacterial superinfection	Antiviral agent oseltamivir or zanamivir, plus a cefotaxime or ceftriaxone or a respiratory fluoroquinolone[5]
Inpatient	
Non-ICU	A respiratory fluoroquinolone alone or macrolide plus a β-lactam[9]
ICU	
Pseudomonas infection is not an issue	Cefotaxime, ceftriaxone, or ampicillin-sulbactam plus either azithromycin or a respiratory fluoroquinolone[5]
Pseudomonas infection is not an issue but patient has a β-lactam allergy	A respiratory fluoroquinolone,[5] with aztreonam
Pseudomonas infection is an issue[10]	Either (1) an antipseudomonal agent[11] plus ciprofloxacin or levofloxacin, or (2) an antipseudomonal agent plus an aminoglycoside[12] plus a respiratory fluoroquinolone[5] or azithromycin
Pseudomonas infection is an issue but the patient has a β-lactam allergy	Substitute aztreonam for any β-lactam antipseudomonal agent[11]
Nursing home	
Receiving treatment in nursing home	A respiratory fluoroquinolone[5] alone or amoxicillin-clavulanate plus an advanced macrolide
Suspicion or MRSA	Add vancomycin or linezolid to any suggested regimens

DRSP = drug-resistant *Streptococcus pneumoniae*; ICU = intensive care unit.

[1]Erythromycin, azithromycin, or clarithromycin.

[2]Chronic heart, lung, liver, and/or renal disease, diabetes, malignancy, or immunosuppressive medication and/or conditions.

[3]That is, the patient was given a course of antibiotic(s) for treatment of any infection within the past 3 months, excluding the current episode of infection. Such treatment is a risk factor for drug-resistant *Streptococcus pneumoniae* and possibly for infection with gram-negative bacilli. Depending on the class of antibiotics recently given, one or other of the suggested options may be selected. Recent use of a fluoroquinolone should dictate selection of a nonfluoroquinolone regimen, and vice versa.

[4]Risk factors for β-lactam-resistant *S. pneumoniae* include age <2 or >65 years, recent antimicrobial therapy (within previous 3 months, and especially to repeated courses of same antibiotic class), alcoholism, comorbidities, immunosuppressive illness or therapy, and exposure to child care centers.

[5]Moxifloxacin, levofloxacin, or gemifloxacin.

[6]Azithromycin or clarithromycin.

[7]Dosage, 1 g P.O. 3 times/day.

[8]Dosage, 2 g P.O. twice daily.

[9]Cefotaxime, ceftriaxone, ampicillin (or ampicillin-sulbactam), or ertapenem; ertapenem was recently approved for such use (in once-daily parenteral treatment), but there is little experience thus far. **Note:** The 2007 CAP guidelines excluded ampicillin-sulbactam in favor of the single agent without the lactamase inhibitor. While this may be useful in specific situations, the prevalence of beta-lactamase-producing *H. influenzae* should be a concern, and thus the use of ampicillin-sulbactam may be more appropriate for empiric use.

[10]The antipseudomonal agents chosen reflect this concern. Risk factors for *Pseudomonas* infection include severe structural lung disease (eg, bronchiectasis), and recent antibiotic therapy or stay in hospital (especially in the ICU). For patients with CAP in the ICU, coverage for *S. pneumoniae* and *Legionella* species must always be assured. Piperacillin-tazobactam, imipenem, meropenem, and cefepime are excellent β-lactams and are adequate for most *S. pneumoniae* and *Haemophilus influenzae* infections. They may be preferred when there is concern for relatively unusual CAP pathogens, such as *Pseudomonas aeruginosa*, *Klebsiella* species, and other gram-negative bacteria.

[11]Piperacillin-tazobactam, imipenem, meropenem, or cefepime.

[12]Data suggest that elderly patients receiving aminoglycosides have worse outcomes.

References

Bartlett JG, Breiman RF, Mandell LA, et al, "Community-Acquired Pneumonia in Adults: Guidelines for Management. The Infectious Diseases Society of America," *Clin Infect Dis*, 1998, 26(4):811-38.

Mandell LA, Bartlett JG, Dowell SF, et al, "Update of Practice Guidelines for the Management of Community-Acquired Pneumonia in Immunocompetent Adults," *Clin Infect Dis*, 2003, 37(11):1405-33.

Mandell LA, Wunderink RG, Anzueto A, et al, "Infectious Diseases Society of America/American Thoracic Society Consensus Guidelines on the Management of Community-Acquired Pneumonia in Adults," *Clin Infect Dis*, 2007, 44(Suppl 2):S27-72.

DEPRESSION

Medications That May Precipitate Depression

Anti-inflammatory & analgesic agents	Indomethacin, pentazocine, phenacetin, phenylbutazone
Antimicrobial agents	Cycloserine, ethambutol, ribavirin, sulfonamides, select gram-negative antibiotics
Cardiovascular/ antihypertensive agents	Amiodarone, B-adrenergic antagonists, clonidine, digitalis, diuretics, guanethidine, hydralazine, indapamide, methyldopa, prazosin, procainamide, propranolol, reserpine
CNS-agents	Alcohol, amantadine, amphetamine & derivatives (withdrawal), barbiturates, benzodiazepines, carbamazepine, chloral hydrate, cocaine (withdrawal), haloperidol, L-dopa, levetiracetam, phenothiazines, succinimide derivatives
Hormonal agents	ACTH, corticosteroids, estrogen, melatonin, oral contraceptives, progesterone
Miscellaneous	Antineoplastic agents, cimetidine, disulfiram, isotretinoic acid organic pesticides, mercury, physostigmine

Medical Disorders and Psychiatric Disorders Associated With Depression

Cardiovascular disease	Cardiomyopathy, cerebral arteriosclerosis, chronic bronchitis, congestive heart failure, emphysema, ischemic heart disease, myocardial infarction, paroxysmal dysrhythmias
Collagen disorders	Rheumatoid arthritis, systemic lupus erythematosus
Deficiency states	Pellagra, pernicious anemia, severe anemia, vitamin deficiencies, Wernicke's encephalopathy
Endocrine diseases	Acromegaly, Addison's disease, Cushing's disease, diabetes mellitus, hyper-/hypoparathyroidism, hyper-/hypothyroidism, insulinoma, pheochromocytoma, pituitary dysfunction
Infections	AIDS, encephalitis, fungal infections, influenza, meningitis, mononucleosis, neurosyphilis, pneumonia, toxoplasmosis, tuberculosis, viral hepatitis
Inflammatory disorders	Chronic liver disorders, collagen-vascular diseases, irritable bowel syndrome
Malignant disease	Breast, gastrointestinal, lung, pancreas, prostate
Metabolic disorders	Electrolyte imbalance, hepatic encephalopathy, hypokalemia, hyponatremia, Pick's disease, uremia, Wilson's disease
Neurologic disorders	Alzheimer's disease, amyotrophic lateral sclerosis, brain tumors, chronic pain syndrome, complex partial seizures, Creutzfeldt-Jakob disease, epilepsies, Huntington's disease, multiple sclerosis, myasthenia gravis, Parkinson's disease, poststroke, sleep apnea, trauma (postconcussion)
Psychiatric disorders	Alcoholism, anxiety disorders, eating disorders, schizophrenia

DIABETES MELLITUS MANAGEMENT, ADULTS

OVERVIEW

Diabetes represents a significant health care problem in the United States and worldwide. Of the nearly 23.6 million Americans (7.8% of the population) with diabetes, the majority (90% to 95%) have type 2 diabetes. Of this number, nearly one-quarter are undiagnosed. The incidence of type 2 diabetes is increasing around the world. There is strong evidence to support an interaction between a genetic predisposition and behavioral or environmental factors, such as obesity and physical inactivity, in the development of this disease. In individuals at high risk of developing type 2 diabetes, it has been shown that the development of diabetes may be prevented or delayed by changes in lifestyle or pharmacologic intervention.

Within the United States, type 1 diabetes is estimated to comprise 5% to 10% of those with diabetes, and therefore represents the minority of individuals with diabetes. In addition to type 1 and type 2 diabetes, approximately 7% of pregnancies are complicated by the development of gestational diabetes. Gestational diabetes mellitus is defined as the first onset or recognition of glucose intolerance during pregnancy. Women who have had gestational diabetes are at an increased risk for later development of type 2 diabetes. In addition to the causes noted above, diabetes may result from genetic syndromes, surgery (pancreatectomy), chemicals and/or drugs, recurrent pancreatitis, malnutrition, and viral infections.

Additional information available at: http://care.diabetesjournals.org/content/34/Supplement_1

COMPLICATIONS OF DIABETES

Diabetes was listed as the seventh leading cause of death in the United States in 2007. Complications of diabetes are often contributing factors in the death of these patients; the most frequently reported diabetes complications on the death certificates of patients with diabetes in 2004 were heart disease and stroke, which were listed as contributing factors in 68% and 16% of diabetes-related deaths, respectively.

In addition to cardiovascular effects, diabetes is the leading cause of new blindness in people 20-74 years old, and diabetic nephropathy is the most common cause of end-stage renal disease. Mild to severe forms of diabetic neuropathy are common. Neuropathy and circulatory insufficiency combine to make diabetes the most frequent cause of nontraumatic lower-limb amputations (60% of cases). The rate of impotence in diabetic males over 50 years old has been estimated to be as high as 35% to 50%. Control of hyperglycemia may significantly decrease the rate at which diabetic complications develop; this provides compelling justification for early diagnosis and management of this disorder.

DIAGNOSIS

Diabetes

Diagnosis of diabetes in nonpregnant adults is made by any of the four criteria described below. In the absence of unequivocal hyperglycemia with acute metabolic decompensation, these criteria should be confirmed by repeat testing on a different day. New in the 2010 American Diabetes Association (ADA) Standards of Medical Care is the recommendation for the use of Hb A_{1c} for the diagnosis of diabetes; the method used should be certified by the National Glycohemoglobin Standardization Program (NGSP) and standardized to the Diabetes Control and Complications Trial (DCCT) assay. Screening should be considered in overweight adult patients (BMI ≥25 kg/m^2) who have at least one risk factor for diabetes (eg, physical inactivity, first-degree relative with diabetes, history of cardiovascular disease, etc). In patients without risk factors, testing should begin at age 45. Repeat testing should occur at least every 3 years in patients with normal test results.

Criteria for Diagnosis

1. Hb A_{1c} ≥6.5%

   OR

2. Fasting plasma glucose (no caloric intake for at least 8 hours) ≥126 mg/dL (7 mmol/L)
   OR

3. Casual plasma glucose concentration≥200 mg/dL (11.1 mmol/L) in patients with symptoms of hyperglycemia (polydipsia, polyuria, unexplained weight loss) or hyperglycemic crisis. **Note:** Casual plasma glucose is defined as any time of day without regard to time of last meal.
   OR

4. A 2-hour plasma glucose ≥200 mg/dL (11.1 mmol/L) during an oral glucose tolerance test (OGTT) in accordance with the standards set forth by the World Health Organization (WHO) using a 75 g anhydrous glucose load (or equivalent) dissolved in water. **Note:** OGTT is not recommended for routine clinical use.

Note: In the absence of unequivocal hyperglycemia, criteria 1, 2, and 4 should be confirmed by repeat testing.

Categories of Increased Risk for Diabetes

Patients with impaired fasting glucose (IFG), impaired glucose tolerance (IGT), or an intermediately high Hb A_{1c} are considered to be in a group whose glucose levels do not meet the criteria for diabetes, yet are higher than normal. Patients who meet any of the following criteria are considered to be at high risk for developing diabetes and cardiovascular disease, and are referred to as having "prediabetes":

1. IFG: Fasting plasma glucose (no caloric intake for at least 8 hours) 100-125 mg/dL (5.6-6.9 mmol/L)
   OR
2. IGT: A 2-hour plasma glucose 140-199 mg/dL (7.8-11 mmol/L) during an oral glucose tolerance test (OGTT) in accordance with the standards set forth by the World Health Organization (WHO) using a 75 g anhydrous glucose load (or equivalent) dissolved in water.
   OR
3. Hb A_{1c}: 5.7% to 6.4%; **Note:** Patients with an Hb A_{1c} >6% should be considered at very high risk for diabetes and receive intensive interventions and monitoring.

The International Expert Committee consisting of members of the ADA, the European Association for the Study of Diabetes (EASD), and the International Diabetes Federation (IDF) recently recommended that the clinical states "prediabetes," IFG, and IGT be phased out as the Hb A1c becomes the preferred diagnostic test (International Expert Committee, 2009).

GOALS

The goals of diabetes treatment include normalization of hyperglycemia, avoidance of hypoglycemia, and slowing the development of diabetic complications. The following is a summary of recommendations for nonpregnant adults with diabetes.

2011 ADA Summary of Recommendations for Adults With Diabetes

Glycemic control	
Hb A_{1c}	<7%[1]
Preprandial capillary plasma glucose	70-130 mg/dL
Peak postprandial capillary plasma glucose[2]	<180 mg/dL
Blood pressure[7]	<130/80 mm Hg
Lipids[3]	
LDL[4]	<100 mg/dL
Triglycerides	<150 mg/dL
HDL	Male: >40 mg/dL Female: >50 mg/dL
Non-HDL chloesterol[5]	<130 mg/dL
Apolipoprotein B[6]	<90 mg/dL

[1]Referenced to a nondiabetic range of 4% to 6% using a DCCT-based assay. **Note:** The Hb A_{1c} goal for patients in general is <7%; an even lower goal may be appropriate for selected individuals (eg, short duration of diabetes, long life expectancy, and no significant cardiovascular disease) so long as a lower goal can be achieved without significant hypoglycemia or other adverse effects. Conversely, a less stringent goal may be appropriate in certain patients (eg, history of severe hypoglycemia, limited life expectancy, advanced micro- or macrovascular complications, extensive comorbid conditions, longstanding diabetes in whom the general goal is difficult to attain despite appropriate diabetes management).

[2]Postprandial glucose measurements should be made 1-2 hours after the beginning of the meal, generally peak levels in patients with diabetes.

[3]Current NCEP/ATP III guidelines suggest that in patients with triglycerides ≥200 mg/dL, the non-HDL cholesterol (total cholesterol minus HDL) be used. The goal is <130 mg/dL.

[4]In patients with overt CVD or cardiometabolic risk factors (eg, central obesity, insulin resistance, hypertension), a lower LDL goal of <70 mg/dL is an option.

[5]In patients with overt CVD or cardiometabolic risk factors (eg, central obesity, insulin resistance, hypertension) with an LDL goal of <70 mg/dL, the non-HDL cholesterol goal is <100 mg/dL

[6]In patients on a statin with an LDL goal of <70 mg/dL or patients with cardiometabolic risk factors (eg, central obesity, insulin resistance, hypertension), the apolipoprotein B goal is <80 mg/dL

[7]Higher or lower systolic blood pressure targets may be appropriate based on individual patient characteristics and response to therapy.

Key concepts in setting glycemic goals:

- Hb A_{1c} is the primary target for glycemic control.
- Goals should be individualized.
- Certain populations (children, pregnant women, and elderly) require special considerations.

- Less intensive glycemic goals may be indicated in patients with severe or frequent hypoglycemia.
- A lower glycemic goal (eg, Hb A_{1c} <6%) may further reduce the risk of microvascular complications at the cost of an increased risk of hypoglycemia (particularly in those with type 1 diabetes). However, recent studies (eg, ACCORD and VADT) have highlighted certain patient populations in which the risks of intensive glycemic control may outweigh the benefits, including patients with a very long duration of diabetes, history of severe hypoglycemia, advanced atherosclerosis, and advanced age or frailty.
- Postprandial glucose may be targeted if Hb A_{1c} goals are not met despite reaching preprandial glucose goals.

MANAGEMENT

Multidisciplinary approach necessary. Patient education:

- Wearing appropriate identification of disease
- Foot care
- Eye care
- Acute illness management
- Hypoglycemia recognition and management
- Weight monitoring and management, including diet and exercise and bariatric surgery options (BMI >35 kg/m^2)

TYPE 1 DIABETES DRUG TREATMENT

Intensive insulin therapy: ≥3 injections/day of basal and prandial insulin or continuous subcutaneous infusion. If hypoglycemia is problematic, the use of insulin analogs may be helpful.

Monitoring

Self-monitoring of blood glucose (SMBG) should be carried out three or more times daily for patients using multiple insulin injections or insulin pump therapy. For patients using less frequent insulin injections, noninsulin therapies, or medical nutrition therapy (MNT) alone, SMBG may be useful as a guide to the success of therapy. To achieve postprandial glucose targets, postprandial SMBG may be appropriate.

Continuous glucose monitoring (CGM) in conjunction with intensive insulin regimens can be a useful tool to lower A1C in selected adults (age ≥25 years) with type 1 diabetes. CGM may be a supplemental tool in those with hypoglycemia episodes.

Insulin

Insulin therapy is required in type 1 diabetes, and may be necessary in some individuals with type 2 diabetes. The general objective of insulin replacement therapy is to approximate the physiologic pattern of insulin secretion which is characterized by two distinct phases. Phase 1 insulin secretion suppresses hepatic glucose production and phase 2 insulin secretion occurs in response to carbohydrate ingestion. This requires a basal level of insulin throughout the day (such as intermediate- or long-acting insulin or continuous insulin infusion administered via an external SubQ insulin infusion pump), supplemented by additional insulin at mealtimes (eg, short- or rapid-acting insulin).

Multiple daily doses guided by blood glucose monitoring are the standard of diabetes care. Combinations of insulin are commonly used. The number and size of daily doses, time of administration, and diet and exercise require continuous medical supervision. In addition, specific formulations may require distinct administration procedures/timing (refer to individual monographs).

There is solid scientific documentation of the benefit of tight glucose control, either by insulin pump or multiple daily injections (4-6 times daily). However, the benefits must be balanced against the risk of hypoglycemia, the patient's ability to adhere to the regimen, and other issues regarding the complexity of management. Diabetes self-management education (DSME) and medical nutrition therapy (MNT) are essential to maximize the effectiveness of therapy. In addition to the educational issues outlined above, patients should be instructed in insulin administration techniques, timing of administration, and sick-day management.

The initial dose of insulin in type 1 diabetes is typically 0.5-1 units/kg/day in divided doses. Conservative initial doses of 0.2-0.4 units/kg/day are often recommended to avoid the potential for hypoglycemia. Generally, one-half to three-fourths of the daily insulin dose is given as an intermediate- or long-acting form of insulin (in 1-2 daily injections). The remaining portion of the 24-hour insulin requirement is divided and administered as a rapid-acting or short-acting form of insulin. These may be given with meals (before or at the time of meals depending on the form of insulin) or at the same time as injections of intermediate forms (some premixed combinations are intended for this purpose). Some patients may benefit from the use of continuous subcutaneous insulin infusion (CSII) which delivers rapid-acting insulin as a continuous infusion throughout the day and as boluses at mealtimes via an external pump device.

Since combinations of agents are frequently used, dosage adjustment must address the individual component of the insulin regimen which most directly influences the blood glucose value in question, based on the known onset and duration of the insulin component (see table). The frequency of doses and monitoring must also be individualized in consideration of the patient's ability to manage therapy.

Types of Insulin	Onset (h)	Peak Glycemic Effect (h)	Duration (h)
Rapid-Acting			
Insulin lispro (Humalog®)	0.25-0.5	0.5-2.5	≤5
Insulin aspart (NovoLog®)	0.2-0.3	1-3	3-5
Insulin glulisine (Apidra®)	0.2-0.5	1.6-2.8	3-4
Short-Acting			
Insulin regular (Humulin® R, Novolin® R)	0.5	2.5-5	4-12 – U-100 Up to 24 – U-500
Intermediate-Acting			
Insulin NPH (isophane suspension) (Humulin® N, Novolin® N)	1-2	4-12	14-24
Intermediate- to Long-Acting			
Insulin detemir (Levemir®)	3-4	3-9	6-23 (duration is dose-dependent)
Long-Acting			
Insulin glargine (Lantus®)	3-4	*	10.8-≥24
Combinations			
Insulin aspart protamine suspension and insulin aspart (NovoLog® Mix 70/30)	0.17-0.33	1-4	18-24
Insulin lispro protamine and insulin lispro (Humalog® Mix 75/25™)	0.25-0.5	1-6.5	14-24
Insulin NPH suspension and insulin regular solution (Novolin® 70/30)	0.5	2-12	18-24

*Insulin glargine has no pronounced peak.

Maintenance Dosing

Typical maintenance insulin doses are between 0.5 and 1.2 units/kg/day in divided doses. Adolescents may require as much as 1.5 units/kg/day during puberty; whereas prepubescent individuals may only require 0.7-1 unit/kg/day.

As stated above, the general objective of insulin replacement therapy is to approximate the physiologic pattern of insulin secretion. This requires a basal level of insulin throughout the day, supplemented by additional insulin at mealtimes. Combination regimens which exploit differences in the onset and duration of different insulin products are commonly used to approximate physiologic secretion. Frequently, split-mixed or basal-bolus regimens are used to approximate physiologic secretion.

Split-mixed regimens: In split-mixed regimens, an intermediate-acting insulin (eg, NPH insulin) is administered once or twice daily and supplemented by short-acting (regular) or rapid-acting (lispro, aspart, or glulisine) insulin. Blood glucose measurements are completed several times daily. Dosages are adjusted emphasizing the individual component of the regimen which most directly influences the blood sugar in question (either the intermediate-acting component or the shorter-acting component). Fixed-ratio formulations (eg, 70/30 mix) may be used as twice daily injections in this scenario; however, the ability to titrate the dosage of an individual component is limited. An example of a "split-mixed" regimen would be 21 units of NPH plus 9 units of regular in the morning and an evening meal dose consisting of 14 units of NPH plus 6 units of regular insulin.

Basal-bolus regimens: Basal-bolus regimens are designed to more closely mimic physiologic secretion. These regimens employ intermediate- to long-acting insulins (eg, glargine, detemir) or a continuous insulin infusion administered via an external SubQ insulin infusion pump to simulate basal insulin secretion. The basal component is frequently administered at bedtime or in the early morning or as a continuous insulin infusion and then supplemented by multiple daily injections of rapid-acting products (lispro, glulisine, or aspart) immediately prior to a meal; thereby, providing insulin at the time when nutrients are absorbed. An example of a basal-bolus regimen would be 30 units of glargine at bedtime and 12 units of lispro insulin prior to each meal.

Adjustment of Insulin Dose

Dosage must be titrated to achieve glucose control and avoid hypoglycemia. In general, dosage is adjusted to maintain recommendations for glycemic control. Since treatment regimens often consist of multiple formulations, dosage adjustments must address the specific phase of insulin release that is primarily contributing to the patient's impaired glycemic control. Treatment and monitoring regimens must be individualized.

Estimation of the effect per unit: A "Rule of 1500" has been frequently used as a means to estimate the change in blood sugar relative to each unit of insulin administered. In fact, the recommended values used in these calculations may vary from 1500-2200 (a value of at least 1800 is recommended for lispro). The higher values lead to more conservative estimates of the effect per unit of insulin, and therefore lead to more cautious adjustments. The effect per unit of insulin (aka, correction factor) is approximated by dividing the selected numerical value (eg, 1500-2200) by the number of units/day received by the patient. The correction factor may be used as a crude approximation of the patient's insulin sensitivity to determine the correction doses of insulin or adjust the current insulin regimen. Each additional unit of insulin added to the corresponding insulin dose may be expected to lower the blood glucose by the value of the correction factor.

To illustrate, in the "basal-bolus" regimen which includes 30 units of glargine at bedtime and 12 units of lispro insulin prior to each meal, the rule of 1800 would indicate an expected change of 27 mg/dL per unit of insulin (the total daily insulin dose is 66 units; using the formula: correction factor = 1800/66 = 27). A patient may be instructed to add additional insulin if the preprandial glucose is >125 mg/dL. For a prelunch glucose of 195 mg/dL (70 mg/dL higher than goal), this would mean the patient would administer the scheduled 12 units of lispro along with an additional "correction dose" of 3 units (70 divided by the correction factor of 27 derived from the formula) for a total of 15 units prior to the meal. If correction doses are required on a consistent basis, an adjustment of the patient's diet and/or scheduled insulin dose may be necessary.

Hypoglycemia

Hypoglycemia is the leading limiting factor in the treatment of diabetes. A patient experiencing an episode of acutely low blood sugar can perceive the event as an inconvenience in milder cases to a real threat of falls, motor vehicle accidents, etc. in severe cases.

Management of hypoglycemia:

- Conscious individual: Oral glucose: 15-20 g (any form of carbohydrate that contains glucose may be used). If a self-measurement of blood glucose (SMBG) 15 minutes after treatment shows continued hypoglycemia, the treatment should be repeated. Once SMBG glucose returns to normal, the individual should consume a meal or snack to prevent recurrence of hypoglycemia.
- Glucagon should be prescribed for all individuals at significant risk of severe hypoglycemia, and caregivers or family members should be instructed in administration.
- Patients with hypoglycemia unawareness or one or more episodes of severe hypoglycemia should be advised to raise their glycemic targets to avoid further hypoglycemia at least for a short period of time.
- Re-enforce education about prevention of hypoglycemia.

TYPE 2 DIABETES DRUG TREATMENT

Insulin therapy

Insulin may be used in type 2 diabetes as a means to augment response to oral antidiabetic agents or as monotherapy in selected patients. According to a consensus statement developed by the ADA and the European Association for the Study of Diabetes, basal insulin (eg, glargine, detemir) should be considered in patients who have failed to achieve their glycemic goals following lifestyle interventions and the administration of the maximal tolerated dose of metformin (ADA, 2009). Furthermore, intensive insulin therapy (eg, basal-bolus regimens) should be considered in patients who have failed to achieve their glycemic goals with an optimized two- or three-drug regimen (ADA, 2009). Augmentation to control postprandial glucose may be accomplished with regular, glulisine, aspart, or lispro insulin. Dosage must be carefully adjusted.

When used as monotherapy, the requirements for insulin are highly variable. An empirically defined scheme for dosage estimation based on fasting plasma glucose and degree of obesity has been published with recommended doses ranging from 6-77 units/day (Holman, 1995). In the setting of glucose toxicity (loss of beta-cell sensitivity to glucose concentrations), insulin therapy may be used for short-term management to restore sensitivity of beta-cells; in these cases, the dose may need to be rapidly reduced/withdrawn when sensitivity is re-established.

Oral Agents

A large number of drugs for oral administration have become available for the management of type 2 diabetes. Oral antidiabetic agents include sulfonylureas, meglitinides, alpha-glucosidase inhibitors, biguanides, thiazolidinediones (TZDs), and dipeptidyl peptidase IV (DPP-IV) inhibitors. The drug classes vary in terms of their magnitude of effect on glycemic control, mechanism of action, and adverse effect profiles. In many cases, the adverse effect profile may influence the selection of a particular drug. The risk of hypoglycemia is higher for drugs which promote insulin secretion (particularly sulfonylureas or insulin secretagogues). Drug selection is based on patient-specific factors and anticipated tolerance of adverse effects.

Metformin is currently the drug of choice if the patient has no contraindications. If lifestyle intervention and the maximal tolerated dose of metformin fail to achieve or sustain the glycemic goals, another medication should be added in several months. Another medication may also be necessary if metformin is contraindicated or not tolerated. Insulin or a sulfonylurea may be considered the next step if metformin and lifestyle changes are not adequate.

Combination therapy may be necessary to achieve glycemic goals. The risk of additive or additional adverse effects must be balanced with the desire to achieve goals of glycemic control as well as normalization of other metabolic parameters. In particular, weight gain and lipid disturbances may complicate drug treatment.

Oral Antidiabetic Agents for Type 2 Diabetes

Generic Name (Brand Name)	Expected Decrease (%) in Hb A_{1c} With Monotherapy	Key Adverse Effects
Alpha-Glucosidase Inhibitors		
Acarbose (Precose®)	0.5-0.8	GI distress, bloating, flatulence
Miglitol (Glyset®)		
Antilipemic Agent (Adjunct Therapy)		
Colesevelam (WelChol®)	0.5-1 (not for use as monotherapy)	Constipation, dyspepsia
Biguanide		
Metformin (Fortamet™; Glucophage® XR; Glucophage®; Glumetza®; Riomet®)	1-2	**Lactic acidosis [BOXED WARNING]**, GI distress, weakness
Dipeptidyl Peptidase IV (DPP-IV) Inhibitors		
Saxagliptin (Onglyza™)	0.4-0.5	Headache, UTI, sinusitis
Sitagliptin (Januvia™)	0.5-0.8	Nasopharyngitis, GI distress, nausea, peripheral edema, hypoglycemia
Dopamine agonists		
Bromocriptine (Cycloset®)	0.1	Nausea, dizziness, somnolence, postural hypotension, headache
Meglitinide Derivatives		
Nateglinide (Starlix®)	0.5-1.5 (repaglinide may be more effective)	Upper respiratory infection, flu-like syndrome, headache, hypoglycemia
Repaglinide (Prandin®)		
Sulfonylurea, 1st Generation		
Chlorpropamide (Diabinese®)	1-2	Hypoglycemia, dizziness, headache, GI distress, SIADH
Tolazamide		
Tolbutamide		
Sulfonylurea, 2nd Generation		
Glimepiride (Amaryl®)	1-2	Hypoglycemia, dizziness, headache, GI distress, SIADH
Glipizide (Glucotrol® XL; Glucotrol®)		
Glyburide (DiaBeta®; Glynase® PresTab®; Micronase®)		
Thiazolidinediones		
Pioglitazone (Actos®)	0.5-1.4	**May cause or exacerbate heart failure [BOXED WARNING]**, hepatic dysfunction, weight gain, edema, lipid changes
Rosiglitazone (Avandia®)		

Injectable Agents (Noninsulin)

In addition to insulin and oral agents, three injectable products are available for the management of diabetes. Exenatide (Byetta®) and liraglutide (Victoza®) are GLP-1 receptor agonists FDA-approved for the treatment of type 2 diabetes. Exenatide is used as an adjunct to diet and exercise to improve glycemic control in patients with type 2 diabetes mellitus. The manufacturer of liraglutide states that it is an injectable prescription medicine that may improve blood sugar in adults with type 2 diabetes when used along with diet and exercise. GLP-1 agonists increase insulin secretion, increase B-cell growth/replication, slow gastric emptying, and may decrease food intake.

Pramlintide (Symlin®) is FDA approved for the treatment of type 1 and type 2 diabetes. In type 1 diabetes, it is approved for use in patients who have failed to achieve glucose control despite optimal insulin therapy. When used for type 2 diabetes, pramlintide is approved for use in patients who have failed to achieve desired glucose control despite optimal insulin therapy, with or without concurrent sulfonylurea and/or metformin. Pramlintide is a synthetic analog of human amylin cosecreted with insulin by pancreatic beta cells. It reduces postprandial glucose increases by prolonging gastric emptying time, reducing postprandial glucagon secretion, and reducing caloric intake through centrally-mediated appetite suppression. It should be noted that the concentration of this product is in mcg/mL; patients and healthcare providers should exercise caution when administering this product to avoid inadvertent calculation of the dose based on "units," which could result in a sixfold overdose.

Injectable Agents (Non-Insulin) for Type 2 Diabetes

Generic Name (Brand Name)	Expected Decrease (%) in Hb A_{1c} With Monotherapy	Key Adverse Effects
Glucagon-Like Peptide 1 (GLP-1) Agonist		
Exenatide (Byetta®)	0.5-1	Hypoglycemia, nausea, vomiting, pancreatitis, headache, jittery feeling
Liraglutide (Victoza®)	1	**Thyroid C-cell Tumors [BOXED WARNING]**, nausea, vomiting, diarrhea, constipation, headache, pancreatitis
Amylin Agonists		
Pramlintide (Symlin®)	0.4-0.6	**Coadministration with insulin may induce severe hypoglycemia [BOXED WARNING]**, nausea, vomiting, hypoglycemia, headache, anorexia

Additional Management Issues

Recommendation by the ADA include glycemic control, as well as the following:

- Monitoring: In all patients with diabetes, cardiovascular risk factors should be assessed at least annually.
- Cardiovascular risk management
  - Use an ACEI or ARB in patients with diabetes who have hypertension and micro- or macroalbuminuria to slow the progression of nephropathy, unless contraindicated (eg, pregnancy); additional agents (eg, thiazide or loop diuretics) may be added as needed to achieve blood pressure goals.
  - Consider statin use in all patients with diabetes and cardiovascular disease or in patients with diabetes >40 years old without cardiovascular disease but have at least one other cardiovascular disease risk factor, irrespective of lipoprotein levels (exception: Statin use is contraindicated in pregnancy). For patients without overt CVD and <40 years old, statin therapy may be considered if LDL remains >100 mg/dL with lifestyles changes or in those with multiple cardiovascular risk factors. In individuals with overt CVD, lower LDL goals (<70 mg/dL) are suggested.
  - Use of low-dose aspirin (75-162 mg daily) is reasonable for primary prevention in all patients with diabetes at increased cardiovascular disease (CVD) risk (10-year risk >10%), including most men >50 years old and most women >60 years old who have at least one additional risk factor (eg, hypertension, smoking, family history of CVD, dyslipidemia, albuminuria), unless contraindicated. Low-dose aspirin may be considered for those at intermediate CVD risk (younger patients with ≥1 risk factor, older patients without risk factors, or patients with 10-year CVD risk of 5% to 10%). Aspirin is not recommended for primary prevention in patients with lower risk for CVD (eg, men <50 years old and women <60 years old without additional risk factor; 10-year CVD risk <5%). In secondary prevention, all patients with a history of CVD should receive aspirin (75-162 mg daily). Given the risk of Reye syndrome with the use of aspirin in patients <21 years old, aspirin is not recommended in this population for primary or secondary prevention. In patients unable to take aspirin (eg, documented allergy), the use of clopidogrel is considered a reasonable alternative.
  - Coronary heart disease (CHD): In patients with known cardiovascular disease (CVD), ACE inhibitor therapy and aspirin and statin therapy (if not contraindicated) should be used to reduce the risk of cardiovascular events. In patients with a prior myocardial infarction, beta-blockers should be continued for at least 2 years after the event. Avoid thiazolidinedione (TZD) treatment in patients with symptomatic heart failure. Metformin may be used in patients with stable congestive heart failure (CHF) if renal function is normal; however, it should be avoided in unstable or hospitalized patients with CHF.
- Other preventative actions
  - Immunize against pneumococcal disease ≥2 years old. One time revaccination is recommended for individuals >64 years old if they were <65 years old when previously immunized >5 years ago.
  - Influenza immunization annually for all diabetic patients ≥6 months old.
  - Patients should be advised not to smoke.
  - Patients should be advised to perform at least 150 minutes/week of moderate-intensity aerobic physical activity (50% to 70% of maximal heart rate). In the absence of contradictions, patients with type 2 diabetes should be encouraged to perform resistance training 3 times/week.
  - Eye care: To reduce the risk or slow the progression of retinopathy, optimize glycemic and blood pressure control. Adults and children ≥10 years old with type 1 diabetes should have an initial dilated and comprehensive eye examination within

5 years after the onset of diabetes (if type 2, exam should occur shortly after the diagnosis of diabetes). Subsequent examinations should be repeated annually. Promptly refer patients with any level of macular edema, severe nonproliferative diabetic retinopathy (NPDR), or any proliferative diabetic retinopathy (PDR) to an ophthalmologist who is knowledgeable and experienced in the management and treatment of diabetic retinopathy.

- Nephropathy: To reduce the risk or slow the progression of nephropathy, optimize glucose and blood pressure control. In the treatment of the nonpregnant patient with micro- or macroalbuminuria, either ACE inhibitors or ARBs should be used (if one class is not tolerated, the other should be substituted). When estimated GFR (eGFR) is <60 mL/minute/1.73 m^2, evaluate and manage potential complications of CKD. Consider referral to a physician experienced in the care of kidney disease when there is uncertainty about the etiology of the disease (heavy proteinuria, active urine sediment, absence of retinopathy, rapid decline in GFR), difficult management issues, or advanced kidney disease.
- Neuropathy: All patients should be screened for distal symmetric polyneuropathy (DPN) at diagnosis and at least annually thereafter, using simple clinical tests. Screening for signs and symptoms of cardiovascular autonomic neuropathy should be instituted at diagnosis of type 2 and 5 years after the diagnosis of type 1 diabetes.
- Foot care: Perform general foot self-care education to all patients with diabetes. For all patients with diabetes, perform an annual comprehensive foot examination. The foot examination should include inspection, assessment of foot pulses, and testing for loss of protective sensation (10 g monofilament, plus testing any one of: Vibration using a 128-Hz tuning fork, pinprick sensation, ankle reflexes, or vibration perception threshold).
- Thyroid: TSH concentrations should be measured after metabolic control has been established. If normal, they should be rechecked every 1-2 years or if the patient develops symptoms of thyroid dysfunction, thyromegaly, or an abnormal growth rate.

REFERENCES

Action to Control Cardiovascular Risk in Diabetes Study Group, "Effects of Intensive Glucose Lowering in Type 2 Diabetes," *N Engl J Med*, 2008, 358(24):2545-59.

ADVANCE Collaborative Group, "Intensive Blood Glucose Control and Vascular Outcomes in Patients With Type 2 Diabetes," *N Engl J Med*, 2008, 358(24):2560-72.

American Diabetes Association, "Diagnosis and Classification of Diabetes Mellitus," *Diabetes Care*, 2011, 34(Suppl 1):S62-9.

American Diabetes Association, "Standards of Medical Care in Diabetes - 2011," *Diabetes Care*, 2011, 34(Suppl 1):S11-61.

Brunzell JD, Davidson M, Furberg CD, et al, "Lipoprotein Management in Patients With Cardiometabolic Risk: Consensus Statement From the American Diabetes Association and the American College of Cardiology Foundation," *Diabetes Care*, 2008, 31(4):811-22.

Centers for Disease Control (CDC), "National Diabetes Fact Sheet: 2007 General Information," Available at: http://www.cdc.gov/diabetes/pubs/pdf/ndfs_2007.pdf. Accessed January 9, 2009.

Colhoun HM, Betteridge DJ, Durrington PN, et al, "Primary Prevention of Cardiovascular Disease With Atorvastatin in Type 2 Diabetes in the Collaborative Atorvastatin Diabetes Study (CARDS): Multicentre Randomised Placebo-Controlled Trial," *Lancet*, 2004, 364(9435):685-96.

Dailey G, "New Strategies for Basal Insulin Treatment in Type 2 Diabetes Mellitus," *Clin Ther*, 2004, 26 (6):889-901.

DeFronzo RA, "Pharmacologic Therapy for Type 2 Diabetes Mellitus," *Ann Intern Med*, 1999, 131 (4):281-303.

DeFronzo RA, "Pharmacologic Therapy for Type 2 Diabetes Mellitus," *Ann Intern Med*, 2000, 133 (1):73-4.

Duckworth W, Abraira C, Moritz T, et al, "Glucose Control and Vascular Complications in Veterans With Type 2 Diabetes," *N Engl J Med*, 2009, 360(2):129-39.

Holman RR and Turner RC, "Insulin Therapy in Type II Diabetes," *Diabetes Res Clin Pract*, 1995, (28 Suppl):S179-84.

International Expert Committee, "International Expert Committee Report on the Role of the A1C Assay in the Diagnosis of Diabetes," *Diabetes Care*, 2009, 32(7):1327-34.

Kitabchi AE, Umpierrez GE, Murphy MB, et al, "Hyperglycemic Crises in Diabetes," *Diabetes Care*, 2004, 27(Suppl 1):S94-102.

Nathan DM, Buse JB, Davidson MB, et al, "Medical Management of Hyperglycemia in Type 2 Diabetes: A Consensus Algorithm for the Initiation and Adjustment of Therapy: A Consensus Statement of the American Diabetes Association and the European Association for the Study of Diabetes," *Diabetes Care*, 2009, 32(1):193-203.

National Institute of Diabetes and Kigestive and Kidney Diseases, "Erectile Dysfunction," available at http://kidney.niddk.nih.gov/kudiseases/pubs/pdf/ErectileDysfunction.pdf. Accessed January 9, 2009.

Oiknine R, Bernbaum M, and Mooradian AD, "A Critical Appraisal of the Role of Insulin Analogues in the Management of Diabetes Mellitus," *Drugs*, 2005, 65(3):325-40.

Pignone M, Alberts MJ, Colwell JA, et al, "Aspirin for Primary Prevention of Cardiovascular Events in People With Diabetes: A Position Statement of the American Diabetes Association, a Scientific Statement of the American Heart Association, and an Expert Consensus Document of the American College of Cardiology Foundation," *Circulation*, 2010, 121(24):2694-701.

Scheife RT (editor), "Liraglutide: A New Option for the Treatment of Type 2 Diabetes Mellitus," *Pharmacotherapy*, 2009, 29(12 part 2): 23s-67s.

Sherifali D, Nerenberg K, Pullenayegum E, et al, "The Effect of Oral Antidiabetic Agents on A1C Levels: A Systematic Review and Meta-Analysis," *Diabetes Care*, 2010, 33(8):1859-64.

Silverstein J, Klingensmith G, Copeland K, et al, "Care of Children and Adolescents With Type 1 Diabetes: A Statement of the American Diabetes Association," *Diabetes Care*, 2005, 28(1):186-212.

The Diabetes Control and Complications Trial Research Group, "The Effect of Intensive Treatment of Diabetes on the Development and Progression of Long-Term Complications in Insulin-dependent Diabetes Mellitus," *N Engl J Med*, 1993, 329(14):977-86.

Tuomilehto J, Lindstrom J, Eriksson JG, et al, "Prevention of Type 2 Diabetes Mellitus by Changes in Lifestyle Among Subjects With Impaired Glucose Tolerance," *N Engl J Med*, 2001, 344(18):1343-50.

UK Prospective Diabetes Study Group, "Intensive Blood Glucose Control With Sulphonylureas or Insulin Compared With Conventional Treatment and Risk of Complications in Patients With Type 2 Diabetes (UKPDS 33)," *Lancet*, 1998, 352(9131):837-53.

DIABETES MELLITUS AND PREGNANCY

OVERVIEW OF DIABETES

Diabetes represents a significant health care problem in the United States and worldwide. Of the nearly 23.6 million Americans (7.8% of the population) with diabetes, the majority (90% to 95%) have type 2 diabetes. Of this number, nearly one-quarter are undiagnosed and the incidence is increasing. There is strong evidence to support an interaction between a genetic predisposition and behavioral or environmental factors, such as obesity and physical inactivity, in the development of this disease. In individuals at high risk of developing type 2 diabetes, it has been shown that the development of diabetes may be prevented or delayed by changes in lifestyle or pharmacologic intervention.

Within the United States, type 1 diabetes is estimated to comprise 5% to 10% of those with diabetes, and therefore represents the minority of individuals with diabetes. In addition to type 1 and type 2 diabetes, approximately 7% of pregnancies are complicated by the development of gestational diabetes. Diabetes may also result from genetic syndromes, surgery (pancreatectomy), chemicals and/or drugs, recurrent pancreatitis, malnutrition, and viral infections.

Approximately 1% of women have diabetes prior to pregnancy (pregestational diabetes). Gestational diabetes mellitus (GDM) has been traditionally defined as the first onset or recognition of glucose intolerance during pregnancy. GDM makes up ~90% of diabetes cases encountered in pregnant women. Women who have had gestational diabetes are at an increased risk for later development of type 2 diabetes. Women at high risk for the development of diabetes, and then diagnosed with diabetes at their first prenatal visit, are considered to have overt diabetes (ACOG, 2005; ADA, 2011).

Women of child bearing potential diagnosed with diabetes prior to pregnancy should understand the need for good glucose control and participate in family planning (ADA, 2008).

COMPLICATIONS OF DIABETES

Diabetes was listed as the seventh leading cause of death in the United States in 2007. Complications of diabetes are often contributing factors in the mortality of these patients; the most frequently reported diabetes complications that were reported as contributing factors in diabetes-related deaths were heart disease (68%) and stroke (16%) (data from 2004). In addition to cardiovascular effects, diabetes is the leading cause of new blindness in people 20-74 years of age and diabetic nephropathy is the most common cause of end-stage renal disease. Control of hyperglycemia may significantly decrease the rate at which diabetic complications develop and provides compelling justification for early diagnosis and management of this disorder.

In pregnant women, diabetes can adversely affect the mother, the fetus, and the newborn, especially if the disease is poorly treated.

- Poorly-treated pregestational diabetes may cause end-organ damage to the mother that may in turn negatively affect obstetric outcomes. Retinopathy can progress acutely during pregnancy, especially in women with hypertension or pre-eclampsia. Diabetic nephropathy and chronic hypertension occur in ~5% to 10% of pregnancies in women with diabetes. Pre-eclampsia occurs in ~15% to 20% of women with type 1 diabetes; the rate is higher with concomitant nephropathy or in women with hypertension. Spontaneous labor and delivery by cesarean section are also more common in women with pregestational diabetes (ACOG, 2005).
- The risk of congenital malformations is increased when the first trimester Hb A_{1c} is 7% or fasting plasma glucose is >120 mg/dL (>6.7 mmol/L) (Metzger, 2007). Cardiac defects, CNS anomalies (anencephaly, spina bifida), and skeletal malformations are most common and the risk may be decreased with good preconception management of diabetes in the mother. When maternal glucose levels are elevated in later trimesters, the risk of excessive fetal growth, intrauterine fetal death, shoulder dystocia with vaginal delivery, macrosomia, neonatal hypoglycemia, respiratory distress, and hyperbilirubinemia in the infant are increased. Macrosomia and hyperbilirubinemia are events more commonly observed in infants of women diagnosed with GDM (ACOG, 2005; ADA, 2011; Metzger, 2007). Increased birth weight and fetal hyperinsulinemia (as measured by cord-blood serum C-peptide) may also be associated with maternal hyperglycemia at levels below those diagnostic of GDM (HAPO Study Cooperative Research Group, 2008; IADPSG, 2010). To prevent adverse fetal events, prior to conception and throughout pregnancy the maternal Hb A_{1c} should be kept close to normal but without causing significant hypoglycemia (ADA, 2011; Kitzmiller, 2008). Women with a preconception Hb A_{1c} of ~5% to 6% have a fetal malformation rate similar to pregnancies of nondiabetic women (2% to 3%). In women with a preconception Hb A_{1c} of 10%, the anomaly rate is increased to 20% to 25% (ACOG, 2005).
- Children of women with poorly controlled diabetes are more likely to be obese, glucose intolerant, and have diabetes in late adolescence or young adulthood (ACOG, 2005; ADA, 2004).

Pre-existing conditions (eg, hypertension, diabetic nephropathy) should be evaluated prior to pregnancy. Medications used to treat diabetes or related conditions should also be reviewed in order to evaluate their safety during pregnancy. In order to avoid complications, glycemic control should be as close to normal as possible (without significant hypoglycemia) prior to pregnancy and effective contraception should be used until glycemic control is achieved (Kitzmiller, 2008).

DIAGNOSIS

The diagnosis of diabetes in nonpregnant adults is made by any of the four criteria described below. New in the 2010 American Diabetes Association (ADA) Standards of Medical Care is the recommendation for the use of Hb A1c for the diagnosis of diabetes; the method used should be certified by the National Glycohemoglobin Standardization Program (NGSP) and standardized to the Diabetes Control and Complications Trial (DCCT) assay.

Diagnosis of Diabetes in Adults

1. Hb A_{1c} ≥6.5%
   OR
2. Fasting plasma glucose (no caloric intake for at least 8 hours) ≥126 mg/dL (7 mmol/L)
   OR
3. Casual plasma glucose concentration ≥200 mg/dL (11.1 mmol/L) in patients with symptoms of hyperglycemia (polydipsia, polyuria, unexplained weight loss) or hyperglycemic crisis. **Note:** Casual plasma glucose is defined as any time of day without regard to time of last meal.
   OR
4. A 2-hour plasma glucose ≥200 mg/dL (11.1 mmol/L) during an oral glucose tolerance test (OGTT) in accordance with the standards set forth by the World Health Organization (WHO) using a 75 g anhydrous glucose load (or equivalent) dissolved in water. **Note:** OGTT is not recommended for routine clinical use.

Note: In the absence of unequivocal hyperglycemia, criteria 1, 2, and 4 should be confirmed by repeat testing.

Screening for and Diagnosis of Gestational Diabetes Mellitus

Screening: In women at 24-28 weeks gestation not previously diagnosed with overt diabetes, perform a 75 g oral glucose tolerance test (OGTT), obtaining plasma glucose levels while fasting and at 1 and 2 hours. **Note:** The OGTT should be performed in the morning after an overnight fast of at least 8 hours.

Diagnosis: The diagnosis of Gestational Diabetes Mellitus is made when any of the following plasma glucose (PG) values are exceeded:

- Fasting PG ≥92 mg/dL (5.1 mmol/L)
- 1 hour PG ≥180 mg/dL (10.0 mmol/L)
- 2 hour PG ≥153 mg/dL (8.5 mmol/L)

The following thresholds proposed by IADPSG can be used at the *first prenatal visit*:

- **To diagnose GDM:** Following a 75 g OGTT, one or more of the following plasma glucose values must be found (IADPSG consensus thresholds):
  - FPG ≥92 mg/dL (5.1 mmol/L) but <126 mg/dL (7 mmol/L); **Note:** If FPG is <92 mg/dL (5.1 mmol/L), test again at 24-28 weeks gestation.
  - 1 hour: ≥180 mg/dL (10 mmol/L)
  - 2 hour: ≥153 mg/dL (8.5 mmol/L)
- **To diagnose overt diabetes in pregnancy:** Following a 75 g OGTT, one or more of the following plasma glucose values must be found (IADPSG consensus thresholds):
  - FPG: ≥126 mg/dL (7 mmol/L)
  - Hb A_{1c}: ≥6.5% (DCCT/UKPDS standardized)
  - Random plasma glucose: ≥200 mg/dL (11.1 mmol/L) **plus** confirmation with FPG or Hb A_{1c}

  If results indicate overt diabetes, treat and follow for preexisting diabetes.

GOALS

The goals of diabetes treatment include normalization of hyperglycemia, avoidance of hypoglycemia, and slowing the development of diabetic complications. For additional information on the goals of treatment in nonpregnant patients, visit the ADA website at http://care.diabetesjournals.org/content/34/Supplement_1.

In women with pregestational diabetes, Hb A_{1c} should be kept as close to normal as possible without significant hypoglycemia. Self-monitoring of blood glucose with the fingerstick method is best during pregnancy. Goals for glycemic control:

- Premeal, bedtime, and overnight glucose: 60-99 mg/dL (3.3-5.4 mmol/L)
- Peak postprandial glucose: 100-129 mg/dL (5.4-7.1 mmol/L)
- Hb A_{1c}: <6.0% (measure monthly until target achieved, then every 2-3 months)

Less intensive glycemic goals may be indicated in patients unaware of hypoglycemia or not able to adhere to intensified management (Kitzmiller, 2008).

MANAGEMENT OF DIABETES

Current ADA recommendations emphasize a multidisciplinary approach to the management of diabetes, with an emphasis on the participation of the patient and/or caregivers in the monitoring and management of the disease. Consultation with a diabetes educator and dietitian may help to prepare the patient to manage her disease and adjust to the necessary changes in diet and lifestyle. Patients must be educated about disease monitoring procedures, including blood glucose self-monitoring equipment and tests. Patients should be encouraged to wear or carry appropriate identification to inform health care providers of their disease in the event of an emergency. It is extremely important to educate patients concerning the recognition and management of hypoglycemic symptoms. The management of diabetes is constantly adapting to new information, techniques, and technologies. For additional information on the management of diabetes in nonpregnant patients, visit the ADA website at http://care.diabetesjournals.org/content/34/Supplement_1.

Recommendations by the ADA include glycemic control, as well as the following for pregnant women with diabetes (Kitzmiller, 2008):

- Women should receive individualized medical nutrition therapy in order to support a healthy pregnancy.
- Assess prepregnancy BMI and target weight gain based on BMI group, energy intake, physical activity, fetal growth, and desire to prevent excess maternal weight gain and postpartum weight retention.
- Individualize daily diet to promote optimal glycemic control and avoid hypoglycemia and ketonemia. Promote a healthy, balanced diet.
- Use supplemental minerals, trace elements, and vitamins to achieve appropriate intake for pregnancy.

DRUG TREATMENT

Insulin

Insulin therapy is considered the drug of choice for the control of all types of diabetes mellitus during pregnancy.

The general objective of insulin replacement therapy is to approximate the physiologic pattern of insulin secretion which is characterized by two distinct phases – phase 1 insulin secretion suppresses hepatic glucose production and phase 2 insulin secretion occurs in response to carbohydrate ingestion. This requires a basal level of insulin throughout the day (such as intermediate- or long-acting insulin or continuous insulin infusion administered via an external SubQ insulin infusion pump), supplemented by additional insulin at mealtimes (eg, short- or rapid-acting insulin).

Multiple daily doses guided by blood glucose monitoring are the standard of diabetes care. Combinations of insulin are commonly used. The number and size of daily doses, time of administration, and diet and exercise require continuous medical supervision. In addition, specific formulations may require distinct administration procedures/timing (refer to individual monographs).

There is solid scientific documentation of the benefit of tight glucose control. However, the benefits must be balanced against the risk of hypoglycemia, the patient's ability to adhere to the regimen, and other issues regarding the complexity of management. Diabetes self-management education (DSME) and medical nutrition therapy (MNT) are essential to maximize the effectiveness of therapy. In addition to the educational issues outlined above, patients should be instructed in insulin administration techniques, timing of administration, and sick-day management.

Since combinations of agents are frequently used, dosage adjustment must address the individual component of the insulin regimen which most directly influences the blood glucose value in question, based on the known onset and duration of the insulin component (see table on next page). The frequency of doses and monitoring must also be individualized in consideration of the patient's ability to manage therapy.

In pregnant women with pre-existing type 1 diabetes, NPH insulin is preferred over insulin detemir or insulin glargine. Transition to NPH should take place prior to pregnancy or at the first prenatal visit. Rapid-acting insulin (eg, insulin lispro, insulin aspart) may be used instead of premeal regular insulin. Insulin requirements may decrease at 10-14 weeks gestation, then increase gradually until ~35 weeks gestation, where they may level off or decline (Kitzmiller, 2008).

In women with pre-existing type 2 diabetes, transition to insulin should take place prior to pregnancy and acceptable glucose control should be achieved prior to conception. Women with type 2 diabetes who become pregnant while taking oral agents should be transitioned to insulin as soon as possible. Initial total daily doses of 0.7-1.0 units/kg are often effective; higher doses may be needed in women who are obese (Kitzmiller, 2008).

Insulin is also recommended for women diagnosed with GDM (ADA, 2004).

Insulin should be injected into the abdomen or hips (Kitzmiller, 2008).

Types of Insulin	Onset (h)	Peak Glycemic Effect (h)	Duration (h)
Rapid-Acting			
Insulin lispro (Humalog®)	0.25-0.5	0.5-2.5	≤5
Insulin aspart (NovoLog®)	0.2-0.3	1-3	3-5
Insulin glulisine (Apidra®)	0.2-0.5	1.6-2.8	3-4
Short-Acting			
Insulin regular (Humulin® R, Novolin® R)	0.5	2.5-5	4-12 – U-100 Up to 24 – U-500
Intermediate-Acting			
Insulin NPH (isophane suspension) (Humulin® N, Novolin® N)	1-2	4-12	14-24
Intermediate- to Long-Acting			
Insulin determir (Levemir®)	3-4	3-9	6-23 (duration is dose-dependent)
Long-Acting			
Insulin glargine (Lantus®)	3-4	*	10.8-≥24
Combinations			
Insulin aspart protamine suspension and insulin aspart (NovoLog® Mix 70/30)	0.17-0.33	1-4	18-24
Insulin lispro protamine and insulin lispro (Humalog® Mix 75/25™)	0.25-0.5	1-6.5	14-24
Insulin NPH suspension and insulin regular solution (Novolin® 70/30)	0.5	2-12	18-24

* Insulin glargine has no pronounced peak.

For a general discussion of maintenance dosing and dosing adjustments in nonpregnant patients, visit the ADA website at http://www.diabetes.org/.

Insulin Therapy During Labor

In women with pregestational diabetes, insulin may not be needed during active labor. In patients who use continuous subcutaneous insulin infusion (CSII), the basal insulin component may be continued during labor (ACOG, 2005).

When labor is induced, the usual dose of intermediate insulin may be given at bedtime the evening before. Hold the morning dose of insulin and begin an I.V. infusion with normal saline. Monitor glucose hourly. Once active labor begins or glucose concentrations are <70 mg/dL (3.9 mmol/L), change NS infusion to D_5W and infuse at a rate of 2.5 mg/kg/minute to reach a glucose concentration of ~100 mg/dL (~5.6 mmol/L). If glucose concentrations are >100 mg/dL (5.6 mmol/L), administer regular insulin I.V. at a rate of 1.25 units/hour (ACOG, 2005).

Following delivery, insulin requirements will decrease rapidly. Once food intake has started, approximately one-half of the predelivery dose may be initiated and titrated as needed (ACOG, 2005).

Oral Agents

The use of oral antihyperglycemic agents in pregnant women with type 2 diabetes or GDM is controversial (Kitzmiller, 2008; Metzger, 2007). Insulin therapy is required in type 1 diabetes. Until additional safety and efficacy data are obtained, the use of oral agents is generally not recommended as routine management of GDM or type 2 diabetes mellitus during pregnancy. Insulin is the drug of choice for the control of diabetes mellitus during pregnancy.

Glyburide: Glyburide was not found to significantly cross the placenta *in vitro* and was not found in the cord serum infants of mothers taking glyburide for GDM. The manufacturer recommends that if glyburide is used during pregnancy, it should be discontinued at least 2 weeks before the expected delivery date. Although studies have shown positive outcomes using glyburide for the treatment of GDM, use may not be appropriate for all women.

Metformin: Metformin has been found to cross the placenta in levels which may be comparable to those found in the maternal plasma. Pharmacokinetic studies suggest that clearance of metformin may be increased during pregnancy and dosing may need adjusted in some women when used during the third trimester. Fetal, neonatal, and maternal outcomes have been evaluated following maternal use of metformin for the treatment of GDM and type 2 diabetes. Available information suggests that metformin use during pregnancy may be safe as long as good glycemic control is maintained; however, many studies used metformin during the second or third trimester only.

Postpartum Considerations

Breast-feeding is encouraged for all women, including those with type 1, type 2, or GDM (ACOG, 2005; ADA, 2004). An increase in caloric intake is required and small snacks before feeds may help decrease the risk of hypoglycemia in women with pregestational diabetes (ACOG, 2005). In women with GDM, breast-feeding for >3 months was shown to decrease the child's risk of becoming overweight by 45% at 2-8 years of age (Metzger, 2007). All types of insulin may be used while breast-feeding and some oral agents may be acceptable for use as well.

For women diagnosed with GDM, most will have normal glucose tolerance after delivery. Serum glucose should be evaluated prior to discharge (1-3 days after delivery) and elevated concentrations should be confirmed and treated. For women diagnosed with GDM and normal glucose concentrations following delivery, the 75 g OGTT should be repeated at 6-12 weeks postpartum, 1 year postpartum, and then every 3 years. Fasting plasma glucose should be monitored yearly. Prior to future pregnancies, the 75 g OGTT should also be performed (Metzger, 2007).

PATIENT-RELATED INFORMATION

"Diabetes and Pregnancy." Informational Fact Sheet from OTIS (Organization of Teratology Information Specialists). Available at: http://www.otispregnancy.org/files/diabetes.pdf.

"Diabetes in Pregnancy." Information from the CDC: http://www.cdc.gov/Features/DiabetesPregnancy/.

"For Women with Diabetes: Your Guide to Pregnancy." Available from the National Diabetes information Clearing House (NDIC): http://diabetes.niddk.nih.gov/dm/pubs/pregnancy/#top.

"It's Never too Early to Prevent Diabetes." Pamphlet for women who had GDM in a previous pregnancy; available from the National Diabetes Education Program: http://ndep.nih.gov/media/NeverTooEarly_Tipsheet.pdf.

REFERENCES

American College of Obstetricians and Gynecologists, "ACOG Practice Bulletin. Clinical Management Guidelines for Obstetrician-Gynecologists. Number 60, March 2005. Pregestational Diabetes Mellitus," *Obstet Gynecol*, 2005, 105(3):675-85.

American Diabetes Association, "Diagnosis and Classification of Diabetes Mellitus," *Diabetes Care*, 2011, 34(Suppl 1):S62-9.

American Diabetes Association, "Gestational Diabetes Mellitus," *Diabetes Care*, 2004, 27(Suppl 1): S88-90.

American Diabetes Association, "Standards of Medical Care in Diabetes - 2011," *Diabetes Care*, 2011, 34(Suppl 1):S11-61.

Centers for Disease Control (CDC), "National Diabetes Fact Sheet: 2007 General Information," Available at: http://www.cdc.gov/diabetes/pubs/pdf/ndfs_2007.pdf. Accessed April 1, 2010.

HAPO Study Cooperative Research Group, Metzger BE, Lowe LP, et al, "Hyperglycemia and Adverse Pregnancy Outcomes," *N Engl J Med*, 2008, 358(19):1991-2002.

International Association of Diabetes and Pregnancy Study Groups Consensus Panel, "International Association of Diabetes and Pregnancy Study Groups Recommendations on the Diagnosis and Classification of Hyperglycemia in Pregnancy," *Diabetes Care*, 2010, 33(3):676-82.

International Expert Committee, "International Expert Committee Report on the Role of the A1C Assay in the Diagnosis of Diabetes," *Diabetes Care*, 2009, 32(7):1327-34.

Kitzmiller JL, Block JM, Brown FM, et al, "Managing Preexisting Diabetes for Pregnancy: Summary of Evidence and Consensus Recommendations for Care," *Diabetes Care*, 2008, 31(5):1060-79.

Metzger BE, Buchanan TA, Coustan DR, et al, "Summary and Recommendations of the Fifth International Workshop-Conference on Gestational Diabetes Mellitus," *Diabetes Care*, 2007, 30(Suppl 2): S251-60.

HEART FAILURE (SYSTOLIC)

INTRODUCTORY COMMENTS

This summarizes the pharmacotherapy of patients with systolic heart failure with respect to treating mild-to-moderate exacerbations and chronic therapy. A more detailed discussion is available at http://content.onlinejacc.org/cgi/content/full/j.jacc.2008.11.013.

It should be recognized that the most common cause for exacerbations of patients' heart failure is poor adherence to therapy (medications and diet restriction). Healthcare providers need to educate patients about the importance of adherence to medical regimens.

For many years, therapy of heart failure focused on correcting the hemodynamic imbalances that occurred in heart failure. It is now recognized that heart failure triggers the release of several neurohormones that, in the short-run, help the patient; but, in the long-run, are detrimental. Newer pharmacotherapeutic approaches address counteracting the actions of these harmful neurohormones as well as address hemodynamic issues.

DIURETICS

Although data have yet to demonstrate that diuretics reduce the mortality associated with heart failure, they relieve symptoms seen in heart failure. Diuretics should only be used in patients experiencing congestion with their heart failure. Although not usually the case, some patients do have heart failure without congestion. In such rare instances, diuretic therapy is not indicated since they further stimulate the deleterious neurohormonal responses seen.

Although some heart failure patients with congestion can be controlled with thiazide diuretics, most will require the more potent loop diuretics, either because a strong diuretic effect is needed or renal function is compromised (thus limiting the effectiveness of the thiazide diuretic). When patients with heart failure are discovered to have mild-to-moderate worsening congestion, they often can be controlled by adjusting their oral loop diuretic dose or, if applicable, initiating a loop diuretic regimen. If a more aggressive diuresis is indicated, especially if the patient is suffering from pulmonary congestion, intravenous loop diuretics would be indicated. When loop diuretics are given intravenously, before any diuretic effect occurs, they benefit the patient by dilating veins and reducing preload, thus relieving pulmonary congestion. Intravenous loop diuretics may also be considered in a patient where concerns exist about the ability to absorb orally administered medication.

If already on an oral loop diuretic, the dosage should be increased (generally, 1.5-2 times their current regimen) in an effort for the patient to lose about 1-1.5 liters of fluid per day (about equivalent to 1-1.5 kg of weight per day). If the patient had yet to be started on a diuretic or was previously receiving a thiazide diuretic, initiating furosemide at 20-40 mg once or twice daily is a reasonable consideration. If the initial increase (or initiation) in dosage fails to induce a diuretic response, the dosage may be increased. If the initial increase (or initiation) does induce a diuretic response but the patient fails to lose weight or is not losing more fluids than taking in, the frequency of giving the loop diuretic may be increased. When an effective regimen is achieved, this regimen should be continued until the patient achieves a goal "dry" weight. Once this weight is attained, a decision needs to be made on how to continue the patient on diuretic therapy. If the patient had not been on a diuretic at home, continuation of the loop diuretic at a reduced dose is a worthy consideration. If the exacerbation was related to nonadherence with the diuretic or diet, the previous home dose might be continued with education on adherence to the prescribed diet and medication use. If the exacerbation was caused by an inadequate pharmacotherapeutic regimen (such as vasodilator was not being use), the previous home dose might be continued in conjunction with a more complete pharmacotherapeutic regimen. If the patient was compliant and on an acceptable pharmacotherapeutic regimen, the patient's original diuretic dose would be increased to some dosage greater than their home regimen, yet generally less than what was just used to achieve their dry weight.

The use of loop diuretics can lead to hypokalemia and/or hypomagnesemia. Electrolyte disturbances can predispose a patient to serious cardiac arrhythmias particularly if the patient is concurrently receiving digoxin. Fluid depletion, hypotension, and azotemia can also result from excessive use of diuretics. In contrast to thiazide diuretics, a loop diuretic can also lower serum calcium concentrations. For some patients, despite higher doses of loop diuretic treatment, an adequate diuretic response cannot be attained. Diuretic resistance can usually be overcome by intravenous administration (including continuous infusion), the use of 2 diuretics together (eg, furosemide and metolazone), or the use of a diuretic with a positive inotropic agent. When such combinations are used, serum electrolytes need to be monitored even more closely.

When loop diuretics are used in patients with renal dysfunction, to achieve the desired diuretic response, dosages typically will need to be greater than what is used in patients with normal renal function.

Due to its long existence and inexpensive price, furosemide tends to be the loop diuretic most commonly used. Bumetanide and torsemide are now available as generics and their use, especially bumetanide, has increased. The oral bioavailability of bumetanide and torsemide are nearly 100%; whereas, furosemide's oral bioavailability averages about 50%. A useful rule of thumb for conversion of intravenous loop diuretics is 40 mg of furosemide is equal to 1 mg bumetanide is equal to 20 mg torsemide. A few patients have allergies to diuretics because many contain a sulfur element. The only loop diuretic that lacks a sulfur element is ethacrynic acid.

VASODILATORS

Combination Hydralazine and Isosorbide Dinitrate

Vasodilator therapy, specifically the combination of hydralazine and isosorbide dinitrate, was the first pharmacotherapeutic treatment demonstrated to enhance survival of heart failure patients. The use of hydralazine 75 mg (which reduces afterload) and isosorbide dinitrate 40 mg 4 times a day (which reduces preload) demonstrated enhanced survival compared to placebo and prazosin. Unfortunately, many patients were unable to tolerate this regimen (primarily due to headaches and gastrointestinal disturbances) and the magnitude of benefit in survival dissipated with time.

The African-American Heart Failure Trial (A-HeFT) demonstrated mortality benefit with the use of a fixed combination of hydralazine and isosorbide dinitrate in combination with standard heart failure therapies, including ACE inhibitors, in self-identified African-American heart failure patients. The use of the commercially available combination of hydralazine and isosorbide dinitrate may be cost prohibitive in some patients; therefore, the use of the individually separate products is justifiable.

ACE Inhibitors

A series of investigations demonstrated that enalapril (which reduces both afterload and preload) enhances the survival of heart failure patients. Dosages used in these trials averaged about 10 mg twice daily. Since these trials, other ACE inhibitors were proven to benefit heart failure patients. This led to the question – which is superior, ACE inhibitor or the combination of hydralazine and isosorbide dinitrate? In a comparative trial, using doses described above, enalapril was superior to the combination of hydralazine and isosorbide dinitrate, making an ACE inhibitor the vasodilator of choice in heart failure patients. An ACE inhibitor can alleviate symptoms, improve clinical status, and enhance a patient's quality of life. In addition an ACE inhibitor can reduce the risk of death and the combined risk of death or hospitalization.

Adverse effects associated with ACE inhibitors include hyperkalemia, rash, dysgeusia, dry cough, and (rarely) angioedema. Patients sometime develop renal dysfunction with the initiation of ACE inhibitors. This is not due to direct nephrotoxicity but is related to the ACE inhibitor dilating the efferent renal artery of the kidney, thus shunting blood away from being filtered in the glomerulus. The risk for renal dysfunction is increased when the ACE inhibitor is introduced to a patient who is hypovolemic, is being aggressively diuresed, is on an NSAID (which should be avoided in heart failure patients), or has bilateral renal artery stenosis (unilateral if only one kidney is present). ACE inhibitors should be avoided in patients with known renal artery stenosis. Monitor renal function and serum potassium within 1-2 weeks of initiation of therapy and routinely thereafter especially in patients with pre-existing hypotension, hyponatremia, diabetes, azotemia, or those taking potassium supplements. Some patients will have an exaggerated hypotensive response following the initial doses (especially the first dose) of an ACE inhibitor.

Angiotensin Receptor Blockers

A major limitation to using ACE inhibitors treatment in heart failure can be the dry cough that some patients develop. Lowering the ACE inhibitor dose sometimes can control it, but this may limit the effectiveness of the ACE inhibitor treatment. The development of angiotensin receptor blockers (ARBs) has helped address this issue. ARBs were demonstrated to enhance survival of heart failure patients. Although they are not the vasodilator of first choice in heart failure, they are a reasonable alternative in patients who cannot tolerate an ACE inhibitor due to the cough or some other adverse effect (with the exception of hyperkalemia and renal dysfunction; ARBs can induce as well). ARBs do not cause an accumulation of kinins as ACE inhibitors do.

Can ARBs be used in patients who suffer angioedema with ACE inhibitors? Reports are available in the literature describing patients who experienced angioedema with both ACE inhibitors and ARBs. These cases do not indicate the safety of an ARB when used in a patient who has experienced ACE inhibitor-induced angioedema. The CHARM-Alternative trial confirmed that only one of 39 patients (~2.6%) who experienced angioedema with an ACE inhibitors also experienced it with an ARB.

Concurrent Use of an ACE Inhibitor and an ARB

In Val-HeFT, valsartan added to conventional treatment (included ACE inhibitor treatment) did not impact survival but did reduce morbidity. Of note, a subgroup analysis of this trial suggested the combination of valsartan and an ACE inhibitor may be detrimental to patients also receiving a beta-blocker. In CHARM-Added, candesartan added to ACE inhibitor therapy was of benefit to heart failure patients (modest reduction in hospitalization; increased risk of hyperkalemia and renal dysfunction), even for those receiving a beta-blocker. As a result, the ACCF/AHA Practice Guidelines do not speak against using the combination of ACE inhibitors and ARBs. However, few patients in these trials were receiving an aldosterone blocker (such as spironolactone), which is now known to be of benefit to heart failure patients. Since there is enhanced risk for hyperkalemia and outcome data are currently unknown, the ACCF/AHA Practice Guidelines for heart failure do not advocate the combined use of ACE inhibitors, ARBs, and an aldosterone inhibitor.

In summary, vasodilator therapy should initially consist of an ACE inhibitor. If such therapy cannot be tolerated due to renal failure or hyperkalemia, the combination of hydralazine and isosorbide dinitrate may be considered as ARBs can also cause renal failure and hyperkalemia. If the ACE inhibitor cannot be tolerated due to adverse effects such as dry cough, an ARB may be considered. If an ACE inhibitor and beta-blocker have been maximized yet heart failure symptoms persist, consider adding hydralazine and isosorbide dinitrate. This approach, in fact, has been demonstrated to enhance the survival of African-American patients with heart failure. Another approach may be to add an ARB to the ACE inhibitor; but caution should occur, due to the risk of hyperkalemia.

BETA-BLOCKERS

Despite being negative inotropes, beta-blockers have been demonstrated to enhance the survival of systolic heart failure patients. Their benefit is attributed to their ability to protect the myocardium from the "bombardment" of catecholamines present in heart failure that can lead to ventricular remodeling. Bisoprolol, metoprolol succinate (extended release), and carvedilol have been demonstrated in trials to improve survival. Carvedilol is also available as a once-a-day extended-release preparation; but, its daily cost is considerably greater than generically-available immediate-release carvedilol that is given twice a day. At present, superiority of a particular beta-blocker over another has not been definitively demonstrated. For patients to be able to tolerate this therapy, beta-blocker treatment needs to be initiated at low doses and titrated slowly (generally, the dose is double every two weeks). Following the initiation of treatment and increase in dosage, patients may feel that their disease is worsening but this should dissipate after a few days. If this ill feeling continues beyond a few days, consideration should be given to regimen adjustments. If the patient is congested, increase the diuretic dosage. If the patient's discomfort is related to hypotension, staggering the beta-blocker dose with the vasodilator dose and/or lowering the vasodilator dosage may be helpful. If these approaches are ineffective or cannot explain the patient's ill feeling, consideration should be given to lowering the beta-blocker dosage and attempt a dose titration increase later on. Sometimes, a patient may not be able to tolerate "goal" doses of both beta-blockers and concurrent vasodilator treatment due to hypotension. It is the consensus opinion that a reduced dose of each agent is better than a goal dose of just one agent. Beta-blockers are not necessarily contraindicated but need to be used cautiously in patients with bronchospastic disease, peripheral arterial disease, or diabetes mellitus.

ALDOSTERONE BLOCKERS

It has been demonstrated, especially in the more severe forms of heart failure, that spironolactone, at an average dose of 25 mg daily, enhances the survival of heart failure patients. In patients who suffer hyperkalemia at this relatively low dosage, lowering the dose to 25 mg every other day may be attempted. In patients who remain symptomatic with their heart failure and have maximized the other proven treatments of heart failure and whose potassium concentrations can tolerate increases, the spironolactone dose may be increased to 50 mg daily.

Obviously, hyperkalemia is a concern with this treatment, especially since patients generally will also be receiving an ACE inhibitor or ARB. It has been demonstrated that the number of emergency visits related to hyperkalemia in heart failure has increased with the introduction of aldosterone blocking therapy in treating heart failure. About 10% of patients will experience endocrinological effects with spironolactone. In men, breast tenderness and gynecomastia may occur. In women, menstrual irregularities may be seen. In such instances, the use of eplerenone may be considered. Eplerenone is less apt to induce endocrinological effects but it is more expensive. A typical dose is 25-50 mg daily. Eplerenone has been demonstrated to enhance survival of post-MI patients with reduced ejection fractions. Spironolactone has not been studied in this patient group.

These medications should not be started in patients with renal insufficiency. These medications should be avoided if the serum creatinine exceeds 2.5 mg/dL in men (2 mg/dL in women) or if baseline potassium ≥5 mEq/L.

DIGOXIN

The value of digoxin in heart failure has crossed the spectrum. In the late 1980s, further investigation with digoxin suggested that indeed it may have a role in heart failure treatment, but the methods of these trials were not ideal (digoxin was taken away from stabilized patients to see if the condition of patients worsened – it did). Finally, digoxin was studied in a prospective manner where patients were on known optimal heart failure treatment at the time and randomized to placebo or digoxin. The digoxin dosage used resulted in digoxin steady-state concentrations of 1 mcg/L. This trial revealed that digoxin did not impact survival but reduced the number of patient hospitalizations, suggesting digoxin has a morbidity benefit. Many are of the opinion that digoxin's benefit is unrelated to its positive inotropic activity but related to inhibiting neurohormonal activity. Healthcare providers may consider adding digoxin in patients with persistent heart failure symptoms as a fourth line agent.

Digoxin is primarily renally eliminated; therefore, renal function of patients should be closely monitored and the dose adjusted. Digoxin does become difficult to use in patients whose renal function is unstable. In the DIG trial, effective digoxin steady-state concentrations ranged between 0.7-1 mcg/L. Concentrations much beyond 1 mcg/L were associated with worsened outcomes, especially in women. Since digoxin's benefit is long-term, a loading dose is not necessary. When checking a digoxin serum concentration, the sample should not be obtained until 12 hours after a dose, especially if it was oral, since digoxin has a relatively long distribution phase. It should also be assured that the patient is at steady-state (recall that the half-life of digoxin in a patient with normal renal function is approximately 36 hours and that patients with heart failure generally have worsened renal function).

Hypokalemia, hypomagnesia, hypercalcemia, and hypothyroidism can precipitate digoxin toxicity in the presence of a therapeutic digoxin concentration. This toxicity can be alleviated by correcting the electrolyte abnormality. In acute digoxin overdoses, hyperkalemia can occur since digoxin inhibits the sodium-potassium ATPase pump. For this reason, one should not assume potassium is given to just **any** patient with digoxin toxicity. Digoxin toxicity can present as bradyarrhythmias, heart blocks, ventricular tachyarrhythmias, and atrial tachyarrhythmias (PAT with block is pathognomonic). Other toxic manifestations include visual disturbances (including greenish-yellowish vision and halos around lights), gastrointestinal disturbances, anorexia, and altered mental status.

Many medications elevate digoxin concentrations and a patient's regimen should be assessed for potential interactions.

OTHER HEART FAILURE THERAPEUTIC CONSIDERATIONS

- If a calcium channel blocker is desired, amlodipine or felodipine are preferred choices.
- To treat arrhythmias, amiodarone and dofetilide are best documented to lack significant proarrhythmic propensity in heart failure patients. Dronedarone, a newer antiarrhythmic agent structurally similar to amiodarone, is contraindicated in patients with NYHA Class IV heart failure or Class II-III heart failure with recent decompensation requiring hospitalization or referral to a specialized heart failure clinic.
- In heart failure patients with diabetes mellitus, metformin should not be used and "glitazones" should not be used in severe heart failure (NYHA III and IV) and used cautiously, if at all, in mild-to-moderate heart failure.
- The use of cilostazol, because it has type III phosphodiesterase-inhibiting properties, is contraindicated in heart failure. This is because the chronic use of *oral* milrinone and inamrinone, also type III phosphodiesterase inhibitors, resulted in enhanced mortality in heart failure patients (and therefore, these two agents were never FDA-approved for oral use).
- NSAID use should be avoided or used minimally as these agents antagonize the effects of diuretics and ACE inhibitors.
- Retrospective data suggests that daily aspirin may also negate the effects of ACE inhibitors but this has yet to be definitively proven in prospective trials. Using the lowest possible aspirin dose with the highest possible ACE inhibitor dose has been suggested as a way to best circumvent this issue.
- Routine intermittent intravenous infusions of positive inotropes are not recommended; but their use may be considered as palliative therapy in end-stage disease when ordinary therapy is insufficient.

CLASS I RECOMMENDATIONS FOR THE HOSPITALIZED PATIENT WITH ACUTE DECOMPENSATED HEART FAILURE

- Patients presenting to the hospital with fluid overload should be treated immediately with intravenous loop diuretics (eg, furosemide) since earlier treatment may be associated with better outcomes. If chronically receiving oral loop diuretic therapy, the initial intravenous dose should equal or exceed their chronic oral daily dose and titrated to relieve symptoms and reduce fluid excess. If this is inadequate, use of higher doses of loop diuretics, adding a second diuretic (eg, intravenous chlorothiazide), or a continuous infusion of the loop diuretic may improve diuresis.
- If evidence of hypotension with associated hypoperfusion and elevated cardiac filling pressures (eg, increase JVP) exists, intravenous inotropic support (eg, dobutamine) or vasopressor drugs (eg, dopamine) should be administered. Use of intravenous inotropes in patients without evidence of hypoperfusion is not recommended.
- In the absence of hemodynamic instability or contraindications, the use of therapies known to improve outcomes (eg, ACE inhibitors or ARBs, and beta-blockers) should be continued during the hospital stay. When appropriate, these agents should be initiated or reinitiated to stabilized patients prior to hospital discharge. Beta-blockers should only be initiated upon successful discontinuation of intravenous diuretics, vasodilators, and inotropic agents in the stabilized patient; initiate at a low dose and use caution in those patients who required inotropic support during their hospital course.

Dosing of ACE Inhibitors in Heart Failure[1]

ACEI	Initial Dose	Maximum Dose[2]
Captopril	6.25 mg tid	50 mg tid
Enalapril	2.5 mg bid	10-20 mg bid
Fosinopril	5-10 mg daily	40 mg daily
Lisinopril	2.5-5 mg daily	20-40 mg daily
Perindopril	2 mg daily	8-16 mg daily
Quinapril	5 mg bid	20 mg bid
Ramipril	1.25-2.5 mg daily	10 mg daily
Trandolapril	1 mg daily	4 mg daily

[1]From ACCF/AHA Guidelines.

[2]Maximum/target dose recommendation may vary between guidelines (also see Heart Failure Society of America, 2010)

Dosing of ARBs in Heart Failure[1]

ARB	Initial Dose	Maximum Dose[2]
Candesartan	4-8 mg daily	32 mg daily
Losartan	25-50 mg daily	50-100 mg daily
Valsartan	20-40 mg bid	160 mg bid

[1]From ACCF/AHA Guidelines.

[2]Maximum/target dose recommendation may vary between guidelines (also see Heart Failure Society of America, 2010)

Initial and Target Doses for Beta-Blocker Therapy in Heart Failure[1]

Beta-Blocker	Starting Dose	Target Dose	Comment
Bisoprolol	1.25 mg daily	10 mg daily	β_1-Selective blocker Inconvenient dosage forms for initial dose titration
Carvedilol	3.125 mg bid	25 mg bid (≤85 kg) 50 mg bid (>85 kg)	β-Nonselective blocker α_1-Blocking properties
Carvedilol phosphate, extended release	10 mg daily	80 mg daily[2]	
Metoprolol succinate, extended release	12.5-25 mg daily	200 mg daily	β_1-Selective blocker

[1]From ACCF/AHA Guidelines.

[2]Equivalent to carvedilol immediate release 25 mg twice daily

Conversion From Immediate Release to Extended Release Carvedilol (Coreg CR®)

Carvedilol Immediate Release Dose	Carvedilol Phosphate Extended Release Dose
3.125 mg twice daily	10 mg once daily
6.25 mg twice daily	20 mg once daily
12.5 mg twice daily	40 mg once daily
25 mg twice daily	80 mg once daily

REFERENCES

Brater DC, "Diuretic Therapy," *N Engl J Med*, 1998, 339(6):387-95.

Granger CB, McMurray JJ, Yusuf S, et al, "Effects of Candesartan in Patients With Chronic Heart Failure and Reduced Left-Ventricular Systolic Function Intolerant to Angiotensin-Converting-Enzyme Inhibitors: The CHARM-Alternative Trial," *Lancet*, 2003, 362(9386):772-6.

Heart Failure Society of America, Lindenfeld J, Albert NM, et al, "HFSA 2010 Comprehensive Heart Failure Practice Guideline," *J Card Fail*, 2010, 16(6):e1-194.

Hunt SA, Abraham WT, Chin MH, et al, "2009 Focused Update Incorporated Into the ACC/AHA 2005 Guidelines for the Diagnosis and Management of Heart Failure in Adults A Report of the American College of Cardiology Foundation/American Heart Association Task Force on Practice Guidelines Developed in Collaboration With the International Society for Heart and Lung Transplantation," *J Am Coll Cardiol*, 2009, 53(15):e1-e90.

McMurray JJ, Ostergren J, Swedberg K, et al, "Effects of Candesartan in Patients With Chronic Heart Failure and Reduced Left-Ventricular Systolic Function Taking Angiotensin-Converting-Enzyme Inhibitors: The CHARM-Added Trial," *Lancet*, 2003, 362(9386):767-71.

Taylor AL, Ziesche S, Yancy C, et al, "Combination of Isosorbide Dinitrate and Hydralazine in Blacks With Heart Failure," *N Engl J Med*, 2004, 351(20):2049-57.

HELICOBACTER PYLORI TREATMENT

Medication Regimen	Dosages	Duration of Therapy
First Line Therapies (Option 1)		
H_2-Receptor antagonist (H_2RA) **or** proton pump inhibitor (PPI)	Standard dose of H_2RA or PPI[1]	10-14 days
plus		
Bismuth subsalicylate	525 mg 4 times/day	10-14 days
plus		
Metronidazole	250 mg 4 times/day	10-14 days
plus		
Tetracycline	500 mg 4 times/day	10-14 days
First Line Therapies (Option 2)		
PPI	Standard dose[1]	10-14 days
plus		
Clarithromycin	500 mg 2 times/day	10-14 days
plus		
Amoxicillin	1000 mg 2 times/day	10-14 days
First Line Therapies (Option 3)		
PPI	Standard dose[1]	10-14 days
plus		
Clarithromycin	500 mg 2 times/day	10-14 days
plus		
Metronidazole	500 mg 2 times/day	10-14 days
Salvage Therapy for Persistent Infection (Option 1)		
PPI (once daily), bismuth, metronidazole, and tetracycline (4 times/day) for 7-14 days		
Salvage Therapy for Persistent Infection (Option 2)		
PPI (standard dose[1]), levofloxacin 500 mg (once daily), and amoxicillin 1000 mg (2 times/day) for 10 days		

[1]Standard proton pump inhibitor dose: Esomeprazole = 40 mg once daily; Lansoprazole = 30 mg 2 times/day; Omeprazole = 20 mg 2 times/day; Rabeprazole = 20 mg 2 times/day

REFERENCES

Chey WD, Wong BC, and Practice Parameters Committee of the American College of Gastroenterology, "American College of Gastroenterology Guideline on the Management of *Helicobacter pylori* Infection," *Am J Gastroenterol*, 2007, 102(8):1808-25.

Saad RJ, Schoenfeld P, Kim HM, et al, "Levofloxacin-Based Triple Therapy Versus Bismuth-Based Quadruple Therapy for Persistent *Helicobacter pylori* Infection: A Meta-Analysis," *Am J Gastroenterol*, 2006, 101(3):488-96.

HYPERLIPIDEMIA MANAGEMENT

MORTALITY

There is a strong link between serum cholesterol and cardiovascular mortality. This association becomes stronger in patients with established coronary artery disease. Lipid-lowering trials show that reductions in LDL cholesterol are followed by reductions in mortality. In general, each 1% fall in LDL cholesterol confers a 2% reduction in cardiovascular events. The aim of therapy for hyperlipidemia is to decrease cardiovascular morbidity and mortality by lowering cholesterol to a target level using safe and cost-effective treatment modalities. The target LDL cholesterol is determined by the number of patient risk factors (see the following Risk Factors and Goal LDL Cholesterol tables). The goal is achieved through diet, lifestyle modification, and drug therapy. The basis for these recommendations is provided by longitudinal interventional studies, demonstrating that lipid-lowering in patients with prior cardiovascular events (secondary prevention) and in patients with hyperlipidemia but no prior cardiac event (primary prevention) lowers the occurrence of future cardiovascular events, including stroke.

Major Risk Factors That Modify LDL Goals

Positive risk factors	Male ≥45 years
	Female ≥55 years
	Family history of premature coronary heart disease, defined as CHD in male first-degree relative <55 years; CHD in female first-degree relative <65 years
	Cigarette smoking
	Hypertension (blood pressure ≥140/90 mm Hg) or taking antihypertensive medication
	Low HDL (<40 mg/dL [1.03 mmol/L])
Negative risk factors	High HDL (≥60 mg/dL [1.6 mmol/L])[1]

[1]If HDL is ≥60 mg/dL, may subtract one positive risk factor.

Adult Treatment Panel (ATP) III LDL-C Goals and Cutpoints for Therapeutic Lifestyle Changes (TLC) and Drug Therapy in Different Risk Categories

Risk Category	LDL-C Goal	Initiate TLC	Consider Drug Therapy[1]
High risk: CHD[2] or CHD risk equivalents[3] (10-year risk >20%)	<100 mg/dL (optional goal: <70 mg/dL)[4]	≥100 mg/dL[5]	≥100 mg/dL[6] (<100 mg/dL: Consider drug options)[1]
Moderately high risk: ≥2 risk factors[7] (10-year risk 10% to 20%)[8]	<130 mg/dL[9]	≥130 mg/dL[5]	≥130 mg/dL (100-120 mg/dL: Consider drug options)[10]
Moderate risk: ≥2 risk factors[7] (10-year risk <10%)[8]	<130 mg/dL	≥130 mg/dL	≥160 mg/dL
Lower risk: 0-1 risk factor[11]	<160 mg/dL	≥160 mg/dL	≥190 mg/dL (160-189 mg/dL: LDL-lowering drug optional)

[1]When LDL-lowering drug therapy is employed, it is advised that intensity of therapy be sufficient to achieve at least a 30% to 40% reduction in LDL-C levels.

[2]CHD includes history of myocardial infarction, unstable angina, stable angina, coronary artery procedures (angioplasty or bypass surgery), or evidence of clinically significant myocardial ischemia.

[3]CHD risk equivalents include clinical manifestations of noncoronary forms of atherosclerotic disease (peripheral arterial disease, abdominal aortic aneurysm, and carotid artery disease [transient ischemic attacks or stroke of carotid origin or >50% obstruction of a carotid artery]), diabetes, and 2+ risk factors with 10-year risk for hard CHD >20%.

[4]Very high risk favors the optional LDL-C goal of <70 mg/dL, and in patients with high triglycerides, non-HDL-C <100 mg/dL.

[5]Any person at high risk or moderately high risk who has lifestyle-related risk factors (eg, obesity, physical inactivity, elevated triglyceride, low HDL-C, or metabolic syndrome) is a candidate for therapeutic lifestyle changes to modify these risk factors regardless of LDL-C level.

[6]If baseline LDL-C is <100 mg/dL, institution of an LDL-lowering drug is a therapeutic option on the basis of available clinical trial results. If a high-risk person has high triglycerides or low HDL-C, combining a fibrate or nicotinic acid with an LDL-lowering drug can be considered.

[7]Risk factors include cigarette smoking, hypertension (BP ≥140/90 mm Hg or on antihypertensive medication), low HDL cholesterol (<40 mg/dL), family history of premature CHD (CHD in male first-degree relative <55 years of age; CHD in female first-degree relative <65 years of age), and age (men ≥45 years; women ≥55 years).

[8]Electronic 10-year risk calculators are available at www.nhlbi.nih.gov/guidelines/cholesterol.

[9]Optional LDL-C goal <100 mg/dL.

[10]For moderately high-risk persons, when LDL-C level is 100-129 mg/dL, at baseline or on lifestyle therapy, initiation of an LDL-lowering drug to achieve an LDL-C level <100 mg/dL is a therapeutic option on the basis of available clinical trial results.

[11]Almost all people with zero or 1 risk factor have a 10-year risk <10%, and 10-year risk assessment in people with zero or 1 risk factor thus not necessary.

Any person with elevated LDL cholesterol or other form of hyperlipidemia should undergo evaluation to rule out secondary dyslipidemia. Causes of secondary dyslipidemia include diabetes, hypothyroidism, obstructive liver disease, chronic renal failure, and drugs that increase LDL and decrease HDL (progestins, anabolic steroids, corticosteroids).

Elevated Serum Triglyceride Levels

Elevated serum triglyceride levels may be an independent risk factor for coronary heart disease. Factors that contribute to hypertriglyceridemia include obesity, inactivity, cigarette smoking, excess alcohol intake, high carbohydrate diets (>60% of energy intake), type 2 diabetes, chronic renal failure, nephrotic syndrome, certain medications (corticosteroids, estrogens, retinoids, higher doses of beta-blockers), and genetic disorders. Non-HDL cholesterol (total cholesterol minus HDL cholesterol) is a secondary focus for clinicians treating patients with high serum triglyceride levels (≥200 mg/dL). The goal for non-HDL cholesterol in patients with high serum triglyceride levels can be set 30 mg/dL higher than usual LDL cholesterol goals. Patients with serum triglyceride levels <200 mg/dL should aim for the target LDL cholesterol goal.

ATP classification of serum triglyceride levels:

- Normal triglycerides: <150 mg/dL
- Borderline-high: 150-199 mg/dL
- High: 200-499 mg/dL
- Very high: ≥500 mg/dL

NONDRUG THERAPY

Dietary therapy and lifestyle modifications should be individualized for each patient. A total lifestyle change is recommended for all patients. Dietary and lifestyle modifications should be tried for 3 months, if deemed appropriate. Nondrug and drug therapy should be initiated simultaneously in patients with highly elevated cholesterol (see LDL Cholesterol Goals and Cutpoints for Therapeutic Lifestyle Changes and Drug Therapy in Different Risk Categories table). Increasing physical activity and smoking cessation will aid in the treatment of hyperlipidemia and improve cardiovascular health.

Note: Refer to the National Cholesterol Education Program reference for details concerning the calculation of 10-year risk of CHD using Framingham risk scoring. Risk assessment tool is available on-line at http://hin.nhlbi.nih.gov/atpiii/calculator.asp?usertype=prof, last accessed March 14, 2002.

Total Lifestyle Change (TLC) Diet

	Recommended Intake
Total fat	25%-35% of total calories
Saturated fat[1]	<7% of total calories
Polyunsaturated fat	≤10% of total calories
Monounsaturated fat	≤20% of total calories
Carbohydrates[2]	50%-60% of total calories
Fiber	20-30 g/day
Protein	~15% of total calories
Cholesterol	<200 mg/day
Total calories[3]	Balance energy intake and expenditure to maintain desirable body weight/prevent weight gain

[1] *Trans* fatty acids (partially hydrogenated oils) intake should be kept low. These are found in potato chips, other snack foods, margarines and shortenings, and fast-foods.

[2] Complex carbohydrates including grains (especially whole grains, fruits, and vegetables).

[3] Daily energy expenditure should include at least moderate physical activity.

DRUG THERAPY

Drug therapy should be selected based on the patient's lipid profile, concomitant disease states, and the cost of therapy. The following table (on next page) lists specific advantages and disadvantages for various classes of lipid-lowering medications. The expected reduction in lipids with therapy is listed in the Lipid-Lowering Agents table. Refer to individual drug monographs for detailed information.

Advantages and Disadvantages of Specific Lipid-Lowering Therapies

	Advantages	Disadvantages
Bile acid sequestrants	Good choice for ↑ LDL, especially when combined with a statin (↓ LDL ≤50%); low potential for systemic side effects; good choice for younger patients	May increase triglycerides; higher incidence of adverse effects; moderately expensive; drug interactions; inconvenient dosing
Niacin	Good choice for almost any lipid abnormality; inexpensive; greatest increase in HDL	High incidence of adverse effects; may adversely affect type 2 DM (with high dose >1.5 g/day) and gout; sustained release niacin may decrease the incidence of flushing and circumvent the need for multiple daily dosing; sustained release niacin may not increase HDL cholesterol or decrease triglycerides as well as immediate release niacin
HMG-CoA reductase inhibitors	Produces greatest ↓ in LDL; generally well-tolerated; convenient once-daily dosing; proven decrease in mortality	Expensive
Fibric acid derivatives	Good choice in patients with ↑ triglycerides where niacin is contraindicated or not well-tolerated	Variable effects on LDL
Ezetimibe	Additional cholesterol-lowering effects when combined with HMG-CoA reductase inhibitors	Effects similar to bile acid sequestrants

Lipid-Lowering Agents

Drug	Dose / Day	Effect on LDL (%)	Effect on HDL (%)	Effect on TG (%)
HMG-CoA Reductase Inhibitors				
Atorvastatin	10 mg 20 mg 40 mg 80 mg	-39 -43 -50 -60	+6 +9 +6 +5	-19 -26 -29 -37
Fluvastatin	20 mg 40 mg 80 mg	-22 -25 -36	+3 +4 +6	-12 -14 -18
Lovastatin	10 mg 20 mg 40 mg 80 mg	-21 -24 -30 -40	+5 +7 +7 +9.5	-10 -10 -14 -19
Pitavastatin	1 mg 2 mg 4 mg	-32 -36 -43	+8 +7 +5	-15 -19 -18
Pravastatin	10 mg 20 mg 40 mg 80 mg	-22 -32 -34 -37	+7 +2 +12 +3	-15 -11 -24 -19
Rosuvastatin	5 mg 10 mg 20 mg 40 mg	-45 -52 -55 -63	+13 +14 +8 +10	-35 -10 -23 -28
Simvastatin	5 mg 10 mg 20 mg 40 mg 80 mg	-26 -30 -38 -41 -47	+10 +12 +8 +13 +16	-12 -15 -19 -28 -33
Bile Acid Sequestrants				
Cholestyramine	4-24 g	-15 to -30	+3 to +5	+0 to +20
Colesevelam	6 tablets 7 tablets	-15 -18	+3 +3	+10 +9
Colestipol	7-30 g	-15 to -30	+3 to +5	+0 to +20
Fibric Acid Derivatives				
Fenofibrate	67-200 mg	-20 to -31	+9 to +14	-30 to -50
Gemfibrozil	600 mg twice daily	-5 to -10[1]	+10 to +20	-40 to -60

Lipid-Lowering Agents *(continued)*

Drug	Dose / Day	Effect on LDL (%)	Effect on HDL (%)	Effect on TG (%)
Niacin	1.5-6 g	-5 to -25	+15 to +35	-20 to -50
2-Azetidinone				
Ezetimibe	10 mg	-15 to -20	+1 to +4	-5 to -8
Omega-3-Acid Ethyl Esters	4 g	+44.5	+9.1	-44.9
Combination Products				
Ezetimibe and simvastatin	10/10 mg 10/20 mg 10/40 mg 10/80 mg	-45 -52 -55 -60	+8 +10 +6 +6	-23 -24 -23 -31
Niacin and lovastatin	1000/20 mg 1000/40 mg 1500/40 mg 2000/40 mg	-30 -36 -37 -42	+20 +20 +27 +30	-32 -39 -44 -44
Niacin and simvastatin	1000/20 mg 1000/40 mg 2000/20 mg 2000/40 mg	-12 -7 -14 -5	+21 +15 +29 +24	-27 -23 -38 -32

[1]May increase LDL in some patients.

Progression of Drug Therapy in Primary Prevention

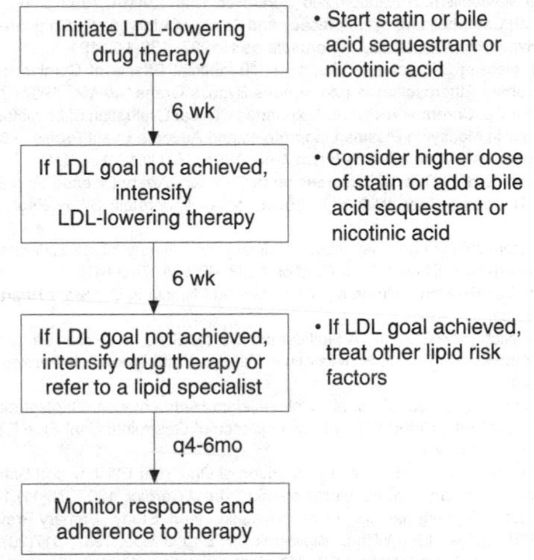

DRUG SELECTION

Lipid Profile	Monotherapy	Combination Therapies
Increased LDL with normal HDL and triglycerides (TG)	Resin Niacin[1] Statin	Resin plus niacin[1] or statin Statin plus niacin[1,2]
Increased LDL and increased TG (200-499 mg/dL)[2]	Intensify LDL-lowering therapy	Statin plus niacin[1,3] Statin plus fibrate[3]
Increased LDL and increased TG (≥500 mg/dL)[2]	Consider combination therapy (niacin,[1] fibrates, statin)	
Increased TG	Niacin[1] Fibrates	Niacin[1] plus fibrates
Increased LDL and low HDL	Niacin[1] Statin	Statin plus niacin[1,2]

[1]Avoid in diabetics.

[2]Emphasize weight reduction and increased physical activity.

[3]Risk of myopathy with combination.

Resins = bile acid sequestrants; statins = HMG-CoA reductase inhibitors; fibrates = fibric acid derivatives (eg, gemfibrozil, fenofibrate).

COMBINATION DRUG THERAPY

If after at least 6 weeks of therapy at the maximum recommended or tolerated dose, the patient's LDL cholesterol is not at target, consider optimizing nondrug measures, prescribing a higher dose of current lipid-lowering drug, or adding another lipid-lowering medication to the current therapy. Successful drug combinations include statin and niacin, statin and bile acid sequestrant, or niacin and bile acid sequestrant. At maximum recommended doses, LDL cholesterol may be decreased by 50% to 60% with combination therapy. This is the same reduction achieved by atorvastatin 40 mg twice daily. If a bile acid sequestrant is used with other lipid-lowering agents, space doses 1 hour before or 4 hours after the bile acid sequestrant administration. Statins combined with either fenofibrate, gemfibrozil, or niacin increase the risk of rhabdomyolysis. In this situation, patient education (muscle pain/weakness) and careful follow-up are warranted.

References

Guidelines

American Diabetes Association, "Standards of Medical Care in Diabetes - 2010," *Diabetes Care*, 2010, 33(Suppl 1):S11-61.

Brunzell JD, Davidson M, Furberg CD, et al, "Lipoprotein Management in Patients With Cardiometabolic Risk: Consensus Statement From the American Diabetes Association and the American College of Cardiology Foundation," *Diabetes Care*, 2008, 31(4):811-22.

Grundy SM, Cleeman JI, Merz CN, et al, "Implications of Recent Clinical Trials for the National Cholesterol Education Program Adult Treatment Panel III Guidelines," *J Am Coll Cardiol*, 2004, 44 (3):720-32.

National Cholesterol Education Program, "Third Report of the Expert Panel on Detection, Evaluation, and Treatment of High Blood Cholesterol in Adults (Adult Treatment Panel III)," *JAMA*, 2001, 285 (19):2486-97.

Others

Berthold HK, Sudhop T, and von Bergmann K, "Effect of a Garlic Oil Preparation on Serum Lipoproteins and Cholesterol Metabolism: A Randomized Controlled Trial," *JAMA*, 1998, 279(23):1900-2.

Bertolini S, Bon GB, Campbell LM, et al, "Efficacy and Safety of Atorvastatin Compared to Pravastatin in Patients With Hypercholesterolemia," *Atherosclerosis*, 1997, 130(1-2):191-7.

Blankenhorn DH, Nessim SA, Johnson RL, et al, "Beneficial Effects of Combined Colestipol-Niacin Therapy on Coronary Atherosclerosis and Venous Bypass Grafts," *JAMA*, 1987, 257(23):3233-40.

Bradford RH, Shear CL, Chremos AN, et al, "Expanded Clinical Evaluation of Lovastatin (EXCEL) Study Results. I. Efficacy in Modifying Plasma Lipoproteins and Adverse Event Profile in 8245 Patients With Moderate Hypercholesterolemia," *Arch Intern Med*, 1991, 151(1):43-9.

Brown G, Albers JJ, Fisher LD, et al, "Regression of Coronary Artery Disease as a Result of Intensive Lipid-Lowering Therapy in Men With High Levels of Apolipoprotein B," *N Engl J Med*, 1990, 323 (19):1289-98.

Capuzzi DM, Guyton JR, Morgan JM, et al, "Efficacy and Safety of an Extended-Release Niacin (Niaspan®): A Long-Term Study," *Am J Cardiol*, 1998, 82(12A):74U-81U.

Coronary Drug Project Research Program, "Clofibrate and Niacin in Coronary Heart Disease," *JAMA*, 1975, 231(4):360-81.

Dart A, Jerums G, Nicholson G, et al, "A Multicenter, Double-Blind, One-Year Study Comparing Safety and Efficacy of Atorvastatin Versus Simvastatin in Patients With Hypercholesterolemia," *Am J Cardiol*, 1997, 80(1):39-44.

Davidson MH, Dillon MA, Gordon B, et al, "Colesevelam Hydrochloride (Cholestagel): A New Potent Bile Acid Sequestrant Associated With a Low Incidence of Gastrointestinal Side Effects," *Arch Intern Med*, 1999, 159(16):1893-900.

Davidson M, McKenney J, Stein E, et al, "Comparison of One-Year Efficacy and Safety of Atorvastatin Versus Lovastatin in Primary Hypercholesterolemia," *Am J Cardiol*, 1997, 79(11):1475-81.

Frick MH, Heinonen OP, Huttunen JK, et al, "Helsinki Heart Study: Primary-Prevention Trial With Gemfibrozil in Middle-Aged Men With Dyslipidemia," *N Engl J Med*, 1987, 317(20):1237-45.

Garber AM, Browner WS, and Hulley SB, "Clinical Guideline, Part 2: Cholesterol Screening in Asymptomatic Adults, Revisited," *Ann Intern Med*, 1995, 124(5):518-31.

Johannesson M, Jonsson B, Kjekshus J, et al, "Cost-Effectiveness of Simvastatin Treatment to Lower Cholesterol Levels in Patients With Coronary Heart Disease. Scandinavian Simvastatin Survival Study Group," *N Engl N Med*, 1997, 336(5):332-6.

Jones P, Kafonek S, Laurora I, et al, "Comparative Dose Efficacy Study of Atorvastatin Versus Simvastatin, Pravastatin, Lovastatin, and Fluvastatin in Patients With Hypercholesterolemia," *Am J Cardiol*, 1998, 81(5):582-7.

Kasiske BL, Ma JZ, Kalil RS, et al, "Effects of Antihypertensive Therapy on Serum Lipids," *Ann Intern Med*, 1995, 122(2):133-41.

Lipid Research Clinics Program, "The Lipid Research Clinics Coronary Primary Prevention Trial Results: I. Reduction in Incidence of Coronary Heart Disease," *JAMA*, 1984, 251(3):351-64.

Mauro VF and Tuckerman CE, "Ezetimibe for Management of Hypercholesterolemia," *Ann Pharmacother*, 2003, 37(6):839-48.

Multiple Risk Factor Intervention Trial Research Group, "Multiple Risk Factor Intervention Trial: Risk Factor Changes and Mortality Results," *JAMA*, 1982, 248(12):1465-77.

Pitt B, Waters D, Brown WV, et al, "Aggressive Lipid-Lowering Therapy Compared With Angioplasty in Stable Coronary Artery Disease. Atorvastatin Versus Revascularization Treatment Investigators," *N Engl J Med*, 1999, 341(2):70-6.

Ross SD, Allen IE, Connelly JE, et al, "Clinical Outcomes in Statin Treatment Trials: A Meta-Analysis," *Arch Intern Med*, 1999, 159(15):1793-802.

Sacks FM, Pfeffer MA, Moye LA, et al, "The Effect of Pravastatin on Coronary Events After Myocardial Infarction in Patients With Average Cholesterol Levels," *N Engl J Med*, 1996, 335(14):1001-9.

Scandinavian Simvastatin Survival Study, "Randomized Trial of Cholesterol Lowering in 4444 Patients With Coronary Heart Disease: The Scandinavian Simvastatin Survival Study (4S)," *Lancet*, 1994, 344 (8934):1383-9.

Schrott HG, Bittner V, Vittinghoff E, et al, "Adherence to National Cholesterol Education Program Treatment Goals in Postmenopausal Women With Heart Disease. The Heart and Estrogen/Progestin Replacement Study (HERS)," *JAMA*, 1997, 277(16):1281-6.

Shepherd J, Cobbe SM, Ford I, et al, "Prevention of Coronary Heart Disease With Pravastatin in Men With Hypercholesterolemia, The West of Scotland Coronary Prevention Study Group," *N Engl J Med*, 1995, 333(20):1301-7.

Stein EA, Davidson MH, Dobs AS, et al, "Efficacy and Safety of Simvastatin 80 mg/day in Hypercholesterolemic Patients. The Expanded Dose Simvastatin U.S. Study Group," *Am J Cardiol*, 1998, 82 (3):311-6.

HYPERTENSION

The optimal blood pressure for adults is <120/80 mm Hg. Consistent systolic pressure ≥140 mm Hg or a diastolic pressure ≥90 mm Hg, in the absence of a secondary cause, defines hypertension. Hypertension affects approximately 25% (50 million people) in the United States. Of those patients on antihypertensive medication, only one in three have their blood pressure controlled (<140/90 mm Hg).

Controlling systolic hypertension has been much more difficult than controlling diastolic hypertension. Educating patients in lifestyle management, cardiovascular risk reduction, and drug therapy aids in improving the morbidity and mortality of patients with hypertension.

The Seventh Report of the Joint National Committee (JNC VII) is an excellent reference and guide for the treatment of hypertension (Chobanian AV, Bakris GL, Black HR, et al, "The Seventh Report of the Joint National Committee on Prevention, Detection, Evaluation, and Treatment of High Blood Pressure: The JNC 7 Report," *JAMA*, 2003, 289(19):2560-71). For adults, hypertension is classified in stages (see following table).

Adult Classification of Blood Pressure

Category	Systolic (mm Hg)		Diastolic (mm Hg)
Normal	<120	and	<80
Prehypertension	120-139	or	80-89
Hypertension			
Stage 1	140-159	or	90-99
Stage 2	≥160	or	≥100

Adapted from Chobanian AV, Bakris GL, Black HR, et al, "The Seventh Report of the Joint National Committee on Prevention, Detection, Evaluation, and Treatment of High Blood Pressure: The JNC 7 Report," *JAMA*, 2003, 289(19):2560-71.

Normal Blood Pressure in Children

Age (y)	Girls' SBP / DBP (mm Hg)		Boys' SBP / DBP (mm Hg)	
	50th Percentile for Height	75th Percentile for Height	50th Percentile for Height	75th Percentile for Height
1	104/58	105/59	102/57	104/58
6	111/73	112/73	114/74	115/75
12	123/80	124/81	123/81	125/82
17	129/84	130/85	136/87	138/88

SBP = systolic blood pressure.

DBP = diastolic blood pressure.

Adapted from the report by the NHBPEP Working Group on Hypertension Control in Children and Adolescents, *Pediatrics*, 1996, 98(4 Pt 1):649-58.

PATIENT ASSESSMENT

- **Cardiovascular Risk Factors:** Hypertension, cigarette smoking, obesity (BMI ≥30), inactive lifestyle, dyslipidemia, diabetes mellitus, microalbuminuria or estimated GFR <60 mL/minute, age (>55 years for men, >65 years for women), family history of premature cardiovascular disease (men <55 years or women >65 years).

  Components of metabolic syndrome include hypertension, obesity, dyslipidemia, diabetes mellitus.
- Identify causes of high BP.
- Assess target-organ damage and CVD.

Target-Organ Disease

Organ System	Manifestation
Cardiac	Clinical, ECG, or radiologic evidence of coronary artery disease; prior MI, angina, post-CABG; left ventricular hypertrophy (LVH); left ventricular dysfunction or cardiac failure, prior coronary revascularization
Cerebrovascular	Transient ischemic attack or stroke
Peripheral vascular	Absence of pulses in extremities (except dorsalis pedis), claudication, aneurysm, peripheral arterial disease
Renal	Serum creatinine ≥130 μmol/L (1.5 mg/dL); proteinuria (≥1+); microalbuminuria, chronic kidney disease
Eye	Hemorrhages or exudates, with or without papilledema; retinopathy

Adapted from Chobanian AV, Bakris GL, Black HR, et al, "The Seventh Report of the Joint National Committee on Prevention, Detection, Evaluation, and Treatment of High Blood Pressure: The JNC 7 Report," *JAMA*, 2003, 289(19):2560-71.

BLOOD PRESSURE MEASUREMENT

At an office visit, patients should be seated quietly for ≥5 minutes in a chair with feet on the floor and arm supported at heart level. At least two measurements should be made. Patients should be given their results and their goal BP.

Ambulatory BP monitoring is useful in evaluating "white coat hypertension" (no end-organ damage), drug resistance, hypotensive symptoms, episodic hypertension, and autonomic dysfunction. Ambulatory BP monitoring correlates better with end-organ damage than office measurements.

Having patients monitor their own BP helps to improve compliance and provides information on response to therapeutic interventions.

Based on these initial assessments, treatment strategies for patients with hypertension are stratified based on their blood pressure and comorbidities (compelling indications).

Management of Blood Pressure

	Management: Based upon highest BP category		
BP Classification	**Lifestyle Modification**	**Initial Therapy Without Compelling Indication**	**Initial Therapy With Compelling Indication[1]**
Normal	Encourage	None	None
Prehypertensive	Yes	None	Treat patients with chronic kidney disease or diabetes to BP goal of <130/80 mm Hg
Hypertension			
Stage 1	Yes	Thiazide-type diuretic for most; consider ACEI, ARB, β-blocker, CCB, or combination	Drugs for the compelling indications; other antihypertensives as needed
Stage 2	Yes	Two drug combos (typically a thiazide-type diuretic and ACEI or ARB or β-blocker or CCB). Use combo cautiously in patients at risk for orthostasis.	Drugs for the compelling indications; other antihypertensives as needed

[1]Compelling Indication: Conditions for which specific classes of antihypertensive drugs have proven beneficial.

Adapted from Chobanian AV, Bakris GL, Black HR, et al, "The Seventh Report of the Joint National Committee on Prevention, Detection, Evaluation, and Treatment of High Blood Pressure: The JNC 7 Report," *JAMA*, 2003, 289(19):2560-71.

ACHIEVING BLOOD PRESSURE CONTROL

Treatment of hypertension should be individualized. Lower blood pressure (goal <130/80 mm Hg) should be achieved in patients with diabetes or chronic renal disease. The following Hypertension Treatment Algorithm may be used to select specific antihypertensives based on compelling indications.

Special consideration for starting combination therapy should be made in each patient.

Starting drug therapy at a low dose and titrating upward if blood pressure is not controlled is recommended.

Most patients with hypertension will require two or more drugs to achieve their BP goals.

Adding a second drug from a different class will help when a single drug at reasonable doses has failed to achieve the goal.

If the untreated BP is >20/10 mm Hg away from the goal, consider initiating therapy with two drugs. Use caution in those at risk for orthostasis (eg, diabetics, geriatrics, and those with autonomic dysfunction).

Low-dose aspirin therapy should be considered when BP is controlled; use in uncontrolled hypertension can increase the risk of hemorrhagic stroke.

Lifestyle modification and risk reduction should always be reviewed and reinforced.

MONITORING THERAPY

Generally, monthly follow-up is recommended until BP control is reached.

More frequent monitoring is required for those patients with Stage 2 hypertension or those with complications.

Serum potassium and serum creatinine should be monitored at least twice yearly.

When BP is at goal and stable, follow-up can be maintained every 3-6 months. Treat other cardiovascular risk factors if present.

Hypertension Treatment Algorithm

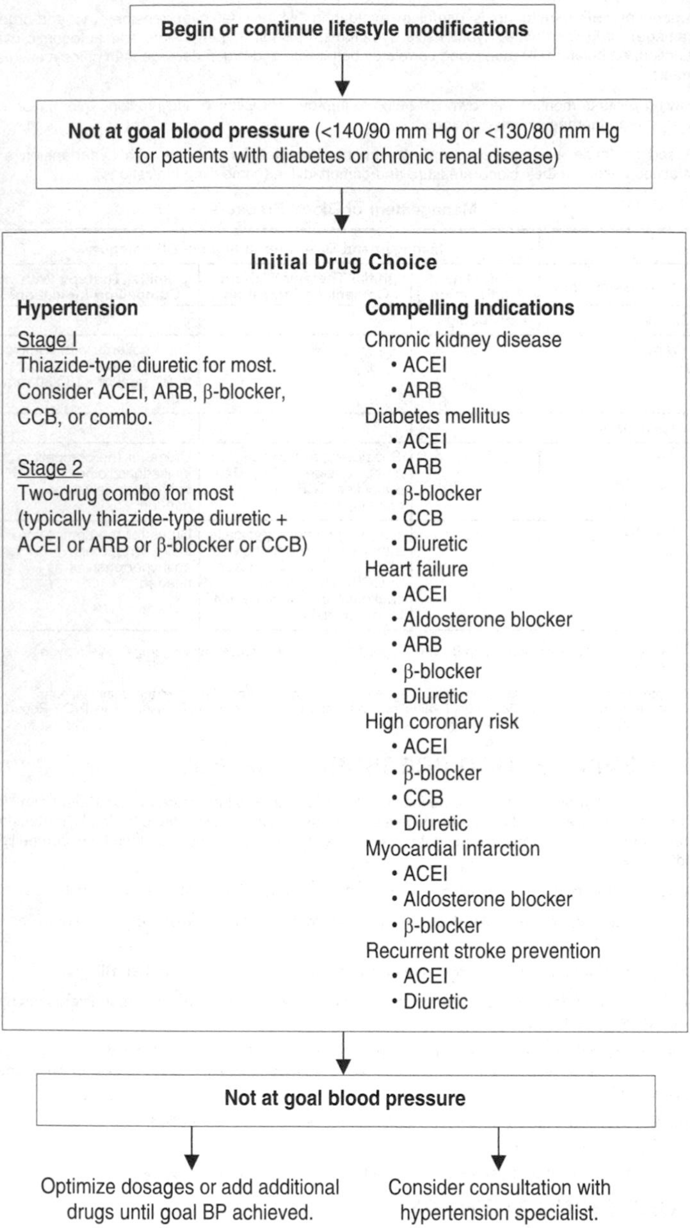

Begin or continue lifestyle modifications

↓

Not at goal blood pressure (<140/90 mm Hg or <130/80 mm Hg for patients with diabetes or chronic renal disease)

↓

Initial Drug Choice

Hypertension

Stage I
Thiazide-type diuretic for most. Consider ACEI, ARB, β-blocker, CCB, or combo.

Stage 2
Two-drug combo for most (typically thiazide-type diuretic + ACEI or ARB or β-blocker or CCB)

Compelling Indications

Chronic kidney disease
- ACEI
- ARB

Diabetes mellitus
- ACEI
- ARB
- β-blocker
- CCB
- Diuretic

Heart failure
- ACEI
- Aldosterone blocker
- ARB
- β-blocker
- Diuretic

High coronary risk
- ACEI
- β-blocker
- CCB
- Diuretic

Myocardial infarction
- ACEI
- Aldosterone blocker
- β-blocker

Recurrent stroke prevention
- ACEI
- Diuretic

↓

Not at goal blood pressure

↓ Optimize dosages or add additional drugs until goal BP achieved.

↓ Consider consultation with hypertension specialist.

Additional Considerations for Specific Therapies

Indication	Drug Therapy
Atrial tachyarrhythmias	β-blocker, CCB (non-DHP)
Chronic kidney disease	
Cl_{cr} <60 mL/min or albuminuria	ACEI or ARB
Cl_{cr} <30 mL/min	Increase loop diuretic
Diabetes	Thiazide diuretic, β-blocker, ACEI, ARB, CCB
Nephropathy	ACEI, ARB
Essential tremor	β-blocker (noncardioselective)
Heart failure	
Ventricular dysfunction (asymptomatic)	ACEI, β-blocker
Ventricular dysfunction (symptomatic)	ACEI, β-blocker, ARB, aldosterone blocker, loop diuretic
Hypertensive women who are pregnant	Methyldopa, β-blocker, vasodilator
Ischemic heart disease	
Angina	β-blocker, CCB (long-acting)
Acute coronary syndromes	β-blocker, ACEI
Migraine	β-blocker (noncardioselective), CCB (long-acting, non-DHP)
Osteoporosis	Thiazide diuretic
Perioperative hypertension	β-blocker
Prostatism (BPH)	Alpha-adrenergic blocking agent
Raynaud syndrome	CCB
Thyrotoxicosis	β-blocker

Note: ACEI = angiotensin-converting enzyme inhibitor; ARB = angiotensin receptor blocker; CCB = calcium channel blocker; DHP = dihydropyridine.

May Have Unfavorable Effects on Comorbid Conditions

Condition	Drug Therapy to Avoid
Angioedema	ACEI
Bronchospastic disease	β-blocker
Gout	Thiazide diuretic
Heart block (second or third degree)	β-blocker, CCB (non-DHP)
Hyponatremia	Thiazide diuretic
Potassium >5 mEq/L before treatment	Potassium sparing diuretic, aldosterone antagonist
Pregnancy or those likely to become pregnant	ACEI, ARB

Note: ACEI = angiotensin-converting enzyme inhibitor; ARB = angiotensin receptor blocker; CCB = calcium channel blocker; DHP = dihydropyridine.

HYPERTENSIVE EMERGENCIES AND URGENCIES

General Treatment Principles in the Treatment of Hypertensive Emergencies

Principle	Considerations
Admit the patient to the hospital, preferably in the ICU. Monitor vital signs appropriately.	Establish I.V. access and place patient on a cardiac monitor. Place a femoral intra-arterial line and pulmonary arterial catheter, if indicated, to assess cardiopulmonary function and intravascular volume status.
Perform rapid but thorough history and physical examination.	Determine cause of, or precipitating factors to, hypertensive crisis if possible (remember to obtain a medication history including Rx, OTC, and illicit drugs). Obtain details regarding any prior history of hypertension (severity, duration, treatment), as well as other coexisting illnesses. Assess the extent of hypertensive end organ damage. Determine if a hypertensive urgency or emergency exists.
Determine goal blood pressure based on premorbid level, duration, severity and rapidity of increase of blood pressure, concomitant medical conditions, race, and age.	Acute decreases in blood pressure to normal or subnormal levels during the initial treatment period may reduce perfusion to the brain, heart, and kidneys, and must be avoided except in specific instances (ie, dissecting aortic aneurysm). Gradually establish a normal (or reasonable) blood pressure over the next 1-2 weeks.
Select an appropriate antihypertensive regimen depending on the individual patient and clinical setting.	Initiate a controlled decrease in blood pressure. Avoid concomitant administration of multiple agents that may cause precipitous falls in blood pressure. Select the agent with the best hemodynamic profile based on the primary treatment goal. Avoid diuretics and sodium restriction during the initial treatment period unless there is a clear clinical indication (ie, CHF, pulmonary edema). Avoid sedating antihypertensives in patients with hypertensive encephalopathy, CVA, or other CNS disorders in whom mental status must be monitored. Use caution with direct vasodilating agents that induce reflex tachycardia or increase cardiac output in patients with coronary heart disease, history of angina or myocardial infarction, or dissecting aortic aneurysm. Preferably choose an agent that does not adversely affect glomerular filtration rate or renal blood flow and also agents that have favorable effects on cerebral blood flow and its autoregulation, especially for patients with hypertensive encephalopathy or CVAs. Select the most efficacious agent with the fewest adverse effects based on the underlying cause of the hypertensive crisis and other individual patient factors.
Initiate a chronic antihypertensive regimen after the patient's blood pressure is stabilized	Begin oral antihypertensive therapy once goal blood pressure is achieved before gradually tapering parenteral medications. Select the best oral regimen based on cost, ease of administration, adverse effect profile, and concomitant medical conditions.

Oral Agents Used in the Treatment of Hypertensive Urgencies

Drug	Dose	Onset	Cautions
Captopril[1]	P.O.: 25 mg, repeat as required	15-30 min	Hypotension, renal failure in bilateral renal artery stenosis
Clonidine	P.O.: 0.1-0.2 mg, repeated every hour as needed to a total dose of 0.6 mg	30-60 min	Hypotension, drowsiness, dry mouth
Labetalol	P.O.: 200-400 mg, repeat every 2-3 h	30 min to 2 h	Bronchoconstriction, heart block, orthostatic hypotension

[1]There is no clearly defined clinical advantage in the use of sublingual over oral routes of administration with these agents.

Recommendations for the Use of Intravenous Antihypertensive Drugs in Selected Hypertensive Emergencies

Condition	Agent(s) of Choice	Agent(s) to Avoid or Use With Caution	General Treatment Principles
Hypertensive encephalopathy	Nitroprusside, labetalol	Methyldopa, reserpine	Avoid drugs with CNS-sedating effects.
Acute intracranial or subarachnoid hemorrhage	Nicardipine,[1] nitroprusside	β-blocker	Careful titration with a short-acting agent.
Cerebral infarction	Nicardipine,[1] nitroprusside, labetalol	β-blocker, minoxidil	Careful titration with a short-acting agent. Avoid agents that may decrease cerebral blood flow.
Head trauma	Esmolol, labetalol	Methyldopa, reserpine, nitroprusside, nitroglycerin, hydralazine	Avoid drugs with CNS-sedating effects, or those that may increase intracranial pressure.
Acute myocardial infarction, myocardial ischemia	Nitroglycerin, nicardipine[1] (calcium channel blocker), labetalol	Hydralazine, minoxidil	Avoid drugs which cause reflex tachycardia and increased myocardial oxygen consumption.
Acute pulmonary edema	Nitroprusside, nitroglycerin, loop diuretics	β-blocker (labetalol), minoxidil, methyldopa	Avoid drugs which may cause sodium and water retention and edema exacerbation.
Renal dysfunction	Hydralazine, calcium channel blocker	Nitroprusside, ACE inhibitors, β-blocker (labetalol)	Avoid drugs with increased toxicity in renal failure and those that may cause decreased renal blood flow.
Eclampsia	Hydralazine, labetalol, nitroprusside[2]	Diuretics	Avoid drugs that may cause adverse fetal effects, compromise placental circulation, or decrease cardiac output.
Pheochromocytoma	Phentolamine, nitroprusside, β-blocker (eg, esmolol) only after alpha blockade (phentolamine)	β-blocker in the absence of alpha blockade, methyldopa, minoxidil	Use drugs of proven efficacy and specificity. Unopposed beta-blockade may exacerbate hypertension.
Dissecting aortic aneurysm	Nitroprusside and beta-blockade	Hydralazine, minoxidil	Avoid drugs which may increase cardiac output.
Postoperative hypertension	Nitroprusside, nicardipine,[1] labetalol, clevidipine		Avoid drugs which may exacerbate postoperative ileus.

[1]The use of nicardipine in these situations is by the recommendation of the author based on a review of the literature.

[2]Reserve nitroprusside for eclamptic patients with life-threatening hypertension unresponsive to other agents due to the potential risk to the fetus (cyanide and thiocyanate metabolites may cross the placenta).

Selected Intravenous Agents for Hypertensive Emergencies

Drug	Dose[1]	Onset of Action	Duration of Action	Adverse Effects[2]	Special Indications
Vasodilators					
Sodium nitroprusside	0.25-10 mcg/kg/min as I.V. infusion[3] (max: 10 min only)	Immediate	1-2 min	Nausea, vomiting, muscle twitching, sweating, thiocyanate and cyanide intoxication	Most hypertensive emergencies; caution with high intracranial pressure or azotemia
Nicardipine hydrochloride	5-15 mg/h I.V.	5-10 min	1-4 h	Tachycardia, headache, flushing, local phlebitis	Most hypertensive emergencies except acute heart failure; caution with coronary ischemia
Clevidipine butyrate	1-21 mg/h I.V.	2-4 min	5-15 min	Atrial fibrillation, nausea, insomnia, fever	Most hypertensive emergencies; caution with lipid disorder
Fenoldopam mesylate	0.1-0.3 mcg/kg/min as I.V. infusion	<5 min	30 min	Tachycardia, headache, nausea, flushing	Most hypertensive emergencies; caution with glaucoma
Nitroglycerin	5-100 mcg/min as I.V. infusion[3]	2-5 min	3-5 min	Headache, vomiting, methemoglobinemia, tolerance with prolonged use	Coronary ischemia
Enalaprilat	1.25-5 mg every 6 hours I.V.	15-30 min	6 h	Precipitous fall in pressure in high-renin states; response variable	Acute left ventricular failure; avoid in acute myocardial infarction
Hydralazine hydrochloride	10-20 mg I.V. 10-50 mg I.M.	10-20 min 20-30 min	3-8 h	Tachycardia, flushing, headache, vomiting, aggravation of angina	Eclampsia
Adrenergic Inhibitors					
Labetalol hydrochloride	20-80 mg I.V. bolus every 10 min; 0.5-2 mg/min as I.V. infusion	5-10 min	3-6 h	Vomiting, scalp tingling, burning in throat, dizziness, nausea, heart block, orthostatic hypotension	Most hypertensive emergencies except acute heart failure
Esmolol hydrochloride	250-500 mcg/kg/min for 1 min, then 50-100 mcg/kg/min for 4 min; may repeat	1-2 min	10-20 min	Hypotension, nausea	Aortic dissection, perioperative
Phentolamine	5-15 mg I.V.	1-2 min	3-10 min	Tachycardia, flushing, headache	Catecholamine excess

[1]These doses may vary from those in the *Physicians' Desk Reference* (51st edition).

[2]Hypotension may occur with all agents.

[3]Require special delivery system.

References

Guidelines

"1999 World Health Organization-International Society of Hypertension Guidelines for the Management of Hypertension. Guidelines Subcommittee," *J Hypertens*, 1999, 17(2):151-83.

Chobanian AV, Bakris GL, Black HR, et al, "The Seventh Report of the Joint National Committee on Prevention, Detection, Evaluation, and Treatment of High Blood Pressure: The JNC 7 Report," *JAMA*, 2003, 289(19):2560-72.

National High Blood Pressure Education Program Working Group on Hypertension Control in Children and Adolescents, "Update on the 1987 Task Force Report on High Blood Pressure in Children and Adolescents: A Working Group Report From the National High Blood Pressure Education Program," *Pediatrics*, 1996, 98(4 Pt 1):649-58.

National High Blood Pressure Education Program Working Group, "1995 Update of the Working Group Reports on Chronic Renal Failure and Renovascular Hypertension," *Arch Intern Med*, 1996, 156 (17):1938-47.

"The Sixth Report of the National Committee on Detection, Evaluation, and Treatment of High Blood Pressure (JNC-VI)," *Arch Intern Med*, 1997, 157(21):2413-46.

Others

Appel LJ, Moore TJ, Obarzanek E, et al, "A Clinical Trial of the Effect of Dietary Patterns on Blood Pressure. The DASH Collaborative Research Group," *N Engl J Med*, 1997, 336(16):1117-24.

Epstein M and Bakris G, "Newer Approaches to Antihypertensive Therapy: Use of Fixed-Dose Combination Therapy," *Arch Intern Med*, 1996, 156(17):1969-78.

Estacio RO and Schrier RW, "Antihypertensive Therapy in Type II Diabetes: Implications of the Appropriate Blood Pressure Control in Diabetes (ABCD) Trial," *Am J Cardiol*, 1998, 82(9B):9R-14R.

Flack JM, Neaton J, Grimm RJ, et al, "Blood Pressure and Mortality Among Men With Prior Myocardial Infarction. The Multiple Risk Factor Intervention Trial Research Group," *Circulation*, 1995, 92 (9):2437-45.

Frishman WH, Bryzinski BS, Coulson LR, et al, "A Multifactorial Trial Design to Assess Combination Therapy in Hypertension: Treatment With Bisoprolol and Hydrochlorothiazide," *Arch Intern Med*, 1994, 154(13):1461-8.

Furberg CD, Psaty BM, and Meyer JV, "Nifedipine: Dose-Related Increase in Mortality in Patients With Coronary Heart Disease," *Circulation*, 1995, 92(5):1326-31.

Glynn RJ, Brock DB, Harris T, et al, "Use of Antihypertensive Drugs and Trends in Blood Pressure in the Elderly," *Arch Intern Med*, 1995, 155:1855-60.

Gradman AH, Cutler NR, Davis PJ, et al, "Combined Enalapril and Felodipine Extended Release (ER) for Systemic Hypertension. The Enalapril-Felodipine ER Factorial Study Group," *Am J Cardiol*, 1997, 79(4):431-5.

Grimm RH Jr, Flack JM, Grandits GA, et al, "Long-Term Effects on Plasma Lipids of Diet and Drugs to Treat Hypertension. The Treatment of Mild Hypertension Study (TOMHS) Research Group," *JAMA*, 1996, 275(20):1549-56.

Grimm RH Jr, Grandits GA, Cutler JA, et al, "Relationships of Quality-of-Life Measures to Long-Term Lifestyle and Drug Treatment in the Treatment of Mild Hypertension Study. The TOMHS Research Group," *Arch Intern Med*, 1997, 157(6):638-48.

Grossman E, Messerli FH, Grodzicki T, et al, "Should a Moratorium Be Placed on Sublingual Nifedipine Capsules Given for Hypertensive Emergencies and Pseudoemergencies?" *JAMA*, 1996, 276 (16):1328-31.

Hansson L, Zanchetti A, Carruthers SG, et al, "Effects of Intensive Blood Pressure Lowering and Low-Dose Aspirin in Patients With Hypertension: Principal Results of the Hypertension Optimal Treatment (HOT) Randomized Trial. HOT Study Group," *Lancet*, 1998, 351(9118):1755-62.

Kaplan NM and Gifford RW Jr, "Choice of Initial Therapy for Hypertension," *JAMA*, 1996, 275 (20):1577-80.

Kasiske BL, Ma JZ, Kalil RSN, et al, "Effects of Antihypertensive Therapy in Serum Lipids," *Ann Intern Med*, 1995, 122(2):133-41.

Kostis JB, Davis BR, Cutler J, et al, "Prevention of Heart Failure by Antihypertensive Drug Treatment in Older Persons With Isolated Systolic Hypertension. SHEP Cooperative Research Group," *JAMA*, 1997, 278(3):212-6.

Lazarus JM, Bourgoignie JJ, Buckalew VM, et al, "Achievement and Safety of a Low Blood Pressure Goal in Chronic Renal Disease: The Modification of Diet in Renal Disease Study Group," *Hypertension*, 1997, 29(2):641-50.

Lindheimer MD, "Hypertension in Pregnancy," *Hypertension*, 1993, 22(1):127-37.

Materson BJ, Reda DJ, Cushman WC, et al, "Single-Drug Therapy for Hypertension in Men: A Comparison of Six Antihypertensive Agents With Placebo. The Department of Veterans Affairs Cooperative Study Group on Antihypertensive Agents," *N Engl J Med*, 1993, 328(13):914-21.

Miller NH, Hill M, Kottke T, et al, "The Multi-Level Compliance Challenge: Recommendations for a Call to Action; A Statement for Healthcare Professionals," *Circulation*, 1997, 95(4):1085-90.

Neaton JD and Wentworth D, "Serum Cholesterol, Blood Pressure, Cigarette Smoking, and Death From Coronary Heart Disease: Overall Findings and Differences by Age for 316,099 White Men. The Multiple Risk Factor Intervention Trial Research Group," *Arch Intern Med*, 1992, 152(1):56-64.

Neaton JD, Grim RH, Prineas RJ, et al, "Treatment of Mild Hypertension Study. Final Results. Treatment of Mild Hypertension Study Research Group," *JAMA*, 1993, 270(6):713-24.

Oparil S, Levine JH, Zuschke CA, et al, "Effects of Candesartan Cilexetil in Patients With Severe Systemic Hypertension," *Am J Cardiol*, 1999, 84(3):289-93.

Peacock WF, Varon J, Garrison N, et al, "I.V. Clevidipine for Hypertension: Safety, Efficacy, and Transition to Oral Therapy," *Ann Emerg Med*, 2007, 50(3 Suppl):S8-9.

Perloff D, Grim C, Flack J, et al, "Human Blood Pressure Determination by Sphygmomanometry," *Circulation*, 1993, 88(5 Pt 1):2460-7.

Perry HM Jr, Bingham S, Horney A, et al, "Antihypertensive Efficacy of Treatment Regimens Used in Veterans Administration Hypertension Clinics. Department of Veterans Affairs Cooperative Study Group on Antihypertensive Agents," *Hypertension*, 1998, 31(3):771-9.

Preston RA, Materson BJ, Reda DJ, et al, "Age-Race Subgroup Compared With Renin Profile as Predictors of Blood Pressure Response to Antihypertensive Therapy," *JAMA*, 1998, 280(13):1168-72.

Psaty BM, Smith NL, Siscovick DS, et al, "Health Outcomes Associated With Antihypertensive Therapies Used as First-Line Agents. A Systemic Review and Meta-analysis," *JAMA*, 1997, 277 (9):739-45.

Radevski IV, Valtchanova SP, Candy GP, et al, "Comparison of Acebutolol With and Without Hydrochlorothiazide Versus Carvedilol With and Without Hydrochlorothiazide in Black Patients With Mild to Moderate Systemic Hypertension," *Am J Cardiol*, 1999, 84(1):70-5.

Setaro JF and Black HR, "Refractory Hypertension," *N Engl J Med*, 1992, 327(8):543-7.

SHEP Cooperative Research Group, "Prevention of Stroke by Antihypertensive Drug Treatment in Older Persons With Isolated Systolic Hypertension: Final Results of the Systolic Hypertension in the Elderly Program (SHEP)," *JAMA*, 1991, 265(24):3255-64.

Sibai BM, "Treatment of Hypertension in Pregnant Women," *N Engl J Med*, 1996, 335(4):257-65.

Singla N, Warltier DC, Gandhi SD, et al, "Treatment of Acute Postoperative Hypertension in Cardiac Surgery Patients: An Efficacy Study of Clevidipine Assessing Its Postoperative Antihypertensive Effect in Cardiac Surgery-2 (ESCAPE-2), a Randomized, Double-Blind, Placebo-Controlled Trial," *Anesth Analg*, 2008, 107(1):59-67.

Sowers JR, "Comorbidity of Hypertension and Diabetes: The Fosinopril Versus Amlodipine Cardiovascular Events Trial," *Am J Cardiol*, 1998, 82(9B):15R-19R.

Sternberg H, Rosenthal T, Shamiss A, et al, "Altered Circadian Rhythm of Blood Pressure in Shift Workers," *J Hum Hypertens*, 1995, 9(5):349-53.

"The Hypertension Prevention Trial: Three-Year Effects of Dietary Changes on Blood Pressure. Hypertension Prevention Trial Research Group," *Arch Intern Med*, 1990, 150(1):153-62.

Trials of Hypertension Prevention Collaborative Research Group, "Effects of Weight Loss and Sodium Reduction Intervention on Blood Pressure and Hypertension Incidence in Overweight People With High-Normal Blood Pressure: The Trials of Hypertension Prevention, Phase II," *Arch Intern Med*, 1997, 157(6):657-67.

Tuomilehto J, Rastenyte D, Birkenhager WH, et al, "Effects of Calcium Channel Blockade in Older Patients With Diabetes and Systolic Hypertension," *N Engl J Med*, 1999, 340(9):677-84.

Veelken R and Schmieder RE, "Overview of Alpha-1 Adrenoceptor Antagonism and Recent Advances in Hypertensive Therapy," *Am J Hypertens*, 1996, 9(11):139S-49S.

White WB, Black HR, Weber MA, et al, "Comparison of Effects of Controlled Onset Extended Release Verapamil at Bedtime and Nifedipine Gastrointestinal Therapeutic System on Arising on Early Morning Blood Pressure, Heart Rate, and the Heart Rate-Blood Pressure Product," *Am J Cardiol*, 1998, 81 (4):424-31.

LATEX ALLERGY

The incidence of clinically significant latex allergy is increasing. This increase has been suggested to be due in part to the implementation of universal precautions by the CDC in 1987 secondary to the AIDS epidemic. **Because of the increased incidence of latex allergy, all patients need a complete history including risk factor evaluation and previous evidence of clinical signs and symptoms suggesting contact dermatitis or urticaria.** For example, patients should be questioned about the presence of swelling or itching of the hands or other areas after contact with rubber gloves, condoms, diaphragms, toys, or other rubber products and about itching or swelling of the lips or mouth after dental exams, blowing up balloons, or after eating bananas, chestnuts, and avocados.

It is important today for health care institutions to have a comprehensive plan (including a perioperative component) in place for dealing with latex allergic patients and healthcare personnel. In cardiovascular medicine, the high proportion of procedures and imaging modalities heightens exposure to latex allergens, usually related to rubber gloves. This is a potentially life-threatening problem, both for the patient and healthcare personnel, in situations such as the cardiac catheterization laboratory. Some institutions have avoided use of latex products throughout the hospital environment.

Hypersensitivity Reactions Caused by Latex

Latex-containing products can produce type I and type IV hypersensitivity reactions.

The type I (IgE-mediated) hypersensitivity reaction is the true "allergic" reaction seen with latex products. Proteins found in the latex promote the production of an antibody of the IgE class which attaches to basophils and mast cells. When the antigen (protein) is encountered again, histamine and other physiologically active mediators are released from mast cells and basophils. The clinical manifestations can include single or multiple system involvement, be mild or severe, ranging from itching to edema, and from mild hypotension to shock. It has been estimated that 10% of the true anaphylactic reactions during anesthesia are due to latex allergy. These reactions are usually seen 5-30 minutes after induction of anesthesia and start of surgery. Seventy-nine percent of of type I patients previously had type IV symptoms.

In the type IV (delayed type) reaction, a contact dermatitis is seen. The preservatives, stabilizers, accelerators, and antioxidants used in the latex manufacturing process serve as the antigens for T-cell lymphocytes. The dermatitis produced can be uncomfortable but is not life-threatening and usually occurs over a 24-hour period; limited to site of contact. Not all patients with type IV symptoms will progress to type I reactivity.

Routes of Exposure to Latex Proteins

It is important to consider the route of exposure of the latex protein in allergic patients as this can be a determinant of the type of reaction produced. The following table summarizes major routes of exposure.

Type of Exposure	Reaction
Direct skin contact	Localized or generalized urticaria
Mucous membrane	Rhinitis, conjunctivitis, stomatitis, angioedema; severe anaphylactic reactions and death reported
Inhalation of airborne starch-protein particles	Wheezing, bronchospasm, reduced lung compliance, episodes of desaturation and/or severe hypoxemia
Intravascular absorption of water soluble latex particles from surgical gloves	Sudden tachycardia, severe hypotension, cardiorespiratory collapse

High-Risk Patients

Several groups have been identified as "high-risk" for allergic reactions to latex. Special consideration should be given these individuals.

Patients having multiple surgical procedures (eg, spina bifida patients/patients with congenital urologic abnormalities). A 30% to 70% incidence of latex allergy has been reported for spina bifida patients. These patients are routinely exposed to latex-containing urinary catheters.

Healthcare providers. Latex sensitivity may be as high as 17%. Approximately 70% of adverse events reported to FDA regarding latex involve healthcare workers.

Workers with occupational exposure to natural rubber latex (eg, hairdressers, greenhouse workers, latex manufacturers).

Patients with a history of atopy, hay fever, rhinitis, asthma, or eczema. Atopy is one of the significant predisposing risk factors for latex allergy.

Patients with history of food allergy to tropical fruits (eg, avocado, kiwi, bananas), chestnuts, stone fruits, and additional specific foods. These plants contain several proteins similar/identical to those found in latex.

Individuals with severe or anaphylactic responses to latex should consider having an Epi-Pen® available at all times, and having a Medic-Alert® bracelet to alert healthcare workers to the potential for life-threatening allergic reactions.

Treatment of Anaphylactic Reaction

Management of an anaphylactic reaction which is thought to be due to latex allergy must be immediate. Initial therapy should consist of the following.

- Stop administration of offending agent.
- Removal of all latex products (switch to nonlatex gloves and latex-free intravenous tubing). Latex-free precautions must accompany the patient throughout the perioperative and hospital stay (PACU, ICU, general floor, and discharge unit).
- Discontinue all antibiotic and blood administration.
- Maintain airway with 100% oxygen.
- Intubate the trachea (as indicated).
- Intravascular volume expansion with crystalloid or colloid.
- Epinephrine administration (see Epinephrine (Systemic, Oral Inhalation) monograph).
- Discontinue all anesthetic agents if appropriate.
- Consider use of Military Anti-Shock Trousers (MAST).
- Display prominent signs to identify latex allergy.
- When appropriate, administer antihistamines (eg, diphenhydramine), corticosteroids (eg, hydrocortisone), catecholamine infusions (eg, norepinephrine), inhaled bronchodilators (eg, albuterol) for bronchospasm, and sodium bicarbonate (guided by arterial blood gas results). Patients should be admitted to the ICU for 24 hours following an anaphylactic reaction because of the possibility of recurrent "late-phase" reactions. To confirm a latex allergy, RAST or AlaSTAT test may be performed.
- Details of any allergic reaction should be clearly documented in the patient's chart and reported to FDA MedWatch program.
- Contact dermatitis and type IV reactions:
  - Avoid irritating skin cleansers.
  - Topical corticosteroids can be applied locally.

Perioperative Management of a Latex Allergic Patient

No evidence exists to demonstrate that prophylaxis before surgery prevents latex-induced anaphylactic reactions. In spite of this, prophylaxis has been used in patients with a positive history of allergy; one suggested regimen uses diphenhydramine P.O. or I.V. every 6 hours at 13, 7, and 1 hours before surgery, prednisone P.O. every 6 hours at 13, 7, and 1 hours before surgery (hydrocortisone I.V. may be substituted), and ranitidine P.O. or I.V. every 12 hours at 13 and 1 hours before surgery. This regimen is continued for 12 hours after surgery.

The key to the hospital management of the latex allergic patient is to provide a latex-free environment. To accomplish this, the following actions should be taken.

- Substitute all items with nonlatex alternatives when possible; if there is a question concerning the latex content of a product, the manufacturer should be called.
- Gloves made of neoprene or other polymers should be used.
- Latex-based adhesives should be eliminated.
- Stopcocks should be used for drug administration instead of injection ports on I.V. tubing.
- Syringes not containing rubber tips on the plunger should be used.
- Drug products in glass ampuls should be used whenever possible; if a vial must be used, utilize a vial stopper remover so the stopper does not have to be punctured or puncture only once.
- To reduce exposure to aerosolized glove powder which is a known carrier of latex proteins, schedule the surgery as the first case of the day. Some institutions have reserved an O.R. suite for latex allergic patients.

Testing for Latex Allergy

Testing for latex allergy is recommended for high-risk patients. Both *in vitro* and *in vivo* tests are available as seen in the following table.

Test	Type	Description
Skin prick (SPT)	*in vivo*	Sensitive method to confirm IgE-mediated latex hypersensitivity; correlates well with clinical presence of allergy; high sensitivity (100%), high specificity (99%)
Patch	*in vivo*	Test for type IV hypersensitivity reaction; test performed with 1 inch square of rubber glove; skin observed for contact dermatitis after 48 hours
Radioallergosorbent (RAST)	*in vitro*	Performed on the serum of patients with natural latex as the antigen; used to detect and quantify allergen specific IgE in patient's serum; positive RAST response correlates strongly with *in vivo* allergic response; sensitivity 67% to 82%
Enzymeallergosorbent (EAST)	*in vitro*	Enzyme-linked immunometric assay used to measure latex-specific IgE antibodies; can be false negatives

REFERENCES AND RECOMMENDED READING

Dakin MJ and Yentis SM, "Latex Allergy: A Strategy for Management," *Anaesthesia*, 1998, 53 (8):774-81.

Hancock DL, "Latex Allergy. Prevention and Treatment," *Anesthesiol Rev*, 1994, 21(5):153-63.

Katz JD, Holzman RS, Brown RH, et al, "Natural Rubber Latex Allergy: Considerations for Anesthesiologists," American Society of Anesthesiologists (ASA), 2005. Available at: http://www.asahq.org/publicationsAndServices/latexallergy.pdf. Last accessed December 6, 2007.

Senst BL and Johnson RA, "Latex Allergy," *Am J Health Syst Pharm*, 1997, 54(9):1071-5.

Steelman VM, "Latex Allergy Precautions. A Research-Based Protocol," *Nurs Clin North Am*, 1995, 30 (3):475-93.

Sussman G and Gold M, "Guidelines for the Management of Latex Allergies and Safe Latex Use in Health Care Facilities." Available at: http://www.acaai.org/public/physicians/latex.htm.

OBESITY TREATMENT GUIDELINES

SUMMARY OF CLINICAL PRACTICE GUIDELINES

ADULTS

ASSESSMENT

Assessment of weight involves evaluating body mass index, waist circumference, and the patient's risk factors.

A. Body Mass Index (BMI)

1. BMI should be calculated for all adults (see table). Those with normal BMI should be reassessed in 2 years. A very muscular person may have a high BMI without the additional health risks. A BMI calculator is available through Lexi-CALC™.

2. Normal BMI is within the range of 18.5-24.9 kg/m^2. Overweight is defined as a BMI of 25-29.9 kg/m^2.

3. Obesity is defined as a BMI of ≥30 kg/m^2. There are 3 classes of obesity: Class I (BMI 30-34.9), Class II (BMI 35-39.9), Class III (BMI ≥40).

B. Abdominal Fat

1. Measuring waist circumference is most beneficial in patients who have a normal weight or are considered overweight.

2. Excess abdominal fat, not proportional to total body fat, is an independent predictor for relative disease risk.

3. Waist circumference for men >40 inches or women >35 inches is associated with an increased risk of dyslipidemia, heart disease, hypertension, and type 2 diabetes for those with a BMI of 25-34.9.

4. Waist circumference should be measured for patients with a BMI <35 kg/m^2 at the initial obesity assessment and during weight loss.

C. Risk Factors and Comorbidities

1. Coronary heart disease, hypertension, stroke, or other atherosclerotic diseases, type 2 diabetes, gallbladder disease, osteoarthritis, sleep apnea, and other respiratory problems are associated with a very high risk of developing disease complications and higher mortality in an obese individual.

2. Obesity is also associated with complications of pregnancy, menstrual irregularities, stress incontinence, and psychological disorders (eg, depression).

3. **Cardiovascular Risk Factors:** Hypertension, cigarette smoking, obesity (BMI ≥30), inactive lifestyle, dyslipidemia, diabetes mellitus, microalbuminuria or estimated GFR <60 mL/minute, age (>55 years for men, >65 years for women), family history of premature cardiovascular disease (men <55 years or women >65 years).
Weight loss is recommended for those who are obese (BMI ≥30 kg/m^2) and for those who are classified as overweight (BMI 25-29.9 kg/m^2) or have a high waist circumference and ≥2 risk factors (eg, coronary heart disease, atherosclerotic disease, type 2 diabetes, or sleep apnea).

Body Mass Index (BMI), kg/m^2

Height (feet, inches)

Weight (lb)	5'0"	5'3"	5'6"	5'9"	6'0"	6'3"
140	27	25	23	21	19	18
150	29	27	24	22	20	19
160	31	28	26	24	22	20
170	33	30	28	25	23	21
180	35	32	29	27	25	23
190	37	34	31	28	26	24
200	39	36	32	30	27	25
210	41	37	34	31	29	26
220	43	39	36	33	30	28
230	45	41	37	34	31	29
240	47	43	39	36	33	30
250	49	44	40	37	34	31

TREATMENT

Patients who are overweight or obese, but are not candidates for a weight loss program (eg, those with serious psychiatric illness) or do not wish to lose weight, should be counseled to avoid further weight gain. Women who are overweight or obese at the onset of pregnancy are advised to gain less total weight during pregnancy.

A. Goals of Treatment

1. Prevent further weight gain.
2. Reduce body weight. The initial goal is to reduce body weight by 10% from baseline over the suggested time period of 6 months.
3. Maintain a lower body weight, long term.

B. Nonpharmacologic treatment should include:

1. An individually-planned diet which includes a decrease in fat as well as total calories. Generally, women may be maintained on 1000-1200 calories/day and men may be maintained on 1200-1600 calories/day.
2. An increase in physical activity. Physical activity should be gradually increased to a goal of 30 minutes per day of moderate-intensity activity.
3. Behavior therapy, which should include tools to help overcome individual barriers to weight loss.

C. Drug Therapy
Select patients with BMI ≥30, or BMI ≥27 with other risk factors (eg, hypertension, diabetes, dyslipidemia), who did not lose weight (after 6 months of nonpharmacologic treatment) or maintain weight loss, may be initiated on drug therapy in combination with dietary therapy, physical activity, and behavior therapy.

D. Surgery
Patients with severe clinical obesity, BMI ≥40 or BMI ≥35 with coexisting conditions, can be considered for weight loss surgery when other methods have failed. Lifelong surveillance after surgery is necessary.

Medications Approved for Long-Term Use in the Treatment of Obesity

Generic (Trade) Name	Therapeutic Category / Mechanism of Action	Usual Dosage
Orlistat (Xenical®)	Lipase inhibitor; a reversible inhibitor of gastric and pancreatic lipases thus inhibiting absorption of dietary fats by 30% (at doses of 120 mg 3 times/day)	≥12 years of age: 120 mg 3 times/day with each main meal containing fat (during or up to 1 hour after the meal); omit dose if meal is occasionally missed or contains no fat.
Orlistat (Alli™; OTC)		≥18 years of age: 60 mg 3 times/day with each meal containing fat (during or up to 1 hour after the meal); omit dose if meal is occasionally missed or contains no fat.
Sibutramine (Meridia®)	Anorexiant; blocks the neuronal uptake of norepinephrine and, to a lesser extent, serotonin and dopamine	≥16 years of age: Initial: 10 mg once daily; after 4 weeks may titrate up to 15 mg once daily as needed and tolerated

CHILDREN

ASSESSMENT

Assessment of weight involves body mass index (BMI), CDC growth charts, and patient risk factors. The goal of identifying overweight or obese children is to prevent or improve obesity-related comorbidities.

A. Body Mass Index (BMI)

1. BMI, in addition to the CDC-derived growth charts, should be used for diagnosing overweight or obese children and adolescents (CDC-derived growth charts found at: www.cdc.gov/growthcharts/clinical_charts.htm).
2. BMI for children and adolescents is based on weight and height, as well as age and gender (Pediatric BMI calculator found at: http://apps.nccd.cdc.gov/dnpabmi/).
3. Overweight is defined as a BMI in the 85th percentile but <95th percentile.
4. Obesity is defined as a BMI ≥95th percentile.
5. Children with a BMI ≥85th percentile should be evaluated for comorbidities.

B. Risk Factors and Comorbidities

1. The presence of cardiovascular risk factors associated with childhood overweight and obesity may lead to an increased prevalence of cardiovascular morbidity and mortality in adulthood.

2. Pediatric comorbidities: Type 2 diabetes, dyslipidemia, metabolic syndrome, acanthosis nigricans, hyperandrogenemia, hyperinsulinism, blood pressure changes, gallstones

TREATMENT

A. Age appropriate recommendations for the treatment of overweight and obese children should be provided to the patient and the entire family.

B. Nonpharmacologic treatment should include:

1. Healthy eating habits (including the avoidance of calorie-dense food [eg, juice, sweetened drinks, soda, sports drinks, and fast food]) are recommended.
2. An increase in moderate-to-vigorous physical activity to 60 minutes daily.
3. Healthcare professionals should educate and encourage parents and families to become more involved in guiding children toward healthy habits in diet and proper exercise routines.

C. Drug Therapy
If lifestyle modifications have failed to prevent weight gain or change the comorbidities in obese children, drug therapy (with continued lifestyle modifications) may be considered. Drug therapy in overweight children should not be considered unless severe comorbidities exist, including a strong family history of type 2 diabetes or cardiovascular risk factors.

D. Surgery
Bariatric surgery is not recommended for preadolescent children; patients with eating disorders, untreated psychiatric disorder, or Prader-Willi syndrome; patients who continue unhealthy dietary and activity habits; adolescents who are pregnant, breast-feeding, or planning to become pregnant within 2 years of surgery.

References

August GP, Caprio S, Fennoy I, et al, "Prevention and Treatment of Pediatric Obesity: An Endocrine Society Clinical Practice Guideline Based on Expert Opinion," *J Clin Endocrinol Metab*, 2008, 93 (12):4576-99.

Centers for Disease Control and Prevention (CDC), "Healthy Weight – It's Not a Diet, It's a Lifestyle!" Available at: http://www.cdc.gov/healthyweight/index.html. Accessed on March 2, 2010.

McTigue KM, Harris R, Hemphill B, et al, "Screening and Interventions for Obesity in Adults: Summary of the Evidence for the U.S. Preventive Services Task Force," *Ann Intern Med*, 2003, 139(11):933-49.

National Heart, Lung, and Blood Institute Obesity Education Initiative, "Clinical Guidelines on the Identification, Evaluation, and Treatment of Overweight and Obesity in Adults. The Evidence Report," NIH Publication No. 98-4083. Bethesda, MD: U.S. Department of Health and Human Services, Public Health Service, National Institutes of Health, National Heart, Lung, and Blood Institute, 1998.

Snow V, Barry P, Fitterman N, et al, "Pharmacologic and Surgical Management of Obesity in Primary Care: A Clinical Practice Guideline From the American College of Physicians," *Ann Intern Med*, 2005, 142(7):525-31.

OSTEOPOROSIS MANAGEMENT

PREVALENCE

Osteoporosis affects more than 10 million Americans. An additional 34 million Americans have low bone density of the hip. An osteoporosis-related fracture will occur in approximately one out of every two Caucasian females at some point in her lifetime, and will occur in approximately one in five men.

CONSEQUENCES

Fractures and the complications resulting from fractures are the clinically significant sequelae of osteoporosis. Fractures may result in pain, physical limitations, lifestyle changes, and decreased quality of life. In particular, hip fractures result in a 10% to 20% excess mortality in one year. In the U.S., osteoporosis-related fractures result in heavy economic burden caused by the >432,000 hospitalizations, almost 2.5 million medical office visits, and ~180,000 nursing home admissions that occur annually as a result.

RISK FACTORS

Conditions, Diseases, and Medications

- Postmenopausal women and men ≥50 years of age
- Endocrine disorders, such as adrenal insufficiency, Cushing's disease, diabetes mellitus, hyperparathyroidism, thyrotoxicosis
- Excessive alcohol intake (≥3 drinks/day)
- Excessive vitamin A intake
- Falls
- Parental history of hip fracture
- Genetic factors, due to conditions such as cystic fibrosis, Ehlers-Danlos, Gaucher's disease, glycogen storage diseases, hemochromatosis, homocystinuria, hypophosphatasia, idiopathic hypercalciuria, Marfan syndrome, Menkes steely hair syndrome, osteogenesis imperfecta, porphyria, Riley-Day syndrome
- Gastrointestinal disorders, such as celiac disease, gastric bypass, GI surgery, inflammatory bowel disease, malabsorption, pancreatic disease, primary biliary cirrhosis
- Hematologic disorders, such as hemophilia, leukemia/lymphoma, multiple myeloma, sickle cell disease, systemic mastocytosis, thalassemia
- High caffeine and/or sodium intake
- Hypogonadal states, due to conditions such as androgen insensitivity, anorexia, athletic amenorrhea, hyperprolactinemia, panhypopituitarism, premature ovarian failure, Turner's and Klinefelter's syndrome
- Low calcium and/or vitamin D intake
- Medications: Aluminum-containing antacids (excessive use), anticoagulants (heparin), anticonvulsants, aromatase inhibitors, barbiturates, chemotherapy, cyclosporine A, depo-medroxyprogesterone, glucocorticoids (≥5 mg/day of prednisone or equivalent for ≥3 months), gonadotropin-releasing hormone agonists, heparin, lithium, parenteral nutrition, tacrolimus
- Miscellaneous conditions/diseases, including amyloidosis, chronic metabolic acidosis, depression, emphysema, end-stage renal disease, epilepsy, heart failure, idiopathic scoliosis, multiple sclerosis, muscular dystrophy, post-transplant bone disease, sarcoidosis
- Previous fracture as an adult
- Rheumatic/autoimmune diseases, such as ankylosing spondylitis, lupus, rheumatoid arthritis
- Sedentary lifestyle or immobilization
- Smoking (active or passive)
- Thinness (low body mass index)

DIAGNOSIS / MONITORING

- Bone mineral density (BMD) measurement using Dual-energy x-ray absorptiometry (DXA) bone density scan[1]
- U.S.-adapted WHO Fracture Risk Algorithm (FRAX®; www.nof.org and www.shef.ac.uk/FRAX)[2]

[1]BMD measurement by DXA at the hip or spine is used to establish or confirm an osteoporosis diagnosis.

[2]US-FRAX® is designed to calculate the 10 year probability of a hip fracture and the 10 year probability of a major osteoporotic fracture (vertebral, hip, forearm, or humerus fracture). Application of Frax™ is intended for postmenopausal women and men ≥50 years of age (not for younger adults or pediatrics) and results apply only to previously untreated patients.

Definition of Osteoporosis[1]

Normal: T score at -1.0 and above
Low bone mass or "osteopenia": T score between -1.0 and -2.5
Osteoporosis: T score at -2.5 or below

[1]Based on World Health Organization (WHO) established definition of osteoporosis using BMD measurements by DXA devices at the spine, hip or forearm. T-score values are based on standard deviations (SD) below that of a "young normal" adult. The WHO diagnostic classification only applies to postmenopausal women and men ≥50 years of age; not applicable for premenopausal women, men <50 years of age or pediatrics.

Bone mineral density (BMD) testing

Recommend for the following patients:

- All women ≥65 years and men ≥70 years
- High risk postmenopausal women and men aged 50-69 years
- Women in menopausal transition if increased fracture risk present (eg, low body weight, prior low-trauma fracture, receiving high risk medication)
- Patients with a history of a fracture (occurring after age 50)
- Adults with a predisposing condition associated with low bone mass or loss (see Risk Factors)
- Any patient being considered for pharmacologic therapy for osteoporosis or receiving treatment for osteoporosis (monitoring typically performed every 2 years unless more frequent testing warranted)
- Any patient not receiving therapy but evidence of bone loss would lead to treatment

Consider for the following patients:

- Postmenopausal women discontinuing estrogen

PREVENTION / TREATMENT

- Fall prevention (eg, visual/hearing checks, minimizing pharmacologic agents that contribute to fall risk, checking environment for safety hazards)
- Weight-bearing exercise (eg, walking) and muscle strengthening, as tolerated
- Avoidance of tobacco use and excessive alcohol intake
- Adequate intake of at least 1200 mg **elemental** calcium daily in the form of dietary calcium or calcium supplementation, particularly women ≥50 years of age. Intakes exceeding 1200-1500 mg offer limited additional benefit and may increase the risk for cardiovascular disease or kidney stones. Also refer to table located at the end of appendix piece for selected calcium supplement information.
- Adequate intake of at least 800-1000 int. units of vitamin D for adults ≥50 years of age. Measuring serum vitamin D concentrations may be warranted, particularly in those at greatest risk for deficiency, to allow for the administration of vitamin D replacement. **Note:** Certain patients at risk for vitamin D deficiency (eg, elderly, diseases associated with malabsorption, chronic renal insufficiency) may require higher intakes.

Pharmacologic Therapy

Consider using FDA approved pharmacologic therapy in postmenopausal women and men ≥50 years with a hip or vertebral fracture **or** those with a T score ≤ -2.5 at the femoral neck or spine (after excluding secondary causes) **or** those with low bone mass (T score between -1.0 and -2.5 at the femoral neck or spine) in combination with a 10-year hip fracture probability of ≥3% or a 10-year osteoporosis-related major fracture probability of ≥20% (based on the U.S.-adapted WHO algorithm)

1. Bisphosphonates: Oral bisphosphonates should be administered ≥30 minutes before first food or drink (except water) with 6-8 ounces tap water (**not** mineral water) and patients should remain upright (or raise head of bed to at least a 30° angle) to avoid ulcerative esophagitis. Consult individual monographs for details regarding use, precautions, and dosing and administration of any of the specific drugs mentioned below.

   Osteoporosis prevention: Postmenopausal females:

   - Alendronate: Oral: 5 mg once daily or 35 mg once weekly
   - Ibandronate: Oral: 2.5 mg once daily or 150 mg once per month
   - Risedronate: Oral: 5 mg once daily or 35 mg once weekly or one 75 mg tablet once daily on two consecutive days per month (total of 2 tablets/month) or 150 mg once per month
   - Zoledronic acid (Reclast®): I.V.: 5 mg infused over at least 15 minutes every 2 years

Osteoporosis treatment:

- Alendronate: Males and Postmenopausal females: Oral: 10 mg once daily or 70 mg once weekly
- Ibandronate: Postmenopausal females:
  - Oral: 2.5 mg once daily or 150 mg once per month
  - I.V.: 3 mg every 3 months
- Risedronate:
  - Postmenopausal females: Oral: 5 mg once daily or 35 mg once weekly or one 75 mg tablet once daily on two consecutive days per month (total of 2 tablets/ month) or 150 mg once monthly
  - Males: Oral: 35 mg once weekly
- Zoledronic acid (Reclast®): Males and Postmenopausal females: I.V.: 5 mg infused over at least 15 minutes every 12 months

Glucocorticoid-induced osteoporosis prevention:

- Risedronate: Oral: 5 mg once daily
- Zoledronic acid (Reclast®): I.V.: 5 mg infused over at least 15 minutes every 12 months (in patients initiating or continuing prednisone ≥7.5 mg/day [or equivalent] and expected to remain on glucocorticoids for at least 12 months)

Glucocorticoid-induced osteoporosis treatment:

- Alendronate: Oral: 5 mg once daily; Postmenopausal women not receiving estrogen: 10 mg once daily
- Risedronate: Oral: 5 mg once daily
- Zoledronic acid (Reclast®): I.V.: 5 mg infused over at least 15 minutes every 12 months (in patients initiating or continuing prednisone ≥7.5 mg/day [or equivalent] and expected to remain on glucocorticoids for at least 12 months)

2. Estrogen agonist/antagonist (previously known as selective estrogen receptor modulators)
   Osteoporosis prevention and treatment: Postmenopausal females:
   - Raloxifene: Oral: 60 mg once daily; may be taken any time of the day without regard to meals but should be stopped 72 hours prior to or during immobilization due to risk of thromboembolic events.

3. Estrogens/hormone therapy: Should not be considered first agents for preventing osteoporosis due to increased risk of breast cancer, heart disease, stroke, and deep-vein thrombosis (DVT) found in the Women's Health Initiative study. Estrogens, as well as various combination therapies, including ethinyl estradiol and norethindrone (femhrt®) and estradiol and norgestimate (Prefest™), have been approved for the prevention of osteoporosis. The FDA recommends that approved nonestrogen treatments should be considered before the use of estrogen/hormone therapy for the sole purpose of prevention of osteoporosis.
   Note: In women with an intact uterus, administer estrogen with oral progesterone; unopposed estrogen can cause endometrial cancer.

4. Calcitonin: Adequate dietary or supplemental calcium and vitamin D are essential.
   Osteoporosis treatment: Postmenopausal females (>5 years postmenopause):
   - Calcitonin (Miacalcin®): I.M., SubQ: 100 units every other day (I.M. route is preferred if volume exceeds 2 mL)
   - Calcitonin (Fortical®, Miacalcin®): Intranasal: 200 units (1 spray) in one nostril daily, alternate right and left nostril daily

5. Parathyroid hormone: Initial administration of teriparatide should occur under circumstances in which the patient may sit or lie down, in the event of orthostasis
   Osteoporosis treatment: Postmenopausal women at high risk of fracture or treatment of primary or hypogonadal osteoporosis in men at high risk of fracture:
   - Teriparatide: SubQ: 20 mcg once daily

   Glucocorticoid induced osteoporosis treatment: Men and women:
   - Teriparatide: SubQ: 20 mcg once daily

Calcium Type	Elemental Calcium	Equivalent Elemental Calcium	Example Brands
Acetate	25%	667 mg = 169 mg	Phos-Lo®
Carbonate	40%	364 mg = 145.6 mg	Florical®
		500 mg = 200 mg	Tums® chewable tablets
		1000 mg = 400 mg	Tums® Ultra chewable tablets
		1500 mg = 600 mg	Calcarb 600, Caltrate® 600, Nephro-Calci®
Citrate	21%	950 mg = 200 mg	Citracal®
Glubionate	6.5%	1.8 g/5 mL = 115 mg/5 mL	Various OTC and generic brands available
Gluconate	9%	500 mg = 45 mg	
Lactate	13%	650 mg = 84.5 mg	
Phosphate (tribasic)	39%	1565.2 mg = 600 mg	Posture®

References

Ashworth L, "Focus on Alendronate. A Nonhormonal Option for the Treatment of Osteoporosis in Postmenopausal Women," *Formulary*, 1996, 31:23-30.

Barrett-Connor E, Grady D, Sashegyi A, et al, "Raloxifene and Cardiovascular Events in Osteoporotic Postmenopausal Women: Four-Year Results From the MORE (Multiple Outcomes of Raloxifene Evaluation) Randomized Trial," *JAMA*, 2002, 287(7):847-57.

Hully S, Grady D, Bush T, et al, "Randomized Trial of Estrogen Plus Progestin for Secondary Prevention of Coronary Heart Disease in Postmenopausal Women. Heart and Estrogen/Progestin Replacement Study (HERS) Research Group," *JAMA*, 1998, 280(7):605-13.

Johnson SR, "Should Older Women Use Estrogen Replacement," *J Am Geriatr Soc*, 1996, 44(1):89-90.

NIH Consensus Development Panel on Optimal Calcium Intake, *JAMA*, 1994, 272(24):1942-8.

National Osteoporosis Foundation, "Clinician's Guide to Prevention and Treatment of Osteoporosis," Washington, DC: National Osteoporosis Foundation, 2010, 1-44. Available at http://www.nof.org/sites/default/files/pdfs/NOF_ClinicianGuide2009_v7.pdf.

Rossouw JE, Anderson GL, Prentice RL, et al, "Risks and Benefits of Estrogen Plus Progestin in Healthy Postmenopausal Women: Principle Results From the Women's Health Initiative Randomized Controlled Trial,"*JAMA*, 2002, 288(3):321-33.

PHARMACOTHERAPY OF URINARY INCONTINENCE

Incontinence Type	Drug Class	Drug Therapy	Adverse Effects and Precautions	Comments
Urge incontinence	Anticholinergic agents (antimuscarinic effects)	**Oxybutynin** (2.5 mg 2-3 times/day, extended release 5-30 mg once daily, or transdermal 1 patch twice weekly delivering 3.9 mg/day, or topical gel 1 g daily), **propantheline** (15-30 mg 3-5 times/day), **dicyclomine** (10-20 mg 3 times/day), **tolterodine** (1-2 mg twice daily; extended release capsule: 2-4 mg once daily), **trospium** (20 mg twice daily, extended release 60 mg daily), **solifenacin** (5-10 mg once daily), **darifenacin** (7.5-15 mg once daily), **fesoterodine** (4-8 mg once daily)	Dry mouth, blurred vision, constipation, dry skin, decreased cognitive function	Anticholinergics are the first-line drug therapy. Propantheline and dicyclomine are not considered drugs of choice in older adults. Darifenacin and solifenacin may cause less anticholinergic side effects. Trospium may cause less CNS effects.
	Tricyclic antidepressants (TCAs)	Imipramine (10-25 mg 1-4 times/day)	Not recommended for older patients because of anticholinergic and orthostatic effects.	May be used in women with mixed incontinence.
Stress or combined urge/ stress incontinence	Estrogen	Topical, intravaginal, dissolving tablets in postmenopausal women; administered with varying dosing intervals (twice weekly to once daily)	Should not be used if suspected or confirmed breast or endometrial cancer, active or past thromboembolism with past oral contraceptive, estrogen, or pregnancy	Medications may not play a strong role in treatment of stress incontinence. Oral estrogen should not be prescribed for this indication; may worsen incontinence.
	Tricyclic antidepressants (TCAs)	Imipramine (10-25 mg 1-4 times/day)	May worsen cardiac conduction abnormalities, postural hypotension, anticholinergic effects	TCAs are generally reserved for patients with an additional indication (eg, depression, neuralgia) at an initial dose of 10-25 mg 1-4 times/day.
Overflow	Alpha-adrenergic antagonists	**Terazosin** (1 mg at bedtime with first dose in supine position and increase by 1 mg every 4 days to maximum 10 mg/day); **doxazosin** (1 mg at bedtime with first dose in supine position and increase by 1 mg every 7-14 days to maximum 8 mg/day); **tamsulosin** (0.4 mg-0.8 mg daily); **alfuzosin** (10 mg daily); **silodosin** (8 mg daily)	Postural hypotension, headache, dizziness	Effective in men with overactive bladder symptoms associated with benign prostatic hypertrophy.

References

Chapple C, Khullar V, Gabriel Z, et al, "The Effects of Antimuscarinic Treatments in Overactive Bladder: A Systematic Review and Meta-Analysis," *Eur Urol*, 2005, 48(1):5-26.

Herbison P, Hay-Smith J, Ellis G, et al, "Effectiveness of Anticholinergic Drugs Compared With Placebo in the Treatment of Overactive Bladder: Systematic Review," *BMJ*, 2003, 326(7394):841-4.

Resnick NM, "Urinary Incontinence," *Lancet*, 1995, 346(8967):94-9.

Rossouw JE, Anderson GL, Prentice RL, et al, "Risks and Benefits of Estrogen Plus Progestin in Healthy Postmenopausal Women: Principal Results From the Women's Health Initiative Randomized Controlled Trial," *JAMA*, 2002, 288(3):321-33.

PROPHYLAXIS FOR PATIENTS EXPOSED TO COMMON COMMUNICABLE DISEASES

Disease	Exposure	Prophylaxis / Management
Anthrax	Postexposure inhalational	Doxycycline and ciprofloxacin; 60-day (oral and intravenous) regimens have been recommended.
Invasive *Haemophilus influenzae* disease	Close contact with an infected child for more than 4 hours	**Treatment with oral rifampin:** Children <12 years of age: 20 mg/kg once daily for 4 days Adults: 600 mg daily for 4 days Contraindication: Pregnant contacts
Hepatitis A	Direct contact with an infected child, or sharing of food or utensils	Give 0.02 mL/kg immune globulin (IG) within 7 days of exposure. Single dose of vaccine if not previously immunized
Hepatitis B	Needlestick (used needle) Mucous membrane exposure with blood or body fluid Direct inoculation of blood or body fluid into open cut, lesion, or laceration	**Known source and employee status unknown: Test patient for HB_sAg and employee for anti-HB_s.** Hepatitis B immune globulin: 0.06 mL/kg I.M. If patient is HB_sAg-negative and the patient does not have non-A, non-B hepatitis, do nothing. If patient is HB_sAg-negative and has non-A, non-B hepatitis, **offer** ISG (optional). If patient is HB_sAg-positive, give HBIG and hepatitis B vaccine within 48 hours of exposure. Employee antibody status may not be available for up to a week, so the above should be given as soon as patient's antigen status is known. Occasionally, the patient's antigen status will be unavailable for more than 24 hours. In these cases, HBIG should be given if the patient is high-risk (ie, Asian immigrants, institutionalized patients, homosexuals, intravenous drug abusers, hemodialysis patients, patients with a history of hepatitis). If the employee is anti-HB_s-negative, give the second and third doses of hepatitis B vaccine. **Known source and employee documented anti-HB_s positive:** If source has non-A, non-B hepatitis, offer ISG (optional). If employee is believed to be anti-HB_s-positive due to vaccination, has received 3 doses of vaccine, and has not had an anti-HB_s test done, draw serum for anti-HB_s.
Measles	15 minutes or more in the same room with a child with measles from 2 days before the onset of symptoms to 4 days after the appearance of the rash	Children who have not been vaccinated and have not had natural infection should be isolated from the seventh through the 18th day after exposure and/or for 4 days after the rash appears. Those who have not been vaccinated should be vaccinated within 72 hours of exposure if no contraindication exists, or receive immune globulin (IG) 0.25 mL/kg I.M. for immunocompetent individuals and 0.5 mL/kg (maximum: 15 mL) for immunosuppressed individuals. Children who are younger than 15 months of age should be revaccinated at 15 months of age but at least 3 months after receipt of vaccine or IG. Older individuals who have received IG should be vaccinated 3 months later. Vaccine and IG should not be given concurrently.
Meningococcal disease	Household contact or direct contact with secretions	Household, day care center, and nursery school children should receive rifampin prophylaxis for 2 days. Dosages are given every 12 hours for a total of 4 doses. Dosage is 10 mg/kg/dose for children ages 1 month to 12 years (maximum: 600 mg/dose), 5 mg/kg/dose for infants <1 month of age, and 600 mg/dose for adults. Alternatively, ciprofloxacin 500 mg orally, ofloxacin 400 mg orally, or ceftriaxone 250 mg I.M. as single doses may be used in adults. Contraindication: Pregnant contacts **Because prophylaxis is not always effective, exposed children should be monitored for symptoms.** **Employee exposure: Anyone who develops a febrile illness should receive prompt medical evaluation. If indicated, antimicrobial therapy should be administered.**
Pertussis	Housed in the same room with an infected child or spent 15 minutes in the playroom with the infected child	**Prophylaxis:** Contacts <7 years old who have had at least 4 doses of pertussis vaccine should receive a booster dose of DTP, unless a dose has been given within the past 3 years, and should receive erythromycin 40-50 mg/kg/day orally for 14 days. Contacts <7 years old who are not immunized or who have received less than 4 doses of DTP should have DTP immunization initiated or continued according to the recommended schedule. Children who have received their third dose 6 months or more before exposure should be given their fourth dose at this time. Erythromycin should also be given for 14 days. Alternatively, clarithromycin for 7 days or azithromycin for 5 days may be used. Contacts 7 years of age and above should receive prophylactic erythromycin (maximum: 1 g/day) for 10-14 days. All exposed patients should be watched closely for respiratory symptoms for 14 days after exposure has stopped because immunity conferred by the vaccine is not absolute and the efficacy of erythromycin in prophylaxis has not been established.

continued

Disease	Exposure	Prophylaxis / Management
Tuberculosis	Housed in the same room with a child with contagious tuberculosis (tuberculosis is contagious if the child has a cough plus AFB seen on smear plus cavitation on CXR)	Administer PPD immediately and 10 weeks after exposure. Start on INH. Consult Infectious Diseases if seroconversion occurs.
Varicella-zoster	1 hour or more in the same room with a contagious child from 24 hours before vesicles appear to when all vesicles are crusted, which is usually 5 to 7 days after vesicles appear. In household exposure, communicability is 48 hours before vesicles appear.	Oka (varicella) vaccine is effective in preventing illness or modifying severity if administered to unvaccinated persons who have other evidence of immunity within 3-5 days of exposure to rash. **Immunocompetent** children who have not been vaccinated or had natural infection should have titers drawn only if they will still be hospitalized for more than 10 days after exposure. If titers are negative, they should be isolated from 10-21 days after exposure and/or until all lesions are crusted and dry. If VariZIG (varicella-zoster immune globulin) was given the child should be isolated from 10-28 days after exposure. **Immunocompromised** children who have not been vaccinated or had natural infection should first have titers drawn, and then receive VariZIG **1 vial/10 kg I.M.** up to a maximum of 5 vials as soon as possible but at most 96 hours after exposure (preferably within 72 hours). Fractional doses are not recommended. If titers are positive, nothing further need be done. If titers are negative, the child should be isolated from 10-28 days after exposure and should be monitored very carefully for the appearance of vesicles so that treatment can be initiated. VariZIG is available from the Blood Bank. Prophylactic antiviral treatment regimens are recommended for high-risk patients who are ineligible for vaccine or beyond the 96-hour window after direct contact. Therapy should be started 7 days after intense exposure (when host is midway into incubation period).

TREATMENT OF ELEVATED INR DUE TO WARFARIN

Eighth ACCP Consensus Conference on Antithrombotic Therapy: Recommendations on Managing Elevated INR In Patients Taking Warfarin

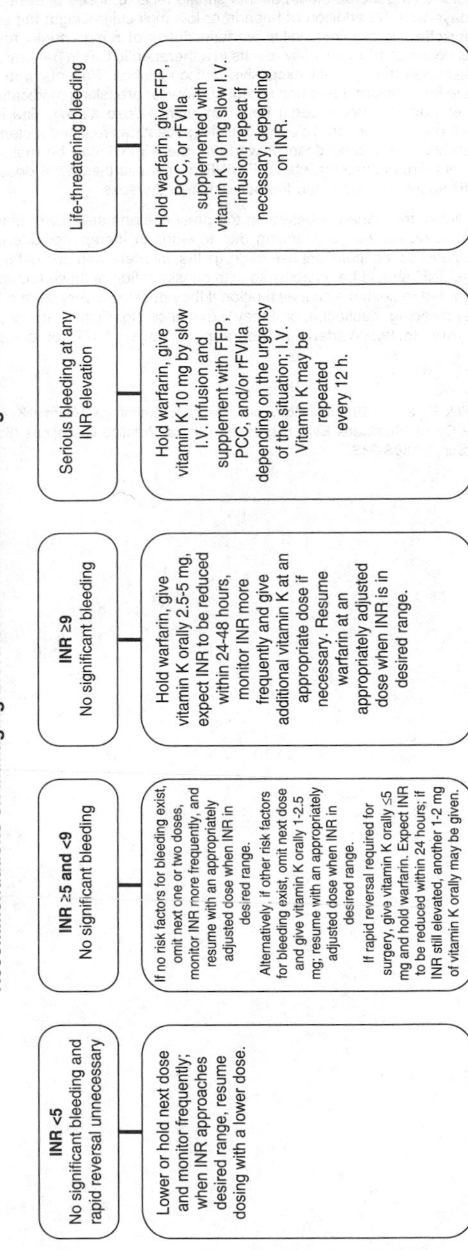

FFP = fresh frozen plasma; INR = international normalized ratio; PCC = prothrombin complex concentrate; rFVIIa = recombinant factor VIIa

Note 1: If mild-moderate INR elevation without major bleeding occurs, give vitamin K orally instead of subcutaneously.

Note 2: Use of high doses of vitamin K (eg, 10-15 mg) may cause warfarin resistance for ≥1 week. During this period of resistance, heparin or low molecular weight heparin may be given until INR responds.

Note 3: PCC may contain II, IX, X; Factor VII is not currently contained in U.S. products.

WARFARIN THERAPY

Patients should **not** receive loading doses of warfarin (ie, doses >10 mg) as the steady-state INR is not achieved more quickly. In general, most patients should receive doses between 5 mg and 10 mg for the first 1-2 days with the addition of heparin or low molecular weight heparin when a more rapid anticoagulant effect is required. Initial warfarin doses of 5 mg usually results in an INR>2 in 4-5 days. Initial doses of 10 mg usually results in a therapeutic INR in 3-4 days; however, 10 mg doses may be associated with more excessive anticoagulation. Patients who are debilitated, malnourished, have heart failure, have had recent surgery, or are taking medications known to increase the effects of warfarin should begin treatment with a dose ≤5 mg. The intensity of anticoagulation therapy should be monitored closely until the patient has reached a stable PT/INR. Once the patient is stabilized on a fixed dose of warfarin, the PT/INR can be monitored on a monthly basis if the patient demonstrates a stable PT/INR on chronic therapy. If dosage adjustments are made, PT/INR should be evaluated in approximately 2 weeks.

Supratherapeutic INR values are managed based on the presence and severity of bleeding (see chart on previous page). Determinants of bleeding due to warfarin therapy include intensity of treatment, patient characteristics, concomitant use of drugs that interfere with hemostasis, and the length therapy. The target INR should be established with consideration of these factors. Patients on warfarin should be warned to seek medical evaluation if they develop a very severe headache, abdominal pain, unusual bleeding, backache, or if they experience significant trauma, particularly head injuries. Please refer to the Warfarin monograph on page 1877 for complete drug information.

Reference

Ansell J, Hirsh J, Hylek E, et al, "Pharmacology and Management of the Vitamin K Antagonists: American College of Chest Physicians Evidence-Based Clinical Practice Guidelines (8th Edition)," *Chest*, 2008, 133(6 Suppl):160S-98S.

NOTES

NOTES

NOTES

Other Products Offered by Lexicomp

Anesthesiology & Critical Care Drug Handbook

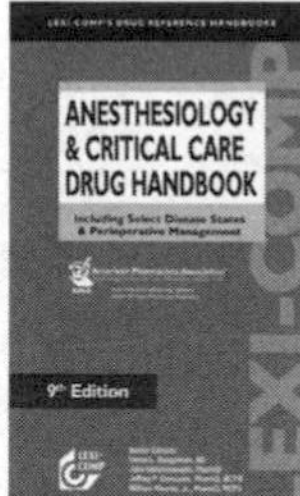

Designed for anesthesiologists, critical care practitioners, and all healthcare professionals involved in the treatment of surgical or ICU patients.

Includes: Comprehensive drug information to ensure appropriate clinical management of patients; Intensivist and Anesthesiologist perspective; Over 2000 medications most commonly used in the preoperative and critical care setting; Special Topics/Issues addressing frequently encountered patient conditions.

Drug Information Handbook

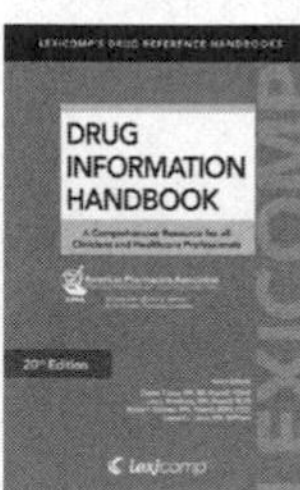

An easy-to-use reference for pharmacists, physicians, or other healthcare professionals requiring fast access to comprehensive drug information. This handbook presents over 1400 drug monographs, each with up to 35 fields of information. A valuable appendix includes hundreds of charts and reviews of special topics such as guidelines for treatment and therapy recommendations. A pharmacologic category index is also provided.

Drug Information Handbook with International Trade Names Index

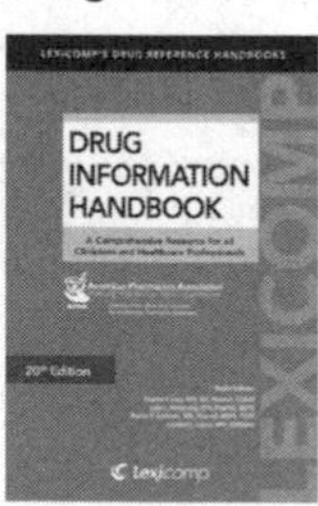

The *Drug Information Handbook with International Trade Names Index* includes the content of our *Drug Information Handbook*, plus international drug monographs for use worldwide! This easy-to-use reference is complied especially for the pharmacist, physician, or other healthcare professional seeking quick access to comprehensive drug information.

Drug Information Handbook for Nursing

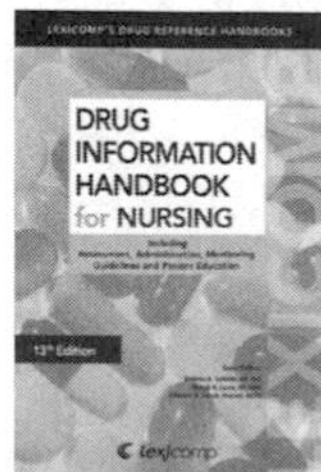

Designed for registered professional nurses and upper-division nursing students requiring dosing, administration, monitoring and patient education information.

Includes: Over 4800 generic and brand name drugs, cross-referenced by page number; drug names and specific nursing fields highlighted in RED for easy reference, Nursing Actions field includes Physical Assessment and Patient Education guidelines.

Other Products Offered by Lexicomp

Drug Information Handbook for Oncology

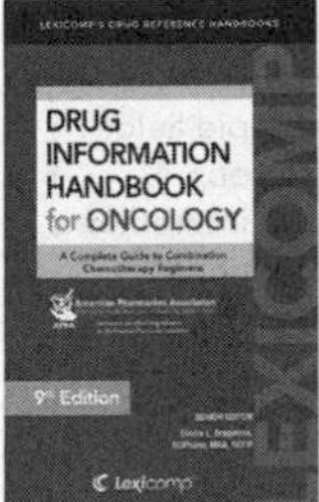

Designed for oncology professionals requiring information on combination chemotherapy regimens and dosing protocols.

Includes: Monographs containing warnings, adverse reaction profiles, drug interactions, dosing for specific indications, vesicant, emetic potential, combination regimens and more; where applicable, a special Combination Chemotherapy field links to specific oncology monographs; Special Topics such as Cancer Treatment Related Complications, Bone Marrow Transplantation and Drug Development.

Drug Information Handbook for Psychiatry

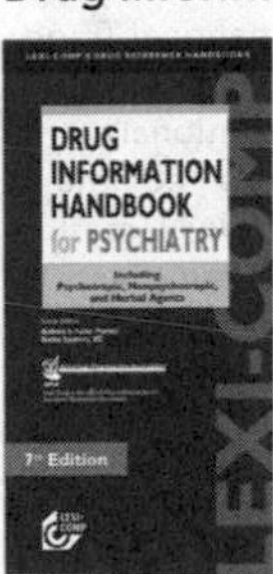

Designed for any healthcare professional requiring quick access to comprehensive drug information as it relates to mental health issues.

Includes: Drug monographs for psychotropic, nonpsychotropic and herbal medications; Special fields such as Mental Health Comment (useful clinical pearls), Medication Safety Issues, Effects on Mental Status and Effects on Psychiatric Treatment.

Geriatric Dosage Handbook

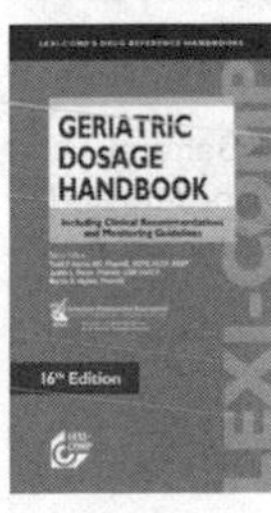

Designed for healthcare professionals managing geriatric patients.

Includes: Complete adult and geriatric dosing; Special geriatric considerations; Up to 41 key fields of information in each monograph, including Medication Safety Issues; Extensive information on drug interactions, as well as dosing for patients with renal/hepatic impairment.

Pharmacogenomics Handbook

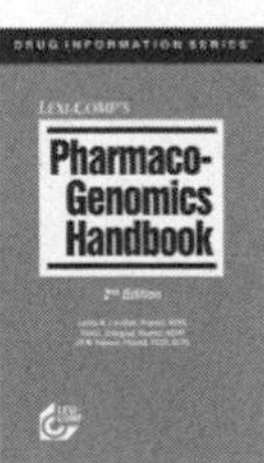

Ideal for any healthcare professional or student wishing to gain insight into the emerging field of pharmacogenomics.

Includes: Information concerning key genetic variations that may influence drug disposition and/or sensitivity; brief introductions to fundamental concepts in genetics and genomics. A foundation for all clinicians who will be called on to integrate rapidly-expanding genomics knowledge into the management of drug therapy.

To order, call Customer Service at 866-397-3433 or visit www.lexi.com.
Outside of the U.S., call +1-330-650-6506 or visit www.lexi.com.

Other Products Offered by Lexicomp

Pediatric Dosage Handbook

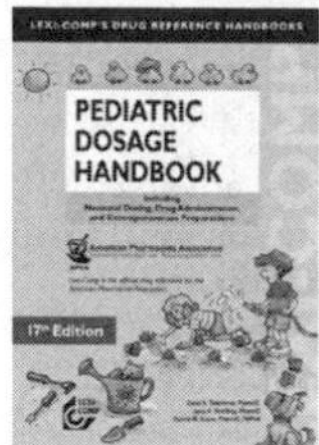

This book is designed for healthcare professionals requiring quick access to comprehensive pediatric drug information. Each monograph contains multiple fields of content, including usual dosage by age group, indication and route of administration. Drug interactions, adverse reactions, extemporaneous preparations, pharmacodynamics/pharmacokinetics data and medication safety issues are covered.

Also available:
Manual de Prescripción Pediátrica (Spanish version)

Pediatric Dosage Handbook with International Trade Names Index

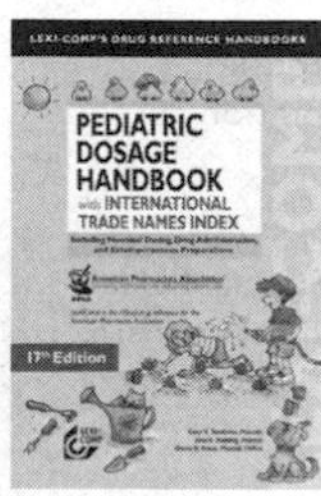

The *Pediatric Dosage Handbook with International Trade Names Index* is the trusted pediatric drug resource of medical professionals worldwide. The International Edition contains all the content of Lexicomp's *Pediatric Dosage Handbook,* plus an International Trade Names Index including trade names from over 100 countries.

Rating Scales for Mental Health

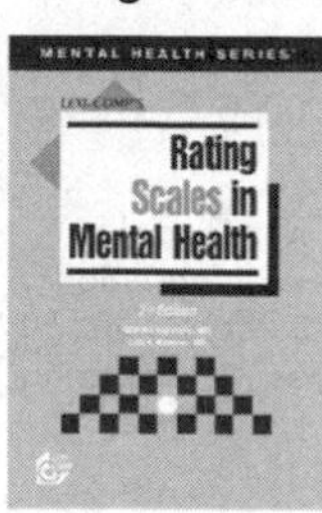

Ideal for clinicians as well as administrators, this book provides an overview of over 100 recommended rating scales for mental assessment.

Includes: Rating scales for conditions such as General Anxiety, Social/Family Functioning, Eating Disorders and Sleep Disorders; Monograph format covering such topics as Overview of Scale, General Applications, Psychometric Properties and References.

To order, call Customer Service at 866-397-3433 or visit www.lexi.com.
Outside of the U.S., call +1-330-650-6506 or visit www.lexi.com.

Other Products Offered by Lexicomp

Lexicomp Online™

Eight of the top 10 hospitals in *U.S. News and World Report's* 2010-11 Honor Roll ranking utilize Lexicomp's clinical databases and technology. These include Johns Hopkins, Massachusetts General, Cleveland Clinic, UCLA and others.

Lexicomp Online™ integrates industry-leading databases and enhanced searching technology to bring you time-sensitive clinical information at the point-of-care. Our easy-to-use interface and concise information eliminate the need to navigate through multiple pages or make unnecessary mouse clicks.

Lexicomp Online includes multiple databases and modules covering the following topic areas:

- Core drug information with specialty fields
- Pediatrics and Geriatrics
- Interaction Analysis
- Pharmacogenomics
- Infectious Diseases
- Laboratory Tests and Diagnostic Procedures
- Natural Products
- Patient Education
- Drug Identification
- Calculations
- I.V. Compatibility: *King® Guide to Parenteral Admixtures®*
- Toxicology

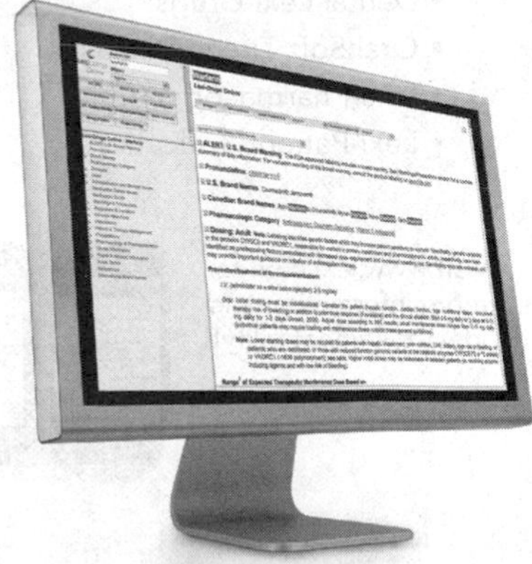

Register for a FREE 45-day trial

Visit www.lexi.com/institutions

Academic and Institutional licenses available.

To order, call Customer Service at 866-397-3433 or visit www.lexi.com.
Outside of the U.S., call +1-330-650-6506 or visit www.lexi.com.